Body Mass Index

	Normal						Overweight					Obese										Extreme Obesity														
BMI	19	20	21	22	23	24	25	26	27	28	29	30	31	32	33	34	35	36	37	38	39	40	41	42	43	44	45	46	47	48	49	50	51	52	53	54
Height (inches)	Body Weight (pounds)																																			
58	91	96	100	105	110	115	119	124	129	134	138	143	148	153	158	162	167	172	177	181	186	191	196	201	205	210	215	220	224	229	234	239	244	248	253	258
59	94	99	104	109	114	119	124	128	133	138	143	148	153	158	163	168	173	178	183	188	193	198	203	208	212	217	222	227	232	237	242	247	252	257	262	267
60	97	102	107	112	118	123	128	133	138	143	148	153	158	163	168	174	179	184	189	194	199	204	209	215	220	225	230	235	240	245	250	255	261	266	271	276
61	100	106	111	116	122	127	132	137	143	148	153	158	164	169	174	180	185	190	195	201	206	211	217	222	227	232	238	243	248	254	259	264	269	275	280	285
62	104	109	115	120	126	131	136	142	147	153	158	164	169	175	180	186	191	196	202	207	213	218	224	229	235	240	246	251	256	262	267	273	278	284	289	295
63	107	113	118	124	130	135	141	146	152	158	163	169	175	180	186	191	197	203	208	214	220	225	231	237	242	248	254	259	265	270	278	282	287	293	299	304
64	110	116	122	128	134	140	145	151	157	163	169	174	180	186	192	197	204	209	215	221	227	232	238	244	250	256	262	267	273	279	285	291	296	302	308	314
65	114	120	126	132	138	144	150	156	162	168	174	180	186	192	198	204	210	216	222	228	234	240	246	252	258	264	270	276	282	288	294	300	306	312	318	324
66	118	124	130	136	142	148	155	161	167	173	179	186	192	198	204	210	216	223	229	235	241	247	253	260	266	272	278	284	291	297	303	309	315	322	328	334
67	121	127	134	140	146	153	159	166	172	178	185	191	198	204	211	217	223	230	236	242	249	255	261	268	274	280	287	293	299	306	312	319	325	331	338	344
68	125	131	138	144	151	158	164	171	177	184	190	197	203	210	216	223	230	236	243	249	256	262	269	276	282	289	295	302	308	315	322	328	335	341	348	354
69	128	135	142	149	155	162	169	176	182	189	196	203	209	216	223	230	236	243	250	257	263	270	277	284	291	297	304	311	318	324	331	338	345	351	358	365
70	132	139	146	153	160	167	174	181	188	195	202	209	216	222	229	236	243	250	257	264	271	278	285	292	299	306	313	320	327	334	341	348	355	362	369	376
71	136	143	150	157	165	172	179	186	193	200	208	215	222	229	236	243	250	257	265	272	279	286	293	301	308	315	322	329	338	343	351	358	365	372	379	386
72	140	147	154	162	169	177	184	191	199	206	213	221	228	235	242	250	258	265	272	279	287	294	302	309	316	324	331	338	346	353	361	368	375	383	390	397
73	144	151	159	166	174	182	189	197	204	212	219	227	235	242	250	257	265	272	280	288	295	302	310	318	325	333	340	348	355	363	371	378	386	393	401	408
74	148	155	163	171	179	186	194	202	210	218	225	233	241	249	256	264	272	280	287	295	303	311	319	326	334	342	350	358	365	373	381	389	396	404	412	420
75	152	160	168	176	184	192	200	208	216	224	232	240	248	256	264	272	279	287	295	303	311	319	327	335	343	351	359	367	375	383	391	399	407	415	423	431
76	156	164	172	180	189	197	205	213	221	230	238	246	254	263	271	279	287	295	304	312	320	328	336	344	353	361	369	377	385	394	402	410	418	426	435	443

Source: Adapted from National Heart, Lung, and Blood Institute: Clinical Guidelines on the Identification, Evaluation, and Treatment of Overweight and Obesity in Adults: the Evidence Report.
See http://www.nhlbi.nih.gov/guidelines/obesity/bmi_tbl.pdf

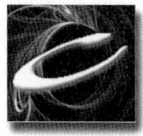

CONN'S
CURRENT THERAPY
2026

CONN'S CURRENT THERAPY 2026

RICK D. KELLERMAN, MD

Professor and Chair Emeritus
Department of Family and Community Medicine
University of Kansas School of Medicine-Wichita
Wichita, Kansas

JOEL J. HEIDELBAUGH, MD

Professor
Department of Family Medicine
University of Michigan Medical School
Ann Arbor, Michigan

ERNESTINE M. LEE, MD, MPH

Associate Professor
Department of Family Medicine
Loma Linda University School of Medicine
Advent Health Orlando Campus
Winter Park, Florida

ELSEVIER

Elsevier
1600 John F. Kennedy Blvd.
Ste 1800
Philadelphia, PA 19103-2899

CONN'S CURRENT THERAPY 2026   ISBN-13: 978-0-443-12182-1

Notice

Practitioners and researchers must always rely on their own experience and knowledge in evaluating
and using any information, methods, compounds or experiments described herein. Because of rapid
advances in the medical sciences, in particular, independent verification of diagnoses and drug dosages
should be made. To the fullest extent of the law, no responsibility is assumed by Elsevier, authors, editors
or contributors for any injury and/or damage to persons or property as a matter of products liability,
negligence or otherwise, or from any use or operation of any methods, products, instructions, or ideas
contained in the material herein.

Senior Content Strategist: Lauren Boyle
Content Development Manager: Meghan Andress
Senior Content Development Specialist: Kevin Travers
Publishing Services Manager: Catherine Albright-Jackson
Senior Project Manager: Doug Turner
Design Direction: Renee Duenow

Printed in Canada

Last digit is the print number: 9 8 7 6 5 4 3 2 1

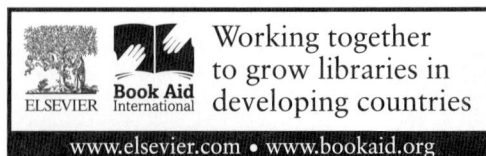

Contributors

Mustafa Abdul-Hussein, MD, MSCR
Gastroenterology and Hepatology, Sarah Bush Lincoln Health Center, Mattoon, Illinois
Gastroesophageal Reflux Disease (GERD)

Sunil Abhyankar, MD
Professor, Internal Medicine, University of Kansas Medical Center, Kansas City, Kansas
Stem Cell Therapy

Rodney D. Adam, MD
Professor, Pathology and Medicine, Aga Khan University, Nairobi, Kenya
Giardiasis

T.M. Ayodele Adesanya, MD, PhD
Assistant Professor, Family and Community Medicine, The Ohio State University College of Medicine, Columbus, Ohio
Premature Beats

Nelson Iván Agudelo Higuita, MD
Associate Professor, Internal Medicine, University of Oklahoma Health Sciences Center, Oklahoma City, Oklahoma
Plague

Mehwish Ahmed, MD
Fellow, Gastroenterology and Hepatology, University of Michigan Medical School, Ann Arbor, Michigan
Inflammatory Bowel Disease: Crohn's Disease and Ulcerative Colitis

Lee Akst, MD
Director, Laryngology, Department of Otolaryngology, Johns Hopkins Medical Institutes, Baltimore, Maryland
Hoarseness and Laryngitis

Ethan Alexander, MD
Assistant Professor, Endocrinology, Diabetes, Metabolism, Clinical Pharmacology, University of Kansas Medical Center, Kansas City, Kansas
Diabetes Mellitus in Adults

Patrick L. Allen, MD
Clinical Assistant Professor, Family and Community Medicine, University of Kansas School of Medicine-Wichita, Wichita, Kansas
Brucellosis

Mohamed AlShamrani, MD
Stroke Fellow, Cumming School of Medicine, University of Calgary, Calgary, Alberta, Canada; Stroke Specialist, Neuroscience Centre, King Faisal Specialist Hospital, Riyadh, Saudi Arabia
Intracerebral Hemorrhage

Alvaro Cervera Alvarez, MD, PhD
Consultant Neurologist, Neurology, Royal Darwin Hospital, Darwin, Northern Territory, Australia
Ischemic Cerebrovascular Disease

Kelley P. Anderson, MD
Clinical Adjunct Professor, Medicine; Researcher Emeritus, Marshfield Clinic Research Institute, University of Wisconsin School of Medicine and Public Health, Marshfield, Wisconsin
Heart Block

Paul Andre, MD
Assistant Professor, Internal Medicine, University of New Mexico School of Medicine, Albuquerque, New Mexico
Tachycardias

Gregory Anstead, MD, PhD
Staff Physician, Medicine, Audie L. Murphy Memorial Veterans Affairs Hospital; Professor, Medicine, University of Texas Health, San Antonio, Texas
Coccidioidomycosis

Ann M. Aring, MD
Associate Program Director, Family Medicine OhioHealth Riverside Family Medicine Program, Columbus, Ohio
Drug Hypersensitivity Reactions; Rhinosinusitis

Cheryl A. Armstrong, MD
Professor, Dermatology, University of Colorado School of Medicine, Aurora, Colorado; Dermatology Division Chief, Medicine, Denver Health Medical Center, Denver, Colorado
Viral Diseases of the Skin

Arash Arshi, MD
Interventional Cardiologist, Cardiology, OhioHealth, Columbus, Ohio
Valvular Heart Disease

Cecilio R. Azar, MD
Gastroenterologist and Hepatologist, Clinical Associate, Gastroenterology, American University of Beirut Medical Center, Beirut, Lebanon
Bleeding Esophageal Varices

Jihoon Baang, MD
Associate Clinical Professor, Internal Medicine, University of Michigan Medical School, Ann Arbor, Michigan
Toxoplasmosis; Histoplasmosis

Zachary Baeseman, MD, MPH
Associate Chief Medical Officer, Leadership Development and Clinical Transformation, ThedaCare Physicians, ThedaCare, Neenah, Wisconsin; Adjunct Professor, Family Medicine, Medical College of Wisconsin, Milwaukee, Wisconsin
Vaginal Bleeding in Pregnancy

Justin Bailey, MD
Associate Professor, Family Medicine, University of Washington School of Medicine; Director, Procedures Institute, Family Medicine Residency of Idaho, Boise, Idaho
Gaseousness, Indigestion, Nausea, and Vomiting; Palpitations

Juliana Bakk, MD
Fellow, Maternal Fetal Medicine, University of Kansas Medical Center, Kansas City, Kansas
Hypertensive Disorders in Pregnancy

Dana M. Bakula, PhD
Pediatric Psychologist, Children's Mercy Kansas City; Assistant Professor, Pediatrics, University of Missouri-Kansas City School of Medicine, Kansas City, Missouri
Infant and Children Feeding Problems

Federico Balagué, MD
Physician, Rheumatology, HFR Fribourg-Hôpital Cantonal, Fribourg, Switzerland
Spine Pain

Bradley E. Barth, MD
Professor, Emergency Medicine, University of Kansas Medical Center, Kansas City, Missouri
Burns

Gina M. Basello, DO
Medical Director, Graduate Medical Education & Designated Institutional Official Medical Education, Medisys Health Network, Jamaica, New York; Assistant Clinical Professor, Family and Social Medicine, Albert Einstein College of Medicine, Bronx, New York
Fever

Renee Bassaly, DO
Associate Professor, Female Pelvic Medicine and Reconstructive Surgery, University of South Florida College of Medicine, Tampa, Florida
Urinary Incontinence

Adel Bassily-Marcus, MD
Associate Professor, Surgery, Mount Sinai Medical Center, New York, New York
Targeted Temperature Management (Therapeutic Hypothermia)

Julie M. Baughn, MD
Consultant, Sleep Medicine, Mayo Clinic, Rochester, Minnesota
Pediatric Sleep Disorders

Aleksandr Belakovskiy, MD
Assistant Professor, Family Medicine, University of Michigan Medical School, Ann Arbor, Michigan
Erectile Dysfunction

Ronen M. Ben-Ami, MD
Head, Infectious Diseases Department, Tel Aviv Sourasky Medical Center, Tel Aviv, Israel
Cat Scratch Disease

David I. Bernstein, MD
Professor Emeritus of Medicine, Immunology, Allergy, and Rheumatology, University of Cincinnati College of Medicine, Cincinnati, Ohio
Hypersensitivity Pneumonitis

Caroline Beyer, MD
Family Physician, Los Angeles LGBT Center, Los Angeles, California
Palpitations

Kaamya Bhandari, MD
Fellow Physician, Pulmonary and Critical Care, Medical University of South Carolina, Charleston, South Carolina
Sarcoidosis

Kristin Schmid Biggerstaff, MD
Associate Professor, Ophthalmology, Baylor College of Medicine; Glaucoma Staff, Eye Care Line, Michael E. DeBakey Veterans Affairs Medical Center, Houston, Texas
Glaucoma

Mitchell C. Birt, MD
Assistant Professor, Orthopedic Surgery, University of Kansas Health System, Kansas City; Kansas; Faculty, Orthopedic Surgery, Kansas City VA Medical Center, Kansas City, Missouri
Osteomyelitis

Lora Black, MD, PhD
Assistant Professor, Psychiatry and Behavioral Health, The Ohio State University Wexner Medical Center, Columbus, Ohio
Fibromyalgia

Yooni Blair, MD
Assistant Professor, Urology, University of Michigan Medical School, Ann Arbor, Michigan
Trauma to the Genitourinary Tract

Natalie Blonien, DPT
Physical Therapist, Department of Physical Therapy University of Wisconsin Madison School of Medicine and Public Health, Madison, Wisconsin
Rehabilitation of the Stroke Patient

Diana Bolotin, MD, PhD
Professor, Dermatology, University of Chicago Pritzker School of Medicine, Chicago, Illinois
Nonmelanoma Cancer of the Skin

Rachel A. Bonnema, MD, MS
Professor, Internal Medicine, UT Southwestern Medical Center, Dallas, Texas
Contraception

Meelie Bordoloi, MD
Assistant Professor, Psychiatry, University of Missouri, Columbia, Missouri
Autism Spectrum Disorder

David Borenstein, MD
Clinical Professor, Rheumatology, The George Washington University Medical Center; Partner, Arthritis and Rheumatism Associates, Washington, District of Columbia
Spine Pain

Nicole Boschuetz, MD
Assistant Clinical Professor, Gastroenterology and Hepatology, University of Wisconsin Hospital and Clinics, Madison, Wisconsin
Metabolic Dysfunction-Associated Steatotic Liver Disease (MASLD)

Christopher Bossart, MD
Associate Professor, Emergency Medicine, University of New Mexico School of Medicine, Albuquerque, New Mexico
Osteoarthritis

Matthew Boyte, MD
Assistant Professor, Psychiatry, UAB Heersink School of Medicine, University of Alabama-Birmingham, Birmingham, Alabama
Obsessive-Compulsive Disorder

Dee Ann Bragg, MD
Associate Professor, Family and Community Medicine, University of Kansas School of Medicine-Wichita Family Medicine Residency Program at Via Christi Hospitals, Wichita, Kansas
Rubella and Congenital Rubella

Scott Bragg, PharmD
Professor, Clinical Pharmacy and Outcomes Science, Family Medicine, Medical University of South Carolina, Charleston, South Carolina
Osteoporosis

Allyson M. Briggs, MD
Assistant Professor, Emergency Medicine, University of Kansas Medical Center, Kansas City, Kansas
Burns

John Brill, MD, MPH
Vice President, Population Health, Advocate Aurora Health, Milwaukee, Wisconsin
Gonorrhea

Sarah Burns, DO, MS
Associate Professor, Hospital Medicine–Internal Medicine, University of New Mexico School of Medicine, Albuquerque, New Mexico
Acute Kidney Injury

Kenneth Byrd, DO
Assistant Professor, Internal Medicine–Hematologic Malignancies and Cellular Therapeutics, University of Kansas Medical Center, Kansas City, Kansas
Disseminated Intravascular Coagulation

Diego Cadavid, MD
Chief Medical Officer, Clinical Development, Verge Genomics, South San Francisco, California; Affiliate Instructor, Neurology, UMass Chan Medical School, Worcester, Massachusetts
Relapsing Fever

Lizbeth Cahuayme-Zuniga, MD
Assistant Clinical Professor, Internal Medicine; Service Chief, Division of Infectious Diseases, University of Michigan Medical School, Ann Arbor, Michigan
Tuberculosis and Other Mycobacterial Diseases

Juana Nicoll Capizzano, MD
Associate Professor, Family Medicine, University of Michigan Medical School, Ann Arbor, Michigan
Pleural Effusion and Empyema

Thomas R. Caraccio, PharmD
Clinical Pharmacist/Toxicologist, Pharmacy Department, NYU Winthrop Hospital, Mineola/New York, New York
Medical Toxicology

Peter Carek, MD, MS
Professor and Chair, Family Medicine, Prisma Health, Greenville, South Carolina
Osteoporosis

Carlos Anthony Casillas, MD, MPH
Fellow, Hospital Medicine, Cincinnati Children's Hospital Medical Center, Cincinnati, Ohio
Viral Meningitis

Amanda S. Cass, PharmD
Clinical Pharmacist Specialist, Thoracic Oncology, Pharmaceutical Services, Vanderbilt University Medical Center, Nashville, Tennessee
Lung Cancer

William E. Cayley Jr., MD, MDiv
Adjunct Clinical Professor, Family Medicine and Community Health, University of Wisconsin School of Medicine and Public Health, Eau Claire, Wisconsin; Family Physician, Prevea Family Medicine Residency Program–Augusta, Augusta, Wisconsin
Chest Pain

Kristine L. Cece, MD, PhD
Assistant Professor, Family Medicine, Michigan Medicine, Ann Arbor, Michigan
Hiccups

Sonia Cerquozzi, MD
Clinical Assistant Professor, Internal Medicine, Hematology, University of Calgary Cumming School of Medicine, Calgary, Alberta, Canada
Polycythemia Vera

Filomena Cetani, MD, PhD
Physician, Endocrinology, University Hospital of Pisa, Pisa, Italy
Hyperparathyroidism and Hypoparathyroidism

Andrea L. Chadwick, MD, MSc
Associate Professor, Anesthesiology, Pain, and Perioperative Medicine, University of Kansas School of Medicine, Kansas City, Kansas
Fibromyalgia

Rachel Chamberlain, MD
Program Director, Sports Medicine Fellowship; Assistant Professor, Family and Community Medicine, University of New Mexico School of Medicine, Albuquerque, New Mexico
Osteoarthritis

Monica Chamorro, MD
Assistant Professor, Family Medicine and Geriatrics, University of Louisville, Glasgow, Kentucky
Keloids and Hypertrophic Scars

Miriam Chan, PharmD
Program Director of Quality and Safety, Medical Education, OhioHealth; Adjunct Assistant Professor, Family Medicine, The Ohio State University College of Medicine, Columbus, Ohio, Adjunct Clinical Assistant Professor, Pharmacology, Ohio University, Athens, Ohio
Drug Hypersensitivity Reactions; Popular Herbs and Nutritional Supplements

Divya Chandramohan, MD
Assistant Professor, Infectious Diseases, UT Health-San Antonio, San Antonio, Texas
Coccidioidomycosis

Zenas Chang, MD
Assistant Professor, Clinical Obstetrics and Gynecology, Gynecologic Oncology, Indiana University School of Medicine, Indianapolis, Indiana
Ovarian Cancer

Jimmy Chen, MD
Pediatric Hospitalist, Pediatrics, University of Florida College of Medicine-Jacksonville, Jacksonville, Florida
Parenteral Fluid Therapy for Infants and Children

Lin Yee Chen, MBBS, MS
Professor, Medicine/Cardiology, University of Minnesota Medical School, Minneapolis, Minnesota
Atrial Fibrillation

Shingo Chihara, MD
Physician, Infectious Disease, Virginia Mason Medical Center, Seattle, Washington
Anthrax

Meera Chitlur, MD
Professor, Pediatric Hematology/Oncology, Central Michigan University/Children's Hospital of Michigan; Barnhart-Lusher Hemostasis Research Endowed Chair, Pediatrics, Wayne State University School of Medicine, Detroit, Michigan
Hemophilia and Related Conditions

Saima Chohan, MD
Clinical Assistant Professor, Rheumatology, University of Arizona College of Medicine, Phoenix, Arizona
Gout and Hyperuricemia

Jacob Christensen, DO
Physician, Primary Care Sports Medicine, University of Idaho, Moscow, Idaho
Osteoarthritis

Kuang-Yuh Chyu, MD, PhD
Associate Director, Coronary Intensive Care Unit, Cardiology, Cedars-Sinai Medical Center; Health Science Clinical Professor, Medicine, David Geffen School of Medicine at UCLA, Los Angeles, California
Acute Myocardial Infarction

Joaquin E. Cigarroa, MD
KCVI Institute Director, Division Head of Cardiology, Professor, Medicine, Knight Cardiovascular Institute, Oregon Health and Sciences University, Portland, Oregon
Congenital Heart Disease

Paul Cleland, MD
Clinical Assistant Professor, Family and Community Medicine, University of Kansas School of Medicine-Wichita, Wichita, Kansas
Heat Illness

Matthew K. Cline, MD
Affiliate Professor, Family Medicine, Medical University of South Carolina, Charleston, South Carolina
Antepartum Care

Laura C. Coates, MBChB, PhD
Associate Professor, Nuffield Department of Orthopaedics, Rheumatology and Musculoskeletal Sciences, University of Oxford, Oxford, United Kingdom
Psoriatic Arthritis

August Colenbrander, MD
Affiliate Senior Scientist, Rehabilitation Engineering Research Center, Smith-Kettlewell Eye Research Institute, San Francisco, California
Vision Rehabilitation

Jeanette R. Comstock, MD
Assistant Professor, Dermatology, University of Wisconsin School of Medicine and Public Health, Madison, Wisconsin
Cutaneous T-Cell Lymphoma, Including Mycosis Fungoides and Sézary Syndrome

Christine Conageski, MD
Associate Professor, Obstetrics and Gynecology, University of Colorado School of Medicine, Aurora, Colorado
Vulvar Neoplasia

John M. Conly, MD
Medical Officer, Infection Prevention and Control, Foothills Medical Center; Professor, Medicine; Medical Director, Ward of the 21st Century, Cummings School of Medicine; Co-Director, Snyder Institute for Chronic Diseases, University of Calgary, Calgary, Alberta, Canada
Methicillin-Resistant Staphylococcus aureus

Ashley Cooper, MD
Associate Professor, Pediatrics, Children's Mercy Kansas City; University of Missouri-Kansas City School of Medicine, Kansas City, Missouri
Juvenile Idiopathic Arthritis

Stacy Cooper, MD
Associate Professor, Oncology, Johns Hopkins University School of Medicine, Baltimore, Maryland
Acute Leukemia in Children

Allison Cormier, MD
Physician, Infectious Disease, South Louisiana Medical Associates, Houma, Louisiana
Human Immunodeficiency Virus: Treatment and Prevention

Burke A. Cunha, MD
Physician, Infectious Disease, NYU Winthrop Hospital, Mineola, New York
Babesiosis; Viral and Mycoplasmal Pneumonias

Cheston B. Cunha, MD
Medical Director, Antimicrobial Stewardship; Assistant Professor, Infectious Disease, Warren Alpert Medical School of Brown University, Providence, Rhode Island
Babesiosis; Viral and Mycoplasmal Pneumonias

Thomas Curran, MD, MPH
Associate Professor, Surgery, Medical University of South Carolina, Charleston, South Carolina
Tumors of the Colon and Rectum

Amy Curry, MD
Clinical Associate Professor, Family and Community Medicine, University of Kansas School of Medicine-Wichita, Wichita, Kansas
Pelvic Inflammatory Disease

Cori L. Daines, MD
Professor and Division Chief, Pediatric Pulmonary and Sleep Medicine, Pediatrics, University of Arizona College of Medicine, Tucson, Arizona
Cystic Fibrosis

Beth Damitz, MD
Professor, Family and Community Medicine; Associate Program Director, All Saints Family Medicine Residency Program, Medical College of Wisconsin, Milwaukee, Wisconsin
Immunization Practices

Nandini Datta, PhD
Clinical Instructor, Child and Adolescent Psychiatry, Stanford University School of Medicine, Stanford, California
Eating Disorders

Natalie C. Dattilo, PhD
Director of Psychology, Psychiatry, Brigham and Women's Hospital, Boston, Massachusetts
Generalized Anxiety Disorder; Posttraumatic Stress Disorder

Raul Davaro, MD
Associate Professor, Clinical Medicine, University of Massachusetts Medical School, Worcester, Massachusetts
Smallpox; Whooping Cough (Pertussis)

John Davis, MD
Fellow, Medicine, University of Wisconsin School of Medicine and Public Health, Madison, Wisconsin
Sepsis

Joshua Davis, MD
Assistant Medical Director, Emergency Medicine, Vituity; Clinical Instructor, Medicine, University of Kansas School of Medicine-Wichita, Wichita, Kansas
Acute Diarrhea

Alexei O. DeCastro, MD
Associate Professor, Family Medicine, Medical University of South Carolina, Charleston, South Carolina
Osteoporosis

Matthew Decker, MD, JD
Assistant Professor, Community and Family Medicine, University of Missouri-Kansas City, Kansas City, Missouri
COVID-19

Katharine C. DeGeorge, MD, MS
Associate Professor, Family Medicine, University of Virginia School of Medicine, Charlottesville, Virginia
Bacterial Pneumonia

Kristina M. Deligiannidis, MD
Professor, Psychiatry, Molecular Medicine and Obstetrics & Gynecology, Donald and Barbara School of Medicine at Hofstra/ Northwell; Director, Women's Behavioral Health, Department of Psychiatry, Zucker Hillside Hospital, Glen Oaks, New York; Professor, Feinstein Institute for Medical Research, Manhasset, New York
Premenstrual Dysphoric Disorder

Thomas G. DeLoughery, MD
Professor, Hematology, Oregon Health & Science University, Portland, Oregon
Hemolytic Anemias

Joanne Dempster, MD, MHA
Assistant Professor, Family Medicine; Attending, Family Medicine, Columbia University; Medical Director, Family Medicine, Ambulatory Care Network-New York Presbyterian Hospital, New York, New York
Vulvovaginitis

Atul A. Deodhar, MD
Professor of Medicine, Arthritis, and Rheumatic Diseases, Oregon Health & Science University, Portland, Oregon
Axial Spondyloarthritis

Sanjal Desai, MD
Assistant Professor, Hematology, Oncology, and Transplantation, University of Minnesota, Minneapolis, Minnesota
Hodgkin Disease

Clio Dessinioti, MD, PhD
Dermatologist, A. Sygros Hospital, Athens, Greece
Parasitic Diseases of the Skin

Mahua Dey, MD
Director of Surgical Neuro-oncology, Neurosurgery, University of Wisconsin School of Medicine and Public Health, Madison, Wisconsin
Central Nervous System Neoplasms

Michael P. Diamond, MD
Senior Vice President for Research, Obstetrics/Gynecology, Augusta University Medical College of Georgia, Augusta, Georgia
Infertility

Christopher Dion, DO
Senior Associate Consultant, Department of Emergency Medicine, Mayo Clinic, Phoenix, Arizona
Venomous Snakebite

Margaret Dobson, MD
Assistant Professor, Family Medicine, University of Michigan Medical School, Ann Arbor, Michigan
Pruritus

Colleen A. Donahue, MD
Assistant Professor, Surgery, Medical University of South Carolina, Charleston, South Carolina
Tumors of the Colon and Rectum

Geoffrey A. Donnan, MD
Professor of Neurology, Director, The Florey Institute of Neuroscience and Mental Health, The University of Melbourne, Melbourne, Australia
Ischemic Cerebrovascular Disease

John N. Dorsch, MD
Professor Emeritus, Family and Community Medicine, University of Kansas School of Medicine-Wichita, Wichita, Kansas
Red Eye

Michael Dougan, MD, PhD
Associate Professor, Medicine/Gastroenterology, Massachusetts General Hospital, Boston, Massachusetts
Monoclonal Antibodies

Chad Douglas, MD, PharmD
Assistant Professor, Family and Preventive Medicine, University of Oklahoma Health Sciences Center, Oklahoma City, Oklahoma
Erythema Multiforme; Fungal Infections of the Skin

Shannon Dowler, MD
Adjunct Associate Professor, Family Medicine, University of North Carolina School of Medicine Asheville, Asheville, North Carolina
Nongonococcal; Urethritis

Douglas A. Drevets, MD
Regents' Professor, Chief, Infectious Diseases, Medicine, University of Oklahoma Health Sciences Center, Oklahoma City, Oklahoma
Plague

Samuel Dudley, MD, PhD
Professor, Medicine, University of Minnesota Medical School, Minneapolis, Minnesota
Atrial Fibrillation

Peter R. Duggan, MD
Clinical Associate Professor, Medicine, University of Calgary Cumming School of Medicine, Calgary, Alberta, Canada
Polycythemia Vera

Ila Durkin, MD
Assistant Professor, Department of Psychiatry, University of Missouri, Columbia, Missouri
Depressive (Major) and Bipolar Disorders

Leigh M. Eck, MD
Professor, Medicine, University of Kansas Medical Center, Kansas City, Kansas
Thyroiditis

Louito Edje, MD, MHPE
Senior Associate Dean for Medical Education, Office of the Dean, Learning Health Science, Family Medicine, University of Michigan Medical School, Ann Arbor, Michigan
Acute Facial Paralysis

Sarah Edwards, DO
Pediatric Gastroenterologist, Pediatrics, Children's Mercy Kansas City, University of Missouri-Kansas City School of Medicine, Kansas City, Missouri
Infant and Children Feeding Problems

Wissam El Atrouni, MD, MSc
Associate Professor, Internal Medicine, University of Kansas School of Medicine, Kansas City, Kansas
Osteomyelitis

Dirk M. Elston, MD
Professor and Chair, Department of Dermatology, Medical University of South Carolina, Charleston, South Carolina
Diseases of the Hair

John M. Embil, MD
Professor, Medicine, University of Manitoba College of Medicine, Winnipeg, Manitoba, Canada
Blastomycosis

Scott K. Epstein, MD
Professor, Medicine, Tufts University School of Medicine, Boston, Massachusetts
Acute Respiratory Failure

Susan Evans, MD
Assistant Professor, Family Medicine, University of Nebraska Medical Center, Omaha, Nebraska
Iron Deficiency Anemia

Andrew M. Evens, DO, MBA, MSc
Associate Director, Rutgers Cancer Institute of New Jersey, Rutgers University; Associate Vice Chancellor, Clinical Innovation & Data Analytics, Rutgers Health Rutgers University, New Brunswick, New Jersey
Non-Hodgkin Lymphoma

Mark Fairweather, MD, PhD
Associate Surgeon, Brigham and Women's Hospital; Assistant Professor, Surgery, Harvard Medical School, Boston, Massachusetts
Tumors of the Stomach

Marni J. Falk, MD
Professor, Division of Human Genetics, Department of Pediatrics Children's Hospital of Philadelphia and University of Pennsylvania Perelman School of Medicine, Philadelphia, Pennsylvania
Mitochondrial Disease

Francis A. Farraye, MD, MS
Director, Inflammatory Bowel Disease Center, Mayo Clinic, Jacksonville, Florida
Inflammatory Bowel Disease: Crohn's Disease and Ulcerative Colitis

Anthony J. Faugno III, MD
Assistant Professor, Pulmonary, Critical Care and Sleep, Tufts Medical Center, Boston, Massachusetts
Acute Respiratory Failure

Hilary Faust, MD
Assistant Professor, Medicine, University of Wisconsin School of Medicine and Public Health, Madison, Wisconsin
Sepsis

Kinder Fayssoux, MD
Faculty, Center for Family Medicine, Eisenhower Medical Associates, La Quinta, California
Bacterial Infections of the Urinary Tract in Women

Katherine Fell, MD
Clinical Assistant Professor, Cardiology, University of Michigan Medical School, Ann Arbor, Michigan
Angina Pectoris

Ian D. Ferguson, MD
Associate Professor, Pediatrics, Yale School of Medicine, New Haven, Connecticut
Post-COVID-19 Multisystem Inflammatory Syndrome in Children

Terry D. Fife, MD
Director, Otoneurology and Balance Disorders, Barrow Neurological Institute; Professor, Neurology, University of Arizona College of Medicine, Phoenix, Arizona
Ménière's Disease

Jonathon Firnhaber, MD, MAEd, MBA
Professor and Residency Program Director, Family Medicine, East Carolina University Brody School of Medicine, Greenville, North Carolina
Diseases of the Nail

Lynn Fisher, MD
Associate Professor, Family and Community Medicine, University of Kansas School of Medicine-Wichita, Wichita, Kansas
Red Eye

William E. Fisher, MD
Professor, Michael E. DeBakey Department of Surgery, Baylor College of Medicine, Houston, Texas
Acute and Chronic Pancreatitis

Maria Fleseriu, MD
Professor, Medicine and Neurological Surgery, Oregon Health & Science University; Director, Pituitary Center, Portland, Oregon
Adrenocortical Insufficiency; Hypopituitarism

Donald C. Fletcher, MD
Adjunct Associate Professor, Ophthalmology, University of Kansas School of Medicine, Kansas City, Kansas; Medical Director, Low Vision Rehabilitation, Envision, Wichita, Kansas; Senior Scientist, Smith-Kettlewell Eye Research Institute; Medical Director, Frank Stein and Paul S May Center for Low Vision Rehabilitation, Ophthalmology, California Pacific Medical Center, San Francisco, California
Vision Rehabilitation

Jennifer Frank, MD
Family Physician, Aurora Family Medicine, Neenah, Wisconsin
Syphilis

David A. Frenz, MD
Adjunct Clinical Assistant Professor, Family Medicine and Community Health, University of Minnesota Medical School, Minneapolis, Minnesota
Alcohol Use Disorder

Ruchi Gaba, MD
Associate Professor, Endocrinology, Diabetes and Metabolism, Baylor College of Medicine, Houston, Texas
Hyperaldosteronism

Virgilio V. George, MD
Director, Division of Colorectal Surgery, Medical University of South Carolina, Charleston, South Carolina
Tumors of the Colon and Rectum

Marc G. Ghany, MD, MHSc
Senior Investigator, Liver Diseases Branch, National Institute of Diabetes and Digestive and Kidney Diseases, National Institutes of Health, Bethesda, Maryland
Hepatitis A, B, D, and E

Muhammad Ahmad Ghazi, MD
Consulting Associate, Family and Community Medicine, Duke University School of Medicine, Raleigh, North Carolina
Pruritus Ani and Vulvae

Geoffrey T. Gibney, MD
Co-Leader, Melanoma Program, Lombardi Comprehensive Cancer Center, Medstar Georgetown University Hospital, Washington, District of Columbia
Melanoma

Karissa Gilchrist, MD
Assistant Professor, Family and Community Medicine, University of Kansas School of Medicine-Wichita, Wichita, Kansas
Bacterial Diseases of the Skin

Erin A. Gillaspie, MD, MPH
Assistant Professor, Thoracic Surgery; Head of Thoracic Surgery Robotics, Vanderbilt University Medical Center, Nashville, Tennessee
Lung Cancer

Tarvinder Gilotra, MD
Consultant Physician, Infectious Disease, Catholic Health, Buffalo, New York
Intestinal Parasites

Mark T. Gladwin, MD
John Z. and Akiko K. Bowers Distinguished Professor and Dean, Medicine, University of Maryland School of Medicine, Vice President for Medical Affairs, University of Maryland, Baltimore, Baltimore, Maryland
Sickle Cell Disease

Stephen J. Gluckman, MD
Emeritus Professor of Medicine, University of Pennsylvania Perelman School of Medicine; Clinical Director, Penn Global Medicine; Medical Director, Travel Medicine Clinic, Philadelphia, Pennsylvania
Myalgic Encephalomyelitis/Chronic Fatigue Syndrome

Andrew W. Goddard, MD
Professor, Psychiatry, University of California San Francisco Fresno, Fresno, California
Generalized Anxiety Disorder

Kyle Goerl, MD
Associate Professor, Family Medicine, University of Colorado Aschutz School of Medicine, Aurora, Colorado; Team Physician, CU Athletics, Boulder, Colorado; Head Sports Medicine, Physician, Colorado Avalanche, Denver, Colorado
Tendinopathy and Bursitis

Mark S. Gold, MD
Professor, Psychiatry, Washington University, St. Louis, Missouri
Drug Use Disorders

David B.K. Golden, MD
Associate Professor, Medicine, Johns Hopkins University, Baltimore, Maryland
Anaphylaxis

Amy Goldstein, MD
Associate Professor, Pediatrics, University of Pennsylvania Perelman School of Medicine; Clinical Director, Mitochondrial Medicine Frontier Program, Division of Human Genetics, Department of Pediatrics, Children's Hospital of Philadelphia, Philadelphia, Pennsylvania
Mitochondrial Disease

Gregory Goodwin, MD
Assistant Professor, Pediatrics, Harvard Medical School; Senior Associate Physician in Pediatrics, Boston Children's Hospital, Boston, Massachusetts
Diabetes Mellitus in Children

Daniel Gorelik, MD
Resident Physician, Otolaryngology-Head and Neck Surgery, Houston Methodist Hospital, Houston, Texas
Rhinitis; Obstructive Sleep Apnea

Aidar R. Gosmanov, MD, PhD, DMSc
Section Chief, Endocrinology, Stratton VA Medical Center; Professor, Endocrinology, Albany Medical College, Albany, New York
Diabetic Ketoacidosis

Timothy P. Graham, MD, MHPE
Chief Medical Officer, Mount Carmel St. Ann's, Westerville, Ohio
Hypertension

Jane M. Grant-Kels, MD
Professor and Founding Chair Emeritus, Vice Chair and Founding Director, Cutaneous Oncology Center and Melanoma Program, Dermatology, University of Connecticut Health Center, Farmington, Connecticut; Adjunct Professor, Dermatology, University of Florida College of Medicine, Gainesville, Florida
Nevi

Kevin W. Gray, MD
Associate Professor, Community and Family Medicine, University of Missouri-Kansas City, Kansas City, Missouri
Asthma in Children

Kristine K. Grdinovac, MD
Associate Professor, Endocrinology, Metabolism, and Genetics; Director, Cray Diabetes Self-Management Center, University of Kansas Medical Center, Kansas City, Kansas
Diabetes Mellitus in Adults

Jenna Greenberg, MD
Assistant Professor, Family Medicine, University of Michigan Medicine Medical School, Ann Arbor, Michigan
Pericarditis

Leslie A. Greenberg, MD
Associate Professor, Family and Community Medicine, University of Nevada Reno School of Medicine, Reno, Nevada
Chronic Diarrhea

William M. Greene, MD
Associate Professor, Psychiatry, University of Florida College of Medicine, Gainesville, Florida
Drug Use Disorders

Joseph Greensher, MD
Professor, Pediatrics, Renaissance School of Medicine at Stony Brook University, Stony Brook, New York; Medical Director and Associate Chair, Department of Pediatrics, Long Island Regional Poison and Drug Information Center, Winthrop-University Hospital, Mineola, New York
Medical Toxicology

David S. Gregory, MD
Professor, Family and Community Medicine, Virginia Tech Carilion School of Medicine, Roanoke, Virginia
Resuscitation of the Newborn

Chad M. Gridley, MD
Assistant Professor, Urology, Duke University School of Medicine, Durham, North Carolina
Benign Prostatic Hyperplasia

Rebat M. Halder, MD
Professor Emeritus and Chairman Emeritus, Dermatology, Howard University College of Medicine, Washington, District of Columbia
Pigmentary Disorders

Alan M. Hall, MD
Associate Professor, Internal Medicine and Pediatrics, University of Kentucky College of Medicine, Lexington, Kentucky
Parenteral Fluid Therapy for Infants and Children

Kari R. Harris, MD
Professor, Pediatrics, University of Kansas School of Medicine-Wichita, Wichita, Kansas
Adolescent Health

Taylor B. Harrison, MD
Associate Professor, Neurology, Emory University School of Medicine, Atlanta, Georgia
Myasthenia Gravis

Adam L. Hartman, MD
Program Director, Division of Clinical Research, National Institute of Neurological Disorders and Stroke, National Institutes of Health, Rockville, Maryland
Epilepsy in Infants and Children

Erin Hayes, MD
Clinical Assistant Professor, Child and Adolescent Psychiatry, Medical University of South Carolina, Charleston, South Carolina
Attention-Deficit/Hyperactivity Disorder

Tara Heagle, PhD, RN
Assistant Professor, Hunter-Bellevue School of Nursing, Hunter College, New York, New York
Home Disaster Preparedness

Joel J. Heidelbaugh, MD
Professor, Department of Family Medicine, University of Michigan Medical School, Ann Arbor, Michigan
Erectile Dysfunction; Medical Toxicology

Molly A. Hinshaw, MD
Vice Chair, Clinical Operations, Professor, Dermatology, Affiliate Professor, Pathology, Section Chief of Dermatopathology, Director of Dermatology Nail Clinic, University of Wisconsin School of Medicine and Public Health, Madison, Wisconsin
Connective Tissue Disorders; Cutaneous Vasculitis

Brandon Hockenberry, MD
Head Team Physician, University of Health Sports Medicine, University of Nevada-Reno, Reno, Nevada
Sports-Related Head Injuries

Ray J. Hohl, MD, PhD
Director, Penn State Cancer Institute; Professor, Medicine and Pharmacology, Milton S. Hershey Medical Center, Penn State University, Hershey, Pennsylvania
Thalassemia

Therese Holguin, MD
Assistant Professor, Dermatology, University of New Mexico School of Medicine, Albuquerque, New Mexico
Fungal Infections of the Skin

Michael J. Holland, MD
Assistant Professor, Pediatrics, Children's Mercy Kansas City, Kansas City, Missouri
Juvenile Idiopathic Arthritis

Sarah A. Holstein, MD, PhD
Professor, Internal Medicine, University of Nebraska Medical Center, Omaha, Nebraska
Thalassemia

Michael Holyoak, DO
Physician, Idaho Endocrinology, Meridian, Idaho
Thyroid Cancer

Gretchen Homan, MD
Professor, Pediatrics, The University of Kansas School of Medicine-Wichita, Wichita, Kansas
Pediatric Failure to Thrive

Kevin Hommema, BSME
Principal Research Scientist, Battelle, Columbus, Ohio
Biologic Agents Reference Chart; Toxic Chemical Agents Reference Chart

Laurie A.M. Hommema, MD
Associate Program Director, Family Medicine Residency, Riverside Methodist Hospital; Medical Director, Well-Being, Quality and Patient Safety, OhioHealth, Columbus, Ohio
Biologic Agents Reference Chart; Toxic Chemical Agents Reference Chart

Justin L. Hoskin, MD
Assistant Professor, Neurology, Barrow Neurological Institute; Assistant Professor, Neurology, University of Arizona College of Medicine; Assistant Professor, Neurology, Creighton University, Phoenix, Arizona
Ménière's Disease

Ahmad Reza Hossani-Madani, MD
Dermatologist, Kaiser Permanente, Upper Marlboro, Maryland
Pigmentary Disorders

Steven A. House, MD
Professor, Family and Geriatric Medicine, University of Louisville/Glasgow Family Medicine Residency Program, Glasgow, Kentucky
Pain; Palliative and End-of-Life Care

Sarah Houssayni, MD
Medical Site Director, AltaMed, Goodrich Clinic, Los Angeles, California
Encopresis

Bethany Howlett, MD, MHS
Assistant Professor, Family Medicine and Community Health, University of Wisconsin School of Medicine and Public Health, Madison, Wisconsin
High-Altitude Illness

Richard Huettemann, MD
Chairman, Department of Pediatrics, Children's Medical Group Providence Hospital, Mobile, Alabama
Tumors of the Colon and Rectum

Alison N. Huffstetler, MD
Medical Director, Health Services Research, Robert Graham Center; Assistant Professor, Family Medicine, Georgetown University School of Medicine, Washington, District of Columbia; Assistant Professor, Family Medicine and Population Health, Virginia Commonwealth University School of Medicine, Richmond, Virginia
Bacterial Pneumonia

Anthony Hunter, MD
Assistant Professor, Hematology and Medical Oncology, Winship Cancer Institute of Emory University, Atlanta, Georgia
Acute Leukemia in Adults

Jacqueline Huynh, MD
Associate Program Director, Family and Community Medicine, Dignity Health East Valley Family Medicine Residency Program, Gilbert, Arizona
Chronic Diarrhea

Oyetokunbo Ibidapo-Obe, MD
Assistant Professor, Director Women's Health, Family Medicine, University of Texas Medical Branch at Galveston, Galveston, Texas
Infective Endocarditis

Gretchen Irwin, MD, MBA
Professor and Chair, Family and Community Medicine, University of Kansas School of Medicine-Wichita, Wichita, Kansas
Otitis Media

Daniel Isaac, DO
Assistant Professor, Medicine, Michigan State University College of Human Medicine, East Lansing, Michigan
Chronic Leukemias

Muaid Ithman, MD
Professor and Vice Chair for Clinical Operations, Psychiatry, University of Missouri, Columbia, Missouri
Depressive (Major) and Bipolar Disorders

Alan C. Jackson, MD
Adjunct Clinical Professor, Department of Clinical Neurosciences, Section of Neurology, Cumming School of Medicine, University of Calgary, Calgary, Alberta, Canada
Rabies

Caitlin Jackson-Tarlton, MD
Assistant Professor, Medicine, Dalhousie University Faculty of Medicine; Neurologist, Medicine; Assistant Director, Multiple Sclerosis Clinic, Nova Scotia Health, Halifax, Nova Scotia, Canada
Multiple Sclerosis

Kurt M. Jacobson, MD
Associate Professor, Cardiovascular Medicine, University of Wisconsin School of Medicine and Public Health, Madison, Wisconsin
Mitral Valve Prolapse

Jose A. Jaller, MD
Assistant Professor, Dr. Phillip Frost Department of Dermatology & Cutaneous Surgery, University of Miami Miller School of Medicine, Miami, Florida
Venous Ulcers

W. Ennis James, MD
Associate Professor, Pulmonary and Critical Care Medicine, Medical University of South Carolina, Charleston, South Carolina
Sarcoidosis

Lauren J. Jeang, MD
Assistant Professor, Ophthalmology, University of Florida College of Medicine, Gainesville, Florida
Dry Eye Syndrome

Deanna Jewell, DO
Assistant Professor, Pediatrics, University of Wisconsin School of Medicine and Public Health, Madison, Wisconsin
Rehabilitation of the Stroke Patient

Abhishek Jha, MBBS
Visiting Postdoctoral Fellow, Medical Neuroendocrinology, Eunice Kennedy Shriver National Institute of Child Health and Human Development, National Institutes of Health, Bethesda, Maryland
Pheochromocytoma

Joshua S. Jolissaint, MD
General Surgeon, Brigham and Women's Hospital, Harvard Medical School, Boston, Massachusetts
Pancreatic Cancer; Atelectasis

Alicia Julovich, MD
Associate Residency Program Director, Family Medicine Battle Creek; Assistant Professor, Family and Community Medicine, Homer Stryker MD School of Medicine, Western Michigan University, Kalamazoo, Michigan
Premalignant Skin Lesions

Tamilarasu Kadhiravan, MD
Professor, Medicine, Jawaharlal Institute of Postgraduate Medical Education and Research, Puducherry, India
Typhoid Fever

Sagar Kamprath, MD
Associate Professor, Family Medicine, University of Texas Medical Branch at Galveston, Galveston, Texas
Post-Acute COVID Syndrome

Jessica Rachel Kanter, MD
Shady Grove Fertility, Atlanta, Georgia
Infertility

Rudruidee Karnchanasorn, MD
Associate Professor, Internal Medicine, University of Kansas Medical Center, Kansas City, Kansas
Thyroid Cancer

Andreas Katsambas, MD, PhD
Emeritus Professor, Dermatology-Venereology, University of Athens; Professor, Dermatology, Hygeia Hospital, Athens, Greece
Parasitic Diseases of the Skin

Ben Z. Katz, MD
Professor, Pediatrics, Northwestern University Feinberg School of Medicine; Attending Physician, Division of Infectious Diseases, Ann & Robert H. Lurie Children's Hospital of Chicago, Chicago, Illinois
Infectious Mononucleosis

Rebecca Katzman, MD
Clinical Assistant Professor, Family Medicine, University of Washington School of Medicine, Seattle, Washington
Palpitations

Andrew M. Kaunitz, MD
Professor and Associate Chairman, Obstetrics and Gynecology, University of Florida College of Medicine-Jacksonville, Jacksonville, Florida
Menopause

Rick D. Kellerman, MD
Professor and Chair Emeritus, Department of Family and Community Medicine, University of Kansas School of Medicine-Wichita, Wichita, Kansas
Chikungunya; Mpox; Zika Virus Disease

Scott Kellermann, MD, MPH
Adjunct Professor, Public Health and Tropical Medicine, Tulane University School of Medicine, New Orleans, Louisiana; Clinical Professor, Clinical Sciences, California Northstate College of Medicine, Elk Grove, California; Adjunct Professor, Clinical Sciences, University of San Francisco School of Medicine, San Francisco, California
Chikungunya; Mpox; Zika Virus Disease

Christina M. Kelly, MD
Associate Professor, Family Medicine, Uniformed Services University of the Health Sciences, Bethesda, Maryland
Ectopic Pregnancy

Sheevaun Khaki, MD
Associate Professor, Pediatrics, Oregon Health & Science University, Portland, Oregon
Infant Hyperbilirubinemia

Morteza Khodaee, MD, MPH
Professor, Family Medicine and Orthopedics, University of Colorado School of Medicine, Denver, Colorado
Lung Abscess

Amelia Khoei, MD, MPH
Resident, Urology, University of Michigan Medical School, Ann Arbor, Michigan
Trauma to the Genitourinary Tract

Patrick Kicker, DO
Assistant Professor, Internal Medicine, Texas Tech University Health Sciences Center-El Paso, El Paso, Texas
Pulmonary Hypertension

Arthur Y. Kim, MD
Associate Professor, Medicine, Harvard Medical School, Boston, Massachusetts
Hepatitis C

Haejin Kim, MD
Senior Staff Allergist, Allergy and Clinical Immunology, Henry Ford Health System; Clinical Assistant Professor, Wayne State University School of Medicine, Detroit, Michigan
Hypersensitivity Pneumonitis

Jami A. Kinnucan, MD
Senior Associate Consultant, Chair, GI Clinical Practice, Gastroenterology & Hepatology, Mayo Clinic, Jacksonville, Florida
Inflammatory Bowel Disease: Crohn's Disease and Ulcerative Colitis

Robert S. Kirsner, MD, PhD
Chair and Harvey Blank Professor, Dr. Phillip Frost Department of Dermatology and Cutaneous Surgery, University of Miami Miller School of Medicine, Miami, Florida
Venous Ulcers

Sonam R. Kiwalkar, MBBS
Assistant Professor, Rheumatology, Washington State University; Associate Program Director, Legacy Salmon Creek; Rheumatologist, The Vancouver Clinic, Vancouver, Washington
Axial Spondyloarthritis

Christopher Klouzek, MD
Assistant Professor, Family and Preventive Medicine, The University of Oklahoma Health Sciences College of Medicine, Oklahoma City, Oklahoma
Constipation

Janice E. Knoefel, MD, MPH
Professor, Neurology and Internal Medicine (Geriatrics), University of New Mexico School of Medicine, Albuquerque, New Mexico
Alzheimer's Disease

Bhanu Prakash Kolla, MD
Center for Sleep Medicine, Mayo Clinic, Rochester, Minnesota
Sleep Disorders

Frederick Korley, MD
Robert E. Meyerhoff Assistant Professor of Emergency Medicine, The Johns Hopkins University School of Medicine; Staff, Johns Hopkins Medicine, Baltimore, Maryland
Disturbances Due to Cold

Mark Kraemer, MD
Neurosurgery, Swedish Health Services, Seattle, Washington
Central Nervous System Neoplasms

Megan Krause, MD
Associate Professor, Allergy, Clinical Immunology, and Rheumatology, University of Kansas School of Medicine, Kansas City, Kansas
Rheumatoid Arthritis

Lakshmanan Krishnamurti, MD
Chief of Pediatric Hematology, Oncology, and Bone Marrow Transplant, Yale School of Medicine, New Haven, Connecticut
Sickle Cell Disease

Kumar Krishnan, MD
Assistant Professor, Internal Medicine, Harvard Medical School, Boston, Massachusetts
Dysphagia and Esophageal Obstruction

Laura Kruger, MD
Clinical Assistant Professor, Family Medicine, University of Michigan Medical School, Ann Arbor, Michigan
Medical Toxicology

Zachary Kuhlmann, DO
Clinical Professor, Program Director, Obstetrics and Gynecology, University of Kansas School of Medicine-Wichita, Wichita, Kansas
Endometriosis

Roshni Kulkarni, MD
Professor and Director Emerita, MSU Center for Bleeding and Clotting Disorders, Pediatrics and Human Development, Michigan State University College of Human Medicine, East Lansing, Michigan
Hemophilia and Related Conditions

Seema Kumar, MD
Professor, Pediatric and Adolescent Medicine, Mayo Clinic, Rochester, Minnesota
Obesity in Children

Shaji Kumar, MD
Professor, Hematology, Mayo Clinic, Rochester, Minnesota
Multiple Myeloma

Sarah Kurz, MD
Clinical Assistant Professor, Internal Medicine, University of Michigan Medical School, Ann Arbor, Michigan
Q-Fever

Mary R. Kwaan, MD, MPH
Health Sciences Clinical Professor, Surgery, David Geffen School of Medicine at UCLA, Los Angeles, California
Hemorrhoids, Anal Fissure, and Anorectal Abscess and Fistula

Matthew Lambert, MD
Clinical Instructor, Infectious Disease, University of Wisconsin School of Medicine and Public Health, Madison, Wisconsin
Travel Medicine

Lucius M. Lampton, MD
Clinical Associate Professor, Family and Community Medicine, Tulane University School of Medicine, New Orleans, Louisiana, Clinical Professor, Family Medicine, William Carey University, Hattiesburg, Mississippi
Yellow Fever

Richard A. Lange, MD, MBA
President, Department of Medicine; Dean, Paul L. Foster School of Medicine, Texas Tech University Health Sciences Center El Paso, El Paso, Texas
Congenital Heart Disease

Fabienne Langlois, MD
Professor, Medicine, Endocrinology, Centre Hospitalier Universitaire de Sherbrooke, Sherbrooke, Quebec, Canada
Adrenocortical Insufficiency; Hypopituitarism

Christine L. Lau, MD
George Minor Professor of Surgery, University of Virginia Health System, Charlottesville, Virginia
Atelectasis

Susan Lawrence-Hylland, MD
Clinical Assistant Professor, Rheumatology, University of Wisconsin Hospital and Clinics, Madison, Wisconsin
Connective Tissue Disorders; Cutaneous Vasculitis

Jake Lazaroff, MD
Meramec Dermatology, Sunset Hills, Missouri
Nonmelanoma Cancer of the Skin

Dennis K. Ledford, MD
Ellsworth and Mabel Simmons Professor of Allergy and Immunology, Department of Internal Medicine, Morsani College of Medicine, University of South Florida, Tampa, Florida
Anaphylaxis

Lydia U. Lee, MD
Clinical Lecturer, Family Medicine, University of Michigan Medical School, Ann Arbor, Michigan
Postpartum Depression

Jerrold B. Leikin, MD
Consultant, Illinois Health and Hospital Association, Illinois Poison Center, Chicago, Illinois; Professor, Medicine, Rosalind, Franklin University/Chicago Medical School, North Chicago, Illinois
Disturbances Due to Cold

Scott Leikin, DO
Assistant Professor, Anesthesia and Critical Care Medicine, Baylor College of Medicine, Houston, Texas
Targeted Temperature Management (Therapeutic Hypothermia); Disturbances Due to Cold

Alexander K.C. Leung, MBBS
Clinical Professor, Pediatrics, University of Calgary Cumming School of Medicine; Pediatric Consultant, Pediatrics, Alberta Children's Hospital, Calgary, Alberta, Canada
Nocturnal Enuresis

Grace Levy-Clarke, MD
Associate Professor, Ophthalmology, West Virginia University School of Medicine, Morgantown, West Virginia
Uveitis

Ming Li, MD, PhD
Staff Physician, Medicine, Phoenix VA Medical Center; Clinical Assistant Professor, Medicine, University of Arizona College of Medicine, Phoenix, Arizona
Hyperlipidemia; Hyperprolactinemia

Tyler K. Liebenstein, PharmD
Clinical Pharmacist, Pharmacy, William S. Middleton Memorial Veterans Hospital, Madison, Wisconsin
Human Immunodeficiency Virus: Treatment and Prevention

Albert P. Lin, MD
Assistant Professor, Ophthalmology, Baylor College of Medicine; Staff Physician, Eye Care Line, Michael E. DeBakey Veterans Affairs Medical Center, Houston, Texas
Glaucoma

Jeffrey A. Linder, MD, MPH
Professor and Chief, General Internal Medicine, Northwestern University Feinberg School of Medicine, Chicago, Illinois
Influenza

Lauren Loeb, MD
Fellow, Gastroenterology, Mayo Clinic Florida, Jacksonville, Florida
Inflammatory Bowel Disease: Crohn's Disease and Ulcerative Colitis

M. Chantel Long, MD
Clinical Assistant Professor, Family and Community Medicine, University of Kansas School of Medicine-Wichita; Staff Physician, Concierge Primary Care Clinic, Ascension Via Christi, Wichita, Kansas
Condylomata Acuminata; Warts (Verrucae)

Colleen Loo-Gross, MD, MPH
Associate Professor, Family and Community Medicine, University of Kansas School of Medicine-Wichita, Wichita, Kansas
Amenorrhea

Julia R. Lubsen, MD
Associate Professor, Family Medicine and Community Health, University of Wisconsin School of Medicine and Public Health, Madison, Wisconsin
Pyelonephritis

Ronda Lun, MD
Clinical Assistant Professor, Neurology, The Ottawa Hospital, Ottawa, Ontario, Canada
Intracerebral Hemorrhage

Matthew Macaluso, DO
Professor and Vice Chair, Psychiatry, UAB School of Medicine, University of Alabama-Birmingham, Birmingham, Alabama
Depressive (Major) and Bipolar Disorders; Obsessive-Compulsive Disorder

David A. Mahvi, MD
Assistant Professor, Surgery, Harvard Medical School, Beth Israel Deaconess Medical Center, Boston, Massachusetts
Tumors of the Stomach

RosaMarie Maiorella, MD
Assistant Professor, Pediatrics, University of Cincinnati College of Medicine, Cincinnati, Ohio
Viral Meningitis

Jonathan Maldonado, MD
Assistant Professor, Urology, Kansas University Medical Center, Kansas City, Missouri
Hematuria

Uma Malhotra, MD
Clinical Professor, Infectious Diseases, University of Washington School of Medicine, Seattle, Washington
Ebola Virus Disease

Emily Manlove, MD
Associate Program Director, Elizabeth Family Medicine, Atrium Health, Charlotte, North Carolina
Cough

JoAnn E. Manson, MD, DrPH
Chief, Division of Preventive Medicine, Bringham and Women's Hospital; Professor of Medicine and the Michael and Lee Bell Professor of Women's Health, Harvard Medical School, Boston, Massachusetts
Menopause

Meghna P. Mansukhani, MD
Professor, Center for Sleep Medicine, Mayo Clinic, Rochester, Minnesota
Sleep Disorders

Claudio Marcocci, MD
Professor, Endocrinology, Clinical and Experimental Medicine, University of Pisa, Pisa, Italy
Hyperparathyroidism and Hypoparathyroidism

Jason E. Marker, MD, MPA
Associate Director, Memorial Family Medicine Residency, Memorial Hospital, South Bend, Indiana
Neurofibromatosis (Type 1)

Paul Martin, MD
Chief, Gastroenterology/Hepatology, University of Miami Miller School of Medicine, Miami, Florida
Cirrhosis

Kristin Matson, MD, MPH, CTropMed
Clinical Professor, Division of Infectious Disease, University of Wisconsin Hospital and Clinics, Madison, Wisconsin
Travel Medicine

Mark A. Matza, MD, MBA
Clinical Director, Rheumatology, Massachusetts General Hospital; Instructor in Medicine, Harvard Medical School, Boston, Massachusetts
Polymyalgia Rheumatica and Giant Cell Arteritis

Pinckney J. Maxwell IV, MD
Associate Professor, Colon and Rectal Surgery, Medical University of South Carolina, Charleston, South Carolina
Tumors of the Colon and Rectum

Danica May, MD
Assistant Professor, Urologic Oncology and Urology, University of Kansas Medical Center, Kansas City, Kansas
Malignant Tumors of the Urogenital Tract

Marshall Mazepa, MD
Associate Professor, Hematology, Oncology, and Transplantation, University of Minnesota Medical School, Minneapolis, Minnesota
Porphyrias

Molly McClain, MD, MPH
Associate Professor, Program Director, Family and Community Medicine, University of New Mexico School of Medicine, Albuquerque, New Mexico
Gender-Affirming Care

Christopher McGrew, MD
Professor, Family and Community Medicine, Orthopedics and Rehabilitation, Sports Medicine, University of New Mexico Health Sciences Center, Albuquerque, New Mexico
Sports-Related Head Injuries

†Michael McGuigan, MD
Professor, Pediatrics and Pharmacology, University of Toronto Faculty of Medicine; Medical Director, Ontario Poison Control Center, Toronto, Ontario, Canada
Medical Toxicology

Stephanie Trentacoste McNally, MD
Director, OB/GYN Services, North Shore University Hospital, Manhasset, New York
Premenstrual Dysphoric Disorder

Meetal Mehta, MD
Nutrition Support Service Attending, Surgery; Obesity Medicine Physician, Endocrinology, Diabetes, and Hypertension, Brigham and Women's Hospital, Boston, Massachusetts
Parenteral Nutrition in Adults

Mick S. Meiselman, MD
Director, Advanced Therapeutic Endoscopy, Gastroenterology; Dignity Health Central Coast, San Luis Obispo, California
Calculous Biliary Disease

Moises Mercado, MD
Director, Endocrine Research Unit, Hospital de Especialidades, Centro Medico Nacional S.XXI, IOMSS; Professor, Medicine, Faculty of Medicine, Universidad Nacional Autónoma de Mexico, Mexico City, Mexico
Acromegaly

William Michael, MD
Assistant Professor, Family Medicine and Community Health, University of Wisconsin School of Medicine and Public Health, Madison, Wisconsin
Peripheral Arterial Disease

Brian J. Miller, MD, PhD, MPH
Professor, Psychiatry and Health Behavior, Augusta University Medical College of Georgia, Augusta, Georgia
Schizophrenia

Moben Mirza, MD
Professor, Urology, University of Kansas Medical Center, Kansas City, Kansas
Hematuria; Malignant Tumors of the Urogenital Tract

†Deceased.

Kriti Mishra, MD
Central Dermatology Center, Chapel Hill, North Carolina
Fungal Infections of the Skin

Howard C. Mofenson, MD
Professor, Pharmacology and Toxicology, New York College of Osteopathic Medicine, Old Westbury, New York; Professor, Pediatrics and Emergency Medicine, Renaissance School of Medicine at Stony Brook University, Stony Brook, New York
Medical Toxicology

Kris M. Mogensen, MS
Team Leader Dietitian Specialist, Nutrition, Brigham and Women's Hospital, Boston, Massachusetts
Parenteral Nutrition in Adults

Vincent Morelli, MD
Associate Professor, Family and Community Medicine; Director, Sports Medicine Fellowship, Meharry Medical College, Nashville, Tennessee
Artificial Intelligence and Primary Care

Michael L. Moritz, MD
Professor, Pediatrics, UPMC Children's Hospital of Pittsburgh, Pittsburgh, Pennsylvania
Parenteral Fluid Therapy for Infants and Children

Cathleen E. Morrow, MD
Associate Professor, Community and Family Medicine, Dartmouth Hitchcock Medical Center, Lebanon, New Hampshire
Female Sexual Concerns

Rami Mortada, MD
Physician, Endocrine Center of Kansas, Wichita, Kansas
Diabetes Insipidus

Salama Mostafa, MBBCh
Fellow, Pediatric Endocrinology, Mayo Clinic, Rochester, Minnesota
Obesity in Children

Judd W. Moul, MD
James H. Semans, MD, Professor, Urologic Surgery, Duke University School of Medicine, Durham, North Carolina
Benign Prostatic Hyperplasia

Martha Muller, MD
Professor, Pediatrics, University of New Mexico School of Medicine, Albuquerque, New Mexico
Bacterial Meningitis

Natalia Murinova, MD
Clinical Professor; Director, Headache Clinic, Neurology, University of Washington School of Medicine, Seattle, Washington
Migraine

Michael Murphy, MD
Professor and Dermatopathologist, Dermatology, UConn Health, Farmington, Connecticut
Nevi

Arjun Muthusubramanian, MD, MPH
Medical Director, Enterprise Clinical Services, Optum, Richmond, Virginia
Bacterial Pneumonia

Kyle Myers, DO
Assistant Professor, Endocrinology, University of Kansas, Kansas City, Kansas
Hyperthyroidism

Alykhan S. Nagji, MD
Assistant Professor, Thoracic Surgery, University of Kansas Medical Center, Kansas City, Kansas
Atelectasis

Brian James Nagle, MD, MPH
Assistant Professor, Neurology, University of Wisconsin School of Medicine and Public Health, Madison, Wisconsin
Parkinson Disease

Rabab Nasim, MD
Attending Physician, Pulmonary and Critical Care Medicine, University of Wisconsin School of Medicine and Public Health, Madison, Wisconsin
Sepsis

Matthew A. Nazari, MD
Clinical Researcher, Eunice Kennedy Shriver National Institute of Child Health and Human Development, National Institutes of Health, Bethesda, Maryland
Pheochromocytoma

Moniba Nazeef, MD
Assistant Professor, Hematology and Oncology, University of Wisconsin School of Medicine and Public Health, Madison, Wisconsin
Venous Thromboembolism

Viswanathan K. Neelakantan, MD
Consultant in Internal Medicine, Faculty of Medicine, Kovai Medical Centre Hospital and Research Institute, Coimbatore, Tamil Nadu, India; Former Senior Professor of Medicine, Consultant in Tropical Medicine, Faculty of Medicine, Sri Manakula Vinayagar Medical College Hospital, Pondicherry, India
Foodborne Illnesses

Donald A. Neff, MD
Associate Professor, Urology, University of Kansas School of Medicine, Kansas City, Kansas
Urinary Tract Infections in the Male

Tara J. Neil, MD
Associate Professor, Family and Community Medicine, University of Kansas School of Medicine-Wichita, Wichita, Kansas
Postpartum Care

William G. Nelson, MD, PhD
Professor and Director, Sidney Kimmel Comprehensive Cancer Center, Johns Hopkins University School of Medicine, Baltimore, Maryland
Prostate Cancer

David G. Neschis, MD
Clinical Associate Professor, Surgery, The Maryland Vascular Center, University of Maryland Baltimore Washington Medical Center, Glen Burnie, Maryland
Aortic Disease: Aneurysm and Dissection

Theresa Nester, MD
Professor, Laboratory Medicine and Pathology, University of Washington Medical Center; Medical Director of Integrated Transfusion Services, Bloodworks Northwest, Seattle, Washington
Blood Component Therapy and Transfusion Reactions

Tam T. Nguyen, MD
Clinician and Instructor, Family Medicine, Washington Township Medical Group, Fremont, California
Papulosquamous Eruptions

Deirdre Nolfi-Donegan, MD
Assistant Professor, Pediatrics, University of Pittsburgh School of Medicine, Pittsburgh, Pennsylvania
Platelet-Mediated Bleeding Disorders

Crystal M. North, MD, MPH
Physician, Pulmonary and Critical Care Medicine, Massachusetts General Hospital; Assistant Professor, Medicine, Harvard Medical School, Boston, Massachusetts
Monoclonal Antibodies

Enrico M. Novelli, MD
Associate Professor, Medicine, University of Pittsburgh School of Medicine, Pittsburgh, Pennsylvania
Sickle Cell Disease

Lauren Nye, MD
Associate Professor, Medical Oncology, University of Kansas, School of Medicine, Kansas City, Kansas
Benign Breast Disease; Breast Cancer

Andrea T. Obi, MD
Assistant Professor, Surgery, University of Michigan Medical School, Ann Arbor, Michigan
Venous Thrombosis

Marie Claire O'Dwyer, MBBCh, BAO, MPH
Clinical Assistant Professor, Family Medicine, University of Michigan Medical School, Ann Arbor, Michigan
Pleural Effusion and Empyema

Linda K. Oge, MD
Section Chief, Family Medicine, Ochsner Lafayette General Medical Center, Lafayette, Louisiana
Acne Vulgaris

Jeffrey Paul Okeson, DMD
Professor and Dean, Oral Health Science, University of Kentucky, Lexington, Kentucky
Temporomandibular Disorders

Carlos R. Oliveira, MD, PhD
Assistant Professor, Pediatrics, Yale School of Medicine; Assistant Professor, Biostatistics, Yale School of Public Health, New Haven, Connecticut
Post-COVID-19 Multisystem Inflammatory Syndrome in Children

Peck Y. Ong, MD
Associate Professor, Pediatrics, USC/Children's Hospital Los Angeles, Los Angeles, California
Atopic Dermatitis

Maria Theresa Opina, MD
Assistant Professor, Internal Medicine, Texas Tech University Health Science Center-El Paso, El Paso, Texas
Pulmonary Hypertension

Daniel Stephen Oram, MD
Adjunct Assistant Professor, Family Medicine, University of Michigan Medical School, Ann Arbor, Michigan
Postpartum Depression

David D. Ortiz, MD
Academic Director, Medical Residency Programs, National Health Institute, Asunción, Paraguay
Leg Edema and Venous Stasis

Sabah Osmani, MD
Resident, Dermatology, University of North Carolina School of Medicine, Chapel Hill, North Carolina
Fungal Infections of the Skin

Brady Otten, MD
Pulmonary and Critical Care Medicine, Cleveland Clinic, Cleveland, Ohio
Sarcoidosis

Bulent Ozgonenel, MD
Associate Professor, Pediatric Hematology Oncology, Children's Hospital of Michigan, Detroit, Michigan
Hemophilia and Related Conditions

Karel Pacak, MD, PhD, DSc
Chief, Section on Medical Neuroendocrinology, Eunice Kennedy Shriver National Institute of Child Health and Human Development, National Institutes of Health, Bethesda, Maryland
Pheochromocytoma

Andrew Pap, MD
Cardiovascular Fellow, Cardiology, University of Wisconsin Hospitals and Clinics, Madison, Wisconsin
Mitral Valve Prolapse

Jose A. Padin-Rosado, MD
Associate Professor, Neurology; Medical Director, Neurodiagnostic Laboratory, University of New Mexico School of Medicine, Albuquerque, New Mexico
Seizures and Epilepsy in Adolescents and Adults

Tanyatuth Padungkiatsagul, MD
Associate Professor, Ophthalmology, Faculty of Medicine, Ramathibodi Hospital, Mahidol University, Bangkok, Thailand
Optic Neuritis

Heather L. Paladine, MD, MEd
Assistant Professor, Medicine, Columbia University Medical Center, Center for Family and Community Medicine, Columbia College of Physicians and Surgeons; New York, New York
Vulvovaginitis

John E. Pandolfino, MD
Hans Popper Professor of Medicine, Northwestern University Feinberg School of Medicine, Chicago, Illinois
Dysphagia and Esophageal Obstruction

Bumsoo Park, MD, PhD
Clinical Assistant Professor, Family Medicine and Urology, University of Michigan Medical School, Ann Arbor, Michigan
Tetanus

Marc Parrish, DO
Professor, Obstetrics and Gynecology; Division Director, Maternal-Fetal Medicine; Fellowship Director, Maternal-Fetal Medicine, University of Kansas Medical Center, Kansas City, Kansas
Hypertensive Disorders in Pregnancy

Deval Patel, MD
Pediatric Hospitalist, Hospital Pediatrics, Nemours Children's Specialty Care; Associate Program Director, Department of Pediatrics, University of Florida College of Medicine-Jacksonville, Jacksonville, Florida
Parenteral Fluid Therapy for Infants and Children

Hirenkumar Patel, MD
Assistant Professor, Pediatric Neonatology, Virginia Tech Carilion School of Medicine; Assistant Medical Director, Pediatric Neonatology, Pediatrix Medical Group, Roanoke, Virginia
Resuscitation of the Newborn

Simon Patton, MD
Clinical Associate Professor and Assistant Residency Program Director, Obstetrics and Gynecology, University of Kansas School of Medicine-Wichita; Female Pelvic Medicine and Reconstructive Surgery, Ascension Via Christi, Wichita, Kansas
Urinary Incontinence

Gerson O. Penna, PhD
Medical and Senior Researcher of the Tropical Medicine Center, University of Brazil, Brasilia, Brazil
Leprosy

Maria Lucia Penna, MD, PhD
Professor, Epidemiology and Biostatistics, Universidade Federal Fluminense, Niteroi, Rio de Janeiro, Brazil
Leprosy

Jamie Peregrine, MD, MS
Clinical Assistant Professor, Obstetrics and Gynecology, Division of Reproductive Endocrinology and Infertility, University of Kansas School of Medicine-Wichita, Wichita, Kansas
Uterine Leiomyoma

Allen Perkins, MD, MPH
Professor and Chair, Family Medicine, University of South Alabama College of Medicine, Mobile, Alabama
Marine Poisonings, Envenomations, and Trauma

Michael Persinger Jr., MD
Resident Physician, Family Medicine, University of Colorado Anschutz School of Medicine, Aurora, Colorado
Lung Abscess

Hanna Phan, PharmD
Clinical Associate Professor, Clinical Pharmacy, University of Michigan; Clinical Pharmacist Specialist, Pediatric Pulmonary, Pharmacy Innovations and Partnerships, C.S. Mott Children's, Michigan Medicine; Faculty Affiliate, Susan B. Meister Child Health Evaluation and Research Center, University of Michigan, Ann Arbor, Michigan
Cystic Fibrosis

Mark Pietroni, MD, MBA
Medical Director, Medical Directorate, Gloucestershire Hospitals NHS FT, Gloucester, United Kingdom
Cholera

Gregory A. Plotnikoff, MD, MTS
Founder and Medical Director, Internal Medicine and Pediatrics, Minnesota Personalized Medicine, Minneapolis, Minnesota
Genomic Testing

Jennifer K. Poon, MD
Professor, Pediatrics, Augusta University Medical College of Georgia, Augusta, Georgia
Attention-Deficit/Hyperactivity Disorder

Andrew S.T. Porter, DO
Director of Sports Medicine Fellowship; Clinical Associate Professor, Family and Community Medicine, University of Kansas School of Medicine-Wichita, Wichita, Kansas
Common Sports Injuries

Charles Powell, MD
Associate Professor, Urology, Indiana University School of Medicine, Indianapolis, Indiana
Prostatitis

Margaret Pusateri, MD
Sports Medicine, Emergency Medicine, Pittsburgh, Pennsylvania
Sports-Related Head Injuries

James M. Quinn, MD
Associate Program Director, Allergy/Immunology, San Antonio Uniformed Service Health Education Consortium, San Antonio, Texas; Professor, Medicine, Uniformed Services University of the Health Sciences, Bethesda, Maryland
Allergic Reactions to Insect Stings

Peter S. Rahko, MD
Professor, Medicine, University of Wisconsin School of Medicine and Public Health; Director, Adult Echocardiography Laboratory, University of Wisconsin Hospital, Madison, Wisconsin
Mitral Valve Prolapse

S. Vincent Rajkumar, MD
Edward W. and Betty Knight Scripps Professor of Medicine, Hematology, Mayo Clinic, Rochester, Minnesota
Multiple Myeloma

Anand Rajpara, MD
Professor and Founding Chair, Department of Dermatology, University Health/University of Missouri School of Medicine-Kansas City, Kansas City, Missouri
Autoimmune Bullous Diseases; Pyoderma Gangrenosum

Kalyanakrishnan Ramakrishnan, MD
Professor, Family and Preventive Medicine, University of Oklahoma Health Sciences Center, Oklahoma City, Oklahoma
Necrotizing Skin and Soft-Tissue Infections

Rajan Ramanathan, MD
Staff Urologist, Urology, Department of Surgery, Chalmers P Wylie VA Ambulatory Care Center, Columbus, Ohio
Nephrolithiasis

Jatin Rana, MD
Associate Professor, Hematology/Oncology, Michigan State University College of Human Medicine, East Lansing, Michigan
Chronic Leukemias

Matthew A. Rank, MD
Professor, Allergy, Asthma, and Clinical Immunology, Mayo Clinic, Scottsdale, Arizona
Asthma in Adolescents and Adults

Alwyn Rapose, MD
Chief, Infectious Diseases, Reliant Medical Group; Assistant Professor, Medicine, UMass Chan Medical School, Worcester, Massachusetts
Toxic Shock Syndrome

Rachel E. Rau, MD
Associate Professor, Pediatrics, Baylor College of Medicine, Houston, Texas
Acute Leukemia in Children

Anita Devi K. Ravindran, MD
Physician, Microbiology, Manipal University College Melaka, Melaka Tengah, Malaysia
Foodborne Illness

Robert L. Redner, MD
Professor, Malignant Hematology and Medical Oncology, UPMC Hillman Cancer Center, University of Pittsburgh School of Medicine, Pittsburgh, Pennsylvania
Megaloblastic Anemias

Jared Regehr, MD
Assistant Professor, Family and Community Medicine, University of Kansas School of Medicine-Wichita, Wichita, Kansas
Fatigue; Hypothyroidism

Ian R. Reid, MBChB, MD
Distinguished Professor, Medicine, University of Auckland Faculty of Medical and Health Sciences, Auckland, New Zealand
Paget's Disease of Bone

Elissa Rennert-May, MD, MSc
Assistant Professor, Infectious Diseases, Medicine, University of Calgary Cumming School of Medicine, Calgary, Canada
Methicillin-Resistant Staphylococcus aureus

Karl T. Rew, MD
Clinical Associate Professor, Family Medicine and Urology, University of Michigan Medical School, Ann Arbor, Michigan
Erectile Dysfunction

Joanna M. Rhodes, MD, MSCE
Director, Lymphoma Program, Rutgers Robert Wood Johnson Medical School, Rutgers University, New Brunswick, New Jersey
Non-Hodgkin Lymphoma

Amanda Rhyne, MD
Clinical Assistant Professor, Family and Community Medicine, University of Kansas School of Medicine-Wichita, Salina, Kansas
Serum Sickness

Martha E. Riese, MD
Clinical Assistant Professor, Family and Community Medicine, University of Kansas School of Medicine-Wichita, Salina, Kansas
Varicella (Chickenpox)

Sophie Robert, PharmD
Clinical Pharmacy Specialist, Psychiatry; Affiliate Faculty, Psychiatry and Behavioral Sciences, Medical University of South Carolina, Charleston, South Carolina
Attention-Deficit/Hyperactivity Disorder

Amy Robertson, PharmD
Assistant Professor, Pharmacy Practice, University of Arkansas–Northwest Campus; Clinical Pharmacist, Family Medicine, UAMS Health Family Medical Center Fayetteville, Fayetteville, Arkansas
Serum Sickness

Malcolm K. Robinson, MD
Associate Professor, Surgery, Harvard Medical School; Attending Physician, Metabolic Support Service, Brigham and Women's Hospital, Boston, Massachusetts
Parenteral Nutrition in Adults

William P. Roche, MD
Neurology Associates, Macon, Georgia
Myasthenia Gravis

Tanya Rodgers, MD
Clinical Instructor, Family Medicine, University of Michigan Health, Ann Arbor, Michigan
Salmonellosis

Tessa E. Rohrberg, MD
Associate Professor, Family and Community Medicine, University of Kansas School of Medicine-Wichita, Wichita, Kansas
Delirium

Candice E. Rose, MD, MS
Assistant Professor, Internal Medicine, The University of Kansas Health System, Kansas City, Kansas
Diabetes Mellitus in Adults

Stephen Ross, MD
Professor and Vice Chair, Neurology, Penn State University, Hershey, Pennsylvania
Nonmigraine Headache

Alan R. Roth, DO
Chairman, Family Medicine and Ambulatory Care, Jamaica Hospital Medical Center, Jamaica, New York; Assistant Professor, Family and Social Medicine, Albert Einstein College of Medicine, Bronx, New York; Professor, Family Medicine, NYIT College of Osteopathic Medicine, Old Westbury, New York; Chief, Integrative Pain and Palliative Care, Medisys Health Network, Jamaica, New York
Fever

Anne-Michelle Ruha, MD
Chief, Medical Toxicology, Banner–University Medical Center Phoenix; Professor, Internal Medicine and Emergency Medicine, University of Arizona College of Medicine, Phoenix, Arizona
Spider Bites and Scorpion Stings; Venomous Snakebite

Arlene M. Ruiz de Luzuriaga, MD, MPH, MBA
Associate Professor, Medicine, Biological Sciences Division, University of Chicago, Chicago, Illinois
Melanoma

Kristen Rundell, MD, MS
Professor and Chair, Department of Family and Community Medicine, University of Arizona College of Medicine, Tucson, Arizona
Drug Hypersensitivity Reactions; Mumps

Adnan Said, MD, MS
Professor, Medicine, Gastroenterology and Hepatology, University of Wisconsin School of Medicine and Public Health, Madison, Wisconsin
Metabolic Dysfunction-Associated Steatotic Liver Disease (MASLD)

Tomoko Sairenji, MD, MS
Associate Professor, Family Medicine, University of Washington School of Medicine, Seattle, Washington
Acute Bronchitis and Other Viral Respiratory Infections

Susan L. Samson, MD, PhD
Professor and Chair, Medicine/Endocrinology, Mayo Clinic, Jacksonville, Florida
Hyponatremia

Carlos E. Sanchez, MD
Faculty, Interventional Cardiology and Advanced Structural Heart Disease, Internal Medicine, Riverside Methodist Hospital, Columbus, Ohio
Valvular Heart Disease

Sunny Sandhu, MD
Clinical Assistant Professor, Gastroenterology and Hepatology, Stanford Digestive Health Center, Stanford Medicine, Pleasanton, California
Cirrhosis

Sandeep Sangodkar, DO
Cardiologist, Cardiology Specialists Medical Group; Assistant Clinical Professor, Internal Medicine/Cardiology, University of California, Riverside, School of Medicine, Riverside, California; Clinical Assistant Professor, Internal Medicine/Cardiology, Western University, Pomona, California
Hypertrophic Cardiomyopathy

Ravi Sarode, MD
Director, Division of Transfusion and Hemostasis, Professor of Pathology, UT Southwestern Medical Center, Dallas, Texas
Thrombotic Thrombocytopenic Purpura

Michael Schatz, MD, MS
Physician, Allergy, Kaiser Permanente; Clinical Professor, Medicine, University of California San Diego School of Medicine, San Diego, California
Asthma in Adolescents and Adults

Alex Schevchuck, MD, MS
Associate Professor, Internal Medicine/Cardiology, University of New Mexico School of Medicine, Albuquerque, New Mexico
Congestive Heart Failure; Tachycardias

Lawrence R. Schiller, MD
Chair, Institutional Review Boards, Baylor Scott & White Research Institute, Baylor University Medical Center; Clinical Professor, Medical Education, Texas A&M School of Medicine, Dallas Campus, Dallas, Texas
Malabsorption

Darren Schmidt, MD
Assistant Professor, Medicine; Clinical Nephrologist, University of New Mexico Health Sciences Center, Albuquerque, New Mexico
Chronic Kidney Disease

Sarina Schrager, MD, MS
Professor, Family Medicine, University of Wisconsin School of Medicine and Public Health, Madison, Wisconsin
Abnormal Uterine Bleeding

Dan Schuller, MD
Professor, Medicine, Texas Tech University Health Science Center; Chair, Department of Medicine-Transmoutain, Texas Tech University Health Sciences Center, El Paso, Texas
Lung Abscess; Pulmonary Hypertension

Teresa Sciortino, MD
St. Lukes Endocrinology Specialists, Saint Luke's Health System, Kansas City, Missouri
Thyroid Cancer

Brian Scott, DO
Assistant Professor, Infectious Diseases, The University of Oklahoma Health Sciences Center, Oklahoma City, Oklahoma
Plague

Cassie Scripter, MD
Assistant Professor, Family and Community Medicine, University of Kansas School of Medicine-Wichita, Wichita, Kansas
Rosacea

Justin Seashore, MD
Physician, Pulmonary and Critical Care, Kaiser Permanente, Vacaville, California
Post-Acute COVID Syndrome

Wafik George Sedhom, MD
Assistant Professor, Hematology/Oncology, Northwestern University Feinberg School of Medicine, Chicago, Illinois
Myelodysplastic Syndromes

†Steven Seifert, MD
Professor, Emergency Medicine, University of New Mexico School of Medicine; Medical Director, New Mexico Poison and Drug Information Center, University of New Mexico Health Sciences Center, Albuquerque, New Mexico
Venomous Snakebite

Jeffery D. Semel, MD
Physician, Infectious Diseases, Medicine, NorthShore University Healthsystem, Evanston, Illinois; Associate Professor, Clinical Medicine, University of Chicago Pritzker School of Medicine, Chicago, Illinois
Clostridioides difficile Colitis

Saeed Kamran Shaffi, MD, MS
Senior Associate Consultant, Internal Medicine/Nephrology, University of New Mexico School of Medicine, Albuquerque, New Mexico
Primary Glomerular Disease

Beejal Shah, MD
Endocrinologist, Bay Pines VA, Bay Pines, Florida
Hyponatremia

Meera Shah, MBChB
Assistant Professor, Endocrinology, Diabetes, and Nutrition, Mayo Clinic, Rochester, Minnesota
Obesity in Adults

Prediman K. Shah, MD
Professor, Medicine, University of California Los Angeles Cedars-Sinai Medical Center; Shapell and Webb Chair in Clinical Cardiology, Director of Oppenheimer Atherosclerosis Research Center and Atherosclerosis Prevention and Treatment Center, Smidt Heart Institute, Cedars-Sinai Medical Center, Los Angeles, California
Acute Myocardial Infarction

Jamile M. Shammo, MD
Professor, Medicine, Hematology, Oncology, and Stem Cell Transplant, Rush University Medical Center, Chicago, Illinois
Myelodysplastic Syndromes

Eugene D. Shapiro, MD
Professor, Pediatrics, Epidemiology of Microbial Diseases and Investigative Medicine, Yale School of Medicine, New Haven, Connecticut
Lyme Disease and Post-Treatment Lyme Disease Syndrome

†Deceased.

Ala I. Sharara, MD
Professor, Internal Medicine, American University of Beirut Medical Center, Beirut, Lebanon
Bleeding Esophageal Varices

Sonal Sharma, MD
Attending Physician, Mitochondrial Medicine Frontier Program, Children's Hospital of Philadelphia, Philadelphia, Pennsylvania
Mitochondrial Disease

John P. Sheehan, MD
Professor, Medicine/Hematology-Oncology, University of Wisconsin School of Medicine and Public Health; Medical Director, UW Health Comprehensive Bleeding Disorders Program, University of Wisconsin Hospital and Clinics; Medical Director, UWHC Special Coagulation Laboratory, UW Health, Madison, Wisconsin
Venous Thromboembolism

Kamille S. Sherman, MD
Associate Professor, Family and Community Medicine, University of North Dakota School of Medicine and Health Sciences, Grand Forks, North Dakota
Sunburn

Carol Shetty, MD
Assistant Professor, Family Medicine, Michigan Medicine, Ann Arbor, Michigan
Leishmaniasis

Sable Shew, MD
Urologist, Parkview Health, Fort Wayne, Indiana
Urethral Stricture Disease

Victor S. Sierpina, MD
Professor, Family and Integrative Medicine, University of Texas Medical Branch at Galveston, Galveston, Texas
Post-Acute COVID Syndrome

Karlynn Sievers, MD
Associate Program Director, Family Medicine, St. Mary's Family Medicine Residency, Grand Junction, Colorado
Trigeminal Neuralgia

Hugh Silk, MD, MPH
Professor, Family Medicine and Community Health, UMass Chan Medical School, Worcester, Massachusetts
Trigeminal Neuralgia; Diseases of the Mouth

Lisa Simon, MD, DMD
Assistant Professor, Department of Medicine, Brigham and Women's Hospital, Boston, Massachusetts
Diseases of the Mouth

Aaron D. Sinclair, MD
Associate Professor, Family and Community Medicine, University of Kansas School of Medicine-Wichita, Wichita, Kansas
Diverticula of the Alimentary Tract

Dawd S. Siraj, MD, MPHTM
Professor, Infectious Diseases, University of Wisconsin School of Medicine and Public Health, Madison, Wisconsin
Travel Medicine

Jeannina Smith, MD
Professor, Clinical Health Sciences, University of Wisconsin School of Medicine and Public Health, Madison, Wisconsin
Sepsis

Rupal Soder, PhD
Project Director, Midwest Stem Cell Therapy Center, University of Kansas Medical Center, Kansas City, Kansas
Stem Cell Therapy

John Sojka, MD
Associate Professor, Director of Orthopedic Trauma, Orthopedic Surgery, University of Kansas Health System, Kansas City, Kansas
Osteomyelitis

Robert Solomon, MD
Physician, Cardiology, University of Michigan Health, Ann Arbor, Michigan
Congestive Heart Failure

Mihae Song, MD
Assistant Professor, Gynecologic Oncology, City of Hope, Duarte, California
Ovarian Cancer

Timothy Sowder, MD
Assistant Professor, Pain Medicine, University of Kansas Health System, Kansas City, Kansas
Fibromyalgia

Chandler Sparks, DO, MPH
Faculty Physician, Family Medicine, AdventHealth Family Medicine Residency, Orlando, Florida
Cancer of the Uterine Cervix

Linda Speer, MD
Professor, Family Medicine, University of Toledo College of Medicine and Life Sciences, Toledo, Ohio
Dysmenorrhea

Stephanie Spivack, MD
Assistant Professor of Medicine, Internal Medicine, Temple University Hospital, Philadelphia Pennsylvania
Malaria; Psittacosis

Erik Kent St. Louis, MD
Professor, Neurology and Medicine, Mayo Clinic, Rochester, Minnesota
Sleep Disorders

Todd Stephens, MD, DTMH
Clinical Associate Professor, Family and Community Medicine, University of Kansas School of Medicine-Wichita, Wichita, Kansas
Genital Ulcer Disease: Chancroid, Granuloma Inguinale, and Lymphogranuloma

Melissa Stiles, MD
Professor, Family Medicine, University of Wisconsin School of Medicine and Public Health, Madison, Wisconsin
Pyelonephritis

Constantine A. Stratakis, MD, PhD
Scientific Director, Eunice Kennedy Shriver National Institute of Child Health and Human Development, National Institutes of Health, Bethesda, Maryland
Cushing Syndrome

Daniel Stulberg, MD
Professor and Chair, Family and Community Medicine, Western Michigan University Homer Stryker M.D. School of Medicine, Kalamazoo, Michigan
Premalignant Skin Lesions

Masayoshi Takashima, MD
Professor and Chair, Otolaryngology–Head and Neck Surgery, Houston Methodist Hospital, Houston, Texas
Rhinitis; Obstructive Sleep Apnea

Varun Takyar, MD
Staff Gastroenterologist/Hepatologist, Sutter Health East Bay Medical Foundation, Berkeley, California
Hepatitis A, B, D, and E

Carolina Talhari, MD, PhD
Adjunct Professor, Dermatology, State University of Amazonas; Dermatologist, Alfredo da Matta Foundation, Manaus, Brazil
Leprosy

Jie Tang, MD
Associate Professor, Kidney Diseases and Hypertension, Warren Alpert Medical School of Brown University, Providence, Rhode Island
Hypokalemia and Hyperkalemia

Laura Tatpati, MD
Professor and Dean, University of Kansas School of Medicine-Wichita, Wichita, Kansas
Uterine Leiomyoma

Emma Taylor-Salmon, MD
Associate Research Scientist, Epidemiology of Microbial Diseases, Yale School of Medicine, New Haven, Connecticut
Lyme Disease and Post-Treatment Lyme Disease Syndrome

Kimberly Templeton, MD
Professor, Orthopedic Surgery, University of Kansas Medical Center, Kansas City, Kansas
Osteomyelitis

Joyce M.C. Teng, MD, PhD
Professor, Dermatology and Pediatrics, Stanford University School of Medicine, Stanford, California
Urticaria and Angioedema

Jill Thein-Nissenbaum, DSc
Professor, Sports Medicine Physical Therapy, Staff Physical Therapist, University of Wisconsin Athletics, University of Wisconsin, Madison, Wisconsin
High-Altitude Illness

Claire Yun Kyoung Ryu Tiger, MD, PhD
Assistant Professor of Medicine, Rutgers Robert Wood Johnson Medical School; Medical Oncologist, Rutgers Cancer Institute of New Jersey, Rutgers University, New Brunswick, New Jersey
Non-Hodgkin Lymphoma

Daniel R. Tilden, MD, MPH
Assistant Professor, Endocrinology, Diabetes, and Clinical Genetics, University of Kansas Medical Center, Kansas City, Kansas
Diabetes Mellitus in Adults

William Tillett, MBChB, PhD
Rheumatologist, Royal National Hospital for Rheumatic Diseases; Senior Lecturer, Pharmacy and Pharmacology, University of Bath, Bath, United Kingdom
Psoriatic Arthritis

Katharine Tippins, MD
Resident, Internal Medicine, University of Wisconsin School of Medicine and Public Health, Madison, Wisconsin
Metabolic Dysfunction-Associated Steatotic Liver Disease (MASLD)

Kenneth Tobin, DO
Clinical Assistant Professor, Cardiovascular Disease, University of Michigan Medical School, Ann Arbor, Michigan
Angina Pectoris

Katherine Turner, MD
Clinical Assistant Professor, Family Medicine, University of Michigan Medical School, Ann Arbor, Michigan
Pruritis

Sebastian H. Unizony, MD
Associate Physician, Rheumatology, Allergy, and Immunology, Massachusetts General Hospital, Harvard Medical School, Boston, Massachusetts
Polymyalgia Rheumatica and Giant Cell Arteritis

Mark Unruh, MD
Chair, Department of Internal Medicine, University of New Mexico School of Medicine, Albuquerque, New Mexico
Chronic Kidney Disease

Locke Uppendahl, MD
Clinical Assistant Professor, Obstetrics and Gynecology, Gynecologic Oncologist, University of Kansas School of Medicine-Wichita, Wichita, Kansas
Cancer of the Endometrium

Colin Vale, MD
Assistant Professor, Hematology and Medical Oncology, Emory University School of Medicine, Atlanta, Georgia
Acute Leukemia in Adults

George Van Buren II, MD
Professor of Surgery, Michael E. DeBakey Department of Surgery, Baylor College of Medicine, Houston, Texas
Acute and Chronic Pancreatitis

Elena V. Varlamov, MD
Associate Professor, Medicine and Neurological Surgery, Oregon Health & Science University, Portland, Oregon
Adrenocortical Insufficiency; Hypopituitarism

Christopher Vélez, MD
Associate Program Director, Advanced Fellowship in Functional and Gastrointestinal Motility Disorders, Center for Neurointestinal Health, Division of Gastroenterology, Department of Medicine Massachusetts General Hospital Boston, Massachusetts
Dysphagia and Esophageal Obstruction

Gregory M. Vercellotti, MD
Professor, Medicine, University of Minnesota Medical School, Minneapolis, Minnesota
Porphyrias

Kyle B. Vincent, MD
Clinical Associate Professor, Surgery, University of Kansas School of Medicine-Wichita, Wichita, Kansas
Gastritis and Peptic Ulcer Disease

Donald C. Vinh, MD
Director, Center of Excellence for Genetic Research in Infection and Immunity, McGill University Health Center; Associate Professor, Clinician-Scientist, Medical Microbiology, McGill University Health Center, Montreal, Quebec, Canada
Blastomycosis

Jatin M. Vyas, MD, PhD
Professor, Medicine, Massachusetts General Hospital, Harvard Medical School, Boston, Massachusetts
Rat-Bite Fever

Tamara Wagner, MD
Associate Professor, Pediatrics, Oregon & Health Science University, Portland, Oregon
Bronchiolitis

Thomas W. Wakefield, MD
Professor Emeritus, Vascular Surgery, University of Michigan Medical School, Ann Arbor, Michigan
Venous Thrombosis

Arnold Wald, MD
Professor, Gastroenterology and Hepatology, University of Wisconsin School of Medicine and Public Health, Madison, Wisconsin
Irritable Bowel Syndrome

Ellen R. Wald, MD
Professor, Pediatrics, University of Wisconsin School of Medicine and Public Health; Physician, Infectious Diseases/Pediatrics, American Family Children's Hospital, Madison, Wisconsin
Urinary Tract Infections in Infants and Children

Robin A. Walker, MD
Clinical Assistant Professor, Family and Community Medicine, University of Kansas School of Medicine-Wichita, Wichita, Kansas
Epididymitis and Orchitis

Ernest Wang, MD
Clinical Professor, Emergency Medicine; Assistant Dean for Medical Education, Office of Academic Affairs, NorthShore University HealthSystem, Evanston, Illinois
Disturbances Due to Cold

Jennifer Wang, DO
Physician, Institute for Critical Care Medicine, Surgery, Mount Sinai Hospital, New York, New York
Targeted Temperature Management (Therapeutic Hypothermia)

Koji Watanabe, MD, PhD
Professor, Division of Host Defense Mechanism, Tokai University School of Medicine, Isehara, Japan; Visiting Associate Professor, The Joint Research Center for Human Retrovirus Infection, Kumamoto University, Kumamoto, Japan
Amebiasis

Alexis Waters, PA
Physician Assistant, Hospital Medicine, UW Health, Madison, Wisconsin
Chronic Obstructive Pulmonary Disease

Cheryl Wehler, MD
Assistant Professor, Psychiatry and Behavioral Sciences, University of Kansas School of Medicine-Wichita, Wichita, Kansas
Panic Disorder

Alice C. Wei, MD, MSc
Attending Surgeon, Memorial Sloan Kettering Cancer Center;
Associate Professor, Surgery, Weill Medical College of Cornell
University, New York, New York
Pancreatic Cancer

Jane A. Weida, MD
Professor, Family, Internal, and Rural Medicine, University of
Alabama, Tuscaloosa, Alabama
Measles (Rubeola)

David N. Weissman, MD
Director, Respiratory Health Division, National Institute for
Occupational Safety and Health, Morgantown, West Virginia
Pneumoconiosis: Asbestosis and Silicosis

Robert C. Welliver Sr., MD
Senior Scientist, Heartland Vaccines LLC, Stillwater, Oklahoma;
Emeritus Professor, Pediatric Infectious Diseases, SUNY at
Buffalo and Children's Hospital, Buffalo, New York
Viral Respiratory Infections

Rebecca M. Wester, MD
Adjunct Associate Professor, Family Medicine-Geriatrics,
University of Nebraska Medical Center, Omaha, Nebraska
Pressure Injury

Randell Wexler, MD, MPH
Professor and Academic Vice Chair, Family Medicine, The Ohio
State University College of Medicine, Columbus, Ohio
Premature Beats

Katarzyna Wilamowska, MD, PhD
Research Assistant Professor, Center for Memory and Aging,
University of New Mexico School of Medicine, Albuquerque,
New Mexico
Alzheimer's Disease

Kimberly Williams, MD
Assistant Professor, Family and Community Medicine, University
of Kansas School of Medicine-Wichita, Salina, Kansas
Otitis Externa

Tracy L. Williams, MD
Associate Professor, Family and Community Medicine, University
of Kansas School of Medicine-Wichita, Wichita, Kansas
Chlamydia Trachomatis

Stacy Willner, DO
Physician, Cardiovascular Disease, Advanced Heart Failure,
University of Michigan Health, Ann Arbor, Michigan
Congestive Heart Failure

J. Lane Wilson, MD
Associate Professor, Community and Family Medicine,
University of Missouri-Kansas City, Kansas City, Missouri
Pharyngitis

Boris Winterhoff, MD
Associate Professor, Gynecologic Oncology, University of
Minnesota Medical School, Minneapolis, Minnesota
Cancer of the Endometrium

Jennifer Wipperman, MD, MPH
Associate Professor, Family and Community Medicine,
University of Kansas School of Medicine-Wichita, Wichita,
Kansas
Dizziness and Vertigo

Mark Wirtz, MD
Assistant Professor, Family Medicine and Community Health,
University of Wisconsin School of Medicine and Public Health,
Madison, Wisconsin
Pyelonephritis

Robert Wittler, MD
Professor, Pediatrics, University of Kansas School of Medicine-
Wichita, Wichita, Kansas
*Tickborne Rickettsial Diseases (Rocky Mountain Spotted Fever
and Other Spotted Fever Group Rickettsioses, Ehrlichioses, and
Anaplasmosis)*

Gary S. Wood, MD
Professor Emeritus and Founding Chair, Dermatology, University
of Wisconsin School of Medicine and Public Health; Physician,
Medicine (Dermatology), Middleton VA Medical Center,
Madison, Wisconsin
*Cutaneous T-Cell Lymphomas, Including Mycosis Fungoides and
Sézary Syndrome*

Scott Worswick, MD
Clinical Professor, Dermatology, USC Keck School of Medicine,
Los Angeles, California
Stevens-Johnson Syndrome and Toxic Epidermal Necrolysis

Dominic J. Wu, MD
Clinical Assistant Professor, Dermatology, University of
Missouri-Kansas City; Kansas City Skin and Cancer Center,
Kansas City, Missouri
Autoimmune Bullous Diseases; Pyoderma Gangrenosum

Kiersten A. Wulff, DNP
Faculty Instructor, Community and Family Medicine, Geisel
School of Medicine, Dartmouth College, Hanover, New
Hampshire; Family Nurse Practitioner, Primary Care, Dartmouth
Hitchcock Medical Center, Lebanon, New Hampshire
Female Sexual Concerns

Hadley Wyre, MD
Associate Professor, Urology, University of Kansas School of
Medicine, Kansas City, Kansas
Urethral Stricture Disease

Cathy Xie, DO
Assistant Professor, Family Medicine, University of Texas
Medical Branch at Galveston, Galveston, Texas
Post-Acute COVID Syndrome

Marita Yaghi, MD
Research Fellow, Dermatology, University of Miami Miller
School of Medicine, Miami, Florida
Venous Ulcers

Steven I. Yakubov, MD
Director, Advanced Structural Heart Disease, Cardiology,
Riverside Methodist Hospital, Columbus, Ohio
Valvular Heart Disease

Yul W. Yang, MD, PhD
Consultant, Dermatology, Mayo Clinic, Scottsdale, Arizona
Contact Dermatitis

Kenneth S. Yew, MD, MPH
Program Director, Parkview Health Family Medicine Residency,
Fort Wayne, Indiana
Tinnitus

James A. Yiannias, MD
Associate Professor, Dermatology, Mayo Clinic, Scottsdale, Arizona
Contact Dermatitis

Natawadee Young, MD
Affiliate Professor, Clinical Director, Family Medicine, AnMed Health Family Medicine Residency Program, Anderson, South Carolina
Antepartum Care

Aiman Zafar, MBBS
Assistant Professor, Endocrinology, University of Kansas Medical Center, Kansas City, Kansas
Thyroiditis

Alonso G. Zea Vera, MD
Attending Physician, Neurologist, Children's National Hospital, Washington, District of Columbia
Gilles de la Tourette Syndrome

Shiwei Zhou, MD
Clinical Assistant Professor, Internal Medicine, University of Michigan Medical School, Ann Arbor, Michigan
Legionellosis (Legionnaire's Disease and Pontiac Fever)

Heinz Zoller, MD
Professor, Hepatology; Head, Christian Doppler Laboratory on Iron and Phosphate Biology, Medical University of Innsbruck, Innsbruck, Austria
Hemochromatosis

Preface

The first edition of *Conn's Current Therapy* was published in 1948, and starting with that first edition, the goal of Conn's has been to provide a personal and evidence-based approach to management of medical conditions. Each chapter is "the method of" the author(s)—a curbside consult, if you will. Conn's, with each of its chapters, represents thousands upon thousands of hours of cumulative clinical expertise. A quarter of the way through the 21st century, Conn's continues to be a trusted and comprehensive resource. The authors, editorial team, and production staff are committed to continued excellence and accuracy of each edition.

As the workforce in medicine and society has become more globally connected and conscious, we are pleased to note that Conn's has not only changed with the medical times but also with the changes in demography. Current authors hail from across the United States and abroad, from academic institutions, community programs, and private practice. Authors represent a vast array of backgrounds and experiences.

Speaking of global, Conn's continues to update chapters on the rapidly evolving epidemiology of zoonoses and infectious diseases such as Lyme disease, babesios, Mpox, and dengue fever. As many children born during the COVID-19 pandemic began kindergarten in 2025, we could not help but consider the reemergence of vaccine-preventable infectious diseases, some of which most practicing clinicians in the United States have not encountered in their practice. The first vaccine for rubeola did not come into wide use until 1968, 20 years after the first edition of Conn's was published. After years of being essentially eradicated as a public health threat, the reemergence of rubeola in the United States is a sobering fact.

Throughout its 78-year history, Conn's has continued to evolve to meet the needs of our readers. In the 2026 edition, our newest chapter is "Home Disaster Preparedness." Other chapters added in the last few years include "Artificial Intelligence," "Genomic Testing," "Monoclonal Antibodies," "Venomous Snakebite," "Gender-Affirming Care," "COVID-19," "Post-COVID Syndrome," "Post-COVID-19 Multisystem Inflammatory Syndrome," and "Mpox."

As we noted in last year's preface, the rapid expansion of artificial intelligence (AI) requires a brief note. Elsevier, the publishers of Conn's, has a policy on the use of AI, part of which states that authors are not permitted to use AI to create content. However, AI can be used to improve readability, and authors are required to note if this has been done in their chapter. The policy can be accessed here: https://www.elsevier.com/about/policies-and-standards/the-use-of-generative-ai-and-ai-assisted-technologies-in-writing-for-elsevier.

The Preface also serves as a chance for us to share acknowledgments and gratitude to the entire team that makes Conn's possible. It indeed takes a team to bring Conn's to fruition each and every year. We'd like to first thank the hundreds of authors from across medical specialties who have a wide variety of experiences. Their work to write and edit their chapters so they remain accurate and timely each year is indispensable.

Our gratitude certainly goes out to the one and only exceptional Pharmacy Editor, Miriam Chan, Pharm D. Dr. Chan has been part of the team since 2001. She reviews every drug dose and mention in the text for FDA status and accuracy.

The team at Elsevier is organized and outstanding. Lauren Boyle is the Senior Content Editor. Doug Turner is the Senior Project Manager who makes sure we bring the final product in on time to meet our deadline. Renee Duenow is the Senior Book Designer who develops the cover design. We are so grateful to the copyeditors who review the chapters and 1500 pages of an annual publication. And last but certainly not least from the Elsevier team is Kevin Travers, Content Development Specialist. Kevin is the "spreadsheet master"! Throughout the year Kevin keeps us all on track to meet the author and editing deadlines. He continually manages communications between the editing team and the authors and makes sure that nothing is missed. He is extremely effective and a team player.

The editors dedicate this edition to the authors and our readers. Authors, thank you for your continued dedication and high-quality contributions. And to our readers, thank you for your trust in the accuracy and approach of Conn's throughout the years.

Rick D. Kellerman, MD, Editor
Joel J. Heidelbaugh, MD, Editor
Ernestine M. Lee, MD, MPH, Associate Editor

Contents

SECTION 6
Hematology

SECTION 7
Head and Neck

SECTION 8
Infectious Diseases

Contents

xxxi

Contents

xxxvi

Conn's Current Therapy 2026 uses a standardized system of footnotes:
1. Not FDA approved for this indication.
2. Not available in the United States.
3. Exceeds dosage recommended by the manufacturer.
4. Not yet approved for use in the United States.
5. Investigational drug in the United States.
6. May be compounded by pharmacists.
7. Available as dietary supplement.
8. Orphan drug in the United States.
9. Available as homeopathic remedy.
10. Available in the United States from the Centers for Disease Control and Prevention.

† Deceased.

1

Symptomatic Care Pending Diagnosis

CHEST PAIN

Method of
William E. Cayley Jr., MD, MDiv

CURRENT DIAGNOSIS

- Initial evaluation of chest pain should include evaluation of clinical stability, a concise history and physical examination, and a chest x-ray and electrocardiogram (ECG) unless the cause is clearly not life threatening.
- Chest pain described as exertional, radiating to one or both arms, similar to or worse than prior cardiac chest pain, or associated with nausea, vomiting, or diaphoresis indicates high risk for acute coronary syndrome. ECG identifies ST-elevation myocardial infarction (STEMI); cardiac biomarkers are essential for further evaluation of suspected chest pain in the absence of STEMI.
- The Wells, Geneva, and Pisa clinical prediction rules and the pulmonary embolism (PE) rule-out criteria can help stratify a patient's risk of PE.
- Aortic dissection is an uncommon cause of chest pain, but patients with abrupt or instantaneous chest pain that is ripping, tearing, or stabbing should be evaluated for dissection with chest x-ray, computed tomography (CT), or magnetic resonance imaging.
- Chest pain associated with dyspnea or painful inspiration and tachycardia or friction rub on auscultation may indicate pericarditis or myocarditis.
- Esophageal rupture may be suspected in patients with pain, dyspnea, and shock after a forceful emesis, and prompt imaging with CT or esophagography is essential.
- Patients who have suspected tension pneumothorax and who are clinically stable should have a chest x-ray for confirmation before needle decompression is attempted.

CURRENT THERAPY

- Patients with ST-elevation myocardial infarction (STEMI) require urgent reperfusion, and those with unstable angina or non-STEMI require admission for further monitoring and evaluation.
- Most patients with pulmonary embolism require admission for monitoring and anticoagulation, although outpatient treatment may be possible for low-risk patients after initial evaluation and anticoagulation.
- Prompt surgical consultation is required for patients with confirmed or suspected aortic dissection or esophageal rupture.
- Clinically unstable patients with suspected tension pneumothorax need immediate needle decompression.

Epidemiology

Chest pain is the chief complaint in 1% to 2% of all outpatient primary care visits. More than 50% of emergency department (ED) visits for chest pain are for serious cardiovascular conditions such as acute coronary syndrome (ACS) or pulmonary embolism (PE), but these account for <15% of outpatient primary care encounters for chest pain, and up to 15% of chest pain episodes never reach a definitive diagnosis. Other potentially life-threatening etiologies for chest pain include PE, dissecting aortic aneurysm, esophageal rupture, and tension pneumothorax. In outpatient primary care, the most common causes of chest pain are musculoskeletal, gastrointestinal, angina caused by stable coronary artery disease (CAD), anxiety or other psychiatric conditions, and pulmonary disease.

Initial Assessment

In the initial evaluation of chest pain, it is important to obtain a clear history of the onset and evolution of the pain, especially details such as location, quality, duration, and aggravating or alleviating factors. Initial physical examination should include vital signs, assessment of the patient's overall general condition, and examination of the heart and lungs. If there are any clinical signs of instability (altered mental status, hypotension, marked dyspnea, or other signs of shock), initial stabilization and diagnosis must be addressed simultaneously, consistent with current guidelines for emergency cardiovascular care. Unless the history and physical examination suggest an obviously nonthreatening cause of chest discomfort, most adults with chest pain should at least have basic diagnostic testing with an electrocardiogram (ECG) and a chest x-ray. Several clinical prediction rules are available to help confirm or exclude some common causes of chest pain (Box 1).

Diagnosis and Treatment
Acute Coronary Syndrome

ACS includes acute myocardial infarction (MI) (ST-segment elevation and depression, and Q wave and non–Q wave) and unstable angina. Findings on the history and physical examination that increase the likelihood of ACS include radiation of pain to the right arm or shoulder, to both arms or shoulders, or to the left arm; pain associated with exertion, diaphoresis, nausea, or vomiting; pain described as pressure or as "worse than previous angina or similar to a previous MI"; or the presence of hypotension or an S3 on cardiac auscultation. Elements of the history and examination that decrease the likelihood of ACS are pleuritic, positional, or sharp chest pain; pain in an inframammary location; pain not associated with exertion; pain lasting just seconds or lasting >24 hours; or chest pain reproducible with palpation. A low-risk score on the Marburg Heart Score (MHS) or the INTERCHEST Clinical Prediction Rule can help exclude CAD in primary care patients with chest pain, and use of the MHS when evaluating primary care patients with chest pain has been shown to improve clinical diagnostic accuracy (Table 1). Recent studies have demonstrated that the presence or absence of typical cardiac risk factors (e.g., gender, diabetes, hypertension, smoking, high cholesterol, family history) have little diagnostic value

Acute Coronary Syndrome
- Diagnosing cardiac ischemia with exercise treadmill testing: Duke Treadmill score: https://www.mdcalc.com/duke-treadmill-score
- Assessing the risk of a major cardiac event in the next 6 weeks: HEART score: https://www.mdcalc.com/heart-score-major-cardiac-events
- Assessing the risk of ACS in someone with chest pain: Marburg Heart Score: https://www.mdcalc.com/marburg-heart-score-mhs
- Assessing the risk of ACS in someone with chest pain: INTERCHEST Clinical Prediction Rule: https://www.mdcalc.com/interchest-clinical-prediction-rule-chest-pain-primary-care
- Assessing long-term risk in those with ACS: GRACE ACS risk calculator: https://www.mdcalc.com/calc/1099/grace-acs-risk-mortality-calculator
- Estimating mortality for patients with unstable angina and NSTEMI: TIMI Risk Score: https://timi.org/calculators/timi-risk-score-calculator-for-ua-nstemi/

Pulmonary Embolism
- Geneva score for predicting risk of PE: https://www.mdcalc.com/geneva-score-revised-pulmonary-embolism
- Pisa clinical model for predicting the probability of PE: https://ebmcalc.com/PulmonaryEmbRiskPisaCXR.htm
- Wells scoring system for risk of PE: https://www.mdcalc.com/wells-criteria-pulmonary-embolism
- Pulmonary embolism rule-out criteria: https://www.mdcalc.com/perc-rule-pulmonary-embolism

Thoracic Aortic Dissection
- Aortic Dissection Detection Risk Score (ADD-RS): https://www.mdcalc.com/aortic-dissection-detection-risk-score-add-rs

Pneumonia
- Diagnostic rule for pneumonia in adults with acute cough: https://mobile.fpnotebook.com/Lung/Exam/DhrRlTDgnsPnmn.htm

---

TABLE 1   Marburg Heart Score*

FINDING	POINTS
Women >64 years, men >54 years	1
Known CAD, cerebrovascular disease, or peripheral vascular disease	1
Pain worse with exercise	1
Pain not reproducible with palpation	1
Patient assumes pain is cardiac	1

*Approximately 23% of patients with an MHS score of ≥3 will have CAD. Approximately 97% of patients with an MHS score of ≤2 will not have CAD.
CAD, Coronary artery disease.
Modified from Haasenritter J, Bösner S, Vaucher P, et al: Ruling out coronary heart disease in primary care: external validation of a clinical prediction rule. *Br J Gen Pract* 62(599):e415–e421, 2021.

---

for determining the likelihood of ACS in patients older than 40 years, and the absence of risk factors should not preclude further cardiac evaluation in patients with concerning symptoms.

An ECG should be obtained promptly for any patient with suspected ACS. ST segment elevation in two or more contiguous leads or a presumed new left bundle branch block is diagnostic of ST-elevation myocardial infarction (STEMI) and requires urgent revascularization with thrombolysis or angioplasty at an appropriate facility. Ischemic ST-segment depression of >0.5 mm in leads V2 to V3 or >1 mm in all other leads, dynamic T-wave inversion with chest discomfort, or transient ST segment elevation of ≥0.5 mm is classified as unstable angina or non–ST-elevation myocardial infarction (NSTEMI). However, none of these findings is sensitive enough that its absence can exclude MI, and patients whose chest pain is not low risk still require further assessment for ACS.

In patients with high-risk chest pain but without STEMI, elevated cardiac troponin (cTn) I or T levels distinguish NSTEMI from unstable angina. High-sensitivity cardiac troponin assays (hs-cTn I or hs-cTn T) have higher sensitivity and better negative predictive values than standard troponin measurements. Initial management of NSTEMI includes hospital admission for antiplatelet, antithrombin, and antianginal therapy. Patients with unstable angina should also be hospitalized for observation, and those with either NSTEMI or unstable angina require risk stratification using the Thrombolysis in Myocardial Infarction Study Group (TIMI) or Global Registry of Acute Coronary Events (GRACE) risk scores (see Box 1).

Patients with chest pain suspicious for CAD but no definite initial diagnosis of STEMI or NSTEMI on initial presentation are often admitted to the hospital for overnight observation and serial cardiac biomarker measurements to "rule out MI." However, numerous clinical decision pathways have been developed integrating history, ECG findings, and cardiac biomarkers to determine who is at sufficiently low risk of major adverse cardiac events (MACEs) to allow discharge for close follow-up. hs-cTn assays may be used to guide disposition of chest pain with repeat sampling at 1, 2, or 3 hours from ED arrival using the pattern of rise or fall (i.e., delta) and the repeat value itself, based on assay-specific diagnostic thresholds; however, when using conventional cTn assays, the sampling time frame is extended to 3 to 6 hours from ED arrival. Recent evidence suggests that the HEART score may outperform TIMI and GRACE in determining which patients are at low risk (see Box 1). The combination of a low-risk HEART score (0 to 3) plus a single normal troponin value may predict sufficiently low risk of ACS to allow discharge from the ED with short-term outpatient follow-up, and a recent retrospective observational study of 1989 patients seen in EDs for chest pain found that those with intermediate-risk HEART scores (4–6) may be at sufficiently low risk of MACE to allow discharge if clinical follow-up can be arranged within 1 week.

Patients at low risk for ACS or MI can usually defer further testing unless there are other risk factors in their family or past medical history markedly increasing the likelihood of CAD. Current recommendations are that all other patients with chest pain suggestive of CAD should have further noninvasive testing within 7 days. However, a retrospective analysis of 7988 ED patients with chest pain who were discharged to complete diagnostic testing found no difference in MACE between those who had testing within 3 days and those who had testing between 4 and 30 days from discharge.

Patients who can exercise and have no left bundle branch block, preexcitation, or significant resting ST-segment depression on an ECG can be evaluated with an exercise stress ECG, and the Duke Treadmill Score (DTS) can then be used to further quantify cardiac risk (see Box 1). The ability to attain a low-risk DTS (≥5) and the ability to achieve 10 metabolic equivalents of exercise are both associated with very low rates of cardiovascular death or nonfatal MI. Patients with baseline ECG abnormalities should have perfusion imaging performed along with a stress ECG, and those who cannot exercise may be evaluated with a pharmacologic stress or vasodilator test (e.g., dobutamine [Dobutrex][1] or adenosine [Adenocard]). Patients at high risk for CAD or those with NSTEMI should generally proceed directly to angiography, which enables definitive assessment of the coronary artery anatomy.

---

[1]Not FDA approved for this indication.

TABLE 2	Simplified Wells Scoring System for Pulmonary Embolism	
CLINICAL FINDING		**SCORE**
Symptoms of DVT		3.0
No alternative diagnosis more likely than PE		3.0
Heart rate >100 beats/min		1.5
Immobilization >3 days or surgery in past 4 weeks		1.5
Previous objectively diagnosed DVT or PE		1.5
Hemoptysis		1.0
Malignancy		1.0
Probability of PE: <2 points = low, 2–6 points = moderate, >6 points = high		

DVT, Deep vein thrombosis; *PE,* pulmonary embolism.
Modified from Miniati M, Bottai M, Monti S: Comparison of 3 clinical models for predicting the probability of pulmonary embolism. *Medicine (Baltimore)* 84(2):107–114, 2005; Torbicki A, Perrier A, Konstantinides S, et al: Guidelines on the diagnosis and management of acute pulmonary embolism: the Task Force for the Diagnosis and Management of Acute Pulmonary Embolism of the European Society of Cardiology (ESC). *Eur Heart J* 29(18):2276–2315, 2008.

TABLE 3	Pulmonary Embolism Rule-Out Criteria
Criteria (excludes PE if all criteria are met and pretest probability is estimated at <15%)
Age <50 years
Heart rate <100 beats/min
Pulse oximetry on room air >95%
No unilateral leg swelling
No hemoptysis
No surgery or trauma in the last 4 weeks
No prior DVT or PE
No hormone use

DVT, Deep vein thrombosis; *PE,* pulmonary embolism.
Modified from Kline JA, Mitchell AM, Kabrhel C, et al: Clinical criteria to prevent unnecessary diagnostic testing in emergency department patients with suspected pulmonary embolism. *J Thromb Haemost* 2(8):1247–1255, 2004.

Pulmonary Embolism

There are no individual symptoms or physical examination findings that reliably diagnose or exclude PE, but four clinical prediction rules have all been validated for use in determining the likelihood of PE and therefore whether further testing is needed (see Box 1). The Pisa rule may be the most accurate, but it is also the most mathematically complicated and depends on clinical, ECG, and x-ray findings. The Geneva rule requires blood gas and chest x-ray findings. The Wells rule (Table 2) is based on the simplest combination of history and examination findings, and a comparison between the Wells and Geneva rules found that the Wells rule has a lower failure rate. With the Wells and Geneva prediction rules, the likelihood of PE is approximately 10% in the low-probability category, 30% in the moderate-probability category, and 65% in the high-probability category. If a patient is clinically suspected to be at low risk for PE (<15% pretest probability) and meets all of the PE rule-out criteria (Table 3), the risk of PE is <2%, and no further testing is needed.

Routine tests done for patients with chest pain are not particularly helpful in diagnosing or excluding PE. The chest x-ray may be abnormal, but findings that typically occur with PE (atelectasis, effusion, or elevation of a hemidiaphragm) are nonspecific. ECG signs of right ventricular strain (S wave in lead I, Q wave, and inverted T wave in lead III) may be helpful if present, but their absence does not exclude PE. Hypoxia may be present, but up to 20% of patients with PE have a normal alveolar-arterial oxygen gradient.

Additional tests recommended for evaluating patients with suspected PE include D-dimer testing, compression ultrasonography, and pulmonary imaging with ventilation-perfusion (VQ) scintigraphy or computed tomography (CT) angiography. Although CT may be more sensitive than VQ scanning, CT is also associated with higher radiation doses; for younger patients with suspected PE and a normal chest x-ray, VQ scanning may be preferable to limit overall radiation exposure. The use of adjusted D-dimer levels based on age or clinical setting has been studied, but none of these approaches has been standardized. Patients with suspected high-risk PE (i.e., those with shock or hypotension) should have immediate imaging and treatment for PE if the imaging is positive, although an echocardiographic finding of right ventricular overload may be used to justify treatment for PE in the unstable patient with high clinical suspicion for PE when imaging is not available. Patients who have suspected PE and are not at high risk (i.e., no shock or hypotension) and have a high clinical probability (based on Wells, Geneva, or Pisa scoring) should also proceed directly to imaging, with appropriate treatment if the scan is positive. Patients with a low clinical probability of PE (based on one of the validated clinical prediction rules) do not need further D-dimer testing or imaging. Patients with intermediate clinical probability should initially have D-dimer testing; further testing or treatment for PE is unnecessary if the D-dimer is negative, and imaging should be performed if the D-dimer is positive.

Anticoagulation, with thrombolysis in high-risk patients, is the foundation of treatment for PE. Patients with shock or hypotension are at high risk and require hemodynamic and respiratory support, thrombolysis, or embolectomy, followed by appropriate attention to anticoagulation. Normotensive patients with echocardiographic evidence of right ventricular dysfunction or serologic evidence of myocardial injury (elevated cTn I or T) have intermediate risk and should be admitted for anticoagulation. Normotensive patients who have normal results on echocardiography and testing for myocardial injury are at low risk and often may be discharged early for management at home after initiation of anticoagulation. Anticoagulation for PE should be started at the time of diagnosis. Apixaban (Eliquis) or rivaroxaban (Xarelto) may be used without prior oral anticoagulation; alternatively, unfractionated heparin, low-molecular-weight heparin, or fondaparinux (Arixtra) may be started and continued for 5 to 10 days with simultaneous initiation of dabigatran (Pradaxa), edoxaban (Savaysa or Lixiana), or warfarin (Coumadin) titrated to maintain an international normalized ratio between 2.0 and 3.0.

Thoracic Aortic Dissection

Thoracic aortic dissection is a much less common cause of chest pain; prevalence estimates are 2.0 to 3.5 cases per 100,000 person-years. Up to 40% of patients die immediately, and 5% to 20% die during or shortly after surgery. Risk factors for acute thoracic aortic dissection include hypertension, presence of a pheochromocytoma, cocaine use, weightlifting, trauma or a rapid deceleration event, coarctation of the aorta, and certain genetic abnormalities. Pain caused by acute aortic dissection is perceived as abrupt and severe in 84% to 90% of cases, and >50% of patients describe the pain as sharp or stabbing. No physical findings are sensitive or specific for detecting aortic dissection because approximately equal percentages of patients are hypertensive or normotensive or have hypotension or shock. The most common physical findings (a murmur of aortic insufficiency or a pulse deficit) occur in less than one-half of patients.

In any patient with severe chest pain that is abrupt or instantaneous in onset or has a ripping, tearing, or stabbing quality, acute thoracic aortic dissection should be suspected. Physical examination should assess for a pulse deficit, a systolic pressure differential between limbs of >20 mm Hg, a focal neurologic deficit, or a new aortic regurgitation murmur. It is also important to ask about a family history of connective tissue disease (including Marfan syndrome), about any family or personal history of aortic dissection or thoracic aneurysm, and about any known aortic valve disease or recent aortic interventions. D-dimer testing has been proposed as a way to screen for aortic dissection, but it is more important to obtain prompt imaging and surgical intervention for those in whom dissection is confirmed. A low-risk aortic dissection detection risk score (see Box 1) can help exclude the diagnosis of aortic dissection, whereas patients with a high-risk score require further evaluation.

An ECG should be obtained in all patients with suspected aortic dissection to exclude STEMI (which can present with similar symptoms). In all low- and intermediate-risk patients, a prompt chest x-ray can help by either confirming an alternative diagnosis or confirming the presence of thoracic aortic disease. High-risk patients should have prompt imaging with CT or magnetic resonance imaging, and those who are in shock or clinically unstable may be evaluated by bedside transesophageal echocardiography. If thoracic aortic dissection is confirmed on imaging, urgent surgical consultation is required. Medical therapy should be started with intravenous β-blockers. Patients with dissection of the ascending aorta require urgent surgery, whereas those with descending thoracic aortic dissection may be managed medically unless hypotension or other complications develop.

Pericarditis and Myocarditis

Acute pericarditis is an inflammatory syndrome of the pericardium (with or without effusion), and myocarditis is an inflammation of the myocardium; some patients may have an inflammatory myopericarditis. Viral infections are the most common identified cause of pericarditis (although most cases are idiopathic). Myocarditis may also be caused by a viral infection (including COVID-19) or secondary to systemic disease (e.g., rheumatoid arthritis or sarcoidosis) or toxin exposure (e.g., alcohol). Pericarditis or myocarditis should be suspected in patients with acute substernal chest pain that is associated with dyspnea or painful inspiration and tachycardia or friction rub on auscultation; myocarditis should also be suspected in any patient with heart failure and no clear underlying cause. Diagnostic testing should include ECG, cTn, and echocardiography. Supportive care and electrocardiographic monitoring are important for any patient with hemodynamic compromise. Pericarditis is typically treated with nonsteroidal antiinflammatory drugs (NSAIDs) plus colchicine,[1] whereas treatment of myocarditis generally involves addressing treatment of any identified causes.

Esophageal Rupture

Esophageal rupture, or Boerhaave syndrome, has a high mortality rate. Esophageal rupture is rare; the most common cause is endoscopically induced injury, but it can happen in other settings as well. Common misdiagnoses include perforated ulcer, MI, PE, dissecting aneurysm, and pancreatitis. The "classic" presentation has been described as pain, dyspnea, and shock associated with forceful emesis, but the history and physical examination are commonly nonspecific. Up to 45% of patients with Boerhaave syndrome have no history of vomiting, and esophageal perforation can develop with any cause of sudden increased intraesophageal pressure, including childbirth, seizure, prolonged coughing or laughing, or extreme exertion. Diagnosis most commonly is made by contrast esophagography or CT of the chest.

Patients whose rupture is diagnosed <48 hours after symptom onset are typically treated surgically (especially if sepsis is present) or endoscopically; however, nonoperative management may be considered in patients with evidence of a contained leak within the cervical esophagus or mediastinum. Those who present >48 hours after symptom onset may be considered for conservative treatment with hyperalimentation, antibiotics, and nasogastric suction.

[1] Not FDA approved for this indication.

TABLE 4	Signs and Symptoms

FINDING	POINTS
Rhinorrhea	−2
Sore throat	−1
Night sweats	1
Myalgia	1
Sputum all day	1
Respiratory rate >25 breaths/min	2
Temperature >100°F	2

Interpretation

SCORE	PROBABILITY OF PNEUMONIA
−3	5
−1	12
0	21
1	30
3	37

Modified from Cayley WE Jr: Diagnosing the cause of chest pain. *Am Fam Physician* 72(10):2012–2021, 2005.

Tension Pneumothorax

Tension pneumothorax is relatively rare among patients presenting with chest pain, but it is potentially life threatening if not treated properly. Common symptoms and physical findings include chest pain, respiratory distress, decreased ipsilateral air entry, and tachycardia; hypoxia, tracheal deviation, and hypotension are less common.

Emergency needle decompression is usually recommended if tension pneumothorax is suspected, but this is ineffective in some cases and is associated with risks to the patient of pain, bleeding, infection, and cardiac tamponade. However, waiting for radiographic confirmation of the diagnosis is associated with up to a fourfold increase in mortality because of delay in decompression of the pneumothorax, and prompt needle decompression is associated with a 9% absolute risk reduction of mortality at 24 hours in trauma patients with tension pneumothorax. Patients most likely to benefit from an immediate attempt at needle decompression are those with an oxygen saturation <92% while on oxygen, a decreased level of consciousness while on oxygen, a systolic blood pressure <90 mm Hg, or a respiratory rate <10 breaths/min. Patients without signs of instability may be better managed by waiting for chest imaging to confirm or exclude the presence of a pneumothorax. Although plain chest x-rays have typically been used for diagnosing pneumothorax, pleural ultrasonography may have higher sensitivity. For clinically stable patients with spontaneous pneumothorax, there may be no difference in clinical success rates between conservative and interventional treatment.

Other Causes of Chest Pain

A patient with chest pain and cough, fever, egophony, or dullness to percussion might have pneumonia, but none of these individual findings is specific enough to confirm the diagnosis. However, adults with an acute respiratory infection who have normal vital signs and a normal pulmonary examination are very unlikely to have community-acquired pneumonia. A large study in 1984 developed a decision rule (Table 4) using seven clinical findings to predict the likelihood of pneumonia. There is ongoing debate over the reliability of pneumonia diagnosis based solely on history and physical examination; chest x-ray is usually considered the reference standard. However, a 2013 Cochrane review found two trials suggesting that routine chest radiography does not affect the clinical outcomes in adults and children whose presentations are suggestive of a lower respiratory tract infection. Thus at least for clinically stable outpatients, treatment for pneumonia based on appropriate clinical findings alone may be reasonable.

Heart failure alone is an uncommon cause of chest pain, but it may accompany ACS or cardiac valve disease. A displaced apical impulse and a prior history of CAD support this diagnosis, and because virtually all patients with heart failure have exertional dyspnea, its absence is very helpful in excluding this diagnosis. An abnormal ECG and cardiomegaly on chest x-ray can increase the likelihood of heart failure among patients with chest pain, and B-natriuretic peptide (BNP) or N-terminal pro-BNP are now commonly used for detecting heart failure in patients presenting with acute dyspnea. Point-of-care ultrasonography may have high sensitivity and specificity for diagnosing acute cardiogenic pulmonary edema.

Panic and anxiety are a common cause of chest pain in those at low risk for heart disease. There is good evidence that psychological interventions, such as cognitive behavioral therapy and breathing exercises, can improve chest pain symptoms for patients with nonspecific chest pain who do not have CAD. However, even in patients with possible panic disorder, further cardiac testing should be done if there are significant cardiac risk factors.

Gastrointestinal disease can cause chest pain, but the history and physical examination are relatively inaccurate for diagnosing or excluding serious gastrointestinal pathology. However, if life-threatening cardiovascular or pulmonary causes of chest pain have been excluded, it is appropriate to try a short course of a high-dose proton pump inhibitor (omeprazole [Prilosec] 40 mg daily, lansoprazole [Prevacid] 30 mg daily, or esomeprazole [Nexium] 40 mg daily) to evaluate for undiagnosed gastroesophageal reflux disease (GERD) as the cause of chest pain (even for patients without typical GERD symptoms).

Chest wall pain can usually be diagnosed by history and examination if other etiologies have been excluded, and such pain is more likely if the patient's pain is reproducible by palpation. Measurement of the sedimentation rate is not generally helpful in making the diagnosis, although in unusual situations radiography may be helpful. Typical management options include heat, NSAIDs, topical lidocaine, physical therapy, and acupuncture.

References

Ammirati E, Moslehi JJ: Diagnosis and treatment of acute myocarditis: a review, *JAMA* 329(13):1098–1113, 2023. https://doi.org/10.1001/jama.2023.3371. PMID: 37014337. https://jamanetwork.com/journals/jama/fullarticle/2802856.

Barton EC, Walker SP: The medical management of spontaneous pneumothorax: a concise review, *Br J Hosp Med (Lond)* 85(9):1–13, 2024. https://doi.org/10.12968/hmed.2024.0047. PMID: 39347673. https://pubmed.ncbi.nlm.nih.gov/39347673/.

DeVivo A, Sheng AY, Koyfman A, Long B: High risk and low prevalence diseases: esophageal perforation, *Am J Emerg Med* 53:29–36, 2022. https://doi.org/10.1016/j.ajem.2021.12.017. Epub 2021 Dec 18. PMID: 34971919. https://pubmed.ncbi.nlm.nih.gov/34971919/.

Gulati M, et al: 2021 AHA/ACC/ASE/CHEST/SAEM/SCCT/SCMR guideline for the evaluation and diagnosis of chest pain: a report of the American college of Cardiology/American heart association joint committee on clinical practice guidelines, *Circulation* 144(22):e368–e454, 2021. https://doi.org/10.1161/CIR.0000000000001029. Epub 2021 Oct 28. Erratum in: *Circulation.* 144(22):e455, 2021. PMID: 34709879. https://pubmed.ncbi.nlm.nih.gov/34709879/.

Hameed I, Cifu AS, Vallabhajosyula P: Management of thoracic aortic dissection, *JAMA* 329(9):756–757, 2023. https://doi.org/10.1001/jama.2023.0265. PMID: 36795378. https://pubmed.ncbi.nlm.nih.gov/36795378/.

Katz PO, Dunbar KB, Schnoll-Sussman FH, Greer KB, Yadlapati R, Spechler SJ: ACG clinical guideline for the diagnosis and management of gastroesophageal reflux disease, *Am J Gastroenterol* 117(1):27–56, 2022. https://doi.org/10.14309/ajg.0000000000001538. PMID: 34807007; PMCID: PMC8754510. https://pubmed.ncbi.nlm.nih.gov/34807007/.

McConaghy JR, Sharma M, Patel H: Acute chest pain in adults: outpatient evaluation, *Am Fam Physician* 102(12):721–727, 2020.

Mott T, Jones G, Roman K: Costochondritis: rapid evidence review, *Am Fam Physician* 104(1):73–78, 2021. PMID: 34264599.

Nohria R, Viera AJ: Acute coronary syndrome: diagnosis and initial management, *Am Fam Physician* 109(1):34–42, 2024. PMID: 38227869. https://pubmed.ncbi.nlm.nih.gov/38227869/.

Peterson TA, Turner SP, Dolezal KA: Acute pericarditis: rapid evidence review, *Am Fam Physician* 109(5):441–446, 2024. PMID: 38804758. https://pubmed.ncbi.nlm.nih.gov/38804758/.

Raja AS, Greenberg JO, Qaseem A, et al: Clinical Guidelines Committee of the American College of Physicians. Evaluation of patients with suspected acute pulmonary embolism: best practice advice from the clinical guidelines committee of the American College of Physicians, *Ann Intern Med* 163(9):701–711, 2015.

CONSTIPATION

Christopher Klouzek, MD

CURRENT DIAGNOSIS

- Constipation is a common complaint whose diagnosis can be complicated by subjective symptom interpretation and a multifactorial cause.
- Red flag symptoms should be identified and used as guidance to progress to more advanced diagnostic techniques.
- Chronic medication regimens should be evaluated as a possible cause and considered when choosing treatment modalities because drug interactions may result.

CURRENT THERAPY

- When anatomic abnormalities are not suspected, conservative therapy including insoluble fiber supplementation and moderate physical activity should be initial therapy.
- Osmotic laxatives should be used for more severe cases, and short-term use of promotility agents can be safely incorporated into a rescue therapy.
- Management with enemas or suppositories should aim toward electrolyte-neutral agents and away from those that may be irritating to the intestinal tract.

Epidemiology

Constipation in its various forms is a common condition in North America. It seems to increase in prevalence with age and is found in women almost twice as often as in men. The number of patients self-reporting symptoms of constipation increases drastically after the age of 65 and seems to be related to decreased calorie intake. Individuals with a more sedentary lifestyle are also more likely to express symptoms of constipation.

Pathophysiology

Constipation can have structural and/or functional components depending on the presentation and symptoms. Functional constipation is a much more common condition and may result from decreased anal and rectal sensation or tone. Although it is not uncommon to have a section of distal colon that may become spastic, complete absence of normal peristaltic motion is not common. When tested, many patients who complain of constipation often have normal intestinal peristalsis. Structural constipation can be the result of a partial or complete obstruction in the bowel tract due to endogenous, abnormal tissue growth such as cancer or the presence of a foreign body.

Prevention

When managing constipation, prevention is significantly superior to treatment. Behavioral techniques such as timed defecation after meals and frequent mild to moderate ambulatory exercise can be used to improve gastrointestinal motility and stool transit. The use of bulking agents such as insoluble fiber, specifically in dietary form, can maintain a healthy bowel and normal stool transit (see Table 3).

Clinical Manifestations

Patients suffering from constipation will often present with that chief complaint. They often acknowledge abdominal bloating, discomfort, or cramping. Some patients will complain of rectal pain, and in some cases, patients will acknowledge they are not aware of the timing of their last bowel movement. These symptoms are not present in every case, however.

Diagnosis

The diagnosis of constipation can be complicated. When asked to self-report, patients may have significantly different ideas about what personal symptoms indicate a condition of constipation. Normal bowel function can vary widely between individuals, and it is often more important to know what an individual patient's normal state may look like when considering diagnosis.

The Rome III criteria have been set forth to assist in the diagnosis of functional constipation. To use these criteria, patients should have symptoms for at least 6 months with the most recent 3 months being evaluated using the criteria. Patients should have at least two positive criteria without a better explanation (Table 1).

The process of diagnosing constipation is a stepwise approach. With many patients it is appropriate to start conservative therapy when functional constipation is believed to be the most likely possibility and certain red flag symptoms are not present before endoscopy or imaging. Red flag symptoms include unintentional weight loss, significant increases in abdominal pain, new-onset rectal bleeding, emesis (particularly of feculent material), or a complete loss of flatulence. For many patients with advanced age, chronic medications are a good place to start the evaluation for the cause of constipation. The list of common medications that can cause these symptoms is lengthy (Table 2 contains an abbreviated list).

If the patient has concerning findings or does not respond to conservative therapy, further evaluation can be performed, including colonoscopy, computed tomography (CT) scan of the abdomen and pelvis, motility studies, manometry, evaluation of both the somatic and autonomic nervous systems, and lab work to include a metabolic panel and thyroid function testing.

Treatment

Treatment of constipation is largely based on its severity and cause. For functional constipation in the mild category, the use of bulking agents and proosmotic agents can produce improved stool motility without many side effects. Osmotic agents including sorbitol, lactulose (Constulose), polyethylene glycol (Mira-LAX), and hypertonic solutions can be used. When choosing the appropriate substance, it is important to consider the effects on electrolyte balance that some hypertonic solutions may have. Some studies have indicated using the substances at frequencies greater than daily does not seem to have any extra benefit. The choice of which agent to use may be largely based on availability, tolerance, and price. Long-term use of osmotic agents can cause abnormalities in fluid balance, as well as electrolytes as mentioned above.

Mild to moderate constipation can also be treated with promotility agents. Although there have not been many studies performed on the efficacy of these medications or their side effects, the studies that have been performed seem to indicate short-term use is safe and effective. These medications function through stimulation of peristaltic activity primarily in the colon and through modification of electrolyte mobilization in

TABLE 1	Rome III Criteria for Diagnosing Constipation
Two positive findings and final two criteria are true
Straining during ≥25% of bowel movements
Lumpy or hard stools during ≥25% of bowel movements
The sensation of incomplete evacuation during ≥25% of bowel movements
The sensation of anal or rectal obstruction during ≥25% of bowel movements
The use of manual maneuvers to assist defecation in ≥25% of bowel movements
Fewer than three bowel movements per week
Diagnostic criteria for irritable bowel syndrome are not met
Loose stools are not present without the use of a bowel regimen

TABLE 2	Commonly Used Medications That Can Cause Constipation
Antihistamines
Antidiarrheals
Antipsychotics
Antidepressants
Oral iron supplements
Aluminum-containing antacids
Antihypertensives
Calcium channel blockers

TABLE 3	Medications to Treat Chronic Functional Constipation	
MEDICATION	**DOSE**	**TIME TO ONSET OF ACTION**
Bulking: Psyllium (Metamucil)	1 Tbsp TID	12–72 hrs
Bulking: Methylcellulose (Citrucel)	2 g TID	12–72 hrs
Bulking: Wheat dextrin (Benefiber)	1–3 g up to TID	24–48 hrs
Surfactant softener: Docusate sodium (Colace)	100 mg BID	24–72 hrs
Osmotic: Polyethylene glycol (MiraLAX)	8.5–34 g in 8 oz liquid	1–3 days
Osmotic: Lactulose (Constulose)	10–20 g every other day to twice per day	24–48 hrs
Osmotic: Sorbitol 70%	30 mL daily	24–48 hrs
Osmotic: Glycerin	2- to 3-g suppository daily	15–60 min
Osmotic: Magnesium sulfate	2–4 tsp in 8 oz water up to twice daily, four hrs apart	30 min to 3 hrs
Osmotic: Magnesium citrate	200 mL daily	30 min to 3 hrs
Stimulant: Bisacodyl (Dulcolax)	10- to 30-mg³ tablet daily 10-mg suppository	6–10 hrs (tablet), 15–60 min (suppository)
Stimulant: Senna (Ex-Lax, Senokot)	16–34 mg daily, may divide dose	6–12 hrs

³Exceeds dosage recommended by the manufacturer.
BID, Twice per day; *Tbsp,* tablespoon; *TID,* three times per day; *tsp,* teaspoon.

the intestine. Currently available data do not seem to support or refute claims of dependence on these medications after long-term use (Table 3).

For more severe cases of constipation or when a distal stool bolus is noted, the patient may benefit from manual disimpaction. If a static bolus of stool cannot be identified on rectal exam, the patient may benefit from a diatrizoate (Gastrografin) enema as part of the diagnostic workup. If stool can be disimpacted, the patient may benefit from follow-up with an osmotic enema. It is worth noting that electrolyte balance can be heavily affected by the enema fluid chosen. Soap suds enemas should be used infrequently or avoided altogether due to their potential irritating effect on the colonic mucosa.

Monitoring

During the acute setting and upon follow-up after successful management, patients with constipation should get in the habit of keeping a daily stool log. This documentation can help take the subjectivity out of complaints of constipation and help patients anticipate worsening symptoms before they occur. During the treatment of an acute exacerbation, these logs can help patients identify which medications are most effective and when they last took their dose. Any structural abnormalities identified during the initial workup should be followed with appropriate endoscopic evaluation and/or CT scan.

References

American College of Gastroenterology Chronic Constipation Task Force: An evidence-based approach to the management of chronic constipation in North America, *Am J Gastroenterol* 100(Suppl 1):S1, 2005.

Chang L, Chey WD, Imdad A, et al: American Gastroenterological Association-American College of Gastroenterology Clinical Practice Guideline: Pharmacological Management of Chronic Idiopathic Constipation, *Am J Gastroenterol* 118:936, 2023.

Mendoza J, Legido J, Rubio S, Gisbert JP: Systematic review: the adverse effects of sodium phosphate enema, *Aliment Pharmacol Ther* 26:9, 2007.

Rao SS, Meduri K: What is necessary to diagnose constipation? *Best Pract Res Clin Gastroenterol* 127–140, 2011, https://doi.org/10.1016/j.bpg.2010.11.001. PMID: 21382584; PMCID: PMC3063397.

Rao MD, PhD, FACG, AGAF, FRCP (Lon) Satish SC, Meduri MD Kalyani: Best practice & research, *Clin Gastroenterol* volume 25(Issue 1):127–140, 2011.

Schuster BG, Kosar L, Kamrul R: Constipation in older adults: stepwise approach to keep things moving, *Can Fam Physician* 61(2):152–158, 2015. PMID: 25676646; PMCID: PMC4325863.

COUGH

Method of
Emily Manlove, MD

CURRENT DIAGNOSIS

- Acute cough
  - Noninfectious
    - Chronic obstructive pulmonary disease exacerbation
    - Asthma exacerbation
    - Congestive heart failure exacerbation
    - Pulmonary embolism
  - Infectious
    - Viral rhinosinusitis (the common cold)
    - Acute bacterial sinusitis
    - Acute bronchitis (chest cold)
    - Pneumonia
    - COVID-19
    - Pertussis (whooping cough)
    - Bronchiolitis (infants)
- Chronic cough
  - First, evaluate/rule out
    - Tobacco smoking and risk for lung cancer
    - Angiotensin-converting enzyme (ACE) inhibitor–associated cough
  - Next, evaluate for the three most common etiologies
    - Chronic upper airway cough syndrome
    - Cough variant asthma/nonasthmatic eosinophilic bronchitis
    - Gastroesophageal reflux disease (GERD)
  - Last, consider other causes and more advanced testing (bronchoscopy, high-resolution computed tomography [CT], referral), and consider earlier if history, physical examination, or chest x-ray suggests an alternative diagnosis
    - Oral pharyngeal dysphagia
    - Lung tumors
    - Interstitial pulmonary diseases
    - Bronchiectasis
    - Occupational and environmental exposures
    - Sarcoidosis
    - Tuberculosis
    - Somatic cough syndrome
    - Tic cough

CURRENT THERAPY

- Acute cough caused by viral rhinosinusitis
  - Dextromethorphan (Delsym) 30 mg PO every 6 to 8 hours × 1 week
  - Diphenhydramine (Benadryl) 25 mg PO every 4 hours × 1 week
  - Nasal saline irrigation twice daily × 1 week
- Acute or subacute cough caused by *Bordetella pertussis*
  - Azithromycin (Z-Pak)[1] 500 mg PO on day 1 followed by 250 mg PO daily on days 2 to 5
- Treatment of unexplained chronic cough
  - Multimodality speech pathology therapy
  - Gabapentin (Neurontin) 300 mg PO daily, can be titrated up to a maximum daily dose of 1800 mg a day in two divided doses (off-label use)

[1]Not FDA approved for this indication.

Acute Cough

Acute cough is a cough that lasts fewer than 3 weeks. It is a common presenting complaint in the primary care physician's office and also in the emergency department. The key goal is to differentiate between patients whose cough has a benign cause and those who may be at risk for more serious illness. Infectious causes of cough are most common, but noninfectious causes should also be considered. Exacerbations of preexisting pulmonary conditions such as asthma and chronic obstructive pulmonary disease (COPD) can be associated with cough, therefore a thorough medical history should be obtained. Cough can also be associated with decompensated heart failure; in fact, cough is present in 70% of congestive heart failure (CHF) exacerbations. Also, 30% to 40% of patients with acute pulmonary embolism (PE) have a new cough at presentation of symptoms, and the classic signs and symptoms of chest pain, dyspnea, and hypoxia may not always accompany the cough.

Upper respiratory tract infections are a common cause of benign acute cough. Viral rhinosinusitis (the common cold) is probably the most common cause of acute cough. The lung examination is normal. If fever is present, it is low grade and is only present on the first or second day of illness. Most symptoms begin to resolve by 7 to 10 days, but cigarette smokers may be ill for twice as long. Symptomatic treatment is the mainstay of therapy. Antihistamine-decongestant-analgesics can provide some symptomatic benefit but may also cause side effects. Second-generation antihistamines are not effective in the treatment of cough associated with viral rhinosinusitis; it is likely that first-generation antihistamines are effective because of their anticholinergic properties. Other treatments that may be helpful include nasal saline irrigation, nasal glucocorticoids, and nasal decongestants. It is necessary to distinguish viral rhinosinusitis from acute bacterial rhinosinusitis, which may also be associated with cough. Less than 2% of all rhinosinusitis has a bacterial cause. Acute bacterial rhinosinusitis should not be diagnosed in the first week of symptoms unless the patient displays severe symptoms such as high fever. Sinus imaging studies are unlikely to be helpful, as both viral and bacterial sinusitis will have radiologic evidence of inflammation.

It is also necessary to distinguish acute cough caused by an upper respiratory tract infection from that caused by a lower respiratory tract infection. Furthermore, it is necessary to distinguish between acute bronchitis, which almost always has a viral cause, versus pneumonia, which may be bacterial. Both illnesses often have a presenting symptom of cough, which may be productive. If there is any derangement in vital signs or evidence of pulmonary consolidation on the lung examination, a chest x-ray should be performed. Influenza and COVID-19 should also be considered for patients who have fever and cough. An elevated procalcitonin level may help guide the physician in his or her decision to prescribe antibiotics. Inhaled beta agonists should not be routinely used to alleviate cough in acute viral bronchitis, but they may be helpful to alleviate wheezing and are more likely to benefit patients with airflow obstruction at baseline.

In pediatric patients younger than 2 years old, bronchiolitis should be considered as a cause of cough and fever. It is the most common cause of hospitalization in those younger than 1 year of age. Laboratory testing (including viral swabs), radiographic imaging, and treatment with beta agonists, epinephrine, or glucocorticoids do not change the course of illness. Exclusive breastfeeding for the first 6 months of infancy can decrease the morbidity of respiratory infections. *Bordetella pertussis* can cause severe illness with cough and apnea in infants. Adults have subtle symptoms and lack the classic "whooping cough" and posttussive emesis seen in children. The physician should have suspicion for pertussis in adult patients who have a cough lasting longer than 2 weeks and paroxysms of coughing; the cough can last up to 2 months. The diagnosis can be confirmed with polymerase chain reaction (PCR). Antibiotics do not alter the course of illness but reduce the spread of infection; azithromycin (Zithromax)[1] should be given for 3 to 5 days. Pregnant women should be vaccinated with each pregnancy, and other adults should replace 1 dose of Td at the earliest convenience.

Chronic Cough

A chronic cough is a cough lasting more than 8 weeks. Patients may have a presenting symptom of a cough that has been present for more than 3 weeks but fewer than 8 weeks; this is considered a subacute cough. In this case, the physician should illicit a history of respiratory infection; the patient is likely suffering from a postinfectious cough, which is related to inflammation of the airway epithelium, mucus hypersecretion, and/or increased cough reflex sensitivity. Inhaled corticosteroids may provide some benefit. If there is no history of recent infection, then the cough should be managed as a chronic cough. Chest x-ray can be considered during this time frame, but if no red flags are present (fever, unintended weight loss, night sweats, dysphagia, odynophagia, hemoptysis), the physician and patient together can decide to wait on radiography.

Chronic cough must be approached in a systematic manner, which is more likely to identify the causative agent of the cough and provide alleviation of symptoms. All of the common causes of chronic cough (see later) must be considered as the associated symptoms and the patient's description of the cough do not alter the diagnostic algorithm. It is important to confirm compliance throughout the treatment course and identify barriers to compliance with the patient. Failure to respond to empiric treatment does not necessarily rule out a diagnosis as the patient may have two diagnoses. Therefore it is prudent to continue any partially effective treatment for chronic cough.

First, it must be determined if the patient smokes. If so, the differential diagnosis is altered. The physician must determine if

the cough is a simple smoker's cough, chronic bronchitis, or possibly lung cancer; cough is the most common presenting symptom of lung cancer. Smokers are less likely to seek help for a cough and may not see a physician until a more serious problem has advanced. It is possible for a cough to worsen initially after smoking cessation, but a cough persisting more than 1 month after cessation should be investigated. Any change in a smoker's cough, a new cough, and cough with hemoptysis should be investigated. Physicians should consider low-dose CT scanning as screening for lung cancer in qualifying smokers. The second factor to rule out in all chronic cough cases is cough induced by an angiotensin-converting enzyme (ACE) inhibitor. All patients with chronic cough should stop taking an ACE inhibitor. The medication is more likely to cause a cough if it was started in the prior year, and the cough should resolve within 1 month after cessation of the ACE inhibitor. The next step to determining the cause of a chronic cough is to obtain a chest x-ray to identify any obvious causative factors. Last, the clinician should work to rule out the three most common causes of cough (see next).

Upper Airway Cough Syndrome

Upper airway cough syndrome (UACS), previously called *postnasal drip syndrome,* is likely caused by activation of cough receptors in the hypopharynx or larynx and increased sensitivity of these receptors. It is likely the most common cause of chronic cough. UACS is almost always associated with rhinosinusitis, which can be caused by a number of factors (allergic rhinitis, postinfectious rhinitis, perennial nonallergic rhinitis, rhinitis resulting from chemical irritants, rhinitis medicamentosa, pregnancy-associated rhinitis, bacterial sinusitis, allergic fungal sinusitis). The patient may complain of frequently needing to clear the throat or a sensation of "dripping" in the back of the throat; however, absence of these symptoms does not rule out UACS, nor does a history of wheezing. The physical examination may reveal mucus in the posterior oropharynx and cobblestoning of the mucosa. If the cause of rhinitis is obvious, it should be specifically treated. Otherwise, a trial of a first-generation antihistamine should be started; improvement should be seen in 2 weeks. If the side effects of this therapy are intolerable, a nasal antihistamine, nasal anticholinergic, or nasal corticosteroid can be used. If the diagnosis of UACS is highly suspected but the patient does not respond to empiric therapy, sinus CT imaging may be necessary to guide diagnosis and treatment.

Cough Variant Asthma and Nonasthmatic Eosinophilic Bronchitis

Cough-variant asthma and nonasthmatic eosinophilic bronchitis (NAEB) both primarily present with a cough, and the patient may have few other symptoms. Patients with cough-variant asthma will have abnormal spirometry, whereas those with NAEB will not. When spirometry is performed, bronchoprovocation testing with methacholine should be performed as it increases the negative predicative value of the test. If spirometry is negative, the sputum should be evaluated for eosinophils, which are present in both diseases. Both diseases are treated as asthma; an inhaled corticosteroid should be started and long-acting beta agonists and leukotriene receptor antagonists can be considered as adjunctive therapy. A positive response should be expected within 2 weeks.

Gastroesophageal Reflux Disease

Gastroesophageal reflux disease (GERD) is common, but not all patients with GERD have an associated cough; therefore, the presence of GERD does not ensure that it is the source of the patient's cough. However, patients whose cough is clearly not caused by UACS, cough-variant asthma, or NAEB are very likely to have a GERD-induced cough. Cough can be caused by acidic and non-acidic reflux, so a proton pump inhibitor (PPI) may not always be beneficial in alleviating the cough. A pH probe can be performed in cases when it is unclear whether reflux is occurring. All patients should utilize lifestyle changes to attenuate reflux, such as smoking cessation, avoidance of alcohol and acidic foods, weight loss, and

---

[1] Not FDA approved for this indication.

treatment of sleep apnea. It may take 3 to 6 months of treatment to see improvement in cough. If the patient does not improve and GERD is highly suspected, referral to a surgeon may be necessary for fundoplication.

Other Causes of Chronic Cough

In patients who still suffer from chronic cough and the above causes have been ruled out, further investigation should be sought. Referral to a pulmonologist may be necessary in addition to high-resolution CT scanning and bronchoscopy. Causative factors may include oral pharyngeal dysphagia, lung tumors, interstitial pulmonary diseases, bronchiectasis, occupational and environmental exposures, sarcoidosis, and tuberculosis. Somatic cough syndrome (previously referred to as *psychogenic cough*), tic cough (previously termed *habit cough*), and cough hypersensitivity syndrome (previously known as *overactive cough reflex*) may be considered in some patients. Treatment options include speech language pathology intervention, empiric gabapentin, and/or referral to a cough clinic.

References

Chung KF, Pavord ID: Prevalence, pathogenesis, and causes of chronic cough, *Lancet* 371(9621):1364–1374, 2008.
Côté A, Russell RJ, Boulet LP, et al: Managing chronic cough due to asthma and NAEB in adults and adolescents: CHEST guideline and expert panel report, *Chest* 158(1):68–96, 2020.
De Sutter AI, Eriksson L, van Driel ML: Oral antihistamine–decongestant–analgesic combinations for the common cold, *Cochrane Database Syst Rev* 1(1):CD004976, 2022.
Gibson P, Wang G, McGarvey L, et al: Treatment of unexplained chronic cough: CHEST guideline and expert panel report, *Chest* 149(1):27–44, 2016.
Irwin RS, French CL, Chang AB, et al: Classification of cough as a symptom in adults and management algorithms: CHEST guideline and expert panel report, *Chest* 153(1):196–209, 2018.
Irwin RS, Madison JM: Unexplained or refractory chronic cough in adults, *NEJM* 392(12):1203–1214, 2025.
Michaudet C, Malaty JJ: Chronic cough: evaluation and management, *Am Fam Physician* 96(9):575–580, 2017.
Ralston SL, Lieberthal AS, Meissner HC, et al.: Clinical practice guideline: the diagnosis, management, and prevention of bronchiolitis, *Pediatrics* 134(5):e1474–1502, 2014.

DIZZINESS AND VERTIGO

Method of
Jennifer Wipperman, MD, MPH

CURRENT DIAGNOSIS

- Benign paroxysmal positional vertigo
  - Repeated, brief episodes lasting less than 1 minute
  - Triggered by changes in head position
  - Positive Dix-Hallpike or Supine Roll Test
- Vestibular neuritis
  - Single, severe, constant episode lasting days
  - Subacute onset
  - Positive head impulse test
  - Nystagmus is unidirectional and horizontal
- Vestibular migraine
  - Recurrent episodes lasting hours to days
  - Includes features of migraine headache
  - Responds to traditional migraine treatment
- Ménière's disease
  - Recurrent episodes of vertigo lasting hours
  - May have hearing loss, tinnitus, or ear fullness
- Red flags for stroke include:
  - Sudden onset
  - Risk factors for stroke
  - Bidirectional or purely vertical nystagmus
  - Abnormal HINTS exam
  - Focal neurologic signs
  - Inability to walk

CURRENT THERAPY

- Benign paroxysmal positional vertigo
  - The canalith repositioning procedure (Epley maneuver) is the most effective treatment.
  - Avoid vestibular suppressant medications
  - Observation with close follow-up is optional if a patient will not tolerate the canalith repositioning procedure and if symptoms are mild
- Vestibular neuritis
  - Brief symptomatic care with benzodiazepines, antiemetics, and antihistamines
  - Early vestibular rehabilitation speeds recovery.
  - Use of corticosteroids is controversial.

The "dizzy" patient is often a frustrating phenomenon in clinical medicine. However, after a careful history and physical examination, most patients can be diagnosed and serious causes excluded. Peripheral causes of vertigo are usually benign and include vestibular neuritis and benign paroxysmal positional vertigo (BPPV). Life-threatening central causes include stroke, demyelinating disease, and an intracranial mass. The first step in evaluating vertigo is differentiating among the four types of dizziness: near syncope or lightheadedness, disequilibrium, psychogenic dizziness, and true vertigo. True vertigo is a false sense of motion, and patients often report that "the room is spinning." This chapter will focus on the two most common causes of episodic vertigo: BPPV and vestibular neuritis.

Epidemiology

Vertigo is a common office complaint. Every year, millions of Americans are evaluated for dizziness in ambulatory care settings, and approximately 50% of these cases are vertigo. BPPV and vestibular neuritis are two of the most common causes of vertigo seen in the office setting.

Risk Factors

BPPV is seven times more likely in individuals over age 60, and it is also more common in women. A history of prior head trauma and other vestibular disorders increases risk of BPPV. There are no identified risk factors for vestibular neuritis.

Pathophysiology

BPPV is thought to occur when calcium carbonate debris (otoconia) are dislodged and float freely in the semicircular canals of the inner ear. The posterior canal is most often involved. During head movement, loose otoconia move in the canal and cause a continued sense of motion for a few seconds until they settle. The pathophysiology of vestibular neuritis is uncertain. Limited evidence supports a viral infection, which causes inflammation of the eighth cranial nerve. When hearing loss accompanies vertigo, the condition is called *acute labrynthitis*.

Clinical Manifestations

The history and physical examination are fundamental in the evaluation of vertigo. Key questions include the frequency and duration of attacks, triggers such as positional or pressure changes, prior head trauma, associated neurologic symptoms, hearing loss, and headache. A personal history of diabetes, hypertension, and hyperlipidemia are risk factors for stroke. BPPV, stroke, and migraine can have a familial preponderance. Many medications, including anticonvulsants and antihypertensives, cause dizziness.

BPPV causes brief, recurrent episodes that last less than 1 minute and are brought on by changes in head movement or position. Nausea and vomiting may be associated. Vestibular neuritis usually has a subacute onset over several hours, peaks in intensity for 1 to 2 days, and then gradually subsides over the next few weeks. Symptoms of vertigo are constant, and nausea and vomiting can be severe during the first few days. Patients with vestibular neuritis may

TABLE 1	Differentiating Peripheral and Central Causes of Vertigo		
	PERIPHERAL CAUSES		
	BPPV	**VESTIBULAR NEURITIS**	**CENTRAL CAUSES**
History	Brief, recurrent attacks of vertigo lasting less than 1 minute Triggered by positional changes No vertigo between attacks	Subacute onset Constant and severe vertigo lasting days Nausea and vomiting may be severe	Sudden onset Risk factors for stroke May have severe headache
Nystagmus	Up-beating and torsional	Horizontal and unidirectional	Bidirectional Pure vertical Pure torsional
Gait	Unaffected between episodes	May veer towards affected side	Unable to walk
Specialized physical examination tests	Positive Dix-Hallpike or Positive supine roll test	Positive head impulse test Visual fixation stops nystagmus	HINTS exam abnormal Visual fixation does not stop nystagmus
Additional neurologic signs	Rare	Rare	Common (e.g., dysarthria, aphasia, incoordination, weakness, or numbness)

Abbreviation: BPPV = benign paroxysmal positional vertigo.

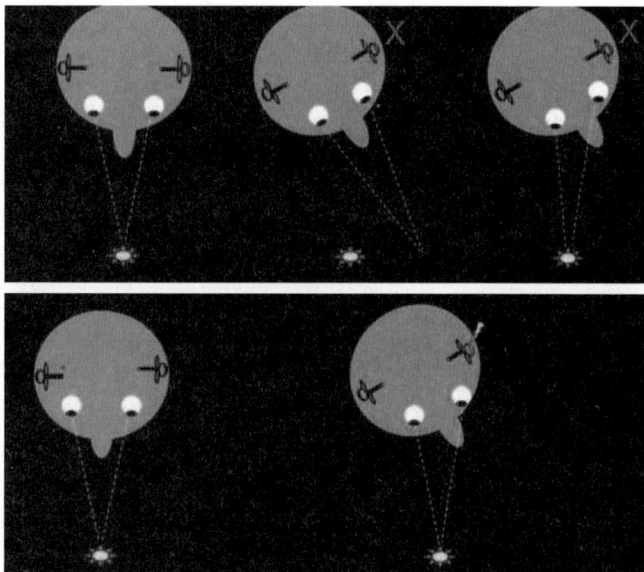

Figure 1 Head impulse test. Top panel shows a positive head impulse test. The examiner moves the patient's head quickly 10 degrees to the side, in this case to the patient's left. A catch-up saccade is observed when the patient looks away and then refixes on the visual target, indicating a peripheral lesion on the left. Lower figure shows a normal head impulse test. The patient maintains visual fixation during head movement. Adapted from Seemungal BM, Bronstein AM. A practical approach to acute vertigo. *Pract Neurol* 2008; 8:211–21.

have difficulty standing and veer toward the affected side. Although changes in position worsen the vertigo in vestibular neuritis, vertigo is always present at baseline. In BPPV, patients have no vertigo between attacks.

General physical examination should include a thorough cardiovascular, ear, nose, throat, and neurologic examination. The neurologic examination can differentiate between benign (peripheral) and life-threatening (central) causes based on the ability to walk, type of nystagmus, results of the head impulse test, and presence of associated neurologic signs (Table 1).

Patients with vestibular neuritis may have difficulty walking, but the inability to walk is a red flag for a central lesion. Nystagmus is unidirectional (always beats in the same direction) and horizontal in vestibular neuritis, and is suppressed by visual fixation. Having a patient focus on an object in the room will stop

the nystagmus, which reappears if a blank sheet of paper is placed a few inches in front of the patient's face. Nystagmus in central causes is not suppressed by visual fixation and may be direction-changing (nystagmus beats to the right when the patient looks right, and beats to the left when the patient looks left) or purely vertical. The head impulse test (Figure 1) is positive in peripheral causes like vestibular neuritis. The examiner holds the patient's head while the patient fixes her eyes on the examiner's nose, and then the examiner quickly moves the patient's head 10 degrees to the right and left. If a saccade (the eyes look away and then re-fixate on the examiner's nose) is found, this indicates a peripheral lesion on the side that the head is turned toward. Central lesions will not cause saccades, and the head impulse test will be negative. HINTS (Head Impulse test, Nystagmus, Test of Skew), which combines three physical examination findings, has been found to have a high sensitivity and moderate specificity for a central cause of vertigo in the acute setting and to be more accurate than MRI in the initial 24 hours after symptom onset. If one or more of the tests indicate a central cause, (e.g., a negative head impulse test, direction-changing horizontal nystagmus, or vertical eye misalignment grossly observed or detected on cover-uncover test), then the HINTS test is considered positive for a central cause and imaging should be obtained. A negative HINTS exam is an excellent rule-out test for stroke, with a negative likelihood ratio of 0.02.

The Dix-Hallpike maneuver is diagnostic of posterior canal BPPV (Figure 2). The patient should be warned that nausea and vomiting may occur. After the patient is placed in the head-hanging position, there is a 5- to 20-second latency period before the nystagmus and symptoms appear. Both the nystagmus and vertigo will increase in severity and then resolve within 60 seconds. The nystagmus observed is up-beating and torsional. If nystagmus is constant for as long as the head is in the hanging position, the patient should be evaluated for a central cause. The maneuver should be repeated with the head held to the opposite side. The side that elicits the symptoms and nystagmus diagnoses BPPV in the ipsilateral ear. If both sides elicit symptoms, the patient may have bilateral BPPV. If the test is negative and BPPV is strongly suspected, the patient should lie supine and the examiner can turn the head to each side (supine roll test; Figure 3). This maneuver will cause vertigo and nystagmus in patients with horizontal canal BPPV.

Diagnosis

BPPV and vestibular neuritis are diagnosed clinically. Further diagnostic testing is indicated if the diagnosis is uncertain or a central cause is suspected. Audiometry may be abnormal in Ménière's disease. MRI is the best imaging test for central lesions because it

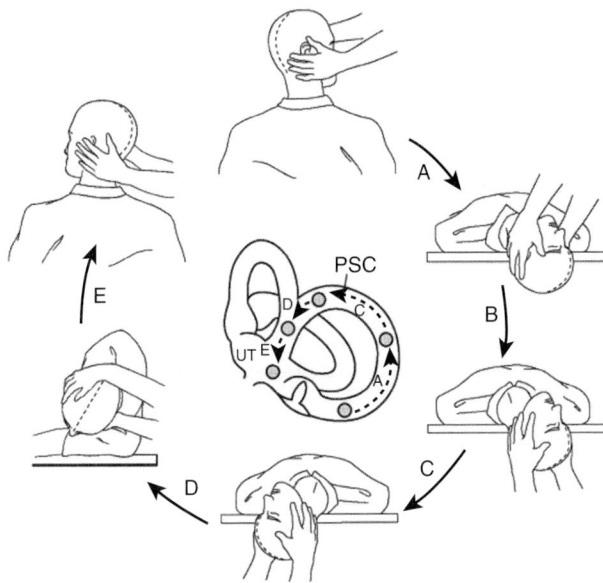

Figure 2 Treatment maneuver for posterior canal benign paroxysmal positional vertigo affecting the right ear. To treat the left ear, the procedure is reversed. The drawing of the labyrinth in the center shows the position of the particle as it moves around the posterior semicircular canal (PSC) and into the utricle (UT). The patient is seated upright, with head facing the examiner, who is standing on the right. **A,** The patient is rapidly moved to head-hanging right position (Dix-Hallpike test). This position is maintained until the nystagmus ceases. **B,** The examiner moves to the head of the table, repositioning hands as shown. **C,** The head is rotated quickly to the left with right ear upward. This position is maintained for 30 seconds. **D,** The patient rolls onto the left side while the examiner rapidly rotates the head leftward until the nose is directed toward the floor. This position is then held for 30 seconds. **E,** The patient is rapidly lifted into the sitting position, now facing left. The entire sequence should be repeated until no nystagmus can be elicited. After the maneuver, the patient is instructed to avoid head-hanging positions to prevent the particles from reentering the posterior canal. Reprinted with permission from Rakel RE. *Conn's Current Therapy 1995.* Philadelphia, WB Saunders, 1995, p 839.

includes the posterior fossa and is most sensitive for stroke. Vestibular function testing is useful if the diagnosis is unclear or in cases of refractory vertigo. Vestibular function testing evaluates the ocular and vestibular response to position changes and caloric stimulation. Video-oculographic recordings of nystagmus can magnify the eye and allow for repeated viewings for further study. Some patients with BPPV may have additional vestibular disorders causing vertigo that vestibular function testing can elucidate.

Differential Diagnosis

Ménière's disease is suspected in patients with the triad of tinnitus, fluctuating hearing loss, and vertigo. Episodes usually last hours, are disabling, and are recurrent over years, over time leading to permanent dysfunction. Migrainous vertigo features episodes lasting hours to days in patients with other migraine symptoms such as headache, photophobia, phonophobia, or aura. Central lesions such as stroke or intracranial mass are most concerning. Red flags for stroke include sudden onset, risk factors for stroke, associated neurologic signs, inability to walk, abnormal HINTS exam, severe associated headache, and characteristic nystagmus. Posttraumatic vertigo may occur in patients after head trauma who present with vertigo, tinnitus, and headache. A perilymphatic fistula is rare, but may be suspected in a patient with episodic vertigo after head trauma, heavy lifting, or barotrauma. Pressure changes with sneezing or coughing trigger vertigo attacks. Postural hypotension should be ruled out in all patients. An acoustic neuroma presents with slowly progressive, unilateral sensorineural hearing loss and tinnitus. Many patients may have an unsteady gait, but true vertigo is rare.

Treatment

Posterior canal BPPV is best treated with the *canalith repositioning procedure (CRP)*, such as the Epley maneuver (Figure 2). Studies have shown the procedure is safe and effective with an odds ratio of 4.2 (95% CI. 2.3-11.4) for symptom resolution. Patients should be warned that nausea or vomiting may occur during the procedure, and may be pretreated with an antiemetic medication. The procedure can be repeated immediately if unsuccessful, and the majority of patients will respond after three attempts. Posttreatment activity restrictions are unnecessary. Horizontal canal BPPV can be treated with the barbeque roll maneuver (Figure 4). Patients

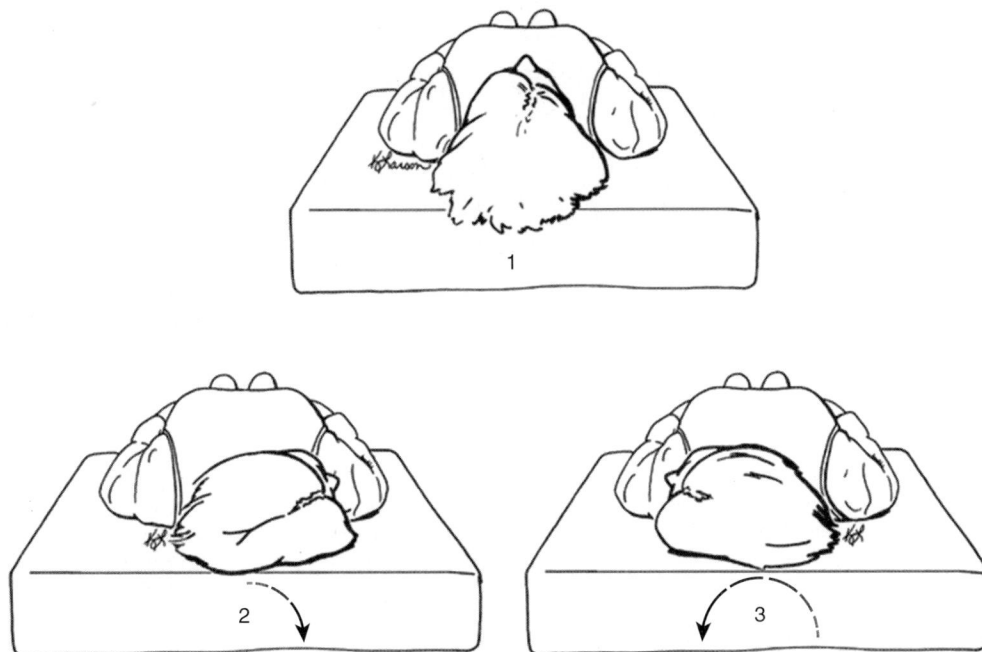

Figure 3 Supine roll test. Patient begins lying supine facing upward. The patient's head is rotated to one side laterally 90 degrees and the examiner observes for nystagmus and vertigo. Once symptoms resolve, the patient's head is rotated back to midline. Next, the patient's head is rotated 90 degrees laterally to the opposite side and the examiner observes for nystagmus and vertigo. The side with the worst symptoms indicates the involved ear. (From Kerber KA, et al: Benign paroxysmal positional vertigo in the acute care setting. NCL, Elsevier, 2015.)

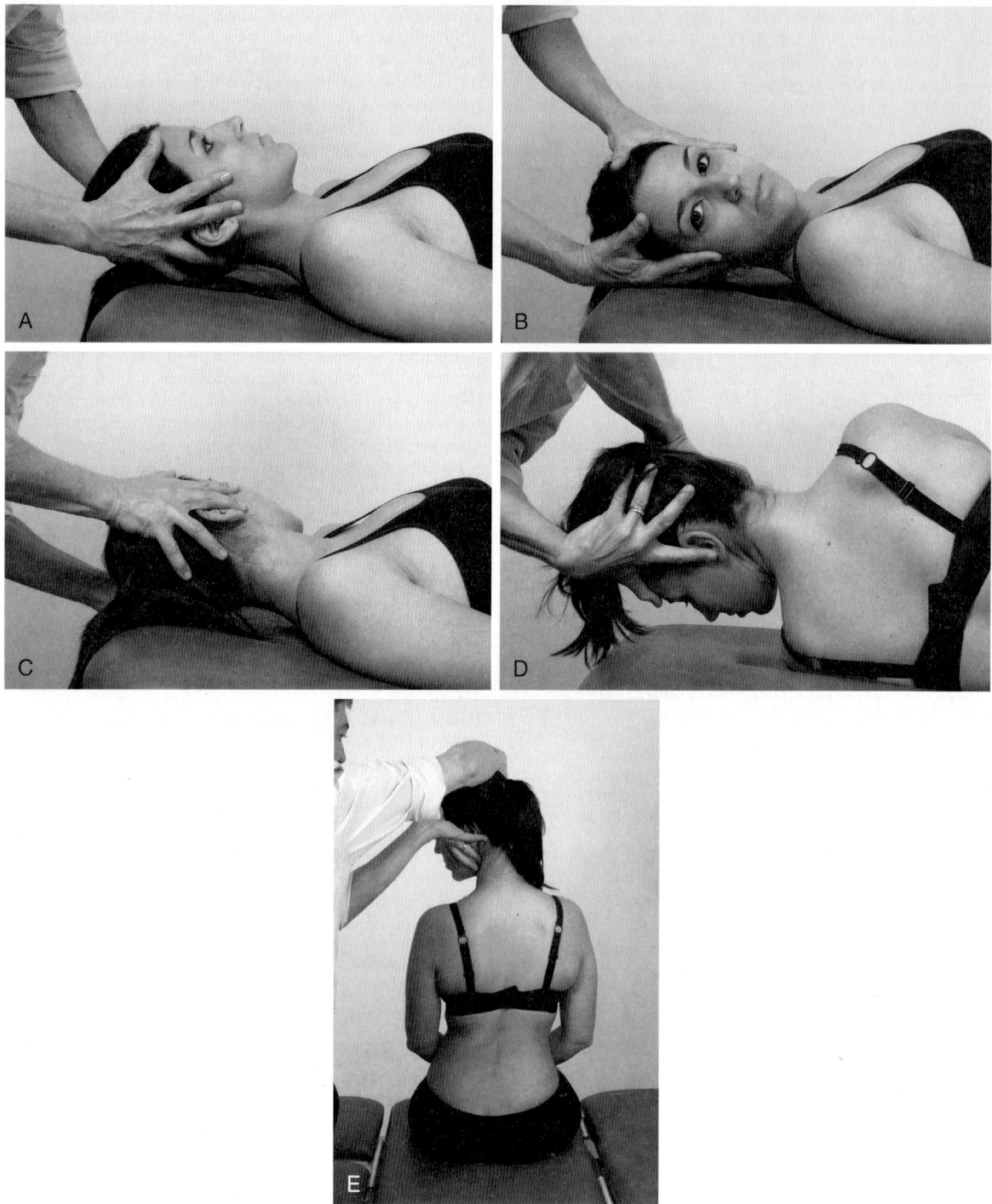

Figure 4 Barbecue roll (Lempert maneuver). Patient begins lying supine facing upward (A). Head is rotated laterally 90 degrees toward the affected ear (B). Next, the head is rotated another 90 degrees laterally back to midline (B). Next, the head is rotated laterally 90 degrees toward the opposite side (C). Next, the head is rotated laterally 90 degrees in the same direction (D). Finally, with the patient's head in the same position, the patient is brought into a seated position (E). Each position is held 30 to 60 seconds, long enough for symptoms to occur and then resolve. Once resolved, the patient is moved into the next position. (From Moseley L, Cueco RT: Essential guide to the cervical spine - Volume 2: Clinical Syndromes and Manipulative Treatment. Elsevier, 2016.)

who do not tolerate a CRP may be referred to vestibular rehabilitation for further evaluation and treatment. Observation is an option if symptoms are mild and if a patient will not tolerate the canalith repositioning procedure. However, time to resolution with observation is 1–3 months, and recurrence rates are higher compared to treatment with CRP. Vestibular-suppressant medications such as antihistamines and benzodiazepines are discouraged because they increase fall risk and treatment with CRP is effective. Surgery is rarely needed for BPPV, but may be helpful in refractory cases.

Vestibular neuritis is primarily treated with rest, vestibular suppressant medications, and vestibular rehabilitation. Patients may

initially be hospitalized if symptoms, such as nausea and vomiting, are severe or if stroke is suspected. Treatment with antihistamines (dimenhydrinate [Dramamine][1] 50 mg every 6 hours), antiemetics (promethazine [Phenergan][1] 25 mg every 6 hours), or benzodiazepines (lorazepam [Ativan][1] 1 to 2 mg every 4 hours) may be used to treat severe symptoms. However, these should not be continued for more than 2 to 3 days because they inhibit central compensation. In vestibular neuritis, patients' vertigo improves not due to return of vestibular nerve function, but due to central

---

[1]Not FDA approved for this indication.

compensation for the peripheral deficit. Using vestibular suppressants blocks central compensation and lengthens the course of the disease. The use of corticosteroids is controversial due to the lack of high quality evidence to support symptomatic improvement. Finally, antiviral medications have not been proven effective for vestibular neuritis.

For patients with vestibular neuritis, vestibular rehabilitation should be started as soon as symptoms improve and a patient can tolerate the exercises. Exercises include balance and gait training as well as coordination of head and eye movements. Vestibular rehabilitation hastens recovery and improves balance, gait, and vision by increasing central compensation for vestibular dysfunction. Exercises may be home-based for compliant patients with mild symptoms, whereas formal referral may be more beneficial for patients with severe symptoms, or for the elderly.

Monitoring
Patients diagnosed with BPPV should be reassessed in 1 month regardless of treatment. Failure to improve warrants further evaluation for other etiologies, including central causes. Similarly, patients with vestibular neuritis should slowly improve over several weeks, and failure to do so suggests alternative diagnoses.

Complications
Patients with BPPV are at increased risk for falls. Thirty percent of elderly patients with BPPV have multiple falls in a year. Thus patients should be assessed for fall risk, functional mobility, and balance. Home safety evaluation and home supervision should be considered. BPPV often recurs, with an estimated rate of 15% per year. Counseling patients about recurrence can lead to earlier recognition, earlier treatment, and avoidance of falls. Patients with vestibular neuritis are at increased risk for BPPV and Ménière's disease. Vestibular neuritis rarely recurs.

References
Bhattacharyya N, Gubbels SP, Schwartz SR, et al: Clinical practice guideline: benign paroxysmal positional vertigo (update), *Otolaryngol Head Neck Surg* 156(Supp 3):S1–S47, 2017.
Chan Y: Differential diagnosis of dizziness, *Otolaryngol Head Neck Surg* 17:200–203, 2009.
Epley JM: The canalith repositioning procedure: for treatment of benign paroxysmal positional vertigo, *Otolaryngol Head Neck Surg* 107:399–404, 1992.
Fishman JM, Burgess C, Waddell A: Corticosteroids for the treatment of idiopathic acute vestibular dysfunction (vestibular neuritis), *Cochran Database Syst Rev* 5, CD008607, 2011. Review.
Gottlieb M, Peksa GD, Carlson JN. Head impulse, nystagmus, and test of skew examination for diagnosing central causes of acute vestibular syndrome. *Cochrane Database Syst Rev*, 2023, 11(11):CD015089.
Hilton MP, Pinder DK: The Epley (canalith repositioning) manoeuvre for benign paroxysmal positional vertigo, *Cochrane Database Syst Rev* 12, CD003162, 2014.
Kerber KA: Vertigo and dizziness in the emergency department, *Emerg Med Clin North Am* 27:39–50, 2009.
McDonnell MN, Hillier SL: Vestibular rehabilitation for unilateral peripheral vestibular dysfunction, *Cochrane Database Syst Rev* 1, CD005397, 2015.
Seemungal BM, Bronstein AM: A practical approach to acute vertigo, *Pract Neurol* 8:211–221, 2008.

FATIGUE

Method of
Jared Regehr, MD

CURRENT DIAGNOSIS

- It is important to evaluate for potential causes of fatigue with a thorough history and physical exam. Basic lab work is also important to evaluate for organic etiologies of fatigue.
- Most cases of fatigue do not have an identifiable underlying etiology.
- A broad differential is important as clinicians evaluate patients with fatigue.

CURRENT THERAPY

- Identifying the underlying cause of fatigue is the most important step in treatment, and any discovered cause should be treated promptly.
- Good sleep hygiene, physical activity, regularly scheduled follow-up visits, and cognitive behavioral therapy have all been shown to improve symptoms of fatigue.
- Short naps are proven performance enhancers.

Epidemiology
Fatigue is a common concern for patients and is the primary complaint for 5% to 10% of patient encounters in the primary care setting. Certain risk factors predispose patients to fatigue. Female sex (1.5 times more likely to report fatigue than males), increased age, and coexisting depression are all associated with higher rates of fatigue. While fatigue can be a normal physiologic response to prolonged activity or stressors, pathologic fatigue has a significant negative impact on patients each year. Individuals with fatigue report decreased quality of life, along with social and emotional dysfunction. Furthermore, it is estimated that fatigue costs US employers $126 billion each year due to decreased production and lost work days.

Prevention
Prevention of fatigue is very similar to the treatment of fatigue. Good sleep hygiene, regular physical exercise, and stress reduction all help with preventing fatigue. Additionally, regularly scheduled follow-up for health maintenance examinations with primary care physicians helps patients avoid comorbidities that may exacerbate fatigue.

Clinical Manifestations
Patients with fatigue often present with lack of energy, delayed recovery after activity, poor muscle endurance, mental exhaustion, and nonrestorative sleep. There is a wide spectrum of severity of disease from a general nuisance to debilitating symptoms.

Diagnosis
Fatigue can be classified based on duration: recent (<1 month), prolonged (1–6 months), and chronic (>6 months). Notably, these timeframes are arbitrary based on the continuous nature of fatigue. For most clinicians, having a broad differential is more helpful in identifying a cause than categorizing fatigue based on time. Even so, identifying the underlying etiology of fatigue can be a challenging and frustrating diagnosis for primary care physicians to make because of vague symptoms and the overlap with comorbidities. A thorough history and physical examination along with appropriate laboratory tests can aid in the diagnosis. There is much debate about the extent of initial laboratory workup, but a reasonable approach includes a complete blood count, basic metabolic panel, hepatic function testing, erythrocyte sedimentation rate, thyroid-stimulating hormone, ferritin, pregnancy test in women of childbearing age, and screening for HIV and hepatitis C in at-risk populations. These tests are useful to help identify "can't miss" diagnoses, but results of laboratory studies only affect management in about 5% of cases. Therefore the importance of a thorough history and physical examination is paramount. It is essential to remember that the information collected from the patient does not need to be limited to the time spent together in the office; a symptom diary with close follow-up can be an extremely beneficial tool as the physician–patient dyad works to find a cause.

The causes of fatigue are extensive and oftentimes coexisting. The most common causes are encompassed in the mnemonic DEAD TIRED (Table 1). Most of these categories have multiple subcategories. As with all chief complaints, it is imperative to allow patients the opportunity to lead the physician to the diagnosis by letting

TABLE 1	Common Causes of Fatigue: DEAD TIRED
D	Depression
E	Endocrine
A	Anemia, apnea
D	Diabetes
T	Thyroid, tumors
I	Infection, insomnia
R	Rheumatologic
E	Endocarditis/cardiovascular
D	Drugs

them speak without interruption. Depression is a common cause of fatigue. Medically unexplained symptoms of fatigue are associated with depressive disorders in 50% to 75% of patients, and patients are nearly 11 times more likely to have a lifetime diagnosis of depression than nonfatigued individuals. Importantly, fatigue may be the first presenting symptom for patients who do not yet meet the *Diagnostic and Statistical Manual of Mental Disorders* (DSM) criteria for depression, so close monitoring for other depressive symptoms is vital for prompt recognition and treatment. In most of these cases, there are often other lifestyle factors that contribute to patients' feelings of fatigue. It is important to ask about sleep hygiene, physical exercise, and home/social stressors, as suboptimal functioning in these areas can exacerbate symptoms of fatigue.

Other common secondary causes of fatigue include anemia, endocrine abnormalities, sleep apnea, and medication use. If anemia is noted on initial laboratory evaluation, further workup is usually patient-specific. Markers such as mean corpuscular volume (MCV), ferritin, iron profile, B12, folate, lactate dehydrogenase, and haptoglobin can help guide decision making as clinicians consider causes of anemia. Gastrointestinal bleeding secondary to ulcers, colon cancer, inflammatory bowel disease, or diverticulosis are critical to rule out. Lack of sufficient dietary vitamin intake may be a simple reason for anemia. Endocrine abnormalities that can lead to fatigue include thyroid dysfunction, diabetes mellitus, and adrenal insufficiency. If patients describe persistent daytime sleepiness, evaluation for obstructive sleep apnea is useful, especially in the setting of risk factors (obesity, snoring, hypertension). Additionally, medication usage can cause fatigue. An in-depth review of the legion of medications that can cause fatigue is beyond the scope of this article, but prescription, over-the-counter, and illicit drugs should be considered in the evaluation of fatigue.

Infection is a cause of fatigue, and the most frequent infectious etiology associated with fatigue is of viral origin. Any one of several viruses can cause fatigue, including hepatitis A, B, and C; Epstein-Barr virus; human immunodeficiency virus; and as of recently, COVID-19. Certainly not every patient presenting with fatigue necessitates laboratory evaluation for each of these causes, but if the history or examination suggests an infectious cause, further workup is prudent. Even after recovery from COVID-19, 72.8% of patients report persistent fatigue, by far the most common long-term symptom reported by survivors of COVID-19. This is an important consideration even months after patients have otherwise recovered from the disease. Postinfluenza asthenia refers to the prolonged fatigue some patients experience after a bout of influenza.

Finally, rheumatologic, cardiovascular, and neoplastic causes should be considered when appropriate in the evaluation of fatigue. Although there are innumerable reports of fatigue in patients with rheumatologic, cardiovascular, oncologic, and hematologic disorders, isolated fatigue as the presenting complaint is not well documented in current medical literature. Additionally, multiple neurologic and autoimmune disorders can have associated fatigue. If the rest of the history and examination

warrants further workup for these causes, then evaluation should be pursued. However, an extensive workup based on an isolated complaint of fatigue is not likely to yield beneficial results.

Therapy

Treatment for fatigue should be directed at managing the underlying cause of fatigue when an etiology can be identified based on the history, physical, and laboratory evaluation. However, when no organic cause is identified, there are still ways to help patients get relief. Importantly, ordering more tests is not one of them. In a systemic review of patients with fatigue in which there was a low level of clinical concern for serious illness, the degree of patient reassurance was not increased with additional laboratory testing. Instead, the clinician should start with having an honest conversation with the patient regarding ways to move forward. It is imperative to acknowledge the patient's symptoms and the negative effects on the patient's life, discuss consistent follow-up, and discuss assessment of any new symptoms that may develop. Additionally, there is evidence that sleep hygiene, physical activity, and cognitive behavioral therapy may be helpful in these settings of nondiagnostic fatigue. Short naps have also proven to be helpful and may be a possible solution for some patients.

Monitoring

Monitoring patients with persistent fatigue in the primary care setting can be accomplished by administering a Fatigue Severity Scale (FSS). This method assesses the impact of fatigue on patients' daily lives with a nine-item survey that incorporates a Likert-type rating scale. The FSS has been validated in multiple studies as a reliable tool to assess fatigue. Although there is no generally agreed upon timing for frequency of monitoring, it is reasonable to start with monthly assessments and utilize shared decision making with each patient to individualize a management plan.

References

Corfield E, Martin N, Nyholt D: Co-occurrence and symptomatology of fatigue and depression, *Compr Psychiatry* 71:1–10, 2016.

Finsterer J, Zarrouk-Mahjoub S: Fatigue in health and diseased individuals, *Am J Hosp Palliat Med* 31(5):562–575, 2014.

Friedberg F, Napoli A, Coronel J, et al: Chronic fatigue self-management in primary care: a randomized trial, *Psychosom Med* 75(7):650–657, 2013.

Kamal M, Abo Omirah M, Hussein A, Saeed H: Assessment and characterisation of post–COVID-19 manifestations, *Int J Clin Pract*, 2020. Available at: https://doi-org.proxy.kumc.edu/10.1111/ijcp.13746. Accessed December 31, 2020.

Morelli V: Toward a comprehensive differential diagnosis and clinical approach to fatigue in the elderly, *Clin Geriatr Med* 27(4):687–692, 2011.

O'Connor K, Wright J: Fatigue, *Med Clin North Am* 98(3):597–608, 2014.

Rosenthal T, Majeroni B, Pretorius R, Malik K. Fatigue: an overview. *Am Fam Physician*. 15;78(10):1173–1179

Valko P, Bassetti C, Bloch K, Held U, Baumann C: Validation of the fatigue severity scale in a swiss cohort, *Sleep* 31(11):1601–1607, 2008.

Zhang XY, Huang HJ, Zhuang DL, et al: Biological, clinical and epidemiological features of COVID-19, SARS and MERS and AutoDock simulation of ACE2, *Infect Dis Poverty* 9, 2020. Available at: https://doi.org/10.1186/s40249-020-00691-6. Accessed December 31, 2020.

▌FEVER

Method of
Alan R. Roth, DO; and Gina M. Basello, DO

CURRENT DIAGNOSIS

- Numerous endogenous and exogenous factors play a role in determining body temperature. Current standards define *fever* as an oral temperature of ≥100.4°F (≥38°C).
- Though temperature varies with measurement technique, in clinical practice, most recommendations refer to oral, rectal, and axillary temperature measurements, with rectal temperature being the standard of care in infants and young children.

- Tympanic thermometers should not be used in young children.
- Fever is not an illness. It is the body's physiologic response to a disease process and has beneficial effects in fighting infection.
- All neonates with a fever should be admitted to the hospital for a sepsis evaluation. For infants between 1 and 3 months of age, evidence-based guidelines, along with clinical evaluation, determine the diagnostic and therapeutic approach.
- For well-appearing term infants 29 to 60 days of age with fever ≥38.0°C and no evident infection source, diagnostic testing should include urinalysis, blood cultures, and inflammatory markers (e.g., procalcitonin and absolute neutrophil count [ANC]).
- With widespread immunization use, the incidence of bacteremia and bacterial meningitis in young infants has significantly decreased, and UTI is now the most prevalent bacterial infection, with the most common etiologic pathogen being *E. coli* for both.
- The possibility of infection with the SARS-CoV-2 virus must be considered in all patients presenting with fever and tested for appropriately. Global health considerations may necessitate additional testing in returning travelers (e.g., monkeypox, polio).
- Urine leukocyte esterase has emerged as a highly accurate diagnostic test for UTI in febrile infants with greater than 95% sensitivity.
- FUO requires a systematic, thoughtful, and thorough evaluation based on the age of the patient and the existing clinical evidence, with repeated clinical assessments being essential.
- Hyperthermia is an unregulated, significant elevation of core body temperature above the normal diurnal range due to failure of thermoregulation from a hypothalamic insult, not a pyogenic source, and is considered a medical emergency. It is not synonymous with fever and often requires immediate intervention to avoid deleterious central nervous system (CNS) effects.

CURRENT THERAPY

- Treating a fever significantly increases the patient's level of comfort, activity, and oral feeding and fluid intake, in addition to decreasing the body temperature.
- Multiple randomized, controlled trials reveal that treating fever does not shorten or prolong the overall duration of illness or reduce the occurrence of febrile seizures.
- Many clinical recommendations state that a temperature less than 102.2°F (39°C) in healthy children does not require treatment. Antipyretics are known to provide comfort to children and their caregivers.
- Antipyretic treatment for children includes acetaminophen (Tylenol) 10 to 15 mg/kg every 4 to 6 hours or ibuprofen (Advil, Motrin) 10 mg/kg every 6 hours.
- Ibuprofen and acetaminophen have both been shown to reduce fever effectively and safely. Combination therapy has been shown in some studies to have an added benefit in both reduction of temperature and comfort without an increase in side effects, though caution should be taken to avoid dosing errors.
- Antipyretic therapy for adults and adolescents includes acetaminophen 650 to 1000 mg orally (PO) every 6 hours to a maximum of 3 g per day, ibuprofen 200 to 400 mg PO every 6 hours, or aspirin (ASA) 325 to 650 mg every 6 hours as needed (PRN) for fever.
- ASA should not be used in children due to the risk of Reye's syndrome.
- Sponge bathing should be done with tepid water and no alcohol. Recommendation: sponge bathing and other home remedies should not be used as sole treatment.

Fever is one of the most common clinical presentations encountered by primary care physicians and the most common complaint of acute visits for children in the ambulatory or emergency department setting. Fever is a symptom and one of the most reliable signs of illness rather than a disease process itself. Most causes of fever are secondary to acute viral illnesses such as upper respiratory infections (URIs), which account for 50 million visits to primary care providers annually. Less commonly, bacterial infections may cause pharyngitis, otitis, sinusitis, pneumonia, and urinary tract infections (UTIs). A cost-effective, evidence-based approach using clinical protocols, guidelines, and consensus recommendations to the diagnosis and management of febrile illness, including the appropriate use of antibiotic therapy, is the cornerstone of quality medical care for this presentation. Fever produces significant anxiety for patients, parents, and health care providers, which can lead to overtreatment. Typically, fever is transient and only requires treatment to provide patient comfort.

Definitions

The definition of fever is dependent on numerous endogenous and exogenous factors that play a role in determining body temperature, including age, time of day, site, and measuring device, as well as operator variables. Fever is an elevation of body temperature due to the adjustment of the hypothalamic-pituitary set point. This usually occurs in response to a pathologic stimulus. Fever is a beneficial physiologic mechanism that helps to promote an augmented immunologic response.

Despite individual variability, core body temperature is maintained at about 98.6°F (37°C). Diurnal variation results in lower body temperatures in the early morning and a temperature higher in the late afternoon or early evening, which is consistent with what is encountered in clinical practice.

In adults, a morning oral temperature of 98.9°F (37.2°C) or higher, or an evening temperature of 99.9°F (37.7°C) or higher defines a fever. Rectal temperatures are generally considered to be 0.7°F (0.4°C) higher than oral readings.

In infants and young children, rectal temperatures are still considered the standard of care and a rectal temperature greater than 100.4°F (38°C) is considered a fever.

Axillary temperatures of greater than 98.6°F (37°C) are regarded as a fever, though this measurement site is generally considered less accurate. An accurate measurement of body temperature is dependent on site, measuring device, and the clinical skills of the operator. Site selection should be determined by the age of the patient.

Young infants and older adults often have a diminished febrile response due to physiologic factors, thereby warranting the use of other clinical factors to guide diagnosis.

Recent technologic advances, including electronic devices, tympanic membrane scanning, and temporal artery scanning, have replaced the older mercury-in-glass thermometers. These devices offer faster results and minimal inconvenience to the patient and are becoming increasingly reliable. Chemical content or liquid crystal thermometers applied to the skin are neither accurate nor cost-effective.

Hyperthermia is an uncontrolled elevation of core body temperature that exceeds the body's ability to lose heat. In hyperthermia, the setting of the hypothalamic thermoregulatory center is unchanged, in contrast to fever. Hyperthermia requires urgent medical intervention because it could be rapidly fatal and does not respond to antipyretics. Common etiologies include heat stroke, neuromalignant syndrome, serotonin syndrome, malignant hyperthermia, endocrinopathy, and CNS damage.

Classic *fever of unknown origin* (FUO) is defined as a disorder with temperatures ≥100.9°F (38.3°C) that have persisted for at least 3 weeks, with no definitive cause elucidated after initial comprehensive inpatient or outpatient workup. The etiologies of FUO generally fall into four diagnostic categories: infectious, autoimmune or inflammatory, neoplastic, and miscellaneous.

Pathophysiology

Fever occurs as part of an inflammatory response to an inciting stimulus. The response includes the production of various cytokines that ultimately increase the production of prostaglandin E_2 (PGE_2), which resets the hypothalamic thermoregulatory set point at a higher level. Important pyogenic cytokines include interleukin-1 (IL-1), interleukin-6 (IL-6), tumor necrosis factor α (TNF-α), interferon-β (IFN-β), and interferon-γ (IFN-γ).

Risks and Benefits of Fever

Fever is known to enhance the immunologic response while suppressing the growth and replication of bacterial and viral infections. Though often uncomfortable for patients, caregivers, and health care providers, evidence supports the notion that fever is beneficial and ultimately protects against the development of asthma and other allergic disorders. In most instances, fever is not harmful. It does increase cardiac demand and metabolic needs, resulting in the common associated signs and symptoms of tachycardia, tachypnea, shivering, malaise, and diaphoresis.

The use of antipyretic agents has not been shown to either prolong or shorten the duration of illness. Febrile seizures cause significant anxiety for parents. They occur most commonly in children between the ages of 6 months and 6 years. Most febrile seizures are uncomplicated and have not been shown to be associated with significant bacteremia or to lead to the development of seizure disorder in older children. Antipyretic agents have not been shown to decrease the incidence of febrile seizures.

Diagnostic Evaluation of Fever

In most cases, the etiology of a febrile illness is a self-limiting viral infection. From 5% to 10% of fevers may be associated with a more serious bacterial infection such as pneumonia, UTI, bacteremia, meningitis, or bone and joint infections. At times, these conditions may be challenging to distinguish, and a thoughtful, systematic, evidence-based approach to the diagnostic evaluation will be most cost-effective while avoiding the inappropriate use of antibiotics.

Although the most common clinical presentation of COVID is fever with respiratory symptoms, a significant proportion of patients will present with fever alone or atypically. Considering this, COVID testing is indicated for all patients presenting with fever.

All infants less than 28 days old with a fever should be admitted to the hospital for a full sepsis workup and empiric intravenous antibiotic therapy.

Young infants, 1 to 3 months of age, with a febrile illness can be especially challenging. Numerous studies addressing this challenging population have led to the development of multiple guidelines and clinical protocols that utilize risk stratification criteria. The use of these age-specific stratification criteria, along with clinical treatment guidelines, helps guide the clinician in the evaluation of febrile illness. Clinical judgment remains the cornerstone of good clinical care.

With the widespread use of *Haemophilus influenzae* type B (Hib) and pneumococcal vaccinations, the incidence of bacteremic illness has decreased significantly. UTI has emerged as the most prevalent bacterial infection. The increased use of rapid viral testing in the office and emergency department settings may alleviate the need for more invasive testing and antibiotic use because the risk of concurrent bacterial infection has been reported to be negligible.

In this age group, an initial workup that reveals a white blood cell (WBC) count of less than 5000 or greater than 15,000 indicates an increased likelihood of a significant bacterial illness (SBI). Blood cultures, urinalysis, urine culture, and cerebrospinal fluid (CSF) evaluation should then be obtained and accompanied by intravenous antibiotic therapy. When considering the use of inflammatory markers diagnostically, lactate, procalcitonin, C-reactive protein, absolute neutrophil count, and white blood cell count are the common markers utilized. Incorporating urine concentration when interpreting urine analyses can help in the differentiation of infants at higher risk of UTI.

Children age 3 to 36 months, who appear well and do not have any underlying medical history, require only a comprehensive clinical evaluation and do not warrant antibiotic therapy or diagnostic testing in most instances. Septic or ill-appearing children need a more aggressive evaluation, including complete blood count (CBC), inflammatory markers, urinalysis, urine culture, blood cultures, and a chest x-ray. High-risk children in this age group require empiric antibiotic therapy, and clinical judgment should guide the decision to hospitalize.

Classic FUO is defined as a disorder with temperatures greater than 100.9°F (38.3°C) that has persisted for at least 3 weeks with no clear etiology determined after 3 days of hospital evaluation or three outpatient visits. Common etiologic categories include infectious, neoplastic, inflammatory, and miscellaneous causes, of which drug fever has been shown to be the most prevalent.

The initial approach includes a thorough history, physical examination, and appropriate laboratory testing. The initial choice of imaging should be guided by clinical findings and most commonly includes a chest x-ray and a CAT scan of the abdomen and pelvis. If the etiology remains elusive, positron emission tomography (PET) scanning or invasive diagnostic testing should then be considered.

Differential Diagnosis

When exploring the etiology of a patient's fever, the main objective in all age groups is to differentiate serious treatable infections and other states from more self-resolving febrile illnesses.

The differential diagnosis for the source of fever remains quite broad, but infections remain the most common source for fever, with a self-limiting viral illness accounting for most cases of fever.

Noninfectious categories of fever include malignancies, systemic rheumatic diseases, medications, and drug reactions, as well as numerous other miscellaneous conditions. The duration, fever pattern exhibited (e.g., the relapsing pattern seen in malaria), presence or absence of other symptoms and risk factors such as decreased immunocompetence or geographic setting (among other individual factors) should guide a determination of "pretest" probability for certain considerations before embarking upon a diagnostic workup.

Because core body temperature demonstrates individual variability, clinicians use standard threshold values for defining a fever, depending on the clinical context. Caution must be taken with older adults as it is well known that they have an impaired ability to develop fever and a lower baseline core temperature relative to younger patients so that temperatures in older adults that are lower than the established thresholds for fever may still reflect fever and a potentially serious infection.

Additionally, patients who feel "feverish" or have chills based on an inflammatory response but do not exhibit an actual elevation of temperature are encountered commonly. This can occur early in the course of an infection such as tuberculosis, a skin abscess, or influenza and can be seen in early sepsis. Hormonal changes may account for feverish symptoms without elevated temperature in menopause or hypothyroidism and may also be experienced by patients with anxiety in response to major stressors, though anxiety responses also may lead to temperature elevations. Therefore the absence of fever should never deter the additional evaluation of a patient with other signs or symptoms that suggest an infection or other illness.

Hyperthermia is an unregulated, significant elevation of core body temperature above the normal diurnal range due to failure of thermoregulation from a hypothalamic insult, not a pyogenic source, and is considered a medical emergency. It is not synonymous with fever and often requires immediate intervention to avoid deleterious CNS effects. Since the hypothalamic set point remains unchanged, antipyretics are ineffective in hyperthermia. The most common etiology is the inability to regulate or dissipate excess body heat. Hyperthermia is a medical emergency that requires immediate treatment to prevent excessive morbidity and mortality.

Treatment

Though controversy exists regarding the necessity of lowering fever, antipyretics have been shown to effectively and safely reduce temperature and improve symptoms with minimal side effects. Acetaminophen (Tylenol) is available in many formulations. Dosing should be based on body weight and not age of the patient. The dose is 10 to 15 mg/kg every 4 to 6 hours, not to exceed 3 g daily or 2 g in patients with renal or hepatic impairment. Ibuprofen (Advil, Motrin) is a nonsteroidal antiinflammatory drug (NSAID) that has both antiinflammatory and antipyretic effects. Dosing is 10 mg/kg every 6 to 8 hours in children and 200 to 400 mg every 6 hours in adolescents and adults. Ibuprofen is also available in multiple formulations, including a newer intravenous preparation (ibuprofen [Caldolor]) that may be beneficial in oral-intolerant hospitalized patients. Some studies suggest that ibuprofen may be a more effective antipyretic agent than acetaminophen.

In adults, aspirin (ASA) remains a therapeutic alternative for lowering fever at a dose of 325 to 650 mg every 4 to 6 hours. It should not be used in children with a febrile illness due to the risk of Reye's syndrome.

A combination of acetaminophen and ibuprofen in alternating doses has been shown in some studies to have an added benefit in both reduction of temperature and comfort without an increase in side effects, though caution should be taken to avoid dosing errors.

Nonpharmacologic therapies such as sponge bathing with tepid water and other environmental measures to control temperature, including adjusting room temperatures and sipping cool fluids to avoid dehydration, are used commonly and do provide symptom relief and comfort. These measures should never be used as the sole therapy for fever reduction.

References

Betrains A, Moreel L, De Langhe E, et al: Rheumatic disorders among patients with fever of unknown origin: a systematic review and meta-analysis, *Semin Arthritis Rheum* 56:152066, 2022.

Betrains A, Mulders-Manders CM, Aarntzen EH, et al: Update on imaging in fever and inflammation of unknown origin: focus on infectious disorders, *Clin Microbiol Infect* 30(3):288–295, 2024.

Dang R, Patel AI, Marlow J, et al: Frequency and consequences of routine temperature measurement at well-child visits, *Pediatrics* 1;149(1):e2021053412, 2022.

Dorney K, Bachur RG: Febrile infant update, *Curr Opin Pediatr* 29(3):280–285, 2017.

Olie SE, Staal SL, Ter Horst L, van Zeggeren IE, et al: Diagnostic accuracy of inflammatory markers in adults with suspected central nervous system infections, *J Infect* 88(3):106117, 2024.

Pantell RH, Roberts KB, Adams WG, et al: Subcommittee on Febrile Infants: Evaluation and management of well-appearing febrile infants 8 to 60 days old, *Pediatrics* 148(2):e2021052228, 2021.

Pantell RH, Roberts KB, Greenhow TL, Pantell MS: Advances in the diagnosis and management of febrile infants: challenging tradition, *Adv Pediatr* 65(1):173–208, 2018.

Ryan K: Fever of unknown origin, *Med Clin North Am* 108(1):79–92, 2024.

Struyf T, Deeks JJ, Dinnes J, et al: Cochrane COVID-19 Diagnostic Test Accuracy Group: Signs and symptoms to determine if a patient presenting in primary care or hospital outpatient settings has COVID-19 disease, *Cochrane Database Syst Rev* 7;7(7):CD013665, 2020.

Trapani S, Fiordelisi A, Stinco M, Resti M: Update on fever of unknown origin in children: focus on etiologies and clinical approach, *Children (Basel)* 24;11(1):20, 2023.

Wouthuyzen-Bakker M, Glaudemans AWJM: Molecularimaging of fever of unknown origin: an update, *Semin Nucl Med* 53(1):4–17, 2023.

Wright WF, Betrains A, Stelmash L, et al: Development of aconsensus-based list of potential quality indicators for fever and inflammation of unknown origin, *Open Forum Infect Dis* 11;11(2):ofad671, 2024.

GASEOUSNESS, INDIGESTION, NAUSEA, AND VOMITING

Method of
Justin Bailey, MD

Nausea is a vague, subjective feeling that vomiting (forceful expulsion of gastric contents) is imminent. Dyspepsia (based on Rome III criteria) can include postprandial fullness, early satiety, epigastric pain, burning, and reflux (return of gastric content to the lower esophagus or mouth, accompanied by a sour taste or "heartburn" sensation). Gaseousness can present with a variety of complaints, including belching, bloating, abdominal pain, or flatulence.

Epidemiology

Nausea and vomiting (ICD-10 Code R11.2) is one of the top reasons patients see a primary care provider. Infectious diseases causing nausea and vomiting, gastroenteritis, diarrhea, and dehydration are leading causes of death in developing countries, and of sick days and reduction of employee productivity in the United States. Nausea and vomiting postoperatively and during cancer chemotherapy add significant costs, pain, and discomfort to hospital and ambulatory treatment. Dyspepsia occurs in an estimated 25% of the US population every year, many of whom do not seek care. Gaseousness is ubiquitous in the population and is troubling to a small portion.

Risk Factors

Previous gastrointestinal (GI) surgery, certain medications, chemotherapeutic regimens, substance abuse, pregnancy, infectious diseases, medical conditions, and central nervous system disorders increase the risk for nausea and vomiting symptoms. Dyspepsia risk is increased significantly with ingestion of nonsteroidal antiinflammatory drugs (NSAIDs), tobacco use, *Helicobacter pylori* infection, obesity, anxiety, somatization, neuroticism, depression, and unemployment. Increased upper GI gaseousness can be seen with air swallowing from gum chewing and eating quickly, as well as consumption of foods that relax the lower esophageal sphincter (e.g., chocolate, fats, mints). Ingestion of lactose, fructose, sorbitol, undigested starches (e.g., bran), and carbonated beverages can all increase the risk of bloating and flatulence.

Pathophysiology

The pathophysiologic regulation of nausea and vomiting is complex and incompletely understood. Multiple neurotransmitters are involved, including acetylcholine, dopamine, histamine, and serotonin. The therapeutic action of antiemetics is often based on blocking the action of these neurotransmitters. Neurologic regulation of nausea and vomiting involves the chemoreceptor triggers in the fourth ventricle, the nucleus tractus solitarius in the medulla, motor nuclei that control the vomiting reflex, and vagal afferent nerves from the GI tract. The sympathetic and parasympathetic nervous systems are involved in conjunction with the smooth muscle cells and the enteric brain within the wall of the stomach and intestine.

The pathophysiology of dyspepsia is unclear but probably has multiple causes. Delayed gastric motility can occur in up to 30% of patients with dyspepsia. In addition, decreased gastric compliance, alteration in gut microbiome, duodenal inflammation, and psychosocial dysfunction can also be associated with dyspeptic patients.

Sensations of lower tract gaseousness result from one of three different mechanisms: excess gas production, abnormal intestinal transit, and increased visceral sensitivity. Gas production caused by carbohydrate maldigestion, (e.g., lactose intolerance, poorly absorbed starches) results in bloating and a sensation of fullness. High-fiber diets, celiac disease, and small intestine bacterial overgrowth can increase gas production. Dysmotility associated with diabetes mellitus, scleroderma, amyloidosis, and endocrine disease may result in gastroparesis and chronic intestinal pseudo-obstruction. In addition, previous Nissen fundoplication, fat intolerance, and various familial conditions may cause dysmotility. Increased visceral sensitivity is thought to be a main cause of pain and fullness in patients with functional bowel disorders such as irritable bowel syndrome (IBS) and functional dyspepsia.

Prevention

Once the diagnosis has been established, appropriate treatment of the underlying cause of the symptoms can be instituted. When the cause of nausea and vomiting is related to medication, the dose can be adjusted or the medication changed as appropriate.

TABLE 1 Key Symptoms and Differential Vomiting, Dyspepsia, and Bloating

SYMPTOMS	DIFFERENTIAL
Abdominal Pain ± N/V • RUQ • Epigastric • RLQ • LLQ • Pelvic	Organic etiologies • Cholelithiasis, cholecystitis • Dyspepsia, pancreatitis, GERD, gastritis, MI • Appendicitis • Diverticulitis • PID, ovarian torsion, ectopic pregnancy
Abdominal pain + distention + N/V	Bowel obstruction
Abdominal distention associated with foods (lactose, wheat-based products, bran, legumes)	Lactose intolerance Celiac disease Carbohydrate malabsorption, Oligosaccharide fermentation (legumes)
Vomiting several hours after eating + succussion splash + N/V	Gastric obstruction Gastroparesis
Heartburn ± N/V	GERD, dyspepsia
Early morning + N/V	Pregnancy
Feculent vomiting + N/V	Intestinal obstruction Gastrocolic fistula
Vertigo + nystagmus + N/V	Vestibular neuritis
Dental erosions, parotid gland enlargement, lanugo-like hair, callus on dorsal surface of hands	Bulimia
Positional N/V	Neurogenic
N/V relieved with hot shower or bath	Cannabis hyperemesis

GERD, Gastroesophageal reflux disease; *LLQ*, left lower quadrant; *MI*, myocardial infarction; *N/V*, nausea and vomiting; *PID*, pelvic inflammatory disease; *RLQ*, right lower quadrant; *RUQ*, right upper quadrant.

TABLE 2 Physical Examination: Nausea, Vomiting, Dyspepsia, and Gaseousness

FINDINGS	POSSIBLE ETIOLOGY
Fever	Infectious
Tachycardia, hypotension	Dehydration, volume depletion, sepsis (infectious), ectopic pregnancy, myocardial infarction, aortic aneurysm
Exophthalmos	Hyperthyroid
Papilledema	Increased intracranial pressure (tumors, subdural hemorrhage)
Bulging tympanic membrane	Otitis media, effusion
Thyromegaly	Hypothyroid
Lymphadenopathy	Infection, malignancy
Dry mucous membranes	Dehydration, volume depletion
Dental erosions	Bulimia
Abdominal distention	Obstruction, ileus, gastroparesis, irritable bowel, hepatic/splenic flexure syndrome, postoperative gas-bloat syndrome
Absent bowel sounds	Ileus, perforation
Sense of abdominal distention without bloating	Irritable bowel syndrome
Abdominal bloating	Irritable bowel syndrome, obstruction
RUQ abdominal pain/guarding	Cholecystitis, cholelithiasis
RLQ/LLQ abdominal pain/guarding	Appendicitis (RLQ), ovarian torsion, diverticulitis, ectopic pregnancy
Cervical motion tenderness	Pelvic inflammatory disease, endometriosis
Bladder tenderness	Urinary tract infection
Testicular pain	Torsion, epididymitis
Abnormal rectal examination	Fecal impaction, prostatitis, appendicitis, ovarian tumor, ectopic pregnancy, endometriosis
Delayed cap refill, poor skin turgor	Dehydration
Jaundice	Gallbladder disease, biliary obstruction

LLQ, Left lower quadrant; *RLQ*, right lower quadrant; *RUQ*, right upper quadrant.

Upper GI bloating and fullness is almost exclusively caused by excess air swallow and can be improved with altering behaviors such as gulping food and gum chewing. Lower GI symptoms can be prevented by avoiding problem foods such as milk products in patients with lactose intolerance.

Clinical Manifestations

Nausea and vomiting are extremely common and are associated with many conditions. Associated symptoms are helpful in sorting out causes. Many common historical associations are listed in Table 1.

The diagnosis of dyspepsia is based mainly on clinical symptoms. The Rome III criteria are listed in the opening paragraph. Alarm symptoms that should raise suspicions for gastric cancer include unintended weight loss, persistent vomiting, progressive dysphasia, odynophagia, unexplained anemia, iron deficiency, hematemesis, palpable abdominal mass, lymphadenopathy, family history of gastric cancer, previous gastric surgery, or jaundice.

Gaseousness usually presents with abdominal fullness and bloating. Pain associated with the fullness is often relieved with eructation or flatulence (see Table 1).

Diagnosis

The first step in the assessment of patients with abdominal complaints is complete history of the duration of symptoms, the frequency of episodes, work environment, recent travel, household member illness, association of symptoms with certain foods or beverages (i.e., pain relief or worsening with food), and determination of the success or failure of what the patient has tried

to alleviate the symptoms, all of which may offer diagnostic clues. Focused inquiries into surgeries, sexual activity, and other elements of a review of symptoms may be helpful. A complete review of medication usage, with particular attention to GI-irritating medications such as NSAIDs and over-the-counter medications, illicit drugs, and herbal products is important. Physical examination and diagnostic work-up can help isolate the cause (Table 2).

In patients with acute (<24 hours) nausea and vomiting, a laboratory work-up is often unnecessary. Patients with the most commonly identified acute causes, such as acute gastroenteritis, vestibular neuritis, chemotherapy, medication, and alcohol ingestion, and those who are postoperative, can be started on symptomatic therapy. For persistent symptoms of nausea and vomiting,

TABLE 3	Differential Diagnosis for Nausea and Vomiting

Central Nervous System	Psychiatric
Multiple sclerosis, tumor, intracranial bleeding, infarction, abscess, meningitis, trauma, labyrinthitis, Ménière disease, vestibular neuritis, motion sickness	Anorexia, anxiety, bulimia, depression
	Medication Related
	Acetaminophen (Tylenol)
Migraine headaches, seizure disorders	Acyclovir (Zovirax)
	Alcohol abuse
Gastrointestinal Disorders	Antibiotics: azithromycin (Zithromax), sulfasalazine (Azulfidine), erythromycin, metronidazole (Flagyl), sulfonamides (e.g., sulfamethoxazole-trimethoprim [Bactrim]), tetracycline
Appendicitis, gastric bypass, gastroparesis, hepatobiliary disease, cholecystitis, hepatitis, neoplasia	
Ileus	
Crohn disease, ulcerative colitis	
Irritable bowel syndrome	Antidepressants: Selective serotonin reuptake inhibitors (SSRIs)
Ischemia: mesenteric, small bowel	
Obstruction: scarring/adhesions from previous surgeries, small bowel obstruction, esophageal spasm	Antihypertensives: β-blockers (atenolol [Tenormin], metoprolol [Lopressor]), calcium channel blockers, diuretics (hydrochlorothiazide)
Pancreatitis	Cannabis
Peptic ulcer disease: esophagitis, gastritis, gastroesophageal reflux	Chemotherapeutic agents: cisplatinum (Cisplatin [Platinol]), cyclophosphamide (Cytoxan), nitrogen mustard (Mustargen), dacarbazine (DTIC-Dome), methotrexate (Trexall), vinblastine (Velban)
Peritonitis	
Endocrine	
Addison disease, diabetes (ketoacidosis, gastroparesis), hyperthyroidism, hypothyroidism, hyperparathyroidism, hypoparathyroidism, porphyria	Diabetes treatment: metformin (Glucophage), sulfonylureas
	Digoxin (Lanoxin)
	Ergotamines: dihydroergotamine (Migranal), methysergide (Sansert)[2]
Genitourinary	Ferrous gluconate, ferrous sulfate
Nephritis, nephrolithiasis, torsion (ovary, testicle), uremia, kidney stone	Gout treatment: allopurinol (Zyloprim)
Infectious Etiologies	Hormones: estrogen, progesterone, and oral and injected contraceptives
Bacterial: Campylobacter, Salmonella, Shigella, Enterogenic Escherichia coli	
Viral: rotavirus, influenza	Levodopa (L-dopa), carbidopa (Lodosyn)
Otitis media: bacterial or viral	
Sexually transmitted infection: cervicitis, epididymitis, pelvic inflammatory disease, prostatitis, urethritis; multiple organisms including gonorrhea and chlamydia	Nicotine (patch, gum, smokeless tobacco, cigarette/pipe/cigar)
	Nonsteroidal antiinflammatory: aspirin, ibuprofen (Motrin), naproxen (Naprosyn)
Urinary tract infection: lower (cystitis) or upper (pyelonephritis)	Opioids: codeine, heroin, hydrocodone, oxycodone, morphine, buprenorphine/naloxone (Suboxone)
	Prednisone
Pregnancy	Seizure medications: phenobarbital, phenytoin (Dilantin)
Morning sickness, hyperemesis gravidarum, intrauterine and ectopic pregnancies	Theophylline (Uniphyl)

[2]Not available in the United States.

TABLE 4	Differential Diagnosis of Dyspepsia

Gastrointestinal Disorders	Medications
Functional or nonulcer (most common)	NSAIDs
	Antibiotics (macrolides and metronidazole)
Peptic ulcer disease	Corticosteroids
Gastroesophageal reflux	Digoxin
Gastritis	Narcotics
Pancreatitis	Theophylline
Gastroparesis	**Respiratory**
Gastric cancer	Pneumonia
Intestinal ischemia	**Cardiac**
Esophageal rupture	Myocardial ischemia or pericarditis
Malabsorption	
Lactase deficiency	**Musculoskeletal**
Celiac	Abdominal hernia
Infectious	**Psychiatric**
Parasite infection	Physical sexual abuse
Helicobacter pylori	
Pregnancy	

NSAIDs, Nonsteroidal antiinflammatory drugs.

TABLE 5	Differential Diagnosis of Bloating and Gaseousness

Upper Gastrointestinal	Gas-Producing Foods
Air swallowing	Beans, peas, lentils, broccoli, Brussels sprouts, cauliflower, cabbage, parsnips, leeks, onions, beer, coffee, pork
Small Bowel	
Pneumatosis cystoides intestinalis	
Carbohydrate Malabsorption	
Lactase deficiency	**Infectious**
Legumes (indigestible oligosaccharides)	Parasites
	Helicobacter pylori
Fructose malabsorption	Bacterial overgrowth
Undigested starch (bran)	**Malabsorption**
Irritable Bowel Syndrome	Celiac
	Crohn disease

laboratory work-up is guided by the history and physical examination and can include a complete blood count and differential, serum chemistries, renal function, liver function tests, serum protein and albumin, thyroid-stimulating hormone, amylase or lipase, drug screen, and a pregnancy test in women of childbearing age. Imaging should not be routine but should be directed by the history and physical findings as well as pertinent laboratory results. Useful studies may include acute abdominal series (chest x-ray, flat and upright views of the abdomen), abdominal computed tomography (CT), and abdominal ultrasound.

Similarly, in patients with dyspeptic symptoms, laboratory tests should be obtained based on the history and physical examination. Many therapies, such as discontinuing offending medications (e.g., NSAIDs) or acid suppression in patients without alarm symptoms, may be started without a laboratory work-up. Blood count chemistries and *H. pylori* testing can be considered if warranted. Alarm symptoms may warrant further imaging or direct visualization with esophagogastroduodenoscopy (EGD).

In gaseousness and bloating, the most sensitive work-up is the history and physical examination. Further work-up should be directed by initial findings. Patients with alarm symptoms such as weight loss, diarrhea, abdominal pain, distention, and anorexia may benefit from a malabsorption work-up including lactose tolerance test, stool fat, ova and parasites, stool culture, *Clostridium difficile*, acute abdominal series, or EGD. A hydrogen breath test may be beneficial in selected patients to assess the relationship between specific foods and symptoms. Other blood work, tests, and imaging, such as CT, magnetic resonance imaging (MRI), and EGD are guided by availability of testing and the history, examination, and laboratory findings.

Differential Diagnosis
Tables 3, 4, and 5 summarize the wide differential diagnoses of nausea and vomiting, dyspepsia, and gaseousness.

Treatment
Antiemetics, hydration, and dietary changes are the first line treatments for acute episodes of nausea and vomiting. Controlling the symptoms is often all that is necessary in acute, self-limited bouts of nausea and vomiting symptoms. If patients are dehydrated, oral rehydration can be accomplished by encouraging the patient to take small amounts (6 ounces or less) of cool water or electrolyte solutions on a frequent basis. If patients are unable to accomplish this, parenteral rehydration and antiemetics may be warranted.

Table 6 lists the common antiemetics agent, indications, dosages, side effects, and relative cost of medications.

I Symptomatic Care Pending Diagnosis

TABLE 6	Medications for Nausea and Vomiting

DRUG	USE	SIDE EFFECTS	DOSAGE
Anticholinergics Act as antimuscarinic agents		Sedation, dry mouth, dizziness, hallucinations, confusion, exacerbate narrow angle glaucoma, blurred vision.	
Scopalamine	Nausea associated with motion sickness		1–1.5 mg patch TD q3d
Antihistamines		Sedation, dry mouth, confusion, urinary retention, blurred vision	
Diphenhydramine (Benadryl)	Nausea associated with motion sickness		50 mg PO q6h or 10–50 mg IV or IM
Doxylamine (Unisom)[1]	Nausea associated with pregnancy		5–10 mg PO qd
Hydroxyzine (Vistaril)[1]	Nausea associated with motion sickness		25–100 mg q6h
Meclizine (Antivert)	Nausea associated with motion sickness		25–50 mg q6h
Promethazine (Phenergan)	Nausea associated with motion sickness		12.5–25 mg (PO, IM, IV, PR) q4–6h
Benzamides: Prokinetic agents; work on peripheral and central dopamine, weak hydroxytryptamine type 3 (5-HT$_3$)		Sedation, hypotension, extrapyramidal effects, diarrhea, neuroleptic syndrome, supraventricular tachycardia, CNS depression	
Metoclopramide (Reglan)	Second line therapy for chemotherapy-induced nausea		10 mg (PO, IM, IV) q6h
Trimethobenzamide (Tigan)[1]	Chemotherapy-induced nausea		300 mg PO q6h
Butyrophenones: Dopamine antagonists		Sedation, hypotension, extrapyramidal effects, tachycardia, dizziness, QT prolongation and torsades de pointes, neuroleptic malignant syndrome	
Droperidol (Inapsine)	Postoperative nausea/vomiting		0.625–1.25 mg (IM, IV) q4h
Haloperidol (Haldol)[1]			0.5–5 mg (PO, IM, IV) q8h
Phenothiazines: Dopamine antagonists		Sedation, hypotension, extrapyramidal effects, neuroleptic malignant syndrome, cholestatic jaundice	
Chlorpromazine (Thorazine)	Generalized nausea		10–25 mg (PO, IM, PR) q6h
Prochlorperazine (Compazine)	Generalized nausea		10 mg (PO, IM, IV) q6h; 25 mg q12h PR
5-HT3: Serotonin Antagonists		Fever, constipation, diarrhea, dizziness, sedation, nervousness, altered liver function tests, headache, fatigue	
Dolasetron (Anzemet)	Chemotherapy-induced nausea		100 mg (PO, IV) q24h
Granisetron (Kytril)	Chemotherapy-induced nausea		2 mg (PO, IV) q24h
Ondansetron (Zofran)	Chemotherapy-induced nausea		4–8 mg (PO, IV) q8–12h
Palonosetron (Aloxi)	Prevention of chemotherapy-induced nausea		0.5 mg PO or 0.25 mg IV ×1
Neurokinin Receptor Antagonists		Headache, site reaction	
Aprepitant capsule (Emend)	Prevention of postoperative nausea and vomiting (POV)		40 mg PO × 1 prior to anesthesia
Fosaprepitant (Emend IV)	Prevention of chemotherapy-induced nausea		115 mg IV × 1, 125 mg PO ×1[3]
Steroids		GI upset, anxiety, euphoria, flushing, insomnia	

TABLE 6	Medications for Nausea and Vomiting—cont'd		
DRUG	**USE**	**SIDE EFFECTS**	**DOSAGE**
Dexamethasone (Decadron)[1]	Prophylaxis of chemotherapy-related nausea and vomiting		4 mg–10 mg (PO, IM, IV) q6–12h
Methylprednisolone (Medrol)[1]			40–100 mg (PO, IM, IV) q24h
Cannabinoids		Vertigo, xerostomia, hypotension, dysphoria	
Dronabinol (Marinol)	Chronic or chemotherapy-induced nausea and vomiting		5 mg/m^2 PO q2-4h; 4–6 doses per day
Miscellaneous			
Erythromycin[1]	Nausea associated with gastroparesis		250 mg PO q8h × 5–7 d
Ginger[7]	Nausea associated with pregnancy		250 mg PO q6h or 1 g qd
Pyridoxine (vitamin B6)[1]	Nausea associated with pregnancy (traditionally combined with doxylamine)		10 mg q6h
Aromatherapy-Isopropyl Alcohol[1]	Nausea	None	Swab held under nose and inhaled.

CNS, central nervous system; *IM*, intramuscular; *IV*, intravenous; *PO*, by mouth; *PR*, per rectum
[1]Not US Food and Drug Administration (FDA) approved for this indication.
[3]Exceeds dosage recommended by the manufacturer.
[7]Available as dietary supplement.

TABLE 7	Medications for Treatment of Gaseousness and Bloating	
MEDICATION	**INDICATION**	**DOSE**
Rifaximin (Xifaxan)[1]	Bloating (flatulence) from suspected bacterial overgrowth	200 mg PO tid × 7 days
Probiotics (multi-component)[7]	Bloating (flatulence)	Varies by preparation
Alpha-galactosidase (Bean-o)	Bloating associated with gas-producing foods	300–1200 mg with meals high in fermentable carbs
Simethicone	Bloating (flatulence) (indicated but not found to be effective)	80–120 mg qid prn
Bismuth subsalicylate	Odor from flatus	525 mg PO qid prn
Odor-neutralizing devices (briefs, pillows)	Odor from flatus	prn

[1]Not US Food and Drug Administration (FDA) approved for this indication.
[7]Available as dietary supplement

Location of the cause with directed treatment is most effective for gaseousness. If no cause is found, it can be difficult to treat. Avoiding foods that are contributory, such as those containing lactose, fructose, sorbitol, high fiber, and starches, may be all that is necessary. Symptoms associated with increased sensitivity to normal levels of gas (i.e., IBS) can be difficult to treat. Therapeutic relationships, education, and dietary modification are the mainstays of IBS treatment. For moderate to severe symptoms, short-term treatment with antispasmodics, tricyclic antidepressants, and antidiarrheal agents may have some benefit. Medical treatments for bloating are listed in Table 7.

For most patients with dyspepsia, information can be powerful. Validation of symptoms and working toward a goal of management rather than cure are therapeutic. In patients with dyspepsia in which a concern for *H. pylori* exists, a test-and-treatment strategy can be effective. In other patients, proton pump inhibitors, H-2 receptor antagonists, prokinetic agents, and peppermint oil are all effective short-term therapies.

Monitoring

For patients who have complications related to nausea and vomiting, monitoring serum electrolytes, renal function, nutritional status, and other parameters may be necessary until hydration improves, electrolytes are replaced, and laboratory results and clinical status return to normal.

Further testing is needed in patients with dyspepsia and alarm symptoms; however, in patients without alarm symptoms, no further testing is needed.

Complications

The complications of prolonged nausea and vomiting are dehydration, electrolyte disturbances (e.g., hypokalemia, hypophosphatemia, and hypomagnesemia), depletion of vitamins and trace elements, metabolic alkalosis, and malnutrition. Usually these can be corrected with oral or intravenous hydration, correction of electrolyte deficiencies, and treatment of the underlying cause. In patients whose nausea and vomiting are accompanied by gastroenteritis, symptoms and clinical status may not return to baseline unless all electrolytes such as potassium, magnesium, phosphorus, and trace elements such as zinc are replaced.

Dyspeptic patients without alarm symptoms rarely have complications. In patients with chronic bloating, complications are uncommon.

References

Abraczinskas D: Intestinal gas and bloating. Available http://www.uptodate.com, December 2018. [Accessed 3 February 2020].

ACOG Practice Bulletin No: 189: American College of Obstetrics and Gynecology: nausea and vomiting in pregnancy, *Obstet Gynecol* 131:e15–e30, 2018.

Bailey J: Effective management of flatulence, *Am Fam Phys* 79:1098–1100, 2009.

Flake ZA, Linn B, Hornecker J: Practical selection of antiemetics in an ambulatory care setting, *Am Fam Phys* 91(15):293–296, 2015 Mar 1.

Kraft R: Nausea and vomiting. In Bope ET, Rakel RE, Kellerman R, editors: *Conn's Current Therapy 2010*, Philadelphia, 2010, Saunders, pp 5–9.

Lacy B, Parkman H, Camilleri M: Chronic Nausea and Vomiting, Evaluation and Treatment, *Am J Gastroenterology* 113:647–659, 2018.

Longstreth GF: Functional dyspepsia in adults. Available at http://www.uptodate.com, December 2019. [Accessed 3 February 2020].

Longstreth GF: Approach to the patient with dyspepsia. Available at http://www.uptodate.com, December, 2019. [Accessed 3 February 2020].

Owings S: Gaseousness and dyspepsia. In Bope ET, Rakel RE, Kellerman R, editors: *Conn's Current Therapy 2010*, Philadelphia, 2010, Saunders, pp 9–11.

Talley NJ, Vakil NB, Moayyedi P: 2005 American Gastroenterological Association technical review on the evaluation of dyspepsia, *Gastroenterology* 125:1756–1780, 2005.

HEMATURIA

Method of
Jonathan Maldonado, MD; and Moben Mirza, MD

CURRENT DIAGNOSIS

- Hematuria is defined as the presence of red blood cells in the urine.
- Hematuria can be gross (readily visible) or microscopic (detected by dipstick or microscopy).
- In the adult population, any unexplained hematuria should be presumed to be of malignant origin until proven otherwise.
- Urologic evaluation of the upper and lower urinary tract is compulsory for patients with gross hematuria.
- Patients with asymptomatic microscopic hematuria (≥3 RBC/HPF) should have a careful history and physical examination performed to rule out benign causes of hematuria as well as to assess overall risk of urologic malignancy.
- Following patient risk stratification, further diagnostic evaluation with repeat urinalysis, cystoscopy, and upper tract imaging (renal ultrasound or multiphasic computed tomography) may be indicated.
- Concurrent nephrologic evaluation should occur in select cases.

Epidemiology

Hematuria is a common clinical finding in adults. The prevalence of hematuria ranges from 2.4% to 31.1%. Prevalence varies based on age, gender, frequency of testing, threshold used to define hematuria, and study group characteristics. Transient microscopic hematuria may occur in up to 40% of patients; however, persistent microscopic hematuria in greater than three evaluated urine samples is limited to 2% of the population. A wide range of causes can result in hematuria. Transient hematuria may be caused by vigorous exercise, sexual intercourse, mild trauma, menstrual contamination, and instrumentation. Patients with underlying urinary tract disease can have transient or persistent hematuria. The presence of gross hematuria carries a higher likelihood of significant pathology compared with microscopic hematuria. For example, approximately 5% of patients with microscopic hematuria in contrast to 40% of patients with gross hematuria are found to have urologic malignancy on evaluation. The most common cause of gross hematuria in adults older than age 50 is bladder cancer.

Risk Factors

Given the wide range of etiologies for hematuria, the risk factors are dependent on the etiology itself. The most concerning etiology of hematuria is urothelial malignancy. Smoking is the best-established and the most significant risk factor for the development of urothelial malignancies of the kidney, ureter, and bladder.

Pathophysiology

The presence of blood in the urine can be separated into glomerular and nonglomerular origin. Normal urine contains less than three red blood cells per high-power field. The kidney does not excrete red blood cells under physiologic conditions. Therefore, the presence of blood in the urine is due to pathology at the glomerulus (glomerular hematuria), allowing excretion of red blood cells into the urine or pathology in the urinary tract distal to the glomerulus (nonglomerular hematuria), which results in blood mixing into the already excreted urine. Nonglomerular hematuria can be further divided into medical and surgical disorders. Except for renal tumors, nonglomerular hematuria of medical/renal origin is due to tubulointerstitial, renovascular, or systemic disorders. Surgical nonglomerular hematuria or essential hematuria includes urologic tumors, stones, and urinary tract infections.

The urine dipstick, commonly used for the detection of blood in the urine, is dependent on the peroxidase-like activity of hemoglobin, which catalyzes the reaction and causes oxidation of the chromogen indicator. False positives can occur in states of hemoglobinuria and myoglobinuria, and microscopic examination of the urine for red blood cells can distinguish hematuria. Glomerular hematuria is suggested when dysmorphic erythrocytes, red blood cell casts, and proteinuria are present. Nonglomerular hematuria can be distinguished from glomerular hematuria in the presence of circular erythrocytes and the absence of erythrocyte casts. In the surgical and medical subcategories of nonglomerular hematuria, surgical hematuria is suggested by the absence of significant proteinuria.

Anticoagulation at normal therapeutic levels does not predispose patients to hematuria. Therefore patients who have hematuria while receiving either anticoagulation or antiplatelet therapy should undergo evaluation similarly to patients who are not receiving these therapies. In fact, supratherapeutic anticoagulation may serve to unmask underlying pathology.

Prevention

As previously mentioned, hematuria can be caused by a spectrum of causes. Prevention can be achieved by the avoidance of what results in the pathologic state. For example, smoking is a modifiable risk factor in urothelial malignancy. Patients who have never smoked are at low risk for bladder cancer. Smoking cessation can also reduce the risk of developing bladder cancer. Liberal fluid intake and balanced sodium and protein intake can help prevent urolithiasis. Urinary tract infections can also be prevented by good voiding habits, facilitation of complete bladder emptying, and use of vaginal estrogen cream[1] in postmenopausal women.

Clinical Manifestations

The presentation of hematuria is often dependent on the cause. Certain characteristics of the presentation can help in the investigation. Is the hematuria gross or microscopic? Is the hematuria associated with pain? Are there any irritative voiding symptoms? Is there a presence of blood clots? Is it related to exercise? Is there any family history? Is there a presence of rash, arthritis,

---

[1] Not FDA approved for this indication

TABLE 1 Differential Diagnosis and Findings in Etiologies of Hematuria

DIAGNOSIS	FINDINGS	OTHER
Glomerular		
Familial hematuria	Abnormal urinalysis	Family history
Systemic lupus erythematous	Elevated C3, C4, ANA	Rash, arthritis
Goodpasture syndrome	Microcytic anemia	Hemoptysis, bleeding tendency
Poststreptococcal glomerulonephritis	Elevated ASO titer, C3	Recent upper respiratory infection, rash
IgA nephropathy	Normal ASO and C3, renal biopsy positive for IgA, IgG	Related to exercise
Nonglomerular Medical		
Exercise-induced hematuria	Abnormal urine analysis	After strenuous exercise
Papillary necrosis	Gross hematuria, absence of urolithiasis on CT	Flank pain, African American, analgesic abuse, diabetes
Medullary sponge kidney, polycystic kidney disease	Abnormal CT	Family history of renal cystic disease
Renovascular disease	Renal artery embolus, vein thrombus, AV fistula	Atrial fibrillation, dehydration, bruit
Nonglomerular Surgical		
Urinary tract infection	Urine dip with LCE, Nit. positive urine culture, elevated WBC	Dysuria, fever
Urolithiasis (renal, ureteral, or bladder stone)	Demonstrated on imaging such as CT, ultrasound, KUB	Flank pain, pelvic pain, vomiting, infection, renal obstruction
Urologic tumor (kidney, ureter, bladder, urethra)	Demonstrated on CT, cystoscopy, ureteropyeloscopy	Constitutional, irritative symptoms, pain if obstructed, blood clots
Enlarged prostate or benign prostatic hyperplasia	Enlarged prostate on examination or cystoscopy	Irritative and obstructive voiding symptoms
Radiation cystitis	Generally gross hematuria, friable tissue on cystoscopy	Irritative voiding symptoms, history of pelvic radiation
Urothelial strictures (ureter or urethra)	Demonstrated on ureteroscopy, pyelography, cystoscopy, or urethrography	Flank pain, renal insufficiency, bladder outlet obstruction

ANA, Antinuclear antibodies; *ASO,* antistreptolysin O; *AV,* atrioventricular; *CT,* computed tomography; *Ig,* immunoglobulin; *KUB kidney, ureter, bladder radiograph, LCE leukocyte esterase, WBC,* white blood cell.

hemoptysis, upper respiratory infection, or skin infection? Is there a history of radiation, diabetes, or analgesic abuse? Is there a history of smoking or occupational exposures? Table 1 highlights findings in etiologies of hematuria. Patients with bladder cancer generally present with gross painless hematuria.

Diagnosis

The diagnosis and evaluation of hematuria starts with a careful history, physical examination, and microscopic urinalysis. The cause in an adult patient is urologic malignancy until proven otherwise. Some important questions are outlined in the section, Clinical Manifestations. The physical exam should first focus on blood pressure and a cardiovascular examination. An abdominal examination should evaluate for the presence of a palpable mass or costovertebral angle tenderness, followed by a complete genitourinary examination including a prostate examination in males and a vaginal examination in the females. The assessment should help rule out causes such as infection, menstruation, vigorous exercise, medical renal disease, viral illness, trauma, or recent urologic procedures.

A urine specimen should be collected as a midstream sample, and patients should be instructed to discard the initial 10 mL. The sample should be collected in a sterile cup after gently cleaning the urethral meatus with a sterilization towelette. Uncircumcised men should retract the foreskin before collection. Female patients should be asked to spread the labia adequately to allow cleansing of the urethral meatus and avoid introital contamination.

The following patients may require catheterization for collection: menstruating women, obese patients, patient with a nonintact urinary tract, patients who do intermittent catheterization, or have an indwelling urinary catheter (Foley or suprapubic tube). Additionally, a urine sample with excessive squamous cells is a sign of contamination, and catheterization may be required for an adequate specimen. A urine dipstick can be performed in the office setting, but all samples should be sent for microscopic analysis. As mentioned previously, attention should be paid to dysmorphic erythrocytes, red blood cell casts, and the presence of protein. A urine culture should be performed based on the clinical presentation and findings of urinalysis. Urine cytology should not be used in the initial evaluation of microscopic hematuria but may have clinical utility in evaluating patients with irritative voiding symptoms or persistent microhematuria after a comprehensive urologic evaluation. The laboratory workup should include an evaluation of the serum creatinine. Additional helpful tests are serum electrolytes and a complete blood count.

Patients with a urinary tract infection should be treated appropriately and should have a urinalysis repeated in 2 to 6 weeks after treatment. Patients with an identified etiology such as urolithiasis should have a reevaluation of urine after the stone has been passed or treated.

A urologic evaluation of the upper and lower urinary tract is compulsory for patients with gross hematuria. Given the high prevalence of asymptomatic microscopic hematuria ($\geq$3 RBC/HPF) and lower rate of malignancy in this population, risk stratification should be performed to guide diagnostic evaluation and limit the

TABLE 2	Microhematuria Risk Stratification		
RISK FACTOR	**LOW RISK**	**INTERMEDIATE RISK**	**HIGH RISK**
Number of criteria	ALL of the following	One or more of the following	One or more of the following
Age for women	<60 years	≥60 years	Women should not be categorized as high risk solely based on age
Age for men	<40 years	40–59 years	≥60 years
Smoking history	Never smoked or <10 pack-years	10–30 pack-years	>30 pack-years
Degree of hematuria	3–10 RBC/HPF on one UA	11–25 RBC/HPF on one UA	>25 RBC/HPF on one UA or prior history of gross hematuria
Prior microhematuria	No prior episodes of microscopic hematuria	Previously low risk, no prior evaluation, and 3–25 RBC/HPF on repeat UA	Previously low risk, no prior evaluation, and >25 RBC/HPF on repeat UA
Presence of additional risk factors	No additional risk factors for urothelial cancer*	Any additional risk factors for urothelial cancer*	One or more additional risk factor plus any High Risk feature

*Irritative voiding symptoms, history of cyclophosphamide or ifosamide chemotherapy, family history of renal cell carcinoma, urothelial carcinoma or Lynch syndrome, occupational exposures to benzene chemicals or aromatic amines, history of chronic indwelling foreign object in urinary tract
UA, Urinalysis.
Adapted from Barocas DA, Lotan Y, Matulewicz RS, et al: Updates to microhematuria: AUA/SUFU Guideline, J Urol 213(5):547–557, 2025.

potential for patient harm. This microhematuria risk stratification has been found to be clinically meaningful and helps differentiate the need for more aggressive diagnostic work-ups based on the likelihoods of bladder cancer within each risk group. Patients should be categorized as low, intermediate, or high risk based on factors in Table 2. Low-risk patients should undergo repeat urinalysis within 6 months to assess for persistence of the microscopic hematuria. An abnormal repeat urinalysis should prompt reclassification as intermediate or high risk and full evaluation should be performed. Cystoscopy and renal ultrasound (intermediate risk) or multiphasic computed tomography (high risk) are indicated for the evaluation of these risk groups. While contrasted computed tomography is preferred for evaluation of the upper tracts, a contraindication may exist for some patients due to allergy or renal insufficiency. In this scenario, a urologist can determine whether magnetic resonance imaging or retrograde pyelography is appropriate.

Differential Diagnosis
The differential diagnosis of hematuria includes glomerular diseases, nonglomerular medical diseases, and nonglomerular surgical diseases. Table 1 shows a differential diagnosis for hematuria.
Hematuria is considered to be from a malignant source until proven otherwise.

Therapy, Monitoring, and Complications
Therapy, monitoring, and complications for hematuria are dependent on the etiology. It is important that hematuria not be ignored even when treated empirically. For example, it is important to recheck a urinalysis after a course of antibiotics for a presumed urinary tract infection. Often, the transient nature of hematuria misleads clinicians into thinking that an intervention or observation without the appropriate workup is adequate. Unfortunately, this can result in significant morbidity from the progression of disease, especially in the case of urothelial malignancies.

References
Barocas DA, Lotan Y, Matulewicz RS, et al: Updates to microhematuria: AUA/SUFU guideline (2025), J Urol 213(5):547–557, 2025.
Davis R, Jones SJ, Barocas D, et al: Diagnosis, evaluation and follow-up of asymptomatic microscopic hematuria (AMH) in adults. AUA guideline, J Urol 188(Suppl 6):2473, 2012.
Gerber GS, Brendler CB: Evaluation of the urologic patient: History, physical, and urinalysis. In Wein Campbell-Walsh Urology, ed 10, Philadelphia, 2011, Saunders, pp 73–98.
Khadra MH, Pickard RS, Charlton M, et al: A prospective analysis of 1,930 patients with hematuria to evaluate current diagnostic practice, J Urol 163:524, 2000.
Masahito J: Evaluation and management of hematuria, Prim Care 37:461, 2010.
Sudakoff GS, Dunn DP, Guralnick ML, et al: Multidetector computerized tomography urography as the primary imaging modality for detecting urinary tract neoplasms in patients with asymptomatic hematuria, J Urol 179:862, 2008.
Woldu SL, Ng CK, Loo RK, et al: Evaluation of the new American Urological Association guidelines risk classification for hematuria, J Urol 205(5):1387–1393, 2021.

HICCUPS

Kristine L. Cece, MD, PhD

CURRENT DIAGNOSIS

- Hiccups result from involuntary contractions of the diaphragm and intercostal muscles, forcing rapid inspiration that is interrupted by the closure of the glottis. This pathway is mediated by a poorly understood reflex arc, with central processing taking place in the midbrain (medulla).
- Hiccups lasting longer than 48 hours are considered to be persistent, and those lasting longer than 1 month are labeled as intractable.
- Hiccups are a symptom of another underlying diagnosis; a thorough history, physical examination, basic laboratory workup, and chest x-ray are indicated in most patients with intractable hiccups. Advanced imaging and diagnostic procedures are warranted on a case-by-case basis depending on the suspected etiology.

CURRENT THERAPY

- Nonpharmacologic treatment including oropharyngeal stimulation (intranasal vinegar, ingestion of ice water, use of smelling salts), vagal maneuvers, and self-induced hypercapnia via paper bag breathing may be useful for treatment of transient hiccups.
- Hiccups are commonly seen in patients with gastroesophageal reflux disease, and therefore a trial of omeprazole (Prilosec)[1] is reasonable first-line therapy.
- Although few high-quality studies have examined use of these medications, the available data support use of baclofen (Lioresal),[1] gabapentin (Neurontin),[1] and metoclopramide (Reglan)[1] for treatment of hiccups.

Pathophysiology

Hiccups (Lat. *singultus*) are a common occurrence that result from involuntary and repetitive contractions of the inspiratory musculature including the diaphragm and intercostal muscles. Rapid inspiration of air is then interrupted by closure of the glottis, generating the characteristic "hic" sound for which this disorder is named. The pathophysiology behind these involuntary contractions is poorly understood but is generally thought to be related to stimulation of a reflex arc that includes peripheral pathways and central midbrain modulation. The afferent component of the reflex arc includes phrenic, vagus, and sympathetic nerves that transmit somatic and visceral sensory information to the midbrain (medulla). Multiple neurotransmitters play a role regulating rhythmic breathing in the midbrain, including dopamine, glutamate, glycine, gamma-aminobutyric acid (GABA), and serotonin. The efferent component of the reflex arc includes motor nerves that communicate via the phrenic nerve to the diaphragm and intercostals. Stimulation of this pathway can occur via many mechanisms including but not limited to neoplastic processes, vascular disease, gastroesophageal reflux disease (GERD), medications, procedural instrumentation, and infection. Hiccups are not thought to serve a physiologic purpose.

Prevention

There are currently no reliable preventative measures for hiccups.

Clinical Manifestations

Virtually all people will experience hiccups during their lifetime. For many, this is a brief and self-limited nuisance. For others, hiccups can be long-lasting and lead to serious morbidity, including insomnia, exhaustion, malnutrition, dehydration, and wound dehiscence. Hiccups can occur 4 to 60 times per minute. Transient hiccups tend to last minutes to hours and are often triggered by eating quickly or in excess, spicy foods, carbonated drinks, or ingesting hot or cold food or beverages. Hiccups lasting longer than 48 hours are considered to be persistent, whereas those lasting more than 1 month are labeled intractable.

Hiccups are observed in utero, most frequently in the third trimester, and are thought to be a mechanism of training the inspiratory muscles for respiration after birth. Intractable hiccups occur more commonly in men (91%) than women, and the incidence increases with age (most often in those over age 50). Hiccups are also frequently experienced by patients with gastrointestinal and central nervous system disorders, including 10% of patients with GERD and 20% of patients with Parkinson disease.

Diagnosis

Hiccups are a symptom of another underlying diagnosis that can be organic, psychogenic, or idiopathic. Persistent and intractable hiccups warrant further workup to identify their etiology, though there is no strong consensus on what that workup entails. A basic evaluation should include a thorough history, physical examination, and laboratory/diagnostic studies.

History

When taking the patient's history, it is important to identify any triggers or comorbid disease processes such as gastrointestinal or neurologic disorders. Understanding frequency, duration, and palliative treatments or maneuvers can also be helpful. Additionally, a thorough medication review is essential, as many common medications have been associated with persistent or intractable hiccups, including aripiprazole (Abilify), antibiotics including azithromycin (Zithromax) and sulfonamides, donepezil (Aricept), benzodiazepines including chlordiazepoxide (Librium) and diazepam (Valium), steroids, barbiturates, opioids, methyldopa, L-dopa, dopamine, and cisplatin. Alcohol has also been identified as a hiccup inducer. In cases in which a medication is the cause of hiccups, symptoms typically resolve once the offending agent is stopped.

Physical Examination

A head-to-toe physical examination looking for signs of neoplasm or infection is warranted. A thorough neurologic exam to rule out stroke or temporal arteritis, a cardiovascular exam to evaluate for pericardial friction rub, and an abdominal exam to identify epigastric tenderness are also helpful. Additionally, foreign body irritation of the tympanic membrane can induce hiccups, so a head, eyes, ears, nose, and throat exam should be performed.

Laboratory/Diagnostic Workup

Basic laboratory studies should include a metabolic panel to look for electrolyte imbalances and uremia, a complete blood cell count to look for infection, an electrocardiogram, and a chest x-ray. Advanced imaging and endoscopy may also be warranted on a case-by-case basis.

Treatment

Nonpharmacologic Interventions

Physical maneuvers are considered first-line for treatment of transient hiccups and can be effective at shortening acute attacks. These maneuvers include nasopharyngeal stimulation by intranasal application of vinegar, use of smelling salts, or ingestion of ice water. Vagal stimulation can also help resolve symptoms, including application of a cold compress to the face, carotid massage, Valsalva, and induced fright or vomiting. Finally, respiratory maneuvers including breath holding, paper bag rebreathing (inducing hypercapnia), and continuous positive airway pressure can be used as well, though clinical trial data on all of these approaches are lacking. None of these maneuvers is thought to be helpful for treatment of persistent or intractable hiccups.

Pharmacologic Interventions

The approach to pharmacologic management of persistent or intractable hiccups should first consider treatment of all identified reversible causes. If no etiology is identified after the history, physical exam, and diagnostic testing discussed above, it is reasonable to start with empiric treatment for GERD given the prevalence of the disease (an estimated 20% of adults in Western culture) and association with hiccups as a prominent symptom. A trial of a proton pump inhibitor such as omeprazole[1] (Prilosec, 20–40 mg once or twice daily) should be initiated for a minimum of 7 days. If no response, other pharmacologic treatments can be considered.

Although data are limited and large-scale studies have not been conducted, pharmacologic therapies shown to be most efficacious in treating intractable hiccups act on dopamine and GABA-ergic receptors. There are two medications that are supported by data from randomized controlled trials: baclofen (Lioresal)[1] and metoclopramide (Reglan).[1] Baclofen, a GABA$_B$ agonist, administered at a dosage of 10 mg three times daily for 5 days, was shown to be effective in treating persistent hiccups in stroke patients compared with placebo. Although this study reported no adverse side effects to baclofen use, this medication is known to cause muscle weakness, confusion, and sedation in some patients, and particular care must be taken in patients with renal impairment to avoid accumulation and toxicity. Metoclopramide, a dopamine receptor antagonist and serotonin agonist, was also shown in a small randomized controlled trial to improve hiccup symptoms at

[1]Not FDA approved for this indication.

a dose of 10 mg every 8 hours for 15 days. Although no adverse effects were observed in this study, one must weigh the known risks of tardive dyskinesia associated with metoclopramide use, which renders this medication more of a second-line therapy.

Several case series have reported use of gabapentin (Neurontin)[1] alone or in conjunction with other medications such as omeprazole as an effective treatment for hiccups, particularly in cases where a central etiology is suspected. These studies looked at doses ranging from 300 to 600 mg three times daily, and durations of therapy from 1 day to indefinite. The side effect profile is generally acceptable, with sedation, dizziness, and vision changes most commonly reported. Other antiepileptics are sometimes used to treat hiccups as well, though evidence to support their use is lacking and they are associated with weight gain, mood, and neurologic disturbance. These include carbamazepine[1] (Tegretol, 100–300 mg three times daily), phenytoin[1] (Dilantin, 100 mg three times daily), and valproic acid[1] (Depakote, 20 mg/kg/day).

Antipsychotic medications have historically been widely used for treatment of hiccups since the 1950s, though have fallen out of favor in more recent years due to their modest benefit and unfavorable side effect profile. Interestingly, chlorpromazine (Thorazine, 10–50 mg three times daily) is the only medication that has been FDA approved for treatment of hiccups. Haloperidol[1] (Haldol, 1–4 mg every 24 hours) is another common antipsychotic that is reached for in cases of intractable hiccups. Both medications act as dopamine receptor antagonists in the brain and should be used with extreme caution due to the risk of sedation, hypotension, dystonia, and tardive dyskinesia.

The use of benzodiazepines is generally not recommended for treatment of intractable hiccups, and, in fact, this class of medications can actually trigger episodes of hiccups when given at low doses. One exception is the use of midazolam (Versed)[1] in patients with terminal illness. Several case reports describe the use of midazolam (10–60 mg every 24 hours subcutaneously) at the end of life to effectively suppress the hiccup reflex.

Limited data from a small case series support the use of nifedipine (Adalat)[1] at doses of 20 to 60 mg/day, which partially or totally resolved intractable hiccups in five of seven patients studied. There was a noted high recurrence rate after stopping the medication. Known side effects of nifedipine use include hypotension and reflex tachycardia.

Amitriptyline (Elavil),[1] which is a tricyclic antidepressant, has been shown to be effective in a small number of patients at doses of 25 to 100 mg nightly. Although amitriptyline is known to increase the neurotransmitters serotonin and norepinephrine in the neuronal synapses, its mechanism of action in reducing hiccup symptomatology is not well understood, though may relate to its sodium channel–blocking properties.

Other medications that have been suggested as potential therapeutic agents for hiccups despite a lack of consistent data supporting their efficacy include lidocaine (Xylocaine),[1] methylphenidate (Ritalin),[1] and ondansetron (Zofran).[1] Interestingly, ondansetron has been noted to worsen hiccups in some cases.

Physical Interventions

Case reports of ultrasound-guided phrenic nerve blockade of the efferent limb of the reflex arc have shown some promise in the treatment of persistent hiccups in cases that were refractory to pharmacologic therapy. In a case where phrenic nerve blockade was unsuccessful, afferent vagal blockade was shown to have some efficacy in alleviating symptoms. Ultrasound-guided ablation of the phrenic nerve can also be effective; however, this runs the risk of respiratory complications.

A common home remedy for hiccups is paper bag rebreathing, which induces hypercapnia. One study reported that use of an airtight plastic bag was more efficacious because CO_2 levels need to increase substantially for suppression of the hiccup reflex arc.

Other physical maneuvers are patient specific; for example, in hiccups that are thought to be due to abdominal distension, placement of a nasogastric tube for decompression may help alleviate symptoms. In patients who are ventilated, inducing a mechanical Valsalva maneuver by increasing positive end-expiratory pressure may be helpful.

Finally, acupuncture may be helpful as an adjunct to medical therapy in patients suffering from intractable hiccups, though, again, data from randomized controlled trials are lacking.

Monitoring

No ongoing monitoring for recurrence of hiccups is necessary as patients will undoubtedly be aware of a return of symptoms. Posttreatment monitoring after pharmacologic therapy should primarily focus on adverse reactions to the medications discussed above. In cases in which phrenic or vagus nerve block or phrenic nerve destruction have been performed, the patient should be monitored for respiratory compromise.

Complications

Complications of untreated intractable hiccups include malnutrition, weight loss, sleep deprivation, wound dehiscence, and depression.

References

Brañuelas Quiroga J, Urbano García J, Bolaños Guedes J: Hiccups: a common problem with some unusual causes and cures, *Br J Gen Pract* 66(652):584–586, 2016.

Chang FY, Lu CL: Hiccup: mystery, nature and treatment, *J Neurogastroenterol Motil* 18(2):123–130, 2012.

Jeon YS, Kearney AM, Baker PG: Management of hiccups in palliative care patients, *BMJ Support Palliat Care* 8(1):1–6, 2018.

Nausheen F, Mohsin H, Lakhan SE: Neurotransmitters in hiccups, *Springerplus* 5(1):1357, 2016.

Obuchi T, Shimamura S, Miyahara N, et al: CO_2 retention: the key to stopping hiccups, *Clin Respir J* 12(8):2340–2345, 2018.

Polito NB, Fellows SE: Pharmacologic interventions for intractable and persistent hiccups: a systematic review, *J Emerg Med* 53(4):540–549, 2017.

Steger M, Schneemann M, Fox M: Systematic review: the pathogenesis and pharmacological treatment of hiccups, *Aliment Pharmacol Ther* 42(9):1037–1050, 2015.

▮ HOARSENESS AND LARYNGITIS

Method of
Lee Akst, MD

CURRENT DIAGNOSIS

- The general term to describe vocal difficulty is dysphonia. Hoarseness is a specific term for rough voice quality, which is one type of dysphonia. Laryngitis signifies laryngeal inflammation, which is one possible cause of dysphonia.
- An accurate history and physical examination guide the diagnosis of voice complaints. Although many portions of the examination for dysphonia can be done in a general setting, videostroboscopy is often necessary for diagnosis and may be available only in specialized laryngology offices.
- The most common cause of acute hoarseness is viral laryngitis. Symptoms are self-limited and usually resolve within 2 weeks.
- Dysphonia persisting for longer than 2 weeks suggests the possibility of another diagnosis, such as vocal cord paralysis, neoplasm, phonotraumatic lesion, or chronic laryngitis.
- Indications for referral of a patient with voice complaints to an otolaryngologist include dysphonia that persists for longer than 2 weeks, that is of acute onset during voicing, or that is accompanied by other symptoms such as otalgia, dysphagia, or difficulty breathing.

---

[1]Not FDA approved for this indication.

- Appropriate treatment of voice complaints depends on accurate diagnosis.
- Supportive therapy is all that is necessary for most cases of acute laryngitis associated with viral upper respiratory tract infections.
- Laryngopharyngeal reflux is a common cause of chronic laryngitis, and appropriate therapy often requires twice-daily administration of proton pump inhibitors for at least 2 months.
- Microlaryngeal phonosurgery may be indicated for some patients with benign phonotraumatic lesions.
- Vocal cord medialization can rehabilitate the voice in a patient with unilateral vocal cord paralysis.
- Many patients with dysphonia benefit from voice therapy, alone or in combination with other treatment strategies.

Voice is an essential component of communication. Vocal difficulty is very distressing to patients and can have a negative impact on physical, social, and emotional qualities of life. To understand the pathophysiology, evaluation, and treatment of voice complaints, it is important to understand the anatomy and physiology of normal voice production. Looking first at how good voice quality is achieved makes it readily apparent how alterations in vocal fold vibration, symmetry, or closure can lead to various vocal difficulties.

To aid discussion of voice complaints, clarification of terminology is necessary. Although "hoarseness" is a term that most patients use to describe any type of voice complaint and "laryngitis" is the presumptive explanation that many patients provide for their symptoms, each of these terms has a more precise meaning. Dysphonia is the general term for vocal difficulty. Hoarseness implies a rough or raspy change in voice quality and is one type of dysphonia. Other categories include limited vocal projection, strained vocal effort, and change in pitch—each of which may occur with or without vocal roughness. The term "laryngitis" specifically describes inflammation of the larynx. This inflammation may be acute or chronic, and again it describes some but certainly not all cases of dysphonia. This distinction will be made clear as the evaluation and management of dysphonia are described.

Normal Laryngeal Function

The larynx plays a central role in voice production by serving as a vibrating instrument that turns airflow from the lungs into sound. The sound is shaped into intelligible speech through the resonating and articulating functions of the pharynx and oral cavity. The ability of the larynx to create vibration and serve as a sound source is a function of its complex, layered microanatomy. The deeper layers of the vocal fold include the thyroarytenoid muscle and the vocal ligament, which position the more superficial layers of the superficial lamina propria and epithelium during phonation. Compared with the fibrous nature of the vocal ligament, the superficial lamina propria is a loose gelatinous layer whose pliability allows for voice production.

During inspiration (Figure 1A), the vocal folds are abducted so that air can move past the larynx without resistance. During phonation (Figure 1B), the vocal folds are held in an adducted position while the lungs drive air toward the larynx. Air pressure builds in the subglottis, beneath the vocal folds, until it overcomes the forces of vocal fold closure, pushes past the vocal folds, and generates negative pressure in its wake as it moves past the larynx. A combination of the vocal folds' intrinsic viscoelasticity and the negative pressure created through Bernoulli's effect draws the vocal fold edges back together, allowing subglottic pressure to rebuild and the cycle to repeat. Repeated cycles of opening and closing at the level of the vocal fold edges generate a so-called mucosal wave, which travels from the inferior edge of each vocal fold up across the medial and superior edges (Figure 1C). These waves may repeat hundreds of times each second, depending on pitch. This cycled opening and closing of the vocal folds during phonation imparts pressure waves to the air column that moves the vocal folds, generating sound. The ability of vocal folds to vibrate easily and symmetrically in this very rapid fashion allows for clear, smooth voicing.

Evaluation of Dysphonia

Central to the evaluation of dysphonia is the understanding that any disruption of vocal fold closure, symmetry, or vibration impairs the ability of the vocal folds to generate a clear sound source. Most voice complaints arise from anatomic or functional limitations in glottal closure or mucosal wave formation, although other parts of the respiratory tree are also responsible for components of the voice. General points concerning evaluation of dysphonia are discussed in this section, with specific causes discussed afterward.

History

A careful history can provide many clues that point toward the proper diagnosis in patients with dysphonia. Although many patients offer the complaint of "hoarseness" as a general term, a careful historian distinguishes between complaints related to voice quality, vocal projection, vocal effort or strain, vocal fatigue, and so on. Two questions that can help a patient organize his or her own thoughts related to poor voice are "What abnormal things does your voice do now that it did not do before?" and "What normal things did your voice do before that it no longer can do?" The acuteness of onset, duration, severity, and progression of any complaint should be determined.

The history should also determine what other factors or events might have caused or exacerbated the dysphonia. Recent sources of laryngeal inflammation might include intubation, excessive voice use, or upper respiratory tract infection. Baseline conditions that foster chronic laryngeal inflammation include environmental allergies, rhinitis, and laryngopharyngeal reflux. Laryngopharyngeal reflux can exist in the absence of heartburn, with reflux-associated inflammation of the larynx and pharynx providing symptoms of globus pharyngeus, throat clearing, nonproductive cough, effortful swallowing, and even mild dysphagia in association with dysphonia.

Concerning the possibility of laryngeal malignancy, any patient with dysphonia should be asked about smoking and alcohol use, because these are risk factors for squamous cell carcinoma. Another important question in distinguishing inflammatory dysphonia from a mass lesion of the vocal fold concerns whether there are any periods of normal voice or the dysphonia is constant—inflammation may wax and wane, but dysphonia associated with mass lesions is usually progressive and unremitting. Finally, the history should elicit other possible head and neck complaints, including dyspnea, stridor, dysphagia, odynophagia, otalgia, sore throat, and pain with speaking (odynophonia). If hoarseness is associated with some of these symptoms for longer than 2 weeks, the suspicion of malignancy is increased.

Physical Examination

The physical examination for patients with dysphonia includes a complete head and neck evaluation with focus on the larynx and laryngeal function. Although much of the head and neck examination can be performed in a general setting, some portions of the laryngeal examination require specialized equipment found only in some otolaryngology offices that specialize in voice care. Routine head and neck evaluation should include systematic examination of the ears, nose, oral cavity, oropharynx, and neck.

Complaint of otalgia in the setting of an unremarkable ear examination suggests a possibility of referred pain from a lesion of the larynx or pharynx, and is concerning for possible malignancy. Edematous and erythematous nasal mucosa suggests rhinitis, with the possibility of postnasal drip contributing to laryngeal inflammation. Tremor of the tongue or palate might suggest neurologic disorder, whereas pharyngeal erythema and exudate suggest possible acute infection. Pachydermia (cobblestoning) of the

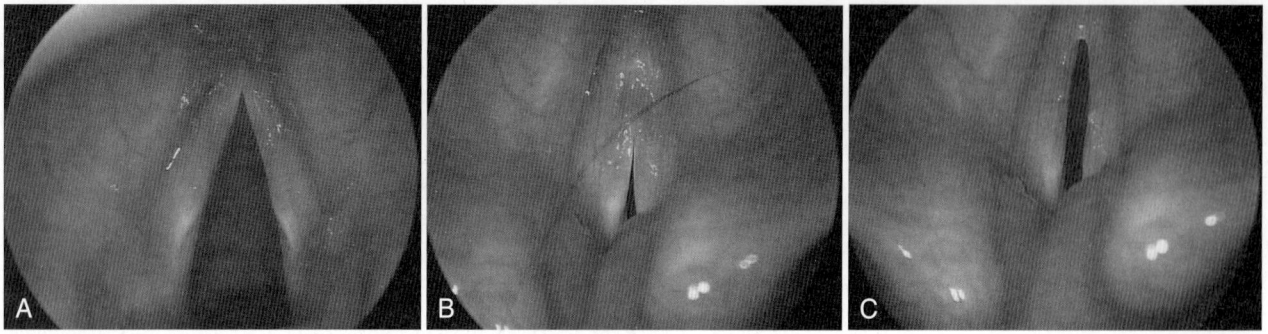

Figure 1 A, Normal vocal folds in abducted position for inspiration. B, Normal vocal folds in adducted position for phonation. C, Displacement of the vocal fold medial edges creates mucosal wave propagation during phonation and produces voice.

posterior pharyngeal wall suggests the possibility of laryngopharyngeal reflux. Tenderness with manipulation of the hyoid bone suggests tension of the strap muscles and correlates closely with complaint of odynophonia and the possibility of muscle tension dysphonia. A neck mass might represent either metastatic lymphadenopathy from a laryngeal malignancy or a primary lesion which itself compresses the recurrent laryngeal nerve and causes paralytic dysphonia. Surgical scarring along the neck suggests the possibility that prior thyroid surgery, carotid endarterectomy, or anterior approach to the cervical spine might have led to vocal fold paralysis.

Laryngeal Examination

Beyond a general examination of the head and neck, there should be directed evaluation of the larynx and laryngeal function. The examiner should listen to the voice carefully, because vocal characteristics such as roughness, breathiness, strain, vocal breaks, and diplophonia (pitch instability, with two different pitches present simultaneously) can help guide the differential diagnosis of dysphonia. Visual examination of the larynx has many forms, ranging from mirror examination to flexible fiberoptic laryngoscopy to videostrobolaryngoscopy.

Mirror examination offers an adequate view of the vocal folds in many patients but may be limited by patient tolerance, physician inexperience, and the inherently limited ability of this technique to brightly illuminate the larynx or record the examination for later review. Flexible laryngoscopy is routinely available in almost all otolaryngology offices, is well tolerated by patients, and offers good views of the larynx that can be recorded with appropriate equipment. Mirror examination and flexible laryngoscopy are limited to observation of vocal fold motion and anatomy but cannot observe laryngeal function because they do not visualize vibration of the vocal folds. To examine vocal fold vibration, videostroboscopy uses a strobe light to create the impression of slow-motion analysis of mucosal waves. Stroboscopy is typically available only in selected otolaryngology practices in which laryngologists specialize in the treatment of voice disorders.

Other Testing

Videostroboscopic evaluation, combined with a thorough history and routine physical examination, can establish the diagnosis for almost all patients with voice complaints, but further testing is sometimes indicated. For instance, electromyography is used by some laryngologists for further evaluation of vocal fold paralysis or paresis. More commonly, radiographic studies are used for further evaluation of some voice complaints. Computed tomography (CT) scans are ordered most often in the evaluation of suspected laryngeal neoplasms and for patients with vocal fold paralysis.

In the case of neoplasm, CT scanning is useful to assess the extent of the primary lesion and to evaluate possible metastatic cervical lymphadenopathy. In patients with laryngeal malignancy, chest radiography is also important to assess for pulmonary metastases. For patients with vocal fold paralysis who do not have a clear history of surgical injury of the recurrent laryngeal nerve, a CT scan from skull base to thoracic inlet identifies

possible lesions along the course of the recurrent laryngeal nerve. Central problems are less likely, but if they are suspected as a cause of vocal fold paralysis, then magnetic resonance imaging of the brain may be indicated as well.

Types of Dysphonia

Although not comprehensive, the conditions discussed here account for the vast majority of voice complaints. Some patients with voice complaints have more than one condition, and not every patient will fit neatly into a single category. Nevertheless, understanding how each of these conditions creates dysphonia, and knowing which particular history and physical examination findings might be associated with each cause, can help a physician to appropriately diagnose and manage voice complaints.

Acute Laryngitis

Acute laryngitis is the most common cause of hoarseness and dysphonia. It is most often viral in nature, and onset of laryngeal symptoms may be associated with other symptoms of upper respiratory tract infection, including fever, myalgia, sore throat, and rhinorrhea. Viral inflammation of the vocal folds leads to diminished and more effortful vocal fold vibration, yielding a voice characterized by increased effort and a harsh, strained quality with decreased projection. Characteristic findings on laryngoscopy include vocal fold edema and erythema with decreased amplitude of the mucosal wave. Treatment of acute viral laryngitis is supportive, with counseling for hydration, humidification, and mucolytics. Symptoms generally are self-limited and resolve within 2 weeks. During this time, patients should be instructed to use the voice in a comfortable fashion, rather than straining or pushing to get loudness, because pushing behaviors may lead to the development of persistent muscle tension dysphonia.

Bacterial or fungal infections also cause acute laryngitis in rare cases. With appropriate physical findings and in the right clinical setting, antibiotic or antifungal therapy may be used to treat these conditions. Amoxicillin-clavulanate (Augmentin) is often the antibiotic of choice, and fluconazole (Diflucan) is a commonly used antifungal agent.

Chronic Laryngitis

Chronic laryngitis is the nonspecific condition of prolonged laryngeal inflammation; the term itself does not indicate an etiology for the inflammation. Among the many possible sources for this inflammation are mechanical irritation from traumatic coughing or prolonged speaking, chemical irritation from environmental irritants (e.g., smoking, inhaled medications), and irritation from postnasal drip or laryngopharyngeal reflux. More than one cause may exist simultaneously. Issues related to cigarette use, excessive voice use, medication effect, and rhinitis can be identified with careful history taking. Laryngopharyngeal reflux is a very common source of chronic laryngitis. It may manifest with several nonspecific symptoms, such as throat irritation, globus pharyngeus, frequent throat clearing, and nonproductive cough, with or without accompanying heartburn. Because vocal fold inflammation increases with continued mechanical trauma, the hoarseness of chronic laryngitis typically gets worse with prolonged voice use and improves with voice rest. Examination findings in chronic laryngitis include generalized laryngeal edema and erythema, and careful inspection may also reveal interarytenoid hyperplasia, subglottic edema, laryngeal ventricular obliteration, and an increase in thick glottic secretions.

Treatment of chronic laryngitis is tailored to the cause of the inflammation. Vocal hygiene with moderate voice use and instructions to reduce throat clearing and coughing may diminish mechanical irritation, and smoking cessation is recommended to any smoker with laryngeal complaints. Several studies have suggested that an appropriate trial of proton pump inhibitors for treatment of laryngopharyngeal reflux includes twice-daily therapy for at least 2 months, in contrast to the once-daily dosing often used for typical heartburn complaints. Lifestyle counseling to limit consumption of caffeine, carbonation, alcohol, and acidic foods can improve reflux, and attention to hydration and humidification decreases the viscosity of glottic secretions. For patients who are troubled by vocal difficulties associated with chronic laryngitis, referral to a speech–language pathologist for voice therapy can improve compliance with suggested lifestyle changes and help foster vocal improvement.

Vocal Fold Paralysis

The dysphonia in cases of vocal fold paralysis usually relates to poor vocal fold closure (Figure 2). The result is a breathy voice with limited projection and increased vocal effort. The farther from midline the immobile vocal fold, the more air leaks through the incompetent glottal valve without being turned into sound. Patients whose immobile vocal fold sits in a lateral position may have severely weak and breathy voices, whereas patients whose immobile vocal fold sits near midline may have a perceptually near-normal conversational voice and complain only of mild increase in effort, vocal fatigue, or problems with loud projection. Because of their glottal insufficiency, patients may complain of "running out of air" with prolonged speech. Impaired glottal closure may also decrease airway protection during swallowing, so patients with vocal fold paralysis need to be questioned about aspiration as well. Whereas rehabilitation of poor voice may be elective, patients with increased aspiration risk need prompt therapy.

Evaluation of vocal fold paralysis includes identification of the cause of paralysis. Surgical injury to the recurrent laryngeal nerve accounts for almost half of all cases of unilateral vocal fold paralysis, and cervical or thoracic neoplasm and idiopathic paralysis account for most of the remaining cases. In a patient without a clear surgical history explaining the paralysis, CT scanning from skull base to mediastinum can identify any possible lesions along the course of the recurrent laryngeal nerve. In those patients whose histories suggest other possible causes (e.g., central neurologic injury, Lyme disease), further investigations, such as magnetic resonance imaging of the brain or blood work may be indicated as well. Some physicians perform laryngeal electromyography to help with the prognosis of paralysis or to differentiate neurologic injury from cricoarytenoid joint fixation; however, this study is neither standardized nor routine in many practices. Although flexible laryngoscopy alone may be satisfactory to document vocal fold immobility, stroboscopy can be added to investigate the impact of glottal insufficiency on vocal cord vibration and possible vocal fold flutter.

Treatment of vocal fold paralysis might include any combination of voice therapy, injection laryngoplasty, transcervical medialization laryngoplasty, and laryngeal reinnervation. Depending on the cause of the paralysis, some patients experience gradual recovery with synkinetic reinnervation or recovery of purposeful vocal fold motion over a period of several months. Based on the degree of voice and swallowing handicap, treatment of patients with vocal fold paralysis may be optional rather than necessary. Voice therapy can help teach patients to produce a stronger voice despite the paralysis, but by itself will not help a paralyzed vocal cord to recover motion. Various medialization techniques have been developed to help reposition an immobile vocal fold in the midline, where the contralateral mobile vocal fold can provide

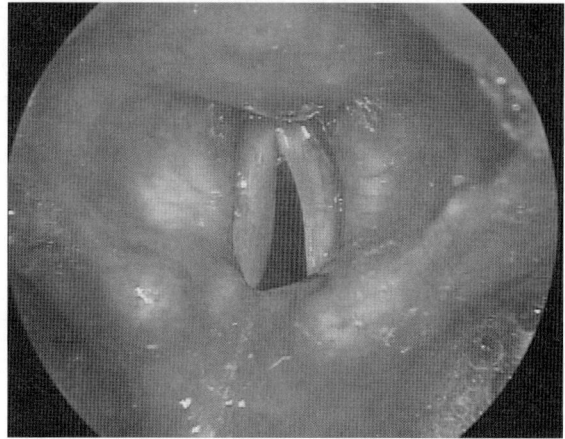

Figure 2 Vocal fold paralysis prevents the right vocal fold from closing to midline and creates dysphonia.

for complete glottal closure and lead to improved voice and swallowing. Injection medialization can be performed in the office or in the operating room, with temporary or permanent materials; if recovery of vocal fold motion is thought possible, then temporary injection is preferred. Transcervical medialization is a permanent but reversible surgical technique performed by otolaryngologists that repositions an immobile vocal fold in the midline. Laryngeal reinnervation offers the possibility of midline positioning of the immobile vocal fold with restored tone and bulk of the vocal fold musculature; however, because results may not mature for several months, this technique is less commonly performed than either injection or transcervical medialization.

Phonotraumatic Lesions: Nodules, Polyps, and Cysts

During vibration, vocal folds are subject to the shearing stresses of vibration. Although vocal fold structure is designed to accommodate these stresses in most circumstances, patients with vocal abuse or excessive voice use are at risk for development of lesions as the result of cumulative phonotrauma. Depending on the location and nature of these lesions, they are categorized as nodules, polyps, or cysts.

Vocal fold nodules are areas of fibrovascular scarring that are located just beneath the epithelium, at the level of the basement membrane and superficial lamina propria. They are typically bilateral and symmetrical, sitting at the junction of the anterior one third and the posterior two thirds of each vocal fold. Polyps are typically unilateral lesions that may be edematous or fibrous in nature and may contain hemorrhage (Figure 3). They usually are exophytic and extend outward from the vocal fold epithelium, although the fibrous base of a polyp may extend into the superficial lamina propria of a vocal fold. In contrast to an epithelial-based lesion such as a polyp, a vocal fold cyst is a subepithelial encapsulated lesion that sits entirely within the vocal fold; its size may exert a mass effect that deforms the medial edge of the involved vocal fold. These cysts are occasionally noted as congenital lesions in children, but in adults they are more often caused by traumatic occlusion of the ducts of the seromucinous glands within the larynx.

Nodules, polyps, and cysts cause dysphonia by disturbing vocal fold vibration, leading to rough voice quality. These lesions get larger as traumatic voice use accumulates, and vocal roughness usually becomes more severe and more constant as the lesions progress. Because vibration is more easily disturbed at high pitch, performers with these lesions may notice that high pitch is affected first. Effort of phonation often increases, but projection remains intact. Lesions large enough to limit vocal fold closure may also cause a slightly breathy voice quality. Because patients with excessive voice use are at risk for these lesions, a history of social and occupational voice demands is valuable in cases of suspected phonotrauma.

Treatment for these lesions always begins with voice therapy designed to modify the patient's voice use so as to diminish trauma. Voice therapy may be all that is necessary to allow

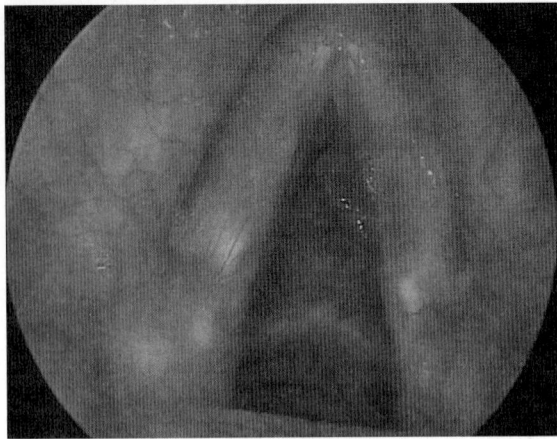

Figure 3 A large right hemorrhagic polyp, which can impair vocal fold vibration.

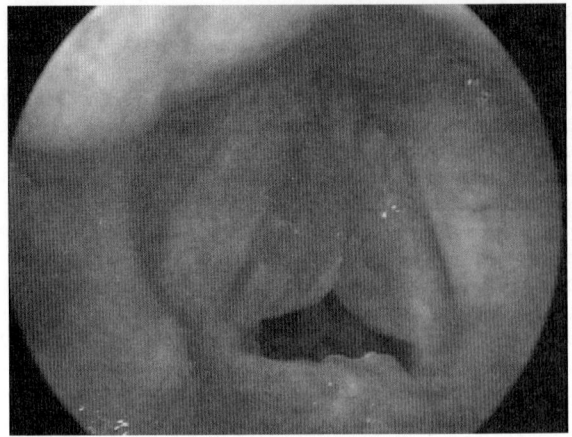

Figure 4 Symmetrical polypoid degeneration of the bilateral vocal folds, characteristic of Reinke's edema.

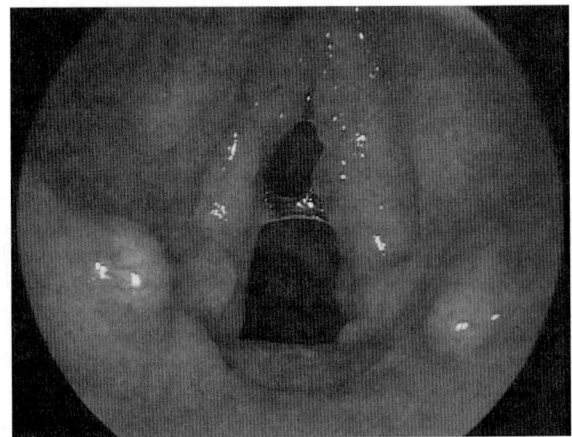

Figure 5 Recurrent respiratory papillomatosis, whose presence along each vocal fold medial edge disrupts sound production.

resolution of some early traumatic changes, particularly in the case of edematous nodules. If dysphonia persists despite voice therapy and other conservative measures, surgery may be considered. Surgery with the goal of voice preservation and restoration (phonosurgery) is typically performed by otolaryngologists who specialize in the care of persons with vocal difficulties. The goal of phonosurgery for these lesions is to remove the lesion that impairs vibration while preserving as much of the remaining, pliable superficial lamina propria as possible, so that vocal fold vibration can be restored.

Reinke's Edema

Reinke's edema, also known as polypoid corditis, is a benign swelling of the vocal folds that is most commonly seen in patients with a long-term smoking history. The edema, a reaction to long-term irritation, accumulates within the superficial lamina propria. The edema is most often bilateral and occurs diffusely along the entire length of the vocal fold, rather than being limited to a more discrete area, as is seen with phonotraumatic polyps (Figure 4). As vocal fold mass increases with disease progression, the pitch of the voice decreases, and this is the change in voice most associated with Reinke's edema. A classic presentation of this condition is a female in her fifth or sixth decade of life who provides a long history of smoking and progressive deepening of her voice. In rare circumstances, the vocal folds gradually accumulate enough edema to compromise the airway, so breathing complaints should be evaluated as well.

Because a significant smoking history is also a risk factor for vocal fold leukoplakia and malignancy, good visualization of the vocal folds is necessary to evaluate for other lesions in these patients. If benign edema of the vocal folds is truly the only lesion noted, management depends on the degree to which voice quality is disturbing to the patient or the degree to which the airway is narrowed. Smoking cessation can lead to stabilization of pitch at its current level, and phonosurgery to remove excess vocal fold mass can help lead to normalization of pitch and improve the airway. Phonosurgery may be performed with cold instruments or with the pulsed photoangiolytic lasers, an emerging therapy; in either case, there is a risk of creating a vocal fold scar that might limit vocal fold vibration even as vocal fold contours are improved.

Recurrent Respiratory Papillomatosis

Recurrent respiratory papillomatosis (Figure 5) is a benign laryngeal neoplasm that is caused by the human papilloma virus. It is the most common source of hoarseness in children, although adults also may be affected. As the lesions grow on the laryngeal epithelium, they create hoarseness and sometimes effortful voice by disrupting vocal fold vibration, particularly if the lesions are located along the medial edge of either vocal fold. Large and bulky lesions may lead to airway compromise, and advanced disease may spread throughout the mucosa of the upper aerodigestive tract rather than being limited to the larynx. Although accurate diagnosis depends on histopathologic analysis, a diagnosis of benign papilloma can be suspected from the characteristic appearance of the vascular fronds, which can be seen under magnified visualization in the office or in the operating room.

Treatment of recurrent respiratory papillomatosis is surgery, which is performed with a carbon dioxide laser, microdebrider, cold instruments, or the emerging technology of pulsed potassium titanyl phosphate (KTP) laser. As its name implies, the condition is recurrent: Even though surgery may reduce or remove the papilloma temporarily, the tissue continues to harbor the papilloma virus, and the disease usually grows back. Because repeated surgeries are expected, the goal of any single procedure is to remove as much disease as possible while limiting surgical scarring of the vocal folds. Scarring created as a result of surgery is cumulative, and over time patients develop persistent dysphonia caused as much by repeated surgeries as by recurrence of the disease. An ability to treat epithelial lesions while limiting scarring at the level of the superficial lamina propria is one main advantage of pulsed laser photoangiolysis; that these pulsed laser procedures can be performed in the office as well as the operating room is another. To help limit the need for repeated surgical procedures, adjunct medical therapies such as interferon and cidofovir are sometimes used for treatment of advanced disease.

Vocal Cord Cancer

In 2008, an estimated 12,250 new cases of laryngeal cancer and 3,670 deaths attributable to laryngeal cancer occurred in the United States. The annual incidence of laryngeal cancer is 6.4 cases per 100,000 for men and 1.3 cases per 100,000 for women. Smoking is the single largest risk factor for laryngeal cancer, and excessive alcohol use has a synergistic effect as a risk factor as well. Survival rates for laryngeal cancer depend on the stage of the tumor at the time of diagnosis, which is a function of tumor size and possible tumor spread to the cervical lymph nodes or distant metastatic sites. Cancers that occur on the medial edge of the vocal fold produce dysphonia while still small, and many laryngeal cancers are diagnosed early.

The dysphonia associated with laryngeal cancer is constant, progressive, and unremitting, without the intermittent vocal improvement that may occur in inflammatory conditions. The presence of dysphagia, odynophagia, otalgia, hemoptysis, or unexplained weight loss further increases the index of suspicion for malignancy. Cervical lymphadenopathy is associated with advanced tumors. Diagnosis may be suspected on the basis of laryngeal examination and is confirmed with biopsy. The presence or absence of mucosal waves on the involved vocal fold on videostroboscopic examination can help predict the depth of the lesion. Both a CT scan of the neck and chest radiographs are indicated to assess for tumor size and spread. Early cancers are treated with surgery or radiation therapy, with similar cure rates. Emerging technologies such as pulsed photoangiolytic lasers may allow for surgical treatment of early disease with better preservation of surrounding normal tissue. More advanced tumors are usually treated with a combination of radiation therapy and surgery or chemotherapy.

Leukoplakia, or a raised white plaque on the epithelial surface, is a visual marker for the likely presence of dysplasia or carcinoma in situ. As a very early lesion, vocal fold leukoplakia may manifest with mild dysphonia or may be found incidentally on head and neck examination performed for other reasons. This early disease may take many years before progressing to invasive carcinoma, and recognition of leukoplakia presents an opportunity for early treatment to prevent progression of disease. Pulsed laser photoangiolysis has emerged as a state-of-the-art therapy for treatment of this epithelial lesion with preservation of the underlying vocal fold pliability.

Neurologic Disorders and the Voice

Neurologic conditions that affect the voice usually do so by causing poor coordination of vocal fold motion. Spasmodic dysphonia, for instance, leads to involuntary spasms that bring the vocal folds either tightly together (adductor spasmodic dysphonia) or apart (abductor spasmodic dysphonia) during phonation. These spasms lead to vocal breaks that are strained or breathy, respectively. Although the cause of spasmodic dysphonia is thought to lie within the central nervous system, the gold standard treatment of botulinum toxin is targeted at the end organ. Injection of botulinum toxin (Botox)[1] into appropriate laryngeal muscles can weaken these muscles and diminish the spasm.

Vocal fold tremor is a neurologic disorder that is distinct from spasmodic dysphonia. Its hallmark is tremulous voice quality caused by tremor of the larynx, which may occur both during phonation and at rest. Vocal fold tremor may exist alone or as part of systemic tremor. Botulinum toxin[1] can decrease the amplitude of the tremor but may exacerbate the loss of projection that many tremor patients also have as a complaint. Medications such as anxiolytics or β-blockers that are used to treat systemic tremor may also improve the voice in patients with vocal fold tremor without worsening hypophonia.

Functional Voice Disorders

Functional dysphonia may exist by itself or in combination with an anatomic or neurologic source of dysphonia. The most common form of functional voice disorder is muscle tension dysphonia, which describes inappropriate hyperfunction of

---

[1]Not FDA approved for this indication

the supraglottic muscles. This hyperfunction often occurs in response to another source of hoarseness, as the patient tries to force out a strained voice with improved projection rather than accept the limited voice quality that may accompany the other disorder. The hyperfunction may then become an entrenched habit separate from the original pathology. In this sense, a classic scenario for muscle tension dysphonia is a patient who strains to speak more loudly during an acute laryngitis episode and whose strained, squeezed voice pattern persists even after the acute laryngitis has resolved. Patients with muscle tension dysphonia may complain of odynophonia as tension in the involved supraglottic muscles leads to muscular pain with prolonged speaking. Once other lesions have been evaluated, the treatment of muscle tension dysphonia is expert voice therapy with an emphasis on decreased hyperfunction.

Presbylaryngis

Presbylaryngis is the term that is used to describe the aging voice. It typically manifests in the seventh or eighth decade but can develop earlier. Acoustically, presbylaryngis results in a characteristic thinned voice, often with decreased projection and increased vocal strain. The condition occurs as cumulative voice use leads to traumatic thinning of the superficial lamina propria, particularly at the mid-cord level. This loss of superficial lamina propria leads to deficiency at the medial edge of each vocal fold, and a spindle-shaped defect in glottal closure may be noticed with close evaluation. Many patients with a complaint of presbylaryngis find that appropriate voice therapy to address breath support and vocal projection leads to satisfactory improvement in the voice without altering the vocal fold anatomy. For those patients who remain unsatisfied with their voice after therapy, vocal fold medialization procedures can restore straight vocal cord edges and may lead to improved projection; however, currently available injectables and implants that address contour defects cannot restore pliability.

Conclusion

Understanding the anatomy and physiology of normal voice production provides a framework through which dysphonia can be evaluated. Application of this knowledge during the history and physical examination guides the diagnosis of hoarseness and allows clinicians to distinguish among conditions as varied as acute laryngitis, benign phonotraumatic lesions, vocal fold paralysis, and laryngeal cancer as part of a differential diagnosis. Videostrobolaryngoscopy allows evaluation of vocal fold function as well as structure and can confirm diagnosis. As with any condition, accurate diagnosis directs appropriate therapy. Because no further evaluation or management is necessary for acute viral laryngitis, many patients with hoarseness require no more than a careful history and physical examination. However, if dysphonia persists for longer than 2 weeks or is accompanied by other laryngopharyngeal symptoms that are not thought to be related to an upper respiratory tract infection, referral should be made to an otolaryngologist for further evaluation.

References

Koufman JA, Aviv JE, Casiano RR, et al: Laryngopharyngeal reflux: Position statement of the committee on speech, voice, and swallowing disorders of the American Academy of Otolaryngology-Head and Neck Surgery, *Otolaryngol Head Neck Surg* 127:32–35, 2002.

Merati AL, Heman-Ackah YD, Abaza M, et al: Common movement disorders affecting the larynx: A report from the neurolaryngology committee of the AAO-HNS, *Otolaryngol Head Neck Surg* 133:654–665, 2005.

Swibel Rosenthal LH, Benninger MS, Deeb RH: Vocal fold immobility: A longitudinal analysis of etiology over 20 years, *Laryngoscope* 117:1864–1870, 2007.

Wilson JA, Deary IJ, Millar A, et al: The quality of life impact of dysphonia, *Clin Otolaryngol* 27:179–182, 2002.

Zeitels SM, Casiano RR, Gardner GM, et al: Management of common voice problems: Committee report, *Otolaryngol Head Neck Surg* 126:333–348, 2002.

Zeitels SM, Healy GB: Laryngology and phonosurgery, *N Engl J Med* 349:882–892, 2003.

LEG EDEMA AND VENOUS STASIS

Method of
David D. Ortiz, MD

CURRENT DIAGNOSIS

- Chronic, lower extremity pitting edema due to increased venous pressure
- Usually bilateral; can be unilateral and asymmetric
- Must be differentiated from congestive heart failure, edema due to hypoproteinemia from hepatic or renal disease, lymphedema, cellulitis, deep venous thrombosis (DVT) and lipedema

CURRENT THERAPY

- Compression stockings and walking exercises
- Horse chestnut seed extract[7] 600 mg daily to reduce venous stasis symptoms
- Topical emollients and short courses of topical steroids for stasis dermatitis
- Compression bandages, noncompression bandages with zinc oxide paste (Unna boot), and pentoxifylline[1] 400 mg three times daily for venous ulcers
- Surgical treatment (sclerotherapy, stripping and ligation, endovenous ablation) for saphenous vein incompetence, nonhealing venous ulcers, and more severe disease

[7]Available as dietary supplement.
[1]Not FDA approved for this indication.

Pathophysiology

The clinical manifestations of venous stasis in the lower extremities are caused by venous hypertension, which is a result of venous valve reflux, venous obstruction, or both. Normally, the combination of functioning venous valves and lower extremity skeletal muscle contraction causes a decrease in venous pressure throughout the venous system. In patients with nonfunctioning or incompetent venous valves, venous reflux occurs, transmitting higher venous pressure to the superficial veins and to the skin microcirculation. This produces edema due to leakage caused by increased hydrostatic pressure, stasis dermatitis, and staining of the skin resulting from hemosiderin deposition. The fluid leakage and increased venous pressure on the vascular endothelium leads to inflammatory mediator release into the surrounding tissue, which can lead to venous wall and valvular damage, remodeling, and valve incompetence

Prevention

Risk factors for chronic venous disease include advancing age, family history, sedentary lifestyle, prolonged standing, smoking, high estrogen states, pregnancy, obesity, lower extremity trauma, and a history of venous thrombosis (postthrombotic syndrome). Therefore an active lifestyle, smoking cessation, maintaining a normal body-mass index, and reducing the risk of venous thrombosis (following evidence-based guidelines) during travel, hospitalization, surgery, and hormonal treatment can reduce the probability of developing chronic venous disease. For patients who have been diagnosed and treated for DVT, the use of compression stockings reduces the risk of developing postthrombotic syndrome.

Clinical Manifestations

The clinical manifestation of venous stasis in the lower extremities include discomfort, swelling, varicose veins, skin changes, nocturnal cramps, and ulceration. Leg edema seen in venous stasis is usually pitting, begins at the ankle and ascends into the legs, worsens with prolonged standing, and is relieved by leg elevation. Varicose veins are dilated, bulging superficial veins that may be asymptomatic, though patients are usually concerned about their cosmetic appearance. The skin changes seen in venous stasis are skin hyperpigmentation caused by hemosiderin deposition, stasis dermatitis, and venous ulceration.

Stasis dermatitis is characterized by irritated reddish-brown colored skin on the ankles and lower legs. Plaques, fissures, and ulcers may be present. Symptoms may include itching and pain. Stasis dermatitis may be confused with cellulitis and a number of other dermatologic conditions, and cellulitis and secondary infection may be a complication.

Diagnosis

A comprehensive history and physical examination should be performed to evaluate for other causes of leg edema. The history should include questions about chronic diseases, medications, personal and family history of clotting disorders, previous surgeries, trauma, and any history of malignancy and/or radiation treatment. Acute (<72 hours) swelling is characteristic of DVT, infections, or trauma, while chronic swelling is more likely a result of venous insufficiency or chronic medical conditions. Bilateral leg edema may be caused by congestive heart failure, hypoalbuminemia (either from renal losses or hepatic disease), myxedema from hypothyroidism, bilateral venous insufficiency, or pulmonary hypertension. Unilateral swelling is more suggestive of primary or secondary venous or lymphatic compromise. Chronic venous disease can present as both unilateral or bilateral leg edema, and it may be symmetric or asymmetric. Leg edema may also be caused by medications, such as calcium-channel blockers. The physical examination should include an evaluation of the heart, lungs, and abdomen for signs of heart failure (jugular-venous distention and lung crackles) and evidence of liver disease (ascites, scleral icterus) as well as a detailed examination of the lower extremities. Localized swelling of the calf may indicate DVT, infection, or trauma, while diffuse swelling is more likely a result of a systemic process. Lipedema (fat deposition that causes nonpitting leg edema) can be differentiated from other cases of leg edema because it does not involve the feet. Lymphedema resulting from lymphatic fluid buildup can be diagnosed by a positive Stemmer sign, which is the inability of the examiner to pinch the skin of the dorsum of the foot. Skin changes such as dryness, ulcers, erythema, and warmth should be noted. Pitting, the indentation remaining in the swollen area after pressure is applied, should be documented.

A thorough pulse examination of the lower extremities should be performed. In patients with signs and/or symptoms of peripheral artery disease (PAD) and in patients with venous ulcers, the ankle-brachial index (ABI) should be measured.

If an obvious cause is not found on the initial physical examination, diagnostic testing can be helpful to elicit the underlying diagnosis or to confirm a suspected diagnosis and guide treatment. A complete blood count and an evaluation of hepatic enzymes, renal function, thyroid function, albumin level, brain natriuretic peptide (in suspected heart failure), and albuminuria/proteinuria should be performed. A D-dimer level can be helpful in ruling out DVT in the appropriate clinical context. If congestive heart failure or pulmonary hypertension is suspected, an echocardiogram should be performed, and in patients with signs or symptoms of sleep apnea, a polysomnogram should be performed as well. In patients with lower limb swelling without a clear etiology, duplex ultrasonography is the imaging modality of choice to assess for vascular and nonvascular causes of leg edema. If ultrasonography does not reveal a cause and a vascular etiology is still suspected, magnetic resonance angiography (MRA) or computed tomography angiography (CTA) should be considered.

Therapy (or Treatment)

Conservative management should be the initial treatment for patients diagnosed with venous stasis. Weight reduction, exercise, and smoking cessation should be encouraged. Compression stockings with graduated compression along with walking exercise are the mainstay of conservative management. Stockings with compression pressures of 20 to 30 mm Hg are recommended for patients with mild to moderate disease. Higher-pressure stockings (30 to 40 mm Hg and 40 to 50 mm Hg) are recommended for patients with more severe disease and venous ulcers. Knee-length stockings are better tolerated by most patients than thigh-length stockings, and the former should be recommended as first-line treatment as studies have not shown any difference in outcomes between thigh-length and knee-length stockings.

Horse chestnut seed extract (escin),[7] at a dose of 300 mg once or twice daily (equivalent to 50 to 100 mg of escin daily) has been shown to improve the symptoms of venous stasis. Phlebotonics, such as diosmin,[7] micronized purified flavonoid fraction (MPFF),[7] calcium dobesilate,[2] and rutosides,[7] may reduce the edema in venous stasis, as well as improve pain, leg heaviness, and night cramps.

For patients with saphenous vein incompetence, more severe disease, or persistent symptoms despite conservative management, referral for surgical treatment should be considered. Sclerotherapy, ligation, stripping of the veins, and endovenous ablation may improve cosmetic symptoms and promote venous ulcer healing in patients in whom first-line therapy has not been effective.

Monitoring

In patients with a history of venous ulceration, regular follow-up is recommended to monitor for ulcer recurrence, promote continued lifestyle modifications, provide patient education, and ensure treatment compliance. Cardiovascular risk factors should be monitored and treated according to current guidelines.

Complications

In chronic venous disease, the most common complications are stasis dermatitis and venous ulcerations. For venous ulcers, compression bandages using higher pressures (40 mm Hg) and nonelastic compression bandages using a zinc oxide paste (Unna boot) have been shown to improve ulcer healing rates. Silver-based dressings may also be more effective than other types of dressings for the healing of venous ulcers. Pentoxifylline[1] 400 mg three times daily, used along with compression, improves ulcer healing rates. Simvastatin (Zocor, generic)[1] 40 mg once daily, in addition to standard therapy, has also been shown to improve ulcer healing rates.

Stasis dermatitis may be treated with skin emollients and short courses of topical steroids. Topical antibiotics are not indicated for stasis dermatitis unless there is evidence of infection.

---

[2] Not available in the United States.
[7] Available as dietary supplement.
[1] Not FDA approved for this indication.

References

Flores TM: Lower extremity pain and swelling. In Paulman PM, Paulman AA, Harrison JD, Nasir LS, Bryan SK, editors: *Signs and Symptoms in Family Medicine*, Philadelphia, 2012, Elsevier, pp 387–388.

Gasparis AP, Kim PS, Dean SM, Khilnani NM, Labropoulos N: Diagnostic approach to lower limb edema, *Phlebology* 35(9):650–655, 2020 Oct. Available at: https://www.ncbi.nlm.nih.gov/pmc/articles/PMC7536506/. Accessed January 3rd, 2022.

Gloviczki P, Lawrence PF, Wasan SM, et al.: The 2023 Society for Vascular Surgery, American Venous Forum, and American Vein and Lymphatic Society clinical practice guidelines for the management of varicose veins of the lower extremities. Part II: Endorsed by the Society of Interventional Radiology and the Society for Vascular Medicine, *J Vasc Surg Venous Lymphat Disord* 12(1):101670,2024. Erratum in: *J Vasc Surg Venous Lymphat Disord*, 12(5):101923, 2024.

Martinez-Zapata MJ, Vernooij RWM, Simancas-Racines D, et al.: Phlebotonics for venous insufficiency. *Cochrane Database of Systematic Reviews*. Issue 11. Art. No.: CD003229. Available at: https://www.cochranelibrary.com/cdsr/doi/10.1002/14651858.CD003229.pub4/full, 2020. Accessed January 4th, 2022.

Norman G, Westby MJ, Rithalia AD, Stubbs N, Soares MO, Dumville JC: Dressings and topical agents for treating venous leg ulcers, *Cochrane Database of Systematic Reviews*, 2018. Issue 6. Art. No.: CD012583. Available at: https://www.cochranelibrary.com/cdsr/doi/10.1002/14651858.CD012583.pub2/full. Accessed January 4th, 2022.

O'Donnell Jr TF, Passman MA, Marston WA, et al.: Society for Vascular Surgery; American Venous Forum: Management of venous leg ulcers: clinical practice guidelines of the Society for Vascular Surgery and the American Venous Forum, *J Vasc Surg* 60(2 Suppl):3S–59S, 2014 Aug. Available at: www.jvascsurg.org/article/S0741-5214(14)00851-9/fulltext.

Pittler MH, Ernst E: Horse chestnut seed extract for chronic venous insufficiency, *Cochrane Database Syst Rev*(11)11, 2012 Nov 14. Available at: https://www.cochranelibrary.com/cdsr/doi/10.1002/14651858.CD003230.pub4/full.

Trayes KP, Studdiford JS, Pickle S, Tully AS: Edema: diagnosis and management, *Am Fam Physician* 88(2):102–110, 2013 Jul 15. Available at: https://www.aafp.org/afp/2013/0715/p102.html. Accessed January 15th, 2022.

Wittens C, Davies AH, Baekgaard N, et al: Management of chronic venous disease, *Eur J Vasc Endovasc Surg* 49:678e–737, 2015. Available at: www.ejves.com/article/S1078-5884(15)00097-0/fulltext. Accessed January 10th, 2022.

Youn YJ, Lee J: Chronic venous insufficiency and varicose veins of the lower extremities, *Korean J Intern Med* 34(2):269–283, 2019 Mar. Available at: https://www.kjim.org/journal/view.php?doi=10.3904/kjim.2018.230. Accessed January 4th, 2022.

PAIN

Method of
Steven A. House, MD

CURRENT DIAGNOSIS

- Always use history and physical examination and consider imaging or laboratory studies to rule out life- or function-threatening pathologies before merely providing symptomatic treatment.

Acute Pain
- Acute pain has a sudden onset, is usually nociceptive (somatic, visceral) in nature, and likely is due to apparent injury or medical condition.
- It can be acute (<1 month) or subacute (1–3 months) and can demonstrate hypersympathetic signs of tachycardia, elevated blood pressure, dilated pupils, or diaphoresis.

Chronic Pain
- Chronic pain is usually gradual in onset, lasts more than 3 months, and rarely serves any purpose. It can manifest with hyperalgesia (hurts more than it should) or allodynia (hurts when it should not, e.g., light touch).
- Vegetative symptoms such as depression, fatigue, or anorexia may be present.
- A significant neuropathic component may be present.
- Psychiatric and social or socioeconomic issues may be exacerbating factors.
- Examples can include headaches, low back pain, osteoarthritis, and fibromyalgia.
- While opioids might be appropriate for some conditions or situations, in general, they are proving to be neither as safe nor as effective for chronic, non-cancer pain as had been believed.

Quality
- Quality of the pain (e.g., sharp, dull, radiating, deep, superficial, lancinating, tingling, burning) is an important factor in determining the best management modalities.
- Quality plays a role in ruling in or ruling out severe disease that can require urgent surgical or other interventions rather than analgesics or adjunctive medications or therapies.

Severity
- Severity of the pain can be rated on a variety of scales such as numerical (0 to 5, 0 to 10), analogue (marked on a line with a range from no pain to the worst possible pain), or facial expression (smiles to grimaces, available for children and the elderly or patients with dementia).
- Functional scales (fully satisfactory function to debilitated) may be more helpful in determining the impact of the pain on the person's life.

CURRENT THERAPY

- Acute pain commonly responds to simple analgesics of the nonopioid, opioid, or combination varieties. Rest, ice, compression, and elevation (RICE) are helpful for acute inflammatory conditions and injuries.
- Chronic pain, because of its complexity, often requires multiple modalities. Pharmacologic options include nonopioid, opioid, adjuvant, or botanical medications. Nonpharmacologic options include physical therapy, chiropractic care, transcutaneous electrical nerve stimulation (TENS) unit, acupuncture, or surgical or anesthesia interventions.
- Adjuvant medications are drugs that are used for pain but do not have pain treatment as their primary indication, and they are often the most effective agents in neuropathic and/or chronic pain.
- Opioids are sometimes safer for long-term use, but the individual's risk for falls must be considered in the elderly, as opioids can increase this risk, and the risks of overdose and other adverse effects rise with increasing age and duration of exposure. For many chronic conditions such as low back pain, the evidence supporting the use of opioids is lacking, with efficacy often superseded by nonopioid medications. The risk of addiction MUST be considered before starting opioids on any patient. The Centers for Disease Control and Prevention (CDC) reported in 2011 that opioid pain relievers were involved in 73.8% of the 20,044 prescription drug overdose deaths. By 2021, drug overdose deaths increased to 106,699, with 80,411 (75.4%) involving opioids.
- Nonsteroidal antiinflammatory drugs (NSAIDs) carry a risk for GI and cardiac complications, especially in the elderly and those with a history of CAD or GI ulcers or gastritis.
- The patient *must* be involved in and cooperative with the treatment plan. Honesty and trust are necessary components of a therapeutic physician-patient relationship.
- Do not underestimate the placebo effect. If the patient feels that a harmless treatment is beneficial, take advantage of it.
- If the patient is not improving adequately, consult a surgeon if the source of pain is an operable condition, or consult a pain specialist if surgical intervention is not appropriate.

Epidemiology

Although estimates vary, approximately 50 million Americans experience chronic pain and incur costs and overall economic impact is estimated as high as $635 billion per year. Pain is the most common symptom that causes patients to pursue medical evaluation and management. The prevalence of several common pain syndromes including headaches, facial pain, abdominal pain, pelvic pain, and low back pain is slightly higher in women than in men because there are gender variations in the perception, coping, and reporting of pain. Pain tends to be undertreated in women, people of color, children, and the elderly, and it is underreported in nonverbal or cognitively impaired children and adults.

Risk Factors

Traumatic injury is a cause of acute pain and a risk factor for chronic pain. Patients who have mastectomy, laminectomy, thoracotomy, or amputations are at risk for pain syndromes. Chronic musculoskeletal conditions such as arthritis, spinal stenosis, degenerative disk disease, or fibromyalgia; infectious diseases including HIV or varicella zoster; neuropathies from diagnoses such as diabetes, B_{12} deficiency, or multiple sclerosis; treatment with certain chemotherapies or isoniazid (INH) without adequate vitamin B_6; psychiatric disorders such as depression,

anxiety, or posttraumatic stress disorder (PTSD), especially as a consequence of domestic violence; or autoimmune disorders including lupus and rheumatoid arthritis can predispose the individual to chronic pain. Although the risk of pain increases with age, pain should not be considered a usual part of aging until it is appropriately evaluated. A motor vehicle accident or work-related injury or other condition where secondary gain is a possibility, especially if there is no apparent injury, raises the consideration of malingering.

Pathophysiology

Injury or potential injury is detected by nociceptors in the peripheral nervous system, and the signal is then transmitted through the dorsal horn of the spinal cord up to the brain for processing. The three primary classes of opioid receptors are the mu, kappa, and delta receptors, which are located in areas throughout the central and peripheral nervous system. Upon binding these receptors, opioids block calcium channels and modulate the nociceptive pathways. The hyperstimulation of chronic pain (often via the N-methyl-D-aspartate [NMDA] receptor and the resultant increase in intracellular calcium are neurotoxic due to lowering the neuronal firing threshold and increasing firing frequency. This neurotoxicity can lead to ongoing pain in the absence of physical insult. Additionally, NMDA receptor activation can increase pre- and post-synaptic substance P while downregulating the mu receptors. This can decrease the efficacy of mu-agonists, as there are fewer receptors to bind. Neuropathic pain can result from chronic pain or from physical or pathophysiologic injury or changes to the nerve, as in diabetic neuropathy or other neuropathies.

Prevention

The best prevention is a safe and healthy lifestyle. The combination of healthy diet and exercise has been demonstrated to improve pain in osteoarthritis better than either intervention alone, and maintaining a healthy weight can help prevent the arthritis in the first place. Smoking and obesity (odds ratio increasing with BMI) have been associated with chronic pain. Relative to people of normal weight, rates of recurring pain were 20% higher in the overweight, 68% greater with class I obesity, 136% more in class II obesity, and 254% more in the morbidly obese.

Regarding safety, wearing seat belts while driving or using appropriate safety equipment at work and during recreational activities can help reduce the severity of injuries should they occur. Proper body mechanics are important as well.

Clinical Manifestations

Manifestations of pain depend on the location and underlying cause. In the acute setting, the patient can have tachycardia, elevated blood pressure, or diaphoresis, whereas chronic pain can manifest with vegetative symptoms of depression, fatigue, anorexia, or insomnia.

Diagnosis

Pain is most commonly a symptom rather than a disease in and of itself, so it behooves the provider to pursue treatable causes, especially red flag conditions, in addition to providing symptomatic treatment. The history regarding onset (shorter or longer than 3 months), exacerbating or remitting factors, quality, radiation, severity, and timing of the pain (constant versus intermittent), in addition to any associated signs or symptoms such as fever, nausea, vomiting, or diarrhea, can help the provider in that regard. The physical examination is a key component in ruling out life- or function-threatening disorders. Is there tenderness, swelling, bruising, erythema, or deformity? Are strength, reflexes, and sensation intact? Does the patient demonstrate a consistent demeanor (grimace or other signs of pain) and gait (antalgic versus normal) when moving from the waiting area to the examination room and out to the parking lot? The choice to use laboratory studies or imaging is determined by the location of the pain and the structures or organs that might be in that area. When determining severity, "What does the pain keep you from doing?" (which uses function as the measure of impairment and treatment efficacy rather than a subjective pain score to guide therapy) may be a much more helpful question than "How bad is your pain?" If function is not improving, that could be considered a treatment failure, and medications and therapy should be adjusted rather than continuing the same regimen.

Differential Diagnosis

The differential diagnosis for all types of pain is far too extensive for the brevity of this chapter, but in addition to the plethora of physical diagnoses to be considered, the provider must consider that chronic fatigue, depression, and domestic abuse can manifest as a chronic pain syndrome.

Treatment
Nonpharmacologic

Physical therapy for chronic pain (for recent-onset low back pain, relief was statistically but not clinically significant as compared to usual care), TENS units, chiropractic care, and regular exercise have shown benefit in certain conditions. Cognitive behavioral therapy (CBT) and mindfulness training improve function more than pain, and CBT, acupuncture, and mind-body therapies (e.g., yoga, tai chi, mindfulness-based stress reduction) provide safer options that may be both beneficial and cost-effective. Surgery may be required, and interventions such as nerve blocks or epidural injections may also be of benefit. Kyphoplasty and vertebroplasty have fallen out of favor. Aerobic exercise and water therapy are helpful for fibromyalgia, but the patient must not overexert because this can exacerbate the pain.

Pharmacologic
Nonopioid Analgesics

Acetaminophen (Tylenol) is generally a safe and effective medication provided the total daily dose for adults remains less than 3 g/day. For osteoarthritis of the hips and knees, acetaminophen provides modest short-term benefit, but it is not generally effective for the management of low back pain. However, due to its relative safety as compared to other medications, it is certainly worth a try. Chronic use can increase the likelihood of transaminase elevations 4-fold, so this is a consideration when patients are using other potentially hepatotoxic medications. There is an IV preparation available (Ofirmev), but the only benefit of the IV over the oral preparations is shorter onset of action. Both the absorption and the action of acetaminophen are augmented by caffeine, so caffeine is utilized in multiple over the counter (OTC) and prescription medications (e.g., Excedrin or Fioricet).

Numerous NSAIDs are available (see Chapter 13, Table 1) but none has been shown to be superior to another except for the convenience of dosing daily versus every 6 hours. All are generally safe in the acute setting but should be used with caution if needed long term, and they should be avoided altogether for long-term use in the elderly or patients with cardiovascular, renal, or peptic ulcer disease. This caution includes the cyclooxygenase (COX)-2-specific drugs. Naproxen and diclofenac seem to have the best cardiac profile while the COX-2 drugs tend to have the best GI profile. Misoprostol (Cytotec) or proton pump inhibitors can be used for GI prophylaxis.

Topical agents such as diclofenac (Flector 1.3% Patch, Voltaren 1% Gel), menthol, camphor, lidocaine, and capsaicin (Zostrix Cream, Qutenza 8% Patch) are effective in some patients. A new nonopioid analgesic on the market in 2025 is suzetrigine (Journavx), a selective voltage-gated sodium channel (NaV1.8) inhibitor that blocks the transmission of pain signals via peripheral nociceptive nerves. It is in a new class of medications and only indicated for the treatment of moderate to severe acute pain in adults.

Opioids (Table.1)

For patients with inadequate response to the nonopioid analgesics, opioids are an option (see Table 1). However, the proven efficacy for cancer pain and palliative care as well as some acute pain conditions cannot be extrapolated to chronic pain syndromes. The benefits of opioids in some conditions (e.g., chronic low back pain), and the overall safety of opioids have been called into question due to the dramatic increase in opioid abuse and opioid overdose deaths. Recent research has demonstrated a 2- to 3-fold increase in all-cause mortality with chronic opioid use and up to 11-fold increase if using more than 200 mg/day morphine equivalent dose (MED) and/or sustained-release or long-acting (methadone) preparations. More recently, a 2023 Cochrane review stated that treating chronic nonmalignant pain with >200 mg MED in clinical practice cannot be supported by any evidence-based arguments. Additionally, risk of overdose death is increased to 3.7- to 4.6-fold at doses of 50 to 100 mg/day MED and as high as 9-fold increased risk for MED >100 mg/day as compared to MED of less than 20 mg/day. These risks are further escalated by co-administration of benzodiazepines or gabapentinoids. A prescription for naltrexone should be considered if the patient is using >50 mg MED per day, and it is highly recommended if using >100 mg MED per day. A useful calculator to calculate MED can be found at https://www.mdcalc.com/calc/10170/morphine-milligram-equivalents-mme-calculator.

According to the CDC, 106,699 drug overdose deaths occurred in the United States in 2021 (up from 91,799 in 2020), with 75.4% (up from 74.8% in 2020) of these deaths attributed to opioids and 88% of those due to synthetic opioids (except methadone). Opioids might be a safer option in the elderly as compared to NSAIDs, but they can increase the risks of falls and cognitive impairment. They should be avoided in patients with untreated sleep apnea because of increased risk for complications, especially in combination with benzodiazepines. This risk increases with age with as much as an eightfold increase for those older than 80 years of age. The risk of postoperative respiratory depression also increases with age. The risks of using chronic opioids likely outweigh the benefits in the management of headache, fibromyalgia, and chronic low back pain, according to a 2014 position paper from the American Academy of Neurology.

The risks and the adverse outcomes (abuse, addiction, overdose, and death) related to this class of medications culminated in the release of guidelines with twelve recommendations from the CDC in March 2016 for the prescribing of opioids for chronic pain. Since approval, some of these guidelines have been treated as "absolutes" by various states' legislatures and third-party payers. Multiple unintended consequences of the resultant rapid-tapering of patients' dosages of opioids have come to light, including worsened mental health and increased risk of overdose and suicide. Additionally, some patients have suffered needlessly. As a result, the CDC revised the guidelines in 2022, and they do not apply to pain related to sickle cell disease, cancer, or palliative/end-of-life care. The guideline includes twelve recommendations, grouped into four areas:

1. Determining the need for opioids.
   a. Nonopioid therapies are as effective as opioids for many common types of acute pain, so clinicians should maximize nonpharmacologic and nonopioid therapies and use opioids only after discussing realistic benefits and known risks of opioid therapy.
   b. Nonopioid therapies are preferred for subacute and chronic pain. Opioids should only be used if benefits outweigh the risks and nonpharmacologic and nonopioid therapies have been insufficient.
2. Selecting the best opioid at the correct dose.
   c. Start with immediate release [IR] opioids rather than extended release or long-acting [ER/LA] opioids.
   d. Use the lowest effective dose of IR opioids, especially for the opioid naive.
   e. For patients already using opioids, maximize nonopioid therapies and weigh the risks and benefits before increasing the dose.

TABLE 1 Opioid Analgesics, Equianalgesic Table

OPIOID	ADMINISTRATION		PROPERTIES
	PARENTERAL	**ORAL**	
Buprenorphine			
Butrans transdermal patch: 5, 7.5, 10, 15, 20 µg/h weekly patches Subutex* SL tab and film: 2, 8 mg Belbuca buccal strip: 75, 150, 300, 450, 600, 750, 900 µg per strip, dosed every 12 to 24 hours (see detailed prescribing instructions) Buprenex injection: 0.3 mg/mL	0.3 mg (IV) Patch: MED <30 mg/day= 5 µg/h patch 30–80 mg/day = 10 µg/h patch; >80 mg/day: do not use	Oral buprenorphine, with or without naloxone (Suboxone, Subutex) and long-acting injection (Sublocade) are limited to treatment of opiate addiction Requires training, but the DEA "X-waiver" is no longer required.	Partial agonist Can cause QT prolongation C-III FDA warning regarding dental problems with the SL tabs, films, patches. Possibly less respiratory depression than full agonists.
Codeine			
Tablet: 15, 30, 60 mg Oral solution: 15 mg/5 mL	130 mg	180 mg	Prodrug converted by liver to morphine About 10% of population cannot convert, and some are rapid metabolizers, resulting in increased levels of morphine Ceiling dose is 60 mg/dose
Fentanyl			
Duragesic 72 h patch: 12, 25, 37.5, 50, 62.5, 75, 87.5, 100 µg/h	~100 µg/h	—	Patch for those who cannot swallow Patient *must* have subcutaneous fat, because drug is lipophilic
Actiq or Oralet lozenge: 200, 400, 600, 800, 1200, 1600 µg Fentora buccal tab or Abstral SL tab: 100, 200, 300, 400, 600, 800 µg Subsys sublingual spray: 100, 200, 400, 600, 800 µg/spray. Lazanda nasal: 100, 300, 400 mcg/spray. Fentanyl injection: 50 mcg/mL.	No conversion for lozenges or buccal tabs; various formulations are not bioequivalent, so use caution when switching from one formulation to another; *must* start at lowest dose and titrate	~½ × daily morphine dose, disregarding units, e.g., 200 mg morphine PO/day = 100 µg/h patch	Lozenge or buccal tab for transmucosal use No cheap forms available Buccal formulations *only* indicated for breakthrough cancer pain in the opioid tolerant; can be rapidly fatal in opioid naïve patients.
Hydrocodone			
Tab: 2.5, 5, 7.5, 10 mg with a max of 325 mg APAP per tablet (Norco) or with 200 mg ibuprofen (Vicoprofen 7.5/200; Ibudone 5/200, 10/200; Reprexain 2.5/200, 5/200, 10/200); Zohydro ER: 10, 15, 20, 30, 40, 50 mg/cap q 12 h; Hysingla ER: 20, 30, 40, 60, 80, 100, 120 mg tabs q 24 h; Solution: with APAP 7.5/325, 10/325 per 15 mL.	N/A	20 mg	C-II as of 2014, so refills and phone orders are no longer allowed. Metabolized to hydromorphone and others
Hydromorphone (Dilaudid)			
Tab: 2, 4, 8 mg Liquid: 1 mg/mL Suppository: 3 mg SR† 24-h tab (Exalgo): 8, 12, 16, 32 mg Injection: 1, 2, 4, 10 mg/mL pre-filled syringes and 1, 2, 4 mg/mL vials.	1.5 mg	7.5 mg	Good alternative to morphine, especially if using SC by continuous infusion (>20 mg/h) Active glucuronide metabolites
Methadone (Dolophine)			
Tab: 5, 10, 40 mg Oral liquid: 1, 2, 10 mg/mL* 40 mg dispersible tab (Methadose)—restricted use in United States, mostly for detox or addiction maintenance dosing		Variable conversion ratios (see Table 2): converted by oral morphine equivalent dose	At least 3 mechanisms: mu agonist, NMDA receptor antagonist, norepinephrine–serotonin reuptake inhibition The longest-acting opioid Cheap: ~ 1¢ /mg Can cause QT prolongation Torsades de pointes is more likely with IV dosing STRONGLY consider risks before prescribing. Safety guidelines available from the American Pain Society.

Continued

TABLE 1 Opioid Analgesics, Equianalgesic Table—cont'd

OPIOID	ADMINISTRATION		PROPERTIES
	PARENTERAL	ORAL	
Morphine			
Tab: 15, 30 mg Liquid: 10, 20, or 100 mg/5 mL (Roxanol) SR[†] 12-h tab (MS Contin): 15, 30, 60, 100, 200 mg SR[†] 24-h cap (Kadian): 10, 20, 30, 50, 60, 80, 100, 200 mg Suppository: 5, 10, 20, 30 mg Epidural or Intrathecal routes only (Mitigo): 200 mg/20 mL (10 mg/mL) or 500 mg/20 mL (25 mg/mL)	10 mg	30 mg	Numerous routes; very cheap, readily available; active metabolites, morphine-6-glucuronide 10 × more potent than morphine Avinza and Kadian capsules may be opened and beads sprinkled in applesauce, but the beads should not be crushed Avinza may be opened into apple juice and injected via gastric tube Kadian may be opened into water and given by gastric tube
Oxycodone			
Tab: 5, 10, 15, 20, 30 mg Liquid: 5 mg/5 mL or 20 mg/mL (OxyFast) ER 12-h cap w/ abuse-deterrant (Xtampza ER): 9, 13.5, 18, 27, 36 mg SR[†] 12-h tab (generic, OxyContin): 10, 15, 20, 30, 40, 60, 80 mg Multiple combinations w/APAP (Percocet, Endocet, Tylox)	N/A	20 mg	Equal potency but a little more bioavailable than morphine Caution in liver disease: T½ extends up to 4 × normal. Metabolized to oxymorphone: 40 × more potent than oxycodone ER/LA. Opioids require REMS. Xtampza ER cannot be interchanged mg for mg with other ER oxycodone products.
Oxymorphone			
Tab: 5, 10 mg (Opana); in opioid-naïve patients, starting dose > 20 mg/day is not recommended ER 12-h Tab: 5, 7.5, 10, 15, 20, 30, 40 mg (Opana ER)	1 mg	10 mg	Potentiated by cimetidine (Tagamet), MAOIs, and other CNS depressants 10% bioavailability Caution with CrCl < 50 or with liver impairment Take 1 h before or 2 h after food (food increases absorption)

*Only approved in the United States for the treatment of opioid dependence.
[†]Sustained-release formulations should never be crushed.
APAP, Acetaminophen (*N*-acetyl-*p*-aminophenol); *bid*, two times per day; *CNS*, central nervous system; *CrCl*, creatinine clearance; *IM*, intramuscular; *IV*, intravenous-*MAOI*, monoamine oxidase inhibitor; *MED*, morphine equivalent dose; *NMDA*, N-methyl-D-aspartate; *po*, by mouth; *pr*, per rectum; *prn*, as needed; *q4h*, every four hours; *q6h*, every 6 hours; *q8h*, every 8 hours; *qAC*, before meals; *qd*, daily; *qHS*, at bedtime; *SC*, subcutaneous; *tid*, three times per day.

Pain

37

3. Determining the duration of the initial opioid prescription and scheduling appropriate follow-up.
   f. Clinicians should prescribe only enough opioid for acute pain to last the expected duration of that pain.
   g. Clinicians should evaluate benefits and risks within 1-4 weeks of starting or increasing the dose of opioids for subacute or chronic pain.
4. Assessing and mitigating risks of opioid use.
   h. Clinicians should evaluate patients for opioid risks and related harms intermittently and mitigate risk by offering naloxone.
   i. Review the patient's history and opioid risk and use the state's prescription drug monitoring program [PDMP].
   j. Monitor the use of prescribed and nonprescribed controlled substances with urine toxicology.
   k. Avoid prescribing opioids in combination with benzodiazepines or other CNS depressants.
   l. Offer or arrange treatment for patients with opioid use disorder.

Additionally, there are five guiding principles to be applied across the twelve recommendations to aid in the individualization of the treatment plan for a given patient.
1. Pain should be appropriately assessed and treated whether or not opioids are used.
2. Recommendations are voluntary and are intended to support, not supplant, individualized, person-centered care.
3. A multimodal and multidisciplinary approach to pain management should be implemented in the context of the patient's overall health and expected outcomes. Refer to a pain management specialist when necessary.
4. Special attention should be given to avoid misapplying this clinical practice guideline beyond its intended use.
5. Attend to health inequities in ensuring access to an appropriate, affordable, and effective pain management regimen for all persons.

In addition to these steps, multiple drugs have been formulated with "abuse-deterrent" properties. Preparations that meet the FDA's Guidance for Industry regarding abuse-deterrent opioids include: OxyContin (oxycodone), Targiniq ER[2] (oxycodone/naloxone), Hysingla ER (hydrocodone), MorphaBond ER (morphine), Xtampza ER (oxycodone), and Arymo ER (morphine). Unfortunately, there are no generic opioids with FDA-approved abuse-deterrent labeling.

Tramadol (Ultram, ConZip) is a weak mu-agonist and an inhibitor of norepinephrine and serotonin uptake, a quality that gives it a niche in the treatment of neuropathic and radicular pain.[1] It is the only opioid studied for fibromyalgia in a randomized trial. While it was found to be beneficial, this is likely due to its inhibition of serotonin and norepinephrine uptake rather than its weak mu-agonism. A study has demonstrated an increased risk for hypoglycemia, notably in the first 30 days of treatment with tramadol.

[1]Not FDA approved for this indication.
[2]Not available in the United States.

Codeine is a prodrug that must be converted to morphine to be effective, and about 10% of the population lacks the cytochrome P450 2D6 enzyme that makes the conversion, resulting in poor analgesic response. Owing to the need for conversion, doses exceeding 60 mg do not increase benefit because the enzyme system is saturated. Avoid prescribing codeine to children, as deaths have been reported, even with the use of age- and weight-appropriate dosages, as a result of the hypermetabolism of codeine to morphine.

Morphine is the prototype for the opioids. It is extremely versatile, it can be given via almost any route, and it is available in multiple dosages and preparations ranging from liquid to daily sustained release. Hydromorphone (Dilaudid, Exalgo) shares similar qualities but is more potent. Hydrocodone is only available in a sustained-release oral form (Zohydro ER, Hysingla ER), and in combination with acetaminophen (Norco). It was rescheduled by the DEA to schedule II in 2014. It had been the number-one prescribed medication in the United States for several years until the rescheduling, which led to >20% reduction in prescriptions and >16% reduction in tablets dispensed.

Methadone (Dolophine) is the longest acting of the opioids at a half-life of 23 hours, although the duration of action can be variable. It is active as an NMDA receptor antagonist, inhibits norepinephrine and serotonin uptake, and is an agonist at the mu receptor. Therefore, methadone can be effective when other opioids fail, especially in the case of chronic or neuropathic pain, where the NMDA receptor is more of a factor in pain control. It must be used with caution (Table 2) because it can prolong the QT interval and has an increased dose-dependent risk of respiratory depression as compared to other opioids.

The mu agonists, other than codeine, meperidine, and tramadol, do not technically have a ceiling dose; however, the dose should be limited to the lowest effective dose (ideally <50 mg morphine equivalents per day), keeping in mind the possible adverse effects and increased risk of death with higher doses. In a 2020 study in the journal *Pain*, opioid dose escalation was not associated with improvements in chronic musculoskeletal pain. In the purely palliative or hospice patient, the dosage may be titrated to effect until the pain is relieved or side effects limit the dosage.

The mixed agonist-antagonists such as nalbuphine (Nubain), pentazocine (Talwin), and butorphanol (Stadol) tend to have a higher incidence of hallucination and confusion, and because they are agonists at kappa and delta receptors and antagonists at the mu receptor, they can produce withdrawal symptoms in patients who are routinely taking mu agonists. The partial agonist buprenorphine (Butrans patch, Subutex, Buprenex) is being used in some acute and chronic pain scenarios, and it is a little less likely to cause respiratory depression.

Patients who are taking opioids on a chronic basis should use a stimulant laxative such as senna with or without docusate, because fiber and dietary modification are usually inadequate for opioid-induced constipation, and fiber can aggravate the problem. Lubiprostone (Amitiza) can be used for opioid-induced constipation at the 24 mcg twice-daily dose. Naloxegol (Movantik), naldemedine (Symproic), and methylnaltrexone (Relistor) are peripheral rather than central mu antagonists, so they are indicated for managing opioid-induced constipation without negatively impacting pain control. Bisacodyl should not be used chronically due to its potential to damage the myenteric plexus of the gut and cause severe and permanent impairment of colonic motility; however, for PRN use, it can be quite effective with the suppository having quicker onset of action than the tablet.

Adjuvant Drugs

Adjuvant medications are drugs that are useful in the management of pain but do not have pain treatment as an indication. Some adjuvant medications such as duloxetine (Cymbalta) and pregabalin (Lyrica) have received an FDA indication for diabetic peripheral neuropathic pain. Tricyclic antidepressants are useful for chronic pain and they have the benefit, unlike duloxetine, of

TABLE 2	Morphine and Methadone Equivalents	
MORPHINE (DAILY REQUIREMENT)	**METHADONE EQUIVALENT**
<500 mg	5:1
500–1000 mg	10:1
>1000 mg	20:1

Acute pain: methadone = morphine (1:1). Chronic pain: The above conversion is for illustration of the complexity of methadone use. A more detailed table should be referenced before prescribing, and methadone should be used with extreme caution because of the risk for cardiac complications and respiratory depression. Many sources recommend starting at 10% of the calculated equianalgesic dose of methadone.

working at the lowest doses rather than having to titrate to the maximum dose to gain benefit.

Several anticonvulsants have demonstrated efficacy in the management of pain, most notably gabapentin (Neurontin)[1], pregabalin (Lyrica), and carbamazepine (Tegretol)[1]. Others have been tested in trials, but these three have the most evidence to support their use. Gabapentin and pregabalin have the benefit of not requiring monitoring of blood levels or for marrow, liver, or renal toxicities. Gabapentin (Neurontin)[1] has been beneficial using a single dose of 1200 mg preoperatively, notably in combination with celecoxib (Celebrex)[1], in reducing postoperative opioid requirements in mastectomy, laminectomy, and thoracotomy patients. The benefits of the gabapentinoids, a.k.a. α-2-δ-ligand calcium channel blockers, in peripheral neuropathies have been inappropriately extrapolated to pain related to radiculopathy. Significant benefits in lumbar and cervical radiculopathy have not been demonstrated in randomized trials.

Corticosteroids can be beneficial in inflammatory conditions, nerve or spinal cord compression, or increased intracranial pressure due to neoplasms. Any can help, but blood pressure elevations and fluid retention can be problematic in all but dexamethasone (Decadron)[1], which lacks mineralocorticoid activity. Steroids also have the downside of elevating blood glucose and, in long-term use, causing osteoporosis and a host of other problems, including Cushing syndrome.

Muscle relaxants may be beneficial if muscle spasm is a source of pain, but there is insufficient evidence to determine relative efficacy or safety. Of these, two stand out: metaxalone (Skelaxin), which lacks the black-box warning for the operation of heavy equipment, and tizanidine (Zanaflex), which can antagonize α_1 receptors in the spinal cord to provide additional pain relief. In chronic use, the patient will need to be monitored for anemia and leukopenia with metaxalone and for liver abnormalities with tizanidine. Cyclobenzaprine (Flexeril) plus naproxen was not superior to naproxen alone for low back pain.

Calcitonin (Miacalcin)[1] has shown very modest benefit for pain due to osteoporotic vertebral compression fractures, but it shows no benefit for compression fractures due to bone metastasis.

Ziconotide (Prialt) has demonstrated benefit as well as safety for long-term pain management, but it is limited to only intrathecal use owing to gastrointestinal side effects.

Caffeine can modulate pain via action upon adenosine receptors that are involved in nociception. It is found in several over-the-counter analgesics, notably for migraine treatment. Regarding alternative medications, riboflavin,[7] butterbur,[7] and coenzyme Q10 (CoQ10)[7] are effective for migraine prophylaxis. Glucosamine,[7] S-adenosylmethionine (SAM-e)[7], methylsulfonylmethane (MSM),[7] and willow bark[7] are likely effective for arthritic and low-back pain.

---

[1]Not FDA approved for this indication.
[7]Available as a dietary supplement

Controlled Substances Agreement Template

1. This agreement is provided to prevent misunderstandings about policies regarding medications designated by the DEA as "controlled substances" that you will be taking for pain management or other medical conditions.

2. I understand that my provider is consenting to treat me based on this Agreement.

3. I understand that if I break this Agreement, my provider might stop prescribing these medications, whether by tapering my medication, discontinuing the medication and prescribing another medication to treat the withdrawal symptoms, or discontinuing the medication and referring me to a detoxification program.

4. I will communicate fully and honestly with my provider about the character and intensity of my pain, the effect that my pain has on my daily life and how well the medication is helping to relieve my pain. I will take the medication ONLY as prescribed and for the treatment of my associated diagnosis as opposed to treating emotional or psychological distress (i.e., to get high).

5. My physician may prescribe other medications (adjuvant medications) or non-pharmacological therapies (physical therapy, TENS unit, etc.) to help with certain aspects of pain such as muscle spasm, burning, tingling or radiating pain. I will comply with this treatment with the same diligence as is expected for my controlled medication.

6. I will not use ANY illegal substances or any legal medication not prescribed to me. Additionally, I understand that alcohol, although legal, should not be used in conjunction with my medication as the combination could be fatal.

7. I will not share, sell or trade my medications with anyone.

8. I will use only one provider and one pharmacy for my medications unless otherwise agreed upon with my provider.

9. I am responsible for my own prescriptions and medications. I will safeguard my medications from loss or theft, understanding they will not be replaced. I will secure my medication in a lock box or safely out of the reach of children at all times.

10. I understand that refills of my prescriptions will be made at the time of an office visit or during regular office hours and never during evenings or weekends when the office is closed.

11. I expect my provider and my pharmacy to cooperate fully with any city, state, and/or federal law enforcement agency in the investigation of any possible misuse, sale or other diversion of my medications.

12. I agree to submit to random blood, urine, or saliva tests, if requested by my provider, in order to determine my compliance with my medication program.

13. I understand that the use of these medications may adversely affect my ability to drive, operate machinery, or perform certain tasks, and I agree not to attempt these tasks under the influence of medication. Additional risks include low testosterone, depression, sleep disturbances, constipation, respiratory depression, and death.

14. I will strive toward smoking cessation, a healthy diet, and exercise as my condition allows, as they can aid in controlling my pain.

15. I agree to these guidelines, and they have been fully explained to me. All of my questions and concerns regarding treatment have been adequately answered.

I agree to use _____ pharmacy, *and only this pharmacy*, for my prescriptions for controlled substances.

This Agreement entered on this date: _____

Patient / Parent / Guardian signature:_____

Provider signature:_____

Figure 1 Controlled substances agreement.

Acetyl-L-carnitine (ALC)[7] had demonstrated efficacy in diabetic neuropathy at 2 to 3 g/day. Capsaicin 0.075% cream (Zostrix) and 8% patch (Qutenza) have demonstrated benefit for peripheral neuropathy,[1] post-herpetic neuralgia, and HIV-associated neuropathy.[1]

Numerous medications in multiple drug classes have been studied for fibromyalgia, but many of the trials are small and/or of poor quality. Of these drugs, duloxetine (Cymbalta), pregabalin (Lyrica), and milnacipran (Savella) have received an FDA indication for fibromyalgia; gabapentin (Neurontin)[1], ondansetron (Zofran)[1], and naltrexone (Depade, Revia)[1] demonstrated modest benefit. The greatest benefit seems to be achieved by duloxetine and tricyclic antidepressants.

The use of cannabinoids has become legal in some states; however, their use for the management of pain is somewhat controversial, as the studies evaluating these drugs are often of low quality. Several systematic reviews and meta-analyses have failed to demonstrate significant reductions in pain, especially when cannabinoids are compared to standard care rather than placebo. A 2015 systematic review and meta-analysis showed mild reductions in pain, but the comparison groups were placebo rather than standard care. Additionally, cannabinoids are not without adverse effects, including impacts on cognition, motivation, reaction time, and psychosis in a 2016 review. Negative impacts could be even greater as unintended consequences of medical and/or recreational use come to light. The cannabinoids do show some promise due to the complexity of the endocannabinoid system, but they need to be studied further and subjected to the same scientific rigor as any other medication in the FDA approval process. A 2020 systematic review and meta-analysis did not demonstrate a benefit of adding cannabinoids to opioids for the management of pain related to advanced cancer. This was supported in a 2025 clinical guideline from the American College of Physicians that reports harms generally outweigh the benefits in the management of chronic, noncancer pain.

Monitoring

Controlled-substance agreements are beneficial in setting the boundaries for the use of opioid pain relievers (Figure 1). Routine visits are necessary to document ongoing need for and adequate response to the prescribed regimen. Routine drug screening is beneficial for monitoring compliance with the opioid as well as nonopioid medications. However, the provider needs to be aware of the metabolites of the different drugs. Hydromorphone (Dilaudid) and oxymorphone (Opana) are metabolites of hydrocodone (Norco) and oxycodone (Percocet, Endocet, OxyContin), respectively. Random pill counts can be incorporated into office workflow as well. As of October 2021, all states have prescription-monitoring programs that allow providers to monitor for the use of multiple providers and pharmacies to obtain controlled medications. Rules governing the prescribing and use of controlled substances vary among states, so the provider should be knowledgeable of local regulations as well as federal DEA requirements.

Complications

The Centers for Disease Control and Prevention (CDC) reported in 2011 that opioid pain relievers were involved in 73.8% of the 20,044 prescription drug overdose deaths. By 2022, drug overdose deaths peaked at 111,029 (84,181; 75.8% opioids) and in 2023 fell, for the first time since 2018, to 107,543 overdose deaths (81,083; 75.4% opioids). The corresponding death rates fell from 32.6/100,000 in 2022 to 31.3/100,000 in 2023. Medicaid populations are at greater risk of opioid overdose than non-Medicaid populations, and prescription drug overdose death rates are higher in the more rural and impoverished counties. A 2020 study demonstrated that more than 25% of opioid overdoses in the United States involve children and adolescents.

Nonmedical use of opioids in 2008 represented up to $78.5 billion in healthcare costs, lost productivity, addiction management, and legal and law enforcement involvement in 2008. By 2017, this cost had increased to $471 billion for opioid use disorder and $550 billion for fatal opioid overdoses for a total of $1.021 trillion. Even more astoundingly, this total only included 39 of the 51 U.S. jurisdictions. Drug addiction is very real, and about 15% of patients may be genetically predisposed to addiction; therefore, clinicians should strongly consider this in their risk/benefit analysis before exposing a patient to these powerful medications. About 25% of opioid-managed chronic pain patients misuse the medications, and about 10% develop opioid use disorders. Using a tool such as the Opioid Risk Tool may be helpful in determining the risk of addiction in a particular individual.

Long-term safety of opioids has not been demonstrated, and chronic use has been associated with sleep disorders, adrenal suppression, and hypogonadism (and secondary erectile dysfunction and depression) among other problems. Conversely, the rapid tapering of opioids can cause needless suffering, both mentally and physically. Like any potentially harmful medication, the risks and benefits of that drug for a particular individual must be considered, using guidelines and the best available evidence to help achieve our goals.

References

Baratloo A, Rouhipour A, Forouzanfar MM, et al: The role of caffeine in pain management: a brief literature review, *Anesth Pain Med* 6(3):e33193, 2016, Published online March 26, 2016.

Boland EG, Bennett MI, Allgar V, Boland JW: Cannabinoids for adult cancer-related pain: systematic review and meta-analysis, *BMJ Support Palliat Care* 10:14–24, 2020.

Center for Behavioral Health Statistics and Quality (CBHSQ): *2017 National Survey on Drug Use and Health: Detailed Tables*, Rockville, MD, 2018, Substance Abuse and Mental Health Services Administration. 05.24.2019 https://www.samhsa.gov/data/nsduh/reports-detailed-tables-2017-NSDUH.

Chou R, Peterson K, Helfand M: Comparative efficacy and safety of skeletal muscle relaxants for spasticity and musculoskeletal conditions, *J Pain Sympt Manage* 28:140–175, 2004.

Dowell D, Ragan KR, Jones CM, Baldwin GT, Chou R: CDC Clinical Practice Guideline for Prescribing Opioids for Pain – United States, 2022, *MMWR Recomm Rep* 71(RR-3):1–95, 2022, https://doi.org/10.15585/mmwr.rr7103a1

Franklin GM: Opioids for chronic noncancer pain: a position paper of the American Academy of Neurology, *Neurology* 83:1277–1284, 2014.

Fritz JM, Magel JS, McFadden M, et al: Early physical therapy vs usual care in patients with recent-onset low back pain: a randomized clinical trial, *JAMA* 314(14):1459–1467, 2015.

Garnett MF, Miniño AM: Drug overdose deaths in the United States, 2003–2023. NCHS Data Brief, no 522. Hyattsville, MD: National Center for Health Statistics. 2024. https://dx.doi.org/10.15620/cdc/170565.

Jones CM, Lurie PG, Throckmorton DC: Effect of US Drug Enforcement Administration's rescheduling of hydrocodone combination analgesic products on opioid analgesic prescribing, *JAMA Intern Med* 176(3):399–402, 2016, https://doi.org/10.1001/jamainternmed.2015.7799.

Kansagara D, Hill KP, Yost J, et al.: Cannabis or cannabinoids for the management of chronic noncancer pain: best practice advice from the American College of Physicians, *Ann Int Med* 178(5):714–724, 2025.

Morasco BJ, Smith N, Dobscha SK, et al: Outcomes of prescription opioid dose escalation for chronic pain: results from a prospective cohort study, *Pain* 161:1332–1340, 2020.

Okifuji A, Hare BD: The association between chronic pain and obesity, *Journal of Pain Research* 8:399–408, 2015. https://doi.org/10.2147/JPR.S55598.

Oliva EM, Bowe T, Manhapra A, Kertesz S, et al: Associations between stopping prescriptions for opioids, length of opioid treatment, and overdose or suicide deaths in US veterans: observational evaluation, *BMJ* 368:m283, 2020. doi: 10.1136/bmj.m283.

Rich RL: Prescribing opioids for chronic pain: unintended consequences of the 2016 CDC guideline. *Am Fam Physician* 101(8):458–459, 2020.

Volkow ND, Swanson JM, Evins AE, et al: Effects of cannabis use on human behavior, including cognition, motivation, and psychosis: a review, *JAMA Psychiatry* 73(3):292–297, 2016.

Vowles KE, McEntee ML, Julnes PS, Frohe T, Ney JP, van der Goes DN: Rates of opioid misuse, abuse, and addiction in chronic pain: a systematic review and data synthesis, *Pain* 156(4):569–576, 2015, https://doi.org/10.1097/01.j.pain.0000460357.01998.f1.

Whiting PF, Wolff RF, Deshpande S, et al: Cannabinoids for medical use: a systematic review and meta-analysis, *JAMA* 313(24):2456–2473, 2015.

PALLIATIVE AND END-OF-LIFE CARE

Method of
Steven A. House, MD

CURRENT DIAGNOSIS

- Any symptom can be in the realm of palliative care. Rapid identification and aggressive management of symptoms are important in maintaining the patient's quality of life.
- Palliative care is treatment that is focused on pain and symptom management, as well as quality of life for patients and their families. It can be rendered at any point in the course or treatment of illness, whether that illness is life limiting/threatening or not.
- Hospice is a philosophy and method of care that is completely focused on symptom management, quality of life for patients and families, and the transition at the end of life.

CURRENT THERAPY

- Recommend that all adult patients, regardless of current health status, execute advance directives (living will, power of attorney for healthcare, healthcare surrogate, etc.) to help ensure that their treatment wishes and end-of-life care goals are met.
- For patients with life-threatening (e.g., progressing cancer) or life-limiting (e.g., patients with severe chronic obstructive pulmonary disease [COPD] or heart failure, requiring dialysis, or residing in a nursing home) illness, consider a Physician Order for Life-Sustaining Treatment (POLST) or Medical Order for Scope of Treatment (MOST) form (the name varies by state). These forms are used to convert the salient points of advance directives into medical orders so that they are immediately actionable by nurses or emergency medical services if the situation arises.
- Advance care planning discussions are billable under Medicare: 99497 for the first 30 minutes and 99498 for each additional 30 minutes.
- The best palliative care involves an interdisciplinary approach by physicians, nurses, counselors, chaplains, and others for the optimal management of symptoms (whether the suffering is physical, emotional, spiritual, existential, practical, or a combination of these to comprise "total pain" that can lead to allostatic overload) and family support.
- Early addition of palliative care to the overall treatment plan can improve survival and quality of life.
- Cancer pain is an indication for opioid therapy because opioids have proven efficacy in this scenario. For detailed information on opioids, see **Table 1** in chapter titled "Pain". Multiple modalities may be required for optimal pain control.
- For patients using opioids chronically, initiate a stimulant laxative such as sennosides (Senokot, Ex-Lax) or lubiprostone (Amitiza) as the opioid's companion. Peripheral mu antagonists such as methylnaltrexone (Relistor), naldemedine (Symproic), or naloxegol (Movantik) are indicated for refractory opioid-induced constipation. Docusate was not demonstrated to be any better than placebo for stool softening.
- Control nausea because it can contribute to anorexia, weight loss, and functional decline. The antiserotonergic drugs (e.g., ondansetron [Zofran, Zuplenz], granisetron, granisetron transdermal [Sancuso], palonosetron [Aloxi], or the combinations netupitant/palonosetron [Akynzeo] or fosnetupitant/palonosetron [Akynzeo IV] are superior to the other classes of antiemetics in the settings of chemotherapy administration and postanesthe-

sia. For uncomplicated nausea, prochlorperazine (Compazine) was found to be superior to promethazine (Phenergan).
- Dyspnea can be improved by providing a fan, a cooler room, and a view to the outside and avoiding confined spaces. Opioids, benzodiazepines, and/or other agents, depending on the situation, might be required. Thoracentesis can be palliative when an effusion is the source of dyspnea.
- Delirium must be evaluated for potential causes. Delirium with or without agitation can occur in up to 80% of patients, depending on the underlying condition. Medications are common causes, but pain and multiple other conditions can cause it as well. Medications such as haloperidol (Haldol)[1], chlorpromazine,[1] or olanzapine (Zyprexa, Zyprexa Zydis)[1] can be helpful in many patients, but haloperidol is by far the cheapest alternative and a good place to start.
- Chlorpromazine is the only medication with the US Food and Drug Administration (FDA) indication for hiccups, but baclofen[1] has good evidence as well.
- Feeding tubes do not improve outcomes in late-stage dementia and can contribute to suffering.

[1]Not FDA approved for this indication

Epidemiology

There were 3,279,857 deaths in the United States in 2022, the most recent year for which mortality data are available, and cardiovascular disease is the top cause of death, followed by all cancers combined, unintentional injuries, COVID-19, stroke, chronic obstructive pulmonary disease (COPD), Alzheimer's Disease, diabetes, influenza and pneumonia, chronic kidney disease, and chronic liver disease and cirrhosis, among others. Any of these disease processes can have a significant symptom burden that worsens with disease progression.

Life has 100% mortality, so individuals should take the time to plan for it. The consequences of failing to plan for the transition to end-of-life care include increased psychological distress, medical treatments that are inconsistent with individual preferences, increased utilization of healthcare resources that have little therapeutic benefit while being very costly in dollars, as well as quality of life, and a more difficult bereavement for survivors.

Cardiopulmonary resuscitation has poor outcomes under the best of circumstances (~15%), but it is even worse in patients with late-stage cancer, with only approximately 2% surviving to hospital discharge. Outcomes are also poor for the other noncardiac diseases listed previously and decline further with age and comorbidities.

Risk Factors

Factors associated with worse pain or less symptom control are being female, elderly, or a child and race other than white. Historically, these groups have received less pain medication than white males for very similar diagnoses. These trends should be reversing. Lacking advance directives and failing to have such discussions with family members are related to receiving excessive and/or unbeneficial interventions/treatments.

Pathophysiology

A patient's symptoms can be caused by the underlying disease itself, mechanical encroachment on other organs and structures (e.g., bowel obstruction, neuropathic pain from nerve destruction, bone metastasis), becoming more sedentary or bedbound, medications, and/or tumor necrosis factor, neurokinin-1, and other inflammatory cytokines. Therefore symptoms may have different etiologies and pathophysiology depending on the underlying disease state. Such a review would be far too extensive for this section.

Prevention

Encourage all adult patients, regardless of current health status, to execute advance directives (living will, power of attorney for healthcare, healthcare surrogate, etc.) to help ensure that their

TABLE 1 Coanalgesic and Adjuvant Treatments for Pain: Adult Dosages

Nonsteroidal Antiinflammatory Drugs

Celecoxib (Celebrex) 200 mg PO daily or 100–200 mg PO bid; maximum: 400 mg/d
Diclofenac sodium (Voltaren, Voltaren XR) 50–75 mg PO bid; injection (Dyloject) 37.5 mg IV q6h prn; maximum: 150 mg/d; Diclofenac
    epolamine topical (Flector patch 1.3%); apply 1 patch to most painful area bid
Ibuprofen (Motrin, Advil) 400–800 mg PO tid; maximum: 3200 mg/d
Ketorolac Nasal (Sprix) 15.75 mg/spray
    <65 years old and <50 kg: 1 spray in one nostril q6h prn. Maximum: 4 sprays/d ×5 days
    <65 years old and ≥50 kg: 1 spray in each nostril q6h prn. Maximum: 8 sprays/d ×5 days
Ketorolac (oral and injection)
    10 mg PO q4h prn. Maximum: 40 mg/day ×5 days
    Single dose: 30–60 mg IM or 15–30 mg IV
    Multiple dose: if <65 years old and >50 kg, 30 mg IM/IV q6h prn. Maximum: 120 mg/d ×5 days
    Or if >65 years old or <50 kg, 15 mg IM/IV q6h prn up to 60 mg/d ×5 days
Naproxen (Naprosyn, EC-Naprosyn) 250–500 mg PO bid prn; maximum: 1500 mg/d
Naproxen sodium (Aleve, Anaprox) 220–550 PO q12h prn: maximum: 1650 mg/d

Voltage-Gated Sodium Channel (NaV1.8) Blockers

Suzetrigine (Journavx)* 50 mg tabs. Take two tabs (100 mg) on first dose then one tab q12h for the shortest treatment course required.
    Only indicated for acute pain; should be given at least 1 hour before or 2 hours after food; should not be crushed or chewed.

Bisphosphonates—Usually Provide Analgesia Within a Week and Last Up to 3 Months

Pamidronate (Aredia)
    Malignant hypercalcemia: 60–90 mg (depending on the severity of hypercalcemia) IV ×1
    Osteolytic lesions (multiple myeloma) or bone metastases: 90 mg IV monthly
Zoledronic acid (Zometa)
    Malignant hypercalcemia: 4 mg IV ×1
    Osteolytic lesions (multiple myeloma) or bone metastases: 4 mg IV q3–4 weeks

Radiopharmaceuticals—usually provide analgesia within 1–2 weeks and lasting 1–6 months. Dosing determined by radiation oncologist.

Antidepressants

Tricyclics (start low and titrate as needed; use with caution in the elderly)
Amitriptyline (Elavil)[1] 25–100 mg qhs. Can increase to 150 mg daily for pain.
Nortriptyline (Pamelor)[1] 25–100 mg qhs. Up to 150 mg/d.

Serotonin and Norepinephrine Reuptake Inhibitors

Duloxetine 60 mg/d; >60 mg rarely more effective for pain, but can titrate higher for comorbid anxiety and/or depression if needed
Venlafaxine (Effexor)[1] 37.5–225 mg daily. Start low and titrate.
    Selective norepinephrine reuptake inhibitors—can be used to improve coexisting anxiety and/or depression.

Antiepileptic Drugs

Gabapentin (Neurontin)[1] 300–1200 mg tid. Maximum: 3600 mg/d. Start 300 mg qhs ×2–3 days, then bid ×2–3 days, then tid. May start with
    100 mg qhs in the elderly.
Pregabalin (Lyrica) 50–300 mg bid. Maximum: 600 mg/d. Start low and titrate for effect, using the lowest effective dose.

General Anesthesia/Sedation

Ketamine (Ketalar)[1] 0.1–0.2 mg/min IV (no bolus). This dosage is an adjunct to opioid therapy for severe uncontrolled pain and NOT intended
    to achieve general anesthesia. However, the clinician should seek assistance from anesthesiology or palliative care specialists. Hospital policies
    may vary.

[1]Not FDA approved for this indication.
bid, Two times per day; *IM*, intramuscular; *IV*, intravenous; *q4h*, every four hours; *q6h*, every 6 hours; *q8h*, every 8 hours; *qAC*, before meals; *qd*, daily; *qHS*, at bedtime;
    po, by mouth; *pr*, per rectum; *prn*, as needed; *SC*, subcutaneous; *tid*, three times per day.

treatment wishes and end-of-life care goals are met. These discussions are billable under Medicare using CPT 99497 for the first 30 minutes face to face with patient, family members, and/or surrogate and 99498 for each additional 30 minutes. For patients with life-threatening (e.g., progressing cancer) or life-limiting (e.g., severe COPD or heart failure, dialysis-dependent, or nursing home residents) illness, consider a Physician Order for Life-Sustaining Treatment (POLST) or a Medical Order for Scope of Treatment (MOST) form (forms vary by state). They are used to convert the salient points of advance directives into medical orders so that they are immediately actionable by nurses, emergency medical services, and others if the situation arises.

Ascertain the patient's/family's goals of care, and assess whether those goals are realistic under the circumstances. Evaluate whether a particular intervention will help achieve that goal. For example, if a patient's goal is to take a child on a special vacation, this cannot be achieved if the patient remains in the hospital receiving chemotherapy that is not working. Another example is a nursing home resident with dementia whose family just wants them "to be kept comfortable" but is considering feeding tube placement. Placing a feeding tube in advanced dementia does not improve outcomes and might require physical restraints to keep the patient from removing the tube. Therefore feeding tube placement will negatively impact the goal of comfort.

When maintaining comfort and improving quality of life become the primary goals, assist patients and their families with the transition to hospice care. (The National Cancer Institute has an excellent free resource at https://www.cancer.gov/about-cancer/advanced-cancer/planning/end-of-life-hp-pdq.) Hospice is grossly underused, with median and average lengths of service of only 18 days and 97 days, respectively, in 2020 for Medicare beneficiaries (NHPCO data). Referrals are too often made excessively late, with 25% of patients having five or fewer days of service; therefore all of the benefits of hospice cannot always be fully realized in such a short time.

Palliative and end-of-life care, like all medical care, needs to be influenced by all four major aspects of medical ethics: autonomy (patient/surrogate has the right to pursue aggressive treatment, as well as to refuse treatment, even if that treatment could be considered life sustaining), beneficence (do "good" for the patient), nonmaleficence ("do no harm"), and justice (appropriate distribution of finite resources to do the most good for the most people). These four ethics can come into conflict at times, especially with the emphasis on autonomy above the other three in the healthcare system in the United States. Hospitals and other medical facilities should have specific policies regarding medical futility, and ethics committees can be helpful in difficult or unusual cases.

Clinical Manifestations

Common symptoms in palliative care include pain, nausea with or without vomiting, dyspnea, delirium, constipation, dysphagia (cannot swallow food, fluids, or medications), and general functional decline (i.e., requiring more assistance with transfers, toileting, and self-care). Anorexia and lack of thirst are very common, notably in the last few hours to days of life, but anorexia can also be a side effect of medications. Intervening with intravenous (IV) fluids or nasogastric feeding can exacerbate symptoms (secretions, dyspnea, pain, nausea) and worsen outcomes. Weight loss is commonly observed. Medications for diabetes and other disorders can often be discontinued at this stage to help avoid side effects, drug interactions, and adverse reactions (e.g., hypoglycemia).

As patients enter the last hours of life, they might experience decreased level of consciousness, agitated delirium, mottling of the extremities beginning distally and moving proximally, changes in breathing (Cheyne-Stokes, rapid and shallow, Kussmaul, or agonal), decreased or absent oral intake, and/or skin cool to touch.

Diagnosis

Diagnosis and prognosis will vary widely depending on the underlying disease processes, but in palliative care, much of the diagnosis (symptom identification) is based on history. Any patient with symptom burden is a candidate for palliative care, whether the symptoms are physical, psychological, spiritual, or existential. The Edmonton Symptom Assessment Scale (https://www.centralhealthline.ca/healthlibrary_docs/ESASrevised.pdf) rates each of 11 different symptoms on a scale of 0 to 3, for a total score of 0 to 33. This scale gives an idea of overall symptom burden. The Karnovsky and Palliative Performance Scales (http://www.nprc.org/files/news/karnofsky_performance_scale.pdf) range from 0% (deceased) to 100% (fully functional) rated on ambulation, activity and evidence of disease, self-care, oral intake, and level of consciousness. A score of approximately 40% is often associated with appropriateness for hospice. Hospice eligibility in the United States is solely based on a life expectancy of 6 months or less if the disease progresses on its expected course. The National Hospice and Palliative Care Organization (NHPCO; https://www.nhpco.org/) has devised some prognostic criteria for a variety of diagnoses including dementia, amyotrophic lateral sclerosis (ALS), acquired immune deficiency syndrome (AIDS), congestive heart failure, end-stage liver or kidney disease, COPD, and so on. Although not fully validated, the criteria can help to guide the clinician in discussions with patients/families. "Hospice" is commonly associated with cancer; however, according to the NHPCO, dementias accounted for 20.9% of Medicare hospice decedents in 2019, followed by respiratory diseases (7.1%), cardiovascular disease (6.4%), and cancer (4.9%). The median length of stay is still quite poor at 18 days, essentially unchanged over the past several years, while the average length of stay has increased by 6 days over the same time frame. There are various prognostic scoring systems for different disease states, and the Palliative Prognosis Score can help to determine the prognosis for patients with terminal cancer. In addition, the American Cancer Society (https://www.cancer.org/) has 5-year survival rates for various stages of numerous cancers on its website.

Differential Diagnosis

Because this chapter discusses management of symptoms for a plethora of different diseases, the differential diagnosis of all symptomatic disease processes is far beyond its scope. However, when assessing various symptoms, treatment options can be selected based on the probable source. Is the pain new or in a new location, or is it in the same area, radiating, or worsening? Are the nausea/vomiting due to chemotherapy, anesthesia, metabolic disorders, bowel obstruction, anxiety, increased intracranial pressure, or something else? Is the constipation opioid induced, due to poor intake, a result of using fiber without adequate fluid intake, or caused by another issue altogether? Is the dyspnea due to pleural effusion (may respond to thoracentesis far better than it would respond to medications), anxiety (could use selective serotonin reuptake inhibitors [SSRIs], hydroxyzine [Vistaril], benzodiazepine, cognitive behavioral therapy), airway obstruction (might use bronchoscopy, suction, or bronchodilators rather than other medications), excessive secretions (could treat with anticholinergic medications such as glycopyrrolate [Robinul][1] or scopolamine[1]), or other cause?

Therapy

To meet the needs of all forms of suffering (physical, emotional/psychological, spiritual, existential), an interdisciplinary approach using physicians, nurses, chaplains, counselors, social workers, and others is essential. For all patients entering palliative care, and especially hospice care, all of their medications should be evaluated for risk and benefit and then prioritized based on the goals of care. In one study, patients with a life expectancy of less than 1 year taking a statin for primary or secondary prevention were randomized to continue or stop the statin. The average number of days until death was 229 after discontinuation versus 190 for continuation; thus survival and quality of life improved at a lower cost. Consider discontinuing statins, some oral hypoglycemic agents (notably sulfonylureas due to risk of hypoglycemia), or oral anticoagulants such as warfarin (Coumadin), apixaban (Eliquis), or dabigatran (Pradaxa) if risks now outweigh benefits. As the end of life approaches, discontinue other medications that are not essential for symptom control or quality of life, have more risks than benefits, or contribute to symptom burden (e.g., cholinesterase inhibitors) at this advanced stage of the disease.

Clinicians might withhold or withdraw treatments, but they should never withdraw "care." Providers can change from "doing everything possible to cure a patient" to "doing everything possible to maintain comfort and quality of life." This is more than semantics. Consider turning off the defibrillator component of a pacer-defibrillator to avoid unnecessary shocks. The pacer can remain on because it can improve some symptoms while not prolonging life.

Pain

For a detailed review of medications used for pain, especially opioids, see chapter titled "Pain." This section will focus on cancer pain and end-of-life pain.

Pain of All Types

Opioids have demonstrated efficacy for cancer-related pain in numerous clinical trials. Methadone (Dolophine) can be effective when other opioids have failed, but it should be used with caution and by those familiar with its use due to variable pharmacokinetics and an increased risk of respiratory depression as compared to other opioids. Multiple recent systematic reviews and meta-analyses have not demonstrated a benefit of adding cannabinoids to opioids for the management of pain related to advanced cancer. Additionally, medical cannabis did not improve insomnia in adults with chronic pain. However, the endocannabinoid system is quite complex. Ideally, as cannabis becomes more available for research, some high-quality, randomized, controlled trials can be conducted to evaluate efficacy, appropriate dose ranges, the best THC:CBD ratios, and safety. Acupuncture and/or accupressure were associated with improved pain scores and reduction of opioid requirements in cancer patients.

---

[1] Not FDA approved for this indication

Bone Pain

The bone pain due to metastatic lesions is partly due to prostaglandin release; thus coanalgesics such as nonsteroidal antiinflammatory drugs or adjuvant medications such as corticosteroids, (e.g., dexamethasone[1] or prednisone[1]) can be particularly helpful. Bisphosphonates such as zoledronic acid (Zometa) and pamidronate (Aredia) usually provide analgesia within a week that lasts up to 3 months. Monthly dosing may be required. In addition, radiopharmaceuticals such as strontium-89 (Metastron), samarium-153 (Quadramet), and phosphorus-32 (Phosphocol P-32) may be helpful for cancer-related bone pain, with analgesia usually beginning within 1 to 2 weeks and lasting 2 to 6 months. Their benefit is derived from significant uptake by areas of high bone turnover to provide internal, localized radiation. Radium-223 (Xofigo; indication limited to castration-resistant prostate cancer with bone metastasis) emits alpha radiation rather than the beta radiation of the three aforementioned agents, and it is more selective for metastatic lesions. External-beam radiation treatment (EBRT) achieves pain relief in more than 75% of patients with analgesia beginning in 1 to 2 weeks and lasting 2 to 6 months. The appropriateness and dosing of radiopharmaceuticals and EBRT are determined by a radiation oncologist. The radiation oncologist might choose a single large fraction of EBRT rather than multiple small fractions if survival is expected to be greater than 3 months or if prolonged treatment will present too much hardship (transportation, increased suffering, time off work for caregivers, etc.) on the patient/family.

Neuropathic Pain

Neuropathic pain can have multiple causes, such as nerve invasion/compression, medication toxicities, human immunodeficiency virus (HIV), and complications of diabetes. Adjuvant medications that have proven efficacy, but not necessarily an indication for use by the US Food and Drug Administration (FDA), include antidepressants such as amitriptyline (Elavil)[1], duloxetine (Cymbalta), and venlafaxine (Effexor)[1], anticonvulsants such as pregabalin (Lyrica) and gabapentin (Neurontin)[1], or, for highly refractory cases (due to significant risk, side effects, and/or legality), ketamine (Ketalar)[1] or cannabinoids[1]. Topical agents such as capsaicin (Capzasin-HP, Salonpas Gel Patch Hot) have evidence to support their use in diabetic neuropathy. Highly active antiretroviral therapy can decrease viral load and improve symptoms of AIDS, including those of HIV-related neuropathy.

Visceral Pain

Octreotide (Sandostatin) can be used for the severe abdominal cramping and diarrhea associated with carcinoid tumors (can overproduce serotonin) or VIPomas (overproduce vasoactive intestinal peptide) or off-label for abdominal pain and other symptoms related to malignant bowel obstruction. An interventional radiologist or pain specialist could provide additional options, such as celiac plexus blocks or thoracoscopic splanchnicectomy, for refractory abdominal pain, notably in patients with pancreatic cancer.

Dyspnea

Dyspnea is a sensation of breathlessness, and the only measure is a patient's self-report. It does not correlate well with respiratory rate, blood gas measurements, or pulse oximetry. The potential causes are many, and they should be considered before merely managing the symptom. The cause can determine the therapy. Anxiety can be managed with SSRIs or benzodiazepines. Airway obstruction could be relieved by suction or bronchoscopy. Hypoxemia has numerous causes that would have to be considered, but supplemental oxygen could help. Pleural or pericardial effusions could be drained. Pneumonia can be treated with antibiotics, pulmonary edema can be managed with diuretics and opioids, and pulmonary embolus can respond to anticoagulants. Transfusions can be helpful for dyspnea due to significant anemia (hemoglobin <7 g/dL) resulting from hemorrhage or myelosuppression. Bronchospasm usually responds to inhaled β_2 agonists. If underlying causes are addressed,

---

| BOX 1 | Nonpharmacologic Interventions for Dyspnea |

- Reassure, work to manage anxiety.
- Behavioral approaches: relaxation, distraction, hypnosis.
- Limit the number of people in the room.
- Open window.
- Eliminate environmental irritants.
- Keep line of sight clear to outside.
- Reduce room temperature, but avoid chilling the patient.
- Introduce humidity.
- Reposition, elevate the head of the bed, keep patient turned.
- Educate and support the family.

either by management or recognizing that treatment would not achieve the goals of care, symptom control is appropriate. The use of pharmacologic interventions such as opioids, benzodiazepines, or other medications for breathlessness in advanced cancer is not supported by the evidence; however, for patients who have tried other options without relief, a trial of medications is appropriate. Nebulized morphine[1] is no better than saline. Excessive secretions can be managed with scopolamine[1] or glycopyrrolate.[1] The latter is preferred in the elderly because it does not cross the blood-brain barrier. For nonpharmacologic interventions, see Box 1.

Nausea/Vomiting

The treatment of nausea and vomiting depends on the underlying cause. For chemotherapy-related nausea/vomiting, the 5HT3 receptor antagonists are far more effective than other classes of antiemetics. The 5HT3 class includes ondansetron (Zofran), granisetron (Sancuso, Sustol), dolasetron (Anzemet), and palonosetron (Aloxi). In addition, there is a combination of netupitant/palonosetron (Akynzeo), which combines a 5HT3 antagonist for acute-phase nausea/vomiting and a substance P/neurokinin-1 receptor antagonist (NK1RA) for the delayed phase, and it should be given with dexamethasone (Decadron)[1]. Its only indication is for prophylaxis of chemotherapy-related nausea/vomiting, especially with highly emetogenic chemotherapy. The combination demonstrated superiority over palonosetron alone. Rolapitant (Varubi), another NK1RA, has a longer half-life than netupitant, with fewer drug interactions. Aprepitant (Emend) is an NK1RA with fosaprepitant (Emend injection) as its IV alternative. Olanzapine (Zyprexa)[1] was more effective than aprepitant and noninferior to fosaprepitant in the setting of highly emetogenic chemotherapy, whereas it is far more cost-effective than either NK1RA and serves as a better acute antiemetic than metoclopramide (Reglan). Prochlorperazine (Compazine) was found to be superior to promethazine (Phenergan) for uncomplicated nausea/vomiting (Table 2).

Constipation

Constipation is quite common in palliative care, and it is easier to prevent than to treat. It is one of the primary side effects of opioids that does not attenuate with time. For routine constipation, almost any laxative will do. Polyethylene glycol 3350 (MiraLax, GlycoLax) daily with as-needed sennosides (Senokot) or bisacodyl (Dulcolax) is one example of a simple regimen. If the patient is taking medications that have constipation as a side effect, such as anticholinergic medications or calcium channel blockers, they should be discontinued if possible. Opioid-induced constipation is due to the interaction of opioids with the mu receptors in the gut, thus leading to poor motility. It can be prevented for the most part if a stimulant laxative is initiated simultaneously with the opioid. Senna is safe for long-term use, but bisacodyl can damage the myenteric plexus over time. The chloride-channel activator lubiprostone (Amitiza) and the guanylate cyclase activator linaclotide (Linzess)[1] increase intestinal fluid secretion and motility, and the peripheral mu antagonists methylnaltrexone (Relistor), naldemidine (Symproic), and

---

TABLE 2 Antiemetics

Antipsychotics/Dopamine Antagonists

Chlorpromazine (Thorazine) 10–25 mg PO q4h prn. Can use 25–50 mg IM q3h prn, but change to PO as soon as possible. Also available as 25 mg or 100 mg (can be halved) suppositories that can be given every 6 hours as needed.
Haloperidol (Haldol) 0.5–5 mg PO/IV bid–tid prn (off-label for nausea/vomiting); maximum 100 mg/d, but use lowest effective dose. Good choice when also managing delirium.
Metoclopramide (Reglan) 5–10 mg PO/IV q6h prn (contraindicated in bowel obstructions)
Olanzapine (Zyprexa) 5–10 mg PO daily–bid prn (off-label for nausea/vomiting)
Prochlorperazine (Compazine) 5–10 mg PO/IM/IV q6h prn; maximum 10 mg/dose, 40 mg/d. Suppository, 25 mg PR q12h prn

Antihistamines

Hydroxyzine (Atarax, Vistaril) 25–100 mg PO q6h prn or IM q4h prn
Meclizine (Antivert, Bonine) 25–100 mg/d PO divided bid–tid prn (off-label)
Promethazine (Phenergan) 12.5–25 mg PO/PR/IM/IV q4h prn. Use with caution IV: can cause necrosis and gangrene.

Antiserotonin (5HT3 Antagonists)

Granisetron (Granisol, Sancuso [transdermal], Sustol [sustained release SC injection]) 2 mg PO ×1 or 1 mg PO q12h ×2 doses given within an hour before chemotherapy. If IV, 10 mcg/kg IV ×1 within 30 min before chemotherapy. Transdermal, apply 1 patch (3.1 mg/24 h) ×1 24 h before chemotherapy and leave on for up to 7 days. If SC, 10 mg SC q 7 days (give with dexamethasone [Decadron][1]).
Ondansetron (Zuplenz, Zofran, Zofran ODT) 8 mg PO q8h for nausea/vomiting; 24 mg PO ×1 30 min before highly emetogenic chemotherapy.
Palonosetron (Aloxi) 0.25 mg IV ×1 or 0.5 mg PO[2] ×1 30 min before chemotherapy.

Antineurokinin (NK1 RA)

Aprepitant oral (Emend) 125 mg PO ×1 day 1 of chemotherapy, then 80 mg PO daily × 2 days. Aprepitant IV (Cinvanti) 130 mg IV on day 1, 30 minutes before chemotherapy, or 100 mg IV on day 1, 30 minutes before chemotherapy, then oral aprepitant 80 mg on days 2 and 3.
Fosaprepitant (Emend injection, Focinvez) 150 mg IV ×1, 30 min before chemotherapy.
Netupitant/palonosetron (Akynzeo), fosnetupitant/palonosetron (Akynzeo IV) 300/0.5 mg, 1 capsule 1 h before highly emetogenic chemotherapy or 235 mg/0.25 mg IV x 1 dose, 30 min before chemotherapy (use w/corticosteroid).
Rolapitant (Varubi) 180 mg PO ×1, 1–2 h before chemotherapy.
All NK1RAs should be given with an HT3RA and dexamethasone[1] before highly emetogenic chemotherapy.

Cannabinoid Receptor Agonists

Dronabinol (Marinol, Syndros) 2.5–10 mg PO bid prn. Syndros is available as a 5 mg/mL solution.
Dronabinol is indicated for chemotherapy-related nausea/vomiting refractory to other drugs and AIDS-associated anorexia and weight loss. Significant psychiatric adverse events are possible.

Unknown Mechanism

Trimethobenzamide (Tigan) 300 mg PO or 200 mg IM q6h prn

[1]Not FDA approved for this indication.
[2]Not available in the United States.
bid, Two times per day; *IM*, intramuscular; *IV*, intravenous; *q4h*, every four hours; *q6h*, every 6 hours; *q8h*, every 8 hours; *qAC*, before meals; *qd*, daily; *qHS*, at bedtime; *po*, by mouth; *pr*, per rectum; *prn*, as needed; *SC*, subcutaneous; *tid*, three times per day.

naloxegol (Movantik) are indicated for use by the FDA to treat refractory opioid-induced constipation. Alvimopan (Entereg)[1] is another peripheral mu antagonist, but its primary indication is for ileus, especially postoperatively. Fiber and bulking agents should be avoided because they can worsen the problem (Table 3). Docusate has not been shown to be superior to placebo for softening stool.

Anxiety

There are numerous reasons for patients receiving palliative care to be anxious, whether undergoing painful/unpleasant but curative interventions, suffering uncontrolled pain or dyspnea, or progressing toward hospice. Fear and uncertainty about the future are common causes, and they can be related to physical, psychological, social, spiritual, or practical (finances, managing home responsibilities) issues. Excessive alcohol or caffeine use can exacerbate anxiety, which may present with agitation, insomnia, restlessness, sweating, tachycardia, hyperventilation, panic disorder, worry, tension, and/or psychosomatic symptoms. For patients with expectation of cure or longer survival, SSRI or serotonin and norepinephrine reuptake inhibitor (SNRI) antidepressants can be beneficial. Venlafaxine (Effexor ER) has the shortest half-life, and steady state can be reached in 4 to 7 days. Benzodiazepines are helpful for shorter life expectancy, or they can be used until the antidepressants take effect. Diazepam (Valium) has a

long duration of action due to numerous active metabolites, but it is slower in onset, as is clonazepam (Klonopin)[1]. Alprazolam (Xanax) has very rapid onset but short duration of action. Lorazepam (Ativan) strikes a happy medium between speed of onset and duration of action. Counseling and cognitive behavioral therapy are effective, especially in combination with medications.

Delirium

Delirium is a waxing/waning state of confusion that can be characterized by anxiety, disorientation, cognitive dysfunction, and hallucinations. There is also a catatonic variety of delirium. This condition can be caused by many things, but a short list would include constipation/impaction, hypoxemia, infection, electrolyte abnormalities, medications (including benzodiazepines and opioids), and pain. If a cause is identified and corrected but the patient is still symptomatic, haloperidol (Haldol)[1], chlorpromazine (Thorazine)[1], or olanzapine (Zyprexa)[1] can be helpful; however, haloperidol is by far the cheapest alternative and a good place to start. It can be given intravenously or orally, or it can be given subcutaneously (off-label).

Hiccups

Hiccups (singultus) is a common nuisance that can become quite distressing, especially if persistent (>48 hours) or intractable

[1]Not FDA approved for this indication

[1]Not FDA approved for this indication

TABLE 3 Laxatives

Osmotic

Lactulose (Kristalose) 10 g per 15 mL; 15–30 mL daily or BID, maximum 60 mL/day (40 g/day)
Magnesium citrate (1.745 g/30 mL) 195–300 mL/d PO daily or divided bid; maximum: 300 mL/d
Magnesium hydroxide (milk of magnesia), 400 mg/5 mL; 30–60 mL (2400–4800 mg) PO daily PRN. Maximum 60 mL/day, can be divided 2–4 doses per day.
Polyethylene glycol 3350 (MiraLax), 17 g in 8 oz. liquid PO daily

Stimulant

Bisacodyl (Dulcolax) 5 mg tabs 1–3 PO daily prn or 10 mg suppository PR daily prn
Sennosides (Senna) 8.6 mg tabs; 2–4 tabs PO bid; maximum: 4 tabs PO bid

Secretory

Linaclotide (Linzess)[1] 145 mcg PO daily. Stimulates cGMP production to increase intestinal fluid secretion and motility.
Lubiprostone (Amitiza) 24 mcg PO bid. Activates chloride channel to increase intestinal fluid secretion and motility.
Plecanatide (Trulance)[1] 3 mg PO daily. Stimulates cGMP production to increase intestinal fluid secretion and motility.

Peripheral Mu-Receptor Antagonists

Methylnaltrexone (Relistor) 8–12 mg SC qod prn (or 0.15 mg/kg SC qod prn). Maximum: 1 dose/24 h
Naldemedine (Symproic) 0.2 mg PO daily
Naloxegol (Movantik) 25 mg PO daily

[1]Not FDA approved for this indication.
*It is only indicated for acute pain and should be given at least 1 hour before or 2 hours after food. It should not be crushed or chewed.
bid, Two times per day; *IM*, intramuscular; *IV*, intravenous; *q4h*, every four hours; *q6h*, every 6 hours; *q8h*, every 8 hours; *qAC*, before meals; *qd*, daily; *qHS*, at bedtime; *po*, by mouth; *pr*, per rectum; *prn*, as needed; *SC*, subcutaneous; *tid*, three times per day.

(>1 month). For patients with pain in the chest or abdominal regions, hiccups can make pain difficult to control in addition to being a bothersome symptom that can significantly decrease quality of life. Chlorpromazine, at 25 to 50 mg PO up to four times per day prn, is the only FDA-approved medication for hiccups, but haloperidol[1] is a viable and much cheaper alternative, as is metoclopramide (Reglan)[1]. Gabapentin (Neurontin)[1] and phenytoin (Dilantin)[1] have been used with some success, notably in cases with a central nervous system etiology. Many other medications, including baclofen (Lioresal)[1], have been tried without much success (i.e., some improvement in symptoms but did not eliminate the hiccups). Nonpharmacologic methods (e.g., breath holding, hyperventilation, gargling) are worth trying, but evidence is lacking for any particular intervention.

Monitoring

Patients should be reevaluated routinely for the adequacy of pain and symptom control, as well as for their ability to cope with the underlying disease, symptom burden, and functional decline. The family needs to be assessed for additional stressors and coping mechanisms, as the family's adjustment, or lack thereof, can be detrimental to the patient's condition. If opioids or benzodiazepines are being used, the supply needs to be monitored for any signs of aberrant use by the patient and/or the family and visitors. In addition, patients can be monitored for excessive sedation or respiratory depression, especially when using methadone with or without a benzodiazepine. The FDA has issued a warning regarding coadmistration of benzodiazepines or gabapentinoids with opioids as a cause of worsened respiratory depression, so these patients in particular should be monitored.

Palliative Sedation

For symptoms refractory to all other measures and with a life expectancy of less than 2 weeks, palliative sedation can be considered, after informed consent, without hastening death according to two studies in palliative care and oncology journals.

Physician-Assisted Suicide

Although this practice has been legalized in several states, the American Medical Association's Council on Ethical and Judicial Affairs has determined that physician-assisted suicide (PAS), as opposed to "aid in dying," is the most accurate description of the practice and that the AMA's current policy forbidding PAS should be upheld. Similarly, in 2017 the American College of Physicians (ACP) also determined that PAS is contradictory to the physician's role in the physician–patient relationship. The Hospice & Palliative Nurses Association (HPNA) takes the position that PAS is not part of palliative care. The NHPCO issued a statement opposing all forms of "Legally Assisted Death" in November 2018 (and updated in June 2021), citing numerous reasons for their rationale. Notable among these is that PAS does not meet the World Health Organization (WHO) definition of palliative care (i.e., "intends to neither hasten nor postpone death"). Conversely, the American Academy of Family Physicians (AAFP) and the American Academy of Hospice and Palliative Medicine (AAHPM) have taken a neutral stance.

Complications

Emergencies do exist within the palliative care and hospice settings. Spinal cord compression, hypercalcemia, superior vena cava syndrome, seizures, airway obstruction, hemorrhage, or acute worsening or crisis in pain or other symptom are examples. Management will depend on the patient's goals of care and stage of illness; however, uncontrolled symptoms should always be addressed. Dark-colored linens and towels are good to have on hand for patients at risk for hemorrhage, because the blood does not appear as dramatic or traumatic for the patient and family as it would on white or light-colored materials.

References

NHPCO Facts and Figures, 2023 Edition. December 2023. Available at: https://www.nhpco.org/wp-content/uploads/NHPCO-Facts-Figures-2023.pdf.

Bao Y, Zhang H, Bruera E, et al.: Medical marijuana legalization and opioid- and pain-related outcomes among patients newly diagnosed with cancer receiving anticancer treatment, *JAMA Oncol* 2023;9(2):206–214, 2023.

Bath C. ASCO 2014: Stopping statins is safe and can improve quality of life for patients with cancer near the end of life. Available at: http://www.ascopost.com/News/16304. Posted 6/11/14.

Boland EG, Bennett MI, Allgar V, Boland JW: Cannabinoids for adult cancer-related pain: systematic review and meta-analysis, *BMJ Support Palliat Care* 10:14–24, 2020.

Camartin C, Björkhem-Bergman L: Palliative sedation—the last resort in case of difficult symptom control: a narrative review and experiences from palliative care in Switzerland," *Life* 2022; 12(2):298, 2022.

[1] Not FDA approved for this indication

Davis MP: New therapies for antiemetic prophylaxis for chemotherapy, *J Community Support Oncol* 14:11–20, 2016.

Davis MP: What can a systematic review of cannabis trials tell us? *J Pain Sympt Manage* 64(5):e285–e288, 2022.

Doppen M, Kung S, Maijers I, et al.: Cannabis in palliative care: a systematic review of current evidence, *J Pain Symptom Manage* 64:e260–e284, 2022.

Dowling R: Bill end-of-life discussion codes correctly, Med Econ March 10, 2016. Available at: http://medicaleconomics.modernmedicine.com/medical-economics/news/how-bill-end-life-discussion-codes-correctly.

Ebell MH: Determining prognosis for patients with terminal cancer, *Am Fam Physician* 72:668–669, 2005.

Farmer C. Fast facts and concepts #81. Management of hiccups, 4th ed,. Updated February 2023. Available at: https://www.mypcnow.org/blank-mkw97.

Feliciano JL, Waldfogel JM, Sharma R, Zhang A, et al: Pharmacologic interventions for breathlessness in patients with advanced cancer: a systematic review and meta-analysis, *JAMA Network Open* 4(2):e2037632, 2021.

He Y, Guo X, May BH, Zhang AL, et al: Clinical evidence for association of acupuncture and acupressure with improved cancer pain: a systematic review and meta-analysis, *JAMA Oncol* 6:271–278, 2019.

Kochanek KD, Murphy SL, Xu JQ, Arias E. Mortality in the United States, 2022. NCHS Data Brief, no 492. Hyattsville, MD: National Center for Health Statistics. 2024. DOI: https://dx.doi.org/10.15620/cdc:135850.

McRorie JW, Petrey ME, Sloan KJ, Gibb RD: Docusate is not different from placebo for stool softening: a comprehensive review, *Am J Gastroenterology* 116(1): s85, 2021.

NCCN clinical practice guidelines in oncology: *antiemesis, version 1*, National Comprehensive Care Network, 2015. AE2–6.

Planning the transition to end-of-life care in advanced cancer–health professional version (PDQ). Available at: https://www.cancer.gov/about-cancer/advanced-cancer/planning/end-of-life-hp-pdq.

Reisfield GM, Wilson GR: Fast facts and concepts #116. Radiopharmaceuticals for painful osseous metastases, Available at: https://www.mypcnow.org/blank-qfwwm. June 2015.

Rutter C, Johnstone C, Weissman DE. Fast facts and concepts #66. Radiation for palliation – part 1. Updated April 2016. Available at: https://www.mypcnow.org/blank-r9t7g.

Rutter C, Weissman DE: Fast facts and concepts #67. Radiation for palliation – part 2, ed 2. Available at: https://www.mypcnow.org/fast-fact/radiation-for-palliation-part-2/.

"NHPCO Statement on Medical Aid in Dying." June 16, 2021. Available at: https://www.nhpco.org/wp-content/uploads/Medical_Aid_Dying_Position_Statement_July-2021.pdf.

Weinstein E, Arnold R: Fast facts and concepts #113. Bisphosphonates for bone pain, Available at: https://www.mypcnow.org/blank-ux03d; June 2015.

Yang J, Wahner-Roedler DL, Zhou X, et al: Acupuncture for palliative cancer pain management: systematic review, *BMJ Supportive & Palliative Care*. Epub ahead of print: January 13, 2021.

PALPITATIONS

Method of
Rebecca Katzman, MD; Justin Bailey, MD; and Caroline Beyer, MD

CURRENT DIAGNOSIS

- History and physical examination
- Electrocardiogram
- Complete blood count (CBC)
- Thyroid-stimulating hormone (TSH)
- Complete metabolic panel

CURRENT THERAPY

- Dependent on underlying etiology. See Table 5.

Palpitations are the unpleasant sensation or awareness of one's own heartbeat. Patients may feel a racing heart, skipped heartbeats, or pounding in the chest or neck. Palpitations have been described as a "flip-flop" or "fluttering" in the chest. Palpitations may be due to cardiac arrhythmia, nonarrhythmic cardiac disease, drugs, other medical conditions, or psychiatric disease. Cardiac arrhythmias and anxiety account for a majority of cases. Palpitations may be completely benign or a manifestation of a potentially fatal arrhythmia.

Epidemiology

Palpitations (ICD-10-CM R00.2) are a common presenting complaint in a primary care office or the emergency department. They affect all genders and ages. Up to 16% of patients in general medical settings report palpitations, and up to 18% of cardiology outpatient visits are for cardiac arrhythmias. The most common etiologies of palpitations are cardiac arrhythmias (43%) and anxiety/psychiatric (31%). In outpatient clinics psychiatric etiologies are slightly more common; in emergency department settings cardiac causes are increasingly likely. The underlying cause of palpitations in 15% of patients cannot be identified.

Nearly 90% of patients who have palpitations have recurrent symptoms. Overall, 1-year mortality does not appear to be significantly increased, but patients report a moderate impact on their quality of life.

Although arrhythmias are frequently found to be the underlying cause of palpitations, it is important to note that many patients with arrhythmias do not have any symptoms.

Differential Diagnosis

The differential for palpitations is broad but can generally be broken down into cardiac versus noncardiac causes. Cardiac causes may be further divided into structural or arrhythmic causes. Noncardiac causes include medications and drugs, high-output states, and certain medical conditions. Gastroesophageal reflux or esophageal spasm may present as a brief intermittent episode of tightness or pounding in the chest. See Table 1 for a full listing of causes.

Psychiatric causes may account for up to one-third of presentations; palpitations can occur with panic attacks, generalized anxiety, depression, and somatization. However, it is important to note that psychiatric illness can coexist with cardiac or other medical causes.

Cardiac arrhythmias often present as palpitations. Nearly any arrhythmia or change from a sinus rhythm can produce this sensation. A less common condition in otherwise healthy patients is inappropriate sinus tachycardia (IST), demonstrated by an elevated resting heart rate, an exaggerated heart rate response to exercise, or both. IST is thought to be due to abnormal autonomic control and response. Long-QT syndrome, both congenital/familial and medication-induced, may predispose to ventricular tachyarrhythmias, including the often-fatal torsades de pointes.

Risk Factors

Structural cardiac disease, including valvular disease, may predispose patients to arrhythmias and palpitations. Box 1 lists symptoms and risk factors that indicate an increased likelihood that palpitations are due to an underlying arrhythmia.

Pathophysiology

An arrhythmia is caused by the disruption of the normal electrical impulse that originates at the sinoatrial node and is conducted to the atrioventricular node, then through the His-Purkinje system to depolarize the ventricles. Disruption may occur anywhere along this pathway. Underlying structural disease, prior ischemia, congenital abnormalities in myocytes, or electrical pathways affect a normal electrical conduction pathway. Palpitations that are due to supraventricular or ventricular tachyarrhythmias often result from sympathetic stimulation and catecholamine surges.

Palpitations involving skipped or premature beats are often a sensation that results from the following episode of systole when stroke volume is increased secondary to the prolonged length of the preceding diastole and increased ventricular inotropy.

Clinical Assessment

The keys to evaluation are a history and physical, a 12-lead electrocardiogram (ECG), and a basic laboratory evaluation including an evaluation of the thyroid gland. Clinicians must identify which patients are more likely to have underlying arrhythmia and require further evaluation. A good clinical history includes age of onset, description of palpitations, frequency, duration, timing, position, and associated symptoms, including dizziness, presyncope, and syncope. The clinical history should include a thorough

TABLE 1 Differential Diagnosis for Palpitations

	CARDIAC		NONCARDIAC
Arrhythmias	Atrial fibrillation	*Medications*	Digoxin [Lanoxin]
	Atrial flutter		Beta agonists (e.g., albuterol [Proventil])
	Benign ectopy (premature ventricular contractions, premature atrial contractions)		Vasodilators
	Nonsustained ventricular tachycardia		Anticholinergics
	Supraventricular tachyarrhythmias (e.g., atrioventricular reentrant tachycardia)		Hydralazine
	Inappropriate sinus tachycardia		Over-the-counter nasal decongestants (e.g., pseudoephedrine [Sudafed])
	Long-QT syndrome	*Substances*	Caffeine
	Torsades de pointes		Alcohol
Structural abnormalities	Mitral regurgitations		Cocaine
	Aortic insufficiency		Amphetamines
	Mitral valve prolapse		Nicotine
	Hypertrophic obstructive cardiomyopathy	*Systemic conditions*	Hyperthyroidism
Other	Pericarditis		Pheochromocytoma
	Pacemaker-mediated tachycardia		Anemia
	Vasovagal syncope		Hypoglycemia
			Mastocytosis
			Gastroesophageal reflux
			Esophageal spasm
		High output states	Fever
			Pregnancy
			Paget's disease
			Extracardiac shunt
			Exercise
			Stress
		Psychiatric conditions	Panic attack
			Generalized anxiety
			Depression
			Somatization

BOX 1 Indicators of Arrhythmic Etiology of Palpitations

Increased Likelihood of Underlying Arrhythmia
Known structural or valvular cardiac disease
Visible neck pulsations
Palpitations that affect sleep
Palpitations that occur at work
Subjective feeling of irregular heart rate
Duration of palpitations more than 5 min
Male gender
Older age

Decreased Likelihood of Underlying Arrhythmia
Family history of panic disorder
Duration of palpitations less than 5 min

medication review, including over-the-counter medications, alcohol and tobacco use, and illicit substance use. An increasing number of medications are being found to cause QT prolongation, especially when used in combination, and may predispose the patient to ventricular arrhythmias (see Table 2 and Box 2). A physical examination should be performed but may be limited, as clinicians rarely have the opportunity to examine a patient during an episode of palpitations.

Diagnostic Testing
A 12-lead ECG should be performed in all patients. It is appropriate to do limited laboratory evaluation with a complete blood count (CBC), thyroid-stimulating hormone (TSH), and complete metabolic panel (CMP or Chem-14) to identify anemia, thyroid disease, and electrolyte abnormalities that predispose to arrhythmias. Etiology can be determined in 40% of patients from this limited evaluation (see Tables 3 and 4).

TABLE 2	History and Physical Examination Clues to the Etiology of Palpitations	
CLUES FROM HISTORY OR EXAMINATION	**SUGGESTED DIAGNOSIS**	
Onset in childhood or adolescence	• AV nodal reentrant tachycardia • Wolff-Parkinson-White syndrome • Idiopathic ventricular tachyarrhythmia	
Onset in older adult Description of irregular rate	Atrial fibrillation	
Feeling of "fluttering"	Prolonged tachyarrhythmia	
Pounding in the neck Exaggerated "a" wave in jugular venous pulse	AV dissociations	
Midsystolic click followed by late systolic murmur	Mitral valve prolapse	
Holosystolic murmur along left sternal border that increases with Valsalva	Hypertrophic obstructive cardiomyopathy Left ventricle outflow tract obstruction	
Pale conjunctiva	Anemia	
Exophthalmos Goiter	Thyrotoxicosis	
Gravid abdomen	Pregnancy	

AV, Atrioventricular.

BOX 2	Medications That Cause QT Prolongation

- Cardiac Antiarrhythmics
  - Amiodarone (Cordarone)
  - Disopyramide (Norpace)
  - Procainamide
  - Quinidine
  - Sotalol (Betapace)
  - Diuretics
  - Sympathomimetics
  - Vasodilators
- Antibiotics
  - Fluoroquinolones
  - Macrolides
- Psychiatric
  - Phenothiazines
    ◦ Chlorpromazine (Thorazine)
    ◦ Promethazine (Phenergan)
    ◦ Prochlorperazine (Compazine)
    ◦ Fluphenazine (Prolixin)
    ◦ Trifluoperazine (Stelazine)
  - Selective serotonin reuptake inhibitors
  - Tricyclic antidepressants
  - Haloperidol (Haldol)
  - Amphetamines
  - Anticholinergics
  - Antihistamines
  - Protease inhibitors
  - Methadone (Dolophine)

Traditionally, ambulatory cardiac monitoring has been done via a Holter monitor. Patients keep a diary of the time and characteristics of their symptoms. This method is appropriate for patients who have daily palpitations. The monitor is worn for 24 to 48 hours. If symptoms are not present during the time the monitor is being worn, the test will be unrevealing. In addition, Holter monitoring may uncover arrhythmias (most commonly benign ectopy) that are unrelated to patient symptoms.

TABLE 3	ECG Findings Suggestive of Diagnosis of Palpitations
ECG FINDINGS	**SUGGESTED DIAGNOSIS**
Irregularly irregular rhythm Absent P waves	Atrial fibrillation
Delta wave Short PR interval Widened QRS	Wolff-Parkinson-White syndrome
Short PR	AV nodal reentrant tachycardia
QT interval >460 m/s in women, >440 m/s in men	Predisposition to ventricular tachyarrhythmias, including torsades de pointes
Left ventricular enlargement with left atrial abnormality	May be a focus for atrial fibrillation

AV, Atrioventricular, ECG, electrocardiogram.

TABLE 4	Diagnostic Considerations in the Evaluation of Palpitations
FINDINGS	**FURTHER EVALUATION**
Arrhythmia or predisposition to arrhythmia seen on ECG	Echocardiogram to look for structural heart disease
Palpitations brought on by exertion	Exercise stress test (avoid dobutamine if suspect arrhythmia)
Suspected arrhythmia, but none identified on ECG	Ambulatory cardiac monitoring • Holter monitor (24–48 h) • Continuous loop event recorder • Patch recorder • Implantable loop recorder
Associated dizziness, syncope, presyncope	Referral to cardiologist for electrophysiology study
Known cardiac dysfunction, structural or valvular abnormality	Referral to cardiologist for electrophysiology study
Family history of sudden cardiac death	Referral to cardiologist for electrophysiology study

If arrhythmia is suspected in a patient but 24 to 48 hours is insufficient time to record an event, it is recommended that the patient be evaluated with an event (loop) monitor or a patch monitor for at least 2 weeks. These ambulatory monitors record continuously but only save data from the specific interval when the patient or program settings activate the monitor (e.g., 2 min before and after an episode of palpitations). Some of these monitors transmit real-time information to a central monitoring system and others store data on the device itself for analysis after completion of the recording period. In patients with infrequent palpitations but known severe heart disease, an implantable loop recorder is an option. These monitors are implanted subcutaneously, typically in the left pectoral region, and usually are left in place for 1 year. As with other loop event recorders, they save data when activated by the patient or the device settings and transmit the information to an external system.

Panic disorder or anxiety is a diagnosis of exclusion. A patient with anxiety or other psychiatric illness may have a significant underlying arrhythmia. The catecholamine increase in patients with psychiatric disorder in times of stress or intense emotional experience may be proarrhythmogenic. These patients should

TABLE 5 Treatment of Specific Causes of Palpitations

CAUSE OF PALPITATIONS	TREATMENT
Medication or drug	Stop offending agent
Premature atrial contractions	Decrease caffeine and alcohol Tobacco cessation Beta blockers may reduce symptoms of PAC
Ectopy (PVCs)	Beta blockers • *Metoprolol Succinate* [Toprol XL][1] 50 mg PO daily • *Atenolol* [Tenormin][1] 50 mg PO daily Nondihydropyridine calcium channel blockers • *Verapamil* [Calan SR][1] 240 mg/day PO • *Diltiazem* [Cardizem CD][1] 120 mg/day PO Antiarrhythmic agents have been shown to reduce PVCs but may increase mortality especially in patients with previous myocardial infarction.
AVNRT Orthodromic AVRT SVT of unknown etiology	Vagal maneuvers (carotid massage, Valsalva, dive reflex) *Adenosine* [Adenocard] 6 mg IV bolus over 1–2 s, increased up to 12 mg IV every 1–2 min as needed for two doses If ineffective can reasonably consider: • *Verapamil* [Isoptin] 5–10 mg IV over 2 min, repeated in 30 min as necessary, then infusion at 0.005 mg/kg/min *Diltiazem* [Cardizem], 0.25 mg/kg IV over 2 min, repeat bolus of 0.35 mg/kg 15 min later if first dose is tolerated but does not produce desired reduction in heart rate. Can then be run as a continuous infusion at a rate of 5–15 mg/h • *Metoprolol Tartrate* [Lopressor][1] 2.5–5 mg IV bolus over 2 min, repeated at 5 min intervals up to three doses *Esmolol* [Brevibloc] 500 mcg/kg IV bolus over 1 min, followed by 50 mcg/kg/min continuous infusion. Can titrate up in 50 mcg/kg/min increments every 4 min to maximum 200 mcg/kg/min with repeat bolus doses between each rate change.
Antidromic AVRT	*Procainamide*[1] 20–50 mg/min up to total 17 mg/kg
Focal atrial tachycardia or multifocal atrial tachycardia	*Metoprolol Tartrate* [Lopressor]1 2.5–5 mg IV bolus over 2 min, repeated at 5 min intervals up to three doses *Verapamil* [Isoptin] 5–10 mg IV over 2 min, repeated in 30 min as necessary, then infusion at 0.005 mg/kg/min
Atrial fibrillation/flutter with rapid ventricular response	*Metoprolol Tartrate* [Lopressor]1 2.5–5 mg IV bolus over 2 min, repeated at 5 min intervals up to three doses *Esmolol* [Brevibloc] 500 mcg/kg IV bolus over 1 min, followed by 50 mcg/kg/min continuous infusion. Can titrate up in 50 mcg/kg/min increments every 4 min to maximum 200 mcg/kg/min with repeat bolus doses between each rate change. *Verapamil* [Isoptin] 5–10 mg IV over 2 min, repeated in 30 min as necessary, then infusion at 0.005 mg/kg/min *Diltiazem* [Cardizem], 0.25 mg/kg IV over 2 min, repeat bolus of 0.35 mg/kg 15 min later if first dose is tolerated but does not produce desired reduction in heart rate. Can then be run as a continuous infusion at a rate of 5–15 mg/h
Preexcited atrial fibrillation	*Procainamide*[1] 20–50 mg/min up to total 17 mg/kg *Ibutilide* [Corvert] 0.01 mg/kg (<60 kg) or 1 mg (≥60 kg) IV over 10 minutes
Ventricular Tachycardia	Synchronized cardioversion

[1]Not FDA approved for this indication. AVNRT, Atrioventricular nodal reentry tachycardia; IV, intravenous; PAC, premature atrial contraction; PVC, premature ventricular contraction; PO, per os (by mouth); SVT, supraventricular tachycardia.

undergo evaluation for arrhythmia, especially in the presence of risk factors, before having all of their symptoms attributed to their psychiatric illness.

Patients who have palpitations associated with dizziness, presyncope, or syncope in whom the diagnosis is not apparent should be referred for evaluation by a cardiologist. This sort of palpitation is the kind most likely to be associated with ventricular tachycardia or other serious arrhythmia.

Palpitations may occur more frequently during pregnancy, which is a high-output state. Postpartum cardiomyopathy is a structural disease that is unique to this population. Because pregnant women also have an increased risk of new arrhythmias, including atrial fibrillation, persistent palpitations should be evaluated thoroughly.

Treatment

Treatment should be focused toward the underlying cause of the palpitation.

Discussion of the management of specific causes of palpitations, including anemia, thyrotoxicosis, and hypoglycemia, can be found elsewhere. Chronic management of atrial fibrillation is also beyond the scope of this article.

Table 5 outlines the treatment of specific causes of palpitations.

Referral to a cardiologist is appropriate for patients with supraventricular tachyarrhythmias, long-QT syndrome, or palpitations associated with syncope/presyncope, as these are more likely to be ventricular arrhythmias.

Patients with potentially malignant ventricular tachyarrhythmias (e.g., frequent premature ventricular depolarizations, up to 3–10 per hour with some repetitive forms) are at increased risk for sudden cardiac death, but there is little evidence that treating with antiarrhythmics decreases mortality; in fact, some evidence suggests that these drugs actually increase mortality via proarrhythmic mechanisms. In these patients, consider a referral to a cardiologist for evaluation for an implantable cardiac defibrillator.

References

Abbott AV: Diagnostic approach to palpitations, *Am Fam Physician* 71:743–750, 2005.

Chan T, Worster A: The clinical diagnosis of arrhythmias in patients presenting with palpitations, *Ann Emerg Med* 57:303–304, 2011.

Crawford MH, Bernstein SJ, Deedwania PC, et al: ACC/AHA guidelines for ambulatory electrocardiography: executive summary and recommendations, *Circulation* 100:886–893, 1999.

Tayal U, Dancy M: Palpitations, *Medicine* 41:118–124, 2013.

Weber BE, Kapoor WN: Evaluation and outcomes of patients with palpitations, *Am J Med* 100:138–148, 1996.

Wexler AK, Pleister A, Raman S: Outpatient approach to palpitations, *Am Fam Physician* 84:63–69, 2011.

PHARYNGITIS

Method of
J. Lane Wilson, MD

CURRENT DIAGNOSIS

- Patients at intermediate or high risk for group A β-hemolytic streptococcal (GABHS) pharyngitis using a clinical decision rule should undergo rapid antigen detection testing. Low-risk patients should forgo testing.
- Children with negative rapid antigen detection testing for GABHS should have follow-up throat culture. Adults should not.
- Suspected infectious mononucleosis should initially be worked up with a complete blood count and heterophile antibody test (monospot). Children under 5 years and those in the first week of illness have high rates of false-negative heterophile antibodies.
- Nucleic acid amplification tests are recommended over antigen testing for suspected COVID-19.
- Pharyngitis lasting longer than 14 days should prompt evaluation for a noninfectious etiology, such as gastroesophageal reflux or allergic disease.

CURRENT THERAPY

- Group A β-hemolytic streptococcal (GABHS) pharyngitis first-line treatment is with oral or intramuscular penicillin. Oral amoxicillin is an acceptable alternative. For patients with penicillin allergy, first-generation cephalosporins, clindamycin,[1] and azithromycin are suitable alternatives.
- Antibiotics should not be prescribed without microbiologic evidence of GABHS or *Neisseria gonorrhea*.
- Infectious mononucleosis is treated supportively and with activity restriction to minimize the risk of splenic rupture.
- Decision to treat with antivirals for both COVID-19 and influenza in the outpatient setting is based upon risk factors and disease severity.
- Corticosteroids are not routinely recommended for symptomatic pharyngitis.

[1]Not FDA approved for this indication.

Introduction

The primary goal of the diagnostic approach to pharyngitis is to identify patients who need intervention other than supportive care. Most commonly, this will be identifying patients with group A β-hemolytic streptococcus (GABHS), or "strep throat." Gonococcal pharyngitis, coronavirus disease 2019 (COVID-19), infectious mononucleosis, influenza, herpes simplex infection, acute human immunodeficiency virus (HIV) infection, Kawasaki disease, and deep throat infections also have treatment considerations beyond supportive care and should be considered with certain clinical presentations and risk factors.

Epidemiology

Up to 2% of all outpatient visits are due to "sore throat." Most cases of pharyngitis are viral and self-limited. A wide range of viruses account for these cases including rhinovirus, adenovirus, coronavirus, enterovirus, coxsackievirus, influenza, and herpes simplex. Bacterial causes are less frequent but often the focus of the diagnostic process.

Up to 15% of adults and 35% of children presenting with sore throat have GABHS. GABHS is uncommon in children 3 years of age or younger or in adults 45 years and older unless they have a known close contact. It most commonly occurs in children aged 5 to 15 years in the late winter or early spring.

Gonococcal pharyngitis is increasingly recognized in sexually active patients. Most data regarding its incidence come from sexually transmitted infection clinics in which up to 7% of patients test positive. Receptive oral sex is the major risk factor associated with the infection.

Epstein-Barr virus (EBV) infection is ubiquitous, but only a small fraction of people will develop the clinical syndrome from primary infection known as infectious mononucleosis, commonly referred to as "mono." About half the population acquires the infection by age 5 years, and most of these cases are asymptomatic or have nonspecific symptoms. The older the patient during primary infection, the more likely they are to develop infectious mononucleosis. If primary infection is not contracted until adolescence or young adulthood, infectious mononucleosis develops up to 80% of the time. By age 20 years, more than 90% of the population has been infected.

Incidence of COVID-19 has varied greatly since the onset of the pandemic in 2020 over time and by variant. Similarly, rates of severe disease and critical illness have varied over time by variant and as vaccination rates have changed. A constant since the pandemic's onset has been advancing age as a risk factor for developing symptomatic and severe illness. Attention to local and regional epidemiologic data regarding current transmission and infection rates is critical to incorporate into diagnostic suspicion and practice.

Similarly, incidence of influenza varies year to year by strain of the virus circulating and by the effectiveness of the annual influenza vaccine. Seasonal epidemics tend to occur every 1 to 3 years. Advanced age, chronic pulmonary disease, immunosuppression, and pregnancy are risk factors for severe disease.

Clinical Manifestations

Group A β-Hemolytic Streptococcus

Patients with GABHS classically present with anterior cervical adenitis, tonsillitis with gray-white exudates, and fever. Nausea, vomiting, and abdominal pain may be features in children. Strawberry tongue, palatal petechiae, and scarlatiniform skin rash may also been seen. When present, the rash classically has a "sandpaper" feel and is more pronounced in skin creases (Pastia's lines). It spares the face, fades after 3 to 4 days, and subsequently desquamates. Presence of upper respiratory symptoms such as cough, coryza, rhinorrhea, hoarseness, conjunctivitis, or diarrhea suggest an alternative viral diagnosis.

Gonococcal Pharyngitis

Gonococcal pharyngitis may be asymptomatic or present with cervical adenopathy, oropharyngeal erythema, and exudate. It typically does not present with systemic symptoms. These patients may also present with symptoms or concerns for other sexually transmitted infections. A history of receptive oral sex is nearly ubiquitous.

Infectious Mononucleosis

Infectious mononucleosis classically presents in adolescence or early adulthood with the triad of fever, sore throat, and cervical lymphadenopathy. Fatigue, headache, myalgia, and upper respiratory symptoms are common. Less commonly, patients can present with abdominal discomfort in the left upper quadrant. Severe left upper quadrant pain with or without radiation to the left shoulder could signal splenic rupture. On examination, tonsillar exudates similar to those seen with GABHS infection and palatal petechiae may be observed. Splenomegaly is variably detected by physical examination but almost always present ultrasonographically. Patients who have taken a previously prescribed beta-lactam antibiotic for suspected GABHS may present with a nonspecific diffuse maculopapular rash. Children are more likely to present initially with rash, even without antibiotic exposure.

Acute HIV

Acute HIV infection may present similarly to both GABHS and infectious mononucleosis with fever, pharyngitis, cervical adenopathy, headache, and myalgia. Adenopathy may be present at other sites as well. Gastrointestinal symptoms including nausea, vomiting, and diarrhea may also present. Painful oral ulcers and a nonspecific exanthem are common. Like GABHS and infectious mononucleosis, respiratory symptoms other than pharyngitis are usually lacking.

COVID-19

COVID-19 may present with a wide range of severity and spectrum of symptoms. They typically develop 2 to 14 days after exposure and can include fevers, cough, shortness of breath, sore throat, loss of taste or smell, sinus pain, myalgias, headache, nausea, vomiting, diarrhea, headache, and rash that may take on a variety of forms. Anosmia and dysgeusia are more specific symptoms of COVID-19 compared with alternative diagnoses, and their presence should raise suspicion. Up to 80% of patients have mild symptoms (defined as lacking viral pneumonia and hypoxemia) or no symptoms at all.

Influenza

Influenza in adults is characterized by rapid onset of fevers, myalgias, cough, headache, nausea, coryza, pharyngitis, and eye pain upon lateral gaze within 2 days of exposure. Children present similarly but are more likely to have cervical adenopathy, conjunctivitis, and gastrointestinal symptoms.

Coxsackie Virus Infections

Coxsackie virus infections can produce a variety of clinical syndromes, most often in children under 10 years. Herpangina is distinguished by a painful enanthem of the soft palate and posterior oropharynx. The lesions begin as erythematous macules and go on to develop into vesicles that eventually ulcerate. Fever, often high grade, and cervical adenopathy are common as well. In hand-foot-and-mouth disease, painful vesicles that ulcerate are also present on the palms, soles, buttocks, and sometimes trunk. Both syndromes generally resolve within 7 days.

Herpes Gingivostomatitis

Primary oral herpes simplex infection can manifest in young children with ulcerating vesicles of the mouth accompanied by fever. In contrast to herpangina and hand-foot-and-mouth disease, the acute gingivostomatitis has lesions that are limited to the anterior mouth and lips as opposed to the oropharynx and can last up to 2 weeks.

Diagnosis

The diagnostic approach to the patient with pharyngitis is first centered on ruling in or ruling out GABHS. This is due to a combination of its prevalence, response to antibiotics and need for antibiotic stewardship, and need to prevent complications of GABHS. There are several clinical decision rules available to aid in the diagnostic testing decision for GABHS. The McIsaac criteria (also known as the modified Centor criteria) and FeverPAIN criteria are detailed in Table 1. Patients scoring in the low-risk group do not need GABHS testing and should not receive antibiotics. Intermediate and high-risk groups should undergo diagnostic testing with rapid antigen detection tests (RADTs) or rapid nucleic acid amplification tests (NAATs). If the RADT result is negative in a pediatric patient, throat culture should be performed. The negative predictive value for RADT is much higher in adults because of the low incidence of GABHS in that population. This, in combination with the low subsequent risk of rheumatic fever for untreated GABHS in adults, makes follow-up throat culture unnecessary in adults unless clinical suspicion is very high.

Patients with an exudative tonsillitis, cervical adenopathy, and fever with a negative streptococcal RADT should have infectious mononucleosis considered. Additional features that should raise the suspicion of infectious mononucleosis include the presence of posterior cervical adenopathy and/or splenomegaly on examination. Laboratory testing should follow clinical suspicion. Initial testing should include a complete blood count and heterophile antibody latex agglutination test (monospot). Great than 10% of atypical lymphocytes on peripheral blood smear is suggestive of infectious mononucleosis with increasing odds as the percent of atypical lymphocytes rises. Monospot testing has a 25% false-negative rate in the first week of symptoms in adults and very high false-negative rates in children 5 years and below. If monospot testing is negative and there are no atypical lymphocytes on peripheral smear, the diagnosis is unlikely. For cases with negative testing but high suspicion, viral capsid antigen IgG and IgM testing can be performed. It is both more sensitive and specific than monospot testing but takes longer to result. Similarly, IgM testing for cytomegalovirus (CMV) can be considered at that time as CMV mononucleosis can produce a nearly identical clinical syndrome to EBV, although it is much less common.

For patients with negative RADT who have a history of receptive oral sex, polymerase chain reaction (PCR) swab for gonorrhea should be considered. Culture on Thayer-Martin media may also be obtained but is not as sensitive as PCR tests that are now widely available. Gonococcal pharyngitis may also be suspected in the absence of systemic symptoms and very mild or no symptoms. Testing for other sexually transmitted infections, particularly

TABLE 1	Decision Rules for Group A β-Hemolytic Streptococcal Pharyngitis				
	McIsaac		**FeverPAIN**		
Viral symptoms	Absence of cough	1	Absence of cough or coryza	1
Lymphadenopathy	Anterior cervical adenopathy	1		
Fever	Temperature >38°C (100.4°F)	1	Feverishness within 24 hours	1
Tonsillar examination findings	Tonsillar exudate or swelling	1	Intensely inflamed tonsils	1
			Purulent tonsils	1
Duration			Presentation within 3 days of onset	1
Age	Age 3–14 years	1		
	Age 15–44 years	0		
	Age 45 years and older	−1		
RISK SCORE	**LIKELIHOOD OF STREP**		**LIKELIHOOD OF STREP**	
Low risk 0–1 points	7.6%–13.1%		1%–10%	
Intermediate risk 2–3 points	20.8%–33.6%		11%–35%	
High risk 4–5 points	50.7%–69.3%		51%–53%	

chlamydia coinfection and genital infections, should be considered for any patient in which gonococcal pharyngitis is suspected.

Acute HIV infection should be suspected in patients with negative RADT, negative heterophile antibody, and risk factors. The presence of painful oral ulcers, nonspecific exanthem, and adenopathy beyond the cervical chains are additional clues that could prompt testing. Often, seroconversion has not yet occurred at the time of presentation, and HIV antibodies are negative if tested. The earliest detection method is via HIV RNA NAAT. The HIV p24 antigen test may detect infection at or beyond 10 to 15 days after infection. This test generally combines p24 antibody testing with it, which would not be positive during acute infection. A positive p24 antigen or antibody should be followed up with confirmatory HIV RNA testing.

Suspicion for COVID-19 and influenza is often dependent upon local circulating incidence. Respiratory symptoms point away from a bacterial pharyngitis and acute HIV infection and toward viral etiology. Symptoms of anosmia or dysgeusia should specifically raise concern for COVID-19, whereas the classic abrupt onset of systemic symptoms points toward influenza. Many patients with either illness will have a known sick contact that may help guide testing. When there are high community levels and a known contact, a clinical diagnosis may be appropriate. Often, COVID-19 and influenza testing is available from a single nasopharyngeal NAAT swab. Rapid influenza diagnostic tests (RIDTs) that detect influenza antigens are poorly sensitive but highly specific. Nasal antigen testing for COVID-19 is similarly poorly sensitive; therefore a negative antigen test should be followed by NAAT. If NAAT is not available, repeat antigen testing every 48 hours increases sensitivity. Asymptomatic patients with a COVID-19 exposure should not be tested using antigen tests. Because many patients with either COVID-19 or influenza will be managed supportively, testing should be reserved for when the result will affect subsequent management.

Vesicles or ulcerations of the oral mucosa are indicative of viral etiologies. Herpangina, hand-foot-and-mouth disease, and primary herpes simplex gingivostomatitis are typically diagnosed clinically. If needed, PCR or viral culture may be obtained from an ulceration to confirm herpes simplex viral infection.

Deep throat infections should be suspected in patients with a toxic appearance, unilateral tonsillar involvement, dysphonia ("hot potato" voice), or evidence of airway obstruction. Epiglottis may present with drooling and stridor. Peritonsillar abscess may generally be recognized on physical exam due to extreme tonsillar asymmetry. Retropharyngeal abscesses are most common in children and associated with bacterial upper respiratory infections or recent oropharyngeal instrumentation.

Kawasaki disease is an inflammatory disease of important consideration on the differential, particularly for children 5 years and younger, who present with fever, cervical adenopathy, and pharyngitis. Children with Kawasaki disease typically have fever above 39°C (102.2°F) and remain febrile for at least 5 days if not treated. Cervical adenopathy is pronounced and at least one lymph node should measure greater than 1.5 cm. Features that should prompt consideration of Kawasaki disease include bilateral conjunctivitis, oral mucosa changes including cheilitis and strawberry tongue, nonspecific maculopapular or polymorphic rash, and extremity changes that include swelling and erythema of the palms and soles. Eventually the rash desquamates in the convalescent phase. Because of the skin changes and strawberry tongue, it can be misdiagnosed as scarlet fever. Presence of conjunctivitis, negative testing for or lack of response to treatment to GABHS, and age less than 3 years should raise suspicion for Kawasaki disease.

Patients who present with sore throat for more than 14 days likely have a noninfectious etiology such as gastroesophageal reflux or allergic disease.

Treatment
Group A β-Hemolytic Streptococcus
GABHS is universally sensitive to penicillins, and efforts should be made to keep the antibiotic spectrum narrow. First-line treatment is therefore penicillin or amoxicillin. Penicillin may be given orally or as a single intramuscular injection. If liquid formulations are needed, amoxicillin is more palatable than penicillin. Alternatives for patients with nonanaphylactic allergies to penicillin include first-generation cephalosporins such as cephalexin. For those with anaphylactic reactions to penicillins and/or other beta-lactam antibiotics, macrolides or clindamycin[1] may be used (Table 2). Because nonpenicillin therapies are associated with higher failure rates, culture with antibiotic susceptibility testing should be obtained to help guide treatment changes if necessary. Microbiologic evidence of GABHS should be present before initiation of antibiotic therapy. Occasionally, group B, group C, or group G streptococcus will be isolated from throat culture. These isolates do not need treatment with antibiotics as they are not associated with immunologic complications and resolve within 4 days untreated. If treated for symptomatic relief, the same antibiotic selection preferences for GABHS apply.

Gonococcal Pharyngitis
Gonococcal pharyngitis is treated with a single dose of intramuscular ceftriaxone based upon weight (see Table 2). Sexual partners should also be treated, and sexual contact should be avoided for at least 7 days after treatment. A test of cure is recommended at 7 to 14 days posttreatment. Alternative therapies to ceftriaxone have significant limitations but include spectinomycin[2], gentamicin[1], and high-dose azithromycin.[1] If an alternative therapy to ceftriaxone is indicated either due to drug resistance or severe allergy, infectious disease consultation is indicated.

Infectious Mononucleosis
Infectious mononucleosis is treated supportively. Antivirals and corticosteroids are not routinely recommended. However, activity restriction of at least 3 weeks (and up to 8 weeks) is an important recommendation to reduce the risk of rare but potentially fatal complication of splenic rupture. The optimal duration of activity limitation is not known.

Acute HIV Infection
Acute HIV symptoms are generally self-limited and treated supportively. Antiretroviral therapy (ART) should be initiated as soon as possible after diagnosis and once genotypic resistance testing has been obtained. Specific antiretroviral regimens are subsequently tailored to those results.

COVID-19
COVID-19 is treated supportively for low-risk patients with mild disease (defined as lacking viral pneumonia and hypoxemia). Patients who are at high risk for hospitalization may be treated with a 5-day course of oral nirmatrelvir/ritonavir (Paxlovid) with initiation of therapy as soon as possible and within 5 days of symptom onset. Interactions with a large number of other medications can limit its application. If contraindications to nirmatrelvir/ritonavir exist, oral molnupiravir (Lagevrio)[1] is an available alternative within the same time frame. Alternatively, if at an equipped institution, intravenous remdesivir (Veklury) may be administered for 3 days as soon as possible and within 7 days of symptom onset (see Table 2). Monoclonal antibody therapy is not currently recommended.

For patients who are hospitalized, whether they require supplemental oxygen dictates much of their treatment decisions. For those not requiring oxygen, thromboprophylaxis should be administered unless contraindicated due to risk of coagulopathy. Remdesivir intravenously for 4 days has benefit, particularly if started within 10 days of symptom onset.

Patients requiring supplemental oxygen should be treated with corticosteroids in addition to a longer 10-day course of remdesivir (or until discharge). Dexamethasone[1] is the most studied agent and may be given orally or intravenously. Therapeutic

---

[1] Not FDA approved for this indication.
[2] Not available in the United States.

TABLE 2 Treatment for Selected Causes of Pharyngitis

DISEASE	FIRST LINE	SECOND LINE	OTHER CONSIDERATIONS
Group A β-hemolytic streptococcus	Penicillin V, oral 250 mg 2–3 times daily for 10 days for children 500 mg twice daily for 10 days in adults or adolescents Penicillin G benzathine, intramuscular (Bicillin LA) 600,000 units once if <27 kg 1.2 million units once if >27 kg Amoxicillin, oral 50 mg/kg (up to 1000 mg) once daily for 10 days 25 mg/kg (up to 500 mg) twice daily for 10 days	Cephalosporins, oral Cephalexin 20 mg/kg (up to 500 mg/dose) twice daily for 10 days Cefadroxil 30 mg/kg (up to 1000 mg/dose) once daily for 10 days Clindamycin,[1] oral 7 mg/kg (up to 300 mg/dose) 3 times daily for 10 days Macrolides, oral Azithromycin 12 mg/kg (up to 500 mg) once daily for 5 days Clarithromycin 7.5 mg/kg (up to 250 mg/dose) twice daily for 10 days	GABHS is universally sensitive to penicillin. Second-line therapies should only be used in penicillin allergic patients.
Gonococcal pharyngitis	Ceftriaxone, intramuscular 500 mg once for patients <150 kg 1 g once for patients >150 kg	Gentamicin,[1] ertapenem (Invanz);[1] recommend infectious disease consultation	If chlamydial coinfection not excluded: Doxycycline 100 mg orally twice daily if nonpregnant Azithromycin[1] 1 g orally once if pregnant
COVID-19 (outpatient)	Nirmatrelvir/ritonavir (Paxlovid) 300 mg/100 mg orally twice daily for 5 days	Remdesivir (Veklury) 200 mg intravenously on day 1 followed by 100 mg intravenously on days 2 and 3 Molnupiravir (Lagevrio)[1] 800 mg orally twice daily for 5 days	Should be started within 5 days of symptom onset (up to 7 for remdesivir)
Influenza (outpatient)	Oseltamivir (Tamiflu), oral, 5-day course If <1 year of age, 3 mg/kg/dose twice daily ≤15 kg, 30 mg twice daily >15–23 kg, 45 mg twice daily >23–40 kg, 60 mg twice daily >40 kg children or adults, 75 mg orally twice daily Zanamivir (Relenza), inhaled, 7 years and older, 5-day course 10 mg (2 inhalations) twice daily Baloxavir (Xofluza), oral, 5 years and older, single dose <20 kg, 2 mg/kg 20–80 kg, 40 mg >80 kg, 80 mg		Greatest benefit if given within 48 hours
Herpetic gingivostomatitis, primary	Acyclovir,[1] oral, 7 days 15 mg/kg acyclovir up to 200 mg/dose 5 times daily	For children 12 years and older: Valacyclovir (Valtrex),[1] oral 1 g twice daily for 5 days, or 2 g orally twice daily for one day Famciclovir, oral 500 mg twice daily for 7 days	For recurrence, treatment ideally starts within an hour of first noticing symptoms. Acyclovir dosing is the same. Valacyclovir may be dosed the same as well but the shorter course may be preferable.

[1]Not FDA approved for this indication.

anticoagulation is indicated in the absence of contraindications if D-dimer levels are abnormal.

For patients requiring high-flow or noninvasive ventilation, immunomodulatory therapy is indicated. Preferred agents are baricitinib (Olumiant) or tocilizumab (Actemra). All patients requiring invasive ventilation should have immunomodulatory therapy. If previously started, remdesivir may be continued, and if not previously started, it may be considered in addition to baricitinib or tocilizumab. If previously on anticoagulation doses of heparin and without evidence of thrombotic complications, de-escalation to prophylactic dosing is appropriate after moving to the intensive care unit (ICU).

Influenza
Antiviral therapy given within 48 hours of symptom onset (and possibly up to within 5 days) can reduce morbidity and mortality in hospitalized patients and high-risk outpatients. In the general adult outpatient population, they may reduce symptoms by one-half to one day. Patients are considered high-risk if less than 2 years or older than 65 years; have chronic cardiovascular, respiratory, renal, or other disease; are immunosuppressed; are pregnant or within 2 weeks of delivery; are obese; or live in a nursing home or other long-term care facility.

For adults and children, a 5-day course of oral oseltamivir (Tamiflu) is most commonly used. Inhaled zanamivir (Relenza) may be used in patients 7 years and older. Peramivir (Rapivab) is an intravenous antiviral option for inpatients. Baloxavir (Xofluza) was FDA-approved in 2018 and has the advantage of being given in a single oral dose (see Table 2).

Corticosteroids should be avoided in patients with influenza.

Herpetic Gingivostomatitis
Herpetic gingivostomatitis may be treated in young children with 15 mg/kg acyclovir[1] up to 200 mg 5 times daily for 7 days.

[1] Not FDA approved for this indication.

Children 12 years and older may alternatively be treated with valacyclovir (Valtrex)[1] 1 g orally twice daily for 5 days or 2 g orally twice daily for one day (see Table 2). All formulations are most effective when given as soon as possible in the course of illness.

Monitoring

For GABHS, follow-up testing after treatment with antibiotics is not indicated unless there is not resolution with adequate therapy. For patients with microbiologically confirmed recurrent GABHS, referral to otolaryngology for consideration of tonsillectomy is recommended after 7 or more confirmed infections in a year, 5 or more infections per year over 2 years, or 3 or more infections per year over 3 years.

For gonococcal pharyngitis, testing for other sexually transmitted infections, including chlamydia, syphilis, and HIV, should be performed. A test of cure is recommended 7 to 14 days after treatment. Sexual partners should also be offered treatment and monitored.

Repeat testing is not recommended for viral etiologies of pharyngitis.

Complications

Group A β-Hemolytic Streptococcus

Complications of GABHS can be divided into suppurative and nonsuppurative conditions. Suppurative conditions include otitis media, sinusitis, mastoiditis, lateral or retropharyngeal abscess, cervical lymphadenitis, and Lemierre's syndrome (although most commonly caused by *Fusobacterium necrophorum*, it can be caused or preceded by other oropharyngeal pathogens, including GABHS). Failure of GABHS to respond to antibiotics and/or worsening unilateral neck pain should prompt the consideration of Lemierre's syndrome. Recognition of and treatment of GABHS with appropriate antibiotics reduces the risk of these suppurative complications.

Nonsuppurative complications are immunologic in nature and include rheumatic fever, poststreptococcal glomerulonephritis, and poststreptococcal reactive arthritis. Acute rheumatic fever may develop after 2 to 3 weeks of GABHS pharyngitis and is prevented by antibiotic therapy when given within 9 days of symptoms. In contrast, poststreptococcal glomerulonephritis and reactive arthritis may follow pharyngitis or skin infections and is not prevented via the use of antibiotics. Pediatric Autoimmune Neuropsychiatric Disorder Associated with group A Streptococcal Infection (PANDAS) is a rare and controversial diagnosis characterized by the acute onset of motor tics or obsessive-compulsive disorder after streptococcal infection.

Gonococcal Pharyngitis

Complications of gonococcal pharyngitis include co-occurring gonococcal infections such as cervicitis or pelvic inflammatory disease in women, epididymitis in men, urethritis, proctitis, conjunctivitis, and, rarely, disseminated gonococcal infection. Reactive arthritis, which may include clinical manifestations of conjunctivitis, aseptic oligoarthritis, and skin and/or mucosal lesions, may follow infection in 1 to 6 weeks. It is self-limited and treated supportively.

Infectious Mononucleosis

The most important complication of EBV infectious mononucleosis is splenic rupture. Although rare, it has a high mortality rate. It usually occurs within 3 weeks of illness but may occur as far out as 7 weeks. Most cases occur spontaneously, but a significant proportion follow a known injury. Hematologic complications are common if sought but generally of little consequence. This can include pancytopenia, thrombocytopenia, and hemolytic anemia. More seriously they may manifest as aplastic anemia, thrombotic thrombocytopenic purpura, hemolytic uremic syndrome, or disseminated intravascular coagulation. Hepatitis or cholestatic liver disease, usually mild, may be present during illness.

Neurologic complications, such as meningitis or transverse myelitis, are uncommon. Persistent fatigue may last more than a month after infection.

COVID-19

COVID-19 has wide range of complications. Although most of these follow moderate to severe disease, mild cases may also develop complications. Acute respiratory distress syndrome (ARDS) is among the most common complications and is an important cause of COVID-related mortality. Coagulopathy may manifest itself as venous thromboembolism, stroke, and, rarely, disseminated intravascular coagulation. These are most common in severe cases or patients admitted to the ICU, and all hospitalized patients should receive thromboprophylaxis to reduce the risk of developing thrombotic complications. Cardiac complications can include myocardial infarction, myocarditis, arrhythmias, and cardiomyopathy. Neurologic complications may present as meningitis or encephalitis, Guillain-Barré syndrome, myositis, acute disseminated encephalomyelitis, ataxia, and deficits of global cognition. Loss of taste or smell are the most common neurologic effects and generally resolve within 90 days.

A rare but important complication of COVID-19 is multisystem inflammatory syndrome in children (MIS-C) and more rarely in adults (MIS-A). It develops days or weeks after COVID-19 and can affect the heart, lungs, kidneys, brain, gastrointestinal system, skin, or eyes and is associated with high inflammatory markers. Treatment is largely supportive with some evidence for the use of intravenous immunoglobulin and steroids as antiinflammatory measures.

Long COVID is defined by persistence of symptoms from acute COVID-19 beyond 4 weeks after onset. Its symptoms are as varied as that of acute COVID-19 and its complications, and there is no specific diagnostic criteria or laboratory test to diagnose it. Its incidence is reported to be as low as 5% and as high as 30%. Diagnosis is made clinically by ruling out other conditions and the temporal relationship to acute COVID-19 infection. It is treated supportively.

Influenza

Complication rates of influenza vary by strain. In children, acute otitis media is the most common complication. Influenza is a common precipitant of febrile seizure in young children. Other neurologic complications, including encephalopathy, transverse myelitis, Guillain-Barré syndrome, and acute disseminated encephalomyelitis, can occur in both children and adults. Viral pneumonia and influenza-associated bacterial pneumonia, most commonly due to *Streptococcus pneumonia* or *Staphylococcus aureus*, can lead to severe illness in children and adults, particularly in those with chronic medical conditions. Myocarditis and pericarditis occur at low rates in both children and adults but tend to be more severe in children.

References

Bhimraj A, Morgan RL, Shumaker AH, et al: Infectious diseases society of America guidelines on the treatment and management of patients with COVID-19, *Clin Infect Disciac724*, 2022.

Centers for Disease Control. *Multisystem Inflammatory Syndrome (MIS)*. Available at https://www.cdc.gov/mis/index.html. [accessed 4/23/24].

Gaitonde DY, Moore FC, Morgan MK: Influenza: diagnosis and treatment, *Am Fam Physician* 100(12):751–758, 2019.

Hamilton JL, McCrea Ii L: Streptococcal pharyngitis: rapid evidence review, *Am Fam Physician* 109(4):343–349, 2024.

Mustafa Z, Ghaffari M: Diagnostic methods, clinical guidelines, and antibiotic treatment for group A streptococcal pharyngitis: A narrative review, *Front Cell Infect Microbiol* 10:563627, 2020.

Sykes EA, Wu V, Beyea MM, Simpson MTW, Beyea JA: Pharyngitis: approach to diagnosis and treatment, *Can Fam Physician* 66(4):251–257, 2020.

Sylvester JE, Buchanan BK, Silva TW: Infectious mononucleosis: rapid evidence review, *Am Fam Physician* 107(1):71–78, 2023.

Usatine RP, Tinitigan R: Nongenital herpes simplex virus, *Am Fam Physician* 82(9):1075–1082, 2010.

Workowski KA, Bachmann LH, Chan PA, et al: Sexually transmitted infections treatment guidelines, 2021, *MMWR Recomm Rep* 70(4):1–187, 2021.

Yonke N, Aragón M, Phillips JK: Chlamydial and gonococcal infections: screening, diagnosis, and treatment, *Am Fam Physician* 105(4):388–396, 2022.

---

[1] Not FDA approved for this indication.

PRURITIS

Method of
Katherine Turner, MD; and Margaret Dobson, MD

CURRENT DIAGNOSIS

- Chronic itching can be as disruptive to quality of life as chronic pain.
- History and physical examination often reveals the cause for pruritis.
- Pruritis without visible skin changes should raise concern for an underlying systemic etiology.
- Consider a skin biopsy if the etiology is not evident by history and clinical examination.

CURRENT THERAPY

- Acute pruritis may be easier to treat than chronic pruritis, but targeted treatment is most successful regardless of the time course.
- General guidance for pruritis due to xeroderma is regular use of emollients and to avoid prolonged hot showers or baths.
- Antihistamines are often first-line therapy for pruritis because many etiologies are histamine mediated.
- Many nonhistamine-mediated etiologies of chronic pruritis may be well managed with neuropathic agents because nerves transmitting the itch sensation also transmit pain.
- Systemic immune modulators are directed at specific causes of pruritis, often after biopsy confirmation.

Pathophysiology

Pruritis, the sensation of itchiness that leads to scratching, has multiple physiologic causes. Pruritis can originate in the skin and have direct correlation with a dermatologic condition. Alternatively, it can be a result of a more generalized condition of which pruritis may be one of multiple symptoms. Pruritis is thought to originate from both histamine sensitive and nonhistamine-sensitive nerve pathways through type C and type Aδ nerve fibers. These nerves transmit itch, pain, and temperature sensations. Histamine is released after mast cell degranulation and attaches to H1 and H4 receptors on the histaminergic nerves. There are multiple pathways through which the nonhistaminergic nerves are activated, which include cytokines, proteases, neuropeptides released from type 2 helper T cells, eosinophils, macrophages, mast cells, and keratinocytes. The activated nerves transmit their impulse through the dorsal nerve root ganglia to the thalamus via the contralateral spinothalamic tract, and then on to the somatosensory cortex, leading to the sensation and localization of itch. The response to antihistamines is variable because of the multiple pathways of pruritis. Generally, the wheal and flare of urticaria and the atopic dermatitis groups are histamine sensitive. The nerve pathways for acute and chronic itching are distinct, with chronic pruritis and itching developing a neuropathic-type presentation.

Clinical Manifestations

Pruritis can present at any age, but it is more common with advanced age. This is expected as many of the underlying causes of pruritis (e.g., certain cancers, spinal nerve compression) are more common with advanced age. Some patients with pruritis present with skin changes but some do not have skin changes.

Classification

Pruritis can be classified as either acute or chronic. The International Federation of the Study of Itch uses 6 weeks to distinguish acute pruritis from chronic pruritis. Unfortunately, there have not been further standardized classifications for the etiologies of pruritis. This text has chosen to classify pruritis as:
1. Group 1: Pruritis of primary inflamed, diseased skin
2. Group 2: Pruritis of primary noninflamed, nondiseased skin
3. Group 3: Pruritis with chronic secondary scratch lesions

Differential Diagnosis

A detailed history and examination are essential in finding the etiology of pruritis. Location, characteristics, associated symptoms, chronic medical diagnoses, use of medications and supplements, skin examination, focused general examination, and review of available prior investigations can help narrow the differential diagnosis. An abnormal dermatologic examination does not exclude a systemic etiology because the itch-scratch cycle can damage skin and/or nerves. Acute pruritis may have a readily identifiable cause, whereas chronic pruritis can be more difficult to diagnose and manage. Initial investigations for pruritis of unknown etiology should include comprehensive metabolic panel, complete blood count (CBC) with platelets, and thyroid-stimulating hormone. Abnormalities in hemoglobin, renal function, hepatic function, or thyroid function can help suggest the etiology.

Prevention

The standard approach to preventing pruritis is to avoid dryness of the skin. Specific preventive measures should be directed at the underlying cause.

Therapy

Treatment of pruritis depends on the underlying etiology if known. For general management, and for unknown etiology, avoid development of dry skin by using a minimal amount of hypoallergenic soap, showering in warm (not hot) water, limiting the time immersed in water or in the shower, frequent application of a neutral hydrating emollient, and limiting hot or spicy foods. Table 1 summarizes conditions, clinical clues, diagnostic measures, and management by the grouping classification mentioned above.

Topical Therapies
Corticosteroids
Topical corticosteroids aid in improvement of pruritis by decreasing the localized inflammation at the area of application. They do not have inherent antipruritic properties. Strength of corticosteroids should be targeted to the primary etiology of pruritis. Topical corticosteroids are most beneficial for pruritis due to group 1 conditions. Overuse of topical steroids can lead to skin atrophy, hypopigmentation, and rebound symptoms.

Capsaicin
Topical capsaicin[1] provides antipruritic treatment by antagonizing histamine receptors at peripheral nerves. It is most beneficial for neuropathic pruritis. It often requires multiple applications per day at higher doses for efficacy. This, as well as local skin irritation, often limits use. It should be avoided in actively inflamed skin because of the irritation it can cause.

Coolants
Topical coolants such as methanol and camphor activate afferent cooling nerves and thus provide antipruritic effects. They can be particularly beneficial for neuropathic itch and can help with infectious pruritis. They can cause skin irritation.

---

[1] Not FDA approved for this indication.

TABLE 1 Causes of Pruritis

GROUP 1: PRURITIS OF PRIMARY INFLAMED, DISEASED SKIN

CONDITION	CLINICAL CLUES	DIAGNOSTIC MEASURES	MANAGEMENT
Inflammatory: dry skin, atopic dermatitis, contact dermatitis, psoriasis, lichen planus, drug reactions	Physical exam consistent with disease, exposures to common contact allergens (cosmetics, plants, fragrances, jewelry), medication use	Auspitz sign (scraping reveals punctate bleeding, points to psoriasis or AK), punch biopsy	Antihistamines, topical corticosteroids, topical doxepin (Prudoxin, Zonalon), topical calcineurin inhibitors, oral corticosteroids, immunosuppressants Referral to dermatology often appropriate if not responsive to initial measures
Infections: scabies, mosquito bite, parasites, viral or bacterial infection, fungal infections	Exposure suggested in history suggests exposure, appearance of lesion	Can perform scraping with microscopy or send sample to pathology for evaluation	Antiinfective agents directed at infectious etiology Symptomatic pruritis treated with antihistamines, coolants, topical corticosteroids
Autoimmune: bullous dermatoses, dermatomyositis	Cutaneous findings consistent with diagnosis; muscle weakness, pain; known or suspected malignancy	Punch biopsy	Topical corticosteroids, topical calcineurin inhibitors, immunosuppressants, dermatology referral for consideration of immune modulator
Dermatoses of pregnancy: polymorphic eruption of pregnancy, pemphigoid gestationis, pustular psoriasis of pregnancy, atopic eruption of pregnancy	Pregnant patients with cutaneous findings consistent with diagnosis	Often not necessary for diagnosis, may consider punch biopsy if diagnosis is uncertain	Topical corticosteroids Pustular psoriasis of pregnancy associated with adverse pregnancy outcomes, requiring oral corticosteroids or immunosuppressants, dermatology referral (if uncertain diagnosis), and maternal-fetal medicine referral (for associated monitoring)

GROUP 2: PRURITIS OF PRIMARY NONINFLAMED, NONDISEASED SKIN

CONDITION	CLINICAL CLUES	DIAGNOSTIC STUDY	MANAGEMENT
Endocrine and metabolic diseases: chronic renal failure, chronic liver disease, hyperthyroidism, malabsorption, perimenopausal pruritis	Systemic symptoms: confusion, jaundice, palpitations, hot flashes, menstrual changes	CMP (uremia, transaminitis, hypoalbuminemia, electrolyte disturbances), TSH	Topical anesthetics, anticonvulsants, SSRIs
Hematologic diseases: polycythemia, Hodgkin and non-Hodgkin lymphoma, iron deficiency, lymphoproliferative diseases	Unintentional weight loss, thrombosis, dyspnea, chronic cough, sleep apnea, smoking	CBC with differential	Anticonvulsants, antidepressants
Infectious diseases: HIV, parasites, helminths	Systemic symptoms: nausea, diarrhea, unintentional weight loss, cough, fevers History: travel, exposure, multiple sex partners, IV drug use	CBC (lymphopenia, eosinophilia), CMP (transaminitis, hypoalbuminemia)	Topical corticosteroids, coolants, antihistamines
Neoplasms: cervix, colon, prostate, carcinoid syndrome	Unintentional weight loss; abnormal uterine bleeding; melena or hematochezia, constipation or diarrhea, urinary hesitancy; flushing, palpitations	Routine screening up to date with additional testing based on history Pap smear/HPV testing; colonoscopy; PSA; urinary 5-hydroxyindoleacetic acid	Treat underlying cancer; for pruritic symptoms: capsaicin, topical anesthetics, SSRIs, mirtazapine (Remeron), anticonvulsants
Pregnancy: pruritis of pregnancy, ICP	Xeroderma; pruritis, particularly of palms and soles, without cutaneous findings	Bile acids, CMP	Ursodeoxycholic acid (ursodiol) for ICP; cholestyramine (Questran), if refractory ICP is associated with adverse fetal outcomes, so referral to maternal-fetal medicine may be appropriate
Drug-induced pruritis: opioids, ACE inhibitors, amiodarone, hydrochlorothiazide, estrogens, simvastatin, allopurinol, trimethoprim-sulfamethoxazole, calcium-channel blockers, heparin	Exposure to offending medication	Often not necessary for diagnosis	Switch offending agent

TABLE 1 Causes of Pruritis—cont'd

GROUP 3: PRURITIS WITH CHRONIC SECONDARY SCRATCH LESIONS			
CONDITION	**CLINICAL CLUES**	**DIAGNOSTIC STUDY**	**MANAGEMENT**
Neurogenic origin: multiple sclerosis, postherpetic neuralgia, cerebral infarcts, spinal infarcts, vulvodynia, neuropathy	Neurologic deficits; prior dermatologic infection; vulvar pain, dyspareunia	Often not necessary for diagnosis	Topical anesthetics, capsaicin, coolants, anticonvulsants, antidepressants
Somatoform pruritis: psychogenic itch, obsessive-compulsive disorder	Psychiatric history, hallucinations	Often not necessary for diagnosis	Behavioral therapy, anticonvulsants, antidepressants

ACE, Angiotensin-converting enzyme; *AK,* actinic keratosis; *CBC,* complete blood cell count; *CMP,* comprehensive metabolic panel; *HPV,* human papilloma virus; *ICP,* intrahepatic cholestasis of pregnancy; *IV,* intravenous; *PSA,* prostate-specific antigen; *SSRIs,* selective serotonin reuptake inhibitors; *TSH,* thyroid-stimulating hormone.

Doxepin

Doxepin 5% (Prudoxin, Zonalon) cream provides pruritis relief as an antihistamine. Its benefit has been demonstrated clinically for atopic dermatitis. In the elderly, it can cause drowsiness with widespread application of more than 10% of body surface area.

Calcineurin Inhibitors

The topical calcineurin inhibitor tacrolimus (Protopic) can improve pruritis by decreasing local inflammation. The efficacy of calcineurin inhibitors has been documented for dermatologic conditions such as some eczema, psoriasis, and seborrheic dermatitis. The most common side effect is a burning sensation, which can improve with continued use.

Anesthetics

Topical anesthetics, including lidocaine, prilocaine, and pramoxine, are useful for uremic and neuropathic itch. Pramoxine is more effective if stored in a cool area. Anesthetics work by antagonizing sodium channels in the nerves. Vectors for administration include creams, patches, and lotions.

Systemic Therapies
Antihistamines

Both first- and second-generation antihistamines can provide pruritis relief by blocking histamine receptors. They are also most effective in acute itch with urticaria because that etiology is primarily mediated by histamine. First-generation antihistamines are more effective than second generation for chronic itch because their sedating effects can help alter neurotransmission in the somatosensory cortex. Long-term use of antihistamines can increase dementia risk. Their use should be limited in the elderly due to their anticholinergic properties.

Immunosuppressants

A variety of immunosuppressive agents (methotrexate, mycophenolate [CellCept],[1] azathioprine [Imuran],[1] cyclosporine [Neoral], prednisone) have demonstrated efficacy in the treatment of primary dermatologic conditions such as atopic dermatitis, psoriasis, dermatomyositis, lupus, and scleroderma. Choice of agent should be directed at the underlying cause. Their use is limited in patients with pruritis of unknown origin but could be beneficial for those with greater than 4% eosinophils on CBC differential. Medications can cause gastrointestinal side effects, myelosuppression, hepatotoxicity, and stomatitis and can increase risks for infections. Patients with acute infections should not take immunosuppressants. Use of medications is limited in patients with underlying hepatic dysfunction, hypersensitivity, immunodeficiency, or underlying blood dyscrasias. Patients whose condition would benefit from the use of immunosuppressants should be referred to a dermatologist.

Anticonvulsants

The gamma-aminobutyric acid inhibitors gabapentin (Neurontin)[1] and pregabalin (Lyrica)[1] improve pruritis by decreasing the pruritis sensation at the dorsal root ganglia and spinal cord. Their sedating side effects often limit use. There have been some documented benefits in treatment of pruritis of unknown origin, neuropathic pruritis, paraneoplastic pruritis, and uremic pruritis. Use with caution in the elderly because of sedating properties and ataxia.

Antidepressants

The tricyclic antidepressants amitriptyline[1] and doxepin[1] are beneficial for neuropathic or psychogenic pruritis. They have antihistamine properties, which help treat pruritis. However, their anticholinergic side effects limit use, particularly in the elderly. Several selective serotonin reuptake inhibitors such as fluoxetine (Prozac),[1] fluvoxamine,[1] paroxetine (Paxil),[1] and sertraline (Zoloft)[1] also may help with psychogenic, paraneoplastic, or cholestatic pruritis. Serotonin acts as a neurotransmitter in the skin to trigger the sensation of pruritis. Mirtazapine (Remeron)[1] may also help with pruritis from malignancy or nocturnal pruritis.

Monitoring

Assess response to therapy and consider further treatment options or diagnostic workup.

Complications

Severe itching can result in disruption of the skin integrity and can lead to complex, chronic itching–related skin conditions including prurigo nodularis or extensive excoriations at risk for infection and cellulitis. Chronic itching can be emotionally debilitating, affecting quality of life similar to chronic pain.

[1] Not FDA approved for this indication.

References

Abu Hassan F, Hafiz S, Dweik A, Alhussain E, Walker J: Decompensated heart failure presenting as severe pruritis, *Am J Med Sci,* 2023.

Cho J, Chiou D, Patil P, Hyder S: Pruritis & dysphagia: gastrointestinal manifestations of lichen planus, *Am Coll Gastroenterol,* 2020.

Grabnar M, Tiwari M, Vallabh J: Brachioradial pruritis due to cervical spine pathology, *JMIR Dermatology* 5(3):e39863, 2022.

Huang AH, Kaffenberger BH, Reich A, Szepietowski JC, Ständer S, Kwatra SG: Pruritus associated with commonly prescribed medications in a tertiary care center, *Medicines (Basel)* 6(3):84, 2019.

Kini SP, DeLong LK, Veledar E, McKenzie-Brown AM, Schaufele M, Chen SC: The impact of pruritus on quality of life: the skin equivalent of pain, *Arch Dermatol* 147(10):1153–1156, 2011.

Sutaria N, Adawi W, Goldberg R, et al: Itch: pathogenesis and treatment, *J Am Acad Dermatol* 86:17–34, 2022.

Yosipovitch G, Bernhard J: Chronic pruritis, *N Engl J Med* 368:1625–1634, 2013.

Voicu C, Tebeica T, Zanardelli M, et al: Lichen simplex chronicus as an essential part of the dermatologic masquerade, *Open Access Maced J Med Sci* 5(4):556–557, 2017. https://www.itchforum.net/general-info/itch/.

[1] Not FDA approved for this indication.

RHINITIS

Method of
Masayoshi Takashima, MD; and Daniel Gorelik, MD

Introduction

Rhinitis is defined as inflammation of the nasal mucous membranes. Despite the definition of rhinitis, there are both inflammatory and noninflammatory forms of rhinitis. Rhinitis presents as one or more of the symptoms of nasal congestion, sneezing, itching, rhinorrhea, and/or postnasal drainage. It can be divided into allergic rhinitis (AR) and nonallergic rhinitis (NAR). Often patients will have a mixed rhinitis, which has components of both allergic and nonallergic disease. AR is nasal inflammation that is mediated by immunoglobulin (Ig)E to environmental allergens. NAR is defined by non–IgE-mediated perennial symptoms. NAR shares symptoms with AR but is only distinguishable by negative allergy tests. NAR includes a broad group of diseases including vasomotor rhinitis, gustatory rhinitis, NAR with eosinophilia syndrome (NARES), occupational rhinitis, hormonal rhinitis, drug-induced rhinitis, atrophic rhinitis, and infectious rhinitis.

Most research still classifies AR according to its seasonality or its perennial nature. Seasonal AR is commonly caused by pollen allergens; perennial AR is mainly caused by dust mites and animal dander. AR can be further classified as mild or moderate/severe. Mild rhinitis is rhinitis that does not impair work, school, daily functioning, or sleep. Moderate to severe rhinitis interferes with activities of daily living, quality of life, and/or sleep. Episodic AR occurs with sporadic inhalant aeroallergen exposure not typically encountered by the patient's usual indoor and outdoor environments. Both AR and NAR can also be classified based on symptom frequency, intermittent (<4 days/week or <4 consecutive weeks/year) versus persistent (>4 days/week and >4 consecutive weeks/year).

Local allergic rhinitis (LAR) is a newly defined entity found in nonatopic patients. LAR is characterized by local inflammatory reactions including local eosinophils and localized IgE in response to aeroallergens. LAR does not show significant skin-prick testing reactions, and patients have negative systemic IgE reactions to aeroallergens.

Rhinitis may be viewed by some as a trivial disease, but it places a significant financial burden on society. The estimated direct and indirect costs to society of rhinitis were around $11.58 billion in 2002. There is a significant loss of work and school days and decreased productivity and school performance. It is estimated at least 20% to 33% decrease in productivity when patients with AR have an exacerbation of their symptoms. Patients also report significant decreased quality of life related to their rhinitis symptoms including disturbed sleep, daytime somnolence, fatigue, irritability, depression, impairment of physical and social functioning, impairment of attention and memory, and learning deficits. Appropriate recognition, diagnosis, and treatment can help alleviate these economic and societal costs.

Epidemiology/Risk Factors

The National Health and Nutrition Survey (NHANES II and III) suggests that the overall prevalence of IgE sensitivity might be increasing. Of the patients evaluated for rhinitis in the United States, 43% (58 million people) have allergic disease, 23% (19 million people) have nonallergic disease, and 34% (26 million people) have mixed rhinitis. It is estimated the prevalence of physician-diagnosed AR is up to 20% of the population and 17% to 52% for NAR. Seventy percent of allergic patients develop the disease in childhood (20 years and younger) as opposed to NAR patients, 70% of whom develop disease in adulthood. Approximately two-thirds of NAR patients have vasomotor rhinitis, and one-third have NARES. NAR has a female predominance.

Pathophysiology

Allergic

Allergic rhinitis is the result of an IgE-mediated, type I hypersensitivity allergic reaction in response to an inhaled allergen. Allergens are proteins derived from airborne particulate matter, including dust mite feces, pollens, animal dander, and cockroach particles. Antigen presenting cells (APCs) engulf allergens, break them down, and then present these peptides to T cells (THO). These cells differentiate into the TH2 subtype and generate cytokines that regulate B lymphocytes and sequester inflammatory cells (including eosinophils). B lymphocytes produce IgE, which attach to mast cells and basophils and render them sensitized. When mast cells and basophils are exposed to the specific allergen, they degranulate and release a host of inflammatory mediators including histamine and prostaglandin. Histamine stimulates histamine type I (H1) receptors on nerve endings that cause pruritus, sneezing, and increased secretions, which constitute the early phase response of AR (minutes to 1 hour).

Eosinophils produce interleukin (IL)-5, which acts to promote activation and survival of other eosinophils. Eosinophils also produce toxic products, which damages the mucosal cells and causes nasal congestion. This damage occurs several hours after allergen exposure and constitutes the late phase.

Nonallergic Rhinitis

The nasal mucosa has two major functions: One is trapping inhaled particles through mucus production and the second is humidifying inhaled air through a complex vascular system. The mucus glands and the vascular system are regulated by the parasympathetic and the adrenergic nervous systems. Sensory nerves are stimulated by irritants in the nose through the use of a sensory receptor called a nociceptor. The nociceptive signal generates a neural reflex in the central nervous system (CNS) controlling sympathetic and parasympathetic tone in the nasal mucosa. Parasympathetic stimulation results in mucus production. Sympathetic stimulation causes vasoconstriction, which empties venous cavities. Lack of sympathetic tone causes venous engorgement and nasal congestion.

Symptomatic NAR is an exaggeration of a normal defensive mechanism. Inflammation in the nose causes an upregulation of this neural activity, resulting in the exaggerated response (also known as neural hyperresponsiveness). Hyperresponsive parasympathetic efferent nerves trigger glandular activation in the nasal mucosa, leading to vasodilation and mucus production. Excessive mucus production anteriorly causes rhinorrhea and posteriorly causes postnasal drip. This hyperresponsiveness can be due to structural or functional components of the nasal mucosa altered through genetic or pathologic factors. NAR is often associated with hyperreactivity of the nasal mucosa but the exact mechanisms is often different based on the specific type of NAR. Broadly speaking, NAR is defined as rhinitis independent of an IgE-mediated mechanism.

Infectious Rhinitis

Most infectious causes of rhinitis occur as a viral upper respiratory infection. Viruses may account for more than 95% of acute rhinitis infections, but it can be difficult to distinguish viral from bacterial infections. Viral rhinitis infections often cause nasal mucosal edema, impairment of the ciliary movement, and often obstruction of the sinonasal cavities. Duration of symptoms greater than 7 to 10 days is used clinically to distinguish viral from bacterial rhinitis/rhinosinusitis.

Clinical History

The best diagnostic tool in the evaluation of rhinitis is the clinical history. Information regarding previous evaluation and treatment should be elicited. A positive family history of rhinitis points toward allergic disease. The history of symptoms should include questions regarding congestion; sneezing; rhinorrhea; sore throat; dry throat; cough; itchy, red, or tearing eyes; voice changes; sinus symptoms of drainage; pressure or pain; snoring; ear pain or loss of hearing; and smelling difficulty.

When gathering the details of each symptom, evaluate the onset (such as those in childhood), frequency (episodic vs. persistent), pattern (seasonality), characteristics of secretions, triggers, severity (to include quality of life evaluation), and associated geographic location or environment (home vs. work). Once a trigger

TABLE 1	Clinical Manifestations of Rhinitis
TYPE OF RHINITIS	**CLINICAL FINDINGS**
Allergic rhinitis	• Symptoms of palatal itching, nasal itching, ocular symptoms, or sneezing • Allergic shiners, allergic salute, bluish boggy turbinates, mucosal stranding
Vasomotor rhinitis	• Predominantly intermittent nasal obstruction and rhinorrhea • Symptoms triggered by temperature, exercise, and environmental stimuli (odors, smoke, and dust).
NARES	• More intense symptoms, paroxysms of flares including sneezing, watery rhinorrhea, nasal itching, congestion, and hyposmia • Eosinophils on a nasal smear, but lack other allergic evidence by skin-prick testing
Gustatory rhinitis	• Nasal congestion and rhinorrhea associated with ingestion of foods and, sometimes, alcoholic beverages
Atrophic rhinitis	• Nasal crusting, dryness, and fetor due to glandular cell atrophy • Patients may have abnormally wide nasal cavities with associated squamous metaplasia
Occupational rhinitis	• Symptoms of nasal congestion and rhinorrhea triggered by an occupational exposure • Symptoms improve when away from occupation • Common substances leading to symptoms include irritating chemicals, grain dust, ozone, laboratory animal antigens, and wood
Hormonal rhinitis	• Symptoms of nasal congestion and rhinorrhea associated with pregnancy and/or menstrual cycle • Resolves 2 weeks postdelivery
Drug-induced rhinitis	• Symptoms of rhinorrhea and congestion caused by certain medications including ACE inhibitors, phosphodiesterase-5 selective inhibitors, alpha-receptor antagonists, and phentolamine
Rhinitis Medicamentosa	• Symptoms of severe rebound nasal congestion caused by prolonged and repetitive use of topical nasal decongestants
Infectious rhinitis	• Symptoms of acute-onset nasal congestion and rhinorrhea most often caused by virus. Bacterial overgrowth from virus-induced inflammation can lead to bacterial rhinosinusitis

ACE, Angiotensin-converting enzyme; *NARES,* nonallergic rhinitis with eosinophilia syndrome.

is identified, history needs to be gathered even further to evaluate the possibility of modifying the exposure.

Physical Examination

As with any disease process, the physical examination provides clues into the diagnosis (Table 1). Although the physical examination in rhinitis patients should focus on the nasal mucosa, other body areas should be examined to rule out other processes. For example, the tympanic membranes should be examined for mobility, retraction, erythema, and Eustachian tube dysfunction. Examination of the eyes in AR might show conjunctival edema, erythema, and/or cobblestoning with excessive lacrimation. Patients with AR may also have darkening of the skin of the lower eyelids, which is also called "allergic shiners."

A nasal examination is essential for the diagnosis of rhinitis. Otolaryngologists will often use nasal endoscopy to evaluate the sinonasal cavity, but it is not necessary to diagnose different forms of rhinitis. Allergic and nonallergic nasal mucosa often will have a similar appearance with boggy, enlarged, and erythematous inferior turbinates. Bluish turbinates with allergic stranding are more common in AR. Evidence of excessive watery-clear mucus and postnasal drainage are also common findings to rhinitis. Other examination findings, which can occur in conjunction with rhinitis, are nasal polyps, sinusitis, septal deviation, septal perforation, and crusting. Looking for elongated facies, mouth breathing, and a high arch in the palate may provide a clue to the severity of the nasal obstruction in children. The tonsils and adenoids should be examined for enlargement. Posterior nasal drainage and cobblestoning in the oropharynx are common findings in rhinitis patients.

The skin examination provides useful information in the patient with AR. Atopic dermatitis or urticaria may be findings associated with allergic disease. The skin should be evaluated for dermatographism because these patients will not be able to be evaluated for allergic disease using skin-prick testing.

Diagnosis

The diagnosis of AR, NAR, and infectious rhinitis is based largely on history and physical examination. Other diagnostic testing can be performed to aid in providing a more definitive diagnosis or to rule out other causes.

AR is confirmed by IgE reactivity to environmental allergen sensitivity through skin-prick testing. When skin-prick testing is difficult to interpret or if it is not feasible, serum–allergen-specific IgE testing can be used. Nasal smears looking for eosinophils are not recommended for routine use in the diagnosis of AR. Other testing available for evaluation of rhinitis includes nasal endoscopy and radiologic imaging. Nasal endoscopy is reserved for those with atypical symptoms or an inadequate response to treatment. Radiologic imaging, such as computed tomography (CT) and magnetic resonance imaging (MRI), is used to evaluate anatomic structure and for evidence of concomitant rhinosinusitis but it is not recommended for the diagnosis of AR. If a provider suspects a cerebrospinal fluid (CSF) leak, the rhinorrhea can be evaluated for beta transferrin protein, which is present only in CSF.

Differential Diagnosis

The differential for chronic rhinitis symptoms includes AR, NAR and the many subtypes described earlier, and mixed rhinitis. Many different pathologic conditions can present similarly to rhinitis including chronic sinusitis with and without nasal polyps; ciliary dyskinesia syndrome; anatomic abnormalities such as deviated septum or septal perforation; sinonasal tumors; nasal turbinate hypertrophy; cerebrospinal fluid rhinorrhea; pharyngonasal reflux; systemic disorders such as vasculitis, sarcoidosis, and autoimmune disorders; aspirin intolerance, and other medication side effects.

Treatment

Overall

Current guidelines in treatment of rhinitis do not take cost into consideration. However, the individual treatment goals should be based on factors such as age, route of administration preference (i.e., nasal vs. oral), severity, seasonality, side effects, cost, benefit to comorbid conditions, and onset of action. For example, onset of action is an important consideration for an individual who has more episodic symptoms. Also, individual patients respond differently to treatment regimens within a given group.

Avoidance

Due to the lack of high-quality evidence, implementation of avoidance measures is largely based on panel recommendations. In addition, the ubiquitous nature of allergens may limit the effectiveness of the avoidance measures. For dust mites, encasing pillows and bedding in dust mite–resistant materials may be beneficial. Pollen is seasonal and can be minimized by keeping the windows closed, using air conditioning, and limiting outdoor exposure. Using particulate filters in the home can also assist in reducing overall allergen load of pollens and dust. Avoiding basements and lowering household humidity may reduce the amount of mold exposure patients receive. Pet avoidance can only be reached by ridding the house of the pet altogether. Other, less effective measures include limiting exposure of the pet to the house and/or bedroom.

Oral Medications

Oral Antihistamine
Oral antihistamines block H1 receptors, thereby reducing nasal and palatal itching, rhinorrhea, sneezing, conjunctivitis, and urticaria. They are recommended in the treatment of AR. However, nasal congestion is not treated well with oral antihistamines. First-generation oral antihistamines are poorly selective for H1 receptors. The sedative effects of these antihistamines result from crossing the blood–brain barrier; they have been linked to industrial accidents and contribute to loss of function at work and school. Given there is no evidence of increased efficacy over second-generation antihistamines, it is not recommended to use these medications. Second-generation H1 antagonists (e.g., cetirizine [Zyrtec, generic], levocetirizine [Xyzal, generic], fexofenadine [Allegra, generic], loratadine [Claritin, generic], desloratadine [Clarinex, generic]) have excellent evidence for therapeutic efficacy and are considered first line in the treatment of AR. They particularly help the systemic symptoms associated with AR. These medications may have some role in the treatment of NAR because of their anticholinergic properties, but consideration must be given to these systemic properties, including dry mucous membranes, blurry vision, constipation, tachycardia, and urinary retention. A combination of intranasal corticosteroid treatment with oral antihistamines may be effective for sneezing and rhinorrhea in NARES.

Leukotriene Receptor Antagonists
Currently leukotriene receptor antagonists (LTRAs) are not recommended as first-line treatment for AR and are only recommended if other first-line treatments have failed. These medications were originally found to have benefits in the treatment of asthma and thus are prescribed for concomitant asthma and AR. Montelukast (Singulair, generic) is the only US Food and Drug Administration (FDA) approved form of LTRA that is clinically efficacious in perennial and seasonal AR and asthma. Montelukast is approved for children 6 months and older and has a pregnancy category B rating. However, because of the potential rare neuropsychiatric side effects including sleep disturbances, depression, anxiety, aggression, psychotic reactions, and suicidal behavior this class of medications are used as second line. Currently LTRAs have no role in the treatment of NAR.

Oral Decongestants
Oral decongestants such as pseudoephedrine reduce nasal congestion and can temporarily relieve symptoms. They can cause significant side effects including insomnia, anorexia, irritability, palpitations, and elevation in blood pressure. They are not routinely used for the treatment for AR and NAR but can help temporarily alleviate symptoms of nasal congestion in severe disease in conjunction with oral antihistamines.

Systemic Corticosteroids
Systemic corticosteroids are only recommended for the treatment of severe or intractable AR. A short 5-to 7-day course is recommended in severe cases to help decrease inflammation to allow better penetration via intranasal therapy and improve symptoms. A prolonged course greater than 3 weeks can lead to serious side effects including adrenal suppression. They have no role in the treatment of NAR.

Intranasal Medications
Intranasal Corticosteroid. Intranasal corticosteroids (INCs) are first-line treatment for moderate to severe AR and most NAR conditions. They penetrate the nasal mucosa with the result of decreased neutrophil chemotaxis, decreased eosinophil chemotaxis, reduced mast cell mediator release, and reduced basophil mediator release. Fluticasone (Flonase, generic) and beclomethasone (Beconase AQ) are the only two topical INCs approved by the FDA for NAR. In general, this class of medications are well tolerated with minimal systemic side effects.

INC side effects include irritation, bleeding, and perforation of the nasal septum; rarely, local candidiasis is seen with INC use. No single INC preparation is more efficacious than, or has any relevant difference from, any other. INC has negligible hypothalamic-pituitary-adrenal axis suppression, and systemic burden is clinically insignificant.

Intranasal Antihistamine. Azelastine (Astepro, generic) and olapatadine (Patanase, generic) are nasal sprays approved by the FDA for AR and NAR. Azelastine, considered a first-line treatment for AR, is available in 0.1% and 0.15% formulations and is thought to improve symptoms because of its antiinflammatory properties. This medication has been shown to diminish eosinophil activation and adhesion molecule expression and suppresses generation of inflammatory cytokines. Azelastine may also reduce neurogenic excitation from olfactory stimuli. These medications have a faster onset of action than INCs and are as effective in the treatment of nasal symptoms. They are more effective and have a faster onset of action than oral antihistamines for the treatment of nasal symptoms associated with AR. Intranasal antihistamine (INA) does not produce a significant amount of sedation, but side effects include headache, epistaxis, bitter taste, and nasal irritation.

Combination Intranasal Antihistamine and Intranasal Corticosteroids. The combined use of INCs and intranasal topical antihistamines is considered to be an effective treatment for both AR and NAR. It is more effective than either medication alone. The combination of the two medications can be given separately or through a combined spray with azelastine (137 mcg) and fluticasone propionate (50 mcg) called Dymista. It is currently recommended to use combination INAs and INCs for moderate to severe AR or NAR[1] that is resistant to monotherapy. The combination therapy is more effective in relieving total nasal symptom score including nasal congestion and obstruction than either drug alone.

Intranasal Anticholinergic. Ipratropium bromide (Atrovent) is the only FDA approved intranasal anticholinergic that inhibits parasympathetic function in the nasal mucosa. The parasympathetic blockade reduces the output of secretions from seromucous glands in the nose. It is mainly used in the treatment of anterior watery rhinorrhea but has a very limited role in reducing postnasal drip, nasal congestion, or sneezing. This medication is especially helpful in gustatory rhinitis and vasomotor rhinitis where there is a specific trigger for the onset of rhinorrhea. Patients can take this medication prophylactically prior to exposure of the known trigger or irritant to help control symptoms.

Nasal Cromolyn. Cromolyn (NasalCrom, generic) is a mast cell stabilizer and inhibits the release of mast cell mediators that promote IgE-mediated AR. It should be given prophylactically prior to allergen exposure in order to reduce symptoms of AR from episodic allergen exposure. It has a favorable safety profile and is considered if first-line treatments are not effective. Cromolyn has very limited usefulness for NAR conditions.

Nasal Saline. Using nasal saline to irrigate the nasal cavities helps remove mucus, enhance ciliary movement, remove allergic and irritant particles, and moisturize the dry nasal passages. There are multiple delivery methods including nose spray, bottle, pump, irrigation, or nebulizer. However, the delivery method, volume, and isotonic or hypertonic use has not been established for the treatment of AR. There is evidence that saline irrigation for AR may reduce patient-reported disease severity compared with no saline irrigation at 3 months of treatment.

Topical Decongestants. Topical decongestants reduce congestion but have no effect on itching, sneezing, or rhinorrhea. Oxymetazoline (Afrin, generic), a common topical decongestant, causes nasal vasoconstriction and can be used as a rescue medication for severe nasal congestion symptoms. There is risk for rebound congestion with prolonged use greater than 2 to 3 days and is not routinely recommended for the treatment of AR and NAR.

---

[1]Not FDA approved for this indication.

Surgery and Procedures for Allergic and Nonallergic Rhinitis

The role of surgery in the treatment and management of both AR and NAR is to improve symptoms that occur as a result of the disease processes rather than treat the underlying disease. Patients with symptoms of nasal obstruction and congestion will get improvement with septoplasty (if deviated and causing obstruction) and turbinate reduction. There are multiple methods to reduce the inferior turbinate, which include minimally invasive radiofrequency ablations to partial resection of the turbinate. Recently there is evidence that reduction of enlarged nasal septal swell body and nasal vestibular swell bodies can improve symptoms of nasal congestion.

Traditionally, patients with vasomotor rhinitis can also be treated with endoscopic Vidian or posterior nasal neurectomy, which improves rhinorrhea and nasal obstruction in 90% of patients. There are risks involved in this surgery including dry eye and cheek and palate numbness, which usually resolve within 6 months of the procedure. This surgery has fallen out of favor to newer in-office techniques including cryoablation and radiofrequency ablation of the posterior nasal nerve (Clarifix and Rhinaer). These procedures can be done under local anesthesia and have shown to significantly improve total nasal symptom score including nasal congestion and rhinorrhea. They are FDA approved for the treatment of chronic rhinitis and vasomotor rhinitis. There is a growing body of evidence that in-office posterior nasal nerve ablation is effective for the treatment of allergic rhinitis. It is important to consider nasal anatomy, given the differences in efficacy due to anatomic variations in nasal structures and the extensive branching of the posterior nasal nerves.

Anti-IgE Therapy

Omalizumab (Xolair) is a monoclonal antibody available for the treatment of poorly controlled asthma, but it might have a role in the treatment of AR.[1] Omalizumab binds to IgE, hindering its relationship with inflammatory cells. Omalizumab only binds to circulating IgE and not bound IgE. Due to its high cost, reports of anaphylaxis, and its injectable-only formulation, omalizumab has a limited role in AR treatment.

Immunotherapy

Allergen extract immunotherapy has been used in the treatment of respiratory allergic disease since 1911, and its efficacy has been documented since the 1970s. The amount of allergen in each immunotherapy dose is slowly increased with each dose until a maintenance phase is reached. Immunotherapy is an effective treatment for AR and is the only treatment proven to alter the course of allergic disease. Debate exists regarding which form of immunotherapy is superior (subcutaneous vs. sublingual). Contraindications to immunotherapy include beta blocker use, due to complications in treating anaphylaxis, and uncontrolled underlying diseases, such as uncontrolled asthma.

Subcutaneous immunotherapy uses the injectable form of allergen extract. Adequate treatment usually consists of a 3- to 5-year course of immunotherapy. Subcutaneous immunotherapy is indicated in those patients for whom medications and avoidance measures are inadequate, as well as those with only a few relevant allergens. The inherent risk of subcutaneous immunotherapy is systemic anaphylaxis; therefore it is dosed in the physician's office. The rate of local reactions in subcutaneous immunotherapy is 0.6% to 58% and systemic reactions is 0.06% to 0.9%. Subcutaneous immunotherapy is covered by most insurance plans.

Studies for local-route immunotherapy (noninjected), many of which were carried out in Europe, have only been undertaken in adults. Local routes of immunotherapy include sublingual, local nasal, oral, and bronchial.

Sublingual immunotherapy was approved by the FDA in April 2014. The risk profile is low and therefore can be dosed at home. The rate of local reactions with sublingual immunotherapy is 0.2% to 97% and systemic reactions is 0.056%. Multiple large meta-analyses have found noninferiority when comparing sublingual to subcutaneous immunotherapy. Some medical allergy providers use subcutaneous extracts (aqueous) as sublingual therapy, but this is an off-label use.

Alternative Treatments

Acupuncture. Acupuncture aims to address AR symptoms, including nasal congestion, and is widely offered as a complementary therapy to pharmacotherapy. This is considered a safe therapy with minimal adverse reactions, although multiple sessions are required for effect. Electroacupuncture involves directing small electrical pulses through needles and can interfere with implantable devices, so this needs to be considered. The mechanism of action for acupuncture remains poorly understood despite its widespread use, but it may have a role in modulating IgE and IL-10 levels. Several systematic reviews have reported equivocal data as to the true effect of acupuncture, but given its low-risk profile, it is supported as an adjunct option to existing therapies.

Monitoring

The provider should consider stepping down treatment when the patient's symptoms have been controlled. The Total Nasal Symptom Score (TNSS) is a subjective assessment of the patient's specific symptoms, including rhinorrhea, nasal congestion, sneezing, and pruritus, and can be used to assess effectiveness of medications. The Rhinoconjunctivitis Quality of Life Questionnaire can also be used. Consideration for referral to an allergist might be extended to patients who have had a prolonged course, secondary infections, polyps, or other comorbid conditions including chronic sinusitis and asthma, or if immunotherapy is a consideration.

References

Brinkhaus B, Witt CM, Jena S, Liecker B, Wegscheider K, Willich SN. Acupuncture in patients with allergic rhinitis: a pragmatic randomized trial. *Ann Allergy Asthma Immunol.* 101(5):535–543, 2008.

Brozek J, Bousquet J, Baena-Cagnani C, et al: Allergic rhinitis and its impact on asthma (ARIA) guidelines: 2010 revision, *J Allergy Clin Immunol* 126:466–476, 2010.

Chaaban M, Corey J: Pharmacotherapy of rhinitis and rhinosinusitis, *Facial Plast Surg Clin North Am* 20:61–71, 2012.

Cox L, Compalati E, Canonica W: Will sublingual immunotherapy become an approved treatment method in the United States? *Curr Allergy Asthma Rep* 11:4–6, 2011.

Davies C, Gorelik D, Lane AP, Takashima M, Ahmed OG. Is posterior nasal nerve ablation effective in treating symptoms of allergic rhinitis?. *Laryngoscope.* 132(12):2295–2298, 2022.

Dykewicz M: Management of rhinitis: guidelines, evidence basis, and systematic clinical approach for what we do, *Immunol Allergy Clin North Am* 31:619–634, 2011.

Dykewicz MS, Wallace DV, Amrol DJ, et al: Rhinitis 2020: a practice parameter update, *J Allergy Clin Immunol* 146(4):721–767, 2020, https://doi.org/10.1016/j.jaci.2020.07.007. Epub 2020 Jul 22. Review.

Fan T, Chandna M, Gorelik D, et al. Correlation between middle turbinate insertion in relation to sphenopalatine foramen and failure rates of cryotherapy and radiofrequency treatment for chronic rhinitis. *Int Forum Allergy Rhinol.* 13(1):88–91, 2023.

Greiner A, Meltzer E: Overview of the treatment of allergic rhinitis and nonallergic rhinopathy, *Proc Am Thorac Soc* 8:121–131, 2011.

Hellings PW, Klimek L, Cingi C, et al: Non-allergic rhinitis: position paper of the European Academy of Allergy and Clinical Immunology, 72:1657–1665, 2017.

Meltzer EO, LaForce C, Ratner P, et al: MP29-02 (a novel intranasal formulation of azelastine hydrochloride and fluticasone propionate) in the treatment of seasonal allergic rhinitis: a randomized, double-blind, placebo-controlled trial of efficacy and safety, 33:324–332, 2012.

Rondon C, Campo P, Galindo L, et al: Prevalence and clinic relevance of local allergic rhinitis, *Allergy* 67:1282–1288, 2012, https://doi.org/10.1111/all.12002.

Seidman MD, Schwartz SR, Bonner JR, et al: Clinical practice guideline: allergic rhinitis, *Otolaryngol Head Neck Surg* 152(1 Suppl):S1–S43, 2015.

Sertel S, Bergmann Z, Ratzlaff K, Baumann I, Greten HJ, Plinkert PK. Acupuncture for nasal congestion: a prospective, randomized, double-blind, placebo-controlled clinical pilot study. *Am J Rhinol Allergy.* 23(6):e23–e28, 2009.

Settipane R, Charnock D: Epidemiology of rhinitis: allergic and nonallergic, *Clin Allergy Immunol* 19:23–34, 2007.

Sin B, Togias A: Pathophysiology of allergic and nonallergic rhinitis, *Proc Am Thorac Soc* 8:106–114, 2011.

van Cauwenberge P, Bachert C, Passalacqua G, et al: Consensus statement on the treatment of allergic rhinitis. European Academy of Allergology and Clinical Immunology, *Allergy* 55:116–134, 2000.

Wallace D, Dykewicz M: The diagnosis and management of rhinitis: an updated practice parameter, *J Allergy Clin Immunol* 122:S1–S84, 2008. Young-Yuen.

Wise SK, Damask C, Roland LT, et al. International consensus statement on allergy and rhinology: allergic rhinitis - 2023 [published online ahead of print, 2023 Mar 6]. *Int Forum Allergy Rhinol.* 2023.

Wu A: Immunotherapy: vaccines for allergic disease, *J Thorac Dis* 4:198–202, 2012.

Yan CH, Hwang PH: Surgical management of nonallergic rhinitis, *Otolaryngol Clin North Am* 51(5):945–955, 2018.

---

[1]Not FDA approved for this indication.

SPINE PAIN

Method of
David Borenstein, MD; and Federico Balagué, MD

CURRENT DIAGNOSIS

- Most spine pain is mechanical in origin in 95% or more of patients.
- Symptoms of mechanical acute spine pain resolve in most patients in 1 to 8 weeks.
- Most patients with spine pain do not require laboratory tests or radiographs to achieve resolution of their symptom of spine pain.

CURRENT THERAPY

- Localized neck or low back pain
  - Encouragement to remain active out of bed
  - Patient education about the natural history to improvement
  - Reassurance about the incidence of resolution
  - Effective oral drug therapy: nonsteroidal antiinflammatory drugs (NSAIDs), analgesics, muscle relaxants
  - Physical therapy with exercise program
- Radicular pain
  - Encouragement to remain active out of bed
  - Patient education about the potential for improvement
  - Efficacy of oral drug therapy: NSAIDs, analgesics, muscle relaxants, corticosteroids, antiseizure medication, epidural corticosteroid injections
  - Physical therapy: Mackenzie exercises for disk herniation (https://sportsrehab.ucsf.edu/sites/sportsrehab.ucsf.edu/files/Mckenzie%20Back%20Protocol.pdf)
  - Surgical decompression for cauda equina, progressive motor weakness, or intractable pain

Spine pain is a common symptom that is diagnosed and treated by a wide variety of healthcare professionals. The interest in this medical problem is not limited to its incidence as a patient problem but also stems from the likelihood of spine pain being experienced by the treating physician as well. The good news about spine pain is that the vast majority of patients (about 90%) improve over 2 months with minimal intervention, but relapses are frequent. The bad news is that the smaller number of patients who develop chronic spine pain use more than the majority of health resources expended on this expensive medical problem. The goal of therapy is to relieve spine pain while it is acute so that chronic pain does not develop.

The axial skeleton may be divided into cervical, thoracic, lumbar, sacral, and coccygeal locations. The lumbar and cervical areas are the most mobile and at greatest risk for damage. These two areas will be the primary subjects of this article.

Epidemiology

Spine pain is the most common musculoskeletal complaint worldwide and produces direct and indirect costs of hundreds of billions of dollars each year in the United States. More than 80% of the world's population at some time during their lives will have an episode of low back pain. An estimated 20% of the US population has back pain every year. Neck pain occurs at a variable rate ranging from 0.055/1000 person-years (disk herniation with radiculopathy) to 213/1000 person-years (self-reported neck pain). Thoracic spine pain is relatively rare compared with the incidence of pain in the other two locations in the axial skeleton.

Persons of all ages develop spine pain. Younger people are at risk for developmental problems (idiopathic scoliosis, spondylolysis,

spondylolisthesis), and older patients develop disorders associated with degeneration of spinal structures (osteoarthritis, spinal stenosis).

Risk Factors

Psychosocial factors are stronger predictors of incident low back pain than mechanical factors in adolescent populations. In adults, psychosocial difficulties are risk factors for chronicity more strongly related to outcome than any clinical or mechanical variables. Previous episodes of spine pain are strong predictors of future ones.

Studies of cohorts of twins have shown that nonspecific low back pain is more than 60% genetically determined, and work and leisure-time physical activities play a minor role. Other environmental factors, such as smoking and obesity, have not been shown to be a predictor of the development of spine pain on a consistent basis.

Pathophysiology

Most of the structures of the axial skeleton receive sensory input. The presence of anatomic alterations in these structures is not sufficient to predict the presence of pain. In general, spine pain is referred to as nonspecific because no definite pain generator can be identified. The nociceptive inputs generated by musculoskeletal structures are referred to as *somatic pain*.

In the first few decades of life, muscular sprains and strains of the paraspinous muscles in the lumbar and cervical regions are the most likely source of spinal pain. These muscular injuries occur when lifting in a position that places stress on paraspinous structures. Often the spine is in an awkward position and is mechanically disadvantaged. The subsequent muscle injury results in reflexive muscular contraction that can recruit muscles in the same myotome. Tonic contraction approximates the damaged components of the muscle but results in relative anoxia that causes the production of anaerobic metabolites that stimulate nociceptors. The number of recruited muscles may be extensive, manifested by severe spinal stiffness and limitation of motion. Most of these soft-tissue injuries to the muscle heal spontaneously without any long-term structural alterations.

Simultaneously, as people age, intervertebral disks become flatter as the nucleus pulposus loses its absorbency and the annulus fibrosus fissures and degenerates. The process results in the loss of disk integrity. Degeneration of normal biomechanical and biochemical disk properties results. Biomechanical insufficiency inevitably results in a transfer of stresses posterior to the facet joints and ligaments that are ill suited to assume compressive, tensile, and shear loads. Osteophytes form in response to these abnormal pressures, compromising the space for the neural elements. Disk degeneration itself might not be a painful process until alterations in facet joint alignment result in the onset of articular pain.

Spondylolysis is a developmental abnormality associated with a stress fracture in the growth plate of the pars interarticularis. This abnormality may be discovered as a radiographic abnormality in an asymptomatic patient. An increased risk of low back pain occurs with spondylolisthesis, the abnormality associated with instability of spinal elements in the setting of spondylolysis.

Pain generation in the axial skeleton may be somatic or neuropathic in origin. The joints, ligaments, muscles, fascia, blood vessels, and disks can be the source of localized somatic spine pain. Somatic pain, when it does radiate, tends to be less focused in distribution and exacerbated by specific positions of the spine.

Neuropathic or radicular pain is the sensation generated by damage of neural elements. Intervertebral disk herniation with compression of spinal nerve roots causes neural inflammation resulting in neuropathic and radicular pain. Radicular pain follows the path of the corresponding spinal nerve root. In addition to pain, sensory deficits and muscle weakness can occur, depending on the intensity of the nerve compression. In the setting of chronic low back pain, the role of the central nervous system in

TABLE 1 Mechanical Low Back Pain

FEATURE	MUSCLE STRAIN	HERNIATED NUCLEUS PULPOSUS	OSTEOARTHRITIS	SPINAL STENOSIS	SPONDYLOLISTHESIS	SCOLIOSIS
Age (year)	20–40	30–50	> 50	> 60	20	30
Pain Pattern						
Location	Back (unilateral)	Back/leg (unilateral)	Back (unilateral)	Leg (bilateral)	Back	Back
Onset	Acute	Acute (previous episodes)	Insidious	Insidious	Insidious	Insidious
Standing	↑	↓	↑	↑	↑	↑
Sitting	↓	↑	↓	↓	↓	↓
Bending	↑	↑	↓	↓	↑	↑
Straight leg	–	+	–	+ (stress)	–	–
Plain radiograph*	–	–	+	+	+	+

↑, Increased; ↓, decreased; +, present; –, absent.
*Possibility of seeing the abnormality, not a recommendation to get radiographs.
Reprinted with permission from Mechanical low back pain. In Borenstein DG, Wiesel SW, Boden SD (eds): Low back and neck pain, 3rd ed., Philadelphia, Saunders, 2004.

mediating persistent symptoms has been highlighted increasingly in the medical literature.

Prevention

Since the turn of the century, epidemiologic studies in adolescents have reported nonspecific spine pain at an incidence similar to that in adult populations. This finding suggests that primary prevention must be given at a very early age to have any chance of efficacy.

Among papers reporting on primary prevention, only exercise has shown effectiveness, with effect sizes ranging from 0.39 to 0.69. Other techniques, such as stress management, shoe inserts, back supports, education, and reduced lifting, were found ineffective. Some evidence in favor of occupational interventions (exercise with or without educational component) has been recently reported.

Clinical Manifestations

The most common symptoms of spinal disorders are regional pain and decreased range of motion associated in a minority of patients with radiating pain. For the majority of patients, pain has mechanical characteristics: Its intensity increases with physical activity, movements, or some postures and decreases with rest. However, it has been demonstrated that nocturnal pain is not uncommon in the absence of serious, specific spinal disorders. The precise topography of pain is often difficult for the patient to describe, and its interpretation is difficult owing to the overlap of the cutaneous projections between adjacent spinal levels and the similarities between dermatomes, myotomes, and sclerotomes.

Diagnosis

The diagnosis of spine pain is based upon the patient's history and physical examination. The history and physical examination should include a description of the pain that is as detailed as possible (e.g., past episodes, precise location, beginning of symptoms, factors increasing or decreasing pain intensity, radiating pain, neurologic symptoms, systemic symptoms), patient's medical history (e.g., past spinal surgery, neoplasia, corticosteroid treatments), and a limited physical examination focused on the posture of the spine, range of motion, muscle contraction, pain on palpation or percussion, and a brief neurologic examination.

Besides the high rate of false-positive results and financial costs, imaging studies have a negative effect on a patient's quality of life. Therefore unless there is a clear-cut surgical indication or a suspicion of an underlying life-threatening disorder, no imaging studies should be ordered on the first encounter for a patient with acute nonspecific low back or neck pain. Similarly,

laboratory testing is not required unless a patient presents with clinical symptoms that suggest a systemic illness (e.g., fever, weight loss).

Differential Diagnosis

A number of guidelines are available in the literature to help a clinician in the diagnosis and treatment of patients with spine pain. The purpose of these approaches is to differentiate the vast majority of patients with mechanical disorders who will improve with noninvasive therapy without the need for radiographic or laboratory investigation from the small minority with a specific cause of spinal pain.

Traditionally, red flags have been used to identify patients with a systemic disorder causing spine pain. The red flags have included questions regarding prior history of cancer, weight loss, prolonged morning stiffness, bladder dysfunction, and bowel dysfunction. The presence of these findings suggests a diagnosis of malignancy, infection, spondyloarthropathy, or cauda equina syndrome, respectively. A study has reported that red-flag disorders occur so infrequently and have so many false-positive findings as not to be helpful in the primary care setting at the initial visit. The one exception was spine pain associated with osteoporotic vertebral compression fractures.

Despite the findings of this one report, clinicians need to be mindful of patients who would be harmed to a significant degree by delayed therapy. The disorders that require expeditious evaluation and treatment are intraabdominal vascular disorders with tearing pain and hemodynamic instability (expanding aortic aneurysm); cauda equina syndrome with bilateral sciatica; saddle anesthesia; bladder or bowel incontinence (lumbar space-occupying compressive lesions); and cervical myelopathy with balance difficulties, autonomic dysfunction, and hyperreflexia with spasticity and Babinski's sign (cervical space-occupying compressive lesions). These disorders require expeditious vessel repair or decompression surgery.

The differential diagnosis of mechanical low back pain (Table 1) and mechanical neck pain (Table 2) includes disorders ranging from muscle strain and herniated disk to scoliosis and whiplash injuries. The age of patients, pain pattern with exacerbating and mitigating factors, tension signs, and findings of plain radiographs can help differentiate among these common causes of spine pain.

Nonspecific is a term used commonly to describe the pain associated with mechanical disorders. On occasion, physicians have confused the use of "nonspecific" as meaning an absence of pathology causing pain associated with mechanical disorders. The "nonspecific" designation refers to the inability to identify the specific pain-generating anatomic structure, not the absence of somatic pain.

TABLE 2 Mechanical Neck Pain

FEATURE	NECK STRAIN	HERNIATED NUCLEUS PULPOSUS	OSTEOARTHRITIS	MYELOPATHY	WHIPLASH
Age (year)	20–40	30–50	> 50	> 60	30–40
Pain Pattern					
Location	Neck	Neck/arm	Neck	Arm/leg	Neck
Onset	Acute	Acute	Insidious	Insidious	Acute
Flexion	+	+	–	–	+
Extension	–	+/–	+	+	+
Plain radiograph*	–	–	+	+	–

+, Present; –, absent.
*Possibility of seeing the abnormality, not a recommendation to get radiographs.
Reprinted with permission from Mechanical neck pain. In Borenstein DG, Wiesel SW, Boden SD (eds): Low back and neck pain, 3rd ed., Philadelphia, Saunders, 2004.

BOX 1 Management of Low Back Pain

Acute (3–6 Weeks)
First consultation: gather information on core outcome domains.
Rule out pain of nonspinal origin.
Rule out specific causes (red flags).
No routine imaging.
Inform and reassure the patient. Advise to stay active and continue daily activities, if possible, including work.
Prescribe analgesia, if necessary. First choice: acetaminophen; second choice: NSAIDs.
Consider adding muscle relaxants (short course) or referring for spinal manipulation.
Avoid overmedicalizing, especially in patients with favorable outcome.
Be aware of yellow flags: inappropriate attitudes and beliefs about back pain, inappropriate pain behavior, emotional problems.
Subacute (6–12 Weeks) Reassessment
Bear in mind minimum clinically important difference of core outcome tools.
Consider patients' expectations.
Consider yellow flags if outcome is not favorable.
Reassess regularly by valid outcome tools to evaluate response to treatment.
Focus on function.
Give priority to active treatments.
Consider multidisciplinary program in occupational setting for workers with subacute low back pain and sick leave (>4–8 weeks).

Chronic (3–12 Weeks)
Repeat thorough clinical examination.
In cases of low impairment and disability, simple evidence-based therapies (e.g., exercises, medication, brief interventions) might be sufficient.
In cases of more-severe disability or chronicity, give priority to multidisciplinary approaches (biopsychosocial).

NSAID, Nonsteroidal antiinflammatory drug.
From Balagué F, Mannion AF, Pellisé F, Cedraschi C: Clinical update: Low back pain. Lancet 369(9563):726–728, 2007.

Therapy

Many mechanical disorders of the spine are self-limited in duration, with a vast majority of patients improving gradually over time (Box 1). This progression to "natural healing" makes placebo look efficacious in many clinical trials investigating therapies for spine pain. This situation results in evidence-based reviews of spine pain therapies revealing very few categories that have a clinically significant impact on improvement. Nonetheless, physicians need to make therapeutic choices for their patients despite this relative paucity of evidence. Therapy for spine pain includes controlled physical activity, nonsteroidal antiinflammatory drugs (NSAIDs), skeletal muscle relaxants, local and epidural corticosteroid injections, and long-term pain therapy. Surgical intervention is reserved for patients who have surgically correctable abnormalities and who have cauda equina syndrome, increasing motor weakness, spasticity, or intractable pain.

The treatment of an individual patient has to be tailored based on the patient's expectations and preferences. Goals of the treatment should be clearly defined, and the patient should be informed about the expected benefits and side effects of the treatment at the first encounter. A short trial limited to a few days may be a good start.

Self-management with education of the patient about maintaining physical activities as tolerated has been encouraged for neck and low back pain. Information on nonpharmacologic pain-management strategies and daily life activities may be provided by healthcare providers, but patients adhere more to the former than to the latter.

Exercises are slightly effective for pain and function in patients with chronic low back pain. No specific form of exercise is clearly better than others. Simply walking has shown an efficacy similar to exercising.

The use of manipulative physical techniques in the care of patients with spine pain remains controversial. The absence of clear-cut distinctions between manipulative techniques with or without thrust adds to the confusion when one analyzes the efficacy of manual therapy treatments. Overall there is some clinical trial evidence in favor of spinal manipulation for acute low back pain.

NSAIDs have short-term efficacy for both acute and chronic low back pain; however, the effect sizes are not very large. The efficacy of these drugs for patients with radicular pain has not been evaluated well enough to make general recommendations. No single class of NSAIDs has superiority to another. Cyclooxygenase 2 (COX-2) inhibitors have a better gastrointestinal (GI) safety profile but no greater efficacy. A patient's response cannot be predicted, and a trial-and-error approach is often necessary.

Opiates have not demonstrated any favorable influence in the outcome of low back pain patients. Side effects are quite common and the risk of addiction is real. When these kinds of drugs are effective, the improvement is more important in pain intensity than in terms of function. Muscle relaxants do have some efficacy for acute and chronic low back pain, but the effect size is limited. Long-term use of muscle relaxants can effect cognitive function due to their strong anticholinergic effects.

Antidepressants are not generally prescribed owing to an inconsistent improvement of patients. For patients with chronic low back pain and depression, an optimized antidepressant treatment shows a better effect on depression than on pain and functional capacity. Duloxetine (Cymbalta), a serotonin and norepinephrine reuptake inhibitor, is approved by the US Food and Drug Administration for the indication of chronic low back pain.

Evidence is lacking to support the prescription of systemic corticosteroids. However, corticosteroids have the advantage of not being toxic to the kidneys. Oral corticosteroids may be considered in patients with radicular pain from a herniated disk or spinal stenosis where epidural injections are relatively contraindicated (chronic warfarin therapy).

Some patients will have persistent neuropathic pain despite surgical decompression or as a result of postsurgical fibrosis. Opioid therapy is ineffective in many patients with chronic neuropathic pain. Antiseizure medicines, such as gabapentin (Neurontin)[1] and pregabalin (Lyrica), have efficacy in peripheral neuropathic pain. These same medicines are prescribed in patients with chronic neuropathic radicular pain with the hope that the mechanisms that work with peripheral neuropathy will also work for spine pain patients. Although the evidence of benefit for nonperipheral neuropathy pain has been limited. Other medicines including antidepressants (duloxetine [Cymbalta],[1] tricyclic antidepressants) have been tried when other drugs have been ineffective.

Epidural, selective nerve root, or facet joint injections have not shown adequate efficacy to be recommended on a regular basis. However, a limited number (two or three) of spinal injections may be attempted for patients with radicular pain who do not improve with oral medication.

Spinal surgery is indicated for disk herniation with radicular compromise, cervical or lumbar spinal stenosis with myelopathy or neurogenic claudication, and unstable spondylolisthesis. Controversy remains, however, concerning the relative benefit of surgical versus medical therapy for radiculopathy. Diskectomy significantly shortens (by about 8 weeks) the acute phase of pain associated with radiculopathy. However, studies with longer follow-up periods have never shown a clear difference between conservative and surgical therapies. Some studies have shown that intensive, multidisciplinary, conservative programs can be compared with surgical fusion procedures for patients with spinal instability.

For the most chronically disabled spine pain patients only, intensive multidisciplinary programs including, among others, physical reconditioning and cognitive-behavioral methods, have shown effectiveness.

Monitoring

From the standpoint of monitoring the efficacy of the treatment, five main dimensions have been recommended to evaluate the outcome of patients with spine pain. The intensity of pain is relevant but so is the perceived functional capacity, generic health status, work disability, and satisfaction with treatment. Many tools are available for the evaluation of each specific dimension. The clinician who decides to start using any specific tool needs to know, among other information, the minimal clinically meaningful changes for each tool, because differences that may be statistically significant when comparing two groups of patients may be irrelevant at the individual patient level. For example, in terms of intensity of pain, the threshold usually accepted is 3.5 to 4.7 and 2.5 to 4.5 out of 10 for patients with acute and chronic pain, respectively.

Precisely evaluating several domains with specific tools is rather time consuming. However, for busy clinicians, there are brief instruments (core set of measures) with roughly seven or eight questions that include all the previously mentioned dimensions and that have been properly validated. One example is the Core Outcome Measure Index (COMI).

Complications

The clinician should inform the patient about the possible side effects of therapies as they are initiated. At subsequent visits, specific questions regarding the potential side effects are asked. For example, the presence of hypertension, peripheral edema, and

hepatic and renal dysfunction need to be evaluated in patients who are taking chronic NSAID therapy.

In addition, a majority of NSAIDs have potential GI toxicity including mild mucosal irritation, ulcers, and perforations. Hematologic and neurologic toxicity are quite variable depending on the prescribed drug. Cardiovascular toxicity may clearly be an issue, particularly for long-term treatments. The benefit of persistent use of NSAIDs for patients with chronic spine pain needs to be weighed against the increased risk of toxicities.

Besides the risks of addiction or death, the use of opiates induces constipation and urinary retention that may be a serious problem for some patients. These drugs can also produce drowsiness, headache, nausea, or vomiting.

Antidepressants also produce drowsiness and anticholinergic symptoms during the first couple of weeks of use. These drugs have specific side effects including tachycardia, weight gain, or sexual problems.

References

Borenstein D: Mechanical low back pain—a rheumatologist's view, *Nat Rev Rheumatol* 9:643–653, 2013.

Borenstein D, Balague F: Low back pain in adolescent and geriatric populations, *Rheum Dis Clin N Am* 47:149–163, 2021.

Bulloch L, Thompson K, Spector L: Cauda equina syndrome, *Orthop Clin N Am* 53:247–254, 2022.

Chou R, Deyo R, Friedly J, et al: Systematoic pharmacologic therapies for low back pain: a systematic review for an American College of Physicians Clinical Practice Guideline, *Ann Intern Med* 166:480–492, 2017.

Cohen SP: Epidemiology, diagnosis and treatment of neck pain, *Mayo Clin Proc* 90:284–299, 2015.

Coombs DM, Machado GC, Richards B, et al: Clinical course of patients with low back pain following an emergency department presentation: a systematic review, *Emerg Med J* 2020. https://doi.org/10.1136/emermed-2019-20929.

Deyo RA, Mirza SK: Herniated lumbar intervertebral disk, *N Engl J Med* 374:1763–1772, 2016.

Enomoto H, Fujikoshi S, Funa J, et al: Assessment of direct analgesic effect of duloxetine for chronic low back pain: post hoc path analysis of double-blind, placebo-controlled studies, *J Pain Res* 10:1357–1368, 2017.

Fritz JM, Lane E, McFadden M, et al: Physical therapy referral from primary care for acute back pain with sciatica: a randomized controlled trial, *Ann Intern Med* 174:8–17, 2021.

Jones CMP, Day RO, Koes BW, Latimer CG, et al: Opioid analgesia for acute low back pain and neck pain (the OPAL trial): a randomised placebo-controlled trial, *Lancet* 402:304–312, 2023.

Karikaran AK, Carroll AH, Benn L et al.: Cauda equina syndrome: a review of classification, diagnosis, treatment, and best practices, *JBJS Reviews* 13(2):e24.00156, 2025.

Karran EL, McAuley JH, Traeger AC, et al: Can screening instruments accurately determine poor outcome risk in adults with recent onset low back pain? A systematic review and meta-analysis, *BMC Med* 15(1):13, 2017. Erratum reported in BMC Med. 2017 Feb 17;15(1):44.

Katz JN, Zimmerman BS, Mass H, Makhni MC: Diagnosis and management of lumbar spinal stenosis: a review, *JAMA* 327:1688–1699, 2022.

Liu C, Ferreira GE, Shaheed CA, et al. Surgical versus non-surgical treatment for sciatica: systematic review and meta-analysis of randomized controlled trials. BMJ2023;381:e070730.

Maher C, Underwood M, Buchbinder R: Non-specific low back pain, *Lancet* 389(10070):736–747, 2017.

Murphy KP, Sander C, Rabatin AE: Evaluation and treatment of the child with acute back pain, *Pediatr Clin N AM* 70:545–574, 2023.

Qaseem A, Wilt TJ, McLean RM, et al: Noninvasive treatments for acute, subacute, and chronic low back pain: a clinical practice guideline from the American College of Physicians, *Ann Intern Med* 166:514–530, 2017.

Rubinstein SM, de Zoete A, van Middelkoop M, et al: Benefits and harms of spinal manipulative therapy for the treatment of chronic low back pain: systematic review and meta-analysis of randomised controlled trials, *BMJ* 364:l689, 2019. https://doi.org/10.1136/bmjl689.

Seneviratne U, McLaughlin K, Reilly J, et al: Nine recommendations for the emergency department for patients presenting with low back pain based on management and post-discharge outcomes in an Australian, tertiary emergency department, *Emerg Med Australas* 2023 Dec 6. 10.111/1742-6723.14354.

Sowah D, Boyko R, Antle D, et al: Occupational interventions for the prevention of back pain: overview of systematic reviews, *J Safety Res* 66:39–59, 2018.

Steffens D, Maher CG, Pereira, et al: Prevention of low back pain: a systematic review and meta-analysis, *JAMA Intern Med* 176:199–2087, 2016.

Theodore N: Degenerative cervical spondylosis, *N Engl J Med* 383:159–168, 2020.

Tsiang JT, Kinzy TG, Thompson N, et al: Sensitivity and specificity of patient-entered red flags for lower back pain, *Spine J* 19(2):293–300, 2019.

Vanti C, Andreatta S, Borghi S, et al: The effectiveness of walking versus exercise on pain and function in chronic low back pain: a systematic review and meta-analysis of randomized trials, *Disabil Rehabil* 41(6):622–632, 2019.

William J, Roehmer C, Mansy L, Kennedy DJ: Epidural steroid injections, *Phys Med Rehabil Clin N Am* 33:215-231, 2022.

[1]Not FDA approved for this indication.

TINNITUS

Kenneth S. Yew, MD, MPH

CURRENT DIAGNOSIS

- Tinnitus is most commonly associated with hearing loss or exposure to loud noise.
- In addition to history and examination, most patients will benefit from an audiogram.
- Unilateral or pulsatile tinnitus, focal neurologic or otologic findings, and tinnitus with vertigo warrant imaging and further evaluation.
- Patients should be evaluated for distress from tinnitus, insomnia, depression, and anxiety.

CURRENT THERAPY

- Although no cure exists for tinnitus, education and support at initial diagnosis will help alleviate fears, dispel misconceptions, and guide expectations of treatment.
- Hearing amplification for patients with significant hearing loss can frequently resolve tinnitus.
- Cognitive behavioral therapy—either online or in person—can relieve distress in patients with chronic tinnitus.
- Tinnitus distress should be monitored, and comorbid insomnia, depression, and anxiety should be treated.

Definition and Epidemiology

Tinnitus is defined as a perceived sound without an external cause. It can be classified in several ways. By a traditional method of classification, the most common type of tinnitus is subjective, defined as tinnitus without a corresponding sound on auscultation. Objective tinnitus, on the other hand, can be heard by the examiner and the patient. The 2014 American Academy of Otolaryngology–Head and Neck Surgery Foundation (AAO-HNSF) tinnitus guideline classifies tinnitus as primary or idiopathic if, after investigation, no cause other than the presence of sensorineural hearing loss (SNHL) can be determined and secondary if it is "associated with a specific underlying cause (other than SNHL) or an identifiable organic condition." Both the traditional and AAO-HNSF classifications see tinnitus from the perspective of the examiner or investigator. Another common classification is dual, based on whether the patient has nonpulsatile or pulsatile tinnitus. Tinnitus that can be modulated by movement of the head, neck, jaw, or a limb is considered to have a somatosensory component, which is detectable in up to 83% of patients with tinnitus.

Prevalence of "any tinnitus" in adults is 14.4% (95% confidence interval [CI], 12.6% to 16.5%). The estimate for children and adolescents (≤17 years) is similar at 13.6% (95% CI, 8.5% to 21.0%) but more uncertain because of variability in how studies asked children about their symptoms. Prevalence increases from 9.7% in young adulthood (18–44 years) to 13.7% in middle age (45–64 years) and to 23.6% in older age (≥65 years). Prevalence of severe tinnitus is similar in adults and children at 2.3% and 2.7%, respectively, but increased to 6.9% in people 65 and older. In the largest review to date, tinnitus prevalence did not vary by sex. Limited adult data suggest a 9.8% prevalence of chronic tinnitus and annual tinnitus incidence of 1%. Pulsatile tinnitus represents less than 10% of all presentations, most commonly in women in their fifth decade of life.

Risk Factors and Etiologies

The most common causes of subjective tinnitus are SNHL and occupational noise exposure. Other etiologies of subjective tinnitus include the following:

- Otologic—Conductive hearing loss, cholesteatoma, Ménière disease, vestibular schwannoma (VS), otitis media, traumatic cerumen removal
- Somatic—Temporomandibular joint (TMJ) dysfunction
- Medications or substances—Antiinflammatory agents (aspirin, nonsteroidals), antimalarials (quinine, chloroquine), antimicrobials (aminoglycosides, macrolides, tetracyclines, others), antineoplastic agents, loop diuretics, local anesthetics, cannabis use, and others
- Genetic—Moderate genetic component noted in chronic tinnitus
- Autoimmune—Systemic sclerosis
- Infectious
- Metabolic/cardiovascular—No association with hyperlipidemia, hypertension, diabetes mellitus, or obesity in most recent epidemiologic data
- Neurologic—Multiple sclerosis, vestibular migraine, tension headache, type I Chiari malformation, spontaneous intracranial hypotension, and brainstem stroke
- Psychiatric—Stress: association between chronic tinnitus and depression found by most studies; greater likelihood of depression and/or anxiety associated with more severe tinnitus; neither depression nor anxiety demonstrated to cause tinnitus. (Data partially adapted from Yew, 2014.)

The most common causes of pulsatile tinnitus include idiopathic, neoplasms, arterial, venous, and middle ear pathology. Specific causes include the following:

- Neoplasm—Paraganglioma, VS, meningioma, dermoid tumor
- Arterial—Dural arteriovenous fistula, arteriovenous malformation, tortuosity or aneurysm, atherosclerotic plaque, congenital abnormality, dissection, fibromuscular dysplasia
- Venous—Idiopathic intracranial hypertension, sigmoid sinus dehiscence or diverticulum, superior semicircular canal dehiscence, jugular or sigmoid sinus venous thrombosis, venous hum
- Otologic—Superior canal dehiscence, patulous eustachian tube, otosclerosis
- Myoclonus—Stapedius, tensor tympani or palatal muscles
- Hyperdynamic states or increased bone vascularity—pregnancy, anemia, thyrotoxicosis, Paget disease, bone-invading tumors or hemangiomas
- Somatosensory

Pathophysiology

Tinnitus is thought to arise from an intricate interaction between peripheral and central mechanisms. Although the inciting event for tinnitus may be hearing loss or cochlear damage, the actual generation and maintenance of tinnitus occurs centrally, involving both auditory and nonauditory pathways. Decreased input from the peripheral auditory system alters the excitatory/inhibitory balance within the central auditory processing system. This, in turn, may cause signal hyperactivity and increased synchrony between neural centers as the brain tries to maintain its pre–hearing loss state, a process called "homeostatic plasticity." These processes may account for a phenomenon called *central gain*, in which the central auditory system becomes hypersensitive. Human and animal studies suggest a role for the brain's emotional/cognitive areas—including the temporal, parietal, sensorimotor, and limbic cortices—in the pathogenesis of tinnitus. Limbic nonauditory and auditory pathway interactions have been found in tinnitus patients using multiple functional imaging modalities, but not all investigators have confirmed differences between patients with and without tinnitus. Frontostriatal circuits appear to be critical in the development and maintenance of both tinnitus and chronic pain, consistent with the view that tinnitus, phantom limb pain, and central pain sensitization may share common pathways. The perception of tinnitus also seems to reside in somatic memory.

The medial geniculate body in the thalamus is posited as the site of connection between sound perception, the auditory cortex, and the limbic system. A number of theoretical models of tinnitus psychopathology exist, but as yet none has been found to account for all findings in patients with tinnitus.

Prevention

Hearing conservation and careful use of ototoxic drugs should help prevent tinnitus. As industrial hearing conservation programs are well established, leisure time noise exposure is now estimated to be associated with more hearing loss than occupational exposure. The use of hearing protection while firing weapons and using power tools should be encouraged. Personal listening devices (PLDs) represent the greatest current risk to hearing. A recent systematic review of studies examining short- and long-term hearing effects in PLD users found evidence of significantly poorer hearing thresholds in long-term PLD users compared with nonusers. Keeping volume settings to no more than 60% or 70% of maximum should comply with current World Health Organization guidelines to limit leisure noise to less than 70 dB for continuous exposure and less than 85 dB for up to 2 hours/day, respectively.

Clinical Manifestations

Patients report an abrupt or insidious onset of a sound in one or both ears that is continuous or intermittent. The sound may be a ringing, buzzing, roaring, or clicking; it may be high or low pitched. The tinnitus may have a pulsatile quality. Its severity and persistence may vary from transient and mild to chronic and severe. If sought carefully, the pitch or loudness of the tinnitus may be modulated by moving the head, neck, or jaw. Other otologic symptoms include preexisting hearing loss, hearing loss or ear fullness during tinnitus, vertigo, noise annoyance, or ear pain. How bothersome tinnitus is to patients varies by its severity and the presence of coexisting depression or anxiety symptoms.

Diagnosis

The evaluation of patients presenting with tinnitus in a primary care setting includes a thorough history and focused examination. Most patients need an audiogram, and some will require imaging or standardized tinnitus impact investigations.

History

- Description—Onset, pitch, quality, unilateral/bilateral, loudness, continuous/intermittent, pulsatile/nonpulsatile
- Associated symptoms—Hearing loss, vertigo, otalgia, ear fullness, hyperacusis, headache, neck or TMJ pain, visual disturbance, gait problem, weakness, or paresthesia
- Provocative/palliative factors—Stress; change in tinnitus with head, neck, or jaw movement or tinnitus severity varying with severity of neck or jaw discomfort
- Past history—Prior tinnitus; hearing loss; occupational/leisure noise exposure; prior head, neck, or ear injury; bruxism; current or recent medications; or medical history
- Family history—Chronic tinnitus, Ménière disease, or otosclerosis
- Impact—Degree of tinnitus distress, insomnia, or lifestyle interference

Examination

- General—Blood pressure, body mass index
- Head—Masticatory muscle, TMJ or suboccipital tenderness; tinnitus changed by head, neck, or jaw movement or contraction
- Eye—Nystagmus if vertigo history and papilledema if headache history
- Ear—Cerumen impaction, otorrhea, cholesteatoma, retrotympanic mass (refer for microscopic otologic exam before imaging if retrotympanic mass suspected)
- Neck—Neck mass, tenderness
- Neurologic—Cranial nerves; neurologic exam if neurologic symptoms, headache, vertigo, or pulsatile tinnitus

- Psychologic—Screen for depression and anxiety if mood symptoms or bothersome tinnitus
- For pulsatile tinnitus
  - Palpate pulse—Ask patient to tap out the tinnitus frequency
  - Pulse asynchronous—Consider patulous eustachian tube or myoclonic etiologies
  - Pulse synchronous—Auscultate for bruits over mastoid, preauricular area, temples, orbits, carotids, and for cardiac murmurs, which can suggest an arterial cause. Assess the effect of light compression of the ipsilateral jugular vein by the examiner or patient. Reduction or cessation of tinnitus can suggest a venous cause.

Although SNHL is the most common etiology for tinnitus, it is important to evaluate for other etiologies during the initial evaluation. Brief, intermittent, nonpulsatile tinnitus without associated headache, neurologic symptoms, hearing loss, or vertigo may be observed without further evaluation. Patients with recent onset of nonbothersome pulsatile tinnitus without history of hypertension, obesity, new vision changes, ipsilateral subjective or objective hearing loss, and normal otoscopic findings may be considered for a month or two of observation. If symptoms persist or worsen, pursue imaging and/or specialty referral. Recent loud noise exposure or use of an ototoxic medication can inform the diagnosis and guide both therapy and prognosis. Headache should prompt a careful search for findings suggestive of vestibular migraine, idiopathic intracranial hypertension, or spontaneous intracranial hypotension. Unilateral tinnitus with vertiginous symptoms with or without hearing loss suggests vestibular migraine, Ménière disease, or VS. An abrupt onset is more often seen in somatosensory tinnitus, migraine, Ménière disease, and brainstem stroke or transient ischemic attack.

Tinnitus with a somatosensory component is suggested if the patient also has neck or jaw symptoms. Patients with both tinnitus and neck/jaw pain in whom the severity of both symptoms vary in concert at least some days are likely to have a somatosensory component to their tinnitus with a prevalence of 84%, and up to 90% if patient endorses suboccipital muscle tension most or all days.

An audiogram should be obtained for patients with unilateral or pulsatile tinnitus, suspicion of hearing loss, or tinnitus lasting over 6 months. It is an option for patients with tinnitus of less than 6 months. A criterion for asymmetric hearing loss to optimize sensitivity for VS is an average 10 dB difference over the frequencies 1 to 8 kHz.

No reviewed guideline recommends laboratory testing to evaluate patients with tinnitus. Laboratory investigation in patients presenting with tinnitus can be guided by clinical suspicion and existing preventive services screening guidelines.

Table 1 lists imaging options for patients with tinnitus. Specialty consultation is helpful to evaluate the myriad causes of pulsatile tinnitus. Magnetic resonance imaging may be uncomfortable for patients with tinnitus with noise sensitivity. In such cases, contrast-enhanced computed tomography is an alternative.

Patients should be asked how bothered they are by their tinnitus. If bothersome tinnitus is endorsed, then it is helpful to learn how the tinnitus is interfering with the patient's sleep, work, concentration, mood, and quality of life. This understanding will guide subsequent education, support, evaluation, and therapy. Validated questionnaires to assess tinnitus impact and monitor therapeutic response include the Tinnitus Handicap Inventory (THI), screening THI, and Tinnitus Functional Index (TFI). The National Institute for Health and Care Excellence tinnitus guideline highlights the TFI as it assesses global tinnitus impact, hearing acuity, sleep, anxiety, and depression. The TFI is available at https://tinnitustherapy.org.uk/tinnitus-functional-index/.

Differential Diagnosis

Brief spontaneous tinnitus, also called "transient ear noise," is a benign, fleeting, high-pitched, unilateral sound of unknown cause

TABLE 1 Imaging for Patients With Tinnitus

PRESENTATION OF TINNITUS	IMAGING CHOICE	COMMENT
Uncomplicated, bilateral, and nonpulsatile	None	Hearing loss symmetric if present. No other indications for imaging, such as stroke/TIA symptoms, acute vestibular syndrome, focal neurologic exam, or retrotympanic mass.
Bilateral and nonpulsatile with asymmetric hearing loss by audiogram or unilateral and nonpulsatile	MRI of head and IAC without and with IV contrast	VS risk ~2% if asymmetric hearing loss by audiogram and <1% if unilateral tinnitus without asymmetric hearing loss.
Pulsatile	Carotid bruit—Carotid duplex ultrasound Orbital or periauricular bruit—CTA/V head or MRA/V of head and IAC Improved with ipsilateral jugular vein compression—High resolution CTTB and CTA/V head or MRA/V of head and IAC No exam findings—CTA/V head	CTA protocols available for arterial and venous imaging during a single study. If ongoing concern for arterial or venous etiologies after negative noninvasive imaging, consider referral for further evaluation including DSA. MRV may be more sensitive for IIH. MRI more sensitive for neoplasms.
Pulsatile with suspicion of retrotympanic mass by microscopic examination or temporal bone disease	High resolution CTTB	IV contrast unnecessary if retrotympanic mass suspected

CT, Computed tomography; *CTA/V,* CT angiogram and venogram; *CTTB,* CT temporal bone; *DSA,* digital subtraction angiography; *IAC,* internal auditory canal; *IIH,* idiopathic intracranial hypertension; *MRA/V,* magnetic resonance angiogram and venogram; *MRI,* magnetic resonance imaging; *MRV,* magnetic resonance venography; *TIA,* transient ischemic attack; *VS,* vestibular schwannoma.

TABLE 2 Treatment for Patients With Chronic Tinnitus

TREATMENT	COMMENT
Support and education—teaching at time of evaluation provided in addition to printed or online materials	Help patients understand what tinnitus is and that it is typically benign. Explain that tinnitus is a result of, not a cause for, hearing loss. Reassure that it may persist but can improve over time. Discuss the potential for medications to cause or worsen tinnitus. Discuss prevention of tinnitus. Discuss no cures at present but management helpful to relieve distress. Review beneficial treatments and treatments unlikely to benefit.
Amplification	Offer amplification for hearing loss affecting communication and consider for hearing loss without communication difficulties. Real ear technique fitting more effectively reduces tinnitus. Consider cochlear implants for those who are candidates. Do not offer without documented hearing loss.
Sound therapy—via an in-ear or wearable device, music therapy, environmental sound, smartphone, etc.	Option to offer, but limited current evidence of efficacy.
Medications	Avoid medications. Currently there is no evidence for efficacy of any medication to improve tinnitus. Medication may help with insomnia, depression, or anxiety, if present.
Psychological therapies	CBT is the most effective therapy for reducing tinnitus distress and severity. The NICE guideline suggests a stepped approach beginning with online CBT, then group therapy, then individual CBT.
Combination therapies—tinnitus retraining therapy with amplification, with or without sound therapy	Current evidence does not support additional efficacy of this widely practiced approach beyond usual care.
Neuromodulation—rTMS, tDCS, tVNS, acoustic neuromodulation therapy, bimodal stimulation, and others	Neuromodulation requires further study.
Other therapies—acupuncture, herbal, vitamins, minerals, and other dietary supplements	Other therapies are ineffective or inconclusive.
Treatments for somatosensory tinnitus	Evidence for oromyofacial therapy, dental occlusal splints, physical therapy, and relaxation training.

AAO-HNSF, American Academy of Otolaryngology–Head and Neck Surgery Foundation; *CBT,* cognitive behavioral therapy; *NICE,* National Institute for Health and Care Excellence; *rTMS,* repetitive transcranial magnetic stimulation; *tDCS,* transcranial direct current stimulation, *tVNS,* transcutaneous vagal nerve stimulation.
Data from NICE, AAO-HNSF, and European tinnitus guidelines.

sometimes accompanied by a sensation of hearing loss. The tonal quality of tinnitus must be distinguished from the voices or music heard in an auditory or musical hallucination. Musical hallucinations can be experienced by people with SNHL or more rarely as a manifestation of epilepsy.

Treatment

Goals for treating patients with tinnitus are to help them understand that tinnitus is common, normally benign, and can improve over time; if it is chronic, therapies exist to help such patients live well with it. Table 2 lists evidence-based tinnitus

TABLE 3	Education Resources for Patients
SPONSORING ORGANIZATION	**INTERNET ADDRESS**
American Tinnitus Association—podcasts, tinnitus education and support	https://www.ata.org Tinnitus Patient Navigator: https://www.ata.org/managing-your-tinnitus/tinnitus-patient-navigator
Tinnitus UK—a wealth of information and support for people with tinnitus	https://www.tinnitus.org.uk
Progressive Tinnitus Management 2.0: Living Better With Tinnitus Workbook—handbook produced by the U.S. Veterans Administration incorporating sound therapy and cognitive behavioral therapy	https://www.healthquality.va.gov/guidelines/CD/tinnitus/CST-02-PTM-WorkBook-11172024-Final-Draft-508-Compliant.pdf

therapies. Observation with support and education after negative diagnostic workup can be sufficient if tinnitus is not bothersome. In an observational study of patients with intrusive tinnitus, the provision of a standardized bundle of tinnitus information to all patients was associated with nearly a fourfold drop in patients who requested further formal treatment for their tinnitus. Patient interview studies document that tinnitus support and education is beneficial at every stage of care. However, as many as 82.6% of patients with tinnitus surveyed worldwide felt that their tinnitus was managed "not very effectively" or "not at all." As there is still no cure for tinnitus, part of this dissatisfaction may stem from their expectations of therapy. When U.S. audiologists and their patients were asked about treatment goals, audiologists endorsed reduced tinnitus awareness, stress, and anxiety, whereas their patients wanted reduced tinnitus loudness or its elimination. Accurate, supportive education about tinnitus and its treatment is essential to help patients develop informed expectations. Table 3 lists selected patient education resources for tinnitus.

Aside from hearing amplification and cognitive behavioral therapy (CBT), no other therapy has proven effectiveness for tinnitus. Patients can be educated that hearing aids accurately verified using a real ear technique, ideally via an internal probe ear microphone, produce twice the reduction in tinnitus distress at 1 year compared with those not fit by real ear measurements. Sound or music therapy to help distract from or mask tinnitus may be helpful for individual patients, but evidence of its overall efficacy is limited. Tinnitus retraining therapy (TRT) classically combines sound-enrichment therapy and directive counseling. It can be combined with amplification. Although its individual components may be beneficial, combined TRT has not proven superior in reducing tinnitus distress compared with usual care. Many medications and mineral and herbal supplements have been studied for the treatment of tinnitus, but none have proven beneficial. Available studies of acupuncture for tinnitus treatment are limited by methodologic flaws, precluding its recommendation as an effective tinnitus therapy. Neuromodulation approaches hold promise to reduce tinnitus by targeting its abnormal neurophysiology; however, studies of a variety of techniques have not shown efficacy for any of these therapies. Patients with a somatosensory component to their tinnitus may benefit from physical or dental splint therapies.

CBT targets thoughts and emotions to affect behavior. Drawing attention to inaccurate thoughts and thought patterns aided by a skilled therapist can help patients develop a more beneficial response to their tinnitus. Other cognitive-based approaches that have been studied for tinnitus include mindfulness-based CBT and acceptance and commitment therapy (ACT). All of these therapies have been shown to decrease the severity and distress of tinnitus but have not improved quality of life or mitigated tinnitus annoyance or loudness, depression, anxiety, or sleep. The exceptions are ACT, which decreases tinnitus-associated depression, and CBT for insomnia, which improved insomnia related to tinnitus in one trial. Limited access to CBT therapists is an issue for many patients. Online CBT and ACT effectively reduces tinnitus severity and distress, although in-person therapy tends to have a larger effect.

Monitoring
Response to therapy can be assessed by clinical impression or a validated instrument like the TFI. As tinnitus can be associated with depression, use of a depression screening instrument such as the PHQ-9 and inquiring about suicidal ideation is recommended, especially for patients with at least moderately distressing tinnitus. Monitor hearing acuity in patients with chronic tinnitus as they are at higher risk for ongoing hearing loss. Patients with both distressing tinnitus and moderate-severe hearing loss are at highest risk for depression. If distress from tinnitus is not improving or worsens, review the completeness of the workup and discuss with the patient a referral for CBT or tinnitus specialty evaluation. Fortunately, although the severity of tinnitus may fluctuate, over time it tends not to worsen and may improve.

Complications
Carefully monitoring the level of a patient's distress from tinnitus, diagnosing treatable etiologies, and recognizing and treating comorbid conditions such as depression, insomnia, and anxiety will help avoid most complications. Care to ensure follow-up and consultation for patients presenting with pulsatile tinnitus is important, as up to one-third of them can have an underlying neoplasm or vascular etiology with potential for complications including vision loss, stroke, or hemorrhage. Tinnitus was not associated with increased risk to develop dementia when hearing loss and other risk factors for dementia were controlled in the best quality study to date.

References
Biswas R, Genitsaridi E, Trpchevska N, et al: Low evidence for tinnitus risk factors: a systematic review and meta-analysis, *J Assoc Res Otolaryngol* 24(1):81–94, 2023. Available at https://link.springer.com/content/pdf/10.1007/s10162-022-00874-y.pdf.

Cavarocchi C, Wong K, Cao AC, et al: Toward a diagnostic imaging algorithm for undifferentiated pulsatile tinnitus, *Otol Neurotol* 45(8):895–900, 2024.

Cima RFF, Mazurek B, Haider H, et al: A multidisciplinary European guideline for tinnitus: diagnostics, assessment, and treatment, *HNO* 67(Suppl 1):10–42, 2019.

Haider HF, Bojic T, Ribeiro SF, et al: Pathophysiology of subjective tinnitus: triggers and maintenance, *Front Neurosci* 12:866, 2018. Available at https://www.ncbi.nlm.nih.gov/pmc/articles/PMC6277522/pdf/fnins-12-00866.pdf.

Hassaan A, Trinidade A: The tinnitus patient information pack: usefulness in intrusive tinnitus, *Int J Health Care Qual Assur* 32(2):360–365, 2019.

Hoare DJ, Shorter GW, Shekhawat GS, et al: Neuromodulation treatments targeting pathological synchrony for tinnitus in adults: a systematic review, *Brain Sci* 14(8):748, 2024. Available at https://www.mdpi.com/2076-3425/14/8/748.

Jain V, Policeni B, Juliano AF, et al: ACR Appropriateness Criteria® Tinnitus: 2023 update, *J Am Coll Radiol* 20(11S):S574–s591, 2023. Available at https://www.jacr.org/article/S1546-1440(23)00604-X/pdf.

Jarach CM, Lugo A, Scala M, et al: Global prevalence and incidence of tinnitus: a systematic review and meta-analysis, *JAMA Neurol* 79(9):888–900, 2022. Available at https://jamanetwork.com/journals/jamaneurology/articlepdf/2795168/jamaneurology_jarach_2022_oi_220043_1667512347.25045.pdf.

Marks E, Hallsworth C, Vogt F, et al: Cognitive behavioural therapy for insomnia (CBTi) as a treatment for tinnitus-related insomnia: a randomised controlled trial, *Cogn Behav Ther* 52(2):91–109, 2023. Available at https://www.tandfonline.com/doi/epdf/10.1080/16506073.2022.2084155?needAccess=true&role=button.

Michiels S: Somatosensory Tinnitus: recent developments in diagnosis and treatment, *J Assoc Res Otolaryngol* 24(5):465–472, 2023.

Reisinger L, Weisz N: Chronic tinnitus is associated with aging but not dementia, *Hear Res* 453:109135, 2024. Available at: https://www.sciencedirect.com/science/article/pii/S0378595524001886?via%3Dihub.

Scherer RW, Formby C, Group TRTTR: Effect of tinnitus retraining therapy vs standard of care on tinnitus-related quality of life: a randomized clinical trial, *JAMA Otolaryngol Head Neck Surg* 145(7):597–608, 2019.

Tinnitus: assessment and management (NG155): *National Institute for Health and Care Excellence*, 2020. Available at: https://www.nice.org.uk/guidance/ng155. [Accessed 4 January 2020].

Trevis KJ, McLachlan NM, Wilson SJ: A systematic review and meta-analysis of psychological functioning in chronic tinnitus, *Clin Psychol Rev* 60:62–86, 2018.

Tunkel DE, Bauer CA, Sun GH, et al: Clinical practice guideline: tinnitus, *Otolaryngol Head Neck Surg* 151(2 Suppl):S1–S40, 2014.

Waechter S, Jönsson A: Hearing Aids Mitigate Tinnitus, but does it matter if the patient receives amplification in accordance with their hearing impairment or not? A meta-analysis, *Am J Audiol* 31(3):789–818, 2022.

Yew KS: Diagnostic approach to patients with tinnitus, *Am Fam Physician* 89(2):106–113, 2014.

You S, Kong TH, Han W: The effects of short-term and long-term hearing changes on music exposure: a systematic review and meta-analysis, *Int J Environ Res Public Health* 17(6):2091, 2020. Available at: https://www.mdpi.com/1660-4601/17/6/2091.

ALLERGIC REACTIONS TO INSECT STINGS

James M. Quinn, MD

CURRENT DIAGNOSIS

Classify reaction based upon clinical manifestations
- Local reactions
  - Uncomplicated "usual" local reaction—mild redness, pain, and swelling limited to area of sting
  - Large local reaction—redness, pain, and swelling extending beyond area of sting
- Systemic reactions
  - Cutaneous only—flushing, urticaria, angioedema (excluding tongue, throat, larynx)
  - Anaphylaxis (e.g., cutaneous symptoms and/or respiratory symptoms, gastrointestinal symptoms, cardiovascular symptoms, uterine cramping)

CURRENT THERAPY

- Local reactions
  - Uncomplicated local reaction
    - H1 antihistamines, analgesics, cold compress
    - Discuss avoidance measures
  - Large local reaction
    - H1 antihistamines, analgesics, cold compress, avoidance measures
    - Discuss avoidance measures
    - Further evaluation, testing, epinephrine administration devices (autoinjectors, nasal sprays) optional
- Systemic reactions
  - Cutaneous only
    - Based upon clinical situation and prior history
    - H1 antihistamines, epinephrine in some circumstances
    - Discuss avoidance measures
    - Further evaluation, testing, epinephrine administration devices (autoinjectors, nasal sprays) optional
  - Anaphylaxis
    - Epinephrine intramuscularly or intranasally (using Neffy nasal spray)
    - Consider adjunctive therapy—antihistamines, bronchodilators, intravenous fluids, vasopressors, oxygen, other supportive measures.
    - Provide epinephrine administration devices (autoinjectors or nasal sprays)
    - Discuss avoidance measures
    - Consider further evaluation, testing, consideration of immunotherapy

Pathophysiology

The pathophysiology of insect sting reactions varies based upon the classification. Uncomplicated local reactions are due to direct toxic effects of the venoms. Venom components include enzymes, vasoactive amines, peptides, and other contents that directly lead to local cell death, tissue destruction, vasodilatation, altered hemostasis, and inflammation.

Fire ant stings initially follow the pattern of the uncomplicated local reactions described. Fire ant venom is unique in containing highly basic pH piperidine alkaloids. Piperidine alkaloids lead to local tissue necrosis and a pathognomonic sterile pseudopustule at the center of an otherwise uncomplicated local reaction.

Large local reactions result from an immunologic response rather than simply direct toxic effects. The reaction is a broader and more sustained immunologic late-phase response to specific antigens in the venom. It is often (up to 80% of cases) associated with and possibly mediated by venom-specific immunoglobulin E (IgE).

Systemic reactions are characterized by signs and symptoms occurring distantly from the sting site. Onset is generally rapid and can include cutaneous, respiratory, cardiovascular, gastrointestinal, and/or other symptoms. Systemic reactions are the result of mast cell degranulation from venom-specific IgE binding. Mast cells release a wide array of vasoactive amines, prostaglandins, leukotrienes, platelet activating factor, and other cytokines. These lead to vasodilatation, capillary leak, edema, bronchospasm, and so on.

There are clinical situations when patients should be suspected of having an underlying mast cell disorder as a pathophysiologic contributor. These include very severe anaphylaxis, hypotension, severe anaphylaxis without cutaneous symptoms, and patients without detectable IgE.

Prevention

Prevention focuses on avoidance of stings. General strategies that may be effective include using professional exterminators for known nests with periodic reinspections; wearing fully closed-toe shoes or sandals outdoors (include socks for fire ant prevention); use of caution when or avoidance of eating or drinking outdoors, especially drinking from closed or opaque containers or straws; vigilance in wooded areas, around flowering plants, and garbage; and wearing shoes, socks, long pants, long sleeves, and hats when gardening or performing other "at-risk" outdoor activity. If the history of the sting or diagnostic testing identifies the suspected insect, teach patients about the habits and nesting of the specific insect.

Stinging insects are the Hymenoptera order and include the Apidae (bee) family of honeybees and bumblebees; the Vespidae (wasp) family of hornets, yellow jackets, and paper wasps; and the Formicidae (ant) family of the imported fire ant. Honeybees and bumblebees are generally not aggressive. They feed on nectar from flowering plants and will sting only in self-defense such as stepping barefoot on a bee in a field or with an accidental close encounter. Bees will also sting after a direct threat to their nests. Bee nests can be found in commercial hives, tree hollows, old logs, or, less commonly, in the walls of buildings. Africanized honeybees, found primarily in the southern third of the United States, differ only in that they are far more aggressive in defense of their hives. Massive and persistent retaliation can result simply from the vibration of lawn equipment several yards from their hive. The stingers of bees are barbed and often result in retention of the stinger and venom sac at the sting site. A retained stinger can occur, although less commonly, with wasps.

Yellow jackets are scavengers, seeking food wherever available—at picnics, around garbage containers, in soda cans, and so on. They are highly aggressive and may sting even if unprovoked. Their nests are found underground, in rotted wood, or in wall spaces. In many areas of the country, yellow jackets are the most common cause of stings.

Hornets and paper wasps generally are not aggressive and do not sting unless defending their nests. Paper wasp nests are classically thin, paper-like honeycomb structures found under the eaves of homes, windowsills, and railings. Hornet nests are typically grayish paper mâché structures hanging from tree limbs. There are several species of hornets and wasps that have black and yellow coloring that can make them difficult to distinguish from yellow jackets and bees, making simple visual identification unreliable.

Imported fire ants are extremely aggressive, especially in defense of their nest. Fire ants are endemic to the southern United States. Fire ant nests are built underground and generally capped by a mound of overlying loose soil. Individual ants can sting multiple times and the disturbed mound easily spills out hundreds to thousands of workers prepared to sting in defense of the nest.

Clinical Manifestations

Classification of insect sting reactions based upon the clinical manifestations is important to the diagnostic and therapeutic approach. Most insect sting reactions can be classified as local or systemic. Local reactions are further subdivided as uncomplicated local reactions or as large local reactions. Systemic reactions can be further subdivided as cutaneous only or as anaphylaxis.

Uncomplicated local reactions are the expected usual reaction and are characterized by mild redness, pain, itching, and swelling limited to the area of sting generally not larger than 5 to 10 cm. These local reactions begin immediately after the sting and generally resolve over several hours but may linger up to 48 hours. Uncommonly, the pain, burning, or itch of an isolated fire ant sting goes unnoticed, but the sterile pseudopustule appears within 24 hours of the sting.

Large local reactions occur in approximately 5% to 15% of insect stings. These reactions are generally defined as larger than 10 cm or a patient's palm and can progress, involving an entire limb. Large local reactions generally begin within 6 to 12 hours, peak within 24 to 48 hours, and resolve within 3 to 10 days. Large local reactions commonly recur with repeat stings.

Systemic reactions occur in approximately 1% to 7% of stings. Systemic cutaneous-only reactions are limited to flushing, urticaria, and angioedema (excluding the airway—tongue, throat, larynx). Most systemic reactions in children are cutaneous only, whereas most systemic reactions in adults are anaphylactic.

Systemic anaphylaxis occurs in 1% to 3% of stings. Anaphylaxis is defined as the acute onset (minutes to several hours) of symptoms after a sting and include two or more of the following organ systems: cutaneous (pruritus, flushing, urticaria, angioedema), respiratory (shortness of breath, chest tightness, cough, stridor, wheezing), cardiovascular (light headedness, syncope, tachycardia, hypotension), or gastrointestinal (abdominal pain, nausea, vomiting, diarrhea). In addition, anaphylaxis can be defined as the acute onset of hypotension after exposure to a known allergen for the patient.

Toxic reactions can occur due to large numbers of stings (>20–50 flying Hymenoptera stings in an adult). Toxic signs and symptoms are often delayed and can include myalgia, fevers/chills, headache, rhabdomyolysis, renal failure, hemolysis, diffuse intravascular coagulation, acute respiratory distress syndrome, and death. The lethal dose for a 60-kg adult has been estimated at more than 1100 honeybee stings.

There are also unusual and rare reactions of unknown pathophysiology that include glomerulonephritis, Guillain-Barré syndrome, seizures, and serum sickness.

Diagnosis

Categorizing the type of reaction is essential for risk assessment, diagnostic evaluation, and treatment planning. History of the event, signs and symptoms, and response to therapy are important and will allow the reaction to be accurately categorized as uncomplicated local, large local, systemic cutaneous-only, or systemic anaphylaxis.

Patients experiencing uncomplicated local reactions are not at increased risk of anaphylaxis and do not require additional diagnostic evaluation.

Patients experiencing large local reactions generally do not require additional diagnostic evaluation because they have a small relative risk of future anaphylaxis. Despite the common occurrence of venom-specific IgE, only 4% to 10% of patients with a history of large local reactions go on to develop a systemic reaction, and less than 5% go on to develop anaphylaxis after repeat stings.

Patients with systemic cutaneous-only reactions generally do not require additional diagnostic evaluation because they also have a small relative risk of future anaphylaxis. Only 10% to 15% of children with systemic cutaneous-only reactions have recurrent cutaneous-only reactions, and less than 3% go on to have anaphylaxis. For adults with cutaneous-only reactions, there is a less than 3% to 5% risk of progression to anaphylaxis after resting.

There may be special situations when patients with large local or systemic cutaneous-only reactions are at increased risk and would benefit from referral to consider additional diagnostic testing, epinephrine administration devices (autoinjectors or nasal sprays), and possible immunotherapy. Special situations include frequent stings, high-risk medical conditions, at-risk medications (β-blockers, angiotensin-converting enzyme [ACE] inhibitors), impaired quality of life, and/or imported fire ant stings. Data regarding future risk of repeat fire ant stings are not robust, and multiple sting attack rates are high. In these patients, the decision regarding evaluation and therapy is based on a risk-benefit discussion with the patient.

Patients with systemic anaphylaxis after stings should undergo referral for further diagnostic testing. Patients with systemic reactions to stings have a 25% to 75% chance of another systemic reaction with the highest rates of recurrence seen with more severe reactions. Systemic anaphylaxis to insect stings can be fatal. Insect stings account for up to 20% of all fatalities due to anaphylaxis, and estimates are that 40 (and likely more) patients die annually from insect sting anaphylaxis in the United States.

Additional diagnostic testing may commonly include prick and intradermal skin testing, serologic assessment of specific IgE, and serum tryptase.

Therapy and Monitoring

Uncomplicated local reaction should be cleaned and any retained stinger carefully removed. Symptomatic therapy with antihistamines, analgesics, and cold compresses can be administered. Patients should also be given advice regarding avoidance measures to prevent future stings. In the case of fire ant stings, the pseudopustule is sterile and bacteriostatic; it should not be unroofed or opened.

Large local reactions should be approached similarly to uncomplicated local reactions with symptomatic therapy. For patients with frequent painful and/or debilitating large local reactions, the unstudied method of a short burst of oral corticosteroids for 3 to 7 days is sometimes used. Efficacy with immunotherapy for large local reactions has been demonstrated in early trials, but further study is needed. Unneeded antibiotic therapy for cellulitis should be avoided. Cellulitis is unlikely at 24 to 48 hours when patients commonly present. Later presentations of large local reactions can make distinguishing cellulitis more difficult. However, after 48 hours, many large, local reactions are plateauing or improving while infection would be expected to worsen. In addition, presence of fever would suggest infection.

Systemic cutaneous-only reactions (flushing, urticaria, angioedema not involving the airway) may require a more nuanced approach. Because of the low risk of developing additional symptoms, patients with a history of prior cutaneous-only reactions can be appropriately treated with antihistamines and close observation if they present again with cutaneous-only reactions. On the other hand, patients with a history of anaphylaxis who may initially present with cutaneous-only symptoms should immediately be treated with epinephrine because of the significant risk that additional symptoms will develop.

Those patients with large local reactions or systemic cutaneous-only reactions and in whom special situations exist may be given epinephrine administration devices (autoinjectors or nasal sprays), recommended to wear medical identification information, and referred to an allergist/immunologist for consideration of further evaluation.

Systemic anaphylaxis to insect stings should be treated acutely in the same way as anaphylaxis from any cause. The primary medication for this is epinephrine, which should be promptly injected into the outer thigh muscle. The recommended dose for individuals weighing 30 kg or more is 0.3 to 0.5 mg of the 1 mg/mL (1:1000) concentration. For those weighing less than 30 kg, the dose is 0.01 mg/kg up to a maximum of 0.3 mg. Another option now available for treating anaphylaxis is an intranasal epinephrine spray (Neffy). For individuals weighing 30 kg or more, the dose is one spray (2 mg/0.1 mL) in one nostril. For those weighing 15 kg to less than 30 kg, the dose is one spray (1 mg/0.1 mL) in one nostril. Transport to a fully capable emergency medical facility should be undertaken as soon as practicable. As available, adjunctive therapies with antihistamines, bronchodilators, intravenous fluids, vasopressors, oxygen, and other supportive measures can be considered after the administration of epinephrine based on the clinical scenario. These adjunctive therapies should not be used as a substitute for possible repeat doses of epinephrine if additional epinephrine is available and indicated. Epinephrine administration should not be delayed because delayed use of epinephrine has been associated with fatal reactions in humans. In addition, animal models demonstrate that advanced anaphylaxis can become refractory to epinephrine. Patients with a rapid and complete response to initial therapy should generally be observed for 3 to 6 hours. Prolonged observation or admission should be considered for patients with severe, prolonged, or refractory symptoms.

After acute treatment but before discharge, patients should be given an epinephrine administration device (autoinjector [Auvi-Q, EpiPen] or Neffy nasal spray) and instructed in the proper technique for use. Patients should be instructed in basic avoidance strategies to prevent future stings and offered medical identification information. Patients should understand the significant risk of recurrence and the need to follow up for additional testing and consideration for immunotherapy. If additional evaluation identifies specific IgE to the stinging insect, immunotherapy can be offered. Immunotherapy to stinging insects is quite effective in reducing the risk of a systemic reaction while on immunotherapy and provides longer-lasting risk reduction for many years after completing 3 to 5 years of immunotherapy.

References

Freeman TM: Hypersensitivity to Hymenoptera stings, *N Engl J Med* 351:1978–1984, 2004.
Golden DBK: Large local reactions to insect stings, *J Allergy Clin Immunol* 3:331–334, 2015.
Golden DBK, Demain J, Freeman TM, et al: Stinging insect hypersensitivity: a practice parameter update 2016, *Ann Allergy Asthma Immunol* 118:28–54, 2017.
Jacobson RS: Entomological aspects of insect sting allergy. In Freeman TM, Tracy JM, editors: *Stinging insect allergy*, Switzerland, 2017, Springer, pp 17–42.
Rueff F, Przybilla M, Bilo MB, et al: Predictors of severe systemic anaphylactic reactions in patients with Hymenoptera venom allergy: importance of baseline serum tryptase, *J Allergy Clin Immunol* 124:1047–1054, 2009.
Sampson HA, Munoz-Furlong A, Campbell RL, et al: Second symposium on the definition and management of anaphylaxis: summary report, *J Allergy Clin Immunol* 117:391–397, 2006.
Tracy JM, Demain JG, Quinn JM, et al: The natural history of the exposure to the imported fire ant (*Solenopsis invicta*), *J Allergy Clin Immunol* 95:824–828, 1995.

ANAPHYLAXIS

Method of
David B.K. Golden, MD; and Dennis K. Ledford, MD

CURRENT DIAGNOSIS

- Onset within minutes to 60 minutes after triggering event
- Systemic symptoms and signs with erythema of skin and urticaria most common
- At least two organ systems involved with cardiovascular (hypotension) and respiratory (wheezing or laryngeal edema) most important as responsible for fatality and morbidity
- Syndrome without sine qua non
- Documented mast cell mediator release, particularly serum tryptase increase of 1.2 × baseline + 2 ng/mL, 1.374 × baseline, or 1.685 × baseline tryptase within 30 minutes to 2 hours of onset, may help retrospectively confirm diagnosis but not required to prove diagnosis
- Infants and toddlers manifest urticaria with one or more alternative presentations including change in affect or facies, reduced activity, throat clearing or cough, vomiting, and decreased muscle tone
- National Institute of Allergy and Infectious Diseases anaphylaxis diagnosis criteria are validated with 95% sensitivity and 71% specificity

CURRENT THERAPY

- The only treatment to reduce mortality is immediate epinephrine administration, 0.01 mg/kg IM (1 mg/mL solution, maximum dose 0.5 mg for adults) or 2 mg/actuation intranasal for adults and children over 30 kg, 1 mg/actuation for children 4 years and older and 15 to 30 kg (Neffy).
- Corticosteroids are not effective and not indicated
- Antihistamine therapy may improve itching but is unlikely to affect the outcome
- Hypotension requires leg elevation and may benefit from infusion of intravenous colloid 500 to 1500 mL over 30 minutes in adults and 20 mL/kg over 5 to 10 minutes in children
- Observation for 12 to 24 hours after initial episode is a consideration for biphasic reactions if multiple doses of epinephrine required for initial episode and/or drug causation in children
- Discharge from medical observation safe after all but cutaneous symptoms and signs are resolved for more than 1 hour and low risk for biphasic reaction

Definition and Pathophysiology

Anaphylaxis, also previously termed *anaphylactic* or *anaphylactoid reaction*, is a syndrome characterized by the rapid (usually in minutes, occasionally a few hours) development of potentially fatal, multiorgan dysfunction due to mast cell and basophil mediator release. The mast cell/basophil degranulation may be due to a specific, immunologic trigger (e.g., the activation of specific IgE on the surface of the cells by a specific allergen [allergic anaphylaxis]) or to a nonallergic trigger by activation of nonspecific receptors unrelated to IgE (e.g., Mas-related G-protein coupled receptor member X2 [MRGPRX2]) by vancomycin. Activation leads to rapid release (within minutes) of preformed or rapidly synthesized mediators with multiple end organ effects, including histamine, leukotrienes, prostaglandins, and tryptase, and is followed within hours by cytokines that contribute to a proinflammatory cascade.

TABLE 1	Factors Associated With More Severe Anaphylaxis

Delay in administration of epinephrine
Advanced age
Cardiovascular disease
Injected antigen
Increased mast cell number or increased mast cell susceptibility to
degranulation
- Atopy
- Mastocytosis
- Clonal or nonclonal mast cell activation syndrome
- Hereditary alpha-tryptasemia
Beta blocker therapy
Angiotensin pathway inhibition therapy
Menstruation
Dehydration
Ethanol ingestion
Nonsteroidal antiinflammatory drug therapy
Rapid onset of signs/symptoms after culprit/trigger exposure
Absence of cutaneous anaphylaxis manifestations

TABLE 2	Factors Associated With Biphasic* Anaphylaxis

More severe initial episode of anaphylaxis
  Wider pulse pressure during initial episode
  Multiple doses of epinephrine required for treatment of initial
    episode
Cutaneous manifestations during initial anaphylaxis
Unknown trigger
Drug allergy anaphylaxis (children)

*Recurrence of anaphylaxis 4–48 hours after resolution of initial episode and with-
out additional allergen/trigger exposure
Shaker MS, Wallace DV, Golden DBK, et al: Anaphylaxis—a 2020 practice parameter update, systematic review, and Grading of Recommendations, Assessment, Development and Evaluation (GRADE) analysis, *J Allergy Clin Immunol*
145:1082–1123, 2020.

TABLE 3	Causes of Anaphylaxis

IgE-MEDIATED REACTIONS	NON–IgE-MEDIATED OR MIXED REACTIONS*
Food	Radiocontrast media
Peanut	Medications
Tree nut	NSAIDs
Crustaceans	Muscle paralytics used for
Fish	surgery
Seeds (sesame)	Opioids
Alpha-galactose-D-galactose	Vancomycin
(mammalian meat)	Mastocytosis/mast cell activation
Insect stings	syndromes
Medications	Exercise dependent
Beta-lactam antibiotic	Idiopathic
Other antibiotics	Biologics and most
Chlorhexidine	chemotherapeutics
Muscle paralytics used for	Hereditary alpha-tryptasemia
surgery	
Protamine used for heparin	
reversal	
Platins (chemotherapy)	
Latex	
Allergy immunotherapy	
Food-dependent exercise induced	

*Allergy testing or immunologic desensitization not likely to be helpful; pretreat-
ment with antihistamines and corticosteroids and reduction in rate of administration more likely to be helpful.
NSAIDs, Nonsteroidal antiinflammatory drugs.

Intravenous (IV) or intramuscular (IM) allergen exposure is typically associated with a more rapid onset of anaphylaxis, but even anaphylaxis from oral ingestion of a food allergen may be very rapid. However, oral-induced anaphylaxis can be delayed for up to several hours (3–6 hours after ingestion by sensitized individuals of galactose-α-1,3-galactose (alpha-gal) in noncatarrhine mammalian meat such as pork, mutton, and beef). Insect sting anaphylaxis is also generally rapid in onset, but some reactions occur 4 to 12 hours after the sting. However, anaphylaxis does not occur days after trigger exposure. Cutaneous manifestations, typically urticaria, are the most frequent signs of anaphylaxis and usually the first to develop. Anaphylaxis mortality is due to cardiovascular collapse or respiratory dysfunction due to laryngeal swelling or bronchospasm or both. Mortality is infrequent, approximately 0.1% to 1.0% but up to 7% to 10% in perioperative anaphylaxis. These estimates are limited by the inability to reliably determine the total number of anaphylaxis episodes. Factors associated with severity or fatality are listed in Table 1.

Systemic hypersensitivity reactions are generalized responses, usually limited to the skin, that may or may not progress to anaphylaxis. Systemic hypersensitivity reactions do not reliably portend more severe anaphylaxis with subsequent exposure. In contrast with systemic hypersensitivity reactions, two or more organs are typically involved in anaphylaxis.

One of the most disturbing aspects to patients is the seemingly unpredictable timing of anaphylaxis. The first reaction is always unexpected and may occur after many uneventful prior exposures to the trigger. Recurrent reactions may occur despite attempted avoidance because of hidden and unexpected exposures. In patients with idiopathic anaphylaxis, every reaction is unexpected. However, with early recognition and prompt use of epinephrine, almost all anaphylactic reactions will clear rapidly.

Biphasic anaphylaxis is the recurrence of anaphylaxis 1 to 48 hours after resolution of the initial manifestations. The mechanism for this phenomenon is not understood but is distinct from late-phase allergic reactions associated with intradermal or inhaled allergen exposure in sensitized subjects. The severity of biphasic anaphylaxis may differ from the severity of the initial episode; specifically, biphasic anaphylaxis may be more (or less) severe than the initial phase. Factors associated with biphasic reactions include severity of the initial episode of anaphylaxis, delayed epinephrine use for the initial event, need for more than one dose of epinephrine, and others shown in Table 2. The presence of one or more of these elements may prompt the decision to keep a patient under longer observation before discharge after treating anaphylaxis (see the "Monitoring" section).

Epidemiology and Causes

Estimating the prevalence of anaphylaxis is difficult in part because of the varying definitions and criteria for the diagnosis, and because many patients do not seek medical attention during or after the reaction. Remarkably, anaphylactic reactions are not fatal in >99% of cases and usually subside within hours, even without medical treatment. The cause may be initially overlooked because very commonly there were previous exposures with no reaction (e.g., amoxicillin treatment, insect stings, shellfish ingestion). Anaphylaxis can be life threatening even on the first reaction (e.g., insect stings, drug reactions, some foods).

The population prevalence of anaphylaxis is reported to be in the range of 1.6% to 5.1%, but the known prevalence related to each of the identified causes of anaphylaxis suggests that the lifetime prevalence from all causes may be as great as 10%. The incidence of anaphylaxis has been growing for more than 3 decades, with increasing numbers of emergency department visits, hospitalizations, and intensive care unit (ICU) admissions, but without an increase in mortality.

The most frequent causes of anaphylaxis in adults and children are listed in Table 3. Identification of the cause is often challenging, may be unclear until after repeated reactions or even supervised challenge, and remains idiopathic in a substantial number of cases. The most common cause in children is foods, and less often insect stings or drugs. In adults, insect stings and drugs are more prominent. Anaphylaxis can also be caused by exercise alone or with concomitant specific food ingestion, by biologic therapies, or by vaccines. Unexplained or "idiopathic anaphylaxis" is common despite efforts to identify culprits.

TABLE 4	Manifestations of Anaphylaxis	
MANIFESTATIONS	**FREQUENCY (ADULTS)**
Urticaria/Flushing/Pruritus	~85%
Respiratory Manifestations	~60%
Laryngeal edema	
Oral edema	
Bronchospasm	
Nasal congestion	
Cardiovascular Manifestations	~50%
Hypotension with wide pulse pressure	
Tachycardia or other arrhythmia	
Vasodilation initially, vasoconstriction late	
Increased vascular permeability with third space vascular volume loss	
Cardiosuppression	
Gastrointestinal Manifestations	~25%–30%
Nausea/vomiting*	
Abdominal cramping	
Diarrhea	
Sense of Impending Doom	?
Vaginal Pruritus	?
Change in Affect*	?
Decreased Skeletal Muscle Tone*	?

*More common in infants and toddlers.

Clinical Manifestations

The manifestations of anaphylaxis are multisystem and highly variable from one person to another but are usually reproducible in the same individual. The most common manifestations are listed in Table 4. These are derived from retrospective data and clinical experience as anaphylaxis usually occurs unexpectedly, and not in situations that lead to accurate documentation of each manifestation. The unique, placebo-controlled study of venom immunotherapy included insect sting challenges of placebo-treated (and whole-body extract immunotherapy–treated) subjects. The observations of stung patients provide probably the best set of human data of anaphylaxis in a research setting. The more frequent use of food challenge to confirm IgE-mediated food allergy has also provided a significant increase in details of anaphylaxis, although in these settings the challenge is interrupted early in the process and epinephrine administered, significantly modifying the clinical manifestations. It is possible that anaphylaxis after an insect sting or food ingestion under medical supervision may not reflect the presentation of anaphylaxis from all triggers and in all circumstances.

A point of emphasis is anaphylaxis manifestations in infants and toddlers is quite disparate from that of adults. Often young children will show a change in facies and behavior without other complaints, except perhaps throat clearing or cough. Infants often experience vomiting and generalized skeletal muscle hypotonia.

Cardiovascular manifestations include tachycardia, increased pulse pressure with hypotension, decreased vascular volume, and reduced venous cardiac filling. Stroke volume is decreased due to both hypovolemia and suppression of cardiac contractility. Bradycardia may occur, particularly in those who are treated with beta blockers.

Respiratory manifestations include one or a combination of the following: inspiratory stridor, uvula or tongue edema, garbled speech, change in voice, dysphagia, chest wheezing, hypoxia, and inspiratory intercostal muscle retractions associated with a paradoxical pulse (>10 mm Hg decrease in systolic blood pressure with inhalation). Associated anxiety with the acute onset of symptoms with suspected anaphylaxis makes the common sensation of "throat tightness" of no diagnostic value unless accompanied by other objective findings.

Diagnosis

The diagnosis of a syndrome is problematic as there is no specific defining sign, laboratory test, or symptom; rather, a constellation of findings is necessary. Thus a variety of clinical definitions have been developed, with two being the most accepted at this point. The National Institute of Allergy and Infectious Diseases and Food Allergy and Anaphylaxis Network (NAIAD/FAAN) criteria are well established and validated with 92% to 97% sensitivity and 82% specificity. The 2020 updated World Allergy Organization (WAO) modified criteria are simplified but have not yet been validated. The two sets of criteria do not agree in every case and may be complementary. The challenge is that anaphylaxis is a multisystem phenomenon with variable presentation and pace. Early recognition and treatment reduce the likelihood of more severe, life-threatening anaphylaxis. Thus treatment with epinephrine should be considered before specific criteria are met if anaphylaxis is suspected. The American Academy of Allergy Asthma and Immunology/American College of Allergy Asthma and Immunology Joint Task Force for Practice Parameters (JTFPP) 2024 Anaphylaxis Parameter suggests that meeting criteria for the diagnosis of anaphylaxis is not necessary for the administration of epinephrine.

Typically, cutaneous manifestations are expected with urticaria, pruritus, and flushing. However, more severe anaphylaxis (e.g., perioperative anaphylaxis and anaphylaxis from insect stings in subjects with mastocytosis) may not have cutaneous manifestations.

Other features are wheezing due to bronchial constriction (usually a problem in patients with asthma) or respiratory distress due to laryngeal edema. An increase in paradoxical pulse may be a useful sign if breath sounds are decreased and stridor is not heard due to reduced air movement. Many patients describe a vague sense of doom or serious threat, though this can be difficult to assess in the context of anxiety. Vaginal, palmar, plantar, scalp, or axillary itching are suggestive of anaphylaxis, as urticaria without anaphylaxis does not typically cause itching in these locations. Vasodilation coupled with vascular volume depletion, due to vascular leakage with third space vascular fluid loss, results in postural hypotension and lightheadedness, usually without vertigo.

The differential diagnosis of anaphylaxis is inherently broad due to its multisystem involvement. Table 5 lists potential considerations. Many of these conditions cannot be completely excluded in the acute setting. Throat tightness without change in voice and without stridor is a common complaint of anxiety. Inducible laryngeal obstruction/paradoxical vocal cord dysfunction may suggest laryngeal edema. Tachycardia with anxiety is a challenge, and this will worsen if parenteral epinephrine is used. It is important to recognize that in a situation with a heightened expectation of a possible reaction, the frequency of presumed reactions is greatly increased. This occurred with the introduction of mRNA COVID vaccines where the majority of the reactions diagnosed as anaphylaxis were later determined to be subjective (with no objective findings); they did not recur with administration of a second dose. A similar finding occurs with placebo-controlled food or drug challenges, where nocebo reactions (i.e., adverse reactions to placebo) are quite common; and although mostly subjective, nocebo reactions can even include objective findings such as urticaria. Thus a confirmatory diagnostic test would be of great value.

TABLE 5	Differential Diagnosis of Anaphylaxis				

ANAPHYLAXIS SYNDROMES	**VASOPRESSOR REACTIONS**	**MAST CELL MEDIATOR RELEASE**
• Exercise	• Flush syndromes (**carcinoid**, menopause)	• Systemic mastocytosis
• Cold, heat, sunlight	• Medullary carcinoma thyroid	• Urticaria pigmentosa
• Idiopathic	• Autonomic epilepsy	• Leukemia
	• Vasovagal reaction	• Hydatid cyst rupture
		• Mast cell activation syndromes
		• Hereditary alpha tryptasemia

NONORGANIC DISEASE	**MISCELLANEOUS**	**MISCELLANEOUS**
• Panic/anxiety	• Hereditary (bradykinin-mediated) angioedema	• Other forms of shock
• VCD/ILO	• Pheochromocytoma	• Seizure
• Munchausen stridor	• Red person syndrome	• Transfusion reaction
• Globus hystericus	• Capillary leak	
• Nocebo* effect		

*Nocebo is the physiologic effects of placebo due to expectations or anxiety.
VCD/ILO, Vocal cord dysfunction/inducible laryngeal obstruction.

Laboratory tests have limited value for initial, acute management because results will not be available in time to inform clinical diagnosis and decision making. However, a blood sample for measurement of acute serum total tryptase is often helpful in subsequently confirming the diagnosis and in postevent assessment. The JTFPP recommends obtaining blood for serum tryptase levels within 1 to 2 hours of onset of anaphylaxis or suspected anaphylaxis in all patients. Tryptase is one of the more stable mast cell mediators released during activation and will be increased in blood for up to 2 hours after anaphylaxis, and even longer with a greater number of mast cells involved. Tryptase does not increase in all cases of anaphylaxis, so the lack of an increased tryptase does not rule out the diagnosis. The acute value should be compared with a baseline tryptase, with an increase of 1.2 × baseline + 2 ng/mL having a sensitivity of 78% and specificity of 91% for the diagnosis of anaphylaxis in one published cohort. An acute tryptase of at least 1.685 times the basal value had a sensitivity and specificity of 94% in individuals with a baseline tryptase of >4.1 ng/mL. Mateja and colleagues suggested a variable tryptase criterion based upon pretest probability of anaphylaxis: ≥1.868 × baseline if suspicion of anaphylaxis is low and ≥1.374 × baseline if suspicion is high. Blood tryptase may increase after death, thus postmortem collections are of questionable reliability to diagnose anaphylaxis. Measurements of other mast cell mediators (histamine, prostaglandins, or leukotrienes) have generally not been of clinical use, though research studies sometimes include urinary studies to confirm anaphylaxis or mast cell disorders. Blood histamine has a half-life of 2 to 4 minutes, which limits its utility, but N-methyl histamine in a spot urine sample has become more available and can be measured after the event, preferably within 5 hours.

Prevention

Avoidance of known triggers is the primary strategy to prevent anaphylaxis; the approach should be tailored specifically for the causative allergen or agent. In addition to avoiding exposure to known triggers, there are many factors (e.g., cofactors, augmentation factors) that may increase the severity of anaphylaxis. Identification and avoidance of these factors may reduce the risk of severe reactions. Retrospective evaluations of individuals with anaphylaxis consistently show associations with delay in the administration of epinephrine and more severe, life-threatening outcomes. Thus the treatment of systemic, immediate hypersensitivity reactions with epinephrine is an important strategy for limiting the severity of anaphylaxis or potential anaphylaxis. However, epinephrine is not indicated before onset of symptoms or signs after exposure to a suspected trigger. Other factors that are associated with more severe anaphylaxis are listed in Table 1. Anaphylaxis is a syndrome without a sine quo non; therefore factors associated with severity may incorrectly be correlated with

susceptibility or prevalence, as it is more likely that severe anaphylaxis will be recognized and diagnosed. The ethical barrier to performing double-blind studies of human anaphylaxis limits the confidence of the evidence.

Pharmacotherapy for prevention of anaphylaxis usually is not helpful; specifically, antihistamine and corticosteroid therapy has not reduced the occurrence of anaphylaxis except in four situations. First is anaphylaxis after high-ionic, high-osmolarity radiocontrast infusion. In contradistinction, however, there is no evidence that such pretreatment is of benefit in reactions to the currently used low-ionic, low-osmolarity radiocontrast or to MRI contrast. The second is non–IgE-mediated reactions to IV infusions of chemotherapy or oncologic biologics, which are prevented or mitigated by preinfusion treatment with antihistamines and corticosteroids. Third, individuals with mastocytosis, mast cell activation disorders, and an inherited gene duplication of the mast cell tryptase gene (hereditary alpha-tryptasemia [HαT] affecting 5% to 7% of the general population) are at increased risk of anaphylaxis compared with the general population. Chronic antihistamine therapy, primarily with histamine-1 receptor (H1) antihistamines as there is less evidence for benefit of histamine-2 receptor (H2) antihistamines, may reduce the occurrence or the severity of anaphylaxis in these individuals. Finally, anaphylaxis occurring with rush or accelerated allergen immunotherapy protocols, with multiple allergen injections on a single day, is probably reduced with antihistamine and/or corticosteroid pretreatment. Antihistamine therapy before a standard schedule immunotherapy injection reduces local reactions, but its role in reducing anaphylaxis is not established.

Allergen immunotherapy reduces the risk of anaphylaxis from stinging insects and food ingestion. Maintenance injection therapy for stinging insects reduces the risk of a sting reaction from approximately a 40% to 70% risk of sting anaphylaxis to a 2% to 15% risk. This risk mitigation can be accomplished within weeks to months, although a rush strategy achieves maintenance dosing and protection within days. After 3 to 5 years of treatment, insect venom immunotherapy may be discontinued in most patients and sustained unresponsiveness is maintained, perhaps for a lifetime. In contrast, oral or sublingual food immunotherapy reduces the risk of anaphylaxis with food ingestion or raises the threshold ingestion amount required for anaphylaxis, but sustained unresponsiveness is not commonly achieved. Both insect and food immunotherapy treatments are associated with systemic reactions or anaphylaxis during the treatment, but the reactions occur under more controlled conditions, contrasted with random insect stings or inadvertent food ingestion.

Reduction or elimination of reactivity by a process of allergen desensitization, used with drugs such as beta-lactam antibiotics and aspirin, will also prevent anaphylaxis during immediate therapeutic use of the culprit drug after achieving nonreactivity. Desensitization is a process of attaining an inactive state related to exhaustion of specific-IgE and/or mediators via repeated dosing of the culprit drug, starting with doses below the threshold sufficient to trigger anaphylaxis and gradually increasing over a period of hours. This is generally only effective for IgE-mediated drug reactions (although aspirin hypersensitivity is an exception as it is not generally IgE mediated), and the desensitized state is temporary; that is, the reactive state returns within days or weeks of stopping the drug. The desensitization process must be repeated for future use of the drug.

There is evidence that non–IgE-mediated anaphylaxis (e.g., the majority of vancomycin and chemotherapy/biologic therapy reactions) may be prevented or mitigated by giving the therapy at a slower rate. Pretreatment before chemotherapy and biologics is often helpful as noted earlier. Pretreatment or modification of rate of infusion is not likely helpful for IgE-mediated reactions to chemotherapeutics such as platins.

Other measures that may minimize the severity of but not eliminate anaphylaxis include hydration and avoidance of ethanol, exercise, and nonsteroidal antiinflammatory drug ingestion in proximity to trigger exposure. Therapeutics that reduce mast cell number or mast cell activation may prevent anaphylaxis, though none is approved for this indication. These include omalizumab ([Xolair][1], a monoclonal antibody that reduces both free IgE and mast cell/basophil IgE receptors), tyrosine kinase inhibitors that interfere with intracellular mast cell signaling (e.g., avapritinib [Ayvakit, Ayvakyt][1] and midostaurin [Rydapt][1]), and inhibitors of stem cell factor's interaction with the cell surface receptor KIT (CD 117) that reduce mast cell number (e.g., barzolvolimab[5] and briquilimab[5]).

Discontinuation of chronic angiotensin pathway inhibitors or beta blockers in individuals with a history of anaphylaxis, with the goal of preventing future reactions, is controversial. The long-term benefits of these therapies are much greater than the incremental absolute risk of a reaction, which remains small. These observations resulted in the most recent JTFPP anaphylaxis document recommending that angiotensin pathway inhibitors and beta blocker therapies not need be routinely discontinued in individuals at risk of anaphylaxis. Rather, there should be a documented, shared decision-making discussion with the patient and prescriber to evaluate the available data on the relative benefits and potential harms of either giving or not giving the medications or proposed intervention, and any other potential risk factors, in the context of the patient's values and preferences.

Therapy

Therapy focuses on cardiovascular and respiratory support while eliminating, if possible, additional exposure to the anaphylaxis cause or trigger. Epinephrine is the only pharmacologic treatment with efficacy for the life-threatening features of anaphylaxis (Table 7). The dose is based upon historical experience and is 0.1 to 0.5 mg IM (0.01 mg/kg of 1-mg/mL solution, up to 0.5 mg per dose for adults and up to 0.3 mg per dose for children), preferably in the lateral thigh as inadvertent injection into subcutaneous fat is less likely in this location. The recommendation of IM administration is based upon studies showing more rapid and consistent absorption with this parenteral delivery, though studies vary. During the development of intranasal epinephrine products, nasal epinephrine (Neffy) was compared with IM epinephrine by autoinjector (EAI) or manual (needle and syringe) injection. High variability in the IM epinephrine pharmacokinetic data was documented between EAI and manual injection, among EAI devices, and even with the same device in different patient cohorts. Subcutaneous (SQ) injections were recommended historically until the 1980s, and it is unclear if IM is definitely more effective than SQ. However, IM remains the recommended route of administration. IV epinephrine administration is preferred by anesthesiologists for perioperative anaphylaxis at a dose of 0.1 mg by slow push[1] over 3 to 5 minutes. The risk of cardiac arrhythmia makes this a nonpreferred option unless the patient can be monitored very closely and continuously, as in the

perioperative setting. Early administration of epinephrine, ideally before the development of severe hypotension, is more effective as the treatment is initiated before significant third space vascular volume loss and before compensatory increase in vascular resistance develops. Thus, if anaphylaxis is suspected, epinephrine should not be delayed until sufficient manifestations are evident to "prove" anaphylaxis. The timing of epinephrine (i.e., early use) is likely more important than the dose. IM or nasal epinephrine (Neffy only) is very safe when administered at the specified dose, and the treatment should be repeated in 5 to 15 minutes depending on the clinical response. Cumulative, intermittent IM doses greater than 2 mg for a single event should be avoided due to potential cardiac adverse effects unless accompanied by large-quantity IV volume replacement (see later). Lower epinephrine doses are likely more effective when administered early in anaphylaxis. However, as stated earlier, epinephrine should not be used before any manifestations of anaphylaxis after a potential exposure to known or suspected trigger. The value of antihistamine therapy before the development of signs or symptoms after exposure to a potential trigger is unknown.

Other treatments are summarized in Table 6. H1 antihistamine therapy (e.g., PO or IV diphenhydramine) improves itch but has little, if any, effect on the overall outcome. H2 antihistamine therapy (e.g., PO or IV famotidine[1]) is often used as well, but there is little or no evidence of clinical value. Corticosteroid therapy (e.g., IV methylprednisolone) is often employed, with the mistaken impression this may minimize biphasic anaphylaxis or accelerate improvement of the immediate episode; however, there is no evidence of benefit from corticosteroid therapy for anaphylaxis, and it may cause harm. Large-volume solution therapy with normal saline with 5% dextrose, normal saline, or lactated Ringer solution is recommended for hypotension; nebulized or inhaled beta agonist is useful for wheezing; nebulized racemic epinephrine 0.5 mL has been used, with limited evidence of benefit, for suspected laryngeal angioedema; and oxygen supplementation should be used if oximetry is reduced. Secure venous access with large-bore needle(s) capable of delivering 1 to 2 L of IV solution in 30 to 60 minutes for adults is needed if epinephrine does not restore the blood pressure. Intraosseous administration of fluid resuscitation is a consideration in children or adults without IV access. In the presence of hypotension, it is critical for the patient to remain in a supine position with legs elevated to maximize cardiac venous return and avoid "empty ventricle syndrome" with sitting or standing, which can be fatal.

Continuous administration of IV vasoconstrictors with monitored infusions of epinephrine, norepinephrine, dopamine, or dobutamine[1] are recommended if hypotension persists despite IM epinephrine and IV solute replacement (Table 6). Fluid resuscitation should precede use of continuous vasoconstrictors due to increased vascular permeability and reduced vascular volume from third space losses. Intractable hypotension may respond to IV methylene blue[1] at a dose of 1 to 2 mg/kg over 20 minutes followed by 0.5 to 1 mg/kg/h in adults and 1 mg/kg over 20 minutes with hourly repeat doses in children. The rationale is a reduction of the vasodilator nitric oxide.

Bradycardia may occur with anaphylaxis, potentially (and erroneously) suggesting a vasovagal reaction. Like anaphylaxis, vasovagal reactions also have an immediate onset but are associated with cutaneous vasoconstriction and initial diaphoresis, in contrast to the warm, erythematous, dry, and pruritic skin initially with anaphylaxis. Bradycardia with anaphylaxis is more likely if the patient is chronically treated with a beta blocker. Atropine 0.3 to 0.5 mg SQ, IM, or IV (0.02 mg/kg in children with maximum dose of 0.5 mg) is a treatment for bradycardia. If anaphylaxis rather than a vasovagal reaction is suspected, epinephrine should be administered for bradycardia, as it is more effective than atropine for the other manifestations of anaphylaxis. IV glucagon[1] 3 mg by slow push followed by infusion at 0.3 to 0.9 mg/hour

[1] Not FDA approved for this indication.
[5] Investigational drug in the United States.

[1] Not FDA approved for this indication.

TABLE 6 Treatments of Anaphylaxis

THERAPY	ADULT DOSE	PEDIATRIC DOSE	ROUTE	POTENTIAL COMPLICATIONS
Adrenergic Agents				
Epinephrine (1 mg/mL IV solution)	0.3–0.5 mg	0.01 mg/kg	IM (may repeat dose 5–15 min if needed)	Arrythmia/tachycardia
			IV injection (use 1 mg/mL solution; may repeat 5–15 min if needed)	
Epinephrine nasal spray (Neffy: 2 mg/0.1 mL/spray or 1 mg/0.1 mL/spray)		>30 kg: 1 spray (2 mg/spray) into one nostril once 15 kg to <30 kg: 1 spray (1 mg/spray) into one nostril once	Intranasal May repeat a second dose in the same nostril in 5 min if needed	Epistaxis Systemic: Tremor, tachycardia, jitteriness
			Nasal spray (2 mg/0.1 mL) (1 mg/0.1 mL) (second dose in the [Neffy] in one nostril in one nostril same nostril after 5 min if needed)	Tremor, anxiety
Epinephrine (slow IV bolus[1] in refractory cases)	0.1 mg	0.01 mg/kg	SP using 0.1 mg/mL solution (further diluted in 10 mL NS)	Coronary vasospasm
			IV injection (only in refractory cases) (use 0.1 mg/mL solution)	
Norepinephrine	2–12 µg/min (0.02–1 µg/kg/min), start at 0.1–0.5 µg/kg/min and titrate	0.02–1 µg/kg/min (start 0.05–0.1 µg/kg/min and titrate)	IV infusion	Arrhythmia/tachycardia Tremor/anxiety
Dopamine	2–20 µg/kg/min	2–20 µg/kg/min	IV continuous	Arrhythmia/tachycardia
Dobutamine[1]	2–20 µg/kg/min (maximum 40 µg/kg/min) for both adults and children	2–20 µg/kg/min	IV continuous	Arrythmia, anxiety
Albuterol	180 µg (90 µg/puff)	180 µg (90 µg/puff)	Metered dose inhaler	Cough, tremor
	2.5–10 mg over 15–60 min Repeat 20 min	2.5 mg	Nebulizer over 15–60 min, may repeat in 20 min	Paradoxical bronchospasm
Racemic epinephrine	0.5–1.0 mL (11.25–22.5 µg) in 2.5 mL NS Repeat 20 min	0.05 mL/kg (max 0.5 mL) in 2.5 mL NS	Nebulizer (2.25% solution mixed with 2.5 mL NS)	Tremor, tachycardia
Fluid Resuscitation/Vascular Volume Expansion				
IV solution*	500–1500 mL over 15–30 min	20 mL/kg over 5–10 min Repeat × 3	IV/interosseous	Fluid overload Edema
Antihistamines				
H1 Antihistamine				
Diphenhydramine	25–50 mg	1–2 mg/kg	IV	Tachycardia Seizure, sedation
Cetirizine[1]	10 mg	2.5–10 mg	IV/PO	
H2 Antihistamine				
Famotidine[1]	20 mg	0.25 mg/kg (max 20 mg)	IV/PO	
Other Therapies				
Oxygen	2–5 L/min	2–5 L/min	Nasal cannula Mask	
Glucagon[1]	1–5 mg	0.03–0.15 mg/kg	Slow IV bolus	Nausea, vomiting
	0.3–0.9 mg/h	0.07 mg/kg/h	IV infusion	

TABLE 6 | Treatments of Anaphylaxis—cont'd

THERAPY	ADULT DOSE	PEDIATRIC DOSE	ROUTE	POTENTIAL COMPLICATIONS
Methylene blue[1]	1–2 mg/kg over 20 min	1 mg/kg over 20 min, may repeat hourly	IV	Nausea Headache
	Followed by 0.5–1 mg/kg/h		IV	
Atropine	0.3–1.0 mg	0.02 mg/kg (max 0.5 mg)	IV infusion	Tachycardia Dry mouth Urinary retention Blurred vision

[1]Not FDA approved for this indication.
*IV solution: Normal saline with 5% dextrose, normal saline, lactated Ringer solution.
IM, Intramuscular; *IV*, intravenous; *NS*, normal saline; *PO*, oral ingestion; *SP*, slow IV push over several minutes; *SQ*, subcutaneous.

is a consideration in patients treated with beta blockers. The rationale is a reduction of ongoing mast cell mediator release by an increase in intracellular mast cell cyclic adenosine monophosphate (cAMP) via an adrenergic independent mechanism. In patients treated with beta blockers, epinephrine is initially recommended as stated earlier, before considering glucagon therapy. Nausea and vomiting is frequent after IV glucagon; the airway should be protected before administration.

Monitoring

Initial monitoring of anaphylaxis necessitates frequent vital signs and subjective evaluation, particularly focusing on oxygen saturation, blood pressure and evidence of tissue perfusion, state of cognition, and airway protection. Elimination of additional exposure to the likely cause is also important. Culprit factors with a longer half-life or delayed absorption may cause more prolonged anaphylaxis. The response to anaphylaxis treatment is usually within minutes with timely use of epinephrine. Discharge from a health facility and medical monitoring is reasonable 1 hour after resolution of signs and symptoms, though residual cutaneous manifestations (erythema, mild pruritus, mild urticaria) are acceptable at discharge. The risk of biphasic anaphylaxis (discussed previously) is a potential concern, and factors that predict a greater chance of biphasic anaphylaxis should prompt longer observation, perhaps 12 to 36 hours (Table 2).

Protracted anaphylaxis, a reaction persisting for >4 hours, also requires prolonged monitoring, usually in an ICU setting. Refractory anaphylaxis is another reason for extended medical observation. Refractory anaphylaxis is persistent manifestations despite multiple doses of epinephrine, which occurs in about 2% of cases. This prevalence is based upon registry data, but the denominator (i.e., the total number of anaphylaxis episodes in the population) is generally not known, making the estimate imprecise. A European registry from 90 medical centers in 10 countries with over 11,000 subjects reported that drug etiologies, particularly perioperative anaphylaxis, and honeybee insect sting anaphylaxis were associated with protracted anaphylaxis in adults. Consistent with the increased frequency of food-triggered anaphylaxis in children, food allergy was most associated with protracted or refractory anaphylaxis in the pediatric population. Hen's eggs and cow's milk were the culprits in children younger than 2 years, hazelnut and cashew for preschool children, and peanut for all pediatric age ranges.

Complications

Anaphylaxis is potentially life threatening, but as stated earlier, mortality is uncommon and likely less than 1%. Advanced age and impaired ability to compensate physiologically to cardiovascular changes are major contributors to mortality. Thus older age is a major risk factor for fatality, although food allergy is a more frequent cause of fatality in adolescents, likely due to increased risk-taking behavior. Mortality in the perioperative setting is an order of magnitude greater, approaching 10%. In addition, there are morbidities from hypoxia and hypotension resulting in more

than 15% to 25% of surviving subjects having permanent ischemic sequelae after perioperative anaphylaxis. Finally, there are psychological and quality of life complications after anaphylaxis. The episodic nature of the condition with potential of severe symptoms often results in chronic anxiety. The burdens of avoiding substances or activities that likely caused or contributed to the condition are a lifetime limitation. Keeping self-administered epinephrine readily available at all times is another burden. After the event, referral to an allergy/immunology specialist is important to assist in possibly confirming the diagnosis, potentially identifying the cause of anaphylaxis, discussing avoidance strategies, and addressing anxiety and quality of life issues.

References

Baretto RL, Beck S, Heslegrave J, et al: Validation of international consensus equation for acute serum total tryptase in mast cell activation: a perioperative perspective, *Allergy* 72:2031–2034, 2017.

Elkhalifa S, Elbashir H, Abuzakouk M: When allergies have no name: is idiopathic anaphylaxis driven by co-factors? *Front Allergy* 18:146845, 2024.

Francuzik W, Dölle-Bierke S, Knop M, et al: Refractory anaphylaxis: data from the European anaphylaxis registry, *Front Immunol* 10:1–8, 2019.

Golden DBK, Carter MC: Anaphylaxis: bench to bedside, *J Allergy Clin Immunol Pract* 11:2049–2050, 2023.

Golden DBK, Wang J, Waserman S, et al: Anaphylaxis: a 2023 practice parameter update, *Ann Allergy Asthma Immunol* 132:124–176, 2024.

Grabenhenrich LB, Dölle S, Moneret-Vautrin A, et al: Anaphylaxis in children and adolescents: the European anaphylaxis registry, *J Allergy Clin Immunol* 137:1128–1137, 2016.

Kaminsky LW, Aukstuolis K, Petroni DH, Al-Shikhly T: Use of omalizumab for management of idiopathic anaphylaxis: a systematic review and retrospective case series, *Ann Allergy Asthma Immunol* 127:481–487, 2021.

Košnik M, Zugan L, Rijavec M: Prevention of anaphylaxis episodes in idiopathic anaphylaxis by omalizumab, *Int Arch Allergy Immunol* 185(8):761–766, 2024.

Mateja A, Wang Q, Chovanec J, et al: Defining baseline variability of serum tryptase levels improves accuracy in identifying anaphylaxis, *J Allergy Clin Immunol* 149:1010–1017, 2022.

Nicolas F, Villers D, Blanloeil Y: Hemodynamic pattern in anaphylactic shock with cardiac arrest, *Crit Care Med* 12:144–145, 1984.

Oya S, Nakamori T, Kinoshita H: Incidence and characteristics of biphasic and protracted anaphylaxis: evaluation of 114 inpatients, *Acute Med Surg* 1:228–233, 2014.

Pouessel G, Deschildre A, Dribin TE, et al: Refractory anaphylaxis: a new entity for severe anaphylaxis, *J Allergy Clin Immunol Pract* 11:2043–2048, 2023.

Pumphrey RSH: Fatal anaphylaxis in the UK 1992-2001. *Anaphylaxis: novartis foundation symposium*, Vol 257. Chichester UK, 2004, John Wiley & Sons, Ltd.

Shaker MS: Anaphylaxis: definition and criteria, *Journal of Food Allergy (USA)* 6:26–31, 2024.

Shaker MS, Oppenheimer J, Wallace DV, et al: Making the GRADE in anaphylaxis management: toward recommendations, integrating values, preferences, context, and shared decision making, *Ann Allergy Asthma Immunol* 124:526–535, 2020.

Shaker MS, Wallace DV, Golden DBK, et al: Anaphylaxis-a 2020 practice parameter update, systematic review, and Grading of Recommendations, Assessment, Development and Evaluation (GRADE) analysis, *J Allergy Clin Immunol* 145:1082–1123, 2020.

Simons FE, Sampson HA: Anaphylaxis: unique aspects of clinical diagnosis and management in infants (birth to age 2 years), *J Allergy Clin Immunol* 135:1125–1131, 2015.

Suresh RV, Dunnam C, Vaidya D, et al: A phase II study of Bruton's tyrosine kinase inhibition for the prevention of anaphylaxis, *J Clin Investig* 15:e172335, 2023.

Tanno LK, Demoly P: Biologicals for the prevention of anaphylaxis, *Curr Opin Allergy Clin Immunol* 21:303–308, 2021.

Voelker D, Pongdee T: Biomarkers in diagnosis of mast cell activation, *Curr Opin Allergy Clin Immunol* 25:27–33, 2025.

DRUG HYPERSENSITIVITY REACTIONS

Method of
**Miriam Chan, PharmD, MHA; Ann M. Aring, MD; and
Kristen Rundell, MS, MD**

CURRENT DIAGNOSIS

- Detailed history should include past medical history; current diagnosis; previous and current medication use, including over-the-counter drugs and herbals as well as other nonprescribed medications; duration of the medication use; any similar reactions in the past.
- Physical examination should include vitals, temperature, and skin examination for rash.
- Laboratory testing should be conducted based on symptoms that may include complete blood count (CBC) with differential, eosinophils, sedimentation rate, liver enzymes, international normalized ratio (INR), C-reactive protein (CRP), and diagnostic skin biopsy or testing.

CURRENT THERAPY

- For life-threatening anaphylaxis reaction, start basic life support using pneumonic CAB-D (compression, airway, breathing, defibrillate) and give epinephrine immediately.
- Discontinue the offending drug if medically possible. Try drug substitution if warranted.
- An alternative option is to reduce the dose or frequency of the drug.
- Start symptomatic treatment based on the type of reaction and the offending medication.
- Some reactions may respond to treatment with antihistamines, H_2 blockers, or steroids.

Epidemiology

Drug hypersensitivity reactions are one of the many different types of adverse drug reactions (ADRs). ADRs are common, yet the more severe reactions have been estimated to cause 3% to 6% of hospital admissions. More than 100,000 deaths annually are caused by serious ADRs, making these reactions one of the leading causes of death in the United States. Early detection of all ADRs can potentially improve patient outcomes and lower health care costs.

Classifications

An ADR is a broad term that refers to any predictable or unpredictable reaction to a medication. A predictable (type A) reaction is dose dependent and is related to the known pharmacologic properties of the drug. Predictable reactions account for about 80% of all ADRs. An example of a type A reaction is gastritis that results from taking nonsteroidal antiinflammatory drugs (NSAIDs). The remaining 20% of ADRs are caused by unpredictable (type B) reactions. Type B reactions occur in susceptible individuals. These are hypersensitivity reactions that are different from the pharmacologic actions of the drug; they are results of interactions between the drug and the individual human immune system. Type B reactions can be further divided into drug intolerance, drug idiosyncrasy, drug allergy (immunologically mediated), and pseudoallergic reactions (anaphylactoid reactions). This chapter will focus on these type B drug hypersensitivity reactions.

Pathophysiology

Several mechanisms may play a role in the underlying etiology of immunologic drug reactions. The Gell and Coombs classification system was the original system to describe four predominant immune mechanisms. These four reaction types are listed as type I reactions (IgE medicated), type II reactions (cytotoxic), type III reactions (immune complex), and type IV reactions (delayed, cell mediated). Table 1 provides a detailed description of this classification. Type I and IV reactions are more common than type II and III reactions. Most drugs cause one type of reaction, whereas certain drugs, such as penicillin, can induce all four types of reactions.

The Gell and Coombs classification has recently been revised to reflect the functional heterogeneity of T cells. Under the new system, type IV reactions are further subclassified into four categories: IVa (macrophage activation), IVb (eosinophils), IVc (CD4+ or CD8+ T cells), and IVd (neutrophils). Nevertheless, many common hypersensitivity reactions cannot be classified in this system because of the lack of knowledge of their immune mechanism or a mixed mechanism.

A new concept of drug interaction with immune receptors has recently been developed by Pichler and colleagues. It is called the *p-i concept* (pharmacologic interaction with immune receptors). In this concept, a drug binds noncovalently to a T-cell receptor and stimulates an immune response, which can cause inflammatory reactions of different types. The stimulation of the T cell is enhanced by the additional interaction with the major histocompatibility complex molecule. This is direct stimulation of memory and effector T cells, and no sensitization is required. The skin has a high concentration of effector memory T cells, which can be rapidly stimulated by antigen penetration. The skin also possesses a dense network of dendritic cells that act as antigen-presenting cells and increase hypersensitivity reactions. As a result, clinical symptoms by p-i drugs may appear more rapidly. Some severe reactions—such as Stevens-Johnson syndrome (SJS), toxic epidermal necrolysis (TEN), the drug rash with eosinophilia and systemic symptoms (DRESS) syndrome, or hypersensitivity syndrome—are believed to be p-i related. Examples are abacavir (Ziagen) hypersensitivity syndrome and SJS/TEN from carbamazepine (Tegretol).

Risk Factors for Hypersensitivity Drug Reactions

The chemical structure and molecular weight of the drug may help predict the type of hypersensitivity reaction. Larger drugs with greater structural complexity are more likely to be immunogenic. However, drugs with small molecular weight (< 1000 Da) can elicit hypersensitivity reactions by coupling with carrier proteins to form hapten-carrier complexes. Other drug-related factors include the dose, route of administration, duration of treatment, repetitive exposure to the drug, and concurrent illness. Topical and intravenous drug administrations are more likely to cause hypersensitivity reactions than are oral medications.

Patient risk factors include age, female gender, HIV and other immunocompromised state (or status), atopy, specific genetic polymorphisms, previous drug hypersensitivity reactions, and inherent predisposition to react to multiple unrelated drugs. A recent case-control study of 60 hospitalized patients suggests that severe vitamin D deficiency may be a risk factor for developing severe cutaneous adverse reactions.

Clinical Manifestations

Drug hypersensitivity reactions can manifest in a great variety of clinical symptoms and diseases. While some reactions are mild and often unnoticed, others, such as anaphylaxis, can be severe and even fatal. Dermatologic symptoms are the most common physical manifestation of allergic drug reactions. Drug hypersensitivity reactions can also affect various internal organs, causing diseases such as hepatitis, nephritis, and pneumonitis. To differentiate the different clinical manifestations, it is important to also consider the timing of the identified rash to the drug exposure. The noncutaneous physical findings are generally nonspecific and may not be helpful and even delay the diagnosis and management decisions.

Dermatologic Symptoms

The most common allergic drug reactions affect the skin and can cause a variety of different exanthems. The most common skin reaction is the classic "drug rash," which is a morbilliform

TABLE 1 Classification of Drug Hypersensitivity Reactions

TYPE	MECHANISM	CLINICAL FEATURES	TIMING OF REACTIONS	EXAMPLES
Type 1 (IgE mediated)	Drug-IgE complex binds to mast cells	Urticaria, angioedema, bronchospasm, pruritus, GI symptoms, anaphylaxis	Immediate (minutes to hours after drug exposure, depending on the route of administration)	β-lactam antibiotic
Type II (cytotoxic)	Specific IgG or IgM antibodies directed at drug-hapten–coated cells	Hemolytic anemia, neutropenia, thrombocytopenia	Variable	Penicillin (hemolytic anemia), heparin (thrombocytopenia)
Type III (immune complex)	Antigen-antibody complexes	Serum sickness, vasculitis, drug fever	1–3 weeks after drug exposure	Penicillin (serum sickness), sulfonamides (vasculitis), azathioprine (drug fever)
Type IV (delayed, cell mediated)	Activation and expansion of drug-specific T cell	Prominent skin findings: Contact dermatitis, morbilliform eruptions	2–7 days after exposure	Topical antihistamine, penicillin, sulfonamides

eruption originating on the trunk. Other dermatologic symptoms include urticaria, angioedema, acne, bullous eruptions, fixed drug eruptions, erythema multiforme, lupus erythematosus, photosensitivity, psoriasis, purpura, vasculitis, and pruritus. The most severe forms of cutaneous drug reactions are Stevens-Johnson syndrome (SJS), toxic epidermal necrolysis (TEN), and drug rash with eosinophilia and systemic symptoms (DRESS) syndrome.

Stevens-Johnson Syndrome

SJS is a systemic disorder that has cutaneous manifestations. SJS was previously thought to be synonymous with erythema multiforme major. There are now criteria that separate the two disorders. In contrast to erythema multiforme, the target lesions associated with SJS have only two rings. The inner ring may have urticaria, pustules, or necrotic lesions surrounded by macular erythema. It is a T-cell–mediated toxic reaction to the basement membrane of the epidermal cells. There is massive and widespread apoptosis, for which there are several associated cytokines. The recent theories suggest that there are two pathways, one that consists of granule-medicated exocytosis (perforin and granzyme B), and one that consists of Fas-Fas ligand interaction associated apoptosis for the keratinocytes. More recent data suggest that granulysin, which is a cationic cytolytic protein released by T lymphocytes, may play a role as well.

Interestingly, HLA genotype may predispose patients to SJS or TEN. Those patients with the HLA-B1502 found among the Han Chinese population may be associated with increased risk for developing SJS/TEN and use of carbamazepine.

SJS and TEN are on the same continuum. The definition of epidermal detachment and desquamation of epidermal cells is less than 10% of the body surface area for SJS and more than 30% for TEN. There is an overlapping diagnosis of SJS/TEN for the 10% to 30% category. To help differentiate from other ADRs, there is often a prodromal period in which a patient may have a cough and a fever. The lesions may occur 1 to 4 weeks after exposure to the drug. In addition, the lesions may be limited to the trunk; however, they more commonly involve the palmar surface of the hands and the dorsum of the feet, as well as the mucous membranes.

The most common drug classes associated with SJS and TENs are sulfonamides, cephalosporins, imidazole agents, and oxicam derivatives. Drugs such as carbamazepine, phenytoin (Dilantin), valproic acid (Depakote), lamotrigine (Lamictal), allopurinol (Zyloprim), nevirapine (Viramune), peramivir (Rapivab), and quinolones have been reported to cause SJS/TEN. In a retrospective chart review of 64 patients who had a diagnosis of SJS/TEN, Miliszewski et al. identified allopurinol as the single most common offending agent (20% of cases). According to the US Food and Drug Administration (FDA) Safety Alerts in 2013, acetaminophen has been associated with SJS,

TEN, and acute generalized exanthematous pustulosis (AGEP). The evidence supporting causality primarily comes from a small number of cases reported in the medical literature.

The treatment is immediate cessation of the culprit drug and symptomatic treatment. Glucocorticoids are controversial and depend on the course and extent of the disease.

Toxic Epidermal Necrolysis

As previously stated, TEN is the cell-mediated disorder that involves more than 30% of the body surface. Similar to SJS, the onset of the rash is 1-3 weeks after drug exposure. This is the more-severe form of the ADR: the mortality rates may be as high as 50%, mostly from sepsis. Patients are usually admitted to the burn unit for electrolyte and infection management. Glucocorticoids are contraindicated. There have been mixed results using IV immunoglobulin (IVIG)[1] in these patients. The IVIG is believed to inhibit the Fas-Fas ligand, which is the underlying mechanism for the basement membrane separation.

Drug Rash with Eosinophilia and Systemic Symptoms

DRESS syndrome or drug-induced hypersensitivity syndrome (DIHS) is a rare, life-threatening drug-induced reaction with a mortality rate of 5%–10%. Therefore it is important to recognize the signs and symptoms early to initiate treatment. Most patients will have fever, lymphadenopathy (75%), eosinophilia, and an erythematous morbilliform rash on the face and body in addition to liver and multiorgan damage. The symptoms can occur 2 to 6 weeks after the drug administration. There are many drugs that can cause DRESS syndrome such as allopurinol, vancomycin, sulfonamides, and psychotropic medications. Based on literature review, DRESS syndrome is increasingly being recognized by psychiatrists. Carbamazepine is the most frequently reported etiology; however, DRESS syndrome is also seen with lamotrigine, phenytoin, valproate, and phenobarbital. The treatment is drug withdrawal, systemic corticosteroids, topical treatment for lesions, and supportive care, often in the ICU or burn unit. Glucocorticoid-sparing drugs and targeted biologic treatments are emerging as alternative therapeutic options to systemic steroids.

Acute Generalized Exanthematous Pustulosis

Acute generalized exanthematous pustulosis (AGEP) is a rare ADR that presents as a fever and small nonfollicular pustules on a widespread erythematous background. AGEP may closely mimic pustular psoriasis clinically. The presence of acanthuses and papillomatosis and a personal or family history of psoriasis favor a diagnosis of pustular psoriasis. Exposure to medication, especially antibiotics with a short latency from the initiation of

---

[1]Not FDA approved for this indication.

the drug, favors AGEP. The eruption usually occurs within 24-48 hours of the initiation of the drug, and healing occurs quickly after the discontinuation of the drug. Lesions heal within 2 weeks of discontinuation without scarring. The exact mechanism of drug-specific T lymphocytes is unknown, yet IL-3 and IL-8 may be the trigger for neutrophil-activating cytokines in the skin.

Acute Interstitial Nephritis

Acute interstitial nephritis (AIN) is an important cause of acute kidney injury (AKI). More than two thirds of AIN cases are caused by drug hypersensitivity reactions. Drugs most commonly associated with AIN include antibiotics (particularly β-lactam, fluoroquinolones, and rifampicin), NSAIDs, proton pump inhibitors, phenytoin, allopurinol, and 5-aminosalicylates.

The clinical presentation of drug-induced AIN is highly variable and depends on the class of drug involved. Patients with AIN may be asymptomatic with elevation in creatinine or blood urea nitrogen or abnormal urinary sediment. When present, symptoms are nonspecific. The "classic" triad of fever, rash, and eosinophilia is present in less than 5% to 10% of patients. Each individual component of the triad also occurs at various rates.

A diagnosis of AIN should be considered in any patients with unexplained AKI, clinical manifestations of a hypersensitivity reaction, and a history of exposure to any drug associated with AIN. A definitive diagnosis of AIN is established by kidney biopsy. AIN is characterized by interstitial inflammation, tubulitis, edema, and, in some cases, eventual interstitial fibrosis. The precise disease mechanism is unclear, but the presence of T lymphocytes in the inflammatory infiltrate suggests a type IV hypersensitivity response.

Early recognition is crucial as patients can ultimately develop chronic kidney disease. The mainstay of therapy is timely discontinuation of the causative agent. If AIN persists, corticosteroids may be used to improve kidney function. However, available data on corticosteroids are inconclusive, and randomized controlled trials are needed to confirm the benefits of corticosteroids in the treatment of AIN.

Evaluation

Because the history is essential for determining whether a patient is experiencing a drug hypersensitivity reaction, it is important to review all medications and the timeline of exposure. This includes any over-the-counter medications, herbal supplements, or occasional-use medications. Occasional-use medications may include NSAIDs, acetaminophen, cold medications, and so forth. It is important to establish a temporal relationship to the onset of the medication and the initiation of the symptoms. Oftentimes, the medication may have been discontinued before the appearance of the first symptom, so a review of medications from several weeks before the symptoms is also important. In addition, because the host immune response plays a role in some of the IgE-mediated reactions, it is important to review any immunocompromising chronic or acute illnesses or states that the patient may have or is currently experiencing. This includes HIV, chronic obstructive pulmonary disease (COPD), asthma, chemotherapy, and pregnancy. For some ADRs, HLA type may be important. A patient's known genetic predisposition needs to be taken into account as well. A thorough history will also need to include any organ system or symptom that may be related to the suspected ADR.

A physical examination should augment and help to establish the working diagnosis of the type of ADR and the potentially offending drug. This should include vital signs of temperature, respiratory, and hydration status. The skin examination is important, as are appropriate evaluation and documentation of the type of lesion or lesions present. An examination of the oral mucosa and the conjunctiva of the eye should be done. Any lymphadenopathy, petechiae, or pallor should be noted.

Laboratory testing may be obtained to confirm or rule out a diagnosis. This may include a chest x-ray, CBC with differential, possible skin biopsy, liver function testing, creatinine, and electrolyte testing. A sedimentation rate and CRP testing may also be useful. Although additional autoimmune or antibody testing may

be done, caution is suggested. There may not be a high yield on these tests, and they can be quite costly for patients.

Management

Anaphylaxis

Anaphylaxis can be a fatal drug hypersensitivity reaction because of its rapid onset. It is often underrecognized and undertreated because it can mimic other conditions and is variable in its presentation. Most cases occur at home, school, or restaurants. Respiratory compromise and cardiovascular collapse are of greatest concern, because they are the most common causes of death. Urticaria and angioedema are the most common manifestations but may be delayed or absent. Anaphylaxis typically occurs within hours after exposure to the offending agent. The more quickly anaphylaxis occurs, the more likely the reaction is to be severe and potentially life threatening. Anaphylaxis can also occur anytime during a drug treatment. According to the FDA Adverse Event Reporting System database and published case reports, glatiramer acetate (Copaxone, Glatopa) was associated with 82 cases of anaphylaxis that occurred between December 1996 and May 2024. The majority of these patients experienced anaphylaxis within 1 hour of taking the drug, but about 25% of the cases occurred more than 12 months after the drug was started.

Most anaphylaxis episodes are IgE-mediated reactions resulting in a sudden mast cell and basophil degranulation. This sudden release of mediators affects the cutaneous, pulmonary, cardiac, GI, vascular, and neurologic systems. Medications are a common trigger of anaphylaxis in adults. Most cases of IgE-mediated drug anaphylaxis in the United States are due to penicillins and cephalosporins. Antibiotics are also the most common cause of perioperative anaphylaxis because skin eruptions may be missed in patients who are draped during surgery. Some anaphylaxis reactions involve other immunologic mechanisms. Administration of blood products (e.g., IVIG, animal antiserum) can cause an anaphylactoid reaction due, at least in part, to complement activation. Activation of the complement cascade can cause mast cell/basophil degranulation. Anaphylaxis episodes can also occur independently of any immunologic mechanism. Certain drugs, such as opioids, dextrans, and protamine, can cause a direct release of histamine and other mediators from mast cells and basophils. Finally, there are acute systemic reactions without any obvious triggers or mechanisms (idiopathic anaphylaxis).

Anaphylaxis is a clinical diagnosis with a short window of treatment time available. Therefore laboratory testing is limited and may not be of much value. Initially, the patient will describe flushing, pruritus, and a sense of impending doom. Some patients will have dyspnea, dizziness, syncope, or GI symptoms of diarrhea and abdominal cramping. Most patients will have cutaneous symptoms of flushing, urticaria, or angioedema. Some patients will progress to respiratory or cardiovascular complications.

The goal of therapy should be early recognition and treatment with epinephrine to prevent a progression to life-threatening respiratory or cardiovascular failure. The immediate intervention should include stopping the offending drug if possible, epinephrine injection, basic life support, high-flow oxygen, cardiac monitoring, and IV access. Epinephrine is the drug of choice for anaphylaxis. The therapeutic actions of epinephrine include α-1-adrenergic vasoconstrictor effects (decreases mucosal edema, thereby relieving upper airway obstruction, and increases blood pressure to prevent shock), β-1 adrenergic effects (increases rate and force of cardiac contractions), and β-2 effects (increases bronchodilation and decreases the release of mediators of inflammation from mast cells/basophils). Delayed epinephrine administration has been associated with fatalities. There is no absolute contraindication to epinephrine in the setting of anaphylaxis. Intramuscular epinephrine in the thigh results in high-plasma concentrations and is preferred in the setting of anaphylaxis. The recommended dose of epinephrine is 0.01 mg/kg of a 1:1000 (1 mg/mL) solution, up to a maximum of 0.3 mg for children and 0.5 mg for adults. Patients in shock should receive epinephrine by slow IV infusion at 2 to 10 mcg/min with the rate titrated according to response and the presence of continuous hemodynamic monitoring. Patients taking beta-blockers may be resistant to treatment with epinephrine. In this case, glucagon[1] 1 to 5 mg IV over 5 minutes should be administered because its cardiac effects are not mediated through beta-receptors.

In light of the fact that most of the anaphylaxis occurs outside the health care setting, epinephrine autoinjectors (EAIs) should be prescribed to patients at risk for anaphylaxis. The patients and their caregivers should be counseled about carrying and using EAIs. This is important because many community settings do not have epinephrine readily available. EAIs are available in dosage forms of 0.3 mg (Auvi-Q, EpiPen) for patients ≥30 kg, 0.15 mg (Auvi-Q, EpiPen Jr) for patients 15 to 30 kg and 0.1 mg (Auvi-Q) for patients 7.5 to 15 kg. Since the 0.1 mg EAI is not universally available, the American Academy of Pediatrics and Joint Task Force on Practice Parameters support the use of 0.15 mg EAIs for children less than 15 kg[3]. Epinephrine should be administered at the first sign of anaphylaxis. After EAI is given, EMS activation is required for slow or incomplete symptom resolution. In addition, EMS should be called if symptoms return or worsen.

The FDA recently approved a new epinephrine nasal spray (Neffy) to treat anaphylaxis in adults and pediatric patients age ≥4 years who weigh 15 kg. The recommended dose is one spray (1 mg/0.1 mL) into one nostril for patients 15 to <30 kg and one spray (2 mg/0.1 mL) into one nostril for patients ≥30 kg. If response is inadequate, administer a second dose in the same nostril with a new nasal spray 5 minutes after the first dose. A prescription for Neffy should consist of two single-dose nasal spray devices.

Adjunctive therapies for the treatment of anaphylaxis include antihistamines and corticosteroids. Consider an inhaled beta-agonist if wheezing. Diphenhydramine (Benadryl), an H_1 antihistamine, may be given intravenously at the dose of 25 to 50 mg. If an H_2 blocker is considered, give famotidine[1] (Pepcid) 20 mg IV over 2 minutes. Corticosteroids are used to prevent a potential late-phase reaction that may occur in up to 23% of adults with anaphylaxis. There is no proven best dose or route of steroid therapy. The most common dosage is prednisone 20 to 60 mg daily for 3 to 5 days.

Angioedema

Angioedema is characterized by a deep dermal, subcutaneous, mucosal swelling. Many patients present with both urticaria and angioedema. Angioedema can progress rapidly from a mild swelling of the oral mucosal to a life-threatening laryngeal edema. With this rapid sequence of events, the most important part of treatment is obtaining and maintaining a patent airway. Epinephrine 0.3 mg IM every 10 minutes should be administered to patients who present with anaphylaxis, respiratory distress, or severe laryngeal edema. Once the airway is patent, the patient should be treated with H_1 antihistamines, H_2 blockers, and steroids. The milder cases may be treated similarly to other allergic reactions. H_1 antihistamines such as diphenhydramine and hydroxyzine (Atarax) are effective in relieving pruritus but can cause significant sedation. Therefore second-generation H_1 antihistamines[1] (loratadine [Claritin], cetirizine [Zyrtec], desloratadine [Clarinex], fexofenadine [Allegra]) are often chosen for outpatient therapy. Doxepin (Sinequan),[1] a tricyclic antidepressant with potent H_1 and H_2 blocker activities, can be used as an alternative to H_1 antihistamines. However, it should not be used as first-line treatment for acute urticaria and angioedema because of its significant side effects of severe sedation, dry mouth, and weight gain. Corticosteroids are used in patients who are not responsive to antihistamines. For most patients, a short course of oral prednisone is adequate.

In drug-induced angioedema, the offending drug should be stopped and avoided. Further trial of the medication is not recommended, because the patient will respond more quickly and with more severe symptoms on reintroduction. The patient should be counseled, and epinephrine 0.3 mg in an auto-injectable device (EpiPen, Auvi-Q, Adrenaclick) may be prescribed in case of recurrence in the future.

Specific Drugs

Almost all drugs can cause a drug hypersensitivity reaction. However, certain drugs are more frequently associated with specific types of reactions. Some of the more commonly used drugs are discussed here in more detail.

Antibiotics
Penicillin

Penicillin allergy is the most well-known drug allergy and also the most costly ADR. Although most drugs usually have type I and type IV reactions, penicillin may cause all four types of allergic drug reactions. The rate of penicillin-induced anaphylaxis after intravenous administration is approximately 1 to 2 per 10,000 treated patients.

Only about 10% of patients who report a penicillin drug allergy actually have a true immunologic response. IgE antibodies in patients with documented IgE-mediated acute penicillin reaction decline with time, resulting in 80% patients tolerating penicillin after 10 years. Patients with a penicillin allergy label are more likely to be treated with broad-spectrum or second-line antibiotics. Inappropriate use of antibiotics is linked to increased antibiotic resistance and adverse health outcomes. There is an increasing focus on penicillin allergy delabeling as an integral part of antimicrobial stewardship. Algorithms are available to clarify a patient's allergy status and expedite the evaluation for true penicillin allergy. Trubiano et al. recently developed a clinical decision tool, PEN-FAST, to aid risk stratification of patients with penicillin allergy and facilitate appropriate delabeling and prescribing strategies.

Penicillin skin testing is the best method for diagnosing an IgE-mediated penicillin allergy. A commercially available product, PRE-PEN, contains benzylpenicilloyl polylysine (PPL), which is a major antigenic determinant of penicillin. Minor determinants are metabolic derivatives of penicillin that may also produce an immune response. The current recommendations for penicillin skin testing are to administer both the major determinant (PPL) and the minor determinants (penicillin G). These two tests identify approximately 90% to 97% of the currently allergic patients. Patients with a history of penicillin allergy but negative skin test should be given an oral 250-mg amoxicillin challenge and observed for 1 hour following the skin test. If the skin test and oral challenge are both negative, the risk for Ig-E-mediated anaphylaxis is almost zero.

In general, patients who report symptoms consistent with an immediate or type I reaction or are skin-test positive to penicillin should not receive penicillin. Desensitization should be considered if penicillin is the treatment of choice for an infection and no acceptable nonpenicillin alternatives are available. Patients should be desensitized in a hospital setting. Desensitization involves administering incremental doses of oral penicillin every 15 minutes for a total of 4 to 12 hours, after which time the first dose of penicillin is given. For intravenous desensitization, three drug concentrations of penicillin are infused in 12 steps. Penicillin desensitization protocols are available in the review article by Castells et al. Desensitization is temporary and only lasts for two dosing intervals of the drug before the desensitization needs to be repeated.

Penicillin and Cephalosporin Cross-Reactivity

The rate of cross-reactivity between penicillin and cephalosporins has been historically cited to be as high as 10%. Recent data suggest that the rate may be much lower. The degree of cross-reactivity is highest between penicillins and first-generation cephalosporins, which have identical R-group side chains. In this case amoxicillin would be cross-reactive with cefadroxil (Duricef) and cefprozil (Cefzil), whereas ampicillin would be with cefaclor and cephalexin. Because of the differences in the chemical structures, second- and third-generation cephalosporins (cefdinir [Omnicef], cefuroxime [Ceftin], cefpodoxime [Vantin], and ceftriaxone [Rocephin]) are unlikely to be associated with cross-reactivity with penicillin. According to the latest guidelines for acute otitis

---

[1] Not FDA approved for this indication.
[3] Exceeds dosage recommended by the manufacturer.

media from the American Academy of Pediatrics and American Academy of Family Physicians, alternative initial antibiotics in patients with penicillin allergy include cefdinir, cefuroxime, cefpodoxime, or ceftriaxone.

Patients with penicillin allergy who have a negative skin-test result to penicillin (major and minor determinants) may safely receive cephalosporins. Cephalosporin treatment of patients with penicillin allergy who did not have a severe or recent penicillin reaction history shows a reaction rate of 0.1%. Use cephalosporin with caution in patients who report an immediate or accelerated penicillin allergy or those with a positive skin test to penicillin.

Sulfonamides (Sulfa Drugs)

Beside penicillins, sulfonamide antibiotics are the second most common cause of drug-induced allergic reactions. They commonly cause a delayed maculopapular/morbilliform eruption. Acute urticarial reactions (IgE mediated) to sulfamethoxazole (SMX) or trimethoprim (TMP) are relatively infrequent; the incidence of skin rash resulting from SMX-TMP (Bactrim) in healthy subjects is estimated to be 3%. Sulfonamides are also the most common cause of SJS and TEN.

Patients with HIV have the greatest risk of sulfonamide-induced allergic reactions. The typical reaction to SMX-TMP in patients with HIV is a generalized maculopapular eruption that occurs during the second week of treatment and is usually accompanied by pruritus and fever. Because SMX-TMP is the drug of choice for a number of HIV-associated infections such as *Pneumocystis carinii* pneumonia and spontaneous bacterial peritonitis, several methods of desensitization have been devised to administer SMX-TMP to patients with HIV with a history of allergic reaction to the drug.

There are three classes of sulfonamides based on chemical structure: sulfonylarylamines (including sulfa antibiotics),

nonsulfonylarylamines, and sulfonamide-moiety-containing drugs. A sulfonylarylamine has a sulfonamide moiety directly attached to a benzene ring with an amine ($-NH_2$) moiety at the N4 position. A nonsulfonylarylamine also has a sulfonamide moiety attached to a benzene ring, but it does not have an amine group at the N4 position. A sulfonamide-moiety–containing drug has a sulfonamide group that is not connected to a benzene ring. Table 2 presents a list of sulfonamide-containing drugs based on their chemical structure.

The N4 amine is critical for the development of delayed reactions to sulfa antibiotics. Given the important chemical differences between drugs containing sulfa antibiotics and sulfa in nonantibiotics, the risk of cross-reactivity is extremely unlikely. A retrospective cohort study by Strom and colleagues showed that approximately 90% of patients with sulfa antibiotic allergy did not have a reaction to a sulfonamide nonantibiotic. Patients with allergic reactions to sulfa antibiotics are also more likely to experience allergic reactions to the other types of sulfonamides, but this is not because of cross-sensitivity. There is no reliable skin test to rule out or confirm sulfa allergy. Some experts recommend avoiding all classes of sulfonamides in patients with serious reactions such as SJS, TEN, or anaphylaxis to any one sulfonamide.

Most diuretics are sulfonamide derivatives. The only diuretics that are not in this group are the potassium-sparing diuretics (triamterene [Dyrenium], spironolactone [Aldactone], amiloride [Midamor]) and ethacrynic acid (Edecrin). Dapsone is a sulfone that is chemically unrelated to sulfonamides. *It should also be noted that sulfates, sulfur, and sulfites are chemically unrelated to sulfonamides and do not cross-react.*

Angiotensin-Converting Enzyme Inhibitors

Angiotensin-converting enzyme inhibitors (ACEIs) have two major adverse effects: cough and angioedema. The cough is typically dry and nonproductive. The incidence of ACEI-induced cough has been reported to be 5% to 35%. Cough occurs more commonly in women, African-Americans, and Asians. The onset of cough ranges from within hours of the first dose to months after the initiation of therapy. The diagnosis is confirmed by the resolution of cough, usually within 1 to 4 weeks after discontinuation of the ACEI; however, the cough can linger for up to 3 months. The cause for ACEI-induced cough is unclear but might be related to bradykinin, substance P, or another mechanism. Angiotensin II receptor blockers (ARBs) are not associated with an increased incidence of cough and can be used as an alternative to ACEIs. Because the cough may persist for several months after stopping the ACEI, starting the ARB is not a contraindication at this time, yet the cough may persist through the initiation of the new drug.

The incidence of angioedema with ACEIs is approximately 0.1% to 0.7%. With the widespread use of ACEIs, angioedema has become a growing problem. ACEI-induced angioedema is more common in patients who are over age 65, black, or female. Angioedema frequently involves swelling of the face or upper airway and can be life threatening or fatal. It can occur within days, months, or even years after the start of treatment. However, nearly 60% of cases occur within the first week of therapy. ACEIs cause angioedema by direct interference with the degradation of bradykinin, thereby increasing bradykinin levels and leading to increased vascular permeability, inflammation, and activation of nociceptors. Bradykinin is also a prominent mediator in hereditary angioedema. Therefore ACEIs are contraindicated in patients with hereditary angioedema.

ARBs directly inhibit the angiotensin receptor and do not interfere with bradykinin degradation. Theoretically, they can be relatively safe alternatives for patients with a previous history of ACEI-associated angioedema. However, some reports of ARB-induced angioedema have recently been published. The mechanism of how ARBs cause angioedema is unclear. A meta-analysis suggests that for patients who developed angioedema when taking an ACEI, the risk of persistent angioedema when subsequently switched to an ARB is less than 10%. Therefore

TABLE 2	Classification of Sulfonamides Based on Chemical Structure

Drug

Sulfonylarylamines

Antibiotics:	*Antiinflammatory:*
Sulfadiazine	Sulfasalazine (Azulfidine)
Sulfamethoxazole	Protease Inhibitors:
Sulfisoxazole	Darunavir (Prezista)
Sulfapyridine	Fosamprenavir (Lexiva)

Nonsulfonylarylamines

Carbonic Anhydrase Inhibitors:	*Sulfonylureas:*
Acetazolamide (Diamox)	Chlorpropamide
Brinzolamide (Azopt)	Glimepiride (Amaryl)
Dorzolamide (Trusopt)	Glipizide (Glucotrol)
Methazolamide (Neptazane)	Glyburide (Diabeta)
Cyclooxygenase 2 (COX-2) Inhibitors:	Tolbutamide
Celecoxib (Celebrex)	Tolazamide (Tolinase)
Loop Diuretics:	Other Agents:
Bumetanide (Bumex)	Mafenide (Sulfamylon)
Furosemide (Lasix)	Probenecid
Torsemide (Demadex)	Tamsulosin (Flomax)
Thiazides Diuretics:	Tipranavir (Aptivus)
Chlorothiazide (Diuril)	
Chlorthalidone	
Hydrochlorothiazide	
Indapamide (Lozol)	
Metolazone (Zaroxolyn)	

Sulfonamide-Moiety-Containing Drugs

5-HT Agonists:	*Other Agents:*
Naratriptan (Amerge)	Ibutilide (Corvert)
Sumatriptan (Imitrex)	Simeprevir (Olysio)
	Sotalol (Betapace)
	Topiramate (Topamax)
	Zonisamide (Zonegran)

ARBs may be an alternative only for patients with a high therapeutic need for angiotensin inhibition. ARB treatment should be started with observation. Patients should be educated on the signs of angioedema and provided with proper emergency instructions on how to proceed if angioedema should occur.

The direct renin inhibitor aliskiren (Tekturna) does not alter local or circulating bradykinin and is believed to be an alternative in patients with ACEI- and ARB-related angioedema. However, cases of angioedema have been reported with aliskiren. As with ARBs, renin inhibitors should be used with caution in patients who previously experienced angioedema to ACEIs. ACEIs and beta-blockers (BB) were previously considered contraindicated in patients at high risk for anaphylaxis because of an increased risk of severe anaphylaxis. According to recent studies, the risk of these medications is small. For most medical conditions, the risk of stopping or changing treatment with ACEI or BB may exceed the risk of more severe anaphylaxis if the ACEI or BB is continued. For patients with insect sting allergy who take ACEIs or BBs, consider venom immunotherapy. Patients may continue receiving maintenance-dose allergen immunotherapy when on ACEI/BB.

Aspirin and NSAIDs

Aspirin (ASA) and NSAIDs can cause several types of hypersensitivity reactions. The four most-common types of reactions are based on the drug pathways. Aspirin-exacerbated respiratory disease (AERD) is a serious reaction induced by ASA and NSAIDs in patients with asthma and chronic rhinosinusitis. AERD does not fit precisely into a specific type of ADR and is often referred to as a type of pseudoallergic reaction. AERD affects up to 20% of adults with asthma. It is more common in women. The usual age of onset is around 30 years. The pathophysiology of AERD is related to aberrant arachidonic acid metabolism. Patients with AERD also have increased respiratory tract expression of cysteinyl leukotriene 1 receptor and heightened responsiveness to inhaled leukotriene E_4. Administration of aspirin or an NSAID to these patients leads to inhibition of cyclooxygenase 1 (COX-1), resulting in a decrease in prostaglandin E_2 levels. Prostaglandin E_2 normally inhibits 5-lipooxygenase. As a result of decreased prostaglandin E_2 levels, arachidonic acid is preferentially metabolized in the 5-lipooxygenase pathway, leading to increased production of cysteinyl leukotrienes.

Patients with AERD typically have both rhinoconjunctivitis and bronchospasm within minutes of ingestion of a dose of ASA or NSAID. The bronchospasm can be severe and result in respiratory failure, which may require intubation and mechanical ventilation. Management of patients with AERD involves treatment of the patient's asthma and chronic rhinosinusitis and avoidance of aspirin and NSAIDs. Desensitization is available in cases when the patient has a specific therapeutic need for regular ASA or NSAID therapy. Grimaldi et al. reviewed aspirin desensitization strategies for patients with true ASA hypersensitivity in the setting of acute coronary syndrome. In nonacute situations (e.g., elective percutaneous coronary intervention or aortic valve replacement), the authors recommended consulting with the immuno-allergologists for an appropriate desensitization protocol. Selective COX-2 inhibitors very rarely cause reactions in patients with AERD and can be taken safely.

The second type of ASA and NSAID hypersensitivity reaction is an exacerbation of urticaria or angioedema in patients with chronic idiopathic urticaria. Approximately 20% to 40% of patients with chronic urticaria may have this drug-induced reaction. The mechanism of this reaction is related to COX-1 inhibition. The exacerbating effects are usually dose dependent. All drugs that inhibit COX-1 cross-react to cause this reaction. Selective COX-2 inhibitors are generally considered safe to take in patients with chronic idiopathic urticaria.

The third type of hypersensitivity reaction is an anaphylactic or immediate urticarial reaction or angioedema appearing soon after the intake of a specific NSAID. Other NSAIDs from other groups or even an NSAID from the same group with a slightly different chemical structure is tolerated by the patient. An IgE-mediated mechanism is implicated only in some instances. The diagnosis is made mainly by exclusion. Further research is needed in this topic.

The fourth type of hypersensitivity reaction is urticaria or angioedema caused by ASA or any NSAID that inhibits COX-1 in patients without chronic urticaria. These reactions may be either drug specific or cross-reactive to other NSAIDs. Rarely, patients may have combined respiratory and cutaneous reactions that cannot be classified into one of the four reaction types described.

Corticosteroids

Corticosteroids are the most frequently used drugs for the treatment of allergic conditions, yet they can also induce hypersensitivity reactions. Most hypersensitivity reactions to steroids can be classified into type I (immediate, IgE-mediated) and type IV (delayed, cell-mediated) mechanisms. Type I reactions are characterized by the presence of urticaria and anaphylaxis. Type IV reactions can be presented as maculopapular exanthema and delayed urticaria.

Allergic contact dermatitis (type IV reaction) caused by topical administration of steroids is the most common type of allergic reaction induced by this class of drugs, occurring at the rate of 3% to 6%. Usually this is seen as a failure to improve or a worsening of an existing dermatitis that is being treated with topical steroid. Keep in mind that the reaction can also be due to other constituents of the creams, such as neomycin or cetostearyl alcohol. The diagnosis can be done using patch testing, which detects more than 90% of allergic patients. The topical steroids most frequently involved are nonfluorinated, such as hydrocortisone and budesonide.

Inhaled and intranasal steroids can induce both local and systemic reactions. Local reactions include contact dermatitis, pruritus, nasal congestion, erythema, and dry cough and are quite often irritant in nature. Systemic reactions include eczematous lesions, particularly on the face, exanthema, and urticaria. The most frequently involved steroid is budesonide. The actual mechanism of this reaction is not clear, but it may be a T-cell–mediated reaction.

Hypersensitivity reactions to systemically administered steroids seldom occur. Most of the data come from case reports. Both immediate and delayed reactions have been described, ranging from urticaria to sudden cardiovascular collapse and death. Most immediate reactions are caused by intravenous methylprednisolone and hydrocortisone. In a few cases, the reactions can be induced by salts, such as succinate, or rarely by certain diluents such as carboxymethylcellulose or metabisulfite. Nonimmediate reactions are mainly mild, such as delayed urticaria or maculopapular exanthema. The drug involved most often is betamethasone.

Cross-reactivity between steroids is difficult to assess. Based on corticosteroid patch test results and their chemical structure, Coopman and colleagues divided the steroids into four groups: A (hydrocortisone type), B (triamcinolone acetonide type), C (betamethasone type), and D (hydrocortisone-17-butyrate type). Group D can be subdivided into D1 and D2 depending on the presence or absence of a C16 methyl substitution and/or halogenations on the C9 of the B ring. Table 3 provides the listing of the four groups. High cross-reactivity exists between corticosteroids in each group, as well as between group D2 and groups A and B, with group D1 exhibiting quite low cross-reactivity with the other groups.

Local Anesthetics

The most common immunologic reaction to local anesthetic is allergic contact dermatitis (type IV). IgE-mediated reactions (type I) to local anesthetics are very rare. Most adverse reactions are due to nonallergic factors such as vasovagal response, anxiety, dysrhythmias, and toxic reactions resulting from inadvertent IV epinephrine effects.

Any patient who presents with a history of an allergic reaction to local anesthetics should be carefully evaluated. Skin testing and graded challenge can be performed in patients who present with a history suggestive of a possible IgE-mediated allergic reaction to these drugs. A local anesthetic that does not contain epinephrine or other additives, such as parabens or sulfites, is preferred in this situation.

GROUP	TYPE	DRUGS
TABLE 3	Coopman Classification of Cross-Reactivity in Corticosteroids	
A	Hydrocortisone	Hydrocortisone (acetate, succinate, phosphate) Methylprednisolone (acetate, succinate, phosphate) Prednisolone, prednisolone acetate Tixocortol pivalate*
B	Triamcinolone acetonide	Amcinonide (Cyclocort) Budesonide (Pulmicort, Rhinocort, Entocort) Desonide (Desonate, DesOwen) Flunisolide Fluocinolone acetonide (Synalar) Fluocinolone Halcinonide (Halog) Triamcinolone Triamcinolone acetonide (Kenalog)
C	Betamethasone	Betamethasone (Celestone) Desoxymethasone Dexamethasone Paramethasone* Fluocortolone*
D1	Hydrocortisone-17-butyrate	Beclomethasone dipropionate (QVAR) Betamethasone valerate Betamethasone dipropionate Clobethasone 17-butyrate* Clobetasol 17-propyonate (Clobex)
D2	Hydrocortisone-17-butyrate	Fluticasone (Flonase) Mometasone Prednicarbate (Dermatop) Hydrocortisone 17-butyrate (Locoid) Hydrocortisone 17-propionate* Methylprednisolone aceponate*

*Not available in the United States.
From Torres and Canto (2010).

It is necessary to identify the type of local anesthetics to be used. Local anesthetics are classified as esters or amides based on their chemical structure. Drugs in the esters group include benzocaine (Americaine, Dermoplast, Lanacane, Hurricaine), chloroprocaine, cocaine, procaine (Novocaine), proparacaine (Alcaine, Opthaine), and tetracaine (Tetcaine). Most allergic reactions reported in the literature have been caused by agents in the esters group, which are derivatives of para-aminobenzoic acid (PABA), a known allergen. Cross-reactivity occurs among members of the ester group, but the esters do not cross-react with the amides. Agents in the amides group include bupivacaine (Marcaine), lidocaine, mepivacaine (Polocaine), prilocaine (Citanest), and ropivacaine (Naropin). Amide local anesthetics generally do not cross-react with other amides or with the esters.

Radiocontrast Media

There are two types of radiocontrast media (RCM): ionic high osmolality and nonionic low osmolality. Both of these agents contain iodine. The nonionic RCMs are much more widely used today than the ionic agents.

Allergic reactions to RCM are common and can range from mild to life threatening. Anaphylactoid reactions and severe life-threatening reactions occur in 1% to 3% and 0.22% of patients who receive ionic RCM, respectively. Less than 0.5% and 0.04% of patients who receive nonionic agents have anaphylactoid reactions and severe reactions, respectively. The fatality rate is approximately 1 to 2 per 100,000 procedures, and it is similar for both ionic and nonionic agents. RCM reactions are typically not mediated by IgE antibodies. RCM acts directly on mast cells and basophils, resulting in the release of histamine and other systemic mediators, which cause the anaphylactoid reactions. Patients at greater risk for more serious anaphylactoid reactions include females; those with asthma, heart disease, and a history of previous anaphylactoid reaction to RCM; and those taking beta-blockers. People who have seafood allergy are not at increased risk for reactions to RCM compared with the general population. The pathogenesis of anaphylactoid reactions is also not related to iodine.

Management of patients with previous RCM reactions include the use of a nonionic, low-osmolarity agent and a pretreatment regimen. One common regimen consists of prednisone (50 mg PO at 13, 7, and 1 hour before the procedure), diphenhydramine (50 mg at 1 hour before the procedure), and a histamine H_2-receptor antagonist (1 hour before the procedure).

Delayed reactions to RCM occur 1 hour to 1 week after RCM administration. Approximately 2% of patients have delayed reactions to RCM. These reactions are generally mild, self-limited cutaneous eruptions. The mechanism is usually T-cell mediated. Rarely, more serious and life-threatening delayed reactions such as SJS, TEN, and DRESS syndrome have been reported.

Other Medications

Antibiotics, antiepileptics, allopurinol, and NSAID medications are known to be associated with severe cutaneous adverse reactions (SCARs). Using data from the US Food and Drug Administration (FDA) Adverse Event Reporting System (FAERS), Godfrey et al updated and stratified a list of medications with significant reporting odds ratios (ROR) of SCARs. They reported that the prototypical medication classes accounted for the majority of reported cases of SJS, TEN, AGEP, and DRESS. In addition, they updated the list of drugs implicated in SCARs to include previously undescribed medications that have significant ROR signals. They identified acetylcysteine and fluconazole for SJS, and furosemide, spironolactone, fluconazole, amphotericin B and acetylcysteine for TEN. For AGEP, they identified acyclovir, valacyclovir, and enoxaparin. For DRESS, vemurafenib, acyclovir, abacavir, raltegravir, and valacyclovir were identified to have strong RORs. When evaluating a suspected SCAR, clinicians may refer to the updated list. They may also refer to the FAERS quarterly data for additional information.

Chlorhexidine

Chlorhexidine gluconate is an antiseptic agent. It is commonly available in OTC products as a skin and wound disinfectant (e.g., Betasept, Hibiclens). Hypersensitivity reactions to chlorhexidine include contact dermatitis, pruritus, urticaria, dyspnea, and anaphylaxis. Prescription chlorhexidine gluconate mouthwashes and oral chips used for gum disease contain a warning about the rare but serious allergic reactions in their labels. According to a recent FDA Drug Safety Communication, the number of reports of serious allergic reactions to chlorhexidine-containing products has increased over the last several years. As a result, an anaphylaxis warning is now added to the OTC product labels under Drug Facts.

Several case reports have suggested that some patients with prior exposure to chlorhexidine and patients with chlorhexidine-induced contact dermatitis may be susceptible to anaphylaxis caused by chlorhexidine sensitization. Since chlorhexidine is the standard skin disinfectant used before surgery or invasive procedures, the exposure to the agent becomes more widespread. Even though severe anaphylaxis to chlorhexidine has been estimated to be rare, the actual rate may be higher than reported. Such reports remind clinicians to be vigilant about chlorhexidine as a hidden allergen, especially in surgical patients.

Herbal Supplements

There is a perception that herbal supplements are "natural" and therefore safe. In fact, severe allergic reactions including asthma and anaphylaxis have been well documented in patients using bee pollen products and echinacea. Echinacea is an herb belonging to a group of flowering plants known as Asteraceae. Asteraceae-derived pollens are an important cause of hay fever and asthma.

Asteraceae may cause contact allergic dermatitis. Cross-reactivity exists between members of the Asteraceae family, such as ragweed, dandelion, daisy, chamomile, echinacea, feverfew, and milk thistle.

A lack of quality control has been a major concern in the herbal supplement industry. Chinese herbal products may be adulterated with synthetic medications not listed on the label. Contaminated supplements may be a potential risk for systemic contact dermatitis in nickel- and mercury-allergic patients. Because of the widespread use of herbal supplements and the underreporting of adverse events to herbs, all patients should be questioned about the use of herbal supplements when being evaluated for hypersensitivity reactions.

Conclusion

Drug hypersensitivity reactions are common; fortunately, severe and often fatal reactions are not. It is important for the clinician to have a working knowledge of common drug-induced hypersensitive reactions as well as the ability to identify and document common dermatologic findings. With that background knowledge, a thorough history and physical examination should enable the clinician to diagnose the majority of these types of reactions. A timely and appropriate management plan can then be implemented. As always, it is important to educate patients regarding their drug hypersensitivity history and the potential for future reactions.

References

American Academy of Pediatrics: Clinical practice guideline: The diagnosis and management of acute otitis media, *Pediatrics* 131:e964–e969, 2013.
Bommersbach TJ, Lapid MI, Leung JG, et al: Management of psychotropic drug-induced DRESS syndrome: A systematic review, *Mayo Clin Proc* 91(6):787–801, 2016.
Castells M, Khan DA, Phillips EJ: Penicillin allergy, *N Engl J Med* 381:2338–2351, 2019.
CDC: Sexually transmitted disease treatment guidelines 2021, *MMWR* 70(4):1–192, 2021.
Fernando SL: Acute generalized exanthematous pustulosis, *Australas J Dermatol* 53:87–92, 2012.
Godfrey H, Jedlowski P, Thiede R: Medication associations with severe cutaneous adverse reactions: A case/non-case analysis using the FDA Adverse Event Reporting System, *J Cutan Med Surg* 28(1):51–58, 2024.
Golden DBK, Wang J, Waserman S, et al: Anaphylaxis: A 2023 Practice Parameter Update, *Ann Allergy Asthma Immunol* 132:124–176, 2024.
Grimaldi S, Migliorini P, Puxeddu I, Rossini R, De Caterina R: Aspirin hypersensitivity: a practical guide for cardiologists, *Eur Heart J* 21;45(19):1716–1726, 2024.
Harr T, French L: Toxic epidermal necrolysis and Stevens-Johnson syndrome, *Orphanet J Rare Dis* 5:39, 2010. Available at http://www.ojrd.com/content/5/1/39.
Haymore BR, Yoon J, Mikita CP, et al: Risk of angioedema with angiotensin receptor blockers in patients with prior angioedema associated with angiotensin-converting enzyme inhibitors: A meta-analysis, *Ann Allergy Asthma Immunol* 101:495–499, 2008.
Husain Z, Reddy BY, Schwartz RA: DRESS syndrome, part I. Clinical perspectives, *J Am Acad Dermatol* 68:693.e1–693.e14, 2013.
Inomata N: Recent advances in drug-induced angioedema, *Allergol Int* 61:545–557, 2012.
Jaroenpuntaruk V, Gray A: Deadly drug rashes: early recognition and multidisciplinary care, *Cleve Clin J Med.* 90(6):373–381, 2023.
Khan DA, Solensky R: Drug allergy, *J Allergy Clin Immunol* 125:S126–S137, 2010.
Kroshinsky D, Cardones ARG, Blumenthal KG: Drug reaction with eosinophilia and systemic symptoms, *N Engl J Med* 391:2242–2254, 2024.
Miliszewski MA, Kirchhof MG, Sikora S, et al: Stevens-Johnson syndrome and toxic epidermal necrolysis: An analysis of triggers and implications for improving prevention, *Am J Med* 129(11):1221–1225, 2016.
Moka E, Argyra E, Siafaka I, Vadalouca A: Chlorhexidine: Hypersensitivity and anaphylactic reactions in the perioperative setting, *J Anaesthesiol Clin Pharmacol* 31(2):145–148, 2015.
Murata J, Abe R: Soluble Fas ligand: Is it a critical mediator of toxic epidermal necrolysis and Stevens-Johnson syndrome? *J Invest Dermatol* 127:744–745, 2007.
Perazella MA, Markowitz GS: Drug-induced acute interstitial nephritis, *Nat Rev Nephrol* 6(8):461–470, 2010.
Philips JF, Yates AB, Deshazo RD: Approach to patients with suspected hypersensitivity to local anesthetics, *Am J Med Sci* 334:190–196, 2007.
Pholmoo N, Thaiwat S, Klaewsongkram J: Severe vitamin D deficiency increases the risk of severe cutaneous adverse reactions, *Exp Dermatol* 33, 2024:e14980.
Pichler WJ: Consequences of drug binding to immune receptors: Immune stimulation following pharmacological interaction with immune receptors (T-cell receptor for antigen or human leukocyte antigen) with altered peptide-human leukocyte antigen or peptide, *Dermatol Sin* 31:181–190, 2013.
Ponka D: Approach to managing patients with sulfa allergy. Use of antibiotic and nonantibiotic sulfonamides, *Can Fam Physician* 52:1434–1438, 2006.
Shenoy ES, Macy E, Rowe T, Blumenthal KG: Evaluation and management of penicillin allergy: a review. *JAMA* 321:188–99, 2019.
Torres MJ, Canto G: Hypersensitivity reactions to corticosteroids, *Curr Opin Allergy Clin Immunol* 10:273–279, 2010.
Trubiano JA, Vogrin S, Chua KY, et al: Development and validation of a penicillin allergy clinical decision rule, *JAMA Intern Med* 180(5):745–752, 2020.

SERUM SICKNESS

Method of
Amy Robertson, PharmD; and Amanda Rhyne, MD

CURRENT DIAGNOSIS

- Identified by: fever, rash, joint pain (in combination or isolated)
- 7–14 days after exposure to offending agent
- Most frequently in the adult female population
- There are no disease defining labs, although complement tests may be elevated

CURRENT THERAPY

- Identify and discontinue offending agent
- Symptomatic relief with analgesics and antihistamines, as needed
- Those with severe disease may be treated with oral or intravenous corticosteroids for 10–14 days
- If symptoms reappear after discontinuation of corticosteroid, reinitiate with a slow taper

Pathophysiology

Serum sickness is classified as a type III delayed immune-complex–mediated hypersensitivity reaction. It was first noted by Von Pirquet in the early 1900s after administration of equine antisera. The mechanism consists of exposure to an antigen (often a large protein) that leads to formation of an antigen-antibody complex. The immune complex load becomes too high to be appropriately excreted from the body, causing deposition in joints, tissues, and vascular endothelium. It also leads to activation of the complement pathway, which prompts mast cell and basophil degranulation with vasoactive amine release. The deposition of immune complexes and release of inflammatory mediators (histamine, serotonin) leads to the common symptoms of urticarial rash, joint pain, and fever.

Serum sickness–like reaction is not as well defined as true serum sickness. It is postulated that a non-protein drug binds to a serum protein to make a complete antigen. The newly formed antigen goes on to become an antigen-antibody complex. These complexes mimic the inflammatory cascade and symptomatic response of a true serum sickness reaction.

Epidemiology

Serum sickness is most common in the adult female population. A systematic review involving 33 cases of rituximab (Rituxan)-induced serum sickness (RISS) showed 76.7% female predominance with a mean age of 39.1 years. The majority of cases occurred in patients with an autoimmune condition, specifically immune thrombocytopenic purpura and Sjogren. Due to a lack of clear diagnostic tools and varying symptoms that can closely mimic a flare of an underlying rheumatologic illness, these reactions are often poorly documented or not identified. A study of Australian snake antivenom showed that the incidence of serum sickness was 29% (N = 32/109). Further research will need to be done to determine current incidence with the increasing treatment of rheumatologic disorders with immunologic medications.

Risk Factors
Risk factors for serum sickness include parenteral and cutaneous administration of chemicals, especially those with large molecular weights (e.g., proteins, serum). Heterologous (animal-derived) proteins, in particular, are associated with a high risk for a delayed immune response. Historically, equine-derived antisera and antitoxins were common causes and now includes murine and chimeric monoclonal antibodies such as rituximab (Rituxan) and infliximab (Remicade). Fewer adverse events have been reported with adalimumab (Humira), a humanized monoclonal antibody. Additional risk factors include administration of large doses, repeated dosing, and longer administration times. Patients with autoimmune disorders, circulating histamine-releasing factors, and atopy are also at an increased risk.

Serum sickness–like reactions are associated with a wider variety of molecules, including non-protein medications (e.g., antibiotics), vaccines, allergy extracts, hormones, and enzymes. See Table 1 for a list of agents commonly associated with serum sickness and serum sickness–like reactions.

Clinical Manifestations
Common manifestations of serum sickness include fever, pruritic rash (not involving mucosal membranes), and arthralgia of the metacarpophalangeal joints, knees, wrists, ankles, and shoulders. The timing of these symptoms occurs 7 to 14 days after exposure to the offending agent and can happen more promptly if there has been previous exposure. Urticaria has been reported as the most prominent symptom, present in 90% of cases. In a study of 33 cases of RISS: 78.8% presented with fever, 72.7% with arthralgia, and 69.7% with rash. The triad of fever, rash, and arthralgia were present in 48.5% of the cases. There are many less prominent manifestations of serum sickness, including headache, gastrointestinal (GI) bloating, cramps, diarrhea, and nephropathy.

Diagnosis
Recommended workup includes complete blood count (CBC), erythrocyte sedimentation rate (ESR), C-reactive protein (CRP), urinalysis (UA), and comprehensive metabolic panel (CMP). Although lab work can help to differentiate from other causes, diagnosis is made clinically. Attempts have been made to link serum sickness to elevated levels of rheumatoid factor, complement, and antibody levels without success.

Differential Diagnosis
The differential diagnoses for serum sickness include: serum sickness–like reaction, other hypersensitivity reactions, viral illness, rheumatologic disease, tick-borne disease, reactive arthritis, Stevens-Johnson syndrome, rheumatic fever, and lupus.

Treatment
Treatment of serum sickness and serum sickness–like reactions are similar. Discontinuation and avoidance of the offending agent is recommended and usually leads to spontaneous resolution within several weeks. Due to the self-limiting nature and generally mild presentation, treatment is symptom driven. Low-grade fever and/or arthralgias can be treated with analgesics (e.g., acetaminophen [Tylenol]) or nonsteroidal anti-inflammatory drugs. Antihistamines and corticosteroids are commonly used, but there are limited data to support their efficacy. Antihistamines may be used to treat urticarial symptoms. Those with more severe disease (e.g., temperature >38.5°C, severe arthralgias, extensive rashes) can be treated with a short course of corticosteroids (e.g., prednisone [Deltasone] 40 to 60 mg by mouth daily). Generally oral corticosteroids are sufficient, but intravenous agents may be appropriate for some patients (e.g., methylprednisolone [Solu-Medrol] 1 to 2 mg/kg in one or two divided doses intravenously). A systematic review revealed intravenous methylprednisolone (Solu-Medrol) as the most common treatment of RISS. Other treatment options identified were intravenous betamethasone (Celestone Soluspan), intravenous hydrocortisone (Solu-Cortef), oral prednisone (Deltasone), and oral prednisolone (Millipred). This study demonstrated a mean treatment duration of 9 days with complete resolution of symptoms in all cases. Some studies recommend tapering corticosteroids over 2 weeks to avoid rebound symptoms. There are currently no evidence-based guidelines available to guide dosing or duration of therapy.

Plasmapheresis or plasma exchange is another treatment option used to eliminate immune complexes. One study reports the use of plasmapheresis in five patients post–renal transplant who experienced anti-thymocyte globulin–induced serum sickness with no improvement after administration of oral prednisone (Deltasone) 1 mg/kg/d or intravenous prednisolone (Millipred) 2 mg/kg/d. This treatment method is generally reserved for refractory cases that do not respond to corticosteroid therapy due to limited evidence of its safety and efficacy.

References
de Silva HA, Ryan NM, de Silva HJ: Adverse reactions to snake antivenom, and their prevention and treatment, *Br J Clin Pharmacol* 81(3):446–452, 2015.
Erffmeyer JE: Serum sickness, *Ann Allergy* 56:105–109, 1986.
Karmacharya P, Poudel DR, Pathak R, et al: Rituximab-induced serum sickness: a systematic review, *Semin Arthritis Rheum* 45:334–340, 2015.
Lawley TJ, Bielory L, Gascon P, et al: A prospective clinical and immunologic analysis of patients with serum sickness, *N Engl J Med* 311:1407–1413, 1984.
Lin RY: Serum sickness syndrome, *Am Fam Physician* 33(1):157–162, 1986.

TABLE 1 Medications Associated With Serum Sickness and Serum Sickness–Like Reactions

Serum Sickness
Heterologous (animal-derived) proteins:
- Antivenom for snake bites: Crotalidae polyvalent immune fab, North and South American snake antivenom (CroFab)
- Chimeric (murine/human) monoclonal antibodies: rituximab (Rituxan), infliximab (Remicade)
- Equine serum heptavalent botulism antitoxin
- Equine-derived antivenom for spider bites
- Equine-derived diphtheria antitoxin
- Murine monoclonal antibodies
- Polyclonal antibodies: equine or rabbit anti-thymocyte globulin (Atgam, Thymoglobulin)

Homologous (human-derived) proteins:
- Anti-D (Rho[D]) immune globulin (RhoGAM)
- Humanized monoclonal antibodies: adalimumab (Humira), omalizumab (Xolair), natalizumab (Tysabri), alemtuzumab (Lemtrada)
- Intravenous immune globulin (Carimune NF, Gamunex-C)

Serum Sickness–like Reactions
- Allopurinol (Zyloprim)
- Antimicrobials
  - Cephalosporins (especially cefaclor [Ceclor])
  - Ciprofloxacin (Cipro)
  - Griseofulvin (Gris-PEG)
  - Isoniazid (Nydrazid, INH)
  - Minocycline (Minocin)
  - Penicillins (Pen-Vee K)
  - Streptomycin (Agri-mycin-17, Agrept)
  - Sulfonamides
- Barbiturates
- Bupropion (Wellbutrin)
- Captopril (Capoten)
- Hydantoins
- Hydralazine (Apresoline)
- Iodides
- Methyldopa (Aldomet)
- Phenytoin (Dilantin)
- Procainamide (Pronestyl, Procan-SR, Procanbid)
- Quinidine (Cardioquine)
- Thiouracils (e.g., methimazole [Tapazole])

Lundquist AL, Chari RS, Wood JH, et al: Serum sickness following rabbit antithymocyte-globulin induction in a liver transplant recipient: case report and literature review, *Liver Transpl* 13:647–650, 2007.

Naguwa SM, Nelson BL: Human serum sickness, *Clin Rev Allergy* 3:117–126, 1985.

Ryan NM, Kearney RT, Brown S, et al: Incidence of serum sickness after the administration of Australian snake antivenom (ASP-22), *Clin Toxicol* 54(1):27–33, 2016.

Solensky R, Khan DA, et al: Drug allergy: an updated practice parameter, *Ann Allergy Clin Immunol* 105:259–273, 2010.

Tatum AJ, Ditto AM, Patterson R: Severe serum sickness-like reaction to oral penicillin drugs: three case reports, *Ann Allergy Asthma Immunol* 86:330–334, 2011.

Tanriover B, Chuang P, Fishbach B, et al: Polyclonal antibody-induced serum sickness in renal transplant recipients: treatment with therapeutic plasma exchange, *Transplantation* 80:279–281, 2005.

Serum Sickness

3 Cardiovascular System

ACUTE MYOCARDIAL INFARCTION

Method of
Kuang-Yuh Chyu, MD, PhD; and Prediman K. Shah, MD, MACC

CURRENT DIAGNOSIS

- Patients are encouraged to seek medical evaluation as soon as possible when chest pain or angina-equivalent symptoms occur.
- Early presentation leads to early recognition, diagnosis, and treatment of acute myocardial infarction (AMI).
- The diagnosis of AMI relies on detailed history, ECG changes consistent with myocardial ischemia, and elevation of serum biomarkers.
- Although echocardiogram is not essential to diagnose AMI, it is useful in diagnosing complications such as left/right ventricular dysfunction with congestive heart failure or mechanical complications from AMI and guiding management.

CURRENT THERAPY

- Timely reperfusion of occluded coronary artery is essential in managing ST-elevation myocardial infarction (STEMI).
- Early reperfusion therapy (percutaneous coronary intervention or coronary artery bypass grafting) in non-STEMI patients with high-risk features such as congestive heart failure, dynamic ECG changes such as ST-segment depression, arrhythmia, and refractory angina is beneficial.
- Medical therapy and lifestyle modification strategies are important to reduce long-term atherosclerotic cardiovascular events.

Acute coronary syndrome (ACS) is an acute manifestation of atherosclerotic coronary artery disease (CAD). Based on the presenting symptoms, characteristic electrocardiogram (ECG) changes, and cardiac biomarkers (e.g., high-sensitivity troponin), ACS can be further subdivided into unstable angina (USA), non–ST-elevation myocardial infarction (NSTEMI), or ST-elevation myocardial infarction (STEMI). Most patients with ACS have similar underlying pathophysiology: atherosclerotic plaque formation leading to narrowing of coronary arteries with plaque rupture or erosion and superimposed thrombus formation causing an acute presentation. A small portion of ACS cases can be due to conditions such as coronary artery spasm, spontaneous coronary artery dissection, coronary embolization, or cocaine use. Stress-induced acute cardiomyopathy, without angiographic signs of severely occlusive disease, can closely simulate atherothrombotic STEMI.

Although the three ACS entities share similar pathophysiology, their presentations vary widely. The initial recognition, diagnostic testing, and management strategies for these entities are similar and applicable to all patients with ACS. Diagnostically,

patients with STEMI as a whole reflect a more homogeneous group of patients compared with patients with USA or NSTEMI, and patients with STEMI carry the highest risk regarding acute morbidity and mortality. The major difference in managing these three groups of patients lies in the decision for and timing of acute reperfusion of occluded coronary arteries.

In the past three decades, there has been a steady decline in the incidence of STEMI and significant improvement in the outcomes of patients with STEMI with the introduction of early coronary reperfusion strategies. Improved adjunctive pharmacologic therapies and adoption of guideline-directed treatments such as lipid lowering, optimal control of hypertension and diabetes mellitus, and cigarette smoking cessation have all contributed to the improved outcomes. Currently, the in-hospital mortality of STEMI has reached as low as 7%.

Diagnosis
Electrocardiogram
ECG is the most important diagnostic test to detect STEMI because clinical features, physical examination, and CAD risk factor profile only have modest sensitivity and specificity in diagnosing STEMI. Current guidelines define ST elevation at the J point in at least two continuous leads of ≥2 mm in men or ≥1.5 mm in women in leads V2 to V3 and/or ≥1 mm in other contiguous chest leads or the limb leads in the absence of left ventricular (LV) hypertrophy or left bundle branch block (LBBB). However, ECG abnormalities such as paced rhythm, drug or electrolyte (hyperkalemia) effects, or Brugada syndrome also reduce the sensitivity and specificity of STEMI ECG interpretation.

Some patients present with ECG changes, although not with typical ST elevation, indicating equivalent clinical risk to STEMI, and should be treated as having a true STEMI. These STEMI-equivalent ECG patterns include (1) isolated ST depression in two or more precordial leads (V1 to V4), indicating true posterior wall STEMI; (2) ST depression in multiple leads with ST elevation in aVR, indicating left main or triple-vessel CAD; (3) Wellens sign with symmetric deep T-wave inversions in anterior precordial leads V2 and V3; (4) LBBB or paced ventricular beats meeting Sgarbossa, modified Sgarbossa, or Barcelona criteria; (5) de Winter sign showing ST depression and peaked T waves in the precordial leads; and (6) N wave, defined as a notch or deflection in the terminal QRS complex in leads II, III and aVF or I and aVL, indicating acute occlusion of the left circumflex artery. Occasionally, patients with acute left circumflex artery occlusion can present with a normal or near-normal ECG.

Some patients with ACS may present with no or minimal changes on their initial ECG. This can occur for several reasons: (1) early presentation in the course of ACS, before significant ECG changes have developed; (2) ischemia occurring in an area that is less visible on a standard 12-lead ECG, such as the territory supplied by the left circumflex artery; (3) transient ischemic changes that resolve before the ECG is performed; (4) spontaneous recanalization of the infarct-related artery (IRA) before presentation, which may normalize the ECG; or (5) the presence of collateral circulation that compensates for reduced blood flow in the occluded coronary artery. Hence, if clinical suspicion for ACS is not low, it is prudent to repeat ECGs preferably every 15 minutes to avoid delaying diagnosis of ACS. The clinical history, risk factors, and presenting symptoms should always guide decision making, as a normal ECG does not exclude ACS, especially in high-risk patients.

Serum Biomarkers

Serum biomarkers of myocardial necrosis, such as cardiac-specific high-sensitivity troponin T and I levels, are complementary to diagnosing STEMI. In clinical practice, STEMI is often diagnosed with ECG alone before the laboratory result of biomarkers is available. The troponin level typically rises 4 to 6 hours after the onset of symptoms and peaks within 12 to 24 hours if reperfusion therapy succeeds in reperfusing the occluded coronary artery and patients present early in the course of STEMI; its level tends to peak after 24 hours if reperfusion therapy fails or in patients who receive no reperfusion therapy. After STEMI, successfully reperfused or not, the troponin level remains elevated for 7 to 10 days.

For patients suspected of having recurrent ACS within a week after the index STEMI, given the troponin level remains elevated, creatine kinase (CK) and the MB isoform of CK (CK-MB) levels can be used as biomarkers to establish additional myocardial necrosis from a recurrent event because CK and CK-MB levels usually return to normal 48 to 72 hours after the initial index event. For patients with symptoms of ACS but without ST elevation on ECG, normal levels of serial high-sensitivity troponin using 0/3-hour algorithm has a negative predictive value of approximately 99% to exclude ACS. Shorter 0/1-hour or 0/2-hour algorithms have also been validated and included in the 2020 European Society of Cardiology NSTEMI guideline.

Imaging

STEMI is commonly accompanied with wall motion abnormalities on echocardiogram, but echocardiogram is not essential to diagnose STEMI. Echocardiogram is extremely useful in managing patients with STEMI, especially when they present with acute complications such as left/right ventricular dysfunction, acute congestive heart failure, acute mitral regurgitation, free wall or ventricular septal rupture, pericardial effusion, cardiogenic shock, or LV thrombus.

Management of STEMI

The principal concept of managing STEMI is "time is muscle"; hence, it is important for patients to recognize symptoms for early presentation and for the medical community to administer suitable reperfusion therapy in a timely manner.

Prehospital Phase

Current guidelines recommend that patients with STEMI receive reperfusion therapy as soon as possible but within 12 hours of symptom onset to achieve optimal myocardial salvage to reduce mortality and morbidity. In daily clinical practice, a substantial number of patients still present late and miss the golden window of reperfusion. Common reasons for late presentation include (1) patients' lack of knowledge to recognize symptoms, (2) patients' reluctance to seek medical care, (3) patients' lack of access to medical care, and (4) atypical symptoms that lead patients or medical care providers to consider noncardiac problems.

Patients with suspicious myocardial ischemic symptoms are encouraged to call emergency medical services (EMS) immediately for help with the following benefits: (1) patients can receive early treatment, (2) patients can receive immediate resuscitation should STEMI complications such as cardiac arrest occur en route to the hospital, and (3) an early prehospital ECG and communication with a hospital capable of percutaneous coronary intervention (PCI) by EMS significantly reduce reperfusion time and improve outcomes. A recent Lifeline STEMI Accelerator Study reported only 55% of STEMI patients were transported via EMS. Improving this requires public education to enhance recognition of symptoms, implementation of an efficient EMS system, and infrastructures with standardized treatment algorithms for STEMI.

Initial management by EMS or outpatient clinic usually includes pain relief by morphine, administration of nitroglycerin,[1] oxygen, and nonenteric-coated aspirin (162–325 mg) unless contraindicated. The role of routine oxygen supplementation to patients with STEMI studied in a randomized clinical trial (Air Versus Oxygen in Myocardial Infarction [AVOID] trial) suggested that supplemental oxygen therapy (8 L/min via face mask) in patients with STEMI without hypoxia (oxygen saturation >94%) may increase early myocardial injury and is associated with larger myocardial infarction (MI) size at 6 months.

Once STEMI is identified by a prehospital ECG performed by EMS, an assessment of candidacy for and availability of reperfusion therapy is an important next step of management to ensure immediate reperfusion and administration of its adjunctive therapy to maintain culprit coronary artery patency, limit infarct size and adverse LV remodeling, and improve outcome. To achieve the best outcome from reperfusion therapy, patients with STEMI should receive suitable reperfusion therapy within 12 hours of symptom onset—the earlier the better. Current reperfusion therapy options for STEMI include primary percutaneous coronary intervention (PPCI) or fibrinolysis.

PPCI is the treatment of choice for STEMI because it confers a beneficial reduction in mortality and recurrent ischemia compared with fibrinolysis. Hence, current guidelines recommend EMS to transport patients to a PCI-capable hospital and PPCI as the preferred method of reperfusion therapy with a system goal of <90 minutes from first medical contact (FMC) to device time. Such timely reperfusion is even more important for STEMI patients with cardiogenic shock but without out-of-hospital cardiac arrest, because every 10-minute treatment delay between 60 to 180 minutes from the FMC leads to 3.3 additional deaths per 100 PCI-treated patients (FITT-STEMI trial).

Not every hospital is capable of performing PCI. If a patient is sent to or arrives at a non–PCI-capable hospital, guidelines recommend transferring the patient to a PCI-capable hospital for PPCI with a system goal of <120 minutes from FMC to device time. If there is an anticipated delay of FMC to device time of ≥120 minutes, a fibrinolytic agent can be given within 30 minutes of hospital arrival if the patient has no contraindications for fibrinolysis (Box 1). Prehospital fibrinolysis, administered by EMS with physician supervision, has been shown to be feasible and safe, with a shortened reperfusion time and reduced mortality. Such strategy, however, is not used in the United States.

In real-world clinical practice, sometimes it is not possible to achieve strict time goals because of uncertainty of the initial diagnosis, necessity to treat concomitant comorbidities or complications, patient preference or consent issues, and local factors delaying treatment or transport. Therefore emphasis should be to deliver reperfusion therapy to eligible patients as rapidly as possible.

In-Hospital Reperfusion Strategy

Primary Percutaneous Coronary Intervention

PPCI performed in a high-volume hospital by experienced operators achieves a higher patency rate of IRA and lower rate of recurrent ischemia, reinfarction, hemorrhagic stroke, and death compared with fibrinolysis. In particular, PPCI has the greatest benefit in high-risk patients, such as those with cardiogenic shock. Hence, PPCI is the preferred method of reperfusion whenever possible with the system goal of 90 to 120 minutes.

The reperfusion technique used in PPCI has evolved greatly in the past few decades, from balloon angioplasty, bare-metal stent (BMS), and drug-eluting stent (DES) to bioresorbable vascular scaffold (BVS). Compared with balloon angioplasty, BMS used in PPCI confers reduced risk for subsequent target vessel revascularization but does not reduce the mortality rate. Compared with BMS, DES used in PPCI decreases the restenosis rate and need for reintervention without reduction in reinfarction and

---

[1] Not FDA approved for this indication.

death. BVS is a new stent technology, with a hope of better restoration of vasomotion, less lumen loss, and reduction of target lesion revascularization in the stented vessels compared with metallic DES. However, polymer-based ABSORB BVS failed to demonstrate such benefits; instead it caused a concerning hazard of device thrombosis. A newer generation of metallic BVS (Magmaris, Biotronik) also increased late lumen loss and target lesion revascularization in STEMI patients compared with sirolimus-eluting stent in a recently published MAGSTEMI trial.

Fibrinolysis

The currently available intravenous fibrinolytic agents are tenecteplase (TNKase), reteplase (Retavase), and alteplase (Activase) (Table 1). A fibrinolytic agent should be administered to eligible patients without contraindication within 30 minutes of arrival at the emergency department. It is important to evaluate the risk/benefit ratio for each individual patient before administering fibrinolytic therapy because it carries a small but fatal risk of hemorrhage stroke (about 1%). The ideal patient to receive a fibrinolytic agent would be with symptom onset within 1 to 2 hours, low bleeding risk, and age younger than 65 years.

Although fibrinolysis achieves a reasonable patency rate of IRA (see Table 1), a substantial portion of patients fail to achieve successful reperfusion as defined by the following clinical criteria: (1) resolution of chest pain, (2) reduction of >50% of the initial ST-segment elevation pattern on follow-up ECG 60 to 90 minutes after initiation of fibrinolysis, and (3) occurrence of reperfusion arrhythmia (accelerated idioventricular rhythm [AIVR]). If fibrinolysis does not achieve resolution of ST elevation by at least 50% in the worst lead at 60 to 90 minutes, rescue PCI (with transfer to PCI-capable hospital if necessary) should be strongly considered.

Percutaneous Intervention After Fibrinolysis

Approximately 40% of STEMI patients who receive fibrinolysis fail to achieve successful reperfusion and require emergent rescue PCI. Other indications for rescue PCI include severe heart failure, cardiogenic shock, persistent chest pain, or electrical instability. Hence, these patients should be transferred to a PCI-capable hospital immediately if fibrinolysis has been administered in a non-PCI capable hospital.

Otherwise, stable patients after successful fibrinolysis can undergo coronary angiography with an intent to revascularize as soon as logistically feasible, ideally between 3 and 24 hours after fibrinolysis (pharmaco-invasive strategy). In patients older than 75 years, if a pharmaco-invasive strategy is chosen as the reperfusion strategy, a fibrinolytic agent at half dose (such as the half dose of tenecteplase used in the STREAM trial) should be used to reduce bleeding risks because patients will receive concomitant antiplatelets and anticoagulants for PCI. The EARLY-MYO trial confirmed the efficacy of a pharmaco-invasive strategy using half-dose alteplase followed by PCI within 3 to 24 hours with noninferiority to primary PCI in 30-day rates of total death, reinfarction, heart failure, or major bleeding but with a higher rate of minor bleeding. Very early PCI after successful fibrinolysis (<2 to 3 hours) is not recommended.

BOX 1	Contraindications and Cautions for Fibrinolytic Therapy in STEMI*

Absolute Contraindications
- Any prior ICH
- Known structural cerebral vascular lesion (e.g., arteriovenous malformation)
- Known malignant intracranial neoplasm (primary or metastatic)
- Ischemic stroke within 3 months except acute ischemic stroke within 4.5 h
- Suspected aortic dissection
- Active bleeding or bleeding diathesis (excluding menses)
- Significant closed-head or facial trauma within 3 months
- Intracranial or intraspinal surgery within 2 months
- Severe uncontrolled hypertension (unresponsive to emergency therapy)
- For streptokinase, prior treatment within the previous 6 months

Relative Contraindications
- History of chronic, severe, poorly controlled hypertension
- Significant hypertension on presentation (SBP >180 mm Hg or DBP >110 mm Hg)
- History of prior ischemic stroke >3 months
- Dementia
- Known intracranial pathology not covered in absolute contraindications
- Traumatic or prolonged CPR (>10 min)
- Major surgery (<3 weeks)
- Recent (within 2–4 weeks) internal bleeding
- Noncompressible vascular punctures
- Pregnancy
- Active peptic ulcer
- Oral anticoagulant therapy

*Viewed as advisory for clinical decision making and may not be all-inclusive or definitive.
CPR, Cardiopulmonary resuscitation; DBP, diastolic blood pressure; ICH, intracranial hemorrhage; SBP, systolic blood pressure; STEMI, ST-elevation myocardial infarction.

TABLE 1	Comparison of Fibrinolytic Agents

	ALTEPLASE (t-PA) (ACTIVASE)	RETEPLASE (r-PA) (RETAVAS)	TENECTEPLASE (TNK-TPA) (TNKase)
Dose	Up to 100 mg in 90 min (weight based)	10 U + 10 U IV boluses given 30 min apart	30–50 mg based on weight as a single bolus
Bolus administration	No	Yes	Yes
Antigenic	No	No	No
Allergic reaction	No	No	No
Fibrin specificity	++	++	++++
90-min TIMI 2 or 3 patency rate (%)	73–84	84	85
TIMI 3 flow (%)	54	60	63

TIMI, Thrombolysis in myocardial infarction.
Modified from 2013 ACCF/AHA STEMI guideline.

Patients With STEMI and Multivessel Coronary Artery Disease

About 40% to 65% of patients with STEMI undergoing PPCI for culprit IRA have multivessel CAD. Significant multivessel CAD, if left unrevascularized, is associated with a worse clinical prognosis. For patients with STEMI with multivessel CAD and cardiogenic shock, the CULPRIT-SHOCK trial showed that initial revascularization of the culprit vessel only by PCI resulted in a lower 30-day risk of death or renal-replacement therapy compared with a strategy of immediate multivessel PCI.

For stable patients, randomized clinical trials have demonstrated the feasibility of performing multivessel PPCI in acute settings. This approach has the following advantages: complete revascularization leading to improved LV function and prognosis, decreased vascular complications from repeated procedures, and reduced length of stay and medical costs. However, the procedure will be longer with higher radiation exposure, larger contrast load leading to higher risk for contrast nephropathy, risk of compromising viable myocardium supplied by the nonculprit coronary artery owing to procedure complications, and unnecessary stenting to the nonculprit artery without objective evidence of ischemia.

Many guidelines published by the professional cardiology societies in North America and Europe support multivessel PCI, either at the time of PCI to the STEMI culprit vessel or as a staged procedure in selected hemodynamically stable patients. A recent COMPLETE trial further confirmed the efficacy of reducing new MI or ischemia-driven revascularization in the complete revascularization group than in the culprit lesion PCI group but without mortality benefit. Interventional cardiologists should integrate clinical data, characteristics of lesions and procedures, clinical risks, and complications from procedures to determine the best timing and strategy to achieve the optimal benefit.

Patients With ACS Older Than 75 Years

Patients older than 75 years are usually underrepresented in STEMI clinical trials; however, revascularization with PCI still confers beneficial clinical outcomes compared with no revascularization despite age, frailty, and comorbidities. Hence, PCI as a revascularization strategy for STEMI in the elderly is encouraged whenever patients' conditions allow. In the United States, the use of PCI for patients with STEMI older than 70 years has increased from 11% in 1998 to 35.7% in 2013 based on data from the National Inpatient Sample Database.

The After Eighty Study showed the invasive strategy (early coronary angiography and revascularization + optimal medical therapy) significantly improved event-free survival compared with conservative strategy (optimal medical therapy) in NSTEMI patients older than 80 years.

When taking care of this group of patients, cardiologists need to pay particular attention to minimize bleeding complication by using radial access; monitoring patients' nonverbal responses as many patients have difficulty communicating with caregivers effectively; and identifying and treating comorbid conditions early given many elderly patients lack functional reserves in many organ systems and are prone to adverse effects of drug interactions.

Patients With STEMI Who Present Later Than 12 Hours After Symptom Onset

Irrespective of time of presentation, patients with STEMI who present with hemodynamic or electrical instability should undergo coronary angiography with an intent to revascularize the jeopardized myocardium as soon as possible.

Patients with STEMI who present between 12 hours and 2 days after symptom onset without unstable symptoms or signs are no longer eligible for fibrinolysis but are still eligible for PPCI to salvage myocardium, which confers the benefit of reduced infarct size compared with conventional therapy guided by a predischarge symptom-limited exercise test or unplanned PCI guided

by clinical instability as demonstrated in the Beyond 12 Hours Reperfusion Alternative Evaluation (BRAVE-2) trial. For patients with STEMI who present >48 hours after symptom onset without clinical instability, a strategy of symptom-limited stress test first or coronary angiography first to delineate high-risk features of coronary anatomy is reasonable with an intent to revascularize high-risk coronary anatomy. If patients are clinically stable without high-risk coronary anatomy noted by angiography and present between 3 and 28 days after symptom onset, PCI to open the occluded IRA does not confer clinical benefits in reducing mortality, congestive heart failure, or nonfatal MI compared with medical therapy as demonstrated in the Occluded Artery Trial (OAT).

Figure 1 summarizes current pathways of managing patients with STEMI based on their time of presentation, their clinical status, and availability of reperfusion therapy.

Adjunct Therapy
Antiplatelet Therapy
Aspirin

Unless contraindicated, 162 to 325 mg of aspirin should be administered as a loading dose immediately followed by at least 81 to 325 mg daily in all patients with STEMI, with 81 mg being the preferred maintenance dose. Patients with a history of aspirin allergy can be given clopidogrel (Plavix) instead.

$P2Y_{12}$ Receptor Inhibitors

Clopidogrel is a second-generation thienopyridine and irreversibly blocks the platelet $P2Y_{12}$ receptor to inhibit platelet activation and aggregation. Current guidelines support the use of clopidogrel during fibrinolysis or PPCI. For patients undergoing fibrinolytic therapy, a loading dose of 300 mg followed by a maintenance dose of 75 mg daily has been recommended for patients younger than 75 years. For patients older than 75 years, only the maintenance dose of 75 mg should be given. Prasugrel (Effient) and ticagrelor (Brilinta)[1] have not been studied and, hence, are not recommended in the setting of fibrinolysis as reperfusion therapy. For patients undergoing PPCI, depending on whether they are receiving a fibrinolytic agent and the timing of subsequent PCI, a different dosing regimen of clopidogrel may be recommended (Figure 2).

Prasugrel is a third-generation thienopyridine $P2Y_{12}$ receptor inhibitor. It is metabolized to its active form more quickly than clopidogrel and hence confers a more potent effect. In a subset of patients with STEMI in the TRITON-TIMI 38 trial, prasugrel was more efficacious in preventing composite endpoints of cardiovascular (CV) death, MI, and stroke compared with clopidogrel, but it had a higher major bleeding rate. Prasugrel is also contraindicated in patients older than 75 years, with body weight <60 kg, or with prior history of stroke or transient ischemic attack.

Ticagrelor is a direct reversible $P2Y_{12}$ receptor inhibitor with a more potent, faster-acting property compared with clopidogrel or prasugrel. In the Platelet Inhibition and Patient Outcomes (PLATO) trial, ticagrelor lowered composite CV death, MI, and stroke compared with clopidogrel but with an increase in non–procedure-related bleeding.

Biotransformation of clopidogrel into active metabolites requires CYP2C19, whereas prasugrel mainly relies on CYP3A4 and CYP2B6, and to a lesser extent CYP2C19, to form active metabolites. Ticagrelor is an active $P2Y_{12}$ inhibitor, and its metabolite via CYP3A4 carries equal antiplatelet potency. About 30% of the US population carries one or two CYP2C19 loss-of-function alleles, rendering them less responsive to the antiplatelet effect of clopidogrel. Hence, genotyping CYP2C19 polymorphism could potentially affect the selection of $P2Y_{12}$ receptor inhibitor. In STEMI populations, a recent study demonstrated that genotype-guided strategy—in which patients without loss of function of CYP2C19 were treated with clopidogrel whereas patients with loss of function received ticagrelor or prasugrel—is

---

[1] Not FDA approved for this indication.

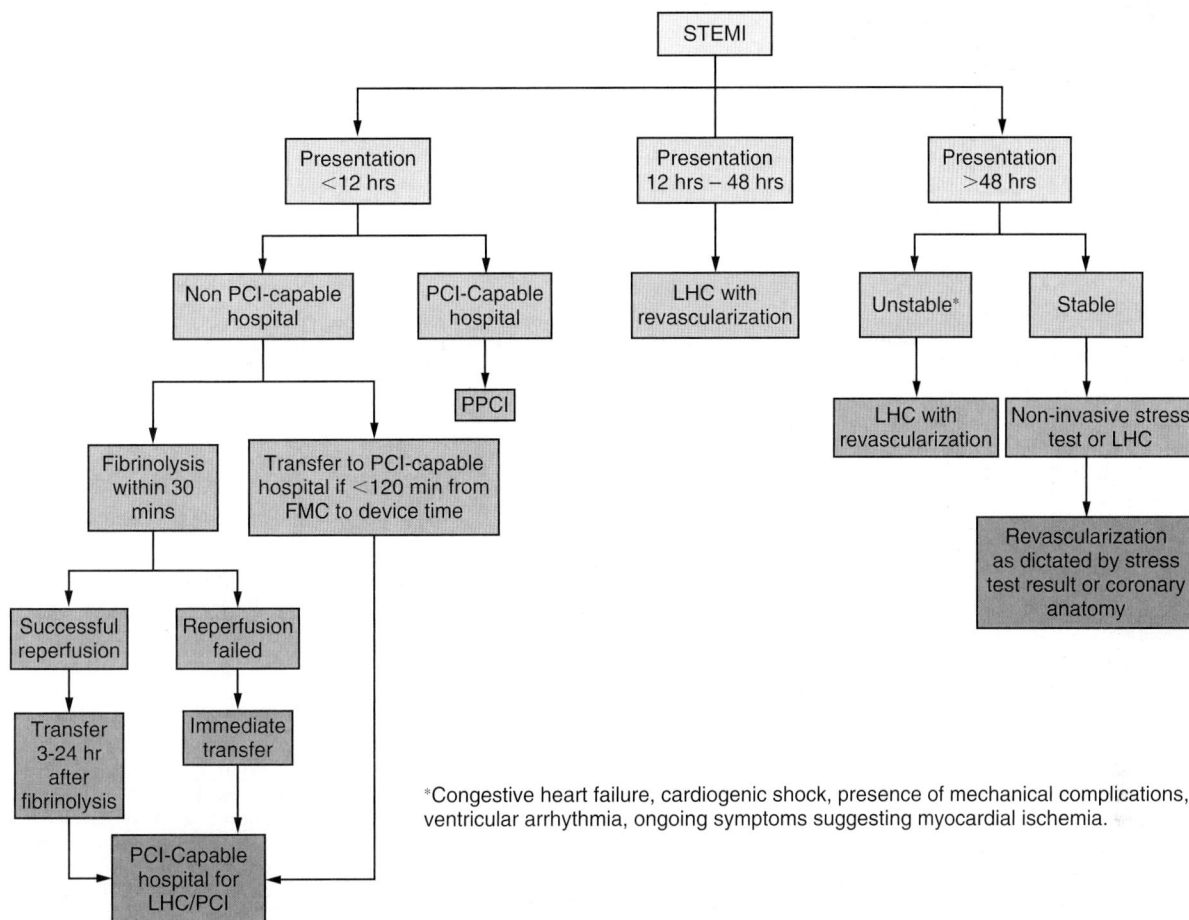

Figure 1 Pathways of managing ST-elevation myocardial infarction *(STEMI)*. *FMC,* First medical contact; *LHC,* Left heart catheterization; *PCI,* percutaneous intervention; *PPCI,* primary percutaneous coronary intervention.

not inferior to a standard treatment with ticagrelor or prasugrel in the control group with respect to thrombotic events at 12 months. However, genotype-guided strategy was associated with lower risk of bleeding.

Clopidogrel, prasugrel, and ticagrelor require several hours to achieve maximal platelet inhibition. Additionally, in the setting of STEMI, the bioavailability of these oral agents may be hampered by clinical factors such as nausea, vomiting, and cardiogenic shock, leading to poor GI absorption and leaving patients not adequately protected by platelet inhibition during immediate PPCI. Cangrelor (Kengreal) is a fast-acting, reversible adenosine diphosphate receptor inhibitor that is administered intravenously to achieve $P2Y_{12}$ inhibition within 2 minutes. Its plasma half-life is 3 to 6 minutes, and platelet function returns to normal within 60 minutes after discontinuation of infusion. The FDA has approved cangrelor to be used as an adjunct therapy during PCI to reduce repeat coronary revascularization and stent thrombosis in patients who have not been pretreated with an oral $P2Y_{12}$ inhibitor and are not receiving a glycoprotein (GP) IIb/IIIa receptor antagonist. How to transition from cangrelor to an oral $P2Y_{12}$ inhibitor after PCI depends on which oral $P2Y_{12}$ inhibitor a patient is being transitioned to. Based on the CHAMPION PHOENIX trial, to transition to clopidogrel, 600 mg clopidogrel loading is necessary immediately after discontinuation of cangrelor infusion. Based on pharmacodynamic data, prasugrel 60 mg should be administered immediately after stopping cangrelor infusion, whereas ticagrelor 180 mg can be given anytime during cangrelor infusion or immediately after infusion ends.

Use and Duration of Antiplatelet Therapy. Current guidelines recommend to give aspirin and one of the potent $P2Y_{12}$ inhibitors (ticagrelor or prasugrel) before primary PCI for STEMI patients. When potent $P2Y_{12}$ inhibitors are not available or

contraindicated, clopidogrel can be given instead. For NSTEMI patients, it is recommended against to routinely administer $P2Y_{12}$ inhibitors in patients in whom coronary artery anatomy is not known and an early invasive management is planned. This recommendation is based on the aggregated results from several clinical trials and registries including ACCOAST, ISAR-REACT 5, DUBIUS, ARIAM-Andalucia, and SCAAR. Once coronary anatomy is defined and PCI deemed necessary, $P2Y_{12}$ inhibitor can be administered. This approach has the benefit of reducing unnecessary bleeding risk in patients whose NSTEMI diagnosis is disproved by coronary angiogram, reducing the wait time for patients with suitable coronary anatomy for bypass surgery.

Current American and European guidelines recommend 12 months of dual antiplatelet therapy (DAPT) in patients with ACS (STEMI or NSTEMI) after stent implantation. If bleeding risk is high (such as PRECISE DAPT ≥25), duration of DAPT can be shortened to 6 months followed by discontinuation of $P2Y_{12}$ inhibitor (American guideline) or aspirin (European guideline). Shorter duration of DAPT (3 months) followed by aspirin may be considered in patients with high bleeding risk (European guideline). Continuation of DAPT beyond 12 months is reasonable in patients who tolerate DAPT, do not have bleeding complications, and are not at high bleeding risk (prior bleeding on DAPT, coagulopathy, or oral anticoagulant use).

The use and duration of DAPT becomes more complicated in patients taking oral anticoagulation therapy for a variety of reasons. Guidelines and consensus documents from North America recommend the default approach of administering triple therapy (DAPT + anticoagulation) during PCI procedure and in hospital for up to 1 week followed by clopidogrel and oral anticoagulant for 12 months. If patients are at high risk for an ischemic event, the default approach is modified to use triple therapy for 1 month

STEMI

ASA 162-325 mg

Fibrinolysis | **Primary PCI**

Clopidogrel 300 mg loading if <75 years old; (No loading, 75 mg qd only if >75 years old)

Clopidogrel 600 mg loading, 75 mg qd for maintenance

Prasugrel 60 mg loading, 10 mg qd for maintenance

Ticagrelor 180 mg loading, 90 mg bid for maintenance

Yes | **No**

PCI 3-24 hrs after fibrinolysis

Timing of PCI

Clopidogrel 75 mg qd for maintenance

<24 hrs | >24 hrs | >24 hrs after fibrin-specific fibrinolysis or >48 hrs after fibrin-nonspecific fibrinolysis

Clopidogrel 300 mg loading, 75 mg qd for maintenance

Clopidogrel 600 mg loading, 75 mg qd for maintenance

Prasugrel 60 mg loading, 10 mg qd for maintenance

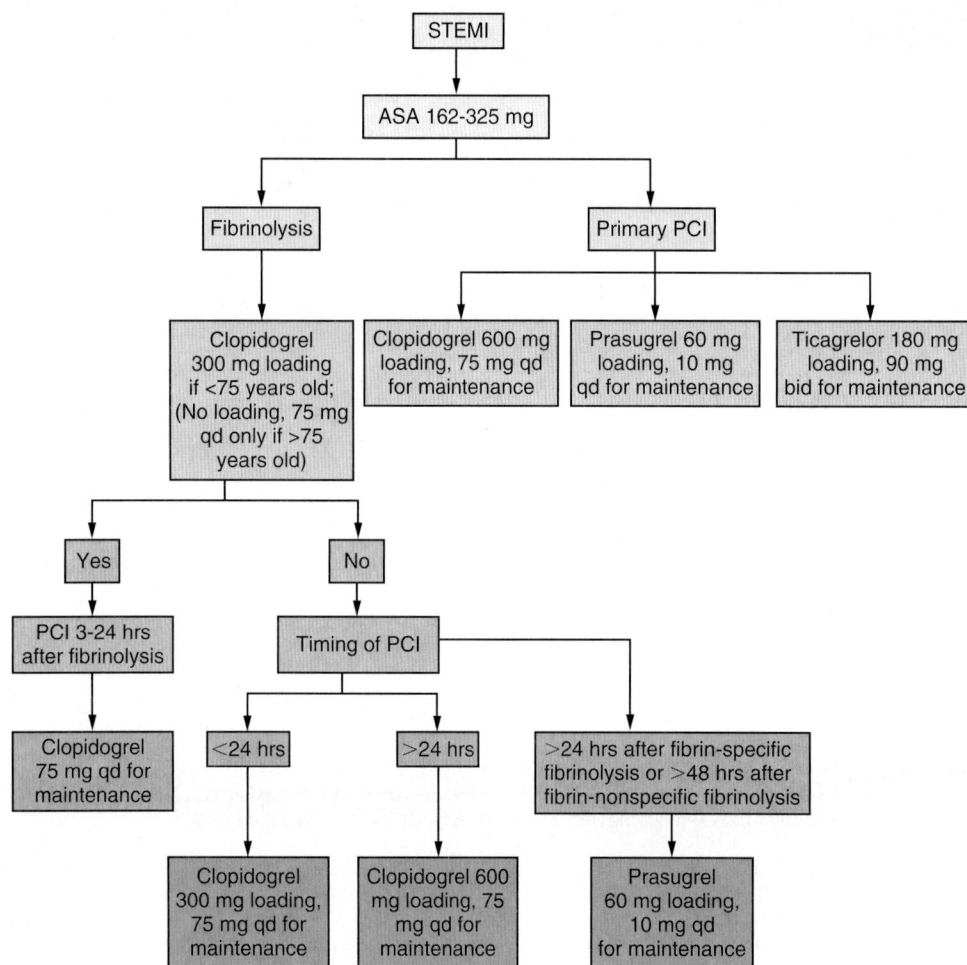

Figure 2 Oral regimen of different P2Y$_{12}$ receptor inhibitors based on reperfusion strategies. *ASA*, acetylsalicylic acid; *PCI*, Percutaneous intervention; *STEMI*, ST-elevation myocardial infarction. Modified from 2013 ACCF/AHA STEMI guideline.

and discontinue aspirin afterward. If patients are at high bleeding risk, the default approach is modified to use triple therapy for up to 1 week followed by oral anticoagulant and clopidogrel with discontinuation of clopidogrel after 6 months. Non–vitamin K antagonist oral anticoagulants (NOACs) are preferred to vitamin K antagonists as oral anticoagulants unless clinical condition prohibits the use of NOACs. Oral anticoagulant alone can be used after 12 months of treatment with an additional single antiplatelet agent based on individual clinical circumstance. Other strategies, including use of the radial artery approach as vascular access, use of proton pump inhibitors, avoidance of GP IIb/IIIa inhibitors unless for periprocedural complications, and avoidance of NSAIDs, should also be used.

Glycoprotein IIb/IIIa Receptor Antagonists
GP IIb/IIIa receptor antagonists include abciximab (ReoPro, a chimeric monoclonal antibody), eptifibatide (Integrilin, a synthetic peptidic inhibitor), and tirofiban (Aggrastat, a nonpeptidic inhibitor). The benefit of intravenous GP IIb/IIIa receptor antagonists in patients with STEMI was largely established before the era of oral DAPT. With current use of DAPT, contemporary trials fail to show benefit with upstream administration of GP IIb/IIIa receptor antagonists before PPCI with either unfractionated heparin (UFH)[1] or bivalirudin (Angiomax). Current US and European guidelines recommend using GP IIb/IIIa receptor antagonists for bailout situations after a large thrombus burden, no reflow or slow flow, or inadequate P2Y$_{12}$ receptor antagonist loading during PCI.

Anticoagulants
UFH[1], low-molecular-weight heparin with enoxaparin (Lovenox) as prototype, fondaparinux (Arixtra)[1], and bivalirudin (Angiomax)

are widely used in reperfusion therapy to limit thrombus propagation, reduce reocclusion and reinfarction, and improve vessel patency unless contraindicated. The choice of individual agent and its dose and duration of use depends on the choice of reperfusion therapy, concomitant use of other antiplatelet agents, and renal function (Table 2).

Given that PPCI is the preferred method of reperfusion and occurs early after presentation, and given physicians' familiarity with UFH, intravenous UFH is the preferred anticoagulant agent for PPCI. In patients with high bleeding risk, bivalirudin with DAPT is a reasonable alternative to UFH (whether the patient was pretreated with UFH) when avoidance of GP IIb/IIIa receptor antagonists is desired during PPCI.

For patients with STEMI who receive fibrinolysis as initial reperfusion therapy, UFH, enoxaparin, and fondaparinux[1] all receive a class I recommendation based on American College of Cardiology/American Heart Association (ACC/AHA) guidelines. UFH is preferred because a pharmaco-invasive strategy is common or for patients who may need rescue PCI. Bivalirudin may be used after fibrinolysis in patients who develop heparin-induced thrombocytopenia and require continued anticoagulation.

Guideline-Directed Medical Therapy
Beta Blockers
Beta blocker therapy decreases myocardial oxygen demand and improves myocardial remodeling with the benefits of reducing angina, infarct size, and mortality. Current guidelines recommend initiating oral beta blockers in the first 24 hours in patients with STEMI who are without contraindications such as congestive heart failure, evidence of a low output state, increased risk for cardiogenic shock, heart block, or reactive airway disease. If not given in the first 24 hours owing to contraindications, physicians need to reevaluate patients to determine their subsequent

---

[1] Not FDA approved for this indication.

TABLE 2 Dosage of Anticoagulants in Reperfusion Therapy for STEMI

	REPERFUSION THERAPY	
	FIBRINOLYSIS	**PRIMARY PCI**
Unfractionated heparin	• IV bolus of 60 U/kg (maximum 4000 U) followed by an infusion of 12 U/kg/h (maximum 1000 U) initially, adjusted to maintain aPTT at 1.5–2.0 times control (approximately 50–70 s) for 48 h or until revascularization	• With GPI planned, 50–70 U/kg IV bolus, to achieve ACT 200–250 s • Without GPI planned, 70–100 U/kg IV bolus to achieve ACT 250–300 s with HemoTec or 300–350 s with Hemochron
Low-molecular-weight heparin (enoxaparin [Lovenox])	• If age <75 years: 30-mg IV bolus, followed in 15 min by 1 mg/kg subcutaneously every 12 h (maximum 100 mg for the first 2 doses) • If age ≥75 years: no bolus, 0.75 mg/kg subcutaneously every 12 h (maximum 75 mg for the first 2 doses) • Regardless of age, if CrCl <30 mL/min: 1 mg/kg subcutaneously every 24 h • Duration: For the index hospitalization, up to 8 days or until revascularization	No information
Bivalirudin (Angiomax)	No information	• With or without prior heparin: 0.75 mg/kg bolus, 1.75 mg/kg/h infusion to the end of PCI. Additional bolus of 0.3 mg/kg if needed • Reduce infusion to 1 mg/kg/h if estimated CrCl <30 mL/min • Prefer over heparin and GPI in high-risk cases of bleeding
Fondaparinux (Arixtra)	• Initial dose 2.5 mg IV, then 2.5 mg subcutaneously daily starting the next day, for the index hospitalization up to 8 days or until revascularization • Contraindicated if CrCl <30 mL/min	Not recommended as sole anticoagulant

ACT, Activated clotting time; *aPTT*, activated partial thromboplastin time; *CrCl*, creatinine clearance; *GPI*, glycoprotein IIb/IIIa inhibitors; *PCI*, percutaneous intervention; *STEMI*, ST-elevation myocardial infarction.
Modified from 2013 ACCF/AHA STEMI guideline.

eligibility. Oral beta blockers should be continued for 3 years after MI as recommended by the ACC/AHA secondary prevention guideline, and longer if there are other indications (such as systolic LV dysfunction). Commonly used beta-blocker regimens are (1) metoprolol tartrate (Lopressor) 25 to 50 mg every 6 to 12 hours orally, transitioned over the next 2 to 3 days to twice-daily dosing of metoprolol tartrate or to daily metoprolol succinate (Toprol XL), and then titrated to a daily dose of 200 mg as tolerated; and (2) carvedilol (Coreg)[1] 6.25 mg twice daily, titrated to 25 mg twice daily as tolerated.

Current guidelines recommend intravenous beta blocker only for patients with refractory hypertension or ongoing ischemia without contraindications. Several small randomized clinical trials have suggested that early use of intravenous metoprolol tartrate in selected patients with STEMI with Killip class I to II and no atrioventricular (AV) block before PPCI may reduce infarct size with a higher LV ejection fraction (LVEF) or reduce the incidence of malignant arrhythmia in the acute phase without an excess of adverse events.

Angiotensin-Converting Enzyme Inhibitors or Angiotensin II Receptor Blockers

Angiotensin-converting enzyme inhibitors (ACEIs) and angiotensin II receptor blockers (ARBs) reduce afterload and decrease myocardial remodeling. Either ACEIs or ARBs should be started within 24 hours if there are no contraindications such as worsening renal function, advanced kidney disease, bilateral renal artery stenosis, hyperkalemia, or hypotension. These agents have the largest benefit in patients with anterior STEMI, congestive heart failure, or LVEF <40%. ACEIs may be given routinely to all patients without contraindication, whereas ARBs are an alternative for patients intolerant to ACEIs. There is no additional benefit, only more harm if ACEIs and ARBs are given concomitantly.

Commonly used ACEI regimens are (1) captopril 6.25 to 12.5 mg three times per day to start, titrated to 25 to 50 mg three times per day as tolerated; (2) lisinopril (Prinivil) 2.5 to 5 mg/day to start, titrated to 10 mg/day or higher as tolerated; (3) ramipril (Altace) 2.5 mg twice daily to start, titrated to 5 mg twice daily as tolerated; and (4) trandolapril (Mavik) test dose 0.5 mg, titrated up to 4 mg daily as tolerated. A commonly used ARB regimen is valsartan (Diovan) 20 mg twice daily to start, titrated to 160 mg twice daily as tolerated.

Angiotensin Receptor-Neprilysin Inhibitor

Valsartan/sacubitril (Entresto) has been shown to confer mortality and heart failure admission benefit in symptomatic heart failure patients with ejection fraction (EF) <40% compared with enalapril in the PARADIGM-HF trial. However, its use in patients with acute myocardial infarction and pulmonary congestion and EF <40% did not confer similar benefit compared with ramipril in a recent PARADISE-MI trial. In clinical practice, as an initial guideline-directed medical therapy strategy, it is reasonable to start and titrate an ACEI or ARB, beta blocker, and mineralocorticoid receptor antagonist for patients with an EF <40% as tolerated in the acute post-STEMI phase while trying to avoid hypotension or acute renal failure. Once the patient is hemodynamically stable, the ACEI or ARB can be replaced with an angiotensin receptor-neprilysin inhibitor in the subacute or chronic phase.

3-Hydroxy-3-Methylglutaryl Coenzyme A Reductase Inhibitors (Statins)

Treatment with statins after ACS lowers the risk of CV mortality, recurrent MI, stroke, and the need for coronary revascularization. All ACS patients should have nonfasting lipid panel obtained as early as possible with lipoprotein(a) level to be included if not known previously for overall risk assessment and high-intensity statins to be initiated as early as possible to improve compliance. Although current guidelines do not endorse a specific low-density lipoprotein cholesterol (LDL-C) level as a treatment goal, it is recommended to reduce the LDL-C level at least 50% from baseline with a goal LDL-C <55 mg/dL.

Statin use needs to be combined with diet and therapeutic lifestyle therapies. A commonly used high-intensity statin regimen is atorvastatin (Lipitor) 40 to 80 mg or rosuvastatin (Crestor) 20 to 40 mg daily as tolerated. Statins need to be used cautiously with drugs metabolized via CYP3A4 and fibrates, with frequent monitoring for myopathy and hepatic toxicity. In patients who cannot achieve an LDL-C level <70 mg/dL on adequate statin treatment, addition of proprotein convertase subtilisin kexin type 9 (PCSK9) antibody such as alirocumab (Praluent) or evolocumab (Repatha) to the statin can further reduce LDL-C level and risk of recurrent CV events. This stepwise approach is now being questioned because observational data indicated there are few dose adjustments or lipid-lowering agents prescribed, leading to LDL-C goals not being met in the majority of patients. A recent European consensus statement advocates dual lipid-lowering agents (high intensity statin + ezetimibe [Zetia]) to be initiated as early as possible, even before coronary angiography. Based on the reduction of lipid levels and improvement of coronary plaque morphology demonstrated in multiple trials, a concept of starting PCSK9 inhibitors in hospital after ACS is emerging. Whether such an approach improves clinical outcomes remains to be demonstrated. For patients with additional CAD high-risk features such as multivessel CAD, polyvascular disease, familial hypercholesterolemia, premature CAD, or recurrent events, it is also reasonable to add PCSK9 inhibitors in the acute phase of ACS.

Aldosterone Antagonists

Eplerenone (Inspra) improves myocardial remodeling and may reduce all-cause and CV mortality and rehospitalization. The 2013 ACC/AHA STEMI guideline recommends starting this medication 3 to 14 days after STEMI in eligible patients (creatinine ≤2.5 mg/dL in men and ≤2.0 mg/dL in women, potassium ≤5.0 mEq/L) with heart failure, with LVEF <35% to 40%, and already on adequate doses of beta blockers and ACEIs or ARBs. However, earlier administration (<7 days) is preferable to achieve mortality and rehospitalization benefits as suggested by a post hoc analysis of the Eplerenone Post-Acute Myocardial Infarction Heart Failure Efficacy and Survival Study (EPHESUS) trial.

Implantable Cardioverter-Defibrillator

Patients who develop ventricular tachycardia (VT) or fibrillation >48 hours after STEMI have the highest risk of sudden cardiac death (SCD) and, hence, are eligible for an implantable cardioverter-defibrillator (ICD) as a secondary prevention measure for SCD. For primary prevention, multiple trials have established the efficacy of prevention of SCD by ICD implantation in patients with LVEF <35% and New York Heart Association (NYHA) class II or III symptoms (or LVEF <30% with NYHA class I symptoms) despite optimal medical therapy 40 days after index STEMI and expectation of at least 1 year survival.

Other Medical Therapy
Morphine

Morphine is a time-honored medication used to reduce pain and anxiety, especially in patients with pulmonary edema during the acute presentation of STEMI. However, analysis of results from several clinical trials and a large meta-analysis involving >69,000 ACS patients suggests that a morphine/P2Y$_{12}$ inhibitor interaction exists, which could lead to adverse clinical consequences. Several pharmacokinetic studies in healthy volunteers have shown that intravenous morphine administration can reduce the level of active metabolites of clopidogrel and delay the maximal inhibition of platelet aggregation. A similar effect of morphine on ticagrelor was also reported. Given the current trend of using oral P2Y$_{12}$ receptor inhibitors before PPCI for STEMI, careful selection of patients and judicious administration of morphine with P2Y$_{12}$ receptor inhibitors deserves careful consideration.

Nitrate

Nitroglycerin reduces LV preload, increases coronary blood flow, and relieves chest pain symptoms. However, it plays no role in decreasing myocardial injury from coronary artery occlusion in STEMI. Its use in STEMI is mostly for congestive heart failure, hypertension, or rare cases of coronary spasm. It is contraindicated in patients with hypotension (systolic blood pressure [SBP] <90 mm Hg or SBP >30 mm Hg below baseline), right ventricular infarction from right coronary artery occlusion, or use of phosphodiesterase-5 inhibitors within 24 to 48 hours.

Major Complications of STEMI
Cardiogenic Shock

Cardiogenic shock is defined as an SBP <90 mm Hg for longer than 1 hour that is (1) not responsive to fluid administration alone, (2) secondary to cardiac dysfunction, or (3) associated with signs of hypoperfusion or cardiac index <2.2 L/min per m^2 and pulmonary capillary wedge pressure >18 mm Hg. It occurs in fewer than 10% of STEMI patients (2.4% in 1986 GISSI-1 trial; 6.5% in Germany ALKK-PCI registry as reported in 2013).

Almost 75% to 80% of cases of cardiogenic shock are due to severe LV systolic dysfunction. Right ventricular infarction, mechanical complications from ventricular septal rupture, acute mitral regurgitation, and free wall rupture leading to tamponade account for the rest. Other uncommon causes of shock from noncardiac etiology after STEMI are bleeding, systemic inflammatory response syndrome, infection, bowel ischemia, or iatrogenic (e.g., due to medication).

Cardiogenic shock due to mechanical complications after STEMI occurs in a bimodal fashion, with most cases occurring within 24 hours. Risk factors for mechanical complication include female sex, old age, and late or no reperfusion in the infarcted territory. Careful monitoring with serial physical examination and an early echocardiogram is extremely helpful to delineate the etiology of cardiogenic shock to guide subsequent definitive treatment. Cardiogenic shock carries a high in-hospital mortality, approaching 50%, and is higher in patients older than 75 years. These high-mortality patients require immediate stabilization to prevent end-stage organ damage followed by emergency coronary angiography and revascularization (Box 2).

In managing post-STEMI cardiogenic shock, mechanical circulatory support is often necessary. A recent randomized clinical trial demonstrated that in a selected group of post-STEMI patients with cardiogenic shock, routine use of a microaxial flow pump reduced mortality risk at 180 days but had a higher incidence of adverse events. In clinical practice, intraaortic balloon pump is more readily available but should not be used as a routine measure for this group of patients.

Electrical Complications
Ventricular Arrhythmia

Lethal ventricular arrhythmia, VT, or ventricular fibrillation (VF), is the most common cause of out-of-hospital cardiac arrest in STEMI. For hospitalized patients, VT/VF occurs in fewer than 10% of cases in the era of reperfusion therapy, and most cases occur within 48 hours of presentation. VT/VF is often associated with congestive heart failure, cardiogenic shock, or failed reperfusion of an occluded coronary artery. Hence, correction of electrolyte and acid-base disturbance, adequate reperfusion to reduce myocardial ischemia, and treatment of heart failure or shock are important preventive measures. Early administration of beta blockers within 24 hours to patients without contraindications reduces the incidence of VF. If VT/VF occurs, treatment includes immediate defibrillation or cardioversion and an antiarrhythmic agent such as amiodarone (Cordarone). Isolated premature ventricular contractions, nonsustained VT without hemodynamic instability, and AIVR do not generally require specific treatment.

Supraventricular Arrhythmia

Common supraventricular arrhythmias after STEMI include atrial fibrillation, atrial flutter, and sinus tachycardia. They are usually the consequence of or triggered by congestive heart failure, atrial infarction, pericarditis, hypoxia, or other underlying systemic problems (e.g., chronic obstructive pulmonary disease, bleeding, anemia, or infection). Treatment is directed to the underlying causes. For atrial fibrillation/flutter, physicians should pay special attention to anticoagulation use given the frequent concomitant use of DAPT and antithrombotics and the rate versus rhythm control strategy.

Bradycardia and Heart Block

Sinus bradycardia may occur after inferior STEMI. Because it is generally mediated through increased vagal tone, close monitoring usually suffices. High-grade AV block (second or third degree) can occur after inferior or anterior STEMI, with a worse prognosis after anterior STEMI owing to a greater degree of myocardial injury. High-grade AV block after inferior STEMI usually is transient and with a narrow complex escape rhythm, which subsides within 2 weeks. Occasionally, temporary pacemaker placement may be necessary if bradycardia causes hemodynamic instability. High-grade AV block from anterior STEMI usually requires placement of a prophylactic temporary pacing system because it is commonly associated with hemodynamic instability.

References

Berg ES, Tegn NK, Abdelnoor M, et al: Long-term outcomes of invasive vs conservative strategies for older patients with Non-ST-segment elevation acute coronary syndrome, *J Am Coll Cardiol* 82(21):2021–2030, 2023.

Canonico ME, Hess CN, Cannon CP: In-hospital use of PCSK9 inhibitors in the post ACS patient: what does the evidence show? *Curr Atheroscler Rep* 25(7):381–389, 2023.

Capodanno D, Angiolillo DJ: Timing, selection, modulation, and duration of P2Y12 inhibitors for patients with acute coronary syndromes undergoing PCI, *JACC Cardiovasc Interv* 6(1):1–18, 2023.

Capodanno D, Huber K, Mehran R, et al: Management of antithrombotic therapy in atrial fibrillation patients undergoing PCI: JACC state-of-the-art review, *J Am Coll Cardiol* 74(1):83–99, 2019.

Collet JP, Thiele H, Barbato E, et al: 2020 ESC Guidelines for the management of acute coronary syndromes in patients presenting without persistent ST-segment elevation: the Task Force for the management of acute coronary syndromes in patients presenting without persistent ST-segment elevation of the European Society of Cardiology, *Eur Heart J* 42(14):1289–1367, 2021.

Damluji AA, Forman DE, van Diepen S: Older adults in the cardiac intensive care unit: factoring geriatric syndromes in the management, prognosis, and process of care. A scientific statement from the American Heart Association, *Circulation* 141:e6–e32, 2020.

Frampton F, Devries JT, Welch TD: Modern management of ST-segment elevation myocardial infarction, *Curr Probl Cardiol* 45(3):100393, 2020.

Guedeney P, Collet JP: Diagnosis and management of acute coronary syndrome: what is new and why? Insight from the 2020 European society of cardiology guidelines, *J Clin Med* 9(11):3474, 2020.

Krychtiuk KA, Ahrens I, Drexel H, et al: Acute LDL-C reduction post ACS: strike early and strike strong: from evidence to clinical practice. A clinical consensus statement of the association for acute CardioVascular care (ACVC), in collaboration with the European association of preventive cardiology (EAPC) and the European society of cardiology working group on cardiovascular pharmacotherapy, *Eur Heart J Acute Cardiovasc Care* 11(12):939–949, 2022.

Mehta SR, Wood DA, Storey RF: Complete revascularization with multivessel PCI for myocardial infarction, *N Engl J Med* 381(15):1411–1421, 2019.

Pfeffer MA, Claggett B, Lewis EF, et al: Angiotensin receptor-Neprilysin inhibition in acute myocardial infarction, *N Engl J Med* 385(20):1845–1855, 2021.

ANGINA PECTORIS

Method of
Katherine Fell, MD; and Kenneth Tobin, DO

CURRENT DIAGNOSIS

- Optimal lifestyle and medical therapy is the cornerstone of management and includes smoking cessation, lipid management, antiplatelet agents, hypertension control, and blood sugar assessment.
- High-risk patients (e.g., unstable angina) often benefit from early invasive strategies combined with optimal medical therapy.
- Diagnosis of angina relies on clinical assessment of cardiovascular risk factors and symptoms.
- Classic angina presents as left-sided chest pressure or discomfort, often radiating to the jaw or arm, triggered by exertion and relieved by rest or nitroglycerin.
- Initial testing (ECG, labs, chest x-ray) is often normal; further evaluation with noninvasive imaging or coronary angiography should be guided by risk assessment and symptom burden.
- Noninvasive testing defines ischemic burden and guides treatment decisions.

CURRENT THERAPY

Stable Angina Pectoris
- First-line therapies include β-blockers, nitrates, and calcium channel blockers for relief of anginal symptoms.
- If symptoms persist, consider adding ranolazine (Ranexa) or ivabradine (Corlanor, Lancora)[1] as second-line agents for additional control.

---

[1]Not FDA approved for this indication.

While acute coronary syndrome (ACS) requires prompt evaluation and management, chronic coronary disease (CCD) is typically managed in the outpatient setting in a stepwise approach aimed at excluding noncardiac causes of chest pain and improving a patient's quality of life and symptoms. Ischemic chest discomfort, known as angina pectoris, is the cardinal symptom of chronic stable myocardial ischemia and occurs when the myocardial oxygen supply is unable to meet the metabolic demand of the myocardium. Chronic stable angina is the initial presentation of ischemic heart disease in approximately 50% of patients. In the United States the prevalence of stable angina is estimated at 4.0%, affecting approximately 11 million individuals. Despite an overall decline in death from coronary heart disease since the 2010s, ischemic heart disease continues to remain the leading cause of death in the United States and worldwide.

Stable angina is characterized by predictable chest discomfort that occurs with various levels of exertional activity and reliably resolves with rest or sublingual nitroglycerin. Whereas exertion (e.g., walking, climbing stairs, cleaning) is the most common precipitant, anxiety and stress also can elicit anginal symptoms. In contrast, unstable angina is an acute ischemic event defined by new-onset cardiac chest pain, angina at rest, or a worsening pattern of previously stable anginal symptoms. The pattern of angina is critical to defining a chronic versus unstable ischemic syndrome. Any change in chronic angina pattern, either occurring at rest or angina with progressively less exertion, requires a more urgent evaluation as it may indicate a conversion to an unstable ischemic syndrome.

The clinical sensation of angina pectoris arises from stimulation of chemosensitive and mechanosensitive receptors of unmyelinated nerve cells in the myocardium and coronary vessels. This occurs during periods of local lactic acidosis, when lactate, serotonin, bradykinin, histamine, reactive oxygen species, and adenosine are released into the coronary circulation. Afferent nerve signals then travel via sympathetic ganglia, primarily between the C7 and T4 spinal levels, explaining the typical radiation of anginal pain to the chest, neck, jaw, and left arm.

The most common cause of angina pectoris is coronary atherosclerosis. In the early stages, positive remodeling preserves the vessel lumen despite plaque accumulation, preventing significant luminal narrowing. However, once this compensatory mechanism reaches its limit, luminal narrowing occurs. Myocardial perfusion can still be maintained if the distal coronary segments retain adequate vasodilatory capacity. When a critical threshold of flow-limiting stenosis is reached and coronary vasodilator reserve is exhausted, myocardial oxygen supply can no longer meet demand, resulting in ischemia and anginal symptoms.

Although atherosclerosis is the most common cause of ischemia, other mechanisms including microvascular disease, vasospasm, and congenital anomalies or nonatherosclerotic valvular injury can also contribute.

Clinical Features
The diagnosis of angina pectoris begins with a careful clinical assessment and history. Through this process, many conditions that mimic angina can be effectively excluded (Table 1). Most patients can identify the specific levels of exertion that reliably trigger their symptoms. Environmental situations such as cold exposure, psychological stress, or heavy meals can also precipitate angina. Although the quality of angina symptoms may vary, it is commonly described as a pressure, heaviness, tightness, or squeezing sensation in the chest, often retrosternal and sometimes radiating to the jaw, neck, or left arm. Some patients may describe other locations, such as epigastric discomfort, or experience no chest pain at all. All patients should be closely questioned regarding changes in their functional status and whether their activities have been reduced to prevent symptom onset.

While chest discomfort is the most common symptom of CCD, many patients will not present with characteristic anginal symptoms, with the symptoms varying by age, sex, race, socioeconomic class, and geographic location. In contemporary studies, only 10% to 25% of patients with suspected CCD report typical anginal symptoms with clear aggravating and relieving factors. Some patients may instead report exertional dyspnea, diaphoresis,

TABLE 1	Differential Diagnosis of Chest Pain

Cardiac ischemia
- Stable angina
- Unstable angina
- Myocardial infarction

Vasospastic angina

Pericarditis

Aortic dissection

Pulmonary embolism

Esophageal spasm

Gastroesophageal reflux disease

Musculoskeletal pain

Biliary colic

Acute pneumonia

fatigue, or arrhythmias. Prior studies had suggested that women were less likely to experience classic anginal symptoms; however, the PROMISE study demonstrated that women present with chest pain symptoms with similar frequency to men but are more likely to report additional symptoms such as palpitations, jaw and neck pain, and back pain. Importantly, the absence of angina does not exclude significant Coronary artery disease (CAD), especially in patients with diabetes with autonomic neuropathy or sedentary elderly individuals.

Angina severity is commonly classified using the Canadian Cardiovascular Society (CCS) grading system. Angina is graded on a range from class I (angina with strenuous activity) to class IV (angina at rest or with minimal exertion). This classification system is valuable for risk stratification and for monitoring treatment response over time.

Diagnostic Testing
A baseline electrocardiogram (ECG) is often one of the initial tests obtained in a patient presenting with chest pain. Although a normal resting ECG does not rule out ischemic heart disease, it can reveal findings, such as pathologic Q waves or left ventricular (LV) hypertrophy, which increase the likelihood of significant CAD and warrant further evaluation and confirmatory testing (e.g., echocardiography). Initial laboratory assessment should include a fasting lipid panel, HbA1c, and renal function to help characterize the patient's cardiovascular risk profile.

In patients with angina who are at intermediate to high risk for CAD, further noninvasive testing is often warranted. The choice of diagnostic testing should be guided by site expertise, test availability, patient characteristics, and any contraindications to specific testing approaches.

Stress Testing
Stress testing is an appropriate screening tool for evaluating suspected or known CCD and assessing the burden of ischemia. When feasible, exercise-based testing is preferred over pharmacologic stress testing due to the additional prognostic information it provides. This includes degree of symptoms, blood pressure and heart rate response, heart rate recovery, achieved workload (metabolic equivalents [METS]), and ECG changes.

Exercise stress testing is most appropriate for patients who:
- Are physically capable of achieving ≥5 METS.
- Do not have disabling comorbidities (e.g., severe obesity [body mass index (BMI) > 40 kg/m²], peripheral arterial disease, orthopedic limitations, chronic obstructive pulmonary disease, or frailty).
- Do not have baseline ECG abnormalities that limit interpretation (e.g., ST depression ≥0.5 mm, left bundle branch block

[LBBB], paced rhythm, Wolff-Parkinson-White pattern, digitalis effect, or significant LV hypertrophy).

The diagnostic accuracy of exercise ECG testing varies, with a sensitivity and specificity of 60% to 77%. However, baseline ECG abnormalities, such as LBBB or paced rhythm, reduce the test specificity and render the test inconclusive for identifying ischemia. In such cases, exercise stress testing may still be valuable for assessing functional capacity and hemodynamic response, even if ischemia interpretation is limited.

Stress test accuracy is markedly improved by the addition of an imaging modality, including exercise or pharmacologic stress echocardiography, nuclear perfusion imaging (single-photon emission computed tomography or pharmacologic positron emission tomography [PET]), or cardiac magnetic resonance. Stress echocardiography and nuclear imaging each offer a sensitivity and specificity of approximately 85% to 90%. Stress echocardiography is generally considered more specific, whereas stress nuclear imaging is more sensitive. Stress echocardiography also provides additional information on valvular function and an estimate of right ventricular pressure. Although stress testing provides valuable information on overall cardiopulmonary health, most stress testing modalities, with the exception of PET, primarily detect hemodynamically significant coronary lesions. Given that many acute coronary events arise from nonobstructive plaques, this limitation helps explain why a patient with a negative stress test may still develop ACS.

Anatomic Testing

Coronary computed tomography angiography (CCTA) provides detailed visualization of both obstructive and nonobstructive CAD, including assessment of plaque burden, composition, and high-risk features. The extent of atherosclerosis identified on CCTA correlates stepwise with clinical risk, with greater risk observed in patients with obstructive lesions (≥50% stenosis), particularly involving the left main or left anterior descending (LAD) arteries.

The SCOT-HEART trial demonstrated that in patients with suspected angina, an initial diagnostic strategy of using CCTA compared with standard of care more frequently led to initiation and intensification of preventive and antiischemic therapies. This strategy was also associated with a significant reduction in cardiovascular events, driven primarily by a decrease in nonfatal and fatal myocardial infarctions (MIs).

CCTA may be particularly advantageous in patients under 65 years of age given its ability to detect early or nonobstructive disease. In contrast, stress testing may be preferred in patients older than 65 years old, who have a higher likelihood of ischemia and obstructive CAD.

Risk Factor Management

Hypertension

Hypertension is a commonly occurring and well-established cardiovascular risk factor. Among individuals with CCD, coexisting hypertension is associated with an increased risk of morbidity and mortality compared with normotensive counterparts. Initial management should prioritize lifestyle modification. Weight reduction to achieve a stable and healthy BMI (<25 kg/m² and waist circumference <94 cm in men and <80 cm in women) can significantly improve hypertension control. Additional measures include reducing dietary salt intake to ≤2 g/day, adopting a heart-healthy diet—such as the Mediterranean diet or the Dietary Approaches to Stop Hypertension (DASH) diet—and engaging in regular physical activity through a structured exercise program.

Evidence shows that cardiovascular risk progressively increases at blood pressures above 115/75 mm Hg. A meta-analysis of over 1 million adults found that for each 20 mm Hg increase in systolic pressure, the risk of cardiovascular death doubled, with the greatest risk observed in older adults (80–89 years old). Even modest reductions in blood pressure yielded significant benefit. A reduction of 4 mm Hg systolic and 3 mm Hg diastolic blood pressure was shown to reduce cardiovascular risk by 15%.

The SPRINT trial further demonstrated that intensive blood pressure control (systolic blood pressure <120 mm Hg) in high-risk nondiabetic patients reduced major cardiovascular events by 25% compared with a standard target of systolic blood pressure <140 mm Hg. Intensive treatment was also shown to slow progression of kidney disease and cognitive decline. The trial was halted early because of the significant benefits seen in the intensive blood pressure arm. A post hoc analysis of SPRINT showed an increase in adverse cardiovascular events if the diastolic blood pressure is lowered to ≤55 mm Hg. Therefore caution is advised in decreasing diastolic blood pressure to <60 mm Hg in any patient with CAD or diabetes or in patients >60 years old. After the publication of SPRINT, the 2017 multisociety guideline on management of hypertension proposed a compromise with recommendations for goal of treatment as <130/80 mm Hg. More lenient targets (e.g., 140/90 mm Hg) can be considered in older patients (≥85 years of age) or patients with pretreatment symptomatic orthostatic hypotension. In hypertensive patients with a history of MI, angiotensin-converting enzyme inhibitors, angiotensin-receptor blockers, or β-blockers are recommended as first-line therapy. In patients with symptomatic angina, β-blockers and/or calcium channel blockers (CCBs) can be considered.

Hyperlipidemia

Dyslipidemia is a major modifiable risk factor for atherosclerotic cardiovascular disease (ASCVD), and reduced low-density lipoprotein cholesterol (LDL-C) is strongly associated with decreased cardiovascular event rates. The current guidelines published by the American College of Cardiology/American Heart Association (ACC/AHA) recommend using high-intensity 3-hydroxy-3-methylglutaryl coenzyme reductase inhibitors (statins) for patients with CCD to reduce LDL cholesterol levels by ≥50%, with goal LDL-C <70 mg/dL (or non-HDL-C <100 mg/dL). In cases where there is very high risk of future ASCVD events (Table 2), a threshold of LDL-C >55 mg/dL (non-HDL-C >85 mg/dL) can guide decisions about intensifying lipid-lowering therapy. Statins are generally well tolerated and offer additional nonlipid lowering benefits, including antiinflammatory and plaque-stabilizing effects.

Randomized controlled trials (RCTs) of lipid-lowering therapies have consistently demonstrated that greater reductions in LDL-C levels are associated with greater reductions in ASCVD, supporting the "lower is better" hypothesis. The most recent European Society of Cardiology and European Atherosclerosis Society recommended aggressive LDL-C targets: <70 mg/dL for patients at high risk of ASCVD, <55 mg/dL for patients at very high risk or those with established ASCVD, and <40 mg/dL for patients at very high risk of a second vascular event within 2 years were recommended.

Statins are the cornerstone of lipid-lowering therapy for reducing cardiovascular mortality. The Cholesterol Treatment Trialists' meta-analysis demonstrated a 12% reduction in all-cause mortality and a 21% reduction in major vascular events per 1 mmol/L (38.6 mg/dL) LDL-C reduction for patients on high-intensity statins compared with moderate-intensity statins. These benefits were consistent across age, sex, and baseline LDL-C levels. Key trials such as the Heart Protection Study showed a target LDL-C < 100 mg/dL was associated with reduced cardiovascular events in high-risk individuals, regardless of initial LDL-C levels. Subsequent studies such as TNT (Treating to New Targets) study demonstrated intensive lipid-lowering therapy and attaining LDL-C level reductions of ≥50% was beneficial in the treatment of CCD. In TNT, intensive lipid lowering with atorvastatin (Lipitor) 80 mg daily compared with 10 mg daily in patients with CCD reduced the primary endpoint of CAD death, nonfatal MI, resuscitation from cardiac arrest or stroke with no overall difference in total mortality. The mean LDL-C level achieved with 80 mg daily atorvastatin was 77 mg/dL versus 101 mg/dL with 10 mg atorvastatin.

Based on this evidence, current guidelines recommend high-intensity statins—atorvastatin 40 to 80 mg or rosuvastatin

TABLE 2 Very High Risk of Future ASCVD Events

Definition of Very High Risk

History of multiple major ASCVD events
or
One major ASCVD event *and* ≥2 major high-risk conditions

Major ASCVD Events

Recent ACS (within the past 12 months)
History of MI (other than recent ACS events listed above)
History of ischemic stroke
Symptomatic peripheral artery disease (history of claudication with ABI < 0.85, or previous revascularization or amputation)

High-Risk Conditions

Age ≥65 years
Familial hypercholesterolemia
History of previous coronary artery bypass graft surgery or percutaneous intervention outside of the major ASCVD event(s)
Diabetes
Hypertension
Chronic kidney disease (eGFR 15–59 mL/min/1.73 m^2)
Current tobacco smoking
Persistently elevated LDL-C ≥ 100 mg/dL despite maximally tolerated statin therapy and ezetimibe
History of congestive heart failure

ABI, Ankle-brachial index; *ACS,* acute coronary syndrome; *ASCVD,* atherosclerotic cardiovascular disease; *eGFR,* estimated glomerular filtration rate; *LDL-C,* low-density lipoprotein cholesterol; *MI,* myocardial infarction.

(Crestor) 20 to 40 mg—for patients with established CAD to achieve ≥50% LDL-C reduction. Although high-dose simvastatin (80 mg daily) has been associated with increased risk of myopathy, other high-intensity statins are generally well tolerated and have favorable pleiotropic effects.

Although statins are the primary pharmacologic therapy for primary and secondary prevention of ASCVD, up to 20% of patients may report intolerance. The numbers may be even higher if medication adherence is included. Muscle symptoms are commonly cited in this group, but this may result from patient expectation that such symptoms will occur (nocebo effect) or unrelated musculoskeletal conditions. Statin-related myopathy is more likely when new-onset, bilateral, symmetric, proximal muscle pain or weakness develops within 1 to 2 weeks of starting or intensifying therapy and resolves within 1 to 2 weeks of discontinuation.

For patients who do not achieve adequate LDL-C on statin therapy alone, a combination of lipid-lowering drug therapy is recommended to reach LDL-C targets. Additional FDA-approved cholesterol lowering options include ezetimibe (Zetia), proprotein convertase subtilisin kexin type 9 (PCSK9) inhibitors, or bempedoic acid (Nexletol). Ezetimibe works via the Niemann-Pick C1-like 1 transport, reducing intestinal cholesterol absorption, and is recommended as the first-line nonstatin therapy in patients on maximally tolerated statin therapy with LDL-C ≥ 70 mg/dL. The IMPROVE-IT trial demonstrated that adding ezetimibe to simvastatin in patients with recent ACS led to a 20% to 25% further LDL-C reduction and a modest but significant decrease in major cardiovascular events compared with statin monotherapy.

Bempedoic acid is an oral cholesterol synthesis inhibitor that upregulates LDL-C receptor expression and enhances LDL-C clearance. Used alone, bempedoic acid lowers LDL-C by approximately 20%; when combined with ezetimibe, reductions of up to 35% can be achieved. In the CLEAR OUTCOMES trial, the combination of bempedoic acid and ezetimibe in statin-intolerant patients with ASCVD significantly reduced LDL-C levels and improved major adverse cardiovascular events (MACEs) compared with placebo. Based on these findings, bempedoic acid can be considered in combination with ezetimibe for statin-intolerant patients who have not achieved their LDL-C targets

with ezetimibe alone. Although bempedoic acid may be used with statins, it should be avoided with simvastatin (Zocor) doses >20 mg daily or pravastatin >40 mg daily due to increased statin serum concentrations. Notable adverse effects of bempedoic acid include elevated uric acid levels and, rarely, tendon rupture.

PCSK9 inhibitors (alirocumab [Praluent] and evolocumab [Repatha]) are highly effective LDL-C–lowering therapies that can be used alone or in combination with statin therapy. PCSK9 is a protein that decreases hepatic LDL-C receptor availability; PCSK9 inhibition increases receptor expression, enhancing LDL-C clearance. Clinical trials, including FOURIER and ODYSSEY OUTCOMES, both demonstrated that adding a PCSK9 inhibitor to maximally tolerated statin therapy (with or without ezetimibe) significantly reduced nonfatal cardiovascular events in patients at very high ASCVD risk with LDL-C ≥ 70 mg/dL. These agents further lower LDL-C by an additional 43% to 64%.

Despite PCSK9 inhibitor efficacy, high cost remains a significant barrier to widespread use. Currently, PCSK9 inhibitors are FDA approved for patients with familial hypercholesterolemia as part of primary and secondary prevention of ASCVD in patients who have not achieved adequate LDL-C reduction with statins and ezetimibe or are intolerant to these therapies.

Omega-3 Fatty Acids

Omega-3 fatty acids, including eicosapentaenoic acid (EPA) and docosahexaenoic acid (DHA), have been studied for cardiovascular risk reduction. In the REDUCE-IT trial, high-risk patients receiving icosapent ethyl ([Vascepa], purified EPA formulation) had a significant reduction in ischemic events compared with placebo, although the benefit was not directly linked to triglyceride levels. However, the use of mineral oil as the placebo raised concerns, as it was associated with increases in LDL-C and inflammatory biomarkers in the control group. These changes have led to questions about whether the observed benefit of EPA may have been overstated and whether results would have been as favorable with a more inert comparator.

In contrast, the STRENGTH trial evaluated a combination of EPA and DHA versus a corn oil placebo in a similar high-risk population. Although triglyceride levels were reduced, there was no significant cardiovascular benefit observed in the overall study population or subgroups.

Based on current evidence, icosapent ethyl may be considered for secondary prevention in patients on maximally tolerated statin therapy with LDL-C < 100 mg/dL and persistent fasting triglycerides of 150 to 499 mg/dL, after addressing secondary causes. It is important to note, however, that icosapent ethyl is associated with an increased risk of atrial fibrillation or atrial flutter requiring hospitalization, particularly among patients with a prior history of these arrhythmias. Over-the-counter omega-3 supplements are not recommended for cardiovascular event protection, as they have not been shown to reduce cardiovascular events.

Metabolic Syndrome

Compared with individuals with normal weight, patients with obesity experience CCD events at an earlier age, live with cardiovascular disease for a greater proportion of their life, and have a shorter average life span. Metabolic syndrome represents a combination of interrelated risk factors that together increase a person's risk of developing diabetes and cardiovascular disease. The syndrome includes three of the following: elevated waist circumference (≥40 inches in men and ≥35 inches in women), elevated fasting triglycerides (≥150 mg/dL), low high-density lipoprotein cholesterol (HDL-C) (<40 mg/dL in men and <50 mg/dL in women), elevated blood glucose (≥100 mg/dL), and elevated blood pressure (>130/80 mm Hg). Metabolic syndrome doubles the risk of future ASCVD events and carries a fivefold risk of developing diabetes. Lifestyle modification with weight loss improves obesity-related cardiovascular comorbidities. Although a 5% to 7% reduction in body weight is achievable with lifestyle changes alone, maintaining this weight loss is often difficult. Pharmacologic therapy may be necessary for additional weight reduction. Glucagon-like peptide-1 (GLP-1) receptor agonists and sodium-glucose cotransporter 2 (SGLT2) inhibitors were initially developed as glucose-lowering medications for patients with type 2 diabetes; however, contemporary trials have established that these drugs lower ASCVD risk and confer cardiovascular benefits beyond their glucose-lowering potential.

GLP-1 receptor agonists are effective when used in conjunction with dietary and physical activity counseling. These agents slow gastric emptying and act on the hypothalamus to reduce appetite and food cravings, promoting early satiety and decreased caloric intake. They additionally enhance insulin secretion, suppress glucagon release, increase peripheral glucose uptake, and reduce hepatic glucose production.

In the STEP8 trial, patients without diabetes experienced significant weight loss after 68 weeks. The mean weight reduction was 15.8% with semaglutide (Wegovy), 6.4% with liraglutide (Saxenda), and 1.9% with placebo. Further, in the SELECT trial, a double-blind placebo-controlled study of adults with established ASCVD and a BMI > 27 kg/m^2 without diabetes, semaglutide use was associated with a 20% reduction in cardiovascular death. Based on these findings, GLP-1 receptor agonists are now recommended by both US and European guidelines for patients with CCD who are overweight or obese, even in the absence of diabetes, to reduce the risk of cardiovascular events and mortality.

SGLT2 inhibitors result in increased urinary glucose excretion. The exact mechanism by which SGLT2 inhibitors improve CVD outcomes remains largely unknown. The benefits may relate more to cardiorenal hemodynamic effects than to atherosclerosis. A recent meta-analysis demonstrated a 9% reduction in MACE, a benefit that was maintained across a diverse patient population, including those with or without established ASCVD, diabetes, or heart failure at baseline, and across a broad spectrum of kidney function. Based on these findings, European guidelines recommend SGLT2 inhibitors in patients with type 2 diabetes and CCD to reduce cardiovascular events, independent of baseline or target hemoglobin A1c.

The cardiovascular safety of other weight-loss drugs has not been established and remains controversial. Other obesity medication including orlistat (Alli, Xenical), lorcaserin (Belviq)[2], naltrexone/bupropion (Contrave), extended release topiramate/phentermine (Qsymia), diethylpropion, and benzphetamine have not been shown to improve cardiovascular outcomes and have significant adverse effects.

In patients who have severe obesity and weight loss goals that have not been met, bariatric surgery can be considered. In patients who are felt to be an acceptable risk, bariatric surgery is a safe and effective intervention for further and sustained weight loss with beneficial metabolic consequences and cardiovascular risk reduction.

Smoking

Cigarette smoking is a major modifiable risk factor for cardiovascular disease. Smokers have a twofold to fourfold higher incidence of CAD compared with nonsmokers. The atherogenic effects of smoking are mediated through mechanisms such as platelet activation, endothelial dysfunction, smooth muscle proliferation, and reduced HDL-C levels. Smoking cessation should be prioritized for all patients with CAD.

Evidence supports the effectiveness of brief clinical interventions, behavioral counseling, and pharmacologic therapies—including nicotine replacement products, varenicline (Chantix), and bupropion (Zyban)—in increasing the likelihood of successful cessation. While each approach is effective independently, the combination of counseling and pharmacotherapy is more effective than either alone. Clinicians are strongly encouraged to consistently provide advice on tobacco cessation and offer

[2] Not available in the United States.

treatment. Importantly, the elevated cardiovascular and all-cause mortality associated with smoking declines substantially after quitting.

Diet

Lifestyle changes for patients with CAD should emphasize heart-healthy dietary habits. A plant-based, Mediterranean-style diet has been shown to reduce cardiovascular risk, while diets high in saturated fats are associated with adverse cardiac outcomes. Patients should be encouraged to adopt a diet that prioritizes fruits, vegetables, nuts, whole grains, and lean protein (e.g., fish) while limiting red meat, saturated fats, refined carbohydrates, and added sugars. Currently, there is insufficient evidence to support the use of nonprescription vitamins or dietary supplements for cardiovascular risk reduction.

Other Lifestyle Changes

Exercise should be encouraged in patients with stable angina once appropriate diagnostic testing has been completed and the patient is on a stable medical regimen. Enhancing aerobic capacity reduces myocardial oxygen demand at a given workload, which can improve exercise tolerance and decrease anginal symptoms. Regular aerobic activity also strengthens endothelial function and favorably affects autonomic balance by improving baroreflex sensitivity and heart rate variability in patients with CAD.

Exercise also confers significant psychological benefits. It stimulates endorphin release, which can improve mood and promote muscle relaxation. Exercise has also been associated with improved sleep quality and reduced cortisol levels, helping to mitigate perceived stress and anxiety. Given these wide-ranging physical and emotional benefits, structured exercise programs are a key component of secondary prevention in patients with stable angina.

Psychosocial factors are important determinants of cardiovascular outcomes. Major depression affects approximately 25% of individuals recovering from MI, and an additional 40% experience mild depressive symptoms. In the Heart and Soul study, depression was associated with a twofold increase in recurrent cardiovascular events in patients with stable CAD. Importantly, patients experiencing depression, anxiety, or psychosocial stress are less likely to adhere to dietary, exercise, and medication recommendations. Therefore routine assessment of psychosocial risk factors should be part of the comprehensive evaluation of patients with angina and CCD.

Approach to Treatment
Medical Therapy

Medications used to treat angina pectoris and typical dosages are listed in Table 3.

Nitrates

Nitrates act as exogenous donors of nitric oxide, promoting smooth muscle relaxation and inhibiting platelet aggregation. Their antianginal effects primarily result from reduced myocardial oxygen demand via systemic and coronary vasodilation. As potent venodilators, nitrates decrease preload, which in turn lowers LV wall stress and oxygen demand. At high doses, they also induce arterial dilation, further contributing to afterload reduction. Additionally, dilation of stenotic coronary arteries and enhancement of intracoronary collateral flow improves myocardial oxygen supply. Collectively, these effects help prevent recurrent anginal episodes and enhance exercise tolerance.

Several nitrate formulations are available, differing primarily in their route of administration, onset of action, and duration of effect. Sublingual or sprays provide rapid relief of acute anginal symptoms. Longer-acting preparations, such as oral or transdermal nitrates, are often used in combination with other antianginal agents to help control chronic symptoms. Tolerance can develop with continuous use; to minimize this, a 10- to 12-hour nitrate-free interval is recommended. Although long-acting nitrates are effective for symptom relief, they have not been shown to improve survival or reduce the incidence of MACE.

TABLE 3	Medications Used for the Treatment of Angina Pectoris

NAME	DOSAGE
β-Blockers	
Atenolol (Tenormin)	50–100 mg PO qd
Metoprolol tartrate (Lopressor)	50–200 mg bid
Metoprolol succinate (Toprol XL)	100–400 mg qd
Carvedilol (Coreg)[1]	6.25–25 mg PO bid
Propranolol (Inderal)	80–320 mg/d, divided bid or tid
Nitrates	
Isosorbide dinitrate (Isordil)	10–40 mg PO bid or tid
Isosorbide mononitrate (Imdur)	30–120 mg qd
Nitroglycerin (Nitrostat)	0.4 mg SL q5min
Nitroglycerin transdermal (Nitro-Dur)	0.2–0.8 mg/h 12–14 h patch
Calcium Channel Blockers	
Dihydropyridines	
Amlodipine (Norvasc)	2.5–10 mg PO qd
Felodipine (Plendil)[1]	2.5–10 mg PO qd
Nifedipine (Procardia XL)	30–90 mg PO qd
Nondihydropyridines	
Verapamil (Calan)	80–120 mg PO tid
Verapamil (Calan SR)	120–480 mg PO qd
Diltiazem (Cardizem)	120–360 mg/d PO, divided tid or qid
Diltiazem (Cardizem LA)	180–360 mg PO qd
Other	
Ranolazine (Ranexa)	500-1000 mg bid as needed, based on clinical symptoms twice daily as needed, based on clinical symptoms

[1]Not FDA approved for this indication.

β-Blockers

β-blockers are a cornerstone of antianginal therapy, particularly in patients with stable CAD, prior MI, or coexisting conditions such as hypertension or arrhythmias. They improve symptoms by reducing myocardial oxygen demand through negative chronotropic and inotropic effects and by lowering LV wall stress. Clinical benefits include reduced frequency of anginal episodes and improved exercise tolerance.

When β-blockers are used for angina, a target resting heart rate of 55 to 60 beats per minute (bpm) is recommended. While prior guidelines endorsed extended long-term β-blocker therapy for all patients with CCD, updated recommendations now limit their use to those with a MI within the past year, reduced LV ejection fraction (LVEF) (≤ 50%), ongoing angina, or other compelling indications, such as hypertension, arrhythmia, or recurrent angina. Recent studies have called into question the routine use of β-blockers beyond 1 year post MI, given mixed data on long-term benefit and potential adverse effects, including fatigue, depression, and drug interactions.

β-blockers act by competitively inhibiting catecholamines binding to β-adrenergic receptors, which over time leads to receptor upregulation. As a result, abrupt withdrawal can trigger transient catecholamine hypersensitivity, potentially precipitating angina or MI. Although cardioselective agents preferentially block β1 receptors, the selectivity diminishes at higher doses, resulting in β2 cross-reactivity. Caution is advised in patients with resting bradycardia, reactive airway disease, severe peripheral vascular disease, or Raynaud phenomenon. Atenolol, which is renally excreted, requires dose adjustment in older adults and those with impaired renal function.

Calcium Channel Blockers

CCBs are classified into two categories: dihydropyridines (e.g., amlodipine [Norvasc], felodipine [Plendil][1], nifedipine [Procardia], and nicardipine [Cardene]) and nondihydropyridine (e.g., diltiazem [Cardizem] and verapamil [Calan]). These agents improve myocardial oxygen balance by promoting coronary and peripheral arterial vasodilation, thereby enhancing oxygen supply and reducing oxygen demand. In addition, nondihydropyridine exerts negative chronotropic and inotropic effects, further decreasing myocardial oxygen requirements.

Early studies raised concerns about the use of short-acting nifedipine for angina, as it was associated with increased MI risk, likely due to rapid afterload reduction and reflex sympathetic activation. However, sustained-release formulations of nifedipine and other dihydropyridines have since been shown to be both safe and effective in patients with cardiovascular disease. Among the CCBs, amlodipine and felodipine[1] are generally well tolerated in patients with LV systolic dysfunction, whereas other agents, particularly those with negative inotropic effects, should be avoided in this population.

Ranolazine

Ranolazine (Ranexa), a late sodium channel blocker, has been approved for patients who remain symptomatic despite standard antianginal therapy or as a substitute when other medications are not tolerated or contraindicated (e.g., hypotension or bradycardia limiting combination therapy). It is contraindicated in patients with severe hepatic impairment, prolonged QT interval, and when used in combination with strong CYP3A inhibitors (e.g., diltiazem, verapamil, macrolide antibiotics). Common side effects include dizziness, constipation, and nausea.

Ivabradine

Ivabradine (Corlanor) is a selective inhibitor of the I_f (funny) current in the sinus node, which regulates spontaneous diastolic depolarization and controls heart rate. It lowers heart rate without affecting myocardial contractility, coronary vasomotor tone, central aortic pressure, or ventricular repolarization. By slowing the heart rate, ivabradine prolongs diastolic perfusion time and reduces myocardial oxygen demand.

Ivabradine[1] may be considered in patients with ongoing anginal symptoms not controlled on β-blocker or CCB therapy. It can also serve as an alternative when traditional agents are contraindicated or poorly tolerated. Because it is metabolized by the cytochrome P450 3A4 (CYP3A4), coadministration with nondihydropyridine CCBs (e.g., verapamil, diltiazem) is not recommended.

The heart rate–lowering effect of ivabradine is most pronounced in patients with elevated baseline resting heart rates. However, it should not be used in patients with stable angina without heart failure or in those with preserved LV function (LVEF > 40%). In the SIGNIFY trial, ivabradine improved anginal symptoms compared with placebo (24% vs. 18.8%) in patients with stable coronary disease without heart failure but was associated with increased rates of bradycardia, cardiovascular death, and nonfatal MI. Based on these findings, ivabradine is not recommended patients without clinical heart failure or in those with preserved LV systolic function.

Medication Combinations

Many patients with chronic stable angina require combination therapy with multiple antianginal medications to achieve adequate

[1]Not FDA approved for this indication.

symptom control. US guidelines recommend β-blockers, CCBs, or long-acting nitrates as initial therapy, with the addition of a second agent from a different class based on symptom burden.

Because no head-to-head trials have demonstrated the superiority of one antianginal class over another, the selection of therapy should be individualized. Key factors include resting heart rate, LV function, heart failure status, comorbidities (e.g., hypertension), and potential side effects.

- Elevated heart rate (>70 bpm): β-blockers or nondihydropyridine CCB are preferred.
- Low resting heart rate (<55 bpm): Dihydropyridine CCBs and nitrates are preferred, as they may cause reflex sympathetic activation and modest increases in heart rate.
- Combination therapy precautions: β-blockers should not be used in combination with nondihydropyridine CCBs (e.g., verapamil or diltiazem) due to the risk of high-grade atrioventricular (AV) block and worsening LV function. Dihydropyridine CCBs (e.g., amlodipine) do not exert AV nodal effects and are generally safer in combination with β-blockers. Nitrates can be safely combined with either class.

Regular reassessment of anginal symptom is essential, typically every 2 to 3 months. If symptoms persist despite one or two antianginal agents, particularly at submaximal doses, treatment should not be considered optimized unless dose escalation is limited by side effects, intolerance, or contraindications. Ongoing symptom burden warrants reevaluation of the regimen and consideration of additional therapy.

Antiplatelet Therapy

The most common etiology leading to an acute ischemic syndrome is a platelet-rich thrombus occurring at the site of ruptured atherosclerotic plaque within a significantly stenosed coronary artery. Antiplatelet therapy has consistently been shown to reduce morbidity and mortality across a broad spectrum of cardiovascular disease patients. A meta-analysis demonstrated that in patients with stable cardiovascular disease, low-dose aspirin therapy (50–100 mg daily) is as effective as higher doses (>300 mg). In this population, aspirin therapy reduced the risk of MI by 26%, with a number needed to treat of 83 to prevent one event.

The Antiplatelet Trialists' Collaboration confirmed that antiplatelet therapy significantly reduces the risk of MI, stroke, and death in high-risk patients. Consensus guidelines recommend indefinite low-dose oral aspirin (75–100 mg daily) for the secondary prevention in all patients with chronic angina or established ASCVD.

Clopidogrel (Plavix), a thienopyridine derivative and irreversible P2Y12 receptor inhibitor, has been evaluated as an alternative to aspirin. In the CAPRIE trial, clopidogrel demonstrated a slightly greater reduction in ischemic events compared with aspirin in patients with prior ASCVD. Data from the 2021 HOST-EXAM trial demonstrated that in patients with prior percutaneous intervention (PCI) who have completed 6 to 18 months of dual antiplatelet therapy, long-term clopidogrel monotherapy may be associated with fewer cardiovascular events and reduced bleeding compared with aspirin. Consequently, aspirin or clopidogrel monotherapy should be considered in patients with CCD and prior PCI.

Ticagrelor (Brilinta) and prasugrel (Effient) offer more potent platelet inhibition and have demonstrated superiority over clopidogrel in ACS. However, due to their increased bleeding risk, they are not routinely recommended for long-term monotherapy in patients with CCD.

Oral Anticoagulation

The use of vitamin K antagonists in patients with stable ischemic heart disease has shown some benefit in reducing cardiovascular events, although this is offset by an increased risk of bleeding. With the introduction of direct oral anticoagulants, there has been renewed interest in targeting the coagulation cascade to improve outcomes in stable atherosclerotic disease.

The COMPASS trial evaluated rivaroxaban (Xarelto), a factor Xa inhibitor, alone or in combination with aspirin, versus aspirin monotherapy in patients with stable atherosclerotic vascular disease. Patients received either rivaroxaban 5 mg twice daily, rivaroxaban 2.5 mg twice daily plus aspirin 100 mg daily, or aspirin alone. The combination of rivaroxaban 2.5 mg and aspirin significantly reduced the primary composite endpoint of cardiovascular events compared with aspirin monotherapy but at the cost of increased bleeding. Notably, the observed benefit was largely driven by a 49% relative risk reduction in ischemic stroke, while the reduction in MI was more modest at 14%. Although patients with atrial fibrillation or prior use of systemic anticoagulation were excluded, the possibility of subclinical atrial fibrillation in this population cannot be entirely ruled out.

At present, there is no compelling evidence to support standard antiplatelet therapy with antithrombotic therapy in patients with stable ischemic heart disease. However, an antithrombotic agent may be considered in patients who are intolerant to antiplatelet therapy, have a low bleeding risk, or have a coexisting long-term indication for oral anticoagulation, such as atrial fibrillation.

Invasive Assessment

The decision to pursue an invasive approach varies significantly between patients with chronic stable angina and those with ACS. In both groups, accurate risk stratification is essential to determine who may benefit from coronary angiography and possible PCI. In ACS, a routine invasive strategy has been shown to reduce recurrent events and is recommended in patients with refractory ischemia, elevated cardiac biomarkers, or new ST-segment changes on ECG. In contrast, patients with stable angina represent a broader and more heterogenous population. The key clinical debates focus on when to initiate invasive therapy versus optimal medical therapy (OMT), and when to transition from a conservative to an invasive approach.

Over the past two decades, multiple RCTs have sought to clarify the role of revascularization in the management of CCD. Many of these earlier trials had limitations, including being conducted during eras of less advanced percutaneous technologies and suboptimal medical therapy. The BARI 2D, for instance, compared revascularization (via PCI or coronary artery bypass graft [CABG]) plus OMT versus OMT alone. It found no difference in mortality or major cardiovascular events overall, although CABG showed greater long-term benefit than PCI in reducing repeat interventions and disease progression among those selected for revascularization.

More recently, the ISCHEMIA trial randomized patients with moderate-to-severe ischemia, preserved LVEF (≥35%), and no left main disease to either an initial invasive strategy (coronary angiography and revascularization when feasible) plus OMT or OMT alone. Results showed no significant difference in all-cause mortality or composite cardiovascular outcomes. However, invasive treatment was associated with greater improvements in angina symptoms and quality of life. This was reinforced by findings from ORBITA-2, which demonstrated that patients with stable angina on minimal or no antianginal therapy and objective evidence of ischemia had greater improvement in angina symptoms after PCI compared with a sham procedure.

The CLARIFY registry further supported a conservative strategy, showing many patients with CCD and angina experienced spontaneous improvement in symptoms over time without the need for revascularization or changes in therapy, while still achieving good clinical outcomes. Based on current available evidence and clinical guidelines, initial conservative medical therapy remains the preferred strategy for managing CCD with stable angina. This includes antianginal therapy and aggressive risk factor modification: blood pressure, lipid and glucose control, and antithrombotic therapy. Revascularization should be considered in patients with persistent symptoms despite OMT, or those with high-risk features, such as left main or three-vessel disease or severely reduced LVEF, where a prognostic benefit has been established.

A unique subset of CCD patients have chronic total occlusions (CTOs), defined as complete arterial blockage (Thrombolysis in myocardial infarction [TIMI] 0 flow) lasting more than 3 months. A CTO impairs coronary flow reserve and can limit compensatory collateral circulation, contributing to recurrent angina.

CTO lesions are encountered in clinical practice at a frequency of 16% to 18%; however, PCI is attempted in only 5% to 10% of cases. Historically, technical complexity and procedural risk associated with CTO intervention limited its widespread adoption. Considerable progress in interventional techniques and operator experience has significantly improved procedural success, with success rates >80% in the hands of skilled operators. There has additionally been a reduction in complication rate, with a roughly 1% risk of stroke, heart attack, or death and 4.8% risk of perforations occurring in the case. Nevertheless, these procedures remain complex and are also associated with increased radiation, contrast use, and procedural time compared with standard diagnostic and percutaneous coronary interventions.

While CTO PCI has demonstrated benefits in angina relief and quality of life, no large trial has shown mortality or MI reduction. Therefore the decision to pursue CTO revascularization should be individual, weighing the symptomatic benefit against procedural risks and the patient's overall clinical context.

Novel Therapies
Enhanced External Counterpulsation
In patients with CCD who have CCS class III or IV refractory angina despite appropriate pharmacotherapy and coronary revascularization, enhanced external counterpulsation (EECP) may be considered for symptomatic relief. EECP uses pneumatic cuffs on the legs that inflate in early diastole (synchronized with the ECG) to increase coronary perfusion, reduce afterload, and enhance venous return. Treatments are typically administered for 1-hour intervals, 5 days per week, for 6 to 7 weeks.

Although the exact mechanism is unclear, potential benefits include improved endothelial function, coronary collateral recruitment, angiogenesis, and enhanced myocardial perfusion, with a possible placebo effect contributing. Although mortality benefits are unproved, small studies and a meta-analysis of 13 observation studies (949 patients) found that 86% experienced at least a one-class improvement in CCS angina. Contraindications include severe aortic regurgitation, aortic aneurysm, acute heart failure, and severe peripheral arterial disease.

Coronary Sinus Reducer Device
The coronary sinus reducer is a stainless-steel device implanted percutaneously to narrow the coronary sinus, thereby increasing coronary sinus pressure and enhancing myocardial perfusion in the LAD territory. In a meta-analysis that included one RCT and eight small registries, use of a coronary sinus reducer led to an improvement of ≥1 CCS class in 76% of patients and an improvement of ≥2 CCS class in 40% of patients. Several RCTs are currently underway to further evaluate its efficacy, including the COSIRA-II trial (NCT05102019). Additional evidence is needed to clarify the role of the coronary sinus reducer and its efficacy in patients with refractory angina despite OMT and prior revascularization.

Spinal Cord Stimulation
For patients whose angina is refractory to medical therapy and who are not candidates for revascularization, spinal cord stimulation with placement of the device and stimulation at the C7–T1 level to help reduce pain sensation has been tried. At present, more research is needed to assess the utility of neuromodulation and thoracic spinal stimulation.

Angina With Nonobstructive Coronary Arteries
Angina with nonobstructive coronary arteries (ANOCA) is increasingly recognized and is observed in more than 50% of patients undergoing elective coronary angiography for suspected ischemic heart disease. When epicardial obstructive CAD is not identified in patients with documented ischemia, this should prompt further investigation for potential ANOCA subtypes.

In ANOCA, myocardial oxygen supply-demand imbalance may result from mechanisms such as coronary microvascular dysfunction (CMD), epicardial and microvascular coronary vasospasm, myocardial bridging, and other coronary abnormalities. Patients with angina and documented ischemia but nonobstructive coronary arteries on angiography tend to be younger and more frequently women. The underlying reason for this sex disparity remains poorly understood but is likely related to differences in vascular biology and hormonal influences.

It has become increasingly clear that nonobstructive CAD is not a benign condition in symptomatic individuals. Compared with age- and sex-matched asymptomatic individuals, nonobstructive CAD is associated with a higher risk of adverse cardiovascular outcomes, reduced quality of life, greater likelihood of disability, and increased healthcare usage. Furthermore, the finding of nonobstructive CAD leads to repeat testing to search for a missed obstruction or noncardiac conditions to explain the continuing episodes of chest pain. Given the challenges in establishing a diagnosis, patients with ANOCA frequently experience invalidation, leading to poor mental health. Symptoms are generally stable and often persist for over 3 months, with many patients experiencing them for years before receiving a formal diagnosis. This delay often coincides with a gradual decline in physical function and exercise capacity.

For patients with refractory angina and a poor quality of life due to suspected or confirmed ANOCA, a comprehensive evaluation of coronary function—including both microvascular and epicardial components—is recommended. This helps define the specific ANOCA subtype and guide targeted treatment. Optimal management requires an accurate diagnosis and therapy tailored to the underlying abnormality.

Treatment should include personalized counseling on lifestyle modifications aimed at addressing risk factors, alleviating symptoms, and improving quality of life and prognosis. Controlling traditional cardiovascular risk factors—such as hypertension, dyslipidemia, smoking, and diabetes—is essential. Exercise training and cardiac rehabilitation have demonstrated benefits in improving exercise tolerance, delaying the onset of angina, and enhancing quality of life. Weight loss may also contribute to symptom relief. Additionally, relaxation techniques and meditation have been associated with reduced chest pain and improved psychological well-being in ANOCA patients.

Pharmacologic management of anginal symptoms in ANOCA is challenging due to the heterogeneity of underlying mechanisms and the limited availability of robust randomized clinical trial data. Therapeutic strategies should be individualized and as specifically targeted as possible to the identified pathophysiologic substrate.

Coronary Vasospasm
Prinzmetal angina was traditionally defined by rest-related chest pain and transient ST elevation but has since evolved into the broader concept of coronary artery spasm (CAS). CAS now includes vasospasm-related angina triggered by stress or occurring spontaneously, often with ST depression, and may involve both epicardial and microvascular vessels.

CAS can present as stable angina, ACS, arrhythmias, or sudden cardiac death. Triggers include circadian variation (often midnight to early morning), alcohol, hyperventilation, smoking, sympathomimetics (e.g., cocaine, ephedrine), cold exposure, and exertion.

Diagnosis is made during angiography by demonstrating ≥90% transient constriction with ischemic ECG changes, either spontaneously or after provocation (e.g., acetylcholine). Acute episodes are treated with nitroglycerin; long-term management includes CCB and long-acting nitrates. Refractory cases may require high-dose CCBs or even a combination of nondihydropyridine with dihydropyridine CCBs. β-Blockers have the potential to increase coronary vasomotor tone owing to unopposed α-adrenergic activity and should be used with caution in patients with coronary spasm.

Coronary Microvascular Dysfunction

CMD is a subtype of ANOCA involving structural and functional abnormalities of the coronary microcirculation. It often coexists with cardiovascular risk factors and contributes to ischemia with prognostic significance.

Cardiac PET is the most accurate noninvasive method to assess CMD, allowing quantification of myocardial blood flow and myocardial flow reserve (MFR)—the latter reflecting the capacity of the microvasculature to increase blood flow during maximal vasodilation (e.g., with adenosine [Adenoscan] or regadenoson [Lexiscan]). Because microvascular resistance determines MFR, it serves as a surrogate for small vessel function. MFR < 2 is considered abnormal and is associated with increased risk of adverse cardiovascular events, including heart failure and mortality. Invasive tools such as coronary flow reserve, index of microcirculatory resistance, and vasoreactivity testing are useful when noninvasive methods are inconclusive.

Although no CMD-specific guidelines exist, management typically includes β-blockers, statins, and other antianginal therapies tailored to symptoms.

Summary

Management of patients with angina should begin with a comprehensive assessment and aggressive treatment of all modifiable cardiovascular risk factors. All patients should be prescribed appropriate doses of statins and antiplatelet therapy, unless contraindicated. Noninvasive testing plays a key role in establishing the initial diagnosis and guiding decisions about further invasive evaluation. Adherence to current clinical guidelines is essential to ensure optimal outcomes.

References

2017 ACC/AHA/AAPA/ABC/ACPM/AGS/APhA/ASH/ASPC/NMA/PCNA guideline for the prevention, detection, evaluation, and management of high blood pressure in adults: a report of the American College of Cardiology/American heart association task force on clinical practice guidelines.

Allan BS, Krumholz HM; SM reviewing the SPRINT research group: N Engl J Med 2015 Nov 9 Chobanian AV., N Engl J Med, 2015 Nov 9.

Anderson JL, Adams CD, Antman EM: ACC/AHA 2007 guidelines for the management of patients with unstable angina/non-ST-elevation myocardial infarction: a report of the American College of Cardiology/American Heart Association Task Force on Practice Guidelines, J Am Coll Cardiol 5067:e1–e157, 2007.

Antithrombotic Trialists Collaboration: Collaborative meta-analysis of randomized trials of antiplatelet therapy for prevention of death, myocardial infarction, and stroke in high risk patients, BMJ 324:71–86, 2002.

Berger J, Brown D, Becker R: Low-dose aspirin in patients with stable cardiovascular disease: a meta-analysis, Am J Med 121:43–49, 2008.

Bhatt DL, Steg PG, Miller M: Cardiovascular risk reduction with icosapent ethyl for hypertriglyceridemia, N Engl J Med 380:11–22, 2019.

Blood Pressure Lowering Treatment Trialists Collaboration: Effects of different blood pressure lowering regimens on major cardiovascular events: results of prospectively designed overviews of randomized trials, Lancet 362:1527–1545, 2003.

Boden WE, O'Rourke RA, Teo KK: Optimal medical therapy with or without PCI for stable coronary disease, N Engl J Med 35:1503–1516, 2007.

Borer JS, Fox K, Jaillon P: Antianginal and antischemic effects of Ivrabadine, a novel I(f) inhibitor, in stable angina: a randomized, double-blind, multicentered, placebo-controlled trial, Circulation 107:817–823, 2003.

Bove KB, Nilsson M, Pedersen LR, Mikkelsen N, Suhrs HE, Astrup A, Prescott E: Comprehensive treatment of microvascular angina in overweight women - a randomized controlled pilot trial, PLoS One 15(11):e0240722, 2020.

Cannon CP, Blazing MA, et al: IMPROVE-IT investigators. Ezetimibe added to statin therapy after acute coronary syndromes, N Engl J Med 372(25):2387–2397, 2015.

CAPRIE Steering Committee: A randomised, blinded, trial of clopidogrel versus aspirin in patients at risk of ischaemic events (CAPRIE). CAPRIE Steering Committee, Lancet. 348(9038):1329–1339, 1996.

Cholesterol Treatment Trialists' Collaborators: Efficacy and safety of cholesterol-lowering treatment: prospective meta-analysis of data from 90,056 participants in 14 trials of statins, Lancet 366:1267–1278, 2005.

De Bruyne B, Fearon WF, Pijls NH: Fractional flow reserve-guided PCI for stable coronary artery disease, N Engl J Med 371:1208–1217, 2014.

Eikelboom JW, Connolly SJ, Bosch J, et al: COMPASS Investigators: Rivaroxaban with or without aspirin in stable cardiovascular disease, N Engl J Med 377:1319–1330, 2017.

Fefer P, Knudtson ML, Cheema AN, et al: Current perspectives on coronary chronic total occlusions: the Canadian multicenter chronic total occlusions registry, J Am Coll Cardiol 59:991–997, 2012.

Fihn SD, Gardin JM, Abrams J: 2012 ACCF/AHA/ACP/AATS/PCNA/SCAI/STS guideline for the diagnosis and management of patients with stable ischemic heart disease: a report of the American College of Cardiology foundation/American heart association task force on practice guidelines, and the American College of physicians, American association for thoracic surgery, preventive cardiovascular nurses association, society for cardiovascular angiography and interventions, and society of thoracic surgeons, J Am Coll Cardiol 60:e44–e164, 2012.

Gibbons RJ, Abrams J, Chatterjee K, et al: ACC/AHA 2007 guideline update for the management of patients with chronic stable angina: A report of the American College of Cardiology/American Heart Association Task Force on Practice Guidelines (Committee to Update the 2002 Guidelines for the Management of Patients with Chronic Stable Angina) Reston, VA, American College of Cardiology, American Heart Association. Available at: www.acc.org/qualityandscience/clinical/guidelines/stable/stable_clean.pdf (Accessed August 20, 2014).

Grundy SM, Cleeman JI, Merz NB: Implications of recent clinical trials for the national cholesterol education program adult treatment panel III guidelines, Circulation 110:227–239, 2004.

Gulati M, Khan N, George M, et al: Ischemia with no obstructive coronary artery disease (INOCA): a patient self-report quality of life survey from INOCA international, Int J Cardiol 371:28–39, 2023.

Heart Outcomes Prevention Evaluation Study Investigators: Effects of an angiotensin-converting-enzyme inhibitor, ramipril, on cardiovascular events in high-risk patients, N Engl J Med 342:145–153, 2000.

Hochstadt A, Itach T, Merdler I, Ghantous E, Ziv-Baran T, Leshno M, et al: Effectiveness of coronary sinus reducer for treatment of refractory angina: a meta-analysis, Can J Cardiol 38:376–383, 2022.

James PA, Oparil S, Carter BL: 2014 evidence-based guideline for the management of high blood pressure in adults: report from the panel members appointed to the eighth Joint National Committee (JNC 8), JAMA 311:507–520, 2014.

Jespersen L, Hvelplund A, Abildstrom SZ, Pedersen F, Galatius S, Madsen JK, et al: Stable angina pectoris with no obstructive coronary artery disease is associated with increased risks of major adverse cardiovascular events, Eur Heart J 33:734–744, 2012.

Koo BK, Kang J, et al: HOST-EXAM investigators. Aspirin versus clopidogrel for chronic maintenance monotherapy after percutaneous coronary intervention (HOST-EXAM): an investigator-initiated, prospective, randomised, open-label, multicentre trial, Lancet 397(10293):2487–2496, 2021.

Krist AH, Davidson KW, Mangione CM, et al; US Preventive Services Task Force: Interventions for tobacco smoking cessation in adults, including pregnant persons: US preventive services task force recommendation statement, JAMA 325(3):265–279, 2021.

Lorenzo C, Williams K, Hunt KJ, Haffner SM: The national cholesterol education program - adult treatment panel III, international diabetes federation, and world health organization definitions of the metabolic syndrome as predictors of incident cardiovascular disease and diabetes, Diabetes Care 30(1):8–13, 2007.

Maddox TM, Stanislawski MA, Grunwald GK, et al: Nonobstructive coronary artery disease and risk of myocardial infarction, JAMA 312:1754–1763, 2014.

Mancia G, Kreutz R, Brunström M, et al: 2023 ESH guidelines for the management of arterial hypertension the task force for the management of arterial hypertension of the European society of hypertension: endorsed by the international society of hypertension (ISH) and the European renal association (ERA), J Hypertens 41(12):1874–2071, 2023.

Marzilli M, Crea F, Morrone D, Bonow RO, Brown DL, Camici PG, et al: Myocardial ischemia: from disease to syndrome, Int J Cardiol 314:32–35, 2020.

Mehta SR, Cannon CP, Fox KA: Routine vs selective invasive strategies in patients with acute coronary syndromes: a collaborative meta-analysis of randomized trials, JAMA 293:2908–2917, 2005.

Messerli FH, Mancia G, Conti CR: Dogma disrupted: can aggressively lowering blood pressure in hypertensive patients with coronary artery disease be dangerous? Ann Intern Med 144:884–893, 2006.

Montalescot G, Sechtem U, Achenbach S: Editor's choice: 2013 ESC guidelines on the management of stable coronary artery disease: the Task Force on the management of stable coronary artery disease of the European Society of Cardiology, Eur Heart J 34:2949–3003, 2013.

Mottillo S, Filion KB, Genest J, Joseph L, Pilote L, Poirier P, Rinfret S, Schiffrin EL, Eisenberg MJ: The metabolic syndrome and cardiovascular risk a systematic review and meta-analysis, J Am Coll Cardiol 56(14):1113–1132, 2010.

Nicholls SJ, Lincoff AM, Garcia M, et al: Effect of high-dose omega-3 fatty acids vs corn oil on major adverse cardiovascular events in patients at high cardiovascular risk: the STRENGTH randomized clinical trial, JAMA 324(22):2268–2280, 2020.

Nissen SE, Lincoff AM, Brennan D, et al: CLEAR outcomes investigators. Bempedoic acid and cardiovascular outcomes in statin-intolerant patients, N Engl J Med 388(15):1353–1364, 2023.

Patel MR, Dai D, Hernandez AF, et al: Prevalence and predictors of nonobstructive coronary artery disease identified with coronary angiography in contemporary clinical practice, Am Heart J 167:846–852.e842, 2014.

Petraco R, Al-Lamee R, Gotberg M: Real-time use of instantaneous wave-free ratio: results of the ADVISE in-practice: an international, multicenter evaluation of instantaneous wave-free ratio in clinical practice, Am Heart J 168:739–748, 2014.

Ray K, Cannon C: Optimal goal for statin therapy use in coronary artery disease, Curr Opin Cardiol 20:525–529, 2005.

Rigotti NA, McDermott MM: Smoking cessation and cardiovascular disease: it's never too early or too late for action, J Am Coll Cardiol 74(4):508–511, 2019.

Rubino DM, Greenway FL, et al: STEP 8 investigators. Effect of weekly subcutaneous semaglutide vs daily liraglutide on body weight in adults with overweight or obesity without diabetes: the STEP 8 randomized clinical trial, JAMA 327(2):138–150, 2022.

Sabatine MS, Giugliano RP, Keech AC: Evolocumab and clinical outcomes in patients with cardiovascular disease, N Engl J Med 376:1713–1722, 2017.

Schwartz GG, Steg PG, Szarek M, et al: ODYSSEY OUTCOMES committees and investigators. Alirocumab and cardiovascular outcomes after acute coronary syndrome, N Engl J Med 379(22):2097–2107, 2018.

The SCOT-HEART investigators: CT coronary angiography in patients with suspected angina due to coronary heart disease (SCOT-HEART): an open-label, parallel-group, multicentre trial, *Lancet* 385(9985):2383–2391, 2015.

SEARCH Collaborative Group: Intensive lowering of LDL cholesterol with 80mg versus 20mg simvastatin daily in 12,064 survivors of myocardial infarction: a double-blind randomised trial, *Lancet* 376:1658–1669, 2010.

Stone G, Teirstein P, Rubenstein R: A prospective, multicenter, randomized trial of percutaneous transmyocardial laser revascularization in patients with nonrecanalizable chronic total occlusions, *J Am Coll Cardiol* 39:1581–1587, 2002.

Stone NJ, Robinson J, Lichtenstein AH, et al: 2013 ACC/AHA guideline on the treatment of blood cholesterol to reduce atherosclerotic cardiovascular risk in adults: a report of the American College of Cardiology/American Heart Association Task Force on Practice Guidelines, *Circulation* 129(25 Suppl 2):S1-45, 2014

Taqueti VR, Di Carli MF: Coronary microvascular disease pathogenic mechanisms and therapeutic options: JACC state-of-the-art review, *J Am Coll Cardiol* 72:2625–2641, 2018.

Tendera M, Borer JS, Tardif JC: Efficacy of I(f) inhibition with Ivabradine in different subpopulations with stable angina pectoris, *Cardiology* 114:116–125, 2009.

Tyni-Lenne R, Stryjan S, Eriksson B, Berglund M, Sylven C: Beneficial therapeutic effects of physical training and relaxation therapy in women with coronary syndrome X, *Physiother Res Int* 7(1):35–43, 2002.

Virani SS, Newby LK, Arnold SV, et al: 2023 AHA/ACC/ACCP/ASPC/NLA/PCNA guideline for the management of patients with chronic coronary disease: a report of the American heart association/American College of Cardiology joint committee on clinical practice guidelines, *Circulation* 148(9):e9–e119, 2023.

Vrints C, Andreotti F, Koskinas KC, et al; ESC Scientific Document Group: 2024 ESC Guidelines for the management of chronic coronary syndromes, *Eur Heart J* 45(36):3415–3537, 2024.

Weber MA, Schiffrin EL, White WB: Clinical practice guidelines for the management of hypertension in the community, *J Clin Hypertens* 16:14–26, 2014.

Wenger NK: *Cardiac rehabilitation: a guide to practice in the 21st century*, New York, 1999, Marcel Dekker.

Whooley MA, Jonge P, Vittinghoff E: Depressive symptoms, health behaviors, and risk of cardiovascular events in patients with coronary heart disease, *JAMA* 300:2379–2388, 2008.

Zhao L, Li D, Zheng H: Acupuncture as adjunctive therapy for chronic stable angina: a randomized clinical trial, *JAMA Intern Med* 179(10):1388–1397, 2019.

Zhu Y, Meng S, Chen M, et al: Long-term prognosis of chronic total occlusion treated by successful percutaneous coronary intervention in patients with or without diabetes mellitus: a systematic review and meta-analysis, *Cardiovasc Diabetol* 20:29, 2021.

AORTIC DISEASE: ANEURYSM AND DISSECTION

Method of
David G. Neschis, MD

CURRENT DIAGNOSIS

- Because the majority of patients with abdominal aortic aneurysms are asymptomatic, the majority of abdominal aortic aneurysms are detected on imaging studies performed for other indications.
- Patients older than 50 years who present with abdominal or back pain of unclear etiology should be considered for evaluation of possible abdominal aortic aneurysm.
- Asymptomatic men older than 65 years who have ever smoked are eligible for abdominal aortic aneurysm screening.
- All patients older than 60 years who have a strong family history of abdominal aortic aneurysms should be considered for screening.
- Patients presenting with sudden onset of chest or back pain without clear etiology should be evaluated for dissection.
- Dissection can mimic numerous other conditions.

CURRENT THERAPY

Indications for Repair of Aneurysm
- Fusiform abdominal aortic aneurysms greater than 5.5cm in maximum diameter
- Most saccular aneurysms and pseudoaneurysms
- Thoracic and thoracoabdominal aortic aneurysms of greater than 6cm in maximal diameter
- Aneurysms that are symptomatic or are rapidly enlarging

Indications for Repair of Aortic Dissection
- Dissections involving the ascending aorta
- Dissections involving only the descending aorta are usually managed medically unless complicated by the following: unrelenting pain, end organ ischemia, or significant aneurysmal degeneration to greater than 6cm in maximal diameter

Abdominal Aortic Aneurysms

Epidemiology

A ruptured abdominal aortic aneurysm is a devastating event leading to approximately 15,000 deaths per year, and it is the 13th leading cause of death in the United States. It is the 10th leading cause of death in men. Once rupture occurs, there is an 85% chance of death overall and approximately 50% mortality in the patients who make it to the hospital alive. Clearly, the goal is to identify this life-threatening lesion and repair prior to rupture. Abdominal aortic aneurysms are approximately four times more prevalent in men than in women. The overall incidence in persons older than 60 years is approximately 3% to 4%, with incidence as high as 10% to 12% in an elderly hypertensive population.

Risk Factors

Men are approximately 4 times more likely than women to develop an abdominal aortic aneurysm. Clearly, older persons, particularly those older than 60 years, are at higher risk. Tobacco use is probably the strongest preventable risk factor, with tobacco users being approximately eight times more likely to be affected than nonsmokers. Hypertension is present in approximately 40% of patients with abdominal aortic aneurysms. Family history also plays a significant role. In fact, men who have first-degree female relatives who had aneurysms are approximately 18 times more likely than the general population to develop an abdominal aortic aneurysm. There is also a strong correlation between abdominal aortic aneurysms and other peripheral artery aneurysms. Patients with bilateral popliteal artery aneurysms have an approximately 50% to 60% risk of having an abdominal aortic aneurysm.

Pathophysiology

An aneurysm is a dilatation of a blood vessel that could occur in any blood vessel in the body, even in the veins. Most commonly it is defined as a dilatation of approximately 1.5 to 2 times at that diameter of the adjacent normal vessel.

The definition of a pseudoaneurysm is often misunderstood. The attempt to describe a pseudoaneurysm in terms of the number of layers of the artery wall involved does nothing to help resolve this confusion. A pseudoaneurysm is a walled-off defect in the artery wall. A circular shell of adventitial and surrounding connective tissue contains the blood, preventing free hemorrhage. However, there remains continued flow out and back into the arterial lumen, resulting in a classic to-and-fro pattern on duplex ultrasound. The most common cause of a pseudoaneurysm is iatrogenic, from needle puncture, but it also can be caused by trauma or focal rupture of the artery at the site of an atherosclerotic ulcer.

The etiology of true aneurysms is not clear, although in the past these have been attributed to atherosclerosis. However, it is well known that the majority of patients with abdominal aortic aneurysms do not have associated significant occlusive disease. Biochemical studies have demonstrated decreased quantities of elastin and collagen in the walls of aneurysmal aortas. It is believed that a family of enzymes known as matrix metalloproteinase (MMP), particularly those that have collagenase and elastase activity, are likely involved in development of arterial aneurysms. The propensity for growth and rupture is based on Laplace's law, $T = PR$, where T represents wall tension (or in other words the propensity to rupture), P is the transmitted pressure, and R is the radius. This explains why patients with hypertension and those with larger aneurysms are at higher risk for aortic rupture.

Prevention

Currently the most effective means to prevent aneurysm rupture is early detection and elective repair. Avoidance of smoking and aggressive control of blood pressure would likely be helpful in preventing aneurysmal development and growth. Patients with known abdominal aortic aneurysms that are relatively small and at low risk for rupture are generally serially followed with imaging studies over time. These patients are advised to avoid straining (e.g., heavy lifting), avoid smoking, and keep their blood pressure well controlled.

Investigation is ongoing in efforts to develop a medication that may be helpful in slowing the growth of abdominal aortic aneurysms. It has been known since 1985 that tetracycline antibiotics have activity against MMPs. There had been several animal studies and at least one small human study suggesting that doxycycline (Vibramycin)[1] may be effective at slowing the growth of abdominal aortic aneurysms. Currently, larger human studies are ongoing. At this point, there are no formal recommendations regarding the use of doxycycline for the purpose of slowing aneurysmal growth.

Clinical Manifestations

Approximately 75% of abdominal aortic aneurysms are asymptomatic and discovered incidentally. Unfortunately, physical examination is an unreliable method for detecting aneurysms or determining aneurysm size. In heavier patients it may be simply impossible to adequately palpate the aorta. The majority of aneurysms are incidental findings identified on imaging studies performed for other reasons. Occasionally, an aneurysm is first detected upon operation for another condition.

Unfortunately, when an aneurysm becomes symptomatic, this is usually a sign of impending rupture. Symptoms related to abdominal aortic aneurysms can include abdominal or back pain. The classic triad of findings in the setting of abdominal aortic aneurysm rupture includes abdominal pain, hypotension, and a pulsatile abdominal mass. This triad, however, occurs in only approximately 20% of the patients. Often a high index of suspicion needs to be maintained.

The episode of hypotension associated with aneurysm rupture may be manifested as an episode of syncope or near-syncope before the patient arrives at the hospital. It is quite possible for the patient to have a contained rupture of the abdominal aorta and appear quite stable with a normal blood pressure in the emergency department. Although uncommon, a primary fistula between the aneurysm and gastrointestinal tract can occur and manifest as gastrointestinal bleeding.

Diagnosis

Several imaging modalities are available that can accurately diagnose and measure abdominal aortic aneurysms. Real-time B-mode ultrasound scanning has the advantage of being almost universally available, relatively inexpensive, and essentially risk free. The major disadvantage, however, is that it is technician dependent. Computed tomography (CT) scans can provide a very accurate representation of the aorta in a very short study time (Figures 1 and 2). The use of iodinated contrast is not necessary to obtain a gross size measurement of the aorta. The contrast, however, helps delineate the flow lumen more clearly, and it is quite valuable in planning repair. Disadvantages include the use of ionizing radiation and the use of iodinated contrast material. MRI is also accurate in determining the size of the aneurysm; however, study times are longer, equipment is less widely available, and the expense is considerable. Angiography, while excellent for evaluating the status of important aortic branches and for evaluating occlusive disease, is not an accurate study for the purpose of determining maximal diameter of the aneurysm. Often aneurysms are filled with laminated thrombus, and the flow

---

[1] Not FDA approved for this indication.

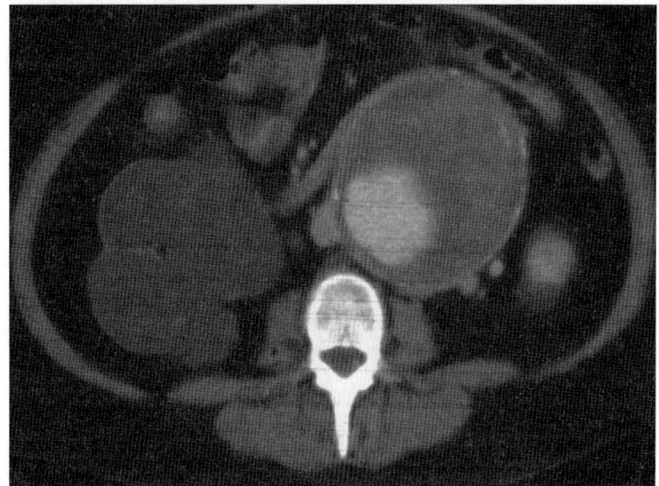

Figure 1 Large abdominal aortic aneurysm. Notice how the majority of this aneurysm is filled with laminated thrombus. The flow lumen is only mildly dilated, and this aneurysm could be missed on angiography alone.

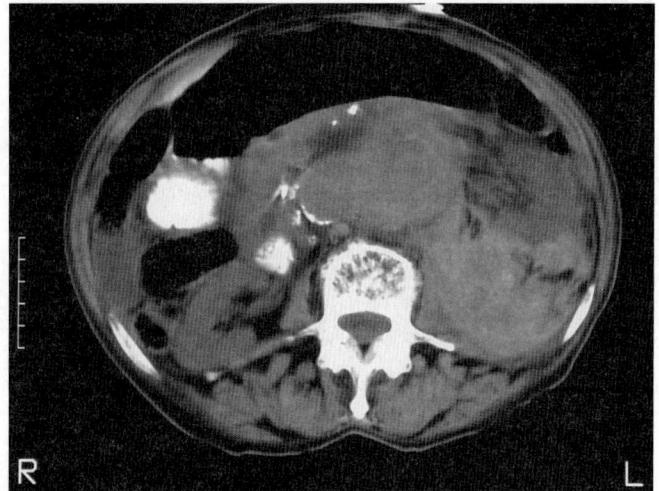

Figure 2 Classic image of a ruptured abdominal aortic aneurysm, which in this case can be seen even without the use of intravascular contrast. Note the lack of symmetry and obliteration of tissue planes in the retroperitoneum on the left.

lumen, which was seen on aortography, is not representative of the true aneurysm size.

Treatment

The decision on when to intervene in an abdominal aortic aneurysm is based on a careful analysis of the patient's risk for rupture versus the risk of operative repair. Historically, open repair can be performed with less than 5% in-hospital mortality. Based on historical studies it was estimated that the risk of rupture for an approximately 5-cm aneurysm was about 1% per year, which increased dramatically to 6.6% for aneurysms between 6 and 7 cm. It has been fairly well established for years that aneurysms larger than 5.5 cm are generally recommended for repair and those less than 4 cm are generally observed over time. There remains a gray area for moderate aneurysms in the 4- to 5.5-cm category.

Two large prospective randomized trials were developed to answer this question. These include the United Kingdom Small Aneurysm Trial and the Department of Veterans Affairs Aneurysm Detection and Management (ADAM) trial. Both these studies randomized patients with moderately sized aneurysms to observation versus open repair. Results of both trials were fairly similar. The rupture rate for aneurysms under observation was

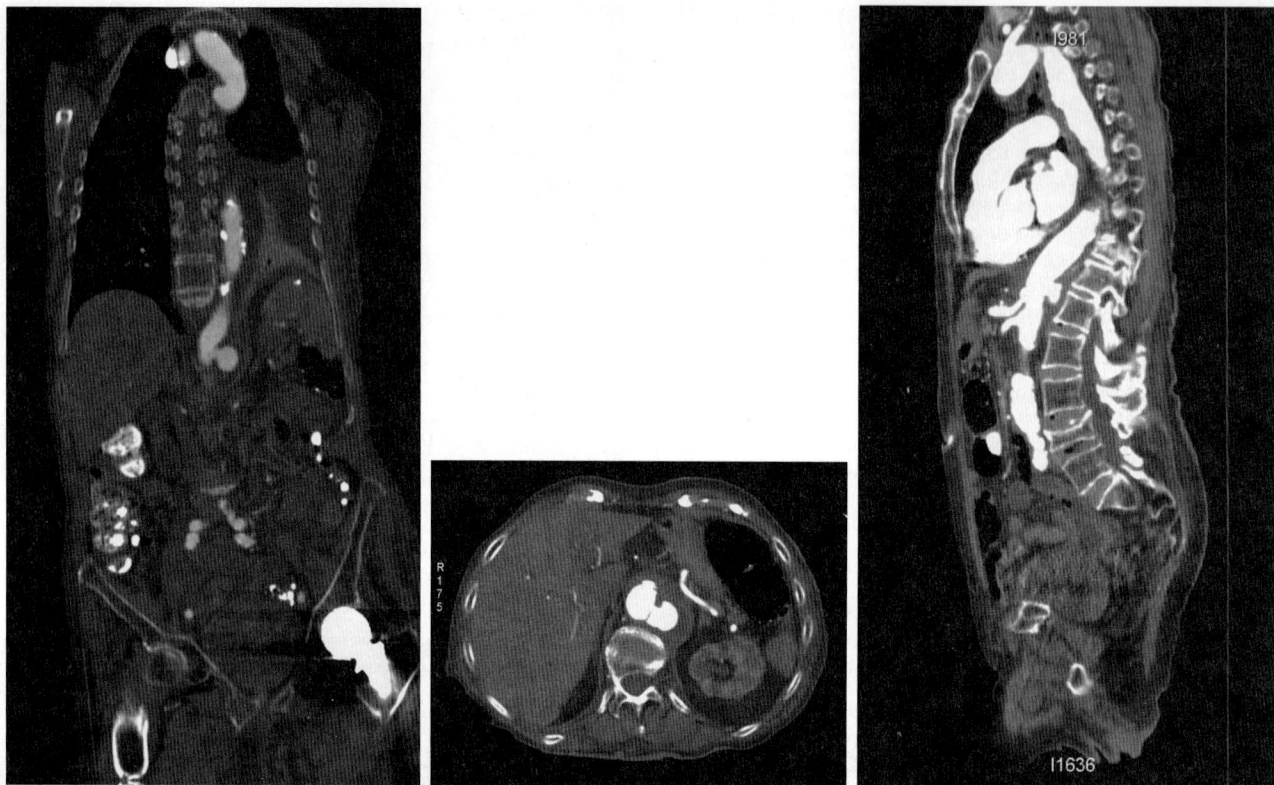

Figure 3 Axial CT slice and reconstructed images of a saccular abdominal aortic aneurysm. This lesion could also be described as a pseudoaneurysm. For these, treatment is recommended because it is thought that the risk of rupture is higher than for a similarly sized fusiform abdominal aortic aneurysm.

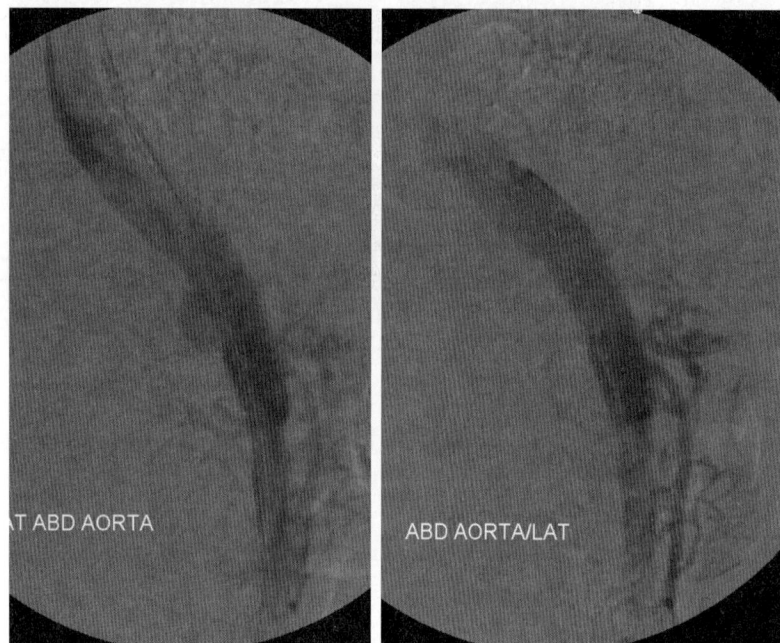

Figure 4 Angiogram of patient in Figure 3, demonstrating aneurysm before and after deployment of an endograft, which successfully excluded the lesion from the circulation.

0.5% to 1% per year, and neither trial showed a difference in long-term survival. Both studies concluded that it was relatively safe to observe patients with aneurysms less than 5.5 cm in diameter, particularly in men who would be compliant with the follow-up regimen. The diameter of the aneurysm, however, should not be the only data point used for a decision on whether to repair.

Women seem to have a higher rupture rate for a particular aneurysm diameter than men, perhaps because they are starting with smaller aortas to begin with. Patients with COPD may be at higher risk for rupture as well. Saccular or eccentric-shaped aneurysms may also have a higher propensity to rupture and should not be subject to diameter recommendations for fusiform aneurysms (Figures 3

and 4). Additionally, rapidly growing aneurysms—growing at a rate faster than approximately 0.5 cm per year—should be considered for repair.

Once it has been determined that repair is indicated, a number of options are available. Traditional open repair involves a relatively large abdominal incision, cross clamping of the aorta, and replacement of the aneurysmal segment with a graft of polyethylene terephthalate (Dacron) or polytetrafluoroethylene (PTFE; Teflon). Often the iliac arteries are involved, and in these cases a bifurcated graft is placed. Open repair is quite durable and very effective at preventing aneurysm-related deaths. Long-term complications are rare, and patients following open repair generally enjoy 95% freedom from issues related to the repair over the course of their lifetime. Disadvantages, however, include the large incision and an approximate 1-week hospital stay. Recovery to a relatively normal level of function occasionally takes months. In the past, many patients were deemed too old or frail to be expected to undergo open surgery.

Endograft repair has revolutionized the practice of vascular surgery. Using small incisions placed at the groin and performing the procedure under fluoroscopic guidance, devices can now be advanced into the aorta from the femoral artery. Using angiography as a guide, the graft typically is deployed below the renal arteries and effectively excludes the aneurysm from the circulation. Advantages include small incisions and very short hospital stays. Patients are typically discharged on the first or second day after aneurysm repair. Recovery to normal activity is also quite rapid, taking approximately 1 to 2 weeks. Use of this modality has allowed treatment of older and frailer patients who previously were denied treatment due to concerns of operative risk.

Endograft repair, however, is clearly not without its disadvantages. Currently, the durability of endograft repair is unknown, and these patients are subject to frequent serial imaging. Also, there is a higher incidence of graft-related complications, which can occur in up to 35% of patients. These include the development of leaks of blood into the aneurysm sac outside the graft device, issues related to graft failure and migration, and graft limb thrombosis. These grafts are also quite expensive.

Two major prospective randomized trials studying traditional open versus endograft repair are often cited. These include the United Kingdom–based EVAR-1 trial (first Endovascular Aneurysm Repair trail) and the Dutch-based DREAM trial (Diabetes REduction Assessment with ramipril and rosiglitazone Medication trial). Both studies randomized patients who were believed to be good risks for open repair to endograft versus traditional open repair. The results of both of these studies were relatively similar in that both studies demonstrated a clear early survival benefit for patients in the endograft group. However, this came at a cost of an increased incidence of graft-related complications in the endograft group and a higher cost for the endograft group. Additionally, at 2 to 4 years, there was no clear difference in long-term survival in either group.

Ultimately, the decision about whether to proceed with open or endograft repair is a decision between surgeon and patient based on the patient's aortic anatomy, overall health, and the patient's and physician's preference. It would appear, however, that older and frail patients with good anatomy should be strongly considered for endograft repair.

Monitoring
Patients with abdominal aortic aneurysms should be evaluated for the presence of femoral and popliteal aneurysms (particularly in men) and for thoracic aortic aneurysms. After open repair, a follow-up CT scan with contrast should be considered approximately 5 years out to evaluate for the integrity of the graft (i.e., pseudoaneurysms), as well as development of new aneurysms. Patients who have undergone endograft repair require more-intensive monitoring. Typical regimens include a contrast-enhanced CT scan approximately 2 weeks after repair, then 6 months after repair, and then based on the perceived stability of the graft, approximately yearly thereafter. Some centers have used duplex ultrasonography for evaluating patients after endograft repair in efforts to reduce the amount of ionizing radiation the patients receive. However, it should be remembered that duplex ultrasound is highly technician dependent, and follow-up of patients with endograft repairs using only duplex ultrasound should be performed in experienced centers.

Thoracic Aortic Aneurysms
Thoracic aortic aneurysms (TAAs) are limited to the chest cavity. Although they are less common than infrarenal abdominal aortic aneurysms, they share similar risk factors. The male-to-female ratio incidence of the TAA is approximately 1:1.

In the past, the threshold for repair was at a diameter greater than 6 cm. This threshold was chosen due to the higher operative

risks associated with repair of the thoracic aorta. Now with the availability of endograft, patients with good anatomy are generally recommended for repair at a diameter similar to those for the infrarenal aorta.

Open repair involves performing a thoracotomy and cross-clamping the aorta. Repair in this location is often performed with the addition of extracorporeal bypass to maintain perfusion to the viscera and spinal cord drain performance of the repair. Although the risk of paraplegia in the treatment of infrarenal aortic is exceedingly low, the risk of paraplegia from a repair of an isolated TAA is approximately 6%. Endograft devices for repair of TAA are now widely available and have reduced the incidence of paraplegia to approximately 3%.

Thoracoabdominal Aortic Aneurysms
By definition, thoracoabdominal aortic aneurysms require entrance to both the thoracic and abdominal cavity to perform repair. These lesions are usually true aneurysms of the aorta and should not be confused with dissection. Repair of thoracoabdominal aortic aneurysms is quite complex and carries risks of death and paraplegia as high as 20% in some settings. These procedures are generally performed at larger institutions with considerable experience with this condition. Unfortunately, endograft devices for the repair of thoracoabdominal aortic aneurysms are limited to a handful of centers in the United States.

Thoracic Aortic Dissection
Thoracic aortic dissection is the most common aortic emergency, even more common than ruptured abdominal aortic aneurysm. This potentially fatal condition is rare in patients younger than 50 years and is approximately two times more common in men than women. Patients at risk include patients with a history of connective tissue disorders and patients with severe, poorly controlled hypertension.

An aortic dissection occurs when there is loss of integrity of the intima and blood dissects into the media. Once in the media, there is a natural plane through which dissection is quite easy.

Although there are various classification systems for aortic dissection, the Stanford classification is perhaps the most widely used and the most useful. In this classification, any dissection that involves the ascending aorta, whether it involves the ascending aorta alone or both the ascending and descending thoracoabdominal aorta, are classified as type A. Dissections that do not involve the ascending aorta are classified as type B. This classification is useful because type A dissections require urgent surgery. Type B dissections are typically managed medically unless they are associated with complications such as unremitting pain, aneurysmal expansion, and end-organ ischemia. By convention, aortic dissections that are evaluated within 14 days after the onset of symptoms are considered acute, and those evaluated beyond 14 days are considered chronic.

Helical CAT scanners with the use of contrast are excellent at defining the location and extent of aortic dissection. However, being alert to the potential for this diagnosis requires a high index of suspicion. Aortic dissection can mimic a variety of common conditions based on the extent of the dissection and the aortic branches involved (Table 1). Uncomplicated type B dissections are typically managed medically. This is usually performed in an intensive care setting with the use of intravenous medications to control contractility and, if necessary, hypertension.

In the past, due to the friability of dissected aortic tissue, the results of operative repair for type B dissections have been particularly poor. Currently, endograft repair with the purpose of excluding the entry point of dissection and reestablishing flow to the true lumen is gaining popularity in the treatment of complex dissection. This at times may be supplemented by stenting of affected aortic side branches and fenestration to establish a connection between the true and false lumen to restore perfusion to certain organs. Once the acute phase has passed and medically treated patients are under good hypertensive control, these patients are then converted to an oral medication regimen and transferred out of the intensive care setting. Patients need to be followed up with serial CT

TABLE 1 Dissection: The Great Mimic

TERRITORY INVOLVED OR AFFECTED BY DISSECTION	MIMICS
Rupture into pericardial sac	Cardiac tamponade
Dissection through aortic valve	Acute aortic insufficiency
Dissection occluding coronary arteries	Myocardial infarction
Involvement of cerebral vessels	Stroke
Involvement of subclavian arteries	Upper extremity ischemia (cold arm)
Dissection running down descending thoracic aorta	Severe back pain and paralysis
Mesenteric artery obstruction	Mesenteric ischemia
Renal artery obstruction	Oliguria and acute renal failure
Iliac artery occlusion	Lower extremity ischemia (cold leg)

imaging after discharge to evaluate for aneurysmal degeneration of the false lumen. This evaluation should occur every 6 months until the patient is stable and then yearly thereafter.

In cases where the total aortic diameter grows to greater than 6 cm, repair for the purpose of preventing rupture is indicated, although this is often technically more complicated than treating a fusiform aneurysm in the absence of a previous dissection. Patients should strictly adhere to their blood pressure medication regimen for life.

References

Blankensteijn JD, de Jong SE, Prinssen M, et al: Two-year outcomes after conventional or endovascular repair of abdominal aortic aneurysms, *N Engl J Med* 352(23):2398–2405, 2005.
Crawford ES, Crawford JL, Safi HJ, et al: Thoracoabdominal aortic aneurysms: Preoperative and intraoperative factors determining immediate and long-term results of operations in 605 patients, *J Vasc Surg* 3(3):389–404, 1986.
Daily PO, Trueblood HW, Stinson EB, et al: Management of acute aortic dissections, *Ann Thorac Surg* 10(3):237–247, 1970.
EVAR Trial Participants: Endovascular aneurysm repair versus open repair in patients with abdominal aortic aneurysm (EVAR trial 1): Randomised controlled trial, *Lancet* 365(9478):2179–2186, 2005.
EVAR Trial Participants: Endovascular aneurysm repair and outcome in patients unfit for open repair of abdominal aortic aneurysm (EVAR trial 2): Randomised controlled trial, *Lancet* 365(9478):2187–2192, 2005.
Lederle FA, Wilson SE, Johnson GR, et al: Immediate repair compared with surveillance of small abdominal aortic aneurysms, *N Engl J Med* 346(19):1437–1444, 2002.
Lee ES, Pickett E, Hedayati N, et al: Implementation of an aortic screening program in clinical practice: Implications for the Screen For Abdominal Aortic Aneurysms Very Efficiently (SAAAVE) Act, *J Vasc Surg* 49(5):1107–1111, 2009.
Nevitt MP, Ballard DJ, Hallett Jr: Prognosis of abdominal aortic aneurysms. A population-based study, *N Engl J Med* 321(15):1009–1014, 1989.
Nienaber CA, Rousseau H, Eggebrecht H, et al: Randomized comparison of strategies for type B aortic dissection: The INvestigation of STEnt Grafts in Aortic Dissection (INSTEAD) trial, *Circulation* 120(25):2519–2528, 2009.
Rentschler M, Baxter BT: Pharmacological approaches to prevent abdominal aortic aneurysm enlargement and rupture, *Ann N Y Acad Sci* 1085:39–46, 2006.

ATRIAL FIBRILLATION

Method of
Lin Yee Chen, MBBS, MS; and Samuel Dudley, MD, PhD

CURRENT DIAGNOSIS

- History taking and physical examination for atrial fibrillation) should focus on determining symptom severity (to decide on treatment strategy), risk of thromboembolic stroke, and associated cardiovascular risk factors.

- Symptoms include palpitations, chest discomfort, shortness of breath, and reduced exercise capacity. Some patients have no symptoms.
- Investigations include a 12-lead electrocardiogram for confirmation; transthoracic echocardiogram to evaluate left atrial size and left ventricular ejection fraction and rule out valvular abnormalities; and blood tests for thyroid, renal, and hepatic function.

CURRENT THERAPY

- Rate control: Achieve average ventricular rate of less than 110 beats/min by using atrioventricular node (AVN) blockers or catheter ablation of AVN.
- Rhythm control: Prevent atrial fibrillation (AF) recurrence by using antiarrhythmic drugs or catheter ablation (pulmonary vein isolation).
- Stroke prophylaxis: Achieve risk stratification and stroke prevention by oral anticoagulation or left atrial appendage closure
- Risk-factor management or lifestyle modification: Prevent AF by weight management, intensive blood pressure reduction, and exercise training

Epidemiology

Atrial fibrillation (AF) is the most common sustained arrhythmia in the adult general population. Globally, the estimated number of individuals with AF in 2020 was 50 million. Between 1990 and 2010, the global estimated age-adjusted prevalence rate of AF increased from 569.5 to 596.2 per 100,000 men and from 359.9 to 373.1 per 100,000 women. This increase in prevalence was accompanied by a substantial increase in health burden: disability-adjusted life-years increased by 18.8% in men and 18.9% in women from 1990 to 2010. Finally, the lifetime risk for development of AF in adults at age 40 is 1 in 4.

Risk Factors and Pathophysiology

Table 1 shows the known risk factors of AF; many of these are also risk factors for atherosclerotic disease. Traditional cardiovascular risk factors such as diabetes, hypertension, and obesity can lead to AF by the following pathway: cardiovascular risk factors → left ventricular diastolic dysfunction → structural and functional alterations in the atria (enlargement, impaired function, fibrosis, etc.) → AF. The aforementioned pathway creates the substrate for AF; premature atrial contractions and supraventricular ectopic beats are the trigger for AF. Other pathophysiologic pathways include inflammation and increased oxidative stress, leading to electrical remodeling and, consequently, AF.

Clinical Manifestations

Common symptoms of AF include palpitations, irregular heartbeat sensation, lightheadedness, dyspnea, chest discomfort, and fatigue. Some patients may have no symptoms at rest but report poor stamina or easy fatigability with physical activity. Other patients, particularly among the elderly, may be asymptomatic.

Diagnosis

The absence of distinct P waves with irregularly irregular RR interval on the electrocardiogram (ECG) are the sine qua non for diagnosing AF. Rhythm documentation can be obtained via the standard 12-lead ECG, Holter monitors that can record up to 48 hours, leadless patch monitors that can record up to 2 weeks, or implantable loop recorders. Newer wearable technologies that can diagnose AF include smartwatches and smartphones with specialized apps.

Paroxysmal AF is defined as AF that terminates spontaneously typically in less than 24 hours and in all cases in less than 7 days.

TABLE 1	Risk Factors of Atrial Fibrillation
Cardiovascular risk factors
Older age
Male sex
Diabetes mellitus
Overweight and obesity
Hypertension
Chronic kidney disease
Structural heart disease
Valvular heart disease
Cardiomyopathy (dilated, restrictive, and hypertrophic)
Congenital heart disease
Coronary heart disease
Left ventricular diastolic dysfunction
Left atrial enlargement
Family history
Genetics (polygenic and monogenic inheritance)
Inflammation
Low serum magnesium
Heavy alcohol consumption
Poor cardiorespiratory fitness
Low physical activity
Premature atrial contractions or supraventricular ectopy

AF that continues for more than 7 days and requires cardioversion for conversion to sinus rhythm is termed persistent AF. Longstanding persistent AF is AF that has been continuous for more than 1 year. Permanent AF exists when both patient and physician have decided not to pursue further attempts to maintain sinus rhythm. Apart from the previous nomenclature, it is also important to consider AF burden, which encompasses both frequency and duration and refers to the amount of AF that an individual has.

Differential Diagnosis
These include other supraventricular arrhythmias such as atrial tachycardia, atrial flutter, long runs of premature atrial contractions, and multifocal atrial tachycardia.

Treatment
Rate Control
The goal of rate control is to prevent excessive ventricular rate response. This is a reasonable treatment strategy given data from randomized controlled trials (RCTs) that did not show any difference in cardiovascular outcomes between rate-control and rhythm-control strategy.

The Atrial Fibrillation Follow-up Investigation of Rhythm Management (AFFIRM) trial found no difference in mortality or stroke rates between patients assigned to rhythm-control and ventricular rate-control strategies. Similarly, the Rate Control versus Electrical Cardioversion for Persistent Atrial Fibrillation (RACE) trial found that rate control was not inferior to rhythm control for prevention of death.

The RACE II study showed that lenient ventricular rate control targeting a heart rate of lower than 110 beats/min was not inferior to stricter rate control of less than 80 beats/min. Lenient rate control is more convenient and requires fewer outpatient visits and fewer medications.

Other than pharmacologic agents (Table 2), catheter ablation of the atrioventricular node (AVN) is effective in controlling ventricular rate in patients with AF. AVN ablation is indicated if patients fail to achieve adequate ventricular rate control despite maximum doses of AVN blockers.

Rhythm Control
Although AF is associated with an increased risk of stroke and mortality, current evidence indicates that there is no difference in the rates of these cardiovascular outcomes between rhythm- and rate-control strategies. In the Catheter Ablation vs Antiarrhythmic Drug Therapy for Atrial Fibrillation (CABANA) trial, based on intention-to-treat analysis, there was no significant difference between catheter ablation and drug therapy with respect to a primary composite outcome of death, disabling stroke, serious bleeding, or cardiac arrest. However, in selected younger patients with paroxysmal AF, rhythm control may be a better approach. Additionally, catheter ablation to maintain sinus rhythm in selected patients with symptomatic AF and heart failure with reduced left ventricular ejection fraction may reduce mortality rate and hospitalization for heart failure. Furthermore, new evidence has emerged to indicate that early initiation of rhythm control is associated with lower risk of adverse cardiovascular outcomes. Finally, in patients who continue to have symptoms despite an adequately controlled ventricular rate, rhythm control is an appropriate next step.

Rhythm control can be achieved by the use of antiarrhythmic drugs (Table 3) or catheter ablation. In patients with paroxysmal and persistent AF who have failed at least one antiarrhythmic drug, catheter ablation by pulmonary vein isolation is indicated to maintain sinus rhythm. In persistent AF, the Substrate and Trigger Ablation for Reduction of Atrial Fibrillation Trial Part II (STAR AF II) showed that performing additional linear ablation or ablation targeting complex fractionated electrograms does not improve rhythm control compared with pulmonary vein isolation alone. The optimal approach to ablate persistent AF remains to be defined.

Stroke Prophylaxis
Stroke prevention is a two-stage process: determination of thromboembolic stroke risk and selection of prevention strategy. The most commonly used risk-stratification scheme for stroke prevention is the CHA_2DS_2-VASc score (https://www.mdcalc.com/cha2ds2-vasc-score-atrial-fibrillation-stroke-risk) (Table 4). Oral anticoagulation is recommended for CHA_2DS_2-VASc score of 2 or greater in men or 3 or greater in women. Aspirin should not be used for stroke prevention in AF.[1]

Oral Anticoagulants
These include vitamin K antagonists (warfarin [Coumadin]) and non–vitamin K oral anticoagulants or novel or direct oral anticoagulants (DOAC) (Table 5). Compared with warfarin, DOACs are as effective in preventing thromboembolic stroke in AF. The risk of intracranial hemorrhage from the use of DOACs is 33% to 60% less than that with warfarin. Other advantages of DOACs over warfarin include the facts that there are fewer interactions with food and there is no need for monitoring the international normalized ratio.

Left Atrial Appendage Closure
The Watchman device is approved by the US Food and Drug Administration (FDA) for stroke prevention in patients with AF with a contraindication to long-term oral anticoagulation and who are at risk of thromboembolic stroke. Patients must be able to take oral anticoagulants for at least 6 weeks after implantation of the device.

Risk Factor Management and Lifestyle Modification
Recent compelling evidence underscores the importance of a fourth pillar of AF management: risk-factor and lifestyle modifications.

---

[1] Not FDA approved for this indication.

TABLE 2 Pharmacologic Agents for Rate Control

DRUG	INTRAVENOUS ADMINISTRATION	USUAL ORAL MAINTENANCE DOSE	MAJOR SIDE EFFECTS
β Blockers			
Metoprolol (Lopressor)[1]	2.5–5 mg IV bolus; up to 3 doses	100–200 mg (long acting) daily	Bradycardia, hypotension, heart block, asthma, heart failure
Atenolol (Tenormin)[1]	N/A	25–100 mg qd	
Esmolol (Brevibloc)	50–200 µg/kg/min IV	N/A	
Propranolol (Inderal)	1–3 mg IV	10–40 mg tid	
Carvedilol (Coreg)[1]	N/A	3.125–25 mg bid	
Nondihydropyridine Calcium Channel Antagonists			
Verapamil (Calan)	5–10 mg bolus	80 mg tid or up to 360 mg (long acting) daily	Hypotension, heart block, heart failure
Diltiazem (Cardizem)	0.25–0.35 mg/kg	60 mg tid or up to 360 mg (long acting) daily	
Digitalis Glycosides			
Digoxin (Lanoxin)	0.25–0.5 mg	0.125–0.25 mg qd	Digitalis toxicity, bradycardia, heart block

[1]Not FDA approved for this indication.
bid, Twice daily; *IV,* intravenous; *N/A,* not available; *qd,* daily; *tid,* three times daily.

TABLE 3 Pharmacologic Agents for Rhythm Control

DRUG	USUAL ORAL MAINTENANCE DOSE	MAJOR SIDE EFFECTS
Flecainide (Tambocor)	50–200 mg bid	Hypotension, atrial flutter with high ventricular rate
Propafenone (Rythmol)	150–300 mg tid	
Propafenone Extended Release (Rythmol SR)	225–425 mg bid	
Sotalol (Betapace)	80–160 mg bid	Bradycardia, hypotension, QT prolongation, torsades de pointes
Dofetilide (Tikosyn)	125–500 µg bid	QT prolongation, torsades de pointes
Amiodarone (Pacerone)[1]	100–200 mg qd	Hypotension, bradycardia, QT prolongation
Dronedarone (Multaq)	400 mg bid	QT prolongation

[1]Not FDA approved for atrial fibrillation.
bid, Twice daily; *qd,* daily; *tid,* three times daily.

TABLE 4 CHA₂DS₂-VASc Score

RISK FACTOR	SCORE
Congestive heart failure, left ventricular dysfunction	1
Hypertension	1
Age ≥75 years	2
Diabetes mellitus	1
Stroke, transient ischemic attack, or thromboembolism	2
Vascular disease (myocardial infarction, peripheral arterial disease, complex aortic plaque)	1
Age 65–74 years	1
Sex category: female	1

TABLE 5 Non–Vitamin K Oral Anticoagulants

DRUG	USUAL DOSE	COMMENTS
Direct Thrombin Inhibitor		
Dabigatran (Pradaxa)	150 mg bid	Reversal agent (Idarucizumab [Praxbind]) FDA approved; interacts with P-glycoprotein inhibitors and inducers
Factor Xa Inhibitor		
Apixaban (Eliquis)	5 mg bid	Interacts with P-glycoprotein and CYP3A4 inhibitors and inducers
Edoxaban (Savaysa)	60 mg qd	Avoid if CrCl >95 mL/min due to increased rate of stroke
Rivaroxaban (Xarelto)	20 mg qd	Interacts with P-glycoprotein and CYP3A4 inhibitors and inducers; should be taken with evening meal

bid, Twice daily; *CrCl,* creatinine clearance; *FDA,* US Food and Drug Administration; *qd,* daily; *tid,* three times daily.

Weight Loss

An RCT has shown that weight reduction with intensive risk-factor management results in a reduction of AF symptom burden and severity and reversal of cardiac remodeling.

Intensive Blood Pressure Lowering

Blood pressure reduction targeting a systolic blood pressure of 120 mm Hg is associated with lower incidence of AF compared with 140 mm Hg.

Exercise Training

A small RCT showed that, compared with nonexercise control patients, high-intensity interval training reduced AF burden and improved atrial contractile function. This time-efficient form of exercise can potentially overcome the lack-of-time problem—an oft-quoted reason for poor compliance with regular aerobic exercise.

Complications

Other than thromboembolic stroke, heart failure, and death, AF is also associated with greater cognitive decline and risk of dementia. More recently, AF has been reported to be associated with a higher risk of sudden cardiac death in the general population. Apart from stroke prevention and rate and rhythm control to prevent heart failure, we currently lack effective prevention strategies for dementia and sudden cardiac death.

Special Considerations

Subclinical Atrial Fibrillation

Subclinical AF is commonly detected from interrogation of cardiac implantable electronic devices. For patients with device-detected atrial high-rate episodes lasting 24 hours or longer and with a CHA_2DS_2-VASc score of 2 or greater or equivalent stroke risk, it is reasonable to initiate oral anticoagulation within a shared-decision making framework.

References

Abed HS, Wittert GA, Leong DP, et al: Effect of weight reduction and cardiometabolic risk factor management on symptom burden and severity in patients with atrial fibrillation a randomized clinical trial, *JAMA* 310:2050–2060, 2013.

Chen LY, Bigger JT, Hickey KT, et al: Effect of intensive blood pressure lowering on incident atrial fibrillation and p-wave indices in the ACCORD Blood Pressure Trial, *Am J Hypertens* 29:1276–1282, 2016.

Chen LY, Norby FL, Gottesman RF, et al: Association of atrial fibrillation with cognitive decline and dementia over 20 years: the ARIC-NCS (Atherosclerosis Risk in Communities Neurocognitive Study), *J Am Heart Assoc* 7(6).

Chen LY, Sotoodehnia N, Bůžková P, et al: Atrial fibrillation and the risk of sudden cardiac death: the Atherosclerosis Risk in Communities (ARIC) Study and Cardiovascular Health Study (CHS), *JAMA Intern Med* 173:29–35, 2013.

Chugh SS, Havmoeller R, Narayanan K, et al: Worldwide epidemiology of atrial fibrillation: a Global Burden of Disease 2010 Study, *Circulation* 129:837–847, 2014.

January CT, Wann LS, Calkins H, et al: 2019 AHA/ACC/HRS focused update of the 2014 AHA/ACC/HRS guideline for the management of patients with atrial fibrillation: a report of the American College of Cardiology/American Heart Association Task Force on Clinical Practice Guidelines and the Heart Rhythm Society, *Circulation* 140(2):e125–e151, 2019.

Joglar JA, Chung MK, Armbruster AL, et al: 2023 ACC/AHA/ACCP/HRS guideline for the diagnosis and management of atrial fibrillation: a report of the American College of Cardiology/American Heart Association Joint Committee on Clinical Practice Guidelines, *Circulation* 149:e1–e156, 2024.

Lloyd-Jones DM, Wang TJ, Leip EP, et al: Lifetime risk for development of atrial fibrillation—The Framingham Heart Study, *Circulation* 110:1042–1046, 2004.

Malmo V, Nes BM, Amundsen BH, et al: Aerobic interval training reduces the burden of atrial fibrillation in the short term a randomized trial, *Circulation* 133:466–473, 2016.

Marrouche NF, Brachmann J, Andresen D, et al: Catheter ablation for atrial fibrillation with heart failure, *N Engl J Med* 378:417–427, 2018.

Okin PM, Hille DA, Larstorp ACK, et al: Effect of lower on-treatment systolic blood pressure on the risk of atrial fibrillation in hypertensive patients, *Hypertension* 66:368–373, 2015.

Packer DL, Mark DB, Robb RA, et al: Effect of catheter ablation vs antiarrhythmic drug therapy on mortality, stroke, bleeding, and cardiac arrest among patients with atrial fibrillation: the cabana randomized clinical trial, *JAMA* 321:1261–1274, 2019.

Van Gelder IC, Groenveld HF, Crijns HJGM, et al: Lenient versus strict rate control in patients with atrial fibrillation, *N Engl J Med* 362:1363–1373, 2010.

Van Gelder IC, Hagens VE, Bosker HA, et al: A comparison of rate control and rhythm control in patients with recurrent persistent atrial fibrillation, *N Engl J Med* 347:1834–1840, 2002.

Verma A, Jiang CY, Betts TR, et al: Approaches to catheter ablation for persistent atrial fibrillation, *N Engl J Med* 372:1812–1822, 2015.

Wyse DG, Waldo AL, DiMarco JP, et al: A comparison of rate control and rhythm control in patients with atrial fibrillation, *N Engl J Med* 347:1825–1833, 2002.

CONGENITAL HEART DISEASE

Method of
Richard A. Lange, MD, MBA; and Joaquin E. Cigarroa, MD

CURRENT DIAGNOSIS

- Examine blood pressures in arms and legs, pulse oximetry, mucous membranes and nail beds, respiratory rate, and peripheral pulses.
- In addition to listening over the precordium for heart sounds and murmurs, palpate for thrills and evidence of right or left chamber enlargement.
- Ancillary testing should include chest radiography, electrocardiography, and echocardiography.
- Consult a cardiologist if the physical examination or ancillary tests suggest congenital heart disease.

CURRENT THERAPY

- All congenital heart disease patients should have long-term follow-up for possible complications.
- Endocarditis prophylaxis is recommended for subjects with:
  - Unrepaired cyanotic congenital heart disease
  - Recently repaired congenital heart disease (<6 months after surgical or percutaneous repair)
  - Repaired congenital heart disease with residual defects
- Closure of defects with large left-to-right shunts (i.e., atrial septal defect, ventricular septal defect, atrioventricular canal, or patent ductus arteriosus) is recommended unless pulmonary vascular obstructive disease is far advanced.
- Patients with bicuspid aortic valves should be monitored for aortic root dilation.
- Pregnancy should be avoided in women with cyanotic congenital heart disease because of high maternal and fetal morbidity and mortality rates.

Congenital heart disease affects 0.4% to 0.9% of live births. Nowadays, most survive to adulthood because of improved diagnosis and treatment. Congenital cardiac defects can be categorized according to the presence or absence of cyanosis (due to right-to-left shunting) and the amount of pulmonary blood flow (Box 1).

Acyanotic Conditions

Atrial Septal Defect

Atrial septal defect (ASD) occurs in female patients two to three times as often as in male patients. Although most result from spontaneous genetic mutations, some are inherited.

The physiological consequences of ASD result from the shunting of blood from one atrium to the other; the direction and magnitude of shunting are determined by the size of the defect and the relative compliances of the ventricles. A small defect (<0.5 cm in diameter) is associated with a small shunt and no hemodynamic sequelae, whereas a sizable defect (>2 cm in diameter) usually is associated with a large shunt and substantial hemodynamic consequences. In most patients with ASD, the right ventricle is more compliant than the left; as a result, left atrial blood is shunted to the right atrium, causing increased pulmonary blood flow and dilation of the atria, right ventricle, and pulmonary arteries (Figure 1). Eventually, if the right ventricle fails or its compliance declines, the magnitude of left-to-right shunting diminishes.

In a patient with a large ASD, a right ventricular or pulmonary arterial impulse may be palpable, and wide, fixed splitting of the second heart sound is present. A systolic ejection murmur, audible in the second left intercostal space, is caused by increased

BOX 1 Categorization of Congenital Heart Disease

Acyanotic Cardiac Defects
Increased pulmonary blood flow
• Atrial septal defect
• Ventricular septal defect
• Atrioventricular canal defect
• Patent ductus arteriosus
Normal pulmonary blood flow
• Aortic stenosis
• Pulmonic stenosis
• Aortic coarctation

Cyanotic Cardiac Defects
Normal pulmonary blood flow
• Ebstein's anomaly
Decreased pulmonary blood flow
• Tetralogy of Fallot
• Eisenmenger syndrome

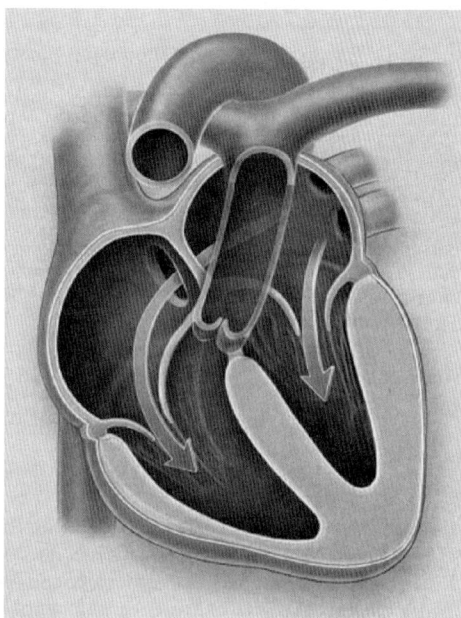

Figure 2 Ventricular septal defect. When the left ventricle contracts, it ejects some blood into the aorta and some across the ventricular septal defect into the right ventricle and pulmonary artery *(arrow)*, resulting in left-to-right shunting. (Reprinted with permission from Brickner ME, Hillis LD, Lange RA: Congenital heart disease in adults. First of two parts. N Engl J Med 2000;342:256–263.)

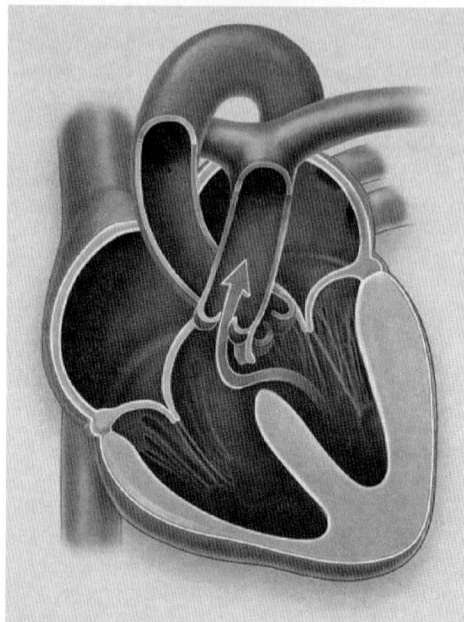

Figure 1 Atrial septal defect. Blood from the pulmonary veins enters the left atrium, after which some of it crosses the atrial septal defect into the right atrium and ventricle *(longer arrow)*. Thus left-to-right shunting occurs. (Reprinted with permission from Brickner ME, Hillis LD, Lange RA: Congenital heart disease in adults. First of two parts. N Engl J Med 2000;342:256–263.)

blood flow across the pulmonic valve; flow across the ASD itself does not produce a murmur.

Because ASDs initially produce no symptoms or striking physical examination findings, they are often undetected for years. Small defects with minimal left-to-right shunting cause no symptoms or hemodynamic abnormalities, so they do not require closure. Even patients with moderate or large ASDs (characterized by a ratio of pulmonary to systemic blood flow of 1.5 or more) often have no symptoms until the third or fourth decade of life. Over the years, the increased blood volume flowing through the right heart chambers usually causes right ventricular dilation and failure. Obstructive pulmonary vascular disease (Eisenmenger syndrome) occurs uncommonly in adults with ASD.

The symptomatic patient with an ASD typically reports fatigue or dyspnea on exertion. Alternatively, the development of supraventricular tachyarrhythmias, right heart failure, paradoxical embolism, or recurrent pulmonary infections might prompt the

patient to seek medical attention. Although an occasional patient with an unrepaired ASD survives to an advanced age, those with sizable shunts often die of right ventricular failure or arrhythmias in their 30s or 40s.

Echocardiography can reveal atrial and right ventricular dilation and identify the ASD's location. The sensitivity of echocardiography may be enhanced by injecting microbubbles in solution into a peripheral vein, after which the movement of some of them across the defect into the left atrium can be visualized.

An ASD with a pulmonary-to-systemic flow ratio of 1.5 or more should be closed (surgically or percutaneously) to prevent worsening right ventricular dysfunction. Prophylaxis against infective endocarditis is not recommended for patients with ASD (repaired or unrepaired) unless a concomitant valvular abnormality is present.

Ventricular Septal Defect

Ventricular septal defect (VSD) is the most common congenital cardiac abnormality, with similar incidence in boys and girls. Approximately 25% to 40% of them close spontaneously by 2 years of age.

The physiological consequences of a VSD are determined by the size of the defect and the relative resistances in the systemic and pulmonary vascular beds. A small defect causes little or no functional disturbance, because pulmonary blood flow is only minimally increased. In contrast, a large defect causes substantial left-to-right shunting, because systemic vascular resistance exceeds pulmonary vascular resistance (Figure 2). Over time, however, the pulmonary vascular resistance usually increases, and the magnitude of left-to-right shunting declines. Eventually, the pulmonary vascular resistance equals or exceeds the systemic resistance; the shunting of blood from left to right ceases; and right-to-left shunting begins (e.g., Eisenmenger physiology).

A small, muscular VSD can produce a high-frequency systolic ejection murmur that terminates before the end of systole (when the defect is occluded by contracting heart muscle). With a moderate or large VSD and substantial left-to-right shunting, a holosystolic murmur, loudest at the left sternal border, is audible and is usually accompanied by a palpable thrill. If pulmonary hypertension develops, the holosystolic murmur and thrill diminish in magnitude and eventually disappear as flow through the defect decreases.

Echocardiography is usually performed to confirm the presence and location of the VSD and to delineate the magnitude and direction of shunting. With catheterization, one can determine the magnitude of shunting and the pulmonary vascular resistance.

The natural history of VSD depends on the size of the defect and the pulmonary vascular resistance. Adults with small defects and normal pulmonary arterial pressure are generally asymptomatic, and pulmonary vascular disease is unlikely to develop. In contrast, patients with large defects who survive to adulthood usually have left ventricular failure or pulmonary hypertension (or both) with associated right ventricular failure.

Closure of VSDs (surgically or percutaneously) is recommended if the pulmonary vascular obstructive disease is not severe. Prophylaxis against infective endocarditis is recommended for patients with unrepaired VSD and those with a residual shunt despite surgical or percutaneous closure.

Atrioventricular Canal Defect

The endocardial cushions normally fuse to form the tricuspid and mitral valves, as well as the atrial and ventricular septa. Atrioventricular (AV) canal defects are caused by incomplete fusion of the endocardial cushions during embryonic development. They are the most common congenital cardiac abnormality in patients with Down syndrome. Such cushion defects include a spectrum of abnormalities, ranging from ASD with a cleft anterior mitral valve leaflet to a common AV canal defect in which a single AV valve in association with a large ASD and VSD is present.

A common AV canal defect permits substantial left-to-right shunting at both the atrial and ventricular levels, which leads to excessive pulmonary blood flow and resultant pulmonary congestion within months of birth. Eventually, the excessive pulmonary blood flow leads to irreversible pulmonary vascular obstruction (e.g., Eisenmenger physiology).

In the patient with an AV canal defect and left-to-right intracardiac shunting, the physical examination reveals a loud holosystolic murmur audible throughout the precordium. As pulmonary vascular resistance increases, the holosystolic murmur diminishes in intensity and duration, eventually disappearing as flow through the defect decreases.

AV canal defects require surgical repair if the magnitude of pulmonary vascular obstructive disease is not prohibitive. Although such patients might initially benefit from medical treatment with diuretics and afterload reduction, the onset of heart failure symptoms is generally the point at which surgery is considered. Prophylaxis against infective endocarditis is recommended for patients with repaired and unrepaired AV canal defects.

Patent Ductus Arteriosus

The ductus arteriosus connects the descending aorta (just distal to the left subclavian artery) and the left pulmonary artery. In the fetus, it permits pulmonary arterial blood to bypass the unexpanded lungs and to enter the descending aorta for oxygenation in the placenta. Although it normally closes spontaneously soon after birth, it fails to do so in some infants, so that continuous flow from the aorta to the pulmonary artery (i.e., left-to-right shunting) occurs (Figure 3). The incidence of patent ductus arteriosus (PDA) is increased in pregnancies complicated by persistent perinatal hypoxemia or maternal rubella infection as well as among infants born prematurely or at high altitude.

A patient with PDA and a moderate or large shunt has bounding peripheral arterial pulses and a widened pulse pressure. A continuous "machinery" murmur, audible in the second left intercostal space, begins shortly after the first heart sound, peaks in intensity at or immediately after the second heart sound (thereby obscuring it), and diminishes in intensity during diastole. If pulmonary vascular obstruction and hypertension develop, the murmur decreases in duration and intensity and eventually disappears.

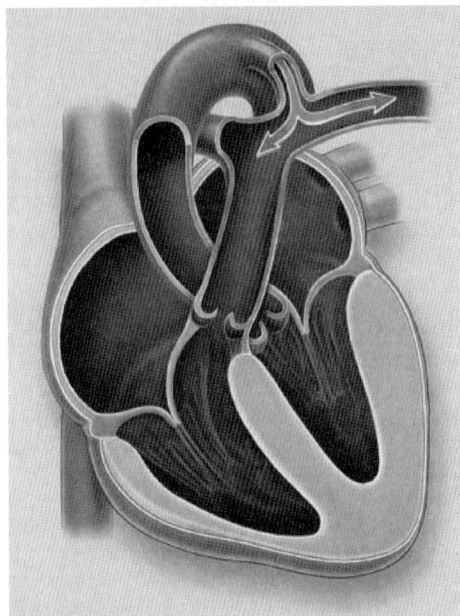

Figure 3 Patent ductus arteriosus. Some of the blood from the aorta crosses the ductus arteriosus into the pulmonary artery *(arrows)*, with resultant left-to-right shunting. (Reprinted with permission from Brickner ME, Hillis LD, Lange RA: Congenital heart disease in adults. First of two parts. N Engl J Med 2000;342:256–263.)

With echocardiography, the PDA can usually be visualized, and Doppler studies demonstrate continuous flow in the pulmonary trunk. Catheterization and angiography allow one to quantify the magnitude of shunting and the pulmonary vascular resistance and to visualize the PDA.

The subject with a small PDA has no symptoms attributable to it and a normal life expectancy. However, it is associated with an elevated risk of infective endarteritis. A PDA of moderate size might cause no symptoms during infancy; during childhood or adulthood, fatigue, dyspnea, or palpitations can appear. Additionally, the PDA can become aneurysmal and calcified, with subsequent rupture. Larger shunts can precipitate left ventricular failure. Eventually, pulmonary vascular obstruction can develop; when the pulmonary vascular resistance equals or exceeds the systemic vascular resistance, the direction of shunting reverses.

One third of patients with an unrepaired moderate or large PDA die of heart failure, pulmonary hypertension, or endarteritis by 40 years of age, and two thirds die by 60 years of age. Because of the risk of endarteritis associated with unrepaired PDA (about 0.45% annually after the second decade of life) and the safety of surgical ligation (generally accomplished without cardiopulmonary bypass) or percutaneous closure, even a small PDA should be ligated surgically or occluded percutaneously. Once severe pulmonary vascular obstructive disease develops, ligation or closure is contraindicated.

Aortic Stenosis

A bicuspid aortic valve is found in 2% to 3% of the population and is four times more common in males than in females. The bicuspid valve has a single fused commissure and an eccentrically oriented orifice. Although the deformed valve is not typically stenotic at birth, it is subjected to abnormal hemodynamic stress, which can lead to leaflet thickening and calcification. In many patients, an abnormality of the ascending aortic media is present, predisposing the patient to aortic root dilation. Twenty percent of patients with a bicuspid aortic valve have an associated cardiovascular abnormality, such as PDA or aortic coarctation.

In patients with severe aortic stenosis (AS), the carotid upstroke is usually delayed and diminished. The aortic component of the second heart sound is diminished or absent. A systolic crescendo–decrescendo murmur is audible over the aortic area and often radiates to the neck. As the magnitude of AS worsens, the murmur peaks progressively later in systole.

In most patients, echocardiography with Doppler flow permits an assessment of the severity of AS and of left ventricular systolic function. Cardiac catheterization is performed to assess the severity of AS and to determine if concomitant coronary artery disease is present.

The symptoms of AS are angina pectoris, syncope or near syncope, and those of heart failure (dyspnea). Asymptomatic adults with AS have a normal life expectancy. Once symptoms appear, survival is limited. The median survival is 5 years once angina develops, 3 years once syncope occurs, and 2 years once symptoms of heart failure appear. Therefore patients with symptomatic AS should undergo surgical or percutaneous valve replacement.

Pulmonic Stenosis

Pulmonic stenosis (PS) is the second most common congenital cardiac malformation (after VSD). Although typically an isolated abnormality, it can occur in association with VSD.

The patient with PS is usually asymptomatic, and the condition is identified by auscultation of a loud systolic murmur. When it is severe, dyspnea on exertion or fatigue can occur; less often, patients have retrosternal chest pain or syncope with exertion. Eventually, right ventricular failure can develop, with resultant peripheral edema and abdominal swelling.

In patients with moderate or severe PS, the second heart sound is widely split, with its pulmonic component soft and delayed. A crescendo-decrescendo systolic murmur that increases in intensity with inspiration is audible along the left sternal border. If the valve is pliable, an ejection click often precedes the murmur. On echocardiography, right ventricular hypertrophy is evident; the severity of PS can usually be assessed with measurement of Doppler flow.

Adults with mild PS are usually asymptomatic and do not require a corrective procedure. In contrast, patients with moderate or severe PS should undergo percutaneous balloon dilation.

Aortic Coarctation

Aortic coarctation typically consists of a diaphragm-like ridge extending into the aortic lumen just distal to the left subclavian artery (Figure 4), resulting in an elevated arterial pressure in both arms. Less commonly, the coarctation is located immediately proximal to the left subclavian artery, in which case a difference in arterial pressure is noted between the arms. Extensive collateral arterial circulation to the lower body through the internal thoracic, intercostal, subclavian, and scapular arteries often develops in patients with aortic coarctation. Aortic coarctation, which is two to five times as common in males as in females, can occur in conjunction with gonadal dysgenesis (e.g., Turner's syndrome), bicuspid aortic valve, VSD, or PDA.

On physical examination, the arterial pressure is higher in the arms than in the legs, and the femoral arterial pulses are weak and delayed. A harsh systolic ejection murmur may be audible along the left sternal border and in the back, particularly over the coarctation. A systolic murmur, caused by flow through collateral vessels, may be heard in the back.

On chest radiography, increased collateral flow through the intercostal arteries causes notching of the posterior third through eighth ribs. The coarctation may be visible as an indentation of the aorta, and one may see prestenotic and poststenotic aortic dilation, producing the "reversed E" or "3" sign. Computed tomography, magnetic resonance imaging, and contrast aortography provide precise anatomic delineation of the coarctation's location and length.

Most adults with aortic coarctation are asymptomatic. When symptoms are present, they are usually those of hypertension: headache, epistaxis, dizziness, and palpitations. Complications of aortic coarctation include hypertension, left ventricular failure, aortic dissection, premature coronary artery disease, infective endocarditis, and cerebrovascular accidents (due to rupture of an intracerebral aneurysm). Two thirds of patients older than 40 years who have uncorrected aortic coarctation have symptoms of heart failure. Three fourths die by the age of 50 years and 90% by the age of 60 years.

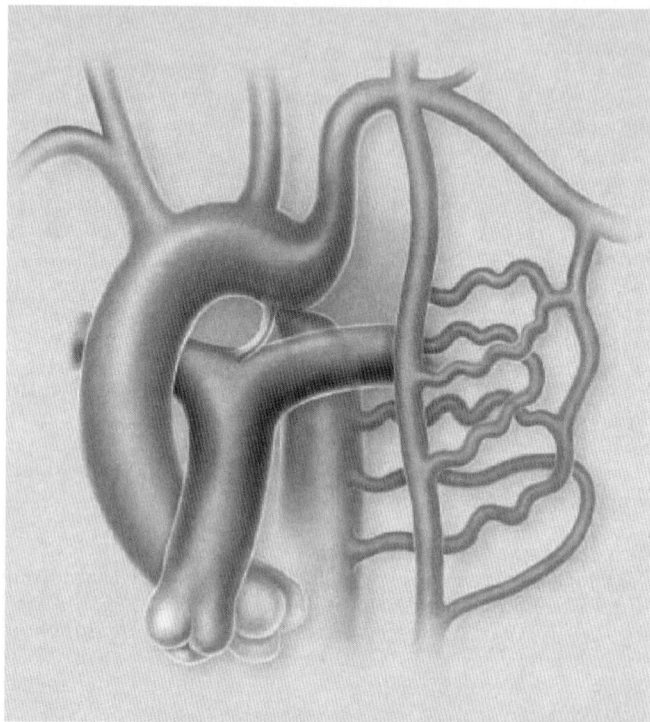

Figure 4 Coarctation of the aorta. Coarctation causes obstruction to blood flow in the descending thoracic aorta; the lower body is perfused by collateral vessels from the axillary and internal thoracic arteries through the intercostal arteries. (Reprinted with permission from Brickner ME, Hillis LD, Lange RA: Congenital heart disease in adults. First of two parts. N Engl J Med 2000;342:256–263.)

Surgical repair or intraluminal stenting should be considered for patients with a transcoarctation pressure gradient greater than 30 mm Hg, with the choice of procedure influenced by the age of the patient, anatomic considerations of the coarctation, and the presence of concomitant cardiac abnormalities. Persistent hypertension is common despite surgical or percutaneous intervention, and recurrent coarctation or aneurysm formation at the repair site may occur.

Cyanotic Conditions

Ebstein's Anomaly

With Ebstein's anomaly, the tricuspid valve's septal leaflet and often its posterior leaflet are displaced into the right ventricle, and the anterior leaflet is usually malformed and abnormally attached or adherent to the right ventricular free wall. As a result, a portion of the right ventricle is atrialized, in that it is located on the atrial side of the tricuspid valve, and the remaining functional right ventricle is small (Figure 5). The tricuspid valve is usually regurgitant, but it may be stenotic. Eighty percent of patients with Ebstein's anomaly have an interatrial communication (ASD or patent foramen ovale) through which right-to-left shunting of blood can occur.

The severity of the hemodynamic derangements in patients with Ebstein's anomaly depends on the magnitude of displacement and the functional status of the tricuspid valve leaflets. On the one extreme, patients with mild apical displacement of the tricuspid valve leaflets have normal valvular function; on the other extreme, those with severe leaflet displacement or abnormal anterior leaflet attachment, with resultant valvular dysfunction, have an elevated right atrial pressure and right-to-left shunting if an interatrial communication is present.

The clinical presentation of subjects with Ebstein's anomaly ranges from severe right heart failure in the neonate to the absence of symptoms in the adult in whom it is discovered incidentally. Older children with Ebstein's anomaly often come to medical attention because of an incidental murmur, whereas adolescents and adults may be identified because of a supraventricular arrhythmia.

On physical examination, the severity of cyanosis depends on the magnitude of right-to-left shunting. The first and second heart

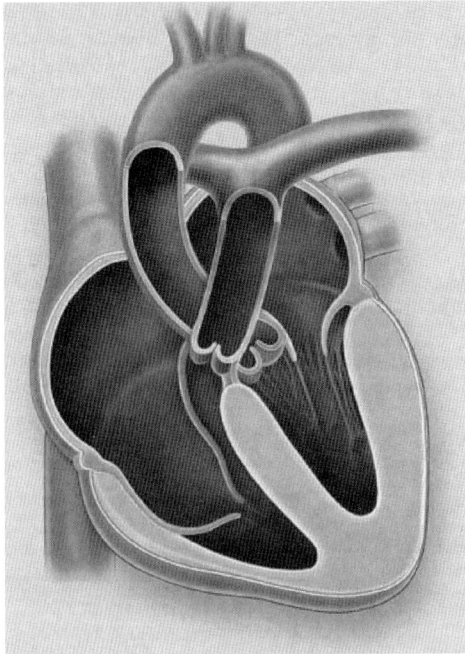

Figure 5 Ebstein's anomaly. With Ebstein's anomaly, the tricuspid valve is displaced apically, a portion of the right ventricle is atrialized (i.e., located on the atrial side of the tricuspid valve), and the functional right ventricle is small. (Reprinted with permission from Brickner ME, Hillis LD, Lange RA: Congenital heart disease in adults. Second of two parts. N Engl J Med 2000;342:334–342.)

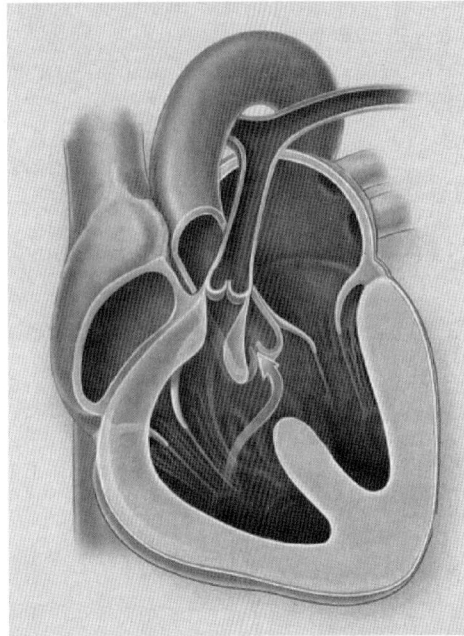

Figure 6 Tetralogy of Fallot. Tetralogy of Fallot is characterized by a large ventricular septal defect, obstruction of the right ventricular outflow tract, right ventricular hypertrophy, and an aorta that overrides the left and right ventricles. With right ventricular outflow tract obstruction, blood is shunted through the ventricular septal defect from right to left *(arrow)*. (Reprinted with permission from Brickner ME, Hillis LD, Lange RA: Congenital heart disease in adults. Second of two parts. N Engl J Med 2000;342:334–342.)

sounds are both widely split, and a third or fourth heart sound is often present, resulting in triple or even quadruple heart sounds. A systolic murmur caused by tricuspid regurgitation is usually present at the left lower sternal border.

Echocardiography is used to assess the presence and magnitude of right atrial dilation, anatomic displacement and distortion of the tricuspid valve leaflets, and the severity of tricuspid regurgitation or stenosis.

Prophylaxis against infective endocarditis is recommended. Patients with symptomatic right heart failure should receive diuretics. Tricuspid valve repair or replacement in conjunction with closure of the interatrial communication is recommended for older patients with severe symptoms despite medical therapy and those with less severe symptoms who have cardiac enlargement.

Tetralogy of Fallot

Tetralogy of Fallot is characterized by a large VSD, an aorta that overrides both ventricles, obstruction to right ventricular outflow (subvalvular, valvular, supravalvular, or in the pulmonary arterial branches), and right ventricular hypertrophy (Figure 6).

Most patients with tetralogy of Fallot have substantial right-to-left shunting through the large VSD because of increased resistance to flow in the right ventricular outflow tract; the magnitude of right ventricular outflow tract obstruction determines the magnitude of shunting. Because the resistance to flow across the right ventricular outflow tract is relatively fixed, changes in systemic vascular resistance affect the magnitude of right-to-left shunting: A decrease in systemic vascular resistance increases right-to-left shunting, whereas an increase in systemic resistance decreases it.

Patients with tetralogy of Fallot typically have cyanosis from birth or beginning in the first year of life. In childhood, they might have sudden hypoxic spells, characterized by tachypnea and hyperpnea, followed by worsening cyanosis and, in some cases, loss of consciousness, seizures, cerebrovascular accidents, and even death. Such spells do not occur in adolescents or adults. Without surgical intervention, most patients die in childhood.

On physical examination, patients with tetralogy of Fallot have cyanosis and digital clubbing. A right ventricular lift or tap is palpable. The second heart sound is single, because its pulmonic component is inaudible. A systolic ejection murmur, audible along the left sternal border, is caused by the obstruction to right ventricular outflow. The intensity and duration of the murmur are inversely related to the severity of right ventricular outflow obstruction; a soft, short murmur suggests that severe obstruction is present.

Laboratory examination reveals arterial oxygen desaturation and compensatory erythrocytosis. Echocardiography can be used to establish the diagnosis and to assess the location and severity of right ventricular outflow tract obstruction.

Complete surgical repair (closure of the VSD and relief of right ventricular outflow tract obstruction) is recommended to relieve symptoms and to improve survival; it should be performed when patients are very young. Those with tetralogy of Fallot (repaired or unrepaired) are at risk for endocarditis and therefore should receive antibiotic prophylaxis before dental or elective surgical procedures.

Patients with repaired tetralogy of Fallot require careful follow-up, because they can subsequently develop atrial or ventricular arrhythmias, pulmonic regurgitation, right ventricular dysfunction, or recurrent obstruction of the right ventricular outflow tract.

Eisenmenger Syndrome

With substantial left-to-right shunting, the pulmonary vasculature is exposed to increased blood flow under increased pressure, often resulting in pulmonary vascular obstructive disease. As the pulmonary vascular resistance approaches or exceeds systemic resistance, the shunt is reversed (right-to-left shunting develops), and cyanosis appears (Figure 7).

Most patients with Eisenmenger syndrome have impaired exercise tolerance and exertional dyspnea. Palpitations are common and most often result from atrial fibrillation or flutter. As erythrocytosis (due to arterial desaturation) develops, symptoms of hyperviscosity (visual disturbances, fatigue, headache, dizziness, and paresthesias) can appear. Patients with Eisenmenger syndrome can experience hemoptysis, bleeding complications, cerebrovascular accidents, brain abscess, syncope, and sudden death.

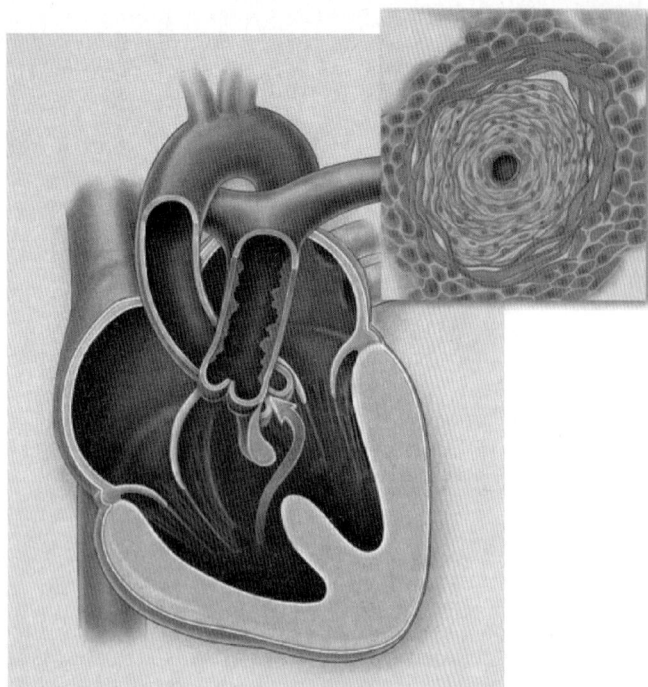

Figure 7 Eisenmenger syndrome. In response to substantial left-to-right shunting, morphologic alterations occur in the small pulmonary arteries and arterioles *(inset)*, leading to pulmonary hypertension and the resultant reversal of the intracardiac shunt *(arrow)*. In the small pulmonary arteries and arterioles, medial hypertrophy, intimal cellular proliferation, and fibrosis lead to narrowing or closure of the vessel lumina. With sustained pulmonary hypertension, extensive atherosclerosis and calcification often develop in the large pulmonary arteries. (Reprinted with permission from Brickner ME, Hillis LD, Lange RA: Congenital heart disease in adults. Second of two parts. N Engl J Med 2000;342:334–42.)

Eisenmenger syndrome patients typically have digital clubbing and cyanosis, a right parasternal heave (due to right ventricular hypertrophy), and a prominent pulmonic component of the second heart sound. The murmur caused by a VSD, PDA, or ASD disappears when Eisenmenger syndrome develops.

The chest x-ray reveals normal heart size, prominent central pulmonary arteries, and diminished vascular markings (pruning) of the peripheral vessels. On transthoracic echocardiography, evidence of right ventricular pressure overload and pulmonary hypertension is present. The underlying cardiac defect can usually be visualized, although shunting across the defect may be difficult to demonstrate by Doppler because of the low jet velocity.

Even though patients with Eisenmenger syndrome have severe pulmonary hypertension, they have a favorable long-term survival: 80% at 10 years after diagnosis, 77% at 15 years, and 42% at 25 years. Death is usually sudden, presumably caused by arrhythmias, but some patients die of heart failure, hemoptysis, brain abscess, or stroke.

Phlebotomy with isovolumic replacement should be performed in patients with moderate or severe symptoms of hyperviscosity; it should not be performed in asymptomatic or mildly symptomatic patients regardless of the hematocrit. Repeated phlebotomy can result in iron deficiency, which can worsen the symptoms of hyperviscosity, because iron-deficient erythrocytes are less deformable than iron-replete ones. Anticoagulants and antiplatelet agents should be avoided, because they exacerbate the hemorrhagic diathesis.

Patients with Eisenmenger syndrome should avoid intravascular volume depletion, high altitude, and the use of systemic vasodilators. Because of high maternal and fetal morbidity and mortality, pregnancy should be avoided. Patients with Eisenmenger syndrome who are undergoing noncardiac surgery require meticulous management of anesthesia, with attention to maintenance of systemic vascular resistance, minimization of blood loss and intravascular volume depletion, and prevention of

iatrogenic paradoxical embolization. In preparation for noncardiac surgery, prophylactic phlebotomy (usually of 1 to 2 units of blood, with isovolumic replacement) is recommended for patients with a hematocrit greater than 65% to reduce the likelihood of perioperative hemorrhagic and thrombotic complications.

Lung transplantation with repair of the cardiac defect or combined heart–lung transplantation are options for patients with Eisenmenger syndrome who are deemed to have a poor prognosis (as reflected by the presence of syncope, refractory right heart failure, a high New York Heart Association [NYHA] functional class, or severe hypoxemia). Because of the somewhat limited success of transplantation and the reasonably good survival among patients treated medically, careful selection of patients for transplantation is imperative. Although pulmonary vasodilators improve exercise capacity, they have not been proved to improve survival.

References

Bhatt AB, Foster E, Kuehl K, et al: on behalf of the American Heart Association Council on Clinical Cardiology: Congenital heart disease in the older adult: a scientific statement from the American Heart Association, *Circulation* 131:1884–1931, 2015.
Brickner ME, Hillis LD, Lange RA: Congenital heart disease in adults. First of two parts, *N Engl J Med* 342:256–263, 2000.
Brickner ME, Hillis LD, Lange RA: Congenital heart disease in adults. Second of two parts, *N Engl J Med* 342:334–342, 2000.
Lange RA, Hillis LD, Vongpatanasin WP, Brickner ME: The Eisenmenger syndrome in adults, *Ann Int Med* 128:745–755, 1998.
Neidenbach R, Niwa K, Oto O, et al: Improving medical care and prevention in adults with congenital heart disease—reflections on a global problem—part II: infective endocarditis, pulmonary hypertension, pulmonary arterial hypertension and aortopathy, *Cardiovasc Diagn Ther* 8(6):716–724, 2018.
Stout KK, Daniels CJ, Aboulhosn JA, et al: 2018 AHA/ACC guideline for the management of adults with congenital heart disease: executive summary: a report of the American College of Cardiology/American Heart Association Task Force on Clinical Practice Guidelines, *Circulation* 139:e637–e697, 2019.

CONGESTIVE HEART FAILURE

Method of
Robert Solomon, MD; and Stacy Willner, DO

Defining Heart Failure

Technological advancements have given providers a variety of different tools to use in the evaluation of cardiac dysfunction including blood biomarkers, imaging modalities, and invasive techniques. However, despite their usefulness, at its essence heart failure (HF) is a clinical diagnosis based on the interplay of various pathophysiologic processes. Identifying signs of intravascular congestion (sometimes accompanied by evidence of decreased end organ perfusion) is key when it comes to making an accurate diagnosis. This congestion can be from either systolic or diastolic dysfunction, often manifesting as shortness of breath, chest pain (due to elevated ventricular filling pressures decreasing coronary perfusion pressure), decreased exertional capacity, fatigue, and edema. Recognition of these symptoms, along with evidence of congestion, allows one to formally diagnose HF according to its current universal definition.

It is important to understand that cardiomyopathy and HF are two distinct entities. Cardiomyopathy refers to a disease of the myocardium (e.g., ischemic, hypertrophic, dilated, restrictive, peripartum, stress), while HF refers to the inability of that muscle to adequately meet the demands of the body. While cardiomyopathy has the ability to produce HF, it is not necessarily required. Additionally, a low ejection fraction (EF) does not imply a diagnosis of HF if the aforementioned criteria are not met. Ultimately, HF is a spectrum that over time can progress through various stages based on the presence of different features (Table 1).

Epidemiology

While HF is estimated to impact over 56 million people across the globe, in the United States, according to data from the 2017 to 2020 National Health and Nutrition Examination Survey, 6.7 million adults had congestive heart failure (close to 2.6% of the

TABLE 1 ACC/AHA Stages of Heart Failure

STAGE A (AT RISK)	STAGE B (PRE-HF)	STAGE C (SYMPTOMATIC HF)	STAGE D (ADVANCED HF)
• Risk factors (e.g., hypertension, diabetes) for HF but with no prior or current signs or symptoms • There is no biomarker or structural evidence of cardiac disease	• Evidence of structural heart disease, but with no prior or current HF signs or symptoms • Evidence can come in the form of positive cardiac biomarkers, increased filling pressures, or other forms of cardiac dysfunction	• Prior or current signs or symptoms of HF in the setting of structural heart disease	• Severe symptomatic HF • This can be seen with patients requiring hospitalizations despite medical optimization, those needing advanced therapies like transplantation or mechanical circulatory support, and those appropriate for palliative care

ACC/AHA, American College of Cardiology/American Heart Association; *HF,* heart failure.

population). Projections point toward this number increasing above 8 million by 2030. The incidence of HF will only continue to rise as lifespans extend thanks to advancements in medical knowledge and disease management. This assuredly will promote further burden on healthcare systems, estimated to cost nearly $70 billion in the United States alone by 2030.

When it comes to demographics, HF is more common in males. Although about 50% of cases are heart failure with reduced ejection fraction (HFrEF), trends point toward heart failure with preserved ejection fraction (HFpEF) clearly overtaking it to become the most common form of dysfunction in the future. These HFpEF patients tend to be older and female, often with hypertension, obesity, or atrial fibrillation. Risk scores have been developed to aid in HF prognostication, largely influenced by factors like comorbidities and hospitalizations. Though data varies depending on the study, for the most part HFpEF seems to have a better prognosis compared with its counterpart. While HF mortality data can differ based on the study and population observed, in general rates remain high, outlining the ongoing need to dedicate resources toward its management.

Classifying Heart Failure

Classifying HF based on left ventricular ejection fraction (LVEF) has evolved over the years. While in the past it was common for practitioners to only focus on two groupings, HFrEF and HFpEF, since the mid-2010s various societies have come to appreciate the complexity of HF and expand their naming systems to recognize additional types of pathology. Specifically, those with an EF between 41% and 49% (heart failure with mildly reduced ejection fraction, HFmrEF) and those whose EF has recovered (heart failure with recovered ejection fraction, HFrecEF) are now acknowledged with more frequency (Table 2). These classifications are important not only due to their association with distinct prognostic data, but also because they may require different treatment regimens. An example of such is HFmrEF, a group that could have characteristics of HFrEF or HFpEF depending on the clinical picture.

Clinicians should remember that like all methodologies in science, cardiac imaging is not exact. Due to several factors, some degree of variability can exist when it comes to EF quantification with echocardiography, and this should be considered when evaluating patients. For example, a documented drop in EF from 43% to 39% may simply represent variability in technique or acquisition, rather than true clinical deterioration requiring an escalation in care. Use of more precise imaging tests like a multigated acquisition (MUGA) scan or cardiac MRI may be worthwhile in the appropriate clinical context, such as when the EF could determine whether a patient meets criteria for a lifesaving device like an implantable cardioverter-defibrillator (ICD).

Functional capacity is often described with the New York Heart Association (NYHA) classification system. Outlined in Table 3, this system helps standardize a HF patient's clinical status, which can be especially useful when making management decisions. It should be recognized that EF is not necessarily correlative with functional status, as one could have an EF of 10% or 60% and

TABLE 2 Heart Failure Classification Based on Ejection Fraction

HF CLASS	ABBREVIATION	LVEF
HF with reduced ejection fraction	HFrEF	≤40%
HF with mildly reduced ejection fraction	HFmrEF	41%–49%
HF with preserved ejection fraction	HFpEF	≥50%
HF with recovered ejection fraction	HFrecEF	Prior ≤40%, recovered to >40% with at least a 10% increase

HF, Heart failure, *LVEF,* left ventricular ejection fraction.

still be NYHA III, for example. The four NYHA classes have prognostic value and is something that should be assessed at each medical encounter when treating someone with HF.

Left Ventricular Physiology and Hemodynamics

Three components are critical in determining the efficiency of cardiac function: preload, afterload, and contractility. Preload refers to the degree of myocardial stretching before ventricular systole, with left ventricular end diastolic pressure (LVEDP) often being used as a surrogate when referencing left ventricular preload. Afterload is the resistance force the left ventricle contracts against, many times referred to as the systemic vascular resistance (SVR). Contractility (also called inotropy) references the ability of cardiac muscle cells to generate force and can be influenced by a variety of different pathologies and pharmacotherapies.

The Frank-Starling law demonstrates how stroke volume will proportionally increase with preload until it reaches its physiologic limit, the point where further stretching will not increase contraction and may in fact be deleterious. This curve can also be influenced by afterload, which has an inverse relationship with stroke volume (its reduction can lead to increased cardiac output). Furthermore, increased inotropy leads to a more forceful contraction, and its influence on the curve is largely seen in how it shifts it upward due to increased stroke volume (and vice versa). Ultimately the relationship between these forces dictates cardiac output and can create one of four standard hemodynamic profiles typically used to offer quick clinical assessments of HF patients (Table 4).

Heart Failure's Impact on Neurohormonal and Sympathetic Systems

As HF is a general state of reduced cardiac output, the body understandably attempts to correct this by activating several physiologic pathways in an effort to maintain cardiovascular equilibrium. However, this ultimately has adverse effects. These pathways include the renin-angiotensin-aldosterone

TABLE 3	NYHA Functional Class
NYHA CLASS	**DESCRIPTION**
I	Not limited. Can perform ordinary physical activities without symptoms.
II	Slightly limited. May have mild symptoms and limitations with ordinary activity.
III	Significantly limited. Can have notable symptoms and limitations with ordinary activities. Often only comfortable when resting.
IV	Severely limited. Any degree of physical activity causes symptoms, which can even be present at rest.

NYHA, New York Heart Association.

TABLE 4	Hemodynamic Profiles	
	NORMAL/LOW LVEDP	**HIGH LVEDP**
Normal cardiac output	Warm and dry	Warm and wet
Decreased cardiac output	Cold and dry	Cold and wet

LVEDP, Left ventricular end diastolic pressure.

TABLE 5	Common Clinical Findings in Heart Failure

- Jugular venous distension
- Lower extremity edema
- Pulmonary edema
- Pulmonary rales
- Third heart sound (S$_3$)
- Orthopnea/paroxysmal nocturnal dyspnea (PND)
- Cardiomegaly
- Dyspnea on exertion
- Tachycardia
- Hepatojugular reflux
- Hepatomegaly
- Pleural effusion

system (RAAS) and sympathetic nervous system (SNS), both typically used to aid end organ perfusion. The RAAS is activated when the kidneys detect decreased perfusion pressure, starting a hormonal cascade triggering various consequences including sodium and water retention, vasoconstriction, and other effects that can cause cardiac remodeling (e.g., hypertrophy, fibrosis). Similarly, the SNS is activated to offer a form of compensation in the setting of cardiac deterioration but can induce deleterious effects by increasing catecholamine levels and overly enhancing sympathetic tone. While offering acute benefits (increased heart rate and cardiac contractility), chronic activation contributes to detrimental changes via peripheral vasoconstriction, increased cardiac afterload, and ventricular remodeling. Appreciating the mechanisms of these pathways has helped aid in the development of various guideline-directed medical therapy (GDMT) agents that are used as the current standard of care in HF patients due to their proven morbidity and mortality benefits.

Diagnosis

There are several basic signs and symptoms that, when seen together, increase the likelihood of HF (Table 5). A few of the most well-known findings include jugular venous distension (JVD), pulmonary rales, a third heart sound (S$_3$), shortness of breath, and edema (abdominal, lower extremity). Several tools can be used to help solidify the diagnosis of HF. An electrocardiogram (ECG) can identify signs suspicious for structural change, electrical conduction errors, or myocardial abnormalities (e.g., chamber enlargement, bundle branch blocks, ischemia, amyloidosis, hypertrophic cardiomyopathy).

Echocardiography can be used to better assess heart anatomy including ventricular systolic function, cardiac chamber size, and valvular integrity while also estimating pressures, identifying shunts, and offering other forms of quantification (e.g., diastolic function, myocardial hypertrophy, pericardial effusions). Nuclear MUGA scans are often used to provide more exact measurements of EF, especially in clinical situations that may require cardiac implantable electronic devices (CIED). Though sometimes not as easily obtainable and more expensive, cardiac MRI gives perhaps the best evaluation of the aforementioned while also providing more detail on things like thrombi, infiltration, inflammation, and scars. Both left and right heart catheterization offer more invasive ways of identifying the etiologies (e.g., ischemia, pulmonary hypertension, severe valvular disease) and comprehending the hemodynamic consequences (e.g., elevated fillings pressures, cardiogenic shock) of HF.

Laboratory and Diagnostic Tests

When dealing with a decompensated HF patient, several laboratory tests should be ordered on the initial encounter, including a complete metabolic panel (CMP), complete blood count (CBC), thyroid-stimulating hormone (TSH), and lactic acid, as well as brain natriuretic peptide (BNP) and N-terminal pro-B type natriuretic peptide (NT-pro BNP). These tests are especially helpful when the patient has a known history of HF and the extent of decompensation needs to be determined. An elevated lactic acid level is indicative of shock and is an ominous sign that should prompt expedited workup and treatment.

When a patient presents with a new diagnosis of HF, the scope of laboratory and diagnostic testing should be increased to assess for the potential cause, including evaluation for acute coronary syndrome (ACS), HIV, rheumatologic disorders, hemochromatosis, amyloidosis, viral infections, substance abuse, postpartum state, or arrhythmia.

Of the aforementioned testing, BNP and NT-pro BNP are essential as these biomarkers are released from the myocytes when they are overstretched, causing these levels to elevate in acute and potentially chronic HF. These circulating peptides have a vasodilatory and natriuretic response. BNP is the biologically active form and is inactivated by the enzyme neprilysin. As will be discussed later, this enzyme is one of the targets for sacubitril-valsartan (Entresto), an essential part of HF GDMT. Assessing BNP and/or NT-pro BNP levels can be helpful in multiple settings. As an outpatient, it can help better define the etiology of unclear dyspnea, while in the inpatient setting it can be used to quickly rule out HF given that normal levels make a diagnosis of HF much less likely. Though there is no formalized role for serial testing, it can be helpful in terms of prognostication. For example, elevated levels on hospital discharge could potentially mean a worse outcome compared with a patient whose levels have normalized.

When it comes to other diagnostic testing, an ECG, chest x-ray (CXR), and echocardiogram should also be obtained. A Swan-Ganz catheter is often not needed for diagnosis but can be helpful when the overall clinical picture is unclear and the exact etiology of shock needs to be determined (e.g., septic vs. cardiogenic).

Therapy for HFrEF

Diuretics (High-Dose IV Diuretics Are Important)

Loop diuretics continue to be the mainstay of therapy to relieve congestion in patients with both HFrEF and HFpEF. Of the loop diuretics, furosemide (Lasix), bumetanide (Bumex, Burinex), and torsemide (Demadex, Soaanz) are all generally effective and well tolerated. In terms of bioavailability, furosemide is about 50% with substantial interpatient and intrapatient variability ranging from 10% to 90%. Alternatively, the bioavailability of torsemide and bumetanide are greater at around 80% to 100%. This is important to keep in mind when furosemide does not seem to be working for a patient, as considering a substitute may be worthwhile.

When starting a loop diuretic in the inpatient setting for a decompensated HF patient, it is a good rule of thumb to increase the home dose by 2 to 2.5 times. If escalation of the loop diuretic alone does not seem to be effective, addition of a thiazide diuretic, such as metolazone (Zaroxolyn), should be considered. It is important to remember that due to its mechanism of action, the thiazide diuretic should be given 30 minutes before the loop diuretic. This allows the thiazide to start blocking sodium reabsorption in the distal convoluted tubule (where thiazides primarily act), before the increased sodium load from the loop diuretic reaches that area. This allows for a sequential nephron blockade, maximizing sodium and water excretion. These medications should be titrated accordingly to keep the patient in a euvolemic state.

Four Pillars of GDMT
Renin-Angiotensin-Aldosterone System Inhibitors
Angiotensin receptor–neprilysin inhibitors (ARNI), angiotensin-converting enzyme inhibitors (ACEI), and angiotensin receptor blockers (ARB) make up one of the four pillars of GDMT for HFrEF therapy. The preferable agent among the three is an ARNI, or sacubitril-valsartan (Entresto), as this has been shown to be superior when it comes to reducing cardiovascular death and hospitalizations (elucidated from the PARADIGM-HF study). This has primarily been attributed to sacubitril-valsartan's unique method of action, which involves inhibiting the breakdown of beneficial peptides, which in combination with valsartan relaxes the blood vessels, improves overall blood flow, and reduces the workload of the heart. The initiation of sacubitril-valsartan can potentially be limited by baseline hypotension (e.g., systolic blood pressure <90–100 mm Hg), as well as cost. In either of these cases an ACEI or ARB should be initiated, with consideration of an ARNI in the future. If a patient is already on an ACEI or ARB, then transition to an ARNI should be initiated. However, it is important to remember that an ACEI will need a 36-hour washout period before ARNI initiation to reduce the risk of unwanted drug interactions.

Mineralocorticoid Receptor Antagonists
Aldosterone antagonists include spironolactone (Aldactone) or eplerenone (Inspra)[1] and are another pillar of GDMT for HFrEF patients. These medications have been studied in randomized controlled trials and shown to reduce the risk of mortality in selected groups of HFrEF patients. It is important to note that this class of medications has the potential to cause hyperkalemia.

Beta Blockers
Beta blockers are another pillar of GDMT for HFrEF therapy. The three agents that have been shown to reduce morbidity and mortality are metoprolol succinate (Toprol XL), carvedilol (Coreg) and bisoprolol (Zebeta)[1], although it is worth mentioning bisoprolol is only FDA approved for hypertension and is used off-label for HFrEF therapy. Before initiating a beta blocker, one should be sure the patient is not in cardiogenic shock and does not have signs of new congestion. For this reason, beta blockers are often started after a hospital stay for decompensated HF, while in the outpatient setting.

Sodium-Glucose Cotransporter-2 Inhibitors
Sodium-glucose cotransporter-2 (SGLT2) inhibitors are the last of the four pillars of GDMT for HFrEF. This class of medications was added after randomized trials showed that HFrEF patients already on mineralocorticoid receptor antagonists (MRAs), RAAS-neprilysin inhibitor, and beta blocker, who had subsequent treatment with an SGLT2 inhibitor, further reduced the risk of mortality and rehospitalization compared with placebo. The agents specifically studied were dapagliflozin (Farxiga) and empagliflozin (Jardiance).

---

[1] Not FDA approved for this indication.

Adjunctive and Optional Therapies
Hydralazine and Isosorbide Dinitrate Combination
Hydralazine, in combination with isosorbide dinitrate, works as a vasodilator. It can be prescribed together as a combination pill (BiDil) or taken separately. This is considered an add-on therapy for patients, especially African Americans, with persistent symptoms and systolic blood pressure >110 mm Hg, or who are hypertensive, despite optimal GDMT as outlined previously. It can also be used in patients who cannot tolerate ACEI/ARB/ARNI but should never be used as a replacement in patients who can tolerate it.

Ivabradine
Ivabradine (Corlanor) can be used as an adjunct in patients with HFrEF who are without a pacemaker and have a sinus rate >70 beats per minute. This therapy is most appropriate when patients are already on an optimized beta blocker regimen and are not in decompensated HF.

Soluble Guanylate Cyclase Inhibitor
Vericiguat. The addition of vericiguat (Verquvo) can be considered in HFrEF patients who are already being optimally treated with all four pillars of GDMT, as well as vasodilatory therapy. Overall, clinical experience with vericiguat is largely limited to patients who have had a recent HF decompensation.

Cardiac Glycoside
Digoxin. Digoxin, an inotrope, is now rarely used in modern practice primarily due to its narrow therapeutic window and overall unclear efficacy.

Device Therapy
For patients with HFrEF, device therapy includes ICDs and cardiac resynchronization therapy (CRT). ICDs are recommended for primary prevention of sudden cardiac death (SCD) in patients who are at least 40 days out from a myocardial infarction (MI) with an EF of ≤30% and NYHA class I symptoms, while receiving GDMT, who have a reasonable expectation of meaningful survival >1 year. CRT is recommended in patients who have an EF of ≤35%, normal sinus rhythm, left bundle branch block (LBBB) with a QRS duration of ≥150 ms and NYHA class II, III, or ambulatory class IV symptoms on GDMT. In this situation, CRT has been shown to reduce total mortality, reduce hospitalizations, and improve symptoms and quality of life.

Therapy for HFpEF
When treating patients with HFpEF, it is important to remember that the goal of treatment is to reduce HF severity and increase overall functional status. Several chronic conditions often accompany HFpEF, including hypertension, atrial fibrillation, coronary artery disease, hyperlipidemia, anemia, diabetes mellitus, obesity, chronic kidney disease, and obstructive sleep apnea. It is important to treat and manage these conditions, along with HFpEF, to optimize outcomes.

Initial pharmacotherapy involves SGLT2 inhibitors, as these have been shown to be beneficial specifically with NYHA class II to III symptoms and an EF >50%. Another class of medications to consider is MRAs. Newly approved in this class is finerenone (Kerendia), which has been found to lower the rate of acute HF episodes. Again, providers should be mindful of the potential for hyperkalemia.

In HFpEF patients with obesity, therapy should be initiated with a glucagon-like peptide (GLP-1) receptor agonist and counseling on healthy diet and lifestyle modifications. RAAS inhibitors are thought to likely have benefit in HFpEF, but they are normally not used as initial treatment unless the patient has uncontrolled hypertension.

Advanced Heart Failure
Stage D, or advanced HF, describes those who have symptoms at rest or with very minimal exertion. They often have recurrent hospitalizations and refractory symptoms despite optimal GDMT. In those

TABLE 6 I-NEED-HELP: Identifying Patients Needing Referral to a Heart Failure Specialist for Advanced Therapy

I	Inotropes	Previous or ongoing requirement for dobutamine, milrinone, or dopamine
N	NYHA class/Natriuretic peptides	Persisting NYHA class III or IV and/or persistently high BNP or NT-pro BNP
E	End organ dysfunction	Worsening renal or liver dysfunction in the setting of HF
E	Ejection fraction	<20%
D	Defibrillator shocks	Recurrent appropriate defibrillator shocks
H	Hospitalizations	More than 1 hospitalization with HF in the last 12 months
E	Edema/Escalating diuretics	Persistent fluid overload and/or increasing diuretic requirement
L	Low blood pressure	Consistently low BP with SBP <90–100 mm Hg
P	Prognostic medication	Inability to uptitrate, or need to decrease or stop GDMT

BNP, Brain natriuretic peptide; *BP*, blood pressure; *GDMT*, guideline-directed medical therapy; *NT-pro BNP*, N-terminal pro-B type natriuretic peptide; *HF*, heart failure; *NYHA*, New York Heart Association; *SBP*, systolic blood pressure.

patients who would be amenable, ideally before they reach stage D, a referral should be made to an advanced HF specialist to determine candidacy for cardiac transplantation or durable mechanical support, such as a left ventricular assist device (LVAD). See Table 6 for a helpful mnemonic on when a patient should be referred.

References

Becher PM, et al: *An update on global epidemiology in heart failure*, 2022, pp 3005–3007.
Gogikar A, Nanda A, Janga LSN, et al: Combination diuretic therapy with thiazides: a systematic review on the beneficial approach to overcome refractory fluid overload in heart failure, *Cureus* 15(9):e44624, 2023.
Heidenreich PA, Bozkurt B, Aguilar D, et al: 2022 AHA/ACC/HFSA guideline for the management of heart failure: a report of the American College of Cardiology/ American Heart Association joint committee on clinical practice guidelines, *J Am Coll Cardiol* 79(17):e263–e421, 2022.
Lam CSP, et al: Epidemiology and clinical course of heart failure with preserved ejection fraction, *Eur J Heart Fail* 13(1):18–28, 2011.
Maddox TM, Januzzi JL, Allen LA, et al: 2024 acc expert consensus decision pathway for treatment of heart failure with reduced ejection fraction: a report of the American College of Cardiology solution set oversight committee, *J Am Coll Cardiol* 83(15):1444–1488, 2024.
Martin SS, Aday AW, Allen NB, Almarzooq ZI, Anderson CA, Arora P, American Heart Association Council on Epidemiology and Prevention Statistics Committee and Stroke Statistics Committee: 2025 heart disease and stroke statistics: a report of US and global data from the American heart association, *Circulation*, 2025.
Ostrominski JW, Solomon SD, Vaduganathan M: Heart failure with preserved ejection fraction therapy: combining sodium-glucose co-transporter 2 inhibitors and glucagon-like peptide-1 receptor agonists, *Eur Heart J* 45(30):2748–2751, 2024.
Ponikowski P, Voors AA, Anker SD, et al: 2016 ESC Guidelines for the diagnosis and treatment of acute and chronic heart failure: the Task Force for the diagnosis and treatment of acute and chronic heart failure of the European Society of Cardiology (Esc)Developed with the special contribution of the Heart Failure Association (Hfa) of the ESC, *Eur Heart J* 37(27):2129–2200, 2016.
Varghese TP, Tazneem B: Unraveling the complex pathophysiology of heart failure: insights into the role of renin-angiotensin-aldosterone system (RAAS) and sympathetic nervous system (SNS), *Curr Probl Cardiol* 49(4):102411, 2024.
Yan T, et al: Burden, trends, and inequalities of heart failure globally, 1990 to 2019: a secondary analysis based on the global burden of disease 2019 study, *J Am Heart Assoc* 12(6):e027852, 2023.

HEART BLOCK

Method of
Kelley P. Anderson, MD

CURRENT DIAGNOSIS

- Assess risk for heart block in the absence of symptoms or heart block on electrocardiogram (ECG).
  - Review cardiac or systemic disorders associated with cardiac conduction disease (CCD), ECG pattern, family history, maternal antibodies, cardiac interventions, and surgery.
- Evaluate documented asystole or bradycardia due to heart block.
  - Classify heart block: transient, recurrent, progressive, permanent.
  - Grade signs and symptoms: none, mild, severe.
- Evaluate signs or symptoms of possible transient heart block with no documentation.
  - Establish temporal pattern: recent versus remote onset, solitary versus recurrent, daily, weekly, monthly, yearly.
  - Grade signs and symptoms: none, mild, severe.
  - Document rhythm during symptoms: telemetry monitoring, Holter monitor, external loop recorder, implantable recorder.

CURRENT THERAPY

- Methods of heart rate support:
  - Immediate: intravenous catecholamines, atropine, or aminophylline[1]; transcutaneous pacing
  - Short term: transvenous temporary pacing
  - Long term: permanent pacemakers
- Pacemaker configuration:
  - Number of leads: 1, 2, 3, 4 or leadless
  - Lead locations: right atrial appendage, Bachman's bundle, right ventricular apex, outflow tract, left ventricle, coronary sinus, His bundle, left bundle branch area
  - Programming to minimize ventricular pacing: manufacturer dependent, biventricular pacing, His bundle pacing, left bundle branch area pacing

[1]Not FDA approved for this indication.

Heart block refers to block or delay of electrical propagation between the atria and ventricles. It is a form of cardiac conduction disease (CCD), which applies more generally to disorders of electrical impulse formation or propagation anywhere along the cardiac conduction system from the sinus node to the ventricular myocardium. Heart block or CCD may present as a syndrome, as an electrocardiographic (ECG) pattern, or as a mechanism of serious signs and symptoms such as sudden death or syncope. Pacemaker therapy is an effective treatment, but it is associated with significant short- and long-term complications. This underscores the importance of recognizing preventable and reversible causes of heart block for accurate targeting of permanent pacing. Risk stratification of patients with heart block, assessment of the benefits and risks of the therapeutic options, and patient education and guidance are largely in the domain of heart rhythm specialists. However, heart block may be encountered unexpectedly in any patient during any clinical encounter. Furthermore, some patients may require evaluation in the absence of known cardiac disease because of increased risk of CCD, or increased risk of CCD in family members or future children. A basic understanding of heart block may be useful to initiate emergency treatment and to recognize patients who warrant further evaluation or specialist referral.

Epidemiology

The prevalence and incidence of heart block are difficult to establish because they are strongly dependent on the demographic and clinical characteristics of the population sample. The prevalence is higher among the elderly and those with cardiovascular disease. First-degree heart block, defined as prolongation of the PR interval >200 ms on ECG, occurs in the population setting with prevalence of 0.7% to 2% in the young and up to 14% in the elderly. Higher degrees of heart block can be expected to be less common but similarly associated with age and underlying cardiovascular disease. In a study of the Framingham population, the prevalence of first-degree heart block was 1.6% and was associated with an incidence of pacemaker implantation of 59 per 10,000 person-years in persons with a PR interval >200 ms compared to 6 per 10,000 person-years in persons with a PR interval <200 ms. Approximately 36% of the pacemakers were for high-grade block.

In 1420 elderly subjects with common risk factors randomized to continuous monitoring by implanted loop recorder (ILR group, mean monitoring duration 39 months) versus 4503 controls in usual care, 4.1% demonstrated first-degree or low-grade second-degree heart block (95.1% asymptomatic) compared with 0.8% in controls. High-grade second-degree block or complete block was observed in 3.1% of the ILR group (28.3% asymptomatic) and in 1.5% of controls. More patients in the ILR group underwent pacemaker implantation with no demonstrable improvements in outcomes. This study suggests that detection of conduction disturbances is increased by longer periods of monitoring, that heart block in elderly patients is infrequent but not rare, that many subjects with incident heart block are asymptomatic, and that pacemaker implantation does not necessarily improve outcomes based on the nearly 6 years of observation in the subjects enrolled in this study.

Risk Factors

Patients with genetic or acquired CCD and patients subject to trauma or surgical procedures that can damage the conduction system are at increased risk for developing symptomatic advanced heart block. In the Framingham population, subjects with first-degree AV block had an increased risk of mortality, atrial fibrillation, and pacemaker implantation. However, the vast majority with risk factors never develop symptomatic heart block and have not been shown to benefit from intense monitoring or prophylactic pacemaker placement. The few possible exceptions are discussed below.

Pathophysiology

The function of the cardiac conduction system is to initiate and coordinate cardiac contraction to circulate blood according to physiological needs. Electrical activation is initiated by pacemaker cells of the sinus node regulated by the autonomic nervous system. Unlike conduction in common electrical circuits in which electrons flow along a conductor according to the voltage gradient, electrical activity in cardiac cells propagates from segment to segment of the cell membrane in cardiac myocytes (myocardial cells) and in specialized cardiac conduction cells. Energy-requiring ion pumps maintain an electrochemical gradient across the insulating cell membrane. Electrical activity opens voltage-sensitive ion channels causing regenerative

TABLE 1	Mechanisms of Conduction Disturbances (Examples)

- Prolonged refractory period (vagal activity, drugs, ischemia)
- Sarcolemmal ion gradient disturbances (hyperkalemia, hypokalemia)
- Sodium channel dysfunction (SCN5A mutations, sodium channel blocking drugs such as lidocaine, procainamide, flecainide [Tambocor], amiodarone [Cordarone], and imipramine [Tofranil])
- Calcium channel dysfunction (verapamil [Isoptin], diltiazem [Cardizem], mutations)
- Energy deprivation (ischemia, cyanide)
- Cell dysfunction (inflammation, barotrauma, thermal injury)
- Cell death (apoptosis, ischemic necrosis, inflammatory necrosis, surgical trauma, ablation)
- Congenital structural defects (endocardial cushion defects)
- Gap junction disturbances (fibrosis, edema, inflammation, genetic defects)
- Genetic defects (SCN5A and NKX2.5 mutations)

electrical activity as ions shift along their electrochemical gradient. Electrical activity in a single cell excites several adjacent cells via gap junctions. This cascade effect makes it possible for a single cell impulse to spread rapidly throughout the myocardium to enhance synchronous contraction. This also provides a safety mechanism in that each myocardial cell can be activated by many electrical paths. In addition, specialized conduction cells exhibit automaticity (impulse formation). Although normally latent because normal activation inhibits spontaneous discharge, when the normal impulse is blocked, discharges from these subsidiary physiological pacemakers provide vital heart rate support.

Block of electrical activation can occur due to failure of any step in the process, for example, lack of metabolic energy, electrolyte imbalance, inflammatory disruption of the membrane, block of ion channels by drugs, or interference with gap junction function due to infiltration of fibrous tissue (Table 1). Because of the extensive redundancy and interconnectivity and because of the capacity to compensate for injury by electrical and anatomic remodeling, there may be extensive damage before signs or symptoms of heart block occur. Regions of the heart where there are fewer alternative paths for electrical activation, such as proximal portions of the His-Purkinje system where all conducting fibers are confined to a relatively small area, are more vulnerable to complete block. Subsidiary pacemakers sometimes fail to provide adequate rate support when heart block occurs because of preexisting injury. If the patient survives an episode of heart block, there is a possibility for recovery due to remodeling. However, remodeling can be maladaptive and result in an adverse long-term outcome by further conduction system damage, by left ventricular dysfunction, and by bradycardia-induced ventricular tachyarrhythmias (VTAs). The mechanisms of bradycardia-induced VTAs are not known, but bradyarrhythmias precipitate torsades de pointes, a specific form of VTA, in the presence of drugs that block potassium channels, electrolyte disturbances, certain genetic abnormalities of ion channel function, heart failure, and myocardial hypertrophy. A comprehensive list of drugs that may account for bradyarrhythmia-related ventricular arrhythmias is available at www.torsades.org.

Although there are many potential causes of heart block, the pathophysiology is not known for the vast majority of cases because there are no tests that allow detailed structural or functional examination in patients. By the time of death, morphologic examination may reveal only nonspecific changes such as fibrosis. Instead, most etiologies are inferred by history of recent or past exposures (e.g., trauma or radiation), concomitant disorders (e.g., muscular dystrophy, cardiac sarcoidosis), abnormal test results (e.g., Lyme disease) or family history (e.g., SCN5A sodium channel mutations) (Table 2). Because most etiologies cannot be verified, the clinician must

TABLE 2 Etiologies of Heart Block

- Frequently permanent or progressive (examples)
  - Alcohol septal ablation (acute, delayed)
  - Cardiomyopathies (hypertrophic, idiopathic, mitochondrial)
  - Catheter ablation (atrioventricular nodal reentry, accessory atrioventricular connections)
  - Congenital heart block (neonatal lupus)
  - Congenital heart disease (endocardial cushion defects)
  - Genetic disorders (SCN5A sodium channel mutations, gap junction gene mutations, fatty acid oxidation disorders, PRKAG2 mutations, LMNA gene mutations)
  - Hypertension
  - Idiopathic fibrosis and calcification (Lev's disease, Lenegre's disease)
  - Infectious disorders—destructive (endocarditis)
  - Infiltrative disorders (amyloidosis)
  - Myocardial infarction
  - Neuromyopathic disorders (myotonic dystrophy, Erb's dystrophy, peroneal muscular atrophy)
  - Noninfectious inflammatory disorders (HLA-B27–associated disorder, sarcoidosis)
  - Tumors (mesothelioma, metastatic cancer)
  - Valvular heart disease
- Frequently transient or reversible (examples)
  - Blunt trauma (baseball)
  - Cardiac surgery (valve replacement)
  - Cardiac transplant rejection
  - Central nervous system
  - Drugs (antiarrhythmics, digoxin [Lanoxin], edrophonium [Enlon])
  - Electrolyte disturbances (hyperkalemia)
  - Metabolic disturbances (hypothermia, hypothyroidism)
  - Increased vagal activity
  - Infectious disorders—nondestructive (Lyme disease)
  - Myocardial ischemia
  - Myocarditis (Chagas disease, giant cell myocarditis)
  - Rheumatic fever

remain open to alternative explanations and accept the likelihood of multiple contributors.

Some patients, usually young, otherwise healthy individuals, present with prolonged asystole due to heart block but have no other detectable abnormalities and have excellent outcomes in the absence of intervention beyond counseling. This suggests that autonomic influences alone can cause prolonged heart block and suppression of subsidiary pacemakers. It is not known whether such responses result from an abnormality or an exaggerated normal reflex. However, the identification of such patients is important because most can be managed without pacemakers.

Prevention

Prevention of heart block is a challenge for the future. Some instances can be prevented by treatment of inflammatory disorders that cause heart block, such as Lyme disease or cardiac sarcoid. Other individuals who should be identified are those with conditions that place them, their relatives, or their unborn children at risk for heart block. This includes patients and family members with genetic disorders associated with heart block. Genetic testing and counseling may be appropriate in some patients with a family history of CCD. Pacemaker therapy may be indicated in some patients with neuromuscular disorders, in particular myotonic dystrophy or Kearns-Sayre syndrome, in the presence of CCD that would be considered low-grade in other individuals. Neonatal lupus syndrome is a rare disorder with a high mortality rate and risk of permanent complete heart block in survivors. This occurs in pregnant women with anti-Ro/SSA or anti-La/SSB antibodies. Some such women have autoimmune disorders such as systemic lupus erythematosus and Sjögren's syndrome, but many are symptom free. Members of this group may benefit from counseling and anticipatory evaluation and treatment of offspring. Although controversial, fetal monitoring of pregnant women with anti-Ro/SSA and/or anti-La/SSB antibodies and treatment of those with signs of fetal conduction system involvement have been recommended. It should be recognized that with current methods the vast majority of heart block events cannot be predicted or prevented, and the vast majority of persons with risk factors never develop symptomatic heart block.

Clinical Manifestations

Most of the symptoms experienced by patients with heart block are common and nonspecific, including syncope, lightheadedness, fatigue, and dyspnea. Asystole or profound bradycardia may cause syncope, death, or other manifestations of hypoperfusion. Rarely, first-degree AV block results in significant symptoms (e.g., fatigue, palpitations, chest fullness), probably due to atrial contraction against a partially closed mitral valve.

Diagnosis

Because various arrhythmias and other cardiac and noncardiac disorders may be responsible for similar symptoms, it is important to identify the cause. An ECG recording of asystole or bradycardia due to heart block at the time of symptoms strongly suggests a causal relationship, but this is usually difficult to accomplish because the symptoms are often transient and infrequent. Absence of arrhythmias at the time of symptoms is also helpful in excluding heart block as the cause. Asymptomatic heart block is not infrequent. Cardiac conduction disturbances are classified by the pattern of ECG complexes. A normal 12-lead ECG lessens the probability of conduction disturbances due to structural changes but it does not eliminate the possibility of transient third-degree block due to reversible functional effects such as intense vagal activity or ischemia. Significant disease of the His bundle may be electrocardiographically silent, but more often concomitant distal disease is evident in the form of fascicular or bundle branch block or a nonspecific intraventricular conduction delay. In a patient with syncope, the presence of bifascicular block raises the possibility of transient third-degree block as the mechanism and of progression to permanent complete block. Most patients with conduction disorders are not symptomatic and do not progress to complete block. However, the combination of right bundle branch block (RBBB) and left posterior fascicle block has a greater tendency to progress to complete block than the more common RBBB and left anterior fascicle block. Nevertheless, conduction disturbances of the His-Purkinje system should not be assumed to be responsible for syncope or cardiac arrest because they are relatively common in patients with cardiovascular disorders that cause syncope or cardiac arrest due to other mechanisms. Conduction disturbances can cause dyssynchronous contraction and result in adverse remodeling. In addition, they can mask or mimic the ECG signs of myocardial infarction. Alternating bundle branch block refers to a changing ECG pattern in which both RBBB and left bundle branch block are observed or when the bifascicular block pattern switches between the anterior and posterior fascicle involvement. This pattern is considered a harbinger of complete block and warrants continuous monitoring and evaluation for permanent pacemaker implantation.

Differential Diagnosis

The challenge in second- and transient third-degree AV block is distinguishing between block in the AV node, which is often functional and reversible, and infranodal block, which often progresses to permanent complete heart block. ECG clues that block is in the AV node include normal QRS duration (<100 ms), type I (Wenckebach) pattern, PR prolongation before blocked impulses and PR shortening after pauses, occurrence during enhanced vagal activity (e.g., sleep), narrow QRS escape complexes, and no factors favoring infranodal block. ECG clues for infranodal block include prolonged QRS duration (≥120 ms), type II pattern, and escape QRS complexes broader than intrinsic complexes. Type II second degree AV block is almost always due to block in the His-Purkinje system. Other second-degree AV block ECG patterns have poor sensitivity and specificity for site of block.

Unsustained polymorphic ventricular tachycardia is an ominous sign in any context and may result from a variety of cardiac, metabolic, and autonomic abnormalities. However, in the presence of heart block it suggests that heart rate support may be necessary to prevent sustained VTA. QT prolongation and postpause U-wave accentuation should be sought as other harbingers of bradycardia-related VTA.

The importance and value of ECG documentation of heart block cannot be overemphasized. ECGs are subject to artifact and may be misleading when standards for acquisition and analysis are not followed. Multiple tracings of suspicious events should be obtained in multiple leads when possible. A 12-lead simultaneous rhythm recording mode is available on most modern ECG machines and should be used when continuous recordings are obtained to document arrhythmias.

Clinicians encounter heart block in three general contexts. For the patient with documented heart block, the clinician selects therapy based, in part, on whether the arrhythmia is permanent or likely to recur. There are currently no tests that provide direct information about the pathologic state of the AV conduction system. Instead, these outcomes must be inferred from functional assessment, that is, from the ECG or electrophysiological testing. Other indirect sources such as coronary angiography, magnetic resonance imaging, nuclear imaging, and myocardial biopsy, as well as a large number of specific laboratory tests, are often helpful for identifying disorders that may be causative or associated with heart block and that may affect the choice of treatment.

Another common context is the patient with symptoms for whom the objective is to verify or exclude heart block as the mechanism by correlating the cardiac rhythm with symptoms. Real-time monitoring (e.g., in-patient telemetry) is used for patients who might require immediate access to drugs or pacing devices to prevent or terminate asystole or bradycardia-dependent VTA. Holter monitoring is useful for patients who have very frequent events (at least 1 every 24 hours), and they are useful for capturing asymptomatic rhythm disturbances. External recorders are applied for a month or longer and are very helpful to associate rhythm abnormalities with symptoms and to rule out a rhythm disorder as the cause of symptoms in patients with at least one event per month. Patients with infrequent events may be candidates for implantable loop recorders, which monitor for greater than a year. Modern monitors will provide a permanent record of arrhythmias on activation by the patient or by a detection algorithm.

Electrophysiological studies allow precise measurements of AV node and His-Purkinje system function and can provide definitive information regarding the site of block if the conduction disturbance occurs during the study. Additional tests have been developed that "stress" the AV conduction system, including rapid atrial and ventricular pacing and administration of drugs such as procainamide and disopyramide (Norpace). The provocation of heart block is assumed to indicate a propensity for spontaneous AV block. Unfortunately, the sensitivity is low and a negative test does not imply a low risk of future episodes. Electrophysiological studies have the additional advantage of providing immediate test results, as well as providing the results of programmed stimulation for provocation of supraventricular and VTAs, which may be included in the differential diagnosis.

Therapy

The object of the evaluation and management for heart block is to prevent death and morbidity by (1) heart rate support in patients with poorly tolerated bradycardia; (2) monitoring and standby heart rate support in patients at high risk for asystole or severe bradycardia; (3) identifying and treating reversible causes of heart block; (4) identifying patients at high risk for sudden death, syncope, or recurrent symptoms; and (5) selecting and implanting the appropriate rate support system as soon as safety permits.

Advanced cardiac life-support guidelines apply to the patient who is unresponsive or severely compromised by heart block. However, heart block is rarely the primary problem. Therefore evaluation and treatment of other disorders should continue while efforts to obtain the appropriate heart rate are underway.

The initial evaluation should include a detailed history and physical examination and review of current and previous ECGs and rhythm strips to determine whether heart block is present or occurred in the past and whether there were symptoms or other evidence of hemodynamic compromise. Basic laboratory tests (electrolytes, metabolic panel, cardiac biomarkers, thyroid function, blood count, and coagulation studies) and basic imaging (chest x-ray and echocardiography) are usually appropriate. The patient should then be stratified for the appropriate level of care: (1) the unstable patient who requires ongoing evaluation and treatment in an intensive care setting, (2) the stable patient at high risk for asystole or complications who needs temporary transvenous pacing or other invasive procedures, (3) the patient at moderate risk who requires continuous monitoring and standby noninvasive heart rate support measures, (4) the patient at low risk who requires rapid but not immediate access to heart rate support measures that hospital monitoring provides, and (5) the patient at low risk who can be evaluated and managed as an outpatient. Additional testing and procedures may be necessary to determine the etiology of heart block and to determine whether there is a significant risk of future adverse events.

Determination of the need for long-term heart rate support, as well as other issues that may affect implantable device selection (e.g., risk for VTAs), should be accomplished as soon as possible because the risk of complications and anxiety associated with temporary heart rate support measures increases over time. Major societies have developed guidelines for implantable rhythm management devices (http://www.cardiosource.org/Science-And-Quality/Practice-Guidelines-and-Quality-Standards.aspx; http://www.escardio.org/guidelines-surveys/esc-guidelines/Pages/GuidelinesList.aspx). The reasons for the selected therapy, including the rationale for any deviation from established guidelines, should be documented and provided to the patient. This will reduce future confusion or misunderstanding about the original rationale for implantation that can affect management of patients with device complications, recalls (safety alerts), and those with a compelling need for device upgrade or explantation.

Patients with acute coronary syndromes require special consideration. The incidence of heart block in patients with myocardial infarction based on creatine phosphokinase as the marker of necrosis is approximately 10%. Although the incidence is probably lower using more sensitive markers such as troponin, heart block is still likely to be associated with increased in-hospital mortality due to larger infarct size. Tachycardia and high blood pressure increase myocardial oxygen consumption. Therefore overcorrection of heart rate and blood pressure should be avoided and ischemia should be relieved by reperfusion as soon as possible. Studies in the prethrombolytic era did not demonstrate a benefit in mortality with prophylactic temporary transvenous pacing, and complications were frequent. The risks of transvenous insertion may be higher in patients requiring administration of thrombolytics and other anticoagulants. Catheter-based revascularization methods should be given strong consideration because of established effectiveness, the possible avoidance of thrombolytic drugs, and because transvenous temporary pacing, if needed, is readily and safely accomplished during the procedure. Suggestions for standby temporary pacing (Table 3) should take into consideration the risks of transvenous pacing based on local circumstances (experience, fluoroscopic guidance, insertion site, use of anticoagulants, etc.). Most conduction

TABLE 3	Suggestions for Temporary Pacing in Acute Myocardial Infarction

- Transvenous pacing
  - Asystole or poorly tolerated bradycardia unresponsive to atropine or aminophylline
  - Persistent third-degree AV block
  - Alternating RBBB and LBBB, or RBBB and alternating LAFB and LPFB
  - Bifascicular block, new
  - Second-degree AV block (any type) and QRS >110 ms
  - Any indication listed below at time of cardiac catheterization if performed
- Standby transcutaneous pacing
  - Any indication listed above until transvenous pacing system inserted
  - Transient asystole or poorly tolerated bradycardia
  - Bifascicular block, uncertain time of onset, or old
  - Second-degree AV block (any type) and QRS <110 ms
  - New first-degree AV block

Abbreviations: AV = atrioventricular; LAFB, LPFB=left anterior, left posterior fascicle block; LBBB, RBBB=left, right bundle branch block.

disturbances associated with myocardial ischemia or infarction resolve quickly but can persist for days or weeks. The need for permanent pacemaker implantation as a consequence of myocardial infarction is rare, and prophylactic pacemaker implantation in high-risk subsets has not been shown to reduce mortality. Guidelines for temporary and permanent pacing in acute myocardial infarction have been published (http://www.cardiosource.org/Science-And-Quality/Practice-Guidelines-and-Quality-Standards.aspx; http://www.escardio.org/guidelines-surveys/esc-guidelines/Pages/GuidelinesList.aspx).

Selection of the correct therapeutic approach balances the risks and benefits of therapy against the risks of heart block for both immediate and long-term management. Catecholamines (dobutamine, dopamine, epinephrine, isoproterenol [Isuprel]) are useful for emergency, temporary, and standby heart rate support. The standby mode is accomplished by a prepared infusion at the bedside. To avoid underdoses or overdoses at the time of sudden symptomatic heart block, the optimal dose can be established in advance by test doses starting at low infusion rates. Atropine (0.5 mg every 3–5 minutes, with a maximum dose of 0.04 mg/kg or total of 3 mg) may be useful for treatment or pretreatment of patients who develop heart block at the level of the AV node in the context of elevated vagal tone (e.g., in association with nausea or endotracheal tube suction). Atropine should be avoided in patients with infranodal AV block because prolonged asystole sometimes occurs due to more frequent His-Purkinje system depolarization from increased sinus rate. Vagal activity inhibits sympathetic activity; therefore, reduction of vagal tone by atropine disinhibits sympathetic activity and may account for the unpredictable effects of atropine on heart rate. Elevations in heart rate after atropine can persist for hours and cannot be readily reversed. Aminophylline[1] (2.5–6.3 mg/kg IV) is reported to reverse heart block resistant to atropine and epinephrine by antagonizing adenosine. Stimulation of β-adrenergic receptors increases sinus node and subsidiary pacemaker rates, AV node and His-Purkinje system conduction velocities, and myocardial contractility. The effective refractory period shortens in most tissue but this effect varies with dose and specific tissue type. Dobutamine[1] (2–40 μg/kg/min) is a useful β-receptor agonist because it increases cardiac output and lowers filling pressures without excessive rise or fall of blood pressure. Dopamine[1] (2–20 μg/kg/min IV) stimulates β_1-adrenergic receptors and increases heart rate by enhancing impulse formation and

conduction, as well as myocardial contractility. At higher doses (10–20 μg/kg/min) dopamine causes vasoconstriction by α_1-receptor stimulation. Isoproterenol (0.02–0.06 mg IV bolus, 0.5–10.0 μg/min IV infusion) stimulates β_1- and β_2-adrenergic receptors and enhances vasodilation more than the other catecholamines. This can result in unwanted hypotension in some circumstances but it is also less likely to cause a reflex increase in vagal tone than drugs that cause vasoconstriction. Epinephrine (1 mg IV boluses for cardiac arrest, 0.2–1 mg subcutaneously, 0.5–10 μg/min IV) stimulates both α- and β-adrenergic receptors. It is recommended for asystolic cardiac arrest in part because it increases myocardial and cerebral flow. However, the increase of systemic vascular resistance may be detrimental by augmenting metabolic acidosis and decreasing cardiac performance in patients with poor left ventricular function. The suggested dose ranges are broad because the response to β-adrenergic stimulants such as improved AV conduction varies widely and may be affected by β-adrenergic receptor down-regulation in patients with chronic elevations in sympathetic activity such as patients with long-standing heart failure.

Temporary pacing includes primarily transcutaneous and transvenous approaches. Transthoracic, transesophageal, and transgastric approaches are rarely used. Transcutaneous pacing provides noninvasive heart rate support, as well as immediate access to countershock, but it is often so painful that most patients require sedation. For these reasons its principal uses are for short-term pacing during cardiopulmonary resuscitation and standby pacing in patients at risk for bradyarrhythmias. Capture is not achieved in some patients. Therefore users should be ready to continue mechanical cardiopulmonary support and seek alternative methods. If used in standby applications, ventricular capture should be verified in advance. Capture is often difficult to ascertain because transcutaneous stimuli cause large deflections on the ECG, and pectoral muscle stimulation can be confused with a pulse. Capture should be verified by careful ECG analysis at subthreshold and suprathreshold stimulus amplitudes and confirmed by appropriately timed femoral artery pulses, Korotkoff sounds, or arterial pressure waveforms.

Transvenous insertion of an electrode catheter is the method of choice for most patients who require temporary pacing. This approach is reliable and safe when performed by competent staff with strict aseptic technique, fluoroscopic guidance, and appropriate catheters. Small studies suggest that long-term (>5 days) temporary pacing can be accomplished with active-fixation permanent pacemaker leads attached to an external pulse generator (not approved by the US Food and Drug Administration [FDA]). Tunneling the lead may enhance stability and reduce the risk of infection.

Monitoring

Patients with high-grade or symptomatic heart block require close monitoring until the process is reversed by treatment or a pacemaker is implanted. All patients who receive pacemakers require lifelong follow-up by a trained team of physicians, nurses, and ancillary personnel using standard procedures guided by practice guidelines and manufacturer recommendations.

Complications

Catecholamines used to increase heart rate may precipitate tachyarrhythmias by electrophysiological effects mediated by adrenergic receptors or by myocardial ischemia, and they may worsen hemodynamic status. The adverse effects of catecholamines increase with duration of exposure. Ischemia and receptor-mediated electrophysiologic effects occur immediately after administration; changes in gene expression of ion channels begin as early as several hours; and long-term changes such as myocardial hypertrophy, apoptosis, and fibrosis occur within 24 hours and may progress over much longer periods. This suggests that the duration and dose of catecholamine

[1] Not FDA approved for this indication.

infusions should be minimized. Complications of temporary transvenous pacing include inadequate pacing or sensing thresholds, vascular complications, pneumothorax, myocardial perforation, infection, and dislodgment. Permanent pacemakers are highly effective, safe, and cost-effective with few contraindications. Although the complications are rarely life threatening, they should be carefully considered and acknowledged. Septicemia or endocarditis has been reported in 0.5% of patients. In patients with pacemaker-related endocarditis, the in-hospital mortality rate is reported to be over 7% with a 20-month mortality rate over 25%. The rate of significant complications has been reported to be 3.5%. About 10% of pacemakers will become infected or develop some other type of failure that may require extraction. In a recent series the rate of major complications associated with extraction was 1.4%. There is a long-term continuous risk of infection, thrombosis, and erosion. In young persons there is a periodic need to replace generators and leads. Abandoned leads block venous access and extractions are associated with significant risks. Perhaps of greater consequence is the constant inconvenience of lifelong follow-up, electromagnetic interference, and false alarms from electronic surveillance devices, as well as exclusion from important procedures, such as magnetic resonance imaging of the thorax. Conventional pacing, that is, from the right ventricular apex, is now known to be detrimental and may cause adverse ventricular remodeling, atrial fibrillation, heart failure, and premature death. Although it has been shown that patients with reduced left ventricular function are at greater risk for adverse effects, it is not known how to identify other patients at risk. Strategies for reducing the adverse effects of conventional pacing are under study, and recommendations are evolving. Because the decision for pacemaker implantation includes selection of lead configuration, lead locations, and pacing mode, patient guidance and education are complex.

Conclusions

Heart block remains a challenge because the cellular mechanisms responsible are poorly understood, prediction of symptomatic heart block (who and when) is unreliable, treatments that restore normal conduction do not exist for most conditions, and pacemaker therapy can have significant long-term adverse consequences. Fortunately, innovations and technological advances such as leadless pacemakers and conduction system pacing have expanded options for personalized therapy, and remote monitoring has enhanced early detection of problems and has reduced the inconvenience of device monitoring. Ongoing clinical trials will provide guidance in pacemaker configurations and programming that will minimize adverse effects. In the future, achievements in molecular biology will elucidate mechanisms and produce treatments that will relegate artificial pacemakers to museum pieces.

References

Diederichsen SZ, Xing LY, Frodi DM. Prevalence and prognostic significance of bradyarrhythmias in patients screened for atrial fibrillation vs usual care: post hoc analysis of the LOOP randomized clinical trial. *JAMA Cardiol.* 8(4):326-334, 2023.
Glikson M, Nielsen JC, Kronborg MB, et al. 2021 ESC Guidelines on cardiac pacing and cardiac resynchronization therapy. *Eur Heart J.* 42:3427, 2021.
Groh WJ, Bhakta D, Tomaselli GF, et al. 2022 HRS expert consensus statement on evaluation and management of arrhythmic risk in neuromuscular disorders. *Heart Rhythm.* 19: e61, 2022.
Kusumoto FM, Schoenfeld MH, Barrett C, et al. 2018 ACC/AHA/HRS guideline on the evaluation and management of patients with bradycardia and cardiac conduction delay. *J Am Coll Cardiol.* 74: 932, 2019.
Priori SG, Wilde AA, Horie M, et al., HRS/EHRA/APHRS expert consensus statement on the diagnosis and management of patients with inherited primary arrhythmia syndromes. *Heart Rhythm.* 10: 1932, 2013.
Shah MJ, Silka MJ, Silva JNA, et al. 2021 PACES expert consensus statement on the indications and management of cardiovascular implantable electronic devices in pediatric patients. *Heart Rhythm.* 18:1888, 2021.

HYPERTENSION

Method of
Timothy P. Graham, MD

CURRENT DIAGNOSIS

- Screening should begin at 18 years of age for the general population per U.S. Preventive Services Task Force (USPSTF) recommendations. The screening interval for those 18 to 39 years of age without other risk factors is every 3 to 5 years. For those older than 40 years of age or those with risk factors, annual screening is recommended.
- Stage 1 hypertension is established at blood pressures of 140 mm Hg systolic and 90 mm Hg diastolic if measured in the office, but 135 mm Hg systolic and 85 mm Hg diastolic if based on ambulatory monitoring per Eighth Joint National Committee (JNC 8) and International Society of Hypertension (ISH) guidelines. The AHA/ACC defines stage I hypertension as at or above 130 mm Hg systolic and at or above 80 mm Hg diastolic.
- Stage 2 hypertension is established at blood pressures of 160 mm Hg systolic and 100 mm Hg diastolic per JNC 8 and ISH guidelines. The American College of Cardiology/American Heart Association (ACC/AHA) defines stage 2 hypertension as at or above 140 mm Hg systolic and at or above 90 diastolic.
- Secondary causes of hypertension should be explored and identified to optimize treatment when there is suboptimal response to treatment, worsening hypertension control, no family history of hypertension, onset of hypertension in patients less than 20 years or older than 50 years.

CURRENT THERAPY

- Initial interventions, regardless of stage, should include lifestyle modifications, including low-sodium diet and exercise.
- Optimal pharmacologic therapy should be tailored to account for age, race, and the presence or absence of chronic kidney disease.
- For individuals 60 years of age and older, consider initiation of pharmacotherapy when systolic blood pressure is 150 mm Hg and diastolic blood pressure is 90 mm Hg.
- For individuals younger than 60 years of age but at least 18 years of age, pharmacotherapy should be initiated when systolic blood pressure is 140 mm Hg and diastolic blood pressure is 90 mm Hg.
- First-line agents for nonblack individuals should include thiazide-type diuretics, calcium channel blockers, angiotensin-converting enzyme inhibitors (ACEIs), or angiotensin receptor blockers (ARBs).
- First-line agents for black individuals should include thiazide-type diuretics or calcium channel blockers.
- Individuals with chronic kidney disease should have therapy that includes ACEIs or ARBs.

Epidemiology

Hypertension is one of the most common conditions encountered in primary care offices. According to the AHA/ACC definition of hypertension, hypertension affects 47% of adults in the United States, which represents approximately 116 million people (cdc.gov). The most commonly affected individuals are black adults, with approximately 56% affected.

In the pediatric population, the prevalence of hypertension in the United States is approximately 2.6% (representing nearly 800,000 children), with nearly one-half of this number being classified as obese (body mass index [BMI] >95%).

Risk Factors

Diet and Sodium Intake

Diet is a clear target for nonpharmacologic management of hypertension. Diets that are high in sodium and fat can put individuals at risk for suboptimal blood pressure control. Limiting sodium to less than 2400 mg per day confers some health benefit to individuals at risk for hypertension. Limiting sodium even further to 1500 mg or less is more ideal and typically results in a significant improvement in both systolic and diastolic blood pressure. Additionally, putting limits on the consumption of sweets, red meat, and soda as well as other sugar-sweetened beverages can help weight reduction and overall health.

Sedentary Lifestyle and Obesity

Lack of physical activity is another important risk factor contributing to poor overall health and obesity. Current recommendations endorse engaging in at least 150 minutes of moderate-intensity activity per week. If patients are unable or unwilling to commit to that level of physical activity, then encouraging any physical activity is prudent, as it will convey at least some health benefit. Participation in physical activity results in absolute reduction in chronic comorbidities including hypertension, stroke, heart disease, diabetes, and metabolic syndrome. Resultant weight loss also results in significant improvement in blood pressure. It is noted that a weight loss of 22 pounds has the potential to reduce systolic blood pressure by 5 to 20 mm Hg.

For children and adolescents, elevated BMI is the greatest risk factor for the development of hypertension.

Alcohol Intake

Although moderate alcohol intake is thought to actually reduce cardiovascular risk, heavier consumption is a risk factor for hypertension. Limiting alcohol intake to no more than two drinks per day (with a *drink* defined as 12 oz. of beer, 5 oz. of wine, or 1 oz. of liquor) for men and no more than one drink per day for women (or lightweight men) is beneficial for overall health.

Smoking

Along with the myriad other reasons that tobacco smoking is not a good choice (e.g., cancer risk, chronic obstructive pulmonary disease, stroke, coronary artery disease), it is also a risk factor for hypertension. This is believed to be at least in part caused by a resultant increase in sympathetic nervous system activity, which leads to an increase in myocardial oxygen demand. Additionally, smoking is the leading modifiable cause of death in the United States.

Of note, the use of marijuana results in an increased risk of hypertension-related death. The magnitude of this increase is estimated to be 3.42-fold higher in marijuana users than in non-users. Risk also further increases with each year of use.

Sleep Apnea

Obstructive sleep apnea is a well-known secondary cause of and independent risk factor for hypertension. Statistically, at least one-half of individuals with sleep apnea also have hypertension.

Age

Age is a nonmodifiable risk factor for cardiovascular disease. Risk is higher in men 55 years of age or older and women 65 years of age or older.

Gender

Gender is another nonmodifiable risk factor. Men are at greater risk for hypertension before 45 years of age. After 45 years of age and until 64 years of age, the risk for men and women is approximately equivalent. At 65 years of age and older, women have a higher hypertensive risk than men.

Race

Black individuals have a prevalence of hypertension than non-black individuals. Statistics from 2019 demonstrated that approximately 56.8% of black men and 57.6% of black women have hypertension compared with approximately 52.7% of white men and 45.4% of white women. Asians had a lower prevalence, at approximately 49.4% of men and 43.6% of women. Hispanic/Latino individuals had an even lower prevalence than white individuals at 46% of men and 35.4% of women.

Family History

Family history is another nonmodifiable risk factor for cardiovascular disease. Individuals with family history of premature cardiovascular disease (men younger than 45 years of age and women younger than 55 years of age) are at increased risk themselves.

Pathophysiology

The pathophysiology of hypertension is a matter of debate. *Essential hypertension*, which is defined as hypertension without a clear secondary cause, makes up the majority of cases. Two primary mechanisms have been proposed for essential hypertension: neurogenic and renogenic (or nephrogenic). The neurogenic model suggests that hypertension is the result of a chronic increase in sympathetic nervous system activity. This is in contrast with the renogenic model, which attributes blood pressure increase to renal origins either through decreased renal blood flow or through renal parenchymal disease.

Prevention

Prevention of hypertension involves optimization of modifiable risk factors. Maintaining a healthy body weight, avoiding smoking, and moderating alcohol use are all key factors in minimizing risk. Additionally, engaging in regular, moderate-intensity cardiovascular exercise and eating a healthy diet without excessive sodium or fat can help significantly reduce cardiovascular risk and optimize health. These risk factors were discussed in detail in the preceding section.

Clinical Manifestations

Hypertension may have very few symptoms or none at all. If symptoms are present, they can include headaches, visual changes, dizziness, nausea, or chest pain. Oftentimes, however, there are no symptoms, and individuals can function for years without being diagnosed.

Diagnosis

Screening

As noted previously, hypertension is oftentimes an asymptomatic condition. As such, screening plays a critical role in early detection to minimize the end-organ damage that could result from untreated, long-standing hypertension. The U.S. Preventive Services Task Force (USPSTF) recommends screening for hypertension in adults who are 18 years of age or older (grade A recommendation). Adults 40 years of age and older and those with increased risk of hypertension should be screened annually. A review of the existing evidence demonstrated minimal harm in screening and a significant resultant benefit in the form of a reduction in cardiovascular disease–related events. Adults 18 to 39 years of age with no additional risk factors should be screened every 3 to 5 years. Recommended screening techniques include measurement of blood pressure in the office setting with either a manual or automatic cuff and ambulatory or home blood pressure measurement. Office measurement should be done with the patient seated and after at least 5 minutes of the patient arriving in the room. Home measurement may be beneficial after the initial screening for confirmation purposes.

For children and adolescents, the USPSTF indicates that the current evidence is insufficient to assess the risk versus benefit of screening in asymptomatic individuals (grade I evidence). The predictive value of childhood hypertension for adult hypertension is modest, with a risk for false-positive readings.

Clinical Diagnosis

Hypertension is classified into two stages based on degree of elevation. In stage 1 hypertension, systolic blood pressure is greater than or equal to 140 mm Hg to 159 mm Hg, and diastolic blood pressure is greater than or equal to 90 mm Hg to 99 mm Hg. Stage 2 hypertension is reached when systolic blood pressure is 160 mm Hg or greater and diastolic blood pressure is 100 mm Hg or greater. Per the 2021 International Society of Hypertension (ISH) guidelines, the setting where the blood pressure is measured affects the threshold for the diagnosis of hypertension. According to the ISH, the above threshold of 140/90 mm Hg applies to the office setting, whereas for home readings, 135/85 should be used. If relying on 24-hour ambulatory monitoring, the thresholds are 130/80 mm Hg when looking at 24-hour average readings, 135/85 mm Hg for daytime average, and 120/70 mm Hg for nighttime average. Also of note, the AHA released a statement in 2017 recommending a change in definition for stage 1 hypertension to greater than or equal to 130/80 mm Hg. The classification and definition is important as the approach to treatment differs for each category, as will be discussed later.

Primary (Essential) Hypertension

Primary hypertension encompasses persistent blood pressure elevation without a discernible cause (idiopathic or of unknown cause). The majority of cases of hypertension will have no discernible cause and fall into this category.

Secondary Hypertension

Secondary hypertension is persistent blood pressure elevation that is the result of some other underlying cause. About 10% of all cases of hypertension will fall into this category. If another cause can be identified, in many cases it may be correctable.

Looking for Secondary Causes

Identifying these underlying causes can be a challenge. Using a systematic method of investigating potential etiologies can simplify this process and improve the chances of identifying a source that with treatment can improve outcomes. One such approach is the *ABCDE* mnemonic. The letter *A* in this mnemonic stands for *accuracy* (making sure the reading is correct—such as checking the cuff for appropriate sizing and measurement technique—and repeating readings that are obtained on automatic cuffs manually). Readings on home monitors may be different from office-based readings for a variety of reasons, such as the effects of "white coat hypertension," *apnea* (considering the presence of obstructive sleep apnea, which is a known contributor to difficult-to-control hypertension), and *aldosteronism* (investigating for the presence of primary hyperaldosteronism through urinary potassium excretion and an elevation in plasma aldosterone level to plasma renin activity). The letter *B* stands for *bruits* (looking for renovascular sources of hypertension/renal artery stenosis, which often presents with renal bruits upon auscultation) and *bad kidneys* (hypertension resulting from renal parenchymal disease). The letter *C* stands for *catecholamines* (elevation that can contribute to "white coat" hypertension as well as overproduction with pheochromocytoma or associated with other conditions such as obstructive sleep apnea and acute stress reactions), *coarctation* (of the aorta), and *Cushing syndrome* (with mineralocorticoid effects of excess glucocorticoids in this setting). The letter *D* represents both *drugs* (including nonsteroidal antiinflammatory drugs, decongestants, estrogens, immunosuppressive agents, as well as nicotine and alcohol) and *diet* (particularly excess sodium intake). The final letter in the mnemonic, *E*, stands for *erythropoietin* (high endogenous levels—such as in chronic obstructive pulmonary disease—or exogenous levels) and *endocrine disorders* (hypothyroidism or hyperparathyroidism). Utilizing a methodical and organized approach to considering potential causes of hypertension can assist with maximizing the chances of optimally controlling blood pressure.

Differential Diagnosis

The differential diagnosis for hypertension coincides with the array of potential secondary causes that were noted earlier (see the "Looking for Secondary Causes" section earlier in this chapter). It is important to rule out potentially treatable secondary causes in the initial phases of hypertension management.

Treatment Approaches

Approaching treatment of a patient with hypertension can be challenging. Many factors must be considered when making these decisions, including reflection on patient age, race, gender, and comorbidities. Each of these factors can influence what the optimal treatment strategy might be. Figure 1 provides a stepwise strategy to blood pressure management.

Initial treatment should always include lifestyle modification as discussed previously, and this modification must be continued throughout the remainder of any management strategies.

JNC 8 Guidelines

In 2014, the Eighth Joint National Committee (JNC 8) released recommendations regarding the treatment of hypertension. These guidelines were a divergence from the prior JNC 7 recommendations, effectively loosening the goals and the levels at which treatment is initiated. The following is a summary of the eight treatment recommendations from JNC 8. (Please note that the strength of recommendation that is referenced corresponds to the following: grade A—strong recommendation based on evidence; grade B—moderate recommendation based on evidence; grade C—weak recommendation with moderate certainty of a small benefit; grade D—recommendation against; grade E—expert opinion with insufficient or conflicting evidence; grade N—no recommendation for or against).

Recommendation 1

Individuals 60 years of age or older in the general population should have pharmacologic treatment initiated at a systolic blood pressure level of 150 mm Hg or a diastolic blood pressure of 90 mm Hg with treatment goals of less than 150 mm Hg systolic and less than 90 mm Hg diastolic. (Strength of recommendation: grade A.)

An additional aspect of this recommendation is that if the pharmacologic treatment results in adequate blood pressure reduction and there is no adverse effect on quality of life or patient health, then the treatment can be continued without alteration. (Strength of recommendation: grade E.)

Recommendation 2

Individuals younger than 60 years of age in the general population should have pharmacologic treatment initiated at a diastolic blood pressure of 90 mm Hg with a treatment goal of less than 90 mm Hg. (Strength of recommendation: grade A for 30 to 59 years of age, grade E for 18 to 29 years of age.)

Recommendation 3

Individuals younger than 60 years of age in the general population should have pharmacologic treatment initiated at a systolic blood pressure of 140 mm Hg with a treatment goal of less than 140 mm Hg. (Strength of recommendation: grade E.)

Recommendation 4

Individuals 18 years of age or older with chronic kidney disease should have pharmacologic treatment initiated at a systolic blood pressure of 140 mm Hg or a diastolic blood pressure of 90 mm Hg with treatment goals of less than 140 mm Hg systolic and less than 90 mm Hg diastolic. (Strength of recommendation: grade E.)

Recommendation 5

Individuals older than 18 years of age with diabetes should have pharmacologic treatment initiated at a systolic blood pressure of 140 mm Hg or a diastolic blood pressure of 90 mm Hg with a treatment goal of less than 140 mm Hg systolic and less than 90 mm Hg diastolic. (Strength of recommendation: grade E.)

Recommendation 6

The treatment of nonblack individuals in the general population (including those with diabetes) who require pharmacologic treatment should include thiazide-type diuretics, calcium channel blockers,

Stage 1 Hypertension
(blood pressure, 140–159/90–99 mm Hg)

Stage 2 Hypertension
(blood pressure, ≥160/100 mm Hg)

Step 1

Lifestyle modification
Alcohol restriction
DASH diet
Exercise
Salt reduction
Weight control

Two-drug regimen for most
patients plus lifestyle
modification
ACE inhibitor
ARB
β-blocker
Calcium-channel blocker
Diuretic

Step 2

Single drug treatment
ACE inhibitor
ARB
Calcium-channel blocker
Diuretic

Add third drug of different class
Assess adherence
Optimize doses

Control other
cardiovascular disease
risk factors

Step 3

Add second drug of different class
ACE inhibitor
ARB
β-blocker
Calcium-channel blocker
Diuretic

Add fourth drug of different class
Assess alcoholic excess
Assess salt retention

Step 4

Add third drug of different class
Assess adherence
Optimize doses

Evaluate for secondary hypertension

Compelling indications	Drug treatment
Post-myocardial infarction	ACE inhibitor, β-blocker
Angina pectoris	β-blocker, calcium-channel blocker
Heart failure	ACE inhibitor, ARB, β-blocker, diuretic, aldosterone antagonist
Chronic renal disease	ACE inhibitor, ARB
Diabetes	ACE inhibitor, ARB, and others
High coronary heart disease risk	ACE inhibitor, ARB, β-blocker, calcium-channel blocker, diuretic

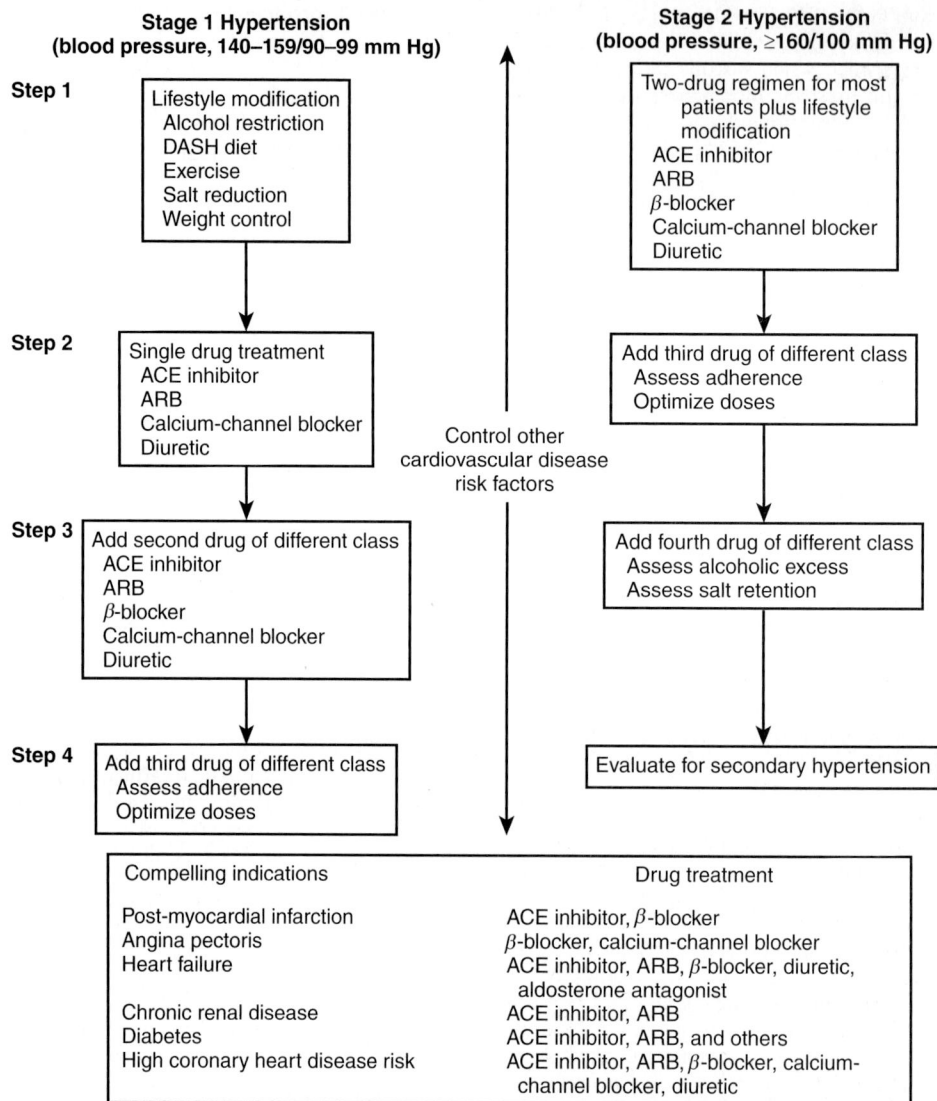

Figure 1 Algorithm for management of hypertension. *ACE*, Angiotensin-converting enzyme; *ARB*, angiotensin receptor blocker; *DASH*, Dietary Approaches to Stop Hypertension. (From Chobanian AV. Shattuck Lecture. The hypertension paradox—More uncontrolled disease despite improved therapy. *N Engl J Med* 2009;361:878–887.

angiotensin-converting enzyme inhibitors (ACEIs), or angiotensin receptor blockers (ARBs). (Strength of recommendation: grade B.)

Recommendation 7
The treatment of black individuals (including those with diabetes) should include thiazide-type diuretics or calcium channel blockers. (Strength of recommendation: grade B for the general population, grade C for patients with diabetes.)

Recommendation 8
The treatment of individuals older than 18 years of age with chronic kidney disease should include, either as initial or add-on treatment, ACEIs or ARBs to improve renal outcomes. (Strength of recommendation: grade B.)

Recommendation 9
The goal of hypertension treatment is to reach and maintain blood pressure goals consistent with the previous recommendations. If goals are not reached within 1 month of starting pharmacologic treatment, the dose of the initial agent should be increased, or a second agent from recommendation 6 should be added. Blood pressure should continue to be assessed until the goal blood pressure is achieved. If blood pressure goals are not achieved with two agents, a third agent should be added.
- ACEIs and ARBs should not be used together.
- If necessary, other classes of agents can be used if more than

three agents are required or if there are contraindications to the agents in recommendation 6.
- Referral to a hypertension specialist should be considered for patients whose blood pressure goals cannot be met with the previous strategies or patients who are more complicated. (Strength of recommendation: grade E.)

ACC/AHA 2017 Hypertension Guidelines
In late 2017, the ACC/AHA released an updated hypertension guideline. This guideline provided a different approach to hypertension management, particularly around blood pressure goals. Hypertension stages have tighter cut points than under the JNC 8 guidelines. Under the ACC/AHA guidelines, normal blood pressure is defined as less than 120/80 mm Hg. Blood pressure is considered elevated when systolic blood pressure is in the 120 to 129 mm Hg range and when diastolic blood pressure remains under 80 mm Hg. Stage 1 hypertension is defined as systolic blood pressure between 130 and 139 mm Hg and diastolic blood pressure between 80 and 90 mm Hg. Stage 2 hypertension is defined as blood pressures that are greater than 140/90. This classification is a deviation from the set points within the JNC 8 recommendations.

Nonpharmacologic
For stage 1 hypertension (140 to 159 mm Hg systolic/90 to 99 mm Hg diastolic), the first treatment step is aggressive lifestyle

TABLE 1	Effect of Lifestyle and Diet Modifications on Systolic Blood Pressure		
MODIFICATION	**AMOUNT**	**REDUCTION IN SBP (mm Hg)**	
Dietary sodium restriction	< 30–50 mmol/day	2–8	
Moderation of daily alcohol intake	150–200 mL	2–4	
Increased physical activity	30 min 3 × per week	4–9	
Reduction in body weight	10 kg or 22 lb	5–10	
Adoption of DASH eating plan (high potassium)		8–14	

DASH, Dietary Approaches to Stop Hypertension; *SBP*, systolic blood pressure.

modification. This includes targeting both diet and exercise. These nonpharmacologic strategies should continue, even if pharmacologic treatment is found to be necessary. The relative effects of lifestyle modification on systolic blood pressure reduction are noted in Table 1. ACC/AHA guidelines also recommend lifestyle changes as initial intervention for individuals with stage 1 hypertension without other cardiovascular risk factors and with an atherosclerotic cardiovascular disease (ASCVD) risk of less than 10%; however, as noted earlier, the definition of stage 1 hypertension is at a lower blood pressure level (130 to 139 mm Hg systolic/80 to 90 mm Hg diastolic).

Diet. Dietary modifications include salt restriction to a level of less than 2400 mg per day, but ideally less than 1500 mg per day. Suggested dietary interventions also include the use of the DASH (Dietary Approaches to Stop Hypertension) framework. This nutritional framework includes recommendations such as increased consumption of fruits and vegetables, preferential use of complex carbohydrates, and consumption of low-fat dairy products. The DASH diet emphasizes the intake of whole grains, fish, poultry, legumes, nuts, and nontropical vegetable oils. This diet also endorses decreasing higher-fat foods.

Exercise. Current exercise recommendations suggest that engaging in a minimum of 150 minutes of moderate-intensity exercise on a weekly basis confers the greatest health benefits. Exercise at this level of intensity reduces the risk of multiple chronic conditions including cardiovascular disease and type 2 diabetes as well as overall all-cause mortality.

Other Lifestyle Modifications. In addition to diet and exercise, other lifestyle interventions can optimize health. Smoking cessation is an important modifiable risk factor and is the single leading cause of preventable death in the United States. Smoking increases the risk of cardiovascular morbidity and mortality, including myocardial infarction.

Alcohol consumption is another important lifestyle modification that can have a significant impact on overall health. The effects of alcohol consumption, unlike smoking, depend on quantity. It has been shown that at moderate levels of consumption, alcohol can actually decrease blood pressure (defined as no more than two drinks per day for men and no more than one drink per day for women). However, when consumed in greater quantity, alcohol can increase blood pressure, contributing to hypertension. It is emphasized that alcohol consumption should not be promoted in nondrinkers simply for the purpose of decreasing blood pressure.

Stress reduction is another lifestyle change that can have effects on blood pressure control. The mechanism of this reduction is not clear, but it is hypothesized that it may be related to decreasing autonomic nervous system output. Studies suggest that activities such as transcendental meditation can lead to modest blood pressure reduction. As such, inclusion of these activities in patient treatment plans may provide additional nonpharmacologic options.

Patients frequently ask about the utility of dietary supplements or other natural alternatives for blood pressure management. There is some evidence for select supplements in the management of hypertension, although such effects appear to be small. Examples of natural substances that may convey a small benefit include garlic and cocoa. Evidence is lacking for other agents including vitamin C, coenzyme Q10, omega-3 fatty acids, and magnesium.

Pharmacologic

In cases in which hypertension is more significant or nonpharmacologic methods have failed to adequately reduce blood pressure, initiation of medications is indicated (Table 2). The selection of an agent or agents is based on a number of factors including race and comorbidities. As noted earlier, the JNC 8 guidelines provide a stepwise, evidence-based approach to blood pressure management including recommended cut points where pharmacologic intervention is appropriate.

One of the points of emphasis of the JNC 8 guidelines is that the point of intervention for individuals 60 years of age or older is higher than for those younger than 60 years of age. One should also balance the side effects or risks of medications with the benefits of intervention in this age group. The cut points for individuals with chronic kidney disease and diabetes do not differ from the general population. The choice of agent according to JNC 8 recommendations does not differ based on the presence or absence of diabetes, but it does differ based on race (see recommendations 6 and 7 earlier in this chapter). Individuals with chronic kidney disease also should have an ACEI or ARB included in their treatment regimen (either as a lone agent or an add-on). In practice, decisions will need to be tailored to individual patient needs and also should consider other factors including whether or not the patient is a reproductive-age female (as ACEIs and ARBs are contraindicated in pregnancy). This is where our role as family physicians becomes increasingly important—embracing our ability to look at the whole patient when making treatment decisions.

The ACC/AHA recommends initiation of pharmacologic therapy in adults with high cardiovascular risk or preexisting cardiovascular disease and stage 1 or greater hypertension. Patients with both diabetes and hypertension are also assumed to fall into the high-risk category. Again, the defined level of blood pressure classified as stage 1 hypertension under the ACC/AHA guidelines (130 to 139 mm Hg systolic/80 to 90 mm Hg diastolic) is lower than the JNC 8 criteria, as noted earlier. The ACC/AHA recommendations also emphasize the need to balance comorbidities as well as preferences, life expectancy, and clinical judgment when making decisions regarding antihypertensive initiation and titration in older adults (65 years of age and older).

A recent trial (Hygia Chronotherapy Trial) published in 2019 investigated whether timing of antihypertensive medication administration affected blood pressure control and overall outcomes. This study demonstrated that for patients on one or more antihypertensive medications, administration of at least one agent at bedtime rather than upon awakening resulted in better ambulatory blood pressure readings as well as an overall decrease in cardiovascular disease–related events. The results of this study are strongly suggestive that prioritizing bedtime dosing of antihypertensive agents for hypertensive patients leads to greater net benefit.

TABLE 2 | Antihypertensive Classes

DIURETICS

GENERIC	BRAND NAME	CLASSIFICATION	MECHANISM OF ACTION	DOSING
Chlorthalidone	Thalitone	Thiazide	Inhibits sodium and chloride reabsorption in distal tubules	25 mg by mouth once daily. May increase to a maximum of 100 mg once daily.
Hydrochlorothiazide	Microzide	Thiazide	Inhibits sodium and chloride reabsorption in distal tubules	25 mg by mouth once daily to a maximum of 50 mg in single or divided doses.
Metolazone	Zaroxolyn	Thiazide	Inhibits sodium and chloride reabsorption in distal tubules	Individualize. 2.5–5 mg once daily.
Triamterene/ hydrochlorothiazide	Dyazide	Potassium-sparing/ thiazide	Inhibits sodium reabsorption in distal tubules	1–2 capsules by mouth once daily (37.5-/25-mg capsules).
Furosemide	Lasix	Loop	Inhibits sodium and chloride reabsorption in ascending loop of Henle	40 mg twice daily by mouth initially. If adding to another antihypertensive, reduce the other agent's dose by 50%
Torsemide	Demadex	Loop	Inhibits sodium and chloride reabsorption in ascending loop of Henle	5 mg once daily by mouth initially. May increase to 10 mg once daily after 4–6 weeks.

Angiotensin-Converting Enzyme (ACE) Inhibitors

Mechanism of action: Suppress the renin-angiotensin-aldosterone system

GENERIC	BRAND NAME	CLASSIFICATION	SPECIAL NOTE	DOSING
Fosinopril	Monopril	ACE inhibitor	Only ACE excreted by both renal and hepatic routes	Initially 10 mg once daily. Usual maintenance is 20–40 mg daily in single or 2 divided doses. Max 80 mg per day. If on a diuretic, suspend diuretic for 2–3 days before starting if possible and resume diuretic if pressure is not controlled with fosinopril alone. If diuretic cannot be discontinued, give 10 mg and monitor carefully.
Captopril	Capoten	ACE inhibitor		Take 1 hour before meals. 25 mg two to three times daily by mouth. May increase to 50 mg two to three times daily by mouth. Maximum 450 mg per day.
Ramipril	Altace	ACE inhibitor		2.5 mg once daily by mouth. May increase to a maximum of 20 mg in 1–2 divided doses by mouth.
Enalapril	Vasotec	ACE inhibitor	If on diuretics or if CrCl <30mL/min: suspend diuretic for 2-3 days if possible. Initially 2.5 mg daily and can titriate to maximum of 40 mg daily in divided doses. If not in above category, start at 5 mg daily. Usual range 10-40 mg in 1-2 divided doses.	2.5 mg daily by mouth initially. Typical dose range is 10–40 mg by mouth daily (may be divided doses).
Lisinopril	Prinivil, Zestril	ACE inhibitor	If renal impairment (CrCl 10-30 mL/min): initially 5 mg once daily. On hemodialysis or CrCl <10mL/min: initially 2.5 mg once daily.	10 mg by mouth daily initial dose. Usual dose range 20–40 mg daily. Doses above 40 mg are not shown to have greater effect. If on diuretics, start 5 mg once daily.

TABLE 2 Antihypertensive Classes—cont'd

GENERIC	BRAND NAME	CLASSIFICATION	SPECIAL NOTE	DOSING
Quinapril	Accupril	ACE inhibitor		10–20 mg daily by mouth initial dose if not on diuretics. Usual maintenance 20–80 mg daily in 1–2 divided doses. If on diuretics, suspend diuretics if possible for 2–3 days before starting and resume if blood pressure not controlled on quinapril alone. Initial dose if on diuretics and CrCl 30–60 mL/min 5 mg. If CrCl 10–30 mL/min, then initially 2.5 mg. If elderly, start 10 mg once daily.

Angiotensin II Receptor Blockers (ARBs)

Mechanism of action: Block binding of angiotensin II to angiotensin I receptors with a resultant inhibition of angiotensin II–mediated vasoconstriction, sodium retention, and release of aldosterone

GENERIC	BRAND NAME	CLASSIFICATION	SPECIAL NOTE	DOSING
Losartan	Cozaar	ARB	If mild to moderate hepatic impairment, start at 25 mg once daily.	50 mg daily by mouth initial dose (25 mg initial dose if also on diuretics). May titrate to a maximum dose of 100 mg daily.
Valsartan	Diovan	ARB	Adding a diuretic has greater effect than dose increases over 80 mg daily.	80–160 mg daily by mouth initial dose. May titrate to a maximum dose of 320 mg daily.
Olmesartan	Benicar	ARB		20 mg daily by mouth initial dose. May titrate to a maximum dose of 40 mg daily after 2 weeks. If volume-depleted (on a diuretic), consider lower initial dose.
Azilsartan	Edarbi	ARB		80 mg once daily by mouth. If on diuretics, start at 40 mg once daily.

BETA BLOCKERS

GENERIC	BRAND NAME	CLASSIFICATION	MECHANISM OF ACTION	DOSING
Atenolol	Tenormin	Beta-1 selective		50 mg once daily by mouth. May increase to 100 mg once daily after 1 week. Max dose 200 mg daily. May need to lower dose for elderly or if renal impairment.
Metoprolol	Lopressor	Beta-1 selective		Immediate-release formulations: 100 mg in single or divided doses. Maximum 450 mg per day.
	Toprol XL	Beta-1 selective		Extended-release formulations: 25–100 mg daily in a single dose. May increase at 1-week intervals. Maximum 400 mg per day.
Propranolol	Inderal	Beta-1 noncardioselective		Immediate-release formulations: 40 mg by mouth twice daily initial dose. Typical dosing 120–240 mg daily. Maximum 640 mg daily.
	Inderal LA, InnoPran XL	Beta-1 noncardioselective		Extended-release formulations: 80 mg once daily at bedtime initial dose. May increase to 120 mg.

Continued

TABLE 2 Antihypertensive Classes—cont'd

BETA BLOCKERS

GENERIC	BRAND NAME	CLASSIFICATION	MECHANISM OF ACTION	DOSING
Bisoprolol	Zebeta	Beta-1 selective	More beta-1 specific than other beta blockers	5 mg by mouth once daily initial dose (2.5 mg if patient has bronchospastic disease such as asthma, chronic obstructive pulmonary disease, or renal or hepatic impairment). May titrate to a maximum dose of 20 mg per day.
Timolol		Beta-1 noncardioselective	CAUTION: Avoid abrupt discontinuation as may exacerbate ischemic heart disease	10 mg twice daily by mouth initially. Increase weekly if needed. May titrate to a maximum dose of 60 mg per day in 2 divided doses. Usual maintenance 20–40 mg daily.
Labetalol	Trandate	Alpha and beta antagonist		100 mg twice daily by mouth initially. May titrate in 2–3 days by 100-mg twice-daily increments. Maximum dose 2400 mg per day. Usual maintenance dose 200–400 mg twice daily.

CALCIUM CHANNEL BLOCKERS

GENERIC	BRAND NAME	CLASSIFICATION	MECHANISM OF ACTION	DOSING
Nifedipine, extended release	Adalat CC, Procardia XL	Dihydropyridine	Binds to L-type calcium channels in sinoatrial (SA) and atrioventricular (AV) node, as well as myocardium and vasculature	30–60 mg by mouth once daily initially. Titrate over 7–14 days. Maximum 90 mg daily. Swallow whole.
Diltiazem, extended release	Cardizem CD, Cardizem LA, Cartia XT, Dilacor XR	Nondihydropyridine	Binds to L-type calcium channels in SA and AV node (primarily), as well as myocardium and vasculature	180–240 mg by mouth once daily initially. May titrate at 1–2 week intervals. Maximum dose 360 mg per day.
Verapamil	Calan, Calan SR	Nondihydropyridine	Binds to L-type calcium channels in SA and AV node, as well as myocardium and vasculature	80 mg by mouth every 8 hours initially. Usual max 360 mg/day in divided doses. If elderly or small, start at 40 mg 3 times daily.
Amlodipine	Norvasc	Dihydropyridine	Binds to L-type calcium channels in smooth muscle (vasculature)	5 mg by mouth daily initially. May increase by 2.5 mg every 1–2 weeks. Maximum 10 mg per day. For small, elderly, fragile, or hepatic impaired patients and patients on other antihypertensives, start at 2.5 mg daily.
Felodipine	Plendil	Dihydropyridine	Binds to L-type calcium channels in smooth muscle (vasculature)	5 mg by mouth once daily initially without food or with a light meal. May increase to a maximum dose of 10 mg by mouth once daily. Adjust at 2 week intervals. For elderly patients or hepatic impairment, start at 2.5 mg once daily. Do not crush or chew.

ALDOSTERONE ANTAGONISTS

GENERIC	BRAND NAME	CLASSIFICATION	MECHANISM OF ACTION	DOSING
Spironolactone	Aldactone	Selective aldosterone antagonist	Competes with aldosterone receptor sites. Reduces sodium reabsorption	25–100 mg by mouth once daily or divided twice daily. Titrate at 2 week intervals.

TABLE 2   Antihypertensive Classes—cont'd

ALDOSTERONE ANTAGONISTS

GENERIC	BRAND NAME	CLASSIFICATION	MECHANISM OF ACTION	DOSING
Eplerenone	Inspra	Selective aldosterone antagonist	Competes with aldosterone receptor sites. Reduces sodium reabsorption	50 mg by mouth once daily initially. May increase after 4 weeks to twice daily if needed. (May cause hyperkalemia if doses exceed 100 mg per day.) If on concomitant moderate CYP3A inhibitors such as erythromycin, verapamil, saquinavir, fluconazole, then initially start 25 mg daily with a max of 25 mg twice daily.

Alpha-2 Agonists

Mechanism of action: Stimulate presynaptic aldosterone receptors, decreasing sympathetic nervous activity

GENERIC	BRAND NAME	CLASSIFICATION	MECHANISM OF ACTION	DOSING
Clonidine	Catapres, Catapres-TTS	Centrally acting alpha-2 agonist	Stimulation of alpha-2 adrenoreceptors, reducing sympathetic nervous system output	0.1 mg every 12 hours by mouth. Maximum 2.4 mg per 24 hours. (Usual dose range 0.1–0.3 mg every 12 hours.) If using transdermal formulation, 0.1-mg patch applied once every 7 days. May increase by 0.1 mg /day patch after 1–2 weeks. Maximum 0.6 mg/day.
Methyldopa		Centrally acting alpha-2 agonist	Directly affects peripheral sympathetic nerves through stimulation of central alpha-adrenergic receptors	250 mg by mouth every 8–12 hours initially, then can increase every 2 days. (maximum 3 g per day). Typical maintenance dose is 500–2000 mg/day by mouth divided every 6–12 hours. If also on other antihypertensives (other than thiazides), initial max 500 mg/day.

Alpha Blockers

Mechanism of action: Selectively block postsynaptic alpha-1 adrenergic receptors

GENERIC	BRAND NAME	CLASSIFICATION	MECHANISM OF ACTION	DOSING
Prazosin	Minipress	Alpha-1 blocker	Competitive antagonist, reduces vascular resistance	1 mg by mouth every 8–12 hours initially. Give first dose at bedtime. Increase dose slowly. Maintenance dose typically 6–15 mg divided every 6–8 hours. Typical maximum 20 mg per day in divided doses (although may increase to 40 mg per day in divided doses in some patients). When adding other antihypertensives, reduce dose to 1–2 mg 3 times daily and retitrate.
Terazosin	Hytrin		Selective competitive inhibitor, decreases vascular resistance	1 mg by mouth at bedtime initially. Typical maintenance 1–5 mg daily or in divided dose every 12 hours. Maximum 20 mg per day.
Doxazosin	Cardura		Selective postsynaptic alpha-1 receptor inhibitor, vasodilation	1 mg once daily initially, titrate gradually at 2 week intervals (based on standing BP at 2–6 hours and 24 hours post-dose) to a maximum of 16 mg/day.

*Exceeds dosage recommended by the manufacturer.

Modified from Medscape. Hypertension Medication. Available at: http://www.emedicine.medscape.com/article/241381-medication.

Monitoring

Clinical practice guidelines vary in their recommendations regarding optimal monitoring. It is clear that monitoring in the early stage or during periods of treatment change should be more frequent than during times of stability, somewhere between monthly and every 6 weeks. Once the patient is stabilized, periodic monitoring can occur either every 3 to 6 months for everyone or in a more risk-stratified manner, with lower-risk patients being seen every 6 months and higher-risk patients every 3 months. Monitoring can also be done through home blood pressure monitoring and through the use of telehealth. This method has become more common and is both convenient and easily accessible to patients. There is evidence to support the use of telehealth for hypertension management, particularly in those individuals with difficult-to-treat hypertension and those with medication compliance issues. Ongoing studies work to support the generalizability to other hypertensive patient populations.

JNC 8 recommendations, as previously discussed, suggest that patients with hypertension be monitored on at least a monthly basis until goal blood pressure is achieved, with any necessary adjustments being made at these visits.

Complications

Hypertension is often referred to as *the silent killer*. This menacing name refers to the fact that this condition often presents without any discernible symptoms, which at times can make treatment compliance challenging. One of the greatest concerns with uncontrolled hypertension is the risk of end-organ damage, which is far-reaching.

Uncontrolled hypertension can lead to serious complications including myocardial infarction, stroke, peripheral artery disease, retinopathy, and renal failure. Given that hypertension is at the same time the most common condition we treat as primary care physicians, the opportunities to circumvent these sources of morbidity and mortality present themselves on a daily basis.

References

Al-Ansary L: A systematic review of recent clinical practice guidelines on the diagnosis, assessment and management of hypertension, *PLOS One* 8(1):1–18, 2013.

Bie P, Evans R: Normotension, hypertension and body fluid regulation: brain and kidney, *Acta Physio* 219:288–304, 2017.

Buelt, et al: Hypertension: New Guidelines from the International Society of Hypertension, *Am Fam Physician* 103(12):763–765, 2021 Jun 15.

Carey: Prevention: detection, evaluation, and management of high blood pressure in adults: synopsis of the 2017 American College of Cardiology/American Heart Association Hypertension Guideline, *Ann Intern Med* 168(5):351–358, 2018.

CDC.gov (Accessed 6/18/2022).

Chobanian AV: Guidelines for the management of hypertension, *Med Clin N Am* 101:219–227, 2017.

Garjon J: First-line combination therapy versus firstline monotherapy for primary hypertension (review), *Cochrane Database Syst Rev* 1, 2017.

Goetsch, et al: New Guidance on Blood Pressure Management in Low-Risk Adults with Stage 1 Hypertension, *ACC.org.*, Jun 21, 2021.

Hermida RC, Crespo JJ, Domínguez-Sardiña M, et al: Hygia Project Investigators: Bedtime hypertension treatment improves cardiovascular risk reduction: the Hygia Chronotherapy Trial, *Eur Heart J*, 2019 Oct 22. ehz754. Online ahead of print.

James P, Oparil S, Carter BL: Evidence-based guideline for the management of high blood pressure in adults: report from the panel members appointed to the Eighth Joint National Committee (JNC 8 h), *JAMA* 311(5):507–520, 2014.

Kallioinen A, Hill A, Horswill MS: Sources of inaccuracy in the measurement of adult patients' resting blood pressure in clinical settings: a systematic review, *J Hypertension* 35:421–441, 2017.

Langan R, Jones K: Common questions about the initial management of hypertension, *Am Fam Physician* 91(3):172–176, 2015.

Leeman L: Hypertensive disorders of pregnancy, *Am Fam Physician* 93(2):121–127, 2016.

Mann S: Redefining beta-blocker use in hypertension: selecting the right beta-blocker and the right patient, *J Am Soc Hypertens* 1–12, 2016.

Monthly Prescribing Reference. Available at: www.empr.com. [accessed February 16, 2023].

Omboni S, et al: Telemedicine in Hypertension Management, *Hypertension* 76:1368–1383, 2020.

Onusko E: Diagnosing secondary hypertension, *Am Fam Physician* 67(1):67–74, 2003.

Oza R, Garcellano M: Nonpharmacologic management of hypertension: what works? *Am Fam Physician* 91(11):772–776, 2015.

Prescribers' Digital Reference. Available at: www.pdr.net. [accessed February 16, 2023].

Quyen N: Screening for high blood pressure in adults, *Am Fam Physician* 93(6):511–512, 2016.

Sexton S: Screening for high blood pressure in adults: recommendation statement, *Am Fam Physician* 93(4):300–302, 2016.

Sexton S: Screening for primary hypertension in children and adolescents: recommendation statement, *Am Fam Physician* 91(4), 2015. A–D.

Springer K: Chlorthalidone vs. hydrochlorothiazide for treatment of hypertension, *Am Fam Physician* 92(11):1015–1016, 2015.

Medscape: Hypertension. Available at: http://emedicine.medscape.com/article/241381. [accessed May 9, 2017].

Yankey BA, Rothenberg R, Strasser, et al: Effect of marijuana use on cardiovascular and cerebrovascular mortality: a study using the National Health and Nutrition Examination Survey linked mortality file, *Eur J Prev Cardio*, 2017.

HYPERTROPHIC CARDIOMYOPATHY

Method of
Sandeep Sangodkar, DO

CURRENT DIAGNOSIS

- Echocardiography is a mainstay of clinical diagnosis.
- Cardiac magnetic resonance imaging (MRI) can help with risk stratification for sudden cardiac death to see if an implantable cardiac defibrillator is indicated; it can also be useful to exclude athlete's heart and infiltrative disease.
- Left ventricular outflow tract flow and outflow measurements during echocardiography and cardiac catheterization show a classic dynamic pattern, which can aid in diagnosis.
- Left ventricular wall thickness of 15 mm seen by various methods of imaging can aid in diagnosis.

CURRENT THERAPY

Asymptomatic Disease
- Periodic follow-up to assess symptoms and risk for sudden cardiac death.
- Important to counsel patients regarding potential genetic transmission.
- Patients with concurrent atrial fibrillation should be anticoagulated.

Symptomatic Disease
- β-Blockers and calcium channel blockers are drugs of choice as decreased ionotropic and chronotropic effects allow for increased ventricular filling and decreased outflow obstruction.
- A new class of medication inhibiting actin-myosin interaction is now available and can reduce left ventricular outflow tract obstruction.
- An implantable defibrillator is indicated if the patient has one of more of the following:
  - Hypertrophic cardiomyopathy (HCM) and risk factors such as sudden death in 1 or more first degree relatives younger than 50 years of age
  - massive left ventricular hypertrophy greater than 30 mm
  - recurrent episodes of syncope suspected to be arrhythmic, LV apical aneurysm with transmural scar,
  - LV systolic dysfunction (EF <50%).
- Surgical myectomy may be undertaken in patients who do not respond to pharmacologic therapy.
- Alcohol ablation may be used in patients who are not candidates for surgery.

Definition

Many names, terms, and acronyms (>80) have been used to describe hypertrophic cardiomyopathy (HCM). Common names such as idiopathic hypertrophic, subaortic stenosis, and hypertrophic obstructive cardiomyopathy, popular in the literature in the 1960s and 1970s, imply that left ventricular outflow tract (LVOT) obstruction is a required component of the disease, whereas one-third of patients have no obstruction at rest or exertion. The term *HCM*, first used in 1979, encompasses both the obstructive and nonobstructive hemodynamic variants of this disease and is now considered the formal name.

Epidemiology

Although once thought of as a rare entity, HCM is now recognized as a common inherited cardiovascular disease. Epidemiologic studies from various parts of the world report a similar prevalence, thought of as 1 in 200 to 1 in 500 people, which occurs equally among sexes and ethnic groups. This may, in fact, be underreported because many people with HCM are not clinically diagnosed and achieve normal life expectancy without any HCM-related complications.

Risk Factors

HCM is caused by mutations in genes coding for thin and thick filament proteins of the sarcomere. These mutations are inherited in an autosomal dominant pattern with variable penetrance and expression. At least 11 genes have been identified as responsible for causing HCM, with 70% of successfully genotyped patients found to have mutations in the two most-common genes: β-myosin heavy chain and myosin binding protein C. More than 1500 individual gene variants have been identified, which complicates predicting prognosis for individual patients.

Clinical Manifestations

HCM is seen in populations from pediatric to geriatric. A classic description of a murmur suggestive of HCM is a harsh crescendo-decrescendo systolic ejection murmur that increases in intensity with Valsalva or standing from a squatting position. Most patients with HCM are asymptomatic or only mildly symptomatic, with the most common presenting complaints being dyspnea or chest pain. The most worrisome manifestation is sudden cardiac death owing to ventricular tachyarrhythmia, seen more commonly in younger symptom-free patients. Systolic anterior motion of the mitral valve can cause significant mitral regurgitation. Heart failure with preserved ejection fraction is another manifestation of HCM; however, systolic dysfunction can be present owing to myocardial scarring. In addition, atrial fibrillation is associated with an increased risk of thromboembolism in patients with HCM, and anticoagulation must be considered. Most patients with HCM have normal life expectancy without a need for major intervention.

Pathogenesis

The pathophysiology of HCM stems from multiple abnormalities, including LVOT obstruction, diastolic dysfunction, mitral regurgitation, myocardial ischemia, and arrhythmias. The peak LV outflow gradient is an important factor in determining treatment options. The obstruction was originally thought to be caused by a hypertrophied basal septum that caused ventricular outflow obstruction during systolic contraction. It is now thought mitral valve systolic anterior motion and mitral-septal contact caused by venturi forces on the mitral leaflets and displacement into the outflow tract cause obstruction of LVOT. The increased LV systolic pressure in turn results in elevated diastolic pressures, mitral regurgitation, and, ultimately, decreased cardiac output.

Diagnosis

Clinically, HCM is defined as maximal end diastolic LV wall thickness of at least 15 mm based on echocardiography or cardiac MRI (Figure 1). Patients should have a comprehensive physical and three-generation family history as part of their initial evaluation. A distinction between HCM and physiologic LV hypertrophy from athletic conditioning must be recognized because the athletic hearts may demonstrate enlargement of the cardiac chambers and thickened septum. The likelihood of clinically significant HCM is determined by identification of sarcomere mutations, marked LV thickness (>25 mm), and LVOT obstruction with systolic anterior motion and mitral-septal contact. Provocative testing (exercise or pharmacologic) may elucidate the diagnosis of HCM in symptomatic patients presenting with a normal LVOT gradient at rest. Measurement of outflow gradients by echocardiography and invasive pressures by cardiac catheterization show a characteristic dynamic pattern that can be enhanced by loading conditions.

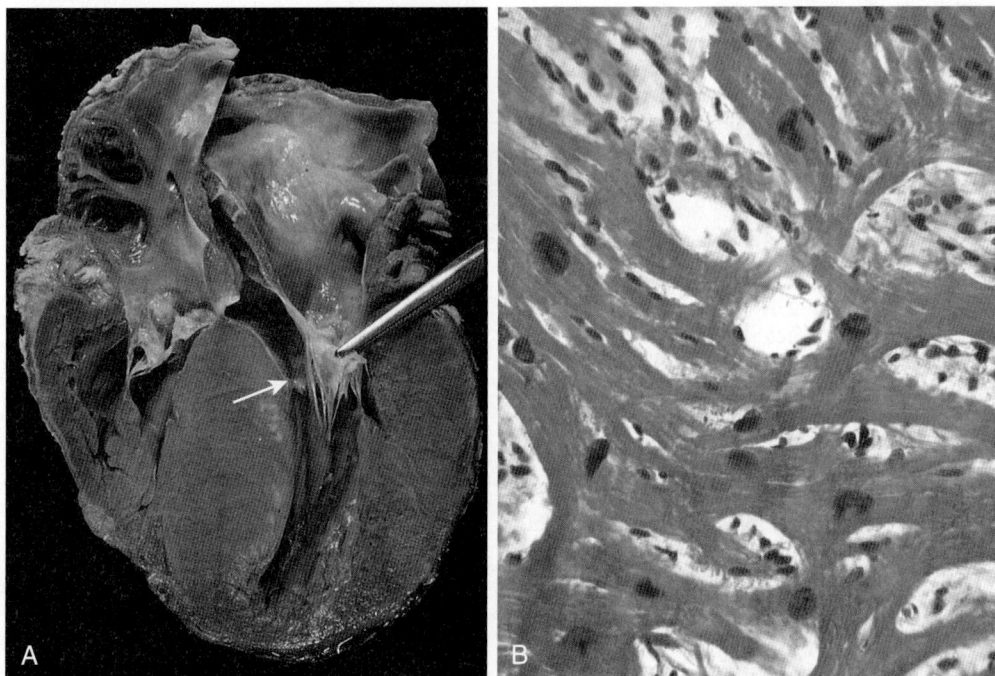

Figure 1 (A) Gross anatomy section of heart demonstrating septal hypertrophy and left ventricular outflow tract obstruction. (B) Microscopic section demonstrating myocyte hypertrophy and disarray.

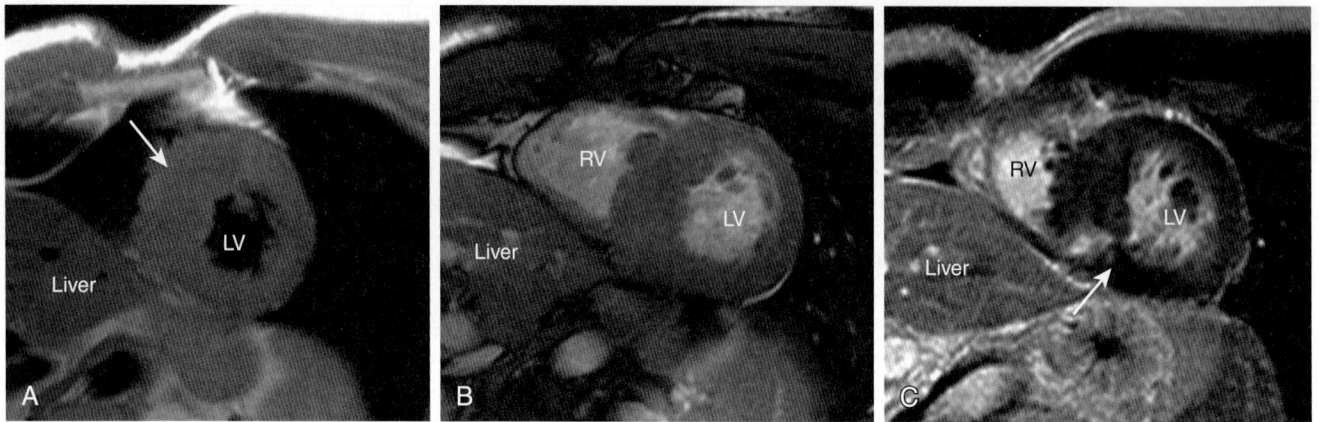

Figure 2 Cardiac MRI demonstrating septal hypertrophy (A, B) and late gadolinium enhancement (C). *Arrow* indicates a thickened LV septum. *LV,* Left ventricle; *RV,* right ventricle.

Imaging

The mainstay of imaging has been held by echocardiography. Transthoracic echocardiography is recommended in the initial evaluation of all patients with suspected HCM and family members of those diagnosed with HCM. Transesophageal echocardiography is used for diagnosis and intraprocedural guidance of surgical myectomy and alcohol septal ablation.

In current practice, cardiac magnetic resonance imaging (CMR) has proven to be an increasingly useful modality in the diagnosis and treatment of HCM (Figure 2). Contrast-enhanced CMR allows imaging of presumed myocardial fibrosis. Late gadolinium enhancement (LGE) is commonly seen in HCM; an extensive percentage of LV mass involvement is associated with higher risk of sudden cardiac death. Consequently, an absence of LGE is associated with a lower risk of sudden cardiac death and can often provide reassurance.

Treatment

Asymptomatic Disease

Given that a large subset of HCM patients are symptom free and will achieve normal life expectancy, it is important to educate patients about the disease process, screen family members, and advise them to avoid strenuous activity. Coronary artery disease has an impact on survival, and thus aggressive modification of risk factors contributing to atherosclerosis (diabetes, hyperlipidemia, and obesity) is recommended. Healthy recreational exercise has not been associated with increased risk of ventricular arrhythmia and is reasonable to allow the patient to maintain fitness. Adequate hydration and avoidance of situations leading to vasodilation are encouraged to minimize exacerbation of an existing LVOT obstruction.

Septal reduction therapy is not indicated in a symptom-free patient with any degree of obstruction.

Symptomatic Disease

Pharmacologic Management

β-Blockade is the mainstay of treatment owing to negative inotropic and negative chronotropic effect. Verapamil (Calan)[1] or diltiazem (Cardizem)[1] are reasonable alternatives to β-blockade. Mavacamten (Camzyos), a cardiac myosin inhibitor, or disopyramide (Norpace)[1] may be added if symptomatic despite these medications (Table 1). An important role in management is to discontinue medications that promote outflow tract obstruction via vasodilatory effects such as dihydropyridine calcium channel blocking agents, angiotensin converting enzyme inhibitors, and angiotensin receptor blockers. Low-dose diuretics may provide symptomatic relief; however, high-dose diuretics should be avoided. Digitalis is potentially harmful in patients without atrial fibrillation. Phenylephrine (Neo-Synephrine)[1] is useful when treating acute hypotension in these patients.

---

[1] Not FDA approved for this indication.

TABLE 1	Pharmacologic Management of Patients With Obstructive Hypertrophic Cardiomyopathy		
		INITIAL DOSE	**TITRATE TO MAX DOSE**
Symptoms Attributable to LVOT Obstruction			
Nonvasodilating β-Blockers	Metoprolol	50 mg/day	400 mg/day
	Atenolol	25 mg/day	100 mg/day
	Propranolol	60 mg/day	240 mg/day
β-Blocker Ineffective or Not Tolerated			
Nondihydropyridine CCB	Verapamil	120 mg/day	480 mg/day
	Diltiazem	120 mg/day	360 mg/day
Severe Symptoms Despite β-Blocker or Nondihydropyridine CCB			
	Mavacamten	5 mg/day	15 mg/day (pending echocardiogram for LVEF and LVOT gradient at scheduled intervals)
	Disopyramide	200 mg BID	300 mg BID

BID, Twice daily; *CCB,* calcium channel blocker; *LVEF,* left ventricular ejection fraction; *LVOT,* left ventricular outflow tract.

For the treatment of atrial fibrillation in HCM, it is recommended to keep a low threshold for initiating prophylactic anticoagulation with a direct-acting oral anticoagulant or vitamin K antagonist caused by a higher risk of thromboembolic stroke.

Invasive Therapies

The major septal reduction therapies are surgical myectomy and alcohol ablation. These should be performed by experienced operators at comprehensive centers in patients with refractory symptoms.

Surgical septal myectomy is considered the most appropriate therapy for eligible patients unresponsive to optimal medical therapy. The most common procedure is a Morrow procedure in which a rectangular trough is created in the basal septum below the aortic valve, which abolishes or reduces the LVOT gradient. Eligible patients include those with severe dyspnea, chest pain, or exertional syncope despite maximal medical therapy. Hemodynamic considerations that determine eligibility consist of an LVOT gradient of at least 50 mm Hg associated with septal hypertrophy and mitral valve systolic anterior motion. Studies have shown that surgical myectomy can reverse heart failure symptoms owing to the fact it permanently removes LVOT obstruction and can reduce mitral regurgitation.

Alcohol septal ablation can benefit adult patients with HCM and LVOT obstruction. This percutaneous procedure involves injection of ethanol into a major septal perforator coronary artery, with the intent of inducing infarction of the basal septal wall near the anterior leaflet contact point. The effectiveness of alcohol septal ablation is not clear in patients with more than 30 mm of septal hypertrophy, and it should not be performed in patients with disease (coronary artery disease, mitral valve repair) that would need surgical correction regardless. Other downsides of septal ablation include an increased risk of complete heart block requiring pacemaker implantation and an undefined risk of arrhythmogenicity owing to scar tissue.

Role of Implantable Devices

Determining which patients with HCM should receive an implantable cardiac defibrillator (ICD) is challenging given the unpredictability of the disease. ICDs are the only treatment to have proven to decrease mortality given their ability to reliably abort life-threatening arrhythmias. All patients with HCM need comprehensive sudden cardiac death risk stratification, with strong consideration for ICD implantation in those with personal history of ventricular fibrillation, sustained ventricular tachycardia, family history of sudden cardiac death, unexplained syncope, abnormal exercise blood pressure response, LGE >15% of LV mass, massive left ventricular hypertrophy (LVH) (>30 mm), or documented nonsustained ventricular tachycardia on Holter monitor. Device-related complications and issues such as inappropriate shocks and multiple generator changes for patients receiving a device at a young age must also be weighed when considering implantation of ICD. Risk scores can be helpful in the processes of shared decision making.

Participation in Sports

HCM has been reported as one of the most common causes of sudden death among competitive athletes; however, SCD is overall a rare event in young people. In the United States, there have been cardiovascular screening initiatives, including history and physical in addition to 12-lead electrocardiograms (ECGs), with limited success. The American College of Cardiology and American Heart Association do not currently recommend a national mandatory cardiovascular screening program.

It is reasonable for most HCM patients to engage in low-intensity competitive sports (golf, bowling) and recreational sporting activities. Whereas previously, patients were discouraged from competitive sports, data in the 2024 guidelines suggest that light (<3 metabolic equivalents [METS], moderate (3–6 METS), and vigorous (>6 METS) exercise are not associated with risk of ventricular arrhythmia. Patients who wish to pursue rigorous exercise training for competition should be evaluated by expert HCM professionals regarding potential risks and benefits in addition to developing an individualized training plan and with schedule for reevaluation. ICD placement should not be implanted for the sole purpose of participating in competitive athletics.

Monitoring

The unpredictability of HCM disease makes regular surveillance a necessity. Patient age has been seen as a predictor of HCM-related events, with sudden death events more common in young patients. With a family history of sudden cardiac death, periodic screening by transthoracic echocardiography (every 12–18 months) is recommended in children by the age of 12 (or younger if the child has signs of early puberty) or if there are plans for intense sports competition. Repeat transthoracic echocardiography is recommended for any change in clinical status or new cardiovascular event. As recognition of the genetic basis of this disease has improved over time, genetic screening and counseling of all first-degree family members of patients with HCM are now recommended.

Future Research

The perception of HCM has evolved from a rare and deadly condition to a more common and treatable disease. Effective use of ICDs for primary prevention and advances in medical therapy and surgical treatment of obstruction now allow most HCM patients to achieve normal quality of life. Although significant progress has been made in elucidating the etiology and pathophysiology of HCM, there is much room for advancement. In addition, the relationship between genetics and environmental influences, as well as the management of family members of genotype positive–phenotype negative patients, is still unclear. Although rapid genetic testing to identify those at risk has become more widespread, further understanding of pathogenic mutations is required. Furthermore, advancement in technology will hopefully lead to therapies that can specifically target these pathways.

References

Cannan CR, Reeder GS, Bailey KR: Natural history of hypertrophic cardiomyopathy. A population based study, 1976 through 1990, *Circulation* 92:2488–2495, 1995.
Elliott PM, Anastasakis A, Borger MA: ESC Guidelines on diagnosis and management of hypertrophic cardiomyopathy, *Eur Heart J* 35:2733–2799, 2014.
Gersh BJ, Maron BJ, Bonow RO: 2011 ACCF/AHA guideline for the diagnosis and treatment of hypertrophic cardiomyopathy, *Circulation* 124:e783–e831, 2011.
Marian AJ: Genetic determinants of cardiac hypertrophy, *Curr Opin Cardiol* 23:199–205, 2008.
Marian AJ: Recent advances in genetics and treatment of hypertrophic cardiomyopathy, *Future Cardiol* 1:341–353, 2005.
Maron BJ: Hypertrophic cardiomyopathy: a systematic review, *J Am Med Assoc* 287:1308–1320, 2002.
Maron B, Ommen S, Semsarian C, et al: State of the art review: hypertrophic cardiomyopathy, *JACC* 64(1).
Ommen S, Ho C, et al: AHA/ACC guideline for management of hypertrophic cardiomyopathy, *JACC* 83(23), 2024.
Ommen S, Mital S, et al: AHA/ACC guideline for the diagnosis and treatment of patients with hypertrophic cardiomyopathy, *JACC* 76(25), 2020.
Robinson AK: Imaging in hypertrophic cardiomyopathy, *JACC* 24, 2018.

INFECTIVE ENDOCARDITIS

Oyetokunbo Ibidapo-Obe, MD

CURRENT DIAGNOSIS

- Infective endocarditis (IE) should be a diagnostic consideration in patients with fever and heart murmur.
- Healthcare related infections account for 25% to 30% of newly diagnosed cases.
- Positive blood cultures are present in approximately 90% of cases. Multiple sets should be obtained prior to initiating antibiotic therapy to improve diagnostic yield.
- Transesophageal echocardiography has the highest sensitivity and specificity in native heart evaluations while alternative imaging techniques can be used in patients with implanted heart valves.
- Complications of disease include heart failure, valvular incompetence, and structural defects such as abscess, perforation, and fistulas.

CURRENT THERAPY

- Empiric therapy for *Staphylococcus aureus* should be initiated after blood cultures have been drawn and before the results are available.
- Antibiotic choice is complex and dependent on culture results and sensitivities of organisms identified.

- Best practices propose a multidisciplinary approach to care for patients with IE and should include specialties such as cardiology, infectious disease/microbiology, and cardiothoracic surgery in cases of complicated IE or if prosthetic valves or a cardiac device is present.
- Neurology or neurosurgery consults should be accessible as up to 30% of patients will experience symptomatic neurologic events during their disease.
- Increasing numbers of patients with IE will require surgical intervention due to complications from disease such as heart failure, embolism, intracardiac abscess, or failure to control infection.
- Outpatient parenteral antibiotic therapy can be considered in a subset of patients based on their culture results and with close follow-up.

Definition

Infective endocarditis (IE) is a microbial infection of the valves or endocardium of the heart.

Epidemiology and Risk Factors

IE remains a rare disease in Western countries with incidence varying by geographic location, predisposing risk factors, and preexisting conditions.

IE has an annual incidence of 3 to 10/100,000 of the North American population with a mortality of about 30% at 30 days and 40% at 1 year.

Over the years, the epidemiology of IE has shifted with a steady increase in healthcare-associated IE accounting for about 25% to 30% of newly reported cases.

Risk factors include advancing age, prosthetic heart valves, congenital heart disease, intracardiac devices, intravenous/parenteral drug use, indwelling venous access lines, diabetes mellitus, or immunosuppression to name a few.

Developing worlds have rheumatic heart disease as a leading risk factor for IE.

Infection with *Staphylococcus aureus* is presently the most prevalent cause of IE accounting for ~26% and overtaking the Strep group, next is *Streptococcus viridans* group at ~19%, other Streptococci at 17.5% and Enterococci at 10.55. The above listed bacteria jointly account for 80% to 90% of all cases of endocarditis.

Pathophysiology

IE occurs as a result of endothelial damage, which invariably exposes the basement membrane on the valve causing a structural abnormality that allows bacteria present in the bloodstream to colonize the initially sterile vegetation (nonbacterial thrombotic endocarditis).

Bacterial involvement and growth enlarge the vegetation, impede blood flow, and cause inflammation with multiple systemic symptoms/signs.

Progressive valve dysfunction can quickly lead to heart failure, and bacterial colonization of the vegetation causes septic emboli into the bloodstream, causing sepsis, and can lead to a metastatic septic site outside of initial vegetation area on the valve.

Prevention

The mainstay of prevention of IE is antimicrobial therapy prior to procedures, which may cause IE. This has been and remains a topic of debate and varies by geographic location worldwide.

The efficacy of antimicrobial therapy as a prophylaxis depends greatly on multiple factors, which include patient's medical conditions in terms of being high risk for IE, the procedure being done, the probability of sending bacteria into the bloodstream as a result of the said procedure, and the evidence backing antibiotic prophylaxis in the patient scenario.

BOX 1 | Antibiotic Regimens for High-Risk Patients and Dental Procedures[1] (Taken 30–60 Minutes Prior to Procedure)

Oral: Amoxicillin 2 g (child 50 mg/kg) PO 30–60 minutes before procedure
Penicillin Allergy: Cephalexin 2 g (child 50 mg/kg) PO 30–60 minutes before procedure or clindamycin 600 mg (child 20 mg/kg)
or azithromycin or clarithromycin 500 mg (child 15 mg/kg)
Unable to tolerate oral: Ampicillin 2 g IM/IV (child 50 mg/kg)
Unable to tolerate oral and PCN allergy: Cefazolin or ceftriaxone 1 g IM/IV (child 50 mg/kg) or clindamycin 600 mg IM/IV (child 20 mg/kg)
Patients that would benefit from antibiotics due to high risk:
- Acquired valvular heart disease with stenosis or regurgitation
- Valve replacement
- Structural congenital heart disease
- Previous endocarditis
- Hypertrophic cardiomyopathy
  Dental procedures to consider antibiotic prophylaxis:
- Manipulation of the gingival or periapical region of the teeth
- Perforation of oral mucosa
- Extractions

All these regimens are not approved by the FDA for this indication.
Adapted from Bonow RO, Carabello BA, Kanu C, et al: ACC/AHA 2006 guidelines for the management of patients with valvular heart disease: A report of the American College of Cardiology/American Heart Association Task Force on Practice Guidelines (writing committee to revise the 1998 Guidelines for the Management of Patients with Valvular Heart Disease): Developed in collaboration with the Society of Cardiovascular Anesthesiologists: Endorsed by the Society for Cardiovascular Angiography and Interventions and the Society of Thoracic Surgeons. *Circulation* 114(5):e84–e231, 2006.

The guidelines have remained dynamic based on review of published literature, most of which seems to favor less use of antibiotics and better patient selection for prophylaxis if needed. See current guidelines in Box 1.

Clinical Manifestations and Diagnosis

The diagnosis of IE is based on findings of bacteremia from an organism associated with IE along with evidence of endocardial involvement. This allows for highly variable presentations of disease. Due to this variability, it is important to perform a detailed history and physical examination to help lead to the diagnosis. Blood cultures should be obtained as discussed below prior to initiating antibacterial therapy to ensure appropriate management of the causative organism. This is especially important in the setting of predisposing conditions or risk factors for IE, including recent invasive procedures, history of structural heart disease, or injection drug use. Because of the insidious nature of the disease process, many patients will present with symptoms within 2 weeks of the inciting event or infection.

The most common presentation includes fever in up to 90% of patients, though it may not be present in immunocompromised patients or those who have received previous antibiotic therapy. This can be seen in postoperative patients after valve replacement or intracardiac devices. Night sweats, fatigue, weight loss, and appetite changes are other nonspecific signs that can indicate an infection and will be present in up to half of patients with IE.

A new or changing regurgitant murmur will also be present on physical examination along with evidence of endocardial involvement. The presentation of such involvement can range from tachycardia and hypotension to embolization of the vegetations causing embolic symptoms. Approximately 25% of patients with IE will present with evidence of embolization. If left untreated, symptoms of heart failure, valvular dysfunction, and destruction of cardiac structures can occur. Other physical exam findings of IE include petechia, splinter hemorrhages, Janeway lesions, Osler nodes, and Roth spots. As these findings can occur in other conditions and have low incidence in proven cases of IE, their diagnostic use is limited.

Differential Diagnosis

There are several conditions that can mimic the symptoms of IE. Consideration of systemic lupus erythematosus, acute rheumatic fever, atrial myxoma, vasculitis, and renal cell carcinoma should be on the differential. Care must be taken to not confuse the complications of IE as the causative etiology for hospitalization. One study found that up to 50% of patients with IE were initially diagnosed with complications of their disease (pneumonia, CNS infection, septic arthritis, heart failure, stroke) before correctly identifying the causative agent. Misdiagnosis was found to significantly increase the risk of comorbidity and in hospital mortality in these patients.

Laboratory Evaluation and Blood Cultures

Blood cultures are one of the major diagnostic criteria used to diagnose IE. They are of utmost importance due to their use in the treatment of IE by identifying the microorganisms involved as well as their antibiotic sensitivities. The continuous bacteremia present in IE means that fever need not be present before ordering blood cultures. In up to 90% of cases, the etiologic agent is identified in the first two blood cultures. It is recommended that three sets of blood cultures be obtained at least 1 hour apart from separate venipunctures for the most sensitive findings (98% of cases successfully identified). Each vial should have at least 10 mL of blood to increase the chances of obtaining an appropriate amount. Alternatively, two sets of three bottles each (two aerobic, one anaerobic—six bottles total) can be drawn if timing of antibiotic therapy is a concern. Unfortunately, the most common cause of negative culture IE is due to prior administration of antibiotic therapy. This results in prolonged, broad coverage antibiotic therapy and increased uncertainty of the diagnosis.

Other lab findings that may be present in IE but are not specific for the disease include a normocytic, normochromic anemia, thrombocytopenia, leukocytosis, and elevations in erythrocyte sedimentation rate (ERS), C-reactive protein, and procalcitonin.

Imaging

Cardiac imaging should be considered if there is a strong clinical suspicion of IE. The inclusion of cardiac imaging of IE has increased the sensitivity of diagnosis (see modified Duke Criteria [Box 2]). Transthoracic echocardiogram (TTE) should be performed if there is clinical suspicion for IE. The echocardiogram should be specifically looking for any oscillating intracardiac mass on the valve or supporting structure which would indicate vegetations. It can also be used to detect abscesses, dehiscence of prostatic valve, or newly identified valvular regurgitations. The sensitivity of detecting vegetations on native valves is approximately 70% with TTE. This is increased to a sensitivity and specificity around 90% if transesophageal echocardiogram (TEE) is used instead. Due to this increased sensitivity, TEE should be used in high-risk patients with a negative TTE. Transesophageal echocardiogram should also be considered in patients with prosthetic valves, those with *S. aureus* bacteremia, and when IE-related complications have occurred such as heart block, cardiac abscess, embolism, or new/worsening murmurs.

Due to the increased number of patients with prosthetic valves or intracardiac devices, TTE and TEE may prove to be unhelpful due to the artifact from these devices. In these cases, additional imaging with F-labeled fluoro-2-deoxyglucose positron emission tomography/computed tomography (F-FDG-PET/CT) or single-proton emission computed tomography-CT (SPECT-CT) should be considered to assess for inflammation around the prosthetic or intracardiac device. These studies have been found to have a sensitivity of 93% in cases of prosthetic valve endocarditis. They

Definite Infective Endocarditis:
- Two major

or
- One major and three minor

or
- Five minor

Possible Infective Endocarditis:
- One major and one minor

or
- Three minor

Major Criteria
Positive blood cultures:
- Typical microorganisms consistent with IE from two separate blood culture: viridans group streptococci, *Streptococcus bovis* group, HACED group, *Staphylococcus aureus*; community acquired enterocci with abscess of primary focus

or
- Microorganisms consistent with IE from persistently positive blood cultures: at least two positive blood cultures drawn more than 12 hours apart; all of three or a majority of positive blood cultures in more than four drawn; or single positive blood culture for *Coxiella burnetii* or phage IgG antibody titer >1:800

Evidence of endocardial involvement:
- Echocardiogram positive for IE showing vegetation, abscess, psuedoaneurysm, intracardiac fistula, valvular perforation or aneurysm, new partial dehiscence of prosthetic valve
- Abnormal activity around site of a prosthetic valve detected by PET/CT assuming >3 months after surgery or radiolabeled leukocyte-SPECT/CT
- Definite paravalvular lesions by cardiac CT

Minor Criteria
- Predisposition: predisposing heart condition or injection drug use
- Fever, temperature >38°C
- Vascular phenomena (including those detected by imaging alone): arterial emboli, septic pulmonary infarcts, myotic aneurysm, intracranial hemorrhage, conjunctival hemorrhage, and Janeway lesions
- Immunologic phenomena: glomerulonephritis, Osler's nodes, Roth's spots, and rheumatoid factor
- Microbiological evidence: positive blood cultures not meeting major criteria above or serologic evidence of infection with organism consistent with IE

CT, Computed tomography; *HACEK, Haemophilus* spp, *Aggregatibacter* spp, *Cardiobacterium* hominis, *Eikenella* corrodens, *Kingella* spp; *IE,* infective endocarditis; *IgG,* immunoglobulin G; *PET,* positron emission tomography; *SPECT,* single-photon emission computed tomography.

have significantly lower sensitivity in cases of native heart disease (22% sensitivity). Thoracic CT scans have significant value in determining presence of perivalvular abscesses, aneurysms, or pseudoaneurysms.

Cerebral magnetic resonance imaging (MRI) should be considered in patients with evidence of embolic neurologic complications as most of these lesions are ischemic in origin.

Treatment

Treatment should be multidisciplinary and involve cardiology, cardiac surgeon, infectious disease, or microbiology. This approach improves outcomes by optimizing appropriate antibiotic regiments and assessments for surgical interventions. Initiating appropriate antibiotic therapy can improve in-hospital survival by 70% to 80%. Recommended antibiotic regimens against common organisms causing IE are listed in

Table 1. These should be adjusted based on the organism and susceptibilities.

Patient with IE will require a prolonged duration of intravenous (IV) antibiotic treatment for up to 6 weeks. This is in order to ensure that all bacteria located in the vegetations are completely eradicated. Blood cultures should be repeated every 24 to 48 hours until resolution of bacteremia is confirmed. If surgery is required, a 4- to 6-week course of antibiotics is still recommended to reduce recurrence of IE.

In addition to IV antibiotic therapy, many patients will also be placed on parenteral therapies. In certain cases, patients may be eligible for transition to oral antibiotic to complete the duration of therapy. The criteria for step down therapy are patients who have no indication for surgery, have completed an initial course of IV antibiotics with no bacteremia, have no concerns for absorption of oral therapy in the gastrointestinal tract, have no psychological or socioeconomic concerns that would cause IV

therapy to be preferred for adherence, and the organism is susceptible to the prescribed oral regiment. Oral therapy is preferred over IV due to the decreased potential for harm.

Due to increasing microorganism resistance, parenteral therapy typically consists of a beta-lactam and aminoglycoside. They should be taken close together to increase the bactericidal effect. Care should be maintained with close observation of renal function.

Complications and Surgical Indications

Infective endocarditis carries a high in-hospital mortality of up to 30% due to the development of potential complications either prior or during effective treatment. Heart failure or pulmonary edema is common, occurring in up to half of patients with IE, and is the most common indication for urgent surgery. Destruction of the valvular tissues creates significant regurgitation leading to volume overload. Conversely, severe vegetations can cause significant stenosis and lead to the same outcome. In rare cases,

TABLE 1 Antimicrobial Regimens Against Typical Infective Endocarditis Organisms

ORGANISM	SUSCEPTIBILITY	REGIMENT	DOSAGE	DURATION (WEEK)
Native Valve				
Streptococcus viridans, Streptococcus bovis	Penicillin	Penicillin G	12–18 MU IV per 24 h continuously or in four to six equally divided doses	4
		or ceftriaxone[1]	2 g IV or IM per 24 h	4
		or vancomycin	30 mg/kg IV per 24 h in two divided doses. Max: 2 g/24 h	4
	Penicillin-relative resistance	Penicillin G	24 MU IV per 24 h continuously or in four to six equally divided doses	4
		or ceftriaxone[1]	2 g IV/IM per 24 h 4	4
		plus gentamicin[1]	3 mg/kg IV/IM per 24 h in one dose	2
		or vancomycin	30 mg/kg IV per 24 h in two divided doses (limit 2 g/24 h)	4
Enterococcus spp	Penicillin	Ampicillin	12 g IV per 24 h in six divided doses	4–6
		or penicillin G[1]	18–30 MU IV per 24 h continuously or in six equally divided doses	4–6
		Plus	gentamicin 3 mg/kg IV or IM per 24 h in three divided doses	2
		or ampicillin	12 g IV per 24 h in six divided doses	6
		plus ceftriaxone[1]	2 g IV every 12 h	6
	Penicillin Resistant	Vancomycin	30 mg/kg IV per 24 h in two divided doses (limit 2 g/24 h)	
Staphylococcus spp	Oxacillin	Nafcillin[1] or oxacillin[1]	12 g IV per 24 h in four to six divided doses	6
		or cefazolin	100 mg/kg IV/IM per 24 h in three equally divided doses	6
			6 g IV per 24 h in three divided doses	6
	Oxacillin resistant	Vancomycin plus gentamicin	30 mg/kg IV per 24 h in two divided doses (goal: 1 h peak concentration 30–45 µg/mL and trough 10–15 µg/mL)	6
Prosthetic Valve				
Staphylococcus spp.	Oxacillin-susceptible	Nafcillin[1] or oxacillin[1]	12 g IV per 24 h in four to six divided doses	6
		plus gentamicin	3 mg/kg IV or IM per 24 h in three divided doses	2
		plus rifampin[1]	900 mg IV or PO per 24 h in three divided doses	6
	Oxacillin-resistant	Vancomycin	30 mg/kg IV per 24 h in two divided doses. Goal: 1 h peak concentration 30–45 µg/mL and trough 10–15 µg/mL	6
		plus gentamicin	3 mg/kg IV or IM per 24 h in three divided doses	2
		plus rifampin[1]	900 mg IV or PO per 24 h in three divided doses	6

[1]Not FDA approved for this indication.

Adapted from Bonow RO, Carabello BA, Kanu C, et al: ACC/AHA 2006 guidelines for the management of patients with valvular heart disease: A report of the American College of Cardiology/American Heart Association Task Force on Practice Guidelines (writing committee to revise the 1998 Guidelines for the Management of Patients with Valvular Heart Disease): Developed in collaboration with the Society of Cardiovascular Anesthesiologists: Endorsed by the Society for Cardiovascular Angiography and Interventions and the Society of Thoracic Surgeons. Circulation 114(5):e84–e231, 2006.

this can lead to cardiogenic shock, which is an immediate indication for surgery (within 24 hours). For those with symptoms of heart failure and worsening hemodynamic response, surgery should be considered within 7 days of identification. Patients with heart failure will typically require surgical intervention as medical therapy alone is insufficient at repairing the damage caused by the infection. It is important to note here that valvular or other surgical interventions for IE may be performed in the acute or active phase of infection as delay can significantly increase the mortality.

Other complications include failure to quickly eradicate infection. This can be due to inability or delays in identifying the causative organism or for severe infections. Severe localized infections can cause paravalvular or aortic root abscesses. These abscess formations usually complicate 30% to 40% of IE cases due to their contiguous spread along the tissue planes. Other risk factors for abscess formation include prosthetic valves or difficult-to-treat organisms such as fungi or multidrug-resistant organisms. For this reason, all IE cases associated with prosthetic valves should have surgical consideration. These cases are typically identified by persistently positive blood cultures despite appropriate antibiotic regiments. Abscesses are identified via TEE or the aforementioned imaging studies in patients with prosthetic valves. Due to the abscess formation and deep infection, surgical debridement or valve replacement is almost always required. Surgical evaluation and debridement is the gold standard of abscess identification.

The third major complication of IE relates to septic emboli from valvular vegetations. While one-third of patients with IE will have signs and symptoms of embolization, another one-third can be found to have silent emboli. Neurologic embolization is the most frequent site (40%), followed by lungs (20%), spleen (20%), peripheral arteries (~15%), and kidneys (10%). Embolization most often occurs prior to the initiation of antibiotic therapy and the risk of embolization is reduced by approximately 65% after 2 weeks of antibiotic therapy. Risk factors include vegetations greater than 10 mm in size and infections associated with *S. aureus* and *Streptococcus bovis*. These embolic events can further complicate treatment by causing metastatic infection sites. Embolic events are an independent risk factor for in-hospital death in IE and as such require surgical evaluation if the vegetations meet certain criteria. Surgery is indicated in valvular vegetations greater than 10 mm with embolic event while on antibiotics, in vegetations greater than 30 mm, and in those with vegetations greater than 10 mm with severe valvular (native and prosthetic) disease who are low operative risk.

Conclusion

Infective endocarditis continues to maintain a relatively high mortality rate even with the advances in both surgical and antibiotic treatment. Prompt diagnosis and targeted antimicrobial therapy are vital to improving outcomes in patients with IE. Surgical evaluation and treatment should be considered relatively early in the disease course. Even with high rates of surgical intervention, in-hospital mortality continues to remain between 15% and 20% in native valves and up to 25% in prosthetic valves. Complications associated with disease progression (heart failure, uncontrolled infections, embolic events) also increase the mortality risk. Therefore a multidisciplinary team should be involved in patients identified with IE to provide best possible outcomes. Additionally, close follow-up after hospitalization should be conducted as up to 30% of patients with IE may require surgery in the first 12 months after diagnosis.

References

Baddour LM, Wilson WR, Bayer AS, et al: On behalf of the American Heart Association Committee on rheumatic fever, endocarditis, and kawasaki disease of the council on cardiovascular disease in the young, council on clinical cardiology, council on cardiovascular surgery and anesthesia, and stroke council. Infective endocarditis in adults: diagnosis, antimicrobial therapy, and management of complications: a scientific statement for healthcare professionals from the American Heart Association, *Circulation* 132:1435–1486, 2015.

Cahill TJ, et al: Challenges in infective endocarditis, *J Am Coll Cardiol* 69(3):325–344, 2017.

Cahill TJ, Harrison JL, Jewell P, et al: Antibiotic prophylaxis for infective endocarditis: a systematic review and meta-analysis, *Heart* 103:937–944, 2017.

Chu VH, Cabell CH, Benjamin Jr DK, et al: Early predictors of in-hospital death in infective endocarditis, *Circulation* 109(14):1745–1749, 2004.

Fowler Jr VG, Miro JM, Hoen B, et al: Staphylococcus aureus endocarditis: a consequence of medical progress, *J Am Med Assoc* 293(24):3012–3021, 2005.

Gaca JG, Sheng S, Daneshmand MA, et al: Outcomes for endocarditis surgery in North America: a simplified risk scoring system, *J Thorac Cardiovasc Surg* 141:98–106, 2011.

Habib G, Lancellotti P, Antunes MJ, et al: 2015 ESC guidelines for the management of infective endocarditis: the Task Force for the Management of Infective Endocarditis of the European Society of Cardiology (ESC). Endorsed by: European Association for Cardio-Thoracic Surgery (EACTS), the European Association of Nuclear Medicine (EANM), *Eur Heart J* 36(44):3075–3128, 2015.

Kang DH, Kim YJ, Kim SH, et al: Early surgery versus conventional treatment for infective endocarditis, *N Engl J Med* 366:2466–2473, 2012.

Kiefer T, Park L, Tribouilloy C, et al: Association between valvular surgery and mortality among patients with infective endocarditis complicated by heart failure, *J Am Med Assoc* 306:2239–2247, 2011.

Li JS, Sexton DJ, Nettles R, et al: Proposed modifications to the Duke criteria for the diagnosis of infective endocarditis, *Clin Infect Dis* 30(4):633–638, 2000.

Liesman RM, Pritt BS, Maleszewski JJ, Patel R: Laboratory diagnosis of infective endocarditis, *J Clin Microbiol* 55:2599–2608, 2017.

Naderi HR, Sheybani F, Erfani SS: Errors in diagnosis of infective endocarditis, *Epidemiol Infect* 146:394–400, 2018.

Nishimura RA, Otto CM, Bonow RO, et al: 2014 AHA/ ACC guideline for the management of patients with valvular heart disease: a report of the American College of Cardiology/American Heart Association Task Force on Practice Guidelines, *J Am Coll Cardiol* 63:e57–e185, 2014.

Rajani R, Klein JL: Infective endocarditis: a contemporary update, *Clin Med (Lond)* 20(1):31–35, 2020.

Spellberg B, et al: Evaluation of a paradigm shift from intravenous antibiotics to oral step-down therapy for the treatment of infective endocarditis: a narrative review, *JAMA Intern Med*, 2020.

Task Force on the Prevention: Diagnosis, and Treatment of Infective Endocarditis of the European Society of Cardiology; European Society of Clinical Microbiology and Infectious Diseases; International Society of Chemotherapy for Infection and Cancer; ESC Committee for Practice Guidelines: Guidelines on the prevention, diagnosis, and treatment of infective endocarditis (new version 2009): the Task Force on the prevention, diagnosis, and treatment of infective endocarditis of the European Society of Cardiology (ESC), *Eur Heart J* 30(19):2369–2413, 2009.

Thornhill MH, Dayer M, Lockhart PB, Prendergast B: Antibiotic prophylaxis of infective endocarditis, *Curr Infect Dis Rep* 19(2):9, 2017.

MITRAL VALVE PROLAPSE

Method of
Kurt M. Jacobson, MD; Peter S. Rahko, MD; and Andrew Pap, MD

CURRENT DIAGNOSIS

- Mitral valve prolapse (MVP) is most commonly an asymptomatic condition. As a result, the physical examination remains crucial to trigger clinical suspicion.
- A midsystolic click is the classic auscultatory finding of MVP, which can be with or without a middle- to late-peaking crescendo systolic murmur indicative of associated mitral regurgitation (MR).
- Transthoracic echocardiographic assessment is critical for the evaluation of MVP when clinical suspicion is present.
- The diagnostic echocardiographic finding of MVP is systolic billowing of the mitral valve leaflets 2 mm above the annulus into the left atrium.
- Particularly relevant features on the echocardiographic evaluation of MVP include the severity of prolapse, the extent of myxomatous thickening, the severity of MR (if present), and the left ventricular size and function.
- The presence of myxomatous thickening of the valve leaflets (>5 mm) separates classic (diffuse myxomatous) MVP from nonclassic (fibroelastic deficiency), which is significant for prognosis, the former having been associated with greater long-term risk.

- Uncomplicated MVP is often a benign condition and can be monitored clinically every 3 to 5 years.
- Complicated MVP (associated with significant MR, left ventricular structural changes, pulmonary hypertension, atrial fibrillation, or stroke) should be observed closely with serial clinical evaluation and echocardiography.
- Surgery should be considered for complicated MVP associated with severe MR. Repair rather than replacement is the procedure of choice and should be performed at surgical centers experienced with mitral valve repair.
- There are currently two mitral transcatheter edge-to-edge repair devices (the MitraClip [Abbott Vascular] and PASCAL [Edwards Lifesciences]) that serve as treatment options for symptomatic patients with moderate-to-severe or severe MR, prohibitive surgical risk, and acceptable anatomy.

Mitral valve prolapse (MVP) has been known by many names, including floppy valve syndrome, Barlow syndrome, click/murmur syndrome, myxomatous mitral valve disease, and billowing mitral cusp syndrome. MVP is a common cardiac valvular abnormality characterized by redundant, floppy mitral valve leaflets; it is often detected initially by characteristic nonejection clicks on physical examination, with or without a middle- to late-peaking crescendo systolic murmur indicative of associated mitral regurgitation (MR).

Pathophysiology

Primary MVP is characterized by idiopathic myxomatous change of the mitral valve leaflets or the chordal structures or both. Secondary MVP is present when underlying conditions such as Marfan syndrome, Ehlers-Danlos syndrome, osteogenesis imperfecta, other collagen vascular disorders, or congenital abnormalities are evident. Common congenital cardiac abnormalities associated with MVP include Ebstein anomaly, aortic coarctation, hypertrophic cardiomyopathy, and ostium secundum atrial septal defects. Familial variants with an autosomal dominant pattern of inheritance have been identified, and work to identify the genes involved is under way. To date, only a few causative genes have been identified, including *FLNA, DZIP1,* and *DCHS1,* which explain a small minority of cases. The reported prevalence of MVP in first-degree relatives is between 30% and 50%.

Macroscopic and microscopic changes can involve both the anterior and posterior leaflets and the chordal structures of the leaflet apparatus. Macroscopically, the surface area of the leaflet is increased, providing the accentuated, billowing appearance of the valve leaflets. Additional notable changes can include thickening of the individual leaflets, increased leaflet length, thinning and stretching of the chordae, and increased circumference of the mitral valve annulus. At the microscopic level (Figure 1), normal mitral valves have three well-defined layers, each containing cells and a characteristic composition and configuration of the extracellular matrix: the fibrosa, composed predominantly of collagen fibers densely packed and arranged parallel to the free edge of the leaflet; the centrally located spongiosa, composed of loosely arranged collagen and proteoglycans; and the atrialis, composed of elastic fibers. In myxomatous mitral valves, the spongiosa layer is expanded by loose, amorphous extracellular matrix that has more proteoglycans but less collagen and more fragmented elastic fibers. What collagen is present appears to be disorganized and fragmented, giving the appearance of a haphazard layering of the spongiosa. It is this thickening that produces the classic macroscopic appearance of the myxomatous valve on two-dimensional echocardiography.

Prevalence

MVP is the most common congenital cause of MR in adults and the most common indication for mitral valve surgery in the United States today. Previously, it was one of the most overdiagnosed conditions within cardiology, with suggested prevalence rates ranging from 5% to 15%. With the use of current diagnostic standards, rates are much lower; the overestimation was a consequence of diverse and nonuniformly accepted two-dimensional echocardiographic diagnostic criteria. Freed and colleagues, using the Framingham study population and applying consistent and more stringent echocardiographic diagnostic criteria, demonstrated a much lower prevalence of MVP (~2.4%). The incidence appeared to be similar among men and women. Sex differences do exist, however. Women tend to have a more benign course, whereas men tend to have more advanced myxomatous disease resulting in a greater chance of more severe MR.

Clinical Manifestations

Most patients with MVP are asymptomatic and will remain so, testifying to the often benign nature of this disease. Previously, a variety of nonspecific symptoms, including fatigue, dyspnea, palpitations, postural orthostasis, anxiety, and panic attacks, were described as an MVP syndrome when present in association with the characteristic auscultatory findings. Other symptoms, including chest discomfort, near-syncope, and syncope, have also been described by patients with MVP. However, in a community-based study, the prevalence of various clinical complaints including chest pain, dyspnea, and syncope was no higher in patients with MVP than in those without evidence of MVP, making such findings nonspecific. In a controlled study that

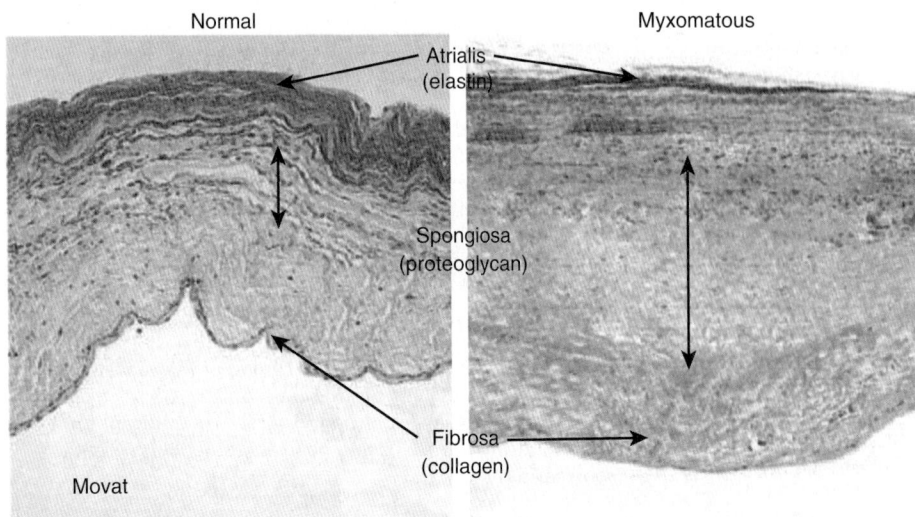

Figure 1 Morphologic features of normal mitral valves *(left)* and valves with myxomatous degeneration *(right)*. Myxomatous valves have an abnormal layered architecture: loose collagen in fibrosa, expanded spongiosa strongly positive for proteoglycans, and disrupted elastin in atrialis *(top)*. Movat pentachrome stain (collagen stains yellow, proteoglycans blue-green, and elastin black). (Modified from Rabkin E, Aikawa M, Stone JR, et al: Activated interstitial myofibroblasts express catabolic enzymes and mediate matrix remodeling in myxomatous heart valves. *Circulation* 104:2525, 2001.)

compared symptomatic MVP patients with first-degree relatives with and without echocardiographic evidence of MVP, there also was no association of MVP with atypical chest pain, dyspnea, panic attacks, or anxiety. There was, however, a significant association of MVP with physical findings of systolic clicks, systolic murmurs, thoracic bony abnormalities, low body weight, and low blood pressure. Congestive heart failure, atrial fibrillation, stroke or transient ischemic attack, hypertension, diabetes, and hypercholesterolemia are no more likely in patients with uncomplicated MVP than in those without MVP.

Although MVP typically remains asymptomatic and benign, development of associated MR can result in symptom development. Symptoms of poor cardiac reserve, such as reduced exercise tolerance, dyspnea on exertion, and fatigue, may reflect the presence of significant MR and warrant clinical concern.

Diagnosis

Given symptoms are typically absent in the setting of uncomplicated MVP, a quality physical examination can serve as the gateway to identification of MVP. Patients with MVP more often have a lower body mass index, a lower waist-to-hip ratio, and are taller. Findings of scoliosis, pectus excavatum, and hyperextensibility are prevalent among patients with MVP.

The auscultatory findings of MVP are best elicited with the diaphragm of the stethoscope. The most important and specific finding on auscultation is the presence of a nonejection midsystolic click or clicks caused by snapping of the valve apparatus as parts of the valve leaflets billow into the atrium during systole. Although these clicks can be heard over the entire precordium, they are best heard at the apex. The click can be misinterpreted as a split S_1, a true S_1 with an S_4, or a true S_1 with an early ejection click from a bicuspid valve. It can be differentiated from an ejection click heard in bicuspid aortic valves by its timing relative to the beginning of the carotid upstroke. Ejection clicks occur as the aortic valve opens and therefore precede the carotid upstroke, whereas the nonejection clicks of MVP occur afterward. Clicks from atrial septal aneurysms are uncommon but can be difficult to distinguish from those of MVP. Ejection clicks and clicks from atrial septal aneurysms are not altered by changes in loading characteristics, allowing them to be differentiated from clicks of MVP. Changes in left ventricle (LV) filling and volume affect the degree of MVP and therefore can alter the relation of the click to the first and second heart sounds. As a result, patients with auscultatory findings concerning for MVP should be examined in several positions: supine (including lateral decubitus), sitting, standing, and, if possible, squatting. Generally, measures that decrease LV volume or increase contractility produce earlier and more prominent systolic prolapse of the mitral leaflets, causing the systolic click to move closer to S_1. For example, in the transition from squatting to standing, LV volume is reduced, and the onset of the click is moved closer to S_1. Conversely, anything that increases LV volume, such as leg-raising, squatting, or slowing

the heart rate (increased diastolic filling), delays the onset of the click (Figure 2).

Often, but not always, a middle- to late-peaking crescendo systolic murmur can be appreciated by itself or after a click. The murmur terminates with closure of the aortic valve (A2). This represents MR, and, in general, the duration of the murmur correlates with the severity of the MR. The earlier in systole the murmur is detected, the more severe the MR. Eventually, with more severe MR, the murmur becomes holosystolic. The MR murmur is impacted by loading conditions in a similar fashion to the click: reduced volume or increased contractility lead to a more prominent murmur, while increased volume leads to a delay in the murmur and diminished intensity and duration. MVP manifestations on examination vary, and they may not always be reproducible, even in the same patient.

In patients for which there is a concern for MVP based on clinical examination, the next step is to acquire a transthoracic echocardiogram. Two-dimensional echocardiography has proved to be the most accurate noninvasive tool for the diagnosis, assessment, and follow-up of MVP. Physical signs of MVP in an asymptomatic patient are an American College of Cardiology/American Heart Association (ACC/AHA) class I indication for use of echocardiography to make the diagnosis of MVP and assess the severity of MR, leaflet morphology, and ventricular size and function. Once the diagnosis is made, follow-up is determined by the severity of MVP. Routine echocardiographic follow-up of asymptomatic patients with MVP is not recommended unless there are significant findings of MR or LV structural changes. Frequency of follow-up in patients with prolapse and MR is determined by the severity of MR and should be at least annual in patients with severe MR.

The diagnostic finding of MVP on 2-dimensional echocardiography is:
- Billowing of one or both mitral valve leaflets or their prolapse superiorly across the mitral annular plane in the parasternal long-axis view by >2 mm during systole

The mitral valve apparatus is saddle shaped; as a result, certain echocardiographic views are more specific than others for determining leaflet prolapse. Most practitioners agree that the parasternal long-axis and apical two-chamber or apical long-axis views are the most accurate for determining prolapse. A finding of prolapse as determined on other views, particularly the apical four-chamber view, is much less specific and frequently leads to a false-positive diagnosis.

After identification of MVP on echocardiography, particular attention is paid to the degree of thickening of the leaflets, which distinguishes classic MVP from nonclassic and has prognostic implications. Classic (aka diffuse myxomatous) MVP has leaflet thickness ≥5 mm. Nonclassic (aka fibroelastic deficiency) MVP has a leaflet thickness <5 mm. In addition to more often being associated with the auscultative findings of the click and murmur, the classic form is more commonly associated with increased risk

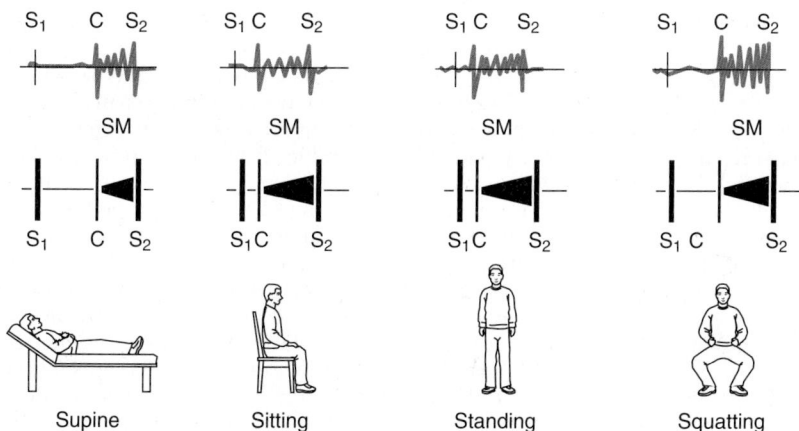

Figure 2 Auscultative findings with changes in position in patients with mitral valve prolapse (MVP). C, Click of MVP; S_1, mitral valve closure; S_2, aortic valve closure. Modified from Devereux RB, Perloff JK, Reichek N, et al: Mitral valve prolapse. *Circulation* 54(1):3–14, 1976.

of endocarditis, stroke, progressive MR, and need for mitral valve repair or replacement.

Therapy—Medical

MVP is ultimately an anatomic problem and thus definitive management, when indicated in the setting of significant concomitant MR, is procedural—either surgical or percutaneously. Fortunately, most patients with MVP remain asymptomatic and require no additional management aside from careful observation over time for the development of significant MR, which is overall uncommon. The estimated occurrence of severe MR in the setting of MVP is ~4%. It is appropriate to provide reassurance that uncomplicated MVP is a non–life-threatening condition and is unlikely to affect longevity. Endocarditis prophylaxis is no longer recommended for patients with MVP unless they have a history of endocarditis or valve replacement. Prophylaxis is recommended for patients who have undergone repair if prosthetic material was used (e.g., in ring repairs). Previous valve guidelines invoked consideration for antiplatelet therapy in certain instances of MVP (complicated MVP). More recent guidelines do not directly address MVP, and antiplatelet therapy remains a topic of debate in the absence of other clear indications (i.e., ischemic neurologic events).

Those who have severe MR and develop either symptoms or LV systolic dysfunction (left ventricular ejection fraction [LVEF] <60%, LV end systolic diameter ≥40mm) require cardiac catheterization and evaluation for mitral valve surgery. Of note, with each contraction in severe MR, a large component (~50%) of blood is moving backward (from the left ventricle to left atrium). Given that LVEF represents the change in LV volume from end diastole to end systole, it is the summation of flow out of the ventricle, both forward and back. Thus, in severe MR a large component of the LVEF is attributable to backward flow. As a result, in severe MR even a minor reduction in LVEF is a marker for significant reduction in LV function. Hence, any LVEF <60% in severe MR is a consideration for intervention. Often the valve can be repaired rather than replaced, with a low operative mortality rate and excellent short- and long-term results when performed at experienced centers. Preservation of the native valve allows for lower risks of thrombosis and endocarditis than prosthetic valve replacement.

Therapy—Surgical

MVP is the most common cause of adult MR requiring mitral valve surgery in the United States. Symptoms of heart failure, severity of MR, presence or absence of atrial fibrillation, LV systolic function, LV end-diastolic and end-systolic volumes, and pulmonary artery pressure (at rest and with exercise) influence the decision to recommend mitral valve surgery. Indications for surgery in patients with MVP and MR mirror those with other forms of nonischemic severe MR. Patient outcomes after mitral valve repair are typically very good, and the surgical risk is lower than for many other forms of cardiac surgery, including mitral valve replacement.

Based on a Cleveland Clinic review of 1072 patients who underwent primary isolated mitral valve repair for MR due to myxomatous disease, the in-hospital mortality rate was 0.3%. The Mayo Clinic reviewed 1173 patients who underwent mitral valve repair for MVP from 1980 to 1999, observing mortality rates of 0.7%, 11.3%, and 29.4% at 30 days, 5 years, and 10 years, respectively.

Because of the remarkably low mortality rates associated with MVP repair, some experts advocate earlier rather than later repair of MVP in asymptomatic patients with severe MR and no evidence of LV dysfunction, pulmonary hypertension, or atrial fibrillation. ACC/AHA recommendations for surgery in patients with chronic primary mitral valve regurgitation are shown in Table 1.

Therapy—Percutaneous Management

In 2013 the FDA approved the MitraClip (Abbott Vascular) for patients with symptomatic degenerative MR who are deemed high risk for mitral valve surgery. The MitraClip technology was the first of its kind, a transcatheter device based on the Alfieri

CLASS	RECOMMENDATION
I	Mitral valve (MV) intervention is recommended for symptomatic patients with chronic severe primary mitral regurgitation (MR) (stage D) irrespective of LV function
	MV intervention is recommended for asymptomatic patients with chronic severe primary MR and left ventricular (LV) dysfunction (left ventricular ejection fraction [LVEF] ≤60% and/or left ventricular end-systolic dimension [LVESD] ≥40 mm, stage C2)
	MV repair is recommended in preference to mitral valve replacement (MVR) when surgical treatment is indicated for patients with chronic severe primary MR due to degenerative disease, if a successful and durable repair is possible
IIa	MV repair is reasonable in asymptomatic patients with chronic severe primary MR (stage C1) with preserved LV function (LVEF ≥60% and LVESD ≤40 mm) in whom the likelihood of a successful and durable repair without residual MR is >95% with an expected mortality rate of <1% when performed at a Heart Valve Center of Excellence
	Transcatheter MV edge-to-edge repair may be considered for severely symptomatic patients (New York Heart Association class III/IV) with chronic severe primary MR (stage D) who have a reasonable life expectancy >1 year and favorable anatomy but a prohibitive surgical risk
IIb	MV repair is reasonable for asymptomatic patients with chronic severe primary MR (stage C1) and preserved LV function (LVEF >60% and LVESD <40 mm) with progressive increase in LV size or decrease in ejection fraction on ≥3 serial imaging studies
III Harm	MVR should not be performed for treatment of isolated severe primary MR limited to less than one-half of the posterior leaflet unless MV repair has been attempted and was unsuccessful

TABLE 1 ACC/AHA Recommendations for Intervention in Patients With Chronic Primary Mitral Valve Regurgitation

Adapted from Otto CM, Nishimura RA, Bonow RO, et al: 2020 ACC/AHA guideline for the management of patients with valvular heart disease: executive summary: a report of the American College of Cardiology/American Heart Association Joint Committee on Clinical Practice Guidelines. *Circulation* 143(5):e35-e71, 2021.

edge-to-edge repair in which the middle segments of the anterior and posterior leaflets are sutured together to create a double-orifice. It is approved for use in patients with New York Heart Association class III or IV heart failure despite medical therapy, chronic moderate-to-severe or severe primary MR, favorable anatomy typically involving the middle segments of the anterior and posterior leaflets, reasonable life expectancy, and prohibitive surgical risk. This approval is based on the results of the Endovascular Valve Edge-to-Edge Repair Study (EVEREST II), which randomized 279 patients to either percutaneous repair or conventional surgery for repair or replacement of the mitral valve with a primary endpoint of freedom from death, from surgery for mitral valve dysfunction, and from grade 3+ or 4+ MR at 12 months. The rates of the combined primary endpoints were 55% in the percutaneous group and 73% in the surgery group (p = 0.007). Rates of death (6% and 6%, respectively) and 3+ or 4+ MR (21% and 20%, respectively) were similar in each group. Major adverse events occurred in 15% of patients in the percutaneous repair group versus 48% in the surgery group at 30 days (p < 0.001). Although the MitraClip was less effective at reducing MR, it was approved on the basis of its superior safety and similar clinical outcomes. In 2022 the FDA approved the second mitral transcatheter edge-to-edge repair device, the PAS-CAL (Edwards Lifesciences). This was based on the result of the randomized clinical trial CLASP IID, which demonstrated non-inferiority in the PASCAL system compared with the MitraClip based on 30-day safety and 6-month efficacy endpoints.

Monitoring

As previously outlined, uncomplicated MVP is generally a benign disease. For these patients, periodic clinical evaluation every 3 to 5 years is reasonable with repeat echocardiographic assessment if there is concern for disease progression, particularly the development of MR.

Patients with complicated MVP (associated with significant MR, left ventricular structural changes, pulmonary hypertension, atrial fibrillation, or stroke) deserve regular clinical follow-up, particularly if MR is present. These patients are more likely to develop moderate or severe MR over time. Patients with mild-to-moderate MR and normal LV function should be clinically evaluated at least annually and should undergo echocardiography every second or third year if stable. Patients with severe MR should have an annual echocardiogram and closer clinical follow-up with particular assessment for features that would be an indication for surgery (i.e., symptoms, impaired LV systolic function).

Complications

The clinical significance of MVP is predominantly related to the risk of developing clinically significant MR. Similarly, the complications of MVP are often a result of associated MR. These complications include heart failure, left atrial dilation, arrhythmias (particularly atrial fibrillation), and infective endocarditis.

References

Bonow R, O'Gara P, Adams D, et al: 2020 focused update of the 2017 ACC expert consensus decision pathway on the management of mitral regurgitation: a report of the American College of cardiology solution set oversight committee, *J Am Coll Cardiol* 75(17):2236–2270, 2020.

Delling FN, Rong J, Larson MG, et al: Evolution of mitral valve prolapse: insights from the Framingham heart study, *Circulation* 133(17):1688–1695, 2016.

Otto CM, Nishimura RA, Bonow RO, et al: 2020 ACC/AHA guideline for the management of patients with valvular heart disease: executive summary: a report of the American College of cardiology/American heart association Joint committee on clinical Practice guidelines, *Circulation* 143(5):e35–e71, 2021.

Vahanian A, Beyersdorf F, Praz F, et al: 2021 ESC/EACTS guidelines for the management of valvular heart disease: developed by the task force for the management of valvular heart disease of the European society of cardiology (ESC) and the European association for cardio-thoracic surgery (EACTS), *Eur Heart J* 43(7):561–632, 2022.

Zahr F, Smith R, Gillam L, et al: 1-Year outcomes from the CLASP IID randomized trial for degenerative mitral regurgitation, *J Am Coll Cardiol Intv* (23)2803–2816, 2023.

PERICARDITIS

Method of
Jenna Greenberg, MD

CURRENT DIAGNOSIS

- Acute pericarditis is an inflammatory condition of the pericardium most commonly due to a viral or idiopathic etiology.
- Diagnosis is made when at least 2 of 4 criteria are met: (1) Pleuritic chest pain, (2) pericardial friction rub, (3) electrocardiogram changes consistent with pericarditis, (4) new or worsening pericardial effusion.
- Markers of inflammation, including erythrocyte sedimentation rate, C-reactive protein, and white blood cell count, are often elevated.
- An echocardiogram should be performed in all patients to assess for an effusion or signs of tamponade. Computed tomography and cardiac magnetic resonance imaging can be used in select cases to provide additional supporting evidence.

CURRENT THERAPY

- Nonsteroidal antiinflammatory drugs (NSAIDs) plus colchicine[1] is the first-line therapy for viral/idiopathic acute pericarditis. Aspirin[1] is the preferred NSAID in patients with a concurrent indication for aspirin.
- Physical activity restriction is recommended until resolution of symptoms or 3 months depending on the degree of activity.
- Treatment should target the underlying etiology when appropriate.
- Corticosteroids can be considered as a second-line treatment in patients who fail NSAIDs/colchicine or have recurrent pericarditis.
- Interleukin-1 inhibitors anakinra (Kineret)[1] and rilonacept (Arcalyst)[1] are used in treatment-resistant recurrent pericarditis or patients who become steroid-dependent.
- Additional steroid-sparing treatment for recurrent pericarditis can include azathioprine (Imuran),[1] methotrexate,[1] mycophenolate mofetil (CellCept)[1] and intravenous immunoglobulin.[1]
- Pericardiectomy is reserved for refractory cases of constrictive pericarditis in unstable patients.
- Cardiac tamponade should be treated urgently with an image-guided pericardiocentesis.

[1]Not FDA approved for this indication.

Pathophysiology

The pericardium is a fibroelastic sac that surrounds the heart and consists of a visceral and parietal layer separated by a potential space. Normally this space contains approximately 50 mL of an ultrafiltrate of plasma from the epicardial and parietal pericardial capillaries. The pericardium performs many essential functions, including (1) acting as a partition from the pulmonary space to decrease the spread of infection, (2) limiting distention of the cardiac chambers in the event of volume overload to prevent anatomic deformities that can worsen mitral and tricuspid regurgitation, and (3) exerting a mechanical pressure on the heart that is responsible for more than 50% of the diastolic pressure in the right atrium and right ventricle.

Acute Pericarditis

Acute pericarditis is the most common pericardial disorder resulting from inflammation of the pericardial sac. Exact incidence data are lacking; however, one study estimated that there are 27 cases per 100,000 persons per year and an incidence of 3.3 hospital admissions per 100,000 persons per year. Acute pericarditis is responsible for 5% of emergency department visits for chest pain. Men aged 16 to 65 have a higher risk of pericarditis than women. Recurrence occurs in 20% to 30% of cases. Up to 50% of patients with one recurrence episode will have additional recurrences. Pericarditis can be acute, incessant, recurrent, or chronic (Table 1).

Diagnosis

Pericarditis is diagnosed when at least 2 of the following 4 criteria are met: (1) Pleuritic chest pain, (2) pericardial friction rub, (3) electrocardiogram (ECG) changes consistent with pericarditis, (4) new or worsening pericardial effusion. Additional supporting evidence can include elevated markers of inflammation (erythrocyte sedimentation rate [ESR], C-reactive protein [CRP], white blood cells [WBCs]) and evidence of pericardial inflammation by computed tomography (CT) or cardiac magnetic resonance (CMR).

Clinical Presentation

Chest pain is the most common clinical presentation of acute pericarditis and present in more than 95% of patients. Typical pain is sudden in onset, sharp, pleuritic, and located over the anterior chest. It is worse with inspiration and improved with sitting up and leaning forward due to decreased pressure on the parietal pericardium. Pain often radiates to the trapezius ridge due to the phrenic nerves passing through the anterior pericardium. Patients may also present with a prodrome of fever, malaise, and myalgias, especially with a viral etiology.

Pericardial friction rub is a highly specific finding (approaching 100% specificity) for pericarditis but has low sensitivity (present in ~33% of cases). A friction rub is a scratching or squeaking sound best heard in the left lower sternal border. It is louder in inspiration, although 35% of cases have no respiratory predilection. The intensity increases with maneuvers that increase the contact between the visceral and parietal pericardium, including firm pressure to the diaphragm, suspended respiration, and leaning forward. The friction rub is often transient and can come and go over hours, so repeated auscultations are important.

ECG changes in pericarditis are due to inflammation of the epicardium and adjacent myocardium and are present in up to 60% of cases. There are 4 stages of ECG changes:

- Stage 1 occurs in the first hours to days with diffuse concave ST elevations and PR depression, which is specific for pericarditis (Figure 1).
- Stage 2 occurs in the first week with normalization of the ST and PR segment.
- Stage 3 is the subacute phase and has diffuse T wave inversions.
- Stage 4 is a normal ECG. Up to 40% of patients will have atypical or nondiagnostic changes. When evaluating ECG changes it is important to differentiate from an acute myocardial infarction (MI), and in pericarditis there will be no reciprocal ST changes or Q waves.

Diagnostic Evaluation

There are no specific biomarkers for pericarditis. Inflammatory markers (ESR, CRP, WBC) are elevated in up to 80% of cases but are not sensitive or specific. Thirty percent of patients will have some degree of troponin-I elevation due to involvement of

TABLE 1 Definitions of Pericarditis Syndromes

PERICARDITIS SYNDROME	DEFINITION
Acute pericarditis	Symptoms resolve within 4–6 weeks
Incessant pericarditis	Symptoms persist >4–6 weeks without remission
Recurrent pericarditis	New symptoms occur after a symptom-free period of 4–6 weeks
Chronic pericarditis	Symptoms present for >3 months

TABLE 2 Pericardial Syndromes and Treatments Summary

PERICARDIAL SYNDROME	TREATMENT	CONSIDERATIONS
Acute pericarditis	NSAIDs	Continue NSAIDs until symptoms resolve and CRP normalizes.
	Colchicine[1]	Continue colchicine for 3 months.
	Physical activity restriction	Physical activity restriction until symptoms resolve or 3 months.
		Treat underlying cause when identified.
Recurrent pericarditis	NSAIDs and colchicine.[1]	NSAIDs until symptoms resolve and CRP normalizes, then taper.
		Colchicine for 6 months.
	Corticosteroids in refractory cases.	Corticosteroids at a low-to-moderate dose until symptoms resolve and CRP normalizes, followed by a slow taper.
	Immunosuppression (IL-1 inhibitors and others) in steroid-dependent patients or those with multiple recurrences.	Immunosuppression for patients who are steroid-dependent and with multiple recurrences.
	Pericardiectomy in refractory cases.	
Constrictive pericarditis	NSAIDs and colchicine[1] if transient/reversible. Treat underlying condition (TB, malignancy). Pericardiectomy if chronic and refractory.	
Cardiac tamponade	Urgent image-guided needle pericardiocentesis. Surgical pericardial window if needle drainage not possible.	No specific treatment is needed of an effusion due to pericarditis in the absence of hemodynamic compromise. It will often resolve with treatment of pericarditis.

[1]Not FDA approved for this indication.
CRP, C-Reactive protein; IL-1, interleukin-1; NSAIDs, nonsteroidal antiinflammatory drugs; TB, tuberculosis.

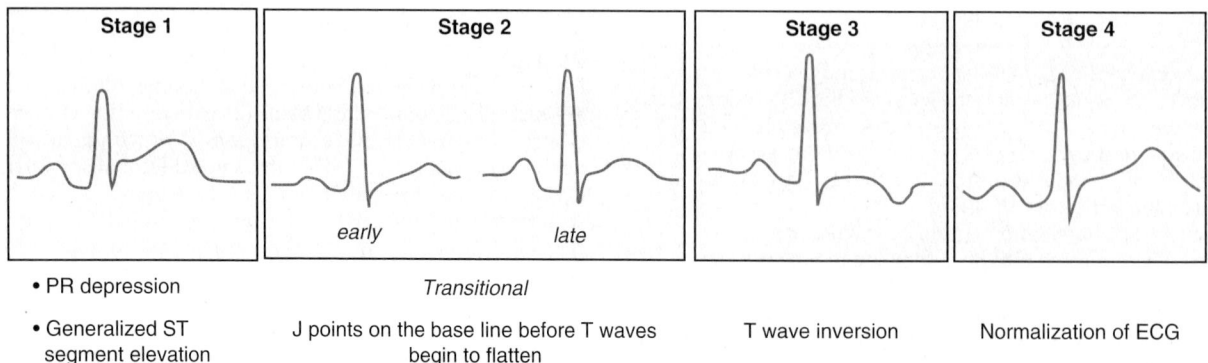

Figure 1 Electrocardiogram *(ECG)* changes in acute pericarditis. (From Chiabrando, J., Bonaventura, A., Veccié, A. et al. [2020]. Management of acute and recurrent pericarditis: JACC state-of-the-art review. *Journal of the American College of Cardiology, 75*[1], 76–92.)

the subepicardium or myocardium and, if elevated, is considered myopericarditis. This can be differentiated from an acute MI due to the lack of ischemic changes on ECG.

Patients presenting with pericarditis should have a chest x-ray performed, which is often normal unless a large pericardial effusion (at least 200 mL) is present, which would enlarge the cardiac silhouette. All patients should have an echocardiogram to evaluate for the presence of an effusion and assess for cardiac tamponade. Sixty percent of patients will have a pericardial effusion. Additional imaging is not necessary in patients with uncomplicated status; however, CT or CMR can be considered if echocardiogram is inconclusive and there is ongoing clinical concern. CT shows pericardial thickening and helps differentiate exudate versus transudate based on attenuation values. It is preferred to evaluate pericardial calcification and coexisting pleuropulmonary disease. CMR can also evaluate pericardial thickening, and enhancement with contrast can confirm active pericardial inflammation and determine severity. It can also show features of a constrictive physiology and evaluate for myocardial inflammation. CMR is preferred over CT to evaluate pericardial and myocardial inflammation and can be used to support the diagnosis of pericarditis in complex or atypical presentations, such as when the objective findings of pericarditis are lacking but clinical suspicion remains high. Pericardiocentesis and pericardial biopsy are low yield and not needed in simple, self-limiting pericarditis. However, in complex cases or cases of cardiac tamponade it can be considered for therapeutic and diagnostic purposes.

Etiology

Acute pericarditis usually has a benign and self-limiting course; therefore, it is not necessary to establish a specific etiology in all cases. In developed countries 80% to 90% of cases have a viral or idiopathic etiology and most idiopathic cases are likely viral. In areas where *Mycobacterium tuberculosis* is endemic, tuberculosis (TB) is the most common causative agent and is often associated with human immunodeficiency virus (HIV) infection.

Many viruses can cause pericarditis, including enteroviruses, herpesviruses (Epstein-Barr virus [EBV], cytomegalovirus [CMV]), adenovirus, parvovirus B19, and hepatitis B and C viruses (HBV and HCV). Bacterial infections are also possible, with *M. tuberculosis* being the most common. Fungal infections (*Histoplasma, Aspergillus, Blastomyces, Candida*) are rare and more common in immunocompromised patients. Parasitic infections (*Echinococcus,*

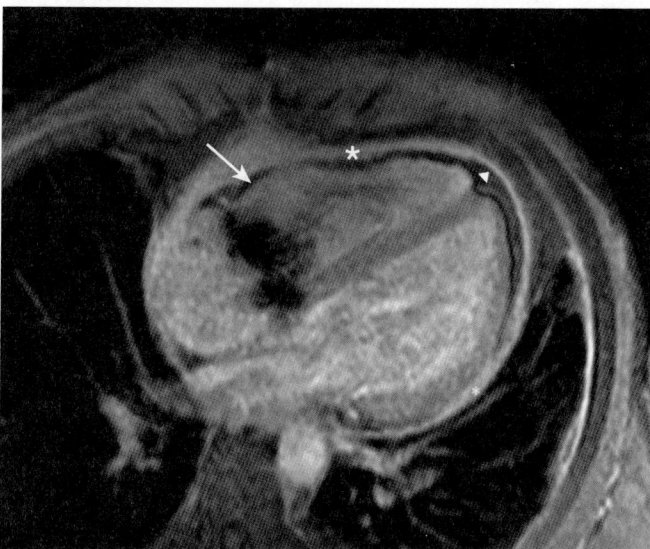

Figure 2 Cardiac magnetic resonance image of acute pericarditis after gadolinium contrast. Enhancement of the pericardium and pericardial thickening indicate inflammation *(asterisk)*. Other findings are pericardial fat *(arrowhead)* and a trace pericardial effusion *(arrow)*. (From Azarbal, A., LeWinter, M., & Kellerman, R. D. [Eds.]. [2024]. *Conn's current therapy* [pp 148–152]. Elsevier.)

Toxoplasma) are exceedingly rare. Autoimmune conditions, including systemic lupus erythematosus (SLE), rheumatoid arthritis, scleroderma, Sjögren syndrome, vasculitis, inflammatory bowel disease, sarcoidosis, mixed connective tissue disorders, familial Mediterranean fever, and tumor necrosis factor receptor–associated periodic fever syndrome are also causes. Pericarditis can be due to malignancy related to metastatic spread from any primary source (most commonly breast cancer, lung cancer, and lymphoma) or rarely a primary malignancy (pericardial mesothelioma). Paraneoplastic pericarditis is also possible.

Post-MI pericarditis can occur with the development of a pericardial effusion on post-MI day 2 to 4 due to a reaction to the necrotic myocardium in up to 25% of patients. Dressler syndrome is pericarditis that occurs weeks to months after an MI due to a late autoimmune reaction stimulated by entry of necrotic myocardial tissue into the circulation, which acts as an antigen. Iatrogenic pericarditis is also an increasing cause related to cardiac procedures such as catheterization, pacemaker placement, and ablations.

Other causes include blunt or penetrating trauma, radiation, and renal failure. Renal failure can cause pericarditis through uremia or associated with dialysis (often due to volume overload and inadequate dialysis). Medications are a rare cause of pericarditis. Procainamide, hydralazine, methyldopa, isoniazid, and phenytoin (Dilantin) can cause drug-induced lupus associated with pericarditis. Penicillins can cause a hypersensitivity pericarditis associated with eosinophilia. Additional causative medications include dantrolene (Dantrium), doxorubicin (Adriamycin), mesalamine (Asacol), and rifampin (Rifadin).

Treatment

Most cases of pericarditis are self-limiting and respond well to outpatient treatment. One study found 85% of cases were low risk and could be managed as an outpatient and resulted in no serious complications. Major risk factors for poor prognosis include high fever (>38°C [>100.4°F]), subacute course (symptoms over several days without a clear onset), large pericardial effusion, cardiac tamponade, and failure to respond to treatment within 7 days. Additional risk factors for poor prognosis include myopericarditis, immunosuppressed state, trauma, and oral anticoagulant use. Any risk factor for poor prognosis is an indication for hospital admission and further evaluation of the underlying cause.

The mainstay of treatment for acute pericarditis is a combination of nonsteroidal antiinflammatory drugs (NSAIDs) and colchicine[1] because most cases are viral/idiopathic. Treatment should target the underlying etiology when a nonviral etiology is suspected. The goal of treatment is to decrease symptoms, resolve the inflammation and/or pleural effusion, and prevent recurrence. Nonpharmacologic management consists of restriction of strenuous activity until symptoms resolve and biomarkers normalize, because exercise-induced tachycardia is thought to increase the shear stress on the pericardium, in turn increasing inflammation. Some experts recommend waiting 3 months to return to competitive sports in all uncomplicated cases. If myopericarditis is present, patients should follow activity restrictions for myocarditis.

NSAIDs are first-line treatment for all patients with acute pericarditis who do not have a contraindication. NSAIDs treat pericarditis by decreasing inflammation through their antiinflammatory effect. No specific NSAID is preferred; however, ibuprofen,[1] indomethacin,[1] naproxen,[1] and aspirin[1] are commonly used. Aspirin is preferred in patients already receiving it for a concurrent condition and for post-MI pericarditis because other NSAIDs can impair scar formation. Recommended NSAID dosing includes ibuprofen (Advil)[1] 600 to 800 mg tid, aspirin[1] 1 g tid, naproxen[1] 500 mg bid, and indomethacin[1] 50 mg tid. NSAIDs should be continued at the initial dose until symptoms resolve and CRP normalizes (usually 1 to 2 weeks) and then tapered over 3 to 4 weeks to prevent recurrence. NSAIDs are well tolerated, but long-term use can be associated with peptic

---

[1] Not FDA approved for this indication.

ulcer disease, gastrointestinal hemorrhage, and renal dysfunction. Gastroprotection with a proton pump inhibitor should be given to patients at risk for gastrointestinal bleeding.

Colchicine[1] should be given with NSAIDs as first-line therapy to all patients with acute pericarditis. Use of colchicine with NSAIDs versus NSAIDs alone has been shown to decrease the risk of recurrence by half and decrease time to symptom resolution. Colchicine has an antiinflammatory effect that differs from NSAIDs and steroids. It inhibits the mobility, phagocytosis, and degranulation of WBCs and also inhibits interleukin-IB (IL-IB) and IL-18. Colchicine should be given at a dose of 0.6 mg bid for 3 months. In patients weighing less than 70 kg or older than 70 consider 0.6 mg/day to decrease side effects. Colchicine has a narrow therapeutic window, and it is important to monitor for drug-drug interactions. It is excreted mainly by the liver, with 10% to 20% excreted by the kidney; dose adjustment may be needed in hepatic and renal impairment. Renal impairment is a significant risk factor for development of colchicine-induced myotoxicity, and renal function should be followed during treatment. Colchicine is generally well tolerated, with the most common side effects being gastrointestinal (nausea, vomiting, and diarrhea). Additional side effects include myalgias, bone marrow depression, and hepatotoxicity.

Glucocorticoids can be used in patients who fail colchicine/NSAIDs or in patients with an absolute contraindication to NSAIDs. Glucocorticoids are not considered first-line therapy because use early in the course is associated with a higher risk of recurrence. Glucocorticoids should be started at a low-to-moderate dose of 0.2 to 0.5 mg/kg/day of prednisone[1] followed by a slow taper over 4 to 6 weeks.

Complications

Recurrent Pericarditis
The diagnosis of recurrent pericarditis is made when symptoms of pericarditis recur after a symptom-free period of 4 to 6 weeks. This occurs in up to 30% of patients with acute pericarditis and is more common in those not treated with colchicine. Diagnosis is made based on the same criteria as the initial episode of acute pericarditis. Initial treatment still consists of NSAIDs and colchicine.[1] However, colchicine should be continued for 6 months in recurrent pericarditis. NSAIDs should still be tapered after symptoms resolve and CRP normalizes. If the patient fails to improve on NSAIDs and colchicine, glucocorticoids should be added at a dose of 0.2 to 0.5 mg/kg/day and tapered over the course of 4 to 6 weeks. Glucocorticoids result in rapid improvement of symptoms, but many patients end up steroid dependent. In resistant cases or inpatients who are glucocorticoid dependent, IL-1 inhibitors anakinra (Kineret)[1] and rilonacept (Arcalyst) are effective and can help patients discontinue steroids. Withdrawal of an IL-1 inhibitor often leads to a recurrence, and they may need to be continued 6 months or longer. Additional steroid-sparing therapy to consider in refractory cases includes azathioprine (Imuran),[1] methotrexate,[1] mycophenolate mofetil (CellCept),[1] and intravenous immunoglobulin.[1] In severe refractory cases pericardiectomy can also be considered. Overall the prognosis of recurrent pericarditis is favorable and is not more significantly associated with outcomes of cardiac tamponade or constrictive pericarditis than the first episode.

Constrictive Pericarditis
Constrictive pericarditis occurs when the pericardium becomes thickened and inelastic, resulting in impaired cardiac filling during diastole. It can occur as a sequela of any pericardial disease process; however, it most commonly occurs in bacterial pericarditis (20% to 30%), with TB as the most causative agent. Constrictive pericarditis rarely follows viral/idiopathic acute pericarditis (<1% of cases) and follows immune-mediated and neoplastic pericarditis in 2% to 5% of cases. Constrictive pericarditis can also occur after cardiac surgery and after radiation.

Signs and symptoms of constrictive pericarditis are related to signs of right heart failure and include fatigue, dyspnea, and peripheral edema. Constrictive pericarditis is diagnosed based on clinical symptoms plus a finding of pericardial thickening with calcifications and impaired diastolic filling on echocardiogram. Chest radiograph will have pericardial calcifications in 25% to 30% of cases. CMR and CT can also be used to evaluate for pericardial thickening and signs of pericardial inflammation when echo is inconclusive. Cardiac catheterization can be used when noninvasive methods are inconclusive and suspicion remains high. On physical examination, 47% of patients have a pericardial knock, which is a high-pitched sound in early diastole resulting from the sudden termination of cardiac filling. Jugular venous distention is often present and Kussmaul's sign of paradoxical rise in jugular venous pressure with inspiration can also be seen. Some cases may have pulsus paradoxus, which is a fall in systolic blood pressure by less than 10 mm Hg during inspiration. ECG findings are nonspecific but can include low voltage.

Treatment depends in part on the type and cause of constrictive pericarditis. Transient constrictive pericarditis is often due to idiopathic/viral acute pericarditis and caused by the inflammation in the pericardium. Treatment with 2 to 3 months of antiinflammatory medication will often resolve the constrictive pericarditis. Effusive constrictive pericarditis is constrictive pericarditis plus the presence of a pericardial effusion. With the constriction even a small amount of fluid can cause tamponade. This is diagnosed when there is a failure of atrial pressure to fall by 50% to below 10 after a pericardiocentesis. Treatment includes pericardiocentesis plus medical therapy and can include surgery for persistent cases. Chronic constrictive pericarditis occurs when symptoms persist 3 to 6 months and treatment for this is pericardiectomy. However, pericardiectomy has a high mortality rate (6% to 12%) so the risks/benefits should be carefully considered.

Pericardial Effusion and Cardiac Tamponade
A pericardial effusion is present in 60% to 80% of patients with acute pericarditis and is diagnosed on echo. The majority (80%) are small, 10% are moderate, and 10% are large. In idiopathic/viral pericarditis the effusion is generally small, but effusions related to malignancy, TB, and hypothyroidism are usually larger. Patients can have muffled heart sounds on examination, and a friction rub may be absent due to the large effusion. Pulsus paradoxus can be present. ECG may show low amplitude and electrical alternans due to movement of the heart within the pericardial fluid.

Cardiac tamponade is a life-threatening complication of a pericardial effusion in which the pericardial fluid compresses all cardiac chambers causing progressive decreases in venous return and stroke volume. It is rare in acute pericarditis (1.2% of cases) and is more common in pericarditis related to TB or malignancy. Patients with cardiac tamponade can exhibit signs of hemodynamic instability, including hypotension, jugular venous distention, and tachycardia. Cardiac tamponade requires immediate treatment with image-guided pericardiocentesis to drain the pericardial fluid contents. Surgical drainage with a pericardial window can be considered when needle drainage is not possible or ineffective.

References
Adler Y, Charron P, et al: 2015 ESC Guidelines for the diagnosis and management of pericardial diseases: The Task Force for the Diagnosis and Management of Pericardial Diseases of the European Society of Cardiology (ESC), *Eur Heart J* 36(42):2921–2964, 2015.

Azarbal A, LeWinter M: *Kellerman. Conn's Current Therapy 2024*, Elsevier, 2024, pp 148–152.

Chiabrando J, Bonaventura A, et al: Management of Acute and Recurrent Pericarditis: JACC State-of-the-Art Review, *J Am Coll Cardio* 75(1):76–92, 2020.

Klein A, Abbara S, et al: American Society of Echocardiography Clinical Recommendations for Multimodality Cardiovascular Imaging of Patients with Pericardial Disease, *J Am Soc Echocardiogr* 26(9):965–1012, 2013.

Lazarou E, Tsioufis P, et al: Acute Pericarditis: Update, *Curr Cardiol Rep* 24(8):905–913, 2022.

---

[1] Not FDA approved for this indication.

PERIPHERAL ARTERY DISEASE

Method of
William Michael, MD

Epidemiology and Risk Factors

Peripheral artery disease (PAD), the third leading cause of atherosclerotic morbidity following coronary artery disease and stroke, is estimated to affect 8.5 million Americans older than 40 years of age and more than 230 million people worldwide. The prevalence ranges from ~5% among individuals 40 to 44 years of age up to ~12% among those 70 to 74 years of age. Although PAD is defined as atherosclerotic disease in any arterial vessel outside of the coronary circulation, the most common sites for the development of PAD are the abdominal aorta and vessels of the lower extremities. Patients at increased risk of PAD are those older than 65 years of age and those with diabetes, a history of smoking, hyperlipidemia, and hypertension. Individuals with a family history of PAD or with known atherosclerotic disease in another vascular bed area are also at increased risk.

Pathophysiology

PAD is related to the development of atherosclerotic plaques of the peripheral arteries that leads to reduction of blood flow to peripheral tissues. Classic claudication involves flow-limiting blockages that present as exertional pain in the lower extremities that is caused by lack of oxygen delivery to the peripheral tissues and improves with rest. More serious manifestations of PAD are termed *critical limb ischemia* (CLI) and involve pain at rest or pain that wakes the patient at night, nonhealing wounds/ulcerations in the distal extremities, or gangrene.

Prevention and Screening Recommendations

Prevention of PAD involves controlling risk factors associated with the development of atherosclerotic disease (e.g., diabetes mellitus, history of smoking, hyperlipidemia, hypertension) and appropriately managing these conditions. The U.S. Preventive Services Task Force (USPSTF) states that the evidence for screening for PAD as part of cardiovascular risk assessment is inconclusive (I rating). However, the American Heart Association (AHA) recommends screening with ankle-brachial index (ABI) in adults at high risk of having PAD (those older than 65 years of age and those 50 to 64 years of age with risk factors for atherosclerotic disease).

Clinical Manifestations

PAD can manifest in a number of different ways, and many individuals are asymptomatic (20% to 50%). Classic intermittent claudication presents with exertional leg pain (often in the calf but also in the buttock, hip, thigh, or foot) that resolves within 10 minutes of rest. However, only 10% to 30% of patients present with classic claudication. The remaining 40% to 50% present with "atypical" leg symptoms that include pain that begins at rest, pain that does not cause the patient to stop walking/activity, or discomfort that does not consistently improve with rest. CLI involves pain at rest, nocturnal pain, nonhealing wounds/ulcers that are located distally (e.g., tips of toes, between toes), and gangrene.

Physical Examination

Physical examination has poor sensitivity in assessing patients with asymptomatic PAD but can be helpful in assessing for and differentiating between claudication and CLI versus presentations that are not related to symptomatic PAD. Lower-extremity pulses should be assessed; pulses are graded on a scale of 0 to 3, with 0 being absent, 1 diminished, 2 normal, and 3 bounding. Absent or diminished pulses are suggestive of PAD and disease at a higher level of the vascular tree than the assessed pulse, making assessment of the dorsal pedal or posterior tibial pulses the most useful. Auscultation for femoral arterial bruit can be helpful but is rare in the primary care setting. Examination of the feet should focus on identification of nonhealing lower-extremity ulceration in a characteristic,

TABLE 1 Ankle-Brachial Index

ABI	MAGNITUDE OF PERIPHERAL ARTERY DISEASE	TREATMENT CONSIDERATIONS
>1.4	Cannot interpret	Consider TBI
1.0–1.4	Normal	None
0.91–0.99	Borderline	If high concern, consider exercise ABI
0.7–0.90	Mild PAD	Treat risk factors, discuss supervised exercise therapy and/or medication management
0.41–0.69	Moderate PAD	Treat risk factors, refer to vascular surgeon
<0.4	Severe PAD	Treat risk factors, refer to vascular surgeon

ABI, Ankle-brachial index; *PAD,* peripheral artery disease; *TBI,* toe-brachial index.

well-demarcated, or "punched-out" pattern and lack of granulation tissue at the base, consistent with arterial ulceration. Careful inspection should be paid to the toes, especially between the toes and the webbing of the toes, as these lesions may not be readily noticed by the patient. The anterior lower leg is also a common place for arterial ulcers as they have less collateral circulation. Other examination findings of the lower extremity that suggest a diagnosis of PAD include elevation pallor and dependent rubor.

Diagnosis

The initial diagnostic workup for patients with suspected PAD involves obtaining a resting ABI or ABI (Table 1). If the resting ABI is normal (1.0 to 1.4 is normal; ≤0.9 is abnormal) but there remains a high clinical suspicion for PAD, an exercise ABI can be obtained. The ABI is less accurate and can be falsely elevated in the presence of medial artery calcification that can stiffen arteries in the ankle, an issue most often encountered in patients with diabetes or end-stage kidney disease. This can result in an ABI >1.4, which is an uninterpretable result. In such cases, a toe-brachial index (TBI) can be considered. An abnormal TBI may predict poor outcomes beyond ABI in such patients (TBI ≤0.7 is diagnostic of PAD). Arterial duplex ultrasonography is also readily available, low risk, and inexpensive, but it is limited in its ability to detect infrapopliteal stenosis, stenosis that exists in the pelvic or abdominal cavities, or in patients with significant arterial calcifications. More advanced noninvasive studies, such as computed tomography angiography (CTA) and magnetic resonance angiography (MRA) can provide more anatomic detail and is often ordered for patients with PAD who fail medical management and/or are candidates for more invasive interventions. These studies are expensive and come with the added risk of contrast-related complications in certain patient populations. Catheter-based angiography remains the gold standard for diagnosing PAD but is reserved for patients receiving endovascular revascularization.

Ankle-Brachial Index

The ABI is an inexpensive way to assess for PAD and can be done within 15 minutes in the primary care setting or ordered to be completed in a vascular laboratory. To obtain an ABI in clinic, the patient should be placed in the supine position with the head, hips, and heels fully supported. The ABI averages 0.35 higher in the seated position than in the supine position. A Doppler probe should be used to obtain both the ankle and brachial pressure. After allowing for a 5- to 10-minute rest period, the Doppler probe is used to auscultate flow, and a pneumatic cuff is inflated until flow ceases. The cuff is then slowly deflated until the flow signal reappears, and the corresponding pressure is recorded as

TABLE 2 Differential Diagnosis for Symptomatic Peripheral Artery Disease

CONDITION	LOCATION	CHARACTERISTIC	EFFECT OF EXERCISE	EFFECT OF REST	OTHER CHARACTERISTICS
Venous claudication	Entire leg, worse in calf	Tight, bursting pain	After walking	Subsides slowly	History of iliofemoral deep vein thrombosis; edema; signs of venous stasis
Popliteal artery entrapment syndrome	Calf muscles	Tight, tearing pain	After moderate to vigorous exercise (jogging)	Subsides slowly	Typically heavy muscular athletes
Spinal stenosis	Often bilateral buttocks, posterior leg	Pain and weakness	May mimic claudication	Variable relief, but can take a long time to recover	Worse with standing and extending spine
Nerve root compression	Radiates down leg	Sharp lancinating pain	Induced by sitting, standing, or walking	Often present at rest	History of back problems; worse with sitting; relief when supine or sitting
Arthritis (hip, foot, or ankle)	Lateral hip, thigh, foot arch, ankle	Aching discomfort	After variable degree of exercise	Not quickly relieved	Symptoms variable; may be related to activity or present at rest

the SBP of that limb. The process is then repeated for each limb, and the higher ankle and higher brachial pressures are used for calculation. The ankle pressure is then divided into the brachial pressure to obtain the ABI. A score between 1.0 and 1.4 is considered normal, and a score ≤0.9 is consistent with mild to moderate PAD. An ABI ≤0.4 is considered severe PAD. An ABI between 0.91 and 0.99 is considered borderline low, and PAD cannot be ruled out. In such cases, exercise ABI or other noninvasive imaging studies can be helpful to further evaluate for PAD.

Differential Diagnosis
PAD can present with symptoms that are similar to those for other vascular pathologies, neurologic conditions, and musculoskeletal etiologies. For example, the terms *pseudoclaudication* and *neuroclaudication* are used because of similarities in the presentation of claudication in PAD to conditions such as lumbar spinal stenosis, sciatica, or structural back disease. Venous claudication, popliteal artery entrapment syndrome, and various arthritides should also be considered in the differential diagnosis. The presence or absence of classic PAD risk factors, the specific location and description of the pain, in addition to the effect of exercise and rest (Table 2) can help differentiate PAD from these other conditions.

Treatment
Risk-Factor Control
Control of preexisting risk factors is crucial in the treatment of PAD. Patients with modifiable risk factors such as smoking must be aggressively counseled on the importance of smoking cessation. Patient with diabetes, hypertension, and hyperlipidemia should be treated per the most up-to-date guidelines published by the American College of Endocrinology (ACE) and the American College of Cardiology/American Heart Association (ACC/AHA). The Edinburgh study suggested that a sedentary lifestyle has also been shown to increase the risk for development of PAD by showing that physical activity was inversely proportional to the development of PAD.

Tobacco Cessation
The risk of developing PAD is double for a smoker compared with a nonsmoker. The risk is related to the number of cigarettes smoked and the age at which an individual started smoking. Although it takes 30 years after quitting for a former smoker's risk for development of PAD to return to that of a nonsmoker, the importance of smoking cessation cannot be overstated. Patients who smoke should be counseled on quitting at every office visit and offered appropriate pharmacotherapy, nicotine replacement, and/or referral to tobacco cessation programs. However, only

one-third of patients with PAD receive these therapeutic recommendations from their primary care team. Patients who successfully quit have lower rates of progression of atherosclerosis in their limbs as evidenced by decreasing rates of decline in their ABIs and lower rates of CLI, amputation, and death.

Glycemic Control
Diabetic patients also carry about double the risk for the development of PAD than do patients without diabetes. Many studies have been designed to look at the role glycemic control should play in reducing both major adverse limb events (MALE) and major adverse cardiovascular events (MACE) in diabetic patients, but the evidence for improved glycemic control in reduction of macrovascular complications for diabetic patients with PAD is lacking, especially in regard to MALE. Multiple studies have demonstrated benefit with sodium glucose transporter 2 inhibitors (SGLT2i) on MACE, heart failure, and overall mortality but did not show a reduction in MALE. In the Canagliflozin Cardiovascular Study (CANVAS), a subgroup analysis suggested that canagliflozin (Invokana) demonstrated up to a twofold increase in risk of amputation in diabetic patients with PAD compared with older insulin management regimens (sulfonylureas, metformin, insulin). The DECLARE-TIMI 58 trial involving dapagliflozin (Farxiga) redemonstrated the overall positive cardiovascular effects of the SGLT2i medications, but the subgroup analysis also demonstrated an increase in amputation risk in diabetic patients with PAD compared with those without PAD. A subsequent subgroup analysis of a study with canagliflozin, the Canagliflozin and Renal Events in Diabetes with Established Nephropathy Clinical Evaluation (CREDENCE) trial, did not show an increase in amputation risk in diabetic patients with PAD, but the concern remains and would benefit from further direct investigation. Trials looking at glucagon-like protein (GLP)-1 receptor agonists suggest a more direct vascular benefit by their mechanism of action and may provide therapeutic advantage over SGLT2i in diabetic patients with PAD. For example, the Liraglutide Effect and Action in Diabetes: Evaluation of Cardiovascular Outcome Results (LEADER) trial demonstrated benefit for diabetic patients in reduction of MACE and MALE in participants with PAD. It should be noted that the reduction in macrovascular complications related to diabetes, such as MACE, heart failure, and diabetic kidney disease provide distinct overall advantages of both the SGLT2i and GLP-1 receptor agonists over older diabetic medications, even in diabetic patients with PAD, despite the potential for increased amputation risk with SGLT2i. However, for the aforementioned reasons, it may be prudent to start with a GLP-1 receptor agonist before deciding to add an SGLT2i in diabetic patients with PAD.

Antithrombic Therapy

The ACC/AHA recommends treatment with once-daily aspirin[1] (81 mg to 325 mg) for patients with PAD based largely on expert opinion. For patients who cannot tolerate aspirin, clopidogrel (Plavix) 75 mg per day is a reasonable alternative. Dual antiplatelet therapy (clopidogrel plus aspirin) may reduce the risk of nonfatal myocardial infarction in patients with PAD and comorbid CAD, but this link is not well established and not generally recommended. However, per the ACC/AHA guidelines, dual antiplatelet therapy may be reasonable to reduce the risk of limb-related events in patients with symptomatic PAD after lower extremity revascularization.

The COMPASS trial looked at patients with symptomatic PAD treated with rivaroxaban (Xarelto) 2.5 mg twice daily and aspirin daily compared with aspirin monotherapy in 7470 patients, and it demonstrated a 46% risk relative risk reduction in MALE and a 24% relative risk reduction in MACE at the expense of a 70% increase in major bleeding events (mainly gastrointestinal), but not a significant difference in fatal bleeding, intracranial bleeding, or bleeding into a critical organ. The VOYAGER trial looked at rivaroxaban 2.5 mg twice daily and aspirin versus aspirin monotherapy in patients who had undergone revascularization for symptomatic PAD and demonstrated similar findings. Based on these trials, rivaroxaban (Xarelto) 2.5 mg twice daily plus aspirin daily is approved by the U.S. Food and Drug Administration (FDA) for the treatment of PAD.

The Warfarin Antiplatelet Vascular Evaluation (WAVE) trial compared warfarin and aspirin to aspirin monotherapy and found no benefit with the combination therapy and a threefold increase in life-threatening and moderate bleed risk compared with aspirin therapy alone. Warfarin is not recommended as part of a PAD treatment plan.

Lipid-Lowering Therapy

PAD is a coronary artery disease equivalent, and as such, patients should be initiated on a high-intensity statin such as atorvastatin (Lipitor) 80 mg or rosuvastatin (Crestor) 40 mg, per ACC/AHA guidelines. The Reduction of Atherothrombosis for Continued Health (REACH) Registry, an observation investigation for subjects at risk for atherothrombotic events, demonstrated that statin use is associated with a reduction in worsening claudication, new CLI, lower extremity revascularization, or amputation.

In the Further Cardiovascular Outcomes Research with PCSK 9 Inhibition in Subjects with Elevated Risk (FOURIER) trial, patients with atherosclerotic disease (with or without PAD) who were maximized on statin therapy and then treated with the proprotein convertase subtilisin/kexin type 9 (PCSK 9) inhibitor evolocumab (Repatha) versus placebo were found to have reduced MALE and MACE at an average 2.2-year follow-up. Although all patients should receive statin therapy, patients with difficult to control low-density lipoprotein and other less commonly used biomarkers such as lipoprotein (a), may help risk-stratify patients who may benefit from therapies such as evolocumab.

Hypertension Therapy

Hypertension should be treated to a goal of <130/80 per current ACC/AHA guidelines. Systolic blood pressure has more of an impact on the development of PAD than diastolic blood pressure. In the Atherosclerosis Risk in the Community (ARIC) study, an increase in the development of PAD was seen in patients with systolic blood pressure over 140 mm Hg (adjusted hazard ratio of 2.6) and between 120 and 139 mm Hg (adjusted hazard ratio of 1.6). Elevated risk for PAD was only observed in patients with diastolic blood pressure above 90 mm Hg. ACC/AHA guidelines can be followed in regard to initiation and management of blood pressure in patients with PAD similarly as to those who do not have PAD.

Cilostazol

Cilostazol (Pletal) is a phosphodiesterase III inhibitor that is used to treat intermittent claudication. Cilostazol increases cyclic AMP, which results in vasodilator activity and antiplatelet effects. A 2021 Cochrane review confirmed a 2014 review and found participants taking 100 mg to 300 mg of cilostazol daily had a significant decrease in claudication symptoms and an increase in distance walked compared with those taking a placebo. The main side effects were headache and diarrhea; dizziness and palpitations were also noted, but the medication was generally well tolerated. Of note, there is a black box warning on cilostazol, and it should not be used in patients with congestive heart failure, regardless of class. Although cilostazol did improve symptom-free walking distance in patients with PAD, there is insufficient evidence about the effectiveness on MALE or MACE. The typical dose of cilostazol is 100 mg twice daily, and the medication takes 2 to 4 weeks to have an effect on walking distance. Cilostazol should be discontinued if there is no improvement in intermittent claudication symptoms after 3 months. Thrombocytopenia and/or leukopenia can occur in patients on cilostazol, and this has the potential to progress to agranulocytosis if the medication is not discontinued immediately.

Exercise Rehabilitation

Supervised exercise programs have been shown to provide improvements in functional status and quality of life that are similar to endovascular interventions and superior to optimized medical therapy alone. The Supervised Exercise, Stent Revascularization, or Medical Therapy for Claudication Due to Aortoiliac Peripheral Artery Disease : The CLEVER study highlighted both the short-term (6 months) and long-term (18 months) benefits of supervised exercise therapy. A Cochrane review published in 2018 investigated supervised versus unsupervised exercise for intermittent claudication and concluded that although supervised exercise was more effective than unsupervised or home-based exercise programs at improving maximal walking distance, there was no difference in patient-reported quality of life or functional impairment outcomes. This is important to note as not all communities will have access to supervised exercise programs. The structure of most of the programs studied involve walking 30 to 45 minutes three times per week for 12 weeks. Participants would rest when claudication symptoms occur until they resolve and then begin walking again.

Revascularization/Vascular Interventions

Patients with symptomatic PAD should be considered for revascularization if they have persistent, lifestyle-limiting symptoms despite maximal medical therapy and trial of an exercise rehabilitation program. Patients with CLI should also be considered for urgent revascularization. For patients in whom interventional therapy is indicated, referral to an appropriate specialist, often a vascular surgeon, is warranted, and imaging with CTA or MRA to identify the specific anatomic location of the atherosclerotic lesion should be considered. Endovascular techniques, such as balloon angioplasty and stenting, are often preferred to surgical revascularization. However, patients with challenging anatomy may benefit from surgical revascularization with endarterectomy or surgical bypass.

Critical Limb Ischemia

Patients with findings consistent with CLI (Table 3) should be managed by an interdisciplinary team that involves vascular surgery, interventionalist (radiology, cardiology), and wound care specialists. The BASIL (Bypass versus Angioplasty in Severe Ischemia of the Leg) trial found that there was no difference in amputation-free survival and overall survival in patients managed with endovascular intervention versus open surgery. The goal in management of such patients is to minimize tissue loss and preserve the function of the foot while also balancing their

---

[1] Not FDA approved for this indication.

TABLE 3	Symptoms Characteristic of Critical Limb Ischemia and Acute Limb Ischemia	
	SYMPTOMS	VASCULAR SURGERY REFERRAL URGENCY
Critical limb ischemia	Ischemic pain at rest >2 weeks (especially at night), tissue loss (typically painful "punched out," sharply demarcated arterial ulcers on toes, foot), gangrene	Urgent
Acute limb ischemia	Paresthesia, Pain, Pallor, Pulselessness, Poikilothermia (cool/cold), and Paralysis (the "6 P's")	Emergent

inherent surgical risk. Although the rate of developing CLI in patients with PAD is low (<10% over 5 years), there is a 20% risk of mortality within 1 year of diagnosis if a patient does develop CLI, and revascularization is generally necessary to avoid amputation.

Acute Limb Ischemia

Acute limb ischemia (ALI) is a medical emergency that requires immediate vascular surgery evaluation. It is characterized by an acute loss of tissue perfusion, as opposed to the more chronically poor limb perfusion characteristic of CLI. Immediate recognition of the signs of ALI (see Table 3) is important as reperfusion may need to occur in <6 hours in some cases to salvage function of the limb and minimize tissue loss. Most commonly, ALI is a result of thromboembolism of a stenotic artery, stent thrombosis, or thrombosis of prior surgical revascularization/bypass graft.

Monitoring

The majority of patients with PAD can be managed with a combination of risk-factor modification and medical management that includes a supervised exercise rehabilitation program. Although it is important to note that disease severity will remain stable over a 5-year period in most patients, up to 20% will progressively worsen in their disease course, and <10% will go on to develop CLI. Patients with PAD should be seen in follow-up at least once per year and potentially more frequently depending on the severity of PAD and other comorbid health conditions.

References

Barraclough JY, Yu J, Figtree GA, et al: Cardiovascular and renal outcomes with canagliflozin in patients with peripheral arterial disease: Data from the CANVAS Program and CREDENCE trial, *Diabetes Obes Metab* 24(6):1072–1083, 2022, https://doi.org/10.1111/dom.14671.
Bhatt DL, Flather MD, Hacke W, et al: Patients with prior myocardial infarction, stroke, or symptomatic peripheral arterial disease in the CHARISMA trial, *J Am Coll Cardiol* 49(19):1982–1988, 2007, https://doi.org/10.1016/j.jacc.2007.03.025.
Bonaca MP, Hamburg NM, Creager MA: Contemporary Medical Management of Peripheral Artery Disease, *Circ Res* 128(12):1868–1884, 2021, https://doi.org/10.1161/CIRCRESAHA.121.318258.
Bonaca MP, Wiviott SD, Zelniker TA, et al: Dapagliflozin and cardiac, kidney, and limb outcomes in patients with and without peripheral artery disease in DECLARE-TIMI 58, *Circulation* 142(8):734–747, 2020, https://doi.org/10.1161/CIRCULATIONAHA.119.044775.
Bradbury AW, Adam DJ, Bell J, et al: Bypass versus Angioplasty in Severe Ischaemia of the Leg (BASIL) trial: An intention-to-treat analysis of amputation-free and overall survival in patients randomized to a bypass surgery-first or a balloon angioplasty-first revascularization strategy [published correction appears in *J Vasc Surg* 2010 Dec;52(6):1751. Bhattachary, V [corrected to Bhattacharya, V]], *J Vasc Surg* 51(5 Suppl):5S–17S, 2010, https://doi.org/10.1016/j.jvs.2010.01.073.
Brown T, Forster RB, Cleanthis M, Mikhailidis DP, Stansby G, Stewart M: Cilostazol for intermittent claudication, *Cochrane Database Syst Rev* 6(6):CD003748, 2021, https://doi.org/10.1002/14651858.CD003748.pub5. Published 2021 Jun 30.
Criqui MH, Matsushita K, Aboyans V, et al: Lower extremity peripheral artery disease: contemporary epidemiology, management gaps, and future directions: a scientific statement from the American Heart Association [published correction appears in *Circulation*. 2021 Aug 31;144(9):e193], *Circulation* 144(9):e171–e191, 2021, https://doi.org/10.1161/CIR.0000000000001005.
Dhatariya K, Bain SC, Buse JB, et al: The impact of liraglutide on diabetes-related foot ulceration and associated complications in patients with type 2 diabetes at high risk for cardiovascular events: results from the LEADER Trial, *Diabetes Care* 41(10):2229–2235, 2018, https://doi.org/10.2337/dc18-1094.
Gerhard-Herman MD, Gornik HL, Barrett C, et al: 2016 AHA/ACC guideline on the management of patients with lower extremity peripheral artery disease: executive summary: a report of the American College of Cardiology/American Heart Association Task Force on Clinical Practice Guidelines [published correction appears in *Circulation*. 2017 Mar 21;135(12):e790], *Circulation* 135(12):e686–e725, 2016, https://doi.org/10.1161/CIR.0000000000000470.
Hageman D, Fokkenrood HJ, Gommans LN, van den Houten MM, Teijink JA: Supervised exercise therapy versus home-based exercise therapy versus walking advice for intermittent claudication, *Cochrane Database Syst Rev* 4(4):CD005263, 2018, https://doi.org/10.1002/14651858.CD005263.pub4. Published 2018 Apr 6.
Huber TS, Commentary Anand, Yusuf Xie, et al: The Warfarin Antiplatelet Vascular Evaluation Trial Investigators. Oral anticoagulation and antiplatelet therapy and peripheral arterial disease, *N Engl J Med* 357:217–227, 2007, https://doi.org/10.1177/1531003508319779. Perspect Vasc Surg Endovasc Ther. 2008;20(4):383-384.
Lu Y, Ballew SH, Tanaka H, et al: 2017 ACC/AHA blood pressure classification and incident peripheral artery disease: The Atherosclerosis Risk in Communities (ARIC) Study, *Eur J Prev Cardiol* 27(1):51–59, 2020, https://doi.org/10.1177/2047487319865378.
Murphy TP, Cutlip DE, Regensteiner JG, et al: Supervised exercise, stent revascularization, or medical therapy for claudication due to aortoiliac peripheral artery disease: the CLEVER study [published correction appears in *J Am Coll Cardiol*. 2015 May 12;65(18):2055], *J Am Coll Cardiol* 65(10):999–1009, 2015, https://doi.org/10.1016/j.jacc.2014.12.043.

PREMATURE BEATS

Method of
Randell Wexler, MD, MPH; and T.M. Ayodele Adesanya, MD, PhD

CURRENT DIAGNOSIS

- The cause of a premature beat may be either atrial (premature atrial contractions or PAC) or ventricular (premature ventricular contractions or PVC) in origin.
- PACs are most often benign but are associated with increased risk of atrial fibrillation.
- PVCs may be benign, but underlying ischemia or structural heart disease is not uncommon and must be ruled out with echocardiography.
- PACs and PVCs are most commonly diagnosed by EKG although Holter or event monitoring may be required.
- A heavier PVC burden is associated with increased development of cardiomyopathy and cardiovascular morbidity and mortality.

CURRENT THERAPY

- PACs are treated if their presence causes the patient symptoms and interferes with daily life.
- Beta blockers are most often used for the treatment of symptomatic PACs.
- In patients with underlying structural heart disease, the treatment of PVCs is directed at the underlying cardiac condition.
- Antiarrhythmics show no benefit in treatment of PVCs in patients with cardiomyopathy and should not be used to suppress their presence post myocardial infarction.
- Patients with a PVC burden of > 15% should see an EPS specialist for evaluation and treatment, as there is an increased risk of a significant cardiac arrhythmia.

It is not uncommon for a patient to present to a primary care physician with the complaint of their "heart pounding," "skipping beats," or having "palpitations." Though often the only symptom, patients may also complain of concomitant dizziness, lightheadedness, or frank syncope. The patient may be young or old, have underlying structural heart disease (or not), or risk factors for heart disease such as hypertension. A patient with such a history may be experiencing one of a number of cardiac arrhythmias, although it is not uncommon to find no underlying etiology at all. No conclusive evidence exists to define the evolving role of wearable devices in assessing such concerns, but abnormal findings may certainly suggest need for further cardiac evaluation.

Normal electrical propagation in the heart begins with the spontaneous electrical discharge at the sinoatrial node, which is then propagated along the right atrial wall to the atrioventricular node and from there to the ventricles via the His-Purkinje System. Disruption anywhere along this pathway may lead to an arrhythmia, which is defined as a rhythm that is not sinus and is accompanied by an abnormal electrical conduction.

If an arrhythmia is present, it is classified by its anatomic location of origin. Common atrial arrhythmias include atrial fibrillation/flutter, paroxysmal supraventricular tachycardia, and premature atrial contractions (PACs). Ventricular arrhythmias are often designated as premature ventricular contractions (PVCs), ventricular tachycardia, and ventricular fibrillation. Other arrhythmias that are often seen include bradycardia, tachycardia, and first-, second-, and third-degree heart block (complex morphology is normal). Age may offer clues as to etiology. As one ages, paroxysmal supraventricular tachycardia and atrial fibrillation/flutter are more likely. This chapter will review arrhythmias commonly referred to as premature beats: PACs, and PVCs.

Premature Atrial Contractions
Epidemiology and Risk Factors
PACs are common and are found in both the general population as well as in those with underlying cardiac disease. Research has established that PACs exist in up to 99% of those over the age of 50 with increasing frequency with each decade of life. It has long been believed that atrial ectopy, especially in a patient with no underlying heart disease, is benign and more of a nuisance than a risk. However, it is now understood that PACs do present an increased risk for atrial fibrillation or ischemic stroke, and although most often benign, are not entirely so.

Underlying structural heart disease (such as mitral valve disease or left ventricular dysfunction) is significantly correlated to the risk of developing PACs. Additional risk factors associated with PACs include: 1) height (potentially due to the relationship between body size and left atrial measurements); 2) those with higher levels of B natriuretic peptide (BNP); as well as 3) those with abnormalities of high-density lipoprotein (HDL) lipid metabolism in which a lower HDL is associated with increased risk of PACs. This inverse relationship has also been reported between PACs and physical activity. The difficulty in determining the clinical significance of PACs is owing to their frequent presence in the population at large.

Pathophysiology
The true etiology of PACs is not well researched and therefore not well understood. Investigation has suggested that normally functioning sino-atrial (SA) and atrio-ventricular (AV) nodes can be impacted by stimuli arising from outside of the atria. It has been proposed that this stimuli leads to reversible nodal remodeling. As a result it has been hypothesized that PACs may occur due to an adversely impacted SA or AV node subsequent to such remodeling. Others have postulated that mechanisms such as reentry and abnormal automaticity initiate PAC transmission but the actual cause is not known.

An electrocardiogram (EKG) provides an electrical account of heart function. Electrical impulses begin in the sinus node and then travel through Bachmann's bundle (the sole specialized atrial conduction system) subsequently diffusing over the atria. The P wave represents atrial electrical activity. A normal P wave as seen on the EKG is smooth and never peaked or sharp. The leads best used to review the P wave are leads II and V1.

A patient may have a left atrial abnormality (LAA), right atrial abnormality (RAA), or both. An LAA results in prolonged atrial activation times, because left atrial activation is later than right atrial activation. Such abnormalities may result in "notched" P waves because of the spatial separation of the left and right atrial peaks. When a patient has a RAA, the P wave tends to have increased amplitude due to the summation of the two peaks. Whenever possible, P wave abnormalities should be labeled left or right in nature.

A PAC will typically be seen on EKG as an abnormal P wave followed by a normal QRS complex. Morphologically, the P wave will be different than a normal (sinus) P wave. If the site of the PAC origin is near the AV node, it will be inverted, whereas if it is more distal, it will be upright. Should the PAC reach the SA node, the resulting finding on the EKG will be a longer interval between sinus beats, but it is not compensatory in nature. PACs may occur singularly or at regular intervals (every other beat is termed bigeminy) or in a group (two sequential PACs are termed a couplet). In addition, a PAC may be blocked (buried in a T wave) or conducted aberrantly (an atypical electrical configuration).

Prevention and Clinical Manifestations
The majority of PACs are idiopathic unless there is underlying heart disease. Potential non-cardiac causes include tobacco use, alcohol consumption, substance abuse, and coffee. Reducing and/or eliminating these substances can be helpful in preventing symptoms. Additionally, certain medications, supplements, or substances of abuse may cause PACs, and therefore in any patient presenting with the complaint of extra beats, a thorough review of all medications, supplements, and elicit substance use should be undertaken.

Although the vast majority of patients who are found to have PACs incidentally will not experience symptoms, patients presenting with the complaint of PACs may state that they feel that their heart is racing, skipping beats, or fluttering, or that they are experiencing palpitations. Though not common, some patients may experience dizziness.

PACs are now known to be precursors to atrial fibrillation or ischemic stroke. Thus the previous belief that atrial ectopy is benign and more of a nuisance has been shown to be incorrect. In fact, some studies suggest that a single PAC on EKG not only predicts atrial fibrillation but may also be a predictor of fatal outcome.

Diagnosis and Differential Diagnosis
The diagnosis of PACs is often made on EKG, especially if the patient is symptomatic at the time of testing. If the EKG does not demonstrate an etiology, a 24-hour Holter monitor, a 30-day event monitor, or mobile cardiac telemetry may also be considered. The diagnoses of a PAC can be made if the P wave has a morphology that is different from and occurs earlier in the cardiac cycle than that of a sinus P wave. Many patients experience palpitations in which the EKG evaluation suggests no underlying etiology. Therefore, in addition to electrocardiography, patients with PACs should have baseline labs drawn to include a thyroid stimulating hormone, complete blood count, magnesium and phosphate, and electrolytes. If drug use is a possible etiology, a toxicology screen can be useful.

Differential diagnosis includes other cardiac arrhythmias such as PVCs, atrial fibrillation, atrial flutter, and paroxysmal supraventricular tachycardia. Underlying disorders that may be the cause include underlying anxiety or thyroid and other metabolic disorder, as well as substance abuse.

Treatment and Monitoring
Echocardiography is helpful in determining if the patient has underlying structural heart disease requiring further evaluation and intervention. If the patient has no underlying structural heart disease, then no treatment is necessary, especially if the individual

is asymptomatic and the PACs are found incidentally. If the patient does have symptomatic PACs to a degree that they interfere with the patient's quality of life, interventions include the use of beta blockers, and if they fail, a trial of type IA, type IC, or type III antiarrhythmic agents may be considered. If the problem is electrophysiological in nature, catheter ablation or pulmonary vein isolation may be helpful. Elimination of tobacco, alcohol, and caffeine should be recommended.

If the patient has underlying structural heart disease, then treatment is directed at the underlying disorder. Frequent PACs can be associated with an increase in cardiovascular mortality. Patients with PACs should be educated as to the association of atrial fibrillation or stroke with instructions to notify their physician or seek attention immediately should symptoms occur. In case reports, normalization of left ventricular function has been reported following ablation.

Premature Ventricular Contractions

Epidemiology and Risk Factors

Premature ventricular contractions (PVCs) are a common cardiac finding, with upward of 40% to 75% of apparently healthy people being affected. As with PACs, they tend to increase with age. Underlying cardiovascular disease, especially ischemic heart disease increases one's risk for PVCs. As such, evaluation should be focused on excluding structural heart disease. Infiltrative cardiomyopathies may be considered, especially if conditions such as sarcoidosis or amyloidosis are present as known comorbidities. It should be noted that PVCs are common in those with inherited channelopathies, so a good family history is important. PVCs are common in well-conditioned athletes due to autonomic tone. Although this may be a normal compensatory mechanism, structural heart disease still needs to be eliminated. PVCs associated with exercise and postexercise recovery portend increased cardiac mortality.

Pathophysiology

After propagation through the atria, the electrical impulse activates the AV node that serves as the sole pathway for electrical transmission between the atria and the ventricles. The terminal portion of the AV junction becomes the bundle of His that propagates the electrical impulse to the bundle branches, which further divide into smaller subdivisions eventually connecting to the Purkinje fibers. From the Purkinje fibers, the electrical impulse diffuses synchronously across the ventricles.

PVCs arise from ectopic foci in the ventricle and occur earlier in the cardiac cycle than expected for a sinus beat. They may be generated by increased automaticity, reentry, or triggered activity. Monomorphic PVCs suggest a triggering component whereas polymorphic PVCs tend to suggest an underlying cardiomyopathy. If the patient has no structural heart disease, the focus is likely to be the right ventricular outflow tract, whereas if the patient has structural heart disease, the left ventricle is most likely to be the site of origin.

PVCs are not preceded by a P wave and demonstrate a prolonged QRS (> 120 ms) with a compensatory pause (as opposed to a noncompensatory pause found with PACs). Conflicting ST and T wave changes are also often seen. ST depression and T-wave inversion tends to occur in R-wave dominant leads, whereas ST elevation and an upright T wave occur in S-wave dominated leads. PVCs may be unifocal or multifocal and their morphology may at times resemble right or left bundle branch blocks. If the PVC occurs with every other beat, it is termed bigeminy (or trigeminy if every third, etc.), or if the PVC is paired with another PVC, it is called a couplet. One may also see an R on T phenomenon whereby the PVC occurs at or near the T wave of the previous QRS complex resulting in the R wave of the PVC blending with the T wave of the preceding beat.

Patients with frequent PVCs will often develop subsequent cardiomyopathy, though the etiology is unknown. There is an increased risk in developing cardiomyopathy the longer one is exposed to PVCs. It is suspected this may be due to a less efficient heartbeat with suboptimal cardiac output similar to bradycardia.

Risk factors for progression to cardiomyopathy have been inconsistently identified but likely include increasing age, high body mass index, and male gender.

Prevention and Clinical Manifestations

Patients with symptoms caused by PVCs often present with palpitations, dizziness, chest pain, syncope, dyspnea, orthopnea, decreased exercise tolerance, and fatigue. If a patient has a cough of unknown etiology, they should be evaluated for PVCs, as PVCs are noted to produce cough as the only symptom. PVCs have also been associated with dysphagia, especially when intermittent, as well as paroxysmal choking or vomiting. As such, PVCs should be considered if a gastroenterological evaluation is normal, or if symptoms persist despite treatment for an underlying gastrointestinal disorder.

PVCs are associated with a multitude of pathologic cardiac processes including heart failure, myocardial ischemia, left ventricular hypertrophy, idiopathic ventricular tachycardia, and right ventricular dysplasia. More recently, PVCs have been demonstrated to increase the risk of new onset atrial fibrillation. Non-cardiac diseases with which PVCs are associated include obstructive sleep apnea, chronic obstructive pulmonary disease, and pulmonary hypertension. On exam patients may present with an irregular pulse or canon A wave. PVCs may also be associated with pulmonary or thyroid disease, the consumption of alcohol, caffeine, and the use of beta agonists. Cocaine, amphetamines, or other illicit drugs may precipitate symptoms as well. Syncope is uncommon with PVCs but, if present, represents a red flag for the presence of malignant arrhythmias.

PVCs are found on 40% to 75% of Holter monitor evaluations and 1% of EKGs. They are defined as frequent if they are seen on an EKG, or are present at a rate of more than 30 an hour on event monitoring. In this instance there is a significantly increased cardiovascular risk as well as mortality. In the athlete, sinus bradycardia is common due to enhanced conditioning. This results in a lengthening of the RR interval and is thought to promote the occurrence of PVCs in this population.

The most important prognostic indicator for PVCs is the presence or absence of structural heart disease. Multifocal PVCs are considered to be risk factors for adverse cardiovascular events.

Potential contributors that are amenable to treatment include electrolyte abnormalities, hypoxia, drugs (including prescription as well as illegal), increased adrenergic drive, or ischemia.

Diagnosis and Differential Diagnosis

A 12-lead EKG is the initial test of choice. Echocardiography is necessary in individuals in which structural heart disease is suspected, or if PVC frequency is high (one or more PVCs on EKG, or more than 30 an hour on event monitoring). This is based on the understanding that the likelihood of underlying structural heart disease increases with PVC burden. In addition, if ischemia is suspected or if PVCs are triggered/evident on exertion, cardiovascular exercise stress testing is recommended. Polymorphic PVCs are more commonly seen in those with underlying cardiomyopathy. Cardiac magnetic resonance imaging may be considered if cardiomyopathy is suspected or if PVC etiology is unclear from baseline EKG and/or echocardiogram.

Differential diagnosis includes ventricular arrhythmias such as ventricular tachycardia and ventricular fibrillation. Cardiac conditions include left ventricular hypertrophy in the setting of hypertension, myocarditis, acute coronary syndrome, heart failure, congenital heart disease, and hypertrophic cardiomyopathy.

Treatment and Monitoring

PVCs have been demonstrated to be an independent risk factor for cardiovascular mortality in heart failure and are associated with ejection fraction and wall motion abnormalities as well. Patients with a family history of frequent PVCs should be evaluated for inherited channelopathies such as catecholaminergic polymorphic ventricular tachycardia. In patients with PVCs but without underlying coronary artery disease or structural heart disease, the clinical course is generally benign. It should be recalled, however, that patients with a history of PVCs can develop coronary artery disease or underlying structural heart disease, so periodic reevaluation of cardiac status is warranted. A sleep study (or titration of current positive airway pressure therapy) may also be advised, given the high association of PVCs with obstructive sleep apnea, which itself confers independent cardiovascular risk.

Treatment for those with symptomatic PVCs may include beta blockers or non-dihydropyridine calcium channel blockers, but treatment is not necessary in asymptomatic patients. Use of antiarrhythmic medication to treat PVCs has not been shown to benefit patients with cardiomyopathy. In addition, treatment is not indicated following myocardial infarction to suppress PVCs that may be present. If the patient has a large PVC burden, considered to be greater than 15%, referral to an EPS specialist for consultation and possible radiofrequency ablation should be considered. If the patient has PVC-induced cardiomyopathy, catheter ablation may be considered, especially if the PVCs are monomorphic. There are limited randomized controlled trials of radiofrequency ablation and anti-arrhythmic drug therapy, but retrospective studies suggest decreased PVC burden in those with radiofrequency ablation. As with all patients, non-anti-arrhythmic medications may have to be adjusted to decrease stimulants, correct electrolyte abnormalities, and reduce cardiovascular risks.

Premature Junctional Contractions

PJCs are less common than either PACs or PVCs and are rarely seen in the setting of a normal heart. These beats arise from the atrioventricular junction. On EKG they are seen as an aberrant beat with underlying sinus rhythm. The P wave may be absent, inverted, or occur following the associated QRS complex that is morphologically normal. Causes include electrolyte and thyroid abnormalities, underlying lung or cardiac disease, or the use of excessive amounts of caffeine, nicotine, or alcohol. Medication toxicity may also be a cause, with digitalis toxicity being the classic example. If patients are asymptomatic, no treatment is required, though structural heart disease needs to be ruled out. In addition, the patient should be observed over time, as PJCs may be a harbinger of progression to a more serious arrhythmia. In the symptomatic patient, treatment is directed at the underlying cause. Supplemental oxygen may be of benefit.

References

Al-Khatib SM, et al: 2017 AHA/ACC/HRS guideline for management of patients with ventricular arrhythmias and the prevention of sudden cardiac death: a report of the American College of Cardiology/American Heart Association Task Force on Clinical Practice Guidelines and the Heart Rhythm Society: Developed in Collaboration With the Heart Failure Society of America, *Circulation*, DOI: https://doi.org/10.1161/CIR.0000000000000549. October 30, 2017.

Farinha JM, Gupta D, Lip GYH: Frequent premature atrial contractions as a signalling marker of atrial cardiomyopathy, incident atrial fibrillation, and stroke, *Cardiovasc Res*, 119(2):429–439, 2023. https://doi.org/10.1093/cvr/cvac054.

Gorenek B, et al: Premature ventricular complexes: diagnostic and therapeutic considerations in clinical practice: A state-of-the-art review by the American College of Cardiology Electrophysiology Council, *J Interv Card Electrophysiol* 57(1): 5–26. https://doi.org/10.1007/s10840-019-00655-3.

Könemann H, Ellermann C, Zeppenfeld K, Eckardt L: Management of ventricular arrhythmias worldwide: comparison of the latest ESC, AHA/ACC/HRS, and CCS/CHRS guidelines: *JACC Clin Electrophysiol* 9(5):715–728, 2023. https://doi.org/10.1016/j.jacep.2022.12.008.

Lee PT, Huang MH, Huang TC, et al: High burden of premature ventricular complex increases the risk of new-onset atrial fibrillation, *J Am Heart Assoc* 12(4):e027674, 2023. Epub 2023 Feb 15.

Lin CY, et al: Prognostic significance of premature atrial complexes burden in prediction of long-term outcome, *J Am Heart Assoc*, 4e002192, 2015. https://doi.org/10.1161/JAHA.115.002192.

Menon T, Ogbu I, Kalra DK: Sleep-disordered breathing and cardiac arrhythmias, *J Clin Med* 13(22):6635, 2024. https://doi.org/10.3390/jcm13226635.

Nguen KT, et al: Ectopy on a single 12-lead ECG, incident cardiac myopathy, and death in the community, *J Am Heart Assoc* 6:e006028, 2017. https://doi.org/10.1161/JAHA.117.006028.

Shoureshi P, et al: Arrhythmia-induced cardiomyopathy: JACC state-of-the-art review, *J Am Coll Cardiol* 4;83(22):2214–2232, 2024. https://doi.org/10.1016/j.jacc.2024.03.416.

Sugumar H, Prabhu S, Voskoboinik A, Kistler PM: Arrhythmia-induced cardiomyopathy, *J Arrhythm* 34(4):376–383, 2018.

TACHYCARDIAS

Method of
Alex Schevchuck, MD, MS; and Paul Andre, MD

CURRENT DIAGNOSIS

- Tachycardia is defined as cardiac rhythm with heart rate >100 bpm.
- 12-lead ECG and hemodynamic assessment are essential in each patient with tachycardia.
- Sustained arrhythmia is an arrhythmia that lasts for more than 30 seconds.
- Narrow complex rhythm (QRS ≤120 ms) favors supraventricular origin, whereas wide complex (QRS >120 ms) could be either supraventricular (with aberrant conduction) or ventricular.
- Every patient with tachyarrhythmia should be promptly assessed for hemodynamic instability and presence of symptoms (palpitations, angina, shortness of breath, lightheadedness, presyncope, syncope, volume overload).

CURRENT TREATMENT

- Vagal maneuvers may be useful for diagnosis and treatment of tachyarrhythmia.
- Direct-current (DC) cardioversion should be considered early if hemodynamic instability is present.
- If uncertain whether arrhythmia is ventricular tachycardia (VT) or supraventricular tachycardia (SVT), VT should be presumed and treated.
- Hemodynamic instability implies medical emergency, and culprit tachyarrhythmia should be treated immediately.
- A subspecialty consultation should be considered for each patient with tachyarrhythmia and high-risk features, such as syncope or family history of sudden cardiac death for diagnostic evaluation, treatment recommendations, and risk stratification.

Definition

Tachycardia is defined as a heart rate greater than 100 beats per min (bpm). This can be a normal response by the heart to the stress on the body (such as sinus tachycardia with exercise or sepsis) or a primary cardiac pathologic condition, such as atrioventricular nodal reentry tachycardia (AVNRT) or ventricular tachycardia (VT). Tachycardia present in the setting of an abnormal cardiac rhythm is defined as tachyarrhythmia.

Classification

Tachycardias classify into two major categories: wide complex (QRS duration >120 ms) or narrow-complex (QRS duration ≤120 ms). This classification is key, as wide-complex tachycardias are usually caused by an arrhythmia arising from the ventricles, such as monomorphic or polymorphic ventricular tachycardia, which are associated with considerable morbidity and mortality. On the other hand, narrow-complex tachycardias reflect ventricular activation by a competent conduction system below the atrioventricular (AV) node, indicating a source of the arrhythmia above the AV node or within the AV node or bundle of His, and are rarely life threatening.

When the tachyarrhythmia originates in the atria or within the conduction system in the AV node, it is described as a supraventricular tachycardia (SVT).

Wide-complex tachycardias include VT, supraventricular tachycardias with aberrant conduction (i.e., presence of a bundle branch block), and some types of pathway-mediated reciprocating tachycardias discussed separately.

Epidemiology

Based on the Marshfield Epidemiological Study Area (MESA) data, the incidence of SVT in the general population is 35/100,000 person-years and the prevalence is 2.25 per 1000 persons. The mean age of onset in the study was 37 years old, and the most likely presenting location was the emergency room.

Prevalence of ventricular arrhythmias is higher in men than in women, increases with age, and is strongly linked to the presence of cardiovascular disease. Fifteen percent to 16% of patients with VT have coronary atherosclerosis; and 8% to 9% have hypertension, valvular disease, or nonischemic cardiomyopathy. Only 2% to 3% of patients with VT do not have cardiovascular disease. Five percent to 10% of patients with acute MI demonstrate VT/VF, most of which occurs during the first 48 hours of hospital admission.

Pathophysiology

There are two major mechanisms of supraventricular tachycardias: automaticity and reentry.

Automaticity involves occurrence of one or multiple ectopic foci of depolarization that are located above or within the AV node. Examples of such tachycardias include focal and multifocal atrial tachycardia and junctional tachycardia.

Reentry mechanism uses a formation of an electrical circuit that may involve the AV node or accessory pathways. These tachyarrhythmias include atrial flutter, AVNRT, and AV-nodal reciprocating tachycardias (AVRT).

Ventricular tachycardias use three major mechanisms: automaticity, triggered activity, and reentry.

Automatic VTs occur from an ectopic focus of depolarization and may originate from either ventricular myocytes or Purkinje fibers. Triggered activity includes early afterdepolarization and delayed afterdepolarization. Early depolarizations occur during the repolarization phase of the membrane, usually in a setting of acquired action potential prolongation (long QT) and serves as a trigger for polymorphic VT or torsades de pointes (Figure 8). Delayed afterdepolarizations occur after a complete cell repolarization and serve as VT triggers in digoxin toxicity, right ventricular outflow tract VT, and catecholaminergic polymorphic VT. Reentry-type VT occurs when an electrical circuit forms around either an anatomic barrier (scar, artificial material in postoperative patients) or an area of a functional block. This mechanism usually results in monomorphic ventricular tachycardia.

Clinical Presentation

Clinical manifestation of tachyarrhythmias may include palpitations or fluttering sensation in the chest and neck, and signs of decreased perfusion, such as hypotension, dizziness, lightheadedness, syncope, hot flushes, altered mentation, and shock. Ventricular tachyarrhythmias in particular may result in acute loss of circulation and sudden cardiac death (SCD). Effects of tachycardia on cardiac output mostly owe to shortened diastole that affects ventricular filling and decreasing preload leading to decreased cardiac output. VTs, in turn, also result in atrioventricular and intraventricular dyssynchrony that may additionally affect cardiac stroke volume and output.

Diagnosis

In the acute setting, prompt and accurate diagnosis of the type of tachycardia is paramount. Every patient with suspected tachyarrhythmia should have a 12-lead electrocardiogram (ECG). Because many tachyarrhythmias may cause hemodynamic compromise, an expedited hemodynamic assessment should be performed (vital signs, oxygen saturation, presence of shock that may manifest as altered mentation or evidence of organ system dysfunction). An unstable patient should be treated emergently with an appropriate antiarrhythmic strategy defined by Advanced Cardiac Life Support (ACLS) algorithms.

History plays an important role in diagnosis of tachycardias. Nature and onset of symptoms, frequency of episodes and possible triggers or predisposing conditions, as well as alleviating factors, should be identified. Past medical history may be helpful in differentiation of different types of tachycardia, such as presence of ischemia or a structural heart disease that may favor VT. History of syncope, specifically if suggesting cardiogenic etiology, may help identify high-risk patients. Family history of arrhythmias or sudden cardiac death may yield important information regarding familial arrhythmias, such as Wolff-Parkinson-White (WPW) or long-QT interval syndromes.

If the patient has an implanted cardiac device, such as permanent pacemaker or a defibrillator, the device interrogation is diagnostic in most cases, especially if an AV system is present that is capable of tracking both atrial and ventricular electrical activity.

Differential Diagnosis for Narrow Complex Tachycardias

Twelve-lead ECG is the first step in differentiating between different types of narrow-complex tachycardia. Analysis of QRS regularity, axis, atrial activity, baseline and relationships between atrial and ventricular activations, and presence of delta-wave (Figure 4) or preexcitation should be performed.

Identification of atrial activity is key in differentiating between subtypes of SVT. When identification of atrial activity is difficult (as during rapid ventricular rate), vagal maneuvers, carotid sinus pressure, or administration of IV adenosine (Adenocard)[1] may assist in diagnosis or potentially terminate the arrhythmia.

Irregular tachyarrhythmia with no identifiable pattern or P waves is diagnostic of atrial fibrillation with rapid ventricular response. Variable baseline that resembles a sawtooth pattern is suggestive of atrial flutter. AV-nodal reentry usually results in a retrograde P wave that may be hidden within QRS complex or follows QRS immediately (short R-P tachycardia). Atrial tachycardia will have one or more P wave morphologies with 1:1 relationship; however, P wave morphology and axis will be different from sinus P waves. Comparison to prior ECG in sinus rhythm may be particularly helpful in this scenario.

An electrophysiology study is the gold-standard diagnostic approach if the mechanism of tachycardia is unclear from the surface ECG.

Differential Diagnosis for Wide Complex Tachycardias

Because SVT with aberrancy and some types of AVRT may result in wide QRS complex, differentiation of such arrhythmia from VT may be challenging even for experts. Orthodromic arrhythmia suggests the electrical impulse travels straight down the normal pathway, and antidromic arrhythmia suggests that the impulse travels in the opposite direction.

Atrial activity is typically not affected by the VT (unless retrograde conduction is present), leading to AV disassociation, when P waves have no relationship to the QRS complexes. This may help differentiate VT from SVT with aberrancy. Fusion and capture beats are other hallmarks of monomorphic VT. Fusion beats occur when atrial activity can conduct through the AV node down the His-Purkinje system and "fuse" with ventricular activity. The resulting QRS complex is a hybrid of the sinus rhythm narrow QRS complex and the widened VT QRS complex. Capture beats occur when atrial activity conducts down the His-Purkinje system and creates a narrow QRS complex, followed by ongoing VT. These findings are very specific for VT, but their absence does not rule it out.

Multiple algorithms have been proposed to assist in differentiating SVT from VT. We will discuss the Brugada algorithm that has excellent sensitivity and specificity (0.978 and 0.965, respectively) for diagnosis of VT. If the answer to any of the following questions is yes, subsequent steps are not necessary and the rhythm is VT (Figure 1).

---

[1]Not FDA approved for this indication.

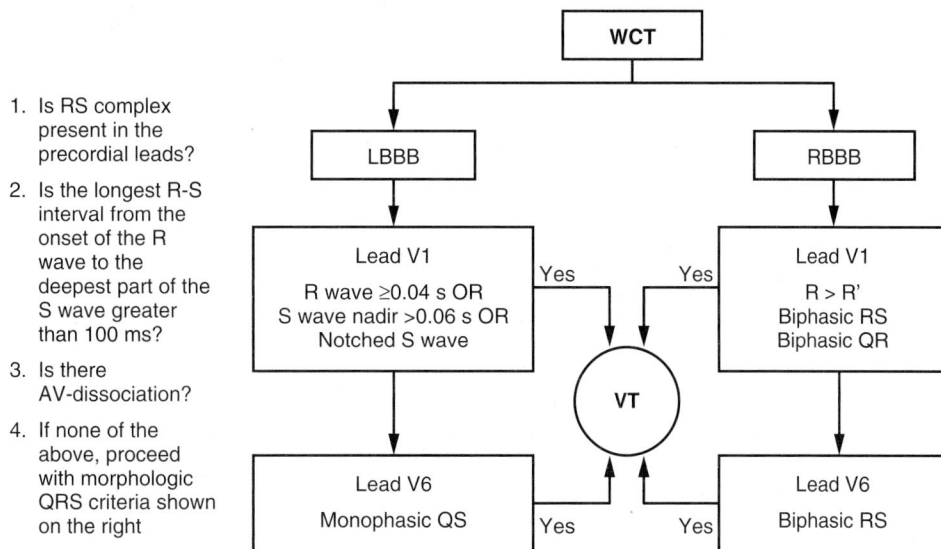

Figure 1 Brugada algorithm for differentiating supraventricular tachycardia from ventricular tachycardia. LBBB, Left bundle branch block; RBBB, right bundle branch block; WCT, wide complex tachycardia.

Specific Tachycardias and Their Treatment

Sinus Tachycardia

Sinus tachycardia is a common narrow-complex tachycardia. It can represent a normal response to stress or a disease process (Table 1). Sinus tachycardia on a 12-lead ECG presents with ventricular rate >100 bpm and sinus P waves that are positive in leads I, II, and III, negative in aVR, and biphasic in lead V_1 with a normal PR interval (120–200 ms). Compared with an ECG in normal sinus rhythm, the P wave axis and morphology should be unchanged. A syndrome of inappropriate sinus tachycardia is a diagnosis of exclusion, when average heart rate exceeds 90 bpm over a 24-hour period and no physiologic or medical cause can be identified.

Atrioventricular-Nodal Reentry Tachycardia

AV-nodal reentry tachycardia results from activation of a dual-pathway conduit (slow and fast) that includes the AV node. This is the most common type of SVT, with a slightly higher prevalence in women. AVNRT manifests as a regular, usually rapid tachycardia with heart rates that may exceed 250 bpm. The patient will usually experience palpitations and symptoms of decreased perfusion, such as lightheadedness, dizziness, hypotension, flushing, and so forth. Syncope is rare but may occur with very rapid heart rates or in subjects with dehydration or underlying heart disease. A distinguishing symptom of AVNRT is neck palpitations. The mechanism of that is the simultaneous atrial and ventricular systole because of excitation origin located within the AV node, which is located between the atria and ventricles. This results in right atrial contraction against the closed tricuspid valve, forcing blood back into the jugular system that is subjectively perceived as palpitations in the neck. Diagnosis of AVNRT is based on a surface electrocardiogram that will classically demonstrate a rapid narrow complex tachycardia with P waves occurring within the QRS complex; therefore they are not immediately discoverable but may cause subtle deflection at the terminal portion of the QRS or immediately after the QRS (short R-P tachycardia, Figure 2). Electrophysiology study yields definitive diagnosis by demonstration of a dual-pathway physiology.

In the acute setting, as soon as AVNRT is suspected, termination of the arrhythmia should be attempted. Vagal maneuvers, such as Valsalva, carotid massage, or application of a cold wet towel to the patient's face may be helpful. Adenosine (Adenocard) has been reported to be effective in greater than 95% of patients with AVNRT. If the type of tachyarrhythmia is uncertain, adenosine may also help make a diagnosis by blocking AV conduction and causing ventricular pause that will unmask the underlying atrial activity, and may reveal arrhythmias, such as atrial tachycardia or atrial flutter. It is important to remember that adenosine has a very short half-life and should be administered as a very rapid IV injection followed by a 20 mL fluid bolus. ACLS recommends the initial dose of 6 mg followed by 12 mg if no response. The 12 mg dose can be repeated one more time. Patients taking theophylline (adenosine antagonist) may require a higher initial dose (12 mg), whereas patients with a heart transplant or on carbamazepine (Tegretol) should be given a lower initial dose (3 mg). A 12-lead ECG recording should be performed in a continuous mode while performing this intervention for more accurate rhythm identification. If these measures are ineffective to terminate the arrhythmia, a brief assessment of hemodynamic status must be made. If patient is hemodynamically unstable, a DC cardioversion should be performed, whereas in a stable patient further treatment may include IV beta blockers, IV verapamil (Calan), or IV diltiazem (Cardizem) (Table 2). IV amiodarone (Pacerone)[1] is recommended as the next line of treatment if all prior measures are ineffective or not feasible. In a stable patient who is not responding to medications, a DC cardioversion should still be performed to restore the sinus rhythm.

Follow-up management of AVNRT should include a specialty consultation for consideration of slow pathway radiofrequency or cryo catheter ablation. The patient may be started on a maintenance oral beta blocker or a nondihydropyridine calcium channel blocker, such as diltiazem or verapamil. An antiarrhythmic medication, such as flecainide (Tambocor), may also be used to control occurrences of tachyarrhythmia; however, ischemic and structural heart disease has to be ruled out before these agents can be used because of their proarrhythmic effects with these conditions.

Pathway-Mediated Tachycardias (Orthodromic AVRT, Antidromic AVRT, WPW Syndrome)

Atrioventricular structures (AV valves and annuli) serve as an insulator, and normally there is no electrical communication between atrial and ventricular myocardium outside the normal conduction system. An accessory pathway is defined as an abnormal extranodal electrical communication between atrial and ventricular myocardium. A pathway that causes ventricular preexcitation pattern on a surface ECG (P-R interval <0.12 and presence of a delta-wave) is called a *manifest pathway*. A pathway that is not detectable on a surface ECG is called *concealed*. Accessory pathways can be located anywhere around AV annuli and may be capable of anterograde, retrograde, or bidirectional conduction. They are responsible for two types of reentry tachycardias: *ORT* that uses the normal conduction

TABLE 1	Common Causes of Sinus Tachycardia		
PHYSIOLOGIC CAUSES	**PATHOLOGIC CONDITIONS**	**MEDICATIONS AND SUBSTANCES**
Exercise	Fever	Caffeine
Stress (fight or flight response)	Substance withdrawal	Nicotine
Anxiety	Hyperthyroidism	Atropine
Emotions	Pulmonary embolism	Dobutamine
Pain	Sepsis	Dopamine
	Dehydration	Pseudoephedrine
	Chronic anemia or acute blood loss	Theophylline
	Pheochromocytoma	Cocaine
	Heart failure	Methamphetamine

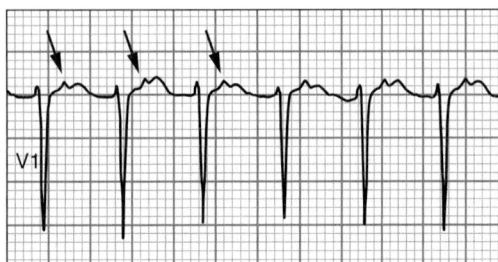

Figure 2 AV-nodal reentry (short R-P) tachycardia. Retrograde P waves are seen (arrows).

system for anterograde conduction and the accessory pathway for retrograde conduction and *ART* that uses the accessory pathway for anterograde conduction and AV node for retrograde conduction.

ORT is the most common type of pathway-mediated SVT and accounts for more than 90% of AVRT cases. Because ORT uses the normal conduction system for ventricular activation, it will demonstrate a normal, narrow QRS morphology, whereas ART leads to direct ventricular activation from pathway-conducting anterograde, which results in a wide-complex QRS morphology (Figure 3).

A WPW syndrome is a bundle of a manifest accessory pathway on a surface ECG in sinus rhythm (preexcitation pattern, Figure 4) and presence of supraventricular tachyarrhythmias.

If a patient with an accessory pathway capable of rapid anterograde conduction develops atrial fibrillation, it may result in a very rapid ventricular response rate and sudden cardiac death. AV blocking agents, such as beta blockers, or calcium channel blockers (CCBs), are contraindicated for treatment of atrial fibrillation in WPW patients, as they suppress the AV node (that competes with accessory pathway for atrioventricular conduction and serves as a rate-control "gate keeper") and further facilitates the conduction down the pathway, increasing the ventricular rate. Instead, procainamide (Pronestyl)[1] should be used to suppress voltage-gated sodium channels of the accessory pathway.

Acute management of AVRT should include assessment of the 12-lead ECG for presence of preexcitation. If no preexcitation is present (ORT), the management is similar to AVNRT, as discussed previously. If preexcitation is detected (ART, WPW), AV blocking agents should be avoided or used with caution. DC cardioversion should be considered early, regardless of hemodynamic status.

For ongoing management, all patients with AVRT should undergo a subspecialty consultation for consideration of a catheter ablation procedure. Patients with a manifest accessory (e.g., WPW) pathway should also undergo risk stratification for sudden cardiac death as soon as diagnosis is made.

Atrial Tachycardias

Atrial tachycardias can be focal or multifocal. Focal atrial tachycardia is usually regular and is characterized by the presence of distinct uniform P waves on the surface ECG. Morphology of these P waves differs from those in sinus rhythm. Multifocal atrial tachycardia will contain three or more different P wave morphologies and is associated with structural heart disease, pulmonary disease, and pulmonary hypertension.

TABLE 2	Doses of Common AV Blocking Agents Used in Acute Setting for SVT Treatment
AGENT	**DOSE**
IV Metoprolol (Lopressor)[1]	2.5–5 mg over 2 min, up to 3 doses
IV Diltiazem (Cardizem)	First dose: 0.25 mg/kg over 2 min, average adult dose, 20 mg; second dose (if first dose is ineffective and tolerated): 0.35 mg/kg in 15–30 min over 2 min, average adult dose is 25 mg
IV Verapamil (Calan)	First dose: 0.075–0.15 mg/kg over 2 min; second dose (if first dose is ineffective and tolerated): 10 mg in 15–30 min over 2 min

[1]Not FDA approved for this indication.

Treatment of atrial tachycardias may be challenging, with limited utility for antiarrhythmic medications and cardioversion that is often ineffective. AV-nodal blockers and ablation procedures have the most established role in treatment of these conditions.

Junctional Tachycardia

Junctional tachycardia is a rapid narrow QRS complex tachyarrhythmia with rates up to 220 bpm that originates within the AV junction and may be regular or irregular. It is more commonly seen in pediatric populations and occurs rarely in adults. In the acute setting, IV beta blockers, nondihydropyridine CCBs, or procainamide[1] can be used. For chronic suppression, oral beta-blockers, verapamil[1], diltiazem[1], or antiarrhythmic drugs may be effective.

Atrial Flutter

Atrial flutter, also known as *macroreentrant atrial tachycardia*, is a reentry arrhythmia that propagates around the tricuspid valve annulus. It most commonly involves the cavotricuspid isthmus (isthmus-dependent) and may be typical, when the signal travels up the intraatrial septum and down the lateral right atrial wall in a counterclockwise fashion around the annulus when observed from the RV apex (Figure 5, panel A), or reverse typical, or clockwise, traveling down the septum and up the atrial wall (see Figure 5, panel B).

Flutter that does not involve the cavotricuspid isthmus is called *atypical*, or *isthmus independent*.

Macroreentrant arrhythmias create a characteristic pattern on the ECG that resembles the "sawtooth" appearance of the electrical baseline, best seen in the inferior leads (Figure 6).

Counterclockwise activation creates positive deflection in lead V_1 (signal travels up the septum toward the lead) and negative deflection in the inferior leads, whereas clockwise demonstrates the opposite. Because the reentrant circle uses a fairly

[1]Not FDA approved for this indication.

consistent anatomic path, the cycle length of reentry is around 220 ms, resulting in an atrial waveform rate around 300 bpm. The AV node will attempt to block the portion of atrial activations, resulting in slower ventricular rates. Two-to-one conduction commonly results in a ventricular rate around 150 bpm, whereas variable conduction may lead to an irregular ventricular response, which, however, usually follows identifiable patterns with R-R intervals multiple to the flutter cycle length, or 220 ms (440 ms, 660 ms, etc.). If the tricuspid annulus is dilated or the patient is receiving an antiarrhythmic medication that slows myocardial conduction (for example, flecainide), it may increase the flutter cycle length, decreasing the flutter rate. This may have an important negative implication. Usually, AV node is able to block fast flutter, decreasing the ventricular response to 2:1. However, when the flutter rate is decreased, it allows the AV node to conduct in 1:1 fashion, leading to very rapid ventricular responses that may result in syncope and ventricular fibrillation. If flecainide is chosen as an antiarrhythmic therapy to control atrial flutter, it is important to always use it in a combination with an AV blocking agent to avoid 1:1 conduction in case of a relapse.

Medical treatment of atrial flutter may be challenging because of weaker ventricular rate responses to AV blocking agents that result in notorious difficulty with the rate-control strategy. One-to-one response should be treated as a medical emergency with a prompt DC cardioversion. For typical flutter, an EP consultation for a radiofrequency catheter ablation procedure should always be considered because of a high success rate and relative simplicity of the procedure. Atypical flutter ablations, however, may be more technically challenging with lower success rates.

Ventricular Tachycardias

Ventricular tachycardia is defined as a cardiac arrhythmia of three or greater beats at a rate of >100 bpm that originates in the ventricles. Sustained VT, just as SVT, is a VT that sustains for >30 seconds. Nonsustained VT terminates spontaneously within 30 seconds after onset.

VT that manifests with uniform beat-to-beat QRS morphology is called *monomorphic* (Figure 7). This type of morphology is more likely to represent structural or functional electrical reentry as the leading mechanism. A common substrate for such arrhythmia is a myocardial scar resulting from chronic ischemic or structural heart disease.

Polymorphic ventricular tachycardia is characterized by the presence of multiform QRS complexes and likely represents unstable myocyte membranes. Such arrhythmia may be seen in multiple conditions, including long-QT syndromes (congenital and acquired). QT should always be assessed as soon as sinus rhythm is restored. When QT prolongation is detected, a reversible cause, such as medication effect or electrolyte abnormality, should be considered and treated. If no cause can be identified, a congenital condition may be suspected.

If polymorphic VT occurs without QT prolongation, acute myocardial ischemia should be considered and promptly evaluated and treated.

Torsades de pointes represents a subtype of polymorphic VT that is usually associated with long-QT syndromes and demonstrates a characteristic ECG pattern with rotating QRS axis appearance (Figure 8).

Of all the arrhythmias seen in clinical practice, ventricular tachycardias are of most concern to practitioners because of the high morbidity and mortality associated with these disorders.

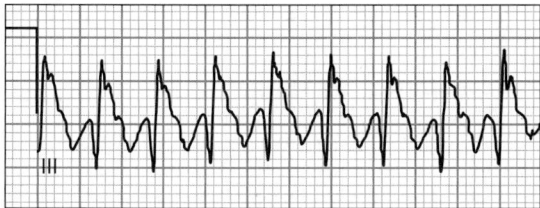

Figure 3 Antidromic reciprocating tachycardia. Wide QRS morphology results from ventricular activation via the accessory pathway. P wave is preceding the QRS complex (long R-P).

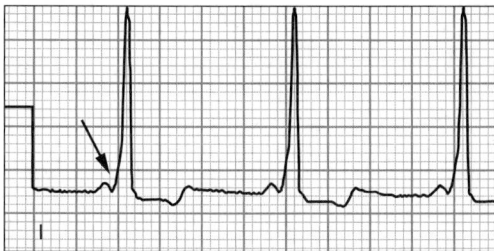

Figure 4 Manifest accessory pathway in a patient with Wolff-Parkinson-White syndrome. A short PR interval and delta-wave (arrow).

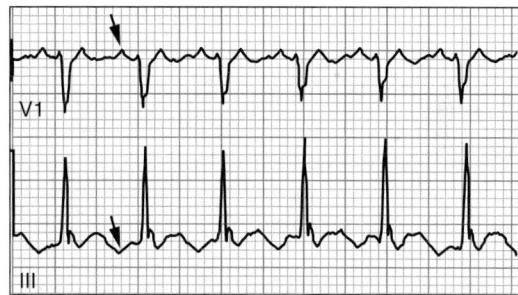

Figure 6 Macroreentrant atrial tachycardia: typical atrial flutter with 2:1 AV-nodal conduction. A variable baseline is seen that resembles a saw-tooth pattern. Positive deflections in lead V_1 and negative in lead III (arrows) indicate counterclockwise signal propagation around the tricuspid annulus.

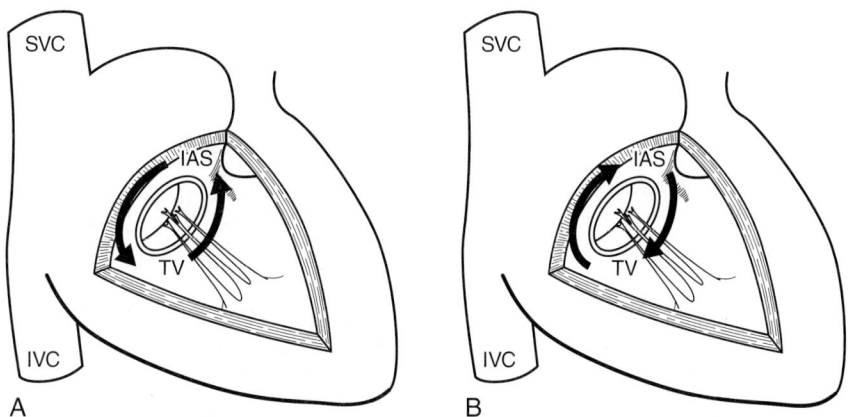

Figure 5 (Panel A) Direction of a typical, counter-clockwise activation in atrial flutter. (Panel B) Direction of a reverse typical, clockwise activation in atrial flutter. IAS, Intraatrial septum; IVC, inferior vena cava; SVC, superior vena cava; TV, tricuspid valve.

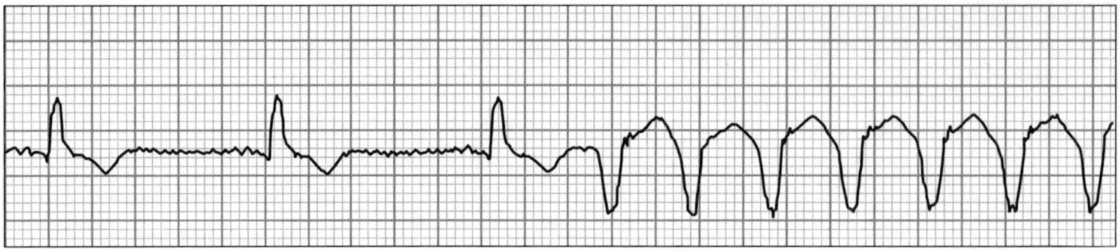

Figure 7 Onset of monomorphic ventricular tachycardia.

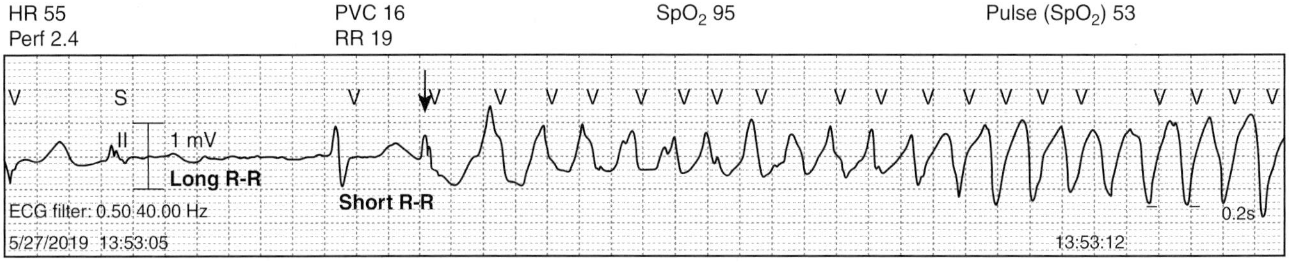

Figure 8 Polymorphic ventricular tachycardia: a premature ventricular complex (PVC, arrow), occurring during relative refractory period ("R on T" phenomenon) triggers the arrhythmia. The QT interval duration in the current R-R cycle is determined by the duration of preceding R-R cycle. A PVC that triggers VT occurs during a prolonged QT interval after a long previous R-R cycle and creates a distinctive "long-short R-R" ECG pattern.

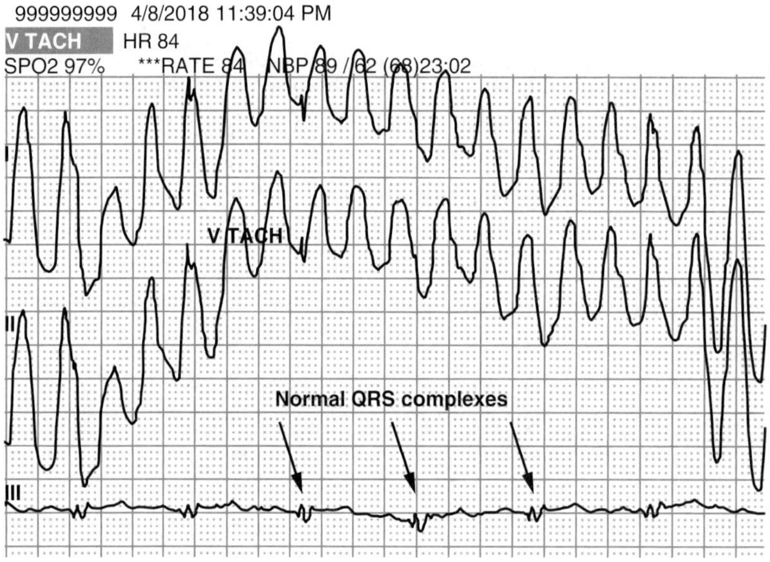

Figure 9 Artifact masquerading as ventricular tachycardia. A diagnosis of wide-complex tachycardia is dismissed by presence of sinus rhythm in lead III.

Although both subtypes require emergent medical attention, polymorphic VT poses particular danger because of the often rapid deterioration of hemodynamics, loss of circulation, and death. Sustained polymorphic VT should be treated immediately with an unsynchronized DC cardioversion.

The approach to monomorphic VT starts with assessment of hemodynamic stability. Faster ventricular rates (>150 bpm) and underlying structural heart disease may be associated with more rapid hemodynamic decline. ACLS algorithms for specific types of VT must be implemented. Each patient with ventricular tachycardia should undergo a prompt specialty consultation and risk stratification for sudden cardiac death.

Artifact

All providers should be aware of telemetry and ECG artifacts that may masquerade as ventricular arrhythmias. If multilead recording is available, all leads should be examined. If sinus rhythm can be found in one or more leads, that indicates the recording is an artifact (Figure 9).

References

Al-Khatib SM, Stevenson WG: *AHA/ACC/HRS Guideline for management of patients with ventricular arrhythmias and the prevention of sudden cardiac death*, 2017.

Aronow WS, Ahn C, Mercando AD, Epstein S, Kronzon I: Prevalence and association of ventricular tachycardia and complex ventricular arrhythmias with new coronary events in older men and women with and without cardiovascular disease, *J Gerontol A Biol Sci Med Sci* 57(3):M178–M180, 2002.

Brady WJ, Mattu A, Tabas J, Ferguson JD: The differential diagnosis of wide QRS complex tachycardia, *Am J Emerg Med* 35(10):1525–1529, 2017.

Brugada P, Brugada J, Mont L, Smeets JLRM, Andries EW: A new approach to the differential diagnosis of a regular tachycardia with a wide QRS complex, *Circulation* 83(5):1649–1659, 1991.

Low PA, Sandroni P: Postural tachycardia syndrome (POTS). Primer on the autonomic nervous system, 2012, Academic Press, pp 517–519.

Meiltz A, Weber R, Halimi F: Permanent form of junctional reciprocating tachycardia in adults: peculiar features and results of radiofrequency catheter ablation, *Europace* 8(1):21–28, 2006.

Orejarena LA, Vidaillet H, DeStefano F: Paroxysmal supraventricular tachycardia in the general population, *J Am Coll Cardiol* 31(1):150–157, 1998.

Page RL: 2015 ACC/AHA/HRS guideline for the management of adult patients with supraventricular tachycardia: a report of the American College of Cardiology/American Heart Association task force on clinical practice guidelines and the Heart Rhythm Society, *J Am Coll Cardiol* 67(13), 2016.

VALVULAR HEART DISEASE

Method of
Carlos E. Sanchez, MD; Steven I. Yakubov, MD; and
Arash Arshi, MD

CURRENT DIAGNOSIS

- The diagnosis of severe aortic valve stenosis is based on an integration of clinical symptoms and hemodynamic echocardiographic criteria.
- Classic symptoms of severe aortic stenosis include fatigue, dyspnea on exertion, angina, near syncope or syncope, and congestive heart failure.
- Chronic mitral regurgitation tends to be a slowly progressive disease and symptoms may not be apparent.
- Cardiac imaging, especially echocardiography, is crucial to the management of patients with valvular heart disease.
- Diagnostic echocardiographic findings of severe aortic stenosis are peak aortic valve velocity of greater than or equal to 4 m/s, transaortic mean gradient of greater than or equal to 40 mm Hg, and aortic valve area less than or equal to 1 cm^2 or aortic valve area index of less than or equal to 0.6 cm^2/m^2.
- Echocardiography should be performed to determine the etiology of and characterize the severity of mitral regurgitation.
- Left ventricular size and function should be assessed in patients with mitral regurgitation.

CURRENT THERAPY

- Medical therapy has not been shown to change hemodynamic progression or clinical outcomes in patients with aortic stenosis.
- Reevaluation for early symptoms and transthoracic echocardiography should be performed every 6–12 months in asymptomatic patients with severe aortic stenosis and normal left ventricular systolic function.
- Transcatheter aortic valve replacement is currently approved in patients with severe symptomatic aortic stenosis with any level of surgical risk.
- The etiology of mitral regurgitation dictates its treatment.
- Primary (degenerative) mitral regurgitation typically requires surgical repair or replacement.
- The management of secondary (functional) mitral regurgitation requires treatment of the underlying cardiomyopathy.
- Mitral transcatheter edge-to-edge repair with MitraClip (Abbott Laboratories, Abbott Park, IL) is currently indicated in secondary mitral regurgitation patients with left ventricular dysfunction who remain symptomatic despite guideline-directed medical therapy.
- The decision-making process in the management of patients with severe aortic stenosis or severe mitral regurgitation is best achieved by a multidisciplinary heart valve team and should include a systematic risk assessment of the patient's comorbidities and estimation of the 30-day cardiac surgical mortality using the Society of Thoracic Surgeons' Predicted Risk of Mortality (STS-PROM) score.

Aortic Stenosis

Aortic stenosis (AS) is the most common form of adult valvular heart disease, becoming more prevalent in the aging population. It is estimated that more than 4% of the U.S. population over age 75 have AS. Aortic valve stenosis is the most common cause of left ventricular (LV) outflow tract obstruction, while less common causes of obstruction may also occur above (supravalvular) or below (subvalvular) the level of the aortic valve and will not be discussed in this chapter.

Etiology

There are three main causes of valvular AS: congenital in origin (which is usually a bicuspid aortic valve), rheumatic valve disease, and degenerative calcification of a normal aortic valve. Congenitally affected aortic valves may be unicuspid or bicuspid and may become stenotic during childhood. In the majority of cases, a congenital bicuspid valve will develop significant calcific stenosis later in life, usually presenting after the fifth decade.

Rheumatic AS is an important cause of aortic valve disease worldwide; however, with the decline of rheumatic fever in developed countries, it is now a rare cause of AS in the United States. Rheumatic valve disease is characterized by commissural fusion, fibrosis, and calcification. Rheumatic AS is also commonly associated with rheumatic involvement of the mitral valve.

Degenerative or calcific AS is now the most common cause of AS in adults in North America. It has been associated with the same risk factors as vascular atherosclerosis including age, smoking, hypertension, diabetes, and hyperlipidemia. Histopathologic data suggest that calcific aortic valve disease is a chronic inflammatory process with lipid deposition and active leaflet calcification leading to restriction of the cusps.

Pathophysiology

In adults with AS, the gradual obstruction of the LV outflow produces a systolic pressure gradient between the left ventricle and aorta. The average time interval of disease progression from nonobstructive valve thickening (aortic sclerosis) to severe AS is 8 years. However, only 16% of individuals with aortic sclerosis will develop any grade of valve obstruction. The average rate of hemodynamic progression once moderate AS is present is an increase in aortic jet velocity of 0.3 m/s per year and mean pressure gradient of 7 mm Hg per year with a decrease in aortic valve area of 0.1 cm^2/year. LV response to chronic pressure overload ultimately leads to concentric wall hypertrophy. This compensatory mechanism helps maintain normal LV contractile function to counteract the gradual increase in afterload at the expense of decreased LV compliance and delayed relaxation resulting in diastolic dysfunction.

Clinical Presentation

The cardinal symptoms of severe AS are angina, syncope, and congestive heart failure. Because symptoms in severe AS may not occur until late in the disease process, usually in the sixth to ninth decades of life, clinicians should obtain a careful history of symptoms during the patient's initial assessment. Particular attention must be directed at early symptoms of fatigue or decreased exercise tolerance as elderly patients may minimize and attribute these symptoms to aging.

Dyspnea on exertion occurs once the pulmonary capillary pressure increases as a result of excessive elevation in LV end-diastolic pressure in a poorly compliant ventricle. Symptoms of angina pectoris in severe AS may occur in a similar manner as in coronary artery disease, with symptoms precipitated by exertion and relieved by rest even in the absence of obstructive epicardial coronary artery disease. Syncope may result from the inability of the heart to increase cardiac output from the stenotic valve in the setting of transient vasodilatation during physical activity, resulting in decreased cerebral perfusion. Other causes of syncope may also be attributable to arrhythmias, either advanced forms of atrioventricular blocks from calcification impinging on the conduction system or tachyarrhythmias causing a sudden decline in cardiac output such as in atrial fibrillation.

Diagnosis and Management

Diagnosis of AS is usually suspected after a systolic ejection murmur is heard during cardiac auscultation. The classic physical findings in patients with severe AS are a loud, late-peaking

TABLE 1	Echocardiographic Stages of Aortic Valve Stenosis and Frequency of Echocardiograms in Asymptomatic Patients With Aortic Stenosis and Normal Left Ventricular Ejection Fraction			
	MAXIMUM AORTIC VELOCITY	MEAN PRESSURE GRADIENT	AORTIC VALVE AREA	TTE FOLLOW-UP IN ASYMPTOMATIC PATIENTS
Mild aortic stenosis	2.0–2.9 m/s	<20 mm Hg	>1.5 cm^2	Every 3–5 years
Moderate aortic stenosis	3.0–3.9 m/s	20–30 mm Hg	1.0–1.5 cm^2	Every 1–2 years
Severe aortic stenosis	≥4.0 m/s	≥40 mm Hg	≤1.0 cm^2	Every 6–12 months
Very severe aortic stenosis	≥5 m/s	≥60 mm Hg	≤1.0 cm^2	

TTE, Transthoracic echocardiogram.

systolic murmur at the base of the heart radiating to the carotid arteries with a delayed and diminished carotid upstroke (*pulsus parvus et tardus*). The latter physical finding may be masked in elderly patients with stiff, inelastic arterial walls. Distinctively, a normally split-second heart sound is the only reliable physical finding to help exclude the diagnosis of severe AS.

A transthoracic echocardiogram (TTE) is recommended as the initial diagnostic test in the evaluation of patients with aortic valve stenosis to determine hemodynamic severity, LV size and function, and prognosis, and to evaluate timing of valve intervention. Echocardiographic valve hemodynamics define the severity of AS (Table 1). Severe AS is characterized by a peak aortic valve velocity of 4 m/s or higher, transaortic mean gradient of 40 mm Hg or higher, and aortic valve area of less than or equal to 1 cm^2 or aortic valve area index of less than or equal to 0.6 cm^2/m^2. In severe symptomatic patients with low-flow, low-gradient severe AS and abnormal LV function (<50%), a dobutamine stress echocardiogram can be used to differentiate between true severe AS and pseudo-severe AS. Low-flow, low-gradient true severe AS is characterized by a severely calcified valve with aortic valve area less than or equal to 1 cm^2 and peak aortic valve velocity less than 4 m/s that increases to 4 m/s or higher with low-dose dobutamine administration. Conversely, in pseudo-severe AS the aortic valve area increases to more than 1 cm^2 and flow normalizes during dobutamine stress echocardiogram.

Patients with asymptomatic AS require frequent monitoring owing to the progressive nature of the disease. The frequency of echocardiograms in asymptomatic patients with AS and normal LV systolic function should be performed every 6 to 12 months for reevaluation in severe AS, every 1 to 2 years for moderate AS, and every 3 to 5 years for mild AS (see Table 1). In seemingly asymptomatic patients with severe AS, exercise testing is safe and helpful to expose symptoms, arrhythmias, or abnormal blood pressure response, defined as an exercise-associated decrease of greater than or equal to 10 mm Hg in systolic blood pressure. Exercise testing should not be performed in symptomatic patients.

Treatment

Indication for intervention in patients with severe AS is dependent on the presence or absence of symptoms, the severity of AS, and LV function. Routine aortic valve replacement in asymptomatic AS is currently not recommended. Importantly, event-free survival at 2 years in asymptomatic patients with severe AS (jet velocity ≥ 4.0 m/s) is 30% to 50%, and as low as 21% in those with very severe AS (jet velocity ≥ 5.0 m/s). Close clinical follow-up to evaluate for early-onset AS symptoms and education regarding the disease course should be performed routinely. Intervention should be considered among asymptomatic patients with very severe AS (V_{max} ≥ 5.0 m/s), serum B-type natriuretic peptide (BNP) >3 times normal, or progression of V_{max} ≥ 0.3 m/s per year.

Medical therapy has not been shown to change hemodynamic progression or clinical outcomes in patients with AS. Clinical data have failed to support the use of statins specifically for the prevention of progression of AS. However, all patients with concomitant coronary artery disease or hypercholesterolemia should be treated per established guidelines. Likewise, concurrent hypertension in patients with severe AS is common and should receive appropriate treatment per standard guidelines starting at a low dose and slowly titrating upward with frequent blood pressure monitoring. Although indicated in the treatment of acute heart failure, diuretics should be used with caution to avoid volume depletion, which may result in marked reduction in cardiac output.

Invasive Treatment

Transcatheter aortic valve replacement (TAVR) has expanded rapidly as an alternative to surgical aortic valve replacement (SAVR) since its approval in 2011. It is currently approved for use in patients with severe symptomatic AS with any level of surgical risk. Recent published clinical trials in low–surgical-risk candidates showed that the risk of death or disabling stroke and new onset atrial fibrillation was lower among the TAVR treated patients compared to SAVR. Additionally, rehospitalization and hospital length of stay was shorter with TAVR.

Recommendations and timing of intervention for aortic valve stenosis by either SAVR or TAVR are summarized in Table 2. Once the patient with AS is considered to meet an indication for aortic valve replacement, an important component when choosing between SAVR and TAVR is the underlying risk assessment for SAVR. In the United States, the Society of Thoracic Surgeons' Predicted Risk of Mortality (STS-PROM) risk score calculator is the initial step in predicting 30-day mortality for SAVR, with three categories: low risk defined as less than 4%, intermediate risk defined as 4% to 8%, and high risk defined as greater than 8% STS mortality risk. This risk calculator, however, does not include certain comorbid conditions that would also increase the surgical mortality risk such as frailty, porcelain aorta, liver cirrhosis, severe pulmonary hypertension, chest wall abnormalities, and hostile mediastinum. If three or more major organ systems are compromised, with severe frailty, or the morbidity and mortality risk is greater than 50%, the patient is considered prohibitive risk for SAVR. In patients with severe AS and a life expectancy less than 1 year, TAVR or SAVR is considered futile despite successful procedure and it is appropriate to avoid any intervention for severe AS. Hence the risk assessment is a combination of the STS-PROM score, frailty, disability, and major cardiovascular and noncardiovascular comorbidities.

The final treatment decision should be individualized with a risk-benefit assessment by a multidisciplinary heart team (including structural interventional cardiologists, imaging specialists, cardiovascular surgeons, and nursing professionals). The heart team assesses potential procedural outcomes based on the patient's individual procedural risk, anatomic considerations, comorbidities, life expectancy, and potential quality-of-life improvement with SAVR or TAVR. The importance of a collaborative and multidisciplinary heart team approach to the evaluation and management of patients with complex AS has been endorsed by professional guidelines to maximize appropriate outcomes.

Once the patient is considered to be a suitable candidate for TAVR, the evaluation of all patients undergoing the procedure

COR	RECOMMENDATION
I	• AVR is recommended for symptomatic patients with severe high-gradient AS who have symptoms by history or on exercise testing • AVR is recommended for asymptomatic patients with severe AS and LVEF <50% • AVR is indicated for patients with severe AS when undergoing other cardiac surgery • For symptomatic patients with severe AS who are >80 years of age or for younger patients with a life expectancy <10 years and no anatomic contraindication to transfemoral TAVR, transfemoral TAVR is recommended in preference to SAVR. • In symptomatic patients with low-flow, low-gradient severe AS with reduced LVEF, AVR is recommended. • In symptomatic patients with low-flow, low-gradient severe AS with normal LVEF (Stage D3), AVR is recommended if AS is the most likely cause of symptoms.
IIa	• AVR is reasonable for asymptomatic patients with very severe AS (aortic velocity ≥ 5.0 m/s) and low surgical risk • AVR is reasonable in asymptomatic patients with severe AS and decreased exercise tolerance or an exercise fall in systolic BP equal to or greater than 10 mm Hg from baseline to peak exercise • In apparently asymptomatic patients with severe AS and low surgical risk, AVR is reasonable when the serum B-type natriuretic peptide (BNP) level is >3 times the normal level • AVR is reasonable in symptomatic patients with low-flow/low-gradient severe AS with reduced LVEF with a low-dose dobutamine stress study that shows an aortic velocity ≥4.0 m/s (or mean pressure gradient ≥40 mm Hg) with a valve area of 1.0 cm^2 at any dobutamine dose • AVR is reasonable for patients with moderate AS (aortic velocity 3.0–3.9 m/s) who are undergoing other cardiac surgery
IIb	• AVR may be considered for asymptomatic patients with severe AS and rapid disease progression and low surgical risk • In asymptomatic patients with severe high-gradient AS and a progressive decrease in LVEF on at least 3 serial imaging studies to <60%, AVR may be considered.

AS, Aortic stenosis; *AVR*, aortic valve replacement by either surgical or transcatheter approach; *BP*, blood pressure; *COR*, class of recommendation; *LVEF*, left ventricular ejection fraction.

Modified from Otto CM, Nishimura RA, Bonow RO, et al: 2020 ACC/AHA guideline for the management of patients with valvular heart disease: a report of the American College of Cardiology/American Heart Association Joint Committee on Clinical Practice Guidelines. *J Am Coll Cardiol.* 2021;77:e25–197.

should include (1) coronary angiography to determine the presence of coronary artery disease; and (2) computed tomography of the chest, abdomen, and pelvis to determine preferred vascular access or contraindications to it and aortic annulus dimension for prosthesis sizing (Figure 1).

The currently available TAVR valves approved by the United States Food and Drug Administration (FDA) include the balloon-expandable Edwards Sapien XT and Sapien 3 (Edwards Lifesciences, Irvine, CA), the self-expandable Medtronic Evolut systems (Medtronic, Minneapolic, MN), and the self-expandable Navitor valve (Abbott, Santa Clara, CA). The choice of valve mostly depends on anatomic considerations and operator preference and experience.

A series of major procedural cardiovascular complications have been described after TAVR, including paravalvular aortic regurgitation, ischemic strokes, conduction disturbances, cardiac perforation, coronary occlusion, and vascular access complications. With the advancement of valve technology and increase in operator experience, the frequency of procedural complications has reduced since the arrival of TAVR procedures. The use of cerebral embolic protection devices during TAVR remains selective, typically reserved for patients at particularly high risk for stroke, such as those with extensive peripheral vascular disease or other significant atheromatous burden. While cerebral protection has gained attention, its impact on reducing clinically meaningful stroke rates remains uncertain. Preprocedure planning by an expert heart team is essential to recognizing and preventing expected complications during and after transcatheter valve implantation.

Currently the optimal antithrombotic regimen following TAVR is daily clopidogrel (Plavix)[1] 75 mg and aspirin[1] 75 to 100 mg for 3 to 6 months followed by daily aspirin alone for life. If there is an indication for chronic anticoagulation, it should follow current guidelines' recommendations for each individual condition (e.g., atrial fibrillation, deep venous thrombosis). The safety of antiplatelet therapy use in conjunction with oral anticoagulation should be individualized based on the patient's bleeding risk.

[1]Not FDA approved for this indication.

Mitral Regurgitation

Mitral regurgitation (MR) is a common valvular disease, and pathology in any of the structures of the mitral valve apparatus may lead to dysfunction of the valve. The base of the leaflets of the mitral valve are attached to the annulus, and the leaflets themselves are attached to the papillary muscles of the left ventricle by the chordae tendineae. The mitral valve is an integral part of both the left atrium and left ventricle, and disorders of these structures affect mitral valve function; likewise, disorders of the mitral valve lead to abnormalities of the left atrium and left ventricle.

Etiology

MR can be divided into primary (degenerative) MR and secondary (functional) MR (Figure 2). Primary MR refers to pathology of the mitral valve leaflets and chordae tendineae that results in valve dysfunction. The most common etiology is mitral valve prolapse, where the underlying pathology is myxomatous mitral valve degeneration that results in redundant leaflets, causing prolapse of the leaflets. A myxomatous mitral valve is also prone to rupture of the chordae tendineae, leading to a flail leaflet or segment of a leaflet. Other common etiologies of MR include rheumatic heart disease and endocarditis. Mitral annular calcification may cause mild to moderate MR, but severe regurgitation is uncommon.

In contrast, in secondary MR, the mitral valve itself has a relatively normal structure. Instead, the pathology is an abnormality of the left ventricle. This most commonly occurs after myocardial infarction, with focal wall motion abnormalities and displacement of the papillary muscle causing tethering of the chordae and leaflets, along with dilatation of the mitral valve annulus, resulting in incomplete coaptation of the mitral valve leaflets during systole. Secondary MR may also occur in a dilated cardiomyopathy.

Clinical Manifestations

The clinical presentation of MR is extremely variable and depends largely on the severity of the regurgitation and its acuity. MR tends to be asymptomatic when mild to moderate, but severe MR frequently results in symptoms. Acute MR occurring from papillary muscle rupture complicating an acute myocardial infarction leads

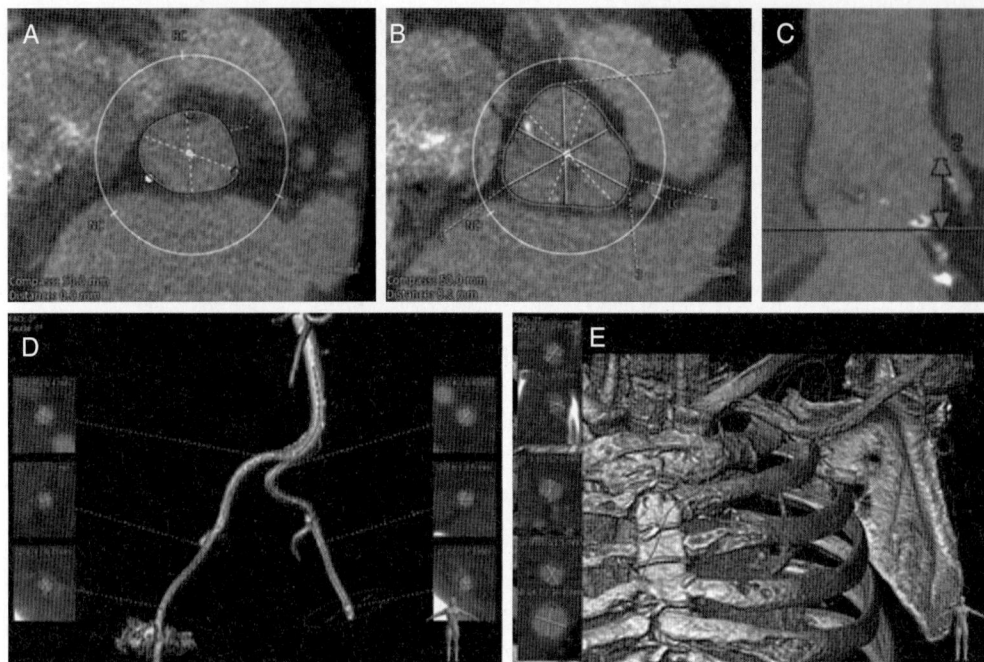

Figure 1 Multidetector computed tomography measurements of the aortic valve complex and peripheral vascular assessment. (A) Aortic annulus perimeter, area, and diameter measurement. (B) The maximum sinus of Valsalva diameters. (C) Height of the left coronary artery from the annular base. (D) Reconstructed view of the iliofemoral anatomy. (E) Left subclavian view with measurement obtained (*left* of image).

to rapid hemodynamic collapse and carries a high risk of mortality. These patients experience pulmonary edema due to the acute volume overload of the left ventricle and left atrium. In contrast, chronic severe MR may have a relatively indolent course, with some patients reporting few symptoms. While chronic MR typically manifests as congestive heart failure, with exertional dyspnea, orthopnea, and lower extremity edema as the hallmark symptoms, owing to the insidious nature of the disease, patients may not always recognize their symptoms. A detailed history with a specific focus on symptoms of congestive heart failure in addition to fatigue and effort intolerance must be elicited. Atrial fibrillation is a common complication of MR and is associated with worse outcomes.

Diagnosis

Physical examination classically may reveal a soft S1 and a holosystolic murmur at the apex that radiates to the left sternal border or to the axilla. However, the intensity of the murmur does not correlate to the severity of disease, nor does the absence of a murmur reliably rule out severe MR. Physical examination is important to assess the patient's volume status, with pulmonary rales and lower extremity edema suggesting congestive heart failure, and an irregularly irregular rhythm indicative of atrial fibrillation.

Cardiac imaging, in particular echocardiography, is crucial in the evaluation of suspected MR. Transthoracic echocardiography can reveal abnormalities of the mitral valve and provide important information on LV size and function and estimation of pulmonary arterial pressure. Given the orientation of the mitral valve and the limits of transthoracic echocardiography, the severity of MR can be grossly underestimated, particularly if the regurgitant jet is eccentric. Transesophageal echocardiography, especially with the availability of three-dimensional imaging, provides higher-quality images of the mitral valve and allows more precise evaluation of the severity and etiology of MR, and has become the gold-standard test in the evaluation of patients with clinically significant MR. Echocardiography with color Doppler can be used to provide a visual estimate of the severity of regurgitation. The presence of reversal of flow into the pulmonary veins during systole suggests severe regurgitation. Quantitative analysis can also be performed to determine the volume of regurgitation and the orifice of the regurgitant jet. There is currently no single echocardiographic parameter to define severe MR, but integration of multiple qualitative and quantitative measurements is recommended. Accurate assessment of LV dimensions and function is important in patients with chronic severe MR. Methods of determining the LV ejection fraction include visual estimation and volumetric analysis. Owing to the volume of blood exiting the left ventricle through both the mitral and aortic valves during systole, the ejection fraction will be increased. In the presence of severe MR, a normal LV ejection fraction approaches 70%, and LV dysfunction is deemed anything less than 60%. Even what would otherwise be considered a mildly reduced ejection fraction may indicate significant myocardial dysfunction in the presence of MR. Left atrial enlargement as a rule is found in chronic severe MR, and its absence should lead to reconsideration of the diagnosis. Exercise echocardiography can play an important role in patients with MR, especially in those with severe MR who report few symptoms, as it is an objective means to assess functional capacity and can also be used to assess changes in pulmonary pressures with exercise. In patients who have mild MR at rest but severe exertional symptoms, exercise echocardiography can identify ischemic MR with concomitant regional wall motion abnormalities.

Cardiac catheterization is performed in many patients with suspected severe MR. Right heart catheterization with measurement of right atrial, right ventricular, pulmonary arterial, and pulmonary capillary wedge pressures and cardiac outputs can help determine volume status and assess for pulmonary hypertension. Attention should be paid to the pulmonary capillary wedge waveform, with large "v" waves, corresponding to ventricular systole, suggestive of severe MR. Left heart catheterization with selective coronary angiography is recommended to identify concomitant obstructive coronary artery disease. Left ventriculography using contrast is commonly performed, and the presence of contrast in the left atrium suggests MR. However, the clinical utility of left ventriculography is limited with the ready availability of echocardiography. The visual estimation of MR by contrast ventriculography is subjective, and the etiology of valve pathology is unable to be defined precisely. Furthermore, in a patient with congestive heart failure, the contrast load may result in acute decompensation.

Magnetic resonance imaging (MRI) is not currently a routinely used test in the evaluation of severe MR but may provide more reproducible quantification of the regurgitant volume and fraction and more accurate measurements of LV size and function. Given the importance of defining the severity of the MR and abnormalities

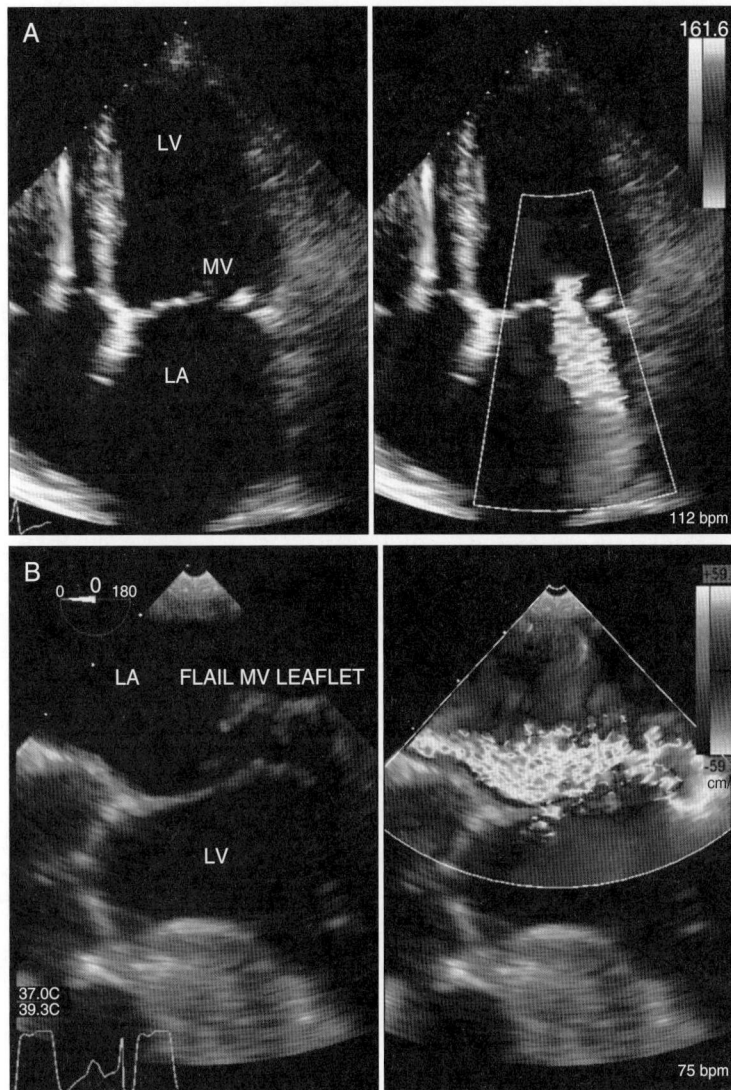

Figure 2 (A) Transthoracic echocardiogram of a patient with a dilated cardiomyopathy with annular dilation resulting in incomplete coaptation of the mitral valve leaflets and severe functional (secondary) mitral regurgitation. The regurgitant jet is central. (B) Transesophageal echocardiogram reveals a markedly myxomatous mitral valve with a large flail segment of the posterior leaflet resulting in severe degenerative (primary) mitral regurgitation. This jet is extremely eccentric. *LA*, Left atrium; *LV*, left ventricle; *MV*, mitral valve.

of LV function in the management of MR, MRI may eventually have a central role in the evaluation of patients and is strongly recommended when echocardiographic data is not satisfactory.

Management and Treatment

The etiology of MR dictates its treatment (Table 3). Primary (degenerative) MR is a mechanical problem of the valve or its apparatus and requires a mechanical solution such as a surgical or percutaneous repair or replacement. Secondary (functional) MR is a problem of the left ventricle and treatment of the underlying ventricular pathology is indicated. Transcatheter edge-to-edge repair with MitraClip (Abbott Laboratories, Abbott Park, IL) in secondary MR is currently indicated in patients with LV dysfunction who remain symptomatic despite guideline-directed medical therapy.

In patients with acute severe MR, the role of medical therapy is to stabilize the patient until surgery. Afterload reduction is the initial treatment strategy, which allows for greater flow through the aortic valve, thereby increasing cardiac output while diminishing the MR. Afterload reduction may be accomplished with intravenous vasodilators such as sodium nitroprusside (Nitropress)[1] or with

TABLE 3	Paradigm for Management of Mitral Regurgitation Based on Etiology and Surgical Risk	
	PRIMARY (DEGENERATIVE)	SECONDARY (FUNCTIONAL)
Low surgical risk	Surgical repair or replacement	CHF therapy TEER or surgery in selected patients
High surgical risk	Percutaneous repair in selected patients	CHF therapy ± TEER with MitraClip

CHF, Congestive heart failure. *TEER*, transcatheter edge-to-edge repair.

an intraaortic balloon pump if the clinical situation requires. The role of medical therapy for chronic severe degenerative MR is less clear, especially in asymptomatic patients with normal LV function. Symptomatic patients with a reduced ejection fraction (<60%) may be treated with heart failure therapy such as angiotensin-converting enzyme (ACE) inhibitors or angiotensin receptor blockers (ARBs), beta-adrenergic blockers, or aldosterone antagonists, in addition to loop diuretics for symptomatic relief while awaiting surgery. Ultimately most patients with severe primary MR will be referred

---

[1]Not FDA approved for this indication.

TABLE 4 Indications for Intervention in Severe Primary (Degenerative) Mitral Regurgitation

SYMPTOMATIC

Recommended if LVEF >30%

May be considered if LVEF ≤30%

TEER may be considered if severely symptomatic with reasonable life expectancy but prohibitive surgical risk

ASYMPTOMATIC

Recommended if LV dysfunction (LVEF 30%–60% or LVESD <40 mm)

Reasonable if preserved LV function (LVEF >60% and LVESD >40 mm) if >95% chance of successful repair with <1% mortality risk

Reasonable if preserved LV function with new-onset atrial fibrillation or PASP >50 mm Hg if high likelihood of successful repair

LV, Left ventricular; *LVEF*, left ventricular ejection fraction; *LVESD*, left ventricular end-systolic dimension; *PASP*, pulmonary arterial systolic pressure; *TEER*, transcatheter edge-to-edge repair.

to surgery (Table 4), and valve repair is preferable to replacement provided the anatomy is amenable to repair. If valve replacement is necessary, options include mechanical and bioprosthetic valves. Mechanical valves provide superior hemodynamic results and durability but are prone to thrombus formation and therefore require lifelong anticoagulation with warfarin (Coumadin). If after consultation with a cardiac surgeon the patient is deemed to be at prohibitive risk for surgery, transcatheter edge-to-edge repair with the MitraClip or Pascal (Edwards Lifesciences, Irvine, CA) device is a reasonable alternative. This procedure is performed under general anesthesia with fluoroscopic and transesophageal echocardiographic guidance, and from the femoral vein via transseptal access, a clip is delivered to the regurgitant orifice of the mitral valve, grasping the anterior and posterior leaflets, thereby improving leaflet coaptation.

For patients with secondary MR, the target for treatment is the left ventricle. Medical therapy for the underlying cardiomyopathy is recommended, with administration of ACE inhibitors or ARBs ± neprilysin inhibitors, aldosterone antagonists, and beta-blockers. If indicated, these patients may require cardiac resynchronization therapy. With medical and device therapy, LV remodeling and function may improve, with reduction in the degree of MR. If severe MR persists despite maximally tolerated medical therapy, percutaneous mitral valve repair with the MitraClip device is the only interventional therapy currently approved that significantly reduces mortality and heart failure rehospitalizations while improving heart failure symptoms. In patients with ischemic cardiomyopathy secondary to obstructive coronary artery disease with severe secondary MR, surgical revascularization and concomitant mitral valve repair is frequently performed if the surgical risk is not prohibitive.

MR can progress over time, as the volume overload can lead to LV dilation and worsening mitral leaflet coaptation. As the disease process may be slow and without sudden worsening of symptoms, patients will require close follow-up. Mild MR can be followed by serial transthoracic echocardiography every 3 to 5 years, and moderate MR every 1 to 2 years. In patients with asymptomatic severe MR who do not undergo surgery, transthoracic echocardiography should be performed at least annually, with special attention to LV dimensions and function.

References

Cosmi JE, Kort S, Tunick PA, et al: The risk of the development of aortic stenosis in patients with "benign" aortic valve thickening, *Arch Intern Med* 162:2345–2347, 2002.

Dal-Bianco JP, Khandheira BK, Mookadam F, et al: Management of asymptomatic severe aortic stenosis, *J Am Coll Cardiol* 52:1279–1292, 2008.

Feldman T, Foster E, Glower DD, et al: Percutaneous repair or surgery for mitral regurgitation, *N Engl J Med* 364:1395–1406, 2011.

Freeman RV, Otto CM: Spectrum of calcific aortic valve disease: pathogenesis, disease progression, and treatment strategies, *Circulation* 111:3316–3326, 2005.

Kapadia SR, Kodali S, Makkar R, et al: Protection against cerebral embolism during transcatheter aortic valve replacement, *J Am Coll Cardiol* 69:367–377, 2017.

Ling LH, Enriquez-Sarano M, Seward JB, et al: Early surgery in patients with mitral regurgitation due to flail leaflets: a long-term outcome study, *Circulation* 96:1819–1825, 1997.

Mack MJ, Leon MB, Thourani VH, et al: Transcatheter aortic-valve replacement with balloon expandable valve in low-risk patients, *N Engl J Med*, 2019. https://doi.org/10.1056/NEJMoa1814052.

Nkomo VT, Gardin JM, Skelton TN, et al: Burden of valvular heart diseases: a population-based study, *Lancet* 368:1005–1011, 2006.

Otto CM, Nishimura RA, Bonow RO, et al: 2020 ACC/AHA guideline for the management of patients with valvular heart disease: a report of the American College of Cardiology/American Heart Association Joint Committee on Clinical Practice Guidelines, *J Am Coll Cardiol* 77:e25–e197, 2021.

Otto CM, Kumbhani DJ, Alexander KP, et al: 2017 ACC Expert Consensus Decision Pathway for Transcatheter Aortic Valve Replacement in the Management of Adults with Aortic Stenosis, *J Am Coll of Cardiol* 69(10):1313–1346, 2017. https://doi.org/10.1016/j.jacc.2016.12.006.

Peltier M, Trojette F, Enriquez-Sarano M, et al: Relation between cardiovascular risk factors and nonrheumatic severe calcific aortic stenosis among patients with a three-cuspid aortic valve, *Am J Cardiol* 91:97–99, 2003.

Popma JJ, Deeb GM, Yakubov SJ, et al: Transcatheter aortic valve replacement with a self-expanding valve in low-risk patients, *N Engl J Med*, 2019. https://doi.org/10.1056/NEJMoa1816885.

Stone GW, Lindenfeld J, Abraham WT, et al: Transcatheter mitral-valve repair in patients with heart failure, *N Engl J Med* 379:2307–2318, 2018.

Wu AH, Aaronson KD, Bolling SF, et al: Impact of mitral valve annuloplasty on mortality risk in patients with mitral regurgitation and left ventricular systolic dysfunction, *J Am Coll Cardiol* 45:381–387, 2005.

Zilberszac R, Gabriel H, Schemper M, et al: Asymptomatic severe aortic stenosis in the elderly, *J Am Coll Cardiol Img* 10:43–50, 2017.

VENOUS THROMBOSIS

Method of

Andrea T. Obi, MD; and Thomas W. Wakefield, MD

CURRENT DIAGNOSIS

- Although clinical assessment and D-dimer levels are useful to rule out thrombosis, there is no combination of clinical findings and biomarker testing at this time that can rule in the diagnosis.
- Duplex ultrasound imaging is the gold standard for the diagnosis of deep venous thrombosis (DVT).
- Spiral computed tomography (CT) scanning, especially higher-resolution multidetector-row CT imaging, is preferred as the initial imaging test to establish the diagnosis of pulmonary embolism.

CURRENT THERAPY

- Initial preventative therapy includes anticoagulation, compression garments, and ambulation.
- The new direct oral anticoagulants (DOACs) are favored over warfarin for acute venous thromboembolism (VTE) treatment and no cancer. Rivaroxaban (Xarelto) and apixaban (Eliquis) are administered as monotherapy whereas dabigatran (Pradaxa) and edoxaban (Savaysa) require a low-molecular-weight heparin (LMWH) bridge. No bridge is needed with rivaroxaban or apixaban.
- When warfarin, dabigatran or edoxaban are used, LMWH should be administered for at least 5 days at the onset of therapy. If warfarin is used, it should be therapeutic (international normalized ratio 2.0–3.0) for 2 consecutive days before stopping LMWH.
- The duration of anticoagulation depends on a number of factors, including the presence of risk factors for thrombosis, the type of thrombosis (unprovoked or provoked), the number of times thrombosis has occurred, and risk factors for bleeding.
- Reduced-dose DOACs lessen VTE recurrences more than placebo or aspirin for long-term treatment after initial anticoagulant therapy is complete.

- Significant iliofemoral DVT may be treated with aggressive pharmocomechanical thrombolysis if a trial of anticoagulation fails to improve moderate to severe symptoms and the patient is ambulatory, has no contraindications to thrombolysis, and places a strong value on reducing the severity of postthrombotic syndrome (PTS) while accepting the inherent bleeding risk. Pulmonary embolism causing hemodynamic deterioration or right heart strain should be treated with thrombolysis.

Epidemiology

Venous thromboembolism (VTE) includes deep venous thrombosis (DVT) and pulmonary embolism (PE). VTE affects up to 900,000 patients per year and results in up to 300,000 deaths per year. The incidence has remained constant and may be increasing since the 1980s and increases with age. The annual VTE rate among persons of European ancestry ranges from 104 to 183 per 100,000 person years. Overall VTE incidence may be higher in Black populations and lower in Asians and Asian- and Native Americans. The increasing prevalence of obesity, cancer, and surgery account in part for the persistent VTE incidence. The lifetime risk of VTE is 8% at age 45, and approximately 20% of VTE patients will die within 1 year (usually due to the provoking conditions associated with the VTE). Worldwide, the VTE incidence is approximately 10 million per year, higher in high-income than low-income countries. Total annual health care budget ranges from €1.5 billion to €3.3 billion and from $7 billion to $10 billion (USD). Treatment of an acute VTE appears to be associated with incremental direct medical costs of $12,000 to $15,000 (2014 US dollars) with subsequent complications to increase cumulative costs up to $18,000 to $23,000 per incident case. Sequelae from VTE including recurrent VTE, postthrombotic syndrome (PTS), ulcers, and varicosities increase the incident cost by an average of 75%.

Risk Factors

Risk factors for VTE include acquired and genetic factors. Acquired factors include increasing age, malignancy, surgery, immobilization, trauma, oral contraceptives and hormone replacement therapy, pregnancy and the puerperium, neurologic disease, cardiac disease, obesity, sepsis, pneumonia, calf muscle pump dysfunction, and inflammatory bowel disease. Genetic factors include antithrombin deficiency, protein C deficiency and protein S deficiency, factor V Leiden, prothrombin 20210A, blood group non-O, abnormalities in fibrinogen and plasminogen, elevated levels of clotting factors (e.g., factors XI, IX, VII, VIII, X, and II), and elevation in plasminogen activator inhibitor-1. When a patient presents with an unprovoked VTE, family history of thrombosis, recurrent thrombosis, or thrombosis in unusual locations, a workup for hypercoagulability, including testing for the conditions noted in the previous sentence, may be indicated, although even in these situations testing is controversial. Routine testing for hypercoagulable states in the setting of a provoked DVT is generally not indicated and in patients with a first time proximal DVT, no difference in recurrence rates or VTE survival has been found with positive hereditary thrombophilia as opposed to negative hereditary thrombophilia. Hematologic diseases associated with VTE include heparin-induced thrombocytopenia and thrombosis syndrome, disseminated intravascular coagulation, antiphospholipid antibody syndrome, myeloproliferative disorders, thrombotic thrombocytopenic purpura, and hemolytic uremic syndrome. There are a number of risk prediction scores that have been advanced, the most widely used being the Caprini risk score (https://www.mdcalc.com/caprini-score-venous-thromboembolism-2005). Using the score, factors that have been found to be associated with VTE are counted and summed, and a score is then calculated, which indicates VTE risk, especially in the context of surgical interventions. Others risk prediction scores include the Roger's score assessing the risk of postoperative VTE among non-cardiac surgery patients, the IMPROVE risk score for hospitalized patients, the Padua score for hospitalized medical patients, and the Khorana score to select ambulatory cancer patients for thromboprophylaxis.

Pathophysiology

Although Virchow's triad of stasis, vein injury, and hypercoagulability has defined the events that predispose to VTE formation since the mid-19th century, the understanding today of events that occur at the level of the vein wall and thrombus, including the inflammatory response on thrombogenesis, thrombus resolution, and the subsequent changes to the vein wall and venous valves, is increasingly becoming apparent and may direct therapy in the future. Recently, Heat shock protein 47 (HSP47) downregulation or ablation in platelets has been found to attenuate immune cell activation, neutrophil extracellular trap (NET) formation, and protection from thrombosis in hibernating bears, spinal cord injury patients, and mice. COVID-19 has also been associated with the development of VTE. Infection with COVID-19 induces overlapping pathways that link the inflammatory response to the coagulation response. The overwhelming inflammatory response in patients with COVID-19 infection leads to a hypercoagulable state, microthrombosis, large vessel thrombosis, and ultimately can lead to death. The endothelium in multiple organs, especially the lungs, appears to play a significant role in the process going from reversible dysfunction to irreversible endothelial dysfunction. In COVID-19 critically ill patients, the rate of VTE has generally been reported between 20% and 40%.

Diagnosis

Deep Venous Thrombosis

The diagnosis of DVT can be ruled out with a clinical scoring system known as the Wells score (https://www.mdcalc.com/wells-criteria-dvt) and a negative D-dimer. Wells has classified patients into a system that emphasizes physical presentation, and the most common physical finding is edema. Characteristics that score points in the Wells system include active cancer, paralysis or paresis, recent plaster/cast immobilization of the lower extremity, being recently bedridden for 3 days or more, localized tenderness along the distribution of the deep venous system, swelling of the entire leg, calf swelling that is at least 3 cm larger on the involved side than on the noninvolved side, pitting edema in the symptomatic leg, collateral superficial veins (nonvaricose), and a history of previous DVT. With extensive proximal iliofemoral DVT there may be significant swelling, cyanosis, and dilated superficial collateral veins. The negative predictive value of a low- or intermediate-risk patient as stratified by Wells score and a negative D-dimer is near 100%. The incidence of DVT over the next 3 months in this patient cohort is 0.0% to 0.6%, suggesting that additional testing is unlikely to improve outcomes.

Duplex ultrasound imaging is the gold standard for ruling in the diagnosis of DVT. Duplex imaging includes both a B-mode image and Doppler flow pattern. Duplex imaging demonstrates sensitivity and specificity rates greater than 95%. According to the grade criteria for the strength of medical evidence, duplex ultrasound is given a 1B level of evidence, depending on the pretest probability for DVT. Even at the level of the calf, duplex imaging is an acceptable technique in symptomatic patients. Duplex imaging is painless, requires no contrast, can be repeated, and is safe during pregnancy. Duplex imaging also identifies other causes of a patient's symptoms. Other tests available for making the diagnosis include magnetic resonance imaging (MRI) (especially good for assessing central pelvic vein and inferior vena cava [IVC] thrombosis) and spiral computed tomography (CT) scanning (especially with chest imaging during examination for PE).

A single complete negative lower extremity duplex scan is accurate enough to withhold anticoagulation with minimal long-term adverse thromboembolic complications. This requires that all venous segments of the leg have been imaged and evaluated. If the duplex scan is indeterminate owing to technical issues or to edema, treatment may be based on factors such as biomarkers, with the duplex repeated in 24 to 72 hours. A recent study to define the role of risk stratification and duplex ultrasound found a negative Wells score and negative D-dimer had a negative predictive value >99% in 2290 patients, while a positive Wells score and positive D-dimer had a positive predictive value of 81.5% in 222 patients. Combining clinical characteristics with a high-sensitivity D-dimer assay can decrease the number of duplex scans performed in the low-risk patient. Although clinical characteristics and D-dimer levels are useful to rule out thrombosis, the converse is not true, and there is no combination of biomarkers and clinical presentation that can rule in the diagnosis. Work is ongoing to establish new biomarkers based on the inflammatory response to DVT. We have data suggesting that a combination of soluble P-selectin and the Wells score can rule in the diagnosis of DVT, whereas D-dimer plus Wells is still the best combination to rule out the diagnosis of DVT.

Conditions that may be confused with DVT include lymphedema, muscle strain, muscle contusion, and systemic problems such as cardiac, renal, or hepatic abnormalities. These systemic problems usually lead to bilateral edema.

Rarely, massive iliofemoral DVT can result in phlegmasia alba dolens (white swollen leg) or phlegmasia cerulean dolens (blue swollen leg). If phlegmasia is not aggressively treated, it can lead to venous gangrene when the arterial inflow becomes obstructed owing to venous hypertension. Alternatively, arterial emboli or spasm can occur and contribute to the pathophysiology. Venous gangrene is often associated with underlying malignancy and is always preceded by phlegmasia cerulea dolens. Venous gangrene is associated with significant rates of amputation and PE and with mortality.

Pulmonary Embolism

The diagnosis of PE historically has involved ventilation-perfusion scanning and pulmonary angiography. However, the most current techniques include spiral CT scanning and MRI, along with assessments of pretest probability and high-sensitivity D-dimer measurements. Age-adjusted D-dimer measurements may increase the diagnostic usefulness of these measurements. CT scanning demonstrates excellent specificity and sensitivity. Emboli down to the subsegmental level can be identified. The sensitivity for isolated chest CT imaging is increased when clinical analysis is added and when adding lower extremity imaging to the chest scan, although with the introduction of higher resolution multidetector-row CT imaging, the need for lower extremity imaging combined with CT is being questioned. Useful alternate techniques when there are contraindications to CT imaging include MRI and ventilation-perfusion imaging.

In low-risk individuals, a score of 0 on the PE Rule-out Criteria (https://www.mdcalc.com/perc-rule-pulmonary-embolism) gives confidence that further testing (D-dimer and CT) is not necessary. The PE Rule-out Criteria include (1) age older than 50 years, (2) pulse less than 100 beats/min, (3) oxygen saturation greater than 95% on room air, (4) absence of unilateral leg swelling, (5) absence of hemoptysis, (6) no recent trauma or surgery, (7) no prior history of VTE, and (8) no exogenous estrogen use.

Axillary and Subclavian Vein Thrombosis

Thrombosis of the axillary and subclavian veins accounts for less than 5% of all cases of DVT. However, it may be associated with PE in up to 10% to 15% of cases and can be the source of significant disability. Upper extremity DVT may be primary (approximately 20%), such as from thoracic outlet syndrome, effort thrombosis, or idiopathic, or secondary (approximately 80%), such as from catheter-related, cancer-associated, surgery-related, or mediastinal tumors. Primary axillary and subclavian vein thrombosis results from obstruction of the axillary vein in the thoracic outlet from compression by the subclavius muscle and the costoclavicular space, the Paget-Schrötter syndrome, noted especially in muscular athletes. Patients with axillary and subclavian vein thrombosis present with arm pain, edema, and cyanosis. Superficial venous distention may be apparent over the arm, forearm, shoulder, and anterior chest wall.

Upper extremity venous duplex ultrasound scanning is used to make the diagnosis of axillary and subclavian vein thrombosis. A secondary DVT (such as related to a central venous catheter or other risk factor) is treated with anticoagulation alone, with the same recommendation regarding anticoagulant type, dose, and duration. If Paget-Schrötter syndrome is suspected, thrombolysis and phlebography are considered as next interventions. If phlebography is performed, it is important that the patient undergo positional phlebography with the arm abducted to 120 degrees to confirm extrinsic subclavian vein compression at the thoracic outlet once the vein has been cleared of thrombus. Because a cervical rib may be the cause of such obstruction, chest x-ray should be obtained to exclude its presence (although its incidence is quite low). Ultimately, decompression of the thoracic outlet with first rib resection (and cervical rib, if present), is necessary to prevent recurrent DVT.

Treatment

Standard Therapy for Venous Thromboembolism

The traditional treatment of VTE is systemic anticoagulation, which reduces the risk of PE, extension of thrombosis, and thrombus recurrence. Because the recurrence rate for VTE is higher if anticoagulation is not therapeutic in the first 24 hours, immediate anticoagulation should be undertaken. For PE, this usually means anticoagulation followed by testing. For DVT, because duplex imaging is rapidly obtained, usually testing precedes anticoagulation. Recurrent DVT can still occur in up to one-third of patients over an 8-year period, even with appropriate anticoagulant therapy.

The first line of therapy in the modern-day treatment of VTE is DOACs. Currently four DOACs are approved by the US Food and Drug Administration (FDA) for the treatment of DVT and one for prophylaxis of VTE. These include rivaroxaban (Xarelto) and apixaban (Eliquis) as oral monotherapy (both require a loading dose period followed by a lower dose) and dabigatran (Pradaxa) and edoxaban (Savaysa), which require a LMWH bridge, and betrixaban (Bevyxxa)[2] for prophylaxis. Alternatively, LMWH or unfractionated heparin is given for 5 days, during which time oral anticoagulation with vitamin K antagonists (warfarin) is begun and LMWH is discontinued as soon as anticoagulation is therapeutic. With warfarin, it is recommended that the international normalized ratio be therapeutic for 2 consecutive days before stopping heparin or LMWH.

The new oral anticoagulants are favored over warfarin for acute VTE and no cancer. Dabigatran targets activated factor II (factor IIa), whereas rivaroxaban, apixaban, and edoxaban target activated factor X (factor Xa). Dabigatran etexilate is FDA approved for stroke and systemic embolization prevention in patients with nonvalvular atrial fibrillation, for treatment and reduction of DVT and PE in patients who have been treated with a parenteral anticoagulant for 5 to 10 days, and for reducing the risk of recurrence of DVT and PE in adult patients who have been previously treated. It is approved for DVT prophylaxis after hip replacement. Dabigatran etexilate has also been approved in oral pellet form for the treatment of venous thromboembolic events (VTE) in pediatric patients 8 to younger than 18 years of age who have been treated with a parenteral anticoagulant for at least 5 days, and to reduce the risk of recurrence of VTE in pediatric patients 8 to younger than 18 years of age who have been previously treated.

Rivaroxaban is FDA approved for VTE prophylaxis in patients undergoing hip or knee replacements, for stroke and systemic embolization prevention in patients with nonvalvular atrial fibrillation, for VTE treatment, and for reduction in the risk of recurrence of DVT and PE. Rivaroxaban has also been approved to prevent VTE in certain adult patients hospitalized for an acute illness and for those patients after discharge who are at higher risk of VTE due to the decreased ability to move without a high risk of bleeding. It has also received two pediatric indications: (1) the treatment of VTE and reduction in the risk of recurrent VTE in patients from birth to younger than 18 years of age after at least 5 days of initial parenteral anticoagulant treatment, and (2) thromboprophylaxis in children age 2 years and older with congenital heart disease who have undergone a Fontan procedure. Apixaban is currently FDA approved for the prevention of complications of nonvalvular atrial fibrillation, for prophylaxis of DVT after hip or knee replacement surgery, for the treatment of DVT/PE, and for the reduction in risk of recurrence of DVT/PE. Edoxaban has been approved for prevention of stroke and non–CNS systemic embolism in patients with nonvalvular atrial fibrillation and for treating DVT and PE in patients who have been treated with a parenteral anticoagulant for 5 to 10 days. Betrixaban[2] is indicated for the prophylaxis of VTE in adult patients hospitalized for an acute medical illness who are at risk for thromboembolic complications due to restricted mobility and other risk factors. When an anticoagulant bridge is required, LMWH is the standard for initial treatment. LMWH is preferred because it is administered subcutaneously, it requires no monitoring (except in certain circumstances such as renal insufficiency or morbid obesity), and it is associated with a lower bleeding potential. Additionally, LMWH demonstrates less direct thrombin inhibition, more factor Xa inhibition, and antiinflammatory properties. Compared with standard unfractionated heparin, LMWH has significantly improved bioavailability, less endothelial cell binding and protein binding, and an improved pharmacokinetic profile. The half-life of LMWH is dose independent. LMWH is administered in a weight-based fashion.

Warfarin (Coumadin), when used, should be started after heparinization is therapeutic to prevent warfarin-induced skin necrosis. For standard unfractionated heparin, this requires a therapeutic activated partial thromboplastin time (aPTT); for LMWH, warfarin is administered after an appropriate weight-based dose of LMWH is administered and allowed to circulate. Warfarin causes inhibition of protein C and S before factors II, IX, and X, leading to paradoxical hypercoagulability at the initiation of therapy. The goal for warfarin dosing is an international normalized ratio between 2.0 and 3.0.

Fondaparinux (Arixtra) is also approved for the treatment of VTE. It is a synthetic pentasaccharide that has an antithrombin sequence identical to heparin and targets factor Xa. Fondaparinux has been additionally approved for thrombosis prophylaxis in patients with total hip replacement, total knee replacement, and hip fracture; in extended prophylaxis in patients with hip fracture; and in patients undergoing abdominal surgery. It is administered subcutaneously and has a 17-hour half-life. Dosage is based on body weight. It exhibits no endothelial or protein binding and does not produce thrombocytopenia. However, no antidote is readily available. For the treatment of VTE, fondaparinux was found equal to LMWH for DVT, and for PE, it was found equal to standard heparin.

In patients with acute proximal DVT of the leg or acute PE, the most recent *Chest* guidelines suggest anticoagulation therapy alone over interventional therapy such as thrombolytic, mechanical, or pharmacochemical therapy. Specifically, DOACs are suggested over vitamin K antagonist therapy and LMWH if the patient does not have cancer.

Patients with cancer have a higher VTE incidence, higher recurrence rate, and a higher mortality rate. Risk factors for cancer VTE include patient-related factors, cancer-related factors, and treatment-related factors. For example, older age, higher-risk cancer types (such as pancreatic adenocarcinoma), or platin-based chemotherapy confer elevated VTE risk. Although LMWH has been the historic standard of care for treating cancer-associated VTE, the DOACS edoxaban[1] and rivaroxaban[1] have been found effective but with a higher risk of bleeding than LMWH. A recent study found that apixaban[1] at therapeutic dose was non-inferior to the LMWH dalteparin (Fragmin) with no increased risk of major bleeding for treatment of cancer-associated VTE. Rivaroxaban and edoxaban were associated with higher risk of GI major bleeding when compared with LMWH in cancer-related VTE; so for those patients with luminal GI malignancies, LMWH or apixaban is preferred. A recent national study of oncology practices found that DOACs were non-inferior to LMWH for preventing recurrent VTE after 6 months.

---

[1]Not FDA approved for this indication.
[2]Not available in the United States.

With significant thrombotic complications with COVID-19, there are many studies ongoing evaluating anticoagulant prophylaxis and treatment in these patients, to treat not only diagnosed macrothrombosis but also microthrombosis with the intent to improve mortality. Regarding prophylaxis, the NIH COVID-19 Treatment Guidelines Panel recently updated their recommendations. The panel does not recommend for or against routine VTE screening for COVID-19 patients without symptoms of VTE. They do recommend beginning therapeutic anticoagulation in patients with high clinical suspicion for thromboembolic disease but where diagnostic imaging may not be possible or available. The guidelines state to approach VTE prophylaxis for COVID-19 patients compared with the usual standard of care for those without COVID-19 and does not recommend ongoing VTE prophylaxis after hospital discharge. Regarding treatment, therapeutic-dose heparin (LMWH preferred) should be used for patients who have a D-dimer above the upper level of normal, require low-flow oxygen, and have no increased bleeding risk (platelet count <50 x 10^9/L, hemoglobin <8g/dL, need for dual antiplatelet medication, known bleeding within the past 30 days, known history of bleeding disorder, or an inherited or active acquired bleeding disorder). Prophylactic dose heparin should be used for those patients who are receiving intensive care unit level of care. Intermediate or therapeutic dose heparin is not recommended in these patients as they do not appear to benefit from therapeutic dose heparin. Several randomized trials have demonstrated that therapeutic anticoagulation does not decrease mortality in these very sick patients but may have a higher risk of bleeding events.

Distal DVT requires its own discussion. Patients with isolated distal DVT without risk factors for extension may undergo serial imaging for 2 weeks. However, if there is significant calf pain or risk factors for extension, anticoagulation for 3 months is indicated. For intermuscular DVT (posterior tibial, anterior tibial, or peroneal) treatment with serial imaging depending on symptoms or ongoing risk factors of thrombus extension is recommended. Factors that favor anticoagulation include active cancer, history of prior venous thromboembolic event, thrombosis that was non-provoked, significant calf pain, immobility, multiple tibial/peroneal vein involvement, or a thrombus within 3 cm of the popliteal vein. Additional factors include if anticoagulation was initially withheld but extension is later visualized on ultrasound or if the patient is more concerned with avoiding DVT extension, PE, or DVT recurrence than the risk of bleeding. For intramuscular DVT (gastroc-soleal), serial imaging and follow-up is indicated.

Duration of Treatment

The recommended duration of anticoagulation after a first episode of provoked VTE is 3 months for both proximal and distal thrombi (if symptomatic) (Table 1). After a second episode of VTE, the usual recommendation is prolonged oral anticoagulation indefinitely, unless the patient is at high bleeding risk (two or more risk factors) or the patient is very young at the time of presentation. VTE recurrence is increased with homozygous factor V Leiden and prothrombin 20210A mutation, protein C or protein S deficiency, antithrombin deficiency, antiphospholipid antibodies, and cancer until resolved. Long-term oral anticoagulation is usually recommended in these situations. However, heterozygous factor V Leiden and prothrombin 20210A do not carry the same risk as their homozygous counterparts, and the length of oral anticoagulation is shortened for these conditions.

Regarding unprovoked DVT, in those with a low bleeding risk, the recommended length of treatment is extended therapy for more than 3 months, provided the patient is at low or moderate risk of bleeding. Patients at high risk of bleeding should be treated for 3 months and reevaluated. Predicted risk of VTE recurrence and patient preference can be used to guide decision making on who should continue anticoagulation therapy. In patients with VTE in the setting of a minor risk factor (admission to hospital for less than 3 days, surgery with general anesthesia for less than 30 min, estrogen therapy, pregnancy, leg injury with reduced mobility) or major transient risk factor (confined to bed for at least 3 days, surgery with general anesthesia for greater than 30 min),

TABLE 1 Case Scenarios for Treatment and Prevention of Venous Thrombosis

INITIAL MANAGEMENT		DECISION POINT	
PRIMARY TREATMENT (3–6 MONTHS)		**SECONDARY PREVENTION**	
CASE	INITIAL MANAGEMENT	PRIMARY TREATMENT	SECONDARY PREVENTION
Provoked DVT of right leg following a prolonged car ride in an otherwise healthy 61-year-old man	Apixaban 10 mg BID for 7 days or rivaroxaban 15 mg daily for 21 days	Apixaban 5 mg BID for 3 months or rivaroxaban 20 mg daily for 3 months	None
PE in 79-year-old man with prostate cancer	Apixaban 10 mg bid for 7 days	Apixaban 5 mg bid	Apixaban 5 mg BID
Pulmonary emboli in a 48-year-old with ESRD	Intravenous heparin	Vitamin K antagonist (Warfarin)	None (secondary to bleeding risk with ESRD)
Unprovoked DVT in a 50-year-old male with factor V Leiden	Apixaban 10 mg BID for 7 days or rivaroxaban 15 mg daily for 21 days	Apixaban 5 mg BID for 3 months or rivaroxaban 20 mg daily for minimum of 3–6 months	Apixaban 2.5 mg BID, rivaroxaban 10 mg daily or low-dose aspirin

BID, Twice daily; *DVT*, deep venous thrombosis; *ESRD*, end-stage renal disease.

anticoagulation therapy beyond 3 months is not recommended. In patients diagnosed with unprovoked VTE or provoked with an ongoing persistent risk factor, continued anticoagulation with a DOAC is recommended while a vitamin K antagonist is recommended for those with contraindications to DOACs. Additional tools that can aid in the decision making to continue or discontinue anticoagulation include thrombosis risk factors, residual thrombus burden, and coagulation system activation. The HERDOO2 score (https://www.mdcalc.com/herdoo2-rule-discontinuing-anticoagulation-unprovoked-vte) has been suggested as a way for identifying women at low risk of recurrent VTE for whom anticoagulation can be stopped. To evaluate both the risk of recurrence and risk of bleeding, the VTE-PREDICT risk score has been proposed. This is a score that uses 15 elements and can be applied to estimate benefits and harms of extended anticoagulation for individual patients without active cancer.

Extended therapy is now recommended with low-dose DOACs when the risk-benefit relationship favors continued treatment. Extended rivaroxaban showed a significant decrease in recurrent VTE without a significant increase in major bleeding compared with aspirin for an additional 6 to 12 months of therapy after initial therapy. Apixaban as extended treatment of VTE has also been found to provide long-term protection against recurrent VTE. After initial treatment, an additional 12 months of apixaban therapy has been compared with placebo. There was a significant decrease in the rate of VTE without an increase in bleeding risk. In patients who cannot continue on DOACs after initial therapy for VTE and who do not have a contraindication, aspirin should be administered to prevent recurrent thrombosis. Bridging has been a complicated issue when patients on chronic anticoagulation with vitamin K antagonists (with long 5–7 days' half-lives) must undergo an operative procedure and the anticoagulation must be stopped and restarted. However, in low- to moderate-risk patients, bridging is associated with no decrease in thrombotic events but with a higher bleeding risk. In fact, bridging is only indicated currently in those patients with atrial fibrillation and a recent stroke, atrial fibrillation and a high CHADS$_2$ score (5–6), a recent VTE within the past 3 months, and mechanical cardiac valves, especially mitral valves. The availability of DOACs, with short half-lives, has dramatically decreased the need for LMWH-based bridging. In most circumstances, DOACs need to be held only for 1 day for minor procedures and 2 days for major procedures and can be started back as soon as it is felt safe from the surgical or procedural perspective.

Complications
Bleeding is the most common complication of anticoagulation and is important as the case fatality rate of bleeding can be approximately 10% for major bleeding. Risk factors for bleeding while on anticoagulation include age >65, previous bleeding, cancer, renal or liver failure, thrombocytopenia, previous stroke,

diabetes, anemia, concurrent antiplatelet therapy, poor anticoagulant control, recent surgery, frequent falls, alcohol abuse, and nonsteroidal antiinflammatory drug use. Presence of zero risk factors (low risk) confers an absolute risk of major bleeding of 0.8% per year. Patients with one risk factor have a risk of 1.6% per year, and those with two or more have a 6.5% risk or higher per year. With standard heparin, bleeding occurs over the first 5 days in approximately 10% of patients. Warfarin is associated with a major bleeding rate of 1% to 2% per year. Even with the new DOACS, bleeding (major plus minor) may occur in 5% to 10% of cases, although the risk of intracerebral bleeding appears to be less than with warfarin. A recent real-world study of non-valvular atrial fibrillation patients suggested that rates of bleeding may be different between DOACs, with ranges between 11% and 16%. Problems specific to the DOACs include the difficulty to reliably reverse their anticoagulant effects and the difficulty with laboratory monitoring. A monoclonal antibody idarucizumab (Praxbind) for the reversal of dabigatran and a recombinant modified human Factor Xa protein andexanet alfa (Andexxa) for the reversal of Factor Xa inhibitors (apixaban or rivaroxaban) have been FDA approved; however, expense may limit their use. For Andexanet alfa, dosage is a bolus follow by an infusion for 2 hours, depending on the dose of the DOAC administered. Aripazine[5] (a Factor Xa inhibitor) is under development for the neutralization of apixaban, rivaroxaban, edoxaban, and dabigatran.

Heparin-induced thrombocytopenia (HIT) occurs in 0.6% to 30% of patients. Although historically morbidity and mortality rates have been high, it has been found that early diagnosis and appropriate treatment have decreased these rates. HIT usually begins 3 to 14 days after unfractionated heparin is begun, although it can occur earlier if the patient has been exposed to heparin in the past. A heparin-dependent antibody binds to platelets, activates them with the release of procoagulant microparticles, leading to an increase in thrombocytopenia, and results in both arterial and venous thrombosis. Both bovine and porcine unfractionated heparin and LMWH have been associated with HIT, although the incidence and severity of the thrombosis is less with LMWH. Even small exposures to heparin, such as heparin coating on indwelling catheters, can cause the syndrome. The diagnosis should be suspected with a 50% or greater drop in platelet count, when the platelet count falls below 100,000/μL, or when thrombosis occurs during heparin or LMWH therapy. The enzyme-linked immunosorbent assay detects the antiheparin antibody in the plasma. This test is highly sensitive but poorly specific. The serotonin release assay is used as a confirmatory test that is more specific but less sensitive than the enzyme-linked immunosorbent assay test.

When the diagnosis is made, heparin must be discontinued. Oral anticoagulation should not be given until an adequate alternative anticoagulant has been established and until the platelet

[5]Investigational drug in the United States.

count has normalized. Because LMWHs demonstrate high cross-reactivity with standard heparin antibodies, they cannot be substituted for standard heparin in patients with HIT. Agents that have been FDA approved as alternatives include the direct thrombin inhibitor argatroban. Fondaparinux (Arixtra)[1] has also been found effective for treatment of HIT in most cases, but it is not FDA approved for this indication.

Nonpharmacologic Treatments

The symptoms of swelling and leg fatigue can be controlled after DVT by the use of compression stockings. Additionally, walking with good compression does not increase the risk of PE, whereas it significantly decreases the incidence and severity of the PTS in small nonrandomized studies. A recent multicenter randomized trial has suggested that stockings do not prevent development of PTS after a first proximal DVT, and for that reason, the ACCP guidelines suggest not using compression stockings to prevent PTS. It must be remembered that the use of strong compression and early ambulation after DVT treatment can significantly reduce the symptoms of pain and swelling resulting from the DVT, even if the development of PTS is not prevented, and a recent study suggests that certain surrogate markers for PTS may be lessened by the application of immediate compression, and it also reduced residual vein obstruction, which correlated with PTS. Thus, the story on the use of compression stockings to prevent PTS is still evolving and a number of trials are ongoing.

Aggressive Therapies for Venous Thromboembolism

The goals of DVT treatment are to prevent extension or recurrence of DVT, prevent PE, and minimize the late sequela of thrombosis, namely chronic venous insufficiency. Standard anticoagulants accomplish the first two goals but not the third goal. The PTS (venous insufficiency related to venous thrombosis) occurs in up to 30% to 50% of patients after DVT and in an even higher percentage of patients with iliofemoral level DVT. It has been hypothesized that reopening the vein will alleviate venous hypertension or prevent PTS. This is known as the "open vein hypothesis." The following evidence suggests more aggressive therapies for extensive thrombosis are indicated: experimentally, prolonged contact of the thrombus with the vein wall increases damage. The thrombus initiates an inflammatory response in the vein wall that can lead to vein wall fibrosis and valvular dysfunction. The longer a thrombus is in contact with a vein valve, the more chance that valve will no longer function.

Venous thrombectomy has proved superior to anticoagulation over 6 months to 10 years as measured by venous patency and prevention of venous reflux. Catheter-directed thrombolysis has been used in many nonrandomized studies and, in small, randomized trials, was more effective than standard therapy. Quality of life was improved with thrombus removal, and results appear to be optimized further by combining catheter-directed thrombolysis with mechanical devices. These devices include but are not limited to a rheolytic catheter, an ultrasound accelerated catheter, and new larger bore extraction devices. With these devices, thrombolysis is hastened, the amount of thrombolytic agent is decreased, and bleeding is thus decreased. New devices now can remove thrombus without the need for thrombolysis. Additionally, the use of venous stents for iliac venous obstruction has been shown to decrease the incidence of PTS, decrease chronic venous insufficiency, and improve disease-specific quality of life at 1, 6, and 24 months after the treatment.

To more fully elucidate the role of aggressive therapy in proximal iliofemoral venous thrombosis, the ATTRACT trial randomized 692 patients with acute proximal DVT to either anticoagulation alone or anticoagulation plus pharmacomechanical thrombolysis. This study found that more aggressive therapy did not decrease the incidence of PTS but did result in more major bleeding. The severity of the PTS was lessened by the pharmacomechanical thrombolysis, suggesting that more aggressive therapy should be offered to patients with significant iliofemoral venous thrombosis, who do not respond appropriately to a course of anticoagulation. This result also suggests that other factors need to be addressed to prevent PTS in addition to opening up the thrombosed vein.

For PE, evidence exists that thrombolysis is indicated when there is hemodynamic compromise from the embolism. It is controversial whether thrombolysis should be used in situations in which there is no hemodynamic compromise, but there is evidence of right heart dysfunction or there are positive biomarkers. For PE, PE response teams (PERTs) have become common, and they allow for a multidisciplinary group of providers to treat PE in a rapid and coordinated fashion. These teams include (for example) noninvasive clinicians, emergency physicians, clinical pharmacists, endovascular proceduralists, and cardiac, thoracic, and/or vascular surgeons. The efficacy of these teams for treatment of PE is an area of active investigation.

Inferior Vena Cava Filters

Traditional indications for the use of IVC filters include failure of anticoagulation, a contraindication to anticoagulation, or a complication of anticoagulation. Protection from PE is greater than 95% using cone-shaped, wire-based permanent filters in the IVC. IVC filters are not recommended as first-line therapy in patients who are treated with anticoagulants. IVC filters can be either permanent or retrievable. If a retrievable filter is left, then it becomes a permanent filter; the long-term fate of these filters has yet to be defined adequately in the literature. Thus great efforts need to be made to remove retrievable IVC filters when the risk period is over. Most filters are placed in the infrarenal location in the IVC. However, they may be placed in the suprarenal position or in the superior vena cava.

Indications for suprarenal placement include high-lying thrombi, pregnancy or women of childbearing age, or previous device failure filled with thrombus. Although some have suggested that sepsis is a contraindication to the use of filters, sepsis has not been found to be a contraindication because the trapped material can be sterilized with intravenous antibiotics. Filters may be inserted under x-ray guidance or using ultrasound techniques, either external ultrasound or intravascular ultrasound.

References

ATTACC Investigators; ACTIV-4a Investigators; REMAP Investigators, et al: Therapeutic anticoagulation with heparin in noncritically ill patients with COVID-19, N Eng J Med 385(9):790–802, 2021.

de Winter MA, Büller HR, Carrier M, et al: Recurrent venous thromboembolism and bleeding with extended anticoagulation: the VTE-PREDICT risk score, Eur Heart J 44(14):1231–1244, 2023.

Heit JA, Ashrani AA, Crusan DJ, McBane RD, Petterson TM, Bailey KR: Reasons for the persistent incidence of venous thromboembolism, Thromb Haemost 117:390–400, 2017.

Kahn SR, Julian JA, Kearon C: Quality of life after pharmacomechanical catheter-directed thrombolysis for proximal deep venous thrombosis, J Vasc Surg Venous Lymphat Disord 8:8–23, 2020.

Khan F, Tritschler T, Kimpton M, et al: Long-term risk for major bleeding during extended oral anticoagulant therapy for first unprovoked venous thromboembolism: A systematic review and meta-analysis, Ann Intern Med 174:1420–1429, 2021.

REMAP-CAP; ACTIV-4a Investigators; ATTACC Investigators; et al: Therapeutic anticoagulation with heparin in critically ill patients with Covid-19, N Eng J Med 385(9):777–789, 2021.

Stevens S, Woller S, Kreuziger L, Bounameaux H, Doerschug K, Geersing G-J, et al: Executive summary: antithrombotic therapy for VTE disease: second update of the CHEST Guideline and Expert Panel Report, Chest 160(6):2247–2259, 2021.

Schafer K, Goldschmidt E, Oostra D, et al: Defining the role of risk stratification and duplex ultrasound in the diagnosis of acute lower extremity deep vein thrombosis, J Vasc Surg Venous Lymphatic Disord 10:1021–1027, 2022.

Schrag D, Uno H, Rosovsky R, et al: Direct oral anticoagulants vs low-molecular-weight heparin and recurrent VTE in patients with cancer: A randomized clinical trial, JAMA 329:1924–1933, 2023.

Tan M, Lurie F, Kim D, et al. Management of Isolated Distal Deep Venous Thrombosis. DOI: 10.1177/02683555231211095/ ID: PHLEB-23-155. Phlebology Oct 2023.

Vedantham S, Goldhaber SZ, Julian JA: Pharmacomechanical catheter-directed thrombolysis for deep-vein thrombosis, N Engl J Med 377:2240–2252, 2017.

Weitz JI, Jaffer IH, Fredenburgh JC: Recent advances in the treatment of venous thromboembolism in the era of the direct oral anticoagulants, F1000Res 6:985, 2017.

[1]Not FDA approved for this indication.

4 Digestive System

ACUTE AND CHRONIC PANCREATITIS

Method of
George Van Buren II, MD; and William E. Fisher, MD

CURRENT DIAGNOSIS

- Acute pancreatitis is usually caused by gallstones, and chronic pancreatitis is usually caused by alcohol abuse.
- Other less common causes of acute and chronic pancreatitis are considered only when gallstones and alcohol are definitively ruled out.
- Pancreatic cancer and chronic pancreatitis can sometimes be difficult to distinguish.

CURRENT THERAPY

- There has been a trend toward conservative and endoscopic medical therapy for acute and chronic pancreatitis, reserving surgery for select patients.
- In acute pancreatitis, try to avoid surgical necrosectomy except in the setting of infected necrosis with organ failure.
- Asymptomatic pseudocysts can generally be observed.
- Persistent symptomatic pseudocysts can often be addressed endoscopically.
- Medical therapy for chronic pancreatitis includes pain management, nutrition, diabetes control, and cessation of drinking alcohol and smoking.
- Surgical treatment for chronic pancreatitis currently favors strict patient selection and consideration of various surgical techniques.

Acute Pancreatitis

Acute pancreatitis is an inflammatory disease of the pancreas that is associated with little or no fibrosis of the gland. It can be initiated by several factors including gallstones, alcohol, trauma, and infections, and in some cases it is hereditary (Box 1). Very often, patients with acute pancreatitis develop additional complications such as sepsis, shock, and respiratory and renal failure, resulting in considerable morbidity and mortality.

Epidemiology

The annual incidence of acute pancreatitis is probably about 50 cases per 100,000 population in the United States. Approximately 3000 of these cases are severe enough to lead to death. Studies worldwide have shown a rising but variable incidence of acute pancreatitis, including large increases in incidence in pediatric populations.

Risk Factors

Biliary tract stone disease accounts for 70% to 80% of the cases of acute pancreatitis. Alcoholism accounts for another 10%, and

the remaining 10% to 20% is accounted for either by idiopathic disease or by a variety of iatrogenic and miscellaneous causes including trauma, endoscopy, surgery, drugs, heredity, infection, and toxins. Medications appear to cause less than 5% of all cases of acute pancreatitis. The drugs most strongly associated with the disorder are azathioprine (Imuran), 6-mercaptopurine (Purinethol), didanosine (Videx), valproic acid (Depakote), angiotensin-converting enzyme inhibitors, and mesalamine (Asacol). Although there has been a concern for increased episodes of pancreatitis with the use of glucagon-like peptide-1 receptor agonists (GLP-1 RAs), it has not shown to be directly related in large population studies. It is difficult to determine whether the drug is responsible. Tobacco use has also been heavily linked to pancreatitis. Meta-analysis has shown cigarette smoking to be associated with acute pancreatitis development in a dose-response manner.

Pathophysiology

Pancreatitis begins with the activation of digestive zymogens inside acinar cells, which cause acinar cell injury. Digestive zymogens are colocalized with lysosomal hydrolase, and cathepsin-B–catalyzed trypsinogen activation occurs, resulting in acinar cell injury and necrosis. This triggers acinar cell inflammatory events with the secretion of inflammatory mediators. Studies suggest that the ultimate severity of the resulting pancreatitis may be determined by the events that occur subsequent to acinar cell injury. These include inflammatory cell recruitment and activation, as well as generation and release of cytokines, reactive oxygen species, and other chemical mediators of inflammation, ultimately leading to ischemia and necrosis. Early mortality in severe acute pancreatitis is caused by a systemic inflammatory response syndrome with multiorgan failure. If the patient survives this critical early period, a septic complication caused by translocated bacteria, mostly gram-negative microbes from the intestine, leads to infected pancreatic necrosis. Late deaths are caused by infected necrosis, leading to septic shock and multiorgan failure.

Prevention

Gallstones are present in about 15% to 20% of patients older than 60 years, but only a fraction become symptomatic. Although

---

BOX 1	Common Causes of Acute Pancreatitis Gallstones

Alcoholism
Hereditary
Hypertriglyceridemia
Trauma (including iatrogenic: ERCP or surgery)
Drugs: azathioprine (Imuran), furosemide, mercaptopurine (Purinethol), opiates, pentamidine (Pentam), steroids, sulfasalazine (Azulfidine), sulindac (Clinoril), tetracycline, trimethoprim-sulfamethoxazole (Bactrim), valproic acid (Depakote)
Tumor
Infection (parasitic and viral)
Idiopathic

ERCP, Endoscopic retrograde cholangiopancreatography.

gallstone pancreatitis can rarely be the first symptom of gallstones, most patients have symptoms of cholecystitis before developing pancreatitis. Thus it is important to make early and prompt referral of patients with symptomatic cholelithiasis for laparoscopic cholecystectomy to prevent life-threatening complications such as acute pancreatitis.

Clinical Manifestations

All episodes of acute pancreatitis begin with severe pain, generally after a substantial meal. The pain is usually epigastric, but it can occur anywhere in the abdomen or lower chest. It has been described as penetrating through to the back, and it may be relieved by the patient's leaning forward. It precedes the onset of nausea and vomiting, with retching often continuing after the stomach has emptied. Vomiting does not relieve the pain, which is more intense in necrotizing than in edematous pancreatitis.

On examination the patient may show tachycardia, tachypnea, hypotension, and hyperthermia. The temperature is usually only mildly elevated in uncomplicated pancreatitis. Voluntary and involuntary guarding can be seen over the epigastric region. The bowel sounds are decreased or absent. There are usually no palpable masses. The abdomen may be distended with intraperitoneal fluid. There may be pleural effusion, particularly on the left side. With increasing severity of disease, the intravascular fluid loss may become life threatening as a result of sequestration of edematous fluid in the retroperitoneum. Hemoconcentration then results in an elevated hematocrit. However, there also may be bleeding into the retroperitoneum or the peritoneal cavity. In some patients (about 1%), the blood from necrotizing pancreatitis can dissect through the soft tissues and manifest as a bluish discoloration around the umbilicus (Cullen sign) or in the flanks (Grey Turner sign). The severe fluid loss can lead to prerenal azotemia, with elevated blood urea nitrogen and creatinine levels. There also may be hyperglycemia, hypoalbuminemia, and hypocalcemia sufficient in some cases to produce tetany.

Diagnosis

The definition of acute pancreatitis is based on the fulfillment of two out of three of the following criteria: clinical (upper abdominal pain), laboratory (serum amylase or lipase >3× upper limit of normal), and/or imaging (computed tomographic [CT], magnetic resonance imaging [MRI], ultrasonography) criteria. Although serum amylase is often elevated in acute pancreatitis, there is no significant correlation between the magnitude of serum amylase elevation and severity of pancreatitis. Other pancreatic enzymes also have been evaluated to improve the diagnostic accuracy of serum measurements. Specificity of these markers ranges from 77% to 96%, the highest being for lipase. Measurements of many digestive enzymes have methodologic limitations and cannot be easily adapted for quantitation in emergency laboratory studies. Because serum levels of lipase remain elevated for a longer time than total or pancreatic amylase, it is the serum indicator of highest probability of the disease.

Abdominal ultrasound examination is the best way to confirm the presence of gallstones in suspected biliary pancreatitis. It also can detect extrapancreatic ductal dilations and reveal pancreatic edema, swelling, and peripancreatic fluid collections. However, in about 20% of patients, the ultrasound examination does not provide satisfactory results because of the presence of bowel gas, which can obscure sonographic imaging of the pancreas. Endoscopic ultrasound (EUS) is an excellent adjunct to evaluate the gallbladder for sludge or microlithiasis that may not be well seen on abdominal ultrasound.

A CT scan of the pancreas is more commonly used to diagnose pancreatitis. CT scanning is used to distinguish milder (nonnecrotic) forms of the disease from more severe necrotizing or infected pancreatitis, in patients whose clinical presentation raises the suspicion of advanced disease (Figures 1 and 2). Pancreatic protocol CT scan of the abdomen and pelvis is recommended when not limited by renal insufficiency: a triphasic thin, multislice CT scan with an arterial, venous, and delayed phase in conjunction with sagittal and coronal views; no oral contrast, instead drink 1000 mL water to opacify the stomach. The scan assesses the degree of pancreatic necrosis, peripancreatic fluid collections,

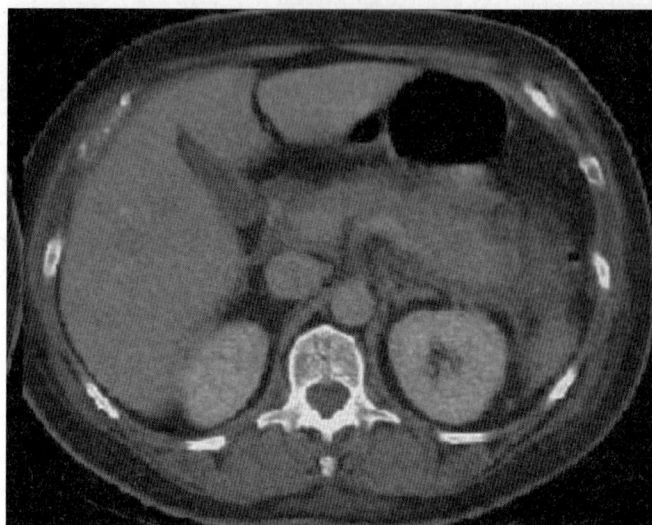

Figure 1 Computed tomographic scan confirming acute edematous pancreatitis.

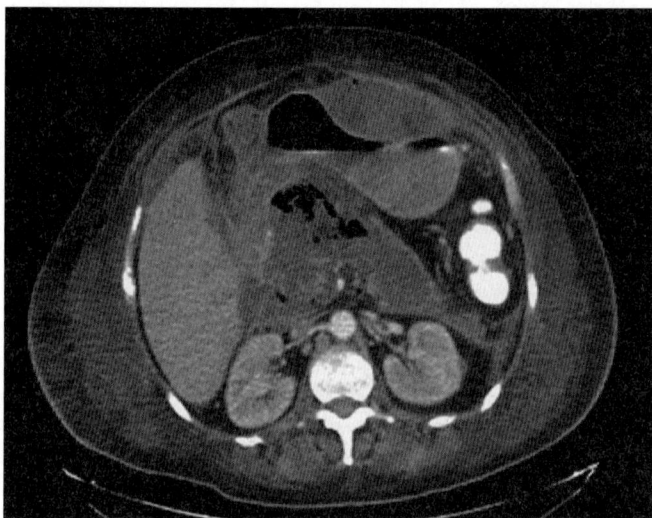

Figure 2 Computed tomographic scan confirming acute necrotizing, emphysematous pancreatitis.

and the surrounding vascular structures. This triphasic scan can also help detect underlying mass lesions.

Magnetic resonance cholangiopancreatography (MRCP) is also of value to assess the pancreatic duct and biliary tree. This can often reveal pancreatic ductal disruption.

Differential Diagnosis

The clinical diagnosis of pancreatitis is one of exclusion. Hyperamylasemia can also occur as a result of conditions not involving pancreatitis. The other upper abdominal conditions that can be confused with acute pancreatitis include perforated peptic ulcer and acute cholecystitis, and occasionally a gangrenous small bowel obstruction. Because these conditions often have a fatal outcome without surgery, urgent intervention is indicated in the small number of cases in which doubt persists. A tumor should be considered in a nonalcoholic patient with acute pancreatitis who has no demonstrable biliary tract disease. Approximately 1% to 2% of patients with acute pancreatitis have pancreatic carcinoma, and an episode of acute pancreatitis can be the first clinical manifestation of a periampullary tumor.

Treatment

The severity of acute pancreatitis covers a broad spectrum of illness, ranging from the mild and self-limiting to the life-threatening necrotizing variety. Some cases are so mild they can be treated in

BOX 2 Treatment of Acute Pancreatitis

Assessment of severity
Fluid resuscitation and oxygenation
Early nasojejunal feeding
Avoid prophylactic antibiotics (reserve antibiotic therapy for specific infections)
Avoid or postpone necrosectomy if possible
Options for necrosectomy
- Open anterior approach with closed lavage
- Open anterior approach with packing and reoperation
- Open retroperitoneal approach
- Laparoscopic anterior approach with closed lavage
- Video-assisted retroperitoneal débridement

BOX 3 Ranson Criteria

There are 11 Ranson signs. Five of the signs are evaluated when the patient is admitted to the hospital, and the remaining six are evaluated 48 hours after admission. The signs are added to reach a score:
- If the score <3, severe pancreatitis is unlikely.
- If the score ≥3, severe pancreatitis is likely.
  or
- Score 0–2: 2% mortality
- Score 3–4: 15% mortality
- Score 5–6: 40% mortality
- Score 7–8: 100% mortality

At Admission
Age in years >55 years
White blood cell count >16,000 cells/mm^3
Blood glucose >11 mmol/L (>200 mg/dL)
Serum AST >250 IU/L
Serum LDH >350 IU/L

At 48 Hours
Calcium (serum calcium) <2.0 mmol/L (<8.0 mg/dL)
Hematocrit fall >10%
Oxygen (hypoxemia Po$_2$ <60 mm Hg)
BUN increased by ≥1.8 mmol/L (≥5 mg/dL) after intravenous fluid hydration
Base deficit (negative base excess) >4 mEq/L
Sequestration of fluids >6 L

AST, Aspartate aminotransferase; *BUN,* blood urea nitrogen; *LDH,* lactate dehydrogenase.

an outpatient setting. However, most cases require hospitalization for observation and diagnostic study. A conservative approach has been advocated in the treatment of acute pancreatitis (Box 2). Severity is assessed with imaging results and clinical parameters and is quantitated with scores such as Ranson criteria (Box 3), the Atlanta classification, and the APACHE II (Acute Physiology and Chronic Health Evaluation) score. Severe acute pancreatitis is defined by associated organ dysfunction. The Atlanta classification is based on an international consensus conference held in Atlanta in 1992 and has been updated. APACHE II was designed to measure the severity of disease for adult patients admitted to intensive care units. Though not specific to pancreatitis, APACHE II can be used in an effort to differentiate patients with mild and severe acute pancreatitis. APACHE II scores of 8 points or more correlate with a mortality rate of 11% to 18%.

Upon confirmation of the diagnosis, patients with severe disease should be transferred to the intensive care unit for observation and maximum support. Adequate fluid resuscitation optimizing organ perfusion and oxygenation is essential. The use of prophylactic intravenous antibiotics in the initial stages of severe acute pancreatitis is not proved to be useful. Two randomized controlled studies failed to show any benefit from antibiotics. Prophylactic antibiotics did not decrease the incidence of infected pancreatic necrosis or lower mortality. Data from these well-designed trials refute prior data from less rigorous studies suggesting prophylactic antibiotics were useful. Additional studies are required, but there is increasing concern that the prolonged use of potent antibiotics might result in an increased prevalence of fungal infections and possibly increased mortality. Currently, antibiotic therapy should be reserved for treatment of specific infections such as positive blood, sputum, and urine cultures or percutaneous or operative cultures of necrotic tissue.

Randomized clinical trials have also shown a benefit from early nasojejunal feeding compared with total parenteral nutrition. Gastric decompression with a nasogastric tube is selectively used in patients with severe ileus and vomiting but is not necessary in a majority of cases. A debate remains regarding the optimal nutritional management in the majority of pancreatitis patients. There has been a trend toward oral enteric feeding in the less severe cases. The benefits of enteric feeding can be significant; however, the patients must be monitored closely as they are trialed on an oral enteric diet.

In biliary pancreatitis, the gallbladder must eventually be removed or recurrent acute pancreatitis will occur in 30% to 60% of cases. The timing of the cholecystectomy depends on the severity of the pancreatitis. Usually, laparoscopic cholecystectomy is performed during the index admission as soon as the attack of acute pancreatitis has resolved. In more severe cases the cholecystectomy is delayed and often combined with interventions for late complications of acute pancreatitis. In cases with severe comorbidity, endoscopic sphincterotomy has been considered as an alternative to cholecystectomy. However, if the patient has a postinflammatory fluid collection, bacteria can be introduced during endoscopic retrograde cholangiopancreatography (ERCP), and sphincterotomy should be delayed.

Currently, there is no role for routine early laparotomy and necrosectomy or resection in the setting of acute necrotizing pancreatitis. If the necrotic pancreas becomes infected and the patient fails to respond to conservative treatment, then necrosectomy may be warranted. Patients with infected necrosis are rarely managed conservatively without eventual surgical intervention. However, even in the setting of infected necrosis, there has been consideration for antibiotic therapy until the acute inflammatory response has subsided, if possible, with the view that surgery that is deferred for several weeks is more easily accomplished with one intervention. Patients who suffer from infected necrosis without having clinical signs of sepsis or other systemic complications might not need immediate surgical necrosectomy.

A nonsurgical alternative for the treatment of infected necrosis is percutaneous catheter drainage. This is considered a temporary measure to allow stabilization of the patient so that a safer surgical necrosectomy can be done at a later time. Multiple large drains are required, and patients frequently undergo repeat CT and revision of the drains. Current recommendations are to postpone surgery for as long as possible, usually beyond the second or third week of the disease or later, when necrotic tissue can be easily distinguished from viable pancreas and débridement without major blood loss can be performed. When surgery is performed, tissue-preserving digital necrosectomy is the usual technique rather than a classic surgical resection of the pancreas (Figure 3).

Necrosectomy can be performed using an open anterior approach with closed lavage or with leaving the abdomen open and packing. The packing is replaced at intervals of 24 to 72 hours. Sometimes a left lateral retroperitoneal approach is helpful. A newer approach is the video-assisted retroperitoneal débridement (VARD). This procedure is a combination of percutaneous drainage and the open lateral retroperitoneal approach. An anterior laparoscopic approach has also been described and mimics the open anterior approach using laparoscopic ports. Surgical necrosectomy is indicated in patients with sepsis caused by infected necrosis and in selected patients with extended sterile necrosis causing severe systemic organ dysfunction and sepsis without a septic focus.

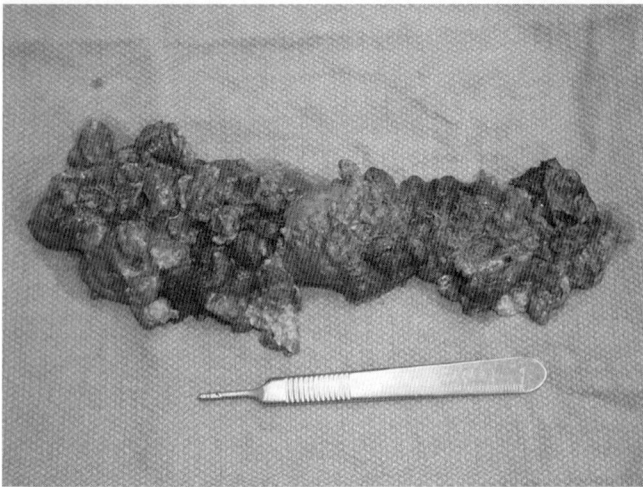

Figure 3 Necrotic material débrided from the retroperitoneum in a case of acute necrotizing pancreatitis.

In some cases, the acute inflammatory process can lead to erosion into retroperitoneal vessels, and acute hemorrhage occurs. This acute emergent complication is best managed with immediate angiography to determine the exact site of bleeding and can often be treated with embolization rather than surgery (Figure 4).

Although previously frowned upon, there has been a move toward enteric drainage of all necrotic collections (even when infected) when technically feasible. This can be initiated through either an endoscopic or surgical approach. Enteric drainage may be done in conjunction with percutaneous drainage if the situation warrants.

Monitoring

Despite a conservative operative approach, endocrine and exocrine insufficiency develop in as many as half of the patients and are determined by the extent of pancreatic necrosis. Therefore patients must be monitored with blood glucose measurements, stabilization of body weight, and proper nutrition.

Complications

The most common complication after successful management of acute pancreatitis is a pseudocyst. The term *pseudocyst* is currently used to broadly categorize most pancreatic and peripancreatic fluid collections (including walled-off pancreatic necrosis [WOPN] and acute peripancreatic fluid collection). The Acute Pancreatitis Classification Working Group recently proposed a revised Atlanta classification that refers to collections within 4 weeks of symptom onset as either acute peripancreatic fluid collections (APFC) or postnecrotic pancreatic fluid collections (PNPFC), depending on the absence or presence of pancreatic/peripancreatic necrosis, respectively. After 4 weeks of the onset of symptoms, persistent collections with discrete walls are referred to as pseudocyst or WOPN, again depending on the absence or presence of necrosis, respectively. In addition, these collections are further classified as sterile or infected, and the term *pancreatic abscess* has been abolished.

The management of pseudocysts has followed a minimally invasive trend. Most pseudocysts resolve spontaneously, even beyond 6 weeks, so asymptomatic pseudocysts are usually observed (70% of pseudocysts will resolve without intervention). Endoscopic cystogastrostomy is the approach of choice for symptomatic fluid-predominant pseudocysts when there is minimal necrosis. If there is significant necrotic debris or a solid-predominant pseudocyst, surgical drainage with laparoscopic cystogastrostomy is preferred (Figure 5). This can also be performed with the traditional open technique. Cystojejunostomy (laparoscopic or open) is used in cases in which the site of the pseudocyst precludes drainage into the posterior aspect of the stomach.

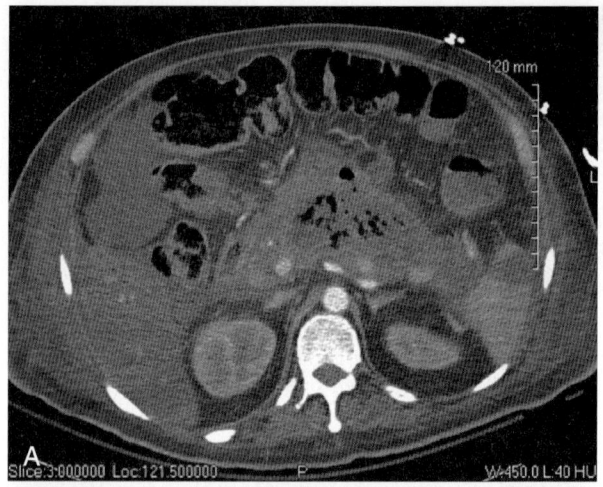

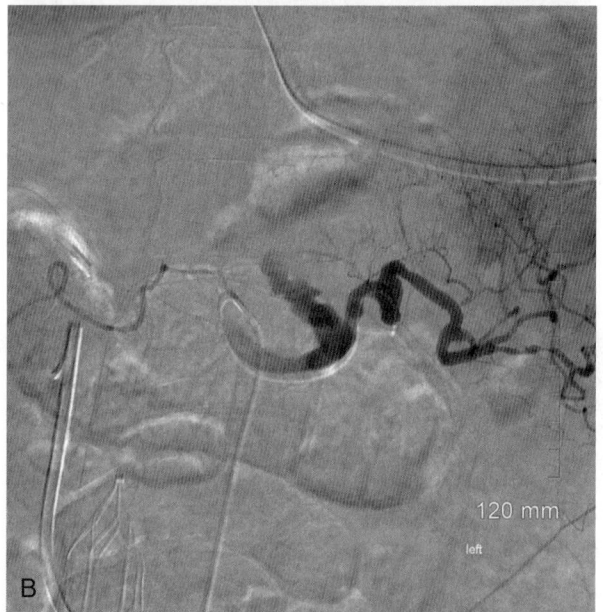

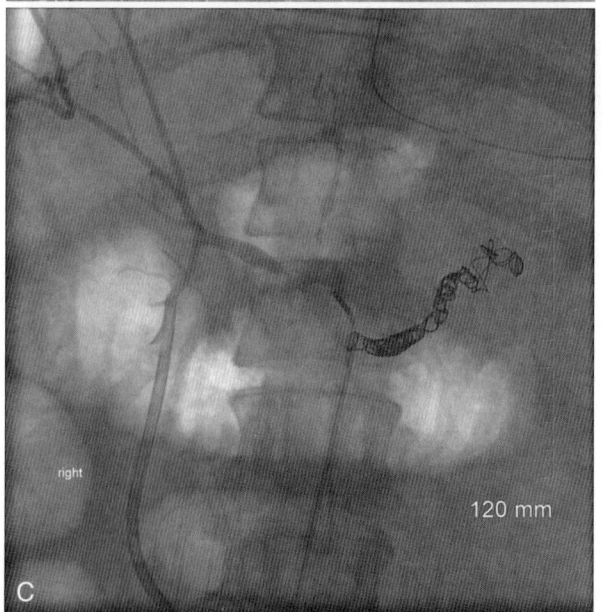

Figure 4 Acute necrotizing pancreatitis. (A) Erosion into the splenic artery as seen on computed tomography. (B) Erosion into the splenic artery as seen on angiogram. (C) This complication of acute pancreatitis is best treated with angiographic embolization.

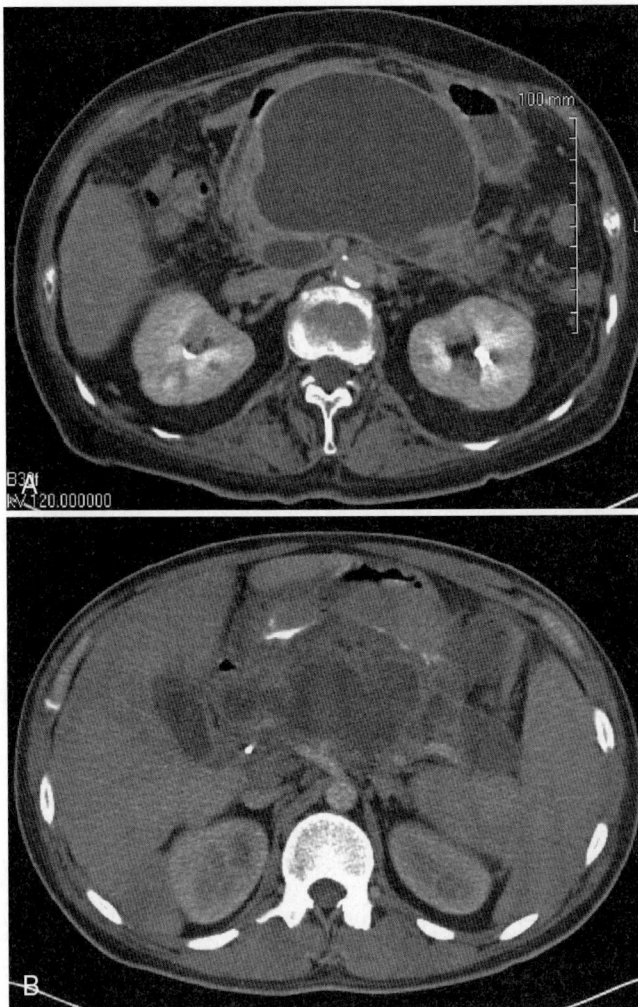

Figure 5 Computed tomographic scan showing fluid-predominant (A) and solid-predominant (B) pseudocysts. The former can be treated with endoscopic cystogastrostomy, and the latter is best treated with laparoscopic cystogastrostomy.

Chronic Pancreatitis

Chronic pancreatitis is a chronic fibroinflammatory disease of the pancreas characterized by irreversible morphologic changes that typically are associated with pain or permanent loss of function, or both.

Epidemiology

Population studies suggest a prevalence of chronic pancreatitis that ranges from 5 to 27 persons per 100,000 population, with considerable geographic variation. Autopsy data are difficult to interpret because a number of changes associated with chronic pancreatitis, such as fibrosis, duct ectasia, and acinar atrophy, are also present in asymptomatic elderly patients. Differences in diagnostic criteria, regional nutrition, alcohol consumption, and medical access account for variations in the frequency of the diagnosis, but the overall incidence of the disease has risen progressively since the 1960s. Chronic pancreatitis in the United States currently results in more than 120,000 outpatient visits and more than 50,000 hospitalizations per year.

Risk Factors

Alcohol consumption and alcohol abuse are associated with chronic pancreatitis in up to 70% of cases. Other major causes include tropical (nutritional) and idiopathic disease, as well as hereditary causes. There is a linear relationship between exposure to alcohol and the development of chronic pancreatitis. The incidence is highest in heavy drinkers (15 drinks/day or 150 g/day). Prolonged alcohol use (four to five drinks daily over a period of more than 5 years) is required for alcohol-associated pancreatitis; the overall lifetime risk of pancreatitis among heavy drinkers is 2% to 5%. The duration of alcohol consumption is definitely associated with the development of pancreatic disease. The onset of disease typically occurs between ages 35 and 40 years, after 16 to 20 years of heavy alcohol consumption. Recurrent episodes of acute pancreatitis are typically followed by chronic symptoms after 4 or 5 years. In most cases, chronic pancreatitis has already developed and the acute clinical presentation represents a flare superimposed on chronic pancreatitis.

Tobacco use has also been heavily linked to pancreatitis. Meta-analysis has shown that both ever and current smokers had higher risks of developing pancreatitis compared with never smokers. This causative relationship was verified by the reduced or eliminated risk after smoking cessation. In comparison with current smokers, the risk of pancreatitis decreased for those who were former smokers.

Pathophysiology

Multiple episodes (or a prolonged course) of pancreatic injury ultimately leading to chronic disease is widely accepted as the pathophysiologic sequence. Abundant data indicate that acute pancreatitis may progress to recurrent acute pancreatitis and then to chronic pancreatitis in a disease continuum. Most investigators believe that alcohol metabolites such as acetaldehyde, combined with oxidant injury, result in local parenchymal injury that is preferentially targeted to the pancreas in predisposed persons. Repeated or severe episodes of toxin-induced injury activate a cascade of cytokines, which in turn induces pancreatic stellate cells to produce collagen and cause fibrosis.

The most common form of chronic pancreatitis is the calcifying type, characterized by the development of intraductal stones; the predominant causative agent is alcohol. Progressive functional impairment can develop from the dilated main pancreatic duct. Furthermore, inflammatory enlargement of the pancreatic head may cause local complications such as stenosis of the pancreatic or bile duct, duodenal obstruction, or compression of retropancreatic vessels.

The pain caused by chronic pancreatitis is thought to be due to increased pressure in the pancreatic ducts and tissue, "parenchymal hypertension" from pancreatic ductal obstruction. Neural and perineural inflammation is also thought to be important in pathogenesis of pain in chronic pancreatitis. Neuropeptides released from enteric and afferent neurons and their functional interactions with inflammatory cells might play a key role.

Prevention

Because alcohol is the cause of most cases of chronic pancreatitis, cessation of alcohol consumption is recommended to prevent progression to chronic pancreatitis. Unfortunately, the majority of patients are not able to recover from alcoholism, and relapse is common.

Clinical Manifestations

Symptoms of chronic pancreatitis may be identical to those of acute pancreatitis, typically midepigastric pain penetrating through to the back. Patients with chronic pancreatic pain typically flex their abdomen and either sit or lie with their hips flexed, or lie on their side in a fetal position. Unlike ureteral stone pain or biliary colic, the pain causes the patient to be still. Nausea or vomiting can accompany the pain, but anorexia is the most common associated symptom. Patients with continuous pain can have a complication of chronic pancreatitis, such as an inflammatory mass, a cyst, or even pancreatic cancer. Other patients have intermittent attacks of pain with symptoms similar to those of mild to moderate acute pancreatitis. The pain sometimes is severe and lasts for many hours or several days.

As chronic pancreatitis progresses, endocrine and exocrine insufficiency begin to appear. Patients describe a bulky, foul-smelling, loose (but not watery) stool that may be pale and float on the surface of toilet water. Patients often describe a greasy or oily appearance to the stool or describe an "oil slick" on the water's surface. In severe steatorrhea, an orange, oily stool is often reported. As exocrine deficiency increases, symptoms of

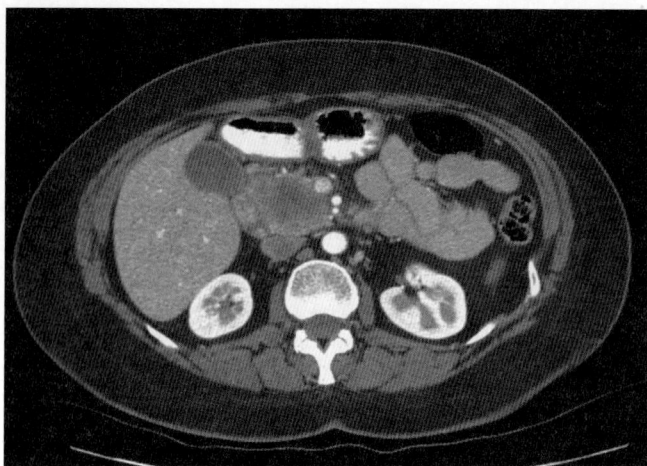

Figure 6 Computed tomographic scan of a patient with autoimmune pancreatitis and an inflammatory mass in the head of the pancreas. Preoperative diagnosis is not always possible, but surgery should be avoided because this disease often responds to steroid therapy.

BOX 4 Treatment of Chronic Pancreatitis

Pancreatic enzyme replacement
Proper nutrition and vitamin supplementation
Blood sugar control
Long-acting narcotic analgesics at lowest effective doses
Cessation of alcohol and tobacco
Endotherapy (pancreatic duct stenting and removal of stones)
Parenchymal preserving surgery (Frey, Beger) in carefully
  selected patients

steatorrhea are often accompanied by weight loss. Patients might describe a good appetite despite weight loss, or they might have diminished food intake due to abdominal pain. The combination of decreased food intake and malabsorption of nutrients usually results in chronic weight loss. As a result, many patients with severe chronic pancreatitis are below ideal body weight. Usually islet cells are spared early in the disease process despite being surrounded by fibrosis, but eventually the insulin-secreting beta cells are also destroyed, gradually leading to diabetes.

Diagnosis

The diagnosis of chronic pancreatitis depends on the clinical presentation, a limited number of indirect measurements that correlate with pancreatic function, and selected imaging studies. Diagnosis is usually simple in the late stages of the disease because of the presence of structural and functional alterations of the pancreas. Early in the disease, the diagnosis is more difficult. Various classification systems have been developed. The Cambridge classification uses imaging tests such as ERCP, CT, and ultrasound to grade severity. The Mayo Clinic system is based on functional and imaging results. Tests of pancreatic function include the secretin-cerulein test, Lundh test, fecal excretion of pancreatic enzymes, and quantitation of fecal fat.

Chronic pancreatitis can be classified as calcifying (lithogenic), obstructive, inflammatory, autoimmune, tropical (nutritional), hereditary, or idiopathic. Autoimmune and hereditary pancreatitis have recently been better understood and diagnosed more than before. Autoimmune pancreatitis is associated with fibrosis, a mononuclear cell (lymphocyte, plasma cell, or eosinophil) infiltrate, and an increased titer of one or more autoantibodies. It is usually associated with autoimmune diseases such as Sjögren syndrome. Increased levels of serum β-globulin or immunoglobulin (Ig)G_4 are often present, but autoimmune pancreatitis can present without these markers. This disease can be mistaken for chronic pancreatitis, with an inflammatory mass in the head of the pancreas suspicious for pancreatic cancer (Figure 6). Diagnosis is important because steroid therapy is uniformly successful in ameliorating the disease, including any associated bile duct compression.

Hereditary pancreatitis first occurs in adolescence with abdominal pain; patients develop progressive pancreatic dysfunction, and the risk of cancer is greatly increased. The disease follows an autosomal dominant pattern of inheritance with 80% penetrance and variable expression. Recent mutational analysis has revealed a missense mutation resulting in an Arg to His substitution at position 117 of the cationic trypsinogen gene, or *PRSS1*, one of the primary sites for proteolysis of trypsin. This mutation prevents trypsin from being inactivated by itself or other proteases, and

it results in persistent and uncontrolled proteolytic activity and autodestruction within the pancreas. Similarly, *PSTI*, also known as *SPINK1*, has been found to have a role in hereditary pancreatitis and some cases of sporadic chronic pancreatitis. *SPINK1* specifically inhibits trypsin action by competitively blocking the active site of the enzyme.

It is likely that many of the "idiopathic" forms of chronic pancreatitis, as well as some patients with the more common forms of the disease, will be found to have a genetic linkage or predisposition.

Differential Diagnosis

There are several clinical conditions from which chronic pancreatitis needs to be distinguished. Other causes of upper abdominal pain, such as peptic ulcer disease, biliary tract disease, mesenteric vascular disease, or malignancy must be excluded. The major difficulty in the differential diagnosis of chronic pancreatitis is distinguishing it from pancreatic ductal adenocarcinoma. Chronic pancreatitis can closely mimic pancreatic cancer, both clinically and morphologically. In addition, chronic pancreatitis is a risk factor for the development of pancreatic cancer. Although in pancreatic resection specimens this problem may be finally resolved, distinguishing these two diseases preoperatively in small (needle) biopsy specimens is a formidable challenge for the pathologist. Therefore especially in the setting of an inflammatory mass in the head of the pancreas, consideration of pancreatic cancer and surgical referral is important. Workup of these patients should include a pancreatic protocol CT scan, an MRCP, and an EUS to evaluate the parenchyma and the ducts of the pancreas.

Treatment

Therapy for chronic pancreatitis is aimed at managing associated digestive dysfunction and relieving pain (Box 4). It is important to first address malabsorption, weight loss, and diabetes. When pancreatic exocrine capacity falls below 10% of normal, diarrhea and steatorrhea develop. Lipase deficiency tends to manifest itself before trypsin deficiency, so the presence of steatorrhea may be the first functional sign of pancreatic insufficiency. As pancreatic exocrine function deteriorates further, the secretion of bicarbonate into the duodenum is reduced, which causes duodenal acidification and further impairs nutrient absorption. Frank diabetes is seen initially in about 20% of patients with chronic pancreatitis, and impaired glucose metabolism can be detected in up to 70% of patients.

The medical treatment of chronic or recurrent pain in chronic pancreatitis requires the use of analgesics, a cessation of alcohol use, oral enzyme therapy, and endoscopic stent therapy. Administration of pancreatic enzyme (e.g., Pancrease MT, Pancrelipase, Creon) serves to reverse the effects of pancreatic exocrine insufficiency and might also reduce or alleviate the pain[1] experienced by patients. Interventional procedures to block visceral afferent nerve conduction or to treat obstructions of the main pancreatic duct are also an adjunct to medical treatment. It has been taught that the pain of chronic pancreatitis decreases with increasing duration of the disease—the so-called burn-out phase, where endocrine and exocrine insufficiency occurs and the pain

---

[1] Not FDA approved for this indication.

decreases. However, some studies have called this concept into question, demonstrating continued pain in patients with chronic pancreatitis despite long-standing disease and pancreatic insufficiency. Cessation of alcohol abuse, if possible, causes the pain to stop in about half of the patients.

Pain relief usually requires the use of narcotics, but these should be titrated to achieve pain relief with the lowest effective dose. Opioid addiction is common, and the use of long-acting analgesics by transdermal patch together with oral agents for pain exacerbations slightly reduces the sedative effects of high-dose oral narcotics. Celiac plexus neurolysis has been an effective form of analgesic treatment in patients with pancreatic carcinoma. However, its use in chronic pancreatitis has been disappointing, with about half of the patients deriving a benefit that lasts 6 months or less.

Pancreatic duct stenting is used for treatment of proximal pancreatic duct stenosis, decompression of a pancreatic duct leak, and drainage of pancreatic pseudocysts that can be catheterized through the main pancreatic duct. Pancreatic duct stones can also be removed endoscopically. Stent therapy in chronic pancreatitis definitely plays a role and can help select patients for successful operative therapy. However, the duration of success with stent therapy for chronic pancreatitis is probably less than with surgical therapy.

There has been significant debate over the years regarding the role and type of surgical therapy in chronic pancreatitis. Progressive functional pancreatic impairment can be delayed by surgical decompression of the dilated main pancreatic duct. Furthermore, inflammatory enlargement of the pancreatic head may cause local complications that require further treatment, such as stenosis of the pancreatic or bile duct, duodenal obstruction, or compression of retropancreatic vessels. Surgery may be superior to conservative or endoscopic treatment in terms of pain relief and preservation of pancreatic function and quality of life. Major pancreatic resections for chronic pancreatitis have a significant complication rate, both early and late. Patients with large duct disease who can have nutrition restored, are working, are not drinking alcohol, and have a supportive family structure fare better with surgical therapies. Failure to carefully select patients for either drainage or resection procedures leads to disappointing results. The surgical management of pancreatic duct stones and stenosis has been shown to be superior to endoscopic treatment in randomized clinical trials. Beger introduced the duodenum-preserving pancreatic head resection (DPPHR) in the early 1980s. Later in the decade, Frey and Smith described the local resection of the pancreatic head with longitudinal pancreaticojejunostomy, which included excavation of the pancreatic head including the ductal structures in continuity with a long ductotomy of the dorsal duct. This operation is basically a hybrid of the Beger and Puestow (Partington-Rochelle modification) procedures and is more popular in the United States (Figures 7 and 8).

Previous randomized prospective studies have compared the Whipple, Beger, and Frey procedures for chronic pancreatitis. Patients who had a Beger procedure had a shorter hospital stay, greater weight gain, less postoperative diabetes, and less exocrine dysfunction than standard Whipple patients over a 3- to 5-year follow-up. Pain control was similar between the two procedures. In a study comparing the pylorus-preserving Whipple to the Frey procedure, there was a lower postoperative complication rate associated with the Frey procedure (19%) compared with the pylorus-preserving Whipple group (53%), and the global quality-of-life scores were better (71% vs. 43%, respectively). Both operations were equally effective in controlling pain over a 2-year follow-up. Operation times, intraoperative blood loss, and transfusion requirements have been shown to be decreased with the Frey and Beger procedures compared with the Whipple procedure. In long-term (>8 years) follow-up, there was no difference between the Beger and Frey procedures in pain relief, pancreatic insufficiency, quality of life, and late mortality. Compared with the Whipple procedure, the Beger and Frey procedures may produce a lower incidence of immediate complications and diabetes

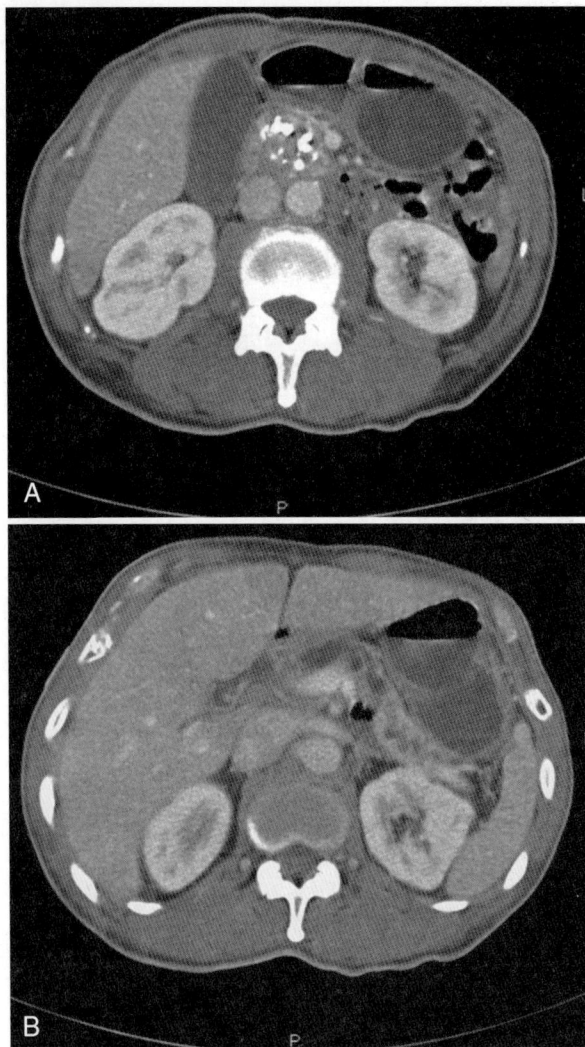

Figure 7 Computed tomographic scan of a patient with chronic calcific pancreatitis and a massively dilated pancreatic duct. (A) Axial view with calcified pancreatic head. (B) Axial view with dilated pancreatic duct.

but no significant differences in pain relief. Although these limited pancreatic procedures have a lower initial rate of endocrine dysfunction, the long-term risk of diabetes is more related to the progression of the underlying disease than to the effects of operation.

A multicenter randomized, controlled, double-blind trial compared DPPHR to partial pancreatoduodenectomy with a primary endpoint of quality of life within 24 months after surgery. The results showed that DPPHR was not superior to partial pancreatoduodenectomy in terms of the primary endpoint, long-term postoperative quality of life. With both resection and drainage procedures offering viable options for treatment, patient selection becomes critical in assuring there is clinical improvement postoperatively.

Recent refinements in the methods of harvesting and preserving pancreatic islets, and standardization of the methods by which islets are infused into the portal venous circuit for intrahepatic engraftment, have improved the success and rekindled interest in islet autotransplantation for chronic pancreatitis. The ability to recover a sufficient quantity of islets from a sclerotic gland depends on the degree of disease present, so the selection of patients as candidates for autologous islet transplantation is important. As success with autotransplantation increases, patients with nonobstructive, sclerotic pancreatitis may be considered for resection and islet autotransplantation earlier in their course, because end-stage fibrosis bodes poorly for transplant success. Patient selection and surgeon experience play a very large role in the outcomes of autotransplantation.

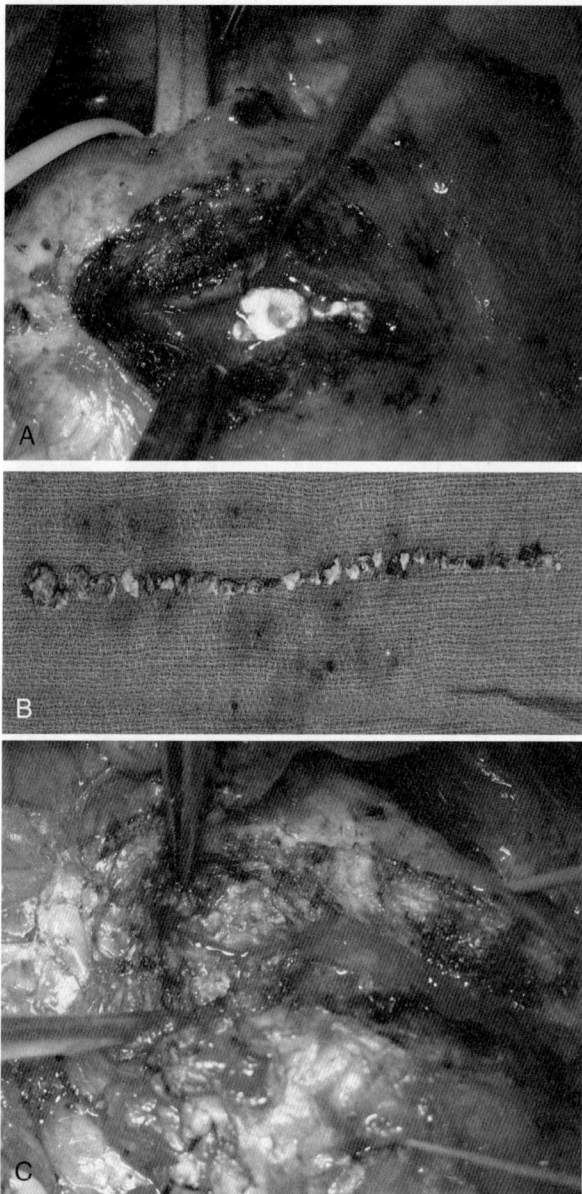

Figure 8 (A) The pancreatic duct is opened to reveal a preoperatively placed pancreatic duct stent. (B) The residual stones removed from the pancreatic duct. (C) In the Frey procedure, the head of the pancreas is cored out in addition to a longitudinal pancreatic ductotomy. The pancreas is drained with a Roux-en-Y limb of jejunum.

Monitoring

Chronic pancreatitis is of course a chronic disease, so continued monitoring and maintenance therapy is essential after an acute exacerbation of chronic pancreatitis. Pain control, proper nutrition, and alcohol and smoking cessation must be maintained as an outpatient. The clinician must also be looking for the development of common complications. An annual physical exam and CT or MRI should be considered in this population to assess for the progression of disease.

Complications

Pseudocysts in the setting of chronic pancreatitis are less likely to resolve without intervention. Often, the pancreatic duct and bile duct are compressed, and the compression might need to be addressed at the same time as the pseudocyst. A trend toward minimally invasive management remains appropriate, with

endoscopic drainage preferred over laparoscopic cystogastrostomy unless additional procedures are required. Resection of a pseudocyst is sometimes indicated for cysts located in the pancreatic tail or when a midpancreatic duct disruption has resulted in a distally located pseudocyst. Distal pancreatectomy for removal of a pseudocyst, with or without splenectomy, can be a challenging procedure in the setting of prior pancreatitis. An internal drainage procedure of the communicating duct, or of the pseudocyst itself, should be considered when distal resection is being contemplated.

Pancreatic ascites results from a disrupted pancreatic duct with extravasation of pancreatic fluid that does not become sequestered as a pseudocyst but drains freely into the peritoneal cavity. Occasionally, the pancreatic fluid tracks superiorly into the thorax, causing a pancreatic pleural effusion. Both complications are seen more often in patients with chronic pancreatitis, rather than after acute pancreatitis. Paracentesis or thoracentesis reveals noninfected fluid with a protein level greater than 25 g/L and a markedly elevated amylase level. Paracentesis is critical to differentiate pancreatic from hepatic ascites.

ERCP is most helpful to delineate the location of the pancreatic duct leak and to elucidate the underlying pancreatic ductal anatomy. Pancreatic duct stenting may be considered at the time of ERCP. Paracentesis and antisecretory therapy with the somatostatin analog octreotide acetate, together with bowel rest and parenteral nutrition, is successful in more than half of patients. Reapposition of serosal surfaces to facilitate closure of the leak is considered a part of therapy, and this is accomplished by complete paracentesis. For pleural effusions, a period of chest tube drainage can facilitate closure of the internal fistula. Surgical therapy is reserved for those who fail to respond to medical treatment.

References

Ayoub M, Chela H, Amin N, Hunter R, Anwar J, Tahan V, Daglilar E: Pancreatitis risk associated with GLP-1 receptor agonists, considered as a single class, in a comorbidity-free subgroup of type 2 diabetes patients in the United States: a propensity score-matched analysis, *J Clin Med* 14(3):944, 2025. https://doi.org/10.3390/jcm14030944. PMID: 39941615; PMCID: PMC11818918.

Acute Pancreatitis Classification Working Group: *Revision of the Atlanta classification of acute pancreatitis*. Available at: http://www.pancreasclub.com/resources/AtlantaClassification.pdf.

Beger HG, Matsuno S, Cameron JL: *Diseases of the pancreas: current surgical therapy*, Berlin, 2008, Springer-Verlag.

Beger HG, Warshaw AL, Buchler MW, et al: *The pancreas: an integrated textbook of basic science, medicine, and surgery*, ed 2nd, Malden, MA, 2008, Blackwell Publishing.

Cunha EF, Rocha Mde S, Pereira FP, et al: Walled-off pancreatic necrosis and other current concepts in the radiological assessment of acute pancreatitis, *Radiol Bras* 47(3):165–175, 2014.

Dellinger EP, Tellado JM, Soto NE, et al: Early antibiotic treatment for severe acute necrotizing pancreatitis: a randomized, double-blind, placebo-controlled study, *Ann Surg* 245:674–683, 2007.

Diener MK, Hüttner FJ, Kieser M, et al: Partial pancreatoduodenectomy versus duodenum-preserving pancreatic head resection in chronic pancreatitis: the multicentre, randomised, controlled, double-blind ChroPac trial, *Lancet* 390(10099):1027–1037, 2017. https://doi.org/10.1016/S0140-6736(17)31960-8.

Fisher WE, Anderson DK, Bell RH, et al: Pancreas. In Brunicardi FC, Andersen DK, Billiar TR, et al: *Schwartz's principles of surgery*, ed 9th, New York, 2010, McGraw-Hill, pp 1167–1243.

Forsmark CE, Vege SS, Wilcox CM: Acute pancreatitis, *N Engl J Med* 375(20):1972–1981, 2016.

Ye X, Lu G, Huai J, Ding J: Impact of smoking on the risk of pancreatitis: a systematic review and meta-analysis, *PLoS One* 16;10(4):e0124075, 2015.

Isenmann R, Runzi M, Kron M, et al: Prophylactic antibiotic treatment in patients with predicted severe acute pancreatitis: a placebo-controlled, double-blind trial, *Gastroenterology* 126:997–1004, 2004.

Working Group IAP/APA Acute Pancreatitis Guidelines: IAP/APA evidence-based guidelines for the management of acute pancreatitis, *Pancreatology* 13(4 suppl 2):e1–15, 2013. https://doi.org/10.1016/j.pan.2013.07.063.

Ye X, Lu G, Huai J, Ding J: *PLoS One* 10(4):e0124075, 2015. https://doi.org/10.1371/journal.pone.0124075, eCollection 2015.

Zaheer A, Singh VK, Qureshi RO, Fishman EK: The revised Atlanta classification for acute pancreatitis: updates in imaging terminology and guidelines, *Abdom Imaging* 38(1):125–136, 2013.

ACUTE DIARRHEA

Method of
Joshua Davis, MD

CURRENT DIAGNOSIS

History
- Onset, duration, frequency, and type of diarrhea
- Associated symptoms (e.g., fever, abdominal pain, vomiting)
- Exposures (sick contacts, contaminated food or water, or antibiotics) or travel
- Medical history and immune status
- Current and new medications or supplements

Examination
- Dehydration assessment
- Abdominal examination

Laboratory Testing
- Not routinely needed
- May include metabolic panel for watery diarrhea with severe dehydration
- Complete blood count and stool testing, preferably by polymerase chain reaction, recommended for bloody diarrhea
- Stool testing also recommended in patients who are immunocompromised or have severe or prolonged (>7 days) illness
- Radiologic imaging and endoscopy are rarely needed

CURRENT THERAPY

Symptomatic Therapy
- Oral rehydration in mild to moderate cases of dehydration
- Parenteral rehydration in severe dehydration
- If no contraindications (e.g., fever, dysentery, possibly *Clostridioides difficile*), loperamide (Imodium) at 4 mg orally, followed by 2 mg orally with each loose stool, up to a maximum of 16 mg per day
- Bismuth subsalicylate (Pepto-Bismol) 524 mg orally four times daily for 3 weeks to prevent traveler's diarrhea[1] or as needed for symptomatic care

Antibiotic Therapy
- Antibiotics should be directed toward detected pathogens identified on testing, when they are indicated.
- Antibiotics are rarely indicated empirically or for patients who are healthy and immunocompetent with mild to moderate illness, regardless of testing results.
- Antibiotic resistance rates worldwide are rising due to overuse of antibiotics leading to resistance, particularly to fluoroquinolones.
- Empiric treatment regimens in adults include azithromycin (Zithromax)[1] 1000 mg orally once (or 500 mg twice daily for 1 to 5 days), ciprofloxacin (Cipro) 500 to 750 mg orally once (or 500 mg twice daily for 1 to 5 days), or levofloxacin (Levaquin)[1] 500 mg orally once (or 500 mg daily for 1 to 5 days).
- Empiric pediatric regimen includes azithromycin[1] 5 to 12 mg/kg orally four times daily for 3 days (max 500 mg/day) or a third-generation cephalosporin for patients younger than 3 months.
- Initial *Clostridioides difficile* treatment should be either vancomycin 125 mg orally four times daily for 10 days or fidaxomicin (Dificid) 200 mg orally twice daily for 10 days
- Probiotics[7] have been shown to prevent antibiotic-associated diarrhea and *C. difficile* infections. The exact best dose and type is not known.

---

[1]Not FDA approved for this indication.
[7]Available as dietary supplement.

Introduction

Gastrointestinal symptoms are a common concern in primary care, leading to up to 18% of primary care visits. Acute diarrhea is the second most commonly reported illness in the United States, next to respiratory infections. Diarrhea is defined as the passage of three or more liquid stools in a day or an increase in baseline for a given patient. Some people consider diarrhea an increase in the number of stools, but stool consistency is really the hallmark. Diarrheal stool will conform to the shape of the container. Acute diarrhea is generally diarrhea lasting less than 14 days, whereas diarrhea lasting more than 14 days is termed *persistent*, and diarrhea lasting more than 30 days is *chronic*. This chapter focuses on acute diarrhea, but it is important to recognize that persistent and chronic diarrhea often start as acute diarrhea. Persistent and chronic diarrhea and recurrent bouts of acute diarrhea require a different evaluation that is outside the scope of this chapter.

Epidemiology

Acute diarrhea is a leading cause of death and disability worldwide. Diarrheal illness is the second leading cause of death for children under the age of 5 years, accounting for 18% of total deaths. This equates to about 5000 deaths per day. In developed countries like the United States, death rates are much lower. But acute diarrhea still accounts for 179 million outpatient visits, about 3% to 18% of all visits, in the United States each year. This leads to about 500,000 hospitalizations and 5000 deaths annually.

Etiology

The two major categorizations of acute diarrhea include watery (i.e., osmotic or secretory) diarrhea and bloody/mucousy diarrhea (i.e., inflammatory).

The more common type of diarrhea encountered in the acute setting in the United States is watery diarrhea. This is further broken down into osmotic and secretory diarrhea. Osmotic diarrhea is caused when a substance prevents normal water reabsorption in the intestine. It is most often seen in causes of chronic diarrhea (e.g., lactose intolerance or celiac disease), but, in the acute setting, is normally caused by medication side effects. Secretory diarrhea, on the other hand, is caused when water and electrolytes are pathologically secreted into the intestine. Secretory diarrhea is normally higher volume (>1 L/day) than osmotic diarrhea. As one would expect, the most common complication from watery diarrhea is dehydration.

Acute bloody or mucousy diarrhea is called inflammatory diarrhea or dysentery. This is normally caused by bacterial pathogens like *Salmonella*, *Shigella*, *Campylobacter*, and *Escherichia coli* or by parasites like *Entamoeba histolytica*. Patients with inflammatory diarrhea are at higher risk of infectious complications like sepsis, hemolytic uremic syndrome, seizures, or abscesses. It is important to differentiate bloody or inflammatory diarrhea from anatomic causes of gastrointestinal bleeding. Inflammatory bloody diarrhea is typically bright red and lower volume. Anatomic gastrointestinal bleeding can be bright red, maroon, dark, or tarry and is typically higher volume. Hemorrhoids will cause hematochezia but typically not diarrhea. Inflammatory diarrhea often requires further testing and laboratory workup compared with watery diarrhea.

The cause of acute diarrhea is often not identified. Viruses, namely norovirus, are the most common cause of acute diarrhea in adults. Bacteria, bacterial toxins, ova, and parasites are rarer but important causes of diarrhea as well (Table 1). In addition to the common infectious causes, noninfectious causes must also be considered. This includes medication side effects (Box 1), food intolerances, anatomic gastrointestinal bleeding, and early presentations of other gastrointestinal conditions.

Viruses

Viruses are the most common cause of acute diarrheal illness. In children, the most common pathogen is rotavirus, and, in

TABLE 1 Common Infectious Causes of Acute Diarrheal Illness

CAUSES	SYMPTOMS	TREATMENTS	RISK FACTORS
Norovirus and rotavirus	Watery diarrhea, fevers, vomiting	Symptomatic only	Contaminated food or water, close living quarters
Enterotoxigenic *Escherichia coli* (ETEC)	Watery diarrhea	Antibiotics rarely needed. Azithromycin,[1] fluoroquinolones, rifaximin, or trimethoprim-sulfamethoxazole	Contaminated food or water
Enterohemorrhagic *E. coli* (EHEC)	Bloody diarrhea, abdominal cramps, rashes, hemolytic uremic syndrome, seizures	Symptomatic only. Antibiotics not recommended	Unpasteurized dairy, uncooked meat, or contaminated water
Shigella	Bloody diarrhea, high fevers, abdominal cramping, rashes, hemolytic uremic syndrome, seizures	Azithromycin[1] or fluoroquinolones; resistance to both has been reported	Contaminated food or water
Clostridioides difficile	High-volume malodorous diarrhea	Oral vancomycin or fidaxomicin	Antibiotic exposure
Vibrio cholera	High-volume watery diarrhea	Fluoroquinolone[1] or tetracycline	Travel to developing nations
Nontyphoid *Salmonella*	Occasionally diarrhea is sometimes bloody, low fevers, abdominal cramping	Rarely needed. Azithromycin,[1] fluoroquinolone, or third-generation cephalosporin[1]	Unpasteurized milk, undercooked eggs or poultry, reptiles
Salmonella typhi	High fever, myalgias, diarrhea not necessarily prominent	Azithromycin (mild)[1] or carbapenems (severe);[1] fluoroquinolones are not recommended	Travel to Southeast Asia, South Asia
Campylobacter jejuni	Watery or bloody diarrhea, fever, abdominal pain, may mimic appendicitis	Rarely needed. Azithromycin[1] or fluoroquinolones; resistance to fluoroquinolones has been reported	
Yersinia enterocolitica	Bloody diarrhea, fever, abdominal pain, occasionally similar to appendicitis	Rarely needed. Trimethoprim-sulfamethoxazole,[1] aminoglycosides, third-generation cephalosporins, fluoroquinolones, or tetracyclines	Undercooked pork, unpasteurized milk, or contaminated water
Entamoeba histolytica	Watery diarrhea and abdominal cramping, rarely dysentery or liver abscess; incubation up to 1 month	Paromomycin +/– metronidazole	Fecal-oral
Cryptosporidium	Prolonged watery diarrhea	Nitazoxanide for immunocompetent patients	Fecal-oral, swimming, found throughout the United States, immunocompromised status
Giardia	Prolonged steatorrhea with flatulence and bloating	Metronidazole,[1] tinidazole, or nitazoxanide	Fecal-oral, found throughout the United States
Cyclospora and *Cystoisospora*	Watery diarrhea, flatulence, and nausea	Trimethoprim/sulfamethoxazole[1]	Travel to tropical regions
Bacillus cereus toxin	Vomiting, with watery diarrhea and abdominal cramping	Symptomatic only	Reheated rice
Staphylococcus aureus toxin	Vomiting, with watery diarrhea and abdominal cramping	Symptomatic only	Mayonnaise, cream-filled bakery products, ham
Clostridium perfringens toxin	Watery diarrhea with abdominal cramping, rarely vomiting	Symptomatic only	Meats and gravies

[1]Not FDA approved for this indication.

Common Medication, Supplement, and Dietary Causes of Diarrhea

- Laxatives (polyethylene glycol [MiraLAX], docusate, senna, lactulose)
- Hyperkalemia medications (sodium polystyrene sulfate [Kayexalate], patiromer [Veltassa], sodium zirconium cyclosilicate [Lokelma])
- Thyroid medications (levothyroxine [Euthyrox, Levoxyl, Synthroid])
- Antiemetics (metoclopramide [Reglan])
- Colchicine
- Antibiotics
- Antidepressants
- Antacids (proton pump inhibitors)
- Metformin
- Cholinesterase inhibitors
- Chemotherapy
- Magnesium supplements
- Fish oil supplements
- Vitamin C supplements
- Fiber
- Coffee/caffeine
- Artificial sweeteners (sorbitol, sugar alcohols)
- Lactose
- Gluten

adults, it is norovirus (also called Norwalk virus). Norovirus is commonly referred to as "cruise ship" diarrhea. Although it can occur in this setting, it also commonly occurs in many other settings. These viruses are typically transmitted via the fecal-oral route. Risk factors include exposure to healthcare settings, close quarters, poor food handling, and daycare centers. It normally occurs 1 to 2 days after exposure and is highly transmissible. It is sometimes associated with fever and vomiting. There is no specific treatment other than supportive care for viral causes of acute diarrhea.

Bacteria

E. coli is the most common worldwide bacterial cause of diarrhea. Although *E. coli* is a part of the normal microbiome, there are many subtypes of *E. coli* that cause diarrheal illness. These include enterotoxigenic *E. coli* (ETEC), enteropathogenic *E. coli* (EPEC), enteroaggregative *E. coli* (EAEC), enteroinvasive *E. coli* (EIEC), and enterohemorrhagic *E. coli* (EHEC or Shiga toxin–producing *E. coli*). The two most well-known types of *E. coli* infection are EHEC and ETEC.

EHEC is a strain of *E. coli* that produces Shiga toxin. Shiga toxin invades the endothelium, leading to bloody diarrhea. It also invades other organs, like the lungs, blood vessels, and kidneys. This invasion of nongastrointestinal sites leads to the many complications of EHEC, including hemolytic uremic syndrome, seizures, and thrombotic thrombocytopenic purpura. The media has focused on EHEC as a cause of diarrheal illness related to meat products caused by the O157:H7 strain of *E. coli*. The infection is spread via consumption of contaminated food, unpasteurized dairy products, and unsanitary water. Symptoms usually appear 3 to 5 days after exposure and last as long as 10 days. EHEC should be reported to local public health authorities. Treatment of EHEC is supportive and directed at rehydration and treating and preventing complications. Antibiotics are not recommended in EHEC as they theoretically increase the release of Shiga toxin and worsen outcomes.

ETEC, on the other hand, produces two types of toxins that cause watery diarrhea. Contaminated food or water is the most common source. It is a common cause of "traveler's diarrhea." Symptoms usually appear 1 to 2 days after exposure and may last from 5 to 7 days. Treatment is generally directed at hydration. Antibiotics have been shown to reduce duration of illness,

but they are rarely necessary, carry their own side effects, and risk increasing resistance. Antibiotic choices include azithromycin (Zithromax),[1] fluoroquinolones, rifaximin (Xifaxan), or trimethoprim-sulfamethoxazole (Bactrim). Single doses for both azithromycin (1000 mg)[1] and a fluoroquinolone (ciprofloxacin 500 to 750 mg) have been shown to be equally effective to multiple-day therapy. Given rising resistance patterns of *E. coli* from antibiotic overuse, in the rare instance where antibiotics are needed for severe ETEC, stool culture and sensitivities might be considered.

Shigella is the most common pathogen associated with dysentery and bloody diarrhea. Associated symptoms include high fevers and abdominal cramping. It is a nationally reportable disease. Similar to Shiga toxin–producing *E. coli*, shigellosis can cause bacteremia, hemolytic uremic syndrome, seizures, and other complications. Treatment is usually indicated and has historically been a fluoroquinolone (e.g., ciprofloxacin 500 mg twice daily for 5 to 7 days). Resistance to both azithromycin[1] and fluoroquinolones has been increasing in Asia and Africa. In 2018 the Centers for Disease Control and Prevention (CDC) announced a health alert that *Shigella* isolates in the United States had been identified with at least one resistance mechanism to fluoroquinolones. Since then, multidrug-resistant *Shigella* species have been reported in the United States. Susceptibility testing should be considered, and suspected treatment failures should be reported to the CDC.

Clostridioides difficile has been classically associated with antibiotic-associated diarrhea. However, community-based cases in patients without antibiotic exposure are on the rise. One study in emergency department patients showed that, when they tested all patients presenting with diarrhea, *C. difficile* rates were as high as 10%, and 30% of these patients had no risk factors or antibiotic exposure. *C. difficile* typically produces large-volume malodorous watery diarrhea. It is occasionally associated with toxic megacolon. There are very high rates of recurrence. *C. difficile* is typically diagnosed via a two-step algorithm involving both toxin testing and either polymerase chain reaction (PCR) nucleic acid amplification (NAAT) or glutamate dehydrogenase testing. Rarely, endoscopic testing is needed to confirm the diagnosis. Traditionally, it was taught that bleach and handwashing with soap and water (instead of alcohol-based products) were necessary to prevent the spread of *C. difficile*. The Infectious Diseases Society of America (IDSA) has backed off this guideline slightly, and now handwashing is preferred over alcohol-based hand sanitizer only in hyperendemic areas or when there is direct fecal or perineal contact. If antibiotic use is associated with *C. difficile*, it should be discontinued as soon as possible. Common antibiotics highly associated with *C. difficile* include clindamycin, fluoroquinolones, and β-lactam antibiotics. Treatment recommendations for *C. difficile* have recently been updated. Metronidazole (Flagyl)[1] monotherapy is no longer recommended unless no other options are available. Fidaxomicin (Dificid, 200 mg twice daily for 10 days) or oral vancomycin (125 mg four times daily for 10 days) is recommended as first-line therapy in an initial episode of *C. difficile*. Severe or fulminant *C. difficile* (defined as presence of shock, ileus, or megacolon) is typically treated in an intensive care setting with oral vancomycin and intravenous (IV) metronidazole.[1] Rectal vancomycin[1] may also be used if ileus is present. Recurrent episodes of *C. difficile* require either prolonged, tapered vancomycin; a fidaxomicin regimen; or fecal microbiota transplant. It is important to note that, while still rare, rates of resistance to vancomycin are on the rise and outbreaks of resistance to fidaxomicin among *C. difficile* isolates have also been reported.

Vibrio cholera, or simply "cholera," is endemic in developing nations and rare in the United States. It leads to profuse, watery diarrhea (classically called "rice-water stools") that usually occurs 1 to 3 days after exposure. Fever is rare. It is a nationally reported disease. Antibiotics are occasionally needed. Options would include

---

[1] Not FDA approved for this indication.

azithromycin,[1] fluoroquinolones,[1] or tetracyclines. An example regimen would be doxycycline (Vibramycin) 300 mg once orally.

Salmonella (nontyphoidal) is the most common bacterial cause of foodborne illness in the United States. It is associated with infected poultry, eggs, and milk. Reptiles, including turtles, are a rare cause of transmission as well. Associated symptoms include fever and abdominal cramping. It is required to report all *Salmonella* infections (both typhoidal and nontyphoidal) to public health authorities in the United States. Rarely, nontyphoidal *Salmonella* can lead to invasive infections like bacteremia or meningitis. *Salmonella* is typically self-limited and requires no treatment. In healthy people with *Salmonella* infection, antibiotics generally do not shorten the duration of illness, diarrhea, or fever. Indications for treatment include immunocompromise, severe disease requiring hospitalization, or extremes of age. Treatment, when needed, is typically either azithromycin, a fluoroquinolone, or a third-generation cephalosporin. An example outpatient regimen would be azithromycin[1] 500 mg once daily for 5 days. An inpatient regimen might consist of ceftriaxone (Rocephin)[1] IV once daily for 5 to 7 days. Antibiotic resistance of (nontyphoidal) *Salmonella* in the United States, though less common than *Shigella*, has been reported most recently regarding the multidrug-resistant Newport strain originating in Mexico.

Salmonella typhi and *Salmonella paratyphi* are special cases of severe *Salmonella* infection that lead to the diseases called typhoid fever and paratyphoid fever, respectively. These infections are typically much more severe than nontyphoidal *Salmonella*, and they often require hospitalization and antibiotic therapy. Associated symptoms include high fever, rigors, myalgias, headache, and, occasionally, a rash. Diarrhea may or may not be a prominent symptom. Typhoid fever and paratyphoid fever are almost exclusively associated with travel to endemic regions, most commonly South and Southeast Asia. Cases are rarely not associated with travel. The incubation period for typhoid fever is typically 6 to 30 days and 1 to 10 days for paratyphoid fever. Diagnosis typically can be done via blood culture, but stool is also acceptable. Urine culture or bone marrow may be needed. Antibiotic resistance is common in the United States. Fluoroquinolones are not recommended as empiric therapy. Oral azithromycin[1] may be used for mild disease, and ceftriaxone[1] (2 g IV daily) or carbapenems (e.g., meropenem [Merrem] 1 g IV three times daily)[1] are recommended for severe disease while awaiting antibiotic sensitivity testing results. Multidrug-resistant isolates have been found in people who have recently traveled to Pakistan, Iraq, and Southeast Asia, and a carbapenem for empiric therapy is recommended. Duration of therapy is based on severity of illness but is typically 10 to 14 days. Case recurrences have been reported when patients stop antibiotics early.

Campylobacter jejuni is another common bacterial cause of diarrhea in the United States. Diarrhea can be watery or bloody. It is often spread by undercooked meat and poultry. Symptoms may present 2 to 5 days after exposure and last up to 1 week. Associated symptoms include abdominal pain, fever, nausea, and vomiting. It can sometimes mimic appendicitis. In addition to foodborne transmission, it has been associated with exposure to the feces of young dogs and cats, including stool that is carried on their fur and paws. Delayed complications include reactive arthritis, rheumatoid arthritis, irritable bowel syndrome, and Guillain-Barré syndrome. *Campylobacter* is typically self-limited, and mild disease in otherwise healthy patients does not require treatment. Azithromycin and fluoroquinolones are commonly used for treatment, but resistance to fluoroquinolones is common. Treatment is associated with prolonged shedding of resistant organisms. When antibiotics are indicated, antimicrobial susceptibility testing can help guide appropriate therapy. Azithromycin[1] 500 mg daily for 3 days would be one potential treatment regimen.

Yersinia enterocolitica is a rare cause of bacterial diarrhea and is more common in children. It can be transmitted by undercooked pork, unpasteurized dairy products, animal contact, or contaminated water. It frequently has associated symptoms of fever and abdominal pain and can sometimes mimic appendicitis. Delayed complications of *Y. enterocolitica* infection include reactive arthritis and erythema nodosum. It is typically self-limited and rarely needs antibiotic therapy. *Y. enterocolitica* isolates are usually susceptible to trimethoprim-sulfamethoxazole,[1] aminoglycosides, third-generation cephalosporins, fluoroquinolones, and tetracyclines. Given how rarely it is needed, there is insufficient evidence to recommend an outpatient regimen. Complicated *Yersinia* infections can be treated with ceftriaxone[1] 2 g IV daily for up to 21 days.

Parasites

Entamoeba histolytica is a parasitic amoeba that is common in tropical regions. It can be contracted via fecal-oral transmission or contact with contaminated foods or surfaces contaminated with eggs. Only about 10% to 20% of patients will become symptomatic when infected. Incubation is quite long and can be up to 1 month. It is known to cause liver abscesses. It is required to be reported to public health authorities. Treatment for asymptomatic individuals is monotherapy with the luminal agent paromomycin monotherapy. For symptomatic carriers, metronidazole is used for the invasive component. Paromomycin (Humatin) can be both nephrotoxic and ototoxic, and its use should be closely monitored. Dose is 25 to 35 mg/kg/day, divided in three daily doses for 5 to 10 days.

Cryptosporidium is a parasitic illness that causes watery diarrhea. It is sometimes associated with fever, nausea, or abdominal cramping. Symptoms of cryptosporidiosis generally begin 2 to 10 days after becoming infected with the parasite and continue 1 to 2 weeks, though symptoms for up to 4 weeks have been reported. It is found throughout the United States. *Cryptosporidium* is typically transmitted via the fecal-oral route, including not only by consuming contaminated foods and water but also by swimming in contaminated locations. It is a nationally reportable disease. It is most well-known for affecting immunocompromised individuals, but it can affect immunocompetent individuals as well. Immunocompetent individuals will often recover without treatment. Nitazoxanide (Alinia, 500 mg twice daily for 3 days) is available and approved for treatment of immunocompetent patients older than 1 year with *Cryptosporidium*. It is not clear if nitazoxanide is effective in immunocompromised individuals.

Giardia is one of the few infectious causes of diarrhea that can cause steatorrhea. It is often associated with flatulence and bloating. Symptoms typically start 1 to 2 weeks after infection and continue 2 to 6 weeks. Other, less common symptoms include fever, itchy skin, hives, and swelling of the eyes and joints. Delayed complications typically occur because of malabsorption, and *Giardia* can lead to lactose intolerance later in life. It is a nationally reportable disease. Like *Cryptosporidium*, it is also spread via the fecal-oral route and found throughout the United States. Treatment options include metronidazole,[1] tinidazole (Tindamax), and nitazoxanide. The simplest regimen is tinidazole 2 g once. Combination therapy may be needed for recurrent infections.

Cyclospora cayetanensis and *Cystoisospora belli* (formerly *Isospora*) are common parasites in tropical regions and are spread by contaminated food and water. Symptoms of *Cyclospora* infection begin an average of 7 days after infection, and untreated disease can last several weeks to months. Associated symptoms include flatulence, nausea, and, rarely, fever. This is a nationally reportable disease. Symptoms in most immunocompetent patients will resolve without treatment, though they may be prolonged or may recur. The mainstay regimen for treatment of both *Cyclospora* and *Cystoisospora* is trimethoprim/sulfamethoxazole[1] 800

[1] Not FDA approved for this indication.

[1] Not FDA approved for this indication.

BOX 2 — History and Physical Examination for Acute Diarrhea

History
- Description of diarrhea (duration, frequency, onset, type)
- Associated symptoms (fever, nausea/vomiting, pain/cramping, rashes, weight loss)
- Previous episodes with similar symptoms
- Medications (see Box 1)
- Recent dietary history (contaminated food or water, poorly prepared food)
- Animal or reptile contacts
- Travel history (endemic regions)
- Sexual history (anal intercourse)
- Vaccination history
- Contact with institutions (hospitals, nursing homes, daycare facilities)
- Employment history (restaurants)
- Immune status (HIV, use of immunosuppressants, congenital illness)

Physical Examination
- Vital signs
- Weight
- Respiratory (hyperventilation may be a sign of acidosis and dehydration)
- Mucous membranes
- Conjunctival pallor
- Skin tenting
- Abdominal palpation (tenderness, rebound, guarding)
- Rectal
- Lymphadenopathy
- Skin (rashes, pallor)

TABLE 2 — Indications for Testing in Acute Diarrhea

FINDING	TESTING
Watery diarrhea	None routinely; consider metabolic panel in severe dehydration
Bloody diarrhea	Blood count and stool testing
Fever	Stool testing
Immunocompromised patients	Stool testing
Prolonged illness >7 days	Stool testing
Severe illness requiring hospitalization	Stool testing, blood counts, and metabolic panel
Suspected *Clostridioides difficile*	Multistep stool testing algorithm for organism and toxin
Fulminant *C. difficile*	Computed tomography imaging for ileus or toxic megacolon
Suspected *Shigella* or enterohemorrhagic *Escherichia coli*	Blood count, metabolic testing, and stool testing
Suspected typhoid or paratyphoid fever	Blood cultures, stool cultures, and blood counts
Symptomatic parasitic infection	HIV testing

mg/160 mg twice daily for 7 to 10 days. No alternative regimen has been shown to be effective for *Cyclospora* infections. Pyrimethamine (Daraprim)[1] or fluoroquinolones may be effective second-line agents for *Cystoisospora* infections. Consultation with an infectious disease specialist is recommended for patients who are immunosuppressed, as dosages and duration of treatment may need to be increased.

Bacterial Toxins

Some forms of diarrhea are caused by preformed bacterial toxins. These are all treated symptomatically. The three most common causes are *Bacillus cereus*, *Staphylococcus aureus*, and *Clostridium perfringens*. *B. cereus* is commonly associated with reheated rice, and vomiting occurs much more frequently than diarrhea. Incubation is 1 to 6 hours. *S. aureus* is commonly associated with mayonnaise, eggs, cream-filled bakery products, and ham. It also causes vomiting much more frequently than diarrhea, and its incubation is 1 to 6 hours. *C. perfringens* has a longer incubation of 6 to 12 hours and is associated with poultry, meat, and gravy, particularly when prepared in large batches or stored improperly. Diarrhea and cramping are common, but vomiting is rare.

Diagnosis

As with most illnesses, a thorough history and physical examination are the keys to diagnosis (Box 2). Occasionally, adjunctive testing may be required (Table 2). There is no single diagnostic test that is required in the evaluation of acute diarrhea, and most cases will not require any testing. Patients with examination findings of dehydration may require a metabolic panel to assess for electrolyte derangements or renal dysfunction. Patients with dysentery may also require a complete blood count and stool testing.

Testing stool for identification of specific pathogens is recommended in patients with severe or prolonged illness, with exposures or risk factors for invasive disease, or who are immunocompromised. The IDSA recommends stool testing in patients with fever or bloody diarrhea. Stool testing is not indicated in otherwise healthy patients with less than 7 days of watery diarrhea. This includes traveler's diarrhea, of which the causative agents are described previously. Some would argue that historical guidelines for diagnostic testing are overly restrictive in the current environment that offers new diagnostic methods for specific identification of infectious agents and enhanced ability to target therapy. When stool testing is indicated, it is generally recommended to use multiplex PCR testing as the first-line test to identify causative agents. National guidelines recommend that stool cultures and ova and parasite examinations should be reserved for patients with prolonged or severe courses of illness after PCR testing is negative or for those with specific risk factors for parasitic disease (e.g., known exposure, untreated HIV, transplant recipients, those on chemotherapy). Tests like fecal leukocytes or lactoferrin have little to no role in the diagnosis of acute infectious diarrhea.

Radiologic imaging is almost never needed for the evaluation of acute infectious diarrhea. It may be considered in patients with severe illness, severe pain, peritoneal findings on physical examination, or persistent fevers. Imaging is used in these cases to identify rare complications like toxic megacolon, mycotic aneurysms, or intestinal perforation. Endoscopic evaluation is also rarely needed for acute diarrhea, with the major exception being immunocompromised patients with prolonged symptoms.

Prevention

Preventing acute diarrheal illness is equally as important as treatment. The most common routes of transmission are fecal-oral and foodborne. Therefore the best preventive measures include hand hygiene, access to clean water, and proper food preparation and storage techniques. Public health reporting of suspected outbreaks is paramount to prevent spread. Worldwide, access to clean water is a key intervention to prevent diarrheal illness. Exclusive breastfeeding for the first 6 months of life has also been shown to reduce the risk of diarrheal illness.

Patients who are traveling should have pretravel counseling. Travelers should be mindful to have access to clean water (and ice) and choose their food sources carefully. Bismuth subsalicylate (Pepto-Bismol) may be used to prevent traveler's diarrhea in patients who can adhere to the frequent dosing regimens (524 mg orally four times daily for 3 weeks).[1] It is associated with black stools and tongue. Prophylactic antibiotics are typically unnecessary, but they may be used selectively for short-term use in patients at high risk who travel to endemic areas. Typically, fluoroquinolones are used (e.g., ciprofloxacin 500 mg daily for 1 week),[1] though alternative regimens include rifaximin 400 mg to 1100 mg daily[1] for 1 week; trimethoprim/sulfamethoxazole 160 mg/800 mg daily for 1 week;[1] azithromycin 250 mg daily for 1 week,[1] or 1000 mg in a single dose;[1] or doxycycline 100 mg daily for 1 to 3 weeks.[1]

Over 30 randomized controlled trials suggest that probiotics reduce the risk of antibiotic-associated diarrhea and prevent *C. difficile* infections. Exactly which type or dose of probiotic is best is not known, but probiotics should routinely be recommended to any patient with any antibiotic prescription. This is particularly important for high-risk antibiotics like clindamycin (Cleocin) and fluoroquinolones.

Routine vaccines exist for both rotavirus and hepatitis A, and these vaccines have reduced the incidence of these viral causes of diarrhea in the adult population. There are also vaccines approved in the United States for *S. typhi* and *V. cholera*, but these are reserved for patients at high risk of traveling to endemic areas.

Therapy

The vast majority of acute diarrhea is infectious in nature and self-limited. Thus symptom control and supportive care are the bedrocks of treatment. Medical interventions and treatments are rarely needed and sometimes even harmful.

The foundation for treatment of any acute diarrhea is supportive care with oral rehydration, antidiarrheal agents, and other symptomatic agents. It is important to use some form of solution containing electrolytes when treating diarrhea with oral rehydration. This can include juice, electrolyte-containing sports drinks (e.g., Gatorade, Powerade), prepackaged rehydration solutions (e.g., Pedialyte, the World Health Organization [WHO] oral rehydration salts), or homemade oral rehydration solution. The latter can be made by dissolving 6 teaspoons of sugar and 0.5 teaspoon salt in 1 L of water.

Occasionally, IV hydration may be needed. This can be done on an inpatient or outpatient basis depending on severity of illness. An isotonic solution should almost always be used for simple hydration. There is ongoing debate about whether balanced IV solutions (e.g., lactated Ringer solution, Hartmann solution, Plasma-Lyte) improve outcomes over 0.9% ("normal") saline solutions in general critically ill patients. Some randomized studies have shown no difference, and some have shown a benefit to balanced solutions. No studies have shown improved outcomes with 0.9% saline compared with balanced solutions.

Zinc supplementation[1] has been shown to reduce duration of diarrhea in children, particularly those who are malnourished. It is recommended by the WHO, but it seems to have limited uptake in developed countries like the United States. Most of the data support its role in countries with a high prevalence of zinc deficiency.

Antimotility agents are another important way to control and reduce symptoms of diarrhea and risk for dehydration. Loperamide (Imodium) is the most common agent used in this respect, and it has been shown to reduce symptoms. Loperamide may be used to reduce diarrhea at 4 mg orally, followed by 2 mg orally with each loose stool up to a maximum of 16 mg/day. It is recommended in traveler's diarrhea being treated with antibiotics to reduce duration of illness. It is advised to avoid loperamide in children under 18 years of age. It is also recommended to avoid loperamide in patients with high fever

or dysentery. Traditionally, loperamide was thought to be contraindicated in patients with *C. difficile* or other bacterial infections as it might lead to delayed clearance and complications like toxic megacolon. More recently, the IDSA notes that addition of an antimotility agent such as loperamide as an adjunct to specific antibacterial therapy for *C. difficile* may be safe, although no prospective or randomized studies are available. Bismuth subsalicylate is another agent that may reduce stool passage rates, particularly for traveler's diarrhea. Studies show it is most effective when taking 524 mg orally four times daily for 3 weeks.

Occasionally, antibiotics are needed for the treatment of acute diarrhea. This should not be routine practice. Instances where antibiotic treatment should be considered empirically before testing results are available include in infants younger than 3 months with suspected bacterial source of diarrhea, in patients with high fevers and suspected *Shigella* (but not EHEC), in patients who have recently traveled internationally and are febrile with signs of sepsis, and in immunocompromised patients with bloody diarrhea and severe illness. Recommendations for specific antibiotics for specific pathogens identified by testing are listed in Table 1. Duration of antibiotic therapy is typically driven by severity of illness, with mild illness requiring 1 to 5 days of antibiotics and more severe illness requiring a 7- to 10-day course.

There has been interest in the use of probiotics[7] in treating acute diarrhea. Despite the well-evidenced role of probiotics in preventing antibiotic-associated diarrhea and *C. difficile*, the most recent 2020 Cochrane review, based on large trials with low risk of bias, suggests that, for treatment of acute diarrhea, probiotics probably make little or no difference in the number of people who have diarrhea lasting 48 hours or longer, and it is uncertain whether probiotics reduce the duration of diarrhea. Similarly, probiotics are not recommended as a stand-alone or adjunct treatment for *C. difficile* infections.

---

[7] Available as dietary supplement.

References

Abrahamian FM, Talan DA, Krishnadasan A, EMERGEncy ID NET Study Group, et al: Clostridium difficile infection among US emergency department patients with diarrhea and no vomiting, *Ann Emerg Med* 70(1):19–27.e4, 2017.

Collinson S, Deans A, Padua-Zamora A, et al: Probiotics for treating acute infectious diarrhoea, *Cochrane Database Syst Rev* 12(12):CD003048, 2020.

Liao W, Chen C, Wen T, Zhao Q: Probiotics for the prevention of antibiotic-associated diarrhea in adults: A meta-analysis of randomized placebo-controlled trials, *J Clin Gastroenterol* 55(6):469–480, 2021.

McDonald LC, Gerding DN, Johnson S, et al: Clinical practice guidelines for Clostridium difficile infection in adults and children: 2017 Update by the Infectious Diseases Society of America (IDSA) and Society for Healthcare Epidemiology of America (SHEA), *Clin Infect Dis* 66(7):e1–e48, 2018.

Meisenheimer ES, Epstein C, Thiel D: Acute diarrhea in adults, *Am Fam Physician* 106(1):72–80, 2022.

Mussell M, Kroenke K, Spitzer RL, Williams JB, Herzog W, Löwe B: Gastrointestinal symptoms in primary care: prevalence and association with depression and anxiety, *J Psychosom Res* 64(6):605–612, 2008.

Nemeth V, Pfleghaar N. Diarrhea. [Updated 2022 Nov 21]. In: StatPearls [Internet]. Treasure Island (FL): StatPearls Publishing.

Redmond SN, Cadnum JL, Jencson AL, et al.: Emergence and spread of Clostridioides difficile isolates with reduced fidaxomicin susceptibility in an acute care hospital, *Clin Infect Dis* 80(5):984–991, 2025.

Riddle MS, DuPont HL, Connor BA: ACG clinical guideline: Diagnosis, treatment, and prevention of acute diarrheal infections in adults, *Am J Gastroenterol* 111(5):602–622, 2016.

Shane AL, Mody RK, Crump JA, et al: 2017 Infectious Diseases Society of America clinical practice guidelines for the diagnosis and management of infectious diarrhea, *Clin Infect Dis* 65(12):1963–1973, 2017.

United States Centers for Disease Control and Prevention Division of Parasitic Diseases and Malaria: *Parasites*, 2022. Available at: https://www.cdc.gov/parasites/index.html.

World Health Organization: *Diarrhoeal Diseases*, 2017. Available at: https://www.who.int/news-room/fact-sheets/detail/diarrhoeal-disease.

---

[1] Not FDA approved for this indication.

BLEEDING ESOPHAGEAL VARICES

Method of
Cecilio R. Azar, MD; and Ala I. Sharara, MD

CURRENT DIAGNOSIS

- Endoscopic screening for esophageal varices is recommended in patients with liver cirrhosis.
- Noninvasive predictors of the presence of large varices, such as splenomegaly and thrombocytopenia, have limited accuracy.
- A combination of clinical and endoscopic findings including the Child-Pugh class, size of varices, and the presence of red wale markings correlates with the risk of first bleeding in patients with cirrhosis.
- Measurement of hepatic venous pressure gradient may be the best indicator of risk and severity of bleeding in patients with varices. It is an invasive test and is not widely available or used routinely in practice.

CURRENT THERAPY

- Nonselective β-blockers and endoscopic band ligation are both effective first-line therapy in the primary prophylaxis of esophageal varices.
- The management of acute variceal hemorrhage consists of prompt resuscitation and correction of coagulation abnormalities, followed by endoscopic and pharmacologic therapy with vasoactive agents. Antibiotic prophylaxis is given to decrease the risk of infection and of rebleeding. Transjugular intrahepatic portosystemic shunt (TIPS) is reserved for refractory, uncontrolled, acute variceal bleeding.
- Strategies for secondary prophylaxis of variceal bleeding include endoscopic band ligation, pharmacologic therapy with nonselective β-blockers with or without nitrates, TIPS, and surgical shunts.
- Comparative cost-effectiveness of secondary prophylaxis strategies is unknown but should take into consideration the cost of failed therapy (e.g., rebleeding, shunt revision) and that of treatment related-complications (e.g., encephalopathy, esophageal stricture).

Epidemiology

Bleeding of esophageal varices is a major complication of portal hypertension, usually in the setting of liver cirrhosis, accounting for 10% to 30% of all cases of upper gastrointestinal hemorrhage. More than any other cause of gastrointestinal bleeding, this complication results in considerable morbidity and mortality, prolonged hospitalization, and increased affiliated costs. Variceal bleeding develops in 25% to 35% of patients with cirrhosis and accounts for up to 90% of upper gastrointestinal bleeding episodes in these patients. About 10% to 30% of these episodes are fatal, and as many as 70% of survivors rebleed following an index variceal hemorrhage. Following such events, the 1-year survival is 34% to 80%, being inversely related to the severity of the underlying liver disease.

Treatment of patients with esophageal varices includes preventing the initial bleeding episode (primary prophylaxis), controlling active variceal hemorrhage, and preventing recurrent bleeding after a first episode (secondary prophylaxis). Data on the optimal management of gastric varices are much more limited, and this topic is not covered in this article.

Pathophysiology

Chronic liver disease leading to cirrhosis is the most common cause of portal hypertension. The level of increased resistance to flow varies with the level of circulatory breach and can be divided into prehepatic, hepatic or sinusoidal, and posthepatic. In cirrhosis, several organ systems are involved in the pathophysiology of portal hypertension. At the splanchnic vascular bed level there is marked vasodilatation and increase in angiogenesis, leading to increase in portal blood flow and formation of collateral circulation, such as gastroesophageal varices, along with decrease in response to vasoconstrictors. At the systemic circulation level, there is an increase in cardiac output, decrease in vascular resistance, and hypervolemia. This hyperkinetic syndrome leads to an effective hypovolemia, with a resultant increase in vasoactive factors to maintain a normal arterial blood pressure.

Varices represent portosystemic collaterals derived from dilatation of preexisting embryonic vascular channels, such as those between the coronary and short gastric veins and the intercostal, esophageal, and azygous veins. In the distal esophagus, over an area extending 2 to 5 cm from the gastroesophageal junction, veins are found more superficially in the lamina propria rather than the submucosa. This results in reduced support from surrounding tissues owing to the predominant intraluminal location of these varices and might explain the predilection for bleeding at this site. The opening and dilation of portosystemic collaterals appears to depend on a threshold portal pressure gradient (measured as hepatic venous pressure gradient [HVPG]) of 12 mm Hg, below which varices do not form. This pressure gradient is necessary but not sufficient for the development of gastroesophageal varices.

Diagnosis

The current consensus states that every patient with liver cirrhosis should undergo an upper endoscopy to detect gastroesophageal varices. The main aim behind screening for gastroesophageal varices is to identify patients requiring prophylactic treatment or further surveillance. Esophageal varices are present in 52% of screened patients and are more prevalent in more advanced disease (43% for Child–Pugh class A versus 72% in Child–Pugh class B or C). On the other hand, gastric varices are present in up to 33% of patients with portal hypertension, with progression rates for both esophageal and gastric varices from small, medium, to large varices of 10% to 15% per year. Several invasive and noninvasive procedures help in detecting portal hypertension and can, with variable accuracy, predict the presence of gastroesophageal varices. Unfortunately, none are sensitive enough to replace endoscopy. A recent meta-analysis showed that transient elastography may be a useful screening tool for the detection of significant liver fibrosis and associated portal hypertension, but it is not useful at predicting the presence or size of esophageal varices. Smaller trials have evaluated the usefulness of spleen and liver MR elastography in assessing portal hypertension and varices, but this modality has not yet found its way into clinical practice. The combination of an elastography value below 20 kPa together and a platelet count above 150,000 nearly excludes the presence of esophageal varices requiring treatment. Endoscopic videocapsule is a new modality introduced for visualizing the esophagus; it allows correct identification of varices in 80% of cases but can have poor accuracy in identifying the presence of hypertensive gastropathy and gastric varices.

Not all esophageal varices bleed; hemorrhage occurs in only 30% to 35% of patients with cirrhosis. Variceal rupture is directly related to physical factors such as the radius, thickness, and elastic properties of the vessel in addition to intravariceal and intraluminal pressure and tension. Endoscopic findings that predict a higher risk of bleeding include larger size of varices and the presence of endoscopic red signs (described as red wale markings) on the variceal wall, indicating dilated intraepithelial and subepithelial superficial veins. A combination of clinical and endoscopic findings, including the Child-Pugh class, size of varices, and the presence or absence of red wale markings, was found to correlate highly with the risk of first bleeding in patients with cirrhosis. Hemodynamic parameters examined as predictors of bleeding include HVPG, azygous blood flow, and direct measurement of intravariceal pressure.

TABLE 1 Summary of Therapy for Esophageal Varices

	FIRST-LINE THERAPY	COMMENTS	ALTERNATIVE THERAPY	COMMENTS
Primary prophylaxis*		In advanced cirrhosis, the best therapy is unclear (probably band ligation) Transplantation should be considered for these patients		The effectiveness of combined β-blockers and band ligation is unknown Neither TIPS nor sclerotherapy is recommended for primary prophylaxis
Active variceal bleeding	Somatostatin,[2] octreotide (Sandostatin),[1] vapreotide (Sanvar),[5] or terlipressin (Glypressin)[2]	Vasoconstrictors should be continued for ≥2 days after endoscopic therapy Band ligation is superior to endoscopic sclerotherapy	Balloon tamponade or SEMS (self-expandable metal stent) TIPS	Tamponade is indicated primarily as a temporizing measure if first-line treatment fails TIPS is reserved for refractory or recurrent early bleeding but should also be considered when basal HVPG >20 mm Hg
	plus Endoscopic therapy	Antibiotic prophylaxis should be initiated	Shunt surgery	Surgery is reserved for patients with compensated liver disease in whom TIPS fails or is not technically feasible
Secondary prophylaxis	β-Blockers ± nitrates *or* Band ligation	The combination of band ligation and β-blockers ± nitrates may be more effective than either alone Nitrates alone are not recommended Patients with advanced liver disease are often intolerant of β-blockers	TIPS Shunt surgery	TIPS is best used after failure of first-line therapy or as a bridge to transplantation in patients with advanced liver disease Shunt surgery is reserved for selected patients with compensated cirrhosis in whom TIPS fails or is not feasible

Abbreviations: HVPG = hepatic venous pressure gradient; TIPS = transjugular intrahepatic portosystemic shunt.
[1]Not FDA approved for this indication.
[2]Not available in the United States.
[5]Investigational drug in the United States.
*Upon documentation of varices, variceal hemorrhage occurs in 25%–30% of patients by 2 years. β-Blockers reduce the risk to 15%–18%, and combination β-blockers plus nitrates reduce the risk to 7.5%–10%.

HVPG, calculated by the gradient of wedged and free hepatic vein pressure (normal value, 5 mm Hg), is used most often and provides reliable measurement of portal pressure in patients with cirrhosis. The extent of elevation of HVPG may be the best indicator of risk of bleeding, severity of bleeding, and survival. A rise in pressure in a patient with known varices increases the risk of bleeding, and the extent of portal pressure elevation has an inverse relationship to prognosis after hemorrhage has occurred. In general, however, a linear relationship between the degree of portal hypertension and the risk of variceal hemorrhage or formation of varices does not exist, so this technique cannot be used routinely to identify individual patients at high risk for bleeding.

Treatment

Primary Prophylaxis

The natural evolution of gastroesophageal varices without treatment is characterized by an increase in size from small to large varices, which eventually rupture and bleed. The progression rate ranges from 5% to 30% per year. The incidence of bleeding from small esophageal varices is estimated to be 4% per year, and it is as high as 15% per year for medium to large varices. In a randomized, controlled trial, the nonselective β-blocker timolol (Blocadren)[1] failed to reduce the development of varices or variceal bleeding in patients without varices. Adverse events were more common in the timolol group. Therefore, it is not recommended to start β-blockers in patients who do not yet have esophageal varices.

Based on prospective studies of cirrhotic patients with varices identified at endoscopy and of untreated groups in randomized controlled trials, the risk of bleeding from esophageal varices has been estimated at 25% to 35% at 1 year. Therapy for primary prophylaxis against variceal bleeding (prevention of a first variceal bleeding) is summarized in Table 1.

Pharmacologic Therapy

The general objective of pharmacologic therapy for variceal bleeding is to reduce portal pressure and consequently intravariceal pressure. Drugs that reduce portocollateral venous flow (vasoconstrictors) or intrahepatic vascular resistance (vasodilators) have been used and include β-blockers, nitrates, β_2-adrenergic blockers, spironolactone (Aldactone), pentoxifylline (Trental),[1] molsidomine (Corvaton),[2] and simvastatin (Zocor).[1] Because varices do not bleed at an HVPG less than 12 mm Hg, reduction to this level is ideal, but substantial reductions in HVPG (i.e., by >20%) are also clinically meaningful.

β-Blockers exert their beneficial effect on portal venous pressure by diminishing splanchnic blood flow and consequently gastroesophageal collateral and azygous blood flow. The effectiveness of β-blockers for primary prophylaxis against variceal bleeding has been demonstrated in several controlled trials. Meta-analyses have revealed a 40% to 50% reduction in bleeding and a trend toward improved survival. The estimated overall response rate is 49%, with bleeding rates of 6% in responders and 32% in nonresponders, with a number needed to treat (NNT) of 10.

The nonselective β-blockers, such as propranolol (Inderal)[1] and nadolol (Corgard),[1] are preferred because of the dual benefit of β_1- and β_2-receptor blockade. In the absence of HVPG determination, β-blockers are titrated to achieve a reduction in resting heart rate

[1]Not FDA approved for this indication.

[1]Not FDA approved for this indication.
[2]Not available in the United States.

to 55 beats/min or 25% of baseline. Propranolol is generally given as a long-acting preparation and titrated to a maximum dose of 320 mg/day. Nadolol is initiated at 80 mg daily up to a maximum daily dose of 240 mg. Carvedilol (Coreg)[1] is initiated at 6.25 mg daily and increased if tolerated to 12.5 mg/day. Carvedilol is superior to propranolol at reducing portal hypertension although available data do not allow a satisfactory comparison of adverse events. The portal pressure–reducing effects of β-blockers are not predictable; the resultant reduction in heart rate or the measurement of drug blood levels are not good indicators of response to therapy. For example, portal venous pressure is reduced in about 60% to 70% of patients who receive propranolol therapy, but only 10% to 30% of these patients show a substantial response (i.e., >20% reduction). Additionally, approximately 20% to 25% of patients have no measurable decline in portal pressure despite increasing dosage of propranolol. Non-selective beta-blockers (NSBB) are effective in preventing first and recurrent variceal hemorrhage both in patients with and without ascites. NSBB-induced reduction in portal pressure is associated with lowering the progression of cirrhosis and even death.

Refractory ascites and spontaneous bacterial peritonitis (SBP) are not absolute contraindications to NSBB as previously thought. However, high-dose NSBB (with resultant decrease in mean arterial pressure) should be used with caution because it can be associated with deleterious outcomes. Hence, careful dosing is necessary in these patients with dose reduction/discontinuation for systolic blood pressure <90 mm Hg.

In addition to β-blockers, a number of vasodilators have been investigated in patients with portal hypertension and in animal models of portal hypertension, most notably isosorbide mononitrate (Imdur).[1] Of note, there is increasing evidence that the use of β-blockers can be deleterious in patients with decompensated liver cirrhosis, refractory ascites, and severe circulatory dysfunction (systolic blood pressure 90 mm Hg, serum sodium <30 meq/fL, or hepatorenal syndrome). The exact mechanism of action of nitrates is unclear but is thought to be mediated primarily by reducing intrahepatic resistance and possibly by splanchnic arterial vasoconstriction induced in response to venous pooling and vasodilation in other regional vascular beds. Monotherapy with nitrates is ineffective in primary prophylaxis and can have detrimental effects, particularly in cirrhotic patients with ascites, and should not be used.

The addition of isosorbide mononitrate to β-blockers, however, has been shown to result in an enhanced reduction in portal pressure in humans. In a randomized, controlled trial involving 42 patients with cirrhosis and esophageal varices, a reduction of greater than 20% in HVPG was documented in only 10% in the propranolol group compared to 50% in the combination therapy group. In patients with Child-Pugh class A and B cirrhosis, the addition of isosorbide mononitrate to nadolol has been shown, in a randomized trial, to result in a greater than 50% additional reduction in variceal bleeding rate when compared with nadolol monotherapy (12% versus 29%). However, a large subsequent double-blind, placebo-controlled study failed to confirm these results. Based on the existing evidence, the combination of β-blockers and isosorbide is not recommended in primary prophylaxis.

Endoscopic Therapy

Endoscopic therapies play a prominent role in treatment of esophageal varices. Endoscopic band ligation (EBL) is the endoscopic procedure of choice in the management of esophageal varices. As of 2010, 16 randomized, controlled trials have compared EBL to β-blockers in the primary prevention of variceal bleeding. These studies suffered from significant heterogeneity, and a large number were published in abstract form. Two meta-analyses of these trials showed a slight advantage of EBL over β-blockers in terms of primary prevention of variceal bleeding, but there were no differences in mortality. A recent Cochrane database systematic review found a beneficial effect of band ligation compared to β-blockers in primary prevention of upper gastrointestinal bleeding

in adult patients with esophageal varices. Again, there was no difference in mortality.

β-Blockers are cheaper and much easier to administer but are associated with issues of noncompliance and a higher incidence of adverse events (e.g., hypotension, impotence, insomnia) than EBL. However, most of these side effects are easy to manage and none require hospitalization or result in direct mortality. On the other hand, adverse events related to EBL, such as bleeding from band-related ulcers, albeit infrequent, are more significant, often requiring hospitalization and blood transfusion, and may rarely be associated with death.

According to the Baveno consensus conference, nonselective β-blockers should be considered as a first choice for preventing first variceal bleeding in high-risk patients who have not bled, and EBL should be provided for patients with contraindications or intolerance to β-blockers. The recent guidelines by the American College of Gastroenterology (ACG) and American Association for the Study of Liver Diseases (AASLD) recommend using β-blockers in low-risk patients who have medium to large varices but suggest both EBL and β-blockers for high-risk patients as first-line therapy. The optimal primary prophylaxis in patients with decompensated cirrhosis remains unclear and is arguably expedited liver transplantation. The combination of pharmacologic plus endoscopic therapy has been investigated in such patients with conflicting results. In one study, EBL plus β-blockers offered no benefit in terms of prevention of first bleeding when compared to EBL alone. In a more recent study, combination therapy significantly reduced the occurrence of the first episode of variceal bleeding and improved bleeding-related survival in a group of cirrhotic patients with high-risk esophageal varices awaiting liver transplantation.

Management of Acute Variceal Hemorrhage

Variceal hemorrhage is usually an acute clinical event characterized by rapid gastrointestinal blood loss manifesting as hematemesis (which can be massive), with or without melena or hematochezia. Hemodynamic instability (tachycardia, hypotension) is common. Although variceal bleeding is common in patients with cirrhosis presenting with acute upper gastrointestinal hemorrhage, other causes of bleeding, such as ulcer disease, must be considered. Urgent initiation of empiric pharmacologic therapy with vasoactive agents is indicated in situations where variceal hemorrhage is likely. Subsequently, direct endoscopic examination is critical to establish an accurate diagnosis and to provide the rationale for immediate and subsequent therapies. The immediate steps in the management of acute variceal bleeding include: volume resuscitation, prevention of complications, ensuring hemostasis, and initiating measures to prevent early and delayed rebleeding.

Using a MELD-based analysis, the overall 6-week mortality is estimated at 16% (5%–20%), with mortality rates worsening with more advanced disease. Recurrence rates are up to 60% within 1 to 2 years if untreated, and mortality rates as high as 33%.

Patients with variceal hemorrhage and ascites are at increased risk for bacterial infections, particularly spontaneous bacterial peritonitis. This risk appears to be increased in the setting of uncontrolled hemorrhage or as a result of transient bacteremia following endoscopic sclerotherapy or variceal ligation. Short-term systemic antibiotics (e.g., third-generation cephalosporins or fluoroquinolones for 4–10 days) have been shown to decrease the risk of bacterial infections and to reduce rebleeding as well as mortality in cirrhotic patients with gastrointestinal bleeding.

A restrictive transfusion strategy should be used, aiming for a hemoglobin of 7 to 8 gm/dL to avoid volume overexpansion and perpetuation of bleeding. The role of platelet transfusion or fresh frozen plasma administration has not been assessed appropriately. The routine administration of fresh frozen plasma in patients with active variceal bleeding may in fact be detrimental because of the resultant volume expansion and should be discouraged. Hypofibrinogenemia should be treated with cryoprecipitate aiming for levels >100 mg/dL. The use of recombinant activated coagulation factor VII (rFVIIa [Novoseven]),[1] which corrects

[1]Not FDA approved for this indication.

[1]Not FDA approved for this indication.

prothrombin time in cirrhotic patients, has been assessed in two randomized, controlled trials. The first trial showed, in a post hoc analysis, that rFVIIa administration might significantly improve the results of conventional therapy in patients with moderate and advanced liver failure (Child-Pugh B and C) without increasing the incidence of adverse events. A more recent trial tested rVIIa in patients with active bleeding at endoscopy and with a Child-Pugh score 8 points or higher. This trial failed to show a benefit of rVIIa in terms of decreasing the risk of 5-day failure, but it did show improved 6-week mortality. In a small prospective study involving cirrhotic patients with acute variceal bleeding and new portal vein thrombosis identified by positive intra-thrombus enhancement on contrast ultrasonography, the use of low molecular weight heparin after hemostasis is achieved by band ligation was shown to be safe, well tolerated, and effective, with complete recanalization of the portal vein within 2 to 11 days and no recurrence of bleeding.

Pharmacologic Therapy

Pharmacologic therapy can be administered early, requires no special technical expertise, and is thus a desirable first-line option for managing acute variceal hemorrhage. Drugs that reduce portocollateral venous flow (vasoconstrictors) or intrahepatic vascular resistance (vasodilators) or both have been used to achieve this effect. Vasoconstrictors work by decreasing splanchnic arterial flow, and vasodilators are used in combination with vasoconstrictors to reduce their systemic side effects, but they can also exert an added beneficial effect on intrahepatic resistance (see Table 1).

Vasopressin and Terlipressin. Vasopressin (Pitressin)[1] is a nonselective vasoconstricting agent that causes a reduction of splanchnic blood flow and thereby a reduced portal pressure. Vasopressin, which is associated with severe vascular complications, has been largely replaced by other vasoconstrictors such as its synthetic analogue, triglycyl-lysine vasopressin (terlipressin [Glypressin]).[2] Terlipressin has fewer side effects and a longer biological half-life, allowing its use as a bolus intravenous injection (2 mg every 4 hours for the initial 24 hours, then 1 mg every 4 hours for the next 24–48 hours). Terlipressin has been shown in numerous placebo-controlled trials to control bleeding in about 80% of cases and is the only pharmacologic therapy proven, as of 2010, to reduce mortality from acute variceal hemorrhage. In patients with esophageal variceal bleeding, a 24-hour course of terlipressin was shown to be as effective as a 72-hour course when used as adjunct therapy to successful variceal band ligation. Terlipressin is not currently available in the United States.

Somatostatin, Octreotide, and Vapreotide. Somatostatin,[2] a naturally occurring peptide, and its analogues, octreotide (Sandostatin)[1] and vapreotide (Sanvar),[1] stop variceal hemorrhage in up to 80% of patients and are generally considered equivalent to vasopressin (Pitressin), terlipressin[2] (Glypressin), and endoscopic therapy for the control of acute variceal bleeding. Their precise mechanism of action is unclear but might result from an effect on the release of vasoactive peptides or from reduction of postprandial hyperemia. Somatostatin is used as a continuous intravenous infusion of 250 µg/hour following a 250-µg bolus injection. Octreotide is used as a continuous infusion of 50 µg/hour and does not require a bolus injection. Side effects are minor, including hyperglycemia and mild abdominal cramps. The addition of octreotide or vapreotide to endoscopic sclerotherapy or banding improves control of bleeding and reduces transfusion requirements, with no change in overall mortality. A continuous infusion of octreotide or vapreotide is therefore recommended for 2 to 5 days following emergency endoscopic therapy.

Endoscopy

Endoscopic sclerotherapy stops variceal hemorrhage in 80% to 90% of cases. Its drawbacks include a significant risk of local complications including ulceration, bleeding, stricture, and perforation. Rare systemic complications have been reported including bacteremia with endocarditis, formation of splenic or brain abscesses, and portal vein thrombosis. Randomized trials in patients with acute variceal bleeding have shown that EBL is essentially equivalent to endoscopic sclerotherapy in achieving initial hemostasis with lesser complications. These include superficial ulcerations, transient chest discomfort, and, rarely, stricture formation. Erythromycin infusion before endoscopy[1] in patients with acute variceal bleeding has been shown to significantly improve endoscopic visibility and to shorten the duration of the procedure.

Balloon Tamponade/SEMS

The use of the Sengstaken-Blakemore or Minnesota tube for hemostasis of variceal bleeding is based on the principle of the application of direct pressure on the bleeding varix by an inflatable—esophageal or gastric—balloon fitted on a rubber nasogastric tube. When properly applied, balloon tamponade is successful in achieving immediate hemostasis in almost all cases. However, early rebleeding following balloon decompression is high. Complications of balloon tamponade include esophageal perforation or rupture, aspiration, and asphyxiation from upper airway obstruction. Balloon tamponade or use of SEMS is generally not recommended and should largely be reserved for rescue of cases of hemorrhage uncontrolled by pharmacologic and endoscopic methods and as a temporary bridge to more definitive therapy. Self-expandable metal stents (SEMS) have recently been shown to be effective in controlling severe bleeding.

Transjugular Intrahepatic Portosystemic Shunt/Variceal Occlusion

Treatment with a transjugular intrahepatic portosystemic shunt (TIPS) consists of the vascular placement of an expandable metal stent across a tract created between a hepatic vein and a major intrahepatic branch of the portal system. TIPS can be successfully performed in 90% to 100% of patients, resulting in hemodynamic changes similar to a partially decompressive side-to-side portocaval shunt while avoiding the morbidity and mortality associated with a major surgical procedure. According to the American Association for the Study of Liver Diseases (AASLD) Practice Guidelines, the indications for TIPS are: (1) as rescue therapy for acute variceal hemorrhage refractory to medical and endoscopic intervention; (2) recurrent variceal hemorrhage despite medical and endoscopic treatment; and (3) an emerging indication is early TIPS within 24 to 72 hours of acute variceal hemorrhage in a select patients (e.g., those with basal HVPG >20 mm Hg). The left gastric vein is frequently embolized (embolotherapy) during TIPS creation. TIPS has been shown to be effective in treating refractory, uncontrolled, acute variceal bleeding. Patients with advanced liver disease and multiorgan failure at the time of TIPS have a 30-day mortality that approaches 100%.

Balloon-occluded retrograde transvenous obliteration (BRTO) is an endovascular technique used as a therapeutic adjunct or alternative to TIPS in the management of gastric varices, particularly in those with prominent infra-diaphragmatic portosystemic venous shunts (e.g., gastrorenal and gastrocaval shunts). It is indicated for patients with gastric variceal hemorrhage and/or those at high risk of hepatic encephalopathy, and is an alternative to endoscopic therapy or TIPS.

Surgery

Surgery is generally considered in the setting of continued hemorrhage or recurrent early rebleeding—uncontrolled by repeated endoscopic or continued pharmacologic therapy—and when TIPS is not available or is not technically feasible. Surgical options include portosystemic shunting or esophageal staple transection alone or with esophagogastric devascularization and splenectomy (Sugiura procedure). Devascularization procedures may be useful in patients who cannot receive a shunt because of splanchnic

[1]Not FDA approved for this indication.
[2]Not available in the United States.

[1]Not FDA approved for this indication.

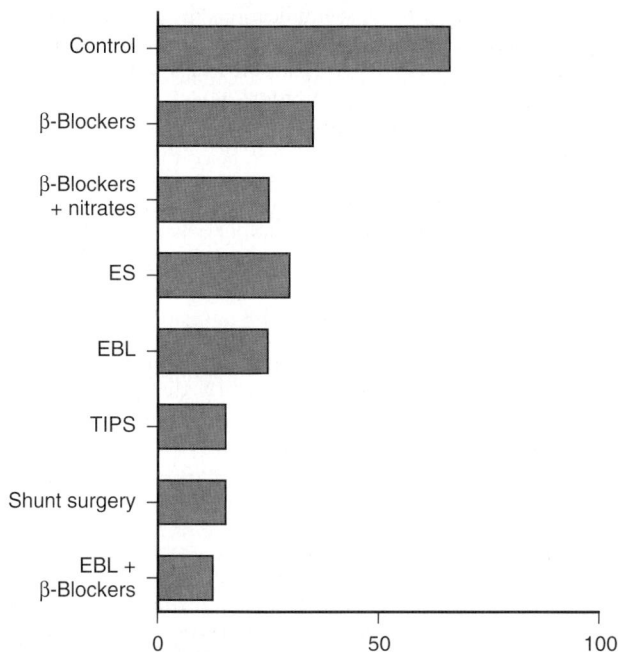

Figure 1 Relative effectiveness of available therapies for preventing recurrent variceal bleeding. The estimates shown are based on the cumulative data available in the literature for recurrent bleeding at 1 year. *Abbreviations:* EBL = endoscopic band ligation; ES = endoscopic sclerotherapy; TIPS = transjugular intrahepatic portosystemic shunt.

venous thrombosis. Regardless of the choice of surgical technique, morbidity is high and the 30-day mortality for emergency surgery approaches 80% in some series. Understandably, rescue liver transplantation is not a practical option in patients with uncontrolled variceal hemorrhage.

Secondary Prophylaxis

Variceal hemorrhage recurs in approximately two thirds of patients, most commonly within the first 6 weeks after the initial episode. Patients with advanced liver disease (MELD [model for end-stage liver disease] score ≥18) have an increased risk of early rebleeding and death. Early rebleeding (within the first 5 days) is reduced by the adjuvant use of octreotide[1] or vapreotide[5]—and possibly terlipressin[2] and somatostatin[2]—after initial endoscopic or pharmacologic control of hemorrhage.

The severity of portal hypertension correlates closely with the severity and risk of rebleeding as well as actuarial probability of survival following an index episode. In a cohort of patients presenting with variceal hemorrhage, those with an initial HVPG greater than 20 mm Hg had a 1-year mortality of 64% compared to 20% for patients with lesser elevations in portal pressure. Given the high risk of recurrent hemorrhage and its associated morbidity and mortality, strategies aimed at prevention should be rapidly instituted following the index episode. The choice of preventive therapy should, therefore, take into consideration the efficacy of therapy, the side effects of the selected treatment, the patient's expected survival, and overall cost. Preventive strategies include pharmacologic, endoscopic, and surgical methods and are listed in Table 1. Relative effectiveness of these strategies is shown in Figure 1.

Pharmacologic Therapy

Reducing the portal pressure by more than 20% from the baseline value pharmacologically results in a reduction in the cumulative probability of recurrent bleeding from 28% at 1 year, 39% at 2 years, and 66% at 3 years to 4%, 9%, and 9%, respectively.

Although adjustment of medical therapy based on portal pressure measurement would be ideal, HVPG determination might not be readily available, and treatment must be adjusted using empiric clinical parameters. Several randomized, controlled trials, including a meta-analysis, have demonstrated that β-blockers prevent rebleeding and prolong survival. The addition of isosorbide mononitrate[1] to β-blockers appears to enhance the protective effect of β-blockers alone for preventing recurrent variceal bleeding but offers no survival advantage and reduces the tolerability of therapy. A recent randomized controlled trial showed that carvedilol[1] is as effective as the combination of nadolol (Corgard)[1] plus isorsorbide-5 mononitrate in the prevention of gastroesophageal variceal rebleeding, with fewer severe adverse events and similar survival. Compared with either sclerotherapy or endoscopic band ligation, combination medical therapy is superior in reducing the risk of recurrent bleeding in patients with esophageal variceal hemorrhage, primarily in patients with Child-Pugh class A and B cirrhosis. Notably, in patients who show a significant hemodynamic response to therapy (defined as a reduction in the hepatic venous pressure gradient to <12 mm Hg or >20% of the baseline value), the risk of recurrent bleeding and of death is significantly reduced.

Endoscopy

Endoscopic therapy has been established over the past decade as a therapeutic cornerstone for preventing esophageal variceal rebleeding. Gastric varices, however, are not effectively treated by sclerotherapy or ligation. Patients with recurrent gastric variceal hemorrhage are best treated by N-butyl-2-cyanoacrylate injection[1] or by nonendoscopic means such as TIPS. On the other hand, EBL is highly effective at obliterating esophageal varices and is considered the endoscopic therapy of choice for secondary prophylaxis.

Combination modality approaches, usually including an endoscopic and pharmacologic treatment, are pathophysiologically attractive and may be more effective than single therapy. Two randomized, controlled trials have shown that adding β-blockers to EBL reduces the risk of rebleeding and variceal recurrence, suggesting that if EBL is used, it should be used in association with β-blockers. One randomized, controlled trial has evaluated whether EBL could improve the efficacy of the combined administration of nadolol[1] plus isosorbide.[1] In this study, adding band ligation to nadolol plus isosorbide was shown to be superior to nadolol plus isosorbide alone in preventing variceal rebleeding, but there were no significant differences in mortality. The combination of the best endoscopic treatment (EBL) and the best pharmacologic treatment (β-blockers plus isosorbide) may be the best choice in preventing rebleeding but needs further studies for confirmation. Statins improve liver generation of NO and hepatic endothelial dysfunction in experimental models of cirrhosis and may also reduce liver fibrosis. Randomized placebo-controlled trials found that simvastatin[1] decreased HVPG and improved liver perfusion and had an additive effect in patients treated with NSBB, and showed survival benefit in patients with early stages of cirrhosis and variceal bleeding.

Transjugular Intrahepatic Portosystemic Shunt

Transjugular shunting is more effective than endoscopic therapy for preventing variceal rebleeding but offers no survival benefit. The cumulative risk of rebleeding following TIPS placement is 8% to 18% at 1 year. The trade-off, however, is that TIPS is associated with a higher incidence of clinically significant hepatic encephalopathy (new or worsened portosystemic encephalopathy was noted in about 25% of patients after TIPS). Advanced liver disease is the main determinant of poor outcome following TIPS. Consequently, in patients with advanced liver disease, TIPS is best used as a bridge to liver transplantation.

TIPS, using bare stents, has been compared with surgical shunts in two studies (8 mm portocaval H-graft shunt in one

---

[1]Not FDA approved for this indication.
[2]Not available in the United States.
[5]Investigational drug in the United State.

---

[1]Not FDA approved for this indication.

and distal splenorenal shunt in the second). Although the first study showed a significantly lower rebleeding rate in the surgical group, the second and larger trial did not find any differences in rebleeding rates, hepatic encephalopathy, or mortality, but it found a significantly higher reintervention rate in the TIPS group. However, the obstruction and reintervention rates are markedly decreased with the recent use of polytetrafluoroethylene (PTFE)-covered stents. According to these data, TIPS using PTFE-covered stents represents the best rescue therapy for failures of medical and endoscopic treatment. In addition to TIPS, balloon-occluded retrograde transvenous obliteration (BRTO) is reserved primarily for prevention of recurrent bleeding, and has recently been included in the AASLD practice guidelines. Typically, it is utilized in patients who are at high risk for TIPS, such as those with elevated MELD (>18), right-sided heart failure, or hepatic encephalopathy. However, a recent prospective study showed that, in patients with Child Turcotte Pugh (CTP) class B >7 and active bleeding or CTP class C 10 to 13, preemptive TIPS (within 72 hours) should be recommended in the absence of contraindications.

Surgery

Portosystemic shunt surgery is the most effective means by which to reduce portal pressure. Although effective at eradicating varices and preventing rebleeding, nonselective portocaval shunts are associated with a significant incidence of hepatic encephalopathy, portal vein thrombosis, and occasionally liver failure. Commonly used shunts include the distal splenorenal shunt and the low-diameter (mesocaval or portocaval) interposition shunt. Rates of recurrent bleeding are on the order of 10%, with the highest risk of bleeding occurring in the first month after surgery. Devascularization procedures (i.e., esophageal transection and gastroesophageal devascularization) are usually considered in patients who cannot receive shunts because of splanchnic venous thrombosis and should be performed only by experienced surgeons. Surgical therapy has been largely supplanted by TIPS.

Cost-Effectiveness of Available Therapies

Data examining the cost of variceal bleeding and the cost-effectiveness of commonly used therapies are limited. The treatment cost of an episode of variceal bleeding has been estimated at $15,000 to $40,000. The cost-effectiveness of diagnostic methods used to guide therapy is unclear. For example, HVPG determination, which can accurately predict pharmacologic response to therapy, is an attractive, although invasive, adjunct in the management of patients with variceal bleeding, but its cost-effectiveness remains in question. Further, screening endoscopy for detecting large varices, while recommended, has not been demonstrated to be cost-effective.

There are areas in which management is controversial and not standardized. For example, given the right expertise, secondary prophylaxis with surgical shunts or TIPS may be more effective than medical or endoscopic therapy in Child-Pugh class A patients. On the other hand, patients with advanced cirrhosis are often intolerant of β-blockers—let alone in combination with nitrates—and therefore the use of combination therapy remains controversial in such patients. Arguably, the preferred treatment for such patients is TIPS as a bridge to early liver transplantation.

Therefore, when choosing a specific treatment plan, the clinician must take into consideration the direct costs of health care utilization, as well as the efficacy and morbidity of therapy. The treatment chosen should be tailored to fit the patient's clinical condition while also taking into account the possibility that the patient's liver disease can progress and thus necessitate transplantation. The cost-effectiveness of various treatment modalities should factor in the cost of failed therapy (e.g., rebleeding, shunt revision) and that of treatment-related complications (e.g., encephalopathy, esophageal stricture).

Summary

Esophageal variceal hemorrhage is a common and devastating complication of portal hypertension and is a leading cause of morbidity and mortality in patients with cirrhosis. Because the clinical outcomes are poor once variceal bleeding has occurred, primary prophylaxis with β-blockers or EBL should be considered in high-risk patients. The treatment of acute variceal hemorrhage is aimed at judicious volume resuscitation and ensuring hemostasis with pharmacologic agents and endoscopic techniques as well as prevention of complications, such as infections by the use of prophylactic antibiotics. Both NSBB and EVL are effective therapeutic options for primary prophylaxis for bleeding. NSBB have additional beneficial effects on the natural course of the disease. EVL is the treatment of choice for patients with contraindication or who are intolerant to NSBB. In patients with small size varices, NSBB is the first-line treatment option. In patients with advanced decompensated cirrhosis (arterial hypotension, hyponatremia, renal dysfunction), NSBB should be used with caution and EVL may be an alternative.

A high risk of rebleeding after an index episode mandates the institution of preventive strategies. Wedge pressure-guided medical therapy may be the preferred mode of secondary prophylaxis in patients with Child Pugh class A or B cirrhosis, but is invasive and not widely available. Patients at high risk for rebleeding, including those with decompensated or advanced liver disease, should be considered for TIPS followed by liver transplantation when applicable. Treatment with a combination of methods is pathophysiologically attractive, but the choice of therapy should ultimately be tailored to fit the patient's clinical condition, risk factors, and prognosis, taking into account issues of risk-to-benefit ratio, compliance, and cost.

References

Abraldes JG, Villanueva C, Aracil C, et al: Addition of simvastatin to standard therapy for the prevention of variceal rebleeding does not reduce rebleeding but increases survival in patients with cirrhosis, *Gastroenterology* 2016 Jan 13. Epub ahead of print.

Azam Z, Hamid S, Jafri W, et al: Short course adjuvant terlipressin in acute variceal bleeding: a randomized double blind dummy controlled trial, *J Hepatol* 56:819–824, 2012.

Bambha K, Kim WR, Pedersen R, et al: Predictors of early rebleeding and mortality after acute variceal haemorrhage in patients with cirrhosis, *Gut* 57:814–820, 2008.

de Franchis R, Baveno VIF: Expanding consensus in portal hypertension: report of the Baveno VI Consensus Workshop: stratifying risk and individualizing care for portal hypertension, *J Hepatol* 63(3):743–752, 2015.

Feu F, Garcia-Pagan JC, Bosch J, et al: Relation between portal pressure response to pharmacotherapy and risk of recurrent variceal haemorrhage in patients with cirrhosis, *Lancet* 346:1056–1059, 1995.

Garcia Pagan JC, De Gottardi A, Bosch J: Review article: the modern management of portal hypertension—primary and secondary prophylaxis of variceal bleeding in cirrhotic patients, *Aliment Pharmacol Ther* 28:178–186, 2008.

Garcia-Pagan JC, Feu F, Bosch J, Rodes J: Propranolol compared with propranolol plus isosorbide-5-mononitrate for portal hypertension in cirrhosis. A randomized controlled study, *Ann Intern Med* 114:869–873, 1991.

Garcia-Tsao G, Abraldes JG, Berzigotti A, Bosch J: Portal hypertensive bleeding in cirrhosis: Risk stratification, diagnosis, and management: 2016 practice guidance by the American Association for the study of liver diseases, *Hepatology* 65(01):310–335, 2017.

Gluud LL, Krag A: Banding ligation versus beta-blockers for primary prevention in oesophageal varices in adults, *Cochrane Database Syst Rev* 8:CD004544, 2012.

Laine L, Cook D: Endoscopic ligation compared with sclerotherapy for treatment of esophageal variceal bleeding. A meta-analysis, *Ann Intern Med* 123:280–287, 1995.

Lo GH, Chen WC, Wang HM, Yu HC: Randomized, controlled trial of carvedilol versus nadolol plus isosorbide mononitrate for the prevention of variceal rebleeding, *J Gastroenterol Hepatol* 27(11):1681–1687, 2012.

Mandorfer M, Bota S, Schwabl P, et al: Nonselective β-blockers increase risk for hepatorenal syndrome and death in patients with cirrhosis and spontaneous bacterial peritonitis, *Gastroenterology* 146:1680–1690, 2014.

Maruyama H, Takahashi M, Shimada T, Yokosuka O: Emergency anticoagulation treatment for cirrhosis patients with portal vein thrombosis and acute variceal bleeding, *Scand J Gastroenterol* 47:686–691, 2012.

Merkel C, Marin R, Sacerdoti D, et al: Long-term results of a clinical trial of nadolol with or without isosorbide mononitrate for primary prophylaxis of variceal bleeding in cirrhosis, *Hepatology* 31:324–329, 2000.

Moitinho E, Escorsell A, Bandi JC, et al: Prognostic value of early measurements of portal pressure in acute variceal bleeding, *Gastroenterology* 117:626–631, 1999.

Nicoară-Farcău O, Han G, Rudler M, et al: Effects of early placement of transjugular portosystemic shunts in patients with high-risk acute variceal bleeding: A meta-analysis of individual patient data, *Gastroenterology* 160(1):193–205.e10, 2021.

North Italian Endoscopic Club for the Study and Treatment of Esophageal Varices: Prediction of the first variceal hemorrhage in patients with cirrhosis of the liver and esophageal varices: A prospective multicenter study, *N Engl J Med* 319:983–989, 1988.

Northup PG, Caldwell SH: Coagulation in liver disease: A guide for the clinician, *Clin Gastroenterol Hepatol* 11:1064–1074, 2013.

Polio J, Groszmann RJ: Hemodynamic factors involved in the development and rupture of esophageal varices: a pathophysiologic approach to treatment, *Semin Liver Dis* 6:318–331, 1986.

Poynard T, Cales P, Pasta L, et al: β-Adrenergic-antagonist drugs in the prevention of gastrointestinal bleeding in patients with cirrhosis and esophageal varices. An analysis of data and prognostic factors in 589 patients from four randomized clinical trials. Franco-Italian Multicenter Study Group, *N Engl J Med* 324:1532–1538, 1991.

Sersté T, Melot C, Francoz C, et al: Deleterious effects of beta-blockers on survival in patients with cirrhosis and refractory ascites, *Hepatology* 52:1017–1022, 2010.

Sharara AI, Rockey DC: Gastroesophageal variceal hemorrhage, *N Engl J Med* 345:669–681, 2001.

Shi KQ, Fan YC, Pan ZZ, et al: Transient elastography: a meta-analysis of diagnostic accuracy in evaluation of portal hypertension in chronic liver disease, *Liver Int* 33:62–71, 2013.

Sinagra E, Perricone G, D'Amico M: Tiné F, D'Amico G, *Systematic review with meta-analysis: the haemodynamic effects of carvedilol compared with propranolol for portal hypertension in cirrhosis. Aliment Pharmacol Ther* 39:557–568, 2014.

Villanueva C, Minana J, Ortiz J, et al: Endoscopic ligation compared with combined treatment with nadolol and isosorbide mononitrate to prevent recurrent variceal bleeding, *N Engl J Med* 345:647–655, 2001.

CALCULOUS BILIARY DISEASE

Method of
Mick S. Meiselman, MD

CURRENT DIAGNOSIS

- True biliary colic is characterized by the abrupt onset and cessation of severe mid-epigastric or, less commonly, right upper quadrant pain.
- Pain commonly starts 1 to 2 hours after eating and can be localized or radiate to the back, right shoulder, or chest.
- The onset of biliary colic commonly occurs during sleep.
- Nausea and vomiting commonly follow the onset of pain.
- Elevations of total and conjugated bilirubin, ALP, and GGT with modest elevations in AST and ALT support a suspected diagnosis of choledocholithiasis.
- A normal serum biochemistry profile has a negative predictive value of 97% for ruling out choledocholithiasis.
- Transabdominal ultrasonography is a useful and cost-effective test for diagnosing cholelithiasis; however, it has significantly lower utility for choledocholithiasis.
- For intermediate-risk patients with suspected choledocholithiasis, examination of the common bile duct with magnetic resonance cholangiopancreatography (MRCP) or endoscopic ultrasonography (EUS) is warranted.

CURRENT THERAPY

- The treatment of choice for symptomatic cholelithiasis is laparoscopic cholecystectomy. Elective laparoscopic cholecystectomy should only be performed for true biliary colic. Vague symptoms such as bloating, dyspepsia, and atypical abdominal pain are not commonly related to gallstone disease and thus are not an indication for gallbladder removal.
- Laparoscopic cholecystectomy should generally take place within 72 hours of presentation for acute cholecystitis in appropriate surgical candidates.
- Laparoscopic cholecystectomy is recommended in pregnant patients with symptomatic cholelithiasis and acute cholecystitis. This is best done by experienced surgeons in the second or early third trimesters.
- Patients who should undergo preoperative ERCP for choledocholithiasis include those with high risk stratification and those deemed intermediate risk in whom a common bile duct stone is identified on MRCP or endoscopic ultrasonography.

Cholelithiasis

Epidemiology

Gallstone disease is common in Western populations, affecting 10% to 15% of adults. It is estimated that 6.3 million men and 14.2 million women in the United States have gallstones. Although the vast majority of patients remain asymptomatic throughout their lifetime, roughly one third develop symptoms or complications.

Pathophysiology

Gallstones can be categorized based on their composition. Of patients with gallstone disease in the Western world, 80% to 90% have cholesterol stones or cholesterol-predominant stones (mixed stones). Pigment gallstones account for the remaining 5% to 10%. Patients with hemolytic disorders are prone to pigment stone formation, and therefore the correspondence with disorders such as sickle cell anemia, hereditary spherocytosis, and Gilbert's syndrome is high.

Risk Factors

Risk factors for gallstone disease include female sex, age greater than 40 years, white, Latin American, and Native American descent, family history, obesity, rapid weight loss, starvation, total parenteral nutrition, bariatric surgery, diabetes mellitus, and hypertriglyceridemia.

Clinical Manifestations

The typical symptomatic presentation of gallstone disease is biliary colic. This is described as severe pain located in the mid-epigastrium or, less commonly, the right upper quadrant, that begins and ceases abruptly. The pain is typically constant, occurring 1 to 2 hours after a meal, and can either be localized or radiate to the back or right shoulder. Often the onset of pain occurs during sleep. Nausea and vomiting commonly accompany biliary pain, and, as with most surgical entities, pain typically precedes the onset of these symptoms. Biliary colic can also manifest as chest pain and is occasionally mistaken for cardiac angina. Prolonged episodes of pain localized to the right upper quadrant often herald cholecystitis rather than biliary colic. A clinical history containing the cardinal features of biliary colic carries a high diagnostic accuracy.

Diagnosis

Transabdominal ultrasonography is the preferred initial imaging test for cholelithiasis. The sensitivity for detecting the presence of gallstones within the gallbladder lumen on ultrasonography is 97%.

Biliary Sludge

Biliary sludge is often diagnosed on transabdominal ultrasonography. It appears as low-amplitude nonshadowing echoes that layer in dependent portions of the gallbladder. The clinical course of biliary sludge varies from patient to patient. Some patients remain symptom free, and others develop overt biliary colic. A fraction of patients demonstrate resolution of biliary sludge on repeat imaging. Symptomatic biliary sludge should be treated the same as cholelithiasis. Similarly, patients with asymptomatic biliary sludge should be managed expectantly.

Treatment

In patients with symptomatic cholelithiasis, treatment should be aimed at acute pain control and prevention of recurrent episodes. In patients without contraindications, cholecystectomy is the preferred choice for treatment of symptomatic uncomplicated cholelithiasis. This is preferably done via laparoscopy, which offers lower rates of complications and postoperative pain along with better cosmetic results when compared with open cholecystectomy.

Because of the high incidence of cholelithiasis, true biliary colic should be identified before a decision is made to proceed with laparoscopic cholecystectomy. Vague symptoms such as bloating or atypical abdominal pain are not typical of gallstone disease and thus often persist after surgery. In cases of asymptomatic uncomplicated cholelithiasis, elective cholecystectomy is not recommended unless the patient is diabetic or is undergoing an operation such as gastric bypass surgery, after which there is an increased risk of gallstone formation.

There is a very limited role for medical management of gallstone disease. Nonoperative management of symptomatic cholelithiasis involves bile dissolution with ursodeoxycholic acid (Actigall). The use of medical therapy is limited based on poor efficacy and high rates of recurrence and thus should be reserved only rarely for nonsurgical candidates.

Analgesia is an important adjunct in the treatment of symptomatic cholelithiasis. In patients with severe symptoms requiring narcotic pain medication, meperidine (Demerol) is preferred over morphine because it has less effect on the sphincter of Oddi. Nonsteroidal antiinflammatory drugs (NSAIDs) are another mainstay of therapy. Parenterally administered ketorolac (Toradol) is perhaps the most commonly used agent for biliary colic in the acute care setting. Studies have shown that NSAIDs are beneficial in the management of pain due to gallstones, and at least one study has suggested that early administration of NSAIDs might decrease the progression to acute cholecystitis.

Complications

Complications that can potentially arise from cholelithiasis include acute cholecystitis, cholangitis, pancreatitis, obstructive jaundice, and, rarely, gallstone ileus.

Choledocholithiasis

Choledocholithiasis often manifests concomitantly with symptomatic gallstone disease and is a finding in 5% to 10% of patients undergoing laparoscopic cholecystectomy for symptomatic cholelithiasis. The workup for suspected choledocholithiasis combines history, physical examination, laboratory data, and various imaging modalities. If the clinical history and physical examination are suggestive, the clinician should obtain serum liver biochemistry tests including alanine aminotransferase (ALT), aspartate aminotransferase (AST), total and fractionated bilirubin, alkaline phosphatase (ALP), and γ-glutamyl transpetidase (GGT).

The typical pattern of serum biochemistry is one of cholestasis. A conjugated hyperbilirubinemia along with high levels of GGT and ALP are seen often in the setting of modest elevation of the transaminases. ALP is usually elevated out of proportion to the transaminases; however, extreme levels of AST and ALT have been described. Transaminase levels greater than 1000 U/L, although rare in gallstone disease, should not dissuade the clinician from a diagnosis of choledocholithiasis. Serum biochemistries provide the most utility in ruling out common bile duct stones. A normal biochemical profile has a negative predictive value of 97%. Clinical predictors for assessing the likelihood of choledocholithiasis in patients with symptomatic cholelithiasis are listed in Box 1.

Diagnosis

A variety of modalities are available for diagnosing choledocholithiasis. Perhaps the least expensive and most widely available test is transabdominal ultrasound. Although the sensitivity for cholelithiasis is quite high with transabdominal ultrasound, identifying stones in the common bile duct (Figure 1) is more difficult. Prospective studies have reported sensitivities ranging from 22% to 55% for detecting common bile duct stones; however, in our clinical experience the sensitivity is much lower. Other indirect indicators of choledocholithiasis such as common bile duct dilation (77%–88% sensitivity) can provide additional diagnostic clues. Based on the high false-negative rates for common bile duct stones and dilation, a negative transabdominal ultrasound scan cannot rule out choledocholithiasis. CT scanning has a higher sensitivity for choledocholithiasis than transabdominal ultrasound. Levels of radiation and cost have limited its use as a first-line diagnostic tool.

Three nonsurgical modalities offer true visualization of the common bile duct with comparable sensitivities: Magnetic resonance cholangiopancreatography (MRCP), endoscopic retrograde cholangiopancreatography (ERCP), and endoscopic ultrasonography (EUS). MRCP has a diagnostic sensitivity of 85% to 92% for detecting choledocholithiasis, and, although it is useful for helping determine which intermediate-risk patients would benefit from preoperative ERCP, small and distal common bile duct stones are often missed.

EUS and ERCP are both minimally invasive techniques useful in the diagnosis and management of choledocholithiasis. Owing to the proximity of the extrahepatic bile duct to the proximal duodenum, EUS provides high sensitivity (89%–94%) for detecting common bile duct stones and is especially useful for detecting stones less than 5 mm in diameter. ERCP provides similar diagnostic sensitivity; however, ERCP offers therapeutic capability. Because of the reasonably high risk of complications including pancreatitis (1.3%–15.1%), infection (0.6%–5.0%), gastrointestinal hemorrhage (0.3%–2.0%), and perforation (0.1%–1.1%), ERCP as an initial modality should be reserved for patients who have a high pretest probability for choledocholithiasis and particularly for those with complications such as acute cholangitis or severe pancreatitis.

Research has evaluated the use of ultrasound-guided ERCP with the goal of avoiding unnecessary bile duct cannulation, and reserving its use for therapeutic purposes only. A systematic review from 2009 showed that compared with ERCP alone, the use of EUS avoided unnecessary ERCP in 67.1% of patients in

---

BOX 1 | Strategy to Assign Risk of Choledocholithiasis in Patients with Symptomatic Cholelithiasis, Based on Clinical Predictors

Predictors of Choledocholithiasis
High Risk
1. Common bile duct stone on ultrasound, CT scan or MRI
2. Total bilirubin >4 mg/dl *and* dilated common bile duct
3. Ascending cholangitis

Intermediate Risk
1. Other abnormal liver chemistry (e.g. total bilirubin 1-8-3.9 mg/dl, elevated AST, ALT, alkaline phosphatase)
2. Age >55 years
3. Dilated common bile duct on imaging

Low Risk
None of the above are present

From ASGE Standards of Practice Committee Buxbaum JL, Abbas SM, Sultan S, et al. ASGE guideline on the role of endoscopy in the evaluation and management of choledocholithiasis. Gastrointest Endosc. 2019;89(6):1075–1105.e15.

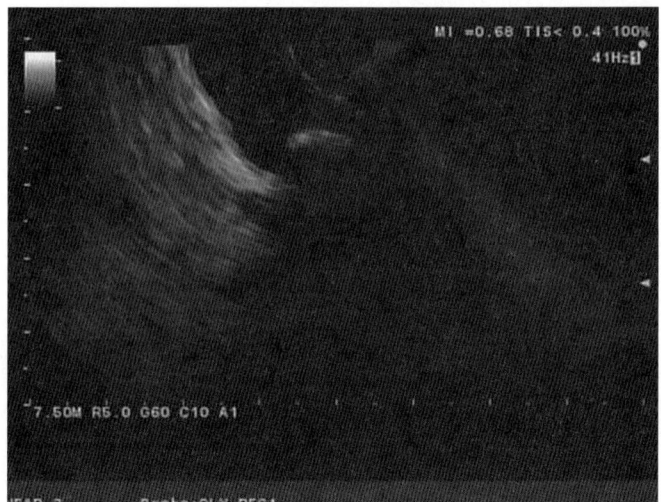

Figure 1 A large gallstone in the common bile duct (CBD) with dilatation of the CBD proximally. The endoscopic ultrasound probe is visualized in the top of the image, and a large cone-shaped shadow is cast distal to the gallstone.

whom no common bile duct stone was identified. As more gastroenterologists become trained in this modality, EUS-guided ERCP might prove to be the preferred diagnostic modality in intermediate-risk patients for the diagnosis and initial therapy of choledocholithiasis.

Treatment

Patients with symptomatic choledocholithiasis should be treated to avoid recurrent symptoms and development of complications. In the instance in which asymptomatic choledocholithiasis is identified, treatment is generally pursued, but current data is not conclusive. Stones can be extracted from the common bile duct via ERCP or laparoscopic cholecystectomy with bile duct exploration. Studies have shown similar efficacies without significant differences in morbidity or mortality; however, clinical expertise varies widely with the laparoscopic approach. Ultimately, cholecystectomy should be performed to prevent recurrence in surgical candidates. In patients undergoing laparoscopic cholecystectomy for suspected choledocholithiasis, perioperative management differs based on the risk stratification of the patient (see Box 1). High-risk patients should proceed directly to ERCP before surgery for attempted stone extraction. In intermediate-risk patients, a preoperative MRCP or EUS should be performed, and, if the results are positive, the patient should undergo ERCP as a prelude to surgery. For suspected choledocholithiasis in low-risk patients, surgery should be performed without further imaging of the common bile duct.

Complications

The two most common adverse complications of choledocholithiasis are gallstone pancreatitis and acute cholangitis. Gallstone pancreatitis develops in 3% to 7% of patients with gallstones and is the most common cause of acute pancreatitis in the United States. The diagnosis and management of acute pancreatitis is discussed in a separate chapter.

Acute cholangitis is caused by obstruction and stasis of the biliary tract with complicating bacterial infection. The syndrome is characterized by fever, jaundice, and abdominal pain, also known as Charcot's triad. Patients who develop hypotension and changes in mental status (Reynold's pentad) have a poorer prognosis. Elderly patients often do not demonstrate the classic signs of acute cholangitis, but they can develop a delayed-sepsis–like syndrome, of which hypotension is the most pronounced feature. High biliary pressures promote the translocation of bacteria from the portal circulation into the biliary tree. The most common bacterial organism seen in acute cholangitis is *Escherichia coli* (25%–50%), followed by *Klebsiella, Enterobacter,* and *Enterococcus* species.

Treatment for acute cholangitis should focus on antimicrobial therapy and biliary drainage. Empiric antibiotic regimens should provide adequate activity against gram-negative and anaerobic organisms. Common regimens include monotherapy with ampicillin and sulbactam (Unasyn), ceftriaxone (Rocephin), and piperacillin and tazobactam or combination therapy with a fluoroquinolone plus metronidazole (Flagyl).

Patients without hypotension or mental status changes commonly show initial improvement after empiric antibiotics are administered, and thus biliary drainage can be done nonurgently. In patients demonstrating signs of sepsis or severe infection, emergency biliary drainage via ERCP is warranted. Patients who are not candidates for ERCP may undergo percutaneous transhepatic biliary drainage as an alternative.

Acute Cholecystitis

Acute cholecystitis is a syndrome defined by right upper quadrant pain, fever, and leukocytosis in the setting of gallbladder inflammation. Nausea and vomiting often occur as concurrent symptoms. Patients commonly have a positive Murphy's sign on physical examination, which is defined as abrupt cessation of inspiration on deep palpation of the gallbladder fossa, just beneath the liver edge. Approximately 95% of patients with acute cholecystitis have gallstones. In these instances, cholecystitis is

thought to be precipitated by obstruction of the cystic duct and by local irritation of the gallbladder wall. Local inflammation is followed by release of pro-inflammatory prostaglandins. Superimposed bacterial infection might or might not complicate acute cholecystitis. As with cholangitis, the main bacteria responsible for infections during acute cholecystitis are *E. coli* and *Klebsiella, Enterobacter,* and *Enterococcus* species.

Diagnosis

The diagnosis of acute cholecystitis can often be made on physical examination alone. The most common laboratory finding in acute cholecystitis is leukocytosis. Mild elevations in AST and ALT can also be seen. Elevations of bilirubin and ALP are typical of biliary obstruction and are not commonly seen in acute cholecystitis. These abnormalities, if present, should raise suspicion for other conditions such as choledocholithiasis, cholangitis, or Mirizzi's syndrome. Mirizzi's syndrome is a rare cause of obstructive jaundice characterized by an impacted cystic duct stone that causes mass effect and compression of the common bile duct or common hepatic duct.

The initial imaging study of choice for acute cholecystitis is transabdominal ultrasound. Findings suggestive of cholecystitis include cholelithiasis, pericholecystic fluid (Figure 2), and a sonographic Murphy's sign (Figure 3). Thickening of the gallbladder wall supports a diagnosis of acute cholecystitis, but it is a nonspecific finding. Transabdominal ultrasound has a sensitivity of 88% for diagnosing acute cholecystitis. Hepatobiliary cholescintigraphy (HIDA scan) (Figure 4) is recommended if the suspicion of cholecystitis remains after a negative transabdominal ultrasound. MRCP and CT scan are typically not necessary for the diagnosis, although CT scan can be useful if complications from cholecystitis such as perforation are suspected.

Treatment

The treatment for acute cholecystitis involves supportive care, analgesia, antibiotics, and either surgery or percutaneous gallbladder drainage. If treatment is delayed or inadequate, numerous potential complications can result. These include emphysematous or gangrenous cholecystitis and gallbladder perforation. All patients with acute cholecystitis should be admitted to the hospital and given supportive care including intravenous fluids. NSAIDs and opioid analgesics are typically used for pain control.

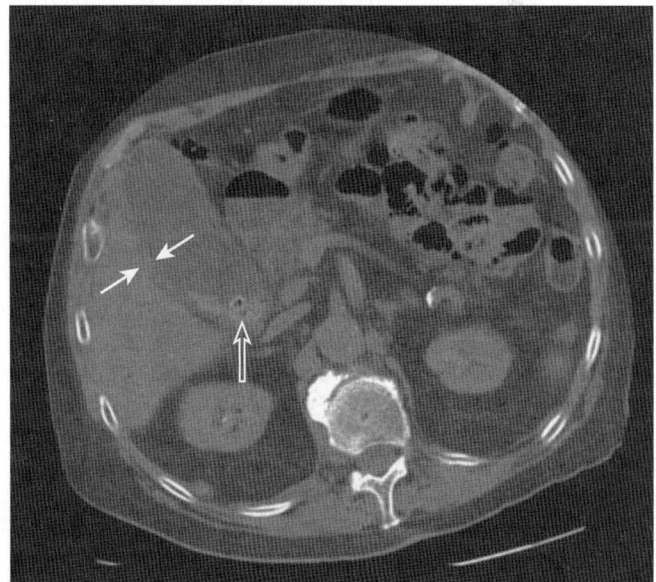

Figure 2 Computed tomography (CT) scan demonstrating acute cholecystitis. The ***outline arrow*** indicates gallstones within the gallbladder lumen. The two ***solid arrows*** highlight mural thickening of the gallbladder wall and small amounts of pericholecystic fluid. Image courtesy of Richard M. Gore, MD, Department of Radiology, NorthShore University Health System, Evanston, IL.

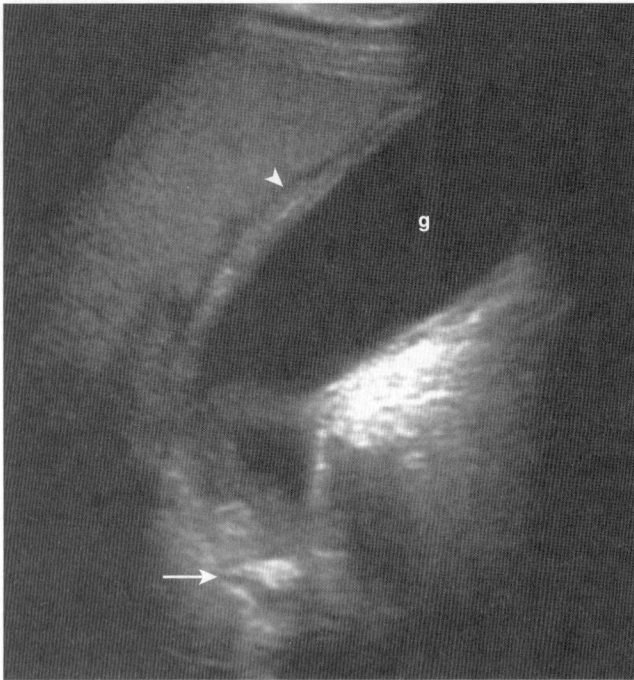

Figure 3 Acute cholecystits: ultrasound. Gallbladder *(g)* is distended, with mural thickening *(arrowhead)* and a stone in the gallbladder neck *(arrow)*. Positive sonographic Murphy sign was present.

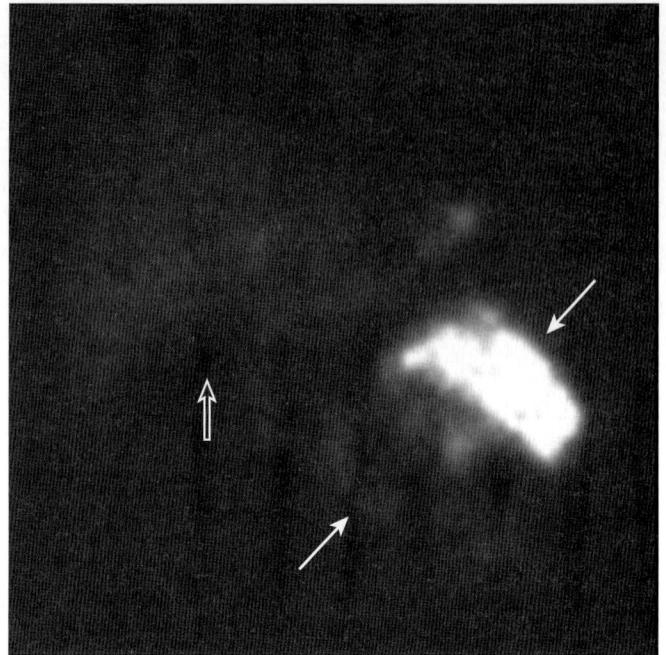

Figure 4 Hepatobiliary iminodiacetic acid (HIDA) scan demonstrating acute cholecystitis. There is nonfilling of the gallbladder *(outline arrow)*, with isotope noted in the stomach and duodenum *(solid arrows)*. Image courtesy of Richard M. Gore, MD, Department of Radiology, North-Shore University Health System, Evanston, IL.

Although bacterial etiologies complicate less than half of all episodes, empiric antibiotics are commonly administered to patients with acute cholecystitis. Appropriate antibiotic regimens are the same as those used in the setting of acute cholangitis (see the discussion of complications of choledocholithiasis).

In patients who are adequate surgical candidates, cholecystectomy should be performed within 72 hours of initial presentation. Numerous prospective trials and a Cochrane Database review have evaluated early versus delayed (6–12 weeks) cholecystectomy. There is overwhelming consensus that early surgery carries no increase in complications or perioperative morbidity and is associated with shorter hospital stays. Furthermore, early laparoscopic cholecystectomy eliminates the risk of recurrent episodes of acute cholecystitis. In patients who are not surgical candidates, percutaneous cholecystostomy is generally considered. Recently, endoscopic ultrasound-guided gallbladder drainage has emerged as an acceptable alternative to percutaneous cholecystostomy in the high-risk population.

Acute Acalculous Cholesystitis

An estimated 5% to 10% of cases of acute cholecystitis develop without the presence of gallstones. Acute acalculous cholecystitis is often seen in the setting of serious medical illness, complicated surgery, severe blunt trauma, and burn injuries. Other conditions such as diabetes mellitus, vasculitis, AIDS, and congestive heart failure have also been implicated as risk factors. Acute acalculous cholecystitis carries major risks of gangrene (50%) and perforation (10%), and mortality ranges from 30% to 50%. Numerous organisms have been associated with acute acalculous cholecystitis, including bacterial, viral, fungal, and parasitic infections.

The diagnosis is difficult. Patients are often critically ill and unable to elicit their symptoms. Transabdominal ultrasound is the best modality to evaluate acute acalculous cholecystitis in the critically ill patient owing to its availability, cost, and ease of performance. Hepatobiliary iminodiacetic acid (HIDA) and computed tomography (CT) scanning can have a role in difficult-to-diagnose acute acalculous cholecystitis and should be considered if ultrasound is nondiagnostic. Whereas false-positive test results can occur, a normal HIDA scan has a high negative predictive value in evaluating acute acalculous cholecystitis.

Because of the high rate of gangrene and perforation, early cholecystectomy should be performed in patients who are surgical candidates. In patients too ill to undergo surgery, biliary drainage with percutaneous cholecystostomy or EUS-guided biliary drainage should be considered.

Gangrenous Cholecystitis, Emphysematous Cholecystitis, and Gallbladder Perforation

Gangrenous cholecystitis is most often seen in elderly patients and diabetics along with patients who delay seeking medical treatment for their symptoms. It is the most common complication of acute cholecystitis and carries a high mortality. Emphysematous cholecystitis is caused by gas-forming bacteria that infect the gallbladder. *E coli* and *Clostridium* species are most commonly implicated. Gas in the gallbladder may be seen on imaging, particularly CT or magnetic resonance imaging (MRI). Patients with gangrenous or emphysematous cholecystitis are at an elevated risk for gallbladder perforation. Early empiric antibiotics and cholecystectomy are crucial in the management of these complications to minimize mortality and prevent perforation of the gallbladder, a condition that carries a mortality rate of 42% to 60%.

Gallbladder Disease in Pregnancy

Pregnancy is a major risk factor for cholesterol gallstone formation. Because of anatomic changes secondary to the gravid uterus, biliary colic can be difficult to delineate from other causes of abdominal pain. Pregnant patients often have gallstones on transabdominal ultrasound, and thus a detailed history and physical examination are needed to diagnose a patient's abdominal pain as biliary. Patients with other symptoms including bloating or dyspepsia should be evaluated for other etiologies.

In pregnant patients with recurrent symptomatic cholelithiasis, laparoscopic cholecystectomy remains the treatment of choice. The second and early third trimesters are the best times to perform cholecystectomy owing to ease and lower rates of complications. Nonsurgical management of gallstones is limited in pregnancy. NSAIDs are generally avoided late in pregnancy owing to the risk of premature closure of the ductus arteriosis, especially after 30 to 32 weeks of gestation.

After appendicitis, acute cholecystitis is the second most common nonobstetric surgical emergency during pregnancy. As with nonpregnant patients, pregnant women with acute cholecystitis should be treated with cholecystectomy in addition to medical management. Early surgery for pregnant patients with acute cholecystitis has been found to decrease relapse rates and hospital readmissions. No differences in maternal or fetal morbidity and mortality have been found in patients treated conservatively versus surgically for acute cholecystitis during pregnancy.

References

Abboud PA, Malet PF, Berlin JA, et al: Predictors of common bile duct stones prior to cholecystectomy: A metaanalysis, *Gastrointest Endosc* 44:450–455, 1996.

Akriviadis EA, Hatzigavriel M, Kapnias D, et al: Treatment of biliary colic with diclofenac: a randomized, double-blind, placebo-controlled study, *Gastroenterology* 113:225–231, 1997.

ASGE Standards of Practice Committee, Buxbaum JL, Abbas fehmi SM, Sultan S, et al: ASGE guideline on the role of endoscopy in the evaluation and management of choledocholithiasis, *Gastrointest Endosc* 89(6):1075–1105.e15, 2019.

Barie PS, Eachempati SR: Acute acalculous cholecystitis, *Gastroenterol Clin North Am* 39:344–357, 2010.

Dhupar R, Smaldone GM, Hamad GG: Is there a benefit to delaying cholecystectomy for symptomatic gallbladder disease during pregnancy? *Surg Endosc* 24:108–112, 2010.

Everhart JE, Khare M, Hill M, Maurer KR: Prevalence and ethnic differences in gallbladder disease in the United States, *Gastroenterology* 117:632–639, 1999.

Freitas ML, Bell RL, Duffy AJ: Choledocholithiasis: Evolving standards for diagnosis and management, *World J Gastroenterol* 12:3162–3167, 2006.

Gore RM, Thakrar KH, Newmark GM, et al: Gallbladder imaging, *Gastroenterol Clin North Am* 39:265–267, 2010.

Gurusamy KS, Samraj K: Early versus late laparoscopic cholecystectomy for acute cholecystitis, *Cochrane Database Syst Rev* 18: CD005440.

Papi C, Catarci M, Ambrosio D, et al: Timing of cholecystectomy for acute calculous cholecystitis: A meta-analysis, *Am J Gastroenterol* 9:147–155, 2004.Omnimodis

CHRONIC DIARRHEA

Method of
Jacqueline Huynh, MD; and Leslie A. Greenberg, MD

CURRENT DIAGNOSIS

- Comprehensive history is key. Determine any precipitating factors.
- Obtain labs: complete blood cell count, comprehensive metabolic panel, thyroid-stimulating hormone, celiac screening (total immunoglobulin [Ig]A and tissue transglutaminase IgA), and C-reactive protein.
- If inflammatory bowel disease is suspected, perform stool testing: fecal calprotectin or fecal lactoferrin. The fecal immunochemical test is also recommended to assess for presence of blood.
- If unable to narrow the differential, stool analysis (stool osmolality, stool pH, fecal calprotectin, fecal elastase) to categorize the diarrhea as watery, inflammatory, or fatty can help.
- Red flag symptoms are unexplained weight loss, rectal bleeding, anemia, or progressive abdominal pain, and patients should receive urgent evaluation.

CURRENT THERAPY

- Treatment of chronic diarrhea depends on the underlying etiology.
- Perform medication and supplement history. Over 700 medications are known to cause diarrhea. Discontinue offending agents if appropriate.

- Patients with irritable bowel syndrome–diarrhea (IBS-D) should trial a bile acid sequestrant, as about one-third of patients with IBS-D also have bile acid diarrhea.
- Patients with suspected small intestine bacterial overgrowth are suggested to take empiric antibiotic treatment with 14 days of rifaximin (Xifaxan),[1] the currently favored first-line medication because of its tolerability.

[1]Not FDA approved for this indication.

The World Health Organization defines diarrhea as the passage of three or more loose or liquid stools per 24 hours, or more frequently than is normal for an individual person. Chronic diarrhea is defined as lasting for 30 days or more. Assessing the consistency of stool can be standardized using the validated Bristol stool chart, which categorizes types 5 through 7 as diarrhea. Chronic diarrhea affects about 5% to 7% of the U.S. population and has a broad differential diagnosis. Evaluation and treatment depend on a detailed history and physical examination (Table 1). The American Gastroenterological Association (AGA) last published Clinical Practice Guidelines on the Laboratory Evaluation of Functional Diarrhea and Diarrhea-Predominant Irritable Bowel Syndrome in Adults in 2019, and the British Society of Gastroenterology (BSG) published guidelines in 2018 for the evaluation of chronic diarrhea.

Pathophysiology

Chronic diarrhea may arise from different mechanisms and underlying etiologies and present as watery, bloody, or fatty stools depending on those mechanisms (Table 2). Chronic diarrhea may be organic (e.g., inflammatory bowel disease [IBD], microscopic colitis, or neoplasms), functional (e.g., irritable bowel syndrome), anatomic, postsurgical, or iatrogenic (e.g., adverse drug reactions). Mechanisms include a decrease in absorptive surface leading to malabsorption, decreased bowel transit time, increased bile acid secretion, and maldigestion.

Diagnosis

Assessment of patients with chronic diarrhea requires a detailed history to narrow the differential. The primary diagnostic assessment should include complete blood cell count (CBC), comprehensive metabolic panel (CMP), thyroid-stimulating hormone, C-reactive protein (CRP), and screening for celiac disease (anti–tissue transglutaminase [anti-tTG] immunoglobulin (Ig)A and total IgA level). As patients with IgA deficiency may have a false-negative result for anti-tTG IgA levels, it is important to also check the total IgA level. If the patient has a low total IgA level, it may suggest an IgA deficiency, and therefore anti-tTG IgG or deaminated gliadin peptide IgG levels should be performed. Stool testing for fecal calprotectin or fecal lactoferrin to evaluate for inflammation in the intestines may be helpful. The fecal immunochemistry test evaluates for occult blood in the stool from gastrointestinal malignancy or IBD.

Red flag symptoms of persistent blood in the stool, anemia, unintentional weight loss, or progressive abdominal pain warrant further urgent evaluation. Patients with unexplained new onset of symptoms after age 50, IBD, or family history of colorectal cancer or inflammatory disease should undergo evaluation including endoscopy.

Targeted secondary evaluation is performed based on the differential diagnosis. If unable to narrow the differential, a comprehensive fecal analysis including fecal fat, osmolality, electrolytes, and pH from a 24- to 48-hour stool collection is suggested. Fecal testing can provide hints to the mechanism of action, either as watery, inflammatory, or fatty stool. Table 3 provides a chart to interpret the results of the fecal testing. Table 4 details a comparison of the recommended diagnostic testing by the AGA and BSG. Figure 1 is a flowchart detailing a diagnostic algorithm based on AGA and BSG guidelines.

TABLE 1 Elements of Detailed History in the Evaluation of Chronic Diarrhea

History of present illness	• Stool appearance and odor • Frequency and duration • Presence/absence of blood • Presence/absence of tenesmus, abdominal pain • Nocturnal pain or diarrhea
Family history	• Colorectal cancer or any other malignancy • Inflammatory bowel disease • Celiac disease • Autoimmune diseases

Surgical history	• Upper GI surgery
	  • May damage vagal nerve
	  • Rapid gastric emptying leading to an osmotic effect
	• Resection of ileum/ascending colon
	  • Decreases absorptive surfaces, decreases transit time
	  • May lead to bile acid diarrhea
	• Bypass procedures (e.g., gastric bypass, Roux-en-Y)
	  • May predispose for bacterial overgrowth because of stasis or abnormal motility
	  • Ineffective clearance of food
	• Cholecystectomy (up to 10% of postcholecystectomy patients are affected)
	  • Increased gut transit
	  • Bile acid diarrhea
	  • Increased enterohepatic cycling of bile acids

Medical history	• Pancreatic disease (chronic pancreatitis, alcohol usage, diabetes, pancreatic cancer)
	  • Pancreatic exocrine insufficiency due to impaired enzyme secretion
	• Thyrotoxicosis and hypoparathyroid disease, diabetes mellitus, adrenal disease, systemic sclerosis
	  • Autonomic dysfunction
	  • Small intestine bacterial overgrowth
	  • Endocrine effects
	  • Slow intestinal transit time
	• Medications
	  • Osmotic agents
	  • Secretory
	  • Motility
	  • Malabsorption
	• Recent infections or antibiotic usage
	  • Subsequent Clostridium difficile infection
	  • Postinfectious IBS due to change in intestinal flora and permeability

Diet history	• Alcohol
	  • Decreased pancreatic function
	  • Rapid gut transit
	  • Impairment of intestinal epithelium
	• FODMAPs
	  • Impaired digestion allowing for bacterial fermentation in colon
	• Milk
	  • Lactase deficiency leading to impaired digestion
	• Excessive caffeine (coffee, energy drinks)
	  • Increased gut motility

Travel history	• Endemic infections • Out of country travel • Immigration • Contaminated water sources • Tropical sprue

FODMAPs, Fermentable oligo-, di-, mono-saccharides and polyols; GI, gastrointestinal; IBS, irritable bowel syndrome.

Clinical Manifestations

Assessment for red flag symptoms (persistent blood in stool, anemia, unintentional weight loss, or progressive abdominal pain) should be performed as these suggest malignancy or IBD and require more urgent evaluation. Symptoms lasting for less than 3 months are more likely due to organic pathology than symptoms of longer duration. Table 5 provides a summary of the common causes of diarrhea, clinical features, diagnostic approach, and treatment.

Diarrhea-predominant irritable bowel syndrome (IBS-D) is a common cause of chronic diarrhea and can be diagnosed without further evaluation if symptoms are consistent with Rome IV criteria with normal physical examination, normal initial laboratory results, and no red flag symptoms. Modified Rome IV criteria include recurrent abdominal pain on average at least 1 day/week in the last 3 months, with symptom onset at least 6 months before diagnosis, associated with two or more of the following: (1) related to defecation, (2) associated with a change in the frequency of stool, or (3) associated with a change in the form (appearance) of stool. The British Society of Gastroenterology (BSG) recommends testing for bile acid diarrhea in patients for whom functional diarrhea or IBS-D is being considered. About one-third of patients diagnosed with IBS-D have bile acid diarrhea. However, the recommended selenium homocholic acid taurine test for bile acid diarrhea is not currently approved by the U.S. Food and Drug Administration or available in the United States. In the absence of available testing, a trial with bile acid sequestrants (e.g., cholestyramine [Questran][1] 4 g orally once a day up to a maximum of six times a day) may be beneficial, but an empiric trial before a diagnosis of IBS-D is made is not required. Additional treatment options include low FODMAP (fermentable oligo-, di-, monosaccharides and polyols) diet, tricyclic antidepressants, and cognitive behavioral therapy. The AGA has no recommendation for use of currently available testing to diagnose IBS.

Bile acid malabsorption causes watery secretory diarrhea due to impaired enterohepatic reabsorption of bile acids in the terminal ileum. This happens in nearly 10% of postcholecystectomy patients and can be seen in those with Crohn disease and microscopic colitis. Some patients experience symptom resolution spontaneously, but treatment with bile acid sequestrants can decrease symptoms and help with diagnosis.

Microscopic colitis presents with watery, secretory, nonbloody diarrhea. It is categorized as either lymphocytic or collagenous. Both categories have an increased number of intraepithelial and lamina propria lymphocytes. In addition, the collagenous type has a thickened subepithelial collagen band. There is a female predominance and the average age at presentation is 60 years, though about 25% of patients present before 45 years of age. Microscopic colitis frequently is associated with nocturnal diarrhea and fecal incontinence. It has a prevalence of about 10% of those diagnosed with IBS but may coexist with other systemic conditions such as autoimmune disease, thyroid disease, and celiac disease. Microscopic colitis has also been associated with medications such as nonsteroidal antiinflammatory drugs (NSAIDs), proton pump inhibitors, and sertraline. Diagnosis requires multiple biopsies of both the ascending and descending colon, even if macroscopic examination is normal. Ascending colon biopsies have better yield than rectal biopsies, but distal biopsies from flexible sigmoidoscopy also can be used to diagnose. There is no reliable biomarker for stool or serologic testing. Treatment of active disease includes extended-release oral budesonide (Entocort EC)[1] 6 to 9 mg/day for 6 to 8 weeks.

IBD, Crohn disease and ulcerative colitis, affects 1.3% of U.S. adults, presents between 10 and 35 years of age, and has an increasing prevalence with age. There is a 10-fold increased risk of developing IBD if there is a first-degree relative who has IBD. Rates of IBD are associated with higher intake of artificial sweeteners. IBD can cause secretory diarrhea, malabsorption, and intestinal fistulas. Presenting symptoms may include arthralgias and

---

[1] Not FDA approved for this indication.

TABLE 2	Categorization of Chronic Diarrhea Based on Mechanism of Action		
TYPES OF DIARRHEA		**MECHANISM OF ACTION**	**EXAMPLES**
Watery	Secretory	Reduced water absorption	• Bile acid malabsorption • Brainerd diarrhea • Crohn ileitis • Microscopic colitis • Postsurgical
	Osmotic	Water retention in intestines due to poorly absorbed solutes	• Carbohydrate malabsorption • Celiac disease
	Functional	Rapid intestinal transit that may be aggravated by stress or postinfectious enteritis	• IBS • Nonceliac gluten sensitivity • Functional diarrhea • Overflow (around impaction)
Inflammatory		Alterations of ion transport directly or indirectly from inflammatory cytokines leading to impaired epithelial barrier function and subsequent decreased water absorption	• Colorectal cancer • Inflammatory bowel disease • *Clostridium difficile* colitis (pseudomembranous colitis) • Parasitic infection • Postradiation colitis
Fatty	Malabsorption	Impaired nutrient absorption due to impaired ion transport systems, GI motility, bacterial flora, infection, compromised blood flow or lymphatic drainage	• Small intestine bacterial overgrowth • Structural (e.g., short bowel, gastric bypass, fistula) • Lymphatic damage (e.g., CHF) • Whipple disease • Tropical sprue
	Maldigestive	Impaired nutrient digestion due to compromised enzymatic activity (production or secretion), intestinal motility, or mucosal integrity	• Pancreatic exocrine insufficiency • Hepatobiliary disorder • Inadequate luminal bile acid

CHF, Congestive heart failure; *GI*, gastrointestinal; *IBS*, irritable bowel syndrome.

TABLE 3	Categorization of Diarrhea Based on Fecal Testing Results		
	WATERY	**INFLAMMATORY**	**FATTY**
Fecal Testing			
Fecal leukocytes	Absent	Present	Absent
Fecal lactoferrin or calprotectin	Absent	Present	Absent
Fecal blood	Absent	Present/absent	Absent
Fecal fat	Not elevated	Not elevated	Elevated

erythema nodosum. The evaluation for IBD includes fecal calprotectin or fecal lactoferrin, and CRP if the fecal tests are not available. Diagnosis can be aided by imaging (computed tomography or magnetic resonance imaging) or from macroscopic appearance and microscopic (biopsy) findings on endoscopy. Treatment includes antiinflammatory medications such as budesonide dosed as above for active disease; 5-aminosalicylic acids (mesalamine [Delzicol] 800 mg orally three times daily for 6 weeks for active disease or 800 mg orally twice daily for maintenance; mesalamine [Apriso] 1.5 g orally once daily for maintenance); sulfasalazine (Azulfidine) 500 to 1000 mg orally every 6 hours; immunomodulators; and biologics.

Celiac disease or gluten-sensitive enteropathy can present as malabsorptive fatty diarrhea or osmotic diarrhea from bile acid malabsorption. It has a prevalence of about 1% in the general population and is increasing. The prevalence is about 5% in those with chronic diarrhea. For those with a family history, the prevalence is 5% to 20%. Testing for celiac disease with IgA tTG is recommended for all patients with chronic diarrhea, even those meeting IBS criteria. Confirmation with duodenal biopsies is recommended. If serology is negative but clinical suspicion remains elevated, biopsies should be obtained. Biopsies may be negative if the patient is on a gluten-free diet. Nonceliac gluten sensitivity will have similar symptoms but no celiac specific antibodies, no intestinal changes, and no malabsorption.

Dietary-related diarrhea presents with bloating, abdominal pain, and diarrhea. Poorly digested foods are poorly absorbed in the small intestine and then become fermented by bacteria in the large intestine. FODMAPs are commonly associated with dietary-related diarrhea. High FODMAPs include fructose (e.g., fruits, sweeteners including high-fructose corn syrup), lactose (milk, cheese), fructans (wheat, cereal, onions, cabbage), galactans (legumes), and polyols (sorbitol, artificial sweeteners, stone fruits). Various hydrogen breath tests (lactose, fructose, sorbitol) are options for definitive testing for suspected intolerances and malabsorption, depending on availability. Decreased intake of the offending food often improves symptoms. For those with lactose intolerance due to lactase nonpersistence, over-the-counter lactase supplementation may be beneficial. A low FODMAP diet is difficult to adhere to but may help decrease symptoms.

Infections usually cause acute diarrhea but may also cause chronic diarrhea. *Clostridium difficile* may occur after a recent course of antibiotics and can persist because of failure of initial treatment or relapse. Testing for *C. difficile* should be a two-step approach, first using enzyme immunoassay (EIA), nucleic acid amplification, or polymerase chain reaction (PCR) technology to

TABLE 4 Side-by-Side Summary Comparison of Key Recommendations for Diagnostic Testing in the Evaluation of Chronic Diarrhea by the British Society of Gastroenterology and the American Gastroenterological Association

MEDICAL CONDITION	DIAGNOSTIC TEST	SENSITIVITY/ SPECIFICITY	AGA RECOMMENDATION AND LEVEL OF EVIDENCE	BSG GUIDELINES RECOMMENDATION AND LEVEL OF EVIDENCE
IBD	Fecal calprotectin, cutoff 50 µg/g	Sens 0.81 Spec 0.87	*Conditional recommendation, low-quality evidence*	Recommended to exclude colonic inflammation in those suspected with IBS and age < 40 years *Strong recommendation, LOE 1*
	Fecal lactoferrin, cutoff 7–7.25 µg/g	Sens 0.79 Spec 0.93		
	CRP, cutoff 5–6 mg/L	Sens 0.73 Spec 0.78	Recommends against use of CRP to screen for IBD unless fecal lactoferrin or calprotectin are not available *Conditional recommendation, low-quality evidence*	Recommended as part of initial blood tests
Giardia	*Giardia* antigens or PCR	Sens > 0.95 Spec > 0. 95	Recommends testing for *Giardia* in patients presenting with chronic watery diarrhea and to use antigen test or PCR test *Strong recommendation, high-quality evidence*	If suspect *Giardia*, use stool ELISA
Ova and parasites	Stool ova and parasites (three stool specimens)	Sens 0.6–0.9	In the absence of travel history or recent immigration from high-risk areas, AGA suggests against testing for ova and parasites (other than *Giardia*) *Conditional recommendation, low-quality evidence*	If suspect *Giardia*, order stool ELISA
Celiac disease	IgA tTG (IgA tTG), cutoff 7–15 AU/mL	Sens > 0.9 Spec > 0.9	Recommends testing for celiac disease with IgA tTG, with second test if IgA deficient (IgG tTG and IgG or IgA deaminated gliadin peptides) Confirm with duodenal biopsy *Strong recommendation, moderate-quality evidence*	Recommend screening for celiac disease with serological tests as part of initial screening, in primary care, and IgG EMA or IgG tTG if IgA deficient *Strong recommendations, LOE 1–3, moderate to strong quality evidence*
Bile acid diarrhea	Total bile acids in 48-hr stool collection		Recommends testing if available or empiric trial of bile acid sequestrants *Conditional recommendation, low-quality evidence*	Not available in UK
	SeHCAT		Not available in U.S.	All patients with persistent undiagnosed chronic diarrhea should be investigated for bile acid diarrhea with SeHCAT, or 7α-hydroxy-4-cholesten-3-one or fecal bile acid
IBS	No currently available serologic tests		No recommendation, knowledge gap	If has IBS-D or functional bowel, positive diagnosis of bile acid diarrhea should be made by SeHCAT testing or bile acid precursor 7α-hydroxy-4-cholesten-3-one if available *Strong recommendation, LOE 1*
PEI	Fecal elastase	Sens 0.73–1 Spec 0.8–1		Recommends testing when fat malabsorption is suspected *Strong recommendation, LOE 1, strong quality evidence*
Microscopic colitis	Colonoscopy with biopsies of ascending and descending colon (not rectal)			*Strong recommendation, LOE 1, strong quality evidence*

TABLE 4 Side-by-Side Summary Comparison of Key Recommendations for Diagnostic Testing in the Evaluation of Chronic Diarrhea by the British Society of Gastroenterology and the American Gastroenterological Association—cont'd

MEDICAL CONDITION	DIAGNOSTIC TEST	SENSITIVITY/ SPECIFICITY	AGA RECOMMENDATION AND LEVEL OF EVIDENCE	BSG GUIDELINES RECOMMENDATION AND LEVEL OF EVIDENCE
Clostridium difficile	Combination testing (PCR or EIA) to confirm presence of *C. difficile* and toxin EIA			*Strong recommendation, LOE 2*
SIBO	Culture of small bowel aspirates >10⁵ bacteria/ mL of jejunal fluid (gold standard)			*Weak recommendation* because methods are not standardized and positive results may not reflect clinically significant SIBO, LOE 2
	Hydrogen breath test (glucose or lactulose)	Sens 0.2–0.93 Spec 0.3–0.86	Suggest use of breath test in symptomatic patients with prior luminal abdominal surgery, symptomatic patients with suspected motility disorders, and patients with IBS *Conditional recommendation, very low level of evidence*	Does not recommend either glucose or lactulose breath test due to poor sensitivity and specificity for diagnosis of SIBO *Strong recommendation, LOE 2*

Level of evidence based on Oxford Center for Evidence-Based Medicine. *Level 1:* systematic review with homogeneity, individual RCTs. *Level 2:* systematic reviews of cohort studies, low quality RCTs and outcomes research. *Level 3:* systematic reviews with heterogeneity and individual case control studies. *Level 4:* poor quality cohort or case series. *Level 5:* expert opinion without critical appraisal.

AGA, American Gastroenterological Association; *BSG,* British Society of Gastroenterology; *CRP,* C-reactive protein; *EIA,* enzyme immunoassay; *ELISA,* enzyme-linked immunosorbent assay; *EMA,* endomysial antibodies; *IBD,* inflammatory bowel disease; *IBS,* irritable bowel syndrome; *IBS-D,* irritable bowel syndrome–diarrhea predominance; *IgA,* immunoglobulin A; *IgG,* immunoglobulin G; *LOE,* level of evidence; *PCR,* polymerase chain reaction; *PEI,* pancreatic exocrine insufficiency; *RCT,* randomized controlled trial; *SeHCAT,* selenium homocholic acid taurine test; *SIBO,* small intestinal bacterial overgrowth; *tTG,* tissue transglutaminase.

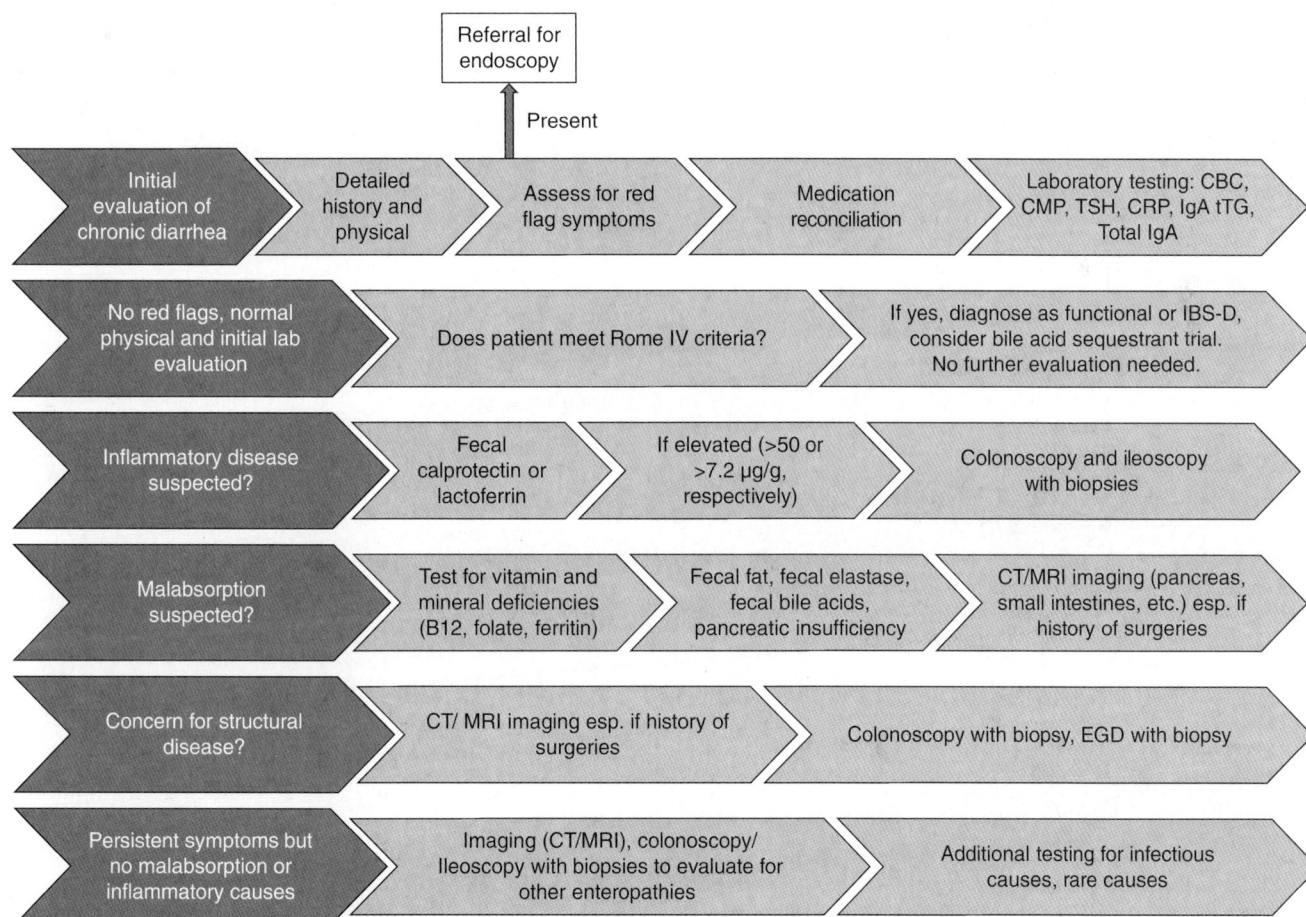

Figure 1 Diagnostic algorithm for evaluation of chronic diarrhea. *CBC,* Complete blood cell count; *CMP,* comprehensive metabolic panel; *CRP,* C-reactive protein; *CT,* computed tomography; *EGD,* esophagogastroduodenoscopy; *EMA,* endomysial antibodies; *IBS-D,* diarrhea-predominant irritable bowel syndrome; *IgA,* immunoglobulin A; *MRI,* magnetic resonance imaging; *TSH,* thyroid-stimulating hormone; *tTG,* tissue transglutaminase. Adapted from Gómez-Escudero O, Remes-Troche JM. Approach to the adult patient with chronic diarrhea: a literature review. *Rev Gastroenterol Mex (Engl Ed).* 2021;86:387-402.

TABLE 5 Summary of Common Causes of Chronic Diarrhea, Key Clinical Features, Diagnostic Testing, and Treatment

ETIOLOGY	KEY CLINICAL FEATURES	DIAGNOSTIC TESTING	TREATMENT OPTIONS EXAMPLES	ADDITIONAL COMMENTS
Colorectal cancer	Unintentional weight loss, change in stool appearance Abdominal pain and/or mass Family history New onset of symptoms age > 50 years	Colonoscopy	Surgical intervention Chemotherapy or radiation for the primary neoplasm if indicated	Common cause
Functional diarrhea or IBS-D	Rome IV criteria, normal physical exam, no red flag symptoms	CBC, CMP, CRP, anti-tTG IgA, total IgA (normal results)	Dietary changes, probiotics[7], tricyclic antidepressants (e.g., amitriptyline[1] 10 mg PO daily), rifaximin (Xifaxan) 550 mg tid for 14 days, loperamide (Imodium) 4–16 mg PO	Before diagnosing, consider trial of bile acid sequestrants (e.g., cholestyramine [Questran][1] 4 g PO once a day up to 4 g PO 6 times a day Very common cause
Bile acid malabsorption diarrhea	Similar to IBS-D Evaluate for surgical scars	48-hr fecal bile acids SeHCAT if available Trial of bile acid sequestrants FGF-19 if available	Dietary changes, bile acid sequestrants like cholestyramine (Questran)[1] 4 g PO once a day up to 4 g PO 6 times a day	Common cause Can be seen in 10% of patients who are postcholecystectomy
Microscopic colitis	Similar to IBS-D	Colonoscopy with biopsies of ascending and descending colon	Dietary changes Extended-release oral budesonide (Entocort EC)[1] 6–9 mg/day PO for 6–8 weeks for active disease	Has been associated with NSAIDS, PPIs, SSRIs Also associated with autoimmune disease, thyroid disorders, and celiac disease Common cause
IBD, includes Crohn disease and ulcerative colitis	Fever, weight loss, fatigue, anemia Bloody stool (hematochezia/melena) Abdominal pain Family history Physical exam: rectal ulcers, anal fissures, dermatitis, arthralgias	CBC, fecal calprotectin or lactoferrin, colonoscopy with biopsies, ileoscopy	Crohn disease: Extended-release oral budesonide (Entocort EC) 6–9 mg/day PO for 6–8 weeks for active disease Ulcerative colitis: 5-aminosalicylic acids – mesalamine (Delzicol) 800 mg PO tid for 6 weeks for active disease or 800 mg PO bid for maintenance – mesalamine (Apriso) 1.5 g PO once daily for maintenance Sulfasalazine (Azulfidine) 500–1000 mg PO every 6 hr Immunomodulators and biologics	Fatigue may be result from malabsorption/anemia, especially if involvement of terminal ileum Common cause
Celiac disease	Sensitivity to gluten Family history Type 1 diabetes Iron-deficiency anemia Dermatitis herpetiformis Systemic symptoms possible	Duodenal biopsies, tTG IgA and total IgA	Gluten-free diet	If patient has IgA deficiency, do IgG tTG If diagnostic evaluation is negative, patient may have nonceliac gluten sensitivity Common cause
Dietary related	Food triggers Family history Postprandial bloating, flatulence, diarrhea	Breath tests Trial of avoidance	Dietary changes (low-FODMAP diet) and avoidance of offending item	Common cause Example: lactase nonpersistence (lactose intolerance)
Clostridium difficile infection (pseudomembranous colitis)	Recent antibiotic use Healthcare stay Immunocompromise	Two-step approach to first use EIA, NAA, or PCR to detect the organism followed by testing for active toxin production with a toxin EIA	Nonfulminant: oral vancomycin 125 mg PO every 6 hr for 10 days Fulminant: oral vancomycin 500 mg PO every 6 hr with metronidazole (Flagyl)[1] 500 mg IV every 8 hr for 10 days Fecal transplant	1 in 6 patients may relapse within 2–8 weeks Infrequent cause
Giardia and other protozoan infection	Travel history or poor sanitation/unsafe water	Three stool samples for ova and parasites *Giardia* antigen, PCR or EIA	Metronidazole (Flagyl)[1] 250 mg PO three times a day for 5–7 days or 2000 mg PO once[3], tinidazole 1–2 g PO once or 300 mg PO daily for 7 days	Infrequent cause

ETIOLOGY	KEY CLINICAL FEATURES	DIAGNOSTIC TESTING	TREATMENT OPTIONS EXAMPLES	ADDITIONAL COMMENTS
HIV	Immunocompromised	HIV	Antiretroviral therapy with integrase inhibitor	50% of newly diagnosed HIV patients have chronic diarrhea
SIBO	History of surgery (especially with resection or blind loop like Roux-en-Y) Evaluate for surgical scars	Hydrogen breath tests Small bowel aspiration cultures with colonies >10⁵/mL	Rifaximin (Xifaxan)[1] 550 mg PO tid for 14 days or 10-day courses of amoxicillin/clavulanate (Augmentin)[1] 875 mg PO bid, ciprofloxacin[1] 500 mg PO bid, TMP-SMX (Bactrim DS)[1] 160/800 mg PO bid, metronidazole[1] 250 mg PO tid, or doxycycline[1] 100 mg PO daily or bid	Empirical treatment is appropriate Infrequent cause
Medication induced	May correlate with new medication or timing of doses	No specific tests	Medication reconciliation; trial off medication if appropriate	Common cause Laxative abuse or factitious diarrhea is rare but may occur; BSG recommends testing should be done on urine and stool periodically, in a specialist setting
PEI	History of chronic pancreatitis, diabetes, alcohol use disorder, cystic fibrosis Steatorrhea Weight loss	Fecal elastase-1, CT imaging	Dietary changes Pancreatic enzymes	Infrequent cause
Neuroendocrine tumors	Carcinoid syndrome (watery diarrhea, flushing, hypotension, right-sided heart failure) or asymptomatic	CT/MRI Lab tests for VIP, gastrin, glucagon if high clinical suspected	Surgical resection of tumor	Very rare

[1]Not FDA approved for this indication.
[3]Exceeds dosage recommended by the manufacturer.
[7]Available as dietary supplement.
bid, Two times daily; *BSG*, British Society of Gastroenterology; *CBC*, complete blood cell count; *CMP*, comprehensive metabolic panel; *CRP*, C-reactive protein; *CT*, computed tomography; *EIA*, enzyme immunoassay; *ELISA*, enzyme-linked immunosorbent assay; *FGF-19*, fibroblast growth factor 19; *FODMAP*, fermentable oligo-, di-, mono-saccharides and polyols; *HIV*, human immunodeficiency virus; *IBD*, inflammatory bowel disease; *IBS-D*, irritable bowel syndrome–diarrhea; *IgA*, immunoglobulin A; *IgG*, immunoglobulin G; *IV*, intravenously; *MRI*, magnetic resonance imaging; *NAA*, nucleic acid amplification; *NSAID*, nonsteroidal antiinflammatory drug; *PCR*, polymerase chain reaction; *PEI*, pancreatic exocrine insufficiency; *PO*, orally; *PPI*, proton pump inhibitor; *SeHCAT*, selenium homocholic acid taurine test; *SIBO*, small intestinal bacterial overgrowth; *SSRI*, selective serotonin reuptake inhibitor; *tid*, three times daily; *TMP-SMX*, trimethoprim/sulfamethoxazole; *tTG*, tissue transglutaminase; *VIP*, vasoactive intestinal peptide.

detect the organism and then testing for active toxin production with a toxin EIA. PCR testing alone may not account for symptoms because postinfectious IBS has been recognized to occur not just after acute gastroenteritis but also after *C. difficile* infections due to changes in intestinal flora and permeability. Nonfulminant *C. difficile* infections are treated with vancomycin 125 mg orally every 6 hours for 10 days, whereas fulminant *C. difficile* infection may be treated with vancomycin 500 mg orally every 6 hours plus metronidazole (Flagyl)[1] intravenously every 8 hours for 10 days. One in six patients will have a recurrence, which can be treated with vancomycin 125 mg orally every 6 hours for 14 days, then 125 mg orally every 12 hours for 7 days, then 125 mg daily for 7 days, followed by 2 to 8 weeks of 125 mg orally every 2 to 3 days. Good hand hygiene, contact precautions, and usage of spore-killing disinfectants will prevent the spread of infection. Advising patients to take probiotics[7] with their antibiotics may decrease the likelihood of *C. difficile* infection.

Protozoan infections, such as *Giardia*, can occur in patients who have had a recent travel history or potential exposure to poor sanitation and unsafe water. Testing *Giardia* in the stool requires enzyme-linked immunosorbent assay technology. Treatment is

with metronidazole (Flagyl) 250 mg orally three times a day for 5 to 7 days or 2000 mg orally once[3], tinidazole 1 to 2 g orally once or 300 mg orally daily for 7 days. If suspecting other protozoan infections, three stool specimens for ova, cysts, and parasites are recommended for diagnosis, with a 60% to 90% chance of detection.

In immunocompromised patients with chronic diarrhea, the BSG recommends testing for the human immunodeficiency virus (HIV). Chronic diarrhea is among the most common symptoms in a patient with newly diagnosed HIV and so needs to be excluded.

Small intestine bacterial overgrowth (SIBO) is an infrequent cause of chronic diarrhea, can be seen in patients with gastric bypass surgeries with a blind loop, and is diagnosed by noninvasive hydrogen breath testing or cultures from a proximal small bowel aspirate. The BSG finds insufficient evidence to recommend hydrogen breath testing but does recommend empiric treatment with antibiotics. Factors that increase the likelihood of SIBO are prior gastric surgery, intestinal pseudoobstruction, diverticula or strictures of the small bowel, or systemic disease like diabetes or scleroderma. Treatment with empiric antibiotics is appropriate,

[1]Not FDA approved for this indication.
[7]Available as dietary supplement.

[1]Not FDA approved for this indication.
[3]Exceeds dosage recommended by the manufacturer.

TABLE 6 Commonly Used Classes of Medications That Can Cause Chronic Diarrhea

- 5-aminosalicylic acids (e.g., mesalamine, sulfasalazine)
- Angiotensin-converting enzyme inhibitors
- Antibiotics (cephalosporins, fluoroquinolones, macrolides)
- Antihyperglycemic medications (acarbose, dipeptidyl peptidase IV inhibitors, metformin, sulfonylureas)
- Antineoplastic agents
- H2 histamine receptor antagonists
- Lipase inhibitor (orlistat [Xenical, Alli])
- Magnesium-containing antacids
- Nonsteroidal antiinflammatory drugs
- Osmotic agents and laxatives
- Proton pump inhibitors
- Selective serotonin reuptake inhibitors
- Thyroid hormones

and current first-line therapy is rifaximin (Xifaxan)[1] 550 mg orally three times daily for 14 days because of its tolerability. Other antibiotic regimens include 10-day courses of amoxicillin and clavulanate (Augmentin)[1] 875 mg orally twice daily, ciprofloxacin[1] 500 mg orally twice daily, trimethoprim/sulfamethoxazole (Bactrim DS)[1] 160/800 mg orally twice daily, metronidazole[1] 250 mg orally three times daily, or doxycycline[1] 100 mg orally every day or twice daily.

Medication-induced diarrhea accounts for up to 4% of chronic diarrhea cases. More than 700 medications have diarrhea as a reported side effect. Medications can induce diarrhea through osmotic, secretory, or malabsorptive mechanisms. Commonly used classes of medications (Table 6) that can cause diarrhea include NSAIDs; magnesium-containing antacids; H2 histamine receptor antagonists; proton pump inhibitors; aminosalicylates (e.g., mesalamine); antibiotics (penicillins, macrolides, fluoroquinolones, cephalosporins); selective serotonin reuptake inhibitors; antihyperglycemic medications (acarbose, sulfonylureas, dipeptidyl peptidase IV inhibitors, metformin); angiotensin-converting enzyme inhibitors; osmotic agents and laxatives; antineoplastic agents; thyroid hormone; and lipase inhibitor (orlistat [Xenical, Alli])

Overflow diarrhea is a common cause of chronic diarrhea and can present or be confounded with fecal incontinence. Overflow diarrhea results when severe fecal rectal loading causes paradoxical leakage around impacted stool. Risk factors include a history of constipation, opiate usage, older age, hemorrhoids, anal fissures, and dementia. Impacted stool may be found during digital rectal exam or anoscopy. Treatment involves digital disimpaction and management of constipation.

Pancreatic exocrine insufficiency (PEI) is an infrequent cause of chronic fatty diarrhea (steatorrhea) and occurs when lipase secretion is less than 10% of normal levels or if there are other enzyme deficiencies. PEI causes maldigestion of foods in the small intestine and fermentation by bacteria of the foods in the large intestine. It may develop 10 to 15 years after the onset of chronic pancreatitis and should be suspected in patients with a history of pancreatic carcinoma, chronic pancreatitis, or pancreatic surgery. Diagnosis involves a single stool sample test for fecal elastase (normal is 200 to 500 μg/g; mild to moderate pancreatic exocrine insufficiency is 100 to 200 μg/g, severe deficiency is <100 μg/g). The fecal elastase biomarker has 73% to 100% sensitivity and 80% to 100% specificity for moderate to severe PEI. The test may not be useful for mild pancreatic insufficiency and may not reliably distinguish pancreatic insufficiency from nonpancreatic malabsorption.

Neuroendocrine tumors are rare causes of chronic diarrhea, with a prevalence of 10 per million population. Neuroendocrine tumors include vasoactive intestinal peptide-secreting tumors (VIPomas), gastrinomas, and glucagonomas and can present with a wide variety of symptoms. Diagnosis requires testing for and demonstrating elevated serum hormone concentrations (VIP, gastrin, glucagon). Up to 50% of patients with carcinoid syndrome will have diarrhea. When patients present with chronic diarrhea as a result of carcinoid syndrome, it almost always occurs in the context of hepatic metastasis. Carcinoid syndrome accounts for about 20% of midgut neuroendocrine tumors. Elevated 24-hour urinary 5-hydroxy-indoleacetic acid has a high sensitivity and specificity for carcinoid syndrome, but testing may be affected by the patient's dietary intake.

Treatment

Treatment of chronic diarrhea is based on the underlying etiology. Treatment options include avoidance of the offending medication or food, antibiotics if appropriate, and antidiarrheal medications. Antidiarrheal therapy with antimotility or antisecretory agents can reduce stool frequency but should be avoided if the patient has bloody diarrhea or high fever. Loperamide (Imodium) 4 mg orally once then 2 mg orally after each loose stool (maximum 16 mg/day) to decrease gut peristalsis can be used. Bile acid sequestrants bind bile acids and decrease the secretory effects of bile acids on the colon. Clonidine is an alpha-2-adrenergic agonist (0.3 mg every day or twice daily) which slows the intestinal tract and is useful for diarrhea in IBS[1], chemotherapy-induced diarrhea[1], and diarrhea due to loss of noradrenergic innervation in patients with diabetes[1] but may have strong antihypertensive side effects.

Complications

Because of the fluid losses from frequent stooling, dehydration, subsequent renal injury, and electrolyte abnormalities may occur. A CMP should be obtained and monitored. Depending on the etiology, patients with chronic diarrhea may be at risk for malabsorption of nutrients and should be evaluated for anemia (iron deficiency, folate deficiency, B12 deficiency) and other deficiencies.

---

[1] Not FDA approved for this indication.

References

Arasaradnam RP, Brown S, Forbes A, et al: Guidelines for the investigation of chronic diarrhoea in adults: British Society of Gastroenterology, 3rd edition, *Gut* 67:1380–1399, 2018. Available at. https://gut.bmj.com/content/gutjnl/67/8/1380.full.pdf. Accessed December 14, 2022.

Center for Disease Control and Prevention. Brainerd Disease. Available at https://www.cdc.gov/ncezid/dfwed/diseases/brainerd-diarrhea/index.html. Accessed 20/12/2022.

Center for Disease Control and Prevention. Inflammatory Bowel Disease (IBD). Available at https://www.cdc.gov/ibd/. Accessed 20/12/2022.

Gomez-Escudero O, Remes-Troche JM: Approach to the adult patient with chronic diarrhea: a literature review, *Rev Gastroenterol México*(86)387–402, 2021. Available at http://www.revistagastroenterologiamexico.org/en-approach-adult-patient-with-chronic-articulo-S2255534X21000876. Accessed March 1, 2023.

Lacy BE, Patel NK: Rome criteria and a diagnostic approach to irritable bowel syndrome, *J Clin Med* 6(11):99, 2017. Available at https://www.ncbi.nlm.nih.gov/mc/articles/PMC5704116/. Accessed January 11, 2023.

Pimentel M, Saad RJ, Long MD, Rao SSC: ACG clinical guideline: small intestinal bacterial overgrowth, *Am J Gastroenterol* 00:1–14, 2020. Available at https://pubmed.ncbi.nlm.nih.gov/32023228/. Accessed December 20, 2022.

Resourcepharm. Drug Induced Diarrhoea. Available at https://www.resourcepharm.com/pre-reg-pharmacist/drug-induced-diarrhoea.html. Accessed 01/03/2023.

Sachdev AH, Pimentel M: Gastrointestinal bacterial overgrowth: pathogenesis and clinical significance, *Ther Adv Chronic Dis* 4(5):223–231, 2013. Available at https://www.ncbi.nlm.nih.gov/pmc/articles/PMC3752184/. Accessed December 14, 2023.

Shane AL, Mody RK, Crump JA, et al: 2017 Infectious Diseases Society of America clinical practice guidelines for the diagnosis and management of infectious diarrhea, *Clin Infect Dis* 65(12):e45–e80, 2017. Available at https://www.idsociety.org/practice-guideline/infectious-diarrhea/. Accessed December 12, 2022.

Singh P, Mitsuhashi S, Ballou S, et al: Demographic and dietary associations of chronic diarrhea in a representative sample of adults in the United States, *Am J Gastroenterol* 113(4):593–600, 2018. Available at https://pubmed.ncbi.nlm.nih.gov/29610515. Accessed December 14, 2022.

Tangri V, Chande N: Use of budesonide in the treatment of microscopic colitis, *Saudi J Gastroenterol* 16(3):236–238, 2010. Available at https://www.ncbi.nlm.nih.gov/pmc/articles/PMC3003217/. Accessed 1 March 2023.

---

[1] Not FDA approved for this indication.

CIRRHOSIS

Method of
Sunny Sandhu, MD; and Paul Martin, MD

CURRENT THERAPY

- Management of the various complications of cirrhosis can be complex and often involves evaluation by a hepatologist and, in some cases, a multidisciplinary team.
- Nonselective β-blockers have been shown to increase decompensation-free survival in patients with compensated advanced chronic liver disease and are being increasingly used.
- Liver transplantation remains a lifesaving intervention for patients with end-stage liver disease.

CURRENT DIAGNOSIS

- Cirrhosis remains a histopathologic diagnosis; however, the diagnosis can be inferred by noninvasive testing and/or clinical manifestations.
- Recently, noninvasive liver disease assessment modalities have emerged, including serum tests, vibration-controlled transient elastography (VCTE), and magnetic resonance elastography.
- Diagnosis of clinically significant portal hypertension (CSPH) can now be performed utilizing non-invasive methods, including VCTE.

TABLE 1	Etiologies of Cirrhosis
ETIOLOGY	**EXAMPLES**
Infectious	Hepatitis B Hepatitis C Hepatitis D
Autoimmune and cholestasis	Autoimmune hepatitis Biliary atresia Primary biliary cholangitis Primary sclerosing cholangitis Secondary biliary cirrhosis Secondary sclerosing cholangitis
Toxins	Alcohol Arsenic Drugs
Metabolic	Metabolic dysfunction-associated steatohepatitis α_1-Antitrypsin deficiency Hemochromatosis Wilson disease Glycogen storage diseases Lysosomal storage diseases Galactosemia
Vascular	Cardiac cirrhosis Budd-Chiari syndrome Sinusoidal obstruction syndrome
Granulomatous	Sarcoidosis Tuberculosis Syphilis
Cryptogenic	Unrecognized metabolic-associated fatty liver disease, infections, or drugs

Cirrhosis, although a histopathologic diagnosis characterized by significant liver remodeling, with development of regenerative nodules and fibrous septa, can be inferred by imaging and/or clinical manifestations. The development of cirrhosis reflects chronic hepatic necroinflammatory activity with an incomplete and disorganized repair process resulting in regenerative nodules and extensive fibrosis with replacement of normal hepatic parenchyma and disturbance of normal hepatic physiology. Activation of hepatic stellate cells into myofibroblasts and matrix deposition are key steps in the pathogenesis of cirrhosis. Cirrhosis can result from various etiologies of chronic liver disease (Table 1). Recently the term *advanced chronic liver disease* (ACLD) has been introduced to more accurately reflect the later stages of chronic liver disease, which is now viewed as part of a continuous spectrum, extending from extensive fibrosis to end-stage cirrhosis. This term has gained growing acceptance with the development of noninvasive tests (NITs), such as liver stiffness measurements (LSMs) and various proprietary and nonproprietary blood tests.

Epidemiology

The prevalence of cirrhosis varies in different regions of the world. The estimated global prevalence of cirrhosis is 4.5% to 9.5% in adults; however, this is likely an underestimate as cirrhosis is often not recognized in asymptomatic individuals. Similarly, it is difficult to obtain accurate estimates of mortality related to cirrhosis, but countries in Central and South America and southern Europe report the highest mortality rates, particularly in males. Epidemiologic trends of cirrhosis have evolved. For instance, widespread immunization against hepatitis B virus (HBV) has markedly reduced the incidence, prevalence, and associated burden of liver disease, including cirrhosis due to chronic HBV infection. In contrast, global alcohol consumption has increased in recent years with a rise in hospitalizations for alcohol-related liver disease in younger adults, most notably since the COVID-19 pandemic. Elsewhere in the world with increased prosperity alcohol consumption has risen, with a corresponding increase in liver disease. A quarter of deaths due to cirrhosis are estimated to be alcohol related. In contrast, successful treatment of hepatitis C virus (HCV) results in reduction of hepatic dysfunction, liver-related and all-cause mortality, and complications of cirrhosis, such as hepatocellular carcinoma (HCC) and portal hypertension. The growing prevalence of metabolic dysfunction-associated steatotic liver disease (MASLD), previously known as nonalcoholic fatty liver disease, is reflected in its current prominence as a major cause of cirrhosis. MASLD has become the most frequent cause of chronic liver disease and cirrhosis in many countries. The development of cirrhosis can be accelerated by the presence of concomitant risk factors, for example, metabolic syndrome in combination with alcohol excess.

Clinical Findings

In the absence of hepatic decompensation, the majority of individuals with cirrhosis are asymptomatic and may exhibit only subtle clinical findings. Clues to the presence of cirrhosis can include elevated serum aminotransferases and/or bilirubin, decreased albumin, and prolongation of the prothrombin time. Approximately 10% to 17% of individuals with unexplained elevation of aminotransferases have unrecognized cirrhosis. Thrombocytopenia in the absence of a primary hematologic explanation is an important clue to the presence of cirrhosis and primarily reflects hypersplenism due to portal hypertension but also diminished production of thrombopoietin, a platelet growth and development factor synthesized by the liver. A platelet count below $160 \times 10/\mu L$ provides the highest diagnostic accuracy for cirrhosis among routine blood tests (sensitivity 74%, specificity 88%, positive likelihood ratio 6.3, negative likelihood ratio 0.29). Thrombocytopenia is also a component of noninvasive scoring systems that predict fibrosis, such as the aspartate aminotransferase to platelet ratio index (APRI) and Fibrosis-4 (FIB-4).

Physical examination may reveal somewhat diminished liver span by percussion and a firm liver edge on palpation.

TABLE 2 Stages of Cirrhosis Based on Clinical Complications and 1-Year Outcome Probabilities

CIRRHOSIS	D'AMICO STAGE	COMPLICATIONS	PROBABILITY OF ADVANCING TO NEXT STAGE	1-YEAR MORTALITY
Compensated	Stage 1	(–) varices (–) ascites	7%	1%
	Stage 2	(+) varices (–) ascites	6.6%	3.4%
Decompensated	Stage 3	(+) ascites (+) varices	7.6%	20%
	Stage 4	(+) variceal hemorrhage (+) ascites	–	57%

From D'Amico G, Garcia-Tsao G, Pagliaro L: Natural history and prognostic indicators of survival in cirrhosis: a systematic review of 118 studies, *J Hepatol* 44:217–231, 2006.

Splenomegaly is suggested by dullness to percussion in the left upper abdominal quadrant or a palpable spleen tip. Cutaneous manifestations of cirrhosis include palmar erythema, spider nevi, facial telangiectasia, decreased chest and/or axillary hair, inversion of the normal male pubic hair pattern, Terry nails ("ground glass" appearance of nails with absent lunula), and Muehrcke nails (paired, white, transverse bands separated by normal color). Finger clubbing may also be present in individuals with cirrhosis, particularly if complicated by the hepatopulmonary syndrome. Dupuytren contracture is relatively common in alcohol-related cirrhosis, but its pathogenesis is not well understood. Palmar erythema due to altered sex hormone metabolism is more evident on the thenar and hypothenar eminences and typically spares the central portion of the palm. Hypogonadism in both sexes and gynecomastia and testicular atrophy in males can be detected, reflecting altered sex hormone metabolism (increased production of androstenedione, enhanced aromatization to estrone, and increased conversion to estradiol). The catabolic effects of advanced cirrhosis often result in marked sarcopenia, which adversely affects quality of life and survival and is also associated with poorer outcomes after liver transplantation.

Various noninvasive methods for evaluation of liver fibrosis are now available for staging of hepatic fibrosis and diagnosis of cirrhosis. In addition to APRI and FIB-4, a variety of serum tests have been developed to estimate the extent of fibrosis in chronic liver disease and are typically available through reference laboratories. Other technologies to evaluate fibrosis include vibration-controlled transient elastography (FibroScan), acoustic radiation force impulse, shear wave and point quantification elastography, and magnetic resonance elastography.

Natural History of Cirrhosis and Prognostic Models

Cirrhosis has typically been divided into two distinct phases, regardless of etiology: compensated and decompensated. Compensated cirrhosis implies the absence of complications, such as jaundice, ascites, hepatic encephalopathy (HE), or gastroesophageal variceal hemorrhage. Hepatic decompensation indicates a more advanced phase of the disease, typically progressive and characterized by development of one or more complications and diminished hepatocellular function with prolongation of the prothrombin time and hypoalbuminemia. Characterizing cirrhosis as compensated or decompensated is simple and reproducible and offers useful prognostic information for clinical practice (Table 2).

More recently, the term ACLD has been introduced to reflect the continuum within the spectrum of cirrhosis, which is a shift away from requiring a histologic or radiologic diagnosis of cirrhosis for initial patient risk stratification. There are two main stages of ACLD: compensated advanced chronic liver disease (cACLD) and decompensated advanced chronic liver disease (dACLD), after the development of at least one decompensating event (Table 3). cACLD typically progresses slowly through a

TABLE 3 Diagnosis of Clinically Significant Portal Hypertension with NIT

Rule out CPSH (>90%)	LSM ≤15 kPa and platelet ≥150 × 10⁹/L SSM ≤40 kPa
Probable CSPH (60%)	LSM 15–20 kPa and platelet count <110 × 10⁹/L
Rule in CSPH (>90%)	LSM ≥25 kPa LSM >20 kPa and platelet <150 × 10⁹/L SSM >40 kPa

CSPH, Clinically significant portal hypertension; *LSM*, liver stiffness measurement; *NIT*, noninvasive testing; *SSM*, splenic stiffness measurement.

relatively slower and asymptomatic stage for a median duration of about 10 years. However, if the etiology of chronic liver disease remains untreated, such as chronic viral hepatitis, ongoing liver fibrosis and structural changes result in increases in portal pressure, reflected in the hepatic venous pressure gradient (HVPG), and the development of dACLD.

Two stages of cACLD have been described based on HVPG. The first stage, which is characterized by the absence of portal hypertension (HVPG <5 mm Hg) or mild portal hypertension (HVPG 5 to 9 mm Hg), has an overall good prognosis with a mortality rate of ~1% per year. The second stage, which is characterized by clinically significant portal hypertension (CSPH) with HVPG ≥10 mm Hg, progresses with development of portosystemic collaterals, varices, and hyperdynamic changes (such as increased cardiac output and blood volume, and splanchnic and systemic vasodilation). In this stage, patients are at a higher risk of developing decompensation (at a rate of about ~5% per year). Further progression of portal hypertension with HVPG levels of >15 mm Hg is associated with increased mortality. As an alternative to invasive HVPG measurement, cACLD can also be clinically diagnosed and staged as CSPH with endoscopic or imaging findings of varices of any size, portosystemic collaterals, or reversal of portal blood flow on Doppler ultrasound. Notably, CSPH may be present in nearly 50% of patients without varices.

Decompensated ACLD signifies progression of CSPH and is characterized by the development of an index complication such as ascites, variceal bleed, or HE. Ascites is the most common decompensating event, with a 5-year cumulative incidence up to 25%, while variceal bleeding and encephalopathy occur at rates of 5% and 3%, respectively. The development of decompensation is of ominous significance, as a single decompensating event implies a 1-year mortality rate of about 10% compared with about 30% in those with multiple decompensating events. The development of further decompensation drastically increases risk of mortality.

A severe subtype of dACLD is acute-on-chronic liver failure (ACLF), which is characterized by abrupt deterioration, multiorgan failure, and a high risk of short-term mortality. Although

TABLE 4	Child-Turcotte-Pugh Classification		
CLINICAL AND LABORATORY CRITERIA	**POINTS**		
	1	**2**	**3**
Albumin (g/dL)	>3.5	2.8–3.5	<2.8
Ascites	None	Mild to moderate (diuretic responsive)	Severe (diuretic refractory)
Bilirubin (mg/dL)	<2	2–3	>3
Encephalopathy	None	Mild to moderate (grade 1 or 2)	Severe (grade 3 or 4)
Prothrombin time Prolongation in seconds International normalized ratio	<4 <1.7	4–6 1.7–2.3	>6 >2.3

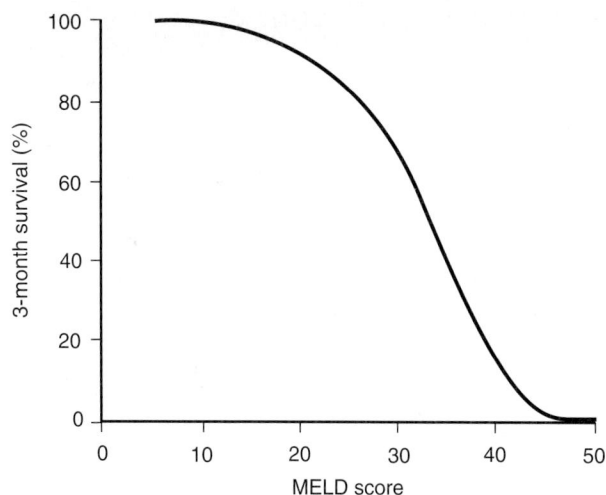

Figure 1 Relationship between Model for End-Stage Liver Disease *(MELD)* score and survival at 3 months. (From Carrion AF, Martin P: *Sleisenger and Fordtran's gastrointestinal and liver disease,* ed 11, Philadelphia, 2021, Elsevier, p. 1538.)

several definitions exist, the American Association for the Study of Liver Diseases (AASLD) suggests the following minimal criteria: (1) acute onset with rapid clinical deterioration, (2) presence of liver failure (defined by elevated INR and bilirubin) in a patient with chronic liver disease with or without cirrhosis, and (3) failure of at least another organ system (neurologic, circulatory, respiratory, renal). ACLF has a 28-day mortality rate of up about 50% depending on the number of organ systems involved. An inciting event is often implicated, which can be primarily hepatic (e.g., alcohol-associated hepatitis) or nonliver related, with infection being most commonly implicated. Although several scoring systems have been developed including the NACSELD ACLF, CLIF-C ACLF score, and CLIF-SOFA score, they share similar components. The management of ACLF typically involves critical care management of multiorgan failure, addressing the precipitating event, and consideration for liver transplantation if feasible.

Prognostic models in cirrhosis such as the Child-Turcotte-Pugh (Table 4) and the Model for End-Stage Liver Disease (MELD) are widely used, the latter the most accurate predictor of short-term mortality in cirrhosis and serving as the basis for the current organ allocation system for liver transplantation in the United States and elsewhere (calculator available at https://optn.transplant.hrsa.gov/data/allocation-calculators/meld-calculator/). The MELD score has undergone several modifications over time; the current version (MELD 3.0) includes serum creatinine, bilirubin, international normalized ratio (INR), serum sodium, albumin, age, and sex. Incorporation of the serum sodium in the MELD formula increases its prognostic accuracy in patients with relatively low scores and hyponatremia. Compared with earlier versions, which did not take into account sex, the most recent MELD score provides more accurate prediction of mortality for women as their lower muscle mass results in lower creatine and hence creatinine production.

Specific etiology of cirrhosis may help determine its prognosis. For instance, persistent viremia in individuals with chronic HBV or HCV infection is implicated in the development of decompensated cirrhosis. Effective antiviral therapy can abort progression of chronic viral hepatitis to cirrhosis and decompensation.

Although cirrhosis per se is not an indication for liver transplantation, an index complication of cirrhosis such as gastroesophageal variceal hemorrhage, ascites, or HE is an indication to consider liver transplantation. The MELD score provides objective and reproducible prognostication of short-term survival without liver transplantation (Figure 1). Liver transplantation is associated with improved survival in individuals with MELD scores >17.

Major Complications of Cirrhosis
Portal Hypertension
Although portal hypertension can be inferred by clues such as splenomegaly with thrombocytopenia in a patient with cirrhosis,

it is defined by an HVPG >5 mm Hg. This gradient is calculated by subtracting the measured free hepatic vein pressure from the wedged hepatic venous pressure (a measurement that reflects portal venous pressure by using the same hemodynamic principle as the wedged pulmonary capillary pressure to assess left atrial pressure). As stated earlier, CSPH typically occurs when the HVPG is ≥10 mm Hg; above this threshold, gastroesophageal varices and ascites develop. Unfortunately, accurate noninvasive measurement of portal pressure is not routinely available, limiting use of HVPG in clinical practice as it requires passage of a transjugular catheter. In the United States, these measurements are typically performed by an interventional radiologist.

Increased intrahepatic resistance to portal venous flow aggravated by increased splanchnic blood flow in cirrhosis leads to portal hypertension. In addition to cirrhosis, which is the most common cause of portal hypertension in Western countries (hepatic schistosomiasis is the leading cause in areas where this infection is common), other disorders may result in prehepatic or posthepatic portal hypertension. Portal vein thrombosis is a common cause of prehepatic portal hypertension. Cardiomyopathy, constrictive pericarditis, Budd-Chiari syndrome, and inferior vena cava webs may result in posthepatic portal hypertension. Ascites and gastroesophageal variceal hemorrhage are the two most common complications of portal hypertension in cirrhosis. Less common but clinically significant complications include portal hypertensive gastropathy, hepatic hydrothorax, hepatopulmonary syndrome, portopulmonary hypertension (PoPH), and hepatorenal syndrome (HRS).

More recently, there has been increasing use of NITs to identify patients with CSPH in cACLD (Table 5). Numerous studies have supported the use of vibration-controlled transient elastography to predict CSPH and risk of hepatic decompensation. The presence of LSM by transient elastography of ≥25 kPa has been found to be highly specific and can be used to rule in CSPH, whereas a liver stiffness of ≤15 kPa and platelet count of >150 × 10⁹/L has been found to be accurate in excluding CSPH and can obviate the need for a screening endoscopy for varices as recommended in the Baveno VII criteria. Similar recommendations are also made in the AASLD guidance, with LSM ≥25 kPa or LSM >20 kPa and platelet count <150 × 10⁹/L as indicators of CSPH. Noninvasive blood-based testing such as the enhanced liver fibrosis and FIB-4 tests are also accurate in predicting decompensation in cACLD.

Gastroesophageal Variceal Hemorrhage
Portal hypertension leads to formation of multiple portosystemic collaterals, including gastroesophageal varices. Formation of gastroesophageal varices typically occurs when the HVPG is ≥10 mm

TABLE 5 Stages of Advanced Chronic Liver Disease

SUBTYPE OF ACLD	HVPG RANGE	CLINICAL FEATURES
Compensated ACLD with absence of portal hypertension	HVPG <5 mm Hg	Early cirrhosis Asymptomatic or mild symptoms
Compensated ACLD with mild portal hypertension	HVPG 5–9 mm Hg	Portal pressures are mildly elevated but still well compensated
Compensated ACLD with CSPH	HVPG ≥10 mm Hg	Development of varices, portosystemic collaterals, or hepatofugal flow on imaging Further development of hyperdynamic circulation Increased risk of decompensation and HCC Goal of therapy: prevent development of clinical decompensation (NSBB)
Decompensated ACLD with advanced portal hypertension	HVPG ≥12 mm Hg	Increased risk of variceal bleeding
	HVPG ≥16 mm Hg	Increased risk of rebleeding and refractory ascites Associated with increased mortality
	HVPG ≥20 mm Hg	Very high-risk population Associated with failure to control active bleeding, early rebleeding and death

ACLD, Advanced chronic liver disease; *CSPH,* clinically significant portal hypertension; *HCC,* hepatocellular carcinoma; *HVPG,* hepatic venous pressure gradient; *NSBB,* nonselective beta blocker.

TABLE 6 Recommendations for Primary Prophylaxis Against Esophageal Variceal Hemorrhage

SIZE OF VARICES	RISK OF HEMORRHAGE	SURVEILLANCE INTERVAL	PRIMARY PROPHYLAXIS
No varices	CTP class A	EGD every 2 years if ongoing liver injury (i.e., obesity or alcohol abuse) or every 3 years if liver injury is quiescent (i.e., viral eradication or alcohol abstinence)	None
	CTP class B/C	EGD yearly	None
Small esophageal varices	CTP class A	EGD yearly if ongoing liver injury (i.e., obesity or alcohol abuse) or every 2 years if liver injury is quiescent (i.e., viral eradication or alcohol abstinence)	BB may be used
	CTP class B/C	EGD yearly; if BB are used, repeat EGD unnecessary	BB recommended
Large esophageal varices	CTP class A/B/C	If BB are used, repeat EGD unnecessary; if no BB, repeat EGD for EVL every 2–8 weeks until variceal eradication, then once in 3–6 months, and regularly every 6–12 months	Either BB or EVL recommended

Child-Turcotte-Pugh class obtained by adding points for each variable.
Class A: 5 to 6 points (compensated cirrhosis); class B: 7 to 9 points (decompensated cirrhosis); class C: 10 to 15 points (decompensated cirrhosis).
BB, Beta blocker; *CTP,* Child-Turcotte-Pugh; *EGD,* esophagogastroduodenoscopy; *EVL,* endoscopic variceal ligation.

Hg, with the risk of variceal hemorrhage increasing once HVPG is >12 mm Hg. Gastroesophageal varices are present in approximately 50% of patients with cirrhosis and commonest in patients with overt hepatic decompensation (Child-Turcotte-Pugh class C). Variceal hemorrhage is the most dramatic complication of cirrhosis and occurs at a rate of 5% to 15% per year. Risk factors for variceal hemorrhage include larger variceal size, more advanced hepatic decompensation, and identification of vascular "red wale" signs during endoscopic evaluation. Esophageal varices are classified according to their size as small (≤5 mm) or large (>5 mm).

Screening for gastroesophageal varices with esophagogastroduodenoscopy (EGD) has previously been recommended when cirrhosis is suspected; however, as discussed earlier the presence of LSM <15 kPa and platelet count of >150 × 10^9/L may obviate the need for a screening endoscopy. Management strategies for patients with esophageal varices that have not previously bled (primary prophylaxis) are summarized in Table 6.

Management of esophageal varices that have previously bled (secondary prophylaxis) includes a combination of a nonselective β-blocker with endoscopic variceal ligation (EVL). The dose of the nonselective β-blocker should be titrated to the maximal tolerated dose (resting heart rate of 55 to 60 beats/min or 25% decrease from baseline), and EVL should be repeated frequently (every 2 weeks or so) until complete variceal obliteration. Carvedilol (Coreg)[1] is the agent of choice due to its anti–α_1-adrenergic activity, which diminishes intrahepatic resistance in addition to nonselective cardiac β-blockade with reduction of portal pressure. Recurrence of esophageal varices may occur after EVL; thus surveillance EGD is recommended. Repeat EGD should be performed 3 to 6 months after variceal obliteration and then at 6- to 12-month intervals.

Gastric varices can be classified according to their relationship to esophageal varices and location (Table 7). The role of endovascular interventions such as transjugular intrahepatic portosystemic shunt (TIPS), retrograde transvenous obliteration (RTO), or endoscopic ultrasound (EUS)-guided therapies for primary prophylaxis of gastric variceal bleeding remains controversial and should be decided on a case-by-case basis.

Acute variceal hemorrhage occurs at a yearly rate of 5% to 15% and is associated with high mortality (at least 20% at 6 weeks). Adequate resuscitation is crucial in acute variceal hemorrhage with some additional precautions. Patients with variceal hemorrhage are at high risk for aspiration, and endotracheal intubation for airway protection should be considered before

---

[1] Not FDA approved for this indication.

TABLE 7	Classification of Gastroesophageal and Gastric Varices and Recommendations for Primary Prophylaxis		
TYPE OF VARICES	**CHARACTERISTICS**		**PRIMARY PROPHYLAXIS**
Gastroesophageal varices type 1 (GOV1)	Extension of esophageal varices along the lesser curvature into the gastric cardia		Similar to esophageal varices
Gastroesophageal varices type 2 (GOV2)	Extension of the esophageal varices along the greater curvature into the gastric fundus		BB can be used, although data not as strong as for esophageal varices
Isolated gastric varices type 1 (IGV1)	Gastric varices localized in the fundus		If high risk, consider BB or cyanoacrylate injection
Isolated gastric varices type 2 (IGV2)	Gastric varices localized in the antrum		No data, consider BB if high risk

BB, Beta blocker.

endoscopy. Overly aggressive expansion of blood volume should be avoided because it may result in increased portal venous pressure. A target hemoglobin level between 7 and 9 g/dL is appropriate. Current guidelines recommend against correcting the INR by use of fresh frozen plasma or recombinant factor VIIa (NovoSeven RT)[1] because this has not shown a clear benefit in individuals with acute variceal hemorrhage. There are no data to support or recommend against transfusion of platelets in this situation. Prophylactic broad-spectrum antibiotics (i.e., intravenous ceftriaxone [Rocephin][1]) reduce bacterial infections, risk of rebleeding, and mortality. Administration of vasoactive drugs such as octreotide (Sandostatin)[1] or terlipressin (Terlivaz)[1] results in increased rates of initial endoscopic control of bleeding, reduced 7-day mortality, and lower transfusion requirements. EGD is recommended within 12 hours, and EVL is the endoscopic treatment of choice for management of esophageal varices. Balloon tamponade (i.e., Sengstaken Blakemore, MN, or Linton-Nachlas tubes) or esophageal stenting are effective rescue therapies when variceal hemorrhage cannot be controlled with standard endoscopic therapy. The role of TIPS has expanded from a salvage intervention for individuals with recurrent variceal hemorrhage after EVL to an early "preemptive" intervention in carefully selected individuals at high risk for treatment failure (Child-Turcotte-Pugh class B with active bleeding or Child-Turcotte-Pugh class C, but with MELD scores ≤13) after EVL, as it appears to result in better outcomes than β-blocker plus EVL. Patients who survive an episode of variceal hemorrhage should receive secondary prophylaxis with a combination of a nonselective β-blocker and repeated EVL until complete obliteration of the varices is achieved. Endovascular interventions such as TIPS or RTO and EUS-guided cyanoacrylate and/or endovascular coil injection are the treatments of choice for management of gastric variceal hemorrhage.

Ascites

Ascites is pathologic accumulation of fluid in the peritoneal cavity (>25 mL) and is the commonest complication of cirrhosis. Portal hypertension is required for development of cirrhotic ascites, as individuals with HVPG <12 mm Hg do not develop this complication. Importantly, sinusoidal hypertension appears to be a requirement for development of ascites, because prehepatic portal hypertension does not typically result in its development. Other relevant mechanisms include splanchnic vasodilatation and its consequences, such as humorally mediated sodium retention and diminished free-water excretion by the kidneys, hypoproteinemia and reduced oncotic pressure, and disruption of normal lymphatic drainage in the liver due to extensive fibrosis.

Ascites can be detected on physical examination when its volume is >1500 mL, although ultrasonography can detect as little as 100 mL. Clinical signs include flank dullness on percussion, shifting dullness, and, if the amount of ascites present is large, demonstration of a fluid wave. A diagnostic paracentesis is mandatory in the following settings: new-onset ascites and/

or change in clinical status, including any hospitalization of a patient with previously diagnosed ascites or evidence of infection (such as diminished renal function or abdominal pain) in a cirrhotic patient with ascites to exclude spontaneous bacterial peritonitis (SBP). The following tests on the fluid are indicated: leukocyte count with differential, culture (on two blood culture bottles inoculated at the bedside), total protein, and albumin. The appearance of the ascitic fluid may yield important clinical clues (Table 8). The serum-to-ascites albumin gradient, obtained by subtracting the ascitic fluid albumin value from the serum albumin value, helps make a distinction between transudative and exudative ascites. A gradient of ≥1.1 g/dL confirms portal hypertension as the etiology of ascites, whereas a value <1.1 g/dL suggests etiologies other than portal hypertension. The absolute number of polymorphonuclear (PMN) cells in the ascitic fluid is an important clue to SBP.

Ascites can be classified according to the amount of fluid accumulation and/or response to treatment. Grade 1 or mild ascites is only detectable by ultrasonography and responds to diuretic therapy with or without moderate dietary sodium restriction. Grade 2, or moderate, ascites is characterized by moderate abdominal distention and recurs on at least three occasions within a 12-month period despite adequate diuretic therapy and moderate sodium restriction. Grade 3, or large-volume, ascites causes marked, usually tense, abdominal distention, is refractory to medical therapy (diuretics and sodium restriction), and recurs after large-volume paracentesis (LVP).

Management of ascites grades 1 and 2 is centered on sodium restriction rather than free-water restriction, and the use of diuretics. Total dietary intake of sodium should be <2000 mg (88 mmol)/day, and compliance with this intervention can be documented by monitoring urinary sodium concentrations. A sodium-to-potassium concentration ratio >1 on a random urine sample correlates well with a 24-hour sodium excretion >78 mmol/day and implies compliance with sodium restriction. Nevertheless, dietary restriction of sodium is efficacious in only 10% of patients, and enhanced natriuresis is typically needed to provide adequate control of ascites. Combining diuretics that work at different nephron sites is more effective than using a single agent. Aldosterone is upregulated in cirrhosis owing to diminished effective arterial blood volume and consequential increased renin and angiotensin activity, resulting in enhanced renal sodium and free water retention. Spironolactone (Aldactone) competitively inhibits aldosterone-dependent sodium–potassium exchange in the distal convoluted renal tubule and the collecting ducts. The recommended initial dose of spironolactone for patients with ascites due to portal hypertension is 100 mg/day PO. Administration of a loop diuretic usually furosemide (Lasix) is recommended in addition to spironolactone, because it potentiates natriuresis. The recommended initial dose for furosemide is 40 mg/day PO. Further increases in doses of diuretics should be made maintaining this 100:40 ratio to a maximum dose of 400 mg/day PO of spironolactone and 160 mg/day PO of furosemide to prevents hypokalemia or hyperkalemia. Renal function and electrolytes must be monitored regularly, particularly after dose modification. Tender

---

[1] Not FDA approved for this indication.

TABLE 8	Characteristics of Ascitic Fluid and Differential Diagnosis	
FLUID APPEARANCE	**DIFFERENTIAL DIAGNOSIS**	**BIOCHEMICAL HINTS ON FLUID ANALYSIS**
Clear	Uncomplicated transudative ascites due to cirrhosis	WBC <500 cells/µL, PMN <250 cells/µL, SAAG ≥1.1
Turbid/cloudy	Infection	PMN ≥250 cells/µL
Bloody	Traumatic paracentesis, hemoperitoneum	RBC >10,000 cells/µL
Milky	Chylous ascites due to obstruction or trauma of lymphatic vessels or thoracic duct	Triglycerides >200 mg/dL

PMN, Polymorphonuclear cells; *RBC,* red blood cell; *SAAG,* serum-to-ascites albumin gradient; *WBC,* white blood cell.

gynecomastia is an unpleasant side effect of spironolactone, and some patients may need to discontinue it, in which case amiloride (Midamor)[1] (10 to 20 mg/day PO) can be used. Two outcomes may occur in patients with ascites that is not adequately controlled with diuretics: (1) diuretic-resistant ascites, or persistent ascites despite maximum diuretic doses and sodium restriction, which typically recurs rapidly after LVP; or (2) diuretic-intractable ascites, or the inability to increase diuretic doses owing to symptomatic hypotension or deterioration in renal function as evidenced by increasing serum creatinine levels.

Grade 3 ascites requires repeated LVP. Removal of >5 L of ascitic fluid per session combined with intravenous albumin infusion (6 to 8 g of albumin per liter of ascitic fluid removed during or immediately after LVP) is a safe and effective intervention to treat refractory ascites; however, mortality within 6 months is 20% once this develops, reflecting the severity of the underlying liver disease, and thus patients should be referred for liver transplantation. Continued dietary restriction of sodium is necessary to avoid overly frequent LVP, and continuation of diuretics should be assessed on a case-by-case basis, taking into consideration potential benefits and adverse reactions. Expansion of plasma volume during LVP is endorsed by current guidelines and supported by data demonstrating reduced postparacentesis circulatory dysfunction and improved survival. Insertion of an indwelling peritoneal catheter is not recommended for cirrhotic ascites due to risk of introducing infection.

Insertion of TIPS offers an attractive alternative for amelioration of refractory ascites in selected patients instead of repeated LVP. TIPS is a minimally invasive technique in which an endovascular stent is used to create an intrahepatic portocaval shunt and has replaced surgical shunts. Transplant-free survival is superior with TIPS compared with repeated LVP. Careful cardiac evaluation is recommended before TIPS as significant hemodynamic changes occur after the creation of the portosystemic shunt that can result in post-TIPS heart failure in individuals with underlying systolic or diastolic dysfunction.

The MELD score is a prognostic model that was initially developed to assess risk of death after TIPS placement, and data demonstrate that patients with a MELD score >18 are at high risk of mortality. TIPS results in HE in a high proportion of patients, but pharmacologic therapy typically provides adequate amelioration.

Hyponatremia is present in almost half of patients with cirrhosis and ascites and reflects expanded volume rather than dehydration. Mild hyponatremia (126 to 135 mEq/L) can be managed by free water restriction and frequent monitoring. Moderate (120 to 125 mEq/L) or severe (<120 mEq/L) hyponatremia requires intervention. Acute hyponatremia can usually be corrected without concern for osmotic demyelinating syndrome (ODS), but severe chronic hyponatremia requires gradual correction to minimize the risk of ODS. Treatment is centered on discontinuation of diuretics and laxatives, free water restriction, and administration of intravenous albumin and vasopressin receptor agonists such as tolvaptan (Samsca). Hypertonic saline may be used in selected cases in the short term to correct symptomatic or severe hyponatremia or for patients with imminent liver transplant.

Spontaneous Bacterial Peritonitis

Cirrhosis and portal hypertension are associated with abnormal intestinal permeability leading to bacterial translocation resulting in SBP. The most commonly isolated microorganisms implicated in SBP are *Escherichia coli* (43%), *Klebsiella pneumoniae* (11%), *Streptococcus pneumoniae* (9%), other streptococcal species (19%), Enterobacteriaceae (4%), *Staphylococcus* (3%), and miscellaneous organisms depending on the region of the world (10%). A small-volume diagnostic paracentesis (30 to 60 mL) rather than LVP (which can increase the risk of HRS if SBP is present) is mandatory for confirmation of SBP before administration of antibiotic therapy. Aerobic and anaerobic blood culture bottles should be inoculated at the bedside to avoid contamination and increase diagnostic yield. Diagnosis of SBP is supported by the presence of ≥250 PMN/µL in the ascitic fluid without an obvious source of infection. Based on the PMN count and the microbiologic analysis of the ascitic fluid, four clinical scenarios summarized in Table 9 may be encountered.

Treatment of SBP is by broad-spectrum empiric antibiotics with bactericidal activity against the most likely infecting bacteria. Third-generation cephalosporins such as cefotaxime (Claforan) 2 g IV every 8 hours or ceftriaxone (Rocephin) 2 g IV daily offer appropriate antimicrobial coverage and are initial agents of choice for treatment of SBP when multidrug-resistant organisms (MDRO) are not suspected. For patients allergic to β-lactams, alternatives include fluoroquinolones such as levofloxacin (Levaquin)[1], although this agent exhibits less penetration into the ascitic fluid compared with a third-generation cephalosporin. In settings of high prevalence of MDRO, broader-spectrum antibiotics such as piperacillin/tazobactam (Zosyn) and daptomycin (Cubicin)[1] or meropenem (Merrem) should be used.

Current guidelines recommend repeat paracentesis 48 hours after initiating antibiotics to assess response (decrease in PMN count >25% from baseline). Lack of response should lead to broadening antibiotic coverage and exclusion of secondary peritonitis.

Plasma volume expansion with albumin[1] is an important adjunct to antibiotic therapy in patients with SBP to decrease the incidence of acute kidney injury (AKI) and reduces mortality. The physiologic effects of intravenous infusion of albumin include increased oncotic pressure with consequential expansion of the effective arterial blood volume, as well as its ability to bind a wide range of endogenous and exogenous ligands, including bacterial lipopolysaccharides, reactive oxygen species, nitric oxide and other nitrogen reactive species, and prostaglandins, thus modulating the inflammatory response. The recommended dosage of albumin 25% is 1.5 g/kg of body weight within 6 hours of establishing the diagnosis of SBP and a second dose of 1 g/kg on day 3.

After an episode of SBP, recurrence occurs in 69% of individuals within 1 year; thus secondary prophylaxis is indicated and current guidelines recommend long-term use of ciprofloxacin (Cipro)[1] 500 mg/day PO or trimethoprim-sulfamethoxazole

---

[1] Not FDA approved for this indication.

[1] Not FDA approved for this indication.

| | TABLE 9 | Spontaneous Bacterial Peritonitis and Associated Conditions Based on Characteristics of the Ascitic Fluid |

CLINICAL ENTITY	POLYMORPHONUCLEAR CELL COUNT	CULTURE RESULTS	ANTIBIOTICS RECOMMENDED
Spontaneous bacterial peritonitis	≥250 cells/μL	Positive, single organism	Yes
Culture-negative neutrocytic ascites	≥250 cells/μL	Negative	Yes
Monomicrobial nonneutrocytic bacterascites	<250 cells/μL	Positive, single organism	Yes
Polymicrobial bacterascites	<250 cells/μL	Positive, multiple organisms	Yes

(Bactrim DS)[1] one double-strength tablet PO daily. Risk factors for recurrent SBP include ascitic fluid total protein concentration <1 g/dL and gastroesophageal variceal hemorrhage. Recommended antibiotic prophylaxis for patients hospitalized with gastroesophageal variceal hemorrhage include ceftriaxone[1] 1 g/day intravenously; once the patient is able to tolerate oral antibiotics, this may be changed to ciprofloxacin (Cipro)[1] 500 mg/day PO for a total of 7 days of antibiotic therapy. Importantly, some data suggest an increased risk for SBP in patients with cirrhosis and ascites taking proton pump inhibitors; thus unnecessary use of these agents should be avoided. The exact mechanism by which acid suppression increases the risk of SBP in cirrhosis is unclear, but intestinal bacterial overgrowth, increased intestinal permeability, and altered intestinal immune response may play a role.

Hepatorenal Syndrome

The ominous significance of impaired renal function as a predictor of mortality in patients with cirrhosis is reflected by inclusion of the serum creatinine level in the MELD score. Renal dysfunction is commonly encountered in patients with cirrhosis, particularly in those with hepatic decompensation. Some studies report AKI in approximately 20% of hospitalized patients with cirrhosis. The differential diagnosis of AKI in patients with cirrhosis is broad and includes common etiologies such as acute tubular necrosis and nephrotoxicity, but specific glomerulopathies associated with HBV and HCV must be considered (i.e., membranous and membranoproliferative glomerulonephritides) in infected patients. In addition, metabolic dysfunction-associated steatohepatitis is characterized by a high prevalence of type 2 diabetes mellitus and systemic hypertension; thus patients are at increased risk for diabetic and hypertensive nephropathies. HRS is one of several potential causes of AKI that occurs in patients with cirrhosis and portal hypertension but also has been recognized in patients with acute liver failure (ALF). Importantly, HRS is a diagnosis of exclusion. The pathophysiology of HRS includes splanchnic vasodilatation causing a decline in renal perfusion with consequent reductions in the glomerular filtration rate and renal excretion of sodium (typically <10 mEq/L).

There are two distinct phenotypes of HRS depending on the acuity and severity of renal dysfunction. HRS-AKI, previously known as type I HRS, is characterized by rapid deterioration of renal function with at least a twofold increase in serum creatinine to a level >2.5 mg/dL and is often precipitated by SBP, acute alcoholic hepatitis, or gastrointestinal hemorrhage. Criteria for diagnosis of HRS-AKI includes (1) cirrhosis with ascites; (2) diagnosis of AKI according to the International Club of Ascites–AKI criteria (increase in serum creatinine by ≥0.3 mg/dL within 48 hours or increase in serum creatinine to ≥1.5 times baseline within 7 days); (3) absence of shock; (4) no sustained improvement of renal function (serum creatinine <1.5 mg/dL) after at least 2 days of diuretic withdrawal and volume expansion with albumin at 1 g/kg/day up to 100 g/day; (5) no current or recent exposure to nephrotoxic agents; and (6) absence of parenchymal renal disease as defined by proteinuria <0.5 g/day, no microhematuria (<50 red cells/high-power field), and normal renal ultrasonography. HRS–chronic kidney disease (CKD), previously referred to as type II HRS, is

more indolent and is associated with less profound renal impairment, typically resulting in ascites resistant to diuretics. Prognosis also differs significantly for both types of HRS, with the median survival in the absence of liver transplantation being 2 weeks for HRS-AKI and 6 months for HRS-CKD.

Discontinuation of all diuretics and nephrotoxic agents is critical in patients with HRS. Plasma volume expansion with administration of 25% albumin[1] IV at a dose of 1 g/kg of body weight (up to a maximum of 100 g/day) to increase renal perfusion is recommended. HRS is characterized by absent or minimal proteinuria (<500 mg/day) and normal urine sediment reflecting the lack of intrinsic renal disease. Renal ultrasonography is also recommended to exclude parenchymal changes that suggest preexisting chronic renal disease and rules out obstructive nephropathy.

Patients with HRS require either improvement in hepatocellular function or liver transplantation for renal recovery. Pharmacotherapy can be used as a bridge to liver transplantation. Based on the pathophysiology of HRS-AKI, vasoconstriction with α-adrenergic agonists (i.e., midodrine [Amatine][1] or norepinephrine [Levophed][1]) or vasopressin analogs (i.e., terlipressin [Terlivaz]) are therapies of choice along with plasma volume expansion achieved with intravenous albumin infusion. Terlipressin is now licensed for use in the United States. The combination of the somatostatin analog octreotide[1] along with oral midodrine[1] and IV albumin infusion[1] also has beneficial effects in HRS-AKI. Data from a meta-analysis support the efficacy of vasoconstrictor therapy (terlipressin, octreotide + midodrine, or norepinephrine) in combination with IV albumin in reducing short-term mortality in patients with type I HRS. The largest randomized clinical trial (RCT) to date evaluating terlipressin in combination with albumin versus placebo plus albumin confirmed the efficacy of terlipressin in reversal of HRS-AKI. Renal replacement therapy may be needed for patients with HRS not responding to pharmacologic therapy awaiting liver transplantation; however, mortality is exceedingly high and hypotensive episodes commonly occur during hemodialysis. After liver transplantation, renal function improves in approximately 60% of patients with HRS. However, in patients who develop renal failure within 1 year of liver transplantation, current US allocation protocols allow for prioritization of kidney transplantation as a safety net to improve survival rates after liver transplantation.

Hepatic Encephalopathy

HE is a clinical syndrome of reversible neuropsychiatric impairment of varying severity. There is continuing controversy about its exact pathogenesis, but gut-derived toxins, including ammonia, are clearly implicated. Features of HE may be subclinical (covert) or clinically evident (overt) and include a wide range of neuropsychiatric signs and symptoms. The prevalence of HE varies depending on the clinical subtype and the severity of liver disease, with cumulative prevalence rates of up to 80% for covert HE and 30% to 40% for overt HE in patients with cirrhosis. Although the West Haven criteria are widely used for grading severity of HE (Table 10), current guidelines recommend using three additional axes to classify HE based on the etiology, time course, and presence or absence of a precipitating factor (Table 11).

---

[1] Not FDA approved for this indication.

[1] Not FDA approved for this indication.

TABLE 10	West Haven Criteria for Grading Hepatic Encephalopathy		
GRADE	LEVEL OF CONSCIOUSNESS	INTELLECT AND BEHAVIOR	NEUROLOGIC FINDINGS
0	Normal	Normal	Normal examination, abnormal neuropsychiatric testing
1	Mild lack of awareness	Shortened attention span	Impaired addition or subtraction, mild asterixis
2	Lethargy	Mild-moderate disorientation, inappropriate behavior	Severe asterixis, slurred speech
3	Somnolence but arousable	Severe disorientation, inexplicable behavior	Clonus, hyperreflexia, muscular rigidity
4	Coma	Coma	Decerebrate posture

TABLE 11	Classification of Hepatic Encephalopathy Based on Four Different Axes			
TYPE OF HEPATIC ENCEPHALOPATHY	GRADE		TIME COURSE	SPONTANEOUS/PRECIPITATED
A (acute liver failure)	MHE	Covert	Episodic (1 episode in 6 months)	Spontaneous: no precipitating factor discovered
B (portosystemic bypass)	1	Covert	Recurrent (>1 episode in 6 months)	
	2	Overt	Persistent (no return to normal baseline)	Precipitated by one or more specific factors
C (cirrhosis)	3	Overt		
	4	Overt		

MHE, Minimal hepatic encephalopathy.
From Patidar KR, Bajaj JS: Covert and overt hepatic encephalopathy: diagnosis and management, *Clin Gastroenterol Hepatol,* 13:2048–2061, 2015.

Covert HE is considered preclinical and encompasses minimal HE (features of HE that are only diagnosed by specialized neuropsychiatric testing) and grade 1 HE by West Haven criteria. In contrast, overt HE is characterized by clinical findings of HE ranging from subtle changes in orientation and presence of asterixis to hepatic coma (grades 2 to 4 per West Haven criteria).

Specialized testing is necessary to establish a diagnosis of covert HE. The psychometric HE score is regarded as the gold standard, but additional assessments include the number connection test, computerized tests such as the inhibitory control test, the cognitive drug research battery, and electroencephalogram. These tests, however, are not applicable in routine clinical practice and usually require consultation with a specialist. A smartphone application that evaluates psychomotor speed and cognitive alertness has been developed and validated as a point-of-care screening tool for covert HE: EncephalApp Stroop.

The diagnosis of overt HE is clinical and supported by the presence of a wide spectrum of global neurologic deficits. Severe HE, grades 3 and 4 West Haven criteria, should prompt airway protection by endotracheal intubation.

There are no laboratory markers that can be accurately used to diagnose overt HE. Blood ammonia levels lack sensitivity and specificity and correlate poorly with the severity of encephalopathy. Furthermore, a normal ammonia level does not preclude the presence of HE, and venous ammonia levels are influenced by several other factors, including phlebotomy technique and handling of the blood specimen. Efforts must be directed at identifying potential precipitants for HE, such as compliance with treatment of HE, new medications, gastrointestinal bleeding, AKI, electrolyte imbalance, and infection.

Management of covert and overt HE is centered on the use of nonabsorbable disaccharides and antibiotics. Lactulose (Enulose, Generlac) is the most widely used nonabsorbable disaccharide. Although the exact mechanism responsible for its therapeutic efficacy is still unclear, this agent is degraded by colonic microbiota to short-chain organic acids, resulting in acidification of the intestinal lumen and increased conversion of absorbable ammonia to nonabsorbable ammonium. The initial dose for lactulose depends on the acuity and severity of HE but must be titrated to achieve two to three soft bowel movements per day. For patients who cannot tolerate oral administration (i.e., high risk for aspiration or coma), lactulose can be administered as an enema (300 mL of lactulose solution 10 g/15 mL in 700 mL of saline or water). The cathartic effects of nonabsorbable disaccharides may result in profuse diarrhea, dehydration, and hypernatremia. Rifaximin (Xifaxan) is a broad-spectrum antibiotic with activity against gram-positive, gram-negative, and anaerobic enteric bacteria that can be used in addition to lactulose for prevention of recurrent episodes of HE. Data from clinical trials show marked reductions in HE-related hospitalization and significant improvements in health-related quality of life in patients treated with a combination of lactulose and rifaximin without an increased rate of adverse events.

The efficacy and safety of other pharmacologic therapies such as probiotics[7], branched-chain amino acids[7], L-ornithine L-aspartate (LOLA)[7], ammonia scavengers, and other laxatives (i.e., polyethylene glycol [MiraLAX][1]) need further evaluation. Because of concerns about ototoxicity and nephrotoxicity, neomycin is no longer used.

Portosystemic shunt creation, now usually with TIPS, for management of complications of portal hypertension is associated with a 13% to 36% incidence of overt HE. Careful patient selection before insertion of TIPS and medical therapy with nonabsorbable disaccharides with or without additional rifaximin remain standard therapy; however, despite compliance, approximately 3% to 7% of patients have recurrent or persistent overt HE post-TIPS. For these patients, endovascular techniques aimed at decreasing the size of the shunt should be considered.

Liver transplantation offers definitive therapy for patients with end-stage liver disease, resulting in restoration of hepatic synthetic function and resolution of neurologic complications associated with portal hypertension. However, in some patients, a degree of residual cognitive impairment may persist or newly develop after liver transplantation, adversely affecting health-related quality of life.

---

[7] Available as dietary supplement.
[1] Not FDA approved for this indication.

Hepatocellular Carcinoma

HCC is the most common primary hepatic malignancy in adults, and is the fifth most common cancer and the second leading cause of cancer-related death worldwide. The epidemiology of HCC varies significantly by region and ethnicity. The majority of patients with HCC in Western populations (95%) have underlying cirrhosis (predominantly due to chronic HCV infection, alcohol-related liver disease, and metabolic dysfunction-associated steatohepatitis), thus limiting applicability of surgical resection (see later) as curative therapy. In contrast, only 60% of patients with HCC in Eastern populations have cirrhosis, largely reflecting the high prevalence of chronic HBV infection and its oncogenic potential. Regions of the world with intermediate-to-high incidence of this malignancy (>3 cases per 100,000 persons per year) include Asia, sub-Saharan Africa, and Western Europe. North and South America have been typically considered low-incidence regions; however, over the past 2 decades there has been a steady increase in the incidence of HCC, particularly in the United States.

Current guidelines endorse implementation of surveillance strategies for early diagnosis of HCC in at-risk individuals with use of ultrasonography with or without serum alpha-fetoprotein (AFP) levels every 6 months. Populations at risk for HCC that may benefit from surveillance include those with cirrhosis of any etiology, Asian males with chronic HBV over age 40, Asian females with chronic HBV over age 50, patients with chronic HBV and family history of HCC, African/North American Black populations with chronic HBV, and individuals with stage 4 primary biliary cholangitis.

HCC can be accurately diagnosed without the need for liver biopsy by contrast-enhanced multiphase cross-sectional imaging modalities such as computed tomography (CT) or magnetic resonance imaging (MRI) based on specific patterns of contrast enhancement of the tumor in relation to the hepatic parenchyma. Key diagnostic characteristics for HCC on CT or MRI are contrast enhancement of the tumor during the early arterial phase and "washout" of contrast from the tumor during the portal venous and delayed phases. Additional features include presence of a capsule and interval growth of the lesion on serial imaging. Biopsy of the tumor carries a small risk for tumor seeding in the biopsy needle tract (~3%) and is rarely required to diagnose HCC due to the diagnostic accuracy of CT and MRI. Results from a recent meta-analysis demonstrate that the use of serum AFP in addition to ultrasound increases the sensitivity of HCC detection. AFP levels >200 ng/mL are highly specific for HCC, and longitudinal follow-up of serum levels permits evaluation of response to therapeutic interventions. Additional serologic markers for HCC include the L3 isoform of AFP (AFP-L3) and des-gamma carboxy prothrombin; however, further validation of these tests for surveillance of individuals at risk for HCC is still required.

The Barcelona Clinic Liver Cancer (BCLC) staging system can be used to categorize patients with HCC and to assist with therapeutic decisions (Figure 2). Surgical resection of HCC is reserved for patients with a single lesion and an absence of portal hypertension. Locoregional therapies include several ablative modalities such as radiofrequency ablation, transarterial chemoembolization (TACE), radioembolization with Y90, cryoablation, and microwave ablation. These modalities are typically used for patients with very early, early, and intermediate stages (BCLC stages 0, A, and B, respectively). TACE is favored for patients with multinodular disease (BCLC stage B). Liver transplantation is an effective treatment for patients with cirrhosis and HCC within the so-called Milan criteria: a single lesion ≤5 cm or no more than three lesions with the largest one being <3 cm and in the absence of portal venous invasion or metastatic disease. Liver transplantation for HCC within these limits results in long-term survival equivalent to that seen in patients with cirrhosis but no HCC. Under the current organ allocation policy in the United States, patients with HCC within Milan criteria are listed for liver transplantation with their biologic MELD score (calculated by the MELD formula and without exception points)

for 6 months, after which time they automatically accrue MELD exception points based on the median MELD score at transplant of all recipients within a specified geographic area in relationship to the candidate's listing transplant center. MELD exception points are granted to patients with HCC ≥2 cm in an effort to balance risk of death that is not adequately represented by the degree of hepatic dysfunction. For patients with HCC listed for liver transplantation, the use of locoregional therapies is recommended to prevent tumor progression that may result in dropout from the waiting list. Furthermore, active surveillance is recommended to evaluate for tumor recurrence or progression, development of new lesions, and metastatic disease while awaiting liver transplantation.

The number of systemic treatments licensed for use in patients with HCC has expanded significantly in recent years, with multiple options now available for first- and second-line therapy, including immunotherapies, checkpoint inhibitors, tyrosine kinase inhibitors, and monoclonal antiangiogenic antibodies. Adverse reactions, tolerability, and potential benefits must be carefully weighed and individualized according to overall health and performance status, as well as severity of hepatic dysfunction. The survival benefit of these agents is modest.

Portopulmonary Hypertension

Pulmonary artery hypertension in a patient with established portal hypertension is indicative of PoPH, in the absence of another explanation. The prevalence of PoPH varies depending on the severity of liver disease and has been reported in 0.7% of patients with cirrhosis but can be as high as 12.5% in patients undergoing evaluation for liver transplantation.

The exact pathophysiology of PoPH remains enigmatic, but increased exposure to humoral vasoconstrictors in the pulmonary vasculature due to portosystemic shunting and hyperdynamic circulation is among the most widely accepted hypothesis. Histologic findings in the pulmonary vasculature of patients with PoPH are indistinguishable from those found in idiopathic pulmonary arterial hypertension and include medial hypertrophy with remodeling of the pulmonary artery walls and occasional in situ microthrombosis.

The majority of patients with PoPH remain largely asymptomatic for extended periods of time. Symptoms associated with PoPH are similar to those of other types of pulmonary arterial hypertension and include dyspnea on exertion, syncope, chest pain, fatigue, hemoptysis, and orthopnea. Physical examination may demonstrate jugular venous distention and lower extremity edema, the latter typically being out of proportion to the severity of ascites. Cardiopulmonary auscultation usually reveals normal clear breath sounds throughout both lung fields, an accentuated pulmonic component of the second heart sound, and a systolic murmur located along the left sternal border that is accentuated with inspiration (tricuspid regurgitation). Chest radiographs may demonstrate right ventricular enlargement and a prominent pulmonary artery.

The diagnostic workup for PoPH should begin with transthoracic echocardiography, which provides an estimate of right ventricular and pulmonary arterial pressures and excludes left ventricular dysfunction. An estimated right ventricular systolic pressure ≥45 mm Hg is typically used as a threshold to obtain more accurate direct hemodynamic measurements through right heart catheterization. Hemodynamic criteria used to diagnose PoPH include mean pulmonary artery pressure (mPAP) >20 mm Hg, pulmonary capillary wedge pressure ≤15 mm Hg, and pulmonary vascular resistance of ≥160 dyn · s · cm^{-5} (2 Wood units) by right heart catheterization.

Pharmacologic therapy includes endothelin receptor antagonists (bosentan [Tracleer][1] and ambrisentan [Letairis][1]), phosphodiesterase inhibitors (sildenafil [Revatio][1] and tadalafil [Adcirca, Alyq, Tadliq][1]), and prostacyclin analogs (epoprostenol

---

[1] Not FDA approved for this indication.

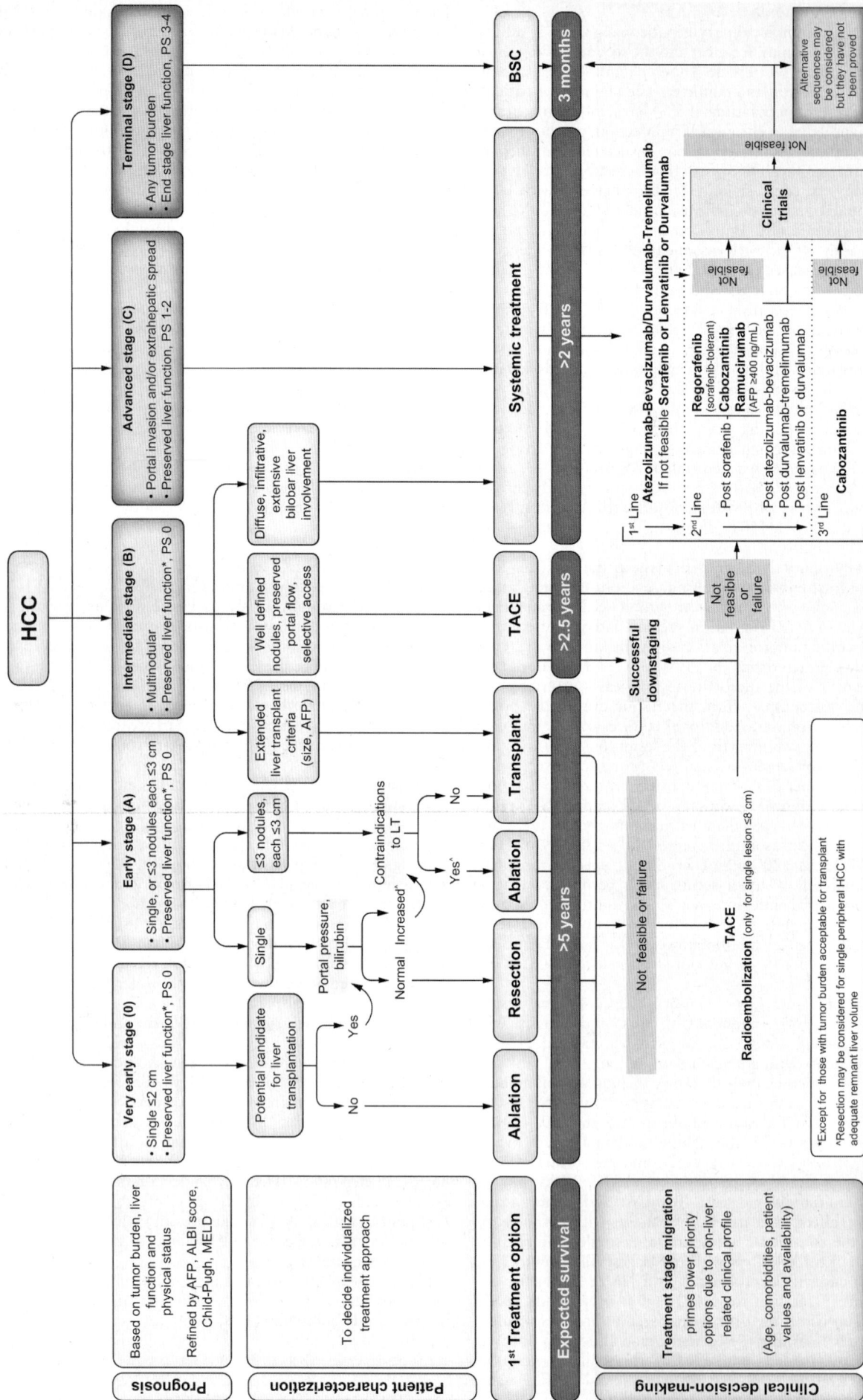

Figure 2 Updated Barcelona Clinic Liver Cancer staging system for hepatocellular carcinoma (HCC). AFP, Alpha-fetoprotein; ALBI, albumin-bilirubin; BSC, best supportive care; ECOG-PS, Eastern Cooperative Oncology Group performance status; LT, liver transplantation; MELD, Model for End-stage Liver Disease; TACE, transarterial chemoembolization. (From Reig M, Forner A, Rimola J, et al: BCLC strategy for prognosis prediction and treatment recommendations: the 2022 update, J Hepatol 76[3], 681–693, 2022.)

[Flolan][1], treprostinil [Orenitram, Remodulin, Tyvaso][1], selexipag [Uptravi][1], and iloprost [Ventavis][1]). All patients with PoPH should be warned not to smoke (tobacco and marijuana) or vape, and exercise as tolerated. In general, β-blocker prophylaxis should be avoided because to avoid reduction of right ventricular cardiac output and increase pulmonary vascular resistance. Calcium channel blockers should also be avoided in patients with PoPH due to lack of vasoactive response in the majority of patients and significant systemic hemodynamic side effects, including hypotension.

Survival in PoPH correlates with the severity of right ventricular dysfunction, and the safety and efficacy of liver transplantation reflects the severity of pulmonary arterial hypertension. Liver transplant may be offered to selected patients with PoPH but is typically contraindicated in those with mPAP >35 mm Hg despite medical management, particularly if right ventricular dysfunction is present, due to considerable perioperative mortality. Resolution of PoPH after liver transplantation is variable.

Hepatopulmonary Syndrome

Hepatopulmonary syndrome (HPS) is characterized by hypoxemia due to intrapulmonary vascular dilatations with right-to-left shunting in the setting of cirrhosis and portal hypertension. Although intrapulmonary vasodilatation is encountered in over 50% of patients with cirrhosis undergoing evaluation for liver transplantation, only 15% to 30% have hypoxemia and true HPS. The most widely accepted pathophysiologic mechanism responsible for HPS is increased pulmonary synthesis of nitric oxide. Similar to PoPH, the majority of patients with HPS are largely asymptomatic.

Clinical manifestations include dyspnea of insidious onset and two characteristic clinical findings: platypnea and orthodeoxia (worsening dyspnea and hypoxemia in upright posture, respectively). Other, more obvious but nonspecific clinical findings include spider angiomata, digital clubbing, and cyanosis. Screening for HPS relies on point-of-care oximetry indicating peripheral arterial oxygen saturation (SpO_2) <96% at rest and at sea level. Hypoxemia must be confirmed by arterial blood gas analysis demonstrating an arterial partial pressure of oxygen (PaO_2) <70 mm Hg and a widened alveolar–arterial oxygen gradient of 15 mm Hg (or ≥20 mm Hg for patients ≥65 years of age). Importantly, blood for arterial gas analysis should be obtained with the patient sitting upright, at rest, and breathing ambient air. After establishing a diagnosis of hypoxemia, documentation of pulmonary vascular dilatations with right-to-left blood shunting is necessary. Two-dimensional contrast-enhanced transthoracic echocardiography offers high sensitivity and is widely available. Agitated saline to produce microbubbles is injected intravenously as contrast, and under normal cardiopulmonary physiology the gas bubbles are rapidly seen in the right atrium and ventricle but then diffuse into alveoli during normal flow through the pulmonary capillaries. In patients with HPS, the presence of intrapulmonary right-to-left shunting due to vascular dilatations results in the presence of the microbubbles opacifying the left heart chambers at least three heartbeats after being seen in the right ventricle. Intracardiac right-to-left blood shunting (i.e., atrial or ventricular septal defects, patent foramen ovale) should be suspected if contrast is seen in the left heart within three heartbeats. Radionuclide lung perfusion scintigraphy using technetium-labeled macroaggregated albumin particles is less sensitive than contrast-enhanced echocardiography for diagnosis of HPS but is more specific and permits accurate quantification of the intrapulmonary shunt fraction, even in the presence of coexisting intrinsic lung disorders. Shunt fractions >6% confirm the diagnosis of HPS in the appropriate clinical setting.

HPS is associated with increased mortality and diminished quality of life compared with patients with cirrhosis but no HPS. After the diagnosis of HPS, median survival is 10.6 months; thus patients with HPS should undergo prompt liver transplant evaluation. Under current organ allocation policies by the United Network for Organ Sharing (UNOS), patients with HPS and PaO_2 <60 mm Hg are eligible for standard MELD exception score of 22 points at the time of listing, regardless of their calculated (biologic) MELD score, and a 10% mortality equivalent increase in points every 3 months. Liver transplantation remains the definitive therapy for HPS based on marked improvement or even resolution of hypoxemia in >85% of transplant recipients; however, clinically meaningful changes may be slow and take up to 1 year after transplantation.

Hepatic Hydrothorax

Hepatic hydrothorax is a transudative process leading to accumulation of >500 mL of fluid in the pleural space in patients with cirrhosis and portal hypertension in the absence of primary cardiopulmonary disease. Hepatic hydrothorax is thought to result from passage of ascitic fluid from the peritoneal cavity into the pleural spaces (typically on the right in ≤85% of patients) via subcentimeter defects and/or microscopic fenestrations in the tendinous portion of the diaphragm and is facilitated by negative intrathoracic pressure generated during inspiration. Clinical features include dyspnea, nonproductive cough, pleuritic chest pain, and even hypoxemia and hypotension in cases of tension hydrothorax. Fluid analysis demonstrates chemical characteristics similar to those of ascites: high serum-to-pleural fluid albumin gradient (>1.1 g/dL) and low total protein concentration (<2.5 g/dL).

Management of noninfected hepatic hydrothorax follows the same principles as those for ascites: sodium restriction, diuretics, repeated thoracenteses, and placement of TIPS for refractory cases. Importantly, indwelling pleural catheters should be avoided because of the high risk for complications, including severe infections that may jeopardize possible liver transplant candidacy in the future.

In patients with fevers and worsening pleuritic chest pain, spontaneous bacterial empyema (SBE) must be excluded. Similar to the diagnostic criteria for SBP, a diagnosis of SBE is established by a PMN count >250 cells/μL in the absence of a parapneumonic effusion. Microorganisms responsible for this infection are also similar to those responsible for SBP; thus third-generation cephalosporins remain the antibacterial agents of choice for empiric therapy. Although the term *empyema* may imply the need for drainage, a chest tube should not be inserted for management of SBE.

Medical Therapies to Prevent Decompensation

There has been an increasing recognition that early use of nonselective beta blockers (NSBBs) increases decompensation-free survival in cirrhosis, mainly by reducing the risk of ascites in those with cirrhosis and CSPH. NSBBs such as nadolol[1] and propranolol[1] have a well-established role in decreasing portal pressures through their mechanism of beta-1 adrenergic blockade (reduction in heart rate and cardiac output) and beta-2 adrenergic blockade (splanchnic vasoconstriction via unopposed alpha-adrenergic tone) and remain the standard of care for prevention of bleeding in cirrhosis and high-risk varices. Current guidelines recommend consideration of NSBB as primary prophylaxis to prevent decompensation in cACLD. Carvedilol (Coreg)[1], an NSBB with an additional mechanism of alpha-1 adrenergic blockade (decreases intrahepatic vascular resistance), is now the preferred NSBB owing to its greater efficacy in reducing portal pressures than the older NSBBs and should be gradually titrated up to goal dose of 12.5 mg PO daily with goal systolic blood pressure maintained >90 mm Hg.

Statins have recently been recognized to have multiple beneficial effects in patients with cirrhosis, including antiinflammatory and antifibrotic properties, as well as improving liver endothelial function. Predominantly retrospective data has shown that the use of statins in cACLD has been associated with reductions in HVPG and lower risk of decompensation, ACLF, hospitalization

---

[1] Not FDA approved for this indication.

TABLE 12 Medical Conditions That Qualify for Standard MELD Exception Points

CONDITIONS	REMARKS
Hepatocellular carcinoma	T2 lesions (at least 2 cm in diameter) within Milan criteria
Hepatopulmonary syndrome	Pao$_2$ <60 mm Hg on ambient air
Portopulmonary hypertension	Mean pulmonary arterial pressure <35 mm Hg with treatment
Familial amyloid polyneuropathy	Confirmed by DNA analysis and histology
Primary hyperoxaluria	Need simultaneous liver-kidney transplant
Cystic fibrosis	Forced expiratory volume in 1 s (FEV$_1$) <40%
Hilar cholangiocarcinoma	Stage I or II, liver transplantation center must have a UNOS-approved protocol
Hepatic artery thrombosis	Within 14 days of liver transplantation, not meeting criteria for status 1A

MELD, Model for End-Stage Liver Disease; *UNOS,* United Network for Organ Sharing.

for infection, development of HCC, and up to 30% reduction in all-cause mortality. The potential benefits may be greatest with lipophilic statins. However, prospective studies including initial small RCTs thus far have not consistently supported significant differences, and further ongoing trials should provide more definitive information. Nonetheless, statins are proven to be safe and very well tolerated in cirrhosis and should be started when medically indicated.

Malnutrition, Frailty, and Sarcopenia in Cirrhosis

Malnutrition is frequent in cirrhosis and occurs from an imbalance (either deficiency or excess) of nutrients, which in turn affects tissue body form or function, and/or clinical outcomes. Notably, malnutrition can exist in a spectrum ranging from underweight to obese. In cirrhosis, malnutrition often manifests as sarcopenia and frailty and increases morbidity and mortality.

Frailty in cirrhosis is defined as the clinical manifestation of decreased physiologic reserve and impaired muscle contractile function, which commonly presents as decreased physical function, decreased functional performance, and disability. Tools studied to assess frailty in cirrhosis include the activities of daily living, Karnofsky Performance Scale, and the Liver Frailty Index. The prevalence of frailty has been reported up to 43% in ambulatory patients with cirrhosis and increases with liver disease severity. Several studies have confirmed an association between frailty and mortality, with up to twofold increases in risk of death in frail patients, whereas improvement in frailty scores pretransplant are associated with lower waitlist mortality. Furthermore, frailty is implicated in accidental falls, depression, and diminished global health-related quality of life.

Sarcopenia in cirrhosis is defined as a progressive and generalized skeletal muscle disorder associated with an increased likelihood of adverse outcomes including falls, fractures, disability, and mortality. Sarcopenia is common in cirrhosis and affects up to 70% of patients with end-stage liver disease, with the degree of muscle loss often correlating with the severity of liver disease. Several methods to assess muscle mass in cirrhosis have been described, including CT imaging (conventionally reported as the "skeletal muscle index"), total psoas muscle area, assessment of fat-free mass, dual-energy x-ray absorptiometry (DEXA) scanning and anthropometrics. The term *sarcopenic obesity* refers to the state of decreased muscle mass with increased fat mass and represents a challenge as fat mass can mask underlying muscle wasting. Sarcopenia has been associated with several outcomes

including pre- and posttransplant mortality, hepatic decompensation, reduced quality of life, increased infections, and prolonged hospitalizations.

Management of frailty and sarcopenia includes effective screening, management of concomitant factors (e.g., HE and ascites), and interventions including nutrition/dietary support and physical therapy. Current guidelines recommend a weight-based daily caloric intake of ≥35 kcal/kg/day. In those with obesity, a BMI-adjusted energy uptake goal can be implemented such as 25 to 35 kcal/kg/day (for BMI 30–40 kg/m^2) and 20 to 25 kcal/kg/day (for BMI ≥40 kg/m^2). Current guidelines also recommend a protein intake of 1.2 to 1.5 g/kg/day for all adults with cirrhosis. Restricting protein intake in those with HE should be avoided, as it does not worsen HE. Timing of nutritional intake is important and prolonged periods of fasting should be avoided, with evidence supporting improvements in muscle mass with an early morning breakfast, late evening snack (of ~700 kcal), and intake of small frequent meals every 3 to 4 hours while awake. Finally, maintaining adequate physical activity with a combination of aerobic and resistance exercises should be recommended, with specific regimens tailored based on baseline and ongoing assessments.

Liver Transplantation

Liver transplantation is effective in salvaging patients with ALF and decompensated cirrhosis, as well as selected patients with HCC (see earlier), with excellent short- and long-term outcomes. Survival after 1 and 5 years after liver transplantation is approximately 80% to 90% and 60% to 75%, respectively. Cirrhosis per se is not an indication to initiate evaluation for liver transplantation, because it is not associated with survival benefit in patients with low MELD scores. Consequently, patients should be referred for liver transplantation evaluation when the MELD score is ≥15 or when an index complication of cirrhosis such as ascites or variceal hemorrhage occurs. Organ allocation in the United States and many other countries is based on disease severity as reflected by the MELD score for patients ≥12 years of age and the Pediatric End-Stage Liver Disease score for patients <12 years of age (includes INR, bilirubin, albumin, and growth failure). Some etiologies of cirrhosis result in diminished survival that is not accurately predicted by the MELD score or is associated with extremely poor quality of life; thus MELD exceptions exist. Standardized MELD exception criteria are summarized in Table 12. For patients with complications related to liver disease and associated increased morbidity and mortality not adequately reflected by the MELD score and not qualifying for standard MELD exceptions, additional points may be petitioned by the transplant center to the National Liver Review Board on a case-by-case basis with no guarantee that they will be granted. Some examples of conditions that may receive additional MELD points include recurrent bacterial cholangitis in patients with primary sclerosing cholangitis, intractable and debilitating pruritus in patients with primary biliary cholangitis, ascites refractory to maximum-tolerated doses of diuretics, HE refractory to medical therapy, and recurrent variceal hemorrhage despite adequate therapy.

Contraindications to liver transplantation continually evolve over time. Relative contraindications are usually associated with suboptimal outcomes after liver transplantation and vary widely across different transplant centers. Absolute contraindications imply that a successful outcome after liver transplantation is unlikely; thus it should not be pursued (Table 13).

ALF is an uncommon but important indication for liver transplantation owing to the high mortality associated with this condition. Although a significant proportion of patients with ALF may have spontaneous recovery, its clinical course is usually unpredictable and early referral for liver transplantation is recommended, regardless of the etiology. Patients with ALF have the highest priority for organ allocation if they meet specific criteria for UNOS status 1A (Table 14).

Evaluation for liver transplantation is a multidisciplinary process carried out over multiple encounters aimed to unveil additional medical, surgical, behavioral, social, and economic issues that may affect liver transplantation candidacy and/or outcomes.

TABLE 13	Absolute Contraindications to Liver Transplantation

Uncontrolled sepsis

Acquired immunodeficiency syndrome

Active alcohol or substance abuse

Advanced cardiac or pulmonary disease

Intrahepatic cholangiocarcinoma

Hepatic hemangiosarcoma

Hepatocellular carcinoma with metastasis

Extrahepatic malignancy

Anatomic abnormalities that preclude liver transplantation

Lack of social support

Persistent nonadherence to medical care

TABLE 14	Criteria for Status 1A Designation in Patients With Acute Liver Failure

Age >18 years

Life expectancy <7 days without liver transplantation

Onset of encephalopathy within 8 weeks of first symptom of liver disease

Absence of preexisting liver disease

Admission to intensive care unit and one of the following:
- Ventilator dependence
- Requirement of renal replacement therapy
- International normalized ratio >2

Fulminant Wilson disease

Primary graft nonfunction

Hepatic artery thrombosis

TABLE 15	Advantages and Disadvantages of Living-Donor Liver Transplantation

ADVANTAGES	DISADVANTAGES
Thorough donor screening process	Only offered in selected liver transplantation centers
Elective timing of liver transplantation permitting optimization of therapies	Donor morbidity and mortality
Diminished wait time with consequent reduction in dropout from the waiting list	Higher risk for biliary complications in the donor and recipient
Minimal cold ischemia time	

References

Ahluwalia V, Wade JB, White MB, et al: Liver transplantation significantly improves global functioning and cerebral processing, *Liver Transplant* 22:1379–1390, 2016.

Angeli P, Volpin R, Gerunda G, et al: Reversal of type 1 hepatorenal syndrome with the administration of midodrine and octreotide, *Hepatology* 29:1690–1697, 1999.

Arguedas MR, Singh H, Faulk DK, et al: Utility of pulse oximetry screening for hepatopulmonary syndrome, *Clin Gastroenterol Hepatol* 5:749–754, 2007.

Arroyo V, Garcia-Martinez R, Salvatella X: Human serum albumin, systemic inflammation, and cirrhosis, *J Hepatol* 61:396–407, 2014.

Bajaj JS, Heuman DM, Sterling RK, et al: Validation of EncephalApp, smartphone-based Stroop test, for the diagnosis of covert hepatic encephalopathy, *Clin Gastroenterol Hepatol* 13:1828–1835.e1, 2015.

Bass NM, Mullen KD, Sanyal A, et al: Rifaximin treatment in hepatic encephalopathy, *N Engl J Med* 362:1071–1081, 2010.

Bernardi M, Caraceni P, Navickis RJ, et al: Albumin infusion in patients undergoing large-volume paracentesis: a meta-analysis of randomized trials, *Hepatology* 55:1172–1181, 2012.

Biggins SW, Angeli P, Garcia-Tsao G, et al: Diagnosis, evaluation, and management of ascites, spontaneous bacterial peritonitis and hepatorenal syndrome: 2021 practice guidance by the American association for the study of liver diseases, *Hepatology* 74(2):1014–1048, 2021, https://doi.org/10.1002/hep.31884.

Blachier M, Leleu H, Peck-Radosavljevic M, et al: The burden of liver disease in Europe: a review of available epidemiological data, *J Hepatol* 58:593–608, 2013.

Bureau C, Thabut D, Oberti F, et al: Transjugular intrahepatic portosystemic shunts with covered stents increase transplant-free survival of patients with cirrhosis and recurrent ascites, *Gastroenterology* 152:157–163, 2017.

Carrion AF, Martin P: Renal dysfunction in patients with cirrhosis, *Am J Gastroenterol* 114:1407–1410, 2019.

D'Amico G, Garcia-Tsao G, Pagliaro L: Natural history and prognostic indicators of survival in cirrhosis: a systematic review of 118 studies, *J Hepatol* 44:217–231, 2006.

Dasarathy S, Merli M: Sarcopenia from mechanism to diagnosis and treatment in liver disease, *J Hepatol* 65:1232–1244, 2016.

de Franchis R, Bosch J, Garcia-Tsao G, Reiberger T, Ripoll C; Baveno VII F. Baveno VII - renewing consensus in portal hypertension. *J Hepatol*. 2022 Apr;76(4):959–974. doi: 10.1016/j.jhep.2021.12.022. Epub 2021 Dec 30. Erratum in: *J Hepatol*. 2022 Jul;77(1):271. doi: 10.1016/j.jhep.2022.03.024. PMID: 35120736; PMCID: PMC11090185.

Duarte-Rojo A, Taouli B, Leung DH, et al: Imaging-based noninvasive liver disease assessment for staging liver fibrosis in chronic liver disease: a systematic review supporting the AASLD Practice Guideline, *Hepatology* 81(2):725–748, 2025, https://doi.org/10.1097/HEP.0000000000000852.

Escorsell À, Pavel O, Cárdenas A, et al: Esophageal balloon tamponade versus esophageal stent in controlling acute refractory variceal bleeding: a multicenter randomized, controlled trial, *Hepatology* 63:1957–1967, 2016.

Flemming JA, Kim WR, Brosgart CL, et al: Reduction in liver transplant wait-listing in the era of direct-acting antiviral therapy, *Hepatology* 65(3):804–812, 2017.

Garcia-Pagan JC, Caca K, Bureau C, et al: Early use of TIPS in patients with cirrhosis and variceal bleeding, *N Engl J Med* 362:2370–2379, 2010.

Ge PS, Runyon BA: Serum ammonia level for the evaluation of hepatic encephalopathy, *J Am Med Assoc* 312:643–644, 2014.

Gluud LL, Christensen K, Christensen E, et al: Systematic review of randomized trials on vasoconstrictor drugs for hepatorenal syndrome, *Hepatology* 51:576–584, 2010.

Goel GA, Deshpande A, Lopez R, et al: Increased rate of spontaneous bacterial peritonitis among cirrhotic patients receiving pharmacologic acid suppression, *Clin Gastroenterol Hepatol* 10:422–427, 2012.

Grace JA, Angus PW: Hepatopulmonary syndrome: update on recent advances in pathophysiology, investigation, and treatment, *J Gastroenterol Hepatol* 28:213–219, 2013.

Humbert M, Kovacs G, Hoeper MM, et al: 2022 ESC/ERS Guidelines for the diagnosis and treatment of pulmonary hypertension, *Eur Respir J* 61(1), 2023:2200879 https://doi.org/10.1183/13993003.00879-2022f, Published 2023 Jan 6.

Kaplan DE, Ripoll C, Maja T, et al: AASLD practice guidance on risk stratification and management of portal hypertension and varices in cirrhosis, *Hepatology* 79:1180–1211, 2024.

Once the patient's candidacy is deemed appropriate, formal listing occurs with UNOS. Blood type is the major determinant for organ compatibility, and appropriate size (based on body weight) must be taken into consideration.

Living-donor liver transplantation was developed as an alternative owing to ongoing shortage of deceased-donor organs; however, living donation carries important risks for the donor that must be carefully taken into consideration. The advantages and disadvantages of living-donor liver transplantation are summarized in Table 15.

Efforts to expand the liver donor pool by including donors previously deemed unsuitable continue to be a key strategy in addressing shortages. These efforts involve donation after circulatory death donors, donors over the age of 70, donors with viral infections like HBV and HCV, as well as split liver transplants.

Adequate long-term immunosuppression prevents graft rejection and is currently centered on the use of calcineurin inhibitors (tacrolimus [Prograf] primarily, and less often cyclosporine [Neoral]) with or without concomitant antimetabolite agents such as mycophenolic acid (Myfortic) or its prodrug mycophenolate mofetil (CellCept). Additional agents include inhibitors of the mammalian target of rapamycin such as everolimus (Zortress).

Long-term care of liver transplant recipients should not by any means focus exclusively on graft function and prevention of rejection, but rather be comprehensive and aimed at maintaining an overall good state of health by instituting preventive health strategies and monitoring for other complications that may ensue, such as diabetes mellitus, hypertension, dyslipidemia, renal dysfunction, obesity, and alcohol relapse, among many others.

Kim WR, Mannalithara A, Heimbach JK, et al: The model for end-stage liver disease update for the modern era, *Gastroenterology* 161:1887–1895, 2021.

Kristina Tzartzeva K, Obi J, Rich NE, et al: Surveillance imaging and alpha fetoprotein for early detection of hepatocellular carcinoma in patients with cirrhosis: a meta-analysis, *Gastroenterology* 154:1706–1718.e1, 2018.

Kronborg TM, Schierwagen R, Trošt K, et al: Atorvastatin for patients with cirrhosis. A randomized, placebo-controlled trial, *Hepatol Commun* 7(12), 2023:e0332https://doi.org/10.1097/HC9.0000000000000332, Published 2023 Dec 1.

Krowka MJ, Plevak DJ, Findlay JY, et al: Pulmonary hemodynamics and perioperative cardiopulmonary-related mortality in patients with portopulmonary hypertension undergoing liver transplantation, *Liver Transplant* 6:443–450, 2000.

Kurokawa T, Zheng YW, Ohkohchi N: Novel functions of platelets in the liver, *J Gastroenterol Hepatol* 31:745–751, 2016.

Lai JC, Tandon P, Bernal W, et al. Malnutrition, frailty, and sarcopenia in patients with cirrhosis: 2021 practice guidance by the American association for the study of liver diseases [published correction appears in *Hepatology.* 2021 Dec;74(6):3563. doi: 10.1002/hep.32224.]. *Hepatology.* 2021;74(3):1611-1644. doi:10.1002/hep.32049.

Lim YS, Kim WR: The global impact of hepatic fibrosis and end-stage liver disease, *Clin Liver Dis* 12:733–736, 2008.

Lin ZH, Xin YN, Dong QJ, et al: Performance of the aspartate aminotransferase-to-platelet ratio index for the staging of hepatitis C-related fibrosis: an updated meta-analysis, *Hepatology* 53:726–736, 2011.

Llovet JM, Ricci S, Mazzaferro V, et al: Sorafenib in advanced hepatocellular carcinoma, *N Engl J Med* 359:378–390, 2008.

Marik PE, Wood K, Starzl TE: The course of type 1 hepato-renal syndrome post liver transplantation, *Nephrol Dial Transplant* 21:478–482, 2006.

Mazzaferro V, Regalia E, Doci R, et al: Liver transplantation for the treatment of small hepatocellular carcinomas in patients with cirrhosis, *N Engl J Med* 334:693–699, 1996.

Merion RM, Schaubel DE, Dykstra DM, et al: The survival benefit of liver transplantation, *Am J Transplant* 5:307–313, 2005.

Mullen KD, Sanyal AJ, Bass NM, et al: Rifaximin is safe and well tolerated for long-term maintenance of remission from overt hepatic encephalopathy, *Clin Gastroenterol Hepatol* 12:1390–1397.e2, 2014.

Ohlsson B, Nilsson J, Stenram U, et al: Percutaneous fine-needle aspiration cytology in the diagnosis and management of liver tumours, *Br J Surg* 89:757–762, 2002.

Patidar KR, Bajaj JS: Covert and overt hepatic encephalopathy: diagnosis and management, *Clin Gastroenterol Hepatol* 13:2048–2061, 2015.

Pereira K, Carrion AF, Martin P, et al: Current diagnosis and management of post-transjugular intrahepatic portosystemic shunt refractory hepatic encephalopathy, *Liver Int* 35:2487–2494, 2015.

Runyon BA, Committee APG: Management of adult patients with ascites due to cirrhosis: an update, *Hepatology* 49:2087–2107, 2009.

Runyon BA, Squier S, Borzio M: Translocation of gut bacteria in rats with cirrhosis to mesenteric lymph nodes partially explains the pathogenesis of spontaneous bacterial peritonitis, *J Hepatol* 21:792–796, 1994.

Salerno F, Merli M, Riggio O, et al: Randomized controlled study of TIPS versus paracentesis plus albumin in cirrhosis with severe ascites, *Hepatology* 40:629–635, 2004.

Sharpton SR, Loomba R: Emerging role of statin therapy in the prevention and management of cirrhosis, portal hypertension, and HCC, *Hepatology* 78(6):1896–1906, 2023, https://doi.org/10.1097/HEP.0000000000000278.

Singal AG, Llovet JM, Yarchoan M, et al: AASLD practice guidance on prevention, diagnosis and management of hepatocellular carcinoma, *Hepatology* 78:1922–1965, 2023.

Sort P, Navasa M, Arroyo V, et al: Effect of intravenous albumin on renal impairment and mortality in patients with cirrhosis and spontaneous bacterial peritonitis, *N Engl J Med* 341:403–409, 1999.

Sterling R, Patel K, Duarte-Rojo A, et al: AASLD practice guidance on blood-based non-invasive liver disease assessments of hepatic fibrosis and steatosis, *Hepatology*, 2024, Epub ahead of print.

Turco L, Taru MG, Vitale G, et al: Beta-blockers lower first decompensation in patients with cirrhosis and enduring portal hypertension after etiological treatment, *Clin Gastroenterol Hepatol* 30, 2024. https://doi.org/10.1016/j.cgh.2024.08.012, Published online August.

Udell JA, Wang CS, Tinmouth J, et al: Does this patient with liver disease have cirrhosis? *J Am Med Assoc* 307:832–842, 2012.

Villanueva C, Albillos A, Genescà J, et al. β blockers to prevent decompensation of cirrhosis in patients with clinically significant portal hypertension (PREDESCI): a randomised, double-blind, placebo-controlled, multicentre trial [published correction appears in *Lancet.* 2019 Jun 22;393(10190):2492. doi: 10.1016/S0140-6736(19)31404-7.]. *Lancet.* 2019;393(10181):1597-1608. doi:10.1016/S0140-6736(18)31875-0

Villanueva C, Colomo A, Colomo A, et al: Transfusion strategies for acute upper gastrointestinal bleeding, *N Engl J Med* 368:11–21, 2013.

Villanueva C, Tripathi D, Bosch J: Preventing the progression of cirrhosis to decompensation and death, *Nat Rev Gastroenterol Hepatol* 27, 2025https://doi.org/10.1038/s41575-024-01031-x, Published online January.

Wang FS, Fan JG, Zhang Z, et al: The global burden of liver disease: the major impact of China, *Hepatology* 60:2099–2108, 2014.

Wells M, Chande N, Adams P, et al: Meta-analysis: vasoactive medications for the management of acute variceal bleeds, *Aliment Pharmacol Ther* 35:1267–1278, 2012.

Williams Jr JW, Simel DL: The rational clinical examination. Does this patient have ascites? How to divine fluid in the abdomen, *J Am Med Assoc* 267:2645–2648, 1992.

Wong F, Pappas SC, Curry MP, et al: Terlipressin plus albumin for the treatment of type 1 hepatorenal syndrome, *N Engl J Med* 384:818–828, 2021.

Zaiac MN, Walker A: Nail abnormalities associated with systemic pathologies, *Clin Dermatol* 31:627–649, 2013.

DIVERTICULA OF THE ALIMENTARY TRACT

Method of
Aaron D. Sinclair, MD

CURRENT DIAGNOSIS

- Endoscopy or barium swallow study may be used in the evaluation of most upper alimentary tract diverticula.
- Symptomatic small intestinal diverticula are difficult to diagnose and require a high index of suspicion and radiographic examination (nuclear medicine scans, capsule endoscopy, or computed tomography scans).
- Diverticulitis of the colon is most accurately identified and the treatment planned with computed tomography of the abdomen and pelvis.
- Diverticulitis of the colon that is slow to resolve may require additional imaging or direct visualization with endoscopy to identify an alternative diagnosis.

CURRENT THERAPY

- Most asymptomatic diverticula are identified incidentally and may require only monitoring.
- Surgical management of symptomatic diverticula may require surgical resection.
- Early in the disease process, uncomplicated diverticulitis of the colon may be managed on an outpatient basis with a conservative no-intervention approach or oral antibiotics.
- Complicated diverticulitis of the colon should be managed in conjunction with a surgeon and in the hospital with intravenous antibiotics.

A diverticulum is an abnormal saccular protrusion from the wall of the alimentary tract. Diverticula may be classified as either true or false. The wall of the alimentary tract is composed of submucosal, mucosal, and muscular layers. A false diverticulum is a protrusion of the submucosa and mucosa through a defect in the muscular wall of the alimentary tract. A true diverticulum is a protrusion of all layers of the alimentary tract wall. Many diverticula are asymptomatic and require no treatment. Some diverticula cause symptoms depending on their anatomic location or associated pathophysiologic complications (e.g., obstruction, infection, inflammation, or bleeding). This chapter categorizes alimentary canal diverticula by their location.

Esophagus

Zenker Diverticulum

Zenker diverticulum is a false diverticulum that develops in the upper posterior esophagus in an area known as Killian triangle, located between the inferior pharyngeal constrictors and the cricopharyngeal muscles. Zenker diverticulum typically presents after age 60 and has a male predominance for reasons that are unclear. It affects only 2 per 100,000 patients per year. Although it can be asymptomatic for years before the development of symptomatology, patients may experience dysphagia, aspiration, and regurgitation of undigested food. The exact cause is unclear, but proposed mechanisms suggest a dysfunction in coordinated swallowing muscle movement and increased intraluminal pressure in the esophagus. There may be an additive component of long-term upper esophageal sphincter irritation from acid reflux.

Diagnosis is primarily made through barium swallow, although small diverticula may be missed (Figure 1). Consider investigating endoscopically diverticula of the esophagus on initial radiologic discovery to rule out associated neoplasm or mass effect. Although endoscopic direct visualization is possible, caution should be

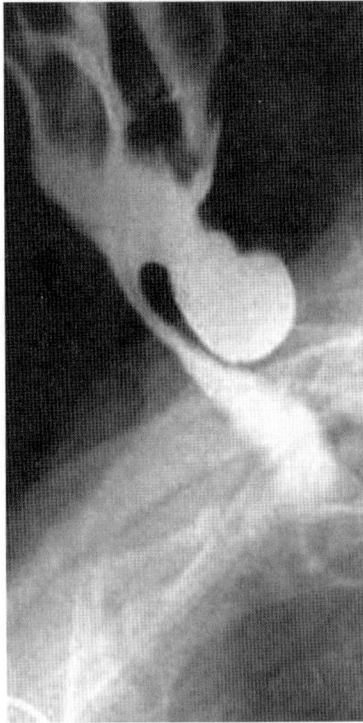

Figure 1 Zenker diverticulum. (Image courtesy Gastrolab—The Gastrointestinal Site. http://www.gastrolab.net [Accessed August 25, 2014].)

exercised owing to the risk of perforation. Small asymptomatic diverticula can be monitored. Regardless of size, Zenker diverticulum that are symptomatic should be surgically evaluated and repair considered. Methods for closure include endoscopic (flexible and rigid) diverticulostomy and myotomy or traditional surgical resection. Due to higher morbidity and mortality rates, treatment has moved away from traditional open surgical resection and toward less invasive endoscopic approaches. Additional studies show rigid endoscopic repair tends to have higher complication rates, longer hospital lengths of stay, and longer procedure times compared with flexible endoscopic repairs. When looking at outcomes, rigid versus flexible endoscopic repairs have similar initial success rates and longer-term failure rates. Emerging technologies have resulted in different techniques (harmonic scalpel, stapler, laser, etc.) used during endoscopic repair. Procedure risk factors appear to be multifactorial based on surgeon, type of procedure, size of diverticulum, and postprocedural diverticulum length.

Traction Diverticulum

Traction diverticula are the only true diverticula of the esophagus. Traction diverticula are rare. Their size tends to stay less than 2 cm. Owing to the proposed mechanism of formation, traction diverticula are isolated to the middle third of the esophagus. It is not fully clear how traction diverticula form. One proposed mechanism is related to a precedent pulmonary infection, most commonly tuberculosis or histoplasmosis, with resultant mediastinal lymph node formation. After the active infection subsides, resultant fibrosis and scarring between the tissues surrounding the mediastinal lymph nodes and esophagus occur. Initially, a small diverticulum develops from this fibrosis, which produces "traction" or a lack of mobility. Diverticular progression results when age-related changes from the dysfunction of coordinated swallowing muscle movement and increased intraluminal pressure in the esophagus develop. Surgical management is rarely needed unless these diverticula become symptomatic or complications, such as fistulas, occur.

Epiphrenic Diverticulum

Epiphrenic diverticula are false diverticula of the distal esophagus affecting only 0.015% of the general population. They are thought to arise secondary to mucosal injury from gastroesophageal reflux and muscle dysmotility. They occur within 10 cm of the gastroesophageal junction, and symptoms include dysphagia, spasmodic chest pain, and gastroesophageal reflux. There does not appear to be a correlation with between diverticular size and symptomatology. With progression of diverticular size, obstruction can become a potential complication. Diagnostic measures typically start with barium swallow. Consider investigating with endoscopy following initial diagnosis to rule out associated neoplasm or mass effect.

Management depends on patient symptoms and size of the diverticulum. If small (<5 cm) and asymptomatic, routine clinical and endoscopic surveillance is permissible. However, any symptomatology necessitates consideration for surgical evaluation and repair. Surgical options include endoscopic, open resection and laparoscopy or possibly a combination of techniques. Partial fundoplication may be indicated, depending on the severity of gastroesophageal reflux present as indicated by ancillary testing of a 24-hour pH probe and esophageal manometry. Less invasive endoscopic myotomy procedures, successfully used to treat Zenker diverticulum, are judiciously being used to treat epiphrenic diverticulum.

Stomach
Gastric Diverticula
Gastric diverticula are rare, with an endoscopic incidence of 0.01%. Gastric diverticulum may be either true or false in nature. True gastric diverticulae (70% to 75%) are typically congenital and situated along the dorsal wall of the fundus within 2 to 3 cm of the gastroesophageal junction. False diverticulae, which are less common and typically acquired, are located around the antrum of the stomach. Most are asymptomatic and small (<3 cm). Symptomatology is not correlated to size of the diverticulum. Symptoms may include epigastric pain, dyspepsia, and emesis. Rarely, ulcerations, perforations, or bleeding can occur. Diagnosis involves endoscopy, barium swallow, or contrast-aided computed tomography (CT) scan. After diverticula of the stomach are initially identified on imaging, endoscopic evaluation should be considered to exclude an associated neoplasm or mass effect. If symptomatic, typical treatment includes a proton pump inhibitor and monitoring for symptom improvement. Additional treatment options include preprandial mineral oil, antispasmodics, or anatacids.[1] Continued symptoms should prompt endoscopic evaluation with biopsies of suspicious lesions with raised or irregular borders. Gastric cancers have been reported in and around gastric diverticulum. Persistent symptoms may necessitate gastrectomy of the diverticulum, especially if concerns about cancer exist. The majority of surgical removals of gastric diverticulum are performed laparoscopically. Caution should be used when approaching the decision of surgical intervention. In one study of 29 patients who underwent surgical removal of a gastric diverticulum, only 15 had resolution of symptoms.

Small Intestine
Duodenal Diverticula
Diverticula located in the duodenum are relatively common, affecting up to 22% of the general population (Figure 2). Duodenal diverticula may be either true or false diverticula. The most common location is the second portion of the duodenum. Although usually asymptomatic, ulcerative bleeding, perforation, infection, or intermittent obstruction, particularly after eating, may occur. The size and position of the diverticula may lead to complications such as obstruction of the sphincter of Oddi and/or impingement of hepatobiliary tree drainage. This impingement may result in jaundice, right upper quadrant pain, or infection signs/symptoms similar to cholecystitis. Obstruction of the bile duct leading to cholangitis is referred to as Lemmel syndrome.

Duodenal diverticula may be identified on barium swallow, contrast-enhanced CT, magnetic resonance imaging, or endoscopy. Duodenal diverticula found incidentally do not require

___
[1] Not FDA approved for this indication.

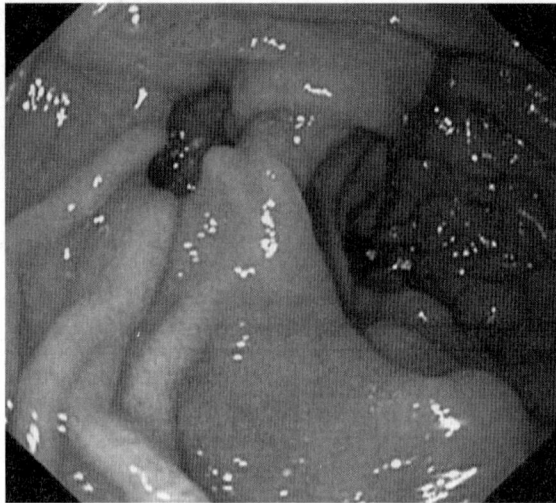

Figure 2 Duodenal diverticulum. (Image courtesy Gastrolab—The Gastrointestinal Site. http://www.gastrolab.net [Accessed August 25, 2014].)

treatment. If symptoms arise, endoscopic evaluation and surgical resection should be considered. Surgical resection decisions should be approached cautiously as mortality rates range from 3% to 31%. Because the second and third portions of the duodenum are retroperitoneal, surgical resection requires an open approach. This has led to the Hinchey classification to help classify duodenal diverticulitis. For lower classified infections, treatment with antibiotics is encouraged. For more complicated infections, invasive intervention is more likely to be required. Advanced interventions to consider initially include endoscopic guided or CT-guided percutaneous drainage. More invasive surgical interventions may be required if the patient does not improve.

Jejunal and Ileal Diverticula

Jejunal and ileal diverticula occur throughout the length of the small intestine in 1% to 2% of the population. There does not appear to be any statistically significant relationship with morbidity or mortality of these types of diverticula with respect to location, gender, size, number, and so forth. These false diverticula are located predominantly where the blood vessels penetrate the muscular wall of the mesenteric side of the bowel. Most are noted incidentally on radiographic studies, but some manifest with symptoms secondary to bleeding, obstruction, or infection. These symptoms are believed to be due to bacterial overgrowth that may occur within the cavity of the diverticulum. Diagnosis can be made with capsule endoscopy or a small bowel barium contrast follow through study, although some may be noted on MRI with intravenous contrast and/or CT with intravenous and oral contrast. Advanced endoscopic procedures such as push enteroscopy and double balloon endoscopy can be used to further evaluate symptomatic diverticula.

Asymptomatic jejunal and ileal diverticula should not be resected. Bacterial overgrowth symptoms may respond to antibiotic treatment and intestinal promotility drug therapy. If diverticulitis is seen radiographically, intravenous antibiotics and bowel rest should be initiated. Surgical intervention with small bowel resection is indicated if symptomatic diverticula persist despite conservative management.

Meckel Diverticulum

Meckel diverticulum is a true diverticulum—a congenital anomaly that occurs owing to incomplete closure of the vitelline duct. This duct typically obliterates during the ninth week of gestational age. Owing to the embryologic origin of the diverticulum, it is almost always located within 2 feet of the ileocecal valve. Meckel diverticulum has a prevalence of 1% to 2% of the population, with a 2:1 male predominance. Approximately 2% of all existing Meckel diverticula will become symptomatic.

Symptomatic diverticula most commonly cause nausea, vomiting, and abdominal pain. The sign most commonly associated with Meckel diverticulum is intussusception. This occurs owing to residual fibrous attachments to the umbilicus causing a lead point for the proximal bowel to involute onto the distal bowel. It most commonly presents with bloody mucoid stools, abdominal pain, and vomiting in children younger than 6 years of age, most commonly within the first 2 years of life. However, other symptoms may occur if ectopic tissue exists in the diverticulum. Gastric ectopic tissue may cause abdominal pain and bloody stools from ulceration of the underlying ileal tissue. Duodenal and pancreatic tissues have been identified in Meckel diverticulum but are very rare and do not typically cause symptoms.

Diagnosis in adults requires a high level of suspicion and is aided by the use of a technetium 99m (^{99m}Tc) scan to identify ectopic gastric mucosa in those patients with bleeding and symptoms of ulceration. For children with obstructive signs or symptoms, the diagnosis may be aided by ultrasound and/or computed tomographic scans. Plain film radiographs of the abdomen have low sensitivity and specificity for the diagnosis of intussusception. The sensitivity of the Meckel scan for the pediatric population is 85% to 97% but is much lower in the adult population at 62%. The choice of imaging procedure is dictated by the experience of the radiologic personnel performing the procedure.

Symptomatic Meckel diverticulum should be surgically resected. Up to 90% of intussusception secondary to Meckel diverticulum may be reduced using diagnostic ultrasonography with saline or pneumatic enema. Treatment of Meckel diverticulum largely depends on age and symptomatology because operating on asymptomatic Meckel diverticulum has been shown to have a fivefold increase in complications, such as postoperative bowel obstruction, leaks, ileus, and infection. Many experts have advocated that incidental, asymptomatic Meckel diverticulum should not be resected. Some experts advocate for selective surgical resection of asymptomatic patients with an incidentally noted Meckel diverticulum for the following: healthy young children, healthy adults younger than 50 years of age with palpable abnormalities suggestive of heterotrophic tissue, size longer than 2 cm, or a broad base wider than 2 cm.

Colon
Diverticulosis

The colon is where most diverticula occur in the alimentary tract. Owing to this predominance, this condition is commonly termed *diverticulosis* or *diverticular disease*. Diverticulum of the colon is of the false type. The incidence increases with age. The incidence of left-sided diverticulosis approaches 5% at age 40 and increases to greater than 60% at age 80. Diverticulosis is most commonly located in the sigmoid colon.

The exact pathogenesis of diverticulosis is unclear. The proposed mechanism of colonic diverticular formation places an emphasis on intraluminal pressure buildup. The pressure across the colonic wall increases as the radius of the wall decreases. Accordingly, the radius is the smallest in the sigmoid colon and thus the most likely location of diverticulosis. Normally, pressure is constant throughout the colon. However, as diverticular disease develops, abnormal pressure segmentations occur, resulting in pressure gradient changes in the colon. With increased pressure, the integrity of collagen and elastin in the wall muscle changes, the circular muscles thicken, colonic segments shorten, and the lumen narrows, leading to propagation of the disease. Several risk factors have been associated with the development of diverticular disease: smoking, lack of physical activity, and obesity. By increasing the amount of dietary fiber, it is theorized that the resultant bulking of the stools may decrease the pressure in the colon lumen and prevent diverticular disease progression. Yet, mixed results have been noted on studies of fiber intake and diverticular development and progression of disease. There is no associated risk with the ingestion of caffeine, alcohol, popcorn, seeds, or nuts and the development of diverticulosis, diverticular bleeding, or diverticulitis.

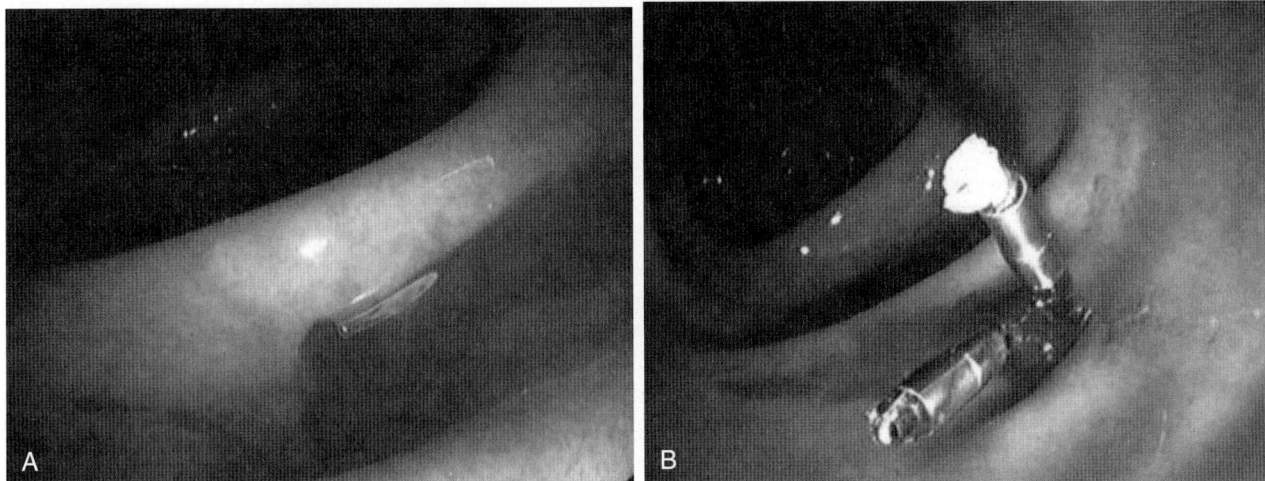

Figure 3 Colonoscopy in a patient with hematochezia from the source isolated to a diverticulum (A) and hemostasis noted after placement of two hemoclips (B). (Courtesy Janak Shah. From Feldman M. *Sleisenger and Fordtran's Gastrointestinal and Liver Disease*. 9th ed. Philadelphia: Elsevier; Figure 117.8.)

Colonic Diverticular Bleeding

Diverticula tend to develop where an arteriole penetrates the circular muscle layer of the colon. This results in vessels arching over the dome of the diverticulum. This leaves fragile vessels in a vulnerable position of a relatively thin mucosal layer prone to trauma and resultant diverticular bleeding. Bleeding typically manifests as hematochezia—a darkish to bright red bleeding that is typically characterized as brisk and acute in nature. Diverticulosis is attributed to 30% to 50% of all hematochezia. Fifteen percent of patients will experience at least one episode of bleeding in their lifetime, with a recurrent bleeding risk of up to 38%. Most patients presenting with diverticular bleeding are asymptomatic, but some may experience bloating or cramping.

Selection of the diagnostic modality depends largely on the degree of bleeding and the cardiovascular stability of the patient. Endoscopy is the preferred treatment modality for stable patients owing to its potential for diagnosis and treatment options. Up to 80% of diverticular bleeding can be isolated with direct endoscopic visualization (Figure 3).

Endoscopic failure to identify or control diverticular bleeding may occur in the patient with massive or intermittent bleeding. Depending on the patient's cardiovascular stability and degree of bleeding, the typical evaluative progression if the site of bleeding is not identified is endoscopy, followed by tagged red blood cell scan, and then angiography. Hemodynamically unstable patients may have a high complication risk from the bowel preparation, sedation, or the procedure. Radionuclide imaging can be considered in unstable patients, nondiagnostic endoscopy, or bleeding recurrence. Radionuclide imaging requires that bleeding be active (at least 0.05 to 0.1 mL/min) to accurately isolate the location of the diverticulum. Radionuclide imaging using ^{99m}Tc sulfur colloid (shorter half-life, thus used for acute bleeding) or ^{99m}Tc pertechnetate (longer half-life more useful for intermittent bleeding)-labeled autologous red blood cells can be used to isolate the location of obscure gastrointestinal bleeding. However, numerous studies have produced highly variable sensitivities (26% to 91%). Many advocate for radionuclide imaging to be used as an ancillary test for directing more definitive treatments such as surgery or angiography-directed therapies. Angiography can be used if bleeding is active (at least 0.5 mL/min) and can isolate the bleeding location with a diagnostic yield of 40% to 78%. Angiography can be combined with embolization and/or vasopressin infusion to achieve hemostasis; however, complications may occur, including bowel infarction, rebleeding, and contrast-induced nephrotoxicity.

Diverticulitis

Diverticulosis is largely asymptomatic. Only approximately 4% will develop inflammation and infection known as diverticulitis.

The disease severity and complications occur along a spectrum. The proposed mechanism of diverticulitis may be a blocked diverticulum or increased intraluminal pressure inducing. Subsequent vascular compromise and microperforation may occur, leading to localized infection and inflammation. These microperforations are usually sequestered and may lead to small localized abscess formation. This process is generally referred to as uncomplicated diverticulitis. Complicated diverticulitis is classified when a localized abscess or infection infiltrates into adjacent organs or viscera causing macroperforations, fistulas, obstructions, or enlarged abscesses.

The clinical presentation often begins with mild left lower abdominal pain, fever, and leukocytosis. Patients who seek care later in the disease process may present with sepsis or diffuse peritonitis. Initial diagnosis should be accomplished with history, physical examination, radiographic imaging, and laboratory evaluation. Abdominal radiography has limited utility but may reveal severe complications of diverticulitis such as bowel perforation or bowel obstruction. Ultrasonography and magnetic resonance imaging can be used with high levels of sensitivity and specificity in centers with demonstrated expertise. Ultrasonography has sensitivities and specificities of 92% and 90% for the detection of diverticulitis, respectively. With sensitivities and specificities of 94% and 99%, respectively, CT appears to be the imaging test of choice. This is especially true, as an alternative diagnosis was more likely to be identified with CT than with ultrasonography (50% to 100% vs. 33% to 78%). Those patients with a past medical history of diverticulitis may be empirically treated without imaging, although imaging may be needed if no clinical improvement is noted within 48 hours.

New trials indicate no added benefit with antimicrobial therapy in select patients with uncomplicated diverticulitis. Factors such as pain control, hospitalization rates, and revisits were found to be similar between patients randomized to conservative management and antibiotic administration plus conservative measures. Thus patients may be treated with a liquid diet, analgesics, and close clinical follow-up without antibiotics. Outpatient management is reasonable if the diagnosis is made early in the disease process. Complicated diverticulitis occurs in 25% of all diverticulitis diagnoses, requiring a surgical evaluation and intervention. Optional antibiotic regimens for gram-negative coverage and anaerobic coverage are listed in Table 1. Inpatient management is recommended with any high-risk comorbid conditions, immunosuppression, high-grade fever, leukocytosis, inability to tolerate oral fluids, and/or for elderly patients. Patient improvement should be seen within 48 hours. Those who do not improve should undergo additional evaluation such as repeat imaging or endoscopy. This is done to evaluate for underlying pathology

TABLE 1 Antibiotic Therapy for Diverticulitis

OPTIONAL REGIMENS	DOSAGE (ADULT)
Uncomplicated Diverticulitis	
Outpatient (10–14 days)	
Ciprofloxacin (Cipro) and Metronidazole (Flagyl)	500 mg PO bid 500 mg PO tid
Amoxicillin-clavulanate (Augmentin)[1]	875 mg PO bid
Moxifloxacin (Avelox)	400 mg PO daily
Complicated Diverticulitis ***Inpatient Transitioning to Outpatient (10–14 Days Total)***	
Piperacillin-tazobactam (Zosyn)[1]	3.375–4.5 g IV every 6 h
Imipenem-cilastatin (Primaxin)	500 mg IV every 6 h
Levofloxacin (Levaquin)[1] and Metronidazole	500 mg IV every 24 h 500 mg IV every 8 h
Ceftriaxone (Rocephin) and Metronidazole	1 g IV every 24 h 500 mg IV every 8 h

[1]Not FDA approved for this indication.
Clindamycin (Cleocin) may be substituted in metronidazole intolerance/allergy.
   Antibiotics continued in complicated diverticulitis cases until negative cultures,
   clinical improvement, or sensitivities obtained on any surgical specimens.
bid, Twice a day; *tid*, three times a day.
Modified from Jacobs DO. Clinical practice: diverticulitis. *N Engl J Med.*
   2007;357:2057–2066.

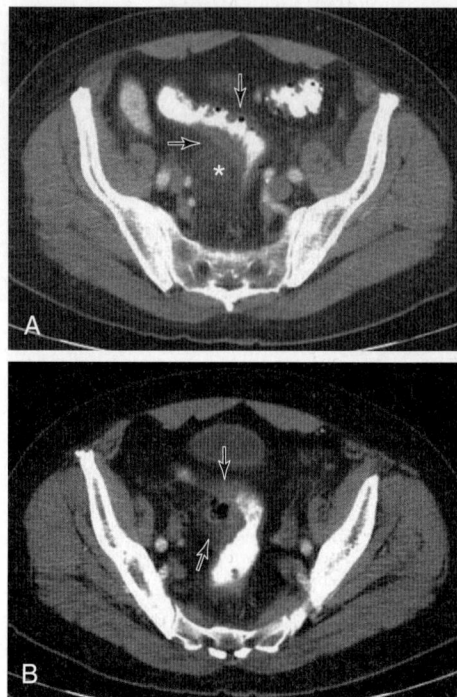

Figure 4 Diverticulitis. (A) Computed tomography (CT) image demonstrates thickened wall of the sigmoid colon *(arrows)* with stranding in the adjacent fat *(*)* indicative of diverticulitis. Fat stranding refers to abnormally increased attenuation of fat from edema and engorgement of lymphatics. (B) CT image slightly more caudal demonstrates an air-filled abscess cavity *(arrows)* with adjacent thickened sigmoid colon wall. (From McNally PR. GI/Liver Secrets Plus, 4th ed. Noninvasive Gastrointestinal Imaging: *Ultrasound, Computed Tomography, Magnetic Resonance Imaging.* Philadelphia: Mosby Elsevier; 2010, Figure 70–16.)

such as cancer or inflammatory bowel disease, which would change the management strategy.

Follow-up scanning should also be considered for cases of slow-resolving diverticulitis. In the past, up to 10% of CT scans in which diverticulitis was the primary diagnosis, cancer could not be fully excluded. As CT scanner resolution has improved, newer studies have demonstrated only a small number of underlying cancers or indeterminate findings. A colonoscopy should be performed to evaluate the extent of diverticular disease and to rule out other comorbid pathology in all patients. Colonoscopy is typically recommended 6 weeks after diverticulitis symptoms have resolved, if one has not been done within the last year. Introduction of stool softeners and a high-fiber diet should begin immediately and continued indefinitely for all patients to help decrease the intraluminal pressure within the colon.

Diverticulitis that is complicated with abscess formation should be evaluated by a surgeon or radiologist for percutaneous drainage using CT or ultrasonography (Figure 4). Depending on location, aspiration or drainage tubes may be used to facilitate drainage. A general recommendation exists for consideration of drainage, preferably with interventional radiology localization, for any abscess measuring greater than 3 to 4 cm.

New research to prevent recurrent diverticulitis with medical management is emerging. Rifaximin (Xifaxan)[1] may help prevent recurrent episodes of diverticulitis. Probiotics[7] have not been shown to prevent recurrence. Fiber may be used as a beneficial supplement for the prevention of recurrent diverticulitis. Recent research has shifted to examine the effects of nutrition and exercise on prevention of diverticulitis. When compared with typical Western diets, male patients with diets high in fruits, vegetables, and whole grains were associated with lower risks of diverticulitis. Similarly, diverticulitis risks were lower in men with increased physical activity, lower red meat consumption, higher dietary fiber intakes, nonsmokers, and a normal BMI. More studies are needed to further investigate these factors and their applicability to women with diverticulitis. Debate exists regarding elective segmental colectomy for patients who have experienced recurrent episodes of diverticulitis. Current recommendations suggest

surgical consultation with discussion of the benefits and risks of surgery compared with the risks of recurrent diverticulitis. This discussion should consider the diverticulitis frequency and severity, the impact on the patient's lifestyle, and the patient's other comorbid conditions. This consultation should at a minimum occur after the fourth recurrence of diverticulitis in patients older than age 50. There is insufficient evidence to advise a patient who has experienced fewer than four recurrent cases of diverticulitis or who is younger than age 50 on the benefit of a segmental colectomy.

References

Aguirre D, Hourneaux de Moura D, Hirsch B, et al: Flexible endoscopy versus rigid endoscopy or surgery for the management of Zenker's diverticulum: a systematic review and meta-analysis, *Cureus* Aug 15(8):e43021, 2023.

Chait J, Galli L, Clark C: Indications for operative management of complicated duodenal diverticula: a review, *Am Surg* 89(7):3043–3046, 2023.

Choi JJ, Ogunjemilusi O, Divino CM: Diagnosis and management of diverticula in the jejunum and ileum, *Am Surg* 79(1):108–110, 2013.

Delavux M: Diverticular disease of the colon in Europe: Epidemiology, impact on citizen health and prevention, *Aliment Pharmacol Ther* 18(Suppl 3):71–74, 2003.

Fry RD, Mahmoud NN, Maron DJ, et al: Colon and rectum. In Townsend Jr CM, Beauchamp D, editors: *Sabiston Textbook of Surgery,* 19th ed, Philadelphia, 2012, Saunders, pp 1309–1314.

Greene CL, McFadden PM, Oh DS, et al: Long-term outcome of the treatment of Zenker's diverticulum, *Ann Thorac Surg* 100:975–978, 2015.

Ishaq S, Sultan H, Siau K, et al: New and emerging techniques for endoscopic treatment of Zenker's Diverticulum: State-of-the-art review, *Digestive Endoscopy* 30:449–460, 2018.

Jacobs DO: Clinical practice, Diverticulitis, *N Engl J Med* 357:2057–2066, 2007.

Janes SE, Meagher A, Frizelle FA: Management of diverticulitis, *BMJ* 332:271–275, 2006.

Kilic A, Schuchert MJ, Awais O, et al: Surgical management of epiphrenic diverticula in the minimally invasive era, *JSLS* 13:160–164, 2009.

Lameris W, van Randen A, Bipat S: Graded compression ultrasonography and computed tomography in acute colonic diverticulitis: Meta-analysis of test accuracy, *Eur Radiol* 18:2498–2511, 2008.

Lin S, Suhocki PV, Ludwig KA, et al: Gastrointestinal bleeding in adult patients with Meckel's diverticulum: The role of technetium 99m pertechnetate scan, *South Med J* 95:1338, 2002.

---

[1]Not FDA approved for this indication.
[7]Available as a dietary supplement.

Maish MS: Esophagus. In Townsend Jr CM, Beauchamp D, editors: *Sabiston Textbook of Surgery*, 19th ed, Philadelphia, 2012, Saunders, pp 1023–1025.

Martinez-Cecilia D, Arjona-Sanchez A, Gomez-Alvarez M, et al: Conservative management of perforated duodenal diverticulum: A case report and review of the literature, *World J Gastroenterol* 14:1949–1951, 2008.

Mohan P, Ananthavadivelu M, Venkataraman J: Gastric diverticulum, *CMAJ* 182:E226, 2010.

Mora-López L, Ruiz-Edo N, Estrada-Ferrer O, et al: Efficacy and safety of nonantibiotic outpatient treatment in mild acute diverticulitis (DINAMO-study): a multicentre, randomised, open-label, noninferiority trial. *Ann Surg.* 274(5):e435, 2021

Morris P, Allaway M, Mwagiru D, et al: Gastric diverticulum: a contemporary review and update in management, *ANZ J Surg* 93(12):2828–2832, 2023.

Morris AM, Rogenbogen SE, Hardiman KM, et al: Sigmoid diverticulitis: A systematic review, *JAMA* 311:287–297, 2014.

Mulder CJ, Costamagna G, Sakai P: Zenker's diverticulum: Treatment using a flexible endoscope, *Endoscopy* 33:991–997, 2001.

Oukachbi N, Brouzes S: Management of complicated duodenal diverticula, *J Visceral Surg* 150:173–179, 2013.

Park JJ, Wolff BG, Tollefson MK, et al: Meckel diverticulum: The Mayo Clinic experience with 1476 patients (1950–2002), *Ann Surg* 241:529–533, 2005.

Sacks O, Hall J: Management of diverticulitis: a review, *JAMA Surg* 159(6):696–703, 2024.

Sartelli M, Catena F, Ansaloni L, et al: WSES Guidelines for the management of acute left sided colonic diverticulitis in the emergency setting, *World J Emerg Surg* 11:37, 2016.

Shabanzadeh DM, Wille-Jørgensen P: Antibiotics for uncomplicated diverticulitis, Nov 14, *Cochrane Database Syst Rev* 11, 2012. https://doi.org/10.1002/14651858.

Shah J, Patel K, Sunkara T, et al: Gastric diverticulum: a comprehensive review, *Inflamm Intest Dis* 3:161–166, 2018.

Shahedi K, Fuller G, Bolus R, et al: Long-term risk of acute diverticulitis among patients with incidental diverticulosis found during colonoscopy, *Clin Gastroenterol Hepatol* 11(12):1609–1613, 2013.

Sinha CK, Pallewatte A, Easty Met al, et al: Meckel's scan in children: A review of 183 cases referred to two paediatric surgery specialist centres over 18 years, *Pediatr Surg Int* 29:511–517, 2013.

Strate LL: Lower GI, bleeding: Epidemiology and diagnosis, *Gastroenterol Clin North Am* 34:643–664, 2005.

Verdonck J, Morton RP: Systematic review on treatment of Zenker's diverticulum, *Eur Arch Otorhnolaryngol* 272:3095–3107, 2015.

Weizman AV, Nguyen GC: Diverticular disease: epidemiology and management, *Can J Gastroenterol* 25:385–389, 2011.

Young-Fadok TM: Diverticulitis, *N Engl J Med* 379, 2018. 1635-164.

Zani A, Eaton S, Rees CM: Incidentally detected Meckel diverticulum: To resect or not to resect? *Ann Surg* 247:276–281, 2008.

DYSPHAGIA AND ESOPHAGEAL OBSTRUCTION

Method of
Christopher Vélez, MD; John E. Pandolfino, MD; Kumar Krishnan, MD

CURRENT DIAGNOSIS

- The evaluation of dysphagia begins with a careful history, though additional diagnostic testing is often required.
- Oropharyngeal dysphagia is best initially evaluated with a video fluoroscopoic examination, whereas esophageal dysphagia is best evaluated with endoscopy.
- Esophageal dysphagia with negative endoscopy and biopsy should be evaluated next with esophageal physiological testing (esophageal manometry or endoscopic functional lumen imaging probe EndoFLIP).

CURRENT THERAPY

- Underlying neuromuscular conditions such as amyotrophic lateral sclerosis, myasthenia gravis, or Guillain-Barré syndrome should be treated accordingly.
- Endoscopic therapy with dilation (often multiple) is the mainstay of treating fibrotic esophageal strictures regardless of etiology.
- Achalasia can be treated surgically or with dilation, which are equally effective. Minimally invasive endoscopic therapy for achalasia is now a well established alternative treatment approach.

Dysphagia is a symptom generated by the perceived sensation of difficulty or inability to swallow. It ranges in severity from mild difficulty with no associated clinical sequelae, to a complete inability to swallow with aspiration and severe malnutrition. Dysphagia can coexist with and must be distinguished from odynophagia, which is pain when swallowing, with associated swallowing aversion. The etiology of dysphagia is protean and includes two main categories, mechanical obstruction and motor dysfunction.

Epidemiology
Dysphagia is a common condition. In studies of outpatients, 22.6% of patients have reported dysphagia at least several times per month. Only half of these patients had discussed their symptoms with their physician. Elderly patients and women were more likely to note symptoms of dysphagia.

Pathophysiology
Effective swallowing and transfer of food bolus into the stomach requires multiple steps. These steps can be broadly placed into two phases: the oropharyngeal phase and the esophageal phase. The oropharyngeal phase of swallowing ultimately transforms the hypopharynx from a respiratory organ to a digestive organ. It requires five main coordinated steps to occur: (1) elevation of the soft palate and closure of the nasopharynx, (2) relaxation of the upper esophageal sphincter (UES), (3) traction opening of the UES, (4) closure of the laryngeal vestibule and, hence, airway protection, and (5) propulsion of the food bolus by the tongue and pharyngeal constrictors. This process is a carefully coordinated neuromuscular phenomenon with both autonomic and volitional components.

The esophageal phase of swallowing begins when a food bolus passes through the UES. During swallowing, the rapidity of bolus transit into the stomach is accomplished primarily by gravity. Esophageal peristalsis is a secondary contributor that functions to strip the bolus and clear the esophagus. Primary peristalsis is associated with oropharyngeal swallowing and propagates down through the predominantly striated muscle of the esophagus via a sequential activation pattern originating from the brainstem. This propagation then involves the esophageal smooth muscle where it also engages the intrinsic enteric nervous system to promote peristalsis through a similar but distinct mechanism. Secondary peristalsis is stimulated by distention of the proximal esophagus and will generate a propagating peristaltic contraction similar to primary peristalsis without a swallow-induced trigger. The strength, propagation velocity, and order of peristaltic contractions can be altered, with perturbations potentially leading to motor abnormalities associated with dysphagia.

Diagnosis
Dysphagia is never a normal symptom and always requires additional investigation. The first step in the diagnostic evaluation of dysphagia begins with a careful history to distinguish true dysphagia from other associated conditions such as odynophagia and globus sensation. Odynophagia can coexist with dysphagia; however, the predominant symptom is pain during swallowing. Globus is a sensation of a lump in the throat. It is likely a pharyngeal hypersensitivity that may coexist with other esophageal diseases or occur alone as a functional disorder. Unlike dysphagia, the symptoms in globus persist between swallows and may actually improve during the swallow.

After the above conditions have been ruled out, the next step focuses on distinguishing oropharyngeal dysphagia from esophageal dysphagia. Asking patients if their difficulty swallowing is "above-the-gulp" can differentiate oropharyngeal dysphagia. Unfortunately, patients have a difficult time communicating their symptoms because localization of the point of perceived obstruction is hampered by poor discriminant capacity and may be masked by compensatory mechanisms. Localization of dysphagia to the throat or sternal notch is unreliable because the point of obstruction may be further down in the body. However, localization in the midchest or below is more reliable that the obstruction is esophageal in origin.

As a result, the most useful and underused test for distinguishing oropharyngeal and esophageal dysphagia focuses on observing the patient swallow sips of water in the office. Often this allows the distinction between oropharyngeal and esophageal dysphagia to become apparent. Patients with oropharyngeal dysphagia will have difficulty almost immediately after initiating a swallow, such as coughing, choking, and nasal regurgitation. Patients who can initiate a swallow without difficulty, but note symptoms soon after the swallow, are likely to have esophageal dysphagia. Furthermore, this exercise may be able to elicit associated odynophagia or regurgitation.

Physical examination plays a minor role in evaluating dysphagia outside of assessing the patient's baseline status to rule out malnutrition and dehydration because this will determine whether an expedited evaluation is required. A careful assessment of the oropharynx and a careful neck examination may unmask a mass lesion (i.e. of the thyroid), and a neurologic examination should be performed if oropharyngeal dysphagia is suspected. Additionally, a skin examination and assessment of the oropharyngeal mucosa may be helpful in assessing for potential dermatologic diseases that are associated with esophageal dysphagia. Regardless of findings, most patients will ultimately be referred for diagnostic testing, and this is dependent on the anatomic zone of interest—oropharyngeal versus esophageal (Figure 1).

Diagnostic Testing
Oropharyngeal Dysphagia
Once a distinction is made that the patient is experiencing oropharyngeal dysphagia, the next step in the evaluation should be referral for a video fluoroscopic swallowing examination, also known as a modified barium study. Standard upper endoscopy is of limited value given the general inability to evaluate lesions in the hypopharynx and the upper esophageal sphincter. Video fluoroscopic swallow examinations have the added benefit of providing functional information in addition to anatomic information. They differ from a standard fluoroscopic examination (i.e., esophogram) by offering the patient various radiopaque food items of different consistency and are often performed by a speech pathologist. They can evaluate delay in initiation of pharyngeal swallowing, aspiration of solids and liquids, retrograde flow of ingested bolus, and residual pharyngeal contents.

If there is a suspicion for a malignancy or mechanical obstruction, a referral to otolaryngology is required. Direct laryngoscopy is used to evaluate for anatomic lesions in the nasopharynx and hypopharynx. In addition to anatomic abnormalities, function can be assessed by having the patient drink liquids with the nasal

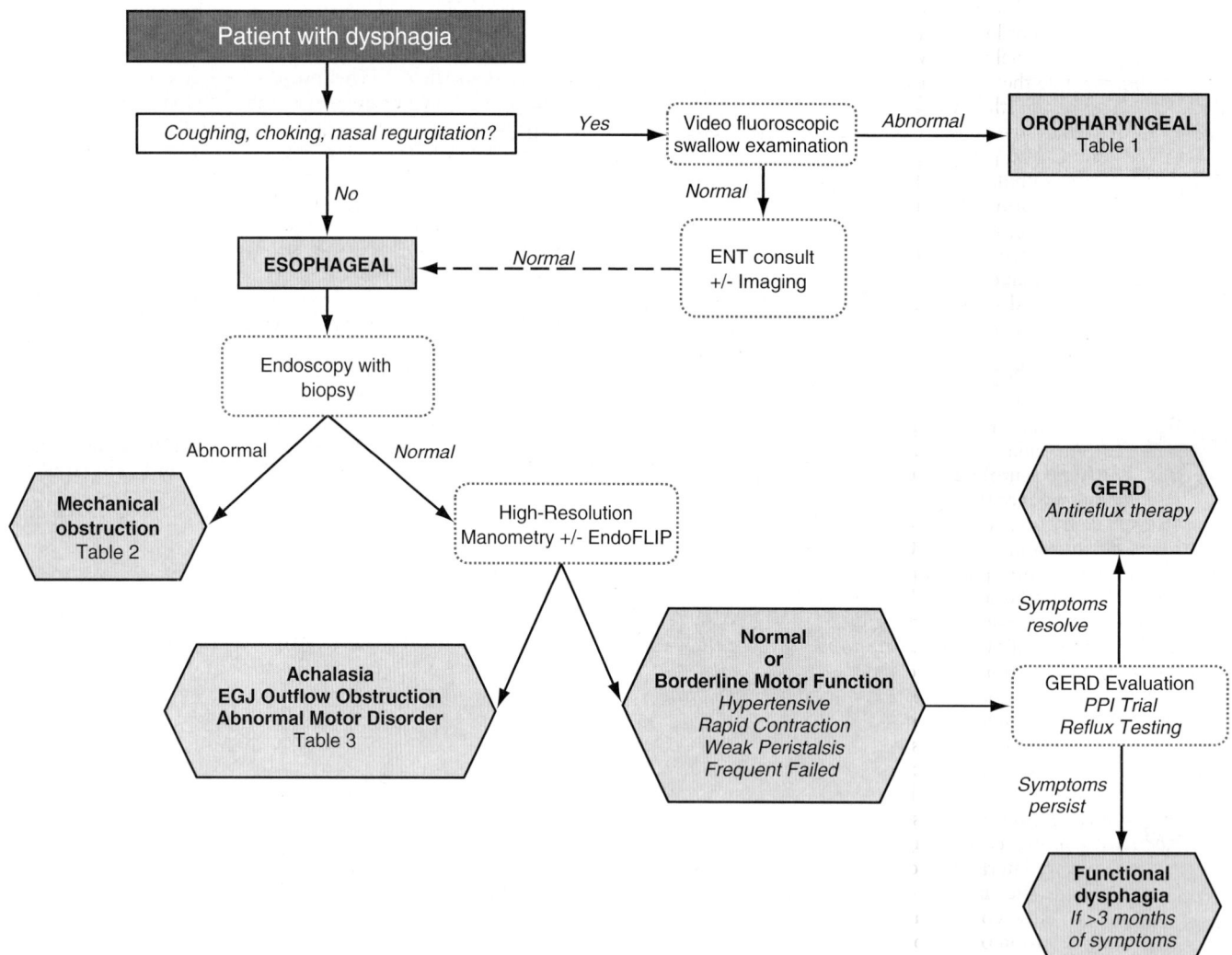

Figure 1 The workup of dysphagia and esophageal obstruction. The first step in the workup of dysphagia focuses on distinguishing oropharyngeal from esophageal dysphagia, which can be done with a history and careful assessment of swallowing during liquid swallows. The workup once this distinction is made is very different. Oropharyngeal dysphagia is typically evaluated by speech pathology and otolaryngology (ENT) based on the results of a video fluoroscopic swallow evaluation. Esophageal dysphagia is evaluated primarily with endoscopy because biopsies and interventions are often required. The primary indication for manometry is to rule out a major motor disorder in patients with a negative endoscopy. Alternatively, the functional lumen imaging probe (FLIP) can be utilized at the time of endoscopy to assess for a primary motor disorder. If a major motor abnormality is not seen on manometry or FLIP, a diagnosis of functional dysphagia should be considered; however, underlying GERD must also be addressed.

endoscope positioned in the hypopharynx. Oropharyngeal pooling of liquid indicates ineffective hypopharyngeal clearance and can suggest a high aspiration risk. Cross-sectional imaging is often an adjunct to the functional assessment of videoscopic imaging or direct laryngoscopy when an obstruction is noted without a clear lesion noted on direct examination.

Esophageal Dysphagia

If oropharyngeal dysphagia is excluded on history, the evaluation of dysphagia should proceed to upper endoscopy to rule out a mechanical obstruction. Although an esophogram can be used to assess for obstruction, most patients will eventually require endoscopy to obtain biopsies to rule out malignancy or eosinophilic esophagitis. Additionally, endoscopy has the added benefit of being therapeutic in some circumstances, and thus it is more cost-effective to begin the evaluation with endoscopy. If the endoscopy is negative, the next step is to evaluate for an underlying esophageal motor disorder. This is traditionally done by performing esophageal manometry. Recently, a novel method of assessing esophageal motor function has been developed. The functional lumen imaging probe (FLIP) is a catheter that can be placed at the time of endoscopy. Using a variety of sensors positioned along the length of the probe, it measures diameter and pressure along the esophagus. This information can be used to evaluate for contractility of the esophageal body and esophageal distensibility at the EGJ, thus providing a comprehensive assessment of esophageal motility that is complementary to esophageal manometry and can help resolve borderline cases of motility abnormality prior to the recommendation of potentially invasive surgical or endoscopic therapy. If these studies are negative, a careful evaluation for the presence of gastroesophageal reflux disease (GERD) should be performed and if suspected, the patient may benefit from ambulatory reflux testing or an empiric trial of proton pump inhibitors. Patients with no evidence of obstruction, abnormal esophageal motor function, or evidence of GERD may be classified as having functional dysphagia and they benefit from the use of neuromodulation (with agents used to treat functional gastrointestinal disorders such as tricyclic antidepressants) to improve sensory function.

Oropharyngeal Dysphagia

Differential Diagnosis

The etiology of oropharyngeal dysphagia can be broadly separated based on neuromuscular causes and anatomic causes (Table 1). The most common neurologic cause is cerebrovascular accident (CVA), with an incidence reported between 20% and 80%. CVAs involving the cerebrum, cerebellum, and brainstem can each lead to swallow dysfunction. Cerebral CVA can lead to impairment in mastication and the oral phase of swallowing and can interrupt normal pharyngeal peristalsis. CVA involving the brainstem can lead to disruption of the sensory afferents in the pharynx that help trigger pharyngeal swallow, and can also lead to motor dysfunction of laryngeal elevation, glottic closure, and cricopharyngeal relaxation/opening. Tumors in these areas can also produce similar effects. While difficulty swallowing liquids can be associated with oropharyngeal dysphagia, distinguishing between liquid versus solid food dysphagia is not a reliable way to differentiate this type of dysphagia from esophageal dysphagia.

A variety of neuromuscular disease can lead to bulbar symptoms, which manifest as dysphagia. This includes myasthenia gravis, amyotrophic lateral sclerosis (ALS), and Guillain-Barré syndrome (GBS). Clinicians need to be able to identify systemic manifestations of these conditions because dysphagia can often be the first manifestation of neuromuscular disorders.

The most common structural abnormalities of the hypopharynx associated with dysphagia are hypopharyngeal diverticula and cricopharyngeal bars. Acquired hypopharyngeal diverticula are most common in men after age 60 and typically present with symptoms of dysphagia, halitosis, post-swallow regurgitation, or even aspiration of material from the pharyngeal pouch. Hypopharyngeal diverticula are the result of a restrictive myopathy

associated with diminished compliance of the cricopharyngeus muscle. The treatment of hypopharyngeal diverticula is cricopharyngeal myotomy with or without a diverticulectomy. Good or excellent results can be expected in 80% to 100% of Zenker's patients treated by transcervical myotomy combined with diverticulectomy or diverticulopexy. Small diverticula may spontaneously disappear following myotomy.

Other anatomic causes associated with oropharyngeal dysphagia that should be considered are cervical osteophytes and head and neck cancers. Cervical osteophytes are associated with cervical spine arthritis and may be confused with a cricopharyngeal bar because the dysphagia is structural and localized to the area of the upper esophageal sphincter. It is easily differentiated on contrast studies because the cervical osteophyte can be seen impinging on the upper sphincter. Additionally, head and neck lesions of the larynx, tonsil, tongue, oral cavity, vocal cord, and nasopharynx may also impair bolus transit into the esophagus. Rapid weight

TABLE 1   Oropharyngeal Dysphagia

Iatrogenic

- Medication side effects (chemotherapy, neuroleptics, etc.)
- Postsurgical muscular or neurogenic
- Radiation
- Corrosive (pill injury, intentional)

Infectious

- Diphtheria
- Botulism
- Lyme disease
- Syphilis
- Mucositis (herpes, cytomegalovirus, candida, etc.)

Metabolic

- Amyloidosis
- Cushing's syndrome
- Thyrotoxicosis
- Wilson's disease

Myopathic

- Connective tissue disease (overlap syndrome)
- Dermatomyositis
- Myasthenia gravis
- Myotonic dystrophy
- Oculopharyngeal dystrophy
- Polymyositis
- Sarcoidosis
- Paraneoplastic syndromes

Neurologic

- Brainstem tumors
- Head trauma
- Stroke
- Cerebral palsy
- Guillain-Barré syndrome
- Huntington's disease
- Multiple sclerosis
- Polio
- Postpolio syndrome
- Tardive dyskinesia
- Metabolic encephalopathies
- Amyotrophic lateral sclerosis
- Parkinson's disease
- Dementia

Structural

- Cricopharyngeal bar
- Zenker's diverticulum
- Cervical webs
- Oropharyngeal tumors
- Osteophytes and skeletal abnormalities
- Congenital abnormalities (cleft palate, diverticula, pouches, etc.)

loss in a patient with oropharyngeal dysphagia warrants further evaluation for malignancy; however, it is often difficult to distinguish weight loss resulting from malignancy from weight loss secondary to dysphagia. Constitutional symptoms (night sweats, fever, etc.) associated with oropharyngeal dysphagia should raise the suspicion for lymphoma.

Management

The management of oropharyngeal dysphagia is dependent on the underlying cause. Neuromuscular conditions such as stroke may respond to speech therapy and rehabilitation. Systemic neuromuscular dysfunction from conditions such as myasthenia gravis, GBS, or ALS will require treatment of the underlying condition. Patients who cannot safely take oral nutrition may need a temporary enteral feeding tube until swallow function is intact.

Management of dysphagia in patients with head and neck cancers requires a multidisciplinary approach and treatment of the underlying malignancy. Some patients are able to take adequate nutrition with dietary modification (soft or full liquid diet) while undergoing therapy. Patients who are losing weight, are dehydrated, or are unable to meet nutritional requirement by dietary modification alone may require enteral nutrition in the form of a gastrostomy tube. Although endoscopic gastrostomy tube placement is typically safe, and routinely performed in patients with head and neck cancer, there are reports of seeding the gastrostomy tube tract with malignant cells from the pharynx. In such circumstances, a direct gastrostomy tube placed by a radiologist may be preferable.

Esophageal Dysphagia

Esophageal dysphagia can be easily separated into mechanical causes and motor abnormalities after upper endoscopy is performed. Mechanical causes can be further separated into malignant and benign causes of dysphagia, and motor disorders can be conceptualized as primary motor abnormalities versus borderline motor abnormalities. Patients who have symptoms in the context of a normal endoscopy (negative biopsies for eosinophilic esophagitis) and no evidence of a primary motor disorder may also have underlying GERD or functional dysphagia (see Figure 1).

Differential Diagnosis: Mechanical Obstruction (Table 2)
Stricture

Fibrotic esophageal strictures are common and can be caused by erosive esophagitis (peptic stricture), radiation therapy, surgical anastomosis, eosinophilic esophagitis, and desquamating lesions (pemphigus, lichen planus, etc.). Peptic strictures are common and are the result of long-standing erosive esophagitis. They typically occur in the distal esophagus. Such patients often have underlying physiologic derangements that favor aggressive reflux (weak lower esophageal sphincter, hiatal hernia, poor esophageal clearance). Postsurgical anastomotic strictures are an unfortunate consequence of surgical therapy for esophageal disease, but these lesions are often amenable to endoscopic therapy.

Eosinophilic Esophagitis

Eosinophilic esophagitis (EoE) requires some focused discussion because its prevalence in patients presenting with dysphagia is increasing. EoE is a condition characterized by marked eosinophilic infiltrate within the esophageal epithelium. This infiltrate results in characteristic endoscopic findings of esophageal rings, furrows, exudate, and eventually stricture formation. The most common symptom in patients with EoE is dysphagia, which often leads to food bolus impaction. Patients are typically young Caucasians and there is a clear male predominance. Atopic conditions are more prevalent in patients with EoE. Patients should initially be treated with proton pump inhibitor (PPI) therapy because there is an overlap between GERD and EoE. Patients with persistent eosinophilia on PPI therapy can be treated by swallowing inhaled formulations of steroids

TABLE 2 Esophageal Dysphagia (Mechanical)

Mucosal disease
  GERD (peptic stricture)
  Esophageal rings
  Esophageal cancer
  Caustic injury (e.g., lye ingestion, pill esophagitis, sclerotherapy)
  Radiation injury
  Infectious esophagitis
  Eosinophilic esophagitis
  Anastomotic stricture
  Submucosal disease
  Gastrointestinal stromal tumor
  Sarcoidosis
  Invasive carcinoma (primary or secondary)
Mediastinal disease
  Tumors (lymph nodes, lung cancer)
  Infection (histoplasmosis, tuberculosis)
  Vascular compression
  Dysphagia lusoria
  Dysphagia aortica

(fluticasone [Flovent],[1] budesonide [Pulmicort][1]) or a food elimination diet (avoid: soy, nuts, wheat, eggs, dairy, seafood) to reduce the inflammatory component of the disease. Additional therapy with dilation will be required in many patients because histologic improvement does not always result in regression of fibrotic strictures. The esophageal body is more prone to fracture in EoE, and deep mucosal tears are often associated with dilation therapy; thus these lesions may require a more gradual and careful dilation protocol.

Rings/Webs

Esophageal webs can exist along the length of the esophagus and lead to dysphagia. The classic triad of proximal esophageal web, iron deficiency anemia, and dysphagia is Plummer-Vinson syndrome. The etiology of this condition is not entirely known; however, it is thought that iron deficiency leads to a decrease in iron-dependent oxidative enzymes, which results in degradation of esophageal tissue, resulting in web formation. Interestingly, iron supplementation alone may result in resolution of symptoms. Whereas Plummer-Vinson syndrome is a rare condition, esophageal webs are relatively common and should prompt an evaluation for caustic pill injury if localized to the transition zone along the aortic impression or distal esophagus. Medications that can be associated with pill esophagitis include NSAIDs, tetracycline, iron, bisphosphonates, potassium, and quinidine.

Malignancy

Dysphagia is often the presenting symptom in a patient with esophageal cancer. There are two subtypes of mucosal cancer in the esophagus, squamous cell and adenocarcinoma. In general, esophageal cancer has a male predominance and is slightly more prevalent among African Americans. The racial disparity is largely due to squamous cell carcinoma, which has noted a sharp decline since the 1960s. Adenocarcinoma tends to be a disease of white men (SEER database). Squamous cell carcinoma typically occurs in the mid esophagus, whereas adenocarcinoma is localized to the distal esophagus where it is associated with intestinal metaplasia (Barrett's esophagus).

Management for Esophageal Obstruction

Endoscopic dilation therapy is the most common therapeutic intervention for patients with nonmalignant mechanical dysphagia. This can be done with a single, large-diameter dilating balloon or semirigid bougie over a guide wire. There has not been any convincing data to demonstrate superiority of

---

[1]Not FDA approved for this indication.

balloon dilators over bougie dilators. In cases of membranous webs or Schatzki rings, the goal of endoscopic therapy is to tear the lesion with a single, large-diameter dilation. In the case of a Schatzki ring, postdilation PPI therapy is associated with decreased recurrence rates.

When treating fibrotic strictures (peptic, anastomotic, radiation, EoE), the goal should be gradual stretching of the stricture. The choice of initial dilation size is based on an estimate of the diameter of the stricture. The extent to which a stricture can be dilated is expressed by the endoscopic axiom of the "rule of threes." This refers to the approach whereby the diameter of the stricture is approximated, and no more than three subsequent dilations are performed at 1-mm intervals once resistance is noted. Although there is no controlled trial for support, this approach is used to minimize the most serious risks of dilation therapy, perforation, and bleeding.

In patients with refractory strictures despite dilation therapy, several therapies have been attempted with variable efficacy. Temporary self-expanding stents have been placed to maintain lumen patency. When placed across a stricture, stents serve two purposes. First, they relieve symptoms of dysphagia by maintaining a patent lumen. In addition, the self-expanding nature of the stent provides ongoing radial force, which gradually stretches the lumen. The main disadvantage of stents is their tendency to migrate.

An alternative endoscopic approach is incisional therapy with an electrocautery knife. This is used to make incisions in the mucosa and fibrotic submucosa. This approach has been best studied in the setting of refractory anastomotic strictures; however, no head-to-head comparisons have been made between incisional therapy and other modalities.

Treatment of malignant etiologies for dysphagia will ultimately depend on the tumor type and extent of disease. Benign tumors and early-stage lesions can be treated with endoscopic resection or surgery. Endoscopic therapy using stents is also an important component of the treatment of malignancy and may be used during the treatment phase of malignant disorders or as a palliative technique for later-stage disease.

Differential Diagnosis: Motility Disorders (Table 3)

Esophageal motor disorders are defined based on patterns of contractile vigor, propagation, and the presence of deglutitive relaxation. The most common classification scheme is the "Chicago classification," at the time this chapter was written currently in its fourth version. This scheme takes advantage of advanced high-resolution manometry with modifications based on refining disorders into clinically relevant phenotypes compared to earlier classification iterations.

Achalasia

The diagnosis of achalasia is made by esophageal manometry and requires two main manometric criteria: (1) inability of the lower esophageal sphincter to relax and (2) absence of peristalsis. Recently achalasia has been subdivided into three different phenotypes using high-resolution manometry, which are associated with varying clinical outcomes. Patients typically describe both solid and liquid dysphagia. Other common symptoms are regurgitation (especially nocturnal), chest pain, and aspiration. Weight loss and malnutrition may be dominant symptoms as the disease progresses. Given that there is no treatment to reverse absent peristalsis, the treatment is focused on improving esophagogastric junction (EGJ) opening by disrupting the poorly relaxing lower esophageal sphincter. Currently, three modalities exist to treat achalasia: (1) pneumatic dilation with rigid balloons ranging in size from 3 to 4 cm; (2) surgical myotomy paired with or without a fundoplication; (3) per-oral endoscopic myotomy or POEM. It appears that the three treatment approaches are associated with good outcomes with surgery having a more durable single intervention success rate, pneumatic dilation typically requiring multiple sessions and POEM combining the benefit of one treatment session with a non-surgical approach. Botulinum toxin type A

TABLE 3	Esophageal Dysphagia (Abnormal Motor Function)
Achalasia	
EGJ outflow obstruction	
Absent peristalsis	
Spasm	
Jackhammer	

(Botox)[1] injected into the lower esophageal sphincter has been shown to reduce EGJ pressure and improve symptoms; however, this treatment only provides temporary relief and should only be reserved for poor surgical candidates or patients unwilling to undergo surgery, dilation, or endoscopic myotomy. Occasionally, esophageal dilatation may progress to a point where EGJ-directed treatment is not adequate and esophagectomy must be performed to prevent severe complications, such as aspiration and severe malnutrition. At times, dysphagia can recur after EGJ-directed therapy; EndoFLIP can help identify patients requiring re-treatment.

Esophagogastric Junction Outflow Obstruction

This pattern of motor disturbance is associated with preserved peristalsis and evidence of high pressures through the EGJ during swallowing. This may be an achalasia variant or could be associated with a subtle obstruction at the distal esophagus not evident on endoscopy. Thus recognition of this pattern should prompt an evaluation for an infiltrating tumor or other potential etiology of obstruction. Treatment is focused on the underlying cause of the obstruction. If distensibility is normal on EndoFLIP, then watchful waiting is appropriate.

Absent Peristalsis

Absent peristalsis is defined as complete absence of contractile activity on all swallows in the context of a normal or low EGJ relaxation pressure. This pattern was previously categorized as scleroderma esophagus if it was found in the context of a hypotensive lower esophageal sphincter; however, this has been abandoned because this pattern may be found in patients with severe GERD without scleroderma. Treatment is focused on aggressive antireflux therapy and lifestyle modifications to reduce dysphagia and caustic injury to the esophagus.

Distal Esophageal Spasm

Distal esophageal spasm is a rare primary motor disorder that can provoke dysphagia and is associated with premature contraction of the esophageal body. Treatment for this disorder is extremely difficult and focuses on medical management with smooth muscle relaxants, such as calcium channel blockers,[1] nitrates,[1] and 5-phosphodiesterase inhibitors.[1]

Jackhammer

Jackhammer esophagus is an extreme form of nutcracker esophagus associated with contractile vigor not encountered in asymptomatic controls or under normal conditions. Previous definitions for hypertensive esophagus had a significant overlap with data from cohorts of asymptomatic controls, and thus the clinical significance of these disorders was unclear. This pattern is associated with dysphagia and chest pain and is typically treated similar to distal esophageal spasm. This motor pattern can also be seen with distal esophageal obstruction, and this should be considered in the differential diagnosis because it would alter management to focus on the obstruction.

[1]Not available in the United States.

Borderline Motor Abnormalities

Borderline motor abnormalities are those associated with ineffective esophageal motility and mild abnormalities of peristaltic propagation (rapid contraction) or hypertensive contraction. These disorders are not considered to be primary motor disorders, and secondary cause for symptoms, such as GERD and visceral sensitivity, should be considered and treated.

Monitoring

Patients with dysphagia or esophageal obstruction should be monitored for three important complications:

- Evidence of aspiration and nocturnal regurgitation because these can be associated with severe complications, such as chemical pneumonitis and aspiration pneumonia.
- Malnutrition and dehydration because this may prompt more aggressive therapy or consideration of non-oral feeding methods.
- Progressive symptoms because this could lead to progression of the disease and early therapy may avoid the above complications.

Acknowledgment

This work was supported by R01 DK079902 (JEP) from the U.S. National Institutes of Health.

References

Bredenoord AJ, Fox M, Kahrilas PJ, et al: Chicago classification criteria of esophageal motility disorders defined in high resolution esophageal pressure topography, *Neurogastroenterol Motil* 24(Suppl. 1):57–65, 2012.

Cook IJ, Kahrilas PJ: AGA technical review on management of oropharyngeal dysphagia, *Gastroenterology* 116:455–478, 1999.

Drossman DA: The functional gastrointestinal disorders and the Rome III process, *Gastroenterology* 130:1377–1390, 2006.

Egan JV, Baron TH, Adler DG, et al: Esophageal dilation, *Gastrointest Endosc* 63:755–760, 2006.

Francis DL, Katzka DA: Achalasia: update on the disease and its treatment, *Gastroenterology* 139:369–374, 2010.

Liacouras CA, Furuta GT, Hirano I, et al: Eosinophilic esophagitis: updated consensus recommendations for children and adults, *J Allergy Clin Immunol* 128:3–20, 2011, e26; quiz 21–2.

Pandolfino JE, Kahrilas PJ: AGA technical review on the clinical use of esophageal manometry, *Gastroenterology* 128:209–224, 2005.

Pandolfino JE, Kwiatek MA, Nealis T, et al: Achalasia: a new clinically relevant classification by high-resolution manometry, *Gastroenterology* 135:1526–1533, 2008.

Spechler SJ: AGA technical review on treatment of patients with dysphagia caused by benign disorders of the distal esophagus, *Gastroenterology* 117:233–254, 1999.

Wilkins T, Gillies RA, Thomas AM, et al: The prevalence of dysphagia in primary care patients: a HamesNet Research Network study, *J Am Board Fam Med* 20:144–150, 2007.

GASTRITIS AND PEPTIC ULCER DISEASE

Method of
Kyle B. Vincent, MD

CURRENT DIAGNOSIS

- Diagnosis of gastritis and peptic ulcer disease (PUD) is based on history of dyspepsia and elimination of other conditions.
- *Helicobacter pylori* and nonsteroidal antiinflammatory drugs (NSAIDs) are the most common cause of ulcer disease. Hypersecretory conditions, such as Zollinger-Ellison syndrome, are rare.
- If testing for *H. pylori* is indicated (test-and-treat strategy), IgG antibody, urea breath test, and fecal antigen test are available, and nonserologic testing is favored.

- Young patients with no "warning signs" can usually be managed on an outpatient basis without immediate endoscopy.
- Patients older than 55 years with bleeding, anemia, loss of more than 10% of body weight, dysphagia, odynophagia, early satiety, history of previous malignancy, lymphadenopathy, abdominal mass, or a previously documented ulcer should undergo upper endoscopy promptly.

CURRENT TREATMENT

- The two principal strategies are empiric treatment or test and treat.
- In areas with an *H. pylori* infection rate of less than 10%, a 4- to 8-week course of proton pump inhibitors (PPIs) given empirically is appropriate.
- In patients who fail empiric PPI treatment or in areas with an *H. pylori* infection rate of greater than 10%, a test-and-treat strategy should be employed. A verified noninvasive *H. pylori* test should be used.
- Patients with active or past PUD, low-grade gastric mucosa-associated lymphoid tissue (MALT) lymphoma, increased risk of gastric cancer (hereditary, first-degree relative, autoimmune gastritis, or history of endoscopic resection of early gastric cancer), idiopathic (autoimmune) thrombocytopenic purpura, unexplained iron deficiency anemia, or household members of individuals who have positive nonserologic tests for *H. pylori* should also be tested and treated.
- First-line treatment of *H. pylori* consists of bismuth subcitrate[2] (120–300 mg) or subsalicylate[1] (300 mg) four times daily (QID), tetracycline[1] 500 mg QID, metronidazole[1] 500 mg three times daily (TID) or QID, and standard-dose PPI twice daily (BID) for 14 days.
- Nonserologic tests of cure should be undertaken in all patients treated for *H. pylori*.
- NSAIDs should be discontinued or standard-dose PPI for ulcer prophylaxis used in patients taking NSAIDs.

[1]Not FDA approved for this indication.
[2]Not available in the United States.

Epidemiology

An estimated four million Americans have active gastric ulcers with 350,000 new cases diagnosed each year. The lifetime prevalence of this condition is around 10%. The incidence was previously higher in men but is currently equal in men and women. Familial clustering is now believed to result from the transmission of *Helicobacter pylori* from person to person or a genetic predisposition to infection with *H. pylori* rather than a genetic predisposition to gastric ulcers.

Risk Factors

Most gastric and duodenal ulcers can be attributed to *H. pylori*, NSAID use, severe physiologic stress, or hypersecretory conditions. In America, 10% of young adults harbor *H. pylori* infections, and this incidence increases with age. Lower socioeconomic status and recent immigration from areas with high rates of infection also increase the incidence of *H. pylori* infection. Hypersecretory conditions, such as Zollinger-Ellison syndrome, are rare, estimated to be responsible for only 0.1% of all ulcers. These conditions should not be routinely considered except in refractory or recurrent cases or in patients who have multiple ulcers.

Pathophysiology

The low pH of gastric acid is required to kill ingested bacteria and to promote proteolysis and activation of pepsin. Postprandial gastric acid production is stimulated by expression of gastrin from G cells and is inhibited in a negative feedback loop by somatostatin from antral D cells. Contrary to previous beliefs, peptic ulcer disease (PUD) is not simply due to excessive acid production. Almost all patients with gastric ulcers have normal acid production, and only one-third of patients with duodenal ulcers have evidence of increased acid production. The protective mechanisms of the mucosa play an important role in maintaining mucosal integrity.

The gastric and duodenal mucosa form a gelatinous layer that is impermeable to gastric acid and pepsin. Mucosal blood flow and the production of mucus and bicarbonate secretion are largely regulated by E-type prostaglandins (PGE). Anything that can disrupt the balance between acid production and the protective barrier has the potential to cause loss of mucosal integrity and tissue exposure to gastric acid and pepsin with subsequent inflammation and potential ulceration.

Two major mechanisms contribute to gastritis and/or ulcer formation. *H. pylori* is a gram-negative curved rod that produces ammonia to control the surrounding pH. Ammonia is toxic to epithelial cells, causing gastritis or duodenitis and damaging mucosal integrity. Many patients with gastritis also have a marked decrease in the number of somatostatin-secreting antral D cells, leading to diminished feedback to control acid secretion during gastrin stimulation.

Prevention

The US Preventative Services Task Force does not currently recommend routine screening for *H. pylori* in asymptomatic individuals. Prevention is based on avoidance or minimization of risk factors. Long-term NSAID use should be avoided. Prophylactic antisecretory medication should be considered when prolonged NSAID use is necessary. Proton pump inhibitors (PPIs) have better protective efficacy than histamine receptor antagonists (H2RAs) when prolonged NSAID use is necessary. Patients with a previous history of ulcer disease who use steroids or are older than 65 years should strongly be considered for prophylaxis with an antisecretory medication. Because of the high risk of gastric ulceration, prophylaxis is recommended for patients experiencing severe physiologic stress, such as mechanical ventilation for longer than 48 hours, hypoperfusion, high-dose corticosteroids, and large surface area burns (>35% total body surface area). H2RAs such as famotidine (Pepcid)[1], cimetidine (Tagamet)[1], and ranitidine (Zantac)[1] or PPIs are recommended. No agent has been shown to be clearly superior for prophylaxis in patients on steroids or undergoing physiologic stress.

No immunization against *H. pylori* is currently available, but early-stage animal trials are in progress.

Clinical Manifestations

Dyspepsia is defined by the American College of Gastroenterology as chronic or recurrent pain or discomfort centered in the upper abdomen. Discomfort is defined as a subjective negative feeling that is not painful. Discomfort can incorporate a variety of symptoms including early satiety or upper abdominal fullness. A thorough history alone is usually sufficient to establish the diagnosis and to differentiate gastritis and peptic ulcers from other common conditions, though gastritis and PUD are difficult to differentiate from each other. Patients with PUD tend to have symptoms that are more pronounced with food intake. A patient with a duodenal ulcer usually reports increased pain 2 to 3 hours after a meal; conversely, a patient with a gastric ulcer tends to have pain precipitated or exacerbated by food intake. However, these classical findings are not reliable diagnostic indicators. Physical examination is important to rule out serious complications from PUD. Patients with a rigid abdomen, rebound tenderness, or guarding should be evaluated with imaging and by a surgeon to rule out perforation. The most common physical finding in PUD is tenderness in the epigastrium.

Differential Diagnosis

The differential diagnosis for gastritis and PUD is broad given its nonspecific nature but can be narrowed down quickly by a good

initial history. The differential diagnosis includes gastroesophageal reflux disease (GERD), cardiac disease, gastric cancer, pancreatitis, pancreatic neoplasm, biliary disease including cholelithiasis or cholecystitis, delayed gastric emptying, or bowel ischemia. Patients presenting with a predominant complaint of heartburn or abdominal pain with heartburn more than once per week should be considered to have GERD until proven otherwise. Any symptoms associated with dyspnea or chest pressure should raise concern for a cardiac etiology. Biliary pain often radiates to the right shoulder and is associated with fatty or greasy foods. Patients with pancreatitis usually describe a severe boring-type pain in the epigastrium. They may also get relief from leaning forward.

Diagnosis

While most dyspepsia symptoms can be treated on a nonurgent basis, specific "warning signs" should prompt referral or performance of upper endoscopy. These include age 55 or older, bleeding, anemia, loss of more than 10% of body weight, dysphagia, odynophagia, early satiety, history of previous malignancy, lymphadenopathy, abdominal mass, or a previously documented ulcer.

H. pylori testing is a cornerstone of managing dyspepsia. However, most other laboratory studies are usually not helpful in establishing the diagnosis in uncomplicated PUD or gastritis but may be helpful in eliminating other conditions in the differential diagnosis.

Noninvasive Testing

Antibody test: Serum IgG antibodies are typically present at 21 days after the onset of *H. pylori* infection but can persist long after active infection. Antibody testing has a sensitivity of 85% and specificity of 79%. The positive predictive value is greatly influenced by the prevalence of the organism in the community; therefore it is less useful in areas with lower rates of *H. pylori* infection. The excellent negative predictive value makes IgG testing a good screening test. However, given that the IgG antibodies can persist for up to a year or longer after infection, it is not as helpful in the acute phase.

Urea breath test: This test identifies infection through urease activity. The patient ingests urea labeled with either ^{13}C or ^{14}C. In the presence of *H. pylori*, urease activity produces labeled CO_2 that is expired and can be collected and measured. Sensitivities and specificities of this test exceed 95%. It maintains a strong positive and negative predictive value despite the prevalence of *H. pylori*, but the test is not universally available.

Fecal antigen test: This assay uses either polyclonal or monoclonal antibodies to identify *H. pylori* antigens in the stool. The sensitivity and specificity exceed 90% in most studies. Like the breath test, it is unaffected by prevalence; however, both tests are affected by previous exposure to bismuth, antibiotics, and PPIs.

Treatment

The treatment of dyspepsia was revolutionized in the 1990s after the discovery of the role of *H. pylori* in pathogenesis. For patients who present with dyspepsia but no warning signs, two separate and approximately equivalent treatment strategies are recommended. The test-and-treat option recommends using a validated noninvasive test for *H. pylori* and treatment of positive tests. The empiric acid suppression option recommends treating with a PPI for 4 to 8 weeks without testing for *H. pylori*. The test-and-treat strategy is recommended for populations where the *H. pylori* infection rate is higher than 10%, in patients with active or past PUD, low-grade gastric mucosa-associated lymphoid tissue (MALT) lymphoma, increased risk of gastric cancer (hereditary, first-degree relative, autoimmune gastritis, or history of endoscopic resection of early gastric cancer), idiopathic (autoimmune) thrombocytopenic purpura, unexplained iron deficiency anemia, or household members of individuals who have positive nonserologic tests for *H. pylori*. As the US prevalence varies from 10% to 40% in different communities, either strategy may be appropriate. The test-and-treat strategy is more appropriate for most urban areas and in communities with a high immigrant

---

[1] Not FDA approved for this indication.

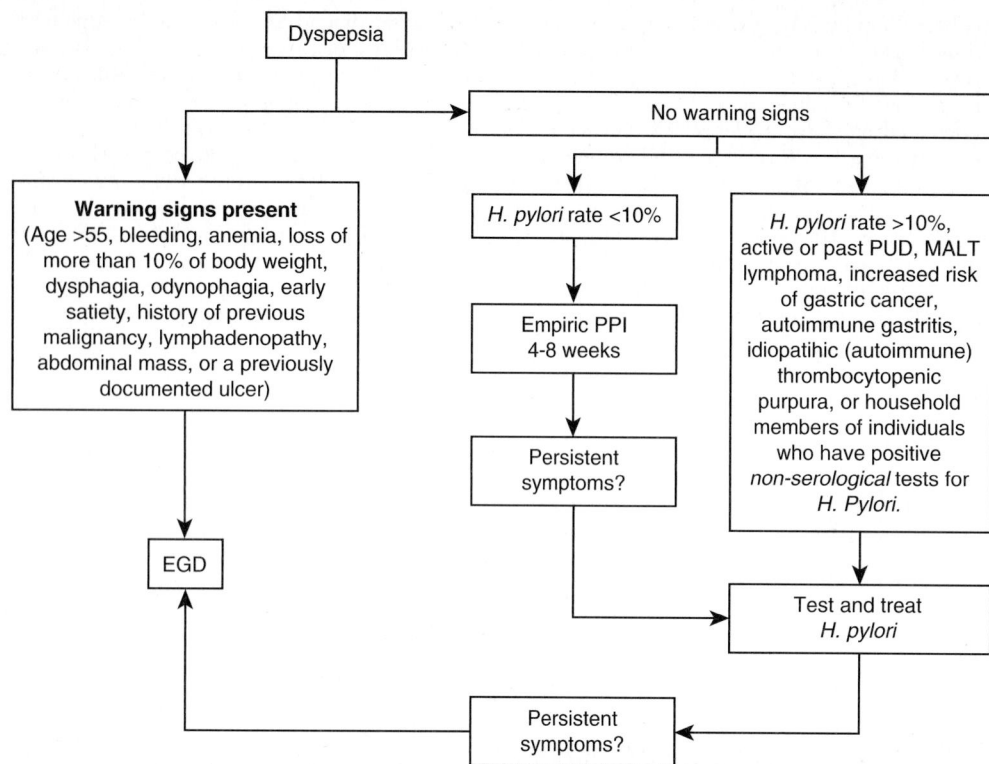

Figure 1 The treatment of dyspepsia. *EGD,* Esophagogastroduodenoscopy; *MALT,* mucosa-associated lymphoid tissue; *PPI,* proton pump inhibitor; *PUD,* peptic ulcer disease.

population or known high rates of *H. pylori* infection. In populations with low *H. pylori* prevalence, such as high socioeconomic areas, empiric acid suppression is an appropriate first strategy, followed by *H. pylori* testing in those patients who have continued symptoms (Figure 1).

The recommendations for eradication of *H. pylori* were updated by the American College of Gastroenterology in 2024. The newest recommendations were made as new data on antibiotic resistance has emerged, new antibiotics were released, and a new class of acid-reducing medications has been released. All regimens are now recommended for 14 days and, as in previous regimens, standard- or double-dose PPI of choice is suggested. Optimized bismuth quadruple therapy (OBQT) is now the first-line recommended therapy for all patients[1]. This includes bismuth subcitrate[2] (120–300 mg) or subsalicylate[1] (300 mg) four times daily (QID), tetracycline[1] 500 mg QID, metronidazole[1] 500 mg three times daily (TID) or QID, and standard-dose PPI twice daily (BID). This regimen has been found to have higher eradication rates than the traditional triple therapy that was previously recommended. There is the added benefit of avoiding any penicillin derivatives. Caution does have to be taken in women of childbearing years with the tetracycline and with photosensitivity. There are three other first-line regimens, which are listed in Table 1. Two of these regimens include the relatively new class of acid-controlling medications, potassium-competitive acid blockers (PCABs).

In patients who have "treatment experience," the American College of Gastroenterology 2024 guidelines recommend the optimized bismuth quadruple therapy as the first line as they have often been treated with an older regimen or one with higher resistance rates. Salvage regimens can be found in Table 2. Both traditional antibiotic susceptibilities testing from cultures and modern molecular techniques for gene mutations are becoming more widespread but are not universally available. In patients who are treatment experienced, susceptibility testing is recommended if available. Treatment regimens that include clarithromycin and levofloxacin[1] should only be considered if antibiotic susceptibility is confirmed.

Monitoring

The recommendations for routine testing for eradication of *H. pylori* were updated in 2024 as well. Directly quoted from the guidelines: "All patients who are treated for *H. pylori* infection should undergo a test of cure with an appropriately conducted urea breath test, fecal antigen test, or biopsy-based test at least 4 weeks after completion of therapy." Patients requiring follow-up endoscopy, such as for an ulcer or MALT lymphoma, should undergo endoscopic testing for eradication. Patients who are not undergoing endoscopy can be tested for eradication with fecal antigen or urea breath testing. The serum antibody test is unreliable for follow-up as it can remain positive for quite some time after successful treatment.

The most common causes of treatment failure are poor compliance with the medications and antibiotic resistance by the organism. Patients should be counseled on the side effects of their regimen and the importance of compliance. About 10% of patients report headaches and diarrhea with PPI use. Clarithromycin (Biaxin) can cause diarrhea, gastrointestinal upset, and altered taste. Similar effects can be seen with amoxicillin and metronidazole. Metronidazole also has disulfiram-like effects if taken with alcohol. Tetracycline should be avoided in women considering getting pregnant. Numerous systemic reviews have failed to show any statistical benefit in either tolerance to treatment or eradication rates with probiotics[7]. Bacterial resistance is continuing to rise with multicenter US data showing resistance rates to be 69.2% for metronidazole, 22.2% for clarithromycin, 37.6% for levofloxacin, and 1.2% for amoxicillin.

Patients who continue to have dyspepsia after successful eradication of *H. pylori* or who have persistent symptoms after a negative test and acid suppression should be considered for upper endoscopy.

Complications

PUD can have severe complications that almost always require hospital admission. The most significant complications are gastric bleeding, perforation, and outlet obstruction.

---

[1] Not FDA approved for this indication.
[2] Not available in the United States.

[7] Available as dietary supplement.

TABLE 1 Treatment Regimens for Treatment-Naïve Patients With *Helicobacter pylori* Infection

REGIMEN	ANTIBIOTIC			ANTACID
Bismuth quadruple therapy[a] (Pylera is a combination of bismuth subcitrate 140 mg, metronidazole 125 mg, and tetracycline 125 mg per capsule. It is FDA approved for treatment of *H. pylori* with omeprazole 20 mg BID. The dose is 3 caps QID × 10 days.)	Tetracycline (Sumycin)[1] 500 mg QID	Metronidazole (Flagyl)[1] 500 mg TID or QID	Bismuth subcitrate[2] 120–300 mg or subsalicylate (Pepto-Bismol)[1] 300 mg QID	PPI (standard dose) BID
Rifabutin triple therapy (Talicia is a combination of rifabutin 12.5 mg, amoxicillin 250 mg, and omeprazole 10 mg per capsule. It is FDA approved for treatment of *H. pylori* infection. The dose is 4 caps TID × 14 days.)	Amoxicillin 1 g TID	Rifabutin (Mycobutin)[1] 50 mg TID		Omeprazole (Prilosec) 40 mg TID
PCAB dual (Voquezna Dual Pak)	Amoxicillin 1 g TID			Vonoprazan 20 mg BID
PCAB triple (Voquezna Triple Pak)	Amoxicillin 1 g BID		Clarithromycin (Biaxin) 500 mg BID	Vonoprazan 20 mg BID

[a]Not FDA approved for this treatment regimen.
[1]Not FDA approved for this indication.
[2]Not available in the United States except in combination drug Pylera.
BID, Twice daily; *PCAB*, potassium-competitive acid blocker; *PPI*, proton pump inhibitor; *QID*, four times daily; *TID*, three times daily.

TABLE 2 Salvage Treatment Regimens for Treatment-Experienced Patients with *Helicobacter pylori* Infection

REGIMEN	ANTIBIOTIC			ANTACID
Optimized Bismuth Quadruple Therapy[a]	Tetracycline (Sumycin)[1] 500 mg QID	Metronidazole (Flagyl)[1] 500 mg TID or QID	Bismuth subcitrate[2] 300 mg or subsalicylate (Pepto-Bismol[1]) 300 mg QID	PPI (standard dose) BID
Rifabutin triple	Amoxicillin 1 g BID or TID	Rifabutin (Mycobutin)[1] 50–300 mg QD, BID, or TID		PPI (standard dose) BID
Levofloxacin triple[a]	Amoxicillin 1 g or metronidazole (Flagyl)[1] 500 mg BID	Levofloxacin (Levaquin)[1] 500 mg daily		PPI (standard dose) BID
PCAB triple (Voquezna TriplePak)	Amoxicillin 1 g BID	Clarithromycin (Biaxin) 500 mg BID		Vonoprazan 20 mg BID
High-dose dual therapy	Amoxicillin 1 g TID			Vonoprazan 20 mg or PPI (double dose) BID

[a]Not FDA approved for this treatment regimen.
[1]Not FDA approved for this indication.
[2]Not available in the United States except in combination drug Pylera.
BID, Twice daily; *PCAB*, potassium-competitive acid blocker; *PPI*, proton pump inhibitor; *QD*, daily; *QID*, four times daily; *TID*, three times daily.

237

Gastrointestinal bleeding is the most common cause of death in patients with PUD. Most cases of massive hemorrhage are due to erosion of a posterior ulcer into the gastroduodenal artery. Although the most common site of such hemorrhage is proximal to the ligament of Treitz, profuse bleeding can result in bright red blood from the rectum.

Approximately 5% of peptic ulcers cause perforation. This usually occurs anteriorly through the duodenum or lesser curve of the stomach. These patients often present in extremis with fever, tachycardia, dehydration, and abdominal findings of rigidity and rebound due to chemical peritonitis. Free air is commonly present under the diaphragm. Perforation almost always requires surgical management.

Gastric outlet obstruction can occur acutely due to inflammation from PUD or more chronically secondary to inflammation and healing that lead to scarring and fibrosis of the duodenum. These patients can present with severe hypochloremic hypokalemic alkalosis due to the loss of hydrogen, potassium, and chloride from gastric secretions. Electrolyte derangements must be corrected before any attempted surgery. Initial treatment with balloon dilation can be attempted, especially in cases with newly diagnosed *H. pylori*. If the patient is negative for *H. pylori* or has successfully eradicated the organism, the long-term outcomes of dilation do not compare well to surgery.

References

Chey WD, Howden CW, Moss SF, et al: ACG clinical guideline: treatment of helicobacter pylori infection, *Am J Gastroenterol* 119:1730–1753, 2024.

Chey WD, Leontiadis GI, Howden CW, et al: ACG clinical guideline: treatment of helicobacter pylori infection, *Am J Gastroenterol* 112:112–238, 2017.

Chey WD, Wong BC: The practice parameters committee of the American college of gastroenterology: american college of gastroenterology guideline on the management of *helicobacter pylori* infection, *Am J Gastroenterol* 102:1808–1825, 2007.

Helicobacter pylori and peptic ulcer disease: FDA approved drug regimens. Available at. http://www.cdc.gov/ulcer/keytocure.htm.

Mercer DW, Robinson EK: Stomach. In *Sabiston textbook of surgery*, ed 18, Philadelphia, 2008, Saunders, pp 1223–1277.

Nordenstedt H, Graham DY, Kramer JR, et al: *Helicobacter pylori*—negative gastritis prevalence and risk factors, *Am J Gastroenterol* 108:65–71, 2013.

Surgical critical care evidence based-medicine guidelines: Stress ulcer prophylaxis. Available at. http://www.surgicalcriticalcare.net/Guidelines/stress%20ulcer%20prophylaxis%202011.pdf.

Talley NJ, Vakil NB: The practice parameters committee of the American college of gastroenterology: guideline for the management of dyspepsia, *Am J Gastroenterol* 100:2324–2337, 2005.

GASTROESOPHAGEAL REFLUX DISEASE (GERD)

Method of
Mustafa Abdul-Hussein, MD, MSCR

Gastroesophageal reflux disease (GERD) is a motility disorder of the lower esophageal sphincter (LES). The definition of this disease has evolved over time, reflecting better understanding of the roles that transient LES relaxations and acid/pepsin contact with esophageal mucosa play, as well as the ability to identify these events. The diagnosis of GERD has changed from identification of a hiatal hernia, to identification of erosive esophagitis, to the currently accepted patient-centered definition: any symptom or injury to esophageal mucosa resulting from reflux of gastric contents into the esophagus. GERD should not be confused with physiologic gastroesophageal reflux, which is not associated with symptoms or esophageal mucosal injury.

The prevalence of GERD is difficult to ascertain, although several studies have indicated it to be as high as 50% of adults in Western countries, with 10% to 18% experiencing heartburn on a daily basis. Studies using healthcare utilization data may underestimate the prevalence because of self-treatment by individuals in the community, whereas population surveys may overestimate it because of inaccurate assessment of symptoms and absence of objective data. Regardless of the real number, the management of this disease costs more than $10 billion annually in the United States. GERD has been called a disease of White males, although recent data suggest increasing prevalence in Asia and Pacific regions. Recent studies assessing the global prevalence of GERD show that the overall burden of GERD has been worsening, with the prevalent cases increasing by 77.53% from 1990 to 2019.

Pathophysiology

GERD is a motility disorder of the LES characterized by inappropriate or transient relaxations that allow gastric contents to reflux into the esophagus. The LES is a tonically contracted ring of smooth muscle fibers innervated by the vagus nerve. Vagal stimulation during swallowing produces physiologic LES relaxation and is a likely source for transient LES relaxations. Gastroesophageal reflux occurs most frequently during postprandial periods, at a rate of six reflux episodes per hour, but averages two episodes per hour over the entire day. Increasing frequency of reflux in the postprandial period results from gastric distention after a meal and stimulation of tension receptors in the proximal stomach leading to transient LES relaxations (Box 1). A chronically hypotensive LES is not a major mechanism for GERD in most patients but can be seen in cases of severe erosive esophagitis.

Reflux of acidic gastric contents can lead to injury of the esophageal mucosa, including inflammation, ulceration, stricturing, Barrett metaplasia, and adenocarcinoma. Peristaltic clearance, tissue resistance, and salivary bicarbonate make up host defense mechanisms that work by clearing reflux and neutralizing the acid residue on the mucosa. Erosive esophagitis or strictures result in the most severe form of GERD, which includes nocturnal reflux with longer acid contact times, decreased salivary production, and lower frequency of swallowing during sleep.

Complications

Acid reflux can lead to significant morbidity if it is not recognized and treated appropriately. Habitual contact of acid and activated pepsin with the stratified squamous epithelium, along with impaired defense mechanisms, results in tissue injury (Box 2). The end result of this process can be ulceration, fibrosis with stricture formation, Barrett esophagus (BE), or adenocarcinoma. These complications can produce alarm symptoms (Box 3). Patients presenting with alarm symptoms should undergo immediate diagnostic evaluation with an esophagogastroduodenoscopy (EGD).

> ### BOX 1 — Factors That Modulate Transient Lower Esophageal Sphincter Relaxation
>
> **Stimulants**
> - Gastric distention
> - Pharyngeal intubation
> - Upright orientation
> - Foods (fatty foods, caffeine, alcohol)
> - Tobacco
>
> **Inhibitors**
> - Recumbency
> - Lateral decubitus (left side)
> - Anesthesia
> - Sleep

> ### BOX 2 — Esophageal Tissue Defense Mechanisms
>
> **Preepithelial**
> - Mucous layer
> - Unstirred water layer
> - Surface bicarbonate concentration
>
> **Epithelial Structures**
> - Cell membranes
> - Intercellular junctional complexes (tight junctions, glycoconjugates/lipid)
>
> **Cellular**
> Epithelial transport (Na^+/H^+ exchanger, Na^+-dependent Cl^-/$HCO3^-$-$HCO3^-$ exchanger)
> - Intracellular and extracellular buffers
> - Cell restitution
> - Cell replication
>
> **Postepithelial**
> - Blood flow
> - Tissue acid-base status

> ### BOX 3 — Alarm Symptoms of Gastroesophageal Reflux Disease
>
> Presence of any of the following symptoms requires immediate evaluation:
> - Dysphagia
> - Odynophagia
> - Weight loss
> - Spontaneous resolution of symptoms
> - Iron deficiency anemia
> - Gastrointestinal bleeding

Erosive Esophagitis

The endoscopic finding of erosive esophagitis is seen in fewer than 50% of patients with heartburn. The severity is stratified according to the Los Angeles Classification of Esophagitis. Treatment with a proton pump inhibitor (PPI) for 4 to 12 weeks heals erosive esophagitis in 78% to 95% of cases. The healing effect of antisecretory therapy, and particularly PPIs, demonstrates the important role of acid reflux in causing tissue injury. The recurrence rates for erosive esophagitis are high after discontinuation of PPI maintenance therapy (75%–92%), necessitating continuation of gastric acid suppression.

Strictures

Most strictures caused by GERD are peptic in origin and are located at the squamocolumnar junction. Patients with GERD and strictures, compared with those without strictures, are more likely to have a hypotensive LES, abnormal peristalsis, and prolonged acid clearance time. Stricture formation decreases the luminal diameter, resulting in solid food dysphagia. Dysphagia in these patients is often a combination of decreased luminal diameter and dysmotility of the distal esophageal body with low-amplitude peristalsis. Patients with GERD who develop dysphagia should have immediate barium radiography and an endoscopic evaluation.

Barrett Esophagus

BE is a premalignant condition that may evolve into esophageal adenocarcinoma. The histologic abnormality involves intestinal-like metaplasia of the stratified squamous epithelium. Epidemiologic studies show BE to be more common among Whites, males, and the elderly (mean age, 60 years). The incidence of esophageal adenocarcinoma (EAC) in patients with BE varies based on the degree of dysplasia and, in general, is estimated to have an annual incidence of 0.2 to 0.7. Despite the prevalent use of PPIs in the treatment of GERD, the incidence of adenocarcinoma has been increasing. Current guidelines encourage endoscopic surveillance for patients with BE, yet there are sparse data showing the cost-effectiveness or mortality benefit of this strategy.

Adenocarcinoma

Approximately 50% of esophageal cancers are adenocarcinomas. Since the 1970s, the incidence has been rising for reasons that are still unknown. GERD is a risk factor for EAC, and the risk increases with the duration and severity of GERD symptoms. There is a suggestion that cagA strains of *Helicobacter pylori* are protective against development of BE and adenocarcinoma. The declining incidence of *H. pylori* may be a possible explanation for the rising incidence of adenocarcinoma.

Diagnosis

GERD is largely a clinical diagnosis under the current definition (i.e., any symptom or tissue injury resulting from reflux of gastric contents into the esophagus). Patients with the typical symptoms of heartburn and regurgitation most often associated with meals have a high pretest probability of having GERD. A well-obtained history and symptom questionnaire are usually sufficient to form a presumptive diagnosis and are more cost-effective than ambulatory reflux testing or EGD. An empiric trial of PPI therapy that leads to a significant reduction or resolution of symptoms likely confirms the diagnosis.

The pathophysiology of GERD is much more complex than previously thought. It involves more than acid reflux, because nonacid reflux with a pH greater than 4 can be a common source of symptoms. This entity is unmasked when PPI therapy is found to control gastric acid secretion and impedance-pH testing identifies a temporal relationship between symptoms and episodes of nonacid reflux.

Direct-to-consumer marketing and the availability of over-the-counter PPI medications (e.g., Prilosec OTC) have led to self-treatment of GERD-type symptoms and a consequent change in the type of patients seeking medical care for their symptoms. Patients with typical GERD symptoms that do not completely respond to therapy with PPIs, including over-the-counter and prescription PPIs, warrant a more detailed evaluation of their symptoms. A separate population requiring earlier diagnostic evaluation includes patients with exclusively atypical GERD symptoms such as cough, hoarseness, throat clearing, asthma attacks, and chest pain. Less commonly, patients presenting with signs or symptoms of tissue injury, such as solid food dysphagia, should also be more rigorously tested for GERD (Box 4).

Patients who have symptoms associated with GERD, whether typical or atypical, are frequently treated empirically with PPI therapy.

Partial responders and nonresponders to PPI therapy should undergo ambulatory reflux testing using combined multichannel intraluminal impedance (MII)-pH or standard pH. MII-pH

> **BOX 4** Clinical Spectrum of Gastroesophageal Reflux Disease–Related Symptoms and Tissue Injury
>
> **Esophageal**
> *Symptomatic Syndromes*
> - Typical reflux syndrome
> - Reflux chest pain syndrome
>
> *Syndromes With Tissue Injury*
> - Reflux esophagitis
> - Reflux stricture
> - Barrett esophagus
> - Adenocarcinoma
>
> **Extraesophageal**
> *Established Association*
> - Reflux cough
> - Reflux laryngitis
> - Reflux dental erosions
>
> *Proposed Association*
> - Sinusitis
> - Reflux asthma
> - Pulmonary fibrosis
> - Pharyngitis
> - Recurrent otitis media

---

catheters measure both esophageal pH changes and impedance changes that occur as an ion-rich refluxate passes a pair of ring electrodes, resulting in a drop in the resistance to a low-voltage current between the electrodes. The change in impedance can detect gastroesophageal reflux regardless of the acid content and can distinguish reflux types as liquid, gas, or mixed.

The goals of ambulatory reflux testing are to determine whether the esophageal acid contact time is abnormal, whether there is an abnormal number of reflux episodes, and whether a relationship between reflux and symptoms exists. The advantage of combined MII-pH is its ability to identify both acid and non-acid reflux, so that testing can be done while the patient is on acid-suppression therapy and the artifact of acidic food or beverage ingestion is eliminated; pH-only testing is affected by both of these conditions. The major disadvantage is that MII-pH testing is less available than conventional pH testing.

EGD is specific for detecting reflux-related tissue injury but is not sensitive, because fewer than 50% of patients with GERD-related heartburn have endoscopic findings of reflux. If erosive esophagitis or BE is found on endoscopy, aggressive antisecretory therapy with a PPI is warranted.

A barium esophagram is unlikely to add useful diagnostic information in patients with GERD symptoms without dysphagia. It is a useful tool in distinguishing obstructive from nonobstructive dysphagia and may even be more sensitive than EGD in detecting causes of obstructive dysphagia. Achalasia is often mistaken for GERD during the onset of symptoms, and early use of esophagography may help make this diagnosis.

Management

GERD is predominantly a postprandial event involving transient LES relaxations. The primary focus in management of this disease is to eliminate or improve symptoms, prevent tissue injury, and prevent complications. In most patients with recurrent GERD symptoms, this can be accomplished by controlling gastric acid secretion with antisecretory therapy. PPIs are the most effective pharmacologic therapy for improving symptoms and preventing tissue injury from acid reflux. Individuals with only occasional heartburn may successfully treat symptoms with a combination of lifestyle modifications and over-the-counter antacids, histamine 2 receptor antagonists, or a PPI.

Patients presenting with typical symptoms and a history consistent with GERD should be given a trial of PPI once daily for at least 4 weeks. A validated GERD symptom assessment questionnaire such as the Reflux Disease Questionnaire should be used as an initial screening tool, because symptom response is the primary outcome measure, and subsequent questionnaire responses are useful in comparison with the initial responses for measuring treatment efficacy. If symptoms have not responded or have responded only partially after this trial, then the dosing or frequency of the PPI should be increased over another 4-week period. If the response is still unsatisfactory, diagnostic testing with ambulatory combined MII-pH or pH-only monitoring is indicated.

PPIs are an effective maintenance therapy for most patients with GERD. Both dose and frequency may be adjusted based on clinical response, but GERD is a chronic condition with a high recurrence rate of symptoms without some form of maintenance therapy. This creates a large population of patients on antisecretory therapy for a disease with a low mortality rate, which raises the question of drug safety. There are insufficient data available that would warrant a recommendation against long-term PPI therapy. Clinical judgment in specific patient populations should be used to determine the optimal PPI regimen.

At present, pharmacologic reflux reduction therapy consists solely of the use of baclofen (Lioresal),[1] which has been shown to reduce transient LES relaxations and associated gastroesophageal reflux. The drawback of this medication is its unwanted side effects, which include somnolence and dizziness, limiting its tolerability and clinical utility as a standalone therapy.

Antireflux surgery is another alternative that is effective in limiting GERD symptoms in patients with a positive reflux-symptom relationship. Candidates for surgery include younger patients who do not want to continue chronic PPI therapy and patients with symptomatic nonacid reflux. Today, most antireflux surgery is performed laparoscopically with a 360-degree Nissen fundoplication. The associated mortality rate is small (0.5% to 1%), and this approach is preferred to open laparotomy. Traditional predictors for surgical success have included the presence of typical symptoms (heartburn and regurgitation), symptom response to a trial of PPIs, and an abnormal ambulatory pH study. These criteria exclude the important group of patients with atypical symptoms or symptoms related to nonacid reflux. However, such patients should be considered candidates for antireflux surgery if a positive reflux-symptom relationship can be demonstrated.

In recent years, several endoscopic therapeutic procedures have been developed for the treatment of GERD. Among these procedures, transoral incisionless fundoplication and Stretta are well-studied and viable options. Stretta is the delivery of radiofrequency energy to the gastroesophageal junction (GEJ). Stretta efficacy lies in increasing thickness of LES, decreasing compliance of GEJ without fibrosis, and decreasing transient LES relaxations. Randomized trials showed improvement in GERD symptoms compared with sham procedure, though follow-up periods in these trials were only 6 to 12 months. A metaanalysis of 18 studies and 1441 patients concluded that Stretta is safe, well tolerated, effective in GERD symptom relief, and significantly reduces acid exposure to the esophagus, though it did not consistently normalize pH. In a recent metaanalysis of 28 studies of 2468 patients with mean follow-up time of 25.4 months, Stretta improved quality-of-life scores and heartburn scores. However, 49% of the patients were still using PPIs at follow-up.

Patients with alarm symptoms and those who are partial responders to PPI therapy should also undergo EGD to aid in determining the cause of the symptoms, such as obstructive dysphagia from peptic strictures, adenocarcinoma, and bleeding esophageal ulcers (which can cause anemia). EGD findings that suggest GERD are a result of acid reflux. However, the incidence of these findings has declined with the use of PPIs.

Nonerosive reflux disease is increasingly common as more patients are converted from acid refluxers to non-acid refluxers with PPI therapy. By definition, these patients have no findings on endoscopy to suggest ongoing GERD. Absence of endoscopic findings does not exclude GERD, however, because tissue injury can occur at the microscopic and macroscopic levels. Patients with either erosive esophagitis or nonerosive reflux disease have dilated intercellular spaces on electron microscopy.

As previously discussed, patients with GERD may develop BE. The metaplastic transformation from normal stratified squamous epithelium to an intestinal-type, columnar-lined epithelium creates a premalignant lesion with a 0.5% per year risk of progression to adenocarcinoma. Screening for BE remains controversial. There is no evidence that screening results in a mortality benefit due to early detection of esophageal adenocarcinoma. Screening of all patients with GERD for BE is clearly not cost-effective, but it is reasonable to target the highest-risk populations, such as White men older than 50 years of age with chronic reflux symptoms. Current American College of Gastroenterology guidelines recommend surveillance endoscopy in patients with known BE at intervals determined by the degree of dysplasia.

References

Bonino J, Sharma P: Barrett's esophagus, *Curr Opin Gastroenterol* 21:461–465, 2005.

Castell DO, Richter JE: *The esophagus*, ed 4, Philadelphia, 2003, Lippincott Williams & Wilkins.

Corley DA, Katz P, Wo JM, et al: Improvement of gastroesophageal reflux symptoms after radiofrequency energy: a randomized, sham-controlled trial, *Gastroenterology* 125:668–676, 2003.

Fass R, Cahn F, Scotti DJ, et al: Systematic review and meta-analysis of controlled and prospective cohort efficacy studies of endoscopic radiofrequency for treatment of gastroesophageal reflux disease, *Surg Endosc* 31(12):4865–4882.

Frye J, Vaezi M: Extraesophageal GERD, *Gastroenterol Clin N Am* 37:845–858, 2008.

Hila A, Agrawal A, Castell D: Combined multichannel intraluminal impedance and pH esophageal testing compared to pH alone for diagnosing both acid and weakly acidic gastroesophageal reflux, *Clin Gastroenterol Hepatol* 5:172–177, 2007.

Hvid-Jensen F, Funch-Jensen P, et al: Incidence of adenocarcinoma among patients with Barrett's esophagus, *N Engl J Med* 365:1375–1383, 2011.

Katz PO, Gerson LB, Vela MF: Guidelines for the diagnosis and management of gastroesophageal reflux disease, *Am J Gastroenterol* 108:308–328, 2013.

Mainie I, Tutuian R, Agrawal A, et al: Combined multichannel intraluminal impedance-pH monitoring to select patients with persistent gastro-oesophageal reflux for laparoscopic Nissen fundoplication, *Br J Surg* 93:1483–1487, 2006.

Mainie I, Tutuian R, Castell D: Comparison between the combined analysis and the DeMeester score to predict response to PPI therapy, *J Clin Gastroenterol* 40:602–605, 2006.

Mainie I, Tutuian R, Shay S, et al: Acid and non-acid reflux in patients with persistent symptoms despite acid suppressive therapy: amulticentre study using combined ambulatory impedance-pH monitoring, *Gut* 55:1398–1402, 2006.

Perry KA, Banerjee A, Melvin WS: Radiofrequency energy delivery to the lower esophageal sphincter reduces esophageal acid exposure and improves GERD symptoms: a systematic review and meta-analysis, *Surg Laparosc Endosc Percutan Tech* 22:283–288, 2012.

Savarino E, Zentilin P, Tutuian R, et al: The role of nonacid reflux in NERD: lessons learned from impedance-pH monitoring in 150 patients off therapy, *Am J Gastroenterol* 103:2685–2693, 2008.

Vakil N: Review article: test and treat or treat and test in reflux disease, *Aliment Pharmacol Ther* 17(Suppl. 2):57–59, 2003.

Vakil N, Van Zanten SV, Kahrilas P, et al: The Montreal definition and classification of gastroesophageal reflux disease: a global evidence-based consensus, *Am J Gastroenterol* 101:1900–1920, 2006.

Verbeek RE, Siersema PD, et al: Surveillance and follow-up strategies in patients with high-grade dysplasia in Barrett's esophagus: a Dutch population-based study, *Am J Gastroenterol* 107:534–542, 2012.

Wang KK, Sampliner RE: Updated guidelines 2008 for the diagnosis, surveillance and therapy of Barrett's esophagus, *Am J Gastroenterol* 103:788–797, 2008.

Zhang D, Liu S, Li Z, Wang R: Global, regional and national burden of gastroesophageal reflux disease, 1990–2019: update from the GBD 2019 study, *Ann Med* 54(1):1372–1384, 2022.

---

[1] Not FDA approved for this indication.

HEMORRHOIDS, ANAL FISSURE, AND ANORECTAL ABSCESS AND FISTULA

Method of
Mary R. Kwaan, MD, MPH

CURRENT DIAGNOSIS

- Although most anorectal complaints are caused by a benign process, it is important to be mindful that the etiology can be a malignancy or other serious medical condition, such as anorectal Crohn's disease.
- A thorough, focused history is often the most helpful diagnostic tool for patients with anorectal complaints.
- In patients in whom no etiology for bleeding is found or there has been a change in bowel movements, a further diagnostic workup should be performed.
- Pain is the predominant symptom with anal fissure, thrombosed external hemorrhoids, and anorectal abscess but is not prominently featured with internal hemorrhoids.

CURRENT THERAPY

- External thrombosed hemorrhoids are treated with evacuation in their early development (<72 hours) but with expectant, supportive management only in their subacute phase.
- Most internal hemorrhoids can be treated with outpatient treatments, including measures to normalize bowel movements and hemorrhoidal banding or injection therapy.
- Anal fissures are treated conservatively with medical therapy but require operative therapy in a minority of cases.
- Anal fistula repair techniques have variable success rates and may require multiple procedures to treat effectively.

A number of conditions cause anorectal symptoms, but the majority of patients present with a complaint of "hemorrhoids." Most anorectal conditions can be diagnosed with a focused history and physical examination. Treatment is aimed at the relief of symptoms, education of the patient, and prevention of further symptoms. Although most anorectal complaints are caused by a benign process, it is important for clinicians to be mindful that in some cases the etiology can be a malignancy or other serious medical condition, such as anorectal Crohn's disease.

History

A thorough, focused history is often the most helpful diagnostic tool for patients with anorectal complaints. Clinicians should inquire about pain, itching, discharge, extra tissue or a lump, and bleeding. It is particularly important to understand the patient's bowel habits with respect to constipation or diarrhea as well as any change in defecatory habits. Other relevant history items include previous anorectal procedures and related medical conditions such as Crohn's disease, malignancy, sexually transmitted diseases, or immunosuppression.

Pain is an important symptom to elicit from patients. In most cases, pain is the predominant symptom with anal fissure, thrombosed external hemorrhoids, and anorectal abscess. Although discomfort from internal hemorrhoids can cause aching, burning, or itching in the setting of tissue prolapse, internal hemorrhoid disease is most often painless. In contrast, external hemorrhoids that are acutely thrombosed cause pain that is severe, constant, and associated with a lump. Fissure pain is often described as a tearing sensation or the feeling of "razor blades" during bowel movements that can continue for more than 1 hour following defecation. Patients with anal fissures might also express a fear of having bowel movements because of pain. Anorectal abscess is often associated with pain, and patients can also present with an acute lump and occasionally a fever. Anal fistula typically is not associated with much pain; rather, patients describe irritation and drainage.

Anal discharge and difficulty with anorectal hygiene are also common complaints. The discharge associated with prolapsing internal hemorrhoids might contain mucus or fecal smearing. In contrast, an anorectal fistula or abscess can spontaneously drain with associated purulent and blood-tinged output.

When a patient has bleeding, specific details to inquire about include color (bright red versus dark blood), amount, frequency, and length of time. When no etiology for bleeding is found, a flexible sigmoidoscopy or colonoscopy should be performed to evaluate for a proximal source. Even if patients are found to have some hemorrhoids, endoscopic evaluation should be strongly considered in patients older than 40 years of age. Although uncommon, the incidence of colorectal malignancy has increased in this age group. Furthermore, patients who are 45 years of age and older should initiate colorectal cancer screening regardless of symptoms based on updated 2021 U.S. Preventive Services Task Force (USPSTF) guidelines. Stool-based screening modalities identify blood in the stool. Therefore patients with anal bleeding should be encouraged to proceed with colonoscopy for screening.

Diagnosis

Although the prone jackknife position allows the greatest exposure, the left lateral decubitus position with the knees up is preferred by patients and usually allows adequate exposure for the anorectal examination. It is critically important to have adequate lighting with a headlight as well as appropriate instrumentation to perform the anoscopy. An adjunctive test that can also be helpful in patients where mucosal (hemorrhoidal) or full-thickness rectal prolapse is suspected is to have patients bear down on the commode and then to examine externally.

The perianal skin is the skin immediately surrounding the anal verge (Figure 1). Perianal inspection includes careful examination of the surrounding skin for excoriation, an external draining orifice in the case of an anorectal fistula, lichenified skin with chronic irritation, other dermatitis, and the presence of perianal lesions. A low-lying anal fistula can be palpated as a fibrotic tract that heads from the external draining site to the anus. The anal verge is the entrance to the anal canal and is defined by the intersphincteric groove. There is frequently a clear demarcation between hair-bearing and non–hair-bearing skin in this location. Careful separation of the anoderm can help visualize an anal fissure located at the anal verge and extending into the anal canal.

A digital rectal examination is helpful for assessing resting and squeeze anorectal tone, palpating the prostate in men, assessing

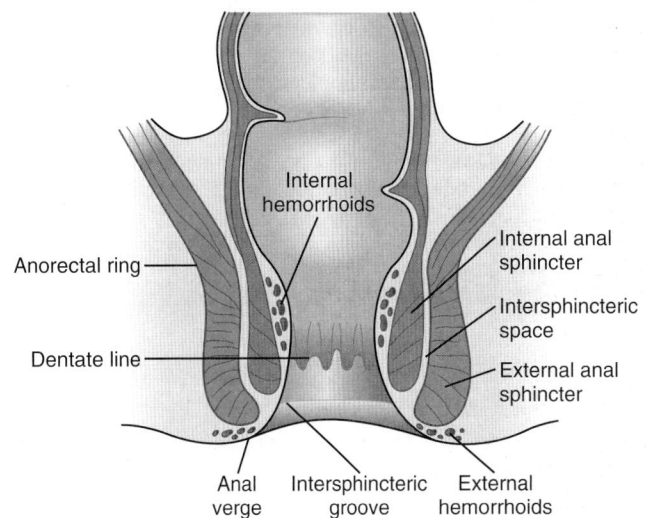

Figure 1 Anatomy of the anal canal.

for rectocele in women, detecting any palpable anorectal lesions, and evaluating for tenderness within the anal canal or at the level of the levator ani muscles at the anorectal ring. Internal hemorrhoids, however, are not usually palpable as they readily compress with digital pressure and are not associated with fibrosis. Anoscopy is used to visually examine the anal canal, which is between 4 and 5 cm in length starting at the anal verge and extending to the top of the anorectal ring (top of external sphincter and levator ani muscles). Within the anal canal is the dentate line, which acts as a landmark anatomically and is located approximately 2 cm from the anal verge. The dentate line represents the transition from the squamous epithelial lining of the anus to the columnar epithelial lining of the rectum. Sensation above the dentate line is mediated by autonomic fibers and results in a relative lack of sensation compared with the highly sensitive, somatically innervated tissue below the dentate line. The dentate line is also the location of the crypt anal glands from which anorectal abscesses and fistulas originate.

Hemorrhoids

Hemorrhoids are anal vascular cushions that are present as normal structures in everyone. In the case of internal hemorrhoids, these cushions are arteriovenous channels that have overlying mucosa, submucosal smooth muscle, and supportive fibroelastic connective tissue. It is believed that internal hemorrhoids function by aiding with fine control of fecal continence of liquids and gases. Internal hemorrhoids enlarge and become symptomatic as fixation by submucosal smooth muscle and connective tissue becomes disrupted and loosens. This results in a sliding or prolapsing of the anal canal lining and further engorgement of the internal hemorrhoid tissues. Common exacerbating factors include constipation, diarrhea, aging, and increased abdominal pressure that can occur with chronic straining, pregnancy, heavy lifting, and decreased venous return. Internal hemorrhoids are not palpable on digital rectal examination and instead must be observed on anoscopy. Internal hemorrhoids are typically staged on a scale from I to IV based on the extent of prolapse (Table 1).

Internal hemorrhoids, when symptomatic, most commonly present with painless bright red bleeding or prolapsing tissue (Figure 2). Patients describe bleeding with or after bowel movements. Other symptoms include itching and leakage of mucus in the setting of tissue prolapse. Pain is rarely a prominent symptom except in the case of mixed hemorrhoid disease, when there is a thrombosed external component, or in the case of grade IV incarcerated hemorrhoids.

The central principles for conservative treatment of internal hemorrhoids and for long-term prevention of worsening symptoms are the normalization of bowel habits and avoidance of straining. Ideal bowel habits include having regular, soft, and formed stool resulting in minimal straining with elimination. An ideal diet should have high fiber content along with sufficient fluid intake. A total of at least 30 g of fiber per day is generally recommended. For most patients, this is most easily achieved with the addition of a fiber supplement such as psyllium. Other medical treatment of hemorrhoids includes local anesthetic topical ointments, such as lidocaine gel or ointment, which relieve symptoms but do not improve the hemorrhoids, and steroid ointments, which should only be prescribed for a defined short course

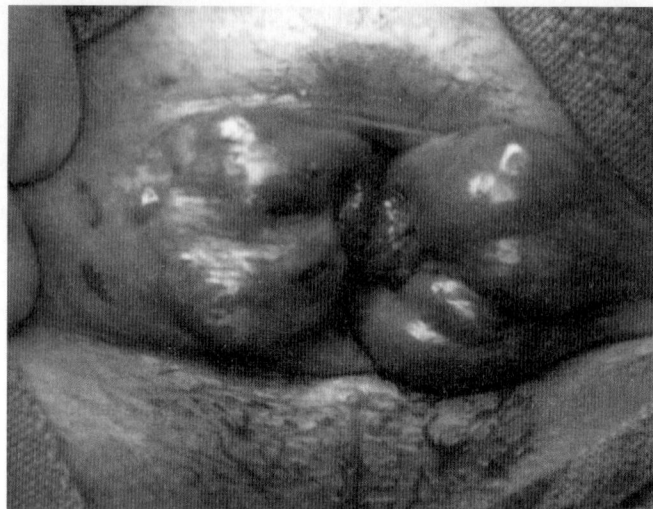

Figure 2 Prolapsing (grade III) hemorrhoids showing a prominent external component *(right)* and two sites of recent bleeding *(left)*.

for symptoms of itching and irritation. Topical hydrocortisone can thin and atrophy the overlying tissue if used regularly.

Internal hemorrhoids might benefit from further treatment in the setting of persistent prolapse or bleeding. Injection sclerotherapy works through shrinking and scarring the internal hemorrhoid by injecting a sclerosing agent (most commonly 5% phenol in oil [Haemorol]).[1,2] Sodium morrhuate is a sclerosing agent approved only for obliteration of varicosed veins. Alternatively, infrared coagulation may be administered at the apex of the hemorrhoid. Both procedures have moderate effectiveness but are considered less effective than rubber-band ligation, which is widely used in the office setting with favorable results.

Rubber-band ligation, an office procedure, requires the use of a rubber-band ligator (either suction type or a ligator with a clamp) and is performed by placing a rubber band around excess hemorrhoidal tissue at the apex of the hemorrhoid. Rubber-band ligation works by strangulating and cutting off blood flow to the hemorrhoid and by creating a scar that helps fix tissue into place. The band must be placed well above the dentate line to prevent pain. Most patients experience a sensation of pressure with the procedure. Rarely, this procedure can cause significant pain, bleeding, or a vasovagal reaction. In general, only one or two band applications are performed in the same setting to prevent excessive pain or a vasovagal reaction. Multiple rounds of hemorrhoid banding can be used to improve the patient's quality of life and has been shown to be more cost effective than hemorrhoid surgery, which is reserved for more severe prolapse.

Surgical treatment for hemorrhoidal disease should be considered in patients with grade III or IV internal hemorrhoids. Grade IV hemorrhoids, especially associated with dusky prolapsed rectal mucosa, urinary retention, or significant pain should be evaluated urgently by a surgeon, as necrotic tissue requires operative debridement. Surgery is also a consideration in cases in which office procedures and conservative treatment have been ineffective or when internal hemorrhoids are circumferential. In the United States, most hemorrhoidectomies continue to be performed using a closed technique in which the hemorrhoid is excised and the defect sutured closed. Stapled hemorrhoidectomy (also known as a *procedure for prolapsed hemorrhoids* (PPH) or *hemorrhoidopexy*) is used for patients who have more circumferential disease and is performed by excising the rectal mucosa and disrupting blood flow, thereby shrinking hemorrhoidal tissue and lifting the prolapsing tissue into the anal canal. Although stapled hemorrhoidectomy has been demonstrated to be effective and on average less painful, it

TABLE 1	Staging of Hemorrhoidal Disease
GRADE	**DESCRIPTION**
I	Protrude only inside the lumen; seen only with an anoscope
II	Protrude during defecation; reduce spontaneously
III	Protrude during defecation; require manual reduction
IV	Permanently prolapsed and irreducible

---

[1] Not FDA approved for this indication.
[2] Not available in the United states.

does not address external hemorrhoids, costs significantly more, and has been associated with rare but severe complications, including pelvic sepsis, rectal perforation, and rectovaginal fistula.

External hemorrhoids are generally painless, except in the case of thrombosis, and they normally appear as more prominent external perianal tissue or painless skin tags. Thrombosed external hemorrhoids, in contrast, are associated with severe pain and a prominent external lump but not with bleeding or fever. On examination, an external thrombosed hemorrhoid appears as a prominent, blue, and firm perianal lump. Patients who present within 72 hours of onset of symptoms benefit from excision of the hemorrhoid rather than evacuation of the thrombosed clot (Figure 3). In contrast, patients who present after 72 hours should be treated expectantly with conservative supportive care, including sitz baths, normalization of bowel habits with fiber or stool softener, and pain management. The natural history in these cases is for the thrombosed clot to gradually be reabsorbed within several weeks. In many cases, a residual skin tag is noted by the patient and can interfere with anal hygiene.

Anal Fissure

An anal fissure is a tear in the anoderm extending proximally into the anal canal and initially resulting from a traumatic bowel movement. Fissures typically occur in the setting of constipation or diarrhea. Most acute fissures will heal, but some patients have prolonged symptoms, causing them to seek medical attention. The pathophysiology of anal fissures is still not completely understood but is related to local ischemia caused by hypertonia of the internal sphincter. Most anal fissures are located at the posterior midline; some also occur at the anterior midline (Figure 4). Lateral fissures are rare and can be associated with anal malignancy, anorectal Crohn disease, HIV, syphilis, or tuberculosis. In these cases, a biopsy should be strongly considered to confirm the diagnosis.

Patients who present with anal fissure most often have a tearing pain that is associated with bowel movements and continues after defecation along with bright red bleeding with bowel movements. Physical examination demonstrates a tear in the anoderm with an exposed internal sphincter on separation of the anus. Chronic cases

also demonstrate a sentinel tag overlying the distal aspect of the fissure.

Conservative treatment for acute anal fissures includes normalization of bowel habits to minimize recurrent trauma to the anoderm and sitz baths for comfort. In cases in which the fissure is chronic or unresponsive to conservative treatment, topical therapy to relax the internal sphincter (i.e., a *chemical sphincterotomy*) is prescribed. Classically, nitroglycerin ointment (0.4% [Rectiv]) has been used but is associated with headaches and lightheadedness. Diltiazem ointment (2%)[1,6] is a commonly used alternative without associated side effects. Either ointment can be applied topically two to three times per day for approximately 8 weeks. Application before bowel movements works best to help with pain on defecation. Reported healing rates are similar and range from 40% to 100%. An alternative agent that can be used for chemical sphincterotomy is botulinum toxin A (Botox)[1], which can be injected in the office or operating room with a single application into the internal sphincter. Although botulinum toxin A appears to be as effective as topical therapy, it is significantly more expensive.

Surgical lateral internal sphincterotomy is the most effective treatment to resolve anal pain associated with fissures and to expedite healing, but it is associated with a small risk of fecal incontinence. This procedure is performed in the outpatient setting and should be considered in cases in which topical medication has failed. This procedure can be performed with an open approach (incising mucosa and exposing muscle) or a closed approach (using landmarks and then dividing muscle by palpation) and can be full thickness (entire internal sphincter) or tailored (partial thickness and length). Most surgeons perform a tailored sphincterotomy from the level of the top of the fissure distally, with partial division of the internal sphincter muscle to decrease the risk of postoperative fecal incontinence.

Anorectal Abscess and Fistula

Anorectal abscess is most commonly a self-limiting process thought to result from obstruction and infection of anal glands located in

---

[1] Not FDA approved for this indication.
[6] May be compounded by pharmacists.

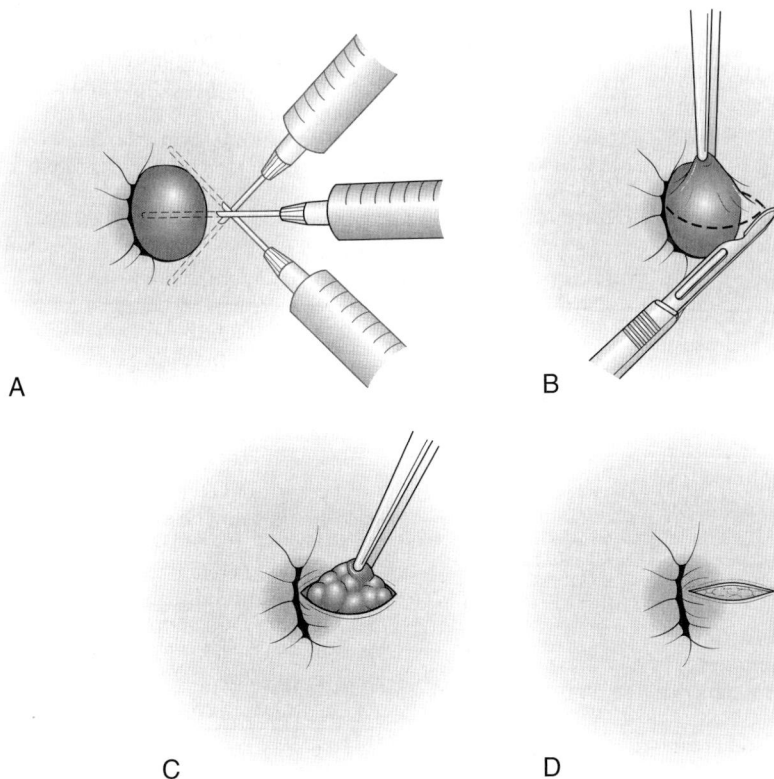

A

B

C

D

Figure 3 Excision and evacuation of an external thrombosed hemorrhoid. **A,** A local anesthetic is injected into the subcutaneous surrounding tissue and at the base of the hemorrhoid. **B,** The skin over the hemorrhoid is lifted, and a small elliptical excision of skin is made. **C,** The thrombotic clot is evacuated. Additional dissection is sometimes needed in the subcutaneous tissue to extract the clot. **D,** The appearance of the evacuated area. The incision is left open, and the skin heals by secondary intention.

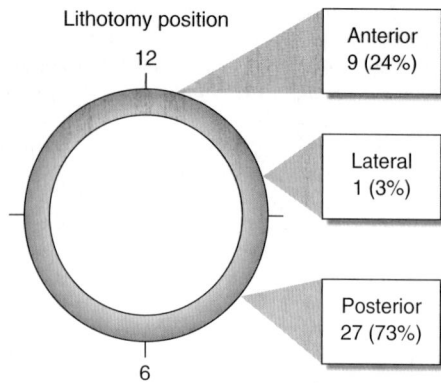

Lithotomy position

12

Anterior
9 (24%)

Lateral
1 (3%)

Posterior
27 (73%)

6

Figure 4 Distribution of the location of anal fissures.

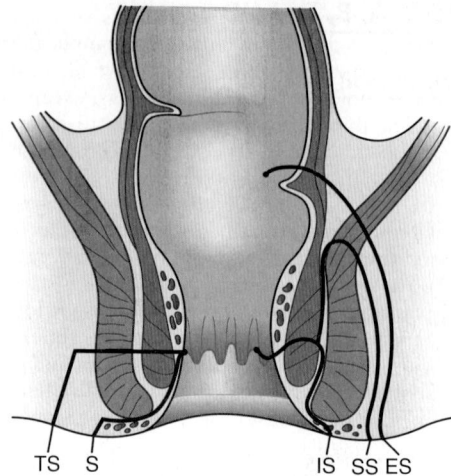

TS S   IS SS ES

Figure 5 Classification of anal fistulas. *ES*, Extrasphincteric; *IS*, intersphincteric; *S*, superficial; *SS*, suprasphincteric; *TS*, transsphincteric.

the crypts along the dentate line. Clinicians should be aware that perianal Crohn's disease, trauma, and malignancy can cause an anorectal abscess or fistula. Anorectal abscesses typically manifest with acute pain in the perianal area, acutely painful defecation, an indurated painful area, or fever. Most anorectal abscesses manifest with pain and swelling either superficially at the anal verge or deeper within the ischiorectal fossa. These patients have obvious tenderness, induration, or fluctuance on external and/or digital examination. In contrast, patients with intersphincteric abscesses have severe pain but minimal findings on external examination and are only suspected on digital rectal examination.

The mainstay of therapy is surgical drainage. Superficial abscesses can be drained using local anesthesia, but more extensive infections typically require general anesthesia. When the abscess is fluctuant and appears easily accessible, an incision and drainage with a local anesthetic can be considered in a motivated patient. Important principles in draining an anorectal abscess include keeping the patient comfortable, using aspiration with a large-bore (14- or 16-gauge) needle to help in the event of difficult localization, using a cruciate incision to ensure adequate drainage, and keeping the incision near the anus to keep any potential fistula tract as short as possible. After the abscess is drained, the area is allowed to heal by secondary intention. Patients are given analgesics and encouraged to take sitz baths. When the abscess is large and extensive, sometimes drainage tubes, débridement, or additional dressing changes are required.

In most patients, drainage of the anorectal abscess is sufficient. However, in one-third of patients, these do not heal and form a fistula with the external opening beyond the anal verge and the internal opening within an infected crypt gland at the dentate line. A recent, small randomized trial suggested that 7 to 10 days of antibiotics after abscess drainage could decrease the risk of fistula formation. Patients developing a fistula can have what appears to be a nearly healed wound but continue to intermittently drain purulent material from the external opening, and some patients continue to have signs and symptoms of infection. Anorectal fistulas are defined by their anatomy and path relative to the sphincter muscles and are classified typically as superficial, intersphincteric, transsphincteric, suprasphincteric, and extrasphincteric, as classically described by Parks (Figure 5). In most cases, patients can proceed directly to the operating room for initial definition of the anatomy and placement of a seton (a length of suture or soft plastic vessel loop that is looped through the fistula), which allows drainage of infection within the tract, prevents recurrent infection, and allows the fistula to mature. Recurrent and complex fistulas may be better defined anatomically with the use of magnetic resonance imaging or endorectal ultrasonography.

Superficial, intersphincteric, or low transsphincteric fistulas can be treated with simple fistulotomy, which opens up the fistula tract and allows the tissue to heal by secondary intention. This, however, can result in impaired fecal continence, particularly if the fistula involves a significant amount of sphincter muscle.

If the fistula is too deep for a fistulotomy because of concern about transsecting too much sphincter muscle, a variety of methods can be used to repair the fistula. One classic technique is the use of a cutting seton, where a taut seton is progressively tightened over several weeks or months to form a scar in place of the fistula and muscle. A cutting seton may be painful, and the scar is associated with impaired continence in some cases. Fibrin glue and fistula plugs have been proposed as a method to repair a fistula, but the recurrence rate with long-term follow-up is high (>85%). Endorectal advancement flaps are the most well-established method to repair an anal fistula. With this technique, the internal orifice is closed, and healthy tissue is brought down over the internal fistula opening to allow the area to heal. This procedure can be technically difficult: failure most commonly results from ischemia of the flap, and repeat flap procedures are often not anatomically feasible because of scarring and fibrosis. Success rates have been reported between 50% and 80%.

The ligation of intersphincteric fistula tract (LIFT) has been investigated for transsphincteric and suprasphincteric fistulas and shows modest success with the benefit of avoiding any sphincter division. In this procedure, the fistula tract is ligated and partially excised through an intersphincteric approach. Although long-term results are still unknown, reports are favorable (on the order of 60% to 80%) for the short-term success of this technique.

References

Bleier JI, Moloo H, Goldberg SM: Ligation of the intersphincteric fistula tract: An effective new technique for complex fistulas, *Dis Colon Rectum* 53:43–46, 2008.

Coughlin OP, Wright ME, Thorson AG, Ternent CA: Hemorrhoid Banding: A Cost-Effectiveness Analysis, *Dis Colon Rectum* 62:1085–1094, 2019.

Davis BR, Lee-Kong SA, Migaly J, Feingold DL, Steele SR: The American Society of Colon and Rectal Surgeons Clinical Practice Guidelines for the Management of Hemorrhoids, *Dis Colon Rectum* 61:284–292, 2018.

Ghahramani L, Minaie MR, Arasteh P, et al: Antibiotic therapy for prevention of fistula in ano after incision and drainage of simple perianal abscess: A randomized single blind clinical trial, *Surgery* 162:1017–1025, 2017.

Hong KD, Kang S, Kalaskar S, Wexner SD: Ligation of intersphincteric fistula to treat anal fistula: a systematic review and meta-analysis, *Tech Coloproctol* 18:685–691, 2014.

Jayaraman S, Colquhoun PH, Malthaner RA: Stapled versus conventional surgery for hemorrhoids, *Cochrane Database Syst Rev* 4:CD005393, 2006.

Nelson R: Nonsurgical therapy for anal fissure, *Cochrane Database Syst Rev* 4:CD003431, 2006.

Nelson RL: Operative procedures for fissure in ano, *Cochrane Database Syst Rev* 1:CD002199, 2010.

Parks AG, Gordon PH, Hardcastle JD: A classification of fistula-in-ano, *Br J Surg* 63:1–12, 1976.

Shanmugam V, Thaha MA, Rabindranath KS, et al: Rubber band ligation versus excisional haemorrhoidectomy for haemorrhoids, *Cochrane Database Syst Rev* 3:CD005034, 2005.

US Preventive Services Task Force: Screening for Colorectal Cancer, *JAMA* 325(19):1965–1977, 2021.

HEPATITIS A, B, D, AND E

Method of
Varun Takyar, MD; and Marc G. Ghany, MD

CURRENT DIAGNOSIS

Hepatitis A
- Typical prodromal symptoms are nonspecific (e.g., fever, anorexia, nausea, vomiting, diarrhea, abdominal pain, weight loss). In about one-half of patients, prodromal symptoms are followed by icterus (i.e., jaundice, pruritus, and dark urine) lasting 2 weeks.
- Serum aminotransferase levels increase to 10 to 20 times the upper limit of normal during the prodromal phase. Total serum bilirubin increases but rarely exceeds 10 mg/dL during the icteric phase. Biochemical recovery usually occurs within 3 months.
- Acute hepatitis A virus (HAV) infection is diagnosed by the presence of anti-HAV immunoglobulin M (IgM). Anti-HAV IgG appears in the convalescent phase and remains detectable for life. Anti-HAV IgG positivity with the absence of anti-HAV IgM antibodies reflects past exposure or vaccination. The antibody test for HAV usually includes total antibodies (IgM and IgG); thus diagnosis of acute hepatitis A requires specific anti-HAV IgM testing.

Hepatitis B
- Acute hepatitis B virus (HBV) infection may be asymptomatic or present with nonspecific symptoms of anorexia, nausea, and fever with development of icterus, pruritus, right upper quadrant pain, or, rarely, acute liver failure. Globally, it is a major cause of chronic hepatitis.
- Serum alanine aminotransferase (ALT) levels peak with the onset of symptoms.
- Suspected acute HBV infection is diagnosed by the detection of hepatitis B surface antigen (HBsAg), hepatitis B e-antigen (HBeAg), IgM antibody to hepatitis B core antigen, and HBV DNA in serum in the appropriate clinical setting. Anti-HBc IgM is detected during acute HBV infection and may be detected during reactivation of chronic HBV infection.
- Chronic infection is defined as the persistence of serum HBsAg for greater than 6 months. If HBsAg is present, serum HBeAg, antibody to hepatitis B e-antigen, HBV DNA, and serum ALT are used to determine the four phases of chronic infection (immune tolerant, HBeAg-positive and HBeAg-negative immune active, and inactive carrier).

CURRENT THERAPY

Hepatitis A
- Treatment is predominately supportive. Avoid hepatotoxic medications and drugs metabolized by the liver. Acute liver failure with encephalopathy and impaired synthetic function occurs rarely and is more common in patients older than 50 years of age and/or those who have coexisting chronic hepatitis B virus (HBV) or hepatitis C virus (HCV) infections.
- Prevention includes administration of the inactivated or attenuated vaccine for children at 1 year of age and older and for at-risk populations (e.g., intravenous drug users, travelers to regions with high or intermediate hepatitis A virus [HAV] rates, men who have sex with men, patients with chronic liver disease or clotting factor disorders).

- Preexposure passive immunization with pooled human anti-HAV immunoglobulin may be used for those at high or intermediate risk of hepatitis A virus exposure.
- Postexposure passive immunization with pooled human anti-HAV immunoglobulin may be used for close personal contacts of an individual with laboratory-confirmed HAV infection, staff and attendees of childcare centers if one or more children and/or staff are diagnosed with HAV infection, and food handlers during a common-source exposure. Concurrent immunization with inactivated or attenuated vaccines for these at-risk contacts is also warranted.

Hepatitis B
- Acute HBV infection in an adult generally only requires supportive care because of high rates of spontaneous recovery. For people with evidence of acute liver failure, prompt institution of antiviral therapy with a potent nucleos(t)ide analog and referral to a transplant center is recommended. Peginterferon alfa-2a (Pegasys)[1] is contraindicated in persons with acute liver failure.
- The treatment goal of chronic hepatitis B is sustained suppression of HBV DNA to prevent the development of cirrhosis, hepatocellular carcinoma, and liver-related mortality. Cure of chronic HBV infection is currently not possible. Treatment recommendations for chronic HBV differ depending on the phase of infection but are generally indicated for immune-active HBeAg-positive patients with confirmed HBV DNA greater than 2000 to 20,000 IU/mL and serum alanine aminotransferase (ALT) two or more times the upper limit of normal; for immune-active HBeAg-negative patients with HBV DNA greater than or equal to 2000 IU/mL and serum ALT two or more times the upper limit of normal; and patients with liver biopsy–proven moderate to severe inflammation and/or moderate fibrosis. Treatment decisions outside these parameters should be individualized based on the risk for complications (e.g., older age [>40 years], family history of cirrhosis or hepatocellular carcinoma, presence of cirrhosis) and the risk of therapy (e.g., chronic kidney disease, previous treatment history). Four agents are considered first line—peginterferon alfa-2a (Pegasys), entecavir (Baraclude), tenofovir (Viread), and tenofovir alafenamide (Vemlidy)—based on their safety, effectiveness, and low rates of antiviral resistance. Peginterferon is generally recommended for those who prefer a finite course of treatment and who have clinical and laboratory features predictive of a response to peginterferon (high ALT, low HBV DNA, young age, female sex, and HBV genotype A or B). Peginterferon is contraindicated in persons with decompensated cirrhosis, compensated cirrhosis with clinically significant portal hypertension, autoimmune illnesses, or active psychiatric illness, and during pregnancy. Nucleos(t)ide analogs are more potent inhibitors of HBV DNA replication, generally better tolerated than peginterferon, and usually administered long-term. The ideal endpoint of treatment is loss of HBsAg, though it is rarely observed with any therapy.
- Prevention includes completion of a three-dose HBV vaccination series for all children by 18 months of age, with the first dose administered within 24 hours of birth. Infants whose mothers are HBsAg positive or whose HBsAg status is unknown should receive the last dose by 6 months of age. Vaccination is also recommended for adolescents younger than 19 years of age who have not been vaccinated, all adults ages 19 through 59 years, and adults age 60 years or older with risk factors for hepatitis B infection. A two-dose HBV vaccine is available for adults.
- Hepatitis B immune globulin (HyperHEP B) and HBV vaccination are recommended at birth for infants whose mothers are HBsAg positive. In mothers with viral loads greater than 200,000 IU/mL, antiviral therapy with tenofovir (Viread), telbivudine[2], or lamivudine (Epivir HBV) in gestational week 28 should be initiated.

- Five viruses, hepatitis A to E, account for the majority of cases of acute and chronic viral hepatitis. Chronic hepatitis is arbitrarily defined as the persistence of elevated serum aminotransferase levels for 6 or more months. Complications of chronic hepatitis (predominantly cirrhosis and hepatocellular carcinoma) account for the majority of morbidity and mortality caused by viral hepatitis. Effective vaccines are available for the prevention of hepatitis A, B, and D infections. A vaccine for hepatitis E has been developed but currently is only available in China. In addition, safe and effective therapy is available for treatment of chronic hepatitis B and C. Therefore it is important to screen individuals who are at high risk for chronic viral hepatitis, to provide them access to care, reduce complications, and offer counseling to prevent transmission of infection.

[1] Not FDA approved for this indication.
[2] Not available in the United States.

Hepatitis A

Introduction

Hepatitis A virus (HAV) is a positive-sense, single-stranded RNA virus of the *Hepatovirus* genus belonging to the Picornaviridae family. Its genome encodes four structural and seven nonstructural proteins. Four genotypes have been identified, but there is only one serotype. Therefore exposure to one HAV genotype confers immunity to all genotypes.

Natural History

HAV is a cause of acute hepatitis and acute liver failure but not chronic hepatitis (Table 1). In about 5% of cases, a prolonged cholestasis lasting more than 3 months may occur, and, in about 10% of cases, a relapsing hepatitis has been observed up to 6 months after the acute illness with recrudescence of symptoms and flare of hepatitis. Cases of relapsing hepatitis continue to remain infectious with fecal shedding of the virus. These atypical presentations of acute hepatitis A should not be mistaken for evolution to chronic hepatitis, as resolution is the rule. Recovery of HAV is associated with development of lifelong immunity.

HAV replication occurs in hepatocytes, and the virus is shed into the intestine via the biliary system. Viral levels peak during the asymptomatic period, and virus shedding continues until around 2 weeks into the icteric phase. HAV is detectable in the blood, but levels are 1000-fold higher in the feces. Children may shed the virus longer than adults.

The incubation period usually lasts 14 to 28 days. This is followed by the onset of symptoms. The presence and severity of symptoms are variable and age related. Generally, more than 70% of adult patients have a symptomatic illness, compared with only 10% of children younger than the age of 10 years. Typical symptoms are nonspecific and include fever, anorexia, nausea, vomiting, diarrhea, abdominal pain, and weight loss. This prodromal phase is followed by an icteric phase in 40% to 70% of patients with jaundice, pruritus, and dark urine. Physical examination findings are usually unremarkable, but hepatomegaly may be observed. Extrahepatic manifestations are uncommon and may include an evanescent rash and arthralgias.

Laboratory studies during the prodromal phase reveal elevated serum aminotransferase levels greater than 10 to 20 times the upper limit of normal. During the icteric phase, total serum bilirubin increases but generally does not exceed 10 mg/dL. In most patients, jaundice lasts 2 weeks, and a complete clinical and biochemical recovery can be expected in 2 to 3 months.

Epidemiology

Hepatitis A occurs throughout the world (Figure 1), either sporadically or in epidemics. The prevalence of HAV correlates with the level of sanitation and hygiene of a region. In developing countries, more than 90% of children are infected before 10 years of age. In developed countries, including the United States, infection rates are low. Lack of exposure at a young age leads to higher susceptibility in certain high-risk adults, including travelers to endemic areas, injection drug users, and men who have sex with men.

In the United States, HAV infection rates have declined by 95% since the introduction of mandatory childhood vaccination in 1995. There was a seven-fold increase in cases of hepatitis A between 2015 and 2020 due to person-to-person outbreaks among homeless persons and persons who use injection drugs. The incidence began to decline in 2020. The overall incidence rate in 2022 was 0.7 per 100,000 persons, which represents a 59% decrease in cases from the reported rate of 1.7 cases per 100,000 during 2021. HAV is spread primarily by the fecal-oral route through the ingestion of contaminated food or water. Humans are the only known reservoir of the virus.

TABLE 1 Hepatitis A, B, D, and E Characteristics

	HEPATITIS A	HEPATITIS B	HEPATITIS D	HEPATITIS E
Classification	Picornavirus, ssRNA(+)	Hepadnavirus, dsDNA	Deltavirus, ssRNA(−)	Hepevirus, ssRNA(+)
Source	Stool	Blood	Blood	Stool
Transmission	Enteric	Percutaneous/permucosal	Percutaneous/permucosal	Enteric
Acute infections (per 1000/year) in the United States	125–200	140–320	6–13	Unknown
Epidemics	Yes	No	No	Yes
Incubation period	15–45 days	30–180 days	30–180 days	15–60 days
Risk of chronic hepatitis	No	Yes	Yes	Yes
Risk of HCC	No	Yes	Yes	No
Acute liver failure	0.10%	0.1%–1%	5%–20%	1%–2%*
Prevention	Pre-/postexposure immunization	Pre-/postexposure immunization	Pre-/postexposure immunization[2]	Preexposure immunization[2]

*Higher in pregnancy at 5%–20%.
[2] Not available in the United States.
dsDNA, Double-stranded deoxyribonucleic acid; *HCC*, hepatocellular carcinoma; *ssRNA*, single-stranded ribonucleic acid.

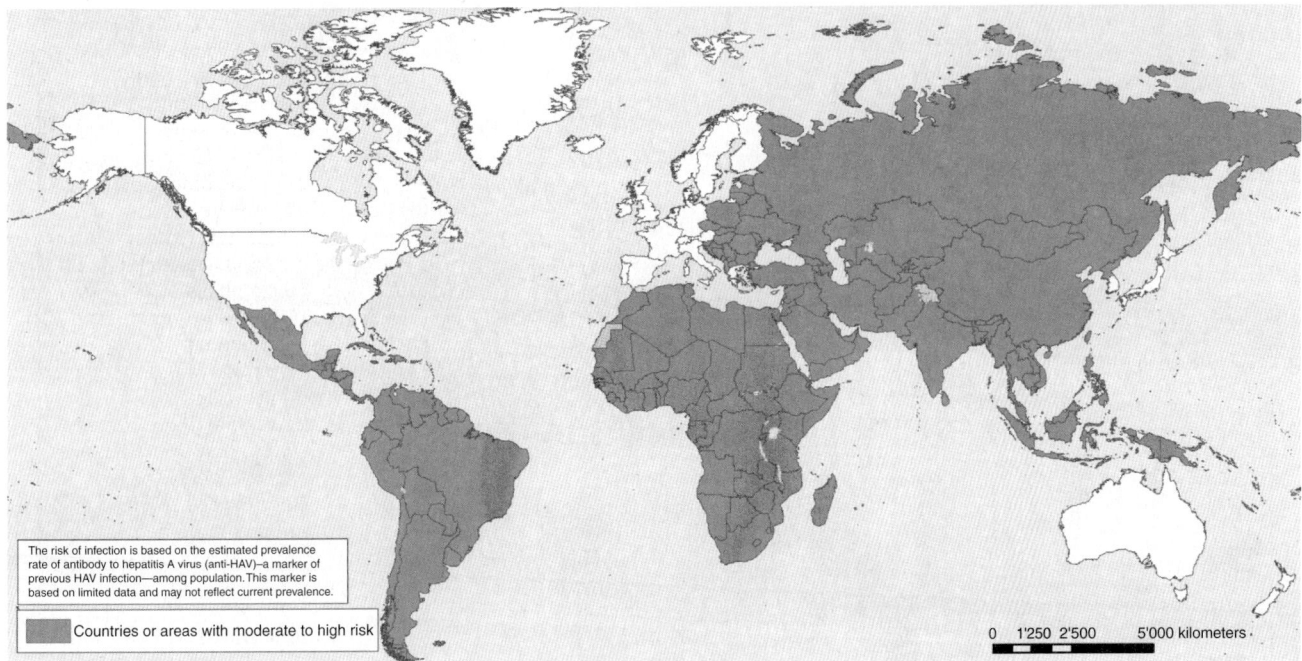

Figure 1 Global prevalence of hepatitis A and infection risk. Hepatitis A has a worldwide prevalence. Prevalence is related to regional income, sanitation, and hygiene. High-income areas (e.g., North America, Western Europe, Australia, New Zealand, Japan, the Republic of Korea, and Singapore) have low levels of hepatitis A virus *(HAV)* endemicity and subsequently a high proportion of susceptible adults. Low-income regions (sub-Saharan Africa and parts of South Asia) have high endemicity levels and very few susceptible adolescents and adults. Middle-income regions have a mix of intermediate and low endemicity levels. *Note:* Map lines delineate study areas and do not necessarily depict accepted national boundaries.

Diagnosis

Serologic testing for antibody to HAV can confirm the diagnosis of acute infection, past exposure, and immunity to the virus. Acute HAV infection is diagnosed by the presence of anti-HAV immunoglobulin M (IgM). Anti-HAV IgG appears in the convalescent phase of infection and remains detectable for life. Past exposure or vaccination confers immunity and is reflected by anti-HAV IgG positivity with the absence of anti-HAV IgM antibodies. The antibody test for HAV usually includes total antibodies (IgM and IgG). Thus to diagnose acute hepatitis A, it is important to order anti-HAV IgM.

Treatment

Given the self-limiting nature of acute hepatitis A, treatment is predominately supportive. Caution should be taken when using hepatotoxic medications or medications metabolized predominately in the liver. Rarely, acute liver failure with encephalopathy and impaired synthetic function can occur. The patients at highest risk for this complication are generally older than 50 years of age and may have coexisting chronic HBV or hepatitis C virus (HCV) infections. Individuals presenting with acute liver failure are more appropriately managed at a liver transplant center.

Prevention

Both inactivated and attenuated vaccines have been licensed against HAV. Inactivated vaccines include HAVRIX (GlaxoSmithKline), VAQTA (Merck), TWINRIX (a combined hepatitis A and B vaccine from GlaxoSmithKline), AVAXIM (Sanofi Pasteur)[2], EPAXAL (Crucell)[2], and HEALIVE (Sinovac)[2]. The only live attenuated vaccine is BIOVAC-A (Pukang)[2]. The World Health Organization (WHO) recommends routine childhood vaccination for HAV in areas with intermediate infection rates. In the United States the Advisory Committee on Immunization Practices (ACIP) recommends that all children be vaccinated at 1 year of age. Other at-risk populations for whom vaccination is recommended include intravenous drug users, travelers to regions with high or intermediate HAV rates, men who have sex with men, persons in close contact with new adoptees from countries

of high or intermediate hepatitis A endemicity, and patients with chronic liver disease or clotting factor disorders.

Passive immunization with immunoglobulin may also be used for preexposure protection among individuals who are at high or intermediate risk of HAV exposure. Pooled human anti-HAV immunoglobulins (GamaSTAN [IGIM]) decrease the HAV infection risk by 90% for up to 3 months. Passive immunization is also recommended for postexposure protection in cases of close personal contacts to an individual with laboratory-confirmed HAV infection, to staff and attendees of childcare centers if one or more children and/or staff are diagnosed with HAV infection, and to food handlers during a common-source exposure. Concurrent immunization for HAV in these at-risk contacts is also warranted.

Hepatitis E

Introduction

Hepatitis E virus (HEV) is a nonenveloped, single-stranded, positive-sense RNA virus of approximately 7300 bases in length and the sole member of the Hepeviridae family. Its genome contains three overlapping open reading frames (ORF). ORF1 encodes four nonstructural proteins, ORF2 encodes the capsid protein, and ORF3 encodes a protein of unknown function. Human infection has been reported with the Orthohepevirus A (HEV-A) and Orthohepevirus C (HEV-C) species of HEV. HEV-A has eight distinct genotypes of which five (genotypes 1, 2, 3, 4, and 7) infect humans. HEV-C, genotype 1 (C-1), which predominantly infects rats, may cause acute and chronic infection in immunosuppressed individuals. Similar to HAV, only one serotype exists, and infection with one strain confers immunity to all others. HEV is likely a zoonosis with multiple nonhuman vectors.

Natural History

HEV is a cause of acute hepatitis and acute liver failure (see Table 1). It can cause chronic hepatitis in immunocompromised individuals. The majority of acute HEV infections are asymptomatic or minimally symptomatic. The incubation period is between 15 and 60 days, and if symptoms arise, they generally consist of anorexia, nausea, vomiting, diarrhea, and abdominal pain. Acute HEV infection rarely causes jaundice, and most symptoms resolve

---

[2] Not available in the United States.

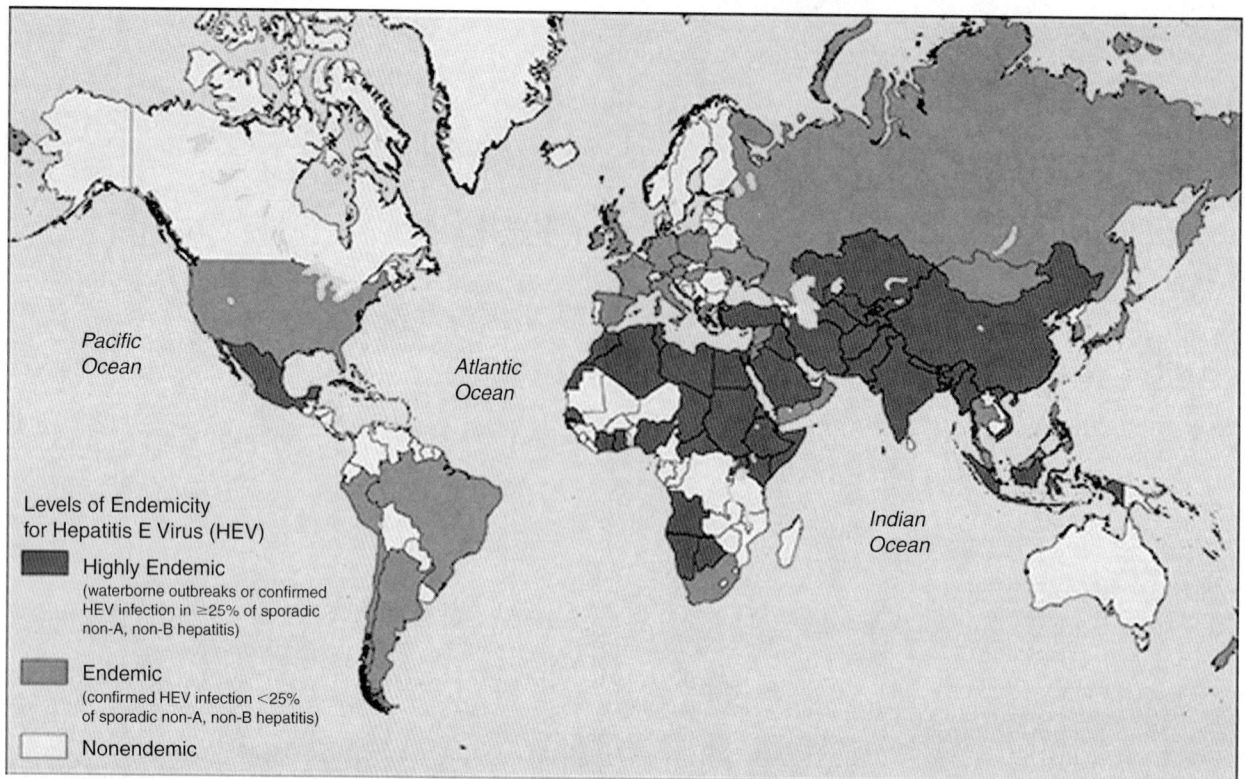

Figure 2 Global prevalence of hepatitis E virus. Hepatitis E is found worldwide. Highly endemic areas, defined by greater than or equal to 25% prevalence of sporadic non-A, non-B hepatitis, include parts of Central America and Mexico, Africa, the Middle East, and most of Asia. Endemic areas, defined as less than 25% prevalence of sporadic non-A, non-B hepatitis, include the United States, Europe, Russia, and parts of South America. Remaining regions are regarded as nonendemic. *Note:* Map lines delineate study areas and do not necessarily depict accepted national boundaries.

within 6 weeks from onset. A notable exception to the generally favorable outcome is an increased risk of acute liver failure among pregnant women during the second and third trimesters in endemic regions. This leads to a high maternal mortality rate of 15% to 25% and poorer maternofetal outcomes in third-trimester infections. Acute HEV infection may also be associated with lymphocytic destructive cholangitis.

Chronic HEV infection is defined as the presence of HEV RNA in the serum or stool for more than 6 months. It is uncommon and has been observed in solid-organ transplant recipients, HIV-positive subjects, and other immunocompromised hosts. Chronic HEV infection has only been reported with HEV-A genotype 3 infections. It is unknown if other HEV genotypes can cause chronic HEV infection. Development of cirrhosis has been described as a consequence of chronic infection.

Epidemiology

HEV is found worldwide and can be divided into three distinct geographic patterns: highly endemic, endemic, and nonendemic (sporadic) (Figure 2). Large waterborne epidemics in highly endemic regions are caused by infection with HEV-A genotypes 1 and 2 in Central America, Africa, and Asia. Sporadic cases of HEV in developed countries (Europe, North America, and Far East Asia) are caused by HEV-A genotypes 3 and 4. The reservoir for autochthonous HEV is unknown but thought to be domestic swine. Sporadic cases may occur in travelers to endemic areas. Interestingly, males are more affected than females in sporadic infections, but this gender bias is not observed during epidemics. HEV is spread by the fecal-oral route, usually through ingestion of contaminated water.

Diagnosis

There are no commercially licensed tests for HEV detection in the United States. Testing is limited to research laboratories and can be obtained through the Centers for Disease Control and Prevention (CDC).

The diagnosis of acute HEV is made by detection of anti-HEV IgM in serum or HEV RNA in stool or serum. Anti-HEV IgG has limited utility in diagnosis of HEV infections and may be a serologic marker for past infection. In immunocompromised patients, antibody testing can be falsely negative, making HEV RNA the more reliable marker of acute and chronic infection. Chronic HEV is diagnosed when HEV RNA is present in sera or stool for more than 6 months in suspected cases.

Treatment

Treatment is generally supportive because most acute HEV infections are mild. Patients who develop acute liver failure should be managed at a liver transplant center. The initial approach to management of chronic HEV infection in posttransplant recipients is to reduce the level of immunosuppression. If this is unsuccessful, then off-label use of antiviral therapy with peginterferon alfa-2a (Pegasys)[1] or ribavirin (Rebetol)[1] may be considered. In immunocompromised individuals, therapy with peginterferon alfa-2a[1] or ribavirin[1] or ribavirin and sofosbuvir (Sovaldi)[1] may be considered.

Prevention

Prevention of hepatitis E relies principally on good sanitation and the availability of clean drinking water. Prevention of transmission in travelers to endemic areas includes avoiding consumption of tap water, street foods, raw vegetables, and raw or undercooked meats such as pork and seafood. A commercially available vaccine for HEV, HECOLIN[2] (Xiamen Innovax Biotech), has been available in China since 2012.

Hepatitis B

Introduction

HBV is a partially double-stranded DNA virus of approximately 3200 bases belonging to the Hepadnaviridae family. HBV consists

---

[1] Not FDA approved for this indication.
[2] Not available in the United States.

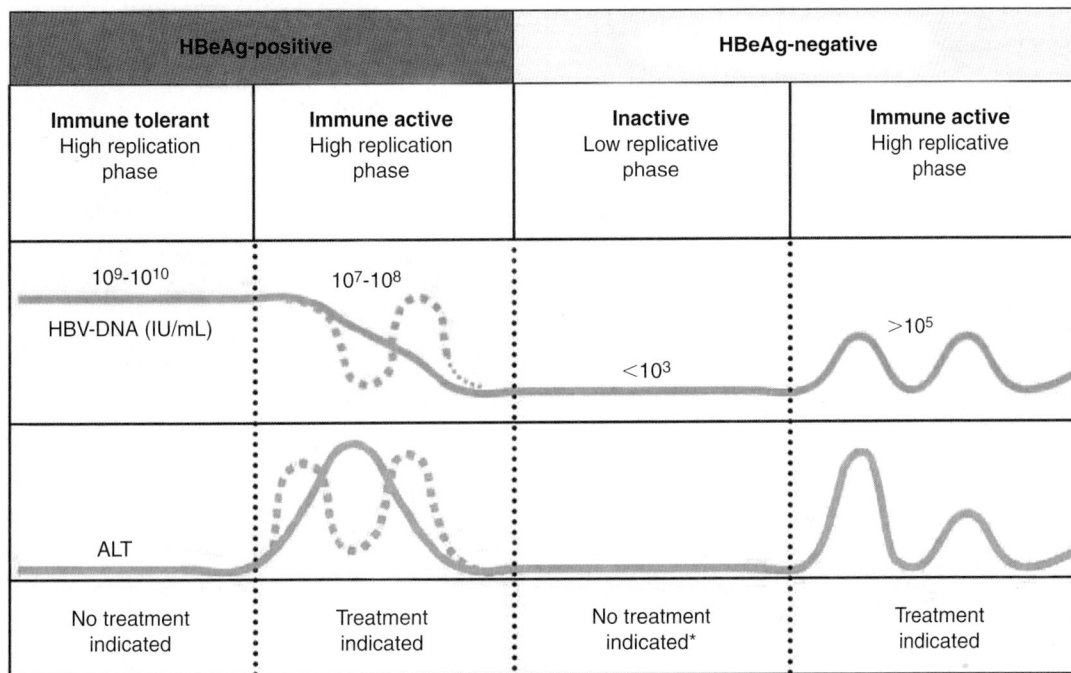

HBeAg-positive		HBeAg-negative	
Immune tolerant High replication phase	**Immune active** High replication phase	**Inactive** Low replicative phase	**Immune active** High replicative phase
10^9-10^{10} HBV-DNA (IU/mL)	10^7-10^8	$<10^3$	$>10^5$
ALT			
No treatment indicated	Treatment indicated	No treatment indicated*	Treatment indicated

Figure 3 Phases of chronic hepatitis B virus *(HBV)* infection. Chronic hepatitis B can be viewed in phases defined by hepatitis B e-antigen *(HBeAg)* status and serum HBV DNA and alanine aminotransferase *(ALT)* levels. The initial phase is the immune-tolerant phase, characterized by HBeAg positivity, high HBV DNA level (>10^7 IU/mL), and persistently normal ALT levels. This is seen only in persons who acquire the infection at birth or infancy and that persists for two to three decades of life. The next phase is the immune-active phase, defined by continued HBeAg positivity, high HBV viral load (>10^5 IU/mL), and elevated ALT levels. The next phase is characterized by loss of HBeAg and development of anti-HBe and heralds a transition from a phase of high viral replication to one of low replication. The viral load is typically less than 10^3 IU/mL, and serum ALT is normal. This phase is termed the *inactive carrier phase*. A proportion of individuals develop raised HBV DNA and ALT levels after HBeAg seroconversion. These persons are said to have transitioned to the immune-escape or HBeAg-negative immune-active phase.

of an outer lipid shell that surrounds a nucleocapsid consisting of the viral DNA, core protein, and polymerase. HBV has four overlapping reading frames (core, surface, polymerase, and x), which encode for seven viral proteins. Hepatitis B surface antigen (HBsAg) is the marker of infection, and hepatitis B e antigen (HBeAg) is a marker of high viral replication and infectivity. The virus is classified into 10 major genotypes (A to J) that have a distinct geographic distribution. Four major serotypes have been described. Humans and Old World primates (e.g., chimpanzees) are the only known hosts.

Natural History
Hepatitis B virus is a cause of acute hepatitis and acute liver failure (see Table 1). Globally, it is a major cause of chronic hepatitis. Infection with HBV is notable for a long incubation period ranging from 1 to 6 months. The majority (two-thirds) of persons with acute HBV infection are asymptomatic, one-third have an icteric presentation, and less than 1% present with acute liver failure. Symptoms of acute HBV are nonspecific and include anorexia, nausea, pruritus, and right upper quadrant pain. Symptoms usually resolve in about 1 to 3 months. Serum ALT levels peak with the onset of symptoms. The outcome of acute hepatitis B is strongly influenced by age at exposure. Resolution of acute infection occurs in 95% of persons exposed as adults, but chronic infection ensues in more than 90% of persons exposed as infants.

The natural history of chronic HBV infection depends on a complex interplay between the virus and the host immune response. Chronic HBV infection is often viewed in four phases (as shown in Figure 3) based on HBeAg status and serum HBV DNA and ALT levels. This classification is useful for providing advice on prognosis and need for treatment. Approximately 25% to 40% of persons with chronic infection will be at risk for development of cirrhosis. The 5-year cumulative incidence of cirrhosis in untreated chronic HBV infection is 8% to 20%. Once cirrhosis develops, the 5-year cumulative incidence of decompensated liver disease (ascites, variceal hemorrhage, hepatic encephalopathy) is

approximately 20%, and the annual risk of hepatocellular carcinoma is 2% to 5%. Persons who have resolved chronic infection (cleared HBsAg) should be counseled at risk for viral reactivation with use of chemotherapy or other immunosuppressive therapies.

Epidemiology
An estimated 2 billion people worldwide have evidence of past HBV infection, and of these an estimated 254 million have chronic HBV infection. The prevalence of HBV infection is declining worldwide because of the availability of an effective vaccine and implementation of successful vaccination programs. Nevertheless, an estimated 1.5 million new infections occur annually. The prevalence of HBsAg, the serologic marker of chronic infection, is highest (≥8%) in sub-Saharan Africa and Central Asia (Figure 4) and lowest (<2%) in Western Europe, Australia, Canada, and the United States (except Alaska) (see Figure 4). HBV is transmitted vertically, sexually, or through percutaneous routes and is more infectious than human immunodeficiency virus or hepatitis C virus. Individuals considered at high risk for acquiring HBV infection should be screened for chronic hepatitis B by testing for HBsAg (Table 2). In 2023 the CDC recommended that all adults aged 18 years and older should be screened for hepatitis B at least once in their lifetime. The screening panel should include testing for HBsAg, anti-HBs, and antibody to core antigen (anti-HBc).

Diagnosis
A number of serologic markers (viral antigens and antibodies to the viral antigens) and nucleic acid tests are available to diagnose acute and chronic HBV infection. Cases of suspected acute HBV infection are diagnosed by detection of HBsAg, HBeAg, IgM anti-HBc, and HBV DNA in serum in the appropriate clinical setting. Although anti-HBc IgM is detected during acute HBV infection, it is not specific for acute hepatitis B and may be seen during reactivation of chronic HBV infection.

Chronic infection is defined as persistence of HBsAg for greater than 6 months in serum. If HBsAg is present, it is advised to check

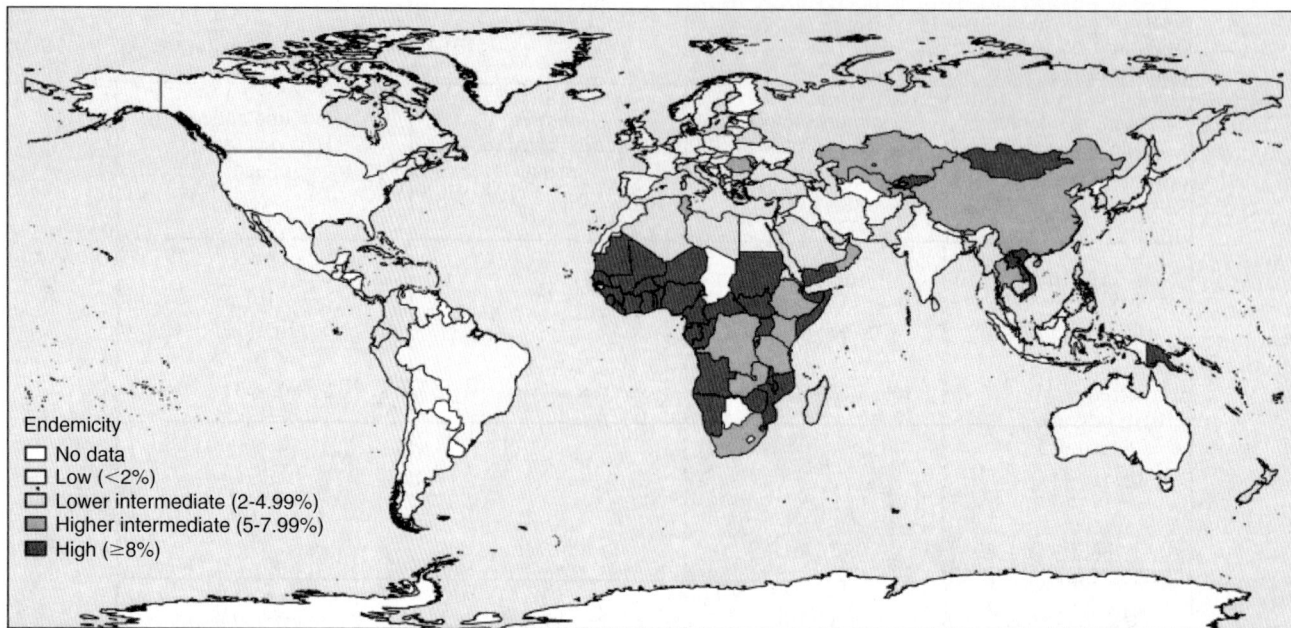

Figure 4 Global prevalence of chronic hepatitis B virus (HBV). Hepatitis B is found worldwide with varying geographic prevalence. High-prevalence areas, defined as a prevalence of hepatitis B surface antigen (HBsAg) greater than or equal to 8%, include western sub-Saharan Africa and Mongolia. Regions of high intermediate prevalence, defined as HBsAg prevalence of 5% to 7%, include China, Southeast Asia, and the remainder of sub-Saharan Africa. Regions of low to intermediate prevalence, defined as HBsAg prevalence of 2% to 4%, include the Mediterranean region, India, the Middle East, Australia, and Japan. Regions with low prevalence, defined as HBsAg prevalence of less than or equal to 2%, include North America and Western Europe. Overall, the prevalence of HBV is declining worldwide. *Note:* Map lines delineate study areas and do not necessarily depict accepted national boundaries.

TABLE 2	Centers for Disease Control and Prevention Guidelines for Hepatitis B Virus Screening

POPULATIONS RECOMMENDED OR REQUIRED FOR ROUTINE TESTING FOR CHRONIC HBV INFECTIONS

Infants born to HBsAg-positive mothers

Persons born in regions of high and intermediate HBV endemicity (HBsAg prevalence >2%)

U.S.-born persons not vaccinated as infants whose parents were born in regions with high HBV endemicity (>8%)

Injection drug users

Individuals incarcerated in a jail, prison or other detention setting

Men who have sex with men

Individuals with sexually transmitted infections or multiple sex partners

Household, needle-sharing, or sex contacts of persons known to be HBsAg positive

Persons with elevated alanine aminotransferase/aspartate aminotransferase of unknown etiology

Donors of blood, plasma, organs, tissues, or semen

Patients on maintenance dialysis, including in-center or home hemodialysis and peritoneal dialysis

All pregnant women

Persons needing immunosuppressive therapy

Persons with hepatitis C virus infection

HIV-positive persons

Persons who request HBV testing

HBsAg, Hepatitis B surface antigen; *HBV,* hepatitis B virus.
Modified from Centers for Disease Control and Prevention: Recommendations for identification and public health management of persons with chronic hepatitis B virus infection, *MMWR Morb Mortal Wkly Rep* 57(RR-8):10–11, 2008.

HBeAg, anti-HBe, HBV DNA, and serum ALT to determine the phase of infection.

Treatment

Acute HBV infection in an adult is associated with a high rate of spontaneous recovery, and antiviral treatment is rarely required. Supportive care is advised. For persons with evidence of acute liver failure, prompt institution of antiviral therapy with a potent nucleos(t)ide analog and referral to a transplant center is recommended. Peginterferon alfa-2a (Pegasys)[1] is contraindicated in persons with acute liver failure.

The goal of treatment of chronic HBV is sustained suppression of HBV DNA to prevent the development of cirrhosis, hepatocellular carcinoma, and liver-related mortality. Cure of chronic HBV infection is currently not possible because of persistence of covalently closed circular DNA within the hepatocyte nucleus and integrated HBV DNA. Treatment recommendations differ among regional guidelines, but treatment is generally indicated for HBeAg-positive patients with confirmed HBV DNA greater than 2000 to 20,000 IU/mL and serum ALT two or more times the upper limit of normal, and for HBeAg-negative patients with HBV DNA greater than or equal to 2000 IU/mL and serum ALT two or more times the upper limit of normal and/or liver biopsy–proven moderate to severe inflammation and/or moderate fibrosis. The decision to treat persons outside these parameters should be individualized based on their risk for complications and risk of therapy. Eight agents are approved for the treatment of chronic HBV infection: four agents are considered first line—peginterferon alfa-2a (Pegasys), entecavir [Baraclude], tenofovir [Viread], and tenofovir alafenamide [Vemlidy]—based on their safety, efficacy, and low rates of antiviral resistance. Peginterferon alfa-2a is generally recommended in persons who would prefer a finite course of treatment and who have clinical and laboratory features predictive of a response to peginterferon (high ALT, low HBV DNA, young age, female sex, and HBV genotype A or B). Peginterferon alfa-2a is contraindicated in persons with decompensated cirrhosis, cirrhosis with clinically

---

[1] Not FDA approved for this indication.

significant portal hypertension, autoimmune illnesses, or active psychiatric illness and during pregnancy. Nucleos(t)ide analogs are more potent inhibitors of HBV DNA replication and generally better tolerated than peginterferon alfa-2a. They are usually administered long-term. The ideal endpoint of treatment is HBsAg loss, but this is rarely observed with any therapy (<10% with interferon and after 5 years of therapy with nucleos(t)ide analogs).

Prevention

Vaccination is the primary method of prevention. An effective vaccine against HBV has been available since 1981. In the United States the ACIP has recommended that all infants complete the series of three vaccinations by 18 months of age, with the first dose administered within 24 hours of birth. Infants whose mothers are HBsAg positive or whose HBsAg status is unknown should receive the last dose by 6 months of age. Hepatitis B immune globulin (HyperHEP B) and HBV vaccination is recommended at birth for infants whose mothers are HBsAg positive to prevent maternal-infant transmission of HBV. In mothers with viral loads greater than 200,000 IU/mL, antiviral therapy with tenofovir disoproxil fumarate (Viread), tenofovir alafenamide (Vemlidy), should be initiated by gestational week 28 to reduce the risk of maternal-to-infant transmission. Entecavir (Baraclude) and peginterferon alfa-2a use are contraindicated during pregnancy. Vaccination is recommended for all persons younger than 19 years. In 2022 the ACIP recommended vaccination for adults 19 to 59 years of age and adults 60 years or older with risk factors for hepatitis B. Postexposure prophylaxis is recommended for anyone who is exposed to HBV and is considered susceptible to HBV infection and consists of hepatitis B vaccination and/or hepatitis B immune globulin depending on the HBsAg status of the exposure source.

Hepatitis D
Introduction

Hepatitis D virus (HDV) is a viroid that is dependent on HBV for its life cycle. The genome consists of a negative-sense, single-stranded circular RNA virus of approximately 1600 bases, classified as the genus Deltavirus. The virus has an outer lipoprotein envelope, HBsAg derived from HBV, and is attached to a single structural protein, the HDV antigen (HDAg). There are eight known genotypes. Immunity to HBV prevents HDV infection.

Natural History

Hepatitis D virus is a cause of acute hepatitis, acute liver failure, and chronic hepatitis (see Table 1). Hepatitis D virus infection can occur either simultaneously with HBV (referred to as *coinfection*) or as an infection in a patient with chronic HBV infection (referred to as *superinfection*). The outcome of HBV/HDV coinfection depends on the course of acute hepatitis B infection and is generally self-limiting with a low risk of chronicity (~5%). In contrast, HDV superinfection of a chronic HBV carrier results in chronic HDV infection in more than 90% of cases. Acute liver failure is observed more commonly with coinfection than with superinfection. Chronic HDV infection has a variable course, from an asymptomatic carrier to cirrhosis and decompensated liver disease. In general, HDV infection is associated with more rapid progression to cirrhosis and decompensated liver disease and a higher rate of hepatocellular carcinoma compared with HBV monoinfection.

Epidemiology

In developed countries, the prevalence of HDV has decreased as a consequence of widespread vaccination against hepatitis B. Chronic HDV infection is predominately seen in intravenous drug users or hemophiliacs requiring frequent transfusions. HDV is prevalent in the Amazon basin, Africa, the Mediterranean basin, Central Asia, Mongolia, and Russia (Figure 5). HDV genotype 1 can be found worldwide, but all other genotypes are restricted to specific geographic areas.

HDV is spread by the same routes as HBV infection and is efficiently transmitted by parenteral and sexual exposure. In contrast with HBV, vertical transmission is not a common mode of transmission. Transmission cannot occur in the absence of HBsAg.

Diagnosis

Testing for hepatitis D should be considered in persons presenting with acute hepatitis B who have additional risk factors for HDV, including a history of injection drug use; persons from endemic regions who present with a severe or protracted hepatitis; patients with chronic hepatitis B who develop an acute hepatitis of undetermined origin; and persons with HBsAg-positive chronic hepatitis B from endemic regions. Total anti-HDV (IgM and IgG) and anti-HDV IgM are the only commercially available assays in the United States; none is approved by the U.S. Food and Drug Administration (FDA). Initial testing for HDV should be with total anti-HDV. Chronic infection should be confirmed by a reverse transcriptase polymerase chain reaction assay for HDV RNA.

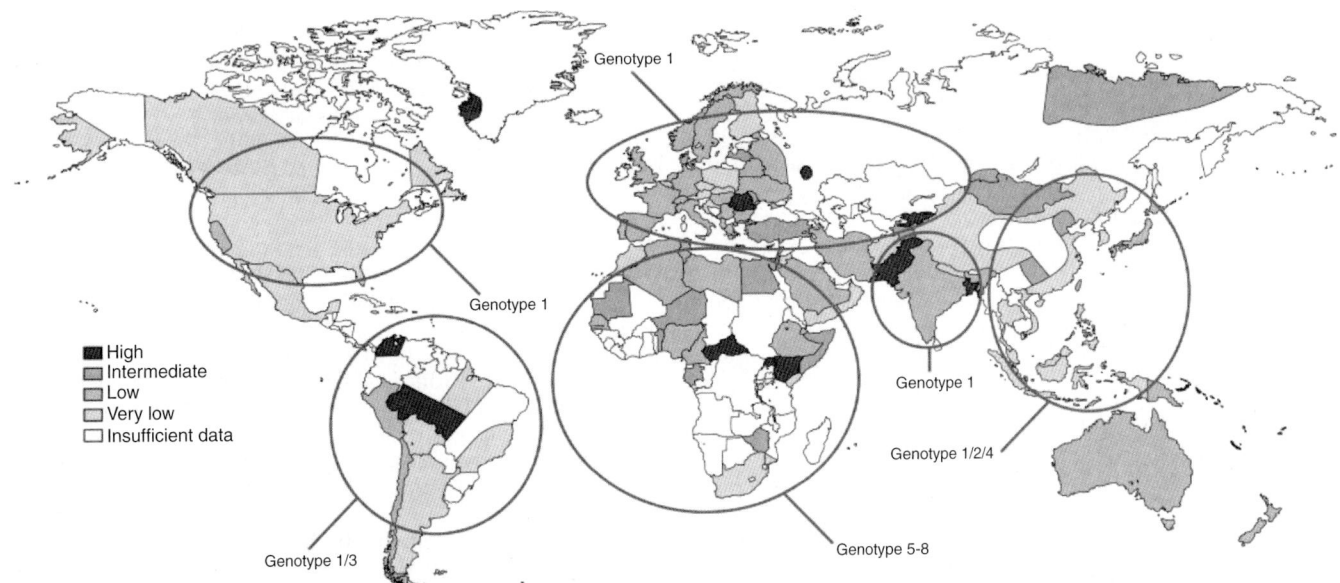

Figure 5 Global prevalence of hepatitis D virus. Hepatitis D is found globally, but prevalence varies among geographic regions. The highest prevalence is observed in Central Africa, Central Asia, and the Amazon. Intermediate-prevalence regions include West Africa and Eastern Europe. Low-prevalence regions include North America, most of Western Europe, and Australia. *Note:* Map lines delineate study areas and do not necessarily depict accepted national boundaries.

Treatment

The goals of treatment are long-term suppression of both HDV and HBV to prevent the development of cirrhosis, hepatocellular carcinoma, and liver-related death. There is no approved effective treatment for HDV in the United States. Peginterferon alfa-2a[1] has been used off-label for treatment of HDV. The most effective dose and duration of treatment have not been established. Peginterferon alfa-2a[1] administered for 48 to 72 weeks results in sustained HDV RNA suppression after 6 months of therapy in 17% to 43% of patients. Bulevirtide (Hepcludex)[5], an entry inhibitor, is approved by the European Medicines Agency (the European equivalent of the U.S. FDA). The combination of bulevirtide and peginterferon alfa-2a administered for 48 weeks was shown to be more effective at suppressing HDV RNA in the immediate 6 months after discontinuation of treatment. Liver transplantation with the use of hepatitis B immune globulin[1] is an option for patients with decompensated liver disease. Novel agents blocking viral entry in combination with a small interfering RNA that blocks the production of HBV proteins are currently being investigated in clinical studies.

Acknowledgments

This work is supported by the Intramural Research Program of the National Institute of Diabetes and Digestive and Kidney Diseases, National Institutes of Health.

Financial Disclosure

The authors are employees of the U.S. government and have no financial conflicts of interest to disclose.

References

Asselah T, Rizzetto M: Hepatitis D virus infection, *N Engl J Med* 389(1):58–70, 2023.
Dusheiko G, Agarwal K, Maini MK: New approaches to chronic hepatitis B, *N Engl J Med* 388(1):55–69, 2023.
Hoofnagle JH, Nelson KE, Purcell RH, Hepatitis E: *N Engl J Med* 367(13):1237–1244, 2012.
Matheny SC, Kingery JE, Hepatitis A: *Am Fam Physician* 86(11):1027–1034, 2012.

[1] Not FDA approved for this indication.
[5] Investigational drug in the United States.

HEPATITIS C

Method of
Arthur Y. Kim, MD

CURRENT DIAGNOSIS

- Hepatitis C virus (HCV) is a common infection in the United States, with major morbidity and mortality.
- The incidence of HCV is rising, linked to the opioid epidemic.
- Given the asymptomatic presentation and long period before complications, screening is warranted: one-time routine opt-out testing for adults age 18–79 is recommended, as is periodic repeat testing for increased risk, especially in people who inject drugs (Table 1).
- Diagnosis is made with two-stage testing: initial screening for anti-HCV antibodies followed by HCV RNA testing to confirm the presence of virus.

CURRENT THERAPY

- Novel therapeutic approaches that are safe and highly effective have revolutionized the care of HCV.
- The goal of therapy is cure of virus, which prevents liver-related complications and further transmission.
- Regimens of combination antivirals typically given for 8–12 weeks can cure over 95% of those living with HCV infection.

TABLE 1	Recommendations for One-Time Screening

All adults aged 18–79 years without prior ascertainment of risk

Risk factor–based screening

Risk behaviors

- Injection drug use (current or ever, including those who injected only once)
- Intranasal drug use

Risk exposures

- Persons on long-term hemodialysis (ever)
- Persons with percutaneous/parenteral exposures in an unregulated setting
- Health care, emergency medical, and public safety workers after needlesticks, sharps, or mucosal exposures to HCV-infected blood
- Children born to HCV-infected women
- Prior recipients of transfusions or organ transplants, including
  - Persons who were notified that they received blood from a donor who later tested positive for HCV infection
  - Persons who received a transfusion of blood or blood components or underwent an organ transplant before July 1992
  - Persons who received clotting factor concentrates produced before 1987
- Persons who were ever incarcerated

Other considerations

- HIV infection
- Sexually active persons about to start preexposure prophylaxis for HIV
- Unexplained chronic liver disease and/or chronic hepatitis, including elevated alanine aminotransferase levels
- Solid-organ donors (deceased and living)
- Pregnant women

HCV, Hepatitis C virus.
Modified from http://hcvguidelines.org.

The diagnosis, management, and therapeutic approaches for patients living with HCV have been dramatically transformed in recent years. Most people (over 95%) living with HCV infection can be cured after 8 to 12 weeks of safe oral regimens involving combined antiviral agents. The availability of novel therapies enhances the effectiveness of screening patients for HCV infection who may otherwise be unaware of infection owing to its asymptomatic presentation.

Virology, Pathogenesis, and Natural History

HCV is a single-strand RNA virus whose genome encodes several viral proteins, including nonstructural proteins (NS3/4A, termed protease; NS5A and NS5B, termed polymerase) that may each be specifically targeted by medications. There are seven known families of virus, commonly known as genotypes 1 through 7, many with subtypes (e.g., genotype 1a or 1b).

After acute infection in the majority of individuals, the virus establishes a chronic lifelong infection characterized by high levels of viremia easily detected in plasma; in a minority, the virus is spontaneously cleared. In the latter scenario, HCV is permanently eradicated, as the polymerase is an RNA-RNA polymerase and there is no DNA intermediate to establish latency in the host. Those who achieve clearance of virus, whether spontaneously or via treatment, are susceptible to reinfection if exposed again.

Both the acute and chronic phases of HCV infection are largely asymptomatic. A minority of those with acute infection may present with nonspecific symptoms such as abdominal pain and malaise, with less than 10% presenting with jaundice. Rarely, those with chronic infection may experience extrahepatic manifestations of HCV infection, such as cryoglobulinemic vasculitis, proteinuria or glomerulonephritis, or lymphoma. Otherwise, alanine transaminase (ALT) levels may be persistently or intermittently elevated but may also be within normal range in up to 20% of infected individuals; thus, ALT is considered an imperfect screening test for HCV.

After establishment of chronic HCV infection, fibrosis occurs at a variable rate and may progress to cirrhosis in about 15% to 20% over a 20-year period. Fibrosis may be accelerated by other liver insults, such as alcohol use, nonalcoholic steatohepatitis, and coinfection with HIV or hepatitis B virus (HBV). Those with HCV-related cirrhosis may experience significant morbidity and mortality from various complications; screening for varices and hepatocellular carcinoma is recommended (see chapter on cirrhosis).

Epidemiology

HCV is estimated to infect at least 58 million people worldwide. In the United States, it is the leading bloodborne pathogen and infects over 3 million Americans. The highest-risk groups are those born between 1945 and 1965 (so-called baby boomers), people who inject drugs, and HIV-positive men who have sex with men. In the United States, the incidence reached a peak in the 1970s and 1980s and then steeply declined; in the past decade there has been a resurgence of new incident cases linked to a widespread opioid epidemic.

Owing to the high number of infections that occurred decades ago, a large number of Americans within the baby-boomer cohort are now at risk for unidentified long-standing HCV infection, cirrhosis, and death. HCV-related cirrhosis remains a leading indication for liver transplantation.

Risk Factors

HCV is most efficiently transmitted via exposure to contaminated blood or its components. In the United States, injection drug use (IDU) is the most common mode of transmission. Nosocomial exposure to contaminated blood or blood products and poorly sterilized or reused contaminated medical equipment remains an important risk, especially if strict universal precautions are not instituted. Mother-to-child transmission is not efficient, as only about 5% of children born to HCV-infected women are infected, with higher rates if HIV/HCV coinfection is present. Sexual transmission is considered very rare in the context of heterosexual relationships but does occur at higher rates in men who have sex with men, particularly with HIV and/or practices that result in exposures to blood.

Diagnosis

Two tests are used for the diagnosis of HCV infection: testing for anti-HCV antibodies and measuring HCV RNA. The suggested algorithm is initial serologic testing to assess exposure, followed by HCV RNA testing to determine current or cleared infection. Currently available anti-HCV testing is highly sensitive (>99%) but may be falsely negative in the earliest stages of infection (typically the first 4 to 12 weeks) or in the setting of immunosuppression (such as dialysis or HIV if CD4 cell counts are below 200/mm³). HCV RNA testing may be utilized to confirm current HCV RNA infection after an initial positive anti-HCV test or in settings when anti-HCV may be falsely negative. There are two types of HCV RNA tests: qualitative HCV RNA tests, which do not quantify the level of viral replication, and quantitative HCV RNA tests. Quantitative testing has improved in recent years and exhibits sensitivity similar to that of qualitative testing; therefore it is preferred in most situations.

Those with confirmed current HCV infection (positive HCV RNA) should also be tested for HIV and HBV (the latter typically by hepatitis B surface antigen [HBsAg]). Follow-up evaluation includes the HCV genotype, which defines therapeutic options.

Discovery of advanced fibrosis or cirrhosis may affect the specifics of recommended antiviral regimens but also has prognostic implications. The likelihood of cirrhosis is dependent on various factors, including advancing patient age, duration of infection, and cofactors such as significant alcohol use or HIV. Noninvasive assessment with serologic testing (such as Fibrosure) or with novel imaging technologies (such as transient elastography) has largely replaced liver biopsies.

Prevention

Prevention of HCV infection should be targeted to the highest-risk groups. For people who inject drugs, clean injecting equipment—including needles, syringes, and other components of drug preparation—is paramount. Risk reduction should also be achieved after viral clearance to prevent reinfection.

Prevention of fibrosis progression includes minimization or abstinence from regular alcohol use, avoidance of fatty liver, and avoidance of primary infection with or control of coexisting viruses (HIV or HBV). For individuals who are not immune, vaccination against hepatitis A virus and HBV is recommended. Patients with coexisting substance use disorder should be referred for appropriate care.

Therapy

Antiviral treatments for hepatitis C have been revolutionized with combination regimens of direct-acting antivirals (DAAs). These new drugs are used in combination with the goal to eradicate HCV. Cure is known as a sustained virologic response (SVR), defined as a negative HCV RNA test 12 or more weeks after cessation of therapy. This definition represents a durable cure in the absence of reinfection. Benefits of SVR include a significant reduction in future liver-related events, especially for those with advanced fibrosis or cirrhosis. Additional benefits include abrogation of further HCV transmission, amelioration of extrahepatic manifestations (if present), and improvement in quality of life. Virtually all patients with current HCV infection are candidates for therapy.

Agents may be classified by the viral protein they target. The following are NS3/4A protease inhibitors: simeprevir, paritaprevir (which requires pharmacologic boosting with ritonavir), glecaprevir, and grazoprevir. NS5A inhibitors include daclatasvir, elbasvir, ledipasvir, ombitasvir, and pibrentasvir; the NS5A nonnucleoside inhibitor dasabuvir; and the NS5B nucleotide polymerase inhibitor sofosbuvir. Simeprevir (Olysio), daclatasvir (Daklinza), and sofosbuvir (Sovaldi) were developed as single agents, but the majority are parts of combination regimens, as described in Table 2. The Infectious Diseases Society of America (IDSA) and American Association for the Study of Liver Diseases (AASLD) maintain guidelines for providers at http://www.hcvguidelines.org, which provides updates with approval of novel agents and as new data become available.

One major consideration in choosing a regimen is the genotype of the virus, although certain regimens such as glecaprevir/pibrentasvir (Mavyret) and sofosbuvir/velpatasvir (Epclusa) are able to treat all genotypes (termed pangenotypic). Other potential influences include presence of cirrhosis, the potential for concomitant drug interactions (including those with HIV coinfection on antiretrovirals), prior treatment experience, and adherence to therapy. Certain regimens such as glecaprevir/pibrentasvir (Mavyret) have been tested for those with advanced renal impairment. Insurance formulary preferences may also dictate the choice. One regimen in particular, elbasvir/grazoprevir (Zepatier), requires testing of genotype 1a virus for resistance-associated substitutions (RASs) associated with decreased response; if these are present, the duration should be increased and ribavirin (Ribasphere) added. In general, almost all patient groups can be offered a regimen with a rate of SVR at or above 95%.

These combinations have favorable safety profiles, with phase III trials reporting very low discontinuation rates. The most common side effects of these regimens are headache and fatigue. At times, ribavirin may be added to the regimen, particularly

GENOTYPE	COMBINATION	USE OF RIBAVIRIN (RBV)	DURATION (WEEKS)	NOTES
1	Elbasvir 50 mg/grazoprevir 100 mg FDC (Zepatier) qd	Add RBV and extend to 16 weeks if baseline NS5A RASs present (genotype 1a only)	12–16	Safe in advanced chronic kidney disease; not recommended in decompensated cirrhosis
	Glecaprevir 300 mg/ pibrentasvir 120 mg FDC (Mavyret) qd	Consider in select re-treatment circumstances	8–16	8 weeks for treatment naive; 12–16 weeks for certain treatment-experienced patients
	Ledipasvir 90 mg/sofosbuvir 400 mg FDC (Harvoni) qd	Add RBV if both interferon-experienced and cirrhosis (12 weeks)	8–24	Antacids reduce absorption; 8 weeks consideration only for naive patients with F0-2 and HCV RNA less than 6M IU/mL
	Sofosbuvir 400 mg/velpatasvir 100 mg FDC (Epclusa) qd	Consider in select re-treatment circumstances	12–24	Antacids reduce absorption
2	Glecaprevir 300 mg/ pibrentasvir 120 mg FDC (Mavyret) qd	Consider in select re-treatment circumstances	8–12	8 weeks for treatment naive; 12 weeks for certain treatment-experienced patients
	Sofosbuvir/velpatasvir FDC (Epclusa) qd	Consider in select re-treatment circumstances	12	Antacids reduce absorption
3	Glecaprevir 300 mg/ pibrentasvir 120 mg FDC (Mavyret) qd	Consider in select re-treatment circumstances	8–16	8 weeks for treatment naive; 12–16 weeks for certain treatment-experienced patients
	Sofosbuvir/velpatasvir FDC (Epclusa) qd	Consider in select circumstances, including cirrhosis + NS5A Y93H mutation	12–24	Antacids reduce absorption
4	Elbasvir/grazoprevir (Zepatier) qd	Consider adding RBV for cirrhosis, prior nonresponder	12–16	
	Ledipasvir/sofosbuvir FDC (Harvoni) qd	Consider for previous SOF failure	12	
	Glecaprevir 300 mg/ pibrentasvir 120 mg FDC (Mavyret) qd	Not proven	8–16	8 weeks for treatment naive; 12–16 weeks for certain treatment-experienced patients
	Sofosbuvir/velpatasvir FDC (Epclusa) qd	Consider in select circumstances	12	Antacids reduce absorption

RBV may be added in select re-treatment situations; refer to https://www.hcvguidelines.org/ for details
FDC, Fixed-dose combination; *NS5A*, nonstructural protein 5A; *RASs*, resistance-associated substitutions; *RBV*, ribavirin; *SOF*, sofosbuvir.

in the cases of relapse after previous treatment and/or cirrhosis (especially if the patient is decompensated or was previously decompensated).

Drug-drug interactions are also potentially problematic. Sofosbuvir-containing regimens should not be coadministered with amiodarone (Cordarone) owing to reports of symptomatic bradycardia with poor outcomes. Medications may significantly decrease the absorption of HCV antivirals, especially rifampin (Rifadin), carbamazepine (Tegretol), oxcarbazepine (Trileptal), and St. John's wort.[7] For the combinations of ledipasvir/sofosbuvir (Harvoni) and sofosbuvir/velpatasvir (Epclusa), care must be taken if they are coadministered with medications that decrease gastric pH. The involvement of clinical pharmacists may be very useful, along with resources such as the website maintained at the University of Liverpool: http://hep-druginteractions.org.

Monitoring

Compared with previous regimens that were associated with more side effects and complications, current treatments are far more tolerable. Clinical visits or phone calls to monitor for side effects and to promote adherence are optional for patients eligible for simplified therapy (see hcvguidelines.org). Certain regimens may require more intensive monitoring in the presence of cirrhosis, as cases of decompensation have been reported. Those with active HBV replication who are untreated are at risk for reactivation of this virus once HCV is suppressed, with rare cases of liver failure reported; cotreatment of both viruses or very close monitoring is recommended for this subgroup. At this time there are few data for the use of these agents in pregnancy or during breastfeeding.

References

Edlin BR, Eckhardt BJ, Shu MA, et al: Toward a more accurate estimate of the prevalence of hepatitis C in the United States, *Hepatology* 62(5):1353–1363, 2015.

Ghany MG, Morgan TR; AASLD-IDSA Hepatitis C Guidance Panel: Hepatitis C guidance 2019 update: AASLD-IDSA recommendations for testing, managing, and treating hepatitis C virus infection, *Hepatology* 71(2):686–721, 2020.

Kim A: Hepatitis C virus, *Ann Intern Med* 165(5):ITC33–ITC48, 2016.

Ly KN, Hughes EM, Jiles RB, Holmberg SD: Rising mortality associated with hepatitis C virus in the United States, 2003- 2013, *Clin Infect Dis* 62(10):1287–1288, 2016.

Suryaprasad AG, White JZ, Xu F, et al: Emerging epidemic of hepatitis C virus infections among young nonurban persons who inject drugs in the United States, 2006-2012, *Clin Infect Dis* 59(10):1411–1419, 2014. 2006-2012.

[7]Available as dietary supplement.

INFLAMMATORY BOWEL DISEASE: CROHN'S DISEASE AND ULCERATIVE COLITIS

Method of
Lauren Loeb, MD; Mehwish Ahmed, MD; Francis A. Farraye, MD, MSc; and Jami A. Kinnucan, MD

CURRENT DIAGNOSIS

- Inflammatory bowel disease (IBD) includes Crohn's disease (CD) and ulcerative colitis, which are classified as immune-mediated chronic intestinal diseases.
- The pathogenesis of IBD is thought to be related to a dysregulated immune response.
- Clinical features of IBD include chronic diarrhea, abdominal pain, and fatigue. There can also be weight loss, bloody stools, fevers, fistulae (CD), or other extraintestinal manifestations.
- The diagnosis of IBD is made with a combination of symptom history, lab work, stool testing, imaging, endoscopic findings, and histology.

CURRENT THERAPY

- IBD is most optimally managed with a "treat-to-target" strategy.
- Medical therapies for the treatment of IBD are divided into induction therapy and maintenance therapy.
- Classes of medications include 5-aminosalicylates, corticosteroids, immunomodulators, biologics, and small molecules.
- The choice of therapy depends on the type of IBD, disease location, extent of disease, severity of disease, disease prognosis, comorbidities, and patient preference. Special considerations should be given to the aging population and patients who are pregnant.
- Preventive health maintenance should be a routine component of IBD care.

Introduction and Epidemiology

Inflammatory bowel disease (IBD) includes Crohn's disease (CD) and ulcerative colitis (UC), which are classified as immune-mediated chronic intestinal diseases. IBD can present at any age, with the most common age at presentation being young adulthood, followed by adults older than aged 60 years. The incidence of IBD has been rising over the last few decades. It is more prevalent in Western populations, although the incidence has risen throughout the world.

The pathogenesis of IBD is thought to be related to a dysregulated immune response. There is a genetic predisposition, with children and first-degree relatives of patients with IBD having an increased risk. However, only 10% to 20% of patients with IBD have first-degree relatives with the disease. Although genetic loci have been found, they explain only a small fraction of the disease risk and phenotype. Environmental factors play a role in disease pathogenesis.

Clinical Manifestations

Clinical features of IBD vary based on disease location and include chronic diarrhea, abdominal pain, and fatigue. Patients can exhibit weight loss, bloody stools, fevers, fistulae (CD), and other extraintestinal manifestations. Extraintestinal manifestations include inflammatory arthritis, skin involvement (erythema nodosum or pyoderma gangrenosum), eye involvement (uveitis, iritis, episcleritis), and liver disease including primary sclerosing cholangitis (PSC). Table 1 compares the clinical features of CD and UC.

Natural History and Complications of Disease
Crohn's Disease

CD is a transmural inflammatory disease that can involve any segment of the gastrointestinal (GI) tract from the mouth to the anus. If left untreated, CD can lead to significant complications. Although most patients do not have penetrating disease initially, up to 50% will develop intestinal complications including strictures, abscesses, or fistulae within 20 years of diagnosis. Risk factors for an aggressive disease course include early age at diagnosis, extensive involvement of bowel or penetrating disease at presentation, ileal involvement, and perianal disease. Chronic inflammation of the bowel increases the risk of both colonic and small bowel cancers and inflammatory or fibrotic strictures potentially leading to bowel obstruction, fistulae with other organs or skin, intra-abdominal abscesses, and micronutrient deficiencies due to malabsorption. Figure 1 demonstrates the natural history of CD with and without tight control and disease management.

Ulcerative Colitis

UC is a chronic inflammatory disease of the colonic mucosa of varying disease severity (proctitis to extensive/pancolitis). It has a

TABLE 1	Clinical Features of Inflammatory Bowel Disease	
	ULCERATIVE COLITIS	**CROHN'S DISEASE**
Symptoms	Rectal bleeding Diarrhea Mucoid stool Urgency Tenesmus Fatigue Weight loss Fever Extraintestinal manifestations	Abdominal pain Diarrhea Fatigue Weight loss Fever Extraintestinal manifestations
Disease features	Colon involvement (various extent) Backwash ileitis Periappendiceal red patch	Patchy intestinal involvement most common: ileal, ileum and right colon Can involve anywhere from mouth to anus Rectal sparing Deep ulcers Fistulae Strictures Granulomas Perianal inflammation
Disease severity criteria	Truelove and Witts Mayo Score	Crohn's Disease Activity Index Harvey Bradshaw Index

peak onset in early adulthood. About 15% of patients have severe disease, and 20% of these patients require hospitalization. The colectomy risk at 5 to 10 years of disease is 10% to 15%. Predictors of an aggressive disease course include young age at diagnosis, extensive disease, severe endoscopic features with large or deep ulcers, extraintestinal manifestations, elevated inflammatory markers, and need for steroids early in the course of disease. Toxic megacolon is a potentially life-threatening complication of severe UC and can lead to intestinal perforation and need for emergency surgery. Colon cancer risk is higher than the general population and especially higher in patients with concomitant PSC.

Defining Disease Severity and Prognosis
Crohn's Disease

In the setting of CD, there are multiple phenotypical expressions, including stricturing, penetrating, inflammatory (without stricturing or penetrating disease), and perianal disease. The clinical severity of CD is defined by the Crohn's Disease Activity Index (CDAI), which has a range of 0 to 600. Remission is defined as a score of less than 150, mild to moderate activity is 150 to 220, and moderate to severe activity is 220 to 450. Any score greater than 450 is severe. The scoring system is based on the severity of abdominal pain, number of bowel movements, general well-being, body weight, presence of an abdominal mass on physical exam, use of antidiarrheals, hematocrit (normalized for sex), and extraintestinal symptoms (arthritis/arthralgia, mucocutaneous findings, iritis/uveitis, perianal disease, fistulae, and fever). Another scoring system for the severity of CD is the Harvey Bradshaw Index (HBI), which includes many of the same components as the CDAI. Those with mild disease tend to have minimal impact on quality of life indices and are overall functional with minimal weight loss and good nutrition. Those with more severe disease may have significant weight loss and complications such as bowel obstruction or abscesses with more severe symptoms and impact on quality of life.

Ulcerative Colitis

Mild UC is defined by the Truelove and Witts criteria as the presence of fewer than four stools a day with intermittent blood in the stool and normal temperature, pulse, hemoglobin, and erythrocyte sedimentation rate (ESR). Acute severe ulcerative colitis (ASUC) is defined by the Truelove and Witts criteria as the presence of more than six bloody bowel movements a day, accompanied by at least one systemic sign of toxicity (heart rate >90 beats/min,

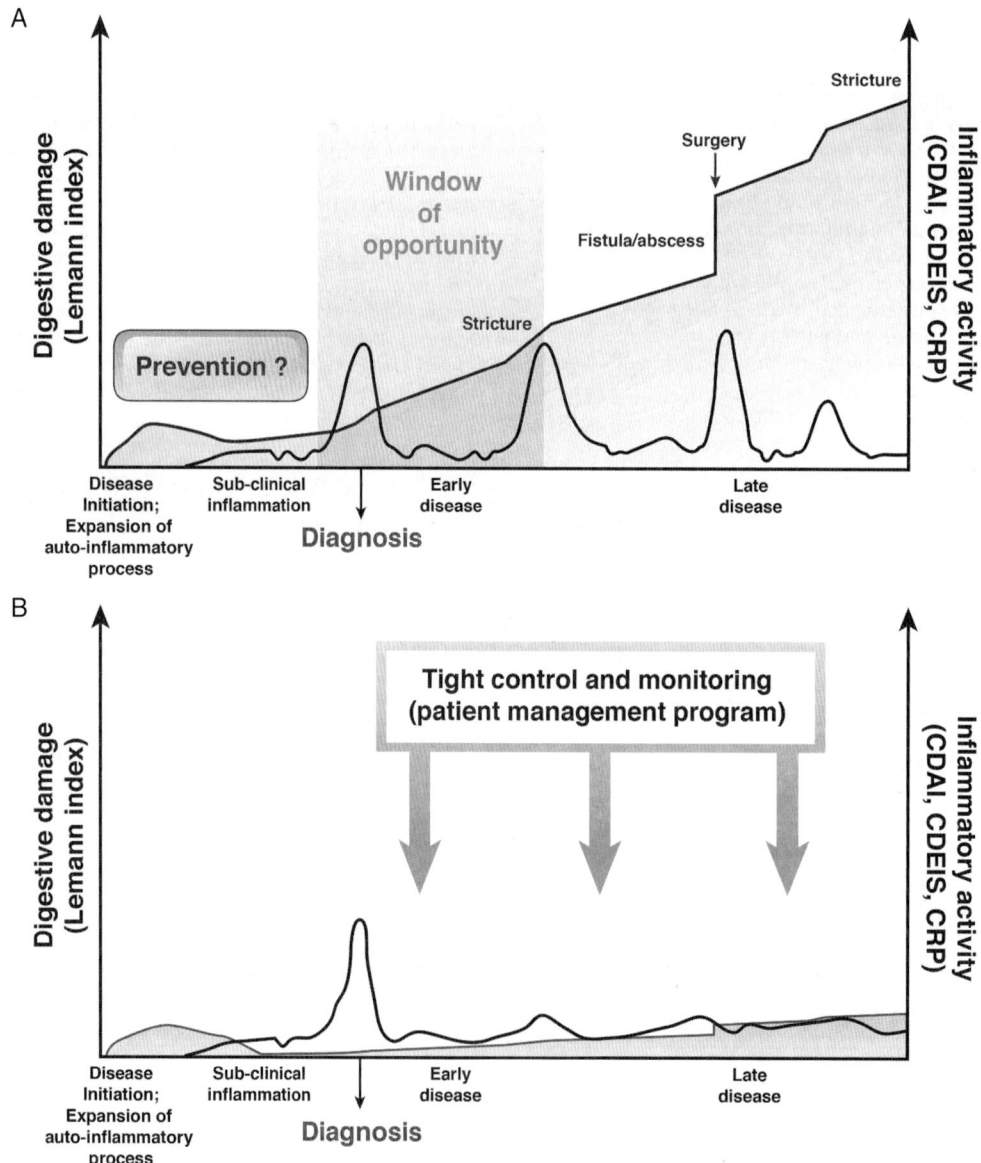

Figure 1 The natural history of Crohn's disease if left untreated (A) and with treatment (B). *CDAI*, Crohn's Disease Activity Index; *CDEIS*, Crohn's Disease Endoscopic Index of Severity; *CRP*, C-reactive protein. (Reprinted with permission from Colombel J-F, Narula N, Peyrin-Biroulet L: Management strategies to improve outcomes of patients with inflammatory bowel diseases, *Gastroenterology* 152:351-361.e5, 2017.)

temperature >37.8° C, hemoglobin <10.5 g/dL, and/or ESR >30 mm/hr). Patients who are hospitalized with ASUC have short-term colectomy rates of 25% to 30%. The Mayo Score for UC activity is another scoring system for UC that includes stool frequency, rectal bleeding, findings on endoscopy (Mayo Endoscopic Score), and physician global assessment. The clinical Mayo Score excludes endoscopic findings.

Diagnosis

History and Physical

A history obtained from patients with IBD should include assessment of symptoms, extraintestinal manifestations, features of high-risk disease, complications of disease, and effects of disease on work and functionality, as well as on mental health. The history should include the number and character of bowel movements, including nocturnal bowel movements, amount of bleeding, abdominal pain, cramping, tenesmus, and urgency. A reproductive history, including plans for pregnancy in both female and male patients, should be assessed to guide treatment. Environmental risk factors, such as cigarette smoking, should be assessed. Family history of IBD or malignancies should also be obtained.

Weight loss, body mass index (BMI), and delay in growth and puberty (pediatric patients) should be assessed at every visit. The assessment tools of CDAI or HBI (CD) and the Truelove and Witts criteria or Mayo Score (UC) can be used to help assess disease activity. Physical exam can help to identify abdominal tenderness or mass; perianal complications; extraintestinal dermatologic, rheumatologic, or ocular manifestations; and signs of malnutrition.

Diagnostics

A diagnosis of IBD is made with a combination of symptom history, lab work, imaging, endoscopic findings, and histology. Fecal calprotectin can be used in patients with clinical features concerning for IBD, to monitor disease activity and response to treatment, and have greater sensitivity in IBD with colonic involvement. Serum inflammatory markers, such as C-reactive protein and ESR, are useful when making an initial diagnosis and monitoring disease activity. However, some patients do not develop elevation of serum inflammatory serum markers despite other objective evidence of active inflammation.

Other lab testing should include assessment for anemia and malnutrition with complete blood count (CBC), liver and renal function tests, iron studies, and vitamin D and B12 levels. Isolated alkaline phosphatase elevation should raise suspicion for possible PSC; however, this can be a nonspecific finding, and further diagnostic imaging should be considered. Infectious causes of diarrhea, especially *Clostridioides difficile,* should be ruled out when evaluating for IBD.

Patients with suspected IBD should have a colonoscopy with terminal ileum intubation and segmental ileal and colon biopsies for diagnosis. Video capsule endoscopy can also be considered to assess and monitor for small bowel involvement of CD. The most common endoscopic finding in patients with CD is involvement of the terminal ileum with or without right colon inflammation. The histology of CD shows chronic inflammation with lymphoid aggregates and irregular crypt architecture. Noncaseating granulomas are pathognomonic for CD; however, they are seen in only 20% to 30% of patients. UC endoscopically appears as inflammation, characterized by any of the following features of erythema: altered vascularity, superficial erosions, ulcerations, and friable mucosa beginning in the rectum and extending proximally in a continuous fashion of various extents. Notably, patients with UC may also have an isolated cecal patch of inflammation (periappendiceal patch), and some patients with pancolitis can have mild ileal inflammation (backwash ileitis). On histology, UC appears as chronic inflammation and architectural distortion.

Radiological studies are useful to determine the extent of disease involvement and complications of disease, especially in patients with CD. They do not replace endoscopic evaluation and can be used concomitantly. Computed tomography enterography (CTE) uses oral and intravenous (IV) contrast to identify thickened bowel wall and has a sensitivity of around 90% for CD. Magnetic resonance enterography is an alternative to CTE to avoid cumulative radiation exposure in patients who require frequent disease assessment with imaging. Magnetic resonance imaging is more effective than computed tomography at detecting perianal fistulae. Transabdominal ultrasound can be helpful in assessing for disease activity in both CD and UC, allowing visualization of strictures, bowel wall thickness, and postoperative recurrence of disease. In UC, a plain abdominal film in hospitalized patients may be useful to assess for toxic megacolon; however, imaging does not have as much of a role in evaluation of UC unless in the evaluation of severe abdominal pain.

Differential Diagnosis

It is important to consider differential diagnoses when evaluating patients with acute or chronic GI symptoms. Table 2 lists both infectious and noninfectious IBD mimickers.

Management of Disease

IBD is most optimally managed with a "treat-to-target" strategy. Various targets have been identified by the STRIDE I and II initiatives of the International Organization for the Study of Inflammatory Bowel Diseases (IOIBD). There has been a focus on clinical, endoscopic, histologic, imaging, biomarker, and patient-reported outcomes as potential targets. In Figure 2, from STRIDE II, targets are divided into short-term, intermediate, and long-term for patients with IBD. Figure 3 defines these targets. As of 2021, histologic remission and transmural healing do not have enough evidence to support escalating therapy to achieve these parameters but can be helpful adjunctive data to assess the depth of remission. In 2025 there is anticipation of updates from the IOIBD group with STRIDE III guidance around treat-to-target strategy.

Medical Management

Medical therapies for the treatment of IBD are divided into *induction therapy* to bring the inflammation under control in the acute setting and *maintenance therapy* to allow for sustained

TABLE 2	Inflammatory Bowel Disease Mimickers
GI infections	*Clostridium difficile*
	Salmonella
	Shigella
	Escherichia coli
	Campylobacter
	Giardia
	Yersinia
	Amebiasis
	Cytomegalovirus colitis (in patients who are immunosuppressed)
	Tuberculosis
Sexually transmitted infections	Chlamydia
	Herpes
	Neisseria gonorrhea
	Treponema pallidum
Noninfectious mimickers	Microscopic colitis
	Diverticulitis
	Segmental colitis associated with diverticulosis
	Ischemic colitis
	Medication associated colitis or enteritis (NSAIDs)
	Solitary rectal ulcer syndrome
	Systemic vasculitis (polyarteritis nodosa, Henoch-Schönlein purpura, Behcet syndrome)
	Celiac disease
	Intestinal lymphoma
	Diversion colitis (in patients with intestinal surgical diversion)

GI, Gastrointestinal; *NSAIDs,* nonsteroidal anti-inflammatory drugs.

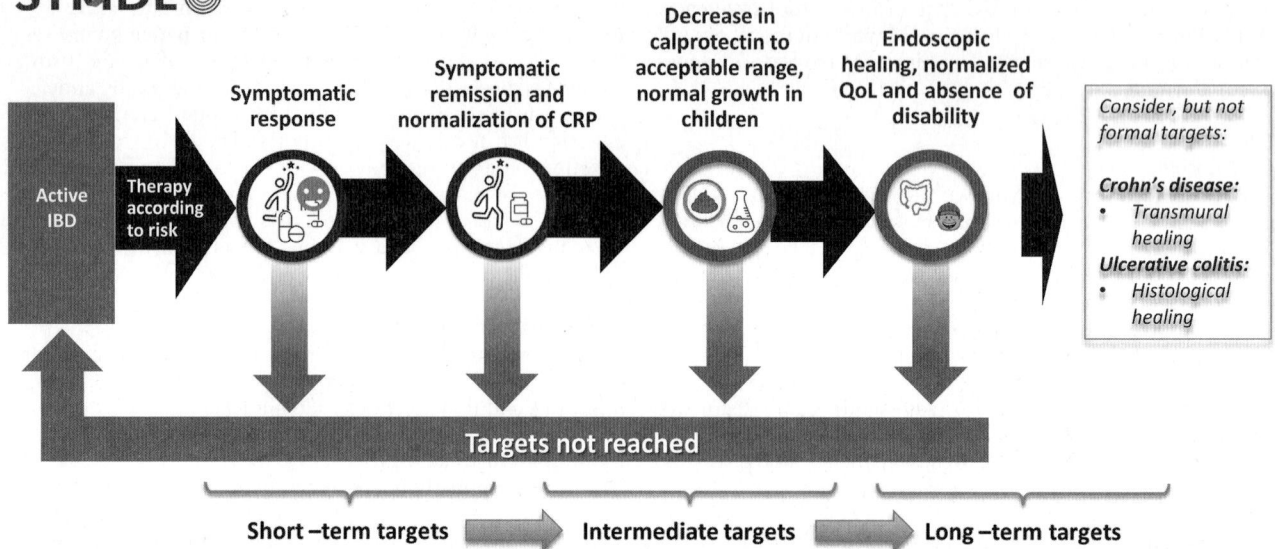

Figure 2 Stride II treatment targets for UC and CD. *CRP,* C-reactive protein; *IBD,* inflammatory bowel disease; *QoL,* quality of life. (Reprinted with permission from Turner D, Ricciuto A, Lewis A, et al: STRIDE-II: an update on the Selecting Therapeutic Targets in Inflammatory Bowel Disease (STRIDE) initiative of the International Organization for the Study of IBD (IOIBD): determining therapeutic goals for treat-to-target strategies in IBD, *Gastroenterology* 160:1570-1583, 2021.)

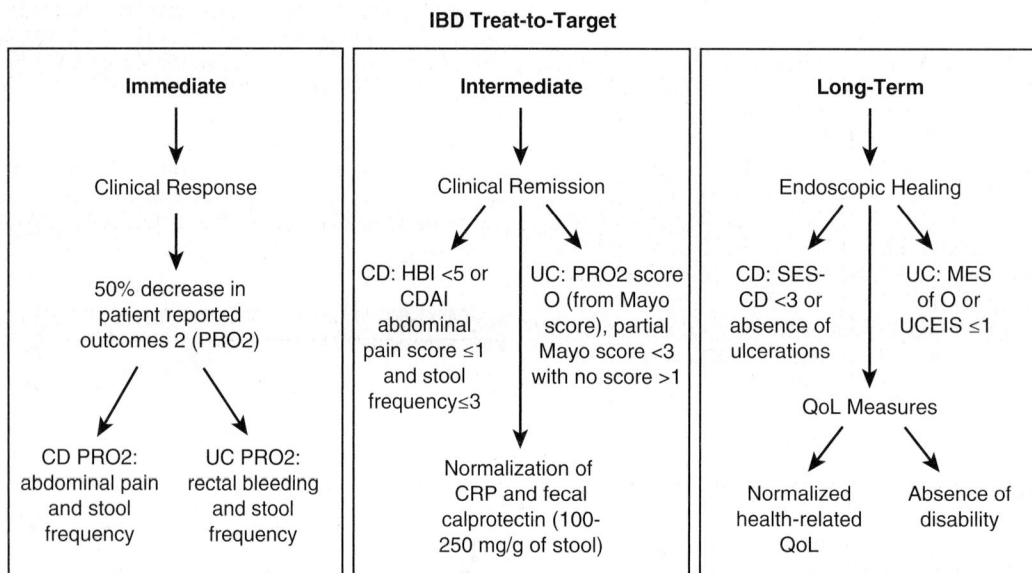

Figure 3 Stride II Treat-to-Target goals for UC and CD. *CD,* Crohn's disease; *CDAI,* Crohn's Disease Activity Index; *CRP,* C-reactive protein; *HBI,* Harvey Bradshaw Index; *MES,* Mayo Endoscopic Score; *QoL,* quality of life; *SES-CD,* Simple Endoscopic Score for Crohn's Disease; *UC,* ulcerative colitis; *UCEIS,* Ulcerative Colitis Endoscopic Index of Severity.

inflammation control. In most situations the medical therapies used for induction can also be used for chronic maintenance therapy. The choice of therapy depends on the type of IBD, disease location, extent of disease, severity of disease, disease prognosis, comorbidities, and patient preference. Table 3 provides a reference for IBD therapies, including formulations, indications, adverse effects, and monitoring. In addition to the medications reviewed later, there are multiple other drugs in Phase II and III trials being studied for the treatment of IBD.

5-Aminosalicylates
5-Aminosalicylates (5-ASAs) are used as first-line therapy for induction and maintenance of remission of mild to moderate UC.

5-ASA use is limited in CD, although sulfasalazine (Azulfidine)[1] can be considered in patients with mild Crohn's colitis. 5-ASAs work by topical contact, exerting anti-inflammatory effects. Rectal formulations are first-line treatments for proctitis (suppositories) and left-sided UC (enemas) up to the splenic flexure. For mild extensive colitis (beyond the splenic flexure), oral 5-ASA is recommended in addition to rectal therapies. For any extent of disease failing to respond to 5-ASA, escalation of therapy is indicated. Once daily dosing is just as effective as divided dosing. If switching to an advanced therapy (biologic or small molecule), there is no indication to continue the 5-ASA to maintain remission.

---

[1] Not FDA approved for this indication.

TABLE 3 Pharmacologic Therapies for Inflammatory Bowel Disease

MEDICATION CLASS	MEDICATION NAME	INDICATIONS	ADVERSE EFFECTS	MONITORING
5-ASA	Mesalamine rectal suppository (Canasa) Mesalamine enema (Rowasa) Mesalamine extended-release capsule (Pentasa) Mesalamine delayed-release (Apriso, Lialda, Asacol HD) Sulfasalazine (Azulfidine), olsalazine (Dipentum), and balsalazide (Colazal)	Mild to moderate UC (induction and maintenance)	Nausea, vomiting, headache, diarrhea, abdominal pain, interstitial nephritis	Urinalysis and renal function yearly
Corticosteroids	Prednisone Methylprednisolone Budesonide Budesonide-MMX (Uceris extended-release tablet) Rectal hydrocortisone (suppository, foam, or enema) Rectal budesonide foam (Uceris Rectal)	UC and CD (induction, use <3 months)	Osteoporosis, adrenal insufficiency, impaired glucose tolerance, infection, fluid retention, hypertension, osteonecrosis, mood and sleep disturbance	DEXA scan if >3 months of systemic use
Biologics				
Anti–TNF-α	Infliximab (Remicade or biosimilar) Adalimumab (Humira or biosimilar) Golimumab (Simponi) (UC only) Certolizumab pegol (CD only)	UC and CD (induction and maintenance)	Infusion reactions, immune-mediated reactions, infections, malignancy (lymphoma, melanoma) Avoid in heart failure, demyelinating disease, or active malignancy	Yearly skin exam TB and hepatitis B
Anti–integrins	Vedolizumab (Entyvio) Natalizumab (Tysabri)	Vedolizumab: UC and CD (induction and maintenance) Natalizumab: CD only (induction and maintenance)	PML (natalizumab), nasopharyngitis	JC virus (natalizumab) TB and hepatitis B
Anti–IL-12/23	Ustekinumab (Stelara)	UC and CD (induction and maintenance)	Nasopharyngitis, other infections, headache, arthralgia	TB and hepatitis B
Anti–IL-23	Risankizumab (Skyrizi) Mirikizumab (Omvoh) Guselkumab (Tremfya)	Risankizumab: UC and CD (induction and maintenance) Mirikizumab: UC and CD (induction and maintenance) Guselkumab: CD and UC (induction and maintenance)	DILI, nasopharyngitis, upper respiratory tract and other infections, headache, arthralgia, rash, injection site reactions, anemia (Guselkumab only)	Liver enzymes TB and hepatitis B
Small Molecules				
JAK inhibitors	Tofacitinib (Xeljanz) Upadacitinib (Rinvoq)	Tofacitinib: UC (induction and maintenance) Upadacitinib: UC and CD (induction and maintenance)	Hyperlipidemia, lymphopenia, blood clots, infection, herpes zoster, GI perforation	CBC Lipid panel Liver enzymes TB and hepatitis B
S1P receptor modulator	Ozanimod (Zeposia) Etrasimod (Velsipity)	UC (induction and maintenance)	Herpes zoster, lymphopenia, bradycardia, HTN, macular edema, elevated liver enzymes	Baseline CBC Liver enzymes ECG Ocular exam Skin exam
Immunomodulators				
Thiopurines	Azathioprine (Imuran) 6-Mercaptopurine (6-MP)	Monotherapy: UC[1] and CD[1] (maintenance) Combination therapy: UC[1] and CD[1] (induction and maintenance)	Hepatotoxicity, leukopenia, lymphoma, pancreatitis, non–melanoma skin cancers, infections	TPMT before initiation CBC and liver enzymes
Methotrexate	Methotrexate (oral, subcutaneous or intramuscular)	Monotherapy: CD[1] (maintenance) Combination therapy: both UC[1] and CD[1] (induction and maintenance)	Myelosuppression, hepatotoxicity, pulmonary fibrosis, teratogenicity	CBC Liver enzymes

Continued

MEDICATION CLASS	MEDICATION NAME	INDICATIONS	ADVERSE EFFECTS	MONITORING
Cyclosporine	Cyclosporine	Induction in acute severe UC[1]	Seizures, nephrotoxicity, neurotoxicity, infections	Not used in maintenance

[1]Not FDA approved for this indication.

5-ASA, 5-Aminosalicylates; *CBC*, complete blood count; *CD*, Crohn's disease; *DILI*, drug-induced liver injury; *ECG*, electrocardiogram; *GI*, gastrointestinal; *HTN*, hypertension; *IL*, interleukin; *JAK*, Janus kinase; *PML*, progressive multifocal leukoencephalopathy; *S1P*, sphingosine-1-phosphate; *TB*, tuberculosis; *TMPT*, thiopurine methyltransferase; *TNF-α*, tumor necrosis factor–α; *UC*, ulcerative colitis.

5-ASA side effects include nausea, vomiting, diarrhea, headache, and abdominal pain. Sulfasalazine may also cause low sperm counts. A small group of approximately 0.5% to 6.5% of patients on 5-ASA may experience worsening of intestinal symptoms consistent with a hypersensitivity reaction. Another rare side effect is interstitial nephritis, which occurs in less than 0.3% of patients. To monitor for this, clinicians should monitor renal function several weeks after starting therapy and then yearly.

Corticosteroids

Corticosteroids are anti-inflammatory medications that are typically used at the time of diagnosis and during relapses but are not recommended to be used for maintenance of remission because of their extensive adverse side effect profile with long-term use. Ultimately, the treat-to-target strategy focuses on achieving treatment targets using steroid-sparing therapies. Budesonide with controlled-release formulations for either ileal (Entocort EC) or colonic (Uceris) disease is an option for clinical relapse with fewer systemic side effects. Per rectum steroids are available as hydrocortisone suppositories, foam formulations, or enemas. These can be used as initial therapy in mild to moderate left-sided colitis or proctitis, although rectal mesalamine is preferred as the initial agent given their higher effectiveness and avoidance of systemic absorption of topical steroids.

Adverse effects of steroids include mood and sleep disturbances, impaired glucose tolerance, metabolic bone disease, adrenal insufficiency, infections, fluid retention, hypertension, and osteonecrosis of the femoral head. If a patient has required systemic steroids for over 3 months, they should undergo a dual-energy X-ray absorptiometry (DEXA) scan to evaluate for osteopenia.

Biologics

Biologic therapies, first introduced in 1998, have transformed the landscape of IBD care. Biologics are recommended to be initiated early in the treatment of patients with moderate to severe UC or CD as they lead to better outcomes, prevention of disease complications, and a higher likelihood of achieving and maintaining a steroid-free remission. These medications are used both for induction and maintenance of remission.

Anti–Tumor Necrosis Factor–α agents

Anti–tumor necrosis factor–α (TNF-α) therapies block TNF-α, which is a cytokine that mediates inflammation in IBD. They can be used for induction and maintenance for CD and UC. Before initiation of anti–TNF-α agents, screening for latent or active tuberculosis (TB) and hepatitis B must be performed. Infliximab (Remicade or biosimilar) is administered as an IV formulation, whereas adalimumab (Humira or biosimilar) is a subcutaneous formulation. These are both approved for UC and CD. The U.S. Food and Drug Administration (FDA) approved infliximab-dyyb (Zymfentra), which is a subcutaneous formulation approved for maintenance therapy. Other formulations include golimumab (Simponi), which is only approved for UC, and certolizumab pegol (Cimzia), which is only approved for CD. Data have also shown that the efficacy of anti–TNF-α agents improves when used in combination with immunomodulators, such as azathioprine (Imuran),[1] 6-mercaptopurine (Purinethol),[1] or methotrexate.[1]

This is thought to be due to prevention of anti–drug antibody formation and higher serum drug levels.

Adverse effects of anti–TNF-α agents include infusion reactions (infliximab), which can be acute or delayed, immune-mediated adverse effects, infections, and rarely, treatment-related malignancy. Other immune-mediated adverse effects include drug-induced lupus-like reactions and psoriasiform reactions that usually resolve with drug discontinuation.

Those on anti–TNF-α therapy are at increased risk for infection, including opportunistic infections and reactivation of TB and hepatitis B. Although rare, treatment-related malignancy is a risk with anti–TNF-α agents, especially when used in combination with immunomodulators. Although there is no significant risk of development of solid organ tumors, there is an increased risk of non–Hodgkin lymphoma and melanoma though it is hard to separate disease-related malignancy versus medication-associated malignancy. Anti–TNF-α therapies are contraindicated in patients with decompensated heart failure and demyelinating neurologic disease.

Anti-integrins

Anti-integrin agents affect leukocyte trafficking. α4 Integrins are cell adhesion molecules that control the migration of leukocytes across the vascular endothelium and play a significant role in intestinal inflammation.

Natalizumab (Tysabri) is an antibody to α4β1 integrin, and vedolizumab (Entyvio) is a selective α4β7 integrin inhibitor. As natalizumab is associated with a rare but often fatal disease called progressive multifocal leukoencephalopathy, its use clinically has been limited since the approval of vedolizumab (Entyvio). Vedolizumab has recently received approval for maintenance subcutaneous formulation in both UC and CD.

Vedolizumab is gut specific and is approved for induction and maintenance of remission in both CD and UC. It has a favorable safety profile with minimal systemic side effects, minimal risk of systemic infections, and no evidence of risk of development of lymphoproliferative disorders.

Anti–IL-12/23

Ustekinumab (Stelara or biosimilar) binds to the p40 subunit of both interleukin (IL)-12 and IL-23 and is approved for induction and maintenance of remission in both CD and UC. The induction dose is a single infusion followed by injections every 8 weeks. The most frequently reported adverse events are nasopharyngitis and upper respiratory tract infections. Ustekinumab has a lower immunogenicity risk relative to anti–TNF-α agents.

Anti–IL-23

There are several treatments in the anti-IL-23 class of treatment. Risankizumab (Skyrizi) targets the p19 subunit of IL-23. It has been shown to be effective in the induction and maintenance of remission in patients with moderate to severe CD and UC. The initial induction dosing with three infusions is followed by maintenance therapy using an on-body subcutaneous injector that can be administered at home every 8 weeks. The most common adverse events include nasopharyngitis, headache, and arthralgia. Serious infections, including herpes zoster and other opportunistic infections, can occur. There is an association with liver injury; therefore it is important to check liver enzymes before initiation and periodically thereafter.

---

[1]Not FDA approved for this indication.

Mirikizumab (Omvoh) is a humanized immunoglobulin G4 variant monoclonal antibody that also binds to subunit p19 of IL-23. It has been shown to be effective in the induction and maintenance of remission and is approved for treatment in patients with moderate to severe UC and CD. The initial induction dosing with three infusions is followed by maintenance therapy using subcutaneous injections that can be administered by the patient every 4 weeks. The most common adverse reactions include upper respiratory tract infections and arthralgia. Rash, injection site reactions, headache, and herpes viral infections have also been reported. Liver enzymes and bilirubin levels should be monitored before and during treatment due to reports of drug-induced liver injury. Patients should be evaluated for TB prior to and during treatment due to increased risk of TB infection.

Guselkumab (Tremfya) is a dual-acting, human IgG1, IL-23p19 subunit inhibitor that neutralizes IL-23 and can bind to CD64, a receptor on myeloid cells, which are one of the cell types that produce IL-23 in addition to other cytokines. It has been shown to be effective in the induction and maintenance of remission and is approved for treatment in patients with moderate to severe UC and CD. In the induction phase, patients receive three doses intravenously at weeks 0, 4, and 8. This is followed by maintenance therapy using subcutaneous injections that can be administered by the patient either every 4 weeks or every 8 weeks. For CD, a self-injection only induction and maintenance option is available. The most common adverse reactions include anemia, headache, arthralgia, injection site reactions, and upper respiratory tract infection. Patients should be evaluated for hepatitis B before treatment and TB before and during treatment due to increased risk of TB infection.

Biosimilars
Biologic agents are large complex molecules of which exact replicas cannot be made. Biosimilars, such as infliximab-dyyb (Zymfentra, Inflectra), infliximab-axxq (Avsola), and infliximab-abda (Renflexis), are very similar in structure to the original molecule but have varying glycosylation patterns that lead to differences in parts of the molecule that are not clinically active. There are multiple adalimumab biosimilars available in the United States including adalimumab-atto (Amjevita), adalimumab-adbm (Cyltezo), and adalimumab-adaz (Hyrimoz). Switching between reference and biosimilar products has not been shown to be inferior to continuing with the original product.

Small Molecules
Small molecule therapies are given orally; have a simple, well-defined structure; and have a favorable pharmacokinetic profile due to lack of immunogenicity.

JAK Inhibitors
Tofacitinib (Xeljanz) and upadacitinib (Rinvoq) are oral medications for IBD that inhibit the Janus kinase (JAK) signaling pathway. Tofacitinib targets JAK 1, 2, and 3, whereas upadacitinib is a selective JAK 1 inhibitor. Both tofacitinib and upadacitinib can be used for induction and maintenance of remission. Tofacitinib has approval for use in moderate to severe UC, and upadacitinib has approval for use in both moderate to severe UC and CD. JAK inhibitors appear to have a role in the induction of remission in hospitalized patients with ASUC as concomitant therapy with IV steroids for those who are at high risk of failure of steroid therapy, such as patients who have previously failed anti–TNF-α agents, recently failed IV steroids, or have failed outpatient steroids of 40 mg daily or higher. These therapies are only approved for use in patients with prior exposure to anti–TNF-α therapies.

Adverse effects of this class include an increase in herpes zoster, TB and other infections, blood clots (pulmonary embolism), elevated creatine phosphokinase level, lymphopenia, neutropenia and anemia, and elevated lipid levels. Because of the high risk of zoster infections, it is recommended that all patients receive the recombinant herpes zoster vaccine. CBC and lipid panels should be monitored for patients on JAK inhibitors. GI perforation has also been reported as a rare serious adverse event for tofacitinib. Based on an oral surveillance study in rheumatoid arthritis, patients 50 years of age and older with at least one cardiovascular risk factor have an increased risk of major cardiovascular events such as heart attack, stroke, or death with tofacitinib use. This risk is higher in patients with a current or past smoking history. While this led to an FDA label change requiring patients to have had an inadequate response or intolerance to treatment with an anti–TNF-α agent prior to prescribing a JAK inhibitor, follow-up studies in patients with IBD have not shown similar outcomes.

Sphingosine-1-Phosphate Receptor Modulator
Ozanimod (Zeposia) and etrasimod (Velsipity) are oral sphingosine-1-phosphate receptor modulators that promote sequestration of lymphocytes within lymph nodes, preventing lymphocyte accumulation in the GI tract. These are oral agents that have been shown to be effective and are approved for use in moderately to severely active UC for induction and maintenance. These drugs are ideally positioned after 5-ASA failures and currently being studied in phase III clinical trials for moderate to severe CD.[1]

Adverse effects include increased risk of infections, including herpes zoster, lymphopenia, bradycardia, elevated liver enzymes, macular edema, and hypertension. Liver enzymes and CBC should be monitored for patients on ozanimod. Prior to starting ozanimod or etrasimod patients required an electrocardiogram, ocular examination and skin examination.

Immunomodulators
Thiopurines
Thiopurines consist of azathioprine (Imuran)[1] and 6-mercaptopurine (Purinethol).[1] Because of delayed onset of action, thiopurines are not recommended for induction of remission; however, they can be used for maintenance of remission for both CD and UC as either monotherapy or as combination therapy with anti–TNF-α agents. Before initiation of a thiopurine, thiopurine methyltransferase enzyme activity along with NUDT15 polymorphism should be checked. Those with low activity may benefit from a lower dose, whereas those with absent activity should not be started on a thiopurine.

Patients on thiopurines are at increased risk of infections, pancreatitis, nonmelanoma skin cancers, and lymphoma (especially non–Hodgkin lymphoma). Hepatosplenic T-cell lymphoma (HSTCL), which is a rare and aggressive form of lymphoma, has been associated with both monotherapy and biologic combination therapy with anti–TNF-α agents. Often these cases of HSTCL have occurred in younger men. Thiopurines also have risk of hepatotoxicity and leukopenia. CBC and liver enzymes should be monitored at least every 3 to 4 months.

Methotrexate
Methotrexate works by interfering with DNA synthesis by inhibiting dihydrofolate reductase, a key enzyme in the purine production pathway, thus leading to decreased inflammation. Studies have shown that intramuscular or subcutaneous methotrexate has been effective in the treatment of patients with CD,[1] though data have not shown efficacy in patients with UC[1] as monotherapy. Methotrexate may also be used as adjunctive therapy to biologics to reduce immunogenicity. Methotrexate can cause myelosuppression, hepatotoxicity, and pulmonary fibrosis. It is also a teratogen and should be avoided in women of reproductive age unless used with birth control. It is recommended that women discontinue methotrexate at least 3 months before attempting pregnancy.

---

[1] Not FDA approved for this indication.

Cyclosporine

Cyclosporine is an inhibitor of calcineurin, which is an enzyme that is required for the activation of T cells. Its use in IBD is limited to use as a salvage therapy to induce remission in hospitalized patients with ASUC[1] that is not responsive to steroids. It is an alternative agent to infliximab, which can also be used in ASUC. Cyclosporine is solely used as induction therapy when there is a plan to transition to an alternative agent for maintenance therapy, such as azathioprine monotherapy or biologic therapy. Side effects include seizures, nephrotoxicity, neurotoxicity, and infections. Cyclosporine requires close monitoring and should not be used unless administered by an experienced clinician.

Surgical Management

The preferred surgical treatment for UC is total proctocolectomy with ileal pouch–anal anastomosis (IPAA). An alternative operation would be total proctocolectomy and end ileostomy. Around 10% to 20% of patients that have UC will require a colectomy by 20 years of diagnosis. Of patients who undergo IPAA, approximately 50% develop an episode of pouch inflammation (pouchitis) that is often responsive to antibiotics.

In CD, about 60% of patients will require surgical intervention for active disease or complications. The most common surgery performed for CD is ileocecal resection with primary anastomosis. Other surgical strategies may include small bowel resection, stricturoplasty, segmental colectomy, and total proctocolectomy with end ileostomy. Most patients who undergo surgery for CD will have a recurrence of inflammation and will require postoperative monitoring and, in high-risk individuals, postoperative treatment to prevent recurrence. With the increased use of advanced therapies, surgical rates for both CD and UC have been decreasing, attesting to the effectiveness of these medications.

Supplemental Therapies

Nutrition and Diet

Patients with IBD are prone to development of micronutrient deficiencies and malnutrition due to malabsorption or history of surgical resection. Patients with ileal disease or resection of the ileum are more likely to have fat-soluble vitamin and vitamin B12 deficiencies. In patients with known stricturing disease, a low-fiber and low-residue diet is currently recommended. Many diets have been evaluated for efficacy in IBD with elemental diets proving efficacious in inducing remission of CD in pediatric patients. In most patients with IBD, a Mediterranean diet is recommended. To improve symptoms, dietary modifications are a helpful adjunct to medical therapy. Patients can work with a nutritionist to evaluate which type of diet is best for their quality of life and symptom pattern.

Pain Management

Many patients with IBD struggle with acute and chronic abdominal pain. Pain in IBD can be difficult to treat, especially if the pain is not related to active inflammation. Disease activity should be assessed when patients have worsening abdominal pain, but other etiologies to consider include visceral hypersensitivity, mechanical obstruction due to stricture, fistulae formation, abdominal infection, or abscess.

Chronic use of nonsteroidal anti-inflammatory drugs (NSAIDs) has been thought to increase the risk for active inflammation in IBD, though they appear to be safe when used in short courses. Chronic narcotic use has been associated with worse outcomes in patients with IBD. Their use should be minimized and only for acute pain. For chronic pain, neuromodulators and antispasmodics are beneficial. Psychosocial factors play a large role in the pain pathways. Addressing underlying depression, anxiety, and stressors may help pain control. Medication options to consider for acute pain include acetaminophen, tramadol, opiates, NSAIDs, or antispasmodics. For noninflammatory etiologies of pain, tricyclic antidepressants, gabapentin (Neurontin),[1] pregabalin (Lyrica),[1]

selective serotonin reuptake inhibitors, serotonin and norepinephrine reuptake inhibitors, and bupropion (Wellbutrin)[1] can be pharmacological options. The use of cannabis[1] has become an area of research interest and has some evidence for use in pain management for patients with IBD. However, there are no convincing data that cannabis decreases inflammation in patients with IBD. Additionally, its use is limited by current federal illegal status.

Special Populations

Pregnancy

A history of IBD has not been shown to affect fertility rates except for those who have undergone IPAA. In women who have active disease at conception, pregnancy can have varying effects on disease activity, with some patients worsening and others improving. In women who are in remission when they conceive, their disease tends to remain in remission throughout pregnancy but still requires monitoring. It is recommended that female patients with IBD remain on medical therapy during pregnancy to maintain remission. There are very few therapies that should be avoided in patients with IBD who are pregnant; these include metronidazole, methotrexate, tofacitinib, upadacitinib, ozanimod, etrasimod, and certain antibiotics.

Adverse outcomes in pregnancy for women with well-controlled IBD are similar to women without IBD. Active IBD in pregnancy has been associated with preterm birth, spontaneous abortion, and infants small for gestational age. Venous thromboembolism is increased in patients with IBD, especially in those with severe active disease. Vaginal delivery is safe in patients with IBD apart from those with active perianal disease.

Aging IBD Population

About 15% of new diagnoses of IBD occur in patients over the age of 60. Patients in this population tend to have more comorbidities and are more prone to infection, venous thromboembolic events, and malignancy. Functional status, frailty, comorbidities, and treatment goals should also be assessed to determine an optimal treatment plan. All routine vaccines should be administered including influenza, pneumococcal, respiratory syncytial virus, COVID-19, and herpes zoster, especially in this subset of patients. Other comorbidities should be optimally managed to enhance overall health and nutrition and prevent poor outcomes.

Preventive Care

Preventive health maintenance should be a routine component of IBD care. Patients with IBD are at increased risk of infections. Regardless of their immunosuppressive status, patients with IBD should receive the influenza vaccine yearly and the pneumococcal vaccinations based on guidance from the Centers for Disease Control and Prevention. Subsets of women on immunosuppressive medication for IBD are at increased risk of cervical cancer and therefore should have regular cervical cancer screening. All men and women under the age of 26 should receive the human papillomavirus vaccine. Patients on anti–TNF-α agents, thiopurines, and JAK inhibitors are at increased risk of skin cancer and should have periodic skin exams. Those with more than one-third of their colon involved with IBD and who have had IBD for over 8 years should have colonoscopic surveillance every 1 to 5 years. Patients with IBD and PSC should begin annual colonoscopy screening at the time of diagnosis with IBD. DEXA scans should be done in patients who have been treated with steroids for over 3 months to assess for osteopenia or osteoporosis. All patients should be screened for tobacco use and counseled on cessation if currently smoking. Depression and anxiety are common in patients with IBD and should be screened for annually. Table 4 provides a summary of preventive care in adult patients with IBD.

As the prevalence of IBD rises, it has become increasingly important for primary care physicians to be acquainted with the diagnosis, natural history of disease, medication adverse effects, lifestyle recommendations, reproductive counseling, and healthcare maintenance of affected patients.

---

[1] Not FDA approved for this indication.

TABLE 4	Adult Inflammatory Bowel Disease Health Maintenance

SCREENING	WHO	WHEN
Cervical Pap smear	All women (starting at age 21) on systemic immunosuppression	Every 1–3 years*
Dermatologic skin exam	All on systemic immunosuppression	Annually*
Colonoscopy	All with at least one-third colon involved after 8 years of diagnosis	Every 1–5 years
DEXA scan	Steroid use >3 months or other high-risk patients	At least 2 years apart
Depression	All patients	Annually
Smoking	All patients	Annually
Vaccinations		
Influenza (inactivated)	All patients	Annually
COVID-19	All patients 6 months and older	Follow CDC recommendations
Pneumococcal	Immunocompromised patients aged ≥19 years and all patients aged ≥65 years	PCV naïve or unknown status: 1 dose of PCV 20 or PCV15 followed by PPSV23 given at least one year later** Previously received PPSV23 only: 1 dose of PCV20 or PCV15 ≥ 1 year Previously received PCV13 only***: PPSV23 at least 8 weeks after or in 5 years if < age 65 or booster in 5 years from last dose and after age 65 Previously received PCV13 and PPSV23: PPSV23 booster in 5 years if < age 65 or booster in 5 years after age 65
Zoster (recombinant vaccine [Shingrix]) series	Immunocompromised patients aged ≥18 years and patients aged 19–49 years at risk for immunosuppression, as well as all patients aged >50 years	Once
Hepatitis A series	Immunocompromised patients and patients aged 40 and older	Once if traveling to an area with high or intermediate endemicity
Hepatitis B series	Immunocompromised patients aged ≥19 years	Once
Meningococcal	At risk (college students, military recruits) regardless of immunosuppression	Once
HPV vaccine series	All aged 9-26 and at-risk individuals, at risk individuals 27-45 years regardless of immunosuppression	Once
Tdap	All adults, regardless of immunosuppression	Every 10 years
Varicella (live)	If nonimmune; however, can only be given >4 weeks before starting advanced therapies	Once (total of two doses)
MMR (live)	If nonimmune; however, can only be given >4 weeks before starting advanced therapies	Once (total of two doses)
RSV (recombinant vaccine [Abrysvo], recombinant adjuvanted [Arexvy]), mRNA [mResvia])	Women 32-36 weeks pregnant (Abrysvo only), and all adults aged 60–74 years old who are at increased risk of severe RSV disease and all adults 75 years and older (per current ACIP recommendation)	Single dose between weeks 32–36 of pregnancy (Abrysvo only). Single dose for all adults aged 60–74 years old who are at increased risk of severe RSV disease and all adults 75 years and older.

[3]Exceeds dosage recommended by the manufacturer.
*Based on risk factors and with input from gynecology and dermatology.
**A minimum interval of 8 weeks between PCV15 and PPSV23 can be considered for adults with who are immunocompromised.
***For adults who have received PCV13 but have not completed their recommended pneumococcal vaccine series with PPSV23, 1 dose of PCV20 may be used if PPSV23 is not available. If PCV20 is used, their pneumococcal vaccinations are considered complete.
DEXA, Dual x-ray absorptiometry; *HPV*, human papillomavirus; *MMR*, measles, mumps, and rubella; *PCV*, pneumococcal conjugate vaccine; *PPSV*, pneumococcal polysaccharide vaccine; *RSV*, respiratory syncytial virus; *Tdap*, tetanus, diphtheria, and acellular pertussis.

References

Abreu MT, Rowbotham DS, Danese S, et al: Efficacy and safety of maintenance ustekinumab for ulcerative colitis through 3 years: UNIFI long-term extension, *J Crohns Colitis* 16:1222–1234, 2022.

Ananthakrishnan AN, Nguyen GC, Bernstein CN: AGA clinical practice update on management of inflammatory bowel disease in elderly patients: expert review, *Gastroenterology* 160:445–451, 2021.

Ananthakrishnan AN, Xavier RJ, Podolsky DK: *Inflammatory bowel diseases: a clinician's guide*, Chichester, West Sussex, UK; Hoboken, NJ, 2017, John Wiley & Sons, Inc.

Cohen NA, Rubin DT: New targets in inflammatory bowel disease therapy: 2021, *Curr Opin Gastroenterol* 37:357–363, 2021.

Crosby S, Schuh MJ, Becker M, et al: New pneumococcal vaccines for prevention of invasive pneumococcal disease in adult patients with inflammatory bowel disease, *Inflamm Bowel Dis* 29(4):661–664, 2023.

D'Haens G, Dubinsky M, Kobayashi T, et al: Mirikizumab as induction and maintenance therapy for ulcerative colitis, *N Engl J Med* 388(26):2444–2455, 2023.

Docherty MJ, Jones RCW, Wallace MS: Managing pain in inflammatory bowel disease, *Gastroenterol Hepatol* 7:592–601, 2011.

Drugs for inflammatory bowel disease, *Med Lett Drugs Ther* 60:107–114, 2018.

Farraye FA, Melmed GY, Lichtenstein GR, Kane SV: ACG clinical guideline: preventive care in inflammatory bowel disease, *Am J Gastroenterol* 112:241–258, 2017.

Ferrante M, Panaccione R, Baert F, et al: Risankizumab as maintenance therapy for moderately to severely active Crohn's disease: results from the multicentre, randomised, double-blind, placebo-controlled, withdrawal phase 3 FORTIFY maintenance trial, *Lancet* 399:2031–2046, 2022.

Feuerstein JD, Ho EY, Shmidt E, et al: AGA clinical practice guidelines on the medical management of moderate to severe luminal and perianal fistulizing Crohn's disease, *Gastroenterology* 160:2496–2508, 2021.

Feuerstein JD, Isaacs KL, Schneider Y, et al: AGA clinical practice guidelines on the management of moderate to severe ulcerative colitis, *Gastroenterology* 158:1450–1461, 2020.

Knowles SR, Drucker AM, Weber EA, et al: Management options for patients with aspirin and nonsteroidal antiinflammatory drug sensitivity, *Ann Pharmacother* 41(7):1191–1200, 2007.

Ko CW, Singh S, Feuerstein JD, et al: AGA clinical practice guidelines on the management of mild-to-moderate ulcerative colitis, *Gastroenterology* 156:748–764, 2019.

Lichtenstein GR, Loftus EV, Isaacs KL, Regueiro MD, Gerson LB, Sands BE: ACG clinical guideline: management of Crohn's disease in adults, *Am J Gastroenterol* 113:481–517, 2018.

Mahadevan U, Robinson C, Bernasko N, et al: Inflammatory bowel disease in pregnancy clinical care pathway: a report from the American gastroenterological association IBD parenthood project working group, *Gastroenterology* 156:1508–1524, 2019.

Nelson NP, Weng MK, Hofmeister MG, et al: Prevention of hepatitis a virus infection in the united states: recommendations of the advisory committee on immunization practices, 2020, *MMWR Recomm Rep* 69(RR-5):1–38, 2020.

Rubin DT, Ananthakrishnan AN, Siegel CA, Sauer BG, Long MD: ACG clinical guideline: ulcerative colitis in adults, *Am J Gastroenterol* 114:384–413, 2019.

Sandborn WJ, Feagan BG, D'Haens G, et al: Ozanimod as induction and maintenance therapy for ulcerative colitis, *N Engl J Med* 385:1280–1291, 2021.

Sandborn WJ, Rebuck R, Wang Y, et al: Five-year efficacy and safety of ustekinumab treatment in Crohn's disease: the IM-UNITI trial, *Clin Gastroenterol Hepatol* 20:578–590.e4, 2022.

Sehgal P, Colombel JF, Aboubakr A, et al: Systematic review: safety of mesalazine in ulcerative colitis, *Aliment Pharmacol Ther* 47(12):1597–1609, 2018.

Syal G, Serrano M, Jain A, et al: Health maintenance consensus for adults with inflammatory bowel disease, *Inflamm Bowel Dis* 27:1552–1563, 2021.

Turner D, Ricciuto A, Lewis A, et al: STRIDE-II: an update on the selecting therapeutic targets in inflammatory bowel disease (STRIDE) initiative of the international organization for the study of IBD (IOIBD): determining therapeutic goals for treat-to-target strategies in IBD, *Gastroenterology* 160:1570–1583, 2021. , .

Weng MK, Doshani M, Khan MA, et al: Universal hepatitis b vaccination in adults aged 19–59 years: updated recommendations of the advisory committee on immunization practices — United States, 2022, *MMWR Morb Mortal Wkly Rep* 71:477–483, 2022.

INTESTINAL PARASITES

Method of
Tarvinder Gilotra, MD

CURRENT DIAGNOSIS

Signs and Symptoms

- Watery diarrhea—Most protozoal infections: *Giardia, Blastocystis, Dientamoeba, Cryptosporidium, Cyclospora, Cystoisospora, Microsporidia*
- Dysentery—Most commonly *Entamoeba histolytica;* less commonly *Balantidium coli, Trichuris trichiura* (whipworm)
- Eosinophilia—Throughout chronic infection: *Strongyloides,* schistosomiasis, *Cystoisospora;* usually only in early infection: *Ascaris,* hookworm, whipworm
- Prolonged or severe diarrhea in HIV infection—Spore-forming protozoal infections: *Cryptosporidium, Cyclospora, Cystoisospora, Microsporidia*
- Visible worms passed in stool—*Ascaris, Taeniasis, Diphyllobothrium*

Diagnosis of Parasitic Infections

- Stool antigen assay: *Entamoeba histolytica, Giardia, Cryptosporidium*
- Serology*: *Strongyloides,* schistosomiasis
- Stool microscopy for ova and parasites: All intestinal parasites. Sensitivity is increased with repeat examinations if necessary. Concentration, preservation, and staining improve diagnosis of certain pathogens.
- Molecular tests: Traditional polymerase chain reaction (PCR), both nested and multiplexed, real-time PCR, and newer gene amplification technologies including loop-mediated isothermal amplification (LAMP) and Luminex-based assays are gaining popularity in detecting some parasitic infections, especially in low parasite load specimens.
- Proteomics: Mass spectrometry technique. Surface-enhanced laser desorption/ionization–time-of-flight (SELDI-TOF) mass spectrometry, which is based on matrix-assisted laser desorption/ionization time of-flight (MALDI-TOF) mass spectrometry, has been used to identify biomarkers associated with some parasitic diseases such as African trypanosomiasis, Chagas disease, cysticercosis, and fascioliasis.
  Note: Key features of intestinal parasitic infection may overlap with other conditions, including nonparasitic infections, and extraintestinal parasites.

*Optimal method of diagnosis in returned travelers and immigrants from endemic to nonendemic areas. Does not distinguish between active and resolved infections.

Intestinal parasites are a diverse group of pathogens with local and global significance. Immigration, international adoption, travel, and the frequency of HIV/AIDS and other immune-compromising conditions (e.g., malignancy, organ transplantation) have all contributed to a need for ongoing or increased awareness of parasitic infections in the United States. Persons who reside in chronic care facilities, children in daycare, and persons whose sexual practices increase the likelihood of fecal–oral contact are also at risk for acquiring intestinal parasitic infection.

Globally, intestinal parasites are responsible for an enormous burden of disease. Although these pathogens are rarely fatal, ongoing exposure to intestinal parasites among persons in endemic areas exacerbates malnutrition, carries multiple morbidities, and causes stunting of growth and development in children, all of which have far-reaching consequences.

Patients who present with diarrheal illness (especially prolonged or travel-associated), unexplained eosinophilia, or expulsion of worms should be evaluated for intestinal parasites. In such cases, a careful history should focus on the patient's country of origin, detailed travel and recreational activities, dietary habits and new or unusual food exposures, occupation, sexual history, sick contacts, and risks for or known immunodeficiency. Some specialists advocate obtaining a complete blood count with differential to assess eosinophil count in all international adoptees and immigrants from areas where parasitic infections are common. If eosinophilia is present, antibody testing for schistosomiasis and strongyloidiasis—two chronic parasitic infections with potentially serious consequences—should be performed, and appropriate therapy should be administered if infection is discovered. For key features of common intestinal parasitic infections, see the Current Diagnosis box.

Diagnosis of intestinal parasites has improved recently with the advent of quick, simple, and accurate stool antigen tests for some major pathogens, such as *Entamoeba, Giardia,* and *Cryptosporidium* species. However, the fecal examination for ova and parasites is still the mainstay of diagnosis in many cases. Whenever possible, stool specimens should be sent to a laboratory with clinical expertise in parasitology, where wet preparation, concentration, or staining can identify most pathogens. Evaluation of fresh specimens and repeated examinations improve diagnostic sensitivity. Key diagnostic points are summarized in the Current Diagnosis box.

This review focuses on basic understanding, recognition, diagnosis, and treatment of common intestinal parasites in the United States and throughout the world. Within each section, parasites are listed in order of relative clinical significance.

Protozoa: Amoebae, Flagellates, and Ciliates

Entamoeba histolytica

Entamoeba histolytica, the cause of amoebic dysentery and amebic liver abscess, is a worldwide pathogen of major clinical significance. Approximately 10% of the world's population and up to 60% of children in highly endemic areas show serologic evidence of infection, and *E. histolytica* is estimated to cause 100,000 deaths per year globally. In the United States, infection is almost exclusively found among returned travelers, immigrants from endemic areas (especially Mexico and Central and South America), men who have sex with men (MSM), and institutionalized persons. *Entamoeba dispar, Entamoeba bangladeshi,* and *Entamoeba moshkovskii* are morphologically indistinguishable from *E. histolytica*. Although these species are usually considered nonpathologic species, there have been increasing reports of *E. moshkovskii* infections associated with gastrointestinal symptoms in humans in endemic areas. Other *Entamoeba*, including *Entamoeba hartmanni, Entamoeba coli, Entamoeba polecki,* and others, can be individually identified on microscopy. Again, these organisms are of uncertain pathogenicity and generally considered as commensal organisms, however *E. polecki, Dientamoeba fragilis,* and *Iodaamopeba bütschlii* have occasionally been associated with diarrheal illness.

E. histolytica exists in two forms: the hardy cyst (infective form) characterized by four nuclei and the trophozoite (responsible for invasive disease), which has a single nucleus and survives poorly outside the human body. *E. histolytica* infection is acquired by ingestion of cysts in contaminated water or food or by sexual transmission through fecal-oral contact. Acquisition of the parasite can result in asymptomatic infection (most common), diarrheal illness, or extraintestinal infection, the latter most commonly manifesting as amebic liver abscess. An appropriately robust layer of colonic mucin may be protective against symptomatic infection, whereas trophozoite attachment to the intestinal epithelium results in penetration of the organism into the submucosal layer, where extensive tissue destruction can take place in the form of apoptosis and lysis of cells, hence the name *histolytica*.

Symptoms of classic amebic dysentery usually begin insidiously over 1 to 3 weeks after infection. Diarrhea is almost universal and typically consists of numerous small-volume stools that can contain mucus, frank blood, or both. Stools are almost always heme positive if not grossly bloody. Abdominal pain and tenesmus are common; fever is present in approximately 30% of cases. Some patients have a chronic course characterized by weight loss, intermittent loose stools, and abdominal pain. Rare presentations of amebic dysentery include amebomas, which can mimic malignancy, and perianal ulcerations or fistulae. Severe disease can occur in the form of fulminant colitis or toxic megacolon; the latter almost universally requires colectomy. Young age, pregnancy, corticosteroid use, malignancy, malnutrition, and alcoholism predispose to severe infection. Although persons with HIV infection or AIDS can develop invasive disease, *E. histolytica* does not appear to be a common opportunistic infection, and infection is curable in this population.

Amebic liver abscess is the most common extraintestinal complication of *E. histolytica* that traffics to the liver via the portal venous system. Cerebral and ocular amebiasis have also been reported. Amebic liver abscess affects children of both sexes equally, but it is up to 7 to 10 times more common in men, indicating that a hormonal milieu likely plays a role. Amebic liver abscess almost always manifests within 3 to 5 months of initial infection, but it can surface years later. Illness is characterized by fever and right upper quadrant abdominal pain that worsens over several days to weeks. Weight loss, jaundice, and cough from diaphragmatic irritation can also occur. Symptoms of dysentery usually are not present, and diarrhea is reported in

less than one-third of cases. Hepatomegaly and point tenderness over the liver is present in about 50% of cases. Rupture of the abscess can occur into the abdomen or pleuropulmonary space, manifesting as acute abdomen or empyema. Laboratory abnormalities include leukocytosis without eosinophilia, transaminitis, elevated alkaline phosphatase, and elevated sedimentation rate. Abscess is usually identified as a well-circumscribed hypoechoic mass on ultrasonography, a low-density mass with enhancing borders on computed tomography (CT), and hypointense on T1 and hyperintense on T2-weighted magnetic resonance imaging (MRI). Chest radiograph often demonstrates elevation of the right hemidiaphragm, and pleural effusion may be present. Radionuclide uptake liver scans can help distinguish amebic abscesses as "cold" compared with pyogenic abscesses that are usually "hot."

Diagnosis of intestinal *E. histolytica* infection has classically relied on stool microscopy, and this remains the only available method in most parts of the world. At least three stool specimens should be examined to improve sensitivity. Cysts visualized in stool cannot differentiate active disease from colonization, and *E. dispar, E. moshkovskii,* and *E. histolytica* species. Presence of trophozoites with ingested red blood cells (hematophagous trophozoites) on stool preparation and/or mobile amebae seen on fresh biopsy material stained with iron hematoxylin and/or Wheatley's trichrome are diagnostic of invasive intestinal amebic disease. Contrary to the common belief, presence of hematophagous trophozoites on stool microscopy is not pathognomonic of *E. histolytica*, as they can be seen with *E. dispar* infections as well.

Serology can distinguish between *E. histolytica* (generates antibodies) and *E. dispar* (does not generate antibodies) infection with good sensitivity in detecting antibodies within 5 to 7 days of infection. Positive serostatus, however, does not discriminate between acute and past infection, but negative serology is quite sensitive in endemic countries. Indirect hemagglutination serology remains the most sensitive test in non-endemic settings.

Diagnosis and species distinction of *Entamoeba* infection has improved greatly with the advent of antigen tests, now available as enzyme-linked immunosorbent assays (ELISAs), radioimmunoassays, and immunofluorescent probes. The Techlab ELISA *E. histolytica* stool antigen test is highly sensitive and specific if used on fresh stool specimens. It becomes positive with onset of symptomatic disease and resolves on treatment of infection.

Parasite DNA/RNA PCR, RT-PCR, multiplex PCR (can detect multiple pathogens), and LAMP fecal probes are highly sensitive and can differentiate *Entamoeba* species.

Aspirate of liver abscess may be necessary to distinguish from pyogenic liver abscess or when empiric therapy fails. Aspirated specimens consist mainly of necrotic hepatocytes ("anchovy paste"), and trophozoites are only seen in less than 20% of cases. Nested multiplex PCR tests on hepatic aspirates might be useful, although sensitivities range from 75% to 100%. As simultaneous colitis and amebic liver abscess are rare, negative stool microscopy and PCR for *E. histolytica* does not preclude amebic liver abscess. In a patient at high risk for amebic liver abscess (e.g., young male immigrants), an adequate response to a trial of antimicrobial therapy can help confirm the diagnosis as well.

All patients who have confirmed *E. histolytica* infection and reside in nonendemic areas should be treated regardless of whether they are symptomatic because invasive disease can develop in the future. Asymptomatic cyst passers may be treated with an intraluminal agent alone, such as paromomycin (Humatin) or diiodohydroxyquin (iodoquinol [Yodoxin]).[2] In the United States, the most readily available effective treatment for patients with amebic colitis or liver abscess is metronidazole (Flagyl). It can be given intravenously for patients who are unable to tolerate oral medications. Recommended management is at least a 10-day course of the metronidazole (or tinidazole [Tindamax]) followed by an intraluminal agent (paromomycin for 7 days, or diiodohydroxyquin[2] for 20 days, or diloxanide furoate[2] for 10 days) for all cases of invasive *E. histolytica*. See Table 1 for medications and doses.

TABLE 1	Pharmacologic Treatment of Major Protozoan Infections.			
CLINICAL SITUATION	**DRUG**	**ADULT DOSE**	**PEDIATRIC DOSE**	**COMMENTS**
Amebiasis				
(Entamoeba histolytica)				
Asymptomatic	Paromomycin* or	25–35 mg/kg/d in 3 doses × 7 d	25–35 mg/kg/d in 3 doses × 7 d	
	Iodoquinol[†,2] or	650 mg tid × 20 d	30–40 mg/kg/d (max 2 g) in 3 doses × 20 d	
	Diloxanide furoate‡[,2]	500 mg tid × 10 d	20 mg/kg/d in 3 doses × 10 d	
Mild to moderate intestinal disease	Metronidazole or	500–750 mg tid × 7–10 d	35–50 mg/kg/d in 3 doses × 7–10 d	Treatment should be followed by a course of iodoquinol or paromomycin in the dosage used to treat asymptomatic amebiasis.
	Tinidazole[1,§]	2 g once daily × 3 d	≥3 y: 50 mg/kg once daily (max 2 g) × 3 d	
Severe intestinal or extraintestinal disease	Metronidazole or	750 mg tid × 7–10 d	35–50 mg/kg/d in 3 doses × 7–10 d	Treatment should be followed by a course of iodoquinol or paromomycin in the dosage used to treat asymptomatic amebiasis.
	Tinidazole[§]	2 g once daily × 5 d	≥3 y: 50 mg/kg once daily (max 2 g) × 5 d	
Balantidiasis				
(Balantidium coli)				
Symptomatic and asymptomatic disease	Recommended: Tetracycline[1,‖]	500 mg qid × 10 d	40 mg/kg/d (max 2 g) in 4 doses × 10 d	
	Alternatives: Metronidazole[1] or	500–750 mg PO tid × 5 d	35–50 mg/kg/d in 3 doses × 5 d	
	Iodoquinol[2,†]	650 mg tid × 20 d	30–40 mg/kg/d (max 2 g) in 3 doses × 20 d	
Blastocystis hominis				
Symptomatic disease only				Organism's pathogenicity is uncertain.[¶]
Cryptosporidiosis				
(Cryptosporidium)				
Immunocompetent	Nitazoxanide	500 mg bid × 3 d	1–3 y: 100 mg bid × 3 d 4–11 y: 200 mg bid × 3 d ≥12 y: adult dose	FDA approved as a pediatric oral suspension for treating *Cryptosporidium* in immunocompetent children <12 y and for *Giardia*. It might also be effective for mild to moderate amebiasis. Nitazoxanide is available in 500-mg tabs and an oral suspension; it should be taken with food.
Immunocompromised	No optimal therapy available			All HIV-infected patients with cryptosporidiosis should receive HAART whenever possible. Nitazoxanide,[1] paromomycin,[1] or paromomycin + azithromycin[1] may have a role in decreasing diarrhea in chronic cases of HIV-infection.

CLINICAL SITUATION	DRUG	ADULT DOSE	PEDIATRIC DOSE	COMMENTS
Cyclosporiasis				
(Cyclospora cayetanensis)				
	Recommended: TMP-SMX (Bactrim, Septra)[1]	160 mg TMP, 800 mg SMX (1 DS tab) bid × 7–10 d	5 mg/kg TMP, 25 mg/kg SMX bid × 7–10 d	In immunocompetent patients, usually a self-limiting illness. Immunosuppressed patients might need higher doses, longer duration (TMP-SMX qid × 10 d, followed by bid × 3 wk) and long-term maintenance.
	Alternative: Ciprofloxacin[1]	500 mg PO bid × 7 d	(No recommended pediatric dose)[1]	
Dientamoebiasis				
(Dientamoeba fragilis)				
Symptomatic disease only	Iodoquinol[2,†] *or*	650 mg tid × 20 d	30–40 mg/kg/d (max 2 g) in 3 doses × 20 d	
	Paromomycin[1,*] *or*	25–35 mg/kg/d in 3 doses × 7 d	25–35 mg/kg/d in 3 doses × 7 d	
	Metronidazole[1]	500–750 mg tid × 10 d	35–50 mg/kg/d in 3 doses × 10 d	
Giardiasis				
(Giardia lamblia)				
All symptomatic disease and asymptomatic carriage in nonendemic areas	Recommended: Metronidazole[1] *or*	250 mg tid × 5–7 d	15 mg/kg/d in 3 doses × 5 d	
	Nitazoxanide *or*	500 mg bid × 3 d	1–3 y: 100 mg bid × 3 d 4–11 y: 200 mg bid × 3 d	
	Tinidazole[§]	2 g once	50 mg/kg (max 2 g) once	Treatment should be followed by a course of iodoquinol[2] or paromomycin in the dosage used to treat asymptomatic amebiasis.
	Alternatives: Quinacrine[2,**] *or*	100 mg tid × 5 d	6 mg/kg/d (max 300 mg/d) tid × 5 d	Albendazole,[1] 400 mg daily × 5 d alone or in combination with metronidazole[1] may also be effective. Combination treatment with standard doses of metronidazole and quinacrine[2] × 3 wk is effective for a small number of refractory infections. In one study, nitazoxanide was used successfully in high doses to treat a case of *Giardia* resistant to metronidazole and albendazole.
	Furazolidone[2] *or*	100 mg qid × 7–10 d	6 mg/kg/d in 4 doses × 10 d	
	Paromomycin[1]	25–35 mg/kg/d in 3 doses × 7 d	25–35 mg/kg/d in 3 doses × 7 d	Nonabsorbed luminal agent; may be useful for treating giardiasis in pregnancy

Continued

TABLE 1	Pharmacologic Treatment of Major Protozoan Infections.—cont'd			
CLINICAL SITUATION	**DRUG**	**ADULT DOSE**	**PEDIATRIC DOSE**	**COMMENTS**
Cystoisosporiasis				
(Cystoisospora belli)				
	TMP-SMX[1]	160 mg TMP, 800 mg SMX bid × 7–10 d	5 mg/kg TMP, 25 mg/kg SMX bid × 7–10 d	In immunocompetent patients, usually a self-limiting illness. Immunosuppressed patients might need higher doses, longer duration (TMP-SMX[1] qid × 10 d, followed by bid × 3 wk) and long-term maintenance. For isosporiasis in sulfonamide-sensitive patients, pyrimethamine[1] 50–75 mg qd in divided doses (*plus* leucovorin[1] 10–25 mg/d) is effective.
Microsporidiosis				
Enterocytozoon bieneusi				
Intestinal disease	Fumagillin[2+]	20 mg PO TID × 14 d		Oral fumagillin (Sanofi Recherche, Gentilly, France) is effective in treating *E. bieneusi* but is associated with thrombocytopenia and neutropenia. HAART can lead to microbiologic and clinical response in HIV-infected patients with microsporidial diarrhea. Octreotide (Sandostatin)[1] has provided symptomatic relief in some patients with large-volume diarrhea.
	Albendazole[1]	400 mg PO bid × 21 d	15 mg/kg/d in 2 doses (max 400 mg/dose)	
Encephalitozoon intestinalis				
Diarrheal or disseminated disease	Albendazole[1]	400 mg bid × 21 d	15 mg/kg/d in 2 doses (max 400 mg/dose)	

[1]Not FDA approved for this indication.
[2]Not available in the United States.
*Should be taken with meals.
†Should be taken after meals.
‡The drug is not available commercially, but may be available through compounding pharmacies.
§A nitroimidazole similar to metronidazole, tinidazole is FDA approved and appears to be as effective and better tolerated than metronidazole. It should be taken with food to minimize GI adverse effects. For children and patients unable to take tablets, a pharmacist may crush the tablets and mix them with cherry syrup. The syrup suspension is good for 7 d at room temperature and must be shaken before use. Ornidazole, a similar drug, is also used outside the United States. Dosing recommendations are only available for children ≥3 years of age.
ˡContraindicated in pregnant and breastfeeding women and children <8 years of age.
¶Clinical significance of these organisms is controversial; metronidazole 750 mg tid × 10 d, iodoquinol 650 mg tid × 20 d, or TMP-SMX11 double-strength tab bid × 7 d are effective. Metronidazole resistance may be common. Nitazoxanide is effective in children.
**Should be taken with liquids after a meal.
DS, Double strength; *GI,* gastrointestinal; *HAART,* highly active antiretroviral therapy; *max,* maximum; *tab,* tablet; *TMP-SMX,* trimethoprim-sulfamethoxazole.
Modified from World Health Organization. Drugs for parasitic infections, *Med Lett Drug Ther.* 2010;8(Suppl).

Giardiasis

Giardia duodenalis, previously known as *Giardia lamblia* or *Giardia intestinalis,* is the most commonly identified diarrheal parasitic infection in the United States, with an estimated 100,000 to 2.5 million cases per year. It is globally distributed and found in fresh water throughout mountainous regions of the United States and Canada. The organism is a flagellated aerotolerant anaerobe that exists in cyst and trophozoite form. Cysts can survive for several weeks in cold water. Contaminated food and water are the most common sources of infection, but the organism can also be passed by person-to-person contact. In the United States, giardiasis is primarily diagnosed among international travelers, persons with recreational water exposure, institutionalized persons and children in day care, and persons with anal-oral sexual practices.

Illness can result from ingestion of as few as 10 to 25 cysts, which transform into trophozoites in the small intestine and attach to and damage the small bowel wall. Symptomatic disease begins insidiously over approximately 2 weeks in 25% to 50% of persons who ingest *Giardia* cysts. Others become asymptomatic cyst passers (5% to 15%) or have no signs of infection (35% to 50%). Hallmarks of infection are watery diarrhea, bloating, flatulence, abdominal pain, and weight loss; less commonly, patients have nausea, vomiting, or low-grade fever. Steatorrhea and malabsorption, particularly secondary to *Giardia*-induced lactase deficiency, is frequently observed. Chronic *Giardia* infection should be considered in the differential diagnosis for a longstanding diarrheal illness, especially if there is history of exposure to possibly contaminated water. Patients with common variable immune deficiency, X-linked agammaglobulinemia, and IgA deficiency syndromes are at risk for fulminant and sometimes incurable disease, suggesting a significant role for humoral immunity in control of infection. Patients with HIV infection or AIDS usually have a similar presentation as in non-HIV patients, can remain asymptomatic, and can be typically cured of infection with standard therapy. However, profound immunosuppression can be associated with more severe, atypical, disseminated and refractory disease requiring combination therapy with quinacrine[2] and metronidazole.[1]

Diagnosis of giardiasis is made by examination of fresh or preserved stool or by stool antigen assays. Stool microscopy can be specific but has low sensitivity because of intermittent shedding of *Giardia* cysts. Trophozoites may be directly visualized in fresh liquid stool; semiformed and preserved stool are likely to contain only cysts and should be stained with polyvinyl alcohol and/or formalin preparation. Antigen detection assays including immunochromographic assays, direct immunofluorescence assays, and ELISAs have higher sensitivity with rapid turnaround time. Many assays are commercially available including the ImmunoCard STAT! Cryptosporidium/Giardia Rapid Assay (Meridian Bioscience, Cincinnati, Ohio) that tests for both pathogens simultaneously. Multiplex nucleic acid amplification tests (NAATs) are frequently used to detect various bacterial, viral, and parasitic pathogens as a workup for infectious diarrhea. Although it is rarely necessary, the diagnosis can sometimes be made on duodenal biopsy.

For details of treatment options, see Table 1. Tinidazole (Tindamax) and nitazoxanide (Alinia) are now the preferred agents for initial treatment of giardiasis. Metronidazole[1] is no longer the first-line therapy because of its adverse effects including metallic taste, nausea, gastrointestinal discomfort, and headache. Patients who fail first-line therapy might have a persistent source of infection (contaminated water source, close contact with an infected person), immune deficiency predisposing to difficult eradication, or persistence of cysts. Once possible sources of reinfection have been investigated and eliminated, relapsed infections should either be retreated with a longer course of therapy (21 to 28 days) or treated with a different agent. Quinacrine[2] is reserved for refractory cases but is contraindicated in pregnancy. Paromomycin[1] is an alternative in those with contraindications to other agents such as in pregnancy. Patients who fail more than one course of therapy should undergo immunologic workup.

Prevention of *Giardia* infection, as with other parasitic infections, involves primarily close attention to personal hygiene, hand washing, and avoidance of ingestion of fresh unfiltered water. Boiling water or use of a 0.2- to 1-μm water filter offer optimal protection against *Giardia* and other parasitic pathogens, although such filters still might not protect against *Cryptosporidium*.

Blastocystis

Blastocystis, formerly considered a yeast, has now been related to *E. histolytica* and is thought to be an anaerobic protozoan. The pleomorphic nature and karyotype diversity of this organism, its worldwide distribution, and varying diagnostic techniques have led to challenges in its identification and taxonomy. Although it has a worldwide distribution, its prevalence is higher in developing countries and is most commonly isolated in tropical regions. In temperate regions, *Blastocystis (B. hominis)* is detected at a high rate among MSM. It is a commensal of humans and several other animals. It appears to be transmitted via the fecal-oral route, possibly from waterborne sources. *Blastocystis* was long thought to cause only asymptomatic colonization, but there is some evidence to suggest a role in human disease, although this remains controversial. *Blastocystis* has marked morphologic variability and has been known to exist in at least four forms: vacuolated, amoeba-like, granular, and cystic, the latter of which is likely to be the infectious form. Ongoing molecular analysis has identified at least 17 subtypes of *B. hominis* (hence now referred to as *Blastocystis* spp., formerly identified as *Blastocystis hominis*) with varying degrees of pathogenicity in humans.

As suggested previously, the majority of infections appear to be entirely asymptomatic, and number of organisms does not appear to accurately predict severity of illness. Symptoms consist mainly of watery diarrhea, bloating, flatulence, abdominal cramps, urticaria, and fatigue. There are typically no pathologic findings on colonoscopy, and there are no reports of invasive disease. Infection is diagnosed by stool microscopy with use of a trichrome or hematoxylin-stained preserved specimen. Fecal leucocytes are generally not found. PCR techniques have also been developed with excellent sensitivity and are available worldwide. The organism is susceptible in vitro to numerous antimicrobials. Asymptomatic detection does not need treatment. Metronidazole[1] and tinidazole[1] are preferred agents for treating symptomatic disease. Trimethoprim-sulfamethoxazole (TMP-SMX, Bactrim)[1] and paromomycin[1] are alternative agents with good efficacy; details are listed in Table 1.

Dientamoeba fragilis

Dientamoeba fragilis was originally classified as an amoeba, but it is more closely related to the flagellates such as *Trichomonas vaginalis*. It is distributed globally, including in the Western nations; however, it is generally more prevalent in areas of the world with limited public sanitation. *D. fragilis* has only recently been recognized as a clinically significant pathogen, possibly because it is difficult to visualize without specific staining techniques. Illness has commonly been found in travelers and MSM, but it can affect anyone. Some studies suggested a coinfection of *D. fragilis* with *E. vermicularis* as trophozoites were believed to survive in *E. vermicularis* eggs. However, this association has not been consistently demonstrated.

Similar to most other intestinal parasites, *D. fragilis* is now known to exist in both trophozoite and cystic form, although it was known to only have a trophozoite phase for a long time. Despite its genetic relationship to the flagellates such as *Trichomonas*, *D. fragilis* does not have a flagellum and is immotile. Trophozoites range in size from 7 to 20 μm and can be binucleate. Cysts and precystic forms have recently been identified from human fecal specimens, suggesting a fecal-oral mode of transmission.

Most patients are asymptomatic; however, numerous case reports and small series describe patients with no other organisms identified to cause their symptoms who improve significantly after treatment and documented clearance of *D. fragilis* from their stool. Illness is typically subacute to chronic and is characterized by abdominal pain, watery diarrhea, anorexia, fatigue, and malaise. Unlike most other enteric parasites, *D. fragilis* is associated with marked peripheral eosinophilia and can masquerade as allergic colitis. Diagnosis can be challenging because the trophozoites are fragile and usually missed on direct microscopy. If *D. fragilis* is suspected, stool should be preserved with

---

[1] Not FDA approved for this indication.
[2] Not available in the United States.

---

[1] Not FDA approved for this indication.

polyvinyl alcohol and quickly stained with iron–hematoxylin and trichrome. PCR-based assays are very sensitive and being increasingly used for diagnosis.

Metronidazole[1] remains the drug of choice and has been efficacious in eradication of *D. fragilis* with a 10-day course. Other nitroimidazoles such as tinidazole[1] (better tolerated than metronidazole), secnidazole (Solosec),[1] and ornidazole[2] have been tested with good efficacy, but data are limited. Paromomycin[1] appears to be efficacious but is only backed up by limited data. Iodoquinol (Yodoxin)[2] has been successfully used very commonly in the past; however, its availability has now declined. See Table 1 for medications and doses.

Balantidium coli

Balantidium coli is the largest protozoan that infects humans and is the only ciliate. Balantidiasis is a relatively rare cause of illness and is found primarily in rural agrarian communities in Southeast Asia, Central and South America, and Papua New Guinea. *B. coli* is highly associated with animal farming, in particular, pigs and primates; humans are incidental hosts. The parasite is transmitted by direct contact with animals or on ingestion of water or food contaminated by animal excrement. Persons with malnutrition or immune deficiency are particularly susceptible to infection.

B. coli invades the intestinal mucosa from the terminal ileum to the rectum. About one-half of infections are asymptomatic; the other half result in a subacute or chronic diarrheal illness with abdominal cramping, nausea, vomiting, weight loss, and occasional low-grade fever. Fewer than 5% of patients present with severe or even fulminant dysentery, and rare cases of colonic penetration with peritonitis, mesenteric lymphadenitis, or hepatic infection have been reported.

Diagnosis is made by visualization of trophozoites in fresh stool specimens or preserved and permanently stained samples. The trophozoite is relatively large (40 to 200 microns) and ciliated; cysts are difficult to distinguish. It displays a distinct spiraling motility that can be seen under low power. On stained sample, visualization of *B. coli*'s characteristic bean-shaped macronucleus and spiral micronucleus can help confirm the diagnosis. All patients should be treated regardless of symptoms. Tetracycline[1] (Sumycin and others) is the therapy of choice; alternative agents include metronidazole,[1] tinidazole[1] and paromomycin[1]; see Table 1 for medications and doses.

Spore-Forming Protozoa and Microsporidia

Cryptosporidium

Cryptosporidium is an intracellular pathogen with worldwide distribution that has been increasingly reported in the United States and other countries including Nordic countries, Denmark, England, and Scotland in the past decade. Humans are most commonly infected by the recently reclassified *Cryptosporidium hominis* (formerly *C. parvum* genotype 1), but *Cryptosporidium parvum* (previously *C. parvum* genotype 2), primarily a bovine pathogen, also causes human disease. *Cryptosporidium* is known to be an important parasitic cause of diarrhea globally; however, it is more frequently associated with overcrowded and poor sanitary environments. In the United States and other developed countries, the incidence is higher in children than in adults. *Cryptosporidium* infections have been reported as sporadic outbreaks of diarrhea and malnutrition syndrome in children from developing countries and as chronic and severe illness in immunocompromised hosts (especially with HIV infection). It is primarily a waterborne illness and has caused multiple outbreaks in the United States secondary to recreational water exposure (e.g., swimming pools, water parks). The best-known outbreak occurred from contamination of the drinking water supply in Wisconsin in 1993 that was thought to be secondary to runoff from the cattle pastures versus contaminated water from melting ice entering water treatment plants through Lake Michigan. It resulted in 403,000 documented cases of cryptosporidiosis and contributed to the deaths of dozens of persons with advanced HIV infection or malignancy.

Cryptosporidium is a coccidian spore-forming protozoa obligate intracellular parasite with a complex life cycle that matures and reproduces both asexually and sexually entirely within human hosts, thereby enabling infection to occur both from environmental sources and by direct person-to-person contact. Its oocysts, the source of infection on ingestion, are markedly hardy; they can withstand heavy chlorination, survive for months in cold water, and are small enough to occasionally evade even the smallest available water filtration systems. As few as 100 oocysts can cause infection, which results when the parasite penetrates small bowel epithelium and replicates just beneath its surface. Villous flattening and small bowel wall edema are seen on pathologic examination from infected persons.

Cryptosporidium infection can be asymptomatic, or it can manifest as mild diarrhea to severe enteritis with or without biliary involvement. Mild illness is usually self-limiting in 10 to 14 days without treatment in immunocompetent patients, although a substantial percentage of patients report a relapse of symptoms after initial improvement. It can have a protracted course with more severe symptoms in immunocompromised hosts. Fulminant and chronic infection has been frequently reported in those with HIV infection (especially those with CD4 <50), malignancy, and in malnourished children. The incubation period ranges from 3 to 28 days following the ingestion of oocysts and appears to be associated with the number of ingested oocysts. The hallmark of infection is explosive watery diarrhea, which can be so voluminous as to resemble cholera and can cause significant dehydration and electrolyte imbalance. Abdominal discomfort, nausea, vomiting, fever, malaise, and myalgia can also be present, and weight loss is common. Extraintestinal manifestations including biliary tract (cholecystitis, cholangitis, pancreatitis) and lung involvement have been reported, particularly in patients with HIV infection.

Diagnosis of *Cryptosporidium* has improved dramatically in recent years with the advent of antigen tests, which are highly sensitive and specific and can be used on a single sample of fresh stool. The ImmunoCard STAT! Cryptosporidium/Giardia Rapid Assay is useful because it can detect both pathogens. PCR is also available, has more sensitivity than direct microscopy, and can differentiate between various genotypes. When such tests are not available, stools submitted for examination should be fixed in formalin and stained for trophozoites or cysts; availability of multiple stool specimens improves the diagnostic sensitivity. Luminal fluid or biopsy specimens obtained during endoscopy can also reveal the organism.

Infection with *Cryptosporidium* is typically a self-limiting illness in otherwise healthy persons, but symptoms can be improved and the course shortened with the antiparasitic nitazoxanide. If nitazoxanide is not available or tolerated, paromomycin can be used, although it is not specifically indicated for this infection. *Cryptosporidium* remains an extremely challenging and potentially devastating infection in immunocompromised patients, especially those with HIV and a low CD4 count (counts <200 increase risk of severe illness, and counts <50 markedly increase risk). Although anticryptosporidial therapies in this population have shown very limited efficacy, restoration of immune function with highly active antiretroviral therapy (HAART) often effects cure. Limited data suggest that a trial of nitazoxanide may be reasonable in this circumstance as well. Appropriate supportive measures are also crucial in all patients with *Cryptosporidium*, including fluid and electrolyte replacement; avoiding lactose products is likely to be beneficial during the first 2 weeks after infection as the brush border regenerates. Appropriate treatment doses for nitazoxanide (Alinia) are listed in Table 1.

Prevention of *Cryptosporidium* infection requires a highly developed public water purification system including flocculation, sedimentation, and filtration. Use of 0.2- to 1-μm personal

---

[1] Not FDA approved for this indication.
[2] Not available in the United States.

water filters for campers and hikers greatly reduces but does not eliminate the risk of infection, whereas boiling water before drinking kills oocysts. Close attention to hygiene and avoidance of fecal-oral contact is the mainstay of prevention in the settings of institutional and community outbreaks. Patients should avoid swimming in public pools for 2 weeks after diarrhea resolution.

Cyclospora

Cyclospora cayetanensis is a coccidian with a structure similar to that of *Cryptosporidium*. *C. cayetanensis* is distributed worldwide, most commonly in the tropics and subtropics including Latin America (Guatemala, Peru, Mexico), the Indian subcontinent, and Southeast Asia. Outbreaks in the United States have been associated with import of contaminated produce such as raspberries and snow peas from Guatemala in 1996 and 2004, respectively. Similar outbreaks were attributed to contaminated lettuce and basil from Peru and to cilantro and prepackaged salad from Mexico. It has also become increasingly recognized as a cause of infectious diarrhea in return travelers. Unlike *Cryptosporidium*, *C. cayetanensis* oocysts are shed in the stool as unsporulated oocysts (uninfected) and require a few days of humid environmental conditions to become sporulated infective oocysts, therefore close person-to-person contact as a means of acquiring the infection is unlikely.

All persons are susceptible to infection, but those with HIV are at risk for more severe and prolonged disease, as seen with cryptosporidiosis and isosporiasis. Symptomatic disease appears to be most common in adults who do not have previous exposure to *Cyclospora*, such as travelers or persons who have relocated to endemic areas. Illness begins about 1 week after ingestion of sporulated oocysts and is characterized by watery diarrhea, abdominal cramping, bloating, anorexia, and weight loss. Low-grade fever can occur; marked fatigue is common and can last for weeks or even months, and untreated infections can relapse after apparent resolution. Biliary involvement can occur in patients with HIV coinfection, as with cryptosporidiosis. Cyclosporiasis, similar to infection with other coccidians, causes damage to the small bowel epithelium, with resultant crypt flattening, edema, and inflammatory infiltrate. Lactose deficiency can remain for months after initial infection.

Diagnosis is made by stool examination. As with diagnosis of other parasitic infections, multiple stool specimens improve sensitivity. In the case of *Cyclospora*, concentration of the stool specimen also increases yield. If cyclosporiasis is suspected, specific testing should be requested because the organism exhibits unique properties. Similar to *Cryptosporidium*, organisms can be stained and visualized with Kinyoun acid-fast stain, but they are about two times the size of *Cryptosporidium* (8 to 10 μm in diameter). The cell wall of their oocysts also maintains its autofluorescence under ultraviolet microscopy, and *Cryptosporidium* does not. The commonly used BioFire FilmArray multiplex antigen detection test (BioFire Diagnostics, Salt Lake City, UT) includes *C. cayetanensis*. Various conventional and real-time PCR techniques have been developed with good sensitivity. No serologic tests are available yet.

Cyclosporiasis is best treated with trimethoprim-sulfamethoxazole (Bactrim)[1]; nitazoxanide and ciprofloxacin may be effective for patients who have a sulfa allergy. Patients with HIV infection can require longer courses of treatment or chronic suppressive therapy; appropriate antiretroviral therapy is also important in the treatment of severe or relapsing infections. See Table 1 for details.

Cystoisospora

Cystoisospora belli, formerly *Isospora belli*, is a large coccidian distributed worldwide; however, infections are more frequent in tropical and subtropical areas. In the United States, infections are largely identified in travelers from endemic areas and foreign-born HIV-positive patients. This is the most common parasitic cause of diarrhea in HIV-infected patients in India. Similar to *Cyclospora*, it requires a period of maturation (sporulation)

outside the human body and therefore cannot be spread directly from person to person.

It appears to cause largely asymptomatic or mild infection in tropical areas to which it is endemic; the exception is among patients coinfected with HIV and particularly those with AIDS, in whom it is a very common cause of chronic diarrhea in the Caribbean and Central America. Currently in wealthy countries it is found primarily in travelers returning from endemic areas. Illness is typically mild and self-limiting, consisting primarily of watery diarrhea. However, some immunocompetent persons can develop a chronic spruelike syndrome with malabsorption, and those with HIV infection or AIDS often have severe and prolonged diarrhea. *Cystoisospora* can invade to the lamina propria and can cause eosinophilia, which is different from other protozoan infections.

Diagnosis is made by observation of cysts in stool. As with *Cyclospora* and *Cryptosporidia*, they are usually not detected on routine stool ova and parasite examinations, hence acid-fast staining or ultraviolet microscopy techniques should be requested for high suspicion. Stool may also contain Charcot-Leiden crystals. No antigen detection tests are yet available. PCR tests have been developed; however, they are not widely available.

Illness is usually self-limiting in immunocompetent hosts, hence antimicrobial therapy is only indicated when symptoms do not resolve spontaneously in 5 to 7 days. Symptomatic HIV-positive and other immunocompromised patients should always be treated. Trimethoprim-sulfamethoxazole (Bactrim)[1] is the treatment of choice. Ciprofloxacin (Cipro)[1] or pyrimethamine (Daraprim)[1] may be used in cases of sulfa allergy. See Table 1 for medications and doses.

Microsporidia

Microsporidia are eukaryotic organisms that have been recently reclassified as fungi based on molecular genotyping. They are distributed globally, and more than 100 genera have been identified, seven of which contain species known to be pathogenic in humans: *Encephalitozoon*, *Enterocytozoon*, *Trachipleistophora*, *Pleistophora*, *Nosema*, *Vittaforma*, and *Microsporidium*. These pathogens cause a wide variety of systemic and focal illness throughout the world.

Many immunocompetent patients in wealthy nations exhibit positive serology for certain types of microsporidial infections without a history of disease or travel. Microsporidia are most commonly associated with systemic infection in immunosuppressed persons, particularly those with HIV and a CD4 count of less than 100 or patients with organ transplants. The mode of transmission is not entirely clear, but the pathogen likely is spread both from water sources and possibly from close household contact.

Encephalitozoon intestinalis and *Enterocytozoon bieneusi* are responsible for intestinal microsporidial infections. *E. bieneusi* has been associated with self-limiting diarrheal illness; *E. intestinalis* is commonly found in stool specimens throughout the developing world, but its pathogenicity is often not certain. Symptomatic infections, most often in patients coinfected with HIV, typically include a gradual onset of watery diarrhea, which may be worse in the morning and after oral intake. Significant volume and electrolyte depletion can occur, as well as fatigue, anorexia, weight loss, and malabsorption. *E. intestinalis* can disseminate and cause acute abdomen with peritonitis, cholangitis, nephritis, and keratoconjunctivitis, and *E. bieneusi* infection can result in cholangitis and nephritis as well as rhinitis, bronchitis, and wheezing. Other microsporidia are implicated in disseminated disease with a wide variety of extraintestinal manifestations including ocular, pulmonary, cerebral, renal, and muscular, both in previously healthy and immunosuppressed hosts.

Diagnosis of microsporidiosis is attained by visualization of spores in stool or in tissue specimens. As suggested by their name, microsporidial spores are much smaller than those produced by spore-forming protozoal infections; most are approximately 1 μm in length and can easily be confused with bacteria or debris on slides. Special staining

Intestinal Parasites

271

---

[1] Not FDA approved for this indication.

[1] Not FDA approved for this indication.

techniques have been described, but electron microscopy is required for species identification. PCR assays have been increasingly used for highly sensitive identification and speciation. Indirect immunofluorescence assays (IFA) are also available for *Encephalitozoon* spp. and *E. bieneusi*. Albendazole (Albenza)[1] is the treatment of choice for *E. intestinalis*. Treatment of *E. bieneusi* is more challenging. Although some response to albendazole has been reported, oral fumagillin[2] may have more efficacy. Unfortunately, it is not currently commercially available in the United States. Use of appropriate antiretroviral therapy is perhaps the most important treatment for patients with HIV infection or AIDS and chronic microsporidial infections. See Table 1 for medications and doses.

Helminths
Nematodes
Nematodes (roundworms) are cylindrical nonsegmented organisms that are found throughout the world both as free-living species and as human and animal pathogens. Nematodes are the most common type of human parasitic infestation, found in approximately one-fourth of the world's population; often, susceptible hosts carry multiple different pathogenic nematodes. There are at least 60 species that have been shown to infect humans and 10 times that many that cause disease in other animals, but a few pathogens account for the bulk of human infections, in particular *Ascaris*, hookworm, and whipworm. These three organisms all require a period of maturation outside the human body—typically in warm, moist soil—underscoring the fact that repeated contact with fecally contaminated soil or food and water is necessary to sustain the cycle of infestation. *Strongyloides* and *Enterobius* are unique in that they can both complete their life cycle on or within human hosts and therefore can cause chronic infection and be transmitted directly by close person-to-person contact where there is the possibility of fecal-oral contamination.

Ascaris
Ascaris lumbricoides, the most common human helminthic infection, is estimated to affect 20% to 25% of the world's population. Up to 80% of community members are infected in heavily endemic areas, namely in Africa, Asia, and Central and South America. Cases of *Ascaris* infestation are also seen in rural areas in the southeastern United States. *A. lumbricoides* are white to pinkish worms that range from 10 to 40 cm in length. Transmission in humans occurs most commonly by ingestion of infectious human or pig eggs that are oval white bodies with an adherent mucopolysaccharide capsule that clings to multiple surfaces and aids in transmissibility of the parasite. Eggs are also remarkably durable, capable of surviving up to 6 years in moist soil, and able to weather brief droughts and periods of freezing. Another means of transmission is by ingesting uncooked pig or chicken liver containing *Ascaris suum* larvae.

Fecal contamination of water, food, and environmental surfaces such as doorknobs and countertops provides the means of transmission for *Ascaris,* and recurrent infection occurs as long as living conditions that predispose people to infection remain unchanged. Lack of adequate public sanitation, use of human feces as fertilizer (night soil), and frequent contact with soil or shared contaminated surfaces among close household members are risk factors for infection. Persons who move to environments with improved sanitation typically lose their infection within 2 years as all of the adult worms die. Eggs excreted by an infected person must mature outside the human body for approximately 2 weeks. On ingestion by a susceptible host, mature eggs hatch in the small intestine and release larvae, which penetrate the intestinal wall and travel through the venous circulation to the lungs, where they are coughed up and swallowed. They then undergo maturation into adult worms in the intestine and produce eggs by 2 to 3 months after initial infection. The eggs are excreted in the feces and mature outside the body to continue the cycle.

Most persons with *Ascaris* infection are asymptomatic. Approximately 15% of infected people have morbidity, which is associated with young age, large burden of worms, coinfection with other intestinal parasites, and genetic predisposition. In children, infection contributes to malabsorption of protein, fat, and vitamins A and C, and treatment of heavily infected children can improve their nutritional status. *Ascaris* infection can also cause intestinal, pancreatic, or biliary obstruction as a result of worm mass or worm migration. Despite the low incidence of obstructive complications per infected person, the *Ascaris*-related acute abdomen is a significant problem on a global level given the enormous number of people infected. Some patients with intestinal *Ascaris* infection report vague abdominal complaints, such as abdominal discomfort, nausea, vomiting, or diarrhea, but these are relatively rare. Pulmonary migration of a large quantity of worms can produce Loeffler syndrome, or eosinophilic pneumonitis.

Diagnosis is easily attained with standard saline stool preparation, and large numbers of eggs are typically seen. Larvae or worms can also sometimes be seen in sputum or stool samples. In cases of intestinal obstruction, worms may be visualized on upper gastrointestinal series, CT, and even ultrasonography. Multiplex PCR assays are highly sensitive at identification and quantification but are currently not routinely used. Peripheral eosinophilia with *Ascaris* infection is found only during the larval migratory phase, but not at all times. Chronic eosinophilia in an at-risk person suggests another parasitic infection, often *Strongyloides*. Sputum eosinophilia and Charcot-Leyden crystals can be seen, although this is common with many parasitic eosinophilic pulmonary infections.

All persons documented to carry *Ascaris* who have migrated to nonendemic areas should be treated to prevent complications in the future; in endemic areas, adults need only be treated if they are symptomatic. Children have been shown to benefit from intermittent anthelminthic therapy in heavily affected areas of the world. For patients with intestinal obstruction, bowel rest and intravenous hydration are usually sufficient to relieve the obstruction, at which time anthelmintic therapy can be administered. In such cases, gastroenterology consultation should be obtained. In rare cases, surgical intervention is required. Treatment of pulmonary infection is controversial; however, most experts recommend steroid therapy for severe infections followed 2 to 3 weeks later (at the time full-grown worms will have migrated to the intestine) by administration of anthelmintic therapy. *Strongyloides* infection should be ruled out before corticosteroid administration as the latter can induce *Strongyloides* hyperinfection syndrome. The benzimidazoles (mebendazole [Emverm, Vermox], albendazole [Albenza],[1] levamisole[2]) exhibit excellent activity against *Ascaris*. Ivermectin (Stromectol)[1] and nitazoxanide (Alinia)[1] are suggested as reasonable alternatives. Doses and other options are listed in Table 2. Pregnant women should be treated with pyrantel pamoate (Pin-Away) as albendazole and mebendazole carry a pregnancy class B label. Pyrantel pamoate is a depolarizing neuromuscular blocking agent that causes paralysis in helminths, which prevents them from invading the intestinal wall, eventually resulting in their natural expulsion from the intestinal lumen. Because no consistent teratogenic effects have been demonstrated with albendazole use in late pregnancy, the World Health Organization (WHO) has allowed the use of albendazole to treat mass infections in the second and third trimesters.

Sanitary conditions that allow for proper management of human feces are crucial in control and prevention of *Ascaris* infection; boiling water kills the eggs.

Whipworm (Trichuris)
Trichuris trichiura has become recognized in recent years as a worldwide pathogen and is frequently found as a coinfection with *A. lumbricoides* as they share a similar scope and environmental conditions.

[1] Not FDA approved for this indication.
[2] Not available in the United States.

[1] Not FDA approved for this indication.
[2] Not available in the United States.

CLINICAL SITUATION	DRUG	ADULT DOSE	PEDIATRIC DOSE	COMMENTS
Anisakiasis				
(Anisakis spp., *Pseudoterranova decipiens)*	No recommended medical therapy	—	—	Successful treatment of a patient with anisakiasis with albendazole[1] has been reported.
	Surgical or endoscopic removal of worm			
Ascariasis				
(Ascaris lumbricoides)	Albendazole (Albenza)[1,*] *or*	400 mg once	400 mg PO once	
	Mebendazole[†] (Vermox) *or*	100 mg bid × 3 d or 500 mg once	100 mg bid × 3 d or 500 mg once	
	Ivermectin[1,†] (Stromectol)	150–200 µg/kg once	150–200 µg/kg once	In heavy infection, therapy may be given for 3 d.
Enterobiasis				
(Enterobius vermicularis)	Mebendazole[†] *or*	100 mg once, repeat in 2 wk	100 mg once, repeat in 2 wk	Because all family members are usually infected, treatment of the entire household is recommended.
	Albendazole[1,*] *or*	400 mg once, repeat in 2 wk	400 mg once, repeat in 2 wk	
	Pyrantel pamoate[‡]	11 mg/kg base (max 1 g) once; repeat in 2 wk	11 mg/kg base (max 1 g) once; repeat in 2 wk	
Hookworm				
(Ancylostoma duodenale, Necator americanus)	Albendazole[1,*] *or*	400 mg once	400 mg once	
	Mebendazole *or*	100 mg bid × 3 d or 500 mg once	100 mg bid × 3 d or 500 mg once	
	Pyrantel pamoate[‡,1]	11 mg/kg (max 1 g) × 3 d	11 mg/kg (max 1 g) × 3 d	
Schistosomiasis				
Schistosoma haematobium, Schistosoma mansoni	Praziquantel[§] *or*	40 mg/kg/d in 2 doses × 1 d	40 mg/kg/d in 2 doses × 1 d	
S. mansoni only	Oxamniquine[1,2]	15 mg/kg once	20 mg/kg/d in 2 doses × 1 d	Praziquantel is first line, but oxamniquine may be effective in some patients in whom praziquantel is less effective. Contraindicated in pregnancy
Schistosoma japonicum, Schistosoma mekongi	Praziquantel[§]	60 mg/kg/d in 2 or 3 doses × 1 d	60 mg/kg/d in 3 doses × 1 d	
Strongyloidiasis				
Strongyloides stercoralis	Recommended: Ivermectin[†]	200 µg/kg/d × 2 d	200 µg/kg/d × 2 d	In immunocompromised patients or in patients with disseminated disease, it may be necessary to prolong or repeat therapy or use other agents.

Continued

CLINICAL SITUATION	DRUG	ADULT DOSE	PEDIATRIC DOSE	COMMENTS
				Veterinary parenteral and enema formulations of ivermectin are used in severely ill patients who are unable to take oral medications.
	Alternative: Albendazole[1],*	400 mg bid × 7 d	400 mg bid × 7 d	
Tapeworm				
(*Diphyllobothrium latum* [fish], *Taenia saginata* [beef], *Taenia solium* [pork], *Dipylidium caninum* [dog])				
	Praziquantel[1] or	5–10 mg/kg PO once	5–10 mg/kg PO once	
	Niclosamide[¶,2]	2 g once	50 mg/kg once	Available in the United States only from the manufacturer
Trichuriasis				
(*Trichuris trichiura*)				
	Recommended: Mebendazole	100 mg bid × 3 d or 500 mg once	100 mg bid × 3 d or 500 mg once	
	Alternatives: Albendazole[1],* or	400 mg daily × 3 d	400 mg daily × 3 d	
	Ivermectin[†,1]	200 µg/kg daily × 3 d	200 µg/kg daily × 3 d	

[1]Not FDA approved for this indication.
[2]Not available in the United States.
*Should be taken with a fatty meal.
[†]Safety of ivermectin in young children (<15 kg) and pregnant women is not yet established. Ivermectin should be taken on an empty stomach with water.
[‡]Limited availability; can be mixed with juice or water to improve palatability.
[§]Should be taken with liquids during a meal.
[∥]Limited or no availability in the United States.
[¶]Available in the United States only from the manufacturer. Must be chewed or crushed thoroughly and swallowed with a small amount of water. Limited or no availability in the United States.
Modified from World Health Organization. Drugs for parasitic infections, *Med Lett Drug Ther.* 2010;8(Suppl).

Almost 90% of individuals from endemic regions are infected. Sanitary conditions that predispose to ingestion of food and water contaminated with human feces place people at risk for infection.

The adult organism is a small worm about 4 cm in length with a unique whiplike structure that allows its thin tail to become embedded in colonic crypts. Infection is acquired by ingesting *Trichuris* eggs that have undergone embryonation in the soil for 2 to 4 weeks after excretion from a previous host. Larvae emerge from eggs in the intestine and migrate into crypts, where they begin to mature. Egg production begins approximately 3 months later.

Most persons with whipworm carry few worms (approximately 20) and are asymptomatic. As with many other intestinal parasites, children are at greater risk for symptomatic infection, which can cause failure to thrive, anemia, clubbing, inflammatory colitis, and rectal prolapse. Adults with a high worm burden can also experience inflammatory colitis characterized by frequent—often bloody—diarrhea and tenesmus. Infection has been shown to result in production of tumor necrosis factor (TNF)-α by lamina propria cells in the colon, which can contribute to poor appetite and wasting that can be seen with significant infection.

Diagnosis is made by standard stool microscopy without a need to concentrate stool because large numbers of eggs are excreted. Whipworm eggs have a characteristic barrel shape with mucous (hyaline) plugs at either end. Worms can also be seen on colonoscopy, or they can be visualized grossly in cases of rectal prolapse. PCR tests are now available with improved but variable sensitivity for species identification. Peripheral eosinophilia may be seen.

Treatment of symptomatic infections can be accomplished with mebendazole (Emverm, Vermox), albendazole (Albenza),[1] or ivermectin (Stromectal)[1]; see Table 2 for details.

[1]Not FDA approved for this indication.

Hookworm

Like other helminthic infections, hookworm affects a substantial portion of the world's population, particularly in rural subtropical and tropical communities where human feces is used as a component of fertilizer. Infection results primarily from parasite penetration into the skin; therefore persons with an agrarian lifestyle and significant soil contact are at greatest risk.

Two species are responsible for the majority of human hookworm: *Necator americanus* and *Ancylostoma duodenale*. *N. americanus* is a smaller and less aggressive pathogen with a longer life span than *A duodenale*. Both parasites are found in warm climates throughout the world; *A. duodenale* exists in smaller pockets in Mediterranean countries, Iran, India, Pakistan, and the Far East, whereas *N. americanus* is widely distributed throughout impoverished rural areas of the tropics in the Americas, Asia, and Africa. *Ancylostoma ceylanicum*, a hookworm of dogs and cats, has been identified as one of the human zoonotic infections in Southeast Asia, tropical Australia, and the Melanesian Pacific Islands. *Ancylostoma braziliense*, a canine intestinal pathogen, causes cutaneous larval migrans in humans because the pathogen cannot penetrate the human dermis.

Hookworms are small helminths, between 0.5 and 1 cm in length. Infection results from larval penetration of the skin on contact with contaminated soil. An intensely pruritic, erythematous, papulovesicular rash called *ground itch* can develop at the site of entry. Parasites then enter the venous or lymphatic circulation and travel to the lungs, at which point an urticarial rash with cough can develop. The larvae are swallowed and migrate to the small intestine, where they attach to the bowel wall with teeth or biting plates and take a continuous blood meal by sucking with strong esophageal muscles. As the larvae lodge in the small intestine, peripheral eosinophilia peaks, and gastrointestinal discomfort with or without diarrhea can result. Large oral ingestion of *A. duodenale* can cause Wakana syndrome, characterized by cough, shortness of breath, nausea, vomiting, and eosinophilia. The most important clinical manifestation of hookworm infection is iron-deficiency anemia, which can be mild or severe and may be accompanied by malabsorption of protein in hosts with heavy burden of disease. Infants and pregnant women can become extremely ill or even die as a result of the anemia.

Hookworm may be difficult to diagnose because light infections often do not produce enough eggs to be readily seen on stool examination; stool should therefore be concentrated if infection is suspected. Eggs do not appear in stool until approximately 2 months after dermal penetration of *N. americanus* and up to 38 weeks from cutaneous entry of *A. duodenale*, hence patients with pulmonary complaints will not yet have a positive stool examination. Multiplex PCR assays that detect *A. lumbricoides, T. trichiura,* and hookworm have higher sensitivity than direct microscopy; however, these are not as widely available yet.

Hookworm infection can be eradicated with benzimidazole anthelmintics; see Table 2 for details. Prevention of hookworm infection, as with other parasites, lies in improved sanitary conditions; wearing shoes is especially important because the majority of infections are acquired through the skin. Mass anthelmintic treatment campaigns have shown some efficacy in reducing disease in children; however, reinfection and concern for development of resistance continue to present significant challenges. Candidate vaccines are currently under investigation.

Toxocara

Human infection is most commonly from the dog ascarid, *Toxocara canis,* and rarely from the cat ascarid, *Toxocara cati.* Humans are infected by embryonated eggs shed by a definitive host (dogs, cats) in contaminated soil or food, and direct contact with a definitive host is usually not a classical mode of transmission. Eggs then hatch into larvae that penetrate the intestinal wall to enter the circulation and embed in various tissues, leading to both visceral larva migrans (VLM), which affects the lungs, liver, heart, muscle, and brain, and ocular larva migrans, which affects the eyes. VLM usually presents as hepatitis (nodular lesions) and pneumonitis (typically with bilateral peribronchial infiltration). Pericarditis, myocarditis, Loeffler endocarditis, heart failure, cardiac tamponade, eosinophilic meningo-encephalitis, cerebral vasculitis, and myelitis have been rarely reported. Ocular larva migrans (OLM) results from a granulomatous inflammatory response to embedded larva that typically presents as a whitish elevated granuloma but red eye from scleritis or uveitis. Visual impairment leading to blindness from retinal detachment are more serious complications.

ELISA immunoglobulin G (IgG) serology in the appropriate clinical setting is the most commonly used diagnostic modality but cannot differentiate active from past infections. Sensitivity of ELISA for OLM is lower than that for VLM. PCR testing is commercially not available yet. Definite diagnosis is established with biopsy that is rarely indicated.

The treatment of choice is albendazole (Albenza),[1] which is preferred over mebendazole (Emverm, Vermox),[1] especially in neurologic disease and OLM because the latter does not cross the blood-brain barrier. Antiinflammatory corticosteroids are used as adjunctive therapy for cardiac, neurologic, and severe vision-threatening illness.

Strongyloides

Strongyloides stercoralis is a global pathogen that is estimated to affect as many as 100 million people, mostly in tropical regions of the world. In recent years, it has become more commonly recognized in the United States among immigrants as a cause of chronic eosinophilia as well as symptomatic infection.

Strongyloides infection results when filariform larvae dwelling in fecally contaminated soil penetrate the skin or mucous membranes of a susceptible host. Larvae move to the lungs and subsequently to the trachea, where they are coughed up and swallowed. Females, about 2 cm in length, lodge in the lamina propria of the duodenum and proximal jejunum, where they begin to oviposit. Rhabditiform larvae (noninfectious form) emerge from these eggs and either transform into infectious filariform larvae (infectious form) that can repenetrate the intestinal wall (autoinfection; unique to *S. stercoralis* among other helminths) or are passed into the feces, at which point they can begin a free-living cycle and reproduce sexually or can molt directly into an infectious form ready to enter a subsequent susceptible host.

Persons infected with *Strongyloides* are typically asymptomatic. Those who have symptoms might report abdominal discomfort, diarrhea alternating with constipation, or, rarely, blood-tinged stool. Severe intestinal infections can occur and are manifest by chronic watery or mucous diarrhea. In such cases, colonoscopy reveals excessive bowel wall thickening and copious secretions, or edema (catarrhal enteritis or edematous enteritis). Parasite migration through the dermis can manifest as pathognomonic serpiginous, erythematous, and pruritic patches along the buttocks, perineum, and thighs, known as *larvae currens ("running" larvae).*

Strongyloides appear to attain a balanced state in their host, with similar numbers of adult worms throughout the many years of infection. During periods of host immunocompromise, particularly in patients taking corticosteroids, *Strongyloides* can enter into a state of rapid autoinfection and rampant reproduction called *hyperinfection syndrome,* which results in devastating illness. Persons with HIV infection do not seem to be at particular risk for symptomatic disease or hyperinfection, but hyperinfection has been linked to human T-lymphotropic virus type 1 (HTLV-1) infection. *Strongyloides* has also caused hyperinfection in organ transplant patients whose donor had been infected asymptomatically with the parasite. Although it has long been thought that steroid-induced immune compromise was the major trigger for hyperinfection, growing evidence suggests that steroids themselves may be the culprit by directly inducing the accelerated life cycle in the parasite.

The hyperinfection syndrome is characterized by systemic illness with fever, cough, hypoxia, patchy or diffuse pulmonary infiltrates with alveolar microhemorrhages, and dermatitis; it can include myocarditis, hepatitis, splenic abscess, meningitis and cerebral abscess, and endocrine organ involvement. Larvae migrating out of the intestines can drag bacteria with them, resulting in gram-negative or polymicrobial sepsis. The prognosis of *Strongyloides* hyperinfection syndrome is grave, even with highly effective anthelmintic treatment given the diffuse nature of this disease. However, earlier recognition and intensive supportive care result in cure.

Diagnosis of uncomplicated *Strongyloides* infection in endemic areas can be challenging because few larvae are passed in stool, and numerous examinations may be necessary to detect them. ELISA IgG serologies to filariform larvae are highly sensitive, but positive results cannot distinguish between active and past infections. Moreover, serologies can be falsely negative in immunocompromised hosts. It is, however, the test of choice for persons who have migrated to nonendemic areas, and all persons in this setting should be treated. Ivermectin (Stromectol) is the treatment of choice; albendazole (Albenza)[1] has some activity again *S. stercoralis* and can be tried as an alternative; see Table 2 for medications and doses. During the first days of treatment, patients can experience intense dermal pruritus as parasites die. Eosinophilia and positive ELISA results can persist for months, even after effective therapy.

Enterobius

Human pinworm infection, caused by the threadlike nematode *Enterobius vermicularis,* is found throughout the world and continues to be diagnosed commonly in the United States, especially

---

[1] Not FDA approved for this indication.

[1] Not FDA approved for this indication.

in children 5 to 10 years of age. It is the most common helmintic infection in the United States and Europe. Its persistence is likely related to the fact that pinworm does not require a period of maturation outside the human body, and autoinfection or transmission by very close contact sustains the parasite within communities. *E. vermicularis* is at maximum 1 cm long with a tapered tail, and it dwells in the cecum, appendix, and adjacent colon. At night, female worms travel to the anus and lay small (25 to 50 μm), double-walled oval eggs in the perianal skin. Within 6 hours, the eggs embryonate within their capsule and are infectious. In scratching the perianal area and subsequently bringing his or her hand to the mouth, the host ingests the embryos, which then hatch in the bowel about 2 months later and continue the cycle of infection. Embryonated eggs can also attach to bedclothes, thereby placing other household members with close contact at risk for infection. In family groups, infection is associated with close living quarters, poor hand washing, and infrequent washing of clothes and sheets. It can also be prevalent among institutionalized persons.

Infection is often asymptomatic, but it can cause perianal itching, which helps facilitate persistent infection by encouraging frequent touching of the perianal area. Rarely, worms migrate into ectopic foci and produce painful genitourinary tract disease with granulomatous inflammation; pinworm infection rarely results in pain that mimics acute appendicitis.

Pinworm infestation is best diagnosed by the classic Scotch tape test, which involves placing and immediately removing a piece of sticky tape firmly across the perianal area early in the morning when the eggs have been deposited. The tape can then be brought into a physician's office or laboratory, where it is placed sticky-side down for microscopic examination to detect the eggs. Sensitivity can be increased by examining at least three specimens. Eggs are small (25 × 50 microns) with a characteristic "bean-shaped" appearance. It is also sometimes possible to see the white small female worms directly on the perianal region, although they are so small (8 to 13 mm in length) that they may easily be mistaken for residual bits of toilet paper. Although *E. vermicularis* is susceptible to standard albendazole[1] or mebendazole (see Table 2), pyrantel pamoate (Pin-Away, OTC) is most frequently used in the United States as it is cheap and effective. All household contacts should be empirically treated with the same regimen to avoid reintroducing infection from family members who may be asymptomatically carrying the parasite. Careful laundering of all bedclothes is recommended as well.

Anisakiasis

Anisakiasis is a descriptive term for human infection with parasites of two distinct genera: *Anisakis* and *Pseudoterranova*. Humans are incidental hosts for these roundworms that inhabit multiple species of fish and other marine animals (tuna, mackerel, hake, cod, sardines, and cephalopods) as intermediate hosts, and marine mammals such as whales, seals, sea lions, and walruses as final hosts. Humans acquire the parasite in its larval stage by eating undercooked or raw fish (e.g., sushi, ceviche), therefore the condition predominates in cultures in which uncooked fish is consumed. Cases are most commonly reported from Japan but are seen throughout the world in other coastal nations and among restaurateurs.

On consumption of fish with anisakid larvae embedded in its musculature, humans can experience immediate symptoms in the form of itching or burning in the throat, which can provoke coughing that expels the parasite. If the parasite is swallowed, the larva attempts to embed in the gastric musculature at the pylorus. This can produce acute, short-lived epigastric abdominal pain and possibly immediate vomiting, at which point the parasite might again be ejected. If the larva does manage to penetrate gastric tissue, it dies because it is incapable of further tissue invasion in humans. An intense inflammatory response to the dead pathogen can then result, with gastric pain, nausea, and occasionally diarrhea with blood or mucus if a gastric ulcerative lesion

has resulted. Eosinophilic enterocolitis, ileitis, appendicitis, and focal peritonitis and abscess formation from penetration of larva into the peritoneum are also rarely reported. Bronchoconstriction, angioedema, and anaphylaxis have been described mimicking seafood allergy. *Pseudoterranova* appears to cause milder symptoms and less tissue invasion, and the worm might simply be vomited several days after initial ingestion and presented to a physician, often by an alarmed patient. Because the vast majority of infections are caused by a single organism, vomiting of the parasite results in a definitive cure, and patients can be reassured. Diagnosis in patients with ongoing symptoms related to an embedded parasite is ultimately endoscopic. Effective cure results on endoscopic or surgical removal of the worm. Albendazole[1] as an effective therapy is reported; however, data are limited.

Trematodes

Schistosoma

Schistosomes are freshwater pathogens that are found in areas of endemicity in Africa, South America, Southeast Asia, and parts of the Middle East. These small trematodes cause varied, often chronic infections that can carry significant morbidity, although some species cannot invade beyond the dermis in humans and result strictly in cercarial dermatitis or swimmer's itch. There are five species of schistosomes known to cause disease in humans: *Schistosoma haematobium*, found through much of Africa and parts of the Middle East; *Schistosoma mansoni*, also native to Africa and the Middle East as well as Latin America; *Schistosoma japonicum*, present in China, Southeast Asia, and the Philippines; *Schistosoma mekongi*, found only in the Mekong River basin in Laos and Cambodia; and *Schistosoma intercalatum*, endemic only in West Africa.

All persons who come in contact with schistosomes are at risk for infection, even with brief exposure to fecally contaminated freshwater in which the intermediate hosts of the pathogen (snails) reside. Frequency and degree of infection tend to be highest in children in endemic areas and then level off in the early teenage years, likely secondary to level of environmental exposure and possibly to host immunity. *S. haematobium* causes disease in the genitourinary system; the others cause intestinal, hepatic, and sometimes pulmonary diseases.

Infection is acquired rapidly on contact with freshwater (including brief swims or by repeated splashing, as can occur during river rafting), when free-living fork-tailed schistosomal larvae (cercariae) penetrate human skin and lose their tail. These schistosomulae can cause intense itching and a papulovesicular, pruritic rash at the site of penetration, swimmer's itch. Invasive schistosomulae then enter the venous bloodstream and reach the liver through portal venules, where they mature into adults. Adult worms then migrate against the portal venous flow to the mesenteric venules of the gut (*S. mansoni*, *S. japonicum*, *S. intercalatum*, *S. mekongi*) and vesical venous plexus (*S. hematobium*), where male and female forms mate for life. Females begin to oviposit, and the resultant inflammatory response to the eggs can cause either acute illness or chronic fibrosis and granulomatous inflammation of the tissues in which they reside.

Acute illness, called *Katayama fever*, is more common among hosts who have not been previously exposed to the organism and can be quite severe and even fatal. Katayama fever begins 3 to 8 weeks after infection, with acute onset of fever, chills, myalgias, cough, urticaria, angioedema, abdominal pain, hepatomegaly, and lymphadenopathy. Eggs might not yet be present in stool at the time of diagnosis. Chronic schistosomiasis is a slowly progressive illness presenting chiefly with intermittent abdominal pain, diarrhea, and anorexia. Colonic ulceration with gastrointestinal bleeding and iron-deficiency anemia from huge parasitic burden has been described. Hepatosplenic schistosomiasis can be caused by granulomatous inflammation surrounding the eggs, eventually leading to periportal fibrosis (Symmers pipestem fibrosis), portal hypertension, and splenomegaly. Portal

---

[1] Not FDA approved for this indication.

[1] Not FDA approved for this indication.

hypertension can then lead to portosystemic collateral vessel development along with deposition of eggs in the pulmonary vasculature. Granulomatous inflammation in the pulmonary tissues eventually causes endarteritis, fibrosis, pulmonary hypertension, and cor pulmonale. *S. haematobium* infection can manifest as gross or microscopic hematuria, irritative urinary symptoms, and chronic bacterial urinary tract infections; ultimately ureteral fibrosis, hydronephrosis, and granulomatous genital lesions also can ensue. Neuroschistosomiasis can cause both myelopathy and intracerebral lesions and can have varied presentation including seizures, focal deficits, encephalopathy, and rapidly progressive transverse myelitis.

Diagnosis of schistosomiasis is by observation of eggs in stool (intestinal disease), urine (urinary tract disease), or biopsy specimens, or by serum antibody testing. Concentration of stool may be necessary to detect the pathogen. The eggs of the three most common species of schistosomes can be readily identified microscopically: *S. haematobium* has an inferior spine, *S. mansoni* has an inferolateral spine, and *S. japonicum* lacks a spine. Quantification of eggs is important as the parasitic burden is proportional to the risk of complications and is usually reported as light (up to 100 eggs/gram), moderate (100 to 400 eggs/gram), and severe (>400 eggs/gram) in stool specimens. Eosinophilia is a hallmark of chronic infection and is a common cause of asymptomatic eosinophilia among immigrants from endemic regions of the world. Serology is useful, particularly in return travelers with low parasitic burden; however, it can be negative in early infection as it takes 6 to 12 weeks after exposure to become positive. It is highly specific but cannot distinguish acute, chronic, or cleared infection. Antigen testing targeting specific schistosomal glycoproteins, circulating cathodic antigen (CCA, genus specific) and circulating anodic antigen (CAA, more specific to *S. mansoni*) is more sensitive than microscopy and can lead to rapid diagnosis, particularly in specimens with low parasitic burden. Highly sensitive PCR assays have been developed to be used on blood, stool, and urine specimens; however, these are not as widely available. Histopathology is better than microscopy, particularly in ectopic manifestations, but is usually not required.

All patients with schistosomiasis should be treated, and those with chronic manifestations might experience significant regression of even late-stage organ-specific disease. Treatment of choice is praziquantel (Biltricide); see Table 2 for details.

Prevention of schistosomiasis involves improving access to treated water and exploration of avenues to eliminate the intermediate snail hosts. Host immunity does appear to occur, and efforts are underway to better understand and induce such immunity in the form of a vaccine.

Cestodes
Taenia
Human tapeworm infection has long been implicated in North American oral folklore as a cause of insatiable appetite and excessive weight loss. In reality, despite their impressive size of up to 12 meters, tapeworm infection tends to be minimally symptomatic.

Taenia solium, pork tapeworm, and *Taenia saginata*, beef tapeworm, are the two most common flatworm infections of humans (humans are the only definitive hosts) worldwide and occur in any setting in which raw or undercooked meat is served and cattle and pigs have access to feed contaminated with human feces. *T. saginata* is still found in areas of North America and Europe as well as in Central and South America and Africa; *T. solium* is common throughout Mexico, Central and South America, Africa, China, and the Indian subcontinent. Although humans are the definitive hosts for both parasites, *T. solium* is best known for its pathogenicity in the form of cysticercosis. Cysticercosis is not an intestinal parasitic infection.

Domesticated animals acquire infection on ingestion of eggs or gravid proglottids excreted by humans; the eggs mature in their musculature and develop a scolex. When humans consume infected meat, the scolex attaches to the small intestine, and the adult tapeworm develops over approximately 2 months. Adult tapeworms are made up of hundreds to thousands of gravid proglottids and can live for up to 25 years with intermittent shedding in the stool.

Symptoms ditend to be mild or absent but can include nausea, abdominal pain, loose stools, anal pruritus, and occasionally weakness or increased appetite, especially in children. Serious illness rarely results when tapeworm proglottids become lodged in the appendix or the biliary or pancreatic duct or are coughed up and aspirated. Some patients come to medical attention when the worm is noted emerging from the anus or on extrusion of proglottids in the stool.

Diagnosis of taeniasis can be made on visualizing the round eggs with hooks and double wall with characteristic striations, however the species cannot be determined unless their proglottids are examined (*T. saginata* has 12 or more uterine branches, whereas *T. solium* has <10). Because the eggs and proglottids are shed intermittently, the sensitivity of microscopy is poor. Serum antibody and antigen tests as well as stool PCR have been developed for diagnosis but are not widely used in clinical practice. Eosinophilia and elevated immunoglobulin E (IgE) levels may be present. Single-dose praziquantel (Biltricide)[1] (see Table 2) is curative in almost all cases, but infectious eggs can still be released in the feces for some time after worm eradication; ingestion of these could result in subsequent development of cysticercosis, so patients should be counseled to avoid fecal-oral contact.

Proper cooking of meat is the mainstay of prevention; disposal of human waste away from animals would also be effective in interrupting the life cycle.

Diphyllobothrium
Diphyllobothrium latum (fish tapeworm) is the longest parasite known to infect humans (10 to 12 m). It is found in freshwater lakes in areas of the Americas, Northern Europe, Africa, China, and Japan and has a complex life cycle involving two intermediate hosts: crustaceans and small fish. Humans and other fish-eating mammals are the definitive hosts and acquire the infection on ingestion of raw fish or roe.

Eggs and proglottids are intermittently shed in human stool that embryonate in the water. Coracidiae hatch from the eggs and are ingested by small crustaceans, the first intermediate hosts. Coracidiae mature into procercoid larvae in the crustaceans that are then ingested by the small freshwater fish (the second intermediate host). Procercoid larvae develop into plerocercoid larvae (sparganum) that are then passed onto the large predator fish (later intermediate host) that is then consumed by humans (definitive host). Sparganum develops into the adult worm inside the human intestine.

The mature adult tapeworm attaches within the small intestine, and hosts are usually asymptomatic. Infected persons might complain of increased appetite, nausea, or abdominal discomfort. Many patients present after passage of portions of the tapeworm in stool, as with taeniasis. In others, diagnosis is incidental on stool examination performed for other purposes or during screening colonoscopy. As with other worms, the parasite occasionally migrates into biliary ducts or causes intestinal obstruction. Attachment of the parasite higher in the intestine competes the host for vitamin B_{12} absorption and can result in vitamin B_{12} deficiency (pernicious anemia).

Diagnosis is made either by visualizing eggs with an operculum (lidlike opening) in an unconcentrated stool or by encountering the adult worm. Proglottids can be differentiated from those in taeniasis by the presence of a rosette-shaped uterus. Eosinophilia is present in a minority of cases. Treatment with praziquantel[1] is curative; see Table 2. Vitamin B_{12} supplementation is necessary in cases of severe or symptomatic deficiency, but it will not recur once the tapeworm is eliminated. Prevention involves not ingesting undercooked fish.

---

[1] Not FDA approved for this indication.

References

Abubakar I, Aliyu SH, Hunter PR, Usman NK: Prevention and treatment of crypto-sporidiosis in immunocompromised patients, *Cochrane Database Syst Rev* (1), CD004932.

Bethony J, Brooker S, Albonico M, et al: Soil-transmitted helminth infections: Ascariasis, trichiurasis, and hookworm, *Lancet* 367(9521):1521–1532, 2006.

Boggild A, Yohanna S, Keystone J, Kain K: Prospective analysis of parasitic infections in Canadian travelers and immigrants, *J Travel Med* 13:138–144, 2006.

Boulware DR, Stauffer WM, Hendel-Paterson RR, et al: Maltreatment of strongyloides infection: Case series and worldwide physicians-in-training survey, *Am J Med* 120:545.e1– 545.e8, 2007.

Concha R, Hartington Jr W, Rogers AI: Intestinal strongyloidiasis: Recognition, management, and determinants of outcome, *J Clin Gastroenterol* 39(3):203–211, 2005.

Drugs for Parasitic Infections: *Treatment Guidelines from the Medical Letter*, 2013, pp e1–e31 (11).

Goodgame RW: Understanding intestinal spore-forming protozoa: Cryptosporidia, microsporidia, isospora, and cyclospora, *Ann Intern Med* 124(4):429–441, 1996.

Guerrant R, Walker D, Weller P, editors: *Tropical infectious diseases: principles, pathogens, and practice*, Philadelphia, 1999, Churchill Livingstone.

Huang DB, White AC: An updated review on Cryptosporidium and Giardia, *Gastroenterol Clin North Am* 35:291–314, 2006.

Mandell G, Bennett J, Dolin R, editors: *Mandell, douglas and bennett's principles and practice of infectious diseases*, 5th ed, Philadelphia, 2005, Churchill Livingstone.

Pardo J, Carranza C, Muro A, et al: Helminth-related eosinophilia in African immigrants, Gran Canaria, *Emerg Infect Dis* 12(10):1587–1589, 2006.

Stark D, Beebe N, Marriott D, et al: Dientamoebiasis: Clinical importance and recent advances, *Trends Parasitol* 22(2):92–96, 2006.

IRRITABLE BOWEL SYNDROME

Method of
Arnold Wald, MD

CURRENT DIAGNOSIS

- Fulfilling diagnostic criteria for irritable bowel syndrome (IBS) using Manning or Rome criteria is mandatory but not sufficient, as some organic diseases may also meet these criteria.
- Against the diagnosis of IBS is new onset in old age, a steady progressive course, frequent awakening by abdominal pain or urge to defecate, and weight loss not attributed to depression.
- The diagnostic approach to patients with IBS symptoms with no "alarm signs" includes a complete blood count; stool testing for occult blood or calprotectin; C-reactive protein and colonoscopy if patient is >45 years of age, has positive stool, or aforementioned blood test results; or if there is a poor response to treatment.
- After a diagnosis of IBS is established with confidence, repeated testing is counterproductive unless there is a distinct change in clinical symptoms or new alarm signs develop.

CURRENT THERAPY

- A robust patient–healthcare provider relationship is perhaps the most important determinant of outcome and reduction of healthcare usage in patients with irritable bowel syndrome (IBS).
- There is significant support for the use of a low-FODMAP (fermentable oligosaccharides, disaccharides, monosaccharides, and polyols) diet in patients with IBS. Gluten restriction is part of this diet and will cover those patients who believe that they are gluten intolerant in the absence of celiac disease.
- Pharmacologic agents can be divided into those for IBS with predominant constipation or IBS with predominant diarrhea, or in any patient with IBS to ameliorate abdominal pain. The evidence to support these agents varies in quality and strength, and none is effective in the majority of patients who have been tested.
- Cognitive-behavioral therapy can be very effective in IBS with unrelenting symptoms but may also be effective for any patient with IBS who exhibits poor stress management.

Introduction and Definitions

Irritable bowel syndrome (IBS) is a chronic functional disorder of the gastrointestinal (GI) tract characterized by chronic abdominal pain and altered bowel habits in the absence of an organic disease. In the absence of a biologic disease marker, the diagnosis has traditionally been based on a cluster of symptoms. The earliest was the so-called Manning criteria, which was based most stringently on the presence of three or more characteristic symptoms (Table 1).

Subsequently, there have been various iterations of IBS criteria created by the Rome study groups that are currently used for research purposes (see Table 1). When evaluating the relevant literature for IBS, it is important to note that various studies have used different criteria that may result in variable data concerning prevalence and economic costs considerations.

From a clinical standpoint, subtypes of IBS have been defined as follows:

- IBS with predominant constipation (IBS-C): Patient reports that abnormal bowel movements are usually constipation (types 1 and 2 in the Bristol Stool Form Scale [BSFS]).
- IBS with predominant diarrhea (IBS-D): Patient reports that abnormal bowel movements are usually diarrhea (types 6 and 7 in the BSFS).
- IBS with mixed bowel habits (IBS-M): Patient reports that abnormal bowel movements are usually both constipation and diarrhea (more than one-fourth of all the abnormal bowel movements are constipation, and more than one-fourth are diarrhea) using the BSFS.
- IBS Unclassified (IBS-U): Patients who meet diagnostic criteria for IBS but cannot be accurately categorized into one of the other three subtypes.

Epidemiology

Prevalence

Numerous surveys have reported the prevalence of IBS in the community. The majority of these studies have used accepted diagnostic criteria, and some have used more than one definition within the same population. In one meta-analysis, 23 studies used the Manning criteria, 24 used Rome I criteria, 36 used Rome II criteria, and 5 used Rome III criteria. The prevalence ranged from 5% to 10% (United States, China) to 15% to 20% (Canada, Brazil, Russia). There were little or no data from Africa, Central America, and large parts of South America.

The majority of studies did not report the predominant stool pattern in IBS. Of the nine that included IBS-U subtypes as well, there was an even distribution, ranging from 22% to 24% mean prevalence for each of the four subgroups. In general, the pooled prevalence was higher in women than in men (14%, range 11%–6% vs. 9%, range 7.3%–10.5%) with significant heterogeneity between studies. There appeared to be no relationship between socioeconomic status in the four studies that reported it and no strong influence of age as well.

It is important to note that the meta-analysis was restricted to studies based on the general population and excluded those based on convenience samples. This makes the data more generalizable to community individuals with IBS.

TABLE 1	Criteria for Irritable Bowel Syndrome
MANNING CRITERIA	**ROME IV CRITERIA***
Looser stools with onset of pain More frequent bowel movements at onset of pain Visible distension Feeling of distension Mucus per rectum Feeling of incomplete emptying (often) Strict criteria >3 of the above Less strict criteria >2 of the above	Recurrent abdominal pain on average at least 1 day per week in the past 3 months associated with two or more of the following: • Related to defecation • Associated with a change in stool frequency • Associated with change in form of stool (appearance)

*Criterion fulfilled for the past 3 months with onset of symptoms at least 6 months before diagnosis.

Causality: A Biopsychosocial Model of Functional Gastrointestinal Disorders Such as IBS

The ability to study causality in a disorder with no biologic disease markers is fraught with difficulties. This is certainly the case with IBS as a representative of functional GI disorders. Many hypotheses have been advanced and found wanting. The current (and in my opinion most relevant) conceptual model is the biopsychosocial construct, as shown in Figure 1.

Figure 1 indicates that predeterminants such as early life experiences together with psychosocial factors may interact with altered gut physiology via the brain-gut axis. This concept infers that these factors are bidirectional and mutually interactive and therefore influence both the clinical presentation and clinical outcomes of the disorder. Among the physiologic processes that may lead to GI symptoms are abnormal gut motility, visceral hypersensitivity, immune dysregulation, inflammation and barrier dysfunction, the intestinal microbiome, diet, and the brain-gut axis. No one factor alone accounts for the symptoms of IBS, and all must be considered in the management of affected patients. The recognition of these interactions has led to the reclassification of functional gastrointestinal disorders to disorders of gut-brain interaction. This becomes apparent when considering treatment approaches (see later).

Impact on Population Health

Although there is no mortality associated with IBS, symptoms are long lasting, and there are no curative therapies available. As a chronic illness, the economic impact of this disorder is considerable.

In a 2015 survey conducted by the American Gastroenterological Association (AGA), IBS patients reported that their symptoms interfered with work productivity on an average of 9 days per month and missed work on an average of 2 days per month. Indirect costs (e.g., loss of work and reduced productivity) have been estimated to be up to $20 billion annually in the United States, with an estimated annual cost per patient of $9933 (in 2021 US dollars).

In a recent study of indirect costs, impairment experienced at work (presenteeism) accounted for approximately 75% of the total annual indirect costs for respondents with IBS, far in excess of absenteeism from work. Compared with controls, IBS respondents missed significantly more work (5.1% vs. 2.9%), experienced higher levels of presenteeism (17.9% vs. 11.3%), and had greater overall work productivity loss (20.7% vs. 13.2%) and higher daily activity impairment.

Direct Healthcare Costs

Almost 30 years ago, it was estimated that up to 25% of all visits to gastroenterologists in the United States were for IBS, with additional others for other functional GI disorders. This accounted for 3.5 million visits to healthcare practitioners in 1991 and undoubtedly is much higher today. Earlier studies showed that IBS patients made twice as many health visits per year as did age-matched controls and that 78% of the excess visits were for non-GI complaints. A subsequent analysis of this phenomenon suggests that comorbidity in IBS may be a consequence of the psychological trait for somatization, defined as the tendency to amplify the intensity and overinterpret the significance of any somatic sensation. This excess comorbidity is the primary determinant of excess healthcare costs associated with IBS, although it does not apply to all patients with IBS.

Recent attempts to identify factors leading to high users with IBS have been made. The investigators used a conceptual framework for accessing healthcare services that holds that a decision to use healthcare is related to (1) predisposition to use services; (2) ability to use services; and (3) need for services. The important conclusion was that decisions to use healthcare are not simply influenced by symptom-specific factors but by a variety of lifestyle and (most importantly) economic factors such as health insurance coverage.

Evaluation of Patients With Suspected Irritable Bowel Syndrome

The diagnosis of IBS should be made based on the clinical history, physical examination, minimal laboratory testing, and colonoscopy or other appropriate tests when clinically indicated. Fulfilling diagnostic criteria is, of course, mandatory but insufficient, as some organic diseases may also meet these criteria. The prevalence of organic disease is lowest in IBS-C and highest in IBS-D, followed by IBS-M; the most common consideration would be Crohn's disease. Against the diagnosis of IBS include new onset in old age, a steady progressive course, frequent awakening by pain or need to defecate, and weight loss not attributed to depression. Additional features that would increase concern about organic disease would include a positive family history of colorectal cancer or inflammatory bowel disease, as well as rectal bleeding or anemia associated with iron or vitamin B_{12} deficiency.

In the absence of "alarm signs," a consensus diagnostic approach to patients with IBS symptoms is listed in Table 2 (Rome IV).

Tests of Unproven Value

A high prevalence of small intestinal bacterial overgrowth (SIBO) has been claimed by some centers leading to the frequent usage of either lactulose or glucose breath tests. This hypothesis is based

Biopsychosocial Conceptual Model

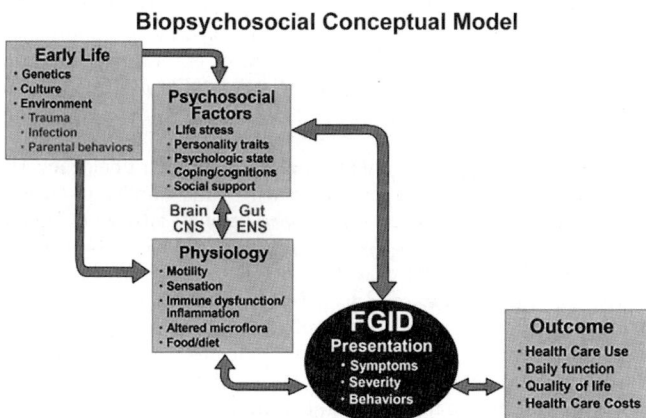

Figure 1 Predeterminants such as early life experiences, together with psychosocial factors, may interact with altered gut physiology via the brain-gut axis. This concept infers that these factors are bidirectional and mutually interactive and therefore influence both the clinical presentation of the disorder and the clinical outcomes. Among the physiologic processes that may lead to GI symptoms are abnormal gut motility, visceral hypersensitivity, immune dysregulation, inflammation and barrier dysfunction, the intestinal microbiome, diet, and the brain-gut axis. No one factor alone accounts for the symptoms of IBS, and all must be considered in the management of affected patients. This becomes apparent when considering treatment approaches. *CNS,* Central nervous system; *ENS,* enteric nervous system; *FGID,* functional gastrointestinal disorder. Reprinted with permission from Drossman DA: Functional gastrointestinal disorders: history, pathophysiology, clinical features and Rome IV, *Gastroenterology,* 150:1262–1279, 2016.

TABLE 2	Diagnostic Approach to Patients With IBS Symptoms (No "Alarm Signs")
Complete blood count	
Stool for occult blood	
Routine colon cancer screening at ages >45 years	
C-reactive protein (inflammatory marker)*	
Fecal calprotectin/lactoferrin (indicators of inflammation)*	
Stool for *Giardia**	
Celiac serologies*	
Diagnostic colonoscopy <45 years of age (if poor response to Rx)	

*For IBS with predominant diarrhea.
IBS, Irritable bowel syndrome.

TABLE 3	Low-FODMAP Diet		
AVOID OR REDUCE THESE FOODS			
FRUCTOSE	**LACTOSE**	**OLIGOS**	**POLYOLS**
Fruits: Apple, mango, pear, watermelon, juice, dried fruit	Milk: Milk from cows/goats/sheep; custard; ice cream; yogurt; eggnog	Vegetables: Beets, broccoli, brussels sprouts, cabbage, fennel, garlic, onion, chicory root	Fruits: Apricot, avocado, blackberry, cherry, nectarine, peach, plum, prune, fig
Other: Asparagus, honey, high-fructose corn syrup, molasses	Cheese: Soft, unripened cheese	Other: Barley, beans, chickpeas, couscous, inulin, lentils, pistachios, rye, soy milk, wheat (pasta, bread), veggie burgers	Vegetables: Cauliflower, corn, mushroom, sweet potato Sweeteners: Ending in "ol" (e.g., xylitol, sorbitol), isomalt

FODMAP, Fermentable oligosaccharides, disaccharides, monosaccharides, and polyols.

on poor methodology and erroneous conclusions. The original studies have not been reproduced by other centers using either similar and/or better techniques. This has led to the frequent use of expensive antibiotics that can be effective in some patients with bloating and IBS but not because these patients have SIBO.

Food allergy testing is not routinely recommended. Stool for ova/parasites is not recommended unless the patient has traveled to an undeveloped area. Finally, after a diagnosis of IBS has been established with confidence, repeated testing is counterproductive unless there is a distinct change in clinical symptoms or new alarm signs develop. This is especially so if endoscopy procedures have already been performed.

Treatment

A validated standardized algorithm for the treatment of IBS does not exist. Treatment therefore depends on the type and severity of symptoms and the nature of associated psychosocial issues in an individual patient. A strong guiding principle is that a robust patient–healthcare provider relationship is an important determinant of outcome and reduction of healthcare usage. Treatments may generally be divided into dietary and lifestyle modifications, pharmacologic agents, and behavioral therapies, all of which have been validated by randomized controlled studies.

Dietary Modifications

Although fiber supplements are widely recommended for IBS, a meta-analysis of seven high-quality studies failed to find significant benefit, although some benefits might occur with soluble fiber (psyllium) versus insoluble fiber (bran) in IBS-C. Unfortunately, fiber supplements may exacerbate symptoms such as abdominal bloating and discomfort.

Other dietary interventions such as gluten-free and low-FODMAP (fermentable oligosaccharides, disaccharides, monosaccharides, and polyols) diets have become increasingly popular. Several studies support the benefit of gluten-free diets in a subset of IBS patients in the absence of celiac disease. It remains uncertain whether the clinical benefits are a consequence of gluten withdrawal, elimination of other wheat proteins and highly fermentable short-chain fatty acids, or a placebo effect. Adding a gluten-free diet to patients who are already on a low-FODMAP diet offers no additional benefits. Monash University has a number of resources including an app that are helpful to patients (https://www.monashfodmap.com/).

There is accumulating evidence from prospective controlled studies that dietary FODMAP restriction is associated with significant symptom improvement in many patients with IBS (Table 3). It appears that restriction of both fructose and fructans is most beneficial. Significant symptom improvement was noted in IBS patients compared with a standard Australian diet and also a National Institute for Health and Care Excellence (England) diet.

Response to a low FODMAP diet is usually assessed after about 2 weeks. Responders are then asked to engage in a structured reintroduction of restricted foods to allow the individual to tailor their diet. It is optimal to involve a properly trained dietitian or nutritionist in the care of these patients.

Pharmacologic Agents

Pharmacologic approaches to IBS may be divided into medications for IBS-C, patients with IBS-D, and for any patient with IBS to ameliorate abdominal pain (Table 4).

Most drugs work through different pathophysiologic mechanisms. For example, for patients with IBS-C, linaclotide (Linzess), plecanatide (Trulance), and lubiprostone (Amitiza) increase intestinal chloride and water secretion to combat constipation, whereas PEG (polyethylene glycol 3350 [MiraLAX])[1] does so through a hyperosmolar effect. Tenapanor (Ibsrela) is a new agent that inhibits sodium absorption to increase water secretion. For IBS-D, rifaximin (Xifaxan) is an antibiotic, loperamide (Imodium)[1] is a peripheral μ-opioid agonist, alosetron (Lotronex) works through the serotonin 3 receptor, and eluxadoline (Viberzi) has effects on all three opioid receptors in the gut (mu, kappa, and delta). Tricyclic antidepressants (TCAs) presumably work via central neurochemical changes, and antispasmodics (dicyclomine [Bentyl], encapsulated oil of peppermint[7]) work largely through peripheral anticholinergic pathways. The large and diverse number of drugs is indicative of the lack of fundamental understanding of IBS. Moreover, few drugs are effective in the majority of IBS patients, and there is no more than a 10% to 15% improvement over placebo in most published studies.

The AGA guidelines published in 2014 incorporated the Grading of Recommendations Assessment, Development and Evaluation methodology and best practices as outlined by the Institute of Medicine. Recommendations are either strong or conditional (weak). The evidence that provides the basis for recommendation is rated high, moderate, or low quality. A similar grading system was used in the recently published American College of Gastroenterology guidelines in 2021.

Of the pharmacologic agents for IBS-C, linaclotide (Linzess) received a strong recommendation with high-quality evidence, lubiprostone (Amitiza) received a conditional recommendation on moderate-quality evidence, and PEG[1] was given a conditional recommendation based on weak evidence. The first two agents showed modest benefit over placebo, whereas there are no data to support the use of PEG. For all three agents, adverse effects were relatively few, and diarrhea is perhaps the major side effect. Both linaclotide and lubiprostone are costly (as are eluxadoline [Viberzi] and plecanatide [Trulance]) and may involve high out-of-pocket expenses for patients.

For IBS-D, both rifaximin (Xifaxan) and alosetron (Lotronex) received conditional recommendations based on moderate-quality evidence. The latter is approved by the US Food and Drug Administration (FDA) only for women who have failed all other treatments. There is a very small risk (approximately 1 case/1000 patient-years) for ischemic colitis with alosetron. Although loperamide (Imodium)[1] has very low-quality evidence to support its use, it can be very effective if used in a proactive fashion.

---

[1] Not FDA approved for this indication.
[7] Available as dietary supplement.

TABLE 4 Pharmacologic Agents for IBS

INDICATION	DRUG	DOSE
IBS-C	Linaclotide (Linzess)	72–290 mcg/d[3]
	Plecanatide (Trulance)	3 mg/d24 mcg bid[3]
	Lubiprostone (Amitiza)	8 mg bid
	PEG-3350 (MiraLAX)[1]	8.5–17 g/d
	Tenapanor (Ibsrela)	50 mg bid
IBS-D	Rifaximin (Xifaxan)	550 mg tid × 2 wk
	Alosetron (Lotronex)	1 mg qd to bid
	Eluxadoline (Viberzi)	75–100 mg/d
	Loperamide (Imodium)[1]	2–16 mg/d
IBS-All	Dicyclomine (Bentyl)	20–40 mg qid
	Desipramine (Norpramin)[1]	10–100 mg/d (desipramine)

[1]Not FDA approved for this indication.
[3]Exceeds dosage recommended by the manufacturer. Per Amitiza's manufacturer package insert, the recommended dose for IBS-C is 8 mcg bid.
IBS, Irritable bowel syndrome; *IBS-C,* irritable bowel syndrome with predominant constipation; *IBS-D,* irritable bowel syndrome with predominant diarrhea.

The case for TCAs and antispasmodics is based on low-quality evidence, but both agents can be very effective for abdominal pain and, in the case of TCAs, for reducing diarrhea in IBS patients.

Behavioral Therapy

For patients with unrelenting IBS symptoms, cognitive-behavioral therapy (CBT) and gut-directed hypnosis have been found to be beneficial. Such therapies should be performed by experienced and well-trained behavioral specialists who are an integral part of the medical team that treats patients with functional GI disorders. The most robust data for efficacy are for CBT. One potential drawback is that these treatments are provider-intensive approaches, but recent studies suggest that CBT can be as effective when given in a shortened course as the traditional method.

References

Buono JL, Carson RT, Flores NM: Health-related quality of life, work productivity, and indirect costs among patients with irritable bowel syndrome with diarrhea, *Health Qual Life Outcomes* 15(1):35, 2017.
Camilleri M: Diagnosis and treatment of irritable bowel syndrome: a review, *JAMA* 325:865, 2021.
Chey WD, et al: AGA Clinical Practice Update on the role of diet in irritable bowel syndrome. Expert review, *Gastroenterology* 162:1737–1745, 2022.
Drossman DA: Functional gastrointestinal disorders: history, pathophysiology, clinical features and Rome IV, *Gastroenterology* 150:1262–1279, 2016.
Eswaran S, Farida JP, Green J, Miller JD, Chey WD: Nutrition in the management of gastrointestinal diseases and disorders: the evidence for the low FODMAP diet, *Curr Opin Pharmacol* 37:151–157, 2017.
Gudleski GD, Satchidanand N, Dunlap LJ, Tahiliani V, Li X, Keefer L, Lackner JM; IBSOS Outcome Study Research Group: Predictors of medical and mental health care use in patients with irritable bowel syndrome in the United States, *Behav Res Ther* 88:65–67, 2017.
Lacey BL, Pimentel M, Brenner DB, et al: ACG Clinical Guideline: management of irritable bowel syndrome, *Am J Gastroenterol* 116:17–44, 2021.
Lembo A, et al: AGA clinical practice guidelines on the pharmacologic management of IBS with diarrhea, *Gastroenterology* 163:137–151, 2022.
Lovell RM, Ford AC: Global prevalence of and risk factors for irritable bowel syndrome: a meta-analysis, *Clin Gastroenterol Hepatol* 10(7):712–721, 2012.
Massey BT, Wald A: Small intestinal bacterial overgrowth: a guide to the use of breath testing, *Dig Dis Sci* 66:338–347, 2021.
Nellesen D, Yee K, Chawla A, Lewis BE, Carson RT: A systematic review of the economic and humanistic burden of illness in irritable bowel syndrome and chronic constipation, *J Manag Care Pharm* 19(9):755–764, 2013.
Radziwon CD, Lackner JM: Cognitive behavioral therapy for IBS: how useful, how often, and how does it work? *Curr Gastroenterol Rep* 19(10):49, 2017.
Rao SS, Yu S, Fedewa A: Systematic review: dietary fiber and FODMAP restricted diet in the management of constipation and IBS, *Aliment Pharm Ther* 41:1256–1270, 2015.
Skodje GI, Sarna VK, Minelle IH, et al: Fructan, rather than gluten, induces symptoms in patients with self-reported non-celiac gluten sensitivity, *Gastroenterology* 154(3):529–539, 2018.
Weinberg DS, Smalley W, Heidelbaugh JJ, Sultan S: American gastroenterological association Institute guideline on the pharmacological management of irritable bowel syndrome, *Gastroenterology* 1146–1148, 2014.

MALABSORPTION

Method of
Lawrence R. Schiller, MD

CURRENT DIAGNOSIS

- Recognize the presence of generalized malabsorption by the combination of typical symptoms: diarrhea, greasy stools, flatulence, weight loss, fatigue, edema.
- Recognize the presence of malabsorption of specific nutrients by associated symptoms and those symptoms particular to deficiency states of the malabsorbed substance: flatus, diarrhea, anemia, dermatitis, glossitis, neuropathy, paresthesias, tetany, ecchymosis.
- Documentation of generalized malabsorption is best done by stool analysis demonstrating steatorrhea and acid stools (reflecting carbohydrate malabsorption). Diagnosis depends on visualization of the small bowel by endoscopy or radiography and small bowel biopsy. Additional tests may be needed.
- Documentation of specific malabsorption is best done by demonstrating low blood levels of the malabsorbed substance or by tests designed to measure absorption of that substance. Diagnosis depends on studies designed to identify the likely diagnosis for a given situation.

CURRENT THERAPY

- Once a diagnosis is reached, therapy can be directed toward that specific problem:
  - Gluten-free diet for celiac disease
  - Antibiotics for bacterial overgrowth
  - Pancreatic enzymes for exocrine pancreatic insufficiency
  - Lactose-free diet for lactase deficiency

Every day the average human being consumes 2000–3000 kcal of food, much of it in the form of polymers or other complex molecules that must be digested and absorbed by the gut. The processes of digestion and absorption are complex and are readily disturbed by pathologic processes. More than 200 conditions have been described that can adversely affect nutrient absorption.

Strictly speaking, *maldigestion* refers to impaired hydrolysis of nutrients, usually due to lack of luminal factors, such as bile acids and pancreatic enzymes, and *malabsorption* refers to impaired mucosal transport. For clinical purposes, "malabsorption" is used to describe both processes.

Malabsorption can be generalized (panmalabsorption) or limited to a specific category of nutrients. Generalized malabsorption is usually due to maldigestion or to extensive mucosal dysfunction. Specific malabsorption occurs when a single transport mechanism is disabled.

The causes of malabsorption can be divided into three categories: impaired luminal hydrolysis, impaired mucosal function (mucosal hydrolysis, uptake, packaging, and excretion), and impaired removal of nutrients from the mucosa (Box 1).

Diagnosis
Symptoms and Signs

Most patients with panmalabsorption have changes in their stools (Box 2). Steatorrhea (excess fat in stools) is characterized by pale color, bulkiness, greasiness, and a tendency to float (probably because of incorporated gas). Occasionally patients with malabsorption present with watery stools due to the osmotic effects of unabsorbed carbohydrates and short-chain fatty acids.

BOX 1 · Causes of Malabsorption or Maldigestion

- Impaired luminal hydrolysis or solublization
  - Bile acid deficiency
  - Impaired mucosal hydrolysis, uptake, or packaging
  - Pancreatic exocrine insufficiency
  - Postgastrectomy syndrome
  - Rapid intestinal transit
  - Small bowel bacterial overgrowth
  - Zollinger-Ellison syndrome
- Brush border or metabolic disorders
  - Abetalipoproteinemia
  - Glucose-galactose malabsorption
  - Lactase deficiency
  - Sucrase-isomaltase deficiency
- Mucosal diseases
  - Amyloidosis
  - Crohn's disease
  - Celiac sprue
  - Collagenous sprue
  - Eosinophilic gastroenteritis
  - Immunoproliferative small intestinal disease (IPSID)
  - Lymphoma
  - Nongranulomatous ulcerative jejunoileitis
  - Drug-induced enteropathy (e.g., olmesartan enteropathy)
  - Radiation enteritis
  - Systemic mastocytosis
- Infectious diseases
  - AIDS enteropathy
  - *Mycobacterium avium-intracellulare*
  - Parasitic diseases
  - Small bowel bacterial overgrowth
  - Tropical sprue
  - Whipple's disease
- After intestinal resection
- Chronic mesenteric ischemia
- Impaired removal of nutrients
  - Lymphangiectasia

BOX 2 · Symptoms and Signs of Malabsorption or Maldigestion

- Changes in stool characteristics
  - Floating stools
  - Pale, bulky, greasy stools
  - Watery diarrhea
- Increased colonic gas production
  - Abdominal distention
  - Borborygmi, increased flatus
- Vitamin and mineral deficiencies
  - Anemia
  - Cheilosis
  - Glossitis
  - Dermatitis
  - Neuropathy
  - Night blindness
  - Osteomalacia
  - Paresthesia
  - Tetany
- Ecchymosis
- Fatigue, weakness
- Edema
- Weight loss, muscle wasting

BOX 3 · Systemic Diseases Associated with Malabsorption or Maldigestion

Endocrine Diseases
- Addison's disease
- Diabetes mellitus
- Hypoparathyroidism
- Hyperthyroidism, hypothyroidism

Collagen-Vascular and Miscellaneous Diseases
- AIDS
- Amyloidosis
- Scleroderma
- Vasculitis (systemic lupus erythematosus, polyarteritis nodosa)

Abdominal distention and excess flatus also commonly occur due to fermentation of unabsorbed carbohydrate by colonic bacteria. This can occur not only with panmalabsorption but also with malabsorption of specific carbohydrates (e.g., lactase deficiency).

Weight loss is typical with severe panmalabsorption, but it might not be very prominent with lesser degrees of malabsorption due to compensatory hyperphagia. Weight loss is most prominent early in the course of the illness, but body weight usually stabilizes as calorie absorption and body weight come into balance again. This is in contrast to illnesses like cancer or tuberculosis that produce continuing weight loss. If a patient with malabsorption has continuing weight loss, inflammatory bowel disease or lymphoma should be considered.

Abdominal pain is usually not present with malabsorption, although some cramping may be associated with diarrhea. Severe pain should bring chronic pancreatitis, Zollinger-Ellison syndrome, lymphoma, Crohn's disease, or mesenteric ischemia to mind.

Constitutional symptoms of fatigue and weakness commonly occur, even early in the course. In contrast, appetite is impaired only late in the course of most malabsorption states. Edema is uncommon until late in the course unless protein-losing enteropathy is present.

Vitamin and mineral deficiencies can lead to several symptoms or signs. Glossitis and cheilosis are common in patients with water-soluble vitamin deficiencies. Florid beriberi, pellagra, and scurvy are not commonly seen unless malabsorption has been particularly severe or long-lasting. Fat-soluble vitamin deficiencies also are unlikely to develop except when malabsorption has been long-standing because of substantial body stores.

Miscellaneous findings occasionally seen in patients with malabsorption can provide clues to the diagnosis. Aphthous ulcers in the mouth may be seen with celiac disease, Behçet's syndrome, or Crohn's disease. Hyperpigmentation is seen in Whipple's disease, and dermatitis herpetiformis (pruritic, blistering skin lesions) is seen in celiac disease. Scleroderma can manifest with tight skin, digital ulceration, nail changes, and Raynaud's phenomenon. Chronic sinusitis, bronchitis, and recurrent pneumonia suggest cystic fibrosis or IgA deficiency. Several systemic diseases can be associated with malabsorption syndrome (Box 3).

Tests

Routine Laboratory Tests

Routine laboratory tests (Box 4) commonly are abnormal in patients with established malabsorption syndrome. Anemia is common but not universal. Iron deficiency anemia may be the only finding in some patients with celiac disease. Microcytic anemia may be present in Whipple's disease (due to occult blood loss) and in lymphomas manifesting with malabsorption. Macrocytic anemia due to folate or vitamin B_{12} deficiency can occur in short bowel syndrome, small bowel bacterial overgrowth, or ileal disease. Lymphopenia may be present in patients with AIDS or lymphangiectasia.

Electrolyte abnormalities may be due to a combination of poor intake and excess loss in stool. Renal function usually is well

Complete Blood Count
- Hemoglobin/hematocrit
- Platelet count
- WBC differential count

Biochemistry Tests
- Blood urea nitrogen
- Prothrombin time
- Serum albumin
- Serum calcium
- Serum creatinine
- Serum potassium

Blood Levels of Potentially Malabsorbed Substances
- Serum iron, vitamin B_{12}, folate, 25-OH vitamin D, carotene

Fat absorption
- Qualitative fecal fat (Sudan stain)
- Quantitative fecal fat (Timed collection)

Protein Absorption and Protein-Losing Enteropathy
- α_1-Antitrypsin clearance
- Fecal nitrogen excretion

Carbohydrate Absorption
- Osmotic gap in stool water
- Quantitative excretion (anthrone)
- Stool pH <5.5
- Stool reducing substances
- D-Xylose absorption test
- Oral glucose, sucrose, and lactose tolerance tests
- Breath hydrogen tests

Vitamin B_{12} Absorption
- Serum B_{12} level

Bile Acid Malabsorption
- Fecal bile acid excretion
- Serum 7α-hydroxy-4-cholesten-3-one (C4)
- ^{75}SeHCAT retention

Small Bowel Bacterial Overgrowth
- ^{14}C-xylose breath test
- Glucose breath hydrogen test
- Quantitative culture of jejunal aspirate

Exocrine Pancreatic Insufficiency
- Secretin/CCK test
- Stool elastase or chymotrypsin concentration

Serologic Testing for Celiac Disease
- Anti-tissue transglutaminase antibody (IgA)
- Anti-endomysial antibody (IgA)

Abbreviations: CCK = cholecystokinin; SLE = systemic lupus erythematosus; ^{75}SeHCAT = selenium-75-labeled taurohomocholic acid; WBC = white blood cell.

Assays are available for several potentially malabsorbed substances, including iron, vitamin B_{12}, folate, 25-hydroxyvitamin D, and β-carotene. Malabsorption tends to lower blood levels, but substantial body stores of many of these can mitigate the reduction in concentration that otherwise might occur. Thus, the sensitivity and specificity of these assays for malabsorption are poor.

Tests for Malabsorption

Fat Malabsorption. The simplest test for fat malabsorption is a qualitative microscopic examination of stool using a fat-soluble stain, such as Sudan III. The finding of more than five stained droplets per high-power field is abnormal and correlates well with quantitative measurement of fecal fat excretion. The test is subject to false-positive results with some drugs and food additives, such as mineral oil, orlistat, and olestra.

A more precise estimate of fat absorption is obtained by a quantitative analysis of a timed stool collection (48 or 72 hours). During the collection, a diary of dietary intake should be maintained so that fat excretion can be assessed as a percentage of intake. Normal fat excretion is <7% of intake when stool weight is normal, but it can be twice as high due to voluminous diarrhea without indicating defective mucosal transport of fat. Thus, fat excretion must be judged against stool weight. Stool fat concentration (grams of fat per 100 grams of stool) also is of value. Pancreatic exocrine insufficiency is associated with high fecal fat concentration (>10 g/100 g stool) because, unlike hydrolyzed fat, unhydrolyzed fat does not stimulate colonic water and electrolyte secretion that would dilute fecal fat concentration.

Protein Malabsorption. Fecal nitrogen excretion can be employed as a marker of protein malabsorption, but is not often used in clinical medicine because it adds little to the evaluation. If protein-losing enteropathy is suspected, an α_1-antitrypsin clearance study can be done. In this study, fecal excretion of α_1-antitrypsin, a serum protein that is relatively resistant to hydrolysis by luminal enzymes, is divided by serum concentration of α_1-antitrypsin, and the volume of serum leaked into the lumen can be calculated. Values of more than 180 mL/day are associated with hypoalbuminemia.

Carbohydrate Malabsorption. Carbohydrate malabsorption is difficult to measure directly because fermentation of malabsorbed carbohydrate by colonic bacteria reduces the amount of intact carbohydrate that can be recovered in stool. Indirect estimates of carbohydrate malabsorption can be made by examining fecal pH (<5.5 with carbohydrate malabsorption) or fecal osmotic gap (> 100 mOsm/kg with osmotic diarrhea) based on chemical analysis of stool water. Oral carbohydrate tolerance tests may be used to evaluate absorption of sugars, such as lactose or fructose. Following an oral load of a given sugar, blood glucose levels are monitored; failure of blood glucose to increase suggests malabsorption.

Another test for carbohydrate malabsorption is the D-xylose absorption test. In this test, a 25-gram dose of D-xylose is given orally; blood xylose levels are measured 1 and 3 hours later, and urinary excretion of xylose is measured for 5 hours. Failure of blood xylose to rise above 20 mg/dL at 1 hour or above 22.5 mg/dL at 3 hours or failure of urinary excretion to exceed 5 g in 5 hours suggests malabsorption. In addition, because xylose does not require pancreatic enzymes or bile acids for absorption, an abnormal D-xylose test suggests a mucosal problem as the cause for malabsorption. The results of this test can be misleading if the patient is dehydrated or has ascites, if renal function is compromised, or if bacterial overgrowth is present in the upper small bowel.

Breath hydrogen testing is another method to assess carbohydrate absorption. If substrates such as lactose or sucrose are not absorbed in the small intestine, they pass into the colon, where bacterial fermentation produces hydrogen gas. The hydrogen is absorbed into the bloodstream and then is exhaled. The concentration of hydrogen in exhaled breath can be measured easily; a rise of more than 10 to 20 ppm after ingestion of a specific substrate is consistent with malabsorption.

maintained in malabsorption syndrome, but blood urea nitrogen may be low due to poor protein absorption, and serum creatinine concentration may be low due to depletion of muscle mass. Serum calcium levels may be low due to malabsorption, vitamin D deficiency, or intraluminal complexing of calcium by fatty acids. Hypomagnesemia can produce hypocalcemia or hypokalemia that is resistant to intravenous repletion. Serum phosphorus, cholesterol, and triglyceride levels may be reduced due to poor intake or malabsorption. Liver tests may be abnormal due to fatty liver. Serum protein and albumin levels are well preserved in patients with malabsorption unless protein-losing enteropathy or an acute illness is present.

Prothrombin time is normal unless vitamin K malabsorption (typically associated with steatorrhea), anticoagulant therapy, antibiotic therapy, or colectomy is present.

False-positive results can be seen in patients with small bowel bacterial overgrowth, and false-negative results can be seen in patients who lack hydrogen-producing flora or who have been on antibiotics recently.

Vitamin B$_{12}$ Malabsorption. Although the Schilling test has been used to measure Vitamin B$_{12}$ absorption, commercial testing kits are no longer available in the United States. Instead, serum B$_{12}$ levels are measured: low levels are consistent with B$_{12}$ malabsorption, but normal levels do not exclude it because enough B$_{12}$ is stored in the liver to maintain serum levels for several years.

Bile Acid Malabsorption. Direct measurement of fecal bile acid excretion in a timed stool specimen can be used to evaluate bile acid malabsorption in the United States. Retention of a radioactive taurocholic acid analogue (SeHCAT, selenium-75-labeled taurohomocholic acid) is used in Europe to assess bile acid malabsorption. Serum 7α-hydroxy-4-cholesten-3-one (C4) reflects bile acid synthesis; higher levels reflect increased synthesis in patients with bile acid malabsorption. The combination of serum C4 and stool bile acid content (from a single stool) has better performance characteristics than either test alone.

Small Bowel Bacterial Overgrowth. The gold standard method used to test for small bowel bacterial overgrowth in the upper intestine is quantitative culture of jejunal fluid. The sample can be obtained during endoscopy and sent to the laboratory with instructions to quantitate the aerobic and anaerobic flora. Finding more than 10^5 bacteria per mL confirms bacterial overgrowth. Breath tests using glucose, ^{14}C-xylose, and lactulose also have been described for this purpose.

Pancreatic Exocrine Insufficiency. Tests for pancreatic exocrine insufficiency are not commonly used. The gold standard test is a secretin test. This study requires duodenal intubation, injection of secretin, and measurement of bicarbonate output. Measurement of fecal chymotrypsin or elastase activity is only moderately useful in predicting the presence of exocrine pancreatic insufficiency. For most situations, a therapeutic trial using a high dose of pancreatic enzymes with monitoring of the effect on steatorrhea is the best that can be done.

Evaluation of Suspected Malabsorption

When malabsorption is suspected because of the history, physical findings, and setting, the physician must decide if the malabsorption involves just carbohydrates or represents a generalized process (Figure 1). If the malabsorption seems to be limited to carbohydrates because stool pH is less than 5.5 and no steatorrhea is present, a diet and symptom diary, breath tests using the presumptively malabsorbed substrate, and stool pH to identify acid stools seen with carbohydrate malabsorption are reasonable diagnostic maneuvers.

Suspected generalized malabsorption requires a more intense evaluation. If steatorrhea is confirmed, serology for celiac disease (IgA anti–tissue transglutaminase, and IgA level to exclude IgA deficiency) should be obtained and the small bowel should be visualized with either capsule endoscopy or radiography (small bowel follow-through examination, magnetic resonance enterography, or computed tomography) and biopsied from above by enteroscopy and from below by colonoscopy. During enteroscopy, an aspirate of small bowel contents can be obtained for quantitative culture to look for small bowel bacterial overgrowth. An alternative method to detect small bowel bacterial overgrowth is breath testing (see earlier). Stool samples also should be examined with microscopy or immunoassay for the presence of parasites that may be associated with malabsorption.

This sequence of evaluation often leads to a specific diagnosis. When it does not, empiric trials of high-dose pancreatic enzyme replacement, low-dose bile acid supplementation, or antibiotics can lead to a presumptive diagnosis of pancreatic exocrine insufficiency, bile acid deficiency, or small intestinal bacterial overgrowth.. Hard endpoints (e.g., reduction in quantitative fat excretion) should be used to assess the effectiveness of these empiric trials.

Specific Disorders Associated With Malabsorption
Malabsorption of Specific Nutrients
Disaccharidase Deficiency

Ingested disaccharides such as lactose and sucrose and starch-digestion products such as maltotriose and α-limit dextrins must be hydrolyzed by brush border enzymes into monosaccharides for absorption by the mucosa. If these brush border enzymes are not active or if the brush border is damaged, malabsorption of the specific carbohydrate substrate results. This can result in gaseousness or osmotic diarrhea when those substrates are ingested. This rarely occurs on a congenital basis, but it commonly occurs as an acquired disorder.

Lactase deficiency is the most common acquired disaccharidase deficiency. Infant mammals all rely on lactose as the carbohydrate source in milk, but lactase activity is shut off after weaning in most species. Most human populations lose lactase activity during adolescence as a normal part of maturation. Members of the northern European gene pool typically maintain lactase activity into adult life, but lactase activity declines gradually in many. At some point the amount of lactose ingested might exceed the ability of the remaining enzyme to hydrolyze it, resulting in lactose malabsorption and symptoms. This also can occur with acute conditions such as gastroenteritis that can disturb the mucosa and temporarily reduce lactase activity. Patients might not recognize lactose ingestion as a cause of their problem because they have not had difficulty tolerating lactose in the past. Restriction of lactose in the diet (or use of products that have predigested lactose) mitigates symptoms. Use of exogenous lactase as a tablet may only be partially effective because of incomplete hydrolysis of ingested lactose.

In an analogous way, an acquired lack of sucrase-isomaltase activity might lead to digestive symptoms often interpreted as irritable bowel syndrome. This condition can be diagnosed by breath testing and treated with a restrictive diet and sacrosidase, a yeast enzyme with sucrase activity.

Transport Defects at the Brush Border

Glucose-galactose malabsorption is a rare congenital disorder resulting from an inactive hexose transporter in the brush border. Hydrolysis of lactose is intact, but transport across the apical membrane of the enterocyte fails to occur. Fructose absorption, which is mediated by a different carrier, is unaffected.

In all human beings, the ability to absorb fructose is limited by the availability of carriers in the brush border and may be overwhelmed when excess fructose is ingested. This can occur relatively easily nowadays, because high-fructose corn syrup is used frequently as a sweetener in commercial products such as soda pop. Limiting the amount of fructose ingested will reduce symptoms.

Abetalipoproteinemia is a rare condition that prevents absorption of long-chain fatty acids due to failure to form chylomicrons. Use of medium-chain triglycerides that do not require transport in chylomicrons can bypass this defect.

Pernicious anemia develops when failure to secrete intrinsic factor in the stomach prevents vitamin B$_{12}$ absorption by the ileal mucosa. Parenteral replacement with cyanocobalamin by injection (Cyanoject) or nasal spray (Nascobal) is necessary.

Generalized Malabsorption
Celiac Disease

Celiac disease (also known as celiac sprue) is a disorder in which the mucosa of the small bowel is damaged due to activation of the mucosal immune system by ingestion of gluten, a protein component found in wheat, barley, and rye. People who have HLA-DQ2 or DQ8 are susceptible to this condition because these specific antigen-presenting proteins produce particularly strong reactions by interacting with a unique peptide digestion product of gluten. Tissue transglutaminase, an enzyme produced in the mucosa, is an important cofactor in pathogenesis by amplifying the immunogenicity of gluten peptide fragments and is the target of autoantibodies that are characteristic of this disease. The condition produces generalized malabsorption by destroying the villi of the small intestine, reducing the surface area available for absorption.

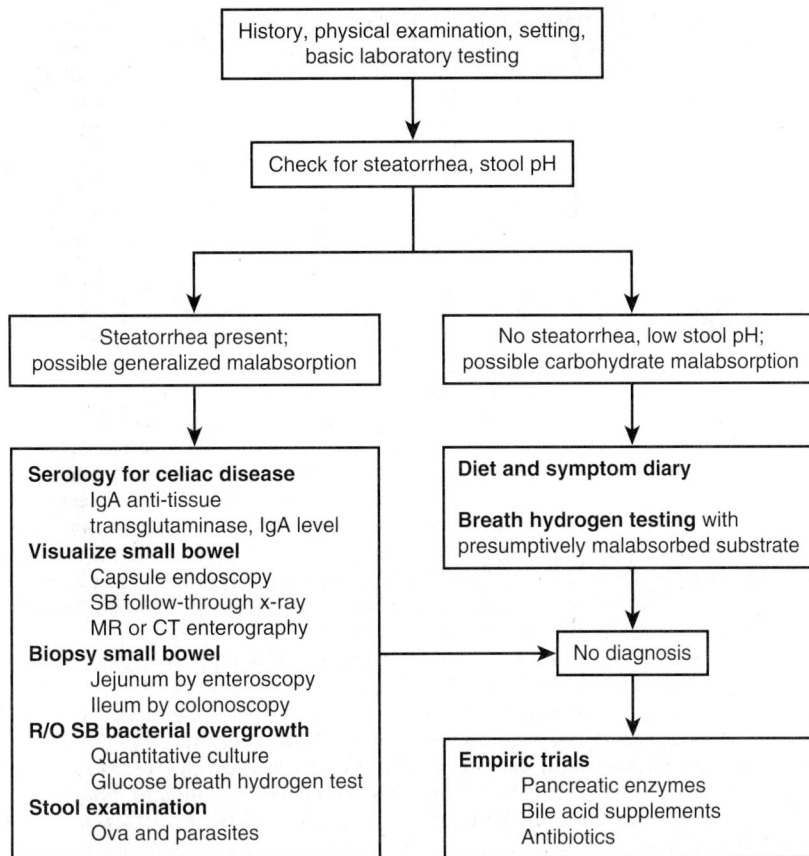

Figure 1 Flow chart for evaluation of malabsorption or maldigestion. *Abbreviations:* CT = computed tomography; MR = magnetic resonance; R/O = rule out; SB = small bowel.

In addition to malabsorption syndrome with diarrhea and weight loss, celiac disease can produce a host of nonspecific symptoms, including abdominal pain, fatigue, muscle and joint pains, and headaches and seemingly unrelated problems such as iron deficiency anemia, abnormal liver tests, and osteoporosis. These protean manifestations mean that celiac disease must be considered in the differential diagnosis of many conditions. The clinical course is quite variable, with symptoms coming and going. Symptoms can develop during childhood and produce growth retardation or first become manifest in adulthood.

Testing for celiac disease has been simplified by the development of an assay for anti–tissue transglutaminase antibodies. This test largely supplants measurement of antigluten antibodies, although these remain of some use in evaluating adherence to a gluten-free diet. IgA antibodies are the most useful for diagnosis, but IgA deficiency is common enough that an IgA level should be measured concomitantly.

Although serologic tests have high sensitivity and specificity, the implications of adhering to a gluten-free diet are so extreme that the diagnosis of celiac disease should be confirmed whenever possible by small bowel mucosal biopsy, now obtained routinely by endoscopy. An empiric trial of a gluten-free diet may be difficult to interpret because many persons with gastrointestinal symptoms improve with dietary carbohydrate restriction. Wheat starch is particularly hard to digest; ordinarily 20% of wheat starch is not digested and absorbed by the small bowel, and enters the colon where it can produce symptoms.

Treatment of celiac disease at present involves strict lifetime exclusion of gluten from the diet. This is a difficult regimen that excludes most processed foods. Assistance of a dietitian is most helpful. The prognosis with effective treatment is very good. Symptoms should respond to the diet within weeks; failure to do so should prompt an examination of compliance with the diet or reconsideration of the diagnosis. Failure to respond may be seen when lymphoma or

adenocarcinoma complicate the course of celiac disease or in cases of "refractory sprue" or "collagenous sprue," which can have a different autoimmune basis from classic celiac disease and which might respond to immunosuppressive drugs such as corticosteroids or azathioprine (Imuran).[1] Persistent diarrhea may be observed in patients with celiac disease who have concomitant microscopic colitis, another condition that is linked to HLA-DQ2 and HLA-DQ8.

Olmesartan (Benicar) and perhaps other angiotensin II receptor blockers can produce enteropathies resembling celiac disease clinically, but which are not related to gluten ingestion. Diarrhea and malabsorption resolve with discontinuing the medication.

Inflammatory Diseases

Diseases that produce extensive mucosal damage by inflammation cause generalized malabsorption by reduction of mucosal surface area, by promotion of small bowel bacterial overgrowth, by ileal dysfunction, or by development of enteroenteral or enterocolic fistulas. Examples include jejunoileitis due to Crohn's disease, nongranulomatous ulcerative jejunoileitis, radiation enteritis, and chronic mesenteric ischemia. With Crohn's disease, previous resection can add to the problem (see later). Therapy aimed at the underlying process can improve absorption; in some cases (e.g., radiation enteritis), no effective therapy is available for the underlying problem, and symptomatic management is all that is possible. This includes use of antidiarrheal drugs to prolong contact time between luminal contents and the small bowel mucosa, ingestion of a reduced-fat diet to reduce steatorrhea, and use of vitamin and mineral supplements to prevent deficiency states.

Infiltrative Disorders

Several conditions involve infiltration of the intestinal mucosa with cells or extracellular matrix that impede absorption or

---

[1]Not FDA approved for this indication.

modify mucosal function by secretion of cytokines and other regulatory substances. These include eosinophilic gastroenteritis, systemic mastocytosis, immunoproliferative small intestinal disease (IPSID), lymphoma, and amyloidosis. These conditions are diagnosed by mucosal biopsy, but special stains might have to be employed to identify the infiltrating cells or matrix accurately.

Treatment of the underlying processes can improve absorption, but it is not uniformly effective. For eosinophilic gastroenteritis, a hypoallergenic (elimination) diet and corticosteroids may be useful. Mild systemic mastocytosis is treated with the mast cell-stabilizer sodium chromoglycate, H_1- and H_2-receptor antagonists, and low-dose aspirin.[1] More advanced disease might respond to interferon or cytotoxic chemotherapy. IPSID initially is treated with antibiotics, because small bowel bacterial overgrowth may be a causative factor. Once malignant change has occurred, it is treated like lymphoma with cytotoxic chemotherapy. Amyloidosis affecting the gut is not amenable to therapy and is usually fatal.

Infectious Diseases

Small Bowel Bacterial Overgrowth. Small bowel bacterial overgrowth in the jejunum can produce generalized malabsorption. It can occur whenever the mechanisms that reduce overgrowth are compromised. These situations include achlorhydria or hypochlorhydria, motility disorders of the small intestine (e.g., diabetes mellitus or scleroderma), and anatomic alterations (e.g., diverticulosis, gastrocolic fistula, or blind loops postoperatively). Fat malabsorption is attributed to bacterial deconjugation of bile acid. Bacterial toxins or free fatty acids can produce patchy mucosal damage, leading to less efficient carbohydrate and protein absorption. Bacteria also can compete with the mucosa for uptake of certain nutrients such as vitamin B_{12}.

Diagnosis of small bowel bacterial overgrowth can be difficult (see earlier). Treatment consists of antibiotic therapy unless a surgically correctable anatomic defect is discovered. Tetracycline is no longer uniformly effective; amoxicillin–clavulanic acid (Augmentin), cephalosporins, ciprofloxacin (Cipro), metronidazole (Flagyl), and rifaximin (Xifaxan)[1] may be employed. Therapy should be given for 1 to 2 weeks initially and then discontinued. It should be restarted when symptoms recur. If this occurs quickly, longer treatment periods should be considered. Continuous antibiotic therapy is needed rarely.

Tropical Sprue. Tropical sprue is a progressive, chronic malabsorptive condition occurring in both the indigenous population and in visitors residing in certain tropical countries for extended periods. The prevalence of tropical sprue seems to be decreasing for uncertain reasons. The disease starts as an acute diarrheal disease that becomes a persistent diarrhea associated with substantial weight loss and typically megaloblastic anemia. Villi become shortened and thickened (partial villous atrophy), but the flat mucosa of celiac disease is not usually present. Enterocytes have disrupted brush borders and can have megaloblastic changes; the submucosa has a chronic inflammatory infiltrate. Intestinal biopsy is required for diagnosis.

Currently, tropical sprue is believed to represent a form of bacterial overgrowth with organisms that secrete enterotoxins. Most patients have evidence of excessive gram-negative bacterial colonization of the jejunum. The declining prevalence of tropical sprue may be due to improved nutrition, better sanitation, or prompt treatment of acute diarrhea with antibiotics. Treatment consists of pharmacologic doses of folic acid (folate) (5 mg daily[3]), injection of cyanocobalamin (if deficient), and antibiotic therapy for 1 to 6 months. Tetracycline 250 mg four times a day or sulfonamide is the treatment of choice. Newer antibiotics have not been tested extensively in this condition. Improvement should be noted after a few weeks. The prognosis with treatment is excellent; without treatment, tropical sprue can be fatal. Recurrence can occur.

Whipple's Disease. Whipple's disease is a rare chronic bacterial infection with multisystem involvement. The small bowel typically is heavily infiltrated with foamy macrophages containing periodic acid–Schiff (PAS)-positive material, distorting the villi. Small bowel biopsy with special stains or electron microscopy or a specific polymerase chain reaction (PCR) is diagnostic. Foamy macrophages and bacteria can be found outside the intestine in lymph nodes, spleen, liver, central nervous system, heart, and synovium. Accordingly, symptoms are protean. The bacterium has been identified as *Tropheryma whipplei*, a relative of *Acinetobacter*. It does not appear to be very contagious, and no direct person-to-person transmission has been demonstrated. Presumably, differences in host resistance allow proliferation within macrophages without clearance of the bacteria.

Whipple's disease occurs mainly in older white men, but women and all ethnic groups are susceptible. Patients can present with malabsorption syndrome or with symptoms related to the extraintestinal disease (arthritis, endocarditis, fever, dementia, headache, or muscle weakness). Gross or occult gastrointestinal bleeding can occur. Protein-losing enteropathy may be present.

Treatment with any of several antibiotics (penicillin, erythromycin, ampicillin, tetracycline, chloramphenicol, or trimethoprim-sulfamethoxazole [TMP-SMX]) produces excellent symptomatic responses within days to weeks, but it should be continued for months to years. Even with protracted courses, relapses are common.

Other Infections. *Mycobacterium avium–intracellulare* is another chronic bacterial infection that can cause malabsorption, particularly in patients with AIDS. Mucosal biopsy with special stains to distinguish it from Whipple's disease is essential. Antibiotic therapy can reduce the intensity of infection; clearance depends on immunologic reconstitution with antiretroviral therapy. Clarithromycin (Biaxin) and ethambutol (Myambutol) are recommended as initial therapy.

Parasitic diseases can produce malabsorption by competing for nutrients and causing mechanical occlusion of the absorptive surface and epithelial damage. Protozoa that may be associated with malabsorption include *Giardia lamblia*, *Cystoisospora belli*, *Cryptosporidium*, and *Enterocytozoon bieneusi*. Tapeworms associated with malabsorption include *Taenia saginata* (beef tapeworm), *Hymenolepis nana* (dwarf tapeworm), and *Diphyllobothrium latum* (fish tapeworm).

Tapeworms compete with their hosts for nutrients in the lumen. Diphyllobothrium latum can produce vitamin B_{12} deficiency. The others can result in more extensive nutritional deficiencies. Diagnosis is based on stool examination, and treatment depends on the particular organism identified.

Giardia lamblia is a cosmopolitan parasite acquired from contaminated water or from another person by fecal-oral transmission. Cysts are relatively hardy, and ingestion of as few as 10 cysts is sufficient to establish infection. Patients with dysgammaglobulinemia (especially IgA deficiency) are likely to become infected. Diagnosis depends on finding the organism (cysts or trophozoites) in stool by microscopy (sensitivity ~50% for a single specimen), or detection of giardia antigens by immunologic testing of stool (sensitivity >90%), multiplex PCR testing (sensitivity >95%), or discovery of the organism on small bowel biopsy.

Therapy consists of a single dose of tinidazole (Tindamax) (2 g), metronidazole (Flagyl)[1] (250 mg three times a day for a week), nitazoxanide (Alinia) (500 mg twice a day for three days), or quinacrine[2] (100 mg three times a day for a week).

Cystoisospora and *Cryptosporidium* spp. are coccidia, protozoa that disrupt the epithelium by intracellular invasion (*Cystoisospora*) or by attaching to the brush border, destroying microvilli (*Cryptosporidium*). Stool examination or small bowel biopsy can identify the organism. *Cryptosporidium* can be discovered by antigen immunoassay or multiplex PCR testing on stool with excellent sensitivity. *Cystoisospora* can be treated with

---

[1]Not FDA approved for this indication.
[3]Exceeds dosage recommended by the manufacturer.

---

[1]Not FDA approved for this indication.
[2]Not available in the United States.

trimethoprim/sulfamethoxazole (TMP-SMX)[1] or furazolidone.[2] *Cryptosporidium* can be treated by nitazoxanide.

Microsporidia are intracellular organisms now believed to be most closely related to fungi and are implicated in diarrhea and malabsorption in patients with AIDS and other immunodeficiency states. Small bowel biopsy can show partial villous atrophy, and electron microscopy displays characteristic changes. Stool examination occasionally is helpful. No treatment is of proven value.

Luminal Problems Causing Malabsorption

Pancreatic Exocrine Insufficiency. Pancreatic exocrine insufficiency is the most common luminal problem that results in maldigestion. Patients develop symptoms of malabsorption when pancreatic enzyme secretion is reduced by >90%. There are several clinical features that distinguish pancreatic exocrine insufficiency from mucosal disorders, such as celiac disease. When fat is not digested, it is transported through the gastrointestinal tract as intact triglyceride, which can appear as oil in the stool. In contrast, if fat is digested but not absorbed, it is in the form of fatty acids that can produce secretory diarrhea in the colon, resulting in more voluminous, even watery stools. This has two important ramifications: Fecal fat concentration is lower with mucosal disease (typically <9% by weight), and hypocalcemia due to formation of soaps (calcium plus 2 fatty acids) is seen with mucosal disease but not with pancreatic exocrine insufficiency. In addition, patients with mucosal disease tend to have more problems with water-soluble vitamin deficiencies than those with pancreatic exocrine insufficiency. In some patients with pancreatic exocrine insufficiency, carbohydrate malabsorption can produce substantial bloating, flatulence, and watery diarrhea.

Tests to document pancreatic exocrine insufficiency are not widely available or are nonspecific (see earlier), and so diagnosis usually hinges on a consistent history, demonstration of anatomic problems in the pancreas (calcification or abnormal ducts), and documentation of a response of steatorrhea to empiric treatment with a large dose of exogenous enzymes.

Bile Acid Deficiency. Bile acid deficiency is a less common cause of maldigestion, and malabsorption in this setting is limited to fat and fat-soluble vitamins. The usual setting is a patient with an extensive ileal resection (see later), but this also occurs in certain cholestatic conditions in which bile acid secretion by the liver is markedly compromised, such as advanced primary biliary cholangitis or complete extrahepatic biliary obstruction. As with pancreatic exocrine insufficiency, stools tend to have high fat concentrations (>9% by weight) when bile acid secretion is limited by hepatic or biliary disorders.

Zollinger-Ellison Syndrome. Zollinger-Ellison syndrome produces several abnormalities that can affect absorption. High rates of gastric acid secretion produce persistently low pH in the duodenum, which precipitates bile acid and inactivates pancreatic enzymes. In addition, excess acid can damage the absorptive cells directly.

Postoperative Malabsorption

Substantial malabsorption can result from bariatric or other gastric surgeries. Weight loss can result from inadequate intake due to early satiety or symptoms of dumping syndrome. Malabsorption can result from impaired mechanical disruption of food, mismatching of chyme delivery and enzyme secretion, rapid transit, or small bowel bacterial overgrowth due to loss of the gastric acid barrier. In addition, gastric surgery sometimes brings out latent celiac disease.

Short intestinal resections are well tolerated, but more extensive resections produce diarrhea and malabsorption of variable severity. When these symptoms are associated with weight loss or dehydrating diarrhea, short bowel syndrome is said to exist. In general, nutrient absorptive needs can be met if at least 100 cm of jejunum are preserved, but fluid absorption will be insufficient and diarrhea may be profuse. The process of intestinal adaptation permits improved absorption with time; it depends on exposure of the absorptive surface to nutrients. Absorption of specific substances, such as bile acids or vitamin B_{12}, is reduced permanently by resection of the terminal ileum.

Malabsorption in short bowel syndrome is not due solely to loss of absorptive surface area. Gastric acid hypersecretion, bile acid deficiency, rapid transit (due to loss of the ileal brake), and bacterial overgrowth may be present. These conditions are amenable to treatment and therapy with antisecretory drugs, exogenous bile acids, opiate antidiarrheals, or antibiotics can produce substantial improvement. Injection of teduglutide (Gattex), a glucagon-like peptide-2 intestinal growth factor, or growth hormone in combination with glutamine and a special diet have been approved as treatments for short bowel syndrome; they can reduce the volume of parenteral fluid or nutrients required. Results with small bowel transplantation are improving with the use of better immunosuppressive regimens, and it remains the only cure for select patients with postresection malabsorption.

Attention to nutrition is vital in any patient with malabsorption. If adequate nutrition cannot be maintained by oral intake, nutritional therapy is needed. Because of impaired bowel function, success with enteral nutrition may be impossible; parenteral nutrition may be needed. It is important to distinguish between the need for supplemental fluid and electrolytes and the need for nutrients; total parenteral nutrition is not a good choice for patients who only require fluids and electrolytes.

References

Boumaza A, Azzouz EB, Arrindell J, et al.: Whipple's disease and Tropheryma whipplei infections: from bench to bedside, *Lancet Infect Dis* 22:e280–e291, 2022.

Bushyhead D, Quigley EMM: Small intestinal bacterial overgrowth—pathophysiology and its implications for definition and management, *Gastroenterology* 163:593–607, 2022.

Fernandez-Bañares F: Carbohydrate malabsorption and intolerance, *Nutrients* 14:1923, 2022.

Ito S, Ishiyama Y, Amiki M: Prognostic factor of patients with short bowel syndrome due to non-Crohn disease: a single institutional observational study, *Medicine (Baltimore)* 103(35):e39460, 2024.

Lenti MV, Hammer HF, Tacheci I, et al.: European consensus on malabsorption-UEG & SIGE, LGA, SPG, SRGH, CGS, ESPCG, EAGEN, ESPEN, and ESPGHAN: Part 2: Screening, special populations, nutritional goals, supportive care, primary care perspective, *United European Gastroenterol J* 13(5):773–779, 2025.

Lupianez-Merly C, Dilmaghani S, Camilleri M: Recent developments in diagnosing bile acid diarrhea, *Expert Rev Gastroenterol Hepatol* 17:1185–1195, 2023.

Omer E, Chiodi C: Fat digestion and absorption: normal physiology and pathophysiology of malabsorption, including diagnostic testing, *Nutr Clin Pract* 39 (Suppl 1):S6–S16, 2024.

Pop A, Popa SL, Pop DD, et al.: Self-perceived lactose intolerance versus confirmed lactose intolerance in irritable bowel syndrome: a systematic review, *J Gastrointest Liver Dis* 2024. https://doi.org/10.15403/jgld-5836.

Rubio-Tapia A, Hill ID, Semrad C, et al.: American College of Gastroenterology guidelines update: diagnosis and management of celiac disease, *Am J Gastroenterol* 118:59–76, 2023.

Whitcomb DC, Buchner AM, Forsmark CE: AGA clinical practice update on the epidemiology, evaluation, and management of exocrine pancreatic insufficiency: expert review, *Gastroenterology* 165:1292-1301, 2023.

METABOLIC DYSFUNCTION-ASSOCIATED STEATOTIC LIVER DISEASE (MASLD)

Method of
Katharine Tippins, MD; Nicole Boschuetz, MD; and Adnan Said, MD, MS

CURRENT DIAGNOSIS

- Suspected in patients with steatosis noted on imaging or elevated liver enzymes (alanine aminotransferase, aspartate aminotransferase, γ-glutamyl transferase) in the setting of one or more cardiometabolic risk factors*

---

[1]Not FDA approved for this indication.
[2]Not available in the United States.

- Rule out other causes of steatotic liver disease
  - Quantify alcohol use by history
  - Hepatitis C antibody and hepatitis B surface antigen should be negative
  - Review medications that can cause steatosis (methotrexate [Trexall], tamoxifen [Nolvadex], diltiazem [Cardizem], amiodarone [Pacerone], steroids)
  - Check serum ferritin, iron saturation (hemochromatosis)
  - Check serum ceruloplasmin and unbound copper (Wilson disease)
  - Check autoantibodies (antinuclear antibody, antismooth muscle antibody) (autoimmune hepatitis)
- Liver biopsy gold standard
  - Not essential for diagnosis
  - Useful for diagnosis of metabolic dysfunction–associated steatohepatitis (MASH) and fibrosis
  - Useful in excluding other conditions (if the preceding tests raise suspicion)
- Noninvasive serum tests (more useful for diagnosis or exclusion of advanced fibrosis and potentially in decision of whom to biopsy or perform elastography)
  - Nonalcoholic fatty liver disease fibrosis score
  - Fibrosis-4 index
- Noninvasive imaging tests for diagnosis of steatosis
  - Transient elastography with controlled attenuation parameter score
  - Right upper quadrant ultrasound
  - MRI liver with proton density fat fraction
- Noninvasive imaging tests for diagnosis of fibrosis
  - Transient elastography with FibroScan
  - Magnetic resonance elastography

*Cardiometabolic risk factors include BMI ≥ 25 kg/m^2 or waist circumference >94 cm (men) or >80 cm (women) or ethnically adjusted equivalent; fasting serum glucose ≥100 mg/dL or 2-hour post load glucose levels ≥40 mg/dL or type 2 diabetes mellitus (T2DM) or treatment for T2DM or HbA1c ≥5.7%; blood pressure ≥130/85 or use of antihypertensive drug treatment; plasma triglyceride ≥150 mg/dL or use of lipid-lowering agent; and plasma high-density lipoprotein <40 mg/dL or use of lipid-lowering agent.

CURRENT THERAPY

Lifestyle Modifications Mainstay of Therapeutic Plan
- Goal is to lose 7% to 10% of body weight gradually over 6 to 12 months
- Lose no more than 1 to 2 lbs/week

Dietary Modification
- Reduce calories by 30% (500–1000 kcal/day)
- Reduce sugars, simple carbohydrates, fructose-enriched foods, or sugar-sweetened beverages
- Reduce consumption of processed foods and saturated fat
- Coffee consumption (>3 cups/day, avoid adding sugar, syrups) has been shown to be beneficial

Exercise
- 150 to 200 minutes per week divided over 3 to 5 days
- Moderate-to-vigorous intensity (swimming, biking, jogging, playing tennis, weights)

Pharmacotherapeutics
- Resmetirom (Rezdiffra) is FDA approved and can be used for diabetic or nondiabetic metabolic dysfunction–associated steatohepatitis (MASH) with fibrosis to reduce hepatic fat content and decrease fibrosis
- Pioglitazone (Actos)[1] can be used for diabetic or nondiabetic MASH but causes weight gain and does not treat fibrosis
- Vitamin E (800 IU/day)[7] can be used for nondiabetic MASH but does not treat fibrosis

Surgery
- Bariatric surgery can be considered if indicated for morbid obesity, complications of metabolic syndrome, and may reverse MASH

[1]Not FDA approved for this indication.
[7]Available as dietary supplement.

New Nomenclature

In 2023 the American Association for the Study of Liver Diseases (AASLD) in conjunction with other international societies released a new consensus statement for a change in the nomenclature of fatty liver disease, now called steatotic liver disease (SLD) to reduce the stigma associated with the previously used terms such as "fatty" and "nonalcoholic" and to more accurately capture the etiology of the liver disease. Nonalcoholic fatty liver disease (NAFLD) should now be referred to as metabolic dysfunction–associated steatotic liver disease (MASLD). MASLD is defined as the presence of hepatic steatosis and at least one cardiometabolic risk factor (CMRF) (BMI ≥25 kg/m^2 or waist circumference >94 cm (men) or >80 cm (women) or ethnically adjusted equivalent; fasting serum glucose ≥100 mg/dL or 2-hour post load glucose levels ≥40 mg/dL or type 2 diabetes mellitus (T2DM) or treatment for T2DM or hemoglobin A1c (HbA1c) ≥5.7%; blood pressure ≥130/85 or use of antihypertensive drug treatment; plasma triglyceride ≥150 mg/dL or use of lipid-lowering agent; and plasma high-density lipoprotein <40 mg/dL or use of lipid-lowering agent). Similarly, metabolic dysfunction–associated steatohepatitis (MASH) has replaced the term *nonalcoholic steatohepatitis* (NASH). These changes have made MASLD now a "positive" diagnosis that can be diagnosed by meeting defined criteria instead of a diagnosis of exclusion. The umbrella of SLD also includes alcohol-related liver disease (ALD) and a new category of MASLD with alcohol use (MetALD). MetALD has been introduced to include patients who previously would be excluded from the categories of NAFLD, NASH, or ALD due to low or moderate alcohol use in the setting of metabolic risk factors. There are other causes of SLD, including medications and monogenic conditions not discussed in this chapter.

While much of the data discussed in this chapter rely on the previously defined NAFLD/NASH, studies published in the 2020s since the adoption of the new nomenclature have shown high concordance rates between MASLD and NAFLD when applied to previous cohort populations, including a 99% concordance in a US population cohort. Given these high concordance rates, MASLD and NAFLD can be used interchangeably, and the previous data and studies on patients with NAFLD remain true. As such, NAFLD will be referred to as MASLD throughout this chapter even if the studies were performed before the adoption of the new nomenclature.

Metabolic Dysfunction–Associated Steatotic Liver Disease

MASLD is defined as the presence of hepatic steatosis (hepatic fat accumulation), on imaging or liver biopsy, in the presence of at least one CMRF. (The CMRF are defined in the "New Nomenclature" section and in the "Current Therapy" box footnote.) Additionally, other causes of SLD should be ruled out, such as excessive alcohol consumption, hepatitis B or C, or certain medications. MASLD is the most common cause of chronic liver disease worldwide.

MASLD is a spectrum of disease spanning from isolated steatosis to more advanced liver disease such as MASH (Figure 1). MASH signifies steatosis with inflammation and hepatocyte injury and has a higher likelihood of progression to cirrhosis, liver failure, and occasionally liver cancer. Besides liver disease, MASLD is also closely associated with cardiovascular disease and malignancy.

Epidemiology of MASLD

The global prevalence of MASLD has surged from 25.3% (1990–2006) to 38.2% (2016–2019), reflecting an almost 50% rise

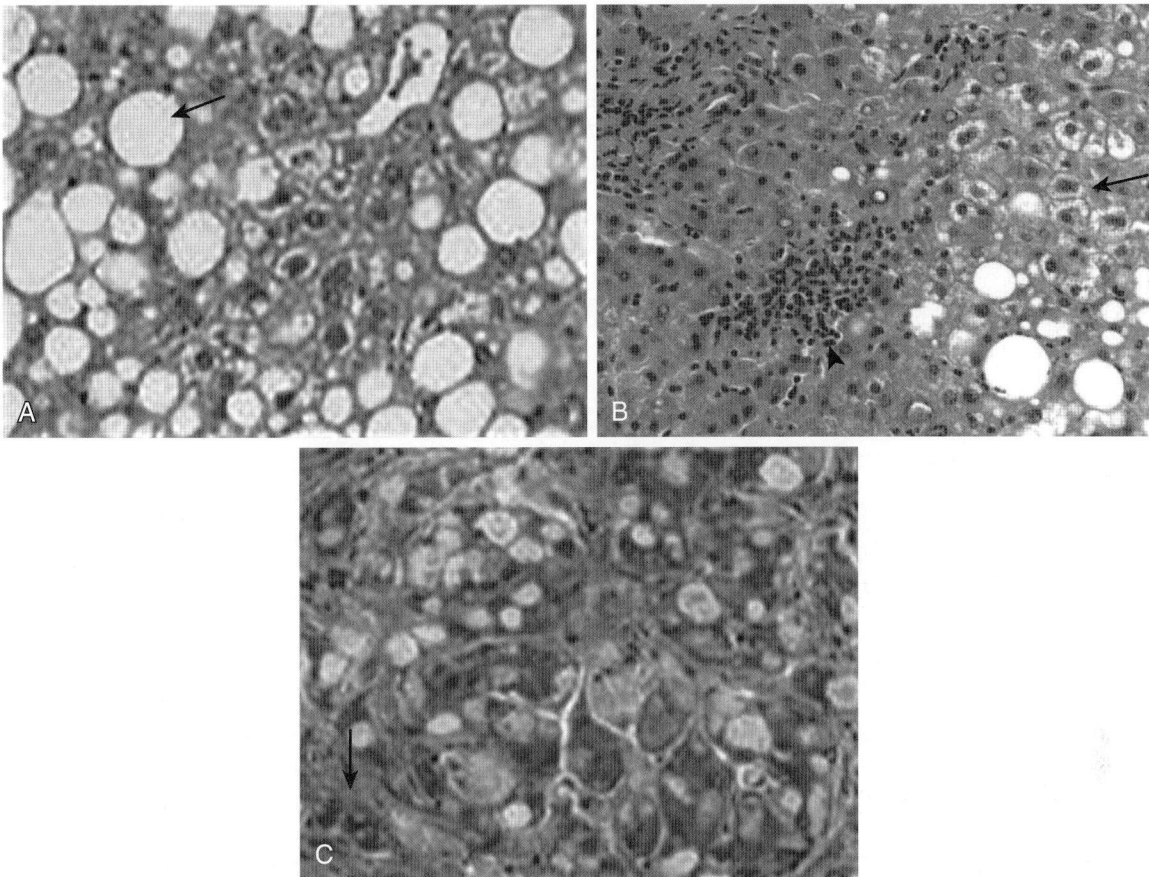

Figure 1 Histology of metabolic dysfunction–associated steatotic liver disease. (A) Hepatic steatosis. *Arrow* points to macrovesicular steatosis in hepatocytes. (B) Metabolic dysfunction–associated steatohepatitis (MASH). *Arrow* points to ballooned hepatocytes. *Arrowhead* points to lobular inflammation. (C) MASH with cirrhosis. *Arrow* points to fibrosis bands (collagen). Trichrome stain.

over the past 30 years, and it has become the leading cause of chronic liver disease worldwide. This dramatic rise has occurred in parallel with rising global prevalence of other metabolic syndromes. Additionally, MASLD is emerging as the fastest-growing contributor to liver-related health complications, including cirrhosis, liver failure, and hepatocellular carcinoma (HCC). Alarmingly, the prevalence in North America was reported to be 48% with the National Health and Nutrition Examination Survey (NHANES) data from 2017 to 2018 demonstrating a prevalence of up to 59% in the United States. Other notable rates include 32% in Asia and 33% in Europe. There are limited recent studies from the 2020s for South America and Africa, though previous rates have been estimated to be 30% and 14%, respectively.

In the United States the prevalence of MASLD is highest in Hispanic Americans (22%–45%), followed by non-Hispanic White Americans (15%–33%) and African Americans (13%–24%). A significant contribution to this ethnic difference can be explained by genetic differences, particularly a single nucleotide polymorphism (SNP) in a gene *(PNPLA3)* that is involved in triglyceride (lipid) hydrolysis in the liver and the ethnic prevalence of which mirrors the ethnic differences in frequency of MASLD.

MASLD prevalence increases with age, with a range from 22% to 30% from age 30 to a peak in the sixth decade. Very few studies report on MASLD prevalence after age 70, but one 2024 Australian study demonstrated that 33% of individuals over 70 had persistent MASLD, though incidence did decline with age after that point. Pediatric MASLD is on the rise paralleling childhood obesity trends, but population data are scant, with estimated population prevalence of 7% to 8% in the United States. An autopsy study of 742 children (ages 2–19 years) who died of unnatural causes used liver histology as the gold standard and demonstrated a MASLD prevalence of 9.6% adjusted for age, sex, race, and ethnicity. Pediatric obesity clinic studies have shown MASLD

prevalence of 34.2% in a meta-analysis. Differences in sex prevalence also exist with some studies reporting the prevalence of MASLD in men significantly higher than women (40% vs. 26%).

Although the prevalence of infectious hepatitis has remained stable and even declined, the prevalence of MASLD has been rising in the global and US adult and pediatric populations, growing in parallel with the epidemic of obesity and metabolic syndrome. In higher-risk populations, such as patients with diabetes, the prevalence of MASLD is as high as 80% in some regions. In patients with morbid obesity attending bariatric surgery clinics, the prevalence of MASLD has been reported at 95%.

Risk Factors for MASLD

MASLD is a complex disease that has genetic predispositions and is affected by various environmental factors. The degree of contribution of each of the risk factors requires further study and may vary depending on region of the world.

MASLD is regarded as the hepatic manifestation of the metabolic syndrome (presence of at least three of the following: abdominal obesity, hypertriglyceridemia, low high-density lipoprotein levels, hypertension, and high fasting glucose levels). Obesity (defined as waist circumference >102 cm in men or >88 cm in women or simplified to BMI ≥30) and T2DM are two of the primary associated risk factors for MASLD. Underpinning the rising prevalence of these associated conditions and MASLD are societal and individual trends in unhealthy eating habits (proliferation of high-calorie processed foods and diets with a high content of sugar, high fructose corn syrup, and fat) and decreased physical activity levels. The industrialization of food production, as well as deficiencies in neighborhood planning with poor walkability and public transport system availability, are partly to blame for this epidemic. This underscores the broader association between general societal disadvantage and development of this disease.

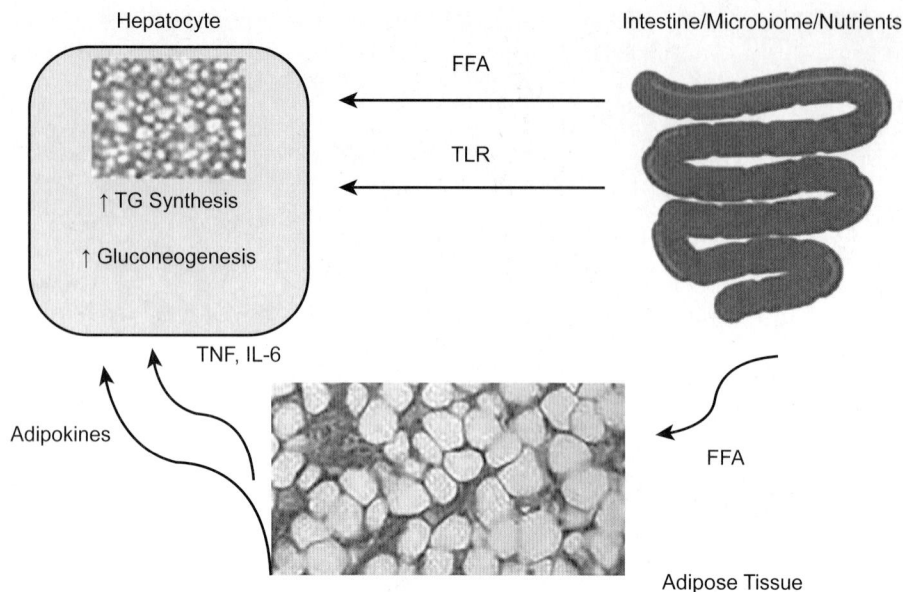

Figure 2 Pathophysiology of metabolic dysfunction–associated steatotic liver disease. An interaction between intestine, adipose tissue, and hepatocytes. *FFA*, Free fatty acids; *IL*, interleukin; *TG*, triglyceride; *TLR*, Toll-like receptor; *TNF*, tumor necrosis factor.

Being overweight in childhood and adolescence, especially weight gain during school years, is a significant risk factor for development of MASLD by late childhood and adulthood.

Several genetic risk factors have been reported, with nonsynonymous SNPs in certain genes, with *PNPLA3* (patatin-like phospholipase domain-containing protein 3), *TM6SF2* (transmembrane 6 superfamily member 2), and *MBOAT7* (membrane bound O-acyltransferase domain containing 7) being the most consistently validated. The prevalence of the *PNPLA3* SNP is highest in the Hispanic population and leads to the higher prevalence of MASLD in this population. The *I148M PNPLA3* genetic mutation has consistently been shown to be the most common genetic determinant of MASLD and correlates with hepatic steatosis, as well as severity of liver disease and risk of cirrhosis and liver cancer in MASLD. Studies conducted since the mid-2010s found that loss of function variants in *HSD17B13* (hydroxysteroid 17-beta dehydrogenase 13) and *CIDEB* are protective against MASLD and MASH.

Heavy alcohol intake and obesity have been shown to act synergistically in increasing the risk of liver disease. The effect of more moderate alcohol consumption on MASLD is being further investigated, though data from 2018 cited in the 2023 American Association for the Study of Liver Diseases (AASLD) practice guidelines on the clinical assessment and management of nonalcoholic fatty liver disease suggests that moderate alcohol use lowers odds of MASH resolution and increases risk of malignancy. Because of this, a new category of SLD has been introduced, termed MetALD, which encompasses patients with MASLD and alcohol use. MetALD includes a group of patients who previously would have been excluded from a diagnosis of NAFLD (due to alcohol use of >20 g [female] or >30 g [male] alcohol per day). These patients can further be categorized as MASLD or ALD predominant depending on the amount of alcohol consumption. Any alcohol use should be avoided completely in those with clinically significant hepatic fibrosis. There are population data suggesting that low levels of alcohol use (≤1 drink per day), wine in particular, may be associated with lower risk of developing MASLD compared with those who drink more or do not drink at all, although these data are of low quality.

MASH, which has a higher chance of progression to fibrosis and cirrhosis, is independently associated with diabetes, age, and BMI, as well as genetic polymorphisms in *PNPLA3*.

Pathophysiology of MASLD

The hallmark finding of MASLD is accumulation of triglyceride (TG) in the cytoplasm of hepatocytes.

This is caused by an imbalance between lipid buildup (fatty acid uptake and de novo lipogenesis [DNL]) and removal (mitochondrial fatty acid oxidation [FAO] and export as a part of very-low-density lipoprotein [VLDL] particles). Further factors contributing to transition from a healthy liver to MASLD include adipose tissue dysfunction, hepatic insulin resistance, dysbiosis of the gut microbiome, toxic metabolites, and genetic factors (Figure 2).

Along with storage of TGs, adipose tissue is involved in the secretion of hormones, cytokines, and chemokines, called adipokines. Overnutrition and/or sedentary lifestyle causes obesity and adipose tissue dysfunction, which likely plays a pivotal role in the development of insulin resistance (IR) and MASLD. Obesity, especially visceral adiposity associated with unhealthy intraabdominal adipose tissue, results in excess free fatty acids (FFAs) entering the liver through the portal circulation, which can increase lipid synthesis and gluconeogenesis. Increased levels of circulating FFAs also lead to peripheral IR along with inflammation and induction of cytokine production, thereby contributing to MASLD. In MASH, liver cell injury occurs (ballooning hepatocytes, inflammation) along with steatosis and varying degree of fibrosis.

Clinical Manifestations of MASLD

MASLD patients are typically asymptomatic until the condition progresses to cirrhosis. Early in the course of disease, it is often found incidentally on abdominal imaging including ultrasound, CT, or MRI (hepatic steatosis). Hepatomegaly may be the presenting symptom in some patients. Vague right upper abdominal discomfort, malaise, and/or fatigue can occur in patients with MASH but is very nonspecific.

The other common presentation of MASLD is with elevation of liver enzymes with mild to moderate elevations in aspartate aminotransferase (AST) and alanine aminotransferase (ALT). However, even advanced MASLD can present with normal liver enzyme levels in up to 30% of individuals, and MASH cannot be excluded based on normal liver enzymes alone.

MASLD patients frequently have comorbidities including hyperlipidemia, obesity, metabolic syndrome, hypertension, and T2DM. Associated conditions also include hypothyroidism, obstructive sleep apnea, and less commonly hypopituitarism, hypogonadism, polycystic ovarian syndrome, pancreaticoduodenal resection, and psoriasis, among others.

In a community study following MASLD patients for over 7 years, there was excessive risk of mortality compared with the general population-based age- and sex-matched controls (standardized mortality ratio [SMR] 1.34, 1.003–1.76). Given the commonality of risk factors for MASLD and cardiovascular disease (CVD), cardiac disease is a leading cause of mortality in these patients. A meta-analysis of observational studies also confirmed the increased risk of CVD in MASLD (OR 1.64, 1.26–2.13) and MASH (OR 2.58, 1.78–3.75). Obesity, diabetes, and metabolic syndrome are also risk factors for carcinogenesis, and a multitude of cancers are increased in patients with MASLD including liver cancer, breast cancer, kidney cancer, and colon cancer, among others. Liver disease mortality from cirrhosis and liver cancer is the third most common risk of mortality in these patients.

MASLD is an increasingly common reason for decompensated cirrhosis and liver cancer. Over their lifetime, 5% to 10% of patients with MASLD progress to cirrhosis. Isolated hepatic steatosis without evidence of hepatocellular injury carries a minimal risk of progression to cirrhosis (<2%). Patients who are older or have T2DM are at higher risk for progressing to MASH and fibrosis. On the other hand, MASH has a higher likelihood of progress to cirrhosis (5%–12%), liver failure, and occasionally liver cancer. Additionally, those with MASH who are identified to have stage 2 fibrosis or higher carry a significantly higher lifetime risk of liver-related mortality and morbidity. In these patients, liver disease mortality predominates the clinical picture. Complications of cirrhosis including variceal hemorrhage, ascites, hepatic encephalopathy, and liver failure can occur.

MASLD is the second most common indication of liver transplantation in the United States after alcohol-related liver disease and is the most common indication of liver transplantation in women. In the US general population, MASLD is already one of the most common reasons for developing liver cancer, with the risk of developing liver cancer in patients with MASLD-related cirrhosis being 1% to 2% per year. HCC in MASH, like in most other chronic liver diseases, occurs predominantly in the setting of cirrhosis. Age, obesity, diabetes, and *I148M PNPLA3* SNP are risk factors for HCC in these patients. MASLD-associated HCC is the third most common cause of HCC in the United States, and the incidence of MASLD-associated HCC is increasing the fastest at a 9% annual incidence rate compared with other causes of HCC.

Diagnosis of MASLD

The diagnosis of MASLD (Figure 3) is made by confirming the presence of hepatic steatosis on either imaging or liver biopsy, in the presence of one or more CMRF (see footnote under the "Current Therapy" box). Diagnosing MASLD based on elevated liver enzymes alone (without imaging or biopsy) is not recommended. Not only is elevation of liver enzymes nonspecific, but they are also frequently normal in patients with MASLD including in those with advanced liver disease.

Alternate causes of steatosis that should be excluded before diagnosing MASLD include the following:
- Alcohol excess (typically defined as >21 standard drinks of alcohol per week in men and >14 drinks per week in women)
- Hepatitis B/C infection
- Medications that cause steatosis (amiodarone [Pacerone], tamoxifen [Nolvadex], methotrexate [Trexall], diltiazem [Cardizem], and prednisone)
- Hemochromatosis
- Wilson disease
- Autoimmune hepatitis

These conditions are easily screened for by history and serologies for these conditions. Excess alcohol use alone may lead to hepatic steatosis and steatohepatitis; however, many patients with MASLD may also drink low or moderate amounts of alcohol. These two causes of hepatic steatosis may work synergistically and contribute to a faster progression of fibrosis, so a thorough alcohol use history should be obtained. These patients may now fall under the category of MetALD. During serologic workup in patients with suspected MASLD, it is common to find elevated ferritin. This is due to MASLD itself in the majority of cases. In patients with significantly elevated ferritin and transferrin

saturation, serum testing for mutations in the hemochromatosis gene *(HFE)* should be performed, and if there are heterozygous or homozygous mutations in this gene, then a liver biopsy should be performed for iron quantification. It is also common to find autoantibodies in MASLD that are often elevated in autoimmune hepatitis (antinuclear antibodies >1:160, antismooth muscle antibodies >1:40). These are often epiphenomena, but if the level of liver enzymes is significantly elevated (greater than fivefold above normal), then a liver biopsy can be done to exclude autoimmune hepatitis.

MASLD is usually diagnosed in one of two common scenarios:
1. Patients with unsuspected hepatic steatosis detected on imaging done for other indications (ultrasound or CT)
2. Patients with unexplained abnormal liver chemistries (liver enzymes); these patients should be assessed for associated cardiometabolic risk factors

Routine screening for MASLD in high-risk groups attending primary care, diabetes, or obesity clinics was previously not recommended. AASLD practice guidelines from 2023, however, now suggest targeted screening for patients at increased risk for advanced liver disease to identify clinically significant fibrosis (stage 2 or greater), including those with T2DM and medically complicated obesity. For these patients, it is recommended that noninvasive screening should be considered every 1 to 2 years (discussed later).

It is essential to emphasize that a diagnosis of MASLD includes the determination of whether progressive liver disease, MASH, and/or fibrosis are present to tailor treatment and monitoring. The state of comorbidities including dyslipidemia, obesity, insulin resistance, diabetes, hypothyroidism, polycystic ovary syndrome, and sleep apnea is important to evaluate at the initial evaluation to recommend specific treatment for these associated disorders.

Role of Liver Biopsy in MASLD

Historically, the gold standard for establishing a diagnosis of MASLD and staging fibrosis is liver biopsy. Current AASLD recommendations suggest reserving liver biopsy for when noninvasive methods are inconclusive and in patients with risk factors for advanced fibrosis or suspicion of other concomitant liver disease. In MASLD, liver histology typically shows steatosis graded as mild (<33% of hepatocytes involved), moderate (33%–66%) or severe (>66%). Other findings seen in MASH include lobular inflammation and hepatocyte ballooning indicative of hepatocyte injury, as well as varying degrees of fibrosis from none (stage 0 fibrosis) to cirrhosis (stage 4 fibrosis).

Although liver biopsy is not essential for diagnosing hepatic steatosis, liver biopsy should be considered in the following patients with MASLD:
1. Those at increased risk of having steatohepatitis (MASH) and/or advanced fibrosis because no serum or radiologic marker thus far can reliably differentiate MASH from isolated steatosis. Thus patients who are older (>50), have long-standing metabolic syndrome, or noninvasive evaluations that suggest advanced fibrosis should undergo biopsy for better characterization of their liver disease. These noninvasive studies (discussed later) would include NAFLD fibrosis score, Fibrosis-4 (FIB-4) scores, liver stiffness measured by imaging techniques such as vibration-controlled transient elastography (VCTE), or MRI-based elastography (MRE).
2. Liver biopsy should also be considered when presence and/or severity of coexisting chronic liver diseases cannot be excluded without a liver biopsy. This may include patients with serum antibodies in whom coexistent autoimmune hepatitis cannot be excluded or patients with significantly elevated ferritin and iron saturation.

Despite the useful information obtained in some patients with MASLD, liver biopsy has several limitations including sampling error and intraobserver and interobserver variability in interpretation. It is costly, invasive, and carries risks of mortality (up to 0.1%), pain, intraperitoneal bleeding, bile leaks, and infection.

Primary care evaluation of elevated LFTs or incidental steatosis on imaging

Review/evaluate for potential etiologies of liver injury:
- Alcohol intake
  - Men >21 drinks/wk
  - Women >14 drinks/wk
- Hepatitis B/C
- Medications
  - Amiodarone
  - Tamoxifen
  - Methotrexate
  - Diltiazem
  - Steroids
- Hemochromatosis
- Wilson's disease
- Autoimmune hepatitis

Primary risk assessment for advanced fibrosis via FIB-4 score

<1.3

Repeat FIB-4:
- Every 1–2 yrs if T2DM or ≥2 metabolic risk factors
- Every 2–3 yrs if no T2DM or <2 risk factors

1.3 – 2.67

Secondary risk assessment via VCTE or ELF

>2.67

Referral to hepatology and consider dedicated imaging including MRE

Metabolic risk factors
- Obesity
- Dyslipidemia (TG > 150 +/− HDL <40 men; <50 women)
- Insulin resistance
- Hypertension (>130/80)

	VCTE	ELF
Low risk	< 8 kPa	< 7.7
Intermediate risk	8 – 12 kPa	7.7 – 9.8
High risk	> 12 kPa	> 9.8

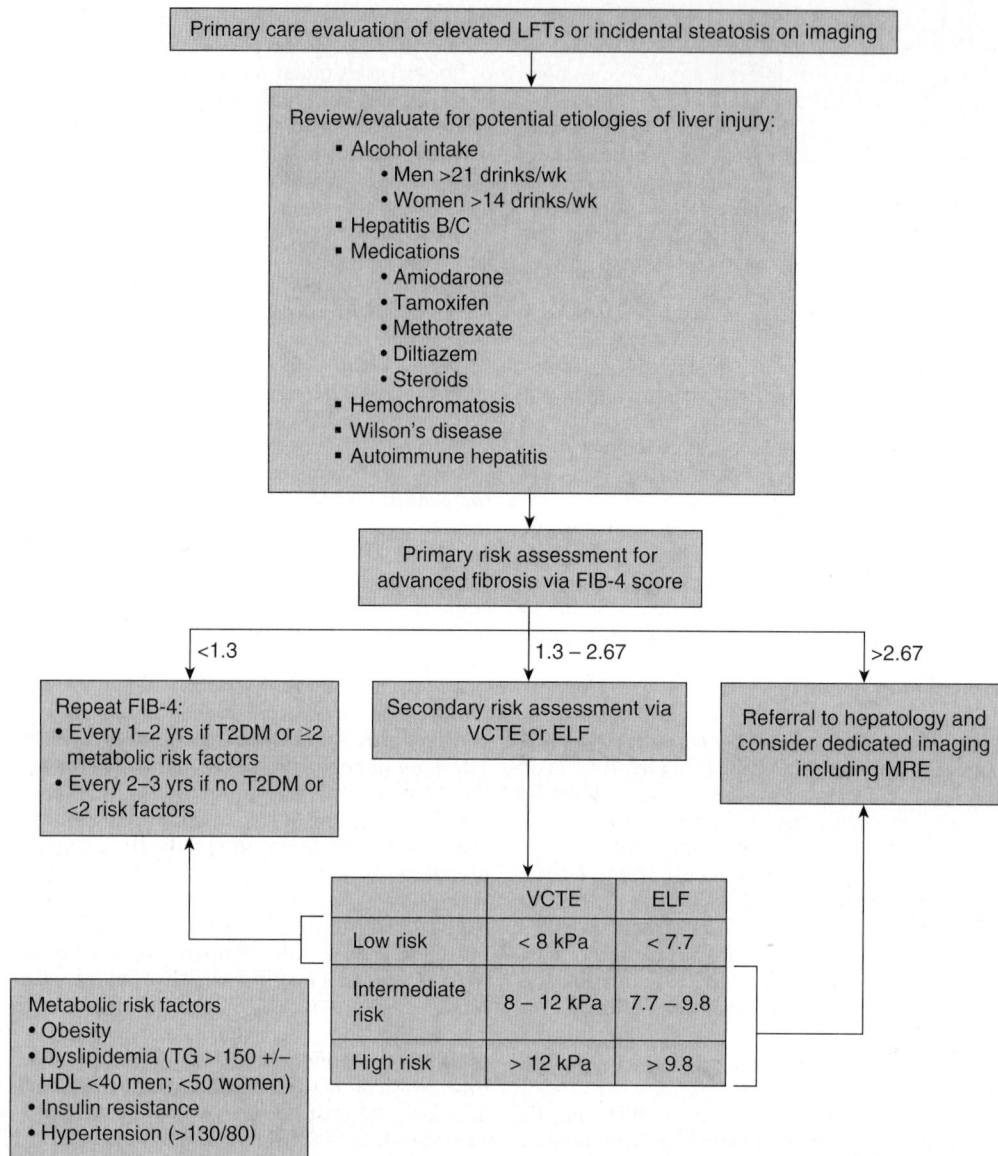

Figure 3 Diagnostic evaluation for suspected metabolic dysfunction–associated steatotic liver disease. *ELF*, Enhanced Liver Fibrosis score; *FIB-4*, Fibrosis-4 score; *HDL*, high-density lipoprotein; *LFTs*, liver function tests; *MRE*, MRI-based elastography; *TG*, triglyceride; *T2DM*, type 2 diabetes mellitus; *VCTE*, vibration-controlled elastography.

As a result, it is not practical for screening millions of at-risk individuals and for frequent repeated assessments. Noninvasive approaches to diagnosis of MASLD are thus used widely in clinical practice.

Noninvasive Testing in MASLD
Hepatic Steatosis
Abnormal hepatic steatosis is defined by a liver fat content of ≥5%. The most accurate noninvasive method to quantify liver fat content is magnetic resonance spectroscopy. However, this modality requires special expertise, is time-consuming, and is not readily available clinically. A good alternative is MRI that uses proton density fat fraction (MRI-PDFF), which provides an accurate estimate of liver fat content, as well as spatial imaging of the liver. Conventional ultrasonography (CUS) remains the most commonly used imaging modality to diagnose hepatic steatosis. It is widely available and cheaper than MRI but has limited accuracy, especially in obese individuals. Additionally, it is not sensitive in detecting mild steatosis (<33%) with lower specificity than MRI for fibrosis.

Transient elastography based techniques are increasingly used to diagnose steatosis and estimate the degree of hepatic fibrosis. Fat and fibrosis affect shear wave propagation through tissue, and this property can be used to measure liver attenuation (steatosis) and velocity (fibrosis) using a specialized ultrasound (FibroScan). This machine uses an ultrasonic probe placed over the skin in the right upper quadrant to produce shear waves of 50 MHz that pass through the liver. Measurements of shear wave attenuation called controlled attenuation parameter (CAP) assess for presence and grade of hepatic steatosis. CAP has been shown to be less accurate than MRI-PDFF in diagnosing steatosis but is cheaper and a point-of-care quantitative modality.

Currently there are many widely available serum-based diagnostic panels for MASLD that use a mix of serum tests and other demographic/anthropometric measures that are combined in single measurements for diagnosis of MASLD. Examples include Fatty Liver Index (triglycerides, BMI, γ-glutamyl transferase, waist circumference) and NAFLD Liver Fat Score (metabolic syndrome, T2DM, fasting insulin, ALT, AST). These panels have been found to have sensitivities and specificities in the 70% range and show reasonable accuracy for predicting steatosis. These tests are not as accurate as imaging or biopsy tests; therefore they are less often used clinically and more often used as research tools in epidemiologic research.

Assessing Fibrosis

Fibrosis is highly correlated with outcomes in liver disease and a marker of worse outcomes. Fibrosis histologically is categorized (staged) as follows on liver biopsy:

- F0: no fibrosis
- F1: portal fibrosis without septa
- F2: portal fibrosis with few septa, extending outside of portal areas
- F3: bridging fibrosis or numerous septa without cirrhosis
- F4: cirrhosis

F3 and F4 are categorized as advanced fibrosis, and F0 and F1 are considered none-to-minimal fibrosis.

Clinical decision aids such as the NAFLD fibrosis score (biomarkers evaluated: age, glucose level, BMI, platelet count, albumin, and AST/ALT ratio) or the FIB-4 index (biomarkers include age, AST, platelet count, ALT) use a combination of serum and clinical variables to predict the presence of advanced fibrosis or cirrhosis. The Enhanced Liver Fibrosis (ELF) test is a serologic test that calculates a score based on serum levels of hyaluronic acid (HA), type III procollagen peptide (PIIINP), and tissue inhibitor of matrix metalloproteinase 1 (TIMP-1). It is approved for prognostication when advanced fibrosis is suspected. When used with the FIB-4 score, the sensitivity and specificity are in the 90% range for predicting advanced fibrosis. These tests are most useful in distinguishing patients who may have advanced fibrosis from those without fibrosis and thus may aid in clinical decision making including referral to a hepatologist and further workup.

Imaging-based techniques such VCTE (FibroScan) or MRE can be used to identify those at low or high risk for advanced fibrosis (bridging fibrosis or cirrhosis) with more accuracy than serum-based markers. However, MRE is costly and limited by availability of scanners and reading radiologists. On the other hand, VCTE is increasingly available and can widely be used as point-of-care tests in liver clinics for fibrosis assessment. However, the accuracy of these results are limited in settings of significant obesity, ascites, and acute inflammation. As noted earlier, the ELF test and FIB-4 score can be used in settings where image-based tests such as the FibroScan are not available.

A suggested algorithm for screening for and diagnosing MASLD/MASH and advanced fibrosis is shown in Figure 3.

Therapy of MASLD

Treatment of MASLD (Table 1) entails treatment of the liver disease and the associated cardiometabolic risk factors.

Lifestyle Modifications in MASLD

Lifestyle modifications are integral in the treatment of MASLD at any stage and are the principal intervention for patients with isolated steatosis and MASH without fibrosis. Patients are advised to lose ≥7% of body weight if overweight or obese (3%–5% weight loss will improve steatosis; 7%–10% is needed to improve histopathological features of MASH and fibrosis).

This weight loss is best achieved gradually (losing no more than 1–2 lbs per week) and sustained through a combination of diet and exercise.

Basic principles of diet include reducing calories (by at least 30% or by 750–1000 kcal/day for an average US adult) and reducing consumption of simple carbohydrates and saturated fat. Reduction of sugar-sweetened beverages and of fructose-enriched food and drinks is recommended. In general, using fresh fruits and vegetables and lean meats and minimizing processed foods is recommended. Although many different diets have been studied and shown to be beneficial (Mediterranean diet), studies have also shown that any diet that follows these basic principles and results in weight loss achieves the benefits of reversing MASH.

Significant alcohol use can exacerbate steatohepatitis, and limiting consumption of alcohol (≤1 drink/day for women and ≤2 drinks/day for men) is recommended in patients with MASH. For patients with liver fibrosis stage 2 or greater, complete abstinence from alcohol is strongly recommended. There is no safe level of alcohol use at that stage.

TABLE 1	Therapy of Metabolic Dysfunction–Associated Steatotic Liver Disease

Assessment of Steatosis and Fibrosis Staging
Consider pharmacotherapy or investigational agents for more advanced liver disease in addition to lifestyle modifications

Lifestyle Modifications Aimed at Weight Loss
Goals
- Lose 7%–10% of body weight
- Gradual weight loss, no more than 2 lbs per week till at goal

Diet Changes
- Reduce calories by 30% (750–1000 kcal/day)
- Reduce simple sugars, saturated fat, sugar-sweetened beverages and foods, including fructose-enriched foods

Exercise
- 150–200 minutes per week spaced over 3–5 days
- Moderate-to-vigorous intensity (e.g., jogging, playing tennis, swimming laps, biking)

Treatment of Associated Metabolic Factors as per Best Practices
Diabetes
- No particular agent proven beneficial as primary treatment for MASLD, although pioglitazone (Actos)[1] may benefit histologic MASH. Be aware of potential weight gain
- Metformin (Glucophage)[1] and DPP-4 inhibitors no proven benefit for MASH
- Insulin can cause weight gain and insulin resistance associated with MASH

Dyslipidemia
- Treat per standard guidelines
- Statins are safe to use if indicated (except in decompensated cirrhosis)

Pharmacotherapy for MASH
Resmetirom (Rezdiffra)
- Reduces hepatic fat content, histologic benefits in MASH, and decreases fibrosis
- Common side effects include nausea and vomiting

Pioglitazone (Actos)[1]
- Histologic benefits in diabetic and nondiabetic MASH except for fibrosis
- Can cause weight gain

Vitamin E[7]
- Histologic benefits in nondiabetic MASH except for fibrosis
- Concerns for long term use—small risk in all-cause mortality, increased risk of prostate cancer

GLP-1 receptor agonists (Liraglutide [Victoza, Saxenda][1], semaglutide [Ozempic[1], Wegovy], and tirzepatide [Mounjaro, Zepbound][1])
- Recommended in diabetic MASH as adjunctive therapy to lifestyle interventions

Investigational trials (generally for biopsy-proven MASH)
Semaglutide and tirzepatide
- Phase 3 trial: Semaglutide: decreases fibrosis without worsening of steatohepatitis, improves resolution of steatohepatitis with no worsening of liver fibrosis
- Phase 2 trial: Tirzepatide: decreases fibrosis without worsening of steatohepatitis

Efruxifermin[5]
- Phase 2 trial: Reduces hepatic fat fraction and improvement of >1 fibrosis stage

[1]Not FDA approved for this indication.
[7]Available as dietary supplement.
[5]Investigational drug in the United States.
DPP-4, Dipeptidyl peptidase-4; *GLP-1,* glucagon-like peptide-1; *MASH,* metabolic dysfunction–associated steatohepatitis; *MASLD,* metabolic dysfunction–associated steatotic liver disease.

A preponderance of epidemiologic data also shows that consumption of coffee (≥3 cups) per day is associated with reduced prevalence of MASLD. If coffee is consumed, it should be caffeinated with no addition of sweetened syrups, sugar, and/or large servings of milk/other calories that may negate any beneficial effects.

Recommendations for physical activity include at least 150 to 200 minutes of moderate-to-vigorous physical activity per week (e.g., moderate jogging, weight training, and sports such as tennis, swimming, or biking). For patients who do not exercise at baseline, a gradual buildup to this level is recommended. Limited data suggest that the combination of diet and exercise may be more beneficial than either in isolation.

Bariatric surgery may be considered for patients with BMI >40 kg/m^2 or >35 kg/m^2 and comorbidities such as diabetes, hypertension, and hyperlipidemia. MASLD is increasingly being considered a metabolic comorbidity. Bariatric surgery, malabsorptive procedures in particular, has been shown to resolve MASH, improve fibrosis, and sustain significant weight loss in addition to other health benefits. A 5-year follow-up of 180 patients undergoing bariatric surgery with biopsy-proven MASH at the time of surgery found resolution of MASH in 84.4% of patients without worsening of fibrosis and improvement in fibrosis in 70.2%. These improvements were associated with higher amounts of weight loss.

Pharmacotherapeutics in MASLD

In the MAESTRO trial published in 2024 and referenced in the current AASLD guidelines, resmetirom, a thyroid hormone receptor beta activator, was found to cause >1 stage improvement in fibrosis without worsening of MASH and MASH resolution without worsening fibrosis in 26% and 30% of patients, respectively, at the 100-mg dose. Resmetirom (Rezdiffra) was FDA approved for the treatment of MASH in 2024. By acting as a thyroid hormone receptor–beta agonist, resmetirom exerts its action by improving lipid metabolism resulting in reduced intrahepatic triglycerides and overall liver fat content. It has also been shown to modify inflammatory pathways, suppressing proinflammatory signaling that is implicated in the inflammatory and fibrotic pathophysiology of MASH.

There are several additional pharmacologic treatments aimed at different components of metabolic syndrome that can be used off-label for MASLD-related liver disease based on controlled studies and published guidelines. These agents, when used for MASLD, should generally be limited to those with biopsy-proven MASH and fibrosis.

Pioglitazone (Actos)[1] is an insulin sensitizing agent used in diabetes (peroxisome proliferator–activated receptors [PPAR]-γ agonist) and can be used to treat patients with and without T2DM with biopsy-proven MASH. It has been shown to improve histologic changes in MASH but not fibrosis.

For nondiabetic adults with biopsy-proven MASH, Vitamin E[7] administered at a daily dose of 800 IU/day can be used as well and can cause similar histologic improvements as pioglitazone. It must be noted that trials of these agents in MASH were generally limited to 24 months or less and longer-term benefits are not known.

Side effect profiles should also be considered with these therapies. Pioglitazone can cause weight gain, has been associated with osteoporosis, and has been known to exacerbate heart failure in susceptible individuals. Vitamin E has some concerns regarding increased all-cause mortality, potentially small increased risk of hemorrhagic stroke, and in a large trial, increased risk of prostate cancer. If medications are started for treatment of MASH, ALT should be monitored every 6 to 12 months with medications discontinued if there is <20% improvement in ALT from baseline or fibrosis progresses.

There are numerous pharmacologic agents in phase 1 and phase 2 trials and a few in phase 3 trials for MASLD. Some of these agents work on glucose or lipid metabolism in the liver whereas others are antifibrotic or antioxidant.

Glucagon-like peptide-1 (GLP-1)-receptor agonists have been approved for the treatment of diabetes and obesity and are recommended by the AASLD for their potential benefits in MASLD via direct therapy against these metabolic comorbidities. While not recommended as a specific treatment for MASLD itself, data from phase 2 and 3 randomized, placebo-controlled clinical trials published in 2024 showed that certain GLP-1 agonists are associated with improved steatosis and resolution of MASH. The ongoing phase 3 ESSENCE trial has demonstrated that weekly semaglutide injection (Ozempic[1], Wegovy) shows statistically significant improvement in hepatic fibrosis regression without worsening of steatohepatitis in individuals with precirrhosis MASH compared with placebo. In the same population, semaglutide (Wegovy) was also shown to significantly improve resolution of steatohepatitis with no worsening of liver fibrosis. Wegovy (semaglutide) is currently the only GLP-1 agonist product that carries FDA approval for noncirrhotic MASH with moderate to advanced liver fibrosis. Tirzepatide (Mounjaro, Zepbound)[1], a GLP-1/glucose-dependent insulinotropic polypeptide receptor agonist, is additionally being shown to decrease hepatic fibrosis without worsening of steatohepatitis in an ongoing phase 2 study.

Efruxifermin[5], a fibroblast growth factor 21 analog, has had promising results in a phase 2 trial, significantly decreasing the MRI hepatic fat fraction (HFF) at 12 weeks compared with placebo with an improvement of >1 stage of fibrosis in 55% of the treatment group whose HFF decreased by >30%. While it remains an investigational therapy, efruxifermin has also demonstrated significant potential in reversing cirrhotic morphology among patients with MASH. In one phase 2 trial, 39% of patients experienced reversal of cirrhosis on therapy without worsening of MASH, compared with 15% in the placebo group.

Currently, the following drugs are not recommended as specific treatment for MASLD as they have shown no specific benefit for MASH: metformin (Glucophage)[1] and dipeptidyl peptidase-4 (DPP-4) inhibitors are agents that can be used for diabetes including in patients with MASLD. However, they have no beneficial effect specifically on MASH. Ursodeoxycholic acid (ursodiol [Actigall])[1] and omega-3 fatty acids[7] can be considered for hypertriglyceridemia concurrent with MASLD but do not specifically improve MASLD.

Patients with MASLD are at high risk for cardiovascular morbidity and mortality, and aggressive modification of CVD risk factors should be considered in all MASLD patients. Statins can be used to treat dyslipidemia in patients with MASLD, MASH, and MASH cirrhosis but should be avoided in patients with decompensated cirrhosis.

Prevention of MASLD

Prevention of MASLD is imperative and is a societal challenge that should focus on reducing obesity and the metabolic syndrome. Early education and focus on healthy nutrition and childhood physical activity are key initiatives, as is neighborhood planning for improving access to healthy foods and healthy spaces.

Monitoring of MASLD

Patients with MASH, especially those with significant fibrosis, are at the greatest risk for increased progression to cirrhosis and mortality. Patients with MASH and F0 or F1 fibrosis are monitored annually for liver disease progression via blood work (liver enzymes and function tests, platelet counts) and physical examinations. Evaluation of fibrosis progression in these patients can be done via noninvasive serum testing (e.g., FIB-4 score), and if there is evidence of progression of serum fibrosis, then further testing through liver biopsy or noninvasive testing such as FibroScan or

---

[1] Not FDA approved for this indication.
[7] Available as dietary supplement.

---

[1] Not FDA approved for this indication.
[5] Investigational drug in the United States.
[7] Available as dietary supplement.

MR elastography can be done approximately 5 years after diagnosis; however, with high interindividual variation in fibrosis progression, the timeline of testing is tailored to each individual.

For patients with more advanced fibrosis (F2 or higher) at MASH diagnosis, severity of fibrosis governs management. Once F3 or F4 fibrosis occurs, the risk of liver-related illness and death increases significantly, making closer follow-up appropriate.

Patients with MASH cirrhosis should be screened for gastroesophageal varices (upper endoscopy) and considered for HCC screening (AASLD guidelines recommend ultrasound of the liver and serum alpha-fetoprotein [AFP] measurements every 6 months). Patients with MASH cirrhosis should be referred to specialty care with a gastroenterologist/hepatologist. All patients with MASLD/MASH should be screened for immunity to hepatitis A and B and vaccinated if not immune.

References

Chen V, Morgan T, Rotman Y, Patton H, Cusi K, Kanwal F, Kim W: Resmetirom therapy for metabolic dysfunction-associated steatotic liver disease: October 2024 updates to AASLD practice guidance, Hepatology 81(1):312–320, 2025. https://doi.org/10.1002/hep.33001.

Clayton-Chubb D, Kemp WW, Majeed A, et al: Metabolic dysfunction-associated steatotic liver disease in older adults is associated with frailty and social disadvantage, Liver Int 44(1):39–51, 2024. https://doi.org/10.1111/liv.15725.

Diehl AM, Day C: Cause, pathogenesis, and treatment of nonalcoholic steatohepatitis, N Engl J Med 377(21):2063–2072, 2017.

Lassailly G, Caiazzo R, Ntandja-Wandji LC, et al: Bariatric surgery provides long term-resolution of nonalcoholic steatohepatitis and regression of fibrosis, Gastroenterology, 2020.

Le P, Tatar M, Dasarathy S, Alkhouri N, Herman M, Taksler G, Zein N: Estimated burden of metabolic dysfunction–associated steatotic liver disease in US adults, 2020 to 2050, JAMA Netw Open 8(1):e2454707, 2025. https://doi.org/10.1001/jamanetworkopen.2024.54707.

Lindenmeyer CC, Mccullough AJ: The natural history of nonalcoholic fatty liver disease-an evolving view, Clin Liver Dis 22(1):11–21, 2018.

Loomba R; Role of imaging-based biomarkers in NAFLD: recent advances in clinical application and future research directions, J Hepatol 68(2):296–304, 2018.

Loomba R, Hartman ML, Lawitz EJ, Vuppalanchi R, Boursier J, Bugianesi E, et al: Tirzepatide for metabolic dysfunction–associated steatohepatitis with liver fibrosis, N Engl J Med 391(4):299–310, 2024. https://doi.org/10.1056/NEJMoa2401943.

Miao L, Targher G, Byrne CD, Cao Y-Y, Zheng M-H: Current status and future trends of the global burden of MASLD, Trends Endocrinol Metab 35(8):697–707, 2024. https://doi.org/10.1016/j.tem.2024.02.007.

Phase 3 ESSENCE Trial: Semaglutide in metabolic dysfunction–associated steatohepatitis, Gastroenterol Hepatol 20(12 suppl 11):6–7, 2024 Dec. PMID: 39896971; PMCID: PMC11784563.

Rinella ME, Lazarus JV, Ratziu V, et al: On behalf of the NAFLD Nomenclature consensus group. A multisociety Delphi consensus statement on new fatty liver disease nomenclature, Hepatology 78(6):1966–1986, 2023. https://doi.org/10.1097/HEP.0000000000000520.

Rinella ME, et al: AASLD Practice Guidance on the clinical assessment and management of nonalcoholic fatty liver disease, Hepatology 77(5):1797–1835, 2023. https://doi.org/10.1097/HEP.0000000000000323. Epub 2023 Mar 17. PMID: 36727674; PMCID: PMC10735173.

Said A, Akhter A: Meta-analysis of randomized controlled trials of pharmacologic agents in non-alcoholic steatohepatitis, Ann Hepatol 16(4):538–547, 2017.

Tapper EB, Lok AS: Use of liver imaging and biopsy in clinical practice, N Engl J Med 377(8):756–768, 2017.

Tsai E, Lee TP: Diagnosis and evaluation of nonalcoholic fatty liver disease/nonalcoholic steatohepatitis, including noninvasive biomarkers and transient elastography, Clin Liver Dis 22(1):73–92, 2018.

Riazi K, et al: "The prevalence and incidence of NAFLD worldwide: a systematic Review and meta-analysis", Lancet Gastroenterol Hepatol 7(9):851–861, 2022. https://doi.org/10.1016/s2468-1253(22)00165-0.

Younossi Z, Anstee QM, Marietti M, et al: Global burden of NAFLD and NASH: trends, predictions, risk factors and prevention, Nat Rev Gastroenterol Hepatol 15(1):11–20, 2018.

Younossi ZM, Loomba R, Anstee QM, et al: Diagnostic modalities for non-alcoholic fatty liver disease (NAFLD), non-alcoholic steatohepatitis (NASH) and associated fibrosis, Hepatology, 2017.

Younossi ZM, Paik JM, Stepanova M, et al: Clinical profiles and mortality rates are similar for metabolic dysfunction-associated steatotic liver disease and non-alcoholic fatty liver disease, J Hepatol 27(24):S0168–8278, 2024. https://doi.org/10.1016/j.jhep.2024.01.014. Epub ahead of print. PMID: 38286339.

Younossi ZM, Ratziu V, Loomba R, et al: Obeticholic acid for the treatment of non-alcoholic steatohepatitis: interim analysis from a multicentre randomized, placebo-controlled phase 3 trial, Lancet 394:2184–2196, 2019.

Younossi ZM, et al: "Performance of the enhanced liver fibrosis test to estimate advanced fibrosis among patients with nonalcoholic fatty liver disease", JAMA Netw Open 4(9), 2021. https://doi.org/10.1001/jamanetworkopen.2021.23923.

Zhai M, Liu Z, Long J, Zhang X, Xu C, Chen L, Fan JG: Global and national prevalence of nonalcoholic fatty liver disease in adolescents: an analysis of the Global Burden of Disease Study 2019, Hepatology Communications 7(4):e2259, 2023. https://doi.org/10.1002/hep4.2259.

PANCREATIC CANCER

Method of
Joshua S. Jolissaint, MD, MSc; and Alice C. Wei, MD, MSc

CURRENT DIAGNOSIS

- Pancreatic cancer remains a lethal diagnosis. The majority of patients present with advanced stage disease, and although survival has improved over the last 2 decades, 5-year survival remains poor at 12.5%.
- Patients with pancreatic cancer can present with painless jaundice, malaise, fatigue, weight loss, and abdominal pain.
- Routine screening for pancreatic cancer for patients at average risk is not recommended. For high-risk patients, screening may be considered on a case-by-case basis.
- Diagnostic workup should include a contrast-enhanced, multiphase, pancreas-protocol CT scan; serum carbohydrate antigen 19-9 (CA 19-9); and staging CT scan of the chest.
- Histologic diagnosis is confirmed with endoscopic ultrasound–guided fine-needle aspiration/biopsy or percutaneous/operative biopsy.

CURRENT THERAPY

- Surgical resection is the only potentially curative treatment; however, only 20% of patients will have localized disease without vascular involvement or metastases at presentation.
- Patients with a localized tumor but with vascular involvement (borderline resectable or locally advanced disease) may be candidates for neoadjuvant chemotherapy and/or radiation. If neoadjuvant therapy is effective at stabilizing or downsizing the tumor, these patients may then be eligible for resection.
- Systemic chemotherapy is the mainstay of therapy for unresectable patients.
- Palliation of symptoms may require endoscopic or surgical management for both extrahepatic biliary obstruction and gastric outlet obstruction, or radiation for local tumor control.

Epidemiology

In 2023 there were an estimated 64,050 new cases of pancreatic cancer in the United States. Although pancreatic cancer accounts for only 3.3% of all new cancer diagnoses, it is the third leading cause of cancer-related deaths, contributing to 8.3% of cancer-associated mortality and carrying a 5-year survival of 12.5%. Survival varies based on stage at presentation, with a 5-year survival for patients with early-stage disease of 44.3%, compared with 3.1% for those with metastatic disease. The incidence of pancreatic cancer has been relatively stable over the last decade, at approximately 13.3 cases per 10,000 males and females per year. Incidence increases with age, peaking between 65 and 74 years, with a median age at diagnosis of 70 years; it is higher in males than in females (15 vs. 11.7 per 100,000 persons per year). Non-Hispanic Black Americans have the highest incidence of any single ethnic group at 15.9 per 100,000 persons per year.

Types of Pancreatic Cancer

Cancer of the exocrine pancreas comprises 93% of pancreatic cancer cases, with pancreatic ductal adenocarcinoma (PDAC) the most common histologic subtype. Less common subtypes include acinar cell carcinoma, adenosquamous carcinoma, and colloid carcinoma. Tumors of the endocrine pancreas,

SYNDROME	GENE	ESTIMATED CUMULATIVE RISK OF PANCREATIC CANCER*	ESTIMATED RISK COMPARED WITH THE GENERAL POPULATION*
Peutz-Jeghers syndrome	*STK11*	11%–36% by age 65–70 years	132-fold
Familial pancreatitis	*PRSS1, SPINK1, CFTR*	40%–53% by age 70–75 years	26- to 87-fold
Melanoma–pancreatic cancer syndrome	*CDKN2A*	14% by age 70 years 17% by age 75 years	20- to 47-fold
Lynch syndrome	*MLH1, MSH2*	4% by age 70 years	9- to 11-fold
Hereditary breast-ovarian cancer syndrome	*BRCA1, BRCA2*	1.4%–1.5% (females) and 2.1%–4.1% (males) by age 70	2.4- to 6-fold
Familial pancreatic cancer	Unknown in most families (one family with a mutation in the *palladin [PALLD]* gene has been identified)	≥3 first-degree relatives with pancreatic cancer: 7%–16% by age 70 2 first-degree relatives with pancreatic cancer: 3% by age 70	≥3 first-degree relatives with pancreatic cancer: 32-fold Two first-degree relatives with pancreatic cancer: 6.4-fold One first-degree relative with pancreatic cancer: 4.6-fold

*See the associated reference for individual sources of data.

pancreatic neuroendocrine tumors, and islet cell tumors constitute the remaining 7% of pancreatic malignancies.

Risk Factors for Pancreatic Ductal Adenocarcinoma

Multiple genetic and modifiable risk factors for PDAC have been identified. Smoking is the strongest risk factor and is associated with approximately one-fourth to one-third of diagnoses. Some studies have associated smoking with double the risk of an individual developing PDAC. Heavy alcohol use (three or more drinks per day) increases the risk of PDAC in a dose-dependent manner. Obesity and both types 1 and 2 diabetes mellitus (DM) are also associated with an increased risk; however, the mechanistic relationship between these metabolic factors is unclear. Similarly, studies have demonstrated an increased risk of PDAC with obesity in early adulthood in addition to a greater risk associated with hyperglycemia, insulin resistance, and low levels of physical activity. Chronic pancreatitis may confer more than a sevenfold increased relative risk of PDAC, and the mechanism may be modifiable (e.g., alcohol-related pancreatitis) or hereditary.

Approximately 10% of PDAC cases have a hereditary/genetic component, and genetic testing is recommended once a diagnosis is established (Table 1). The *BRCA1* and *BRCA2* genes encode proteins involved in DNA repair, and germline loss-of-function mutations in these genes are highly penetrant, significantly increasing the risk of breast and ovarian cancer, as well as pancreatic cancer in female carriers. Notably, *BRCA2* mutants carry an approximately threefold increased relative risk, and 4% to 7% of patients with PDAC will harbor a germline *BRCA1/2* mutation.

Other hereditary syndromes, such as Lynch syndrome or hereditary nonpolyposis colorectal cancer (*MLH1, MSH2, MSH6*, or *PMS2* genes), familial adenomatous polyposis (*APC* gene), Peutz-Jeghers syndrome (*STK11* gene), and familial atypical multiple mole melanoma (*CDK2NA* gene), also confer an increased risk of PDAC. Mutations in the *ATM* gene and non-O blood groupings have also been associated with an increased risk of pancreatic cancer. In addition, having a single first-degree relative with PDAC increases a patient's risk of developing PDAC by more than fourfold; however, approximately 80% of patients with a family history of PDAC have no known predisposing genetic mutation or cause. Last, 68% to 80% of hereditary pancreatitis is attributed to germline mutations in the *PRSS1* gene, which are inherited in an autosomal dominant fashion and are highly penetrant (approximately 80%). Both the *SPINK1* and *CFTR* genes are also associated with familial pancreatitis. Patients who develop symptoms of pancreatitis in this setting have an increased risk of PDAC that increases with age. By the age of 75 years, patients may have a greater than 50% cumulative incidence of pancreatic cancer.

Screening

Currently, there is no role for routine screening for pancreatic cancer for patients at average risk. The U.S. Preventive Services Task Force has issued a grade D rating (moderate or high certainty that these diagnostic methods have no benefit or that the harm outweighs the risk) for abdominal ultrasonography, abdominal palpation, or serologic markers. For high-risk patients, those with multiple first-degree relatives with PDAC, or individuals with certain germline mutations (see "Risk Factors for Pancreatic Ductal Adenocarcinoma"), screening may be considered on a case-by-case basis. Some authors have suggested the use of endoscopic ultrasound (EUS) or magnetic resonance cholangiopancreatography, although the efficacy of these modalities as screening tools is still unknown. CA 19-9 is a serum biomarker used to track disease progression or recurrence in established diagnoses of PDAC; however, CA 19-9 testing should not be used as a screening tool in otherwise healthy patients.

Presentation and Diagnosis

The presentation of patients with PDAC is variable. The most common presenting symptoms are painless jaundice and conjugated hyperbilirubinemia due to biliary tract obstruction, both of which are seen more commonly in tumors of the pancreatic head. Nonspecific complaints can include malaise, fatigue, weight loss, steatorrhea, dyspepsia, and abdominal pain radiating to the back. A new diagnosis of DM (<24 months duration) in patients 50 years of age or older, particularly if it is refractory to lifestyle modification and pharmacologic intervention, may also indicate the presence of underlying pancreatic cancer. New-onset DM compared with long-standing DM may convey a greater than twofold increase in risk.

If a diagnosis of PDAC is suspected, the initial diagnostic workup should include a contrast-enhanced multiphase pancreas protocol CT scan and measurement of serum CA 19-9. Early multidisciplinary consultation is encouraged to optimize symptom management and establish the best course of multimodal treatment. Patients with jaundice due to biliary obstruction should be referred to both a gastroenterologist capable of performing endoscopy and a surgeon in an expedited fashion. Endoscopic intervention has the potential to be both diagnostic and therapeutic, particularly in cases of cholangitis or intense pruritis from symptomatic jaundice. To obtain a tissue diagnosis, EUS-guided fine-needle aspiration/biopsy can be performed, followed by endoscopic retrograde cholangiopancreatography with common bile duct stent placement (see "Managing Symptoms and Complications"). Staging should be completed with cross-sectional imaging of the chest to evaluate for distant metastases. MRI and positron emission tomography may be useful adjuncts in characterizing the tumor or ruling out distant metastatic disease.

Treatment

Surgical resection is the only potentially curative treatment. Tumors of the pancreatic head may be removed by pancreaticoduodenectomy (i.e., the Whipple procedure), whereas tumors of the pancreatic tail may require a distal pancreatectomy with or without splenectomy. More central or larger tumors may require a central pancreatectomy or total pancreatectomy. These operations may be performed in the traditional open fashion; however, there has been increased interest in minimally invasive approaches, particularly with implementation and dissemination of robotic surgery. Proponents of minimally invasive approaches suggest improvements in functional recovery, length of stay, and decreased recovery. Results from the recently published DIPLOMA (distal pancreatectomy) and EUROPA (Whipple) trials have shown that in the least, minimally invasive approaches have noninferior oncologic and postoperative outcomes compared with traditional open approaches, but further study is ongoing. Unfortunately, only approximately 20% of patients with PDAC will have localized disease without mesenteric or portovascular involvement (termed "resectable"). Patients who do have vascular involvement but no evidence of distant metastases are classified as either borderline resectable (BR) or locally advanced (LA).

Resectable

For resectable patients, upfront surgical resection is the most common initial treatment; however, there is currently significant interest in neoadjuvant chemotherapy before consideration of surgery for PDAC. Systemic chemotherapy is a mainstay in the treatment with sequenced multimodal disease management. Chemotherapy may be given before (neoadjuvant) or after (adjuvant) surgery, or as induction treatment in cases of LA or unresectable disease. Neoadjuvant chemotherapy has a higher rate of treatment completion (compared with adjuvant), the theoretical benefit of treating micrometastatic disease early, and assisting in improving patient selection and sparing patients a morbid operation who would otherwise develop early recurrence. Although the phase III PREOPANC trial comparing preoperative gemcitabine (Gemzar)-based chemoradiation to upfront resection did not demonstrate a difference in the primary endpoint of overall survival (OS), investigators did note a 1.4-month, statistically significant, median improvement in OS when reporting long-term results. This study has been criticized for not using contemporary chemotherapeutic regimens. Conversely, the recently published phase II NORPACT-1 trial comparing neoadjuvant FOLFIRINOX (see full dosing in "Borderline Resectable and Locally Advanced") followed by resection to upfront resection failed to show a survival benefit for this chemotherapy-first approach, however there was a higher rate of R0 resection and N0 status in the per-protocol analysis. Randomized clinical trials, including the Alliance A021806 phase III trial comparing preoperative to adjuvant FOLFIRINOX, are currently ongoing in an effort to better answer this question (NCT04340141). As such, both upfront resection and preoperative chemotherapy are currently practiced, and this nuanced decision is best made in a high-volume multidisciplinary setting.

Borderline Resectable and Locally Advanced

For BR/LA PDAC, National Comprehensive Cancer Network Pancreatic Adenocarcinoma guidelines recommend neoadjuvant

chemotherapy with consideration of resection, depending on the patient's tolerance of chemotherapy, their fitness, and the stage of the disease. Currently accepted systemic neoadjuvant chemotherapy regimens include FOLFIRINOX-based regimens (14-day cycles of 85 mg/m^2 oxaliplatin[1], 400 mg/m^2 leucovorin[1], 180 mg/m^2 irinotecan [Camptosar][1], and 400 mg/m^2 5-fluorouracil [Adrucil] bolus followed by 2400 mg/m^2 infusion over 46 hours), mFOLFIRINOX (without 5-fluorouracil bolus) or gemcitabine (1,000 mg/m^2), and N-albumin-bound (nab) paclitaxel (Abraxane) (125 mg/m^2) (biweekly for 4 weeks). Preoperative chemoradiation may improve local control; however, it has not demonstrated a survival benefit. The optimal duration of neoadjuvant therapy has not been established; however, most clinicians repeat imaging after 2 to 3 months of chemotherapy to restage the patient and reevaluate the potential for resection.

Adjuvant Therapy

For patients who undergo resection, adjuvant chemotherapy improves both overall and disease-free survival after surgery. Current preferred regimens include FOLFIRINOX (see "Borderline Resectable and Locally Advanced") or gemcitabine plus capecitabine (Xeloda) (1660 mg/m^2/day on days 1–21 every 4 weeks) based on the phase III ESPAC4 trial and improved median OS compared with capecitabine alone (28.0 vs. 25.5 months, $P = .032$). Other regimen options include gemcitabine plus nab-paclitaxel, gemcitabine monotherapy, or 5-fluorouracil plus leucovorin for patients who do not tolerate other regimens because of side effects or overall fitness. Systemic chemotherapy dosing and recommendations for patients who previously received neoadjuvant chemotherapy and/or progress/fail to respond on a certain regimen, are varied and dependent on clinical considerations.

Radiation

Radiation therapy (RT) may be offered for all stages of disease in the neoadjuvant, adjuvant, unresectable, or palliative settings. Neoadjuvant radiation in 36 to 54 Gy has the goal of sterilizing high-risk areas before attempted resection or increasing the likelihood of R0 resection; however, data are inconclusive about its efficacy. In the adjuvant setting, RT in 45 to 50.5 Gy may be recommended in the setting of a positive margin to reduce the risk of local recurrence. In cases of unresectable disease, RT to the primary, specifically in ablative doses of 98-Gy biologically effective dose, can provide durable local tumor control and favorable OS.

Unresectable Disease

Most patients will present with unresectable or metastatic disease. For these patients, FOLFIRINOX or gemcitabine plus nab-paclitaxel are the preferred regimens for those with a good performance status (European Cooperative Oncology Group [ECOG] status 0–1). For patients with ECOG performance status of 2, gemcitabine alone is recommended, whereas for patients with a performance status equal to or greater than 3, emphasis should be placed on palliation, with cancer-directed therapy administered on a case-by-case basis.

Advanced Therapies

Routine testing of tumor tissue for genetic alterations, including actionable somatic findings such as fusions, mutations, amplifications, and copy number alterations, is recommended. In certain patients with actionable mutations, treatment with targeted therapy may be warranted. For example, for patients with mismatch repair deficiency, high levels of microsatellite instability, or tumor mutation burden index ≥ 10 mut/Mb, the programmed cell death protein 1 inhibitor pembrolizumab (Keytruda) is recommended for patients with LA/metastatic disease. Patients with germline *BRCA1/2* mutations who have metastatic but stable or

---

[1] Not FDA approved for this indication.

responsive disease after 4 to 6 months of platinum-based chemotherapy, the poly (ADP ribose) polymerase inhibitor olaparib (Lynparza) (300 mg twice daily), is currently recommended as maintenance therapy based on the results of the phase III POLO trial, which showed improvement in progression-free survival. Of note, olaparib maintenance therapy was not associated with an improvement in OS.

Managing Symptoms and Complications

Once a diagnosis of pancreatic cancer has been established, all patients should be evaluated for symptomatology, physical function, and fitness. The active treatment of symptoms and introduction of palliative care services should be considered early. Modern palliative care is not synonymous with hospice, and palliation has been shown to both improve quality of life and decrease the use of aggressive care measures at the end of life.

Pain can be a predominant symptom in patients with pancreatic cancer and may be described as a midepigastric pain radiating to the back. This can be often managed by traditional multimodal analgesia, including opioid/narcotic analgesia; however, consideration can be given to celiac plexus nerve block or palliative radiation for refractory pain due to local tumor invasion. As described earlier, many patients will also present with **jaundice** due to extrahepatic biliary tract obstruction. Decompression can be achieved with endoscopic, surgical, or percutaneous interventions. Endoscopic stent placement is considered the first line of treatment. Although endoscopically placed stents may be associated with higher rates of readmission for in-stent occlusion or recurrent biliary obstruction, these modalities are generally associated with lower rates of adverse events than percutaneous stent placement. Current guidelines recommend placing a self-expanding metal stent (SEMS) when feasible and only after a histologic diagnosis has been made. Fully covered SEMS can be removed or exchanged and are preferred for patients receiving neoadjuvant chemotherapy; however, the migration rate for non-covered SEMS is lower. Plastic stents are acceptable for patients with a short life expectancy. The decision as to whether to place a plastic, covered metal, or uncovered metal stent is nuanced and should be assessed by a multidisciplinary team, factoring in the full course of multimodal therapy and prognosis. If endoscopic or percutaneous interventions are unavailable or if unresectable disease is discovered at the time of surgery, surgical biliary bypass in the form of choledochojejunostomy may be performed. This may be accompanied by a gastrojejunostomy for the treatment or prevention of **gastric outlet obstruction** (also known as a "double bypass") (Figure 1). As many as 20% of patients with PDAC of the pancreatic head will develop symptomatic gastric outlet obstruction. If not discovered intraoperatively or in patients with short prognoses or limited functional status, endoscopically placed duodenal stents can provide adequate relief of obstructive symptoms.

Pancreatic cancer is generally regarded as one of the highest risk states that predispose patients to **venous thromboembolism** (VTE), conferring a four- to sevenfold higher risk than that faced by the general population. All patients should be counseled about signs and symptoms that may indicate the presence of VTE—either deep venous thrombosis or pulmonary embolism. Current guidelines recommend the use of low-molecular-weight heparin (enoxaparin [Lovenox]) in lieu of warfarin for patients who develop a cancer-related VTE. Routine prophylactic anticoagulation has not been widely adopted because of a lack of survival benefit despite a reduction in VTE events.

Finally, patients with pancreatic cancer may develop **pancreatic exocrine insufficiency** due to pancreatic resection, tumoral destruction of the parenchyma, or blockage of the pancreatic duct. Symptoms include steatorrhea, weight loss, abdominal pain, and malnutrition due to malabsorption of fat-soluble nutrients. Pancreatic enzyme replacement may be started empirically at a dose of 25,000 to 75,000 units of pancrelipase (Creon or Zenpep) per meal with 10,000 to 25,000 units per snack (off-label dosing).

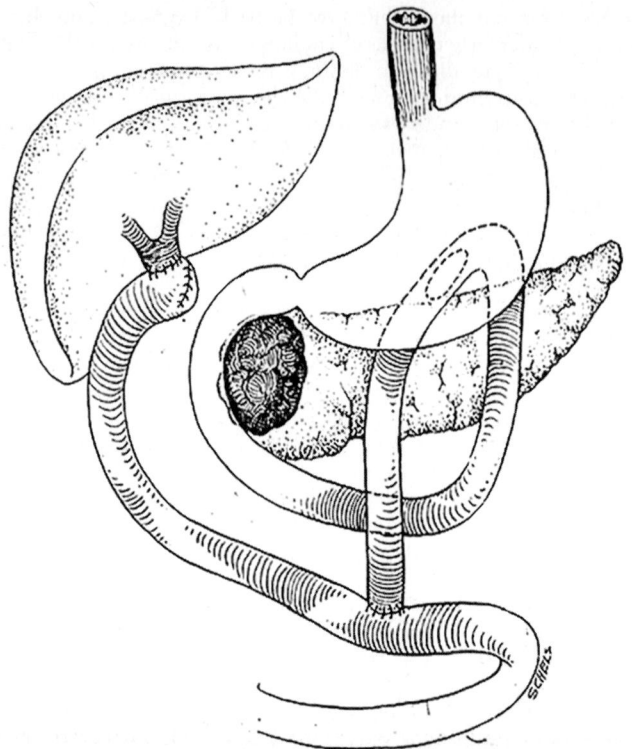

Figure 1 Double bypass showing choledochojejunostomy and gastrojejunostomy with an intact pancreatic head tumor. Reproduced with permission from Scott, E. N., Garcea, G., Doucas, H., Steward, W. P., Dennison, A. R., & Berry, D.P. [2009]. Surgical bypass vs. endoscopic stenting for pancreatic ductal adenocarcinoma. *HPB JOxford], 11*[2], 118–124. Referenced with permission from the NCCN Clinical Practice Guidelines in Oncology [NCCN Guidelines] for Pancreatic Adenocarcinoma V.1.2024. © National Comprehensive Cancer Network, Inc. 2023. All rights reserved. Accessed April 2, 2024. To view the most recent and complete version of the guideline, go to NCCN.org.

Summary

Pancreatic cancer remains a lethal disease. Most patients are not candidates for resection, and appropriate emphasis should be placed on the palliation of symptoms. Improvements in chemotherapy over the last decade have increased both survival and rates of resectability.

References

Becker AE, Hernandez YG, Frucht H, Lucas AL: Pancreatic ductal adenocarcinoma: risk factors, screening, and early detection, *World J Gastroenterol* 20(32):11182–11198, 2014.

Golan T, Hammel P, Reni M, et al: Maintenance Olaparib for Germline BRCA-Mutated Metastatic Pancreatic Cancer, *N Engl J Med* 381(4):317–327, 2019, https://doi.org/10.1056/nejmoa1903387.

Heestand GM, Murphy JD, Lowy AM: Approach to patients with pancreatic cancer without detectable metastases, *J Clin Oncol* 33(16):1770–1778, 2015.

Khorana AA, Mckernin SE, Berlin J, et al: Potentially curable pancreatic adenocarcinoma: ASCO clinical practice guideline update, *J Clin Oncol* 37(23):2082–2088, 2019.

Klotz R, Mihaljevic AL, Kulu Y, et al: Robotic versus open partial pancreatoduodenectomy (EUROPA): a randomised controlled stage 2b trial, *Lancet Reg Health Eur* 39, 2024:100864, https://doi.org/10.1016/j.lanepe.2024.100864.

Korrel M, Jones LR, van Hilst J, et al: Minimally invasive versus open distal pancreatectomy for resectable pancreatic cancer (DIPLOMA): an international randomised non-inferiority trial, *Lancet Reg Health Eur* 31, 2023, https://doi.org/10.1016/j.lanepe.2023.100673.

Kruse EJ: Palliation in pancreatic cancer, *Surg Clin North Am* 90(2):355–364, 2010.

Labori KJ, Bratlie SO, Andersson B, et al: Neoadjuvant FOLFIRINOX versus upfront surgery for resectable pancreatic head cancer (NORPACT-1): a multicentre, randomised, phase 2 trial, *Lancet Gastroenterol Hepatol* 9(3):205–217, 2024, https://doi.org/10.1016/S2468-1253(23)00405-3.

Neoptolemos JP, Palmer DH, Ghaneh P, et al: Comparison of adjuvant gemcitabine and capecitabine with gemcitabine monotherapy in patients with resected pancreatic cancer (ESPAC-4): a multicentre, open-label, randomised, phase 3 trial, *Lancet* 389(10073):1011–1024, 2017, https://doi.org/10.1016/S0140-6736(16)32409-6.

Oettle H, Neuhaus P, Hochhaus A, et al: Adjuvant chemotherapy with gemcitabine and long-term outcomes among patients with resected pancreatic cancer: The CONKO-001 randomized trial, *JAMA* 310(14):1473–1481, 2013, https://doi.org/10.1001/jama.2013.279201.

Pannala R, Basu A, Petersen GM, Chari ST: New-onset diabetes: a potential clue to the early diagnosis of pancreatic cancer, *Lancet Oncol* 10(1):88–95, 2009, https://doi.org/10.1016/S1470-2045(08)70337-1.

Rebours V, Lévy P, Ruszniewski P: An overview of hereditary pancreatitis, *Dig Liver Dis* 44(1):8–15, 2012.

Reyngold M, O'Reilly EM, Varghese AM, et al: Association of Ablative Radiation Therapy With Survival Among Patients With Inoperable Pancreatic Cancer, *JAMA Oncol* 7(5):735–738, 2021, https://doi.org/10.1001/jamaoncol.2021.0057.

SEER*Explorer: An interactive website for SEER cancer statistics [Internet]: *Surveillance Research Program*, National Cancer Institute, 2023. [updated: 2023 Nov 16; cited 2024 Apr 2]. Available from: https://seer.cancer.gov/statistics-network/explorer/. Data source(s): SEER Incidence Data, November 2022 Submission (1975-2020), SEER 22 registries.

Sohal DPS, Kennedy EB, Khorana A, et al: Metastatic pancreatic cancer: ASCO clinical practice guideline update, *J Clin Oncol* 36(24):2545–2556, 2018.

Versteijne E, Suker M, Groothuis K, et al: Preoperative Chemoradiotherapy Versus Immediate Surgery for Resectable and Borderline Resectable Pancreatic Cancer: Results of the Dutch Randomized Phase III PREOPANC Trial, *J Clin Oncol* 19(02274), 2020, https://doi.org/10.1200/jco.19.02274.

Versteijne E, Van Dam JL, Suker M, et al: Neoadjuvant Chemoradiotherapy Versus Upfront Surgery for Resectable and Borderline Resectable Pancreatic Cancer: Long-Term Results of the Dutch Randomized PREOPANC Trial, *J Clin Oncol* 40:1220–1230, 2022, https://doi.org/10.1200/JCO.21.

TUMORS OF THE COLON AND RECTUM

Method of
Richard Huettemann, MD; Colleen A. Donahue, MD; Thomas Curran, MD, MPH; Virgilio V. George, MD; and Pinckney J. Maxwell IV, MD

CURRENT DIAGNOSIS

- Screening of asymptomatic average-risk patients should begin at 45 years of age.
- Colonoscopy should be performed if any screening test results are positive.
- Colonoscopy should be performed on any patient with signs or symptoms of colorectal cancer
- Screening of high-risk patients, those with inflammatory bowel disease (IBD), familial adenomatous polyposis (FAP), hereditary nonpolyposis colorectal cancer (HNPCC), or a significant positive family history, should begin at an earlier age and occur more frequently.

CURRENT THERAPY

- Patients with FAP should undergo early prophylactic colon resection. Patients with HNPCC should be counseled regarding prophylactic total colectomy.
- Colon tumors should be treated with segmental laparoscopic or open resection.
- Chemotherapy is offered for colon cancers with locally advanced, nodal (stage III), or metastatic (stage IV) disease. It may also be considered in stage II patients with high risk features on pathology.
- Rectal tumors that are small (<3 cm), <25% of the rectal circumference, superficial (Tis or T1), lack nodal involvement, and have favorable pathologic characteristics should be removed by transanal techniques.
- Rectal tumors may be treated using open or minimally invasive techniques by performing a total mesorectal excision.
- Combination chemotherapy and radiation therapy is offered for advanced (stage II), nodal (stage III), or metastatic (stage IV) rectal cancer. All rectal cancers should be screened for microsatellite instability prior to initiating treatment.
- Postoperative surveillance includes frequent office evaluations, carcinoembryonic antigen (CEA) levels, endoscopy, and imaging.

Background, Epidemiology, and Etiology

Colorectal cancer is the third most common cancer in men and women, after prostate and lung/bronchus in men and breast and lung/bronchus in women. The American Cancer Society (ACS) expects an estimated 106,970 new diagnoses of colon cancer and an estimated 46,050 new diagnoses of rectal cancer in 2023. The overall incidence of colorectal cancer has been decreasing since the mid-1980s, with a more dramatic decrease in the past decade. This decrease is likely related to an increase in screening with removal of precancerous polyps. However, despite an overall decrease in incidence in colorectal cancer, there has been an increase in incidence of colorectal cancer of those under 50 years of age. The ACS expects an estimated 52,550 deaths from colorectal cancer in 2023, which accounts for 8.6% of all cancer deaths. There has been a similar decrease in mortality since the mid-1980s, again with a sharper decline in the past decade likely related to improved screening as well. Colorectal cancer is a highly treatable and frequently curable malignancy when detected early, with a 91% 5-year survival for localized (stage I and II) disease highlighting the need for better screening.

The development of colorectal cancer is related to a number of factors, including age, diet, activity, environmental exposures, family history, and genetics. Ninety percent of colorectal cancers are diagnosed after 50 years of age, and fewer than 5% of cases are diagnosed before 40 years of age. The peak incidence of diagnosis is in the seventh decade of life. Dietary factors play a role in carcinogenesis as well. Western diets, consisting of high-fat and low-fiber, and the intake of red or processed meats and alcohol have been associated with increased rates of colorectal cancer. It is likely that this low-fiber Western diet slows transit time, leading to increased exposure to carcinogens. Activity level also can play a role in carcinogenesis, as studies have shown an increase in cancer among those with sedentary jobs and a decreased incidence among those with regular exercise. Exposure to cigarette smoke increases the risk of colorectal adenomas and cancers. The ACS Cancer Prevention Study II revealed that 12% of colorectal cancer deaths in the general U.S. population can be attributed to smoking. Family history and genetics also play a significant role in carcinogenesis, as approximately 10% of patients diagnosed have a first-degree relative with colorectal cancer.

Adenomatous Polyps

The progression from normal mucosa to an adenomatous polyp to an invasive colorectal cancer proceeds through a well-defined process, over many years. Aberrant crypt foci develop into microadenomas and then into adenomatous polyps. Dysplastic cells develop within the polyp, continue to multiply, become a tumor, and then break through the subepithelial barrier and invade through the layers of the bowel wall, eventually spreading to pericolic tissues or to lymph nodes and distant sites. A number of genes have been implicated in carcinogenesis, including proto-oncogenes *(K-ras, src, c-myc)*, tumor-suppressor genes *(APC, DCC, p53, MCC, DPC4)*, and DNA mismatch repair genes *(MLH1, PMS2, MSH2, MSH6, EPCAM)*. Sporadic colorectal cancers generally develop as a result of several cumulative genetic insults involving these genes (Figure 1).

Familial Colorectal Cancer Syndromes

Familial adenomatous polyposis (FAP) is an inherited, non–sex-linked, Mendelian-dominant disease that accounts for approximately 1% of all colorectal cancers. The high penetrance of FAP means that there is a 50% chance of development within affected families. However, 25% of FAP patients have no family history, likely representing a new, spontaneous mutation. The disorder is caused by mutations in either the tumor-suppressor *APC* gene, which is located on chromosome 5 (5q21–q22), or in the *MUTYH* gene, which is located on chromosome 1 (1p34.3–p32.1). FAP is characterized by the progressive development of hundreds to thousands of adenomatous polyps located throughout the entire colon. The clinical diagnosis is based on the histologic confirmation of at least 100 adenomas. All patients will eventually develop colorectal

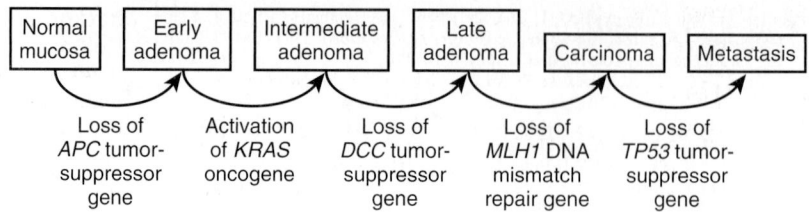

Figure 1 Adenoma to carcinoma sequence.

BOX 1   Diagnosis of Hereditary Nonpolyposis Colon Cancer

Amsterdam I Criteria, 1990
- Three or more family members with histologically verified colorectal cancer, one of whom is a first-degree relative (parent, child, sibling) of the other two
- Two successive affected generations
- One or more colon cancers diagnosed before 50 years of age
- Familial adenomatous polyposis has been excluded

Amsterdam II Criteria, 1999
- Three or more family members with histologically verified HNPCC-related cancers (endometrium, ovary, stomach, small intestine, hepatobiliary, upper urinary tract, brain, and skin), one of whom is a first-degree relative (parent, child, sibling) of the other two
- Two successive affected generations
- One or more colon cancers diagnosed before 50 years of age
- Familial adenomatous polyposis has been excluded

Revised Bethesda Guidelines, 2002
- Colorectal cancer diagnosed in a patient who younger than 50 years of age
- Presence of a synchronous, metachronous colorectal, or other HNPCC-related malignancy, regardless of age
- Colorectal cancer with the *MSI-H* histology diagnosed in a patient younger than 60 years of age
  - Presence of carcinoma-infiltrating lymphocytes, Crohn's-like lymphocytic reaction, mucinous/signet-ring differentiation, or medullary growth pattern
  - No general consensus based on this age
- Colorectal cancer diagnosed in one or more first-degree relatives with an HNPCC-related neoplasm
  - With one or more neoplasm being diagnosed before 50 years of age
- Colorectal cancer diagnosed in two or more first- or second-degree relatives With HNPCC-related malignancies, regardless of age

HNCC, Hereditary nonpolyposis colorectal cancer.

---

cancer. Adenomas generally appear by the mid-20s, and cancers generally appear by the late-30s. An attenuated form of FAP is recognized in which fewer adenomas (12–100) are identified, with cancer developing between 50 and 70 years of age. FAP also exhibits extracolonic manifestations including gastric/duodenal/small bowel polyps, osteomas and desmoid tumors (Gardner syndrome), eye lesions (congenital hypertrophy of retinal pigment epithelium [CHRPE]), papillary thyroid cancer (up to 12% of FAP patients), epidermoid cysts, and brain neoplasms (Turcot syndrome).

Hereditary nonpolyposis colon cancer (HNPCC), also called *Lynch syndrome*, is an inherited, non–sex-linked, Mendelian-dominant disease with virtually complete penetrance. HNPCC is caused by a defect in any of a number of DNA mismatch repair genes *(MLH1, MSH2, MSH6, EPCAM, PMS2)*, which leads to microsatellite instability *(MSI-H)*. A number of criteria have been generated for the diagnosis of HNPCC, including the Amsterdam I and II criteria and the Bethesda guidelines (Box 1). According to the EPICOLON study, the revised Bethesda guidelines are the most discriminating set of clinical parameters for diagnosing HNPCC. However, the use of clinical guidelines alone for Lynch syndrome screening has been shown to underestimate the number of patients with Lynch syndrome. Therefore, in 2009, the NCCN recommended universal Lynch syndrome screening for all colorectal or endometrial cancers.

HNPCC is subdivided into Lynch syndrome types I and II. Lynch type I refers to site-specific nonpolyposis colon cancer, and Lynch type II (formerly called *familial cancer syndrome*) refers to cancers that develop in the colon and related organs such as the endometrium, ovaries, stomach, pancreas, and proximal urinary tract, among others.

Lynch syndrome differs from sporadic colorectal cancer in a number of important ways. It has an autosomal dominant inheritance, a predominance of proximal lesions (75% are found in the right colon), an excess of multiple primary colorectal cancers (18%), an early age of onset averaging 44 years, a significantly improved survival rate of right-sided lesions when compared with family members with distal colorectal cancer (53% vs. 35% 5-year survival), and an increased risk of development of metachronous lesions (24%). Lynch syndrome is the most common herditary form of colon cancer and affects approximately 1/300 people. Increased surveillance for patients with Lynch syndrome has been shown to reduce cancer-related deaths. Patients and family members of those diagnosed with HNPCC and FAP should undergo genetic testing to aid in future diagnosis and treatment options.

Inflammatory Bowel Disease

Both Crohn's disease (CD) and ulcerative colitis (UC) confer an increased risk of colorectal cancer, with UC approximately double the risk of CD. The duration and severity of CD and the duration and extent (left-sided colitis vs. pancolitis) of UC contribute to cancer risk in inflammatory bowel disease (IBD). Cancer in CD can occur in any segment with inflammation, but is more likely to occur in a stricture or bypass segment given the inability to surveil these areas. Importantly, neoplasia in UC does not follow the adenoma-carcinoma sequence of sporadic colorectal cancer. This change has important screening and treatment implications.

Screening the Average-Risk Patient

Patients with no personal history of colorectal polyps or cancers, no personal history of IBD, no symptoms suspicious for colorectal cancer, no family history of colorectal polyps or cancers, and no evidence of a familial or genetic syndrome can be screened as average risk. Two main categories of screening tests include those that detect adenomatous polyps and cancer (flexible sigmoidoscopy, colonoscopy, double-contrast barium enema, and computed tomography [CT] colonography) and those that primarily detect cancer (fecal occult blood testing [FOBT], fecal immunohistochemical testing [FIT], and stool DNA testing). The goal of screening is to reduce mortality by reducing the incidence of advanced disease. It seems intuitive that tests detecting polyps, the premalignant phase of colorectal cancer, would be preferred to tests detecting only cancers. However, testing for polyps and cancer is generally procedure related, requiring access to care, while testing for cancers can be conducted on stool studies alone and done at home. Screening with simple stool samples has the potential to more easily increase overall screening, but is not preventive without the ability for endoscopic polyp removal.

BOX 2   Screening the High Risk Patient for Colorectal Cancer

Risk Category	Age to Begin	Recommendation	Comment
Personal history of <3 adenomas with low- grade dysplasia	5–10 years after the initial polypectomy	Colonoscopy	Examination interval should be based on other clinical factors such as prior examination findings, family history, or preferences of the endoscopist or patient.
Personal history of 3–10 adenomas, or 1 adenoma >1 cm, or any adenoma with villous features or high-grade dysplasia	3 years after the initial polypectomy	Colonoscopy	Adenomas require compete excision. If the follow-up is normal, the next examination should be in 5 years. More than 10 adenomas should raise suspicion of a familial syndrome.
Personal history of colorectal cancer	1 year after resection	Colonoscopy	Patients should undergo high- quality preoperative clearing. Follow-up after normal examinations should be extended to 3 years and then to 5 years
Family history of adenomas or cancer in a first-degree relative <60 years of age or in two first-degree relatives at any age	40 years of age or 10 years before the youngest case	Colonoscopy	Every 5 years
Family history of adenomas or cancer in a first-degree relative >60 years of age or in two second-degree relatives with cancer	40 years of age	Colonoscopy	Screening should be initiated at an earlier age. Intervals based on findings or by the average-risk patient
FAP or suspected FAP	10–12 years of age	Annual FS, counseling for genetic testing if showing polyps	Colectomy should be considered for positive genetic testing/after puberty
HNPCC or risk of HNPCC	20–25 years of age or 10 years before the youngest case	Colonoscopy, counseling for genetic testing	Every 1–2 years. Genetic testing should be offered to first-degree relatives of persons with a known DNA mismatch repair gene, or with one of the first three Bethesda criteria
IBD, Crohn's, or chronic UC	8 years after the onset of pancolitis, or 12–15 years after the onset of left- sided colitis	Colonoscopies with random 4 quad biopsies every 10 cm for dysplasia	Screening should be offered every 1–2 years, and patients are best referred to a center with experience in the surveillance and management of IBD.

FAP, Familial adenomatous polyposis; *FS*, flexible sigmoidoscopy; *HNPCC*, hereditary nonpolyposis colorectal cancer; *IBD*, inflammatory bowel disease.

Regardless of the method employed, testing in the average-risk, asymptomatic patient should begin at 45 years of age based on the most recent updated guidelines because of the increasing disease burden in people younger than 50 years of age. A complete colonoscopy is only required every 10 years, but it requires an oral bowel preparation and carries a small risk of perforation of approximately 1 in 1000. A flexible sigmoidoscopy is required every 5 years when combined with FOBT annually, and this is the only colorectal cancer screening method that has been studied in a randomized control trial. The testing is more frequent, but it requires only enemas for preparation and carries a lower risk of perforation. Air-contrast barium enemas can be used for screening every 5 years, but they also require an oral bowel preparation and are only diagnostic. CT colonography is an evolving method for screening every 5 years and has the opportunity for more accessible screening; however, there are limitations on the identification of polyps less than 1 cm. It also requires an oral bowel preparation and is only diagnostic; thus it is used in conjunction with flexible sigmoidoscopy and FIT. FOBT and FIT require annual testing. The U.S Food and Drug Administration (FDA) has also approved a FIT-fecal DNA test that is performed at 3-year intervals; however, it is less specific and less cost-effective than FIT, making it unlikely to replace FIT. The most complete screening test, allowing removal of precancerous lesions if identified, remains complete colonoscopy,

and importantly, the patient should undergo full endoscopic evaluation if any other screening test is positive.

Screening the High-Risk Patient

High-risk patients include those with a personal history of colorectal polyps or cancers, a family history of colorectal cancer in a first-degree relative, those with Crohn's disease or UC, and those with a personal or family history of FAP or HNPCC. Screening in these patients has been adjusted for changes in incidence and age of onset of neoplasia (Box 2).

Symptoms and Diagnosis

Symptoms of colorectal cancer include bleeding (85%), a change in bowel habits, abdominal pain, malaise, and obstruction. Frequently, anemia may be the only sign a patient exhibits. Patients with symptoms suspicious for colorectal cancer should undergo colonoscopy. An anorectal source of bleeding should not preclude a complete colonic evaluation.

Preoperative Management

Before operative intervention, a complete evaluation should occur, including a careful history and physical examination, routine laboratory testing, and a carcinoembryonic antigen (CEA) level. A complete evaluation of the colon is essential and utilizes colonoscopy with biopsy or barium enema or CT colonography if colonoscopy is incomplete. Bowel preparation with antibiotics is indicated as a routine preoperative measure for colonic surgery per the latest guidelines from the American Society of Colon and Rectal Surgeons (ASCRS).

Preoperative staging should be undertaken for colorectal cancers. This includes CT of the abdomen and pelvis with contrast and CT scan of the thorax to rule out intrathoracic metastatic disease. CT scanning of the abdomen and pelvis are indicated to aid in the evaluation of the extent of localized or metastatic disease and the presence of enlarged lymph nodes. Staging of rectal cancers includes determining the distance from the anal verge (frequently utilizing a rigid proctoscope), the depth of invasion, and the presence of enlarged lymph nodes (utilizing magnetic resonance imaging). Metastatic disease mandates neoadjuvant chemotherapy in the absence of acute symptoms of obstruction or exsanguination. Rectal cancers with locally advanced disease (T3-4, N1-2) or evidence of enlarged metastatic lymph nodes benefit from neoadjuvant chemotherapy and radiation. Preoperative staging allows for the application of neoadjuvant therapy in selected candidates, which can downstage and downsize tumors and can decrease rates of local recurrence in rectal cancer. Neoadjuvant therapy can also allow for sphincter-preserving procedures for previously bulky or very low rectal tumors.

Surgery for Colonic Tumors

The primary therapy for tumors of the colon is operative. The basic principles of surgery for colon cancer include the following:

- Exploration: adequate visual, tactile, and potentially intraoperative hepatic ultrasound staging at the time of primary resection to evaluate for peritoneal, mesenteric, or hepatic disease
- Removal of the entire cancer with enough bowel proximal and distal to encompass the possibility of submucosal lymphatic tumor spread. At least 5-cm margin proximal and distal for colon and upper rectal cancers is recommended. Any negative margin is acceptable in low rectal cancers.
- Removal of regional mesenteric pedicle, including draining lymphatics, based on the predictable lymphatic spread of the disease and the potential for regional mesenteric involvement without concurrent distant involvement
- En bloc resection of involved structures (T4 tumors)
- Segmental colonic resections (right, transverse, left, or sigmoid colectomy) based on the tumor location and blood supply with lymphatic drainage, specifically the ileocolic, middle colic, and left colic arteries. These resections define both a convenient anatomic boundary for standard colonic resection and also provide for adequate regional lymph node clearance because the major draining lymphatics follow these blood vessels in the mesentery. Locally invasive tumors (T4) require en bloc resection of involved structures. Metastatic colonic tumors (M1) may require neoadjuvant chemotherapy before resection or palliation.

Numerous studies have proven that minimally invasive surgery is appropriate and perhaps preferred for colon cancer in experienced hands. There is evidence showing decreased length of stay for minimally invasive surgery without a decrease in oncologic outcomes; reduction in homeostatic insults likely leads to more favorable overall outcomes. The application of minimally invasive techniques for rectal cancer resection is still controversial but is gaining popularity.

Surgery for Rectal Tumors

Two different approaches for rectal tumors include local excision and formal oncologic rectal resection. Local excision is the treatment of choice for a select, small group (3%–5%) of all patients diagnosed with rectal cancer. Tumors amenable to transanal excision are small (<3 cm), <25% of the rectal circumference, confined to the mucosa or submucosa (Tis or T1), lack nodal involvement by preoperative imaging, and have favorable pathologic characteristics (well or moderately differentiated with no lymphovascular invasion). Tumors in the lower or middle third of the rectum are accessible by simple transanal excision, but tumors of the upper rectum require the use of transanal endoscopic microsurgery (TEMS) or transanal minimally invasive surgery (TAMIS) techniques for resection. Local excision requires a 1-cm normal margin, but the defect generally does not require closure.

Tumors staged at T2 or greater require a formal resection, the type of which depends on the location of the tumor. Upper and middle rectal tumors can generally be managed with a low or very low anterior resection. Lower rectal tumors frequently require a proctectomy with coloanal anastomosis or an abdominoperineal resection (APR) depending on sphincter involvement and patient-related quality-of-life factors. The goal of resection is to obtain a 5-cm distal margin; however, lower tumors can be managed with a 2-cm distal margin. Very low tumors or those involving the sphincter mechanism require an APR. Rectal tumors with a greater depth of rectal wall invasion (T3), evidence of fixation or local invasion (T4), or evidence of lymph nodal (N1–N2) or metastatic (M1) disease mandate neoadjuvant chemoradiation therapy and more recently, total neoadjuvant therapy which includes chemoradiation as well as chemotherapy in the neoadjuvant setting. Proctectomy requires a tumor-specific total mesorectal excision (TME). This involves complete excision of all mesorectal tissue located behind the rectum and no carcinoma at the lateral or circumferential margins. The goal of the TME is to remove all malignant tissue to reduce or eliminate the possibility of locally recurrent disease. Locally advanced rectal tumors may preclude an effective or safe resection. Some indications for likely inoperability include extensive pelvic disease, invasion of ileofemoral vessels, extensive lymphatic involvement or significant lower extremity lymphedema, bony involvement, or life expectancy less than 3 to 6 months.

Minimally invasive surgical techniques are similarly being performed for rectal malignancies. Studies are underway to verify the efficacy and safety of these methods in rectal resection compared with traditional open resection. It has gained widespread popularity and is very commonly used. Given the complexity and constantly evolving management for rectal cancer, we recommend all patients be presented at a multidisciplinary tumor board and referred to a high volume rectal cancer center or rectal cancer center of excellence.

Complicated Disease

Colorectal tumors may present with complications including obstruction, perforation, or significant bleeding. These presentations are generally related to more advanced disease and may preclude a complete staging workup or potential neoadjuvant therapy. Unless patients are unstable or critically ill or the tumor is unresectable, an oncologic resection should be performed. An ostomy is generally performed, whether as an end ostomy or as a proximal loop diversion for a primary anastomosis. Colonic stenting is an attractive option for obstructing lesions as either palliation or as a bridge to resection after medical stabilization and staging for potential neoadjuvant therapy.

Surgery for High-Risk Conditions

High-risk conditions for the development of colorectal malignancies include FAP, HNPCC, and chronic UC. Surgical management may be prophylactic or possibly therapeutic after a malignancy has been diagnosed. The mainstay of operative management in FAP and chronic UC is a total proctocolectomy. Reconstructive options include an ileal pouch-anal anastomosis, a continent ileostomy (Kock pouch), or an end ileostomy. A total abdominal colectomy with ileorectal anastomosis may be performed for temporary preservation of rectal function in selected cases of chronic UC with rectal sparing and FAP with few rectal polyps, but this requires aggressive surveillance of the remaining rectal mucosa's risk of malignancy. Patients with HNPCC should be counseled regarding the increased risk of metachronous cancers and therefore consider subtotal colectomy with ileorectal anastomosis, and a total hysterectomy with bilateral salpingoophorectomy should be offered because of the preponderance of associated gynecologic malignancy at the age of 40 years or after child bearing.

Pathologic Staging and Adjuvant Therapy

Excellent pathologic sampling and review of the operative specimen provides important prognostic and therapeutic information. Current standards recommend at least 12 lymph nodes be removed for adequate staging of colon cancer. The decision for adjuvant chemotherapy and/or radiation therapy is based on pathologic staging. This information also provides prognostic information in terms of survival to the patient and their family. A number of staging systems have been developed, however the TNM system is most commonly used in the United States (Box 3).

Chemotherapy is offered for colorectal cancers with locally advanced, nodal (stage III), or metastatic (stage IV) disease. There may be a subset of patients with stage II disease and high risk pathologic features who may be recommended for chemotherapy and should be discussed at a multidisciplinary conference. The combination of chemotherapy and radiation therapy for advanced rectal cancer (stages II to IV) has decreased local recurrence and increased survival. The current guidelines recommend total neoadjuvant therapy with both radiation and chemotherapy in the preoperative setting. Additional adjuvant chemotherapy is dependent on the final pathology and extent of chemotherapy received preoperatively. Numerous protocols are available for treatment, with the standard of care being FOLFOX: 5-fluorouracil (5-FU), leucovorin, and oxaliplatin (Eloxatin). Older adult patients or those with multiple comorbidities who may not be able to tolerate full-dose chemotherapy may be candidates for capecitabine (Xeloda) or 5-FU and leucovorin. Numerous study protocols are available at specialized centers evaluating other medications. Newer technologies continue to evolve, such as anti-angiogenesis agents and immunomodulatory agents. The latest development is the use of PDL-1 inhibitors in microsatellite unstable colon and rectal cancers in place of chemotherapy. Therefore, it is highly recommended

that all patients are tested for microsatellite instability or mismatch repair deficiency prior to initiating treatment.

Metastatic Disease

Surgical therapy is also available for metastatic disease in certain situations. Metastatic liver lesions amenable to resection can be addressed either at the time of colon resection or after the patient has healed from the colectomy. The lesions could be resected or treated using radiofrequency ablation (RFA), a newer technology allowing in-situ destruction of liver lesions. Similarly, selected pulmonary metastases can be resected, possibly using minimally invasive thoracoscopic techniques. The majority of deaths from colorectal cancer are from metastatic disease; over 20% of patients have widespread disease at diagnosis. A multidisciplinary approach to patients with metastatic disease should be undertaken to discern if it is resectable and what intervention should be pursued.

Surveillance

Surveillance for colon and rectal cancer is a lifelong process. Patients are seen and examined in the office every 3 months for 2 years, then every 6 months for 3 years, and then yearly. CEA levels are routinely obtained as a marker for tumor recurrence. Endoscopy should be performed at 1 year postoperatively, given a high-quality preoperative study to clear the entire colon. Normal examinations allow subsequent colonoscopies to occur at 3 years and then every 5 years. Similarly, annual imaging utilizing chest radiography and CT of the abdomen and pelvis are obtained. Patients with increased or rising CEA levels or with evidence of recurrent disease can be evaluated using positron emission tomography (PET). Newer testing for surveillance and treatment response in colorectal cancer is on the horizon, such as circulating tumor DNA; however, these studies are still in process and are not yet part of the national guidelines for surveillance.

References

American Cancer Society: *Cancer facts and figures 2022*, Atlanta, GA, 2022, American Cancer Society. Available at: https://www.cancer.org/content/dam/cancer-org/research/cancer-facts-and-statistics/annual-cancer-facts-and-figures/2022/2022-cancer-facts-and-figures.pdf.

Beart RW, Steele Jr GD, Menck HR, Chmiel JS, Ocwieia KE, Winchester DP: Management and survival of patients with adenocarcinoma of the colon and rectum: a national survey of the commission on cancer, *J Am Coll Surg* 181:225–236, 1995.

Bentrem DJ, Okabe S, Wong WD, et al: T1 adenocarcinoma of the rectum: transanal excision or radical surgery? *Ann Surg* 242:472–479, 2005.

The Clinical Outcomes of Surgical Therapy Study Group: A comparison of laparoscopically assisted and open colectomy for colon cancer, *N Engl J Med* 350:2050–2059, 2004.

Floyd ND, Saclarides TJ: Transanal endoscopic microsurgical resection of pT1 rectal tumors, *Dis Colon Rectum* 49:164–168, 2005.

Lan Y-T, Lin J-K, Li AF-Y, et al: Metachronous colorectal cancer: necessity of postoperative colonoscopic surveillance, *Int J Colorectal Dis* 20:121–125, 2005.

Maetani I, Tada T, Ukita T, et al: Self-expandable metallic stent placement as palliative treatment of obstructed colorectal carcinoma, *J Gastroenterol* 39:334–338, 2004.

Patel SG, May FP, Anderson JC, et al: Updates on age to start and stop colorectal cancer screening: recommendations from the U.S. multi-society task force on colorectal cancer, *Gastroenterology* 162(1):285–299, 2022 Jan, https://doi.org/10.1053/j.gastro.2021.10.007. Epub 2021 Nov 15. PMID: 34794816.

Pinol V, Castells A, Andreu M, et al: Accuracy of revised bethesda guidelines, microsatellite instability, and immunohistochemistry for the identification of patients with hereditary nonpolyposis colorectal cancer, *JAMA* 293:1986–1994, 2005.

Rex DK, Boland CR, Dominitz JA, et al: Colorectal cancer screening: recommendations for physicians and patients from the U.S. multi-society task force on colorectal cancer, *Am J Gastroenterol* 112(7):1016–1030, 2017 Jul, https://doi.org/10.1038/ajg.2017.174. Epub 2017 Jun 6. PMID: 28555630.

Sauer R, Becker H, Hohenberger W, et al: For the german rectal cancer study group. preoperative versus postoperative chemoradiotherapy for rectal cancer, *N Engl J Med* 351:1731–1740, 2004.

Steel SR, Hull TL, Hyman N, Maykel JA, Read TE, Whitlow CB: *The ASCRS textbook of colon and rectal surgery*, ed 4, Springer Nature Switzerland AG, 2022.

Stipa F, Chessin DB, Shia J, et al: A pathologic complete response of rectal cancer to preoperative combined-modality therapy results in improved oncological outcome compared with those who achieve no downstaging on the basis of preoperative endorectal ultrasonography. *Ann Surg Oncol* 13(8): 1047–1053.

TUMORS OF THE STOMACH

Method of
David A. Mahvi, MD; and Mark Fairweather, MD

CURRENT DIAGNOSIS

- Screening programs exist in countries with a very high incidence of gastric adenocarcinoma and can be considered elsewhere for individuals at high risk.
- Esophagogastroduodenoscopy with biopsy is the gold standard for diagnosis of stomach tumors.
- Staging workup for adenocarcinoma includes computed tomography (CT) of the chest, abdomen, and pelvis to evaluate for metastatic disease. Fluorodeoxyglucose position-emission tomography/computed tomography (FDG-PET/CT) is indicated for locally advanced disease, and endoscopic ultrasonography (EUS) is recommended for suspected early-stage disease.

CURRENT THERAPY

Adenocarcinoma

- All treatment decisions for gastric adenocarcinoma should be made by multidisciplinary teams.
- Universal testing for microsatellite instability (MSI) is recommended for all patients. HER2, PD-L1, and claudin 18.2 testing is recommended if patients have advanced or metastatic disease.
- Patients with T1a tumors and no evidence of nodal or metastatic spread can be candidates for endoscopic or surgical resection.
- Patients with T1b tumors without nodal involvement or metastatic disease should undergo upfront surgical resection.
- Patients with T2 or higher disease or any nodal involvement should receive perioperative chemotherapy, with the FLOT regimen (5-fluorouracil, leucovorin[1], oxaliplatin[1], and docetaxel[1]) being first-line treatment.
- Surgery consists of either a distal gastrectomy or total gastrectomy depending on tumor location and should include at least 15 lymph nodes for accurate staging. Less frequently a proximal gastrectomy or esophagogastrectomy can be considered for proximal stomach adenocarcinoma.

Gastrointestinal Stromal Tumors

- All tumors greater than 2 cm should be considered for resection. Gastrointestinal stromal tumors less than 2 cm in size without high-risk features can be considered for surveillance.
- No lymphadenectomy is required, and grossly negative margins are sufficient.
- Imatinib (Gleevec), a tyrosine kinase inhibitor, should be offered after surgery to patients with a high risk of tumor recurrence (either a primary tumor >5 cm or a mitotic rate >5 per 50 high-power field).
- Imatinib can be given to patients before surgery if preoperative tumor shrinkage is needed[1].

Neuroendocrine Tumors

- Type 1 and type 2 tumors can undergo endoscopic resection if they are less than 2 cm in size, are not poorly differentiated, and do not invade beyond the submucosa.
- Surgical resection should be performed for all type 3 tumors, as well as for type 1 and 2 tumors that have positive margins, recur, or have the worrisome features listed earlier.
- Patients can develop carcinoid syndrome with liver metastases, which can be treated with somatostatin analogs, surgical cytoreduction, or liver-directed therapies.

Gastric Lymphoma

- Mucosa-associated lymphoid tissue (MALT) lymphomas often respond to *Helicobacter pylori* eradication.
- Other lymphomas are treated with chemotherapy, with surgery being reserved for patients with complications such as bleeding or perforation.

[1]Not FDA approved for this indication.

Gastric Adenocarcinoma

Gastric adenocarcinoma is the fourth leading cause of cancer-related death worldwide, accounting for an estimated 768,000 deaths in 2020. Gastric cancer is the fifth most common cancer worldwide, with just over 1 million new cases annually. The highest incidence rates are in Eastern Asia, Eastern Europe, and the Andean region of South America. The annual burden is predicted to increase to 1.8 million new cases and 1.3 million deaths by the year 2040. In the United States gastric cancer is less prevalent, with the predicted 16th highest incidence and 17th highest mortality rate estimated in 2025.

Classification

Historically, gastric adenocarcinomas have been divided into two main subtypes by the Lauren classification system: intestinal and diffuse. Intestinal-type gastric cancers are similar to adenocarcinomas elsewhere in the gastrointestinal tract, appearing in glandular or tubular formations. Intestinal-type gastric adenocarcinomas are more likely to occur in male and older adult patients and have a more favorable prognosis. The diffuse subtype lacks cohesive molecules, specifically E-cadherin, and will invade without gland formation. The diffuse subtype has a worse prognosis.

Risk Factors

There are a number of risk factors for gastric adenocarcinoma. Although most cancers are sporadic, 1% to 3% are caused by a genetic mutation (most commonly *E-cadherin/CDH1* mutations). Numerous dietary factors have been linked to subsequent gastric cancer development, including salt and salt-preserved foods, dietary nitrites, and processed foods. Additional factors include obesity and cigarette use. Men are also more likely to develop the disease than women.

A history of *H. pylori* infection or chronic atrophic gastritis also increases a patient's risk of developing subsequent stomach cancer. The International Agency for Research on Cancer has designated *H. pylori* as a group 1 carcinogen and estimates that *H. pylori* solely attributes to 36% of gastric cancers in developed countries and 47% in developing countries. Both intestinal and diffuse subtypes of gastric adenocarcinoma are associated with *H. pylori*. *H. pylori* strains with the *cagA* gene have a poorer prognosis. The purported mechanism is that chronic inflammation associated with the infection and subsequent development of atrophic gastritis can lead to intestinal metaplasia.

Screening

National screening programs have been established in Japan and South Korea, both of which have a relatively high incidence of gastric cancer. In Korea, screening is recommended every 2 years starting at 40 years of age. In Japan, screening is performed every 2 to 3 years starting at 50 years of age. Both countries have shown diagnosis at earlier cancer stages improved with use of their screening programs. The relative utility and cost-effectiveness of national gastric cancer screening with either upper endoscopy or upper gastrointestinal series has not been established in countries with a lower relative incidence of gastric cancer. Individualized screening can be considered for those with high-risk genetic syndromes, such as *CDH1* mutation, Lynch syndrome, Peutz-Jeghers syndrome, and familial adenomatous polyposis. Patients with a pathogenic variant of *CDH1* should be referred to expert centers for discussion of risk-reducing total gastrectomy and high-risk endoscopic surveillance with biopsies according to the Bethesda protocol. Screening can also be considered in patients with a strong family history of gastric cancer or who have previously established atrophic gastritis or intestinal metaplasia.

Clinical Manifestations

Patients with gastric adenocarcinoma often have vague symptoms that may not be present until they develop more advanced disease. Epigastric abdominal pain (52%) and weight loss (62%) are the most common symptoms, but early satiety, decreased appetite, and nausea can also occur. New-onset heartburn or reflux can be a presenting symptom and warrants further workup, especially in older adults. Melena and anemia can be seen in tumors that are bleeding. A rare subset of patients may have systemic manifestations of gastric cancer. These paraneoplastic syndromes include the Leser-Trélat sign, which is characterized by sudden onset of multiple seborrheic keratoses, and acanthosis nigricans, which appears as dark pigmentation in skin folds. However, these manifestations are not specific to gastric cancer and can be associated with benign processes as well.

Diagnosis

Esophagogastroduodenoscopy (EGD) with biopsy is the gold standard for gastric cancer diagnosis. This allows for tissue diagnosis and anatomic localization of the primary tumor. Of note, per the American Joint Committee on Cancer (AJCC) and the Union for International Cancer Control (UICC) TNM classification, 8th edition, esophagogastric junction tumors with an epicenter less than 2 cm into the proximal stomach are classified as esophageal cancers for the purposes of staging; those more than 2 cm into the stomach are staged as gastric cancers. The location of the tumor in the stomach and the distance from the esophagogastric junction for proximal tumors should be documented.

Gastric adenocarcinomas usually appear as friable ulcerated masses endoscopically. However, it should be noted that the gastric mucosa can appear normal in linitis plastica (an aggressive form of diffuse-type adenocarcinoma), with the only endoscopic finding being poor stomach distensibility. Deep biopsies beyond the superficial mucosa must be obtained to evaluate for these lesions. Any suspicious lesion should have multiple biopsies taken to improve the diagnostic yield. For example, a single biopsy has a 70% sensitivity for diagnosis compared with 98% with seven biopsies. For this reason, six to eight biopsies are recommended for each suspicious lesion.

For lesions less than 2 cm in size, endoscopic mucosal resection (EMR) or endoscopic submucosal dissection (ESD) can be considered in experienced hands, which can be both diagnostic and therapeutic depending on the pathology of the specimen. The pathology report of the biopsy should include presence of lymphovascular invasion, histologic subtype (intestinal or diffuse), and tumor depth of invasion. Unfortunately, in the United States the vast majority of tumors present at later stages of disease and are not candidates for curative endoscopic resection given the increased risk of nodal disease at the T1b and greater tumor stages.

Staging

Once adenocarcinoma is diagnosed on endoscopic biopsy, patients should undergo CT of the chest, abdomen, and pelvis to evaluate for regional and metastatic disease. For suspicious lesions in the common sites of metastatic disease, such as the liver and lung, a biopsy should be performed for tissue confirmation. If ascitic fluid is seen on staging CT scan, it may be sampled by paracentesis and sent for cytologic and chemical analysis. Involvement of abdominal lymph nodes outside the standard lymphadenectomy resection (i.e., pancreatoduodenal, peripancreatic, middle colic, para-aortic) are classified as distant metastasis.

In patients without evidence of nodal or metastatic disease on CT, EUS is recommended to assess the T stage. EUS can also identify enlarged nearby lymph nodes, which can be biopsied using fine-needle aspiration. If there is high clinical suspicion of

TABLE 1	8th Edition AJCC Staging of Gastric Adenocarcinoma		
AJCC STAGE	T-STAGE	N-STAGE	M-STAGE
IA	T1	N0	M0
IB	T1	N1	M0
IB	T2	N0	M0
IIA	T1	N2	M0
IIA	T2	N1	M0
IIA	T3	N0	M0
IIB	T1	N3a	M0
IIB	T2	N2	M0
IIB	T3	N1	M0
IIB	T4a	N0	M0
IIIA	T2	N3a	M0
IIIA	T3	N2	M0
IIIA	T4a	N1 or N2	M0
IIIA	T4b	N0	M0
IIIB	T1 or T2	N3b	M0
IIIB	T3 or T4a	N3a	M0
IIIB	T4b	N1 or N2	M0
IIIC	T3 or T4a	N3b	M0
IIIC	T4b	N3a or N3b	M0
IV	Any T	Any N	M1

metastasis but initial CT is unrevealing or equivocal, positron emission tomography (PET)/CT may be considered. Diagnostic staging laparoscopy is an outpatient surgical procedure that is useful in detecting occult disease in patients with T1b or higher locoregional disease. Staging laparoscopy is superior to cross-sectional imaging for identifying peritoneal spread and allows for peritoneal fluid sampling for cytologic analysis. A complete blood count and comprehensive metabolic profile should be obtained to evaluate for anemia and electrolyte derangements.

The most recent AJCC/UICC TNM staging classifications were published in 2017 (Table 1). An important update in the new classification system is separate staging for patients with and without neoadjuvant therapy. Early gastric adenocarcinoma is defined as cancers that do not invade past the submucosa (T1), T1a tumors involve the mucosa, and T1b tumors involve the submucosa. T2 tumors involve the muscularis propria, T3 tumors penetrate to the subserosa, and T4 tumors invade beyond the serosa (T4a) or invade adjacent structures (T4b). Regional nodal classification is N1 for 1 to 2 lymph node metastases, N2 for 3 to 6 nodes, N3a for 7 to 15 nodes, and N3b for 16 or more involved nodes. The M1 stage indicates the presence of metastatic disease.

Treatment

It is recommended that treatment decisions for all patients diagnosed with gastric cancer be discussed by a multidisciplinary team including medical oncology, radiation oncology, surgical oncology, gastroenterology, radiology, and pathology. Complete surgical resection of the cancer and adjacent lymph nodes offers the best opportunity for long-term survival when possible. Indicators of surgical unresectability include presence of metastatic disease or involvement of a major vascular structure such as the aorta, celiac axis, or hepatic artery. Multivisceral resection of adjacent organs can be considered in locally advanced cases but should be done in centers of expertise and only after adequate preoperative therapy.

Patients with either Tis or T1a disease (tumor that does not invade past the submucosa) may be candidates for either endoscopic or surgical resection given the lower risk of nodal spread. Patients with T1b cancers (a tumor that invades the submucosa) should undergo upfront surgical resection after a staging diagnostic laparoscopy confirms no peritoneal disease. Patients with T2 or higher disease or any nodal involvement are recommended to undergo perioperative chemotherapy. Radiation therapy can be considered, especially in cases of locally advanced disease or for palliation of bleeding gastric tumors. Patients who are not candidates for curative surgical resection or with metastatic disease should be considered for palliative treatment in addition to systemic chemotherapy.

Surgery

Endoscopic resection with either EMR or ESD can be considered adequate therapy for gastric tumors less than 2 cm in size that (1) are well-differentiated or moderately differentiated, (2) do not penetrate past the submucosa, and (3) do not have evidence of lymphovascular invasion. Endoscopic resection of gastric tumors requires advanced endoscopic techniques and should be done in high-volume centers.

Surgical resection typically consists of either a distal/subtotal or total gastrectomy depending on where the tumor is located in the stomach. Tumors in the proximal third of the stomach typically require total gastrectomy, while a subtotal distal gastrectomy can be performed in the distal two-thirds. A proximal gastrectomy can be considered for proximal gastric cancers in select situations. There is no survival difference between total and distal gastrectomy for distal tumors, and the quality of life in patients has been shown to be superior with partial gastrectomy. Patients undergoing surgery should be considered for a diagnostic laparoscopy to detect the possible presence of occult metastatic disease before committing to curative surgery. Diagnostic laparoscopy should be done on a separate day before gastrectomy surgery to allow time for peritoneal washing cytology to be performed. A 5-cm proximal margin should be obtained with at least a 2-cm distal margin on the duodenum. T4b tumors require en bloc resection of nearby involved organs or structures. Retrieval of at least 15 lymph nodes is necessary for accurate nodal staging.

Minimally invasive gastrectomy, when technically feasible, has been shown to be noninferior oncologically to open surgery. Additionally, minimally invasive gastrectomy has been shown to have fewer wound complications, decreased postoperative pain, and shorter length of stay. This can be performed laparoscopically or robotically when technically feasible.

The appropriate extent of lymphadenectomy for gastric cancer has been well studied. A D1 lymphadenectomy involves removal of the perigastric lymph nodes alone, with D2 lymphadenectomy involving additional removal of lymph nodes around the left gastric, common hepatic, celiac, and splenic arteries. More extensive lymphadenectomy has been used in Eastern countries since the 1960s, but it has not been routinely adopted in Western countries, A seminal randomized trial from the Netherlands compared D1 to D2 lymphadenectomy. While the initial report showed significantly higher perioperative mortality in the D2 lymphadenectomy group, this was largely driven by pancreatectomy and splenectomy in that group. Additionally, the long-term gastric cancer survival was superior in the D2 lymphadenectomy group. Current guidelines recommend D2 lymphadenectomy with an emphasis on this surgery needing to be performed by experienced surgeons in high-volume centers and without routine pancreatectomy. D3 lymphadenectomy (para-aortic lymph nodes), however, is associated with increased morbidity without evidence of oncologic benefit and is not presently recommended.

In cases that require reconstruction after a distal gastrectomy, options include Roux-en-Y gastrojejunostomy, Billroth I gastroduodenostomy, and Billroth II gastrojejunostomy depending on a technical intraoperative assessment by the surgeon.

Reconstruction after total gastrectomy is performed with a Roux-en-Y esophagojejunostomy. Placement of a jejunal feeding tube can be considered at the time of operation, especially if a patient is likely to receive adjuvant therapy or their nutritional status is poor, though their use is not standardized.

Chemotherapy

The efficacy of perioperative chemotherapy in resectable gastric adenocarcinoma has been established in multiple randomized trials. The first major trial (MAGIC) randomized 503 patients with resectable adenocarcinoma of the stomach, gastroesophageal junction, or lower esophagus to surgery alone versus surgery with perioperative ECF (epirubicin [Ellence][1], cisplatin[1], 5-fluorouracil). Chemotherapy consisted of three preoperative and three postoperative cycles. Perioperative ECF resulted in improved 5-year overall survival (36% compared with 23% for patients who received surgery alone). In 2019 a randomized phase 2/3 trial of 716 patients with resectable stage II or III gastric or gastroesophageal junction adenocarcinomas was conducted to compare perioperative ECF and perioperative FLOT (fluorouracil, leucovorin[1], oxaliplatin[1], and docetaxel [Taxotere]). Survival was significantly improved with FLOT, with a median overall survival of 50 months compared with 35 months with ECF.

In patients who are medically fit and thereby recommended to receive perioperative chemotherapy, the FLOT regimen is recommended. Patients who are unable to tolerate this more aggressive chemotherapy regimen may undergo treatment with a fluoropyrimidine and oxaliplatin[1] or fluorouracil and cisplatin[1]. The ECF regimen is no longer first-line therapy.

For patients who do not receive neoadjuvant therapy, treatment recommendations are guided by the pathologic tumor classification, operative margins, and extent of lymphadenectomy. Those whose final surgical pathology reveals T3, T4, or any N-positive disease should be offered adjuvant chemotherapy. Those with T2N0 disease may be offered either adjuvant chemotherapy or surveillance. All patients with positive operative margins should be considered for adjuvant chemoradiation. Adjuvant chemotherapy is fluoropyrimidine-based. In patients who received less than a D2 lymphadenectomy, fluorouracil or capecitabine (Xeloda)[1] is recommended before and after fluoropyrimidine-based regimens. For patients who did have a D2 lymphadenectomy, oxaliplatin[1] and fluorouracil or capecitabine[1] is recommended.

Immunotherapy

Approximately 3% to 7% of gastric adenocarcinomas are mismatch repair deficient (MMRd). There are currently ongoing clinical phase trials of various immunotherapy agents in the treatment of gastric adenocarcinoma. For example, the NEONIPIGA study is a phase II trial of patients with resectable MMRd gastric adenocarcinoma. Of the 29 patients who underwent surgery, the pathologic complete response rate to neoadjuvant ipilimumab (Yervoy)[1] and nivolumab (Opdivo) was 58%. The phase III KEYNOTE-585 study used cisplatin-based doublet chemotherapy with or without pembrolizumab (Keytruda). The pathologic response was significantly improved with pembrolizumab; however the event-free survival was statistically similar. The chemotherapy regimen for KEYNOTE-585 was transitioned to FLOT, and results of this arm are yet to be reported at this time. The MATTERHORN phase III trial randomized 948 patients to FLOT perioperative chemotherapy with or without durvalumab (Imfinzi)[1]. Pathologic response was again significantly improved, but longer-term survival data has not yet been presented. Perioperative immunotherapy in addition to chemotherapy may be of benefit but should be considered investigational as we await long-term survival data from ongoing randomized trials.

---

[1] Not FDA approved for this indication.

Radiotherapy

The benefits and indications for radiotherapy are less well established for noncardia gastric adenocarcinoma. Preoperative chemoradiotherapy is beneficial in patients with esophageal, gastroesophageal junction, and gastric cardia tumors as shown in the CROSS trial, but its role specifically in gastric cancer is less clear. Furthermore, the majority of the survival benefit in the CROSS trial was in patients with squamous cell carcinoma, not adenocarcinoma. Additionally, the ESOPEC randomized trial more recently reported superior survival outcomes for esophageal adenocarcinoma treated with perioperative FLOT chemotherapy compared with the CROSS chemoradiation regimen. The INT-0116 trial randomized patients with resectable gastric adenocarcinoma to surgery plus adjuvant chemotherapy and chemoradiation versus surgery alone and showed a survival benefit with adjuvant therapy. Two studies published in 2024 and 2021 have sought to ascertain the benefit of radiation separate from systemic chemotherapy for gastric cancer. The TOPGEAR randomized phase III trial compared perioperative chemotherapy with or without preoperative radiation before gastrectomy. There was no survival benefit with the addition of preoperative radiation. The ARTIST II study in Korea randomized patients who had undergone surgery with D2 lymphadenectomy and were node-positive to adjuvant chemotherapy versus adjuvant chemoradiation. Similarly, there was no additional survival benefit with radiotherapy. Radiation therapy is no longer recommended either in the preoperative or postoperative setting in most patients. NCCN guidelines do recommend adjuvant chemoradiotherapy for patients with positive surgical margins after gastrectomy. Radiotherapy can be considered as an adjunct in multidisciplinary discussions for patients with locally advanced disease or for palliation of symptoms for patients with unresectable or metastatic disease.

Palliation

The most common indications for palliative procedures in gastric cancer are gastric outlet obstruction, bleeding, and perforation. Choosing among the various palliative options involves consideration of the risks and benefits specific to each patient's case, as well as the patient's goals of care. For patients with an obstructing tumor, especially in the prepyloric or antral regions, surgical or endoscopic interventions may be beneficial. For a patient whose life expectancy is greater than 6 months and who is medically fit, surgical gastrojejunostomy may be preferred if technically feasible in either an open or laparoscopic/robotic fashion. If the patient is not a surgical candidate or has a shorter life expectancy, endoscopic stent placement or endoscopic gastrojejunostomy may be considered. Finally, a venting gastrostomy tube is another alternative. However, the patient will no longer be able to eat if this is the only therapy offered, and a feeding jejunostomy tube should also be considered for enteral nutrition.

Patients who present with uncontrollable bleeding may initially undergo endoscopic treatment, but this is associated with a high likelihood of recurrent bleeding. Angiographic embolization or radiation therapy are potential alternatives. In rare circumstances when these more conservative measures are unsuccessful, palliative resection can be considered, but these treatment decisions should be made within a multidisciplinary team. Should a patient pursue palliative operative intervention, lymph node dissection is not required. If patients present with gastric perforation and surgery is within the patient's goals of care, urgent palliative resection may be attempted.

Surveillance

Patients with stage I disease successfully treated with endoscopic resection should undergo a thorough history and physical examination every 3 to 6 months after treatment for the first 1 to 2 years, and then every 6 to 12 months for 3 to 5 years, followed by annual follow-up thereafter. EGD should be performed every 6 months for 1 year and then annually for up to 5 years. CT scans should be performed as clinically indicated by symptoms.

Patients with stage I disease treated by surgery should undergo a history and physical examination every 3 to 6 months after treatment for 1 to 2 years, and then every 6 to 12 months for 3 to 5 years, followed by annual follow-up thereafter. They should have EGD and/or CT scans as clinically indicated by symptoms. These patients must additionally be monitored for nutritional deficiencies, especially involving B_{12} and iron.

Patients with stage II or III disease who received surgery should undergo a history and physical examination every 3 to 6 months after treatment for 1 to 2 years, and then every 6 to 12 months for 3 to 5 years, followed by annual follow-up thereafter. EGD may be performed as clinically indicated. CT of the chest/abdomen/pelvis should be performed every 6 to 12 months for the first 2 years and then annually up to 5 years. PET/CT should be considered as clinically indicated when suspicion for disease recurrence and/or metastasis is high. These patients must also be monitored for nutritional deficiencies.

Complications

In the early postoperative period, patients can develop peritonitis from an anastomotic leak or duodenal stump perforation. Bowel obstructions can also develop. It should be noted that acute afferent limb obstruction in patients who had a Billroth II reconstruction should be treated differently than other small bowel obstructions in that they typically require immediate operative intervention with either surgical revision of the gastrojejunostomy, conversion to a Roux-en-Y anastomosis, or a Braun's enteroenterostomy.

Clinically significant dumping syndrome is seen in approximately 20% of patients after distal gastrectomy. Early dumping, which occurs within 1 hour of eating, is associated with abdominal pain, cramping, nausea, diaphoresis, palpitations, and flushing. Late dumping occurs hours after eating and is caused by hypoglycemia after the postprandial insulin peak. Most patients can be managed conservatively with small, frequent meals and avoidance of exacerbating foods. Octreotide (Sandostatin)[1] can be a useful adjunct in patients with persistent symptoms. Rarely, surgical revision to a Roux-en-Y gastrojejunostomy is required.

Gastrointestinal Stromal Tumors

Gastrointestinal stromal tumors (GISTs) are mesenchymal subepithelial neoplasms. The incidence of GISTs is 7 to 15 cases per 1 million, and the most common tumor location is the stomach. GISTs account for 1% to 3% of stomach neoplasms. GISTs are thought to arise from the interstitial cells of Cajal and are identified histologically by their overexpression of CD117 (KIT) and DOG1 (Discovered on GIST-1). The most common presenting symptom is gastrointestinal bleeding, though they are increasingly being diagnosed incidentally on cross-sectional imaging or upper endoscopy. The prognosis for GISTs has greatly improved after the discovery of imatinib (Gleevec), a receptor tyrosine kinase inhibitor that specifically targets c-KIT.

Surgery is the only curative option for patients with gastric GIST. All GISTs >2 cm should be considered for resection. Grossly negative margins are sufficient, and no lymphadenectomy is required given the very low rates of lymph node metastases in these tumors. Care should be taken to preserve the tumor capsule as intraoperative rupture increases the risk of recurrence. Neoadjuvant imatinib can be considered in patients with locally advanced or borderline resectable disease or in whom preoperative tumor shrinkage[1] would potentially reduce surgical morbidity.

Imatinib (Gleevec) is an oral medication taken at a dose of 400 mg daily. Adjuvant imatinib should be offered to patients with a high risk of recurrence, although there is no consensus cutoff for what disease recurrence risk should select for therapy. Tumor recurrence increases with increasing size and mitotic rate. Gastric GISTs that are >5 cm and have >5 mitoses per 50 high-power field (HPF) are considered high risk per the College of American

---

[1] Not FDA approved for this indication.

Pathologists. Gastric GISTs that are 2 to 5 cm in size with >5 mitoses or that are >10 cm in size with ≤5 mitoses are moderate risk. The phase III ACOSOG Z9001 established the significant improvement in recurrence-free survival with 1 year of adjuvant therapy compared with placebo (98% vs. 83% at 1 year, $P < 0.0001$). Further, the Scandinavian Sarcoma Group XVIII phase III trial showed that 3 years of adjuvant imatinib was superior to 1 year in both recurrence-free survival (65.6% vs. 47.9% at 5 years) and overall survival (92.0% vs. 81.7% at 5 years). However, recurrences are not uncommon soon after discontinuation of imatinib, and further studies are ongoing to establish if a longer regimen may be more beneficial. For tumors resistant to imatinib, second-line therapy is sunitinib (Sutent), another tyrosine kinase inhibitor. Sunitinib is first line for succinate dehydrogenase (SDH)-deficient GIST. For GISTs with a *PDGFRA* exon 18 mutation, avapritinib (Ayvakit) is the preferred first-line therapy.

Neuroendocrine Tumors

Gastric neuroendocrine tumors (gNETs) arise from enterochromaffin-like cells and were previously referred to as *carcinoid tumors*. The incidence of gNETs increased 15-fold from 1973 to 2012 as a result of increased awareness of the disease, an increased number of upper endoscopies, and possibly increased use of proton pump inhibitors (PPIs). There are three distinct subtypes of gNET. Type 1 gNETs are the most common (70%–80%) and are associated with pernicious anemia and atrophic gastritis. Type 2 gNETs account for 5% to 10% and are associated with Zollinger-Ellison syndrome and multiple endocrine neoplasia type 1. Type 3 gNETs have normal gastrin and stomach acid levels, are solitary lesions, and are more aggressive and tend to metastasize. Neuroendocrine carcinomas are sometimes referred to as type 4 lesions and are poorly differentiated tumors that behave similarly to gastric adenocarcinoma.

Upper endoscopy and biopsy are indicated for diagnosis. The mitotic rate and Ki-67 proliferation index should be measured from the specimen to allow for tumor grading. Patients with type 3 gNETs or with worrisome features (size >2 cm, high grade) should undergo multiphasic abdominal CT or MRI for a complete staging workup.

Type 1 gNETs less than 1 cm can undergo endoscopic resection or surveillance. If they are greater than 1 cm in size, not high grade, and EUS shows no invasion beyond the submucosa, endoscopic resection can be considered in experienced centers. If they are poorly differentiated, have invasion beyond the submucosa, or have positive margins after endoscopic resection, surgical resection should be performed. If there is persistent or recurrent disease after surgery, an antrectomy can be considered.

For type 2 tumors, gastrinoma resection or high-dose PPI therapy should be initiated. If tumor size is less than 2 cm without worrisome features on biopsy, endoscopic resection can be performed; otherwise surgical resection is recommended.

Type 3 tumors, given their more aggressive behavior, should undergo anatomic surgical resection with lymphadenectomy.

If there is metastatic disease to the liver, carcinoid syndrome can occur. A transthoracic echocardiogram should be obtained to assess for cardiac involvement. The most common systemic therapy uses somatostatin analogs (octreotide [Sandostatin] or lanreotide [Somatuline Depot]). If there is disease progression on somatostatin therapy, cytotoxic chemotherapy (i.e., etoposide [Toposar][1] with carboplatin [Paraplatin][1] or cisplatin[1]), everolimus (Afinitor), or interferon-alpha-2b (Intron A)[1] can be given as second-line agents. Peptide receptor radionuclide therapy (PRRT) delivers radiation therapy via binding of the somatostatin receptor by 177-Lu-Dotatate and may be considered in locally advanced or metastatic gNETs. Surgical cytoreduction or liver-directed therapies can be offered. Given the complexity of management and multiple treatment options, patients with metastatic GIST and carcinoid syndrome should be managed by expert multidisciplinary teams.

Gastric Lymphomas

The stomach is the most common extranodal site of lymphoma. Gastric lymphomas account for approximately 3% of gastric malignancies and 10% of lymphomas. The most common presenting symptom is epigastric pain, followed by anorexia, weight loss, nausea, and bleeding. Fever and night sweats are seen in 12% of patients. Diagnosis is established by endoscopic biopsy. The two most common subtypes in the stomach are diffuse large B-cell lymphoma and marginal-zone B-cell lymphoma of mucosa-associated lymphoid tissue (MALT). MALT lymphomas of the stomach often respond to *H. pylori* eradication. Patients with persistent or recurrent disease can undergo radiotherapy or chemotherapy. Surgery is only indicated in patients with complications from their disease such as significant bleeding or perforation.

---

[1]Not FDA approved for this indication.

References

Al-Batran SE, Homann N, Pauligk C, et al: Perioperative chemotherapy with fluorouracil plus leucovorin, oxaliplatin, and docetaxel versus fluorouracil or capecitabine plus cisplatin and epirubicin for locally advanced, resectable gastric or gastro-oesophageal junction adenocarcinoma (FLOT4): a randomised, phase 2/3 trial, *Lancet* 393(10184):1948–1957, 2019.

André T, Tougeron D, Piessen G, et al: Neoadjuvant nivolumab plus ipilimumab and adjuvant nivolumab in localized deficient mismatch repair/microsatellite instability–high gastric or esophagogastric junction adenocarcinoma: the GERCOR NEONIPIGA phase II study, *J Clin Oncol* 41(2):255–265, 2023.

Cunningham D, Allum WH, Stenning SP, et al: Perioperative chemotherapy versus surgery alone for resectable gastroesophageal cancer, *N Engl J Med* 355:11–20, 2006.

DeMatteo RP, Ballman KV, Antonescu CR, et al: Placebo-controlled randomized trial of adjuvant imatinib mesylate following the resection of localized, primary gastrointestinal stromal tumor (GIST), *Lancet* 373(9669):1097–1104, 2009.

Joensuu H, Eriksson M, Sundby Hall K, et al: One vs three years of adjuvant imatinib for operable gastrointestinal stromal tumor: a randomized trial, *JAMA* 307(12):1265–1272, 2012.

Noh SH, Park SR, Yang HK, et al: Adjuvant capecitabine plus oxaliplatin for gastric cancer after D2 gastrectomy (CLASSIC): 5-year follow-up of an open-label, randomised phase 3 trial, *Lancet Oncol* 15(12):1389–1396, 2014.

Raderer M, Kiesewetter B, Ferreri AJM: Clinicopathologic characteristics and treatment of marginal zone lymphoma of mucosa-associated lymphoid tissue (MALT lymphoma), *CA Cancer J Clin* 66(2):153–171, 2016.

Sok C, Ajay P, Tsagkalidis V, et al: Management of gastric neuroendocrine tumors: a review, *Ann Surg Oncol* 31(3):1509–1518, 2024.

5

Endocrine and Metabolic Disorders

ACROMEGALY

Method of
Moises Mercado, MD

CURRENT DIAGNOSIS

Clinical
- Headaches, visual field defects
- Coarse features, increased size of hands (rings) and feet (shoes)
- Thick, oily skin, skin tags, acanthosis nigricans
- Arthralgias, osteoarthritis
- Paresthesias, carpal tunnel syndrome
- Hypertension, arrhythmia, heart failure
- Glucose intolerance, diabetes, hypertriglyceridemia
- Snoring, sleep apnea
- Risk of colon polyps or colon cancer
- Risk of thyroid cancer

Biochemical
- Glucose-suppressed growth hormone >0.4 ng/mL by ultrasensitive assays or >1 ng/mL by old radioimmunoassays
- Elevated age-adjusted insulin-like growth factor 1

Imaging
- Magnetic resonance imaging

CURRENT THERAPY

- If a pituitary surgeon is available: Transsphenoidal surgery for microadenomas, intrasellar macroadenomas, and debulking or decompressing surgery in invasive macroadenomas
- Depot Somatostatin analogues (SA) (lanreotide autogel [Somatuline Depot] or octreotide LAR [Sandostatin LAR Depot]) as secondary treatment for patients failing surgery or waiting for radiotherapy effect to occur and as a primary treatment for patients with inaccessible lesions, contraindications for surgery, or preference. An effective, orally available octreotide (Mycapssa) has recently been approved by the FDA. The second generation SA pasireotide (Signifor LAR) seems to be somewhat more effective than octreotide or lanreotide. Paltusotine[5] is an orally administered non-peptidic SA that effectively reduces GH and IGF-1 levels.
- Dopamine agonists: Cabergoline (DOSTINEX)[1] is effective alone or in combination with somatostatin analogues in 15% to 30% of patients
- Growth hormone receptor antagonists: Pegvisomant (Somavert) for patients resistant or intolerant to somatostatin analogues and who have tumors >5 mm from the optic chiasm
- Radiotherapy for patients resistant or intolerant to pharmacologic therapy, with clinically and biochemically active disease and a tumor remnant on MRI

[1]Not FDA approved for this indication.
[5]Investigational drug in the United States.

Acromegaly is a disorder resulting from an excessive secretion of growth hormone (GH), with a prevalence of 40 to 60 cases per million and an annual incidence of 3 to 4 per million.

Physiology, Biochemistry, and Regulation of the GH/IGF-1 Axis

GH secretion is regulated at the hypothalamus (Figure 1). The pulsatile secretion of GH-releasing hormone (GHRH) stimulates somatotroph proliferation and GH gene transcription, whereas somatostatin, which is secreted tonically, inhibits GH synthesis. These two hypothalamic signals result in the pulsatile secretion of pituitary GH, with most pulses occurring during the night. GH is also stimulated by ghrelin, a hypothalamic and gastrointestinal orexigenic hormone that binds specific receptors in the somatotroph known as GH-secretagogue receptors. GH exerts its actions through a specific membrane receptor located predominantly in the liver and cartilage, but ubiquitously present in all tissues. One molecule of GH interacts with two molecules of GH receptor, resulting in functional dimerization and conformational changes that lead to the phosphorylation of several kinases and eventually the interaction with target genes such as the insulin-like growth factor (IGF)-1 gene.

IGF-1 is closely related to proinsulin and circulates in plasma bound to six binding proteins (IGFBPs) that are synthesized and released by the liver. IGFBP3 is the most important of these binding proteins and is also GH dependent; it forms a heterotrimeric complex composed of BP3, IGF-1, and the acid-labile subunit (ALS). IGF-1 is responsible for most of the trophic and growth-promoting effects of GH. Blood levels of IGF-1 are increased during puberty, coinciding with the acceleration of somatic growth, and decline with aging. Malnutrition, poorly controlled type 1 diabetes, hypothyroidism, and liver failure all result in diminished IGF-1 concentrations. IGF-1 is the main player in GH negative feedback regulation and it acts at both the pituitary and the hypothalamic levels. Glucose regulates GH release by increasing (hyperglycemia) or decreasing (hypoglycemia) somatostatin synthesis in the hypothalamus. Exercise and amino acids such as arginine also stimulate GH secretion.

Etiopathogenesis of Growth Hormone–Secreting Tumors

The molecular pathogenesis of pituitary tumors includes the inactivation of tumor suppressor genes, the activation of oncogenes, and the trophic effect of factors such as the hypothalamic releasing hormones. Less than 5% of acromegaly cases occur in a syndromic or hereditary context, including type 1 multiple endocrine neoplasia (MEN1), due to inactivating mutations of the gene encoding the tumor suppressor gene menin, MEN4 due to inactivating mutations of CDKN1B (p27), the Carney complex due to mutations of PRKAR1A, the paraganglioma/pheochormocytoma/pituitary adenoma due to a variety of mutations of the genes encoding the different isoforms of succinate dehydrogenase, the familial pituitary adenoma syndrome (FIPA), due to inactivating mutations of the gene encoding the Aryl-hydrocarbon receptor interacting protein (AIP) and X-linked acrogigantism due to duplications of the gene encoding the G-protein receptor 101. Patients with isolated familial somatotrophinomas are younger and usually have more aggressive tumors than subjects with sporadic acromegaly. Approximately 40% of GH-producing tumors in Caucasians harbor somatic point mutations of the α subunit stimulatory G protein coupled to the GHRH receptor (GSPα mutations or

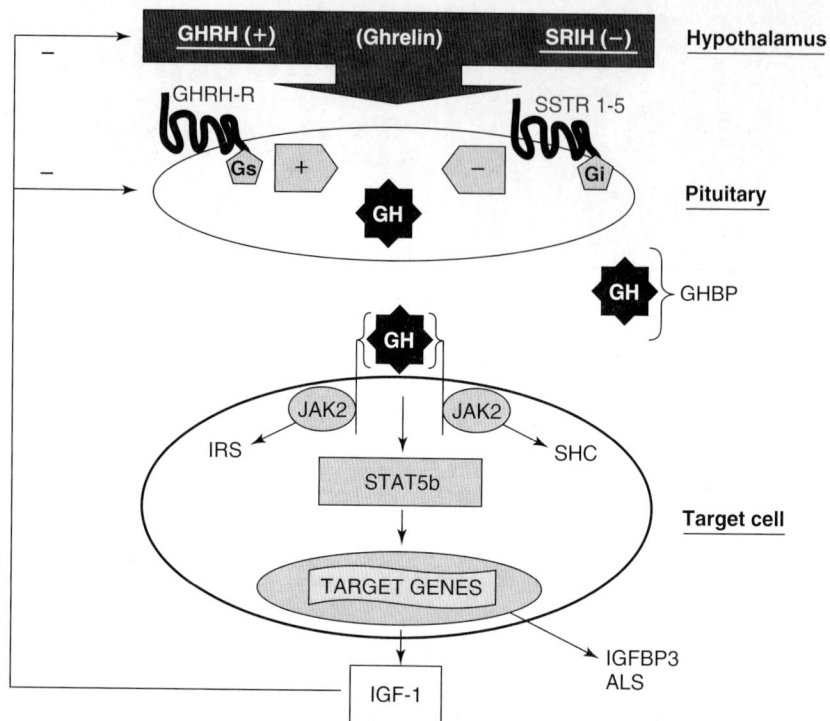

Figure 1 GH is regulated positively by GHRH and negatively by somatostatin. Fifty percent of circulating GH is bound to the GH binding protein, which represents the extracellular portion of the GH receptor. One molecule of GH dimerizes two molecules of GH receptor, and the ensuing signal transduction results in IGF-1 synthesis and secretion, which exerts negative feedback on GH secretion at the hypothalamic and pituitary levels. *Abbreviations:* ALS = acid-labile subunit; GH = growth hormone; GHRH = growth hormone–releasing hormone; IGF = insulin-like growth factor; IGFBP3 = insulin-like growth factor binding protein 3; IRS = insulin receptor S; JAK2 = Janus kinase 2; SRIH = somatostatin; SSTR = somatostatin receptor.

GNAS oncogene). This molecular alteration causes constitutive activation of the GHRH receptor, resulting in an increased transcription of the GH gene and the promotion of somatotroph proliferation. Patients with acromegaly whose tumors harbor GNAS mutations usually have a more benign clinical course and appear to respond better to somatostatin analogues. Nonwhite populations with acromegaly, including persons of Japanese, Korean, and Mexican heritage, have a much lower prevalence of *GNAS* mutations. *GNAS* mutations occurring in a post-zygotic manner are responsible for the McCune-Albright syndrome, which not infrequently includes prolactin (PRL) and to a lesser extent GH-secreting adenomas.

Other molecular events should be present in GSPα-negative somatotrophinomas. Menin is a protein encoded by a tumor suppressor gene located on the short arm of chromosome 11. Inactivating mutations of menin are the molecular basis of type 1 multiple endocrine neoplasia (MEN1); however, GH-secreting tumors occurring out of this context do not have such genetic abnormalities. Inactivating mutations of other putative tumor-suppressor genes located relatively close to the menin locus have been described in several kindreds with familial acromegaly; however, they do not seem to play an important oncogenic role in the sporadic form of the disease. Other genetic alterations such as underexpression of GADD 45γ (growth arrest and DNA damage-inducible protein) and overexpression of the securin molecule PTTG (pituitary tumor transforming gene) have also been shown to be involved in the molecular pathogenesis of acromegaly. Although hereditary acromegaly is rare (less than 2% of the cases), familial somatotrophinomas account for 30% of the tumors seen in the syndrome of familial isolated pituitary adenomas. Patients with isolated familial somatotrophinomas are younger and usually have more aggressive tumors than subjects with sporadic acromegaly. Affected members do not show any molecular alterations in the MEN1 gene. However, 15% of 73 tested families harbor inactivating, germline mutations of the AIP (aryl hydrocarbon interacting protein) gene located on chromosome 11q13.3.

In more than 90% of cases, acromegaly is caused by a sporadic pituitary adenoma. In approximately 70% of these patients, these benign epithelial neoplasms are larger than 1 cm in diameter and are known as *macroadenomas*, whereas one-third of the patients harbor lesions smaller than 1 cm or *microadenomas*. One-third of the patients have tumors that cosecrete GH and prolactin (PRL) (mammosomatoroph cell adenomas). Real pituitary GH-secreting carcinomas, with documented metastasis as the irrefutable malignancy criterion, are exceedingly rare. On rare occasions, acromegaly results from GHRH-secreting neuroendocrine tumors, usually located in the lungs, thymus, or endocrine pancreas. In this scenario, the ectopically produced GHRH leads to hyperplasia of the somatotroph, with the consequent excessive production of GH. Even less common are GH-secreting tumors arising in ectopic pituitary tissue, usually located in the sphenoid sinus. A case of GH-secreting lymphoma has been reported.

Clinical Manifestations

Acromegaly develops insidiously over many years. An 8- to 10-year delay in diagnosis has been estimated from the beginning of the first symptom. Clinical characteristics are often attributed to aging. Symptoms and signs can be divided into those resulting from the compressive effects of the pituitary tumor and those that are a consequence of the GH and IGF-1 excess.

Local Tumor Effects

Headache results from an increase in intracranial pressure and from the effects of GH itself; it is usually described as a dull pain that persists throughout the day. Occasionally, large tumors invading laterally into the cavernous sinuses give rise to cranial nerve syndromes, usually third and sixth. Visual field defects are relatively common with macroadenomas extending superiorly and compressing the optic chiasm. This usually results in different combinations of bitemporal homonymous hemianopia or quadrontopia.

Consequences of the GH/IGF-1 Excess
Skeletal Growth and Skin Changes
A GH excess developing before the pubertal closure of epiphyseal bone leads to an acceleration of linear growth, and this results in gigantism. Once the patient is in adulthood, the GH/IGF-1 excess results in acral enlargement, which is manifested by increases in ring and shoe sizes as well as enlargement of the nose, supracilliary arches, frontal bones, and mandible (Figure 2). There is thickening of soft tissues of the hands and feet; hands are fleshy and bulky and the heel pad is increased. The skin is thickened due to the deposition of glycosaminoglycans and excessive collagen production. Hyperhidrosis and seborrhea occur in 60% of patients; skin tags (previously associated with colon cancer) and acanthosis nigricans are common.

Musculoskeletal System
Generalized arthralgias are present in the majority (80%) of patients. Degenerative osteoarthritis is more common than in

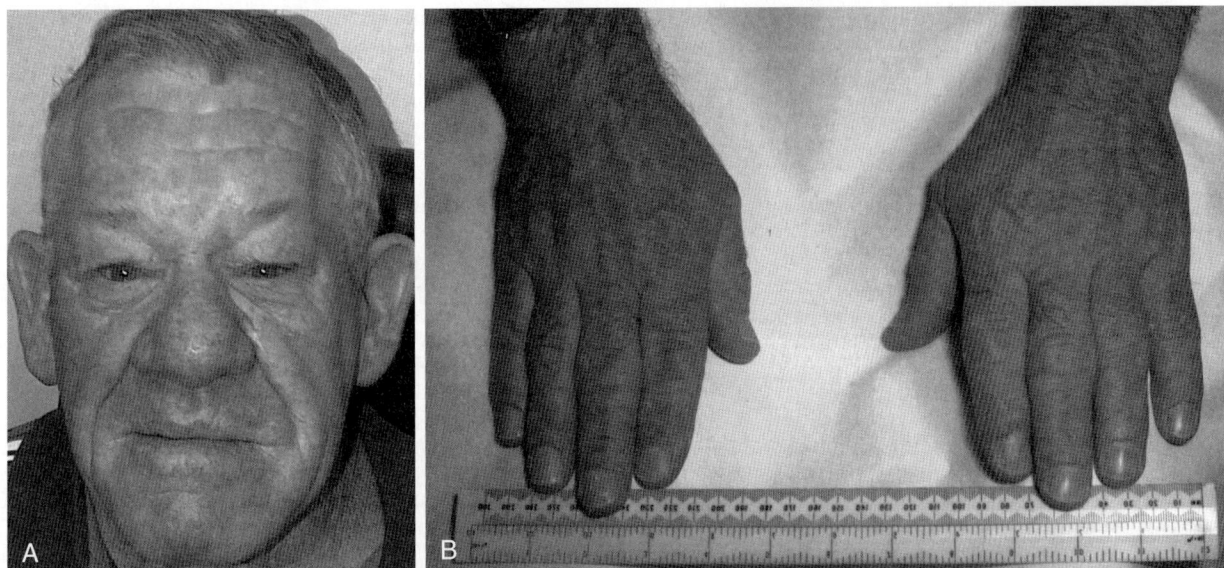

Figure 2 A and B, Skeletal growth and skin changes in acromegaly. (From Salmon JF: *Kanski's Clinical Ophthalmology*, 9th edition. Elsevier, 2020.)

the general population. Paresthesias of the hands and feet and a proximal painful myopathy are often reported. Nerve entrapment syndromes such as the carpal tunnel syndrome occur in nearly half of patients.

Cardiovascular System

Arterial hypertension is found in 30% of patients, and when associated with diabetes, it contributes to the increased mortality rate of the disease. Hyperaldosteronism with low renin levels and the resulting sodium retention play an important role in the pathogenesis of hypertension, but other contributors such as an increased sympathetic tone are also present. Echocardiographic findings include left ventricular and septal hypertrophy with varying degrees of diastolic dysfunction. Symptomatic cardiac disease develops in 15% of patients and is usually due to coronary artery disease, heart failure, and arrhythmias. Although the existence of an acromegalic cardiomyopathy is still controversial, there are patients without hypertension and with angiographically normal coronaries, who develop severe congestive heart failure, in whom histologic evidence of subendocardial, subepicardial, and myocardial fibrosis and necrosis has been documented.

Respiratory Abnormalities

The majority of patients with acromegaly are affected by loud snoring. A significant fraction of these have sleep apnea (with both central and obstructive components) with significant drops in oxygen saturation, which can be complicated by arrhythmias, daytime somnolence, and chronic fatigue.

Abnormalities in Glucose Metabolism

Chronic GH hypersecretion creates a state of insulin resistance, and glucose intolerance has been reported in 30% to 50% of patients with acromegaly; the percentage with fasting hyperglycemia can be close to 30%, depending on the population. Hyperglycemia has correlated with GH concentrations in some studies and with IGF-1 levels in others. Although successful treatment of acromegaly, be it by surgical, pharmacological, or radiotherapeutical interventions, results in significant improvements in metabolic control, the prevalence of diabetes remains higher than in the general population.

Abnormalities in Lipid Metabolism

The classic lipid profile consists of diminished total cholesterol, along with elevated triglyceride concentrations. Intermediate-density lipoprotein (IDL) particles and lipoprotein(a) might also be elevated, and there is a higher percentage of the more atherogenic type II low-density lipoprotein (LDL).

Bone and Calcium Metabolism

Acromegaly is associated with hypercalciuria and hyperphosphatemia. High serum 25-hydroxyvitamin D_3 and urinary levels of hydroxyproline can be found, reflecting a state of increased bone turnover. Cortical bone mineral density is elevated, whereas trabecular bone mass is diminished.

Neoplasia

Retrospective studies suggested that colonic adenomatous polyps and adenocarcinoma were more frequent in patients with acromegaly than in the general population. Prospective studies have demonstrated that the risk, albeit smaller than previously thought, is real and probably justifies a screening colonoscopy in these patients. Patients with uncontrolled acromegaly have a higher risk of recurrence of premalignant polyps and a higher mortality rate from colon cancer compared with subjects with biochemically controlled disease and the general population. Recently, an increased incidence of well-differentiated thyroid carcinoma has been documented.

Associated Endocrine Abnormalities

A euthyroid goiter is often found but seldom requires specific treatment. Hypopituitarism occurs variably, depending on the size and extension of the tumor and whether the patient has undergone surgery or radiation therapy. Hypogonadotropic hypogonadism is the most common pituitary deficiency, occurring in 20% of patients. A decreased libido is a common presenting complaint in both male and female patients with acromegaly; women often have menstrual and ovulatory disturbances and men complain of impotence.

Although an elevated PRL is common, it does not always reflect cosecretion of this hormone by the somatotrophinoma, but rather an interruption of the descending dopaminergic tone by the tumor compressing the pituitary stalk. Central hypocortisolism and hypothyroidism are less common.

GH-secreting pituitary adenomas are the second, after prolactinomas, pituitary tumor occurring in the context of MEN1 (multiple parathyroid adenomas, pituitary adenoma, and pancreatic islet cell tumors). Acromegaly can also develop in patients with the McCune-Albright syndrome (polyostotic fibrous dysplasia, café au lait spots, and endocrinopathies such as sexual precocity and autonomous thyroid nodules), and occurs in the context of the Carney complex.

Mortality

Life expectancy in patients with acromegaly is decreased by about 10 to 15 years, and the standardized mortality ratio is 1.5 to 2. Most patients die of cardiovascular causes, followed by cerebrovascular events, respiratory abnormalities, and neoplastic diseases. Hormonal control has a definite impact on survival. Lowering serum GH to less than 2.5 ng/mL results in reduction of the mortality rate to levels comparable with the general population. These safe GH levels were obtained using old radioimmunoassays, and there are no equivalent studies using ultrasensitive GH assays. IGF-1 levels have not been as good as GH as independent predictors of mortality. Other factors associated with an increased mortality include advanced age and the presence of hypertension and diabetes. Mortality rate in acromegaly can be reduced to that seen on the general population when patients are treated using a multidisciplinary approach not only aiming at controlling the GH and IGF-1 levels but also focusing on the management of comorbidities.

Biochemical Diagnosis

Due to the pulsatile nature of GH secretion, random determinations of this hormone are not useful in the diagnosis of acromegaly. The gold standard for the diagnosis is the measurement of GH after an oral glucose load of 75 g; current guidelines state that suppression to less than 0.4 ng/mL (using ultrasensitive assays) reliably excludes the diagnosis. Situations associated with decreased suppression of GH by glucose include puberty, pregnancy, use of oral contraceptives, uncontrolled diabetes, and renal and hepatic insufficiency.

IGF-1 levels reflect the integrated concentrations over 24 hours of GH and correlate well with clinical activity. Blood IGF-1 concentrations decrease with age, reflecting the parallel decline of the somatotropic axis. There is a gender difference in IGF-1 (premenopausal women have lower levels than age-matched male subjects). Other conditions that lower IGF-1 levels include malnutrition, uncontrolled diabetes, and hepatic and renal failure. Normal ranges for IGF-1 should be established in each particular center based on age. The determination of other GH-dependent peptides such as IGFBP3 and ALS has not proved to be superior to IGF-1.

Imaging

Pituitary magnetic resonance imaging (MRI) with gadolinium enhancement allows visualization of lesions as small as 2 or 3 mm in diameter. Hypointense lesions on T2 MRI sequences appear to respond better to treatment with SAs. High-resolution computed tomography (CT) is a reasonable alternative, although it is much less sensitive. An ectopic source of GHRH should be suspected when the MRI is completely normal. In these rare cases, serum GHRH should be measured and the ectopic tumor should be sought, usually with high-resolution CT of the chest and abdomen.

Treatment

The decision as to what therapeutic modality should be used has to take into account medical issues (cardiopulmonary comorbidities, size, and extension of the tumor) as well as the local characteristics of the treating center. The latter refers to the availability of pituitary surgeons and radiotherapeutic technologies as well as the economic feasibility of pharmacologic therapy.

Surgery

Transsphenoidal surgery has been the traditional treatment for acromegaly and achieves biochemical cure (achievement of a post-glucose GH <1 ng/mL and normalization of IGF-1) in 80% to 90% of microadenomas. According to the latest published acromegaly consensus, biochemical cure is defined as a glucose-suppressed GH of 0.4 ng/mL as well as a normal age-adjusted IGF-1. Cure rates for macroadenomas are much lower (40%–50%), and invasive lesions have a very slight chance (<10%) of being cured by surgery. Even though surgery often fails to achieve a full biochemical cure, debulking the pituitary adenoma relieves optic chiasm compression and can result in a sufficient decrement of tumor mass (and therefore of GH production) to allow better results with either pharmacologic or radiotherapeutic regimens.

Pharmacologic Therapy

Somatostatin analogues (SAs) are the most commonly used medical treatment for acromegaly. Somatostatin inhibits GH secretion and somatotroph cell growth via its interaction with five different somatostatin receptor (SSTR) subtypes. The development of long-acting SAs such as octreotide (Sandostatin) and lanreotide (Somatuline) overcame the pharmacologic difficulties of native somatostatin (short half-life, rebound GH secretion, and need for IV administration) and resulted in a more potent inhibition of GH secretion. The most commonly used preparations are intramuscular octreotide LAR (long-acting repeatable) (Sandostatin LAR Depot) and subcutaneous lanreotide autogel (Somatuline Depot), which are administered every 4 weeks. Doses of octreotide-LAR range from 10 to 40 mg and those of lanreotide autogel from 60 to 120 mg, both administered every 4 weeks, although in specific patients the interval of injection can be increased to every 6 or even 8 weeks, thus diminishing the cost of therapy. Octreotide and lanreotide have very high affinities for SSTR-2 and to a lesser extent SSTR-5, which are precisely the most commonly expressed somatostatin receptors in GH-secreting adenomas.

When used after surgery has failed, SAs can achieve a safe and a normal IGF-1 in 25% to 35% of patients. Primary treatment with SAs is increasingly being used in patients with invasive tumors, when cardiopulmonary contraindications are present, and more recently as a result of the patient's or treating physician's preference. In these settings, biochemical success rates (achievement of a GH <2.5 ng/mL and normalization of IGF-1) have ranged between 30% and 80%, and more than 80% report significant relief of symptoms. More recent trials performed in unselected populations reveal that the real success rate lies between 25% and 35%. Tumor shrinkage occurs in 70% of primarily treated patients. Overall, treatment success is directly related to the abundance of SSTR-2 and SSTR-5 in the tumor. Lower pretreatment GH levels are also associated with a better response to SAs. Side effects of SAs, including nausea, abdominal pain, alopecia, and biliary sludge, occur in 20% of subjects. The currently recommended biochemical targets when treating patients with SAs are the achievement of a GH of 1 ng/mL and an IGF-1 level within the normal age-adjusted range patients with SAs is 1 ng/mL.

Pegvisomant (Somavert) is a GH mutant that prevents functional dimerization of the GH receptor, thus acting as an antagonist. Its use results in normalization of IGF-1 in more than 70% of patients, while increasing GH levels. Concern about adenoma growth due to the abolition of IGF-1 negative feedback on the tumoral somatotroph prevents its use in patients with very large lesions in close proximity to the optic chiasm. Transient elevations of liver aminotransferases can occur, although this seldom requires drug discontinuation. Pegvisomant does not compromise insulin secretion, as SAs do. GH-receptor antagonists are expensive and should not be used as primary treatment; they are currently indicated in patients who are intolerant or have failed SA therapy.

Few patients respond marginally to difficult-to-tolerate large doses of bromocriptine.[1] Newer dopamine agonists, such as cabergoline,[1] are better tolerated and achieve biochemical control in 20% to 30% of patients. Combination treatment with cabergoline and octreotide appears to be promising in cases resistant to SAs.

Radiation Therapy

Both external-beam radiotherapy and radiosurgery are indicated in patients with persistent disease and a demonstrable tumor remnant who are either intolerant or resistant to pharmacologic treatment. Biochemical success occurs in 20% to 60% and requires many years to become apparent. Hypopituitarism, involving at least two axes, develops in more than 50% of patients within 10 years. Serious adverse effects such as brain necrosis and optic nerve damage seldom occur with the

---

[1]Not FDA approved for this indication.

currently used techniques that minimize radiation to the normal surrounding tissues. With the currently available radiation techniques, radiotherapy is an effective and safe treatment alternative. The two major drawbacks of radiotherapy are the time it takes to achieve biochemical control and the almost unavoidable induction of hypopituitarism.

Novel pharmacologic therapies are being developed, some of which will likely become useful particularly in patients who do not respond to current SAs. These include the so-called "universal" SA pasireotide (Signifor LAR), which is capable of interacting not only with the SSTRs 2 and 5, but also with subtypes 1 and 3. Pasireotide seems to be slightly more effective than octreotide in achieving GH and IGF-1 targets; however, its major drawback is the worsening of hyperglycemia. Dopastatin[5] is a recently developed chimeric compound that behaves both as an analog and as a dopamine agonist; clinical trials had to be discontinued at early stages due to lack of efficacy. Oral octreotide capsules are a new preparation of octreotide acetate attached to a transient permeability enhancer, which selectively allows the translocation of the SA through the paracellular tight junctions. Oral octreotide (Mycapssa Delayed Release capsule), which was granted FDA approval in June 2020, has been shown to be as efficacious as the parenteral preparation in at least three phase III trials, including two open label non-inferiority studies and a more recent placebo-controlled trial. Paltusotine is a nonpeptidal small molecule with high affinity for SSTR2. This orally administered SA is effective in maintaining GH and IGF-1 control in patients previously treated with first generation SAs, but it has not been approved by the FDA. On a more experimental level, antisense oligonucleotides that target the GH receptor mRNA inhibiting the translation of its protein have been evaluated in phase II studies but are not yet available for clinical use.

---

[5]Investigational drug in the United States.

References

Espinosa E, Ramirez C, Mercado M: The multimodal treatment of acromegaly: current status and future perspectives, *Endocr Metab Immune Disord Drug Targets* 14:169–181, 2014.

Espinosa-de-Los-Monteros AL, González B, Vargas G, et al: Clinical and biochemical characteristics of acromegalic patients with different abnormalities of glucose metabolism, *Pituitary* 14:231–235, 2011.

Espinosa de los Monteros AL, Gonzalez B, Vargas G, et al: Octreotide LAR treatment of acromegaly in "real life": long term outcome at a tertiary care center, *Pituitary* 18:290–296, 2015.

Espinosa-de-Los-Monteros AL, Sosa E, Cheng S, et al: Biochemical evaluation of disease activity after pituitary surgery in acromegaly: a critical analysis of patients who spontaneously change disease status, *Clin Endocrinol* 64:245–249, 2006.

Fleseriu M, Deval A, Bondat 1, et al: Maintenance of response to oral octreotide compared with injectable somatostatin receptor ligands in patients with acromegaly: a phase 3, multicenter randomized controlled trial, *Lancet Diabetes Endocrinol* 10:102–111, 2022.

Fleseriu M, Langlois F, Lim DST, et al.: Acromegaly: pathogenesis, diagnosis, and management, *Lancet Diabetes Endocrinol* 10:804–826, 2022.

Gadelha MR, Kasuki L, Lim DST, Fleseriu M: Systemic complications of acromegaly and the impac of the current treatment landscape: an update, *Endocr Rev* 40:268–332, 2019.

Gadhelha M, Gordon MB, Doknic, et al.: ACROBAT Edge. Safety and efficacy of swithcing injected SRL to oral paltusotine in patients with acromegaly. *J Clin Endocrinol Metab* dgac643, 2022.

Garcia Guzman B, Portocarrero Ortiz L, Dorantes Argandar A: Hereditary pituitary tumor syndromes: Genetic and clinical aspects, *Rev Invest Clin* 72:8–18, 2020.

Giustina A, Chanson P, Bronstein MD: A consensus on criteria for cure of acromegaly, *J Clin Endocrinol Metab* 95:3141–3148, 2010.

Giustina A, Chanson P, Kleinberg D, et al: Expert consensus document: a consensus on the medical treatment of acromegaly, *Nat Rev Endocrinol* 10:243–248, 2014.

Gonzalez-Virla B, Vargas-Ortega G, Martinez-Vazquez KB, Espinosa de los Monteros AL, Sosa-Eroza E, López-Felix B, Mendoza-Zubieta V, Mercado M: Efficacy and safety of fractionated conformal radiation therapy in acromegaly: A long-term follow-up study, *Endocrine* 65:386–392, 2019.

Holdaway IM, Rajasoorya RC, Gamble GD: Factors influencing mortality in acromegaly, *J Clin Endocrinol Metab* 89:667–674, 2004.

Kopchick JJ, Parkinson C, Stevens EC, Trainer PJ: Growth hormone receptor antagonists: discovery, development, and use in patients with acromegaly, *Endocr Rev* 23:623–646, 2002.

Madan A, Markison S, Betz SF, et al.: Paltusotine, a novel oral once-daily nonpeptide SST2 receptor agonist, suppresses GH and IGF-1 in healthy volunteers, *Pituitary* 25(2):328–339, 2022.

Mercado M, Abreu C, Vergara-López A, et al: Surgical and pharmacological outcomes in acromegaly: real-life data from the Mexican Acromegaly Registry, *J Clin Endocrinol Metab* 105:dga664, 2020.

Mercado M, Espinosa E, Ramirez C: Current status and future directions of pharmacological therapy for acromegaly, *Minerva Endocrinol* 41:351–365, 2016.

Mercado M, Gonzalez B, Vargas G, et al: Successful mortality reduction and of comorbidities in patients with acromegaly followed at a highly specialized multidisciplinary clinic, *J Clin Endocrinol Metab* 99:4438–4446, 2014.

Mercado M, Ramirez-Rentería C: Metabolic complications of acromegaly, *Front Horm Res* 49:20–28, 2018.

Potorac I, Petrossians P, Daly AF, et al.: T2-weighted MRI signal predicts hormone and tumor responses to somatostatin analogs in acromegaly, *Endocr Relat Cancer* 23(11):871–881, 2016.

Portocarrero-Ortiz LA, Vergara-Lopez A, Vidrio-Velazquez M, et al: The Mexican Acromegaly Registry: clinical and biochemical characteristics at diagnosis and therapeutic outcomes, *J Clin Endocrinol Metab* 101:3997–4004, 2016.

Trainer PJ, Newell-Price JDC, Ayuk J, et al.: A randomised, open label, parallel group, phase 2 study of antisense oligonucleotide therapy in acromegaly, *Eur J Endocrinol* 179:97–108, 2018.

ADRENOCORTICAL INSUFFICIENCY

Method of
Fabienne Langlois, MD; Elena V. Varlamov, MD; and Maria Fleseriu, MD

CURRENT DIAGNOSIS

- An initial diagnosis of adrenocortical insufficiency (AI) is based in most cases on an evaluation of morning cortisol level(s), measured at 8 AM in patients who have a normal circadian rhythm.
- A morning cortisol level less than 3 µg/dL to 5 µg/dL supports an AI diagnosis, and a value greater than 15 µg/dL effectively rules out AI.
- To confirm the diagnosis, especially in cases with intermediate cortisol values, a high-dose (250 µg) cosyntropin (Cortrosyn) stimulation test is suggested with a normal cutoff peak cortisol greater than 18 µg/dL to 20 µg/dL at 30 or 60 minutes.
- Primary AI is characterized by elevated endogenous adrenocorticotropic hormone (ACTH) levels and absence of mineralocorticoid hormones in addition to glucocorticoid (GC) deficiency; antibody screening and/or adrenal imaging is indicated.
- Secondary AI is characterized by an inappropriately normal or low endogenous ACTH level and low cortisol with preserved mineralocorticoid hormones. If an exogenous GC source/use is ruled out, pituitary hormone testing and magnetic resonance imaging (MRI) of the pituitary sella is appropriate.

CURRENT THERAPY

- Oral hydrocortisone (Cortef) is the preferred form of steroid to attain physiologic replacement. Doses are usually 15 mg to 20 mg divided into two or three daily doses, with the highest dose in the morning.
- In case of physiologic stress—such as fever, severe infection, or minor surgery—doses should be doubled or tripled (depending on the type of stress or procedure) for the duration of the event.
- In patients with primary AI, fludrocortisone (Florinef), a mineralocorticoid, should be added to the treatment regimen, with a typical dose between 0.05 mg and 0.1 mg daily.
- For adrenal crisis in patients with known AI, administer bolus hydrocortisone injection (Solu-Cortef) 100 mg followed by 50 mg to 100 mg IV every 6 hours to 8 hours or continuous infusion of 200 mg/24 h along with substantial volumes of saline.
- Patients should wear a medical alert bracelet or necklace and have frequent education regarding AI, its treatment, and the prevention of adrenal crisis.

Epidemiology

Primary adrenocortical insufficiency (AI) has a prevalence of 100 to 140 cases per million persons. More than 90% of primary AI in the developed world is secondary to autoimmune adrenalitis, also known as Addison disease, and is more common in women. Secondary AI caused by withdrawal of therapeutic glucocorticoid (GC) administration is the most prevalent; pituitary tumors and surgeries and opioid use are other common etiologies.

Risk Factors

Primary Adrenocortical Insufficiency

A personal or family history of autoimmune disease (e.g., type 1 diabetes, Hashimoto disease, vitiligo, pernicious anemia) is a risk factor for autoimmune adrenalitis. In the context of acute AI in the hospital, thrombosis and secondary adrenal hemorrhage must be ruled out and the possibility of heparin-induced thrombocytopenia (HIT) elicited if the patient is receiving parenteral anticoagulation. Miliary tuberculosis is the most frequent cause of primary AI in endemic regions. Bilateral infiltration in the context of malignancy is often due to a known metastatic cancer; other infiltrative diseases are rare.

Secondary Adrenocortical Insufficiency

The most common risk factor for secondary AI is prolonged use of exogenous GC. In general, patients taking more than 5 mg of prednisone or the equivalent for longer than 3 weeks are at risk for secondary AI. Patients receiving chronic CG will experience adrenal insufficiency symptoms acutely if GC are suddenly stopped. In some patients with GC receptor hypersensitivity, even smaller doses of GC other than oral (topical, injected, or inhaled) can also suppress the hypothalamic-pituitary-adrenal axis. Immunotherapy-related hypophysitis, most often related to inhibition of cytotoxic T-lymphocyte antigen-4 (CTLA-4), but also programmed cell death protein 1 (PD-1), and/or its ligand (PD-L1) induce AI, which is usually irreversible. Chronic opioid use, especially long-acting opioids, can also suppress ACTH and induce secondary AI.

Patients with tumors of the hypothalamic-pituitary region or a history of treatment of such tumors with surgery and/or radiation are at significant risk. Pituitary apoplexy occurs due to hemorrhage or infarction of the pituitary tumor and causes acute secondary AI. Autoimmune lymphocytic hypophysitis is more common in women and usually occurs in the third pregnancy trimester or postpartum. Pituitary ischemia due to severe blood loss postpartum is known as Sheehan syndrome. Patients with traumatic brain injury may experience transient or permanent AI in both the acute and/or recovery phase.

Pathophysiology

Primary AI is characterized by complete loss of the adrenal cortex function, usually due to an infiltrative, autoimmune or a genetic cause, inducing deficits in all hormones: GC, mineralocorticoid, and androgens. With loss of cortisol feedback inhibition, ACTH will be markedly elevated. Secondary AI is characterized by low GC production and reduced adrenal androgens; it is due a defect at the pituitary or hypothalamus level and results in low (or inappropriately normal) ACTH. Mineralocorticoid activity is maintained in secondary AI as it is controlled by the renin-angiotensin-aldosterone system.

Prevention

There is no clinically practicable strategy for preventing primary AI. Opioids and GC-associated secondary AI may be prevented through judicious use of systemic GC and opioids, with efforts made to limit administration to the lowest effective dose for the shortest possible time.

Clinical Manifestations

Primary Adrenocortical Insufficiency

The presentation of primary AI is sometimes dramatic, with a constellation of weakness, fatigue, anorexia, weight loss, nausea, abdominal pain, salt craving, and orthostatic hypotension. Symptoms start as subtle and nonspecific in some patients but may evolve rapidly in adrenal crisis, especially if concomitant stress occurs. The skin and buccal mucosa are often hyperpigmented owing to the effect of excess ACTH on cutaneous melanocortin receptors. Hyponatremia and hyperkalemia (as a result of mineralocorticoid deficiency) are often present.

Secondary Adrenocortical Insufficiency

The presentation of secondary AI is more insidious, with weight loss, fatigue, nausea, and malaise as presenting features. This often leads to a delay in diagnosis. The production of mineralocorticoid is relatively intact in secondary AI, and as such potassium levels are usually normal. Hyponatremia may be present due to an increase in antidiuretic hormone. Hyperpigmentation is not present, reflecting normal or low ACTH levels. Other laboratory abnormalities are less common but hypoglycemia is occasionally observed, especially with concomitant growth hormone deficiency (GHD). Isolated ACTH deficiency in pituitary tumors is rare, and signs and symptoms of other pituitary hormone abnormalities—such as hyperprolactinemia, central hypogonadism, GHD, or central hypothyroidism—may be present.

Diagnosis

Morning cortisol levels (within 2 hours of waking up) of 3 µg/dL to 5 µg/dL or less has a relatively high predictive value for AI; a morning cortisol level greater than 15 µg/dL effectively rules out AI. To confirm the diagnosis of AI, a cortisol stimulation test is performed. Insulin tolerance testing has largely been replaced by stimulation testing with synthetic cosyntropin (ACTH—Cortrosyn, Synacthen). ACTH stimulation testing of cortisol is a reliable method of evaluating adrenal reserve. However, it should not be used in cases of acute secondary AI (less than 6 weeks), such as apoplexy or after recent pituitary surgery, because adrenal atrophy must have occurred for the adrenal response to cosyntropin to be blunted. In high-dose ACTH testing, a cortisol level is checked before and at 30 and 60 minutes after 250 µg of cosyntropin has been administered intravenously. A peak cortisol level greater than 18 µg/dL to 20 µg/dL at 30 or 60 minutes defines a normal response. The low-dose (1 µg) test[1] measures cortisol 20 to 30 minutes after cosyntropin administration and may be more sensitive for the diagnosis of secondary AI. However, the high-dose (250 µg cosyntropin) test remains the standard. The above-mentioned cortisol cutoffs are based on laboratory methods using polyclonal antibody immunoassays. Newer assays (liquid chromatography mass spectrometry [LC-MS/MS]) and some monoclonal antibody immunoassays) have reduced cross-reactivity with cortisol precursors and therefore result in 10% to 20% lower total cortisol levels. For example, lower stimulated cutoffs of 14 µg/dL to 17 µg/dL have been proposed with those more specific methods. Additionally, one must consider total serum cortisol level, as this can be affected by diurnal rhythm and binding proteins, which are elevated in hyperestrogenic states and low in hypoalbuminemia. If the clinical picture is not concordant with the investigation, an endocrinology consult should be sought.

Once a diagnosis has been confirmed, a low or normal plasma ACTH level will indicate secondary AI; however, care must be taken with the methodology of the test, as some immunoassays for ACTH can give falsely low results if preanalytic precautions are not respected. An elevated ACTH level (more than twofold the upper limit of normal) typically indicates primary AI, and hyperkalemia, high plasma renin, and simultaneously low aldosterone levels will confirm associated mineralocorticoid deficiency. After the diagnosis of primary versus secondary AI has been established, an etiology should be sought (Boxes 1 and 2). Serology for antiadrenal (anti 21-hydroxylase) antibodies or evidence of other autoimmune diseases is useful in primary AI, given the very large fraction of these patients with autoimmune adrenalitis. In cases with absent antibodies, adrenal computed tomography imaging is indicated. Enlarged adrenal glands with high-density areas or calcification can suggest granulomatous disease or neoplasm. Acute hematoma or fluid collections around the adrenals during an acute adrenal crisis can indicate adrenal hemorrhage. Secondary AI is most often associated with

---

[1]Not FDA approved for this indication.

BOX 1 — Causes of Primary Adrenocortical Insufficiency

Autoimmune
Isolated
Autoimmune polyglandular syndromes 1 and 2

Infectious
Fungal
  Tuberculosis
  Histoplasmosis
Viral
  Human immunodeficiency virus
  Cytomegalovirus
Parasitic
Syphilis
Rarely bacterial

Bilateral Adrenal Infarction
Hemorrhage
  Anticoagulation
  Sepsis (e.g., meningococcemia)
  Trauma
  COVID-19 infection or vaccination
Thrombosis
  Thrombophilic condition (e.g., antiphospholipid antibody
    syndrome)
  Heparin-induced thrombocytopenia

Neoplastic
Metastatic cancer
  Breast
  Colon
  Melanoma
  Lymphoma
  Non–Small Cell Lung Cancer

Infiltrative Diseases
Hemochromatosis
Primary amyloidosis
Sarcoidosis

Bilateral Adrenalectomy
For bilateral tumors or intractable Cushing syndrome

Familial or Genetic
Classical congenital adrenal hyperplasia
Adrenoleukodystrophy
Familial glucocorticoid deficiency
Adrenocorticotropic hormone insensitivity syndromes
X-linked adrenal hypoplasia (associated with DAX-1 mutation,
  may be of late onset)
Triple-A or Allgrove syndrome (alacrimia, achalasia, adrenal
  insufficiency)

Drugs
Steroidogenesis inhibitors (osilodrostat [Isturisa], meryrapone
  [Metopirone], ketoconazole, levoketoconazole [Recorlev],
  mitotane [Lysodren])
Cancer immunotherapy

BOX 2 — Etiologies of Secondary Adrenocortical Insufficiency

Iatrogenic/Medication
Chronic steroid therapy, most often oral or parenteral, but
  could also be inhaled, topical, or injected
Chronic opioid therapy
Immunotherapy (CTLA-4 and PD-1/PDL-1 inhibitors)
Drugs used for treatment of Cushing syndrome
  Pituitary tumor directed drugs (pasireotide)
  Glucocorticoid receptor blockers (Mifepristone)

Pituitary Injury
Posttranssphenoidal or transcranial surgery
Radiation to the sella
Infarction/hemorrhage (pituitary apoplexy, Sheehan
  syndrome)
Traumatic brain injury

Tumors of the Sella
Pituitary adenoma
Craniopharyngioma
Meningioma
Rathke cleft cyst
Metastatic cancer

Infiltrative/Inflammatory Diseases
Sarcoidosis, tuberculosis, or other granulomatous diseases
Lymphocytic hypophysitis
Idiopathic adrenocorticotropic hormone deficiency

Congenital
Genetic mutations in transcription factors (PROP-1, PIT-1, etc.)
Midline defect
Septo-optic dysplasia

and septic shock. Fever can be part of an AI crisis, but an infectious process must be ruled out as the precipitating cause.

Treatment

GC replacement is recommended with oral hydrocortisone two or three times daily for primary AI and once or twice daily for secondary AI. One-half to two-thirds of the daily dose is given upon waking, and the dosage is roughly 15 mg to 20 mg/day (or 10 mg/m^2 to 12 mg/m^2 body surface area per day), typically 10 mg or 15 mg in the morning and 5 mg in the afternoon. Once-daily modified-release hydrocortisone is available in Europe and may better mimic the physiologic circadian rhythm of cortisol, but it is not yet available in the United States. Longer-acting GCs (prednisone, dexamethasone [Decadron]) may be used in patients who remain severely symptomatic in the evenings or early morning hours or who are unable to comply with a multidose hydrocortisone regimen. However, in such cases the risk of overreplacement is much higher.

Patients should be instructed to increase this dosage according to physiologic stress, as doses should be doubled or tripled for the duration of the fever or intercurrent systemic illness. Day-to-day emotional stress does not require an increment in dosing. For surgery, GC parenteral doses should be administered according to the level of surgical stress, such as 25 mg for minor stress (e.g., cataract surgery), 50 mg to 75 mg for moderate stress (e.g., cholecystectomy), and 100 mg to 150 mg daily in divided doses for major stress (e.g., heart surgery).

Patients should wear a medical alert bracelet or necklace and should be dispensed hydrocortisone or dexamethasone injection with instructions for home self-administration in case of vomiting and inability to take oral doses. If symptoms do not improve within hours after injection, patients should seek urgent medical evaluation.

Mineralocorticoid replacement is indicated in most patients with primary AI, and fludrocortisone (Florinef) is the recommended medical therapy, with a typical dose between 0.05 mg and 0.1 mg once daily.

If a patient with known AI presents in adrenal crisis, hydrocortisone (Solu-Cortef) 100 mg bolus followed by 150 mg to 250 mg/day,

chronic GC therapy but may be caused by a number of other diseases affecting the hypothalamic-pituitary region. If exogenous GC administration has been excluded, pituitary magnetic resonance imaging (MRI) and testing of the other pituitary axes are appropriate.

Differential Diagnosis

Presentation of AI can be subtle (especially in secondary AI), and differential diagnosis is broad and includes a number of illnesses associated with fatigue, weight loss, and malaise as well as occult malignancies, renal or hepatic dysfunction, and electrolyte disturbances. In acute AI crisis, differential diagnosis includes other systemic illnesses associated with orthostatic hypotension and electrolyte abnormalities, including dehydration and distributive

TABLE 1 Stress Dose Glucocorticoid Dosage Recommendations for Patients With Adrenal Insufficiency*,†

CLINICAL CONTEXT	MANAGEMENT
Minor surgical or medical stress, for example: Mild fever, colonoscopy, mild gastroenteritis, dental procedures	Hydrocortisone twice the usual maintenance dose on days of stress (min 25 mg/day)
Moderate surgical or medical stress, for example: Cholecystectomy, pneumonia, severe gastroenteritis	Hydrocortisone 50–75 mg/day for 1–2 days followed by twice usual dose for 1–2 days, then resume the usual dose
Major surgical or medical stress, for example: Cardiopulmonary bypass, pancreatitis, vaginal delivery	Hydrocortisone 100–150 mg/day for 1–3 days followed by twice to thrice usual dose for 2–7 days, then resume usual dose
Adrenal crisis or critical illness, for example: Septic shock, hemodynamic instability	Hydrocortisone 100 mg bolus followed by 50–100 mg every 6–8 hours OR continuous infusion of 200 mg/24 h (or 0.18 mg/kg/day)

*For an uncomplicated course, the glucocorticoid dosage should always be individualized according to patient's clinical status.

†Patients with primary adrenal insufficiency may require slightly higher doses compared with patients with secondary adrenal insufficiency and may benefit more from additional intravenous fluids to compensate for the lack of mineralocorticoids.

divided every 6 to 8 hours or as a continuous 200 mg/24 hours intravenous (IV) infusion, is an appropriate initial therapy, with the dose tapered to an appropriate oral dose as the patient's condition improves. Aggressive hydration with a saline solution will help increase the intravascular volume, and high-dose GCs have some mineralocorticoid activity; thus mineralocorticoids are not required in the treatment of acute adrenal crisis.

In critical illness, the treatment of AI should not be delayed if diagnosis cannot be established and the patient is unstable. Baseline cortisol and ACTH levels should preferably be drawn prior to the initiation of treatment and should be interpreted as a stress value (i.e., should be >18 μg/dL). If in doubt, high-dose stress GCs are administered until testing is complete and cosyntropin stimulation testing may be delayed until the patient's condition improves because hydrocortisone has to be suspended at least 24 hours before testing. The controversial entity of suboptimal cortisol response during acute stress may be associated with worse outcomes, but no consensus exists for its diagnosis and treatment. Refer to Table 1 for GC dosage recommendations.

The replacement of dehydroepiandrosterone (DHEA) is controversial and not recommended for all patients by present guidelines. However, a trial may be warranted in selected cases of women with primary AI and persistent symptoms, including low libido and low energy. DHEA is available only as a dietary supplement and has not been approved by the US Food and Drug Administration (FDA).

Patients with GC-induced AI are candidates for tapering and discontinuation of GCs if their underlying disease no longer requires GCs. Recovery of hypothalamic-adrenal-pituitary (HPA) axis can be assessed by obtaining a morning serum cortisol level once the patient is receiving no more than a physiologic dose of GCs (equivalent to 15–25 mg of hydrocortisone or prednisone 5 mg daily). A morning cortisol of >10 mcg/dL 24 hours after the last GC dose usually indicates that GCs can be stopped. An ACTH stimulation test can be performed to assess for HPA axis recovery in cases when a morning cortisol is not reliable (e.g., shift workers) or in cases of clinical uncertainty.

Monitoring

Patients should be interviewed and examined routinely for indicators of excess GC replacement, such as weight gain, striae, facial plethora, osteoporosis, or glucose intolerance; they should also be checked for under replacement if symptoms of AI persist. Cortisol

levels and ACTH are not helpful in monitoring GC doses. Monitoring of mineralocorticoid status should include volume status, electrolytes, blood pressure, and occasionally serum renin levels. The development of hypertension, edema, or hypokalemia could mandate a dose reduction.

Complications

Adrenal crisis is the most severe and life-threatening manifestation of both primary and secondary adrenal insufficiency. In patients with known AI, it occurs at a rate of approximately six cases per 100 patient-years and contributes to approximately 10% deaths; it is more common in primary than secondary AI.

Adrenal crisis is characterized by profound weakness, nausea, vomiting, abdominal pain, and fever and, if not properly treated with GC, can result in cardiovascular collapse resistant to administration of fluids and vasopressors. Precipitating causes of adrenal crisis are mainly gastrointestinal and other infections, acute illness, trauma, surgery, severe emotional distress, and pregnancy. Adrenal crisis usually develops in the setting of lack of GC replacement or failure to administer stress doses of GC during illness or severe physiological stress. Iatrogenic Cushing syndrome can develop if the dose of GC replacement is supraphysiologic long term.

Acknowledgments

The authors thank Shirley McCartney, PhD, for editorial assistance.

References

Annane D, Pastores SM, Rochwerg B, et al: Guidelines for the diagnosis and management of critical illness-related corticosteroid insufficiency (CIRCI) in critically ill patients (Part I): Society of Critical Care Medicine (SCCM) and European Society of Intensive Care Medicine (ESICM) 2017, Crit Care Med 45:2078–2088, 2017.

Beuschlein F, Else T, Bancos I, Hahner S, et al.: European Society of Endocrinology and Endocrine Society joint clinical guideline: diagnosis and therapy of glucocorticoid-induced adrenal insufficiency, J Clin Endocrinol Metab 109(7):1657–1683, 2024.

Husebye ES, Pearce SH, Krone NP, Kämpe O: Adrenal insufficiency, Lancet 13 397(10274):613–629, 2021.

Bornstein SR, Allolio B, Arlt W, et al: Diagnosis and treatment of primary adrenal insufficiency: an Endocrine Society clinical practice guideline, J Clin Endocrinol Metab 101:364–389, 2016.

Charmandari E, Nicolaides NC, Chrousos GP: Adrenal insufficiency, Lancet 383:2152–2167, 2014.

Dillard T, Yedinak CG, Alumkal J, Fleseriu M, et al: Anti-CTLA-4 antibody therapy associated autoimmune hypophysitis: serious immune related adverse events across a spectrum of cancer subtypes, Pituitary 13(1):29–38, 2010.

Dorin RI, Qualls CR, Crapo LM: Diagnosis of adrenal insufficiency, Ann Intern Med 139:194–204, 2003.

Elhassan YS, Iqbal F, Arlt W, et al.: COVID-19-related adrenal haemorrhage: multicentre UK experience and systematic review of the literature, Clin Endocrinol (Oxf) 98(6):766–778, 2023.

Fleseriu M, Christ-Crain M, Langlois F, Gadelha M, Melmed S: Hypopituitarism, Lancet, 403(10444):2632–2648, 2024.

Fleseriu M, Hashim IA, Karavitaki N, et al: Hormonal replacement in hypopituitarism in adults: an Endocrine Society clinical practice guideline, J Clin Endocrinol Metab 101:3888–3921, 2016.

Husebye ES, Allolio B, Arlt W, et al: Consensus statement on the diagnosis, treatment and follow-up of patients with primary adrenal insufficiency, J Intern Med 275:104–115, 2014.

Isidori AM, Venneri MA, Graziadio C, et al: Effect of once-daily, modified-release hydrocortisone versus standard glucocorticoid therapy on metabolism and innate immunity in patients with adrenal insufficiency (DREAM): a single-blind, randomised controlled trial, The Lancet Diabetes & Endocrinology 6:173–185, 2018.

Javorsky BR, Raff H, Carroll TB, Algeciras-Schimnich A, Singh RJ, Colón-Franco JM, et al: New cutoffs for the biochemical diagnosis of adrenal insufficiency after ACTH stimulation using specific cortisol assays, Journal of the Endocrine Society, 2021. https://doi.org/10.1210/jendso/bvab022. bvab022.

Kazlauskaite R, Evans AT, Villabona CV, et al: Corticotropin tests for hypothalamic-pituitary-adrenal insufficiency: a metaanalysis, J Clin Endocrinol Metab 93:4245–4253, 2008.

Martin-Grace, J., Tomkins, M., O'Reilly, M.W. et al. Iatrogenic adrenal insufficiency in adults. Nat Rev Endocrinol 20:209–227, 2024. https://doi.org/10.1038/s41574-023-00929-x.

Ngaosuwan K, Johnston DG, Godsland IF, et al.: Increased mortality risk in patients with primary and secondary adrenal insufficiency, J Clin Endocrinol Metab, 106(7):e2759–e2768, 2021.

Rushworth RL, Torpy DJ, Falhammar H: Adrenal crisis, N Engl J Med 29(9):852–861, 2019. 381.

Woodcock T, Barker P, Daniel S, et al: Guidelines for the management of glucocorticoids during the peri-operative period for patients with adrenal insufficiency—guidelines from the Association of Anaesthetists, the Royal College of Physicians and the Society for Endocrinology UK, Anaesthesia 75(5):654–663, 2020.

CUSHING SYNDROME

Method of
Constantine A. Stratakis, MD, PhD

CURRENT DIAGNOSIS

- Cushing syndrome remains one of the most challenging diagnoses in endocrine medicine.
- Cushing disease is caused by corticotropin (ACTH)-producing pituitary adenomas (corticotropinomas) and constitutes the most common cause of endogenous Cushing syndrome, although its prevalence varies across different age groups.
- Growth failure in children, facial plethora and rounded face, central fat deposition, supraclavicular fat accumulation, buffalo hump, purple striae, thin skin, and proximal myopathy are relatively sensitive clinical features of Cushing syndrome.
- Ectopic ACTH syndrome occasionally has an unusual presentation of rapid onset, severe weakness, and hypokalemia without classic symptoms of Cushing syndrome.
- A urinary free cortisol test is the most cost-effective and reliable outpatient screening test.
- A 1-mg overnight dexamethasone screening test is less useful and more expensive than the urinary free cortisol test, but it provides a good alternative for patients in whom urinary collection is impossible or unreliable.
- Midnight salivary cortisol levels greater than 3.6 nmol/L (0.13 µg/dL) have a sensitivity and specificity of approximately 95% for the diagnosis of Cushing syndrome.
- Undetectable ACTH levels (<1 pmol/L or <5 pg/mL) indicate a primary autonomous adrenocortical disease. For patients with mild autonomous adrenocortical Cushing syndrome ACTH levels may be as high as 30 pg/mL but not higher.
- Postcontrast spoiled gradient-recalled acquisition (SPGR) magnetic resonance imaging (MRI) is superior to conventional MRI for the localization of corticotropinomas in children and adults.
- Computed tomography (CT) is used to investigate adrenal disease in patients with ACTH-independent Cushing syndrome. Usually, conventional MRI is less useful owing to motion artifacts.

CURRENT THERAPY

- The initial therapy of choice for patients with Cushing disease is transsphenoidal surgery of the pituitary gland to remove the responsible adenoma.
- Transsphenoidal surgery has a success rate greater than 80% in most experienced centers. Lower success rates and higher incidence of relapse are recorded in less experienced centers.
- Laparoscopic adrenalectomy has become the treatment of choice for benign adrenal lesions with a diameter of less than 6 cm.
- In stages I to III adrenocortical carcinoma, complete tumor resection offers the best chance for cure.
- Mitotane (Lysodren), an adrenolytic agent, is used in the treatment of metastatic adrenocortical carcinoma and as an adjuvant for tumors with a high risk of recurrence.
- Medical treatment with ketoconazole[1], metyrapone[1], aminoglutethimide (Cytadren)[2], and mitotane[1] may be used to control hypercortisolism in preparation for surgery; medical adrenalectomy may also be used in cases of cyclic Cushing syndrome.

- Levoketoconazole (Recorlev) is now available for the treatment of Cushing syndrome and is an alternative to ketoconazole.
- Osilodrostat (Isturisa) blocks the activity of 11-β-hydroxylase specifically and has recently become available for the treatment of endogenous Cushing syndrome in adults.
- Pasireotide (Signifor) and mifepristone (Korlym) may be used for the treatment of Cushing disease that cannot be cured by surgery and/or irradiation.
- The most effective treatment option for ectopic corticotropin-releasing hormone (CRH) or ACTH syndrome is resection of the causative tumor. However, these tumors are often hard to localize. Recently, gallium-68 Dotatate positron emission tomography (PET) scan has been used with success in localizing these tumors. Somatostatin analogs and various chemotherapeutic regimens have been used in the treatment of metastatic tumors.

[1]Not FDA approved for this indication.
[2]Not available in the United States.

Definition and Epidemiology

Cushing syndrome remains one of the most difficult diagnoses in endocrinology. By definition, Cushing syndrome is a multisystem disorder that develops in response to glucocorticoid excess. Iatrogenic Cushing syndrome is common, but endogenous Cushing syndrome is a rare condition, with an estimated incidence of 0.7 to 2.4 per million population per year. The etiology of Cushing syndrome may be excessive adrenocorticotropic hormone (ACTH) production from the pituitary gland, ectopic ACTH secretion by nonpituitary tumors, or autonomous cortisol hypersecretion from adrenal hyperplasia or tumors (Table 1). Cushing disease refers to the subset of Cushing syndrome cases caused by an ACTH-producing pituitary adenoma. Cushing disease is the most common cause of spontaneous Cushing syndrome in almost all ages, including older children and adolescents. Approximately 20% to 30% (with the exception of very young children) of endogenous Cushing syndrome is caused by primary adrenocortical diseases that are not ACTH dependent. Cushing disease and adrenocortical adenomas occur more commonly in women, with a female-to-male ratio of 3 to 5:1.

Pathophysiology

Cortisol inhibits the biosynthesis and secretion of corticotropin-releasing hormone (CRH) and ACTH in a negative feedback loop that is tightly controlled. The hallmark of Cushing syndrome is the absence of suppression of cortisol levels after low-dose dexamethasone administration owing to autonomous ACTH secretion by a tumor or autonomous glucocorticoid production by a primary adrenocortical disease. It is essential to understand that all diagnostic testing in Cushing syndrome relies on the disturbance of this feedback mechanism, as revealed by dexamethasone, CRH (corticorelin ovine triflutate [Acthrel]), and all related testing.

ACTH-producing pituitary adenomas are typically microadenomas (<1 cm in diameter) in 80% to 90% of cases. Macroadenomas are rare and often invasive, with extension outside of the sella turcica. Chronic ACTH hypersecretion commonly leads to secondary adrenocortical hyperplasia.

Ectopic ACTH secretion is most often associated with small cell lung carcinoma, which accounts for half of the cases in adult patients with Cushing syndrome. The ectopic ACTH syndrome causes severe hypokalemia and is usually underdiagnosed in patients during advanced stages of neoplasia. Other tumors causing the syndrome are bronchial, thymic, and pancreatic carcinoids; medullary thyroid carcinoma; pheochromocytoma; or other rare neuroendocrine tumors, especially in pediatric patients.

Adrenocortical tumors are more often adenomas that are usually smaller than 5 cm. Adrenocortical carcinomas are rare but very aggressive neoplasms; they most commonly occur as large

TABLE 1	Etiology of Cushing Syndrome in Older Children, Adolescents, and Young Adults*	
SYNDROME	**% OF TOTAL**	
ACTH Dependent		
Cushing disease	60–70	
Ectopic ACTH syndrome	5–10	
Ectopic CRH syndrome	<1	
ACTH Independent		
Adrenocortical adenoma	10–15	
Adrenocortical carcinoma	5	
Bilateral adrenocortical disease	5–10	

*In infants and younger children, the distribution is different.
ACTH, Adrenocorticotropic hormone; CRH, corticotropin-releasing hormone.

nonsecreting abdominal masses at diagnosis, and only rarely does Cushing syndrome develop.

Up until 2025, only two types of primary adrenal hyperplasias that are ACTH independent and cause Cushing syndrome were known: primary pigmented nodular adrenocortical disease (PPNAD) and ACTH-independent macronodular adrenocortical hyperplasia.

Table 2 lists six types of bilateral adrenocortical hyperplasias. They are divided into two groups of disorders, macronodular and micronodular hyperplasias, on the basis of the size of the associated nodules. In macronodular disorders, the greatest diameter of each nodule exceeds 1 cm; in the micronodular group, nodules are less than 1 cm. Although nodules less than 1 cm can occur in macronodular disease (especially the form associated with McCune-Albright syndrome), and single large tumors may be encountered in PPNAD (especially in older patients), the size criterion has biologic relevance, because we rarely see a continuum in the same subject: most patients have either macronodular or micronodular hyperplasia. We use two additional basic characteristics in this classification of bilateral adrenocortical hyperplasias: presence of tumor pigment and status (hyperplasia or atrophy) of the surrounding cortex.

Pigment in adrenocortical lesions is rarely melanin; most of the pigmentation in adrenocortical adenomas and bilateral adrenocortical hyperplasias that produce cortisol is lipofuscin. The accumulation of lipofuscin-like material results from the progressive oxidation of unsaturated fatty acids by oxygen-derived free radicals in lysosomes. Lipofuscin pigmentation appears macroscopically as light brown to occasionally dark brown or even black discoloration of the tumor or hyperplastic tissue. Lipofuscin can be seen with a light microscope, but it is better detected by electron microscopy. Massive macronodular adrenocortical disease—better known today as primary bilateral macronodular adrenocortical hyperplasia (PBMAH)—is a bilateral disease and may be caused by abnormal hormone receptor expression or activating mutations of $G_S\alpha$, which lead to stimulation of steroidogenesis. About 30% to 50% of the cases may be caused by ARMC5 mutations. Another cause of ACTH-independent Cushing syndrome is PBMAH due to food-dependent Cushing syndrome, which is caused by KDM1A mutations.

Clinical Manifestations

The clinical presentation of Cushing syndrome is variable and differs in severity (Table 3). Truncal obesity is the most common clinical sign and is usually the initial manifestation in most patients. Growth failure in children is the most reliable sign of Cushing syndrome, especially when combined with continuing weight gain. Other symptoms include central fat deposition, supraclavicular fat accumulation, buffalo hump, plethora,

rounded face, purple striae, thin skin, proximal muscle weakness, hypertension, impaired glucose metabolism, gonadal dysfunction, and hirsutism (see Table 3). Diabetes mellitus and hypertension also develop. Osteoporosis, mood disorders, emotional lability, and cognitive deficits are commonly observed. Proximal myopathy is common, especially in older patients. Ectopic ACTH syndrome caused by small cell lung cancer can have an unusual presentation characterized by rapid onset, severe weakness, and associated hypokalemia without classic symptoms of Cushing syndrome. In contrast, ACTH-secreting carcinoids manifest with typical clinical manifestations.

Diagnosis
Confirmation of the Diagnosis

The initial evaluation should always include a careful clinical history and physical examination. Reliable symptoms and signs of Cushing syndrome (see Table 3) should be present in any patient who undergoes evaluation for Cushing syndrome; patients with no reliable symptoms and signs of Cushing syndrome should not be investigated, as this often leads to unnecessary, extensive, and expensive testing. It is essential to investigate the use of exogenous glucocorticoids and other conditions that may be associated with mild hypercortisolism, such as alcoholism, anorexia nervosa, severe depression, and morbid obesity; these are pseudo-Cushing states and are often difficult to exclude, especially in older or chronically ill patients.

The first task in the workup of any patient is documentation of hypercortisolism. On an outpatient basis, this is typically done through the urinary free cortisol test. This is the most cost-effective and relatively reliable outpatient screening test. We typically recommend collections over two or three consecutive days so that we avoid errors due to over- or undercollection that are not uncommon with single 24-hour studies. The results of the test need to be corrected for body surface area, as long as total creatinine excretion is normal. A 1-mg overnight dexamethasone test is less useful and more expensive, but it provides a good alternative for patients in whom urinary collection is impossible or unreliable. During these screening tests for hypercortisolism, patients should avoid any activation of the hypothalamic-pituitary-adrenal axis by stress, especially physical. The baseline measurements may be repeated as needed, because cyclic hypercortisolism often precedes overt Cushing syndrome (Figure 1).

A 24-hour urinary free cortisol excretion of greater than 250 nmol per 24 hours (90 μg/24 hours measured by radioimmunoassay) is highly specific for the diagnosis of hypercortisolism. However, pseudo-Cushing states are often associated with abnormal levels of 24-hour urinary free cortisol. Administration of 1 mg dexamethasone (15 μg/kg for children) at 11 PM results in suppression of the hypothalamic-pituitary-adrenal axis in normal persons and a fall in plasma and urinary cortisol levels. At 8 AM, serum cortisol should be less than 50 nmol/L (1.8 μg/dL). Unfortunately, dexamethasone is primarily metabolized by the cytochrome P-450 (CYP) system; several drugs, such as phenobarbital, carbamazepine (Tegretol), and rifampicin (Rifadin), which induce the activity of CYP3A4, can lead to false-positive tests. Oral contraceptives also interfere with serum cortisol levels owing to an increase in corticosteroid-binding globulin and by increasing dexamethasone metabolism. The test can only be interpreted if the serum dexamethasone levels reach the expected range; however, this additional requirement can make the test significantly more cumbersome and expensive.

Once hypercortisolism is suspected by the urinary free cortisol or the overnight dexamethasone test, the patient may undergo testing of the cortisol diurnal rhythm. The lack of circadian rhythm of cortisol is the earliest consistent biochemical abnormality of Cushing syndrome, even in situations of cyclic or other atypical forms of Cushing syndrome. Serum or salivary cortisol levels at midnight may be used for this test. Normally, the level of serum cortisol begins to rise at 3 to 4 AM and reaches a peak at 7 to 8 AM, falling during the day. A sleeping midnight serum cortisol level lower than 50 nmol/L (1.8 μg/dL) excludes the diagnosis

TABLE 2 Bilateral Adrenal Hyperplasias Causing Cushing Syndrome

LESION	AGE GROUP	HISTOPATHOLOGY	GENETICS	GENE, LOCUS
Macronodular Hyperplasias (Multiple Nodules >1 cm Each)				
Bilateral macroadenomatous hyperplasia	Middle age	Distinct adenomas (usually 2 or 3) with internodular atrophy	MEN1, FAP, MAS, HLRCS; isolated (AD); other	Menin, *APC, GNAS,* FH, ectopic GPCRs, ARMC5, PRKACA, KMD1A, other
Bilateral macroadenomatous hyperplasia of childhood	Infants, very young children	Distinct adenomas (usually 2 or 3) with internodular atrophy; occasional microadenomas	MAS	*GNAS*
ACTH-independent macronodular adrenocortical hyperplasia, also known as massive macronodular adrenocortical disease or primary bilateral adrenocortical hyperplasia (PBMAH)	Middle age	Adenomatous hyperplasia (multiple) with internodular hyperplasia of the zona fasciculata	Isolated, AD	Ectopic GPCRs; WISP2 and Wnt-signaling; 17q22–24, other; ARMC5, PRKACA, KMD1A, other
Micronodular Hyperplasias (Multiple Nodules <1 cm Each)				
Isolated primary pigmented nodular adrenocortical disease	Children; young adults	Microadenomatous hyperplasia with (mostly) internodular atrophy and nodular pigment (lipofuscin)	Isolated, AD	*PRKAR1A, PDE11A; PDE8B;* 2p16; PRKACA 5; other
Carney complex–associated primary pigmented nodular adrenocortical disease	Children; young and middle aged adults	Microadenomatous hyperplasia with (mostly) internodular atrophy and (mainly nodular) pigment (lipofuscin)	CNC (AD)	*PRKAR1A,* 2p16; other
Isolated micronodular adrenocortical disease	Mostly children; young adults	Microadenomatous, with hyperplasia of the surrounding zona fasciculata and limited or absent pigment	Isolated, AD; other	*PDE11A, PDE8B;* other; 2p12-p16, other

ACTH, Adrenocorticotropic hormone; *AD,* autosomal dominant; *APC,* adenomatous polyposis coli gene; *cAMP,* cyclic adenosine monophosphate; *CNC,* Carney complex; *FAP,* familial adenomatous polyposis; *FH,* fumarate hydratase; *GNAS,* gene coding for the stimulatory subunit alpha of the G-protein (Gsα); *GPCR,* G-protein-coupled receptor; *HLRCS,* hereditary leiomyomatosis and renal cancer syndrome; *MAS,* McCune-Albright syndrome; *MEN1,* multiple endocrine neoplasia type 1; *PDE8B,* phosphodiesterase 8B gene; *PDE11A,* phosphodiesterase 11A gene; *PRKAR1A,* protein kinase, cAMP-dependent, regulatory, type I, alpha gene; *WISP2,* Wnt1-inducible signaling pathway protein 1; *Wnt,* wingless-type MMTV integration site family.

TABLE 3 Clinical Manifestations of Cushing Syndrome

SIGNS AND SYMPTOMS	INCIDENCE (%)
Central obesity	97
Plethora	89
Moon facies	89
Decreased libido	86
Atrophic skin and easy bruising	75
Decreased linear growth	70–80
Menstrual irregularities	80
Hypertension	76
Hirsutism	56
Depression or emotional lability	67
Glucose intolerance/diabetes mellitus	70
Purple striae	60
Buffalo hump	54
Osteoporosis	50
Headache	10

of Cushing syndrome, whereas a midnight serum cortisol higher than 207 nmol/L (7.5 µg/dL) is highly suggestive of Cushing syndrome. This test does require inpatient admission. Salivary cortisol levels have an excellent correlation with serum cortisol levels and offer an easy and convenient outpatient way of evaluating circadian rhythm; saliva is also stable at room temperature (for up to 7 days). Midnight salivary cortisol levels greater than 3.6 nmol/L (0.13 µg/dL) have a sensitivity and specificity of approximately 95% for the diagnosis of Cushing syndrome (see Figure 1).

After the biochemical confirmation of hypercortisolism, the next step is to investigate the source (see Figure 1). Baseline ACTH plasma levels greater than 2 to 5 pmol/L (>20–25 pg/mL) are diagnostic of ACTH-dependent Cushing syndrome. On the other hand, undetectable ACTH levels (<1 pmol/L or 5 pg/mL) indicate a primary autonomous adrenocortical disease. Values in between should be further investigated with dynamic testing.

High-Dose Dexamethasone Testing
Oral dexamethasone is administered as 2 mg every 6 hours for 48 hours or as a single 8-mg (120-µg/kg for children) overnight dose. Urinary and serum cortisol levels are suppressed by more than 50% in most patients with Cushing disease.

Corticotropin-Releasing Hormone Testing
Synthetic ovine CRH (corticorelin ovine triflutate [Acthrel]), an analog of human CRH, is administered intravenously (100 µg), and plasma ACTH and cortisol levels are measured at 15-minute

Figure 1

Screening
- Post-1 mg ON DEX 8 AM serum cortisol >1.8 µg/dL
- 24 h urinary free cortisol >90 µg/24 h (RIA) or 50 µg/24 h (DHPLC/ICMA)
- Midnight salivary cortisol levels >0.13 µg/dL or serum cortisol levels >7.5 µg/dL

↓

Cushing's syndrome

↓

ACTH

- <5 pg/mL ACTH-independent CS
- ACTH = 5–20 pg/mL CRH testing 8 mg ON DEX Liddle's test
- >20 pg/mL ACTH-dependent CS

Adrenal CT

- Pituitary MRI
- CRH test
- 8 mg ON DEX

Normal or micronodules | Single mass or macronodules

Negative MRI or inconclusive testing | Cushing's disease

Liddle's test: Paradoxical stimulation of cortisol or 17OHS

Unilateral | Bilateral

Adenoma carcinoma | MMAD or other bilateral hyperplasias

Inferior petrosal sinus sampling

PPNAD or MAD

No ACTH central-to-peripheral gradient | ACTH central-to-peripheral ratio: basal ≥2 or post CRH or DDAVP ≥3

Chest CT/abdominal MRI/Octreoscan/PET-scan

Cushing's disease

Ectopic ACTH-secreting tumor

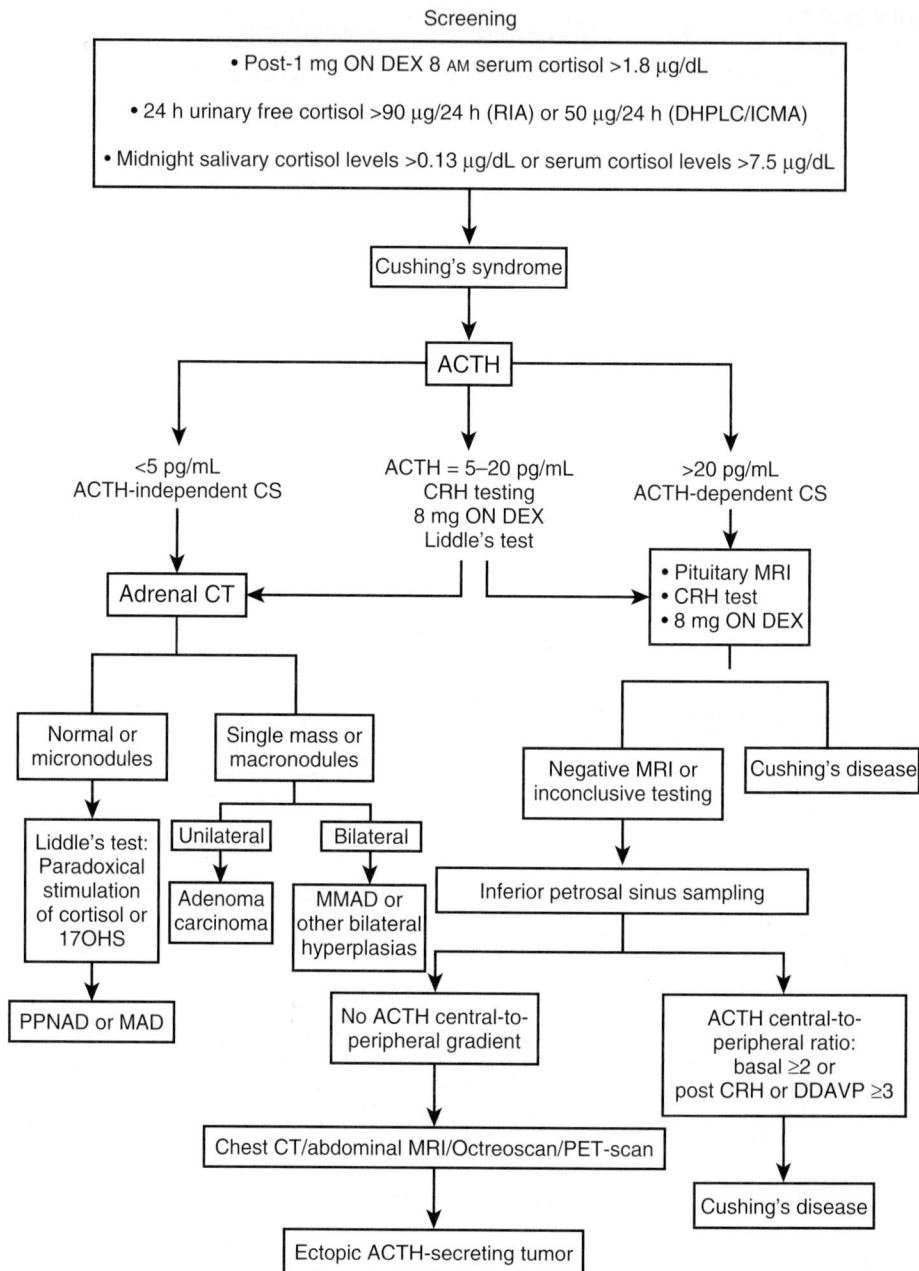

Figure 1 Algorithm for evaluating patients with Cushing syndrome. *ACTH*, Adrenocorticotropic hormone; *CRH*, corticotropin-releasing hormone; *CS*, Cushing syndrome; *CT*, computed tomography; *DDAVP*, desmopressin; *DHPLC*, denaturing high-performance liquid chromatography; *ICMA*, immunochemiluminometric assay; *MAD*, micronodular disease; *MMAD*, massive macronodular adrenocortical disease; *MRI*, magnetic resonance imaging; *17OHS*, 17-hydroxysteroids; *ON DEX*, overnight dexamethasone; *PET*, positron emission tomography; *PPNAD*, primary pigmented nodular adrenocortical disease; *RIA*, radioimmunoassay.

intervals during the next 60 minutes. Patients with Cushing disease typically have an increase in ACTH or cortisol level of 35% and 22%, respectively. This test has a sensitivity of approximately 85% for the diagnosis of Cushing disease, but it is often falsely positive in patients with adrenal, ACTH-independent Cushing syndrome, who do not have a fully suppressed hypothalamic-pituitary-adrenal axis. If CRH is not available, one may use vasopressin; typically, 10 units of lysine vasopressin (Lypressin)[2] produce equivalent stimulation of ACTH levels to that of 100 µg of CRH, and the diagnostic cut-off criteria are identical.

Inferior Petrosal Sinus Sampling

None of the noninvasive tests is 100% accurate in distinguishing pituitary (Cushing disease) from ectopic sources of ACTH. Inferior petrosal sinus sampling (IPSS) is indicated in all cases where an ACTH-dependent source of hypercortisolism is expected but the diagnosis of Cushing disease versus an ectopic source remains uncertain. Typically, IPSS is done when the ovine CRH and dexamethasone tests are in disagreement or when the pituitary

imaging by magnetic resonance imaging (MRI) is negative. An ACTH gradient of central-to-peripheral ACTH levels of 2 or more suggests Cushing disease. When ovine CRH, human CRH, or desmopressin (DDAVP) testing is performed during IPSS, the diagnostic accuracy of IPSS increases. After ovine CRH stimulation, a central-to-peripheral ratio of ACTH levels of 3 or more suggest the diagnosis of Cushing disease with specificity and sensitivity greater than 95%. The test is less useful for suggesting the tumor location (right versus left side of the pituitary gland). Like in the case of the peripheral CRH test, if CRH is not available, one may use vasopressin; 10 units of lysine vasopressin (Lypressin)[2] produce equivalent stimulation of ACTH levels to that of 100 µg of CRH, and the diagnostic cut-off criteria are identical.

Imaging Studies
Pituitary Magnetic Resonance Imaging

Unfortunately, less than 50% of ACTH-producing pituitary adenomas are detectable with MRI, even with the use of contrast enhancement. Typically, we recommend against obtaining an

---

[2] Not available in the United States.

[2] Not available in the United States.

MRI until ACTH dependency is established, because as many as 20% of the patients have an incidental pituitary microadenoma. To avoid false-negative and false-positive imaging, several centers have sought improved methods for MRI detection of ACTH-producing tumors. Our studies demonstrated that postcontrast spoiled gradient-recalled acquisition (SPGR) MRI in addition to the conventional T1-weighted spin echo was superior to conventional MRI for the diagnostic evaluation of corticotropinomas in both children and adults.

Adrenal Imaging

Computed tomography (CT) and MRI are used to investigate adrenal disease in patients with ACTH-independent Cushing syndrome. Adrenal tumors larger than 6 cm are highly suspicious for adrenocortical carcinomas. The fat content contributes to the differentiation between benign and malignant adrenal tumors. Measurement of Hounsfield units (HU) in unenhanced CT is of great value in differentiating malignant from benign adrenal lesions. Adrenal lesions with an attenuation value of more than 10 HU in unenhanced CT or an enhancement washout of less than 50% and a delayed attenuation of more than 35 HU (on 10- to 15-minute delayed enhanced CT) are suspicious for malignancy. MRI with dynamic gadolinium-enhanced and chemical shift technique is as effective as CT in distinguishing malignant from benign lesions. However, MRI is much less useful for detecting adrenal nodularity owing to motion artifacts. Thus especially for detecting small unilateral adrenocortical adenomas or bilateral micronodular hyperplasia, we recommend a dedicated (thin-sliced) adrenal CT rather than MRI.

Ectopic Adrenocorticotropic Hormone Syndrome

High Resolution Chest-CT 7 and abdominal MRI are the recommended imaging procedures in patients with an IPSS that indicates a nonpituitary ACTH-producing source. Additionally, somatostatin receptor scintigraphy is a useful and complementary tool in the evaluation of patients with ectopic ACTH-dependent Cushing syndrome. Recent studies have demonstrated a higher sensitivity of somatostatin receptor scintigraphy in comparison to CT or MRI for diagnosing occult ectopic tumors. Additional methods include positron emission tomography–computed tomography (PET-CT) and fluorodeoxyglucose (FDG) scans.

Treatment

Untreated chronic hypercortisolism is associated with high morbidity and mortality owing to diabetes mellitus, hypertension, cardiovascular disease, thromboembolism, and suppression of the immune system. Cushing syndrome should be treated effectively; patients should be closely monitored to rapidly detect recurrent disease.

Treatment of Pituitary Corticotropinomas
Transsphenoidal Pituitary Surgery

The initial therapy of choice for patients with Cushing disease is transsphenoidal surgery. This procedure is associated with low mortality and morbidity, but complications can include cerebrospinal fluid leaks, meningitis, hypopituitarism, and venous thromboembolism. The success rate for transsphenoidal surgery varies between 60% and 80%, but in experienced centers can be as high as 90% to 95%. Relapses are rare when surgery is performed in an experienced tertiary care center; it can be as high as 30% in less experienced centers. Postoperative morning serum cortisol levels of less than 50 nmol/L (2 μg/dL) are highly predictive of remission and a low recurrence rate of less than 10% at 10 years.

After successful transsphenoidal surgery, glucocorticoid replacement therapy (hydrocortisone at 12–15 mg/m²/day; 20–30 mg daily in adults) is mandatory until the hypothalamic-pituitary-adrenal axis recovers from the chronic exposure to glucocorticoid excess; this usually takes place within a year after surgery. For recurrent disease, the choice of second-line therapy remains controversial. Repeat surgery can be successful when residual tumor

is detectable on MRI imaging, but it carries a high risk of hypopituitarism. Irradiation is recommended in most cases where a tumor is not seen on MRI.

Radiotherapy

Radiotherapy has been used to suppress pituitary secretion of ACTH, but its success rate is variable (50% in some series). It can take as long as 5 years for a full effect; hypopituitarism develops in more than 70% of the patients over a period of 10 to 20 years after the therapy is completed. Stereotactic radiosurgery with gamma knife is associated with a more rapid effect and a lower risk of hypopituitarism, but it has not been extensively studied.

Medical Treatment to Control Secretion of Adrenocorticotropic Hormone

Cushing disease responds to the dopamine agonist cabergoline (Dostinex)[1] with a normalization of cortisol production in as many as 40% of the cases. The peroxisome proliferator-activated receptor γ (PPAR-γ) agonist rosiglitazone (Avandia)[1] was demonstrated to be effective in animal models, but it was unsuccessful in controlling ACTH oversecretion in patients with Cushing disease. SOM-230 (pasireotide [Signifor]) blocks both type 2 and type 5 somatostatin receptors and reduces ACTH secretion in vitro. Mifepristone (Korlym), a glucocorticoid receptor antagonist, is now available for patients who failed surgical or irradiation therapies (see also "Medical Adrenalectomy").

Bilateral Adrenalectomy

Bilateral adrenalectomy offers a definitive treatment that provides immediate control of hypercortisolism, but this surgery should be reserved for patients with Cushing disease who have failed all other treatments. Bilateral adrenalectomy in active Cushing disease often leads to Nelson syndrome, a condition characterized by unabated progression of a corticotropinoma (owing to the lack of negative feedback by cortisol), very high ACTH levels, and high morbidity.

Treatment of Adrenal Disease
Adrenocortical Tumors

For adrenocortical tumors, the recommended treatment is surgical. Laparoscopic adrenalectomy has become the treatment of choice for benign adrenal lesions with a diameter of less than 6 cm. In stages I to III adrenocortical carcinoma, complete tumor removal by a well-trained surgeon offers by far the best chance for cure. Surgery often needs to be extensive, with en bloc resection of invaded organs, and regularly includes lymphadenectomy. Surgery for local recurrences or metastatic disease is accepted as a valuable therapeutic option and was associated with improved survival in retrospective studies. The overall 5-year survival in different series ranged between 16% and 38%. Median survival for metastatic disease (stage IV) at the time of diagnosis is still consistently less than 12 months.

Radiotherapy has been considered ineffective for treatment of adrenocortical cancer, but it can be indicated to control localized disease not amenable to surgery.

Mitotane (o,p'-DDD [Lysodren]) is the only adrenal-specific agent available for treating adrenocortical cancer. Mitotane is indicated in metastatic adrenocortical carcinoma and can also be used as an adjuvant for tumors with a high risk of recurrence. Mitotane exerts a specific cytotoxic effect on adrenocortical cells, leading to focal degeneration of the fascicular and particularly the reticular zone. In most patients, treatment should be initiated with a dose that does not exceed 1.5 g/day; this is then rapidly increased, depending on gastrointestinal symptoms, to 5 to 6 g/day. This high-dose regimen requires measurement of mitotane blood levels 14 days after initiation of therapy. The dose is then adjusted according to the medicine's plasma concentrations (which should be greater than 14 mg/L) and tolerance of the side

---

[1] Not FDA approved for this indication.

MEDICATION	INITIAL DOSE	MAXIMUM DOSE	ADVERSE EFFECTS
Ketoconazole (Nizoral)[1]	100–200 mg bid/tid	1200 mg	Nausea, vomiting, abdominal pain, weakness, hypothyroidism, gynecomastia, hepatotoxicity, hypertriglyceridemia
Metyrapone (Metopirone)[1]	250 mg qid	6000 mg	Headache, alopecia, hirsutism, acne, nausea, abdominal discomfort, hypertension, weakness, leucopenia
Mitotane (Lysodren)[1]	500 mg tid	9000 mg	Nausea, vomiting, anorexia, diarrhea, ataxia, confusion, skin rash, hepatotoxicity
Aminoglutethimide (Cytadren)[2]	250 mg qid	2000 mg/d	Lethargy, nausea, anorexia, hypothyroidism, somnolence
Levoketoconazole (Recorlev)	300 mg bid	1200 mg/d	Nausea, vomiting, abdominal pain, hepatotoxicity
Osilodrostat (Isturisa)	2 mg bid	60 mg/d	Adrenal insufficiency, fatigue, nausea, increased testosterone, hypertension

TABLE 4 Medical Treatment for Hypercortisolism

[1]Not FDA approved for this indication.
[2]Not available in the United States.

effects. Because mitotane treatment induces adrenal insufficiency and increases the metabolic clearance of glucocorticoids, glucocorticoid replacement is indicated, often at higher than normal doses owing to increased clearance.

Cytotoxic Chemotherapy

Cytotoxic chemotherapy includes etoposide (VePesid)[1], doxorubicin (Adriamycin)[1], and cisplatin (Platinol)[1], or streptozocin (Zanosar)[1] plus mitotane. Chemotherapy has limited efficacy for advanced adrenocortical cancer and is associated mainly with partial responses.

Bilateral Adrenal Hyperplasias

The treatment of choice for bilateral adrenal hyperplasias associated with ACTH-independent Cushing syndrome is bilateral adrenalectomy. Patients require lifelong replacement therapy with glucocorticoids and mineralocorticoids, and they should be adequately educated about the risk of acute adrenal insufficiency.

Treatment of Ectopic Corticotropin Syndrome

The choice of treatment for ectopic ACTH syndrome depends on tumor identification, localization, and classification. The most effective treatment option is surgical resection, although this is not always possible in metastatic disease or in the case of occult tumors. Because the ectopic ACTH syndrome is usually severe and occult tumors can become evident at imaging studies only during the follow-up, medical treatment to control hypercortisolism is often necessary. Bilateral adrenalectomy may be an option to be considered when the hypercortisolism cannot be controlled by other treatment options.

Medical Adrenalectomy

Several drugs that inhibit steroid synthesis are often effective for rapidly controlling hypercortisolism in preparation for surgery, after unsuccessful transsphenoidal surgery or removal of an adrenal tumor such as extensive cancer, or while awaiting the full effect of radiotherapy in recurrent Cushing disease (Table 4).

Most experience with inhibitors of steroidogenesis has been with metyrapone (Metopirone)[1] and ketoconazole (Nizoral)[1], two medications that appear to be more effective and better tolerated than aminoglutethimide (Cytadren)[2]. Metyrapone reduces cortisol and aldosterone production by inhibiting 11β-hydroxylation

[1]Not FDA approved for this indication.
[2]Not available in the United States.

in the adrenal cortex. Ketoconazole is a broad-spectrum antifungal drug, which inhibits c17-20 desmolase, cholesterol side-chain cleavage, and 11β-hydroxylation. Ketoconazole is also associated with inhibition of testosterone biosynthesis and gynecomastia. Levoketoconazole (Recorlev) is an enantiomer of ketoconazole and is now approved for the treatment of patients with Cushing syndrome. Like ketoconazole, it inhibits CYP11B1 (11β-hydroxylase), CYP17A1 (17α-hydroxylase/17,20-lyase), and CYP21A2 (21-hydroxylase), but it less potent in inhibiting liver CYP7A1 (cholesterol 7α-hydroxylase) and thus has less hepatotoxicity. Osilodrostat (Isturisa) is yet another medication that became recently available for patients with Cushing syndrome and is a specific inhibitor of CYP11B1 (11β-hydroxylase).

RU-486, or mifepristone (Korlym), is an antagonist of the progesterone and glucocorticoid receptors. Unexpectedly, the treatment of Cushing disease with this glucocorticoid antagonist has been associated with increased ACTH secretion and consequent stimulation of cortisol production. RU-486 may be more useful in ectopic ACTH-producing tumors and in adrenal Cushing syndrome, but its efficacy and potential side effects when administered chronically are currently unknown. More medications like mifepristone are expected to become available for patients with Cushing syndrome with fewer side effects.

References

Allolio B, Fassnacht M: Clinical review: Adrenocortical carcinoma: clinical update, *J Clin Endocrinol Metab* 91:2027–2037, 2006.

Assie G, Libe R, Espiard S, et al: ARMC5 mutations in macronodular adrenal hyperplasia with Cushing's syndrome, *N Engl J Med* 369(22):2105–2114, 2013.

Batista D, Courkoutsakis NA, Oldfield EH, et al: Detection of adrenocorticotropin-secreting pituitary adenomas by magnetic resonance imaging in children and adolescents with Cushing disease, *J Clin Endocrinol Metab* 90:5134–5140, 2005.

Batista DL, Riar J, Keil M, Stratakis CA: Diagnostic tests for children who are referred for the investigation of Cushing syndrome, *Pediatrics* 120:e575–e586, 2007.

Bertagna X, Guignat L, Groussin L, Bertherat J: Cushing's disease, *Best Pract Res Clin Endocrinol Metab* 23:607–623, 2009.

Biller BM, Grossman AB, Stewart PM, et al: Treatment of adrenocorticotropin-dependent Cushing's syndrome: a consensus statement, *J Clin Endocrinol Metab* 93:2454–2462, 2008.

Boscaro M, Arnaldi G: Approach to the patient with possible Cushing's syndrome, *J Clin Endocrinol Metab* 94:3121–3131, 2009.

Feelders RA, Hofland LJ: Medical treatment of Cushing's disease, *J Clin Endocrinol Metab* 98(2):425–438, 2013.

Newell-Price J, Trainer P, Besser M, Grossman A: The diagnosis and differential diagnosis of Cushing's syndrome and pseudo-Cushing's states, *Endocr Rev* 19:647–672, 1998.

Terzolo M, Angeli A, Fassnacht M, et al: Adjuvant mitotane treatment for adrenocortical carcinoma, *N Engl J Med* 356:2372–2380, 2007.

DIABETES INSIPIDUS

Method of
Rami Mortada, MD

CURRENT DIAGNOSIS

- Diabetes insipidus (DI) is a disorder of excess urine production (i.e., "diabetes") that is dilute and tasteless (i.e., "insipidus"). DI contrasts with the concentrated and sweet urine in diabetes mellitus.
- Patients with DI present with polyuria and polydipsia; urine output is usually more than 40 mL/kg/day or more than 3 L/day.
- There are three subtypes of DI:
  - Central DI: due to relative or absolute lack of vasopressin
  - Nephrogenic DI: due to partial or total resistance to the renal antidiuretic effects of vasopressin
  - Dipsogenic DI (also called primary polydipsia): where polyuria is secondary to excessive, inappropriate fluid intake
- Initial labs should include plasma sodium and urine osmolality. Under normal physiologic conditions, the urine osmolality is less than 300 mOsm/L, but if the patient does not have sufficient fluid intake, the urine osmolality can be higher.
- The diagnosis is confirmed by examining urine output and osmolality. It can be followed by an assessment of renal response to the synthetic arginine vasopressin (AVP) analogue desmopressin (DDAVP).
- In primary polydipsia, urine concentration is normal in response to dehydration.
- In central DI, urine concentration does not increase appropriately with dehydration, but does respond to desmopressin (DDAVP). After dehydration in central DI, urine osmolality remains <300 mOsm/kg, and plasma osmolality is >290 mOsm/kg. Urine osmolality rises to >750 mOsm/kg after desmopressin.
- In nephrogenic DI, urine concentration does not increase appropriately with either dehydration or exogenous desmopressin.

CURRENT THERAPY

- The treatment goal is to control polyuria and ensure electrolyte stability.
- In Central DI:
  - The mild form might not require treatment.
  - Significant polyuria can be treated with desmopressin in divided doses: nasal spray 5 to 100 µg/day; tablets 100 to 1000 µg/day; or parenterally 0.1 to 2.0 µg/day.
  - Overtreatment can cause hyponatremia.
- In Nephrogenic DI:
  - Urine output should not be expected to normalize after DDAVP administration.
  - Correct the culprit cause (hypercalcemia or lithium [Eskalith, Lithobid] cessation).
  - Follow a low-sodium, low-protein diet, as tolerated.
  - Hydrochlorothiazide[1] 25 to 50 mg/day may be taken either alone or in combination with indomethacin (Indocin) 25 to 50 mg twice daily.
  - Symptoms may respond partly to high-dose desmopressin (e.g., 4 mcg IM twice daily).
- Primary polydipsia is treated by limiting an excessive fluid intake.

[1]Not FDA approved for this indication.

Physiology of Antidiuretic Hormone

Arginine vasopressin (AVP), also known as antidiuretic hormone (ADH), is a neurohypophysial hormone. It is a peptide hormone that promotes water retention by increasing the permeability of the kidney's collecting duct and distal convoluted tubule to water. It also increases peripheral vascular resistance, which in turn increases arterial blood pressure. In the clinical setting, the terms AVP, ADH, and vasopressin are used interchangeably.

Vasopressin is considered the main hormone involved in the regulation of water homeostasis and osmolality. The regulation and synthesis of vasopressin is under the influence of two systems: osmotic and pressure/volume status. In the case of osmoregulation, a small increase in plasma osmolality produces a parallel increase in vasopressin secretion; a small decrease in plasma osmolality causes a parallel drop in vasopressin.

Vasopressin is one among other hormones and systems that are involved in the regulation of volume and blood pressure. Other factors influence vasopressin production. For example, glucocorticoids inhibit secretion, whereas nausea and vomiting have a stimulatory effect.

Pathophysiology of Diabetes Insipidus

The kidneys exercise one of their urine-concentrating abilities by promoting water retention. If the concentration of vasopressin is decreased, polyuria occurs and diluted urine is excreted. A decrease in total body water results in an increase in the plasma osmolality. If the physiologic response is intact, thirst is stimulated, which leads to an increase in water consumption and the correction of plasma osmolarity. Therefore, unless there is a dysregulation in the thirst mechanisms or water consumption is limited due to a lack of availability (e.g., decreased level of consciousness, immobility, or physical restraints) severe dehydration does not develop.

Clinical Causes

There are three subtypes of diabetes insipidus (DI).

- DI secondary to excess water intake (primary polydipsia)

  Primary polydipsia is a disorder characterized by inappropriate excess fluid intake due to a disordered thirst sensation seen mostly in patients with psychiatric illnesses. A central defect in thirst regulation plays an important role in the pathogenesis of primary polydipsia. Such patients continue drinking even if the plasma osmolality falls below normal. It is not easy to achieve or maintain a low plasma osmolality because vasopressin secretion will normally be suppressed by the fall in plasma osmolality, resulting in rapid excretion of the excess water. If vasopressin regulation is intact, primary polydipsia should not lead to clinically important disturbances in the plasma sodium concentration unless hyposmolar fluid intake overwhelms the kidneys' ability to excrete excess water. Thus the serum sodium concentration is usually normal or slightly reduced in primary polydipsia. These patients may be asymptomatic or present with complaints of polydipsia and polyuria. In rare circumstances where water intake exceeds the kidneys' ability to excrete the water load of about 500 mL/hour, symptomatic severe hyponatremia might result in severe psychosis. Psychosis from hyponatremia in primary polydipsia is most commonly seen in institutionalized patients or in individuals attempting to dilute their urine to avoid a positive urine drug test.

- DI secondary to a decrease in or absence of vasopressin secretion (central DI)

  Central DI may be caused by genetic anomalies of the vasopressin gene (Table 1). Familial neurohypophyseal DI is characterized by the onset of DI with polyuria and polydipsia in childhood or early adulthood. The most common MRI finding in familial neurohypophyseal DI is the progressive disappearance of the posterior pituitary bright spot in children. The normal pituitary bright spot seen on unenhanced T_1-weighted MRI is thought to result from the T_1-shortening effect of the vasopressin stored in the posterior pituitary. The disappearance of the bright spot corresponds to the disappearance of vasopressin stores in the posterior pituitary. Wolfram's syndrome is a rare autosomal recessive syndrome manifested by DI, diabetes mellitus, optic atrophy, and deafness.

TABLE 1	Central Diabetes Insipidus (DI) Etiologies
Idiopathic	Unknown etiology
Genetic	Familial neurohypophyseal DI, Wolfram's syndrome (autosomal recessive)
Mass effect	Craniopharyngiomas, primary germ cell tumors, metastatic tumors
Infiltrative diseases	Lymphoma, leukemia, sarcoidosis, amyloidosis
Autoimmune	Lymphocytic infundibuloneurohypophysitis
Trauma	Motor vehicle accident, closed head trauma
Surgical	Surgical intervention at the pituitary region

Central DI may be caused by mass lesions of the neurohypophysis, such as craniopharyngiomas, and primary germ cell tumors in childhood. DI can be the initial presentation. MRI often shows a thickened pituitary stalk and may show a hypothalamic mass. Metastasis to the pituitary usually is found with widespread metastatic disease and is twice as likely to involve the posterior pituitary than the anterior pituitary. DI can be associated with pituitary infiltration associated with lymphomas and leukemias.

In granulomatous disease that affects the hypothalamic-pituitary axis, there is usually clear evidence of disease elsewhere in the body. MRI shows an absence of the pituitary bright spot and widening of the hypothalamic-pituitary stalk. Lymphocytic infundibuloneurohypophysitis is a new, well-recognized cause of autoimmune DI, characterized by MRI appearance of a thickened hypothalamic-pituitary stalk and large posterior pituitary gland mimicking a pituitary tumor. Pituitary abscess is a rare cause of pituitary mass and DI. In situations where the cause is not easily diagnosed, an autoimmune process should be suspected. In some patients, the cause is idiopathic.

Central DI may be caused by surgery or trauma to the pituitary region. Vasopressin is normally secreted after any kind of surgical stress, and secretion is more pronounced after surgery to the pituitary region. Only a small percentage of patients undergoing pituitary surgery have permanent DI. A triphasic DI can occur after complete hypothalamic-pituitary stalk transection. The first phase is polyuric and appears within the first 24 hours after surgery. It is thought to be secondary to axonal shock with a resultant inability to release prefabricated vasopressin. The second phase is antidiuretic and starts on about day 6, after stalk injury. It is thought to be secondary to the unregulated release of vasopressin stores. The third phase, also polyuric, starts about day 12, after vasopressin stores have been depleted. It may result in permanent or partial DI or resolve to clinically asymptomatic disease.

The same patterns of DI that occur after pituitary surgery can be seen in patients who experience a closed head trauma. Three-quarters of traumatic induced DI are secondary to motor vehicle accidents. Trauma is usually severe and causes unconsciousness. There is a high association of anterior pituitary deficiency in association with DI induced by head trauma, so the possibility of central hypocortisolism should be considered and treated immediately. DI is reported in 50% to 90% of patients with brain death.

- DI secondary to the lack of renal response to vasopressin (nephrogenic DI)

Genetic anomalies resulting in a lack of renal response to vasopressin are caused by either a mutation in the V2 receptors or a mutation of the aquaporin 2 water channels gene. The majority of the cases are X-linked recessive disorders in males. Newborns present with polyuria, vomiting, constipation, and failure to thrive. Symptoms usually occur within the first week of life.

Acquired nephrogenic DI can be caused by a kidney disease that distorts the architecture of the kidney and impairs its urine-concentrating ability (e.g., polycystic kidney disease, sickle cell disease). Decreased function of vasopressin or downregulation of aquaporin 2 channels can be caused by hypokalemia, hypercalcemia, and relief of bilateral urinary tract obstruction. Drugs such as lithium (the most common cause of drug-induced nephrogenic DI) and demeclocycline (used clinically to treat a syndrome of inappropriate ADH secretion) may cause nephrogenic DI.

Clinical Manifestations

Patients with central DI typically present with polyuria, nocturia, and polydipsia. The serum sodium concentration in untreated central DI is often in the high normal range, which provides the ongoing stimulation of thirst that replaces urinary water losses. Moderate to severe hypernatremia can develop when thirst is impaired or if there is a lack of access to free water, such as the postoperative period in patients with unrecognized DI or infants with DI. For uncertain pathophysiologic reasons, patients with central DI may develop decreased bone mineral density at the lumbar spine and femoral neck, even if treated with desmopressin.

Nephrogenic DI in its mild form can be asymptomatic. Patients with moderate to severe nephrogenic DI, as with central DI, typically present with polyuria, nocturia, and polydipsia.

Primary polydipsia is the result of an abnormal compulsion to drink water. This disorder is most often seen in middle-aged women and in patients with psychiatric illnesses. The excessive water intake initially drives the excessive urination.

Diagnosis

Polyuria must be distinguished from simple urinary frequency in the absence of excess urine volume. The initial diagnostic approach should be to confirm polyuria, defined as greater than 30 mL/kg or 3 L/day, with a urine osmolality measuring less than 300 mOsm/L. Simple metabolic causes such as hyperglycemia, uremia, and hypercalcemia should be excluded. A definitive diagnosis of DI requires testing of vasopressin production and action in response to osmolar stress. All forms of DI may be partial or complete. In primary polydipsia, the plasma sodium, blood urea nitrogen (BUN), and uric acid are relatively low. In other forms of DI, the plasma sodium and uric acid are relatively high and the BUN is relatively low.

Central DI usually has an abrupt onset resulting from destruction of more than 80% of vasopressin-secreting hypothalamic neurons. The etiology of polyuria is not always evident after history and laboratory tests are completed. In that case, a water restriction test (e.g., dehydration test or water deprivation test) is completed. The water deprivation test is an indirect assessment of the AVP axis, measuring renal concentrating capacity in response to dehydration. It can be followed by assessment of the renal response to the synthetic AVP analogue desmopressin to determine whether any defect identified in urine-concentrating ability can be corrected with AVP-replacement. Office testing is acceptable unless the patient cannot be watched closely. No food or water is allowed. The patient is watched for signs of dehydration and surreptitious water drinking. Baseline measurements include weight, plasma osmolality, sodium, BUN, glucose, and urine volume and osmolality. Weight, plasma osmolality, and urine osmolality are measured hourly. The test is ended if urine osmolality has not increased to more than 300 mOsm/kg for 3 consecutive hours, plasma osmolality has reached 295 to 300 mOsm/kg, or the patient has lost 3% to 5% of body weight. All initial measurements are repeated at the end of the water restriction test. Then, 5 units of aqueous AVP (Pitressin) is administered or 2 μg of desmopressin is given subcutaneously and the plasma osmolality, sodium, BUN, glucose, and urine volume and osmolality are measured at 30, 60, and 120 minutes.

In primary polydipsia, urine concentration is normal in response to dehydration (Table 2).

TABLE 2	Values Before and After Water Restriction			
	INITIAL PLASMA OSMOLALITY	INITIAL PLASMA SODIUM	POSTTEST URINE/PLASMA OSMOLALITY	POSTTEST URINE/PLASMA OSMOLALITY+ADH
Normal	NL	NL	>1	>1
Central DI	High (high NL)	High (high NL)	<1	>1
Nephrogenic DI	High (high NL)	High (high NL)	<1	<1
Primary polydipsia	Low (low NL)	Low (low NL)	>1	>1

TABLE 3	Treatment Options for Diabetes Insipidus
Central DI	Divide doses of two to three times per day:
	Desmopressin nasal spray 5–100 µg/day
	Desmopressin tablets 0.1–1 mg/day
	Desmopressin injection 0.1–2 µg/day
Nephrogenic DI	Low-salt, low-protein diet
	HCTZ[1] 25 mg one to two times per day
	Indomethacin[1] 25–50 mg bid
	Amiloride[1] 5–10 mg bid
Primary polydipsia	Water restriction to less than 1.5 L/day

[1]Not FDA approved for this indication.

In central DI, urine concentration does not increase appropriately with dehydration, but responds to desmopressin. Urine osmolality remains <300 mOsm/kg, accompanied by plasma osmolality >290 mOsm/kg after dehydration, and urine osmolality rising to >750 mOsm/kg after desmopressin administration.

In nephrogenic DI, urine concentration does not increase appropriately with either dehydration or exogenous desmopressin.

In practice, many results are indeterminate. If central DI is suspected, but the water deprivation test data are inconclusive, a reasonable approach is a therapeutic trial of 10 to 20 µg intranasal desmopressin per day with close monitoring of plasma sodium. If the diagnosis is confirmed, pituitary function testing and cranial MRI should follow.

Treatment

The treatment goal is to improve polyuria and polydipsia symptoms while attempting to treat the etiologic factors (Table 3). This is achieved by appropriate correction of dehydration, if present, and replacing vasopressin or augmenting its effect on the target tissue.

Mild forms of central DI may not require pharmacologic treatment. Desmopressin effectively treats polyuria and polydipsia. Desmopressin comes in different forms, and dosages usually need to be divided.

Hyponatremia from plasma dilution can be avoided by skipping treatment for a short period on a regular basis (e.g., on Sunday). No second dose of desmopressin should be given unless the patient has urine output after the first dose.

Nephrogenic DI may respond to the removal of the offending agent (e.g., lithium) or correction of the underlying electrolyte disturbance (e.g., hypercalcemia or hypokalemia). Drug-induced nephrogenic DI, however, may persist after discontinuation of the drug.

Patients should be instructed to eat a low-sodium, low-protein diet, resulting in a decrease in urine output secondary to the drop in solute excretion. If symptomatic polyuria persists, hydrochlorothiazide[1] can be started. Hydrochlorothiazide presumably acts by inducing mild hypovolemia that induces an increase in proximal sodium and water reabsorption, thereby diminishing water delivery to the vasopressin-sensitive sites in the collecting tubules and reducing the urine output. Indomethacin (Indocin[1]) is an add-on medication if there is not enough response. Given that prostaglandins antagonize the action of vasopressin, indomethacin inhibits renal prostaglandin synthesis and subsequently decreases urine output.

Amiloride (Midamor)[1] might be more effective for lithium-induced nephrogenic DI. This drug closes the sodium channels in the luminal membrane of the collecting tubule cells. These channels constitute the mechanism by which filtered lithium normally enters the collecting tubule cells and interferes with the collecting tubule response to ADH.

The approach to primary polydipsia treatment is reduction in fluid intake. Desmopressin treatment should be avoided due to the risk of hyponatremia.

Monitoring

Primary polydipsia is the most challenging of all types of DI to treat. It requires a multidisciplinary approach that frequently demands medical and psychiatric involvement.

In central DI, patients will require frequent follow-up to adjust desmopressin dosing. Once stable, patients can be seen less frequently to assess symptom control and to check plasma sodium levels to avoid overtreatment resulting in hyponatremia.

In nephrogenic DI, after the precipitating agent has been withdrawn, follow-up is needed to assess the reversibility of polyuria. If acquired nephrogenic DI becomes irreversible, patients might require prolonged pharmacological treatment. In both central and nephrogenic DI, the patient is advised to wear a medical alert bracelet stating the disease and the potential complications.

Acknowledgment

I would like to thank K. James Kallail, PhD, for his contribution to the final editing of this chapter.

[1]Not FDA approved for this indication.

References

Bockenhauer D, Bichet DG: Inherited secondary nephrogenic diabetes insipidus: Concentrating on humans, *Am J Physiol Renal Physiol* 304:F1037–F1042, 2013.

Crowley RK, Sherlock M, Agha A, et al: Clinical insights into adipsic diabetes insipidus: A large case series, *Clin Endocrinol (Oxf)* 66:475–482, 2007.

Fujiwara TM, Bichet DG: Molecular biology of hereditary diabetes insipidus, *J Am Soc Nephrol* 16:2836–2846, 2005.

Hannon MJ, Sherlock M, Thompson CJ: Pituitary dysfunction following traumatic brain injury or subarachnoid haemorrhage, *Best Pract Res Clin Endocrinol Metab* 25:783–798, 2011.

Monnens L, Jonkman A, Thomas C: Response to indomethacin and hydrochlorothiazide in nephrogenic diabetes insipidus, *Clin Sci (Lond)* 66:709–715, 1984.

Oiso Y, Robertson GL, Nørgaard JP, Juul KV: Clinical review: Treatment of neurohypophyseal diabetes insipidus, *J Clin Endocrinol Metab* 98:3958–3967, 2013.

Vande Walle J, Stockner M, Raes A, Nørgaard JP: Desmopressin 30 years in clinical use: A safety review, *Curr Drug Saf* 2:232–238, 2007.

DIABETES MELLITUS IN ADULTS

Method of
Kristine K. Grdinovac, MD; Ethan Alexander, MD; Candice E. Rose, MD, MS; and Daniel R. Tilden, MD

CURRENT DIAGNOSIS

- Established guidelines define diabetes as a fasting blood sugar ≥126 mg/dL, a hemoglobin A1C (HbA1C) of ≥6.5%, or a blood sugar ≥200 mg/dL 2 hours after a 75-g oral glucose load.
- Prediabetes is defined as a blood sugar of 100 to 125 mg/dL or an HbA1C between 5.7% and 6.4%.
- The diagnostic guidelines are derived from inflection points in the risk of acquiring complications at any given glucose elevation.
- People with prediabetes share a similar risk of cardiovascular disease (CVD) as those with diabetes. Thus intervention with weight loss, exercise, and metformin is very beneficial in this population.
- Early detection of complications can slow the progression to end-stage disease. Routine surveillance includes annual dilated eye examinations, foot inspection, measurement of microalbuminuria, and measurements of blood lipids and kidney and liver function.

CURRENT THERAPY

- Treatment should be started early when signs of hyperglycemia appear, including prediabetes. The risks of complications are related to the lifetime duration of hyperglycemia.
- A standard glycemic treatment goal is a hemoglobin A1C (HbA1C) below 7%. It is justified, in a few patients, to set a higher goal when factors such as age, desire to lose weight, and catastrophic risk of hypoglycemia (hypoglycemic unawareness), concurrent disease, and/or other barriers are detected. Time in range (TIR), a statistic from continuous glucose monitoring (CGM) reflecting the time/day capillary glucose is 70 to 180 mg/dL, is an evolving goal. The suggested TIR is 70% or more.
- Because the treatment of diabetes is largely focused on prevention of atherosclerotic disease, aggressive control of blood pressure and lipids is also recommended.
- Treatment of type 2 diabetes mellitus (T2DM) is fundamentally based on diet (weight loss) and exercise with the addition of pharmacologic therapy (or bariatric surgery) when treatment goals are not achieved. No patient should experience uncontrolled hyperglycemia for more than 3 months without the addition of more therapy.
- The ADA now considers glucagon-like peptide-1 (GLP-1) receptor agonists and sodium-glucose cotransporter 2 (SGLT2) inhibitors as first-line drugs for those with atherosclerotic cardiovascular disease (ASCVD), ASCVD risk factors, heart failure, and chronic kidney disease (CKD).
- There are now many options for additional medications that may best fit a patient's disease characteristics, financial resources, and lifestyle. Some of the newer (and more expensive) medications are weight neutral, may promote weight loss, and have been shown to reduce the risk of ASCVD and deterioration in renal function.
- Assessment of glucose control includes periodic measurement of HbA1C, home blood glucose monitoring, and, when appropriate, CGM.
- Treatment with insulin is an option that can be introduced at any time during the course of T2DM. The goal, ideally, is to normalize the blood sugar without significant or frequent hypoglycemia.

Epidemiology

Diabetes has been on the rise both domestically and internationally, and this steady increase presents growing problems for patients and health systems alike. According to the most recent 2024 CDC data, about 38.4 million, or 11.6% of Americans, are known to have diabetes. There are populations that have seen changes in diabetes epidemiology over time. Specifically, both age and gender influence diabetes with prevalence increasing in age and women having a slightly higher rate of diagnosis. Different socioeconomic statuses and racial groups see disproportionate impacts of diabetes. Specifically, people from Asian, Hispanic, and non-Hispanic Black backgrounds have higher rates of the diagnosis. Longitudinally, the socioeconomic status of patients also impacts outcomes through things like nutritional support, medication affordability, and access to care.

Prediabetes (clinically diagnosed when the hemoglobin A1C (HbA1C) lies between 5.7% to 6.4% or as a fasting blood sugar of 100 to 125 mg/dL) has also grown in prevalence and is estimated to be approximately 97.6 million people, or 38% of the US adult population based on the most recent CDC data.

There are well-established predictive factors for the development and progression of diabetes. These risk factors include modifiable risks such as diet, exercise, and sleep. Nonmodifiable risk factors, such as genetic susceptibility, also play a role. One of the most important risk factors that shares a continued rise nationally is obesity. Data from the U.S. National Health Interview Survey highlighted the impact of obesity on acquiring diabetes. With results from nearly 800,000 respondents, the reported lifetime risk of diabetes was approximately 7.6% among men who were underweight. This is starkly contrasted to 70.3% of respondents for those who were very obese. The predictive nature of weight/body mass index (BMI) is sufficient to determine that those with a BMI greater than 30 kg/m^2 have at least a fivefold increase in the risk of acquiring diabetes. All adipose tissue is not created equal, meaning the metabolic impact of different adipose tissues is different. Visceral fat, or intraabdominal accumulation of fat that surrounds organs, is very metabolically active. This type of fat is highly correlated to the development of diabetes. This is juxtaposed to fat depots such as subcutaneous fat, which does not share the same metabolic activity. This sets up a very interesting clinical scenario where individuals may have the same weight and/or BMI, but if their body composition favors visceral fat over subcutaneous fat, their likelihood of developing metabolic syndrome, insulin resistance that can continue to full-blown diabetes, as well as dyslipidemia and hypertension, is higher. Mechanistically, visceral fat produces more free fatty acids whose breakdown products can accumulate intracellularly and impair insulin receptor signaling. Visceral fat also can reduce amounts of hormones such as adiponectin, which is important for insulin sensitivity.

By definition, a BMI between 25 and 30 kg/m^2 places patients in the overweight category, whereas a BMI greater than 30 kg/m^2 is consistent with obesity. These categories have good predictive value for diabetes risk in multiple populations including African Americans and non-Hispanic Whites. Interestingly, among Hispanic and Asian populations, a lower BMI is the set point for increased risk. In the pivotal Diabetes Prevention Program (DPP), a BMI of 22 kg/m^2 as opposed to 25 kg/m^2 identified Asian patients with an increased risk for diabetes.

A wide spectrum of risk factors for the development and progression of diabetes exists. This spectrum includes the lack of physical activity, dyslipidemia, tobacco use, genetic predisposition, and the previously discussed obesity. Regarding physical activity, it is important to highlight even small persistent changes in physical activity can have very positive outcomes for the prevention of diabetes and improve metabolic function. Encouraging people living with diabetes to start small and build up physical activity goals over time is an important part of their longitudinal care. When patients start to see the positive impact that even a 15-minute walk after a large meal has on their blood sugar, they are encouraged to continue to build physical activity goals.

Fundamental genetic understanding of the development of diabetes is extremely complex and continues to be investigated. Despite rigorous investigation, the underlying genetic mechanisms are still poorly understood. Currently, there are over 120 identified gene variants that increase the risk of type 2 diabetes mellitus (T2DM). Despite this understanding, there is currently limited clinical applicability for genetic testing in the endeavor to assess risk for patients.

Diagnosis and Classification of Diabetes and Prediabetes

Widely accepted and standardized definitions for diabetes and prediabetes exist. These are based on laboratory analysis and quantification of hyperglycemia. Rather than a static measurement, these diagnostic criteria should be viewed on the spectrum of dysregulated glucose metabolism that ultimately increases risk for both micro- and macrovascular complications. Diabetes is diagnosed if any of the following criteria are met:

- HbA1C 6.5% or higher
- Fasting plasma glucose of 126 mg/dL or higher
- A 2-hour glucose of 200 mg/dL or higher after a 75-g oral glucose load (oral glucose tolerance test)

Although these modes of diagnosis are widely accepted, all three of these diagnostic criteria may not be met at the time of diagnosis. Extrapolating future micro- and macrovascular complications from the mode of diagnosis is up for debate. There is heterogeneity among diabetologists regarding whether one or more criteria must be met to make the diagnosis of diabetes, but it is the authors' opinion that setting the benchmark for diagnosis at two criteria is unnecessary and likely delays the onset of intervention. It is recommended accepting any one of the three diagnostic criteria is sufficient for a diagnosis of diabetes and thus should prompt intervention with lifestyle changes and possibly pharmacologic therapy.

Diabetes is an amalgamation of the complex interactions between glucose metabolism, resultant hyperglycemia, varying degrees of insulin resistance, and the impact that this pathophysiology has on both micro- and macrovascular complications.

To this end, the complications of diabetes, which are largely separated into microvascular and macrovascular complications, are not as closely linked in a linear fashion to the degree of hyperglycemia itself. It is certainly less than the linear relationship of obesity and the development of diabetes discussed previously. To illustrate this discordance, evidence has shown that the risk of atherosclerotic cardiovascular disease (ASCVD) can be found in patients with "well-controlled" diabetes, as well as in patients with prediabetes. This conundrum continues to be investigated, but the progress made in cardiovascular risk reduction with novel antidiabetic agents such as glucagon-like peptide-1 (GLP-1) receptor agonists and sodium-glucose cotransporter 2 (SGLT2) inhibitors is promising.

Prediabetes is diagnosed when fasting serum blood glucose lies between 100 to 125 mg/dL, HbA1C lies between 5.7% and 6.4%, or if the 2-hour oral glucose tolerance test with a load of 75 grams of sugar reveals a blood sugar between 140 and 199 mg/dL. A diagnosis of prediabetes should sound the alarm bell for intervention to prevent the progression to overt diabetes. This moment provides a key point where counseling in nutritional therapy, exercise, and potentially pharmacologic therapy should be discussed. Metformin has been the foundational pharmacologic intervention and should be considered in adults with high risk of conversion to T2DM. Those risks include ages 29 to 59, BMI greater than 35, HbA1C greater than 6.0%, and those with a history of gestational diabetes (GDM). Metformin is not a perfect medicine, and a multifactorial approach to treating prediabetes should be implemented at the time of diagnosis.

Diabetes Categories

Type 1 Diabetes

The pathophysiology behind the emergence of type 1 diabetes mellitus (T1DM) is an autoimmune destruction of pancreatic beta cells, which are chiefly responsible for insulin production.

This destruction places the patient on a progressive spectrum on insulin deficiency. Antibodies identified as culprits for beta cell destruction include glutamic acid decarboxylase-65 (GAD-65), anti–zinc transporter protein, and anti–islet cell antibodies. Over 90% of patients diagnosed with T1DM will have at least one antibody detected. There is likely some environmental trigger for the development of these antibodies, also in the context of genetic predisposition. Despite a patient having a positive antibody associated with the development of T1DM, this does not mean this patient immediately has insulin deficiency. What this does highlight is that this patient has the propensity, and is highly likely, to develop overt insulin deficiency over time. A common phenomenon called the *honeymoon phase* exists in patients who have positive antibodies for T1DM but still have endogenous insulin secretion and therefore can maintain some semblance of euglycemia. The more antibodies a person has, the more rapid the destruction of the beta cell and the faster the time course to insulin deficiency requiring exogenous insulin therapy.

When it comes to diagnosing a patient with diabetes, it is best to think about diabetes on the spectrum of relative insulin deficiency versus insulin excess/resistance. There are some clinical clues that can help with the diagnosis such as age of diagnosis and BMI, but these markers have been proven to be nonspecific. Patients with T1DM can have obesity and insulin resistance. Also, T2DM diagnoses are occurring earlier in life than in decades past. What once was a key marker for the diagnosis of T1DM, diabetic ketoacidosis (DKA) is no longer a reliable marker to diagnose someone with T1DM. There are patients with T2DM who can present acutely with ketoacidosis, have negative antibodies, and can be successfully treated with oral agents once the ketoacidosis has resolved. This group of patients carries the diagnosis called "Flatbush diabetes," named after a group of patients in Flatbush, New York, who presented to area hospitals with the same clinical picture. This is now more aptly named *ketosis-prone T2DM*.

When working to differentiate between T1DM and T2DM, laboratory investigation including C-peptide (a peptide cleaved from endogenously produced insulin), accompanied by a serum glucose measurement, and obtaining a GAD-65 antibody level, can help differentiate the two. Patients with a low C-peptide in the setting of hyperglycemia and positive T1DM antibodies almost always have T1DM, and prompt insulin administration is recommended.

Whereas traditionally T1DM is considered a pediatric disease, there is a subset of patients who present with diabetes due to autoimmune destruction of pancreatic beta cells (like T1DM) but present much later in life. This phenomenon is termed latent autoimmune diabetes of adulthood (LADA). LADA shares similarities with T1DM regarding a likely underlying environmental trigger to start the autoimmune process. Management of LADA is like T1DM, and patients can have a significant honeymoon phase before developing absolute insulin deficiency and requiring exogenous insulin.

Type 2 Diabetes

T2DM is responsible for over 90% of cases of diabetes both domestically and internationally. In T2DM there is sufficient insulin produced by the pancreas (at least initially), but ultimately peripheral tissues are resistant to the action of this insulin. This sets up a dangerous metabolic cycle of weight gain, increased insulin secretion, increased insulin resistance, increased weight gain (as insulin is an anabolic hormone), and so on. The diagnosis of T2DM historically has occurred later in life, but unfortunately, the epidemic of obesity has not spared pediatric patients. Therefore pediatric T2DM cases are on the rise.

T2DM is progressive in nature over time, and if there is not a multifactorial intervention, severe micro- and macrovascular complications are seen. The underlying driver for this cycle is complex and includes interactions between the waning ability of the pancreas to keep up with the amount of insulin needed to achieve euglycemia and the concomitant resistance to that insulin in peripheral tissue. Other factors such as age and chronic inflammatory states also play a role. A common finding in T2DM is obesity and increased metabolically active visceral adipose tissue. Despite this, there are subsets of patients with T2DM who have normal BMIs. Further work to understand the underlying mechanisms for these outliers is needed.

Gestational Diabetes

GDM is separate and distinct from T2DM as GDM is most commonly diagnosed in the second or third trimester of pregnancy in a patient who did not have preexisting diabetes. A 50-g oral glucose tolerance test is the test of choice to diagnose GDM. The diagnosis of GDM is important for the current pregnancy as risks of fetal macrosomia and preeclampsia increase significantly, but increases in rates of T2DM are also seen in the postpartum period. This understanding should raise suspicion for T2DM in the care of patients who previously had GDM, even from many years before. Intensive intervention is warranted to prevent both maternal and fetal complications. Intervention ranges from dietary changes, metformin[1], or insulin. The care of patients with GDM is often multidisciplinary, including maternal fetal medicine, endocrinology, and general obstetrics.

Specific Types of Diabetes due to Other Causes

Although T2DM and T1DM make up the majority of cases of diabetes, it is important to remember that there are many other disease states and/or medications that can lead to diabetes. Maintaining a wide differential diagnosis list based on the patient's history is imperative. Common causes of medication-induced diabetes include many HIV medications (protease inhibitors), glucocorticoids, and anticancer medications. Specifically, there is much interest in anticancer medications such as checkpoint inhibitors and other immunotherapies and their impact on metabolism and diabetes, but also other endocrinopathies. Other pathologies such as cystic fibrosis, Cushing syndrome, hemochromatosis, and other pancreatic infiltrative disease such as pancreatic adenocarcinoma have the potential to cause diabetes.

As discussed previously, the genetic influence on diabetes is complex. Despite this, there are well-established forms of monogenic diabetes. This spectrum of monogenic diabetes can be seen in pediatric and adult populations. The most common monogenic diabetes form, an autosomal dominant type, is typically diagnosed later in life and is called maturity-onset diabetes of youth (MODY). There is likely a small portion of patients diagnosed with T2DM who actually have MODY. A broad differential diagnosis and high index of suspicion must be had when diabetes is diagnosed in the teens or early adulthood. If the suspicion for MODY is high, genetic testing is available. The care of the patient may change based on this genetic testing as there are MODY subsets that respond very well to sulfonylurea use alone.

Clinical Manifestations of Diabetes

T2DM often has an insidious onset, and individuals can remain asymptomatic for years before the diagnosis is made. Many patients are incidentally diagnosed during routine blood testing. When present, early symptoms of T2DM are often nonspecific and can include fatigue, polyuria, polydipsia, blurred vision, and/or weight loss resulting from glucose catabolism. A subset of patients may present acutely with DKA or a hyperosmolar hyperglycemic state (HHS), both of which are severe metabolic derangements requiring urgent medical attention. This typically occurs in combination with some inciting factor, such as infection, stress, or myocardial ischemia. At the time of diagnosis, patients may already have significant microvascular and/or macrovascular diabetic complications because there is often a long prodrome of hyperglycemia. A delay in diagnosis may increase the risk of complications, underlining the importance of early recognition and management of T2DM.

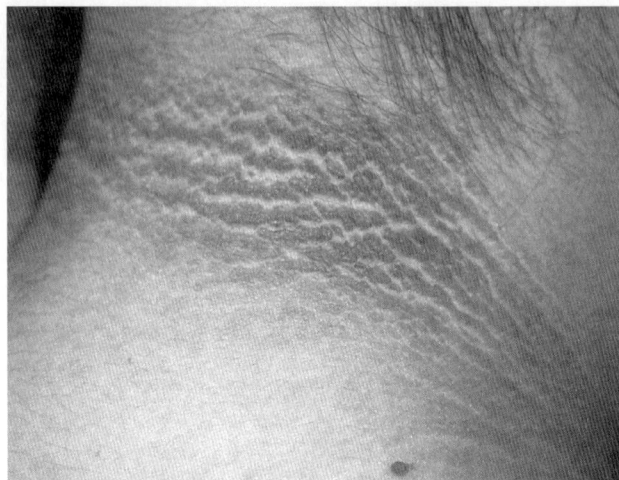

Figure 1 Acanthosis nigricans is a common examination finding of insulin resistance. It presents as a hyperpigmented, velvety, gray-to-brown thickening of the skin folds at the posterior neck and intertriginous folds. (From James, W. D., Elston, D., Treat, J., & Rosenbach, M. [2020]. *Andrews' diseases of the skin: clinical dermatology* [13th ed.]. Elsevier.)

Individuals with components of metabolic syndrome (e.g., hypertension, dyslipidemia, abdominal obesity) are at an increased risk of T2DM. Other common conditions highly correlated with insulin resistance and the development of T2DM include increasing age, sedentary lifestyle, polycystic ovarian syndrome, history of GDM, nonalcoholic fatty liver disease, and sleep apnea. Although the peak incidence of T2DM is in midlife, there is an increase in the incidence of T2DM in children and adolescents, especially in those with obesity or in those belonging to racial and ethnic minorities. Screening these patients can aid in the early diagnosis and management of both metabolic syndrome and diabetes, mitigating the risk of cardiovascular and other complications.

On physical examination, several findings can suggest the presence of T2DM. Obesity, particularly central adiposity, is a common feature. Acanthosis nigricans, characterized by dark velvety patches of skin typically seen along the posterior neck and body folds such as the axilla, can indicate insulin resistance (Figure 1). Skin tags around the base of the neck and intertriginous fold are also recognized as a sign of insulin resistance. Another skin condition associated with T2DM is necrobiosis lipoidica, which presents as well-demarcated, yellow-brown plaques, often on the shins (Figure 2). These lesions can be tender and prone to ulceration. Additionally, examination might reveal signs of peripheral neuropathy such as reduced sensation in a glove-and-stocking distribution, and vascular complications like diminished peripheral pulses or evidence of retinopathy on fundoscopic examination. Such findings underscore the systemic nature of T2DM and the importance of a comprehensive physical assessment in these patients.

Beyond glucose measurements, regular monitoring of renal function and liver enzymes is essential, as T2DM can affect these organs. Lipid profile abnormalities are common, including elevated triglycerides (TGs), low high-density lipoprotein (HDL) cholesterol, and high low-density lipoprotein (LDL) cholesterol. Monitoring these parameters is crucial, as they contribute to the increased cardiovascular risk associated with T2DM. In patients presenting with DKA, laboratory findings typically include elevated blood glucose, ketonemia or ketonuria, and metabolic acidosis. In HHS, profound hyperglycemia, hyperosmolarity, and significant dehydration are the hallmark findings, often with minimal to no ketosis.

Prevention and Reversal of Diabetes

Several large, randomized controlled trials have shown behavior and lifestyle changes are highly effective in preventing T2DM. The strongest evidence comes from the DPP. This trial showed a reduction in incidence of T2DM among prediabetic enrollees by 58% over 3 years. The lifestyle intervention goals of the DPP

---

[1] Not FDA approved for this indication.

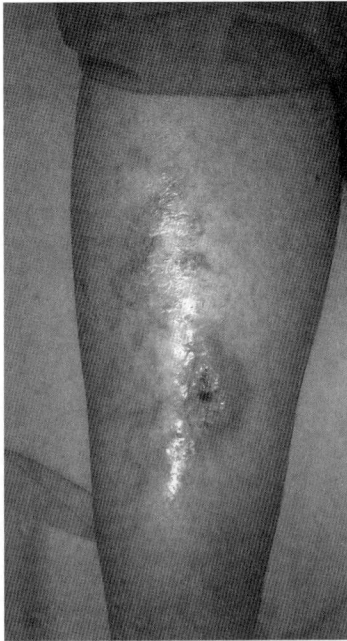

Figure 2 Necrobiosis lipoidica is a granulomatous skin disorder that is prevalent in up to 65% of patients with diabetes. It appears as reddish-brown to yellow-brown oval-shaped plaques with central atrophy and telangiectasias that frequently ulcerate.

were to attain and maintain a weight loss of 7% minimum and 150 minutes of physical activity per week, similar in intensity to brisk walking. Few patients achieved these modest goals, but the benefit was seen among most patients assigned to lifestyle changes alone. Similarly, modest reduction in weight has a significant protective effect on the progression to diabetes. The DPP study also included a metformin-only arm, and these patients also had a reduction in the incidence of diabetes of about 25%. It has been estimated that prediabetic patients following lifestyle suggestions *and* daily metformin[1] may have the lowest risk of diabetes over time compared with control groups and those receiving intensive lifestyle intervention only or daily metformin only. Outcomes of bariatric surgery and significant weight loss among T2DM suggests reversal of the disease occurs in the majority of patients, especially those whose duration of diabetes is less than 10 years.

General Medical Management of Diabetes

Optimal management of T2DM is best accomplished through a patient-centered approach. This involves collaboration between patients and their caregivers to create personalized treatment plans that align with the patient's preferences, lifestyle, existing comorbidities, safety considerations, and socioeconomic and psychosocial contexts.

Comprehensive Management Plan

A comprehensive diabetes management plan integrates various elements to optimize patient outcomes:

- **Lifestyle modifications:** Encouraging a balanced diet and regular physical activity is fundamental. A balanced diet rich in fiber, whole grains, lean proteins, and healthy fats, combined with regular exercise, can significantly improve glycemic control and overall health. Patients should aim for weight loss if they are overweight, as this can improve insulin sensitivity and glycemic control.
- **Blood glucose monitoring:** Regular monitoring of blood glucose levels helps patients and healthcare providers adjust treatment plans as needed. Self-monitoring can provide immediate feedback on how lifestyle choices and medications affect glucose levels.

---

[1] Not FDA approved for this indication.

- **Pharmacologic therapy:** Medications are often necessary to manage blood glucose levels effectively. The choice of pharmacologic agents should consider the patient's individual health profile, including any comorbid conditions, risk of hypoglycemia, and potential side effects.
- **Regular medical checkups:** Ongoing monitoring by healthcare providers is essential to assess the effectiveness of the treatment plan, manage complications, and adjust therapies as required. The American Diabetes Association (ADA) recommends seeing patients with uncontrolled T2DM at 3-month intervals and patients with controlled T2DM at 6-month intervals.
- **Psychosocial support:** Addressing the psychological and social aspects of living with diabetes is crucial. Depression, anxiety, and diabetes distress can adversely affect self-care behaviors and glycemic control. Patients may benefit from counseling, support groups, and other resources that help them cope with the emotional and social challenges of diabetes management.

Patient Education

Patient education, particularly diabetes self-management education and support (DSMES), is critical in empowering individuals with T2DM to manage their condition effectively. DSMES equips patients with the necessary knowledge and skills to engage in diabetes-related self-care and develop effective problem-solving strategies. The ADA recommends patients use DSMES services at multiple points in their care: at diagnosis, annually or when treatment goals are not met, during the emergence of complicating factors, and at times of significant life or care transitions. Research has shown that DSMES can lead to improved outcomes, such as better HbA1C levels and enhanced quality of life. Moreover, DSMES has been associated with reduced healthcare costs by lowering the use of acute care and inpatient services for diabetes management. The ADA also endorses the use of digital coaching and digital self-management tools as effective means of delivering DSMES.

Glucose Measurement and Glycemic Targets
Hemoglobin A1C

HbA1C is the most common tool for monitoring long-term glycemic control in patients with T2DM. This marker is a convenient, simple blood test that reflects average blood glucose levels over the past 3 months, and it allows healthcare providers to track patients' progress over time. However, the HbA1C does not capture short-term fluctuations in blood glucose levels, which may be important in certain clinical scenarios. Additionally, conditions such as anemia or hemoglobinopathies can affect HbA1C accuracy, leading to potential misinterpretation of results.

The ADA recommends a target HbA1C of less than 7% for most nonpregnant adults with T2DM. This goal reflects a balance between reducing the risk of long-term complications and minimizing the risk of hypoglycemia. However, individualization of targets is important, especially in special populations (Table 1). For example, for elderly patients with multiple comorbidities or cognitive impairments, less stringent A1C goals may be appropriate to prevent hypoglycemia and improve quality of life. Conversely, for those with newly diagnosed T2DM at a relatively young age without complications, a more stringent A1C goal may be appropriate.

Patients with well-controlled T2DM should have HbA1C checked at least twice a year, or every 6 months. For those with HbA1C values above goal, HbA1C should be assessed more frequently, every 3 months, until the patient reaches target goals.

Fingerstick Glucose

Self-monitoring of blood glucose (SMBG) through finger sticks and glucometers plays a vital role in the day-to-day measurement of diabetes. The ADA recommends individualized glycemic goals for SMBG based on factors such as age, comorbidities, and treatment regimens. For most nonpregnant adults, fasting blood glucose targets are typically 80 to 130 mg/dL and peak postprandial glucose targets are less than 180 mg/dL. SMBG provides immediate feedback on blood glucose levels, allowing patients to make

TABLE 1	Decision Factors in Selecting Glycemic Goals	
DECISION FACTORS	**HBA1C <7%**	**HBA1C >7%–8%**
Consequences of hypoglycemia	Low risk of severe hypoglycemia, patient senses hypoglycemia, has access to good support system	High risk, hypoglycemia unawareness, lives alone
Duration of diabetes	Short; tight control early in the disease promotes reduction in complications over time	There is little evidence that tight control late in the disease alters outcome
Life expectancy	Long	Short; reduction in macro- and microvascular diseases seen after years or decades of good glycemic control
Life-shortening comorbidities	Absent	Patients with life-limiting comorbidities may justifiably have glycemic goals that avoid extreme highs and lows
Well-established comorbidities such as retinopathy, nephropathy, neuropathy	Absent. However, improvement in retinopathy and delay in progression of neuropathy are recognized benefits of tight control	Many comorbidities such as end-stage renal disease, moderate-severe ischemic vascular disease, severe peripheral or autonomic nephropathy
Patient preferences	Highly motivated, strong support	Prefers less burdensome therapy, voices resistance to treatment; obstacles potentially modifiable over time
Available resources	Readily available, good health insurance, strong social network	Limited resources, including cost of medication, poor social support, and so on. The provider can choose low-cost medications (human insulins, sulfonylureas, metformin) to attempt to reach glycemic goals

timely adjustments to their treatment. It also helps identify patterns and trends in glucose levels, guiding therapeutic decisions.

Frequency of monitoring should be individualized based on various factors, including the type of diabetes management plan, treatment regimen, overall health status, level of glycemic control, and the presence of complications. For example, patients who are newly diagnosed with T2DM may need more frequent monitoring initially to establish baseline levels and determine effectiveness of treatment. For individuals on insulin therapy, blood sugar monitoring is typically more frequent, including before meals, snacks, bedtime, and occasionally during the night. There is inconsistent evidence to recommend daily SMBG for those not on insulin therapy or medications that can predispose to hypoglycemia. However, regular SMBG in these individuals may still be useful during periods of medication adjustments, diet or physical activity, illness, or stress.

Continuous Glucose Monitoring

Continuous glucose monitoring (CGM) systems offer real-time glucose readings throughout the day, providing valuable insights into glucose trends, variability, and patterns (Figure 3). A CGM system measures blood glucose levels through the interstitial fluid. A small sensor is inserted into the skin, and the sensor converts glucose levels into an electrical signal that is sent to a receiver, which can be a smartphone app, an insulin pump, or standalone reader.

The ADA acknowledges the benefits of CGM in improving glycemic control and reducing hypoglycemia in patients with diabetes. These devices offer several advantages over traditional SMBG, including the ability to detect trends and patterns in glucose levels, allowing for more customized medication adjustments, lifestyle modifications, and overall diabetes management strategies to optimize outcomes. There are also alerts for hypo- and hyperglycemia, which can be shared with other individuals. Many of these devices also offer remote monitoring for healthcare providers, improving ease of information sharing. However, challenges such as cost, sensor accuracy, calibration requirements, and patient adherence to wear time can impact the effectiveness of CGM.

The ADA recommends a time in range (TIR) of 70 to 180 mg/dL to be greater than 70% for most adults using CGM systems. Time spent below 70 mg/dL should be less than 5%, whereas time above 180 mg/dL should be less than 25%. Another useful tool on the CGM report is the glycemic management indicator (GMI). The GMI is a metric that provides an estimate of the average blood glucose levels over a 24-hour period based on CGM data. It provides a more comprehensive and real-time assessment of glycemic control compared with the traditional HbA1C test, which provides an average of blood glucose levels over the past 3 months. Research has shown that GMI correlates well with HbA1C levels, allowing healthcare providers to track trends, variability, patterns, and blood glucose levels more accurately and frequently than relying solely on periodic HbA1C measurements.

Comprehensive Medical Management and Risk Reduction
Cardiometabolic Complications

Over the past decade, there has been a convergence of describing multiple metabolic risk factors and grouping them together under the umbrella of cardiometabolic health. As the pathological process of dysregulated glucose metabolism leads to dysregulated lipid metabolism, and both glucose and lipid metabolism are ubiquitous across the body, it makes sense to start to group disorders under the umbrella of cardiometabolic health to care for the whole person with diabetes. The foundational parts of cardiometabolic health are changes in lipid metabolism, which increases the risk of macrovascular complications such as heart attack and stroke, blood pressure management, and the management of fatty liver disease. Fatty liver disease has undergone a nomenclature change in recent years and is also currently known as metabolic dysfunction-associated steatohepatitis (MASH) and metabolic dysfunction–associated steatotic liver disease (MASLD).

Dyslipidemia. The development and progression of ASCVD is the culprit disease process for the leading cause of morbidity in the United States. For patients with diabetes, the atherosclerotic process can be accelerated, and morbidity from major adverse cardiovascular events (MACEs) is more than double that of the general population without diabetes. The driver of the atherosclerotic process is retention of apolipoprotein B (Apo B) containing lipoproteins in the subendothelial space. This drives foam cell development and plaque progression. Therefore the management of dyslipidemia in the patient with diabetes is of paramount importance.

Pharmacologic intervention for dyslipidemia has progressed substantially, with multiple novel agents becoming available in recent years. Although the statin class of medications is the foundational intervention for managing dyslipidemia in diabetes, there are new medications with novel mechanisms that can aid

Example of AGP report

AGP Report

Name _____

MRN _____

Glucose statistics and targets

26 Feb 2019 - 10 Mar 2019   **13 days**
% Time CGM is active   **99.9%**

Glucose ranges	Targets [% of readings (Time/Day)]
Target range 70–180 mg/dL............	Greater than 70% (16hr 48min)
Below 70 mg/dL.............................	Less than 4% (58min)
Below 54 mg/dL.............................	Less than 1% (14min)
Above 250 mg/dL...........................	Less than 5% (1hr 12min)

Each 5% increase in time in range (70–180 mg/dL) is clinically beneficial.

Average glucose   **173 mg/dL**
Glucose management indicator (GMI)   **7.6%**
Glucose variability   **49.5%**
Defined as percent coefficient of variation (%CV): target ≤36%

Time in ranges

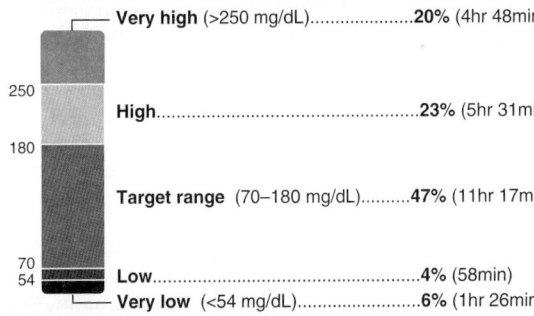

Very high (>250 mg/dL)....................**20%** (4hr 48min)

High..**23%** (5hr 31min)

Target range (70–180 mg/dL)..........**47%** (11hr 17min)

Low..**4%** (58min)
Very low (<54 mg/dL).......................**6%** (1hr 26min)

Ambulatory glucose profile (AGP)

AGP is a summary of glucose values from the report period, with median (50%) and other percentiles shown as if occurring in a single day.

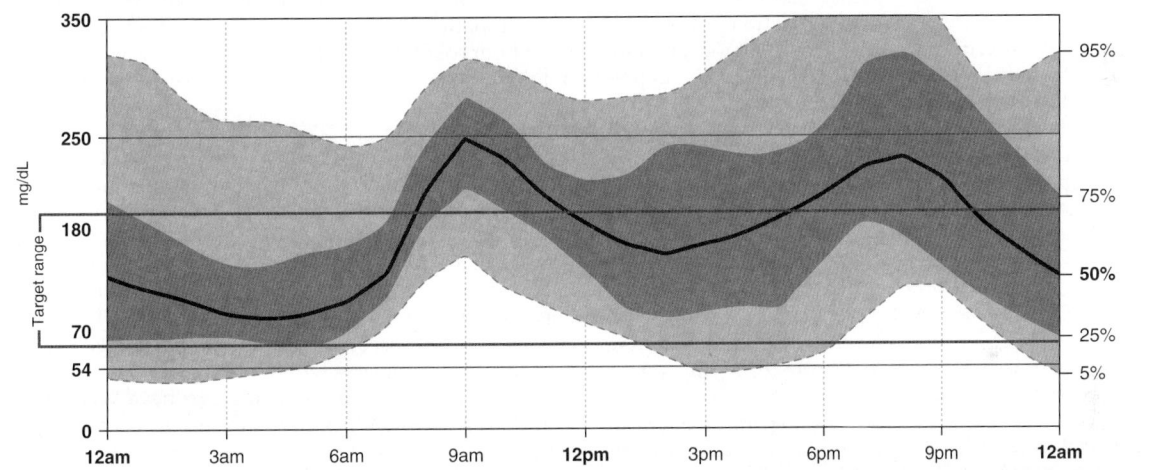

Daily glucose profiles

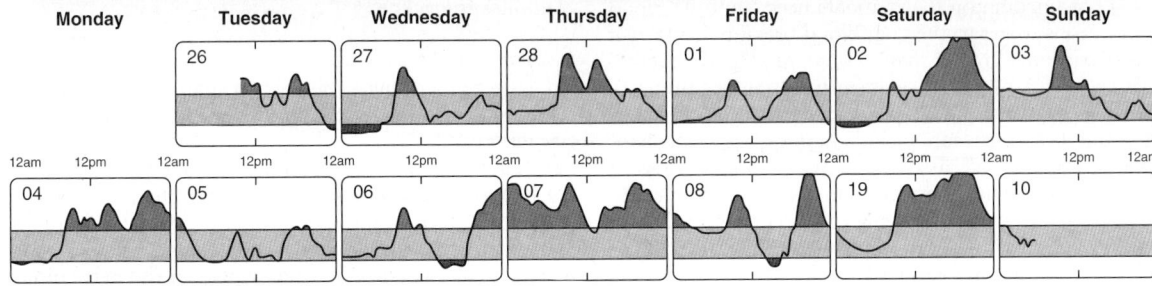

Each daily profile represents a midnight to midnight period.

Figure 3 The report from a continuous glucose monitor *(GCM)* contains valuable information. The time of day is along the *x*-axis, and the blood glucose is along the *y*-axis. The solid line is the median glucose over 2 weeks, and the dark and light shaded areas represent 90% and 95% of the values over the past 2 weeks. On the right, average glucose sensor usage and time and range is documented. The glycemic goals are shown on the graph by two horizontal lines. The glycemic management indicator *(GMI)* of 7.6% shows the computer-generated estimate of HbA1C from the glucose collected over the past ~2 weeks. In this case, the patient experiences postprandial hyperglycemia after breakfast and the evening meal and a tendency towards hypoglycemia around 3:00 PM and overnight.

in management. These include the PCSK9 inhibitors, ezetimibe, bempedoic acid, and icosapent ethyl. The longer-term MACE impact of newer medications such as inclisiran remains to be seen.

Overall, the management of lipoproteins in patients with diabetes is key to improving cardiovascular outcomes, and new therapies help get patients to their goals. Primary prevention using statins should be given to diabetic patients 40 to 75 years of age. The goal is to reduce LDL by 50% or to reach 70 mg/dL or less with diabetes and one or more ASCVD risk factors. High-intensity statin therapy is recommended for all people with diabetes and ASCVD to target an LDL cholesterol reduction of 50% or greater from baseline and an LDL cholesterol goal of less than 55 mg/dL. Addition of ezetimibe or a PCSK9 inhibitor is recommended if this goal is not achieved on maximum tolerated statin therapy.

The pattern of hypertriglyceridemia with concomitant low HDL is common in diabetes. Although hypertriglyceridemia certainly contributes to insulin resistance, a more pressing concern occurs when serum TGs exceed ~1000 mg/dL and the risk of pancreatitis significantly increases. Instituting a short-term fast, ensuring strict glycemic control, statins, and fibric acid derivatives help with acute lowering of TGs to help prevent pancreatitis. TG-specific medications in diabetes have not consistently shown cardiovascular outcome benefit (apart from icosapent ethyl acid demonstrated in the REDUCE-IT trial). Fibric acid derivatives, specifically fenofibrate, have a significant positive impact on microvascular diabetic complications. The fundamental approach to diabetic hypertriglyceridemia is to improve glycemic control, which in turn reduces TG production and hastens clearance of very-low-density lipoprotein, the major TG-containing lipoprotein.

Blood Pressure. Hypertension is a well-known contributor to cardiovascular risk. Patients with diabetes very commonly have concomitant hypertension. Diabetes and hypertension work synergistically to damage the vascular endothelial lining and increase atherosclerotic risk. Multiple large studies have shown treatment of hypertension in patients who have diabetes not only reduces MACEs but can also lower microvascular complications. The ADA concurs with the American Heart Association (AHA) and the American College of Cardiology (ACC) that blood pressure goals should be less than 130/80 mm Hg. Screening for hypertension should occur at every visit for diabetes due to the high prevalence. For patient with diabetes and hypertension, the first step is to examine the lifestyle to see if there are areas of improvement that can also improve blood pressure. Of note, the DASH diet (Dietary Approaches to Stop Hypertension) has been shown to help lower blood pressure. Other lifestyle changes include increasing physical activity, lowering/eliminating alcohol intake, and stopping smoking.

If pharmacologic interventions are needed for patients with persistent blood pressures greater than 130/80 mm Hg despite lifestyle changes, there are four main categories of antihypertensive agents that can be employed. Those agents include angiotensin convertase (ACE) inhibitors (e.g., lisinopril), angiotensin receptor blockers (ARBs) (e.g., losartan), diuretics (e.g., hydrochlorothiazide), and dihydropyridine calcium channel blockers (e.g., amlodipine). Importantly, ACE inhibitors and ARBs are not used concurrently as they reside within the same metabolic chain of events. It is not uncommon that patients need multiple blood pressure medications to get to the goal blood pressure. In fact, if the patient is persistently greater than 150/90 mm Hg, the recommendation is to start a two-drug regimen from the beginning to help get the blood pressure under control faster. Special considerations for treating blood pressure include monitoring electrolytes when using medications such as diuretics that can cause loss of potassium, monitoring renal function, and specific follow-up to ensure that the blood pressure is staying consistently normal.

Liver Disease. An emerging topic of interest within the realm of diabetes and cardiometabolic health is hepatic dysfunction. Previously termed nonalcoholic fatty liver disease (NAFLD), MAFLD/MASH is a chronic metabolic disease process consisting of a continuum of fat accumulation within the liver, progression to inflammatory changes (hepatitis), fibrosis, and ultimately cirrhosis. MASLD is now the most prevalent chronic hepatic disease. Strong associations exist between MAFLD/MASH and obesity, metabolic syndrome, and T2DM. Multiple professional societies agree that screening for MASH in patients with T2DM is beneficial, as anywhere from 30% to 55% of patients with T2DM have MASLD and are at risk of progressing to steatohepatitis without intervention. Screening is typically done with a Fibrosis-4 (FIB-4) score, a calculation done using the patient's age, platelet count, aspartate aminotransferase (AST), and alanine aminotransferase (ALT). Agents such as the GLP-1 receptor agonists, which

allow potent glycemic control, and significant weight loss show promising effects on hepatic steatosis and will hopefully work to stem the tide of this growing complication. As in many cases with patients who have diabetes, a multidisciplinary approach should be the standard with close connection with hepatologists, especially for those with more advanced fibrosis and cirrhosis.

Microvascular Complications

Prolonged elevations in blood glucose can trigger a cascade of biochemical and cellular changes that damage the small blood vessels. This damage predominantly affects the eyes, kidneys, and nerves, leading to significant morbidity. Prevention and early detection through regular medical care, blood glucose control, and healthy lifestyle habits are crucial in reducing the risk and progression of these complications.

Retinopathy

Damage to retinal blood vessels can cause microaneurysms, hemorrhages, exudates, and neovascularization. The condition progresses from nonproliferative retinopathy to proliferative retinopathy, potentially leading to vision loss.

Diabetic retinopathy is strongly correlated with hyperglycemia and length of time since diabetes onset. People with T1DM should have a dilated eye exam within 5 years of diagnosis. Those with T2DM should have a dilated eye exam at the time of diagnosis. Lowering HbA1C quickly can lead to (temporary) worsening of retinopathy. If patients have diabetic macular edema or moderate nonproliferative retinopathy, they should be referred to an ophthalmologist.

Nephropathy

Chronic kidney disease (CKD) occurs in approximately one-third of patients with diabetes, and diabetes is the most common cause of kidney failure in the United States. It most commonly is found 5 to 15 years after diagnosis of T1DM but may be found at the time of diagnosis of T2DM. Early signs include hyperfiltration and microalbuminuria, with progression leading to overt proteinuria, declining glomerular filtration rate (GFR), and eventual end-stage renal disease (ESRD). Blood glucose control and blood pressure control have been proven to prevent CKD and slow its progression. ACE inhibitors and ARBs have been shown to prevent the progression of CKD and prevent cardiovascular events in those with moderate or severe albuminuria. Screening with annual urine albumin lab (spot urine albumin/creatinine ratio) and serum estimated GFR (eGFR) should be obtained. These should be assessed more frequently if kidney function declines or continues to decline.

Neuropathy

Damage to peripheral nerves, primarily due to microvascular injury and metabolic imbalances, causes sensory and motor deficits. This can lead to distal symmetric polyneuropathy (most common), autonomic neuropathy, and focal neuropathies.

Peripheral Neuropathy. Diabetic peripheral neuropathy arises from prolonged exposure to high glucose levels in the blood. Chronic hyperglycemia leads to damage to the peripheral nerves that control sensation and movement in the extremities. Peripheral neuropathy is one of the most common microvascular complications of both T1DM and T2DM and can often lead to lower limb amputations.

Healthcare providers should be vigilant for symptoms such as numbness, tingling, burning pain, or sharp sensations in the extremities, particularly in the feet and hands, commonly referred to as a glove-and-stocking distribution. Patients may also report muscle weakness and difficulties with coordination and balance. Given the progressive nature of diabetic peripheral neuropathy, preventive measures through physical exams and screening are important to circumvent complications such as foot ulcers or infections. Healthcare providers should perform comprehensive foot examinations, assessing foot sensation, checking for any foot deformities or ulcers, and evaluating reflexes during routine

TABLE 2	Diabetic Autonomic Neuropathy (DAN)		
ORGAN SYSTEM	**SIGNS AND SYMPTOMS**	**MONITORING AND PHYSICAL EXAM**	**TREATMENT OPTIONS**
Cardiovascular	• Resting tachycardia • Orthostatic hypotension	• Heart rate variability • Postural blood pressure changes	• Cautious use of β-blockers • Increased salt and fluid intake • Compression stockings • Midodrine (Amatine) and fludrocortisone (Florinef)[1]
	• Silent myocardial ischemia	• ECG	
Gastrointestinal	• Gastroparesis (delayed gastric emptying)	• Gastric emptying study	• Prokinetics: metoclopramide (Reglan) (short-term); erythromycin[1] • Small frequent meals; low-fiber and low-fat diet
	• Diarrhea or constipation	• Symptom assessment with focus on patterns	• Symptom management
Genitourinary	• Bladder dysfunction (neurogenic bladder) • Erectile dysfunction	• Postvoid residual volume • Sexual history	• Scheduled voiding • Intermittent catheterization • Phosphodiesterase type 5 inhibitor (e.g., sildenafil [Viagra])
Metabolic	• Hypoglycemia unawareness	• Assess threshold for signs/symptoms hypoglycemia to be present	• Frequent glucose monitoring • Continuous glucose monitoring • Glucagon (GlucaGen, Gvoke, Baqsimi) • Prescription on hand

[1]Not FDA approved for this indication.

visits. A foot exam is recommended yearly for patients with diabetes at low risk of foot ulcer or neuropathy, and more frequently for those at higher risk. The 10-g monofilament test and physical exam are very useful in determining feet at high risk of ulceration. High-risk feet include those with loss of peripheral sensation, deformities, preulcerative corns or calluses, and prior amputation. People with high-risk feet may benefit from custom shoes or orthotics and consider referral to podiatry.

Treatment options for diabetic peripheral neuropathy are limited and focus on managing symptoms and preventing further nerve damage. Tight glycemic control is important in slowing the progression of diabetic peripheral neuropathy. Pharmacologic management focuses on pain management. First-line agents include anticonvulsants such as gabapentin or pregabalin, although these should be titrated upwards based on efficacy and tolerance due to risk of sedative effects. Serotonin-norepinephrine reuptake inhibitors are also used due to their favorable side effect profiles. Tricyclic antidepressants are effective but may have anticholinergic side effects and are less commonly used. Some patients find relief with topical agents for localized pain relief, such as capsaicin cream or lidocaine patches. Opioids are generally reserved for refractory cases due to potential for dependence and side effects. Physical therapy may also help in maintaining mobility and function period. When other avenues are exhausted, some patients find pain relief with transcutaneous electrical nerve stimulation (TENS).

Autonomic Neuropathy. Diabetic autonomic neuropathy (DAN) is a serious and often underrecognized complication of diabetes mellitus (both type 1 and type 2). The etiology is multifactorial, involving chronic hyperglycemia, metabolic imbalances, and microvascular insufficiency leading to nerve damage. Risk factors include long-standing diabetes, poor glycemic control, and the presence of other diabetic complications such as peripheral neuropathy and retinopathy.

DAN results from damage to the autonomic nerves, which control involuntary bodily functions. Chronic hyperglycemia leads to the accumulation of advanced glycation end-products (AGEs), oxidative stress, and inflammation, which contribute to nerve fiber damage and loss. Microvascular insufficiency exacerbates this damage, leading to impaired blood supply to the nerves. DAN can affect multiple organ systems, leading to a variety of symptoms (Table 2).

Mental Health
The treatment and management of diabetes has wide-reaching effects on the lives of both patients and their loved ones. With these broad impacts, most patients who receive a diagnosis experience some level of psychosocial distress during their time living with the disease. Achieving optimal medical outcomes requires integrating diabetes into all facets of daily life, as well as maintaining often complex medication regimens. Thus the psychosocial well-being of people living with diabetes is a key component of diabetes care in itself, but poor mental health can lead to poor regimen adherence and difficulty achieving optimal glycemic control. Given the importance of this aspect of care, guidelines suggest routinely discussing and assessing the psychosocial well-being of people living with diabetes as a part of diabetes care visits. Specifically, annual depression and anxiety screening, as well as monitoring for evidence of diabetes distress and disordered eating, are recommended with referrals to mental health specialists as indicated. Use of validated screening tools such as the PHQ-9 (depression), BAI (anxiety), and DDS or PAID (diabetes distress) are recommended to increase reliability of monitoring and reduce bias. Special populations among people living with diabetes such as young adults or older adults may require special attention to particular aspects of diabetes care (diabetes distress in young adults), or additional assessments (cognitive testing in older adults) to more accurately assess their psychosocial well-being.

Lifestyle Interventions for Diabetes
Diet
A variety of eating patterns are acceptable for management of T2DM. There is no one preferred eating plan, as it should be individualized for each person. Referral to a registered dietitian nutritionist (RD/RDN) is recommended for all people with diabetes, prediabetes, and GDM to educate and help plan a diet with specific caloric and metabolic goals. Patients with diabetes should have medical nutrition therapy (MNT) with an RD/RDN at the time of diagnosis and as needed throughout their lives.

Reduced overall carbohydrate intake and emphasis on carbohydrates that are high in fiber and minimally processed are recommended. An eating plan emphasizing monounsaturated and polyunsaturated fats and fewer processed foods (Mediterranean-style diet) has been shown to improve glucose metabolism and

TABLE 3 Treatment Options for Overweight and Obesity in Type 2 Diabetes

TREATMENT[a]	BMI CATEGORY (KG/M²)		
	25.0–26.9 (OR 23.0–24.9[b])	27.0–29.9 (OR 25.0–27.4[b])	≥30.0 (OR ≥27.5[b])
Diet, exercise, and behavioral therapy	Yes	Yes	Yes[b]
Pharmacotherapy—weight-loss medications for selected patients	No	Yes	Yes[b]
Metabolic surgery (vertical gastroplasty or modified Roux-en-Y)	No	No	Yes[a,b]

[a]Asian Americans in italics.
[b]For obese patients with comorbidities.
BMI, Body mass index.

lower cardiovascular disease (CVD) risk. A diet that is lower in calories and that the patient enjoys enough to continue can cause weight loss.

Exercise

Vigorous-intensity exercise of 150 minutes per week improves insulin sensitivity, has been shown to reduce body fat, and is recommended for most patients with T1DM or T2DM. Ideally, this activity is spread over at least 3 days, with no more than 2 days in a row without exercise. It has been shown that 200 to 300 minutes per week helps maintain weight loss. Prolonged sitting has negative effects on postprandial blood glucose levels and should be avoided. People with T2DM should decrease the amount of time sitting and other sedentary behaviors. For sedentary activity lasting 30 minutes or longer, a 3-minute (minimum) break of walking, stretching, or isometric exercise is encouraged for improved glycemic control. Resistance training should be done two to three times per week for improved strength and improved glycemic control. Even light activities such as housework, gardening, parking farther away, and taking the stairs all have beneficial effects on weight and blood glucose values.

Weight Loss

BMI should be calculated at least annually, although it is useful to do at each visit. This can be calculated as weight in kilograms divided by height in meters squared (kg/m²) or electronically in the electronic medical record (EMR) or online calculator. BMI should be classified as underweight (<18.5 kg/m²), normal (18.5 to 24.9 kg/m²), overweight (25 to 29.9 kg/m²), or obese (>30 kg/m²). In general, higher BMIs increase the risk of all-cause mortality and CVD and reduce quality of life. Weight-loss goals and intervention strategies should then be discussed (Table 3). Frequent sessions with a trained individual have been shown to help facilitate weight loss. Loss of 5% body weight is recommended for people with T2DM and overweight or obese, and often can be achieved with a deficit of 500 kcal/day. Further weight loss usually leads to further improvements in glycemia and other metabolic measures. Weight loss maintenance is often less successful. Self-monitoring strategies, monthly (or more frequent) check-ins, and high levels of physical activity are recommended to maintain weight loss.

Drugs That Are Associated With Weight Loss

Medications for treatment of diabetes associated with modest weight loss include metformin, Sodium-glucose cotransporter-2 (SGLT2) inhibitors, amylin mimetics, and alpha-glucosidase inhibitors. GLP-1 receptor agonists such as semaglutide, dulaglutide, liraglutide, and exenatide produce, on the average, the greatest amounts of weight loss, averaging about 2 kg per month.

Pharmacotherapy

For people with T2DM and overweight or obese, GLP-1 receptor agonists such as semaglutide, or the dual glucose-dependent insulinotropic polypeptide and glucagon-like peptide 1 receptor (GIP/GLP-1) receptor agonist tirzepatide, is preferred unless contraindications exist. These medications should be started at a low dose and

titrated upward, as nausea and gastrointestinal distress can occur if higher doses are started in naïve patients. These often induce significantly more weight loss than other diabetes medications and have cardiometabolic benefits. SGLT2 inhibitors (the -gliflozins) and dipeptidyl peptidase-4 (DPP-4) inhibitors (the -gliptins) also induce weight loss, but less than the GLP-1 class. Medications causing weight gain should be minimized or exchanged if possible.

Bariatric Surgery

Bariatric surgery should be considered in patients with diabetes and BMI greater than 30 if they are good surgical candidates. Patients should be evaluated for social and living situations, as well as psychological comorbidities that could interfere with health and progress after surgery. There should be a plan in place for long-term support after surgery and monitoring micronutrient, nutritional, and metabolic status.

If postsurgery hypoglycemia occurs, other potential disorders should be evaluated. Management should include education and referral for MNT with a bariatric RD/RDN, as this can often be treated with changing timing and composition of meals and snacks.

Pharmacologic Therapy

Along with lifestyle modifications, pharmacologic therapies may be needed to achieve optimal glycemic control in patients with T2DM. Previously, metformin was the standard first-line agent in diabetes pharmacotherapy. However, the ADA now recommends using either a GLP-1 receptor agonist or SGLT2 inhibitor as the preferred first-line agents for cardiorenal risk reduction in patients with ASCVD, indicators of high-risk ASCVD, heart failure, and/or CKD. This arguably encompasses most patients with T2DM. Metformin is still included in standards of care but has fallen short in its risk reduction of cardiovascular and renal disease compared with the GLP-1 receptor agonists and SLGT2 inhibitors.

For patients not meeting glycemic targets after first-line treatment is initiated, the ADA advises an individualized approach in selecting appropriate pharmacologic therapy and escalation of treatment to achieve glycemic goals for patients with T2DM. Many agents now offer added benefits for protection against ASCVD and progression of diabetic kidney disease (DKD), as well as additional weight-loss effects. A patient-centered approach should guide treatment, considering the potential for additional risk factor reduction, mitigating weight gain, hypoglycemia risk, cost, and patient preference (Figure 4). HbA1C should be checked every 3 months, with escalation of care if targets are not achieved. However, intensification of care, including initiation of insulin, should not be delayed in patients with markedly uncontrolled glycemia.

Noninsulin Agents
Metformin

Metformin is a biguanide that inhibits hepatic glycogenolysis and gluconeogenesis. It improves insulin sensitivity in muscle and fat. It can lower HbA1C by 1.0% to 1.5% on the average, but

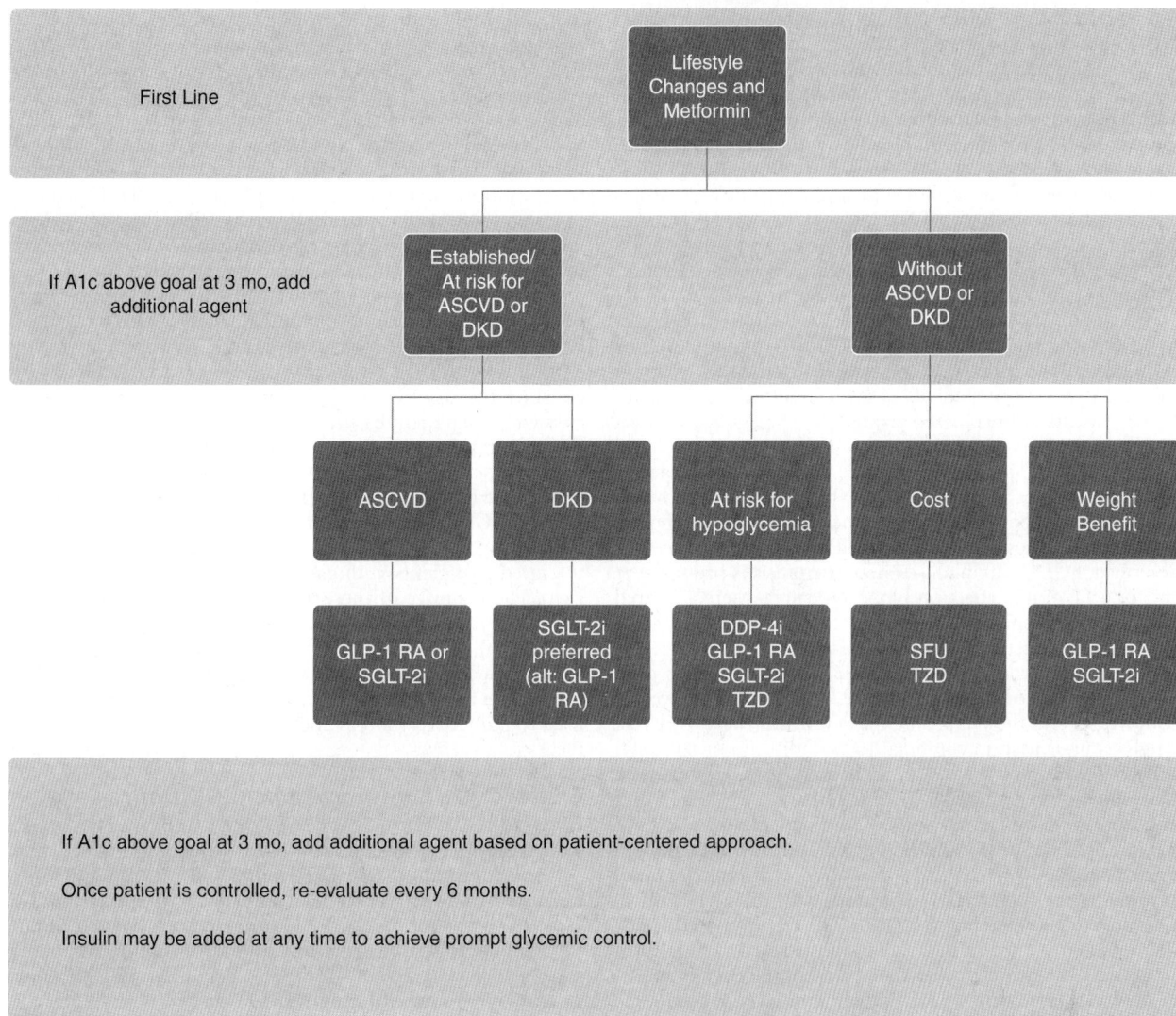

Figure 4 The choice of oral agents is based on many factors including the patient's financial resources and risk or presence of complications. In this figure, we show a decision tree based on the presence or absence of major complications. *ASCVD,* Atherosclerotic cardiovascular disease; *DPP-4i,* dipeptidyl peptidase 4 inhibitor; *DKD,* diabetic kidney disease; *GLP-1 RA,* glucagon-like peptide 1 receptor agonist; *SGLT-2i,* sodium-glucose cotransporter 2 inhibitor; *TZD,* thiazolidinedione. (Modified from the ADA Standards of Medical Care in Diabetes, 2024.)

occasionally it can be very effective, even in new-onset patients with rather high HbA1C levels. Metformin is inexpensive with good efficacy and no risk of hypoglycemia. It is usually weight neutral and may even provide modest weight loss. Metformin has cardiovascular benefits.

Common adverse effects include gastrointestinal upset, which can be minimized by taking metformin with a meal instead of before a meal or by using the extended-release formula. Gradual titration up to full dose also reduces gastrointestinal side effects, especially when taken with meals. Metformin is associated with a reduction in vitamin B_{12} but rarely with a deficiency. Lactic acidosis is a very rare but catastrophic complication of metformin, usually occurring in patients with significant reduction in GFR.

Metformin has often been inaccurately accused of causing renal damage, and there is little to no evidence to support this belief. The FDA has approved metformin for use in patients with eGFR greater than 30 mL/min/1.73 m^2. The authors typically give a reduced dose of metformin for eGFR less than 60 mL/min/1.73 m^2. As metformin is renally cleared, it should be withheld for 48 hours after iodinated contrast administration to avoid contrast-induced nephropathy. Metformin should be avoided in unstable or hospitalized patients with acute heart failure because of the increased risk of lactic acidosis and worsened myocardial dysfunction. Metformin should be continued as long as it is tolerated and there are

no contraindications, even as additional agents including insulin are added. Of note, there is probably little benefit in the use of metformin in T1DM[1], although it may be beneficial for patients with concomitant insulin resistance caused by overweight/obesity.

Sodium-Glucose Cotransporter 2 Inhibitors
SGLT2 is expressed in the proximal renal tubule and mediates reabsorption of the majority of the glucose load filtered through the kidneys. SGLT2 inhibitors block renal glucose reabsorption, thus promoting excretion of glucose and sodium via glucosuria and lowering blood glucose levels in patients with T2DM. The glucose-lowering effects are independent of insulin, beta-cell function, and insulin sensitivity, thus offering an additional pathway for glucose regulation with low risk of hypoglycemia when used without insulin. These agents lower HbA1C by 0.5% to 1.0%. They are now approved for use in individuals with an eGFR of 20 mL/min/1.73m^2 or greater.

Several landmark trials have demonstrated a significant benefit of the SGLT2 inhibitors for both ASCVD risk and DKD. The Cardiovascular Outcome Event Trial in Type 2 Diabetes Mellitus Patients (EMPA-REG OUTCOME) was the first pivotal trial showing reduced composite outcomes for cardiovascular death,

---

[1] Not FDA approved for this indication.

nonfatal myocardial infarction (MI), or nonfatal stroke with the use of empagliflozin (Jardiance). There was a significant relative risk reduction in rates of cardiovascular death by 38%, all-cause mortality by 32%, and hospitalization for heart failure by 35%. As a result of this trial, empagliflozin received FDA approval for reduction of cardiovascular death in adults with T2DM and CVD. The Canagliflozin Cardiovascular Assessment Study (CANVAS) demonstrated reduction in cardiovascular events, but not cardiovascular death, in patients with T2DM at high risk for CVD in the canagliflozin (Invokana) group when compared with the placebo group. Subsequently, the Evaluation of the Effects of Canagliflozin on Renal and Cardiovascular Outcomes in Participants with Diabetic Nephropathy (CREDENCE) trial showed a 30% risk reduction for composite ESRD, doubling of serum creatinine level, or death from renal or cardiovascular causes, as well as a lower risk of cardiovascular events in patients of the canagliflozin group compared with patients in the placebo group. The Dapagliflozin Effect on Cardiovascular Events randomized double-blind controlled (DECLARE-TIMI 58) trial evaluated time to first event for cardiovascular death, MI, or ischemic stroke, which was reduced in the dapagliflozin arm when compared with the placebo arm. Although the mechanisms responsible for these clinical outcomes are not well described, SGLT2 inhibitor–related natriuresis is proposed to account for a favorable effect on blood pressure, whereas altered myocardial metabolism and weight loss could account for additional benefits to reduction in CVD-related mortality.

Along with the cardiovascular and renal benefits of this drug class, SGLT2 inhibitors also contribute to very modest weight loss. Unfortunately, they can be expensive, and there is a risk of hypoglycemia if used in combination with insulin or sulfonylureas. Because they are renally cleared, considerations for renal dose adjustment are required. There is also an FDA black box warning for the risk of amputations with canagliflozin, a finding that has not been uniformly supported in subsequent studies. There is an increased risk of bone fractures with long-term use (canagliflozin), euglycemic DKA, genitourinary and other infections, volume depletion, slight elevation of LDL cholesterol, and Fournier gangrene. The marked benefit in cardiac and renal protection of these drugs must be balanced against the risks of euglycemic DKA, increased urinary tract infections (UTIs) (about 10% in women, >5% in men), and intolerance caused by dehydration. However, 90% to 95% of patients prescribed this class of drugs tolerate them well.

Glucagon-Like Peptide 1 Receptor Agonists

The GLP-1 receptor agonists are, with one exception, injectables that act through several mechanisms, including increased insulin secretion in response to hyperglycemia, reduction of gastric emptying, reduction of inappropriate glucagon secretion, and potentially slowing the loss of beta-cell function over time. On the average, they lower HbA1C by 1.0% to 1.5%. This class of medications promotes significant weight loss by enhancing a sense of early satiety and has a low risk of hypoglycemia when used as monotherapy because of its glucose-dependent mechanism of action.

Like the SGLT2 inhibitors, this class of medications has also demonstrated significant risk reductions in ASCVD and DKD. The Liraglutide Effect and Action in Diabetes: Evaluation of Cardiovascular Outcome Results (LEADER) trial included subjects at risk for CVD and found that liraglutide significantly reduced cardiovascular death, nonfatal MI, or nonfatal stroke, as well as all-cause mortality relative to placebo. Based on the LEADER data, the FDA approved liraglutide for the reduction of major cardiovascular events and cardiovascular deaths in adults with T2DM and CVD. Additional studies have shown benefit of GLP-1 receptor agonists in cardiovascular outcomes. The Trial to Evaluate Cardiovascular and Other Long-Term Outcomes with Semaglutide in Subjects with T2DM (SUSTAIN-6) showed statistically significant reductions in nonfatal MI, nonfatal stroke, or cardiovascular death in the semaglutide group. An additional meta-analysis of seven GLP-1 receptor agonist cardiovascular

outcome trials found this drug class reduced MACEs by 12%, all-cause mortality by 12%, and hospitalization for heart failure by 9%. There was also a 17% reduction in a composite of various renal outcomes.

The most common side effects of these agents include mild injection-site reactions, abdominal cramping, and nausea and vomiting, which are typically transient and lessened by gradual dose uptitration. There is a risk of hypoglycemia if used in combination with insulin or sulfonylureas. This class of medications has been found to increase the incidence of benign and malignant C-cell tumors in rodents and is contraindicated in patients with a personal or family history of medullary thyroid carcinoma or multiple endocrine neoplasia 2A or 2B. There have also been postmarketing reports of acute pancreatitis and cholecystitis in association with GLP-1 receptor agonists, and providers should consider the risks versus benefits of this class of drug and discuss with the patient before prescribing the medication. Although there are reports of increased incidence of pancreatic cancers and neuroendocrine tumors, a causal relationship has not been established, and the FDA cites insufficient evidence to confirm this risk. Like the SGLT2 inhibitors, these medications may be costly, especially for patients without insurance. The drugs may be poorly tolerated in patients with gastroparesis or previous bariatric surgery. The majority of these agents are injectables. Although one preparation has been approved for oral use (semaglutide), there is a loss of efficacy and no trials on ASCVD or CKD outcomes exist when compared with the injected compounds. GLP-1 receptor analogs are not labeled for use in T1DM and are infrequently used to induce weight loss and possibly produce modest improvements in glycemia.

Glucose-Dependent Insulinotropic Polypeptide and Glucagon-Like Peptide-1 Receptor Agonist

Tirzepatide is a novel agent that combines both a glucose-dependent insulinotropic polypeptide (GIP) and a GLP-1 receptor agonists as a once-weekly injection for the treatment of T2DM. The GIP is part of the incretin family of hormones. Its main role is to stimulate insulin secretion, and it also inhibits apoptosis of pancreatic beta cells and promotes proliferation. The combination of GLP-1 and GIP agonists seems to promote greater efficacy in the management of T2DM and significant weight reduction. A multicenter trial demonstrated substantial weight loss in participants over the course of 72 weeks. A 5% weight reduction was achieved by at least 85% of participants. Impressively, at least one-half of the participants achieved a weight loss of 20% body weight with higher doses. Its safety profile is comparable to the GLP-1 receptor agonist class. Tirzepatide is approved by the FDA for the treatment of T2DM in adults. Although currently costly, this medication is an exciting advancement in the treatment of T2DM and obesity.

Dipeptidyl Peptidase-4 Inhibitors

DPP-4 inhibitors work by inhibiting the degradation of incretin hormones (like GLP-1) and thus increasing the half-life to increase insulin secretion in a glucose-dependent manner and decrease glucagon secretion. They lower HbA1C by 0.5% to 1.0%. They are weight neutral and do not contribute to hypoglycemia if used as monotherapy. This class of medications is generally well tolerated, but a few patients complain of upper respiratory symptoms and joint pain. There is a risk of hypoglycemia if used in combination with insulin or sulfonylureas. This class can still be used in renal failure with appropriate dose adjustments. One drug in the class, linagliptin, is hepatically metabolized, and no dose adjustment is needed in patients with poor renal function. Like the more potent GLP-1 receptor agonists, the DDP-4 inhibitors can be associated with pancreatitis. There is no additive benefit with a DDP-4 inhibitor with GLP-1 receptor agonist, and the combination should be avoided, with preference usually for the GLP-1 receptor agonist. Of note, the ADA suggests against the use of saxagliptin and alogliptin in patients with heart failure because they may potentially exacerbate underlying myocardial

TABLE 4 Noninsulin Treatment for Adults with Type 2 Diabetes: Factors to Consider for a Patient-Centered Approach

	EFFICACY	WEIGHT CHANGE	ASCVD BENEFIT	DKD BENEFIT	HYPOGLYCEMIA RISK	COST
Metformin	Intermediate	Neutral/modest loss	Benefit	Benefit	None	Low
SGLT2 inhibitor	High	Loss	Benefit	Benefit	Low	High
GLP1-GIP RA	High	Loss+	?	?	None	High
GLP-1 receptor agonist	High	Loss	Benefit	Benefit	Low	High
DPP-4	Low	Neutral	Neutral	Neutral	Low	High
TZD	High	Gain	Potential benefit	Neutral	None	Low
SFU	Intermediate	Gain	Neutral	Neutral	High	Low

ASCVD, Atherosclerotic cardiovascular disease; *DKD*, diabetic kidney disease; *DPP-4*, dipeptidyl peptidase 4; *GLP-1*, glucagon-like peptide 1 receptor; *SFU*, sulfonylurea; *SGLT*, sodium-glucose cotransporter 2; *TZD*, thiazolidinedione.
Modified from the ADA Standards of Medical Care in Diabetes 2024.

dysfunction. However, there is still an overall role for these agents when there is a compelling need to minimize hypoglycemia, when weight neutrality is desired, or in case of significant renal failure.

Thiazolidinediones

Thiazolidinediones (TZDs) are insulin sensitizers that increase insulin sensitivity in muscle and fat. Pioglitazone and rosiglitazone are currently available. They are potent in lowering HbA1C by 1.0% to 1.5%. They are not associated with hypoglycemia. Pioglitazone may reduce CVD and TGs. These medications may cause weight gain in the form of both volume retention and increase in fat mass. There is an FDA black-box warning against the use of these agents in congestive heart failure (CHF). They are also associated with an increased risk of bone fractures and small relative risk of bladder cancer with long-term use (pioglitazone). Pioglitazone can also raise LDL cholesterol. There is a role for these agents when patients do not want to use an injectable medication, when cost is an issue, or when there is a need to minimize hypoglycemia. However, most clinicians avoid the use of TZDs in patients who are already taking insulin because of the risk of edema and CHF.

Secretagogues

Sulfonylureas stimulate beta-cell insulin secretion from the pancreas. They can lower HbA1C by 1.0% to 1.5%. These medications are initially effective and inexpensive. However, the authors typically do not prescribe these medications unless cost is an issue. Sulfonylureas lose their efficacy because they result in beta-cell loss over time and also cause weight gain, potentially contributing to further insulin resistance. Newer agents, such as the SGLT2 inhibitors and GLP-1 receptor agonists, preserve islet cell function, maintain their efficacy, and have shown both cardiovascular and renal protective benefits. Sulfonylureas also have a risk of hypoglycemia and should be taken with food. Caution should be used with hepatic or renal impairment.

Other Agents

Other less used agents include amylin agonists (pramlintide), bile acid sequestrants (cholestyramine resin, colesevelam), and dopamine receptor agonists (bromocriptine). The authors use these infrequently given their cost, modest impact on glycemia, and relative inconvenience for the patient.

See Table 4 for a summary of prescribing noninsulin medications.

Insulin

Insulin is frequently perceived as the ultimate intervention for managing T2DM. Contrary to this perception, insulin can be introduced at any stage of diabetes management. Insulin therapy is typically considered when lifestyle modifications, oral medications, and GLP-1 agonists fail to achieve glycemic targets. Delaying insulin therapy can increase the risk of future complications due to prolonged hyperglycemia, emphasizing the importance of timely intervention. Insulin regimens (Table 5) whether basal-bolus or combinations of regular and NPH insulin, aim to replicate physiological insulin patterns, providing both postprandial and basal insulin coverage.

Basal Insulin

The most common approach to initiating insulin in T2DM is starting with basal insulin. A starting dose of 0.2 U/kg is recommended, with subsequent titration to achieve fasting blood glucose levels of 80 to 130 mg/dL without causing hypoglycemia. Various titration protocols, known as treat-to-target (TTT), enable patients to adjust their basal insulin dose independently. For insulins such as glargine, increasing the dose by 1 unit daily until fasting targets are met is recommended. Conversely, reducing the dose by 1 unit is recommended if overnight hypoglycemia occurs. For ultra–long-acting insulins like glargine 300 U/mL and degludec, a stronger dose adjustment, such as 2 units, is recommended every 5 days due to their extended pharmacodynamic half-lives.

If glycemic targets are not met with basal insulin alone, a "basal-plus-one" regimen is often the next step. This involves adding a dose of short-acting insulin for the largest meal of the day. The additional dose is initially estimated as one-third of the basal insulin dose. The aim is to keep 2-hour postprandial blood glucose levels below 180 mg/dL.

Multiple Daily Injections and Basal-Bolus Therapy

Multiple daily injections (MDI), or basal-bolus therapy, is standard for many T2DM patients and is essential for T1DM. This regimen can be tailored to a patient's lifestyle and preferences. Typically, short-acting insulin constitutes 40% to 60% of the total daily dose (TDD).

The gold standard for prandial insulin dosing involves carbohydrate counting combined with a correction dose of insulin to also manage any premeal hyperglycemia. This method offers the most flexibility in meal planning but requires the patient to accurately calculate carbohydrate intake and perform premeal blood glucose testing. Collaboration with a nutritionist and using online resources and smartphone apps can facilitate this process.

Steps to calculate doses:
1. Estimate TDD: This is approximately 0.5 U/kg for those with T2DM.
2. Calculate carbohydrate ratio: 500/TDD = grams of carbohydrate covered by 1 unit of insulin.

TABLE 5 Comparison of Various Types of Insulin

TRADE NAME	GENERIC NAME[a]	ONSET	PEAK	DURATION	COST
Rapid Acting					
Admelog	Lispro	15–30 min	30–90 min	3–5h	$$
Apidra	Glulisine	10–20 min	90–120 min	2–4 h	$$
Fiasp	Aspart + niacinamide	15–20 min	30–90 min	5 h	$$
Humalog	Lispro U100 and U200 formulations	10–20 min	60–180 min	3–5 h	$$
Lyumjev	Lispro-aabc U100 and U200 formulations	15–20 min	60 min	5 h	$$
Novolog	Aspart	10–20 min	2.5–5 h	3–5 h	$$
Short Acting					
Humulin R, Novolin R	Regular human	16–30 min	4–8 h	4–12 h	$
Humulin R U500	Concentrated regular human	30 min	4–8 h	18–24 h	$$$$
Intermediate Acting					
Humulin N, Novolin N	NPH (human + protamine)	1–2 h	4–12 h	14–24 h	$
Long Acting					
Basaglar	Glargine	3–4 h	Flat	11–24 h	$$
Lantus	Glargine	3–4 h	Flat	11–24 h	$$
Rezvoglar (Biosimilar glargine)	Glargine-aglr	3–4 h	Flat	11–24 h	$$
Semglee (Biosimilar glargine)	Glargine-yfgn	3–4 h	Flat	11–24 h	$$
Ultra-long acting					
Toujeo (U-300)	U300 glargine		Flat	24–36 h	$$
Tresiba (U100 and U200)	Degludec		Flat	36–42 h	$$
Combinations[b]					
Humulin 70/30, Novolin 70/30	NPH 70%/regular 30%	30 min	50 min–2 h and 6–10 h	18–24 h	$
Novolog Mix 70/30	NPH 70%/aspart 30%	15–30 min	50 min–2 h and 6–10 h	18–24 h	$$
Humalog Mix 75/25	NPH 75%/lispro 25%	15–30 min	50 min-2 h and 6–10 h	12–24 h	$$
Humalog Mix 50/50	NPH 50%/lispro 50%	15–30 min	2–4 h and 6–10 h	12–24 h	$$

[a]Insulins are commonly available in 100 U/mL formulations.

[b]The fixed combination insulins generally have high inter- and intrapatient variability because of their reliance on NPH as a background or late-peaking insulin. With their use, the practitioner is trading convenience in exchange for flexible dosing. Despite these concerns, some studies have found using these combinations in type 2 diabetes mellitus produces acceptable control of glucose with slightly more hypoglycemia than multiple daily injections (separate dosing) of basal insulin plus short-acting premeal insulin.

NPH, Neutral protamine Hagedorn.

3. Determine correction factor: 1600/TDD = mg/dL reduction in blood glucose per unit of insulin. This correction is applied for blood glucose levels above a target, often set at 150 mg/dL but adjustable based on individual circumstances.

These calculations provide initial dosing estimates, with the goal of achieving a 2-hour post meal glucose value of less than 180 mg/dL while avoiding hypoglycemia. Ideally, if the correct dose of prandial insulin was administered for carbohydrate, blood glucose should be within the normal range before the next meal, or 4 hours later. Patients may need to adjust their doses for different meals based on their glycemic responses, activity, and even stress levels.

Carbohydrate counting may be difficult for some patients, especially those new to insulin, and fixed meal dosing may be an option for these individuals. In this regimen, patients receive a fixed dose of insulin before each meal, with an additional correction amount added if needed based on their premeal blood glucose levels. This method is suitable for patients with consistent carbohydrate diets or those who prefer a simpler dosing method. Some may even categorize their meals as *small*, *medium*, or *large* carb meals and dose their prandial insulin accordingly, giving larger doses of short-acting insulin for higher carb meals.

Insulin Pumps

Insulin pumps, although less commonly used in general practice, are essential tools for certain patients. They come in two main types: open-loop and semiautonomous (closed-loop) systems. Open-loop pumps require manual programming to deliver basal insulin and premeal boluses. Closed-loop systems, paired with continuous glucose monitors via Bluetooth, adjust basal insulin automatically to maintain near-normal glycemia, although patient input is still necessary for mealtime dosing.

Other Considerations With Insulin

Physical activity significantly influences glucose utilization and insulin sensitivity. During exercise, muscles increase glucose uptake independently of insulin. Regular exercise enhances glucose transport efficiency, reduces insulin resistance, and improves body composition by increasing lean muscle mass. Patients with T2DM are advised to decrease short-acting insulin before anticipated exercise, typically reducing the dose by 30% to 50% depending on level of intensity. For prolonged or high-intensity exercise, insulin may need to be reduced more substantially or omitted entirely. Education on exercise's impact on glycemia and the need for frequent blood glucose monitoring is important. Patients should also always have a source of rapid-acting carbohydrate on hand to treat hypoglycemia should it occur. Hypoglycemia can occur up to 24 hours postexercise due to ongoing glucose uptake by muscles replenishing glycogen stores.

Another important time for frequent blood glucose monitoring and insulin adjustment are during times of illness. Insulin requirements often increase during illness due to the stress response. Withholding insulin during times of illness can lead to uncontrolled hyperglycemia and metabolic decompensation. The authors advise "sick-day rules" that include checking blood glucose every 4 hours, monitoring urine for moderate to large ketones, adequate hydration, correction boluses of insulin for hyperglycemia, and alerting the provider for uncontrolled hyperglycemia, significant nausea or vomiting, or high ketones.

Insulin Management in Type 1 Diabetes

Insulin therapy in T1DM, although similar to insulin treatment in T2DM, has several important distinctions due to the distinct pathophysiology that underlies each of these conditions. Most notably, whereas controlling fasting blood sugars is an important target for dosing basal insulin, among patients with T1DM, the primary role of basal insulin is to ensure sufficient insulin action during fasting periods to prevent the onset of ketosis. Therefore patients should be made aware that consistent dosing of basal insulin plays a critical role in preventing severe manifestations of T1DM. In addition, in cases where diabetes type is not immediately obvious based on clinical or laboratory data, early initiation of basal insulin alongside non–insulin therapy is recommended while additional laboratory evaluations are pending.

As with short-acting insulins given in T2DM, patients with T1DM should be encouraged to give meal dose insulin 10 to 15 minutes before each meal. Due to minimal residual pancreatic insulin secretion, most patients with T1DM will need to adjust insulin meal doses based on carbohydrate intake to achieve glycemic targets. This is most commonly achieved using an insulin-to-carbohydrate ratio in patients who have been trained to estimate the carbohydrate content of meals, which allows them to determine a premeal insulin dose based on these variables. Insulin-to-carbohydrate ratios are generally empirically determined in collaboration with the patient, provider, and a diabetes-focused dietician or certified diabetes care and education specialist (CDCES). Most patients with T1DM will also use a correction factor to calculate short-acting insulin doses. The correction factor allows patients to determine an additional insulin dose to be added to a calculated meal insulin dose to *correct* for hyperglycemia at the time of the meal. The meal dose and correction dose are typically given together as a single injection before meals after patients have completed the appropriate calculations to determine an estimated dose.

Recent advances in diabetes technology including continuous glucose monitors and their integration into insulin pump systems represent an important step forward in the treatment of T1DM. These so-called automated insulin delivery (AID) systems have significant advantages over typical MDI regimens or previous iterations of insulin pumps. These systems integrate blood sugar data from continuous glucose monitors to predict future changes in blood sugars and can both vary the programmed basal rate and deliver correction boluses to reduce blood sugars without user input. These systems still require user input at meals to input carbohydrate estimates and/or deliver meal boluses, but have been shown to significantly reduce HbA1C compared with other insulin delivery methods.

At this time, the only noninsulin medication approved for the treatment of T1DM is pramlintide. This injectable medication is approved for use before meals and is to be used alongside insulin to reduce meal-time insulin requirements. Due to the cost and additional injection burden of this medication, it is rarely used in routine care. Other medications, most notably SGLT2 inhibitors and GLP-1 receptor agonists, are currently being used off-label by select patients with T1DM and are subject of active study. SGLT2 inhibitor use in T1DM in particular should be approached with caution given the increased risk of euglycemic DKA associated with these medications. Although we do consider using these medications in patients with T1DM, we do this only after extensive discussion of risks and benefits with patients and only in highly motivated patients. We would not recommend routine off-label use at this time although this likely will change as more data become available in the future.

Hypoglycemia

Hypoglycemia is defined as a glucose concentration of less than 70 mg/dL and is further classified into three levels. Level 1 is a glucose value less than 70 mg/dL but greater than or equal to 54 mg/dL. Level 2 is a glucose value less than 54 mg/dL. Level 3 is any event with severe symptoms that require medical assistance for treatment. Hypoglycemia can present with both neurogenic (autonomic) and neuroglycopenic symptoms. Neurogenic symptoms include adrenergic responses such as tremor, palpitations, and/or anxiety, as well as cholinergic responses such diaphoresis, hunger, and paresthesias. Conversely, neuroglycopenic symptoms are those that cause an altered sensorium such as confusion, dizziness, weakness, and drowsiness but can ultimately progress to seizures or coma with severe hypoglycemia. Neuroglycopenic symptoms typically occur with glucose values less than 54 mg/dL.

Studies have suggested significant long-term risks from frequent severe hypoglycemia, including significant cognitive impairment, falls and fractures, and increased mortality. Risk factors for hypoglycemia include advanced age, African American race, longer duration of diabetes, use of sulfonylureas and/or insulin, renal impairment, dementia, alcohol ingestion, and erratic meal timing.

Hypoglycemia is also graded as mild, moderate, or severe. *Mild* is an event in which the patient feels the symptoms and treats the low level on their own. *Moderate* events require assistance but do not involve unconsciousness or the need for glucagon. *Severe* hypoglycemia is defined as a seizure, obtundation, need for emergency department visit, or need to call emergency medical technicians (EMTs). Many patients with well-controlled insulin-treated diabetes experience occasional mild hypoglycemia, and these episodes can be acceptable if they are not too frequent or reach moderate-to-severe levels. Moderate and severe events should be addressed with changes in the regimen and a thorough investigation as to why the event occurred, such as skipping a meal or insulin dose error.

Clinicians should be aware that patients with poorly controlled diabetes with frequent episodes of hypoglycemia can often lose their counterregulatory responses to low blood glucose and develop hypoglycemia unawareness in which blood glucose can drop significantly. It is important to ask patients at which glucose threshold they begin to feel symptoms of hypoglycemia. Patients can, occasionally, regain some sensitivity to hypoglycemia by relaxing blood glucose control for several weeks.

Hypoglycemia should be treated with glucose administration if the patient is alert and able to take in food by mouth. The authors educate their patients on the "Rule of 15" for treating hypoglycemia. Patients should ingest 15 g of rapid-acting carbohydrates (such as 4 oz orange juice, 4 oz regular soda, 8 oz skim milk, 3 to 4 glucose tablets, or 15 jelly beans or hard candies) every 15 minutes until fingerstick blood glucose is greater than 70 mg/dL. For prolonged hypoglycemia, we suggest a snack with complex carbohydrates, fats, and protein. It is important to always evaluate the underlying cause of hypoglycemia and adjust the treatment regimen accordingly.

For severe hypoglycemia in which the patient needs the assistance of another person or medical professional, glucagon can be administered. Glucagon is now available in intramuscular, subcutaneous, or intranasal formulations. The authors always educate patients that use of an emergency glucagon kit warrants evaluation in the emergency department after they have taken it.

Special Populations

Adolescents and young adults with diabetes are a rapidly growing population due to the rising incidences of both T1DM and T2DM. Among all people with T1DM, this age group has the highest average HbA1C, is the most likely to experience acute complications such as DKA, and presents a unique set of challenges to care systems and providers. Adolescents and young adults with diabetes confront additional challenges as they move from pediatric to adult care and encounter gaps in insurance, pharmacy benefits, and other issues navigating within care systems. In addition, depression and/or diabetes distress are common among these patients, all of which present additional barriers to engagement with diabetes care.

Given these barriers, developing comprehensive programs to prepare and support adolescents before, during, and after their transfer to adult care, including assistance to address health systems barriers to care, is critical. Furthermore, addressing psychological concerns before or alongside glycemic control is needed to improve outcomes in this population. Planning and preparation for transfer to adult care should begin early, starting the process as early as age 14. Although there is no established ideal age for transfer to adult care, a shared decision-making approach that accounts for potential life stressors, systems issues such as changes in insurance coverage, and consideration of local regulations to determine the optimal timing for transfer to adult care is needed. Aside from discussions between patient and provider, a provider-to-provider conversation should occur before transfer of care to ensure key clinical details are communicated before the first visit with the new adult-based provider. Resources from the ADA, International Society of Pediatric and Adolescent Diabetes (ISPAD), and the National Alliance to Advance Adolescent Health (https://gottransition.org) are available to help design and plan transition programs to address the many needs of this growing and vulnerable population.

References

American Diabetes Association Professional Practice Committee: 3. Prevention or Delay of Diabetes and Associated Comorbidities: Standards of Care in Diabetes—2024, *Diabetes Care* 47(Supplement_1):S43–S51, 2024, https://doi.org/10.2337/dc24-S003.

American Diabetes Association Professional Practice Committee: 10. Cardiovascular Disease and Risk Management: Standards of Care in Diabetes—2024, *Diabetes Care* 47(Supplement_1):S179–S218, 2024, https://doi.org/10.2337/dc24-S010.

Agarwal R, Filippatos G, Pitt B, et al: FIDELIO-DKD and FIGARO-DKD Investigators: Cardiovascular and kidney outcomes with finerenone in patients with type 2 diabetes and chronic kidney disease: the FIDELITY pooled analysis, *Eur Heart J* 43:474–484, 2022.

Bethel MA, Diaz R, Castellana N, et al: HbA1c change and diabetic retinopathy during GLP-1 receptor agonist cardiovascular outcome trials: a meta-analysis and meta-regression, *Diabetes Care* 44:290–296, 2021.

CDC: National Diabetes Statistics Report, *Diabetes*, 2024. http://www.cdc.gov/diabetes/php/data-research/index.html, .

Colberg SR, Sigal RJ, Yardley JE, et al: Physical activity/exercise and diabetes: a position statement of the American Diabetes Association, *Diabetes Care* 39(11):2065–2079, 2016.

David M, Nathan DM: for the DCCT/EDIC Research Group: the diabetes control and complications trial/epidemiology of diabetes interventions and complications study at 30 years: overview, *Diabetes Care Jan* 37(1):9–16, 2014, https://doi.org/10.2337/dc13-2112.

De Boer IH, Khunti K, Sadusky T, et al: Diabetes management in chronic kidney disease: a consensus report by the American Diabetes Association (ADA) and Kidney Disease: Improving Global Outcomes (KDIGO), *Diabetes Care* 45:3075–3090, 2022.

Diabetes Care 47(Suppl.1):S219–S230, 2024.

Duckworth W, Abraira C, Moritz T, et al: VADT investigators. Glucose control and vascular complications in veterans with type 2 diabetes, *N Engl J Med* 360:129–139, 2009.

El Sayed NA, Aleppo G, Aroda VR, on behalf of the American Diabetes Association, et al: Summary of revisions: standards of care in diabetes—2023, *Diabetes Care* 46(Suppl 1):S5–S9, 2023.

Evert AB, Dennison M, Gardner CD, et al: Nutrition therapy for adults with diabetes or prediabetes: a consensus report, *Diabetes Care* 42:731–754, 2019.

Galiero R, Caturano A, Vetrano E, et al: Peripheral Neuropathy in Diabetes Mellitus: Pathogenetic Mechanisms and Diagnostic Options, *Int J Mol Sci* 24(4):3554, 2023, https://doi.org/10.3390/ijms24043554. PMID: 36834971; PMCID: PMC9967934.

Gerstein HC, Miller ME, Genuth S, et al: ACCORD study group. Long-term effects of intensive glucose lowering on cardiovascular outcomes, *N Engl J Med* 364:818–828, 2011.

Grundy SM, Stone NJ, Bailey AL, et al: 2018 AHA/ACC/AACVPR/AAPA/ABC/ACPM/ADA/AGS/APhA/ASPC/NLA/PCNA guideline on the management of blood cholesterol: a report of the American College of Cardiology/American Heart Association Task Force on Clinical Practice Guidelines, *Circulation* 139(25):e1082–e1143, 2019. Erratum in: Circulation 18;139(25):e1182–e1186, 2019.

Heerspink HJL, Stefansson BV, Correa-Rotter R, et al: DAPA-CKD Trial Committees and Investigators: dapagliflozin in patients with chronic kidney disease, *N Engl J Med* 383:1436–1446, 2020.

Holman RR, Paul SK, Bethel MA, et al: 10-year follow-up of intensive glucose control in type 2 diabetes, *N Engl J Med* 359:1577, 2008.

Jardine MJ, Mahaffey KW, Neal B, investigators CREDENCE study, et al: The Canagliflozin and Renal Endpoints in Diabetes with Established Nephropathy Clinical Evaluation (CREDENCE) study rationale, design, and baseline characteristics, *Am J Nephrol* 46:462–472, 2017.

Jastreboff AM, Aronne LJ, Ahmad NN, et al: Tirzepatide Once Weekly for the Treatment of Obesity, *N Engl J Med*, 2022, https://doi.org/10.1056/NEJMoa2206038.

Newman CB, Blaha MJ, Boord JB, et al: Lipid management in patients with endocrine disorders: an Endocrine Society Clinical practice guideline, *J Clin Endocrinol Metab* 105(12):dgaa674, 2020. 2020. Erratum in: J Clin Endocrinol Metab 13;106(6):e2465, 2021.

Patel A, MacMahon S, Chalmers J, et al: ADVANCE collaborative group. intensive blood glucose control and vascular outcomes in patients with type 2 diabetes, *N Engl J Med* 358:2560–2572, 2008.

Schaper NC, van Netten JJ, Apelqvist J, Bus SA, Hinchliffe RJ, Editorial Board IWGDF: Practical guidelines on the prevention and management of diabetic foot disease, *Diabetes Metab Res Rev* 36(Suppl 1):e3266, 2020.

Skyler JS, Bergenstal R, Bonow RO, et al: Intensive glycemic control and the prevention of cardiovascular events: implications of the ACCORD, ADVANCE, and VA diabetes trials, *Diabetes Care* 32(1):187–192, 2009, https://doi.org/10.2337/dc08-9026.

U.S. Department of Veterans Affairs: U.S. Department of Defense: VA/DoD Clinical practice guideline for the management of type 2 diabetes mellitus in primary care, version 5.0, 2017. Available at: https://www.healthquality.va.gov/guidelines/CD/diabetes/VADoDDMCPGFinal508.pdf, .

U.S. Preventive Services Task Force: Screening for abnormal blood glucose and type 2 diabetes mellitus: U.S preventive services task force recommendation statement, *Ann Intern Med* 163(11):861–868, 2015.

Vinik AI, Maser RE, Mitchell BD, Freeman R: Diabetic Autonomic Neuropathy, *Diabetes Care* 26(5):1553–1579, 2003, https://doi.org/10.2337/diacare.26.5.1553.

Young-Hyman D, de Groot M, Hill-Briggs F, Gonzalez JS, Hood K, Peyrot M: Psychosocial Care for People With Diabetes: A Position Statement of the American Diabetes Association, *Diabetes Care* 39(12):2126–2140, 2016, https://doi.org/10.2337/dc16-2053. Erratum in: Diabetes Care. 2017 Feb;40(2):287. doi: 10.2337/dc17-er02. Erratum in: Diabetes Care. 2017 May;40(5):726. doi: 10.2337/dc17-er05. PMID: 27879358; PMCID: PMC5127231.

Zeitler P, Arslanian S, Fu J, et al: ISPAD clinical practice consensus guidelines 2018: type 2 diabetes mellitus in youth, *Pediatr Diabetes* 19(Suppl 27):28–46, 2018. https://doi-org.proxy.kumc.edu/10.1111/pedi.12719.

▌ DIABETIC KETOACIDOSIS

Method of
Aidar R. Gosmanov, MD, PhD, DMSc

⊘ CURRENT DIAGNOSIS

- Initial evaluation includes physical examination and comprehensive metabolic panel, serum osmolality, blood β-hydroxybutyrate, complete blood count, urinalysis, urine ketones, and arterial blood gases.
- Search for precipitating causes. Omission of insulin, underlying medical illness, cardiovascular events, gastrointestinal disorders, recent surgery, medications, eating disorders, psychological stress, insulin pump malfunction, and infection are potential causes; white blood cell count greater than 25,000 suggests presence of infection.
- β-Hydroxybutyrate of 3.0 mmol/L or greater in adults indicates presence of diabetic ketoacidosis (DKA), even if serum ketones are negative.
- Patients with severe chronic kidney disease (CKD) require careful evaluation of acid-base status.

- Start intravenous fluids early before insulin therapy.
- Potassium level should be more than 3.5 mEq/L before insulin therapy is initiated. Supplement potassium intravenously if needed.
- Initiate continuous insulin infusion at 0.1 U/kg/h and measure bedside glucose every 1 hour to adjust the insulin infusion rate.
- Avoid hypoglycemia during the insulin infusion by initiating dextrose-containing fluids and/or reducing the insulin infusion rate until DKA is resolved.
- Transition to subcutaneous insulin only when DKA resolution is established.

Epidemiology

There were 188,965 hospital discharges for diabetic ketoacidosis (DKA) in 2014 in the United States, compared with 140,000 in 2009 and 80,000 in 1988. The in-hospital fatality rates declined consistently from 2009 to 2014 from 1.1% to 0.4%, although mortality remains high in developing countries. In 2014 the direct and indirect annual cost of DKA hospitalization was $5.1 billion.

Risk Factors

Omission of insulin is the most common precipitant of DKA. Infections, acute medical illnesses involving the cardiovascular system (myocardial infarction, stroke) and gastrointestinal tract (bleeding, pancreatitis), diseases of the endocrine axis (acromegaly and Cushing syndrome), and stress from recent surgical procedures can contribute to the development of DKA by causing dehydration, increase in insulin counterregulatory hormones, and worsening of peripheral insulin resistance. Medications such as diuretics, β-blockers, corticosteroids, second-generation antipsychotics, and anticonvulsants can affect carbohydrate metabolism and volume status; therefore they can precipitate DKA. Other factors that can contribute to DKA include psychological problems, eating disorders, insulin pump malfunction, lower socioeconomic status, and drug abuse. It is now recognized that new-onset type 2 diabetes mellitus can manifest with DKA. These patients are obese, mostly African American or Hispanic, and extremely insulin resistant on presentation. The use of sodium-glucose cotransporter 2 (SGLT-2) inhibitors has been implicated in the development of DKA in patients with both type 1 and type 2 diabetes. Since the mid-2010s, the immune checkpoint inhibitors (ICI) used in patients with advanced malignancy were shown to cause DKA de novo in patients without a prior history of diabetes. The DKA risk is significantly more common with use of programmed cell death protein 1 inhibitors such as nivolumab (Opdivo) compared with cytotoxic T-lymphocyte associated antigen 4 inhibitors such as ipilimumab (Yervoy). Early evidence suggests that coronavirus disease 2019 (COVID-19) infection can trigger DKA in subjects without or with prior diabetes history.

Pathophysiology

Insulin deficiency, increased insulin counterregulatory hormones (cortisol, glucagon, growth hormone, and catecholamines), and peripheral insulin resistance lead to hyperglycemia, dehydration, ketosis, and electrolyte imbalance, which underlie the pathophysiology of DKA. The hyperglycemia of DKA evolves through accelerated gluconeogenesis, glycogenolysis, and decreased glucose utilization, all due to absolute insulin deficiency. Owing to increased lipolysis and decreased lipogenesis, abundant free fatty acids are converted to ketone bodies: acetoacetate and β-hydroxybutyrate (β-OHB). Hyperglycemia-induced osmotic diuresis, if not accompanied by sufficient oral fluid intake, leads to dehydration, hyperosmolarity, electrolyte loss, and subsequent decrease in glomerular filtration.

With a decline in a renal function, glycosuria diminishes and hyperglycemia worsens. With impaired insulin action and hyperosmolar hyperglycemia, potassium uptake by skeletal muscle is markedly diminished, which, along with hyperosmolarity-mediated efflux of potassium from cells, results in intracellular potassium depletion. Potassium is lost via osmotic diuresis, causing profound total body potassium deficiency. Therefore DKA patients can present with a broad range of serum potassium concentrations. A "normal" plasma potassium concentration still indicates that potassium stores in the body are severely diminished, and the institution of insulin therapy and correction of hyperglycemia will result in hypokalemia.

On average, patients with DKA have the following deficit of water and key electrolytes: water 100 mL/kg, sodium 7 to 10 mEq/kg, potassium 3 to 5 mEq/kg, and phosphorus 1 mmol/kg.

Clinical Manifestations

Polyuria, polydipsia, weight loss, vomiting, and abdominal pain usually are present in patients with DKA. Abdominal pain can be closely associated with acidosis and resolves with treatment. Physical examination findings such as hypotension, tachycardia, poor skin turgor, and weakness support the clinical diagnosis of dehydration in DKA. Mental status changes can occur in DKA and are likely related to the degree of acidosis and hyperosmolarity. A search for symptoms of precipitating causes such as infection, vascular events, or existing drug abuse should be initiated in the emergency department. Patients with hyperglycemic crises can be hypothermic because of peripheral vasodilation and decreased utilization of metabolic substrates.

Diagnosis

The DKA diagnosis is made when all of the following criteria are met: (1) blood glucose ≥200 mg/dL or there is prior history of diabetes; (2) venous or capillary blood β-OHB ≥3.0 mmol/L or urine ketone strip 2+ or greater; and (3) pH <7.3 and/or bicarbonate concentration <18 mmol/L. Therefore initial laboratory evaluation should include a comprehensive metabolic panel, arterial or venous arterial blood gases, and/or urinalysis or measurement of blood β-OHB. In early DKA, acetoacetate concentration is low, but it is a major substrate for ketone measurement by many laboratories; therefore ketone measurement in serum by usual laboratory techniques has a high specificity but low sensitivity for the diagnosis of DKA. Conversely, β-OHB is an early and abundant ketoacid that can first signal development of DKA, but its measurement requires the use of a specific assay that is different from ketone measurement.

In patients with chronic kidney disease (CKD) stage 4 or 5, the diagnosis of DKA is challenging because of the presence of chronic metabolic acidosis and the possibility of mixed acid-base disorders on presentation with DKA. An anion gap greater than 20 supports the diagnosis of DKA in such patients. Hyperglycemia is not always present in SGLT-2 inhibitor-induced DKA. These patients not infrequently present with a blood glucose level below 250 mg/dL (i.e., euglycemic DKA). Therefore clinicians should always assess the acid-base status in persons with type 2 diabetes treated with SGLT-2 inhibitors who present with acute illness and/or have new onset of nonspecific symptoms.

Differential Diagnosis

Hyperglycemic hyperosmolar state (HHS) is usually not associated with ketosis, but mixed HHS and DKA can occur. Patients with HHS present with severe hyperglycemia, associated total serum osmolarity greater than 320 mOsm/kg, and mental status changes. A mixed DKA + HHS presentation will be associated with more extreme clinical and biochemical deviations than each pathology alone. Patients with mixed DKA + HHS have more severe ketoacidosis, blood glucose levels exceeding 1000 mg/dL, and more profound dehydration and altered sensorium.

Clinical scenarios that may be accompanied by acidosis are described in Table 1. Pregnancy, starvation, and alcoholic ketoacidosis are not characterized by hyperglycemia greater than 200 mg/dL.

TABLE 1 Laboratory Evaluation of Metabolic Causes of Acidosis

LAB VALUE	DKA	STARVATION KETOSIS	LACTIC ACIDOSIS	UREMIC ACIDOSIS	ALCOHOL KETOSIS	SALICYLATE POISONING	METHANOL OR ETHYLENE GLYCOL POISONING
pH	↓	Normal	↓	Mild ↓	↑↓	↑↓*	↓
Plasma glucose	↑	Normal	Normal	Normal	↓or normal	Normal or ↓	Normal
Plasma ketones†	↑↑	Slight ↑	Normal	Normal	↑	Normal	Normal
Anion gap	↑	Slight ↑	↑	Slight ↑	↑	↑	↑
Osmolality	↑	Normal	Normal	↑ or normal	Normal	Normal	↑↑
Other	—	—	Lactate ↑	BUN ↑	—	Serum level +	Serum level +

*Respiratory alkalosis or metabolic acidosis.
†Acetest and Ketostix (Bayer, Leverkusen, Germany) measure acetoacetic acid only; thus misleadingly low values may be obtained because the majority of "ketone bodies" are β-hydroxybutyrate.
BUN, Blood urea nitrogen; DKA, diabetic ketoacidosis.

With hypotension or a history of metformin (Glucophage) use, lactic acidosis should be suspected. Ingestion of methanol, isopropyl alcohol, and paraldehyde[2] can also alter the anion gap and/or osmolality but are not associated with hyperglycemia.

Treatment

The therapeutic goals of management include optimization of volume status, hyperglycemia and ketoacidosis, electrolyte abnormalities, and potential precipitating factors. DKA management workflow is presented in Figure 1. The efficiency of early DKA therapy can be improved by clustering key diagnostic and therapeutic steps in one protocol that is easy to understand for both nursing staff and physicians. Table 2 provides one example of such a DKA care bundle. Given the complexity of the condition management, provision of a single care bundle/order set allows the fundamentals of DKA treatment to be delivered safely and efficiently while giving the providers guidance on tackling unanticipated issues during DKA care. Special considerations should be given to patients with congestive heart failure and CKD. These patients tend to retain fluids; therefore caution should be exercised during volume resuscitation in these patient groups. Patients with SGLT-2 inhibitor–induced DKA may require longer time for ketoacidosis resolution due to more profound metabolic derangements preceding DKA diagnosis. Finally, use of isotonic intravenous fluids such as 0.9% NaCl solution or lactated Ringer (LR) solution are now equally recommended for volume repletion and maintenance fluid replacement in DKA. Several studies suggested that administration of crystalloid solutions such as LR may lead to better patient outcomes when treating DKA compared with isotonic saline.

Bicarbonate therapy is not indicated in mild and moderate forms of DKA because metabolic acidosis should correct with insulin therapy. The use of bicarbonate in severe DKA is controversial owing to a lack of prospective randomized studies. It is thought that the administration of bicarbonate actually results in peripheral hypoxemia, worsened hypokalemia, paradoxical central nervous system acidosis, cerebral edema in children and young adults, and an increase in intracellular acidosis. Because severe acidosis is associated with worse clinical outcomes and can lead to an impairment in sensorium and a deterioration of myocardial contractility, bicarbonate therapy may be indicated if the pH is 6.9 or less. Therefore the infusion of 100 mmol (2 ampules) of bicarbonate in 400 mL of sterile water mixed with 20 mEq potassium chloride over 2 hours and repeating the infusion until the pH is greater than 7.0 can be recommended pending the results of prospective trials.

A whole-body phosphate deficit in DKA can average 1 mmol/kg. Insulin therapy during DKA will further lower serum phosphate concentration. Prospective randomized studies have failed to show any beneficial effect of phosphate replacement on the clinical outcome in DKA. However, a careful phosphate replacement is sometimes indicated in patients with serum phosphate concentration less than 1.0 mg/dL and in those with cardiac dysfunction, anemia, or respiratory depression who have a serum phosphate level between 1.0 and 2.0 mg/dL. An initial replacement strategy may include infusion of potassium phosphate at the rate of 0.1 to 0.2 mmol/kg over 6 hours, depending on the degree of phosphate deficit (1 mL potassium phosphate solution for intravenous use contains 3 mmol phosphorous and 4.4 mEq potassium). Overzealous phosphate replacement can result in hypocalcemia; therefore close monitoring of phosphorous and calcium levels is recommended. Patients who have renal insufficiency or hypocalcemia might need less aggressive phosphate replacement.

When DKA is resolved, and independent of the patient's ability to tolerate oral intake, transition to subcutaneous insulin must be initiated. Patients are given intermediate neutral protamine Hagedorn (NPH) or long-acting insulin (glargine [Lantus]) 2 hours before termination of intravenous insulin to allow sufficient time for the injected insulin to start working (Table 3). Once the patient can eat, we recommend the addition of short- or rapid-acting insulin for prandial glycemic coverage (see Table 3). This is the basal-bolus insulin regimen and provides physiologic replacement of insulin. It is common to see transition from intravenous to subcutaneous insulin using sliding-scale insulin only. This strategy as a sole approach should be discouraged because it cannot provide the necessary insulin requirement in patients recovering from hyperglycemic crisis and beta-cell failure.

If the patient used insulin before admission, the same dosage can be restarted in the hospital. Insulin-naïve patients require insulin at a total dose of 0.5 to 0.8 U/kg/day divided as 50% basal insulin and 50% as prandial insulin before each meal. Initially, after DKA resolution and given the possibility of fluctuating oral intake, the use of once-daily long-acting insulin such as glargine or detemir to provide basal insulin coverage is encouraged. Long-acting insulin glargine U300 (Toujeo) and insulin degludec (Tresiba), which were approved by the FDA in 2015, as well as biosimilar insulin glargine (Basaglar), which was approved in 2016, have not been studied in hospitalized patients treated for DKA and therefore cannot be recommended for subcutaneous administration immediately after DKA resolution. For patients who are not able to adhere to or afford multiple daily insulin injections, conversion of inpatient basal-bolus insulin regimen before discharge to split-mix insulin preparation (Humulin 70/30, Novolin 70/30, Humalog mix 75/25, Novolog mix 70/30)

---

[2] Not available in the United States.

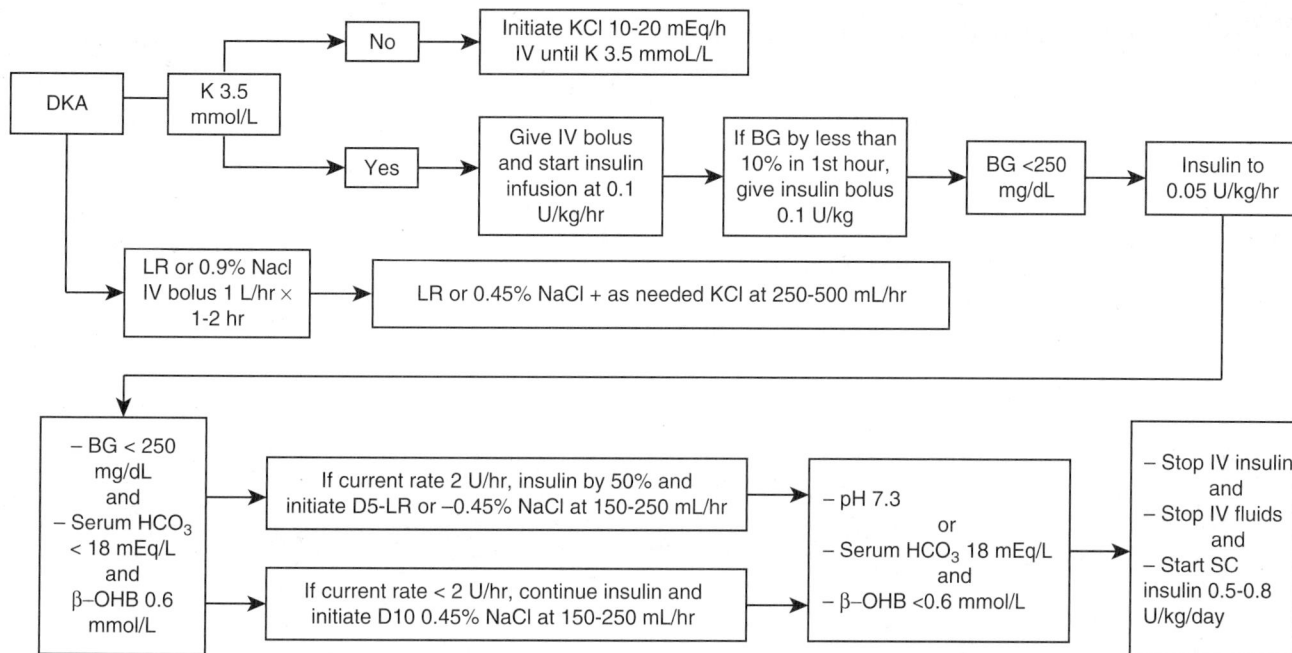

Figure 1 Diabetic ketoacidosis *(DKA)* management protocol. *BG,* Blood glucose; *β-OHB,* β-hydroxybutyrate; *LR,* lactated Ringer solution.

twice a day that contains a mixture of intermediate-acting insulin NPH and short-acting insulin formulations such as regular (Humulin R, Novolin R), aspart (Novolog), or lispro (Humalog) can be considered. Finger-stick glucose measurements before each meal and at night should be taken after discontinuation of intravenous insulin to correct for possible fluctuations in insulin needs while in the hospital.

Monitoring

Serial measurements (every 2–4 hours) of metabolic parameters are required to monitor therapy and then confirm the resolution of DKA. DKA is considered resolved when plasma glucose ideally is less than 200 mg/dL, serum bicarbonate concentration is 18 mEq/L or higher, venous blood pH is greater than 7.3, and β-OHB is less than 0.6 mmol/L. In general, resolution of hyperglycemia, normalization of bicarbonate level, and closure of the anion gap is sufficient to stop insulin infusion. The anion gap is calculated by subtracting the sum of Cl^- and HCO_3^+ from measured (not corrected) Na^+ concentration and can improve even before the restoration of serum bicarbonate owing to hyperchloremia from normal saline infusion. Venous pH is recommended for assessing the degree of acidosis. If plasma glucose is less than 200 mg/dL but β-OHB and bicarbonate or venous pH are not normalized, insulin infusion must be continued and dextrose-containing intravenous fluids started. The latter approach will continue to suppress ketogenesis and prevent hypoglycemia. To prevent hypokalemia, maintain a serum potassium level of 3.5 to 5.0 mmol/L.

Complications

Hypoglycemia is the most common complication and can be prevented by the timely adjustment of insulin dosage and frequent monitoring of blood glucose levels. Hypoglycemia is defined as any blood glucose level below 70 mg/dL. If DKA is not resolved and blood glucose level is below 200 mg/dL, decreases in insulin infusion rate and/or addition of 5% or 10% dextrose to current intravenous fluids may be implemented (see Figure 1). For patients in whom DKA is resolved, strategies to manage hypoglycemia depend on whether the patient is able to eat. For patients who are able to drink or eat, ingestion of 15 to 20 g of carbohydrates (e.g., four glucose tablets or 6 oz orange or apple juice or "regular" soft drink) is advised. In patients who are allowed

nothing by mouth, are unable to swallow, or have an altered level of consciousness, administer 25 mL 50% dextrose IV or give 1 mg glucagon IM if no IV access is present. Blood glucose should be rechecked in 15 minutes; only if the glucose level is less than 80 mg/dL should these steps be repeated.

Non–anion-gap hyperchloremic acidosis occurs from urinary loss of ketoanions, which are needed for bicarbonate regeneration, and preferential reabsorption of chloride in proximal renal tubules secondary to intensive administration of chloride-containing fluids and low plasma bicarbonate. The acidosis usually resolves and should not affect the treatment course. Cerebral edema has been reported in young adult patients. This condition is manifested by the appearance of headache, lethargy, papillary changes, or seizures. Mortality is up to 70%. Mannitol (Osmitrol) infusion and mechanical ventilation should be used to treat this condition. Rhabdomyolysis is another possible complication resulting from hyperosmolality and hypoperfusion. Pulmonary edema can develop from excessive fluid replacement in patients with CKD or congestive heart failure.

Prevention

Discharge planning should include diabetes education, selection of an appropriate insulin regimen that the patient can understand and afford, and preparation of set of supplies for the initial insulin administration at home. Many cases of DKA can be prevented by better access to medical care, proper education, and effective communication with a healthcare provider during an intercurrent illness.

Sick-day management should be reviewed periodically with all patients. It should include specific information on when to contact the healthcare provider, blood glucose goals and the use of supplemental short- or rapid-acting insulin during illness, insulin use during fever and infection, and initiation of an easily digestible liquid diet containing carbohydrates and salt. Most importantly, the patient should be advised never to discontinue insulin and to seek professional advice early in the course of the illness. The patient or family member must be able to accurately measure and record insulin administered, blood glucose, and blood β-hydroxybutyrate with a point-of-care device when blood glucose is higher than 300 mg/dL. Studies performed in outpatient setting demonstrated that β-OHB testing is more effective than urine acetoacetate testing in preventing DKA, which may reduce the costs

TABLE 2 Diabetic Ketoacidosis Order Set

Allergies: ☐ **NKDA or** ☐ **Other (specify):**

Baseline Labs:
☐ CBC w/ Diff, CMP, Magnesium, Phosphorus, venous BG, Fingerstick Blood Glucose, Hemoglobin A1c
☐ Urinalysis ☐ Troponins q6h ×3 ☐ β-hydroxybutyrate ☐ Other (specify):

Follow-up Labs:
☐ Fingerstick Blood Glucose q1h ☐ BMP, Magnesium, Phosphorus q2h ☐ VBG q____h
☐ β-hydroxybutyrate q____h ☐ BMP, Magnesium, Phosphorus q4h ☐ Other (specify):

Consults: ☐ Endocrinology ☐ Diabetes Education

Nursing: ☐ Strict I + O

PHASE I: INITIAL MANAGEMENT

Initial Potassium Replacement for baseline potassium <3.5 mmol/L
☐ Potassium Chloride_____mEq IVPB (infuse at 10mEq/h)

Initial Fluid Replacement
☐ 2 L bolus 0.9% NaCl at 500 mL/h OR ☐_____L bolus 0.9% NaCl at____mL/h (specify)
☐ 2 L bolus LR at 500 mL/h OR ☐_____L bolus LR at____mL/h (specify)

Insulin Therapy:
Do NOT start insulin infusion until K+ ≥ 3.5 mmol/L
☐ Regular Human Insulin Continuous Infusion: (specify below)
☐ 0.1 units/kg/h (_____units/h)
☐ 0.05 units/kg/h (_____units/h) (if end-stage renal disease)

PHASE 2: USE UNTIL BLOOD GLUCOSE <200 mg/dL for the FIRST TIME during insulin therapy

BLOOD GLUCOSE (MG/DL)	INSULIN INFUSION RATE (ROUND UP TO NEAREST WHOLE NUMBER)	FLUID THERAPY
<100	See PHASE 3	
100–200	Decrease current infusion rate by half, MOVE to PHASE 3	D5 ½ NS or LR + as needed KCl 10–20 mEq/L at 200 mL/h
>200 AND: a) Glucose dropped by less than 50 mg/dL in 1 h b) Glucose dropped by 50–100 mg/dL in 1 h c) Glucose dropped by over 100 mg/dL in 1 h	a) Maintain current infusion rate and CALL MD for additional bolus (0.1 units/kg) b) Maintain current infusion rate c) Decrease current infusion rate by half	½ NS or LR + as needed KCl 10–20 mEq/L at 200 mL/h

PHASE 3: USE FOR ALL BLOOD GLUCOSE READINGS AFTER PHASE 2, or if blood glucose is <100 mg/dL at any time

BLOOD GLUCOSE (MG/DL)	INSULIN INFUSION RATE (ROUND UP TO NEAREST WHOLE NUMBER)	FLUID THERAPY
<70	HOLD insulin infusion and give 1 amp D50W IV NOTIFY MD and check fingerstick blood glucose every 15 min until glucose >70, then every 1 h until glucose >100 RESTART insulin at half the previous rate when glucose >100	D5 ½ NS or LR + as needed KCl 10–20 mEq/L at 200 mL/h
70–100	HOLD insulin infusion and give ½ amp D50W IV NOTIFY MD and recheck BG in 15 min RESTART insulin at half the previous rate when glucose >100	D5 ½ NS or LR + as needed KCl 10–20 mEq/L at 200 mL/h
101–200	If current rate ≥2 units/h, decrease rate by half If current rate <2 units/h, continue current rate	D5 ½ NS or LR + as needed KCl 10–20 mEq/L at 200 mL/h
>200	Return to PHASE 2	

ABG, Arterial blood gas; *BMP,* basic metabolic profile; *CBC,* complete blood count; *CMP,* comprehensive metabolic panel; *IVPB,* intravenously per bag; *LR,* lactated Ringer solution; *NKDA,* no known drug allergies; *VBG,* venous blood gas.

of care of patients with insulin-dependent diabetes. COVID-19–positive patients with diabetes outside of a hospital environment should be particularly vigilant in home monitoring of blood glucose and/or β-OHB until the resolution of infection. Most recent studies have convincingly demonstrated that the implementation of intermittently scanned continuous glucose monitoring as part of global care of a type 1 diabetes patient can significantly reduce the risk of new or recurrent DKA episodes. Finally, until further evidence is available, resuming the SGLT-2 inhibitor therapy after an episode of SGLT-2 inhibitor–induced DKA cannot be advised.

Because of the significant cost of repeated admissions for DKA, resources should be directed toward educating primary care providers and school personnel so that they can identify signs and symptoms of uncontrolled diabetes earlier.

TABLE 3	Pharmacokinetics and Pharmacodynamics of Subcutaneous Insulin Preparations				
INSULIN	**ONSET OF ACTION**	**TIME TO PEAK**	**DURATION**	**TIMING OF DOSE**	
Regular (Humulin R, Novolin R)	30–60 min	2–3 h	8–10 h	30–45 min before meal	
Aspart (Novolog)	5–15 min	30–90 min	4–6 h	15 min before meal	
Ultrarapid Aspart (Fiasp)	2.5 min	63 min	5–7 h	Within 0–20 min after meal start	
Glulisine (Apidra)	15 min	30–90 min	5.3 h	15 min before meal	
Lispro (Humalog)	5–15 min	30–90 min	4–6 h	15 min before meal	
NPH (Humulin N and Novolin N)	2–4 h	4–10 h	12–18 h	Twice a day	
Glargine (Lantus)	2 h	No peak	20–24 h	Once a day	
Glargine (Basaglar)	2 h	No peak	20–24 h	Once a day	
Glargine U-300 (Toujeo)	6 h	No peak	24–36 h	Once a day	
Degludec (Tresiba)	1 h	No peak	42 h	Once a day	

References

Benoit SR, Zhang Y, Geiss LS, et al: Trends in diabetic ketoacidosis hospitalizations and in-hospital mortality-United States, 2000-2014, *MMWR Morb Mortal Wkly Rep* 67:362–365, 2018.

Cardoso L, Vicente N, Rodrigues D, et al: Controversies in the management of hyperglycaemic emergencies in adults with diabetes, *Metabolism* 68:43–54, 2017.

Desai D, Mehta D, Mathias P, et al: Health care utilization and burden of diabetic ketoacidosis in the U.S. over the past decade: a nationwide analysis, *Diabetes Care* 41:1631–1638, 2018.

Fadini GP, Bonora BM, Avogaro A: SGLT2 inhibitors and diabetic ketoacidosis: data from the FDA adverse event reporting system, *Diabetologia* 65:1385–1389, 2017.

Hirsch IB: Insulin analogues, *N Engl J Med* 352:174–183, 2005.

Jeyam A, Gibb FW, McKnight JA: Flash monitor initiation is associated with improvements in HbA1c levels and DKA rates among people with type 1 diabetes in Scotland: a retrospective nationwide observational study, *Diabetologia* 60:159–172, 2022.

Kamel KS, Halperin ML: Acid-base problems in diabetic ketoacidosis, *N Engl J Med* 372:546–554, 2015.

Kitabchi AE, Umpierrez GE, Miles JM, et al: Hyperglycemic crises in adult patients with diabetes, *Diabetes Care* 32:1335–1343, 2009.

Li J, Wang X, Chen X, et al: COVID-19 infection may cause ketosis and ketoacidosis, *Diabetes Obes Metab* 22:1935–1941, 2020.

Sheikh-Ali M, Karon BS, Basu A, et al: Can serum beta-hydroxybutyrate be used to diagnose diabetic ketoacidosis? *Diabetes Care* 31:643–647, 2008.

Stamatouli AM, Quandt Z, Perdigoto AL, et al: Collateral damage: insulin-dependent diabetes induced with checkpoint inhibitors, *Diabetes* 67(8):1471–1480, 2018.

Tzamaloukas AH, Ing TS, Siamopoulos KC, et al: Pathophysiology and management of fluid and electrolyte disturbances in patients on chronic dialysis with severe hyperglycemia, *Semin Dial* 21:431–439, 2008.

Umpierrez GE, Davis GM, ElSayed NA, et al: Hyperglycemic crises in adults with diabetes: a consensus report, *Diabetes Care* 47:1257–1275, 2024.

Umpierrez GE, Smiley D, Kitabchi AE: Narrative review: ketosis-prone type 2 diabetes mellitus, *Ann Intern Med* 144:350–357, 2006.

Vellanki P, Umpierrez GE: Increasing hospitalizations for DKA: a need for prevention programs, *Diabetes Care* 41(9):1839–1841, 2018.

GENDER-AFFIRMING CARE

Method of
Molly McClain, MD, MPH

CURRENT DIAGNOSIS

- The diagnosis of gender dysphoria can be made by any clinician trained and licensed to manage behavioral health diagnoses. A team approach to care of gender-expansive people, particularly youth, is optimal. Linking the expertise of primary care, endocrinology, nursing, and behavioral health professionals is preferred though not always possible.

- Primary care is becoming the most appropriate and accessible venue to receive gender care, similar to endocrinologic diagnoses that are routinely addressed in the primary care setting, such as diabetes or thyroid anomalies.

- The diagnostic terminology has changed over time as the understanding of gender has evolved. Gender identity and expression is most accurately represented as a continuum. Diversity in gender is not a pathology. To reflect this, terms such as "transsexualism" or "gender identity disorder of children" are no longer used.

- The current diagnosis "gender dysphoria" is categorized in the *Diagnostic and Statistical Manual of Mental Disorders*, Fifth Edition (DSM-V). The 10th revision of the International Statistical Classification of Diseases and Related Health Problems (ICD-10), frequently used in the United States, uses the same terminology. ICD-11 uses the term "gender incongruence," which is categorized as a sexual health diagnosis. The significance of this shift is that there will no longer be a diagnostic requirement for significant distress or impairment related to a person's gender.

- That gender diversity should require a diagnosis is up for debate. However, the World Health Organization included gender incongruence in the ICD-11 to ensure trans and nonbinary people's access to gender-affirming care, as well as adequate health insurance coverage for these services.

- Box 1 defines commonly used terminology.

CURRENT THERAPY

- There is a paucity of data related to general health and long-term effects of hormone therapy or pubertal blockade for gender-diverse people. The most commonly used guidelines from the World Professional Association of Transgender Health (WPATH), the Endocrine Society, and the University of San Francisco (UCSF) Transgender Center of Excellence are based on available empiric evidence and clinician consensus.

- In addition to the above guidelines, general principles support the creation of an affirming environment for patients. Principles such as informed consent recognize that the medical provider is not a gatekeeper to desired therapies but is an advisor to the patient for the patient's own decision making in the setting of limited empiric data.

- Trauma-informed care, or a healing-centered approach, is based on facilitating a safe environment in which patient empowerment and dignity are supported, recognizing people's inherent strengths and capacities.
- Patient-centered care recognizes that everyone's gender journey is different and there is no "full transition" that has a shared meaning. This requires the provider to follow the lead of patients in terms of their personal gender goals, which may not include medications or surgery.
- Because avoiding harm is an important ethical stance of medical professionals and use of accurate names and pronouns has been shown to dramatically reduce suicidal behavior, using correct names and pronouns are part of the care plan.
- As the political environment evolves, gender-expansive people's health and ability to receive care may be affected. These debates may strengthen long-standing calls for high-quality research studies, particularly related to treatment of trans and nonbinary youth.
- "Detransition," or choosing to live again as one's sex assigned at birth, is safe, rare, and most often related to external pressures rather than regret.
- Withholding of gender-affirming treatments, or access to a physician who can provide them, is not a neutral option given the well-documented evidence of depression, anxiety, substance use, and suicidality in the setting of lack of access to gender-affirming medical therapies.

Epidemiology

The estimates of the number or percentage of those who are gender diverse are based on limited and incomplete data. Per the most recently updated version of the World Professional Association of Transgender Health Standards of Care Version 8 published in 2022, the best estimates or proportions of gender-expansive people vary based on the study design. In health systems–based studies the estimates range from 0.02% to 0.1%, whereas in survey-based studies the numbers are higher. For adults the range was 0.3% to 0.5%, and for children and adolescents the range was 2.5% to 8.4%. The higher rates in survey-based studies may be accounted for by differences of use of diagnostic codes for health systems studies compared with self-report of most surveys. The dearth of data is largely related to the lack of options to select a gender other than male and female on most surveys, census data collection tools, and health system electronic medical records. In addition, the discrimination faced by gender-expansive people results in reduced disclosure of gender in settings when the option to select something other than male or female is available.

Structural Determinants of Health Outcomes

The key determinant of health for gender-expansive people is gender affirmation. The depth and breadth of discrimination against gender-expansive people in families, education, healthcare, housing, and employment creates severe social and economic exclusion. It is this exclusion, not any biologic determinant, that leads to poorer health outcomes compared with cisgender counterparts. An observational study with nearly 28,000 trans and nonbinary respondents found that nearly 60% reported significant rejection from family because of their gender identity or harassment so severe that almost one-sixth reported leaving school in K through 12 or higher education settings. Additionally, 19% were refused medical care because of their gender, and 41% reported attempting suicide (compared with 1.6% of the general population).

On the other hand, data demonstrate that gender affirmation and social/economic inclusion dramatically improves health outcomes. Use of appropriate name and pronouns has been shown to decrease suicide attempts by 56% in one study. Access to medications that suspend puberty or initiate appropriate puberty has been shown to confer lifetime protection against suicide. Even in the face of extensive institutional discrimination, family acceptance has been shown to have the most significant protective effect against homelessness, incarceration, tobacco smoking, drug and alcohol use, anxiety, depression, and suicidal behaviors.

Experts in the neurobiology of trauma describe a lack of gender affirmation as "not being seen or heard." This involves a significantly broader conceptualization of trauma than the diagnostic criteria for posttraumatic stress disorder. Many physical and behavioral health issues that gender-expansive people experience stem from chronically not being seen or heard in regard to their gender. The effects of chronic trauma, or stress, on health have been well-documented. The concept of allostatic load might explain the physiologic link between discrimination and ill health. Short bursts of stress that cause release of cortisol, adrenaline, and other hormones responsible for the fight-or-flight response is adaptive. However, chronic, repeated exposures to stress and the chronic release of cortisol is similar to long-term administration of corticosteroids; no system in the human body is left unaffected. As a result, it is common for gender-expansive people and anyone who has been exposed to chronic stress to experience depression, anxiety, self-harm, suicidal ideation and attempt, and substance use in addition to autoimmune issues (including mast cell activation), autonomic nervous system dysregulation (such as postural orthostatic tachycardia syndrome), chronic pain, increased rates of metabolic disorders, and increased risk of cardiovascular concerns. Recognizing the wide-ranging effects of trauma (in addition to recognition of people's resilience) can support creation of care plans that validate people's medical concerns while also attending to the likely root cause of trauma. Behavioral health professionals skilled in the trauma-informed model, and in the many evidence-based modalities of trauma processing, can be very helpful in the care of all people with an extensive history of discrimination and social exclusion.

Evaluation

It is important to create a clinical environment that is affirming, including intake forms with gender neutral language and inclusive options for patient gender selection. All clinic staff should be trained on the importance of correct name and pronoun use and for all clinic employees to use their own pronouns during introductions.

At the initial visit, healthcare professionals might elicit the individual's history, including the patient's gender as described by the patient, the patient's gender journey, social support, past medical/surgical/behavioral health history, family history, whether the patient is currently engaged in behavioral health counseling, and the goals of care. Goals of care might include primary care, medical therapy for pubertal suppression or hormone therapy, and/or gender confirmation surgeries. There is no single or "correct" way that people engage in their gender journey, and it is the clinician's role to follow each individual's lead and to provide support and assistance in reaching the stated goals. It is important to use the patient's name, gender (as stated by the patient), and pronouns throughout the visit and consistently in documentation. The identification statement might read "25-year-old male (designated female at birth [DFAB], he/him) here to discuss hypertension."

As with any approach to a complex issue in medical care, attention to the whole person, including social context, psychiatric and other medical comorbidities, safety at home and safety outside the home, are vital to elicit in the initial and subsequent visits. All gender-care guidelines align with best practice of providing health care, which is to recognize that gender incongruence is one aspect of people's health that should be understood and addressed in the context of the multitude of other factors that can affect wellness.

The diagnosis of gender dysphoria is based on *Diagnostic and Statistical Manual of Mental Disorders* (DSM)-5 criteria and can be made by any clinician who has been trained and licensed to diagnose and manage behavioral health diagnoses.

The diagnosis supports the consistency (lasting 6 months or longer) and insistence and persistence of one's gender being incongruous with that designated at birth. Commonly, the description

BOX 1   Terminology

Sex: An assignment or designation made at birth (e.g., male, female, or intersex) typically on the basis of external genital anatomy. The appearance of external genital anatomy is the most common method of assigning sex at birth. Other attributes that contribute to sex include sex chromosomes, H-Y antigen, gonadal anatomy, sex hormone levels, and internal and external genitalia. Gender is not based on the appearance of external genitalia. Use of the term "assigned or designated male, female, or intersex at birth" is preferred to "female to male," "male to female," or "transgender man or woman" because these terms are limited to binary gender identities and are less precise. Use of "transgender man or woman" does not clearly indicate true gender nor the gender the individual was assigned at birth.

Gender identity: A person's concept of self as male, female, a blend of both, or neither. One's gender identity can be the same or different from sex assigned at birth. Gender identity results from a complex interaction of biologic traits, environmental factors, self-understanding, and cultural expectations.

Gender expression: The external presentation of one's gender, as expressed through one's name, clothing, behavior, social roles, hairstyle, or voice. This may or may not conform to socially defined behaviors and characteristics typically associated with being masculine or feminine.

Gender diverse/expansive: A term that is used to describe people with gender behaviors, appearances, or identities that do not align with the culturally expected norms assigned to their gender designated at birth. It can be considered an umbrella term for people who identify as transgender, genderqueer, gender fluid, gender creative, gender independent, or agender, as examples.

Transgender: A subset of gender diverse people whose gender identity does not align with their designated gender or sex at birth and is persistent, consistent, and insistent over time.

Cisgender: A term used to describe persons whose gender is congruent with the gender or sex they were assigned at birth.

Agender: A term that people may use when their identity does not align with gender at all.

Nonbinary/gender fluid: A term individuals might use to describe themselves if their gender does not align exclusively with male or female or if their gender identity is dynamic over time.

Gender affirmation or confirmation surgery: A term used for both top and bottom surgeries for those interested in surgery as part of their gender journey.

Sexual orientation: A term that describes an individual's attraction to other people or lack thereof. Sexual orientation and gender identity develop separately and are not linked to each other. There are many terms that people of all genders use to describe their sexual orientation including asexual, pansexual, demisexual, bisexual, gay, straight, and aromantic, to name a few.

Classification of Diseases and Related Health Problems (ICD), have the ability to determine capacity for consent, be knowledgeable in prescribing and monitoring hormone therapies, and stay abreast of the most current recommendations. Similar to other endocrinologic issues seen in primary care, referral to specialists may be warranted in specific cases but can in large part be addressed by primary care healthcare professionals.

Given the extensive discrimination experienced by gender-diverse people, it is helpful for clinicians to have a healing-centered approach in all aspects of care. Healing-centered care orients the care process beyond the effects of trauma that people may have faced and brings focus toward their inherent strength and healing capacity. Creating a therapeutic alliance of safety and respect between the patient and healthcare professional is another foundation of healing-centered care. This concept can be helpful when considering physical examinations.

Many gender-expansive people have experienced negative interactions with medical professionals, including inappropriate physical examinations that are incongruent with the presenting issue. To help people feel more comfortable, clinicians can consider making clear that patients have the right to refuse anything that makes them uncomfortable and that the examination will be based only on the current needs for the visit. It is helpful to ask the patient "Is it ok with you if I listen to your heart and lungs?" and only proceed when consent has been given for each examination. There is little indication for genital examination at the initial visit unless the patient has a stated concern that would warrant it.

Treatment

Preventive Health

Very few studies have addressed preventive health in gender-expansive populations; however, there are general principles that can help the clinician advise the patient in choices regarding health maintenance and preventive care. If an organ is present, follow the same guidelines as for cisgender patients and use gender-affirming or gender-neutral language as much as possible.

Bone health is an important consideration for people who may be status post-gonadectomy and who may have had subphysiologic levels of sex hormones secondary to pubertal suppression or initiation of hormone therapy. The recommendation for all trans and nonbinary people is to start bone density screening at age 65 and for people between 50 and 64 to be considered for bone density screening if other risk factors are present.

Data are mixed on whether people on hormone therapy are at higher risk for cardiovascular disease. Therefore screening for cardiovascular disease is the same as current recommendations for all people. When calculating the atherosclerotic cardiovascular disease (ASCVD) risk score, it may be more accurate to use the patient's predominant hormonal milieu when selecting gender on the risk calculator.

No data exist that people on hormone therapy have higher rates of any type of cancer. For cancer screenings, if an individual has a particular body part or organ and meets criteria for screening based on risk factors or symptoms, the patient should be advised on risks and benefits of that screening regardless of hormone use. For breast cancer screening, if tissue is present, the patient should be advised to follow the same guidelines used for ciswomen. Cervical cancer screening is recommended for anyone with a cervix and guidelines used for ciswomen are appropriate regardless of hormone use. Changes in anatomy of the cervix resulting from use of testosterone leads to a 10-fold higher incidence of unsatisfactory Pap smear cytology results; therefore it is advised to always perform HPV co-testing. Self-swab for HPV alone is an alternative option that can be used by people who find co-testing unacceptable.

Sexually transmitted infection screening is the same for all people as supported by the Centers for Disease Control and Prevention and the U.S. Preventive Services Task Force. Discussion of preexposure and postexposure HIV prophylaxis should be considered for all who meet the criteria. Questions around sexual activity should be limited to the patient's concerns. It is helpful to

of someone's gender journey elicits elements that support the diagnosis. These elements include incongruence of a person's experienced gender, primary and/or secondary sex characteristics, desire to have primary and secondary sex characteristics be more aligned with experienced gender, and desire to treated by others as the person's experienced gender.

It is optimal for gender care to occur in the setting of team-based care consisting of primary care, endocrinology, nursing, behavioral health, and case management. However, expert consensus is consistent with the reality that this type of care is not always accessible. The Endocrine Society recommends that clinicians who diagnose and manage therapies for gender dysphoria be trained in use of the DSM and International Statistical

ask, "What words do you use to describe your genitals?" before discussing anatomy or sexual practices. Attending to sexual health and satisfaction is an important part of whole person care. There is evidence that many people of all genders are reticent to discuss sexual health with clinicians. Inclusion of a question regarding sexual health in the review of systems for all patients during all visits may facilitate comfort in discussing sexual health. For example, "Are you currently sexually active and do you have any questions or concerns?"

Hormone Therapy

Gender goals may include initiation of hormone therapy. The intent of hormone therapy is to express secondary sex characteristics and to feel more internally aligned with one's affirmed gender. Because gender is a spectrum and goals for hormone therapy might include masculinization, feminization, or nonbinary/gender-fluid goals, it is necessary to ask what an individual's gender and goals for therapy include. Although there is mixed evidence about the safety profile of exogenous hormones compared with endogenous hormones, it can be helpful to consider hormone therapy as initiation of an individual's true puberty and then a lifelong continuation of the hormonal milieu of their accurate gender.

Before initiation of hormone therapy, an in-depth evaluation including use of DSM criteria for gender dysphoria, additional consent criteria and evaluation of decisional capacity must be completed. Any untreated psychiatric issues that affect someone's ability to make safe and informed decisions for themselves is a contraindication to initiation of hormone therapy. The clinician should verify absence of hormone-sensitive malignancies and whether the patient has past or current medical issues that may increase the likelihood of side effects from the hormones. It is also imperative that the patient is informed that hormone therapy could irreversibly affect fertility yet does not protect against pregnancy or sexually transmitted illness.

Estradiol-based regimens consist of an antiandrogen (most commonly spironolactone [Aldactone][1] in the United States or gonadotropin hormone–releasing hormone (GnRH) agonist for suppression of all sex hormones) and bioidentical estradiol (Estrace, generic).[1] Before initiation, the medication's effects and possible side effects must be discussed. In addition to the likely effect on fertility, venous thromboembolic events (VTE) can occur while on estradiol, and the patient should have detailed information on signs and symptoms of both deep vein thrombosis and pulmonary embolism. Tobacco use increases this risk, and clinicians can work with their patients on tobacco cessation if indicated. Effects individuals might look forward to are softening of skin, thinning of body hair growth, fat redistribution, decreased muscle mass, decreased sperm production, decreased spontaneous erections, and breast development. Voice timbre is not typically affected by feminizing therapies. The most commonly used formulations are oral tablets (taken daily), patches (switched once or twice weekly), or injectables (once a week). Subcutaneous and intramuscular injections are equally effective. There is no evidence that any formulation has the capacity to cause more feminization than another because they are all the same medication. The effectiveness stems from the consistency of dosing and level of estradiol and testosterone in the serum. Before initiation of hormone therapy, baseline laboratory results should be obtained to evaluate for preexisting issues (chemistry panel, hemoglobin A1c, liver function tests, lipid panel, vitamin D, complete blood count (CBC), and differential, and estradiol and testosterone levels). It is advised to start with a lower dose of antiandrogen and estradiol (50 mg spironolactone daily, and 2 mg PO, injectable at 2.5 mg once a week, or 0.05 mg/day once weekly or twice weekly transdermal patch). Per the Endocrine Society, follow-up should occur every 3 months during the first year of hormone therapy, with previsit laboratory tests (estradiol

and testosterone levels and chemistry panel if on spironolactone). At each visit, doses of both medications can be adjusted based on patient preference and laboratory values. The final goal for estradiol serum level is 100 to 200 pg per mL, and the goal for serum testosterone, if full suppression is desired, is below 50 ng per dL. Some patients may be interested in progesterone. No high-quality studies have been performed on the effects of progesterone. Many people who advocate its use feel that it leads to mood stabilization and more rounded, though not larger, breasts. Bioidentical progesterone (Prometrium)[1] at 100 mg daily is a reasonable starting dose. People should be warned that it can decrease estradiol serum levels, so a 3-month follow-up with sex hormone levels may be helpful.

Testosterone therapy consists of parenteral and topical formulations.[1] The most commonly used formulations are injectable (subcutaneous is equally effective as intramuscular), topical gel (or compounded topicals), and patches. The possible side effects of testosterone must be discussed before initiation and include erythrocytosis and possible VTE secondary to chronic untreated erythrocytosis. Large population analyses have not shown increased risk of cardiovascular outcomes compared with cismales. Concern for metabolic effects should be considered but have not been consistently demonstrated in studies. The effects of masculinizing hormones include acne, increased body hair growth, male-pattern baldness, increased libido, clitoromegaly, vaginal atrophy, and more readily achievable fat loss and muscle gain. As with feminizing hormones, it is advised to start with a lower dose and increase based on laboratory values and patient preference. For optimized masculinization, the goal serum testosterone is between 400 and 1000 ng per dL. Before initiation of hormone therapy, baseline laboratory values should be obtained to evaluate for preexisting medical problems (chemistry panel, hemoglobin A1c, liver function tests, lipid panel, vitamin D, CBC and differential, and estradiol and testosterone levels). A reasonable starting dose is 30 mg injectable testosterone cypionate (Depo-Testosterone)[1] once weekly. Follow-up during the first year is every 3 months with previsit testosterone, estradiol, and hematocrit/hemoglobin levels. Dose change at these visits can be guided by patient preference and serum levels. An increase or decrease by 10 mg may be a reasonable increment at each quarterly visit.

Gender-expansive goals can be achieved by lower doses of hormone therapy or "microdosing." In these cases, all of the previous instructions can be applied. However, the goal serum levels differ. For nonbinary masculinization the serum level of testosterone should be as close to 400 ng/dL as possible. This is easier to achieve with either daily topical testosterone[1] at lower doses or low doses of injectable testosterone administered twice weekly to achieve a decreased range of peak and trough levels. If people on feminizing hormones are interested in nonbinary outcomes and/or maintenance of sexual function, the serum goal for estradiol is still between 100 and 200 pg/mL, and people can choose to use an antiandrogen to achieve the desired effect. Lower doses of spironolactone may lead to decreased feminizing effect, and the patient can balance what is most affirming to them in terms of feminization and maintenance of sexual function. As long as either estradiol or testosterone is within physiologic range, bone health is maintained.

Gender Affirming/Confirmation Surgery

As with hormone therapy, not all gender-expansive people are interested in gender-affirming/confirmation surgeries. The term "sex reassignment surgery" is no longer favored. For those who are interested, access to procedures improves mental health outcomes. Most guidelines suggest that people who undergo gender confirmation surgery be 18 years or older and have been on affirming hormones for at least 12 months. If patients have severe dysphoria and do not meet these criteria, clinicians can still consider supporting the medical necessity of a procedure if

---

[1] Not FDA approved for this indication.

---

[1] Not FDA approved for this indication.

they feel it is indicated. "Top surgery" includes chest reduction or breast augmentation. Top surgery requires evaluation and a letter from a behavioral health professional to verify the diagnosis and the patient's readiness for surgery (notably an additional requirement not necessary for cis-people when undergoing breast reduction or augmentation). "Bottom surgery" includes hysterectomy with or without oophorectomy, orchiectomy, vaginoplasty, phalloplasty, and metoidioplasty. For any procedure that may affect fertility, two letters from behavioral health professionals are required. The choice to undergo hysterectomy is based on patient preference. There is no evidence that hysterectomy is indicated in the setting of long-term masculinizing regimens, nor is there evidence of harms specific to people on testosterone. Those who choose to undergo hysterectomy or orchiectomy should be counseled on the need for lifelong exogenous hormones. Other procedures may include facial feminization, tracheal shave, and gluteal lift.

Insurance coverage differs by insurance carrier and state. In some states the medical and surgical coverage for gender dysphoria must be supplied by insurance carriers; it is helpful for healthcare professionals to have some understanding of the legal context of the state and city they practice in for patient pursuit of surgery. It is also helpful to know what (if any) procedures are available locally and the experience that patients have with local surgeons.

Youth

Affirming care for youth includes provision of developmentally appropriate care focused on recognizing the individual's gender experience, creation of a nonjudgmental partnership with the whole family, and facilitation of discussions regarding risks and benefits of medical treatments if desired. The prevalence of youth who identify as gender diverse may be higher than that of adults. And similar to data for adults, gender-expansive youth have dramatically elevated levels of depression, anxiety, disordered eating, self-harm, substance use, suicidal ideation, and attempts compared with cisgender counterparts. Gender affirmation is the key determinant of health for gender-expansive youth, as it is for adults. Data have shown that although family rejection does little to change the gender identity of youth, family acceptance has the most powerful impact on decreasing the previously mentioned health outcomes. The second most impactful intervention is access to medical therapy if desired. The American Academy of Pediatrics encourages families to seek gender-informed therapy and explore legitimate fears, concerns, and confusion regarding how best to support their gender diverse or gender questioning youth. The care of youth is best provided within the context of multidisciplinary care. However, this is not always available.

Providing affirming primary care and gender care during prepubertal stages of childhood is identical to care of all children with regular well-child visits and acute care visits as needed. When youth begin to experience pubertal changes, they may experience worsening dysphoria. If desired, pubertal suppression using GnRH agonist starting at Tanner stage II or III is indicated. Pubertal suppression allows for cessation of pubertal development, which can decrease dysphoria and allow for continued clarification of gender identity. Although pubertal suppression is described as reversible, the long-term effects on bone health and fertility are currently unknown and families should be informed of this. The Endocrine Society guidelines and the World Professional Association for Transgender Health (WPATH) delineate adolescent eligibility for GnRH agonist treatment that can be helpful for clinicians to use during evaluation of patients who desire pubertal suppression. GnRH agonists can be started if the youth has demonstrated consistent gender incongruence, has decisional capacity, and has been informed of effects and side effects and options to preserve fertility. In addition, the patient and guardians must have given consent, a pediatric endocrinologist or other clinician experienced in pubertal assessment must agree with initiation of pubertal suppression, the patient must be

in Tanner stage G2/B2, and there must be no medical contraindications. It is encouraged, but not necessary, for the youth to be engaged in behavioral health support. The dosing, monitoring, and laboratory schedules for safe administration of GnRH agonists can be found in the Endocrine Society Guidelines of 2017.

The timing of pubertal induction with hormone therapy while on GnRH analogs should be based on patient and family-centered circumstances. There is no empirical evidence to support a particular age of hormone therapy initiation. The recommendation of initiation at age 16 was based on the age cutoff of certain countries regarding medical decision making and is not consistent with average age of endogenous puberty. This can make the decision of when to initiate hormone therapy more complex.

The current political environment that has primarily targeted trans and nonbinary youth has already had an impact on the health and well-being of many young people and their families. However, the increased focus on the paucity of data regarding long-term health effects of gender care may galvanize support for more high-quality research studies.

Other Considerations

Detransitioning

Data demonstrate that "detransition" (opting to return to live in line with sex assigned at birth) is rare. A study of nearly 28,000 trans and nonbinary respondents demonstrated that 13% had opted to detransition and that the vast majority of those individuals (82.5%) had done so secondary to external pressures (such as from family) and effects of social stigma. Detransitioning is safe from a medical perspective and should be normalized during the initial visit with discussion of a plan for safe follow-up if an individual opts to stop medical therapies.

Voice Training

Gender-diverse individuals may want speech therapy to support their gender affirmation. Masculinizing hormones affect voice tenor permanently, but feminizing regimens do little in this regard. Some speech and language pathologists are specialized in voice feminization or masculinization practices, and for those who find this prohibitively expensive (or if this service is not available locally), there are many smartphone applications that can assist people in voice training.

Fertility Counseling, Gamete Preservation, and Contraception

Pubertal suppression and hormone therapy affect fertility; however, there are no data regarding the specifics with which to counsel patients and families. In terms of informed consent, it is most appropriate for people to recognize that the likelihood of having biologic children is drastically reduced, if not impossible. Patients should be counseled to seek gamete preservation if desired. If biologic children are desired, it is safest to postpone initiation of all medications until gamete preservation has been completed. At the same time, none of the medications protect against pregnancy or sexually transmitted infections. Condom use is safe and effective for everyone, and for people on masculinizing hormones more acceptable forms of contraception include progesterone-only birth control pills, Nexplanon, and Mirena IUD.

Hair Removal

Hair removal from face and body may be pursued for aesthetic purposes or in preparation for surgery. It is best to suggest a hair removal specialist who provides affirming care and can offer electrolysis and laser hair removal for a tailored approach. Patients should first query their insurance carrier for possible coverage of hair removal. It is more common that insurance will cover hair removal in the setting of preoperative preparation for vaginoplasty because this is a requirement for that procedure.

Legal Considerations

Legal considerations include legal name change, change of gender, and/or name on legal documents, providing letters of medical necessity for procedures, and addressing possible insurance denials of medical and/or surgical coverage. The process for legal name change, change of name and gender on birth certificates, and other state-based documents such as driver's licenses differs by state. Many states require that a medical provider write a letter demonstrating that someone meet criteria for gender dysphoria to change any legal documents, but some do not require this form of gatekeeping. Typically, if the state does require provider documentation or signatures, the format for any letter should be readily accessible and easy to create. To change federal documents, such as passports, there is a form letter that is easy to find online (https://transequality.org/sites/default/files/docs/resources/ID-Documents-Overview.pdf) that should be adjusted per patient and clinician as indicated, printed on letterhead, and signed in blue ink.

References

Hembree WC, Cohen-Kettenis PT, Gooren L, et al: Endocrine treatment of gender-dysphoric/gender-incongruent persons: an endocrine society clinical practice guideline, *JCEM* 102(11), 2017. Available at https://academic.oup.com/jcem/article/102/11/3869/4157558. [Accessed 24 February 2021], .

National Center for Transgender Equality. U.S. Transgender Survey. Available at https://transequality.org/issues/us-trans-survey. [accessed February/24/2021].

Rafferty J: Ensuring comprehensive care and support for transgender and gender-diverse children and adolescents, *AAP* 142(4), 2018. Available at https://pediatrics.aappublications.org/content/pediatrics/142/4/e20182162.full.pdf. [Accessed 24 February 2021], .

The Lancet. Series on Transgender Health. Available at https://www.thelancet.com/series/transgender-health. [accessed February/24/2021].

Turban, et al: Factors leading to "Detransition" among transgender and gender diverse people in the United States: a mixed-methods analysis, *LGBT Health* 8(4), 2021. Available at https://www.liebertpub.com/doi/10.1089/lgbt.2020.0437. [Accessed 21 May 2024], .

USCF. Guidelines for the Primary and Gender-Affirming Care of Transgender and Gender Nonbinary People. Available at https://transcare.ucsf.edu/guidelines. [accessed February/24/2021].

World Professional Association for Transgender Health. Standards of Care Version 8. Available at https://www.wpath.org/soc8/chapters. [accessed Jan/27/2023].

GOUT AND HYPERURICEMIA

Method of
Saima Chohan, MD

CURRENT DIAGNOSIS

- Gout is the most common inflammatory arthritis in men and is increasing in prevalence.
- A definitive diagnosis of gout requires the demonstration of monosodium urate crystals in synovial fluid or tophi.
- Gouty arthritis often begins in the joints of the lower extremities.
- Septic arthritis, rheumatoid arthritis, and calcium pyrophosphate disease (pseudogout) can mimic gout and should be ruled out.

CURRENT THERAPY

- The goals of successful gout treatment include terminating the acute attack, preventing intermittent attacks, and undertaking long-term therapy to avoid chronic arthritis.
- Indications for the chronic treatment of gout include frequent attacks, recurrent arthritis, and kidney disease.
- A serum urate level of less than 6.0 mg/dL is the goal when urate-lowering therapy is being used.
- Nonpharmacologic treatment includes lifestyle modification and dietary changes.
- The mainstay of urate-lowering therapies remains xanthine oxidase inhibition.

Epidemiology

Gout, or monosodium urate crystal deposition disease, is the most common inflammatory arthritis of men and is an increasingly common problem among postmenopausal women. It is a chronic disorder, affecting more than 5 million people in the United States and increasing in both prevalence and incidence, especially in persons older than 65 years. Gout is often accompanied by serious comorbid disorders (hypertension, cardiovascular disease, chronic kidney disease, and all of the component features of the metabolic syndrome). About 90% of affected persons are managed in primary care practices. Therefore identifying risk factors, optimizing diagnosis, and choosing the appropriate treatment for gout are important skills for a wide array of caregivers.

Pathophysiology and Risk Factors

Uric acid is the end product of purine metabolism in humans. Hyperuricemia, a serum urate concentration exceeding urate solubility (6.8 mg/dL), is an invariable accompaniment of gout, although serum uric acid levels might not be elevated during an acute attack. Hyperuricemia predisposes affected persons to urate crystal formation and deposition, leading to the inflammatory responses underlying the symptoms of gout. Thus, treatment of gout is aimed at reducing and maintaining serum urate concentration at subsaturating levels, usually set at less than 6.0 mg/dL.

Hyperuricemia

Risk factors for hyperuricemia include obesity, hypertension, hyperlipidemia, insulin resistance, renal insufficiency, and the use of diuretics. Diets rich in certain foods are also associated with increased risk for gout. Many studies with large patient cohorts have demonstrated a relationship between hyperuricemia and hypertension, cardiovascular and peripheral vascular disease, chronic kidney disease, and diabetes mellitus. The association of hyperuricemia and metabolic syndrome has also been shown in children and adolescents. Interventional trials of asymptomatic patients with hyperuricemia and high cardiovascular risk must be performed before such treatment can be advocated.

Diagnosis

Acute gout is characterized by an abrupt onset of joint pain, erythema, and swelling, usually of one joint but less commonly of more than one. The arthritis most often occurs first in the joint of a lower extremity, especially the first metatarsophalangeal (MTP) joint at the base of the great toe. The predilection for this site is thought to be secondary to cooler acral temperature or repeated trauma and pressure on this joint.

The gold standard for the diagnosis of gout is the demonstration of monosodium urate crystals by polarized light microscopy either in joint fluid aspirated during an acute attack or between attacks or from material aspirated from suspected tophi. To aspirate the first MTP joint, the joint is first identified by palpating the space at the base of the metacarpal on the dorsal aspect while flexing and extending the toe. The needle is then inserted perpendicularly into the joint space to avoid the extensor hallucis tendon. Synovial fluid from affected joints should immediately be examined under polarized microscopy to confirm the diagnosis of needle-shaped crystals with negative birefringence. If polarized microscopy is unavailable, then fluid should be promptly sent in a sterile tube to an appropriate laboratory for crystal confirmation.

Unfortunately, the equipment and analytical expertise necessary to make this diagnosis are not widely available to primary care physicians. As a result, the diagnosis of acute gout is commonly made on clinical grounds, using the 2015 classification criteria of the American College of Rheumatology and the European League Against Rheumatism. These diagnostic guidelines use a point system and emphasize the presence of signs of inflammation (redness, tenderness, and loss of joint function), abrupt onset, monoarticular involvement, occurrence in the first MTP joint, presence of tophi, and radiographic findings.

The initial symptoms and signs of gout often arise after many years of asymptomatic hyperuricemia. In untreated or inadequately treated patients, the course of the disease often involves acute attacks at increasing frequency, with shortening of asymptomatic periods (called intercritical gout) and, ultimately, the development of chronic joint disease (gouty arthropathy) and tophi (masses of urate crystals in a chronic inflammatory matrix) in bone, joints, skin, and even solid organs (Figure 1).

Indications for Treatment

Early in gout, patients might have attacks that are separated by years and are manageable over the course of a few days with antiinflammatory medications and adjuncts such as joint rest and the application of ice. Over time, the attacks usually become more frequent, prolonged, and disabling, eventually requiring long-term urate-lowering treatment aimed at preventing the deposition of urate crystals and eventually abolishing acute flares and resolving tophi. Indications for urate-lowering (antihyperuricemic) therapy are listed in Box 1.

Treatment

Acute Gout

Gouty arthritis occurs suddenly, and attacks are often very painful and disabling. Patients describe an acute onset of exquisite pain, swelling, erythema, and inability to bear weight on the afflicted joint. Occasionally patients have constitutional symptoms including fever and chills, with an elevated sedimentation rate and white blood cell count. To terminate an attack, NSAIDs, colchicine (Colcrys), or corticosteroids can be offered. If given at full antiinflammatory dosage, NSAIDs have a rapid onset and are quite efficacious in relieving pain and shortening the duration of an attack. The utility of this class of drugs may be limited by renal insufficiency, cardiovascular risk factors, and gastrointestinal bleeding. Although indomethacin (Indocin), sulindac (Clinoril), and naproxen (Naprosyn) are all approved by the FDA for treating acute attacks of gout, nearly every drug in this class and the selective cyclooxygenase (COX)-2 inhibitors also have considerable efficacy. High-dose salicylate therapy lowers serum uric acid by interfering in renal urate transport; low-dose aspirin[1] has the opposite effect but it is often continued in gout patients because of its overriding importance in managing coronary artery disease.

Oral colchicine has been used to treat gout for many years as an unproven drug with no FDA dosage recommendations or prescribing information. In July 2009, however, the FDA approved Colcrys, a single-ingredient colchicine product, for the first day of treatment of acute gout attacks at a low-dose regimen of 1.2 mg followed by 0.6 mg in 1 hour (total 1.8 mg). With this regimen, colchicine can be used to abort an attack if it is taken immediately after the development of the first symptom of gout flare. Higher colchicine doses (0.6 mg every hour until symptoms improve or until gastrointestinal symptoms of diarrhea, nausea, or vomiting develop for a total of 4.8 mg over 6 hours)[3] have traditionally been recommended. A randomized placebo-controlled trial comparing the low- and high-dose regimens showed both approaches to have equivalent efficacy in pain relief at 24 hours (compared with placebo). However, adverse gastrointestinal events were significantly less common with the low-dose regimen. In subjects warranting additional flare treatment, continued use of colchicine 0.6 mg twice daily (reducing to once daily as the flare subsides) is appropriate in persons with normal renal and hepatic function. Oral colchicine is now available in generic form and in two branded versions (Colcrys, Mitigare).

Gastrointestinal symptoms are generally the first clinical signs of colchicine toxicity in patients with normal renal and hepatic function. More serious toxicities do occur and include neuromyopathy, aplastic anemia, and worsening renal and hepatic function. Patients with renal or hepatic impairment should be treated with caution; because of potentially serious drug-drug interactions, colchicine should be avoided in patients receiving cyclosporine (Neoral), clarithromycin (Biaxin), verapamil (Calan), or amlodipine (Norvasc). Intravenous colchicine is not available

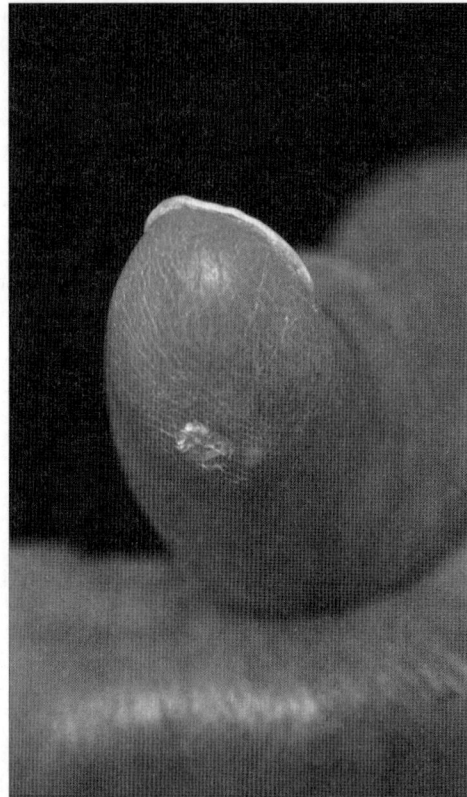

Figure 1 Intradermal urate deposit (tophus). (Reprinted with permission from Mandell, B. F. (2010). Gout and crystal deposition disease. In M. H. Weisman, M. E. Weinblatt, J.S. Louie, & R. Van Vollenhoven (Eds.), *Targeted treatment of the rheumatic diseases* (pp. 293–302). Saunders.)

BOX 1 Indications for Urate-Lowering Therapy

- Frequent and disabling gouty attacks are often defined as two or three flares annually, although this is not evidence based; the decision to treat is based on both number of flares and the disability resulting from flares
- Chronic gouty disease: clinically or radiographically evident joint erosions
- Tophaceous deposits: subcutaneous or intraosseous
- Gout with renal insufficiency
- Recurrent kidney stones
- Urate nephropathy
- Urinary uric acid excretion exceeding 1100 mg/day (6.5 mmol), when determined in men younger than 25 years or in premenopausal women

---

in Europe. The FDA has stopped the marketing of unapproved injectable colchicine products in the United States and discourages the compounding of intravenous colchicine because of reports of preparation errors causing deaths.

Corticosteroids provide a safe alternative for patients with contraindications to NSAIDs or colchicine. For isolated monoarticular attacks, especially of medium or large joints, aspiration of joint fluid and intraarticular injection with triamcinolone acetonide (Kenalog) 20 to 40 mg can quickly terminate an attack. For polyarticular attacks or attacks in smaller joints, systemic corticosteroids (oral or intramuscular) may be used. Oral prednisone starting at 20 mg twice daily with a taper over 10 to 14 days is very effective. Patients can have rebound attacks if oral steroids are terminated too quickly; thus methylprednisolone (Medrol) dose packs should be avoided. If intramuscular injection is required, a single dose of triamcinolone 40 mg may be used.

There is interest in agents blocking the action of interleukin-1 (IL-1), a cytokine thought to play a major role in initiating and

---

[1] Not FDA approved for this indication.

sustaining acute gouty inflammation. Anakinra (Kineret)[1] and canakinumab (Ilaris) are potent injectable IL-1 inhibitors; studies are ongoing to assess the utility of these agents to mitigate acute attacks. In 2013 canakinumab became the first biologic agent approved for acute gout in Europe. It was approved by the European Medicines Agency for symptomatic treatment of adult patients with frequent gouty arthritis attacks in whom NSAIDs and colchicine are contraindicated, are not tolerated, or do not provide an adequate response and in whom repeated courses of corticosteroids are not appropriate. Rilonacept (Arcalyst)[1], which is also in this class, was declined approval for gout by the FDA in 2012 because of concerns about its long-term safety.

Intercritical Gout

After an attack subsides, management is directed at preventing recurrent attacks. During acute attacks of gout, normal serum urate concentration is reported in up to 40% of affected patients, and thus it is not an accurate reflection of the true urate pool. Confirmation of hyperuricemia is best achieved either before the resolution of an attack or 2 to 4 weeks after it to achieve an accurate serum urate concentration. There is a generalizable correlation between the serum urate level and the risk for a recurrent attack.

Prophylaxis of future attacks during early urate-lowering therapy can consist of colchicine at doses of 0.6 mg once or twice a day (based on renal function) or NSAIDs. If chronic NSAIDs are used, acid-reducing medications such as proton pump inhibitors or histamine-2 blockers may be used for patients at risk for gastrointestinal bleeding.

Long-Term Urate-Lowering (Antihyperuricemic) Therapy

The aim of urate-lowering therapy is to reduce and maintain serum urate at concentrations below those at which extracellular fluids are saturated with monosodium urate. In general, an ultimate serum urate concentration of less than 6.0 mg/dL is advised. Urate lowering can be achieved either by increasing urinary excretion or decreasing production of urate.

Nonpharmacologic urate-lowering treatment begins with lifestyle changes. Diet and weight loss must be addressed. Obesity and weight gain are risk factors for gout, and weight loss has been shown to decrease the risk of gout. A purine-restricted diet has often been recommended to patients but is often unpalatable and impractical. Reduction in alcohol intake, namely beer and liquor, can effectively reduce urate levels. Similarly, a reduced intake of red meat and shellfish also lowers the risk of recurrent gouty attacks. Studies have shown an increased frequency of attacks in patients who consume fruit juices and soft drinks containing high-fructose corn syrup, an ingredient not found in diet drinks.

Once the decision is made to institute serum urate–lowering therapy, the duration of treatment is indefinite and must be long-term to be effective. The majority of patients with gout and tophaceous disease will continue to have attacks if therapy is discontinued; thus, education is a key part of the treatment plan. Patients should be instructed that, with initiation of any urate-lowering therapy, they will be at increased risk for a flareup and thus must continue regular use of prophylactic agents as outlined earlier. At least 80% to 95% of cases of hyperuricemia and gout are attributable to impaired urate excretion, which is reflected in diminished urate clearance or fractional excretion of uric acid but not usually in low daily urine uric acid excretion. In practice, 24-hour urine collections are rarely performed. Patients are preferentially treated with xanthine oxidase inhibitors because of the easier dosing schedule, and many patients have contraindications to uricosurics such as renal insufficiency and kidney stones.

Uricosurics

Relative to medications aimed at urate synthesis, uricosurics are relegated to second-line treatment of patients with elevated urate burden or tophaceous disease. The most commonly used uricosuric

agent in the United States is probenecid. This is a very effective drug that concentrates and promotes urinary excretion of urate. Its utility is limited in patients with renal insufficiency, and probenecid is not recommended as first-line therapy in patients with nephrolithiasis or uric acid overexcretion. The maintenance dose of probenecid required to achieve and maintain serum urate concentration at less than 6.0 mg/dL is 0.5 to 3 g/day[3] administered in 2 or 3 daily doses. Once goal serum urate concentration has been achieved with a uricosuric agent, the risk of uric acid calculi is diminished because urinary uric acid excretion becomes normal.

Other drugs found to have uricosuric effects include fenofibrate (Tricor)[1], a fibric acid derivative used to treat hyperlipidemia; atorvastatin (Lipitor)[1], a lipid-lowering agent; and the antihypertensives losartan (Cozaar)[1] and amlodipine (Norvasc).[1] These agents have mild uricosuric properties and may be useful adjuncts to urate-lowering therapy. The ingestion of skim milk has been shown to lower serum urate levels through uricosuric effects. Lower urate levels have also been seen in patients who consume coffee, but the mechanism of action is unknown.

Xanthine Oxidase Inhibitors

Allopurinol (Zyloprim) and febuxostat (Uloric) are the only FDA-approved xanthine oxidase inhibitors for the treatment of gout. Allopurinol, introduced in 1966, is approved in doses of 100 to 800 mg/day. More than 90% of patients with gout treated with urate-lowering medication in the United States are given allopurinol, but dosages of more than 300 mg/day are rarely employed and often patients do not achieve serum urate concentrations of 6.0 mg/dL or less. Appropriate use of allopurinol is limited for several reasons. There are genuine concerns about allopurinol drug interactions, gastrointestinal intolerance, rashes (ranging from mild to life-threatening), and the rare but sometimes fatal hypersensitivity syndrome. Allopurinol should be avoided with the immunosuppressives azathioprine (Imuran) and 6-mercaptopurine (Purinethol) because it can increase the risk of bone marrow toxicity. That can occur because these medications are partially metabolized by xanthine oxidase. Allopurinol should not be taken with ampicillin owing to an increased risk of rash.

Effective dosing of allopurinol is often not achieved because of compliance with published but disputed recommendations for allopurinol dose reduction in states of renal impairment. Allopurinol should be initiated at 100 mg/day in patients with creatinine clearance of 40 mL/min or greater, and it should be titrated in 100-mg increments every 2 to 4 weeks, with the endpoint of dosing determined by achievement of serum urate concentration of 6.0 mg/dL or less.

The FDA approved febuxostat (Uloric) in 2009. Unlike allopurinol, this is a nonpurine analog and selective xanthine oxidase inhibitor that is not incorporated into purine nucleotides and does not appear to affect pyrimidine metabolism. Febuxostat is primarily metabolized by oxidation and glucuronidation in the liver, with little renal excretion; this contrasts with the renal elimination of oxypurinol, the main allopurinol metabolite. The recommended starting dose of febuxostat is 40 mg/day, with an increase to 80 mg/day if serum urate concentrations do not reach goal urate levels in 2 weeks in patients with normal renal function. In Europe, higher dosages (80–120 mg/day)[3] have received approval, and studies have affirmed the efficacy and safety of dosing in this range. In the FOCUS trial, a 5-year study of efficacy and safety, febuxostat was shown to have durable maintenance of serum urate concentration at 6.0 mg/dL or less, nearly complete elimination of gouty flares, and resolution of baseline tophi in subjects. In 2019, a boxed warning was added by the FDA as studies showed that febuxostat was associated with an increased risk of cardiovascular and all-cause mortality compared with allopurinol. Although an advantage of febuxostat over allopurinol is that it can safely be taken by patients with creatinine clearance greater than 30 mL/min, we recommend allopurinol in patients with elevated cardiovascular risk.

[3] Exceeds dosage recommended by the manufacturer.

[1] Not FDA approved for this indication.
[3] Exceeds dosage recommended by the manufacturer.

Pegloticase

Pegloticase (pegylated porcine recombinant uricase [Krystexxa]) was granted FDA approval in 2010 for the treatment of refractory gout. Humans lack the enzyme uricase, which converts uric acid to allantoin, a more soluble purine degradation product. Replacement of this missing enzyme allows direct conversion of urate to allantoin with eventual depletion of increased body urate pools and control of disease, including resolution of tophi. Recombinant uricase therapy profoundly lowers serum urate concentration, as was demonstrated in two large trials. Pegloticase is approved at a dosage of 8 mg IV every 2 weeks. Methotrexate[1] 15 mg/wk should be started 4 weeks before initiation of pegloticase and is used to increase response to treatment and to decrease infusion reactions.

New Therapies

Canakinumab (Ilaris) is a monoclonal antibody that can be used for the treatment of gout flares in adults who have had an inadequate response to treatment or who cannot tolerate NSAIDs, colchicine, or corticosteroids. The dosage is 150 mg in a single subcutaneous injection. Safety concerns include a history of immunosuppression, active or underlying chronic infections such as tuberculosis, pregnancy, breastfeeding, close temporal administration of a live vaccine, and a risk of allergic reactions. Several other novel agents with new therapeutic targets for the treatment of acute and chronic gout are under investigation.

---

[1] Not FDA approved for this indication.

References

Becker MA, Chohan S: We can make gout management more successful now, *Curr Opin Rheumatol* 20:167–172, 2008.

Dalbeth N, Stamp L: Allopurinol dosing in renal impairment: Walking the tightrope between adequate urate lowering and adverse events, *Semin Dial* 20:391–395, 2007.

Macdonald TM, Ford I, Nuki G, et al: Protocol of the Febuxostat versus Allopurinol Streamlined Trial (FAST): a large prospective, randomised, open, blinded endpoint study comparing the cardiovascular safety of allopurinol and febuxostat in the management of symptomatic hyperuricaemia, *BMJ Open* 4(7), 2014:e005354. Epub 2014 Jul 10.

Neogi T, Jansen T, Dalbeth N, et al: 2015 Gout Classification Criteria: An American College of Rheumatology/European League Against Rheumatism Collaborative Initiative, *Arthr Rheum* 67:2557–2568, 2015.

Schumacher HR, Becker MA, Lloyd E, et al: Febuxostat in the treatment of gout: 5-year findings of the FOCUS efficacy and safety study, *Rheumatology* 48:188–194, 2009.

Stamp L, O'Donnell JL, Zhang Met, et al: Using allopurinol above the dose based on creatinine clearance is effective and safe in patients with chronic gout, including those with renal impairment, *Arthritis Rheum* 63:412–421, 2011.

Sundy JS, Becker MA, Baraf HS, et al: Reduction of plasma urate levels following treatment with multiple doses of pegloticase (polyethylene glycol–conjugated uricase) in patients with treatment-failure gout. Results of a phase II randomized study, *Arthritis Rheum* 58:2882–2891, 2008.

Terkeltaub R, Furst DE, Bennett K, et al: High versus low dosing of oral colchicine for early acute gout flare, *Arthritis Rheum* 62:1060–1068, 2010.

Zhu Y, Pandya BJ, Choi HK: Comorbidities of gout and hyperuricemia in the US general population: NHANES 2007-2008, *Am J Med* 125:679–687, 2012.

HYPERALDOSTERONISM

Method of
Ruchi Gaba, MD

CURRENT DIAGNOSIS

- Hyperaldosteronism may be suspected in patients with severe, resistant, or early-onset hypertension and hypertensive patients with family history, hypokalemia, adrenal mass, and obstructive sleep apnea. Evaluation begins with measurement of morning plasma aldosterone concentration (PAC in ng/dL) and plasma renin activity (PRA in ng/mL/h) in a sodium- and potassium-repleted state and off of significantly interfering medications (spironolactone [Aldactone], eplerenone [Inspra], amiloride [Midamor], triamterene [Dyrenium], potassium-wasting diuretics, and licorice-derived products[7]) for at least 4 weeks.
- Elevated PRA and PAC suggest secondary hyperaldosteronism; suppressed PRA and PAC suggest conditions mimicking hyperaldosteronism; suppressed PRA but elevated PAC suggests primary hyperaldosteronism (screening positive if PAC/PRA ratio > 20 to 40 and PAC > 5 to 10 ng/dL).
- Positive screening of primary hyperaldosteronism should be confirmed with one of the following tests: intravenous saline suppression, oral salt loading, fludrocortisone (Florinef)[1] suppression, or captopril (Capoten)[1] challenge test (may skip if spontaneous hypokalemia, renin below the detection limit, and PAC > 20 ng/dL).
- Once primary hyperaldosteronism is biochemically confirmed, computed tomography of the adrenal glands is recommended to exclude adrenocortical carcinoma and help subtype primary hyperaldosteronism.
- If surgical treatment is considered, adrenal vein sampling is indicated to differentiate unilateral versus bilateral lesions (may skip if the patient is <35 years with spontaneous hypokalemia, PAC > 30 ng/dL, and unilateral adenoma). A cortisol-corrected aldosterone ratio from the high to the low side greater than 4:1 with cosyntropin (Cortrosyn) stimulation confirms unilateral aldosterone excess.

---

[1] Not FDA approved for this indication.
[7] Available as dietary supplement.

CURRENT THERAPY

- Laparoscopic adrenalectomy is recommended for unilateral disease. Otherwise, medical treatment with a mineralocorticoid receptor antagonist (MRA; spironolactone [Aldactone] as the primary agent and eplerenone [Inspra][1] as an alternative) is recommended.
- Spironolactone: 12.5 to 25 mg/day titrated to a maximum dose of 400 mg/day to achieve normal blood pressure (BP) and normokalemia. Side effects include increased serum creatinine, hyperkalemia, gynecomastia, and menstrual irregularities.
- Eplerenone: 25 mg once or twice daily titrated to a maximum dose of 100 mg/day to achieve normal BP and normokalemia. Side effects include increased creatinine, hyperkalemia, hypertriglyceridemia, increased liver enzymes, headache, and fatigue.
- Amiloride (Midamor)[1] or triamterene (Dyrenium)[1] (epithelial sodium channel antagonists) can be used in those who cannot tolerate MRAs or are still hypertensive/hypokalemic while on MRAs. Other antihypertensive agents are also added if necessary to control hypertension.

---

[1] Not FDA approved for this indication.

Introduction

Hyperaldosteronism is a state of excessive aldosterone secretion. Primary hyperaldosteronism occurs due to autonomous hypersecretion of aldosterone that is independent of renin and angiotensin II and is relatively nonsuppressible, whereas secondary hyperaldosteronism occurs due to activation of the renin-angiotensin-aldosterone system (RAAS). The pathophysiology and symptoms of primary hyperaldosteronism can manifest at a broad continuum; thus it is best considered as a syndrome rather than a binary disease. Primary hyperaldosteronism not only contributes to cardiovascular, kidney, and metabolic disease but is also the most common cause of secondary hypertension, and recent reports suggest that

5% to 20% of hypertensive patients have primary hyperaldosteronism (as opposed to less than 1%, as previously reported). Secondary hyperaldosteronism includes two different categories: one is compensatory activation of the RAAS due to decreased effective circulating volume, as in congestive heart failure and liver cirrhosis; the other is overactivity of the RAAS accompanied by hypertension, as in renovascular hypertension. There are also several conditions that mimic aldosterone excess through various mechanisms that present with hypertension and other metabolic perturbations. Except for the compensatory activation of the RAAS, these conditions cause secondary hypertension with or without other metabolic consequences, such as hypokalemia and metabolic alkalosis, which bring them to medical attention. This chapter covers the current approaches to hyperaldosteronism for patients suspected of having hypertension secondary to excess aldosterone production.

Pathophysiology

Aldosterone is a steroid hormone produced by the zona glomerulosa in the adrenal gland and contributes to volume and potassium homeostasis via its action primarily on the principal cells in the collecting tubule of the kidney. The main stimuli of aldosterone secretion are angiotensin II and hyperkalemia, which increase synthesis and activity of aldosterone synthase mediated by calcium signaling. Angiotensin II releases calcium from the endoplasmic reticulum, whereas both angiotensin II and hyperkalemia depolarize membrane potential and open voltage-gated calcium channels. Therefore changes in genes regulating ionic homeostasis and membrane potential can affect aldosterone secretion. Aldosterone and angiotensin II are part of the RAAS; plasma renin from the juxtaglomerular apparatus converts angiotensinogen to angiotensin I, and angiotensin-converting enzyme converts angiotensin I to angiotensin II. Subsequently, angiotensin II stimulates secretion of aldosterone. Renin secretion is controlled by renal artery pressure, sodium delivery to the distal nephron, and sympathetic activation (via β1). Increased effective arterial circulating volume from the action of aldosterone decreases renin secretion by negative feedback (Figure 1). Other minor factors involved in aldosterone secretion are adrenocorticotropic hormone (ACTH) and hyponatremia (which increase aldosterone secretion) and atrial natriuretic peptide (which decreases aldosterone secretion).

Aldosterone binds to the nuclear mineralocorticoid receptors. Activation of the mineralocorticoid receptors upregulates the basolateral Na^+/K^+ pumps and the epithelial sodium channels (ENaC), leading to increased reabsorption of Na^+ and Cl^- and secretion of K^+ and H^+. The mineralocorticoid receptors can also be activated by other hormones with mineralocorticoid activity. Cortisol is able to bind to the mineralocorticoid receptors with similar affinity as aldosterone but normally is converted to inactive cortisone by 11β hydroxysteroid dehydrogenase 2 (11β HSD2). Mutations/inhibition of 11β HSD2 or very high cortisol levels above the capacity of 11β HSD2, as in Cushing syndrome (particularly ectopic Cushing syndrome), and glucocorticoid resistance can cause activation of the mineralocorticoid receptors. Aldosterone precursors such as deoxycorticosterone have a weak mineralocorticoid effect but can cause features of hyperaldosteronism when they are present at very high levels, as in some forms of congenital adrenal hyperplasias (11β hydroxylase deficiency or 17α hydroxylase deficiency) or deoxycorticosteroid-secreting tumors. In addition, activating mutations of the ENaCs also cause increased sodium absorption and hypertension mimicking hyperaldosteronism (Liddle syndrome).

With the development of specific antibodies against human CYP11B2 (aldosterone synthase) and its application to immunohistochemistry, diverse histopathological and genetic characteristics of primary hyperaldosteronism have been determined. An international consensus for the nomenclature and definition of adrenocortical lesions from patients with unilateral primary hyperaldosteronism was endorsed by the World Health Organization and includes aldosterone-producing adenoma (APA), aldosterone-producing nodule (APN), aldosterone-producing micronodule (APM) (formerly known as "aldosterone-producing cell cluster"), aldosterone-producing diffuse hyperplasia, and, rarely, aldosterone-producing adrenocortical carcinoma. Multiple aldosterone-producing lesions can occur within a single adrenal gland, and adrenal lesions identified by imaging studies might not necessarily be the source of aldosterone excess. Incidental nonfunctioning adenomas can commonly occur in patients with primary hyperaldosteronism; in these cases, satellite APA or APN/APM in the adjacent or contralateral adrenal tissue may be the source of excess aldosterone production. Multiple APMs appear to be a common histologic feature of idiopathic hyperaldosteronism.

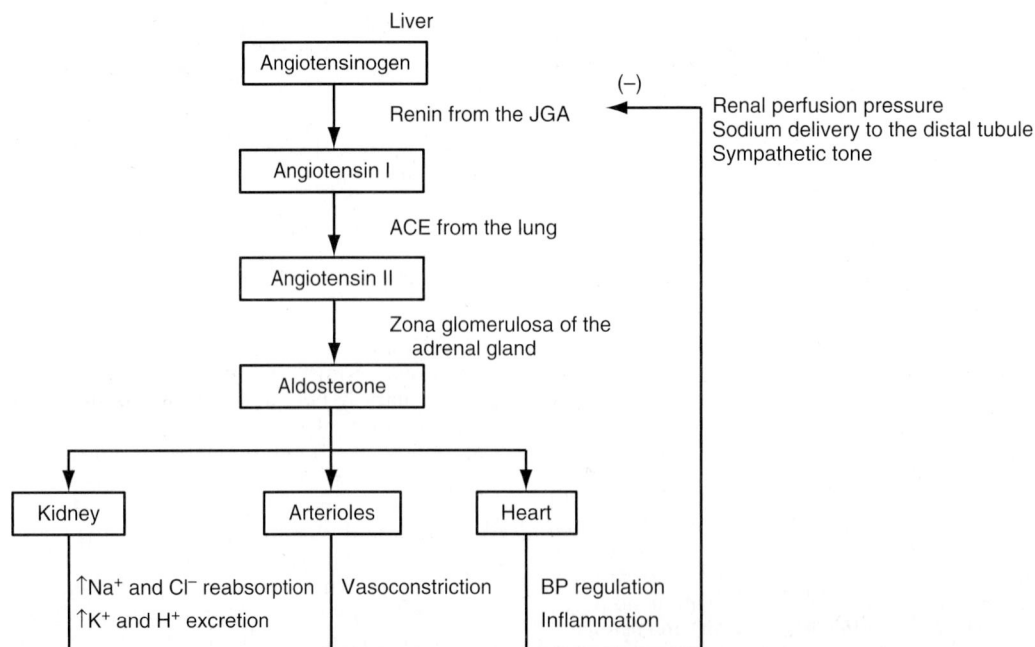

Figure 1 The renin-angiotensin-aldosterone system. *ACE*, Angiotensin-converting enzyme; *BP*, blood pressure; *JGA*, juxtaglomerular apparatus.

Whereas heritable forms are rare, somatic mutations causing primary hyperaldosteronism are common. Next-generation genetic sequencing has resulted in the identification of somatic mutations in approximately 90% of the APAs, which are a major cause of primary hyperaldosteronism. The mutation occurs in one of the aldosterone-driver genes, which include *KCNJ5, ATP1A1, ATP2B3, CACNA1D, CACNA1H,* and *CLCN2,* causes alteration of intracellular ion homeostasis, and enhances aldosterone production. In a small subset of APAs, somatic activating mutations in the *CTNNB1* gene, which encodes β-catenin, have also been detected. Interestingly, race and sex impact the somatic mutation spectrum of APA. Specifically, somatic mutations in the *KCNJ5* gene, encoding an inwardly rectifying K^+ channel, are common in APAs from Asian populations, as well as in women regardless of race.

Clinical Manifestations

The continuum in the pathophysiology of primary hyperaldosteronism translates into a spectrum of symptoms based on severity ranging from mild to overt. Primary hyperaldosteronism usually presents with normokalemic hypertension. Hypokalemia is present only in 9% to 37% of cases and may indicate more severe cases. A few rare patients might present with hypokalemia but have a normal systemic blood pressure (BP). Patients with primary hyperaldosteronism usually do not develop severe volume overload or edema because of aldosterone escape possibly related to atrial natriuretic peptide, pressure natriuresis, or decreased sodium absorption at other nephron segments. Metabolic alkalosis, mild hypernatremia (due to reset osmostat from volume expansion), and hypomagnesemia may be observed. Glomerular filtration rate and urinary albumin excretion can be elevated independent of systemic hypertension. Target organ (heart and kidney) damage and cardiovascular-related morbidity and mortality are higher in primary hyperaldosteronism than in essential hypertension with similar degrees of BP elevation. In fact, milder phenotypes of primary hyperaldosteronism pathophysiology (i.e., renin-independent aldosterone production that lies below the categorical thresholds for overt primary hyperaldosteronism [PA]) are independently associated with the development or progression of cardiovascular and kidney disease. Once hypertension has developed, the magnitude of the pathophysiology is associated with risk for worsening hypertension, incident structural heart disease, adverse cardiovascular events, and death. Thus, even though considered "overt primary hyperaldosteronism," there exists a large and clinically relevant spectrum of milder forms of the disease. Moreover, primary hyperaldosteronism is associated with an increased risk of type 2 diabetes mellitus and metabolic syndrome, which is attributable to both decreased insulin secretion and increased insulin clearance, as well as concurrent cortisol cosecretion. PA frequently co-occurs with obstructive sleep apnea given its association with obesity and its pathophysiology of chronic volume retention with a prevalence of 21% to 34%. Finally, it increases the risk for both osteoporosis and fractures, possibly mediated by hypercalciuria-induced secondary hyperparathyroidism.

Secondary hyperaldosteronism (when it is not from hypovolemia) and other conditions mimicking hyperaldosteronism can present with similar features as primary hyperaldosteronism plus specific manifestations for each disease entity. Depending on the mechanism of disease, more severe volume overload and pulmonary edema may be found (e.g., renovascular hypertension) because aldosterone escape may not work.

Evaluation

Screening

Despite its substantial clinical and public health implications, PA remains highly underdiagnosed. Hyperaldosteronism may be suspected based on severe (BP > 150/100 on three separate occasions) or resistant hypertension (uncontrolled BP despite use of three conventional antihypertensive agents including a diuretic, or well-controlled BP in the presence of four or more antihypertensive

agents), early-onset hypertension without known risk factors, and hypertension with other features such as family history of hyperaldosteronism, early-onset hypertension, cerebrovascular accident at a young age, hypokalemia, adrenal mass, and obstructive sleep apnea. Currently there is no evidence-guided screening strategy. Some experts believe that routine screening for primary hyperaldosteronism is warranted in newly diagnosed hypertension considering its high prevalence, whereas others recommend that targeted screening is more appropriate, such as the Endocrine Society guidelines for primary hyperaldosteronism in 2016 (Box 1).

When a decision is made to screen for excessive mineralocorticoid effect, one should first examine the plasma renin and aldosterone levels (i.e., plasma renin activity [PRA, ng/mL/h] and plasma aldosterone concentration [PAC, ng/dL]). It is important to note that several factors can affect PRA and PAC, such as age, medications, time of day, diet (salt intake), posture, method of blood collection, level of potassium, and level of creatinine (Table 1). Diuretics (both potassium sparing and wasting) and mineralocorticoid antagonists can have a significant effect on PRA and PAC. Angiotensin-converting enzyme inhibitors (ACEIs)/angiotensin receptor blockers (ARBs) and dihydropyridine calcium channel blockers can affect PRA and PAC modestly. Ideally, all medications and other factors that may affect PRA and PAC should be removed; unfortunately, it is not always practical and safe to do this because of the possibility of uncontrolled hypertension. If necessary, antihypertensive agents that affect PRA and PAC only minimally, such as slow-release verapamil (Calan SR), hydralazine (Apresoline), prazosin (Minipress), doxazosin (Cardura), or terazosin (Hytrin), can be used. The Endocrine Society 2016 guidelines recommend certain caveats that optimize the chance for obtaining more easily interpretable PRA and PAC results (Box 2). However, if needed, the screening can occur irrespective of concurrent medications or the time of day to simplify the approach and maximize opportunities to test. If there is renin suppression, defined as a plasma renin activity less than 1.0 ng/mL/h or corresponding plasma renin concentration less than 10 mU/L despite the use of medications that increase renin, it should raise suspicion for presence of nonsuppressible aldosterone.

Patterns of PRA and PAC help differentiate among primary hyperaldosteronism, secondary hyperaldosteronism, and conditions mimicking hyperaldosteronism. Differential diagnoses according to different patterns of PRA and PAC are listed in Box 3. If both PRA and PAC are high, further investigation for causes of secondary hyperaldosteronism should follow. If both PRA and PAC are suppressed, further investigation for conditions that mimic hyperaldosteronism is indicated. Suppressed PRA and elevated PAC suggest primary hyperaldosteronism. The next step is to calculate the aldosterone renin ratio (ARR), and the individual aldosterone and renin values should be individually evaluated. An ARR greater than 20 to 40 is considered screening positive for primary hyperaldosteronism. PAC greater than 15 ng/dL was recommended by some investigators to avoid false-positive ARR

BOX 1 Groups Indicated for Case Detection With Relatively High Prevalence of Primary Hyperaldosteronism

Sustained blood pressure > 150/100 mm Hg on three different occasions
- Drug-resistant hypertension (>140/90 mm Hg despite three medications, including a diuretic)
- Hypertension and hypokalemia (spontaneous or diuretic-induced)
- Hypertension and family history of early-onset hypertension or cerebrovascular accident at a young age (<40 years)
- Hypertension with adrenal incidentaloma
- Hypertensive first-degree relatives of primary hyperaldosteronism patients
- Hypertension with obstructive sleep apnea

TABLE 1	Medical Factors That May Affect Aldosterone and Renin Measurement		
	EFFECT ON ALDOSTERONE	**EFFECT ON RENIN**	**EFFECT ON ALDOSTERONE–RENIN RATIO**
Medications			
β-Blocker	↓	↓↓	↑
Central α$_2$ agonists (clonidine [Catapres], α-methyldopa [Aldomet])	↓	↓↓	↑
NSAIDs	↓	↓↓	↑
K$^+$ wasting diuretics	→↑	↑↑	↓
K$^+$ sparing diuretics	↑	↑↑	↓
ACE inhibitors	↓	↑↑	↓
Angiotensin II receptor blockers	↓	↑↑	↓
Dihydropyridine Ca^{2+} blockers	→↓	↑	↓
Renin inhibitors	↓	↓ plasma renin activity	↑
		↑ direct renin concentration	↓
Potassium Status			
Hypokalemia	↓	→↑	↓
Potassium loading	↑	→↓	↑
Dietary Sodium			
Sodium restricted	↑	↑↑	↓
Sodium loaded	↓	↓↓	↑
Others			
Advanced age	↓	↓↓	↑
Renal impairment	→	↓	↑
Oral contraceptives*	↑	↑ plasma renin activity	→
		↓ direct renin concentration	↑
Pregnancy	↑	↑↑	↓
Renovascular hypertension	↑	↑↑	↓
Malignant hypertension	↑	↑↑	↓

*Premenopausal women have higher aldosterone level during the luteal phase and lower renin level throughout the cycle than men. False-positive aldosterone renin ratio during the luteal phase was reported when direct renin concentration was used.
ACE, Angiotensin-converting enzyme; *NSAIDs,* nonsteroidal antiinflammatory drugs.

from very low renin level, but in many cases PAC can be less than 15 ng/dL, though this occurs more commonly in bilateral adrenal hyperplasia (BAH) than in aldosterone-producing adenoma. More recently, a new approach has been advocated wherein a "high-risk" patient with a suppressed renin should be assumed to have PA until proven otherwise. This approach is distinct from the stepwise approach prescribed by guidelines. By refining the approach to assume PA until proven otherwise in high-risk phenotypes, there is an increase in the probability of making a clinical diagnosis and/or initiating empiric treatment with MRAs for a wider array of PA phenotypes, especially the underrecognized mild ones. Diagnostic flow and subsequent management of hyperaldosteronism are summarized in Figure 2. Of note, there is no consensus on cutoff values for PRA, PAC, or ARR. There exist systematic differences in the calibration of aldosterone assays that have to be taken into account. The measurement of aldosterone by liquid chromatography–tandem mass spectrometry, which is now widespread, is 27% to 87% lower compared with immunoassay-based techniques. Moreover, a single cross-sectional circulating aldosterone level is not a reliable indicator of integrated physiology; an obtained high level can be informative, but a low value is not exclusionary. With aldosterone production and sensitivity being extremely variable and with systematic

differences in measurement, screening tests should be repeated if results are inconclusive or if PA is strongly suspected but the initial screening tests are negative. Confirmatory tests should follow to avoid false positives.

Confirmatory Tests of Primary Hyperaldosteronism

The positive screening test should be followed by one or more confirmatory tests to avoid false positives. The confirmatory tests are designed to physiologically suppress aldosterone levels that would normally occur in the absence of primary hyperaldosteronism. However, some experts believe that some aldosterone-producing lesions are not completely independent of the RAAS, and confirmatory suppression tests can give false-negative results. Other experts think that confirmatory tests are not necessary for those with obvious clinical/biochemical features. Those with spontaneous hypokalemia, renin level below the detection level plus PAC greater than 20 ng/dL may not need further confirmatory tests. Furthermore, there is no gold standard confirmatory. Therefore factors such as cost, accessibility, feasibility, patient compliance, local expertise, and accuracy of assay should be taken into consideration in selecting confirmatory tests. If there is a positive screen with a negative confirmatory testing but the suspicion of the disease stays high, especially with progressive refractory hypertension, then the repetition of the confirmatory testing over time might be beneficial and should be considered. The Endocrine Society guidelines in 2016 state that any of the following four confirmatory tests can be used: oral salt loading test, saline suppression test, fludrocortisone (Florinef)[1] suppression test, and captopril (Capoten)[1] challenge test (Table 2). Finally, there is increasing evidence that cortisol cosecretion can commonly occur in primary hyperaldosteronism with a prevalence range from 4% to 27%. It usually happens in patients with a visible adrenal mass on cross-sectional imaging, as clinically relevant hypercortisolism usually requires some degree of adrenocortical neoplasia and is associated with increased risk for adverse events. Screening can be conducted by measuring a baseline serum dehydroepiandrosterone sulfate and performing a 1-mg overnight dexamethasone[1] suppression test (DST). Cortisol-producing adenoma-related somatic mutations in unilateral primary aldosteronism with concurrent autonomous cortisol secretion have been noted with a prevalence of approximately 36.7%. The presence of these mutations is associated with higher post-DST cortisol levels and larger adenoma size, though no eventual effect on outcomes after surgery has been noted.

Subtype Classification of Primary Hyperaldosteronism

Once primary hyperaldosteronism is biochemically confirmed, subtype classification follows to guide treatment. Lateralization of the source of excessive aldosterone production is crucial as the next step, as unilateral lesions such as APAs can be treated surgically. In contrast, bilateral lesions, such as BAHs, which account for almost 60% to 70% of the cases and in general are a milder disease, are treated medically. Aldosterone-producing carcinoma is rare but should be ruled out. In this regard, computed tomography (CT) of the adrenal glands should be done first to rule out aldosterone-producing carcinoma and obtain anatomic information. However, imaging studies are usually not reliable enough

to lateralize lesions. If surgical treatment is considered, adrenal vein sampling (AVS) should be performed. Most cases of primary hyperaldosteronism are sporadic; about 5% are familial, mostly via autosomal dominant inheritance. Young patients (<20 years of age) and those with family history of primary hyperaldosteronism or strokes at young age (<40 years) should have genetic testing for glucocorticoid remediable aldosteronism (GRA) or familial hyperaldosteronism type I, which is caused by the hybrid gene of 11β hydroxylase and aldosterone synthase (increased aldosterone synthesis by ACTH). Patients with GRA are less likely to be hypokalemic than other patients with primary hyperaldosteronism, perhaps because of the circadian nature of ACTH secretion. In very young patients, *KCNJ5* germline mutations, causing familial hyperaldosteronism type III, should be tested. Familial hyperaldosteronism type II is clinically indistinguishable from nonfamilial hyperaldosteronism and can be caused by gain-of-function mutations in the *CLCN2* (chloride voltage-gated channel 2) gene. Familial hyperaldosteronism type IV generally involves patients with early-onset hypertension and primary hyperaldosteronism before the age of 10. Germline mutations in the *CACNA1H* (calcium voltage-gated channel subunit alpha1H) gene occur in type IV patients who also exhibit mental retardation and developmental disorders, as well as seizures and neurologic abnormalities in some patients.

Imaging

CT and magnetic resonance imaging (MRI) scans of the adrenal glands provide one of five conclusions: normal adrenal glands, unilateral macroadenomas (>1 cm), minimal unilateral adrenal limb thickening, unilateral microadenomas (≤1 cm), and bilateral macroadenomas and/or microadenomas. APAs are typically smaller

[1]Not FDA approved for this indication.

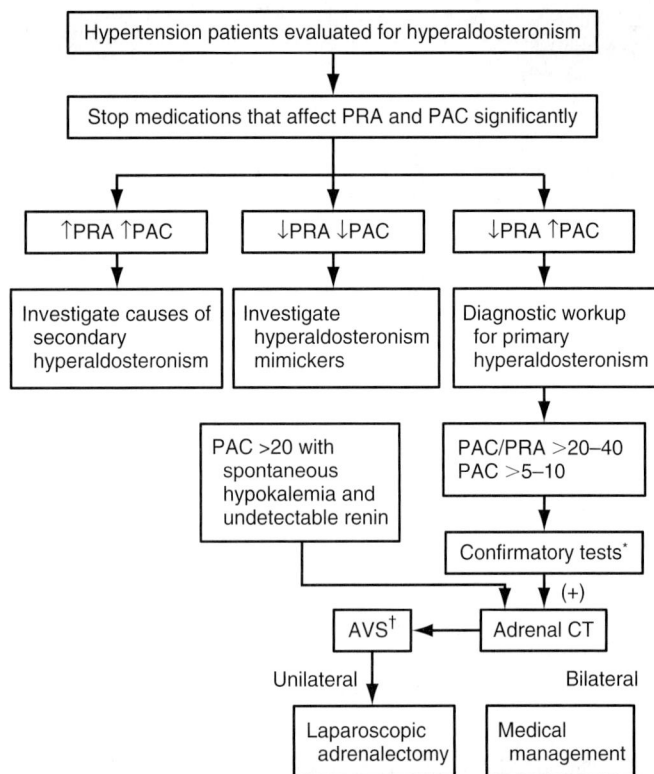

Figure 2 Evaluation of hyperaldosteronism. *AVS,* Adrenal vein sampling; *CT,* computed tomography; *PAC,* plasma aldosterone concentration in ng/dL; *PRA,* plasma renin activity in ng/mL/h. *May skip if spontaneous hypokalemia, renin level below the detection limit, and PAC >20 ng/dL. †If surgical treatment is pursued. May skip if <35 years old, spontaneous hypokalemia, PAC > 30 ng/dL, and unilateral adenoma.

than 2 cm, and BAHs exhibit either normal or nodular changes. Aldosterone-producing adrenal carcinomas are almost always larger than 4 cm in diameter and have imaging characteristics suspicious for malignancy. However, there are limitations: small APAs may be missed, hyperplasia may be misread as adenomas, and nonfunctional tumors are radiologically indistinguishable from APAs. Although several studies suggested imaging criteria for different subtypes, no study has conclusively established specific criteria that differentiate among different subtypes of primary hyperaldosteronism. In fact, CT accurately lateralizes in only about 50% to 70% of cases, and there is no evidence that MRI is superior to CT for subtype classification. Therefore AVS is required to differentiate unilateral from bilateral lesions if surgical resection is being pursued. Patients younger than 35 years with marked hyperaldosteronism with spontaneous hypokalemia and PAC greater than 30 ng/dL and solitary unilateral adenoma may not need AVS, because nonfunctioning tumors are uncommon in this young age group.

Adrenal Vein Sampling

Aldosterone levels are measured from adrenal venous blood samples (Box 4) obtained through adrenal vein cannulation to distinguish between unilateral and bilateral lesions. Unilateral lesions are associated with a marked increase in PAC on the side of the tumor (and suppressed PAC on the other side), whereas bilateral lesions have little difference between the two sides. AVS should be performed only by experienced physicians in part because recognition and successful cannulation of the right adrenal vein especially can be challenging. Complications of AVS include adrenal hemorrhage, adrenal infarction, adrenal vein perforation, and adrenal vein thrombosis, which occur only rarely (<2.5%) in the hands of a physician skilled in the procedure.

The use of cosyntropin stimulation to minimize stress-induced fluctuation in aldosterone level is controversial, and some believe that it has no effect on AVS accuracy. If cosyntropin is not used, then AVS should be done in the morning after overnight recumbency to avoid postural aldosterone changes and reflect circadian aldosterone secretion.

In reality, different centers use different techniques, protocols, and interpretation criteria. The Endocrine Society guidelines in 2016 provide interpretation criteria with and without cosyntropin use. The first step for interpretation is to determine whether the procedure was done correctly. The adrenal vein–to–inferior vena cava cortisol ratio should be greater than 5:1 with cosyntropin given and greater than 3:1 without cosyntropin. If the ratio is significantly lower than these values, improper cannulation is implied. Next, divide the PAC values for the right and left adrenal veins by their respective cortisol values to correct the dilutional effect of the inferior phrenic vein flow into the left adrenal vein; this is termed the *cortisol-corrected aldosterone* (A/C). If cosyntropin is used, an A/C ratio of the high to the low side of greater than 4:1 indicates unilateral aldosterone hypersecretion, whereas an A/C ratio of less than 3:1 suggests bilateral aldosterone hypersecretion. These cutoffs were reported to have sensitivity of 95% and specificity of 100% for unilateral lesions. If the A/C ratio is between 3:1 and 4:1, the results of AVS should be interpreted in the context of CT, clinical findings, and other tests. Without cosyntropin, an A/C ratio of the high to the low side of greater than 2 or an A/C ratio of the high side to the periphery greater than 2.5 plus an A/C ratio of the low side to the periphery of less than 1 (suppressed contralateral aldosterone secretion) is consistent with unilateral aldosterone excess.

Ancillary Tests

Clinical findings and other ancillary tests may help differentiate unilateral APAs from BAHs. BAHs will respond with increase in plasma aldosterone to postural stimulation, whereas APAs will not. Plasma 18-hydroxycorticosterone level tends to be higher in APAs compared with BAHs. Iodocholesterol scintigraphy may be able to show functional correlation of anatomic abnormalities (but is not available at most centers). APA-specific tracers such as (11)C-metomidate for positron emission tomography may be useful. Interpretation criteria of these tests are listed in Table 3. Patients with APAs tend to be younger (<40 years), predominantly female, very hypertensive with marked hypokalemia (<3 mmol/L), and tend to have a very high PAC (>25 mg/dL) compared with those with BAHs.

Treatment

Treatment of secondary hyperaldosteronism and conditions mimicking hyperaldosteronism depends on their etiology. Treatment of primary hyperaldosteronism is discussed here. The goals of treatment of primary hyperaldosteronism are (1) normalization of the serum potassium in hypokalemic patients, (2) normalization of the BP, and (3) reversal of the effects of hyperaldosteronism on the cardiovascular system. When a small group of patients were followed after treatment with adrenalectomy or MRAs, left ventricular mass was reduced (faster with adrenalectomy than MRAs), increase in carotid intima-media thickness and arterial stiffness was reversed, glomerular filtration rate and urinary albumin secretion decreased and became similar to that in essential hypertension, and excessive cardiovascular risk compared with essential hypertension disappeared. Cardiovascular complications were rather related to age, duration of hypertension, and smoking. In addition, there was an improvement in the quality of life at 3 months, which was sustained at 6 months. Therefore timely diagnosis and treatment is essential. For unilateral lesions, surgical resection of the affected adrenal gland is recommended mainly to obviate the need for prolonged medical treatment and side effects. Moreover, adrenalectomy in unilateral PA significantly reduces the risk for cardiovascular events, kidney disease, type 2 diabetes mellitus, and mortality while improving quality of life compared with medical therapy. Even in patients with stage 3 chronic kidney disease, the treatment of PA can be beneficial

	PROTOCOL	INTERPRETATION	REMARKS
Oral sodium loading test	Place the patient on a high-sodium diet (>200 mmol/day) for 3 days. Replace potassium to compensate for the kaliuresis induced by the high-sodium diet. Collect a 24 h urine on the third day for determination of aldosterone, sodium, and creatinine; adequate if the urine sodium >200 mmol/24 h	Confirmed if the 24-h urine aldosterone is >12 mcg (33.3 nmol) to 14 mcg (38.8 nmol). Ruled out if the 24-h urine aldosterone is <10 mcg (27.7 nmol). The test is equivocal if the value falls in between	Do not perform this test in patients with severe uncontrolled hypertension, renal failure, cardiac failure/arrhythmias, or severe hypokalemia
IV saline infusion test*	1. Place the patient supine 1 h before drawing blood for morning baseline fasting levels of renin, aldosterone, cortisol, and potassium 2. Infuse 2 L of 0.9% NaCl over 4 h, keeping the patient supine. Monitor blood pressure and heart rate 3. After 4 h, draw blood for measurement of renin, aldosterone, cortisol, and potassium	Confirmed if the PAC is >10 ng/dL (277 pmol/L). Ruled out if the PAC is <5 ng/dL (139 pmol/L). If the PAC falls between these values, the test is equivocal	Do not perform this test in patients with severe uncontrolled hypertension, renal failure, cardiac failure/arrhythmias, or severe hypokalemia
Fludrocortisone[1] suppression test	Give 0.1 mg fludrocortisone every 6 h for 4 days, with the potassium level checked every 6 h to be sure that it is greater than 4 mmol/L Encourage a liberal sodium diet to keep urinary sodium excretion greater than 3 mmol/kg/day On day 4, draw blood for an upright 7 a.m. plasma cortisol level and 10 a.m. plasma aldosterone, renin, and cortisol levels	Confirmed if the 10 a.m. PAC is >6 ng/dL, as long as PRA is <1 ng/mL/h and the plasma cortisol at 10 a.m. is less than at 7 a.m. (to exclude the ACTH effect)	The test may require hospitalization. Risks include severe hypokalemia, QT changes, worsening of left ventricular function, hypertension, and frequent phlebotomy
Captopril[1] challenge test	Give 25–50 mg captopril after the patient has been sitting or standing for 1 h. The patient remains seated throughout the test. Draw blood for measurement of plasma renin, aldosterone, and cortisol at time 0, at 1 h, and at 2 h	Normally, captopril suppresses PAC by more than 30% from baseline. Confirmed if there is no suppression of PAC and PRA remains suppressed. The false-negative rate for this test is high because suppression occurs in more than 30% of cases. A slight decrease in aldosterone can suggest bilateral adrenal hyperplasia	

*The patient may be seated for 30 minutes before and during the infusion to improve sensitivity, and PAC > 6 ng/dL (170 pmol/L) confirms primary hyperaldosteronism.
[1]Not FDA approved for this indication.
ACTH, Adrenocorticotropic hormone; *IV,* intravenous; *PAC,* plasma aldosterone concentration; *PRA,* plasma renin activity.

Hyperaldosteronism

359

BOX 4 Adrenal Vein Sampling

- After both adrenal veins have been cannulated, draw baseline samples for PRA, PAC, ACTH, and cortisol from the peripheral such as cubital or iliac, right adrenal vein, and left adrenal vein.
- Inject 250 mcg of cosyntropin (Cortrosyn) after cannulation, or infuse 50 mcg cosyntropin per hour beginning 30 min before adrenal vein cannulation. This reduces stress-related fluctuations in aldosterone and cortisol values and augments the biochemical gradients. (This step is controversial.)
- Draw blood for aldosterone and cortisol levels at 5, 15, and 30 min from the peripheral site and from each adrenal vein.

ACTH, Adrenocorticotropic hormone; *PAC,* plasma aldosterone concentration; *PRA,* plasma renin activity.

and useful in preventing renal injury. Interestingly the postoperative reduction in aldosterone corrects the renal hyperfiltration and occasionally might unmask preexisting renal impairment in patients with normal preoperative glomerular filtration rate. More recently, ablative procedures in the treatment of unilateral AP have been attempted, but future clinical trials of ablation versus adrenalectomy are needed to compare their clinical and cost-effectiveness and further define patient populations that are likely to benefit.

For bilateral lesions, medical treatment is recommended because surgical risk outweighs benefits. BP control per se does not reduce risk of cardiovascular complications unless renin activity is restored to normal (>1 ng/mL/h), which can be accomplished by salt restriction or increasing the dose of the MRA. MRAs are a key component of medical treatment and used as a preoperative measure or maintenance treatment (GRA should be treated with the lowest dose of glucocorticoid that can normalize BP and potassium levels rather than MRAs). A low-sodium diet (sodium <100 mEq/day = 2.3 g/day or salt 6 g/day) is also important, because left ventricular hypertrophy is associated with urine sodium excretion in primary hyperaldosteronism but not in essential hypertension. Other lifestyle changes include aerobic exercise, smoking cessation, and weight loss.

Unilateral Hypersecretion

Adrenalectomy, usually laparoscopic, is recommended. MRAs such as spironolactone (Aldactone) and eplerenone (Inspra)[1] can

---

[1]Not FDA approved for this indication.

TABLE 3 Interpretation of Dynamic Testing

TEST	FINDINGS
Screening Test	
PAC/PRA ratio	Positive if >20–40 with PAC >5–10 ng/dL
Confirmatory Tests	
Oral sodium loading test	Positive if 24-h urine aldosterone excretion is >12–14 mcg
Saline infusion test	Positive if PAC after infusion is >10 ng/dL
Fludrocortisone[1] suppression test	Positive if upright PAC is >6 ng/dL on day 4 at 10 a.m.
Captopril[1] challenge test	Positive if PAC does not decrease by 30% and PRA remains suppressed
AVS	
With cosyntropin stimulation	A/C ratio (the high to the low side) >4:1 → unilateral aldosterone excess A/C ratio 3:1–4:1 → unclear A/C ratio <3:1 → bilateral aldosterone excess
Without cosyntropin stimulation	A/C ratio from the high to the low side >2:1 → unilateral aldosterone excess A/C ratio from the high side to the periphery >2.5 and A/C ratio from the contralateral side to the periphery <1 → unilateral aldosterone excess
If Equivocal AVS	
Postural stimulation test	PAC falls or fails to rise by 30%: consistent with APAs PAC increases by at least 33%: consistent with BAHs
Recumbent 18-hydroxycorticosterone	>100 ng/dL is consistent with APAs
NP-59 iodocholesterol scintigraphy	Unilateral early uptake (<5 days): consistent with unilateral aldosterone excess Bilateral early uptake (<5 days): consistent with bilateral aldosterone excess Negative scan does not rule out either etiology
(11)C-metomidate positron emission tomography	Preliminary data showed (11)C-metomidate uptake in APA

[1]Not FDA approved for this indication.

A/C ratio, Cortisol-corrected aldosterone ratio; *APA,* aldosterone-producing adenomas; *AVS,* adrenal vein sampling; *BAH,* bilateral adrenal hyperplasia; *PAC,* plasma aldosterone concentration; *PRA,* plasma renin activity.

be used to control BP in patients awaiting adrenalectomy and also to prevent postoperative hypoaldosteronism. Postoperatively, normal saline is given to maintain volume status, MRAs and potassium supplements are discontinued, and antihypertensive medications may be reduced. To confirm biochemical cure, PAC and PRA should be checked shortly after the operation, though renin levels might not change immediately. Risk factors for persistent hypertension after adrenalectomy include older age, duration of hypertension (>5 years), use of two or more antihypertensive agents preoperatively, BP higher than 165/100 mm Hg, low ARR preoperatively, low urine aldosterone, poor response to spironolactone preoperatively, family history of more than one first-degree relative with hypertension, and elevated serum creatinine level. When patients are unwilling or unable to undergo curative adrenalectomy, MRA therapy should be used as the alternative.

Bilateral Hypersecretion

MRAs and/or ENaC antagonists combined with other antihypertensives are used. One study showed that spironolactone had stronger antihypertensive effect than eplerenone, but there is insufficient evidence to choose one medication over another. When MR antagonist therapy is recommended, patients should be counseled on dietary sodium reduction (<1500 mg per day) as it can result in volume contraction, a rise in renin, and normalization of BP.

Spironolactone is the most widely used MRA. It is very effective in decreasing BP. The medication is initiated at 12.5 to 25 mg/day and can be titrated to 400 mg/day, with most patients requiring at least 200 mg/day. Potassium should be maintained at normal levels without use of potassium supplements. Use of spironolactone can be limited by side effects: antiandrogenic effects can cause gynecomastia in men, and progesterone effect can cause menstrual irregularities in women. There are drug interactions to consider: spironolactone increases the half-life of digoxin (Lanoxin) and salicylates, and other nonsteroidal antiinflammatory drugs may decrease the effectiveness of spironolactone. Serum potassium and creatinine should be closely monitored for the first 4 to 6 weeks, in particular for those with renal insufficiency or diabetes. Spironolactone is not recommended if creatinine clearance is less than 30 mL/min.

Eplerenone[1] is a competitive and selective antagonist of the aldosterone receptors. It has a lower binding affinity to androgen and progesterone receptors than spironolactone. This leads to fewer side effects. Eplerenone is 25% to 50% less potent in antagonizing the aldosterone receptors than spironolactone. Eplerenone has a short half-life and should be taken twice daily. Dosing is started at 25 mg twice daily, with a maximum dose of 100 mg/day. Again, serum potassium and creatinine should be closely monitored for the first 4 to 6 weeks in particular for those with renal insufficiency or diabetes. Other adverse effects include hypertriglyceridemia, increased liver enzymes, headache, and fatigue. Eplerenone is contraindicated if serum potassium is greater than 5.5 mEq/L at initiation, if creatinine clearance is less than 30 mL/min, or if there is concomitant use of strong CYP3A4 inhibitors such as ketoconazole (Nizoral) and itraconazole (Sporanox).

ENaC antagonists, amiloride (Midamor)[1] and triamterene (Dyrenium),[1] can be used in patients who cannot tolerate MRAs or are still hypertensive/hypokalemic while on MRAs. Amiloride is prescribed at 10 to 20 mg/day in divided doses. Side effects include dizziness, fatigue, and impotence. Triamterene is dosed at 100 to 300 mg/day in divided doses, and its side effects are mainly dizziness and nausea. Addition of thiazide diuretics can help control BP by relieving volume overload. If BP remains uncontrolled, other antihypertensive agents such as ACEIs/ARBs or calcium channel blockers may be used.

---

[1]Not FDA approved for this indication.

References

Adler GK, Murray GR, Turcu AF, et al: Primary aldosteronism decreases insulin secretion and increases insulin clearance in humans, *Hypertension* 75, 2020. 1251–125.

Baudrand R, Guarda FJ, Torrey J, Williams G, Vaidya A: Dietary sodium restriction increases the risk of misinterpreting mild cases of primary aldosteronism, *J Clin Endocrinol Metab* 101:3989–3996, 2016.

Bayomy O, Zaheer S, Williams JS, Curhan G, Vaidya A: Disentangling the relationships between the renin-angiotensin-aldosterone system, calcium physiology, and risk for kidney stones, *J Clin Endocrinol Metab* 105:1937–1946, 2020, https://doi.org/10.1210/clinem/dgaa123.

Born-Frontsberg E, Reincke M, Rump LC, et al: Cardiovascular and cerebrovascular comorbidities of hypokalemic and normokalemic primary aldosteronism: results of the German Conn's registry, *J Clin Endocrinol Metab* 94:1125–1130, 2009.

Bouhanick B, Delchier MC, Lagarde S, et al: Radiofrequency ablation for adenoma in patients with primary aldosteronism and hypertension: ADERADHTA, a pilot study, *J Hypertens* 39:759–765, 2021.

Boulkroun S: Old and new genes in primary aldosteronism, *Best Pract Res Clin Endocrinol Metab* 34, 2020.

Brown JM, Siddiqui M, Calhoun DA, et al: The unrecognized prevalence of primary aldosteronism: a cross-sectional study, *Ann Intern Med* 173(1):10–20, 2020, https://doi.org/10.7326/M20-0065. Epub 2020 May 26. PMID: 32449886; PMCID: PMC7459427.

Buffolo F, Pecori A, Reincke M, et al: Long-term follow-up of patients with elevated aldosterone-to-renin ratio but negative confirmatory test: the progression of primary aldosteronism phenotypes, *Hypertension* 81(2):340–347, 2024.

Catena C, Colussi G, Lapenna R, et al: Long-term cardiac effects of adrenalectomy or mineralocorticoid antagonists in patients with primary aldosteronism, *Hypertension* 50:911–918, 2007.

Catena C, Colussi GL, Nadalini E, et al: Cardiovascular outcomes in patients with primary aldosteronism after treatment, *Arch Intern Med* 168:80–85, 2008.

Cohen JB, Cohen DL, Herman DS, Leppert JT, Byrd JB, Bhalla V: Testing for primary aldosteronism and mineralocorticoid receptor antagonist use among U.S. veterans: a retrospective cohort study, *Ann Intern Med* 174(3):289–297, 2021, https://doi.org/10.7326/M20-4873. Epub 2020 Dec 29. PMID: 33370170; PMCID: PMC7965294.

Fujimoto K, Honjo S, Tatsuoka H, et al: Primary aldosteronism associated with subclinical Cushing syndrome, *J Endocrinol Invest* 36:564–567, 2013.

Funder JW: Primary aldosteronism and cardiovascular risk, before and after treatment, *Lancet Diabetes Endocrinol* 6:5–7, 2018.

Funder JW, Carey RM, Mantero F, et al: The management of primary aldosteronism: case detection, diagnosis, and treatment: an Endocrine Society clinical guideline, *J Clin Endocrinol Metab* 101:1889–1916, 2016.

Gordon RD, Gomez-Sanchez CE, Hamlet SM, et al: Angiotensin-responsive aldosterone-producing adenoma masquerades as idiopathic hyperaldosteronism (IHA: adrenal hyperplasia) or low-renin essential hypertension, *J Hypertens* 5:S103–S106, 1987.

Hundemer GL, Curhan GC, Yozamp N, et al: Cardiometabolic outcomes and mortality in medically treated primary aldosteronism: a retrospective cohort study, *Lancet Diabetes Endocrinol* 6:51–59, 2018.

Hundemer GL, Imsirovic H, Vaidya A, et al: Screening rates for primary aldosteronism among individuals with hypertension plus hypokalemia: a population-based retrospective cohort study, *Hypertension* 79(1):178–186, 2022, https://doi.org/10.1161/HYPERTENSIONAHA.121.18118. Epub 2021 Oct 18. PMID: 34657442; PMCID: PMC8664996.

Hundemer GL, Vaidya A: Primary aldosteronism diagnosis and management: a clinical approach, *Endocrinol Metab Clin North Am* 48(4):681–700, 2019, https://doi.org/10.1016/j.ecl.2019.08.002. PMID: 31655770; PMCID: PMC6824480.

Hundemer Gregory L, Vaidya A: "Management of endocrine disease: the role of surgical adrenalectomy in primary aldosteronism." *Eur J endocrinol* 183(6):R185–R196, 2020. Web.

Kempers MJ, Lenders JW, van Outheusden L, et al: Systematic review: diagnostic procedures to differentiate unilateral from bilateral adrenal abnormality in primary aldosteronism, *Ann Intern Med* 151:329–337, 2009.

Kono T, Ikeda Y, Oseko F, Imura H, Tanimura H: Normotensive primary aldosteronism: report of a case, *J Clin Endocrinol Metab* 52(5):1009–1013, 1981, https://doi.org/10.1210/jcem-52-5-1009. PMID: 6262353.

Lechner B, Lechner K, Heinrich D, et al: Therapy of endocrine disease: medical treatment of primary aldosteronism, *Eur J Endocrinol* 181:R147–R153, 2019.

Mete O, Erickson LA, Juhlin CC, et al: Overview of the 2022 WHO classification of adrenal cortical tumors, *Endocr Pathol* 33:155–196, 2022.

Mulatero P, Bertello C, Rossato D, et al: Roles of clinical criteria, computed tomography scan, and adrenal vein sampling in differential diagnosis of primary aldosteronism subtypes, *J Clin Endocrinol Metab* 93:1366–1371, 2008.

Nakano Y, Murakami M, Hara K, et al: Long-term effects of primary aldosteronism treatment on patients with primary aldosteronism and chronic kidney disease, *Clin Endocrinol (Oxf)* 98(3):323–331, 2023.

Nanba K, Rainey WE: Genetics in endocrinology: impact of race and sex on genetic causes of aldosterone-producing adenomas, *Eur J Endocrinol* 185(1):R1–R11, 2021.

Ng E, Gwini SM, Libianto R, et al: Aldosterone, renin, and aldosterone-to-renin ratio variability in screening for primary aldosteronism, *J Clin Endocrinol Metab* 108(1):33–41, 2022. Erratum in: *J Clin Endocrinol Metab.* 2023;108(5):e206.

O'Toole SM, Sze WC, Chung TT, et al: Lowgrade cortisol cosecretion has limited impact on ACTH-stimulated AVS parameters in primary aldosteronism, *J Clin Endocrinol Metab* 105:e3776–e3784, 2020.

Parthasarathy HK, Menard J, White WB, et al: A double-blind, randomized study comparing the antihypertensive effect of eplerenone and spironolactone in patients with hypertension and evidence of primary aldosteronism, *J Hypertens* 29(5):980–990, 2011.

Pimenta E, Gordon RD, Ahmed AH, et al: Cardiac dimensions are largely determined by dietary salt in patients with primary aldosteronism: results of a case-control study, *J Clin Endocrinol Metab* 96:2813–2820, 2011.

Reincke M, Fischer E, Gerum S, et al: Observational study mortality in treated primary aldosteronism: the German Conn's registry, *Hypertension* 60:618–624, 2012.

Rossi GP, Barisa M, Allolio B, et al: The adrenal vein sampling international study (AVIS) for identifying the major subtypes of primary aldosteronism, *J Clin Endocrinol Metab* 97:1606–1614, 2012.

Rossi GP: A comprehensive review of the clinical aspects of primary aldosteronism, *Nat Rev Endocrinol* 7:485–495, 2011.

Rossi GP, Bernini G, Caliumi C, et al: A prospective study of the prevalence of primary aldosteronism in 1,125 hypertensive patients, *J Am Coll Cardiol* 48:2293–2300, 2006.

Rossi GP, Seccia TM, Pessina AC: Adrenal gland: a diagnostic algorithm—the holy grail of primary aldosteronism, *Nat Rev Endocrinol* 7:697–699, 2011.

Rutherford JC, Taylor WL, Stowasser M, Gordon RD: Success of surgery for primary aldosteronism judged by residual autonomous aldosterone production, *World J Surg* 22(12):1243–1245, 1998.

Sawka AM, Young WF, Thompson GB, et al: Primary aldosteronism: factors associated with normalization of blood pressure after surgery, *Ann Intern Med* 135:258–261, 2001.

Scholl UI: Genetics of primary aldosteronism, *Hypertension* 79:887–897, 2022.

Sechi LA, Novello M, Lapenna R, et al: Long-term renal outcomes in patients with primary aldosteronism, *JAMA* 295:2638–2645, 2006.

Stowasser M: Update in primary aldosteronism, *J Clin Endocrinol Metab* 100:1–10, 2015.

Sukor N, Gordon RD, Ku YK, et al: Role of unilateral adrenalectomy in bilateral primary aldosteronism: a 22-year single center experience, *J Clin Endocrinol Metab* 94:2437–2445, 2009.

Takeda M, Yamamoto K, Akasaka H, et al: Clinical characteristics and postoperative outcomes of primary aldosteronism in the elderly, *J Clin Endocrinol Metab* 103:3620–3629, 2018.

Thuzar M, Young K, Ahmed AH, et al: Diagnosis of primary aldosteronism by seated saline suppression test—variability between immunoassay and HPLC-MS/MS, *J Clin Endocrinol Metab* 105:e477–e483, 2019.

Vaidya A, Brown JM, Carey RM, Siddiqui M, Williams GH: The unrecognized prevalence of primary aldosteronism, *Ann Intern Med* 173(8):683, 2020.

Vaidya A, Carey RM: Evolution of the primary aldosteronism syndrome: updating the approach, *J Clin Endocrinol Metab* 105(12):1–3783, 2020.

Vorselaars WMCM, Nell S, Postma EL, et al: Clinical outcomes after unilateral adrenalectomy for primary aldosteronism, *JAMA Surg* 154:e185842, 2019.

Williams TA, Gomez-Sanchez CE, Rainey WE, et al: International histopathology consensus for unilateral primary aldosteronism, *J Clin Endocrinol Metab* 106(1):42–54, 2021.

Wu WC, Peng KY, Lu JY, et al: Cortisol-producing adenoma-related somatic mutations in unilateral primary aldosteronism with concurrent autonomous cortisol secretion: their prevalence and clinical characteristics, *Eur J Endocrinol* 187(4):519–530, 2022.

Yozamp N, Hundemer GL, Moussa M, et al: Intraindividual variability of aldosterone concentrations in primary aldosteronism: implications for case detection, *Hypertension* 77:891–899, 2021.

Zennaro MC, Boulkroun S, Fernandes-Rosa F: An update on novel mechanisms of primary aldosteronism, *J Endocrinol* 224:R63–R77, 2015.

HYPERLIPIDEMIA

Method of
Ming Li, MD, PhD

CURRENT DIAGNOSIS

- Hyperlipidemia is diagnosed by assessing a lipid profile in the context of overall cardiovascular risk (see Table 1). In addition, triglyceride levels greater than 500 mg/dL pose a significant risk of pancreatitis.
- The Pooled Cohort Equation is the most used cardiovascular risk predictor in the United States.
- Borderline-to-intermediate risk scores by PCE can be modified by risk enhancers and the coronary artery calcium score.
- Secondary causes of hyperlipidemia, such as hypothyroidism, alcoholism, uncontrolled diabetes mellitus, kidney disorders, pregnancy, and medications, warrant comprehensive investigation and prompt treatment upon diagnosis.
- Consider the possibility of familial hyperlipidemia based on the lipid profile, family history, and physical examination. It is crucial to recognize that cardiovascular risk may be underestimated and management can present challenges in familial cases. Cascade testing should be carried out in at-risk relatives after an index case is diagnosed.

CURRENT THERAPY

- Therapy should be guided by goals of treatment based on estimated cardiovascular risk.
- When the triglyceride (TG) level is 500 mg/dL or greater, lowering TG to prevent acute pancreatitis is a priority.

- Low-density lipoprotein cholesterol (LDL-C) is a primary target, followed by non–high-density lipoprotein cholesterol (non–HDL-C) as a secondary target, with individualized goals dictated by atherosclerotic cardiovascular disease (ASCVD) risk assessment (see Table 2). TG has also emerged as a target to further reduce residual cardiovascular risk in select patients with high cardiovascular risk.
- A healthy lifestyle is encouraged for all individuals to reduce risk of ASCVD. Lifestyle therapy is especially indicated for patients with hyperlipidemia.
- Weight loss is the most effective lifestyle intervention for hypertriglyceridemia and metabolic syndrome. For patients with severe hypertriglyceridemia (TG ≥ 500 mg/dL), a low-fat or very-low-fat diet should be initiated for prevention of pancreatitis.
- Statins are the cornerstone of cholesterol-lowering therapies, with proven efficacy for both primary and secondary prevention of ASCVD; the intensity of statin therapy should be dictated by the degree of cardiovascular risk.
- Nonstatin therapies for LDL-C lowering can be added to maximally tolerated doses of statins to achieve further cholesterol lowering, as indicated by the patient's ASCVD risk.
- Icosapent ethyl (Vascepa) can be added to statin therapy for patients with high TG levels and either established ASCVD or diabetes with additional cardiovascular risks for further reduction of residual ASCVD risk.
- All other cardiovascular risk factors should be treated aggressively at the same time.

TABLE 1 Classification of Low-Density Lipoprotein, Total Cholesterol, High-Density Lipoprotein Cholesterol, and Triglycerides (mg/dL)

LDL-C (mg/dL)

<100	Optimal
100–129	Near optimal/above optimal
130–159	Borderline high
160–189	High
≥190	Very high

Total Cholesterol (mg/dL)

<200	Desirable
200–239	Borderline high
≥240	High

HDL-C (mg/dL)

<40	Low
≥60	High

Triglycerides (mg/dL)

<150	Normal
150–199	Borderline high
200–499	High
≥500	Very high

HDL-C, High-density lipoprotein cholesterol; *LCL*, low-density lipoprotein; *LDL-C*, low-density lipoprotein cholesterol.
Based on the National Cholesterol Education Program Adult Treatment Panel III guidelines.

Hyperlipidemia is a condition of elevated serum lipids and lipoproteins. Hyperlipidemia is associated with an increased risk of atherosclerotic cardiovascular disease (ASCVD) and, if triglyceride (TG) level is greater than 500 mg/dL, pancreatitis. The primary goals of management of hyperlipidemia are to decrease the risk of ASCVD and pancreatitis. ASCVD, as defined by the *2018 Multisociety Guideline on the Management of Blood Cholesterol*, encompasses acute coronary syndrome; history of myocardial infarction; stable or unstable angina; coronary or other arterial revascularization; stroke; transient ischemic attack; or peripheral arterial disease, including aortic aneurysm; all of these conditions are of atherosclerotic origin. ASCVD is the leading cause of mortality in the United States. Consumption of low-density lipoprotein cholesterol (LDL-C) by vascular macrophages plays a central role in the development of atherosclerosis, and it is well established in epidemiology, genetics, and clinical studies that lower LDL-C levels are closely associated with fewer ASCVD events in a linear relationship, as summarized by the mantra "lower is better." Appropriate treatment of hyperlipidemia is therefore essential in patients with established cardiovascular disease (secondary prevention), whereas detection and treatment of hyperlipidemia are guided by the risk of ASCVD in patients without known clinical ASCVD (primary prevention).

The prevalence of hyperlipidemia varies with the definition of hyperlipidemia (see Table 1) and the population studied. From 2017 to 2020, 86.4 million US adults (>20 years of age) had borderline high or high cholesterol (i.e., total cholesterol [TC] level of ≥200 or 240 mg/dL, respectively). The percentage of US adults with a high TC level (≥240 mg/dL) has continued a long-term trend of decline from 18.3% to 10.5% during the period of 1999 to 2018. The decline is in part attributed to increased use of lipid-lowering medications. This has contributed to a significant drop (>60%) of total cardiovascular mortality since 1968. Unfortunately, the rate of decline has stagnated since 2018, with the improved cholesterol and blood pressure control and reduction in smoking and physical inactivity offset by increases in the prevalence of obesity and diabetes. Hence, effective management of hyperlipidemia remains pivotal in addressing overall cardiovascular risk.

Various societies and professional organizations have published clinical guidelines for hyperlipidemia. The *2018 Multisociety*

Guideline on the Management of Blood Cholesterol is widely endorsed by physician societies in the United States, whereas in Europe, the *2019 European Society of Cardiology and European Atherosclerosis Society (ESC/EAS) Guidelines for the Management of Dyslipidaemias* is the most influential. The two are largely consistent but with notable differences. We mostly adhere to the 2018 Multisociety guideline and incorporate updates in more recent American guidelines, especially the *2021 ACC Expert Consensus Decision Pathway (ECDP) on the Management of ASCVD Risk Reduction in Patients With Persistent Hypertriglyceridemia*, the *2022 ACC ECDP on the Role of Nonstatin Therapies for LDL-Cholesterol Lowering in the Management of Atherosclerotic Cardiovascular Disease Risk*, and recent results of randomized clinical trials yet to be covered in current guidelines.

Pathophysiology

Lipids have two main points of entry into the circulation: the gut (exogenous pathway) and the liver (endogenous pathway). They are carried in the circulation in the form of lipoproteins, in complex with a group of amphipathic proteins known as apolipoproteins (Apos). In addition to serving as carriers for lipids, Apos play important roles in metabolism of the different species of cargo lipids and the eventual clearance of lipoproteins from circulation. Major Apos include Apo AI, AII, AIV, AV, B48, B100, CI, CII, CIII, E and apo(a). Apo B, including both B48 and B100, are the major structural proteins for the lipoproteins in the exogenous and endogenous pathways, respectively. They are both products of the *APOB* gene on chromosome 2. Apo B100 is the full-length protein produced in hepatocytes, whereas Apo B48, the truncated protein product, is produced in the intestine. Apo B48 mRNA differs from Apo B100 mRNA by a single base, the product of a single base conversion whereby a specific cytosine (C) in ApoB mRNA is converted to uracil (U), producing a stop codon and resulting in the production of a truncated Apo B48

TABLE 2 Risk Groups and Treatment Goals (2018 Multisociety Blood Cholesterol Guidelines, 2021 ACC ECDP on Persistent Hypertriglyceridemia, and 2022 ACC ECDP on Nonstatin Therapies)

	RISK CATEGORY	RECOMMENDED STATIN THERAPY TO INITIATE	TREATMENT GOAL	NONSTATIN THERAPY
Secondary prevention	Very high risk*	High-intensity statin	LDL-C reduction ≥50%, LDL-C <55 mg/dL, non–HDL-C <85 mg/dL	Ezetimibe[1] PCSK9 mAbs Bempedoic acid (Nexletol) Inclisiran (Leqvio)[1] Icosapent ethyl (Vascepa)[†]
	Not very high risk	High-intensity statin	LDL-C reduction ≥ 50%, LDL-C <70 mg/dL, non–HDL-C <100 mg/dL	Ezetimibe[1] PCSK9 mAbs Bempedoic acid Inclisiran[1] Icosapent ethyl[†]
Primary prevention	LDL-C ≥190 mg/dL	High-intensity statin	LDL-C reduction ≥50%, LDL-C <100 mg/dL, non–HDL-C <130 mg/dL	Ezetimibe PCSK9 inhibitors Bempedoic acid Inclisiran
	Diabetes mellitus	Moderate-intensity statin if 10-year ASCVD risk‡ <7.5%	LDL-C reduction ≥30%–49%, LDL-C <100 mg/dL, non–HDL-C <130 mg/dL	Ezetimibe after escalating to high-intensity statin
	Diabetes mellitus	High-intensity statin if 10-year ASCVD risk ≥7.5–20%, diabetes specific risk enhancers present,§ or subclinical atherosclerosis present	LDL-C reduction ≥50%, LDL-C <100 mg/dL, non–HDL-C <130 mg/dL	Ezetimibe Icosapent ethyl[†]
	Diabetes mellitus	High-intensity statin if 10-year ASCVD risk ≥20%	LDL-C reduction ≥50%, LDL-C <70 mg/dL, non–HDL-C <100 mg/dL	Ezetimibe Icosapent ethyl[†]
	High risk (10-year ASCVD risk ≥20%)	High-intensity statin	LDL-C reduction ≥50%, LDL-C <70 mg/dL, non–HDL-C <100 mg/dL	Ezetimibe
	Intermediate risk (10-year ASCVD risk ≥7.5–20%)	If risk enhancers‖ present or if CAC score elevated, should initiate moderate-intensity statin	LDL-C reduction ≥30%–49%, LDL-C <100 mg/dL, non–HDL-C <130 mg/dL	
	Borderline risk (10-year ASCVD risk 5% to <7.5%)	If risk enhancers present, may consider moderate-intensity statin	LDL-C reduction ≥30–49%, LDL-C <100 mg/dL, non–HDL-C <130 mg/dL	
	Low risk (10-year ASCVD risk <5%)	Statin deferred		

[1]Not FDA approved for this indication.

*Very high risk defined by a history of multiple major ASCVD events or at least one major ASCVD event plus multiple high-risk conditions (age ≥65 years, heterozygous familial hypercholesterolemia, history of coronary bypass surgery or percutaneous coronary intervention outside of the major ASCVD events, diabetes mellitus, hypertension, chronic kidney disease, current smoking, persistently elevated LDL-C ≥100 mg/dL despite maximally tolerated statin and ezetimibe, or history of congestive heart failure).

[†]If persistent fasting triglycerides (TGs) ≥150 mg/dL with history of ASCVD or diabetes mellitus with age ≥50 years with additional high-risk features.

[‡]10-year ASCVD risk as estimated by the Pooled Cohort Equation.

[§]Diabetes-specific risk enhancers include long duration of disease (type 2 ≥10 years; type 1 ≥20 years), albuminuria ≥30 mcg of albumin/mg creatinine, estimated glomerular filtration rate <60 mL/min/1.73 m², retinopathy, neuropathy, and ankle-brachial index <0.9.

[‖]Risk enhancers include family history of premature ASCVD, chronic kidney disease, metabolic syndrome, inflammatory disease, conditions specific to women (i.e., preeclampsia, premature menopause), ethnicity (i.e., South Asian ancestry), persistently elevated LDL-C ≥160 mg/dL, persistently elevated TGs (≥175 mg/dL), high sensitivity C-reactive protein ≥2.0 mg/L, lipoprotein (a) ≥50 mg/dL or 125 nmol/L, apolipoprotein B ≥130 mg/dL, and ankle-brachial index <0.9. The Endocrine Society recognizes endocrine disorders, including persistent Cushing syndrome and Cushing disease, high-dose chronic glucocorticoid therapy, adult growth hormone deficiency, acromegaly, and hypothyroidism, as additional risk enhancers.

ACC ECDP, American College of Cardiology Expert Consensus Decision Pathway; *ASCVD,* atherosclerotic cardiovascular disease; *CAC,* coronary artery calcium; *LDL-C,* low-density lipoprotein cholesterol; *non–HDL-C,* non–high-density lipoprotein cholesterol; *PCSK9,* proprotein convertase subtilisin/kexin type 9.

protein. Each lipoprotein particle only carries one molecule of Apo B, making the latter a good indicator for the levels of atherogenic lipoprotein particles. The lipoproteins are in constant flux, with lipids being metabolized and products released to target cells, lipid species, and Apos exchanging between lipoproteins while converting one lipoprotein species into another. These activities tightly interconnect the exogenous and endogenous pathways, as well as the reverse cholesterol transport pathway, as outlined in Figure 1.

Exogenous Pathway

Lipids in food undergo emulsification by bile acids and subsequent hydrolysis into fatty acids and cholesterol by pancreatic lipases within the intestinal lumen. These products are then reesterified and packaged with Apo B48 to form chylomicrons. Chylomicrons are secreted into the intestinal lymph and delivered to the systemic circulation. At peripheral tissues, lipoprotein lipase (LPL) hydrolyzes TGs within chylomicrons, releasing free fatty acids for energy or storage. Chylomicron remnants are taken up by the liver via the interaction between Apo E and chylomicron remnant receptors. LPL plays a central role in clearance of both exogenous and endogenous TGs. A deficiency of LPL underlies familial hyperchylomicronemia. LPL is regulated by insulin and thyroid hormone. A deficiency of insulin or thyroid hormone leads to diabetes mellitus and hypothyroidism, respectively, often complicated by secondary hypertriglyceridemia. Apo

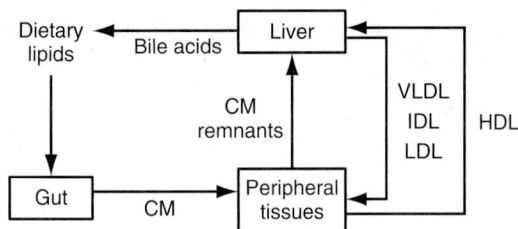

Figure 1 Overview of exogenous and endogenous pathways of lipid metabolism. *CM*, Chylomicrons; *HDL*, high-density lipoproteins; *IDL*, intermediate-density lipoproteins; *LDL*, low-density lipoproteins; *VLDL*, very-low-density lipoproteins.

CII is an essential cofactor for LPL, while Apo CIII and secreted glycoproteins angiopoietin-like 3 (ANGPLT3) and angiopoietin-like 4 (ANGPLT4) are known inhibitors.

Endogenous Pathway

The endogenous pathway begins in the liver with the synthesis of TG-rich very-low-density lipoproteins (VLDLs). Microsomal triglyceride transfer protein (MTP) facilitates the transfer of lipids onto Apo B100 and stabilizes the protein for secretion as VLDLs. VLDLs, as chylomicrons, undergo lipolysis by LPL, releasing free fatty acids, generating smaller particles called intermediate-density lipoproteins (IDLs, also known as VLDL remnants). IDLs are either removed by the liver via interaction between Apo E and remnant receptors, or further processed into cholesterol-rich LDLs. LDLs are taken up into the liver or other cells via the interaction of LDL receptors (LDLRs) with Apo B100, a process regulated by cellular cholesterol requirement. Therefore inhibition of cholesterol synthesis leads to increased expression of LDLR at the cell surface and clearance of LDL-C, which is the major mechanism of action of statins and bempedoic acid (Nexletol) for lowering cholesterol. A secreted protease known as proprotein convertase subtilisin/kexin type 9 (PCSK9) binds to cell surface LDLR and promotes the latter's destruction in lysosome by preventing it from recycling to the cell membrane.

Prolonged clearance from circulation subjects LDL to modifications such as oxidation and acetylation. Within the arterial wall, macrophages avidly ingest these altered LDL particles via scavenger receptors and transform into foam cells, triggering inflammatory reactions by releasing cytokines and recruitment of other inflammatory cells, culminating in the formation of atherosclerotic plaques.

Of note, all Apo B–containing lipoprotein particles enriched with cholesterol from either exogenous or endogenous pathway, including chylomicron remnant and IDL, contribute to atherogenesis.

Reverse Cholesterol Transport

High-density lipoproteins (HDLs) are the major lipoproteins involved in the transport of cholesterol from peripheral tissues back to the liver. HDLs are synthesized by both the hepatocytes and the enterocytes in the form of small discoidal particles containing Apo AI and phospholipids. HDLs acquire additional lipids and Apos from TG-depleted chylomicrons and VLDL remnants. HDLs remove free cholesterol from tissues with the help of Apo AI and esterify it with lecithin cholesterol acyltransferase (LCAT). Cholesteryl esters are then transferred to Apo B 100–containing lipoproteins (VLDLs, IDLs, and LDLs) by cholesteryl ester transfer protein (CETP). HDLs can also be taken up directly by the liver class B, type I scavenger receptors.

Plasma Lipids and Atherosclerosis

Multiple studies have shown that total cholesterol and LDL-C levels contribute to cardiovascular disease risk and that lowering of total cholesterol and LDL-C levels reduces the risk. Non–HDL-C (i.e., total cholesterol – HDL-C = VLDL + IDL + LDL-C) reflects total atherogenic lipoprotein burden and may be a better risk indicator than LDL-C, especially in people with combined

hyperlipidemia, diabetes, metabolic syndrome, and chronic kidney disease. Table 1 shows the classification of lipid profile.

Recent mendelian randomization studies have suggested that TG-rich lipoproteins, including chylomicrons, VLDLs, and their remnants, also have a causal relationship with ASCVD. Therefore not only does hypertriglyceridemia represent an independent cardiovascular risk marker, it is also a significant risk factor and a target for therapy. Currently available TG-lowering therapies vary greatly in efficacy for reducing ASCVD. Although there is no evidence supporting niacin, fibrates (gemfibrozil and fenofibrate), or regular omega-3 fish oil (eicosapentaenoic acid [EPA] and docosahexaenoic acid [DHA]) in preventing ASCVD, icosapent ethyl (Vascepa), which is an EPA-only omega-3 acid ethyl ester, is able to reduce ASCVD in patients with elevated TG and heightened ASCVD risk; however, the cardioprotective effect is not correlated with the degree of TG lowering. Therefore the exact role of TG in contributing to ASCVD remains to be defined.

It is significant that mendelian randomization studies suggest that HDL-C does not have a causal relationship with ASCVD. Moreover, medications that increase HDL-C (i.e., niacin and CETP inhibitors) have largely failed to show efficacy in ASCVD risk reduction in randomized clinical trials. Therefore although HDL-C was shown to be inversely associated with cardiovascular risk, the mechanism of the relationship between HDL-C and ASCVD is not fully understood.

Additionally, the level of lipoprotein (a) [Lp(a)] is progressively associated with ASCVD risk. A mendelian randomization study suggested that elevation of Lp(a) is an independent causal risk factor. It is considered a risk-enhancing factor for ASCVD if greater than 50 mg/dL. Lp(a) is a special type of LDL, with apoB conjugated with Apos (a) [apo(a)]. Apo(a) is structurally similar to plasminogen and promotes atherosclerosis and thrombosis. The Lp(a) level is mostly determined genetically (e.g., with polymorphism of the apo[a] gene) but it can also increase with renal impairment. Lifetime exposure to severely elevated Lp(a) levels can lead to premature ASCVD. Pharmacologic treatments (PCSK9 inhibitors and niacin) and lipoprotein apheresis can effectively lower Lp(a). However, niacin has no proven cardiovascular benefits, and it remains to be determined whether PCSK9 inhibitors and lipoprotein apheresis lower ASCVD risk via lowering Lp(a), independent from their LDL-C lowering effects.

Importantly, ASCVD cannot be viewed as a disease caused solely by a lipid disorder; rather, it is the result of a complex interplay between dyslipidemia, metabolic derangements, inflammation, and endothelial dysfunction. For instance, even mildly elevated TGs (≥150 mg/dL) can suggest metabolic syndrome, an important risk factor for cardiovascular disease. Meanwhile, chronic systemic inflammation has been shown to accelerate atherogenesis, and therapies that target inflammation have been demonstrated in clinical trials to reduce the risk for ASCVD.

Plasma Lipid and Pancreatitis

Hypertriglyceridemia is the third most common cause of acute pancreatitis. In addition, acute pancreatitis associated with hypertriglyceridemia is often more severe. The risk of acute pancreatitis is progressively increased when the TG level is greater than 500 mg/dL and especially so when it is greater than 1000 mg/dL. The exact mechanism whereby severe hypertriglyceridemia triggers pancreatitis is poorly understood but is thought to be related to proinflammatory effects of fatty acids released by pancreatic lipase.

Evaluation
Measurement of Lipid Profiles

Lipid profiles should be measured as a part of global risk assessment, and the frequency of checkup is determined by age, sex, and risk factors for cardiovascular disease. Testing should start in childhood, at least once between 9 and 11 years of age and then again between 17 and 21. Healthy individuals should have a lipid profile tested every 4 to 6 years, and more often if risk factors for ASCVD are present. In patients on lipid-lowering therapy, a lipid panel should be performed after initiation or dose change in therapy; it should also be performed periodically in patients on stable therapy to assess treatment efficacy and medication adherence.

A fasting lipid profile (fasting for 8–12 hours) ensures the most accurate lipid assessment, specifically of TGs (and subsequently LDL-C, if calculated using the Friedewald equation). On the other hand, a strict requirement for fasting may become a barrier to timely risk assessments for many patients. A nonfasting lipid profile for total cholesterol, HDL-C, Apo B, and Apo AI is generally acceptable. Recent studies show that differences in TG levels according to fasting time are small; thus calculated LDL-C is often minimally affected in nonfasting samples. Notably, a nonfasting lipid panel has been accepted by the 2018 Multisociety guideline and other recent guidelines as an option for initial screening or establishing an LDL-C baseline before starting statin treatment, unless a prior lipid panel showed a TG level greater than 400 mg/dL. A fasting lipid profile is still recommended for monitoring adherence to lipid-lowering therapies and identifying cases of metabolic syndrome, severe hypertriglyceridemia, and genetic lipid disorders, including a family history of premature ASCVD.

LDL-C can be either calculated or measured directly. The standard method used to derive LDL-C from other components of the lipid panel is the Friedewald equation (LDL-C = Total cholesterol – HDL-C – TG/5), in which TG/5 is used to calculate VLDL cholesterol (VLDL-C). This equation should be used with caution: it becomes less accurate if TG is 200 mg/dL or greater and is invalid with TG of 400 mg/dL or greater. LDL-C can be underestimated at levels less than 70 mg/dL. A new method, the Martin-Hopkins equation, was found to be more accurate when TGs are between 150 and 400 mg/dL and when non–HDL-C is low. Instead of a fixed factor of 5, as in the Friedewald equation, the Martin-Hopkins method uses an adjustable factor for the TG/VLDL-C ratio. When the TG is greater than 400 mg/dL, an enzymatic assay is available to directly measure LDL-C.

Outside the standard lipid profile, the 2018 Multisociety guideline also considered Apo B and Lp(a) as relatively indicated in assessment of ASCVD risk in select populations. The Apo B level reflects the number of atherogenic lipoprotein particles but measurement is limited by expense and test accuracy. Because the Apo B level is strongly associated with the non–HDL-C level in most situations, it does not seem to add to diagnostic value except in patients with elevated TG levels (≥200 mg/dL). In patients with a family history of premature ASCVD or with personal ASCVD not explained by traditional risk factors, testing of Lp(a) may be considered. Elevation of Lp(a) can be present in up to 20% adult population. Because its levels are mainly genetically determined, it only needs to be tested once in an individual's lifetime for risk assessment. The 2019 ESC/EAS guidelines for the management of dislipidemias has therefore recommended universal Lp(a) testing once in all individuals. Wide adoption of this recommendation is hampered by lack of reliability of the current commercial assays and lack of evidence that Lp(a) directly contributes to ASCVD pathogenesis.

Global Cardiovascular Risk Assessment

Risk assessment is an integral part in the evaluation of patients with hyperlipidemia. Contemporary guidelines from the United States provide detailed algorithms for risk stratification. The 2013 and 2018 cholesterol guidelines identified four subgroups of patients for whom the benefits of statin therapy outweigh the risk. Secondary prevention patients are automatically considered to be at high risk for recurrent ASCVD events and thus would necessitate initiation of lipid-lowering therapy. In the 2018 Multisociety guideline, secondary prevention patients may be further stratified into those at very high risk and those at not very high risk for ASCVD, based on the presence or absence of high-risk features. The value of further delineating risk among secondary prevention patients was, in part, to facilitate the evidence-based use of newer nonstatin therapies (i.e., ezetimibe [Zetia],[1] bempedoic acid [Nexletol], and PCSK9 inhibitors).

---

[1] Not FDA approved for this indication.

Among primary prevention patients, a history of diabetes mellitus or significantly elevated LDL-C (≥190 mg/dL) signifying a likely genetic cause of hypercholesterolemia automatically warrants initiation of lipid-lowering therapy. In primary prevention patients with hyperlipidemia but without these two high-risk features, a global cardiovascular risk score can be used to further stratify a patient. Global risk scores estimate 10-year cardiovascular risk, which combines the effects of well-known risk factors, using one of several risk-calculation tools. Individual tools have been developed based on large epidemiology studies examining a limited number of available risk factors. Traditional risk factors such as age, sex, cigarette smoking, cholesterol, diabetes, and blood pressure are able to predict 80% to 90% of the cardiovascular events in people 40 years or older. However, these tools may not accurately estimate cardiovascular risk in individuals with unaccounted risk factors or those with demographics distinct from the populations used to derive the risk scores. The risk score most commonly used (and endorsed by guidelines) in the United States is the Pooled Cohort Equation (PCE). The PCE is used to estimate a 10-year risk for ASCVD for men and women aged 40 to 79 years of White or Black race, incorporating age, sex, race, HDL and total cholesterol, diabetes, hypertension, and smoking status (https://tools.acc.org/ascvd-risk-estimator-plus/). The 2018 Multisociety guidelines recommend the initiation of statin therapy in patients with intermediate (≥7.5% to <20%) and high (≥20%) 10-year ASCVD risk, with consideration of statins even in select patients with borderline 10-year risk (5% to <7.5%). Of note, the risk stratification system used by the European guidelines, known as the Systematic COronary Risk Evaluation (SCORE) algorithm, considers similar risk factors but gives an estimate of 10-year cardiovascular mortality (https://www.heartscore.org).

Risk-Enhancing Factors

Because the PCE does not consider risk factors with smaller population effect, the 2013 guideline and the 2018 Multisociety guideline recommend that individuals with borderline to intermediate ASCVD risk based on the PCE be assessed for additional risk-enhancing factors (Table 2). These risk enhancers, when present, significantly increased cardiovascular risk in affected individuals. The Endocrine Society's *Clinical Practice Guidelines on Lipid Management for Patients With Endocrine Disorders* describes additional risk-enhancing factors to consider (see Table 2). Presence of these factors in patients with borderline and intermediate 10-year ASCVD risks would favor initiating statin therapy. Additionally, some of these risk-enhancing factors are themselves treatable targets (e.g., hypothyroidism and hypertriglyceridemia).

Risk Reclassifying With Coronary Artery Calcium Score

If the decision to initiate LDL-C–lowering therapy remains uncertain after ASCVD risk assessment (e.g., in patients with borderline to intermediate ASCVD risk), measuring a coronary artery calcium (CAC) score is recommended by the 2018 and later guidelines to reclassify the patient's risk. A CAC score is an indicator of total burden of calcified plaques in coronary arteries as measured by computed tomography. A CAC score of 0 Agatston unit (AU) can downclassify the patient to low risk and justify deferral of statin therapy. A score of 100 AU or greater or in the 75th percentile or greater upclassifies borderline risk patients to intermediate risk, warranting moderate intensity statins. A score between 1 and 99 AU would justify moderate-intensity statin treatment for patients above 55 years old. A score of 300 AU or greater upclassifies patients to the high-risk category, justifying initiation or intensification to high-intensity statins.

Differential Diagnosis of Hyperlipidemia

Lipid levels are influenced by a multitude of factors, including genetics, lifestyle choices (e.g., diet, substance use, and physical activity), medications, and other underlying medical conditions, which may differentially affect the levels of cholesterol and TG. Secondary causes of hyperlipidemia include hypothyroidism, nephrotic syndrome, use of progestin (especially those with androgenic activity), cholestasis, use of protease inhibitors, chronic kidney disease, uncontrolled diabetes, obesity, excessive alcohol intake, use of atypical antipsychotics, use of thiazide or β-blockers, use of corticosteroids, use of oral estrogen (not transdermal), and pregnancy. Their effects on different aspects of the lipid profile are summarized in Table 3. A thorough history and physical examination should be carried out in search of these conditions, aided by screening tests that should minimally include blood glucose, hemoglobin A1c, urinary protein, hepatic and renal functions, and thyroid stimulating hormone. Once recognized, these secondary conditions should be optimally managed.

Hyperlipidemia not explained by secondary conditions, also known as primary hyperlipidemia, is due to genetic causes. The underlying genetic defects can be either monogenic or polygenic. Affected patients typically have severe dyslipidemia, early onset of complications (e.g., ASCVD or pancreatitis), and strong family history and are refractory to standard treatments. Physical examination often reveals hallmarks of these diseases; xanthomas, xanthelasmas, and premature arcus cornealis may suggest familial hypercholesterolemia; eruptive xanthoma and lipemia retinalis may suggest familial hyperchylomicronemia; and familial dysbetalipoproteinemia may exhibit palmar xanthoma in palmar and finger creases. Diagnosis of primary hyperlipidemia can be made clinically with the described findings and can be further confirmed with genetic testing which, however, is not always necessary. As the risk for ASCVD associated with very elevated levels of atherogenic lipoproteins begins to accumulate very early in life, all children should be screened with a lipid profile between 9 and 11 years of age, and once diagnosed, treated aggressively. Once diagnosed, cascade testing of lipid profile should be offered to family members of the index patients who are at high risk. Table 3 summarizes common genetic and secondary causes of hyperlipidemia and dyslipidemia.

Treatment
Overview
Treatment is primarily aimed at lowering LDL-C level, which has been shown to decrease the risk of cardiovascular disease in numerous randomized clinical trials and meta-analyses. Every reduction of LDL-C of 1 mmol/L (~39 mg/dL) is associated with an approximate 22% reduction in cardiovascular risk. The absolute risk reduction by lowering LDL-C is proportional to the global cardiovascular risk; therefore patients with higher baseline LDL-C levels and higher ASCVD risks stand to reap the most benefits in starting lipid-lowering therapy early and adequately. In patients with severe hypertriglyceridemia (i.e., TG ≥500 mg/dL and especially ≥1000 mg/dL), TG should be treated to less than 500 mg/dL to prevent acute pancreatitis.

Treatment Targets
The 2013 American College of Cardiology/American Heart Association (ACC/AHA) guideline departed from the traditions of previous lipid guidelines by not setting hard LDL-C targets and, instead, emphasizing percentage reduction of LDL-C as a primary goal and the use of statins of corresponding strength. In short, the desired LDL-C reduction from baseline is 50% or greater, with high-potency statin for secondary prevention, and between 30% and 49% for primary prevention with moderate-intensity statins, except for patients with higher 10-year ASCVD risk.

Since then, additional nonstatin therapies have become available. In particular, cardiovascular outcome trials for PCSK9 inhibitors show that cardiovascular risk progressively decreases as LDL-C levels are reduced to the lowest achievable level (i.e., <25 mg/dL) without any notable harm. As such, the principle of "lower is better" has been validated for all levels of LDL-C. Considering these findings, the 2018 Multisociety guideline introduced LDL-C thresholds for adding nonstatin therapies for secondary prevention patients with or without high-risk features.

TABLE 3	Differential Diagnosis of Hyperlipidemia and Dyslipidemia			
HYPERTRIGLYCERIDEMIA	**HYPERCHOLESTEROLEMIA**	**INCREASED CHOLESTEROL AND TRIGLYCERIDES**	**LOW HDL**	
Primary Disorders				
LPL deficiency	Familial hypercholesterolemia	Familial combined hyperlipidemia	Familial hypoalphalipoproteinemia	
Apo CII deficiency	Familial defective Apo B100	Dysbetalipoproteinemia	Apo AI mutations	
Familial hypertriglyceridemia	PCSK9 gain-of-function mutations		LCAT deficiency	
	Polygenic hypercholesterolemia		ABCA1 deficiency	
	Sitosterolemia			
Secondary Disorders				
Diabetes mellitus	Hypothyroidism	Diabetes Mellitus	Anabolic steroids	
Hypothyroidism	Cholestasis	Hypothyroidism	Retinoids	
High-carbohydrate diets	Nephrotic syndrome	Glucocorticoids	HIV infection	
Renal failure	Thiazides	Immunosuppressants	Hepatitis C	
Obesity/insulin resistance		Protease inhibitors		
Estrogens		Nephrotic syndrome		
Ethanol		Lipodystrophies		
β-Blockers				
Protease inhibitors				
Glucocorticoids				
Retinoids				
Bile acid sequestrants				
Antipsychotics				
Lipodystrophies				
Thiazides				

ABCA1, Adenosine triphosphate–binding cassette transporter 1; *apo*, apolipoprotein; *HDL*, high-density lipoprotein; *HIV*, human immunodeficiency virus; *LCAT*, lecithin:cholesterol acyltransferase; *LPL*, lipoprotein lipase.
Modified from Semenkovich CF, Goldberg IJ: Disorders of lipid metabolism. In S. Melmed S, Koenig R, C. Rosen C, et al, eds: *Williams textbook of endocrinology E-Book*, ed 14. Philadelphia: Elsevier; 2020.

The *2022 ACC ECDP for Nonstatin Therapies* further lowered these thresholds for secondary prevention patients and set LDL-C thresholds for primary prevention patients as well.

The treatment goals and approaches according to the *2018 Multisociety Cholesterol Guidelines, 2021 ACC ECDP on Hypertriglyceridemia*, and *2022 ACC ECDP on Nonstatin Therapies* are summarized in Table 2. Briefly, these guidelines recognize three separate goals for LDL-C–lowering treatment for different risk groups, including percentage reduction, LDL-C level, and non–HDL-C level. Moderate- and high-intensity statins are the first-line treatment options. Different nonstatin therapies for LDL-C and TG lowering can be added after maximally tolerated statins fail to achieve appropriate goals for the respective risk group.

Lifestyle Therapy

The 2018 Multisociety guideline strongly recommended that all individuals, regardless of lipid status, assume a heart-healthy lifestyle. As accumulative exposure to atherogenic lipoproteins since childhood increases lifetime risk of ASCVD, lifestyle interventions should be initiated as early as possible. Dietary modification to limit intake of lipids is an essential component given that the main source of lipids is dietary fat. Saturated fatty acids and trans unsaturated fatty acids increase LDL-C, whereas dietary fibers and phytosterols decrease LDL-C. Carbohydrates do not affect LDL-C but increase TGs and decrease HDL-C, particularly if they have a high glycemic index. Intake of fructose, a component of sucrose, increases TGs and decreases HDL-C. Body weight reduction, increasing physical activity, and avoidance of a sedentary lifestyle have a small effect on LDL-C, but they reduce TGs, increase HDL-C, and are associated with improved cardiovascular outcome. Alcohol intake has an adverse effect on TGs and therefore should be restricted or avoided in patients with hypertriglyceridemia. Moderate alcohol drinking is associated with higher HDL-C levels, but there is no evidence that any amount of alcohol is cardioprotective.

Individual patients will need different approaches based on their cardiovascular risk and lipid profiles. Generally, total dietary fat is recommended to constitute 25% to 35% of the total calorie intake, mainly as monounsaturated or polyunsaturated fat, limiting saturated fats to less than 7% and trans fats to less than 1% of the total calorie intake. Therapeutic lifestyle changes for lowering LDL-C include diets with emphasis on vegetables, fruits, whole grains, low-fat dairy products, poultry, fish, legumes, nontropical vegetable oils, and nuts, as well as limited intake of sweets, sugar-sweetened beverages, and red meats; further reduction of saturated fats (<5%–6% of the total caloric intake) and avoidance of trans fats; weight reduction; and increased regular physical activity. The amount of cholesterol intake is not well correlated with LDL-C level, and there is no recommended limit for intake. Management of other risk factors, such as smoking cessation and controlling blood pressure in hypertensive patients and blood glucose in diabetics, is also very important.

With severe hypertriglyceridemia (TG ≥500 mg/dL), the capacity of plasma LPL becomes saturated; further fat intake would significantly raise TG level even higher and potentially precipitate acute pancreatitis. Therefore it is important to start a low-fat or very-low-fat diet in patients with severe hypertriglyceridemia. Alcohol and added sugars should be avoided as well. Weight loss is considered the single most effective lifestyle therapy for persistent hypertriglyceridemia and metabolic syndrome and may lead to a 50% to 70% reduction of TG level in the long term. The *2021 ACC ECDP on Persistent Hypertriglyceridemia* made specific recommendations regarding lifestyle therapies for persistent hypertriglyceridemia based on the TG levels, as outlined in Table 4.

Pharmacologic Agents

The currently available lipid-lowering agents can be classified based on their mechanism of action. Statins (3-hydroxy-3-methylglutaryl coenzyme A [HMG-CoA] reductase inhibitors), ezetimibe, bempedoic acid, PCSK9 inhibitors, bile acid sequestrants, MTP inhibitor, and ANGPLT3 inhibitor are used primarily to reduce LDL-C. Fibrates, niacin, and omega-3 fatty acid prescriptions are used primarily for the treatment of hypertriglyceridemia. These classes of agents differ with regard to degree and type of lipid lowering, and agents within the same group may differ in efficacy and side effects. Conventional dosing regimens and common adverse effects are summarized in Table 5. Expected changes in lipid profiles are shown in Table 6. The choice of drug depends on the specific lipid abnormalities, the patient's tolerability to the medication, and concurrent medical conditions. In general, statins are the most effective drugs to lower cardiovascular risk and are the treatment of choice when medications are indicated based on the global cardiovascular risk. If the treatment goal is not achieved by statins or statins are not tolerated, other validated nonstatin therapies (ezetimibe, bempedoic acid, and PCSK9 inhibitors) may be considered, followed by other agents such as bile acid sequestrants. If the primary goal is to lower TGs, fibrates, omega-3 fatty acids, or niacin may be more effective.

Statins

Statins are usually the first drug of choice in patients with high cholesterol levels to reduce cardiovascular risk and have been validated in multiple randomized controlled trials and their meta-analyses. Furthermore, risk reduction was apparent in a wide range of patients in both primary and secondary prevention; in men and women, smokers, patients with diabetes, and those with hypertension. In general, statins result in a high degree of LDL-C reduction. The approximate equipotent dosages of various statins and their cholesterol-lowering effects are listed in Table 7. The 2013 and 2018 cholesterol guidelines recommend moderate- or high-intensity statins (see Table 2) based on the global risk. Statins inhibit HMG-CoA reductase, the rate-limiting enzyme in cholesterol biosynthesis. By blocking cholesterol biosynthesis, statins upregulate the LDLR on the hepatocytes and increase clearance of IDL and LDL. In addition to their direct effects on lipid metabolism, statins have been reported to have pleiotropic effects (e.g., reduced formation of reactive oxygen species, inhibition of platelet reactivity, and decreased vasoconstriction).

TABLE 4	Lifestyle Therapy for Persistent Hypertriglyceridemia *(2021 ACC ECDP on Persistent Hypertriglyceridemia)*		
	TG <500 MG/DL	**TG 500–999 MG/DL**	**TG ≥1000 MG/DL**
Added sugars (% calories)	<6%	<5%	Eliminate
Total fat (% calories)	30%–35%	20%–25%	10%–15%
Alcohol	Restrict	Eliminate	Eliminate
Aerobic activity	At least 150 minutes of moderate intensity or 75 minutes of vigorous intensity aerobic activity each week, or equivalent combinations of both		
Weight loss (% of body weight)	5%–10% weight loss		

ACC ECDP, American College of Cardiology Expert Consensus Decision Pathway; *TG*, triglycerides.

TABLE 5 Major Drugs for Management of Hyperlipidemia

AGENT	STARTING DAILY DOSAGE	DOSAGE RANGE	MECHANISM	SIDE EFFECTS
Statins				
Lovastatin (Mevacor)	20 mg	10–80 mg	Decreased cholesterol synthesis, increased hepatic LDL receptors, decreased VLDL release	Myalgias, arthralgias, high liver enzymes, dyspepsia
Pravastatin (Pravachol)	40 mg	10–80 mg		
Simvastatin (Zocor)	20–40 mg	5–40 mg		
Fluvastatin (Lescol)	40 mg	20–80 mg		
Atorvastatin (Lipitor)	10–20 mg	10–80 mg		
Rosuvastatin (Crestor)	10 mg	5–40 mg		
Pitavastatin (Livalo)	2 mg	2–4 mg		
Cholesterol Absorption Inhibitors				
Ezetimibe (Zetia)	10 mg	10 mg	Deceased intestinal cholesterol absorption	High liver enzymes
Combination Therapies (Single Pill)				
Ezetimibe/Simvastatin (Vytorin)	10/20 mg	10/10–10/40 mg		
ATP Citrate Lyase Inhibitor				
Bempedoic acid (Nexletol)	180 mg		Inhibit cholesterol synthesis, increase LDLR and cholesterol clearance	Uric acid level increase, gout, tendon rupture
Combination Therapies (Single Pill)				
Bempedoic acid/Ezetimibe (Nexlizet)	180/10 mg			
PCSK9 Inhibiting Monoclonal Antibodies (Subcutaneous)				
Alirocumab (Praluent)	75 mg every 2 wk	75–150 mg every 2 wk	Increased hepatic LDL receptors	Injection site reactions, nasopharyngitis, upper respiratory tract infection, influenza, back pain
Evolocumab (Repatha)		140 mg every 2 wk or 420 mg mo		
PCSK9 Inhibiting siRNA (Subcutaneous)				
Inclisiran (Leqvio)	284 mg at baseline and 3 mo, then every 6 mo		Increased hepatic LDL receptors	Injection site reactions, arthralgia, bronchitis
ANGPLT3 Inhibiting Monoclonal Antibody (Intravenous Infusion)				
Evinacumab (Evkeeza)	15 mg/kg every 4 wk		Inhibiting LPL and endothelial lipase	Nasopharyngitis, dizziness
Bile Acid Sequestrants				
Cholestyramine (Questran)	8–16 g	4–24 g	Increased bile acid excretion, increased LDL receptors	Bloating, constipation, elevated TGs
Colestipol (Colestid)	2 g	2–16 g		
Colesevelam (Welchol)	3.75 g	3.75 g		
Fibrates				
Fenofibrate (Tricor)	48–145 mg	48–145 mg	Increased LPL activity, decreased VLDL synthesis	Dyspepsia, myalgia, gallstones, high liver enzymes
Gemfibrozil (Lopid)	1200 mg	1200 mg		
Fenofibric acid (Trilipix)	45–135 mg	45–135 mg		
Niacin				
Immediate release	250 mg	250–3000 mg	Decreased VLDL synthesis	Flushing, high glucose, uric acid, high liver enzymes
Extended release (Niaspan)	500 mg	500–2000 mg		

TABLE 5	Major Drugs for Management of Hyperlipidemia—cont'd				
AGENT	STARTING DAILY DOSAGE	DOSAGE RANGE	MECHANISM	SIDE EFFECTS
Omega-3 Fatty Acid Prescriptions				
Icosapent ethyl (Vascepa)	4 g	4 g		Arthralgia, atrial fibrillation, lower extremity edema
Omega-3 fatty acid ethyl esters (Lovaza)	4 g	4 g		Eructation, dyspepsia, and taste perversion

ATP, Adenosine triphosphate; *LDL*, low-density lipoprotein; *LDLR*, low-density lipoprotein receptor; *PCSK9*, proprotein convertase subtilisin/kexin type 9; *TG*, triglycerides; *VLDL*, very-low-density lipoprotein.

TABLE 6	Metabolic Effects of Each Lipid-Lowering Drug Class		
	LDL-C	HDL-C	TGS
Statins	↓21%–55%	↓2%–10%	↓6%–30%
Fibric acids	↓20%–25%	↑6%–18%	↓20%–35%
Niacin	↓10%–25%	↑10%–35%	↓20%–30%
Bile acid sequestrants	↓15%–25%		May ↑
Cholesterol absorption inhibitors	↓10%–18%		
PCSK9 inhibitors	↓39%–62%	↑4%–7%	↓12%–17%

HDL-C, High-density lipoprotein cholesterol; *LDL-C*, low-density lipoprotein cholesterol; *PCSK9*, proprotein convertase subtilisin/kexin type 9; *TG*, triglycerides.
Modified from Lipoprotein management in patients with cardiometabolic risk, consensus statement from the American College of Cardiology Foundation and the American Diabetes Association (ACC/ADA) (2008), and American Association of Clinical Endocrinologists' (AACE) guidelines for management of dyslipidemia and prevention of atherosclerosis (2012).

TABLE 7	Equipotency and Percentage Reduction in Total Cholesterol According to the Different Types and Doses of Statins				
REDUCTION IN TOTAL CHOLESTEROL (%)	PRAVASTATIN (PRAVACHOL), MG	FLUVASTATIN (LESCOL), MG	SIMVASTATIN (ZOCOR)*, MG	ATORVASTATIN (LIPITOR), MG	ROSUVASTATIN (CRESTOR), MG
6–15	5	10	–	–	–
15–17	10	20	5	2.5	–
22	20	40	10	5	–
27	40[†]	80[†]	20[†]	10[†]	5[†]
32	80[†]	–	40[†]	20[†]	10[†]
37	–	–	(80)	40[‡]	20[‡]
42	–	–	–	80[‡]	40[‡]

*See the text for the FDA warning.
[†]Moderate-intensity statins (reduction of LDL-C 30%–49%).
[‡]High-intensity statins (reduction of LDL-C ≥50%).
FDA, US Food and Drug Administration; *LDL-C*, low-density lipoprotein cholesterol.
Modified from Penning-van Beest, F. J. A., Termorshuizen, F., Goettsch, W. G. et al. (2007. Adherence to evidence-based statin guidelines reduces the risk of hospitalizations for acute myocardial infarction by 40%: a cohort study. *Eur Heart J, 28,* 154–159.

Statins are usually well tolerated. Potential common side effects include myopathy, fatigue, headaches, and nonspecific gastrointestinal symptoms such as dyspepsia. Elevation of liver enzymes occurs in less than 1%. There is also a small but significant association with increase in risk of developing diabetes. Myopathy is one of the most common causes for cessation of statins. Myalgia can occur in about 10% to 20% of patients, which is much more often than reported in the clinical trials. The risk of rhabdomyolysis, however, is very low (0.1–0.2/1000 person-years). Risk for myopathy is increased in patients with advanced age, female sex, small body habitus, hypothyroidism, alcoholism, vitamin D deficiency, medical conditions (particularly liver or kidney disease), major surgery, excessive physical activity, history of myopathy, family history of myopathy, high-dose statins, and interacting medications or food such as grapefruit juice (>1 L/day). Simvastatin (Zocor), lovastatin (Mevacor), and atorvastatin (Lipitor) are primarily metabolized through CYP3A4, which is inhibited by protease inhibitors, cyclosporine (Neoral, Sandimmune), amiodarone (Cordarone, Pacerone), nondihydropyridine calcium channel blockers, fibrates, and other agents. Pravastatin (Pravachol) is metabolized by the kidney, not by the P450 system. Fluvastatin (Lescol) and rosuvastatin (Crestor) are primarily metabolized through CYP2C9. Pitavastatin (Livalo) is marginally metabolized by CYP2C9 and to a lesser extent by CYP2C8. Simvastatin and lovastatin should be avoided in patients receiving protease inhibitors. Statin dosage should be reduced in patients taking cyclosporine. Because of significant risk of myopathy and rhabdomyolysis related to high-dose simvastatin, the US Food and Drug Administration (FDA) recommends that 80 mg/day should not be used. The FDA further recommends that the dose be limited to 20 mg if the patient is also taking amiodarone, amlodipine (Norvasc), or ranolazine (Ranexa), and to 10 mg/day if taking diltiazem (Cardizem), dronedarone (Multaq), or verapamil (Calan). Addition of fibrates increases the risk of myopathy; in patients on a statin, fenofibrate (Tricor) is preferred, whereas gemfibrozil (Lopid), which has a much higher risk of rhabdomyolysis, is contraindicated. Symptoms of statin myopathy are heaviness, stiffness, cramping associated with weakness during exertion, and tendon-associated pain. Location of symptoms can be at the thighs, at the calves, or generalized. Symptoms can be very nonspecific, and differentiating statin-related myopathy from other causes is not easy. Therefore baseline symptoms, physical examination, and assessment of creatinine kinase level before the initiation of statins can be very helpful. Modifiable risk factors for statin-induced myopathy, such as hypothyroidism and vitamin D deficiency, should be optimally managed. Further decisions regarding stopping, dose reduction, or switching medications can be made based on the severity of symptoms, level of creatinine kinase elevation, and presence of rhabdomyolysis. In patients who develop myopathy while on simvastatin or atorvastatin, if the decision is to continue treatment with a statin, one option is to cautiously switch them to pravastatin, fluvastatin, or rosuvastatin, which are less prone to cause myopathy. Alternatively, lower statin dosing or less frequent dosing may be considered. For instance, rosuvastatin has a long duration of action and can be taken once every other day[1] or weekly,[1] if necessary. For patients who cannot tolerate statins, other agents should be used, starting with validated nonstatin agents.

Ezetimibe

Ezetimibe (Zetia, generic) is the first in a new class of pharmaceutical agents that primarily targets the cholesterol transport protein Niemann-Pick C1–like 1 protein in the intestine. Ezetimibe is an efficacious and cost-effective add-on agent in people taking a statin, if the LDL-C goal is not achieved or high doses of statin cannot be tolerated. Ezetimibe was shown to modestly decrease LDL-C and cardiovascular events when added to simvastatin in high-risk patients in the Improved Reduction of Outcomes: Vytorin Efficacy International Trial (IMPROVE-IT) study. Moreover, ezetimibe has become generic in the United States, and its safety profile is well characterized. Elevated liver enzymes have been reported, but the risk of hepatotoxicity seems to be no different from that of placebo.

PCSK9 Inhibitors

The PCSK9 protein plays a major role in regulating the number of LDLRs at the cell surface, including on hepatocytes. Binding of the LDLR by PCSK9 leads to the destruction of the LDLR. Therefore interference with the binding capacity of PCSK9 to LDLR or silencing the expression of the *PCSK9* gene allows more LDLRs to recycle to the cell surface, effecting the removal of more of the circulating plasma LDL. Gain-of-function mutations of the *PCSK9* gene were found to underlie a rare form of autosomal dominant hypercholesterolemia, and conversely, individuals with loss-of-function mutations in the *PCSK9* gene were found to have very low LDL-C levels and protected from coronary heart disease. These discoveries led to the development of pharmacologic agents against *PCSK9* as a novel cholesterol-lowering treatment.

To date, three anti-PCSK9 agents with different mechanisms of action have been approved by the FDA for lowering cholesterol. Two of them are human monoclonal antibodies (alirocumab [Praluent] and evolocumab [Repatha]), whereas the other is small interference ribonucleic acid (siRNA) (inclisiran [Leqvio]). All are administered by subcutaneous injection and have similar efficacy in LDL-C reduction. Both alirocumab and evolocumab have been shown to provide cardiovascular benefit in outcome trials, whereas the cardiovascular outcome trial for inclisiran is currently underway.

In the Further Cardiovascular Outcomes Research With PCSK9 Inhibition in Subjects With Elevated Risk (FOURIER) trial, evolocumab was found to significantly reduce the risk for ASCVD events in patients with clinical ASCVD and LDL-C of 70 mg/dL or greater or a non–HDL-C level of 100 mg/dL or greater who were receiving optimized lipid lowering using a high-intensity statin or at least atorvastatin 20 mg with or without ezetimibe. Similarly, in the Evaluation of Cardiovascular Outcomes After an Acute Coronary Syndrome During Treatment With Alirocumab (ODYSSEY OUTCOMES) trial, alirocumab was shown to significantly reduce the risk for ASCVD events in patients with recent acute coronary syndrome who had a LDL-C of 70 mg/dL or greater, a non-HDL-C of 100 mg/dL or greater, or an apo B level of 80 mg/dL or greater and who were receiving statin therapy at a high-intensity dose or at the maximum tolerated dose. Considering the results, the 2018 Multisociety guidelines and the *2022 ACC ECDP on Nonstatin Therapies* recommended adding PCSK9 inhibitors in secondary prevention patients on maximally tolerated statin and in primary prevention patients with high baseline LDL-C levels of 190 mg/dL or greater not from secondary causes if treatment goals appropriate for the risk are not achieved (see Table 2). Both alirocumab and evolocumab are also indicated for heterozygous and homozygous familial hypercholesterolemia (HeFH and HoFH, respectively) as an adjunct to other LDL-C–lowering therapies.

With lack of cardiovascular outcome results, inclisiran, at this time, should be considered as an alternative to the monoclonal antibodies for PCSK9 if the latter fails to achieve appropriate LDL-C goals. Inclisiran is typically administered in clinic twice annually after initial injections at baseline and 3 months; thus it is particularly useful for patients who have difficulty with self-administering the monoclonal antibodies that are required every 2 weeks or monthly.

PCSK9 inhibitors are powerful LDL-C–lowering agents and enable reduction of LDL-C by up to approximately 60% as a single agent or an adjunct therapy. Moreover, the absolute level of LDL-C achieved may be as low as less than 25 mg/dL. There have been concerns regarding the potential adverse effects that may occur at such low LDL-C levels, such as neurocognitive side effects. However, results from these trials and their subanalyses have not shown a significant signal, although more long-term follow-up analysis is needed. Common side effects associated with PCSK9 inhibitors include injection site reactions, nasopharyngitis, upper respiratory tract infection, influenza, and back pain.

A significant hurdle to more widespread use of PCSK9 inhibitors is their high cost. Since their approval in 2015 by the FDA, the cost of evolocumab and alirocumab has consistently decreased and approached the threshold of cost-effectiveness. As a result, the *2022 ACC ECDP on Nonstatin Therapies* dropped the value statement on PCSK9 inhibitors and lowered the threshold for adding them.

Bempedoic Acid

Bempedoic acid (Nexletol) is a new anticholesterol medication that decreases cholesterol synthesis by inhibiting ATP citrate lyase. It is a prodrug, requiring conversion in the liver by very-long-chain acyl-CoA synthetase, which is absent in muscle and is thus expected to have minimal muscle side effects compared with statins. Bempedoic acid added to maximally tolerated statin therapy led to a mean of 18% further reduction in LDL-C. A fixed-dose combination of bempedoic and ezetimibe (Nexlizet) added to a maximally tolerated dose of statins led to a 38% reduction of LDL-C. It is well tolerated, with the main side effects being an increase in uric acid level and tendon rupture. It is approved for patients with ASCVD or HeFH who require further LDL-C lowering, and the *2022 ACC ECDP on Nonstatin Therapies* suggested that it be added after ezetimibe and PCSK9 inhibitors if further LDL-C lowering is indicated. In the recently finished CLEAR outcome trial, patients with ASCVD or at high risk for ASCVD who did not tolerate or would not take any statins were given bempedoic acid or placebo; after a median follow-up of 40.6 months, patients treated with bempedoic acid had significantly reduced 4-point major adverse cardiovascular events, the study's primary end point. Although this result has yet to be reflected in any guidelines, it would be reasonable to consider

---

[1] Not FDA approved for this indication.

bempedoic acid for both primary[1] and secondary prevention if the desired LDL goal has not been achieved after maximally tolerated statin and ezetimibe. A possible cost-effective algorithm for adding nonstatins could be adding ezetimibe if less than 25% further reduction is needed to reach treatment goal, bempedoic acid/ezetimibe combination (Nexlizet) if 25% to 50% reduction is needed, and PCSK9 inhibitors if 50% or greater reduction is needed.

Bile Acid Sequestrants

Bile acid sequestrants have been in clinical use for many decades. These agents promote fecal excretion of bile acids. The liver responds with increased integration of cholesterol into bile acid synthesis to maintain a stable bile acid pool. The consequent decrease in cholesterol in the liver leads to upregulation of the LDLR and enhanced LDL clearance from the plasma. HMG-CoA synthase activity can increase, so combination therapy with statins would be synergistic, especially in patients with a suboptimal response. Available agents are cholestyramine (Questran), colestipol (Colestid), and colesevelam (Welchol). Most side effects involve the gastrointestinal tract, with constipation and bloating being the most common. These agents may interfere with the absorption of warfarin, phenobarbital, levothyroxine (Synthroid), and digoxin (Lanoxin), among other medications. Patients on multiple medications should be advised to take bile acid sequestrants 1 hour before or 4 hours after taking the other medications. These agents can also cause elevation of TG level and are contraindicated if TG level is greater than 500 mg/dL. Because they are not systemically absorbed, the bile acid sequestrants may be the preferred agents when systemic absorption is to be avoided, such as during pregnancy or lactation.

Fibrates

The effect of fibrates on cardiovascular outcomes is not as favorable as with statins. However, fibrates can be useful in subsets of patients with high TGs and low HDL-C. The Action to Control Cardiovascular Risk in Diabetes (ACCORD) lipid trial showed that addition of fenofibrate to simvastatin in patients with type 2 diabetes with cardiovascular risk factors did not improve cardiovascular outcomes, although there was a trend for better outcomes in a subgroup with TGs greater than 204 mg/dL and HDL-C less than 34 mg/dL. Fibrates have multiple favorable metabolic effects, including activation of peroxisome proliferator-activated receptor-α (contributing to the regulation of both lipid and carbohydrate metabolism), stimulation of LPL (increasing TG hydrolysis), and downregulation of Apo CIII (improving lipoprotein remnant clearance as Apo CIII inhibits LPL). An enhanced VLDL-to-LDL conversion may lead to mild LDL-C elevation in some patients. This effect may decrease over weeks as the LDLRs are upregulated. Interestingly, fenofibrate has been shown to delay the progression of diabetic retinopathy[1] and should be considered in such patients beside standard treatments. Fibrates are generally well tolerated. The most common side effect is dyspepsia. Other side effects include myopathy and hepatic enzyme elevation, particularly when fibrates are added to statins. The use of gemfibrozil (Lopid) should be avoided in patients on statin therapy due to increased risk for muscle-related adverse events. Fibrates increase the risk of gallstones, and patients on warfarin (Coumadin) may need dose adjustment. Monitoring of liver enzymes is recommended, at baseline and within 3 months and then periodically. Creatinine level can be increased through unclear mechanisms.

Niacin

Niacin or nicotinic acid effectively decreases the hepatic production of VLDL and thus LDL-C levels and raises HDL-C levels by reducing cholesterol transfer from HDL to Apo B–containing lipoproteins and HDL clearance by the liver. Niacin is also able to reduce the level of Lp(a) by about 20%; however, this effect on the reduction of cardiovascular events in patients with elevated Lp(a)

is not known. Several trials showed the effect of niacin in preventing cardiovascular disease; however, the benefit of adding niacin to statins has not been proved. Niacin did not improve cardiovascular risk when added to simvastatin in patients with high risk for cardiovascular disease in the Atherothrombosis Intervention in Metabolic Syndrome with Low HDL/High TGs: Impact on Global Health Outcomes (AIM-HIGH) study and the Heart Protection Study 2–Treatment of HDL to Reduce the Incidence of Vascular Events (HPS2-Thrive) study. There were excess adverse events and trends toward signs of harm among the niacin groups. The FDA has recently withdrawn the approval for the coadministration of niacin extended-release tablets (Niaspan) with statins. The most common side effect of niacin is flushing. This can be avoided or minimized by initiating therapy with a low dose of niacin, taking an aspirin 1 hour before niacin, avoiding hot foods or beverages at the time the niacin is taken, or switching to extended-release forms (Niaspan). Hepatotoxicity can occur at any time. Immediate-release forms are less likely to cause hepatotoxicity than sustained-release forms (Slo-Niacin). Extended-release forms can minimally elevate transaminases, but significant hepatotoxicity is rare. They can, however, also cause dose-dependent reversible thrombocytopenia, which can be insidious and severe. When switching to different forms, it is recommended that one should start with low doses and titrate up to achieve desired response. Liver function tests should be monitored regularly, at baseline and every 3 months for the first year, and then periodically. Other side effects include pruritus, increased uric acid levels, and hyperglycemia.

Omega-3 Fatty Acid Prescriptions

Highly purified omega-3 fatty acid preparations containing either a mixture of EPA and DHA (Lovaza) or EPA alone (Vascepa) are effective agents used in the treatment of hypertriglyceridemia, the first FDA-approved indication for these agents. Omega-3 fatty acids are polyunsaturated fatty acids and are essential in humans. A significant proportion of omega-3 fatty acids is consumed in the diet. Major dietary sources of omega-3 fatty acids include nuts, vegetable oils, flax seeds, and leafy vegetables, as well as fish and fish oil. EPA and DHA are the two major types of marine-derived omega-3 fatty acids. The mechanism by which omega-3 fatty acids lower TGs is incompletely understood.

Multiple clinical trials have been examining the efficacy of omega-3 fatty acid in improving cardiovascular outcome. Although trials using lower doses of EPA-DHA mixtures (≤1 g total daily) have shown inconsistent results, findings from recent trials assessing higher doses of pure EPA have been more favorable.

Purified EPA was first shown in the Japan Eicosapentaenoic acid Lipid Intervention Study (JELIS) trial to significantly reduce risk for major coronary events in patients with hypercholesterolemia. Subsequently, the Reduction of Cardiovascular Events With Icosapent Ethyl–Intervention Trial (REDUCE-IT) study, a large, randomized controlled trial, assessed the efficacy and safety of purified EPA ethyl ester, icosapent ethyl (Vascepa) in secondary prevention and high-risk primary prevention patients with reasonably controlled LDL-C but elevated TGs. The REDUCE-IT trial showed that treatment with icosapent ethyl was associated with a significant reduction in ASCVD events. In secondary analyses, icosapent ethyl has also been shown to reduce the risk for total ischemic events (first plus subsequent events). Results from REDUCE-IT suggest that high-risk patients with elevated TGs reap additional cardiovascular benefits from icosapent ethyl, when the latter is added to LDL-C lowering therapies. Finally, the overall rates of adverse events were not significantly different between the treatment and control arms of REDUCE-IT. However, there were increased rates of atrial fibrillation and peripheral edema associated with patients taking icosapent ethyl observed in the trial. On the strength of the REDUCE-IT trial, the FDA has approved icosapent ethyl for reduction of cardiovascular events in high-risk patients with elevated TG levels. Icosapent ethyl has also been incorporated into the *2021 ACC ECDP on Persistent Hypertriglyceridemia*, which recommends icosapent ethyl be added to other cholesterol-lowering

---

[1] Not FDA approved for this indication.

medications in patients with clinical ASCVD or in diabetic patients who are more than 50 years old and who have an additional risk factor, if the fasting TG level is 150 mg/dL or greater.

Evinacumab

Evinacumab (Evkeeza) is a human monoclonal antibody against ANGPLT3, a dual inhibitor for LPL and endothelial lipase. Genetic deficiency of ANGPLT3 was associated with a very low level of LDL-C and TGs and significantly reduced ASCVD risk. The mechanism for LDL reduction with ANGPLT3 inactivation is independent from LDLR; thus evinacumab could be effective for patients with HoFH. In the ELIPSE HoFH trial, evinacumab was shown to reduce LDL-C by approximately 50% in HoFH patients on stable therapy with baseline LDL-C of 70 mg/dL or greater. The treatment was well tolerated, with side effects comparable to the placebo group. Currently, evinacumab is approved by the FDA for treating patients with HoFH who need further LDL-C reduction. It is administered via intravenous infusion every 4 weeks.

References

2019 ESC/EAS guidelines for the management of dyslipidaemias, *Eur Heart J* 41:111–188, 2020.

ACCORD Study Group; ACCORD Eye Study Group, Chew EY, et al: Effects of medical therapies on retinopathy progression in type 2 diabetes, *N Engl J Med* 363:233–244, 2010.

Bhatt DL, Steg PG, Miller M, et al: Cardiovascular risk reduction with icosapent ethyl for hypertriglyceridemia, *N Engl J Med* 380(1):11–22, 2019.

Bhatt DL, Steg PG, Miller M, et al: Effects of icosapent ethyl on total ischemic events: from REDUCE-IT, *J Am Coll Cardiol*, 2019.

Brunzell JD, Davidson M, Furberg CD: Lipoprotein management in patients with cardiometabolic risk: consensus conference report from the ADA and the ACC foundation, *J Am Coll Cardiol* 51:1512–1524, 2008.

Chen SH, Habib G, Yang CJ, et al: Apolipoprotein B-48 is the product of a messenger RNA with an organ-specific in-frame stop codon, *Science* 238:363–366, 1987.

Dullaart RP: PCSK9 Inhibition to reduce cardiovascular events, *N Engl J Med* 376:1713–1722, 2017.

Eckel RH, Jakicic JM, Ard JD, et al: 2013 ACC/AHA guideline on lifestyle management to reduce cardiovascular risk: a report of the American College of Cardiology/American Heart Association task force on practice guidelines, *J Am Coll Cardiol* 63:2960–2984, 2014.

Elam M, Lovato L, Ginsberg H: The ACCORD-Lipid study: implications for treatment of dyslipidemia in Type 2 diabetes mellitus, *Clin Lipidol* 6:9–20, 2011.

Everett BM, Smith RJ, Hiatt WR: Reducing LDL with PCSK9 inhibitors — the clinical benefit of lipid drugs, *N Engl J Med* 373:1588–1591, 2015.

Ginsberg HN, Elam MB, Lovato LC, et al: Effects of combination lipid therapy in type 2 diabetes mellitus, *N Engl J Med* 362:1563–1574, 2010.

Goff Jr DC, Khan SS, Lloyd-Jones D, et al: Bending the curve in Cardiovascular Disease Mortality: bethesda + 40 and beyond, *Circulation* 143:837–851, 2021.

Greenland P, Alpert JS, Beller GA, et al: 2010 ACCF/AHA guideline for assessment of cardiovascular risk in asymptomatic adults: a report of the American College of Cardiology Foundation/American Heart Association Task Force on Practice Guidelines developed in collaboration with the American Society of Echocardiography, American Society of Nuclear Cardiology, Society of Atherosclerosis Imaging and Prevention, Society for Cardiovascular Angiography and Interventions, Society of Cardiovascular Computed Tomography, and Society for Cardiovascular Magnetic Resonance, *J Am Coll Cardiol* 56:e50–e103, 2010.

Grundy SM, Cleeman JI, Merz CNB, et al: Implications of recent clinical trials for the national cholesterol education program adult treatment panel III guidelines, *Circulation* 110:227–239, 2004.

Grundy SM, Stone NJ, Bailey AL, et al: AHA/ACC/AACVPR/AAPA/ABC/ACPM/ADA/AGS/APhA/ASPC/NLA/PCNA guideline on the management of blood cholesterol: executive summary: a report of the American College of Cardiology/American Heart Association Task Force on Clinical Practice Guidelines, *J Am Coll Cardiol* 18:39033–39038, 2018. pii: S0735-1097.

Hlatky MA, Kazi DS: PCSK9 inhibitors: economics and policy, *J Am Coll Cardiol* 70(21):2677–2687, 2017.

Huffman MD, Capewell S, Ning H, et al: Cardiovascular health behavior and health factor changes (1988–2008) and projections to 2020: results from the National Health and Nutrition Examination Surveys (NHANES), *Circulation* 125:2595–2602, 2012.

IMPROVE-IT Investigators: Ezetimibe added to statin therapy after acute coronary syndromes, *N Engl J Med* 372:2387–2397, 2015.

Jellinger PS, Smith DA, Mehta AE, et al: American Association of Clinical Endocrinologists' guidelines for management of hyperlipidemia and prevention of atherosclerosis, *Endocr Pract* 18:1–78, 2012.

Joy TR, Hegele RA: Narrative review: statin-related myopathy, *Ann Intern Med* 150:858–868, 2009.

Kazi DS, Moran AE, Coxson PG, et al: Cost-effectiveness of PCSK9 inhibitor therapy in patients with heterozygous familial hypercholesterolemia or atherosclerotic cardiovascular disease, *JAMA* 316(7):743–753, 2016.

Keaney JF, Curfman GD, Jarcho JA: A pragmatic view of the new cholesterol treatment guidelines, *N Engl J Med* 370:275–278, 2014.

Musunuru K, Kathiresan S: Surprises from genetic analyses of lipid risk factors for atherosclerosis, *Circ Res* 118(4):579–585, 2016.

Newman CB, Blaha MJ, Boord JB, et al: Lipid management in patients with endocrine disorders: an Endocrine Society clinical practice guideline, *J Clin Endocrinol Metab* 105:3613–3682, 2020.

Nissen SE, Lincoff AM, Brennan D, et al: CLEAR Outcomes Investigators. Bempedoic acid and cardiovascular outcomes in statin-intolerant patients, *N Engl J Med* 388(15):1353–1364, 2023.

O'Connell C, Horwood K, Nadamuni M: Correction of refractory thrombocytopenia and anemia following withdrawal of extended release niacin, *Am J Hematol* 91(7):E318, 2016.

Orringer CE, Blaha MJ, Blankstein R, et al: The National Lipid Association scientific statement on coronary artery calcium scoring to guide preventive strategies for ASCVD risk reduction, *J Clin Lipidol* 15(1):33–60, 2021.

Otvos JD, Collins D, Freedman DS, et al: Low-density lipoprotein and high-density lipoprotein particle subclasses predict coronary events and are favorably changed by gemfibrozil therapy in the Veterans Affairs High-Density Lipoprotein Intervention Trial, *Circulation* 113:1556–1563, 2006.

Penning-van Beest FJA, Termorshuizen F, Goettsch WG, et al: Adherence to evidence-based statin guidelines reduces the risk of hospitalizations for acute myocardial infarction by 40%: a cohort study, *Eur Heart J* 28:154–159, 2007.

Phan BAP, Dayspring TD, Toth PP: Ezetimibe therapy: mechanism of action and clinical update, *Vasc Health Risk Manag* 8:415–427, 2012.

Reiner Z, Catapano AL, De Backer G, et al: ESC/EAS guidelines for the management of dyslipidaemias: the task force for the management of dyslipidaemias of the European Society of Cardiology (ESC) and the European Atherosclerosis Society (EAS), *Eur Heart J* 32:1769–1818, 2011.

Reyes-Soffer G, Ginsberg HN, Berglund L, American Heart Association Council on Arteriosclerosis, Thrombosis and Vascular Biology; Council on Cardiovascular Radiology and Intervention; and Council on Peripheral Vascular Disease, et al: Lipoprotein(a): a genetically determined, causal, and prevalent risk factor for atherosclerotic cardiovascular disease: a scientific statement from the American Heart Association, *Arterioscler Thromb Vasc Biol* 42(1):e48–e60, 2022.

Ridker PM, Cook NR: Statins: new American guidelines for prevention of cardiovascular disease, *Lancet* 382:1762–1765, 2013.

Robinson JG, Farnier M, Krempf M, et al: Efficacy and safety of alirocumab in reducing lipids and cardiovascular events, *N Engl J Med* 372:1489–1499, 2015.

Robinson JG, Rosenson RS, Farnier M, et al: Safety of very low low-density lipoprotein cholesterol levels with alirocumab, *J Am Coll Cardiol* 69(5):471–482, 2017.

Sabatine MS, Giugliano RP, Keech AC, et al: Evolocumab and clinical outcomes in patients with cardiovascular disease, *N Engl J Med* 376(18):1713–1722, 2017.

Sabatine MS, Giugliano RP, Wiviott SD, et al: Efficacy and safety of evolocumab in reducing lipids and cardiovascular events, *N Engl J Med* 372:1500–1509, 2015.

Schwartz GG, Steg PG, Szarek M, et al: Alirocumab and cardiovascular outcomes after acute coronary syndrome, *N Engl J Med* 379(22):2097–2107, 2018.

Semenkovich CF, Goldberg IJ: Disorders of lipid metabolism. In Melmed S, Koenig R, Auchus R, Goldfine A, editors: *Williams textbook of endocrinology E-Book*, ed 14, Elsevier - OHCE, 2020.

Stone NJ, Robinson J, Lichtenstein AH, et al: ACC/AHA guideline on the treatment of blood cholesterol to reduce atherosclerotic cardiovascular risk in adults: a report of the American College of Cardiology/American Heart Association task force on practice guidelines, *J Am Coll Cardiol* 63:2889–2934, 2014.

Tall AR, Rader DJ: Trials and tribulations of CETP inhibitors, *Circ Res* 122(1):106–112, 2018.

The AIM-HIGH Investigators: Niacin in patients with low HDL cholesterol levels receiving intensive statin therapy, *N Engl J Med* 365:2255–2267, 2011.

Third report of the National Cholesterol Education Program (NCEP) expert panel on: detection, evaluation, and treatment of high blood cholesterol in adults (Adult treatment panel III) final report, *Circulation* 106:3143–3421, 2002.

Tsao CW, Aday AW, Almarzooq ZI, et al: Heart Disease and Stroke Statistics-2023 Update: A Report From the American Heart Association, *Circulation* 147(8):e93–e621, 2023.

Tsimikas S: A test in context: lipoprotein(a): diagnosis, prognosis, controversies, and emerging therapies, *J Am Coll Cardiol* 69(6):692–711, 2017.

Virani S, Morris P, Agarwala A, et al: 2021 ACC expert consensus decision pathway on the management of ASCVD risk reduction in patients with persistent hypertriglyceridemia, *J Am Coll Cardiol* 78(9):960–993, 2021.

Writing Committee, Lloyd-Jones DM, Morris PB, Ballantyne CM, et al: 2022 ACC expert consensus decision pathway on the role of nonstatin therapies for LDL-cholesterol lowering in the management of atherosclerotic cardiovascular disease risk: a report of the American College of Cardiology Solution Set Oversight Committee, *J Am Coll Cardiol* 80(14):1366–1418, 2022.

Yokoyama M, Origasa H, Matsuzaki M, et al: Effects of eicosapentaenoic acid on major coronary events in hypercholesterolaemic patients (JELIS): a randomised open-label, blinded endpoint analysis, *Lancet* 369(9567):1090–1098, 2007.

HYPERPARATHYROIDISM AND HYPOPARATHYROIDISM

Method of
Claudio Marcocci, MD; and Filomena Cetani, MD

CURRENT DIAGNOSIS

Primary Hyperparathyroidism
- Third most common endocrine disorder and most common cause of hypercalcemia in the general population.
- Diagnosis based on confirmed hypercalcemia (total calcium [albumin corrected] or ionized calcium) associated with elevated or inappropriately normal serum parathyroid hormone (PTH) level.
- Hypercalcemia on routine blood testing or in postmenopausal women investigated for osteoporosis is typically the first clue to the diagnosis.
- Mainly occurs as a solitary disease (90%) but may be part of hereditary syndromes.
- Genetic causes should be searched for in young patients.

Secondary Hyperparathyroidism
- Secondary hyperparathyroidism defines any condition in which the increased PTH secretion occurs as a normal physiologic response, often mediated by a decrease of serum calcium.
- Vitamin D deficiency, as a result of inadequate nutritional intake/sun exposure, malabsorption, liver diseases, or chronic renal failure, is the most common cause.
- At variance with primary hyperparathyroidism, secondary hyperparathyroidism is characterized by low or, more often, low-normal serum calcium and decreased urinary calcium excretion.

Hypoparathyroidism
- Rare disorder.
- Inadvertent removal or damage to the parathyroid gland during thyroid surgery and, much less frequently, autoimmune destruction are the most common causes.
- Diagnosis based on low serum calcium along with undetectable or inappropriately low serum PTH level.

CURRENT THERAPY

Primary Hyperparathyroidism
- Parathyroidectomy is the only definitive therapy.
- Surgery should be considered in all cases and recommended in patients with symptoms and in those who, albeit asymptomatically, meet the surgical criteria.
- Surveillance without surgery can be considered in patients without symptoms who do not meet the surgical criteria.
- Patients not undergoing surgery should be given vitamin D when indicated, and calcium intake should not be restricted.
- Medical treatment can be considered in selected cases: antiresorptive therapy to increase bone mineral density and cinacalcet (Sensipar) to lower serum calcium.

Hypoparathyroidism
- Severe hypocalcemia is a medical emergency, and treatment with intravenous calcium should be promptly instituted and maintained for 24 to 48 hours; oral therapy with calcium and active vitamin D metabolites should be started as soon as practical.

- The goal of chronic treatment is to maintain serum calcium in the low-normal range, avoiding hypocalcemic symptoms and long-term complications.
- Chronic conventional therapy is based on adequate calcium intake (calcium supplement needed in most cases) and active vitamin D metabolites.
- Recombinant full-length parathyroid hormone 1 to 84 (Natpara) has been approved by the US Food and Drug Administration and European Medicines Agency for patients not controlled with conventional therapy.
- An individualized approach is necessary to optimize patient care. Lifelong monitoring is needed to decrease the risk of complications.

Primary Hyperparathyroidism
Epidemiology
Primary hyperparathyroidism (PHPT) is currently the third most common endocrine disorder and the most frequent cause of hypercalcemia in the general population.

The disease was considered rare until the early 1970s, when its incidence in the United States rose dramatically after the introduction of serum calcium in the multichannel autoanalyzer. The incidence varies according to geographic areas and assessment measures; recent data in the United States indicate an incidence of 79.6 per 100,000 person-years in women and 35.6 per 100,000 person-years in men of all races, with the highest rate among Black people. The incidence peaks in the sixth decade of life. The prevalence ranges between 1 and 7 cases per 1000 adults. Most cases occur in women (with a female-to-male ratio of 3:1), but there is no sex difference before the age of 45 years. PHPT is rare in children and adolescents.

Pathogenesis
PHPT mainly occurs as a solitary disease (90%) but may be part of hereditary syndromes (e.g., multiple endocrine neoplasia [MEN] types 1, 2A, 4, and 5; hyperparathyroidism–jaw tumor syndrome; familial isolated hyperparathyroidism) (Table 1). A single, benign adenoma is found in 80% to 85% of cases, multigland involvement in 15% to 20%, and parathyroid carcinoma in <1%. Multigland involvement is more common in hereditary cases, particularly MEN1. In the absence of local infiltration or metastases, the diagnosis of parathyroid carcinoma may be difficult at histology. Genetic studies (*CDC73* gene mutations) and immunohistochemical studies (loss of parafibromin [the protein encoded by the *CDC73* gene] expression) may help in equivocal cases. Predisposing factors are external neck irradiation in childhood and long-term lithium therapy.

PHPT is characterized by excessive parathyroid hormone (PTH) secretion from one or more parathyroid glands, due to the loss of the homeostatic control of PTH synthesis and secretion. Extracellular ionized calcium (Ca^{2+}_o) is the main regulator of PTH secretion. Ca^{2+}_o interacts with the Ca^{2+}-sensing receptor (CaSR) present on the surface of parathyroid cells; there is an inverse sigmoidal relationship between Ca^{2+}_o concentration and PTH release. In adenomas, hypercalcemia is due to the loss of normal sensitivity of the parathyroid cell to the inhibitory action of Ca^{2+}, whereas in parathyroid hyperplasia the increased number of parathyroid cells, which have a normal sensitivity to the inhibitory action of Ca^{2+}, causes hypercalcemia. Serum phosphate, 1,25-dihydroxyvitamin D ($1,25(OH)_2D$), and fibroblast growth factor 23 are also involved in the control of PTH secretion.

Although major progress has been made in the last two decades, the molecular basis of PHPT is still unclear in the majority of cases. The clonality of most parathyroid tumors suggests a defect in the pathways that control parathyroid cell proliferation or the expression of PTH. The genes involved are listed in Table 1. Germline mutations are often found in hereditary forms. On the other hand, somatic mutations may occur in sporadic cases, even

DISORDER	GENE	PATTERN OF INHERITANCE
Multiple endocrine neoplasia type 1	*MEN1*	Autosomal dominant
Multiple endocrine neoplasia type 2A	*RET*	Autosomal dominant
Multiple endocrine neoplasia type 4	*CDKN1B*	Autosomal dominant
Multiple endocrine neoplasia type 5	*MAX*	Autosomal dominant
Hyperparathyroidism–jaw tumor syndrome	*CDC73*	Autosomal dominant
Familial isolated hyperparathyroidism	*MEN1, CDC73, CASR, GCM2, CDKN1B*	Autosomal dominant
Familial hypocalciuric hypercalcemia type 1	*CASR*	Autosomal dominant
Familial hypocalciuric hypercalcemia type 2	*GNA11*	Autosomal dominant
Familial hypocalciuric hypercalcemia type 3	*AP2S1*	Autosomal dominant
Neonatal severe hyperparathyroidism	*CASR*	Autosomal recessive

AP2S1, Adaptor-related protein complex 2 sigma 1 subunit; *CASR*, calcium-sensing receptor; *CDC73*, cell division cycle 73; *CDKN1B*, cyclin-dependent kinase inhibitor 1B; *GCM2*, glial cells missing transcription factor 2; *GNA11*, G protein subunit alpha 11; *MAX*, myc-associated factor x; *MEN1*, multiple endocrine neoplasia type 1; *PHPT*, primary hyperparathyroidism; *RET*, rearranged during transfection.

though germline mutations have also been described in apparently sporadic cases.

Clinical Presentation

In recent years the clinical presentation of PHPT in Western countries has changed from a symptomatic disease, characterized by hypercalcemia and renal (nephrolithiasis and nephrocalcinosis) and skeletal (osteitis fibrosa cystica, fragility fractures) manifestations, to one with subtle and nonspecific clinical manifestations (asymptomatic PHPT). Nephrolithiasis remains the most common classic clinical manifestation (15%–20%), and silent stones are frequently detected at ultrasound. Bone mineral density (BMD) is reduced particularly at sites rich in cortical bone (one-third distal radius). Studies using peripheral high-resolution quantitative computed tomography (CT) have shown involvement of both cortical and trabecular sites, the latter confirmed by the trabecular bone score (TBS) at the lumbar spine. An increased rate of vertebral and nonverbal fractures has also been documented. Nonclassical manifestations, including subtle cardiovascular abnormalities and psychological and cognitive symptoms, have also been reported.

A new variant of PHPT (normocalcemic PHPT) has recently been identified, namely patients with increased serum PTH levels in the absence of hypercalcemia (also by measurement of ionized calcium) or other causes of secondary hyperparathyroidism (SHPT). This condition, called normocalcemic PHPT, has been typically recognized in persons evaluated for low BMD, in whom PTH was measured even in the absence of hypercalcemia. In some cases, this new phenotype may represent an early phase of classical hypercalcemic PHPT, when PTH elevation precedes the occurrence of hypercalcemia.

Evaluation and Diagnosis

The finding of hypercalcemia on routine blood testing or in postmenopausal women investigated for osteoporosis is typically the first clue to the diagnosis of PHPT. Hypercalcemia should be confirmed in repeated testing, preferably evaluating albumin-corrected total calcium (measured total calcium in mg/dL + [0.8 × (4.0 – serum albumin in g/dL)]) or ionized calcium. The next diagnostic step is the measurement of serum PTH. An elevated (or unexpectedly normal) serum PTH in the face of hypercalcemia is virtually diagnostic of PHPT. Serum phosphate is normal or in the low-normal range in mild PHPT and low in severe cases. A low or undetectable PTH level in a patient with hypercalcemia rules out the diagnosis of PHPT. The most common cause of PTH-independent hypercalcemia is malignancy, where hypercalcemia is due to the secretion by the tumor of PTH-related peptide, a molecule that shares with PTH the amino-terminal active part but does not cross-react in the PTH assay, or osteolytic lytic bone metastases. Urinary calcium should also be measured. If hypercalciuria is >400 mg per day, a more extended evaluation of the stone risk profile should be performed. Urinary calcium measurement is also useful to exclude familial hypocalciuric hypercalcemia, which is suggested by the finding of the calcium-to-creatinine clearance ratio of <0.01.

A hereditary form of PHPT, accounting for 5% to 10% of cases, should be sought in patients younger than 30 years at diagnosis, with a family history of hypercalcemia and/or neuroendocrine tumors (see Table 1). In this setting, serum calcium should be measured in first-degree relatives and genetic tests performed. Parathyroid cancer should be suspected in individuals, especially males, with marked hypercalcemia, a palpable neck mass, and serum PTH concentration 3 to 10 times the upper normal value. Some ultrasound features may raise the suspicion for cancer, such as a large (i.e., >3 cm) lobulated hypoechoic/heterogeneous parathyroid gland with irregular borders, thick capsule, suspicious vascularity, and calcifications.

Renal ultrasound should be performed in all patients, even in those with no history of nephrolithiasis, because recent studies have shown that silent kidney stones are common in patients with asymptomatic PHPT. Routine BMD testing by dual-energy x-ray absorptiometry (DXA) at the lumbar spine, hip, and distal forearm is also an essential component of the evaluation. BMD is typically low at the one-third distal radius, a site of enriched cortical bone, but a few patients may show predominant cancellous bone involvement, as documented by vertebral osteopenia or osteoporosis. The involvement of the trabecular compartment is also confirmed by the TBS at the lumbar spine. Vertebral imaging by x-ray or DXA (vertebral fracture assessment [VFA]) should also be routinely performed to detect silent vertebral deformities because vertebral fracture risk is increased in asymptomatic patients.

Neck imaging (ultrasound and sestamibi scanning) has no value in the diagnosis of PHPT, but it is a useful tool for localizing the abnormal parathyroid gland in patients selected for parathyroidectomy (PTx). Sestamibi has the advantage of localizing the ectopic parathyroid gland outside the neck. The 4D CT protocol has emerged as a useful tool. Recently, 18F-fluorocholine positron emission tomography has proven to be useful in the localization of hyperfunctioning parathyroid glands before surgery.

Treatment

The aim of treatment is to remove all hyperfunctioning parathyroid tissue, resolve biochemical abnormalities, improve BMD, and decrease the risk of nephrolithiasis and fractures.

TABLE 2	Guidelines for Surgery for Patients With Asymptomatic PHPT and Monitoring for Those Followed Without Surgery	
PARAMETER	**GUIDELINES FOR SURGERY**	**GUIDELINES FOR MONITORING**
Serum calcium	>1 mg/dL (0.25 mmol/L) above the upper normal limit	Annually
Skeletal	BMD by DXA: T-score less than −2.5 at lumbar spine, femoral neck, total hip, or distal one-third radius Vertebral fractures by x-ray, CT, MRI, or VFA	BMD by DXA every 1–2 years at lumbar spine, total hip, or distal one-third radius Spine x-ray or VFA or TBS when clinically indicated (e.g., back pain or height loss)
Renal	Creatinine clearance <60 mL/min Daily urinary calcium excretion >250 mg in women and >300 mg in men Nephrolithiasis or nephrocalcinosis by x-ray, ultrasound, or CT	Serum creatinine annually If renal stone suspected: 24-hour urinary calcium Renal imaging by x-ray, ultrasound, or CT
Age	<50 years	–

BMD, Bone mineral density; *CT*, computed tomography; *DXA*, dual x-ray absorptiometry; *MRI*, magnetic resonance imaging; *PHPT*, primary hyperparathyroidism; *TBS*, trabecular bone score; *VFA*, vertebral fracture assessment.
Modified from Bilezikian JP et al: Evaluation and management of primary hyperparathyroidism: summary statement and guidelines from the Fifth International Workshop. *J Bone Miner Res*, 37:2293-2314, 2022.

Surgical Treatment

Parathyroid surgery represents the only definitive cure of PHPT. Successful PTx normalizes serum calcium and PTH, improves BMD, and decreases the risk of nephrolithiasis and fragility fractures. Patients selected for surgery should be referred to an experienced parathyroid surgeon. A focused, minimally invasive approach, guided by imaging studies associated with intraoperative monitoring of serum PTH, is the preferred surgical procedure in sporadic PHPT. In experienced hands the rate of surgical cure reaches 95% to 98% with a negligible rate of surgical complications. In hereditary cases the surgical approach (bilateral neck exploration by classical cervicotomy) may differ because multigland involvement is common. An en bloc resection of the parathyroid lesion together with the ipsilateral thyroid lobe with clear gross margins and the adjacent structures is recommended when parathyroid carcinoma is suspected. Particular attention should be paid to avoid seeding of neoplastic parathyroid cells. Surgery should be considered for any patient with a confirmed diagnosis of PHPT and recommended in those with symptomatic disease.

Patients with mild hypercalcemia (serum calcium <12 mg/dL [3 mmol/L]) can proceed directly to surgery. When serum calcium is higher, preoperative treatment with saline infusion eventually followed by loop diuretics, intravenous (IV) bisphosphonates, denosumab (Prolia, Xgeva)[1], or cinacalcet (Sensipar) may be considered to reduce serum calcium levels and decrease the risk of complications, particularly cardiac arrhythmias, which are associated with more severe hypercalcemia.

Surgery is also a reasonable option for patients with asymptomatic PHPT. International guidelines provide guidance to select patients who should be referred for surgery or followed without surgery. The most recent revised (2022) guidelines for surgery or monitoring are reported in Table 2. These guidelines are largely consistent with the previous ones and recommend PTx for all patients with symptomatic PHPT and asymptomatic patients who meet one or more of the indicated criteria. The new indications for surgery in asymptomatic patients include a 24-hour urinary calcium excretion >250 mg/day in women and >300 mg/day in men. According to the guidelines, about 60% of patients with asymptomatic PHPT meet the criteria for surgery. As mentioned before, patients with mild PHPT may have subtle cardiovascular abnormalities and complain of psychological and cognitive symptoms. It is unclear whether and to what extent these abnormalities are reversible after successful PTx; for now they are not considered indications for surgery. Nonetheless, surgery could be considered in a middle-aged patient in whom asymptomatic PHPT is associated with increased cardiovascular risk (metabolic syndrome, hypertension, ischemic heart disease) if the surgical risk is low.

Randomized clinical trials have also shown that patients with sporadic asymptomatic PHPT who do not meet the surgical criteria may benefit from surgery, not only because it normalizes serum calcium and PTH, but also because it improves BMD and quality of life (QoL). On the other hand, surgery could be postponed in hereditary cases with mild hypercalcemia because multigland disease, occasionally with asynchronous involvement of the various parathyroid glands, is not uncommon and carries an increased risk of surgical complications and recurrence/persistence of PHPT.

Therefore individual counseling addressing the benefits and risks of PTx is mandatory, and the preference of the patients should be taken into account. It is well-known that parathyroid surgery, when performed by skilled neck surgeons, is safe, cost-effective, and associated with low perioperative morbidity. On the other hand, it is important to recognize that PTx, particularly if performed by inexperienced surgeons, may be associated with complications that could be invalidating and not acceptable for a patient with mild disease and a good QoL. In this regard, the choice of surgery may be reconsidered in a patient with asymptomatic PHPT in whom parathyroid surgery was initially advised or selected by the patient when preoperative imaging studies are negative. Indeed, in this setting the patient may feel uncomfortable undergoing a blind neck exploration, a surgical procedure more extensive than the minimally invasive approach and carrying the greatest risk of complications. Regarding normocalcemic PHPT, because of limited data, no guidelines for surgery have been recommended.

Nonsurgical Management

As mentioned before, many patients with PHPT do not meet the criteria for surgery. These patients, as well as those who decline surgery or have contraindications to surgery, need to be monitored.

Monitoring. Randomized clinical studies have shown stability over a short period of observation (up to 2 years) in patients with asymptomatic PHPT followed without surgery and benefits in those who underwent PTx even if they did not meet the criteria for surgery. The extension up to 5 years of one of these randomized studies has shown a more frequent occurrence of a vertebral fracture in patients belonging to the observation group than in those cured by PTx. However, this difference was not observed in the extension study up to 10 years. Long-term observational studies indicate that the disease remains stable in the majority for up to 8 to 9 years, but more than one-third of patients show a progression of the disease.

Calcium intake should not be restricted, and an intake appropriate for age and sex as in the general population (preferably with food) should be recommended. Vitamin D–depleted patients should be supplemented with daily doses of 800 to 1000 IU of vitamin D; weekly or monthly doses calculated on this daily dose

[1] Not FDA approved for this indication.

can also be used. A serum level of 25(OH)D >20 ng/mL should be reached, and the attainment of a higher target (>30 ng/mL) is suggested by some guidelines.

General principles for monitoring are reported in Table 2. Serum calcium and creatinine (creatinine clearance preferred over estimated glomerular filtration rate [eGFR]) should be measured annually, and BMD at the lumbar spine, total hip, and distal forearm should be measured every 1 to 2 years. Vertebral morphometry (by x-ray or VFA) or TBS should be performed when clinically indicated (back pain, height loss). Finally, 24-hour urinary collection for biochemical stone risk profile and renal imaging (x-ray, ultrasound, or CT) should be performed if there is a suspicion of renal stones.

Parathyroid surgery should be recommended in patients who are followed without surgery in the following instances: (1) serum calcium concentration >1 mg/dL above the upper normal limit; (2) significant reduction of creatinine clearance; (3) detection of nephrocalcinosis or kidney stones; (4) BMD T-score at any site less than –2.5 or the finding of a significant (greater than the least significant change as defined by the International Society for Clinical Densitometry) decrease of BMD, even if the T-score is not less than –2.5; and (5) clinical fractures or morphometric vertebral fractures, even if asymptomatic.

Medical Treatment. No medical treatment is currently available to cure PHPT. Therefore when PTx is indicated and there are no contraindications for surgery, medical treatment should not be considered a valuable alternative option. Medical treatment may be considered for patients who have contraindications to surgery or are unwilling to undergo PTx, as well as for those who have failed surgery. Treatment should be guided by the aim of therapy.

Calcimimetics. If the aim of treatment is to reduce serum calcium, the calcimimetic cinacalcet (Sensipar) can be effective. The serum calcium typically declines over a few weeks and may normalize in most patients with moderate hypercalcemia. In addition, cinacalcet increases serum phosphate and only slightly reduces PTH concentration but has no effect on BMD. The beneficial effects are sustained over time as long as the drug is used. Adverse events are dose related: modest and transient when low doses of cinacalcet are used (up to 30 mg twice daily), but rather frequent (particularly gastrointestinal) symptoms, occasionally severe enough to require treatment withdrawal, when higher doses are employed. The use of cinacalcet has been approved by the US Food and Drug Administration (FDA) for the treatment of severe hypercalcemia in patients with PHPT who are unable to undergo PTx, and by the European Medicines Agency (EMA) for the reduction of hypercalcemia in patients with PHPT, for whom PTx would be indicated on the basis of serum calcium levels (as defined by relevant guidelines) but in whom surgery is not clinically appropriate or contraindicated. As clearly stated, the EMA indications leave more room for the use of cinacalcet.

Cinacalcet should not be used as an initial treatment or in patients who do not meet the approved criteria for its prescription. The long-term safety of cinacalcet has not been established. Moreover, the rather high cost is another important limit for its long-term use.

Antiresorptive Therapy. If the aim is to increase BMD, antiresorptive therapy can be considered. Alendronate (Fosamax) is the bisphosphonate that has been more extensively used and shown to be effective in reducing bone turnover markers and increasing BMD. Over a short period of time, its effectiveness in increasing BMD is comparable to that observed after successful PTx. No effect has been shown on serum calcium and PTH levels. BMD also improved in a retrospective study that included 50 elderly women treated with denosumab for 2 years.

Combined Therapy With Cinacalcet and Antiresorptive Therapy. As mentioned before, cinacalcet is effective in the control of hypercalcemia but has no effect on BMD. Conversely, bisphosphonates increase BMD, with no effect on serum calcium. Limited data indicate that combination therapy is associated with both the calcium-lowering effect of cinacalcet and the skeletal advantage of bisphosphonates. Therefore if a patient has a low

BMD and serum calcium concentration appropriate for the use of cinacalcet, combined therapy could be of benefit. A recent study has shown that denosumab[1] is effective in increasing BMD and lowering bone turnover irrespective of cinacalcet treatment and might be a valid option for patients in which surgery is undesirable.

Pregnancy and Lactation
PHPT may be diagnosed during pregnancy by the finding of hypercalcemia on routine blood testing. There are some distinctive features that should be considered in the evaluation and management: (1) pregnancy is associated with hemodilution and occasionally hypoalbuminemia, and therefore it would be preferable to measure ionized calcium; (2) the hereditary form should be sought because of the young age of pregnant women; and (3) women with mild elevation of calcium should be managed conservatively, mostly by hydration—in the case of worsening of hypercalcemia PTx in the second trimester and cinacalcet[1] may be considered.

Secondary Hyperparathyroidism
SHPT defines any condition in which the increased PTH secretion occurs as a normal physiologic response, often mediated by a decrease of serum calcium. Vitamin D deficiency, as a result of inadequate nutritional intake/sun exposure, malabsorption, liver diseases, or chronic renal failure, is the most common cause. Other, less common causes include vitamin D resistance (Fanconi syndrome, vitamin D receptor defects), PTH resistance (pseudohypoparathyroidism, hypomagnesemia), drugs (calcium chelators, inhibitors of bone resorption, and drugs that interfere with vitamin D metabolism [phenytoin and ketoconazole]), acute pancreatitis, and osteoblastic metastases (prostate and breast cancer).

SHPT should always be considered and ruled out before making the diagnosis of normocalcemic PHPT. At variance with PHPT, SHPT is characterized by low or, more often, low-normal serum calcium and decreased urinary calcium excretion. An elevation of serum phosphate levels can be a clue to pseudohypoparathyroidism.

A prolonged stimulation of PTH synthesis and secretion, as may occur in end-stage renal failure and severe gastrointestinal diseases, may lead to the emergence of an autonomous clone of parathyroid cells into a single gland, leading to hypercalcemia (tertiary hyperparathyroidism).

Hypoparathyroidism
Hypoparathyroidism (HypoPT) is the clinical spectrum caused by insufficient production of PTH by the parathyroid glands. The major distinguishing feature is hypocalcemia, resulting from inadequate mobilization of calcium from bone and reabsorption of calcium at the distal tubule, and decreased activity of renal 1α-hydroxylase and therefore generation of calcitriol; as a consequence, the intestinal calcium absorption will be reduced.

Epidemiology
HypoPT is a rare condition designated in both the United States and Europe as an orphan disease. The estimated prevalence is 37 and 24 per 100,000 inhabitants in the United States and Europe, respectively.

Pathogenesis
HypoPT can be congenital or acquired (Table 3).

Congenital HypoPT is usually hereditary and may be isolated or combined with organ defects. The autoimmune is the most common form and may be either isolated or part of the autoimmune polyglandular syndrome type 1 (APS1). The other forms are much rarer.

Acquired HypoPT is much more common than the congenital counterpart. Bilateral neck surgery for thyroid or parathyroid

---

[1] Not FDA approved for this indication.

| TABLE 3 | Classification of Hypoparathyroidism* |

Congenital

Isolated
Defective PTH biosynthesis
- Abnormal development of parathyroid glands (GCMB, GCM2, GATA3)
- Autosomal dominant hypocalcemia
- Type 1 (CASR)
- Type 2 (GNA11)

Associated with additional features or organ defects
- Autoimmune
- Isolated
- Polyglandular syndrome type 1 (AIRE)
- Di George syndrome (TBX1)
- Sanjad-Sakati/Kenny-Caffey type 2 (TBCE)
- Kenny-Caffey type 2 (FAM111A)
- Mitochondrial DNA mutations

Defective action of PTH
- Pseudohypoparathyroidism
- Type 1a (GNAS)
- Type 1b (STX16, GNAS; in sporadic form paternal UPD)
- Type 1c (GNAS)
- Type 2 (not yet identified)

Acquired

Destruction or removal of the parathyroid glands
- Postoperative (neck surgery)
- Radiation induced
- Infiltration of the parathyroid glands (metastatic, granulomatous)
- Deposition of heavy metals (iron, copper)

Reversible impairment or PTH secretion or action
- Severe magnesium deficiency
- Hypermagnesemia (e.g., due to tocolytic therapy)
- CaSR-stimulating antibodies

*Mutated genes are indicated in parentheses.
AIRE, Autoimmune regulatory; *CASR,* calcium-sensing receptor; *FAM111A,* family with sequence similarity 111 member A; *GATA3,* GATA-binding protein 3; *GCMB,* glial cell missing gene; *GCM2,* glial cell missing homolog 2; *GNA11,* G protein subunit alpha 11; *GNAS,* GNAS complex locus; *PTH,* parathyroid hormone; *STX16,* syntaxin 16; *TBCE,* tubulin folding cofactor E; *TBX1,* T-Box1; *UPD,* uniparental disomy.

disorders is the most common cause. Postoperative HypoPT can be transient (caused by reversible parathyroid ischemia and resolving within a few weeks) or chronic/permanent (caused by irreversible parathyroid damage such as ischemia, electric scalpel damage, or, rarely, inadvertent removal of parathyroid glands). Its rate largely depends on the experience of the surgeon and the extent of the neck surgery.

Clinical Presentation

The clinical manifestations of HypoPT are largely related to the level of serum calcium and the speed of its fall and may range from asymptomatic cases, when hypocalcemia is mild (corrected calcium ≥7.0 mg/dL [1.75 mmol/L]), to a severe, life-threatening condition that requires hospital admission and intensive treatment. In mild cases signs related to neuromuscular irritability, namely the Chvostek sign (twitching and/or contracture of the facial muscles produced by tapping on the facial nerve just anterior to the ear and just below the zygomatic bone) and Trousseau sign (carpal spasm evoked by inflating a sphygmomanometer cuff above systolic blood pressure for several minutes), may be present at physical examination. Moderate to severe hypocalcemia (corrected calcium <7.0 mg/dL [1.75 mmol/L]) is usually symptomatic, even though there is no strict relationship between the severity of symptoms and the degree of hypocalcemia. In patients with postoperative HypoPT, symptoms usually appear on the first postoperative day, but, in some cases, hypocalcemia may become clinically manifest even after 3 to 4 days. Classical manifestations include paresthesias, carpopedal spasm, tetany,

seizures, positive Chvostek and Trousseau signs, and prolongation of the QT interval on electrocardiography. Papilledema and subcapsular cataract can be present. Pseudohypoparathyroidism is a group of genetic disorders caused by end organ resistance to the action of PTH. Patients with the type 1a variant have a typical phenotype (Albright hereditary osteodystrophy), characterized by short stature, shortened fourth and fifth metacarpals, rounded face, and mild intellectual deficiency. Other endocrine glands, including the thyroid and the gonads, may be dysfunctional. This clinical and endocrine phenotype is also typical of patients with type 1c. Patients with type 1b have PTH resistance and in some cases partial resistance to thyroid-stimulating hormone and mild brachydactyly. Patients with the type 2 variant have PTH resistance in the absence of the aforementioned clinical phenotype.

Evaluation and Diagnosis

The finding of low albumin–corrected serum calcium, high serum phosphate, and inappropriately low or undetectable serum PTH confirms the diagnosis of HypoPT. A recent neck surgery strongly suggests the postoperative form. A family history of hypocalcemia suggests a genetic cause. Coexistence of other autoimmune endocrinopathies (e.g., adrenal insufficiency) or candidiasis prompts consideration of APS1. Immunodeficiency and the presence of other congenital organ defects point to DiGeorge syndrome. Genetic testing may be warranted to confirm the diagnosis of this and other genetic forms. Magnesium should also be measured because magnesium deficiency impairs the secretion of PTH and its action in target tissues. Urinary calcium is usually low because of the low filtered calcium. The 24-hour calcium-to-creatinine clearance ratio is increased in patients with the activating mutation of *CaSR*. A biochemical profile of low serum calcium and high phosphate levels, together with high serum PTH, in the absence of vitamin D deficiency, reflects the PTH-resistant state and suggests a case of pseudohypoparathyroidism.

Treatment

The goal is to control symptoms of hypocalcemia and improve QoL while avoiding side effects and complications. The target serum calcium concentration is in the lower part of the normal range. Treatment relies on the administration of calcium (oral [dietary or supplements] or IV), active vitamin D metabolites, magnesium, and, where available, recombinant human PTH1-84 (Natpara). Thiazide diuretics may help reduce hypercalciuria; a low-phosphate diet and phosphate binders may help control hypophosphatemia and lower the calcium–phosphate product.

Acute Hypoparathyroidism

Acute hypocalcemia typically follows neck surgery and may be favored by a low vitamin D status and magnesium deficiency that, when present, should be corrected before surgery. In patients with high risk (total thyroidectomy, repeated thyroid surgery), perioperative administration of calcitriol (Rocaltrol) decreases the incidence of postoperative hypocalcemia and shortens the hospital stay.

Mild Hypocalcemia. In mild hypocalcemia (corrected calcium ≥7.0 mg/dL [1.75 mmol/L]), oral calcium supplements (usually calcium carbonate, 1–3 g daily in divided doses) alone or combined with active vitamin D metabolites should be administered. Calcitriol is typically initiated at an initial dose of 0.25 to 1.0 μg twice daily; equivalent doses of 1α-calcifediol[2] (1.0–2.0 μg) may also be used (see later [Chronic Hypoparathyroidism, Conventional Therapy] for more details on calcium and active vitamin D therapy) (Table 4). Serum calcium is checked weekly until optimal levels are reached.

Moderate to Severe Hypocalcemia. Patients with moderate to severe hypocalcemia (corrected calcium <7.0 mg/dL [1.75 mmol/L]) are usually admitted to the hospital and treated with IV calcium until an oral regimen can be started. One to two ampules

---

[2]Not available in the United States.

CALCIUM

AGENT	FORMULATION AND DOSE	COMMENTS
Calcium gluconate	One ampule of 10% calcium gluconate contains 93 mg; preferably diluted in 5% dextrose	Tissue necrosis may be caused by elemental calcium; preferably diluted in 5% dextrose extravasation in the adjacent subcutaneous space
Calcium salts		
Calcium carbonate	40% elemental calcium by weight; 1 g calcium carbonate contains 400 mg elemental calcium	Best absorbed with meals in an acidic environment; constipation is a common side effect
Calcium citrate	21% elemental calcium by weight; 1 g calcium citrate contains 210 mg elemental calcium	Well absorbed independent of meal and acid environment; in patients with atrophic gastritis or taking proton pump inhibitors

VITAMIN D METABOLITES

MEDICATION	TYPICAL DAILY DOSE	TIME TO ONSET OF ACTION	TIME TO OFFSET OF ACTION
Calcitriol [1,25(OH)$_2$D]$_3$ (Rocaltrol)	0.25–2.0 µg once or twice	1–2 days	2–3 days
Alfacalcidol[2] [1α(OH)D][2]	0.5–4 µg once	1–2 days	5–7 days
Dihydrotachysterol[2,†,*]	0.3–1.0 mg once	4–7 days	7–21 days
Vitamin D$_2$ (ergocalciferol) (Drisdol)[2] or vitamin D$_3$ (cholecalciferol)[2,†]	25,000–200,000 IU	10–14 days	14–75 days

[2]Not available in the United States.
[†]These compounds could be used in a setting where active vitamin D metabolites are not available and/or are too expensive.
[*]This compound is rapidly activated in the liver to 25(OH) dihydrotachysterol.
Modified from Shoback D: Clinical practice. Hypoparathyroidism. *N Engl J Med*, 359:391-403, 2008.

of 10% calcium gluconate diluted in 50 to 100 mL of 5% dextrose should be infused over a period of 10 to 20 minutes with electrocardiographic and clinical monitoring. The calcium infusion will raise the serum calcium concentration for no more than 2 to 4 hours; thus this initial treatment should be followed by a continuous infusion (50–100 mL/h) of a solution containing 1 mg/mL of elemental calcium (11 ampules of 10% calcium gluconate added to 5% dextrose in a final volume of 1 L). The rate should be adjusted according to corrected serum calcium level, which should be measured initially every 1 to 2 hours and subsequently every 4 to 6 hours and should be maintained at the lower limit of the normal range while the patient is asymptomatic. This calcium infusion protocol maintained for 8 to 10 hours will raise serum calcium by approximately 2 mg/dL. Oral administration of active vitamin D metabolites and calcium should be started as soon as practical. Calcitriol is typically initiated at a dose of 0.5 to 1.0 µg twice daily; oral calcium (1–3 g daily in divided doses) is also added.

If hypocalcemia is due to magnesium deficiency, the previous protocol should be applied while magnesium is being replaced by administering IV magnesium sulfate (initial dose 2 g as a 10% solution over 10 to 20 minutes, followed by 1 g/h in 100 mL) until a normal serum level of magnesium is reached. The only administration of magnesium will be unable to correct hypocalcemia because hypomagnesemia inhibits the secretion of PTH and consequently the renal activation of 25(OH)D and induces a peripheral resistance to the action of PTH.

The rate of calcium infusion should be increased if symptoms of hypocalcemia recur. The IV infusion should be slowly tapered and discontinued when an effective regimen of oral calcium and active vitamin D is reached (up to 24 to 48 hours or longer) and stable desired serum calcium levels are obtained.

Chronic Hypoparathyroidism
The goal of therapy is to maintain serum calcium in the low-normal range, avoid hypocalcemic symptoms and long-term complications, and improve QoL. An individualized approach is

necessary to optimize patient care. Guidelines for the management of chronic HypoPT have only recently been developed by the European Society of Endocrinology, the American Association of Clinical Endocrinologists, the American College of Endocrinology, and a panel of international experts.

Conventional Therapy. An adequate calcium intake from dietary sources (mainly dairy products) should be recommended, but calcium supplements (1–3 g daily in divided doses) are needed in almost all adult patients. Calcium carbonate is generally preferred because fewer pills per day are needed. Calcium carbonate requires an acidic gastric environment to be absorbed and should be taken with meals. Its bioavailability decreases in patients with atrophic gastritis or taking proton pump inhibitors. In these circumstances, calcium citrate, which is well absorbed independent of meal and acid environments, should be preferred. Calcium citrate might also be a preferred option for patients who complain of gastrointestinal side effects using calcium carbonate or who prefer to take calcium supplements outside mealtimes. Calcium carbonate and calcium citrate interfere with levothyroxine absorption; therefore a patient who has had a thyroidectomy should be advised to take levothyroxine well apart from calcium supplements.

Before the availability of synthetic active vitamin D metabolites, supraphysiologic doses (25,000–200,000 IU daily) of either cholecalciferol (vitamin D$_3$) or ergocalciferol (vitamin D$_2$) were used (see Table 4). Nowadays, active 1α-hydroxylated vitamin D metabolites are preferred because patients with HypoPT have impaired renal activation of 25(OH)D. Calcitriol (Rocaltrol) and alfacalcidol (One-Alpha)[2] have a similar time of onset, but the latter has a longer time of offset (5–7 days vs. 2–3 days). Calcitriol is more potent (about 50%) than alfacalcidol when compared in terms of the calcemic effect. The daily dose of calcitriol in adults ranges between 0.25 and 2.0 µg, equal to 0.5 to 4 µg of alfacalcidol. Weight-based dosing (0.01–0.04 µg/kg per day), eventually associated with calcium supplements (20–40 mg/kg per day),

[2]Not available in the United States.

should be used in infants and young children. Adult doses should be used in older children. Another active vitamin D analog, dihydrotachysterol[2], is also available in some countries. Where active vitamin D metabolites are not available or too expensive, large doses of parent vitamin D can still be used, but attention should be paid to the risk of vitamin D toxicity.

A low vitamin D status is not uncommon in patients with HypoPT, and patients with vitamin D deficiency treated with active vitamin D metabolites should be supplemented with vitamin D_2 or D_3, because active vitamin D metabolites do not correct hypovitaminosis D.

Active vitamin D metabolites stimulate intestinal absorption of phosphate, which may cause hyperphosphatemia and an increased calcium–phosphate product, with the risk of soft tissue calcification. In this setting, the intake of phosphate-rich foods should be reduced, and the daily dose of calcium supplements should be increased because calcium binds phosphate.

Hypercalciuria (≥250 mg [6.25 mmol] in women, ≥300 mg [7.5 mmol] in men, or >4 mg [0.1 mmol]/kg body weight in both sexes) is a common feature in patients with chronic HypoPT, because of the lack of PTH-dependent renal tubular reabsorption of calcium. In such instances a low-sodium diet should be advised either alone or combined with the administration of a thiazide diuretic that decreases renal calcium excretion. The combination of thiazide with amiloride[1] may further lower urinary calcium excretion and decrease the risk of hypokalemia. Thiazide diuretics are not advised in autosomal dominant hypocalcemia, a condition caused by mutations of the *CASR*. Magnesium deficiency, when present, should also be corrected.

Lifelong monitoring is needed in patients with chronic HypoPT. No study has evaluated how to best monitor these patients. The target serum calcium concentration is within the low-normal range, with no symptoms of hypocalcemia. In some patients a higher serum calcium level is needed to be symptom-free. A baseline renal imaging should be obtained. The published guidelines of the European Society of Endocrinology and the recent guidelines of the international experts participating in the Fifth International Workshop on the evaluation and management of primary hyperthyroidism suggest measuring ionized or albumin-corrected total calcium, phosphorus, magnesium, and creatinine (eGFR) every 3 to 12 months; 25(OH)D every 6 to 12 months; and 24-hour urinary calcium excretion every 6 to 24 months. They also suggest performing renal imaging when patients have symptoms of nephrolithiasis or increasing serum levels of creatinine. Biochemical monitoring should be performed weekly or every other week when changing the daily dose of calcium or active vitamin D metabolites or introducing a new drug. It is important to note that serum calcium may fluctuate once the therapeutic regimen has been stabilized. Several comorbidities (e.g., gastrointestinal disease, diarrhea, immobilization) and drugs (loop and thiazide diuretics, systemic glucocorticoids, proton pump inhibitors, antiresorptive drugs, cardiac glycosides, and chemotherapeutics) may interfere with calcium homeostasis; therefore patients should be periodically asked about their occurrence or use.

Conventional therapy only partially restores calcium homeostasis, and patients with chronic HypoPT have a reduced QoL and an increased risk of comorbidities, which include nephrocalcinosis, nephrolithiasis, impaired renal function, neuropsychiatric diseases, muscle stiffness and pain, infections, and seizures. An increased rate of intracerebral calcifications and cataracts has been documented in nonsurgical HypoPT. Bone mineral content is increased in patients with chronic HypoPT, but cancellous bone microarchitecture is abnormal.

Parathyroid Hormone. Until recently, HypoPT was the only major hormonal insufficiency state not treated with the missing hormone. The development of the recombinant human N-terminal 1 to 34 fragment (rhPTH$_{1-34}$) molecule has stimulated several studies on its use as replacement therapy, which led to the approval by the FDA of rhPTH$_{1-84}$ (Natpara) for the management of chronic HypoPT.

TransCon PTH is an investigational prodrug consisting of PTH (1-34) transiently conjugated to a polyethylene glycol carrier molecule providing stable PTH concentrations in the physiologic range for 24 hours a day. TransCon PTH was developed as a therapy for the treatment of HypoPT. After subcutaneous injection with exposure to physiologic pH and temperature, the linker is cleaved, releasing PTH (1-34) in a controlled manner.

A phase 3 double-blind, placebo-controlled study (PaTHway Trial) with TransCon PTH 18 µg daily versus placebo recently evaluated safety and efficacy in 84 patients with chronic HypoPT. At 26 weeks, cessation of active vitamin D was possible in 93% of participants while maintaining normal serum calcium. Statistically significant reductions in 24-hour urine calcium were also observed in comparison to placebo. Improvements in QoL were also observed. The ongoing phase 3 and phase 2 open-label extension studies will provide data on the long-term efficacy and safety of TransCon PTH therapy for HypoPT. Recently the results at week 52 of the PaTHway trial have been reported and showed sustained efficacy, safety, and tolerability in adults with HypoPT. The TransCon PTH (palopegteriparatide [Yorvipath]) has been approved by the European Medicines Agency and by the Food and Drug Administration (FDA) as a PTH replacement therapy for adults with chronic HypoPT.

Pregnancy and Lactation

There are limited data to inform treatment strategies in chronic HypoPT in pregnancy and lactation. The guidelines, recently updated, and the expert consensus of the European Society of Endocrinology suggest the use of active vitamin D metabolites and oral calcium as in nonpregnant women. Frequent monitoring (every 2 to 3 weeks) of serum calcium, possibly ionized calcium, is recommended. No studies have addressed the use of rhPTH$_{1-84}$ therapy in pregnant women. The FDA suggests that it should be used "only if the potential benefit justifies the potential risk to the fetus."

References

Arnold A, Levine A: Molecular basis of primary hyperparathyroidism. In Bilezikan JP, et al: *The parathyroids, basic and clinical concept*, London, 2015, Academic Press, pp 279–296.

Bilezikian JP, Bandeira L, Khan A, et al: Hyperparathyroidism, *Lancet* 1:168178, 2018.

Bilezikian JP, Cusano NE, Khan AA, et al: Primary hyperparathyroidism, *Nat Rev Dis Prim* 2:16033, 2016.

Bilezikian JP, Khan A, Potts Jr JT, et al: Hypoparathyroidism in the adult: epidemiology, diagnosis, pathophysiology, target-organ involvement, treatment, and challenges for future research, *J Bone Miner Res* 26:2317–2337, 2011.

Bilezikian JP, Khan A, Silverberg SJ, et al: Evaluation and management of primary hyperparathyroidism: summary statement and guidelines from the fifth international workshop, *J Bone Miner Res* 37:2293–2314, 2022.

Bilezikian JP, Silverberg SJ, Bandeira F, et al: Management of primary hyperparathyroidism, *J Bone Miner Res* 37:2391–2403, 2022.

Bollerslev J, Rejnmark L, Marcocci C, et al: European Society of Endocrinology Clinical Guideline: treatment of chronic hypoparathyroidism in adults, *Eur J Endocrinol* 173:G1–G20, 2015.

Bollerslev J, Rejnmark L, Zahn A, et al: European expert consensus on practical management of specific aspects of parathyroid disorders in adults and in pregnancy: recommendation of the ESE educational program of parathyroid disorders, *Eur J Endocrinol* 186, 2021.

Cetani F, Marcocci C: Parathyroid carcinoma. In Bilezikian JP, editor: *The parathyroids, basic and clinical concepts*, London, 2015, Academic Press, pp 409–422.

Cetani F, Pardi E, Aretini P, et al: Whole exome sequencing in familial isolated primary hyperparathyroidism, *J Endocrinol Invest* 43:231–245, 2020.

Clarke BL, Khan AA, Rubin MR, et al: Efficacy and safety of TransCon PTH in adults with hypoparathyroidism: 52-week results from the phase 3 PaTHway trial, *J Clin Endocrinol Metab*, 2024:dgae693, 2024. https://doi.org/10.1210/clinem/dgae693.

Cusano NE, Silverberg SJ, Bilezikian JP: Normocalcemic primary hyperparathyroidism, *J Clin Densitom* 16:33–39, 2013.

EMA/CHMP/124164/2017 Media and public relations, 2017. http://www.ema.europa.eu/docs/en_GB/document_library/Press_release/2017/02/WC500222215.pdf.

https://www.ema.europa.eu/en/documents/product-information/yorvipath-epar-product-information_en.pdf.

https://www.fda.gov/drugs/news-events-human-drugs/fda-approves-new-drug-hypoparathyroidism-rare-disorder.

---

[1] Not FDA approved for this indication.

Khan AA, Bilezikian JP, Brandi ML, et al: Evaluation and management of hypoparathyroidism summary statement and guidelines from the second international workshop, *J Bone Miner Res* 37:2568–2585, 2022.

Khan AA, Koch C, Van Uum SHM, et al: Standards of care for hypoparathyroidism in adults, *Eur J Endocrinol EJE* 180:1–22, 2019.

Khan A, Rejnmark L, Rubin M, et al: PaTH forward: a randomized, double-blind, placebo-controlled phase 2 trial of TransCon PTH in adult hypoparathyroidism, *J Clin Endocrinol Metab* 107(1):e372–e385, 2021.

Khan AA, Rubin MR, Schwarz P, et al: Efficacy and safety of parathyroid hormone replacement with TransCon PTH in hypoparathyroidism: 26-week results from the phase 3 PaTHway trial, *J Bone Miner Res* 38(1):14–25, 2023.

Leere JS, Karmisholt J, Robaczyk M, et al: Denosumab and cinacalcet for primary hyperparathyroidism (DENOCINA): a randomised, double-blind, placebo-controlled, phase 3 trial, *Lancet Diabetes Endocrinol* 8:407–417, 2020.

Lundstam K, Pretorius M, Bollerslev J, et al: Positive effect of parathyroidectomy compared to observation on BMD in a randomized controlled trial of mild primary hyperparathyroidism, *J Bone Miner Res* 38(32–380), 2023.

Mannstadt M, Bilezikian JP, Thakker RV, et al: Hypoparathyroidism, *Nat Rev Dis Primers* 3:17055, 2017. http://www.ema.europa.eu/docs/en_GB/document_library/Press_release/2017/02/WC500222215.pdf.

Mannstadt M, Clarke BL, Vokes T, et al: Efficacy and safety of recombinant human parathyroid hormone (1-84) in hypoparathyroidism (REPLACE): a double-blind, placebo-controlled, randomised, phase 3 study, *Lancet Diabetes Endocrinol* 1:275–283, 2013.

Marcocci C, Bollerslev J, Khan AA, Shoback DM: Medical management of primary hyperparathyroidism: proceedings of the fourth international workshop on the management of asymptomatic primary hyperparathyroidism, *J Clin Endocrinol Metab* 99:3607–3618, 2014.

Marcocci C, Cetani F: Clinical practice, primary hyperparathyroidism, *N Engl J Med* 365:2389–2397, 2011.

Mazoni L, Matrone A, Apicella M, et al: Renal complications and quality of life in postsurgical hypoparathyroidism: a case-control study, *J Endocrinol Invest* 45:573–582, 2022.

NATPAR. https://www.ema.europa.eu/en/medicines/human/EPAR/natpar.

NATPARA: *Shire-NPS pharmaceuticals*, Inc, 2015. [package insert] https://www.accessdata.fda.gov/drugsatfda_docs/label/2015/125511s000lbl.pdf.

Pretorius M, Lundstam K, Hellström M, et al: Effects of parathyroidectomy on quality of life: 10 years data from a prospective randomized controlled trial on primary hyperparathyroidism (the SIPH-study), *J Bone Miner Res* 36(1):3–11, 2021.

Rubin MR, Bilezikian JP, McMahon DJ, et al: The natural history of primary hyperparathyroidism with or without parathyroid surgery after 15 years, *J Clin Endocrinol Metab* 93:3462–3470, 2008.

Seabrook AJ, Harris LE, Velosa SB, et al: Multiple endocrine tumors associated with dermline MAX mutations: multiple endocrine neoplasia type 5?, *J Clin Endocrinol Metab* 106:1163–1182, 2021.

Sidhu PS, Talat N, Patel P, et al: Ultrasound features of malignancy in the preoperative diagnosis of parathyroid cancer: a retrospective analysis of parathyroid tumours larger than 15 mm, *Eur Radiol*, 2011.

Shoback D: Clinical practice. Hypoparathyroidism, *N Engl J Med* 359:391–403, 2008.

Shoback DM, Bilezikian JP, Costa AG, et al: Presentation of hypoparathyroidism: etiologies and clinical features, *J Clin Endocrinol Metab* 101:2300–2312, 2016.

Treglia G, Piccardo A, Imperiale A, et al: Diagnostic performance of choline PET for detection of hyperfunctioning parathyroid glands in hyperparathyroidism: a systematic review and meta-analysis, *Eur J Nucl Med Mol Imag* 46:751–765, 2019.

Vignali E, Viccica G, Diacinti D, et al: Morphometric vertebral fractures in postmenopausal women with primary hyperparathyroidism, *J Clin Endocrinol Metab* 94:2306–2312, 2009.

HYPERPROLACTINEMIA

Method of
Ming Li, MD, PhD

CURRENT DIAGNOSIS

- Hyperprolactinemia is diagnosed by biochemical tests based on two-site immunoassay, which can be confounded by extreme hyperprolactinemia (hook effect) and biologically inactive macroprolactinemia.
- Hyperprolactinemia can be caused by physiologic, pharmacologic, or pathologic conditions; careful clinical, laboratory, and radiology evaluations are required to identify its underlying cause.
- The most common causes of hyperprolactinemia include medications, prolactinoma, and other pituitary and hypothalamic/pituitary stalk diseases.
- Clinical features of hyperprolactinemia include galactorrhea, menstrual abnormalities (in women), impotence (in men), infertility, and osteoporosis.

- Patients with prolactinoma may also have local compression symptoms including headache, visual disturbance, and hypopituitarism.
- Pituitary magnetic resonance imaging (MRI) is the imaging method of choice for diagnosing prolactinoma and other sellar/parasellar lesions.

CURRENT THERAPY

- For secondary hyperprolactinemia, treatment should be directed at correcting underlying causes.
- Treatment goals for prolactinoma are relief of symptoms and the long-term effects of hyperprolactinemia and of tumor mass effects.
- The dopamine agonists cabergoline (Dostinex) and bromocriptine (Parlodel) are effective in normalizing the prolactin level and shrinking the tumor in patients with prolactinoma.
- Surgery and radiotherapy of prolactinoma are reserved for patients resistant to or intolerant of medical therapy.
- Temozolomide (Temodar)[1] monotherapy is the first-line chemotherapy for aggressive or malignant prolactinomas after failing standard treatments.

[1]Not FDA approved for this indication.

Biochemistry and Physiology of Prolactin

Prolactin is a polypeptide hormone produced by pituitary lactotroph cells. It is also produced locally in a variety of extrapituitary tissues such as mammary glands, decidua, gonads, brain, liver, fat, pancreas, and the immune system, along with its receptors. Prolactin is highly pleiotropic in terms of its functions. Many of its actions collectively support puerperal lactation. Prolactin displays considerable sequence homology to growth hormone (GH) and placental lactogen. The prolactin and GH receptors both belong to the class I cytokine/hematopoietic receptor superfamily. Prolactin is responsible for maturation of the mammary glands during pregnancy, but it plays only a minor role in pubertal mammary development, which requires GH instead. It appears not to be an essential hormone for nonchildbearing individuals. Rare patients deficient in either prolactin or its receptor are largely healthy despite difficulty with fertility and lactation.

Prolactin circulates mainly as a 23-kDa 199-aa polypeptide. Several of its cleavage products exist in blood, which may have functions unrelated to lactation; for example, one 16-kDa cleavage product of prolactin displays antiangiogenic and prothrombotic properties and has been implicated in the development of preeclampsia and peripartum cardiomyopathy. Several forms of prolactin aggregate, known as macroprolactins, also exist in circulation at lower levels. They are formed either by covalent bonding of prolactin monomers or by their nucleating around autoimmune immunoglobulin G. These macroprolactins are not biologically active in vivo and have a prolonged half-life. At times they can build up in the circulation to a level high enough to cause diagnostic difficulties.

Among the major pituitary hormones, prolactin is unique for its predominantly negative mode of regulation by the hypothalamus. It does not have a known hypothalamus-derived releasing hormone. Instead, lactotrophs are under tonic inhibition by dopamine secreted from hypothalamic neurons. Increase in prolactin output is mostly mediated by withdrawing dopaminergic control in response to environmental cues, such as physical activity, stress, and nipple stimuli (Figure 1). Under experimental and pathologic conditions, several factors, including thyrotropin-releasing hormone, vasoactive intestinal peptide, oxytocin, and vasopressin, have been shown to increase prolactin secretion, but these peptides appear to play only minor and insignificant roles for the physiologic regulation of prolactin.

Estrogen is the main driver of prolactin secretion during pregnancy. Stimulated by persistently elevated estrogen, lactotrophs grow in number and size. By term the pituitary gland can reach two to three times its normal size, and prolactin levels increase some 20-fold. Along with placental hormones such as estrogen, progesterone, and placental lactogen, prolactin drives the maturation of the mammary glands. Lactation starts after parturition, when estrogen withdraws from the circulation. Frequent infant suckling maintains physiologic hyperprolactinemia, which is important for sustained milk production. In addition, hyperprolactinemia during this critical period provides a natural although unreliable way of contraception. This is achieved by suppression of the hypothalamus-pituitary-gonad axis. Hyperprolactinemic hypogonadism and parathyroid hormone–related peptide (PTHrP) secreted from mammary epithelial cells help mobilize skeletal calcium store in support of milk production. Through its receptors in liver, intestine, fat, and pancreas, prolactin also adjusts maternal nutrient metabolism to meet the nutrition needs of the fetus during pregnancy and breast-feeding newborns. In the brain, prolactin modifies parental behavior toward closer infant attendance (see Figure 1).

Pathophysiology of Hyperprolactinemia

Physiologic hyperprolactinemia as occurs during pregnancy and nursing is essential for child raising through the actions of prolactin in target organs discussed above. Similar changes in these organs under the influence of persistent pathologic hyperprolactinemia in the absence of pregnancy and lactation, however, are inappropriate and could lead to a variety of undesired long-term consequences.

Mammary Glands

One common symptom of persistent hyperprolactinemia is galactorrhea; that is, milk production not associated with childbirth or breast-feeding. Because puerperal lactation normally ends within 6 months after delivery or weaning, any milk production beyond this point is also considered galactorrhea. Because maturation of mammary glands is completed during pregnancy, galactorrhea typically happens in women between 20 to 35 years of age with previous childbirths. It also occurs in nulligravid women, women postmenopause, and men, although less frequently.

Prolactin is a known mitogen for mammary epithelial cells, and concern has been raised regarding its potential role in the pathogenesis of breast cancer. In a large prospective study by the Women's Health Initiative, there was evidence of a significant increase in breast cancer incidence in women postmenopause with high normal prolactin levels, which is within the highest quartile of the normal range compared with those in the lowest quartile. On the other hand, increased breast cancer risk has not been observed in patients with overt hyperprolactinemia. In fact, early parity and lactation history are strong protective factors against breast cancer. Further research is required to resolve these seemingly discrepant observations.

Female Reproductive System

Persistent hyperprolactinemia significantly diminishes the pulsatile release of gonadotropin-releasing hormone (GnRH). Because GnRH neurons do not themselves express prolactin receptors, prolactin exerts its effects on their afferent neurons instead by suppression of secretion of kisspeptin, a potent secretagogue for GnRH. Prolactin receptors are also found in the gonads, and prolactin has been reported to inhibit folliculogenesis and estrogen production in the ovary directly. However, this likely has only a limited contribution to infertility and hypogonadism associated with hyperprolactinemia, because the hypothalamus-pituitary-gonad axis can be reactivated by administration of GnRH or kisspeptin, with return of ovulation and fertility in subjects with hyperprolactinemia.

Male Reproductive System

As in women, hyperprolactinemia causes secondary hypogonadism and infertility in men by suppression of GnRH pulses and a decrease in luteinizing hormone and follicle-stimulating hormone levels. Patients often have low or low normal testosterone levels, as well as abnormal sperm counts and morphology in semen analysis. Patients usually seek medical attention for diminished libido and impotence. The central nervous system (CNS) actions of prolactin are likely partly responsible for these symptoms, because restoration of testosterone level alone is often inadequate for symptom relief, which occurs only when prolactin levels also return to normal.

Adrenal Glands

Prolactin stimulates the synthesis of androgen in the zona reticularis of the adrenal cortex. Mild elevations in serum levels of adrenal androgens—for example, dehydroepiandrosterone (DHEA) and dehydroepiandrosterone sulfate (DHEA-S)—are

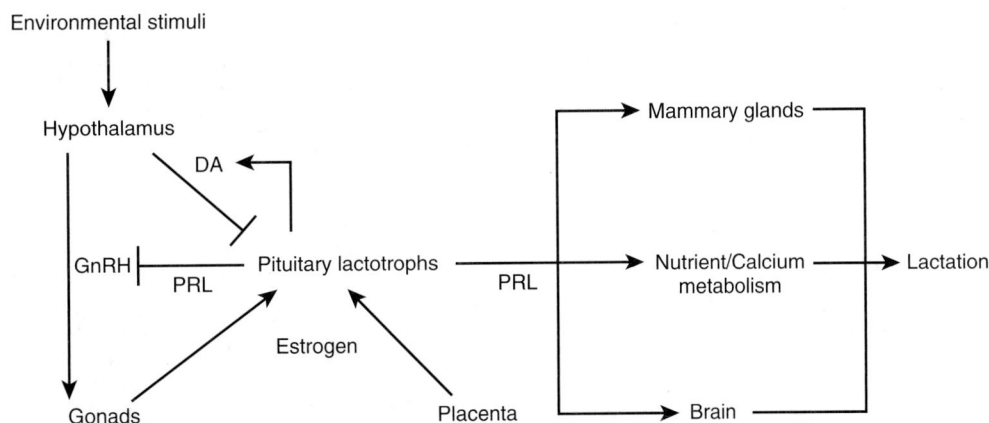

Figure 1 Physiology of prolactin and its regulation. At baseline, prolactin production and secretion are under tonic inhibition by dopamine released from hypothalamic neurons. The hypothalamus controls prolactin production by altering output of dopamine after integrating environmental stimuli and changes in hormonal homeostasis. Prolactin increases hypothalamic dopamine output, providing a negative feedback regulatory loop. Estrogen stimulates prolactin synthesis and secretion during pregnancy. Prolactin supports puerperal lactation via its action on the mammary glands, nutrient/calcium metabolism, and brain. Unlike most other anterior pituitary hormones, feedback regulation of prolactin secretion does not occur via factors produced by a peripheral endocrine target organ. Prolactin also suppresses the hypothalamic-pituitary-gonadal axis by inhibiting GnRH release. *DA,* Dopamine; *PRL,* prolactin.

seen in approximately 50% of women with hyperprolactinemia. Symptoms of clinical hyperandrogenism such as hirsutism and acne are rare in these patients. When present, they are almost always associated with a concurrent increase in testosterone level. Elevation of adrenal androgens in hyperprolactinemia may contribute to the suppression of GnRH release in the hypothalamus and secondary hypogonadism.

Skeletal System
Premenopausal women with hyperprolactinemia have lower bone density and approximately a 4.5 times higher risk for osteoporotic fractures. Hypogonadism associated with hyperprolactinemia is the main cause of bone loss, whereas restoration of sex hormones with either hormone replacement or correction of hyperprolactinemia improves bone density. Bone density is preserved in women with hyperprolactinemia who continue to have regular menses. Nonetheless, not all studies showed a clear correlation between the degree of bone loss and duration of amenorrhea or levels of sex hormones, suggesting involvement of additional processes. For example, the levels of PTHrP were found to be significantly higher in patients with hyperprolactinemia and correlated well with bone density measurements. Correction of hyperprolactinemia by dopamine agonists was shown to normalize PTHrP levels.

Metabolic Effects of Hyperprolactinemia
During pregnancy and nursing, physiologic elevation of prolactin, via signaling in fat, small intestine, pancreas, and liver, regulates maternal nutrient metabolism to meet the needs of the fetus and newborn, leading to hyperphagia, weight gain, insulin resistance, and leptin resistance. Similarly, pathologic hyperprolactinemia is strongly correlated with obesity, insulin resistance, hyperlipidemia, diabetes, and all-cause and cardiovascular mortality, although the clinical presentations vary greatly. Medications blocking prolactin release were reported to improve cardiometabolic risk factors. Bromocriptine (Cycloset) is approved by the U.S. Food and Drug Administration (FDA) as a hypoglycemic agent for treating type 2 diabetes. It remains to be determined what level of prolactin is associated with higher cardiovascular risk; high normal and mildly elevated prolactin levels have been reported as cardioprotective. Hyperprolactinemia has not been formally recognized as a risk enhancer for considering lipid-lowering therapies by the Endocrine Society's recent *Clinical Practice Guidelines on Lipid Management in Patients With Endocrine Disorders*. It would be advisable to screen for and treat established cardiovascular risk factors in patients with hyperprolactinemia and consider testing for coronary calcium score in patients with borderline to intermediate cardiovascular risk, if decisions regarding lipid-lowering therapies remain uncertain.

Etiology of Hyperprolactinemia
Any conditions that affect production or clearance of prolactin can lead to hyperprolactinemia (Table 1). Physiologic hyperprolactinemia is transient and adaptive, whereas persistent hyperprolactinemia from pharmacologic and pathologic causes is often symptomatic with undesired long-term consequences. Pituitary adenomas overproducing prolactin (prolactinomas) are the most important cause of pathologic hyperprolactinemia. In addition to the elevated prolactin levels, prolactinomas produce pathologic local mass effects. Secondary hyperprolactinemia is most commonly related to disruption of dopaminergic control of lactotrophs, secondary to the use of dopamine antagonists or hypothalamic and pituitary stalk lesions.

Epidemiology and Natural History of Prolactinoma
Prolactinoma is the most common type of pituitary adenoma, contributing to approximately 40% to 50% of pituitary tumor cases. Prolactinomas are categorized according to size into microprolactinomas (<1 cm) and macroprolactinomas (>1 cm). Clinically these two conditions behave very differently and can be considered as separate entities. In general, macroprolactinomas tend to grow progressively and are often locally invasive; they are also generally more resistant to treatment and have a higher

TABLE 1	Causes of Hyperprolactinemia
Physiologic	
Pregnancy	
Lactation and breast stimulation	
Neonatal period	
Physical activity	
Stress	
Sexual intercourse	
Pharmacologic	
Dopamine antagonists—antipsychotics and antiemetics	
Tricyclic antidepressants	
Selective serotonin reuptake inhibitors	
Antihistamines (H2)	
Verapamil (Calan)	
Protease inhibitors	
Dopamine synthesis inhibitors	
Pathologic	
Pituitary Diseases	
Prolactinoma	
Plurihormonal adenomas	
Lymphocytic hypophysitis	
Empty sella syndrome	
Macroadenoma with or without suprasellar extension	
Idiopathic hyperprolactinemia	
Hypothalamic/Pituitary Stalk Diseases	
Tumors: meningioma, craniopharyngioma, germinoma, metastasis, etc.	
Granulomas	
Infiltrative diseases	
Irradiation	
Trauma	
NEUROGENIC: chest wall lesions, spinal cord lesions, herpes zoster, and epileptic seizure	
Paraneoplastic syndrome	
Systemic Diseases	
End-stage renal disease	
Cirrhosis	
Adrenal insufficiency	
Pseudocyesis	

Adapted from Bronstein (2016); Melmed et al. (2016).

risk of recurrence. On the other hand, microprolactinomas rarely progress in size (~7% of cases) and have a good chance (~15% of cases) of going into remission on their own.

The prevalence of prolactinoma has been estimated to be 500 cases per million with an incidence of about 27 cases per million per year based on survey of asymptomatic populations. In autopsy series, however, lactotroph neoplasms staining positive for prolactin are much more common, being found in approximately 5% of the subjects. They are predominantly microadenomas. Only a small fraction of these small lactotroph neoplasms develop overt hyperprolactinemia by escaping tonic dopaminergic suppression from the hypothalamus, presumably via down-regulation of dopamine D2 receptor-mediated signaling pathway and/or bypassing the portal system for blood supply. Microprolactinomas predominantly affect women of childbearing age, with a female-to-male ratio of approximately 20:1. Macroprolactinoma, on the other hand, shows no sex predilection. Neoplastic transformation of lactotroph involves accumulation of genetic and epigenetic events. The best understood candidate genes involved include the pituitary tumor–transforming gene (PTTG) and the heparin-binding secretory transforming (HST) gene. Pituitary tumor–transforming gene expression is positively regulated by estrogen.

Most prolactinomas occur sporadically. Most prolactinomas are benign, although they can be locally invasive. Malignant prolactinomas, as defined by the presence of extrapituitary metastases, are extremely rare. Familial cases, such as those associated with multiple endocrine neoplasia I (MEN I) and familial isolated pituitary adenoma (FIPA), typically occur at a younger age and are more often macroprolactinomas that are locally invasive.

Clinical Manifestations

Clinical manifestations of prolactinomas fall under two categories: systemic effects of hyperprolactinemia and local compression symptoms.

Symptoms of Hyperprolactinemia

Persistent hyperprolactinemia inappropriately recapitulates symptoms associated with normal pregnancy and nursing. In extreme cases, hyperprolactinemia has been associated with delusions of pregnancy in susceptible individuals, for example, some women on psychotropic medications.

Menstrual abnormalities and infertility are the most common symptoms associated with hyperprolactinemia in women of childbearing age. These symptoms may be masked by use of oral contraceptive pills, which often delays diagnosis. The mildest cases include women presenting with infertility caused by shortened luteal phase despite preserved regular menses. As the degree of hypogonadism worsens, patients experience menstrual irregularities ranging from anovulatory cycles to oligomenorrhea and amenorrhea. Patients with amenorrhea may also experience psychological stresses and other menopausal symptoms like vaginal dryness and dyspareunia. Of note, high prolactin levels may sometimes mask vasomotor symptoms of women in menopause and perimenopause with prolactinoma, who may develop hot flashes once they are successfully treated with dopamine agonists.

Galactorrhea occurs in up to 80% of cases of hyperprolactinemia. This will need to be differentiated from nipple discharges of other causes, especially those from breast neoplasms. Further evaluation with breast imaging and cytology is indicated when the discharge is unilateral, bloody, or associated with a breast mass. Galactorrhea is by definition milk-like in appearance, and when in doubt, Sudan Black B staining showing fat globules is confirmatory. Although considered a classic sign and symptom for hyperprolactinemia, galactorrhea per se is a poor predictor for hyperprolactinemia in the absence of additional symptoms, because it can be seen in about 10% of healthy women of childbearing age. If amenorrhea is present at the same time, the patient should be assumed to harbor a prolactinoma unless proven otherwise. The degree of galactorrhea is quite variable, from barely expressible to bothersome bra stain and copious free flow, and does not necessarily reflect the severity of hyperprolactinemia. In fact, most patients with galactorrhea and normal menses have normal prolactin levels. On the other hand, in some patients with extremely high levels of prolactin, galactorrhea could be masked by severe hypogonadism.

Men with hyperprolactinemia mainly present with impotence and diminished libido, which is not always corrected with testosterone replacement. As noted in the section on pathophysiology, these symptoms are not all caused by hypogonadism but may involve the central effects of prolactin. Other symptoms and signs of hypogonadism, such as loss of body hair and muscle bulk, are less common. Infertility could also occur with decrease in sperm count and morphology, although hyperprolactinemia is only present in approximately 5% of male patients seeking treatment for infertility.

For both male and female patients, persistent hypogonadism from hyperprolactinemia leads to osteoporosis and increased risk of fracture. This could be effectively treated with either sex hormone replacement or dopamine agonists.

Mass Effects of Prolactinomas

Headache is the most common neurologic symptom caused by pituitary tumors. It can occur even with microadenomas presumably caused by dural stretch. More severe headache results from larger tumors, especially those with extrasellar invasion, and occasionally from apoplexy.

Visual disturbance typically only happens with macroadenomas with suprasellar extension impinging on the optic chiasm, leading to loss of visual acuity and visual field defects. The typical pattern of visual field defect is bitemporal hemianopsia, which usually starts from the upper field and progresses downward as the tumor impinges upward from below. Ophthalmoparesis typically happens in the setting of apoplexy and only rarely results from parasellar invasion of the cavernous sinus and impingement of cranial nerves III, IV, or VI.

By compressing the rest of the pituitary gland, including the stalk, prolactinoma can cause deficiencies of other anterior pituitary hormones including GH, thyroid-stimulating hormone (TSH), and adrenocorticotropic hormone, in addition to hypogonadism from the hyperprolactinemia. The degree of the risk is proportional to tumor size.

Cerebrospinal fluid (CSF) rhinorrhea occurs when a macroprolactinoma invades inferiorly into the sphenoid sinus. Other rare compressive symptoms from giant prolactinomas include epilepsy (temporal lobe involvement), exophthalmos, and hydrocephalus. Life- and vision-threatening emergencies could arise from apoplexy and CNS infection.

Laboratory Evaluation
Prolactin Assay and Pitfalls

Hyperprolactinemia is diagnosed by individual measurements of serum prolactin levels. Patients should be well rested, because physical activity stimulates prolactin secretion. Fasting is normally not needed but can be justified when the initial reading is only mildly elevated, to rule out meal effects. Repeated testing with venous cannulation should be attempted with mildly elevated prolactin levels (<5-fold of upper normal limit), especially if stress associated with venipuncture is suspected, which may lead to 2- to 4-fold higher prolactin secretion. Dynamic tests such as thyrotropin-releasing hormone stimulation do not appear to add to diagnostic value and are not recommended. The level of prolactin may provide valuable diagnostic clues. Secondary hyperprolactinemia rarely exceeds 150 ng/mL. On the other hand, a prolactin level of greater than 100 ng/mL is highly suggestive, and severe hyperprolactinemia of greater than 500 ng/mL is virtually diagnostic for prolactinoma. On rare occasions, secondary hyperprolactinemia can produce prolactin levels in the prolactinoma range. For example, risperidone (Risperdal)-induced hyperprolactinemia could be as high as 250 to 500 ng/mL, and patients with end-stage renal disease who are on antipsychotics or antiemetics can have prolactin levels greater than 1000 ng/mL. The size of the prolactinoma shows a rough correlation with the serum prolactin level. Patients with microprolactinomas usually have prolactin levels in the range of 50 to 300 ng/mL, whereas those with macroprolactinomas have levels of 200 to 5000 ng/mL.

Most clinical laboratories measure prolactin using a two-site immunoassay. A capture antibody first affixes prolactin in the sample to a solid matrix. Subsequently, a second signal antibody is attached to the now-immobilized prolactin. The signal antibody is engineered to carry either a radioisotope or a chemiluminescent enzyme to provide a readout. The assay is accurate within its designed linear range, which is typically under 10,000 ng/mL. Beyond this level, both capture and signal antibodies could be saturated, preventing the signal antibody from attaching. As a result, signal outputs will be falsely diminished. This phenomenon, known as the hook effect, produces a falsely low reading that could lead to the misdiagnosis of a macroprolactinoma as a nonfunctioning pituitary tumor, and should be suspected in pituitary adenomas larger than 3 cm with only mildly increased prolactin levels. This artifact can be circumvented by repeating the assay with a 100-fold diluted sample. Many laboratories also opt for an additional washout step to eliminate excess prolactin before adding the signal antibody, preempting the artifact.

Macroprolactinemia is another potential diagnostic pitfall masquerading as true hyperprolactinemia. Macroprolactins are biologically inactive prolactin aggregates that could accumulate in blood to a high level. Macroprolactinemia does not cause any morbidities but could contribute to analytical difficulties as the antibodies used in prolactin assays cross-react with macroprolactins. Most laboratories rely on polyethylene glycol (PEG) precipitation to determine the proportion of macroprolactins and the true concentration of monomeric prolactin. Up to 25% of monomeric prolactin can be also precipitated by PEG, potentially masking true hyperprolactinemia. Therefore patients with macroprolactinemia may still need to be further evaluated if clinical suspicion is high for true hyperprolactinemia.

Other Supporting Laboratory Tests

After confirming hyperprolactinemia, a simple chemistry panel may reveal or suggest the underlying cause, such as chronic kidney disease and cirrhosis. A pregnancy test (beta human chorionic gonadotropin level) is essential for women of childbearing age, and hypothyroidism needs to be ruled out with a TSH assay. Both pregnancy and hypothyroidism may have presenting symptoms of sellar mass and hyperprolactinemia and therefore be mistaken for prolactinoma.

For established prolactinoma cases, it is important to also assess other pituitary axes. Up to 20% of GH-secreting tumors co-secrete prolactin, and insulin-like growth factor 1 (IGF-1) level is an essential screening test for these cases. If hypogonadism is suspected, levels of luteinizing hormone, follicle-stimulating hormone, and sex hormones (testosterone or estrogen) should be obtained. Screening for central hypothyroidism and secondary adrenal insufficiency should be done with TSH, free thyroxine (T4), and morning cortisol levels, respectively, for patients with pituitary tumors larger than 6 mm.

Neuroimaging

Pituitary imaging should be considered for all patients with unexplained significant hyperprolactinemia, especially if there are signs or symptoms of local compression. Magnetic resonance imaging (MRI) with and without gadolinium contrast with dedicated pituitary protocol is the test of choice. Compared with other modalities, MRI provides superior soft tissue contrast, revealing the tumor's inner structure and its relationship to surrounding tissues, including cavernous sinus, pituitary stalk, and optic chiasm. Computed tomography scan still has a role for patients with metal implants or other contraindications for MRI and is especially useful for revealing bony erosions and tissue calcification; its use is limited by suboptimal soft tissue contrast and exposure to ionizing radiation.

Visual Field Testing

A formal visual field test with a perimeter is recommended when suprasellar extension of a pituitary adenoma brings it close to the optic chiasm. Improvement or worsening in visual field often precedes imaging evidence of tumor shrinkage or expansion during treatment. Therefore visual field testing is an excellent monitoring tool for patients under treatment for macroadenoma and visual impairment.

Diagnosis

Prolactin testing is usually prompted by suggestive signs and symptoms of hyperprolactinemia such as menstrual abnormalities, infertility, and galactorrhea. A careful history, including medication use, physical examination, and routine laboratory evaluation (see preceding sections), is invaluable for uncovering secondary causes. Pituitary imaging should be performed when no other underlying causes are found, especially if the levels of prolactin are higher than 100 ng/mL. A diagnostic algorithm shown in Figure 2 provides a framework for a structured and cost-effective workup of hyperprolactinemia.

Differential Diagnosis

An exhaustive list of etiologies is provided in Table 1. A few entities deserve additional comments.

Drug-induced hyperprolactinemia is common and at times may produce serum prolactin levels matching those in patients with prolactinoma (see prior section on laboratory evaluation).

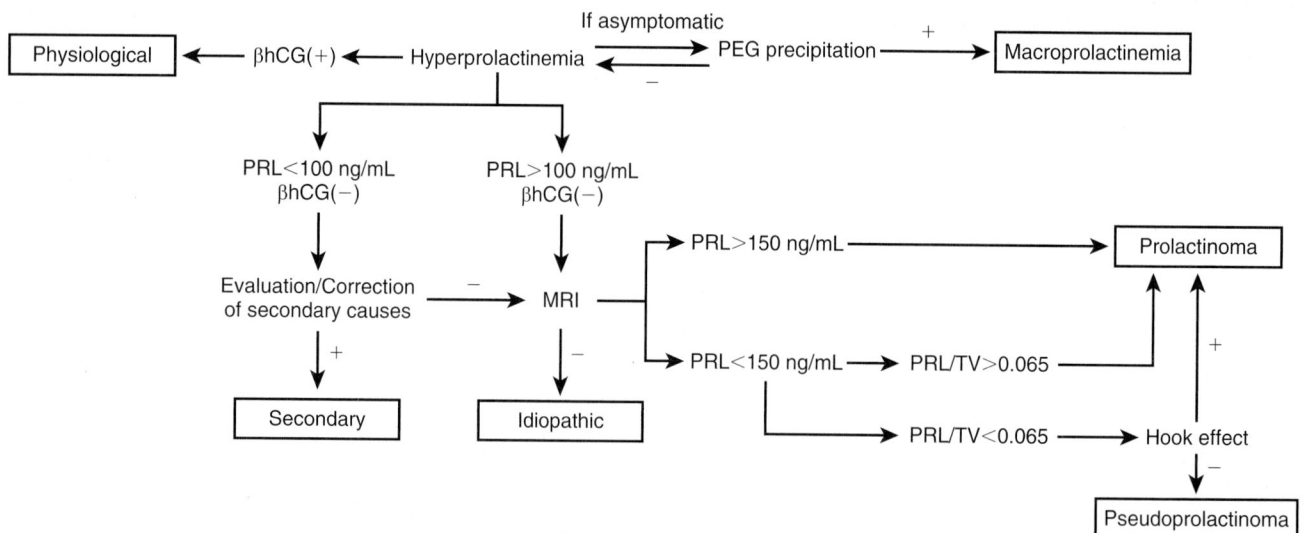

Figure 2 Diagnostic algorithm for hyperprolactinemia. If hyperprolactinemia occurs in the absence of relevant clinical symptoms and signs, one should rule out macroprolactinemia by PEG precipitation. When hyperprolactinemia is confirmed, pregnancy should be ruled out with a βhCG test. In the absence of pregnancy, if the PRL level is higher than 100 ng/dL, the pretest probability for a prolactinoma is high enough to justify a pituitary MRI scan, even if potential secondary causes exist. Regardless of prolactin levels, secondary causes should be carefully evaluated with medication history, physical examination, and laboratory tests such as thyroid function tests and chemistry panel, and appropriately treated. If hyperprolactinemia remains unexplained or persists despite correction of other contributing factors, a pituitary MRI is in order. Patients with negative sellar findings have idiopathic hyperprolactinemia. Patients with sellar mass may have either prolactinoma or pseudoprolactinoma. The latter is suggested by a discordant prolactin level less than 150 ng/mL and prolactin/tumor volume ratio lower than 0.065 (ng/mL)/mm³, after hook effect has been ruled out. *βhCG*, β Human chorionic gonadotropin; *PRL*, prolactin; *PRL/TV*, prolactin level/tumor volume ratio in nanograms per milliliter per cubic millimeter.

A more typical range of prolactin level is 25 to 100 ng/mL for drug-induced hyperprolactinemia. It is not always possible to correlate in time the initiation of the culprit drug with the onset of symptoms or rise of prolactin levels. The way to confirm medication-related hyperprolactinemia is to discontinue the putative offending agent(s) for 3 days before repeating a prolactin assay. Some medications may require a longer period of abstinence, and in such cases the level of prolactin can be retested later if the second value is reduced but still elevated. Before discontinuing psychotropic medications, one should consult with the prescribing psychiatrist to prevent worsening of the patient's mental symptoms.

Pseudoprolactinoma refers to a nonfunctioning sellar or suprasellar mass associated with hyperprolactinemia caused by stalk disruption. The prolactin level is seldom >150 ng/mL for pseudoprolactinomas. Accordingly, the Pituitary Society's 2006 guidelines for the diagnosis and management of prolactinomas use 150 ng/mL as a cutoff for diagnosing prolactinoma. Recent literature, however, has revealed significant overlap of prolactin levels in patients with true prolactinoma and secondary hyperprolactinemia <150 ng/mL. Taking into consideration tumor volume in assessing prolactin levels significantly improves diagnostic accuracy. In patients with prolactin levels ≤150 ng/mL, a prolactin level/tumor volume ratio of 0.065 $(ng/mL)/mm^3$ accurately separates patients with nonfunctional pituitary tumors from true prolactinomas without any overlap. Before making a diagnosis of pseudoprolactinoma, one must exclude hook effect with a 100-fold diluted sample. Prolactin levels are typically normalized within several days after initiation of dopamine agonists, because lactotrophs are still sensitive to dopamine, but local compressive symptoms do not improve. In contrast, patients with true macroprolactinoma experience a more gradual decrease in prolactin levels after they are put on dopamine agonists, but they could expect improvement in compressive symptoms within 12 hours to days and imaging evidence of tumor shrinkage in weeks.

Polycystic ovary syndrome (PCOS) and hyperprolactinemia are among the most common causes of menstrual irregularities and infertility and affect women of similar ages. PCOS has also been associated with hyperprolactinemia. However, multiple studies have shown that the prevalence of hyperprolactinemia in women with PCOS is not significantly higher than that of matched populations. Although mild elevations of DHEA-S or DHEA are common in patients with hyperprolactinemia, hirsutism is rare and, when present, is always associated with an increase in testosterone level, likely reflecting possible coexisting PCOS. Therefore the presence of hyperprolactinemia in patients with PCOS or hirsutism warrants additional evaluation.

Management of Secondary Hyperprolactinemia

Treatment of secondary hyperprolactinemia should focus on correcting the underlying conditions; for example, treating hypothyroidism and resection of nonfunctioning pituitary tumors. For drug-induced hyperprolactinemia, the responsible medications should be removed or replaced with alternatives. Newer antipsychotics such as aripiprazole (Abilify) may be used in place of older agents such as risperidone (Risperdal) because they have better metabolic/hormonal profiles. For irreversible conditions such as end-stage renal disease, hyperprolactinemia can be effectively controlled with dopamine agonists. Ectopic prolactin secretion, which occurs in paraneoplastic syndrome, is a rare exception where dopamine agonists are ineffective, because extrapituitary production of prolactin is driven by alternative promoters, which do not respond to dopamine. Asymptomatic patients with modest hyperprolactinemia may not need treatment, however, and sex hormone replacement may be adequate for correcting hypogonadism if fertility is not desired.

Management of Prolactinoma

The goals for managing prolactinomas are twofold: treating symptomatic hyperprolactinemia and relief of tumor mass effects.

Treatment thus needs to be tailored to the patient's unique clinical picture and the desired outcome. Mass effects are not a concern for microprolactinomas, whereas for patients with giant prolactinomas (defined as >4 cm or >2 cm of suprasellar extension) and extreme hyperprolactinemia, normalization of prolactin levels is less likely, and treatment should focus on reversal or minimization of mass effects and symptomatic relief. The following are appropriate options in specific settings.

Observation

Active surveillance is appropriate for patients with microprolactinoma who are asymptomatic or not troubled by galactorrhea, especially if fertility is not a concern. As long as regular menses are preserved, they seem to be spared any long-term consequences from hyperprolactinemia. Bone mineral density appears to be preserved in these patients. It is noteworthy that a significant fraction of patients may have tumor resolution during surveillance without treatment. Tumor expansion is a rare event, and serial measurements of serum prolactin level are effective for monitoring interval tumor growth. Pituitary imaging is indicated when there is a significant increase in prolactin level or emergence of local compression symptoms.

Hormone Replacement

For patients with microprolactinoma bothered only by symptoms related to hypogonadism including menstrual abnormalities, sexual dysfunction, and osteoporosis but who no longer desire fertility, hormone replacement is a valid alternative to dopamine agonists, especially when the latter are not tolerated or are contraindicated. This can be achieved with oral contraceptive pills in women premenopause or testosterone in men. This approach compares favorably to dopamine agonists in terms of cost and side effects. Patients may experience slight increases in prolactin level, but tumor progression has not been associated with use of oral contraceptive pills for up to 2 years. It would be prudent to use lower doses of estradiol (≤30 μg/day) and closely monitor patients for prolactin level and tumor growth.

Dopamine Agonists

Medical treatment with dopamine agonists has replaced surgery as the first-line treatment for prolactinomas, with excellent efficacy in achieving treatment goals and minimal risk. The therapeutic effects of dopamine agonists are mediated by dopamine D2 receptors in tumor cells, which inhibit prolactin synthesis and secretion, slow cell proliferation, and reduce tumor vascularity. Normalization of prolactin levels and reduction of tumor size can be expected in most patients. A small fraction of prolactinomas is resistant to dopamine agonists, as defined by failure in normalizing prolactin level, reduction in tumor size by 50%, or restoration of gonadal function with standard doses. In general, microprolactinomas are more sensitive to dopamine agonists than macroprolactinomas are, and men are more likely to be drug resistant than are women. Rapid responders experience significant improvement of visual symptoms within 24 to 72 hours; some of them may develop complications resulting from the rapid receding of macroprolactinomas (uncorking); for example, CSF leak, pituitary apoplexy, and optic chiasm hernia. For most patients, however, progressive reduction of tumor size occurs over the course of months to years, although some patients may never experience tumor shrinkage despite normalization of prolactin levels at the highest tolerated doses.

Patients with microprolactinoma may discontinue treatment upon menopause because their treatment goal has been fulfilled. Patients with macroprolactinoma, on the other hand, may require lifelong treatment to prevent tumor regrowth. A meta-analysis showed that a small fraction of patients may enter long-term remission after discontinuing dopamine agonists (21% for microprolactinomas and 16% for macroprolactinomas). The odds are significantly improved if patients have been treated for at least 2 years and tumor size has reduced by ≥50%. The 2011 Endocrine Society practice guidelines suggest that tapering or discontinuing dopamine agonists may be attempted in patients who have been

TABLE 2	Use of Dopamine Agonists in Hyperprolactinemia				
	ROUTE	DOSING FREQUENCY		STARTING DOSE	USUAL DOSE RANGE
Bromocriptine (Parlodel)	PO Intravaginal[1]	Twice a day		1.25 mg after dinner or before bed for 1 week, then twice a day	2.5–10 mg/day
Cabergoline (Dostinex)	PO	Once to twice a week		0.25 mg twice a week or 0.5 mg once a week	0.5–2 mg/week

[1]Not FDA approved for this indication.

treated for at least 2 years and experienced complete biochemical and radiographic resolution. The risk for recurrence after drug discontinuation is related to the size of adenoma at the time of the diagnosis. For tumors larger than 2 cm, especially giant prolactinomas, tapering the dopamine agonists to a lower maintenance dose for lifelong treatment after achieving maximal tumor reduction would be a better strategy for these patients. Tapering or withdrawal of dopamine agonists should be followed by close surveillance of prolactin levels and pituitary MRI when prolactin level increases, especially during the first year.

Three dopamine agonists are currently used for treating hyperprolactinemia, including bromocriptine (Parlodel), cabergoline (Dostinex), and quinagolide (not currently available in the United States). Bromocriptine was the first dopamine agonist available, and it has the best established safety record. It is still the only dopamine agonist approved by the FDA to be used in pregnancy, when indicated. Cabergoline is a more specific agonist of the D2 dopamine receptor and is superior in many respects to bromocriptine because of dosing convenience, tolerability, and treatment efficacy. Many patients not controlled with bromocriptine may achieve normal prolactin levels after switching to cabergoline, which has become the drug of choice for cases not involving pregnancy. The safety data for cabergoline are now substantial during pregnancy, but the FDA has not yet approved its use in pregnant women. Common side effects for this class of drugs include nausea, orthostatic hypotension, fatigue, mental fogginess, and, less frequently, nasal stuffiness, Raynaud phenomenon, constipation, depression, and psychosis. Nausea is more common in patients taking bromocriptine; for these patients the intravaginal route[1] can be tried. Patients receiving higher doses of cabergoline are at risk of developing cardiac valvulopathy. This has so far been a concern for patients with Parkinson's disease, who may require much higher doses. However, the lifelong exposure to high cumulative doses in patients with resistant prolactinoma is considerable, and regular echocardiogram surveillance is recommended for patients taking doses higher than 2 mg/week. Dosing regimens for bromocriptine and cabergoline are listed in Table 2. In general, patients should be started on the lowest doses and titrated upward monthly based on the serum prolactin level until treatment goals are reached.

Surgery

With the availability of the second-generation dopamine agonists, surgery is mostly reserved for the following situations: (1) patients intolerant of, or resistant to, dopamine agonists; (2) women with macroprolactinoma who are planning for conception, to forestall tumor expansion during pregnancy; (3) pituitary apoplexy threatening neurologic and visual functions if not managed urgently. For select patients with access to experienced pituitary surgeons, surgery can be offered for first line treatment for microprolactinomas and well-circumscribed macroprolactinoma (Knosp grade 0 or 1), with benefits including possibility of cure without cost and potential side effects associated with long term medical treatments. In particular, fibrosis of prolactinoma after treatment with dopamine agonists may complicate future surgeries should needs arise. Transsphenoidal tumor resection is the standard surgical approach. Perioperative mortality and morbidity are low in the hands of experienced pituitary surgeons in high-volume centers. Major surgical complications include vision loss, CNS infection, stroke, and oculomotor palsy. Craniotomy is occasionally needed for masses with extrasellar extensions that may be inaccessible by the transsphenoidal route, with higher risk for complications. Postoperatively, patients need to be monitored for signs of diabetes insipidus and secondary adrenal insufficiency, which may be transient or permanent.

Radiotherapy

Radiotherapy is inadequate as a primary treatment for prolactinoma, because its efficacy is poor and latency is long. It is also associated with long-term complications including permanent hypopituitarism, cerebrovascular accidents, and secondary intracranial malignancies. Currently it is reserved mostly for patients with aggressive and malignant prolactinomas failing medical/surgical treatment. Stereotactic radiosurgery is preferred over conventional fractionated radiotherapy for more convenient dosing, better efficacy, and lower rate of complications. However, radiosurgery should not be attempted for tumors in close proximity to the visual apparatus (less than 5 mm of clearance), because it is associated with an unacceptably high rate of vision loss.

Management of Prolactinoma During Pregnancy

Mild hyperprolactinemia is part of normal pregnancy, and there are concerns for the safe use of dopamine agonists in pregnant women. There is convincing evidence that as long as bromocriptine is withdrawn within a week after confirmation of pregnancy, obstetric outcome is not altered. Less robust data to date suggest that continuing bromocriptine treatment until term is also safe. Despite its longer half-life, as long as cabergoline is discontinued in early pregnancy, it also has not been found to be associated with adverse outcomes. Until there is incontrovertible evidence for the absolute safety of these dopamine agonists, however, it is prudent to discontinue these drugs as soon as pregnancy is confirmed. Mechanical contraception should be advised for women not desiring fertility when initiating dopamine agonists. Given its shorter half-life and established safety record, bromocriptine is the preferred agent for fertility induction in women with hyperprolactinemia, although cabergoline would also be acceptable if bromocriptine is not tolerated. If cabergoline is already initiated at the time of fertility planning, most experts prefer reducing cabergoline to a lowest effective dose instead of switching to bromocriptine because of the substantial safety data accumulated for cabergoline in pregnancy and concern of side effects and treatment noncompliance associated with switching to bromocriptine. The major indication to treat prolactinomas medically during pregnancy is the concern for tumor expansion. Such risk is negligible for microprolactinomas. For patients with macroprolactinoma, however, symptomatic tumor expansion during pregnancy can occur in up to about 30% of cases. This risk can be significantly reduced if the patient has been treated with a dopamine agonist for at least a year with evidence of tumor shrinkage or has undergone pituitary surgery or radiotherapy prior to pregnancy. Until these conditions are met, women of childbearing age with macroprolactinomas should be advised to take nonhormonal contraceptive measures. For patients who fail to achieve tumor shrinkage with dopamine agonists or cannot tolerate them, prophylactic surgery prior to pregnancy may be considered, after careful discussion with the patient on surgical risks and the possibility of permanent hypopituitarism, which further impairs fertility. The Endocrine Society practice guidelines recommend against measurement of serum prolactin levels during pregnancy. Instead, the patient should be followed

[1]Not FDA approved for this indication.

clinically for any signs or symptoms of tumor expansion. MRI without gadolinium and visual field testing should be done when clinical suspicion arises. If tumor expansion is confirmed, the patient should be reinitiated on bromocriptine. Debulking surgery is reserved for patients failing or not tolerating medical treatment. Lactation usually does not cause tumor progression, and patients are encouraged to breast-feed their infants with close surveillance. They should not take either bromocriptine or cabergoline, however, because both are secreted in the milk and are effective lactation inhibitors.

Management of Resistant and Malignant Prolactinoma

Several other treatment options are available for patients who fail the highest tolerated doses of dopamine agonists, surgery, and radiation. A small fraction of these patients have malignant prolactinoma, which is defined by extrapituitary metastasis; histopathologically, malignant prolactinomas can appear very similar to aggressive prolactinomas. An alkylating agent, temozolomide (Temodar),[1] has been successfully used in the treatment of aggressive pituitary adenoma and pituitary carcinoma. Monotherapy with temozolomide has been established as the first-line chemotherapy for these conditions, following documented tumor growth despite standard therapies. Selective estrogen receptor modulators, including raloxifene (Evista)[1] and tamoxifen (Temodar),[1] have been found to be useful adjuncts that can reduce prolactin level and inhibit tumor growth.

[1] Not FDA approved for this indication.

References

Ahuja N, Moorhead S, Lloyd AJ, Cole AJ: Antipsychotic-induced hyperprolactinemia and delusion of pregnancy, *Psychosomatics* 49:163–167, 2008.
Andereggen L, Frey J, Andres RH, et al: First-line surgery in prolactinomas: lessons from a long-term follow-up study in a tertiary referral center. *J Endocrinol Invest.* 44:2621–2633, 2021.
Bernard V, Young J, Chanson P, Binart N: New insights in prolactin: pathological implications, *Nat Rev Endocrinol* 11:265–275, 2015.
Bronstein MD: Disorders of prolactin secretion and prolactinomas. In Jameson JL, De Groot LJ, editors: *Endocrinology: adult and pediatric*, ed 7, Philadelphia, 2016, Elsevier.
Casanueva FF, Molitch ME, Schlechte JA, et al: Guidelines of the Pituitary Society for the diagnosis and management of prolactinomas, *Clin Endocrinol (Oxf)* 65:265–273, 2006.
Chanson P, Maiter D: Prolactinoma. In Molmed S, editor: *The pituitary*, ed 4, San Diego, 2017, Elsevier.
Ciccarelli A, Daly AF, Beckers A: The epidemiology of prolactinomas, *Pituitary* 8:3–6, 2005.
Dekkers OM, Lagro J, Burman P, Jorgensen JO, Romijn JA, Pereira AM: Recurrence of hyperprolactinemia after withdrawal of dopamine agonists: systematic review and meta-analysis, *J Clin Endocrinol Metab* 95:43–51, 2010.
Faje A, Jones P, Swearingen B, Tritos NA: The prolactin per unit tumor volume ratio accurately distinguishes prolactinomas from secondary hyperprolactinemia due to stalk effect, *Endocr Pract* 28:572–577, 2022.
Filho RB, Domingues L, Naves L, et al: Polycystic ovary syndrome and hyperprolactinemia are distinct entities, *Gynecol Endocrinol* 23:267–272, 2007.
Glezer A, Bronstein MD: Prolactinomas, cabergoline, and pregnancy, *Endocrine* 47:64–69, 2014.
Grattan DR: 60 years of neuroendocrinology: the hypothalamo-prolactin axis, *J Endocrinol* 226:T101–T122, 2015.
Horseman ND, Gregerson KA: Prolactin. In Jameson JL, De Groot LJ, editors: *Endocrinology: adult and pediatric*, ed 7, Philadelphia, 2016, Elsevier.
Huang W, Molitch ME: Evaluation and management of galactorrhea, *Am Fam Physician* 85:1073–1080, 2012.
Kirsch P, Kunadia J, Shah S, Agrawal N: Metabolic effects of prolactin and the role of dopamine agonists: a review, *Front Endocrinol* 13:1002320, 2022.
Melmed S, Casanueva FF, Hoffman AR, et al: Diagnosis and treatment of hyperprolactinemia: an Endocrine Society clinical practice guideline, *J Clin Endocrinol Metab* 96:273–288, 2011.
Melmed S, Kleinberg D: Pituitary masses and tumors. In Melmed S, et al: *Williams textbook of endocrinology*, ed 13, Philadelphia, 2016, Elsevier.
Miyai K, Ichihara K, Kondo K, Mori S: Asymptomatic hyperprolactinaemia and prolactinoma in the general population: mass screening by paired assays of serum prolactin, *Clin Endocrinol* 25:549–554, 1986.
Molitch ME: Drugs and prolactin, *Pituitary* 11:209–218, 2008.
Newman CB, Blaha MJ, Boord JB, et al: Lipid management in patients with endocrine disorders: an endocrine society clinical practice guideline, *J Clin Endocrinol Metab* 105:3613–3682, 2020.
Petersenn S, Fleseriu M, Casanueva FF, et al.: Diagnosis and management of prolactin-secreting pituitary adenomas: a Pituitary Society international consensus statement, *Nat Rev Endocrinol* 19:722–740, 2023.
Raverot G, Burman P, McCormack A, et al: European Society of Endocrinology Clinical Practice Guidelines for the management of aggressive pituitary tumors and carcinomas, *Eur J Endocrinol* 178:G1–G24, 2018.
Samson SL, Hamrahian AH, Ezzat S: American Association of Clinical Endocrinologists, American College of Endocrinology disease state clinical review: clinical relevance of macroprolactin in the absence or presence of true hyperprolactinemia, *Endocr Pract* 21:1427–1435, 2015.
Schlechte J, Dolan K, Sherman B, et al: The natural history of untreated hyperprolactinemia: a prospective analysis, *J Clin Endocrinol Metab* 68:412–418, 1989.
Stiegler C, Leb G, Kleinert R, et al: Plasma levels of parathyroid hormone-related peptide are elevated in hyperprolactinemia and correlated to bone density status, *J Bone Miner Res* 10:751–759, 1995.
Testa G, Vegetti W, Motta T, et al: Two-year treatment with oral contraceptives in hyperprolactinemic patients, *Contraception* 58:69–73, 1998.
Vartej P, Poiana C, Vartej I: Effects of hyperprolactinemia on osteoporotic fracture risk in premenopausal women, *Gynecol Endocrinol* 15:43–47, 2001.

HYPERTHYROIDISM

Method of
Kyle Myers, DO

CURRENT DIAGNOSIS

- Hyperthyroidism is relatively uncommon, affecting about 2.5% of the general population in iodine-sufficient areas, with Graves disease among the most common etiologies. Toxic nodular goiter and thyroiditis are other common etiologies.
- Symptoms of hyperthyroidism may include heat intolerance, weight loss, tachycardia, palpitations, tremors, anxiety, insomnia, or diarrhea. Many signs and symptoms are driven by β-adrenergic stimulation by thyroid hormone.
- Hyperthyroidism is typically diagnosed biochemically with a low or suppressed thyroid-stimulating hormone (TSH) with elevated free or total thyroxine (T_4) or total triiodothyronine (T_3).
- TSH-receptor antibodies (TRAb) are generally used initially to screen for Graves disease given its prevalence.
- In the presence of negative TRAb, thyroid uptake and scan or scintigraphy can help distinguish etiologies.
- Subclinical hyperthyroidism is defined as a low or suppressed TSH with normal T_4 and T_3 levels. Causes include etiologies similar to those of overt hyperthyroidism, and clinical manifestations are usually mild or asymptomatic.
- Thyroid storm is a rare but severe and life-threatening form of thyrotoxicosis that is usually precipitated by a physiologic stress in the setting of underlying hyperthyroidism from any cause.

CURRENT THERAPY

- Symptomatic management with β-adrenergic blockade is a first-line treatment. For patients with contraindications to β-blockers, calcium channel blockers may be used to control heart rate.
- For the treatment of Graves disease or toxic nodular goiters, antithyroid drugs (ATDs) may be used to reduce thyroid hormone synthesis in most patients. Recent data suggest ATDs may be used long term—many years—in select patients.
- Radioiodine ablation and surgery with total thyroidectomy are definitive management options for some patients and preferred in those with toxic nodular goiter.
- Subclinical hyperthyroidism should be treated in select patients to reduce the risk of complications such as cardiovascular disease or osteoporosis.
- Thyroid storm requires emergent treatment with β-blockers, ATDs, potassium iodide (SSKI)[1] and glucocorticoids, and admission to an intensive care unit for close observation.

[1] Not FDA approved for this indication.

Background

Thyrotoxicosis refers to the clinical manifestations of elevated thyroid hormone in systemic circulation and is typically caused by either hyperthyroidism or thyroiditis. Hyperthyroidism, specifically, refers to overproduction of thyroid hormone T_4 or T_3 by the thyroid gland due to various causes. Thyroiditis refers to inflammation of the thyroid gland resulting in the release of preformed thyroid hormone into the systemic circulation. Differentiating between hyperthyroidism and thyroiditis has unique treatment implications and is an important distinction for the clinician to make.

This chapter will focus primarily on hyperthyroidism. Thyroiditis is covered briefly here and in more detail in a separate chapter.

Hyperthyroidism may be overt or subclinical depending on the degree and severity of biochemical abnormality. Overt hyperthyroidism is diagnosed biochemically with a low or suppressed TSH and elevated free or total T_4 and/or free or total T_3 hormones.

Subclinical hyperthyroidism refers to the biochemical findings of a low or suppressed TSH with normal range free or total T_4 and/or T_3. Overt or subclinical hyperthyroidism could lead to symptomatic thyrotoxicosis, though subclinical is usually milder or asymptomatic. The global prevalence of hyperthyroidism, overt or subclinical, ranges from 0.2% to 3.0%.

Pathophysiology

A list of etiologies of hyperthyroidism can be found in Table 1. The most common causes of hyperthyroidism include Graves disease, toxic adenoma (TA), or multinodular goiter (MNG).

In iodine-sufficient areas, Graves disease is the most common cause of hyperthyroidism. Graves disease is an autoimmune condition defined by autoantibodies that stimulate the TSH receptor, increasing the production of thyroid hormones. Graves disease has an incidence of about 30 cases per 100,000 per year, is seen more commonly in females (with a ratio of ~6 to 9:1, female-to-male), and tends to manifest in the third or fourth decade of life. The predisposition to develop Graves disease is thought to arise from a complex interaction of genetic and environmental factors. Variants in immunoregulatory genes (notably, HLA-B, HLA, DR3, and CD40), play a role. Additionally, there is a strong hereditary component.

TA refers to the autonomous function of a thyroid nodule within the thyroid gland that causes hyperthyroidism through increased thyroid hormone production. Toxic MNG denotes the presence of more than one autonomously functioning nodule. In iodine-sufficient areas, the incidence of toxic nodular goiters is about 6 per 100,000 per year. Toxic nodular goiters are more common in females and tend to manifest after the age of 50, with preexisting nodules developing autonomy over time.

Thyroiditis refers to the inflammation of the thyroid gland from any cause. Thyroiditis causes hyperthyroidism by the release of preformed thyroid hormone from the thyroid gland into the systemic circulation. Common causes of thyroiditis include autoimmune (Hashimoto thyroiditis), medications (e.g., amiodarone, lithium, immune-checkpoint inhibitors), infection, and postpartum.

Amiodarone-induced thyrotoxicosis (AIT) is a common phenomenon seen in up to 11% to 12% of patients on amiodarone. Amiodarone can induce thyrotoxicosis either through increased production of thyroid hormone via the exposure of the high iodine content of the medication (AIT type 1) or via thyroiditis and the release of preformed hormone from the thyroid gland (AIT type 2).

With the rising use of immunotherapy for cancer treatment, endocrinopathies, including thyrotoxicosis, have been more prevalent. Notably, anti–cytotoxic T-lymphocyte antigen 4 (CTLA-4) antibody and anti–programmed cell death 1 (PD-1) antibody treatments have been associated with both hyperthyroidism and destructive thyroiditis.

Exogenous thyroid hormone use can result in hyperthyroidism, by either supratherapeutic doses of thyroid hormone for the treatment of hypothyroidism or factitious use of thyroid hormone for weight loss abuse.

Thyroid storm refers to the rare disorder of life-threatening and severe thyrotoxicosis with multiorgan involvement. It is usually precipitated by an event such as thyroid or nonthyroidal surgery, infection, trauma, acute iodine load, or discontinuation of ATDs. Signs and symptoms of thyroid storm include those of general thyrotoxicosis but are typically more severe. Extreme tachycardia (ventricular rates >140 beats/min), signs of acute heart failure, fever, and neuropsychiatric symptoms (agitation, delirium, psychosis, coma) are typical features of the clinical diagnosis.

Thyroid storm carries increased risk of morbidity and mortality and is diagnosed clinically. Additional diagnostic algorithms may be used, including the Burch-Wartofsky Point Scale or Japanese Thyroid Association scale. Treatment is discussed later.

Prevention

There are no known prevention methods for hyperthyroidism. Patients who are treated for hypothyroidism with levothyroxine can avoid iatrogenic hyperthyroidism by titration of medication dose to maintain a normal-range TSH.

Clinical Manifestations

Thyroid hormones exert effect on nearly all organ systems in the body, basal metabolism, and thermogenesis. Many of the cardiovascular signs and symptoms are mediated by β-adrenergic stimulation by thyroid hormone. Clinical manifestations may include palpitation, tremor, increased anxiety and nervousness, insomnia and sleep difficulties, weight loss, diarrhea, increased sweating, and heat intolerance. A high index of suspicion is warranted for diagnosing hyperthyroidism, given the clinical manifestations are varied and nonspecific. The severity of signs and symptoms are not always correlated to the degree of biochemical thyroid hormone elevation. Younger patients may be more likely to have pronounced symptoms of β-adrenergic stimulation, such

TABLE 1	β-Adrenergic Blocker Options for the Treatment of Symptomatic Thyrotoxicosis		
	DOSE	**FREQUENCY**	**CONSIDERATIONS**
Propranolol[1]	10–40 mg	3–4 times daily	Inhibits conversion of T_4 to T_3 in high doses. Easily titratable. Preferred for nursing or pregnant mothers.
Atenolol[1]	25–50mg	1–2 times daily	Avoid during pregnancy. Increased compliance with once-daily schedule.
Metoprolol[1]	25–50 mg	Every 8–12 hours	Relative β_1 selective
Esmolol[1]	IV; loading dose of 250–500 mcg/kg, followed by infusion at 50–100 μg/kg/min		IV only. Used in the intensive care setting for severe thyrotoxicosis or thyroid storm. Very short duration of action, and reasonable option to trial if β-blocker tolerability is uncertain.

[1]Not FDA approved for this indication.

TABLE 2	Antithyroid Drugs		
	INITIAL DOSING	FREQUENCY	CONSIDERATIONS
Methimazole	10–30 mg daily*	1–2 times daily	Avoid during first trimester. Increased compliance with once-daily schedule.
Propylthiouracil	50–150 mg*	Three times daily	Relative β_1 selective

For MMI: 5–10 mg/d for free T_4 concentrations 1.0–1.5 times the upper limit of normal, 10–20 mg/d for free T_4 1.5–2.0 times the upper limit of normal, and 30–40 mg/d for free T_4 2–3 times the upper limit of normal.
*The starting dose of either thionamide depends on the severity of the hyperthyroidism.

as tachycardia or tremor. A subset of older patients may present with "apathetic" hyperthyroidism with less severe signs or symptoms.

Patients with Graves disease or enlarged goiter may present with compressive symptoms such as difficulty swallowing or vocal hoarseness. Thyroiditis, depending on the cause, may manifest with thyroid pain and tenderness.

Graves ophthalmopathy (GO), or thyroid eye disease, is an inflammatory process that develops in the orbit due to autoimmune processes. GO may occur in up to one-third of patients with Graves hyperthyroidism. Signs or symptoms of GO may include painful eye movements, pain behind the eyes, dry eyes, swelling of the eyelids, decreased visual acuity, or proptosis. All patients diagnosed with Graves hyperthyroidism should undergo ophthalmologic evaluation. Treatment for GO, under the direction of an ophthalmologist, varies depending on severity and ranges from surveillance measures for mild disease to immunomodulatory therapy (e.g., teprotumumab [Tepezza]) in severe cases.

Subclinical hyperthyroidism is more likely to manifest with asymptomatic or mild symptoms, though cardiovascular, metabolic, and neuropsychiatric changes can be present even in milder cases.

Untreated overt and subclinical hyperthyroidism have been associated with an increased risk of cardiovascular disease, atrial fibrillation, osteoporosis, and cognitive decline.

Diagnosis

Serum TSH is the most sensitive and specific test to evaluate thyroid function and should be the initial screening test when hyperthyroidism is suspected. In the normal pituitary-thyroid axis, serum TSH and free T_4 have an inverse relationship. Serum TSH is low or suppressed in cases of hyperthyroidism. The serum thyroid hormones free or total T_4 and/or free or total T_3 are elevated in overt hyperthyroidism or normal in subclinical hyperthyroidism. Rare entities such as a TSH-producing pituitary adenoma or thyroid hormone resistance may be associated with normal or elevated TSH values and elevated T_4 or T_3, though these are uncommon.

After biochemical diagnosis, the etiology should be determined. In some cases, the cause may be apparent, such as a patient with an enlarged, non-nodular goiter and exophthalmos having Graves disease. In patients without a nodular thyroid goiter on examination, measurement of thyrotropin receptor antibodies (e.g., TRAb or thyrotropin-stimulating immunoglobulin [TSI]) is recommended as initial next steps. If positive, the TRAb-receptor antibodies confirm a diagnosis of Graves disease; however, negative antibody testing does not exclude Graves disease entirely, given a small subset of antibody-negative disease.

Antibody-negative hyperthyroidism, or nodular goiters, should be evaluated by thyroid scintigraphy, measuring uptake of radioactive iodine to assess thyroid gland activity. Increased radioiodine (RAI) uptake suggests Graves disease if uptake is seen diffusely, or a toxic nodular goiter if uptake is seen focally with suppression of uptake in the surrounding thyroid tissue. RAI uptake is low or near absent in cases of thyroiditis, iatrogenic thyrotoxicosis, or factitious ingestion of thyroid hormone. RAI imaging is contraindicated in pregnant or breastfeeding patients.

Ultrasound with color Doppler flow, when available at centers with expertise, may also be helpful in suggesting an etiology, particularly when RAI is contraindicated. High blood flow seen on color Doppler imaging has been associated with Graves'

hyperthyroidism, with normal or low blood flow more so associated with painless thyroiditis, though these findings may be less specific. Ultrasound is also helpful to define thyroid nodules found on examination or scintigraphy to evaluate for thyroid malignancy. Biopsy of hyperfunctioning nodules is not routinely recommended, as these are almost always benign.

Therapy

Treatment for hyperthyroidism is twofold: symptom management of thyrotoxicosis and attenuating excessive thyroid hormone synthesis (see Table 1).

Management of Symptomatic Thyrotoxicosis

Symptoms of thyrotoxicosis, regardless of the cause, should be treated to attenuate the adverse cardiovascular and hemodynamic effects of excessive β-adrenergic stimulation by thyroid hormone. This is particularly important in the elderly and patients who are more severely thyrotoxic. β-Blockers are the preferred first-line therapy for symptomatic management and should be titrated to achieve desired heart rate (resting <90 bpm) and blood pressure control.

Preparations and doses of various β-blockers are listed in Table 2.

β-Blockers are generally contraindicated in patients with bronchospastic disease, though they could be cautiously trialed in patients with mild obstructive airway disease if close monitoring of airway status is possible. For patients unable to tolerate higher doses of β-blockade, or in whom β-blockers are contraindicated, calcium channel blockers verapamil[1] and diltiazem[1] may be used for rate control.

In thyroid storm, β-blockers may be contraindicated in patients with acute decompensated heart failure with systolic dysfunction, because the hyperadrenergic state and increased heart rate are important for maintaining cardiac output.

In thyroiditis, β-blockers are typically the only treatment needed given the self-limited nature and absence of increased thyroid hormone production. Glucocorticoids may be used to decrease peripheral T_4 to T_3 conversion in more severe cases.

Decreasing Thyroid Hormone Synthesis

Treatment options for Graves disease and toxic nodular goiter include ATDs, thyroid gland ablation using RAI, or surgical removal of the thyroid gland. The decision should be made based on various patient-specific factors and the underlying etiology. Graves disease has a higher likelihood of either spontaneous or treatment-induced remission, and ATDs are generally preferred. Toxic nodular goiters are unlikely to remit and are more likely to require definitive therapy.

Antithyroid Drugs

ATDs render patients euthyroid quickly and safely in most circumstances. ATDs do not cure underlying Graves disease or toxic nodular goiter, though patients using ATDs for Graves have been shown to have higher rates of remission than those with spontaneous remission.

Relevant ATDs include methimazole (MMI) and propylthiouracil (PTU), with MMI generally preferred over PTU for its safer adverse effect profile and easier dosing schedule. MMI should be

---

[1] Not FDA approved for this indication.

used over PTU in all patients except during the first trimester of pregnancy, where PTU is favored given the higher risk of teratogenic effects with MMI during this period. Patients are generally transitioned back to MMI at the start of the second trimester.

Initial ATD dosing should be based on the severity of hyperthyroidism.

Before starting ATD, patients should have baseline complete blood count (CBC) and liver function testing done and be counseled on potential rare side effects, including agranulocytosis, hepatocellular injury, or cholestatic jaundice. Patients with fever or sore throat should present for immediate medication evaluation, including CBC. Patients should also be counseled to monitor for dark urine, jaundice, abdominal pain. ATDs have also been associated with drug-induced lupus, vasculitis, and rash. The prevalence of any adverse effect with ATD may be as high as 13%.

ATDs are the preferred treatment for patients with a high-likelihood of remission (patients with mild disease and low-titer TRAb), pregnant patients, the elderly or others with comorbidities increasing surgical or RAI risk, patients who need rapid biochemical control of hyperthyroidism, or patients with Graves ophthalmopathy.

Definitive contraindications to ATDs include patients with a documented history of adverse reaction to a specific ATD.

ATDs should be continued for approximately 12 to 18 months, after which patients with normal thyroid function on a stable dose of ATD can have TRAb levels measured to assess the likelihood of remission off therapy. Patients with normal levels have a greater chance of remission. Patients with persistently elevated TRAb may either continue ATD therapy or choose alternative treatments. Long-term use of ATDs over several decades is thought to be a safe and reasonable option for many patients.

Radioactive Iodine

RAI is used to chemically ablate thyroid tissue, rendering the patient hypothyroid in the majority of cases (>80%). Dosing of RAI may either be a fixed dose (typically 10 to 15 millicuries, per American Thyroid Association guidelines) or individualized based on the size of thyroid gland and RAI uptake. RAI may cause a transient worsening of thyrotoxicosis after administration, and, thus, use of β-blockade and/or ATDs before RAI administration may be advised in select patients. Immediately after RAI administration, ATDs and β-blockers should be continued and tapered based on serial laboratory testing until T_4/T_3 reach normal reference range. After RAI, most patients reach euthyroid state within 4 to 6 weeks and the majority go on to develop hypothyroidism, which occurs from 4 weeks on, in most patients.

RAI may be preferred in specific situations such as toxic nodular goiters, patients with contraindication to ATDs, and at high surgical risk or failure to achieve biochemical control on ATD. A small percentage of patients may have persistent hyperthyroidism after RAI, which can be treated with ATDs, surgery, or retreatment with RAI.

RAI is contraindicated in pregnant or breastfeeding women, women planning a pregnancy in less than 6 months out from RAI treatment, coexisting thyroid cancer or suspicion of thyroid cancer, and individuals unable to comply with radiation safety guidelines. RAI may exacerbate eye disease among patients with Graves disease and should be avoided or patients may undergo glucocorticoid pretreatment before RAI administration.

Surgery

Surgery may be preferred in patients with large goiters with compressive symptoms, patients in whom thyroid malignancy is known or suspected, patients with moderate-to-severe Graves ophthalmopathy, or women planning pregnancy in less than 6 months.

If surgery is preferred, patients should be made euthyroid before surgery with ATD. SSKI[1] may be given for moderative-to-severe

---

[1] Not FDA approved for this indication.

BOX 1	Causes and Mechanism of Thyrotoxicosis

Causes of Thyrotoxicosis	Mechanism
Hyperthyroidism	
Graves disease	Excessive thyroid hormone production by TSH-receptor stimulation
TSH-producing pituitary adenoma	
hCG-mediated	
Medication-induced (AIT type 1, immunotherapy, lithium)	
Toxic nodular goiter	Autonomous thyroid hormone production
Thyroiditis	
Subacute granulomatous (de Quervain)	Release of preformed thyroid hormone due to thyroid follicular cell destruction
Painless thyroiditis (silent, lymphocytic)	
Medication-induced (AIT type 2, immunotherapy, lithium)	
Checkpoint-inhibitor induced	
Radiation thyroiditis	
Suppurative thyroiditis	
Postpartum thyroiditis	
Excessive exogenous thyroid hormone	As seen in overtreatment of hypothyroidism or surreptitiously self-administered
Struma ovarii	Paraneoplastic hyperthyroidism

AIT, Amiodarone-induced thyrotoxicosis; *hCG,* human chorionic gonadotropin; *MNG,* multinodular goiter; *TSH,* thyroid-stimulating hormone.

hyperthyroidism before surgery to further block hormone synthesis (e.g., saturated solution of potassium iodine diluted in water, 50 to 100 mg (0.05 to 0.1 mL, 1 to 2 drops) three times daily for 7 to 10 days in the immediate preoperative period). Total thyroidectomy renders patients immediately and permanently hypothyroid, necessitating lifelong thyroid hormone supplementation. Common complications of surgery should be discussed with the patient before surgery, including risk of hypoparathyroidism and injury to recurrent laryngeal nerve among other risks associated with any surgery, such as bleeding or infection.

Contraindications to surgery may include those who are poor surgical candidates or lack of access to a high-volume experienced surgeon. Pregnancy is a relative contraindication, and surgery should be not undertaken in the first or third trimester if at all possible due to teratogenic effects associated with anesthesia.

Thyroid Storm

Treatment of thyroid storm is directed at rapidly reducing circulating T_3 and blunting its β-adrenergic effects. Management necessitates a multifaceted approach, including β-adrenergic blockade; ATD therapy to block new hormone synthesis; inorganic iodine to block the release of stored thyroid hormone; corticosteroid therapy to reduce T_4 to T_3 peripheral conversion and promote vasomotor stability; and bile acid sequestrants to reduce enterohepatic recycling of thyroid hormone. Additionally, support and monitoring in the intensive care setting is essential.

Subclinical Hyperthyroidism

Untreated subclinical hyperthyroidism carries increased risk for cardiovascular disease and osteoporosis, and treatment is recommended in select cases. All individuals over age 65 with TSH less than 0.1 mU/L and any patient with known cardiac risk factors, heart disease, or osteoporosis should undergo treatment.

Treatment of subclinical hyperthyroidism should follow the same principles as for overt hyperthyroidism.

Monitoring

Patients on ATDs should have serum free T_4 and total T_3 monitored every 4 to 6 weeks, depending on severity of hyperthyroidism, until a stable euthyroid state is achieved. Serum TSH may remain low or suppressed for several months and is not a good measure or thyroid status in the initial treatment period. Once a euthyroid state is achieved, the dose of ATD can be tapered gradually, monitoring laboratory test results every 4 to 6 weeks after each dose adjustment. Patients on stable and long-term ATD use can have less frequent laboratory tests, approximately every 4 to 6 months.

After RAI ablation, follow-up should include biochemical monitoring with TSH, free T_4 and total T_3 levels every 4 to 6 weeks through the period of withdrawing ATD and subsequent levothyroxine initiation, until normal thyroid function is achieved. ATDs should be stopped once T_4/T_3 levels have normalized. Levothyroxine should be started once the patient becomes hypothyroid. Repeat RAI administration may be needed if hyperthyroidism persists after 6 months.

Complications

Untreated, hyperthyroidism may increase the risk of complications such as atrial fibrillation, osteoporosis, weight loss, muscle weakness, and neuropsychiatric symptoms. Untreated subclinical hyperthyroidism carries similar risks for osteoporosis and cardiovascular adverse outcomes. Thyroid storm is a medical emergency that must be managed expeditiously and appropriately or else there is increasing risk of cardiovascular and hemodynamic collapse and/or death.

References

Chaker L, Cooper DS, Walsh JP, Peeters RP: Hyperthyroidism, *Lancet*. 403(10428):768–780, 2024, https://doi.org/10.1016/S0140-6736(23)02016-0. Epub 2024 Jan 23. PMID: 38278171.

Hoang TD, Stocker DJ, Chou EL, Burch HB: 2022 Update on Clinical Management of Graves Disease and Thyroid Eye Disease, *Endocrinol Metab Clin North Am* 51(2):287–304, 2022, https://doi.org/10.1016/j.ecl.2021.12.004. Epub 2022 May 11. PMID: 35662442; PMCID: PMC9174594.

Lee SY, Pearce EN: Hyperthyroidism: A Review, *JAMA* 330(15):1472–1483, 2023, https://doi.org/10.1001/jama.2023.19052.

Ross DS, Burch HB, Cooper DS, et al: 2016 American Thyroid Association Guidelines for Diagnosis and Management of Hyperthyroidism and Other Causes of Thyrotoxicosis, *Thyroid* 26(10):1343–1421, 2016.

Tsai K, Leung AM: Subclinical Hyperthyroidism: a review of the clinical literature, *Endocr Pract* 27(3):254–260, 2021.

HYPOKALEMIA AND HYPERKALEMIA

Method of
Jie Tang, MD

CURRENT DIAGNOSIS

- The "initial approach" to the evaluation of dyskalemia is to determine if it is secondary to transcellular shifts (in vitro or in vivo) of potassium (K) or a result of a true change in total body K.
- A thorough history and physical will provide useful information regarding the causes of hypokalemia and hyperkalemia, especially in cases of low or high intake of K, and transcellular shifts.
- Key steps in the diagnostic approach to hypokalemia include assessments of urinary K excretion and acid-base status.
- Key steps in the diagnostic approach to hyperkalemia include assessments of renal function and aldosterone activity.

CURRENT THERAPY

- For both hypokalemia and hyperkalemia, it is critical to assess the underlying transcellular K shift, given the risk of rebound hyperkalemia after K repletion or hypokalemia after K restriction and removal.
- In cases of severe dyskalemia, close cardiac monitoring is needed.
- The aggressiveness of therapy for dyskalemia is directly related to the rapidity with which the condition has developed, the absolute level of serum K, and the clinical evidence of toxicity.
- In severe or symptomatic cases of hypokalemia, both intravenous and oral K repletion are often needed.
- In severe or symptomatic cases of hyperkalemia, supported by electrocardiogram (ECG) abnormalities, both immediate temporizing measures and definitive therapy for K removal are necessary.

Epidemiology

Hypokalemia is defined as a serum K level of 3.5 mmol/L or lower. It is a common electrolyte disorder encountered in clinical practice. According to one study, serum K less than 3.6 mmol/L was found in up to 20% of hospitalized patients. The majority of these patients had serum K concentrations between 3.0 and 3.5 mmol/L, but as many as 25% had values less than 3.0 mmol/L. Even mild or moderate hypokalemia increases the risks of morbidity and mortality in patients with cardiovascular disease. Hyperkalemia is defined as a serum K of 5.5 mmol/L or higher. The prevalence among hospitalized patients not yet on dialysis was reported to be about 3.3%, and among them, up to 10% had significant hyperkalemia (≥6.0 mmol/L). Hyperkalemia also carries a significantly increased risk of mortality.

Risk Factors

People most at risk for hypokalemia are those who are malnourished, with poor oral intake; those who use certain medications, such as diuretics; and those who have uncontrolled vomiting or diarrhea. People most at risk for hyperkalemia are those with reduced kidney function, those who have a history of diabetes mellitus, or those who take certain medications, such as angiotensin-converting enzyme inhibitors.

Pathophysiology

K is the most abundant cation in the human body. It regulates intracellular enzyme function and helps determine neuromuscular and cardiovascular tissue excitability. The total body store is approximately 55 mmol/kg of body weight. Over 98% of total body K is located in the intracellular fluid (primarily in muscle), and less than 2% in the extracellular fluid. A typical Western diet provides 40 to 120 mmol of K per day. Tight control of the serum K is primarily accomplished by the kidney, where approximately 95% of body K is excreted. Under normal circumstances, K losses in stool and sweat are small. In addition, the interplay of several hormonal systems (insulin, catecholamine), serum tonicity, and the internal acid-base environment contribute to the exchange of K between the extracellular fluid and intracellular fluid, which helps keep the serum K concentration tightly controlled. Hypokalemia occurs when there is a significant intracellular K shift or a reduced total body K store from poor intake, or excessive renal or extrarenal loss, whereas hyperkalemia develops when there is a significant extracellular shift, high body K load, or ineffective K elimination (aldosterone resistance/deficiency or reduced renal function).

Prevention

For patients at risk for hypokalemia, adequate dietary K intake is essential. Additional K supplements may be needed for patients taking high doses of diuretics (especially thiazide diuretics) or experiencing prolonged vomiting or diarrhea. For patients with

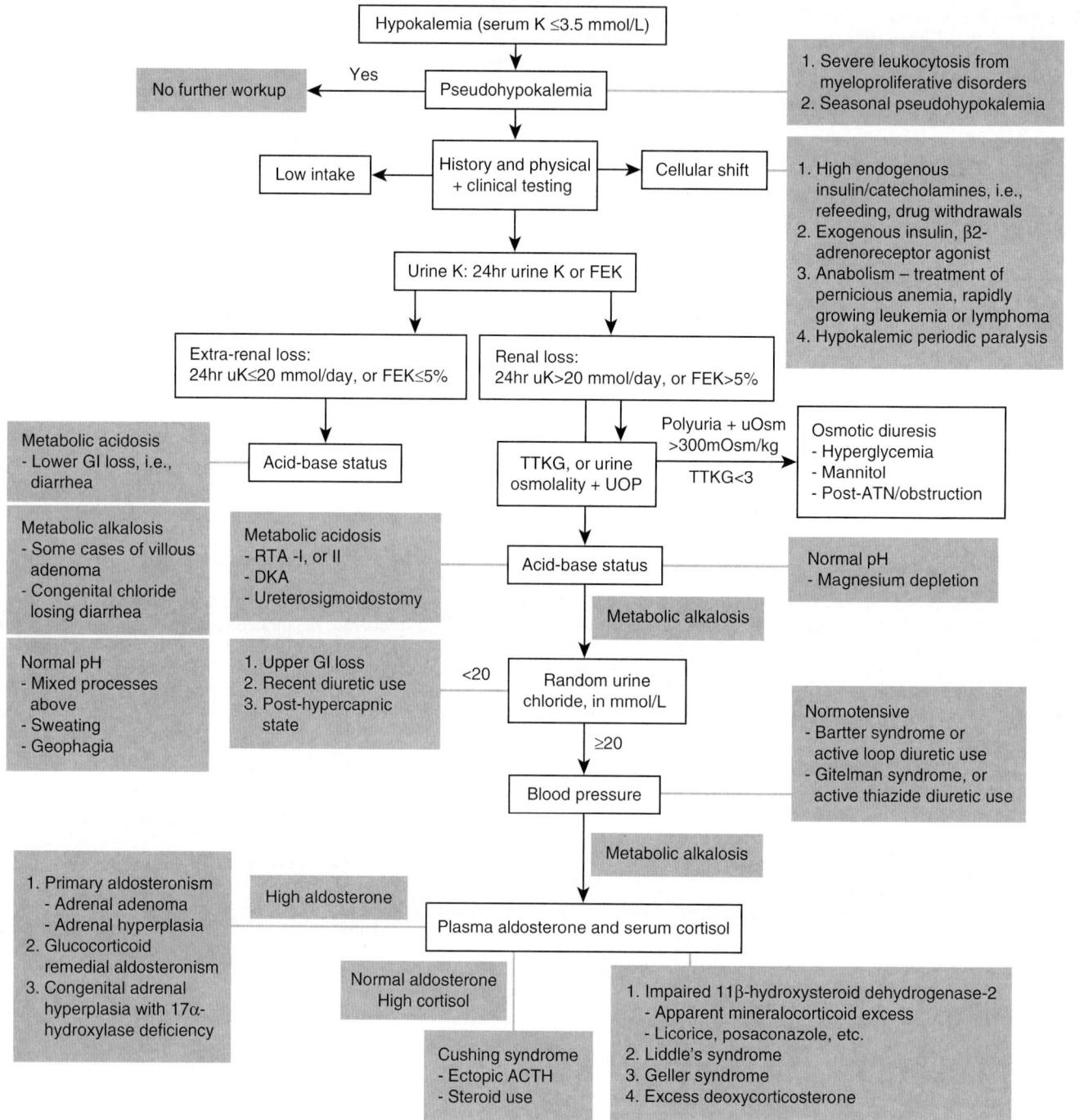

Figure 1 The diagnostic approach to hypokalemia. *ACS*, Acute coronary syndrome; *ATN*, acute tubular necrosis; *DKA*, diabetic ketoacidosis; *FEK*, fractional excretion of K; *GI*, gastrointestinal; *Met*, metabolic; *RTA*, renal tubular acidosis.

hyperkalemia and severe kidney dysfunction, dietary K restriction is critical in maintaining body K balance. Sometimes, the empirical use of K exchange resin is needed to prevent hyperkalemia. Lastly, medications that contribute to hypokalemia or hyperkalemia should be avoided if possible.

Clinical Manifestations

Mild hypokalemia (serum K 3.0 to 3.5 mmol/L) is usually well tolerated. Moderate hypokalemia (serum K 2.5 to 3.0 mmol/L) may cause nonspecific symptoms, such as fatigue, weakness, muscle cramps, and constipation. When the serum K drops to less than 2.5 mmol/L, muscle necrosis and flaccid paralysis with eventual respiratory failure may occur. K depletion also causes supraventricular and ventricular arrhythmias, especially in patients on digitalis therapy. Although severe hypokalemia is more likely to cause complications, even minimal decreases in serum or total body K can be arrhythmogenic in patients with underlying heart disease or who are receiving digitalis therapy. Lastly, increases in systolic and diastolic blood pressures can occur in patients with hypokalemia while they are on a liberal salt diet. Overall, the likelihood of symptoms tends to correlate with the rapidity of the decrease in serum K. As with hypokalemia, patients with hyperkalemia may present with nonspecific complaints such as fatigue and malaise. But the predominant manifestations in more severe hyperkalemia are neuromuscular and cardiac. Neuromuscular symptoms range from muscle weakness to paralysis. Cardiac arrhythmias, including asystole, ventricular tachycardia or fibrillation, and pulseless electrical activity, can also occur in severe hyperkalemia.

Diagnosis

Figures 1 and 2 illustrate the diagnostic approaches to hypokalemia and hyperkalemia. It is important to assess for pseudodyskalemia

Hyperkalemia (Serum K ≥5.5 mmol/L)

Pseudohyperkalemia — Yes → No further workup

- Severe leukocytosis
- Severe thrombocytosis

High K load

Tissue breakdown/cell lysis
- Rhabdomyolysis
- Massive hemolysis
- Resolving hematoma
- Trauma
- Tumor lysis

History and Physical, corresponding tests — Transcellular shift →

Low endogenous insulin/catecholamines

Acidosis

Hyperglycemia

Hyperkalemic periodic paralysis

Medications:
- Mannitol
- β blockers
- Succinylcholine
- Somatostatin
- Octreotide
- Digitalis

1. Acute renal failure or Advanced CKD (GFR <20 mL/min)*
2. Reduced renal tubular flow from low sodium
3. Reduced effective renal blood flow

Reduced renal K excretion

Other medications:
1. Collecting tubule Na/K ATPase blockade
   - Cyclosporin
   - Tacrolimus
2. ENAC blockade
   - Amiloride
   - Triamterene
   - Trimethoprim
   - Pentamidine

TTKG <5

Primary hypoaldosteronism

Secondary hypoaldosteronism
1. Renin deficiency/resistance
   - Diabetes mellitus
   - RTA-4
   - Multiple myeloma
   - Meds: β blocker; direct renin inhibitor; NSAIDs
2. Aldosterone deficiency/resistance
   - Addison disease
   - RTA-4
   - Renal tubulointerstitial disease
   - Hereditary diseases: Gordon syndrome, pseudohypoaldosteronism type 1
   - Medications: ACEI/ARB; heparin; spironolactone; eplerenone

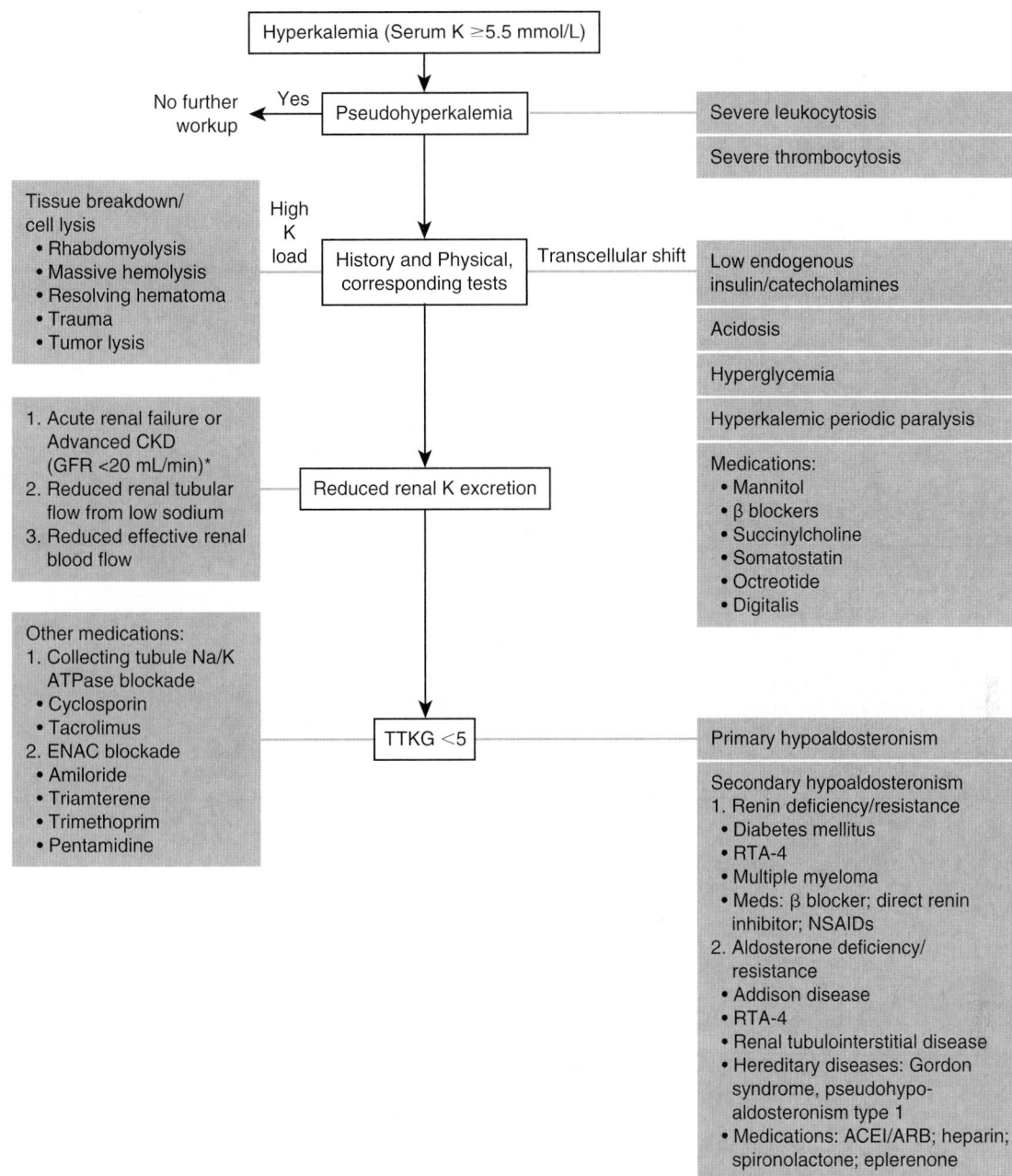

Figure 2 The diagnostic approach to hyperkalemia. *Hyperkalemia may occur with higher GFR if K load is excessive. *ACEI*, Angiotensin-converting enzyme inhibitor; *ARB*, angiotensin receptor blocker; *ENAC*, epithelial sodium channel; *GFR*, glomerular filtration rate; *NSAIDs*, nonsteroidal anti-inflammatory drugs; *RTA*, renal tubular acidosis.

393

(in vitro shift of K) and dyskalemia from in vivo transcellular shift of K because neither is associated with disturbances in total body K balance. Although cellular shift of K and changes in total body K occur as isolated problems, they frequently coexist. In hypokalemia, the assessment of renal K excretion is a key step in the initial diagnostic evaluation, followed by the assessment of acid-base status. In hyperkalemia, medical history and laboratory testing can help identify altered K distribution, reduced urinary K excretion, or an excessive K load from exogenous intake or transcellular leakage. Under normal circumstances, high K intake alone is not sufficient to lead to significant hyperkalemia unless there are other risk factors present such as reduced aldosterone action or significant loss of kidney function. Measurement of the transtubular potassium gradient (TTKG) has been widely used as a diagnostic tool in both conditions. However, recent evidence suggests that the assumption inherent in the calculation of the TTKG lacks validity. That said, I still find it useful in the initial assessment.

Differential Diagnosis

Figures 1 and 2 outline a diagnostic approach, including differential diagnosis, for hyperkalemia and hypokalemia.

Therapy

The treatment of hypokalemia depends on the underlying cause, the degree of K depletion, and the risk of K depletion to the patient. In general, hypokalemia secondary to cell shift is managed by treating underlying conditions. For example, hypokalemia in the setting of catecholamine increases, as in chest pain syndromes, is managed with appropriate treatments for the pain. However, when cell-shift hypokalemia is associated with life-threatening conditions such as paresis, paralysis, or hypokalemia in the setting of myocardial infarction, the administration of K is indicated. With K depletion, replacement therapy depends on the estimated degree of decreases in total body K. For example, decreases in total body K accompanied by a fall in serum K from 3.5 to 3.0 mmol/L are associated with a K deficit of 150 to 200 mmol. Decreases in serum K from 3 to 2 mmol/L are associated with 200- to 400-mmol additional decreases in total body K. K can be administered intravenously but in limited quantities (10 mEq/h into a peripheral vein; 15 to 20 mEq/h into a central vein). Larger K requirements can only be accomplished by oral therapy or with dialysis.

The acute management of hyperkalemia depends on the presence or absence of ECG and neuromuscular abnormalities. In the absence of symptoms or ECG abnormalities, hyperkalemia is treated conservatively—for example, by decreasing dietary K or withdrawing offending drugs. In the presence of ECG abnormalities or symptoms, the goal of therapy is to stabilize cell membranes. First-line therapy includes calcium gluconate, 10 to 30 mL IV as a 10% solution (onset of action 1 or 2 minutes). Although the mechanism remains undefined, calcium "stabilizes" the cardiac membranes. The dose can be repeated after five minutes if the ECG changes persist or recur. Other therapies include 8.4% IV sodium bicarbonate[1], 50 to 150 mEq (onset 15 to 30 minutes), and rapid-acting insulin[1] 5 to 10 units intravenously (onset 5 to 10 minutes). Insulin increases the activity of the Na-K-ATPase pump in skeletal muscle and drives K into cells. Glucose 50%, 25 g intravenously, is given simultaneously with insulin to prevent hypoglycemia. Albuterol given as 0.5 mg in D5W IV or 10–20 mg in 4 mL normal saline by nebulizer (onset 15 to 30 minutes), also activates the Na-K-ATPase and drives K into cells. K driven intracellularly generally begins to move extracellularly again after approximately 6 hours, increasing the serum K concentration. Therefore, therapy to remove K from the body should be started simultaneously. Reductions in total body K may be achieved through a K exchange resin. The primary K resin used is sodium polystyrene sulfonate (Kayexalate). One gram of this medication binds approximately 1 mEq of K and releases 1 to 2 mEq of sodium back into the circulation. This medication may be given orally (onset 2 hours) or by enema with sorbitol to induce diarrhea (onset 30 to 60 minutes).

In 2015, patiromer, a polymer that exchanges calcium for potassium in the gastrointestinal tract, was approved by the Food and Drug Administration (FDA) for the management of hyperkalemia. In 2018, sodium zirconium cyclosilicate (SZC), a novel nonabsorbed, nonpolymer zirconium silicate compound that exchanges hydrogen and sodium for potassium and ammonium was also approved by the FDA for the same indication. Both agents are well tolerated and effective. Patiromer is administered orally at an initial dose of 10 g three times a day for up to 48 hours, followed by a maintenance dose of 10 g daily (maximum daily maintenance dose 15 g/day).

If renal function is adequate, volume expansion with simultaneous diuresis can be attempted. Finally, hemodialysis is very effective in removing excess K.

The chronic management of hyperkalemia starts with dietary K restriction. Other management options include the use of diuretics, cessation or dose reduction of renin-angiotensin-aldosterone system inhibitors, and/or intermittent use of Kayexalate. Both patiromer and SZ are also well tolerated, safe, and effective in the chronic management of hyperkalemia. Just as important, they may allow the optimal use of renin-angiotensin-aldosterone system inhibitors in patients who have been previously untreated, had their dose reduced, or stopped treatment altogether.

Monitoring

Treatment for severe or symptomatic dyskalemia requires close cardiac monitoring and frequent laboratory testing to prevent overcorrection. If insulin and glucose are used in patients with hyperkalemia, blood sugars should be monitored for approximately 6 hours to identify and treat hypoglycemia from the insulin.

Complications

Complications from dyskalemia include cardiac arrhythmias, neuromuscular events, and, rarely, death. There are potential treatment-related complications if pseudodyskalemia or dyskalemia from in vivo transcellular shift is not recognized.

---

[1]Not FDA approved for this indication.

References

Gennari FJ: Hypokalemia, *N Engl J Med* 339:451–458, 1998.
Krishna GG, Kapoor SC: Potassium depletion exacerbates essential hypertension, *Ann Intern Med* 115:77–83, 1991.
Paice BJ, Paterson KR, Onyanga-Omara F, et al: Record linkage study of hypokalaemia in hospitalized patients, *Postgrad Med J* 62:187–191, 1986.
Stevens MS, Dunlay RW: Hyperkalemia in hospitalized patients, *Int Urol Nephrol* 32:177–180, 2000.

HYPONATREMIA

Method of
Beejal Shah, MD; and Susan L. Samson, MD, PhD

CURRENT DIAGNOSIS

- Perform a thorough history and physical examination with focus on the accurate assessment of volume status, neurologic symptoms and signs, current medications, and concurrent illnesses.
- Classify the hyponatremia as hypovolemic, euvolemic, or hypervolemic.
- Determine whether the hyponatremia is acute or chronic, based on the history and the clinical manifestations.
- Order key laboratory tests, including a basic metabolic panel (serum sodium, glucose, blood urea nitrogen, and creatinine), plasma osmolality, urine osmolality, and urine sodium.

CURRENT THERAPY

- Severe and symptomatic hyponatremia should be treated with hypertonic saline (3%) at 1 to 2 mL/kg per hour. Neurologic status and serum sodium should be monitored every 2 to 4 hours. The objective is to raise sodium by 2 mEq/L per hour (or to >125 mEq/L) until deleterious neurologic symptoms improve. After this, the rate of infusion should be titrated to increase the serum sodium by 0.5 to 1.0 mEq/L per hour, with a maximum increase of 6 to 8 mEq/L over 24 hours and no more than 18 mEq/L over 48 hours, to avoid precipitating osmotic demyelination.
- As a general rule, the treatment of hyponatremia should be adjusted for the serum sodium to increase by 0.5 to 1.0 mEq/L per hour with a maximum increase of 6 to 8 mEq/L over 24 hours and no more than 18 mEq/L over 48 hours.
- Acute hyponatremia (<48 hours) with neurologic symptoms should be treated more rapidly than chronic hyponatremia, a 4 to 6 mEq/L increase in serum sodium over 6 hours can reverse severe neurologic symptoms.
- Before a diagnosis of syndrome of inappropriate antidiuresis (SIAD) is made, rule out adrenal insufficiency and hypothyroidism.
- Most cases of euvolemic hyponatremia are caused by the SIAD, which usually can be managed with fluid restriction, salt tablets, and vasopressin receptor antagonists ("vaptans") as indicated.
- Discontinue thiazide diuretics in all cases of hypoosmolar hyponatremia.
- Hypovolemic and hypervolemic hyponatremia require therapy to correct the underlying cause (e.g., heart failure) and restore status to euvolemia.
- Vasopressin receptor antagonists (vaptans) are approved for short term management of euvolemic and hypovolemic hyponatremia. The same parameters apply for rate of sodium correction and monitoring as in conventional therapy.
- Overcorrection of hyponatremia should be recorrected in patients at high risk for osmotic dyemelation.

Homeostasis maintains the concentration of sodium in the serum between 138 and 142 mEq/L (normal, 135–145 mEq/L) despite variations in water intake. Hyponatremia is defined as a serum sodium concentration of less than 135 mEq/L, although normal range values may differ slightly among laboratories, usually to a minimum normal sodium of 133 mEq/L. It is one of the most common electrolyte abnormalities found in the inpatient setting, occurring in up to 2.5% of patients, and it is a significant marker for mortality, associated with a 60-fold higher risk of death. It is not clear whether hyponatremia itself is the cause of a more adverse prognosis or whether it echoes the degree of stress caused by illness. In the outpatient setting, chronic hyponatremia is most prevalent among the elderly and nursing home residents. The approach to management of hyponatremia is highly dependent on the underlying process. Establishing the correct etiology is critical, because inappropriate treatment can worsen hyponatremia. Therapy must be administered judiciously because of the risk of severe neurologic sequelae, including central nervous system demyelination. However, with a systematic approach to the differential diagnosis of hyponatremia, the correct diagnosis can be made and therapy initiated.

Clinical Presentation

Acute hyponatremia is defined as hyponatremia of less than 48 hours in duration. Mild symptoms include headache, nausea, vomiting, confusion, and weakness, which usually occur with a sodium level of less than 129 mEq/L. More severe neurologic manifestations—seizure and coma—are seen usually below a threshold of 120 mEq/L, although there currently is no evidence-based critical sodium level above which neurologic sequelae do not occur. The neurologic manifestations of acute or recurrent symptomatic hyponatremia can be delayed, so continued monitoring is important.

In contrast, patients with chronic hyponatremia more often are asymptomatic or have blunted symptoms. In elderly patients with mild chronic hyponatremia, subtle neurocognitive manifestations can occur, with decreased balance, lowered reaction speed, memory loss, and directed gait. Mild hypoosmolar hyponatremia is not independently associated with increased morbidity and mortality. Even so, the underlying etiology needs to be determined because of the potential for other factors (e.g., new medications, dehydration, occult illness) to contribute to the development of more severe hyponatremia with its potential for neurologic injury.

Regulation of Water Balance

Approximately two thirds of total body water is contained in the intracellular fluid (ICF) and one third as extracellular fluid (ECF). Plasma osmolality is tightly regulated between 280 and 290 mOsm/kg and reflects the osmolality of the ECF. A change in plasma osmolality results in a shift of total body water between the ECF and the ICF to maintain their osmolar equivalence. Because sodium is the major osmole in the ECF, hyponatremia most often is a manifestation of decreased osmolality, so-called hypoosmolar or hypotonic hyponatremia.

Renal Handling of Water

The major osmoregulatory hormone is arginine vasopressin, also called antidiuretic hormone, which is synthesized in the paraventricular and supraoptic nuclei of the hypothalamus. It is transported along axons to the posterior pituitary, where it is processed and stored in vesicles. Vasopressin secretion is regulated by osmotic and nonosmotic stimuli. Secretion occurs with a 1% to 2% rise in osmolality (>288 mOsm/kg), as detected by receptors in the anterolateral walls of the hypothalamus adjacent to the third ventricle. Vasopressin secretion is inhibited when the plasma osmolality is lower than 280 mOsm/kg. The major nonosmotic stimulus is a decrease in effective circulating volume, which is detected by baroreceptors in the aortic arch and carotid sinuses. Although this mechanism requires a large drop (10%–15%) in blood pressure, the secretory response is more robust than for increases in osmolality. As such, acutely lowered blood pressure can override the inhibitory signal of low osmolality because of the need to maintain perfusion. Other physiologic nonosmotic stimuli include catecholamines and angiotensin II, but there is a

long list of hormones and pharmacologic agents that induce or repress vasopressin secretion (Table 1).

The renal site of action of vasopressin is the V_2 receptors on the basolateral membrane of collecting duct cells in the distal nephron. The hormone-receptor interaction initiates intracellular signaling via cyclic adenosine monophosphate–dependent pathways, resulting in translocation of cytoplasmic aquaporon-2 channels to the surface of the collecting duct luminal membrane. These channels allow movement of water back into the cell for later reabsorption into the circulation. This results in a net concentration of urine and decreased plasma osmolality.

Renal Handling of Sodium

In addition to renal water handling, sodium reabsorption and excretion are important for maintenance of water homeostasis. The renin-angiotensin-aldosterone system is activated by reduced arterial perfusion pressure sensed by the juxtaglomerular apparatus of the afferent renal arteriole. Reduced arteriole effective volume (low or perceived) is sensed by the juxtaglomerular apparatus, which secretes renin, activating the renin-angiotensin system. This cascade of events ultimately stimulates aldosterone secretion, which acts at the distal nephron to cause reabsorption of filtered sodium via Na^+,K^+-adenosine triphosphatase (ATPase)–dependent sodium channels.

Central Nervous System Response to Hyponatremia/Hypoosmolality

Osmolar equivalence between the ECF and ICF is closely maintained by shifts in water between the two compartments. The major symptoms and signs of hyponatremia are neurologic in nature and are a clinical manifestation of swelling of the cells in the central nervous system, which results in cerebral edema. The most devastating consequence is herniation due to anatomic limitations on brain volume within the confines of the skull. Premenopausal women are at the highest risk for brain injury from hyponatremia.

A major compensatory mechanism in the central nervous system is the extrusion from the cells of intracellular solutes, which prevents further water influx. In the first few hours, inorganic ions (potassium, sodium, chloride) move out of the cell. After a few days of persistent hypoosmolality, the cells further compensate by extruding organic osmoles (glutamate, taurine, inositol). The clinician must be aware of this protective adaptation, because it necessitates a slower time course of correction during treatment.

TABLE 1 Molecules That Regulate Vasopressin Secretion

STIMULATE VASOPRESSIN RELEASE	INHIBIT VASOPRESSIN RELEASE
Hormones and Neurotransmitters	
Acetylcholine (nicotinic)	Atrial natriuretic peptide
Angiotensin II	γ-Aminobutyric acid
Aspartate	Opioids (κ receptors)
Cholecystokinin	
Dopamine (D_1 and D_2)	
Glutamine	
Histamine (H_1)	
Neuropeptide Y	
Prostaglandin	
Substance P	
Vasoactive inhibitory peptide	
Pharmacologic Agents	
Adrenaline (epinephrine)	Butorphanol (Stadol)
Cyclophosphamide (Cytoxan)	Ethanol
High-dose morphine	Fluphenazine (Prolixin)
Nicotine	Glucocorticoids
Selective serotonin reuptake inhibitors	Haloperidol (Haldol)
Tricyclic antidepressants	Low-dose morphine
Vincristine (Oncovin)	Phenytoin (Dilantin)
	Promethazine (Phenergan)

A rapid rise in plasma osmolality from aggressive treatment causes water to rapidly shift out of the cells, resulting in demyelination of neurons. In the past, this was termed pontine demyelinosis, but it has also been reported for extrapontine neurons and is now referred to as osmotic demyelination. The sequelae are permanent and devastating. There is clinical progression from lethargy to a change in affect, to mutism and dysarthria, and finally to spastic quadriparesis and pseudobulbar palsy.

Classification and Differential Diagnosis of Hyponatremia

Initial evaluation of hyponatremia requires a systematic and sequential approach. First, a thorough history and physical examination are required. It is important to identify any history of brain injury, stroke, mental illness, or chronic illness and the patient's current medication usage. On examination, special attention should be paid to mental status and neurologic abnormalities; manifestations of cardiac, hepatic, or renal disease; and signs of adrenal insufficiency or hypothyroidism. From the assessment of volume status, the hyponatremia should be classified as hypervolemic, euvolemic, or hypovolemic; each of these conditions leads in a different direction for diagnosis and treatment of the underlying cause (Figures 1 and 2). Finally, it should be determined whether the hyponatremia is acute (<48 hours) or chronic, because this can determine the time course of treatment.

For the laboratory work-up, essential basic tests are the serum sodium and potassium levels, renal function tests with blood urea nitrogen (BUN) and creatinine, and liver function tests. It is likely that these tests have already been performed, motivating the assessment of hyponatremia. After this, the plasma osmolality (P_{Osm}), urine osmolality (U_{Osm}), and urine sodium concentration are key diagnostic tests. P_{Osm} is directly measured in the laboratory and also can be calculated. Calculated osmolality is the sum of the concentrations of the known major osmoles—sodium and glucose—in the ECF and the BUN:

$$P_{Osm} = (2 \times Na) + (glucose) + (BUN)$$

The calculation is done in SI units. For sodium, mEq/L is the same as the SI unit, mmol/L; if glucose and BUN values were reported in mg/dL, they must be divided by 18 and 2.8, respectively, to convert to SI units (mmol/L). The directly measured osmolality should be within 10 to 12 mOsm/kg of the calculated value; an increased osmolar gap compared with the calculated value points toward the presence of additional osmoles in the plasma that are causing hypertonicity.

Because hyponatremia usually is a reflection of plasma osmolality, most patients also have a low P_{Osm}, and the clinician often can proceed to the differential diagnosis of hypoosmolar (or hypotonic) hyponatremia after excluding pseudohyponatremia (which usually has normal osmolality) and hyperosmolar hyponatremia. Pseudohyponatremia can occur if the plasma lipid or protein content is greatly increased in the plasma (usually to >6%–8% of volume), as in extreme hypertriglyceridemia and paraprotein disorders. These extra components decrease the aqueous portion of the plasma volume and thereby interfere with the laboratory measurement of sodium by dilutional, indirect methods such as flame photometry. Most laboratories now use direct measurement of sodium to avoid this problem.

Hyperosmolar hyponatremia can occur if there are additional osmoles present that cause water movement from the ICF into the ECF, resulting in ECF expansion and dilutional hyponatremia. Overall, the total body water and total body sodium are unchanged in this situation. An important clinical example occurs with hyperglycemia, and the reported sodium value should be corrected for high glucose by the clinician by adding 1.6 mEq/L to the measured Na for every 100 mg/dL rise in glucose above 200 mg/dL. Because glucose is included in the calculation of osmolality, there will be no significant osmolar gap.

Other osmotically active solutes encountered clinically are mannitol, which is used to manage increased intracranial pressure, and glycine, which is used for irrigation in urologic procedures. Mannitol and glycine are retained in the ECF and are not part of the calculated osmolality, so their presence results in an osmolar gap.

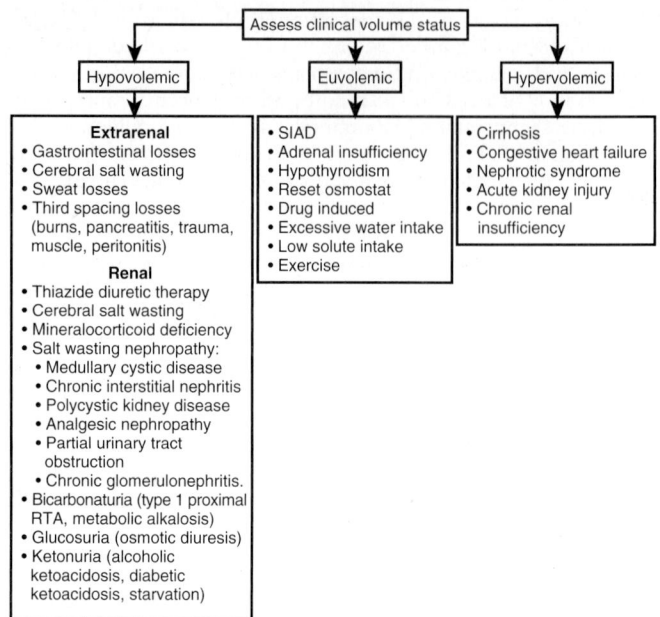

Figure 1 The differential diagnosis of hypoosmolar hyponatremia. *Abbreviations:* RTA = renal tubular acidosis; SIAD = syndrome of inappropriate antidiuresis.

High levels of alcohol or ethylene glycol also increase the osmolality, but these substances are so quickly metabolized that an osmolar gap may not be apparent by the time testing is performed.

Once pseudohyponatremia and hypertonicity have been ruled out, the diagnosis is narrowed to hypoosmolar hyponatremia. The combined physical examination and laboratory results allow classification of the patient as having hypervolemic hyponatremia with excess total body sodium, hypovolemic hyponatremia with a deficit of total body sodium, or euvolemic hyponatremia with near-normal total body sodium.

Hypovolemic Hyponatremia

The causes of hypovolemic hyponatremia can be classified as extrarenal or renal (see Figure 1). Signs of volume contraction are apparent on examination, including poor skin turgor, skin tenting (forehead), decreased or undetectable jugular venous pressure, dry mucous membranes, and orthostatic changes in blood pressure and pulse rate. If the volume status is not completely clear from the examination, laboratory values can be helpful (see Figure 2), but they need to be interpreted in the context of renal function tests. If the urine osmolality is less than maximally concentrated (<500 mOsm/kg), an infusion of 0.5 to 1 L of isotonic saline over 24 to 48 hours may help with differentiation. With hypovolemia, the sodium will begin to correct and the patient should improve clinically. Conversely, if the patient is actually euvolemic, such as with syndrome of inappropriate antidiuresis (SIAD), discussed later, the serum sodium level will remain constant or decrease due to retention of free water with a concomitant increase in urinary sodium.

Extrarenal causes of hyponatremia include gastrointestinal losses and third-space losses such as in severe burns and pancreatitis. In the volume-depleted state, with intact renal function, the urine sodium is low (<10 mEq/L), reflecting a normal response by the kidney to maximally reabsorb sodium in response to volume depletion.

The renal causes of hypovolemic hyponatremia involve the inappropriate loss of sodium into the urine, and this is reflected by a urine sodium concentration of greater than 20 mEq/L.

Thiazide diuretics cause renal sodium loss, so the urine sodium is high. However, they also impair the kidney's diluting capacity, decreasing free water excretion and concentrating the urine. Only certain patients may be susceptible to hyponatremia while on thiazides. These patients may have an abnormally sensitive thirst response to the mild hypovolemia induced by the diuretics, causing increased water intake. Elderly women are the most susceptible,

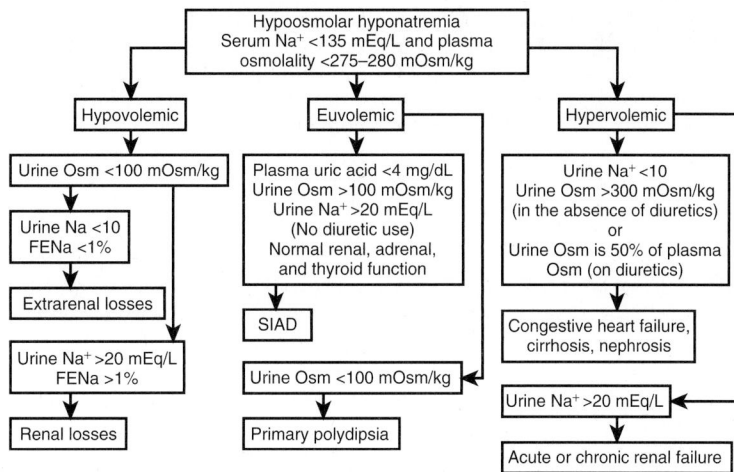

Figure 2 Laboratory findings in hypoosmolar hyponatremia. *Abbreviations:* FENa = fractional excretion of sodium; Osm = osmoles; SIAD = syndrome of inappropriate antidiuresis.

and hyponatremia can occur within days after initiation of thiazide therapy. Additional laboratory results reveal hypokalemia and a metabolic alkalosis. It is appropriate to stop the diuretic and restore potassium levels and volume status. Patients often have a recurrence of hyponatremia if rechallenged with thiazides. Loop diuretics, such as furosemide, are a less frequent cause of hyponatremia, which occurs only after long-term therapy.

In the absence of diuretic use, a urine sodium concentration greater than 20 mEq/L with hypovolemia is evidence for underlying renal pathology. Patients with salt-wasting nephropathy, from a number of causes (see Figure 1), usually have significant renal failure, with a creatinine value in the range of 3 to 4 mg/dL. Because of the large net sodium loss, this condition is treated with salt tablets. Renal tubular acidosis causes bicarbonaturia, which requires a compensatory excretion of urinary cations, mainly Na^+ and K^+, to maintain electroneutrality. Similarly, excretion of ketones into the urine also demands additional electrolyte losses in spite of ECF volume depletion, leading to a loss of sodium.

Cerebral salt wasting (CSW), although it could be considered an extrarenal cause, also involves the renal loss of sodium (>20 mEq/L). The biochemical presentation is very similar to that of SIAD, but the diagnosis of CSW is restricted to cases involving extreme central nervous system pathology. CSW is most commonly associated with subarachnoid hemorrhage but also has been reported with stroke, brain trauma, infection, metastases and after neurosurgery. Onset of CSW is usually within the first 10 days after the neurologic event.

CSW may be a protective mechanism against increased intracranial pressure. The proposed pathophysiologic mechanism of CSW is controversial, but one hypothesis is that the initiating event is a primary natriuresis, with renal loss of sodium, caused by the secretion of natriuretic peptides. Clinical studies have found both increased brain natriuretic peptide and increased atrial natriuretic peptide in neurosurgical patients with hyponatremia. Both hormones are vasodilators that increase the glomerular filtration rate while suppressing the renin-angiotensin system. This increases renal sodium losses, as well as water excretion, resulting in volume depletion. Vasopressin levels rise in response to low volume, so that it becomes biochemically difficult to differentiate CSW from SIAD, with a urine sodium level greater than 20 mEq/L, low uric acid, and high urine osmolality. It is helpful if CSW patients have signs of volume depletion in combination with the laboratory results. Also, the hyponatremia of CSW responds to normal saline, whereas SIAD worsens with normal saline. CSW is relatively rare in most case series, and it is important to rule out other causes for natriuresis.

Hypervolemic Hyponatremia

There are a variety of causes of hypervolemic hyponatremia (see Figure 1), all of which are a result of decreased effective circulating volume. To correct this imbalance, the ECF expands, leading to fluid retention and hyponatremia. In spite of the increased total body water and low serum sodium on testing, all of these patients have some degree of total body sodium excess. In many cases, volume overload is clinically evident from the presence of subcutaneous edema, ascites, elevated jugular venous pressure, or pulmonary edema.

In congestive heart failure (CHF), patients can develop hyponatremia with only 2 to 3 L of fluid intake per day despite normal renal function. The decreased filling pressures and cardiac output of CHF are perceived as volume depletion, detected by the baroreceptors. This stimulates vasopressin secretion, overriding the signal of low osmolality detected by the hypothalamic osmoreceptors. This lack of inhibition of vasopressin secretion is believed to be the most important contributing factor to the development of hyponatremia. In addition, decreased right atrial pressures result in inhibition of secretion of atrial natriuretic peptide, contributing to the water and sodium gain. With the low perfusion pressure, there is a decrease in the glomerular filtration rate, which is sensed by the juxtaglomerular apparatus, causing neurohumoral activation of the renin-angiotensin system and sympathetic nervous system. This leads to increased circulating levels of catecholamines, angiotensin II, and aldosterone, further stimulating tubular sodium and water reabsorption. In the absence of diuretics, the urine sodium level is very low (<10 mEq/L) in patients with CHF because of activation of the renin-angiotensin-aldosterone system and maximal tubular reabsorption of sodium. Also, there is less than maximally dilute urine (usually >300 mOsm/kg) in the absence of diuretic therapy. An elevated brain natriuretic peptide concentration helps to confirm the hypervolemia.

A similar mechanism is at work in cirrhotic patients, in whom the incidence of hyponatremia is even higher and is a strong predictor of poor outcome. In cirrhosis, low albumin results in third-spacing and decreased effective circulating volume. In addition, portal hypertension leads to splanchnic vasodilation, which also decreases the effective circulating volume. This serves to activate vasopressin secretion and the renin-angiotensin-aldosterone system.

Hyponatremia is less common in acute and chronic renal failure, but it can occur with a significant decrease in glomerular filtration rate accompanied by severe hypoalbuminemia. Interpretation of the laboratory results may be confounded by a high urine sodium concentration (>20 mEq/L) that reflects the concomitant presence of tubular dysfunction. Hyponatremia can develop in stage IV or V renal failure when fluid intake is in excess of 3 L/day.

Euvolemic Hyponatremia

Euvolemic hyponatremia is caused by impaired excretion of free water by the kidney. The differential diagnosis is more limited (see Figure 1) and the majority of cases are due to SIAD (Table 2). However, this often is a diagnosis of exclusion, and

TABLE 2   Causes of SIAD

CNS Disorders

Mass lesions (tumors; CNS abscess; intracranial hemorrhage or
    hematoma)
Stroke
CNS infections or inflammatory diseases
Spinal cord lesions
Acute psychosis
Pituitary stalk lesions
Hydrocephalus
Dementia
Guillain-Barré syndrome
Head trauma

Pulmonary Disorders

Viral/bacterial pneumonia
Positive-pressure ventilation
Bronchogenic carcinoma (small cell)
Acute respiratory failure
COPD
Tuberculosis
Aspergillosis
Pulmonary abscess

Medications/Drugs

Vasopressin analogues (desmopressin [DDAVP])
NSAIDs
Tricyclic antidepressants
Phenothiazines
Butyrophenones
SSRIs/SNRIs
Morphine
Opiates
Chlorpropamide (Diabinese)
Clofibrate (Atromid-S)[2]
Cyclophosphamide (Cytoxan)
Vincristine (Oncovin)
Nicotine
Tolbutamide (Orinase)
Barbiturates
Acetaminophen (Tylenol)
ACE inhibitors
Carbamazepine (Tegretol)
Omeprazole (Prilosec)
MDMA (Ecstasy)
Lamotrigine (Lamictal)
Sodium valproate (Depakote)
Monomaine oxidase inhibitors
Ifosfamide (Ifex)
Melphalan (Alkeran, Evomela)
Platinum agents

Other

Pain
Nausea
HIV infection/AIDS
Prolonged exercise (e.g., marathon running)
Idiopathic
Acute intermittent porphyria

[2]Not available in the United States.
Abbreviations: ACE = angiotensin-converting enzyme; AIDS = acquired immunodeficiency syndrome; CNS = central nervous system; COPD = chronic obstructive
pulmonary disease; DDAVP = 1-deamino, 8-D arginine-vasopressin; MDMA
= methylenedioxymethamphetamine; NSAIDs = nonsteroidal antiinflammatory
drugs; SSRIs = selective serotonin reuptake inhibitors.

hypothyroidism and adrenal insufficiency must be ruled out clinically or biochemically in patients with euvolemic hyponatremia.

Hypothyroidism leads to reduced glomerular filtration rate and
decreased flow to the distal nephron, causing maximal reabsorption of water to maintain arterial volume. Hypothyroidism has
to be severe to cause hyponatremia and usually is obvious on
examination. However, in the elderly population, apathetic hypothyroidism may be difficult to diagnose. Hypothyroidism can be

confirmed by the presence of a high level of thyroid-stimulating
hormone and a low level of free T_4 (thyroxine). Treatment
involves thyroid hormone replacement and supportive care.

In primary adrenal insufficiency (Addison's disease), the concomitant aldosterone deficiency results in hyponatremia combined
with hyperkalemia, prerenal azotemia, a urine sodium concentration greater than 20 mEq/L, and a urine potassium level lower
than 20 mEq/L. In secondary or central adrenal insufficiency,
the adrenal zona glomerulosa remains intact for the secretion
of aldosterone. However, glucocorticoid deficiency still causes
impaired water excretion, which can lead to dilutional hyponatremia. Vasopressin release may be stimulated by the nausea,
vomiting, and orthostatic hypotension that occurs with adrenal
insufficiency. Finally, corticosteroids normally inhibit vasopressin
release, so their deficiency leads to enhanced vasopressin release,
causing retention of free water that further contributes to the
hyponatremia. The appropriate diagnostic test is a 250-μg ACTH
(cosyntropin, Cortrosyn) stimulation test, although an extremely
low 8 AM cortisol level (<3 μg/dL) can be diagnostic. Treatment
consists of glucocorticoid replacement.

Syndrome of Inappropriate Antidiuresis

SIAD is the most common cause of euvolemic hypoosmolar hyponatremia. Edema, ascites, and orthostasis are absent, and thyroid, adrenal, and renal functions are normal. Recent diuretic use
should be ruled out. The primary event is the release of vasopressin, which results in water retention. The increased intravascular
volume stimulates a natriuresis, which actually is appropriate,
but the resulting loss of sodium compounds the hyponatremia.
There is an extensive list of causes of SIAD, usually involving
pulmonary or central nervous system pathology (see Table 2). A
number of medications also are known to stimulate vasopressin
release or to potentiate its antidiuretic properties at the level of
the kidney (see Tables 1 and 2).

The diagnosis of SIAD is suggested by a low P_{Osm} (<280 mOsm/
kg) with a high U_{Osm} (>100 mOsm/kg), confirming water retention and an inappropriately concentrated urine. A spot urine
sodium level will be greater than 20 mEq/L, and usually greater
than 30 mEq/L. Other helpful laboratory findings include low
plasma uric acid (<4 mg/dL), which has a positive predictive value
of 73% to 100% for SIAD in this setting. In complicated cases
confounded by use of diuretics, the fractional excretion of uric
acid has a positive predictive value of 100% for SIAD when the
calculated excretion is greater than 12%.

Reset osmostat can be considered a form of SIAD, but the hyponatremia is usually chronic, mild, and asymptomatic. Vasopressin
release continues to be regulated, but at a lower threshold of plasma
osmolality. The thirst threshold may be altered as well. Interventions to raise the sodium usually have short-lived effects, and the
sodium resets at its previous value over time. Therefore, treatment
is not recommended if the sodium level is stable and the patient is
asymptomatic. A physiologic example of reset osmostat is seen in
pregnancy, when the normal sodium range is lowered by 5 mEq/L.

Other Causes of Euvolemic Hypoosmolar Hyponatremia

Primary or psychogenic polydipsia should be considered in patients
presenting with hyponatremia and a history of psychiatric illness
and treatment. Almost 6% to 7% of psychiatric inpatients are at
risk for hyponatremia from increased water intake. The polydipsia
may be related to a lowered osmolar threshold for thirst, below
the threshold of suppression of vasopressin secretion. This can be
further complicated by the side effect of dry mouth caused by many
psychiatric medications, which compounds the increased thirst and
water intake. Because the kidney is capable of excreting up to 15
to 20 L/day of dilute urine, the fact that hyponatremia develops
in these patients may point toward an additional and inappropriate increase in vasopressin release or sensitivity. These patients are
clinically euvolemic because of renal excretion of the excess water
and have otherwise normal laboratory results except for a dilute
urine (<100 mOsm/kg), which is caused by vasopressin suppression
and helps differentiate primary polydipsia from SIAD. However,

some patients have mildly concentrated urine (>100 mOsm/kg), in which case the psychiatric history helps with the diagnosis.

Exercise-induced hyponatremia (e.g., from marathon running) is a form of euvolemic hypoosmolar hyponatremia primarily caused by retention of water relative to fluid lost via sweating or renal excretion. Vasopressin levels are inappropriately increased during exercise-induced hyponatremia. Most importantly, it is an acute hyponatremia, developing in less than 24 hours, and should be treated accordingly.

Vasopressin levels also may be inappropriately high, secondary to pain or the use of NSAIDs, which remove prostaglandin inhibition of vasopressin release. Low solute intake combined with high fluid intake also can cause hyponatremia, as with beer potomania or a low-protein "tea and toast" diet in elderly patients. In both cases, the lack of solute in the urine does not allow retention of water in the filtrate, so the excess water is not excreted.

Hyponatremia also is common after pituitary surgery (transsphenoidal or by craniotomy) and may be a result of damage to the hypothalamic-pituitary tract that causes release of preformed vasopressin from damaged neurons. Hyponatremia can occur as the second phase of the classic triphasic response: transient arginine vasopressin deficiency (AVPD or central diabetes insipidus), transient hyponatremia, followed by permanent AVPD. More commonly, hyponatremia can occur as an isolated event between post-operative days 3 to 10. Sodium monitoring during this time may help to mitigate the severity of hyponatremia with timely interventions, including fluid restriction and salt tablets. More recently, prophylactic fluid restriction (1000–1500 mL) has been implemented by some high volume pituitary centers to prevent severe hyponatremia and readmissions. Contributions by central adrenal insufficiency and hypothyroidism also are considerations after pituitary surgery, although with these conditions there will be obvious clinical manifestations in addition to the hyponatremia.

Management
The major considerations for choosing the type and time course of treatment for hyponatremia are the duration of hyponatremia (acute or chronic) and the presence of neurologic signs and symptoms, especially severe manifestations such as altered mental status or seizure (see Table 2). Treatment options for hyponatremia include fluid restriction, saline infusion (hypertonic or isotonic), vasopressin receptor antagonists and demeclocycline (Declomycin).[1] Also, treatment of the underlying abnormality, such as CHF or salt wasting, and correction of volume status are important for hypovolemic or hypervolemic patients. Autocorrection may occur after initiation of therapy, especially in cases of hypovolemia, adrenal insufficiency, or thiazide use. Once treatment is started, the contribution of the nonosmotic stimulation of vasopressin secretion is removed, and the patient is able to raise the sodium level by 2 mEq/L per hour over 12 hours.

Acute Severe Symptomatic Hyponatremia
Acute severe hyponatremia is defined as a rapid fall in sodium in less than 48 hours to less than 120 mEq/L. Under these circumstances, most patients develop neurologic symptoms because of the rapid fluid shifts between the ECF and the ICF in the brain. If left untreated, it can result in irreversible neurologic damage and death. Because of the acute drop in sodium, initial rapid correction is acceptable and should not lead to osmotic demyelination. Treatment is aimed at raising the sodium enough to resolve the neurologic signs and symptoms. The goal is to raise the serum sodium by 1 to 2 mEq/L per hour or to greater than 125 mEq/L until symptoms resolve. Hypovolemic patients will respond to infusion of isotonic saline (normal saline 0.9%), especially if the urine sodium concentration is less than 30 mEq/L. If the neurologic findings are severe, hypertonic saline (3%) may be infused at rate of 1 to 2 mL/kg per hour, or even up to 4 to 6 mL/kg per hour if the imbalance is life-threatening. A loop diuretic can be combined with the saline

to enhance solute-free water excretion. In exercise-induced hyponatremia, hypertonic (3%) saline is the preferred treatment to prevent cerebral edema due to water shifting into the brain along the osmotic gradient. A hypertonic (3%) saline 100 mL bolus can be given to promptly to decrease the osmotic gradient, which is promoting water entry into cells. Thereafter, in the inpatient setting, hypertonic (3%) saline infusion should be continued to promote correction of hyponatremia. Sodium levels should be monitored every 2 to 4 hours in patients undergoing hypertonic infusion. Once symptoms resolve, the rate of correction should be reduced to 0.5 to 1 mEq/hr, and the total rise in sodium should not exceed 18 mEq in 48 hours. Studies demonstrate a 6 mEq/L increase in serum sodium in 6 to 12 hours can reverse the most severe neurologic symptoms of acute hyponatremia. No benefit has been observed for faster rates of correction of hyponatremia, whether acute or chronic. Useful formulas to determine the rate of infusion for fluids are provided in Figure 3. The formulas can only estimate the rate of correction, and sodium should be measured frequently.

Chronic Hyponatremia
Chronic hyponatremia is defined as a gradual fall in sodium over more than 48 hours. By this time, the brain has begun to compensate for hypoosmolality by extrusion of solutes. However, the patient is at risk of osmotic demyelination if hyponatremia is treated too aggressively. If the duration of hyponatremia is unknown, the recommendation is to assume that it is chronic. However, as with acute hyponatremia, severe neurologic symptoms and signs need to be treated with hypertonic saline until they resolve, after which the rate of correction can be slowed to 0.5 to 1 mEq/L per hour. Most cases of osmotic demyelination occur with correction rates of greater than 12 mEq/L in 24 hours, but there are cases reported with increases of 9 or 10 mEq/day. Asymptomatic hyponatremia can be treated with an infusion of isotonic saline calculated to raise the sodium by 0.5 to 1 mEq/hour. If the patient has a dilute urine (<200 mOsm/kg), water restriction may be sufficient. Data support favorable outcomes for a maximum target rise in serum sodium of 6 to 8 mEq for any 24 hour period.

Syndrome of Inappropriate Antidiuresis
The mainstays of treatment of SIAD are fluid restriction and treatment of the underlying cause. Mild SIAD usually can be controlled with fluid restriction alone.

In most cases of SIAD, the degree of fluid restriction required can be calculated. It is dependent on three factors: the daily osmolar load, the minimum U_{Osm}, and the patient's maximum urine volume. A typical diet has a daily osmolar load of 10 mOsm/kg of body weight. For a 70-kg person, this would be 700 mOsm/day. With SIAD, the urine osmolality is held constant for that particular patient, as revealed by a spot U_{Osm}. If the U_{Osm} is 500 mOsm/kg and the solute load is 700 mOsm, the fluid load has to be less than 700/500 or 1.4 L/day just to maintain the serum sodium level. Fluid intake above this amount will cause the sodium to decrease.

When needed, salt tablets (sodium chloride tablet 1-3 g taken once to three times daily) can help to make up for renal loss of sodium in SIAD. Urea also can be administered (15–30 g/day in divided doses) and is available as a powder to add to a low volume 3- to 4-oz glass of water or juice. Urea causes an osmotic diuresis and increases free water excretion. Preclinical data support that urea may decrease osmotic delyemlination. With symptoms and severe hyponatremia, short-term use of hypertonic saline may also be instituted to restore sodium to the ECF compartment. Loop diuretics (e.g., furosemide [Lasix]) can increase free water clearance when given with solute (e.g., hypertonic saline or salt tablets). In refractory cases, demeclocycline[1] (300–600 mg PO twice daily)[3] can be used. Demeclocycline (Declomycin) antagonizes the actions of vasopressin by inhibiting formation of cyclic adenosine monophosphate in the collecting duct. Long-term use is limited by

---

[1]Not FDA approved for this indication.

---

[1]Not FDA approved for this indication.
[3]Exceeds dosage recommended by the manufacturer.

Parameters for acute or chronic hyponatremia:
Do not increase serum Na by more than 9 mEq in 24 hours and 18 mEq in 48 hours

Symptomatic hyponatremia with severe neurologic symptoms (acute <48 hrs or chronic >48 hrs)
1. Correct serum Na at a rate of 1–2 mEq/l per hour (for 2 to 4 hours) until symptoms have resolved
2. Correct Na at a rate of 6–8 mEq/24h and 18 mEq/48 h

Acute hyponatremia symptoms
1. Correct at rate of 0.5 to 1 mEq/L per hour to a maximum of 6–8 mEq for the first 24 h

Chronic hyponatremia with mild symptoms or asymptomatic
1. Correct at a rate of 0.5 mEq/L per hour with fluid restriction
2. Treat underlying etiology

Calculation of the rate of infusion of saline to correct hyponatremia
1. Change in serum sodium per liter infusate

$$(\Delta Na/L) = \frac{\text{Infusate [sodium]} - \text{Serum [sodium]}}{\text{TBW} + 1}$$

2. Amount of infusate (in L) required in 24 hours

$$L = \frac{\text{desired change in sodium } (\Delta Na) \text{ over 24 hrs}}{\Delta Na/L \text{ (from 1)}}$$

3. Rate of infusate to raise serum Na by desired amount

$$ml/hr = \frac{L \text{ (from 2)} \times 1000 \text{ mL/L}}{24 \text{ hr}}$$

4. (Simplified) Hypertonic saline infused at 1–2 mL/kg per hour

Monitoring:
1. Monitor frequently for clinical improvement or worsening of symptoms
2. If on hypertonic saline or severely symptomatic check sodium q2–4 hrs.
3. If undergoing treatment but asymptomatic, check sodium q6–12 h.

Infusate	Infusate [Na] (mmol/L)
5% sodium chloride in water	855
3% sodium chloride in water	513
Isotonic saline (0.9%)	154
Ringer's lactate solution	130
0.45% sodium chloride in water	77
0.2% sodium chloride in water	34
5% dextrose in water	0

Total Body Water (TBW) is equal to 60% of body weight in young adult men and 50% in young adult women. Older patients have less TBW. In elderly males, TBW is equal to 50% of body weight and in elderly females it is 45%.

Figure 3 Treatment of hyponatremia. *Abbreviation:* TBW = total body water.

the side effect of photosensitivity and by nephrotoxicity in patients with underlying liver disease. Vasopressin receptor antagonists also are important adjunct treatments (see later discussion). A less commonly used treatment is urea (powder or capsules),[1] which causes an osmotic diuresis and increased free water excretion. Preclinical data support that urea may decrease osmotic demyelination.

Cerebral Salt Wasting
Management of CSW involves treatment of the underlying neurologic problem, as well as volume replacement. CSW often is difficult to differentiate biochemically from SIAD, but the rise in vasopressin in CSW is secondary to volume depletion. As a result, CSW responds to volume replacement with isotonic saline, suppressing release of vasopressin, whereas SIAD worsens with this therapy. The recommended correction rate is 0.7 to 1.0 mEq/L per hour, with a maximum of 9 mEq per 24 hours. Salt tablets may also be given to replete total body sodium. Fludrocortisone (Florinef 0.05 to 0.1 mg every 12 hours), an aldosterone receptor agonist, is a third-line treatment to encourage volume expansion and sodium retention, but the potassium concentration and blood pressure should be monitored. Fluid restriction is inappropriate for CSW and should be avoided, especially in patients with subarachnoid hemorrhage, because volume depletion can exacerbate cerebral vasospasm and cause infarction. The duration of CSW is usually 3 to 5 weeks.

Vasopressin Receptor Antagonists
Vasopressin receptor antagonists, or vaptans, are a treatment option for clinically significant euvolemic hyponatremia defined as a serum Na <125 mEq/L or if hyponatremia is symptomatic and resistant to correction with standard therapy. Vaptans also can be used for asymptomatic hypervolemic hyponatremia, but the benefit must clearly outweigh the risk, and the patient should be refractory to standard therapy. There are currently two FDA-approved vaptans, conivaptan (Vaprisol) and tolvaptan (Samsca). Conivaptan is a dual V_{1a}/V_2 arginine vasopressin receptor antagonist and tolvaptan is a selective V_2 arginine vasopressor receptor antagonist with about 29 times the affinity to the V_2 receptor compared to conivaptan. The primary action of both medications is to block the binding of vasopressin to its receptors in the distal nephron which leads to a decrease in translocation of the aquaporin-2 channels to the apical membrane of the collecting duct in the renal tubule. As a result, vaptans cause an increase in excretion of solute-free water resulting in a rise in serum sodium.

Conivaptan is an IV formulation approved for inpatient hospital use for euvolemic and hypervolemic hyponatremia. It is contraindicated for hypovolemic hyponatremia, euvolemic or hypervolemic hyponatremia with moderate to severe central nervous system (CNS) symptoms, and hypervolemic hyponatremia due to cirrhosis. Conivaptan should be used very cautiously in patients with hypervolemic hyponatremia due to heart failure because safety data are limited and efficacy has not been clearly established. Conivaptan is not recommended in those with severe renal impairment CrCl < 30 mL/min. Conivaptan is given intravenously with a bolus of 20 mg over 30 minutes in 100 mL of 5% dextrose in water (D5W) followed by a continuous infusion of 20 mg conivaptan diluted in 250 mL of D5W over 24 hours. After the initial day of treatment, conivaptan can be continued for an additional 1 to 3 days. Sodium is monitored every 2 to 4 hours and the dose may be titrated to 40 mg per 24 hours to obtain an increase in sodium of 0.5 to 1.0 mEq/L per hour. In clinical trials, the average rise in serum Na after 4 days of therapy is about 6 mEq/L. During conivaptan treatment, fluid restriction can be liberal or is not required. Close monitoring of the rate of sodium rise, neurologic status, and hemodynamic stability are required and treatment should be discontinued or resumed at a reduced dose if clinically indicated. The most common side effects of conivaptan are infusion site reactions and to a lesser degree headache, hypotension, nausea, constipation, and postural hypotension.

Tolvaptan is an oral V_2 receptor antagonist that carries the same indications for use as conivaptan. Tolvaptan should be initiated only in the hospital setting for careful monitoring of potassium and the rate of Na rise, and then can be used in the outpatient setting. The starting dose is 15 mg once daily and can be titrated to 60 mg daily after the initial 24 hours. Patients should not be on fluid restriction for the first 24 hours of tolvaptan therapy and be advised to drink based on thirst. Tolvaptan carries a risk of serious liver injury. The FDA recommends that tolvaptan should not be used for durations longer than 30 days or in any patient with underlying liver disease. Monitoring parameters are equivalent to conivaptan the drug should be stopped promptly in patients with abnormal liver tests or symptoms of hepatotoxicity. In clinical

---

[1]Not FDA approved for this indication.

studies, the average rise in serum Na after 4 days of therapy is 4.2 mEq/L and 5.5 mEq/L after 30 days of therapy. The vaptans are a substrate and potent inhibitor of cytochrome P-450 3A4 isoenzyme (CYP3A4). Prior to initiation of therapy drug-drug interactions should be reviewed with the pharmacists and vaptans are contraindicated with other CYP3A4 inhibitors.

Overcorrection of Hyponatremia

If the correction of chronic hyponatremia exceeds our therapeutic limits over the course of 6, 12 or 24 hours, the approach to readjust treatment depends on the risk of osmotic demyelination. In acute hyponatremia, the risk of osmotic demyelination due to overcorrection is lower especially if the etiology is due to water intoxication. The risk for cerebral injury is greatest when hyponatremia is both longer in duration and at lower sodium levels (i.e., <120 mEq/L). Risk factors for osmotic demyelination with correction for chronic hyponatremia are serum sodium less than 105 mEq/L, hypokalemia, alcoholism, malnutrition and advanced liver disease. Overcorrection is prevented by careful monitoring of serum sodium and urine output at least every 4 to 6 hours. If the 24 hour increase has exceeded 8 mEq/L, active therapies to raise serum sodium should be held over the next 24 hours. In high risk patients for ODS where serum sodium correction is above 8 mEq/L over 24 hours, therapeutic re-lowering of serum sodium may be justified. In such cases, 1 to 2 mcg of desmopressin (DDAVP)[1] in combination with 3 mL/kg infusion of 5% dextrose in water given over 1 hour has been effective. A serum sodium should be checked after each infusion and therapeutic re-lowering repeated if indicated. In chronic hyponatremic patients not at high risk for ODS, studies have shown 10 to 12 mEq increases over 24 hours were still safe.

Summary

Hyponatremia is a common electrolyte abnormality and is usually caused by decreased plasma osmolality. Accurate assessment of volume status is a key to determining the underlying cause and choosing the correct treatment approach. The biggest risk of hyponatremia and its treatment is the possibility of severe neurologic sequelae, including fatal cerebral edema and osmotic demyelination. Therefore more aggressive initial treatment is needed in patients with neurologic manifestations (hypertonic saline), but a more conservative approach (e.g., fluid restriction) is needed for less symptomatic patients. Vasopressin antagonists are additional tools for the treatment of euvolemic or hypervolemic hyponatremia refractory to more conservative measures. In patients at high risk for ODS, overcorrection of serum sodium should be avoided and recorrected with holding active therapy or treating with desmopressin and D5W.

---

[1]Not FDA approved for this indication.

References

Andr\'egué, Tucker B, Madias N. Diagnosis and Management of Hyponatremia. *JAMA.* 328:280–291, 2022.
Cerdà-Esteve M, Cuadrado-Godia E, Chillaron JJ, et al: Cerebral salt wasting syndrome: Review, *Eur J Intern Med* 19:249–254, 2008.
Dineen R, Thompson CJ, Sherlock M: Hyponatremia presentations and management, *Clin Med (Lond)* 17:263–269, 2017.
Ellison DH, Berl T: Clinical practice: The syndrome of inappropriate antidiuresis, *N Engl J Med* 356:2064–2072, 2007.
Fenske W, Störk S, Koschker A: Value of fractional uric acid excretion in differential diagnosis of hyponatremia patients on diuretics, *J Clin Endocrinol Metab* 93:2991–2997, 2008.
Gankam Kengne F, Decauz G: Hyponatremia and the Brain, *Kidney Int Rep* 3:24–35, 2018.
Hew-Butler T, Rosner MH, et al: Statement of the Third International Exercise-Induced Hyponatremia Consensus Development Conference, *Clin J Sport Med.* 25:303–320, 2015.
Hoom EJ, Zieste R: Diagnosis and treatment of hyponatremia: Compilation of the guidelines, *J Am Soc Nephrol* 28:1340–1349, 2017.
Jovanovich AJ, Berl T: Where vaptans do and do not fit in the treatment of hyponatremia, *Kidney Int* 83:563–567, 2013.
Sterns RH, Silver AM, Hix JK: Urea for hyponatremia? *Kidney Int* 87:268–270, 2015.
Verbalis J, Goldsmith S, Greenberg, et al: Diagnosis, evaluation, and treatment of hyponatremia: expert panel recommendations, *Am J Med.* 126:S5–S41, 2013.

HYPOPITUITARISM

Method of
Fabienne Langlois, MD; Elena V. Varlamov, MD; and Maria Fleseriu, MD

CURRENT DIAGNOSIS

- Hypopituitarism is rare and occurs most commonly due to sellar tumors and their treatment (pituitary surgery and radiation); less commonly hypopituitarism is due to infiltrative disease, cancer immunotherapy, traumatic brain injury, congenital and other disorders.
- Heightened awareness is required, as clinical manifestations are often nonspecific and insidious, and patients can deteriorate and experience adrenal crisis if hypopituitarism is not detected and treated.
- Diagnosis is based on a combination of low baseline peripheral gland hormones (cortisol, thyroid hormone, insulin-like growth factor-1 [IGF-1], testosterone, and estrogen) and low or inappropriately normal pituitary hormones as well as complementary dynamic testing for adrenal insufficiency (AI) and growth hormone (GH) deficiency.
- Pituitary imaging should be performed when a biochemical diagnosis is confirmed or pituitary disease is suspected based on neurologic symptoms (headaches and peripheral vision loss).

CURRENT THERAPY

- Glucocorticoid (GC) replacement is the most critical of all replacements for hypopituitarism; in such cases hydrocortisone is the preferred medication.
- Physiologic replacement of each pituitary deficiency is individualized and monitored with clinical assessment and/or laboratory measurements.
- Of note: interactions exist between different hormones, thus changes or replacement in one hormonal axis may affect other axes.

Epidemiology

Hypopituitarism results from a partial or complete pituitary hormone deficiency. Current epidemiology is not well known. A 2001 Spanish population study showed a prevalence of 45.5 cases per 100,000 and an incidence of 4.2 per 100,000 individuals per year. This estimate is likely conservative, as clinical awareness, imaging studies, and overall understanding of hypopituitarism pathophysiology have improved over the last decades.

Pathophysiology

The pituitary gland is a small endocrine gland (~1 cm in size) located in sella turcica of the sphenoid bone at the base of the brain; its function is closely linked to the hypothalamus and is controlled by various neurohormonal and nonhormonal inputs. The pituitary secretes hypophyseal hormones into the systemic circulation, stimulating target peripheral glands to produce specific hormones, which in turn feed back to the hypothalamic-pituitary system and maintain a highly regulated homeostasis (Figure 1).

The pituitary is composed of two functionally distinct structures that differ in embryologic development and anatomy: the adenohypophysis (anterior pituitary) and the neurohypophysis (posterior pituitary). The anterior pituitary is responsible for GH, prolactin, ACTH, TSH, LH, and FSH. The posterior pituitary has a neural origin and stores vasopressin (or antidiuretic hormone [ADH]) and

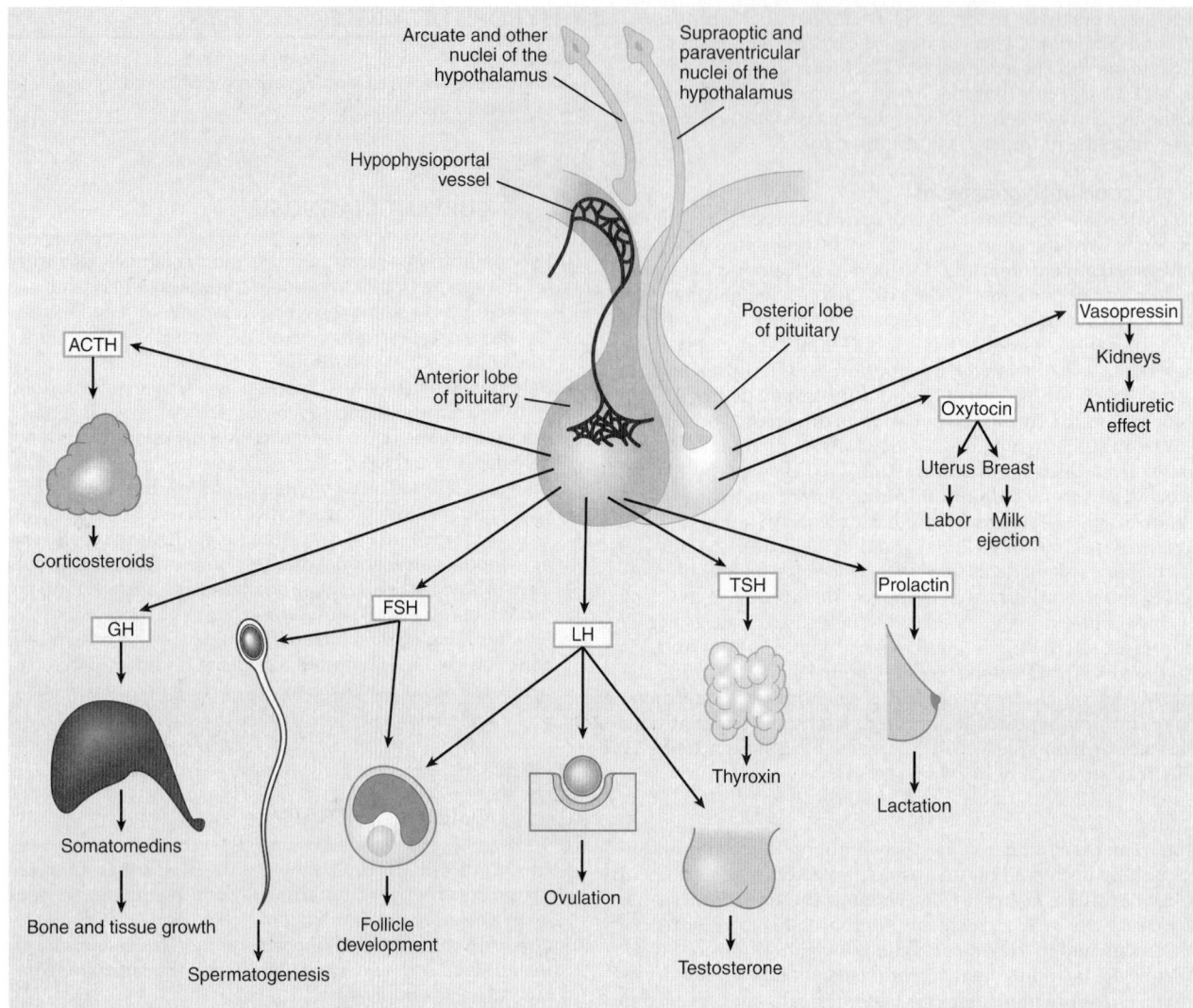

Figure 1 Relationships between hypothalamic hormones, pituitary hormones, and target organs. Numerous hormone-releasing and hormone-inhibiting factors formed in the arcuate and other hypothalamic nuclei are transported to the anterior pituitary by hypophysioportal vessels. In response to hypothalamic hormones, the anterior pituitary secretes the following: corticotropin, which evokes corticosteroid secretion by the adrenal cortex; growth hormone *(GH)*, which elicits production of insulin-like growth factors by the liver; follicle-stimulating hormone *(FSH)*, which stimulates spermatogenesis and facilitates ovarian follicle development; luteinizing hormone *(LH)*, which elicits testosterone secretion by the testes, facilitates ovarian follicle development, and induces ovulation; thyroid-stimulating hormone *(TSH)*, which stimulates thyroxin secretion by the thyroid gland; and prolactin, which induces breast tissue growth and lactation. The posterior pituitary hormones, which are formed in the supraoptic and paraventricular nuclei, are transported by nerve axons to the posterior lobe, where they are released by physiologic stimuli. Oxytocin induces the ejection of milk from the breast and stimulates uterine contractions during labor. Vasopressin increases water reabsorption by the kidneys. *ACTH,* Adrenocorticotropic hormone. From Brenner GM, Stevens CW: *Brenner and Stevens' Pharmacology,* 5th ed., pages 359–365. Elsevier; 2018.

oxytocin, which are produced in the hypothalamus. Therefore any damage to the hypothalamic-pituitary unit can cause an isolated or combined hormonal deficiency (Table 1).

Different etiologies affect various hormonal patterns. In approximately 70% of cases, the anterior pituitary is affected by a locally expanding tumor, causing mass effect. The most frequent pituitary hormonal deficiency related to sellar tumors is growth hormone (GH) deficiency, followed by gonadal axis hormones (luteinizing and follicle-stimulating hormones [LH/FSH]), and thyroid-stimulating hormone (TSH) deficiencies. However, in other etiologies, the pattern of pituitary deficiency differs. For example, in immunotherapy-related hypophysitis, adrenocorticotropic hormone (ACTH) is the first and most common deficiency noted. Lymphocytic hypophysitis preferentially affects the adrenal and gonadal axes. Infiltrative diseases can also manifest as arginine vasopressin deficiency (AVP-D), formerly diabetes insipidus, and/or anterior pituitary dysfunction. Congenital diseases may affect one or more axes and usually present in childhood; for example, an Anosmin-1 (*ANOS1*)

mutation results in isolated hypogonadotropic hypogonadism (Kallmann syndrome) and failure to go through puberty, whereas a *PROP-1* mutation presents with low GH, TSH, and LH-FSH.

In severe illness, functional hypopituitarism may cause low GH, hypogonadism, and central hypothyroidism, which are transient and may recover with acute stress resolution. Traumatic brain injury may cause hypopituitarism in up to 30% to 40% of cases, most commonly as GH deficit with or without gonadal dysfunction. Many deficiencies resolve within a year. Surgery in the pituitary region can lead to one or complete pituitary hormone deficit, including transient or permanent AVP-D.

Prevention

In most cases, hypopituitarism is not preventable. Awareness is most important for early diagnosis, as the development of hormonal deficiencies is often insidious and characterized by nonspecific symptoms such as fatigue or weight changes. Pituitary surgery should be performed by a high-volume pituitary neurosurgeon to decrease the risk of surgery-related hypopituitarism. High-dose or prolonged glucocorticoid (GC) therapy suppresses the hypothalamic-pituitary-adrenal (HPA) axis and may also alter the gonadal and thyroid axes. Prolonged opioid use can also induce hypopituitarism, especially adrenal insufficiency (AI) and hypogonadism. Limiting GCs and opioids to the lowest effective dose and for the shortest possible time allows for a reduction in the risk of HPA axis suppression.

Clinical Manifestations
Signs and symptoms of hypopituitarism vary depending on the type and severity of the pituitary hormones affected and also disease duration.

Signs and symptoms may include the following:
- ACTH deficiency—generalized fatigue, weakness, nausea, loss of appetite, failure to thrive, hypotension, hyponatremia, and hypoglycemia (note that mineralocorticoid secretion is intact; thus hyperkalemia, the hallmark of primary AI, is not present).
- TSH deficiency—fatigue, weight gain, cold intolerance, dry skin, bradycardia, and constipation.
- Gonadotropin deficiency—decreased sex drive; infertility; in women, oligo- or amenorrhea; in men, erectile dysfunction; gynecomastia; muscle atrophy; and decreased exercise capacity.
- GH deficiency—failure to thrive and short stature in children; some adults are symptomatic, experiencing fatigue, abdominal fat deposition, weight gain, and decreased concentration, memory, productivity, and quality of life.
- Prolactin—inability to lactate.
- ADH deficiency—polyuria, polydipsia with excessive thirst, hypernatremia if uncompensated.

Detailed Diagnosis
The diagnosis of hypopituitarism is based on a combination of high clinical suspicion, imaging studies, and demonstration of inappropriate pituitary hormone in the setting of low levels of a target peripheral gland hormone.

In most cases, once a single pituitary hormone deficit is confirmed, other axes should be tested and pituitary magnetic resonance imaging (MRI) performed. In cases of peripheral vision deterioration with or without headaches, imaging should not be delayed.

Corticotropin (Adrenocorticotropic Hormone)
AI is confirmed when low cortisol level is measured early in the morning, before 9 a.m. An early-morning serum cortisol level greater than 15 µg/dL is usually sufficient to rule out AI, and a level below 3 µg/dL to 5 µg/dL is strongly suggestive of AI. Additionally, serum cortisol testing should be repeated and interpreted in the clinical context (e.g., time of day, acute illness status) and also according to levels of cortisol binding proteins (lower in malnutrition and hypoalbuminemia and higher in hyperestrogenic states). If the serum cortisol level is between 5 µg/dL and 15 µg/dL, an ACTH stimulation test should be performed to confirm diagnosis. An ACTH stimulation test evaluates adrenal reserve that is diminished without the presence of adequate ACTH amount. A standard high-dose test involves administering 250 µg of cosyntropin (Cortrosyn) and then measuring serum cortisol levels after 30 and 60 minutes. A cortisol level of higher than 18 µg/dL to 20 µg/dL at 30 or 60 minutes is considered normal. In an alternative low-dose (1 µg) test,[1] cortisol is measured 20 to 30 minutes after cosyntropin administration. This test has been suggested to be more sensitive for the diagnosis of secondary AI. However, technical issues (e.g., improper dilution, delay in blood draw) can lead to inaccurately low results. Of note, lower cortisol cutoffs (14 µg/dL to 17 µg/dL) have been proposed recently for new, more selective assays (liquid chromatography/mass spectrometry and monoclonal rather than polyclonal immunoassays), which have

less cross-reactivity with cortisol precursors; however, these cutoffs need further validation. The serum ACTH level is measured concurrently with baseline cortisol to distinguish between primary and secondary AI. A low or normal ACTH level is consistent with the diagnosis of central AI, while a high ACTH level (typically greater than twice above the upper limit of normal) with primary AI (refer to AI section for further details).

Thyrotropin (Thyroid-Stimulating Hormone)
The key to a diagnosis of secondary (central) hypothyroidism is inappropriately low or normal TSH in the presence of low free T_4. Occasionally, in pituitary or hypothalamic disease, TSH is minimally elevated (usually less than 5 mU/L) and often has lower bioactivity. In contrast, in primary hypothyroidism caused by thyroid gland disorders, TSH is markedly elevated. Therefore TSH levels alone are not sufficient for diagnosis in central hypothyroidism. It is therefore important to measure paired TSH and T_4 levels.

Gonadotropins (Follicle-Stimulating Hormone and Luteinizing Hormone)
In males, central hypogonadism is diagnosed by low testosterone levels when measured between 8 a.m. and 10 a.m. in conjunction with inappropriately normal or low LH and FSH. In premenopausal females, irregular or absent periods (after exclusion of pregnancy) along with low estrogen and low or inappropriately normal gonadotrophins indicate central hypogonadism. Hyperprolactinemia, thyroid dysfunction, and hyperandrogenic states (in females) and hemachromatosis (in males), should be excluded as a cause of gonadal dysfunction. In contrast, in primary hypogonadism and in the postmenopausal state, FSH and LH are markedly elevated.

Growth Hormone
GH secretion is pulsatile, and a single low measurement of GH is not diagnostic of GH deficiency (GHD). Low age-adjusted IGF-1 in adults is suggestive of GHD; however, normal IGF-1 does not rule out GHD. Provocative testing with glucagon (GlucaGen),[1] GH-releasing hormone (GHRH), arginine (R-Gene 10), macimorelin (Macrilen), or insulin tolerance tests are recommended for the diagnosis of GHD in adults. Diagnostic cutoffs differ for different tests and for different body mass indices; therefore careful interpretation is important for accurate diagnosis. When three or more pituitary deficiencies are present along with low IGF-1 levels, confirmatory provocative testing is not required.

Vasopressin (Antidiuretic Hormone)
Hypernatremia in AVP-D may occur due to low ADH, although it is not always present in compensated states if the patient has unlimited access to free water. When hypernatremia is suspected by polyuria and polydipsia, simultaneous measurement of serum and urine osmolality is recommended as an initial test. High serum osmolality (>295 mOsmol/L) and concurrent low urine osmolality (<300 mOsmol/L) are diagnostic of AVP-D. In subtle or unclear cases, a water deprivation test should be performed. Measurement of serum copeptin level at baseline, after water deprivation, hypertonic saline, or with arginine stimulation using specific cutoffs can be helpful in diagnosis. Copeptin is derived from ADH preprohormone and is more stable than ADH; however, copeptin assays may not be available in some countries.

Differential Diagnosis
Hypopituitarism causes secondary endocrine organ failure and should be distinguished from primary failure (primary AI, primary hypothyroidism, and primary hypogonadism), where the corresponding pituitary hormone will be elevated. An ACTH stimulation test can be normal for more than 2 weeks in patients with an acute onset of central AI, such as pituitary apoplexy or after pituitary surgery, because the adrenal cortex is able to respond to stimulation for several weeks until it undergoes atrophy in the presence

---

[1]Not FDA approved for this indication.

[1]Not FDA approved for this indication.

of low ACTH. Critical illness may result in temporary suppression of TSH, GH, and gonadotrophins and does not require hormonal replacement in the acute period. Obesity can be a cause of male hypogonadotropic hypogonadism. Central DI should be distinguished from nephrogenic DI and primary polydipsia by means of a water deprivation test or other confirmation testing.

Treatment

Glucocorticoid Replacement

Oral hydrocortisone (Cortef) is the preferred GC. A typical replacement regimen is 15 mg/day to 20 mg/day as a single or divided dose (e.g., two-thirds in the morning and one-third in the early afternoon) due to its short half-life. Single doses in the morning can also be used in patients with central AI. A once-daily dual-release hydrocortisone formulation has been designed to mimic physiologic cortisol production; this is available in Europe but not in the United States. Of note, GC replacement at physiologic doses does not require treatment for bone protection or gastric ulcer prophylaxis.

Longer-acting GCs (prednisone, dexamethasone [Decadron]) may be used in patients who remain severely symptomatic in the evenings or early morning hours or who are unable to comply with a multidose hydrocortisone regimen. However, in such cases the risk of overreplacement is much higher.

Patients and families should be educated about the "sick day regimen" (i.e., to double or triple their daily dose for 3 days to 5 days according to the degree of physical stress or illness). In cases of repeated vomiting or deterioration of illness, it is recommended that patients administer injectable GC (hydrocortisone [Solu-Cortef] 100 mg IM or dexamethasone [Decadron] 4 mg IM) and seek immediate medical attention.

Minor surgical stress (e.g., cataract removal) requires additional administration of intravenous (IV) 25 mg hydrocortisone on the day of surgery only. The suggested dose for moderate stress (e.g., cholecystectomy) is 50 mg to 75 mg IV in divided doses on the day of surgery and the first postoperative day. Severe stress (e.g., coronary bypass surgery) requires 100 mg to 150 mg IV in divided doses for 2 days to 3 days with a subsequent rapid taper to the daily maintenance dose in an uncomplicated surgery (refer to the earlier section on adrenal insufficiency for further details).

Adrenal crisis and critical illness in adrenally insufficient patients are managed by administering a 100-mg IV bolus of hydrocortisone followed by 50 mg to 100 mg every 6 hours to 8 hours or continuous infusion of 200 mg/24 hours with the dose gradually decreased as the patient's condition improves. Additionally, it is recommended that patients wear a medical bracelet indicating AI diagnosis.

Thyroid Deficiency

Central hypothyroidism is treated by T_4 replacement (levothyroxine [Euthyrox, Levoxyl, Synthroid]). A standard replacement dose for complete central hypothyroidism is 1.6 µg/kg/day; however, lower doses are needed in cases of partial deficiency. TSH should not be used as a marker of adequacy of replacement. Instead, one should adjust the dose to target free T_4 levels in the mid to upper half of the normal range and consider a lower target in elderly patients and in those with comorbidities in an effort to avoid over replacement.

Thyroid replacement should be administered only after corticosteroids have been replaced or adrenal function has been confirmed to be normal. Thyroid replacement in untreated AI can provoke an adrenal crisis.

Sex Hormone Deficiency

Testosterone replacement in men and estrogen (plus progesterone if the uterus is present) replacement in women is appropriate in symptomatic patients without contraindications after a discussion regarding risks and benefits. Combined oral contraceptive or hormone replacement therapy may be offered to premenopausal women. Premenopausal women not receiving estrogen replacement have an increased risk of cardiovascular disease and osteoporosis. Testosterone improves libido, sexual function, anemia, and bone density in men. Prostate, breast, and uterine cancer are contraindications to sex steroid replacement. Patients at high risk for thrombotic and cardiovascular events, including smokers, are poor candidates for hormone replacement.

Growth Hormone Deficiency

GH replacement (somatropin [Genotropin, Humatrope]) is administered as a daily injection; longer-acting formulations are in clinical trial testing for adults. In GH-deficient adults, GH replacement improves body composition, has a modest effect on the maintenance of bone density, and improves quality of life. Although mortality in patients with hypopituitarism is increased, GH replacement has not been shown to improve mortality. Side effects of treatment include worsening of insulin resistance, joint pain, and peripheral edema. Although GH replacement has not been directly linked to cancer development or tumor regrowth, replacement is contraindicated in cases of active cancer.

Arginin Vasopressin Deficiency

Desmopressin (DDAVP) therapy is individualized based on the patient's symptoms (severity or persistence of polyuria and polydipsia) and serum sodium levels especially during the initiation phase of therapy due to risk of hyponatremia from overcorrection. Desmopressin may be administered orally, intranasally (in some countries), or via a sublingual route; in a hospital setting it may be given via an IV or subcutaneous route. A low dose is used at initiation to avoid hyponatremia. Some patients with partial AVP-D are only mildly symptomatic and prefer no treatment while keeping sodium levels normal with adequate water intake.

Monitoring

Patients should be periodically assessed for signs of GC overreplacement (weight gain, facial rounding, hyperglycemia, and osteoporosis) or under-replacement (nausea, fatigue, joint pain) and the GC dose adjusted accordingly.

Monitoring for thyroid, GH, gonadal and AVP deficiencies in patients receiving replacement therapy includes periodic clinical assessment and measurement of hormone levels (free T_4, IGF-1, testosterone, and sodium). Regular follow-up by an endocrinologist is warranted.

Interaction exists between the various hormone replacements. For example, thyroid replacement and GH affect GC metabolism and may cause AI in patients with low adrenal reserve. Higher maintenance hydrocortisone doses may be required in patients who initiate GH or thyroid replacement. Oral estrogen can increase cortisol- and thyroid-binding globulins, resulting in an increase of the total cortisol and thyroxine levels and relative decrease in the bioavailable free hormone; therefore careful interpretation of test results is necessary.

Special Circumstances

Fertility and Pregnancy

New assisted reproductive techniques have led to the increased prevalence of women with hypopituitarism achieving fertility, and birth rates seem to be high in women with hypopituitarism achieving pregnancy. During pregnancy, many continuous adjustments in pituitary hormonal replacement should be considered.

Although GCs, levothyroxine, and desmopressin are safely prescribed during pregnancy, GH treatment regimens vary significantly between countries. GH is not approved for use in pregnancy, but several publications have shown that it can improve outcomes in women pursuing fertility.

In women with hypopituitarism who desire to be pregnant, close monitoring is needed, and such patients will benefit from an evaluation at a pituitary center of excellence.

Complications

Complications arise from a failure to diagnose hypopituitarism, especially in the event of an acute onset or severe illness or trauma, as untreated AI can result in cardiovascular collapse, organ failure, and death. Insufficient chronic replacement can lead to persistent symptoms and poor quality of life, whereas over replacement can result in the development of iatrogenic Cushing syndrome, iatrogenic hyperthyroidism, and other complications.

Conclusion

Early recognition and treatment of hypopituitarism is essential to reduce morbidity and mortality and improve quality of life. Care for patients with multiple pituitary deficiencies is often complex and requires expert management by an endocrinologist in conjunction with a pituitary neurosurgeon when surgical treatment for pituitary lesion is required. Although some pituitary deficiencies except adrenal and thyroid may recover or may not necessitate treatment, most patients require lifelong hormonal replacement and follow-up.

References

Brenner GM, Stevens CW: In *Brenner and Stevens'* pharmacology, ed 5, © 2018, Elsevier.

Carmichael J: Anterior pituitary failure. In Melmed S, editor: *Pituitary*, ed 4, 2007, Elsevier Inc., pp 329–364.

Fleseriu M, Christ-Crain M, Langlois F, Gadelha M, Melmed S: Hypopituitarism, *Lancet* 403(10444):2632–2648, 2024.

Fleseriu M, Hashim IA, Karavitaki N, et al: Hormonal replacement in hypopituitarism in adults: an endocrine society clinical practice guideline, *J Clin Endocrinol Metab* 101(11):3888–3921, 2016.

Higham CE, Johannsson G, Shalet SM: Hypopituitarism, *Lancet* 388(10058):2403–2415, 2016.

Honegger J, Schlaffer S, Menzel C, et al: Diagnosis of primary hypophysitis in Germany, *J Clin Endocrinol Metab* 100(10):3841–3849, 2015.

Molitch ME, Clemmons DR, Malozowski S: Evaluation and treatment of adult growth hormone deficiency: an Endocrine Society clinical practice guideline, *J Clin Endocrinol Metab* 96(6):1587–1609, 2011.

Regal M, Paramo C, Sierra SM, Garcia-Mayor RV: Prevalence and incidence of hypopituitarism in an adult Caucasian population in northwestern Spain, *Clin Endocrinol (Oxf)* 55(6):735–740, 2001.

Vila G, Fleseriu M: Fertility and pregnancy in women with hypopituitarism: a systematic literature review, *J Clin Endocrinol Metab* 105(3):e53–e65, 2020.

Javorsky BR, Raff H, Carroll TB, Algeciras-Schimnich A, Singh RJ, Colón-Franco JM, et al: New cutoffs for the biomechanical diagnosis of adrenal insufficiency after ACTH stimulation using specific cortisol assays, *J Endocr Soc*, bvab022, 2021. https://doi.org/10.1210/jendso/bvab022.

Ueland GA, Methlie P, Oksnes M, Thordarson HB, Sagen J, Kellmann R, et al: The short cosyntropin test revisited: new normal reference range LC-MS/MS, *J Clin Endocrinol Metab* 103(4):1696–1703, 2018.

▮ HYPOTHYROIDISM

Method of
Jared Regehr, MD

⊘ CURRENT DIAGNOSIS

- Common symptoms of hypothyroidism include fatigue, lethargy, cold intolerance, weight gain, and constipation.
- There is considerable overlap of symptoms with other conditions, therefore confirming the diagnosis of hypothyroidism requires biochemical testing.
- Hypothyroidism is significantly more common in women. The risk for developing hypothyroidism also increases with age.
- It is imperative to distinguish between primary and secondary hypothyroidism as this may affect further workup.

⊘ CURRENT THERAPY

- Thyroid hormone replacement with levothyroxine (Synthroid, Levoxyl) remains the standard of care for treating hypothyroidism.
- Elderly patients and patients with heart disease should start at a lower dose of levothyroxine (12.5–50 mcg daily) compared with the general population.

- Patients with hypothyroidism should have their dose of levothyroxine increased by ~30% at the time of pregnancy diagnosis if this had not already been done at preconception counseling.
- Untreated hypothyroidism can lead to life-threatening complications such as myxedema coma.

Epidemiology

Hypothyroidism is one of the most common endocrine disorders in the United States and the incidence only continues to increase. Overt or primary clinical hypothyroidism, defined as an elevated thyroid-stimulating hormone (TSH) and low free thyroxine (T_4), affects roughly 1 in 300 patients in the United States, although some studies have shown up to 1 in 50 people being affected. Subclinical hypothyroidism, defined as an elevated TSH with normal T_4, affects even more people with as much as 5% of the population being diagnosed. Hypothyroidism is 5 to 8 times more common in women than men and is much more common as age increases. It is reported to be more common in White patients, although there is a paucity of data specifically studying differences among ethnic groups. Other factors that are associated with higher rates of hypothyroidism include a family history of thyroid disorders, Down syndrome, previous thyroid surgery or irradiation, lack of iodine, taking certain medications (e.g., amiodarone [Pacerone]), and autoimmune disorders such as type 1 diabetes and rheumatoid arthritis.

Prevention

Despite the frequency with which hypothyroidism is diagnosed, the US Preventive Services Task Force has found insufficient evidence to assess the balance of benefits and harms of routine screening for thyroid dysfunction in asymptomatic adults. However, all patients with symptoms of hypothyroidism should have TSH and free T_4 levels tested.

Pathophysiology

Thyroid hormone exerts an effect on nearly every cell in the body, thus it is important for its level to be maintained near the physiologic level. Synthesis of thyroid hormone is a complex biochemical process involving many steps. Thyrotropin-releasing hormone is released from the hypothalamus to stimulate the release of TSH from the anterior pituitary gland. TSH then binds receptors on the thyroid gland to stimulate release of thyroid hormone. The process of making and releasing normal thyroid hormone at the level of the thyroid gland is an intricate interaction requiring sufficient iodine, the actions of multiple enzymes, and an appropriate negative feedback loop involving the hypothalamic-pituitary axis. A disruption at any of these steps can lead to inadequate daily production and release of thyroid hormone, which could lead to hypothyroidism.

Clinical Manifestations

As noted previously, thyroid hormone affects nearly every cell in the human body. Therefore any deviation from the physiologic level of thyroid hormone can have wide-ranging effects. A deficiency of thyroid hormone can clinically present anywhere along the spectrum from asymptomatic to life threatening; most present between these two extremes. Subclinical hypothyroidism, by its definition, has no clinical symptoms but patients will have an elevated TSH value. Common symptoms of patients who present with clinical hypothyroidism include fatigue, cold intolerance, weight gain, constipation, and dry skin. Hypothyroidism may also be implicated in women experiencing menstrual irregularities. These symptoms are nonspecific and can occur in any number of other pathologies as well. Therefore it is essential for clinicians to recognize signs of hypothyroidism and maintain a high index of clinical suspicion when a patient presents with any

		TABLE 1	Etiologies of Hypothyroidism		

PRIMARY	SECONDARY	IATROGENIC	DRUGS	TRANSIENT
Hashimoto thyroiditis	Pituitary adenoma or pituitary surgery	Radioactive iodine treatment for Graves disease	Amiodarone	De Quervain thyroiditis (viral)
Severe iodine deficiency	Hypothalamus dysfunction	Thyroid surgery	Lithium	Postpartum thyroiditis
Congenital thyroid gland anomalies	Radiation (cerebral)	Radiation (neck)	Tyrosine kinase inhibitors	Subacute lymphocytic thyroiditis
Malignancy	Sheehan syndrome		Monoclonal antibodies	Destructive thyroiditis
Infections (mycoplasma)	Resistance to TSH or TRH receptors		Interferon-alpha	
	Congenital hypopituitarism			

TRH, Thyrotropin-releasing hormone; *TSH,* thyroid-stimulating hormone.

combination of these symptoms, especially considering the high prevalence of this disease.

Due to the heterogeneity of presentations, physical examination for patients with hypothyroidism can vary drastically. It is not uncommon for the physical examination to be entirely normal. It is necessary to examine for dry skin, low blood pressure, weight gain, nonpitting edema, and hair thinning. Examination of the thyroid gland will often reveal a normal thyroid gland with no nodules or tenderness with palpation. If there is pain with manipulation of the thyroid gland, this might be evidence of inflammation within the thyroid gland, which could indicate thyroiditis.

In cases of severe hypothyroidism, patients may present with life-threatening myxedema coma. Potential symptoms include pleural effusion, bradycardia, hypotension, altered mental status, hypothermia, hypoglycemia, and hyponatremia. This dangerous condition is a rare manifestation, but prompt recognition and management are necessary to prevent serious morbidity and mortality. The details of treatment for myxedema coma are discussed later.

Another clinical syndrome to be aware of is euthyroid sick syndrome. This can occur in patients who have severe nonthyroid systemic disease. In this condition, systemic disease causes thyroid hormone values to be abnormal despite a normally functioning thyroid gland. Because of this, testing thyroid levels for inpatients who are acutely ill must be approached with caution and used judiciously, reserved only for specific clinical scenarios with a high likelihood of thyroid dysfunction being the cause of the patient's symptoms.

Diagnosis

Clinical hypothyroidism is diagnosed based on low free T_4 levels, although TSH is the preferred initial marker of thyroid status. There is some variation between labs, but a standard reference range for normal TSH is 0.4 to 4.0 mU/L. When an abnormal TSH is identified, a reflex T_4 should be obtained. An elevated TSH in conjunction with a low T_4 indicates primary clinical hypothyroidism, whereas a T_4 within the normal reference range in the setting of an elevated TSH indicates subclinical hypothyroidism.

There are many causes of primary hypothyroidism (Table 1). After recognition of the role of iodine in thyroid function, many countries developed iodine-fortification programs through public health institutions. Unfortunately, iodine deficiency remains a major cause of hypothyroidism in large swaths of Africa and Asia, along with other subpopulations on other continents. In areas with sufficient iodine, Hashimoto thyroiditis (autoimmune thyroiditis) is the most common cause of hypothyroidism. Testing for thyroid peroxidase (TPO) antibodies can be done to confirm this diagnosis. In addition to these, it is important to closely examine patients' medication lists as several medications can cause hypothyroidism, most notably amiodarone (Pacerone).

There is no role for thyroid ultrasound in the diagnosis of hypothyroidism, but it can be used to evaluate palpable thyroid nodules if any are identified on physical examination.

Subclinical hypothyroidism is diagnosed when TSH is elevated but free T_4 is in the normal range. Patients with subclinical hypothyroidism should have TPO antibodies checked as patients with positive antibodies are at increased risk of disease progression with an average of ~5% per year progressing to clinical hypothyroidism.

Although a low TSH often is found in hyperthyroidism, it can rarely cause hypothyroidism. Secondary (or central) hypothyroidism is diagnosed by a low TSH and a low T_4. This is most commonly due to pituitary gland dysfunction but can be a result of hypothalamus dysfunction or a combination of the two. The most common cause of secondary hypothyroidism is pituitary adenomas, accounting for over half of identified cases. Secondary hypothyroidism may require an endocrinology consult to identify and treat the cause of the dysfunction within the hypothalamus or pituitary gland.

Therapy

The mainstay of treatment for hypothyroidism is replacement of thyroid hormone with oral levothyroxine (Synthroid, Levoxyl). There is no strong evidence that treatment with alternative regimens, including triiodothyronine (T_3, Cytomel), is superior to levothyroxine monotherapy. There are multiple formulations of brand and generic levothyroxine available. There is no convincing evidence to avoid generic preparations, although once thyroid function is stable on a certain formulation patients should not switch between preparations. The usual full replacement dose is ~1.6 µg/kg/day, although most patients start slightly lower than that. It is particularly important to start at lower doses in elderly patients or those with cardiovascular disease. In these patients, it is recommended to start at 12.5 to 25 mcg/day and titrate based on TSH levels. If repeat TSH remains above the upper limit of normal, the daily levothyroxine dose should be increased by 12.5 to 25 mcg. If repeat TSH is below the lower limit of normal, the daily levothyroxine dose should be decreased by 12.5 to 25 mcg. Levothyroxine should be taken once per day at least 30 to 60 minutes before breakfast and at least 4 hours before taking any other medications that can affect absorption or availability (Table 2).

The treatment goals of subclinical hypothyroidism have been a source of debate among experts. There is a lack of strong data proving consistent clinical benefit of treatment for subclinical hypothyroidism, as it has been difficult to prove mildly elevated TSH levels are associated with adverse outcomes when left untreated. Whereas there is some evidence that treatment of subclinical hypothyroidism reduced cardiac events in patients aged 40 to 70, there was no evidence in the same study of any benefit in adults over age 70. Some observational studies have shown TSH levels >4.5

TABLE 2	Medications That Can Impact Levothyroxine Absorption or Availability
Proton pump inhibitors	Calcium carbonate
Ferrous sulfate	Sucralfate (Carafate)
Orlistat (Alli, Xenical)	Sertraline (Zoloft)
Phenobarbital	Carbamazepine (Tegretol)
Phenytoin (Dilantin)	Androgens

mU/L in elderly patients to be associated with decreased mortality, whereas other data suggest that subclinical hypothyroidism in the elderly is associated with increased mortality, particularly in patients with TSH values >10 mU/L. Generally, most patients over the age of 30 with subclinical hypothyroidism do not benefit from thyroid hormone replacement, but one reasonable approach is to treat all patients with TSH values >10 mU/L due to an increased incidence of cardiovascular disease and mortality.

Treatment for secondary hypothyroidism presents a unique challenge because the normal strategy of checking TSH with reflex T_4 is unreliable. In this setting, clinicians will not treat to a target TSH because the TSH is already low. These patients usually require assistance from an endocrinology consultant for treatment.

Pregnancy Considerations

Levothyroxine requirements for pregnant patients being treated for hypothyroidism increase, often before pregnancy is clinically recognized. Therefore some experts recommend increasing levothyroxine dose at preconception counseling visits after discussion of risks and benefits with the patient. The goal TSH for pregnant patients is <2.5 to 3.0 mU/L. The dose requirement for levothyroxine is usually ~30% higher in the first trimester than baseline nonpregnancy dose. Monitoring during pregnancy is required every 4 to 6 weeks to ensure TSH goal is being met. Significant adverse effects for both mother (preterm birth, preeclampsia, gestational diabetes) and baby (neurodevelopmental deficits, low birth weight) can result from untreated or undertreated hypothyroidism during pregnancy.

Monitoring

TSH level should be monitored every 6 to 8 weeks for nonpregnant individuals being treated for hypothyroidism until it is consistently within the normal range on a stable dose of levothyroxine. Once the TSH is at goal, repeat lab measurements can be spaced out to every 6 months and if it remains stable can just be checked annually thereafter unless an indication arises to check it sooner. If a patient develops change in symptoms, change in medications, or change in medical conditions then it might be prudent to recheck TSH sooner than 1 year.

For patients with subclinical hypothyroidism who do not require treatment, TSH level should be checked 6 to 12 months after initial diagnosis due to the rate of progression to clinical hypothyroidism in this population. In some cases, the abnormal TSH level will spontaneously resolve and no further monitoring is necessary unless clinical status changes. For patients with persistently high TSH and normal T_4, it is reasonable to continue checking TSH levels annually.

Although there is no universally agreed upon adjustment of TSH reference ranges for age, the upper limit of normal should generally increase with age as it has been proven that TSH levels increase with age in the general population (including patients without thyroid disease).

Complications

Undertreated or untreated hypothyroidism can present as myxedema coma. Patients diagnosed with myxedema coma must be treated as intensive care patients with particular focus on circulation, airway, and breathing. Other main tenets of treatment of myxedema coma include aggressive ventilation, IV fluids, maintenance of electrolytes and glucose within normal range, thyroid hormone replacement, glucocorticoids, and consultation with endocrinology and nephrology. Levothyroxine should be replaced with 200 to 400 mcg IV one time, followed by 50 to 100 mcg PO daily thereafter. Hydrocortisone 100 mg every 8 hours is administered for at least 48 hours, or until adrenal insufficiency can be excluded. The use of T_3 is controversial. Antibiotics are recommended until sepsis can be definitively ruled out. Prompt recognition and treatment of myxedema coma are essential as mortality rates for myxedema coma have been reported as high as 25% to 60%.

Finally, there are long-term complications associated with hypothyroidism, most notably cardiovascular disease. Patients with untreated hypothyroidism who develop cardiovascular disease have an increased mortality rate. Other conditions associated with hypothyroidism, yet without proven mortality changes, include renal disease, arthritis, liver disease, and diabetes. Additionally, patients with hypothyroidism that is overtreated are at risk for cardiovascular disease (notably atrial fibrillation and ventricular hypertrophy) and osteoporosis. These risks of untreated and overtreated hypothyroidism further illustrate the wide-ranging effects thyroid hormone has on the body's systems.

References

Chaker L, Bianco AC, Jonklaas J, Peeters RP: Hypothyroidism, *Lancet* 390(10101):1550–1562, 2017. https://doi.org/10.1016/S0140-6736(17)30703-1. Epub 2017 Mar 20. PMID: 28336049; PMCID: PMC6619426.

Citterio CE, Targovnik HM, Arvan P: The role of thyroglobulin in thyroid hormonogenesis, *Nat Rev Endocrinol* 15(6):323–338, 2019. https://doi.org/10.1038/s41574-019-0184-8. PMID: 30886364.

Garber JR, Cobin RH, Gharib H, American Association of Clinical Endocrinologists and American Thyroid Association Taskforce on Hypothyroidism in Adults, et al: Clinical practice guidelines for hypothyroidism in adults: cosponsored by the American Association of Clinical Endocrinologists and the American Thyroid Association, *Endocr Pract* 18(6):988–1028, 2012. https://doi.org/10.4158/EP12280.GL. Erratum in: Endocr Pract. Jan-Feb;19(1):175, 2013. PMID: 23246686.

Jonklaas J, Bianco AC, Bauer AJ, American Thyroid Association Task Force on Thyroid Hormone Replacement, et al: Guidelines for the treatment of hypothyroidism: prepared by the American thyroid association task force on thyroid hormone replacement, *Thyroid* 24(12):1670–1751, 2014. https://doi.org/10.1089/thy.2014.0028. PMID: 25266247; PMCID: PMC4267409.

Nussey S, Whitehead S: *Endocrinology: an integrated approach*, Oxford, 2001, BIOS Scientific Publishers, Chapter 3, The thyroid gland. Available from: https://www.ncbi.nlm.nih.gov/books/NBK28/.

Rizzo LFL, Mana DL, Bruno OD, Wartofsky L: Coma mixedematoso [Myxedema coma], *Medicina* 77(4):321–328, 2017. Spanish. PMID: 28825577.

Ross DS: *Myxedema Coma*, UpToDate, 2025. https://www.uptodate.com/contents/myxedema-coma. Accessed 3 April 2025.

Taylor PN, Medici MM, Hubalewska-Dydejczyk A, Boelaert K: Hypothyroidism, *Lancet* 404(10460):1347–1364, 2024. https://doi.org/10.1016/S0140-6736(24)01614-3. PMID: 39368843.

US Preventive Services Taskforce: *Thyroid dysfunction: screening*, 2015. Recommendation: Thyroid Dysfunction: Screening | United States Preventive Services Taskforce. https://www.uspreventiveservicestaskforce.org/uspstf/recommendation/thyroid-dysfunction-screening.

Wilson SA, Stem LA, Bruehlman RD: Hypothyroidism: diagnosis and treatment, *Am Fam Physician* 103(10):605–613, 2021. PMID: 33983002.

OBESITY IN ADULTS

Method of
Meera Shah, MBChB

CURRENT DIAGNOSIS

- The diagnosis of obesity is based on the patient's body mass index (BMI), which is a ratio of weight to height. However, there are recognized limitations to using BMI alone when defining obesity.
- Waist circumference can aid the identification of patients who are not obese by BMI criteria but who are still at heightened metabolic risk.

- Certain ethnic groups, such as Asians, have a higher body fat content at a lower BMI and are therefore defined as being overweight or obese at lower BMI cutoffs.
- Diagnosing obesity early, and recognizing it as a chronic disease, allows for discussion and formulation of a plan to mitigate health risks associated with this disease.

CURRENT THERAPY

- The cornerstone of any weight management program is lifestyle intervention that focuses on calorie restriction, an increase in physical activity, and behavioral modification. A multidisciplinary team approach offers the greatest benefit.
- The most effective pharmacotherapies for obesity modulate appetite regulation.
- Pharmacotherapy for obesity can be considered as an adjunct to lifestyle modification in the appropriate patient, after having a thorough discussion about benefits and associated risks.
- Weight loss procedures can be considered in patients with medically complicated obesity. This tends to be the most effective way of losing weight but is also associated with the highest risk. Therefore appropriate patient selection is key.

Obesity was recognized as a complex, chronic disease by the American Medical Association in 2013. The designation of obesity as a disease recognizes that obesity develops in response to an aberration in physiology, and its designation as a chronic disease recognizes that obesity is often present for a period greater than a year and often requires ongoing medical attention and impairs activities of daily living.

Epidemiology

Obesity is a global phenomenon. At the current rate of growth, it is projected that by the year 2030, almost one in two adults in the United States will have a body mass index (BMI) of greater than 30 kg/m². With a higher prevalence of obesity comes a greater burden of obesity-associated chronic disease and comorbidities. Managing obesity is therefore a public health priority.

Obesity and Health Disparity

Obesity disproportionately affects certain racial, ethnic, and socioeconomic groups. Between 2017 and 2018, non-Hispanic Black adults (49.6%) had the highest age-adjusted prevalence of obesity, followed by Hispanic adults (44.8%), non-Hispanic White adults (42.2%), and non-Hispanic Asian adults (17.4%). Within these racial and ethnic differences, prevalence of obesity was lowest in women with college degrees compared with people with lower educational attainment, and in men there was no observable difference in obesity prevalence based on education level.

Among non-Hispanic White and Hispanic men, obesity prevalence was lower in the lowest and highest income groups compared with the middle-income group. Conversely, obesity prevalence was higher in the highest income group than in the lowest income group among non-Hispanic Black men. Among non-Hispanic White, non-Hispanic Asian, and Hispanic women, obesity prevalence was lower in the highest income group than in the middle and lowest income groups. Obesity prevalence was not affected by income in non-Hispanic Black women.

The reasons for these health disparities in adults with obesity are complex. However, there is widespread recognition of the fundamental importance of preventing childhood obesity because children with obesity are more likely to become adults with obesity.

Diagnosis

The current definition of obesity is based on the BMI. The BMI is defined as follows:

$$\frac{\text{Weight (kg)}}{\text{Height (m}^2)}$$

BMI is a practical measure of an individual's degree of adiposity and generally correlates well with comorbidities. However, it is well recognized that BMI has several limitations with regard to body composition and weight distribution and may therefore be misleading if taken as the only measure of obesity, particularly at lower BMI values.

Waist circumference roughly correlates with visceral adiposity and can be an important adjunct when assessing risk associated with obesity in patients with a BMI less than 35 kg/m². In adults with a BMI of 25 to 34.9 kg/m², waist circumference of greater than 102 cm (40 in.) for men and 88 cm (35 in.) for women is associated with greater risk of developing hypertension, type 2 diabetes, and coronary heart disease. Waist circumference is measured with the measuring tape situated above the iliac crest and snugged up against the skin. There is significant intraoperator variability, which limits the reproducibility and use of this metric in the longitudinal assessment of patients with obesity.

BMI cutoffs (Table 1) are applicable to the general population in the United States. Certain ethnic groups, such as Asians, have a higher body fat content at a lower BMI and are therefore defined as being overweight or obese at lower BMI cutoffs (23–24.9 kg/m² and >25 kg/m², respectively).

Assessing the Patient With Obesity in the Office

Once the patient has been diagnosed with obesity, effort then should turn toward understanding the etiology of the disease in the individual patient and assessing for comorbidities associated with obesity.

The following components in the patient's history should be elicited:
- Age of onset of weight gain
- Weight loss attempts
- Changes in dietary patterns
- History of exercise and activity in general
- A comprehensive medication history

The dietary assessment should ideally be performed by a registered dietitian.

A comprehensive medication history may identify medications that are associated with weight gain. Chief among these are psychotropic medications, antidepressants, antiepileptics, insulin secretagogues, and glucocorticoids. Progestational hormones and implants, antihistamines, and oral contraceptives may contribute to weight gain in some patients. Wherever possible, the potential for weight gain should be considered when starting patients with obesity on a new medication. If a weight-neutral alternative exists, effort should be made to switch the patient from a medication that could be contributing to weight gain as long as the underlying disease process remains adequately managed on the new medication regimen. This can be difficult to achieve particularly

TABLE 1	BMI Classification and Weight
CLASSIFICATION	BODY MASS INDEX, KG/M²
Underweight	≤18.5
Normal weight	18.5–24.9
Overweight	25.0–29.9
Obesity, Class I	30.0–34.9
Obesity, Class II	35.0–39.9
Obesity, Class III	≥40

when dealing with psychotropic medications and requires careful coordination with the patient's other prescribers.

The physical examination of the patient should focus on assessing for a pattern of weight distribution that may confer higher risk (i.e., higher waist circumference than BMI alone would confer), as well as physical findings that may allude to a secondary cause of obesity such as glucocorticoid excess, thyroid dysfunction, or dependent edema.

Comorbidities Associated With Obesity

Type 2 Diabetes

It is estimated that about 85% patients with type 2 diabetes are in the overweight or obese category.

The prevalence of diabetes has increased over the years in line with the increase in population-level obesity. The risk of developing type 2 diabetes in people with obesity increases when there is a strong family history of the disease, a history of gestational diabetes, or a weight distribution that is metabolically unfavorable (i.e., high waist circumference). Certain high-risk groups, such as South Asians, are 30% to 50% more likely to develop diabetes than their White counterparts despite having a lower BMI.

A fasting plasma glucose concentration of 126 mg/dL or greater or hemoglobin A1c of 6.5% or greater on two separate occasions can be used to make a diagnosis of type 2 diabetes.

When considering treatment for patients with type 2 diabetes and obesity, careful attention should be paid to the choice of antihyperglycemic agent. Weight-neutral options or medicines that actively promote weight loss, such as glucagon-like peptide-1 (GLP-1) receptor agonist or sodium-glucose cotransporter-2 (SGLT-2) inhibitors, should be prioritized where possible. Conversely, patients on medications that can promote weight gain, such as sulfonylureas or insulin, should be counseled on alternative regimens. In patients with type 2 diabetes, weight loss of 5% to 10% is associated with hemoglobin A1c reductions of 0.6% to 1.0% and reduced need for diabetes medications.

Prevention of type 2 diabetes is possible with modest weight loss. Participants in the Diabetes Prevention program who were at high risk for developing type 2 diabetes and who were able to lose about 7% body weight through lifestyle intervention delayed development of diabetes by approximately 35%. In overweight and obese adults at risk for type 2 diabetes, average weight loss achieved with lifestyle intervention of 2.5 kg to 5.5 kg over 2 years reduces the risk of developing type 2 diabetes by 30% to 60%.

Thyroid Dysfunction

The 2021 guidelines published by European Society of Endocrinology recommends thyroid function testing in all patients with obesity, even in the absence of a clinical suspicion for hypothyroidism. The guideline is an acknowledgment of a relatively simple diagnostic test, low-risk treatment, and potential for untreated hypothyroidism to adversely affect weight loss efforts. Thyroid-stimulating hormone (TSH) is the first thyroid hormone that should be measured. If this is elevated, free thyroxine (free T_4) should be measured to accurately classify the disease process.

Reproductive Dysfunction

Obesity in women increases the risk for menstrual dysfunction, infertility, and adverse outcomes in pregnancy. Obesity is an independent risk factor for erectile dysfunction in men. Weight loss has been shown to improve several aspects of reproductive function in both men and women.

Cardiovascular Disease

Obesity increases the risk of coronary heart disease, heart failure, and overall cardiovascular mortality. People with obesity have a higher likelihood of developing risk factors such as hypertension and dyslipidemia that lead to cardiovascular disease.

Hypertension is a common chronic disease. Obesity has been shown to worsen hypertension; conversely there is a dose-response relationship between weight loss and improvements in blood pressure. Hence, even modest weight loss of less than 5%

body weight can improve blood pressure in a clinically meaningful way.

Screening for dyslipidemia is best performed with a fasting lipid profile. Treatment guidelines for dyslipidemia are based on underlying comorbidities and calculated risk for developing atherosclerotic cardiovascular disease. Modest weight loss (<3 kg) leads to improvement in serum triglycerides and high-density lipoprotein (HDL) and low-density lipoprotein (LDL) cholesterol. In the presence of obesity, other modifiable risk factors such as smoking, hypertension, and sedentary lifestyle should be aggressively targeted.

Obstructive Sleep Apnea

Obstructive sleep apnea is a common but underrecognized complication of obesity. Patients with obesity who present with clinical features suspicious for sleep apnea or a neck circumference of greater than 17 inches in men or 16 inches in women should be screened for sleep apnea. Untreated sleep apnea has numerous health consequences related to the cardiorespiratory system and may also make it difficult for the patient to successfully lose weight. In addition to sleep apnea, obstructive lung disease, apnea-hypopnea syndromes, and restrictive lung disease are common complications of obesity that improve with weight loss.

Fatty Liver Disease

End-stage liver disease from metabolic dysfunction–associated steatotic liver disease (MASLD) is one of the most common reasons for liver transplantation in the world. The prevalence of MASLD increases as BMI increases, and up to 80% of patients with a BMI greater than 40 kg/m² are estimated to have steatosis. The diagnosis of MASLD is made on imaging (most commonly ultrasound) or biopsy. Weight loss is the first line of treatment for MASLD; 5% to 10% weight loss has been shown to improve liver biochemistries and liver histology.

Mechanical Complications From Weight

Patients with overweight and obesity are at high risk of developing degenerative joint disease in weight-bearing joints. This in turn can promote further weight gain, and a vicious cycle therefore develops. A multidisciplinary approach comprising calorie restriction, behavioral therapy, physical therapy, and pain management is often necessary to achieve successful weight loss in this group of patients.

Gastroesophageal reflux is another mechanical complication from carrying excess weight, resulting from increased intraabdominal pressure from visceral adiposity. Patients who lose weight often see improvements in reflux symptoms.

Risk of Cancer

A number of malignancies are associated with obesity. In 2012 in the United States, about 28,000 new cases of cancer in men (3.5%) and 72,000 in women (9.5%) were associated with overweight or obesity. The risk of developing esophageal, stomach, liver, kidney, gallbladder, pancreas, and colorectal cancers is higher in people who are overweight or obese. Endometrial carcinoma, breast cancer (in postmenopausal women), and ovarian cancer occur more commonly in women who are overweight or obese. Obesity also worsens several aspects of cancer survivorship such as quality of life, recurrence, progression, and prognosis.

Psychosocial Functioning

Patients with obesity frequently face stigma in areas such as education, employment, and healthcare, resulting in inequity and loss of opportunity. Patients with obesity often correlate their mental health and well-being with their ability to lose weight, and this can be a challenging situation to navigate. One condition that has been shown to correlate with obesity is seasonal affective disorder. Patients with this diagnosis are prone to gaining weight in the wintertime.

Treatment

Weight loss can only occur with the creation of an energy deficit in an individual. The cornerstone of any weight management program is lifestyle intervention that focuses on calorie restriction, increase in physical activity, and behavioral modification. Other modalities that can help promote weight loss include pharmacotherapy and weight loss procedures. These can be considered adjuncts to lifestyle intervention if lifestyle intervention alone does not produce the desired outcomes.

Successful management of obesity involves a multidisciplinary team working in partnership with the patient. Before making specific recommendations, the patient encounter should address the following:

1. *Assessing the patient's readiness for change.* The clinician can ask, "How prepared are you to make changes in your diet, to be more physically active, and to use behavior change strategies such as recording your weight and food intake?" A patient who is not ready to engage in changes will not be receptive to counseling on lifestyle changes.
2. *Identification of barriers.* Limitations to activity because of mechanical joint pain or lymphedema are relatively common and specific strategies to manage these may be necessary. Time and financial resources are also common barriers to successful weight loss. Identifying and acknowledging barriers can help build trust and forge a partnership with the patient.
3. *Goal-setting.* Patients are often overwhelmed by the amount of weight they need to lose. Clarifying that small but meaningful weight loss will improve health can be helpful to the patient. Aiming for 5% to 10% weight loss over 6 months is a reasonable initial goal.

Lifestyle Intervention Program

The key components of a lifestyle intervention prescription are listed in Table 2. An individualized lifestyle intervention program, based on the patient's dietary preferences, physical activity ability, and underlying motivation is most likely to result in successful weight loss.

Pharmacotherapy for Weight Loss

Appetite regulation is a complicated process that involves peripheral gut signaling, central coordination of those signals, and modulation by the environment, emotion, and behavior. Pharmacotherapy for weight loss primarily focuses on central appetite regulation and the most effective weight loss medications are appetite suppressants. Thus they can reduce caloric intake while simultaneously reducing cravings and other aspects of hedonic eating.

Current U.S. Food and Drug Administration (FDA)-approved weight loss medications are indicated for individuals with a BMI of 30 kg/m² or greater or BMI of 27 kg/m² or greater with at least one obesity-associated comorbid condition who are motivated to lose weight, as an adjunct to comprehensive lifestyle intervention to help achieve targeted weight loss and health goals.

The FDA-approved weight loss medications, their dosing, and their side effect profiles are listed in Table 3. All current FDA-approved weight loss medications, with the exception of weekly semaglutide (Wegovy) and tirzepatide (Zepbound), have an average reported clinical efficacy of 5% to 10% weight loss over 6 months. Choice of therapy is typically guided by weight loss goals, and the principle of minimizing medication interactions and side effects. All current FDA-approved weight loss medications are category X in pregnancy, and patients should be counseled to avoid pregnancy while taking these medications.

Phentermine (Adipex-P) is a short-acting sympathomimetic that has been approved for short-term weight loss (i.e., 12 weeks). However, phentermine is often used off-label for longer periods in patients who show a response to the medication in both weight loss and weight maintenance phases. Retrospective analyses of phentermine users demonstrated no increase in cardiovascular morbidity and no increase in addictive potential with phentermine use. If phentermine monotherapy is being considered as a long-term weight loss medication, the risks and benefits of this

| TABLE 2 | Components of a Lifestyle Intervention Program |
COMPONENT	INTERVENTION
Diet	*Calorie restriction of 300–500 kcal/day.* Goal for most women: 1200–1500 kcal/day. Goal for most men: 1500–1800 kcal/day. There is no specific dietary macronutrient composition that promotes long-term weight loss. The best predictor of weight loss is dietary adherence; thus patients should be counseled on dietary strategies that are most likely to be sustained.
Physical activity	*Goal: ≥150 minutes a week of moderate-intensity exercise* Patients should be encouraged to increase physical activity wherever possible. The first goal may be to decrease sedentary time. Patients can aim for 10 minutes of activity at a time. Self-monitoring of activity, such as using a step counter, can be helpful. Patients with multiple comorbidities and limitations to activity may benefit from a specific physical activity prescription from a physical therapist.
Behavioral therapy	Behavioral modification is key to ensuring long-term success. Daily monitoring of food and activity can help patients make behavioral changes. Ideally, patients will also be enrolled in a structured behavioral modification curriculum supervised by a behavioral psychologist. Patients benefit from regular feedback and support of their efforts.

Modified from Heymsfield SB, Wadden TA: Mechanisms, pathophysiology, and management of obesity, *N Engl J Med* 376(15):1492, 2017.

approach should be thoroughly discussed with the patient and an appropriate monitoring plan instituted.

Topiramate (Topamax) monotherapy is also used off-label to assist with weight management. Topiramate is a carbonic anhydrase inhibitor that has beneficial effects on appetite suppression and satiety. A meta-analysis on the efficacy and safety of topiramate in weight loss showed that patients on topiramate on average were able to lose an additional 5.3 kg over patients on placebo. The most common side effects with topiramate were noted to be paresthesias (tingling of the fingers), changes in taste, and psychomotor impairment.

Semaglutide is a once-weekly GLP-1 receptor agonist that has been FDA approved for the treatment of obesity (Wegovy) and for type 2 diabetes (Ozempic). In early 2021, a number of phase III randomized, placebo-controlled trials using semaglutide at a dose of 2.4 mg once weekly (weight loss dose) were published. The Semaglutide Treatment Effect in People with Obesity (STEP) randomized controlled trials were designed to study the weight loss effect of high-dose semaglutide in patients with and without type 2 diabetes (STEP 1, 2, 3, and 6) and weight maintenance in patients without type 2 diabetes (STEP 4 and 5). On average, participants taking 2.4 mg semaglutide subcutaneously once weekly were able to achieve 15% weight loss compared with patients on placebo who achieved 2% to 5% weight loss. Overall, the gastrointestinal (GI)-related side effect profile was higher in the semaglutide group (nausea, constipation, diarrhea, gallbladder-related conditions), and treatment discontinuation was seen in approximately 3% of participants in that group.

Tirzepatide is a dual GLP-1/GIP agonist that has been approved by the FDA as a once-weekly injection for the treatment of obesity (Zepbound) and type 2 diabetes (Mounjaro). The SURMOUNT series of randomized placebo-controlled trials report on the effect of tirzepatide on weight loss (SURMOUNT-1, SURMOUNT-2, and SURMOUNT-3), and weight maintenance (SURMOUNT-4).

TABLE 3 FDA-Approved Pharmacologic Agents for Weight Loss

NAME/TRADE NAME	DOSING	COMMON SIDE EFFECTS
Orlistat/Xenical	120 mg tid with meals	Bloating, abdominal cramps, diarrhea, steatorrhea
Phentermine-Topiramate ER/Qsymia	3.75/23 mg daily for 2 weeks, then 7.5/46 mg daily thereafter High-dose therapy is 11.25–69 mg daily for 2 weeks, then 15–92 mg daily thereafter	Phentermine side effects: Constipation, dry mouth, tachycardia, insomnia, hypertension Topiramate side effects: Paresthesias, dizziness, cognitive dysfunction, kidney stones, glaucoma
Naltrexone-SR/ bupropion-SR/ Contrave	Each tablet contains 8 mg naltrexone and 90 mg bupropion Titrate by 1 tablet a week until maximal therapeutic dose of 2 tablets twice daily	Nausea, constipation, dry mouth, headache
Liraglutide/Saxenda	Titrate by 0.6 mg daily every week until maximal therapeutic dose of 3 mg daily subcutaneously	Nausea, abdominal discomfort, constipation, or diarrhea
Semaglutide/Wegovy	Start at 0.25 mg subcutaneously weekly for 4 weeks, then 0.5 mg weekly for 4 weeks, then 1 mg weekly for 4 weeks, then 1.7 mg weekly for 4 weeks, then 2.4 mg weekly (if tolerated). 1.7 mg weekly and 2.4 mg weekly are maintenance doses	Nausea, vomiting, constipation or diarrhea, gallbladder-related symptoms
Tirzepatide/Zepbound	Start at 2.5 mg subcutaneously weekly for 4 weeks, then 5 mg weekly for 4 weeks, then 7.5 mg weekly for 4 weeks, then 10 mg weekly for 4 weeks, then 12.5 mg weekly for 4 weeks, then 15 mg weekly	Nausea, vomiting, constipation or diarrhea, gallbladder-related symptoms

On average, participants taking 15-mg tirzepatide subcutaneously once weekly achieve 21% weight loss over 72 weeks, compared with 3% with placebo. Nausea, diarrhea, and constipation were the most commonly reported side effects, and treatment discontinuation was seen in 2.6% of the group receiving the highest dose of the medication.

Monitoring Patients on Weight Loss Medications

Patients on weight loss medications should be evaluated early and often to ensure continued efficacy of the drug and to monitor for side effects. The best predictor of overall response to a weight loss medication is weight loss achieved in the first 3 months. In general, 5% weight loss in the first 3 months is indicative of a "responder." If a patient with a previously upward weight trend is able to maintain their weight on the new medication after 3 months of use, then that patient may still be considered a responder. Patients who have had significant changes to their health, overall medication regimen, or physical activity routine may not achieve the goal of 5% weight loss over 3 months; in these situations, a longer duration of follow-up might be necessary to determine whether the patient is a responder to the medication.

Except for the scenarios listed previously, patients who do not achieve a 5% weight loss over 3 months have several options. If appetite suppression is inadequate per clinical history, then a higher dose of the drug or a different weight loss medication could be considered. Patients could also benefit from meeting with a dietitian to ensure that their dietary plan is adequately calorie-restricted. If a patient has significant side effects from the medication, an alternative weight loss medication could be considered.

Patients should be seen every 3 to 6 months to assess their weight loss trends and monitor for side effects and the potential for new medication interactions. Patients with a clinically meaningful weight loss can also be retested for improvements in their metabolic profile (e.g., fasting glucose), because this may affect therapeutic decision making.

Weight loss typically slows after about 6 months of therapy, sometimes referred to as a "weight plateau"; this is a physiologic adaptation to weight loss. Specifically, it is estimated that for each kilogram of lost weight, calorie expenditure decreases by about 20 to 30 kcal/day, whereas appetite increases by about 100 kcal/day above the baseline level before weight loss. Hence, the default trend is for weight loss followed by weight regain.

This is an important phenomenon to highlight with patients who can become frustrated that their efforts are not yielding results. Patients may be more willing to engage in modifications to their dietary intake or energy expenditure to overcome this when they understand how metabolic adaptation occurs with weight loss.

Special Considerations for Patients on GLP-1–Based Weight Loss Medications. When counseling patients on weight loss expectations, it is helpful to remember that in the randomized trials of these medications, the average patient continued to lose weight at 52 weeks without reaching a weight plateau. Therefore a longer follow-up time is necessary to see the full therapeutic effect of these medications.

Each dose increment typically results in greater appetite suppression but can also be accompanied by more GI side effects. Patients who cannot tolerate dose increases should be counseled to decrease the dose to the last tolerated dose for at least another month before considering an increase. The magnitude and speed of weight loss seen with these agents also raises concern for disproportionate loss of muscle mass and function. This is an area of research, and guidelines are forthcoming. Current practice is to emphasize the importance of exercise, ideally a regimen that includes weight training or resistance exercise, as well as good quality nutrition that emphasizes adequate protein intake.

Procedural Interventions for Weight Loss
Endoscopic Interventions

Endoscopic weight loss procedures, such as the endoscopic sleeve gastroplasty (ESG) and endoscopic intragastric balloon, are increasing in popularity because of their efficacy and noninvasive nature.

The ESG is a procedure by which the patient's stomach capacity is endoscopically reduced, creating a gastric sleeve the size of a small banana. A systematic review and meta-analysis to evaluate the efficacy and safety of ESG in adults showed the average total body weight loss to be approximately 17%; 2.2% of patients in this cohort experienced side effects, most commonly GI related.

Most patients included in the analysis had a BMI between 30 and 40 kg/m^2; thus this procedure may not yield similar results in patients with class III obesity (BMI >40 kg/m^2). The procedure is also technically challenging and may therefore not be widely available. Patients interested in the ESG should continue to be counseled on making sustainable lifestyle changes after the procedure to ensure long-term weight maintenance.

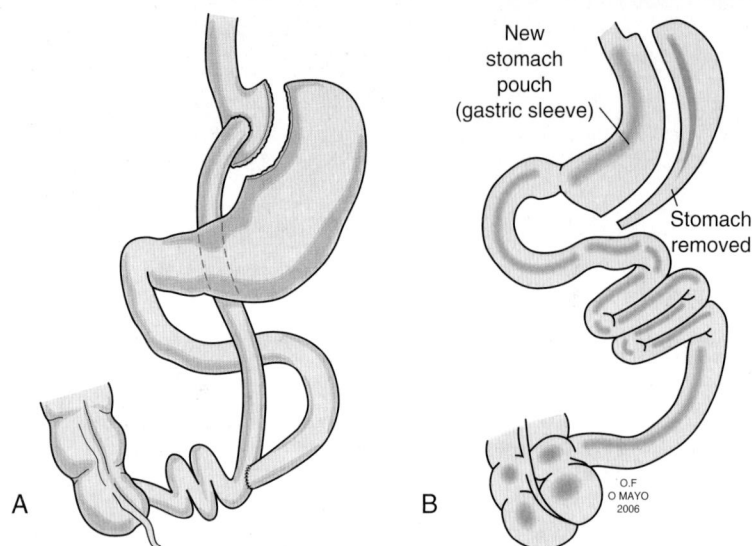

Common bariatric procedures

New
stomach
pouch
(gastric sleeve)

Stomach
removed

A   B

O.F
O MAYO
2006

Figure 1 Techniques commonly used for the surgical treatment of obesity: (A) Roux-en-Y gastric bypass; (B) laparoscopic sleeve gastrectomy.

Intragastric balloon devices are approved to treat obesity in patients with a BMI greater than 30 kg/m^2. In this procedure, a gastric balloon is endoscopically inserted and filled with saline. It remains in place for 6 months, after which it is deflated endoscopically and removed. The intragastric balloon increases satiety and decreases gastric emptying, thus promoting decreased caloric intake and ultimately weight loss. Total body weight loss at 12 months is approximately 10%; patients who lose weight with the balloon in place often see some degree of weight regain after balloon removal. Adverse effects are most commonly seen in the first week after balloon placement and consist of nausea and constipation. Balloons that are left in place for longer than 6 months run the risk of causing gastric erosion.

Bariatric Surgery

Bariatric (or metabolic) surgery results in significant weight loss leading to remission or resolution of several weight-related comorbidities. Compared with usual obesity care, bariatric surgery has also been shown to prolong life expectancy. Bariatric surgery is indicated in patients with a BMI greater than 40 kg/m^2 or in patients with a BMI greater than 35 kg/m^2 with associated weight-related comorbidities. Compelling data indicate that patients with diabetes with a BMI as low as 27 kg/m^2 may benefit from bariatric surgery, but this has not been adapted into practice.

Candidacy for bariatric surgery is determined on medical and psychological grounds. Patients interested in bariatric surgery should be motivated and ready for the significant and lifelong changes that occur after surgery. Psychological contraindications to pursuing surgery include untreated major depression or psychosis and other active psychiatric illnesses, including chemical dependency, binge-eating disorders, and the inability to comply with nutritional requirements and lifelong vitamin supplementation.

There are several types of bariatric surgeries. Here we present the two most common, which are the laparoscopic Roux-en-Y gastric bypass (RYGB) and the laparoscopic sleeve gastrectomy (Figure 1).

Roux-en-Y Gastric Bypass

In this surgery, a small "pouch" is formed from the proximal part of the stomach, which is divided and separated from the distal part of the stomach. The pouch has a capacity of approximately 1 tablespoon at the time of creation. The small intestine is divided approximately 100 cm distal to the pylorus; one end forms the anastomosis with the pouch, and the other end is anastomosed at the jejunum about 75 to 100 cm distal to the pouch. These anatomic alterations result in restriction

of food intake and decreased absorption capacity of the small intestine, thus leading to weight loss. The average weight loss seen after gastric bypass surgery is approximately 30% of total body weight.

Patients who undergo gastric bypass surgery often develop an aversion to high sugar content and fatty foods (i.e., calorie-dense foods). This in turn does help decrease total caloric intake. Patients can often develop lactose intolerance as well, which limits their total dairy consumption.

Guidelines for multivitamin supplementation after RYGB are outlined later (Table 4).

Complications from RYGB can be categorized as either surgical complications or nutritional complications. In the immediate postoperative period, anastomotic ulcerations and strictures may occur, requiring reintervention. Longer-term surgical complications may include the development of intestinal obstruction from internal hernias or adhesions. Overall, the mortality from bariatric surgery is less than 1%. Nutritional deficiencies after RYGB most commonly involve deficiencies of iron, vitamin D, and calcium. This is partly driven by the exclusion of the proximal duodenum, which is the major side of absorption of these specific nutrients.

Sleeve Gastrectomy

The sleeve gastrectomy is the most widely performed bariatric procedure worldwide. In this surgery, approximately 80% of the body of the stomach is removed, leaving behind a tubular structure that resembles a shirtsleeve. The average weight loss seen with the sleeve gastrectomy is approximately 15% to 25% of total body weight. The sleeve gastrectomy is the preferred bariatric procedure in patients who have a need to be consistent with absorption of specific medications, for example antirejection medications after organ transplantation.

Guidelines for multivitamin supplementation after sleeve gastrectomy is outlined later (see Table 4).

Postoperative complications of the sleeve gastrectomy include staple line leak or dilation of the gastric sleeve. Approximately 15% of patients who undergo sleeve gastrectomy can develop new or worsening gastroesophageal reflux symptoms. Patients who have undergone a sleeve gastrectomy often do not develop food aversion and are able to continue eating a wide variety of foods.

Monitoring After Bariatric Surgery
Nutrition

Patients who have undergone bariatric surgery should obtain annual levels of complete blood count, ferritin, 25-hydroxy

TABLE 4	Guidelines for Standard Multivitamin and Mineral Supplementation After Bariatric Surgery
SUPPLEMENT	**DOSING AND SUPPLY**
200% of recommended daily allowance for vitamins and minerals	Two chewable multivitamins daily Patients with renal impairment may need dose adjustment
Elemental calcium	1500–2000 mg daily with meals, in divided doses. If supplements are required, calcium citrate is better absorbed in a low-acid environment such as after gastric bypass
Vitamin D	3000–5000 units of vitamin D_3 daily, total through dietary intake and supplements
B_{12}	1000 mcg deep subcutaneous injection monthly *or* 500–1000 mcg orally daily

vitamin D, fasting glucose, and lipid profile (if indicated). B_{12} levels should be checked if the patient is not taking a parenteral formulation of B_{12} as absorption in the altered GI anatomy can be variable. Patients who have undergone more malabsorptive procedures such as the biliopancreatic diversion/duodenal switch or very long limb RYGB may be screened for deficiencies in vitamin A, zinc, and copper.

Patients who have undergone gastric bypass surgery and other malabsorptive bariatric procedures should also have annual measurements of 24-hour urine volume, calcium, creatinine, and oxalate excretion. This is the most reliable way of ensuring adequate calcium absorption while screening for hyperoxaluria.

An annual dietitian review is strongly recommended to ensure that patients are adhering to nutritional guidelines and meeting their nutritional goals.

Physical Activity
Patients should be encouraged to pursue moderate-intensity physical activity for at least 150 minutes a week (i.e., 30 minutes a day). When advising on the intensity of physical activity, patients can be guided to choose options that result in the following: "Your breathing quickens, but you're not out of breath. You develop a light sweat after about 10 minutes of activity. You can carry on a conversation, but you can't sing."

Data from the National Weight Control Registry show that the majority of nonsurgical weight loss patients engage in a structured and consistent daily physical activity program to successfully maintain their weight.

Weight
In a long-term study of patients who had undergone RYGB, 93% of patients maintained at least a 10% weight loss from baseline, 70% maintained at least a 20% weight loss, and only 40% maintained at least a 30% weight loss after 12 years. Weight regain is therefore a reality that tends to occur after the second postoperative year in a proportion of patients who undergo bariatric surgery. Weight regain may lead to relapse of weight-related comorbidities and can be psychologically difficult for the patient.

When a patient who has undergone bariatric surgery presents with weight regain, a number of factors should be considered. The patient's dietary habits should be evaluated by a dietitian familiar with bariatric surgery. The patient's physical activity habits should also be evaluated, and assistance from a physical therapist can be considered for patients with significant limitations to exercise. Anatomic changes such as dilation of the gastrojejunal anastomosis or the presence of a gastrogastric fistula can contribute to excess calorie intake and weight regain; these can be detected

with an upper GI contrast study. The patient's medication record should be carefully evaluated to identify medications that may predispose to weight gain. Finally, a psychology evaluation may uncover behaviors that may be predisposing to weight regain, for example, graze-eating, nighttime eating, or binge-eating.

Patients who experience weight regain after bariatric surgery should be offered a multidisciplinary approach to management. In addition to dietary and behavioral intervention, patients may also be candidates for antiobesity medications or procedures that revise their postbariatric surgery anatomy.

Specific Complications of Roux-en-Y Gastric Bypass
A number of unique complications that can occur after RYGB as a result of anatomic alterations. Here, we will highlight two: nephrolithiasis and alcohol use disorder.

Nephrolithiasis
The risk for nephrolithiasis after gastric bypass surgery is moderately high, with reported prevalence rates of 7.65% to 13%. Solely gastric restrictive operations such as the gastric sleeve are not associated with higher risk for kidney stone formation beyond that attributed to obesity alone. Nephrolithiasis can present as early as the first year after surgery; thus patients should be counseled on interventions to prevent kidney stone formation soon after surgery. Current guidelines recommend completing a 24-hour urine supersaturation between 6 and 12 months after surgery. This can assess for adequacy of hydration status, calcium ingestion, oxalate excretion, and citrate excretion (low urinary citrate predisposes to kidney stone formation).

Patients with nephrolithiasis should be counseled on adequate fluid intake (1500–2000 mL of urine output per day), a low-fat diet, a low-oxalate diet, and adequate dietary or supplemental calcium with meals. Hypocitraturia may be treated with potassium citrate salts. Patients with nephrolithiasis after gastric bypass may benefit from more frequent visits with a dietitian to help meet the patient's nutrition and hydration goals.

Alcohol Use Disorder
Alcohol use disorder is a rare complication that can occur in the long term after gastric bypass. Changes in the GI anatomy after gastric bypass surgery alter the pharmacokinetics of alcohol metabolism, leading to early and higher blood alcohol concentration peaks accompanied by a greater feeling of drunkenness. Additionally, there is decreased clearance of alcohol through the first-pass mechanism. In practical terms, peak blood alcohol levels achieved after consuming about two drinks in women who have had RYGB surgery resemble that observed after consuming about four drinks in women who have not had surgery.

Large prospective observational studies show that the prevalence of alcohol use disorder after RYGB increases over time since surgery. Risk factors for developing alcohol use disorder after gastric bypass surgery include male sex, younger age, smoking, and any presurgery alcohol consumption. Although baseline alcohol consumption is a risk factor, about 20% of patients diagnosed with alcohol use disorder within 5 years of RYGB reported no alcohol consumption the year before surgery. Patients undergoing gastric bypass surgery should therefore be routinely screened for and counseled on the effects of alcohol use after surgery.

References
Adams TD, Davidson LE, Litwin SE, et al: Weight and metabolic outcomes 12 years after gastric bypass, *N Engl J Med* 377(12):1143–1155, 2017.
Arnold M, Pandeya N, Byrnes G, et al: Global burden of cancer attributable to high body-mass index in 2012: a population-based study, *Lancet Oncol* 16(1):36–46, 2015.
Bhatti UH, Duffy AJ, Roberts KE, Shariff AH: Nephrolithiasis after bariatric surgery: a review of pathophysiologic mechanisms and procedural risk, *Int J Surg* 36(Pt D):618–623, 2016.
Canales BK, Hatch M: Kidney stone incidence and metabolic urinary changes after modern bariatric surgery: review of clinical studies, experimental models, and prevention strategies, *Surg Obes Relat Dis* 10(4):734–742, 2014.
Carlsson LMS, Sjoholm K, Jacobson P, et al: Life expectancy after bariatric surgery in the Swedish obese subjects study, *N Engl J Med* 383(16):1535–1543, 2020.

Centers for Disease Control and Prevention: Prevalence of overweight and obesity among adults with diagnosed diabetes-United States, 1988-1994 and 1999-2002, *MMWR Morb Mortal Wkly Rep* 53(45):1066–1068, 2004.

Clinical guidelines on the identification, evaluation, and treatment of overweight and obesity in adults-the evidence report. National institutes of health, *Obes Res* 6(suppl 2):51S–209S, 1998.

Davies M, Faerch L, Jeppesen OK, et al: Semaglutide 2.4 mg once a week in adults with overweight or obesity, and type 2 diabetes (STEP 2): a randomised, double-blind, double-dummy, placebo-controlled, phase 3 trial, *Lancet* 397(10278):971–984, 2021.

Fabbrini E, Sullivan S, Klein S: Obesity and nonalcoholic fatty liver disease: biochemical, metabolic, and clinical implications, *Hepatology* 51(2):679–689, 2010.

Greenway FL, Aronne LJ, Raben A, et al: A randomized, double-blind, placebo-controlled study of Gelesis100: a novel nonsystemic oral hydrogel for weight loss, *Obesity (Silver Spring)* 27(2):205–216, 2019.

Hagedorn JC, Encarnacion B, Brat GA, Morton JM: Does gastric bypass alter alcohol metabolism?, *Surg Obes Relat Dis* 3(5):543–548, 2007; discussion 8.

Hales CM, Carroll MD, Fryar CD, Ogden CL: Prevalence of obesity and severe obesity among adults: United States, 2017-2018, *NCHS Data Brief* 360:1–8, 2020.

Hedjoudje A, Abu Dayyeh BK, Cheskin LJ, et al: Efficacy and safety of endoscopic sleeve gastroplasty: a systematic review and meta-analysis, *Clin Gastroenterol Hepatol* 18(5):1043–10453 e4, 2020.

Hendricks EJ, Srisurapanont M, Schmidt SL, et al: Addiction potential of phentermine prescribed during long-term treatment of obesity, *Int J Obes (Lond)* 38(2):292–298, 2014.

Heymsfield SB, Wadden TA: Mechanisms, pathophysiology, and management of obesity, *N Engl J Med* 376(15):1492, 2017.

Himpens J, Dobbeleir J, Peeters G: Long-term results of laparoscopic sleeve gastrectomy for obesity, *Ann Surg* 252(2):319–324, 2010.

Jakicic JM, Marcus BH, Lang W, Janney C: Effect of exercise on 24-month weight loss maintenance in overweight women, *Arch Intern Med* 168(14):1550–1559, 2008; discussion 9–60.

Jensen MD, Ryan DH, Apovian CM, et al: 2013 AHA/ACC/TOS guideline for the management of overweight and obesity in adults: a report of the American college of cardiology/American heart association task force on practice guidelines and the obesity society, *J Am Coll Cardiol* 63(25 Pt B):2985–3023, 2014.

King WC, Bond DS: The importance of preoperative and postoperative physical activity counseling in bariatric surgery, *Exerc Sport Sci Rev* 41(1):26–35, 2013.

King WC, Chen JY, Courcoulas AP, et al: Alcohol and other substance use after bariatric surgery: prospective evidence from a U.S. multicenter cohort study, *Surg Obes Relat Dis* 13(8):1392–1402, 2017.

Knowler WC, Barrett-Connor E, Fowler SE, et al: Reduction in the incidence of type 2 diabetes with lifestyle intervention or metformin, *N Engl J Med* 346(6):393–403, 2002.

Kramer CK, Leitao CB, Pinto LC, Canani LH, Azevedo MJ, Gross JL: Efficacy and safety of topiramate on weight loss: a meta-analysis of randomized controlled trials, *Obes Rev* 12(5):e338–e347, 2011.

Kumar RB, Aronne LJ: Iatrogenic obesity, *Endocrinol Metab Clin North Am* 49(2):265–273, 2020.

Lee JW, Brancati FL, Yeh HC: Trends in the prevalence of type 2 diabetes in Asians versus whites: results from the United States national health interview survey, 1997-2008, *Diabetes Care* 34(2):353–357, 2011.

Lieske JC, Mehta RA, Milliner DS, Rule AD, Bergstralh EJ, Sarr MG: Kidney stones are common after bariatric surgery, *Kidney Int* 87(4):839–845, 2015.

Parrott J, Frank L, Rabena R, Craggs-Dino L, Isom KA, Greiman L: American society for metabolic and bariatric surgery integrated health nutritional guidelines for the surgical weight loss patient 2016 update: micronutrients, *Surg Obes Relat Dis* 13(5):727–741, 2017.

Pepino MY, Okunade AL, Eagon JC, Bartholow BD, Bucholz K, Klein S: Effect of Roux-en-Y gastric bypass surgery: converting 2 alcoholic drinks to 4, *JAMA Surg* 150(11):1096–1098, 2015.

Polidori D, Sanghvi A, Seeley RJ, Hall KD: How strongly does appetite counter weight loss? Quantification of the feedback control of human energy intake, *Obesity (Silver Spring)* 24(11):2289–2295, 2016.

Rubino D, Abrahamsson N, Davies M, et al: Effect of continued weekly subcutaneous semaglutide vs placebo on weight loss maintenance in adults with overweight or obesity: the STEP 4 randomized clinical trial, *J Am Med Assoc* 325(14):1414–1425, 2021.

Salminen P, Helmio M, Ovaska J, et al: Effect of laparoscopic sleeve gastrectomy vs laparoscopic Roux-en-Y gastric bypass on weight loss at 5 years among patients with morbid obesity: the SLEEVEPASS randomized clinical trial, *J Am Med Assoc* 319(3):241–254, 2018.

Schauer PR, Bhatt DL, Kashyap SR: Bariatric surgery or intensive medical therapy for diabetes after 5 years, *N Engl J Med* 376(20):1997, 2017.

Shaker M, Tabbaa A, Albeldawi M, Alkhouri N: Liver transplantation for nonalcoholic fatty liver disease: new challenges and new opportunities, *World J Gastroenterol* 20(18):5320–5330, 2014.

Singh S, de Moura DTH, Khan A, et al: Intragastric balloon versus endoscopic sleeve gastroplasty for the treatment of obesity: a systematic review and meta-analysis, *Obes Surg* 30(8):3010–3029, 2020.

Sjostrom CD, Lissner L, Wedel H, Sjostrom L: Reduction in incidence of diabetes, hypertension and lipid disturbances after intentional weight loss induced by bariatric surgery: the SOS Intervention Study, *Obes Res* 7(5):477–484, 1999.

Smith MD, Patterson E, Wahed AS, et al: Thirty-day mortality after bariatric surgery: independently adjudicated causes of death in the longitudinal assessment of bariatric surgery, *Obes Surg* 21(11):1687–1692, 2011.

Sohn CH, Lam RW: Update on the biology of seasonal affective disorder, *CNS Spectr* 10(8):635–646, 2005. quiz 1-14.

Svensson PA, Anveden A, Romeo S, et al: Alcohol consumption and alcohol problems after bariatric surgery in the Swedish obese subjects study, *Obesity (Silver Spring)* 21(12):2444–2451, 2013.

Wadden TA, Bailey TS, Billings LK, et al: Effect of subcutaneous semaglutide vs placebo as an adjunct to intensive behavioral therapy on body weight in adults with overweight or obesity: the STEP 3 randomized clinical trial, *J Am Med Assoc* 325(14):1403–1413, 2021.

Ward ZJ, Bleich SN, Cradock AL, et al: Projected U.S. state-level prevalence of adult obesity and severe obesity, *N Engl J Med* 381(25):2440–2450, 2019.

Wilding JPH, Batterham RL, Calanna S, et al: Once-weekly semaglutide in adults with overweight or obesity, *N Engl J Med* 384(11):989, 2021.

PARENTERAL NUTRITION IN ADULTS

Method of
**Meetal Mehta, MD; Kris M. Mogensen, MS; and
Malcolm K. Robinson, MD**

CURRENT DIAGNOSIS

- Reserve parenteral nutrition (PN) for patients with intestinal dysfunction or failure.
- Reserve PN for conditions such as short-bowel syndrome, severe malabsorption, ileus or intestinal dysmotility, intractable vomiting, and severe diarrhea.
- Always reevaluate the need for PN and work toward a transition to enteral nutrition or an oral diet, if possible, to limit complications associated with PN.

CURRENT THERAPY

- Correct electrolyte abnormalities and hyperglycemia before initiating parenteral nutrition (PN).
- Start with no more than 150 to 200 g dextrose on the first day of PN; start with 100 to 150 g dextrose for patients with diabetes or patients at risk for the refeeding syndrome.
- Advance PN by 100 to 150 g dextrose daily until the goal is achieved.
- Maintain blood glucose less than 180 mg/dL.
- Monitor electrolytes, including phosphate and magnesium, until stable; the frequency of laboratory monitoring can be decreased based on stability.
- Monitor closely for complications associated with PN: electrolyte abnormalities, hyper/hypoglycemia, PN-associated liver disease, and central line infections.

Since the inception of parenteral nutrition (PN) in the 1960s, the science of PN has matured in a number of ways. The initial excitement of being able to feed basic nutrients, vitamins, and trace elements intravenously has been tempered by the realization that indiscriminate use of PN can be harmful. Although PN can still be lifesaving, it is imperative that it be used judiciously and only as long as necessary. This chapter discusses the current use of PN in adult patients.

Indications and Contraindications

Enteral nutrition (EN) is the preferred method of nutrition support, primarily because it is associated with fewer infectious and metabolic complications. However, total PN (TPN), which is the provision of all nutrient requirements intravenously, may be indicated when feeding through the gastrointestinal (GI) tract is not possible. PN may be appropriately initiated in those who cannot receive enteral nourishment and are malnourished or at risk

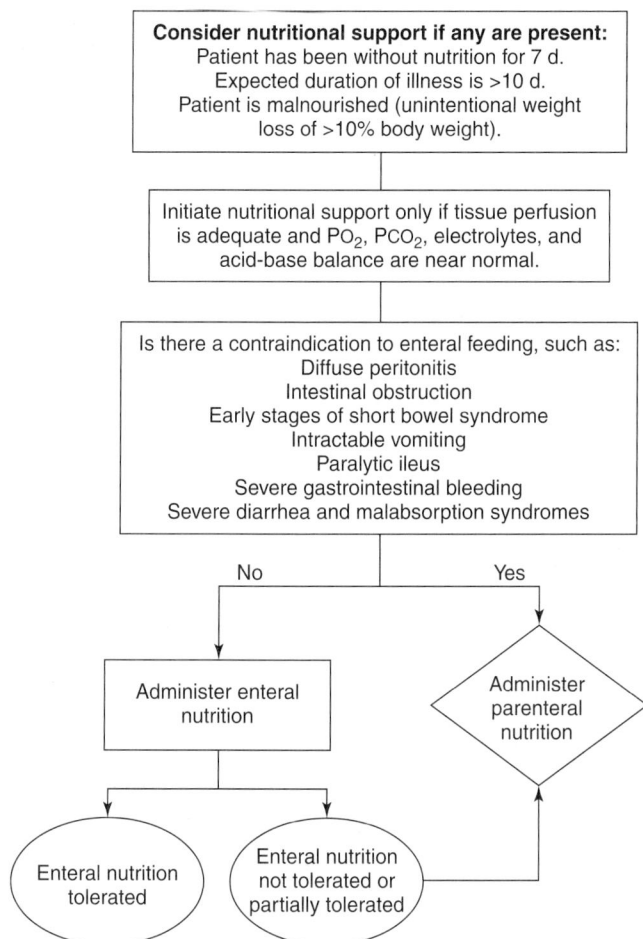

Consider nutritional support if any are present:
Patient has been without nutrition for 7 d.
Expected duration of illness is >10 d.
Patient is malnourished (unintentional weight loss of >10% body weight).

Initiate nutritional support only if tissue perfusion is adequate and PO_2, PCO_2, electrolytes, and acid-base balance are near normal.

Is there a contraindication to enteral feeding, such as:
Diffuse peritonitis
Intestinal obstruction
Early stages of short bowel syndrome
Intractable vomiting
Paralytic ileus
Severe gastrointestinal bleeding
Severe diarrhea and malabsorption syndromes

No → Administer enteral nutrition

Yes → Administer parenteral nutrition

Enteral nutrition tolerated

Enteral nutrition not tolerated or partially tolerated

Figure 1 Determining route of feeding.

BOX 1 Decision-Making Steps When Initiating Parenteral Nutrition

Assess the patient's nutritional status. Nutrition support (PN or EN) should not be initiated in well-nourished patients unless they have received a suboptimal diet for more than 7 days.

Determine whether the patient has extreme energy needs (hypermetabolism) that warrant the early use of nutrition support (PN and/or EN) within 7 days of injury or illness. These are typically critically ill patients who have suffered severe burns or trauma.

Evaluate the function of the GI tract; if it is intact and can be used safely, PN should be avoided. PN support is indicated until enteral access is established and the patient can meet nutrient needs via tube feedings.

Estimate how long the patient will require PN support. If GI function is expected to return within 5 days, there is no known benefit of initiating PN.

EN, Enteral nutrition; *GI,* gastrointestinal; *PN,* parenteral nutrition.

to have malnutrition. Therefore it is imperative to identify patients who have or are at risk for developing protein-energy malnutrition or have specific nutrient deficiencies. A patient's risk of developing malnutrition-related medical complications needs to be quantified, and it is necessary to monitor the adequacy of nutritional therapy.

Nutrition assessment begins with a thorough history and physical examination in conjunction with select laboratory tests aimed at detecting specific nutrient deficiencies in patients who are at high risk for future abnormalities. The nutrition assessment should establish whether the patient will need maintenance therapy or nutrition repletion and should assess the status of the patient's GI tract, especially if nutrition support will be required.

A thorough history includes an assessment of recent weight changes, dietary habits, GI symptoms, and changes in exercise tolerance or physical abilities that would indicate functional capacity deficiencies. Screening for malnutrition risk, using a validated nutrition screening tool (e.g., Mini Nutritional Assessment-Short Form, Malnutrition Screening Tool, Malnutrition Universal Screening Tool, Nutritional Risk Index, Nutrition Risk Screening–2002), may identify these relevant changes. Diagnosis of malnutrition includes further history taking and a physical examination. This includes inspection for subcutaneous fat and muscle wasting, which indicate a loss of body energy and protein stores; edema and ascites, which can also indicate altered energy demands or decreased energy intake; and signs of vitamin and mineral deficits such as dermatitis, glossitis, cheilosis, neuromuscular irritability, and coarse, easily pluckable hair.

Several nutritional biomarkers have traditionally been used to quickly assess nutritional status. The serum proteins prealbumin, transferrin, and retinol-binding protein have a rapid turnover rate and short half-lives and therefore may be used as indicators of recent nutritional intake. However, these proteins are affected by the metabolic responses to stress and illness, as well as other conditions, including iron status (transferrin) and renal status (retinol-binding protein, prealbumin). This can limit their usefulness in acute and chronic inflammatory states.

Prealbumin is least affected by fluctuations in hydration status and by liver and renal function compared with other plasma proteins. However, prealbumin levels drop in acute inflammatory conditions during which the liver prioritizes production of positive acute-phase reactants, decreasing negative acute-phase reactants such as prealbumin. A rise in C-reactive protein, a protein synthesized by the liver as part of the acute-phase response, indicates an active inflammatory state. Thus C-reactive protein, when measured along with prealbumin, can help differentiate a low prealbumin due to nutritional inadequacy versus low prealbumin due to an acute-phase response.

for developing malnourishment. Malnourishment can be defined as unintentional loss of more than 10% of usual body weight or greater than 7 to 10 days of inadequate nutrient intake. The body stores of well-nourished persons are generally sufficient to provide the essential nutrients, resist infection, promote wound healing, and support other necessary physiologic functions for this time period. In patients who are anticipated not to be able to receive adequate EN for longer than 10 days, it is not necessary to wait 10 days before initiating PN. This may include patients with short-bowel syndrome and others who are expected to have prolonged GI dysfunction.

According to the American Society for Parenteral and Enteral Nutrition (ASPEN) guidelines, EN is contraindicated in conditions such as diffuse peritonitis, intestinal obstruction, early stages of short-bowel syndrome, intractable vomiting, paralytic ileus, severe GI bleeding, and severe diarrhea and malabsorption syndromes. Other relative contraindications to EN include severe pancreatitis and enterocutaneous fistulas, although depending on the clinical circumstances, EN may be indicated. PN and EN may be provided concomitantly, although in patients who are critically ill, PN should not be started until all strategies to maximize enteral feeding (such as the use of postpyloric feeding tubes and motility agents) have been attempted. PN support is unlikely to benefit a patient who will be able to take EN within 4 or 5 days after the onset of illness or who has a relatively minor injury (Figure 1).

There are four key steps to consider before initiating PN, including assessing nutritional status, determining energy and protein needs, evaluating GI function, and estimating the length of time a patient will require PN (Box 1).

Assessment of Nutritional Status

Nutrient depletion is associated with increased morbidity and mortality, and up to 60% of hospitalized patients are estimated

Serum albumin, another negative acute-phase reactant, has traditionally been used as an indicator of nutritional status. Although it is a good preoperative predictor of outcome for patients undergoing surgery, its sensitivity to many variables in the acute care setting make it an unreliable marker to assess nutritional status under such conditions or in the immediate postoperative period. Additionally, redistribution of albumin, increases in GI and renal losses, and alterations in tissue catabolism during inflammatory states affect its intravascular concentrations.

Notably these serum markers are affected only after weeks of starvation in noninflammatory states and do not increase with adequate nutritional support, making it a poor initial indicator of nutritional status or muscle mass. However, they may be used to indicate inflammatory status and nutritional risk, instead of nutritional status and muscle mass.

A simple and practical index of malnutrition is the degree of weight loss. Unintentional weight loss of greater than 10% within the previous 6 months indicates protein-energy malnutrition and is a good prognosticator of clinical outcome. Weight can also be compared with an ideal or desirable weight, or an index of body weight relative to height. The body mass index (BMI), reported as weight in kilograms divided by height in meters squared, is the best known such index and can be used to detect both undernutrition and overnutrition. This index is dependent on height, and the same standards apply to both men and women. A BMI of 18.5 to 25 kg/m^2 is considered normal, 25 to 29.9 kg/m^2 is considered overweight, and greater than 30 kg/m^2 is considered obese. Patients with a normal or high BMI can still have nutrient deficiencies and therefore can be malnourished if they have recently lost a significant amount of weight. In addition, a BMI of 18.5 kg/m^2 or less in an adult indicates malnutrition, and a BMI less than 15 kg/m^2 is associated with increased morbidity.

Another practical tool for evaluating nutritional status is the subjective global assessment (SGA) that encompasses historical, symptomatic, and physical parameters. The SGA technique determines whether nutrient assimilation has been restricted because of decreased food intake, maldigestion, or malabsorption; whether any effects of malnutrition on organ function and body composition have occurred; and whether the patient's disease process influences nutrient requirements. The findings of the history and physical examination are subjectively weighted to rank patients as being well nourished, moderately malnourished, or severely malnourished and are used to predict their risk for medical complications (Box 2).

Estimating Nutritional Requirements

Historically, TPN often provided nutrients in excess of actual requirements. This was based on the assumption that patients requiring nutritional intervention were severely depleted and required aggressive repletion; hence, the misnomer "hyperalimentation." Overfeeding is associated with increased CO_2 production and difficulty weaning from a ventilator, as well as metabolic complications, such as hyperglycemia, which can lead to increased infection, morbidity, and mortality. Thus nutritional support should be titrated to match actual metabolic requirements.

In addition, there are times when *underfeeding* calories may be necessary and beneficial. In such cases, this is referred to as "permissive" underfeeding to distinguish it from underfeeding that occurs due to the unintentional inadequate delivery of nutrients. For example, permissive underfeeding of energy may be appropriate for some critically ill patients with obesity who are receiving adequate protein. Such permissive underfeeding with adequate protein delivery for critically ill patients with obesity is now the recommendation of ASPEN and the Society of Critical Care Medicine (SCCM).

Energy Requirements

There are four components of daily energy requirement. The first is the basal metabolic rate (BMR), which is the amount of

---

BOX 2 Subjective Global Assessment

Select the appropriate category with a checkmark, or enter a numeric value where indicated by #.

History
- Weight change
  Overall loss in past 6 months: amount = # _____ kg; % loss = # _____
  Change in past 2 weeks: _____ increase, _____ no change, _____ decrease
- Dietary intake change (relative to normal)
  _____ No change
  _____ Change duration = # _____ week.
  _____ Type: _____ suboptimal solid diet, _____ full liquid diet, _____ hypocaloric liquids, _____ starvation
- Gastrointestinal symptoms (that persisted for >2 weeks)
  _____ None, _____ nausea, _____ vomiting, _____ diarrhea, _____ anorexia
- Functional capacity
  _____ No dysfunction (e.g., full capacity)
  _____ Dysfunction duration = # _____ week
  _____ Type: _____ working suboptimally, _____ ambulatory, _____ bedridden
- Disease and its relation to nutritional requirements
  Primary diagnosis (specify): _____
  Metabolic demand (stress): _____ no stress, _____ low stress, _____ moderate stress, _____ high stress

Physical (for each trait specify: 0 = normal, 1+ = mild, 2+ = moderate, 3+ = severe)
_____ Loss of subcutaneous fat (triceps, chest)
_____ Muscle wasting (quadriceps, deltoids)
_____ Ankle edema
_____ Sacral edema
_____ Ascites

SGA Rating (select one)
_____ A = Well nourished
_____ B = Moderately (or suspected of being) malnourished
_____ C = Severely malnourished

Reprinted with permission from Detsky AS, McLaughlin JR, Baker JP, et al. What is subjective global assessment of nutritional status? *JPEN J Parenter Enteral Nutr.* 1987;11:8–13.

---

energy expended under complete rest shortly after awakening and in a fasting state (12–14 hours). BMR varies with age, sex, and body size; correlates roughly with body surface area; and is proportional to lean tissue mass. This relationship holds true even among persons of different ages and sexes. Resting metabolic rate or resting energy expenditure (REE) represents the amount of energy expended 2 hours after a meal under conditions of rest and thermal neutrality. Although it is often used synonymously with BMR, the REE is typically 10% higher.

The second component of daily energy expenditure is the thermic effect of exercise or the energy used in physical activity. The contribution of this component increases markedly during intense muscular work. However, admission to a hospital generally results in a marked decrease in physical activity. Hospital activity in ambulatory patients accounts for a 20% to 30% increase in BMR. Critically ill patients who are on a ventilator generally have low activity levels (BMR increases by only 5%–10%) because the ventilator performs the work of breathing and they are not ambulatory.

The third component of energy expenditure is diet-induced thermogenesis, the increase in BMR that follows food intake. The digestion and metabolism of exogenous nutrients, whether delivered to the gut or vein, result in an increase in metabolic rate. The magnitude of the thermic effect of food varies depending on the amount and composition of the diet and accounts for approximately 10% of daily energy expenditure.

Finally, acute illness adds an additional stress factor to the daily energy expenditure and correlates with disease severity. For example, a patient's metabolic rate increases by 10% to 30% after a major fracture, from 20% to 60% with severe infection, and from 40% to 110% with a severe third-degree burn. In addition, fever accelerates chemical reactions, and the BMR rises approximately 10% for each degree Celsius increase in temperature. Alternatively, cooling of febrile patients produces a reduction in BMR of approximately 10% per degree Celsius.

The first step of estimating energy requirements is to estimate the BMR. This is usually accomplished using one of several predictive equations. The most commonly used method is based on the predictive equations reported by Harris and Benedict in 1919. The Harris-Benedict equations are as follows:

$$BMR \text{ (men)} = 66.47 + 13.75 \ (W) + 5.0 \ (H) - 6.76 \ (A)$$

$$BMR \text{ (women)} = 655.1 + 9.56 \ (W) + 1.85 \ (H) - 4.68 \ (A)$$

where W is weight in kg, H is height in cm, and A is age in years.

After the BMR is calculated, it is adjusted for the level of stress induced by injury or the disease process and activity level. Activity factors for hospitalized patients are 1.0 to 1.1 for intubated patients, 1.2 for patients confined to bed, and 1.3 for patients out of bed. Stress factors may vary from 1.1 for patients with minimal stress, to 1.3 for patients with moderate stress, to up to 2.0 for patients with severe burns. Therefore the patient's energy requirements (total energy expenditure [TEE]) are finally calculated:

$$TEE = BMR \times Activity \ factor \times Stress \ factor$$

The thermic effect of feeding is generally not included in the calculation of energy requirements for hospitalized patients.

Alternatively, some clinicians estimate energy requirements based on actual body weight, providing about 25 to 30 kilocalories (kcal)/kg administered to critically ill patients. Predicting energy expenditure in patients with obesity can be difficult because using predictive formulas with actual body weight can lead to high TEE and potentially to overfeeding. Determining energy requirements for critically ill patients with obesity is discussed later in this chapter. The Harris-Benedict equation using the average of actual and ideal weight and a stress factor of 1.3 predicts REE in acutely ill patients with a BMI of 30 to 50 kg/m^2.

Indirect calorimetry is a more precise, clinically practical, and individualized method to determine energy expenditure, particularly in patients in whom estimating requirements through predictive equations is difficult, such as those who continue to lose weight despite what appears to be an adequate caloric intake, who are critically ill, or who have rapidly changing energy needs. Indirect calorimetry measures changes in oxygen consumption and CO_2 production to calculate the REE. As indirect calorimetry accounts for the effects of disease state, stress, and trauma, a stress factor is not necessary in calculating energy needs. However, the measurement occurs at rest, and therefore an activity factor of 1.0 to 1.3, depending on whether the patient is intubated, bedridden, or ambulatory, must be applied.

Nutrient Requirements

The recommended daily protein allowance for most healthy persons who are not hospitalized is 0.8 g/kg, or about 60 to 70 g of protein each day. The stressed, critically ill patient generally needs a higher dose of protein in the range of 1.2 to 2.0 g/kg/day. For most patients, providing protein beyond 1.5 g/kg/day is not beneficial. In fact, providing excess protein does not enhance uptake and can lead to increased ureagenesis, which can cause renal injury in some patients.

The calorie-to-nitrogen ratio for most PN solutions is typically about 150:1, with an acceptable range of 100:1 to 180:1. Nitrogen content is used as a marker for protein, and, hence, the two terms are used interchangeably. Usually, 6.25 g of protein is

TABLE 1	Recommended Daily Doses of Parenteral Vitamins and Trace Elements
MICRONUTRIENT	**PARENTERAL DOSE**
Vitamins	
Vitamin A	3300 IU
Vitamin D	200 IU
Vitamin E	10 IU
Vitamin K	150 µg
Ascorbic acid (vitamin C)	200 µg
Folic acid	600 µg
Niacin	40 mg
Riboflavin (vitamin B$_2$)	3.6 mg
Thiamine (vitamin B$_1$)	6 mg
Pyridoxine (vitamin B$_6$)	6 mg
Cyanocobalamin (vitamin B$_{12}$)	5 µg
Pantothenic acid	15 mg
Biotin	60 µg
Trace Elements	
Zinc	2.5–5 mg
Copper	0.3–0.5 mg
Chromium	10–15 µg
Manganese	60–100 µg
Selenium	20–60 µg

Data from American Medical Association, Department of Foods and Nutrition. Multivitamin preparations for parenteral use. A statement by the Nutrition Advisory Group. *JPEN J Parenter Enteral Nutr.* 1979;3:258-262, 1979; Food and Drug Administration. Parenteral multivitamin products: drugs for human use: drug efficacy study implementation: amendment. *Federal Register.* 2000;65(77):21200–21201.

equal to 1.0 g of nitrogen. The conversion factor is slightly higher (6.4) for PN solutions, such as those with higher concentrations of crystalline amino acids.

Vitamin and mineral requirements are altered in certain disease states due to increased losses, greater use, or both. Guidelines for parenteral vitamin and trace elements, developed by the Nutrition Advisory Group of the American Medical Association (AMA), were approved by the U.S. Food and Drug Administration (FDA) in 1979 and amended in 2000 (Table 1).

Composition of Central and Peripheral Venous Solutions

Central venous access is required for providing TPN because of the hypertonicity of the formulas infused (>900 mOsm/L). The infusion of a hypertonic solution into a peripheral vein, known as *peripheral parenteral nutrition* (PPN), can result in thrombophlebitis and venous sclerosis unless the PN is drastically diluted to lower the tonicity. ASPEN clinical guidelines for PN recommend a maximum osmolarity of 900 mOsm/L for PPN solutions. To minimize the hypertonicity of PPN solutions, dextrose is limited to 5% to 10%, and amino acids are limited to 2.5% to 3.5%. Lipids are isotonic and therefore provide a significant portion of the caloric substrate of PPN formulas.

Central venous solutions typically combine carbohydrate in the form of dextrose, protein as crystalline amino acids, and lipids. Lipid emulsions come in many forms, with differing oil sources that provide varying amounts of essential fatty acids and phytosterols. The first lipid emulsion approved for PN uses a polyunsaturated long-chain triglyceride soybean oil base. It provides adequate essential fatty acids but has inflammatory properties

TABLE 2	Central Versus Peripheral Parenteral Nutrition	
PROPERTY	CENTRAL PARENTERAL NUTRITION	PERIPHERAL PARENTERAL NUTRITION
Volume of fluid required (mL)	1500–2500	2500–3500
Duration of therapy (d)	>7–14	5–14
Route of administration	Dedicated central venous catheter	Peripheral vein or multiuse central catheter
Substrate profile	150–600 g/day dextrose	150–300 g/day dextrose (5%–10% of final concentration)
		50–100 g/day amino acid (3% of final concentration)
Osmolarity (mOsm/L)	1300–1800	600–900

because of its high phytosterol and omega-6 fatty acid content, which may play a role in PN-associated liver disease. Newer lipid emulsions have been approved by the FDA that provide different types of oils including a blend of soybean, medium chain triglyceride, olive, and fish oils (SMOFlipid, Fresenius Kabi USA, Melrose Park, IL); soybean and olive oils (Clinolipid, Baxter, Deerfield, IL); and fish oil (Omegaven, Fresenius Kabi USA, Melrose Park, IL; currently only approved for use in children in the United States). Fish oil and mixed lipid emulsions have more favorable, antiinflammatory profiles, and studies suggest that they may prevent or reverse PN associated liver disease. For this reason, these newer lipid emulsions should be considered in patients who are at risk for developing PN-associated liver disease.

Vitamins, electrolytes, and trace elements are added to the formulation as needed. Typical substrate profiles of carbohydrate, protein, and lipids in central PN are shown in Table 2. A usual PN prescription administers 1 to 2 L of a solution each day. Administration of 500 mL of a 20% soybean-oil emulsion 1 day each week is sufficient to prevent essential fatty acid deficiency. Alternatively, if additional energy from lipids are needed on a daily basis, they can be administered as a separate infusion or most commonly as part of the mixture of dextrose and amino acids, a technique known as *triple mix* or *three-in-one*.

Including lipid injectable emulsion into a parenteral admixture changes the conventional nutritional solution into an emulsion. Various electrolytes and micronutrients can adversely influence emulsion stability, and therefore their concentration in three-in-one solutions is limited to prevent "cracking" of the PN solution, in which microscopic or macroscopic precipitates are formed. The higher the cation valence, the greater the destabilizing influence to the emulsifier. Therefore trivalent cations such as ferric ion (iron dextran) are more disruptive than divalent cations such as calcium or magnesium ions, which are more disruptive than monovalent cations such as sodium or potassium. No concentration of iron dextran is safe in triple-mix formulations. In-line filters prevent infusion of precipitates and are necessary for all PN solutions (including triple-mix solutions) because it is impossible to visually detect precipitates until they are grossly incompatible and unsafe for infusion.

Once the basic solution is created, electrolytes are added as needed (Table 3). Sodium or potassium salts are given as chloride or acetate depending on the patient's requirements. Normally, equal amounts of chloride and acetate are provided. However, if chloride losses from the body are increased, which can occur in patients who have nasogastric tubes, then most of the salts should be given as chloride. Similarly, more acetate should be given to patients when additional base is required because acetate generates bicarbonate when it is metabolized. Sodium bicarbonate is incompatible with PN solutions and cannot be added to the mixture. Phosphate may be given as the sodium or potassium salt. Lipid injectable emulsions contain an additional 15 mmol/L of phosphate.

Commercially available preparations of fat-soluble and water-soluble vitamins, minerals, and trace elements are added to the nutrient mix unless they are contraindicated. Adequate thiamine is essential for patients receiving PN and can be provided

TABLE 3	Electrolyte Concentrations in Parenteral Nutrition
ELECTROLYTE	RECOMMENDED PN DOSES
Potassium	1–2 mEq/kg
Sodium	1–2 mEq/kg
Phosphate	20–40 mmol
Magnesium	8–20 mEq
Calcium	10–15 mEq
Chloride	As needed*
Acetate (mEq/L)	As needed*

*Depending on acid-base balance.
PN, Parenteral nutrition.

separately. Vitamin K is now a component of standard intravenous (IV) multivitamin preparations. Trace element preparations that include copper, manganese, selenium, and zinc are added to the PN solution in amounts consistent with the AMA guidelines (Table 1). Manganese accumulation can be toxic, and overexposure can lead to progressive neurodegenerative damage. Manganese is usually supplied in the PN solution at a daily dose of 0.5 mg as part of a multiple trace element additive. Because manganese is primarily eliminated via biliary excretion, patients with biliary obstruction or cholestasis can accumulate potentially toxic levels of manganese. Hence, manganese should be removed from the PN of patients with hyperbilirubinemia. Higher doses (10 to 15 mg/day) of zinc are provided to patients with excessive GI losses.

Iron is not a part of commercial additive preparations because it is incompatible with triple-mix solutions and can cause anaphylactic reactions when it is given intravenously. Patients who need this trace element should receive it orally or by injection. Iron is avoided in patients who are critically ill because hyperferremia can increase bacterial virulence, alter polymorphonuclear cell function, and increase host susceptibility to infection.

PPN is less commonly used than central PN and can be disadvantageous. Because of the low concentration of dextrose, greater volumes (typically >2 L/day) are required to provide sufficient calories, which might not be feasible in fluid-restricted patients. PPN generally does not approximate a patient's energy needs because PPN provides only 1000 to 1500 kcal/day, and a large percentage of the calories (60%) are derived from fat. High-fat infusions are undesirable because they are associated with impaired reticuloendothelial system function and are potentially immunosuppressive. There is no evidence that lipid injectable emulsions improve outcomes or significantly decrease nitrogen losses. Generally, PPN should be avoided unless it is combined with enteral feeding in patients who cannot tolerate full enteral feeding, patients who cannot get a central venous catheter, or patients with low body weights in whom PPN can meet at least two-thirds of estimated needs.

Administration and Venous Access

Typically, central PN solutions are administered into the superior vena cava. Access to this vein can be achieved by cannulation of the subclavian or internal jugular veins. Peripherally inserted central catheters (PICCs), typically inserted via an antecubital vein and advanced into the superior vena cava, are the most commonly used central venous access devices for providing short-term PN. PICC placement offers the advantage of central venous access while avoiding the risks associated with accessing the subclavian or jugular veins, such as hemothorax, pneumothorax, and arterial injury.

Tunneled catheters or catheters with indwelling ports should be considered for patients who will need prolonged central venous nutrition (e.g., >6 weeks). Patients who will be using their catheters solely for daily central PN and who require home IV nutrition may be best served by a tunneled catheter rather than an indwelling port. Tunneled catheters may be more easily used and cared for, which can minimize the risk of infection.

Inserting a dedicated line for infusing hypertonic solutions requires strict aseptic technique and maximal barrier protection: hat, mask, gown, and gloves must be worn. The position of the catheter tip in the superior vena cava is confirmed by chest x-ray before any concentrated solutions are administered. Once the position of the tip has been confirmed, the line should be used exclusively for administering the hypertonic nutrient solution.

Multiple-lumen central venous catheters are most commonly used. Although at least one lumen is dedicated to the infusion of the PN solutions, the other(s) may be used for monitoring, blood drawing, or medication. The rate of catheter sepsis associated with multiple-port catheters may be the same as or slightly greater than the rate associated with the use of single-port catheters. However, multiple-port PICCs are used to infuse PN solutions for a shorter period of time, which can minimize their inherent risk. Multiple-port catheters should be carefully maintained, including dressing changes, maintaining the dedicated lumen, careful handling of the other lumens, and removing the catheter as soon as it is no longer needed.

Infusion and Patient Monitoring

It is advisable to start with 1 L of central PN and increase the volume as needed, depending on the patient's metabolic stability. Blood glucose levels should be closely monitored and maintained at less than 180 mg/dL, tissue perfusion should be adequate, and Po_2, Pco_2, electrolytes (especially potassium, phosphate, and magnesium) and acid-base balance should be near normal before starting or advancing to the goal solution. The solutions should be administered using a volumetric pump set at a constant rate. It is important not to modify the infusion rate during any given day to try to compensate for excess or inadequate administration of the PN solution, such as when the PN solution arrives later than expected. A cyclic schedule (10–16 hours/day) for patients requiring long-term PN can be initiated once the patient is metabolically stable. In situations when the central PN solution must be suddenly discontinued, a 10% dextrose solution may be given at the same infusion rate as was used for the PN unless the patient is severely hyperglycemic. PN solutions may be administered at one-half the infusion rate to patients who are undergoing surgical procedures because circulating glucose and electrolyte levels are easier to control.

In addition to hyperglycemia, metabolic complications include hyper- and hypophosphatemia, hyper- and hypokalemia, hyper- and hypomagnesemia, and hyper- and hypocalcemia. Thus it is important to monitor the patient's serum electrolytes closely, especially when initiating TPN. In the inpatient setting, once the patient stabilizes on the individual nutritional prescription, serum chemistries should be obtained at least twice weekly to measure chloride, CO_2, potassium, sodium, blood urea nitrogen, creatinine, calcium, and phosphate levels and once weekly for a full profile that includes liver function, magnesium, and triglyceride levels. Stable home PN patients may have less frequent chemistry monitoring, typically starting with once per week monitoring, then decreasing to twice per month and then monthly, depending on overall stability and clinical status.

Patients With Special Needs

Glucose Intolerance

Hyperglycemia is the most common metabolic complication related to PN, and glucose regulation may be especially difficult in patients who have diabetes mellitus or who develop insulin resistance in response to severe stress or infection. Control of blood glucose levels is important for all patients who receive PN because uncontrolled hyperglycemia may be associated with complications such as fluid and electrolyte disturbances and increased infection risk due to impairment of host defenses, including decreased polymorphonuclear leukocyte mobilization, chemotaxis, and phagocytic activity. Intensive insulin therapy, maintaining blood glucose concentrations between 80 and 110 mg/dL, was once considered standard practice for critically ill patients. However, more recent literature has demonstrated significant morbidity and mortality with this approach. For hospitalized patients, a target blood glucose of 140 to 180 mg/dL is recommended. Select circumstances may require more stringent blood glucose goals (110–140 mg/dL) if this can be maintained without hypoglycemic episodes.

Patients with difficult glycemic control may best be managed by continuous insulin infusion, which is safe, effective, and more timely than subcutaneous insulin therapy. Hypoglycemia that occurs during this type of infusion generally is short-lived and more easily corrected than hypoglycemia resulting from subcutaneous insulin administration. A separate IV insulin infusion can be used rather than adding incremental doses of insulin to the PN bag every 24 hours in patients for whom glycemic control is difficult. Many intensive care units (ICUs) have an insulin drip infusion protocol in which there are frequent checks of serum glucose and adjustments of the insulin infusion drip (e.g., every 1–2 hours) to maintain target glucose levels. The conventional approach of using sliding scale insulin to cover high blood glucose levels may be unsafe and ineffective, and repetitive doses of subcutaneous insulin in the edematous patient can have a cumulative effect leading to prolonged hypoglycemia. In addition, adjusting insulin in the PN bag every 24 hours might not achieve the desired rapid correction of hyperglycemia deemed appropriate based on the literature, which indicates worse outcomes for those with poor glucose control.

Abrupt discontinuation of PN can lead to hypoglycemia and should be avoided. Instead, it is recommended to decrease the PN infusion rate by one-half for the last hour of infusion before discontinuation to prevent rebound hypoglycemia.

Pancreatitis

Most cases of pancreatitis are mild, and nutritional support is not needed. However, 10% to 20% of patients with pancreatitis develop severe disease that results in a hypermetabolic, hyperdynamic, systemic inflammatory response syndrome that creates a highly catabolic stress state. In an evidence-based report evaluating nutrition support in acute pancreatitis patients, EN delivered to the small intestine (distal to the ligament of Treitz) is preferred over PN; EN patients are less likely to suffer from multiorgan failure, systemic infections, and death.

Initiation of PN should be delayed in patients with acute pancreatitis who cannot tolerate EN even though they might eventually require PN. Providing PN within 24 hours of admission has been shown to worsen outcome, and providing PN after resuscitation and abatement of the acute inflammatory process appears to improve outcome compared with standard therapy. Consequently, if EN is not feasible, the initiation of PN should be delayed for at least 5 days after admission to the hospital, when the peak period of inflammation has abated.

Acute Kidney Injury and Chronic Kidney Disease

Acute kidney injury (AKI) is associated with severe nutritional deficits. Most patients with AKI are catabolic and have energy requirements 50% to 100% greater than resting requirements, likely the result of other coexisting conditions such as sepsis, trauma, and burns. Energy is provided to patients with AKI in sufficient quantities to minimize protein degradation, generally in the range of 20 to 30 kcal/kg/day. Lipid injectable emulsions can be used as a source of concentrated energy in patients who require a fluid restriction.

Protein loss is accelerated and protein synthesis is impaired in patients with AKI. Loss of amino acids in the dialysate and renal replacement therapies add to the protein deficit and increase individual protein needs. Approximately 10 to 12 g of amino acids are lost with each dialysis therapy, depending on the type of dialyzer membrane, blood flow rate, and dialyzer reuse procedure, and approximately 10 to 16 g/day of amino acids are lost through continuous renal replacement therapies (CRRT). The provision of protein at 1.2 g/kg/day and up to 2.5 g/kg/day is recommended for AKI patients receiving hemodialysis and CRRT, respectively.

Protein is provided with a standard solution containing both essential and nonessential amino acids. Although some data suggest essential amino acids alone may be beneficial compared with a mixture of both essential and nonessential amino acids, the efficacy of using essential amino acid solutions remains uncertain. The goal is to provide adequate protein while treating the patient aggressively with dialysis to prevent the accumulation of nitrogenous waste products.

Fluid and electrolyte balance are often impaired in patients with AKI. The amount of fluid from the PN might need to be adjusted daily, depending on the phase of AKI, whether the patient is receiving dialysis, and whether dialysis is continuous or intermittent. Serum potassium and phosphate levels typically rise in patients with AKI until dialysis is initiated, at which time levels might drop, especially with the provision of PN. Potassium, phosphate, and magnesium levels need close monitoring and adjustment to correct imbalances. Acetate salts of potassium or sodium can be administered to help correct a metabolic acidosis.

Standard doses of the water-soluble vitamins and additional folic acid (1 mg/day total) and pyridoxine (vitamin B_6) (10 mg/day) might need to be added to the solution for patients who are being dialyzed because these vitamins are lost from the body in the dialysate bath. Thiamine losses are increased with CRRT, and repletion (100 mg/day) must be provided for patients receiving this therapy. The dose of vitamin C might need to be restricted to 100 mg/day to prevent oxalate deposits. However, additional vitamin C (250 mg/day) should be provided to patients receiving CRRT. The supplementation of fat-soluble vitamins is usually not required, especially in patients who also are eating, because excretion of fat-soluble vitamins is reduced in renal failure. For example, serum vitamin A levels may be elevated in AKI because of enhanced hepatic release of retinol and retinol-binding protein, decreased renal catabolism, and decreased degradation of vitamin A transport protein by the kidneys. Vitamin D levels may be decreased because of impaired activation of 1,25-dihydroxycholecalciferol in the kidneys. In anuric patients, trace elements may be withheld from the PN solution; however, for prolonged PN, trace elements and fat-soluble vitamins should be monitored and replaced accordingly.

Patients with chronic kidney disease (CKD) also have nutritional deficits due to anorexia, amino acid losses into the dialysate, concurrent illness, metabolic acidosis, and endocrine disorders. However, unlike those suffering from AKI, patients with CKD have normal energy requirements. Protein intake generally is restricted in predialysis patients to 0.6 g/kg/day or 0.75 g/kg/day if the patient is malnourished. Protein is required in higher amounts in patients on dialysis, depending on the type of dialysis: 1.2 g/kg/day for hemodialysis; 1.2 to 1.5 g/kg/day for peritoneal dialysis. Predialysis patients who become acutely ill should be given protein 1.2 to 1.5 g/kg/day even if this precipitates the need for dialysis. Starvation from insufficient calories or protein in the patient with renal dysfunction increases the risk of nutritionally related complications and should be avoided in the severely ill patient regardless of the potential need for dialysis.

Intradialytic PN is the provision of IV amino acids, carbohydrates, and fat directly into the venous drip chamber of the hemodialysis unit during treatment. It is a method of providing additional calories and protein in malnourished chronic hemodialysis patients. It is associated with significant increases in body weight and serum albumin in patients with end-stage renal disease (ESRD). However, intradialytic PN is expensive, and the benefits have not been fully elucidated. A typical solution contains about 1100 kcal and 50 g of protein, which is provided three times per week with hemodialysis. For example, in a dialysis patient who requires 2500 kcals and 70 g protein/day, intradialytic PN will provide approximately 20% of the weekly energy and approximately 30% of the weekly protein needs. Thus intradialytic PN is reserved for patients with ESRD on hemodialysis who cannot ingest sufficient nutrients by mouth and who are not candidates for nutritional support via EN or PN because of GI intolerance, venous access problems, or other reasons. Appropriate use of intradialytic PN should be limited to a very small fraction of people who are on hemodialysis.

Hepatic Dysfunction and Liver Failure

Hepatic dysfunction is associated with a variety of abnormalities including metabolic abnormalities, malabsorption, maldigestion, anorexia, and early satiety due to ascites. Dietary restrictions also can contribute to malnutrition.

Protein intake in patients with stable chronic liver disease depends on the patient's nutritional status and protein tolerance. Nutritionally depleted patients can require as much protein as 1.5 g/kg estimated dry weight. In a minority of patients who have protein-sensitive hepatic encephalopathy, protein intake might need to be decreased to 0.5 to 0.7 g/kg/day and gradually increased to 1.0 to 1.5 g/kg/day, as tolerated. These patients have deranged plasma amino acid profiles, with increased concentrations of aromatic amino acids (phenylalanine, tyrosine, and tryptophan) and methionine and decreased branched-chain amino acids (leucine, isoleucine, and valine). Randomized, controlled trials that provided parenteral or enteral formulas enriched with branched-chain amino acids have been inconsistent with regard to improvements in encephalopathy, morbidity, and mortality. These specialty products should be reserved for patients with disabling encephalopathy who do not tolerate standard proteins and have not responded to other therapies, such as lactulose or neomycin administration.

Energy requirements are difficult to predict in patients with liver failure. Whereas most patients have a normal metabolic rate, up to one-third may be hypermetabolic. Although providing 25 to 30 kcal/kg/day is a guideline for providing energy needs, basing requirements on indirect calorimetry is often recommended.

Fluid restriction due to ascites and edema often necessitates increasing the dextrose concentration in the PN so as to maintain sufficient calories in a restricted volume. Sodium is reduced in the formula because patients with liver failure excrete nearly sodium-free urine. Vitamin and mineral deficiencies often occur as a result of suboptimal nutrient intake, decreased absorption, decreased storage, and in some cases alcohol use, which decreases thiamine (vitamin B_1) and folate absorption. Copper and manganese may be contraindicated because a major route of excretion for these substances is the biliary system. Zinc deficiency is common in cirrhotic patients, and supplementation of this mineral may be necessary, especially if there are excessive GI losses.

Acute Respiratory Distress Syndrome

Patients with protein-calorie malnutrition have an increased incidence of pneumonia, respiratory failure, and acute respiratory distress syndrome (ARDS). Nutritional support is indicated in patients with ARDS. Notably, underfeeding and overfeeding can be detrimental to pulmonary function.

Overfeeding calories, and particularly glucose, can lead to increased minute ventilation, increased dead space, and increased CO_2 production and ultimately to difficulty weaning from a ventilator. Hypercapnia from increased CO_2 production is the result of glucose combustion causing more CO_2 production and excess calories triggering lipogenesis. A healthy person increases ventilation in response to increased calories and thus avoids hypercapnia. However, patients with compromised ventilatory status might not be able to compensate with increased ventilation and can develop respiratory distress, acute respiratory failure, and difficulty weaning from mechanical ventilation. Thus the use of indirect calorimetry measurements to determine energy expenditure is imperative in patients with ARDS.

Critically Ill Patients With Obesity

Obesity is a growing problem worldwide, and management of critically ill patients with obesity poses many challenges. These patients are at risk for hyperglycemia, hyperlipidemia, and hypercapnia, all of which can be exacerbated by metabolic changes associated with critical illness. As with any critically ill patient, those with obesity will preferentially use protein and carbohydrate for energy and cannot effectively draw upon adipose tissue for energy. These patients require nutrition support to minimize loss of lean body mass.

The concept of "hypocaloric feeding" has emerged as the preferred way to feed critically ill patients with obesity. Energy delivery is restricted to approximately 60% to 70% of estimated energy requirements, and protein delivery is high (typically >2 g/kg ideal body weight [IBW]). This is to avoid hyperglycemia, hyperlipidemia, and hypercapnia while providing the protein required to spare lean body mass and support recovery. Small-scale studies employing this feeding method have demonstrated that patients can achieve positive nitrogen balance. One study found decreased ICU length of stay, decreased antibiotic days, and a trend toward decreased mechanical ventilation days.

Energy and protein delivery for critically ill patients with obesity is guided by BMI. The ASPEN-SCCM guidelines recommend providing 11 to 14 kcal/kg of actual weight for patients with a BMI of 30 to 50 kg/m² or 22 to 25 kcal/kg IBW for patients with a BMI greater than 50 kg/m². For protein delivery, ASPEN and SCCM recommend protein provision of 2 g/kg or greater IBW for patients with class I and class II obesity (BMI of 30–35 kg/m² and 35–40 kg/m², respectively), and, for patients with class III obesity (BMI > 40 kg/m²), protein provision should be 2.5 g/kg or greater IBW.

Other Conditions and Nutritional Treatments

The catabolic response to major surgery, trauma, burn, and sepsis is characterized by a net breakdown of body protein stores to provide substrates for gluconeogenesis and acute-phase protein synthesis. Adequate nutrition can attenuate whole-body catabolism but rarely, if ever, prevents or reverses the loss of lean body mass during the acute phase of injury. Several strategies to prevent the loss of lean body mass have been investigated, including growth hormone, growth factors, and conditionally essential amino acids, such as glutamine.

Growth hormone is a potent anabolic agent, and administration to humans increases the rate of wound healing, decreases rates of wound infection, and decreases the catabolism and muscle wasting of critical illness. However, a large European trial found increased morbidity and mortality in patients with prolonged critical illness who received high doses of growth hormone. Thus the use of growth hormone in patients who are in the acute phase of critical illness is not recommended.

Alternative anabolic agents such as oxandrolone (Oxandrin)[1] and testosterone[1] are being pursued to induce positive nitrogen balance and enhance wound healing in critically ill patients. These anabolic steroid hormones increase protein synthesis and can reduce the rate of protein breakdown. In a study of patients with alcoholic hepatitis, administration of oxandrolone was associated with lower mortality compared with patients receiving placebo. The patients receiving oxandrolone had improvements

in the severity of their liver injury and the degree of malnutrition. Several studies have demonstrated a benefit of oxandrolone use in the burn patient population. Other anabolic steroid hormones, such as methandienone[2] and nandrolone decanoate (Deca Durabolin),[2] have been shown to increase protein anabolism and nitrogen balance in hospitalized patients.

Hormone treatment should be reserved for patients with major burns and documented impaired healing, patients who have large wounds or enterocutaneous fistulae who have impaired healing, patients with muscle wasting and weakness associated with AIDS or other failure to thrive conditions, and, in general, patients who have not responded to aggressive nutritional support but whose underlying disease processes are controlled. Growth factors have not been shown to decrease length of time on a respirator in ICU patients. In fact, such factors can increase ventilator time and worsen outcome.

Glutamine-supplemented PN solutions administered to trauma or critically ill patients can improve overall nitrogen balance, enhance muscle protein synthesis, improve intestinal nutrient absorption, decrease gut permeability, improve immune function, and decrease hospital stays and costs in some patient populations. A review of 14 randomized trials in surgical and critically ill patients found that glutamine supplementation was associated with reduced mortality, lower rates of infectious complications, and a decreased hospital stay. The greatest benefit was in patients receiving high-dose (>0.29 g/kg/day) parenteral glutamine.

However, a recent randomized trial of glutamine and antioxidant micronutrient supplementation in critically ill patients showed a trend toward increased 28-day mortality and significant in-hospital and 6-month mortality in patients receiving glutamine supplementation. There were limitations in this study in that baseline glutamine levels were not checked for all patients; in a subset of 66 patients with plasma glutamine levels evaluated, all had normal levels at baseline. This suggests that glutamine supplementation may not be appropriate for all critically ill patients. In addition, patients received approximately 50% of goal energy requirements and approximately 45% of goal protein delivery from glutamine. The total amount of glutamine given in this study was significantly higher than the dose of glutamine usually recommended. This raises the possibility that there is an optimal "therapeutic window" for glutamine administration: giving too little glutamine may not be efficacious, and giving too much may be toxic. Further investigation is required before a definitive recommendation can be given based on this study alone.

Patients with intestinal dysfunction requiring PN, such as those with short-bowel syndrome or mucosal damage after chemotherapy and/or radiation therapy, might benefit from glutamine-containing PN. Glutamine-containing PN might also be beneficial in patients with immunodeficiency syndromes, including AIDS, immune-system dysfunction associated with critical illness, and bone marrow transplantation; patients with severe catabolic illness; patients with multiple trauma; and patients with other diseases associated with a prolonged ICU stay. Glutamine-supplemented solutions should not yet be considered routine care and should not be used in patients with significant renal insufficiency or in patients with significant hepatic failure. A recent ASPEN position paper summarizes recommendations for use of both enteral and IV glutamine.

Common Complications and Management
Catheter Sepsis

Catheter-related bloodstream infection (CRBSI) is an infection that originates from the catheter itself and is confirmed by culture. Central line–associated bloodstream infection is a bloodstream infection without another identified focus of infection in a patient with a central line in place for at least 48 hours before

---

[1] Not FDA approved for this indication.

[2] Not available in the United States.

TABLE 4 Possible Etiologies and Treatment of Common Complications of Central Parenteral Nutrition

PROBLEM	POSSIBLE ETIOLOGY	TREATMENT
Glucose		
Hyperglycemia, glycosuria, hyperosmolar nonketotic dehydration, or coma	Excessive dose or rate of infusion, inadequate insulin production, concomitant steroid administration, infection	Decrease the amount of glucose given, increase insulin, administer a portion of calories as fat
Diabetic ketoacidosis	Inadequate endogenous insulin production and/or inadequate insulin therapy	Give insulin Decrease glucose intake
Rebound hypoglycemia	Persistent endogenous insulin production by islet cells after long-term high-carbohydrate infusion	Give 5%–10% glucose before parenteral infusion is discontinued
Hypercarbia	Carbohydrate load exceeds the ability to increase minute ventilation and excrete excess CO_2	Limit glucose dose to 5 mg/kg/min Give greater percentage of total caloric needs as fat (up to 30%–40%)
Fat		
Hypertriglyceridemia	Rapid infusion	Decrease rate of PN infusion
	Decreased clearance	Allow clearance (~12 h) before testing blood
Essential fatty acid deficiency	Inadequate essential fatty acid administration	Administer essential fatty acids in doses of 4%–7% of total calories
Amino Acids		
Hyperchloremia metabolic acidosis	Excessive chloride content of amino acid solutions	Administer Na^+ and K^+ as acetate salts
Prerenal azotemia	Excessive amino acids with inadequate caloric supplementation	Reduce amino acids Increase the amount of glucose calories
Miscellaneous		
Hypophosphatemia	Inadequate phosphorus administration with redistribution into tissues	Give 15 mmol phosphate/1000 IV kcal Evaluate antacid and Ca^{2+} administration
Hypomagnesemia	Inadequate administration relative to increased losses (diarrhea, diuresis, medications)	Administer Mg^{2+} (15–20 mEq/1000 kcal)
Hypermagnesemia	Excessive administration; renal failure	Decrease Mg^{2+} supplementation
Hypokalemia	Inadequate K^+ intake relative to increased needs for anabolism; diuresis	Increase K^+ supplementation
Hyperkalemia	Excessive K^+ administration, especially in metabolic acidosis; renal decompensation	Reduce or stop exogenous K^+ If ECG changes are present, treat with calcium gluconate, insulin, diuretics, and/or sodium polystyrene sulfonate (Kayexalate)
Hypocalcemia	Inadequate Ca^{2+} administration; reciprocal response to phosphorus repletion without simultaneous calcium infusion	Increase Ca^{2+} dose
Hypercalcemia	Excessive Ca^{2+} administration; excessive vitamin D administration	Decrease Ca^{2+} and/or vitamin D administration
Elevated liver transaminases or serum alkaline phosphatase and bilirubin	Enzyme induction secondary to amino acid imbalances or overfeeding	Reevaluate nutritional prescription Cycle TPN Avoid overfeeding calories Consider change to a blended lipid rather than 100% soybean oil-lipid Consider administering carnitine

ECG, Electrocardiographic; *IV*, intravenous; *PN*, parenteral nutrition; *TPN*, total parenteral nutrition.

the development of infection. Central venous CRBSIs range from 3% to 20% in hospitalized patients and are the most common complication of central venous catheters. Colonization of the skin, intraluminal contamination from manipulation of the catheter hub or IV connectors, and seeding of microorganisms from the bloodstream are common sources of infection. Common organisms associated with CRBSIs include *Staphylococcus epidermidis, Staphylococcus aureus, Enterococcus* spp., *Candida albicans, Escherichia coli, Klebsiella* spp., *Pseudomonas* spp., and *Enterobacter* spp., as well as resistant strains such as methicillin-resistant *S. aureus* and vancomycin-resistant enterococci.

Management of patients with catheter infection depends on their clinical condition. In extremely ill patients with high fevers who are hypotensive or who have local signs of infection around the catheter site, the catheter should be removed, its tip cultured, and peripheral and central venous blood cultures should be obtained. In CRBSI, the organisms that grow from the catheter tip are the same those identified in the peripheral blood culture, and typically more than 10^3 organisms are grown from cultures of the catheter tip.

Specific therapy should be initiated against the primary source in patients in whom a source of infection other than the catheter tip is present. Peripheral blood cultures should be obtained. Blood cultures should not be taken from the central venous catheter port dedicated for PN because this increases the risk of contaminating the line. If the infection resolves, central venous feedings can be continued while making sure to maintain euglycemia. If a source is not identified and the symptoms persist,

BOX 3 Management of Parenteral Nutrition-Related Liver Dysfunction

Have the patient eat, if possible.
Avoid administering large amounts of glucose or protein calories.
Supply intravenous fat emulsions (up to 30% of total calories).
Consider addition of blended lipid emulsions with lower concentrations of soybean oil.
Cycle the parenteral nutrition, infusing for 10 to 12 hours/day.
Reevaluate energy needs; reduce energy delivery if liver dysfunction persists.

the catheter should be removed, and its tip should be cultured. If the culture of the catheter tip returns positive or if the index of suspicion is high, empiric antibiotic therapy is initiated and later narrowed to target the specific microorganism once culture and susceptibility data become available. If removal of the catheter is indicated and is not possible because of lack of access sites or high risk of bleeding complications, then salvage therapy (systemic antibiotics plus antibiotic lock therapy or ethanol lock therapy) or, as a last resort, exchange of the catheter over a guidewire with systemic antibiotics and antibiotic lock therapy may be considered, with long-term ethanol lock therapy to prevent further infections. Central venous feedings may be continued during this interval if the patient is stable. It is important to note that changing the site of catheter, rather than salvage therapy or guidewire exchange, is preferred in patients in whom infection is suspected.

Other Complications

Common complications, their etiologies, and treatments are outlined in Table 4. Prolonged administration of PN can result in altered hepatic function and can lead to liver failure. Transaminases may be elevated 1 to 2 weeks after initiating PN, but this often resolves without any change in the composition of PN or rate of administration. However, in patients receiving long-term PN (>20 days), prolonged elevations of alkaline phosphatase followed by elevated levels of serum transaminases can occur, even after therapy is discontinued.

Serum levels of alkaline phosphatase and bilirubin initially remain normal, but they rise in many patients who receive long-term PN. Patients who do not receive lipids in the PN solution have more frequent and severe hepatic abnormalities, most likely due to higher carbohydrate loads. Excess glucose increases insulin secretion, which stimulates hepatic lipogenesis and results in hepatic fat accumulation. Fatty infiltration is the initial histopathologic change; it is readily reversible and might not be accompanied by altered liver function tests.

Longer PN therapy may be associated with cholestasis, cholelithiasis, steatosis, and steatohepatitis and can progress to active chronic hepatitis, fibrosis, and eventual cirrhosis. The management of PN-related liver dysfunction is summarized in Box 3.

Complications are minimized and nutritional therapy maximized when the care of patients who require specialized nutritional support is supervised by a nutrition support team. Ideally, the nutrition support team consists of a pharmacist, dietitian, nurse, and physician.

References

Al-Omran M, Albalawi ZH, Tashkandi MF, Al-Ansary LA: Enteral versus parenteral nutrition in acute pancreatitis, Cochrane Database Syst Rev, 2010. http://dx.doi.org/10.1002/14651858.CD002837.pub2. CD002837.

A.S.P.E.N, Ayers P, Adams S, Boullata J, et al: Parenteral nutrition safety consensus recommendations, JPEN J Parenter Enteral Nutr 38:296–333, 2014.

A.S.P.E.N. Board of Directors: Guidelines for the use of parenteral and enteral nutrition in adult and pediatric patients, JPEN J Parenter Enteral Nutr 26:1SA–138SA, 2002.

Bistrian BR, McCowen KC: Nutritional and metabolic support in the adult intensive care unit: key controversies, Crit Care Med 34:1525–1531, 2006.

Boullata JI, Gilbert K, Sacks G, et al: A.S.P.E.N. Clinical guidelines: parenteral nutrition ordering, order review, compounding, labeling, and dispensing, JPEN J Parenter Enteral Nutr 38(3):334–377, 2014.

Butler SO, Btaiche IF, Alaniz C: Relationship between hyperglycemia and infection in critically ill patients, Pharmacotherapy 25:963–976, 2005.

Evans DC, Corkins MR, Malone A, et al: The use of visceral proteins as nutrition markers: an ASPEN position paper, Nutr Clin Pract 36:22–28, 2021.

Heyland DK, Dhaliwal R, Suchner U, Berger MM: Antioxidant nutrients: a systematic review of trace elements and vitamins in the critically ill patient, Intensive Care Med 31:327–337, 2005.

Heyland D, Muscedere J, Wischmeyer PE, et al: A randomized trial of glutamine and antioxidants in critically ill patients, N Engl J Med 368:1489–1497, 2013.

Li Y, Tang X, Zhang J, Wu T: Nutritional support for acute kidney injury, Cochrane Database Syst Rev, 2010. https://doi.org/10.1002/14651858.CD005426.pub3. CD005426.

McClave SA, Chang W-K, Dhaliwal R, Heyland DK: Nutrition support in acute pancreatitis: a systematic review of the literature, JPEN J Parenter Enteral Nutr 30:143–156, 2006.

McClave SA, Taylor BE, Martindale RG, et al: , Guidelines for the provision of nutrition support therapy in the adult critically ill patient: Society of Critical Care Medicine (SCCM) and American Society for Parenteral and Enteral Nutrition (A.S.P.E.N.), JPEN J Parenter Enteral Nutr. 40:159–211. 40:1200, 2016. Erratum in: JPEN J Parenter Enteral Nutr 2016.

McMahon MM, Nystrom E, Braunschweig C, et al: A.S.P.E.N. Clinical guidelines: nutrition support of adult patients with hyperglycemia, JPEN J Parenter Enteral Nutr 37:26–36, 2013.

O'Grady NP, Alexander M, Burns LA, et al: Guidelines for the prevention of intravascular catheter-related infections, Clin Infect Dis 52:e162–e193, 2011.

Vanek VW, Matarese LE, Robinson M, et al: A.S.P.E.N. Position paper: parenteral nutrition glutamine supplementation, JPEN J Parenter Enteral Nutr 26:479–494, 2011.

Worthington P, Balint J, Bechtold M, et al: When is parenteral nutrition appropriate? JPEN J Parenter Enteral Nutr 41:324–377, 2017.

PHEOCHROMOCYTOMA

Method of
Matthew A. Nazari, MD*; Abhishek Jha, MBBS*; and Karel Pacak, MD, PhD, DSc

CURRENT DIAGNOSIS

- Pheochromocytoma/paraganglioma (PPGL) should be suspected in patients with hypertension and three or more signs and symptoms of catecholamine excess, such as hyperhidrosis, palpitations, pallor, tremor, or nausea, especially if the patient has a body mass index (BMI) <25 kg/m^2 or a heart rate >85 beats per minute.
- A biochemical diagnosis of PPGL should be established with elevated plasma or urinary free metanephrines and plasma methoxytyramine.
- Localize tumors with anatomic imaging (computed tomography [CT] or magnetic resonance [MRI]), followed by, if necessary, specific functional imaging using positron emission tomography (PET) modalities.
- After diagnosis, a thorough medical and family history should be obtained to assess for syndromic clinical presentations of PPGL. If available, all patients with confirmed PPGL should undergo genetic testing.
- If a causative pathogenic variant is identified, the patient's first-degree relatives should be appropriately tested. Positive individuals should be presymptomatically screened with plasma or urinary free metanephrines and imaging as described, if appropriate.

*Share joint first coauthorship.

- Prompt surgical excision remains the primary treatment for PPGL. If feasible, cortical sparing adrenalectomies should be attempted in patients with bilateral or hereditary PPGLs (except succinate dehydrogenase subunit B [*SDHB*]–related disease) to prevent lifelong corticosteroid supplementation.
- One to 2 weeks before the operation, patients with biochemically active tumors (e.g., elevated plasma free metanephrines) should be started on preoperative α- followed by β-adrenoceptor blockade to avoid unopposed α-adrenoceptor stimulation leading to vasoconstriction and hypertensive crisis. At minimum, a normotensive patient should be maintained on low-dose calcium channel blockers.
- After surgery, scheduled clinical follow-up is necessary, particularly in cases of underlying pathogenic variants or large tumors (>5 cm), which are more likely to metastasize.
- Management of metastatic PPGL requires a multidisciplinary approach involving surgical excision alongside pharmacologic, targeted radio-, and chemotherapies.

The 2022 World Health Organization (WHO) Classification of Tumors of Endocrine Organs defines pheochromocytoma (PHEO)[†] as a chromaffin cell tumor arising from the adrenal medulla, or an intraadrenal paraganglioma. Lesions smaller than 1 cm within the adrenal gland are called micropheochromocytomas. Paragangliomas (PGLs) are functionally similar tumors that originate along the extraadrenal ganglia and are further classified as parasympathetic or sympathetic. Predominantly located in the head and neck, parasympathetic PGLs are locally invasive, rarely develop metastases (10%), but are often multifocal and produce dopamine (30%), with a minority (approximately 5% or less) producing and releasing norepinephrine/normetanephrine. In contrast to their parasympathetic counterparts, sympathetic PGLs are concentrated primarily in the abdomen and pelvis, with 2% found in the mediastinum and 1% in the neck. Abdominal PGLs often derive from the organ of Zuckerkandl, a collection of neural crest cells above the bifurcation of the aorta at the origin of the inferior mesenteric artery (Figure 1). Biochemically, PHEOs are characterized by the synthesis, metabolism, storage, and almost always the release of metanephrines/methoxytyramine (in approximately 98% of cases) and usually the release of catecholamines (in approximately 70% of cases).

Epidemiology
Previously, PHEOs were primarily diagnosed at autopsy. However, as the sensitivity of biochemical assays and imaging scans increased, the incidence of PHEO likewise increased. Over the last decade, analyses have demonstrated an increase in incidence of PHEO from 0.19/100,000 per annum before 2000 to 0.58/100,000 per annum after 2010, a trend largely attributed to advancements in diagnosis. While PHEO can occur at any age (including childhood, particularly when associated with germline pathogenic variants), the average age of diagnosis is most commonly in the fifth decade. Although no consistent gender preference has been reported, in the Netherlands, a statistically significant number of PHEOs occurred in females (55%) compared with their male counterparts (45%). The PHEO to PGL ratio is approximately 0.80 to 0.20, respectively. Approximately 30% to 40% of patients with PHEO carry a germline or somatic pathogenic variant, respectively, in one of the 25 known PHEO susceptibility genes (see "Genetics"). The rate of malignancy varies from 0% to 71% depending on genetic background, with succinate dehydrogenase subunit B (*SDHB*)–related disease being the most clinically aggressive.

[†]From this point forward, PHEO represents pheochromocytoma and paraganglioma unless otherwise specified. For example, when both tumors should be emphasized, the term PPGL will be used.

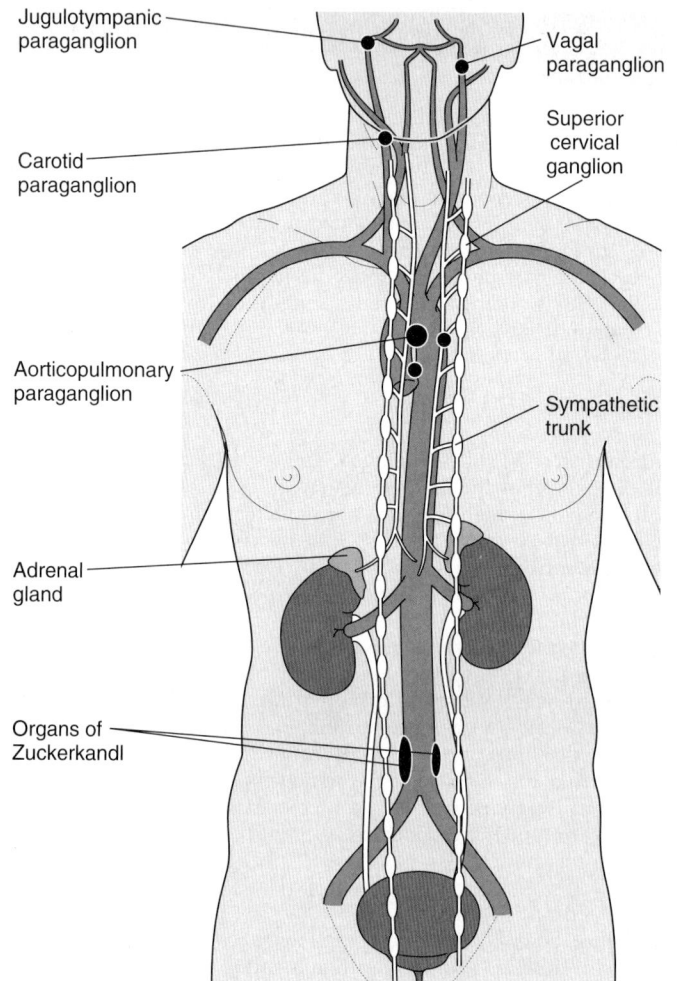

Figure 1 Important anatomic distribution of chromaffin tissue composing paraganglia.

Genetics
While complete consensus is lacking, 30% to 40% of PHEOs are hereditary, with a significant percentage (>20%) of apparently sporadic tumors carrying pathogenic variants. Identification of a genetic alteration allows for appropriate treatment algorithms and management of subsequent endocrinopathies or syndromic neoplasias in the proband and at-risk relatives as well.

At present, at least 25 PHEO susceptibility genes have been discovered, which can broadly be categorized into major and minor contributors, with the major genes representing 85% to 90% of all hereditary tumors. Well-known hereditary pathogenic variants include von Hippel–Lindau tumor suppressor (*VHL*), rearranged during transfection (*RET*) proto-oncogene resulting in multiple endocrine neoplasia (MEN) types 2A and 2B, neurofibromin 1 (*NF1*) tumor suppressor, and the succinate dehydrogenase (*SDHx*) subunits *SDHB* and *SDHD* genes. The minor susceptibility genes, representing 10% to 15% of hereditary tumors, include *SDHA*, *SDHC*, succinate-CoA ligase GDP-forming subunit beta (*SUCLG2*), succinate dehydrogenase assembly factor 2 (*SDHAF2*), fumarate hydratase (*FH*), Myc-associated factor X (*MAX*), hypoxia-inducible factor 2 alpha (*HIF2A*), malate dehydrogenase 2 (*MDH2*), isocitrate dehydrogenase 1 (*IDH1*), isocitrate dehydrogenase 2 (*IDH2*), HRas (*H-RAS*) and KRAS (*K-RAS*) proto-oncogenes, transmembrane protein 127 (*TMEM 127*), cold-shock domain containing E1 (*CSDE1*), mastermind like transcriptional coactivator 3 (*MAML3*) fusion genes, prolyl hydroxylase 1 and 2 (*PHD1/2*), iron regulatory protein 1 (*IRP1*), malate dehydrogenase 2 (*MDH2*), kinesin superfamily member (*K1F1B*), dihydrolipoamide S-succinyltransferase (*DLST*), and DNA methyltransferase 3 alpha (*DNMT3A*). Characteristics of the most important hereditary tumor syndromes are described in Table 1.

	OTHER NAME	PENETRANCE	BILATERAL ADRENAL/ MULTIFOCAL	METASTATIC	PHEO OR PGL	BIOCHEMICAL PHENOTYPE
Cluster 1 Genes						
SDHA	PGL5	<5%	Not well reported	Up to 70%	PGL	Noradrenergic or dopaminergic
SDHB	PGL4	30%–40%	Usually rare as bilateral adrenal, but commonly multifocal	Up to 70%	PGL, less commonly PHEO	Noradrenergic or dopaminergic
SDHC	PGL3	Not well reported	Inconsistent reports	Rare	PGL, less commonly PHEO	Noradrenergic or dopaminergic
SDHD	PGL1	90% if paternally transmitted	Inconsistent reports	15%–20% but more data is needed	PGL, less commonly PHEO	Noradrenergic or dopaminergic silent
FH	—	About 1%–3%	Moderate	More reports needed but usually moderate/high	PHEO and PGL	Noradrenergic
HIF2A (*EPAS1*)	—	If somatic pathogenic variants, none; in those with germline pathogenic variants, more reports are needed	100% for those with somatic pathogenic variants	Over 50% for those with somatic pathogenic variants	PGL, less commonly PHEO	Noradrenergic
VHL	—	10%–30%	50%	5%–7%	PHEO, PGL is rare	Noradrenergic
Cluster 2 Genes						
RET	MEN2A	50%	50%–80%	<5%	PHEO, very rarely PGL	Adrenergic
RET	MEN2B	50%	50%–80%	<5%	PHEO, very rarely PGL	Adrenergic
NF1	—	1%–3%	16%	7%	PHEO, rarely PGL	Adrenergic
H-RAS	—	Not well reported	Low	Unknown	PHEO, less commonly PGL	Adrenergic
Others						
H3F3A	—	Not well reported	Present but very limited reports	Unknown	PHEO, PGL	Unknown

Note that penetrance and the presence of metastatic lesions in percentages are estimates based on several studies and vary greatly based on individual reports published until now.

Adapted from Pacak K: New biology of pheochromocytoma and paraganglioma, *Endocr Pract* 28(12):1253–1269, 2022.

Several well-established PHEO syndromes (Table 1) exhibit characteristic clinical features. Rare PGL-associated syndromes include Carney triad and a syndrome characterized by *SDHB* and *SDHD*-related gastrointestinal stromal tumors (GISTs). As first described in 2012, Pacak-Zhuang syndrome consists of *HIF2A*-associated PPGLs in the setting of polycythemia, duodenal somatostatinomas, and marked, permanent choroidal thickening and tortuous dilated veins in the choroid and retina. Another rare PHEO syndrome, first reported in 2013, is characterized by pheochromocytomas, PGLs, and giant cell tumors of bone associated with a postzygotic *H3F3A* pathogenic variant.

In conjunction with the US Endocrine Society Clinical Practice Guidelines published in 2014, interim publications have also emphasized genetic counseling and subsequent testing in all patients diagnosed with PHEO, regardless of suggestive family history or age at presentation. Within the United States, several commercially available PPGL gene panels screen patients for the most prevalent hereditary genetic syndromes via DNA sequencing and deletion/duplication analysis. However, broad, comprehensive genetic panels covering 10 to 12 genes are expensive and may not be covered by insurance. In patients with a confirmed PHEO, an algorithm (Figure 2) based on family history, syndromic clinical features, and biochemical phenotype could be used to tailor

genetic testing and reduce the financial burden. If genetic testing is positive for hereditary PPGL, all first-degree relatives should undergo genetic evaluation. Asymptomatic carriers should undergo annual biochemical evaluation with plasma metanephrines and whole-body magnetic resonance imaging (MRI) every other year for surveillance. Genetic testing in children (Box 1) should be approached on an individual basis after discussion with parents/guardians, geneticists, and psychiatrists due to the ethical and legal ramifications. Children should only be screened if they will be offered regular surveillance.

Expert consensus statements on the management of patients carrying *SDHD* and *SDHB* pathogenic variants were published in 2021 and 2024, respectively.

Clinical Manifestations

As a result of episodic catecholamine secretion and stimulation of α- and β-adrenoceptors, the clinical manifestations of PHEO are related to hemodynamic and metabolic instability. While the majority of primary clinical indicators (Box 2) for PHEO are nonspecific, when several symptoms are simultaneously present, the diagnosis should be considered. Patients with three or more signs and symptoms of catecholamine excess (hyperhidrosis, palpitations, pallor, tremor, and nausea), especially when combined with a body mass index of

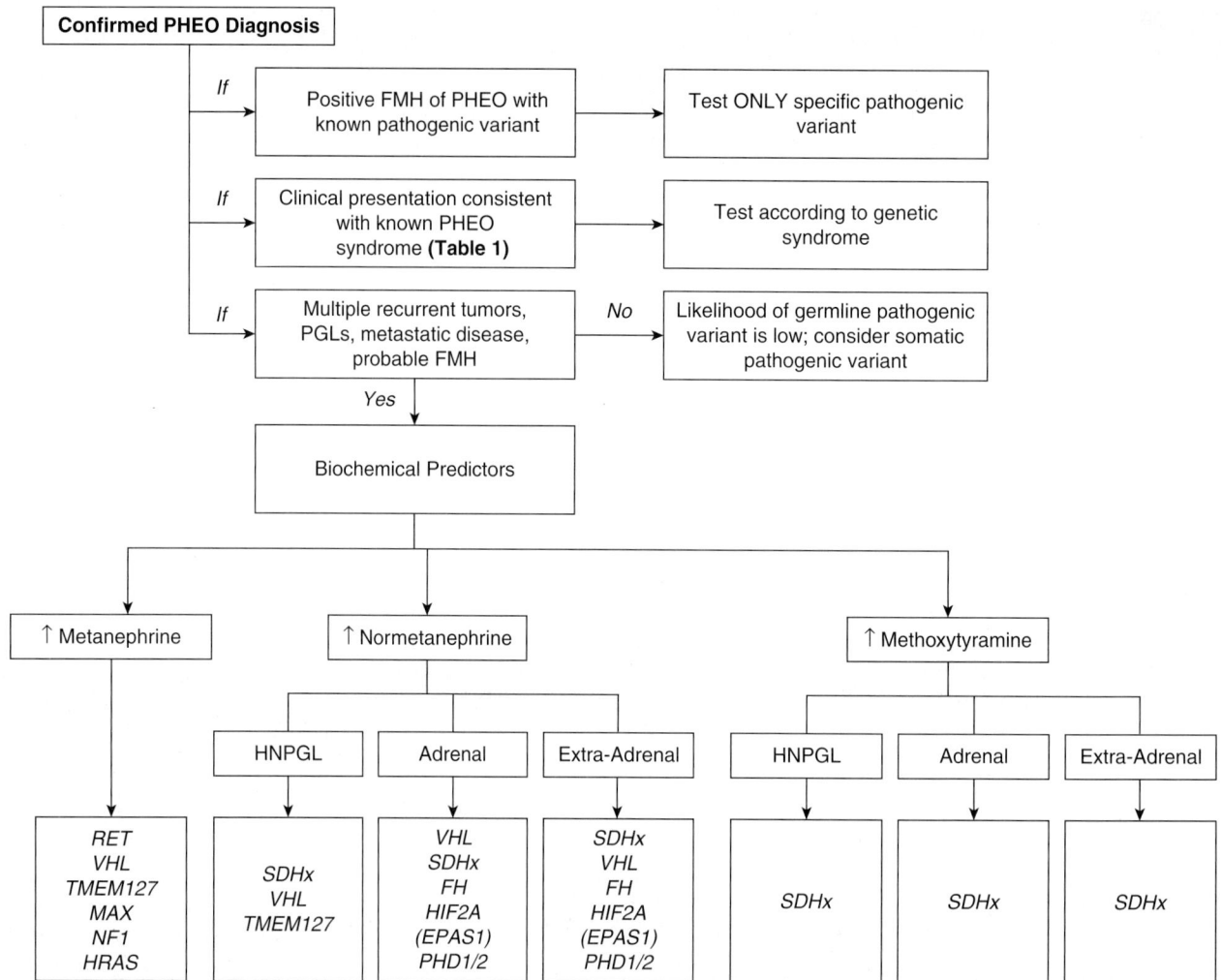

Figure 2 Targeted algorithm for genetic analysis in patients with confirmed pheochromocytoma. If both normetanephrine and methoxytyramine are elevated, follow the algorithm for methoxytyramine. If both normetanephrine and metanephrine are elevated, follow the algorithm for metanephrine. *SDHAF2* pathogenic variant screening should be considered in patients who suffer exclusively from head and neck paragangliomas and who have familial antecedents, multiple tumors, or a very young age of onset and in whom *SDHB/C/D* gene pathogenic variants are negative. Only the most common genes are listed. *FMH*, Family medical history; *PHEO*, pheochromocytoma. Adapted from Karasek D, Shah U, Frysak Z, et al: An update on the genetics of pheochromocytoma, *J Hum Hypertens* 27[3]:141–147, 2013.

BOX 1 Considerations for Pediatric Genetic Testing

- Parent/Guardian should meet with geneticist and/or psychiatrist in the absence of the child to discuss implications for genetic testing and subsequent screening recommendations if positive.
- Parent/Guardian should be given adequate time to reflect on their consultation and develop a plan to discuss why the child is undergoing the testing and the implications of the results.
- Medical providers should work with the family to avoid testing or revealing results close to or falling on birthdays, religious holidays, or important school activities, as this may negatively impact the memory of these events.
- If possible, avoid simultaneously testing multiple siblings given the potential impact of discordant results.
- If positive, genetic counselors should emphasize the importance of "at risk" vs. "being ill" and provide all parties with the appropriate space to express their immediate reactions, ask questions, and process their emotions.

Adapted from Lahlou-Laforet K, Consoli SM, Jeunemaitre X, et al: Presymptomatic genetic testing in minors at risk of paraganglioma and pheochromocytoma: our experience of oncogenetic multidisciplinary consultation, *Horm Metab Res* 44:354–358, 2012.

BOX 2 Clinical Indications to Screen for Pheochromocytoma

- Patients with a known PPGL susceptibility pathogenic variant or a positive family history.
- Patients with triad of headaches, sweating, and tachycardia (regardless of blood pressure).
- Patients with recent onset of uncontrolled hypertension on greater than three to four standard oral therapies.
- Patients with previous history of hypertension, tachycardia, or arrhythmia after anesthesia, surgery, or ingestion of medications known to precipitate symptoms of PPGL.
- Patients with an incidental adrenal mass.

PPGL, Pheochromocytoma/paraganglioma.

<25 kg/m^2 and a heart rate >85 beats per minute, are 7.5-fold more likely to have a PPGL. Symptoms may occur spontaneously or as a result of direct tumor manipulation, anesthesia, or ingestion of tyramine-rich foods, which trigger catecholamine release and subsequent crisis. Unfortunately, patients may not exhibit any signs or symptoms of PHEO, thereby delaying a timely diagnosis. Therefore, if biochemistry or imaging suggests PHEO, the diagnosis may not be excluded based on the patient's asymptomatic state.

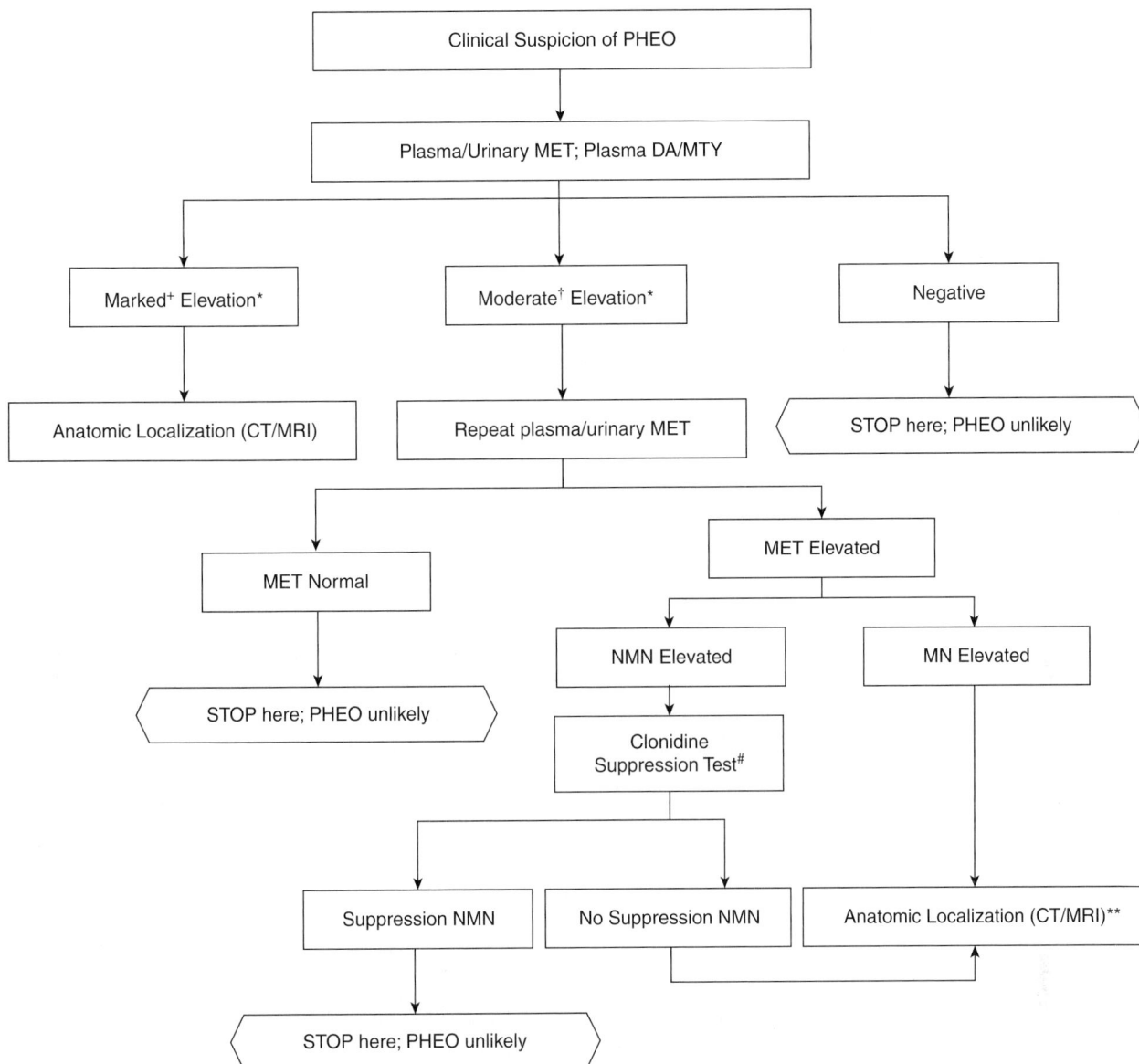

Figure 3 Algorithm for biochemical diagnosis of pheochromocytoma.

[+]Marked: greater than 2x the URL of normal
[†]Moderate; less than 2x the URL of normal
*First rule out any drug-related false elevation of MET/MTY (see Table 2) or renal failure
[#]If suspicion for PHEO is low or interfering drugs cannot be held
**If metanephrine is elevated, anatomic localization should be focused on the adrenal gland
CT: computed tomography; DA: dopamine; MET: metanephrines; MN: metanephrine; MRI: magnetic resonance imaging;
MTY: methoxytyramine; NMN: normetanephrine.

BOX 3	Optimal Conditions for Collection of Plasma Metanephrines/Catecholamines

- Patient should fast from midnight the previous evening.
- Patient should abstain from nicotine, alcohol, and vigorous exercise for 12 hours before collection.
- Establish intravenous access.
- Patient should lie supine in a quiet, dark room without distraction for 20–30 minutes before collection.

Differential Diagnosis

Referred to as the "great mimic," PHEO manifests with a myriad of signs and symptoms that are easily misconstrued for more common disorders, which often prevents a timely diagnosis. Consideration should be given to conditions that also result in sympathomedullary activation, including hyperadrenergic and renovascular hypertension,

panic disorders, menopausal syndrome, temporal lobe epilepsy, and other neuroendocrine tumors that release vasoactive substances. Patients with a presumptive diagnosis of PHEO should be screened biochemically. If results are unequivocal, a normal response to the clonidine suppression test will effectively rule out PHEO.

Biochemical Evaluation

PHEOs are capable of secreting all, none, or any combination of catecholamines—epinephrine, norepinephrine, and dopamine. Plasma metanephrines (the O-methylated metabolites of parent catecholamines) are the current gold standard for evaluating and therefore diagnosing or excluding PHEO. Twenty-four-hour urinary metanephrines are a comparable alternative when plasma is not available. Definitive diagnosis is likely when biochemical evaluation is greater than two times the upper reference limit (URL) (Figure 3). Diagnostic accuracy of plasma metanephrines is enhanced with age-specific URLs correcting for chronic kidney disease. To reliably interpret test results, specific conditions (Box 3) should be

TABLE 2	Diet- and Medication-Induced* Interference of Fractionated Plasma Metanephrines	
	MN	**NMN**
Diet		
Tomatoes, beans, coffee, cheese, wine, fermented foods	↑	↑
Medications		
TCA	-	↑↑
SNRI#	-	↑↑
MAOi##	↑↑	↑↑
Phenoxybenzamine	-	↑
Sympathomimetics+	-	↑↑
Labetalol	-	↑
Cocaine	-	↑↑
β-Adrenoceptor blocker	-	↑
Methyldopa/carbidopa	-	↑
Buspirone	↑↑	↑↑

*All increases are relative and depend on drug dose, duration of treatment, and quantity of food.
#Reported cases of SNRIs potentially leading to elevated NMN level.
##Also elevated MN and methoxytyramine.
+Pseudoephedrine, nicotine, amphetamines.
†Moderate elevation.
††Marked elevation.
Drug interference is not seen with mass spectrometry-based assays.
MAOi, Monoamine oxidase inhibitor; MN, metanephrine; NE, norepinephrine; NMN, normetanephrine; SNRI, selective serotonin reuptake inhibitor; SNRI, serotonin norepinephrine reuptake inhibitor; TCA, tricyclic antidepressants.

ensured throughout the blood draw. Additionally, there are a variety of foods and medications (Table 2) that interact either directly or indirectly with catecholamine measurement and should therefore be avoided for 12 hours before collection. Patients with acute or chronic kidney disease, particularly those on dialysis, commonly have elevated plasma metanephrines (although likely less than three to four times the URL of normal). If necessary, liquid chromatography with tandem mass spectrometry is a quick and cost-effective means to detect and remove potentially interfering substances.

Confirmatory follow-up testing is necessary in almost all cases of PHEO given (some) false-positive rate. Repeat plasma or urinary metanephrines and catecholamines, or the clonidine suppression test, can be used in equivocal cases, as secondary validation, especially in patients in whom interfering drugs cannot be stopped. Before clonidine suppression testing, patients should undergo a complete medication review with consideration to hold antihypertensives given the predilection for profound hypotension in response to clonidine. Additionally, diuretics, antidepressants, and adrenoceptor blockers have been reported to interfere with test results and should be held when appropriate. The patient should be fasting overnight and resting comfortably supine for 20 to 30 minutes before baseline blood draw. Clonidine (Catapres)[1] is administered at a dose of 0.3 mg per 70 kg, with appropriate dose adjustments as necessary (>0.5 mg based on weight), and subsequent repeat blood draw 3 hours after administration.

With an increasing proportion of hereditary PHEO, it is important to distinguish their various biochemical profiles, which can help guide genetic testing. In the last several years, the O-methylated metabolite of dopamine—methoxytyramine—has

[1] Not FDA approved for this indication.

been used to confirm head and neck PGLs, as 30% produce only dopamine and are therefore missed with standardized biochemical analysis. Furthermore, methoxytyramine has become a novel marker for metastatic PPGL, which can be used in conjunction with large tumor size, germline pathogenic variants (particularly SDHx), and the presence of extraadrenal PGLs to indicate a higher likelihood of metastatic disease.

Localization of Pheochromocytoma

Imaging should be pursued after clear biochemical evidence is confirmed. In rare instances, biochemically negative disease can be present. For optimal results, initial anatomic scans should consist of whole-body CT or MRI. T2-weighted MRI is preferred in patients in whom radiation exposure should be limited, those with a CT contrast allergy, and for the detection of skull-based lesions with the presence of known surgical clips. Ultrasound is not recommended for the localization of PHEO but may be used in children and during pregnancy if MRI is unavailable. Anatomic imaging is only sufficient for PHEO confirmation if the adrenal gland is the sole site of involvement (tumors <5 cm in size) and the metanephrine level is elevated—all other patients should proceed with functional imaging, which is also useful in ruling out metastatic disease.

Currently, there are four primary nuclear imaging techniques used to confirm or detect metastatic PPGL (iodine-123 metaiodobenzylguanidine [^{123}I-MIBG], gallium-68 DOTA(0)-Tyr(3)-octreotate [^{68}Ga-DOTATATE], fluorine-18-fluorodihydroxyphenylalanine [^{18}F-FDOPA], and fluorine-18-fluorodeoxyglucose [^{18}F-FDG]). Several algorithms (Figure 4) have been proposed based on tumor location, genetic predisposition, and presence of metastatic disease. While ^{18}F-FDG was previously preferred for comprehensive localization of metastatic disease, subsequent systematic reviews have reported the superiority of ^{68}Ga-DOTATATE in apparently sporadic, SDHx-related, and spinal bone metastatic PPGL. However, for other inherited PHEO (NFI, VHL, RET, MAX) or apparently sporadic PHEO, ^{18}F-FDOPA is the preferred positron emission tomography (PET) radiopharmaceutical. In 2020, copper-64-DOTATATE [^{64}Cu-DOTATATE] was FDA approved and has been found to be comparable to ^{68}Ga-DOTATATE in metastatic PPGL per preliminary results. Given the relatively novel status of ^{68}Ga/^{64}Cu-DOTATATE and ^{18}F-FDOPA, these modalities may not be available at a particular institution. In this case, physicians should proceed with traditional ^{18}F-FDG. The use of ^{123}I-MIBG scintigraphy should be limited to patients with known metastatic PHEO in the evaluation and eligibility for targeted radionuclide therapy with ^{131}I-MIBG.

Radiomics and Artificial Intelligence

With the increasing availability and use of imaging examinations, the number of subclinical pheochromocytomas discovered incidentally is also rising (e.g., detection bias). In such cases, it is necessary to follow established guidelines for the management of adrenal incidentalomas. Specifically, differential diagnosis must distinguish between lipid-poor adenomas, metastases, and carcinomas. Current guidelines recommend unenhanced CT, CT washout protocols, or chemical shift MRI as the primary morphologic imaging tools.

Within the last few years, artificial intelligence (AI), machine learning, and radiomics have emerged as promising tools in medical imaging. Radiomics is based on the computational processing of digital medical images, extracting parameters imperceptible to the human eye, which are then analyzed using machine learning or neural networks. The main advantage of radiomics lies in its ability to quantify intratumoral heterogeneity in a noninvasive, three-dimensional manner, under the theoretical assumption that radiomic features reflect biologic and genetic characteristics.

Most published studies on the use of radiomics in pheochromocytomas (PHEOs) focus on CT-based diagnostics to differentiate PHEOs from other adrenal tumors, particularly lipid-poor adenomas. Although these studies are typically based on smaller, retrospective cohorts, the results have been promising. A 2022

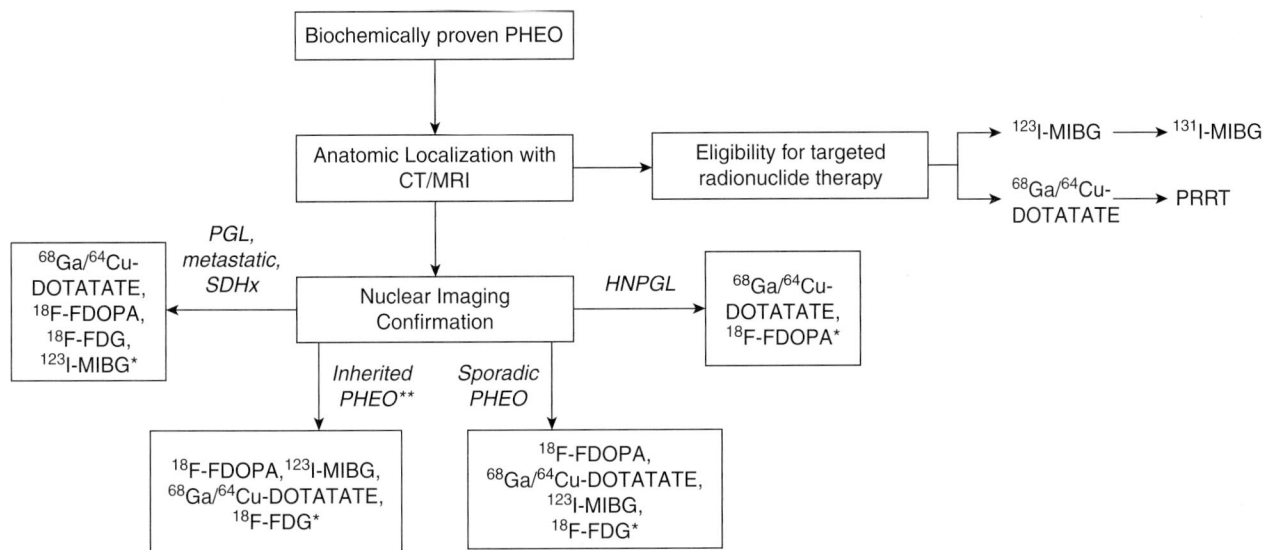

Figure 4 Imaging algorithm for pheochromocytoma localization. (Adapted from Taieb D, Hicks RJ, Hindie E, et al: European Association of Nuclear Medicine Practice Guidelines/Society of Nuclear Medicine and Molecular Imaging Procedure Standard 2019 for Radionuclide Imaging of Pheochromocytoma and Paraganglioma, *Eur J Nucl Med Mol Imaging* 46:2112–2137, 2019; and Taïeb D, Jha A, Treglia G, et al: Molecular imaging and radionuclide therapy of pheochromocytoma and paraganglioma in the era of genomic characterization of disease subgroups, *Endocr Relat Cancer* 26:R627–R652, 2019.)

meta-analysis reported a pooled sensitivity of 80% and specificity of 83% in distinguishing benign from malignant adrenal tumors.

Radiomics also holds potential for predicting various risks and treatment responses. In PHEO, it may help identify high-risk tumors, defined by a Pheochromocytoma of the Adrenal gland Scaled Score (PASS) of ≥4. One study achieved an 80% accuracy in identifying high-risk PHEOs; similar results were observed in a study predicting elevated Grading system for Adrenal Pheochromocytoma and Paraganglioma (GAPP) scores. Furthermore, radiomics has been explored for predicting the risk of metastasis, a concept previously studied in lung and colon cancers. A single study investigating metastatic risk in PHEO achieved an accuracy of 84%.

Additionally, radiomics has been applied to predict perioperative hemodynamic instability in PHEO. A published radiomic model predicted perioperative instability with an accuracy of 86%.

The term *radiogenomics* refers to the use of radiomics to predict genetic pathogenic variants. In the context of PHEO, this primarily involves predicting *SDHx* pathogenic variants. Several studies have used radiomics to identify *SDHx* pathogenic variant carriers using functional nuclear medicine imaging (particularly PET), as well as CT and MRI, with promising results.

However, it is important to acknowledge the challenges associated with radiomics and machine learning, including the quality of input data, lack of methodological standardization, and limited reproducibility. Further work is needed to translate these tools into clinical practice and integrate them into clinical decision support systems for predictive and prognostic purposes.

Treatment

The preferred, localized treatment for PHEO is surgical resection. Even in patients with metastatic disease or where complete excision is not feasible, debulking procedures may be favorable to reduce hormonal secretion and prevent anatomic complications. To ensure patient safety throughout the perioperative period, a multidisciplinary team should include a medical internist/endocrinologist, anesthesiologist, and surgeon, preferably in an experienced center (see "Perioperative Management" for details). For metastatic, systemic treatment options, see "Metastatic Pheochromocytoma."

Preoperative Medical Preparation

Surgical resection bears high perioperative risks and complications, which can be mitigated with appropriate α- and β-adrenoceptor blockade. Multiple case series have called into question the necessity of such medical management. However, the US Endocrine Society Clinical Practices guidelines recommend α-adrenoceptor blockade to ensure the protection of patients, secondary to prolonged circulating catecholamines. While patients are most at risk for a catecholamine and subsequent hypertensive crisis during induction of anesthesia and direct tumor manipulation, daily psychological and physical stressors are just as likely to result in a sudden release of catecholamines. Therefore it is imperative patients be adequately blocked even without a surgical plan.

At minimum, blood pressure should be treated preoperatively for 7 to 14 days barring extenuating circumstances (Figure 5). The most commonly used nonselective α-adrenoceptor blocker is phenoxybenzamine (Dibenzyline). However, this medication may be expensive, poorly covered by insurance, and is associated with nasal congestion, fatigue, and ejaculatory dysfunction—which may be rate limiting for patients. Selective α1-adrenoceptor blockers include doxazosin (Cardura), prazosin (Minipress), and terazosin (Hytrin). Selective adrenoceptor blockers have a shorter duration of action and are more likely to result in first-dose orthostatic hypotension, while the long-acting phenoxybenzamine is associated with postoperative hypotension. In low-risk, normotensive patients, calcium channel blockers and metyrosine (Demser) can be used if available within the institution.

If tachycardia ensues, cardioselective β1-adrenoceptor blockers, such as atenolol (Tenormin) or metoprolol (Lopressor), can be initiated 2 to 3 days after α-adrenoceptor administration. β-Adrenoceptor blockers *cannot* be given before initiation of an α-adrenoceptor blocker as unopposed antagonism can result in severe hypertensive crisis. In patients with persistent tachyarrhythmia, cardioselective calcium channel blockers (diltiazem [Cardizem] or verapamil [Isoptin]) and ivabradine (Corlanor) can be used; however, ivabradine is not approved by the FDA for this indication.

Perioperative Management

As stated previously, appropriate preoperative blockade is a necessity to ensure 24 hours of systolic blood pressure <140 mm

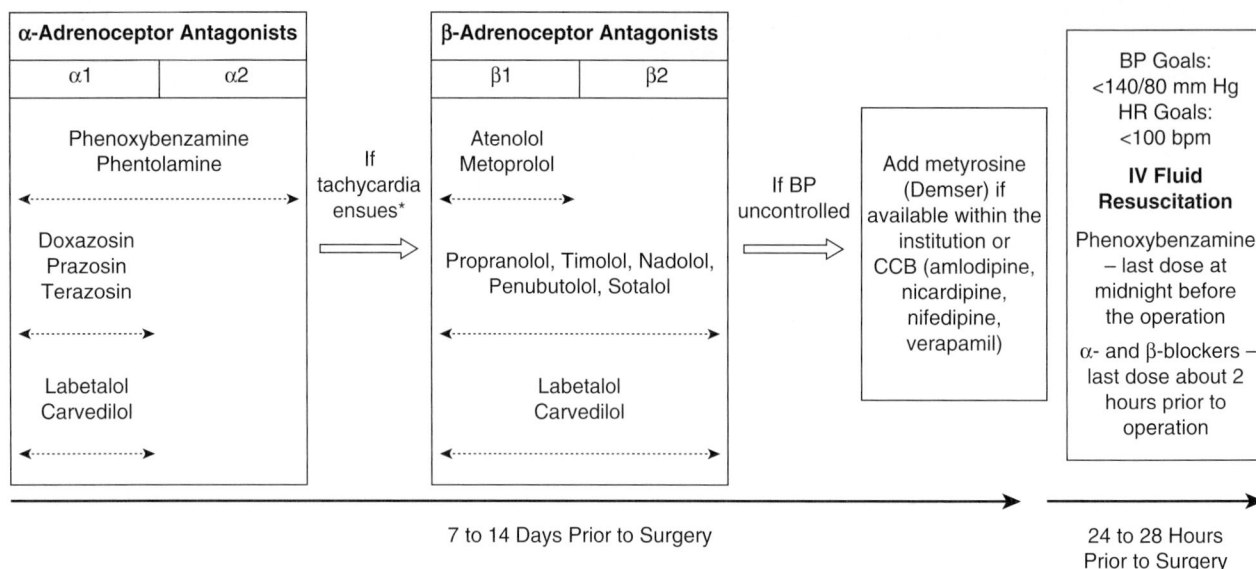

Figure 5 Preferred preoperative treatment regimen for pheochromocytoma. (Adapted from Wolf KI, Santos JRU, Pacak K: Why take the risk? We only live once: The dangers associated with neglecting a preoperative alpha adrenoceptor blockade in pheochromocytoma patients, *Endocr Pract* 25:106–108, 2019.)

Hg before surgery. Orthostatic hypotension is tolerated, but not <90/45 mm Hg. Immediately before surgical intervention, patients should receive 1 to 1.5 L of intravenous crystalloid. Notably, despite blockade, about 70% of patients experience hemodynamic instability (either hypertension or hypotension), which is often associated with or due to a longer duration of preoperative treatment with an α-adrenoceptor blocking agent, elevated urinary epinephrine levels, and greater preoperative heart rate. Operative approach should be decided on an individual basis by the surgeon. When appropriate and feasible, small, nonmetastatic PHEOs and retroperitoneal PGLs should be surgically excised with a minimally invasive technique. Locoregional invasion is difficult to assess preoperatively; therefore suspected cases should initially be explored by laparoscopy with conversion to an open procedure in the face of critical adhesions. In non–SDHB-related bilateral PHEOs, an adrenocortical sparing procedure is recommended to avoid permanent glucocorticoid deficiency.

Intraoperatively, direct communication between the surgeon and anesthesiologist—particularly during tumor manipulation and excision—is imperative to minimize hemodynamic fluctuations secondary to massive catecholamine release or pharmacotherapy. Careful and continued monitoring of postoperative hemodynamic stability is crucial. Common complications include hypertension, hypotension, arrhythmias, adrenocortical insufficiency, and hypoglycemia. Within the immediate (first 24 hours) postoperative period, transient hypertension is likely attributable to pain, volume overload, or autonomic instability, which should be treated symptomatically. However, persistent hypertension should be concerning for incomplete tumor resection, metastatic disease, excess fluid administration, or underlying essential hypertension. Recommended first-line management is with short-acting, easily titratable agents, such as nicardipine (Cardene) or labetalol (Trandate). Attempts to repeat plasma/urinary metanephrine levels to assess for residual disease burden should be delayed for 5 to 7 days after surgery to ensure resolution of operative catecholamine spikes. In a postoperative hypotensive (SBP <90 mm Hg) patient, hemorrhage should be excluded before deliberating a differential. Alternative etiologies include prolonged adrenoceptor blockade action, abrupt cessation of serum catecholamines, chronically low circulating plasma volume, or blood loss. The primary treatment modality is fluid resuscitation or blood transfusion, if needed. Vasopressors should be used sparingly, especially when metyrosine or long-acting β-adrenoceptor blockers were used preoperatively.

Postoperative tachyarrhythmias (>100 beats/min) may be a reflex response in patients with postoperative hypotension or the result of continued catecholamine release, while bradyarrhythmias (<60 beats/min) are due to a variety of concerns. For persistent abnormal rhythms, expert evaluation is recommended. If adrenal insufficiency is expected postoperatively, patients should receive 50 to 100 mg hydrocortisone (Cortef) before induction, followed by 25 to 50 mg every 8 hours thereafter. Barring any postoperative complications, transition to an oral steroid regimen 24 to 48 hours after surgery (glucocorticoid and mineralocorticoid) and provide appropriate education on adrenal crisis, emergency bracelets, and dosage adjustments in times of sickness. In the absence of catecholamine excess, upregulated liver glycogenolysis and inhibition of insulin secretion may cease, leading to postoperative hypoglycemia. Importantly, the classic signs and symptoms may be masked in the immediate postoperative period and should be routinely monitored for the first 24 hours after surgery.

Hypertensive Crisis

The most dangerous PHEO-related complication, a catecholamine-induced hypertensive crisis, can manifest with a severe headache, visual disturbances, myocardial infarction, congestive heart failure, or a cerebrovascular accident. Immediate treatment with 5-mg intravenous boluses of phentolamine (Regitine)—a short-acting, reversible, nonselective α-adrenoceptor agonist—should be repeated every 2 minutes until hypertension is adequately controlled (or initiate a continuous infusion). Phentolamine may be unavailable; thus continuous infusions of nicardipine (Cardene), sodium nitroprusside (Nitropress), or verapamil can be used with appropriate dose de-escalation upon the resolution of hypertension and subsequent symptoms related to the crisis (Figure 6). Belzutifan (Welireg)[1], a novel HIF-2α inhibitor, may be particularly effective in treating hypertension in *HIF2A*-mediated PGL.

The treatment of hypertension may be complicated by hypotension, which often corrects with administration of approximately 1 L of intravenous crystalloid. If hypotension persists, consider potential catecholamine-induced cardiomyopathy and obtain an echocardiogram. In cases of severe persistent hypotension, catecholaminergic vasopressors (e.g., norepinephrine infusion) may be less effective, with arginine vasopressin being more effective.

---

[1] Not FDA approved for this indication.

Management of a CIHC

Either algorithm can be chosen considering provider preference and practical implementation given clinical setting and agent availability

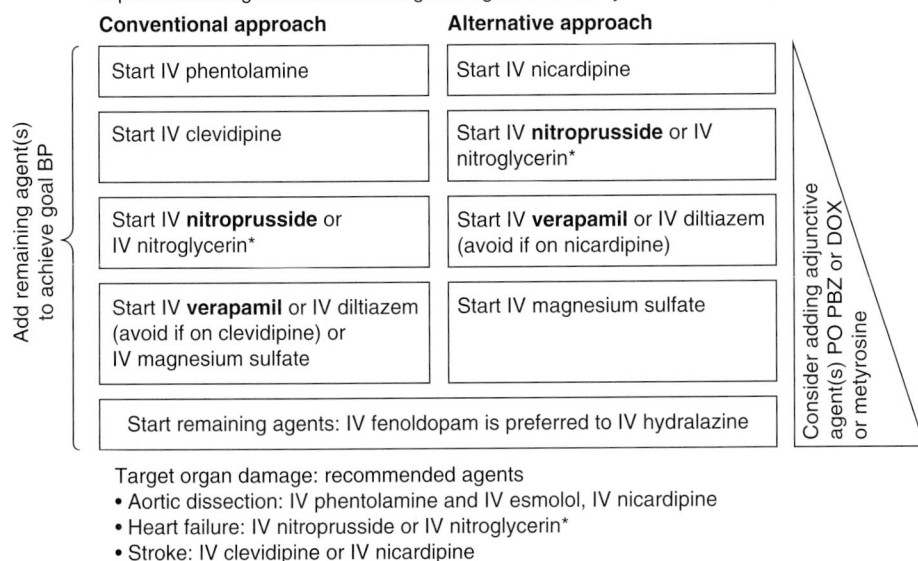

Conventional approach

Start IV phentolamine
Start IV clevidipine
Start IV **nitroprusside** or IV nitroglycerin*
Start IV **verapamil** or IV diltiazem (avoid if on clevidipine) or IV magnesium sulfate
Start remaining agents: IV fenoldopam is preferred to IV hydralazine

Add remaining agent(s) to achieve goal BP

Alternative approach

Start IV nicardipine
Start IV **nitroprusside** or IV nitroglycerin*
Start IV **verapamil** or IV diltiazem (avoid if on nicardipine)
Start IV magnesium sulfate

Consider adding adjunctive agent(s) PO PBZ or DOX or metyrosine

Target organ damage: recommended agents
• Aortic dissection: IV phentolamine and IV esmolol, IV nicardipine
• Heart failure: IV nitroprusside or IV nitroglycerin*
• Stroke: IV clevidipine or IV nicardipine

Figure 6 Management of a catecholamine-induced hypertensive crisis and target organ damage. *Avoid nitrates in preload-dependent states or with concomitant use of phosphodiesterase inhibitors. *BP*, Blood pressure; *CIHC*, catecholamine-induced hypertensive crisis; *DOX*, doxazosin; *IV*, intravenous; *PBZ*, phenoxybenzamine; *PO*, oral. (Adapted from Nazari MA, Hasan R, Haigney M, et al: Catecholamine-induced hypertensive crises: current insights and management, *Lancet Diabetes Endocrinol* 11[12]:942–954, 2023.)

Mechanical circulatory support and extracorporeal membrane oxygenation should be considered early in cases of refractory shock as prognosis is often quite favorable (up to 95% survival).

Metastatic Pheochromocytoma

According to the 2022 WHO report, metastatic PHEO is only established by the presence of chromaffin cells where they are normally absent. PHEO metastasizes via a hematogenous or lymphatic route with the bones and lymph nodes considered the only definitive sites of metastasis. However, in 2024, primary bone PGL arising from the maxillary bone was reported. While the bones, lungs, and liver are also common sites of metastasis, they may also be sites of primary tumor development. Now, almost half of patients with metastatic PHEO present within 1 year of initial diagnosis, while >70% of patients will develop metastatic disease within 5 years of their primary diagnosis. At the time of primary tumor resection, over 75% of metastatic PHEO patients have a tumor >5 cm, with one study reporting a median tumor diameter of 7.0 cm. From a genetic perspective, around half of all patients with metastatic disease do not express a germline pathogenic variant and are apparently sporadic; however, of the remaining 50%, anywhere from 10% to 42% have been associated with *SDHB*-related disease. Biochemically, markedly elevated norepinephrine and/or dopamine/methoxytyramine are associated with the presence of metastases, especially in patients with *SDHx*-related disease, and can be used to monitor disease progression. Current publications indicate that the 5-year overall survival ranges from 62% to 85%, while the median overall survival varies between 6 and 24 years. Location and type of tumor also indicate a higher likelihood of malignancy, with extraadrenal PGLs the most worrisome for metastatic disease. Meanwhile, head and neck PGLs were associated with improved prognosis and very rarely reported cases of rapidly progressive disease.

Management of metastatic PPGL (Figure 7) requires a multidisciplinary approach, consisting of targeted pharmacology, radiotherapy, chemotherapy, and surgery. Surgical debulking procedures continue to be the mainstay of palliative treatment. Delaying any procedures is positively correlated with rapidly progressive metastatic disease and should be avoided whenever possible. Chemotherapy with CVD[1] (cyclophosphamide [Cytoxan][1], vincristine [Oncovin][1], and dacarbazine [DTIC-Dome][1]) is the primary therapeutic modality in patients with rapidly progressive (within 3–6 months) PHEO. While only 30% of the metastatic PHEO population exhibits clinical benefit, the reported advantages in *SDHB*-related disease is as high as 80%. Temozolomide (TMZ [Temodar])[1] is the only other chemotherapeutic agent with significant experience in PHEO patients. In 2024, FIRSTMAPPP, a phase 2 prospective, multicentric, double-blinded, randomized, placebo-controlled trial reported the efficacy of a tyrosine kinase inhibitor (sunitinib [Sutent])[1] in 78 progressive patients (39 in each arm), with 32% of patients carrying a germline *SDHx* pathogenic variant, who had a median follow-up of 29.7 months. A median progression-free survival (PFS) of 8.9 months was reported in patients taking sunitinib (vs. 3.6 months in the placebo group) with a 12-month PFS of 36% (vs. 19% in the placebo group) and an objective response rate of 36.1% (vs. 8.3% in the placebo group). Three deaths were reported in the sunitinib group versus two deaths in the placebo group, with only one death found to be drug-related. The most common grade 3 or 4 adverse events were asthenia (18% vs. 3%), hypertension (13% vs. 10%), and back and bone pain (3% vs. 8%) in the sunitinib and placebo groups, respectively. Thus in patients who progress despite CVD[1] chemotherapy, TMZ[1] or sunitib[1] may be attempted.

Emerging targeted therapies include adjunctive olaparib (Lynparza)[1] in combination with TMZ[1], belzutifan (Welireg)[1] in patients with a causative *HIF2A* pathogenic variant, tyrosine kinase inhibitors (cabozantinib [Cabometyx][1] or anlotinib [Fukewei][5]), and various immunotherapies (including chimeric antigen receptor–expressing T cells or CAR-T-cell therapy).

For patients with slow to moderate progression, eligibility for targeted radionuclide therapy should be considered with ^{131}I-MIBG and peptide receptor radionuclide therapy (PRRT) if they have avid disease on ^{123}I-MIBG and ^{68}Ga/^{64}Cu-DOTATATE, respectively. Targeted radiotherapy with low-specific activity ^{131}I-MIBG should be considered for patients with avidity on ^{123}I-MIBG scintigraphy. Notably, high-specific-activity ^{131}I-MIBG (Azedra) was discontinued in 2024. In a meta-analysis of 243 pooled patients treated with 1 to 12 cycles of low-specific-activity ^{131}I-MIBG using various doses and regimens, 82% of patients achieved a complete partial response or (PR)/stable disease (SD). In contrast, 92% of patients treated with high-specific-activity ^{131}I-MIBG had a PR/SD. Thus low-specific-activity ^{131}I-MIBG remains an

---

[1] Not FDA approved for this indication.

[1] Not FDA approved for this indication.
[5] Investigational drug in the United States.

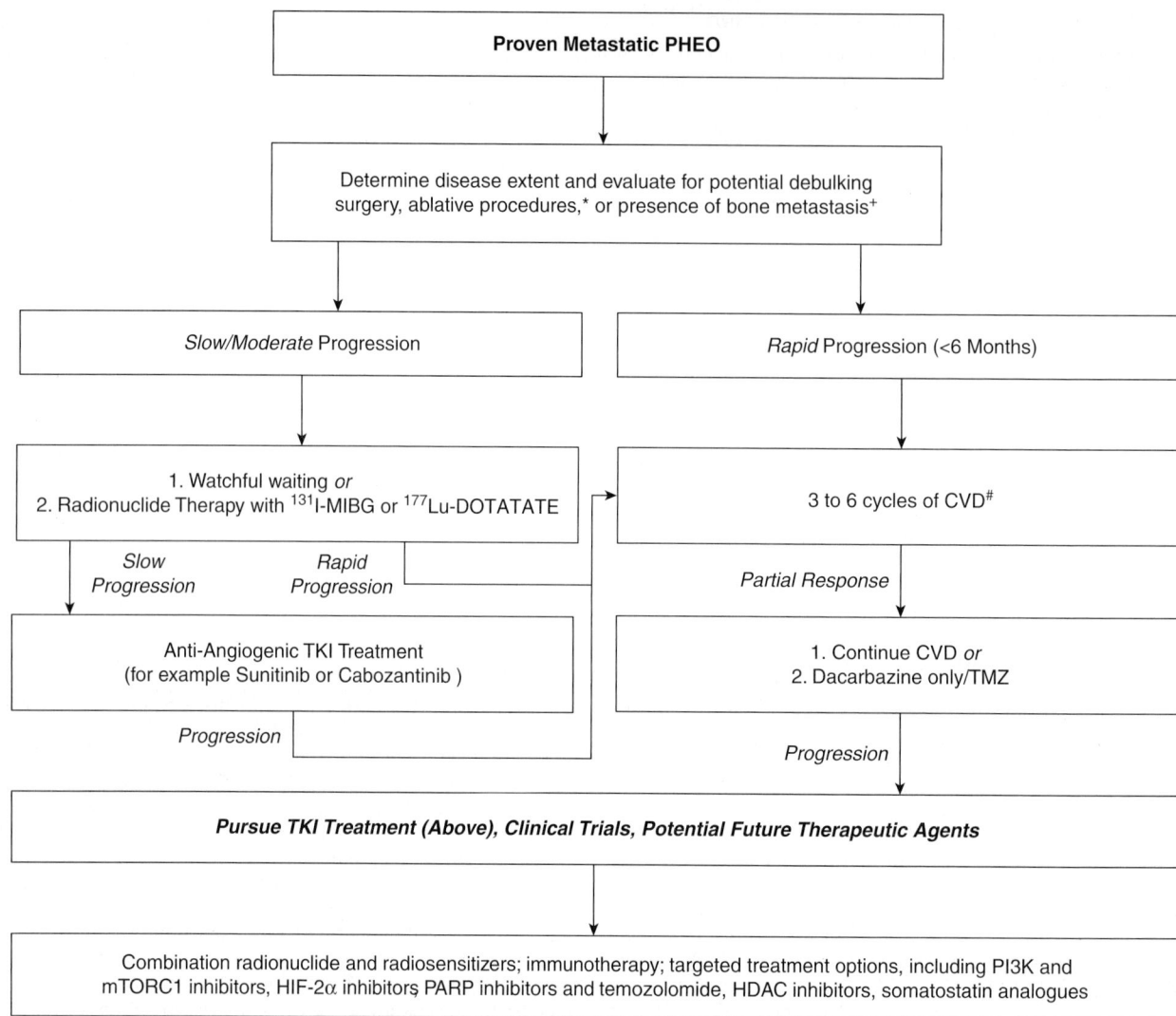

Figure 7 Treatment algorithm for metastatic pheochromocytoma/paraganglioma. (Adapted from Nölting S, Ullrich M, Pietzsch J, et al: Current management of pheochromocytoma/paraganglioma: A guide for the practicing clinician in the era of precision medicine, *Cancers (Basel)* 11:1505, 2019.)

appropriate treatment strategy for metastatic patients. PRRT with lutetium-177/yttrium-90/actinium-225-DOTATATE/DOTATOC (^{177}Lu/^{90}Y/^{225}Ac-DOTATATE/TOC)[1] has been used to treat patients with metastatic or inoperable PPGL[1]. In a meta-analysis of 179 pooled patients treated with 1 to 11 cycles of PRRT using various dose regimens and radiopharmaceuticals, 90% of patients had achieved PR or SD. However, currently, lutetium-177 DOTATATE (^{177}Lu-DOTATATE, Lutathera) is not approved by the FDA for metastatic PPGL in the United States. An ongoing clinical trial with ^{177}Lu-DOTATATE (NCT03206060) released its interim analysis results in 36 (18 each with *SDHx* and apparently sporadic) patients. The progression-free survival at 6 months after the initiation of ^{177}Lu-DOTATATE was 19.1 months, with a duration of 22.7 months in the apparently sporadic cohort and 15.4 months in the *SDHx* cohort. Overall survival was not reached in either cohort. According to RECIST 1.1 criteria, 86.1% of patients exhibited a partial response or stable disease, in contrast to 72.2% of patients with *SDHx* pathogenic variants. The most common severe adverse events were hematologic, occurring in 5% to 10% of cases. In 2021, a study in 9 metastatic PGL patients (7 of whom had previously received ^{177}Lu-DOTATATE, with 3 of these 7 having failed prior treatment) examined the efficacy of ^{225}Ac-DOTATATE (an α-particle–based radiotherapy) along with concomitant capecitabine. The results showed a high

partial response rate of 50% and stable disease in 37.5%, leading to a disease control rate of 87.5%. Importantly, there were no instances of grade 3/4 hematotoxicity, nephrotoxicity, or hepatotoxicity. These findings demonstrate that α-particle–based targeted radiotherapy is both safe and effective in treating metastatic PGLs, providing a viable alternative for patients who are refractory to ^{177}Lu-DOTATATE.

In May 2025, belzutifan, a HIF-2a inhibitor, was FDA approved for the treatment of locally advanced, unresectable, or metastatic PPGL. There are several up-and-coming novel therapeutic agents that will hopefully be approved for treatment of metastatic PPGL after further validation, including alternative HIF-2α, mTOR, and P13K inhibitors, as well as cold somatostatin analogs (octreotide[1] and lanreotide[1]) and immunotherapy.

Prognosis and Monitoring

The long-term survival of patients after surgical excision of a solitary PHEO without evidence of metastasis is the same as age-adjusted normal subjects. A longitudinal follow-up study determined that recurrences are more likely in patients with extraadrenal PGLs and those with germline pathogenic variants. After treatment, 25% of patients continue to have well-controlled hypertension on oral medications. Periodic, lifelong biochemical and/or imaging surveillance is required for all patients, but especially for those with an underlying hereditary disorder. Beware that patients with predominant and persistent elevations in normetanephrine often develop atherosclerosis, while patients with predominant and persistent elevations in metanephrine suffer from cardiomyopathies and arrhythmias. Thus appropriate evaluation by a cardiologist with risk-reductive therapies (e.g., antihyperlipidemic agents) may be prudent. Frequency of follow-up depends on the surgical pathology, presentation at diagnosis, and biochemical profile. Patients with metastatic disease should have routine, scheduled observation with a specialist to ensure proper care.

References

Aggarwal A, et al: Clinical implications of incidentally discovered pheochromocytomas, *J Clin Endocrinol Metab* 108(9):e1421–e1430, 2023.

Al Subhi AR, Boyle V, Elston MS: Systematic review: incidence of pheochromocytoma and paraganglioma over 70 years, *J Endocr Soc* 6, 2022:bvac105.

Alkaissi H, Nazari MA, Hadrava Vanova K, et al: Rapid cardiovascular response to belzutifan in *hif2a*-mediated paraganglioma, *N Engl J Med* 39:1552–1555, 2024.

Alkaissi H, Pacak K: A targetable receptor tyrosine kinase in metastatic pheochromocytoma and paraganglioma: a future journey for anlotinib? *J Endocr Soc* 8, 2024:bvae092.

Amar L, Pacak K, Steichen O, et al: International consensus on initial screening and follow-up of asymptomatic SDHx mutation carriers, *Nat Rev Endocrinol* 17:435–444, 2021.

Baudin E, Goichot B, Berruti A, et al: Sunitinib for metastatic progressive phaeochromocytomas and paragangliomas: results from FIRSTMAPPP, an academic, multicentre, international, randomised, placebo-controlled, double-blind, phase 2 trial, *Lancet* 403:1061–1070, 2024.

Berends AMA, Buitenwerf E, de Krijger RR, et al: Incidence of pheochromocytoma and sympathetic paraganglioma in the Netherlands: a nationwide study and systematic review, *Eur J Intern Med* 51:68–73, 2018.

Bjorklund P, Pacak K, Crona J: Precision medicine in pheochromocytoma and paraganglioma: current and future concepts, *J Intern Med* 280:559–573, 2016.

Carrasquillo JA, Chen CC, Jha A, et al: Imaging of pheochromocytoma and paraganglioma, *J Nucl Med* 62:1033–1042, 2021.

Carrasquillo JA, Chen CC, Jha A, et al: Systemic radiopharmaceutical therapy of pheochromocytoma and paraganglioma, *J Nucl Med* 62:1192–1199, 2021.

Chuki E, Saleh Anaraki K, Jha A, et al: Primary paraganglioma arising from the maxillary bone, *JCEM Case Reports* 2:luae18, 2024.

Crona J, Lamarca A, Ghosal S, et al: Genotype-phenotype correlations in pheochromocytoma and paraganglioma: a systematic review and individual patient meta-analysis, *Endocr Related Cancer* 26:539–550, 2019.

Crona J, Taïeb D, Pacak K: New perspectives on pheochromocytoma and paraganglioma: toward a molecular classification, *Endocr Rev* 38:489–515, 2017.

Darr R, Kuhn M, Bode C, et al: Accuracy of recommended sampling and assay methods for the determination of plasma-free and urinary fractionated metanephrines in the diagnosis of pheochromocytoma and paraganglioma: a systematic review, *Endocrine* 56:495–503, 2017.

Dmitriev PM, Wang H, Rosenblum JS, et al: Vascular changes in the retina and choroid of patients with epas1 gain-of-function mutation syndrome, *JAMA Opthalmol* 138:148–155, 2020.

Eisenhofer G, Pamporaki C, Lenders JWM: Biochemical assessment of pheochromocytoma and paraganglioma, *Endocr Rev* 44:862–909, 2023.

Else T, Marvin ML, Everett JN, et al: The clinical phenotype of SDHC-associated hereditary paraganglioma syndrome (PGL3), *J Clin Endocrinol Metab* 99:E1482–E1486, 2014.

Fassnacht M, et al: Management of adrenal incidentalomas: European Society of Endocrinology Clinical Practice Guideline, *Eur J Endocrinol* 188(5):G1–G26, 2023.

Fu H, et al: A radiomic approach to predict perioperative instability in pheochromocytoma, *J Clin Endocrinol Metab* 109(3):e1125–e1132, 2024.

Geroula A, Deutschbein T, Langton K, et al: Pheochromocytoma and paraganglioma: clinical feature-based disease probability in relation to catecholamine biochemistry and reason for disease suspicion, *Eur J Endocrinol* 181:409–420, 2019.

Gupta G, Pacak K: Precision medicine: an update on genotype/biochemical phenotype relationships in pheochromocytoma/paraganglioma patients, *Endoc Pract* 23:690–704, 2017.

Hadrava Vanova K, Pang Y, et al: Germline SUCLG2 variants in patients with pheochromocytoma and paraganglioma, *J Natl Cancer Inst* 114:130–138, 2022.

Hamidi O, Young Jr WR, Iniguez-Ariza NM, et al: Malignant pheochromocytoma and paraganglioma: 272 patients over 55 years, *J Clin Endocrinol Metab* 102:3296–3305, 2017.

Hescot S, Curras-Freixas M, Deutschbein T, et al: Prognosis of malignant pheochromocytoma and paraganglioma (MAPP-Prono Study): a European network for the study of adrenal tumors retrospective study, *J Clin Endocrinol Metab* 104:2367–2374, 2019.

Ilanchezhian M, Jha A, Pacak K, et al: Emerging treatments for advanced/metastatic pheochromocytoma and paraganglioma, *Curr Treat Options Oncol* 21(85), 2020.

Jha A, de Luna K, Balili Ca, et al: Clinical, diagnostic, and treatment characteristics of *SDHA-related* metastatic pheochromocytoma and paraganglioma, *Front Oncol* 22:53, 2019.

Jha A, Patel M, Ling A, et al: Diagnostic performance of 68Ga-DOTATATE PET/CT, 18F-FDG PET/CT, MRI of the spine, and whole-body diagnostic CT and MRI in the detection of spinal bone metastases associated with pheochromocytoma and paraganglioma, *Eurol Radiol* 34:6488–6498, 2024.

Jha A, Patel M, Carrasquillo JA, et al: Choice is good at times: the emergence of [64Cu]Cu-DOTATATE-based somatostatin receptor imaging in the era of [68Ga]Ga-DOTATATE, *J Nucl Med* 63:1300–1301, 2022.

Jha A, Patel M, Carrasquillo JA, et al: Sporadic primary pheochromocytoma: a prospective intraindividual comparison on six imaging tests (CT, MRI, and PET/CT using 68Ga-DOTATATE, 18F-FDG, 18F-FDOPA, and 18F-FDA), *AJR Am J Roentgenol* 218:342–350, 2022.

Jha A, Taïeb D, Carrasquillo JA, et al: High-specific-activity 131I-MIBG vs 177Lu-DOTATATE therapy: an evolving conundrum in targeted radionuclide therapy of metastatic pheochromocytoma and paraganglioma, *Clin Cancer Res* 27:2989–2995, 2021.

Jochmanova I, Pacak K: Genomic landscape of pheochromocytoma and paraganglioma, *Trends Cancer* 4:6–9, 2018.

Jochmanova I, Wolf KI, King KS, et al: SDHB-related pheochromocytoma and paraganglioma penetrance and genotype-phenotype correlations, *J Cancer Res Clin Oncol* 143:1421–1435, 2017.

Karasek D, Shah U, Frysak Z, et al: An update on the genetics of pheochromocytoma, *J Hum Hypertens* 27:141–147, 2013.

Kim JH, Lee HC, Kim SJ, et al: Perioperative hemodynamic instability in pheochromocytoma and sympathetic paraganglioma patients, *Sci Rep* 11, 2021.

Kunst HP, Rutten MH, de Mönnink JP, et al: SDHAF2 (PGL2-SDH5) and hereditary head and neck paraganglioma, *Clin Cancer Res* 17:247–254, 2011.

Lahlou-Laforet K, Consoli SM, Jeunemaitre X, et al: Presymptomatic genetic testing in minors at risk of paraganglioma and pheochromocytoma: our experience of oncogenetic multidisciplinary consultation, *Horm Metab Res* 44:354–358, 2012.

Lambin P, et al: Radiomics: the bridge between medical imaging and personalized medicine, *Nat Rev Clin Oncol* 14(12):749–762, 2017.

Lang F, Jha A, Meuter L, et al: Identification of isocitrate dehydrogenase 2 (*IDH2*) mutation in carotid body paraganglioma, *Front Endocrinol (Lausanne)* 20, 2021:731096.

Lenders JW, Duh QY, Eisenhofer G, et al: Pheochromocytoma and paraganglioma: an endocrine society clinical practice guideline, *J Clin Endocrinol Metab* 99:1915–1942, 2014.

Lenders JW, Eisenhofer G, Mannelli M, Pacak K: Phaeochromocytoma, *Lancet* 366(9486):665–675, 2005.

Lin F, Carrasquillo J, del Rivero J, et al: Safety and efficacy of Lu-177-DOTATATE in metastatic or inoperable pheochromocytoma/paraganglioma—an interim analysis, *J Nucl Med* 64(Suppl 1), 2023:P1296.

Mamilla D, Araque KA, Brofferio A, et al: Postoperative management in patients with pheochromocytoma and paraganglioma, *Cancers* 11:936, 2019.

Mayo-Smith WW, et al: ACR appropriateness criteria adrenal incidentaloma, *J Am Coll Radiol* 14(5S):S190–S195, 2017.

Muth A, Crona J, Gimm O, et al: Genetic testing and surveillance guidelines in hereditary pheochromocytoma and paraganglioma, *J Intern Med* 285:187–204, 2019.

Nazari MA, Hasan R, Haigney M, et al: Catecholamine-induced hypertensive crises: current insights and management, *Lancet Diabetes Endocrinol* 11:942–954, 2023, Erratum in: Lancet Diabetes Endocrinol. 12:e1, 2024.

Nazari MA, Rosenblum JS, Haigney MC, et al: Pathophysiology and acute management of tachyarrhythmias in pheochromocytoma: JACC review topic of the week, *J Am Coll Cardiol* 76:451–464, 2020.

Neumann HP, Bausch B, McWhinney SR, et al: Germ-line mutations in nonsyndromic pheochromocytoma, *N Engl J Med* 346:1459–1466, 2002.

Nölting S, Ullrich M, Pierzsch J, et al: Current management of pheochromocytoma/paraganglioma: a guide for the practicing clinician in the era of precision medicine, *Cancers (Basel)* 11:1505, 2019.

Nölting S, Bechmann N, Taïeb D, et al: Personalized management of pheochromocytoma and paraganglioma, *Endocr Rev* 43:199–239, 2022.

Pacak K: New biology of pheochromocytoma and paraganglioma, *Endocr Pract* 28:1253–1269, 2022.

Pacak K: Preoperative management of the pheochromocytoma patient, *J Clin Endocrinol Metab* 92:4069–4079, 2007.

Pacak K, Eisenhofer G, Carrasquillo JA, et al: Diagnostic localization of pheochromocytoma: the coming of age of positron emission tomography, *Ann N Y Acad Sci* 970:170–176, 2002.

Pacak K, Taïeb D, Lin FI, et al: Approach to the patient: concept and application of targeted radiotherapy in the paraganglioma patient, *J Clin Endocrinol Metab* 109:2366–2388, 2024.

Pamporaki C, Prejbisz A, Małecki R, et al: Optimized reference intervals for plasma free metanephrines in patients with CKD, *Am J Kidney Dis* 72:907–909, 2018.

Pamporaki C, Prodanov T, Meuter L, et al: Determinants of disease-specific survival in patients with and without metastatic pheochromocytoma and paraganglioma, *Eur J Cancer* 169:32–41, 2022.

Pang Y, Liu Y, Pacak K, Yang C: Pheochromocytomas and paragangliomas: from genetic diversity to targeted therapies, *Cancers* 11:436, 2019.

Patel M, Jha A, Ling A, et al: Performances of functional and anatomic imaging modalities in *succinate dehydrogenase a*-related metastatic pheochromocytoma and paraganglioma, *Cancers* 14:3886, 2022.

Patel M, Jha A, Ling A, et al: Performances of modalities in succinate dehydrogenase A- related metastatic pheochromocytoma and paraganglioma, *Cancers* 14:3886, 2022.

Petrák O, Krátká Z, Holaj R, Zítek M, et al: Cardiovascular complications in pheochromocytoma and paraganglioma: does phenotype matter? *Hypertension* 81:595–603, 2024.

Rao D, Peitzsch M, Prejbisz A, et al: Plasma methoxytyramine: clinical utility with metanephrines for diagnosis of pheochromocytoma and paraganglioma, *Eur J Endocrinol* 177:103–113, 2017.

Shintaro I, Tsukasa Y, Takeshi I, Multicentric giant cell tumor of bone and paraganglioma: a case report, *JBJS Case Connect* 3(1):e23, 2013.

Taieb D, Hicks RJ, Hindie E, et al: European association of nuclear medicine practice guideline/society of nuclear medicine and molecular imaging procedure standard 2019 for radionuclide imaging of pheochromocytoma and paraganglioma, *Eur J Nucl Mol Imaging* 46:2112–2137, 2019.

Taieb D, Jha A, Treglia G, Pacak K: Molecular imaging and radionuclide therapy of pheochromocytoma and paraganglioma in the era of genomic characterization of disease subgroups, *Endocr Related Cancer* 26:R627–R652, 2019.

Taïeb D, Wanna GB, Ahmad M, et al: Clinical consensus guideline on the management of phaeochromocytoma and paraganglioma in patients harbouring germline *SDHD* pathogenic variants, *Lancet Diabetes Endocrinol* 11:345–361, 2023.

Taieb D, Wanna GB, Ahmad M, et al: Clinical guideline on the management of phaeochromocytoma and paraganglioma in patients harboring germline *SDHB* pathogenic variants, *Nat Rev Endocrinol* 20:168–184, 2024.

Tella S, Jha A, Taieb D, et al: A comprehensive review of evaluation and management of cardiac paragangliomas, *Heart* 106:1202–1210, 2020.

Toledo RA, Qin Y, Cheng ZM, et al: Recurrent mutations of chromatin-remodeling genes and kinase receptors in pheochromocytomas and paragangliomas, *Clin Cancer Res* 22:2301–2310, 2016.

Tüdös Z, et al: Radiomics and artificial intelligence in adrenal imaging, *Best Pract Res Clin Endocrinol Metab* 39(1), 2025:101923.

Wang K, Crona J, Beuschlein F, et al: Targeted therapies in pheochromocytoma and paraganglioma, *J Clin Endocrinol Metab* 107:2963–2972, 2022.

Wolf KI, Santos JRU, Pacak K: Why take the risk? We only live once: the dangers associated with neglecting a pre-operative alpha adrenoceptor blockade in pheochromocytoma patients, *Endocr Pract* 25:106–108, 2019.

Yadav MP, Ballal S, Sahoo RK, Bal C. Efficacy and safety of 225Ac-DOTATATE targeted alpha therapy in metastatic paragangliomas: a pilot study, *Eur J Nucl Med Mol Imaging* 49(5):1595–1606, 2022.

Zhang M, et al: Diagnostic accuracy of radiomics in distinguishing adrenal lesions: a meta-analysis, *Front Oncol* 12, 2022:975183.

Zhou F, et al: Predicting metastatic risk in pheochromocytoma using radiomics, *Acad Radiol* 31(1):11–18, 2024.

THYROID CANCER

Method of
Michael Holyoak, DO; Teresa Sciortino, MD; and Rudruidee Karnchanasorn, MD

CURRENT DIAGNOSIS

- Most thyroid cancer will present as incidentally discovered thyroid nodules.
- The vast majority of thyroid nodules are benign, and risk of malignancy can be reliably estimated based on sonographic features.
- Thyroid function should always be assessed if a nodule is discovered. If thyroid stimulating hormone is low, a thyroid uptake and scan should be obtained.
- The American Thyroid Association and the American College of Radiology's Thyroid Imaging Reporting and Data System uses ultrasound features to determine risk of malignancy and the need for fine needle aspiration (FNA).
- Approximately 90% to 95% of thyroid nodules are benign and can be monitored with serial ultrasound. FNA is only indicated for nodules equal to or greater than 1 cm.
- Benign nodules can be monitored with ultrasound at intervals based on their risk of malignancy.
- The vast majority of thyroid cancer is classified as differentiated thyroid cancer. Medullary thyroid cancer is less common and somewhat more aggressive. Anaplastic thyroid cancer is a rare and very aggressive thyroid cancer that typically presents at a more advanced stage.

CURRENT THERAPY

- Although thyroid cancer is relatively common, it is responsible for a very small portion of cancer-related mortality.
- Some experts have expressed concern about potentially unnecessary morbidity associated with overtreatment of very low risk differentiated thyroid cancers (DTCs), particularly micropapillary carcinoma.
- Most patients with thyroid cancer should be managed surgically. Smaller, lower risk differentiated cancers can be treated with lobectomy. Larger or higher-risk tumors should be treated with total thyroidectomy and compartment neck dissections based on the presence of lymphadenopathy.
- Radioactive iodine should be used based on the American Thyroid Association (ATA) risk stratification.
- Patients with DTC should be monitored longitudinally using serum thyroglobulin levels and serial ultrasound.
- Thyroid stimulating hormone suppression is indicated for many patients postoperatively, initially based on their ATA risk and later on their response to therapy.
- Patients with medullary thyroid cancer should undergo surgery and be monitored with serial carcinoembryonic antigen and calcitonin levels in addition to imaging studies.
- Patients with anaplastic thyroid cancer typically require aggressive surgery, often including tracheostomy and management by a multidisciplinary team.

Epidemiology

Thyroid nodules are highly prevalent. Data show that approximately 5% to 10% of patients will have palpable nodules, and approximately 34% of patients will have nodules detectable by ultrasound. The prevalence of nodules increases significantly with age, and they are three to four times more common in women. Only a small portion of thyroid nodules (about 5% to 15%) are malignant. From the early 1980s to mid-2010s, the incidence of thyroid cancer rapidly increased before reaching a plateau and subsequent decline beginning in the late 2010s. Despite the near tripling of new diagnoses during this time period, thyroid cancer mortality has remained relatively low, as the upward trend in diagnosis has been primarily driven by small, early-stage differentiated papillary thyroid carcinomas (PTCs). Many of these indolent, slow-growing cancers would otherwise have gone undetected without advances in ultrasonography and other detection modalities. In one study involving patients with low-risk differentiated thyroid cancers (DTCs) who were monitored without surgery, only 10% were found to have disease progression at a median follow-up interval of 6 years. Clinical guidelines have been modified with the increased understanding of the potential harms of overdiagnosis and treatment, resulting in a leveling off and decreased rate of newly diagnosed cases in more recent years.

Risk Factors

The majority of thyroid cancer cannot be attributed to specific risk factors. Nutritional factors including iodine intake have been associated with an increased risk of thyroid nodularity. Childhood exposure to ionizing radiation is one particularly well-documented risk factor for thyroid cancer. In a large retrospective study, individuals treated with radiation for Hodgkin disease were 27 times more likely to have thyroid nodules than those treated without radiation. Family history is an important risk factor, with one study showing a 10-fold increased risk in first-degree relatives of patients with thyroid cancer. An elevated thyroid stimulating hormone (TSH) level in the setting of thyroid nodularity has been associated with an increased risk of thyroid cancer. Cigarette smoking has been negatively correlated with risk of thyroid cancer.

Pathophysiology

Thyroid cancer may arise from two major parenchymal cell types: thyroid follicular cells giving rise to DTC and parafollicular, or C-, cells giving rise to medullary thyroid cancer (MTC). DTCs are responsible for more than 95% of cases of thyroid cancer (Table 1). DTC includes PTC, follicular thyroid carcinoma (FTC), and the follicular variants, including Hurthle cell cancer. Another related variant of thyroid tumor termed noninvasive follicular thyroid neoplasm with papillary-like nuclear features (NIFTP)

TABLE 1 Overview of Thyroid Tumor Subtypes

SUBTYPE	ORIGIN CELL TYPE	% OF THYROID CANCER	5-YEAR SURVIVAL	COMMON MUTATIONS
PTC	Follicular	~80%	~99%	BRAF, TKR
FTC	Follicular	~15%	~98%	RAS, PAX8-PPARG
NIFTP	Follicular	0.4%–2.6%	N/A	RAS
PDTC	Follicular	~1%	~62%	RAS, P53
MTC	Parafollicular/C-cell	~3%	~90%	RET
ATC	Follicular	~1%	~7%	BRAF, TERT, P53

ATC, Anaplastic thyroid cancer; MTC, medullary thyroid cancer; NIFTP, neoplasm with papillary-like nuclear features; PDTC, poorly differentiated thyroid carcinomas.

has an exceptionally low recurrence rate of less than 1% at 15 years. NIFTP is best described as a benign tumor and does not require completion thyroidectomy or radioactive iodine (RAI). PTC metastasizes via the lymphatic system, typically to cervical lymph nodes. FTC and its variants classically spread hematogenously, which contributes to a less favorable prognosis. The BRAF mutation is the most frequently encountered mutation in non-MTC and is present in 50% to 70% of patients with PTC. TERT mutations are frequently present in high-risk forms of PTC. Mutations in the RAS family of oncogenes are also commonly present in FTC.

Poorly differentiated thyroid carcinomas are high-risk cancers that classically spread hematogenously to lung and bone. These cancers are also derived from follicular cells.

MTC originates from parafollicular or calcitonin-producing C cells. Mutations of the RET protooncogene are thought to be responsible for the majority of cases. RET mutations are classically inherited in an autosomal dominant pattern; however, they can occur sporadically. All patients diagnosed with MTC should be screened for RET mutations. If such testing is positive, first-degree relatives should be screened as well. Specific RET mutations result in specific phenotypes with varying risks of MTC. Knowledge of the specific RET mutation guides the need and timing of prophylactic thyroidectomy; this is of particular importance in the pediatric setting. MTC is part of the classic presentation of patients with multiple endocrine neoplasia type 2 (MEN 2), which also includes a risk of pheochromocytoma and parathyroid adenomas.

Anaplastic thyroid cancer (ATC) is an uncommon (<1%) but aggressive form of cancer. Despite its rarity, ATC is responsible for as much as 50% of thyroid cancer–related mortality. Patients usually present with advanced disease, commonly with symptoms of hoarseness or dysphagia due to local invasion. Approximately 50% of ATCs arise from a known DTC, with the hypothesis of dedifferentiation changes from preexisting DTC to aggressive ATC.

Clinical Manifestations

Most patients with thyroid cancer, particularly with DTCs, present asymptomatically with incidentally discovered thyroid nodularity on imaging. More aggressive forms of thyroid cancer, including poorly differentiated cancers and ATC, can present with symptoms related to regional invasion, including dysphasia, hoarseness-related recurrent laryngeal nerve injury, and tracheal compression.

Diagnosis

All patients suspected of having thyroid nodules should undergo ultrasound and measurement of their serum TSH levels. A TSH below normal should prompt a scintigraphic evaluation with thyroid uptake and scan to assess for functioning or "hot" nodules. Fine needle aspiration (FNA) is not generally indicated for hyperfunctioning nodules because of a low likelihood of malignancy. Thyroid scintigraphy is not needed when serum TSH is normal or elevated. Serum calcitonin measurement used as a screening test for MTC remains controversial because of its low specificity.

Ultrasound is a critical step in evaluating thyroid nodules. It is not only safe and cost-effective but also reliably determines risk of malignancy and therefore need for FNA. Suspicious sonographic features of nodules associated with increased risk of malignancy include hypoechogenicity (darker than normal thyroid parenchyma), microcalcifications, irregular margins, taller than wide shape, and evidence of extrathyroidal extension. Ultrasound of the central and lateral neck compartments is critical to screen for suspicious lymphadenopathy, which can influence the surgical approach. The American Thyroid Association (ATA) recommends FNA using a risk stratification system based on size and sonographic patterns. FNA is recommended for nodules equal to or greater than 1 cm with intermediate (10% to 20% malignancy risk) or high suspicion patterns (>70% to 90% risk), 1.5 cm for low suspicion (5% to 10% risk), and 2 cm for very low suspicion (<3%). Purely cystic nodules are benign and do not need FNA.

The Thyroid Imaging Reporting and Data System (TIRADS) is another validated clinical tool produced by the American College of Radiology (ACR). It uses a points system based on sonographic features to stratify nodules into one of five TIRADS categories: TR1, benign; TR2, not suspicious; TR3, mildly suspicious; TR4, moderately suspicious; and TR5, highly suspicious, with malignancy risks of 0.3%, 1.5%, 4.8%, 9.1%, and 35%, respectively. TR1 and TR2 nodules do not require FNA. FNA is indicated for TR3 nodules starting at 2.5 cm, TR4 at 1.5 cm, and TR5 at 1 cm. Nodules less than 1 cm are too small for FNA based on both the ATA and ACR-TIRADS owing to the slow-growing nature of micropapillary thyroid cancer. In general, the ACR-TIRADS is more selective than the 2015 ATA guidelines in regard to a decision to pursue FNA. Other considerations governing the need for FNA include specific risk factors of thyroid cancer or syndromes associated with thyroid cancer, such as MEN, Cowden syndrome, familial adenomatous polyposis, and Carney complex. In addition, fluorodeoxyglucose-avid nodules are associated with a malignancy rate of about 35%. However, the recommended FNA size of these nodules remains at least 1 cm or greater.

The 2017 Bethesda system has been the standard method of cytology diagnosis of thyroid nodules, consisting of six categories. Category I, nondiagnostic or unsatisfactory, represents a 5% to 10% malignancy risk; in such cases repeat FNA is required unless the lesion is mostly cystic or ultrasound features of very low suspicion. Category II, benign, represents approximately 70% of specimens and a less than 3% risk of malignancy. Both category III, atypia of undetermined significance/follicular lesion of undetermined significance (AUS/FLUS), and category IV, follicular neoplasm or suspicious for follicular neoplasm (FN/SFN), are associated with a slightly higher malignancy risk: 10% to 30% in AUS/FLUS and 25% to 40% in FN/SFN. The management of both categories III and IV is not straightforward, and various molecular assessments can be used to help with decision making. Currently available molecular tests—including the Afirma GSC, RNA seq panel, and ThyroSeq3 112-gene panel—have high sensitivity and specificity, functioning as rule-out and rule-in tests to decrease the number of unnecessary thyroid surgeries. Category V (suspicious for malignancy [SFN]) and category VI (malignant) carry high rates of malignancy (60% to 75% and 97% to 99%, respectively) and should prompt referral for operative management.

Nodules that do not meet the initial threshold for cytologic assessment require continued sonographic surveillance, the recommended interval of which ranges from 6 to 24 months based on sonographic features. FNA should be performed if there is a 50% increase in the tumor volume or 20% increase in nodule diameter (with a minimum increase in two or more dimensions of at least 2 mm) or once nodules reach the threshold size. A nodule with two negative biopsies should be considered benign.

Therapy

Papillary thyroid microcarcinoma (PTMC) is defined as a small PTC equal to or less than 10 mm in size. PTMCs generally grow very slowly and carry an excellent prognosis. Although many individuals are asymptomatic and do not require treatment, an increased rate of detection has likely resulted in overtreatment. It has been shown that PTMCs in young patients are more likely to progress more than those in elderly patients. Active surveillance for most PTMCs has been shown to be safe, and FNA is not recommended for thyroid nodules smaller than 1 cm. Active surveillance should not be considered in the presence of high-risk features such as nodal metastasis or distant metastasis, vocal cord paralysis due to invasion of the recurrent laryngeal nerve, high-grade malignancy on cytology, or in the case of PTMCs attached to the trachea or located along the path of the recurrent laryngeal nerve. Ultrasound-guided percutaneous ethanol ablation (UPEA) by experienced specialists has been shown to be a safe and well-tolerated definitive minimally invasive alternative for PTMC patients who do not wish to have surgery and are uncomfortable with active surveillance, although UPEA is currently available at only a limited number of centers.

Treatment of thyroid cancer is mainly based on individualized risk stratification, accounting for mortality based on TNM (tumor, node, and metastases) staging, the risk of disease recurrence, and the persistence of structural disease.

Although DTC carries a very low risk of mortality compared with other cancers, the TNM staging system remains an accurate predictor of mortality. Recent changes to the system recommend that patients younger than 55 years of age at the time of diagnosis receive only stage I (no distant metastases) or stage II (distant metastases present) classification. Ten-year disease-specific survival rates for stages I to IV were 99.5%, 94.7%, 94.1%, and 67.6%, respectively.

In addition to TNM staging, an individualized risk stratification outlined by the ATA 2015 guidelines is an important milestone for the assessment of risk of thyroid cancer recurrence and persistence of structural disease. The ATA system uses variables such as histology, extent of the first surgery, and postoperative thyroglobulin (Tg) to guide initial postoperative therapy and treatment in follow-up. Patients with tumor sizes less than 4 cm without clinical lymph node metastases or micrometastases measuring less than 2 mm in five or fewer lymph nodes can be classified as ATA low risk. Intermediate-risk disease is defined as DTC with minimal extrathyroidal extension or aggressive histology. High-risk disease includes patients with gross extension, distant metastases, any lymph node metastases greater than 3 cm, as well as FTC with greater than four foci of vascular invasion. In contrast, minimally invasive FTC is considered low risk.

The ATA recommends either total thyroidectomy or lobectomy for low-risk patients with DTC. The decision to proceed with total thyroidectomy or lobectomy primarily depends on tumor size and patient preference. Low-risk patients are not routinely treated with RAI.

Use of RAI after total thyroidectomy is based on individualized risk stratification accounting for extent of tumor, histology type, age, and presence of distant metastases. Radioiodine is typically delayed several months after surgery to allow for complete recovery and assessment of the biochemical response with Tg.

Serum Tg reaches its nadir approximately 4 to 6 weeks postoperatively, and measurement at this point is perhaps the most accurate method of appraising the quality of surgery and probability of cure.

RAI remnant ablation uses a low dose of radioiodine-131 (131-I), around 30 mCi, to destroy any residual thyroid tissue postoperatively. Remnant ablation thus facilitates the interpretation of subsequent serum Tg levels and follow-up RAI whole-body scans to detect any residual or recurrence disease or metastatic foci. Remnant ablation is not routinely recommended in ATA low-risk DTC patients.

Adjuvant treatment uses a higher dose of 131-I (75 to 150 mCi) postoperatively to destroy microscopic thyroid cancer and/or suspected residual disease to potentially decrease recurrence and mortality. RAI adjuvant treatment should be considered in ATA intermediate-risk DTC patients.

Primary treatment with RAI uses 100 to 200 mCi of 131-I to destroy known locoregional and/or distant metastasis with a goal of cure, reduced recurrence and mortality, and/or palliation among high-risk DTC patients.

Serum TSH should be elevated before proceeding with RAI, as TSH potentiates RAI uptake by iodine-avid tissues including normal thyroid tissue and most thyroid cancers. This has historically been accomplished by withdrawing thyroid hormone replacement for approximately 2 weeks until TSH increases to 30 or more. During this time patients should be instructed to consume a low-iodine diet. The use of recombinant human TSH, thyrotropin alfa (Thyrogen), is also a safe and effective alternative to thyroid hormone withdrawal in the detection of recurrent/residual thyroid cancer and facilitation of RAI ablation.

TSH suppression therapy (TST) requires supraphysiologic doses of exogenous thyroid hormone, with the goal of lowering serum TSH. TSH has trophic effects on thyroid tissue, and a subnormal serum TSH may minimize tumor growth and reduce the risk of progression of advanced thyroid cancer. Aggressive TST is not recommended for low-risk patients but may improve survival outcome for those at high risk. Serum TSH levels that were consistently maintained in the subnormal to normal ranges have led to better outcomes in patients at all stages of disease compared with subjects whose serum TSH levels were in the normal to elevated ranges.

Localized treatments with external beam radiation are sometimes needed for gross residual disease or bone metastases. Surgery may be necessary when bone metastases threaten a limb's function.

Systemic treatments for advanced DTC and MTC include tyrosine kinase inhibitors (TKIs). These agents are reserved for patients with progressive or unresectable disease or tumor that is threatening vital structures. TKI-associated adverse effects are common and include hypertension, hand-foot skin reactions, diarrhea, rash, fatigue, and weight loss. The dose of TKI often needs to be titrated based on tolerability.

Most patients with MTC have advanced disease at the time of diagnosis, leading to an unfavorable prognosis. Cure is much more probable if all disease is intrathyroidal at the time of diagnosis. Early identification and complete surgical resection are ideal for the definite treatment of MTC. Calcitonin is a specific serum marker, and its doubling time is the most important prognostic factor for survival and disease progression. Serum carcinoembryonic antigen (CEA) is usually elevated in advanced cases and is often used as a tumor marker in conjunction with calcitonin. The risk of recurrence is low when postoperative calcitonin is undetectable. Patients with low but detectable calcitonin level less than 150 pg/mL likely have persistent or recurrent disease confined to neck lymph nodes and can be followed every 6 to 12 months with physical examination, neck ultrasound, and serial measurement of calcitonin and CEA. If postoperative calcitonin is greater than 150 pg or has a rapid doubling time, additional imaging studies are required to evaluate for distant metastases. If there is concern for disease progression, systemic therapy with vandetanib (Caprelsa) or cabozantinib (Cometriq) should be considered. Before starting this, the possibility of using a local treatment should be evaluated to delay systemic therapy, along with a multidisciplinary team approach.

Patients with ATC usually present with a rapidly enlarging neck mass that can cause compressive neck symptoms and invasion of the adjacent recurrent laryngeal nerve, leading to dysphonia, or compression of the trachea, causing airway obstruction. Ultrasound remains the primary imaging study for ATC, but additional studies, including computed tomography (CT) with contrast of neck, abdomen, and pelvis; positron emission tomography CT, if available; and brain magnetic resonance imaging, can be used. Because of the risk of acute airway compromise, an expeditious diagnosis and management plan by a multidisciplinary team is crucial. Ideally a care team would include a pathologist, head and neck surgeon, medical oncologist, radiation oncologist, and endocrinologist. A palliative care physician should also be involved, given ATC's extremely poor prognosis. Patients with ATC and their families should take part in an in-depth discussion about the natural history of the disease, goals of treatment, treatment toxicities, and expected outcomes. Most untreated patients will die of asphyxiation; therefore, treatment addressing the primary neck disease, even with a goal of only palliation, is a priority. Hospice care could be the best option for patients who do not wish to pursue aggressive therapy. Tracheostomy to prevent airway obstruction as a part of palliative care is controversial but may be appropriate for patients with impending airway compromise. In contrast, patients with limited disease should initially be treated with surgery followed by chemoradiotherapy (intensity-modulated radiotherapy plus taxane-based chemotherapy) as a standard of care when feasible, unless hospice is alternatively elected. Patients with widely metastatic or stage IVC disease should instead be treated with palliative systemic therapy or best supportive care.

Recent studies have indicated improvements in overall survival in early multimodality therapy, especially with recent advancements in systemic therapy including targeted and immunotherapies such as the *BRAF* inhibitor dabrafenib (Tafinlar) and the *MEK* inhibitor trametinib (Mekinist), anti-PD1 monoclonal antibody spartalizumab,[5,8] and newer agents such as the peroxisome proliferator-activated receptor-γ agonist efatutazone,[5] and mammalian target of rapamycin inhibitors, which seem to provide a more efficacious treatment in advanced ATC.

Monitoring

Regardless of the initial risk assessment, patients with DTC should be monitored longitudinally and classified as having either an excellent, indeterminate, or incomplete response, both biochemically and structurally, to therapy. Initial monitoring includes serial neck ultrasounds, TSH, and serum Tg and Tg antibody levels at intervals determined by initial risk assessment. An excellent response (1% to 4% recurrence rate) is defined as no clinical, biochemical, or structural evidence of disease. Serum Tg should be less than 0.2 ng/mL with a suppressed TSH, or less than 1 ng/mL if TSH is stimulated. Patients with an indeterminate response (15% to 20% recurrence rate) will have nonspecific biochemical or structural findings. A biochemical incomplete response (20% recurrence rate) reflects abnormally elevated Tg or Tg antibody levels (serum Tg > 1 ng/mL basal or > 10 ng/mL if TSH is stimulated or increasing Tg antibodies) in the absence of disease. A structural incomplete response (50% to 85% recurrence rate) includes persistent or newly identified locoregional or distant metastasis with or without abnormal Tg or Tg antibodies.

Management of Complications

Immediate surgical complications after thyroidectomy are correlated with low-volume surgeons. High-volume surgeons are also associated with an increased risk of postoperative complications;

however, this is likely attributable to overall greater case complexity. Potential complications include injury of the recurrent laryngeal nerve leading to temporary or permanent hoarseness, airway difficulty due to bilateral vocal cord paralysis, and need for tracheostomy. Total thyroidectomy can lead to transient or permanent hypoparathyroidism with resultant hypocalcemia. Adequate preoperative vitamin D replacement can help maintain normocalcemia. Postoperatively the parathyroid hormone (PTH) level should be checked; calcitriol (Rocaltrol) may be needed in addition to calcium supplementation if the PTH level is low or undetectable. Serial calcium levels should be obtained after discharge.

Long-term TST can result in adverse outcomes such as osteoporosis, fracture, and cardiovascular disease, including atrial fibrillation. In general, daily levothyroxine (Levoxyl, Synthroid) doses of 1.6 to 1.8 μg/kg are the initial treatment after thyroidectomy, whereas doses of 2.0 to 2.2 μg/kg are needed to suppress the serum TSH. The dosage requirements of individual patients are highly variable and depend on multiple factors, including body mass index, the concomitant use of other medications, and patient adherence. The ATA recommends maintaining serum TSH levels between 0.5 and 2 mU/L in low-risk and intermediate-risk patients with an excellent response to treatment. Mild TSH suppression (TSH 0.1 to 0.5 mU/L) should be used for high-risk patients who have had an excellent response (negative imaging and undetectable suppressed Tg). Mild TSH suppression is also recommended in patients with a biochemically incomplete response. More significant TSH suppression (i.e., serum TSH <0.1) is recommended in patients with residual structural disease or a biochemically incomplete response if they are young or at low risk for complications from iatrogenic hyperthyroidism.

Adverse effects of RAI—including radiation thyroiditis, sialadenitis, and tumor hemorrhage or edema—occur in 10% to 30% of patients. The possibility of adverse effects is dose dependent. Long-term risk of secondary malignancies has been reported; however, the risk is considerably lower when the total dose is less than 100 mCi. Immediately after patients have been treated with RAI, an appropriate isolation protocol is required to protect household members, especially women who are pregnant and infants, from radiation exposure. The required duration of isolation is predominantly based on RAI dose and rate of clearance.

Conclusion

Thyroid nodules are very common and are often discovered incidentally. The vast majority of nodules, approximately 90% to 95%, are benign. Thyroid sonography should be obtained for all nodules, as this reliably predicts the risk of malignancy and need for FNA. DTCs are indolent; FNA is not indicated for nodules less than 1 cm in size. Thyroid function should be assessed before proceeding with FNA. Patients with a TSH below normal should undergo thyroid uptake and scan to investigate for an autonomously functioning nodule or nodules. Most nodules can be monitored with ultrasound alone. Guidelines produced by either the ATA or ACR can reliably determine the need for FNA. PTC is the most common type of DTC and typically has a very favorable prognosis. Lower-risk patients with DTC can be managed with lobectomy. Patients with larger tumors (>4 cm), extrathyroidal extension, or higher-risk cytology should be treated with total thyroidectomy and central neck dissection. Lateral compartment neck dissections should be completed if there is FNA-positive disease.

Low-risk patients with DTC do not need treatment with RAI, whereas intermediate- and high-risk cases should receive RAI. All patients should be monitored longitudinally after initial therapy, both radiographically and biochemically, using serum Tg. The ATA categorizes patient response as excellent, indeterminate, or incomplete. Patients should receive appropriate levels of TSH suppression, initially based on their ATA risk and subsequently on their response to therapy. TSH suppression poses multiple risks if continued long-term.

[5] Investigational drug in the United States.
[8] Orphan drug in the United States.

MTC should be considered of higher risk than DTC and is managed surgically. MTC is often detected later and is usually more advanced than DTC. Calcitonin and CEA levels can be monitored longitudinally. Calcitonin doubling time is a particularly important prognostic factor for following these patients.

ATC is a rare but extraordinarily aggressive and rapidly growing form of thyroid cancer. Patients should be managed by a multidisciplinary team with consideration for tracheostomy because of the risk of asphyxiation in the setting of rapid tumor growth. Aggressive resection and prompt chemotherapy are suitable treatment options in appropriately selected patients with less advanced disease.

References

Biondi B, Cooper DS: Thyroid hormone suppression therapy, *Endocrinol Metab Clin North Am* 48(1):227–237, 2019. https://doi.org/10.1016/j.ecl.2018.10.008.

Brito JP, Hay ID: Management of papillary thyroid microcarcinoma, *Endocrinol Metab Clin North Am* 48(1):199–213, 2019. https://doi.org/10.1016/j.ecl.2018.10.006.

Cabanillas ME, Mcfadden DG, Durante C: Thyroid cancer, *The Lancet* 388(10061):2783–2795, 2016. Print.

Chintakuntlawar AV, Foote RL, Kasperbauer JL, Bible KC: Diagnosis and management of anaplastic thyroid cancer, *Endocrinol Metab Clin North Am* 48(1):269–284, 2019. https://doi.org/10.1016/j.ecl.2018.10.010.

Cho A, Chang Y, Ahn J, Shin H, Ryu S: Cigarette smoking and thyroid cancer risk: a cohort study, *Br J Cancer* 119(5):638–645, 2018. https://doi.org/10.1038/s41416-018-0224-5.

Du L, Wang Y, Sun X, et al: Thyroid cancer: trends in incidence, mortality and clinical-pathological patterns in Zhejiang Province, Southeast China, *BMC Cancer* 18(1):291, 2018. https://doi.org/10.1186/s12885-018-4081-7.

Haugen BR, Alexander EK, Bible KC, et al: 2015 American Thyroid Association management guidelines for adult patients with thyroid nodules and differentiated thyroid cancer: the American Thyroid Association guidelines task force on thyroid nodules and differentiated thyroid cancer, *Thyroid* 26(1):1–133, 2016. https://doi.org/10.1089/thy.2015.0020.

Maxwell C, Sipos JA: Clinical diagnostic evaluation of thyroid nodules, *Endocrinol Metab Clin North Am* 48(1):61–84, 2019.

Mayson SE, Haugen BR: Molecular diagnostic evaluation of thyroid nodules, *Endocrinol Metab Clin North Am* 48(1):85–97, 2019. https://doi.org/10.1016/j.ecl.2018.10.004.

Miyauchi A, Ito Y: Conservative surveillance management of low-risk papillary thyroid microcarcinoma, *Endocrinol Metab Clin North Am* 48(1):215–226, 2019. https://doi.org/10.1016/j.ecl.2018.10.007.

Nikiforov YE, et al: Nomenclature revision for encapsulated follicular variant of papillary thyroid carcinoma: a paradigm shift to reduce overtreatment of indolent tumors, *JAMA Oncol* 2(8):10–1029, 2016.

Pal T, Vogl FD, Chappuis PO, et al: Increased risk for nonmedullary thyroid cancer in the first degree relatives of prevalent cases of nonmedullary thyroid cancer: a hospital-based study, *J Clin Endocrinol Metab* 86(11):5307–5312, 2001.

Powers AE, Marcadis AR, Lee M, Morris LG, Marti JL: Changes in trends in thyroid cancer incidence in the United States, 1992 to 2016, *Jama* 322(24):2440–2441, 2019.

Viola D, Elisei R: Management of medullary thyroid cancer, *Endocrinol Metab Clin North Am* 48(1):285–301, 2019. https://doi.org/10.1016/j.ecl.2018.11.006.

Xing M: Genetic-guided risk assessment and management of thyroid cancer, *Endocrinol Metab Clin North Am* 48(1):109–124, 2019. https://doi.org/10.1016/j.ecl.2018.11.007.

THYROIDITIS

Method of
Leigh M. Eck, MD; and Aiman Zafar, MBBS

CURRENT DIAGNOSIS

- Thyroiditis is a term used to describe a diverse group of disorders associated with thyroid inflammation.
- Thyroiditis can be associated with a euthyroid state, thyrotoxicosis, or hypothyroidism.
- The clinical presentation of thyroiditis will direct the evaluation with useful testing to include measurement of thyroid hormone levels, thyroid antibody testing, white blood cell count, erythrocyte sedimentation rate, thyroid scintigraphy, and thyroid ultrasound.

CURRENT THERAPY

- Abnormalities of thyroid hormone levels resulting from thyroiditis may be transient and require no or only short-term therapy.
- If symptomatic thyrotoxicosis is present, beta-blocker therapy should be initiated.
- Thyroiditis associated with persistent hypothyroidism is managed with synthetic thyroxine (levothyroxine, T4 [Levoxyl, Synthroid, Tirosint]).
- Thyroid pain associated with subacute thyroiditis is managed with a nonsteroidal antiinflammatory drug or, if ineffective, glucocorticoid therapy.
- Acute suppurative thyroiditis requires immediate parenteral antibiotic therapy, as well as surgical drainage, if indicated.

Thyroiditis is a term used to describe a diverse group of disorders characterized by inflammation of the thyroid gland (Table 1). Presentation of thyroiditis is variable depending on the etiology. The most common thyroid disorder in the United States, Hashimoto thyroiditis, most often presents with hypothyroidism. Other forms of thyroiditis may present with thyrotoxicosis because of inflammation in the thyroid gland resulting in the release of stored hormone. Painful thyroiditis is seen with subacute, suppurative, and radiation-induced thyroiditis, while other variants are most often painless.

Epidemiology

The most common cause of hypothyroidism in iodine-sufficient areas of the world is *Hashimoto thyroiditis*, also known as *chronic autoimmune thyroiditis*. Elevated serum antithyroid peroxidase antibody concentrations are found in ~5% of adults and ~15% of older women; overt hypothyroidism is seen in up to 2% of the population. A variant of chronic autoimmune thyroiditis, *postpartum thyroiditis*, is a destructive thyroiditis induced by an autoimmune mechanism that occurs within 1 year of parturition. Postpartum thyroiditis occurs in up to 10% of women in the United States. It can also occur after spontaneous or induced abortion. *Silent thyroiditis* is indistinguishable from postpartum thyroiditis, with the exception of lack of temporal relationship to pregnancy. Silent thyroiditis may account for about 1% of all cases of thyrotoxicosis. Many medications are associated with an alteration in thyroid function testing; however, only a few are known to provoke an autoimmune or destructive inflammatory thyroiditis, including amiodarone (Cordarone), lithium, interferon alfa, interleukin-2, tyrosine kinase inhibitors, and checkpoint inhibitor immunotherapy. *Riedel thyroiditis* (RT) is a progressive fibrosis of the thyroid gland. The incidence of RT is estimated at 1.06 cases per 100,000 population, with a higher prevalence in women aged 30 to 50. *Subacute thyroiditis*

TABLE 1	Causes of Thyroiditis

Autoimmune thyroiditis: Hashimoto thyroiditis, postpartum thyroiditis, silent thyroiditis

Subacute thyroiditis, also known as de Quervain thyroiditis or subacute granulomatous thyroiditis

Suppurative thyroiditis, also known as infectious thyroiditis or pyrogenic thyroiditis

Riedel thyroiditis, also known as fibrous thyroiditis

Therapy-induced thyroiditis: amiodarone (Cordarone), interferon-alpha, interleukin-2, lithium, alemtuzumab (Lemtrada), tyrosine kinase inhibitors, radioactive iodine, checkpoint inhibitor immunotherapy

is the most common cause of thyroid pain. A study conducted in Olmsted County, Minnesota, from 1960 to 1997 identified 160 patients with subacute thyroiditis, revealing an age- and sex-adjusted incidence of 4.9 cases per 100,000 per year. In the 1970 to 1997 period, 94 patients were identified with subacute thyroiditis, and their major presenting symptom was pain. Subacute thyroiditis recurred in 4% of patients after 6 to 21 years.

Suppurative thyroiditis, most commonly caused by bacterial infection, is rare because of the thyroid gland's encapsulation, high iodine content, rich blood supply, and extensive lymphatic drainage. *Radiation-induced thyroiditis* occurs in approximately 1% of patients who receive radioactive iodine therapy for hyperthyroidism. It may also be seen after external beam radiation therapy for certain cancers.

Risk Factors

Hashimoto thyroiditis is more common in women, particularly older women. Hashimoto thyroiditis is associated with several gene polymorphisms, suggesting a role for genetic susceptibility. Subacute thyroiditis frequently follows an upper respiratory tract infection, with its incidence highest in summer. Suppurative thyroiditis is most likely to occur in patients with preexisting thyroid disease, those with congenital anomalies such as pyriform sinus fistula, and those who are immunosuppressed. Postpartum thyroiditis is 5.7 times more likely to occur in women with thyroid peroxidase antibodies, and prevalence among women with type 1 diabetes mellitus is 19.6%.

Pathophysiology

Hashimoto thyroiditis, postpartum thyroiditis, and silent thyroiditis all have an autoimmune basis. The antithyroid immune response begins with the activation of thyroid antigen-specific helper T cells. Once helper T cells are activated, they induce B cells to secrete thyroid antibodies; thyroid antibodies most frequently measured are those directed against thyroid peroxidase and against thyroglobulin. The mechanism for autoimmune destruction of the thyroid likely involves both cellular immunity and humoral immunity. RT is the local involvement of the thyroid in a systemic disease, multifocal fibrosclerosis; the etiology remains unclear but is linked to systemic fibrosis or autoimmune processes, possibly involving IgG4. Suppurative thyroiditis is most often associated with a bacterial pathogen; however, fungal, mycobacterial, or parasitic infections may also be the cause. Although rare, radiation-induced thyroiditis may occur after the treatment of hyperthyroidism with radioactive iodine because of radiation-induced injury and necrosis of thyroid follicular cells and associated inflammation. Drug-induced thyroiditis is caused by several drugs such as checkpoint inhibitors (ipilimumab [Yervoy], nivolumab [Opdivo], pembrolizumab [Keytruda]), amiodarone (Cordarone, Pacerone), alemtuzumab (Lemtrada) used for multiple sclerosis, tyrosine kinase inhibitors/multikinase inhibitors (sunitinib [Sutent]), interleukin-2, and interferon alpha. Alemtuzumab is a humanized monoclonal antibody that targets CD52, leading to significant depletion of B and T cells in multiple sclerosis patients. It is associated with a high rate of thyroid autoimmunity. Thyroid dysfunction during immune checkpoint blockade is thought to be related to a reduction in immune self-tolerance. Amiodarone causes destructive thyroiditis by causing a direct cytotoxic effect to thyrocytes. This is referred to as type 2 amiodarone-induced thyroiditis.

Clinical Manifestation

A symmetric, painless goiter is frequently the initial finding in Hashimoto thyroiditis. The usual course of Hashimoto thyroiditis is gradual loss of thyroid function. Among patients with this disorder who have subclinical hypothyroidism, overt hypothyroidism occurs at a rate of about 5% per year. Many studies have shown a relationship between papillary thyroid cancer and autoimmune thyroid disease. The classic presentation of postpartum thyroiditis occurs in only approximately 30% of afflicted women, with the characteristic sequence of hyperthyroidism, followed by hypothyroidism, and then recovery. Persistent hypothyroidism is seen in up to 30% of women after an episode of postpartum thyroiditis.

Silent thyroiditis is marked by a similar characteristic sequence of thyroid hormone dysfunction. However, it is not temporally associated with pregnancy; 20% will have residual hypothyroidism. *Medication-induced thyroiditis* is variable in its presentation. Amiodarone (Cordarone), rich in iodine, is associated with hypothyroidism and hyperthyroidism; type 2 amiodarone-induced thyrotoxicosis is due to a destructive thyroiditis process. Lithium is more commonly associated with hypothyroidism. Interferon-alfa and interleukin-2 can cause both permanent and transient hypothyroidism likely related to the ability of these substances to induce or exacerbate thyroid autoimmune disease. RT presents with neck discomfort or tightness, dysphagia, hoarseness, and a diffuse goiter that is hard, fixed, and often not clearly separable from the adjacent tissues. A systematic review of 212 cases of RT found that common symptoms include neck swelling (89%), dyspnea (50%), neck pain (41%), and hoarse voice (41%), with a median symptom duration of 4 months before seeking medical help. Due to the firm nature of the mass, it can sometimes be clinically mistaken for anaplastic thyroid cancer, thyroid angiosarcoma, or lymphoma. Biochemical abnormalities can also be seen, such as hypothyroidism and hypocalcemia. Subacute granulomatous thyroiditis is characterized by acute thyroid pain, hypermetabolism, a low-grade fever, occasional difficulty swallowing (dysphagia), suppressed levels of thyroid-stimulating hormone (TSH), and an elevated erythrocyte sedimentation rate. A painful thyroid after an upper respiratory tract infection often indicates subacute granulomatous thyroiditis. This is a self-limiting condition that typically resolves on its own, usually without any lasting thyroid function abnormalities. Additionally, there are case reports of this condition developing after SARS-CoV-2 infection. Early transient hypothyroidism is common in subacute thyroiditis. Permanent hypothyroidism is less common, and in the Olmsted County study, only 15% of the patients required T4 therapy after 28 years of follow-up.

Patients with suppurative thyroiditis are usually acutely ill with fever, dysphagia, dysphonia, anterior neck pain with erythema, and a tender thyroid mass. Radiation-induced thyroiditis presents 5 to 10 days after radioactive iodine treatment with neck pain and tenderness. In addition, there can be a transient exacerbation of hyperthyroidism.

Diagnosis and Differential Diagnosis

The diagnostic approach to suspected thyroiditis can be focused based on an association with thyroid pain and circulating thyroid hormone status (Figure 1). Hashimoto thyroiditis is diagnosed when a goiter is found on examination with a subsequently noted elevation of thyroid antibodies or when subclinical or overt hypothyroidism is detected with associated elevated thyroid antibodies. Screening for postpartum thyroiditis with a measurement of TSH and free thyroxine should be undertaken in women presenting with symptoms of thyroid dysfunction in the postpartum period. If hyperthyroidism is present, thyroid scintigraphy (if not contraindicated, e.g., breastfeeding) or measurement of thyroid-stimulating immunoglobulins is helpful in the differentiation of postpartum thyroiditis from Graves disease. The diagnostic approach to silent thyroiditis is similar. The laboratory hallmark of subacute thyroiditis is a markedly elevated erythrocyte sedimentation rate; the leukocyte count is normal or slightly elevated. Thyrotoxicosis may be present; if so, thyroid scintigraphy will reveal a low iodine uptake state. Thyroid antibody testing is typically normal. Thyroid ultrasound is valuable for the initial diagnosis and follow-up of patients with subacute granulomatous thyroiditis. The characteristic ultrasound findings for this condition include an ill-defined hypoechoic area, lacking round or ovoid mass formation across multiple ultrasound planes, and no vascular flow on color Doppler ultrasound. Subacute thyroiditis should be considered in the differential diagnosis for lesions that display these characteristics in the absence of clinical symptoms. In such cases, a follow-up ultrasound examination is recommended instead of immediately performing a fine-needle aspiration biopsy. However, fine-needle aspiration biopsy is essential for lesions that appear as a focal mass, which may mimic thyroid malignancy. Follow-up

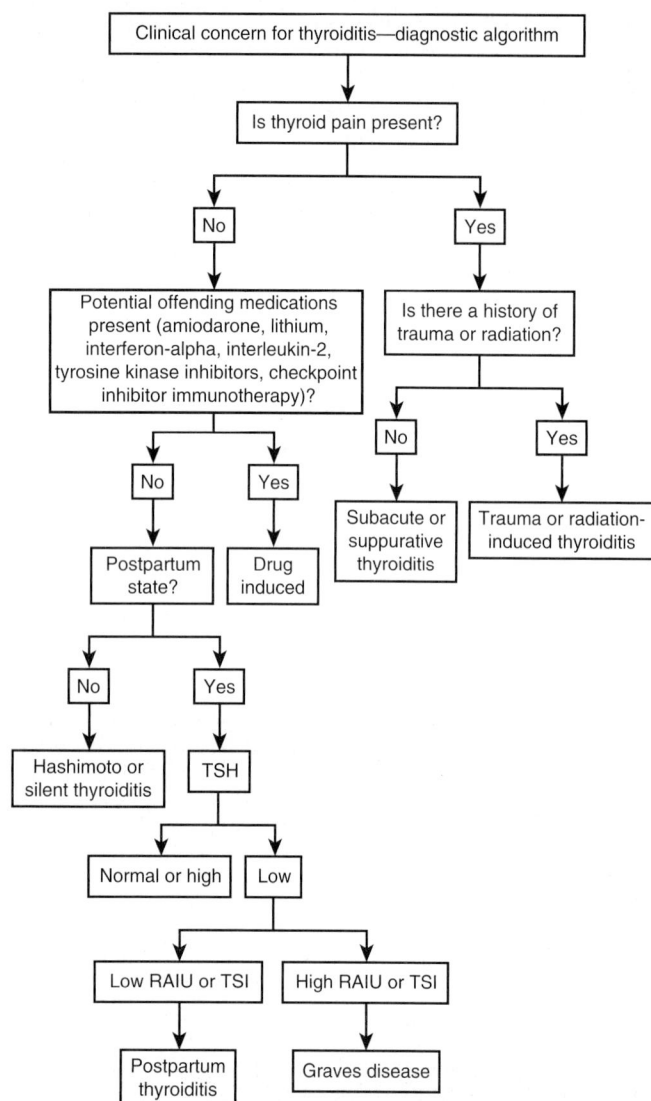

Figure 1 Clinical concern for thyroiditis—diagnostic algorithm. *RAIU*, Radioactive iodine uptake; *TSH*, thyroid-stimulating hormone; *TSI*, thyroid-stimulating immunoglobulins.

thyroxine in adults is approximately 1.6 mcg/kg body weight per day. Adjustment of dosage is undertaken every 6 weeks until a euthyroid status is achieved. The majority of women with post-partum thyroiditis will not need treatment during either the hyper-thyroid or hypothyroid phase. If symptomatic hyperthyroidism is present, beta-blocker therapy can be used; antithyroid medications have no utility in the management of postpartum thyroiditis. Women with symptomatic hypothyroidism should be treated with synthetic thyroxine therapy; in asymptomatic women, initiation of thyroxine therapy should be considered if TSH is >10 mU/L. Management of silent thyroiditis is the same as that for postpartum thyroiditis. Symptoms associated with RT may be relieved with prednisone; a small case series associated improvement and even resolution of the process with tamoxifen (Nolvadex)[1] therapy. Surgery is indicated in RT if compressive symptoms are present. The goal of therapy in subacute thyroiditis is to provide symptom relief. Nonsteroidal antiinflammatory medications are often adequate to control pain; if insufficient, glucocorticoid therapy should be initiated. Corticosteroid therapy may provide symptomatic relief but does not prevent thyroid dysfunction. Beta-blockade therapy can ameliorate symptoms of thyrotoxicosis if indicated. Suppurative thyroiditis is managed with appropriate antibiotics and drainage of any abscess; the disease may prove fatal if diagnosis and treatment are delayed. Pain associated with radiation-induced thyroiditis can be managed with nonsteroidal antiinflammatory therapy or, if ineffective, a short course of glu-cocorticoid therapy. Radiation-induced thyroiditis is a self-limited process and will resolve spontaneously within days to weeks.

Monitoring

In the patient with Hashimoto thyroiditis with a euthyroid state, routine TSH testing should be undertaken given the risk of development of overt hypothyroidism at 5% per year. Any woman who has had postpartum thyroiditis should be monitored very closely for thyroid dysfunction with future pregnancies, as reoccurrence is likely. For women who have fully recovered from postpartum thyroiditis, yearly TSH measurements should be considered because of underlying chronic autoimmune thyroiditis and risk for overt hypothyroidism. Although overall recurrence rates for silent thyroiditis have not been well established, a similar monitoring plan is warranted for this variant of chronic autoimmune thyroiditis. Subacute thyroiditis recurs in only about 2% of patients. Routine monitoring after resolution of process has not been defined.

---

[1] Not FDA approved for this indication.

ultrasound findings for subacute granulomatous thyroiditis typically show a reduction in enlarged thyroid volume and a decrease or absence of the hypoechoic area. Suppurative thyroiditis is typically associated with normal thyroid function. Leukocyte counts and erythrocyte sedimentation rates are elevated. Fine-needle aspiration with Gram stain and culture is the diagnostic test of choice. The diagnosis of RT is complex, often requiring histopathologic confirmation due to the potential for misdiagnosis as thyroid malignancy. Features noted on biopsy include (1) a fibroinflammatory process in the thyroid with extension into surrounding tissue; (2) inflammatory infiltrate containing no giant cells, lymphoid follicles, oncocytes, or granulomas; (3) evidence of occlusive phlebitis; and (4) no evidence of thyroid malignancy. Radiation-induced thyroiditis should be considered if a temporal relationship to radioactive iodine treatment is present. If there is an exacerbation of hyperthyroidism immediately after radiation treatment for the same, consideration of radiation-induced thyroiditis due to the release of preformed thyroid hormone associated with destruction of follicular cells should be considered as an etiology of thyrotoxicosis in addition to the underlying disease process.

Treatment

Once overt hypothyroidism is present in the patient with Hashimoto thyroiditis, treatment with synthetic L-thyroxine (Levoxyl, Synthroid) therapy is indicated. The average replacement dose of

References

Bogazzi F, Bartalena L, Martino E: Approach to the patient with amiodarone-induced thyrotoxicosis, *J Clin Endocrinol Metab* 95:2529–2535, 2010.

Burch HB: Drug effects on the thyroid, *N Engl J Med* 381(8):749–761, 2019. https://doi.org/10.1056/NEJMra1901214. PMID: 31433922.

Cooper DS, Ladenson PW: The thyroid gland. 2011. In Gardner DG, Shoback D, editors: *Greenspan's basic & clinical endocrinology*, ed 9, New York, 2011, McGraw-Hill. Available at http://accessmedicine.mhmedical.com/content.aspx?bookid¼380&Sectionid¼39744047.

De Groot L, Abalovich M, Alexander ED, et al: Management of thyroid dysfunction during pregnancy and postpartum: an endocrine society clinical practice guideline, *J Clin Endocrinol Metab* 97:2543–2565, 2012.

Fatourechi Vahab, Aniszewski Jaroslaw P, Eghbali Fatourechi Guiti Z, Atkinson Elizabeth J, Jacobsen Steven J: Clinical features and outcome of subacute thyroiditis in an incidence cohort: olmsted County, Minnesota, study, *J Clin Endocrinol Metab* 88(5):2100–2105, 2003. https://doi.org/10.1210/jc.2002-021799.

Nicholson WK, Robinson KA, Smallridge RC, Ladenson PW, Powe NR: Prevalence of postpartum thyroid dysfunction: a quantitative review, *Thyroid* 16(6):573–582, 2006.

Park SY, Kim EK, Kim MJ, et al: Ultrasonographic characteristics of subacute granulomatous thyroiditis, *Korean J Radiol* 7(4):229–234, 2006. https://doi.org/10.3348/kjr.2006.7.4.229. PMID: 17143025; PMCID: PMC2667608.

Pearce EN, Farwell AP, Braverman LE: Thyroiditis, *N Engl J Med* 348:2646–2655, 2003.

Samuels MH: Subacute, silent and postpartum thyroiditis, *Med Clin North Am* 96:223–233, 2012.

Zala Aakansha, Berhane Thomas, Juhlin C Christofer, Calissendorff Jan, Falhammar Henrik, Thyroiditis Riedel: *J Clin Endocrinol Metab* 105(9):e3469–e3481, 2020. https://doi.org/10.1210/clinem/dgaa468.

6 Hematology

ACUTE LEUKEMIA IN ADULTS

Method of
Colin Vale, MD; and Anthony Hunter, MD

CURRENT DIAGNOSIS

- Diagnosis of acute leukemia is made based on the presence of myeloid (acute myeloid leukemia [AML]) or lymphoid (T- or B-cell acute lymphoblastic leukemia [ALL]) blasts in blood and/or bone marrow. Acute leukemia may uncommonly have an ambiguous lineage [AUL] or mixed phenotype [MPAL].
- Medical history taking should identify risk factors such as prior exposure to chemotherapy for other malignancies (or nonmalignant disorders), antecedent hematologic disorders, familial hematologic disorders, or other inherited genetic disorders (e.g., Down syndrome).
- Clinical examination should identify extramedullary sites of involvement such as meninges/central nervous system (CNS), active infection, hemorrhage, or disseminated intravascular coagulation.
- AML requires the presence of at least 20% myeloblasts in blood or marrow except in subsets of disease defined by specific cytogenetic or molecular aberrations. These include mutations in the *NPM1* gene, and the chromosomal abnormalities t(8;21)(q22;q22), inv(16)(p13q22) or t(16;16)(p13;q22), and t(15;17)(q22;q12), each of which is associated with more favorable clinical outcomes. Testing for cytogenetic and molecular aberrations is critical for diagnosis, prognosis, and therapy.
- Acute promyelocytic leukemia (APL) is defined by the *PML-RARA* gene fusion, which can be detected by genetic methods or cytogenetics showing t(15;17). APL is a unique entity requiring different therapy, and demonstrates a favorable prognosis.
- ALL is subcategorized based on B- or T-cell lineage; cases with less than 20% blasts constitute lymphoblastic lymphoma, which is treated similarly.
- For B-ALL (also in mixed-phenotype acute leukemia), identification of the Philadelphia chromosome, t(9;22)(q34.1;q11.2), or its *BCR-ABL1* gene fusion is essential for proper diagnosis and treatment. Similar to AML, testing for established chromosomal and molecular aberrations is standard.

CURRENT THERAPY

- Acute myeloid leukemia (AML) is typically treated with intensive initial therapy (induction) followed by repetitive cycles of intensive postremission therapy (consolidation). Induction chemotherapy most commonly consists of anthracycline plus cytarabine (Cytosar). Several acceptable postremission approaches are used; often, these are repetitive high-dose cytarabine–based regimens.

- Acute promyelocytic leukemia (APL) is uniquely treated with all-*trans* retinoic acid (tretinoin [Vesanoid]) and arsenic trioxide (Trisenox), instead of chemotherapy. Cases with elevated white blood cell counts also require the antibody-drug conjugate gemtuzumab ozogamicin (Mylotarg)[1] for cytoreduction.
- Acute lymphoblastic leukemia (ALL) is treated with multidrug regimens for induction and postremission therapies. Postremission therapies include further intensification cycles and prolonged lower-dose maintenance therapy. Central nervous system (CNS)-directed therapy is a critical component of treatment, even in patients without baseline CNS involvement. Most acute leukemias of ambiguous lineage are treated with ALL-type regimens, although clinical outcomes are poor.
- The use of "pediatric-inspired" ALL regimens for adolescents and young adults has improved outcomes.
- Older patients or those with medical infirmities may require less intensive treatment regimens; because of a greater likelihood of adverse risk disease and higher toxicities, such patients fare worse than younger patients. Novel treatment approaches, such as the combination of a hypomethylating agent and venetoclax (Venclexta) in AML, have led to improved outcomes.
- Because of high relapse risk, allogeneic hematopoietic stem cell transplantation (alloHCT) in first remission is an important consideration for eligible patients with AML. However, alloHCT is generally not pursued in patients with favorable-risk disease who achieve measurable residual disease–negative remission, due to high chance of cure with chemotherapy alone. High-risk adult patients with ALL are also offered early transplantation. All patients who relapse should be considered for transplantation if remission is again achieved.
- Several subsets of acute leukemia can be treated by effective therapies that target specific aberrant signaling or enzymatic activities or that are directed to unique biologic targets of disease. Most important among these are the tyrosine kinase inhibitors (TKIs), which are used in treating acute leukemia (typically ALL) with *BCR-ABL1*.
- Advances in immunology have rapidly and dramatically improved the options for treatment, especially for those with B-ALL. Novel antibody constructs and genetically engineered autologous cellular products directed to eliminate B-lymphocytes can induce durable remissions in B-ALL.

[1]Not FDA approved for this indication.

Epidemiology

According to data from the National Institutes of Health and American Cancer Society, the incidence of acute myeloid leukemia (AML) in the United States is 4.1 per 100,000 per year, with an estimate of 22,010 new cases for 2025. AML accounts for approximately 1.0% of all new cancer cases and 33% of all new leukemia diagnoses but is responsible for more than half of all leukemia deaths. AML is far more common than acute lymphoblastic leukemia (ALL) in adults. Although AML affects all age groups, the incidence increases with advancing age, presenting at a median of 69 years of age. ALL is estimated to occur in 6100 cases in the United States in 2025 and has a bimodal distribution across ages, with a peak in early childhood and a smaller second peak around 70 years of age.

Risk Factors

Most cases of acute leukemia in adults have no established cause. Genetic predisposition, drugs, and radiation have been associated with the development of acute leukemia, particularly AML. Several rare genetic syndromes—including Down syndrome, Fanconi anemia, Bloom syndrome, Li-Fraumeni syndrome, neurofibromatosis type I, short telomere syndromes, Shwachman-Diamond syndrome, and ataxia telangiectasia—are associated with an increased risk for developing acute leukemia. AML with germline predisposition represents a less common yet important and underrecognized subset of disease. Germline mutations associated with increased risk of developing a myeloid neoplasm include *CEBPA*, *DDX41*, *RUNX1*, *ANKRD26*, *ETV6*, and *GATA2*. Down syndrome–associated AML and ALL pose an increased risk of toxicity with standard chemotherapy and require dose adjustment (and expert management).

Anticancer drugs are the leading cause of therapy-associated AML. Alkylating agent–associated leukemias typically occur 4 to 6 years after exposure; affected individuals often have multilineage dysplasia and monosomy/aberrations in chromosomes 5 and 7. Topoisomerase II inhibitor–associated leukemias typically occur with shorter latency, 1 to 3 years after exposure; affected individuals often have AML with monocytic features and aberrations involving chromosome 11q23.

Pathophysiology

Acute leukemias are hematologic malignancies arising from hematopoietic stem and progenitor cells in the bone marrow. Clonal immature cells accumulate in the blood, bone marrow, and occasionally in the extramedullary tissues. These malignant cells divide and proliferate, but they do not differentiate into functional cells. Patients with acute leukemia are immunocompromised and have impaired oxygen-carrying capacity (anemia) and bleeding diathesis (because of thrombocytopenia or disrupted coagulation).

Patients experience complications directly from the accumulation of abnormal immature blasts or indirectly from the reduction in functional hematopoietic cells in the marrow and blood. Leukemic involvement of the bone marrow typically results in cytopenias, which may affect all hematopoietic cell lineages. Patients with acute leukemias often have evidence of circulating leukemic blasts in the peripheral blood (sometimes with high white blood cell [WBC] counts consisting entirely of blasts) but may have pancytopenia with no circulating blasts at all. Patients frequently require transfusions of red blood cells and platelets and are at risk of life-threatening infectious complications caused by neutropenia. Infection is the most common cause of death in patients with acute leukemia.

Patients with morphologically similar acute leukemias may experience vastly different clinical outcomes. Increasingly, this is explained by karyotyping and genetic sequencing studies that demonstrate marked heterogeneity in the cytogenetic and molecular profiles among patients with acute leukemia. Several critical cellular pathways are commonly dysregulated on genetic sequencing studies, while a myriad of additional genetic alterations may only occur in small subsets. In adults, most cases of AML ultimately arise against the backdrop of a limited number of mutations that accumulate with advancing age. As noted earlier, cases with an identifiable risk factor, such as germline predisposition or drug exposure, are less common. The Cancer Genome Atlas and other databases have shown that 5% to 10% of healthy individuals older than 70 years of age have blood cells with potentially "premalignant" mutations that are associated with clonal expansion, referred to as *clonal hematopoiesis of indeterminate potential*. There appears to be a variety of "final insults" that transform these expanded clones to AML, but how these genetic aberrations contribute to leukemic transformation remains incompletely understood. Although the number of mutations per cell in AML is relatively small (median of 13 mutations) compared with other

cancers (e.g., melanoma and non–small cell lung cancer may have several hundred mutations per cell), great heterogeneity exists in the mutations identified between individual patients with AML. The same can be said of ALL. Indeed, dramatic differences in mutations/genetic signatures have been observed among patients with childhood, adolescent, young adult, and older adult ALL, respectively, and contribute to stark differences in prognosis among these groups.

Great heterogeneity exists not just among patients with different types of acute leukemia, but within each individual patient. Each patient may have several leukemic clones and subclones with slightly different mutational profiles. The presence of genetically different clones and subclones explains why a patient may achieve remission but then experience relapse with more resistant disease. Sensitive clones are eliminated by chemotherapy, whereas surviving clones are likely to be more resistant to subsequent treatment. Furthermore, clones that persist after treatment may demonstrate clonal evolution. Additional genetic aberrations (clonal cytogenetic abnormalities or gene mutations) can be detected in this setting. Therefore, cytogenetic and molecular analyses should be repeated at relapse because these results affect prognosis and treatment selection.

Clinical Manifestations

Patients with acute leukemias often present with similar symptoms. Typically, the onset of illness is no more than 3 months before diagnosis unless the leukemia is associated with an antecedent hematologic disorder. Most have vague symptoms that are consequences of pancytopenia. Fatigue is common, as are anorexia and weight loss. Fever or infection is also common at presentation, and patients may have evidence of abnormal hemostasis (bleeding, easy bruising). Bone pain, lymphadenopathy, nonspecific cough, headache, and diaphoresis may also occur. Patients with ALL (compared with AML) are more likely to have lymphadenopathy, splenomegaly, or extramedullary involvement at other sites, such as the testis or central nervous system (CNS). However, involvement at any of these sites is not exclusive to ALL and can also be observed in AML patients, particularly in cases with monocytic differentiation. Rarely, patients present with primary symptoms caused by extramedullary leukemia. Extramedullary disease in AML is known as a *myeloid sarcoma* (also called a *granulocytic sarcoma* or *chloroma*). This is a tumor mass consisting of myeloid blasts and is most commonly seen in the skin, lymph nodes, gastrointestinal tract, soft tissue, or testis. Patients who present with isolated myeloid sarcoma typically develop blood or marrow involvement quickly thereafter and require systemic treatment akin to that used in patients with systemic disease (not solely surgical resection or local radiation). CNS involvement at initial presentation (headache, cranial nerve palsies) is uncommon; however, patients with ALL have an increased risk of CNS disease and should thus be given intrathecal chemotherapy as prophylaxis even without detectable CNS involvement at diagnosis.

Severe hemorrhagic complications are relatively infrequent at presentation but are more commonly encountered in acute promyelocytic leukemia (APL). Recognition of this risk at the time of initial presentation is critical, as replacement of fibrinogen and/or clotting factors may be lifesaving. Patients with APL often present with disseminated intravascular coagulation (DIC)-associated hemorrhage and may have intracranial hemorrhage or bleeding at other sites. Appropriate therapy for APL such as all-*trans* retinoic acid (tretinoin [Vesanoid]) should be initiated on suspicion and not withheld while awaiting genetic confirmation of the classic t(15;17) rearrangement. Thrombosis is a less frequent but well-recognized feature of APL. Bleeding associated with coagulopathy may also occur in monocytic AML and with extreme degrees of leukocytosis or thrombocytopenia in other acute leukemias. Retinal hemorrhage caused by thrombocytopenia and extreme leukocytosis is detected in approximately 15% of patients.

Laboratory parameters are quite variable with any type of acute leukemia. The presenting WBC count may be elevated, normal, or low. A minority of patients present with marked leukocytosis and high levels of circulating blasts, with hyperleukocytosis defined as WBC count greater than 100,000/μL. Patients with AML and hyperleukocytosis are at increased risk of developing leukostasis, which manifests with CNS and pulmonary symptoms and requires prompt recognition and management. Alternatively, many patients present with low WBC count or even with no circulating blasts. Typically, review of the peripheral blood smear identifies the classic blast—fine, lacy chromatin with one or more nucleoli and a high nucleus-to-cytoplasm ratio, which is characteristic of immature cells. The presence in blasts of abnormal rod-shaped granules called *Auer rods* on light microscopy indicates myeloid lineage.

Anemia is observed at diagnosis in nearly all patients but may not be severe. Decreased erythropoiesis often results in a reduced reticulocyte (immature red blood cell [RBC]) count, and RBC survival may be shortened by accelerated destruction. Most patients also present with thrombocytopenia (less than the normal lower limit value of 150,000/μL); severe thrombocytopenia (<10,000/μL) can be life threatening and requires immediate platelet transfusion.

Diagnosis

When acute leukemia is clinically suspected, in addition to morphologic and flow-cytometric analyses of bone marrow and blood, cytogenetic and genetic tests are mandatory to aid rapid diagnosis, assess prognosis, and inform the best approach to treatment. Clinical features also influence prognosis and treatment selection. These include a history of antecedent hematologic disorder or prior chemotherapy, advanced age, and a strong family history of acute leukemia or related hematologic disorder (all favoring AML); each of these has an adverse prognosis. In ALL, *KMT2A* rearrangement and complex karyotype are examples of abnormalities associated with adverse prognosis.

Initial assessments should evaluate cardiovascular, pulmonary, hepatic, and renal systems; patients should also be evaluated and treated for infection, tumor lysis syndrome, leukostasis, or DIC. Preparation for transfusion of blood or platelets requires blood type and crossmatch to be determined, and human leukocyte antigen (HLA) testing is required early in the treatment course (before chemotherapy) in consideration of future allogeneic hematopoietic stem cell transplantation (allo-HCT). Cytogenetic analysis typically requires bone marrow. Genetic testing (from blood or marrow) continues to evolve and is critical for successful diagnosis, prognosis, and therapy. Younger patients should be counseled regarding fertility preservation at diagnosis.

The diagnosis of AML is based on a finding of at least 20% myeloid blasts in the blood or bone marrow. However, this 20% threshold is not required for diagnosis in cases of myeloid sarcoma or in cases of AML with defining genetic abnormalities; this includes the classic cytogenetic abnormalities *t*(15;17) (diagnostic of APL), *t*(8;21), inv(16), or *t*(16;16), and mutation of the nucleophosmin *(NPM1)* gene, in addition to several less common genetic entities. In 2022 the International Consensus Classification of Myeloid Neoplasms and Acute Leukemias added a new myelodysplastic syndrome (MDS)/AML categorization for patients with 10% to 19% blasts to reflect the biologic continuum between MDS and AML. Myeloid blasts stain positive for myeloperoxidase; by flow cytometry, myeloid blasts are typically positive for CD13 and CD33. A prognostic schema developed by the European LeukemiaNet assigns prognostic risk based on cytogenetic and genetic features of disease (Table 1). Some morphologic features are associated with specific cytogenetic or molecular findings such as atypical promyelocytes and *t*(15;17) in APL or dysplastic eosinophils and inv(16) or *t*(16;16). The expression of B-cell markers (CD19, PAX5, cytoplasmic CD79a) is not infrequent in *t*(8;21).

The diagnosis of ALL likewise requires at least 20% lymphoid blasts. Cases with primarily nodal or extranodal involvement and less than 20% blasts in the blood and marrow are classified as

TABLE 1	2022 European LeukemiaNet Risk Classification by Genetics at Initial Diagnosis
RISK CATEGORY*	**GENETIC ABNORMALITY**
Favorable	t(8;21)(q22;q22.1)/*RUNX1::RUNX1T1**,† inv(16)(p13.1q22) or t(16;16)(p13.1;q22)/ *CBFB::MYH11**,† Mutated *NPM1**,‡ without *FLT3-ITD* bZIP in-frame mutated CEBPA§
Intermediate	Mutated *NPM1**,‡ with *FLT3-ITD* Wild-type *NPM1* with *FLT3-ITD* (without adverse-risk genetic lesions) t(9;11)(p21.3;q23.3)/*MLLT3::KMT2A**,¶¶ Cytogenetic and/or molecular abnormalities not classified as favorable or adverse
Adverse	t(6;9)(p23.3;q34.1)/*DEK::NUP214*t(v;11q23.3); *KMT2A-rearranged*¶ t(9;22)(q34.1;q11.2)/*BCR::ABL1* t(8;16)(p11.2;p13.3)/*KAT6A::CREBBP* inv(3)(q21.3q26.2) or t(3;3)(q21.3;q26.2)/*GATA2, MECOM(EVI1)* t(3q26.2;v)/*MECOM(EVI1)*-rearranged −5 or del(5q); −7; −17/abn(17p)Complex karyotype,# monosomal karyotype** Mutated *ASXL1, BCOR, EZH2, RUNX1, SF3B1, SRSF2, STAG2, U2AF1,* and/or *ZRSR2*†† Mutated *TP53*§§

*Mainly based on results observed in intensively treated patients. Initial risk assignment may change during the treatment course based on the results from analyses of measurable residual disease.
†Concurrent *KIT* and/or *FLT3* gene mutation does not alter risk categorization.
‡AML with *NPM1* mutation and adverse-risk cytogenetic abnormalities is categorized as adverse risk.
§Only in-frame mutations affecting the bZIP region of *CEBPA*, irrespective of whether they occur as monoallelic or biallelic mutations, have been associated with favorable outcome.
¶Excluding *KMT2A* PTD.
#Complex karyotype: Three or more unrelated chromosome abnormalities in the absence of other class-defining recurring genetic abnormalities; excludes hyperdiploid karyotypes with three or more trisomies (or polysomies) without structural abnormalities.
**Monosomal karyotype: presence of two or more distinct monosomies (excluding loss of X or Y) or one single autosomal monosomy in combination with at least one structural chromosome abnormality (excluding core-binding factor AML).
††"Myelodysplasia-related gene mutations." For the time being, these markers should not be used as an adverse prognostic marker if they co-occur with favorable-risk AML subtypes.
§§*TP53* mutation at a variant allele fraction of at least 10%, irrespective of the *TP53* allelic status (mono- or biallelic mutation); *TP53* mutations are significantly associated with AML with complex and monosomal karyotype.
¶¶The presence of t(9;11)(p21.3;q23.3) takes precedence over rare, concurrent adverse-risk gene mutations.
AML, Acute myeloid leukemia; *bZIP*, basic leucine zipper region; *PTD*, partial tandem duplication.
Modified from Döhner H, Wei A, Applebaum R, et al: Diagnosis and management of AML in adults: 2022 recommendations from an international expert panel on behalf of the ELN, *Blood* 140(12):1345–1377, 2022.

lymphoblastic lymphoma. By immunohistochemical methods, lymphoid blasts stain positive for terminal deoxynucleotidyl transferase; by flow cytometry, lymphoid blasts are typically positive for CD10, CD19, CD22, CD79a, and CD20 (variable) for B-ALL and CD3, CD4, CD7, and CD8 for T-ALL.

Patients may uncommonly present with acute leukemia of ambiguous lineage; this classification includes acute undifferentiated leukemias, which express no lineage-defining antigens, and mixed-phenotype acute leukemias, which express antigens defining more than one lineage. However, more common are AML cases that express an aberrant B-cell or T-cell marker (e.g., CD7 on myeloid blasts), referred to as an *aberrant immunophenotype.* Likewise, B-ALL may aberrantly express CD13 or CD33.

Molecular testing is an important component of diagnosis. For AML, molecular testing is performed by next-generation sequencing and/or polymerase chain reaction (PCR) assays and should, at minimum, include assessment of *FLT3, NPM1,*

CEBPA, IDH1, IDH2, RUNX1, ASXL1, DDX41, BCOR, EZH2, SF3B1, SRSF2, STAG2, U2AF1, ZRSR2, and TP53. The 2022 European LeukemiaNet guidelines recommend additional genes to be tested at diagnosis. For ALL, testing is equally important but is still evolving in terms of commercial availability for important molecular analyses. Critical to the initial assessment of ALL is testing for the *BCR-ABL1* fusion by molecular methods that are widely available; tyrosine kinase inhibitors (TKIs) targeting this lesion are an integral part of treatment of ALL with *BCR-ABL1*. Likewise, testing by interphase fluorescence in situ hybridization for the major recurrent cytogenetic abnormalities seen in ALL—including *ETV6-RUNX1*, *TCF3-PBX1*, and *KMT2A* rearrangements, among others—is mandatory. Testing for the "*BCR-ABL1*-like" genetic signature identifies a subset of patients with adverse prognosis but potential responsiveness to TKI therapies. *BCR-ABL1*–like disease has several common genetic features, including disruption of B-lymphoid transcription factors such as *IKZF1*, *CRLF2*, *JAK2*, and others. Diagnostic testing guidelines for both AML and ALL are delineated and annually updated by the National Comprehensive Cancer Network (https://NCCN.org).

Cytogenetic analysis should be performed on the bone marrow aspirate taken at diagnosis in any patient suspected to have acute leukemia. Prognosis is defined by genetic risk stratification systems that incorporate cytogenetic and molecular analyses. Broadly speaking, patients with AML with t(15;17), known as APL as described earlier, have an excellent prognosis, with cure rates greater than 90% after completion of modern therapies. Patients with AML with t(8;21) or inv(16) also have a favorable prognosis. Patients with no cytogenetic abnormalities (cytogenetically normal AML [CN-AML]) have an intermediate prognosis (classification is further dependent on molecular testing; see later discussion), whereas patients with adverse-risk cytogenetic abnormalities (see Table 1) have a poor prognosis, particularly older adult patients. At least 20 metaphases are necessary to define a normal karyotype. Molecular testing provides valuable additional information, especially in CN-AML. *NPM1* mutations without co-occurring *FLT3* internal tandem duplication and *CEBPA* in-frame mutations affecting the basic leucine zipper region are "favorable risk" molecular features. Conversely, "myelodysplasia-related gene mutations" (see Table 1) and mutations in *TP53* (often but not exclusively observed in the setting of complex karyotype) are associated with adverse risk, with *TP53*-mutated patients demonstrating particularly dismal outcomes. Mutations in genes encoding isocitrate dehydrogenase (IDH) enzymes identify patients who are likely to respond to novel therapies that target these aberrant pathways.

Cytogenetic testing for ALL enables classification into several groups, including, for example, *BCR-ABL1* fusion disease. This fusion, known cytogenetically as t(9;22) and colloquially referred to as the *Philadelphia (Ph) chromosome* (based on the city where it was originally identified), has historically been associated with a poor prognosis. However, the incorporation of TKIs that target the aberrantly active kinase has improved clinical outcomes. Other important ALL subsets include *KMT2A* (formerly *MLL*) rearrangements at chromosome 11q23 (with various translocation partners but often chromosome 4 in B-ALL), which are associated with an unfavorable prognosis. Many other subsets of ALL exist in the World Health Organization (WHO) classification. Favorable risk is seen in patients with B-ALL with hyperdiploidy (51–65 chromosomes) and t(12;21)(p13.2;q22.1), the *ETV6-RUNX1* fusion. T-ALL is characterized by activating mutations in *NOTCH1* (present in about 60% of cases) and deregulation of a number of transcription factors; immunophenotyping showing an early T-cell precursor (ETP-ALL) phenotype (low expression of CD1a, CD8, CD5) has been associated with an adverse prognosis, although the prognostic significance of ETP-ALL is less clear in adolescent and young adults treated with "pediatric-inspired" multiagent chemotherapy regimens.

Historically, the diagnosis and classification of acute leukemia was based on the French American-British morphologic and cytochemical criteria, which assigned patients with AML to one of eight groups designated M0 to M7. Likewise, ALL was classified into L1, L2, and L3 groups. These categories, although still in the vernacular on the clinical wards, have been replaced by modern classification systems. Diagnosis and classification are based instead on the complex morphologic, flow cytometric, cytogenetic, and molecular characterization schemas outlined by the WHO Classification of Haematolymphoid Tumours, with increasing dependence on genetic features.

Differential Diagnosis

The differential diagnosis for acute leukemia includes many bone marrow disorders that present with pancytopenia. However, the presence of excess blasts in the blood or marrow limits the diagnosis to AML, ALL, or acute leukemia of ambiguous lineage. For patients without circulating blasts in the blood, highest in the differential diagnosis of pancytopenia are other hematologic cancers with marrow infiltration or bone marrow failure syndromes such as aplastic anemia. Advanced myeloproliferative neoplasms with bone marrow fibrosis and myelodysplastic syndromes can also present similarly, occasionally with rare circulating blasts. Rarely, the pancytopenia caused by the displacement of hematopoietic bone marrow tissue by fibrosis, tumor, or granuloma (called *myelophthisis*) mimics acute leukemia. Examples include solid organ cancers with extensive marrow involvement and granulomatous diseases such as tuberculosis. However, essentially only acute leukemia is the appropriate diagnosis in patients with high-level circulating blasts visualized on light microscopy.

Treatment of Acute Myeloid Leukemia

Treatment of the newly diagnosed adult patient with AML is usually divided into two phases: (1) induction and (2) consolidation (i.e., postremission management). The aim of induction chemotherapy is complete remission (CR), defined as fewer than 5% blasts on a bone marrow aspirate, with recovery of blood counts (absolute neutrophil count >1000/μL and platelet count >100,000/μL). Additional defining criteria of CR include absent circulating blasts and no detectable extramedullary disease. Achievement of CR (or failure to do so) is the best predictor of long-term clinical outcome. The definition of CR is further refined based on the detection of measurable residual disease (MRD) by flow cytometry and/or molecular testing. Marrow response *without* full blood count recovery meets lesser response definitions (often termed CR with incomplete hematologic recovery); patients with such responses have outcomes inferior to those with CR. Blood count recovery occurs approximately 4 weeks after the initiation of intensive induction chemotherapy. CR is achieved in 60% to 90% of younger patients (depending on molecular risk) and in approximately 2% to 60% of older adult patients (>60 years). Notably, for older adult patients, this estimate is from the subset of patients who are offered intensive therapy; many older patients are not treated intensively because of medical comorbidities or poor performance status. Long-term survival estimates are approximately 60% for younger patients with favorable-risk disease (see Table 1), 40% for intermediate-risk disease, and 20% for adverse-risk disease. Older adult patients do poorly in each group; indeed, there are very few long-term survivors among older patients with adverse-risk disease.

Induction and consolidation therapies are chosen after considering both patient and disease-specific factors, including overall fitness, comorbidities, and cytogenetic/molecular risk. Intensive induction therapy is the norm in younger, medically fit patients (<60 years). In older patients, the benefit of intensive therapy is more controversial in all but those with a favorable risk profile; novel approaches for selecting patients predicted to be responsive to treatment and new therapies remain under investigation. Notably, large data sets have demonstrated that even more infirm older patients with AML benefit from treatment compared with palliative care alone.

Standard induction therapy for AML consists of cytarabine (cytosine arabinoside [Ara-C, Cytosar]), 100 to 200 mg/m²/day administered as a continuous infusion for 7 days, and daunorubicin (Cerubidine), 60 to 90 mg/m²/day for 3 days, commonly known as the *7 + 3* schema. Idarubicin (Idamycin; 12 mg/m²/day) can be used in place of daunorubicin. Resistant disease is more frequent in older adult patients and those with prior hematologic disorders, therapy-related AML, or adverse-risk cytogenetic and molecular abnormalities (which are more frequent in older patients). In older adult patients, the long-term outcome is generally poor because of the higher frequency of resistant disease in this group plus an increased rate of treatment-related mortality. As an alternative to intensive induction, unfit or adverse-risk older patients may instead receive lower intensity therapy with a hypomethylating agent (e.g., decitabine [Dacogen][1] or azacitidine [Vidaza])[1]. For patients older than 75 years of age or those who are not candidates for intensive therapy, the Bcl-2 inhibitor venetoclax (Venclexta) has been approved in combination with hypomethylating agent therapy. A randomized trial demonstrated improved survival and higher remission rates with azacitidine in combination with venetoclax compared with azacitidine alone, and this combination is now considered standard of care in this patient population. All patients should be considered for clinical trials, but those in adverse-risk groups should ideally be offered investigational approaches whenever available.

Induction of first complete remission (CR1) is critical to long-term survival in AML. However, without further therapy, virtually all patients in CR will eventually relapse. Patients are estimated to have 10^{12} leukemic cells at diagnosis, which intensive induction chemotherapy reduces by four to five orders of magnitude. Although this reduces the disease burden by 99.9%, approximately 10^8 residual leukemic cells remain after successful induction therapy. These residual cells may not be measurable at all or may be measurable only by sensitive techniques such as multiparameter flow cytometry or quantitative reverse-transcriptase polymerase chain reaction (RT-PCR); they cannot be detected by morphology alone. Thus postremission therapy is designed to eradicate residual (typically undetectable) leukemic cells to prevent relapse and prolong survival. Similar to induction, the type of postremission therapy in AML is selected for each individual patient based on age, fitness, and cytogenetic/molecular risk.

Postremission treatment options include chemotherapy and/or transplantation. The choice between consolidation with chemotherapy alone or transplantation is complex and based on age, disease risk, and practical considerations. In younger patients receiving chemotherapy, postremission therapy with intermediate/high-dose cytarabine[1] for two to four cycles is standard practice. It is clear that alloHCT is the best relapse-prevention strategy currently available for AML. However, the benefit of alloHCT in reducing relapse risk is offset somewhat by increased morbidity and mortality from transplant-related complications including graft-versus-host disease (GVHD) and infectious complications. Given that relapsed AML is frequently resistant to chemotherapy, alloHCT in CR1 is a favored strategy for patients at high risk for relapse. Transplantation is generally recommended for physically fit patients younger than 75 years of age who do not have favorable-risk disease (see Table 1) and have a suitable donor. Donors are typically HLA matched (related or unrelated) or, increasingly, haploidentical (half-matched sibling, parent, child, or other relative). With the incorporation of novel GVHD prophylaxis regimens, HLA-mismatched unrelated donors are increasingly practical. Prognostic factors help in selecting the appropriate postremission therapy in patients in CR1. In general, patients with favorable-risk AML in CR1 are treated with chemotherapy alone, though MRD status may be used to identify patients more likely to benefit from alloHCT. Patients with adverse-risk disease should proceed to alloHCT at CR1 if possible. The decision for alloHCT versus chemotherapy in CR1 for intermediate-risk patients remains in debate, but transplant is typically favored for young, fit patients.

The U.S. Food and Drug Administration (FDA) has approved several targeted drugs since 2017. For AML patients with *FLT3* mutation, midostaurin (Rydapt, in combination with induction chemotherapy), quizartinib (Vanflyta, in combination with induction chemotherapy), and gilteritinib (Xospata, as monotherapy for relapsed AML) have improved outcomes compared with chemotherapy alone. Likewise, agents targeting mutated IDH enzymes 1 or 2 (in AML patients with *IDH1* or *IDH2* mutations) have been shown to be effective in both relapsed and initial therapy settings. CPX-351 (Vyxeos, a liposomal combination of daunorubicin [an anthracycline] and cytarabine) has been approved in patients with therapy-related AML or AML with myelodysplasia-related changes (including patients with antecedent hematologic disorder). All these drugs, as well as venetoclax and many other novel agents, are currently in additional clinical trials. Menin inhibition has demonstrated notable therapeutic promise in patients with acute leukemias harboring sensitizing molecular alterations, including mutations in *NPM1*. The first-in-class menin inhibitor revumenib (Revuforj) was approved by the FDA in late 2024 for the treatment of relapsed/refractory acute leukemias with *KMT2A* rearrangements.

APL is uniquely treated with all-*trans* retinoic acid (tretinoin [Vesanoid]) and arsenic trioxide (ATO, Trisenox) rather than chemotherapy, although cases with high presenting WBC counts (>10,000/μL) require the addition of the antibody-drug conjugate gemtuzumab ozogamicin (Mylotarg)[1] for cytoreduction. Cases with high WBC counts are at increased risk for fatal hemorrhage and other complications. Low-risk patients (WBC <10,000/μL) have a virtually nonexistent frequency of resistant disease when treated with all-*trans* retinoic acid (tretinoin) and arsenic trioxide. Patients with APL require expert management to address complications of DIC and hemorrhage and the so-called *APL syndrome* (formerly known as *differentiation syndrome* and *retinoic acid syndrome*). APL syndrome is marked by an increasing WBC count, fever, hypoxia, shortness of breath, and fluid accumulation; it occurs up to 3 weeks after treatment initiation. It is common, especially in presentations with higher WBCs, and requires urgent therapy consisting of steroids, diuresis, supportive care, and possibly cytoreduction.

Treatment of Acute Lymphoblastic Leukemia

Standard chemotherapy treatment of ALL is of much more extended duration compared with that for AML. However, the same general principles apply; achievement of CR1 with initial therapy is the critical first step for long-term survival. Postremission therapy in ALL is broken into different segments of various intensity, including consolidation, interim maintenance, delayed intensification, and prolonged (24–36 months) maintenance. CNS-directed therapy (systemic chemotherapy with intrathecal chemotherapy, or cranial radiotherapy) is an important and mandatory feature of ALL treatment because of high rates of CNS relapse in patients who do not receive such therapy. Generally, treatment of younger, fit patients with Ph-negative disease includes variations of a five-drug induction combination of cyclophosphamide (Cytoxan), prednisone[1] or dexamethasone (Decadron)[1], anthracycline (doxorubicin [Adriamycin] or daunorubicin), PEGylated asparaginase (Oncaspar), and vincristine (Oncovin). The principle of therapy for ALL is continuous exposure to multiple chemotherapy/immunotherapy agents with nonoverlapping resistance mechanisms; all protocols use alternating chemotherapy/immunotherapy regimens given over an extended period. Additional agents include rituximab (Rituxan) in CD20-positive disease[1], methotrexate, cytarabine (Cytarabine), 6-mercaptopurine (Purinethol), and others. Examples of common treatment strategies are the Berlin-Frankfurt-Munster (BFM) approach and the hyper-CVAD (hyperfractionated cyclophosphamide, vincristine, doxorubicin, dexamethasone) regimen. Although data are sparse, patients with mixed-phenotype acute leukemias appear to fare

---

[1]Not FDA approved for this indication.

[1]Not FDA approved for this indication.

better with ALL-like treatment approaches compared with those used in AML.

Although children with B-ALL have favorable long-term survival in the 80% to 90% range, adults fare worse. Outcomes in young adults (up to 40 years of age) have improved with the use of "pediatric-inspired" regimens, which typically incorporate PEGylated asparaginase (Oncaspar) in these multiagent schemas. Unfortunately, older adults (>40 years of age) often have difficulty tolerating such approaches. The addition of nelarabine (Arranon) to first-line therapy has improved outcomes in T-ALL.

As noted previously, the identification of the Ph chromosome (t(9;22)) or the *BCR-ABL1* fusion is critical in the initial diagnosis of B-ALL or mixed-phenotype acute leukemia. The introduction of TKIs for Ph-positive patients into multiagent induction and postremission treatment has dramatically improved outcomes and is now standard. Second- or third-generation TKIs such as dasatinib (Sprycel) and ponatinib (Iclusig) are commonly used. AlloHCT in CR1 may not be necessary, especially if a complete molecular remission is rapidly achieved and high-risk genetic features are absent. "Chemotherapy-free" approaches incorporating TKI, corticosteroids, and the bispecific T-cell engager blinatumomab (Blincyto; see later) have been associated with promising outcomes in Ph-positive B-ALL[1].

Additional advances to traditional approaches include the use of CD20 monoclonal antibodies (rituximab [Rituxan][1]) for patients with B-ALL whose lymphoid blasts express this surface marker and nelarabine in T-ALL. Nelarabine (Arranon) is a purine analog with increased activity in T-ALL demonstrating 30% response rates in the relapsed setting; it has been incorporated into front-line multiagent clinical trials. AlloHCT in adult ALL is more controversial than in AML, although most trials offer alloHCT in CR1 for high-risk disease. Increasingly, MRD status at various time points is used to identify patients most likely to benefit from alloHCT. The addition of the bispecific antibody blinatumomab (Blincyto) for patients who remain MRD positive after intensive chemotherapy has improved clinical outcomes. In 2024, blinatumomab was approved in the consolidation phase of Ph-negative disease in MRD-negative first remission after a randomized, controlled trial demonstrated improved overall survival.

Immune-Based Therapies in Acute Leukemia

Beyond the use of alloHCT, recent years have seen remarkable progress in immunologic therapies for acute leukemia (Figure 1). In 2017 the FDA approved exciting engineered cellular therapies for relapsed malignancies of B-lymphocytes: chimeric antigen receptor (CAR) T cells that target CD19 (in B-ALL and non-Hodgkin lymphoma). Tisagenlecleucel (Kymriah) is approved for relapsed or refractory B-ALL in patients 25 years or younger, while brexucabtagene autoleucel (Tecartus) and obecabtagene autoleucel (Aucatzyl) have been approved for all adult patients. In these cases, autologous B cells are collected by apheresis from the patient, genetically engineered ex vivo to target CD19, and then infused back into the patient to treat CD19+ malignancy (after receipt of lymphodepleting therapy). In the process, CD19+ normal B cells are also eliminated. High response rates and long-term remissions have been reported in patients with ALL with highly refractory disease using CAR T-cell therapy; complete response rates in the range of 70% to 90% have been observed in CD19+ cancers: ALL, chronic lymphocytic leukemia, diffuse large B-cell lymphoma, and mantle cell lymphoma. Challenges of CAR T cells include issues with uncontrolled immune cell activation (termed *cytokine release syndrome [CRS]*), neurotoxicity (termed *immune effector cell–associated neurotoxicity syndrome [ICANS]*), killing of normal CD19+ B cells, and resistance caused by loss of CD19 expression on leukemic cells (e.g., CD19– relapse). CAR retargeting to other hematologic targets beyond CD19 remains an area of active investigation; CAR T cells targeting the BCMA antigen

[1] Not FDA approved for this indication.

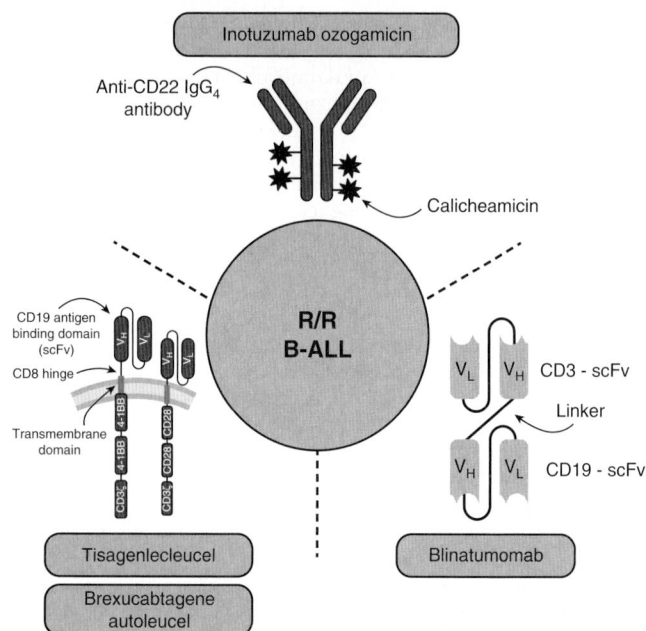

Figure 1 Structures of FDA-approved immune therapies. *B-ALL*, B-cell acute lymphoblastic leukemia; *IgG*, immunoglobulin G; *R/R*, relapsed/refractory; *scFV*, single-chain variable fragment; V_H, immunoglobulin variable heavy domain; V_L, immunoglobulin variable heavy domain. From Kegyes D, Jitaru C, Ghiaur G, et al: Switching from salvage chemotherapy to immunotherapy in adult B-cell acute lymphoblastic leukemia, *Blood Rev* 59:101042, 2023.

have been approved in multiple myeloma since 2021, whereas products targeting CD22 or multiple targets appear promising.

Several novel antibodies have also been approved. Inotuzumab ozogamicin (Besponsa; targeting CD22 in B-ALL) and gemtuzumab ozogamicin (Mylotarg; targeting CD33 in AML) are antibody-drug conjugates that deliver the toxin calicheamicin to lymphoid or myeloid blasts, respectively. Both agents have activity as a monotherapy and may also be incorporated into chemotherapy regimens. Blinatumomab (Blincyto) is a CD3-CD19 bispecific T-cell engager; this class of agents functions by linking immune cells to malignant cells resulting in cytotoxicity. Bispecific agents targeting CD7, CD33, CD123, and CD20 are in ongoing clinical trials.

Monitoring

Measurement of residual disease is an important component of management in ALL. Unsurprisingly, initial responsiveness to chemotherapy is a useful predictor for long-term outcome. Persistence of abnormal karyotype after induction among patients in CR is associated with poor clinical outcomes. For patients in morphologic CR, measurement of MRD is standard in both ALL and AML. More sensitive methods of MRD measurement beyond light microscopy and cytogenetics are increasingly used to aid decision making. Examples of sensitive MRD assessment include immunophenotyping by multiparameter flow cytometry to detect minute populations of blasts or quantitative RT-PCR, as well as other molecular methods to detect leukemia-associated molecular abnormalities, such as next-generation sequencing. Particularly in B-ALL, early clearance of MRD is favorable. In ALL and in APL, MRD assessment is a very useful and reliable tool to refine prognostication, detect early relapse, and direct the initiation of additional therapy. Quantitative measurement of mutated *NPM1* transcript levels during first remission provides important and potentially actionable information in that subset of AML.

Management of Complications

The treatment of acute leukemia involves repeated cycles of myelotoxic or immunosuppressive chemotherapy, requiring intensive supportive care. The emergence of infections with multidrug-resistant organisms is a growing concern. In addition, invasive fungal infections are associated with early death. Standard infection precautions include reverse isolation, air filtration, and prophylactic antimicrobials. Recommendations on the latter are best tailored based on institutional antibiograms; in AML patients undergoing intensive induction therapy, antifungal prophylaxis using agents with broad mold coverage is generally recommended.

Transfusion of red blood cells and platelets is a common and necessary part of treatment. Blood products should ideally be leukoreduced (done by the American Red Cross in the United States) to reduce the risk of febrile transfusion reaction and alloimmunization. Particularly in the multicourse induction and postremission therapies in ALL, optimization of supportive care strategies to facilitate the on-time administration of subsequent therapies whenever possible improves outcomes.

References

Arber D, Orazi A, Hasserjian R: International consensus classification of myeloid neoplasms and acute leukemias: integrating morphologic, clinical, and genomic data, *Blood* 140:1200–1228, 2022.

Brown AL, Churpek JE, Malcovati L, et al: Recognition of familial myeloid neoplasia in adults, *Semin Hematol* 54:60–68, 2017.

Döhner H, Wei A, Applebaum F, et al: Diagnosis and management of AML in adults: 2022 recommendations from an international expert panel on behalf of the ELN, *Blood* 140:1345–1377, 2022.

Heuser M, Freeman S, Ossenkoppele G, et al: Update on MRD in acute myeloid leukemia: a consensus document from the European LeukemiaNet MRD Working Party, *Blood* 138:2753–2767, 2021.

Iacobucci I, Mullighan CG: Genetic basis of acute lymphoblastic leukemia, *J Clin Oncol* 35:975–983, 2017.

Khoury JD, Solary E, Abla O, et al: The 5th edition of the World Health Organization classification of haematolymphoid tumours: myeloid and histiocytic/dendritic neoplasms, *Leukemia* 36:1703–1719, 2022.

Lim WA, June CH: The principles of engineering immune cells to treat cancer, *Cell* 168:724–740, 2017.

Maude SL, Frey N, Shaw PA, et al: Chimeric antigen receptor T cells for sustained remissions in leukemia, *N Engl J Med* 371:1507–1517, 2014.

National Comprehensive Cancer Network (NCCN): Clinical practices guidelines in oncology. Available at: https://www.nccn.org/guidelines/category_1. Accessed March 2025.

Papaemmanuil E, Gerstung M, Bullinger L, et al: Genomic classification and prognosis in acute myeloid leukemia, *N Engl J Med* 374:2209–2221, 2016.

TCGA Research Network, Ley TJ, Miller C, et al: Genomic and epigenomic landscapes of adult de novo acute myeloid leukemia, *N Engl J Med* 368:2059–2074, 2013.

Welch JS, Ley TJ, Link DC, et al: The origin and evolution of mutations in acute myeloid leukemia, *Cell* 150:264–278, 2012.

BLOOD COMPONENT THERAPY AND TRANSFUSION REACTIONS

Method of
Theresa Ann Nester, MD

CURRENT DIAGNOSIS

- Fever greater than 1°C rise during or within 3 hours after transfusion should prompt evaluation of the patient and consideration of a transfusion reaction.
- Fever and pain are the most common manifestations of an acute hemolytic transfusion reaction.
- The point of the transfusion reaction laboratory investigation is to evaluate for hemolysis, either intravascular or extravascular. The majority of reactions are negative for hemolysis.
- The differential diagnosis of a transfusion reaction with respiratory symptoms includes febrile nonhemolytic and circulatory overload (common), allergic or anaphylactic reaction, transfusion-related acute lung injury, acute hemolytic reaction, and bacterial contamination (rare).

CURRENT THERAPY

- The decision to transfuse red blood cells to a patient should depend more on the clinical state of the patient than on an absolute trigger for hemoglobin (Hb) or hematocrit.
- A transfusion trigger of less than 7 g/dL is recommended for hospitalized adult patients who are hemodynamically stable, including critically ill patients. A transfusion trigger of 8 g/dL is recommended for patients undergoing orthopedic or cardiac surgery, as well as those with preexisting cardiovascular disease.
- For severe autoimmune hemolytic anemia, maintenance of Hb at greater than 4 g/dL in younger patients and greater than 6 g/dL in older patients or patients with cardiovascular disease is appropriate.
- Platelets are not typically indicated in thrombotic thrombocytopenic purpura, autoimmune thrombocytopenic purpura, and heparin-induced thrombocytopenia unless the patient has significant bleeding.
- Currently available coagulation tests are not very useful for predicting bleeding in patients with end-stage liver disease. These patients establish a new equilibrium between coagulation, anticoagulation, and fibrinolysis that results in relatively less bleeding than predicted by the international normalized ratio.
- The goal during massive transfusion scenarios should be to prevent marked acidosis, hypothermia, and coagulopathy. The latter is often achieved with replacement of coagulation factors using plasma or cryoprecipitate within the first hour of the resuscitation.
- Cryoprecipitate is useful as a source of concentrated fibrinogen. In a patient who is actively bleeding and has a fibrinogen less than 100 mg/dL, cryoprecipitate is indicated.

Therapeutic Use of Blood Components

The community blood supply depends on two types of donors: whole blood donors and apheresis donors. Units of whole blood are centrifuged and then separated into components within a closed system. Using apheresis techniques, individual components of whole blood can be collected. Citrate is used to keep blood components from clotting.

The decision to transfuse blood to a patient should always include a consideration of the risks versus the benefits. Risks of transfusion-transmitted diseases are small with current testing standards. Transfusion reactions do occur; the most common ones are not life threatening unless the patient cannot tolerate tachycardia or hypertension. Rarely, a patient experiences a life-threatening reaction. Thus it is important to ensure that the need for the blood component outweighs the risks. Additionally, in a bleeding patient, it is important to check coagulation parameters (platelet count, prothrombin time [PT], international normalized ratio [INR], activated partial thromboplastin time [aPTT], fibrinogen) and hematocrit (Hct) to ensure that the component that will best address the bleeding is being used.

Red Blood Cells
Indications
Red blood cells (RBCs) should be given to increase oxygen-carrying capacity. The hemoglobin (Hb) and Hct levels alone should not be used to determine the need for transfusion; instead, the patient's clinical picture should drive the decision to transfuse. The patient's intravascular volume status, cardiopulmonary function, and baseline vital signs in the presence of anemia should all be considered. When anemia has persisted over weeks and months, large volume transfusion is often not indicated because compensatory mechanisms have had time to work.

TABLE 1 Component Therapy: Dosage and Expected Increment

COMPONENT	DOSE	EXPECTED INCREMENT	AVERAGE VOLUME
Red blood cells	1 unit	Hct 3%, Hb 1 g/dL	250 mL
Whole blood platelets	1 unit	Platelet count increased by 5000–10,000/μL	50 mL/unit (1 pool of 6 = 300 mL)
Apheresis platelet	1 unit	Platelet count increased by 20,000–60,000/μL	300 mL/unit
Plasma	10 mL/kg	Factor levels increased by 20%	300 mL/unit
Cryoprecipitate	1 unit	Fibrinogen increased by 5 mg/dL	15 mL/unit
Prepooled cryoprecipitate	1 6-unit pool	Fibrinogen increased by 45 mg/dL	120 mL/pool

Hb, Hemoglobin; *Hct,* hematocrit.

Transfusion Triggers

The 2023 clinical practice guideline from the Association for the Advancement of Blood and Biotherapies (formerly the American Association of Blood Banks) has the following recommendations: in hospitalized adult patients who are hemodynamically stable, including critically ill patients, a transfusion threshold of 7 g/dL is acceptable. In patients undergoing cardiac surgery, a threshold of 7.5 g/dL may be used. For orthopedic surgery and patients with preexisting cardiovascular disease, a transfusion threshold of 8 g/dL is recommended. The recommendations do not apply to patients with acute coronary syndrome, severe thrombocytopenia, or chronic transfusion dependent anemia, because of insufficient evidence.

Dosage

One unit of packed RBCs will increase the Hb by 1 g/dL and Hct by 3% in the patient who is not bleeding or experiencing hemolysis (Table 1).

Autoimmune Hemolytic Anemia
Special Situation

When the autoantibody responsible for autoimmune hemolytic anemia reacts at body temperature, all RBC units can appear incompatible. This is because the antibody binds to an epitope common to all RBCs, such as the band 3 protein. The clinician needs to decide when to transfuse the (apparently) incompatible units. In a patient who has never received a transfusion or been pregnant, there is little possibility of RBC alloantibodies in circulation, and the chance of hemolysis (beyond that being caused by the autoantibody) is low. For the patient who has received a transfusion or who has been pregnant in the past, the risk that a circulating RBC alloantibody is present and is being masked by the autoantibody is higher; special studies are available to reduce the risk of an alloantibody being overlooked. The transfusion trigger depends on whether the anemia is acute or chronic. For acute severe anemia, maintenance of Hb at greater than 4 g/dL in younger patients and greater than 6 g/dL in older patients or patients with cardiovascular disease is appropriate.

Trauma

In the prehospital setting, transfusion may help save the life of a trauma patient who is progressing to hemorrhagic shock.

Whole blood may be used for this purpose. The criteria for this product is to collect from a group O male (to reduce the risk of transfusion-related acute lung injury [TRALI]) previously tested to have low anti-A and anti-B titers (often <256). The product may or may not be leukoreduced (depending on the blood supplier and choice of bags), and is most often RhD positive due to the relative rarity of group O RhD-negative donors. Whole blood has a 21-day shelf life (compared with 42 days for packed RBCs), and studies indicate that the coagulation factors decline below hemostatic levels by about day 15 of storage. It is important to draw the patient's ABO type as soon as possible after arrival to the emergency department so that the patient's native type can still be determined; component therapy with type-specific components can expand the available products available to support the patient.

Platelets

Platelets are required as part of normal clotting. The first stage of clot formation is development of a platelet plug over the site of endothelial injury.

Indications

The indications for platelet transfusion may be divided into prevention of bleeding and treatment of bleeding in the setting of thrombocytopenia or platelet dysfunction.

Transfusion Triggers

Prevention of Bleeding. In a stable patient with normal platelet function, transfusion is appropriate if the platelet count is less than 10,000/μL. One randomized, controlled trial has shown that transfusion at platelet counts of 5000/μL to 10,000/μL prevents bleeding in the stable patient. In a stable patient with other hemostatic abnormalities (e.g., on anticoagulation), transfusion is appropriate with a platelet count less than 50,000/μL.

Before a planned invasive procedure such as open lung biopsy, transfusion is appropriate with a platelet count of less than 50,000/μL. For lumbar puncture, consensus guidelines suggest that a platelet count of 50,000/μL is appropriate, although there are a few large studies suggesting that counts between 20,000 and 50,000/μL may be adequate. A patient undergoing major surgery should receive platelets if the count is less than 50,000 to 100,000/μL. The transfusion should take place as close to the procedure as possible so that the platelets remain in circulation while the procedure is occurring.

Treatment of Bleeding. Platelets may be transfused with a major hemorrhage (e.g., gastrointestinal or genitourinary) and a platelet count less than 30,000 to 50,000/μL. For bleeding with major surgery or trauma, transfusion is appropriate for counts less than 80,000/μL. For bleeding into critical areas (e.g., central nervous system bleeding or diffuse alveolar hemorrhage), platelets may be given for counts less than 100,000/μL.

Dosage

Dosage is determined on the basis of the baseline platelet count, desired platelet count, and estimated blood volume. For a 70-kg patient, 3×10^{11} platelets (4–6 units of pooled whole blood platelets or 1 unit of apheresis platelets) increases platelet count by approximately 30,000 to 50,000/μL in the absence of alloimmunization or excessive consumption. For prophylactic therapy, lower dosages have been shown to be as effective as higher dosages in the prevention of bleeding.

Out of ABO Group Platelet Transfusion

Because platelets can only be stored for a maximum of 7 days after collection, and the community platelet supply is collected from volunteer donors, a platelet product that is identical to the patient's ABO type might not be available (Table 2 and Box 1). Thus it may be necessary to infuse a small volume of incompatible plasma (suspending the platelets) to the patient. Therefore there is a small risk of hemolysis of the patient's RBCs if the isoagglutinin (anti-A or anti-B) titer in the donated plasma is high. Studies of

TABLE 2	ABO Compatibility*		
PATIENT'S ABO	ANTIBODIES IN CIRCULATION	COMPATIBLE PACKED RED BLOOD CELLS	COMPATIBLE PLASMA
O	Anti-A, anti-B	O	O, A, B, AB
A	Anti-B	O or A	A or AB
B	Anti-A	O or B	B or AB
AB	None	O, A, B, AB	AB

*For platelet compatibility, see text.

BOX 1	Rh(D) Compatibility

Rh(D)-negative patients should receive Rh-negative red blood cells and platelet units.*,†

Rh(D)-positive patients can receive Rh-positive or Rh-negative red blood cells and platelet units.

Rh compatibility does not apply to acellular components (plasma and cryoprecipitate).

Only 15% of blood donors are Rh negative.

---

*In times of shortage, it becomes necessary to preserve the Rh(D) negative red blood cell inventory for females of childbearing potential (<50 years old).

†Platelet components contain very few red blood cells; Rho(D) immune globulin (RhoGAM) may be administered if prevention of anti-D formation is deemed appropriate. Consult with a transfusion medicine physician if further discussion is needed.

---

healthy blood donors indicate that these antibody titers are typically low and do not precipitate hemolysis. Transfusion services often have policies that limit the amount of incompatible plasma a patient has received with platelet transfusion. Alternatively, some centers measure the antibody titer in the donated product and give high-titer products only to patients whose RBCs lack the corresponding ABO antigen.

Unresponsiveness to Platelet Transfusion

A number of clinical factors can result in a patient's less-than-optimal response to platelet transfusion. In addition to consumption, some of these factors include splenomegaly, fever, and antifungal therapy. Patients who have been sensitized to foreign human leukocyte antigens through prior pregnancy or transfusion can also have a poor response to platelet transfusion. Transfusion medicine consultation regarding the evaluation of refractoriness to platelet transfusion may be indicated.

Special Situations

Uremia. Patients who are dialysis dependent might have an acquired platelet defect as a result of the uremic environment. Transfusion of platelets into this environment will render the transfused platelets dysfunctional. Thus if optimal platelet function is desired, dialysis should be performed frequently. Consider performing dialysis without heparin if the patient is actively bleeding.

Purpura and Thrombocytopenia. In patients with autoimmune thrombocytopenic purpura (ITP), thrombotic thrombocytopenic purpura (TTP), or heparin-induced thrombocytopenia, platelet transfusion is not indicated unless the patient has significant bleeding. Other therapies, such as steroid administration for ITP and plasma exchange for TTP, should be initiated to address the condition.

Trauma

Cold-stored platelets (CSP) may be produced by the blood supplier to help support trauma patients. This product has a longer shelf life than the standard platelet products. Studies indicate that CSP possess effective hemostatic potential upon transfusion.

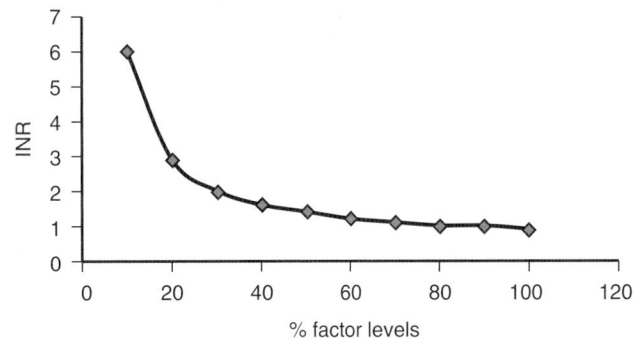

Figure 1 American Association of Blood Banks international normalized ratio (INR) compared with percentage factor levels. (Reprinted with permission from Nester T, AuBuchon, J: Hemotherapy decisions and their outcomes. In Roback JD, editor: *AAB technical manual*, ed 17, 2011, American Association of Blood Banks, p 592.)

However, these platelets will not stay in circulation for more than 24 hours and so they are not a good choice for situations such as chemotherapy or sepsis support. The 2023 FDA Guidance on CSP gives the indication of treatment of active bleeding when conventional platelets are not available or their use is not practical.

Plasma

Plasma contains all of the coagulation proteins needed for clot formation, as well as all of the fibrinolytic proteins that prevent systemic thrombosis. There are currently several kinds of plasma, such as fresh frozen, FP24, thawed, and liquid. All contain hemostatic levels of coagulation factors as long as they are stored appropriately. The effect of plasma transfusion on the PT and INR is 4 to 6 hours, owing to the short half-life of coagulation factor VII. Thus other, longer-lasting means of restoring coagulation factors, such as vitamin K administration, should be undertaken if a more durable response is desired.

When replacing coagulation factors with plasma, it is not necessary to have 100% factor replacement as the goal. Hemostasis is typically able to occur if circulating coagulation factor levels are between 40% and 50%. It is important to understand that the relationship between the INR and the percentage factor level is a logarithmic, rather than a linear, relationship (Figure 1). Thus whether the INR is 9 or 1.8, the initial dosage of plasma should be 10 to 20 mL/kg, with recheck of the laboratory values a few minutes after infusion. The more prolonged the INR, the more significant the effect of the dose on the INR.

Transfusion Triggers

For bleeding or imminent surgery that cannot be corrected in a timely manner by vitamin K administration, use plasma to correct an INR greater than 1.8 to 2.0. The exception is patients with end-stage liver disease (see later).

Dosage

At a dosage of 10 mL/kg, each unit has an average of 300 mL (3–5 units in a 70-kg adult). This dosage should increase circulating coagulation factors by 20% immediately after infusion.

Special Situations

Liver Disease. The INR is a less useful test in patients with end-stage liver disease. The destruction of liver tissue leads to decreased production of coagulation and fibrinolytic proteins such that a new balance is established. Patients with end-stage liver disease have been shown to have normal levels of circulating thrombin and reduced levels of certain anticoagulant proteins (e.g., protein C), which could explain why they do not bleed as often as predicted with the elevation in INR. Thus the prophylactic use of plasma to correct a mildly prolonged laboratory value in the absence of bleeding is not indicated. It will lead to unnecessary plasma infusion, and the risk of volume overload and transfusion reactions outweighs the benefit in these patients.

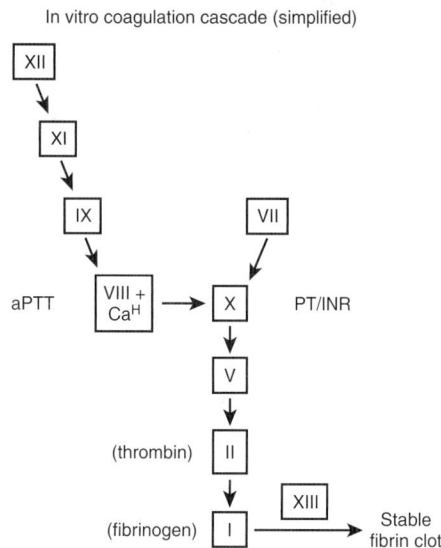

Figure 2 Coagulation cascade. *aPTT*, Activated partial thromboplastin time; *INR*, international normalized ratio; *PT*, prothrombin time.

Massive Transfusion. In trauma patients, patients with ruptured aortic aneurysms and patients with other arterial bleeding, massive transfusion may be necessary. The basic principles of such a scenario include taking steps early into the resuscitation to prevent the patient from becoming too cold, acidotic, or coagulopathic to reverse the situation. Some plasma (and cryoprecipitate, if the fibrinogen is very low) should be infused early into the resuscitation to help prevent coagulopathy. RBCs and plasma should be infused through a blood warmer, if possible.

Isolated Prolonged aPTT. Other than a deficiency in coagulation factor XI, bear in mind that the differential of an isolated prolonged aPTT includes entities that do not typically require plasma (refer to Figure 2). Hemophilia A, hemophilia B, and von Willebrand disease are no longer treated by plasma but can require factor concentrates to prevent bleeding. Systemic administration of heparin must be reversed by protamine if fast reversal is desired. Note that plasma transfusion will not reverse the effect of heparin. One of the most common causes of a prolonged aPTT is a lupus anticoagulant; this is an antibody directed against phospholipids that typically leads to thrombosis rather than hemorrhage.

Intracranial Hemorrhage or Life-Threatening Bleeding. Reversal of anticoagulation in the setting of intracranial hemorrhage or life-threatening bleeding depends on the anticoagulant. For patients taking warfarin (Coumadin), refer to Box 2.

Prothrombin complex concentrates (PCCs) may be used to replenish factors II, VII, IX, and X rapidly. KCentra is a four-factor PCC that has been FDA approved to treat life-threatening hemorrhage in adult patients on warfarin. For reversal of dabigatran (Pradaxa), a direct oral anticoagulant, idarucizumab (Praxbind), is approved by the U.S. Food and Drug Administration (FDA) as a reversal agent. For reversal of apixaban (Eliquis) and rivaroxaban (Xarelto) in life-threatening bleeding, andexanet alfa (Andexxa) is available.

Cryoprecipitate

Cryoprecipitate contains fibrinogen, coagulation factors VIII and XIII, and von Willebrand factor. The most common current use is as a source of concentrated fibrinogen. It may also be used to treat hemorrhage in the rare patient with factor XIII deficiency.

Indications

Clinical scenarios that increase probability for low fibrinogen include any clinical situation in which disseminated intravascular coagulation (DIC) may be present. These include obstetric bleeding, trauma involving head injury or crush injury, and sepsis. Clinical events that can lead to an isolated decrease in serum

fibrinogen concentration include administration of L-asparaginase (Elspar) and surgeries that disrupt bladder or salivary gland endothelium. Fibrinogen concentrates are available for patients who will not accept cryoprecipitate.

Transfusion Triggers

Transfusion is appropriate in patients with low serum fibrinogen, typically less than 100 mg/dL. In cases of massive transfusion, a trigger of 150 mg/dL is considered practical, so that the patient becomes less coagulopathic in the time that it takes to draw and review new laboratory values. A fibrinogen level of less than 300 mg/dL predicts severe postpartum hemorrhage, with a normal postpartum fibrinogen level typically in the 600 mg/dL range. Because component therapy aims to replete coagulation factors to hemostatic (rather than completely normal) levels, consensus guidelines suggest maintaining a fibrinogen level greater than 200 mg/dL during a postpartum hemorrhage.

Dosage

Dosage depends on the type of cryoprecipitate available. If the product requires resuspension in saline before pooling, then 1 unit (average 15-mL volume) will increase fibrinogen by 5 mg/dL. If the product has been pooled in plasma before freezing, then 1 unit will increase fibrinogen by 7 to 8 mg/dL; a 6-unit pool will increase fibrinogen by 45 mg/dL. Check with the transfusion service laboratory regarding which product is available and the expected increment.

Special Situation

DIC is a state where fibrinogen is consumed at a faster rate than other circulating coagulation factors. This is because DIC is typically a thrombin-generating process (thrombin cleaves fibrinogen into fibrin for clot formation). Thus although all coagulation factors are being consumed in DIC, timely repletion of fibrinogen by use of cryoprecipitate can result in more timely cessation of bleeding in a patient with active DIC. The target value is fibrinogen at least 100 mg/dL. If the PT and INR are still prolonged with fibrinogen greater than 100 mg/dL, administration of plasma will replete other coagulation factors being consumed.

TABLE 3	Transfusion Reactions
MOST COMMON REACTIONS	**INCIDENCE**
Allergic reaction of mild severity	1:33–1:100
Febrile nonhemolytic reaction	1:100–1:1000 with leukocyte reduction
Transfusion-related circulatory overload	<1:100

MOST DANGEROUS REACTIONS	**INCIDENCE**
Acute hemolytic reaction	1:38,000–1:70,000
Anaphylactic reaction	1:20,000–1:50,000
Transfusion-related acute lung injury	1:1200–1:190,000
Bacterial contamination of red cell unit with gram-negative organisms	1:1,000,000

Transfusion Reactions

Reactions to transfusion are relatively common; life-threatening reactions are rare (Tables 3 and 4).

Because fever is a feature of both common and dangerous reactions, a transfusion reaction evaluation should be initiated with fever greater than 1°C above patient's baseline temperature at the start of the transfusion. The infusion of product should cease, at least until the laboratory results are known and the patient has responded to treatment. The main point of the laboratory investigation is to evaluate the plasma for abnormal (usually red) color in an effort to detect intravascular hemolysis as quickly as possible. If the clerical check and hemolysis direct antiglobulin tests are negative, one might consider restarting the transfusion with careful surveillance of the patient. A direct antiglobulin test is performed to detect the presence of antibody coating RBCs in circulation; a positive result could indicate extravascular hemolysis, which is not as dangerous as intravascular hemolysis.

Most Common Reactions

Febrile Nonhemolytic Reaction

Presentation. A febrile nonhemolytic transfusion reaction manifests as a fever greater than a 1°C rise above the patient's baseline, often accompanied by rigors. Hypertension, tachypnea, and transient decrease in oxygen saturation can also occur until the symptoms are treated. Evidence of hemolysis will be absent on laboratory evaluation. These reactions can manifest during or 2 to 3 hours after the transfusion.

Pathophysiology. Cytokines produced by white blood cells (WBCs) present in cellular blood components (RBC and platelet units) are responsible for the clinical presentation. Platelets also secrete cytokines; thus leukoreduction of platelet units might not be successful in preventing the reaction.

TABLE 4	Transfusion Reactions With Respiratory Symptoms		
REACTION	**CLASSIC SIGNS**	**RELATIVE FREQUENCY**	**ACUTE MANAGEMENT (TRANSFUSION STOPPED IN ALL CASES)**
Febrile nonhemolytic reaction	Transient tachypnea in the presence of rigors and fever	Common	Antipyretic ± meperidine (Demerol)[1]
Circulatory overload	Hypoxia Crackles in lower lung fields Increased BP Chest radiograph consistent with volume overload	Common	Diuresis
Allergic reaction of moderate severity	Wheezes Possible perioral or periorbital edema Possible hives	Uncommon	IV antihistamines and possibly epinephrine (Adrenalin)
Allergic reaction of marked severity	Wheezes, swollen lips, tongue, uvula Stridor or other signs of airway compromise Very decreased BP	Rare	Epinephrine IV, fluids and airway management Bronchodilators and glucagon (GlucaGen)[1] for patient on β-blockers
Transfusion-related acute lung injury	Tachypnea and hypoxia during or within 6 h of transfusion Persisting for several hours Chest radiograph consistent with bilateral white-out	Rare	Respiratory support of noncardiogenic pulmonary edema
Acute hemolytic reaction	Red urine and red serum Hypotension and diffuse oozing may be present Tachypnea (10% of patients)	Rare	Supportive (possibly ICU) care Administration of crystalloid solution Blood component therapy if DIC is present
Bacterial contamination with gram-negative organism	Very decreased BP Fever Nausea, vomiting Possible tachypnea	Rare	Intensive care for support of gram-negative sepsis

[1]Not FDA approved for this indication.
BP, Blood pressure; *DIC*, disseminated intravascular coagulation; *ICU*, intensive care unit.

Acute Management. Administration of an antipyretic is the routine treatment; meperidine (Demerol)[1] may be required to address severe rigors. Slow IV push of 25 mg as a first dose is recommended; an additional 25-mg dose can be given 10 to 15 minutes later if rigors persist.

Prevention of Febrile Nonhemolytic Transfusion Reactions. Ordering leukoreduced RBCs and platelets (if the hospital inventory is not entirely composed of leukoreduced components) is a preventive measure. For recurring reactions with platelets, volume reduction of the component can reduce the incidence.

Allergic Reaction of Mild Severity

Presentation. Urticaria or flushing occurs during a transfusion. Evidence of hemolysis is absent on laboratory evaluation.

Pathophysiology. Allergic reactions are immunoglobulin (Ig) E–mediated reactions against some allergen in the donor plasma. Because all blood components have some amount of plasma, it is possible to experience an allergic reaction with any blood product.

Acute Management. Slowing the infusion rate may be all that is required to alleviate the reaction. Antihistamine administration also addresses the symptoms.

Prevention of Allergic Transfusion Reactions of Mild Severity. A reaction of this type may be a one-time event. For patients with recurrent reactions, transfusing the blood product more slowly (maximum of transfusion over 4 hours) or premedication with antihistamines will reduce the incidence.

Transfusion-Associated Circulatory Overload

Presentation. The patient has respiratory distress, typically during the transfusion, and increase in blood pressure unless cardiac decompensation occurs. Tachycardia, tachypnea, and decrease in oxygen saturation are often present. Jugular venous distension may be seen. Radiographic findings include pleural effusions, perihilar edema, and increased vascular pedicle width.

Pathophysiology. The reaction results in cardiogenic pulmonary edema.

Acute Management. Diuretic should be administered. Supplemental oxygen may be required temporarily to improve oxygen saturation.

Prevention of Transfusion-Associated Circulatory Overload. Slowing the infusion rate with a maximum time of transfusion over 4 hours can prevent the reaction. Diuretic administration may be necessary in patients with poor heart function.

Most Dangerous Reactions

Acute Hemolytic Transfusion Reaction

Presentation. The most common signs include fever with or without rigors and pain. The more commonly reported sites of pain include flank, back, chest, or abdomen. Nausea and vomiting and dyspnea can also occur. In more severe presentations, hemodynamic instability is present, accompanied by oozing from line sites or petechial hemorrhage if DIC is occurring. Red or cola-colored urine is another manifestation of an acute hemolytic transfusion reaction and represents overwhelming of the renal capacity to recirculate free heme.

Pathophysiology. RBCs have proteins and carbohydrates on the cell surface that are antigenic. These epitopes are categorized into blood groups based on structure and sharing of a parent protein. A patient who lacks particular epitopes can develop antibodies through pregnancy or transfusion. Such RBC alloantibodies then lyse transfused RBCs that possess the cognate antigen. When time allows for pretransfusion testing, the antibodies are identified, and antigen-negative units are provided. The ABO blood group system is unusual in that almost all patients older than 4 months have naturally occurring antibodies to the A and B antigens that they did not inherit. These antibodies are capable of activating complement and causing intravascular lysis when bound to their cognate antigen. Thus it is of utmost importance to avoid transfusing RBCs against the ABO antibody in circulation. Refer to the ABO compatibility table (see Table 1).

Acute Management. Management is largely supportive. The end result of intravascular hemolysis and activation of the complement cascade can be shock, uncontrolled bleeding secondary to DIC, and renal failure. Therefore prompt infusion of IV crystalloid solutions are indicated to maintain blood pressure and renal perfusion. The goal for urine flow rate should be more than 1 mL/kg per hour. Coagulation laboratory values should be obtained to determine whether DIC is present; if so, component therapy to reverse the DIC is indicated. If the reaction is severe, intensive care is appropriate, because inotropic agents and mechanical ventilation may be necessary to support the patient.

Prevention of Acute Hemolytic Transfusion Reaction. An acute hemolytic reaction is one of the most feared complications of transfusion. It is also often one of the most preventable. Great care should be given to the pretransfusion blood sample draw, comparing the label to the patient's unique identifiers and labeling the tube at the patient's bedside as soon as the blood is in the tube. Just before transfusion, the unit label attached to the blood product should be compared with the patient's armband to ensure that the product is intended for this particular patient. To prevent intravascular hemolysis from antibodies directed against non-ABO antigens, pretransfusion testing (antibody screen or crossmatch) should be done in advance of the need for red cell transfusion for any patient whose clinical situation indicates a likelihood of needing blood. The exception is a patient who is hemodynamically unstable because of acute RBC loss, where uncrossmatched RBCs are indicated. If the patient's identity is known, a call to the hospital transfusion service in this situation is warranted; explain that the patient needs uncrossmatched RBCs and ask if there are transfusion records that indicate a need for antigen-negative units.

Allergic Reaction of Marked Severity (Anaphylaxis)

Presentation. Significant drop in blood pressure occurs, typically early into the transfusion. Wheezes, difficulty breathing, and stridor may be present. Tongue or facial edema and hives may be observed.

Pathophysiology. Anaphylaxis is an IgE-mediated reaction against an allergen in the donor plasma. In a patient with absolute IgA deficiency, naturally occurring anti-IgA can precipitate this reaction on binding IgA in the plasma. Antihaptoglobin antibodies can also induce a severe reaction.

Acute Management. Airway and blood pressure support should be provided with the patient recumbent and the lower extremities elevated. The treatment of choice is epinephrine (Adrenalin) 1 mg/mL, also labeled as 1:1000 or 0.1%, using an adult dosage of 0.3 to 0.5 mg per single dose, typically administered intramuscularly to the midquadriceps area. If symptoms persist, the dose may be repeated every 5 to 15 minutes for a maximum of three times, unless palpitations, tremors, or extreme anxiousness occurs. Supplemental oxygen should be administered, and the airway should be maintained. IV fluid administration is also recommended. Bronchodilators such as albuterol can be given as adjunctive treatment for bronchospasm that does not appear to respond to epinephrine. For patients on β-blockers, the addition of IV glucagon (GlucaGen)[1] 1 to 5 mg administered over 5 minutes, followed by infusion of 5 to 15 μg/min, may be required. The addition of glucocorticoids can help prevent the biphasic reaction that occurs in some patients.

Prevention of Allergic Reaction of Marked Severity (Anaphylaxis). Slow administration with careful observation of any transfusion is required. Premedication with IV antihistamines is appropriate. Steroids may be administered, although their effectiveness has not been confirmed through controlled trials. Epinephrine should be available at the bedside. For severe allergic

---

[1] Not FDA approved for this indication

[1] Not FDA approved for this indication.

reactions, a discussion with the transfusion service physician regarding washed components is appropriate.

Transfusion-Related Acute Lung Injury

Presentation. The signs of TRALI are difficulty breathing, tachypnea, and hypoxia during or within 6 hours of a transfusion of any blood component. Ideally, signs of underlying lung disease or circulatory overload are absent. Chest radiograph may show diffuse bilateral opacities (white-out). Diuretic administration does not result in improvement. The hypoxemia can progress to the point that the patient requires mechanical ventilation, and thus the patient should be closely monitored while the reaction is occurring.

Pathophysiology. The factors that result in TRALI are not entirely known. In a portion of cases, antibodies against WBC antigens are present in donor plasma. These antibodies are believed to bind the cognate antigens on the patient's WBCs, leading to degranulation and a capillary leak syndrome involving the lungs. Other theories regarding the pathophysiology of TRALI exist. One such theory implicates biologically active substances, such as lipids and cytokines, in the stored blood products. These substances are believed to prime the patient's granulocytes and activate pulmonary endothelium, setting the stage for an additional trigger to cause acute lung injury. Regardless of the cause of TRALI, the result is an increase in pulmonary vascular permeability and noncardiogenic pulmonary edema. The estimated mortality rate from TRALI is 5% to 8%.

Acute Management. Management consists of supportive care, with particular regard to respiratory support. With adequate supportive care, the process most often reverses over 48 to 96 hours.

Prevention of Transfusion-Related Acute Lung Injury. Marked respiratory compromise is occasionally due to WBC antibodies in the patient, which bind cognate antigens in the donated RBCs or platelet unit ("reverse TRALI"). In these cases, leukoreduction of cellular blood products may reduce the severity of subsequent transfusions, although solid evidence to support this is lacking. For TRALI caused by WBC antibodies in the donated product, there are no preventive measures for the clinician to take. The majority of U.S. blood suppliers provide plasma from only male donors, in an effort to reduce the incidence of TRALI caused by multiparous women with WBC antibodies.

Bacterial Contamination of a Blood Component

Presentation. The most common presentation includes fever and rigors, nausea and vomiting, and possible onset of moderate hypotension during or after a platelet transfusion. Rarely, presentation includes signs of overt septic shock, including marked hypotension, typically early into the transfusion of an RBC or platelet component. Bacterial contamination of plasma or cryoprecipitate is extremely rare.

Pathophysiology. The most common organisms to contaminate a platelet product are skin flora such as *Staphylococcus epidermidis*. These organisms are thought to be introduced into the collection bag via a skin plug that results from phlebotomy using a large-gauge needle when sterilization of the phlebotomy site has been ineffective.

The most common organisms to contaminate an RBC unit are gram-negative, endotoxin-producing organisms such as *Yersinia enterocolitica*. This organism is introduced into the blood product as a result of asymptomatic bacteremia in the donor, from sources such as the gastrointestinal tract. The donor-screening questionnaire and vital sign assessment at the time of donation help make collection from such a donor a very rare event. Transfusion of a bacterially contaminated RBC unit is most often a fatal event. It is important to remember that platelets can also be contaminated by the same gram-negative, endotoxin-producing organisms; in this case, signs of septic shock may manifest.

Acute Management. Blood cultures from the patient should be drawn, and then prompt IV antibiotic administration should begin. Supportive care including inotropic agents and close nursing attention may be required.

Prevention of Bacterial Contamination of a Blood Component. Bacterial contamination is associated with a donor product, and thus preventive measures for the patient do not apply. Blood suppliers perform bacterial detection tests on platelet components or choose to treat platelets with pathogen reduction technology. Transfusion services also have strict policies related to visual inspection of all blood products before they are issued to a patient-care area.

Other Reactions

Delayed Hemolytic Transfusion Reaction

Presentation. The main finding with a delayed hemolytic transfusion reaction is usually an unexplained decrease in Hct within 2 to 7 days after transfusion. The patient often remains symptom free unless the decline in Hb is poorly tolerated. Jaundice can occur, and laboratory values consistent with hemolysis may be positive (elevated indirect bilirubin, elevated lactate dehydrogenase, decreased haptoglobin). Rarely, signs of intravascular hemolysis can occur.

Pathophysiology. The most common source of this reaction is an RBC alloantibody that the patient developed with prior transfusion or pregnancy; the antibody titer wanes over time such that pretransfusion testing does not detect the antibody. A unit of RBCs positive for the cognate antigen is then transfused, and within a few days the patient's memory B cell response produces the antibody again. Transfused cells are then cleared, most often by an extravascular mechanism.

Acute Management. Most transfusion services have a policy to notify the clinician that a serologic delayed hemolytic transfusion reaction is present on testing a new plasma sample from the patient. If the patient's Hct has declined, it may be useful to determine a clinical correlation by obtaining the laboratory values just described. This is of particular importance when the distinction between hemolysis and bleeding will lead to different management strategies for the patient. Although extravascular clearance of Hb is fairly well tolerated by the kidneys, the conservative approach is to increase renal perfusion with IV crystalloid solutions if possible.

Prevention of Delayed Hemolytic Transfusion Reaction. For a patient who routinely receives care through one hospital system, the transfusion service will keep a record of the RBC alloantibody and provide antigen-negative cells for transfusion. The prevention, then, is to plan ahead for transfusion when possible, so that fully compatible units can be provided. Uncrossmatched RBCs may be positive for the cognate antigen.

Allergic Reaction of Moderate Severity

Presentation. The patient has labile blood pressure, either hyper- or hypotension, accompanied by at least one of the following: throat scratchiness, respiratory wheezes, or perioral or periorbital edema. Hives may be present. Gastrointestinal symptoms such as crampy abdominal pain may also be present.

Pathophysiology. This is an IgE-mediated reaction against an allergen in the plasma of the donated product.

Acute Management. Treatment is administration of IV antihistamines. If the respiratory component does not resolve, consider epinephrine administration, and treat similarly to anaphylaxis (see previous section).

Prevention of Allergic Transfusion Reaction of Moderate Severity. Slower infusion of blood products can reduce further episodes of this type of reaction. If the patient is atopic, IV antihistamines may be administered as a premedication. If the patient requires chronic transfusion and experiences this type of reaction on a repeated basis, discussion with the transfusion service regarding washed components may be warranted.

Hypotensive Transfusion Reaction

Presentation. The patient has isolated hypotension (drop in systolic blood pressure >30 but <80 mm Hg) that responds quickly to cessation of the transfusion. The reaction classically occurs within the first 15 minutes of infusion of the blood product.

Pathophysiology. Pathophysiology is unclear. Some research indicates that the patient may have slower ability to metabolize bradykinin compared with other individuals.

Acute Management. Stop the transfusion.

Prevention of Hypotensive Transfusion Reaction. Prevention is unclear. In the author's experience, rate of infusion has a role. Slower infusion may help prevent this type of reaction.

Transfusion-Associated Dyspnea

Presentation. Acute respiratory distress that occurs within 24 hours of cessation of transfusion.

Pathophysiology. Pathophysiology is unclear

Acute Management and Prevention of Transfusion-Associated Dyspnea. Management is supportive and prevention is unclear.

References

Abdel-Wahab OI, Healy B, Dzik WH: Effect of fresh-frozen plasma transfusion on prothrombin time and bleeding in patients with mild coagulation abnormalities, *Transfusion* 46:1279–1285, 2006.

Carson JL, Stanworth SJ, Guyatt G, et al: Red blood cell transfusion, 2023 AABB international guidelines, *JAMA* 330(19):1892–1902, 2023.

Cuker A, Burnett A, Triller D: Reversal of direct oral anticoagulants: Guidance from the anticoagulation forum, *Am J Hematol* 94(6):697–709, 2019.

Francis RO, Stotler BA: Noninfectious complications of blood transfusion. In Cohn C, editor: *AABB technical manual*, ed 21, Bethesda, MD, 2023, American Association of Blood Banks, pp 675–703.

Kaufman RM, et al: Platelet transfusion: a clinical practice guideline from the AABB, *Ann Internal Med* 162(3):205–213, 2015.

Lisman T, Porte RJ: Rebalanced hemostasis in patients with liver disease: evidence and clinical consequences, *Blood* 116:878–885, 2010.

Patel IJ, Rahim S, Davidson JC, et al: Consensus guidelines for the periprocedural management of thrombotic and bleeding risk in patients undergoing percutaneous image guided interventions—Part II, *Recommendations JVIR* 30(8):1168–1184, 2019.

Tummula R, et al: Specific antidotes against direct oral anticoagulants: a comprehensive review of clinical trials, *Int J Cardiol* 214:292–298, 2016.

CHRONIC LEUKEMIAS

Method of
Jatin Rana, MD; and Daniel Isaac, DO

CURRENT DIAGNOSIS

Chronic Myelogenous Leukemia
- Clinical symptoms
  - Constitutional symptoms
  - Splenomegaly (abdominal discomfort, early satiety)
- Laboratory parameters
  - Elevated white blood cell count, ~100,000/μL, with differential consisting of various stages of granulocyte maturation from myeloblasts to mature neutrophils
  - Absolute basophilia
- Genetic parameters
  - Presence of *bcr-abl1* by cytogenetics, fluorescence in situ hybridization, or reverse transcriptase polymerase chain reaction

Chronic Lymphocytic Leukemia
- Clinical symptoms
  - B symptoms (fevers, night sweats, weight loss)
  - Lymphadenopathy and/or organomegaly
  - Recurrent infections
- Laboratory parameters
  - Absolute lymphocytosis
  - Anemia
  - Thrombocytopenia
- Immunophenotypic analysis by flow cytometry
  - Monoclonal population of light-chain–restricted mature B cells that express CD19, CD20(dim), and CD23 and coexpress CD5

CURRENT THERAPY

Chronic Myelogenous Leukemia: Chronic Phase
- First-line therapy
  - Imatinib mesylate (Gleevec) 400 mg daily
  - Dasatinib (Sprycel) 100 mg daily
  - Nilotinib (Tasigna) 300 mg twice daily
  - Bosutinib (Bosulif) 400 mg daily
- Later-line therapy
  - Imatinib mesylate (Gleevec)
  - Dasatinib (Sprycel)
  - Nilotinib (Tasigna)
  - Bosutinib (Bosulif)
  - Ponatinib (Iclusig)
  - Omacetaxine mepesuccinate (Synribo)
  - Asciminib (Scemblix)
- High risk for failure
  - Allogeneic stem cell transplantation

Chronic Lymphocytic Leukemia
- Chemotherapy
  - Fludarabine (Fludara)
  - Cyclophosphamide (Cytoxan)
  - Chlorambucil (Leukeran)
  - Bendamustine (Treanda)
- Immunotherapy (monoclonal antibodies)
  - Rituximab (Rituxan)
  - Ofatumumab (Arzerra)
  - Obinutuzumab (Gazyva)
  - Alemtuzumab (Campath)
- Targeted therapy
  - Idelalisib (Zydelig)
  - Duvalisib (Copiktra)
  - Ibrutinib (Imbruvica)
  - Venetoclax (Venclexta)
  - Acalabrutinib (Calquence)

Chronic Myelogenous Leukemia

Chronic myelogenous leukemia (CML) is a myeloproliferative disorder with malignant clonal expansion and pathogenic leukemogenesis. It is defined by a translocation of chromosomes 9 and 22 (the Philadelphia [Ph] chromosome) with the resultant formation of a fusion gene product *bcr-abl* (Figure 1). In 2001, management of the disease changed dramatically with the approval and clinical use of imatinib mesylate (Gleevec), the first tyrosine kinase inhibitor (TKI) targeting the BCR-ABL1 oncoprotein.

Epidemiology and Risk Factors

The worldwide incidence of CML is 1 to 2 cases per 100,000 adults. In the United States, the disorder accounts for approximately 11% to 15% of all new adult cases of leukemia annually. CML is predominately a disorder of adults with a median age at diagnosis of 55 to 60 years. The disease has a slight predominance to males, with a male-to-female ratio of 1.4 to 1.0. The number of patients living with CML is expected to continually increase as a result of successful management of the disorder with TKI therapy. Other than prior radiation exposure, little is known regarding potential risk factors. No specific genetic or familial predisposition to the pathogenesis of CML has been identified.

Pathogenesis

The reciprocal translocation between chromosomes 9 and 22 giving rise to the Ph chromosome is key to the pathogenesis of CML. There is an exchange of genetic material with a portion of the Abelson murine leukemia *(abl1)* gene on the long arm of chromosome 9 relocating next to the breakpoint cluster region *(bcr)* on the long arm of chromosome 22. The presence of the newly formed Ph chromosome

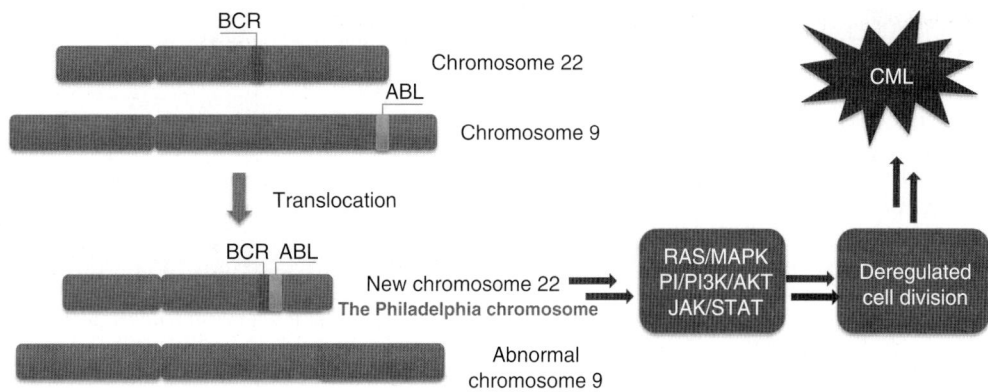

Figure 1 Schematic of the formation of Philadelphia chromosome (the new chromosome 22) and its physiological consequences. (From Chen, et al. *Protein Kinase Inhibitors as Sensitizing Agents for Chemotherapy*, Fig. 2.1. Elsevier, 2019.)

(t9;22)(q34;q11.2) is a characteristic rearrangement seen in approximately 95% of CML cases. This leads to the creation of a hybrid oncogene *bcr-abl1*, which in turn translates into a BCR-ABL1 protein. There are three distinct breakpoint regions in the *BCR* gene, and each one is associated with a unique disease phenotype. The transcript from the most common breakpoint region (major breakpoint cluster region [M-BCR]) is translated into the p210BCR-ABL1 oncoprotein with the molecular consequence of constitutive tyrosine kinase activity. This leads to activation of signal-transduction proteins and upregulation of several key signaling pathways (RAS, JAK/STAT, and PI-3-kinase) with consequential alterations in cellular proliferation, differentiation, adhesion, and survival.

The clinical course of CML can be divided into three distinct phases of the disorder: the chronic phase, in which the vast majority (90% to 95%) of patients are diagnosed, or the more aggressive accelerated and blast phases. The malignant clone acquires additional mutations with time with subsequent progression to the advanced phases of CML. The aberrations most commonly seen at the chromosomal level include trisomy 8, amplification of t(9,22), abnormalities in chromosome 17, trisomy 19, trisomy 21, and monosomy 7, which if present at diagnosis may have a negative prognostic impact on survival. Changes at the molecular level (e.g., *bcr-abl1* kinase domain mutations) are associated with clinical resistance to TKI therapy.

Clinical and Laboratory Characteristics

The malignant disorder of hematopoietic stem cells produces marked myeloid hyperplasia in the bone marrow and resultant uncontrolled proliferation of myeloid cells, erythroid cells, and platelets in the peripheral blood. Up to 50% of CML patients in the United States are asymptomatic at diagnosis and have abnormalities only noted on routine physical examination or with the presence of abnormalities on a complete blood count (CBC). Clinical manifestations seen at presentation include fatigue, weight loss, splenomegaly leading to abdominal fullness and early satiety, malaise, and acute gouty arthritis. Laboratory findings include a markedly elevated white blood cell count (~100,000/μL) with a differential consisting of various stages of granulocyte maturation from myeloblasts to mature neutrophils. There is presence of absolute basophilia and often associated absolute eosinophilia. The findings of an elevated platelet count and anemia can be seen at presentation in approximately 20% to 30% and 50% of patients, respectively. High levels of lactate dehydrogenase (LDH) and uric acid can be seen as a result of increased cellular turnover associated with the disorder.

Without therapy, a patient in the chronic phase of CML will eventually progress to the more aggressive phases in 3 to 5 years. A consensus is lacking on the definition of accelerated phase; however, common features include an increase in the number of peripheral blood myeloblasts and basophils, development of low platelet counts, or discovery of additional clonal cytogenetic abnormalities. The definition of *blast phase* by the International Bone Marrow Transplant Registry (IBMTR) uses criteria of at least 30%

blasts in the peripheral blood or bone marrow, or the presence of extramedullary infiltrates of the clonal leukemic cells. The blast phase of CML presents clinically like acute leukemia (30% having a lymphoid morphology, 60% as acute myeloblastic leukemia, and the remainder as megakaryocytic or undifferentiated) with worsening constitutional symptoms, anemia, and bleeding tendencies.

Diagnosis

Clinical suspicion of a CML diagnosis is made from a patient presenting with the typical laboratory abnormalities with or without any physical manifestations (see the Current Diagnosis box earlier in this chapter). Examination of a peripheral blood smear reveals increased neutrophils and immature circulating myeloid cells, increased basophils and eosinophils, a normal to increased number of platelets, and possible normocytic anemia. Obtaining a bone marrow examination with aspirate is essential in the initial workup of a CML patient to appropriately stage the disorder and to assess for the presence of the Ph chromosome by cytogenetics. The routine cytogenetic study is valuable to evaluate for clonal evolution denoted by the presence of additional karyotypic changes, which may poorly affect prognosis. Utilizing fluorescence in situ hybridization (FISH) or reverse transcriptase polymerase chain reaction (RT-PCR) amplification studies for the detection of the *bcr-abl1* hybrid gene or its transcripts is important both as a baseline confirmatory test for CML and its continued monitoring. FISH analysis has the ability to detect the *bcr-abl1* molecular anomaly using specific probes targeting the chimeric oncogene among interphase nuclei in the peripheral blood. Qualitative RT-PCR can reveal the presence of bcr-abl1 transcripts, whereas continued monitoring of CML patients for the amount of residual disease can be assessed by obtaining quantitative RT-PCR levels. The techniques involving FISH analysis and RT-PCR have both demonstrated high concordance in simultaneous sampling of peripheral blood and bone marrow specimens.

Differential Diagnosis

At presentation, CML can be routinely differentiated from leukemoid reactions, which typically have lower white blood cell counts, absence of basophilia, and presence of Döhle bodies and toxic vacuolation of granulocytes. Temporary extreme neutrophilia and associated left shift can be present after corticosteroid use. The detection of *bcr-abl1* can aid in differentiating CML from other myeloproliferative disorders (essential thrombocytosis, polycythemia vera), chronic neutrophilia leukemia, chronic myelomonocytic leukemia, chronic eosinophilia leukemia, chronic basophilic leukemia, or myelodysplastic syndromes. Rarely, patients can have *bcr-abl1*-negative or atypical CML in which additional mutations (*CSF3R, KRAS/NRAS, SETBP1*) may be present and are associated with a poor outcome.

Prognosis

The introduction of imatinib mesylate and additional TKIs in the 2000s has changed a dismal prognosis of CML into a manageable

	OPTIMAL*	WARNING	FAILURE
Baseline	NA	High-risk ACA, high-risk ELTS score	NA
3 months	≤10%	>10%	>10% if confirmed within 1–3 months
6 months	≤1%	>1%–10%	>10%
12 months	≤0.1%	>0.1%–1%	>1%
Any time	≤0.1%	>0.1%–1%, loss of ≤0.1% (MMR)[†]	>1%, resistance mutations, high-risk ACA

*For patients aiming at treatment-free remission, the optimal response (at any time) is BCR-ABL1 ≤0.01% (MR[4]). A change of treatment may be considered if MMR is not reached by 36 to 48 months.

[†]Loss of MMR (BCR-ABL1 >0.1%) indicates failure after TFR.

[4]Not yet approved for use in the United States.

ACA, Additional chromosome abnormalities in Ph+ cells; *ELTS,* EUTOS long-term survival score; *MMR,* major molecular response; *NA,* not applicable; *TFR,* treatment-free remission.

From Hochhaus A, Baccarani M, Silver RT, et al.: European LeukemiaNet 2020 recommendations for treating chronic myeloid leukemia, *Leukemia* 34(4):966–984, 2020.

TABLE 2	European LeukemiaNet Definitions and Monitoring Recommendations

HEMATOLOGIC RESPONSE	CYTOGENIC RESPONSE	MOLECULAR RESPONSE
Definitions		
Complete: Platelet count <450 × 10⁹/L WBC count <10 × 10⁹/L Differential without immature granulocytes and with <5% basophils Nonpalpable spleen	Complete: Ph+ 0% Partial: Ph+ <35% Minor: Ph+ 36–65% None: Ph+ >95%	Complete: transcript nonquantifiable and nondetectable Major: ≤0.10
Monitoring		
Check every 2 wk until complete response achieved and confirmed, then every 3 mo unless otherwise required	Check at 3 and 6 mo, then every 6 mo until complete response achieved and confirmed; thereafter every 12 mo if molecular monitoring cannot be ensured; check always for occurrence of treatment failure or unexplained cytopenia	Check every 3 mo until major response is achieved; conduct mutation analysis in case of failure, suboptimal response, or increase in transcript level

Ph, Philadelphia chromosome; *WBC,* white blood cell.

From Baccarani M, Saglio G, Goldman J, et al: Evolving concepts in the management of chronic myeloid leukemia: Recommendations from an expert panel on behalf of the European LeukemiaNet, *Blood* 108(6):1809–1820, 2006; Baccarani M, Cortes J, Pane F, et al.: Chronic myeloid leukemia: an update of concepts and management recommendations of European LeukemiaNet, *J Clin Oncol* 27(35):6041–6051, 2009.

chronic disorder with a near-normal lifespan. Before the current TKI-based era, the median survival for patients with CML was 5 to 7 years. Oral chemotherapeutics (hydroxyurea [Hydrea] and busulfan [Busulfex, Myleran]) and injectable interferon alfa (interferon alfa-2b [Intron A][1] and peginterferon alfa-2a [Pegasys][1]) were important in achieving hematologic remissions, reducing thrombotic complications, and increasing median survival. Allogeneic stem cell transplantation (allo-SCT) remains a vital option for patients with advanced phases of CML or following failure of multiple TKIs.

CML prognostic scoring systems (Sokal, Euro) have traditionally used basic hematologic data, spleen size, and age to stratify patients into risk groups. Compared with the prior conventional cytotoxic-based scoring systems (Sokal), the new EUTOS Long Term Survival (ELTS) score considers the current TKI treatment era, and age does not hold such a negative impact in the scoring.

The mainstay of managing CML is continuation of long-term TKI therapy to maintain a remission. This has resulted in most patients achieving a normal life expectancy. More recently, there has been a greater acceptance to the concept of TKI therapy discontinuation in carefully chosen patients, for example, chronic phase patients with a minimum TKI therapy duration of 3 years and sustained deep molecular remission of at least 2 years. In such patients, there is an emphasis on more frequent molecular

testing and monitoring for adverse events associated with discontinuation (TKI withdrawal syndrome). The recent success of maintaining prolonged treatment-free remission (TFR) is promising. Importantly, in patients who lost a major molecular response (MMR), nearly all were able to regain their response with prompt resumption of TKI treatment.

Monitoring Response to Tyrosine Kinase Inhibitor Therapy

First-line TKI use in CML is aimed at achieving a maximal reduction of leukemia burden with the goal of obtaining a complete cytogenetic response within 12 months of therapy initiation. Peripheral CBCs with differential are frequently ordered until a complete hematologic response is achieved. Quantitative RT-PCR (international scale [IS]) is followed every 3 months to assess for residual *bcr-abl1* transcripts relative to *abl1* transcripts and for the degree of molecular response. Cytogenetics and FISH analysis can be helpful in patients with atypical translocations and atypical *bcr-abl1* transcripts and in those with additional chromosome abnormalities. Milestones of hematologic, cytogenetic, and molecular response to therapy and monitoring recommendations are summarized in Tables 1 and 2. Testing for *bcr-abl1* kinase mutations is recommended in patients who fail to achieve a timely optimal response or display resistance/loss of response to a first-line TKI. Salvage therapy consists of alternative TKI use or consideration of allo-SCT for advanced phases of CML.

[1] Not FDA approved for this indication.

Treatment

There are currently four TKIs approved for first-line CML: imatinib (Gleevec), dasatinib (Sprycel), nilotinib (Tasigna), and bosutinib (Bosulif). Each of these TKI therapeutic agents are acceptable options for a patient with newly diagnosed chronic phase CML. The decision of which TKI to choose is dependent on a variety of factors including patient comorbidities, drug toxicity profile, cost, and disease characteristics.

In 2001, the development of imatinib mesylate (Gleevec) changed the treatment landscape for patients with CML. The first-generation TKI was established as the standard of care for first-line patients with chronic phase CML following the International Randomized Study of Interferon Versus STI571 (IRIS) trial. A total of 1106 patients with chronic phase CML were randomized to receive imatinib (400 mg daily) versus interferon alfa (Intron-A)[1] (5 million units/m[2] daily) plus low-dose cytarabine (Cytosar) (20 mg/m[2] daily for 10 days per month). At 18 months, the imatinib arm was found to have superior outcomes including tolerability, hematologic response, complete cytogenetic response (76.2% vs. 14.5%, P <.001), and freedom from progression to advanced phase (accelerated or blast) CML (96.7% vs. 91.5%, P <.001). Long-term outcomes revealed that the imatinib-assigned group had an overall survival rate of 83.3%, a cumulative complete cytogenetic response rate of 83%, and a 10-year MMR rate of 93%. Because of the high crossover rate from the interferon alfa plus cytarabine arm, no comparative survival benefit was seen with use of the TKI.

The suggested starting dose of imatinib is 400 mg once daily taken with a meal. Higher doses (600 mg daily or 800 mg daily) are associated with increased toxicity without proven overall survival benefit. Although well tolerated by most patients, common side effects include superficial edema, muscle cramps, abdominal pain, nausea, rash, and diarrhea. Patients should be routinely assessed for low blood counts (cytopenias), and those with liver or kidney impairment may require closer monitoring and dose adjustments. Since its introduction, the cost of brand-name imatinib has risen from $30,000 per year to an annual price of $140,000, illustrating the financial toxicity associated with potential long-term TKI-based therapy for CML. Since 2015, the availability of generic imatinib has reduced the annual cost in the United States, albeit the price remains higher compared with other regions of the world.

Second-generation TKIs approved for first-line chronic phase CML include dasatinib (Sprycel), nilotinib (Tasigna), and bosutinib (Bosulif). Compared with the use of imatinib, these agents have demonstrated faster and deeper responses as well as less disease progression to the advanced accelerated and blast phases. Thus second-generation TKIs may be the preferred choice for chronic phase CML patients with high-risk disease.

The phase III Evaluating Nilotinib Efficacy and Safety in Clinical Trials—Newly Diagnosed Patients (ENESTnd) trial evaluated the efficacy and safety of nilotinib versus imatinib in 846 newly diagnosed chronic phase CML patients. Patients in the nilotinib (300 mg twice daily) arm were shown to have improved cumulative rates of MMR (77.7% vs. 62.5%, P <.0001) compared with imatinib 400 mg daily, with no difference in 10-year progression-free survival (86.2% vs. 87.2%). There are increased rates of ischemic heart disease, ischemic cardiovascular events, and peripheral artery disease among those treated with nilotinib, especially at a higher dose (400 mg twice daily). Additional adverse events associated with nilotinib therapy include elevation in blood glucose levels, headaches, rash, QTc prolongation, pancreatitis, and increased liver enzyme levels.

The Dasatinib versus Imatinib Study in Treatment-Naïve Chronic Myeloid Leukemia Patients (DASISON) was a randomized trial of 519 patients with first-line chronic phase CML assigned to dasatinib (100 mg daily) or imatinib (400 mg daily).

Treatment with the second-generation TKI demonstrated earlier and more robust MMR rates at 3 months (84% vs. 64%, P <.0001) and deeper molecular response with 4.5-log reduction of *bcr-abl1* transcripts (<0.0032 IS, MR4.5) (42% vs. 33%). Dasatinib therapy is associated with less nausea, rash, and muscle aches. Patients should be monitored for potential low blood counts and the development of pleural effusions. We await longer follow-up for a recent trial, which has shown effective activity of lower-dose dasatinib (50 mg daily) with a more acceptable safety profile.

In the Bosutinib Versus Imatinib for Newly Diagnosed Chronic Myeloid Leukemia (BFORE) randomized trial, the bosutinib (400 mg daily) arm achieved significantly higher MMR rates (47% vs. 37%, P = .02) and complete cytogenetic response rates (77% vs. 66%, P = .007) at 12 months compared with imatinib (400 mg daily) therapy. There were similar rates of 2-year survival with both drugs. Patients taking the second-generation TKI are more likely to experience gastrointestinal adverse effects (diarrhea, liver enzyme elevation), which may necessitate dose reductions and temporary holding of the medication.

The preference of using a second-generation TKI as the initial treatment of chronic phase CML should be performed in the context of the available data, understanding the unique side-effect profile of each drug, assessing the cost-effectiveness of long-term treatment, and appropriate patient selection. The ability to achieve response milestones faster and with a deeper response (MR4.5 rates) displays the potential of using second-generation TKIs for patients in whom eventual TKI discontinuation would be considered. The lack of overall survival benefit of these agents compared with imatinib seen in clinical trials could be secondary to effective salvage therapy.

Continuation of long-term therapy with TKIs can be difficult for the patient and provides additional challenges to the treating physician. Routine monitoring for and managing TKI-associated toxicities is as vital as regular assessment of disease response. Despite many short- and long-term toxicities from TKIs graded as mild, they have resulted in poorer patient-reported quality-of-life scores and often can lead to treatment nonadherence. Newly prescribed medications should also be assessed for potential drug-drug interactions with the TKI, which may require dose adjustments.

Other Therapeutic Options

Patients on first-line TKI who fail to meet treatment response milestones, display intolerance to the medication, or have progression/relapse should be assessed for treatment adherence and evaluated for possible drug interaction affecting TKI metabolism. Bone marrow examination should be performed to ensure that the patient has not progressed to an advanced phase of the disease. Often acquisition of novel point mutations in *bcr-abl1* leads to treatment resistance. Determining the type of mutation guides appropriate switching to an alternative TKI. Most of the mutations displaying resistance to imatinib therapy can be overcome by the use of a second-generation TKI. These have the ability to once again achieve high rates of response, especially when compared with increased doses of imatinib (400 mg twice daily). The *T315I* mutation is a unique alteration that confers resistance to all available second-generation TKIs. Ponatinib (Iclusig), a third-generation TKI, is effective in heavily pretreated CML patients and is approved with activity displayed against the *T315I* mutation. However, the drug at the approved dose (45 mg daily) is associated with considerable risk of vascular occlusive disease, thrombotic events, heart failure, and hepatotoxicity. In an attempt to minimize toxicity, it is recommended to reduce the dose upon achieving *bcr-abl1* ≤1%.

In 2012, omacetaxine mepesuccinate (Synribo) subcutaneous injection was approved for patients with resistance or intolerance to two or more prior TKIs. The drug is dosed based on body surface area (1.25 mg/m[2]) twice daily with an induction and maintenance dosing schedule over 28-day cycles. The approval provided patients with acquired mutations, including *T315I*, an

---

[1] Not FDA approved for this indication.

additional treatment option for their difficult-to-control disease. Treated patients should be monitored for cytopenias, bleeding, and hyperglycemia, which may necessitate dose adjustment. In 2021, asciminib (Scemblix) became the latest approved drug for chronic-phase CML patients previously treated with two or more TKIs or for those with the *T315I* mutation. In the ASCEMBL multicenter, randomized clinical trial, asciminib at a dose of 40 mg twice daily was compared with bosutinib 500 mg once daily in the pretreated specified population. The novel agent showed an improvement in MMR rate (25% vs. 13%, *P* = 0.029) compared with bosutinib in addition to a lower discontinuation rate (7% vs. 25%) as a result of adverse reactions. A second trial showed asciminib's ability to be an effective option for chronic phase CMP patients presenting with the *T315I* mutation. The drug was given at 200 mg twice daily and showed an achievement of MMR at 24 weeks in 42% of the patients with the difficult-to-treat mutation status. Dose adjustments may be necessary for hematologic toxicities, hypertension, hypersensitivity reactions, and pancreatic toxicity.

As the only curative option for patients with CML, an evaluation for allo-SCT candidacy is appropriate if optimal response is not achieved after two or more TKIs as a result of resistance, drug intolerance, or inadequate response to newer agents for those harboring the *T315I* mutation. Patients with accelerated phase CML are treated initially with TKI therapy (second or third generation preferred) and early consideration of allo-SCT based on a lack of optimal response. Blast phase CML requires a more aggressive combined approach using the newer-generation TKIs and intensive chemotherapy, followed by immediate allo-SCT in responders. For the advanced phases of the disease, TKI therapy is typically administered at a higher starting dose: imatinib 600 mg daily for accelerated phase and 800 mg daily for blast phase, dasatinib 140 mg daily, nilotinib 400 mg twice daily, bosutinib 500 or 600 mg daily, and ponatinib 45 mg daily. A list of potential palliative options includes hydroxyurea, hypomethylating agents, cytarabine, and busulfan. Unfortunately, survival in end-phase CML is measured in months.

Chronic Lymphocytic Leukemia

Chronic lymphocytic leukemia (CLL) is a chronic, mature B-cell neoplasm and is the most common type of leukemia in Western countries. CLL is a heterogeneous disease, and not all patients require treatment at the time of diagnosis, as randomized trials have failed to demonstrate a survival advantage with early treatment strategies. Molecular profiling and whole-exome sequencing have led to improved understanding of the pathogenesis of CLL and significant improvements in our therapeutic approach. Historically, therapy for CLL included alkylating agents, purine analogues, and CD20-directed monoclonal antibodies. However, the treatment approach to CLL has rapidly evolved over the past several years with the advent of targeted agents such as Bruton tyrosine kinase (BTK) inhibitors, B-cell leukemia/lymphoma 2 (BCL2) inhibitors, and phosphoinositide 3-kinase (PI3K) inhibitors. The development of such agents has led to significant improvement in outcomes for these patients including those with high-risk genomic aberrations that had historically been resistant to standard chemotherapies.

Epidemiology and Risk Factors

CLL accounts for approximately 30% of all leukemias in the United States. It is a disease of older adults with a median age at diagnosis of 70 years. CLL occurs more commonly in men than in women, with a male-to-female ratio of approximately 1.7 to 1. The incidence of CLL also varies by race, with a higher incidence in Caucasians. Furthermore, the incidence of CLL in Asian countries is quite low. Although the exact reasons racial disparities exist are not clear, it appears that genetic factors are the most likely explanation. CLL does appear to be seen at a higher frequency among those with a first-degree family member with CLL. There are no clearly identified environmental or occupational risk factors. Most cases of CLL are preceded by development of

monoclonal B-cell lymphocytosis (MBL). However, despite the presence of MBL, only a small portion of patients will progress to CLL at a rate of 1% to 2% per year.

Pathogenesis

CLL is a disease of clonal B-cell lymphocytes arrested in B-cell differentiation. The pathogenesis of CLL is complex, and many steps in the developmental pathway have yet to be elucidated. Nevertheless, the development of CLL appears to follow a two-step process in which one first develops MBL due to an unknown event (i.e., gene mutation, epigenetic changes, cytogenetic abnormalities, antigenic stimulation) resulting in proliferation of a clone of B cells. A second event or "hit" occurs (i.e., further cytogenetic changes), leading to accumulation of the malignant clone and subsequent progression to CLL. Malignant cells accumulate as a result of their inability to undergo apoptosis. This is thought to be mediated by overexpression of anti-apoptotic proteins such as BCL2. The exact cell of origin likely differs among cases specifically related to the mutational status of the immunoglobulin variable region genes. FISH detects chromosomal abnormalities in 70% to 80% of patients with CLL, and certain genetic abnormalities are clearly associated with disease prognosis (discussed later in this chapter). Furthermore, it appears that karyotypic abnormalities are acquired throughout the disease course, and such clonal evolution has been associated with progressive disease.

Clinical Manifestations

The clinical manifestations of CLL vary widely, with most patients displaying no clinical symptoms and diagnosis made by routine blood counts showing lymphocytosis. Persistent lymphadenopathy is another common presenting symptom and is present in up to 90% of patients. The spleen is the most commonly enlarged lymphoid organ, and splenomegaly is detected in up to 50% of patients. Splenomegaly can lead to a variety of clinical symptoms including abdominal discomfort or early satiety contributing to poor oral intake and weight loss. Up to 10% of patients may present with "B" symptoms such as unintentional weight loss (10% or more of body weight within previous 6 months), fevers not associated with infection, drenching night sweats, and/or profound fatigue. Importantly, patients with CLL are immunocompromised and can present with recurrent infections. Autoimmune complications of CLL should be considered including hemolytic anemia, immune thrombocytopenia, and pure red cell aplasia, to name a few. Anemia and thrombocytopenia are findings consistent with advanced disease.

Diagnosis

A diagnosis of CLL is suspected when a patient presents with lymphocytosis with an absolute lymphocyte count greater than 5000/µL. Subsequent peripheral blood flow cytometry demonstrates immunophenotypic evidence of a monoclonal B-cell population that coexpresses the T-cell antigen CD5 and B-cell surface antigens CD19, CD20 (usually low/dim expression), and CD23 (Table 3). Typically, there is a low level of surface membrane immunoglobulin (most often IgM) along with a single immunoglobulin light chain, kappa, or lambda, which confirms the clonal nature. The presence of a monoclonal B-cell population with the same immunophenotypic profile but with an absolute lymphocyte count less than 5000/µL is termed *MBL*. Bone marrow aspirate and biopsy are not required for the diagnosis of CLL but may be helpful in certain circumstances.

Differential Diagnosis

Peripheral lymphocytosis can occur in viral or other infectious processes, and immunophenotyping by peripheral flow cytometry is helpful to distinguish between reactive and malignant causes and allows one to establish the diagnosis of CLL. Caution must be taken to differentiate from other low-grade B-cell malignancies (see Table 3). Importantly, one must distinguish mantel cell lymphoma from CLL. As CLL expresses CD23, MCL is typically CD23 negative and is characterized by strong

TABLE 3 Differential Diagnosis of Chronic Lymphocytic Leukemia by Immunophenotype

DISEASE	CD5	CD10	CD20	CD23	SURFACE IMMUNOGLOBULIN	OTHER
Chronic lymphocytic leukemia	+	–	+ (dim)	+	+ (dim)	
B-cell prolymphocytic leukemia	±	–	+	±	+ (bright)	
Mantle cell lymphoma	+	–	+	–	+ (bright)	t(11;14)
Hairy cell leukemia	–	–	+	–	+	CD11c, CD103, CD123 positive
Lymphoplasmacytic lymphoma	– (rarely +)	–	+	±	+	Most have monoclonal IgM paraprotein. Associated with *MYD88* mutations.
Splenic marginal zone lymphoma	±	–	+	±	+ (bright)	

TABLE 4 Rai Staging System for Chronic Lymphocytic Leukemia

RISK	STAGE	CLINICAL DESCRIPTION
Low	0	Lymphocytosis
Intermediate	I	Lymphocytosis + lymphadenopathy
	II	Lymphocytosis + hepatomegaly or splenomegaly (± lymphadenopathy)
High	III	Lymphocytosis + anemia (Hb <11 g/dL)
	IV	Lymphocytosis + thrombocytopenia (<100,000/μL)

expression of cyclin D1. A lymph node biopsy should be pursued when immunophenotyping of the peripheral blood fails to yield a diagnosis.

Prognosis

Although most patients with CLL are diagnosed with early-stage disease, the prognosis and clinical course is highly heterogeneous. Historically, risk stratification using the Rai or Binet clinical staging systems have been the mainstay of predicting prognosis in clinical practice (Tables 4 and 5). Over the past several years, our understanding of the molecular biology and underlying genetic aberrations in CLL have led to complementary prognostic variables to predict survival, which are widely used in clinical practice today. FISH testing to identify cytogenetic aberrations before treatment has allowed for more robust risk stratification. Specifically, deletion of 13q and trisomy 12 are favorable prognostic abnormalities, whereas deletion of 17p and 11q are higher-risk abnormalities. Deletion of 17p and/or aberrations in *TP53* predict an aggressive disease course and refractoriness to conventional chemoimmunotherapy regimens. The mutational status of immunoglobulin heavy-chain variable genes (IGHV) is also associated with survival. Unmutated *IGHV* genes have a more aggressive clinical course and shorter survival compared with those with mutated *IGHV* genes. Other prognostic factors have also been identified such as lymphocyte doubling time, Beta-2 microglobulin levels, expression of CD38 by flow-cytometry, and ZAP-70 expression in addition to clinical factors (i.e., age, sex, performance status). The CLL-IPI score has been validated by several groups and uses five independent prognostic factors: *TP53* deletion and/or mutation, *IGHV* mutational status, serum B2-microglobulin concentration, clinical stage, and age. This has identified four distinct prognostic subgroups with 5-year overall survival rates ranging from 93% in the low-risk group to 23% in the very-high-risk group. More recently, the International

TABLE 5 Binet Staging System for Chronic Lymphocytic Leukemia

STAGE	CLINICAL DESCRIPTION
A	Two or less lymphoid areas enlarged
B	Three or more lymphoid areas enlarged
C	Anemia (<10 g/dL) or thrombocytopenia (<100,000/μL)

Prognostic Score for Early-stage CLL (IPS-E) scoring system has been developed to predict time to first treatment in early-stage, asymptomatic patients. This system identified three covariates independently correlated with time to first treatment including unmutated *IGHV* genes, absolute lymphocyte count greater than 1500/μL, and the presence of palpable lymphadenopathy. However, it should be noted that none of these prognostic scoring systems have yet to affect the decision of when to initiate therapy.

Treatment

Not all patients with CLL require treatment at the time of diagnosis. In fact, recent data suggest that although early therapy for high-risk, asymptomatic patients postpones the development of active disease, there is increased toxicity associated with therapy and no clinical data to suggest that such outcomes lead to improved long-term survival. Thus CLL-directed treatment is only indicated for those with active disease as defined by the International Workshop on Chronic Lymphocytic Leukemia Treatment (i.e., progressive marrow failure, symptomatic splenomegaly, bulky lymphadenopathy, rapid lymphocyte doubling time, and/or constitutional symptoms). Therapy for patients with active disease has rapidly evolved over the past several years. It is important to note, however, that patients with advanced CLL are not cured with conventional therapy, thus treatment is directed at alleviating symptoms, improving quality of life, and prolonging survival. With the incorporation of monoclonal antibodies into standard therapy with purine analogues, we began to see significant improvements in patient outcomes, with prolonged remissions in some patients. Additionally, the development of BTK and BCL2 inhibitors has yielded a significant advancement in the treatment of advanced-stage CLL leading to deep remissions, prolonged progression-free survival, and improved overall survival. Importantly, such therapies have yielded marked improvement in outcomes in patients with high-risk disease who historically do not respond or relapse soon after conventional chemoimmunotherapy. Nevertheless, CLL remains an incurable disease, short of allo-SCT.

First-Line Therapy

The choice of first-line therapy in CLL should be made based on patient characteristics and patient preferences/goals as well as on tumor characteristics. Typically, the preferred initial therapy depends on genetic risk stratification and the patient's ability to tolerate therapy. Genetic risk stratification is typically based on *IGHV* mutational status and the presence of 17p deletion or *TP53* mutation. Patients with *IGHV*-unmutated disease with or without 17p deletion or *TP53* mutations are typically treated with targeted agents such as BTK inhibitors or BCL2 inhibitors with or without monoclonal antibodies. For those with IGHV-mutated disease without 17p deletions or *TP53* mutations, conventional chemoimmunotherapy and targeted therapy remain treatment options, with no single agreed-upon standard treatment.

First-line therapy with fludarabine (Fludara), cyclophosphamide (Cytoxan), and rituximab (Rituxan) (FCR) has historically been the most commonly used chemoimmunotherapy combination. The addition of rituximab (Rituxan) to fludarabine and cyclophosphamide represented significant progress in the treatment of CLL, with an overall response rate approaching 95% and a complete response rate of 70%. FCR remains an acceptable initial treatment option for younger patients with active disease, specifically those with *IGHV*-mutated disease who do not harbor 17p deletions or *TP53* mutations. For older adult patients (>65 years of age) or those who cannot tolerate FCR, the combination of bendamustine (Treanda) and rituximab (Rituxan) (BR) offers similar efficacy with improved tolerability compared with FCR. Again, BR is a reasonable first-line therapy for those with *IGHV*-mutated disease without a 17p deletion or *TP53* mutation only.

BTK inhibitors such as ibrutinib (Imbruvica) and acalabrutinib (Calquence) and the BCL2 inhibitor venetoclax (Venclexta) are highly effective therapies that have been shown to improve progression-free survival and overall survival. In patients with high-risk disease (17p deletion and/or *TP53* mutations or *IGHV* unmutated), treatment with targeted agents are preferred given improved outcomes demonstrated in multiple clinical trials. In those with standard-risk disease (*IGHV*-mutated without 17p deletion or *TP53* mutation), chemoimmunotherapy and targeted agents appear to be similar in efficacy, and the choice of which agent to use must be individualized. There remains a lack of clinical data directly comparing targeted agents, and the choice of which agent to use must be based on patient preferences and comorbidities. Of note, data from a recent phase III study comparing ibrutinib to acalabrutinib (Calquence) in patients with previously treated disease shows similar efficacy but fewer cardiovascular adverse events with acalabrutinib. Based on this, acalabrutinib is approved by the U.S. Food and Drug Administration (FDA) as initial or subsequent treatment for adults with CLL. Thus options include single-agent ibrutinib (Imbruvica) with or without rituximab (Rituxan) or

obinutuzumab (Gazyva) for younger patients or the combination of venetoclax plus obinutuzumab (Gazyva) or acalabrutinib (with or without obinutuzumab). Although the combination of ibrutinib plus venetoclax has shown promise in early studies, this is not yet recommended in routine clinical practice.

Other Therapeutic Options

Treatment of relapsed disease in those who achieve at least a partial remission to first-line therapy requires assessment of time to progression from prior therapy. Early relapse is considered for those who experience disease progression at a shorter interval than the median expected for that treatment (i.e., within 5 to 6 years of targeted therapy and 2 to 3 years of FCR). Targeted therapy with *BTK* inhibitors or *BCL2* inhibitors is the preferred treatment at the time of relapse, with the choice of therapy depending on numerous factors including patient preferences, comorbidities, and first-line therapy received. Additionally, PI3K inhibitors idelalisib (Zydelig) plus rituximab and duvelisib (Copiktra) have gained FDA approval for patients with relapsed CLL after one or two prior lines of therapy, respectively.

Hematopoietic stem cell transplantation remains the only curative therapy for CLL; however, the ideal timing is not clear, and data are limited in nature. Perhaps more important is the associated considerable treatment-related morbidity and mortality. Chimeric antigen receptor T-cell (CAR-T) therapy has been investigated in patients with relapsed or refractory CLL and has shown promising activity in early-phase studies with complete response rates in the largest series of ~28%. Further work is needed to better define the role of CAR-T therapy in patients with relapsed CLL. Patients with relapsed CLL should be encouraged to participate in ongoing clinical trials.

Complications

The most common complications that occur in patients with CLL are related to intrinsic immune dysfunction. Specifically, patients with CLL have abnormal immune responses and thus are at a high risk for infectious complications. Infections are the major cause of mortality in patients with CLL, and patients with recurrent major bacterial infections should be considered for intravenous immunoglobulin therapy (IVIg) (Gammagard S/D). Anemia can be related to direct bone marrow infiltration or hypersplenism. In such circumstances, CLL-directed therapy results in improvement in anemia. Additionally, autoimmune hemolytic anemia and pure red cell aplasia can also occur. Similarly, thrombocytopenia may be related to autoimmune destruction, hypersplenism, or disease burden. CLL transformation to aggressive B-cell lymphomas (most commonly diffuse large B-cell lymphoma), called Richter's transformation, is seen in 5% to 10% of patients. Patients with CLL have a higher risk of secondary malignancies, both hematologic and solid tumors. A retrospective review of the Surveillance, Epidemiology and End Results (SEER) program showed that ~11% of patients with CLL developed a secondary solid tumor. Thus appropriate screening must be undertaken in this population.

References

Condoluci A, Bergamo T, Langereins P, et al: International prognostic score for asymptomatic early-stage chronic lymphocytic leukemia, *Blood*, 2020. https://doi.org/10.1182/blood.2019003453.

Faderl S, et al: The Biology of Chronic Myeloid Leukemia, *N Engl J Med* 341:164–172, 1999.

Hallek M, Shanafelt T, Eichhorst B: Chronic lymphocytic leukemia, *Lancet* 391(10129):14–20, 2018.

Hochhaus A, Baccarani M, et al: European LeukemiaNet 2020 recommendations for treating chronic myeloid leukemia, *Leukemia* 34:966–984, 2020.

Jabbour E, Kantarjian H: Chronic myeloid leukemia: 2020 update on diagnosis, therapy and monitoring, *Am J Hematol* 95:691–709, 2020.

Rawstron AC, Bennett FL, O'Connor SJ, et al: Monoclonal B-cell lymphocytosis and chronic lymphocytic leukemia, *N Engl J Med* 359:575–583, 2008.

Siegel RL, Miller KD, Jemal A: Cancer statistics, Cancer, *CA Cancer J Clin* 70(1):7, 2020.

DISSEMINATED INTRAVASCULAR COAGULATION

Method of
Kenneth Byrd, DO

CURRENT DIAGNOSIS

- Disseminated intravascular coagulation (DIC) is an abnormal activation of the coagulation system that is caused by predisposing conditions such as sepsis, malignancy, and trauma.
- Clinical manifestations include organ injury due to microvascular thrombosis and less commonly macrovascular thrombosis. DIC can alternatively present with severe bleeding.
- Laboratory findings include thrombocytopenia, elevated D-dimer, elevated international normalized ratio (INR) and partial thromboplastin time (PTT), and sometimes decreased fibrinogen.
- The International Society on Thrombosis and Haemostasis (ISTH) scoring system predicts overt DIC if score ≥5.

CURRENT TREATMENT

- Aggressive and prompt treatment of the underlying condition causing DIC is paramount.
- If the patient is bleeding or undergoing a procedure, aggressive transfusion support with platelets and fresh frozen plasma (FFP) or cryoprecipitate is often advised.
- Unless the patient is bleeding or undergoing a procedure, FFP or cryoprecipitate is usually not indicated, and platelets are only transfused if less than 20×10^9/L. The major exception is acute promyelocytic leukemia (APL).
- Prophylactic low-molecular-weight heparin (LMWH) is often indicated in DIC.
- Therapeutic heparin/LMWH is rarely indicated in DIC unless there is clear evidence of a severe prothrombotic state.
- No other treatments are routinely used for DIC, including antithrombin, activated protein C, antifibrinolytics, and thrombomodulin. However, the role of these agents continues to be evaluated.

Introduction

Disseminated intravascular coagulation (DIC) is a complex and often life-threatening manifestation of an acquired disease process. This process is initiated by a strong procoagulant cascade that leads to microthrombi throughout the vasculature. A risk of hemorrhage often follows due to a depletion of platelets, consumption of coagulation factors, and accelerated plasmin formation.

Epidemiology

DIC has been reported in approximately 10% to 20% of critical care admissions. It is an independent predictor of mortality and the risk of death in a patient with sepsis is doubled when accompanied by DIC. Mortality rates vary based on the scoring system used but can be as high as 46%. The mortality rate appears to correlate with the severity of laboratory abnormalities at diagnosis.

Pathophysiology

DIC is primarily a coagulation dysfunction due to excessive procoagulant activity. The overactivation is multifactorial but is mainly due to the generation of excessive thrombin, which is mediated by the extrinsic pathway involving tissue factor and factor VIIa. Thrombin excess leads to increased platelet aggregation and thrombotic occlusion of small and midsize vessels with fibrin. Vascular occlusion leads to the derangement of oxygen supply and tissue demand, which can compromise multiple organs. This effect is compounded by defects in inhibitors of coagulation along with fibrinolytic suppression. Antithrombin activity is diminished due to increased consumption, degradation, and impaired synthesis. Likewise, protein C, tissue factor-pathway inhibitor (TFPI), and thrombomodulin activity are decreased in part due to excess inflammatory cytokines. Fibrinolytic suppression occurs in many instances of DIC due to an increase in plasminogen activator inhibitor-1 (PAI-1), which is the principal inhibitor of the fibrinolytic system.

The excessive activation of the coagulation pathway predictably leads to the depletion of platelets and clotting factors. However, the cause of bleeding in DIC is multifactorial, including consumption of clotting factors, thrombocytopenia, platelet dysfunction, endothelial damage, and excess fibrin degradation products (FDPs) that cause feedback anticoagulant effect.

Clinical Manifestations

The manifestations of DIC are often obscured by the underlying causative etiology. Many times, the diagnosis of DIC is solely laboratory based without any clear clinical manifestations. At other times, DIC may be overtly symptomatic. Recently, it has been suggested that DIC could be divided into clinical subtypes that include asymptomatic, bleeding, and organ failure types. The presentation depends on whether there is a predominance of thrombosis from excessive thrombin activation or bleeding from consumptive coagulopathy.

Overall, the incidence of major bleeding in DIC is 5% to 12%. DIC that presents with acute bleeding is most commonly seen in acute leukemia, obstetric disorders, and trauma. Typical hemorrhagic features of DIC include bleeding from venipuncture sites or indwelling catheters, generalized ecchymosis that develops spontaneously or with minimal trauma, bleeding from mucous membranes, unexpected and major bleeding from around drain sites or tracheostomies, and concealed hemorrhage in serous cavities such as retroperitoneal hemorrhage.

Thrombotic organ failure type of DIC is most commonly seen with sepsis. The incidence of organ involvement secondary to thrombosis is 10% to 40%. This occurs due to thromboses in small and midsize vessels. Many organs can be involved, but it is most commonly seen in the kidneys, lungs, liver, and brain. This can manifest as respiratory distress syndrome, acute kidney injury, confusion, and seizures. The skin can also be involved and present as purpura fulminans or acral ischemia. Macrovascular thrombosis such as venous thromboembolism may present as a later manifestation. COVID-19 frequently presents with a DIC-like coagulopathy. Unlike classic acute DIC, fibrinogen is often elevated and there is excessive thrombotic risk.

Diagnosis

Making the diagnosis of DIC starts with identifying an underlying associated disease state. Table 1 lists the known risk factors for DIC. Once this is established, the diagnosis entails a combination of laboratory values along with an analysis of the clinical presentation. The difficulty with diagnosing DIC is that there is no gold standard and no pathognomonic test. There have been several scoring systems developed for DIC to assist in standardizing the diagnosis. The most commonly utilized is the International Society on Thrombosis and Haemostasis (ISTH) scoring system, which was originally devised in 2001 and has been subsequently validated. The scoring system is outlined in Table 2. A score of ≥5 suggests overt DIC. A score of < 5 indicates a lack of DIC or nonovert DIC (i.e., subtle and compensated hemostatic dysfunction). The ISTH scoring system has a sensitivity of 93% and a specificity of 98%. Most other available scoring systems are more sensitive but less specific for DIC. Importantly, if DIC is suspected but not confirmed, then labs should be repeated to assess trends.

TABLE 1 Risk Factors for Disseminated Intravascular Coagulation (Incidence of Disseminated Intravascular Coagulation Per Etiology)

- Sepsis (35%)
  - Most commonly bacterial
- Severe trauma (up to 50%)
  - Most commonly brain injury or burns
- Malignancy
  - Metastatic cancer (up to 20%)
  - Acute leukemia (15%)
  - Acute promyelocytic leukemia (90%)
  - COVID-19
- Obstetrical
  - Placental abruption
  - Amniotic fluid embolism
  - Postpartum hemorrhage
  - Acute fatty liver of pregnancy
- Vascular malformations
  - Kasabach-Merritt syndrome
  - Large aortic aneurysms
  - Other large vascular malformations
- Severe immunologic reaction
  - Acute hemolytic transfusion reaction
  - Anaphylaxis
- Heat stroke
- Postcardiopulmonary resuscitation

TABLE 2 International Society on Thrombosis and Haemostasis Scoring System

Platelet count × 10⁹/L
- ≥100 = 0
- <100 = 1
- <50 = 2

Fibrin marker levels (D-dimer, fibrin degradation products)
- No increase = 0
- Moderate increase (>ULN but <5× ULN) = 2
- Strong increase (≥5× ULN) = 3

Prothrombin time
- <3 s (*INR <1.3) = 0
- ≥3 but <6 s (*INR 1.3–1.5) = 1
- ≥6 s (*INR ≥1.6) = 2

Fibrinogen
- >100 mg/dL = 0
- ≤100 mg/dL = 1

*Assuming the International Survey Index value of the thromboplastin reagents used is close to 1
- A score of ≥5 points is compatible with overt DIC
- The scoring system is only appropriate in patients with an underlying disorder that can be associated with DIC
- If the score if <5 and DIC is still suspected, then consider repeating labs in 1–2 days

DIC, Disseminated intravascular coagulation; *ULN,* upper limits of normal.

The decreased platelet count in DIC is due to excessive thrombin activation and is almost always less than 100×10^9/L and often trending down. A normal platelet count without a downward trend would essentially rule out DIC. The INR and PTT are often elevated due to consumption of coagulation factors but can be normal in up to 50% of cases. The vast majority of DIC is also marked by an increase in fibrin-related markers due to increased fibrinolysis. Traditionally, FDPs were used but have largely been replaced by D-dimer. Fibrinogen is traditionally decreased in DIC but is often normal as it frequently surpasses compensated consumption only later in the clinic course. It can also be falsely normal or even elevated as it is an acute phase reactant. It is only rarely severely diminished. A fibrinogen level of <100 mg/dL is seen in <50% of DIC and usually reflects the late, severe, consumptive stage of DIC.

Thromboelastography (TEG) and rotational thromboelastometry (ROTEM) testing have been evaluated to assess overall coagulation, including platelet function, and clot dissolving potential. TEG has demonstrated good correlation with clinically important organ dysfunction and survival, although its advantage over usual coagulation assays has not yet been confirmed. The role of these two modalities in DIC is still unclear.

DIC often presents with a small population of schistocytes. If the red blood cell population is > 10% schistocytes, then an alternative diagnosis is more likely (i.e., TMA). Of note, a low ADAMTS13 can be seen in DIC but is usually >30%. There is also frequently a reduction in antithrombin and protein C. These tests are not done routinely and are likely not as sensitive as the ISTH scoring system. Finally, factor VIII can be low in DIC due to consumption, but it can also be elevated at times as it is an acute phase reactant.

The differential diagnosis of DIC is explained in Table 3.

Therapy

The foundation of treatment for DIC is to treat the underlying disorder. If the underlying disorder is reversed, then DIC typically resolves.

During active DIC there may be a need for transfusion support. It is important to note that the following transfusion recommendations are mostly based on low-quality evidence, including expert opinion. In the presence of bleeding, platelet transfusions should be given to keep platelet count greater than 30 to 50×10^9/L. Similarly, in the setting of invasive procedures, platelets should be maintained greater than 20 to 50×10^9/L, depending on the risk of the procedure. Importantly, in the absence of bleeding or procedure, platelets should be transfused only if platelet count is less than 20×10^9/L (a range of 10 to 30 $\times 10^9$/L has been proposed by various sources). The exception to this threshold would be acute promyelocytic leukemia (APL), in which platelets should be maintained greater than 30 to 50 × 10^9/L even in the absence of bleeding (less commonly some suggest a 20×10^9/L threshold).

A similar approach to the replacement of factors is indicated. If the patient is bleeding or undergoing a high risk procedure and fibrinogen is less than 150 mg/dL or PT/PTT is greater than 1.5 upper limits of normal (ULN), then fresh frozen plasma (FFP) or cryoprecipitate is recommended. Keep in mind that FFP contains all factors of the soluble coagulation system, while cryoprecipitate contains a concentrated subset of plasma factors including fibrinogen, factor VIII, von Willebrand factor, and factor XIII. The choice between FFP and cryoprecipitate is made on a case-by-case basis and can often be influenced by fluid status. The recommended dose of FFP is 15 to 30 mL/kg and cryoprecipitate is 5 to 10 units. A less frequently used option is 2 g of fibrinogen concentrate. Factor replacement is not indicated in the absence of bleeding or procedure. An exception to this threshold is APL, in which factor replacement could be considered if fibrinogen is less than 100 to 150 mg/dL, even in the absence of bleeding.

In addition to transfusion support and treatment of the underlying etiology, heparin[1] can be considered in a few circumstances. Most importantly, guidelines recommend prophylactic heparin or low-molecular-weight heparin (LMWH)[1] in the absence of bleeding as long as platelet count is greater than 20 to 30×10^9/L, INR greater than 1.5, and fibrinogen greater than 100 mg/dL. This is especially vital in prothrombotic DIC (i.e., sepsis, solid tumor malignancy). An exception to the general use of LMWH prophylaxis is in hyperfibrinolytic DIC (i.e., APL and prostate cancer), in which more caution is advised with heparin use. Therapeutic heparin is uncommonly advised in DIC, but it can be considered in prothrombotic DIC, as evidenced by thromboembolism, purpura fulminans, or acral ischemia. As heparin can partially inhibit activation of the coagulation, it would make sense that it could help offset DIC. In small studies,

---

[1] Not FDA approved for this indication.

TABLE 3	Differential Diagnosis of Disseminated Intravascular Coagulation		
DISEASE	**SIMILARITIES**	**DIFFERENCES**	**COMMENTS**
Liver disease	Low plt; prolonged PT/PTT; low fibrinogen; increased FDP (DIC > Liver disease)	No schistocytes in liver disease; worsening labs in DIC and more stable in liver disease	Factor VIII not very helpful for differentiation. Normal or elevated in liver disease (not synthesized in liver). However, as an acute phase reactant, often normal or elevated in DIC
Thrombotic microangiopathy (TMA)	Low plt; increased FDP (DIC > TMA); decreased ADAMTS13 (TMA lower than DIC)	MAHA in TMA; normal PT/PTT and fibrinogen in TMA; numerous schistocytes common in TMA, but not DIC	Extremely low plt with normal PT/PTT is common in TMA but unusual in DIC; TMA includes TTP, HUS, secondary TMAs
Heparin-induced thrombocytopenia (HIT)	Low plt, increased FDP	Normal PT/PTT in HIT; low fibrinogen unusual in HIT	Plt <20 × 10⁹/L is uncommon in HIT
Catastrophic antiphospholipid syndrome (CAPS)	Low plt; increased FDP; PTT elevation (false elevation of PTT commonly due to LA)	Normal PT in CAPS; lab diagnosis of APLS in CAPS	Normal plt often seen in CAPS and severe thrombocytopenia is rare; microvascular thromboses in both; macrovascular thrombosis is a more common initial presentation of CAPS than DIC
Hemophagocytic lymphohistiocytosis (HLH)	Low plt; prolonged PT/PTT; low fibrinogen; increased FDP	HLH with very high ferritin, TGs, organomegaly, and often hemophagocytosis	

APLS, Antiphospholipid antibody syndrome; *DIC*, disseminated intravascular coagulation; *FDP*, fibrin degradation products; *LA*, lupus anticoagulant; *MAHA*, microangiopathic hemolytic anemia; *plt*, platelet count; *PT*, prothrombin time; *PTT*, partial thromboplastin time; *TG*, triglycerides; *TTP*, thrombotic thrombocytopenic purpura.

heparin has shown beneficial effects on coagulation parameters. However, improvement in clinically important outcomes in DIC has not been clearly demonstrated.

Other therapies that have been studied in the treatment of DIC include antithrombin concentrate (AT [Thrombate III]),[1] activated protein C (APC), recombinant thrombomodulin, and antifibrinolytics. Currently, these agents are rarely, if ever, indicated for use. AT and APC have been extensively studied in the setting of sepsis. One of the issues in assessing the benefit of AT and APC is that many clinical trials assess the general sepsis population and do not limit analysis to those specifically with DIC. For AT, there has been no significant reduction in mortality in these studies. However, there is a suggestion that there may be significant benefit in the subset of patients with severe sepsis and DIC. This requires prospective validation. APC has also shown promise at times, including improvement in mortality in an early randomized controlled trial (RCT). However, subsequent studies showed an increased risk of serious bleeding and lack of survival benefit. Therefore, the FDA advised to stop using APC for DIC in 2011.

Caution is advised with the use of antifibrinolytics in DIC. Since the excessive fibrin deposition appears in part to be due to insufficient fibrinolysis, further inhibition of the fibrinolytic system would clearly not be appropriate. This is especially the case in sepsis, but there are a few exceptions to this. Antifibrinolytics can be considered in hyperfibrinolytic DIC (i.e., APL or prostate cancer) only in the setting of life-threatening bleeding. The other exception is in acute trauma. A large RCT showed that early use of antifibrinolytics in trauma was beneficial. However, once the acute phase has passed, further thrombin generation eventually predominates, and the balance is tipped toward thrombosis.

Recombinant soluble thrombomodulin continues to be actively evaluated and shows some potential. While efficacy outcomes have been heterogeneous, a 2020 meta-analysis suggested a 28-day mortality benefit of recombinant thrombomodulin[5] in patients with sepsis and coagulopathy. Results of ongoing studies are pending.

Finally, it is worth mentioning that a Cochrane review evaluated recombinant factor VIIa (NovoSeven)[1] and concluded that it does not have proven efficacy in DIC and that there is an increased risk of arterial thrombotic events. Its use is not advised.

---

[1]Not FDA approved for this indication

References

Asakura H, Ogawa H: COVID-19-associated coagulopathy and disseminated intravascular coagulation, *Int J Hematol* 113(1):45–57, 2021.

Bakhtiari K, Meijers JC, de Jonge E, Levi M: Prospective validation of the International Society of Thrombosis and Haemostasis scoring system for disseminated intravascular coagulation, *Crit Care Med* 32(12):2416–2421, 2004.

Bernard GR, Vincent JL, Laterre PF, et al: Efficacy and safety of recombinant human activated protein C for severe sepsis, *N Engl J Med* 344(10):699–709, 2001.

Gando S, Levi M, Toh CH: Disseminated intravascular coagulation, *Nat Rev Dis Primers* 2:16037, 2016.

Levi M: Pathogenesis and diagnosis of disseminated intravascular coagulation, *Int J Lab Hematol* 40:15–20, 2018.

Levi M, Scully M: How I treat disseminated intravascular coagulation, *Blood* 131(8):845–854, 2018.

Sanz MA, Grimwade D, Tallman MS, et al: Management of acute promyelocytic leukemia: recommendations from an expert panel on behalf of the European Leukemianet, *Blood* 113(9):1875–1891, 2009.

Squizzato A, Hunt BJ, Kinasewitz GT, et al: Supportive management strategies for disseminated intravascular coagulation, *ThrombHaemost* 116(05):896–904, 2016.

Valeriani E, Squizzato A, Gallo A, et al: Efficacy and safety of recombinant human soluble thrombomodulin in patients with sepsis-associated coagulopathy: A systematic review and meta-analysis, *J Thromb Haemost* 18(7):1618–1625, 2020.

Wada H, Thachil J, Di Nisio M, et al: Guidance for diagnosis and treatment of disseminated intravascular coagulation from harmonization of the recommendations from three guidelines, *J ThrombHaemost* 11(4):761–767, 2013.

Warren BL, Eid A, Singer P, et al: High-dose antithrombin III in severe sepsis: a randomized controlled trial, *JAMA* 286(15):1869–1878, 2001.

Disseminated Intravascular Coagulation

---

[1]Not FDA approved for this indication
[5]Investigational drug in the United States.

HEMOCHROMATOSIS

Method of
Heinz Zoller, MD

CURRENT DIAGNOSIS

- Consider diagnosis in patients with symptoms of iron overload such as fatigue, grayish-brown discoloration of the skin, arthralgias, diabetes, cardiac arrhythmia, or sexual dysfunction.
- High transferrin saturation (TSAT) and a low unbound iron-binding capacity (UIBC) are the clinical biochemical hallmarks of hemochromatosis.
- In patients with high TSAT, homozygosity for the p.Cys282Tyr (C282Y) in the *HFE* gene confirms hemochromatosis genetically.
- Hemochromatosis can be phenotypically diagnosed when transferrin saturation is high, hepatic iron is increased, and spleen iron content is normal.
- Magnetic resonance imaging (MRI) with R2* sequences allows noninvasive quantification of liver and spleen iron.
- Liver biopsy may be required for disease staging or when MRI is not available.
- Genetic testing beyond *HFE* genotyping by multiple gene sequencing can yield alternative genetic hemochromatosis causes but is not necessary for diagnosis because phenotypic diagnosis is sufficient to initiate treatment.

CURRENT TREATMENT

- Management of hemochromatosis requires disease staging and the assessment of hepatic fibrosis, glucose metabolism, heart function, and arthropathy.
- In patients with onset of hemochromatosis before the age of 20 years, left ventricular function, thyroid function, and pituitary function should be assessed.
- Serum ferritin is a surrogate marker for the severity of iron overload but is also increased by inflammation, alcohol intake, and the metabolic syndrome.
- In patients with hemochromatosis with hepatic fibrosis, endocrine, skeletal, and cardiac complications should be recognized and treated accordingly.
- Patients with hemochromatosis and iron overload should be treated by phlebotomy weekly or every other week to achieve a serum ferritin less than 50 ng/mL while avoiding anemia.
- After a ferritin less than 50 ng/mL has been achieved, phlebotomy frequency should be reduced to maintain ferritin less than 100 ng/mL; most patients will require two to six phlebotomies per year.
- Siblings of patients with hemochromatosis should be tested.

Definition and Pathogenesis

Hemochromatosis is defined as a genetic disease caused by deficiency of the hormone hepcidin, which normally controls plasma iron concentrations. The clinical surrogate for hepcidin deficiency is elevated transferrin saturation or low unbound iron-binding capacity (UIBC). Under physiologic conditions, transferrin saturation is maintained in the range of 15% to 45% by hepcidin, which inhibits iron release from cells, mainly the recycling macrophages in the spleen and resorptive duodenal enterocytes. Consequently, hemochromatosis is associated with high intestinal iron absorption, high liver iron concentrations, and low spleen iron. In hemochromatosis, liver iron is increased because elevated transferrin saturation (>65%) results in *nontransferrin-bound iron* in the plasma. The nontransferrin-bound iron is removed from the circulation by hepatocytes. Tissue damage in hemochromatosis has been proposed to result from excess iron in hepatocytes and from redox-active nontransferrin-bound iron in circulation.

Epidemiology

The prevalence of hemochromatosis in populations of European ancestry is about 1 in 1000. The disease is typically diagnosed between 40 and 60 years of age. Hemochromatosis is about four times more common in males than in females. The most common genotype associated with hemochromatosis, present in about 80% to 95% of patients with phenotypic hemochromatosis, is homozygosity for C282Y in the *HFE* gene. This genotype has a prevalence of approximately 1:400 among populations of Northern European ancestry. This means that cumulative lifetime penetrance of hemochromatosis, defined as elevated transferrin saturation and elevated ferritin in C282Y homozygotes, is less than 40%. The prevalence of the C282Y allele in different European populations is variable, ranging from <1% to 12%, with the highest prevalence in Ireland. Disease penetrance among patients homozygous for C282Y increases with age, is higher in males, and is increased by alcohol and a diet high in red meat.

Clinical Features

Fatigue is a typical but nonspecific symptom of hemochromatosis. Signs associated with hemochromatosis include joint pain, bronze discoloration of the skin or porphyria cutanea tarda, diabetes, and hepatomegaly. Advanced hemochromatosis and other coincident risk factors for liver disease, such as viral hepatitis or increased alcohol consumption, can result in progressive fibrosis and cirrhosis, as well as hepatocellular carcinoma. Iron-induced tissue damage is not restricted to the liver and can also affect the endocrine system, heart, bone, and joints. The most common endocrine manifestation of hemochromatosis in adults is diabetes, which is significantly more common among men with hemochromatosis than in controls. Other common manifestations in adults are osteoporosis and arthropathy, which are often misclassified as rheumatoid arthritis or osteoarthritis. In patients with severe forms of hemochromatosis and early disease onset, cardiomyopathy, hypogonadotropic hypogonadism, and hypothyroidism are more common.

Diagnosis and Disease Staging

In patients with suggestive symptoms or signs of hemochromatosis and siblings of patients with hemochromatosis, the first diagnostic step is determination of transferrin saturation (TSAT) or UIBC and serum ferritin, followed by *HFE* genotyping if TSAT is increased. Iron quantification in the liver and spleen by magnetic resonance imaging (MRI) is recommended in patients with elevated TSAT who are not homozygous for C282Y. Liver biopsy is rarely required because noninvasive methods can be used for fibrosis staging (Figure 1).

Transferrin Saturation or Unbound Iron-Binding Capacity

The pathogenesis and definition of hemochromatosis are based on hepcidin deficiency, which results in elevated TSAT or low UIBC. Studies have shown that TSAT levels are highly variable upon repeat determination. A population-based study has not demonstrated additional value in repeated determination of TSAT, but, in clinical practice, it is recommended to confirm an elevated TSAT in an independent blood sample taken after an overnight fast before further evaluation is pursued in patients with low clinical suspicion of hemochromatosis.

Ferritin

High ferritin is a surrogate marker of iron overload but has limited specificity because alcohol consumption, the metabolic syndrome, and inflammatory and neoplastic diseases can also cause high serum ferritin levels. In patients with hemochromatosis and the absence of any of these conditions, ferritin is correlated with the severity of iron overload. In hemochromatosis, provisional iron overload is defined as the presence of high TSAT and high ferritin levels (males and postmenopausal women >300 ng/mL and women of childbearing potential >200 ng/mL).

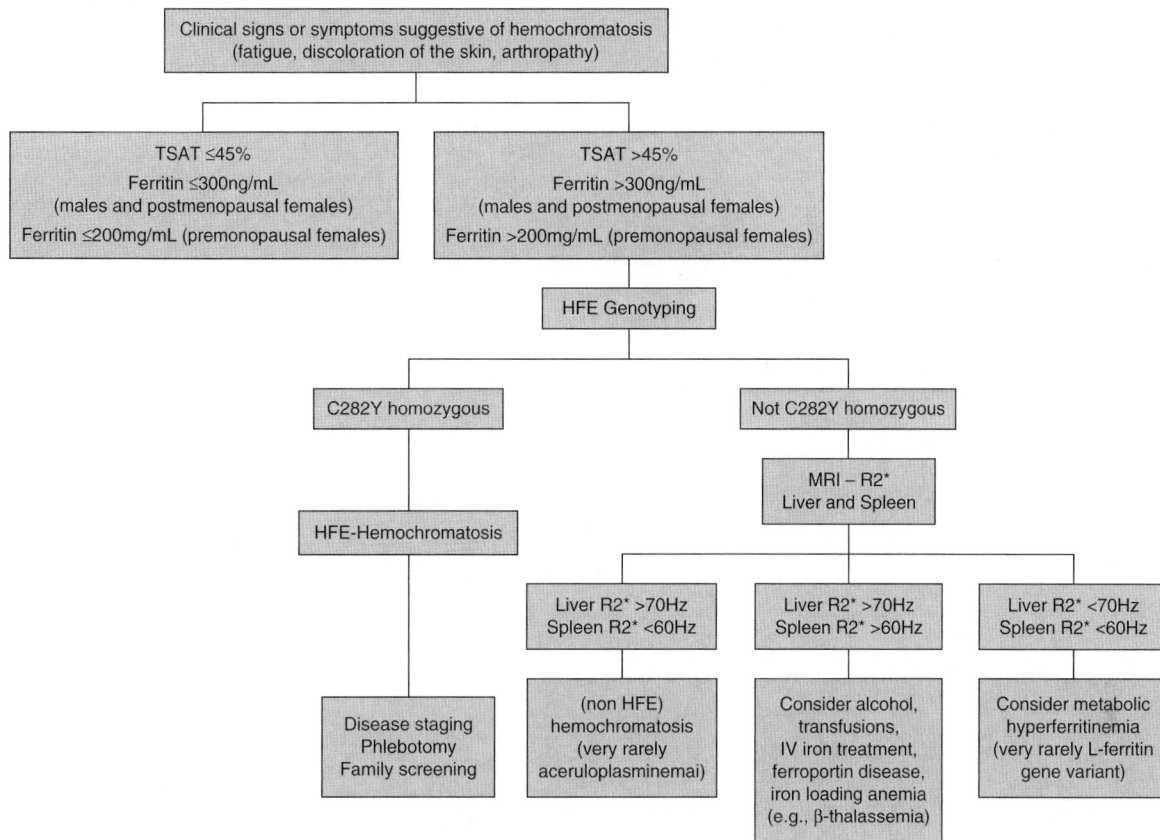

Figure 1 Algorithm summarizing the diagnostic path in patients with suspected hemochromatosis.

The flowchart contains the following boxes:

Clinical signs or symptoms suggestive of hemochromatosis (fatigue, discoloration of the skin, arthropathy)

TSAT ≤45%
Ferritin ≤300ng/mL (males and postmenopausal females)
Ferritin ≤200mg/mL (premenopausal females)

TSAT >45%
Ferritin >300ng/mL (males and postmenopausal females)
Ferritin >200mg/mL (premenopausal females)

HFE Genotyping

C282Y homozygous

Not C282Y homozygous

MRI – R2* Liver and Spleen

HFE-Hemochromatosis

Liver R2* >70Hz Spleen R2* <60Hz

Liver R2* >70Hz Spleen R2* >60Hz

Liver R2* <70Hz Spleen R2* <60Hz

Disease staging Phlebotomy Family screening

(non HFE) hemochromatosis (very rarely aceruloplasminemai)

Consider alcohol, transfusions, IV iron treatment, ferroportin disease, iron loading anemia (e.g., β-thalassemia)

Consider metabolic hyperferritinemia (very rarely L-ferritin gene variant)

Transferrin or Total Iron-Binding Capacity

At physiologic concentrations, iron in circulation is mainly bound to the protein transferrin. Transferrin or total iron-binding capacity is increased in patients with iron deficiency and can be mildly decreased in patients with iron overload. It has limited diagnostic value for the diagnosis of hemochromatosis but is important in the differential diagnosis. In patients with inflammation, alcohol consumption, or end-stage liver disease, the transferrin protein itself can be markedly reduced, resulting in an increased transferrin saturation.

Genetic Testing

Genotyping for the C282Y variant in the *HFE* gene (rs1800562) is recommended in patients with suspected hemochromatosis and repeatedly elevated transferrin saturation. In such patients, homozygosity for the C282Y variant confirms the diagnosis. Because of incomplete penetrance, for patients diagnosed with C282Y homozygosity and with a normal TSAT and normal serum ferritin, a genetic risk for the development of iron overload can be asserted, but the genotype alone is not sufficient for the diagnosis of hemochromatosis. In such individuals, lifestyle modifications (see later) and follow-up are recommended.

A minority of patients with phenotypic hemochromatosis are compound heterozygous for the C282Y and the H63D variant in the *HFE* gene. Because of the high allele frequency of H63D, compound heterozygosity is more common than C282Y homozygosity, though the penetrance of this genotype is much lower than in C282Y homozygotes. Patients with compound heterozygosity with provisional iron overload (elevated TSAT and high ferritin) should be evaluated for the presence of iron overload by MRI and for the coincidence of additional risk factors, including the metabolic syndrome, iron-loading anemias, or alcohol intake. The same applies to patients homozygous for H63D.

Magnetic Resonance Imaging

Quantification of liver and spleen iron can be performed noninvasively by special protocols on MRI. The so-called R2* frequency,

expressed in s^{-1} or Hertz (Hz), is directly proportional to tissue iron concentration, where an R2* value of greater than 70 Hz in the liver and greater than 60 Hz in the spleen indicate iron overload in the respective organ. In patients with provisional iron overload (high ferritin and elevated TSAT) who are not homozygous for the C282Y variant, MRI is recommended (Figure 2). The presence of elevated liver iron in the absence of spleen iron overload confirms the phenotypic diagnosis of hemochromatosis. In patients with elevated liver and spleen iron, other causes of iron overload are typically found, including a history of repeated transfusions, IV iron therapy, or high alcohol intake. A rare genetic cause, important in the differential diagnosis for increased iron concentrations in the liver and spleen, is loss-of-function variants in the cellular iron export pump ferroportin, which is encoded by the SCL40A1 gene. The most common cause of high ferritin with variable TSAT and normal liver iron is the metabolic syndrome. In such patients, hepatic steatosis is present and, in more advanced cases, hepatic and spleen iron can be mildly elevated. An alternative genetic cause for high ferritin with normal liver iron are genetic variants in the 5′ untranslated region of the L-ferritin mRNA.

Fibrosis Assessment

Liver fibrosis is a common complication of hepatic iron overload. In all patients diagnosed with hemochromatosis, the degree of liver fibrosis should be assessed. In the absence of clinically evident cirrhosis, the first step in fibrosis assessment is calculation of the FIB-4 score from patient age, alanine aminotransferase (ALT) level, aspartate aminotransferase (AST) level, and platelet count. A FIB-4 score of less than 1.3 rules out advanced fibrosis, and no further testing is recommended in such patients. As age is an important determinant for the stage of fibrosis, higher cutoff values have been recommended in patients older than 65 years. In patients with hepatomegaly, ferritin greater than 1000 ng/mL and elevated ALT or AST, advanced fibrosis cannot be ruled out. Before elastography became widely available, liver biopsy was recommended. Studies have shown that noninvasive fibrosis assessment by vibration

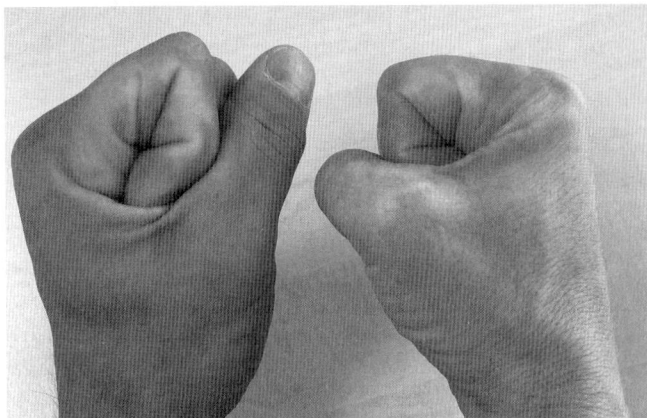

Figure 2 Skin discoloration and impaired flexibility of the second metacarpophalangeal (MCP) joint as typical signs in a hemochromatosis patient (left hand). Normal skin color and normal MCP-joint flexibility in a control person.

controlled transient elastography has a reasonable predictive value for the diagnosis and exclusion of fibrosis. Hence liver biopsy is now only required for disease staging in hemochromatosis patients with a FIB-4 score of greater than 1.3 and indeterminate results on transient elastography, between 6.5 and 12 kPa.

Liver Biopsy and Hepatocellular Carcinoma Surveillance

Introduction of noninvasive iron quantification by MRI and noninvasive fibrosis assessment by FIB-4 followed by elastography have greatly reduced the need for liver biopsy. Liver biopsy is still recommended in patients with contraindications for MRI, indeterminate readings on elastography, or diagnostic uncertainty. In patients with advanced fibrosis on noninvasive fibrosis assessment or cirrhosis on liver biopsy, surveillance for early detection of hepatocellular carcinoma by biannual abdominal ultrasound should be strongly considered. As treatment can be associated with the regression of cirrhosis, fibrosis stage can be reassessed after excess iron has been removed. In patients with regression of cirrhosis, discontinuation of hepatocellular carcinoma surveillance can be considered.

Family Screening

The majority of patients with hemochromatosis are homozygous for C282Y. The autosomal recessive nature of this *HFE*-associated hemochromatosis renders family screening of siblings cost-effective. In families with three or more children, testing the unaffected spouse before testing the children is also cost-effective. In patients with "non-*HFE* hemochromatosis," genetic testing by sequencing of a gene panel that includes but is not limited to *HFE* can be performed but is not required to initiate treatment because in such patients the diagnosis is based on phenotypic criteria. Rarely, hemochromatosis can be caused by autosomal dominant gain-of-function mutations in SCL40A1, which should be included in the gene panel and also prompt family screening.

Treatment

Phlebotomy

In patients with hemochromatosis and iron overload as indicated by elevated ferritin or on liver MRI, iron removal by phlebotomy is recommended. Phlebotomy can reduce fatigue, prevent progression of fibrosis, and may revert cirrhosis in some patients. Hemochromatosis arthropathy, which can currently only be treated symptomatically, typically does not respond to phlebotomy. In the initial treatment phase, phlebotomy should be performed weekly or every other week by removing 500 mL of blood after anemia has been excluded by quantifying the hemoglobin concentration. Serum ferritin should be determined every 3 months during the initial treatment phase or when the patient develops anemia, which should ideally be avoided. The treatment goal during the initial phase is a serum ferritin less than 50 ng/mL while avoiding the development

of anemia. Once this target has been achieved the patient should enter maintenance treatment with increased time intervals between phlebotomies. As phlebotomy does not correct the genetic cause of hemochromatosis, iron can reaccumulate and maintenance treatment is recommended. The rate of iron reaccumulation is highly variable, and treatment intervals must be individualized. The target ferritin during this treatment phase is serum ferritin in the range of 50 to 100 ng/mL. To achieve this goal, serum ferritin should be checked every 3 months because most patients require two to six phlebotomies per year.

Second-Line Treatment

Erythrocyte apheresis has been shown to be effective in reducing fatigue and achieving target ferritin in clinical trials and has been associated with fewer procedures, milder hemodynamic changes, and shorter treatment duration to achieve treatment targets. Apheresis depends on local availability, local expertise, and reimbursement.

Oral iron chelators are not approved for hemochromatosis, but in patients with needle phobia, limited venous access, or poor tolerance of hemodynamic changes associated with phlebotomy, treatment with oral iron chelators can be considered.

Hepcidin mimetics and drugs that indirectly stimulate hepcidin production are under development and could offer additional benefits in the future, especially in patients with increased transferrin saturation despite having achieved the recommended treatment targets for serum ferritin.

Dietary Recommendations

The most important dietary recommendation in patients with hemochromatosis is to minimize or avoid alcohol consumption. Diets high in bioavailable iron, such as red meat, and high in citrus fruits, which enhance iron absorption, should be reduced. Proton pump inhibitors, low-iron diets, and the intake of coffee or tea can reduce the rate of iron reaccumulation but do not replace phlebotomy. Hemochromatosis patients should avoid handling of raw seafood because of the risk of fulminant infections with *Vibrio vulnificus*.

Summary

Hemochromatosis should be diagnosed before arthropathy, cirrhosis, or heart failure have developed. Early initiation of phlebotomy can prevent these complications and normalize life expectancy. Well-defined diagnostic criteria and the availability of genetic testing can guide physicians and patients to early diagnosis and the prevention of disease complications by phlebotomy.

References

Adams PC, Reboussin DM, Barton JC, et al: Hemochromatosis and iron-overload screening in a racially diverse population, *N Engl J Med* 352:1769–1778, 2005.

Adams PC, Reboussin DM, Press RD, et al: Biological variability of transferrin saturation and unsaturated iron-binding capacity, *Am J Med* 120:999 e1–7, 2007.

Allen KJ, Gurrin LC, Constantine CC, et al: Iron-overload-related disease in HFE hereditary hemochromatosis, *N Engl J Med* 358:221–230, 2008.

Bardou-Jacquet E, Morandeau E, Anderson GJ, et al: Regression of fibrosis stage with treatment reduces long-term risk of liver cancer in patients with hemochromatosis caused by mutation in HFE, *Clin Gastroenterol Hepatol* 18:1851–1857, 2020.

Hagstrom H, Ndegwa N, Jalmeus M, et al: Morbidity, risk of cancer and mortality in 3645 HFE mutations carriers, *Liver Int* 41:545–553, 2021.

Le Lan C, Loreal O, Cohen T, et al: Redox active plasma iron in C282Y/C282Y hemochromatosis, *Blood* 105:4527–4531, 2005.

Legros L, Bardou-Jacquet E, Latournerie M, et al: Non-invasive assessment of liver fibrosis in C282Y homozygous HFE hemochromatosis, *Liver Int* 35:1731–1738, 2015.

Pilling LC, Tamosauskaite J, Jones G, et al: Common conditions associated with hereditary haemochromatosis genetic variants: cohort study in UK Biobank, *BMJ* 364:k5222, 2019.

Rombout-Sestrienkova E, Nieman FH, Essers BA, et al: Erythrocytapheresis versus phlebotomy in the initial treatment of HFE hemochromatosis patients: results from a randomized trial, *Transfusion* 52:470–477, 2012.

Vanclooster A, van Deursen C, Jaspers R, et al: Proton pump inhibitors decrease phlebotomy need in hfe hemochromatosis: double-blind randomized placebo-controlled trial, *Gastroenterology* 153:678–680.e2, 2017.

Valenti L, Corradini E, Adams LA, et al. Consensus statement on the definition and classification of metabolic hyperferritinaemia. *Nat Rev Endocrinol* 2023:1-12.

Viveiros A, Schaefer B, Panzer M, et al: MRI-based iron phenotyping and patient selection for next-generation sequencing of non-homeostatic iron regulator hemochromatosis genes, *Hepatology* 74:2424–2435, 2021.

HEMOLYTIC ANEMIAS

Method of
Thomas G. DeLoughery, MD

CURRENT DIAGNOSES

- Suspect hemolysis when anemia is accompanied by signs of red cell breakdown: high low-density lipoprotein (LDH) and indirect bilirubin with a low haptoglobin.
- The reticulocyte count is often high.
- A positive direct antibody test (DAT) confirms the diagnosis of autoimmune hemolytic anemia in the presence of hemolysis.
- In patients with non-immune hemolysis, specific testing is required to make the diagnosis.

At the most basic level, hemolytic anemias are caused by red cell destruction. This destruction can be caused by factors that are either intrinsic or extrinsic to the red blood cell (RBC). The pace of the hemolysis can vary from being only detectable by laboratory abnormalities to fulminant acute severe anemia. A useful way to think about hemolytic anemias is to divide them into hereditary disorders and acquired disorders (Table 1). Defects in any part of the RBC lead to inherited disorders, while acquired disorders are caused by immune-related processes and other etiologies extrinsic to the RBC.

Pathophysiology

Congenital

The major components of the RBC are the membrane, hemoglobin, and enzymes; therefore the three major classes of hereditary hemolytic anemias are caused by defects in any of these three red cell components.

Hereditary spherocytosis is the most common hemolytic anemia caused by membrane defects. This condition is caused by mutation in the proteins that make up the red cell skeleton, which leads to an unstable membrane. The RBCs in hereditary spherocytosis initially have a normal biconcave disc structure, but after repeated passage through the spleen, they gradually lose portions of the membrane and become more spherical as they age (a process known as *splenic conditioning*). These spherocytes are less deformable and because of that are ultimately trapped and destroyed in the spleen. Less common anemias caused by membrane defects are hereditary elliptocytosis and pyropoikilocytosis. The skeletal defects are not as profound in elliptocytosis, so the clinical presentation is usually milder. Most patients with pyropoikilocytosis are homozygous for mutations that cause elliptocytosis and have very unstable red cell membranes; often fragments of RBCs are seen in the circulation.

The most common RBC enzyme defect is glucose-6-phosphate dehydrogenase (G6PD) deficiency. An adequate supply of reduced glutathione (GSH) is necessary to protect the erythrocyte from oxidative damage. G6PD catalyzes the conversion of glucose-6-phosphate to 6-phosphogluconate, in the process reducing NADP to NADPH. NADPH is necessary for the conversion of glutathione (GSSG) to reduced glutathione (GSH). The erythrocyte does not have any other source of NADPH and so is dependent solely on this pathway for reducing power. When G6PD is deficient, this leads to decreased NADPH, which results in decreased GSH. When the RBC undergoes oxidative stress, this lack of reducing power results in damage of red cell proteins, especially hemoglobin. These damaged proteins can aggregate, causing membrane damage and red cell destruction as the crystallized proteins are removed by the spleen.

Pyruvate kinase (PK) deficiency is a hemolytic anemia caused by an enzymatic defect in the glycolytic pathway. Pyruvate kinase catalyzes conversion of phosphoenolpyruvate (PEP) to pyruvate, generating ATP in the same reaction. Deficiency of PK results in decreased levels of erythrocyte ATP. Lack of ATP results in a leaky cell membrane and loss of water and potassium. This leads to cellular dehydration and rigid, nondeformable cells that are susceptible to destruction within the spleen.

By far the most common hereditary hemolytic hemoglobin defect is sickle cell anemia. The abnormal hemoglobin protein forms long polymers that disrupt red cell integrity. There are also very rare defects in hemoglobin that can cause unstable molecules that can crystallize and lead to hemolysis—most often resulting from splenic removal of damaged proteins.

Acquired

Autoimmune hemolytic anemias (AIHAs) can be mediated by either anti–red cell IgG or IgM antibodies. In IgG-mediated disease, the antibody binds to red cell membrane proteins. The antibody-coated RBCs are then phagocytized by macrophages found primarily in the spleen, leading to hemolysis.

In IgM-mediated hemolysis *(cold agglutinin disease)*, the antibody binds to the RBC most often in the periphery of the body. The *cold* appellation comes from the fact that the antibody binds more strongly when below body temperature. Most commonly, complement is fixed only through C3, and then the C3-coated RBCs are taken up by the macrophages. In rare patients, the IgM can fix complement rapidly, leading to intravascular hemolysis by formation of the end product of complement, the membrane attack complex.

Rare patients can develop immune hemolysis induced by medication. There have been three mechanisms proposed for drug AIHA. The hapten mechanism is most often associated with the use of high-dose penicillin. High doses of penicillin lead to drug incorporation into the red cell membrane by binding to proteins. Another mechanism is the formation of an immune complex of drug, antibody, and red cell membrane which leads to hemolysis. Finally, patients taking certain drugs such as methyldopa will develop a positive direct antibody (DAT) after 6 months of

TABLE 1	Hemolytic Anemia: Classification of Common Causes
Congenital	
Membrane defects	
Hereditary spherocytosis	
Hereditary elliptocytosis	
Hereditary pyropoikilocytosis	
Enzymatic defects	
G6PD deficiency	
Pyruvate kinase deficiency	
Hemoglobin defects	
Sickle cell disease	
Unstable hemoglobins	
Acquired	
Autoimmune	
Warm antibody IgG	
Cold antibody IgM	
Drug-induced	
Paroxysmal nocturnal hemoglobinuria	
Mechanical	
Microangiopathic	
Toxins	
Parasites	

therapy and hemolysis that is indistinguishable from warm antibody AIHA.

In paroxysmal nocturnal hemoglobinuria (PNH), RBCs lack the regulatory membrane proteins that inhibit activated complement proteins. These proteins include membrane inhibitor of reactive lysis (CD59) and decay accelerating factor (CD55). The molecular defect in PNH is a mutation of the phosphatidyl inositol glycan complementation group A *(PIG-A)* gene located on the X chromosome. This enzyme is required for synthesis of glycosyl phosphatidylinositol (GPI)-linked proteins. Cells derived from the PNH stem cells are deficient in all proteins that are linked to the membrane by a GPI molecule, including those that inactivate complement. Normally there is baseline activation of complement; it is thought that one of the functions of RBCs is inactivation of these active complement proteins. When activated complement binds PNH RBCs instead of being destroyed, the resulting membrane attack complex leads to lysis of the RBC.

Microangiopathic hemolytic anemias (MAHAs) result from destruction of circulating RBCs. Although MAHA is commonly associated with thrombotic microangiopathies such thrombotic thrombocytopenia purpura (TTP) and hemolytic uremic syndrome (HUS), there are many other possible associated disease states. For example, patients with malignant hypertension can have very severe hemolysis resulting from increased shearing of RBCs traversing damaged glomeruli. There may also be associated thrombocytopenia, which can lead to concern that TTP may be present. Hemolysis associated with malignant hypertension resolves rapidly with control of the blood pressure. Scleroderma renal crisis is often accompanied by a MAHA due to both severe hypertension and renal damage.

Cardiac valvular disease can lead to MAHA. This is seen most commonly after mitral valve repair if there is a small defect at the site where the valve ring is sewn in. Ventricular contraction leads to a small resurgent jet that results in a high shear situation in the jet and red cell destruction. In some cases, this can result in severe hemolysis and a transfusion-dependent anemia.

Ventricular-assist devices (VADs) to support heart failure patients can also lead to hemolysis. This is blood flowing through the device being subjected to high shear rates. Most patients have low levels of hemolysis, but with VAD thrombosis there is an abrupt increase in hemolysis because of higher shear forces; an increasing LDH is an indication to look for VAD thrombosis.

Along with MAHA, there are several other syndromes which may cause mechanical damage to RBCs. *Clostridium* infections can lead to hemolysis by direct damage to red cell membranes. The bacteria secrete an alpha-toxin that has phospholipase activity and leads to the red cell membrane literally dissolving, which causes the hemoglobin to leak out of the cells. In some cases, this can be so severe that the measured hemoglobin may equal the hematocrit. Empty red cell "ghosts" may be seen on the smear.

Wilson disease may cause episodes of hemolysis along with the neurologic and hepatic disease. This is caused by large amounts of hepatic copper entering the circulation and inducing an oxidative hemolysis. The smear can show spherocytes and *bite cells* (RBCs with defects caused by splenic conditioning). The hemolysis is often transient as it is related to high levels of copper in the serum.

Spur cell anemia is a hemolytic process seen in patients with end-stage liver disease. The lipid metabolism alterations induced by severe liver disease lead to cholesterol crystal formation in the red cell membrane. These crystals are removed by the spleen and can lead to both hemolysis and deformed RBCs *(spur cells)*.

Prevention

There are a few supportive steps in patients with hemolysis. Although most food is supplemented with folate, high red cell turnover can increase the need for this vitamin. Patients with hemolysis are often supplemented with folic acid 1 mg daily.[1]

---

[1] Not FDA approved for this indication.

TABLE 2	Drugs That May Precipitate a Hemolytic Crisis with G6PD Deficiency
Acetanilide[4]	
Dapsone	
Furazolidone[2]	
Isobutyl nitrate[4]	
Methylene blue	
Nalidixic acid[2]	
Naphthalene	
Nitrofurantoin (Macrobid)	
Pamaquine[2]	
Phenazopyridine (Pyridium)	
Phenylhydrazine	
Primaquine	
Quinolones	
Sulfacetamide	
Sulfamethoxazole	
Sulfanilamide	
Sulfapyridine	

A key preventive measure for those with G6PD deficiency is avoiding agents that can lead to oxidative stress of RBCs. The most complete list of medications found at https://www.g6pd.org/ and common medications are listed in Table 2. Some rarer red cell enzymatic or hemoglobin defects are also sensitive to oxidative stress, so these medications also should be avoided in those diseases.

Clinical Manifestations

Inherited

The severity of congenital hemolytic anemia varies tremendously. Some children are very symptomatic right after birth, while older patients may only present with mild anemia and subtle laboratory findings. A common presentation is a burst of hemolysis with oxidative or other stressors. Hereditary hemolytic anemias are often more severe right after birth, and severity may decrease with age. Patients with congenital anemia can have presentation with extrahematologic problems. Given that the serum bilirubin is increased and more bilirubin is excreted in the bile, they may present with pigmented gallstones. Patients can present with gallbladder disease in their teens or 20s, and this should raise suspicion of a hemolytic anemia. These patients may be more prone to skin ulcers around the ankle that may not heal well.

Classically patients with congenital hemolytic anemias can develop three types of crises. The first is the *hemolytic crisis*. When patients develop fevers or encounter other stressors, the rate of hemolysis may increase, and any inflammation can suppress erythropoiesis, leading to severe anemia. The second type of crisis is the *megaloblastic crisis* in which patients become folic acid deficient because of high folate demand associated with increased red cell production. With mass supplementation of folate in the food supply, this incidence has decreased. The final crisis is the *aplastic crisis* in which RBC production is temporarily compromised and the reticulocyte count plummets. This is most commonly found with infections with parvovirus B-19. The infection clears in most patients within 1 week, but patients often require transfusion support during this time.

Hereditary spherocytosis is most prevalent in northern European populations and occurs with a frequency of approximately 1 in 5000. The majority of cases (75%) show an autosomal dominant pattern of inheritance. The remainder result from autosomal recessive inheritance and new mutations. Common clinical features of hereditary spherocytosis include anemia, jaundice, reticulocytosis, splenomegaly, and microspherocytes. Anemia later in life is variable and usually mild. Complications include hemolytic crises, leg ulcers, and gallstones.

With hereditary elliptocytosis, the majority of patients are asymptomatic, and the frequent finding of elliptocytes on the blood smear is of no clinical consequence. However, approximately 10% to 15% of patients have significant hemolysis and may develop anemia. Mild hereditary elliptocytosis is inherited in an autosomal dominant fashion. The incidence is higher in African and Asian populations because of its beneficial impact on malarial infection. Patients with pyropoikilocytosis have severe hemolysis.

G6PD deficiency is the most common enzyme defect in humans and affects an estimated 600 million people worldwide. G6PD deficiency is transmitted as an X-linked recessive condition. There have been hundreds of G6PD variants identified. Enzymatic activity varies from normal with no clinical consequences to severe deficiency resulting in chronic hemolysis and shortened red cell life span, even in the absence of stressors. The two most common variants are the G6PD A- variant that has moderate enzyme deficiency (10% to 15% activity), and the G6PD Mediterranean mutation that has almost no detectable enzyme activity. Despite this, patients with the G6PD Mediterranean mutation have a nearly normal erythrocyte life span except under conditions of metabolic or oxidative stress.

The classic presentation of hemolysis with G6PD deficiency is with oxidative stress. For example, certain medications such as sulfonamides can lead to increased oxidative stress. Patients with G6PD deficiency cannot generate enough reducing power to overcome this stress, which leads to oxidative damage to proteins, especially hemoglobin. The patient presents with fulminant hemolysis that can lead to a severe anemia. As a result of membrane damage, the blood smear can show spherocytes and bite cells. Treatment is removing the offending agent and is otherwise supportive. A unique presentation is *favism*. After eating fava beans, an overwhelming hemolysis develops. This can be idiosyncratic and occur even in patients who have safely eaten the beans in the past.

Pyruvate kinase deficiency is inherited as an autosomal recessive condition. Anemia is variable and may range from a presentation in early infancy requiring transfusions to fully compensated hemolysis presenting with jaundice alone. Many patients have moderate anemia, jaundice, and splenomegaly. Patients with this disorder are also susceptible to the crises identified earlier. Splenectomy may be helpful in severe cases, but response is variable.

Acquired

AIHA patients who have IgG as the offending antibody are said to have *warm antibody AIHA*. The name *warm* comes from the fact that the antibody reacts best at body temperature. The incidence varies by series but is about 1 in 100,000 patients per year, and women are more often affected than men.

Warm AIHA can complicate several diseases. Lupus patients can develop warm AIHA as part of their disease complex. Of the malignancies, the one with the strongest association with AIHA is chronic lymphocytic leukemia (CLL). Series show that 5% to 10% of patients with CLL will have warm AIHA. The disease can appear concurrently with CLL or may develop during the course of the disease.

A rare but important variant of warm AIHA is Evan syndrome. This is the combination of AIHA and immune thrombocytopenia (ITP). One to three percent of AIHA is the Evan variant. The ITP can precede, occur concurrently, or develop after the AIHA. The diagnosis of Evan syndrome should raise concern of underlying disorders. In pediatric and young adult patients, immunodeficiencies such as autoimmune lymphoproliferative disease (ALPS) must be considered. In older patients, Evan syndrome is often associated with T-cell lymphomas.

In rare patients with warm AIHA, IgA or IgM antibodies are implicated. Patients with IgM AIHA often have a severe course with a fatal outcome. Plasma may show spontaneous hemolysis and agglutination. The DAT may not be strongly positive or show C3 reactivity. The clinical clues are C3 reactivity with no cold agglutinins and severe hemolysis, sometimes with intravascular hemolysis.

In cold agglutinin disease, patients often note symptoms related to agglutination of RBCs in the peripheral circulation in addition to hemolysis. For example, acrocyanosis will be noted in cold weather. Rare patients will have abdominal pain when eating cold food resulting from ischemia related to agglutination of RBCs in the viscera. Some patients with cold agglutinins can experience exacerbation of their hemolysis with cold exposure.

In young patients, cold AIHA is often post-infectious (such as from viral and mycoplasma infections), and the course is self-limiting. The hemolysis usually starts 2 to 3 weeks after the illness and will last for 4 to 6 weeks. In older patients, the etiology in over 90% of cases is a B-cell lymphoproliferative disorder, usually with monoclonal kappa B cells. The most commonly seen are marginal zone lymphoma, small lymphocytic lymphoma, and lymphoplasmacytic lymphoma.

A unique cold AIHA is paroxysmal cold hemoglobinuria (PCH). This AIHA is most often postviral and affects children; in the past, it complicated any stage of syphilis. The antibody is IgG directed against the P antigen on the RBC. Binding is best in the "cold," but then complement is activated at body temperature. Because this antibody can fix complement, hemolysis can be rapid and severe, leading to extreme anemia.

Drug-induced AIHA is a rare drug reaction with a lower incidence than drug-related immune thrombocytopenia. The rate of severe drug-related AIHA is estimated at 1 in 1 million individuals, but less severe cases may be missed. Most patients will have positive DAT without signs of hemolysis, though rare patients will have relentless hemolysis resulting in death. With hapten-related AIHA, very few patients will have hemolysis; in these cases, the hemolysis will resolve a few days after discontinuation of the offending drug. With immune complex disease, most often the patient will only have a positive DAT, but rare patients will have life-threatening hemolysis upon exposure or reexposure. The onset of this hemolysis is rapid, with signs of acute illness and intravascular hemolysis. The classic associated drug is quinine, but many other drugs have been implicated.

A virulent form of immune complex hemolysis is associated with both disseminated intravascular coagulation (DIC) and brisk hemolysis. Patients who receive certain second- and third-generation cephalosporins (especially cefotetan and ceftriaxone) have developed this syndrome. The clinical symptoms start 7 to 10 days after receiving the drug. Often the patient has only received the antibiotic for surgical prophylaxis. Warm DAT hemolysis with an acute hematocrit decrease as well as hypotension and DIC develops. Patients are often believed to have sepsis and are then often reexposed to the cephalosporin, resulting in worsening of the clinical status. The outcome is often fatal as a result of massive hemolysis and thrombosis.

Hemolysis caused by methyldopa is indistinguishable from warm AIHA, which is consistent with the notion that methyldopa induces an autoimmune hemolytic anemia. The hemolysis often resolves rapidly after discontinuing the methyldopa, though the Coombs test may remain positive for months. This type of drug-induced hemolytic anemia has been reported with levodopa, procainamide, and chlorpromazine.

In MAHA, the course of the presentation is dictated by the underlying cause. In valvular hemolysis, the onset of hemolysis is soon after the cardiac procedure and may require transfusion support. With VAD hemolysis, most patients have only mild hemolysis, but with pump thrombosis, the hemolysis can be severe. Patients with spur cell anemia have findings of severe liver disease: high INRs and bilirubin (mean of 9.5 mg/dL). Spur cell hemolysis is associated with an ominous prognosis and average survival of a few months.

PNH is characterized by episodes of hemolysis and a propensity for thrombosis and pancytopenia. Often patients can have PNH for years before the diagnosis is made. The hemolysis can range from being well-compensated to transfusion-dependent. Patients with PNH often have a severe thrombophilia; the leading cause of morbidity and mortality (before the release of effective therapy) has been thrombosis. The cause of the hypercoagulable state is unknown, but complement-activated platelets have been implicated.

Diagnosis

There are two steps in the diagnosis of hemolytic anemia. The first step is determining the presence of hemolysis, and the second step is finding the cause. Hemolysis is demonstrated by evidence of both red cell breakdown as well as the compensatory increase in red cell production this stimulates. When RBCs undergo hemolysis, their contents, mostly hemoglobin and also the enzyme LDH, are released. Free hemoglobin is bound by haptoglobin, and the heme moiety is broken down, first to bilirubin and then to urobilinogen, which is excreted in the urine.

The following tests are performed to investigate hemolysis:

LDH: Lactic dehydrogenase is an enzyme found in high concentration in the RBC; hemolysis releases this enzyme into the plasma. Most patients with hemolysis will have an elevated LDH, making this a sensitive test. However, many other processes including liver disease, pneumonia, and so on, will also increase serum LDH.

Serum bilirubin: Heme is broken down to produce bilirubin. Initially unconjugated, the bilirubin is delivered to the liver, where it is conjugated and excreted into the bile. In hemolysis, the unconjugated (indirect bilirubin) is increased as opposed to liver disease, in which the conjugated (direct bilirubin) is increased. If a patient has coexisting liver disease with an elevated direct bilirubin, this test is not reliable.

Serum haptoglobin: Haptoglobin binds free serum hemoglobin and is taken up by the liver. Haptoglobin usually falls to very low levels in hemolysis. It is important to remember that haptoglobin is also an acute-phase reactant that can increase with systemic disease or inflammation. However, patients with advanced liver disease will have low haptoglobin as a result of lack of synthesis, and up to 2% of the population may congenitally lack haptoglobin.

Hemoglobinemia: If the hemolysis is very rapid, the amount of free hemoglobin that is released will overwhelm haptoglobin and lead to the presence of free hemoglobin in the plasma. This can be crudely quantified by examining the plasma. Even minute amounts of free hemoglobin will turn the plasma pink. In fulminant hemolysis, the serum will be cola colored.

Urine hemosiderin: When hemoglobin is excreted by the kidney, the iron is deposited in the tubules. When the tubule cells are sloughed off, they will appear in the urine. The urine can be stained for iron; if positive, this is another sign of hemolysis. This is a later sign as it takes a week for enough iron-laden tubule cells to be excreted in detectable quantities.

Mean corpuscular volume (MCV): The MCV may be larger in hemolysis for several reasons. The size of reticulocytes is larger than normal RBCs, so a brisk reticulocytosis will have a higher MCV. In cold agglutinin disease, the aggregation of RBCs will falsely increase the MCV. Finally, hemolysis can lead to folate deficiency and an increase in MCV.

Reticulocyte count: With hemolysis, the breakdown of RBCs is accompanied by an increase in the reticulocyte count as marrow tries to compensate. The reticulocyte percentage must be adjusted for the hematocrit; a correct value above 1.5% is considered increased. Recently, automated complete blood count machines have taken advantage of the fact that reticulocytes will absorb certain stains, and these machines can directly measure the reticulocyte count via flow cytometry. This results in an "absolute" reticulocyte count. This does not have to be corrected for hematocrit, and levels about 90,000/μL are considered elevated. However, the reticulocyte count can also be increased in blood

TABLE 3	Typical Blood Smear Findings in Hemolysis

Bite Cells

Oxidative hemolytic anemia such as G6PD deficiency

Elliptocytes

Heredity elliptocytosis

Schistocytes

Thrombotic thrombocytopenic purpura, valvular hemolysis

Spherocytes

Hereditary spherocytosis, autoimmune hemolytic anemia, Wilson disease, burns

Spur Cells

Severe liver disease

loss or in patients who have other causes of anemia (such as treated iron deficiency). In addition, as many of 25% of patients with AIHA will never have elevated reticulocyte counts for reasons such as nutritional deficiency, autoimmune destruction of red cell precursors, or lack of erythropoietin.

The blood smear provides vital information (Table 3). The finding of abnormal red cell shapes can be a clue to autoimmune hemolysis or red cell membrane defects. For example, spherocytes are seen in autoimmune hemolytic anemia, heredity spherocytosis, Wilson disease, clostridial sepsis, and severe burns. Schistocytes are a sign of microangiopathic hemolytic anemia and should prompt concerns for such disease processes as thrombotic thrombocytopenia purpura, valvular hemolysis, VAD, march hemoglobinuria, among many others.

In hereditary spherocytosis, the blood smear suggests the diagnosis. Confirmation is by demonstrating an increased osmotic fragility, although direct genetic screening for the molecular defects is becoming more common. The blood smear is also critical for diagnosing hereditary elliptocytosis and hereditary pyropoikilocytosis, although there is an increasing role for genetic diagnosis. Patients with hereditary pyropoikilocytosis are usually homozygous or compound heterozygous for one of the mutations causing mild hereditary elliptocytosis.

Diagnosis of G6PD deficiency is made by measuring enzyme activity. This is best performed after the hemolytic episode is over as reticulocytes have higher G6PD levels and can lead to falsely normal enzyme activity levels.

Increasingly genetic sequencing is being used to screen for inherited disorders, but more experience is required for interpretation of mutations.

AIHAs demonstrate either IgG or complement on the RBC. This is done by the direct antibody or Coombs test. IgG bound to RBCs will not agglutinate them. However, if IgM that is directed against IgG or C3 is added, the RBCs will agglutinate, proving that there is IgG and/or C3 on the red cell membrane. The finding of a positive DAT in the setting of a hemolytic anemia is diagnostic of AIHA.

There are several pitfalls to the DAT. One is that a positive DAT can be found in 1 in 1000 patients in the normal population and up to several percent of ailing patients, especially those with elevated gamma globulin such as patients with liver disease or HIV. Administration of IVIG can also create a false-positive DAT. Conversely, patients can have AIHA with a negative DAT. Some patients have a low amount of IgG binding the RBC that is below the detection limit of the DAT reagents. Other patients can have IgA or "warm" IgM as the cause of the AIHA. Specialty laboratories can test for these possibilities. The diagnosis of DAT-negative AIHA should be made with caution, and other causes of hemolysis like hereditary spherocytosis or PNH should be excluded.

The DAT in patients with cold AIHA will show cells coated with C3. The blood smear will often show agglutination of the blood, and if the blood cools before being analyzed, the agglutination will interfere with the analysis. Titers of cold agglutinin can range from 1 in 1000 to 1 in over 1 million. The autoantibodies are most often directed against the I/i antigen system, with 90% against I. The I specificity is typical with primary cold agglutinin disease and also following *Mycoplasma* infection. The i-specific antigen is most typical of Epstein-Barr and CMV infections.

In PCH, the DAT is often weakly positive but can be negative. The diagnostic test is the Donath-Landsteiner test. This complex test is performed by incubating samples in three temperature ranges: one set at 0° to 4°C, one set at 37°C, and one incubated first at 0° to 4°C and then 37°C. The diagnosis of PCH is made if only the third tube shows hemolysis.

For many patients, the first clue to drug-associated AIHA is the finding of a positive DAT in a patient taking a suspect drug (Table 4). Specialty laboratories such as Wisconsin Blood Center or the Los Angeles Red Cross can perform in-vitro studies of drug interactions that can produce a certain diagnosis.

For PNH, the diagnosis had been based on an in vitro demonstration of increased sensitivity of RBCs to complement lysis. Currently, flow cytometry is performed to examine cells for the absence of GPI-anchored proteins (CD55 or CD59 on RBCs, other GPI-anchored proteins on white blood cells).

In patients with microangiopathy, the smear will show abundant schistocytes with a marked elevated LDH.

Therapy

Splenectomy is curative for most cases of hereditary spherocytosis but is reserved for patients with severe symptoms. For patients with hereditary pyropoikilocytosis, splenectomy can also be useful.

Most patients with G6PD deficiency require no special management beyond the avoidance of provocative medications and food. Highly symptomatic patients with pyruvate kinase deficiency may respond to splenectomy, and in clinical trials, a small molecule agent that can increase enzyme activity.

Initial management of warm AIHA is prednisone starting at 1 mg/kg daily. It can take up to 3 weeks to see a response. Once the hematocrit is above 30%, the prednisone is slowly tapered. Eighty percent of patients will respond to steroids, but the steroids can be fully tapered off in only 30%. For patients who can be maintained on 10 mg or less of steroids daily, this may be the most reasonable long-term therapy.

Current data show that adding rituximab (Rituxan)[1] to steroids for warm AIHA will improve overall response and should be considered early in most patients. These responses appear to be durable, and for relapses, repeating treatment is effective. It is important to remember that, for most patients, the response to rituximab is a gradual one over months; one should not expect a rapid response. Most studies have used the "traditional" 375 mg/m^2 dosing weekly for 4 weeks, and another option is 1000 mg repeated once 14 days apart.

Splenectomy is now reserved for patients with warm AIHA who do not respond to steroids or rituximab. Reported response rates in the literature range from 50% to 80%, with 50% to 60% remaining in remission. Timing of the procedure is a balance between allowing time for the steroids to work versus the risk of toxicity of steroids. A patient who is at low risk associated with surgery and has either refractory disease or an inability to be weaned from high doses of steroids should have splenectomy considered early.

For patients who do not respond to either splenectomy or rituximab, therapy is less certain. Although intravenous immune globulin is a standard therapy for immune thrombocytopenia, response rates are low in warm AIHA. Numerous therapies have

TABLE 4	Drugs Implicated in Autoimmune Hemolytic Anemia

Most Common

Cefotetan (Cefotan)

Ceftriaxone (Rocephin)

Piperacillin (Pipracil)

Fludarabine (Fludara)

Other Implicated Drugs

Acetaminophen

Amphotericin B

Beta-lactams (any)

Carboplatin (Paraplatin)

Cephalosporins (any)

Chlorpromazine (Thorazine)

Chlorpropamide (Diabinese)

Cimetidine (Tagamet)

Ciprofloxacin (Cipro)

Diclofenac (Voltaren)

Doxycycline

Enalapril (Vasotec)

Erythromycin

Isoniazid

Levodopa

Melphalan (Alkeran)

Methyldopa

Nonsteroidal antiinflammatory drugs

Omeprazole (Prilosec)

Oxaliplatin (Eloxatin)

Probenciden

Probenecid

Procainamide

Quinidine

Quinine

Rifampin

Sulfa drugs

Teniposide (Vumon)

Tetracycline

Thiazides

Thiopental (Pentothal)

Tolbutamide (Orinase)

Tricyclic antidepressants

been reported in small series, but there is no clear approach. Options include the following:
- Azathioprine (Imuran)[1] 75 to 150 mg/day
- Cyclophosphamide (Cytoxan)[1] 1000 mg monthly bolus IV
- Mycophenolate (CellCept)[1] 500 to 1000 mg bid
- Cyclosporine (Neoral)[1] 5 mg/kg daily divided in two doses
- Danazol (Danocrine)[1] 200 mg tid

---

[1] Not FDA approved for this indication.

---

[1] Not FDA approved for this indication.

Our approach has been to use mycophenolate for patients who require high doses of steroids or need transfusions. Patients who need lower doses of steroids may be good candidates for danazol to help wean them from the steroids.

The sparse literature on Evans syndrome suggests that it can be more refractory to standard therapy, with response rates to splenectomy being in the 50% range. In patients with lymphoma, antineoplastic therapy is crucial. Data is accumulating for patients with ALPS: mycophenolate or sirolimus (Rapamune)[1] starting at 2 mg/m^2, may be effective for splenectomy or rituximab failures.

The importance of diagnosing cold AIHA and differentiating it from warm AIHA is the fact that standard therapy for warm disease steroids is ineffective. C3-coated RBCs are taken up through the reticulo-endothelial system, especially in the liver as well as the spleen, so splenectomy is also an ineffective therapy.

Simple measures to help with cold AIHA should be employed. Patients should be kept in a warm environment and should try to avoid the cold. If transfusions are needed, they should be infused via blood warmers to prevent hemolysis. In rare patients with severe hemolysis, plasma exchange can be considered. Given the culprit antibody is IgM (mostly intravascular), use of plasma exchange can slow the hemolysis to give time for other therapies to take effect.

Therapy of cold AIHA remains difficult. Currently the drug of choice is rituximab.[1] Response can be seen in 45% to 75% of patients but is almost always a partial response; retreatment is often necessary. As with other autoimmune hematologic diseases, there can be a delay in response. There is data to support adding either fludarabine (Fludara)[1] or bendamustine (Treanda)[1] 90 mg/m^2 to rituximab. The response rates are higher, but so are the complications of therapy. Although more toxic, this combination can be considered in patients with aggressive disease. For acute treatment, the monoclonal antibody sutimlimab (Enjaymo) is available.

For most patients with drug-induced AIHA, discontinuing the offending drug is sufficient. It is doubtful that steroids or other autoimmune-directed therapy is effective. For patients with the DIC-hemolysis syndrome, there are anecdotes that plasma exchange may be helpful. Therapy for patients with positive DAT without signs of hemolysis is uncertain. If the drug is essential, then the patient can be observed. If the patient has hemolysis, the drug must be stopped and the patient observed for signs of end-organ damage.

Transfusions can be very difficult in AIHA. The presence of the autoantibody can interfere with typing of the blood and almost always interferes with the cross-match because this final step consists of mixing the patient's serum with donor RBCs. In most patients with AIHA, the autoantibodies will react with any donor cells, rendering a negative cross-match impossible. Without the cross-match, the concern is that underlying alloantibodies can be missed, which can lead to transfusion reactions.

Some of these concerns may be allayed by remembering that patients who have never been transfused or pregnant will rarely have alloantibodies. Secondly, a patient who has been transfused in the remote past may have an amnestic antibody response but not an immediate hemolytic reaction.

When a patient is first suspected of having AIHA, a generous sample of blood should be given to the transfusion service. This will allow for adequate testing of the sample. Secondly, many centers will test the blood not only for blood groups ABO and D but will also perform full Rh typing and check for Kidd, Duffy, and Kell status. This can allow transfusion of phenotypically matched blood to lessen the risk of alloantibody formation.

One difficult issue is timing of transfusion. Clinicians are often hesitant to transfuse patients with AIHA because of fear of reactions. But in frail patients with severe anemia, especially older adults or those with heart disease, transfusion can be lifesaving. In some cases it can take hours to screen for alloantibodies; therefore it is often preferable to transfuse patients with severe anemia while carefully observing for reactions.

The treatment for PNH is complement inhibition, thereby preventing assembly of the terminal complement complex during complement activation. Eculizumab (Soliris), which blocks C5, has been shown to reduce hemolysis and improve anemia, fatigue, and quality of life in patients with PNH. In addition, eculizumab has demonstrated efficacy in reducing thrombosis. Patients who experience breakthrough hemolysis despite treatment with eculizumab may benefit from agents that block the complement cascade more upstream, such as pegcetacoplan (Empaveli).

Management of Complications

The most concerning complication of splenectomy is overwhelming postsplenectomy infection (OPSI). In adults, the spleen appears to play a minimal role in immunity, except for defense from certain encapsulated organisms. Patients will often present with DIC and will rapidly progress to purpura fulminans. Approximately 40% to 50% of patients will die from sepsis, even when detected early. The overall lifetime risk may be as high as 1 in 500. The organism most commonly found in these cases is *Streptococcus pneumoniae*, which is reported in over 50% of cases. *Neisseria meningitidis* and *Haemophilus influenzae* have also been implicated in many cases.

Patients who have undergone splenectomy must be warned about the risk of OPSI and instructed to report to the emergency department immediately if they develop a fever greater than 101°F or shaking chills. Once in the emergency department, blood cultures should be rapidly obtained and the patient started on antibiotic coverage with agents that cover encapsulated organisms. Patients who are planning to have or are being considered for a splenectomy should be vaccinated for pneumococcal, meningococcal, and *H. influenzae* infections. If patients are planning to be treated with rituximab first, they should also be vaccinated because they will not be able to mount an immune response after receiving rituximab.

The major side effects of rituximab are infusion reactions, and they are often worse with the first dose. These can be controlled with antihistamines, steroids, and, for severe rigors, meperidine (Demerol).[1] Rare patients can develop neutropenia (about 1 in 500) that appears to be autoimmune in nature. Infections appear to be only minimally increased with the use of rituximab. One group at higher risk are patients who are chronic carriers of hepatitis B. These patients may have reactivation of the virus that can be fatal in some cases; patients being considered for rituximab must be screened for hepatitis B. Progressive multifocal leukoencephalopathy is a very rare risk that is more common in cancer patients and heavily immunosuppressed patients. The overall risk is unknown but is less than 1 in 50,000.

Eculizumab is well tolerated except for a risk of meningococcal infection, which is estimated at 1 in 500. All patients receiving this agent should be vaccinated and must report to the emergency department with any sign of infection.

[1] Not FDA approved for this indication.

References

Barcellini W, Bruno Fattizzo B: How I treat warm autoimmune hemolytic anemia, *Blood* 137(10):1283–1294, 2021.

Berentsen S: How I treat cold agglutinin disease, *Blood* 137(10):1295–1303, 2021.

Cappellini MD, Fiorelli G: Glucose-6-phosphate dehydrogenase deficiency, *Lancet* 371(9606):64–74, 2008.

Gavriilaki E, Peffault de Latour R, Risitano MA: Advancing therapeutic complement inhibition in hematologic diseases, *PNH and beyond* 139(25):3571–3582, 2022.

Haley K: Congenital Hemolytic Anemia, *Med Clin North Am* 101(2):361–374, 2017.

Hill A, DeZern AE, Kinoshita T, Brodsky RA: Paroxysmal nocturnal haemoglobinuria, *Nat Rev Dis Primers* 3:17028, 2017.

Liebman HA, Weitz IC: Autoimmune Hemolytic Anemia, *Med Clin North Am* 101(2):351–359, 2017.

[1] Not FDA approved for this indication.

HEMOPHILIA AND RELATED CONDITIONS

Method of
Bulent Ozgonenel, MD; Roshni Kulkarni, MD; and Meera Chitlur, MD

CURRENT DIAGNOSIS

- The hemophilias and von Willebrand disease (VWD) account for 80% to 85% of inherited bleeding disorders. Hemophilia A and B are X-linked, whereas VWD and rare bleeding disorders (RBDs) are autosomal disorders.
- The diagnosis of hemophilia and other inherited bleeding disorders should be confirmed by specific laboratory assays because screening tests such as prothrombin time and activated partial thromboplastin time may be normal. Plasma levels of deficient factor determine clinical severity and management.
- Major complications associated with hemophilia are inhibitor development, hemarthrosis, and intracranial hemorrhage. Hemarthrosis is the most common and debilitating complication, and central nervous system bleeding is the most common cause of mortality in hemophilia. Mucosal bleeding and menorrhagia are the most common manifestations of VWD. Bleeding manifestations of RBDs are mild, although homozygotes can present with severe disease.
- Newborns have normal levels of factor VIII; therefore the diagnosis of hemophilia A can be established at birth. Vacuum-assisted delivery should be avoided to prevent head bleeds.
- Females with menorrhagia and no underlying pathology should be investigated for a bleeding disorder.

CURRENT THERAPY

- Currently there is a paradigm shift in the treatment of hemophilia. In addition to the traditional plasma-derived and recombinant concentrates, the new extended half-life recombinant products have reduced the treatment burden by reducing the frequency of intravenous injections. Novel, subcutaneously administered, nonfactor replacement therapy with prolonged hemostatic efficiency has been a game changer for patients both with and without inhibitors. Gene therapy is on the horizon, offering a promise of cure. Even for VWD and RBDs such as deficiencies of factors VII, XI, XIII, X, and fibrinogen, replacement factor concentrates are currently available. Early and effective treatment and prophylaxis can prevent bleeding episodes, including repeated hemarthrosis and joint destruction in persons with hemophilia. Patients should be tested annually for the presence of inhibitors. Cryoprecipitate is not recommended for the treatment of hemophilia because of concerns regarding transmission of bloodborne pathogens.
  - For mild and moderate hemophilia A and VWD, the use of desmopressin (DDAVP) coupled with antifibrinolytics can obviate the use of concentrates. Continued vigilance should be implemented for inhibitory antibodies and new and emerging bloodborne pathogens.
  - All patients with inherited bleeding disorders should be immunized against hepatitis A and B and followed in close collaboration with their local hemophilia treatment center (https://www.cdc.gov/hemophilia/treatment/treatment-centers.html). The National Bleeding Disorders Foundation's (https://www.hemophilia.org) Medical and Scientific Advisory Committee guidelines for updated recommendations and product choice should be followed.

Hemophilia A and Hemophilia B

Hemophilia is an X-linked congenital bleeding disorder caused by a deficiency of factor VIII (hemophilia A) or factor IX (hemophilia B). Hemophilia A is the most common severe bleeding disorder and affects 1 in 5000 males in the United States; hemophilia B occurs in 1 in 30,000 males.

Pathophysiology

The *factor VIII* gene is one of the largest genes and spans 186 kb of genomic DNA at Xq28. Intron 22 of the *factor VIII* gene is particularly large and is therefore susceptible to inversion mutations. Inversions of this intron account for 50% of all severe hemophilia A cases, and inversions of other introns, deletions, point mutations, and insertions account for the remainder.

Hepatic and reticuloendothelial cells are presumed sites of factor VIII synthesis. Factor VIII is synthesized as a single-chain polypeptide with three A domains (A1, A2, and A3), a large central B domain, and two C domains (Figure 1). The binding sites for von Willebrand factor (VWF), thrombin, and factor Xa are on the C2 domain, and factor IXa binding sites are on the A2 and A3 domains. The B domain can be deleted without any consequences. VWF protects factor VIII from proteolytic degradation in the plasma and concentrates it at the site of injury.

The *factor IX* gene is 34 kb long and located at Xq26. It is a vitamin K–dependent serine protease composed of 415 amino acids. It is synthesized in the liver, and its plasma concentration is approximately 50 times that of factor VIII. Gene deletions and point mutations result in hemophilia B.

Role of Factors VIII and IX in Coagulation

Factor VIII circulates bound to VWF. It is a cofactor for factor IX and is essential for factor X activation. In the classic coagulation cascade, activation of the intrinsic or extrinsic pathway of coagulation results in sufficient thrombin generation. The fact that bleeding still occurs in hemophilia despite an intact extrinsic pathway has led to the revised cell-based model of coagulation.

The revised pathway incorporates all coagulation factors into a single pathway initiated by factor VII and tissue factor. The contact factors (XI, XII, kallikrein, and high-molecular-weight [HMW] kininogen) are not essential but serve as a backup. After injury, encrypted tissue factor is exposed and forms a complex with factor VIIa. The tissue factor–factor VIIa complex activates factor IX to IXa (which moves to the platelet surface) and factor X to Xa. This generates small amounts of thrombin that activates platelets, converts platelet factor V to Va and factor XI to XIa, and releases factor VIII from VWF and activates it. The factor XIa activates plasma factor IX to IXa on the platelet surface, which together with factor VIIIa forms the tenase complex (factor VIIIa/IXa) that converts large amounts of factor X to Xa. Factor Xa forms a prothrombinase complex with factor Va and converts large amounts of prothrombin to thrombin, called *thrombin burst*. This results in the conversion of sufficient fibrinogen to fibrin to form a stable clot. In hemophilia, lack of factor VIII or IX produces a profound abnormality. Factor Xa generated by factor VIIa and tissue factor is insufficient because this pathway is inhibited by tissue factor pathway inhibitor (TFPI) as part of a negative feedback, and factors VIII and IX, which are required for amplifying the production of Xa, are absent. The primary platelet plug formation and initiation phases of coagulation are normal. Any clot that is formed (from the initiation phase) is friable and porous.

Clinical Features

The diagnosis of hemophilia is often made after a bleeding episode or because of a family history; however, 50% of cases have no family history. Based on the plasma levels of factor VIII or IX (normal levels are 50%–150%) that correlate with severity and predict bleeding risk, hemophilia is classified as mild (>5%–40%), moderately severe (1%–5%), and severe (<1%) (Table 1). Approximately 65% of persons with hemophilia have severe

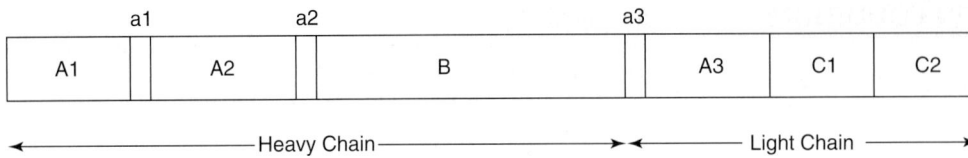

| A1 | | A2 | | B | | A3 | C1 | C2 |

a1 · a2 · a3

←————————————— Heavy Chain —————————————→ ←————— Light Chain —————→

Figure 1 Factor VIII protein structure.

TABLE 1	Hemophilia Severity and Clinical Manifestations		
CHARACTERISTICS	**SEVERE (50%–70%)**	**MODERATE (10%)**	**MILD (30%–40%)**
Factor VIII or IX activity (normal 50%–150%)	<1%	1%–5%	>5%–40%
Age of diagnosis	Birth to 2 years	Childhood or adolescence	Adolescence or adulthood
Bleeding patterns	2–4 per month	4–6 per year	Rare
Clinical manifestations	Hemarthroses, muscle, central nervous system, gastrointestinal bleeding, hematuria	Bleeding into joints or muscle after minor trauma, surgical procedure, dental bleeding Rarely spontaneous	Surgical procedures (including dental) and major trauma

disease, 15% have moderate disease, and 20% have mild disease. Most cases of severe disease manifest by 4 years of age; moderate or mild disease is diagnosed later and often after bleeding secondary to trauma or surgery.

Hemophilia can be diagnosed in the first trimester, using chorionic villus sampling and gene analysis. In the second trimester, fetal blood sampling can be performed. Prenatal diagnosis to determine fetal gender can aid in the management of pregnancy and delivery.

The hallmark of severe hemophilia is hemarthrosis, or bleeding into the joint, that can occur spontaneously or with minimal trauma. The immediate effects of a joint bleed are excruciating pain, swelling, warmth, and muscle spasms, and the long-term effect of recurrent hemarthrosis is hemophilic arthropathy, which is characterized by synovial thickening and chronic inflammation. Repeated hemorrhage results in a target joint. Knees, elbows, ankles, hips, and shoulders are commonly affected. Disuse atrophy of surrounding muscles leads to further joint instability. Limitation of joint range of motion resulting from hemarthrosis often correlates positively with older age, non-White race, and increased body mass index, and it adversely affects quality of life.

Muscle hematomas, another characteristic site of bleeding, can lead to compartment syndrome, with eventual fibrosis and peripheral nerve damage. Iliopsoas bleeds manifest with pain and flexion deformity. Gastrointestinal bleeding and hematuria occur less often.

Central nervous system (CNS) hemorrhage is a rare but serious complication with a 10% recurrence rate, and it is the leading cause of mortality in patients with hemophilia. Although most newborns with severe hemophilia experience an uneventful course after vaginal delivery, vacuum extraction is associated with an increased CNS bleeding risk. The incidence of intracranial hemorrhage in newborns with hemophilia is 1% to 4%.

Diagnosis

Hemophilia A and B are clinically indistinguishable, and specific factor assays are the only way to differentiate and confirm the diagnosis. Both should be differentiated from VWD. The prothrombin time (PT), platelet function analysis (PFA)-100, and fibrinogen activity are normal. (PFA replaces bleeding time because the bleeding time has low sensitivity and specificity and is operator dependent.) The activated partial thromboplastin time (aPTT) is prolonged when the factor levels are <30%. Table 2

shows the characteristics and differences between the hemophilias and VWD.

Female carriers may be asymptomatic except for those with extreme lyonization resulting in low factor VIII or IX levels. Carrier females, whose factor VIII or IX levels are <40%, are therefore also considered to have hemophilia, with the same criteria for severity as males. In fact, the most current terminology reserves the term *carrier* only for females whose factor levels are ≥40%. Carriers are further classified as symptomatic (i.e., with bleeding manifestations) or asymptomatic. It is important to note that carriers may experience bleeding episodes (such as heavy menstrual bleeding, postpartum hemorrhage, or joint bleeding), even with levels of factors VIII or IX in the 40% to 60% range. Often with the onset of menarche, asymptomatic girls may become symptomatic as a result of heavy menstrual bleeding. Factor VIII levels increase throughout pregnancy and drop to prepregnancy levels after delivery, but factor IX levels remain constant throughout pregnancy.

Treatment

There are four types of treatment for hemophilia:
1. Factor therapies
   A. Based on half-life: standard half-life factor products, extended half-life (EHL) factor products, and novel EHL factor products
   B. Based on type of product: plasma derived versus recombinant
2. Nonfactor therapies
   A. Mimetics
   B. Rebalancing agents
3. Gene therapies
4. Adjunctive therapies

Factor Therapies for the Treatment of Hemophilia

The factor treatment for hemophilia consists of replacement therapy with intravenous factor VIII or factor IX concentrates produced by purification of donor plasma (plasma derived) (e.g., factor VIII [human]: Hemofil M, Koate; factor IX [human]: AlphaNine SD, Mononine) or in cell culture bioreactors (recombinant) (e.g., factor VIII [recombinant]: Advate, Afstyla, Kogenate FS, Nuwiq, Xyntha; factor IX [recombinant]: BeneFIX, Ixinity, Rixubis). Careful screening of donors combined with heat treatment and viral inactivation methods have made plasma-derived products safer. Plasma-derived and recombinant products appear to have equivalent clinical

TABLE 2	Hemophilias and von Willebrand Disease: Key Characteristics and Differences		
CHARACTERISTIC	HEMOPHILIA A	HEMOPHILIA B	VON WILLEBRAND DISEASE
Incidence	1:5000	1:30,000	1%–3% of US population
Abnormality	Factor VIII deficiency	Factor IX deficiency	VWF (qualitative and quantitative defect)
Inheritance	X-linked, affects males Gene at the tip of X chromosome	X-linked, affects males Gene at the tip of X chromosome	Autosomal dominant (gene: chromosome 12) Some are recessive or compound heterozygotes
Production site	Unknown, liver endothelium	Liver (vitamin K dependent)	Megakaryocytes and endothelial cells
Function	Cofactor; forms tenase complex with factor IX and activates factor X, leading to a thrombin burst that results in conversion of large amounts of fibrinogen to fibrin	Serine protease (inactive form: zymogen) activated by factor XI or VIIa; forms a tenase complex with factor VIII and activates factor X	Platelet adhesion to site of injury or damaged endothelium Protects factor VIII from proteolysis
Classification (normal levels 50%–150%)	Mild (>5%) Moderate (1%–5%) Severe (<1%)	Mild (>5%) Moderate (1%–5%) Severe (<1%)	Type 1 Type 2 (2A, 2B, 2M, 2N) Type 3
Clinical presentation	Positive family history (30% new mutation) Hemarthroses, hematomas, hematuria, intracranial hemorrhage, gastrointestinal hemorrhage, and so on	Positive family history (30% new mutation) Milder disease, although identical hemorrhage sites as hemophilia A	Positive family history Mucocutaneous bleeding (epistaxis, menorrhagia, postdental bleeding, gastrointestinal bleeding in adults) Type 3 can manifest as hemophilia A
PFA, bleeding time	Normal	Normal	May be prolonged
PT	Normal	Normal	Normal
aPTT	Prolonged	Prolonged	Prolonged or normal
Factor VIII assay	Decreased or absent	Normal	Decreased or normal (absent type 3)
Factor IX assay	Normal	Decreased or absent	Normal
VWF:Ag	Normal	Normal	Decreased or absent (type 3)
VWF:RCo	Normal	Normal	Decreased or abnormal
VWF multimers	Normal	Normal	Abnormal in types 1, 2A, 2B; absent in type 3
Specific treatment	Recombinant factor VIII (preferred) Pathogen-safe plasma-derived concentrates DDAVP for mild cases	Recombinant factor IX Pathogen-safe plasma-derived concentrates DDAVP ineffective	DDAVP (intranasal or intravenous) (FDA approved for type 1) VWF concentrates (pathogen-safe plasma derived or recombinant VWF)
Inhibitor patients	Immune tolerance, recombinant factor VIIa, APCC	Immune tolerance, recombinant factor VIIa	Inhibitors are rare
Adjunct therapy	Antifibrinolytics	Antifibrinolytics	Hormonal therapy (oral contraceptives), antifibrinolytics

APCC, Activated prothrombin complex concentrates; *aPTT,* activated partial thromboplastin time; *DDAVP,* desmopressin; *FDA,* US Food and Drug Administration; *PFA,* platelet function analyzer; *PT,* prothrombin time; *RCo,* ristocetin cofactor; *VWF,* von Willebrand factor; *VWF:Ag,* von Willebrand factor antigen.

efficacy. Cryoprecipitate is no longer recommended because of concerns regarding pathogen safety.

Treatment administered only during bleeding symptoms is known as *episodic therapy,* and periodic administration of factor concentrates to prevent bleeding is known as *prophylactic therapy.* Response to treatment is more effective when it is administered early. Although prophylaxis prevents the development of joint disease, the high cost of factor replacement coupled with the need for venous access makes it expensive, difficult, and out of reach for patients in the developing world.

The goal of treatment is to raise factor levels to approximately 30% or more for minor bleeds (hematomas or joint bleeds) and 100% for major bleeds (CNS or surgery). Administering 1 U/kg of factor concentrate raises plasma factor VIII levels by 2% and

factor IX levels by approximately 1%. The half-life of factor VIII is 8 to 12 hours and that of factor IX is up to 24 hours with standard half-life factor products.

Factor concentrates can also be given by continuous infusion (3–4 U/kg/h). The bolus dose varies from 25 to 50 U/kg depending on the severity, site, and type of bleeding and is dosed to the available vial size because of the cost of the products. Table 3 lists the dosing schedule for various types of bleeds.

For prophylaxis, factor VIII 25 to 40 U/kg administered every other day or factor IX 100 U/kg once weekly for BeneFIX and 40 U/kg once weekly for Rebinyn (because of the longer half-life of factor IX) is aimed at preventing joint disease. Prophylaxis may begin at 1 to 2 years of age and is continued lifelong. Self-infusion before any planned strenuous activity is recommended.

TABLE 3	Treatment of Bleeding Episodes and Desired Plasma Levels in Hemophilias A and B		
TYPE OF BLEEDING	**FACTOR DOSE***	**DURATION OF TREATMENT**	**COMMENTS**
Persistent or profuse epistaxis Oral mucosal bleeding (including tongue and mouth lacerations) Dental procedures Acute hemarthrosis Intramuscular hematomas Physical therapy	Single dose	1–2 days	Local pressure, antifibrinolytics, fibrin glue for local control, WoundSeal Powder for epistaxis Sedation in small children with tongue laceration
Dental procedures	Single dose	1 hour before procedure	Antifibrinolytics for 7–10 days
Acute hemarthrosis, intramuscular hematomas	Single dose	1–3 days	Use lower doses if treated early Non–weight bearing on affected joint
Physical therapy	Single dose	Treat before PT	Consider synovectomy (surgical, radioisotope or chemical) for target joints
Gastrointestinal bleeding	Single dose	2–3 days	May use oral antifibrinolytics
Persistent painless gross hematuria	Single dose	1–2 days	Increase PO or IV fluids with low-dose antifibrinolytics; risk of clotting in the urinary tract with factor replacement
Life-threatening bleeding such as intracranial hemorrhage, major surgery, and trauma	Double dose	10–14 days	Bolus dose followed by continuous infusion (3–4 U/kg/h); may switch to bolus before discharge

Single dose refers to a factor dose that aims to achieve 40%–50% factor level and is ~20–25 U/kg for factor VIII products and ~50 U/kg for factor IX products. *Double dose* refers to a factor dose that aims to achieve 80%–100% factor level and is ~40–50 U/kg for factor VIII products and ~80–100 U/kg for factor IX products. Factor doses are dosed closest to the vial.

PT, Physical therapy.

Because of the complications of central venous catheters (infections, thrombosis, and mechanical), use of a peripheral vein is encouraged.

EHL factor products have increased the half-lives by 1.5-fold in the case of factor VIII products and 2.4- to 4.8-fold in the case of factor IX products. EHL factor products have been developed with an aim to decrease the frequency of infusions and improve quality of life for patients with hemophilia, achieved through PEGylation or fusion of the factor protein to the Fc fragment of an immunoglobulin (Ig) or albumin. The first of these EHL products was approved by the US Food and Drug Administration (FDA) in 2014: factor IX (recombinant), Fc fusion protein (Alprolix) for use in patients with hemophilia B, and factor VIII (recombinant), Fc fusion protein (Eloctate) for use in patients with hemophilia A. Subsequently, PEGylated recombinant factor VIII (Adynovate, Takeda Pharmaceuticals, Palo Alto, CA) was approved in 2015; PEGylated recombinant factor IX (Rebinyn, Novo Nordisk, Plainsboro, NJ) was approved in 2017, but not for prophylaxis; and recombinant albumin fusion factor IX (Idelvion, CSL Behring) was approved in 2016 for use in patients with hemophilia B. Recently, further extension of the half-life of factor VIII was achieved by a novel fusion protein called *BIVV001*, now FDA approved and called Altuviiio, consisting of a single recombinant factor VIII protein fused to a dimeric FC, a D'D3 domain of VWF (factor VIII binding domain), and two XTEN polypeptides. The mean half-life of Altuviiio was three to four times that of recombinant factor VIII (37.6–42.5 hours vs. 9.1–13.2 hours, respectively), thereby allowing weekly dosing.

Nonfactor Therapies for the Treatment of Hemophilia

Mimetics. A novel treatment for hemophilia A with inhibitors is emicizumab (Hemlibra), a chimeric humanized antibody that triggers and propagates thrombin generation by binding to both factor IX and factor X. By binding to these coagulation factors, the antibody mimics the function of factor VIII. The medication is given subcutaneously, making it a preferred drug in young children. Emicizumab (Hemlibra) showed remarkable success in preventing bleeding complications in patients with severe hemophilia A with inhibitors. The FDA initially approved emicizumab in 2017 for routine prophylaxis to prevent or reduce the frequency of bleeding episodes in patients with hemophilia A with inhibitors, but they extended the approval to hemophilia A without inhibitors in 2018 after studies in noninhibitor patients. Emicizumab can be administered subcutaneously once a week, every 2 weeks, or every 4 weeks, and all regimens have been found to be equally effective. In general, emicizumab has been well accepted by hemophilia patients, especially children and those with difficult venous access as its treatment regimen does not require intravenous dosing, and the dose frequency is much easier to manage than prophylaxis with conventional factor VIII products. Emicizumab treatment is safe by itself, but thrombotic microangiopathy and thrombotic complications have been observed in hemophilia A with inhibitor individuals receiving concomitant high doses of activated prothrombin complex concentrates (APCC) for management of breakthrough bleeds while on emicizumab (>100 U/kg of FEIBA [Antiinhibitor Coagulant Complex] for ≥24 hours). Hence it is recommended that recombinant factor VIIa (NovoSeven RT) be used as the first line of treatment for management of breakthrough bleeds in inhibitor patients on emicizumab (Medical and Scientific Advisory Committee document #255).

Rebalancing Agents. Rebalancing agents that inhibit endogenous anticoagulants and restore coagulation are in clinical trials and include small interfering RNA (siRNA) targeting antithrombin (Fitusiran [Qfitlia], Sanofi), anti-TFPI antibody (Concizumab [Alhemo], Novo Nordisk; Marstacimab [Hympavzi], Pfizer), and products targeting the anticoagulant effect of activated prothrombin complex (APC). The advantages are that these rebalancing agents can be given to either hemophilia A or B patients, provide the benefits of prophylaxis, and can be given subcutaneously, thereby eliminating the need for intravenous injection. These agents have been approved by the FDA and are being used in the treatment of both hemophilia A and hemophilia B.

Gene Therapy

Gene therapy offers promise of a cure, and trials of gene therapy for both hemophilia A and B are currently in process. This has been a significant breakthrough in the treatment of hemophilia. In December 2011, Nathwani and colleagues reported that a single injection of factor IX–expressing adeno-associated virus (AAV) vector was effective in treating patients with hemophilia B for

TABLE 4	Treatment Options in Hemophilia*

Factor VIII and factor IX replacement	Standard half-life (SHL) products
	• Plasma-derived
	• Factor VIII: e.g., Alphanate
	• Factor IX: e.g., AlphaNine SD, Bebulin†
	Recombinant (many products)
	• Factor VIII: (First, second, third and fourth generation): e.g., Advate
	• Factor IX: e.g., Benefix
	Extended half-life (EHL) products
	First-generation:
	• EHL factor VIII products:
	  • Recombinant, Fc Fusion: Eloctate/Elocta†
	  • Recombinant, Pegylated: Adynovate/Adynovi†, Jivi, Esperoct
	• EHL factor IX products:
	  • Recombinant, Fc Fusion: Alprolix
	  • Recombinant, Albumin Fusion: Idelvion
	  • Recombinant, Glycopegylated: Rebinyn/Refixia†
	Second-generation
	• Efanesoctocog alfa (Altuviiio): Factor VIII-VWF-XTEN fusion protein (Hemophilia A only)

Nonfactor therapy	Bispecific antibody (Hemophilia A only) • Emicizumab (Hemlibra) Rebalancing agents *Antithrombin RNA interference molecule* • *Fitusiran (Qfitlia)* *Anti–tissue factor pathway inhibitor (A-TFPI)* • *Concizumab (Alhemo)* • *Marstacimab (Hympavzi)* *Anti–protein C* • *SerpinPC[5]*
Adjunctive therapy	Antifibrinolytics • ε-aminocaproic acid (Amicar) • Tranexamic acid (Cyklokapron or Lysteda)[1] • Desmopressin acetate (DDAVP) (Stimate) (Hemophilia A only)
Therapy in patients with inhibitors	Recombinant factor VIIa • NovoSeven and SEVENFACT • Activated prothrombin complex concentrates (e.g., FEIBA) • Recombinant, porcine factor VIII • Obizur (hemophilia A only) • Nonreplacement therapy products
Gene therapy[5]	Hemophilia A • Valoctocogene roxaparvovec (Roctavian) • *Dirloctocogene samoparvovec (SPK-8011)[5]* • *BAY 2599023[5]* • *Giroctocogene fitelparvovec (PF-070554480/SB-525)[5]* Hemophilia B • *AMT-060[5]* • Etranacogene dezaparvovec (Hemgenix) • Fidanacogene elaparvovec (Beqvez) • *Verbrinacogene setparvovec (FLT180a)[5]*

*All non–FDA-approved products are italicized.
†Brand name available in Europe.
[1]Not FDA approved for this indication.
[5]Investigational drug in the United States.

>1 year. Since this breakthrough, more successful gene therapy trials have been currently underway for the treatment of both hemophilia A and B. The trials have incorporated modifications of promoters, transgenes and AAV serotypes, and lentiviral vectors. Results from the initial factor IX gene therapy trials have demonstrated continued factor IX expression at levels shown to decrease bleeding episodes for up to 9 years. In fact, gene therapy has been approved by the FDA for hemophilia B (etranacogene dezaparvovec-drlb [Hemgenix] and fidanacogene elaparvovec-dzkt [Beqvez]). Gene therapy trials in hemophilia A, although

still showing benefits in some patients, have shown lower levels of factor VIII expression in the long term compared with hemophilia B. A major limitation to this therapeutic option has been hepatotoxicity typically occurring 1 to 4 months postdelivery of the vector, resulting in transaminitis followed sometimes by loss of gene expression. The long-term outcomes and safety remain to be determined. Table 4 lists novel and current treatments for hemophilia.

Adjunctive Therapies
Adjunctive therapies are discussed later in this chapter in the section "General Hemostatic Agents."

Complications of Treatment
One of the most serious complications of hemophilia treatment is the development of inhibitors or neutralizing antibodies (IgG) that inhibit the function of substituted factor VIII and factor IX. Five percent to 10% of all patients with hemophilia and up to 30% of patients with severe hemophilia A develop inhibitors. The incidence of inhibitors in hemophilia B is lower (1%–3%). Most factor VIII inhibitors arise after a median exposure of 9 to 12 days in patients with severe hemophilia A. They can be transient or permanent and should be suspected if a patient fails to respond to an appropriate dose of clotting factor concentrate. Inhibitors can exacerbate bleeding episodes and hemophilic arthropathy.

Inhibitor levels, measured using Bethesda units (BUs), are classified as high titer (>5 BU) or low titer (<5 BU). In patients with low-titer inhibitors, higher-than-normal doses of factor VIII or IX may be used to treat bleeding. For those with high-titer inhibitors, agents that bypass factor VIII or factor IX are used. These include recombinant activated factor VII and, in the case of hemophilia A, APCCs or recombinant porcine factor VIII (currently in precensure clinical trials). Immune tolerance induction, a long-term approach designed to eradicate inhibitors, is effective in 70% to 85% of patients with severe hemophilia A; the most important predictor of success of immune tolerance induction is an inhibitor titer of <10 BU at the start of immune tolerance induction.

Although inhibitors are rare in hemophilia B, they can result in anaphylaxis with exposure to factor IX–containing products. Immune tolerance regimens are associated with nephrotic syndrome and are successful in eradicating the inhibitor only in 40% of cases.

Another important complication of treatment is the transmission of bloodborne pathogens such as hepatitis B and C viruses and human immunodeficiency virus (HIV). In the 1970s, lyophilized plasma factor concentrates of low purity resulted in the transmission of HIV, causing the deaths of many people with hemophilia. Currently, donor screening for pathogens coupled with viral attenuation by heat or solvent detergent technology make these products pathogen safe. However, nonenveloped viruses (parvovirus and hepatitis A) and prions can resist inactivation and can be potentially transmitted.

Patients with bleeding disorders should be encouraged to attend the comprehensive hemophilia treatment centers (HTCs), where they are seen by a multidisciplinary team of hematologists, nurses, social workers, geneticists, physical therapists, dental hygienists, nutritionists, and so on, who educate patients and address issues such as self-care, transitions, and quality of life. Patients are trained to self-infuse and calculate dosage, maintain treatment logs, and call for serious bleeding episodes. The mortality rate among patients who receive care at HTCs is lower than among those who do not: 28.1% versus 38.3%, respectively. At the HTCs, hemovigilance for bloodborne and emerging pathogens was maintained through participation in the Centers for Disease Control and Prevention (CDC) Universal Data Collection (UDC) project. The grant cycle of the UDC was completed in 2012, and a new surveillance instrument is currently in use (Community Counts) that incorporates collecting information on comorbidities and complications of bleeding disorders in this population. Routine vaccination against hepatitis A and B is recommended.

von Willebrand Disease

VWD is an inherited (autosomal dominant) bleeding disorder caused by deficiency or dysfunction of VWF, a plasma protein that mediates platelet adhesion at the site of vascular injury and prevents degradation of factor VIII. A defect in VWF results in bleeding by impairing platelet adhesion or by decreasing factor VIII.

VWF is synthesized in endothelial cells and undergoes dimerization and multimerization, forming low, intermediate, and HMW multimers. The HMW multimers are most effective in promoting platelet aggregation and adhesion. Circulating HMW multimers are cleaved by the protease ADAMTS13, which is deficient in patients with thrombotic thrombocytopenic purpura.

VWD is the most common bleeding disorder, affecting ≥1% of the population. It occurs worldwide and affects all races. VWD is classified into three major categories: partial quantitative deficiency (type 1), qualitative deficiency (type 2), and total deficiency (type 3). There are several different variants of type 2 VWD: 2A, 2B, 2N, and 2M based on the phenotype. Approximately 75% of patients have type 1 VWD.

Clinical Presentation

Mucous membrane–type bleeding (e.g., menorrhagia, epistaxis) and excessive bruising are characteristic clinical features in VWD. Bleeding manifestations vary considerably, and in some cases the diagnosis is not suspected until excessive bleeding occurs with a surgical procedure or trauma. Although excessive menstrual bleeding may be the initial manifestation, it takes 16 years for a diagnosis of bleeding disorder. It is for this reason that the American College of Obstetrics and Gynecology recommended screening for hemostatic disorders in all adolescents and females presenting with menorrhagia and no pathology and before hysterectomy for menorrhagia. In infants or small children with type 3 (severe) VWD, excessive bruising and even joint bleeding (caused by very low levels of factor VIII) can mimic hemophilia A.

Diagnosis

Laboratory evaluation for VWD requires several assays to quantitate VWF and characterize its structure and function. Many variables affect VWF assay results, including the patient's ABO blood type. Persons of blood group AB have 60% to 70% higher VWF levels than those of blood group O.

Clinical conditions and disorders with elevated VWF levels include pregnancy (third trimester), collagen vascular disorders, postoperative period, liver disease, and disseminated intravascular coagulation. Low levels are seen in hypothyroidism and the first 4 days of the menstrual cycle.

Symptoms are modified by medications like aspirin or nonsteroidal antiinflammatory drugs (NSAIDs), which can exacerbate the bleeding; oral contraceptives can decrease the bleeding in females with VWD by increasing VWF levels. VWF levels in African American females are 15% higher than in White females.

Clinical symptoms and family history are important for establishing the diagnosis of VWD, and a single test is sometimes not sufficient to rule out the diagnosis.

Initial workup should include a complete blood count, aPTT, PT, fibrinogen level, and thrombin time. These tests do not rule out VWD but help rule out thrombocytopenia or factor deficiency as the cause for bleeding. The closure times on the PFA-100, which has replaced the bleeding time as a screening test in some centers, may be prolonged. The aPTT in VWD is only abnormal when factor VIII is sufficiently reduced.

Specific tests for VWD include ristocetin cofactor assay, a factor VIII activity, and VWF antigen (VWF Ag) assay. The ristocetin cofactor activity measures induced binding of VWF to platelet glycoprotein Ib and is subject to significant intralaboratory and interlaboratory variability, making it an unreliable assay for the diagnosis. In addition, certain mutations in the A1 domain of the VWF, especially the *D1472H* mutation, have been found to attenuate the VWF-ristocetin binding, leading to misdiagnosis of VWD. This has led to the development of the glycoprotein 1bM assay (direct measure of platelet-binding activity of VWF), collagen binding assay (measure of multimeric function), and genotyping (especially for type 2 VWD, which are the new tests available to assist with the diagnosis). Multimer analysis is done by agarose gel electrophoresis using anti-VWF polyclonal antibody and is available at reference laboratories.

In type 1 VWD, the VWF is subnormal in amount, with normal multimer structure. Those with types 2A and 2B VWD lack the HMW multimers. In type 2B, the VWF has a heightened affinity for platelets, often resulting in some degree of thrombocytopenia from platelet aggregation. A useful laboratory test for type 2B is the low-dose ristocetin-induced platelet aggregation (RIPA) assay.

In type 3 (severe) VWD, the affected person has inherited a gene for type 1 VWD from each parent, resulting in very low levels (3%) of VWF (and low factor VIII, because there is no VWF to protect factor VIII from proteolytic degradation). Less commonly, a person with type 3 is doubly heterozygous. Table 5 provides an overview of the laboratory findings in the different variants of VWD.

Treatment

See the "General Hemostatic Agents" section later in this chapter for a discussion on the use of desmopressin (DDAVP) and antifibrinolytic agents.

For type 3 patients and in patients with type 1 VWD who do not respond adequately to desmopressin, an intermediate-purity plasma-derived concentrate rich in the hemostatically effective HMW multimers of VWF (e.g., Humate-P) should be used to treat moderately severe or severe bleeding episodes and before surgery. Prophylaxis with VWF concentrates is effective in reducing the bleeding episodes and joint disease in severe VWD. A recombinant VWF concentrate enriched with HMW multimers,

TABLE 5	Clinical Variants of von Willebrand Disease					
TYPE	**FACTOR VIII**	**VWF AG**	**RISTOCETIN COFACTOR**		**RIPA**	**MULTIMER**
1	↓	↓	↓		↓ or normal	Normal
2A	↓or normal	↓↓	↓		↓↓	Large and intermediate multimers absent
2B	↓or normal	↓↓	↓ or normal		↓ to low dose	Large multimers absent
2M	Variably ↓	Variably ↓	↓		Variably ↓	Normal
2N	↓↓	Normal	Normal		Normal	Normal
3	↓↓↓↓	↓↓↓↓	↓↓↓↓		None	Absent
Platelet type	↓ or normal	↓ or normal	↓		↓ to low dose	Large multimers absent

AG, Antigen; *RIPA,* ristocetin-induced platelet aggregation; *VWF,* von Willebrand factor.

Vonvendi (Baxalta, Illinois City, IL) does not contain any factor VIII and is now available and approved for use only in adults.

As in hemophilia, antifibrinolytics are an effective adjunctive treatment for invasive dental procedures or other bleeding in the oropharyngeal cavity. These may be effective even when used alone in some females with VWD and menorrhagia. For epistaxis, Nosebleed QR, a hydrophilic powder (over-the-counter [OTC] product), can help.

Special Situations

Pregnancy

VWF (and factor VIII) levels increase during the third trimester of pregnancy, and females with type 1 VWD have a decrease in bruising or other bleeding symptoms. However, those with type 2 VWD (abnormal VWF) and type 3 (no VWF) have no change in bleeding tendency. Even in type 1 VWD, VWF levels decrease after delivery, so treatment (with intravenous DDAVP or Humate P) may be needed. Antifibrinolytic agents can be used to prevent/treat postpartum hemorrhage.

Acquired Hemophilia

This is a very rare situation in which inhibitory antibodies develop against factor VIII or factor IX, usually in the setting of an inflammatory condition. The bleeding complications are severe, with patients usually developing extensive hematomas or ecchymoses. Treatment includes porcine factor VIII concentrates or emicizumab[1]; immunosuppression with corticosteroids with or without cyclophosphamide[1]; or rituximab (Rituxan)[1].

Acquired von Willebrand Disease

Acquired VWD occurs in persons who do not have a lifelong bleeding disorder. Conditions associated with acquired VWD include underlying autoimmune disease (lymphoproliferative disorders, myeloproliferative disorders, or plasma cell dyscrasias), valvular and congenital heart disease, Wilms tumor, chronic renal failure, and hypothyroidism. The mechanism of acquired VWD is unknown. Medications such as valproic acid can also cause VWD. Removal of the underlying condition often corrects the VWF. DDAVP, Humate P, recombinant factor VIIa (NovoSeven RT)[1], or plasma exchange may be tried, if necessary, to treat bleeding.

Rare Bleeding Disorders

The RBDs account for 3% to 5% of inherited coagulation deficiencies other than factor VIII, factor IX, or VWF deficiencies. They are mostly autosomal recessive (AR), but a few conditions are autosomal dominant (AD) and thus affect both sexes. The prevalence of RBDs ranges from 1 in 500,000 to 1 in 2,000,000. Bleeding manifestations are restricted to persons who are homozygotes or compound heterozygotes. RBDs are common in countries such as Iran, where consanguineous marriages are customary. Ashkenazi Jews are particularly affected by factor XI deficiency. Deficiency of factor XII is a risk factor for thrombosis but not for bleeding. Most cases of RBDs are identified by abnormal screening tests coupled with specific factor assays.

Factor concentrates (recombinant or plasma derived) are available for some of the deficiencies such as factor VII, X (Coagadex [human]; Bio Products Laboratory, Durham, NC), XIII (Tretten [recombinant], Novo Nordisk; Corifact [human], CSL Behring, King of Prussia, PA), XI (in Europe), and fibrinogen concentrate (human) (Fibryga, Octapharma, Switzerland; RiaSTAP, CSL Behring). The advantages of concentrates are pathogen safety and small volume. The use of antifibrinolytics and fibrin glue as adjunct therapy for bleeding manifestations is encouraged.

Factor I (Fibrinogen) Deficiency

The incidence of factor I deficiency is 1:1,000,000. This deficiency can manifest as afibrinogenemia (AR), dysfibrinogenemia (AD), and hypofibrinogenemia (AD). The bleeding phenotype is generally mild, although it can cause CNS bleeding, umbilical bleeding at birth, or joint bleeding. Dysfibrinogenemia can also cause recurrent miscarriages and paradoxically can give rise to thrombosis.

Laboratory findings include prolonged PT, prolonged aPTT, prolonged thrombin time (TT), and normal liver function tests. Reptilase time is markedly prolonged. In hypofibrinogenemia, both fibrinogen activity and antigen levels are equally low, but in dysfibrinogenemia the activity level is much lower than the antigen level. A ratio of fibrinogen activity to antigen <0.7 suggests dysfibrinogenemia.

Treatment or prophylaxis of bleeding can be achieved by administering FFP 15 to 30 mL/kg or cryoprecipitate 1 bag/5 to 10 kg; or fibrinogen concentrate (RiaSTAP) treatment q3–5d. Vigorous treatment with high doses of any of these may be complicated by the development of thrombosis; therefore the goal of the treatment should be to supplement only enough fibrinogen to maintain hemostasis.

Factor II (Prothrombin) Deficiency

The incidence of factor II deficiency is 1:2,000,000. Type I is characterized by hypoprothrombinemia (AR) and type II is characterized by dysprothrombinemia (AR). The bleeding manifestations include hematomas, hemarthroses, menorrhagia, CNS bleeding, umbilical bleeding, and postpartum hemorrhage.

Laboratory findings include prolonged PT, prolonged aPTT, normal TT, and normal liver function tests.

Treatment or prophylaxis of bleeding can be achieved by administering fresh frozen plasma (FFP) 15 to 20 mL/kg or prothrombin complex concentrate (PCC) 20 to 30 U/kg. Because factor II has a long half-life of 60 hours and low levels of 20% to 40% can be hemostatic, minimal treatment with a single dose of FFP can successfully achieve hemostasis.

Factor V (Labile Factor or Proaccelerin) Deficiency

The other names for this AR bleeding disorder are parahemophilia and Owren disease. Its incidence is 1:1,000,000. The bleeding manifestations include mucosal bleeding, postpartum hemorrhage, and CNS bleeding. Platelet factor V deficiency is more reflective of a bleeding potential.

Laboratory findings include prolonged PT, prolonged aPTT, normal TT, and normal liver function tests. Treatment or prophylaxis of bleeding can be achieved by administering FFP 15 to 20 mL/kg or platelet transfusions. Caution that antiplatelet antibodies can develop with repeated platelet transfusions.

Factor VII Deficiency

Although the estimated incidence of factor VII deficiency is 1:500,000, it may be even more frequent. Factor VII deficiency is considered to be *the most common* rare bleeding disorder. Although this is an AR disorder, the clinical picture shows variability. The bleeding manifestations include menorrhagia; mucosal, muscle, and intracranial bleeds (15%–60%); and hemarthrosis. Some patients have a high-risk bleeding phenotype (factor VII levels <2%, personal history of severe spontaneous bleeding, family history of severe spontaneous bleeding), and some have a low-risk bleeding phenotype (factor VII levels >20%, no personal or family history of severe spontaneous bleeding). The bleeding phenotype may determine the management decisions.

Laboratory findings include prolonged PT, normal aPTT, normal TT, normal fibrinogen, and normal liver function tests. Treatment or prophylaxis of bleeding can be achieved by administering recombinant factor VIIa (NovoSeven, Sevenfact, Aryoseven), 15 to 30 μg/kg q2–6h; FFP 15 to 20 mL/kg or PCC 20 to 30 U/kg. The recombinant factor VIIa has a short half-life of 3 to 6 hours. Note that the recombinant factor VIIa doses used in the

Hemophilia and Related Conditions

[1] Not FDA approved for this indication.

treatment of factor VII deficiency (15–30 µg/kg) are much lower than the bypassing doses used in hemophilia with inhibitors (90 µg/kg), and in fact much smaller doses (down to 10 µg/kg) have been effective in achieving hemostasis.

Factor X Deficiency

The incidence of this AR bleeding disorder is 1:1,000,000. The bleeding manifestations include menorrhagia and also umbilical, joint, mucosal, muscle, and intracranial bleeding.

Laboratory findings include prolonged PT, prolonged aPTT, normal TT, and normal liver function tests.

Treatment or prophylaxis of bleeding can be achieved by administering FFP 15 to 20 mL/kg; PCC 20 to 30 U/kg; or Pd FX (plasma-derived Factor X [Coagadex]).

Factor XI Deficiency

Although the incidence of this AR bleeding disorder is 1:1,000,000, it is more common among Ashkenazi Jews. The bleeding manifestations include posttraumatic bleeding and menorrhagia.

Laboratory findings include normal PT, prolonged aPTT, normal TT, and normal liver function tests.

Treatment or prophylaxis of bleeding can be achieved by administering Hemoleven[2] or FFP 15 to 20 mL/kg. Inhibitors can occur after treatment.

Factor XIII Deficiency

The incidence of this AR bleeding disorder is 1:2,000,000. The bleeding manifestations include intracranial bleeding, joint, umbilical bleeding, delayed wound healing and recurrent miscarriages.

Laboratory findings include normal PT, normal aPTT, and normal TT; suspected patients must have a factor XIII assay done. Treatment or prophylaxis of bleeding can be achieved by administering factor XIII concentrate (Corifact) 35 to 40 IU/kg or q28d to maintain a trough level of 5% to 20%. Tretten, a recombinant factor XIII-A subunit concentrate, can be used in patients with factor XIII-A subunit deficiency at 35 U/kg/mo for prophylaxis. Although cryoprecipitate has been used in the past, it is no longer the first choice.

Combined Factor V and VIII Deficiencies

The incidence of this AR disorder is 1:2,000,000. Its manifestations include mostly mucosal bleeding. Laboratory findings include prolonged PT along with a disproportionately prolonged PTT. Both factor VIII concentrates and FFP can be used in the treatment.

Vitamin K–Dependent Multiple Deficiencies

The incidence of this AR disorder is 1:2,000,000. Clinical manifestations include umbilical stump, intracranial, and postsurgical bleeding. Affected patients may also have skeletal abnormalities or hearing loss. Treatment consists of oral vitamin K, FFP, and PCC.

General Hemostatic Agents

For short-term therapy (before dental procedures and minor bleeding episodes), the synthetic vasopressin analog desmopressin acetate (DDAVP injection, Stimate nasal spray) is useful both in mild hemophilia A and type 1 VWD, and occasionally in type 2A VWD[1]. Some young females with menorrhagia have also benefited from its use at the onset of menses, with a second dose given after 24 hours. The mechanism of action for desmopressin is increase in plasma concentrations of factor VIII and VWF by stimulating release of the endothelial stores of VWF. The levels of both factor VIII and VWF increase threefold to fivefold within 15 to 30 minutes after infusion. A DDAVP trial to determine response is helpful in selecting patients who might benefit from such therapy. For

hemostatic purposes, intravenous (0.3 µg/kg in 50 mL of normal saline infused over 15–30 minutes, max dose 20 µg) or intranasal dose (150 µg) can be used. The intranasal dose is 15 times larger than that recommended for diabetes insipidus. A multidose intranasal spray formulation (Stimate nasal spray in the United States and Octostim nasal spray in Canada; Ferring Pharmaceuticals, Parsippany, NJ) of 1.5 mg/1 mL delivers 150 µg per spray. The recommended dosage is one spray for patients who weigh <50 kg and two sprays (one in each nostril) for those who weigh >50 kg. (Note that Ferring Pharmaceuticals issued a voluntary recall of Stimate in July 2020 because of higher-than-specified doses in the sprays. Stimate brand was discontinued in the United States in 2024. This recall does not affect intravenous doses.) The intravenous route, which was usually used for surgical coverage or for severe bleeding episodes requiring hospitalization, is now the only available route until the intranasal medication is released again.

When necessary, repeat doses may be given at 12- to 24-hour intervals. Tachyphylaxis (diminished response to repeated doses of the medication) occurs as a result of depletion of endothelial VWF stores. Tachyphylaxis is less commonly seen in VWD patients than in hemophilia patients. It is important to monitor free water intake after DDAVP administration because it can cause hyponatremia and seizures.

Desmopressin can also be used in the treatment of bleeding in patients with platelet dysfunction secondary to uremia[1]. Desmopressin seems to be effective in reducing blood loss during cardiac surgery in patients who are taking antiplatelet medications[1]. Because desmopressin requires the presence of either factor VIII or VWF to be able to show its effect, it is ineffective in moderate to severe hemophilia A, type 2M VWD, type 2N VWD, and type 3 VWD (there is no VWF to be released from storage sites). Desmopressin should be used with caution in type 2B VWD[1] as it can exacerbate the thrombocytopenia. Some patients with type 2A VWD may respond to desmopressin[1], and a desmopressin test may be needed to determine benefit. Desmopressin is ineffective in hemophilia B and other coagulation disorders.

Antifibrinolytics such as ε-aminocaproic acid (Amicar; Akorn Inc., Lake Forest, IL) and tranexamic acid (Cyklokapron [Pfizer, New York, NY] or Lysteda [Amring Pharmaceuticals, Berwyn, PA])[1] are used as adjunct therapies in hemophilia, VWD, and other rare bleeding disorders, reducing the need for factor concentrates. The recommended dosage for ε-aminocaproic acid is 50 to 100 mg/kg/dose intravenously or orally (adult dose 4–5 g/dose IV or 5 g/dose PO) every 4 to 8 hours (maximum daily dose 24 g/24 h for children, 30 g/24 h for adults). Most bleeding disorder treatment centers do not exceed 3 g for individual doses. The recommended dosage for tranexamic acid is 10 mg/kg/dose intravenously or 25 mg/kg body weight orally, three times daily (for adolescents and adults 1300 mg tid for a total of 5 days).

General Measures

Aspirin and aspirin-containing compounds should be avoided in patients with bleeding disorders because they interfere with platelet function and can exacerbate bleeding.

References

Aledort LM: Do hemophilia carriers bleed? Yes, *Blood* 108(1):6, 2006.
Arnold WD, Hilgartner MW: Hemophilic arthropathy. Current concepts of pathogenesis and management, *J Bone Joint Surg Am* 59(3):287–305, 1977.
Batty P, Lillicrap D: Gene therapy for hemophilia: current status and laboratory consequences, *Int J Lab Hematol* 43(Suppl 1):117–123, 2021.
Bolton-Maggs PH, Pasi KJ: Haemophilias A and B, *Lancet* 361(9371):1801–1809, 2003.
d'Oiron R, O'Brien S, James AH: Women and girls with haemophilia: lessons learned, *Haemophilia* 27(Suppl 3):75–78, 2021.
Flood VH, Gill JC, Morateck PA, et al: Common VWF exon 28 polymorphisms in African Americans affecting the VWF activity assay by ristocetin cofactor, *Blood* 116(2):280–286, 2010.
Franchini M, Mannucci PM: Non-factor replacement therapy for haemophilia: a current update, *Blood Transfus* 14:1–5, 2018.

---

[1] Not FDA approved for this indication.
[2] Not available in the United States.

---

[1] Not FDA approved for this indication.

Gill JC, Wilson AD, Endres-Brooks J, Montgomery RR: Loss of the largest von Willebrand factor multimers from the plasma of patients with congenital cardiac defects, *Blood* 67(3):758–761, 1986.

Hoffman M, Monroe 3rd DM: A cell-based model of hemostasis, *Thromb Haemost* 85(6):958–965, 2001.

Miller CH, Dilley AB, Drews C, et al: Changes in von Willebrand factor and factor VIII levels during the menstrual cycle, *Thromb Haemost* 87(6):1082–1083, 2002.

Miller CH, Dilley A, Richardson L, et al: Population differences in von Willebrand factor levels affect the diagnosis of von Willebrand disease in African-American women, *Am J Hematol* 67(2):125–129, 2001.

Mulder K, Llinas A: The target joint, *Haemophilia* 10(Suppl 4):152–156, 2004.

National Hemophilia Foundation Medical and Scientific Advisory Council (MASAC): MASAC recommendations concerning the treatment of hemophilia and other bleeding disorders. Available at http://www.hemophilia.org/Researchers-Healthcare-Providers/Medical-and-Scientific-Advisory-Council-MASAC/MASAC-Recommendations.

Pabinger-Fasching I, Pipe S: Innovations in coagulation: improved options for treatment of hemophilia A and B, *Thromb Res* 131(2):S1, 2013.

Pierce GF, Lillicrap D, Pipe SW, Vandendriessche T: Gene therapy, bioengineered clotting factors and novel technologies for hemophilia treatment, *J Thromb Haemost* 5(5):901–906, 2007.

Shapiro A: Development of long-acting recombinant FVIII and FIX Fc fusion proteins for the management of hemophilia, *Expert Opin Biol Ther* 13(9):1287–1297, 2013.

Soucie JM, Nuss R, Evatt B, et al: Mortality among males with hemophilia; relations with source of medical care. The hemophilia surveillance system project investigators, *Blood* 96(2):437–442, 2000.

van Galen KPM, d'Oiron R, James P, et al: A new hemophilia carrier nomenclature to define hemophilia in women and girls: communication from the SSC of the ISTH, *J Thromb Haemost* 19(8):1883–1887, 2021.

Veldman A, Hoffman M, Ehrenforth S: New insights into the coagulation system and implications for new therapeutic options with recombinant factor VIIa, *Curr Med Chem* 10(10):797–811, 2003.

Warrier I, Ewenstein BM, Koerper MA, et al: Factor IX inhibitors and anaphylaxis in hemophilia B, *J Pediatr Hematol Oncol* 19(1):23–27, 1997.

Weyand AC, Pipe SW: New therapies for hemophilia, *Blood* 133(5):389–398, 2019.

HODGKIN DISEASE

Method of
Sanjal Desai, MD

CURRENT DIAGNOSIS

- Painless and persistent supradiaphragmatic lymphadenopathy with or without systemic symptoms is the most common presentation of classic Hodgkin lymphoma (cHL).
- Excisional biopsy of the involved lymph node is the gold standard approach for diagnosis of cHL. Fine needle aspirations are inadequate.
- cHL is positron emission tomography (PET) avid, and PET scan is essential for assessment of stage, response to treatment, and response-adapted therapy.
- Bone marrow biopsy is generally not needed, because PET scan is able to detect bone marrow involvement.

CURRENT THERAPY

- Classic Hodgkin lymphoma (cHL) is potentially curable with systemic therapy in the majority of cases.
- Monitoring for late effects of chemotherapy and/or radiation is the cornerstone of care for cHL survivors.

Introduction and Epidemiology

Hodgkin disease (HD) is a relatively rare B cell lymphoma with approximately 8000 to 9000 new cases diagnosed in the United States every year. HD has a bimodal distribution: the first peak in incidence of HD is seen in young adults (20–30 years) followed by a drop in middle age. A second peak is seen at approximately 65 years. Older adults with HD are more likely to have extensive disease and poor outcomes. HD cases are largely sporadic. There are some familial tendencies identified: for example, siblings of HD patients have a 10-fold higher risk of developing the disease. Infections with Epstein-Barr virus (EBV) and human immunodeficiency virus (HIV) are associated with increased risk of HD, suggesting abnormal immune response to infection as a possible pathophysiologic mechanism. Certain other childhood infections are possibly protective.

HD traditionally has been divided into two subtypes: classic Hodgkin lymphoma (cHL) and nodular lymphocyte predominant Hodgkin lymphoma (NLPHL). The two subtypes differ in pathology, pathophysiology, management, and prognosis. cHL accounts for 95% of total HD cases and runs an aggressive course with frequent involvement of extranodal sites and B symptoms. cHL requires treatment with a multiagent chemotherapy-based regimen in a time-sensitive manner and is potentially curable. NLPHL, on the other hand, accounts for 5% of total HD cases, runs an indolent course, rarely causes extranodal involvement, and is considered incurable with frequent late recurrences. Management of NLPHL is frequently like other indolent lymphomas.

Pathophysiology

cHL histology consists of Hodgkin Reed-Sternberg (HRS) cells scattered among profuse and abundant immune effector cells. HRS cells are positive for CD15 and CD30 and negative for CD20. Immune effector cells are lymphocytes, eosinophils, and histiocytes. The HRS cell is the malignant cell of cHL, and it has its origins in follicular center B cells. HRS cells use multiple pathways to send inhibitory signals to surrounding immune effector cells. These signals suppress immune response to HRS cells and promote their survival. One of the mechanisms that HRS cells use to inhibit surrounding immune effector cells is through the PD1/PDL1 axis. Copy number variation at the 9p24.1 locus on HRS chromosomes leads to enhanced PDL1 (or PDL2) expression on the HRS cell surface. PDL1/PDL2 binds to PD1 on T helper cells and blocks T cell receptor signaling. This inhibits T cell–mediated immune response to HRS cells and promotes their survival. cHL is divided into four subgroups with unique pathologic and clinical features: nodular sclerosis, lymphocyte rich, lymphocyte depleted, and mixed cellularity.

NLPHL is characterized by the presence of large neoplastic cells with folded nuclei, also known as histiocytic cells, that are positive for CD20 and negative for CD15, CD30. Because of CD20 positivity, management of NLPHL is like indolent CD20+ non-Hodgkin lymphomas. NLPHL is now categorized as NLPBL in 2022 International Consensus Classification of Mature Lymphoid Malignancies.

Prevention

Most HD cases occur sporadically. No definite link to genetic or environmental factors are established. Consequently, there is no definite preventive or screening strategy for HD.

Clinical Manifestations

Lymphadenopathy is a core manifestation of cHL. Affected lymph nodes are enlarged, firm, usually painless, and persistent. The most common locations are cervical, anterior mediastinal, and supraclavicular lymph nodes. A subdiaphragmatic presentation, with exclusive involvement of lymph nodes and extranodal sites below the diaphragm, is uncommon and suggests a poor prognosis. Splenomegaly is also seen. Lymph node involvement is the most common presentation, but extranodal involvement of lung, liver, and bone marrow can also be seen. High-grade fevers, chills, drenching night sweats, unintentional weight loss, and appetite loss are common at presentation. Itching that is sometimes mitigated by alcohol consumption is a common presenting symptom of cHL.

The majority of NLPHL patients have early-stage disease. B symptoms, bulky disease, and extranodal involvement are rare.

Diagnosis

Microscopic examination of affected lymph node architecture is necessary to make the diagnosis of HD. Excisional biopsy of affected lymph nodes provides the best opportunity for a thorough examination of lymph node architecture and therefore is

TABLE 1	Ann Arbor Staging System for Classic Hodgkin Lymphoma
Stage I	Involvement of single lymph node region or localized involvement of single extranodal site
Stage II	Involvement of ≥2 lymph node sites on the same side of diaphragm *or* Involvement of single extranodal site with associated regional lymph nodes with or without other lymph nodes on the same side of diaphragm
Stage III	Involvement of ≥2 lymph node sites above and below diaphragm
Stage IV	Multifocal or diffuse involvement of extranodal organs or involvement of extranodal organs with nonregional or distant lymph node sites

Each stage can be labeled as A or B:
A: No B symptoms present
B: Unexplained fevers >38° C, unintentional weight loss >10% in last 6 months, drenching night sweats

The spleen is considered a lymph node site.

TABLE 2	Features Defining Unfavorable Risk in Early-Stage Classic Hodgkin Lymphoma
Age ≥50 years	
ESR >50 or ESR >30 if B symptoms are present	
MMR >0.33	
Involvement of ≥3 lymph node regions	
largest lymph node diameter >10 cm	
Any extranodal lesion	

ESR, Erythrocyte sedimentation rate; *MMR*, mediastinal mass ratio.

TABLE 3	International Prognostic Scoring System (IPSS) for Advanced Stage Hodgkin Lymphoma

IPSS: 1 point for each factor

- Albumin <40 g/L
- Hemoglobin <105 g/L
- Male sex
- Age ≥45 years
- Stage IV disease
- Leukocytosis >15×10^9/L
- Lymphocytopenia with absolute lymphocyte count <0.6×10^9/L or <8% of total white blood cells

0 = low risk
1–3 = intermediate risk
4–5 = high risk

the gold standard approach for diagnosis of HD. When excisional biopsies are not feasible, core needle biopsy can provide a diagnosis in certain cases, but excisional biopsy needs to be done when core needle biopsy is nondiagnostic if lymphoma is clinically suspected. Fine needle aspirations are inadequate for diagnosis of HD. cHL is unique in its feature that malignant HRS cells are the minority of the population. Therefore a small fine or core needle biopsy can fail to include malignant cells and consequently be nondiagnostic. Differentiation between cHL and NLPHL is necessary to determine therapy, and excisional biopsy might be required for that purpose as well.

Hodgkin lymphoma is fluorodeoxyglucose (FDG) avid on positron emission tomography (PET) scan. A PET scan is recommended for initial staging of cHL and subsequent assessment of treatment response. A PET scan can detect bone marrow involvement by HD; therefore bone marrow biopsy is not required for initial staging. An exception to this rule would be a patient with unexplained cytopenia and no FDG avidity of bone marrow on PET scan. It is important to remember that cHL commonly causes anemia of chronic inflammation, which should be assessed for before pursuing bone marrow biopsy.

Other necessary investigations before starting treatment are complete blood counts, metabolic panel with electrolytes, kidney function tests, liver function tests, and erythrocyte sedimentation rate. Screening for cardiomyopathy with an echocardiogram is conducted in all patients before considering anthracycline-based therapy. Screening for chronic and indolent viral illness including hepatitis and HIV should be considered before administering immunosuppressive chemotherapy. If bleomycin-based therapy is being considered, pulmonary function should be evaluated using spirometry. Before beginning chemotherapy, fertility preservation should be offered to individuals of reproductive potential.

Therapy

cHL is an aggressive lymphoma that requires therapy in an urgent manner. Treatment modalities depend on stage, risk, and interim response to employed treatment. Table 1 summarizes the staging system used for Hodgkin and non-Hodgkin lymphoma. Table 2 summarizes all unfavorable risk factors in early-stage disease as described by different research groups. For advanced-stage disease, the International Prognostic Scoring System (IPSS) is used to estimate risk as summarized in Table 3. IPSS does not determine treatment strategy in the current treatment paradigm of advanced-stage cHL.

Patients with early-stage disease are often treated with combined modality treatment. Multiple approaches are available that differ in number of chemotherapy cycles, radiation dose, and utility of interim PET scan. The optimal treatment strategy is a subject of ongoing debate.

For early-stage favorable disease, we usually begin with multiagent chemotherapy with doxorubicin (Adriamycin), bleomycin, vinblastine, and dacarbazine (ABVD). Two cycles of ABVD followed by involved site radiation is an acceptable treatment option for patients with very localized, nonbulky disease without any unfavorable risk factors. Alternatively, a response-adapted approach can be used: if an interim PET scan is negative for residual disease after two cycles, patients can receive radiation only if there are two or fewer nodal sites, no extranodal disease, and no other unfavorable risk features. Multiple studies have underscored importance of radiation in these patients. If patients have more extensive or extranodal disease, one or two more cycles of ABVD are considered. If the interim PET scan is positive after two cycles of ABVD, we generally employ combination of ABVD (two cycles) along with radiation, because these patients are thought to require more treatment.

For early-stage unfavorable disease, treatment begins with two cycles of ABVD. If patients have interim PET-negative status, then a combination of two more cycles of ABVD with radiation is generally accepted. Where radiation is not feasible, four more cycles of ABVD without radiation are acceptable. For PET positive patients, intensification of chemotherapy regimen has been shown to improve outcomes but should be weighed against increased treatment-related toxicities and second malignancies.

For advanced-stage disease, six cycles of chemotherapy is the standard of care. For decades, PET-adapted therapy with ABVD followed by response-adapted escalation to bleomycin, etoposide[1], doxorubicin (Adriamycin), cyclophosphamide, vincristine (Oncovin), procarbazine, and prednisone (BEACOPP) was the standard of care. Patients received two cycles of ABVD followed by interim PET scan. Patients with complete metabolic response will go on to receive four cycles of doxorubicin (Adriamycin), vinblastine, and

---

[1] Not FDA approved for this indication.

dacarbazine (AVD). Patients with partial metabolic response on interim PET scan can receive either four more cycles of (escalated [esc]) BEACOPP or four more cycles of ABVD. Esc BEACOPP increases the likelihood of remission compared with ABVD in these patients, with the potential long-term risk of second cancers, including therapy-related myeloid neoplasms. Furthermore, many patients who relapse after ABVD are salvageable with high-dose chemotherapy and autologous stem cell rescue. So, the practice of escalation to BEACOPP has not been universally accepted in the United States and is even more controversial in the era of novel agents.

In the last decade, there have been notable advances in the management of cHL with the addition of brentuximab vedotin (BV [Adcetris]). BV in combination with AVD (BV + AVD) for six cycles (regardless of interim PET) has shown to improve the likelihood of remission, as well as survival from cHL compared with six cycles of ABVD. Patients who have complete metabolic response after two cycles have better outcomes compared with patients who have partial metabolic response. These results have led to acceptance of BV + AVD as a preferred treatment option for newly diagnosed cHL in the United States. Comparison of this new treatment with PET-adapted escalation of therapy has not been studied yet. In 2023, combination of PD1-antagonist nivolumab (Opdivo) with AVD (N + AVD) has shown to improve the likelihood of remission compared with BV + AVD. Studies incorporating BV and nivolumab in early-stage cHL are being conducted with excellent initial results.

After completion of cancer-directed therapy, a PET scan is conducted to assess disease response. If persistent disease is found, a biopsy is done, and if persistent lymphoma is confirmed, disease is declared refractory to frontline therapy and second-line or salvage therapy is started.

Salvage chemotherapy followed by high-dose chemotherapy and autologous stem cell rescue is the current standard of care for patients who have relapsed after or are refractory to frontline therapy. The advent of BV and PD1 antagonists has improved outcomes in this population as well. For patients who are ineligible for high-dose chemotherapy, treatment is palliative and disease is incurable.

Because NLPHL runs an indolent course, intensive treatments are frequently not required. Patients with single-site involvement with NLPHL can be treated with involved-site radiation. For more advanced disease, asymptomatic patients can be monitored without any treatment. Treatment can be initiated for bulky, symptomatic disease and can range from single agent rituximab (Rituxan)[1] to chemoimmunotherapy options used for other indolent B cell non-Hodgkin lymphoma.

During treatment, patients are at high risk of tumor lysis syndrome. Prophylactic antiuric acid therapy can prevent this complication. Prophylactic antiviral and antibacterial agents are employed to decrease the risk of opportunistic infections. Malignancy produces a hypercoagulable state. Clinical monitoring for arterial and venous thromboembolism should be performed, and prompt treatment should be initiated if thromboembolism is detected. With BV- and nivolumab-based frontline chemoimmunotherapy regimens, granulocyte colony-stimulating factor (GCSF) prophylaxis is used to prevent neutropenia but not with regimens using bleomycin because of an increased risk of bleomycin toxicities in the setting of GCSF use.

Monitoring and Survivorship
Monitoring
Patients with cHL are monitored closely for relapse during the first 2 years after treatment as the likelihood of relapse is highest during that time. Patients are followed with serial history-taking, physical examination, and laboratory testing every 3 months. A computed tomography (CT) scan can be conducted every 6 months to monitor for radiographic signs of relapse for the first 2 years, but they are not imperative and the risk of long-term radiation exposure should be weighed against potential benefit. After 2 years, CT scans can be stopped. Serial clinical examinations

and laboratory testing are continued every 6 months for 5 years. Patients who stay in remission for 5 years are likely cured. These patients should be monitored for late effects of therapy.

Survivorship
Survivors of cHL are at risk of several late effects that require monitoring. Use of anthracycline and bleomycin increase the long-term risk of cardiomyopathy and interstitial lung disease, respectively. Involved site radiation to the chest increases the risk of interstitial lung disease and coronary artery atherosclerosis. Radiation of the spleen or thyroid increases the risk of hyposplenism and hypothyroidism, respectively. Both chemotherapy and radiation increase risk of second cancers in lymphoma survivors, including second skin cancers.

Survivors of cHL should be monitored for these late effects. Many recommendations come from guideline publications. For all patients, an annual blood count, metabolic panel, and fasting glucose, hemoglobin A1c, and annual lipid profile are recommended. Blood pressure should be monitored. All patients should follow vaccination guidelines for cancer survivors. An echocardiogram at 10 years after treatment is indicated to screen for cardiomyopathy. For patients who received neck radiation, carotid ultrasound at 10 years after treatment completion is recommended. If thyroid radiation was given, annual measurement of thyroid-stimulating hormone is recommended to screen for hypothyroidism. If splenic radiation is given, functional hyposplenism can develop and patients require prophylactic vaccination against pneumococcal, meningococcal, and *Haemophilus influenzae* infections, if not given preemptively. Survivors who have received chest or axillary radiation and were assigned female at birth should undergo breast magnetic resonance imaging in addition to mammogram annually starting at age 40 years or 8 years after completion of treatment, whichever is earlier. Others should follow age-appropriate cancer screening guidelines. Annual skin examination is recommended for all lymphoma survivors.

Prognosis
cHL is curable with frontline chemoimmunotherapy in up to 80% to 90% of cases. Of the 10% to 20% of patients who relapse, high-dose chemotherapy and autologous stem cell rescue can cure two-thirds of patients. Patients who are ineligible for autologous stem cell transplant or those who progress after autologous stem cell transplant are treated with single-agent therapies. In the era of novel agents, median survival of these patients approaches 10 years.

NLPHL runs an indolent course. Late relapses are seen occasionally even with chemoimmunotherapy. NLPHL is very treatable and in most cases, does not affect life expectancy.

References
Ansell Stephen M: Hodgkin lymphoma: 2025 update on diagnosis, risk-stratification, and management, *Am J Hematol* 99(12):2367–2378, 2024.
Connors JM, Jurczak W, Straus DJ, et al: Brentuximab vedotin with chemotherapy for stage III or IV Hodgkin's Lymphoma, *N Engl J Med* 378:331–344, 2018.
Desai S, Spinner MA, Sykorova A: Overall survival of patients with cHL who progress after autologous stem cell transplant: results in the novel agent era, *Blood Adv* 7(23):7295–7303, 2023.
Diehl V, Sextro M, Franklin J: Clinical presentation, course, and prognostic factors in lymphocyte-predominant Hodgkin's disease and lymphocyte-rich classical Hodgkin's disease: report from the European Task Force on Lymphoma project on Lymphocyte-Predominant Hodgkin's disease, *J Clin Oncol* 17(3):776–783, 1999.
Herrera AF, Leblanc M, Castellino SM: Nivolumab + AVD in advanced-stage classic Hodgkin's Lymphoma, *N Engl J Med* 391:1379–1389, 2024.
Johnson P, Federico M, Kirkwood A: Adapted treatment guided by interim PET-CT scan in advanced Hodgkin's Lymphoma, *N Engl J Med* 374:2419–2429, 2016.
Mauch P, Ng A, Alenman B, et al: Report from the Rockefeller Foundation-sponsored international workshop on reducing mortality and improving quality of life in long-term survivors of Hodgkin disease, *Eur J Haematol Suppl* (66)68–76, 2005.
Ng Andrea: Current survivorship recommendations for patients with Hodgkin lymphoma: focus on late effects, *Blood* 124(23):3373–3379, 2014.
Nogova L, Reineke T, Brillant C: Lymphocyte-predominant and classical Hodgkin's lymphoma: a comprehensive analysis from the German Hodgkin Study Group, *J Clin Oncol* 26(3):434–439, 2008.
Radford J, Illidge T, Counsell N, et al: Results of a trial of PET-directed therapy for early-stage Hodgkin's Lymphoma, *N Engl J Med* 372:1598–1607, 2015.
Siegel R, Giaquinto AN, Jemal A: Cancer statistics, 2024, *CA Cancer J Clin* 74(1):12–49, 2024.

---

[1] Not FDA approved for this indication.

IRON DEFICIENCY ANEMIA

Method of
Susan Evans, MD

CURRENT DIAGNOSIS

- The presence of symptoms and signs depends on the degree of iron deficiency, the time course of the development of iron deficiency, and the overall physiologic state of the patient. Patients may be asymptomatic. Signs and symptoms are more likely if anemia and/or hemodynamic instability are present.
- Symptoms include fatigue, poor exercise tolerance, weakness, headache, pica, dyspnea, dizziness, vertigo, and angina pectoris.
- Signs include pallor, dry and rough skin, brittle nails, defects of the nail bed (koilonychias), atrophy of the lingual papillae, and cheilosis.
- Systolic heart murmur if anemia is present
- Neonates: delayed growth and development
- Adolescents: learning and behavior problems
- Blood loss is the most common cause of iron deficiency
- Iron deficiency is the most common cause of anemia

Laboratory Findings

- Decreased iron on bone marrow aspirate is the gold standard but is rarely used
- Low serum hemoglobin to diagnose anemia
- Low mean corpuscular hemoglobin: late finding
- Low mean corpuscular volume: late finding
- Low serum iron
- High serum iron-binding capacity
- Low percent transferrin saturation (TSAT)
- Low serum ferritin, but may be normal in the presence of inflammation or infection

CURRENT THERAPY

Oral Replacement

- Ferrous sulfate (or another equivalent iron preparation) 325 mg (65 mg elemental iron) once daily or once daily on alternating days if that is better tolerated.
- Avoid taking with meals to increase absorption.

Parenteral Replacement

- Recommended when blood loss exceeds the ability to replace orally, in the context of malabsorption and if oral iron is not tolerated
  - Ferric carboxymaltose (Ferinject and Injectafer)
  - Ferric gluconate (Ferrlecit)
  - Ferumoxytol (Feraheme)
  - Iron sucrose (Venofer)

Unstable Patient

- If the patient is hemodynamically unstable due to anemia, consider blood transfusion

Treatment Endpoint

- Continue iron replacement for 3 months after anemia is resolved and iron replaced.

Epidemiology

Anemia affects more than one-third of the world's population, or 2 billion people. Iron deficiency continues to be the most common cause of anemia. Iron deficiency is the only micronutrient deficiency that remains a significant problem in both developing and developed countries. Iron deficiency refers to a decrease in iron stores below a normal level and can cause fatigue and decreased exercise intolerance even without anemia. In the case of iron deficiency without anemia, iron stores are still adequate for erythropoiesis. Iron deficiency anemia is a more serious condition in which there is not enough erythroid iron available, leading to anemia. Worldwide levels of iron deficiency are estimated to be twice that of iron deficiency anemia.

Risk Factors

Risk factors for iron deficiency anemia include age, socioeconomic status, female gender, race and ethnicity, diet low in iron, disease, and medical treatment. Several groups of people are at an increased risk of iron deficiency based on age or their stage in life. Infants and children ages 0 to 5 years old are at risk for iron deficiency because of their rapid rate of growth, which necessitates increased iron stores. Based on 2019 World Health Organization information, 39.8% of children aged 6 to 59 months were anemic. Adolescent girls and women of child bearing age are also at risk due to iron loss through menstruation. In 2019, 29.9% of women aged 15 to 49 were anemic. In the United States, Black women of childbearing age are 4 to 7 times more likely to have anemia than White women, and for Hispanic women the prevalence is 2 to 3 times that seen in White women. During pregnancy, a woman's iron needs triple because of the expansion of red cell mass, the placenta, and the growth of the fetus. Worldwide, anemia affects 36.5% of pregnant women and is known to increase the risk of cesarean section and maternal mortality. Elderly people are also at risk for iron deficiency for a number of reasons, including inadequate diet, poor absorption due to disease or antacid medicines, or as a complication of chronic disease. The 2025 Global Nutrition Targets aim to decrease the prevalence by 50%.

Dietary causes of iron deficiency anemia include lack of access to or preference against eating a diet including iron rich foods. While 90% of iron in the body is recycled every day, dietary iron is essential for replacing lost iron, which is mainly excreted in bile. Iron supplementation of common foods such as breads and rice in the United States decreases the risk of dietary iron deficiency. Iron is found naturally in both animal products such as meat and in plant based foods such as green leafy vegetables, sweet potatoes, and legumes. As long as they eat a healthy and well-balanced diet, vegetarians and vegans have not been shown to be at an increased risk for iron deficiency; such diets have many other health benefits.

Any illness or therapy that leads to decreased iron absorption or blood loss may cause iron deficiency. Common causes of blood loss include gastrointestinal diseases such as cancer, inflammatory bowel disease, and ulcer disease. Taking aspirin, nonsteroidal anti-inflammatory drugs (NSAIDs), or anticoagulants also increases the risk of gastrointestinal blood loss. Iron absorption is decreased in the context of celiac disease, post gastric bypass surgery, and *Helicobacter pylori* infection. Chronic diseases associated with iron deficiency include chronic kidney disease, rheumatoid arthritis, cancer, obesity, and chronic heart failure. There are also medical treatments that may cause iron deficiency such as antacid medicines, which decrease iron absorption, dialysis that causes blood loss, and erythropoietin therapy that depletes iron stores through increased erythropoiesis. Frequent phlebotomy, including repetitive blood donation or treatment for polycythemia or hemochromatosis, decrease iron stores. Rarely, there may be a genetic cause for iron deficiency anemia such as iron-refractory iron deficiency anemia.

Pathophysiology

Iron in the body can be broken down into two main types: functional iron and storage iron. Functional iron plays many essential roles in the human body. It is found in hemoglobin, which carries oxygen from the lungs to body tissues, and in muscles as myoglobin, which helps with oxygen use and storage. Iron plays a role in enzymatic reactions, DNA synthesis, mitochondrial energy generation, and cell proliferation. Storage iron is found in ferritin, hemosiderin, and transferrin. Iron homeostasis is very important to the body and is regulated through the diet, gastrointestinal absorption, and the recycling of the iron in red blood cells. Total body iron stores are about 3.5 g for men and 2.5 g for women. Approximately 20 to 25 mg of iron is needed daily for red cell production and body processes. Dietary absorption of iron is limited to about 1 to 2 mg/day; the daily requirement is primarily produced through the recycling of iron in used red blood cells by macrophages.

Dietary iron is found in two forms. Heme iron (Fe^2+) is found in animal products such as meat, poultry and seafood and is more easily absorbed than plant-based iron. Nonheme iron (Fe^3+) is found in plant sources such as beans and lentils, baked potatoes, dark green leafy vegetables, tofu, and cashews. Dietary iron is also found in iron fortified breakfast cereals and enriched breads. Adding foods high in vitamin C to a meal with nonheme iron can increase iron absorption. There are other foods that inhibit the absorption of iron, including polyphenols found in some vegetables, tannins found in tea, and calcium found in dairy products. Dietary iron absorption takes place almost exclusively in the duodenum and upper jejunum.

The recycling of iron from used red blood cells provides about 90% of body iron and is essential for maintaining normal iron levels in the body. Hepcidin, a peptide hormone mainly synthesized in the liver, controls the process of iron absorption and recycling. When serum iron levels are high, hepcidin levels increase in response, which leads to breakdown of the iron transporter called ferroportin. A decrease in ferroportin leaves more iron inside macrophages, enterocytes, and hepatocytes, and the serum iron level decreases. When serum iron levels drop, expression of hepcidin should decrease as well. However, inflammation and infection can cause hepcidin to increase inappropriately; this is one of the ways in which chronic disease contributes to iron deficiency.

Prevention

Prevention plays a large role in the treatment of iron deficiency anemia worldwide and includes both dietary interventions and supplementation. A food-based approach to prevention would include encouraging patients to eat more iron rich foods such as meats and dark green leafy vegetables. A list of iron rich foods is found in Table 1. Heme iron, found in animal sources, is easily absorbed; however, the absorption of nonheme iron from plant sources is affected by the foods with which they are eaten. Foods that can inhibit the absorption of iron include the tannins in tea and coffee and the calcium found in milk. It is best to eat these foods separately from iron rich foods to increase iron absorption. Certain foods increase the absorption of non-heme iron when they are eaten at the same time, including foods that contain heme (such as meat) or foods that contain vitamin C (such as fruit, orange juice, or broccoli). Encouraging iron fortified foods, which in the United States include cereals, rice, pasta, and bread, is another effective way to prevent deficiency. There are some cases when the risk of developing iron deficiency is so high that supplementation with an oral iron supplement is recommended. The World Health Organization recommends universal supplementation for low-birth-weight infants with 2 mg/kg daily from age 2 months to 23 months. They also recommend universal supplementation for pregnant women with 60 mg iron per day. While supplementation for pregnant women is common practice in the United States, the US Preventive Services Task Force states that there is insufficient evidence to show that these practices help prevent adverse maternal health and birth outcomes. According to the US Preventive Services Task Force, evidence is also insufficient to recommend screening children age 6 months to 2 years of age for iron deficiency anemia in the United States.

Clinical Manifestations

Patients with iron deficiency may be asymptomatic. The presence of symptoms and signs of iron deficiency depend on the degree of deficiency, the time course of the development of iron deficiency, and the overall physiologic state of the patient. Common symptoms of iron deficiency include fatigue, weakness, irritability, poor concentration, decreased exercise intolerance, dry mouth, headache, and restless leg syndrome. Severe iron deficiency can cause pica, a craving to eat substances such as ice, dirt, clay, or paint. Signs of iron deficiency include pallor and a systolic heart murmur if anemia is present, hair loss, atrophy of lingual papillae, and nail changes such as koilonychias.

Diagnosis

Normal hemoglobin levels depend on age, gender, pregnancy status, altitude, and smoking, but in general, an adult male is considered anemic with a hemoglobin level less than 13 g/dL and an adult female at less than 12 g/dL. In 2024, the World Health Organization published updated hemoglobin cutoffs to define anemia in individuals and populations as shown in Table 2. Iron deficiency may be present with or without anemia; therefore, measuring hemoglobin level is neither a sensitive nor a specific test for iron deficiency. Absolute iron deficiency occurs when the amount of total body iron is low. Functional iron deficiency occurs

TABLE 1	Iron Rich Foods
IRON TYPE	**DIETARY SOURCES**
Heme Iron	Beef
	Chicken
	Fish
	Organ Meats
	Oysters
Nonheme Iron	Dark Green Leafy Vegetables
	Beans
	Lentils
	Tofu
	Baked Potato
	Cashews
	Fortified Cereals, Breads and Pasta

TABLE 2	Hemoglobin Cutoffs to Define Anemia in Individuals and Populations	
POPULATION	**HEMOGLOBIN CONCENTRATION (g/dL)**	
Children, 6–23 months	<10.5	
Children, 24–59 months	<11.0	
Children, 5–11 years	<11.5	
Children, 12–14 years, nonpregnant girls	<12.0	
Children, 12–14 years, boys	<12.0	
Adults, 15–65 years, nonpregnant women	<12.0	
Adults, 15–65 years, men	<13.0	
Pregnancy First trimester Second trimester Third trimester <110	<11.0 <10.5 <11.0	

Adapted from Guideline on haemoglobin cutoffs to define anaemia in individuals and populations. Geneva: World Health Organization; 2024. Licence: CC BY-NC-SA 3.0 IGO.

when there is not enough iron available to meet the demand of body tissues and processes because iron is sequestered either in macrophages or the reticuloendothelial system.

Diagnosing iron deficiency is not straightforward because serum ferritin level, which is often used as a screening test, is affected by gender, age, inflammation, infection, and chronic diseases such as liver disease and cancer. While a serum ferritin concentration less than 12 µg/L makes iron deficiency very likely, a person with inflammation or chronic disease may have iron deficiency at much higher ferritin levels. Increasing the cutoff for normal ferritin concentration to 30 µg/L has been shown to increase sensitivity for iron deficiency, and an even higher cutoff of 100 µg is recommended by some specialty societies. For this reason, utilizing more than one iron status indicator to make the diagnosis is important. A low iron level (<50 µg/dL) and an elevated total iron binding capacity (TIBC >450 µg/dL) also support the diagnosis of iron deficiency. Other supporting labs include a drop in transferrin saturation (TSAT) to less than 16% or less than 20% if inflammation or disease is present. Low mean corpuscular volume (MCV) may be another sign of iron deficiency, but this is generally a late finding, so MCV may be in the normal range. Low MCV can also be seen in thalassemia. Low mean corpuscular hemoglobin concentration (MCHC) is another late finding in iron deficiency. Decreased iron seen on bone marrow aspiration is still considered the gold standard for diagnosing iron deficiency, but it is rarely done due to both cost and patient discomfort.

Differential Diagnosis

The differential diagnosis of iron deficiency includes causes of fatigue and exercise intolerance such as hypothyroidism, electrolyte disturbances due to diuretic therapy, left ventricular dysfunction, chronic lung disease, malignancies, or liver disease.

Anemia of chronic disease can mimic iron deficiency anemia and may be found concurrently in the same patient. The differential diagnosis for iron deficiency also includes thalassemia, sideroblasitc anemias, and lead poisoning

Treatment

The goal of treatment is to replace iron so that hemoglobin levels normalize and iron stores are replenished. Treatment of iron deficiency must take into consideration the type of patient being treated and the source and amount of iron deficit or blood loss. Patients who are severely anemic and hemodynamically unstable may be candidates for blood transfusion. For people in groups that are at high risk for iron deficiency, such as infants, toddlers, adolescents, and menstruating women, it is reasonable to start with oral supplementation with iron and only proceed with further work-up if that is unsuccessful. However, in patients at low risk for iron deficiency, such as men and post-menopausal women, it is important to determine the underlying cause of iron deficiency. Blood loss is the most common cause of iron deficiency, so this work-up includes evaluation for a source of bleeding. Urinalysis and heme-occult testing are preliminary tests, and upper and lower endoscopy is needed to evaluate for gastrointestinal pathology, including cancer, colitis, or celiac disease. If those tests are inconclusive, consider proceeding to video capsule endoscopy to further evaluate the small intestine. Heavy gynecologic bleeding may require further evaluation and treatment. Persistent blood noted on urinalysis would warrant referral to urology for further testing.

Oral iron supplementation continues to be the first line treatment for iron deficiency anemia. Common forms include ferrous sulfate (Feosol), ferrous gluconate (Fergon), and ferrous fumarate (Ferro-Sequels). A typical dose of ferrous sulfate is 325 mg (65 mg elemental iron) daily. However, there is now evidence that a dose of oral iron increases serum hepcidin, which then decreases iron absorption. Based on these findings, an alternate recommendation would be to give a single dose of iron on alternate days. This dosing schedule may increase iron absorption and adherence to treatment due to simpler regimen with decreased side effects. Iron is best absorbed when taken between meals; however,

this can also worsen side effects. It is best to take iron separate from acid-reducing medicines and foods that inhibit iron absorption. Common side effects of oral iron include diarrhea, nausea, epigastric discomfort, and constipation. Side effects can be lessened by taking iron with food and taking smaller doses such as ferrous gluconate 325 mg (38 mg elemental iron).

Parenteral iron may be indicated when oral therapy is unsuccessful due to malabsorption, when oral iron is not tolerated, or when the rate of absorption with oral supplementation is insufficient due to the rate of blood loss. New forms of parenteral iron are safer, less likely to cause hypersensitivity reactions, and their use is increasing. The dose of IV iron needed can be calculated with the following formula: body weight in kilograms × 2.3 × hemoglobin deficiency (target hemoglobin level – patient hemoglobin level). Add another 500 to 1000 mg iron to replace low iron stores. Parenteral iron preparations licensed for use in the United States include iron sucrose (Venofer), ferumoxytol (Feraheme), ferric carboxymaltose (Ferinject and Injectafer), and ferric gluconate (Ferrlecit). A common dose for iron sucrose is 200 mg IV over 2 to 5 minutes, which is often repeated 5 times or until the target dose of iron is reached. Ferumoxytol has a usual dose of 510 mg IV infusion over at least 15 minutes, which can be repeated 3 to 5 days after the initial dose. For patients who weigh ≥50 kg, the dose of ferric carboxymaltose is 750 mg IV over 15 to 30 minutes, and this can be repeated 7 days after the first dose. Ferric gluconate is generally used for patients on dialysis, and the typical dose is 125 mg IV over 10 minutes or IV infusion over 60 minutes per dialysis session.

Monitoring

The earliest marker for successful iron replacement is an increase in the reticulocyte count, which occurs within 5 to 10 days of initiation of iron replacement. Darkening of stools after 2 or 3 days of starting oral iron replacement is a reliable marker of compliance. A hemoglobin increase of 2 g/dL is considered an appropriate response to oral iron replacement. Reaching a serum ferritin level of 100 µg/L will ensure good iron stores in nearly all patients. Once iron deficiency has been corrected, a complete blood count and labs to evaluate iron stores should be checked monthly for 3 months and then every 3 months for a year. If iron levels are not maintained, then further work up is indicated to discover the cause.

Management of Complications

If properly treated, iron deficiency has few complications in adults. Untreated iron deficiency in infants and small children can lead to cognitive development and growth deficits. Treating iron deficiency without identifying the source and cause of blood loss could result in a delay or failure to diagnose gastrointestinal malignancies or other serious clinical problems.

Plummer–Vinson syndrome is a rare clinical condition characterized by a triad of iron deficiency anemia, post-cricoid esophageal webs, and dysphagia. The pathogenesis of Plummer-Vinson syndrome remains unclear, though iron and other nutritional deficiencies, genetic predisposition, and autoimmunity have all been implicated in the formation of the webs. Treatment includes the correction of iron deficiency and endoscopic dilation of the esophageal webs to relieve dysphagia.

References

Auerbach M, Adamson JW: How we diagnose and treat iron deficiency anemia, *Am J Hematol* 91(1):31–38, 2016 Jan.

Camaschella C, Girelli D: The changing landscape of iron deficiency, *Mol Aspects Med* 2020 Oct;75:100861. https://www.doi.org/10.1016/j.mam.2020.100861. Epub 2020 May 14. PMID: 32418671

Centers for Disease Control. Recommendation to Prevent and Control Iron Deficiency in the United States. Available at https://www.cdc.gov/MMWR/preview/mmwrhtml/00051880.htm. [Accessed April 16, 2019].

Craig WJ, Mangels AR, American Dietetic Association: Position of the American Dietetic Association: vegetarian diets, *J Am Diet Assoc* 109(7):1266–1282, 2009 Jul.

Engebretsen KV, Blom-Hogestol IK, Hewitt S, et al: Anemia following Roux-en-Y gastric bypass for morbid obesity; a 5-year follow-up study, *Scand J Gastroenterol* 53(8):917–922, 2018 Aug.

Guideline on haemoglobin cutoffs to define anaemia in individuals and populations. Geneva: World Health Organization; 2024. Licence: CC BY-NC-SA 3.0 IGO.

Le CHH. The Prevalence of Anemia and Moderate-Severe Anemia in the US Population (NHANES 2003-2012). *PLoS ONE* 11(11):e0166635, 2016.

Lopez A, Cacoub P, Macdougall IC, Peyrin-Biroulet L: Iron deficiency anaemia, *Lancet* 387(10021):907–916, 2016 Feb 27.

Parrott J, Frank L, Rabena R, Craggs-Dino L, Isom KA, Greiman L: American Society for Metabolic and Bariatric Surgery Integrated Health Nutritional Guidelines for the Surgical Weight Loss Patient 2016 Update: Micronutrients, *Surg Obes Relat Dis* 13(5):727–741, 2017 May.

Peyrin-Biroulet L, Williet N, Cacoub P: Guidelines on the diagnosis and treatment of iron deficiency across indications: a systematic review, *Am J Clin Nutr* 102(6):1585–1594, 2015 Dec.

Stoffel NU, Cercamondi CI, Brittenham G, et al: Iron absorption from oral iron supplements given on consecutive versus alternate days and as single morning doses versus twice–daily split dosing in iron–depleted women: two open–label, randomised controlled trials, *Lancet Haematol* 4(11):e524–33, 2017.

World Health Organization: Anaemia in women and children. Available at https://www.who.int/ data/gho/data/themes/topics/anaemia_in_women_and_children. [Accessed 30 March 2022].

MULTIPLE MYELOMA

Method of
S. Vincent Rajkumar, MD; and Shaji Kumar, MD

CURRENT DIAGNOSIS

- Malignant clonal plasma cell disorder
- Characterized by presence of a monoclonal immunoglobulin in the serum or urine in most patients
- Typical manifestations include anemia, osteolytic bone lesions, and renal failure
- Initial work-up should include a bone marrow aspiration and biopsy with fluorescent in situ hybridization studies to determine molecular cytogenetic-type
- Standard risk: myeloma without high risk features
- High risk: del(17p) or p53 mutation; biallelic deletion(1p), gain/amp(1q) plus del(1p), or gain/amp(1q) or del(1p) plus t(4;14), (t14;16) or t(14;20)

CURRENT THERAPY

- Do not begin treatment until symptomatic multiple myeloma develops (CRAB: calcium elevated, renal failure, anemia, bone lesions) or other myeloma defining events are present. Patients with high risk smoldering multiple myeloma are candidates for preventive therapy with daratumumab (Darzalez) for 3 years, or lenalidomide (Revlimid) or lenalidomide plus dexamethasone (Decadron)[1] (Rd) for 2 years.
- Decide whether an autologous stem cell transplant is feasible.
- Initial therapy typically consists of a quadruplet regimen such as daratumumab, bortezomib (Velcade), lenalidomide, and dexamethasone (Dara-VRd) or isatuximab (Sarclisa), bortezomib, lenalidomide, and dexamethasone (Isa-VRd).
- Patients who are candidates for autologous stem cell transplantation should collect stem cells after 3 to 4 cycles of induction. After collection, patients proceed to either early transplantation, or resume initial therapy and postpone transplant until relapse. After transplant, and after initial therapy in patients who delay transplant, patients should receive maintenance therapy.
- Patients who are not stem cell transplant candidates who are treated with Dara-VRd or Isa-VRd receive about 8 to 9 cycles of quadruplet therapy followed by maintenance. Frail

patients can be treated with a triplet regimen such as daratumumab, lenalidomide, dexamethasone (DRd), or isatuximab, lenalidomide, dexamethasone (Isa-Rd), or bortezomib, lenalidomide, dexamethasone (VRd), or if unable to tolerate a triplet, the doublet regimen of Rd.
- Relapsed or refractory myeloma should be treated with one of the active drugs given alone or in combination. Active agents include thalidomide, lenalidomide, bortezomib, carfilzomib (Kyprolis), pomalidomide (Pomalyst), daratumumab (Darzalex), ixazomib (Ninlaro), elotuzumab (Empliciti), isatuximab (Sarclisa), teclistamab (Tecvayli), talquetamab (Talvey), elranatamab (Elrexfio), selinexor (Xpovio), ide-cel (Abecma), cilta-cel (Carvykti), corticosteroids, anthracyclines, and alkylators.

Multiple myeloma is characterized by the neoplastic proliferation of clonal plasma cells. It is typically associated with a monoclonal (M) protein in the serum and/or urine.

Epidemiology

In the United States, multiple myeloma constitutes 1% of all malignant diseases and slightly more than 10% of hematologic malignancies. The annual incidence is 4 to 5 per 100,000; the incidence in African Americans is twice that in whites. The apparent recent increase in rates is probably caused by increased availability and use of medical facilities and improved diagnostic techniques, particularly in the older population. The median age at diagnosis is approximately 70 years.

Risk Factors

The cause of multiple myeloma is unclear. Exposure to radiation might play a role. Persons in agricultural occupations who are exposed to pesticides, herbicides, or fungicides have an increased risk of multiple myeloma. Benzene and petroleum products, hair dyes, engine exhaust, furniture worker products, obesity, and chronic immune stimulation have also been reported as risk factors. The risk of developing multiple myeloma is higher for patients with a first-degree relative with the disease. Clusters of two or more first-degree relatives or identical twins have been recognized.

Clinical Manifestations

Weakness, fatigue, bone pain, recurrent infections, and symptoms of hypercalcemia or renal insufficiency should alert the physician to the possibility of multiple myeloma. Anemia is present in 70% of patients at the time of diagnosis. An M protein is found in the serum or urine in more than 97% of patients with multiple myeloma by immunofixation studies and the serum free light chain (FLC) assay. Lytic lesions, osteoporosis, or fractures are present at diagnosis in 80% of patients and are best detected by whole body low-dose computed tomography (CT) or positron emission tomography (PET)/CT. Magnetic resonance imaging (MRI) and PET/CT are also helpful in patients who have skeletal pain but no abnormality on radiographs or when there are other clinical concerns about the extent of the disease. Conventional radiography is less sensitive and is no longer recommended. Hypercalcemia is present in 15% of patients, and the serum creatinine value is 2 mg/dL or greater in almost 20% of patients at diagnosis.

Diagnosis

If multiple myeloma is suspected, the patient should have, in addition to a complete history and physical examination:
- Determination of values for hemoglobin, leukocytes with differential count, platelets, serum creatinine, calcium, and uric acid
- A radiographic survey of bones, including humeri and femurs using low-dose whole body CT or PET-CT.

| BOX 1 | International Myeloma Working Group Diagnostic Criteria. |

Monoclonal Gammopathy of Undetermined Significance
- Serum M protein <3 g/dL
- Clonal bone marrow–plasma cells <10%
- Absence of end-organ damage (CRAB) attributable to a plasma cell proliferative disorder

Smoldering Multiple Myeloma
- Serum M protein ≥3 g/dL and/or clonal bone marrow–plasma cells 10%–60%
- Absence of myeloma defining events or amyloidosis

Multiple Myeloma
- Presence of clonal bone marrow plasma cells 10% or greater or biopsy-proven plasmacytoma
- Presence of end-organ damage (CRAB) thought to be related to a plasma cell proliferative disorder or other myeloma defining event (clonal bone marrow plasma cells 60% or higher, serum free light chain ratio 100 or more provided involved free light chain level is 100 mg/L or more, more than one focal lesion on magnetic resonance imaging)

CRAB, Calcium elevated, renal failure, anemia, bone lesions; M, monoclonal.
Derived from Rajkumar SV, Dimopoulos MA, Palumbo A, et al. International Myeloma Working Group updated criteria for the diagnosis of multiple myeloma. *Lancet Oncol.* 2014;15:e538–e548.

- Serum protein electrophoresis with immunofixation
- Quantitation of immunoglobulins (Igs), serum FLC assay
- Bone marrow aspirate and biopsy
- Routine urinalysis
- Electrophoresis and immunofixation of an adequately concentrated aliquot from a 24-hour urine specimen
- Fluorescence in situ hybridization (FISH)
- Measurement of β_2-microglobulin, C-reactive protein, and lactate dehydrogenase

Box 1 lists the International Myeloma Working Group updated criteria for diagnosis of myeloma and related disorders. Metastatic carcinoma, lymphoma, leukemia, and connective tissue disorders can resemble multiple myeloma and must be considered in the differential diagnosis. Patients with multiple myeloma must be differentiated from those with monoclonal gammopathy of undetermined significance (MGUS) and smoldering (asymptomatic) multiple myeloma (SMM). Patients with MGUS and low-risk SMM may remain stable for long periods and not require treatment (see Box 1). Patients with high-risk SMM (any two or more of the following: >20% bone marrow plasma cells, >2g/dL serum M protein, >20 serum FLC ratio) should be considered for daratumumab (Darzalex), or lenalidomide (Revlimid)[1] or lenalidomide plus dexamethasone (Decadron)[1] as preventive therapy.

Treatment

Patients with symptomatic multiple myeloma may be classified as having high-risk or standard-risk disease. High-risk disease is defined as the presence of del(17p) or p53 mutation; biallelic deletion(1p), gain/amp(1q) plus del(1p), or gain/amp(1q) or del(1p) plus t(4;14), t(14;16), or t(14;20). Lactate dehydrogenase, circulating plasma cells, and β_2-microglobulin levels are additional important risk factors. Approximately 20% of patients with symptomatic multiple myeloma have high-risk disease.

Initially, patients are classified into those eligible for an autologous stem cell transplant (SCT) versus those not eligible. An autologous SCT adds approximately 1 year of survival on average when compared with patients treated with conventional-dose chemotherapy alone.

Eligibility for autologous SCT in multiple myeloma varies from country to country. In the United States, decisions are made on a patient-by-patient basis depending on the physiologic age rather than the chronologic age. In most institutions, patients older than 70 years or with serum creatinine greater than 2.5 mg/dL, Eastern Cooperative Oncology Group (ECOG) performance status of 3 or 4, or New York Heart Association (NYHA) functional status class III or IV are considered ineligible for autologous SCT. Although patients with kidney failure may have an autologous SCT, the morbidity and mortality are higher.

Initial Therapy for Transplant-Eligible Patients

The approach to treatment of newly diagnosed myeloma in patients eligible for stem cell transplantation is summarized in Figure 1A. Currently we prefer a quadruplet regimen such as daratumumab (Darzalex), lenalidomide, bortezomib, dexamethasone (Dara-VRD) or isatuximab (Sarclisa), bortezomib, lenalidomide, dexamethasone (Isa-VRd) as initial therapy. Quadruplet regimens provide superior progression-free survival in randomized trials compared with triplet regimens. Bortezomib (Velcade), lenalidomide (Revlimid), dexamethasone (Decadon) (VRd) is an alternative to Dara-VRd, especially if daratumumab is not available or is unaffordable. Dexamethasone is administered once weekly. Lenalidomide is given at a dose of 25 mg daily on days 1 to 14 of a 21-day cycle. Bortezomib should be given using the once-weekly subcutaneous schedule to reduce the risk of peripheral neuropathy. Daratumumab, bortezomib, cyclophosphamide (Cytoxan) 300 mg/m² orally once weekly plus dexamethasone 40 mg once weekly (Dara-VCD) is an option for patients presenting with acute renal failure. In all regimens, it is preferable to administer dexamethasone at a dose no greater than 40 mg per week unless there is need for urgent cytoreduction as in patients with acute renal failure and cast nephropathy.

Autologous Stem Cell Transplantation

Following 3 to 4 months of induction therapy with one of the initial regimens, one must collect the stem cells in patients eligible for transplantation. The stem cells must be collected before the patient is exposed to prolonged therapy, especially melphalan (Alkeran). Granulocyte colony-stimulating factor (G-CSF, Neupogen) with or without cyclophosphamide (Cytoxan) is used for mobilizing stem cells. G-CSF plus cyclophosphamide is preferred in patients who are treated with lenalidomide plus dexamethasone induction, who are older than 65 years, or who have received such therapy for over 4 months. Plerixafor (Mozobil) may also be used for mobilization of hematopoietic stem cells. It is advisable to collect 6×10^6 CD34+ cells/kg, which is sufficient for two transplants in patients below 65 years of age.

The timing of autologous SCT takes into account the patient's wishes, and it may be done early (when the patient recovers from stem cell collection) or delayed until relapse. There is no difference in OS even at 8 years of follow up among patients who receive an autologous SCT immediately following collection of stem cells and those who receive it at first relapse. In general, we prefer an early transplant because this provides a better quality of life and time without therapy.

The preferred conditioning regimen for autologous SCT is melphalan (Evolmela) 200 mg/m².[3] Tandem transplantation is not recommended for most patients.

The mortality rate with autologous SCT is approximately 1%. Unfortunately, multiple myeloma is not eradicated, and the autologous peripheral stem cells are contaminated by myeloma cells or their precursors.

Bone marrow transplantation from an identical twin donor (syngeneic) is the treatment of choice if such a donor is available. Results are superior to allogeneic transplantation.

Maintenance Therapy Following Autologous Stem Cell Transplantation

Randomized trials have tested the value of lenalidomide as maintenance therapy following stem cell transplantation. An OS

---

[1]Not FDA approved for this indication.

[3]Exceeds dosage recommended by the manufacturer.

Newly Diagnosed Myeloma: Transplant Eligible

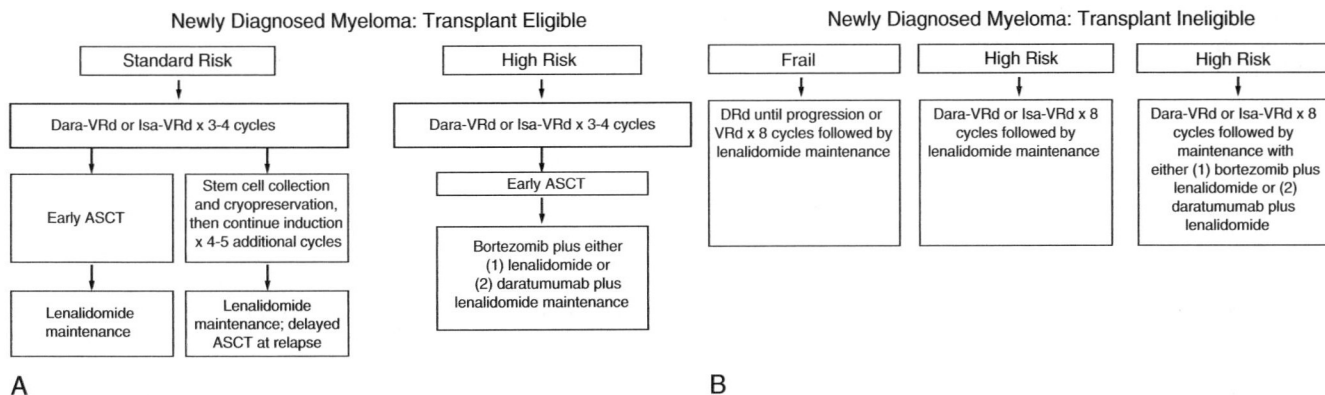

Standard Risk
- Dara-VRd or Isa-VRd x 3-4 cycles
- Early ASCT → Stem cell collection and cryopreservation, then continue induction x 4-5 additional cycles
- Lenalidomide maintenance → Lenalidomide maintenance; delayed ASCT at relapse

High Risk
- Dara-VRd or Isa-VRd x 3-4 cycles
- Early ASCT
- Bortezomib plus either (1) lenalidomide or (2) daratumumab plus lenalidomide maintenance

Newly Diagnosed Myeloma: Transplant Ineligible

Frail
- DRd until progression or VRd x 8 cycles followed by lenalidomide maintenance

High Risk
- Dara-VRd or Isa-VRd x 8 cycles followed by lenalidomide maintenance

High Risk
- Dara-VRd or Isa-VRd x 8 cycles followed by maintenance with either (1) bortezomib plus lenalidomide or (2) daratumumab plus lenalidomide

A   B

Figure 1 Approach to the treatment of newly diagnosed myeloma in patients eligible for stem cell transplantation (A) and approach to the treatment of newly diagnosed myeloma in patients not eligible for stem cell transplantation (B). *ASCT*, autologous stem cell transplantation; *Dara-VRd*, daratumumab, bortezomib, lenalidomide, dexamethasone; *DRd*, daratumumab, lenalidomide, dexamethasone; *Isa-Rd*, isatuximab, lenalidomide, dexamethasone; *Isa-VRd*, isatuximab, bortezomib, lenalidomide, dexamethasone. (Modified from Rajkumar SV. Multiple myeloma: 2024 update on diagnosis, risk-stratification, and management, *Am J Hematol* 99:1802–1824, 2024.)

benefit has been observed in a meta-analysis of three trials. This benefit appears to be mainly restricted to standard-risk patients. An increased risk of second cancers has been noted with lenalidomide maintenance and further follow-up is needed. In another randomized trial improved OS with bortezomib maintenance has been reported, but it is not clear whether the benefit is due to the maintenance therapy or differences in induction therapy between the two groups. We recommend lenalidomide maintenance for standard-risk patients following autologous SCT, and following approximately 12 months of initial therapy in patients not eligible for SCT and in patients who delay SCT. In high-risk patients, we recommend doublet maintenance with either bortezomib plus lenalidomide, or daratumumab plus lenaldiomide.

Allogeneic Transplantation

Allogeneic transplantation is currently not recommended for routine use outside of a clinical trial. An exception to this are young patients with high-risk disease in first relapse after autologous transplantation who are willing to assume the high treatment-related mortality associated with allogeneic SCT.

Initial Therapy for Patients Who Are Ineligible for Autologous Stem Cell Transplantation

The initial therapy for patients not eligible for transplantation now resembles that of transplant-eligible patients. The current approach to treatment of newly diagnosed myeloma in patients not eligible for stem cell transplantation is summarized in Figure 1B. Currently, we prefer either Dara-VRd or Isa-VRd; for frail patients the triplet regimens of daratumumab, lenalidomide, dexamethasone (DRd), isatuximab, lenalidomide, dexamethasone (Isa-Rd), or VRd can be considered.

When using VRd, we continue the initial chemotherapy regimen for approximately 6 to 9 cycles followed usually by lenalidomide maintenance in standard-risk patients and bortezomib plus lenalidomide maintenance in high-risk patients.

Relapsed or Refractory Multiple Myeloma

Almost all patients with multiple myeloma who survive eventually relapse. If relapse occurs more than 6 months after treatment is discontinued, the initial chemotherapy regimen should be reinstituted. Most patients respond again, but the duration and quality of response are usually inferior to the initial response. Recently, several new drugs have been approved for the treatment of multiple myeloma including pomalidomide (Pomalyst), carfilzomib (Kyprolis), daratumumab (Darzalex), elotuzumab (Empliciti), ixazomib (Ninlaro), selinexor (Xpovio), isatuximab (Sarclisa), teclistamab (Tecvayli), talquetamab (Talvey), elranatamab (Elrexfio), idecabtagene vicleucel (ide-cel [Abecma]), and ciltacabtagene autoleucel (ciltacel [Carvykti]).

Thalidomide

Thalidomide (Thalomid) is usually instituted in a dose of 50 to 100 mg daily and, if necessary, escalated to 200 mg daily if tolerated. It is most often used in combinations such as VTD. Side effects include sedation, fatigue, constipation, rash, deep venous thrombosis (DVT), edema, bradycardia, and hypothyroidism. Virtually all patients develop a sensorimotor peripheral neuropathy. The use of thalidomide in pregnancy is contraindicated, and the System for Thalidomide Education and Prescribing Safety (STEPS) program must be followed to prevent teratogenic effects.

Bortezomib

Bortezomib (Velcade) is a proteasome inhibitor that produces a response rate of approximately 35% in patients with relapsed or refractory myeloma. It is most often used in combinations such as VRD, VCD, or VTD to maximize response rates. The most troublesome side effect is peripheral neuropathy, which can occur in 35% to 40% of patients. The neuropathy is often painful but does improve in most patients after discontinuing bortezomib. The risk of neuropathy can be greatly reduced by using bortezomib in a once-weekly subcutaneous schedule.

Lenalidomide

Lenalidomide (Revlimid) as a single-agent produces an objective response in approximately 30% of patients with relapsed or refractory multiple myeloma. The major side effects are cytopenias, and the dose needs to be modified accordingly. The combination of lenalidomide plus low-dose dexamethasone (Rd) is the backbone of several myeloma treatment regimens.

Carfilzomib

Carfilzomib (Kyprolis) is a new proteasome inhibitor approved for the therapy of patients with multiple myeloma who have received at least two prior therapies, including both an immunomodulatory agent and bortezomib, and have disease progression on or within 60 days of the completion of the last therapy. Carfilzomib needs to be administered intravenously twice weekly. In a recent randomized trial, the combination of carfilzomib, lenalidomide, and dexamethasone (KRD) was found to have superior response rate, PFS, and OS compared with Rd.

Pomalidomide

Pomalidomide (Pomalyst) is an analog of lenalidomide and thalidomide. It has shown significant clinical activity in patients who are refractory to both bortezomib and lenalidomide (dual refractory). It is approved for patients with multiple myeloma who received at least two prior therapies, including both lenalidomide and bortezomib, and have disease progression on or within 60 days of the completion of the last therapy. It is administered orally at a dose of 2 to 4 mg daily for 21 days every 28 days. The major side effects are cytopenias and fatigue.

Elotuzumab

Elotuzumab (Empliciti) is a monoclonal antibody that is approved for the treatment of relapsed myeloma. It targets the signaling lymphocytic activation molecule F7 (SLAMF7). In a randomized trial of 646 patients, elotuzumab plus Rd was superior to Rd, median PFS 19.4 months versus 14.9 months, respectively ($P < .001$).

Daratumumab

Daratumumab (Darzalex) is a monoclonal antibody that is approved for the treatment of relapsed myeloma. It targets CD38, a molecule universally expressed on myeloma cells. Daratumumab has a response rate of approximately 30% in heavily pretreated patients. Two randomized trials have found improvement in PFS with the addition of daratumumab to Rd and bortezomib-dexamethasone, respectively.

Ixazomib

Ixazomib (Ninlaro) is an oral proteasome inhibitor approved for the treatment of relapsed myeloma. It is a boronic acid derivative similar to bortezomib. It is administered once weekly orally. Compared with bortezomib, it has a lower risk of peripheral neuropathy.

Selinexor

Selinexor (Xpovio) is an oral drug that acts by binding to nuclear export protein 1 (XPO1) and selectively blocking the transport of various proteins within the cell. It has been approved in combination with low dose dexamethasone for patients with relapsed or refractory multiple myeloma who have received at least 4 prior therapies, and whose disease is refractory to at least 2 proteasome inhibitors, at least 2 immunomodulatory agents, and an anti-CD38 monoclonal antibody. It is administered orally at a dose of 80 mg twice a week. However, due to toxicities, a once weekly regimen is likely more preferable.

Bispecific Antibodies

Three bispecific antibodies have been approved for use in relapsed refractory myeloma in patients who have failed at least 4 prior regimens. Two of these, teclistamab (Tecvayli) and elranatamab (Elrexfio), target the B-cell maturation antigen (BCMA), and one, talquetamab (Talvey), targets GPRC5D. These bispecific antibodies engage T-cells and are potent immunotherapeutic options in myeloma, with single agent response rates of approximately 60%. Cytokine release syndrome, neurotoxicity, and infections are the major side effects.

Chimeric Antigen Receptor T (CAR-T) Cell Therapy

Idecabtagene vicleucel (ide-cel; Abecma) and ciltacabtagene autoleucel (cilta-cel; Carvykti) are CAR-Ts targeting BCMA. They have been approved for patients with relapsed myeloma. Ide-cel is well tolerated, with less than 5% of patients experiencing severe cytokine release syndrome or neurological toxicity. It has a response rate of 73%, with a response duration of approximately 9 months. Cilta-cel is also well tolerated and has a 2-year progression free survival rate of approximately 60%.

Isatuximab

Isatuximab (Sarclisa) is a monoclonal antibody targeting CD38 and is an alternative to daratumumab. It has been approved in combination with pomalidomide and dexamethasone, as well as in combination with carfilzomib and dexamethasone. In certain patients, isatuximab may be significantly less expensive than daratumumab, which may be a consideration.

Other New Drugs

New drugs that are in clinical trials include new bi-specific antibodies such as cevostamab[5] (targeting FcRH5 and CD3). Venetoclax (Venclexta)[1] has shown promise against t11;14 subtype of multiple myeloma. Iberdomide[5] is a new cereblon targeting agent that has also shown promise.

Supportive Therapy
Radiotherapy

Palliative radiation in a dose of 20 to 30 Gy should be limited to patients who have disabling pain and a well-defined focal process that has not responded to chemotherapy. Analgesics in combination with chemotherapy usually can control the pain. This approach is preferred to local radiation because pain often occurs at another site, and local radiation does not benefit the patient with systemic disease. In addition, the myelosuppressive effects of radiotherapy and chemotherapy are cumulative and can restrict future therapy. Radiation is required for spinal cord compression from plasmacytoma. Postsurgical radiation after stabilization of fractures or impending fractures is rarely needed.

Hypercalcemia

Hypercalcemia must be suspected if the patient has anorexia, nausea, vomiting, polyuria, increased constipation, weakness, confusion, stupor, or coma. If it is untreated, renal insufficiency usually develops. Hydration, preferably with isotonic saline and prednisone (25 mg orally four times daily), is effective in many patients with mild to moderate hypercalcemia (calcium < 13 mg/dL). If more-severe hypercalcemia occurs, zoledronic acid (Zometa) at a dose of 4 mg intravenously over 15 minutes or pamidronate (Aredia) 90 mg given intravenously over at least 2 hours is indicated. Calcitonin (Miacalcin) may be used if rapid reduction of calcium levels is needed. Hemodialysis may be necessary for extremely severe hypercalcemia. The dosage of prednisone must be reduced and discontinued as soon as possible.

Renal Insufficiency

Approximately 20% of patients with multiple myeloma have a serum creatinine level of 2.0 mg/dL or more at diagnosis. Myeloma kidney (cast nephropathy) and hypercalcemia are the two major causes. Myeloma kidney is characterized by the presence of large, waxy, laminated casts in the distal and collecting tubules. Some light chains are very nephrotoxic, but no specific amino acid sequence of the nephrotoxic light chain has been identified.

Dehydration, infection, nonsteroidal antiinflammatory agents, and radiographic contrast media can contribute to acute kidney failure. Hyperuricemia or amyloid deposition can produce renal insufficiency. Nephrotic syndrome rarely occurs in multiple myeloma unless amyloidosis is present.

Maintenance of a high fluid intake producing 3 L of urine per 24 hours is important for preventing kidney failure in patients with Bence Jones proteinuria. If hyperuricemia occurs, allopurinol (Zyloprim) in doses of 300 mg daily provides effective therapy.

Acute kidney failure should be treated promptly with appropriate fluid and electrolyte replacement. Patients with kidney failure should be treated with either VCD or VTD to reduce the tumor mass as quickly as possible. A trial of plasmapheresis is reasonable in an attempt to prevent chronic dialysis. Hemodialysis and peritoneal dialysis are equally effective and are necessary for patients with symptomatic azotemia.

Anemia

Almost every patient with multiple myeloma eventually becomes anemic. Increased plasma volume from the osmotic effect of the M protein can produce hypervolemia and can spuriously lower

---

[1]Not FDA approved for this indication.
[5]Investigational drug in the United States.

the hemoglobin and hematocrit values. Patients with significant symptoms should be considered for red blood cell transfusion. If a transfusion is indicated, irradiated leukocyte-reduced red cells are preferred.

In patients with newly diagnosed myeloma, induction chemotherapy is often associated with a prompt improvement in hemoglobin levels, so it is better to avoid the use of erythropoietin. Erythropoietin (Epogen) should be seriously considered in relapsed patients receiving chemotherapy who have a persistent, symptomatic hemoglobin level of 10 g/dL or less.

Erythropoietin reduces the transfusion requirement and increases hemoglobin concentration in more than half of patients. Those with low serum erythropoietin values are more likely to respond. Most physicians proceed with a trial of erythropoietin 150 U/kg three times weekly or 40,000 U once a week. Darbepoetin, a long-lasting erythropoietin (Aranesp), may be given weekly or biweekly. Erythropoietin should be discontinued when the hemoglobin reaches 11 g/dL.

Skeletal Lesions

Bone lesions manifested by pain and fractures are a major problem. A skeletal radiographic survey should be repeated at 6-month intervals or sooner if pain develops. Patients should be encouraged to be as active as possible because confinement to bed increases demineralization of the skeleton. Trauma must be avoided because even mild stress can result in a fracture. Fixation of long bone fractures or impending fractures with an intramedullary rod and methyl methacrylate gives excellent results.

All patients with multiple myeloma who have lytic lesions, pathologic fractures, or severe osteopenia should receive an intravenous bisphosphonate. Pamidronate (Aredia) 90 mg intravenously over 2 hours every 4 weeks or zoledronic acid (Zometa) 4 mg intravenously over 15 minutes every 4 weeks are equally efficacious. The dosage of bisphosphonates should be reduced with renal insufficiency. Because renal insufficiency or nephrotic-range proteinuria can occur, serum creatinine and 24-hour urine protein monitoring is necessary. One should seriously consider stopping the intravenous bisphosphonate in patients who have responsive or stable disease after 2 years of therapy. In other patients, we recommend reducing the dose to once every 3 months. A randomized trial has found that denosumab (Xgeva), a monoclonal antibody targeting RANKL, may be as effective in reducing skeletal events as zoledronic acid and may be an option for selected patients with significant renal impairment.

Bisphosphonates should be resumed upon relapse with new-onset skeletal-related events. Osteonecrosis of the jaw can occur in patients receiving bisphosphonates. Although the relationship is unclear, it is essential to obtain a complete dental evaluation and perform preventive dental treatment before beginning bisphosphonates. The patient should practice good oral hygiene during therapy. Invasive procedures (especially dental extractions) should be avoided during bisphosphonate therapy. Osteonecrosis of the jaw should be managed conservatively.

Vertebroplasty or kyphoplasty may be helpful for patients with an acute compression fracture of the spine. Both have been associated with pain relief. Results appear to be better when the procedure is performed shortly after the compression fracture. Leakage of the methyl methacrylate is a potential adverse event. A choice between vertebroplasty and kyphoplasty depends on the expertise of the physician performing the procedure.

Infections

Bacterial infections are more common in patients with myeloma than in the general population. All patients should receive pneumococcal and influenza immunizations despite their suboptimal antibody response. Substantial fever is an indication for appropriate cultures, chest radiography, and consideration of antibiotic therapy. The greatest risk for infection is during the first 3 months after chemotherapy is initiated, and prophylactic antibiotics (levofloxacin [Levaquin] or cotrimoxazole [Bactrim]) should be considered during this period. Antiviral prophylaxis (acyclovir [Zovirax] 400 mg twice daily or valacyclovir [Valtrex] 500 mg once daily) should be given to all patients receiving bortezomib because of the increased risk of herpes zoster. Intravenous immunoglobulin (IVIg, Gammagard)[1] may be helpful in selected patients who have recurrent serious infections despite the use of prophylactic antibiotics. It is inconvenient, associated with side effects, and very expensive. Consequently, few of our patients receive IVIg.

Hyperviscosity Syndrome

Symptoms of hyperviscosity can include oronasal bleeding, gastrointestinal bleeding, blurred vision, neurologic symptoms, or congestive heart failure. Most patients have symptoms when the serum viscosity measurement is more than 4 cP, but the relationship between serum viscosity and clinical manifestations is not precise. The decision to perform plasmapheresis, which promptly relieves the symptoms of hyperviscosity, should be made on clinical grounds rather than serum viscosity levels. Hyperviscosity is more common in IgA myeloma than in IgG myeloma.

Extradural Myeloma (Cord Compression)

The possibility of cord compression must be considered if weakness of the legs or difficulty in voiding or defecating occurs. The sudden onset of severe radicular pain or severe back pain with neurologic symptoms suggests compression of the spinal cord. MRI or CT of the entire spine must be performed immediately. Radiation therapy in a dose of approximately 30 Gy is beneficial in about one half of patients. Dexamethasone (Decadron)[1] should be administered in addition to radiation therapy. Surgical decompression is necessary only if the neurologic deficit does not improve.

Venous Thromboembolism

Patients with multiple myeloma have an increased risk of venous thromboembolism. This is due to the malignancy itself, as well as therapy with lenalidomide, thalidomide, or pomalidomide. All patients receiving lenalidomide (or thalidomide or pomalidomide) need DVT prophylaxis with aspirin[1] (81 mg or 325 mg daily) or full-dose warfarin (Coumadin)[1] or low-molecular-weight heparin.[1]

Emotional Support

All patients with multiple myeloma need substantial and continuing emotional support. The physician's approach must be positive in emphasizing the potential benefits of therapy. It is reassuring for patients to know that some survive for 10 years or more. It is vital that the physician caring for patients with multiple myeloma has the interest and capacity for dealing with incurable disease over the span of years with assurance, sympathy, and resourcefulness.

---

[1]Not FDA approved for this indication.

References

Anderson K, Ismaila N, Flynn PJ, et al: Role of bone-modifying agents in multiple myeloma: American Society of Clinical Oncology Clinical Practice Guideline Update, *J Clin Oncol*, 2018 Jan 17, JCO2017766402. Available at: 10.1200/JCO.2017.76.6402 [Epub ahead of print].

Attal M, Lauwers-Cances V, Marit G, et al: Lenalidomide maintenance after stem-cell transplantation for multiple myeloma, *N Engl J Med* 366:1782–1791, 2012.

Chari A, Minnema MC, Berdeja JG, et al: Talquetamab, a T-cell–redirecting GPRC5D bispecific antibody for multiple myeloma, *N Engl J Med* 387(24):2232–2244, 2022.

Dimopoulos MA, Oriol A, Nahi H, et al: Daratumumab, lenalidomide, and dexamethasone for multiple myeloma, *N Engl J Med* 375(14):1319–1331, 2016.

Facon T, Dimopoulos MA, Leleu XP, et al.: Isatuximab, bortezomib, lenalidomide, and dexamethasone for multiple myeloma, *N Engl J Med* 391(17):1597–1609, 2024.

Facon T, Kumar S, Piesner T, et al: Daratumumab plus lenalidomide and dexamethasone for untreated myeloma, *N Engl J Med* 380(22):2104–2115, 2019.

Krishnan A, Pasquini MC, Logan B, et al: Autologous haemopoietic stem-cell transplantation followed by allogeneic or autologous haemopoietic stem-cell transplantation in patients with multiple myeloma (BMT CTN 0102): a phase 3 biological assignment trial, *Lancet Oncol* 12:1195–1203, 2011.

Kyle RA, Rajkumar SV: Epidemiology of the plasma-cell disorders, *Best Pract Res Clin Haematol* 20:637–664, 2007.

Lonial S, Lee HC, Badros A, et al: Belantamab mafodotin for relapsed or refractory multiple myeloma (DREAMM-2): a two-arm, randomised, open-label, phase 2 study, *Lancet Oncol* 21:207–221, 2020.

McCarthy PL, Owzar K, Hofmeister CC, et al: Lenalidomide after stem-cell transplantation for multiple myeloma, *N Engl J Med* 366:1770–1781, 2012.

Moreau P, Garfall AL, van de Donk N, et al.: Teclistamab in relapsed or refractory multiple myeloma, *N Engl J Med* 387(6):495–505, 2022.

Munshi NC, Anderson LD, Shah N, et al: Idecabtagene vicleucel in relapsed and refractory myeloma, *N Engl J Med* 384:705–716, 2021.

Rajkumar SV, Jacobus S, Callander NS, et al: Lenalidomide plus high-dose dexamethasone versus lenalidomide plus low-dose dexamethasone as initial therapy for newly diagnosed multiple myeloma: an open-label randomised controlled trial, *Lancet Oncol* 11:29–37, 2010.

Rajkumar SV, et al: International Myeloma Working Group updated criteria for the diagnosis of multiple myeloma, *Lancet Oncol* 15:e538–e548, 2014.

Richardson PG, Jacobus SJ, Weller EA, et al.: Triplet therapy, transplantation, and maintenance until progression in myeloma, *N Engl J Med* 387(2):132–147, 2022.

Rodriguez-Otero P, Ailawadhi S, Arnulf B, et al.: Ide-cel or standard regimens in relapsed and refractory multiple myeloma. *N Engl J Med* 388(11):1002–1014, 2023.

San-Miguel J, Dhakal B, Yong K, et al.: Cilta-cel or standard care in lenalidomide-refractory multiple myeloma, *N Engl J Med* 389(4):335–347, 2023.

Sonneveld P, Dimopoulos MA, Boccadoro M, et al.: Daratumumab, bortezomib, lenalidomide, and dexamethasone for multiple myeloma, *N Engl J Med* 390(4):301–313, 2024.

MYELODYSPLASTIC SYNDROMES

Method of
Wafik George Sedhom, MD; and Jamile M. Shammo, MD

CURRENT DIAGNOSIS

- Myelodysplastic syndromes (MDSs) are diseases of the elderly.
- Chronic unexplained cytopenias should be evaluated to rule out MDSs.
- Bone marrow biopsy with cytogenetic testing is necessary for diagnosis.
- The International Prognostic Scoring System, Revised IPSS, and Molecular IPSS are important tools for risk stratification and choice of therapy.

CURRENT THERAPY

- Myelodysplastic syndromes are broadly divided into two therapeutic categories per the International Prognostic Scoring System (IPSS): low-risk disease (encompassing low and intermediate-1 risk groups), and high-risk disease (encompassing intermediate-2 and high-risk groups).
- The Revised IPSS defines five prognostic groups (very low, low, intermediate, high, and very high risk). Treatment options are also dependent on risk category.
- Patients with low-risk disease should receive supportive care and hematopoietic growth factors or luspatercept (Reblozyl); those with the deletion 5q abnormality should be treated with lenalidomide (Revlimid).
- Patients with high-risk disease should be treated with a hypomethylating agent and should be considered for allogeneic stem cell transplantation.

Epidemiology

Myelodysplastic syndrome (MDS) has an annual incidence of approximately 4 in 100,000 people in the United States. Disease incidence increases with age, with a median age of diagnosis of 76 years. Disease in patients younger than 50 years is rare except in the case of therapy-related MDS (t-MDS). Whites are the most affected at 4.2 cases per 100,000 person-years. Men are nearly twice as likely to be affected as women (5.8 vs. 3.3 per 100,000 per year), except in the case of MDS with isolated del(5q), which is more common in women.

Risk Factors

MDS can be classified as primary or secondary. Primary (or de novo) MDS indicates disease where no inciting exposure can be identified. Secondary MDS occurs from exposure to various substances. t-MDS occurs in patients exposed to certain chemotherapeutics, radiotherapy, or both. The onset of t-MDS varies from 2 to 10 years depending on the agent implicated. Tobacco use and occupational exposure to solvents and agricultural chemicals have also been associated with MDS development. A minority of MDS cases might have evolved from an antecedent hematologic disorder such as aplastic anemia or paroxysmal nocturnal hemoglobinuria (PNH). Several rare and inherited genetic "bone marrow failure syndromes"—such as Fanconi anemia, dyskeratosis congenita, Diamond-Blackfan anemia, and Shwachman-Diamond syndrome—have been associated with a higher risk of developing MDS.

Pathophysiology

Ineffective hematopoiesis and resulting cytopenias are major features of the disease. The first step in MDS development arises from a driver mutation in a hematopoietic stem cell that gives growth and survival advantage over wild type cells in the bone marrow. Over time, this mutated stem cell uses hematogenous spread to reach other bone marrow sites (clonal hematopoiesis of indeterminate potential [CHIP]). Additional mutations that increase proliferation are acquired over time until this clone becomes dominant in the bone marrow. Excessive apoptosis of myeloid progenitors, abnormal responses to cytokines and growth factors, epigenetic aberrations resulting in gene silencing, chromosomal abnormalities, and a defective bone marrow microenvironment have all been described in association with MDS. Our understanding of CHIP and clonal cytopenia of undetermined significance in the development of MDS is evolving.

Clinical Manifestations

Some patients with MDS are asymptomatic, but the majority present with cytopenias. Anemia is the most common cytopenia (usually macrocytic), and patients can develop fatigue, pallor, and dyspnea. If presenting with neutropenia or thrombocytopenia, they can develop infections or bleeding/bruising, respectively. Infection is the cause of death in approximately 20% to 35% of cases. Organomegaly and lymphadenopathy are uncommon. Systemic symptoms, like fevers, chills, or weight loss, are uncommon and may be initial signs of progression to leukemia. MDS can transform to acute myeloid leukemia (AML) in 25% to 30% of cases.

Diagnosis

The diagnosis of MDS can be challenging because of its similarity in clinical manifestations and pathology to disorders such as aplastic anemia, myeloproliferative neoplasms, and acute leukemia. The evaluation for MDS begins with a thorough history of potential exposures, family history of bone marrow failure syndromes, and full physical examination. Complete blood cell count may show cytopenias. Iron studies, vitamin B12, and folate levels should be obtained to identify other causes of cytopenias. Peripheral blood smear may show a pseudo–Pelger-Huet anomaly, blasts, or macrocytic red blood cells (RBCs). Patients with unexplained cytopenia(s) should be referred to a hematologist for further evaluation. The gold standard test is bone marrow biopsy and aspirate to identify myeloid dysplasia. Iron stains on the marrow are needed to identify ring sideroblasts, and cytogenetic analysis will identify chromosomal abnormalities driving the disease (observed in 50% to 60% of patients).

TABLE 1	The WHO 5th Edition Classification of MDS		
CLASSIFICATION	BLASTS	CYTOGENETICS	MUTATIONS
MDS With Defining Genetic Abnormalities			
MDS with low blasts and isolated 5q deletion (MDS-5q)	<5% BM and <2% PB	5q deletion alone, or with 1 other abnormality other than monosomy 7 or 7q deletion	
MDS with low blasts and SF3B1 mutation (MDS-SF3B1)		Absence of 5q deletion, monosomy 7, or complex karyotype	SF3B1
MDS with biallelic TP53 inactivation (MDS-biTP53)	<20% BM and PB	Usually complex	Two or more TP53 mutations, or 1 mutation with evidence of TP53 copy number loss or cnLOH
MDS, Morphologically Defined			
MDS with low blasts (MDS-LB)	<5% BM and <2% PB		
MDS, hypoplastic (MDS-h)			
MDS with increased blasts (MDS-IB)			
MDS-IB1	5–9% BM or 2–4% PB		
MDS-IB2	10-19% BM or 5–19% PB or Auer rods		
MDS with fibrosis (MDS-f)	5–19% BM; 2–19% PB		

BM, Bone marrow; *IB*, increased blasts; *MDS*, myelodysplastic syndrome; *PB*, peripheral blood.
Adapted from Alaggio R, et al.: The World Health Organization Classification of Haematolymphoid Tumours: Lymphoid Neoplasms, ed 5. *Leukemia* 36:1720–1748, 2022.

Bone marrow dysplasia involving at least 10% of the cells of a specific myeloid lineage is the hallmark of MDS. The marrow is usually hypercellular. Next-generation sequencing is a highly sensitive test that identifies mutated genes encoding for splicing factors, epigenetic modifiers, and transcription factors, among others. Examples include *SF3B1*, *TET2*, *ASXL1*, *TP53*, and *RUNX1*. These genes can assist in prognostication (*TP53* in del[5q] MDS) or confirming the diagnosis (*SF3B1* in MDS with ringed sideroblasts [MDS-RS]).

Differential Diagnosis

The differential diagnosis of MDS includes other causes of dysplasia. Nutritional deficiencies of vitamin B12, folate, and copper should be ruled out. Drugs such as ganciclovir (Cytovene), valproic acid (Valproic), zinc, and mycophenolate mofetil (CellCept) have also been implicated in dysplastic marrow. These changes are reversible with discontinuation of the drug. Infections of HIV and parvovirus B19 can contribute to cytopenia and dysplasia as well. Hematopoietic disorders such as large granular lymphocytic leukemia and aplastic anemia also should be ruled out. All these reactive causes of dysplasia should be thoroughly evaluated before the diagnosis of MDS is confirmed.

Classification and Risk Stratification

Beginning in 1982, there have been efforts to classify subtypes of MDS to risk-stratify and guide management. The French-American-British (FAB) classification was the first. Currently, two classification schemes are used most widely: the World Health Organization (WHO) and the International Consensus Classification (ICC).

The WHO fifth edition classification (2022) builds upon the principles made with the fourth edition and further separates distinct clinical entities based on genetics or morphology, reflecting the increasing understanding genetics play in the development, prognosis, and therapy for this disease. Genetic categories include MDS with low blasts and del(5q), MDS with low blasts and *SF3B1* mutation (replacing MDS-RS), and MDS with biallelic *TP53* inactivation (a newly defined subtype). Morphologic categories include MDS with low blasts, hypoplastic MDS, and MDS with increased blasts, which is further divided based on blast percentage (Table 1). The 20% blast cutoff that defines AML is retained.

The ICC classification divides MDS into subtypes based on either cytogenetics, the percentage of blasts, or on the amount of dysplasia present. Cytogenetic categories include MDS with mutated *SF3B1* and MDS with deletion of chromosome 5q. MDS with *TP53* mutation is classified into a separate category of *TP53*-mutated myeloid neoplasms (given the clinical similarities of this mutation). Categories of dysplasia include MDS, not otherwise specified without dysplasia, MDS with single lineage dysplasia, and MDS with multiple lineage dysplasia. MDS with excess blasts defines 5% to 9% blasts in bone marrow, whereas the category MDS/AML encompasses blast counts of 10% to 19% (Table 2).

The International Prognostic Scoring System (IPSS) was introduced in 1997 to address the variability in prognosis within FAB subtypes. It predicts survival and risk of evolution to acute leukemia. The IPSS is calculated by adding scores assigned to three variables: blast cell count, cytogenetics, and number of cytopenias. The IPSS was revised in 2012 (IPSS-R) to incorporate five cytogenetic categories and account for the depth of cytopenias in MDS (Tables 3 to 5). IPSS-M is the latest prognostic scoring system that incorporates molecular data. It has the advantages of being personalized to the molecular profile, easy to interpret (an increase of 1 is equal to doubling of risk), and more accurate than the IPSS-R in prognosticating overall survival and transformation to AML. Although the IPSS-M is emerging as a new predictive model, the IPSS and IPSS-R are still widely used to predict the prognosis and clinical behavior of MDS patients and to guide choice of therapy.

Treatment

The treatment of MDS varies from supportive care to allogeneic stem cell transplantation. The objectives of treatment may be improving quality of life, delaying morbidity, extending overall survival, or cure. The treating physician should determine which of these objectives is right for each patient—a decision made by looking at a patient's age, comorbidities, risk (based on IPSS-R/IPSS-M), and incorporation of patient's goals. Stratification into lower-risk and higher-risk MDS is key to guiding management. There are several medications approved by the U.S. Food and Drug Administration (FDA) for MDS treatment, including recent advances that are sure to change the treatment landscape for years to come.

Supportive Care

Supportive care has been the cornerstone of MDS therapy for decades; it includes RBC transfusion for symptomatic anemia, platelet transfusion to reduce the risk of bleeding or to treat bleeding, and use of hematopoietic growth factors such as erythropoiesis-stimulating agents (ESAs) and colony-stimulating factors such as granulocyte

TABLE 2 | ICC Classification of MDS

CLASSIFICATION	DYSPLASTIC LINEAGES	CYTOPENIAS	CYTOSES*	BM AND PB BLASTS	CYTOGENETICS	MUTATIONS
MDS with mutated SF3B1 (MDS-SF3B1)	Typically ≥1	≥1	0	<5% BM; <2% PB	Any, except isolated del(5q), −7/del(7q), abn3q26.2, or complex	SF3B1 (≥ 10% VAF), without multi-hit TP53, or RUNX1
MDS with del(5q)	Typically ≥1	≥1	Thrombocytosis allowed	<5% BM; <2% PB	del(5q), with up to 1 additional, except −7/del(7q)	Any, except multi-hit TP53
MDS, NOS without dysplasia	0	≥1	0	<5% BM; <2% PB	−7/del(7q) or complex	Any, except multi-hit TP53 or SF3B1 (≥ 10% VAF)
MDS, NOS with single lineage dysplasia	1	≥1	0	<5% BM; <2% PB	Any, except not meeting criteria for MDS-del(5q)	Any, except multi-hit TP53; not meeting criteria for MDS-SF3B1
MDS, NOS with multilineage dysplasia	≥2	≥1	0	<5% BM; <2% PB	Any, except not meeting criteria for MDS-del(5q)	Any, except multi-hit TP53; not meeting criteria for MDS-SF3B1
MDS with excess blasts (MDS-EB)	Typically ≥1	≥1	0	5-9% BM; 2-9% PB	Any	Any, except multi-hit TP53
MDS/AML	Typically ≥1	≥1	0	10-19% BM or PB	Any, except AML-defining	Any, except NPM1, bZIP CEBPA or TP53
MDS with mutated TP53	—	Any	0	0-9% BM or PB	Complex karyotype often with loss of 17p	Multi-hit TP53 mutation or TP53 mutation (VAF >10%)

*Cytoses: Sustained white blood count ≥ 13 × 10⁹/L, monocytosis (≥0.5 × 10⁹/L and ≥10% of leukocytes) or platelets ≥450 × 10⁹/L; thrombocytosis is allowed in MDS-del(5q) or in any MDS case with inv(3) or t(3;3) cytogenetic abnormality.
AML, Acute myeloid leukemia; *BM,* bone marrow; *MDS,* myelodysplastic syndrome; *NOS,* not otherwise specified; *PB,* peripheral blood; *VAF,* variable allele frequency.
Adapted from Arber DA, et al.: International consensus classification of myeloid neoplasms and acute leukemias: integrating morphologic, clinical, and genomic data, *Blood* 140,11: 1200–1228, 2022.

TABLE 3 | IPSS-R Prognostic Score Values

PROGNOSTIC VARIABLE	0	0.5	1	1.5	2	3	4
Cytogenetics	Very Good	-	Good	-	Intermediate	Poor	Very Poor
BM Blast %	≤2	-	>2-<5%	-	5-10%	>10%	-
Hemoglobin	≥10	-	8-<10	<8	-	-	-
Platelets	≥100	50-<100	<50	-	-	-	-
ANC	≥0.8	<0.8	-	-	-	-	-

ANC, Absolute neutrophil count; *BM,* bone marrow.

TABLE 4 | IPSS-R Prognostic Risk Categories/Scores

RISK CATEGORY	RISK SCORE
Very Low	≤1.5
Low	>1.5–3
Intermediate	>3–4.5
High	>4.5–6
Very High	>6

TABLE 5 | IPSS-R Cytogenetic Groups

CYTOGENETIC PROGNOSTIC SUBGROUPS	CYTOGENETIC ABNORMALITIES
Very good	-Y, del(11q)
Good	Normal, del(5q), del(12p), del(20q), double including del(5q)
Intermediate	del(7q), +8, +19, i(17q), any other single or double independent clones
Poor	-7, inv(3)/t(3q)/del(3q), double including -7/del(7q), Complex: 3 abnormalities
Very poor	Complex: >3 abnormalities

From Greenberg PL, Tuechler H, Schanz J, et al. Revised International Prognostic Scoring System (IPSS-R) for myelodysplastic syndromes, *Blood* 120:2454–2465, 2012.

colony-stimulating factor filgrastim (Neupogen)[1] and granulocyte-macrophage colony stimulating factor sargramostim (Leukine)[1]. The last two cytokines have limited efficacy and are not routinely recommended for the treatment of MDS-related neutropenia.

---

[1] Not FDA approved for this indication.

ESAs are generally indicated for symptomatic anemia, transfusion-dependence, or Hgb less than 10 g/dL. Two ESAs are currently available: a recombinant human erythropoietin (rhu-EPO; epoetin alfa [Epogen, Procrit])[1] and a supersialylated form of EPO (darbepoetin alfa [Aranesp])[1]. These are considered the standard of care for the treatment of anemia in patients with low-risk MDS. A predictive model for response to such treatment has been developed by the Nordic MDS study group to guide patient selection. In general, patients with a serum EPO level less than 500 mU/mL and low transfusion burden (<2 units pRBC/month) are likely to respond by improving their hemoglobin level and reducing their need for transfusions.

Thrombopoietin agonists such as romiplostim (N-Plate)[1] and eltrombopag (Promacta)[1] are not yet FDA approved but are sometimes used to alleviate symptomatic thrombocytopenia. Although they have been shown to reduce thrombocytopenia and bleeding rates, they can increase the blast count in some patients. Trials are being conducted to evaluate the efficacy and safety of this intervention.

Immunomodulatory Drugs

The novel class of immunomodulatory drugs includes thalidomide (Thalomid)[1] and lenalidomide (Revlimid). Thalidomide was investigated initially with some success in patients with low-risk disease. However, its use was compromised because of poor tolerability. Lenalidomide has been approved for the treatment of patients with low-risk MDS with deletion 5q because it was shown in clinical trials to result in transfusion independence in about two-thirds of such patients.

Luspatercept (Reblozyl)

A recombinant fusion protein that acts as a ligand trap for transforming growth factor beta superfamily has shown positive results in early phase trials in ameliorating anemia in transfusion-dependent MDS patients. The pivotal MEDALIST trial was a randomized, double-blind, placebo-controlled trial that evaluated the efficacy of luspatercept as defined by the proportion of patients who achieved RBC transfusion independence during any consecutive 8-week period between weeks 1 and 24 of therapy and enrolled 229 transfusion dependent patients with low-risk MDS-RS who were randomized at 2:1 to either luspatercept or placebo. The trial demonstrated that 37.9% of those who were randomized to luspatercept achieved the primary efficacy endpoint compared with 13.2% who received placebo (P < 0.0001). Subsequently, the drug was approved by the FDA in 2020 for the treatment of anemia in transfusion-dependent patients with MDS-RS and MDS with ringed sideroblasts and thrombocytosis (MDS-RS-T). The phase III, randomized COMMANDS trial published in 2023 looked to study luspatercept frontline in ESA naïve low-risk MDS. Its primary endpoint was RBC transfusion independence for at least 12 weeks with a Hgb increase of 1.5 g/dL. Results demonstrated a 59% response with luspatercept versus 31% with ESA alone. This data has pushed luspatercept to first line in a subset of low-risk MDS patients.

Imetelstat

Imetelstat[5] is a telomerase inhibitor that has shown impressive results in the IMerge trial. This double-blind, placebo-controlled trial randomized patients who were refractory or ineligible for ESAs to imetelstat or placebo. For patients reaching the primary endpoint of 8-week transfusion independence, Hgb increased on average 3.6 g/dL with imetelstat compared with placebo, which offers significant improvement in quality of life. Although not yet approved for MDS, it is an exciting new treatment possibility.

Hypomethylating Agents

Two parenteral hypomethylating agents are currently approved for the treatment of MDS: 5-azacitidine (Vidaza) and decitabine (Dacogen). These agents are cytosine analogs known to inhibit and deplete DNA methyltransferase, which adds a methyl group to cytosine residues in newly formed DNA, resulting in the formation of hypomethylated DNA in vitro. The exact mechanism of action in vivo has not yet been identified. Results of randomized clinical trials comparing these agents to best supportive care in patients with MDS have demonstrated a statistically significant improvement in response rate and hematologic improvement. It has been shown for the first time that treatment with 5-azacitidine was reported to result in prolongation of survival in patients with Int-2 and high-risk disease. Both drugs have myelosuppressive properties and comparable response rates. In 2020 an oral hypomethylating agent combining decitabine and cedazuridine (Inqovi) was approved by the FDA for MDS.

Immunosuppressive Therapy

Immunosuppressive therapy with antithymocyte globulin (Thymoglobulin)[1] or cyclosporine (Neoral)[1] or both was evaluated in several clinical trials and was shown to result in durable hematologic responses in a subset of MDS patients—specifically, younger patients with low-risk disease, hypocellular marrows, PNH clone, human leukocyte antigen (HLA)-DR 15 phenotype, and low transfusion need.

Hematopoietic Stem Cell Transplantation

Allogeneic stem cell transplantation is the only curative therapy for MDS patients; this option is feasible for a small subset: typically younger patients with good performance status and an available HLA-matched donor. Approximately 40% of patients can be cured with this modality. The recent introduction of reduced intensity conditioning regimens and nonmyeloablative transplants has resulted in expanding the age limit for performing the procedure, thus reducing transplant-related complications and mortality. However, it has been associated with a higher risk of relapse. Because stem cell transplantation is associated with a high rate of treatment-related death (estimated at 39% at 1 year) and the development of acute and chronic graft-versus-host disease, such treatment is recommended only to patients with high-risk disease. Patients with low-risk MDS may be considered for transplant at disease progression.

Conclusion and Future Direction

MDS is a chronic disease characterized by bone marrow dysplasia with a variable propensity for leukemic evolution. It is curable only by allogeneic stem cell transplantation, which is feasible in only a small subset of patients. For all others, the treatment goal is aimed at improving quality of life and prolonging survival. New drugs are being studied to improve quality of life for patients with MDS, with several exciting changes on the horizon. Meanwhile, a great deal of research is focused on understanding the molecular underpinning of this heterogeneous disorder to enhance our understanding of its biology.

References

Arber DA, Orazi A, Hasserjian RP, Borowitz MJ, Calvo KR, Kvasnicka HM, et al: International consensus classification of myeloid neoplasms and acute leukemias: integrating morphologic, clinical, and genomic data, *Blood* 140(11):1200–1228, 2022.

Bejar R, Stevenson K, Abdel-Wahab O, Galili N, Nilsson B, Garcia-Manero G, et al: Clinical effect of point mutations in myelodysplastic syndromes, *N Engl J Med* 364(26):2496–2506, 2011.

Cazzola M: Myelodysplastic syndromes, *N Engl J Med* 383(14):1358–1374, 2020.

de Swart L, Smith A, Johnston TW, Haase D, Droste J, Fenaux P, et al: Validation of the revised international prognostic scoring system (IPSS-R) in patients with lower-risk myelodysplastic syndromes: a report from the prospective European LeukaemiaNet MDS (EUMDS) registry, *Br J Haematol* 170(3):372–383, 2015.

Fenaux P, Platzbecker U, Mufti GJ, Garcia-Manero G, Buckstein R, Santini V, et al: Luspatercept in patients with lower-risk myelodysplastic syndromes, *N Engl J Med* 382(2):140–151, 2020.

Godley LA, Larson RA: Therapy-related myeloid leukemia, *Semin Oncol* 35(4):418–429, 2008.

Greenberg P, Cox C, LeBeau MM, Fenaux P, Morel P, Sanz G, et al: International scoring system for evaluating prognosis in myelodysplastic syndromes, *Blood* 89(6):2079–2088, 1997.

---

[1] Not FDA approved for this indication.

[5] Investigational drug in the United States.

Hellstrom-Lindberg E, Negrin R, Stein R, Krantz S, Lindberg G, Vardiman J, et al: Erythroid response to treatment with G-CSF plus erythropoietin for the anaemia of patients with myelodysplastic syndromes: proposal for a predictive model, *Br J Haematol* 99(2):344–351, 1997.

Kantarjian H, Issa JP, Rosenfeld CS, Bennett JM, Albitar M, DiPersio J, et al: Decitabine improves patient outcomes in myelodysplastic syndromes: results of a phase III randomized study, *Cancer* 106(8):1794–1803, 2006.

Khoury JD, Solary E, Abla O, Akkari Y, Alaggio R, Apperley JF, et al: The 5th edition of the world health organization classification of haematolymphoid tumours: myeloid and histiocytic/dendritic neoplasms, *Leukemia* 36(7):1703–1719, 2022.

List A, Dewald G, Bennett J, Giagounidis A, Raza A, Feldman E, et al: Lenalidomide in the myelodysplastic syndrome with chromosome 5q deletion, *N Engl J Med* 355(14):1456–1465, 2006.

Ma X, Does M, Raza A, Mayne ST: Myelodysplastic syndromes: incidence and survival in the United States, *Cancer* 109(8):1536–1542, 2007.

Malcovati L, Hellstrom-Lindberg E, Bowen D, Ades L, Cermak J, Del Canizo C, et al: Diagnosis and treatment of primary myelodysplastic syndromes in adults: recommendations from the European LeukemiaNet, *Blood* 122(17):2943–2964, 2013.

Martino R, Iacobelli S, Brand R, Jansen J, van Biezen A, Finke J, et al: Retrospective comparison of reduced-intensity conditioning and conventional high-dose conditioning for allogeneic hematopoietic stem cell transplantation using HLA-identical sibling donors in myelodysplastic syndromes, *Blood* 108(3):836–846, 2006.

Platzbecker U, Della Porta MG, Santini V, Zeidan AM, Komrokji RS, Shortt J, et al: Efficacy and safety of luspatercept versus epoetin alfa in erythropoiesis-stimulating agent-naive, transfusion-dependent, lower-risk myelodysplastic syndromes (COMMANDS): interim analysis of a phase 3, open-label, randomised controlled trial, *Lancet* 402(10399):373–385, 2023.

Rotter LK, Shimony S, Ling K, Chen E, Shallis RM, Zeidan AM, et al: Epidemiology and pathogenesis of myelodysplastic syndrome, *Cancer J* 29(3):111–121, 2023.

Silverman LR, Demakos EP, Peterson BL, Kornblith AB, Holland JC, Odchimar-Reissig R, et al: Randomized controlled trial of azacitidine in patients with the myelodysplastic syndrome: a study of the cancer and leukemia group B, *J Clin Oncol* 20(10):2429–2440, 2002.

Tefferi A, Vardiman JW: Myelodysplastic syndromes, *N Engl J Med* 361(19):1872–1885, 2009.

Zeidan AP U, et al: IMerge: results from a phase 3, randomized, double-blind, placebo-controlled study of imetelstat in patients (pts) with heavily transfusion dependent (TD) non-del(5q) lower-risk myelodysplastic syndromes (LR-MDS) relapsed/refractory (R/R) to erythropoiesis stimulating agents (ESA), *J Clin Oncol* 41(16):7004, 2023.

Zhang Y, Wu J, Qin T, Xu Z, Qu S, Pan L, et al: Comparison of the revised 4th (2016) and 5th (2022) editions of the world health organization classification of myelodysplastic neoplasms, *Leukemia* 36(12):2875–2882, 2022.

NON-HODGKIN LYMPHOMA

Method of
Claire Yun Kyoung Ryu Tiger, MD, PhD; Andrew M. Evens, DO, MBA, MSc; and Joanna M. Rhodes, MD, MSCE

CURRENT DIAGNOSIS

- Non-Hodgkin lymphoma (NHL) has many different clinico-pathologic subtypes—more than 75 types are included in the World Health Organization (WHO) classification of lymphoid neoplasms. The natural history and prognosis of these vary greatly from indolent and slow-growing types (over many years) to highly aggressive types (within weeks).
- Excisional lymph node biopsy is the gold standard procedure in establishing the precise NHL histology. Expert hematopathology review incorporating morphologic, immunophenotypic, and genetic features is essential for an accurate diagnosis.
- The etiology of NHL is not known, although several risk factors and conditions are associated with an increased risk of developing lymphoma, including congenital immunosuppression conditions (ataxia-telangiectasia, Wiskott-Aldrich syndrome, and X-linked lymphoproliferative syndrome), acquired immunodeficiency states (e.g., human immunodeficiency virus [HIV] and after solid organ transplantation), viruses (e.g., human T-lymphotropic virus [HTLV]-1 and hepatitis C virus [HCV]), and autoimmune disorders (e.g., Sjögren syndrome, celiac sprue, and systemic lupus erythematosus).
- Patients most commonly present clinically with enlarged, painless lymph nodes, splenomegaly, and bone marrow involvement, but they may also present with other extranodal disease sites (e.g., stomach, skin, liver, bone, brain).

CURRENT THERAPY

- Indolent lymphomas are low-grade and represent slow-growing NHL that may remain stable with low tumor burden, not warranting therapy for several years. The disease is highly responsive to treatment with a variety of treatment options (remission rates exceeding 90% with combined rituximab (Rituxan)/chemotherapy), although the clinical course is characterized by repetitive relapses. Outside of early-stage disease and therapy with allogeneic stem cell transplantation, low-grade NHLs are not curable.
- Transformation of follicular lymphoma to a high-grade NHL occurs in 2% to 3% of patients each year; it is less common in other indolent subtypes. Transformation is typically heralded by an aggressive change in the patient's clinical condition.
- Diffuse large B-cell lymphoma (DLBCL), the most common aggressive NHL, is curable in all stages in most patients with rituximab (Rituxan)-based chemotherapy. A variety of primary extranodal DLBCL clinical subtypes warrant specialized therapy, such as primary central nervous system (CNS) lymphoma and testicular lymphoma.
- Long-term survivors are at increased risk for second cancers. The highest relative risk of developing a secondary malignancy occurs more than 21 to 30 years after the original diagnosis. Patients who received an anthracycline (e.g., doxorubicin [Adriamycin]) as part of therapy are at a long-term increased risk for cardiovascular disease.

The term *malignant lymphoma* was originally introduced by Billroth in 1871 to describe neoplasms of lymphoid tissue. Generally speaking, lymphomas are neoplasms of the immune system. Traditionally, lymphomas are divided into Hodgkin lymphoma (HL) and non-Hodgkin lymphoma (NHL).

There are many different clinicopathologic subtypes of NHL (>60). By cell of origin, most NHLs are of B-cell origin (85%–90%); T-cell NHLs account for 10% to 15% of lymphomas in the United States, whereas natural killer cell or histiocytic lymphomas are rare (<1%). The NHL subtypes for lymphoid, histiocytic, and dendritic neoplasms as classified by the World Health Organization (WHO) were updated in 2022.

NHLs manifest most commonly clinically with involvement of lymph nodes, spleen, and bone marrow, but they can involve other extranodal sites (e.g., stomach, skin, liver, bone, brain). Peripheral blood involvement uncommonly occurs (leukemic phase of lymphoma). The natural history and prognosis vary greatly among the different subtypes of NHL, from indolent subtypes that are often slow growing (i.e., therapy not warranted for years) to very aggressive and rapidly fatal types (within weeks) if not treated. Most NHL subtypes are highly treatable with initial remission rates greater than 90% using combined rituximab (Rituxan)/chemotherapy; however, indolent NHLs are generally incurable, whereas the goal of treating most aggressive NHLs is cure.

Epidemiology

Currently, NHL represents approximately 5% of all cancer diagnoses, being the seventh most common cancer in women and men. Estimates from the American Cancer Society indicate that in 2023 approximately 80,000 new cases of NHL will be diagnosed in the United States, and approximately 20,000 people will die of the disease. In addition, there are approximately 900,000 people living with NHL in the United States.

Geographic Distribution

The incidence of NHL varies throughout the world, in general being more common in developed countries, with rates in the United States of more than 15 per 100,000 compared with 1.2 per 100,000 in China. In the United States the incidence rates of NHL more than

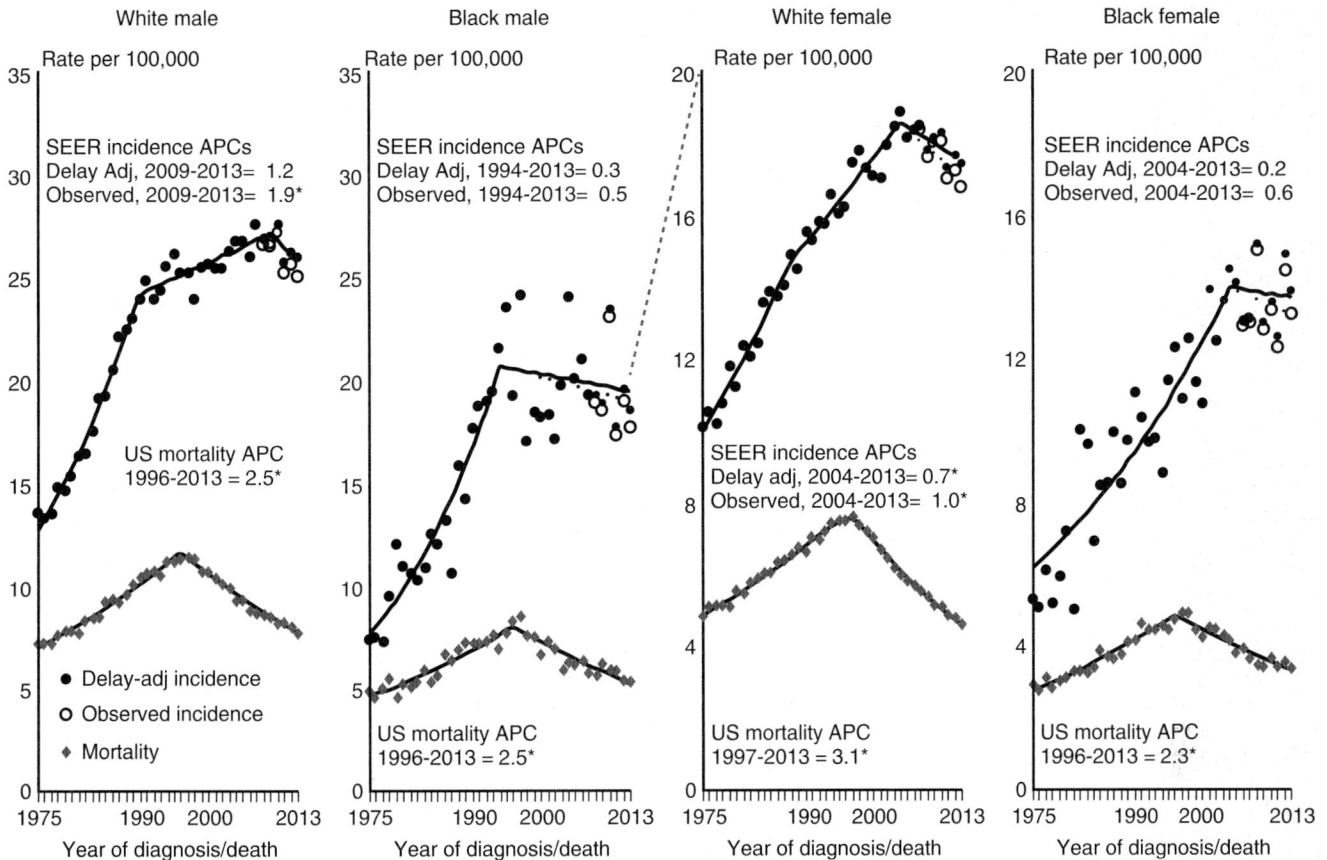

Source: SEER 9 areas and US mortality files (National Center for Health Statistics, CDC).
aRates are age-adjusted to the 2000 US Std population (19 age groups - census P25-1103).
Regression lines and APCs are calculated using the joinpoint regression program version 4.3.0.0. April 2016, National Cancer Institute.
The APC is the annual percent change for the regression line segments. The APC shown on the graph is for the most recent trend.
*The APC is significantly different from zero P < .05.

Figure 1 Surveillance, epidemiology, and end results (SEER) observed incidence, SEER delay-adjusted incidence, and U.S. death rates for non-Hodgkin lymphoma, by race and sex.

doubled between 1975 and 1995, representing one of the largest increases of any cancer. The increases have been more pronounced in White populations, males, older adults, and those with NHL diagnosed at extranodal sites. Similar findings have been reported in other developed countries. The incidence rates of NHL began to stabilize in the late 1990s, although the temporal trends vary by histologic subtype, as well as by race and sex (Figure 1). Some of the increase may be related to improved diagnostic techniques and access to medical care and the increased risk of NHL attributable to human immunodeficiency virus (HIV) infection. However, additional factors are likely responsible for this unexpected increase in incidence.

Age
Overall, NHL incidence rises exponentially with increasing age. In persons older than 65 years, the incidence is 90.9 per 100,000 population compared with 7.1 per 100,000 population for persons aged 20 to 49 years. Except for high-grade lymphoblastic and Burkitt lymphomas (the most common types of NHL seen in children and young adults), the median age at presentation for most subtypes of NHL exceeds 60 years.

Race and Ethnicity
Incidence varies by race and ethnicity, with White people overall having a higher risk than Black people and Asians (incidence increased 50%–60% in White people compared with Black people). Most NHL subtypes are more common in White people than in Black people; however, peripheral T-cell lymphoma (PTCL), mycosis fungoides, and Sézary syndrome occur more often in Black people than in White people.

Etiology and Risk Factors
Chromosomal Translocations and Molecular Rearrangements
Nonrandom chromosomal and molecular rearrangements play an important role in the pathogenesis of many lymphomas and often correlate with histology and immunophenotype. These chromosomal changes often result in oncogenic gene products; for example, t(11;14)(q13;q32) translocation results in overexpression of bcl-1 (cyclin D1) in mantle cell lymphoma (MCL), whereas translocation with 8q24 leads to c-myc overexpression in nearly all Burkitt lymphomas and in 10% to 15% of patients with diffuse large B-cell lymphoma (DLBCL). Research to discover more information regarding the prognostic and pathogenic importance of these oncogenes continues, although they are currently used primarily in clinical practice for diagnostic purposes. In addition, these genes serve as potential targets for novel therapeutics.

Environmental Factors
Environmental factors may also play a role in the development of NHL, including specific occupations (e.g., chemists, painters, mechanics, machinists) and chemicals (solvents and pesticides). Patients who receive chemotherapy or radiation therapy for any indication are also at increased risk for developing NHL as a secondary cancer as discussed later.

Viruses
Several viruses have been implicated in the pathogenesis of NHL, including Epstein-Barr virus, human T-lymphotropic virus (HTLV-1), Kaposi sarcoma–associated herpesvirus (KSHV, also

known as human herpesvirus 8 [HHV-8]), and hepatitis C virus (HCV). Meta-analyses have shown 13% to 15% seroprevalence of HCV in certain geographic regions among persons with B-cell NHL. Furthermore, HCV infection is associated with the development of clonal B-cell expansions and certain subtypes of NHL, particularly in the setting of essential (type II) mixed cryoglobulinemia. HTLV-1 is a human retrovirus that establishes a latent infection through reverse transcription in activated T-helper cells. A minority (5%) of carriers will develop adult T-cell leukemia lymphoma. KSHV-like DNA sequences are often detected in primary effusion lymphomas in patients with HIV infection and those with multicentric (plasma cell variant) Castleman disease.

Bacterial Infections
Gastric mucosa-associated lymphoid tissue (MALT) lymphoma is seen most often, but not exclusively, in association with *Helicobacter pylori* infection. Infection with *Borrelia burgdorferi* has been detected in approximately 35% of patients with primary cutaneous B-cell lymphoma in Scotland. Studies indicate that *Campylobacter jejuni* and immunoproliferative small intestinal disease are related. European reports have noted an association between infection with *Chlamydia psittaci* and ocular adnexal lymphoma. The infection was found to be highly specific and does not reflect a subclinical infection among the general population. Furthermore, remission of NHL to antibiotics has been reported. Attempts to confirm this association in the Western Hemisphere have been unsuccessful.

Immunodeficiency
Patients with congenital conditions of immunosuppression are at increased risk of NHL. These conditions include ataxia-telangiectasia; Wiskott-Aldrich syndrome; X-linked lymphoproliferative syndrome; severe combined immunodeficiency; acquired immunodeficiency states, such as HIV infection; and iatrogenic immunosuppression. Relative risk of NHL is increased 150- to 250-fold among patients with acquired immunodeficiency syndrome (AIDS); patients usually develop high-grade NHLs, such as Burkitt lymphoma or DLBCL. The incidence of posttransplantation lymphoproliferative disorders (PTLDs) after solid organ transplantation ranges from 1% to 3% in kidney transplant recipients to 10% to 12% in heart and multiorgan transplant recipients, the latter of whom require more potent immunosuppressive therapy.

Autoimmunity
An increased incidence of gastrointestinal lymphomas is seen in patients with celiac (nontropical) sprue and inflammatory bowel disease, particularly Crohn disease. An aberrant clonal intraepithelial T-cell population can be found in up to 75% of patients with refractory celiac sprue before overt T-cell lymphoma develops. Sjögren disease is associated with a sixfold increased risk of NHL overall, with risk varying in part on severity of disease (5–200 times); moreover, the risk specifically of parotid marginal zone lymphoma is increased 1000-fold. In addition, systemic lupus erythematosus and rheumatoid arthritis have been associated with a slightly increased risk of B-cell lymphoma.

Genetic Susceptibility
Several studies have implicated a role for genetic variants in the risk of NHL, including genes that influence DNA integrity and methylation; genes that alter B-cell survival and growth; and genes that involve innate immunity, oxidative stress, and xenobiotic metabolism.

Signs and Symptoms
Fever, weight loss, and night sweats, referred to as B symptoms, are more common in advanced and aggressive subtype NHLs, but they may be present at all stages and in any histologic subtype.

Low-Grade or Indolent Lymphomas
Painless, slowly progressive peripheral adenopathy is the most common clinical presentation in patients with low-grade lymphomas. Patients sometimes report a history of waxing and waning adenopathy before seeking medical attention. Spontaneous regression of enlarged lymph nodes can occur, which may cause a low-grade lymphoma to be confused with an infectious condition. Primary extranodal involvement and B symptoms are uncommon at presentation; however, both are more common in advanced or end-stage disease and in particular indolent NHL subtypes (e.g., gastric MALT and nongastric extranodal MALT). Bone marrow is frequently involved, sometimes in association with cytopenias. Splenomegaly is seen in approximately 40% of patients, but the spleen is rarely the only involved site besides the specific subtype of splenic marginal zone lymphoma.

High-Grade or Aggressive Lymphomas
The clinical presentation of high-grade lymphomas is more varied. Although most patients present with adenopathy, more than one-third present with extranodal involvement alone or with adenopathy, the most common sites being the gastrointestinal tract (including Waldeyer ring), skin, bone marrow, sinuses, genitourinary tract, bone, and central nervous system (CNS). B symptoms are more common, occurring in approximately 30% to 40% of patients. Lymphoblastic lymphoma often manifests with an anterior mediastinal mass, superior vena cava syndrome, and leptomeningeal disease. American patients with Burkitt lymphoma often present with a large abdominal mass and symptoms of bowel obstruction. In addition, certain histologic NHL subtypes manifest with symptoms unique to that specific lymphoma subtype; for example, angioimmunoblastic T-cell lymphoma (AITL) in addition to lymphadenopathy presents with disease features including organomegaly, skin rash, pleural effusions, arthritis, eosinophilia, and varied immunologic abnormalities such as positive Coombs test, cold agglutinins, hemolytic anemia, antinuclear antibodies, and polyclonal hypergammaglobulinemia.

Screening
No effective methods are currently available for screening patients or populations for NHL.

Diagnosis
A definitive diagnosis can be made only by biopsy of pathologic lymph nodes or tumor tissue. It is critical in most cases to perform an *excisional* lymph node resection to avoid false-negative results and inaccurate histologic classification; fine-needle aspirations or core biopsies are often insufficient for diagnostic purposes. When clinical circumstances make surgical biopsy of involved lymph nodes or extranodal sites prohibitive, a core biopsy obtained under computed tomography (CT) or ultrasonographic guidance may suffice, but it often requires the integration of histologic examination and immunophenotypic and molecular studies for accurate diagnosis. A formal review by an expert hematopathologist is mandatory. In addition to morphologic review and immunostaining of tissue, other studies such as detailed cellular immunophenotyping and genotyping for relevant oncogenes are often needed to complete the diagnosis.

In addition to a detailed history and physical examination, baseline staging studies are warranted. These consist of blood tests (complete blood count with differential, complete metabolic panel including liver function tests, and lactate dehydrogenase [LDH]); CT of chest, abdomen, and pelvis; and bone marrow biopsy and aspirate in some cases (Box 1). For aggressive NHL histologies, functional imaging is advocated (i.e., fluorodeoxyglucose [18F] positron emission tomography [FDG-PET]), as is assessment of ejection fraction in anticipation of anthracycline-based chemotherapy. Testing for history of hepatitis B virus (HBV) is recommended, especially before starting anti-CD20 antibody therapy; evidence suggests that anti-CD20 antibody therapy (e.g., rituximab [Rituxan]) increases the risk of HBV reactivation above the known rate of chemotherapy-associated reactivation. HIV serology should be obtained in patients with relevant risk factors, especially for DLBCL and Burkitt lymphoma. HTLV-1 serology is recommended in patients who present with cutaneous T-cell lymphoma lesions or adult T-cell leukemia/lymphoma (ATLL), especially if they have hypercalcemia.

Examination of cerebrospinal fluid and consideration of intrathecal chemotherapy prophylaxis or integration of intravenous high-dose methotrexate are applicable for patients with DLBCL with bone marrow, epidural, testicular, paranasal sinus, breast, or multiple extranodal sites (especially in conjunction with elevated LDH). Testing is mandatory for high-grade lymphoblastic lymphoma, Burkitt lymphoma and its variants, and primary CNS lymphoma if there is no evidence of increased intracranial pressure. Upper gastrointestinal endoscopy or gastrointestinal series with small bowel follow-through is recommended in some patients with head and neck involvement (tonsil, base of tongue, nasopharynx) and those with primary gastrointestinal disease. MCL is associated with a high incidence of occult gastrointestinal involvement. In addition, magnetic resonance imaging (MRI) of the complete craniospinal axis and ocular examination is advocated with any brain or leptomeningeal disease involvement to rule out multifocal disease.

Classification

The 1965 Rappaport classification of malignant lymphomas was based solely on architecture and cytology. Since then, with the help of advanced cellular and genetic technologies, numerous new unique NHL entities have emerged. The WHO and ICC classifications were most recently revised in 2022, which continues to emphasize immunophenotyping, genotyping, and clinical features. Another way to group the many different lymphoma histologies is by clinical presentation and prognosis (Table 1).

Prognosis

International Prognostic Index

The International Prognostic Index (IPI) was developed as a prognostic factor model for aggressive NHLs treated with doxorubicin (Adriamycin)-containing regimens (Box 2). In the prerituximab era, persons with no risk factors or one risk factor had a predicted 5-year overall survival (OS) rate of 73%, compared with 26% for high-risk patients with four or five risk factors. In the postrituximab era, the survival rates have improved (see Box 2). A variant of the IPI is also useful in predicting outcome in patients with follicular low-grade lymphoma (FLIPI), MCL (MIPI), and most recently in Burkitt lymphoma (BLIPI; Box 3).

Molecular Profiling

DNA microarray technology for gene expression profiling has identified distinct prognostic subgroups in many NHL subtypes,

including DLBCL and follicular NHL. Patients with germinal center B-like DLBCL have an improved OS compared with other molecular profiles. Additional pivotal work has found that gene expression signatures incorporating mutations in MYD88 (L265P), CD79B, NOTCH1, NOTCH2, EZH2, and translocations in BCL6 and BCL2 predicted responses to immunochemotherapy and survival. Favorable outcomes were seen in cases with simultaneous BCL6 fusions and NOTCH2 mutations and simultaneous BCL2 translocations and EZH2 mutations. Inferior outcomes were seen in cases with the co-occurrence of MYD88 and CD79B mutations, as well as isolated NOTCH1 mutations. Studies in follicular NHL have identified gene expression signatures that also predicted survival. Interestingly, the genes that

TABLE 1	Clinical Prognostic Classification of Adult Immunocompetent Non-Hodgkin Lymphomas	
LYMPHOMA TYPE		**PERCENTAGE OF ALL U.S. NON-HODGKIN LYMPHOMAS**
Indolent or Low-Grade Non-Hodgkin Lymphomas		
Follicular lymphoma		20–25
Small lymphocytic lymphoma		7
MALT-type marginal zone lymphoma		7
Nodal-type marginal zone lymphoma		<2
Lymphoplasmacytic lymphoma		<2
Aggressive or High-Grade Non-Hodgkin Lymphomas		
Diffuse large B-cell lymphoma		30–35
T-cell lymphomas: peripheral or systemic (multiple subtypes)		10–12
Mantle cell lymphoma		6
Lymphoblastic lymphoma		<2
Burkitt lymphoma		<1

Subtypes are listed in order of most to least common.
MALT, Mucosa-associated lymphoid tissue.

BOX 1	Initial Assessment and Workup for Non-Hodgkin Lymphoma

- Excisional tissue biopsy
- Detailed history and physical examination
- CBC with differential, metabolic panel (including liver function), and LDH
- CT scans (chest, abdomen, pelvis)
- Nuclear functional imaging (i.e., FDG-PET)
- Bone marrow biopsy and aspirate
- Heart function (e.g., echocardiogram) if anthracycline therapy anticipated
- Upper endoscopy, colonoscopy, or both
- HIV and HBV testing (with risk factors and/or if monoclonal antibody therapy planned)
- Consider tuberculosis testing (i.e., purified protein derivative with energy panel) with history of exposure
- Assessment of CSF (when applicable or with risk factors)
- Consider early institution of TLS prophylaxis (e.g., intravenous fluids, allopurinol [Zyloprim])

CBC, Complete blood cell count; *CSF,* cerebrospinal fluid; *FDG-PET,* fluorodeoxyglucose positron emission tomography; *HBV,* hepatitis B virus; *LDH,* lactate dehydrogenase.

BOX 2	Enhanced International Prognostic Index Risk Factors and Associated Approximate Cure Rates for Diffuse Large B-Cell Lymphoma

Factors/Scoring
- Age, years
  - >40 to ≤60: 1
  - >60 to ≤75: 2
  - >75: 3
- LDH, normalized
  - >1 to ≤3: 1
  - >3: 2
- Ann Arbor stage III–IV: 1
- Extranodal disease: 1
- Performance status ≥2: 1
- Five-year PFS rates based on score at diagnosis
  - Score 0–1: 91%
  - Score 2–3: 74%
  - Score 4–5: 51%
  - Score ≥6: 30%

LDH, Lactate dehydrogenase; *PFS,* progression-free survival.

defined the prognostic signatures were not expressed in the tumor cells but were expressed by the nonmalignant tumor-infiltrating cells—primarily T cells, macrophages, and dendritic cells.

Treatment

The therapeutic approach for NHL differs for each clinicopathologic subtype. Chemotherapy remains an important modality. However, in some instances, radiation therapy or, rarely, surgical resection plays a role. Biologic approaches, including monoclonal antibodies, bispecific antibodies, antibody-drug conjugates, and cellular therapies have shown significant activity and are currently incorporated into many treatment paradigms. In addition, other novel therapeutics targeting the cell surface of lymphoma cells or varied transcription factors continue to be incorporated into treatment paradigms. Autologous and allogeneic stem cell transplantation are mostly reserved for patients with recurrent or refractory disease, although there are some subtypes in which consolidative autologous transplantation after frontline therapy is considered (e.g., MCL and PTCLs).

Indolent B-Cell Non-Hodgkin Lymphomas

Indolent lymphomas are low grade and represent slow-growing NHLs that may be stable with low tumor burden that may not warrant therapy for several years. The disease is responsive to treatment (remission rates >90% with combined rituximab/chemotherapy), although the clinical course is characterized by repetitive relapses. Outside of early-stage disease and therapy with an allogeneic stem cell transplant, low-grade NHLs are not curable with current treatments. The median survival of patients with advanced-stage follicular lymphoma in the prerituximab era was 9 to 10 years, although that is currently significantly longer (≈16–18 years). Transformation to a high-grade NHL occurs in 2% to 3% of patients each year with follicular lymphoma (less common in other indolent subtypes) and is typically heralded by an aggressive change in the patient's clinical condition (e.g., B symptoms, rapidly rising LDH). Follicular grade 3b is not considered low grade and should be treated in a similar manner as aggressive B-cell lymphoma.

General Principles

Only a minority of patients present with early-stage disease (i.e., stage I or II). Low-dose involved field radiotherapy is a valid treatment option for these patients (especially stage I without central sites of disease), and associated 20-year disease-free survival rates are greater than 50%. Treatment for patients with advanced-stage disease ranges from observation (i.e., watchful waiting) to anti-CD20 monoclonal antibody therapy (rituximab [Rituxan] or obinutuzumab [Gazyva]) with or without chemotherapy. Treatment choice depends in part on tumor burden and the patient's individual disease characteristics and baseline functional status. Treatment with frontline anti-CD20 monoclonal antibody with chemotherapy (outpatient therapy given once every 3–4 weeks typically for six cycles), possibly followed by 2 years

of maintenance therapy with anti-CD20 monoclonal antibody for patients with high tumor burden, is associated with median progression-free survival (PFS) rates of approximately 10 years.

Treatment options for relapsed or refractory (R/R) indolent lymphoma include repeating rituximab with or without a different chemotherapy regimen, radioimmunotherapy, oral lenalidomide (Revlimid) immunomodulatory therapy, CAR-T therapy, bispecific T-cell engager (BITE) therapy, or stem cell transplantation. There is a small subset of patients with follicular lymphoma who experience early progression to first-line therapy (i.e., within 2 years), and survival rates are significantly inferior with conventional therapies. Autologous stem cell transplantation is an option for patients with relapsed disease, especially early progressors, although an improvement in OS is debated. Allogeneic stem cell transplantation is a potential curative modality for patients with R/R disease, although patient selection is critical owing to potential morbidity and mortality related to this therapeutic option.

Special Considerations

Localized gastric MALT lymphoma cases often may be managed with therapy for *H. pylori* infection; radiation is typically reserved for failure to eradicate *H. pylori*. Patients with lymphoplasmacytic lymphoma (Waldenström macroglobulinemia) can present clinically with hyperviscosity or cryoglobulinemia, which may be managed acutely with plasmapheresis, but ultimately systemic therapy similar to that for other indolent NHLs is warranted. More recently, the Bruton tyrosine kinase (BTK) inhibitor ibrutinib (Imbruvica) was used for the treatment of patients with R/R marginal zone lymphoma who require systemic therapy after at least one anti-CD20–based therapy[1], as well as for frontline treatment for Waldenström's macroglobulinemia.

Aggressive or High-Grade Non-Hodgkin Lymphomas

High-grade B- and T-cell NHLs are typically aggressive lymphomas that are fatal in weeks to a few months if not treated. However, many of these NHLs are curable with multiagent chemotherapy.

General Principles

DLBCL, the most common aggressive NHL, is curable in all stages in most patients (60%–70%). A common treatment is anti-CD20 monoclonal antibody combined with anthracycline-based chemotherapy: rituximab–cyclophosphamide, doxorubicin (hydroxydaunorubicin), vincristine (Oncovin), and prednisone (R-CHOP) or polatuzumab (Polivy)-rituximab-cyclophosphamide-doxorubicin-prednisone (Pola-R-CHP). The number of treatment cycles depends on the stage of disease and response to treatment. Standard therapy for advanced-stage disease is six R-CHOP cycles (or Pola-R-CHP), whereas patients with early-stage disease may receive three or four cycles with or without involved field radiation. There are emerging data regarding the prognostic importance of *MYC* rearrangement (from tumor testing) as a single finding and especially in conjunction with *BCL-2* and/or *BCL6* (i.e., double or triple hit) by molecular studies, as well as with immunohistochemical staining. Outcomes with R-CHOP for DLBCL patients with a molecular double hit (e.g., presence of *MYC* and *BCL-2* rearrangements) are modest; more intensive and novel therapeutic options should be considered. Therapy for R/R DLBCL typically includes abbreviated salvage non–cross-resistant chemotherapy followed by autologous stem cell transplantation for patients who have chemotherapy-sensitive disease (relapse >12 months of chemotherapy), which is curative in approximately 35% to 45% of patients. However, recent studies have highlighted the efficacy of CAR-T therapy in patients with R/R DLBCL, importantly in cases relapsing within 1 year of first-line therapy where their use is now standard of care or in patients not eligible for autologous stem cell transplantation.

---

[1] Not FDA approved for this indication.

MCL is a B-cell NHL with initial high remission rates (>90%–95%), but it has more modest long-term outcomes, and it is difficult to cure with current treatments. With standard chemotherapy regimens (e.g., R-CHOP), the median PFS rates are only 18 to 20 months. With more intensive chemotherapy regimens, especially ones incorporating high-dose cytarabine as a component of induction therapy, 5-year PFS rates are near 70%. Some groups advocate induction therapy with aggressive high-dose cytarabine (Cytosar)[1]-based chemotherapy followed by consolidative autologous stem cell transplantation in first remission. As noted later, there has been the integration of several novel therapeutic agents into the treatment paradigm of MCL. Bendamustine (Bendeka, Treanda) in combination with rituximab has also become a widely used and more tolerable induction regimen, especially in older patients with MCL. Recent studies have also shown a benefit with adding ibrutinib (Imbruvica) to initial chemotherapy with or without use as part of maintenance therapy. However, in 2023, ibrutinib's accelerated approval was voluntarily withdrawn for MCL patients. Second-generation (covalent; acalabrutinib [Calquence], Zanubrutinib [Brukinsa]) and third-generation (noncovalent; pirtobrutinib [Jaypirca]) Bruton tyrosine kinase inhibitors (BTKi) are currently FDA approved for MCL.

Burkitt lymphoma and related high-grade NHLs (e.g., lymphoblastic lymphomas) are often rapidly growing malignancies with a doubling time of 24 hours. Prompt initiation of therapy, including aggressive supportive care measures, is often warranted. With aggressive chemotherapy regimens, including prophylactic intrathecal chemotherapy, the majority of Burkitt patients younger than age 40 years are cured (>70%–80%). In addition, there are data showing high efficacy using lower-intensity treatment consisting of infused etoposide (Toposar)[1], doxorubicin, and cyclophosphamide with vincristine, prednisone, and rituximab (EPOCH-R), especially for patients' untreated Burkitt lymphoma without CNS involvement, including HIV related.

Systemic (i.e., noncutaneous) PTCLs are mostly aggressive malignancies. They are treatable; however, cure rates are lower compared with most aggressive B-cell NHLs, and many patients relapse early after initial treatment. Standard therapy had consisted of CHOP-based chemotherapy with or without autologous stem cell transplantation in first remission as consolidation. Recently published data from the ECHELON-2 trial combining the antibody drug conjugate, brentuximab vedotin (Adcetris) with cyclophosphamide, doxorubicin, and prednisone (CHP) chemotherapy versus standard CHOP for untreated CD30+ PTCLs was associated with significantly improved PFS and OS. This regimen (i.e., brentuximab vedotin + CHP) was subsequently FDA approved for this indication. Several additional novel targeted agents have also been FDA approved over the past several years for the treatment of T-cell NHL (see later).

Special Considerations

There are several clinical subtypes of DLBCL that present as primary extranodal manifestations, and the prognosis differs based on the affected organs. Primary gastric DLBCL, for instance, when localized can be typically treated with abbreviated cycles (three to four) of R-CHOP followed by involved field radiation. Diagnosis usually involves endoscopic biopsy in addition to systemic imaging such as CT or PET imaging. Prognosis is usually good. Primary testicular DLBCL, on the other hand, has relatively poor prognosis with relatively high risk of CNS involvement or CNS relapse. Therefore patients with primary testicular DLBCL should receive CNS prophylaxis with either intrathecal chemotherapy or agents such as intravenous high-dose methotrexate[1]. Testicular DLBCL also requires radical orchiectomy and contralateral testicular radiation for prophylaxis.

Primary CNS lymphoma is typically DLBCL; high-dose methotrexate is a key component of therapy. Response rates are high with MATRix (methotrexate, cytarabine[1], thiotepa[1], and rituximab) followed by consolidative autologous transplantation. Therefore consolidative autologous transplantation must be considered for younger fit patients. In older and transplant-ineligible patients, high-dose methotrexate may be combined with rituximab and alkylators (procarbazine [Matulane][1] or temozolomide [Temodar][1]). There is a suggestion of benefit of maintenance therapy in this patient population, but this has not been proven in prospective studies. In very elderly or frail patients, methotrexate should still be considered as first-line therapy, but reduced dosage may be warranted. In patients who are ineligible for methotrexate, BTK inhibitors in combination with rituximab and/or lenalidomide (Revlimid)[1] can be considered. Whole brain radiation therapy can be considered in those who are too frail to undergo any systemic therapy such as palliative therapy, but it is associated with substantial toxicity including cognitive decline.

A long-standing therapeutic maneuver for solid organ transplant–related PTLDs has been reduction of immunosuppression, although, using this approach alone, mortality rates have ranged from 50% to 60% in most series. Evidence of the use of initial rituximab-based therapy together with reduction in immunosuppression suggests improved outcomes in the modern era.

Most AIDS-related NHLs are aggressive or high-grade types: DLBCL or Burkitt lymphoma. Similar therapy as immunocompetent NHL is often recommended. Response to therapy, including cure rate, has improved significantly with better control of opportunistic infections and initiation of highly active antiretroviral therapy (HAART).

Mycosis fungoides and Sézary syndrome are cutaneous T-cell lymphomas that initially might show eczematous lesions. It is often difficult to establish the diagnosis, but eventually the lesions develop into plaques and tumors. Lymph nodes, spleen, and visceral organs may be involved. Sézary syndrome is a variant of mycosis fungoides and shows peripheral blood involvement; patients usually have diffuse erythroderma. Skin-targeted modalities for treatment of early-stage mycosis fungoides include psoralens with ultraviolet A (PUVA) light; narrowband-ultraviolet light; skin electron-beam radiation; and topical steroids, retinoids, carmustine (BCNU) and nitrogen mustard (Mustargen)[1]. Treatment goals in advanced stages are to reduce tumor burden and to relieve symptoms. Treatment options also include monochemotherapy or polychemotherapy, including CHOP; extracorporeal photopheresis; interferons; retinoids; liposomal doxorubicin (Doxil)[1]; monoclonal antibodies; recombinant toxins; histone deacetylase inhibitors; and, most recently, the antibody drug conjugate brentuximab vedotin (Adcetris) and humanized antibody against CCR4, mogamulizumab (Poteligeo).

During therapy for aggressive/high-grade NHLs, attention should be paid to preventing tumor lysis syndrome. Measures to prevent this complication include aggressive hydration, allopurinol (Zyloprim), and frequent monitoring of electrolytes, uric acid, and creatinine. Rasburicase (Elitek), a recombinant urate oxidase enzyme, is an expensive but potent agent for treating hyperuricemia.

Novel Treatment Options and Modalities

Many new agents targeting specific molecular targets have become available for the treatment of lymphoma (Tables 2 and 3). Novel agents in lymphoma include bortezomib (Velcade) and lenalidomide (Revlimid), which are FDA approved for R/R MCL (and lenalidomide also for R/R follicular and marginal zone lymphoma), and histone deacetylase inhibitors, which are approved for cutaneous T-cell lymphoma and peripheral T-cell NHLs as well. In addition, bortezomib is FDA approved for untreated patients with MCL in combination with immunochemotherapy. Other newer agents that are FDA approved for the treatment of patients with chronic lymphocytic leukemia (CLL), including in higher-risk patient populations (e.g., p53 mutated), are the BTK

TABLE 2	Targeted Therapeutics FDA Approved for the Treatment of B-Cell Non-Hodgkin Lymphoma

BTK inhibitors	Mechanism: BTK bound by and downstream signaling pathways initiated by B-cell receptor inhibited by small molecule Notable toxicities: atrial fibrillation, myelosuppression, rash, arthralgias, headache, bleeding, and impaired wound healing (should be held perioperatively and before other invasive procedures)

Drug Name	Indication and Year Approved
Ibrutinib (Imbruvica)	CLL/SLL (2014) Waldenström macroglobulinemia (2015)
Acalabrutinib (Calquence)	Mantle cell lymphoma (2017) CLL/SLL (2019)
Zanubrutinib (Brukinsa)	Mantle cell lymphoma (2019) CLL/SLL Marginal zone lymphoma Waldenstrom's macroglobulinemia R/R follicular lymphoma
Pirtobrutinib (Jaypirca)	Mantle cell lymphoma (2023) CLL/SLL (2023)

Anti-CD20 monoclonal antibodies	Mechanism: Bind to CD20 molecule on B lymphocytes and induce a variety of responses, including antibody-mediated cytotoxicity, complement-mediated cytotoxicity, and apoptosis Notable toxicities: infusion reactions, hypogammaglobulinemia, hepatitis B virus reactivation, progressive multifocal leukoencephalopathy (rare)

Drug Name	Indication and Year Approved
Rituximab (Rituxan)	Relapsed indolent B-cell lymphomas (1997) Untreated DLBCL with CHOP (2006) CLL (2010) Follicular lymphoma maintenance (2011) Waldenström macroglobulinemia[1], with ibrutinib (2018)
Obinutuzumab (Gazyva)	Untreated CLL with chlorambucil (Leukeran) (2013) Relapsed rituximab refractory follicular lymphoma with bendamustine (Bendeka) (2016) Untreated follicular lymphoma with bendamustine (2017) Untreated CLL with ibrutinib (2019)
Ofatumumab (Arzerra)	Relapsed CLL (2016)

Anti-CD79b monoclonal antibody	Mechanism: Binds to CD79b molecule on B lymphocytes; conjugated MMAE then internalized by lymphocyte; tubulin bound by MMAE, resulting in cell cycle arrest Notable toxicities: neuropathy, immunosuppression, fatigue, diarrhea

Drug Name	Indication and Year Approved
Polatuzumab vedotin (Polivy)	Relapsed DLBCL with bendamustine and rituximab (2019) Untreated DLBCL in combination with rituximab, cyclophosphamide, doxorubicin, prednisone in patients with IPI of 2 or higher (2023)

Bispecific T-cell engager	Mechanism: CD20 on B cells and CD3 on cytotoxic T cells bound by anti-CD20/CD3 bispecific antibody Notable toxicities: CRS: fever, hypotension, hypoxia, tachycardia; neurotoxicity (encephalopathy, headache)

Drug Name	Indication and Year Approved
Mosunetuzumab-axgb (Lunsumio)	Relapsed/refractory follicular lymphoma (2022)
Epcoritamab (Epkinly)	Relapsed/refractory DLBCL (2023)
Glofitamab (Columvi)	Relapsed/refractory follicular lymphoma Relapsed/refractory DLBCL (2023)

Immuno-modulators	Mechanism: affect T-cell stimulatory pathways, angiogenesis, and cell proliferation Notable toxicities: myelosuppression, fatigue, rash, thrombosis (prophylactic aspirin or anticoagulants typically advised)

Drug Name	Indication and Year Approved
Lenalidomide (Revlimid)	Relapsed mantle cell lymphoma (2013) Relapsed follicular lymphoma and marginal zone lymphoma (2019)

Anti-CD19 monoclonal antibody	Mechanism: binds to CD19 antigen and mediates B-cell lysis through apoptosis and immune effector mechanisms, including ADCC and antibody-dependent cellular phagocytosis Notable toxicities: neutropenia, fatigue, anemia, diarrhea, thrombocytopenia, cough, pyrexia, peripheral edema, and pleural effusions (loncastuximab)

Drug Name	Indication and Year Approved
Tafasitamab-cxix (Monjuvi) in combination with lenalidomide	Relapsed DLBCL (2020); relapsed FL (2025; in combination with rituximab and lenalidomide)
Loncastuximab tesirine-lpyl (Zynlonta)	Relapsed DLBCL (2021)

EZH2 inhibitors	Mechanism: inhibit EZH2, a histone methyltransferase responsible for repression of tumor suppressor genes. Notable toxicities: fatigue, infection	
	Drug Name	*Indication and Year Approved*
	Tazemetostat (Tazverik)	Follicular lymphoma (2020)
Phosphatidy-linositol-3-kinase (PI3Kδ) inhibitors	Mechanism: are small molecule inhibitors of PI3 kinase, resulting in inhibition of various cellular processes, such as cellular growth, proliferation, and intracellular trafficking. Notable toxicities: pneumonitis, colitis, transaminitis, hypertension, hyperglycemia (copanlisib)	
	Drug Name	*Indication and Year Approved*
	Idelalisib (Zydelig)	Relapsed CLL (2014)
PD-1 inhibitors	Mechanism: block PD-1 on cellular surface, facilitating T-cell–mediated immune killing. Notable toxicities: pneumonitis, colitis, dermatitis, endocrinopathies (hypothyroidism)	
	Drug Name	*Indication and Year First Approved*
	Pembrolizumab (Keytruda)	Relapsed primary mediastinal large B-cell lymphoma (2018)
CAR T-cell therapy	Mechanism: CD19-expressing lymphoma cells targeted by CD19-directed genetically modified autologous T cells. Notable toxicities: cytokine release syndrome (fever, hypotension, organ dysfunction), neurotoxicity (mental status changes, confusion, seizures), cytopenias	
	Drug Name	*Indication and Year Approved*
	Axicabtagene ciloleucel (Yescarta)	Relapsed DLBCL (2017) Chemorefractory large B-cell lymphoma (<12 mo of chemotherapy) after 1 L of therapy (2022) Relapsed follicular lymphoma (2021)
	Tisagenlecleucel (Kymriah)	Relapsed DLBCL (2018) Relapsed follicular lymphoma (2022)
	Brexucabtagene autoleucel (Tecartus)	Relapsed mantle cell lymphoma (2020) Relapsed or refractory B-ALL (2021)
	Lisocabtagene maraleucel (Breyanzi)	Relapsed DLBCL (2021) Chemorefractory large B-cell lymphoma (<12 mo of chemotherapy) (2022) Relapsed/refractory CLL after BTK inhibitor and BCL2 inhibitor therapy (2024)
BCL2 inhibitors	Mechanism: antiapoptotic activities of protein BCL2 inhibited by small molecule. Notable toxicities: tumor lysis syndrome, myelosuppression, fever, diarrhea	
	Drug Name	*Indication and Year Approved*
	Venetoclax (Venclexta)	Relapsed CLL/SLL (2016) Untreated CLL/SLL in combination with obinutuzumab (2019)
Proteasome inhibitors	Mechanism: inhibit proteasomal clearance of multiple molecules, including proapoptotic molecules. Notable toxicities: peripheral neuropathy, fatigue, diarrhea	
	Drug Name	*Indication and Year Approved*
	Bortezomib (Velcade)	Relapsed mantle cell lymphoma (2006) Untreated mantle cell lymphoma with chemotherapy (2014)
Nuclear export inhibitor	Mechanism: actively binds to export protein 1 (XPO1 or CRM1), inhibiting the nuclear export of tumor suppressors, growth regulators, and antiinflammatory proteins. Notable toxicities: fatigue, nausea, diarrhea, appetite decrease, weight decrease, constipation, vomiting, pyrexia; dizziness and mental status changes; thrombocytopenia, neutropenia, anemia, and hyponatremia	
	Drug Name	*Indication and Year Approved*
	Selinexor (Xpovio)	Relapsed DLBCL (2020)
Radioimmunotherapy	Mechanism: targeted radiation to lymphoma cells delivered by monoclonal antibodies. Notable toxicities: cytopenias (delayed), fatigue, MDS	
	Drug Name	*Indication and Year Approved*
	Ibritumomab tiuxetan (Zevalin)	Relapsed follicular lymphoma (2002) Consolidation for follicular lymphoma after initial chemotherapy (2009)

[1]Not FDA approved for this indication.

ADCC, Antibody-dependent cellular cytotoxicity; *BTK*, Bruton tyrosine kinase; *CAR*, chimeric antigen receptor; *CHOP*, cyclophosphamide, doxorubicin, oncovin, prednisone; *CLL/SLL*, chronic lymphocytic leukemia/small lymphocytic lymphoma; *CRS*, cytokine release syndrome; *DLBCL*, diffuse large B-cell lymphoma; *EZH2*, enhancer of zeste homolog 2; *FL*, follicular lymphoma; *IPI*, International Prognostic Index; *MDS*, myelodysplastic syndrome; *MMAE*, monomethyl auristatin E; *PD-1*, programmed cell death-1.

TABLE 3	Targeted Therapeutics FDA Approved for the Treatment of T-Cell Non-Hodgkin Lymphoma	
Histone deacetylase inhibitors	Mechanism: modules acetylation of key targets, including genes involved in cancer-related cellular pathways Notable toxicities: QT prolongation, electrolyte abnormalities, cytopenias (especially thrombocytopenia), nausea, fatigue	
	Drug Name	*Indication and Year Approved*
	Romidepsin (Istodax)	Relapsed CTCL (2009)
	Vorinostat (Zolinza)	Relapsed CTCL (2006)
	Belinostat (Beleodaq)	Relapsed PTCL (2014)
Anti-CD30 monoclonal antibody	Mechanism: binds to CD30 molecule on T lymphocytes; conjugated MMAE then internalized by lymphocyte; tubulin bound by MMAE, resulting in cell cycle arrest. Notable toxicities: peripheral neuropathy, diarrhea, cytopenias, fatigue, pancreatitis	
	Drug Name	*Indication and Year Approved*
	Brentuximab vedotin (Adcetris)	CD30-positive mycosis fungoides and cutaneous anaplastic large cell lymphoma (2017) Untreated CD30-expressing PTCL in combination with CHP chemotherapy (2018)
Anti-CCR4 monoclonal antibody	Mechanism: binds CCR4 and inhibits downstream signal transduction pathways and chemokine-mediated cellular migration and T-cell proliferation Notable toxicities: infusion reactions, infection, rash, fever, edema, nausea, headache, cytopenias	
	Drug Name	*Indication and Year Approved*
	Mogamulizumab (Poteligeo)	Mycosis fungoides (2018) Approved outside United States for adult T-cell leukemia/lymphoma
Folate antagonists	Mechanism: are a folate analog that accumulates in lymphoma cells and impairs DNA synthesis Notable toxicities: mucositis, myelosuppression, nausea, fatigue	
	Drug Name	*Indication and Year Approved*
	Pralatrexate (Folotyn)	Relapsed PTCL (2009)

CCR4, CC chemokine receptor type 4; *CHP*, cyclophosphamide, doxorubicin, and prednisone; *CTCL*, cutaneous T-cell lymphoma; *MMAE*, monomethyl auristatin E; *PTCL*, peripheral T-cell lymphoma.

inhibitors (ibrutinib [Imbruvica], acalabrutinib [Calquence] and zanubrutinib [Brukinsa]) and venetoclax (Venclexta), a BH3 mimetic acting as an inhibitor of BCL2. A 2023 study found that zanubrutinib therapy resulted in longer PFS with fewer toxicities compared with ibrutinib. There are several recently published and a number of ongoing clinical studies to evaluate the optimal sequence and varied combinations for patients with CLL, especially vis-à-vis harnessing frontline targeted therapeutics. A novel class of drugs, EZH2 inhibitors, have also shown promise in R/R lymphomas by modulation of epigenetic pathways. One of these, tazemetostat (Tazverik), has been approved for use in R/R follicular lymphoma after two prior lines of therapy, with higher response rates in patients harboring EZH2 mutations compared with those without.

As mentioned previously, the BTK inhibitor acalabrutinib (Calquence) and zanubrutinib (Brukinsa) are FDA approved for R/R MCL patients who have received at least one prior therapy and pirtobrutinib (Jaypirca) in patients after two lines of prior therapy. The PI3K inhibitor copanlisib [Aliqopa] was previously approved for adult patients with relapsed or refractory follicular lymphoma, but has since voluntarily withdrawn. Antibody drug conjugates contain potent drugs that are conjugated to a monoclonal antibody. These include brentuximab vedotin (Adcetris), which is FDA approved for newly diagnosed CD30-positive T-cell lymphomas and relapsed anaplastic (T-cell) large-cell lymphoma, and the anti-CD79b monoclonal antibody drug complex, polatuzumab vedotin (Polivy), which the FDA approved in combination with rituximab and bendamustine for R/R DLBCL. As noted earlier, polatuzumab vedotin was FDA approved in 2023 as part of combination chemotherapy for newly diagnosed DLBCL in patients with an IPI score of 2 or higher.

These novel therapeutic agents are mostly FDA approved for patients with R/R disease; however, there are a multitude of

TABLE 4	Efficacy of CAR-T in Indolent and Aggressive B-Cell Lymphoma
CAR-T PRODUCT	**RESPONSE RATE**
Lisocabtagene maraleucel (Breyanzi)	73%–87% (54%–74%)
Axicabtagene ciloleucel (Yescarta)	82%–83% (54%–65% CR)
Axicabtagene ciloleucel in R/R indolent lymphoma	96% (74% CR)
Tisagenlecleucel (Kymriah)	53% (39% CR)
Tisagenlecleucel in R/R FL	86% (68%)
Brexucabtagene autoleucel (Tecartus)	61% (38%)

CR, Complete response; *FL*, follicular lymphoma; *R/R*, relapsed or refractory.

ongoing studies in the frontline/untreated setting and in varied sequences and combinations.

There is also great excitement in the continued application of new immunotherapy approaches in NHL such as checkpoint inhibitors (e.g., programmed death-1 [PD-1] inhibitors), as well as chimeric antigen receptor (CAR) T-cell therapy, which involve removal of T cells from patients followed by bioengineered CARs (e.g., CD19) that facilitate T-cell expansion and antigen/tumor recognition when reinfused into the patient. Axicabtagene ciloleucel (Yescarta), tisagenlecleucel (Kymriah), and lisocabtagene maraleucel (Breyanzi) are anti-CD19 CAR T-cell therapies the FDA approved for patients with R/R DLBCL (Table 4). Overall response rates range from 50% to 72%, with complete remission rates of 32% to 51%. Furthermore, 25% to 35% of patients appear to experience

| TABLE 5 | CRS and ICAN Rate With CAR-T Therapy |

CAR-T PRODUCT	ALL GRADE CRS	GRADE ≥3 CRS	MEDIAN TIME TO ONSET OF CRS (DAYS)	MEDIAN DURATION OF CRS (DAYS)	ALL GRADE ICAN	GRADE ≥3 ICAN	MEDIAN TIME TO FIRST ICAN (DAYS)	MEDIAN DURATION OF ICAN (DAYS)
Lisocabtagene maraleucel (Breyanzi)	42%–52%	1%–4 %	4–5	4–5	27%–30%	4%–11%	8	6–12
Axicabtagene ciloleucel (Yescarta)	83%–93%	6%–13%	4–5	4–6	55%–77%	21%–28%	6	12–16
Axicabtagene ciloleucel in R/R indolent lymphoma	82%	7%–8%	4	5–6	59%	19%	7	10–14
Tisagenlecleucel (Kymriah)	57%–74%	23%	3	7	20%–60%	11%–19%	6	13
Tisagenlecleucel in R/R FL	49%–53%	0%	4	4	8%–43%	2%–6%	8	5
Brexucabtagene autoleucel (Tecartus)	91%	18%	5	8	81%	37%	7	15

CRS, Cytokine release syndrome; *FL*, follicular lymphoma; *ICAN*, immune effector cell-associated neurotoxicity syndrome; *R/R*, relapsed or refractory.

longer-term disease remission. In particular, lisocabtagene mara-leucel and axicabtagene ciloleucel are approved for patients with DLBCL relapsed within 12 months of initial therapy or not eligible for autologous stem cell transplant. Tisagenlecleucel (Kymriah) and axicabtagene ciloleucel (Yescarta) and lisocabtagene maraleucel (Breyanzi) are also approved for patients with R/R follicular lymphoma. Brexucabtagene autoleucel (Tecartus) is approved for R/R MCL and B-cell precursor acute lymphoblastic leukemia (ALL). There are a multitude of other CAR T-cell and natural killer-based constructs being studied across several lymphoma subtypes.

Despite the high efficacy of CAR-T cell therapy, relapse remains a challenge. Higher baseline tumor burden decreases CAR-T effectiveness and increases the risk of cytokine release syndrome (CRS) and immune effector cell–associated neuro-toxicity syndrome (ICANS) (Table 5). Bridging therapy before CAR-T cell infusion should be considered for patients with high tumor burden, avoiding agents that could result in T cell depletion, such as bendamustine (Bendeka, Treanda) before CAR-T cell collection

Whereas CAR-T therapy uses ex vivo manipulation of T cells to facilitate lymphoma-directed cytotoxicity, a novel class of monoclonal antibodies known as bispecific antibodies directs cytotoxic T cells to target tumor-specific molecules. Mosunetu-zumab (Lunsumio) and epcoritamab (Epkinly) are bispecific, CD20-directed, CD3 T-cell engagers approved for use in patients with R/R follicular lymphoma after two or more lines of prior therapy. Glofitamab (Columvi) also targets CD3 and CD20 and, with epcoritamab, are approved for R/R DLBCL. The investiga-tional agent odronextamab has a similar mechanism of action and has also shown encouraging results in a variety of B-cell lym-phoma subtypes. Use of bispecific antibodies in combination with chemotherapy or other targeted agents is currently being investi-gated in R/R disease and in the frontline setting.

Follow-Up of Long-Term Survivors

Relapse

Among patients with aggressive lymphomas, such as DLBCL, most recurrences are seen within the first 2 years after the com-pletion of therapy, although later relapses can occur. Physical examination and laboratory testing at 2- to 3-month intervals and follow-up CT scans at 6-month intervals for the first 2 years after diagnosis are recommended; however, there is ongoing debate regarding the potential improvement that postsurveillance scans have on disease outcomes if patients relapse. Detection of recurrent disease is important in part because these patients may be candidates for potentially curative therapy (e.g., cellular thera-pies). Patients with advanced low-grade NHL are at a constant risk for relapse, as discussed before.

Secondary Malignancies

Long-term NHL survivors are at an increased risk for second can-cers. In general, the risk is increased with a history of radiation use, but it is also seen with chemotherapy. In a survey of 28,131 Dutch registry patients with NHL who survived 2 years or lon-ger, significant excesses of second cancers were seen for nearly all solid tumors, as well as acute myelogenous leukemia (AML) and HL. The standardized incidence ratio (SIR) for solid tumors after NHL was 1.65. The SIRs for solid tumors are increased for up to 30 years after NHL diagnosis, with the highest relative risk of developing a secondary malignancy occurring more than 21 to 30 years after original diagnosis.

Late Treatment Complications

There has been more selective use of radiation as part of ther-apy for NHL. Thus the risk of certain radiation-induced com-plications has been reduced in patients treated more recently. Nevertheless, the risk still exists. Transplant recipients are at increased risk for secondary myelodysplasia and AML, regard-less of whether they received radiation. All chemotherapy agents may cause long-term morbidity; in particular, patients who received an anthracycline (e.g., doxorubicin [Adriamycin]) are at a long-term increased risk of cardiovascular disease. Among Dutch and Belgian patients with NHL treated with at least six cycles of doxorubicin-based chemotherapy, cumulative incidence of cardiovascular disease was 12% at 5 years and 22% at 10 years. Risk of coronary artery disease matched that of the general population; however, risk of chronic heart failure was signifi-cantly increased (SIR, 5.4), as was stroke (SIR, 1.8). Risk factors associated with excess risk included younger age at start of NHL treatment (<55 years), preexisting hypertension, any salvage treatment, and use of radiotherapy; risk relating to radiotherapy was dose dependent. Continued studies are needed to develop optimal secondary prevention strategies.

References

Bishop MR, Dickinson M, Purtill D, et al: Second-line tisagenlecleucel or standard care in aggressive B cell lymphoma, *N Engl J Med* 386:629–639, 2022.

Brown JR, Eichhorst B, Hillmen P, et al: Zanubrutinib or ibrutinib in relapsed or refractory chronic lymphocytic leukemia, *N Engl J Med* 388(4):319–332, 2023.

Budde LE, Sehn LH, Matasar M, et al: Safety and efficacy of mosunetuzumab, a bispecific antibody, in patients with relapsed or refractory follicular lymphoma: a single-arm, multicentre, phase 2 study, *Lancet Oncol* 23(80):1055–1065, 2022.

Burger JA, et al: Ibrutinib as initial therapy for patients with chronic lymphocytic leukemia, *N Engl J Med* 373(25):2425–2437, 2015.

Chapuy B, Stewart C, Dunford AJ, et al: Molecular subtypes of diffuse large B cell lymphoma are associated with distinct pathogenic mechanisms and outcomes, *Nat Med* 24:679–690, 2018.

Dickinson MJ, Carlo-Stella C, Morschhauser F, et al: Glofitamab for relapsed or refractory diffuse large B cell lymphoma, *N Engl J Med* 387:2220–2231, 2022.

Dunleavy K, Pittaluga S, Shovlin M, et al: Low-intensity therapy in adults with Burkitt's lymphoma, *N Engl J Med* 369(20):1915–1925, 2013.

Evens AM, Danilov AV, Jagadeesh D, et al: Burkitt lymphoma in the modern era: real world outcomes and prognostication across 30 US Cancer Centers, *Blood* 137:374–386, 2021.

Fischer K, Al-Sawaf O, Bahlo J, et al: Venetoclax and obinutuzumab in patients with CLL and coexisting conditions, *N Engl J Med* 380(23):2225–2236, 2019.

Fowler NH, Dickinson M, Dreyling M, et al: Tisagenlecleucel in adult relapsed or refractory follicular lymphoma: the phase 2 ELARA trial, *Int J Hematol* 28:325–332, 2022.

Gopal AK, Kahl BS, de Vos S, et al: PI3Kδ inhibition by idelalisib in patients with relapsed indolent lymphoma, *N Engl J Med* 370(11):1008–1018, 2014.

Hemminki K, Lenner P, Sundquist J, Bermejo JL: Risk of subsequent solid tumors after non-Hodgkin's lymphoma: effect of diagnostic age and time since diagnosis, *J Clin Oncol* 26(11):1850–1857, 2008.

Horwitz S, O'Connor OA, Pro B, et al: Brentuximab vedotin with chemotherapy for CD30-positive peripheral T-cell lymphoma (ECHELON-2): a global, double-blind, randomised, phase 3 trial, *Lancet* 393(10168):229–240, 2019.

Jacobson CA, Chavez JC, Sehgal AR, et al: Axicabtagene ciloleucel in relapsed or refractory indolent non-Hodgkin lymphoma (ZUMA-5): a single-arm, multicentre, phase 2 trial, *Lancet Oncol* 23(1):91–103, 2022.

Marcus R, Davies A, Ando K, et al: Obinutuzumab for the first-line treatment of follicular lymphoma, *N Engl J Med* 377(14):1331–1344, 2017.

Morschhauser F, Tilly H, Chaidos A, et al: Tazemetostat for patients with relapsed or refractory follicular lymphoma: an open-label, single-arm, multicentre, phase 2 trial, *Lancet Oncol* 21(11):1433–1442, 2020.

Morton LM, Curtis RE, Linet MS, et al: Second malignancy risks after non-Hodgkin's lymphoma and chronic lymphocytic leukemia: differences by lymphoma subtype, *J Clin Oncol* 28:4935–4944, 2010.

Moser EC, Noordijk EM, van Leeuwen FE, et al: Long-term risk of cardiovascular disease after treatment for aggressive non-Hodgkin lymphoma, *Blood* 107:2912–2919, 2006.

Neelapu SS, Locke FL, Bartlett NL, et al: Axicabtagene ciloleucel CAR T-Cell therapy in refractory large B-Cell lymphoma, *N Engl J Med* 377(26):2531–2544, 2017.

Olszewski AJ, Jakobsen LH, Collins GP, et al: Burkitt lymphoma international prognostic index, *J Clin Oncol* 39(10):1129–1138, 2021.

Prince HM, Kim YH, Horwitz SM, et al: Brentuximab vedotin or physician's choice in CD30-positive cutaneous T-cell lymphoma (ALCANZA): an international, open-label, randomised, phase 3, multicentre trial, *Lancet* 390(10094):555–566, 2017.

Roberts AW, et al: Targeting BCL2 with Venetoclax in relapsed chronic lymphocytic leukemia, *N Engl J Med* 374(4):311–322, 2016.

Schmitz R, Wright GW, Huang DW, et al: Genetics and pathogenesis of diffuse large B cell lymphoma, *N Engl J Med* 378:1396–1407, 2018.

Schuster SJ, Bishop MR, Tam CS: Tisagenlecleucel in adult relapsed or refractory diffuse large B-Cell lymphoma, *N Engl J Med* 380(1):45–56, 2019.

Seghal A, Hoda D, Riedell PA, et al: Lisocabtagene maraleucel as second-line therapy in adults with relapsed or refractory large B-cell lymphoma who were not intended for haematopoietic stem cell transplantation (PILOT): an open-label phase 2 study, *Lancet Oncol* 23(8):1066–1077, 2022.

Sehn LH, et al: Tafasitamab plus lenalidomide and rituximab for relapsed or refractory follicular lymphoma: results from a phase 3 study (inMIND), *Blood* 144(suppl 2), 2024, LBA–1.

Shanafelt TD, Wang XV, Kay NE, et al: Ibrutinib-rituximab or chemoimmunotherapy for chronic lymphocytic leukemia, *N Engl J Med* 381(5):432–443, 2019.

Siegel RL, Miller KD, Fuchs HE, et al: Cancer statistics, 2021, *CA Cancer J Clin* 71(1):7–33, 2021.

Swerdlow SH, Campo E, Pileri SA, et al: The 2016 revision of the World Health Organization classification of lymphoid neoplasms, *Blood* 127(20):2375–2390, 2016.

Trappe RU, Dierickx D, Zimmermann H, et al: Response to rituximab induction is a predictive marker in B-cell post-transplant lymphoproliferative disorder and allows successful stratification into rituximab or R-CHOP consolidation in an international, prospective, multicenter phase II trial, *J Clin Oncol* 35(5):536–543, 2017.

Wang ML, Rule S, Martin P, et al: Targeting BTK with ibrutinib in relapsed or refractory mantle-cell lymphoma, *N Engl J Med* 369(6):507–516, 2013.

Woyach JA, Ruppert AS, Heerema NA, et al: Ibrutinib regimens versus chemoimmunotherapy in older patients with untreated CLL, *N Engl J Med* 379(26):2517–2528, 2018.

Zhou Z, Sehn LH, Rademaker AW, et al: An enhanced International Prognostic Index (NCCN-IPI) for patients with diffuse large B-cell lymphoma treated in the rituximab era, *Blood* 123(6):837–842, 2014.

MEGALOBLASTIC ANEMIAS

Method of
Robert L. Redner, MD

CURRENT DIAGNOSIS

- The megaloblastic anemias represent a subset of macrocytic anemias, often characterized by cells with a mean corpuscular volume greater than 110 fl.
- Folic acid deficiency and vitamin B12 deficiency are classic causes of megaloblastic anemia.
- Megaloblastic changes often occur in patients receiving chemotherapy.
- Megaloblastic anemias are caused by asynchrony of nuclear and cytoplasmic maturation. Though usually thought of as a red blood cell problem, megaloblastic changes can affect any dividing cell.
- Folic acid is necessary for synthesis of DNA; B12 is necessary for activation of folic acid to an active form.
- Folic acid deficiency arises from either decreased intake in the diet, or malabsorption in the gastrointestinal (GI) tract. B12 deficiency almost always arises from decreased GI absorption. Pernicious anemia is an immunologic disease in which the absorption of B12 is inhibited by anti–intrinsic factor or anti–parietal cell antibodies.
- Humans contain a 3-month reserve of folic acid but a 3- to 5-year supply of B12. The clinical manifestations of B12 deficiency become manifest several years after decreased B12 absorption begins.
- Serum folic acid levels can be used to monitor folic acid in the outpatient setting. Folate in the diet can mask underlying folate deficiency; in hospitalized patients, it is best to measure red blood cell folate.
- Homocysteine levels rise in either folic acid or B12 deficiency, but elevated methylmalonic acid levels are distinct to B12 deficiency.

CURRENT THERAPY

- Green vegetables are rich in folic acid. Dietary sources of vitamin B12 include meat, liver, shellfish, some cheeses, yeast extract, and root nodules of legumes.
- Folic acid deficiency can be treated with oral or IV folic acid, 1 to 2 mg/day.
- B12 deficiency is treated with parenteral administration of 1000 microgram B12 weekly, followed by slow taper to a maintenance dose of 1000 µg monthly. Because of a low level of passive diffusion of B12 across the gut, high doses of oral B12 (1000–2000 µg/day) can also be effective.
- In the setting of concurrent folic acid and B12 deficiency, B12 deficiency needs to be replaced first, lest the repleted folic acid biochemical pathways deplete limited B12 reserves and exacerbate neurologic deficits.

Introduction and Pathophysiology

Macrocytic anemias are characterized by large red blood cells. The megaloblastic anemias represent a subset of macrocytic anemias, often characterized by cells with a mean corpuscular volume (MCV) greater than 110 fl. Megaloblastic anemias are the result of disrupted nuclear maturation. Because of slowed DNA replication, affected cells transit the cell cycle more slowly. This leads to asynchrony between the slowed nuclear maturation and the unaffected maturation of the cytoplasm. As applied to red cell precursors, the normoblasts in the bone marrow have enlarged immature-appearing nuclei with an abundance of well hemoglobinized cytoplasm. Such abnormal cells are readily identified in the bone marrow. After karyorrhexis and expulsion of the nucleus, the mature red cells have a high MCV and high mean corpuscular hemoglobin (MCH). It is important to note that the megaloblastic precursors have a high apoptotic rate, and megaloblastic marrows often manifest ineffective hematopoiesis and erythropoiesis. Ineffective erythropoiesis, as well as lysis of the enlarged red cells as they pass through the spleen, leads to elevated levels of serum lactic dehydrogenase and bilirubin, often to levels above those seen with hemolytic anemias.

Megaloblastic changes often occur in patients receiving chemotherapy. Most forms of chemotherapy target cells that are rapidly cycling to block their replication without having significant effects on cytoplasmic maturation. Of note, hydroxyurea, commonly used to enhance hemoglobin F expression in sickle cell anemia, similarly induces megaloblastic changes, and an increase in the MCV of patient's red blood cells. Indeed, one of the ways of assessing adherence with a hydroxyurea regimen is to monitor macrocytosis in patients on this drug. As we shall see, folic acid deficiency, and vitamin B12 deficiency, the two most common causes of megaloblastic anemia, follow the same paradigm. Myelodysplastic neoplasms manifest many of the changes seen in megaloblastic anemias, with dysplastic growth of hematopoietic precursors. Potential causes of megaloblastic anemia need to be excluded in patients with suspected myelodysplastic neoplasms.

Clinical Manifestations

The abnormal maturation of megaloblastic cells can occur not only in red cells, but in any dividing cell. Bone marrow myeloid cells, skin and hair follicles, and mucosal cells of the gastrointestinal (GI) tract are most susceptible to megaloblastic changes. In myeloid cells asynchronous nuclear maturation is reflected in abnormal-appearing myeloid precursors in the bone marrow and nuclear hypersegmentation in mature neutrophils. Changes in hair follicles leads to thinning and lightening of hair. In the GI tract, loss of papillation and enlargement of the tongue can be seen (particularly in B12 deficiency); loss of small bowel villi results in malabsorption, which can exacerbate folate or B12 deficiency (see later) to potentially worsen the megaloblastic process.

Folic Acid Deficiency
Pathophysiology
Folic acid deficiency is one of the classic causes of megaloblastic changes. Folic acid is required for two of the critical biochemical pathways that synthesize DNA nucleotides. In a separate reaction, folic acid serves as a cofactor in the conversion of homocysteine to methionine. There is a limited folic acid reserve of less than 3 months in most people. Folic acid is absorbed primarily in the duodenum and jejunum; malabsorptive processes often result in folate deficiency. Green vegetables are rich in folic acid, and the classic "tea and toast" diet of elderly, or the lack of diet in severe alcoholics, can result in folate deficiencies. Conversely, any physiologic or pathologic state characterized by increased DNA synthesis, such as the hyperactive bone marrow that characterizes sickle cell or other hemolytic anemias, synthesis of keratinocytes as in severe psoriasis, fetal growth during pregnancy, or rapidly growing cancers, can all lead to depletion of limited stores of folic acid. Being a water-soluble small molecule, folate is easily dialyzed, and so folate supplementation should always be considered in patients with chronic kidney disease undergoing dialysis.

Diagnosis
Confirmation of suspected folic acid deficiency can be difficult. Although measurement of serum folic acid levels is usually a reliable indicator of the state of folic acid levels in the outpatient setting, measuring serum folic acid levels in hospitalized patients can be misleading. This is because most hospital meals contain a sufficient amount of folic acid to replete serum levels. Eating one or two meals after admission to the hospital will result in normalization of folic acid levels and mask underlying folate deficiency. Thus, in hospitalized patients, it is best to measure red blood cell folate, not serum folate levels. This test involves lysis of the erythrocytes and measurement of the folic acid that is contained within the erythrocyte cytoplasm. The folate within erythrocytes, and within all human cells, differs from the ingested folate in that it has multiple glutamic acid groups attached to it. Each glutamate conveys a negative charge to the molecule; as a result of polyglutamation, folic acid in cells becomes highly negatively charged and is more likely to stay within the confines of the cytoplasm. Because folic acid is needed primarily for DNA replication, as red blood cells mature and lose their nuclei, they lose their need for, and the ability to produce, the enzyme that catalyzes polyglutamation. Thus the folic acid found within enucleate erythrocytes reflects the levels of folic acid that were present when the erythrocyte precursor cells were developing in the marrow. Measuring the polyglutamated folic acid within red blood cells can therefore be interpreted as a sensor for the amount of folic acid that was available in weeks and months past, presumably before the patient was hospitalized and exposed to folate-rich hospital food. Conceptually, this is similar to assessing HbA1c to integrate the levels of blood sugar over time.

In difficult cases, measurement of homocysteine levels can be used to support a diagnosis of folate deficiency. Folic acid provides a methyl group to homocysteine to create methionine. In the absence of folic acid, homocysteine levels rise. As discussed later, homocysteine levels also rise in B12 deficiency: a distinction between folic acid deficiency and B12 deficiency is that methylmalonic acid levels will also rise in B12 deficiency, whereas they will be normal in folic acid deficiency.

Therapy
Once identified, folic acid deficiency can be readily replaced either orally or parenterally at a dose of 1 to 5 mg per day. It is important to recognize that the folic acid administered as a supplement or obtained through the diet is not active, but must be activated by the enzyme dihydrofolate reductase (DHFR). DHFR is also necessary for intracellular recycling of folic acid used in DNA nucleotide synthesis. This critical enzyme is targeted by the chemotherapeutic agent methotrexate, which affects cell replication through inhibition of folic acid metabolism. Similarly the bacterial form of DHFR is inhibited by trimethoprim and pyrimethamine; at high doses these antibiotics can also inhibit human DHFR to cause megaloblastic anemia. Leucovorin (folinic acid) bypasses the steps mediated by DHFR and can be easily modified into the active form of folic acid. Leucovorin can be used as an antidote to ameliorate methotrexate toxicity. Leucovorin can also be used to enhance binding and uptake of fluorouracil (5-FU) to the enzyme thymidine synthase. This combination of leucovorin and 5-FU forms the backbone of the FOLFIRI (leucovorin, fluorouracil, irinotecan) and FOLFOX (leucovorin, fluorouracil, and oxaliplatin) combination chemotherapy regimens used in treatment of GI cancers.[1]

Vitamin B12 Deficiency
Pathophysiology
The mechanism by which B12 deficiency induces megaloblastic anemia is intertwined with folic acid metabolism. B12 is essential for folic acid activation and serves as a cofactor in the activation of folic acid with concomitant transfer of a methyl group to homocysteine to produce methionine. In the absence of B12, an inactive form of folic acid accumulates, leading to depletion of intracellular active folate. Since both B12 and folate are essential cofactors for the conversion of homocysteine into methionine, deficiency of either B12 or folate will result in a rise in measurable homocysteine levels.

In humans, B12 serves as a cofactor in only two known enzymatic reactions—the conversion of homocysteine to methionine with the cognate activation of folic acid, and the conversion of malonyl-CoA to succinyl-CoA in the metabolism of odd-chain fatty acids. In the absence of B12, malonyl-CoA, builds up and is converted to methylmalonic acid, which can be measured in serum or urine as a marker of B12 deficiency. Whereas homocysteine levels are elevated in either B12 deficiency or folate deficiency, elevation of methylmalonic acid is distinct to B12 deficiency and can be useful in distinguishing between these two causes of megaloblastic anemia.

---

[1] Not FDA approved for this indication.

B12 is not synthesized in humans, but only by microorganisms. Dietary sources of B12 include meat, liver, shellfish, some cheeses, yeast extract, and root nodules of legumes. The average daily requirement of B12 is only 2 to 4 μg. Yet, because of its importance in key biologic pathways, the average body store is 1000-fold more—3 to 5 milligrams—mostly stored in the liver. It is very rare to develop B12 deficiency from inadequate nutrition, even in strict vegans. Rather, B12 deficiency is almost always caused by dysfunction in one of the many steps required for B12 absorption in the GI tract.

The first step in B12 absorption begins in the mouth. Most B12 in the diet is bound to proteins, which are degraded by enzymes produced both in the saliva and the stomach. B12 binding proteins (haptocorrins, also known as R-factors) are produced in salivary glands. In the acidic environment of the stomach B12 binds to haptocorrin. Parietal cells in the gastric antrum produce and secrete intrinsic factor, though intrinsic factor does not bind B12 in the stomach; rather, B12 remains complexed to haptocorrins. In the duodenum pancreatic proteases degrade the haptocorrins and, in the presence of alkalotic environment of the duodenum and upper jejunum, B12 is then transferred to intrinsic factor. The B12-intrinsic factor complex transits the jejunum and ileum to the terminal ileum, where specific cellular receptors bind the B12-intrinsic factor complex and initiate endocytosis; lysosomal enzymes degrade intrinsic factor, allowing free B12 to be secreted into the bloodstream, where it binds to transcobalamin and is transported to cells throughout the body.

Interference in any of the steps necessary for B12 absorption will result in B12 deficiency. Decreased salivary production, as occurs in aging or scleroderma, will affect production of salivary proteases and haptocorrins. Interference with acid production in the stomach, as in gastrectomy, atrophic gastritis, or even prolonged use of antacids or proton pump inhibitors, will interfere with binding of B12 to haptocorrins. Decreased stomach protease production will affect release of B12 from ingested food. Disruption in production of intrinsic factor, either due to surgical removal of the gastric antrum or immunologic interference with production of intrinsic factor (the classic cause of pernicious anemia, discussed in greater detail later) affects the ultimate absorption of B12. Chronic pancreatitis can lead to decreased production of the proteases and the alkaline environment necessary for release of B12 from haptocorrins and binding to intrinsic factor. Disruption of the anatomy of the duodenum, as in Roux-en-Y surgical procedures, will affect the alkalotic environment necessary for B12 to bind to intrinsic factor. Similarly, bacterial overgrowth in a blind loop of the duodenum or jejunum can affect stability of the B12 complexes. A rare cause of B12 deficiency is infestation with the parasite *Diphyllobothrium latum,* a tapeworm that can be ingested by consumption of raw freshwater fish, which grows in the jejunum and absorbs B12 directly from the jejunal fluids. Interference with the terminal ileum, as can occur in surgical removal during colectomy, or involvement of the ileum from ulcerative colitis or Crohn disease, will interfere with absorption of intrinsic factor–B12 complexes. One of the unusual causes of B12 deficiency is chronic nitrous oxide inhalation; nitrous oxide irreversibly oxidizes cobalt in the corrin ring of B12, leading to nonfunctional B12. Metformin use has also been associated with B12 deficiency, though the mechanism remains controversial.

Pathophysiology of Pernicious Anemia. Pernicious anemia is an immunologic disease in which production of anti–intrinsic factor antibodies, or anti–parietal cell antibodies, decreases the ability of parietal cells in the gastric antrum to produce intrinsic factor. It is often familial and can be associated with other autoimmune dieses, such as vitiligo, thyroiditis, or Addison disease. The liver contains a 3- to 5-year store of B12, which is released through the enterohepatic circulation in bile. It takes several years to deplete the liver stores, so B12 deficiency may not be recognized for years after development of the underlying pathologic insult that interferes with B12 absorption. This insidious onset of B12 deficiency led to the term pernicious anemia, which now refers specifically to an immunologic cause of B12 deficiency. First recognized in the late 1800s, pernicious anemia was the scourge of hematology 100 years ago. Indeed, development of a treatment for pernicious anemia was of such importance that it garnered the 1934 Nobel Prize in Medicine for Minot, Murphy, and Whipple.

Diagnosis

B12 deficiency should be suspected with a low-normal serum B12 level (usually <300) and diagnosed with B12 level less than 200. Confirmation can be performed by measuring serum or urine methylmalonic acid levels, which should be elevated in B12 deficiency.

Diagnosis of Pernicious Anemia. The diagnosis of pernicious anemia is fairly straightforward with tests for anti-intrinsic factor or anti-parietal cell antibodies.. These tests have high specificities and sensitivities.

Therapy

Treatment for B12 deficiency is usually parenteral B12: 1000 μg intramuscularly (IM) weekly, with a gradual decrease in dosing until a maintenance of 1000 μg monthly is obtained. Approximately 1% of B12 is absorbed passively in the GI tract (this fact may well underly the success of liver therapy first advocated by Minot and Murphy) and some patients may respond to high doses of oral B12 on the order of 1000 to 2000 μg daily. B12 is water soluble, and excess B12 is excreted through the liver and eventually the feces. Toxicity from B12 overdose is almost unheard of, though rare case reports mention acne, palpitation, anxiety, akathisia, headache, and insomnia, which are readily reversible.

Therapy for Pernicious Anemia. Aside from receiving B12 replacement therapy, patients with suspected pernicious anemia should be followed with periodic endoscopies to assess for atrophic gastritis and associated development of gastric cancer.

Complications

B12 deficiency of any cause will give rise not just to a megaloblastic anemia akin to that seen in folic acid deficiency but also neurologic disorders unique to B12 deficiency. The neurologic disorders are likely caused by interruption in the conversion of malonyl-CoA to succinyl-CoA and accumulation of nonphysiologic lipids that accumulate in myelin sheaths of nerves, though the exact mechanism remains unclear. The neurologic abnormalities associated with B12 deficiency can be myriad, ranging from peripheral neuropathies to loss of vibration and position sense (classic subacute combined degeneration of the spinal cord secondary to demyelination of the dorsal and lateral spinal columns) to psychosis or dementia. The presence of any of these in a patient with suspected B12 deficiency should be a signal to immediately start B12 supplementation. Of importance to note, in the presence of concomitant folate deficiency, B12 replacement should always be initiated first. Otherwise, replacement of folic acid could divert B12 to the folic acid/methionine synthesis pathway and deplete B12 from the malonyl-CoA/succinyl-CoA conversion, which could exacerbate neurotoxicity. B12 associated neuropathy can be reversible, but severe neurologic changes may take years to improve.

References

Abuyaman O, Abdelfattah A, Shehadeh-Tout F, Deeb AA, Hatmal MM: Vitamin B12 insufficiency and deficiency: a review of nondisease risk factors, *Scand J Clin Lab Invest* 83(8):533–539, 2023. 38145316.

Creary S, Chisolm D, Stanek J, et al: Measuring hydroxyurea adherence by pharmacy and laboratory data compared with video observation in children with sickle cell disease, *Pediatr Blood Cancer* 67(8):e28250, 2020. 32386106.

Kumar N, Boes CJ, Samuels MA: Liver therapy in anemia: a motion picture by William P. Murphy, *Blood* 107(12):4970, 2006. 16754778.

Minot GR: *The Development of liver therapy in pernicious anemia,* Nobel Lecture, 1934.

Sobczynska-Malefora A, Delvin E, McCaddon A, Ahmadi KR, Harrington DJ: Vitamin B(12) status in health and disease: a critical review. Diagnosis of deficiency and insufficiency - clinical and laboratory pitfalls, *Crit Rev Clin Lab Sci* 58(6):399–429, 2021. 33881359.

Torrez M, Chabot-Richards D, Babu D, Lockhart E, Foucar K: How I investigate acquired megaloblastic anemia, *Int J Lab Hematol* 44(2):236–247, 2022. 34981651.

Zarou MM, Vazquez A, Vignir Helgason G: Folate metabolism: a re-emerging therapeutic target in haematological cancers, *Leukemia* 35(6):1539–1551, 2021. 33707653 PMC8179844.

Zwart NRK, Franken MD, Tissing WJE, et al: Folate, folic acid, and chemotherapy-induced toxicities: A systematic literature review, *Crit Rev Oncol Hematol* 188:104061, 2023. 37353179.

PLATELET-MEDIATED BLEEDING DISORDERS

Method of
Deirdre Nolfi-Donegan, MD

CURRENT DIAGNOSIS

- Platelet-related bleeding typically manifests as mucosal bleeding, menorrhagia, petechiae, purpura, superficial ecchymoses, and immediate bleeding after injury or surgery.
- Bleeding can arise from quantity or function issues of platelets, though bleeding risk generally remains low when counts are above 20 to $30 \times 10^9/L$.
- Available diagnostic methods to evaluate platelet count, function, and structure include a complete blood count; light microscopy review of the peripheral smear; closure times via platelet function analyzer; thromboelastography for global coagulation assessment; light aggregometry for platelet-platelet interactions and milder drug effects; transmission electron microscopy for ultrastructure review; flow cytometry for surface proteins and dense granule release; and genetic testing for inherited platelet disorders and predisposition syndromes.
- Thrombocytopenia is the most common cause of platelet-related bleeding and can occur because of inadequate platelet production, increased platelet destruction, or platelet sequestration.
- Acquired conditions such as renal dysfunction, paraproteinemia, and medication-induced inhibition can lead to platelet dysfunction and bleeding despite normal platelet counts.
- Congenital platelet disorders may encompass disorders of platelet production, surface protein dysfunction, and granule abnormalities.

CURRENT THERAPY

- Treatment for platelet disorders stemming from production issues often involves platelet transfusion when the platelet count drops below $10 \times 10^9/L$ or with bleeding. However, this approach poses the risk of alloimmunization resulting in platelet refractoriness and reduced effectiveness of subsequent transfusions.
- For most mild to moderate platelet disorders, pharmacologic therapies are sufficient to manage symptoms. Desmopressin acetate (DDAVP) stimulates the release of von Willebrand factor, enhancing platelet adhesion and aggregation. Antifibrinolytic agents prevent clot breakdown, whereas hormonal management with estrogen addresses specific manifestations like menorrhagia and uremia. Recombinant human activated factor VIIa (NovoSeven) may be used to promote clot formation, though efficacy varies based on the underlying cause and severity. This treatment is typically reserved for specific scenarios where other options are inadequate or when transfusion is contraindicated.
- Classic autoimmune thrombocytopenia is managed conservatively by observation in the absence of bleeding. Bleeding requires treatment with corticosteroids, intravenous immunoglobulin (IVIG), or anti-D immune globulin (WinRho SDF); refractory cases may require rituximab (Rituxan)[1], other immunosuppressives, thrombopoietin receptor agonists, or splenectomy.
- Other types of immune thrombocytopenia are managed according to their underlying cause; drug-induced immune thrombocytopenia is managed by discontinuing the offending drug; maternal autoimmune thrombocytopenia in neonates is treated with IVIG and platelet transfusion; neonatal alloimmune thrombocytopenia is treated with platelet transfusion often supplemented with IVIG.
- Thrombotic microangiopathies and disseminated intravascular coagulation are largely managed with supportive care; thrombotic thrombocytopenic purpura requires plasmapheresis with or without steroids and rituximab[1] for acquired cases, and ADAMTS13 (Adzynma) replacement for congenital cases.
- Severe platelet dysfunction, bone marrow failure syndromes, and cancer predisposition syndromes warrant consideration for stem cell transplant.
- Managing platelet disorders requires a tailored approach considering the individual's condition, underlying pathology, comorbidities, and treatment risks and benefits.

[1]Not FDA approved for this indication.

Platelet Physiology

Platelets are small anucleate cells that play a crucial role in primary hemostasis, endothelial junctional integrity, innate immunity, angiogenesis, and inflammatory signaling. Mature megakaryocytes (MKs), located primarily in the bone marrow, produce about 150 billion platelets daily in adults. Platelets circulate for 8 to 10 days and are removed by consumption or by apoptosis within the reticuloendothelial system. Thrombopoietin (TPO), produced steadily by the liver, regulates MK and platelet numbers through Mpl receptor adsorption on MKs and platelets. This mechanism adjusts TPO levels based on platelet/MK counts, with TPO decreasing when cell counts are high and increasing when low.

Structurally, platelets possess alpha granules, dense granules, and lysosomes, which fuse with the surface membrane and release their contents in response to specific stimuli. Alpha granules store large molecules including von Willebrand factor (VWF), fibrinogen, and platelet-derived growth factor. Dense granules contain smaller signaling molecules like adenine nucleotides (adenosine diphosphate [ADP] and adenosine triphosphate [ATP]), serotonin, and histamine. Alterations in granule morphology, content, and secretion are present in several congenital platelet disorders as discussed further later. The platelet cytoskeleton and tubular system provides structural support and enables shape change.

Platelets play a pivotal role in primary hemostasis through structural and functional adaptations. Upon endothelial injury or disruption, platelets adhere to exposed VWF and collagen on the vascular subendothelial matrix. They activate, undergo shape change, and degranulate. The granule contents summon additional platelets to the growing plug mainly through ADP's receptors P2Y1 and P2Y12 and thrombin receptors PAR-1 and PAR-4. Simultaneously, fibrinogen binds to platelet surface protein GPIIb/IIIa to stabilize platelet-platelet connections (aggregation). Other granule contents facilitate vasoconstriction and stimulate procoagulant factors necessary for secondary hemostasis while the clot continues to organize.

Clinical Features

Platelet-related bleeding is caused by insufficient platelet quantity, function, or both, and can be either inherited or acquired. Clinical signs of thrombocytopenia or impaired platelet function include immediate bleeding after injury or surgery, mucosal bleeding (including epistaxis and oral bleeding with dental procedures), menorrhagia, petechiae, purpura, and superficial ecchymoses.

Deep muscle hematomas, hemarthroses, and delayed bleeding are uncommon without trauma.

Platelet Testing

A complete blood count (CBC) assesses platelet count and mean platelet volume measures size. Peripheral smear review evaluates granularity, platelet size, and in vitro clumping, or pseudothrombocytopenia. Clumping can arise from phlebotomy difficulties, or from the presence of EDTA-dependent antiplatelet antibodies that react in EDTA tubes in vitro. It should be suspected when bleeding symptoms (or their lack thereof) do not align with the platelet count, and the CBC should be recollected in a sodium citrate tube. Closure times are measured using a platelet function analyzer equipped with a collagen-coated aperture through which whole blood is flowed and the time to aperture closure is recorded. Closure times offer insight into major platelet function defects but typically miss milder ones. Closure times are not specific to any particular platelet disorder and are prolonged in the setting of low hematocrit, drugs with antiplatelet effects, and von Willebrand disease (VWD). Thromboelastography (TEG) is another assay that uses whole blood to provide a global assessment of platelet function, coagulation and fibrinolysis. It is validated to guide blood product replacement in trauma and surgery. TEG can inform the need for platelet transfusion but is not useful for diagnosing platelet disorders. Light aggregometry is the gold standard for platelet function defects. The pattern of the aggregation curve in response to various agonists like ADP, collagen, ristocetin, epinephrine, and thromboxane can be distinct for major platelet disorders (Glanzmann, Bernard-Soulier) but nonspecific in milder ones. Transmission electron microscopy (TEM) assesses platelet structures and helps diagnose platelet granule disorders and corroborates suspected platelet cytoskeletal disorders. It is not performed at many institutions but can be sent out to reference laboratories. Inadvertent platelet activation and morphology changes can occur during collection or transport and may affect interpretation by TEM. Flow cytometry is instrumental for diagnosing platelet disorders related to surface proteins like Glanzmann and Bernard-Soulier, as well as dense granule release. Flow cytometry can target distinct surface proteins for quantification, and the flow cytometry-based mepacrine assay provides a more accurate assessment of dense granule release than older adenine nucleotide release assays. Last, genetic testing has emerged as the definitive testing for not only rarer platelet disorders, but also the platelet disorders associated with systemic syndromes and cancer/myelodysplastic predisposition syndromes.

Functional Disorders

Acquired Functional Disorders

Platelet dysfunction despite normal platelet count is well recognized in renal dysfunction and some myeloproliferative disorders. Uremia is thought to disrupt critical platelet interactions and granule release. Although there is no specific threshold at which circulating urea affects platelets, rising blood urea nitrogen levels and decreasing glomerular filtration rates often correlate with platelet dysfunction. Correction of platelet function is typically unnecessary unless bleeding occurs. Transfusions are generally ineffective because of the acquisition of similar defects by transfused platelets. Treatment strategies focus on addressing the underlying renal dysfunction and supportive care with interventions such as dialysis, desmopressin (DDAVP)[1], estrogen[1] therapy, and correction of anemia using erythropoietin (Epogen) or packed red blood cells. Likewise, disorders associated with paraproteinemia, like multiple myeloma and Waldenstrom macroglobulinemia, disrupt platelet function through adherence of immunoglobulins to the platelet surface, and the removal of the paraprotein improves platelet function.

Several medication classes intentionally inhibit platelet function to treat and prevent cerebrovascular and cardiovascular thromboembolic events. These include agents targeting cyclooxygenase-1/thromboxane A2 formation, such as acetylsalicylic acid (aspirin) and ibuprofen, as well as ADP receptor antagonists (ticagrelor [Brilinta], cangrelor [Kengreal], clopidogrel [Plavix], ticlopidine, and prasugrel [Effient]), and integrin $\alpha IIb\beta 3$ (GPIIb-IIIa) blockers (abciximab [ReoPro][2], eptifibatide [Integrilin], and tirofiban [Aggrastat]). Hold times before major surgery are specific to each agent based on their biologic clearance rates and may be unnecessary for minor procedures. Additionally, many medications and substances not primarily designed for platelet inhibition may also inhibit platelet function in vitro and/or be associated with clinical bleeding. These include some antibiotics

(penicillins, cephalosporins, nitrofurantoin), sildenafil (Revatio, Viagra), caffeine, nitrates, several antihypertensives (β-blockers, angiotensin-converting enzyme inhibitors, calcium channel blockers), statins, antihistamines, tricyclic antidepressants, selective serotonin reuptake inhibitors, phenothiazines, certain anesthetics, garlic, and alcohol. A comprehensive list has been outlined by Scharf (see *Semin Thromb Hemost* 2012;38:865–883). Notably, the ability of a drug to inhibit platelet function in vitro does not always translate to clinically significant hemostasis impairment. Therefore, deciding whether to discontinue an agent should be guided by data regarding its clinical impact on bleeding, as well as the importance to the patient's overall health of continuing the medication.

Thrombocytopenia

Thrombocytopenia is a platelet count below $150 \times 10^9/L$, further classified as mild (100 to $149 \times 10^9/L$), moderate (50 to $99 \times 10^9/L$), or severe ($<50 \times 10^9/L$). Hemostasis remains largely intact above $50 \times 10^9/L$, with "spontaneous" bleeding only occurring below 20 to $30 \times 10^9/L$, and severe bleeding below $10 \times 10^9/L$. Thrombocytopenia occurs due to decreased production, increased destruction, or excessive sequestration of platelets, whereas dilutional thrombocytopenia results from massive blood product transfusion. In general, inadequate platelet production tends to manifest more bleeding symptoms than other types of thrombocytopenia, although platelet count does not correlate with bleeding risk across all platelet disorders.

Thrombocytopenia Due to Increased Destruction

Autoimmune Thrombocytopenia (ITP)

Autoimmune thrombocytopenia (ITP) arises from antiplatelet autoantibodies binding to platelets leading to their premature destruction by the reticuloendothelial system. Classic ITP manifests as isolated macrothrombocytopenia with normal hemoglobin and leukocyte counts. Concurrent cytopenias in other cell lines warrant evaluation for alternative etiologies such as bone marrow failure or infiltration. Acute ITP, defined as ITP persisting for less than 6 months, often follows a viral infection and typically resolves spontaneously in children. Chronic ITP, lasting from 6 to 12 months, can be idiopathic or secondary to conditions like systemic lupus erythematosus (SLE), primary immunodeficiencies, malignancy, or chronic infections, and can exhibit fluctuating levels of thrombocytopenia severity. Idiopathic cases are not linked to any primary systemic disorder. Life-threatening bleeds are rare even at platelet counts less than $10 \times 10^9/L$, thus observation is often appropriate irrespective of platelet number, whereas mucosal involvement or other bleeding necessitates treatment. First-line therapies include corticosteroids, intravenous immunoglobulin (IVIG), or anti-D immune globulin (WinRho SDF) for Rh+ patients with a spleen. Refractory cases may benefit from rituximab (Rituxan)[1], mycophenolate mofetil (CellCept)[1], or other immunosuppressives. Splenectomy remains an option for refractory cases or for emergent bleeds but is now considered a third-line choice because of the rise of TPO receptor agonists.

Special Subsets of ITP

Drug-induced ITP (DITP) has been reported with exposure to drugs like heparin, quinine, sulfas, valproic acid, rarely vaccines, and many others. DITP can be diagnosed by confirming autoantibody binding to the patient's sample in the presence of the suspected drug in vitro. It is managed by discontinuing the offending drug. One of the most common DITPs, heparin-induced thrombocytopenia (HIT), arises from the formation of antibodies against complexes of heparin and platelet factor 4.

Unlike most other immune thrombocytopenias, HIT is linked to a heightened risk of both venous and arterial thrombosis. Managing HIT involves discontinuing all heparin-containing products, including heparin-containing flushes and prothrombin

[1] Not FDA approved for this indication.
[2] Not available in the United States.

[1] Not FDA approved for this indication.

complex concentrates. A subset of HIT does not respond to cessation of heparin, and autoantibody-mediated destruction persists, requiring intervention with IVIG and plasma exchange.

Maternal ITP arises in neonates whose mothers have underlying ITP or SLE. The mother may not necessarily have thrombocytopenia during the pregnancy or the birth, but maternal autoantibodies are present in maternal circulation and cross the placenta to the fetus, resulting in infant platelet consumption that manifests 3 to 5 days post birth. There is low risk of bleeding in the infant even at platelet counts less than 50×10^9/L, although platelet counts less than 20 to 30×10^9/L or bleeding requires treating the infant with IVIG and platelet transfusion. It is important to distinguish neonatal ITP from neonatal alloimmune thrombocytopenia (NAIT) (see later).

Alloimmune Thrombocytopenia

In contrast to autoimmune thrombocytopenia, alloimmune thrombocytopenia is a condition in which antibodies target platelets with foreign human platelet antigens (HPAs). Posttransfusion purpura is a rare but serious condition characterized by severe thrombocytopenia that emerges a few days after exposure to foreign platelets. In this condition, HPA-1a negative recipients generate alloimmune antibodies against an HPA-positive donor transfusion. These antibodies not only target the transfused platelets but also the patient's own platelets for unclear reasons. High-dose IVIG is first-line treatment, whereas long-term management involves transfusion of HPA-1a negative blood products. A similar pathophysiology underlies NAIT, where mothers lacking platelet antigen HPA-1a (or rarely HPA-5b) develop antibodies against their HPA-1a positive fetus. These antibodies cross the placenta, causing severe thrombocytopenia in the infant shortly after birth and potentially lead to severe bleeding including intracranial hemorrhage. Subsequent pregnancies are more severely affected, although NAIT can also occur in first pregnancies. Diagnosis involves detecting circulating alloantibodies in the mother, but treatment for the infant should not wait for maternal results. Management includes transfusion of maternal platelets when available or random donor platelets, often supplemented with IVIG. High-risk obstetric care is crucial for subsequent pregnancies.

Thrombocytopenia Due to Microvascular Consumption

Thrombotic microangiopathies encompass a spectrum of disorders where abnormal endothelial activation causes microvascular thrombosis and resultant thrombocytopenia. It is essential to limit platelet transfusions in these conditions, as it can accelerate the rate of consumption. Hemolytic uremic syndrome (HUS) and atypical HUS (aHUS) present with nonimmune hemolytic anemia, thrombocytopenia, and acute kidney injury. Classic HUS is often linked to Shiga toxin–producing *Escherichia coli*, whereas aHUS results from dysregulated complement activation. Treatment involves antibiotics and dialysis for HUS, and complement inhibition for aHUS. Thrombotic thrombocytopenic purpura (TTP) exhibits similar symptoms to HUS but with less renal involvement and more neurological symptoms. TTP arises from excess of very high-molecular-weight VWF multimers due to low levels of ADAMTS13 (responsible for cleaving large von Willebrand multimers), either from acquired anti-ADAMTS13 antibodies or congenital deficiency of ADAMTS13. The large VWF multimers lead to hyperaggregation and clearance of platelets. Treatment involves plasmapheresis +/– steroids and rituximab[1] for acquired cases, whereas congenital cases require ADAMTS13 (Adzynma) replacement with fresh frozen plasma or recombinant protein.

Disseminated intravascular coagulation (DIC) is the systemic rapid cycling between coagulation and fibrinolysis secondary to an underlying systemic condition, for example sepsis or an oncological process. A special type of DIC called Kasabach-Merritt phenomenon involves thrombocytopenia from localized

coagulation, fibrinolysis, and platelet consumption by kaposiform hemangioendotheliomas and tufted hemangiomas. Additionally, shear stress and turbulent blood flow observed with some intravascular devices such as extracorporeal membrane oxygenation and mechanical heart valves can cause hemolysis and platelet consumption as a kind of localized DIC.

Thrombocytopenia Due to Sequestration

Circulating platelets may become trapped within the reticuloendothelial system in conditions where the spleen enlarges (including liver cirrhosis, portal hypertension, and myeloproliferative diseases). In these instances, the platelet count is often mildly to moderately low and responds suboptimally to platelet transfusions. Definitive treatment targets the underlying cause of the splenomegaly.

Thrombocytopenia Due to Inadequate Production

Platelet production can be suppressed from a variety of causes. Liver disease, for instance, can disrupt TPO levels and impair platelet production. Bone marrow damage or infiltration hampers platelets production by affecting the MK population, as seen in radiation exposure, leukemia, myelodysplasia, and metabolic diseases. Severe deficiencies of essential nutrients such as vitamin B_{12}, folate, and copper can lead to cytopenias across all cell lines, including platelets. Medications, in addition to causing thrombocytopenia through immune-mediated mechanisms as previously mentioned, can induce bone marrow suppression. Well-known myelosuppressive pharmacotherapies include chemotherapy and cytotoxic medications like hydroxyurea. More commonly implicated drugs in marrow suppression include thiazide diuretics, hormones like estrogens, and antiepileptic drugs such as levetiracetam (Keppra) and valproic acid. Likewise, infectious suppression from a number of entities has been widely reported, including mycoplasma, mycobacteria, ehrlichiosis, and malaria. By far, viruses such as mumps, rubella, measles, varicella, cytomegalovirus, Epstein-Barr virus, hepatitis, and parvovirus are the most commonly reported entities associated with infectious suppression.

Unlike the etiologies discussed thus far, which can be transient and reversible, genetically driven thrombocytopenias due to production issues may progress over time. Some inherited disorders feature thrombocytopenia as part of a broader syndrome, and congenital thrombocytopenias are discussed later. Moreover, thrombocytopenia can be the presenting sign of a cancer predisposition syndrome, which encompasses various entities such as ANKRD26-related thrombocytopenia, familial platelet disorder with predisposition to acute myelogenous leukemia (RUNX1), ETV6-related thrombocytopenia (associated with high mean corpuscular volume in erythrocytes), and GATA1-related disorders (involving dyserythropoiesis with or without anemia). Typically, these syndromes present with mild to moderate thrombocytopenia, although GATA1-related disorders can manifest as severe thrombocytopenia.

Congenital Disorders
Congenital Microthrombocytopenias

Congenital microthrombocytopenia comprise conditions such as Wiskott-Aldrich syndrome (WAS) and X-linked thrombocytopenia (XLT). WAS arises from an X-linked mutation of the WAS gene, resulting in severe thrombocytopenia from birth, eczema, recurrent bacterial infections in childhood, and a later predisposition to autoimmune disorders and leukemia/lymphoma. Platelets are small, measuring less than 2 μm, compared with the normal diameter of 2 to 3 μm. Bleeding management involves support with on-demand platelet transfusions and TPO receptor agonists, whereas definitive management targets the underlying immunologic deficits through stem cell transplantation or gene therapy. XLT shares similarities with WAS but lacks the associated immunologic dysfunction.

Congenital Macrothrombocytopenias

Congenital macrothrombocytopenias encompass platelet cytoskeletal protein mutations, surface glycoprotein defects, and alpha granule disorders.

---

[1] Not FDA approved for this indication.

Myosin heavy chain 9 (MYH9)-related thrombocytopenia is the umbrella term for a group of entities formerly separately known as May-Hegglin anomaly, Sebastian syndrome, Fechtner syndrome, and Epstein syndrome. MYH9 is a cytoplasmic myosin essential to the cytoskeletal functions of many cell types including platelets. Bleeding risk is typically mild to moderate, with platelet counts typically ranging from 20 to 130 × 10⁹/L. On peripheral smear, neutrophils in MYH9 disease contain Döhle-like bodies within the cytoplasm. Associated clinical manifestations may include early onset of cataracts, hearing loss, and glomerulonephritis. Treatment of platelet dysfunction involves the use of antifibrinolytics or on-demand platelet transfusions for trauma or procedures.

Bernard-Soulier syndrome is a severe bleeding disorder stemming from a reduced expression or defect of the GPIb/IX/V complex on the platelet surface (part of the VWF receptor), leading to impaired platelet adhesion and reduced platelet survival. Implicated genes include GPIBA, GPIBB, GP9, and GP5. Closure times are extremely prolonged (300 seconds), and the aggregation pattern is distinct: normal aggregation for all agonists except ristocetin, which relies on the VW receptor for agglutination. Aggregation does not correct with the addition of normal plasma as it would for VWD. Flow cytometry reveals decreased surface expression of GPIb-α (VWF receptor). Platelet counts may be anywhere from approximately 30 × 10⁹/L to normal. Notably, patients experience bleeding symptoms beyond the degree of thrombocytopenia due to the presence of the functional defect. Treatment options include on-demand transfusions for bleeding, although there is a risk of refractoriness and alloimmunization to transfusions due to recognition of the missing glycoproteins. Recombinant factor VIIa (NovoSeven) may also be considered for management.

Alpha granule disorders comprise a rare category of macro-thrombocytopenias. Gray platelet syndrome, associated with NBEAL mutations, exhibits reduced or absent α-granules and an average platelet count of approximately 50 × 10⁹/L. Peripheral smear shows large ghost-like platelets lacking purple granules. Aggregation with traditional agonists may be either normal or impaired. Associated clinical features include development of myelofibrosis and splenomegaly. Treatment options include DDAVP[1], transfusion, and splenectomy. Alternatively, Paris-Trousseau and Jacobsen syndrome both present with a mild bleeding diathesis, and thrombocytopenia may or may not be present. They are associated with giant α-granules visible on TEM in some platelets and two morphologically distinct populations of MKs. Diagnosis is typically made based on the combined presence of congenital abnormalities such as developmental delay, and cardiac and craniofacial abnormalities that prompt genetic investigations for the presence of a FLI1 mutation.

Congenital Thrombocytopenia With Normal Platelet Size

Congenital thrombocytopenia presenting with normal platelet size includes disorders such as congenital amegakaryocytic thrombocytopenia (CAMT) and thrombocytopenia with absent radii (TAR). CAMT is characterized by isolated severe thrombocytopenia at birth due to absent MKs, which progresses to severe pancytopenia over the first decade of life. CAMT is associated with mutations in the MPL gene. Short-term treatment involves supportive platelet transfusions, whereas long-term management typically requires a stem cell transplant. In contrast, TAR presents with severe thrombocytopenia at birth that gradually improves over time. TAR is associated with a mutation in the RBM8A gene and is characterized by bilateral absent radii (but normal thumbs), gastrointestinal problems such as cow's milk intolerance, and sometimes skeletal abnormalities of the lower limbs, renal and cardiac anomalies, and facial capillary hemangioma.

Treatment involves supportive transfusions throughout infancy.

Congenital Functional Defects of Normal-Sized Platelets Without Thrombocytopenia

Congenital platelet disorders may present with normal platelet counts and with unremarkable platelet morphology. These include disorders of platelet surface receptors, dense granules, and platelet signal transduction pathways.

Glanzmann thrombasthenia is a severe bleeding disorder stemming from mutations in ITGA2B or ITGB3 genes resulting in a deficiency or absence of platelet surface GPIIb/IIIa necessary for aggregation and clot retraction. It presents with mucocutaneous, gastrointestinal, genitourinary, and postsurgical bleeding. Like Bernard-Soulier, closure times are distinctly prolonged. Unlike Bernard-Soulier, platelet aggregation in Glanzmann is impaired in response to ADP, collagen, thrombin, and adrenaline, but not ristocetin. Definitive diagnosis is made via flow cytometry for GPIIb (CD41) and GPIIIa (CD61). Treatment for bleeding involves judicious use of platelet transfusions because of the high risk of alloimmunization and platelet refractoriness. High-dose recombinant factor VIIa is used in Glanzmann patients who are refractory to platelet transfusions. Bone marrow transplant is an option for patients with recurrent severe bleeding.

Dense granule disorders like Hermansky-Pudlak syndrome (HPS) and Chediak-Higashi syndrome (CHS) share traits of oculocutaneous albinism and reduced granule content, as well as abnormal ADP to ATP ratios or absent ATP release. TEM confirms diminished or absent dense granules. CHS is the more severe of the two and without stem cell transplantation is often fatal within the first decade of life due to lymphoproliferation and infection. CHS is characterized by large peroxidase-positive cytoplasmic granules in neutrophils. HPS typically displays a mild bleeding diathesis, and certain subtypes are prone to additional manifestations such as pulmonary fibrosis, granulomatous colitis, neutropenia, and immunodeficiency.

Disorders involving platelet surface receptors such as P2Y12 and signal transduction pathways are rare and heterogeneous and are best diagnosed through a combination of stepwise platelet function testing and genetic sequencing. They typically present with normal platelet count but reduced aggregation to one or more agonists despite normal platelet nucleotide content and release. Bleeding risk tends to be mild to moderate. Management includes DDAVP[1], antifibrinolytics, and hormonal therapy.

Declaration of AI and AI-Assisted Technology in the Writing Process

During the preparation of this work the author used Chat GPT 3.5 to refine and clarify grammar and improve readability. After using this tool/service, the author reviewed and edited the content as needed and takes full responsibility for the content of the publication.

---

[1] Not FDA approved for this indication.

References

Banerjee S, Angiolillo DJ, Boden WE, Murphy JG, Khalili H, Hasan AA, et al: Use of antiplatelet therapy/DAPT for Post-PCI Patients Undergoing Noncardiac Surgery, *J Am Coll Cardiol* 69(14):1861–1870, 2017.

Bolton-Maggs PH, Chalmers EA, Collins PW, Harrison P, Kitchen S, Liesner RJ, et al: A review of inherited platelet disorders with guidelines for their management on behalf of the UKHCDO, *Br J Haematol* 135(5):603–633, 2006.

Drachman JG: Inherited thrombocytopenia: when a low platelet count does not mean ITP, *Blood* 103(2):390–398, 2004.

Hayashi T, Hirayama F: Advances in alloimmune thrombocytopenia: perspectives on current concepts of human platelet antigens, antibody detection strategies, and genotyping, *Blood Transfus* 13(3):380–390, 2015.

Konkle BA: Acquired disorders of platelet function, *Hematology Am Soc Hematol Educ Program* 2011:391–396, 2011.

Periayah MH, Halim AS, Mat Saad AZ: Mechanism action of platelets and crucial blood coagulation pathways in hemostasis, *Int J Hematol Oncol Stem Cell Res* 11(4):319–327, 2017.

Sharda A, Flaumenhaft R: The life cycle of platelet granules, *F1000Res* 7:236, 2018.

Scharf RE: Drugs that affect platelet function, *Semin Thromb Hemost* 38(8):865–883, 2012.

Villar P, Carreno S, Moro S, Diez Galindo I, Bernardo A, Gutierrez L: Platelet function testing: Update on determinant variables and permissive windows using a platelet-count-based device, *Transfus Apher Sci*, 2024:103930.

Visentin GP, Liu CY: Drug-induced thrombocytopenia, *Hematol Oncol Clin North Am.* 21(4):685–696, 2007. vi.

---

[1] Not FDA approved for this indication.

POLYCYTHEMIA VERA

Method of
Peter R. Duggan, MD; and Sonia Cerquozzi, MD

CURRENT DIAGNOSIS

- Polycythemia vera (PV) should be considered when there is persistent elevation of hemoglobin (>165 g/L in men and >160 g/L in women) or hematocrit (>49% in men and >48% in women).
- *JAK2V617F* mutation testing and erythropoietin levels should be performed when PV is suspected.
- Bone marrow biopsy and aspiration may be necessary in some cases to confirm the diagnosis of PV and to distinguish PV from other myeloproliferative neoplasms (MPNs).
- PV is highly likely when *JAK2V617F* mutation is present and erythropoietin level is subnormal. When *JAK2V617F* mutation is seen with normal erythropoietin level, PV is possible; bone marrow biopsy is recommended to differentiate PV from other MPNs. When *JAK2V617F* is normal and erythropoietin is low, consider *JAK2* exon 12 mutational analysis or alternative diagnosis of congenital polycythemia. Wildtype *JAK2V617F* with normal or high erythropoietin level makes PV very unlikely, and patients should be investigated for secondary causes of polycythemia.
- Investigations for secondary polycythemia that may be indicated include:
  - Chest x-ray
  - Pulse oximetry
  - Arterial blood gas including carboxyhemoglobin and methemoglobin levels
  - Kidney and liver function tests
  - Abdominal imaging studies (ultrasound or computed tomography scan)
  - Oxyhemoglobin dissociation curve
  - Nocturnal polysomnography

CURRENT THERAPY

- All patients should be treated with phlebotomy and/or cytoreductive therapy to target hematocrit less than 45%.
- Low-dose aspirin[1] (acetylsalicylic acid [ASA]) should be used in *all patients* without a contraindication.
- In *high-risk* patients with polycythemia vera (age ≥ 60 years and/or history of thrombosis), cytoreductive therapy should be used in combination with low-dose ASA.
- Alkylating agents should be avoided as cytoreductive therapy owing to the risk of acute leukemia.
- Conventional cardiovascular risk factors (diabetes, hypertension, hyperlipidemia) should be aggressively managed, and cigarette smoking should be discouraged.
- Thromboembolic events should be managed according to accepted management guidelines. Thromboprophylaxis should be used after surgery and in other high-risk situations.

[1]Not FDA approved for this indication.

Polycythemia vera (PV) is a clonal stem cell disorder characterized by an increase in red blood cell production independent of the stimulation by erythropoietin. PV is the most common of the chronic myeloproliferative neoplasms (MPNs), occurring in approximately 2 to 3 people per 100,000 annually. The median age at diagnosis is 70 years, and it is rare in patients younger than 40 years.

A mutation of the tyrosine kinase Janus kinase 2 (*JAK2*) is consistently found in PV. This sheds some light on the pathogenesis of the disease and is useful in the diagnosis of PV and other MPNs. A single acquired mutation (*V617F*) of the gene for the JH-2 domain of *JAK2* can be found in 90% to 95% of patients with PV. The JH-2 domain functions to inhibit *JAK2* activity. In normal erythropoiesis, binding of erythropoietin to its receptor lifts this inhibition and allows *JAK2* stimulation of cell division and differentiation. In mutated *JAK2*, this inhibitory function is absent, leading to constitutive activity of the tyrosine kinase. This mutation is also present in about half of patients with essential thrombocytosis and primary myelofibrosis. The small number of patients with PV who are negative for the common *JAK2V617F* mutation have another functionally similar mutation within *exon 12*.

Presentation

Many patients with PV are asymptomatic, and PV is diagnosed after the incidental finding of an elevated hemoglobin or hematocrit on routine complete blood cell count. Splenomegaly is present in 30% to 40% of patients. Up to half of patients experience nonspecific symptoms such as weight loss, sweating, headache, fatigue, epigastric discomfort, visual disturbances, and dizziness. Many of these symptoms are likely caused by decreased blood flow due to an increased blood viscosity from polycythemia.

Generalized pruritus is often described, often after a warm bath or shower (aquagenic pruritus). Although the cause of this is unknown, it is thought to be due to the degranulation of increased numbers of mast cells in the skin of patients, releasing histamine and other inflammatory mediators. However, the symptom responds poorly to antihistamines, and it does not always resolve with treatment of PV.

Venous and arterial thromboembolic events are a major cause of morbidity and mortality in PV. Thrombosis at presentation occurs in up to 40% of patients. Ischemic stroke, transient ischemic attack, and myocardial infarction are common, especially among elderly patients. These, along with deep venous thrombosis and pulmonary embolus, are the most common thrombotic events and often result in serious morbidity, disability, and even death. Thrombotic events that are considered unusual in the general population, such as Budd-Chiari syndrome; portal, mesenteric, and other abdominal vein thrombosis; and cerebral venous thrombosis, occur more commonly among patients with PV. The possibility of an underlying MPN should be considered when a patient presents with such an event.

PV can manifest with symptoms of peripheral vascular disease. Patients with erythromelalgia describe a painful burning sensation of the hands and feet; pallor, erythema, or cyanosis of the extremities; and sometimes cutaneous ulceration. Erythromelalgia results from microvascular thrombosis and ischemia due to platelet activation and aggregation and responds well to platelet reduction and antiplatelet agents such as aspirin (ASA).[1]

Almost all patients with PV are iron deficient at diagnosis, even before the onset of therapeutic phlebotomy. Other manifestations of PV include acute gouty arthritis, peptic ulcer disease, erosive gastritis, and hypertension.

Diagnosis and Differential Diagnosis

The 2022 World Health Organization (WHO) diagnostic criteria incorporating recent International Consensus Classification changes for PV are shown in Box 1. The *JAK2V617F* mutation is present in about 95% of cases of PV. Erythropoietin level is decreased in more than 90% and is rarely elevated. Few patients with PV carry a mutation of exon 12 (~ 4%) of the *JAK2* gene instead of the more common *JAK2V617F* mutation. A *JAK2* mutation can also be found in about half of patients with essential thrombocytosis and primary myelofibrosis.

Polycythemia Vera

---

[1]Not FDA approved for this indication.

Leukocytosis and thrombocytosis are present in the majority of cases of PV. Red blood cell mass is increased. A nuclear medicine study measuring red blood cell mass and plasma volume is rarely required with the availability of *JAK2* testing, but it may be useful when relative polycythemia is suspected. Bone marrow biopsy and aspiration are not often needed for a diagnosis of PV but have been included as a major criterion within the revised WHO classification. Bone marrow examination can be important for diagnosing PV in the rare cases where *JAK2* is negative and to differentiate PV from other *JAK2*-positive MPNs when the distinction cannot be made based on peripheral blood cell counts.

Erythrocytosis can occur as a result of a number of other conditions in the absence of PV (Box 2). A careful history and physical examination with selected investigations can usually distinguish PV from secondary polycythemia and relative polycythemia (see Current Diagnosis). In relative (apparent, spurious) polycythemia, there is usually only a modest increase in the hematocrit, because of a decrease in plasma volume rather than a true increase in red blood cell mass. Thrombocytosis, leukocytosis, and splenomegaly should be absent. Causes include smoking, dehydration, and use of diuretics, and it is also described in middle-aged, obese, hypertensive men (Gaisböck syndrome).

Red blood cell mass can be elevated owing to increased stimulation of erythropoiesis by high levels of erythropoietin. Erythropoietin can be increased as an appropriate response to chronic hypoxia (sleep apnea, right-to-left cardiac shunts, chronic lung disease, high altitude, smoking, methemoglobinemia), and it can be inappropriately elevated owing to erythropoietin-secreting tumors (renal cell carcinoma, hepatocellular carcinoma, cerebellar hemangioma, uterine fibroids) or decreased kidney perfusion (renal artery stenosis). Familial causes of polycythemia include high-affinity hemoglobins, erythropoietin receptor mutations, and Chuvash polycythemia. Polycythemia occurs in 10% to 15% of patients after kidney transplantation, and this may be due to erythropoietin secretion by the native kidneys or increased sensitivity to erythropoietin. Polycythemia can be drug induced, such as with the use of performance-enhancing drugs (erythropoietin [Epogen], androgens) in athletes and testosterone replacement in men.

Prognosis

Patients with PV have a reduced life expectancy compared with the general population, with a median survival of approximately 14 years or, if younger than 60 years at diagnosis, 24 years.

Despite therapy, thrombosis remains an important cause of mortality. Cardiac disease, ischemic stroke, pulmonary embolus, and other thrombotic events account for 40% of deaths among patients with PV. Nonfatal thrombosis is common, occurring in almost 4% of patients annually. Age and a history of prior thromboembolic events are independent risk factors for thrombosis and can be used to predict a patient's risk of future events (Box 3). Low-risk patients are younger than 60 years and have no history of thrombosis. They experience new events at a rate of 2% per year. For patients older than 60 years or with a past history of thrombosis, this rate is 5% annually, but it can be as high as 11% when both risk factors are present.

The contribution of other cardiovascular risk factors (smoking, diabetes, hypertension, hyperlipidemia) to thrombotic risk in PV has been studied, with inconclusive results. However, because these are major contributors to the development of cardiovascular disease in the general population, they should also be considered when assessing risk in patients with PV. Leukocytosis (white blood cell count > 15 × 10^9/L) has been associated with a higher risk of arterial thrombosis.

Conversely, the risk of major hemorrhage is low, with fatal bleeding responsible for less than 5% of all deaths. However, there is considerable excess mortality from malignancy, in particular transformation to a myelodysplastic syndrome, myelofibrosis, or acute leukemia. The rate of leukemic transformation is less than 10% at 20 years. Risk factors for leukemic transformation include advanced age, leukocytosis, and abnormal karyotype. Approximately 10% of patients transform to myelofibrosis (post-PV myelofibrosis). Risk factors for post-PV myelofibrosis include leukocytosis and *JAK2V617F* allele burden of greater than 50%.

Treatment

The goals of treatment in PV are to lower the risk of thrombosis and improve patient symptoms, while minimizing toxicity. This is achieved by a combination of phlebotomy, ASA, and cytoreductive therapy, such as hydroxyurea (Hydrea) or pegylated interferon (PEG-IFN)-based therapy such as PEG-IFN-α2a (Pegasys) or ropeginterferon alfa-2b (Besremi). The use of these therapies can be individualized based on a patient's risk of developing future thromboembolic events. Risk stratification (Box 3) aims at identifying patients with PV at higher risk of thrombotic events who require cytoreductive therapy. Because cerebrovascular and cardiovascular disease are among the main causes of morbidity and mortality for these patients, careful attention should be paid to the management of conventional cardiovascular risk factors. Hypertension, diabetes, and hyperlipidemia should be controlled with standard measures based on current guidelines, and patients should be encouraged to stop smoking. As the hematocrit increases in PV, there is a dramatic increase in blood viscosity. Phlebotomy is the fastest, most effective way to normalize a patient's hematocrit, and it should be initiated immediately in those with newly diagnosed PV. Blood volume should be reduced as rapidly as possible. Usually, 500 mL of blood is removed every 1 or 2 days until the hematocrit is less than 45%. The frequency of phlebotomy or the volume of blood removed can be decreased in elderly patients, those with cardiovascular disease, or others who do not tolerate this schedule. The optimal target in patients with PV is to maintain a hematocrit less than 45% to lower the risk of major thrombotic events and death from cardiovascular causes. Regular phlebotomy eventually results in iron deficiency, at which point most patients' phlebotomy needs to decrease dramatically. Iron replacement should be avoided.

Aspirin

Previous studies did not support the routine use of ASA to prevent thrombosis in PV. However, high doses of ASA were used in these early studies, resulting in excess bleeding in the treatment arm. The results of a recent large randomized trial show that low-dose ASA (100 mg/day) reduces major thrombotic events (nonfatal myocardial infarction, nonfatal stroke, pulmonary embolism, major venous thrombosis). This was accomplished without an increase in bleeding risk. Although there was a trend suggesting more minor bleeding events in those receiving ASA, the rates of major bleeding were identical for those receiving ASA or placebo. The benefit from ASA was seen, even though this study included many low-risk patients without a prior history of thromboembolism. Low-dose ASA (75 to 100 mg daily)[1] should be started in all patients without a contraindication to the drug (history of bleeding or intolerance). Because of the risk of bleeding from acquired von Willebrand disease that can occur with extreme thrombocytosis, ASA should be held when platelets are more than 1500×10^9/L until the count can be lowered by cytoreduction.

Cytoreductive Therapy

Cytoreductive therapy is recommended for high-risk patients with PV (Box 3). Hydroxyurea (HU) or interferon (IFN)-based therapy are the first line cytoreductive agents most commonly used to treat PV. Aims of cytoreduction are to safely lower blood cell counts. Cytoreduction can also decrease spleen size. When using hydroxyurea[1] a starting dosage of 15 to 20 mg/kg daily (1000–1500 mg daily) is often suggested. Occasional phlebotomy is still required to maintain hematocrit at less than 45%, but the frequency usually decreases with time due to the development of iron deficiency and/or if concomitant cytoreduction is used. Myelosuppression is the main toxicity of HU. The lowest dosage that provides therapeutic effect should be used, and excess myelosuppression should be avoided. The dosage can be titrated to ensure that the white blood cell count remains higher than 3.0 × 109/L, neutrophils are higher than 2.0 × 109/L, and platelets are in the normal range. HU has been associated with leg ulcers and other skin changes, especially after long-term use. HU resistance can occur in up to 11% of patients and is associated with

increased risk of death. Both HU resistance and intolerance are defined according to the European Leukemia Net criteria.

IFN-α2b has been an alternative first-line therapy and is now only available in two controlled-release (pegylated) formulations. It is recommended that patients of childbearing age are prescribed IFN-based therapy due to the teratogenic effects of HU. PEG-IFN-α2a (Pegasys)[1] is given at 45 to 90 μg weekly, up to a dose of 180 μg weekly. Studies have shown its efficacy in controlling blood cell counts in addition to achieving complete hematologic and molecular responses. The inconvenience of its administration and its side effects, including mood disturbance and flu-like illness, have made it a less desirable first-line option. A newer formulation of PEG-IFN is now available, ropeginterferon alfa-2b (Besremi; Ropeg [Europe]). This is a monopegylated, long-acting, interferon administered once every 2 weeks or longer. It was FDA approved for PV at the end of 2021 based on results from the phase 3 PROUD/CONTINUATION-PV clinical trials. In the CONTINUATION-PV trial, which included 171 patients, 61% of patients on ropeginterferon alfa-2b met complete hematologic response (CHR). Over 6 years of follow-up, ropeginterferon improved event-free survival vs. hydroxyurea/best available therapy (BAT). It also achieved higher complete hematologic response (CHR) rates at 72 months (54.5% vs. 34.9%). Molecular responses were markedly higher with the use of Besremi.

National Comprehensive Cancer (NCCN) MPN guidelines were updated in 2023. These guidelines suggested that ropeginterferon alfa-2b (Besremi) be listed as the preferred first-line method for cytoreduction in adults with low-risk, symptomatic PV. Ropeginterferon-alfa-2b is also the preferred treatment option for patients with high-risk PV, with an alternative first-line option being hydroxyurea. The PEGINVERA study showed that, after 7.5 years of treatment with ropeginterferon alfa-2b, 61% of patients with PV achieved a complete hematologic response and a normal spleen size, with 80% of patients having a hematologic response. An approved starting dosing of Besremi is 50 μg subcutaneous every 2 weeks and takes approximately 20 weeks to reach a plateau of maximum dosing of 500 μg. The most common adverse effects are arthralgias, influenza-like illness, fatigue, nasopharyngitis, musculoskeletal pain, pruritus, and depression.

JAK Inhibitors

Ruxolitinib (Jakafi), a *JAK1/2* inhibitor, was originally approved in patients with myelofibrosis, including myelofibrosis evolving from PV. There was a significant reduction in spleen size and constitutional symptoms in almost half of these patients. In the phase III RESPONSE trial, ruxolitinib illustrated its effectiveness in controlling hematocrit (<45%), reducing spleen size (≥35%), and improving symptoms in patients with PV who had HU intolerance or resistance, resulting in its approval as a second-line cytoreductive agent in PV. The most common side effects are anemia, thrombocytopenia, and atypical infection risk.

The MAJIC-PV was an open-label, randomized, phase II clinical trial that compared ruxolitinib vs. best available therapy (BAT) in patients with PV who were resistant or intolerant to hydroxyurea. Among a total of 180 patients (93 to ruxolitinib, 87 to BAT) a complete response (by 12 months) was achieved in 43% of patients on ruxolitinib vs. 26% on BAT ($P = .02$). Event-free survival, including major thrombosis, major hemorrhage, disease transformation, or death, was improved in those receiving ruxolitinib (HR 0.58). The reduction in JAK2 V617F allele burden was more frequent with ruxolitinib, and these molecular responses were associated with improved event-free survival and overall survival.

Other Treatment Issues

Hyperuricemia is common in MPNs and occasionally results in kidney stones or gout. Allopurinol (Zyloprim) can be used to reduce uric acid levels in patients with these complications. For those with intractable pruritus, several agents have been used with variable success. Some patients respond to ASA,[1] hydroxyurea,[1]

---

[1] Not FDA approved for this indication.

cimetidine (Tagamet),[1] cyproheptadine (Periactin),[1] and/or paroxetine (Paxil)[1] 20 mg daily. Both PEG-IFN-α2b[1] and ruxolitinib have been successful.

Less than 60% of pregnancies occurring in patients with PV are successful. First-trimester fetal loss is the most common complication, and third-trimester fetal loss, preterm birth, and intrauterine growth restriction are also common. Phlebotomy should be used to keep the hematocrit at less than 45%. PEG-IFN therapy is recommended for those requiring cytoreductive therapy during pregnancy; other cytoreductive agents are contraindicated owing to possible teratogenic effects. There is some evidence that the use of low-dose ASA[1] throughout pregnancy improves the live birth rate. It is recommended that prophylactic low-molecular-weight heparin (LMWH) be used for 6 weeks postpartum.

Surgery in patients with PV has a high risk of both operative bleeding and postoperative thromboembolism. Elective surgeries should be delayed until cytoreductive measures and phlebotomy can be used to achieve good control of blood cell counts. ASA should be held for 1 week before surgery to reduce the risk of hemorrhage. LMWH should be given after surgery to prevent deep venous thrombosis. Mechanical compression stockings are an option for patients with bleeding that prevents the use of anticoagulation. When thromboembolic events do occur, treatment should be according to current management guidelines. Venous thromboembolism is treated with LMWH, warfarin (Coumadin), and/or direct oral anticoagulants. Indefinite anticoagulation should be considered because of the high risk of recurrent events. Low-dose ASA is indicated in those with a history of arterial events such as stroke and myocardial infarction.

---

[1] Not FDA approved for this indication.

References

Arber DA, Orazi A, Hasserjian R, et al: The 2016 revision to the World Health Organization classification of myeloid neoplasms and acute leukemia, *Blood* 127(20):2391–2405, 2016.

Barosi G, Birgegard G, Finazzi G, et al: A unified definition of clinical resistance and intolerance to hydroxycarbamide in polycythemia vera and primary myelofibrosis: results of a European LeukemiaNet (ELN) consensus process, *Br J Haematol* 148:961–963, 2010.

Finazzi G, Caruso V, Marchioli R, et al: for the ECLAP Investigators: Acute leukemia in polycythemia vera: an analysis of 1638 patients enrolled in a prospective observational study, *Blood* 105(7):2664–2670, 2005.

Gianelli U, Thiele J, Orazi A, et al: International Consensus Classification of myeloid and lymphoid neoplasms: myeloproliferative neoplasms, *Virchows Arch* 482(1):53–68, 2023.

Gisslinger H, Klade C, Georgiev P, et al: Ropeginterferon alfa-2b versus standard therapy for polycythaemia vera (PROUD-PV and CONTINUATION-PV): a randomised, non-inferiority, phase 3 trial and its extension study, *Lancet Haematol* 7(3):e196–e208, 2020.

Gisslinger H, Klade C, Georgiev P, et al.: Event-free survival in patients with polycythemia vera treated with ropeginterferon alfa-2b versus best available treatment, *Leukemia* 37:2129–2132, 2023.

Harrison CN, Fox S, Boucher R, et al. Ruxolitinib versus best available therapy for polycythaemia vera intolerant or resistant to hydroxycarbamide (MAJIC-PV): an open-label, randomised, phase 2 trial, J Clin Oncol 41(14):2531–2542, 2023.

Kiladjian JJ, Cassinat B, Chevret S, et al: Pegylated interferon-alfa-2a induces complete hematologic and molecular responses with low toxicity in polycythemia vera, *Blood* 112:3065–3072, 2008.

Landolfi R, Marchioli R, Kutti J, et al: Efficacy and safety of low-dose aspirin in polycythemia vera, *N Engl J Med* 350:114–124, 2004.

Marchioli R, Finazzi G, Landolfi R, et al: Vascular and neoplastic risk in a large cohort of patients with polycythemia vera, *J Clin Oncol* 23(10):2224–2232, 2005.

Marchioli R, Finazzi G, Specchia G, et al: Cardiovascular events and intensity of treatment in polycythemia vera, *N Engl J Med* 368:22–33, 2013.

National Cancer Comprehensive Network. https://www.nccn.org/professionals/physician_gls/pdf/mpn.pdf.

Them NC, Bagienski K, Berg T, et al.: Molecular responses and chromosomal aberrations in patients with polycythemia vera treated with peg-proline-interferon alpha-2b, *Am J Hematol* 90(4):288–294, 2015.

Passamonti F: How I treat polycythemia vera, *Blood* 120(2):275–284, 2012.

Passamonti F, Rumi E, Caramella M, et al: A dynamic prognostic model to predict survival in post-polycythemia vera myelofibrosis, *Blood* 111(7):3383–3387, 2008.

Quintas-Cardama A, Kantarjian H, Manshouri T, et al: Pegylated interferon alfa-2a yields high rates of hematologic and molecular response in patients with advanced essential thrombocythemia and polycythemia vera, *J Clin Oncol* 27:5418–5424, 2009.

Tefferi A, Barbui T: Polycythemia vera and essential thrombocythemia: 2015 update on diagnosis, risk-stratification and management, *Am J Hematol* 90(2):163–173, 2015.

Tefferi A, Guglielmelli P, Larson DR, et al: Long-term survival and blast transformation in molecularly annotated essential thrombocythemia, polycythemia vera, and myelofibrosis, *Blood* 124(16):2507–2513, 2014.

Tefferi A, Rumi E, Finazzi G, et al: Survival and prognosis among 1545 patients with contemporary polycythemia vera: an international study, *Leukemia* 27:1874–1881, 2013.

Them NC, Bagienski K, Berg T, et al.: Molecular responses and chromosomal aberrations in patients with polycythemia vera treated with peg-proline-interferon alpha-2b, *Am J Hematol* 90(4):288–294, 2015.

Vannucchi AM, Kiladjian JJ, Griesshammer M, et al: Ruxolitinib versus standard therapy for the treatment of polycythemia vera, *N Engl J Med* 372:426–435, 2015.

PORPHYRIAS

Method of
Gregory M. Vercellotti, MD; and Marshall Mazepa, MD

CURRENT DIAGNOSIS

- Making the diagnosis relies on, first, an awareness and index of suspicion for these rare conditions, which manifest as either unexplained abdominal pain and neurologic symptoms, photosensitive skin lesions (some blistering and some not), or both.
- Patients with inexplicable recurrent abdominal pain may request an evaluation for acute intermittent porphyria (AIP), which can be excluded with a spot urine aminolevulinic acid (ALA) and porphobilinogen (PBG) test. Urine ALA and PGB will be extremely elevated at the time of acute attack, which is the ideal time to make the diagnosis, but levels *will remain elevated* (many times the upper limit of normal) for many weeks to months afterward, which can facilitate making the diagnosis in the nonacute setting.
- Porphyria cutanea tarda (PCT), the most common porphyria, is typically acquired concurrent with iron overload, hepatitis C infection, and/or smoking and classically presents with blistering skin lesions on the backs of the hands due to sun exposure.

CURRENT THERAPY

- Patients should avoid alcohol consumption, smoking, hormone therapy, and other drugs known to trigger attacks.
- Treatment of acute neurovisceral pain attacks includes outpatient oral carbohydrate loading or intravenous hemin (Panhematin) for treatment of severe attacks that require hospitalization.
- For patients with an acute hepatic porphyria (AHP) and recurrent severe neurovisceral attacks, givosiran (Givlaari), a small interfering RNA targeting aminolevulinic acid synthase-1 (ALAS-1), is a recently FDA-approved treatment that has been shown to reduce the frequency of attacks.
- For patients with erythropoietic protoporphyria (EPP), afamelanotide (Scenesse), an analog of human α-melanocyte–stimulating hormone (α-MSH) that stimulates melanin production, was recently FDA approved for reduction in EPP-related photosensitivity.

The porphyrias are a family of metabolic disorders of heme synthesis, where symptoms occur due to abnormal accumulation of metabolites, and most are congenital. Porphyria cutanea tarda (PCT) is the exception, which is caused by the acquired inhibition of hepatic uroporphyrinogen decarboxylase (UROD), commonly associated with hepatitis C virus (HCV) infection and iron overload. The porphyrias can be classified by the organ of heme

TABLE 1   Heme Synthesis Pathway

METABOLITES	ENZYME	DISEASE	PATHOLOGY
Succinyl CoA and glycine			
Delta aminolevulinic acid (ALA)	ALA synthase (ALAS-1)	X-linked protoporphyria (XLP)	Gain-of-function mutation in ALA synthase Mimics EPP <10% of erythropoietic porphyrias (EPs) Males > females
Porphobilinogen (PBG)	ALA dehydratase	ALA dehydratase deficiency porphyria (ADP)	Elevated urine ALA
Hydroxymethylbilane	Porphobilinogen deaminase	**Acute intermittent porphyria (AIP)**	Elevated urine ALA and PBG
Uroporphyrinogen III	Uroporphyrinogen synthase	Congenital erythropoietic porphyria (CEP)	Excess erythrocyte, plasma porphyrins, urinary and fecal porphyrins; hemolytic anemia
Coproporphyrinogen III	Uroporphyrinogen decarboxylase (UROD)	**Porphyria cutanea tarda (PCT)**	Elevated plasma and urine uroporphyrins Normal urine ALA and PBG
Protoporphyrinogen IX	Coproporphyrinogen oxidase (CPOX)	Hereditary coproporphyria (HCP)	Elevated urine ALA and PBG Plasma and stool porphyrins to differentiate VP
Protoporphyrin IX	Protoporphyrinogen oxidase (PPOX)	Variegate porphyria (VP)	Elevated urine ALA and PBG Plasma and stool porphyrins to differentiate HCP
Heme	Ferrochelatase	**Erythropoietic protoporphyria (EPP)**	Elevated erythrocyte, plasma, stool porphyrins

precursor overproduction and acuity—the acute and chronic hepatic porphyrias and the acute erythropoietic porphyrias. This new system of classification has largely been driven by the development of new therapies that specifically target the metabolic driver of disease in the acute hepatic porphyrias (AHPs), including the recent FDA approval of givosiran (Givlaari) for AHPs. From a more practical standpoint, we recommend considering classifying the patient's symptoms as either neurovisceral alone, neurovisceral plus dermatologic, or dermatologic alone, because the symptoms inform potential diagnoses and requisite testing.

While there are at least nine porphyrias in total, from a therapy perspective, three porphyrias are the most important to recognize. Acute intermittent porphyria (AIP) is likely the most common AHP. Patients with unexplained recurrent abdominal pain may request an evaluation for this disorder from their primary care doctor or consultant. PCT is likely the most common porphyria overall, and treatment with phlebotomy and avoidance of alcohol and other triggers can lead to profound relief of symptoms. Erythropoietic protoporphyria (EPP) is a very rare porphyria with dermatologic findings only and has a newly FDA-approved therapy to increase melanocyte melanogenesis, which is protective against UV light–associated painful skin manifestations, the first of its kind. Given that these conditions are rare, we suggest coordinating diagnosis and management with an expert. The American Porphyria Foundation (APF) website (https://porphyria foundation.org) provides an important resource for patients and providers alike, including US experts in the field.

Pathophysiology and Clinical Manifestations

The heme synthetic pathway includes eight enzymes and is shown in Table 1. Heme is primarily synthesized in the bone marrow (giving rise to hemoglobin in erythroblasts), and about 20% is synthesized in the liver. While the pathways to synthesize heme are similar in the two organs, regulation of the two pathways differs. Aminolevulinic acid synthase-1 (ALAS-1) regulates heme synthesis in the liver and other organs; ALAS-2 regulates heme synthesis in the bone marrow. Both heme (the end product of the pathway) and glucose downregulate ALAS-1 activity through negative feedback, observations that inform treatment. Conversely, demand for ALAS-1 activity can be increased by many inducers of cytochrome P450 because heme is central to the

function of these enzymes. Hence, drugs that induce cytochrome P450 should be avoided in patients with porphyria.

Clinical manifestations of the porphyrias include neurovisceral and/or dermatologic symptoms. The term *neurovisceral* refers to unexplained generalized abdominal pain plus neurologic symptoms ranging from mild (e.g., paresthesias and weakness) to, rarely, severe neurologic manifestations, including seizures and respiratory failure. Patients commonly describe a prodrome they can recognize over time, and some can abort severe attacks with measures at home such as carbohydrate consumption, rest, and hydration. They may also recognize extreme alcohol intolerance; triggers of attacks from new medications, herbs, or supplements; and, in women, onset of symptoms after puberty and during the luteal phase (premenstrual, when progesterone levels are highest) of their menstrual cycle. Women are more commonly diagnosed with AHPs than men (estimated 4:1). Due to a delay in diagnosis, many patients have had multiple nondiagnostic evaluations or surgical interventions. Hyponatremia may occur during episodes, and prompt treatment should be made to avoid precipitating seizures. Dark or reddish-tinged urine may also be present during an acute episode.

The dermatologic manifestations of the porphyrias includes photosensitivity and either blistering or nonblistering skin lesions on sun-exposed areas. The most common by far is PCT, which has isolated blistering skin findings, classically on the backs of hands and other sun-exposed areas. In erythropoietic porphyrias, skin lesions are nonblistering but extremely painful and have a prodrome of escalating pain with light exposure. Coordination of care with a dermatologist is frequently necessary for diagnosis (as there are many other blistering skin lesions and causes of photosensitivity) and management. Liver damage in the form of cholestatic hepatitis is an uncommon complication, as are porphyrin-contain gallstones.

Diagnosis

The diagnosis of the porphyrias relies on the presence of symptoms (neurovisceral and/or dermatologic) consistent with the diagnosis and biochemical abnormalities to confirm the diagnosis. A careful history of painful episodes, prodrome, exacerbating and alleviating factors including alcohol tolerance, skin rashes or dermatologic evaluations, neurologic manifestations (most commonly weakness) is important. In addition to alcohol and tobacco

TABLE 2 Diagnosis and Treatment of Porphyrias

	SPECIFIC PORPHYRIAS	NEURO-VISCERAL	DERMATOLOGIC	TREATMENT	TREATMENT MECHANISM
Acute hepatic porphyrias	AIP (most common), ADP, HCP, VP	Yes	AIP, ADP—none VP and HCP photosensitive blistering	Hemin (Panhematin)—acute Givosiran (Givlaari)—prophylaxis[1]	Hemin—negative feedback on ALAS-1 Givosiran—direct inhibition of transcription of ALAS-1
Chronic hepatic porphyrias	PCT	No	Photosensitive blistering	1. Phlebotomy plus 2. HCV eradication HIV treatment Alcohol and tobacco cessation	1. Iron reduction 2. Elimination/reduction of susceptibility factors
Erythropoietic porphyrias	EPP, XLP, CEP	No	Photosensitive nonblistering	Sun avoidance Afamelanotide (Scenesse)—EPP only	Prevention of blue light (410 nM) to activate pathogenic metabolites to cause dermatologic damage Afamelanotide—increase melanin to absorb light and improve sunlight tolerance

[1]Not FDA approved for this indication.

ADP, ALA dehydratase deficiency porphyria; *AIP,* acute intermittent porphyria; *ALAS-1,* aminolevulinic acid synthase-1; *CEP,* congenital erythropoietic porphyria; *EPP,* erythropoietic protoporphyria; *HCP,* hereditary coproporphyria; *HCV,* hepatitis C virus; *PCT,* porphyria cutanea tarda; *VP,* variegate porphyria; *XLP,* X-linked protoporphyria.

histories, a careful review of all current and past medications and their associations with attacks should be evaluated. Among the more common inducers of attacks include oral contraceptives and many anticonvulsants. An excellent resource on drug safety in the porphyrias is provided at the APF website (https://porphyriafoundation.org). An account of the most recent painful episode and timing from testing may also be helpful when considering testing.

The linchpin to the diagnosis of the AHPs, and AIP in particular, is the spot urine ALA, PGB, and creatinine test (creatinine normalizes the measurement and negates the need for a 24-hour urine collection). While the time most likely to find extreme elevations in heme metabolites will be during an attack, because testing is now done exclusively at reference labs, it is often impractical to base a diagnosis and treatment plan on acute testing. However, testing should be sent if the diagnosis is being considered during an episode of acute abdominal pain. In the outpatient setting, often there is confusion about the utility of testing outside of an acute episode. Because this is a congenital metabolic disorder, for most porphyrias, including AIP, a spot ALA, PBG, and creatinine test are sufficient to make the diagnosis. The levels of ALA and PBG outside of an acute episode will often remain high for many weeks. Hence, even without acute abdominal pain, levels greater than 4 to 5 times the upper limit of normal will make the diagnosis. Conversely, a common error in diagnosis is to measure levels of *all* porphyrins in the urine. Drugs whose metabolism induces cytochrome P450 (and hence heme synthesis), excess alcohol, and other chronic illnesses can result in relatively minor elevations in downstream porphyrins and lead to confusion about the diagnosis.

The APF website (https://porphyriafoundation.org) is an excellent resource for providers and patients alike. There are a limited number of reference laboratories with proficiency in performing the diagnostic assays for these disorders, which are listed on this website. Most helpful to a specialist is to send the spot urine ALA, PGB, and creatinine test before referral for evaluation of the AHPs.

For PCT, the diagnosis can be suspected by visual inspection of blistering skin lesions, aided by the evaluation by a dermatologist including a skin biopsy and confirmed with biochemical testing. The first step in diagnosis is to measure plasma porphyrins. If elevated, then typically labs will reflexively fractionate the different porphyrins, which reveals elevated uroporphyrin and heptacarboxyl porphyrins. Given that blistering skin lesions are not specific to PCT, a spot urine porphyrin test should also be done concurrently. In PCT, urine ALA and PBG will be normal, in contrast to the HCPs that have blistering skin lesions. After the diagnosis of PCT is made, an evaluation for susceptibility factors that led to the uncovering of PCT (given that 80% are acquired) should also be done, including HCV and HIV infections, alcoholic liver disease, and iron overload. Genetic predisposition to iron overload due to mutations in the *HFE* gene (pathogenic in hereditary hemochromatosis) are frequently found.

For the very rare erythropoietic porphyrias, including EPP, a more specialized approach is needed, including evaluation by a dermatologist. EPP in particular is diagnosed by elevated protoporphyrin in red blood cells (erythrocyte protoporphyrin), plasma, and stool (normal in urine), which shares a phenotype with the very rare X-linked protoporphyria (XLP) but differs in the genetic lesion.

Given that these metabolic disorders are genetic in origin (again, PCT is the exception), there may be a temptation to perform genetic testing over biochemical testing to make the diagnosis. However, genetic testing should only be performed to confirm the diagnosis *after* discovery of biochemical evidence to support the diagnosis. The incomplete penetrance in these disorders has been well established, so starting with genetic testing would likely falsely assign the diagnosis to patients whose symptoms should not be attributed to the disorder.

Management
Acute Hepatic Porphyrias
The main principle of management of all AHPs is *avoidance* of inducers of heme biosynthesis to reduce production of excess toxic metabolites that drive the clinical disease manifestations (Table 2). In AHPs, where neurovisceral and/or skin symptoms are hallmarks, patients should be counseled to avoid alcohol use, smoking, and oral contraceptives (both estrogen and progestins have been associated with attacks), and physicians should carefully prescribe drugs that induce cytochrome P450. The drug database for acute porphyrias created by the Norwegian Porphyria Centers (https://porphyriadrugs.com) has an excellently curated and searchable drug database that should be consulted before starting any new medication. Patients should also be counseled about the risks of over-the-counter medications, herbal medicines, and supplements as potential inducers of attacks. Patients should also be counseled about environmental or situational inducers of attacks that in general would be considered metabolic stressors: physical or emotional stress, infection, fasting (fad diets), pregnancy (also a high-progesterone state), and surgery. For women with attacks that are regularly triggered by menstrual cycles, ovarian suppression with gonadotropin-releasing hormone analog can be used as a preventive measure as well.

When patients experience the prodrome of an acute attack (neurologic symptoms, tachycardia, vague abdominal pain), some are able to abort attacks by oral carbohydrate loading (at least 300 g/day). For those patients who present for medical attention, in addition to withdrawal of any identifiable precipitants of the attack (new medications, supplements, or alcohol), IV dextrose (10% dextrose in 0.45% normal saline) can be used as a temporizing measure if hemin is not available or for treatment of mild attacks. Carbohydrates directly but weakly inhibit ALAS1, so hemin is preferred for treatment of attacks that require more than therapy at home.

Hemin (Panhematin), intravenous heme, rapidly reduces plasma PBG and ALA by reducing ALAS-1 activity through negative feedback. The primary acute toxicity from this therapy is phlebitis, so it is strongly recommended to deliver this therapy by a central catheter. The drug is dosed once per day for 4 consecutive days at a dose of 3 to 4 mg/kg and reconstituted in albumin for better stability. Other supportive measures for an acute attack include antiemetics and analgesics (opioids are commonly required for pain control). While seizures are highly uncommon, management is quite challenging given that the most common anticonvulsants are also strong precipitants of porphyric attacks. Thus electrolyte abnormalities and other precipitants of seizures should be carefully managed.

Some patients with frequent attacks require regular treatment with hemin or preventive hemin infusions. However, because the effect of this therapy is short-lived, this can lead to iron overload and poor quality of life. Givosiran (Givlaari) was recently approved exclusively as a treatment that can prevent attacks for AHPs. This novel therapy is a small interfering RNA therapy that inhibits ALAS1, hence it is a potent inhibitor of hepatic heme synthesis. The most commonly reported toxicities in the trials included injection site reactions, nausea, rash, and elevated transaminases. The phase 3 clinical trial found a significant reduction in attacks when this therapy was given as a once-monthly subcutaneous injection overall by about 70% over placebo, and nearly half had no attacks. Hemin was still effective as a rescue therapy for acute attacks.

Porphyria Cutanea Tarda

Porphyrins may accumulate in the skin due to a deficiency of the enzyme uroporphyrinogen III decarboxylase (UROD), secondary to a mutation of the UROD gene. When exposed to sunlight, the porphyrins are oxidized, resulting in skin damage and blisters. Exacerbating factors include iron overload, tobacco and alcohol use, hepatitis C virus (HCV). HIV infection, and use of estrogen. By treating iron overload with phlebotomy, plus removing or treating underlying triggers such as alcohol and tobacco use, HCV infection, or HIV infection, PCT can be effectively managed. Phlebotomy can be initiated on an every-2-weeks schedule with careful attention to the patient's hemoglobin and symptoms of anemia. While ideally iron deficiency is the target (ferritin <20), a careful balance between symptoms of PCT and symptoms of iron deficiency should be considered. In addition to phlebotomy, skin protection from sun exposure is the other important management strategy, along with supportive care of blistering lesions, including treatment of secondary bacterial infections.

If phlebotomy is poorly tolerated, then hydroxychloroquine (Plaquenil)[1] 100 mg twice weekly is another effective treatment. In a randomized trial, this therapy has been shown to reduce PCT symptoms and plasma porphyrin levels as quickly as phlebotomy (approximately 6 months).

In addition, patients with HCV infection should be considered for eradication therapy and/or screened for cirrhosis and hepatocellular carcinoma. It is not known whether HCV eradication alone will cause remission in PCT, but certainly it is beneficial to reduce the patient's risk of HCV-related complications such as cirrhosis. HIV infection should be treated and smoking cessation should be pursued. Patients often avoid alcohol as they recognize its deleterious effects, but for those with alcohol use disorder,

cutting back on use or abstinence is much more challenging, and management should be coordinated with an addiction specialist. Similarly, tobacco cessation is strongly encouraged.

Erythropoietic Porphyrias

In treatment of erythropoietic porphyrias, where EPP is the more common of these rare diseases, again trigger avoidance is the mainstay of treatment. Patients from a young age can identify the prodrome of an attack during sunlight exposure. Thus avoidance of sunlight exposure is the primary preventive strategy. It should be noted that UV light exposure still occurs through glass, so precautions should be made with an employer if necessary, and a physician letter is necessary to allow for window tinting in a patient's car. In addition, exposure from other sources of UV light, such as fluorescent lights, can cause photosensitivity. For any patient with EPP undergoing surgery, particular attention needs to be paid to avoid excess UV exposure from operating room lights. Transparent sunscreens block UV light only and are not effective for prevention of symptoms in EPP. Regular use of protective clothing and hats were the only treatment for EPP until recently. Avoidance of sunlight also frequently leads to vitamin D deficiency.

Afamelanotide (Scenesse) is a synthetic analog of alpha-melanocyte stimulating hormone. This recently approved drug, the first drug approved for EPP, increases melanin and skin pigmentation, and hence, improves sunlight tolerability. The drug is administered as a SQ bimonthly controlled-release implant. Overall this new therapy is well tolerated and, though it improves sunlight tolerability, it does not affect the underlying cause. Dersimelagon, a selective melanocortin 1 receptor agonist, is currently in clinical trials as an oral therapy for photoprotection in EPP, but it is still an investigational therapy.

Many patients with EPP also develop hepatobiliary disease ranging from elevated liver enzymes to biliary stones that may require cholecystectomy and, rarely (estimated <5%), severe liver injury in the form of acute cholestatic hepatitis or chronic protoporphyric hepatopathy. Those with severe chronic hepatopathy often require liver transplantation. Recent guidelines have been published on the management of these forms of liver disease in EPP. For mild-to-moderate liver disease, experts recommend continued avoidance of alcohol and estrogens but also referral to a center with expertise in EPP liver disease management, where other hepatoprotective therapies can be considered, including ursodeoxycholic acid (Ursodiol)[1], cholestyramine (Questran)[1], colestipol (Colestid)[1], and vitamin E[7], along with close monitoring. For advanced liver disease, again referral to a center with expertise and experience in acute liver disease from EPP is recommended, where therapies such as therapeutic plasma exchange, red blood cell exchange, IV hemin, and ultimately allogeneic stem cell transplantation and/or liver transplantation can be considered.

---

[1] Not FDA approved for this indication.
[7] Available as dietary supplement.

References

Balwani M, Bonkovsky HL, Endeavor Investigators: Dersimelagon in erythropoietic protoporphyrias, *N Engl J Med* 388:1376–1385, 2023.

Bissell MD, Anderson KE, Bonkovsky HL: Porphyria, *N Engl J Med* 377:862–872, 2017.

Langendonk JG, Balwani M, Anderson KE, et al: Afamelanotide for erythropoietic protoporphyria, *N Engl J Med* 373:48–59, 2015.

Levy C, Dickey AK, Wang B, et al: Evidence-based consensus guidelines for the diagnosis and management of protoporphyria-related liver dysfunction in erythropoietic protoporphyria and X-linked protoporphyria, *Hepatology* 79:731–743, 2024.

Porphyria Drug List, available at porphyriadrugs.com. [Accessed 07/04/25].

Sardh E, Harper P, Balwani M, et al: Phase 1 trial of an RNA interference therapy for acute intermittent porphyria, *N Engl J Med* 380:549–558, 2019.

Sarkany RPE, Phillips JD: The clinical management of porphyria cutanea tarda: an update, *Liver Int* 44:2191–2196, 2024.

Singal AK, Kormos-Hallberg C, Lee C, et al: Low-dose hydroxychloroquine is as effective as phlebotomy in treatment of patients with porphyria cutanea tarda, *Clin Gastroenterol Hepatol* 10:1402–1409, 2012.

Wang B, Rudnick S, Cengia B, et al: Acute hepatic porphyrias: review and recent progress, *Hepatol Commun* 3:193–206, 2019.

---

[1] Not FDA approved for this indication.

SICKLE CELL DISEASE

Method of
Enrico M. Novelli, MD; Mark T. Gladwin, MD; and Lakshmanan Krishnamurti, MD

CURRENT DIAGNOSIS

- Sickle cell disease (SCD) is diagnosed by neonatal screening in the United States.
- Persons with congenital hemolytic anemia should be tested for SCD by hemoglobin electrophoresis regardless of their ethnic background.
- Infection with parvovirus B19 should be suspected in children presenting with acute anemia and reticulocytopenia.
- Human leukocyte antigen (HLA) class I and II testing should be performed in all patients with SCD and unaffected siblings to identify candidates for hematopoietic stem cell transplant.
- Transcranial Doppler screening for primary prevention of stroke is standard of care in children with homozygous SCD.
- Acute chest syndrome is diagnosed in patients presenting with fever, hypoxemia, and a radiographic pulmonary infiltrate.
- Screening for kidney disease should be performed by obtaining a spot urine albumin/creatinine or protein/creatinine ratio.
- Screening for iron overload by ferritin, quantitative liver magnetic resonance imaging (MRI), cardiac MRI, or liver biopsy is indicated in all patients who have received more than 10 lifetime transfusions.
- Pulmonary hypertension screening by transthoracic echocardiogram is indicated in all patients with homozygous SCD.

CURRENT THERAPY

- All children with sickle cell disease (SCD) should receive penicillin prophylaxis and penumococcal vaccination.
- High fever should be treated empirically with coverage for *Streptococcus pneumoniae* pending results of blood cultures.
- Children with high transcranial Doppler velocity need to be placed on a chronic transfusion regimen to keep the hemoglobin (Hb) S less than 30%.
- Painful vaso-occlusive episodes warrant prompt treatment with an individualized intravenous opioid regimen, as well as supportive care and incentive spirometry.
- Preoperative transfusion should aim at a target hemoglobin level of 10 g/dL regardless of the HbS percentage and is indicated in all patients with SCD undergoing major surgery.
- Therapy with hydroxyurea (Droxia, Siklos) is indicated in all patients at all ages with HbSS disease and HbSβ-thalassemia, and in patients with HbSC with a severe phenotype on a case-by-case basis.
- Iron chelation is indicated in all patients with findings of iron overload.
- Treatment of acute chest syndrome includes parenteral antibiotics to cover atypical microorganisms and transfusion, with exchange transfusion reserved for the most severe cases.
- Patients with pulmonary hypertension should receive optimal hematologic care (maximal hydroxyurea and/or chronic transfusion therapy) and specific therapy for pulmonary hypertension in severe cases, with coordination and referral to a pulmonary hypertension specialist.
- Stem cell transplantation should be offered to all patients who have a matched donor and display a severe phenotype.

Epidemiology

Sickle cell disease (SCD) affects 70,000 to 100,000 persons in the United States and millions worldwide. The hemoglobin S (HbS) mutation arose in West-Central Africa approximately 7300 years ago and then propagated to vast tropical and subtropical areas due to the selective pressure of malaria infection. It is predominantly found in persons of African, Mediterranean, Arab, or Indian ancestry. In the United States, approximately 1 in 15 African Americans harbors the HbS (sickle hemoglobin) mutation and 1 in 400 is affected by the disease. Most patients with SCD in the United States are homozygous for HbS (SS), with heterozygous HbSC being the second most common abnormality. Conversely, in Mediterranean countries, HbS/β-thalassemia is the most common SCD syndrome, and in the Arab peninsula HbSS in combination with hereditary persistence of fetal hemoglobin (HPFH) is particularly prevalent.

Pathophysiology

SCD consists of a group of inherited hemoglobinopathies characterized by a qualitatively abnormal hemoglobin molecule that affects the structure and integrity of the red blood cells (RBCs). SCD is an autosomal recessive disease due to homozygosity for HbS, characterized by a single base substitution in the β-globin gene of the hemoglobin tetramer, leading to an amino acid substitution (valine to glutamic acid), or coinheritance of HbS with other abnormal hemoglobins such as hemoglobin C, D, E, and O or β-thalassemia.

HbS is less soluble than normal hemoglobin (HbA) in the deoxygenated state and polymerizes when sickle RBCs are exposed to hypoxic conditions in the microcirculation. In the classic pathophysiologic explanation of SCD, sickled RBCs containing HbS polymers are less deformable and remain trapped in the microcirculation, causing end-organ ischemia and necrosis. Compounding this mechanism, more recent literature has emphasized the role of cellular adhesion, abnormal cytokine levels, ischemia-reperfusion injury, oxidative damage, sterile inflammation, and an abnormal endothelial milieu (Figures 1 and 2). HbS polymers also lead to deformity and fragility of the RBC membrane, with resulting intravascular and extravascular hemolysis.

Patients with SCD suffer from severe chronic hemolytic anemia and acute episodes of RBC trapping and destruction in the microvasculature (vaso-occlusive episodes). Vaso-occlusive episodes are the hallmark of SCD and are characterized by more intense episodic vaso-occlusion, often with increasing hemolysis, and are due to exogenous or endogenous factors that acutely alter the rheologic properties of the RBCs. The main determinants of RBC sickling and vaso-occlusion are hypoxemia, RBC dehydration, RBC concentration, high HbS relative to fetal hemoglobin (HbF), and blood viscosity; these can occur in a multitude of clinical settings. Most common clinical inciting events leading to vaso-occlusive episodes are dehydration due to inadequate replacement of fluid losses, thermal changes, surgical stress, exposure to low oxygen tension, infections, and psychological stressors.

Epidemiologic studies indicate that the risk of vaso-occlusive episodes and acute chest syndrome is related to high steady-state hemoglobin levels, leukocytosis, and low HbF levels. These findings are consistent with pathogenic mechanisms of altered red cell rheology, higher viscosity, HbS polymerization, and inflammatory cellular adhesion. Interestingly, the epidemiologic risk factors associated with chronic vascular complications such as pulmonary hypertension (PH), cutaneous leg ulceration, priapism, systemic systolic hypertension, renal failure with proteinuria, and possibly stroke are different and include a low steady-state hemoglobin level, increased hemolytic intensity, iron overload, and markers of low nitric oxide (NO) bioavailability. One hypothesis is that SCD is driven by two overlapping but different mechanisms of disease: on one hand, vaso-occlusion causes vaso-occlusive episodes and acute chest syndrome, and on the other hand, hemolytic anemia leads to endothelial dysfunction and chronic vasculopathy. Both are caused fundamentally by HbS polymerization.

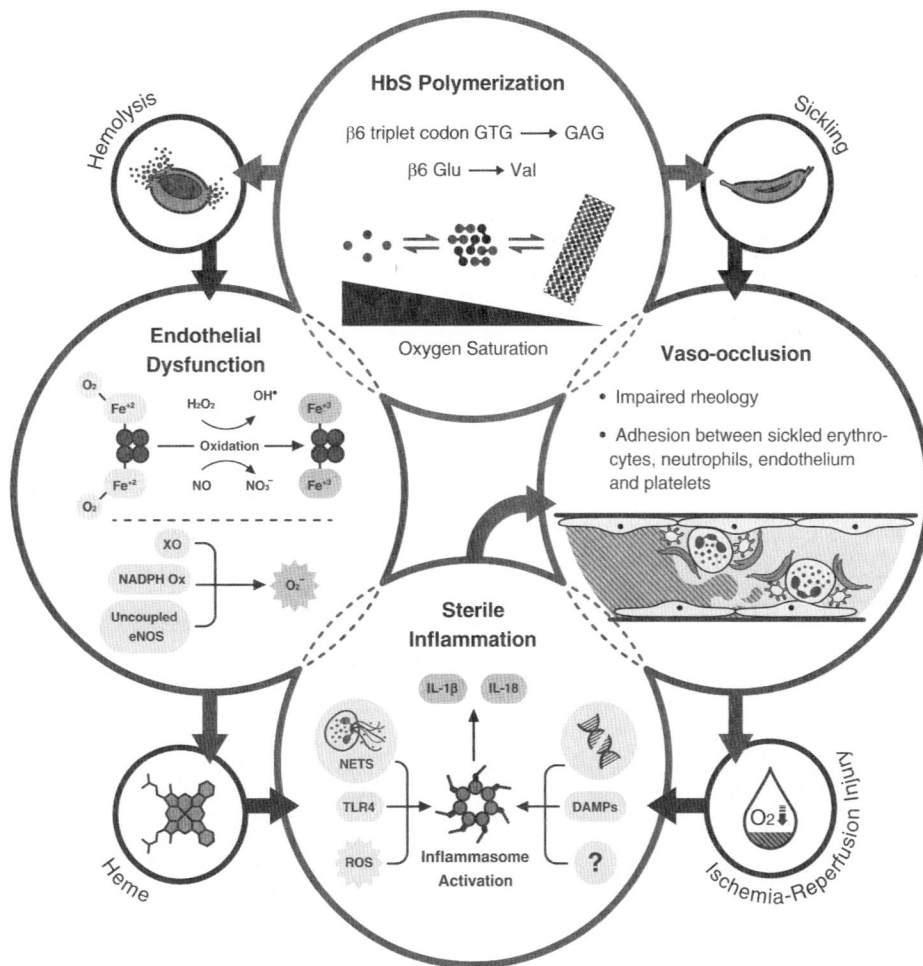

Figure 1 Molecular pathophysiology of SCD. A mutation in the β-globin gene leads to substitution of valine for glutamic acid at the 6th position in the β-globin chain. Following deoxygenation, the mutated hemoglobin (HbS) molecules polymerize to form bundles (top circle). The polymer bundles result in erythrocyte sickling (clockwise), which results in impaired rheology of the blood and aggregation of sickle erythrocytes with neutrophils, platelets and endothelial cells to promote stasis of blood flow referred to as "vaso-occlusion" (right circle). Vaso-occlusion promotes ischemia-reperfusion (I-R) injury (clockwise). Hb polymer bundles (top circle) also promote hemolysis or lysis of erythrocytes (counter-clockwise) that releases cell free Hb into the circulation. Oxygenated Hb (Fe2+) promotes endothelial dysfunction (left circle) by depleting endothelial nitric oxide (NO) reserves to form nitrate (NO3-) and methemoglobin. Alternatively, Hb can also react with H_2O_2 through the Fenton reaction to form hydroxyl free radical (OH·) and methemoglobin (Fe3+). Also, NADPH oxidase (NADPH ox), Xanthine oxidase (XO) and uncoupled endothelial NO synthase (eNOS) generate oxygen free radicals to promote endothelial dysfunction. Methemoglobin (Fe3+) degrades to release cell free heme (counter-clockwise), which is a major eDAMP. Reactive oxygen species (ROS) generation, toll-like-receptor-4 (TLR4) activation, neutrophil extracellular traps (NETs) generation, release of tissue or cell derived DAMPs, DNA and other unknown factors (?) triggered by cell free heme or I-R injury can contribute to sterile inflammation by activating inflammasome pathway in vascular and inflammatory cells to release IL-1β (bottom circle). Finally, sterile inflammation further promotes vaso-occlusion through a feed-back loop by promoting adhesiveness of neutrophils, platelets and endothelial cells. (Reproduced with permission from the Annual Review of Pathology: Mechanisms of Disease, Volume 14 © 2019 by Annual Reviews, http://www.annualreviews.org.)

Prevention

See "Evidence-Based Management of Sickle Cell Disease: Expert Panel Report, 2014" at http://www.nhlbi.nih.gov/health-pro/guidelines/sickle-cell-disease-guidelines for detailed, consensus guidelines on prevention and treatment.

Bacterial Infections

Before the antibiotic era, most patients with SCD succumbed to bacterial sepsis from encapsulated organisms. A landmark multicenter, randomized, double-blind, placebo-controlled clinical trial of prophylaxis with oral penicillin in children with sickle cell anemia published in 1986 showed that bacterial prophylaxis started at birth reduced by approximately 80% the incidence of infection in the penicillin group, as compared with the group given placebo. This study became the foundation for universal neonatal screening of SCD. Results of the Penicillin Prophylaxis in Sickle Cell Study II (PROPS 2) trial show that prophylaxis can be safely discontinued at age 5 years as long as there is no history of prior serious pneumococcal infection or surgical splenectomy and in the setting of appropriate comprehensive care. The

CDC recommends that all children under 5 years old, including those with SCD, receive a routine 4-dose series of pneumococcal conjugate vaccine (PCV15 [Vaxneuvance] or PCV20 [Prevnar20]). Children with SCD who completed a PCV series other than PCV20 should receive one dose of PCV20 or pneumococcal polysaccharide vaccine (PPSV23 [Pneumovax 23]) starting at 2 years of age. Adults with SCD who have not previously received a PCV should receive a single dose of PCV15, PCV20, or PCV21 (Capvaxive). Those who receive PCV15 should also get one dose of PPSV23 at least 1 year after the PCV15 dose. Vaccinations for *Haemophilus influenzae* and *Neisseria meningitidis* are also indicated.

Neurologic Events

Stroke is a devastating complication of SCD and affects predominantly children with HbSS and abnormal transcranial Doppler (TCD) results. Silent cerebral infarcts are magnetic resonance imaging (MRI)-detectable abnormalities that also carry a high risk of morbidity, including overt stroke and cognitive impairment. There is conclusive evidence that chronic

HbS Polymerization

- **Hydroxyurea**
- Metformin
- Sodium butyrate
- Aes-103
- Osivelotor
- Mitapivat
- Etavopivat
- Senicapoc
- PEGylated bovine carboxyhemoglobin

Hemolysis

Sickling

Endothelial Dysfunction

- Haptoglobin
- **Hydroxyurea**
- **L-glutamine**
- **Hemopexin**
- Oral or IV nitrite therapy
- Inhaled NO
- Antioxidants
- Arginine

Vaso-occlusion

- **Hydroxyurea**
- **Crizanlizumab** and rivipansel
- IVIG
- CCP-224
- Tinzaparin, dalteparin, and sevuparin
- Eptifibatide
- NKTT120
- Propranolol
- MEK inhibition
- Prasugrel and ticagrelor

Sterile Inflammation

- Hemopexin
- MP4CO
- Antioxidants
- **L-glutamine**
- TLR4 inhibition
- DNAse-1
- Inflammasome inhibition
- Anakinra and canakinumab
- Montelukast and zileuton
- Simvastatin

Heme

Ischemia-Reperfusion Injury

$O_2\downarrow$

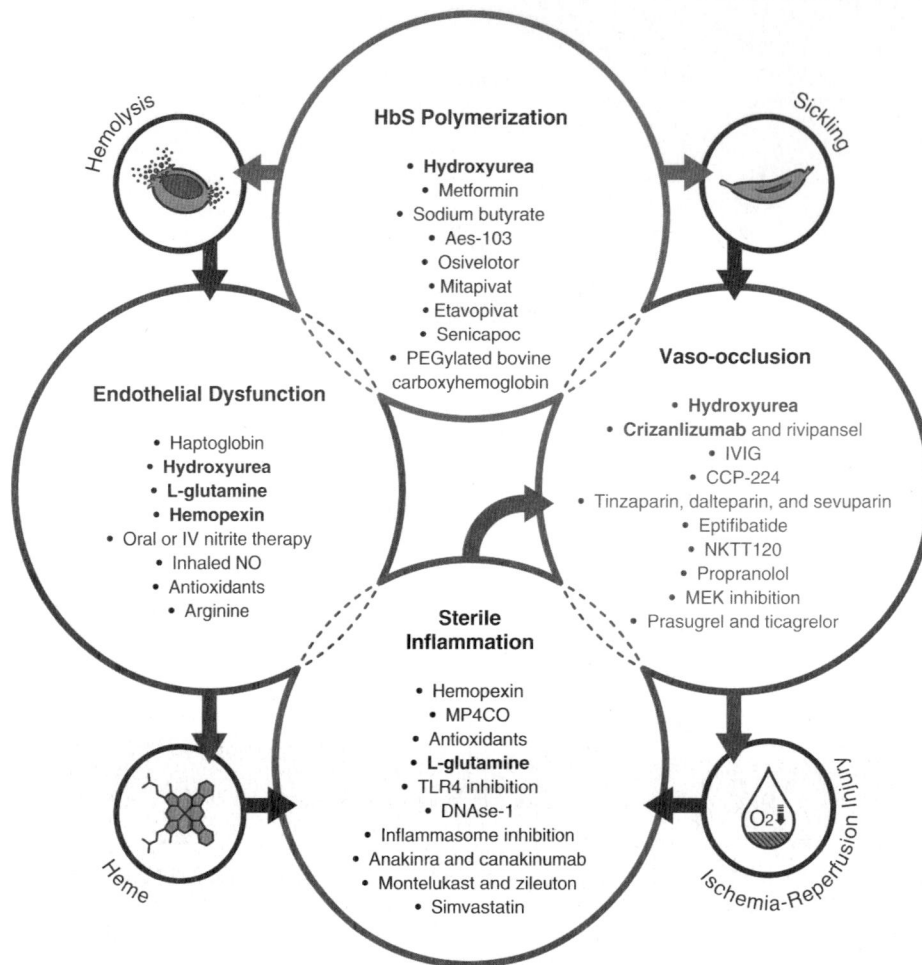

Figure 2 FDA approved and experimental therapies targeting the molecular pathobiology of sickle cell disease. The FDA approved drugs are in bold. (Reproduced with permission from the Annual Review of Pathology: Mechanisms of Disease, Volume 14 © 2019 by Annual Reviews, http://www.annualreviews.org.)

transfusions are effective in the primary and secondary prevention of both overt and silent strokes in SCD. The first landmark trial (STOP) published in 1995 showed that the first stroke can be prevented by placing children with abnormal TCD on prophylactic monthly transfusions with a target HbS of less than 30%. Transfusions were later found to also have a beneficial effect on reducing the incidence of the recurrence of silent cerebral infarcts, as shown by the SIT trial. The importance of continuing transfusions for more than 30 months was underscored by the STOP 2 trial, where TCD abnormalities recurred and the incidence of silent cerebral infarctions on MRI was higher in the transfusion-halted group. The enthusiasm over the beneficial effects of transfusions was tempered by the concerns about the side effects of long-term, possibly indefinite use of this therapeutic strategy. Therefore there has been an interest in exploring whether hydroxyurea (Droxia, Siklos) could represent an alternative to transfusion in high-risk children. Specifically, the SWiTCH trial explored the hypothesis that hydroxyurea and phlebotomy could maintain an acceptable stroke recurrence rate and significantly reduce the hepatic iron burden as compared with a prophylactic chronic transfusion regimen. Unfortunately, the trial was terminated early because of a significantly higher stroke recurrence rate in the hydroxyurea arm compared with the transfusion arm, with equivalent hepatic iron burden in both groups. Thus the issue of when, if ever, it is safe to discontinue transfusions for the secondary prevention of stroke is still unknown. Conversely, as shown by the results of the TWiTCH trial, another study halted prematurely by the National Institutes of Health, hydroxyurea is not

inferior to chronic transfusions in lowering TCD velocities in children at high risk but without a history of stroke, thereby suggesting that this drug may be equally effective in the primary prevention of neurologic complications.

Clinical Manifestations

Multiple genetic and epigenetic factors affect the SCD phenotype. Patients homozygous for HbS (SS) or compound heterozygous for HbS and a nonfunctional β^0-thalassemia allele tend to display the most severe manifestations. On the other end of the spectrum, HPFH, particularly common in Saudi Arabia, or coinheritance of β-thalassemia mitigates the phenotype. Although the net effect of high HbF levels on the phenotype of SCD is beneficial, coinheritance of one or two α-thalassemia alleles has a more complex effect. α-Thalassemia is present in approximately 30% of patients with SCD and is associated with higher hemoglobin, lower mean corpuscular volume (MCV), and decreased rate of hemolysis. These effects are protective toward stroke and leg ulcers but lead to increased rates of vasoocclusive episodes, osteonecrosis, and acute chest syndrome because of increased blood viscosity related to the higher hemoglobin level. Patients with HbSC and HbS/β+-thalassemia have an intermediate severity phenotype (Table 1). Haplotypes of polymorphic sites in the β-globin gene cluster in chromosome 11 have been associated with different disease severity and rates of complications. Other yet unidentified genetic factors predispose certain patients to develop a particularly severe hemolysis with brisk reticulocytosis and a high rate of specific complications that include leg ulcers, priapism, and PH.

TABLE 1	Severity of the Main Sickle Cell Syndromes	
GENOTYPE	CLINICAL SEVERITY	HEMOGLOBIN (G/DL)
HbSS	Usually marked	6–10
HbS-β⁰-thalassemia	Moderate to marked	6–10
HbS-β⁺-thalassemia	Mild to moderate	9–12
HbSC	Mild to moderate	10–15
HbSS-HPFH	Mild	

HbSC, Heterozygous phenotype; *HbSS,* homozygous phenotype; *HPFH,* hereditary persistence of fetal hemoglobin.

Hematology

This section describes the main clinical manifestations of SCD in each organ system (Figure 3 and Table 2).

Baseline or Steady-State Hematologic Abnormalities

Chronic intravascular and extravascular hemolysis causes a chronic anemia of moderate to severe intensity in HbSS and HbS/β⁰-thalassemia, with a hemoglobin range of 6 to 9 g/dL. In HbSC and HbS/β⁺-thalassemia, the anemia may be mild or absent. The anemia of SCD is usually normocytic in HbSS, with anisocytosis and poikilocytosis and a population of small dehydrated dense cells, irreversibly sickled cells, numerous reticulocytes, and schistocytes. Reticulocytosis is common but not compensatory, and nucleated RBCs are seen in acute exacerbations of the anemia such as in splenic or hepatic sequestration. Baseline leukocytosis with neutrophilia is also common and is a poor prognostic sign associated with acute chest syndrome in adults and frequent vaso-occlusive episodes in children. Preclinical studies have shown that leukocytes are not simply a marker of disease activity and acute phase but also have a direct pathogenic role in cellular adhesion and vaso-occlusion. The platelet count is commonly elevated in SCD, particularly in patients who are autosplenectomized as a result of repeated splenic infarction, and platelet activation is increased. In the subset of patients with HbSC and HbS/β⁺-thalassemia who retain a functional spleen and develop splenomegaly, features of hypersplenism may instead be observed with resulting mild pancytopenia.

Hematologic Indices During Vaso-occlusive Episodes

In acute vaso-occlusive episodes the total Hb decreases as a result of hemolysis (by 1.6 g/dL in acute chest syndrome). The lactate dehydrogenase (LDH), reticulocyte count, and other markers of hemolysis such as aspartate transaminase (AST) and indirect bilirubin are elevated in steady state, and in many— but not all—patients are further increased during vasoocclusive episodes. Haptoglobin levels are chronically depressed in SCD and typically not measurable, even in steady state, in patients with HbS homozygosity. In patients with HbSC, vaso-occlusive episodes may be due to increased blood viscosity and RBC sickling, and worsening hemolysis might not be readily appreciated.

Splenic sequestration crises occur mostly in childhood and are characterized by anemia disproportionate to the degree of hemolysis, reticulocytosis, and acute splenomegaly. Splenic sequestration and repeated episodes of splenic infarction eventually lead to autosplenectomy, although some patients develop splenomegaly. Splenic infarction usually manifests with left upper-quadrant pain and may be massive, involving more than 50% of the splenic tissue.

In severe vasoocclusive episodes, massive bone marrow infarction can also occur. In these instances, the peripheral blood smear reveals a leukoerythroblastic picture with immature neutrophilic forms, nucleated RBCs, and teardrop cells. Fat emboli syndrome, a life-threatening complication of vasoocclusive episodes, can then develop as bone marrow fat embolizes to peripheral capillary beds, leading to multiorgan failure.

Red Blood Cell Alloimmunization

RBC alloimmunization is a common complication of transfusional therapy in SCD and occurs in approximately 30% of patients. It is primarily due to the disparate expression of RBC antigens in African Americans as compared with the donor pool, which is mostly composed of whites. Alloimmunization complicates RBC matching and leads to delayed hemolytic transfusion reactions. Alloantigens that become undetectable by indirect Coombs test 2 months after exposure to mismatched blood have the potential to result in future false-negative cross-matching results. A subset of heavily alloimmunized patients with SCD undergoes life-threatening hemolytic reactions upon exposure to mismatched RBC units. In these hyperhemolytic crises, there is intense hemolysis of transfused and nontransfused RBCs and acute anemia. Treatment of hyperhemolytic crises is empirical and includes erythropoietin-stimulating agents (ESAs), parenteral steroids, and intravenous immunoglobulins (Gammagard).[1]

Iron Overload

Hemosiderosis is the other major complication of transfusional therapy in SCD and is characterized by iron deposition in the heart, liver, and endocrine glands, leading to organ failure and significant morbidity and mortality. It commonly occurs in patients who have received more than 10 lifetime transfusions or more than 20 packed RBC units. Liver biopsy is the "gold standard" for diagnosis, but it is an invasive and uncomfortable procedure. Hepatic and myocardial iron quantitation by MRI has supplanted liver biopsy as the preferred test to diagnose iron overload and monitor therapy with iron chelators, although when this is not available diagnosis often rests on the finding of an elevated ferritin and transferrin saturation in the appropriate clinical setting.

Hemostatic Activation and Thrombosis

Numerous studies have shown that arterial and venous thrombosis are common in SCD and include pulmonary embolism, in situ pulmonary thrombosis, and stroke. In SCD, alterations at all levels of the hemostatic system have been described: patients with SCD exhibit increased basal and stimulated platelet activation, increased markers of thrombin generation and fibrinolysis, increased tissue factor activity, and increased von Willebrand factor (vWF) antigen and thrombogenic ultralarge vWF multimers with depressed ADAMTS13 activity. Interestingly, hemostatic activation is amplified during vaso-occlusive episodes, as shown by increases in multiple markers of thrombosis as compared with steady state, suggesting a link between hemolysis and thrombosis.

Neurology

Ischemic stroke is common in SCD, with the highest incidence between 2 and 5 years of age. Patients may develop overt stroke from large vessel occlusion (5% to 8% of patients with HbSS) or silent infarcts from focal ischemia detectable by MRI without symptoms of acute stroke (20% to 35% of patients with HbSS). The pathophysiology of stroke in SCD is unclear, although genetic factors and an unbalance between oxygen demand and supply have been postulated. Multiple epidemiologic studies have shown that the risk factors for ischemic stroke in adult patients include HbSS genotype, severity of anemia, systolic hypertension, male gender, and increasing age. Patients with repeated strokes are at risk for development of anatomic abnormalities and Moyamoya pattern of vascularization, which predisposes to both ischemic and hemorrhagic stroke later in life. The highest incidence of intracerebral hemorrhages occurs in patients older than 20 years.

---

[1]Not FDA approved for this indication.

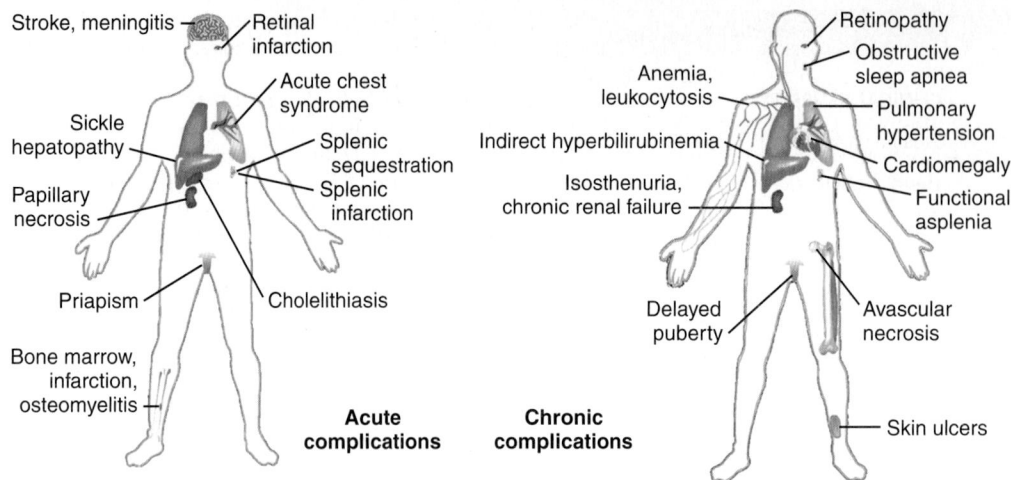

Figure 3 Acute and chronic complications of sickle cell disease.

TABLE 2	Landmark Clinical Trials in Sickle Cell Disease	
YEAR OF PUBLICATION	**TITLE**	**MAIN FINDINGS**
1986	Prophylaxis with oral penicillin in children with sickle cell anemia: A randomized trial	84% reduction in incidence of infection and no deaths from pneumococcal septicemia in the penicillin group
1995	Multicenter Study of Hydroxyurea in Sickle Cell Anemia (MSH)	Reduced incidence of painful crises, ACS, and transfusion in the hydroxyurea group Survival benefit in follow-up study
1995	Preoperative Transfusion in Sickle Cell Disease Study	A conservative transfusion regimen was as effective as an aggressive regimen in preventing perioperative complications in patients with sickle cell anemia
1996	Multicenter investigation of bone marrow transplantation for sickle cell disease	HCT is safe in SCD with survival and event-free survival at 4 years of 91% and 73% and can lead to cure
1998	Stroke Prevention Trial in Sickle Cell Anemia (STOP)	Transfusion reduces the risk of a first stroke by 92% in children with sickle cell anemia who have abnormal results on transcranial Doppler ultrasonography
2005	Optimizing Primary Stroke Prevention in Sickle Cell Anemia (STOP 2)	Discontinuation of transfusion for the prevention of stroke in children with sickle cell disease results in a high rate of reversion to abnormal blood-flow velocities on Doppler studies and stroke
2009	Improving the Results of Bone Marrow Transplantation for Patients with Severe Congenital Anemias	Nine of 10 adults who received nonmyeloablative allogeneic hematopoietic stem cell transplantation for severe sickle cell disease achieved stable, mixed donor–recipient chimerism and reversal of the sickle cell phenotype, without acute or chronic GVHD.
2011	Pediatric Hydroxyurea Phase III Clinical Trial (BABY HUG)	Children ages 9–18 months randomized to receive hydroxyurea irrespective of disease severity for 2 y had decreased pain episodes, dactylitis, ACS, hospitalization, leukocyte count, and transfusion and increased hemoglobin as compared with children receiving placebo.
2014	Silent Infarct Trial (SIT)	Children with silent cerebral infarcts and normal TCD velocity who were randomized to chronic transfusion therapy had a 58% relative risk reduction in the recurrence of silent cerebral infarct or stroke as compared to those in the observation arm.
2017	Sustain Study	Crizanlizumab, a monoclonal antibody that targets P-selectin, reduced the rate of VOE to a median/year of 1.63 compared to 2.98 with placebo and increased the median time to the first and second crisis.
2019	Realizing Effectiveness Across Continents With Hydroxyurea (REACH)	Children 1 to 10 years of age with sickle cell anemia in four sub-Saharan countries had lower rates of vaso-occlusive pain, malaria, transfusion and death on hydroxyurea (Tshilolo, 2019).

ACS, Acute chest syndrome; *GVHD,* graft-versus-host disease; *HCT,* hematopoietic cell transplantation; *SCD,* sickle cell disease; *TCD,* transcranial Doppler; *VOE,* vaso-occlusive crisis.

Data from Walters MC, Kwiatkowski JL, Tisdale JF, et al.: LentiGlobin gene therapy for sickle cell disease, *N Engl J Med* 386(7):617–628, 2022; and Frangoul H, Zettl M, Longo DL, et al.: CRISPR–Cas9 gene editing for sickle cell disease and β-thalassemia, *N Engl J Med* 389(24):2212–2223, 2023.

Both overt and silent strokes have a negative impact on IQ and cause cognitive impairment measurable by psychometric testing. Children and adults with SCD can develop cognitive impairment and subtle signs of accelerated brain aging and vascular dementia even in the absence of focal ischemia by MRI, with a low hematocrit being a predictor of neuropsychological dysfunction. These abnormalities are probably due to chronic and diffuse, as opposed to focal, cerebral anoxia and may be unmasked by psychometric testing.

Ophthalmology

Retinal abnormalities are common in SCD and are often asymptomatic until the occurrence of ophthalmologic emergencies. Retinal disease is due to arteriolar occlusion, with subsequent vascular proliferation, neovascularization, retinal hemorrhage (stage IV), and detachment (stage V). Patients with HbSC are more prone to retinal complications, possibly as a result of increased blood viscosity.

Nephrology

Renal abnormalities are common in SCD and manifest primarily as hematuria, proteinuria, and renal tubular acidosis. Hematuria is usually due to papillary necrosis and is an acute finding that requires supportive care and carries a good prognosis. Rarely, gross hematuria requires urologic consultation. Tubular functional defects include an inability to concentrate the urine (hyposthenuria) and renal tubular acidosis. Hyposthenuria often manifests with enuresis in childhood, and it is clinically relevant because it predisposes patients to an increased risk of dehydration. Renal tubular acidosis similar to type IV renal tubular acidosis is a common finding in SCD and may lead to hyperkalemia, an important consideration in patients already predisposed to hyperkalemia with intravascular hemolysis and whenever therapy with angiotensin-converting enzyme inhibitors is entertained.

Hyperphosphatemia and hyperuricemia are also often observed in SCD. Microalbuminuria may be detected in early adulthood and tends to progress to nephrotic range proteinuria. Focal segmental glomerulosclerosis is the most common glomerular abnormality and it is probably due to glomerular sickling and infarction. There are currently no approved therapies to prevent progression to end-stage renal disease, which occurs in up to 20% of patients and at a median age of 37 years. Renal replacement therapy is often needed in older adults with SCD. Serum creatinine and 24-hour creatinine clearance are not adequate for screening and monitoring of progression of kidney disease, because tubular secretion of creatinine is preserved and glomerular hyperfiltration is common in SCD, leading to a relatively low creatinine and a high glomerular filtration rate even in patients with underlying kidney impairment. Testing for microalbuminuria, plasma cystatin C levels, and hemoglobinuria may instead be used as screening tools for chronic kidney disease.

Leg Ulcers

Leg ulcers occur in 10% to 20% of patients with HbSS and have been associated with a chronically high hemolytic rate. They are usually located over the malleolar areas and are exquisitely painful, debilitating, disfiguring, and nonhealing. Vascular and plastic surgery consultations are recommended and aim at excluding local vascular problems that can complicate management of the ulcers and at providing prompt débridement and skin grafting. Although hydroxyurea is associated with development of leg ulcers in patients with myeloproliferative disorders, there is no such link with leg ulcers in SCD. Although wound healing may be impaired with hydroxyurea use, patients who develop an increase in fetal hemoglobin and have reduced sickling as a result of hydroxyurea therapy might have a net benefit in terms of tissue oxygenation and perfusion. Transfusional therapy, including exchange transfusional therapy, topical nitrates[1], and nutritional zinc[7] or L-arginine[7] supplementation, have shown benefit in anecdotal reports, but the evidence is inconclusive.

Gastroenterology

Nausea, vomiting, and dyspepsia in SCD are related to delayed gastric emptying and gastrointestinal motility disorders, autonomic neuropathy, or medical therapy. Opioids are often responsible for acute nausea and vomiting, whereas other medications such as hydroxyurea and deferasirox (Exjade) are occasionally responsible for chronic symptoms. Gastroparesis may be due to damage of the microvasculature of autonomic nerves (vasa vasorum) from repeated episodes of sickling.

The liver may be episodically affected by hepatic sequestration crises, heralded by direct hyperbilirubinemia, right upper quadrant pain from distention of the hepatic capsule, acute anemia, and reticulocytosis or by sinusoidal vaso-occlusion leading to severe episodes of intrahepatic cholestasis. Supportive therapy and transfusions are indicated for hepatic vaso-occlusive complications. Exchange transfusion may be the preferred modality for hepatic sequestration with the goal of preventing erythrocytosis once the pooled RBCs are released back into the circulation. Elevation of liver injury tests may be drug induced (hydroxyurea, deferasirox) but also related to hepatic sickling, particularly if it occurs during a vaso-occlusive episode.

Infectious Disease

Patients homozygous for HbSS develop functional asplenia during childhood. This is due to repeated episodes of splenic infarction leading to fibrosis and autosplenectomy. As a result, children are susceptible to overwhelming bacterial sepsis from encapsulated organisms such as Streptococcus pneumoniae, H. influenzae, and N. meningitidis. High pediatric mortality from sepsis was therefore common before a landmark study published in 1986 demonstrated the benefit of penicillin prophylaxis instituted at birth. Vaccination for encapsulated organisms is also standard of care in children and adults. In spite of preventive measures, the incidence of life-threatening bacterial infections is increased in SCD, and high fever should be treated empirically as in splenectomized patients, with coverage for penicillin-resistant S. pneumoniae pending blood culture results. Patients with indwelling venous catheters are at risk of catheter-related bacteremia.

Viral infections with bone marrow–tropic viruses such as Epstein-Barr virus, cytomegalovirus, and predominantly parvovirus B19 place patients at risk for myelosuppression, which can further worsen chronic anemia. In children, infections with parvovirus B19 are responsible for transient red cell aplasia and severe aplastic crises, characterized by acute anemia and reticulocytopenia due to intramarrow destruction of erythroid precursors. Treatment of these episodes includes transfusion and intravenous immunoglobulins[1], besides supportive measures.

Individuals with SCD are known to be particularly vulnerable to H1N1 influenza, which has raised concerns about the outcomes of SARS-CoV-2 infection and COVID-19 in SCD. Based on a meta-analysis and a review of electronic medical records from a multisite research group, individuals with SCD are more likely to be hospitalized and develop adverse outcomes due to COVID-19 than Black individuals without SCD/SCT.

Pulmonology

A subset of patients with vaso-occlusive episodes develop acute chest syndrome, the major pulmonary complication of SCD. Acute chest syndrome is a lung injury syndrome defined by fever, pleuritic chest pain, oxygen desaturation, and multilobar radiographic infiltrates associated with severe vaso-occlusive episodes, infection, and bone marrow fat embolization (Figure 4). It usually develops 2 to 3 days after hospitalization for vaso-occlusive episodes and is often misdiagnosed as nosocomial pneumonia or aspiration pneumonia, particularly because it displays a predilection for the lower lobe of the lungs. Although pneumonia often accompanies acute

---

[1]Not FDA approved for this indication.

[7]Available as dietary supplement.

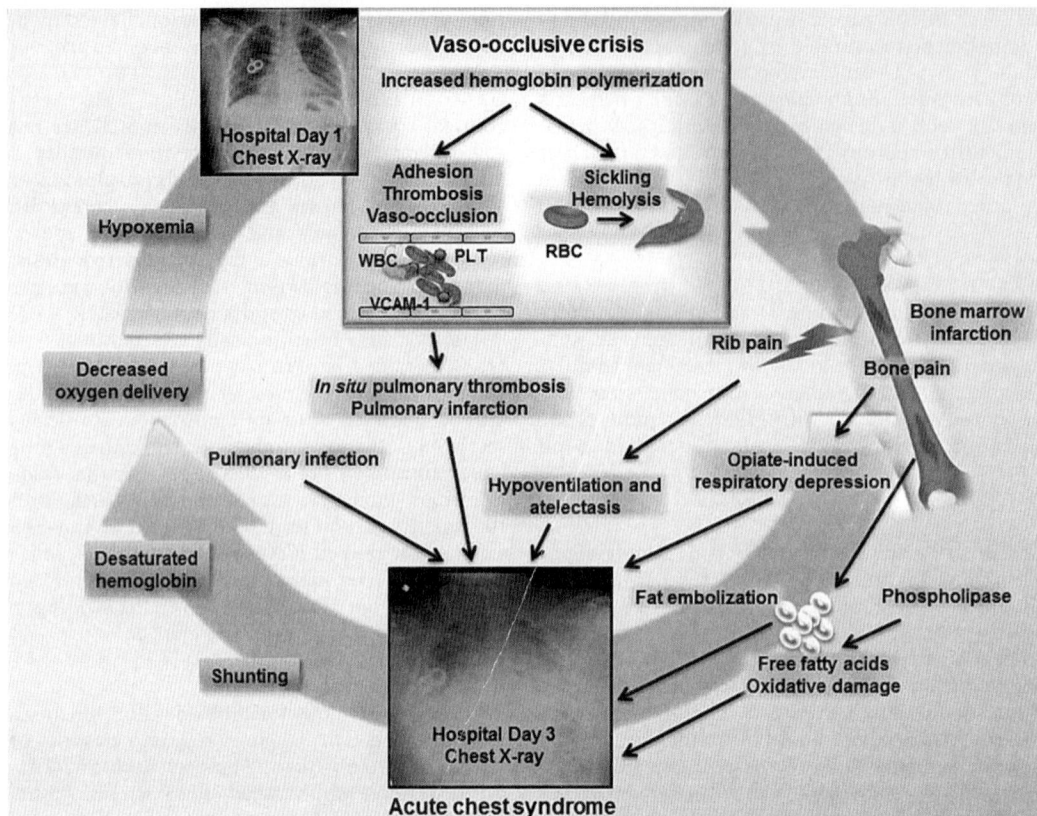

Figure 4 Vicious cycle of acute chest syndrome (ACS). Vaso-occlusive crises are characterized by increased intraerythrocytic polymerization of deoxygenated hemoglobin S, leading to red blood cell sickling, cellular hyperadhesion, hemolysis, and vaso-occlusion in the microvasculature. These processes are responsible for acute pain (pain crisis) and bone marrow necrosis. ACS typically occurs in a subset of patients 2 to 3 days after hospitalization for a vaso-occlusive episode, and radiographically may present as new multilobar, basilar infiltrates on a chest x-ray. Fat embolization from the necrotic marrow is a recognized cause of ACS and is diagnosed by identifying lipid-laden macrophages in the bronchoalveolar lavage. However, pulmonary infection is the most common trigger of ACS and may be superimposed over existing pulmonary infarction. Hypoventilation and molecular pathogens such as reactive oxygen species from ischemia-reperfusion injury and by-products of hemolysis may also play a role in inducing or exacerbating lung injury. Finally, in situ pulmonary thrombosis has been frequently identified as a comorbid condition in patients with ACS and may be caused by endothelial and hemostatic activation. As a result of lung injury, ventilation-perfusion mismatches and shunting ensues, with subsequent hemoglobin desaturation and hypoxemia. Tissue hypoxia in turn triggers further hemoglobin S polymerization and sickling in a vicious cycle.

chest syndrome, proper diagnosis is important because acute chest syndrome warrants simple or exchange transfusion in addition to antibiotic therapy and supportive measures. Common infectious pathogens identified in cases of acute chest syndrome include *Chlamydia pneumoniae*, *Mycoplasma pneumoniae*, and *Legionella pneumophila*, thus dictating inclusion of a macrolide in the antibiotic cocktail. Pulmonary embolism with resulting infarct is also in the differential diagnosis of acute chest syndrome and may occur concurrently in 17% of patients. If not recognized and treated promptly, acute chest syndrome leads to pulmonary failure and carries a high mortality.

Airway hyperreactivity is common in children with SCD and needs to be actively diagnosed and aggressively treated because it is associated with worse SCD outcomes. Children with chronic respiratory symptoms should be tested for bronchial hyperresponsiveness.

Chronic complications of SCD include pulmonary fibrosis and PH. PH is an emergent complication of SCD and is associated with a high morbidity and mortality. Multiple epidemiologic studies have shown that a high baseline hemolysis rate, low hemoglobin, increasing age, a history of leg ulcers, liver dysfunction, iron overload, and kidney failure are risk factors for the development of PH. Three epidemiologic studies and a randomized clinical trial have shown that an elevated tricuspid regurgitant jet velocity (TRV) measured by Doppler echocardiography is a common occurrence in SCD with 30% of the patients having a TRV of 2.5 m/s (2 standard deviations [SDs] above the normal mean) or higher, and 10% of the patients having a TRV of 3.0 m/s (3 SDs above the normal mean) or higher. These have proven to be valuable cutoff values, as a TRV of less than 2.5 m/s, when combined

with an N-terminal pro B-type natriuretic peptide (NT-proBNP) value less than 160 has a high negative predictive value for PH. A TRV of 3.0 m/s or higher confers a positive predictive value for having PH by right heart catheterization (RHC) of 60% to 75% and a relative risk for death of 10.6. Controversy exists on the significance of an intermediate TRV value of 2.5 to 2.9 m/s, because it is unclear how accurately it predicts RHC-diagnosed PH. In three subsequent studies, patients with intermediate or high TRV values had a prevalence of PH by RHC ranging from 25% to 65% depending on what specific cutoff value was used as the criteria to perform an RHC (2.5 vs. 2.8) and on whether patients with evidence of end-organ damage were included or excluded. However, it is worrisome that regardless of the prevalence of PH, patients with an intermediate TRV are as a whole at increased risk of death (relative risk 4.4). One screening approach is to consider RHC in all patients with TRV of 3.0 or higher and in patients with intermediate TRV values of 2.5 to 2.9 m/s if the NT-proBNP is greater than 160 pg/mL or the 6-minute walk is less than 333 m or there is a high clinical pretest probability of having PH (mosaic perfusion pattern on computed tomography [CT] scan, low diffusing capacity of the lung for carbon monoxide (DLCO), significant dyspnea on exertion, etc.). It is likely that intermediate TRV values will need to be combined with other measures of right ventricular function and functional capacity such as NT-proBNP, and 6-minute walk to derive a highly predictive composite biomarker of PH. All studies have been concordant on the high risk of death conferred by PH in SCD whether measured by echocardiography, NT-proBNP, or RHC. Noninvasive transthoracic Doppler echocardiography is recommended by the American Thoracic Society as a screening test in homozygous SCD due to its safety, low cost, and availability. However, the definitive diagnosis of PH requires a confirmatory RHC.

RHC studies of patients with SCD and PH reveal a hyperdynamic state similar to the hemodynamics characteristic of portopulmonary hypertension. It is increasingly clear that pulmonary pressures rise acutely in vaso-occlusive episodes and even more during acute chest syndrome. This suggests that acute PH and right heart dysfunction represent a major comorbidity during acute chest syndrome, and right heart failure should be considered in patients presenting with acute chest syndrome.

Cardiology
Similar to other conditions with chronic anemia, SCD is associated with a hyperdynamic state, low peripheral vascular resistance, and normal blood pressure or hypotension. In this setting, even mild elevation of the blood pressure can indicate relative hypertension and represent a risk factor for stroke. Because there are no studies on the treatment of hypertension in SCD, general guidelines on antihypertensive therapy are applied.

Coronary artery disease is rarely observed in SCD, although many patients complain of chest pain during vaso-occlusive episodes. In these instances, the usual work-up for acute coronary syndrome is recommended. It is possible that myocardial microvascular occlusions are the predominant ischemic event in SCD.

Left-sided heart disease in SCD is primarily due to diastolic dysfunction (present in approximately 13% of patients), although systolic dysfunction and mitral or aortic valvular disease (2% of patients) can also occur. The presence of diastolic dysfunction alone in SCD patients is an independent risk factor for mortality. Patients with both pulmonary vascular disease and echocardiographic evidence of diastolic dysfunction are at a particularly high risk for death (odds ratio, 12.0; 95% confidence interval [CI], 3.8 to 38.1; $P < .001$).

Cardiac dysfunction is a late complication and the major cause of death in patients with iron overload. Heart failure and conduction defects are the most common abnormalities and warrant emergent iron chelation treatment. Among the iron chelators, deferiprone (Ferriprox) appears to be particularly apt at reducing cardiac iron content. Chelators may be used in combination for cases of severe cardiac decompensation from hemosiderosis.

Methadone (Dolophine) is associated with a risk of QTc prolongation, which carries a risk of arrhythmias and sudden death, particularly in the setting of PH and iron overload. Frequent electrocardiographic (ECG) monitoring, as well as dosage reduction or discontinuation, are warranted in this group, particularly if the QTc is greater than 500 ms.

Endocrinology
Iron overload is a common cause of endocrinopathy in SCD and thalassemia, with the hypophysis, gonads, and thyroid glands being particularly affected. Patients with iron overload should therefore undergo screening for endocrine dysfunction as it is mandated in thalassemia.

However, patients with SCD are at risk for specific endocrine problems regardless of their iron status. Delayed growth and puberty are relatively common, presenting in females with delayed age of menarche by 2 to 3 years and in males with small testicular size and hypospermia. Likely pathogenic factors include increased catabolism, chronic hypoxemia, hospitalizations with prolonged immobility, ischemic insults during vaso-oclusive episodes, and chronic use of opioids.

Priapism
Priapism is the most common urogenital complication in patients with the HbSS genotype. It is a sustained, painful erection in the absence of sexual stimulation from occlusion of the penile blood return. It is defined as stuttering if it lasts from minutes to less than 3 hours and as prolonged if it lasts more than 3 hours. The latter is considered a urologic emergency because of the risk of permanent fibrosis and impotence and requires a urologic consultation.

Pseudoephedrine (Sudafed)[1] may lead to detumescence in nonemergency settings, whereas aspiration of the corpus cavernosum is required in the emergency setting and is performed under conscious sedation and local anesthesia. This is usually accompanied by instillation of epinephrine. Other supportive measures, such as intravenous fluids and parenteral opioids, are usually indicated.

Penile shunts are used as a last resort to prevent further episodes of priapism by increasing the cavernous blood flow using native vessels or by creating an arteriovenous shunt. They invariably result in erectile dysfunction, which can be ameliorated by implantation of an inflatable penile prosthesis. There are data showing that sildenafil (Viagra)[1] therapy can prevent priapism by altering vascular smooth muscle tone through inhibition of phosphodiesterase 2 activity.

Diagnosis
SCD can be diagnosed with a multitude of laboratory assays including hemoglobin electrophoresis, high-performance liquid chromatography (HPLC), and isoelectric focusing, which allow detection of most hemoglobin variants. Newer point-of-care tests are gaining traction and offer less costly and more practical testing in resource limited settings. In patients with microcytosis α-globin gene sequencing may reveal coinheritance of an α-thalassemia trait.

Neonatal Screening
Children with SCD have an increased susceptibility to bacteremia due to *S. pneumoniae*, which can occur as early as 4 months of age and carries a case fatality rate as high as 30%. Acute splenic sequestration crises also contribute to mortality in infancy. Diagnosis by newborn screening and immediate entry into programs of comprehensive care, including the provision of effective pneumococcal prophylaxis, can reach infants who might otherwise be lost to the healthcare system and has been demonstrated to decrease morbidity and improve survival. Currently, newborn screening and follow-up of SCD are carried out in all 50 states in the United States, as well as in many high income countries, and initiatives are under way to introduce universal newborn screening in most sub-Saharan African countries.

Late Diagnoses and Misdiagnoses
Rarely, patients who were born before the adoption of universal screening or who were lost at the time of follow-up of positive neonatal screening results are only diagnosed late in life. This occasionally occurs in patients with HbSC who might have normal hemoglobin and hematocrit and a mild disease phenotype. Alternatively, the disease may be misdiagnosed as iron deficiency in patients with HbS/β+-thalassemia on account of their microcytosis, which places them at risk of futile and potentially harmful prolonged trials of iron supplementation. Patients who have a low HbS level (< 40%) due to recent transfusion or who have only mildly decreased hemoglobin (HbSC or HbS/β+-thalassemia) may receive an erroneous diagnosis of sickle cell trait (carrier state).

Treatment
From the original description of SCD in 1910 to the 1970s, there was no efficacious therapy for SCD, and most patients died within the first 2 decades of life, with infectious complications being responsible for the majority of pediatric fatalities. Several preventive and pharmacologic milestones since then, and the realization that care has to occur in a multidisciplinary setting, have profoundly affected the natural history of the disease (Table 3). Median age at death in resource-rich countries was 42 years in male patients and 48 years in female patients with HbSS, according to data from the Cooperative Study of Sickle Cell Disease in the 1980s (a prehydroxyurea setting), thereby still lagging approximately 2 to 3 decades behind that of the general African-American population. The following sections

---

[1]Not FDA approved for this indication.

TABLE 3 Manifestations of Sickle Cell Disease With Key Prevention and Treatment Strategies

MANIFESTATION	PREVENTION	TREATMENT
Pneumococcal sepsis	Penicillin, Prevnar/Pneumovax vaccination	Antibiotic therapy for penicillin-resistant *Streptococcus pneumoniae*
Splenic or liver sequestration	—	Exchange transfusion
Painful vaso-occlusive episode	Hydroxyurea (Droxia), prevention of exposure to triggers	Intravenous fluids, parenteral opioids, supplemental oxygen
Acute chest syndrome	Incentive spirometry during VOE, hydroxyurea	Transfusion, broad-spectrum antibiotics with atypical coverage
Iron overload	Optimization of transfusion therapy	Iron chelation with deferasirox (Exjade) or deferoxamine (Desferal)
RBC alloimmunization	Transfusion with leukoreduced RBCs	—
CVA	Chronic transfusion in children with high transcranial Doppler velocity	Exchange transfusion and thrombolytics in selected cases
Pulmonary hypertension	Hydroxyurea?, treatment of predisposing conditions such as obstructive sleep apnea, hypoxemia, thromboembolism	Hydroxyurea, chronic transfusion therapy, specific therapy
Kidney disease	Antihypertensive therapy?, hydroxyurea?, ACE inhibitors?	ACE inhibitors, renal replacement therapy, kidney transplant
Priapism	Hydroxyurea?	Pseudoephedrine (Sudafed)[1], aspiration of corpus cavernosum, sildenafil (Viagra)[1]
Leg ulcers	Hydroxyurea?, topical sodium nitrite?, voxelotor?	Surgical débridement, surgical grafting

ACE, Angiotensin-converting enzyme; *CVA,* cerebrovascular accident; *RBCs,* red blood cells; *TCD,* transcranial Doppler; *VOE,* vaso-occlusive episode (crisis).
[1]Not FDA approved for this indication.

summarize the therapeutic approach to the most important complications of SCD.

Vaso-occlusive Episodes

Acute pain from vaso-occlusive episodes in SCD is extremely intense, affects both children and adults, and is due to ischemia or necrosis of the vascular beds. Most patients report severe pain in the bones and joints of the extremities, as well as lower back, although acute ischemia and pain can affect unusual sites such as the mandibular area. Infants and young children may experience dactylitis, a painful swelling of the hands from bone marrow infarct in the small bones of the digits. Occasionally, adults may also experience the typical signs of inflammation, such as edema, warmth, and erythema in an affected limb, but a paucity or absence of signs is the norm. Imaging studies such as MRI, positron emission tomography (PET), and bone scan can reveal signs of acute bone marrow infarction in a painful bony area, but they are not routinely used in the work-up of a pain episode, unless osteomyelitis or septic arthritis are suspected.

Intravenous opioids are the mainstay of treatment of a pain episode. Even in opioid-naïve patients with SCD, opioid dosages often exceed those required for other indications. For instance, doses of intravenous hydromorphone (Dilaudid) of 1 to 2 mg are typical in adult patients. However, most patients, are on an oral pain regimen at home and have a history of multiple admissions for vaso-occlusive episodes. In these cases, individualized care based on prior effective regimens and the patient's own perception of the intensity of pain are recommended. After an attempt at controlling the pain with three or four closely spaced opioid boluses is made, patients who are in persistent discomfort or have evidence of underlying complications triggering the vaso-occlusive episode should be admitted and ideally placed on patient controlled analgesia. Nonsteroidal antiinflammatory drugs such as ketorolac (Toradol) have fallen out of favor due to their risks in patients with renal disease and their questionable efficacy. The American Pain Society, the National Heart, Lung and Blood Institute (NHLBI), and the American Society of Hematology have published guidelines for the treatment of acute and chronic pain in SCD.

Common obstacles to prompt and effective care in SCD are the health professional's fear of overdosing the patient, as well as misconceptions about addiction and pseudoaddiction. In general, healthcare professionals tend to overestimate the prevalence of opioid use disorder in SCD and tend to undertreat patients significantly, leading to patients' frustration and anger when their pain demands are not met (pseudoaddiction).

Nonpharmacologic therapies such as biofeedback, relaxation, and localized heat may be effective and should be incorporated into the management of pain episodes whenever possible. Care for vaso-occlusive episodes should also include management of possible precipitating factors: dehydration and hypovolemia should be corrected with hypotonic crystalloids, and an infection work-up should be initiated in patients with fever, hypoxemia, or leukocytosis above baseline. Antiemetics and antipruritus therapy are also usually required.

Prior experiences in multiple institutions have shown that a dedicated facility for effective and rapid management of uncomplicated vaso-occlusive episodes reduces hospitalizations and length of stay and facilitates integration of care—psychological, socioeconomic, and nutritional—in a multidisciplinary approach. This experience is the basis of the concept of the day hospital in SCD and relies on the need to provide prompt assessment and treatment of pain, safe dose titration to relief, monitoring of adverse effects, and adequate disposition (emergency department, inpatient admission, home) in a clinical environment familiar with SCD and the individual patient.

Chronic Pain

Chronic pain is common, and a study using pain diaries compiled by patients shows that most patients with SCD experience pain on an almost daily basis (PiSCES study). Orthopedic problems such as avascular necrosis (AVN) are common and tend to develop early in patients with HbSS disease, thus exposing patients to a lifetime of pain. There is an increasing realization that nociplastic pain and opioid-induced hyperalgesia also play a significant role in chronic pain in SCD. Unfortunately, there is a dearth of safe and effective strategies to manage chronic pain in SCD. At times, short-acting and long-acting opioids are required to empower the patient to manage pain at home and minimize use of the emergency department. Drugs for neuropathic pain, such as gabapentin (Neurontin)[1], may also be used in combination with opioids because neuropathic pain may develop as a result of tissue ischemia and necrosis.

Patients who have successfully transitioned from pediatric to adult care, have a good support system, and are distracted by their work or school schedules tend to cope better and require less pharmacologic support.

Because analgesic care is life-long, consultation with pain specialists is often valuable, particularly in patients for whom more-sophisticated pain regimens are needed. For instance, the mu-opioid receptor partial agonist buprenorphine (Buprenex, Butrans), opioid rotation, and methadone used as analgesic can help to reduce the total opioid requirements. Several States in the United States have approved the use of marijuana for medical purposes for several conditions including SCD. Although controlled studies on the benefits and risks of medical marijuana in SCD are lacking, studies in sickle mice and anecdotal reports hold promise. Urine toxicology screens and written "opioid agreements" are indicated in patients receiving opioids to ensure adherence with the therapy and to minimize the risk of use of illicit substances, particularly at a time of heightened surveillance for opioid abuse in the United States. The ASH guidelines published in 2020 emphasized an individualized approach in the management of chronic pain in SCD due to the lack of extensive evidence on the benefits of opioids for chronic pain in this population. In addition, they recommended "against the initiation of chronic opioid therapy unless pain is refractory to multiple other treatment modalities" in children and adults with chronic pain from SCD. All recommendations on opioids for chronic pain were "conditional" based on very low certainty in the evidence about effects, and reflect a more guarded stance on opioids due to the deeper appreciation of the risks of chronic opioids for noncancer pain that has emerged in the past few years.

Transfusional Therapy

In SCD, the benefits of transfusion in terms of improved hemodynamics and oxygenation need to be balanced with the risks of iron overload, alloimmunization, transfusion reactions, and viral transmission of infectious agents. Leuko-reduced, sickle-negative RBCs with extended phenotypic matching for Rh Cc, Ee, and Kell, which account for 80% of detected antibodies, are required. By using extended phenotypic matching, the rate of alloimmunization decreased from 3% to 0.5% per unit, and the rate of delayed hemolytic transfusion reactions decreased by 90% in the STOP study. In previously immunized patients, a full RBC match also inclusive of matching for the Duffy, Kidd, and S antigens is recommended. Indications for transfusion include hemoglobin less than 5 g/dL or less than 6 g/dL with symptoms and any severe complication such as stroke, aplastic anemia, splenic or hepatic sequestration, or acute chest syndrome.

Prophylactic transfusions have been considered standard of care before surgery (with the exclusion of minor procedures such as intravenous port placement); the benefit of preoperative transfusions in preventing SCD-related complications in HbSS patients has also been confirmed in a small randomized clinical trial (the TAPS study). As to the type of transfusion strategy to be used, a clinical trial published in 1995 showed that a conservative prophylactic transfusion regimen to achieve a target hemoglobin of 10 g/dL and any HbS value was as effective as an aggressive regimen to achieve a hemoglobin of 10 g/dL and a target HbS value of less than 30% in preventing postsurgical complications such as acute chest syndrome.

Exchange transfusion (erythrocytapheresis with RBC exchange) is usually reserved for the most severe complications, which include acute chest syndrome with impending pulmonary failure, acute stroke and its prevention in children, multiorgan failure, and sepsis. Box 1 summarizes the main indications for

---

[1]Not FDA approved for this indication.

No Indication
Chronic steady-state anemia
Uncomplicated painful episode
Infections
Minor surgery without general anesthesia
Aseptic necrosis of hip or shoulder
Uncomplicated pregnancy

Unclear Indication
Intractable or frequent painful episodes
Leg ulcers
Before receiving intravenous contrast dye
Complicated pregnancy
Cerebrovascular accident in adults
Chronic organ failure

Simple Transfusion
Symptomatic anemia
- High output cardiac failure
- Dyspnea
- Angina
- Central nervous system dysfunction
Sudden decrease in hemoglobin
- Aplastic crisis
- Acute splenic sequestration
Severe anemia (hemoglobin ~5 g/dL) with fatigue or dyspnea
Preparation for surgery with general anesthesia

Exchange Transfusion
Acute cerebrovascular accident
Multiple organ system failure
Acute chest syndrome
Hepatic sequestration
Retinal surgery

---

simple and exchange transfusion in SCD, as well as the areas of uncertainty.

Iron Chelation

Patients who have received more than 10 transfusions or 20 units of packed RBCs should be screened for iron overload. Most authorities recommend initiation of iron chelation based on a ferritin level consistently greater than 1000 ng/mL, based on data from the thalassemia literature, although liver iron quantitation by MRI or biopsy should be obtained, when available, prior to therapy and to monitor its effectiveness. In the United States, the oral chelating agents deferasirox (Exjade) and deferiprone (Ferriprox) and the parenteral deferoxamine (Desferal) are available and should be administered until the ferritin level is less than 500 ng/mL for three consecutive measurements. Patients on iron chelation with deferasirox and deferoxamine require monitoring of hepatic, renal, auditory, and visual toxicity, and particular caution has to be exercised in the setting of renal disease, because transient, reversible increases in serum creatinine and rare instances of irreversible acute kidney injury have been reported in patients with underlying renal insufficiency. Deferiprone has been associated with agranulocytosis and neutropenia, mandating close monitoring of the absolute neutrophil count during therapy.

Erythropoietic Stimulating Agents

Although a brisk reticulocytic response is common in SCD, patients who develop renal failure or aplastic crises or who receive therapy with hydroxyurea may experience a relative or absolute reticulocytopenia (<100,000 reticulocytes/mL) and a worsening of their baseline anemia. In these situations, therapy with ESAs may be beneficial.

Because of bone marrow expansion in patients with HbSS, higher starting doses of erythropoietin (Epogen, (Epogen,

Procrit)[1] than in patients without SCD may be considered. For darbepoetin (Aranesp)[1], a reasonable starting dose is 100 to 200 μg/weekly or every 2 weeks. ESAs can be titrated by 20% to 25% increases in dose per week in patients who do not respond adequately. Weekly monitoring of hematocrit is essential to avoid overdosage and relative erythrocytosis, which can lead to hyperviscosity and vaso-occlusive episodes. Clinical trials are ongoing to test the safety and efficacy of ESA for the anemia of SCD.

Nutritional Considerations

Malnutrition, growth retardation, and stunting with findings of low lean and fat body mass are highly prevalent in children and adolescents with SCD, due to their increased caloric demands and a hypermetabolic state. Macronutrient and micronutrient deficiencies are common, and nutritional counseling is warranted. Hypovitaminosis D and low bone mineral density are also prevalent in children and adults. Folic acid[1] is indicated at the dose of 1 mg daily as in other hemolytic diseases, particularly where folate nutritional supplementation programs are absent. Strategies aimed at decreasing iron intake and absorption should be implemented early. There is also growing interest in antioxidant nutraceuticals, particularly in light of the clinical trial showing beneficial effects with L-glutamine (Endari) in SCD; however, evidence on other substances remains limited. The small subset of patients who are overweight or obese is at risk for exacerbating or precipitating common orthopedic problems in SCD such as AVN of the femoral head and its resulting disability. These patients should also receive targeted nutritional counseling.

Hydroxyurea

Since the pediatric hematologist Janet Watson suggested in 1948 that the paucity of sickle cells in the peripheral blood of newborns was due to the presence of increased HbF, there has been interest in developing therapies to modulate the hemoglobin switch from fetal to newborn life and prolong HbF production. Several antineoplastic agents, including 5-azacytidine (Vidaza)[1] and hydroxyurea, became the focus of attention after they were found to increase HbF levels in nonhuman primates and individuals with SCD.

The landmark Multicenter Study of Hydroxyurea in Sickle Cell Disease (MSH) showed that the incidence of painful crises was reduced from a median of 4.5 per year to 2.5 per year in hydroxyurea-treated patients with SCD. The rates of acute chest syndrome and blood transfusion were also reduced significantly. A follow-up for up to 9 years of 233 of the original 299 subjects showed a 40% reduction in mortality among those who received hydroxyurea. This study led to the approval of hydroxyurea (Droxia, Siklos) as the first disease-modifying therapy in adults with SCD. More recent studies showed that hydroxyurea is safe and effective in children and adults with SCD. The recently concluded BABY HUG study showed that children 9 to 18 months with HbSS disease randomized to receive 2 years of hydroxyurea therapy, irrespective of the disease severity, had less dactylitis and fewer pain episodes, hospitalizations, and transfusions than children receiving placebo.

On the molecular and cellular levels, the benefits of hydroxyurea are mostly related to increased intracellular HbF, which prevents the formation of HbS polymers and sickling. In addition to this mechanism, some patients on hydroxyurea who do not adequately increase their HbF levels also display clinical benefits, suggesting that hydroxyurea might have other beneficial rheologic properties.

Although the MSH study only included patients with HbSS, its findings traditionally have been extrapolated to other sickle cell syndromes such as HbSC and HbS/β-thalassemia. A report from Greece, where S/β-thalassemia is highly prevalent, has confirmed that hydroxyurea similarly reduces complications and mortality in patients with HbS/β[0]-thalassemia, with a nonsignificant benefit

also observed in HbS/β[+] thalassemia. Existing guidelines also recommend hydroxyurea in patients with HbSC disease, but there is still no high-level evidence to support this practice.

Hydroxyurea has been indicated at a dosage of 15 mg/kg (7.5 mg/kg in patients with renal disease) in patients with frequent pain episodes, history of acute chest syndrome, other severe vaso-occlusive episodes, or severe symptomatic anemia, although another sensible approach is to prescribe it to all patients with HbSS regardless of their phenotype. End points are less pain, increase in HbF to 15% to 20%, increased hemoglobin level to 7 to 9 g/dL in severely anemic patients, improved well-being, and acceptable myelotoxicity. The dosage can be increased by 500 mg every other day every 8 weeks to a maximum of 35 mg/kg if no toxicity is encountered. Considering the potential myelotoxicity, hepatotoxicity, and nephrotoxicity of this medication, laboratory monitoring needs to be performed every 2 weeks at the time of initiation or escalation and monthly during maintenance therapy. Laboratory studies should include a complete blood cell (CBC) count, differential and reticulocyte count, and serum chemistries. Measurements of HbF can be performed every 3 months. An elevated MCV is a marker of adherence to the therapy.

Criteria for holding hydroxyurea are listed in Figure 5. Patients need to be counseled on the teratogenic potential, as demonstrated in animal studies, as well as the risks of infertility and leukemogenesis, although a growing body of evidence shows that these risks may have been overestimated in patients with SCD.

Other side effects that can affect compliance include, but are not limited to, weight gain, alopecia, skin and nail hyperpigmentation (melanonychia), nausea and vomiting, and mucosal ulcerations. Because of the toxicity concerns, as well as factors intrinsic to long-term preventive therapy, hydroxyurea therapy has had low effectiveness in spite of high efficacy, with underprescribing by healthcare professionals and poor patient compliance being major obstacles to its widespread adoption.

Therapy of Pulmonary Hypertension

Because evidence-based guidelines for managing PH in patients with SCD are not available, recommendations are based upon the pulmonary arterial hypertension literature, case reports, small open-label studies, and expert opinion. For patients with mild PH (tricuspid regurgitant velocity [TRV], 2.5 to 2.9 m/s), it is important to identify and treat risk factors associated with PH such as rest, exercise or nocturnal hypoxemia, sleep apnea, pulmonary thromboembolic disease, restrictive lung disease or fibrosis, left ventricular systolic and diastolic dysfunction, severe anemia, and iron overload. These patients may benefit from aggressive SCD management, including optimization of hydroxyurea dosage and initiation of a chronic transfusion program in those who do not tolerate or respond poorly to hydroxyurea. Consultation with a pulmonologist or cardiologist experienced in PH is also recommended.

For patients with TRV 3 m/s or more, we recommend following the guidelines for TRV 2.5 to 2.9 m/s. In addition, RHC is necessary to confirm diagnosis and to directly assess left ventricular diastolic and systolic function. We would consider specific therapy with selective pulmonary vasodilator and remodeling drugs if the patient has pulmonary arterial hypertension defined by RHC and exercise limitation defined by a low 6-minute walk distance.

US Food and Drug Administration (FDA)-approved drugs for primary pulmonary arterial hypertension include the endothelin receptor antagonists (bosentan [Tracleer] and ambrisentan [Letairis]), prostaglandin-based therapy (epoprostenol [Flolan], treprostinil [Remodulin, Tyvaso, Orenitram], and iloprost [Ventavis]), the phosphodiesterase-5 inhibitors (sildenafil [Revatio]), and riociguat (Adempas), the first member of a new class of drugs, the soluble guanylate cyclase (sGC) stimulators. No published randomized studies in the SCD population exist for any of these agents, although a multicenter placebo-controlled trial of sildenafil for PH of SCD was stopped early

---

[1]Not FDA approved for this indication.

Start therapy if one or more of the following conditions are present:
- frequent pain episodes
- history of acute chest syndrome
- other severe VOE
- severe symptomatic anemia

Starting dose: 15 mg/kg or 7.5 mg/kg if the patient has kidney disease

Endpoints:
- less pain
- increase in HbF to 15%–20%
- increased hemoglobin level to 7–9 g/dL
- improved well-being
- acceptable myelotoxicity

Dose escalation: increase dose by 500 mg every other day every 8 weeks if no toxicity encountered to a maximum of 35 mg/kg

Lab monitoring:
- At time of initiation or escalation: check CBC/differential/reticulocyte count every 2 weeks; serum chemistries every 2–4 weeks, percent HbF every 6–8 weeks
- During maintenance: check CBC/differential/reticulocyte count chemistries monthly, percent HbF every 3 months

Criteria to hold:
- ANC <2000
- Hb <9.0 g/dL and reticulocyte count <80,000 (alternatively start Epo)
- Platelet count <80,000
- Raising creatinine
- 2-fold elevation of AST or ALT over baseline
- 2 months prior to planned conception/pregnancy

Figure 5 Protocol for hydroxyurea treatment.

because of an unexpected increase in hospitalizations for vaso-occlusive crisis in the treatment group receiving sildenafil.

Anticoagulation is indicated in patients who have evidence of pulmonary thromboembolic complications and is supported by evidence of benefit in other populations with PH.

Hematopoietic Stem Cell Transplantation

Despite improvement of supportive care in SCD, life expectancy remains lower than for those not affected. In addition, quality of life for patients with SCD is usually significantly impaired. Although hydroxyurea can decrease acute complications of SCD such as vaso-occlusive episodes and acute chest syndrome, no satisfactory measures exist to prevent the development of irreversible organ damage in adults. Furthermore, therapy with hydroxyurea is lifelong, and only 20% to 30% of eligible patients are prescribed or actually take the drug.

Currently, allogeneic hematopoietic stem cell transplantation (HCT) remains the only curative treatment. Indications for HCT have been empirically determined from prognostic factors derived from studies of the natural history of SCD. The most common indications for which patients with SCD have undergone HCT are a history of stroke, recurrent acute chest syndrome, or frequent vaso-occlusive episodes.

Allogeneic HCT after myeloablative therapy has been performed in hundreds of pediatric and numerous adult patients with SCD. The backbone of the preparative regimens have consisted of busulfan (Busulfex)[1] 14 to 16 mg/kg and cyclophosphamide (Cytoxan)[1] 200 mg/kg. Additional immunosuppressive agents used have included antithymocyte globulin (Atgam)[1], rabbit antithymocyte globulin (Thymoglobulin)[1], antilymphocyte globulin, or total lymphoid irradiation (Figure 6). Cyclosporine A (Neoral)[1], alone or with mercaptopurine (Purinethol)[1] or methotrexate[1], has been used for posttransplant graft-versus-host disease prophylaxis.

The outcome of HCT for patients with SCD from matched siblings is excellent. Of 1000 recipients of human leukocyte antigen (HLA)-identical sibling transplants performed between 1986 and 2013 and reported to the European Blood and Marrow Transplant, Eurocord, and the Center for International Blood and Marrow Transplant Research, the 5-year event-free and overall survival were 91.4% (95% CI 89.6% to 93.3%) and 92.9% (95% CI 91.1% to 94.6%), respectively. Event-free survival was lower with increasing age at transplantation (hazard ratio [HR] 1.09; $P < .001$) and higher for transplantations performed after 2006 (HR 0.95, $P = .013$). Twenty-three patients experienced graft failure; 70 patients (7%) died, the most common cause of death being infection. Stabilization or reversal of organ damage from SCD has been documented after HCT. In patients who have stable donor engraftment, complications related to SCD resolve, and there are no further episodes of pain, stroke, or acute chest syndrome. Patients who successfully receive allografts do not experience sickle-related central nervous system complications and have evidence of stabilization of central nervous system disease by cerebral MRI. However, the impact of successful HCT on reversal of cerebral vasculopathy has been variable. Current research is focused on improving the applicability of HCT to a greater proportion of patients with SCD by the development of novel conditioning regimens minimizing myeloablation (see Figure 6), the use of novel sources of hematopoietic stem cells such as umbilical cord blood, extending HCT to adult recipients and alternate donors such as matched unrelated donors and haploidentical donors. Recent phase 2 trials of haploidentical transplant in adults and children with SCD have shown 1- to 2-year event-free survival >90% and a relatively low incidence of severe GVHD, supporting haploidentical transplant as a viable therapy for SCD patients lacking matched sibling donors. Advancements in conditioning regimens (e.g., the inclusion of thiotepa [Tepadina][1] to reduce rejection) and GVHD prophylaxis have significantly improved outcomes, making this approach a less costly and more accessible alternative to gene therapies.

New and Experimental Therapies

The last few years have witnessed a flourishing of new therapeutic approaches for SCD. New drugs have received FDA approval and have been incorporated in the clinical practice across the United States, and several are in the pipeline or being reviewed in accelerated approval pathways by the FDA. Several decades of preclinical research in sickle mouse models are finally bearing fruit with pathologic pathways identified in sickle mice being harnessed for the development of molecular targeted biologicals. Finally, gene therapy is currently on the horizon with several gene therapy and gene editing approaches being developed simultaneously.

Antioxidant Strategies

In 2018, pharmacologic L-glutamine (Endari) received FDA approval as the second disease-modifying drug in SCD. A randomized, phase III multicenter trial showed that patients in the L-glutamine group had significantly fewer pain crises and hospitalizations than those in the placebo group. Of note, two-thirds of the patients in both arms received concomitant hydroxyurea. Reassuringly, the drug had relatively mild side effects including nausea and fatigue. L-glutamine presumably acts by reducing oxidant stress in the sickle RBCs, although its effects on major disease parameters such as hemolysis are unclear.

Modulation of Cellular Adhesion

Adhesive interactions between RBCs, white blood cells, and platelets, and between cells and endothelium are implicated in the pathogenesis of vaso-occlusive episodes. Recently, several compounds have been developed to target specific adhesion molecules such as E-selectin and P-selectin. This is a particularly promising area of research that has yielded several compounds in advanced phases of development. The P-selectin inhibitor crizanlizumab has shown significant reduction of the rate of crises per year and longer median time to the first crisis and second crisis when given

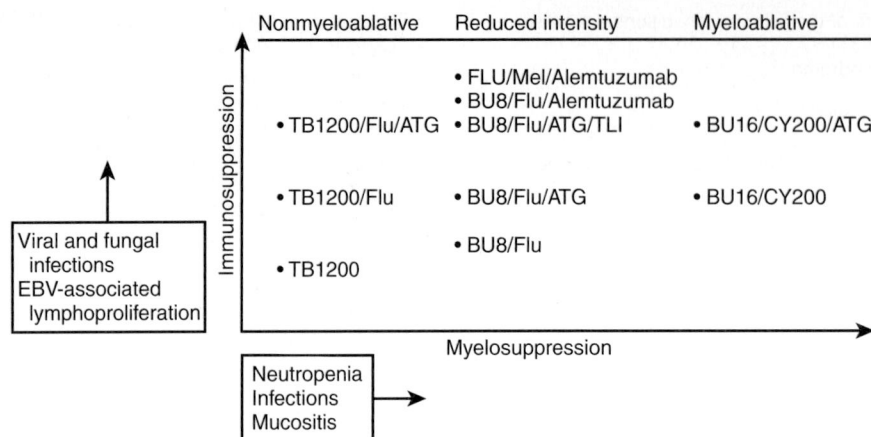

Figure 6 Spectrum of immunosuppression and myelosuppression in preparative regimens in hematopoietic stem cell transplantation (HCT) in sickle cell disease (SCD). Most preparative regimens for HCT in SCD have used a backbone of busulfan (BU) (Busulfex)[1] and cyclophosphamide (CY) (Cytoxan)[1]. Additional immunosuppressive agents include equine antithymocyte globulin (Atgam)[1] or leporine antithymocyte globulin (Thymoglobulin) (ATG)[1], antilymphocyte globulin, total lymphoid irradiation (TLI) or total body irradiation (TBI), fludarabine (Flu) (Fludara)[1], and alemtuzumab (Campath)[1]. Attempts to reduce the intensity of preparative regimens for patients with SCD have been based on one of two approaches. The first is the use of reduced-intensity conditioning regimens to produce less myeloablation. These require donor marrow infusion for hematopoietic recovery. The second is the use of nonmyeloablative regimens, which do not eradicate host hematopoiesis and allow hematopoietic recovery even without donor stem cell infusion. [1]Not FDA approved for this indication. Adapted with permission from Krishnamurti L. Hematopoietic cell transplantation: a curative option for sickle cell disease. *Pediatr Hematol Oncol.* 2007;24:569–575.

as intravenous prophylaxis in a double-blind, randomized, phase II clinical trial. Unfortunately, a global phase 3 clinical trial failed to detect a significant difference between crizanlizumab 5mg/kg or crizanlizumab 7.5mg/kg and placebo in annualized rates of vaso-occlusive episodes, a result that may have been impacted by the low baseline rate of vaso-occlusive episodes in the study population. The FDA approved crizanlizumab (Adakveo) for the prevention of vaso-occlusive episodes in SCD in November 2019. As in the case of *L*-glutamine, crizanlizumab can be used with and without concurrent hydroxyurea therapy. The pan-selectin inhibitor rivipansel[5] had shown promising results in a phase II trial of treatment of vaso-occlusive episodes but failed to meet the primary end point of time to readiness for discharge and other key secondary endpoints in a phase III trial.

Modulation of Hemoglobin Oxygen Affinity

Deoxygenation of HbS leads to polymerization, sickling, and hemolysis. Thus strategies aimed at increasing the oxygen affinity of HbS may be beneficial. Clinical trials in adults and children have shown reduced hemolysis and improved hemoglobin with voxelotor (Oxbryta), a once daily oral drug that increases the oxygen affinity of hemoglobin maintaining it in the oxygenated state and reducing polymerization and sickling. The drug was FDA approved for the treatment of SCD in 2019, but unfortunately it was withdrawn from the market in 2024 owing to safety concerns emerging from postmarketing clinical trials. Voxelotor (Oxbryta) was also approved by the FDA for the treatment of SCD in November 2019.

Another promising strategy to reduce HbS polymerization by modulating oxygen affinity involves the use of pyruvate kinase activators. Both mitapivat (Pyrukynd)[1] and etavopivat[5] are promising pyruvate kinase activators that ameliorate the sickling of SCD RBCs by reduction of 2,3-diphosphoglycerate (2,3-DPG), which in turn increases hemoglobin oxygen affinity. Other, newer generation pyruvate kinase activators are under development.

Modulation of Nitric Oxide

NO is an active biogas and a free radical species that mediates arterial relaxation, cellular adhesion to endothelium, hemostasis, and blood viscosity. In SCD, NO bioactivity is reduced

as a result of decreased production due to endothelial perturbation and NO scavenging by cell-free hemoglobin generated during intravascular hemolysis. Dietary supplementation with *L*-arginine, a precursor of NO, and delivery of exogenous NO or NO bioactivity to the microvasculature in SCD, should promote dilatation of the terminal arterioles where obstruction to flow and tissue damage occurs, improvement of lung ventilation and perfusion is matching, decrease in pulmonary artery pressures, and inhibition of platelet aggregation and cellular adhesion. Although two recent clinical trials on *L*-arginine supplementation and inhaled NO (DeNOVO trial) for vaso-occlusive episodes failed to show a clinical benefit, optimization of timing and dosing and novel strategies to target the NO pathway might lead to valuable NO therapeutics in the future.

Gene Therapy

To date, the FDA has approved two gene therapy products: exagamglogene autotemcel (Casgevy), utilizing a CRISPR-Cas9 gene editing approach; and lovotibeglogene autotemcel (Lyfgenia), based on lentiviral technology. Casgevy induces a mutation in the *BCL11A* gene, a transcription factor that suppresses γ-globin and fetal hemoglobin (HbF) expression, thereby increasing HbF production. Conversely, Lyfgenia introduces a modified, non-sickling beta-globin gene (βA-T87Q-globin). Both therapies demonstrate sustained and significant reductions in vaso-occlusive episodes. As their names suggest, they are ex vivo treatments involving apheresis-derived cells from patients, followed by autologous transplant after myeloablative conditioning.

However, the considerable expense of both treatments (ranging approximately from \$2-3M), alongside recognized toxicity concerns such as side effects from busulfan, the necessity for fertility preservation, and uncertainties regarding long-term risks, such as insertional mutagenesis with Lyfgenia and off-target effects with Casgevy, pose barriers to widespread adoption, particularly in low- and middle-income countries. Additionally, it remains unclear whether either therapy can achieve permanent suppression of HbS polymerization, thus precluding them from being labeled as curative. Furthermore, the development of myelodysplastic syndrome (MDS) and acute myeloid leukemia (AML) in some initial Lyfgenia recipients has led to a black box warning for this product, further heightening concerns.

The ultimate solution for sickle cell disease (SCD) is likely to be a curative, in vivo direct correction of the HbS mutation, which,

[5]Investigational drug in the United States.
[1]Not FDA approved for this indication.

given recent successes in gene therapy for SCD, appears to be increasingly attainable.

Surgical Issues

Preoperative patient optimization includes prophylactic transfusion, close monitoring of pulse oximetry, adequate analgesia based on the patient's opioid tolerance, and monitoring for sickle cell–related complications.

AVN of the femoral heads, and more rarely of the humeral heads, is the most common orthopedic problem in SCD. Surgery is usually deferred until the pain and disability from AVN become intolerable and usually involves total hip or shoulder arthroplasty. This is usually a more involved procedure than in the general population on account of the altered bone anatomy in SCD. Patients with bone marrow expansion may experience thinning of the cortical bone and prosthetic instability, whereas some may suffer from the opposite problem of obliteration of the medullary shaft by sclerotic bone in response to multiple necrotic events.

Patients with SCD tend to develop pigmented gallstones and cholelithiasis. Cholecystectomy is performed in patients with SCD with cholelithiasis, right upper quadrant pain, and a positive hepatobiliary iminodiacetic acid (HIDA) scan. In SCD, the rate of intraoperative complications is higher and so is the rate of reversion from laparoscopic to open cholecystectomy.

Splenectomy has been reserved for patients with massive splenic infarction (>50% of the spleen volume); intractable, recurrent splenic pain; and splenic abscess in the setting of splenic infarction. It is important to limit splenectomy to these few specific circumstances, because overwhelming sepsis and acute PH have been reported in the postsplenectomy period in SCD.

Kidney transplantation has been successfully performed in patients with SCD on chronic renal replacement therapy, although survival at 7 years is lower than in African Americans without SCD (67% vs. 83%). This difference is mostly due to vaso-occlusive complications in the transplanted kidney, possibly exacerbated by the higher hematocrit in the postoperative period from resumption of endogenous erythropoietin production and increased blood viscosity. It is therefore critical to closely monitor ESA therapy in the posttransplantation period to prevent overdosing and relative erythrocytosis. A chronic transfusion program to prevent intrarenal sickling and maximization of hydroxyurea therapy should also be entertained, although its benefits need to be balanced against the risk of HLA alloimmunization and rejection. Combined solid organ and HCT protocols are being developed to overcome these complications. Recently, lung transplantation has been successfully performed in a SCD patient with severe pulmonary arterial hypertension and pulmonary venoocclusive disease.

References

Adams RJ, Brambilla D: Discontinuing prophylactic transfusions used to prevent stroke in sickle cell disease, N Engl J Med 353:2769–2778, 2005.

Adams RJ, Brambilla DJ, Granger S, et al: Stroke and conversion to high risk in children screened with transcranial Doppler ultrasound during the STOP study, Blood 103:3689–3694, 2004.

Ataga KI, et al: Crizanlizumab for the prevention of pain crises in sickle cell disease, N Engl J Med 376:429–439, 2017.

Bunn HF: Pathogenesis and treatment of sickle cell disease, N Engl J Med 337:762–769, 1997.

Charache S, Terrin ML, Moore RD, et al: Effect of hydroxyurea on the frequency of painful crises in sickle cell anemia. Investigators of the Multicenter Study of Hydroxyurea in Sickle Cell Anemia, N Engl J Med 332:1317–1322, 1995.

DeBaun MR, et al: Controlled trial of transfusions for silent cerebral infarcts in sickle cell anemia, N Engl J Med 371(8):699–710, 2014.

Falletta JM, Woods GM, Verter JI, et al: Discontinuing penicillin prophylaxis in children with sickle cell anemia. Prophylactic Penicillin Study II, J Pediatr 127:685–690, 1995.

Gaston MH, Verter JI, Woods G, et al: Prophylaxis with oral penicillin in children with sickle cell anemia. A randomized trial, N Engl J Med 314:1593–1599, 1986.

Gladwin MT, Sachdev V: Cardiovascular abnormalities in sickle cell disease, J Am Coll Cardiol 59:1123–1133, 2012.

Gladwin MT, Sachdev V, Jison ML, et al: Pulmonary hypertension as a risk factor for death in patients with sickle cell disease, N Engl J Med 350:886–895, 2004.

Gladwin MT, Vichinsky E: Pulmonary complications of sickle cell disease, N Engl J Med 359:2254–2265, 2008.

Gluckman E, Cappelli B, Bernaudin F, et al: Sickle cell disease: An international survey of results of HLA-identical sibling hematopoietic stem cell transplantation, Blood 129(11):1548–1556, 2017.

Hoppe CC, Inati AC, Brown C, et al: Initial results from a cohort in a phase 2a study (GBT440- 007) evaluating adolescents with sickle cell disease treated with multiple doses of GBT440, a HbS polymerization inhibitor, Blood 130.

Howard J, Malfroy M, Llewelyn C, et al: The Transfusion Alternatives Preoperatively in Sickle Cell Disease (TAPS) study: A randomised, controlled, multicentre clinical trial, Lancet 381:930–938, 2013.

Hsieh MM, Fitzhugh CD, Weitzel RP, et al: Nonmyeloablative HLA-matched sibling allogeneic hematopoietic stem cell transplantation for severe sickle cell phenotype, JAMA 312(1):48–56, 2014.

Jeong GK, Ruchelsman DE, Jazrawi LM, Jaffe WL: Total hip arthroplasty in sickle cell hemoglobinopathies, J Am Acad Orthop Surg 13:208–217, 2005.

Krishnamurti L, Kharbanda S, Biernacki MA, et al: Stable long-term donor engraftment following reduced-intensity hematopoietic cell transplantation for sickle cell disease, Biol Blood Marrow Transplant 14:1270–1278, 2008.

Lee MT, Piomelli S, Granger S, et al: Stroke Prevention Trial in Sickle Cell Anemia (STOP): Extended follow-up and final results, Blood 108:847–852, 2006.

Little JA, McGowan VR, Kato GJ, et al: Combination erythropoietin-hydroxyurea therapy in sickle cell disease: Experience from the National Institutes of Health and a literature review, Haematologica 91:1076–1083, 2006.

Mehari A, Alam S, Tian X, et al: Hemodynamic predictors of mortality in adults with sickle cell disease, Am J Respir Crit Care Med 187:840–847, 2013.

Merkel KH, Ginsberg PL, Parker JC, Post MJ: Cerebrovascular disease in sickle cell anemia: A clinical, pathological and radiological correlation, Stroke 9:45–52, 1978.

Morris CR, Kato GJ, Poljakovic M, et al: Dysregulated arginine metabolism, hemolysis-associated pulmonary hypertension, and mortality in sickle cell disease, JAMA 294:81–90, 2005.

Noguchi CT, Rodgers GP, Serjeant G, Schechter AN: Levels of fetal hemoglobin necessary for treatment of sickle cell disease, N Engl J Med 318:96–99, 1988.

Novelli EM, Huynh C, Gladwin MT, et al: Pulmonary embolism in sickle cell disease: A case-control study, J Thrombosis and Hemostasis 10:760–766, 2012.

Ohene-Frempong K, Weiner SJ, Sleeper LA, et al: Cerebrovascular accidents in sickle cell disease: Rates and risk factors, Blood 91:288–294, 1998.

Niihara Y, et al: A phase 3 trial of l-glutamine in sickle cell disease, N Engl J Med 379:226–235, 2018.

Platt OS: The acute chest syndrome of sickle cell disease, N Engl J Med 342:1904–1907, 2000.

Platt OS, Brambilla DJ, Rosse WF, et al: Mortality in sickle cell disease. Life expectancy and risk factors for early death, N Engl J Med 330:1639–1644, 1994.

Platt OS, Thorington BD, Brambilla DJ, et al: Pain in sickle cell disease. Rates and risk factors, N Engl J Med 325:11–16, 1991.

Reiter CD, Wang X, Tanus-Santos JE, et al: Cell-free hemoglobin limits nitric oxide bioavailability in sickle-cell disease, Nat Med 8:1383–1389, 2002.

Ribeil J, et al: Gene therapy in a patient with sickle cell disease, N Engl J Med 376:848–855, 2017.

Scheinman JI: Sickle cell disease and the kidney, Nat Clin Pract Nephrol 5:78–88, 2009.

Smiley D, Dagogo-Jack S, Umpierrez G: Therapy insight: Metabolic and endocrine disorders in sickle cell disease, Nat Clin Pract Endocrinol Metab 4:102–109, 2008.

Steinberg MH: Management of sickle cell disease, N Engl J Med 340:1021–1030, 1999.

Steinberg MH, Barton F, Castro O, et al: Effect of hydroxyurea on mortality and morbidity in adult sickle cell anemia: Risks and benefits up to 9 years of treatment, JAMA 289:1645–1651, 2003.

Telen MJ, Wun T, McCavit TL, et al: Randomized phase 2 study of GMI-1070 in SCD: Reduction in time to resolution of vaso-occlusive events and decreased opioid use, Blood 125:2656–2664, 2015.

Tshilolo L, Tomlinson G, Williams TN, et al: Hydroxyurea for children with sickle cell anemia in sub-Saharan Africa, N Engl J Med 380:121–131, 2019.

Vichinsky EP, Neumayr LD, Earles AN, et al: Causes and outcomes of the acute chest syndrome in sickle cell disease, N Engl J Med 342:1855–1865, 2000.

Vichinsky E, Hoppe CC, Ataga KI, et al: A phase 3 randomized trial of voxelotor in sickle cell disease, N Engl J Med 381(6):509–519, 2019.

Walters MC, Patience M, Leisenring W, et al: Bone marrow transplantation for sickle cell disease, N Engl J Med 335:369–376, 1996.

Walters MC, Storb R, Patience M, et al: Impact of bone marrow transplantation for symptomatic sickle cell disease: An interim report. Multicenter investigation of bone marrow transplantation for sickle cell disease, Blood 95:1918–1924, 2000.

Yawn BP, et al: Management of sickle cell disease: Summary of the 2014 evidence-based report by expert panel members, JAMA 312(10):1033–1048, 2014.

THALASSEMIA

Method of
Sarah A. Holstein, MD, PhD; and Ray J. Hohl, MD, PhD

CURRENT DIAGNOSIS

- Complete blood count: anemia (very severe in β-thalassemia major, mild in β-thalassemia minor and α-thalassemia trait), low mean corpuscular volume, variable leukocytosis, thrombocytopenia (secondary to splenomegaly), or thrombocythemia (after splenectomy)
- Peripheral blood smear: hypochromia, microcytosis, anisocytosis, poikilocytosis, target cells, Heinz bodies, nucleated red blood cells
- Evidence of hemolytic anemia: indirect hyperbilirubinemia, elevated lactate dehydrogenase, decreased haptoglobin
- Hemoglobin electrophoresis pattern:
  - β-Thalassemia minor: elevated HbA2 ($\alpha_2\delta_2$)
  - β-Thalassemia intermedia: elevated HbA2, elevated HbF ($\alpha_2\gamma_2$), and decreased HbA ($\alpha_2\beta_2$)
  - β-Thalassemia major: absence of HbA, markedly elevated HbF, and elevated HbA2
  - α-Thalassemia trait: normal
  - Hemoglobin H disease: decreased HbA, presence of HbH (β_4) and HbBart (γ_4)
  - Hemoglobin Barts hydrops fetalis: HbBart, absence of HbA, HbA2, and HbF
- Timing of symptomatic disease:
  - β-Thalassemia minor: asymptomatic
  - β-Thalassemia intermedia: variable
  - β-Thalassemia major: within first year of life
  - α-Thalassemia trait: asymptomatic
  - Hemoglobin H disease: symptomatic at time of birth
  - Hemoglobin Barts hydrops fetalis: death during gestation

CURRENT THERAPY

- Chronic packed red blood cell transfusions for β-thalassemia major (1–3 units of packed leukoreduced erythrocytes every 3–5 weeks) with a target hemoglobin concentration of 9 to 10.5 g/dL; variable transfusion needs for β-thalassemia intermedia and hemoglobin H disease
- Splenectomy with antibiotic prophylaxis and vaccination
- Iron chelation: deferoxamine (Desferal) or deferasirox (Exjade); deferiprone (Ferriprox)
- Osteoporosis management: calcium with vitamin D supplementation; bisphosphonates
- Allogeneic hematopoietic cell transplantation for β-thalassemia major
- Luspatercept (Reblozyl) for transfusion-dependent adults with β-thalassemia
- Betibeglogene autotemcel (Zynteglo) for children and adults with transfusion-dependent β-thalassemia
- Exagamglogene autotemcel (Casgevy) for people 12 years and older with transfusion-dependent β-thalassemia

Globin Gene Arrangements

Thalassemia syndromes encompass a spectrum of hemoglobin disorders that arise from impaired production of globin chains. The genes that encode globins are located in two clusters: the β gene cluster on chromosome 11 and the α gene cluster on chromosome 16 (Figure 1). The β gene cluster includes the adult globin genes (β and δ), as well as the fetal Aγ and Gγ genes and the embryonic ε gene. The arrangement of the 5' to 3' sequence of these genes parallels the order of their developmental expression. Functional hemoglobin is a tetramer that includes two α and two β globin units. The α gene cluster includes two fetal/adult α genes (α_1 and α_2) and the embryonic ζ genes. In the embryo, three hemoglobins are found ($\zeta_2\varepsilon_2$, $\alpha_2\varepsilon_2$, and $\zeta_2\gamma_2$). Fetal hemoglobin (HbF) is composed of two α chains and two γ chains ($\alpha_2\gamma_2$). In adults, the predominant hemoglobin is hemoglobin A (HbA), consisting of two α chains and two β chains ($\alpha_2\beta_2$) (see Figure 1). Hemoglobin A2, consisting of two α chains and two δ chains ($\alpha_2\delta_2$), is a normal variant in adults and typically represents <3% of the total hemoglobin (see Figure 1).

In β-thalassemia, there is diminished production of β globin genes, resulting in an excess of α globin chains. Conversely, in α-thalassemia, there is impaired production of α globin genes, resulting in an excess of β globin chains. This imbalance of globin production is variable, and the degree of accumulation of unpaired globin chains is directly related to the severity of the disease phenotype. The genetic basis of thalassemia is heterogeneous, and several hundred mutations have been identified. These mutations may affect any level of globin gene expression, including arrangement of the globin gene complex, gene deletion, splicing, transcription, translation, and protein stability. In general, β-thalassemia occurs as a result of mutations, whereas α-thalassemia occurs as a result of gene deletion.

It has been estimated that there are 270 million carriers of thalassemia in the world, including 80 million β-thalassemia carriers. The frequency of β-thalassemia carriers is highest in the malarial tropical and subtropical regions of Asia, the Mediterranean, and the Middle East. (The term *thalassemia* is derived from the Greek word *thalassa*, which refers to the Mediterranean Sea.) This distribution is secondary to the selective advantage of heterozygotes against malaria. β-Thalassemia is subdivided into major, intermedia, and minor types (Table 1). α-Thalassemia is classified into four syndromes: α-thalassemia trait 2 (loss of one α globin gene [αα/α–]); α-thalassemia trait 1, also referred to as *α-thalassemia minor* (loss of two α globin genes [αα/– – or α–/α–]); hemoglobin H (HbH) disease (loss of three alleles [α–/– –]); and hemoglobin Barts hydrops fetalis (loss of all four α globin loci [– –/– –]).

Pathophysiology

The clinical manifestations of thalassemia and their severity are a consequence of the relative excess of unpaired globin chains. In particular, excess α globin chains are unstable and insoluble and therefore precipitate inside the red blood cell (RBC). These inclusions (precipitated hemoglobin) may be visualized as Heinz bodies. The accumulation of α globin chains leads to a variety of insults to the erythrocyte, including changes in membrane deformability and increased fragility. Free β chains are more soluble than free α chains and are able to form a homotetramer (HbH). The

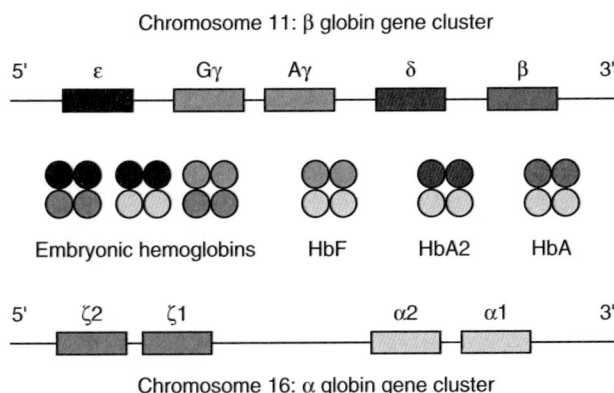

Figure 1 Representation of the β and α globin gene clusters. Also shown are the globin tetramers produced during embryonic development.

TABLE 1	Summary of Hematologic and Clinical Features of the Thalassemias		
TYPE	**HEMATOLOGIC FINDINGS**	**HEMOGLOBIN ELECTRO-PHORESIS PATTERN**	**CLINICAL FEATURES**
β-Thalassemia major	Severe anemia, microcytosis, hypochromia, target cells, nucleated RBCs	Absence of HbA, markedly elevated HbF, elevated HbA2	Splenomegaly, jaundice, skeletal abnormalities, abnormal facies; transfusion dependent
β-Thalassemia intermedia	Mild to moderate anemia, microcytosis, hypochromia	Elevated HbA2, elevated HbF, decreased HbA	Splenomegaly; variable transfusion dependence
β-Thalassemia minor	Mild anemia, microcytosis, target cells	Elevated HbA2	None
Hemoglobin Bart hydrops fetalis	Severe anemia, anisopoikilocytosis, hypochromia, nucleated RBCs	HbBart; absence of HbA, HbA2, and HbF	Death during gestation; fetus with massive hepatosplenomegaly, generalized edema
Hemoglobin H disease	Moderately severe anemia, anisopoikilocytosis, microcytosis, Heinz bodies	Decreased HbA; HbH and HbBart present	Splenomegaly, jaundice; generally transfusion dependent
α-Thalassemia trait 1	Mild anemia, hypochromia, microcytosis, target cells	Normal	None
α-Thalassemia trait 2	Normal	Normal	None

HbA, Hemoglobin A; *HbF*, fetal hemoglobin; *HbH*, hemoglobin H; *RBCs*, red blood cells.

hallmark of thalassemia is an anemia that is a consequence of both increased destruction (i.e., hemolysis) and decreased production (i.e., ineffective erythropoiesis). The bone marrow typically displays erythroid hyperplasia.

Oxidant injury is closely linked with the pathology of thalassemia. Under normal conditions, a small amount of methemoglobin (Fe^{3+}) is formed via oxidation and can then be reduced back to hemoglobin (Fe^{2+}). However, isolated globin chains can be oxidized to hemichromes, some forms of which are irreversibly oxidized. The hemichromes can then generate reactive oxygen species, which can oxidize membrane components, leading to cell injury. There is an increase in membrane rigidity in β-thalassemia, and this appears to be secondary to the binding of partially oxidized α globin chains to components of the membrane skeleton. Increased membrane rigidity in turn leads to decreased membrane deformability and increased destruction. In α-thalassemia, HbH has a left-shifted oxygen disassociation curve and therefore does not readily transport oxygen. HbH erythrocytes have increased rigidity, which is thought to be secondary to interactions between excess β globin chains and the membrane. Unlike with β-thalassemia, HbH erythrocytes have increased membrane stability. Inclusion bodies have been identified in HbH cells, and there appears to be a correlation between RBC age and solubility of HbH. As cells age, the amount of soluble HbH decreases and the level of inclusions increases.

It has also been recognized that there is increased phagocytosis of thalassemia RBCs compared with normal controls. The etiology is not completely understood, but it may be a consequence of reduction in surface levels of sialic acid, increase in surface immunoglobulin G binding, and changes in phosphatidylserine localization.

Despite the pronounced hemolysis and marrow erythroid hyperplasia, patients with thalassemia generally do not display the compensatory reticulocytosis that is indicative of the other basis for anemia, ineffective erythropoiesis. Accumulation of α-chain aggregates is thought to lead to death of erythrocyte precursors. Furthermore, abnormal assembly of membrane proteins in erythroid precursors has been demonstrated.

Iron overload is one of the primary causes of morbidity. Even without transfusion, the long-standing anemia, however mild, leads to increased iron absorption in the gut and eventual chronic iron overload. Excessive iron deposition causes devastating damage to multiple organs, particularly affecting the heart, liver, and endocrine organs.

β-Thalassemia Major

Symptoms of β-thalassemia major are not present at birth because HbF ($\alpha_2\gamma_2$) is present. However, as HbF levels decline over the first year, the signs and symptoms of severe hemolytic anemia begin to manifest. Affected individuals display hepatosplenomegaly from expansion of the reticuloendothelial system, as well as extramedullary hematopoiesis, pallor, growth retardation, and abnormal skeletal development. If left untreated, 80% of children with β-thalassemia major will die before 5 years of age.

Laboratory Features

Thalassemia major is characterized by a severe microcytic anemia. Hemoglobin levels may be as low as 3 to 4 g/dL. The peripheral blood smear is markedly abnormal and is notable for hypochromia, microcytosis, anisocytosis, poikilocytosis, target cells, and teardrop cells. Routine stains show the presence of precipitated α globin chains as Heinz bodies. The reticulocyte count is often low. The white blood cell count is often high but may be artifactually elevated as a consequence of automated inclusion of high numbers of circulating nucleated RBCs. The platelet count is typically normal, but progressive hypersplenism can result in decreased platelet counts. Patients who have undergone splenectomy often have increased white blood cell and platelet counts. Iron studies reveal elevated serum iron, transferrin saturation, and ferritin. Consistent with hemolysis and ineffective erythropoiesis, indirect bilirubin and lactate dehydrogenase levels are increased, and haptoglobin levels are low.

Clinical Features

Unique to β-thalassemia major is the development of extramedullary erythropoiesis. This may be so severe that the masses of bone marrow lead to broken bones and spinal cord compression. Sites of involvement include the sinuses and the thoracic and pelvic cavities. The expansion of the erythroid bone marrow can lead to a number of skeletal changes. In particular, characteristic changes in the facial bones and skull result in frontal bossing, overgrowth of the maxillae, and malocclusion. This has sometimes been referred to as *chipmunk facies*. Other bones are also affected, and premature fusion of the epiphyses results in shortened limbs. Compression fractures of the spine may occur. Even if the disease is managed appropriately with transfusions and iron chelation, patients will still suffer from osteopenia and osteoporosis. Possible mechanisms include changes secondary to hypogonadism or increased bone resorption secondary to vitamin D deficiency.

Hepatomegaly and splenomegaly, secondary to extramedullary erythropoiesis and RBC destruction, are prominent. Injury to Kupffer cells and hepatocytes from chronic overload leads to fibrosis and end-stage liver disease. Hepatic iron overload is probably caused in part by comparatively high levels of transferrin receptors. Iron overload and perhaps other factors increase susceptibility to viral hepatitis. Laboratory studies show indirect hyperbilirubinemia, hypergammaglobulinemia, and elevated liver markers. The chronic hemolysis leads to formation of bilirubin gallstones, although cholecystitis or cholangitis is not common. Splenic dysfunction results in immune dysfunction. The shortened erythrocyte survival time leaves patients susceptible to aplastic crisis induced by parvovirus B19 infection. Extramedullary hematopoiesis may also affect the kidneys, and patients often have large kidneys. Rapid cell turnover leads to hyperuricemia, and children may develop gouty nephropathy.

A number of endocrine abnormalities are commonly seen in β-thalassemia major, including hypogonadism, growth failure, diabetes, and hypothyroidism. These abnormalities occur even in chronically transfused patients and may be in part related to iron overload. Endocrine glands, such as the liver and heart, have high levels of transferrin receptor and therefore are more susceptible to iron overload. The typical growth pattern for a child with β-thalassemia major is relatively normal until 9 to 10 years of age. After that time, the growth velocity slows, and the pubertal growth spurt is either absent or reduced. Although secretion of growth hormone does not appear to be altered in thalassemic patients, a reduction in peak amplitude and nocturnal levels of growth hormone has been observed. Amenorrhea is quite common, with 50% of girls presenting with primary amenorrhea. Secondary amenorrhea also develops, particularly in patients who do not receive regular chelation therapy. In males, impotence and azoospermia are common. Primary hypothyroidism typically appears during the second decade of life. The prevalence of diabetes mellitus and impaired glucose intolerance has been estimated at 4% to 20%. Unlike type 1 diabetes mellitus, diabetes associated with thalassemia is rarely complicated by diabetic ketoacidosis. The risk of diabetic retinopathy is lower, but the risk of diabetic nephropathy is higher. Patients with a high ferritin level (>1800 μg/L) experience faster progression to hypothyroidism, hypogonadism, and other endocrinopathies.

Thalassemic patients suffer from extensive cardiac abnormalities. Chronic anemia causes cardiac dilation. Although long-term transfusion can help prevent cardiac dilation, the resulting iron overload leads to cardiac hemosiderosis. Pericarditis, ventricular and supraventricular arrhythmias, and end-stage cardiomyopathy can develop. Ventricular arrhythmia is a common cause of death. Patients may also develop pulmonary hypertension. The degree of iron overload in the heart has traditionally been assessed by cardiac biopsy, but cardiac magnetic resonance imaging (MRI) is increasingly being used.

Vitamin and mineral deficiencies may occur. Folic acid deficiency may develop in patients, presumably as a consequence of increased cell turnover. Although the cause is unknown, patients with β-thalassemia major often have very low serum zinc levels. Serum levels of vitamin E and vitamin C may also be low.

Management of β-Thalassemia Major
Transfusion
The key intervention for the management of β-thalassemia major is chronic transfusion therapy. In particular, during the first decade of life, regular transfusion results in improvements in hepatosplenomegaly, skeletal abnormalities, and cardiac dilation. Patients typically require 1 to 3 units of packed RBCs every 3 to 5 weeks. The optimal target total hemoglobin level has yet to be determined. Alloimmunization does occur, and some blood centers try to leukodeplete their products, match donors by ethnicity, and limit the donor pool for any particular patient. Although the risk of bloodborne infections is currently quite small, regular transfusion of blood products still carries a risk for infections such as human immunodeficiency virus and hepatitis C.

Splenectomy
The general indication for splenectomy is an increase of >50% in the RBC transfusion requirement over a period of 1 year. Splenectomy may initially yield a decrease in the RBC transfusion requirement. It has been noted that thalassemia patients are at higher risk for infection after splenectomy than patients who are splenectomized for other reasons. The bacteria that most frequently cause infections in these patients include *Streptococcus pneumoniae*, *Haemophilus influenzae*, *Neisseria meningitidis*, *Klebsiella*, *Escherichia coli*, and *Staphylococcus aureus*. The increased susceptibility to infection compared with other splenectomized patients is thought to be a result of greater immune dysfunction secondary to iron overload. In particular, it has been reported that iron-overloaded macrophages lose the ability to kill intracellular pathogens. Antibiotic prophylaxis with penicillin, amoxicillin, or erythromycin is recommended for children up to 16 years of age. In addition, patients should receive immunizations, including the pneumococcal, influenza, and *H. influenzae* vaccines.

Iron Chelation Therapy
Because of increased iron absorption and long-term transfusion therapy, iron overload develops. As noted earlier, iron overload causes damage to multiple organs. Because iron is poorly excreted, removal must be accomplished by phlebotomy (not an option in thalassemic patients) or by chelation therapy. Historically, deferoxamine (Desferal) has been the most widely used chelator. This agent may be administered subcutaneously (SQ), intramuscularly (IM), or intravenously (IV). The dosing for chronic iron overload is 1000 to 2000 mg/day (or 20–40 mg/kg/day) SQ or 500 to 1000 mg/day IM or 40 to 50 mg/kg/day IV. The IV-only route is indicated for patients with cardiovascular collapse. Multiple studies have shown that deferoxamine therapy improves long-term survival. In addition, intensive therapy with deferoxamine has been shown to improve cardiac function in patients with severe iron overload. However, compliance with daily injections has been a particular problem, and unless regular therapy is given, iron will reaccumulate.

Deferiprone (Ferriprox) was the first orally active chelator to be introduced. It is given three times daily (total of 75 mg/kg/day). Studies have indicated that deferiprone may be as effective as deferoxamine in lowering iron levels. A recent Cochrane review concluded that deferiprone is indicated in the treatment of iron overload in thalassemia major if deferoxamine therapy is contraindicated or inadequate. Agranulocytosis associated with deferiprone has been reported, and because of this risk, the drug has a black box warning on its label. The U.S. Food and Drug Administration (FDA) also requires that medication guides be issued to patients when the drug is dispensed. Deferiprone is currently available at selected specialty pharmacies. Deferiprone is available in Europe and Asia. There has also been interest in combined therapy with deferiprone and deferoxamine, and one study showed that the combination was more effective in removing cardiac and hepatic iron but did not further improve cardiac function.

Deferasirox (Exjade) is the first orally active agent approved for use in the United States. Its longer half-life in comparison with deferiprone allows this drug to be given once daily (total of 20–40 mg/kg/day). A phase III trial comparing deferasirox to deferoxamine in patients with thalassemia revealed similar decreases in liver iron concentrations. Side effects include gastrointestinal complaints (abdominal pain, nausea, vomiting, diarrhea) and skin rash. There have been postmarketing reports of acute renal failure, hepatic failure, and cytopenias. It is recommended that serum creatinine, ferritin, and alanine aminotransferase be monitored monthly during therapy. A prospective, randomized study comparing deferiprone and deferoxamine versus deferiprone and deferasirox in 96 patients with β-thalassemia major demonstrated that both regimens reduced iron overload. However, the latter regimen was found to be superior with respect to improving cardiac iron, patient compliance, and patient satisfaction.

The gold standard for measurement of liver iron concentration has been liver biopsy with iron measurement by atomic absorption spectrometry. Increasingly, MRI is being used to measure liver iron levels. In general, iron content determined by MRI methodology correlates with liver iron concentration determined by biopsy. However, the precision of liver MRI measurement appears to be dependent on iron levels, liver fibrosis, and calibration. Hepatic iron concentration has also been measured using a superconducting quantum interference device, although reported consistency has varied, and widespread use of this technique has been limited by expense and complexity.

Novel Agents Targeting Iron Homeostasis

A variety of agents that modulate hepcidin activity are being explored as potential therapies for β-thalassemia. Preclinical data demonstrated that minihepcidins restrict iron absorption. A synthetic hepcidin, LJPC-401, was studied in a phase II trial involving patients with transfusion-dependent thalassemia. However, the study was stopped early as a result of lack of efficacy at an interim analysis. Another phase II study of MTG-300, a hepcidin mimetic, was also stopped. Studies are underway evaluating VIT-2763, an oral ferroportin inhibitor. Finally, approaches that increase hepatic synthesis of hepcidin by suppressing the gene transmembrane protease serine 6 (either via siRNA or antisense oligonucleotides) are currently being evaluated in early-phase trials.

Management of Osteoporosis

Even with calcium and vitamin D supplementation, iron chelation, transfusion therapy, and hormonal therapy, bone loss continues to be a significant problem for thalassemia patients. Several studies have evaluated the potential benefit of bisphosphonates. This class of drugs, which includes clodronate (Bonefos)[2], alendronate (Fosamax), pamidronate (Aredia), zoledronate (Zometa), and neridronate (Nerixia)[2], inhibit osteoclastic bone resorption and have found extensive use in the management of Paget disease, osteoporosis, and skeletal metastases. Small studies performed in thalassemia patients have failed to show benefit with clodronate 100 mg IM every 10 days or 300 mg IV every 3 weeks. A very small study using alendronate (Fosamax)[1] 10 mg orally daily revealed an increase in bone mineral density only at the femoral level. Conversely, in a study involving pamidronate[1] 30 or 60 mg IV every month, there was an increase in bone density only at the lumbar level. The most promising results have been achieved with the most potent member of the class, zoledronate. Several trials demonstrated that zoledronate[1] 4 mg IV every 3 or 4 months results in significant improvement in femoral and lumbar bone mineral density and reduces bony pain. The largest randomized trial involved 118 β-thalassemia patients who received calcium plus vitamin D with or without neridronate[2] (given every 90 days). At 6 and 12 months, there was increased bone mineral density, as well as decreased back pain and analgesic use in the neridronate arm. Larger long-term trials are necessary before this agent finds widespread use in the management of thalassemia-induced osteoporosis.

Hematopoietic Cell Transplantation

Hematopoietic cell transplantation is the only curative strategy for patients with hemoglobinopathies. Patients are assigned to a risk class (Pesaro class) based on adherence to regular iron chelation therapy, presence or absence of hepatomegaly, and presence or absence of portal fibrosis. Those children with no or little hepatomegaly, no portal fibrosis, and regular iron chelation therapy (class I) have a better than 90% chance of cure, whereas those with both hepatomegaly and portal fibrosis (class III) have long-term survival rates of approximately 60% in older studies. More recent reports from the 2010s to 2020s era indicate that class III survival has improved to 80% to 90%.

The use of human leukocyte antigen (HLA)-identical sibling donors has been preferred, because the use of HLA-mismatched donors has produced inferior results and is associated with increased graft rejection, graft-versus-host disease, and infection. However, it is estimated that only one-third of patients will have a matched donor. The use of unrelated donors has been explored, and initial studies showed poorer outcomes. However, data from over the past decade suggest that matched unrelated donors might be a viable option if a suitable sibling donor is lacking, thanks to improved donor selection and transplantation techniques. The use of partially HLA-matched unrelated cord blood has been reported, although 4 of 9 children did not engraft.

Another emerging technique is the use of reduced-intensity conditioning regimens, although long-term success has yet to be achieved. However, no randomized controlled studies have been performed evaluating the role of transplant in thalassemia patients.

Gene Therapy

Globin gene therapy, achieved through manipulation of autologous stem cells, is an attractive alternative to allogeneic transplantation. There are three major scientific hurdles that must be overcome: design of vectors that yield therapeutic levels of globin gene expression, ability to isolate and transduce autologous stem cells, and development of transplantation conditions that will permit host repopulation. In addition, the safety of viral and nonviral transfections is an issue. Initial studies involved ex vivo transduction of autologous hematopoietic stem cells with a lentiviral vector carrying the transgene. This gene therapy has been administered intravenously or via intrabone injection after a myeloablative conditioning regimen. Many of the patients treated to date have achieved transfusion independence, and thus far no unusual toxicities have been observed.

The first gene therapy to obtain regulatory approval was betibeglogene autotemcel (Zynteglo), which was granted conditional approval by the European Commission for patients with transfusion-dependent non-β_0/β_0-thalassemia who are 12 years of age and older. Subsequently the FDA granted approval of betibeglogene autotemcel for children and adults with transfusion-dependent β-thalassemia. Betibeglogene autotemcel therapy involves the ex vivo transduction of autologous CD34+ cells with the gene-encoding βA-T87Q-globin via a BB305 lentiviral vector. After a myeloablative conditioning regimen with busulfan (Busulfex)[1], the transduced CD34+ cells are administered (single dose of 5.0×10^6 CD34+ cells/kg). Two phase III, open-label, single-arm studies of this product enrolled 41 patients aged 4 to 34 years. In the first study, 20 of 22 evaluable patients with a non-β_0/β_0 genotype achieved transfusion independence with a median duration of 20.4 months. The average hemoglobin level was 11.7 g/dL. In the second study, 16 of 18 evaluable patients with a β_0/β_0 or non-β_0/β_0 genotype achieved transfusion independence with a median duration of 38.7 months. Both studies were 24 months in length and then rolled over into a long-term follow-up study.

Exagamglogene autotemcel (Casgevy) was recommended for conditional marketing authorization by the European Medicines Agency, as well as approval by the FDA for individuals 12 years and older with transfusion-dependent β-thalassemia. This therapy uses CRISPR/Cas9-mediated gene editing to yield increased production of HbF, followed by busulfan[1] conditioning and autologous transplantation of the edited stem cells. Hematopoietic stem cells are first mobilized and then edited ex vivo at the erythroid specific enhancer region of the *BCL11A* gene. This gene encodes a transcriptional repressor that regulates globin gene switching from γ globin to β globin in early infancy, thus leading to decreased HbF production and increased HbA production. An open-label, single-group phase 3 study was conducted in patients aged 12

---

[1] Not FDA approved for this indication.
[2] Not available in the United States.

---

[1] Not FDA approved for this indication.

to 35 years with transfusion-dependent β-thalassemia with $β_0/β_0$, $β_0/β_0$-like, or non-$β_0/β_0$ genotype. A prespecified interim analysis of 52 patients was conducted. Of the 35 evaluable patients, 32 achieved transfusion independence with a mean total hemoglobin level of 13.1 g/dL and a mean HbF level of 11.9 g/dL. Additional phase III studies are enrolling for patients with β-thalassemia, as well as a long-term phase IV study.

Pharmacologic Induction of Fetal Hemoglobin

Induction of HbF expression has been proposed as a therapeutic strategy. For β-thalassemia, induced γ globin gene expression would be predicted to decrease globin chain imbalance by complexing with free α chains. Hydroxyurea (Hydrea)[1] is an antimetabolite thought to interfere with DNA synthesis. It is well established in the management of sickle cell disease, where it has been shown to increase levels of HbF. The use of hydroxyurea in β-thalassemia is much less well established. In the United States, hydroxyurea has been approved for use in sickle cell disease but not for thalassemia. Studies published elsewhere in the world have generally shown improvements in hemoglobin levels in thalassemia intermedia patients, with some patients becoming transfusion independent. A 2017 metaanalysis on the use of hydroxyurea in patients with transfusion-dependent β-thalassemia concluded that this agent might offer some benefit but that double-blinded placebo-controlled studies are lacking.

5-Azacytidine (azacitidine [Vidaza])[1], an inhibitor of DNA methyltransferase, has been shown to induce HbF. However, concerns regarding long-term use have prevented further evaluation in thalassemia. Decitabine (Dacogen)[1], an analog of 5-azacytidine, has been shown to increase HbF levels in patients with sickle cell disease refractory to hydroxyurea. A small pilot study of low-dose decitabine in β-thalassemia intermedia patients demonstrated an increase in total hemoglobin and hemoglobin F levels. Butyrate[5], an inhibitor of histone deacetylases, is another agent capable of inducing HbF. However, butyrate and its derivatives (arginine butyrate[5], sodium isobutyramide[5], and sodium phenylbutyrate [Buphenyl][1]) have failed to show significant clinical benefit in thalassemia patients. Therefore no agent has been approved for use in thalassemia patients at this time.

IMR-687 (tovinontrine)[5], a small molecule inhibitor of phosphodiesterase 9, increases intracellular cGMP levels and leads to reactivation of HbF. An interim analysis of a randomized, double-blind, placebo-controlled phase IIb study of this agent in adults with β-thalassemia (transfusion-dependent and non–transfusion-dependent cohorts) reported no meaningful benefits in either transfusion burden or hemoglobin, and the sponsor has discontinued further development of this agent for β-thalassemia.

Novel Agents Targeting Ineffective Erythropoiesis

An alternative strategy that is being investigated involves the targeting of ineffective erythropoiesis. Luspatercept-aamt (Reblozyl) and sotatercept (ACE-011)[5] are activin receptor trap ligands that were developed to treat postmenopausal osteoporosis but were noted to increase Hb levels. Initial phase II studies with these agents in thalassemia patients revealed reductions in transfusion burden, increase in Hb, and reduction in liver iron levels. A phase III study comparing luspatercept plus best supportive care to placebo plus best supportive care revealed that 21.4% of patients receiving luspatercept achieved a reduction in transfusion burden compared with 4.5% in the placebo group. Luspatercept (initial dose 1 mg/kg SQ every 3 weeks; maximum dose 1.25 mg/kg SQ every 3 weeks) is approved by the FDA for the treatment of anemia in adult patients with β-thalassemia who require regular RBC transfusions.

Janus kinase 2 (JAK2) plays a key role in erythropoiesis, and there is interest in the potential use of JAK2 inhibitors in thalassemia. A phase II study with ruxolitinib (Jakafi)[1] showed a reduction in spleen size. However, there was no clinically relevant improvement in pretransfusion hemoglobin, and subsequent phase III studies are not planned.

The pyruvate kinase activator AG-348 (mitapivat [Pyrukynd])[1] increased ATP levels, reduced markers of ineffective erythropoiesis, and improved anemia in mouse models of β-thalassemia. Results from a phase II study of mitapivat recorded an increase in hemoglobin in patients with non–transfusion-dependent thalassemia. A randomized, placebo-controlled phase III study in patients with non–transfusion dependent thalassemia demonstrated significant improvement in hemoglobin response (42% in the mitapivat group vs. 2% in the placebo group), and this agent is being considered for FDA approval for this indication.

Antioxidants

Oxidative damage is believed to be an important cause of tissue damage, and there has been interest in the use of antioxidants in thalassemia patients. A variety of substances have been investigated, including ascorbate[1], vitamin E[1], N-acetylcysteine (Mucomyst)[1], flavonoids, and indicaxanthin[5]. A variety of antioxidant effects have been observed in vitro with these agents, but none has been shown to improve anemia in patients with thalassemia.

β-Thalassemia Intermedia

Given the underlying genetic heterogeneity, it is not surprising that the clinical manifestations of β-thalassemia intermedia are also quite varied. Some patients with more mild forms of β-thalassemia intermedia do not require long-term transfusion therapy. There is no clear consensus about when long-term transfusion should be initiated. Factors that are considered for children include growth patterns, spleen size, and bone development. Transfusion may be necessary during infection-induced aplastic crises. In some instances, transfusions are begun in childhood to help with growth and then discontinued after puberty. Some adults gradually become more anemic and eventually require transfusion. Some authors have argued that starting transfusions early in life is advantageous because the prevalence of alloimmunization appears to increase if transfusion is started after the first few years of life.

Splenomegaly usually develops in all patients, including those who do not require transfusion. With progression of splenomegaly and the accompanying sequestration and hemolysis, there is usually worsening of anemia to the point at which transfusions may be required. Most patients achieve transfusion independence after splenectomy. Gallstones may develop, and a prophylactic cholecystectomy is sometimes performed at the same time as the splenectomy. As with β-thalassemia major patients, thalassemia intermedia patients are at increased risk for infection and should be appropriately vaccinated.

For reasons that are not entirely clear, there is an increased risk of thromboembolic complications in thalassemia intermedia patients compared with thalassemia major patients. An Italian study reported that 10% of thalassemia intermedia and 4% of thalassemia major patients experienced a thromboembolic event. Another study reported that thromboembolism occurred four times more frequently in patients with intermedia versus major disease. This report noted that venous events were more common in the thalassemia intermedia population, whereas arterial events were more common in the thalassemia major population. An even higher rate of venous thrombotic events (29%) was reported in a population of splenectomized patients with thalassemia intermedia. It has been suggested that exposed anionic phospholipids on the surface of damaged RBCs may induce a procoagulant effect. There is no consensus regarding the prophylactic use of antiplatelet agents or anticoagulants in this population.

Patients with thalassemia intermedia may develop iron overload, although it is less severe than in patients with thalassemia major. Even those who are not regularly transfused may develop

[1] Not FDA approved for this indication.
[5] Investigational drug in the United States.
[1] Not FDA approved for this indication.

[5] Investigational drug in the United States.

a degree of iron overload as a result of increased iron absorption. Iron overload may be managed with the iron chelating agents described earlier. Cardiac toxicity, including congestive heart failure, valvular problems, and pulmonary hypertension (leading to secondary right-sided heart failure) resulting from iron overload is not infrequent in the thalassemia intermedia population.

Bone abnormalities and osteoporosis may develop in thalassemia intermedia patients. In a North American study, the prevalence of fractures in these patients was 12%. Leg ulcers involving the medial malleolus are common and are often difficult to treat. Hypogonadism, hypothyroidism, and diabetes may occur, with frequency related to the severity of anemia and iron overload. Pseudoxanthoma elasticum, a syndrome consisting of skin lesions, angioid streaks in the retina, calcified retinal walls, and aortic valve disease, is more common in thalassemia intermedia than in thalassemia major. Currently, no effective therapy exists, although it has been reported that aluminum hydroxide (Alternagel)[1] reduces skin calcification.

β-Thalassemia Minor

Most patients with β-thalassemia minor are asymptomatic. However, they have an abnormal complete blood cell count that may sometimes lead to the misdiagnosis of iron deficiency. Although these patients have a microcytic anemia, it is much less severe than in patients with β-thalassemia major. In general, the hematocrit is >30%. The mean corpuscular volume is typically <75 fL, and the RBC distribution width index is normal, in contrast with iron deficiency in which the degree of microcytosis is less and the distribution width index is usually increased. The peripheral blood smear shows the presence of target cells. Hemoglobin electrophoresis typically reveals an increase in HbA2. The normal anemia experienced during pregnancy may sometimes be exacerbated in patients with β-thalassemia minor, necessitating transfusion. Otherwise, no long-term effects of β-thalassemia minor have been described, and no interventions are required.

α-Thalassemia

Laboratory and Clinical Features

Patients with α-thalassemia trait 2 are symptom free and have normal laboratory values, including complete blood count, peripheral smear, and hemoglobin electrophoresis. Individuals with α-thalassemia trait 1 are symptom free, and the disease resembles β-thalassemia minor. The peripheral smear shows a hypochromic microcytic anemia with the presence of target cells. Hemoglobin electrophoresis is normal.

HbH disease does produce symptoms. Unlike β-thalassemia major, in which HbF production protects the fetus, individuals with HbH disease develop hemolytic anemia during gestation and are symptomatic at birth. This is because α globin production is required for HbF ($\alpha_2\gamma_2$). As with β-thalassemia major, patients with HbH disease suffer from the consequences of chronic hemolytic anemia, although the severity is somewhat less. The transfusion requirements for HbH patients resemble those for patients with β-thalassemia intermedia, with transfusion support initiated in the second and third decades of life. These patients also develop iron overload, necessitating treatment with chelation therapy.

Hydrops fetalis with HbBart is usually fatal in utero. The utter lack of α globin chain production results in absence of HbF. HbBart, a homotetramer consisting of four γ globin genes, is unable to deliver oxygen to tissues. Severe tissue hypoxia develops, leading to widespread tissue ischemia. High cardiac output failure leads to massive edema (hydrops). In most cases, death occurs in the third trimester or late second trimester. There have been reports of live births after intrauterine transfusion, but survival beyond the perinatal period is exceedingly rare. Prenatal diagnosis of HbBart hydrops fetalis may be achieved through DNA-based testing using amniocytes from amniocentesis or chorionic villi sampling.

Noninvasive testing is under development, including methods that isolate circulating fetal DNA in maternal peripheral blood.

Management

Patients with α-thalassemia 1 and 2 traits do not require treatment. The management of HbH disease is similar to that described for β-thalassemia.

References

Algiraigri A, Wright N, Paolucci EO, et al: Hydroxyurea for lifelong transfusion-dependent β-thalassemia: a meta-analysis, *Pediatr Hematol Oncol* 34(8):435–448, 2017.

Arab-Zozani M, Kheyrandish S, Rastgar A, et al: A systematic review and meta-analysis of stature growth complications in β-thalassemia major patients, *Ann Glob Health* 87(1):48, 2021, 1–17.

Bhardawj A, Swe KM, Sinha NK: Treatment for osteoporosis in people with β-thalassaemia, *Cochrane Database Syst Rev* 5(5), 2023.

Bou-Fakhredin R, Motto I, Cappellini MD: Advancing the care of β-thalassaemia patients with novel therapies, *Blood Transfus* 20(1):78–88, 2022.

Kattamis A, Kwiatkowski JL, Aydinok Y: Thalassaemia, *Lancet* 399(10343):2310–2324, 2022.

Langer AL, Esrick EB: β-Thalassemia: evolving treatment options beyond transfusion and iron chelation, *Hematology Am Soc Hematol Educ Program* 2021(1):600–606, 2021.

Porter JB, Garbowski MW: Interaction of transfusion and iron chelation in thalassemias, *Hematol Oncol Clin North Am* 32(2):247–259, 2018.

Sharma A, Jagannath VA, Puri L: Hematopoietic stem cell transplantation for people with β-thalassaemia major, *Cochrane Database Syst Rev* 4(4), 2021.

THROMBOTIC THROMBOCYTOPENIC PURPURA

Method of
Ravi Sarode, MD

CURRENT DIAGNOSIS

- A provisional diagnosis based on unexplained microangiopathic hemolytic anemia and thrombocytopenia in the absence of oliguric renal failure is sufficient to initiate emergent plasma exchange (PLEX) for a suspected diagnosis of autoimmune acquired thrombotic thrombocytopenic purpura (TTP).
- The final diagnosis is usually established by the documentation of a severe deficiency (<10% activity) of ADAMTS13 (*a disintegrin and metalloproteinase with thrombospondin 1 motif, 13th member of the family*).
- These laboratory tests are recommended for patient evaluation:
  - Complete blood count (shows anemia and decreased platelet count, usually <30,000/uL)
  - Peripheral blood smear (shows "schistocytes/fragmented red blood cells," a hallmark of thrombotic microangiopathy)
  - Reticulocyte count (elevated)
  - Haptoglobin (usually undetectable in TTP)
  - Lactate dehydrogenase (usually more than twice the upper limit of normal in TTP)
  - Blood urea nitrogen, serum creatinine (determine nonoliguric renal insufficiency, serum creatinine < 2.5 mg/dL)
  - Liver function tests, including direct and indirect bilirubin
  - Troponin (many patients have an ischemic cardiac injury)
  - Plasma ADAMTS13 activity (<10% is diagnostic of TTP) and inhibitor level (usually detected in 90% of cases of acquired TTP) or ADAMTS 13 antibodies by enzyme-linked immunosorbent assays (almost all acquired TTP)
  - Prothrombin time, partial thromboplastin time, fibrinogen, and D-dimers (to rule out disseminated intravascular coagulopathy)
  - Direct antiglobulin test (to rule out autoimmune hemolytic anemia)
  - Urinalysis

---

[1] Not FDA approved for this indication.

CURRENT THERAPY

- The goal is to normalize ADAMTS 13 levels (>50%).
- Daily plasma exchange (PLEX) uses plasma as a replacement fluid (1.0–1.5 total body plasma volume) until the platelet count is greater than 150,000/μL for 2 days. Thereafter, the frequency of PLEX may be guided more judiciously if ADAMTS13 levels are obtained once or twice a week during hospitalization.
- Caplacizumab (Cablivi, 11 mg intravenous loading dose followed by daily 11 mg subcutaneously), a potent disease modifying agent, is a nanobody that interferes with the binding of von Willebrand factor to the GPIb domain on platelets and disrupts the pathophysiology of the disease; thus, it may prevent deaths and reduce the number of PLEXs needed. It is given daily until ADAMTS13 levels are greater than 10% to 20%.
- Prednisone 1 mg/kg/day is tapered gradually as platelet count remains greater than 150,000/uL.
- Rituximab (Rituxan)[1] (either 100 mg fixed dose or 375 mg/m^2 weekly for 4 weeks) is given upfront as soon as the diagnosis of autoimmune thrombotic thrombocytopenic purpura (TTP) is confirmed (reduces length of stay, number of PLEXs, and exacerbations and relapses, and thus overall cost).
- Plasma (10–15 mL/kg) or cryoprecipitate (one dose = 10 units of pooled cryoprecipitate) infusion is used if PLEX will be delayed more than 6 hours on day 1.
- ADAMTS13 testing is done during follow-up to detect early biologic relapse and preemptive rituximab to avoid clinical relapse and hospitalization.
- For exacerbation or relapsing of TTP, the following therapies are used:
  - Rituximab (Rituxan)[1] (100 mg fixed dose or 375 mg/m^2 once a week for 2 to 4 weeks).
  - Cyclosporine (Neoral)[1] (2–3 mg/kg/day up to 6 months).
  - Vincristine (Oncovin)[1] (1.4 mg/m^2 once a week for 4 weeks).
  - Bortezomib (Velcade)[1] (1.3 mg/m^2 one to two cycles or 1 mg fixed dose once a week for 4 weeks).
  - Splenectomy as a last resort.

[1]Not FDA approved for this indication.

Thrombotic thrombocytopenic purpura (TTP) is a rare (1 to 2 cases per million) but life-threatening thrombotic microangiopathy (TMA) disorder characterized by the presence of microthrombi in the microcirculation of various organs, including the brain, kidneys, heart, and abdominal viscera. Microthrombi consist of platelets and von Willebrand factor (vWF), resulting in microangiopathic hemolytic anemia (MAHA) and thrombocytopenia. MAHA refers to the fragmentation of red blood cells (schistocytes) during their passage through partially occluded arterioles and capillaries by microthrombi. TTP diagnosis requires a high degree of suspicion because a delay in initiating plasma exchange (PLEX), the current standard of care, could result in a poor response or fatal outcome. In the past, diagnosis of TTP was made based on a pentad that included MAHA, thrombocytopenia, neurologic involvement, renal affection, and fever. This pentad was found in patients who had died of TTP, indicating advanced disease; therefore one should not wait for the development of a pentad, which could delay TTP diagnosis and lead to a potentially fatal outcome. Currently, unexplained MAHA and thrombocytopenia in the absence of oliguric renal failure are sufficient to make a working diagnosis of TTP and initiate emergent PLEX. Patients may present with only severe thrombocytopenia and/or with warm autoimmune hemolytic anemia and be managed as nonresponding immune thrombocytopenia/Evans syndrome. However, after a few days, such patients may develop MAHA, establishing a TTP diagnosis. Therefore such patients not responding to standard therapy should have high suspicion of TTP. Similarly, but rarely, a young patient may present with unexplained ischemic stroke without hematologic features and later develop hematologic features.

Pathophysiology

In congenital TTP (Upshaw-Shulman syndrome), ultralarge (UL) multimers of vWF were detected during remission but were absent during relapse. Later, an ADAMTS13 (a disintegrin and metalloproteinase with thrombospondin 1 motif, 13th member of the family), vWF-cleaving protease was identified that was responsible for cleaving UL multimers secreted from endothelium into normal-sized vWF multimers seen in normal plasma. This cleavage occurs under high-shear-rate flow conditions in smaller blood vessels where the UL-vWF undergoes unfolding, exposing the cleavage site for ADAMTS13. ADAMTS13 is severely deficient (<10%) in patients with both congenital and acquired (autoimmune) TTP. Persistence of UL-vWF multimers in the microcirculation results in unfolding of the molecule, enabling it to bind to platelets at GPIb, thus producing platelet-vWF microthrombi in capillaries and arterioles that cause end organ ischemic damage (Figure 1). Elevated lactate dehydrogenase (LDH) reflects not only MAHA but also organ damage; hence very high LDH reflects more severe disease.

Classification

TTP can be divided into (1) a congenital form resulting from a genetic defect in the *ADAMTS13* gene and (2) an acquired form due to an autoantibody against the ADAMTS13 enzyme (Figure 2). Congenital TTP can present in the neonatal period, early childhood, or later in life, when it is usually associated with an inciting trigger in the form of pregnancy, severe infection, surgery, or other stress. Acquired TTP is usually idiopathic without an underlying disorder or secondary when associated with an underlying autoimmune disorder, such as systemic lupus erythematosus, HIV, or use of ticlopidine (Ticlid).[2] Other clinical conditions that present with MAHA and thrombocytopenia with nonsevere ADAMTS13 deficiency are grouped under the broader term TMA.

Clinical Presentation

Autoimmune TTP is a disease of young adults (20–50 years of age, female-to-male ratio 2:1), with the majority being African American. Most patients present in the emergency department with an acute onset of vague, anemia-like symptoms (malaise, fatigue, weakness) and thrombocytopenia (petechiae, bleeding gums). Detailed evaluation reveals that these symptoms had their onset several days before presentation. Up to 70% to 80% of patients have some neurologic features, including severe headaches, visual disturbances, focal neurologic deficits, transient ischemic attacks, memory deficits, unusual behavior, confusion, seizures, paraparesis, stupor, and coma. Mild renal insufficiency is seen in less than 50% and fever in less than 15%. Because of the generalized nature of the disease, any organ system can be affected, and ischemic insult to the heart is common.

Diagnosis

Unexplained MAHA and thrombocytopenia constitute the diagnostic features and are associated with elevated LDH, reticulocytosis, undetectable haptoglobin, elevated bilirubin, and nonoliguric renal insufficiency in some patients. A severe deficiency of ADAMTS13 (<10% activity with a detectable inhibitor in up to 90% of patients and antibodies by enzyme-linked immunosorbent assays in almost all) confirms the diagnosis. Because this test is usually sent to a reference laboratory, this level is unavailable in most hospitals at the time of clinical diagnosis. Therefore based on the initial clinical and laboratory features, PLEX should be initiated emergently because a delay can increase not only morbidity but also mortality. A sample for ADAMTS13 must be drawn before initiating PLEX or plasma/cryoprecipitate infusion to avoid measuring enzyme from transfused products. ADAMTS13 is a stable enzyme; if a sample for ADAMTS13 could not be drawn before plasma therapy, a routine coagulation test sample may be used. In congenital TTP, a persistent severe deficiency of ADAMTS13 (without an inhibitor) is associated with

[2]Not available in the United States.

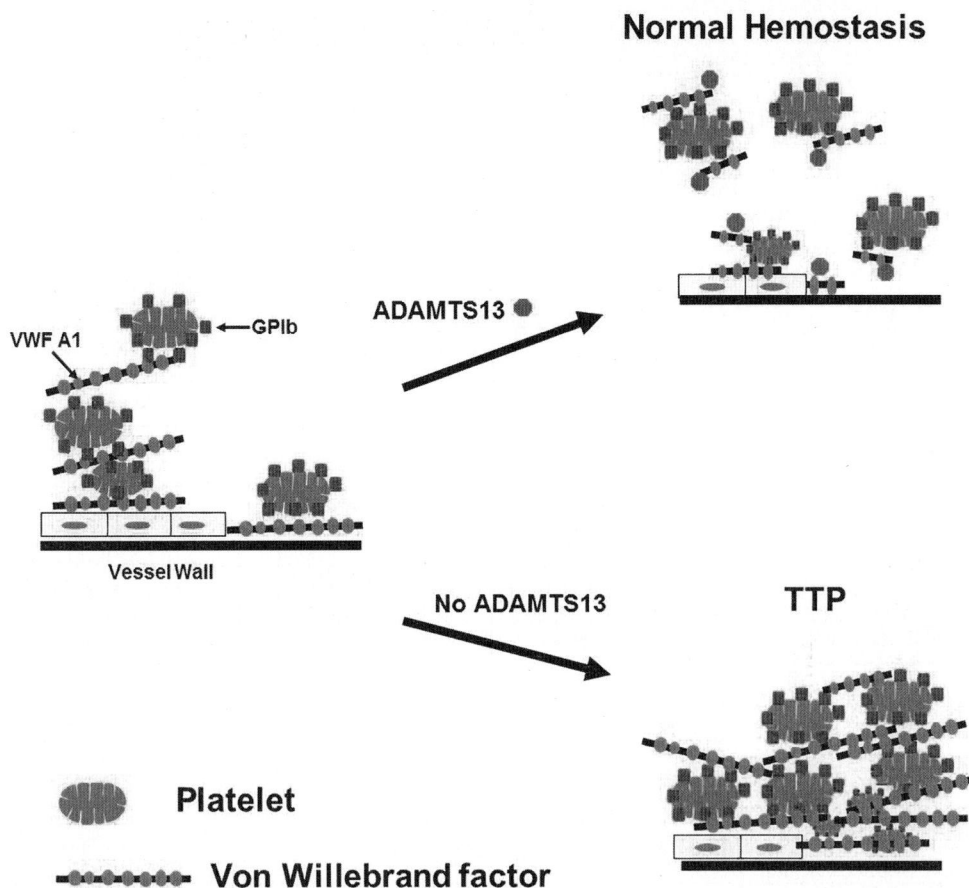

Normal Hemostasis

VWF A1 ←GPIb

ADAMTS13 ●

No ADAMTS13   **TTP**

Vessel Wall

● **Platelet**

●●●●●●● **Von Willebrand factor**

Figure 1 During normal hemostasis, *ADAMTS13* enzyme cleaves ultralarge multimers of von Willebrand factor (vWF) in normal sizes and prevents the formation of platelet-vWF aggregates under high shear rates. However, in the absence of *ADAMTS13* (a disintegrin and metalloproteinase with thrombospondin 1 motif, 13th member of the family) due to congenital deficiency or autoantibodies, vWF persist as ultralarge multimers that unfold under high shear rates in small blood vessels and induce vWF-platelet microthrombi in various organs, causing ischemic damage.

ADAMTS13 gene defect. However, this diagnosis is sometimes made difficult because many patients, especially children and young adults, are often misdiagnosed as having immune thrombocytopenia or anemia of unknown origin or the hemolysis elevated liver enzymes and low platelets (HELLP) syndrome in pregnancy.

Differential Diagnosis

The differential diagnosis of TTP includes clinical conditions that present with MAHA and thrombocytopenia but without severe ADAMTS13 deficiency (i.e., TMA). These conditions include hematopoietic stem cell transplantation, drug toxicities (e.g., mitomycin, clopidogrel [Plavix], cyclosporine A [Neoral]), malignant hypertension (usually mild to moderate thrombocytopenia), HELLP syndrome with severe preeclampsia, mechanical cardiac devices (e.g., left ventricular assist devices, intraaortic balloon pumps, mechanical heart valves), disseminated intravascular coagulation, vasculitis, and both diarrhea-associated and atypical hemolytic uremic syndrome.

Treatment

PLEX is the standard of care therapy. Its use has reduced mortality from more than 90% to less than 20%. Ideally it should be initiated within 4 to 6 hours of suspected diagnosis. The patient's plasma (which contains autoantibody) is selectively removed during PLEX (1.0–1.5 plasma volume processed) and replaced with donor plasma containing ADAMTS13. Neurologic symptoms usually disappear within 24 to 48 hours. The platelet count is the most useful laboratory parameter in the assessment of initial response. Complete clinical response, defined as normalization of platelet count for at least 2 days with near normal LDH, is generally achieved in most patients with seven to nine daily PLEXs. Thereafter, a gradual taper—that is, PLEX every other day in the first week, twice in the next week, and once in the third

week—may be performed. However, the number of PLEXs can be guided by frequent ADAMTS13 measurements to avoid unnecessary PLEXs and reduce exposure to hundreds of plasma donors, thus reducing the risk of transmitting known and unknown pathogens. Another option is to use pathogen-inactivated plasma, such as Octaplas (Octapharma Plasma Centers), which is approved by the U.S. Food and Drug Administration (FDA) for the treatment of TTP. Given the autoimmune nature of the disease, glucocorticoid therapy is often given from the beginning. Approximately 30% to 50% of patients will have an exacerbation of the disease (worsening of clinical or laboratory features after initial response) or relapses (recurrence of the disease 30 days after discontinuation of PLEX). Such patients require additional PLEXs and other immunomodulatory therapies (e.g., rituximab [Rituxan],[1] cyclosporine [Neoral],[1] vincristine [Oncovin],[1] bortezomib [Velcade],[1] or splenectomy as a last resort). Early rituximab use, within the first week, has recently been shown to reduce number of PLEXs, length of stay, and exacerbation/relapse. Preliminary data also suggest that a lower dosage of rituximab (100 mg weekly for 4 weeks) elicits a similar clinical response as a higher dosage (375 mg/m^2 weekly for 4 weeks). However, the former offers the benefits of reduced cost, lower infusion time, and fewer side effects. A dialysis-type catheter is required for PLEX and can be placed with ultrasound guidance in patients with platelet counts as low as 5000/µL. With the exception of a life-threatening bleed, platelet transfusion is contraindicated in TTP because it is a thrombotic disorder of platelet consumption and transfused platelets may worsen the condition (with the appearance of new neurologic symptoms, myocardial infarction, etc.). Most fatalities occur during the first few days of diagnosis, probably because of the

---

[1] Not FDA approved for this indication.

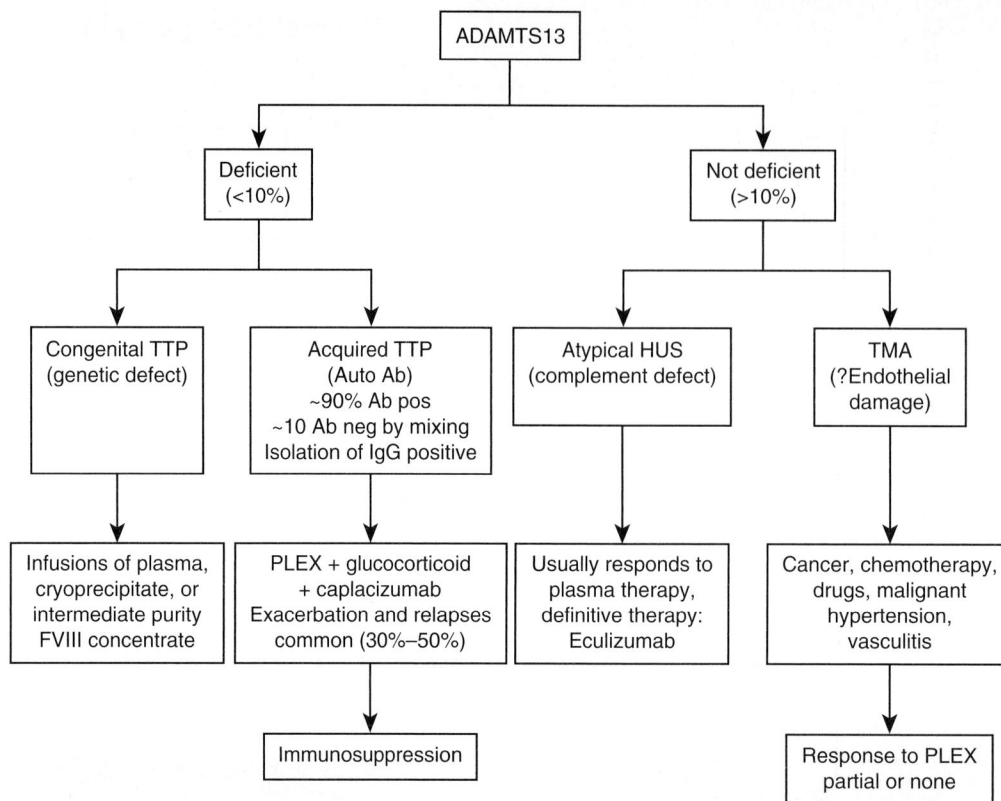

Figure 2 Classification of TTP. *Ab*, Antibody; *ADAMTS13*, a disintegrin and metalloproteinase with thrombospondin motif 1, 13th member of the family; *HUS*, hemolytic uremic syndrome; *MAHA*, microangiopathic hemolytic anemia; *PLEX*, plasma exchange; *TMA*, thrombotic microangiopathy; *TTP*, thrombotic thrombocytopenic purpura.

severity of the disease or delay in the initiation of PLEX. If initiation of PLEX is likely to be delayed, either plasma or cryoprecipitate can be infused temporarily to supplement ADAMTS13.

Caplacizumab (Cablivi), a nanobody that binds to the A1 domain of vWF and blocks its interaction with GPIb/IX/V receptors on platelets, was FDA approved for the treatment of TTP. This is a very potent disease-modifying agent; therefore it should be used in all cases of TTP. A randomized clinical trial showed that caplacizumab given once as an intravenous (IV) bolus (of 11 mg) followed by daily subcutaneous injections (of 11 mg) up to 30 days post-PLEX led to normalization of the platelet count slightly faster and reduced the numbers of PLEXs, disease exacerbations, and possibly deaths but also led to more relapses compared with placebo. It seems that the use of caplacizumab can definitely benefit severe and refractory TTP and may be tailored based on frequent ADAMTS13 testing during the treatment course. Once ADAMTS13 levels are greater than 10% to 20%, caplacizumab should be discontinued to prevent a bleeding tendency due to development of a severe acquired von Willebrand syndrome. Congenital TTP is treated with plasma infusions (10–15 mL/kg); however, cryoprecipitate and intermediate purity Factor VIII concentrate that contain adequate ADAMTS13 have been used successfully to avoid volume overload in susceptible patients. In congenital TTP, a recombinant ADAMTS13 has recently been shown to produce very promising results in a phase I clinical trial.

Monitoring

Considering the relatively high frequency of cardiac involvement, cardiac monitoring should be performed initially. Although PLEX is an otherwise safe procedure, complications related to catheter infection and line thrombosis are not uncommon and should be identified as soon as possible to avoid exacerbation of the disease. Exacerbation of TTP is often related to an infection. There is increasing awareness of delayed long-term psychological and psychosocial effects in up to 50% patients; these are probably related to silent cerebral infarct often documented on imaging in these patients. Therefore a careful follow-up is recommended to identify and manage these issues. Because of recent awareness of silent cerebral infarcts in many patients, use of caplacizumab in all cases seems prudent.

Prognosis

Although PLEX has reduced TTP mortality in the last two decades, most deaths occur within 24 to 48 hours of presentation and are due to delay in the administration of PLEX for a variety of reasons, including a delay in diagnosis or line placement or nonavailability of PLEX at the institution. After one PLEX, survival rates can increase to greater than 90%. Importantly, no clinical or laboratory parameter exists to predict outcome or relapse. Frequent ADAMTS13 monitoring is now used during follow-up to detect early biologic relapse (decrease in activity <30%–50%); preemptive rituximab[1] has been used to prevent overt hematologic and clinical relapse and avoid hospitalization.

References

Fujimura Y, Matsumoto M, Isonishi A, et al: Natural history of Upshaw-Schulman syndrome based on ADAMTS13 gene analysis in Japan, *J Thromb Haemost* 9(Suppl 1):283–301, 2011.

Peyvandi F, Rock GA, Shumak KH, Buskard NA, et al: Comparison of plasma exchange with plasma infusion in the treatment of thrombotic thrombocytopenic purpura. Canadian Apheresis Study Group, *N Engl J Med* 325:393–397, 1991.

Sarode R, Bandarenko N, Brecher ME, et al: Thrombotic thrombocytopenic purpura: 2012 American Society for Apheresis (ASFA) consensus conference on classification, diagnosis, management, and future research, *J Clin Apher*, https://doi.org/10.1002/jca.21302.

Sarode R. Thrombotic thrombocytopenic purpura in caplacizumab era – An individualized approach. *Transfs Apher Sci*, https://doi.org/10.1016/j.transci.2023.103682

Shah N, Rutherford C, Matevosyan K, et al: Role of ADAMTS13 in the management of thrombotic microangiopathies including thrombotic thrombocytopenic purpura (TTP), *Br J Haematol* 163:514–519, 2013.

Tsai HM: Thrombotic thrombocytopenic purpura and atypical hemolytic uremic syndrome—An update, *Hematol Oncol Clin North Am* 27:565–584, 2013.

---

[1] Not FDA approved for this indication.

DRY EYE SYNDROME

Method of
Lauren J. Jeang, MD

CURRENT DIAGNOSIS

- Dry eye disease can manifest as a multitude of symptoms, including dryness, burning, irritation, foreign body sensation, and fluctuating vision.
- Patients of older age are more commonly affected.
- Patients can have a combination of contributing factors that culminate in reduced aqueous tear production and increased tear evaporation.
- Environmental causes include fans, air conditioning, low humidity, and electronic screen use.
- Ocular risk factors include contact lens use, blepharitis, and eyelid malposition.
- Systemic diseases such as Sjögren syndrome, thyroid eye disease, graft-versus-host disease, and mucous membrane pemphigoid should be considered in the differential diagnosis, especially if there are other suggestive signs or symptoms.
- Slit-lamp examination and ocular surface staining provide the most helpful clinical findings. Corneal esthesiometry, Schirmer tests, and tear composition assays are useful as adjunct testing.

CURRENT THERAPY

- Patients should be educated on the chronic nature of dry eye disease.
- Treatment depends on the contributing factors and severity of disease. Multiple simultaneous therapies may be required.
- For mild and moderate disease, initial treatment includes environmental modification and artificial tear lubrication.
- If artificial tears are required more than four times a day, preservative-free artificial tears are recommended to avoid ocular surface irritation from preservatives.
- Other treatment options include prescription anti-inflammatory topical medication, punctal plugs, oral medications, autologous serum tears, and scleral contact lenses. Management of blepharitis should also be considered.
- Cases of eyelid malposition or dysfunction may require surgical intervention.
- Extreme disease can lead to sight- or eye-threatening complications and require more aggressive treatment.

Epidemiology

Dry eye syndrome is a multifactorial disease with a wide range of findings including eye discomfort, burning, irritation, blurry vision, altered tear film, and ocular surface damage. The prevalence of dry eye is unclear because of the broad disease definition and lack of universal diagnostic criteria. It is estimated that 20 million people in the United States suffer from dry eye. Signs and symptoms of dry eye increase by every decade of age. Among older age groups, higher rates of dry eye have been reported in women than in men. Additional terms associated with dry eye include dry eye disease, dry eye syndrome, dysfunctional tear syndrome, and keratoconjunctivitis sicca.

Risk Factors

Multiple risk factors have been associated with dry eye disease. Demographic risk factors include older age (>65 years), female sex, and Asian race. Ocular risk factors include blepharitis, meibomian gland dysfunction, ocular rosacea, contact lens wear, and eyelid malposition such as entropion and ectropion. Systemic diseases strongly associated with dry eye include vitamin A deficiency, mixed connective tissue disorders, Sjogrens disease, androgen deficiency, and hematopoietic stem cell transplantation. Thyroid orbitopathy increases ocular exposure and tear evaporation, while Parkinson disease decreases blink rate. A wide range of medications including antihistamines, antidepressants, anxiolytics, and isotretinoin can induce eye dryness. Environmental risk factors such as prolonged electronic screen time, low humidity, and fan use can increase tear evaporation from the ocular surface.

Blepharitis and meibomian gland dysfunction are often diagnosed in conjunction with dry eye disease. Blepharitis is a chronic inflammation of the eyelid margins, including the eyelashes and meibomian glands. Meibomian gland dysfunction, which is considered a subcategory of blepharitis, is defined by duct obstruction/atrophy or altered glandular secretions. Both blepharitis and meibomian gland disease can cause eye irritation, inflammatory tear film state, and ocular surface changes.

Pathophysiology

Healthy tears are important in maintaining a lubricated ocular surface. The precorneal tear film is classically described as having an inner mucin layer, middle aqueous layer, and outer lipid layer. More recent studies suggest that the tear film may be a complex gel substance containing soluble mucus, water, electrolytes, proteins, and lipids. Mucus from goblet cells protects and hydrates the eye through formation of a glycocalyx on the surface epithelium. Aqueous fluid, protein, and electrolytes are produced by the lacrimal gland. The outer lipid layer is secreted by meibomian glands and prevents rapid tear evaporation of the aqueous layer to the air.

Adequate tear production, maintenance, and clearance is the responsibility of the lacrimal functional unit, which includes the lacrimal glands, cornea, conjunctiva, meibomian glands, eyelids, and their associated sensory and motor nerves. Cranial nerve V1 sensory input from the ocular surface stimulates eyelid blinking, which allows for even distribution of tears across the eye surface and directs excess tears down through the eyelid punctum. Blinking also allows for expression of lipid material into the tear film from the meibomian glands.

Dry eye disease is the result of any condition that affects a component of the tear film or the lacrimal functional unit.

Lacrimal gland secretion inhibition may be caused by lacrimal duct obstruction in sclerosing diseases such as mucous membrane pemphigoid, graft-versus-host disease, ocular burns, or by inflammation of the ductal and acinar epithelial cells in Sjögren syndrome. Systemic medications can reduce tear secretion. Corneal hypoesthesia caused by previous herpes simplex or herpes zoster keratitis, prior laser-assisted in-situ keratomileusis (LASIK) surgery, small incision lenticule extraction (SMILE) surgery, or trigeminal nerve damage can lead to decreased tear production and decreased blinking. Poor eyelid movement from Parkinson disease, Bell's palsy, or increased ocular surface exposure from thyroid eye disease and electronic screen use prevent formation of an even and adequate tear film. Blepharitis and meibomian gland dysfunction prevent adequate meibum secretion and increase inflammatory factors on the ocular surface.

The combination of poor aqueous secretion by the lacrimal gland and increased tear evaporation leads to tear film hyperosmolality, which in turn triggers an inflammatory cascade in the junction between ocular surface epithelial cells. This in turn leads to a loss of epithelial and goblet cells and T-cell recruitment. The resulting loss of corneal epithelium and unstable tear film then propagates this cycle.

Clinical Manifestations

Dry eye can be classified as mild, moderate, or severe. Patients with mild dry eye may have a multitude of complaints including dryness, discomfort, irritation, burning, foreign body sensation, and fluctuating or blurry vision. Vision may improve with blinking or with use of lubricating drops. Worsening vision may be reported with prolonged screen use, upon awakening, or toward the evening. Moderate disease manifests as increasing symptoms and more persistent visual changes. Severe dry eye, especially when caused by an underlying inflammatory condition, may cause sight- or eye-threatening problems such as corneal scarring, thinning, sterile or infectious ulcers, and perforation.

Diagnosis

The diagnosis of dry eye is made clinically. A gross external examination may reveal proptosis, excessive eyelid laxity, trichiasis, entropion, or ectropion. Patients may demonstrate incomplete blinking or lagophthalmos. The skin may demonstrate changes consistent with blepharitis and rosacea, including rhinophyma, erythema, and telangiectasias. Eyelid changes consistent with blepharitis include debris at the eyelash bases, lid margin telangiectasias, and poor meibum flow from the meibomian glands. Slit lamp examination with the aid of fluorescein staining may show evidence of poor tear production and distribution. A drop of saline applied to a fluorescein strip, or a drop of premade 1% or 2% solution is placed on the lower tarsal conjunctiva. Using the cobalt blue filter on the slit lamp, fluorescein may highlight a low tear lake over the lower eyelid (normal is 1 mm), irregular or rapid breakup of the tear film (normal is 10 seconds), and punctate changes representing epithelial cell loss over the cornea. Lissamine Green is another type of stain used to reflect areas of mucin or glycocalyx loss on the conjunctiva. The pattern of staining may suggest the underlying cause. Corneal hypoesthesia is evaluated before the use of any eyedrops. Sensation is evaluated by using a cotton-tip applicator with the fibers twisted to a point or using a Cochet-Bonnet aesthesiometer device.

Schirmer's testing is useful in assessing decreased aqueous tear production. The test can be performed with or without topical anesthesia. A thin strip of filter paper is placed along the lateral one-third of the lower eyelid. The amount of aqueous absorbed after 5 minutes is measured. If topical anesthesia is not used, a value less than 10 mm is considered abnormal. However, there is no established cutoff, and results are poorly reproducible. Therefore the use of Schirmer's testing as a sole diagnostic test is not recommended.

Multiple tear composition assays are available that examine different markers of dry eye including elevated tear osmolality, decreased lactoferrin and lysozyme, and increased matrix metalloproteinase-9 (MMP-9). However, there are conflicting studies on whether or not these markers strongly correlate with symptoms and other examination findings. There is some suggestion that multiple measurements over time may be more useful. Additionally, imaging devices are available to assess the ocular surface. These include devices that can image the meibum glands (meibography) and/or evaluate the tear film. These imaging devices are a relatively new concept and have yet to be widely adopted.

Additionally, the workup should include a careful review of medications and systemic symptoms. Patients with severe or intractable dry eye should raise questions of concurrent dry mouth, arthritis, or history of inflammatory or autoimmune disease. These patients may benefit from evaluation for Sjögren syndrome or another autoimmune condition. Similarly, patients with significant proptosis and lagophthalmos should be examined for possible thyroid disease.

Differential Diagnosis

The differential diagnosis for dry eye disease can be broad because of overlapping signs and symptoms with other ocular diseases. Burning and irritation may be caused by blepharitis or meibomian gland dysfunction without dry eye. Patients presenting with severe dry eye may have another underlying ocular condition such as a thermal or chemical ocular burn, Stevens-Johnson syndrome, graft-versus-host disease, or mucous membrane pemphigoid.

Additional history may elucidate other conditions in the differential diagnoses. Patients with ocular irritation after initiating eye drops may be suffering from topical drug toxicity. Redness, itching, and mucoid discharge can be suggestive of allergic or viral conjunctivitis. Foreign body sensation or eye pain in the setting of recent ocular trauma may be due to a corneal abrasion. Infectious corneal ulceration should also be considered if there is redness, tearing, or decreased vision in a patient with prior ocular trauma or poor contact lens hygiene.

Therapy

Treatment of dry eye disease begins with addressing the underlying cause and educating patients on the nature of this disease. Potential environmental factors should be eliminated first. Air conditioners, heaters, and fans should be avoided or diverted away from the eyes. Patients should be reminded to take short breaks every 20 minutes or consciously blink during prolonged digital screen use. Moisture chamber goggles and humidifiers may help improve periocular humidity. Discontinuation of an offending systemic drug should be considered if medically appropriate.

Basic treatment includes the use of eye lubricants to enhance aqueous volume. Over-the-counter artificial tears dosed two to six times a day is often the first treatment modality. If patients need lubricants more than four times a day, preservative-free artificial tears are recommended over non–preservative-free products. Artificial tear ointments are also available over the counter and are best used at nighttime to avoid blurred vision. Introductory blepharitis management includes warm compresses over the eyelids to soften meibomian gland secretions and eyelid scrubs twice a day to loosen adherent eyelash debris.

Medications can be added in cases of moderate or severe disease. Topical anti-inflammatory medications include cyclosporine (0.05% [Restasis], 0.09% [Cequa], and 0.1% [Vevye]) and lifitegrast 5% (Xiidra) which are dosed BID. Patients should be educated on the side effects of these medications, which include burning and, in the case of lifitegrast, a bitter taste. Topical steroids such as prednisolone, fluorometholone, and loteprednol (Eysuvis) dosed QD to QID are useful in inflammatory dry eye, but should be limited to a few weeks as they can elevate intraocular pressure and promote cataract formation. The FDA recently approved perfluorohexyloctane [Miebo], a water-free lipophilic liquid dosed 4 times/day for treatment of signs and symptoms of dry eye disease.

Topical erythromycin or bacitracin ointment applied to the eyelids multiple times a day or at bedtime for a few weeks has been used for treatment of blepharitis. For patients with suspected *Demodex* blepharitis, tea tree oil[7] in the form of a scrub or a wipe may improve symptoms. Alternatively, lotilaner 0.25% ophthalmic solution [Xdemvy] can be applied topically twice a day to decrease parasitic load. The most common side effect includes stinging with medication application. A novel intranasal formulation of 0.03 mg varenicline (Tyrvaya) was recently introduced as an alternative to topical treatments. This medication, dosed twice a day, increases tear film production through activation of the nasolacrimal reflex. The most common side effects include sneezing and coughing. Additional studies will be required to examine the long-term effects. Oral medications such as doxycycline[1] (20 to 100 mg QOD to BID), minocycline[1] (50 mg QD to BID) and azithromycin[1] (500 mg per day for 3 days in three cycles with 7-day intervals) can been used for their anti-inflammatory properties. Clinicians should keep in mind that tetracyclines are contraindicated in children younger than 8 years of age and in pregnant and nursing patients. Side effects include photosensitivity, gastrointestinal upset, and vaginitis. Azithromycin may cause arrythmias. Initiation of omega-3 and omega-6 supplementation[7] has been suggested to enhance tear film quality, although more studies are required to confirm their efficacy. Patients with Sjögren syndrome or other autoimmune disorders may need more aggressive management of their underlying disorder through oral steroids or disease-modifying antirheumatic drugs (DMARDs).

Punctal occlusion is another option to improve tear volume on the ocular surface once ocular surface inflammation has been controlled. Occlusion can be achieved with dissolvable polymer plugs or more durable silicone plugs. Polymer plugs are positioned deep into the canaliculus to allow for patient comfort, but they require replacement every few months. Silicone plugs are placed over the punctum opening. These are advantageous in that they can last years and be removed at any time. However, if incorrectly sized, they can self-extrude or cause ocular irritation. The largest-diameter plug should be used to avoid dislocation. Permanent punctum occlusion by thermal cautery is reserved for patients who show consistent improvement with plugs or those with severe disease. The biggest side effect of punctal occlusion is epiphora. Therefore it is highly recommended to perform a trial with silicone plugs before performing cautery because of the irreversibility of the procedure.

Various in-office procedures that warm and express the meibomian glands are available. Many involve devices that apply localized heat and massage to the eyelids. Other options include intense pulsed light (IPL) followed by manual gland expression, direct intraductal probing, and microblepharoexfoliation. These procedures can be costly, and data on long-term success are limited. Additional studies are required to confirm their efficacy.

Severe disease states may need "third-tier" treatments. Patients with Sjögren syndrome–associated dry eye disease may benefit from oral secretagogues. Although neither are approved by the U.S. Food and Drug Administration (FDA) for the treatment of dry eye, studies suggest that pilocarpine (Salagen)[1] dosed at 10 to 30 mg a day or cevimeline (Evoxac)[1] may improve symptoms, although perhaps not tear production. Side effects include excessive salivation and sweating.

Another option is autologous serum drops, which are thought to contain anti-inflammatory mediators. They have shown the most benefit in patients with Sjögren syndrome, graft-versus-host-disease, and other dry eye–related ocular surface conditions. Serum drawn from the patient is diluted to various concentrations and is dosed anywhere from four to eight times a day. The need for repeated blood draws, medication refrigeration, and out-of-pocket cost to patients are the biggest drawbacks. This treatment is not formally FDA approved, and more studies are necessary to confirm their general utility.

Scleral contact lenses have been shown to help in refractory or severe cases of dry eye. Scleral lenses are rigid and vaulted over the globe to create a chamber of fluid. This technology protects the corneal surface from eyelid trauma and exposure while constantly hydrating the eye. These lenses require consultation with a specialty-trained optometrist.

Patients with poor eyelid positioning caused by entropion and ectropion may require surgical repair. Patients with severe corneal exposure from poor eyelid closure may need eyelid reconstruction, upper-lid weight placement, tarsorrhaphy (placement of a suture through the eyelids to promote eye closure), or placement of retained amniotic membranes.

Dry eye treatment continues to evolve. There are many promising medications and devices in the pipeline that may expand options for patients in the future.

Monitoring

Patient follow-up depends on the severity of disease and the treatments initiated. Severe disease may require weeks or months of follow-up visits. Patients should be monitored for medication side effects.

Complications

Complications are usually limited to cases of severe dry eye. Persistent corneal epithelial defects may form and cause significant decreased vision. Such compromised corneal epithelium places the eyes at risk for microbial keratitis. Additionally, corneal stromal thinning can occur as a result of prolonged dehydration and uncontrolled inflammation. In some cases, thinning progresses and may result in corneal perforation. Both sterile and infectious keratitis may lead to loss of vision or loss of the eye itself. Therefore urgent ophthalmology referral is warranted in these cases to initiate aggressive dry eye treatment, frequent topical antibiotics, placement of corneal glue, and/or surgical rehabilitation.

References

Amescua G, Ahmad S, Cheung AY, et al: American Academy of Ophthalmology Preferred Practice Pattern Cornea/External Disease Panel. Dry eye syndrome preferred practice pattern, *Ophthalmology* 131(4):P1–P49, 2024.

Amescua G, Akpek EK, Farid M, Garcia-Ferrer FJ, Lin A, Rhee MK, Varu DM, Musch DC, Dunn SP, Mah FS: American Academy of Ophthalmology Preferred Practice Pattern Cornea and External Disease Panel. Blepharitis Preferred Practice Pattern®. *Ophthalmology*. 126(1):P56–P93, 2019.

Craig JP, Nelson JD, Azar DT, Belmonte C, Bron AJ, Chauhan SK, de Paiva CS, Gomes JAP, Hammitt KM, Jones L, Nichols JJ, Nichols KK, Novack GD, Stapleton FJ, Willcox MDP, Wolffsohn JS, Sullivan DA: TFOS DEWS II Report Executive Summary, *Ocul Surf* 15(4):802–812, 2017.

Foulks GN, Forstot SL, Donshik PC, Forstot JZ, Goldstein MH, Lemp MA, Nelson JD, Nichols KK, Pflugfelder SC, Tanzer JM, Asbell P, Hammitt K, Jacobs DS: Clinical guidelines for management of dry eye associated with Sjögren disease, *Ocul Surf* 13(2):118–132, 2015.

Jones L, Downie LE, Korb D, Benitez-Del-Castillo JM, et al: TFOS DEWS II Management and Therapy Report, *Ocul Surf* 15(3):575–628, 2017.

Pflugfelder SC, Stern ME: Biological functions of tear film, *Exp Eye Res* 197:108115, 2020.

GLAUCOMA

Method of
Albert P. Lin, MD; and Kristin Schmid Biggerstaff, MD

CURRENT DIAGNOSIS

Primary Open Angle Glaucoma
- Primary open angle glaucoma is an irreversible optic neuropathy typically associated with elevated intraocular pressure.

---

[1]Not FDA approved for this indication.
[7]Available as dietary supplement.

- Primary open angle glaucoma is the most common form of glaucoma, affecting more than 68 million people worldwide. There are more than 36 million Asians with the condition, accounting for over 50% of all those affected. The disease has the highest prevalence in Africans, affecting more than 4% of the population, while prevalence in other ethnicities ranges from 1% to 2%. It is more common in older adults: 1 to 2% in 50-year-olds compared with 6% to 12% in 80-year-olds.
- Primary open angle glaucoma is diagnosed by a complete ophthalmic examination, including dilated stereoscopic optic nerve examination and formal visual field.
- Untreated primary open angle glaucoma can lead to slow irreversible loss of vision and blindness. Other common causes of slow and progressive vision loss in older adults include cataracts, macular degeneration, and diabetic retinopathy.

Acute Angle Closure Glaucoma

- Pupillary block in susceptible patients leads to block of aqueous drainage and sudden and extreme rise of intraocular pressure. Acute angle closure can damage the optic nerve, resulting in acute angle closure glaucoma.
- About 0.6% of the global population, or 70 million people, are at risk for acute angle closure. It is more common in Inuits and Asians and rare in African Americans. The risk of acute angle closure increases with age. It is also more common in hyperopes.
- Patients can present with blurry vision, red eye, pain, headache, nausea, or vomiting. Acute angle closure is sometimes misdiagnosed as migraines or gastrointestinal illnesses. Patients with conjunctivitis, keratitis, uveitis, and corneal abrasion can also present with the same symptoms.
- Peripheral iridotomy prevents acute angle closure in susceptible patients. High intraocular pressure can result in irreversible damage of the optic nerve within hours, making acute angle closure one of the true ophthalmic emergencies.

CURRENT THERAPY

Primary Open Angle Glaucoma
- Topical eye drops, including β-blockers, selective α_2 agonists, carbonic anhydrase inhibitors, prostaglandin analogues, and rho kinase inhibitors, can be used to reduce intraocular pressure.
- Oral carbonic anhydrase inhibitors are typically used in recalcitrant cases until surgery can be performed.
- Laser trabeculoplasty may be used as first-line or adjunct therapy.
- Glaucoma surgery, including trabeculectomy, tube shunt, and cyclodestruction, may be performed if goal intraocular pressure cannot be reached with medical therapy or in nonadherent patients.

Acute Angle Glaucoma
- All glaucoma eye drops are used to reduce intraocular pressure.
- Oral and intravenous medications are added sequentially to reduce intraocular pressure as needed.
- Laser iridotomy can be performed as prophylactic treatment or acutely to break the pupillary block if the patient is unresponsive to medical intervention.
- Emergency glaucoma incisional surgery is performed if the patient is unresponsive to all other treatments.

Glaucoma is an optic neuropathy with characteristic optic nerve head appearance: narrowing of the neuroretinal rim. The optic nerve is a collection of more than 1 million axons from the retinal ganglion cells. The anterior 1-mm portion of the optic nerve within the globe is referred to as the *optic disk* or simply the disk.

When the disk is examined with direct or indirect ophthalmoscopy, a cup, or a physiologic empty space, is observed centrally. The remainder of the disk, which has a yellow-orange appearance, contains the axons and is referred to as the *neuroretinal rim*. The area of the cup compared to the entire disk is the cup-to-disk ratio, which is normally less than 0.4 (Figure 1A). When patients develop glaucoma, axons are lost from the neuroretinal rim and the size of the cup increases in relation to the disk. Narrowing of the neuroretinal rim and increased cup-to-disk ratio are the hallmarks of glaucomatous optic neuropathy (see Figure 1B).

Glaucoma can result in significant and irreversible loss of vision and is one of the leading causes of blindness in the world. Early in the disease state, glaucoma is asymptomatic; it is sometimes called "the sneak thief of sight." As the disease progresses, the patient develops decreased peripheral vision and eventually loss of the central vision.

Glaucoma is typically associated with increased intraocular pressure (IOP), but it is possible to have normal-tension or low-tension glaucoma. Glaucoma treatment is focused on the reduction of IOP to prevent or slow optic nerve damage and preserve visual function.

Glaucoma is classified in many ways, and it is most useful to approach it clinically based on the status of the angle, the area between the cornea and iris where aqueous humor exits the globe through the trabecular network. We further discuss primary open angle glaucoma, the most common form of glaucoma, and the management of acute angle closure, one of the true ophthalmic emergencies.

Primary Open Angle Glaucoma

Glaucoma is one of the leading causes of blindness in older adults, especially in patients of African descent. Vision loss from glaucoma is irreversible, and the treatment goal is to reduce IOP, slow disease progression, and preserve visual function during the patient's lifetime. Glaucoma is a slowly progressive disease, and progression to blindness often takes more than 10 years, even in untreated patients. Given its slow progression and the fact that central vision loss occurs in late disease, most patients do well with early diagnosis and treatment. Treatment is more difficult in late disease because the rate of disease progression and visual deterioration is accelerated, sometimes despite good control of IOP.

Due to the early asymptomatic nature of the disease, the patient's adherence to and persistence with treatment is often less than optimal. Studies have shown patients who obtain glaucoma information from physicians in addition to their ophthalmologists have a higher rate of medication adherence. Ophthalmologists have the options to use treatment modalities such as laser and surgery to obtain pressure control and decrease or eliminate the need for medication use.

The American Academy of Ophthalmology recommends asymptomatic patients older than 40 years be referred for ophthalmic evaluation once every several years for early detection of glaucoma and other chronic eye diseases. However, the US Preventive Services Task Force found insufficient evidence to recommend for or against screening for glaucoma in adults. Risks, benefits, and cost effectiveness of screening are beyond the scope of this chapter, but symptomatic patients or patients at high risk for glaucoma (African descent and family history) might benefit from ophthalmology consultation. It is possible to diagnose glaucoma by direct ophthalmoscopy, but this is not a substitute for binocular assessment of the disk through dilated pupils and formal visual field testing. If glaucoma is suspected or diagnosed, primary care visits should include inquiries regarding glaucoma medication use, medication side effects, and the time of last eye examination. Primary care physicians can improve glaucoma outcome by promoting adherence to medication and follow-up. Glaucoma patients need to follow up with their ophthalmologists at least biannually, and in severe cases every 3 months, for intraocular pressure checks.

Treatment
Topical Glaucoma Medications
Topical glaucoma medications are administered once or twice daily. Patients should look up, pull down their lower eye lid, drop the medication on the inferior conjunctival cul-de-sac, and keep their eyes

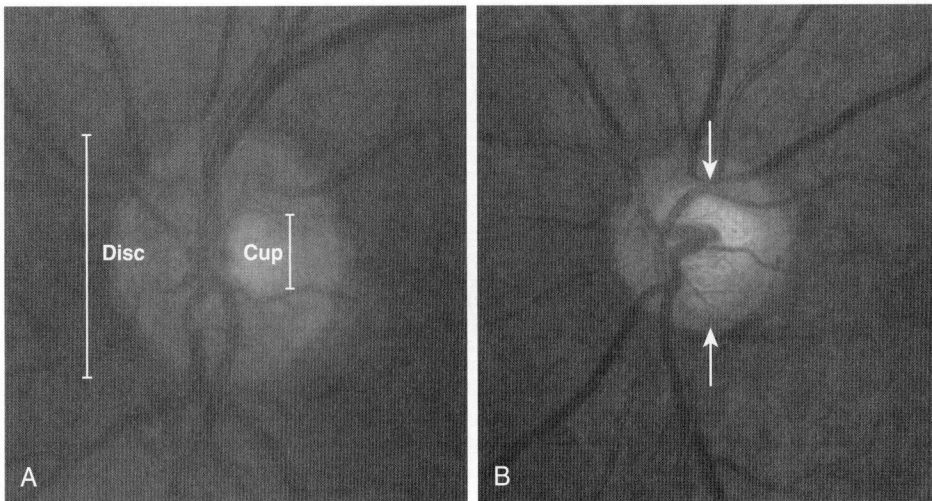

Figure 1 Disk appearance. (A) Normal disk. Cup-to-disk ratio is less than 0.4. (B) Glaucoma. Increased cup-to-disk ratio and narrow neuroretinal rim superiorly and inferiorly (arrows).

closed for at least 1 min. Applying gentle pressure next to the bridge of the nose to occlude the puncta can improve absorption of the medication. Medication bottle caps are color-coded by their class, and patients can usually identify their eye drops by color. Glaucoma medications are not subject to first-pass effect through the liver and can sometimes have significant systemic side effects, especially the β-blockers. Topical glaucoma medications are described later and summarized in Table 1.

Prostaglandin Analogues. Latanoprost (Xalatan), travoprost (Travatan), and bimatoprost (Lumigan) are prostaglandin analogues and are color-coded by teal caps. They are administered once at bedtime but may be administered once at any time during the day to promote adherence. They decrease IOP by increasing uveoscleral outflow. Latanoprostene bunod (Vyzulta) is converted into latanoprost and nitric oxide inside the eye and decreases IOP by promoting aqueous outflow through both the uveoscleral and trabecular meshwork pathways. It is considered a prostaglandin analogue with an additional mechanism of action. Side effects are primarily local and include increased conjunctival hyperemia, increased lash growth, and possible irreversible increase in periocular and iris pigmentation.

β-Blockers. Timolol (Betimol, Istalol, Timoptic), levobunolol (Betagan), and betaxolol (Betoptic) are color-coded by yellow caps. They are administered once or twice daily and decrease IOP by decreasing aqueous production. Side effects include bradycardia, exacerbation of chronic obstructive pulmonary disease (COPD) and asthma, impotence, and decreased serum high-density lipoprotein (HDL) cholesterol. Physicians need to be aware that a topical β-blocker is a potential cause of acute changes in cardiovascular or pulmonary status. There are several reported incidents of death following the use of topical β-blockers mostly due to exacerbation of asthma.

Selective α₂ Agonists. Brimonidine (Alphagan) and is a selective α₂ receptor agonist. It decreases IOP by decreasing aqueous production. Allergic conjunctivitis has been reported in up to 10% of patients. Rarely, it causes dry mouth and chronic fatigue and drowsiness in the elderly.

Carbonic Anhydrase Inhibitors. Dorzolamide (Trusopt) and brinzolamide (Azopt) are color-coded by orange caps and are sulfa-based medications. They are administered twice daily and decrease IOP by decreasing aqueous production. This class of medication has minimal systemic side effects. However, some patients complain about transient stinging and a bitter taste in the mouth after administration. These side effects, if tolerable, are not indications for discontinuing therapy.

Rho Kinase Inhibitors. Netarsudil (Rhopressa) affects actin and myosin contraction and decreases IOP by increasing aqueous outflow through the trabecular meshwork. It is color coded white and administered once daily. Conjunctival hyperemia is reported in up to 50% of the patients. Ophthalmologists have also observed pinpoint conjunctival hemorrhages and corneal verticillata (lipid deposits on the corneal epithelium) because these observations are asymptomatic and generally not reported by the patients. Compared to other medications, rho kinase inhibitor has a unique mechanism of action and is considered to be an excellent adjunct medication to lower IOP when other medications are already in use.

Combined Topical Medications. Timolol and dorzolamide (Cosopt) and timolol and brimonidine (Combigan) are color-coded by blue caps. Brimonidine and brinzolamide (Simbrinza) are color-coded by a light green cap. Netarsudil and latanoprost (Rocklatan) are color-coded by white caps. Combined medications decrease exposure to preservatives and can decrease irritation and problems with dry eyes. Adherence might also be improved.

Oral Carbonic Anhydrase Inhibitors

Oral carbonic anhydrase inhibitors include acetazolamide (Diamox), 250 mg or 500 mg given twice daily, and methazolamide (Neptazane), 25 mg or 50 mg given twice daily. They are sulfa-based medications and decrease IOP by decreasing aqueous production. Oral carbonic anhydrase inhibitors are not commonly used today because effective topical medications are available. They are typically used on a short-term basis to achieve IOP control in acute or refractory cases. Side effects can include aplastic anemia, kidney stones, bitter taste, indigestion, paresthesia of the extremities, tinnitus, and polyuria. Clinicians need to consider the possibility of hypokalemia when patients take other diuretics to control blood pressure (Table 2). Acetazolamide may also be given intravenously.

Laser Trabeculoplasty

Argon or selective laser trabeculoplasty can be used to increase aqueous outflow. Laser trabeculoplasty is noninvasive and safe, and it can be performed in the office in less than 10 minutes. Compared to surgery, IOP reduction is limited, up to 25% as primary treatment, but less as an adjunct modality. It is ineffective or less effective in some patients with light trabecular meshwork pigmentation. The effect of laser decreases over time but may be repeated in the case of selective laser trabeculoplasty.

Surgery

The most commonly performed traditional glaucoma surgeries (TGS) are trabeculectomy, tube shunt, and cyclodestruction. Trabeculectomy and tube shunt are procedures that create an opening in the sclera to increase aqueous outflow. Cyclodestruction destroys the ciliary body and decreases aqueous production. Angle surgeries, such as Trabectome, canaloplasty, iStent, Kahook dual blade, Hydrus, and trabecolotmy (GATT, Trab 360, OMNI) augment the outflow through the eye's existing outflow pathway. There are fewer potential complications with these minimally invasive glaucoma surgeries (MIGS), but they also do not lower the pressure as much as TGS.

TABLE 1 Topical Glaucoma Medications: Carbonic Anhydrase Inhibitors

CLASS	β-BLOCKER	SELECTIVE α₂ AGONIST	CARBONIC ANHYDRASE INHIBITOR	PROSTAGLANDIN ANALOGUE	RHO KINASE INHIBITOR	COMBINATION
Medication	Timolol (Timoptic) Betaxolol (Betoptic) Levobunolol (Betagan)	Brimonidine (Alphagan)	Dorzolamide (Trusopt) Brinzolamide (Azopt)	Latanoprost (Xalatan) Travoprost (Travatan) Bimatoprost (Lumigan) Latanoprostene bunod (Vyzulta)	Netarsudil (Rhopressa)	Timolol/Dorzolamide (Cosopt) Timolol/Brimonidine (Combigan) Brimonidine/Brinzolamide (Simbrinza) Netarsudil/latanoprost (Rocklatan)
Dosing	qd or bid	bid	bid	qhs	qd	bid or qd (Rocklatan)
Cap color	Yellow	Purple	Orange	Teal	White	Blue (Cosopt, Combigan), light green (Simbrinza), white (Rocklatan)
Side effects	Bradycardia, COPD, and asthma exacerbation	Allergic conjunctivitis, dry mouth, and fatigue in elderly	Stinging and bitter taste	Hyperemia, lash growth, and increased pigmentation	Hyperemia	See individual components

COPD, Chronic obstructive pulmonary disease.

TABLE 2 Oral and Intravenous Glaucoma Medications

	ACETAZOLAMIDE (DIAMOX)	METHAZOLAMIDE (NEPTAZANE)	MANNITOL (OSMITROL)	GLYCERIN 50%[1]
Class	CAI	CAI	Hyperosmotic	Hyperosmotic
Dosage	250 or 500 mg bid	25 mg or 50 mg bid	1 g/kg in 30 min	1 g/kg once
Route	PO or IV	PO	IV	PO
Side effects	Bitter taste, indigestion, paresthesia, tinnitus, polyuria, kidney stones, hypokalemia, aplastic anemia, and sulfa allergy		Polyuria, dehydration Exacerbate CHF and diabetes (glycerin)	

CAI, Carbonic anhydrase inhibitor; CHF, congestive heart failure
[1]Not FDA approved for this indication.

Visual Impairment and Blindness

Patients who are visually impaired (Snellen vision of <20/40) or legally blind (Snellen vision of <20/200 or visual field of <20 degrees) may have significantly decreased mobility and ability to function. Continued glaucoma treatment is still important in these patients because even maintenance of count-finger vision can allow the patients some degree of independence. Low-vision devices and services, including high-contrast video magnifiers, audiobooks, eccentric viewers, and mobility training, can allow patients maximal use of their residual vision and improve their confidence and quality of life.

Acute Angle Closure Glaucoma

Pupillary block in susceptible patients blocks aqueous drainage and leads to sudden and extreme rise of intraocular pressure. Acute angle closure can damage the optic nerve, resulting in acute angle closure glaucoma.

About 0.6% of people worldwide are at risk for acute angle closure. It is more common in Inuits and Asians and rare in African Americans. The risk of acute angle closure increases with age. It is also more common in hyperopes (farsightedness).

Mechanism of Acute Angle Closure: Pupillary Block

After aqueous is produced in the ciliary body in the posterior chamber, it travels through the pupil and exits the anterior chamber through the trabecular meshwork located between the iris and the cornea. Pupillary block occurs when the iris contacts the lens and obstructs the flow of aqueous through the pupil. Increased posterior chamber pressure displaces the iris anteriorly against the trabecular meshwork and stops aqueous outflow.

Patients at risk for acute angle closure have narrow occludable angles. These patients have smaller eyes, allowing the lens to contact the iris to initiate papillary block. The distance between the iris and the lens is the shortest when the pupil is mid-dilated. Therefore, patients who present with acute angle closure might have a history of dim light exposure (movies) or use of medications with anticholinergic properties (antihistamines, decongestants, antispasmodics). High IOP causes iris and corneal endothelial cell dysfunction, resulting in nonreactive pupil and hazy cornea, respectively. High IOP also results in inflammation and red eye, as well as severe pain, nausea, and vomiting (Figure 2). Elevated IOP can damage the optic nerve within hours, and acute angle closure needs to be treated on an emergent basis to prevent permanent loss of vision.

Diagnosis

Patients with acute angle closure can present with blurry vision, red eye, pain, headache, nausea, or vomiting. History can include hyperopia, onset after exposure to a dim environment, or taking anticholinergic medications. Examination findings include decreased vision, conjunctival hyperemia, mid-dilated, nonreactive pupil with or without an afferent papillary defect, and increased IOP (by palpation or tonometry). Acute angle closure is sometimes misdiagnosed as migraines or gastrointestinal illness. Patients with conjunctivitis, keratitis, uveitis, and corneal abrasion can also present with the same symptoms.

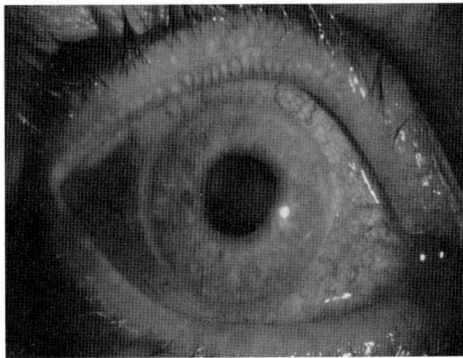

Figure 2 Acute angle closure patient with red eye and mid-dilated and nonreactive pupil.

Treatment

If acute angle closure is suspected, an emergent referral to ophthalmology is indicated. If an ophthalmologist is not immediately available, the goal will be to medically control the IOP as soon as possible. One drop of topical aqueous suppressant—β-blocker, selective α2 agonist, or carbonic anhydrase inhibitor—should be administered (timolol, brimonidine, and dorzolamide) (see Table 1). The maximum dose of oral or intravenous carbonic anhydrase inhibitor is given: acetazolamide 500 mg or methazolamide 50 mg (see Table 2). The patient is placed in the supine position to allow the lens and iris to fall posteriorly. The patient is reassessed in 30 minutes, and if the condition is not improved, topical drops are repeated. If there is no improvement after another 30 minutes, a hyperosmotic, oral glycerin[1] 1 g/kg or intravenous mannitol (Osmitrol) 1 g/kg over 30 minutes, is administered. Hyperosmotics may be contraindicated in patients with congestive heart failure, and glycerin can cause severe hyperglycemia in diabetic patients.

An ophthalmologist can break the pupillary block by medically lowering the IOP or by performing anterior chamber paracentesis, compression gonioscopy, laser peripheral iridotomy, and, in recalcitrant cases, emergent trabeculectomy. Once the pressure is controlled, it is important to perform an iridotomy in both eyes to prevent future episodes. Patients with patent iridotomies may safely take anticholinergic medications. Early cataract surgery has been shown to be effective in the treatment and prevention of acute angle closure glaucoma in older adults, either as an initial modality or in those who do not respond well to laser iridotomy.

References

Allingham RR, Damji KF, Freedman S, et al: *Shield's Textbook of Glaucoma*, ed 7, Philadelphia, 2020, Lippincott Walters Kluwer.

American Academy of Ophthalmology: Available at: Practice guidelines. Preferred practice patterns. Primary angle-closure disease. November 2020. http://www.aao.org/preferred-practice-pattern/primary-angle-closure-ppp. [Accessed April 30, 2023].

American Academy of Ophthalmology: Practice guidelines. Preferred practice patterns. Primary open-angle glaucoma, November 2020. Available at: http://www.aao.org/preferred-practice-pattern/primary-openangle-glaucoma-ppp [accessed April 30, 2023].

Azuara-Blanco A, Burr J, Ramsay C, et al: Effectiveness of early lens extraction for the treatment of primary angle-closure glaucoma (EAGLE): a randomised controlled trial, *Lancet* 388:1389–1397, 2016.

Lin AP, Orengo-Nania S, Braun UK: PCP's role in chronic open-angle glaucoma, *Geriatrics* 64:20–28, 2009.

Nordstrom BL, Friedman DS, Mozaffari E, et al: Persistence and adherence with topical glaucoma therapy, *Am J Ophthalmol* 140:598–606, 2005.

Schwartz GF, Quigley HA: Adherence and persistence with glaucoma therapy, *Surv Ophthalmol* 54:S57–S68, 2008.

Tham YC, Li X, Wong TY, et al: Global prevalence of glaucoma and projections of glaucoma burden through 2040, *Ophthalmology* 121(11):2081–2090, 2014.

US Preventive Services Task Force: Screening for glaucoma, Available at: http://www.uspreventiveservicestaskforce.org/uspstf/recommendation/primary-open-angle-glaucoma-screening; May, 2022. [accessed April 30, 2023].

Zhang N, Wang J, Chen B, et al: Prevalence of primary angle closure glaucoma in the last 20 years: a metaanalysis and systemic review, *Front Med (Lausanne)* 7:624179, 2021.

Zhang N, Wang J, Li Y, et al: Prevalence of primary open angle glaucoma in the last 20 years: a meta-analysis and sysetmic review, *Sci Rep* 2;11(1):13762, 2021.

[1]Not FDA approved for this indication.

MÉNIÈRE'S DISEASE

Method of
Terry D. Fife, MD; and Justin L. Hoskin, MD

CURRENT DIAGNOSIS

- Ménière's disease is characterized by recurrent attacks of severe vertigo, nausea, and vomiting typically lasting 1 to 6 hours.
- Ménière's disease causes tinnitus on the side of the affected ear; the tinnitus can change in pitch and loudness during attacks of vertigo.
- Attacks of vertigo are associated with reduced or muffled hearing on the affected side.
- Fluctuating unilateral hearing loss and low-frequency hearing loss on the side of the affected ear is characteristic.

CURRENT THERAPY

- Initial therapy includes a sodium-restricted diet (preferably <1500 mg of sodium daily) and a diuretic agent (e.g., thiazide diuretics).
- Betahistine,[1] a medication widely used in Europe that may be obtained at compounding pharmacies in the United States, may be helpful in selected patients at a dosage 16 to 48 mg three times daily though some authors have recommended even higher dosages.
- Transtympanic infusion of gentamicin[1] or corticosteroids and endolymphatic sac surgery may be considered as minimally invasive options in patients with serviceable hearing. Gentamicin poses a moderate risk of inducing hearing loss.
- Vestibular nerve sectioning is highly effective in stopping vertigo attacks with a reasonably low risk of causing further hearing loss in the short-term, but it is a more invasive procedure.
- Labyrinthectomy is highly effective in stopping vertigo attacks but causes complete hearing loss, so it is only an option for patients who have already lost all useful hearing.

Patients who have undergone procedures that cause acute loss of vestibular function often have vertigo for a while after the surgery; the vertigo improves more quickly with vestibular rehabilitative therapy.

[1]Not FDA approved for this indication.

Ménière's disease is a disorder of the inner ear that results in recurrent, spontaneous episodes of vertigo, hearing loss, ear fullness, and tinnitus affecting the same ear. The hearing loss often fluctuates early in Ménière's disease, but fluctuating hearing is not always present. Eventually permanent hearing loss occurs, affecting the low frequencies initially but ultimately affecting all frequencies.

Epidemiology

The reported prevalence of Ménière's disease varies from about 50 to 200 per 100,000. Females are somewhat more prone to Meniere's disease than males, with a female/male ratio of about 1.9:1.

Risk Factors

Possible risk factors for later development of Ménière's syndrome include autoimmune disorders, migraine, allergies, syphilitic otitis and viral infection of the inner ear, head trauma, and a family history of Ménière's disease. Despite the emergence of COVID-19, no correlation with Ménière's is evident with infection or following vaccination (Wachova, 2021).

Pathophysiology

The underlying mechanism is generally thought to be due to endolymphatic hydrops, a type of swelling of the endolymphatic compartment that ultimately leads to permanent damage of the inner ear structures. Possible reasons for this periodic swelling of the endolymph compartment include mechanical obstruction of endolymph flow or at least dysregulation of the electrochemical membrane potential between endolymph and perilymph compartments.

Endolymphatic hydrops appears to be the mechanism for a number of conditions that can lead to Ménière's syndrome. When no primary cause is identified, the idiopathic form of the syndrome is called Ménière's disease. When an underlying cause is found, it is referred to as Ménière's syndrome or secondary Ménière's or secondary endolymphatic hydrops. Secondary Ménière's syndrome can result from delayed endolymphatic hydrops in which symptoms come on years after a prior disorder or viral injury of the labyrinth, syphilitic otitis, autoimmune inner ear disease, and trauma.

Prevention

There is no known way of preventing the development of Ménière's disease because it occurs in many people with no risk factors.

Clinical Manifestations

Ménière's disease can manifest with periodic unilateral (or, less commonly, bilateral) hearing loss or isolated attacks of vertigo. Not uncommonly, Ménière's disease has both elements present at its onset, but the vertigo is usually the symptom that gets the most attention. Vertigo usually lasts 1 to 6 hours but can last as little as 30 minutes or as long as all day. Patients prone to motion sickness often report that their dizziness lasts longer because the aftereffect of vertigo lingers longer in those who are motion sensitive. Vertigo attacks in Ménière's disease are often quite severe and generally render patients unable to move around owing to the vertigo, nausea, and recurrent vomiting.

The hearing loss is usually unilateral, and patients might notice fluctuation in hearing accompanied by ear fullness and a low-pitched roaring tinnitus either before or coincident with the vertigo. If audiometry can be performed during this time, low-frequency (250–1000 Hz) hearing loss may be documented and might improve after the attack ceases. This signature fluctuating low-frequency sensorineural hearing loss is very helpful (Figure 1) when found, but getting patients with vertigo attacks in for testing while they are in the acute stage of vertigo is usually not feasible.

Occasionally, patients with Ménière's have sudden random drop attacks in which they abruptly fall without loss of consciousness. These spells, referred to as otolithic crises of Tumarkin, can lead to serious injury and should prompt aggressive treatment. The mechanism is presumed to be related to sudden mechanical deformation or sudden neural discharges related to the otolith structures of the inner ear. Because there is no specific treatment for Tumarkin crises, treatment entails the standard treatments for Ménière's disease in general.

As Ménière's disease progresses, usually over months to years, permanent low-frequency hearing loss develops that gives way to hearing loss at all frequencies. Eventually, the patient can lose all or most hearing on the affected side. Meanwhile, with each vertigo attack, some vestibular function is lost, and so as vertigo attacks continue, vestibular loss ensues, often paralleling the hearing loss. Ménière's occasionally burns out, meaning that enough vestibular function has been lost that acute hydrops no longer produces vertigo. Patients might report less severe dizziness or just a vague feeling of unsteadiness. This usually indicates advanced Ménière's, and unilateral hearing and vestibular loss should be expected.

Bilateral Ménière's disease is present at the time of initial diagnosis in about 10% of cases and by 10 years of symptoms, about 35% have bilateral involvement. Bilateral Ménière's disease has treatment implications because treating one side alone will be unlikely to stop the vertigo attacks, which could be emanating from the untreated side. Surgical treatment of both sides is also problematic because it could leave the patient with bilateral hearing loss, vestibular loss, or both.

Diagnosis

The diagnosis of Ménière's disease is made clinically based on unilateral hearing loss, tinnitus, ear fullness, and episodic vertigo typically lasting 1 to 6 hours. The criteria for definite, probable, and possible Ménière's disease are listed in Box 1. Recent studies using three-dimensional fluid-attenuated inversion recovery (3D-FLAIR) 24 hours after administration of bilateral intratympanic gadolinium (Gd) injection and similar techniques have demonstrated abnormalities consistent with endolymphatic hydrops. The use of MRI is improving and newer techniques are emerging, but so far MRI is not yet established as useful in affirming the diagnosis of Ménière's disease.

Differential Diagnosis

Vestibular neuritis causes a single attack of vertigo, sometimes with acute hearing loss (labyrinthitis), but it can usually be distinguished from Ménière's disease because vestibular neuritis has a lifetime recurrence rate of only 2%, whereas Ménière's vertigo attacks recur multiple times and cause fluctuating and gradual decline in hearing.

When a patient reports episodic vertigo attacks in the absence of unilateral tinnitus, ear fullness, and hearing loss, one must be cautious in diagnosing Ménière's disease because vestibular migraine (basilar-type migraine) can produce a similar pattern. Diagnostic criteria have been published for vestibular migraine.

Benign paroxysmal positional vertigo causes brief recurrent spells of spinning without hearing loss, so it is rarely confused with Ménière's disease.

Vertebrobasilar insufficiency can cause isolated vertigo, but the duration is usually only several minutes and without hearing loss, whereas Ménière's attacks last hours and are associated with unilateral auditory symptoms.

Acoustic neuroma (vestibular schwannoma) typically leads to slowly progressive unilateral sensorineural hearing loss, but vertigo is infrequently a prominent feature because patients compensate gradually as their vestibular function wanes due to compressive effects of the tumor.

Fluctuating unilateral hearing loss, ear fullness, and tinnitus can occur without vertigo and is referred to as cochlear hydrops. Such symptoms can precede the development of vertigo but may be treated as Ménière's nonetheless. Lermoyez's syndrome refers to transiently improved hearing and tinnitus during attacks of vertigo. More commonly, however, hearing declines around and during vertigo spells.

Treatment
Medical Management

Treatment of Ménière's disease is mainly aimed at preventing the vertigo attacks, but no treatments are known that reliably restore or arrest hearing loss or tinnitus. It is presumed that if attacks of vertigo, ear fullness, fluctuating hearing, and tinnitus are all stopped, hearing should stabilize, but this is still a supposition. The management of Ménière's is hierarchical, starting with a low-sodium diet and a diuretic and proceeding to more-invasive or destructive surgical procedures only when initial medical treatment fails. When a patient has very frequent vertigo attacks and is disabled, more-aggressive treatment may be considered sooner.

Dietary sodium should be restricted to 1000 to 1500 mg daily. The average person consumes about 4000 mg daily, and the maximum recommended daily intake of sodium is 2300 mg. Because more than 70% of the daily sodium

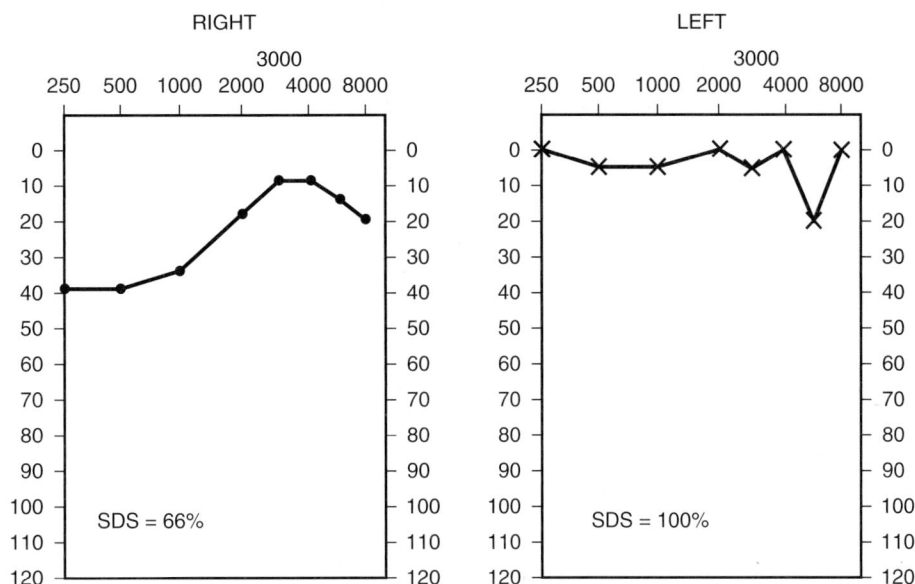

Figure 1 Audiogram showing typical low-frequency hearing trough of Ménière's disease affecting the right ear.

| BOX 1 | Diagnostic Criteria for Ménière's Disease |

Definite Ménière's Disease

1. Two or more spontaneous attacks of vertigo, each lasting 20 minutes to 12 hours
2. Audiometrically documented low- to mid-frequency SNHL in the affected ear on at least 1 occasion before, during, or after 1 of the episodes of vertigo
3. Fluctuating aural symptoms (hearing loss, tinnitus, or ear fullness) in the affected ear
4. Other causes excluded by other tests

Probable Ménière's Disease

1. At least 2 episodes of vertigo or dizziness lasting 20 minutes to 24 hours
2. Fluctuating aural symptoms (hearing loss, tinnitus, or fullness) in the affected ear
3. Other causes excluded by other tests

Basura GJ, Adams ME, Monfared A, et al: Clinical practice guideline: Ménière's disease, *Otolaryngol Head Neck Surg* 162:415–434, 2020.

---

comes from processed foods, this dietary restriction generally requires more than simply stopping the use of table salt, which generally accounts for only about 10% of daily sodium intake for most people.

A diuretic is usually added to the sodium restriction. The most commonly prescribed diuretic is hydrochlorothiazide 25 mg combined with triamterene 37.5 mg (Dyazide)[1] because this combination usually obviates the need for potassium supplementation. Acetazolamide (Diamox)[1] 125 to 250 mg bid or furosemide (Lasix)[1] 10 to 20 mg daily are also options. Patients with severe sulfa allergy can use low-dose ethacrynic acid (Edecrin)[1] 12.5 to 25 mg daily.

An acute attack of vertigo from Ménière's disease can be managed with vestibular suppressants such as dimenhydrinate (Dramamine)[1] 50 mg, meclizine (Antivert) 25 to 50 mg, diazepam (Valium)[1] 2 to 5 mg, or promethazine (Phenergen)[1] 12.5 to 50 mg. Scopolamine in patch form (Transderm-Scōp)[1] is too slow to be useful because it takes hours to be absorbed transdermally. Scopace (oral scopolamine) has been discontinued and is no longer being manufactured in the United States.

Scopolamine tablets[1] may be available in certain compounding pharmacies. Nausea can additionally be managed with prochlorperazine (Compazine) 10 mg orally or 25 mg by suppository, with oral or sublingual ondansetron (Zofran)[1] 4 to 8 mg, or with other antiemetics. Generally, the vertigo attacks subside in several hours even without treatment.

Betahistine hydrochloride or dihydrochloride[2] may also be helpful in Ménière's, although it is not commonly used in the United States. The role of betahistine is not firmly established, although it is widely prescribed for vertigo throughout the world. Betahistine may be helpful when successful medical management with diet and diuretics has helped but is inadequate to stop attacks. Betahistine is a vasodilator, a modest H_1 histamine agonist, and a powerful H_3 histamine receptor antagonist. Its method of action in Ménière's is unknown, though it may influence perfusion of the stria vascularis to reduce pressure in the endolymphatic space. Doses of betahistine may start at 8 mg PO three times daily and may be increased to 48 mg three times daily. It is available outside the United States in many trademarks throughout the world. Betahistine may be made within the United States at compounding pharmacies with a physician prescription[1] and may also be imported from outside the United States for personal use. This is often done using an encapsulated powder form of betahistine dihydrochloride USP (from manufacturers such as Fagron, Inc., St. Paul, MN USA) by weight in capsules with or without filler. Side effects are few, although occasionally patients report some gastrointestinal upset or mild headache. Betahistine is not histamine, and has not been found to cause or aggravate urticaria.

Oral corticosteroids are often used but rarely seem effective except in cases of bilateral Ménière's resulting from autoimmune inner ear disease (AIED). Oral corticosteroids rarely seem to be effective in typical Ménière's disease.

Ménière's attacks have been said to be triggered by caffeine, chocolate, stress, visual stimuli, and dropping barometric pressure. Such triggers should be avoided when possible, but strong associations with these triggers can also occur in migrainous vertigo. Vestibular rehabilitative therapy is not generally helpful in Ménière's because most vertigo attacks remit and the patients have few vestibular symptoms between attacks. However, when vestibular loss has occurred and the patient appears

---

[1]Not FDA approved for this indication.

[2]Not available in the United States.

TABLE 1	Procedures Used in the Management of Ménière's Disease		
METHOD	**TECHNIQUE**	**ADVANTAGES**	**DISADVANTAGES**
Procedures Intended to Spare Serviceable Hearing			
Intratympatic corticosteroids	Injection of steroid through the tympanic membrane to the middle ear to be absorbed in the inner ear	Minimally invasive, few side effects	Effectiveness unclear when compared to placebo
Intratympanic gentamicin (Garamycin)[1]	Injection of gentamicin through the tympanic membrane to the middle ear to be absorbed in the inner ear	Simple office-based procedure, low risk profile	Number of injections is unpredictable; some risk of hearing loss
Endolymphatic mastoid shunt	Placing a shunt from the endolymphatic sac to the mastoid air cells	Effective in 50%–75% of cases; low risk of hearing loss; day procedure	Vertigo can recur; effectiveness depends on surgical experience and technique
Vestibular neurectomy	Surgical sectioning of the vestibular part of cranial nerve VIII, sparing the auditory part of the nerve	Highly effective in eliminating vertigo attacks	Requires general anesthesia; risk of facial weakness, hearing loss
Procedures Expected to Eliminate Residual Hearing			
Labyrinthectomy or cochleosacculotomy	Several methods of removing all or part of the labyrinth	Highly effective in stopping vertigo attacks	Inevitable complete hearing loss

[1]Not FDA approved for this indication.

to have not compensated well for it, vestibular rehabilitation can be helpful.

Bilateral Ménière's Disease

The estimated incidence of bilateral Ménière's disease varies in the literature but is estimated to occur in about 15% of cases and bilateral involvement increases over time. The possibility of bilateral involvement weighs on the decision-making for any procedures that sacrifice hearing or vestibular function because it leaves the patient with only one functioning labyrinth.

Serviceability of Hearing

Serviceable hearing is residual hearing that can be useful to the patient by wearing hearing aids. In general, because hearing loss is permanent, one should avoid sacrificing any serviceable hearing.

Injections and Surgical Treatments

Patients who continue to have disabling vertigo despite a low-salt diet, diuretics, and possibly betahistine are considered to have failed conservative medical therapy. The next step in treatment depends on the age, health status, and residual hearing and vestibular function of the patient and also on the surgeon's opinion and experience with the various options. If spells are infrequent, symptomatic management of vertigo attacks may be the best option. Table 1 outlines some of the additional interventional options.

Intratympanic Gentamicin

Transtympanic gentamicin (Garamycin)[1] administration has become increasingly used as an effective treatment of Ménière's disease. This is partly due to the ease of administration of gentamicin and its relative safety. Gentamicin is a commonly used aminoglycoside antimicrobial agent with activity against gram-negative bacteria that also happens to be ototoxic. It damages hair cells of the labyrinth and preferentially affects hair cells of the vestibular neuroepithelium over that of the cochlea. Even so, transtympanic administration still has some risk of causing hearing loss. Gentamicin is administered by injecting a small amount (usually about 0.5 mL) of gentamicin sulfate (80 mg/2 mL) solution through the tympanic membrane into the middle ear space. To avoid rapid drainage through the

eustachian tube, the injection is done with the patient supine and kept in that position for an hour or so to allow the gentamicin to absorb through the round window into the inner ear. There are many protocols, but commonly an injection is given once, and additional injections can be considered every 3 to 4 weeks until improvement in vertigo attacks is realized. Studies remain mixed on the benefits of intratympanic gentamicin, with further randomized controlled trials needed.

Endolymphatic Sac Surgery

Another option for patients with residual functional hearing is endolymphatic sac shunt or decompression. This procedure eliminates vertigo in 50% to 75% of those treated. Nevertheless, its effectiveness compared with placebo has remained a point of contention based on a number of studies. It has been suggested that the procedure's effectiveness depends on the operative technique and experience of the surgeon.

Intratympanic Steroids

Sometimes, a trial of intratympanic corticosteroids may be offered (Basura, 2020), although its effectiveness in controlled trials is still not compelling. Even so, a trial of corticosteroids administered in this manner poses little risk.

Vestibular Neurectomy

The most definitive procedure for stopping vertigo attacks in Ménière's when the goal is to preserve hearing is vestibular neurectomy. This procedure involves craniotomy and severing the vestibular nerve while preserving the cochlear nerve. This procedure requires overnight hospitalization and general anesthesia, and it does pose some risk to facial nerve function and hearing on the affected side.

Labyrinthectomy

For patients who have unilateral Ménière's disease and no serviceable hearing, labyrinthectomy is a commonly used procedure. This procedure entails the removal of the membranous labyrinth and is highly effective in stopping recurrent vertigo attacks from that ear. In elderly patients or those who are poor surgical candidates, a more limited transtympanic cochleosacculotomy may be performed.

Meniett Treatment

The Meniett device is a portable, low-frequency, pressure-wave delivery system that administers a wave of pressure of about

[1]Not FDA approved for this indication.

12 cm H_2O to the middle ear via a tympanostomy tube for about 0.6 seconds pulsed at 6 Hz for 5 minutes about three to five times daily. Quality randomized trials demonstrating effectiveness of this treatment are lacking, and it is recommended by a recent evidence-based guideline that this treatment should NOT be prescribed (Basura, 2020).

Monitoring

Following patients with Ménière's disease should include monitoring of the frequency and severity of vertigo spells and the fluctuation in hearing, ear fullness, and tinnitus. Periodic audiometry is probably the most sensitive measure of stabilization of the condition. Vestibular testing may be considered when changes might alter the treatment strategy. Brain imaging is only helpful in excluding other disorders, but does not yet have an established role in the management of Ménière's disease.

Complications

Known complications include the progression of unilateral and occasionally bilateral hearing and vestibular function. There may also be complications associated with some of the treatments as described earlier. Owing to the unpredictability of the vertigo attacks, many patients avoid certain activities and might even develop agoraphobic features because the attacks are so severe and disruptive. In most cases, these avoidance behaviors improve if Ménière's disease can be controlled.

Conclusion

The management of Ménière's disease is still part art and part science. Treatment options are many, but patients should be reassured that, in most cases, something can be offered to help improve their vertigo and quality of life.

References

Basura GJ, Adams ME, Monfared A, et al: Clinical practice guideline: Ménière's disease, *Otolaryngol Head Neck Surg* 162:415–434, 2020.
Hoskin JL. Ménière's disease: new guidelines, subtypes, imaging, and more, *Curr Opin Neurol* 35:90–97, 2022.
Luca P, Ralli M, Cassandro C, et al: Surgical Management of intractable Meniere's disease. *Int Tinnitus J* 26(1):50–56, 2022.
Nevoux J, Franco-Vidal V, Bouccara D, et al: Diagnostic and therapeutic strategy in Ménière's disease. Guidelines of the French Otorhinolaryngology-Head and Neck Surgery Society (SFORL), *Eur Ann Otorhinolaryngol Head Neck Dis*, 134(6):441–444, 2017.
Rizk HG, Mehta NK; Qureshi U. et al. Pathogenesis and etiology of Meniere's disease: a scoping review of a century of evidence. *JAMA Otolryngal Head Neck Surg* 148(4):360–368, 2022.
Webster KE, Lee A, Galbraith K, et al: Intratympanic corticosteroids for Ménière's disease. *Cochrane Database Syst Rev.* 2(2):CD015245, 2023.
Wichova H, Miller ME, Derebery MJ: Otologic manifestations after COVID-19 vaccination: the House Ear Clinic experience, *Otol Neurotol* 42:e1213–e1218, 2021.
Yaz F, Ziylan F, Smeeing DPJ, Thomeer HGXM: Intratympanic treatment in Meniere's disease, efficacy of aminoglycosides versus corticosteroids in comparison studies. A systemic review, *Otology and Neurotology* 41(1):1–10, 2020.

OTITIS EXTERNA

Method of
Kimberly Williams, MD

CURRENT DIAGNOSIS

- Pain, itching, or fullness of the ear
- Tenderness of tragus, pinna, or both
- Onset <48 h
- Physical examination findings of erythema, edema, ± drainage and debris

CURRENT THERAPY

- Aural toilet
- Topical antimicrobials
- Analgesic treatment

Otitis externa is an inflammation of the ear canal and can be either acute or chronic. It is often called swimmer's ear.

Epidemiology

Acute otitis externa is a common problem seen in the primary care office. The annual incidence falls between 1:100 and 1:250 with a lifetime incidence approaching 10%. Peak incidence is in children 7 to 12 years old. It does appear to have a genetic link, because it occurs more often in people with blood group type A. Chronic otitis externa affects 3% to 5% of the population.

Risk Factors

Otitis externa is more common in warmer climates with high humidity. Increased water exposure, especially from swimming, places a person at higher risk. Other risk factors include debris from dermatologic conditions such as psoriasis, trauma due to use of hearing aids and ear plugs and abrasions from cleaning of the ear canal. Cerumen helps prevent microbial growth by providing an acidic pH; when cerumen is removed in cleaning, an environment ready for microbial growth is set up.

Pathophysiology

Approximately 95% of acute otitis externa is due to bacterial infection (Figure 1). The other 5% can be attributed to fungal infections or, less commonly, herpes zoster. Fungal infection is more common in chronic otitis externa. Of the bacterial infections, 20% to 60% are due to *Pseudomonas aeruginosa*. *Staphylococcus aureus* is the next major causative organism. Gram-negative organisms account for 2% to 3% of bacterial infections.

Prevention

Prevention is aimed at avoiding water accumulation and retention in the ear canal. Using ear plugs while swimming and using a hair dryer to dry the ear canal after water exposure can be beneficial. The use of acidifying eardrops, such as acetic acid 2% (Vosol), before and after swimming can also help prevent otitis externa. Other preventive measures include stopping the removal of cerumen and avoiding trauma to the ear canal. Finally, proper treatment of dermatologic conditions such as eczema and psoriasis can help reduce debris that can be a risk factor for infection.

Clinical Manifestations

Otitis externa usually develops rapidly over 1 to 2 days. Most patients complain of a feeling of ear pain, fullness, or itching. Hearing loss may be another symptom. Key physical examination findings include tenderness on palpation of the tragus, discomfort with traction on the pinna, edema of the ear canal, and erythema of the canal. Pain may be out of proportion to examination findings. Regional lymphadenitis and cellulitis of the pinna and adjacent skin can also be present.

Diagnosis

The diagnosis of otitis externa is made clinically by history and physical examination. The history should be positive for otalgia, itching, or sense of fullness. The exam should be positive for tenderness if the tragus is palpated or if the pinna is pulled up and out. If the cause is bacterial, purulent drainage is usually present. Otoscopy will show diffuse canal edema, usually present with erythema. Often there will be copious amounts of debris.

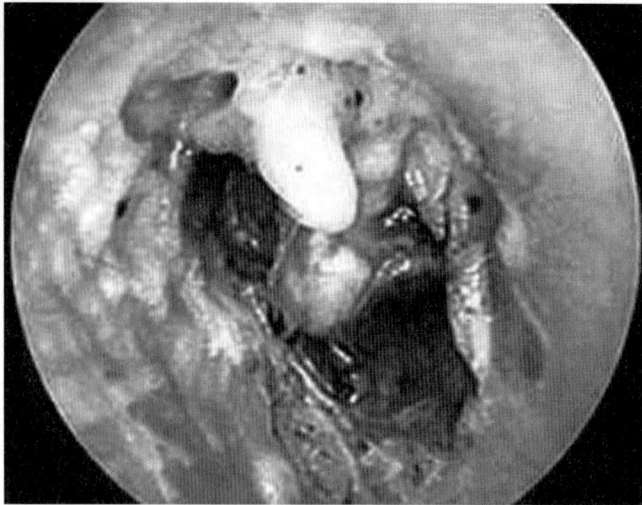

Figure 1 Acute otitis externa with the canal somewhat narrowed from edema and obstructed by desquamating epithelium, soft cerumen, and purulent discharge; this must be removed to visualize the tympanic membrane and to allow ototopical therapy to penetrate to all the superficially infected areas of the canal skin. Reprinted with permission from Osguthorpe JD, Nielsen DR. Otitis externa: review and clinical update. *Am Family Physician.* 2006;74(9):1510–1516.

TABLE 1	Topical Otic Preparations for Treatment of Otitis Externa.		
ACTIVE DRUGE	**BRAND NAME**	**DOSING**	**COMMENTS**
Acetic acid 2% solution with steroid	Vosol HC, Acetasol HC	q4–6h	Can sting/local irritation
Ciprofloxacin/ hydrocortisone	Cipro HC	q12h	Approved if tympanic membrane is perforated
Ciprofloxacin/ dexamethasone	Ciprodex	q12h	Approved if tympanic membrane is perforated
Neomycin, polymyxin B, hydrocortisone	Cortisporin Otic	q6h	Neomycin can cause local irritation, ototoxic potential
Ofloxacin	Floxin Otic	q24h	Can cause local irritation
Tobramycin[1]	Tobrex	q6h	Minimally irritating, ophthalmic preparation, ototoxic potential
Gentamycin[1]	Garamycin	q6h	Ophthalmic preparation, ototoxic potential

[1]Not FDA approved for this indication.

Debris should be cleared to visualize the tympanic membrane. There should be good mobility of the tympanic membrane and the tympanometry curve will be normal unless there is concomitant acute otitis media.

Differential Diagnosis
Middle ear disease should be distinguished from external disease by ensuring that the tympanic membrane is normal. Acute otitis media with perforation of the tympanic membrane may result in purulent middle ear secretions into the external ear canal. Contact dermatitis of the ear canal can mimic otitis externa, and a thorough history of exposure to metals such as nickel and copper, chemicals such as new soaps, topical antibiotics, detergents, cosmetics, and other irritants should be obtained. Fungal infection of the ear canal can mimic bacterial otitis externa. Fungus tends to infect the medial portion of the ear canal and has spores and filaments that can be seen both macroscopically and microscopically. Also in the differential are carcinoma of the external auditory canal, which mimics chronic infection; herpes, which is rare and forms vesicles on the outer ear canal; and radiation therapy.

Therapy
Topical therapy is the treatment of choice in mild to moderate disease in healthy patients. The choice of topical agent is based on cost, ease of administration, and risk of side effects (Table 1). Topical aminoglycoside and fluoroquinolone antibiotics have a response rate of more than 70%. If there is a perforation of the tympanic membrane, ciprofloxacin topical solutions are preferred because of the risk of ototoxicity from aminoglycosides and neomycin. Using a topical steroid in conjunction with topical antibiotic therapy has been shown to shorten duration of ear pain. Duration of topical therapy should be 7 to 10 days. Clotrimazole 1%[1] may be used for superficial fungal infections of the ear canal.

For the topical therapy to be effective, it must be delivered to the tissue of the ear canal. First, the canal must be cleared of debris. This can be done in the physician's office under direct visualization or with lavage of the ear canal using saline or hydrogen peroxide warmed to body temperature. The patient should then be instructed on the proper delivery of the eardrops. Eardrops are administered more effectively if another person delivers the drops. The patient should lie on his or her side with the affected ear up, and drops should be placed in the ear canal until it is filled. The patient should remain on his or her side for 3 to 5 minutes. If greater than 50% of the canal is edematous, a wick made of cellulose material should be placed to facilitate delivery of the drops. The wick may fall out or can be removed by either patient or clinician once the edema has resolved.

Systemic therapy should be used in patients who are immune compromised, including those with diabetes, and in patients with surrounding cellulitis. The systemic therapy chosen should be effective against pseudomonas.

Adequate pain control is another important factor in the treatment of otitis externa. Often this can be achieved with nonsteroidal antiinflammatory medications, but opioid analgesics may be necessary, especially to remove debris. Analgesics should be used early in treatment of the disease.

Monitoring
Patients should respond to therapy in 48 to 72 hours. If therapy fails, the clinician should evaluate adherence to therapy and ability of the drug to be delivered properly. Alternative diagnoses should be considered, including fungal infections, dermatitis, foreign bodies, and middle ear disease with perforation of the tympanic membrane. If the infection has spread outside of the ear canal, systemic therapy should be started.

Complications
One complication of simple otitis externa is malignant otitis externa, an invasive infection of the external auditory canal causing osteomyelitis of the temporal bone. It most commonly occurs in elderly diabetic patients or the immunocompromised. Complications include meningitis, dural sinus thrombosis, cranial abscess, and cranial nerve

[1]Not US Food and Drug Administration approved for this indication.

neuropathy including facial nerve paralysis. Diagnosis may require computed tomography and cultures. Treatment includes systemic antipseudomonal antibiotics and surgical débridement. Contact dermatitis from the topical antimicrobials prescribed for otitis externa may also complicate treatment. This is due to a delayed-type hypersensitivity reaction to one or more of the components of the topical therapy. Neomycin is the most common cause, but hypersensitivity reactions can also occur from other agents including preservatives and fragrances. The reaction is characterized by pruritus, edema, and inflammation of the skin in the auditory canal. It can spread beyond the canal to the pinna and even the skin of the neck. This is treated with topical steroids and by stopping the offending agent.

References

Kaushik V, Malik T, Saeed SR: Interventions for acute otitis externa. *Cochrane Database of Systematic Reviews* 2010, Issue 1. Art. No.: CD004740. https://doi: 10.1002/14651858.CD004740.pub2.

Long M. Otitis externa. *Pediatrics in Review* 2013; 34 (3):133–134.

Rosenfeld RM, Brown L, Cannon CR, et al: Clinical practice guideline: acute otitis externa. *Otolaryngology—Head Neck Surg* 2006; 134:S4.

Schaefer P, Baugh R: Acute Otitis Externa: An update. *Am Fam Physician* 2012; 86(11):1055–1061, 2012.

OTITIS MEDIA

Method of
Gretchen Irwin, MD, MBA

CURRENT DIAGNOSIS

- History of acute onset of symptoms
- Middle ear effusion
  - Bulging tympanic membrane
  - Limited mobility of tympanic membrane or air fluid level visible behind tympanic membrane
- Middle ear inflammation
  - Erythema of tympanic membrane or distinct otalgia

CURRENT THERAPY

- Watchful waiting—appropriate for children:
  - Older than 2 years of age with nonsevere illness
  - Older than 6 months of age with uncertain diagnosis and nonsevere illness
  - Older than 2 years of age with severe illness, but uncertain diagnosis
    - Need close follow-up in 48 hours
    - Consider delayed prescription
- Antibiotics
  - First-line therapy should be amoxicillin (Amoxil) 80 to 90 mg/kg/day[3]
  - Treat 10 days if child younger than 6 years of age, 5 to 7 days if older than 6 years of age
  - Follow up if not improving in 48 hours
- Analgesia
  - Acetaminophen (Tylenol), ibuprofen (Motrin, Advil)
- Antihistamines and decongestants are of no benefit
- Surgery—consider tympanostomy tubes when:
  - First acute otitis media (AOM) episode at younger than 6 months of age and child with two or more episodes in 6 months or three episodes in 24 months
  - First AOM episode at older than 12 months of age and child with three episodes in 6 months, five episodes in 12 months, or seven episodes in 24 months

[3]Exceeds dosage recommended by the manufacturer.

Epidemiology

Acute otitis media (AOM) is a common condition of childhood, with one in four children having at least one episode of AOM by 10 years of age. The majority of cases of AOM occur within the first 5 years of life. Younger children are more likely to be affected, with a peak incidence noted between 6 and 20 months of age, likely because of the relative immaturity of the immune system and eustachian tube function. On average, $5 billion are spent per year on office visits, lost productivity, and diminished parental quality of life as a result of AOM infections. As a result, research has focused on effective strategies both to prevent episodes of AOM and also to efficiently treat episodes that do occur.

Risk Factors

Identifying children at risk for AOM has been an important strategy to attempt to limit instances of AOM. Unfortunately, many of the risk factors associated with AOM are not modifiable, including male sex, Native American ethnicity, presence of siblings within the home, and a family history of recurrent AOM. Additional risk factors include low socioeconomic status, premature birth, attendance at out-of-home daycare, lack of breastfeeding, and history of poor maternal health during pregnancy. Limited studies have suggested that interventions such as avoiding supine feeding or bottle propping, reducing pacifier use after the first 6 months of life, and eliminating passive tobacco exposure can help reduce the incidence; however, the evidence in which these interventions demonstrate clear impact is limited. Public health programs that encourage breastfeeding and optimal maternal health during pregnancy, as well as those focused on reducing tobacco use, have perhaps the best opportunity to affect AOM incidence rates. Not only are these identified risk factors for any episode of AOM, but children with these characteristics are also more likely to have recurrent AOM. Although many children will be affected in their lifetimes, those with recurrent disease are most at risk of complications leading to morbidity or mortality.

Other risk factors specifically for recurrent AOM include an early onset of the first episode and low parental education. Pathophysiologically, AOM has classically been associated with three bacteria, namely, *Streptococcus pneumoniae, Moraxella catarrhalis,* and *Haemophilus influenzae*. The introduction of pneumococcal vaccines has led to a shifting in the frequency with which each pathogen causes disease. In 1999 *S. pneumoniae* was responsible for 40% to 45% of AOM, while *H. influenzae* was responsible for 25% to 30%. In 2017 the bacteria were responsible for 15% to 25% and 50% to 60% of infections, respectively. The frequency of *M. catarrhalis* infections has remained consistent at 12% to 15%. The bacteria responsible for AOM become pathogenic in the setting of eustachian tube dysfunction. A relative obstruction of the eustachian tube develops most commonly secondary to secretions from an antecedent viral upper respiratory infection or allergies, but it may result from neuromuscular conditions or abnormal anatomy. Such relative obstruction creates a negative pressure within the middle ear leading to serous effusion and secondary infection of this collection of interstitial fluid. Thus prevention of AOM is aimed at both reducing the presence of pathogenic bacteria and preventing upper respiratory infections that may create eustachian tube dysfunction. Interestingly, during the COVID-19 pandemic, cases of otitis media in children decreased. This may be a result of infection control measures such as widespread use of masks or avoidance of healthcare as a strategy to avoid contracting COVID-19.

Prevention

The successes of immunization programs in virtually eliminating childhood illnesses such as measles, polio, and varicella have led to great interest in the development of vaccines capable of eradicating the causative agents of AOM. Immunizations targeting the specific bacteria most commonly associated with AOM have had mixed success, however. For example, although the serotypes contained in the 7-valent pneumococcal conjugate vaccine (PCV7, Prevnar7) are responsible for approximately 66%

of pneumococcal-related AOM, only moderate effectiveness has been noted in reducing AOM incidence among vaccinated children. After the introduction of the 7-valent PCV into practice in February 2000, the incidence of AOM decreased only 6% to 7% among vaccinated children. The 9-valent and 11-valent PCVs[2] have been shown to result in a risk reduction of *S. pneumoniae* isolates in children with AOM of 17% and 34%, respectively. An epidemiologic increase in AOM due to serotype 19A has been noted in the last 20 years. Serotype 19A is not covered in the 7-, 9-, or 11-valent PCVs[2] but is included in the 13-valent PCV (Prevnar 13). The 13-valent PCV was incorporated into the recommended childhood immunization schedule in February 2010. Since 2010, there has been a steady decline in otitis media attributable to *S. pneumoniae* with one study reporting a 50% reduction in AOM in children younger than 2 years who have been vaccinated with Prevnar 13. With the advent of pneumococcal vaccines that include more serotypes, such as PCV15, PCV20, and PCV23, immunogenicity data suggests that routine pneumococcal vaccination will only continue to help decrease incidence of AOM. Currently, children are recommended to receive PCV15 or PCV20 between 2 and 15 months with catchup vaccination as needed. Prevnar 20 has a label indication for otitis media prevention for patients 6 weeks to 5 years of age.

Similar vaccines are in development for *H. influenzae* and *M. catarrhalis* as causative agents of AOM. The current *H. influenzae* b vaccine (Hib) has had little impact on AOM because <5% of episodes are caused by the type b strain of *Haemophilus*. Instead, nontypeable *H. influenzae* is a much more common cause of AOM. Although the vaccines targeting specific bacteria that have been shown to cause AOM have been successful, so too has the influenza vaccine been shown to affect the course of AOM. In several studies, children who received seasonal influenza vaccine (Fluzone) were found to have fewer episodes of AOM than unvaccinated children. Furthermore, those who did have an AOM episode were found to use fewer antibiotics and have shorter duration of middle-ear effusion compared with unvaccinated counterparts.

With evidence that reducing the incidence of viral influenza may reduce the occurrence of secondary AOM, several other interventions aimed at reducing viral upper respiratory infection incidence have been studied for their impact on AOM rates. The use of zinc[7] and propolis[7] as agents to prevent viral upper respiratory infections, for instance, has been shown to have mixed benefit in reducing AOM in children. In multiple studies, zinc has been well tolerated with no contraindications to use identified. Zinc as a single agent has been shown to prevent AOM only when used in children younger than 5 years of age who are also malnourished. However, when combined with propolis, zinc was shown to be effective at reducing AOM episodes for children with a history of recurrent AOM. Of note, in several trials zinc did not reduce upper respiratory infection rates; rather, rates of secondary AOM alone were decreased. Although not necessarily effective as a preventive measure for all children, zinc and propolis may be an option for children with recurrent infections.

Similarly, probiotics[7] added to infant formula have been shown to be beneficial for some children. Although breastfeeding has been shown to be most beneficial in preventing AOM compared with formula supplementation, infant formulas supplemented with *Lactobacillus rhamnosus* GG and *Bifidobacterium lactis* BB-12 (Enfamil Premium, Nestlé Good Start) were shown to reduce the incidence of AOM over the first 7 months and the first year. Children who received placebo formula had an incidence of AOM of 50% in the first 7 months, whereas children who received the probiotic-supplemented formula had an incidence of only 22%.

Dietary supplementation to limit AOM is not limited to infant formulas, however. Xylitol,[7] a polyol sugar alcohol found in birch plants, plums, strawberries, and raspberries, has been demonstrated in several studies to be effective at preventing both dental caries and AOM, although its dosage forms make administration difficult. Xylitol is available as a chewing gum, which raises concern as a choking hazard in young children. Similarly, in its oral syrup form, xylitol must be administered five times daily to be effective. Studies of thrice-daily dosing have not been able to demonstrate the same preventive effect as dosing five times daily despite a consistent total daily dose of 10 g/day. Furthermore, emerging evidence suggests that xylitol must be given daily to remain effective at reducing AOM episodes because prophylaxis only during winter months or use only during upper respiratory tract infections is ineffective. Of note, children who have already received tympanostomy tubes receive no prevention benefit from xylitol administration. Research is ongoing to increase physician awareness of xylitol as a possible prophylactic measure because current studies suggest less than one-half of U.S. physicians are aware of xylitol, and less than one-fourth discuss or recommend its use to patients.

Echinacea[7] and osteopathic manipulation have also been cited as potential prophylactic treatments, particularly for children at high risk of recurrence. However, little evidence exists that either are effective. In fact, one large study demonstrated an increased risk of AOM with echinacea use during an upper respiratory tract infection episode and no benefit to manipulation treatment. Ongoing studies are examining the use of these modalities.

Clinical Manifestations

AOM presents with a rapid onset of symptoms that may include fever, chills, ear pain, or ear pulling. In fact, ear pulling and ear rubbing have been demonstrated to be quite sensitive for the diagnosis of AOM in the setting of a history consistent with AOM and middle ear effusion. Often, symptoms may be preceded by upper respiratory symptoms such as rhinorrhea, cough, or congestion. Children who have had tympanostomy tubes placed will likely have a far different presentation, with fever and pain being quite unlikely; rather, a thin, yellow or milky discharge may be the only sign that AOM is present.

Diagnosis

The 2013 update of the guidelines of the American Academy of Pediatrics (AAP) for the diagnosis and treatment of AOM acknowledged that no gold standard exists for the clinical diagnosis of AOM. History and physical examination should be consistent with rapid onset of inflammation in the middle ear. Both pneumatic otoscopy and tympanometry may be useful in the diagnosis of AOM. Tympanic membranes should be evaluated for position, mobility, color, and degree of translucency using pneumatic otoscopy to assess for presence of middle ear effusion or inflammation. Moderate to severe bulging of the tympanic membrane, new onset of otorrhea without other cause, or mild bulging of the tympanic membrane with intense erythema or ear pain should prompt diagnosis of AOM. Furthermore, tympanometry may be useful in determining whether an effusion is present if the diagnosis is otherwise unclear.

One concern of physicians has been accurately diagnosing middle ear inflammation after a child has been vigorously crying. A study of 125 healthy children, age younger than 30 months, assessed the impact of crying on tympanic membrane color by performing otoscopy both before and after administering at least two immunizations. Although crying can cause a pinkening of the tympanic membrane, it should disappear when the child quiets and should be less intense than what is observed with inflammation. True middle ear inflammation results in an angry, red eardrum, not the milder, pink flush seen with vigorous crying. The presence of effusion should also help support a diagnosis of inflammation.

Differential Diagnosis

Otitis media with effusion (OME) is often misdiagnosed as an episode of AOM. Like AOM, OME is common, with 2.2 million

---

[2] Not available in the United States.
[7] Available as dietary supplement.

---

[7] Available as dietary supplement.

TABLE 1 Treatment Options for Acute Otitis Media

AGE OF CHILD	AOM WITH OTORRHEA		AOM WITHOUT OTORRHEA		AOM WITH SEVERE SYMPTOMS*	
	UNILATERAL	BILATERAL	UNILATERAL	BILATERAL	UNILATERAL	BILATERAL
6 months to 2 years	Antibiotics	Antibiotics	Antibiotics or observation	Antibiotics	Antibiotics	Antibiotics
>2 years	Antibiotics	Antibiotics	Antibiotics or observation	Antibiotics or observation	Antibiotics	Antibiotics

*Severe symptoms include toxic-appearing child, persistent otalgia for >48 hours, temperature >39°C in the past 48 hours, or uncertain access to follow-up.
AOM, Acute otitis media.

episodes annually, representing an estimated cost of $4 billion. OME can also occur with a viral upper respiratory infection and may follow or precede an episode of AOM. OME differs from AOM, however, because fluid may be present in the middle ear with OME, but there are no signs of acute infection. Although OME is not associated with acute infection, it is nonetheless critical to diagnose because research has demonstrated that chronic OME is associated with hearing loss and subsequent developmental delay. In fact, OME in infancy has been shown to be associated with, on average, a 7-point reduction in IQ at 7 years of age. The cornerstone of treatment for OME is observation for 2 to 3 months to allow the effusion to clear. Avoidance of allergens and tobacco exposure that may worsen eustachian tube dysfunction is also important. Decongestants and antihistamines are not effective. If an effusion does not clear within 2 months, a single course of amoxicillin (Amoxil) or penicillin may be given.

Audiometry should be performed in all children with OME for longer than 3 months or, in the setting of language delay, learning problems, or suspected hearing loss in a child with OME. If the effusion persists or if a child has multiple episodes of OME or has hearing or learning difficulties as a result of OME, surgical intervention should be considered. Initial surgical intervention for children with persistent OME should be myringotomy with placement of tympanostomy tubes. Tonsillectomy and myringotomy alone are not indicated for treatment of OME. However, adenoidectomy may have a role, particularly in children 4 to 8 years of age. Current recommendations include adenoidectomy only if repeat surgery for OME is needed. However, emerging evidence suggests that adenoidectomy may decrease the need for surgical retreatment, reduce ongoing hearing loss, and be of benefit during initial surgery for older children.

Treatment

The treatment of AOM has been controversial in with the advent of watchful waiting recommendations. Because it is the most common childhood bacterial infection for which antibiotics are prescribed worldwide, debate continues about both the most effective regimen and appropriate time to treat AOM. On average, $2.8 billion is spent per year on antibiotics for episodes of AOM, yet emerging evidence suggests that watchful waiting is appropriate for some children. Despite recommendations for watchful waiting, 85% to 95% of children in the United States receive immediate antibiotics for AOM. However, schema that involve watchful waiting have not been fully embraced by U.S. physicians. Judicious use of antibiotic therapy remains key in the prevention of morbidity and mortality associated with otitis media but is not an appropriate therapy for every child. All children require analgesia of some type, as well as close, scheduled follow-up, but use of observation or an antibiotic varies with severity of illness and age of the child. Treatment options are summarized in Table 1.

Treatment Options
Observation
For some children with AOM, observation has been shown to be an appropriate therapy that avoids the possible side effects of antibiotics, with low risk of complications developing from an untreated otitis media. Evidence suggests that 78% of AOM

episodes will spontaneously resolve within the first few days of infection. In fact, for every 100 otherwise healthy at-risk children with AOM, 80 will improve within 3 days without antibiotic therapy. If the same 100 children were all treated with amoxicillin or ampicillin, 92 would improve, although 3 to 10 would develop a rash and 5 to 10 would develop diarrhea. Thus in a typical family medicine practice, 16 children with AOM would need to be treated with antibiotics to prevent 1 child from experiencing ongoing otalgia, whereas 1 of every 24 children treated will experience harm related to therapy. Hence, the use of antibiotics is not without risk. Multiple studies have demonstrated that even in children as young as 2 months of age, many will improve without antibiotic therapy, and delaying antibiotics may prevent undesirable side effects without exposing the child to undue risk. No studies have demonstrated a resurgence of either mastoiditis or meningitis with implementation of watchful waiting for AOM. If observation is chosen as a management strategy for AOM, it is important to reevaluate the child in 48 to 72 hours to ensure that they are improving and that a rescue antibiotic is prescribed if symptoms are not resolving.

Delayed prescriptions are one strategy that has been effective at reducing antibiotic use, maintaining parental satisfaction, and improving healthcare efficiency. Physicians are often concerned that parental satisfaction will decrease if watchful waiting for an episode of AOM is recommended. Interestingly, satisfaction has been tied to the receipt of an antibiotic prescription, though not necessarily the administration of antibiotics to the child. Declines in satisfaction are noted when parents are advised to return to care in 2 to 3 days if the child is not improving while undergoing watchful waiting. By offering a delayed prescription, the parent can avoid the difficulties associated with needing to be seen again if the child fails to improve, and parental satisfaction is maintained even if the child never receives any medication. Parents should be educated that up to one-third of children who initially are treated with observation will eventually need antibiotic therapy. Although this suggests that up to two-thirds of children can avoid unnecessary antibiotics, parents should be aware that many children will go on to need antibiotic therapy. Clearly, however, not every child is a candidate for observation therapy.

Antibiotic Therapy
Antibiotic therapy may be associated with less duration of pain, less analgesic use, and less absence for both children and parents from school and work, respectively. It should be noted that there is likely little effect on pain in the first 24 hours. The AAP and the American Academy of Family Physicians in a joint position statement have recommended that, when a decision is made to use antibiotics, amoxicillin (Amoxil) be given as a first-line agent at a dose of 80 to 90 mg/kg/day[3]. For penicillin-allergic children, cefdinir (Omnicef), cefpodoxime (Vantin), or cefuroxime (Ceftin) may be used. Although the cross-reactivity of cephalosporins and penicillins is likely lower than previously believed, if concern exists about treating a child with a cephalosporin, clindamycin[1] (30–40 mg/kg/day)[3] may be used. Macrolide antibiotics may

[3] Exceeds dosage recommended by the manufacturer.
[1] Not FDA approved for this indication.

TABLE 2　Antibiotic Selection for Specific Patient Populations

	ANTIBIOTIC OF CHOICE	DOSE (MG/KG/DAY)	ROUTE	DURATION OF THERAPY
AOM in child older than 2 years	Amoxicillin (Amoxil)	80–90[3]	PO	5–7 days
AOM in child younger than 2 years	Amoxicillin	80–90[3]	PO	10 days
AOM in child with allergy to penicillin	Cefdinir (Omnicef)	14	PO	10 days
	Cefpodoxime (Vantin)	10	PO	5 days
	Cefuroxime (Ceftin)	30	PO	10 days
AOM with inability to tolerate oral medications	Ceftriaxone (Rocephin)	50	IV/IM	1 day
AOM with amoxicillin failure	Amoxicillin with clavulanate (Augmentin)	90 of amoxicillin and 6.4 of clavulanate[3]	PO	10 days
	Ceftriaxone (Rocephin)	50	IV/IM	3 days[3]
AOM with amoxicillin/clavulanate failure	Ceftriaxone (Rocephin)	50	IV/IM	3 days[3]
AOM with ceftriaxone failure and tympanocentesis not available	Clindamycin (Cleocin)[1]	30–40[3]	PO	10 days
Perforated tympanic membrane	Amoxicillin	80–90[3]	PO	10 days
Tympanostomy tube in place	Amoxicillin and topical 0.3% ciprofloxacin/0.1% dexamethasone (Ciprodex Otic)	80–90 / 8 drops	PO / Topical bid	10 days / 7 days

[1]Not FDA approved for this indication.
[3]Exceeds dosage recommended by the manufacturer.
AOM, Acute otitis media; *IM,* intramuscular; *IV,* intravenous; *PO,* by mouth.

have limited efficacy. Ceftriaxone (Rocephin) may be used as a single dose for a child who is unable to tolerate oral medications. Although amoxicillin continues to be the preferred first-line agent, 30% to 70% of *S. pneumoniae* strains have become penicillin and macrolide resistant, whereas 20% to 40% of *H. influenzae* has β-lactamase–producing capabilities. Given the various resistance patterns of organisms, a child who fails to improve on amoxicillin should receive amoxicillin with clavulanate (Augmentin) or ceftriaxone as second-line therapy. Clindamycin (Cleocin)[1] or tympanocentesis to identify a causative organism may also be considered. Current evidence continues to suggest that a 10-day course is optimal for children younger than 2 years of age. Less benefit to longer-duration therapy is noted in older children, and therefore a shorter 5- to 7-day course is recommended for those older than 2 years of age. If a child has a perforation of the tympanic membrane, treatment considerations may be slightly different. Oral antibiotics continue to be recommended if perforation is a result of the AOM episode; however, if a child has an episode of AOM with tympanostomy tubes in place, topical 0.3% ciprofloxacin/0.1% dexamethasone (Ciprodex Otic) should be added to oral amoxicillin. Table 2 provides antibiotic dosing recommendations. Regardless of the decision to implement watchful waiting or antibiotic therapy, any child with AOM should be expected to improve within 48 to 72 hours. If improvement is not occurring, the child should be reevaluated.

Surgery

For some children, AOM will not be an isolated event. Instead, the child will have recurrent infections and require multiple antibiotic courses throughout a year, prompting consideration of tympanostomy tube placement. Currently, referral for evaluation for tympanostomy tubes is recommended when a child has had three or more episodes of AOM within a 6-month period or more than four episodes within a 12-month period. Some have argued, however, that this recommendation should be considered within the context of the child's age at first presentation. A child who has the first episode of AOM before 6 months of age is likely to go on to have many more episodes. Ultimately, they will likely meet the criteria for myringotomy and thus may warrant a more aggressive approach from the outset. Conversely, a child who presents with a first episode of AOM as an older child is less likely to have recurrent episodes and can therefore be treated in a more conservative manner. Using an age-stratified approach, children who experience a first episode of AOM before 6 months of age should receive tympanostomy tubes if they have two episodes in a 6- or 12-month time period or three episodes in 24 months. Similarly, children who have a first episode of AOM after 1 year of age should receive tympanostomy tubes only if they have three episodes within 6 months, five within 12 months, or seven within 24 months. Referral may also occur if a child has a history of AOM associated with meningitis, facial nerve paralysis, coalescent mastoiditis, or brain abscess. Tympanostomy tubes are also often placed because of prolonged OME resulting in hearing loss and language delay. Myringotomy without tube placement may be considered for either diagnosis of an infection that has not responded to numerous antibiotics or for relief of severe otalgia. AOM episodes will continue to occur despite tympanostomy tube placement. However, episodes will likely be less severe, of shorter duration, and less frequent. In addition to ongoing AOM episodes, tympanostomy tubes can be problematic if they become clogged. New studies in animal models suggest that applying colchicine[1] in the external ear may prevent this complication.

Analgesia

Regardless of a decision to pursue watchful waiting or antibiotics, analgesics are an important component in the treatment of AOM. Multiple homeopathic interventions and home remedies including application of heat, ice, or mineral oil (Min-O-Ear)[1] have been used for pain control, although no studies exist to verify their effectiveness. Acetaminophen (Tylenol), ibuprofen (Motrin), narcotics, and tympanostomy have all been demonstrated to be effective at reducing pain. However, the side effects of altered mental status, gastrointestinal upset, and respiratory depression with narcotics, as well as the skill needed to perform tympanostomy, limit the usefulness of these interventions in primary care practice. Antihistamines and decongestants have often been prescribed in an attempt to reduce the fluid volume in the middle

[1] Not FDA approved for this indication.

ear and hence provide relief. Unfortunately, use of antihistamines and decongestants has been shown to result in a fivefold to eightfold increase in the risk of side effects with no benefits, including no decreased time to cure, no prevention of surgery or complications, and no increased symptom resolution. Therefore antihistamines and decongestants have not been routinely recommended.

Conclusion

AOM continues to be one of the most costly and common childhood illnesses in developed nations throughout the world. Successful management of this condition requires much more than choosing amoxicillin at an appropriate dose and duration or appropriately timing a surgical referral. Vigilant attention to modifying risk factors when possible, promoting immunization, and limiting the spread of viral illnesses have been shown to prevent AOM instances. Furthermore, adhering to diagnostic criteria to attempt to accurately distinguish between AOM and OME, as well as implementing observation when appropriate, can significantly reduce antibiotic usage, thereby minimizing side effects for patients and the opportunity to develop resistance in pathogens.

References

Monasta L, Ronfani L, Marchetti F, et al: Burden of disease caused by otitis media: systematic review and global estimates, *PLoS One* 7(4):e36226, 2012.

Frost HM, Bizune D, Gerber JS, et al: Amoxicillin versus other antibiotic agents for the treatment of acute otitis media in children, *J Pediatr* 251:98–104.e5, 2022.

de Sévaux JLH, Damoiseaux RA, van de Pol AC, et al: Paracetamol (acetaminophen) or non-steroidal anti-inflammatory drugs, alone or combined, for pain relief in acute otitis media in children. *Cochrane Database Syst Rev* 18;8(8):CD011534, 2023.

Fuji N, Salamone FN, Kaur R, et al: Eighteen-year longitudinal study of uncomplicated and complex acute otitis media during the pneumococcal conjugate vaccine era, 2006–2023, *J Infect Dis* 14;232(2):417–429, 2025.

RED EYE

Lynn Fisher, MD; and John N. Dorsch, MD

CURRENT DIAGNOSIS

- Bacterial, viral, and allergic conjunctivitis can often be distinguished by the course of spread in the eye, the type of ocular discharge present, and associated symptoms.
- Subconjunctival hemorrhage can occur from trauma, increased intrathoracic pressure, anticoagulants, or idiopathically.
- Physicians should consider referring to an ophthalmologist patients with traumatic injury to the eye, loss of vision, extreme pain not explained by pathology, keratitis, suspected uveitis or glaucoma, chemical injury, or nonhealing corneal abrasion.

CURRENT THERAPY

- Do not use eye patches in patients with corneal abrasions.
- Do not use topical anesthetics for the eye outside a clinic or hospital setting because corneal toxicity can occur.
- Patients with corneal abrasions should be reexamined the following day.
- Patients with corneal abrasions from extended-wear contact lenses often become colonized with *Pseudomonas aeruginosa* and should be treated with appropriate antibiotics (quinolones).

In the primary care office, the most common causes of red eye are conjunctivitis, subconjunctival hemorrhage, and corneal abrasions due to a foreign body. Other common causes of red eye include blepharitis and hordeolum. Less common but serious causes of red eye include viral keratitis, uveitis, scleritis, and angle-closure glaucoma. Other usually less serious causes of red eye include episcleritis, pingueculum, and pterygium. All primary care physicians should have expertise in recognizing and treating the common causes of red eye and should recognize and refer patients with higher-stakes diagnoses (Boxes 1 and 2).

Physical Examination

Always check visual acuity in any patient with an eye complaint. Fluorescein strips (Flu-Glo, Fluorets), topical anesthetic drops, and cobalt blue light are used to examine the cornea for abrasions, keratitis, and ulceration. Cotton-tipped applicators are used to evert the upper eyelid and look for a foreign body.

Pupillary reaction is often affected by angle closure glaucoma and uveitis, but it is rarely affected by conjunctivitis, blepharitis, and corneal disorders. The pupil may be irregular in the patient with uveitis.

Patients with uveitis often have pain in the closed affected eye when a bright light is shined in the normal eye or with convergence of the eyes. This is due to consensual reflex of the pupils to light and accommodation.

Examine the conjunctiva by pulling the lower eyelid down with the examiner's finger. If the bulbar or palpebral conjunctivae are inflamed (i.e., hyperemic, edematous, discharge), conjunctivitis is present. Palpable preauricular nodes may be present with viral conjunctivitis and chlamydial conjunctivitis.

Conjunctivitis

Conjunctivitis is the most common cause of red eye encountered by primary care clinicians. Among the etiologies of conjunctivitis, viral conjunctivitis is the most common. Although patients with conjunctivitis might have some minor irritation of the eyes, they usually do not complain of pain in the eye or loss of vision. Ocular discharge is generally considered to be an important diagnostic feature of conjunctivitis (Table 1). Although much has been written about characterizing conjunctivitis by the nature of the discharge, one meta-analysis failed to find evidence of the diagnostic usefulness of clinical signs or symptoms in distinguishing bacterial conjunctivitis from viral conjunctivitis.

Viral Conjunctivitis

Viral conjunctivitis is often seen in epidemics and is most commonly caused by members of the Adenovirus family. Typically, viral conjunctivitis starts in one eye and spreads to the other eye a few days later. The conjunctivae appear red and swollen, with copious watery discharge (Figure 1). The natural course of viral conjunctivitis is self-limiting, lasting 10 to 14 days. Tender preauricular lymph nodes, when present, indicate the presence of viral or chlamydial conjunctivitis. Management should be directed at scrupulous hygiene. Patients must be informed that their infection is highly contagious. They should avoid close contact with other persons (e.g., towels, direct contact, swimming pools) for 2 weeks and wash hands or use hand sanitizer frequently to prevent the spread of their infection. Topical antibiotics have been prescribed to try to prevent bacterial superinfection, but there is no good evidence that they have any significant impact. Symptomatic treatment with cold compresses and topical vasoconstrictors may be helpful.

If a patient has a red eye with burning and watery discharge that is also associated with fever, cough, shortness of breath, fatigue, or loss of taste/smell, coronavirus should be considered as a potential cause. A 2024 systematic review showed that the most common ocular symptom of Covid was conjunctivitis, followed by photophobia, burning, chemosis, itching, and ocular pain. In general, ocular manifestations are typically infrequent in Covid-19 patients. Symptoms are 2-3 times more likely in those

Approach to the Patient with Red Eye

The following questions are often helpful in making the diagnosis in patients with red eyes.
- *Is one eye or are both eyes involved?* Infections, allergy, and systemic illness are more likely to cause bilateral eye involvement.
- *Does the patient have intense eye pain?* If yes, likely diagnoses include acute angle closure glaucoma, uveitis, scleritis, keratitis, foreign body, or corneal abrasion.
- *Does the patient have a foreign body sensation?* If so, consider corneal abrasion, trauma, dry eye, keratitis, and other corneal disorders.
- *Is there a discharge?* If it is very copious and purulent, consider gonococcal conjunctivitis. If it is discolored and purulent, consider bacterial conjunctivitis. Copious watery discharge is typical of viral conjunctivitis. Stringy, mucoid discharge is typical of allergic or chlamydial conjunctivitis.
- *Do the eyes itch?* If so, consider blepharitis or allergy in the differential.
- *Are the eyelids swollen?* Consider allergy or infection.
- *Do the eyelids have lumps?* Hordeolum and chalazion should be considered.
- *Do the eyes burn?* Consider blepharitis or dry eye.
- *Is the eye redness recurrent?* Consider herpes keratitis, uveitis, and allergic conjunctivitis.
- *Does the patient have photophobia?* Corneal problems (abrasions, keratitis) and uveitis should be considered.
- *Is there loss of vision?* Consider corneal ulcer, uveitis, and angle closure glaucoma.
- *Is the patient using ocular medications?* Prolonged use of neomycin and sulfa ophthalmic medications can cause sensitization and redness of the eyes.

BOX 2 Red Eye

Common Causes
- Conjunctivitis: bacterial, viral, allergic
- Subconjunctival hemorrhage
- Corneal abrasion
- Blepharitis

Less Common Causes
Less Serious
- Episcleritis
- Pingueculum
- Pterygium

More Serious
- Viral keratitis
- Uveitis
- Scleritis
- Angle closure glaucoma

TABLE 1 Conjunctivitis

TYPE	COURSE	CHARACTERISTICS	DISCHARGE
Bacterial	Starts in one eye, often spreads to other eye		Purulent
Allergic	Accompanies allergic rhinitis	Itchy eyes	Mucus
Viral	Usually bilateral	Very red eyes	Watery

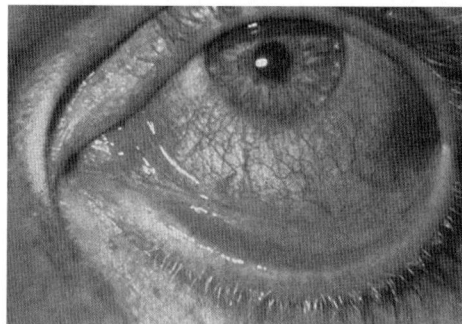

Figure 1 Viral conjunctivitis. Reproduced with permission from the University of Michigan Kellogg Eye Center, https://www.kellogg.umich.edu.

conjunctivitis, but the most common causes are *Staphylococcus aureus*, *Streptococcus pneumoniae*, and *Haemophilus pneumoniae*. Treatment of bacterial conjunctivitis is usually empiric, but conjunctival scraping for smears and cultures should be done in infants, immunocompromised patients, and patients with hyperacute conjunctivitis in which *Neisseria gonorrhoeae* or *Chlamydia trachomatis* infection is suspected. Treatment of bacterial conjunctivitis (excluding gonococcal or chlamydial conjunctivitis) usually consists of a topical antibiotic used four times a day (Table 2). Topical antibiotics are usually prescribed for 5 to 7 days, and resolution of conjunctivitis is expected within that time.

Hyperacute bacterial conjunctivitis has an abrupt onset, copious purulent discharge, and rapid progression, and it is usually associated with gonococcal infection in a sexually active patient. Chemosis (edema of the conjunctivae) may be present.

Chlamydial conjunctivitis is acquired through exposure to infected secretions from the genital tract, either direct or indirect. The infection is usually unilateral (at least initially), and often there is involvement of the preauricular node on the ipsilateral side. Gonococcal and chlamydial infections are treated systemically (Box 3).

Chronic bacterial conjunctivitis is commonly caused by *Staphylococcus aureus* or *Moraxella lacunata*. It is defined by symptoms lasting at least 4 weeks. This often occurs with blepharitis and so there can be crusting and warmth along the eyelid. If suspected, this condition should be referred to an ophthalmologist.

Conjunctivitis of the Newborn

Chlamydial conjunctivitis is the most common cause of infectious conjunctivitis of the newborn in the United States. Onset of conjunctivitis is 3 to 10 days after birth, but it has been reported as late as 2 months after birth. Erythromycin ointment (Ilotycin 0.5%) or tetracycline ointment[2] given shortly after delivery is effective in preventing chlamydial conjunctivitis but not systemic chlamydial infections. *Chlamydia trachomatis* infections, causing pneumonia and otitis media, can be treated either with ethylsuccinate (EryPed Drops) orally 50 mg/kg/day in four divided doses for 14 days or azithromycin (Zithromycin)[1] 20 mg/kg/day orally

with a severe Covid-19 infection compared with a mild infection. Symptoms are usually self-limiting.

With increasing vaccine hesitancy, clinicians should consider vaccine preventable diseases such as rubella and measles virus as a potential cause for conjunctivitis in areas of disease outbreak. These viral illnesses will also usually be accompanied by rash, fever, and cough.

Bacterial Conjunctivitis

Bacterial conjunctivitis typically starts abruptly in one eye and spreads to the other eye in 1 to 2 days. Usually a purulent discharge is present that persists throughout the day. A variety of gram-positive and gram-negative organisms cause bacterial

---

[2]Not available in the United States.
[1]Not FDA approved for this indication.

TABLE 2	Topical Antibiotics Used to Treat Bacterial Conjunctivitis
DRUG	**DOSAGE**
Bacitracin (Ak-Tracin, Bacticin) ointment	Apply 0.5 inch in eye q3–4 h
Ciprofloxacin (Ciloxan) 0.3% ophthalmic solution	1–2 gtt in eye q15 min × 6 h, then q30 min × 18 h, then q1 h × 1 d, then q4 h × 12 d[3]
Gatifloxacin (Zymaxid) 0.5% ophthalmic solution	1 gtt in eye q2 h up to 8 ×/d on day 1, then 1 gtt 2–4 ×/day on day 2–7
Gentamicin (Gentak, Gentasol) 0.3% ophthalmic solution or ointment	Ointment: 0.5 inch applied to eye 2–3 times per day Solution: 1–2 gtt in eye q4 h
Levofloxacin (Quixin) 0.5% ophthalmic solution	1–2 gtt in eye q2 h × 2 d while awake, then q4 h while awake × 5 d
Moxifloxacin (Vigamox) 0.5% ophthalmic solution	1 gtt in eye tid × 7 d
Neomycin/polymyxin B/ gramicidin (Neosporin) ophthalmic solution	1–2 gtt in eye q4 h × 7–10 d
Ofloxacin (Ocuflox) 0.3% ophthalmic solution	1–2 gtt in eye q2–4 h × 2 d, then 1–2 gtt in eye qid × 5 d
Polymyxin B and trimethoprim (Polytrim) ophthalmic solution	1 gtt in eye q3 h × 7–10 d
Sulfacetamide (Isopto Cetamide, Ocusulf-10, Sodium Sulamyd, Sulf-10, AK-Sulf) 10% ophthalmic solution, ointment	Ointment: 0.5-inch ribbon in eye q3–4 h and q h × 7 d Solution: 1–2 gtt in eye q2–3 h × 7–10 d
Tobramycin (AK-Tob, Tobrex) 0.3% ophthalmic solution	1–2 gtt in eye q4 h

[3]Exceeds dosage recommended by the manufacturer.

BOX 3	Treatment of Chlamydial and Gonococcal Conjunctivitis

Chlamydial Conjunctivitis
- Doxycycline (Vibramycin) 100 mg PO bid × 7 days
- Or
- Azithromycin (Zithromax) 1 g PO X 1
- Treat partners

Gonococcal Conjunctivitis
- Ceftriaxone (Rocephin 1 g IM x 1 in patients ≥150 kg, or 500 mg IM x 1 in patients <150 kg)
- Azithromycin (Zithromax) 1 g PO x 1 (when chlamydial infection has not been excluded)

BOX 4	Patient Hygiene Measures for Conjunctivitis

- Do not wear contact lens until the conjunctivitis has cleared and resume wear with a new set. Wear and clean your contact lens as recommended by your eye doctor.
- Avoid touching the eyes and if you do, immediately wash your hands. Use a clean towel or tissue each time you wipe your face and eyes.
- Wash your hands or use hand sanitizer frequently. Always wash them before and after eating, after using bathroom, and after sneezing/coughing.
- Do not use eye makeup while an eye is infected with conjunctivitis. Replace eye makeup if the eye becomes infected and never share makeup.

up to 1 g daily for 3 days. Chlamydial infections of rectal and urogenital sites can only be treated with erythromycin ethylsuccinate orally 50 mg/kg/day in four divided doses for 14 days.

Gonococcal conjunctivitis of the newborn is a hyperacute infection that occurs 2 to 4 days after birth. It can cause corneal ulceration and loss of vision. Gonococcal conjunctivitis can be prevented with silver nitrate drops[2] or erythromycin (Ilotycin) or tetracycline ointment[2] administered shortly after delivery. Silver nitrate commonly causes a self-limited chemical conjunctivitis, which can delay visual bonding of the infant to the parents in the first few hours of life. Gonococcal conjunctivitis of the newborn is treated with Ceftriaxone (Rocephin) 25 to 50 mg/kg up to 125 mg IM/IV.

Conjunctivitis–Otitis Media Syndrome
Conjunctivitis–otitis media syndrome is a common condition in which children with otitis media also have purulent bilateral ocular discharge. It responds to treatment of otitis media; no topical treatment of conjunctivitis is required.

Methicillin-Resistant *Staphylococcus Aureus* Conjunctivitis
Increasing numbers of cases of bacterial conjunctivitis are caused by methicillin-resistant *S. aureus* (MRSA). MRSA conjunctivitis manifests as bacterial conjunctivitis resistant to conventional therapy and is treated with the same drugs used to treat MRSA in other parts of the body (Doxycycline [Vibramycin],[1] vancomycin [Vancocin], sulfamethoxazole-trimethoprim [Bactrim][1]). Cultures should be obtained when MRSA is suspected.

[2]Not available in the United States.

Allergic Conjunctivitis
Allergic conjunctivitis is an immunoglobulin E (IgE)-mediated condition characterized by bilateral eye involvement, itchy eyes, and mucoid discharge. *Seasonal* conjunctivitis is caused by exposure to common allergens (e.g., pollens, dander) and usually accompanies allergic rhinitis. *Perennial* allergic conjunctivitis is similar to seasonal allergic conjunctivitis, but the symptoms are usually less severe. Patients are usually treated with a systemic antihistamine. Ophthalmic (topical) medications include antihistamine or decongestants, mast cell inhibitors, nonsteroidal antiinflammatory drugs (NSAIDs), H_1-antagonists, and various combinations of these (Table 3). Milder cases can be treated with a decongestant-antihistamine combination for about 2 weeks. Moderate to more severe cases can require longer use of these medications or the addition of systemic antihistamines or mast cell inhibitors. Some patients require topical corticosteroids or cyclosporine (Restasis)[1] for severe allergic conjunctivitis, but these should be evaluated by an ophthalmologist because of potential complications of therapy.

Subconjunctival Hemorrhage
In subconjunctival hemorrhage, the redness of the eye is localized and sharply circumscribed, and the underlying sclera is not visible (Figure 2). Conjunctivitis is not present, and there is no discharge. There is typically no pain or visual change. Subconjunctival hemorrhage may be spontaneous, but it can also result from trauma, hypertension, bleeding disorders, or increased intrathoracic pressure (e.g., straining, coughing, retching). No treatment is necessary, but investigation may be warranted if the etiology is in question or the hemorrhage is recurrent. Referral to an ophthalmologist should be considered if the subconjunctival hemorrhage is from trauma or has not resolved within 2 to 3 weeks.

TABLE 3	Topical Medications for Allergic Conjunctivitis		
GENERIC NAME	**BRAND NAME(S)**	**DOSING**	**MODE OF ACTION**
Azelastine 0.05% solution	Optivar	1 gtt in eye(s) bid	H$_1$-antagonist, mast cell inhibitor
Cromolyn 4% solution	Crolom, generic	1–2 gtt in eye(s) 4–6 times per day	Mast cell inhibitor
Emedastine 0.05% solution	Emadine	1 gtt in eye(s) qid	H$_1$-antagonist
Epinastine 0.05% solution	Elestat	1 gtt in eye(s) bid	H$_1$- and H$_2$-antagonist, mast cell inhibitor
Ketorolac 0.5% solution	Acular	1 gtt in eye(s) qid up to 1 week	NSAID
Diclofenac 0.1% solution[1]	Voltaren ophthalmic	1 gtt in eye(s) qid × 2 weeks	NSAID
Lodoxamide 0.1% solution	Alomide	1–2 gtt in eye(s) qid up to 3 months	Mast cell inhibitor
Loteprednol 0.2% susp.	Alrex	1 gtt in eye(s) qd	Corticosteroid
Naphazoline/pheniramine (solution)	• Naphcon-A (OTC) • Opcon-A (OTC) • Visine-A (OTC)	1–2 gtt in eye(s) qd-qid prn	Antihistamine, decongestant
Nedrocomil 2% solution	Alocril	1–2 gtt in eye(s) bid	H$_1$-antagonist, mast cell inhibitor
Olopatadine 0.1% solution	Patanol	1 gtt in eye(s) bid	H$_1$-antagonist, mast cell inhibitor
Olopatadine 0.2% solution	Pataday	1 gtt in eye(s) qd	Mast cell inhibitor

[1]Not FDA approved for this indication.
NSAID, Nonsteroidal antiinflammatory drug.

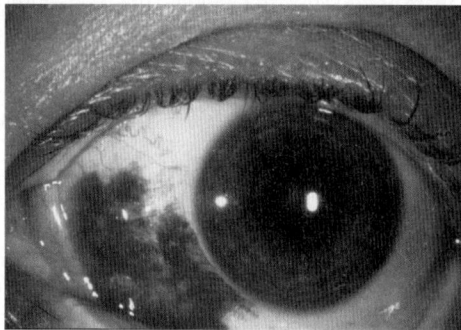

Figure 2 Subconjunctival hemorrhage. Reprinted with permission from American Academy of Ophthalmology: Managing the red eye. eye care skills for the primary care physician series. San Francisco: American Academy of Ophthalmology, 2001.

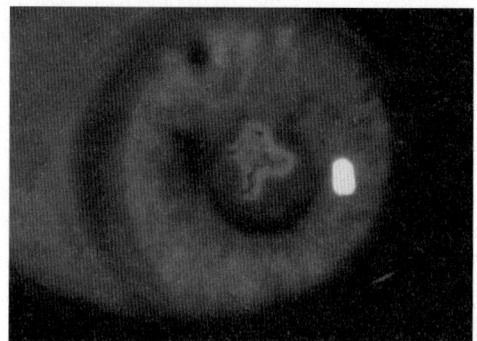

Figure 3 Corneal abrasion with fluorescein stain with cobalt blue light. Reprinted with permission from American Academy of Ophthalmology: Managing the red eye. eye care skills for the primary care physician series. San Francisco: American Academy of Ophthalmology, 2001.

Corneal Abrasion

Corneal abrasions typically result from scratching of the corneal epithelium due to trauma, but they can also occur from extended-wear contact lenses. Patients with corneal abrasions present with pain, excessive tearing from the involved eye, photophobia, a foreign-body sensation (like having sand in the eye), and blurry vision.

Corneal abrasions are identified by staining the cornea with fluorescein and examining under cobalt blue light (Figure 3). The eye should also be examined carefully to check for foreign bodies. Topical anesthetic is administered to make the patient comfortable during the examination, but continued use can cause corneal damage.

Management of corneal abrasions consists of pain relief and prevention of infection. Pain can be relieved with topical NSAIDs such as ketorolac (Acular)[1] and diclofenac (Voltaren),[1] oral over-the-counter analgesics, and occasionally oral narcotics. Topical antibiotics are usually prescribed to prevent infection. Antibiotic ointments are lubricating and soothing to the eye, making them a good option for traumatic corneal abrasions. Topical ophthalmic antibiotic ointments commonly used are bacitracin (Bacticin), erythromycin (Ilotycin), and gentamicin (Gentak).

In patients who have corneal abrasions from contact lens overwear, eyes are commonly colonized with *Pseudomonas aeruginosa.* These patients should be treated with topical antibiotics such as ciprofloxacin (Ciloxan) or ofloxacin (Ocuflux) solutions.

Patching of the eye, though a common practice of the past, has not shown evidence of benefit in recent studies. It was found that eye patching can actually cause harm, so this practice is no longer recommended.

Infrequently, patients have traumatic uveitis accompanying corneal abrasion. Traumatic uveitis usually causes significantly more pain than a corneal abrasion, and, if uveitis is suspected, the clinician should consider referral to an ophthalmologist.

Patients with corneal abrasions should be reexamined in 24 hours. Corneal abrasions typically should be healed or greatly improved in 24 hours. If the abrasion is not completely healed after 24 hours, the patient should be examined again in 2 or 3 days. Referral should be considered if any worsening occurs or if the abrasion does not heal within 5 days. Corneal abrasions can be prevented by using protective eyewear.

Other Causes of Red Eye

Other causes of red eye are somewhat less common.

---

[1]Not FDA approved for this indication.

TABLE 4	Blepharitis		
TYPE	**SITE OF ORIGIN**	**CLINICAL CHARACTERISTICS**	**TREATMENT**
Staphylococcal	Accessory glands of eyelids	Erythema and induration of eyelid; crusting; discharge; loss of eyelashes	• Warm compresses • Baby shampoo scrubs • Erythromycin ointment (Ilotycin)
Seborrheic	Meibomian glands	More chronic, scaling	1. Warm compresses 2. Baby shampoo scrubs 3. Oral tetracycline for resistant cases

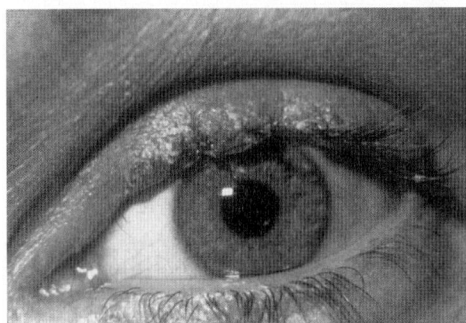

Figure 4 Staphylococcal blepharitis. Reprinted with permission from American Academy of Ophthalmology: Managing the red eye. eye care skills for the primary care physician series. San Francisco: American Academy of Ophthalmology, 2001.

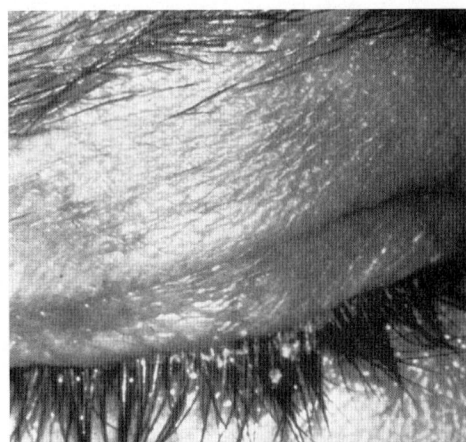

Figure 5 Seborrheic blepharitis. Reprinted with permission from American Academy of Ophthalmology: Managing the red eye. eye care skills for the primary care physician series. San Francisco: American Academy of Ophthalmology, 2001.

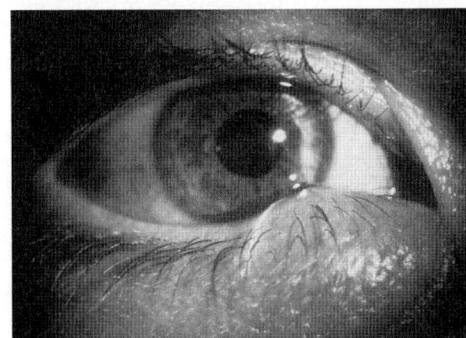

Figure 6 Hordeolum. Reprinted with permission from American Academy of Ophthalmology: Managing the red eye. eye care skills for the primary care physician series. San Francisco: American Academy of Ophthalmology, 2001.

Blepharitis

Blepharitides are inflammatory conditions of the eyelid caused by infection or obstruction of eyelid glands (Table 4). Blepharitis may be accompanied by conjunctivitis. Staphylococcal blepharitis arises from the accessory glands to the eyelashes and causes discharge from the eyelid, often associated with erythema, induration, loss of eyelashes, and crusting of the eyelid (Figure 4). This is treated with hot, moist packs to the eyes, baby shampoo scrubs (3 oz. water and 3 drops baby shampoo used on a washcloth bid), and erythromycin ointment (Ilotycin) at bedtime. Seborrheic blepharitis, a more chronic form of blepharitis, arises from the meibomian glands and causes scaling of the eyelids (Figure 5). Seborrheic blepharitis is often associated with skin disorders such as rosacea, eczema, and seborrheic dermatitis. This is treated with hot, moist packs and baby shampoo scrubs. Resistant cases are treated with oral tetracycline (Sumycin) (or one of its derivatives).

Hordeolum (Stye)

A hordeolum is an acute, painful mass of the eyelid that is caused by inflammation of the glands (Figure 6). It does not usually cause the eye to become red as well. Warm compresses to the eyelid four times a day for 3 to 5 minutes typically causes resolution within 1 week. Because they arise from the same glands, hordeola and blepharitis commonly occur together.

Episcleritis

Episcleritis is a self-limited inflammation of the episcleral vessels and is believed to be autoimmune. It has a rapid onset and usually minimal discomfort. Redness is most often confined to a sector of the eye. Episcleritis usually resolves in 7 to 10 days. Recurrence is not uncommon. Oral NSAID drugs may be prescribed, but treatment is usually not necessary.

Scleritis

Scleritis is, fortunately, much less common than episcleritis. Patients with scleritis experience intense inflammation and deep eye pain. Scleritis is commonly associated with rheumatoid arthritis and inflammatory bowel disease. The patient should be promptly referred to an ophthalmologist if scleritis is suspected.

Acute Angle Closure Glaucoma

Acute angle closure glaucoma is characterized by acute ocular pain and is often accompanied by vomiting, blurred vision, acute photophobia, pupils unreactive to light, and circumcorneal redness (ciliary flush). Treatment of glaucoma with pilocarpine (Isopto Carpine), topical timolol (Timoptic), and acetazolamide (Diamox) should be started, and the patient should be given an urgent referral to an ophthalmologist.

Anterior Uveitis

Uveitis is the inflammation of the iris and ciliary muscle, often associated with autoimmune disease. Trauma can also cause uveitis. Signs of uveitis include ocular pain, ciliary flush, and occasionally irregularity of the pupil. Prompt referral should be arranged for a patient in whom uveitis is suspected.

In general, referral to an ophthalmologist should be considered for the following:

- Traumatic injury to the eye
- Loss of vision
- Extreme eye pain not explained by pathology
- Keratitis
- Suspected uveitis or glaucoma
- Chemical injury (especially alkali)
- Corneal abrasion not healing

References

Ackay B, Kardes E, Kiray G, et al: Evaluation of ocular symptoms in COVID-19 subjects in inpatient and outpatient settings, *International Ophthalmology* 41:1541–1548, 2021.

American Optometric Association: *Optometric clinical practice guideline: Care of the patient with anterior uveitis*, June 23, 1994. Revised March 1999. PDF available at www.aoa.org/documents/CPG-7.pdf. June 23, 1994 [accessed July 10, 2015].

Arbour JD, Brunette I, Boisjoly HM, et al: Should we patch corneal abrasions? *Arch Ophthalmol* 115(3):313–317, 1997.

Au YK, Henkind P: Pain elicited by consensual pupillary reflex: a diagnostic test for acute iritis, *Lancet* 2:1254–1255, 1981.

Avdic E, Cosgrove SE: Management and control strategies for community-associated methicillin-resistant *Staphylococcus aureus*, *Expert Opin Pharmacother* 9(9):1463–1479, 2008.

Boder F, Marchant C, et al: Bacterial etiology of conjunctivitis-otitis media syndrome, *Pediatrics* 76:26–28, 1985.

Bradford CA: *Basic Ophthalmology* San Francisco, ed 8, 2004, American Academy of Ophthalmology.

Centers for Disease Control and Prevention. Zika Virus. Symptoms, diagnosis, and treatment. Available at www.cdc.gov/zika/symptoms. Accessed Feb. 3, 2016.

Centers for Disease Control and Prevention: *Sexually Transmitted Diseases Treatment Guidelines*, 2015. Available at www.cdc.gov/std/tg2015/default.htm. Accessed May 25, 2021.

Centers for Disease Control and Prevention. Conjunctivitis (Pink Eye). Conjunctivitis Information for Clinicians. Accessed March 26, 2024.

De Toledo AR, Chandler JW: Conjunctivitis of the newborn, *Infect Dis Clin North Am* 6(4):807–813, 1992.

Frith P, Gray R, MacLennan S, et al: *The Eye in Clinical Practice*, Oxford, 1994, Blackwell Scientific.

Jackson WB: Blepharitis: Current strategies for diagnosis and treatment, *Can J Ophthalmol* 43(2):170–179, 2008.

Khan J, Mack H: Management of conjunctivitis and other causes of red eye during the COVID-19 Pandemic, *AJGP* 49(10):656–661, 2020.

Kimberlin D, Brady M, Jackson M: *Red Book. Report of the Committee on Infectious Diseases*, ed 31, AAP Committee on Infectious Diseases, 2018.

Liebowitz HM: The red eye, *N Engl J Med* 343(5):345–351, 2000.

Patterson J, Fetzer D, Krall J, et al: Eye patch treatment for the pain of corneal abrasion, *South Med J* 89(2):227–229, 1996.

Prochazka AV: Diagnosis and treatment of red eye, *Primary Care Case Reviews* 4:23–31, 2001.

Rietveld RP, van Weert H, Riet G, Bindels P: Diagnostic impact of signs and symptoms in acute infectious conjunctivitis: systematic literature search, *BMJ* 327(4):789, 2003.

SeyedAlinaghi S, Mehraeen E, Afzalian A, et al: Ocular Manifestations of Covid-19: A systematic review of current evidence, *Preventive Medicine Reports* 38, 2024:102608.

Tarabishy A: Jeng B: Bacterial conjunctivitis: A review for internists, *Cleve Clin J Med* 75(7):507–512, 2008.

Talbot EM: A simple test to diagnose iritis, *BMJ* 295:812–813, 1987.

Trobe JD: *The Physician's Guide to Eye Care*, ed 2, San Francisco, 2001, Foundation of the American Academy of Ophthalmology.

Wilson SA, Last A: Management of corneal abrasion, *Am Fam Physician* 70:123–130, 2004.

Wong AH, Barg SS, Leung AK: Seasonal and perennial allergic conjunctivitis, *Recent Pat Inflamm Allergy Drug Disc* 3(2):118–127, 2009.

RHINOSINUSITIS

Method of
Ann M. Aring, MD

CURRENT DIAGNOSIS

- Because inflammation of the sinuses rarely occurs without concurrent inflammation of the nasal mucosa, *rhinosinusitis* is a more accurate term for what is commonly called sinusitis.
- Most cases of sinusitis are caused by viral infections associated with the common cold. Viral rhinosinusitis improves in 7 to 10 days.

- Four signs and symptoms with a high likelihood ratio for acute bacterial sinusitis are double sickening, purulent rhinorrhea, erythrocyte sedimentation rate (ESR) >10 mm, and purulent secretion in the nasal cavity. A combination of at least three of these four symptoms and signs has a specificity of 0.81 and sensitivity of 0.66 for acute bacterial rhinosinusitis.
- Acute rhinosinusitis lasts up to 4 weeks, subacute rhinosinusitis lasts from 4 to 12 weeks, and chronic rhinosinusitis lasts 12 weeks or longer. Recurrent acute rhinosinusitis is defined as four or more episodes per year with complete resolution between episodes.
- Radiographic imaging in a patient with acute rhinosinusitis is not recommended unless a complication or an alternative diagnosis is suspected. Computed tomography of the sinuses without contrast media is the imaging method of choice.

CURRENT THERAPY

- Mild rhinosinusitis symptoms of less than 7 days' duration can be managed with supportive care including analgesics, saline nasal irrigation, and intranasal corticosteroids.
- Antibiotic therapy is recommended for patients with sinusitis symptoms that do not improve within 7 to 10 days or that worsen at any time.
- First-line antibiotics include amoxicillin with or without clavulanate.
- Macrolides and trimethoprim sulfamethoxazole (Bactrim) are not recommended for empiric therapy owing to high rates of resistance among *Streptococcus pneumoniae* and *Haemophilus influenzae*.
- For adults allergic to penicillin, doxycycline may be used as an alternative regimen for initial empiric therapy for bacterial rhinosinusitis. According to a US Food and Drug Administration (FDA) safety alert, fluoroquinolones such as levofloxacin (Levaquin) and moxifloxacin (Avelox) should be reserved for patients who do not have other treatment options.
- In adults with confirmed acute rhinosinusitis, more than 70% will clinically improve after 2 weeks with or without antibiotic therapy.
- Antibiotic use increases the absolute cure rate by 5% compared with placebo at 7 to 15 days.

Epidemiology of Acute Rhinosinusitis and Predisposing Factors

Each year in the United States, rhinosinusitis affects one in seven adults and is diagnosed in 31 million patients. Rhinosinusitis is the fifth most common diagnosis for which antibiotics are prescribed. Rhinosinusitis has a higher frequency in the winter months and lower frequency in the summer and autumn months.

Predisposing Factors

Predisposing factors for acute rhinosinusitis include viral upper respiratory infections and allergic rhinitis. Anatomic malformations including polyps, deviated nasal septum, foreign bodies, and tumors can also predispose to acute rhinosinusitis.

Pathogenesis and Etiology of Rhinosinusitis

Most cases of acute rhinosinusitis are caused by viral infections associated with the common cold. The most common viruses in acute viral rhinosinusitis are rhinovirus, adenovirus, influenza virus, and parainfluenza virus. Mucosal edema occurs with the viral infection with subsequent obstruction of the sinus ostia. In addition, viral and bacterial infections impair the cilia, which help transport the mucus. The ostia obstruction and slowed mucus transport cause stagnation of secretions and lowered oxygen tension within the sinuses. This environment is an excellent culture medium for both viruses and bacteria, and the infectious particles grow rapidly. The body responds with an inflammatory reaction. Polymorphonuclear leukocytes are mobilized, which results in pus formation. The most common bacteria found in acute community-acquired bacterial rhinosinusitis are *Streptococcus pneumoniae, Haemophilus influenzae, Staphylococcus aureus,* and *Moraxella catarrhalis.* Acute adult rhinosinusitis most commonly involves the maxillary and ethmoid sinuses. More than one of the paranasal sinuses can be affected.

Diagnosis of Acute Rhinosinusitis

Diagnosis of acute bacterial rhinosinusitis requires that symptoms persist for longer than 10 days or worsen after 5 to 7 days. Four signs and symptoms with a high likelihood ratio for acute bacterial sinusitis are double sickening, purulent rhinorrhea, erythrocyte sedimentation rate (ESR) >10 mm, and purulent secretion in the nasal cavity. A combination of at least three of these four symptoms and signs has a specificity of 0.81 and sensitivity of 0.66 for acute bacterial rhinosinusitis. Table 1 lists the sensitivity, specificity, likelihood ratio, and odds ratio of criteria used to diagnose acute rhinosinusitis. If resistant pathogens are suspected or if the patient's immune system is compromised, bacterial culture of the secretions may be used for diagnosis and to direct therapy.

Imaging

For uncomplicated acute rhinosinusitis, radiographic imaging is not recommended. Plain sinus radiography shows air–fluid levels in patients with both viral and bacterial rhinosinusitis. Sinus computed tomography (CT) should not be used for routine evaluation of acute bacterial rhinosinusitis. However, sinus CT without contrast media can be used to identify suspected complications and define anatomic abnormalities.

Differential Diagnosis

The signs and symptoms of acute bacterial rhinosinusitis and prolonged viral upper respiratory infection are similar, which can lead to overdiagnosis of acute bacterial rhinosinusitis. Other conditions that mimic bacterial rhinosinusitis are migraine headache, tension headache, trigeminal neuralgia, and temporomandibular joint disorders.

Treatment of Acute Rhinosinusitis
Symptomatic Treatment

Mild rhinosinusitis symptoms less than 7 days in duration can be managed with supportive care including analgesics, saline nasal irrigation, and intranasal corticosteroids. There are no randomized controlled trials that evaluate the effectiveness of decongestants in patients with sinusitis. Nasal saline is used to soften viscous secretions and improve mucociliary clearance. The mechanical cleansing of the nasal cavity with saline has been shown to benefit patients with rhinosinusitis. Most studies of intranasal corticosteroids are industry sponsored. A Cochrane review found that patients receiving intranasal corticosteroids were more likely to experience symptom improvement after 15 to 21 days compared with those receiving placebo (73% vs. 66.4%; $p < .05$; number needed to treat [NNT] = 15). Antihistamines should not be used for symptomatic relief of acute rhinosinusitis, except in patients with a history of allergic rhinitis.

Antibiotic Treatment

Antibiotic therapy is recommended for patients with sinusitis symptoms that do not improve within 7 to 10 days or that worsen at any time. Amoxicillin with or without clavulanate is recommended as the first-line antibiotic in adults with acute bacterial rhinosinusitis. "High-dose" amoxicillin-clavulanate (Augmentin XR) is recommended for patients with high risk of *S. pneumoniae* resistance, recent antibiotic use, or treatment failure. Macrolides and trimethoprim sulfamethoxazole are not recommended for empiric therapy owing to high rates of resistance among *S. pneumoniae* and *H. influenzae.* Fluoroquinolones are not recommended as first-line antibiotics because they do not demonstrate benefit over β-lactam antibiotics and are associated with a variety of adverse effects. According to an FDA safety alert, fluoroquinolones should be reserved for patients who do not have other treatment options.

Complications and Referral

Complications of acute bacterial rhinosinusitis are estimated to occur in 1 in 1000 cases. Patients with acute bacterial rhinosinusitis who present with visual symptoms (diplopia, decreased visual acuity, disconjugate gaze, difficulty opening the eye), severe headache, somnolence, or high fever should be evaluated with emergency CT with contrast. Sinonasal cancers are uncommon in the United States, with an annual incidence of less than 1 in 100,000 patients. However, cancer should be included in the differential diagnosis. Referral to an otolaryngologist is needed if symptoms persist or progress after maximal medical therapy when CT shows evidence of sinus disease. Table 2 summarizes indications for subspecialist referral in a patient with acute bacterial rhinosinusitis.

TABLE 1	Signs and Symptoms of Acute Bacterial Rhinosinusitis			
SIGN/SYMPTOM	SENSITIVITY (%)	SPECIFICITY (%)	LR +	ODDS RATIO
Symptoms after upper respiratory tract infection	87	27	1.2	2.6
Facial pain on bending forward	72	39	1.2	1.7
Nasal congestion	83	24	1.1	1.5
Purulent rhinorrhea	71	54	1.6	2.9
Maxillary pain, pressure, or fullness	70	20	0.88	1.9
Double sickening	74	41	1.3	2.7
Previous sinusitis	59	27	0.81	0.55
Upper teeth pain	34	80	1.8	2.1
Unilateral facial pain, pressure, or fullness	30	80	1.5	1.9

LR, Likelihood ratio.
From Ebell, MH, McKay, B, Dale A, et al: Accuracy of signs and symptoms for the diagnosis of acute rhinosinusitis and acute bacterial rhinosinusitis, *Ann Fam Med* 17(2):164–172, 2019.

TABLE 2	Indications for Subspecialist Referral for Acute Bacterial Rhinosinusitis
Anatomic defects causing obstruction
Complications such as orbital involvement, altered mental status, meningitis, cavernous sinus thrombosis, intracranial abscess, Pott puffy tumor (osteomyelitis of front bone)
Evaluation of immunotherapy for allergic rhinitis
Frequent recurrences (3–4 episodes per year)
Fungal sinusitis, granulomatous disease, or possible neoplasm
Immunocompromised host
Nosocomial infection
Severe infection with persistent fever >102°F or 39°C
Treatment failure after extended antibiotic courses
Unusual or resistant bacteria

From Aring AM, Chan MM: Current concepts in adult acute rhinosinusitis, *Am Fam Physician* 94(2):97–105, 2016.

References

Aring AM, Chan MM: Current concepts in adult acute rhinosinusitis, *Am Fam Physician* 94(2):97–105, 2016.

Butler FM, Rivera Hernandez D: Acute rhinosinusitis: rapid evidence review, *Am Fam Physician* 111(1):47–53, 2025.

Chow AW, Benninger MS, Brook I, et al: IDSA clinical practice guideline for acute bacterial rhinosinusitis in children and adults, *Clin Infect Dis* 54(8):e72–112, 2012. Epub 2012 Mar 20.

Cornelius RS, Martin J, Wippold 2nd FJ, et al: ACR appropriateness criteria sinonasal disease, *J Am Coll Radiol* 10(4):241–246, 2013.

DeSutter AI, Lemiengre M, Campbell H: Antihistamines for the common cold, *Cochrane Database Syst Rev* CD009345, 2015.

Ebell MH, McKay B, Dale A, et al: Accuracy of signs and symptoms for the diagnosis of acute rhinosinusitis and acute bacterial rhinosinusitis, *Ann Fam Med* 17(2):164–172, 2019.

Hagiwara M, et al: ACR appropriateness criteria sinonasal disease: 2021 update, *J Am Col Radiol* 19(5):S175–192, 2022.

Hayward G, Heneghan C, Perera R, Thompson M: Intranasal corticosteroids in management of acute sinusitis: a systematic review and meta-analysis, *Ann Fam Med* 10:241–249, 2012. https://doi.org/10.1370/afm.1338.

King D, Mitchell B, Williams CP, Spurling GKP: Saline nasal irrigation for acute upper respiratory tract infections, *Cochrane Database Syst Rev* 4, 2015. https://doi.org/10.1002/14651858.CD006821.pub3.

Lemiengre MB, van Driel ML, Merenstein D, et al: Antibiotics for acute rhinosinusitis in adults, *Cochrane Database Syst Rev* 9:CD006089, 2018.

Rosenfeld RM, Piccirillo JF, Chadrasekhar SS, et al: Clinical practice guideline (update): adult sinusitis, *Otolaryngol Head Neck Surg* 152(2S):S1–39, 2015.

U.S. Food and Drug Administration. FDA Drug Safety Communication: FDA updates warnings for oral and injectable fluoroquinolone antibiotics due to disabling side effects. Available at http://www.fda.gov/Drugs/DrugSafety/ucm511530.htm [accessed January 28, 2017].

Zalmanovici Trestioreanu A, Yaphe J: Intranasal steroids for acute sinusitis, *Cochrane Database Syst Rev* 12, 2013.

TEMPOROMANDIBULAR DISORDERS

Method of
Jeffrey Paul Okeson, DMD

Temporomandibular disorder (TMD) is a collective term that includes a number of clinical complaints involving the muscles of mastication, the temporomandibular joints (TMJs) and associated orofacial structures. Other commonly used terms are Costen's syndrome, TMJ dysfunction, and craniomandibular disorders. TMDs are a major cause of nondental pain in the orofacial region and are considered a subclassification of musculoskeletal disorders. In many TMD patients the most common complaint is not with the TMJs but rather the muscles of mastication. Therefore the terms *TMJ dysfunction* or *TMJ disorder* are actually inappropriate for many of these complaints. It is for this reason that the American Dental Association adopted the term *temporomandibular disorder*.

Signs and symptoms associated with TMDs are a common source of pain complaints in the head and orofacial structures. These complaints can be associated with general joint problems and somatization. Approximately 50% of patients suffering with TMDs do not first consult with a dentist but seek advice for the problem from a physician. The family physician should be able to appropriately diagnose many TMDs. In many instances the physician can provide valuable information and simple therapies that will reduce the patient's TMD symptoms. In other instances, it is appropriate to refer the patient to a dentist with training in TMD. The dental profession has a specialty in orofacial pain, and this formal training can be very useful in selecting the best care for the patient.

Epidemiology

Cross-sectional population-based studies reveal that 40% to 75% of adult populations have at least one sign of TMJ dysfunction (e.g., jaw movement abnormalities, joint noise, tenderness on palpation), and approximately 33% have at least one symptom (e.g., face pain, joint pain). Many of these signs and symptoms are not troublesome for the patient, and only 3% to 7% of the population seeks any advice or care. Although in the general population

women seem to have only a slightly greater incidence of TMD symptoms, women seek care for TMD more often than men at a ratio ranging from 3:1 to 9:1. For many patients, acute TMDs are self-limiting or are associated with symptoms that fluctuate over time without evidence of progression. Even though many of these disorders are self-limiting, the healthcare provider can provide conservative therapies that will minimize the patient's painful experience.

Signs and Symptoms

The primary signs and symptoms associated with TMD originate from the masticatory structures and are associated with jaw function (Box 1). Pain during opening of the mouth or during chewing is common. Some persons even report difficulty speaking or singing. Patients often report pain in the preauricular areas, face, or temples. TMJ sounds are often described as clicking, popping, grating, or crepitus and can produce locking of the jaw during opening or closing. Patients commonly report painful jaw muscles, and, on occasion, they even report a sudden change in their bite coincident with the onset of the painful condition.

It is important to appreciate that pain associated with most TMDs is increased with jaw function. Because this is a condition of the musculoskeletal structures, function of these structures generally increases the pain. When a patient's pain complaint is not influenced by jaw function, other sources of orofacial pain should be suspected.

The spectrum of TMD often includes commonly associated complaints such as headache, neckache, or earache. These associated complaints are often referred pains and must be differentiated from primary pains.

As a general rule, referred pains associated with TMDs are increased with any activity that provokes the TMD pain. Therefore, if the patient reports that the headache is aggravated by jaw function, it could very well represent a secondary pain related to the TMD. Likewise, if the secondary symptom is unaffected by jaw use, one should question its relationship to the TMD and suspect two separate pain conditions. Pain or dysfunction due to non-musculoskeletal causes such as otolaryngologic, neurologic, vascular, neoplastic, or infectious disease in the orofacial region is not considered a primary TMD even though musculoskeletal pain may be present. However, TMDs often coexist with other craniofacial and orofacial pain disorders.

Anatomy and Pathophysiology

The TMJ is formed by the mandibular condyle fitting into the mandibular fossa of the temporal bone. The movement of this joint is quite complex as it allows hinging movement in one plane and at the same time allows gliding movements in another plane. Separating these two bones from direct articulation is the articular disk. The articular disk is composed of dense fibrous connective

---

BOX 1 Common Primary and Secondary Symptoms Associated With Temporomandibular Disorders

Primary Symptoms
Facial muscle pain
Preauricular (TMJ) pain
TMJ sounds: jaw clicking, popping, catching, locking
Limited mouth opening
Increased pain associated with function (e.g., chewing, talking)

Secondary Symptoms
Earache
Headache
Neckache

TMJ, Temporomandibular joint.

tissue devoid of any blood vessels or nerve fibers. The articular disk is attached posteriorly to a region of loose connective tissue that is highly vascularized and well innervated, known as the retrodiscal tissue. The anterior region of the disk is attached to the superior lateral pterygoid muscle.

The movement of the mandible is accomplished by four pairs of muscles called the muscles of mastication: the masseter, temporalis, medial pterygoid, and lateral pterygoid. Although not considered to be muscles of mastication, the digastric muscles also play an important role in mandibular function. The masseter, temporalis, and medial pterygoid muscles elevate the mandible and therefore provide the major forces used for chewing and other jaw functions. The inferior lateral pterygoid muscles provide protrusive movement of the mandible, and the digastric muscles serve to depress the mandible (open the mouth).

When discussing the pathophysiology of TMD, one needs to consider two main categories: joint pathophysiology and muscle pathophysiology. Because etiologic considerations and treatment strategies are different for these conditions, they are presented separately.

Pathophysiology of Intracapsular Temporomandibular Joint Pain Disorders

Several common arthritic conditions such as rheumatoid arthritis, traumatic arthritis, hyperuricemia, and psoriatic arthritis can affect the TMJ. These conditions, however, are not nearly as common as local osteoarthritis. As with most other joints, osteoarthritis results from overloading the articular surface of the joint, thus breaking down the dense fibrocartilage articular surface and ultimately affecting the subarticular bone. In the TMJ, this overloading commonly occurs as a result of an alteration in the morphology and position of the articular disc. In the healthy TMJ, the disc maintains its position on the condyle during movement because of its morphology (i.e., the thicker anterior and posterior borders) and interarticular pressure maintained by the elevator muscles. If, however, the morphology of the disc is altered and the discal ligaments become elongated, the disk can be displaced from its normal position between the condyle and fossa. If the disc is displaced, normal opening and closing of the mouth can result in an unusual translatory movement between the condyle and the disc, which is felt as a click or pop. Disc displacements that result in joint sounds might or might not be painful. When pain is present it is believed to be related to either loading forces applied to the highly vascularized retrodiscal tissues or a general inflammatory response of the surrounding soft tissues (capsulitis or synovitis).

Pathophysiology of Masticatory Muscle Pain Disorders

The muscles of mastication are a common source of TMD pain. Understanding the pathophysiology of muscle pain, however, is very complex and still not well understood. The simple explanation of muscle spasm does not account for most TMD muscle pain complaints. It appears that a better explanation would include a central nervous system effect on the muscle that results in an increase in peripheral nociceptive activity originating from the muscle tissue itself. This explanation more accurately accounts for the high levels of emotional stress that are commonly associated with TMD muscle pain complaints. In other words, an increase in emotional stress activates the autonomic nervous system, which in turn seems to be associated with changes in muscle nociception. It is important to appreciate that there are common chronic overlapping pain conditions that are associated with TMD that can complicate diagnosis and management. Such overlapping conditions include fibromyalgia, migraine, lower back pain, and irritable bowel syndrome.

These masticatory muscle pain conditions are further complicated when one considers the unique masticatory muscle activity known as bruxism. Bruxism is the subconscious, often rhythmic, grinding or gnashing of the teeth. This type of muscle activity is considered to be parafunctional and can also occur as a simple static loading of the teeth known as clenching. This activity commonly occurs during sleep but can also be present during the day.

These parafunctional activities are central nervous system induced and can cause tooth wear. This activity is common and not normally associated with pain. Muscle pain seems to be more related to maintaining a prolonged slight increase in muscle tonicity.

Etiology

Because TMD represents a group of disorders, any of several etiologies may be associated. Problems arising from intracapsular conditions (clicking, popping, catching, locking) may be associated with various types of traumas. Gross trauma, such as a blow to the chin, can immediately alter ligamentous structures of the joint, leading to joint sounds. Trauma can also be associated with a slight injury such as stretching, twisting, or compressing forces during eating, yawning, yelling, or prolonged mouth opening.

When the patient's chief complaint is muscle pain, etiologic factors other than trauma should be considered. Masticatory muscle pain disorders have etiologic considerations similar to other muscle pain disorders of the neck and back. Emotional stress seems to play a significant role for many patients. This can explain why patients often report that their painful symptoms fluctuate greatly over time.

Although most acute TMD patients may not have a major psychiatric condition, psychological factors can certainly enhance the pain condition. The clinician needs to consider such factors as anxiety, depression, secondary gain, somatization, and hypochondriasis. Psychosocial factors can predispose certain people to TMD and can also perpetuate TMD once symptoms have become established. A careful consideration of psychosocial factors is therefore important in the evaluation and treatment, especially in patients with chronic TMD. TMDs have a few unique etiologic factors that differentiate them from other musculoskeletal disorders. One such factor is the occlusal relationship of the teeth. Traditionally it was thought that malocclusion was the primary etiologic factor responsible for TMD. Recent investigations, however, do not support this concept. Still, in certain instances occlusal instability of the teeth can contribute to a TMD. This may be true in patients with or without teeth. Poorly fitting dental prostheses can also contribute to occlusal instability. The occlusal condition should especially be suspected if the pain problem began with a change in the patient's bite (e.g., after a dental appointment).

History and Examination

All patients reporting pain in the orofacial structures should be screened for TMD. This can be accomplished with a brief history and physical examination. The screening questions and examination are performed to rule in or out the possibility of a TMD. If a positive response is found, a more extensive history and examination is indicated. Box 2 lists questions that should be asked during a screening assessment for TMD. Any positive response should be followed by additional clarifying questions.

Patients experiencing orofacial pain should also be briefly examined for any clinical signs associated with TMD. The clinician can easily palpate a few sites to assess tenderness or pain, as well as assess for jaw mobility. The masseter muscles can be palpated bilaterally while asking the patient to report any pain or tenderness. The same assessment should be made for the temporal regions, as well as the preauricular (TMJ) areas. While the examiner's hands are over the preauricular areas, the patient should repeatedly open and close the mouth. The presence of joint sounds should be noted along with whether these sounds are associated with joint pain.

A simple measurement of mouth opening should be made. This can be accomplished by placing a millimeter ruler on the lower anterior teeth and asking the patient to open as wide as possible. The distance should be measured between the maxillary and mandibular anterior teeth. It is generally accepted that less than 40 mm is a restricted mouth opening.

It is also helpful to inspect the teeth for significant wear, mobility, or decay that may be related to the pain condition. The clinician should examine the buccal mucosa for ridging and the lateral aspect of the tongue for scalloping. These are often signs of clenching and bruxism. A general inspection for symmetry and alignment of the face, jaws, and dental arches may also be helpful. A summary of this screening examination is shown in Box 3.

Treatment

Most recent studies suggest that TMDs are generally self-limiting, and symptoms often fluctuate over time. Understanding this natural course does not mean these conditions should be ignored. TMD can be a very painful condition leading to a significant decrease in the patient's quality of life. Understanding the natural course of TMD does suggest, however, that therapy might not need to be very aggressive. In general, initial therapy should begin very conservatively and only escalate when therapy fails to relieve the symptoms.

When the physician identifies a patient with a TMD, he or she has two options. The physician can elect to treat the patient or refer the patient to a dentist who specializes in orofacial pain for further evaluation and treatment. The decision to refer the patient should be based on whether the patient needs any unique care provided only in a dental office. The following are some indications for referral to a dentist:

- History of trauma to the face related to the onset of the pain condition
- The presence of significant TMJ sounds during function
- A feeling of jaw catching or locking during mouth opening
- The report of a sudden change in the occlusal contacts of the teeth
- The presence of significant occlusal instability
- Significant findings related to the teeth (e.g., tooth mobility, tooth sensitivity, tooth decay, tooth wear)
- Significant pain in the jaws or masticatory muscles upon awakening
- The presence of an orofacial pain condition that is aggravated by jaw function and has been present for more than several months

The specific therapy for a TMD varies according to the precise type of disorder identified. In other words, masticatory muscle pain is managed somewhat differently than intracapsular pain. Generally, however, the initial therapy for any type of TMD should be directed toward the relief of pain and the improvement of function. This initial conservative therapy can be divided into three general types: patient education, pharmacologic therapy, and physical therapy.

Patient Education

It is very important that patients have an appreciation for the factors that may be associated with their disorder, as well as the natural course of the disorder. Patients should be reassured and if necessary, convinced by appropriate tests, that they are not suffering from a malignancy. Properly educated patients can contribute greatly to their own treatment. For example, knowing that emotional stress is an influencing factor in many TMDs can help the patient understand the reason for daily fluctuations of pain intensity. Attention should be directed toward changing the patient's response to stress or, when possible, reducing exposure to stressful conditions. Patients with pain during chewing should be told to begin a softer diet, chew slower, and eat smaller bites. As a general rule the patient should be told "if it hurts, don't do it." Continued pain can contribute to the cycling of pain and should always be avoided. The patient should be instructed to let the jaw muscles relax, maintaining the teeth apart. This will discourage clenching activities and minimize loading of the teeth and joints.

When pain is associated with a clicking TM joint, the patient should be informed of the biomechanics of the joint. This information often allows the patient to select functional activities that are less traumatic to the joint structures. For example, some patients may report that the pain and clicking are less when they chew on a particular side of the mouth. When this occurs, they should be encouraged to continue this type of chewing.

Pharmacologic Therapy

Pharmacologic therapy can be an effective adjunct in managing symptoms associated with TMDs. Patients should be aware that medication alone will not likely solve or cure the problem. Medication, however, in conjunction with appropriate physical therapy and definitive treatment, does offer the most complete approach to many TMD problems. Mild analgesics are often helpful for many TMDs. Control of pain is not only appreciated by the patient but also reduces the likelihood of other complicating pain disorders such as muscle co-contraction, referred pain, and central sensitization.

Nonsteroidal antiinflammatory drugs are very helpful with many TMDs. Included in this category are aspirin, acetaminophen (Tylenol), and ibuprofen (Motrin, Advil, Nuprin). Ibuprofen is often very effective in reducing musculoskeletal pains. A dosage of 400 to 600 mg three times a day for 3 to 5 days commonly reduces pain and stops the cyclic effects of the deep pain input. For patients with gastrointestinal issues, short-term use of a cyclooxygenase-2 inhibitor such as celecoxib (Celebrex) can also be useful.

Physical Therapy

In many patients with TMD, symptoms are relieved with very simple physical therapy methods. Simple instructions for the use of moist heat or cold can be very helpful. Surface heat can be applied by laying a hot, moist towel over the symptomatic area. A hot water bottle wrapped inside the towel will help maintain the heat. This combination should remain in place for 10 to 15 minutes, not to exceed 30 minutes. An electric heating pad may be used, but care should be taken not to leave it on the face too long. Patients should be discouraged from using the heating pad while sleeping because prolonged use is likely.

Like thermotherapy, coolant therapy can provide a simple and often effective method of reducing pain. Ice should be applied directly to the symptomatic joint or muscles and moved in a circular motion without pressure to the tissues. The patient will initially experience an uncomfortable feeling that will quickly turn into a burning sensation. Continued icing will result in a mild aching and then numbness. When numbness begins the ice should be removed. The ice should not be left on the tissues for longer than 5 minutes. After a period of warming a second cold application may be desirable.

The physician should be aware that many TMDs respond to the use of orthopedic appliances such as occlusal appliances, bite guards, and splints. These appliances are made by the dentist and are custom fabricated for each patient. Several types of appliances are available. Each is specific for the type of TMD present. The dentist should be consulted for this type of therapy.

Other Therapeutic Considerations

Sometimes TMDs become chronic and, as with other chronic pain conditions, might then be best managed by a multidisciplinary approach. If the patient reports a long history of TMD complaints, the physician should consider referring the patient to a trained orofacial pain dentist associated with a team of therapists, such as a psychologist, a physical therapist, and even a chronic pain physician. Generally, patients with chronic TMD are not managed well by the simple initial therapies discussed in this chapter. Often other factors, such as mechanical conditions within the TMJs or psychological factors, need to be addressed. The physician who attempts to manage these conditions in the private practice setting can become very frustrated with the results. It is therefore recommended that if the patient's history suggests chronicity or if initial therapy fails to reduce the patient's symptoms, referral is indicated.

References

Klasser GD, Romero Reyes M: *Orofacial pain: Guidelines for assessment, diagnosis, and management*, ed 7, Chicago, 2023, Quintessence.
Okeson JP: *Management of temporomandibular disorders and occlusion*, ed 8, St. Louis, 2019, Elsevier.
Okeson JP: In *Bell's orofacial pains*, ed 7, Chicago, 2014, Quintessence.
Scrivani SJ, Keith DA, Kaban LB: Temporomandibular disorders, *N Engl J Med* 359(25):2693–2705, 2008.

UVEITIS

Method of
Grace Levy-Clarke, MD

CURRENT DIAGNOSIS

- Uveitis is classified by anatomic location and etiology.
- Most forms of uveitis are due to infectious or immune-mediated disease.
- Drug-induced uveitis and masquerade disorders (neoplasms) must be excluded in diagnostic evaluations.
- Patients with first-time uveitis should have a medical history, physical examination, and targeted laboratory studies, with the possible exception of adults who have a single episode of mild anterior uveitis that responds to therapy and who have no systemic signs or symptoms.
- Diagnostic evaluation must differentiate infectious from noninfectious uveitis.
- Patients who are immunosuppressed are at higher risk of infectious uveitis, and their clinical presentations may be atypical.
- Uveitis in children is uncommon and deserves a thorough medical evaluation at initial presentation.
- Uveitis is managed optimally through a collaborative multidisciplinary approach.

CURRENT THERAPY

- Eradication of infection is the primary objective in infectious uveitis but may require judicious use of local antiinflammatory agents to mitigate structural and functional damage to intraocular tissues.
- The goal of therapy in noninfectious uveitis is to suppress and eliminate inflammation, achieving lasting remission through the stepwise implementation of therapy.
- First-time anterior uveitis in adults with negative medical history and review of systems can be treated with topical corticosteroids and cycloplegic agents and careful clinical monitoring.
- Corticosteroids can be delivered topically, through periocular and intravitreal injection, via sustained release devices implanted in the eye, and systemically.
- Immunomodulating therapy using alkylating agents, antimetabolites, biologic response modulators, or inhibitors of T-lymphocyte signaling are indicated for uveitis not responsive to systemic corticosteroids.
- A thorough history, physical examination, and select laboratory studies are required before initiating immunomodulating therapy. Subspecialty evaluations, when clinically indicated, may also be needed, such as rheumatology, neurology, or infectious disease specialists.

Current Diagnosis

Uveitis describes a heterogeneous group of disorders that have in common inflammation of the uveal tract (i.e., iris, ciliary body, and choroid). Symptoms are nonspecific, usually involving various combinations of blurred vision, ocular discomfort, intolerance to light, and floaters. Onset may be sudden or insidious. Children may have no symptoms. The essential signs of uveitis are the presence of inflammatory cells in the aqueous humor and/or vitreous gel. Sufficient magnification with a slit lamp is required to confidently detect these inflammatory cells and avoid confusion with suspended red blood cells or pigment epithelial cells. Although the uveal tract is the conceptual epicenter of uveal inflammation, there is spillover inflammation in the aqueous humor and vitreous gel, the two anatomic locations used to quantify the severity of inflammation and to monitor response to therapy. Grading schemes for recording the severity of anterior chamber and vitreous inflammatory cell density and protein content (flare) have been published by the Standardization of Uveitis Nomenclature (SUN) Classification Working Group.

Clinical Features and Diagnosis

The anatomic classification of intraocular inflammation into anterior, intermediate, and posterior uveitis and panuveitis guides the diagnostic workup toward the determination of etiology. When the anterior chamber is the principal site of inflammation, the terms iritis or iridocyclitis are often used. When the vitreous is the primary focus of inflammation, the term intermediate uveitis is preferred, but posterior cyclitis or vitritis are commonly used synonyms. Pars planitis is a clinical subtype of intermediate uveitis and is characterized by clumping or a layering of inflammatory cells over the pars plana and anterior retina called "snowballs" or a "snowbank lesion." These characteristic cells may also be seen in sarcoidosis. Posterior uveitis refers to diseases limited to the posterior segment of the eye. Comprehensive anatomical characterization includes retinitis, choroiditis, or neuroretinitis and is clinically described as focal or multifocal. This classification is informative in developing an appropriate differential diagnosis.

Most cases of uveitis are caused by infection or immune-mediated disease. A substantial proportion of immune-mediated disease is a manifestation of systemic disease. Arriving at a diagnosis of infectious or noninfectious uveitis requires exclusion of drug-induced uveitis and so-called masquerade disorders (usually neoplasms) that mimic uveal inflammation. Most undifferentiated idiopathic forms of uveitis are localized immune-mediated disease whose pathogenesis is not yet understood. Immune-mediated and infectious uveitides may have overlapping clinical features. This is important as some diseases are diagnosed based on clinical features with supporting laboratory findings. The diagnostic evaluation for persons with noninfectious uveitis and no known systemic disorders involves a complete history, review of systems, physical examination, and select laboratory tests. There is limited consensus in the uveitis community regarding appropriate laboratory testing for specific uveitic entities; however, the general recommendation is to make case-specific determinations.

The anatomic categories of posterior uveitis and panuveitis have vastly expanded the number of potential diagnoses. The pattern and distribution of inflammatory lesions of the choroid, retina, and optic nerve, along with a host of other clinical findings (e.g., vascular or perivascular involvement, severity of overlying inflammation, color and shape of choroidal and retinal lesions), are critical to narrowing the differential diagnosis. The importance of pattern recognition in the diagnosis of posterior uveitis and panuveitis cannot be overstated. Toxoplasma chorioretinitis, the most common form of posterior uveitis, can usually be confidently diagnosed by clinical ophthalmoscopic appearance of a yellow-white retina with overlying vitreal inflammation adjacent to a hyperpigmented chorioretinal scar. On the other hand, the disorders belonging to the so-called white dot syndromes (acute posterior multifocal placoid pigment epitheliopathy, multifocal chorioretinitis with panuveitis, punctate inner choroidopathy, multiple evanescent white dot syndrome, and birdshot chorioretinopathy) require diagnostic studies such as fluorescein angiography, indocyanine green angiography, optic coherence tomography (OCT), and OCT angiography to elucidate. Most of these disorders, and a few others such as Vogt-Koyanagi-Harada disease and sympathetic ophthalmia, are clinically defined syndromes. Laboratory studies in the context of a clinically defined syndrome are used to exclude conditions that could possibly mimic their appearance.

Uveitis occurs in children substantially less often than adults. Although a majority of the same infectious and noninfectious etiologies that occur in adults also affect children, juvenile idiopathic arthritis has a relatively unique clinical presentation in young patients. All four subtypes of juvenile idiopathic arthritis are associated with anterior uveitis, but the pauciarticular category may present with anterior chamber inflammation and advanced band keratopathy with few or no symptoms. This degree of incongruity between symptoms and clinical findings on slit-lamp examination is unusual in adults.

Current Therapy

The heterogeneous nature of uveitis limits the generalizability of a universal therapeutic algorithm. When the cause of uveitis is infection, the goal of therapy is to eradicate the infectious organism while controlling inflammation during the process. For noninfectious uveitis, the goal of therapy is to suppress and eliminate inflammation and to achieve lasting remission. We know from published retrospective studies that early effective treatment minimizes the disease burden, so the current paradigm is the one used by rheumatologists, which is a treat-to-target approach. The severity and pattern of inflammation at presentation and the perceived risk to vision and ocular integrity guide the initial selection of therapy. Timing of treatment escalation and transition to noncorticosteroid therapy are decisions based on multiple factors, including but not limited to ocular and systemic comorbidities. Simultaneous therapies, particularly local and systemic antiinflammatory agents, are commonly used. Multidisciplinary management is ideally suited to combine the expertise needed to track the ocular response to treatment and to prescribe and monitor many of the systemic mediations.

Anterior Uveitis

Anterior uveitis, the most common subset of uveitis, is usually noninfectious. A minority of cases are attributed to viruses, most often herpes simplex virus (HSV), varicella-zoster virus (VZV), and cytomegalovirus (CMV). Acute anterior uveitis associated with an underlying viral etiology is typically associated with increased intraocular pressure and iris atrophy. The diagnosis of viral anterior uveitis is typically a clinical one; when a diagnostic dilemma exists, then an anterior chamber tap with polymerase chain reaction analysis is recommended. In general, prompt empiric oral therapy will shorten the course, and tailored maintenance therapy may be indicated to decrease recurrences. For HSV or VZV, therapy with oral acyclovir (Zovirax),[1] valacyclovir (Valtrex),[1] or famciclovir (Famvir)[1] is started. After clinical resolution of inflammation, maintenance therapy with an oral antiviral drug is recommended. The optimal treatment for anterior uveitis due to CMV is still being evaluated, with current recommendations for systemic therapy (with oral ganciclovir[2] or intravenous foscarnet [Foscavir][1] or intravenous ganciclovir [Cytovene]).[1] Maintenance therapy with topical ganciclovir (Zirgan)[1] or oral valganciclovir (Valcyte)[1] should be considered. The antiviral therapy is used with concomitant topical therapy discussed in the next section. Duration of maintenance therapies for viral anterior uveitis is a clinical decision and should be individualized.

The vast majority of anterior uveitis is noninfectious, for which the mainstay of treatment is topical corticosteroids with cycloplegics (Table 1). There are nearly 20 different preparations of topical corticosteroid (e.g., dexamethasone sodium phosphate 0.1% solution; prednisolone acetate 1.0% suspension [Pred Forte]) that come in suspension or solution (and some as ointment) and in different concentrations. Dose and duration of use is tailored to the clinical setting.

Topical nonsteroidal antiinflammatory agents (e.g., diclofenac 0.1% [Voltaren][1]; ketorolac 0.4% [Acular];[1] flurbiprofen 0.03% [Ocufen][1]) are less effective than topical corticosteroids in controlling the inflammation of anterior uveitis. Their use in combination with topical corticosteroids may be additive.[1]

Topical cycloplegics provide pain relief, and the mydriasis they produce reduces the risk of iridolenticular scarring. The selection of a long-acting (e.g., atropine sulfate 1% [Isopto Atropine][1] twice daily) versus short-acting cycloplegic agent (e.g., cyclopentolate hydrochloride 0.5%–1.0% [Cyclogyl][1] two or three times a day) is based on clinical features such as severity of inflammation, presence of synechial scarring, age of patient, ability to take topical medications, and so on. Duration of action varies from 1 to 2 weeks for topical atropine to approximately half a day for cyclopentolate.

Noninfectious anterior uveitis is commonly associated with surgical trauma and accidental blunt trauma (concussive injury). They are usually effectively managed with tapering regimens of topical corticosteroids and cycloplegics.

Oral prednisone (1 mg/kg/day) may be needed for severe or recalcitrant anterior uveitis. Strategies for therapeutic escalation beyond oral corticosteroids parallel that of intermediate or posterior uveitis.

Although topical corticosteroids and cycloplegics do not play a primary role in intermediate and posterior uveitis, they are used as adjuvant therapies for comfort and to minimize the formation

---

[1] Not FDA approved for this indication.
[2] Not available in the United States.

TABLE 1 Topical Medications for Anterior Uveitis

DRUG NAME (TRADE NAMES)	FORMULATION	STARTING DOSE SCHEDULE*
Topical Corticosteroids		
Dexamethasone (Decadron phosphate [Maxidex])	0.1% suspension; 0.1% solution; 0.05% ointment[2]	4 times per day
Difluprednate (Durezol)	0.05% emulsion	4 times per day
Fluorometholone alcohol (Flarex, FML)	0.1 and 0.25% suspensions; 0.1% ointment	2–4 times per day; 1–3 times per day
Loteprednol etabonate (Lotemax)	0.5% suspension	4 times per day
Loteprednol etabonate (Alrex)	0.2% suspension[1]	3 times per day
Prednisolone acetate (Pred Forte, Econopred Plus; AK-Tate)	1.0% suspension	4 times per day
Prednisolone sodium phosphate (Inflamase Forte; AK-Pred)	1.0% solution	4 times per day
Prednisolone acetate (Pred Mild; Econopred)	0.12% suspension	4 times per day
Topical Cycloplegic Agents		
Atropine sulfate (Isopto Atropine)	1.0%	Once or twice a day
Cyclopentolate hydrochloride (Cyclogyl)[1]	0.5% and 1.0%	Twice a day
Homatropine hydrobromide (Isopto homatropine)	5.0% (1.0%–2.0%)	Once or twice a day
Scopolamine hydrobromide (Isopto hyoscine)	0.25%	Once or twice a day
Tropicamide (Mydriacyl)[1]	0.5% and 1.0%	2–3 times a day
Topical Nonsteroidal Antiinflammatory Medications		
Bromfenac (BromSite; Prolensa; Xibrom)[1]	0.075%–0.09% solution	Once or twice daily
Diclofenac (Voltaren)[1]	0.1% solution	2 times per day
Flurbiprofen (Ocufen)[1]	0.03% solution	2 times per day
Ketorolac (Acular LS; Acular)[1]	0.4%–0.5%	3 times per day
Nepafenac (Ilevro; Nevanac)[1]	0.1%–0.3% suspension	1–3 times a day, based on formulation

*Frequency of use of corticosteroids is dictated by severity of inflammation and tapered based on clinical response.
[1]Not FDA approved for this indication.
[2]Not available in the United States.

Uveitis

571

of peripheral and posterior synechiae due to associated anterior inflammation/iridocyclitis.

Intermediate Uveitis

Intermediate uveitis, characterized by inflammatory cells in vitreous, peripheral retina, and pars plana, can be associated with systemic disorders such as multiple sclerosis, sarcoidosis, syphilis, toxocariasis (in children), the human leukocyte antigen (HLA)-B27 spondyloarthropathies, and Lyme disease. Vitritis is also a presenting sign of endogenous endophthalmitis and can be mimicked by primary vitreoretinal lymphoma. Once infection, drug-related uveitis, and masquerading conditions are excluded, the approach to therapy for noninfectious forms of intermediate uveitis is similar to the stepladder approach (described later) that typically begins with oral corticosteroids. A treat-to-target approach should be taken, tailored based on disease severity, ocular and systemic comorbidities, and the presence/absence of an underlying systemic rheumatologic disorder. Additionally, known chronic/progressive ocular disorders that historically require early aggressive systemic therapy such as serpiginous or birdshot will require special considerations (Table 2). For pars planitis recalcitrant to medical therapy, options include peripheral ablation of the snowbank lesion with indirect laser photocoagulation and pars plana vitrectomy. Their effectiveness has not been rigorously tested in clinical trials.

Adjunct periocular or intravitreal therapy (i.e., regional therapy) may be an option for noninfectious intermediate, posterior, and panuveitis. Regional therapy delivers medications closer to the site of inflammation. The currently available regional therapeutic options include periocular injections of depot corticosteroids (40 mg triamcinolone acetonide [1 mL of 40 mg/mL Kenalog-40][1]); intravitreal corticosteroid injection through the pars plana (4 mg triamcinolone acetonide suspension [0.1 mL of 40 mg/mL Kenalog-40;[1] Triesence]); and a sustained-release corticosteroid implant embedded to either a biodegradable or nonbiodegradable vehicle to achieve sustained release. The implants are injected into the vitreous or surgically fixed to the sclera. Dexamethasone (Ozurdex, 0.7 mg) has a delivery span of 6 months, and fluocinolone acetonide (Iluvien 0.19 mg,[1] Retisert 0.59 mg, Yutiq 0.18 mg) 18 to 36 months. A suprachoroidal route, XIPERE is 4 mg (0.1 mL of the 40 mg/mL triamcinolone injectable suspension), specifically approved for retinal edema associated with uveitis, and was approved in 2021. In the appropriate clinical setting, these options may be tried before moving to oral prednisone or other systemic immune modulator therapy. The risk of endophthalmitis and the necessity of repeat injections need to be considered.

Posterior Uveitis and Panuveitis

The general diagnostic approach to posterior uveitis and panuveitis begins by excluding infection and drug-induced uveitis and not overlooking the possibility of a masquerade condition. The optimal strategy for laboratory testing to identify a culpable systemic disorder responsible for noninfectious uveitis is

TABLE 2 Treatment of Infectious Uveitis

DIAGNOSIS	INFECTIOUS ORGANISM(S)	TREATMENT	COMMENT
Acute retinal necrosis	Herpes zoster virus (HZV) Herpes simplex virus (HSV) I and II	Acyclovir (Zovirax)[1] 13 mg/kg/dose divided every 8 h IV for 7 days, followed by 800 mg PO 5 times/day for 3–4 months or Famciclovir (Famvir)[1] 500 mg PO q8h or Valacyclovir (Valtrex)[1] 1000–2000 mg PO q8h for induction Ganciclovir (Cytovene)[1] 500 mg IV q12h; maintenance: (duration varies with response) Valganciclovir (Valcyte)[1] 900 mg PO BID for 3 weeks then 450 mg PO BID Ganciclovir[2] 1000 mg PO TID	Adjuvant intravitreal injection options: Ganciclovir (200–2000 µg/0.1 mL)[6] Foscarnet (Foscavir)[1] (1.2–2.4 mg/0.1 mL)[6] Possible role for prednisone (0.5–2.0 mg/kg/day PO for up to 6–8 weeks)
Anterior uveitis, viral	HSV	Valacyclovir[1] 1000 mg PO TID Acyclovir[1] 400 mg PO × 5/day 4 weeks Famciclovir[1] 250 mg PO TID	Topical corticosteroids and cycloplegic recommended. Alternative options include an intravitreal ganciclovir (2 mg/0.05 mL).[6] After active infection eradicated, consider maintenance therapy for HSV and CMV Ganciclovir ophthalmic gel (Zirgan)[1] 0.15% × 5/day (optional)
	HZV	Valacyclovir[1] 1 g PO TID Acyclovir[1] 800 mg PO × 5/day 5–6 weeks Famciclovir[1] 500 mg PO TID 5–6 weeks	
	Cytomegalovirus (CMV)	Ganciclovir[1] 5 mg/kg IV BID 2–3 weeks Valganciclovir[1] 900 mg PO BID × 6 weeks, then 450 mg PO BID × 6 weeks	
Cat-scratch disease	*Bartonella henselae*	Doxycycline (Vibramycin)[1] 100 mg PO BID 2–4 weeks	Children: antibiotic selection based on age, dental maturity
Cytomegalovirus retinitis	Cytomegalovirus	Ganciclovir 5 mg/kg IV BID for 2–3 weeks followed by maintenance 5 mg/kg/day PO Cidofovir (Vistide)[1] 5 mg/kg/week IV for 2 weeks then 5 mg/kg every 2 weeks Valganciclovir 900 mg BID PO, then PO qd for maintenance. Foscarnet 90 mg/kg IV BID × 2 wks; maintenance 90–120 mg/kg IV daily	Immune reconstitution targets cause of immune compromise
Diffuse unilateral subacute neuroretinitis (DUSN)	Possible larva of *Baylisascaris procyonis, Toxocara canis*	Photocoagulation of intraretinal nematode	Destruction of intraretinal larva may preserve vision
Lyme disease	*Borrelia burgdorferi*	Doxycycline[1] 100 mg PO BID × 21 days (adults) Amoxicillin[1] 500 mg PO BID (adult); 50 mg/kg PO in divided doses × 14–21 days (children)	Alternative: cefuroxime axetil (Ceftin) 500 mg PO BID × 14–21 days (adult); 30 mg/day PO (children)
Metastatic endophthalmitis (endogenous)	Numerous bloodborne bacteria and fungi	Sepsis treatment protocol; antibiotic selections based on cultures and sensitivities	Role and timing of intravitreal antibiotics and of vitrectomy less well defined
Onchocerciasis	*Onchocerca volvulus*	Ivermectin (Stromectol) 150 µg/kg single oral dose; repeat at 6 months for the lifespan of adult worm	Corticosteroids to control ocular inflammation; route of administration depends on site of inflammation
Syphilis	*Treponema pallidum*	Aqueous penicillin G 18–24 million units, IV qd divided doses for 10–14 days	Ocular syphilis is considered a subset of neurosyphilis
Toxocariasis	*Toxocara canis* or *Toxocara cati*	Prednisone 1 mg/kg/day PO; timing of anthelminthic therapy unresolved.	Laser ablation and vitrectomy depending on stage of disease. Intraocular larval death incites considerable inflammation

TABLE 2 Treatment of Infectious Uveitis—cont'd

DIAGNOSIS	INFECTIOUS ORGANISM(S)	TREATMENT	COMMENT
Toxoplasmosis	*Toxoplasma gondii*	Pyrimethamine (Daraprim): loading dose 50–100 mg PO; treatment dose 25–50 mg/day PO; and sulfadiazine: loading dose 2–4 g PO; treatment dose 1.0 g PO QID, and prednisone (0.5–1.0 mg/day PO)	Modify doses if pregnant or immune compromised. Some recommend adding clindamycin[1] or azithromycin[1]
		Trimethoprim-sulfamethoxazole (Bactrim DS)[1] 160 mg/80 mg PO BID, plus above regimen of prednisone	
Tuberculosis	*Mycobacterium tuberculosis*	For first-line therapy for active tuberculosis, follow recommendations on CDC website.	

[1]Not FDA approved for this indication.
[2]Not available in the United States.
[6]May be compounded by pharmacists.
BID, Twice a day; *IV*, intravenous; *PO*, by mouth; *TID*, three times a day.

a matter of debate. Many posterior uveitis and panuveitis disorders are clinically defined syndromes. For example, Behçet disease, multifocal choroiditis with panuveitis, acute posterior multifocal placoid pigment epitheliopathy, serpiginous choroiditis, punctate inner choroidopathy, multiple evanescent white dot syndrome, Vogt-Koyanagi-Harada disease, and sympathetic ophthalmia are diagnoses based on clinical findings (e.g., ophthalmoscopy, fluorescein angiography, optical coherence tomography). These syndromes have no confirmatory laboratory tests, other than several with strong HLA haplotype associations (e.g., Behçet disease [HLA-B51] and birdshot chorioretinopathy [HLS-A29]).

Management of inflammation associated with noninfectious posterior uveitis requires systemic medications. Most clinicians initiate oral corticosteroids, understanding that high-dose long-term use is associated with serious and predictable side effects. The risk of systemic side effects may be reduced with judicious use of periocular or intravitreal corticosteroid injections, but those routes of administration also have their own potential adverse effects and complications. These range from elevated intraocular pressure and glaucoma to infectious endophthalmitis.

The optimal time to transition to corticosteroid-sparing immunomodulatory therapy is a clinical decision-making process, focused on limiting the long-term systemic side effects of oral corticosteroids, treating inflammation recalcitrant to oral corticosteroids, and managing specific diseases expected to fare poorly with less aggressive therapies. The guidelines for treatment escalation should be based on a treat to target approach, to minimize disease burden and improve clinical outcomes. A frequently cited reference is the SITE (Systemic Immunosuppressive Therapy for Eye diseases) Cohort Study series, a retrospective cohort study with multiple publications detailing the use of antimetabolites, T-cell inhibitors, alkylating agents, and other immunosuppressives ascertained from medical records of approximately 9250 patients with ocular inflammation. Data are collected with up to 30 years of follow-up from five US tertiary centers and analyzed by fellowship-trained ocular immunologists. Immunomodulatory therapy for the treatment of uveitis falls into four drug categories: antimetabolites, inhibitors of T-lymphocyte signaling, biologic response modifiers, and alkylating agents (Table 3). Their judicious use has been shown to reduce or eliminate the need for systemic corticosteroids, improve long-term visual prognosis, and reduce ocular complications from inflammation. Meaningful clinical responses should occur within 3 months of initiating therapy. After achieving clinical end points, patients should be monitored and the decision to taper

based on input from patients and disease-specific criteria. A thorough history, physical examination, and select laboratory tests and imaging studies should be completed before initiation of therapy, in conjunction with appropriate subspecialty consultation.

The most commonly used antimetabolites for the treatment of noninfectious uveitis are methotrexate (Rheumatrex),[1] azathioprine (Imuran)[1], and mycophenolate mofetil (CellCept).[1] Oral methotrexate, 7.5 to 15 mg once per week with daily folic acid[1] 1 mg, can be increased to 20 to 25 mg/week based on clinical response. Appropriately adjusted intravenous dose can be tried for persons with gastrointestinal intolerance. Intravitreal injection of 400 μg/0.1 mL has been used for refractory inflammation. Oral azathioprine is begun at 1 mg/kg/day. Depending on clinical response, it can be incrementally increased to 2.5 mg/kg/day. Mycophenolate mofetil is started at 1 to 2 g orally per day in divided doses up to 3 g/day. The manifold side effects of antimetabolites necessitate close clinical monitoring.

Most experience in treating noninfectious uveitis with inhibitors of T-lymphocyte signaling, or calcineurin inhibitors, is with cyclosporine (Sandimmune).[1] Given 2.5 to 5 mg/kg/day in divided doses, cyclosporine can cause nephrotoxicity, bone marrow suppression, and hypertension.

Alkylating agents used to treat noninfectious uveitis include cyclophosphamide (Cytoxan)[1] and chlorambucil (Leukeran).[1] These immunomodulating drugs are titrated to keep white blood cell counts in the range of 3000 to 4500 cells per cubic millimeter. Chlorambucil is started at 0.15 mg/kg/day and cyclophosphamide at 1 to 3 mg/kg/day. Regular monitoring for bone marrow suppression and opportunistic infection is needed for both drugs. Risks of hemorrhagic cystitis with cyclophosphamide may be reduced by consuming generous amounts of water daily.

Biologic response modifiers, or "biologics," have expanded the therapeutic arsenal for treating advanced or severe noninfectious uveitis. This family of medications consists of antibodies directed against key cytokines in the immune response pathway. Most experience in treating noninfectious uveitis has been with tumor necrosis factor (TNF)-α inhibitors (infliximab [Remicade][1] and adalimumab [Humira]). Although other biologics have been used to treat advanced or severe noninfectious uveitis, their equivalence or superiority to the drugs already mentioned are under study. Etanercept (Embrel)[1] may increase the risk of anterior uveitis in persons with ankylosing spondylitis.

---

[1]Not FDA approved for this indication.

| TABLE 3 | Immune Modulator Therapy for Uveitis |

GENERIC (TRADE) NAME	DOSE (ROUTE)*,†	COMMENT/INDICATIONS‡
Alkylating Agents		
Chlorambucil (Leukeran)[1]	0.15 mg/kg/day (oral)	Behçet disease; juvenile idiopathic arthritis; pars planitis; sympathetic ophthalmia
Cyclophosphamide (Cytoxan)[1]	1–2 mg/kg/day (oral)	Sclerouveitis; sympathetic ophthalmia
Antimetabolites		
Azathioprine (Imuran)[1]	1–1.5 mg/kg/day (oral) can increase to 2.5 mg/kg/day	Severe anterior uveitis; panuveitis, juvenile idiopathic arthritis; pars planitis, sarcoidosis; sympathetic uveitis; VKH
Methotrexate (Otrexup, Rasuvo, Rheumatrex, Trexall)[1]	7.5–15 mg/week (oral)	Anterior, intermediate, and posterior uveitis; juvenile idiopathic arthritis; sympathetic uveitis
Mycophenolate mofetil (CellCept);[1] Mycophenolate sodium (Myfortic)[1]	Mofetil: 1 g (oral) divided dose/day; sodium: 360 mg (oral)/day	Anterior, intermediate, and posterior uveitis
Calcineurin Inhibitors		
Cyclosporine (Gengraf, Neoral, Sandimmune)[1]	2.5–5 mg/kg/day (oral) divided dose	Often given with prednisone 10–20 mg/day; Behçet disease; birdshot chorioretinopathy; pan uveitis; posterior uveitis; sarcoidosis; sclerouveitis; sympathetic uveitis; VKH
Tacrolimus (Prograf, Astagraf XL, Envarsus XR)[1]	0.15–0.3 mg/kg/day (oral)	Behçet disease; birdshot chorioretinopathy; posterior uveitis
Biologic Response Modifier TNF-α Inhibitor		
Adalimumab (Humira)	40 mg every other week subcutaneous injection	Anterior, intermediate and posterior uveitis; juvenile idiopathic arthritis; sarcoidosis
Infliximab (Remicade)[1]	3 mg/kg/day (intravenous) weeks 0, 2, and 6	Behçet disease; anterior uveitis; juvenile idiopathic arthritis; sarcoidosis
Certolizumab pegol (Cimzia)[1]	400 mg subcutaneous induction 1–3 doses weeks 0, 2, 4; then 200 mg every 2 weeks	Refractory uveitis
Golimumab (Simponi)[1]	50 mg subcutaneous every 4 weeks	Juvenile idiopathic arthritis; Behçet disease
Biologic Response Modifier IL-1 Inhibitor		
Anakinra (Kineret)[1]	100 mg subcutaneous daily	Behçet disease
Canakinumab (Ilaris)[1]	150–300 mg subcutaneous every 4–8 weeks	Behçet disease; juvenile idiopathic arthritis
Biologic Response Modifier Anti–IL-6 Receptor		
Tocilizumab (Actemra)[1]	4–8 mg/kg (intravenous) every 2–4 weeks	Juvenile idiopathic arthritis; Behçet disease; persistent macular edema
Biologic Response Modifier Anti-CD20		
Rituximab (Rituxan)[1]	375 mg/m² intravenous weekly, modify accordingly	Refractory uveitis; juvenile idiopathic arthritis; refractory VKH

*Therapeutic doses and schedules in clinical trials have differed in loading doses and maintenance doses. Cited doses reflect lower ranges.
†Variations in these treatment regimens are actively being studied.
‡Refers to reported success at controlling or eliminating inflammation as a single or as a steroid-sparing agent. Strength of recommendations will vary by level of evidence.
[1]Not FDA approved for this indication.
IL-1, Interleukin-1; *IL-6*, interleukin-6; *TNF-α*, Tumor necrosis factor-α; *VKH*, Vogt-Koyanagi-Harada disease.

Infliximab (Remicade) is given intravenously beginning with two loading doses of 3 to 5 mg/kg each given 2 to 4 weeks apart. Injections are then continued at 4-week intervals. Based on clinical response, the dose can be gradually increased to 10 mg/kg. Side effects include infection from activation of latent tuberculosis or hepatitis, drug-induced autoimmune disease, and demyelinating disease. If non–melanoma skin cancer is excluded, current published data indicate that TNF inhibitors do not increase the risk for solid malignancies. Adalimumab (Humira) is given subcutaneously starting at 40 mg/kg every 2 weeks. Children are started at a reduced dose. The adverse risk profile of adalimumab is similar to that of infliximab.

Other biologics used to treat noninfectious uveitis such as anti–CD20 monoclonal antibody (Rituximab [Rituxan][1]) have clinically established utility in the treatment of specific disease entities such as severe scleritis, peripheral ulcerative keratitis, ocular mucous membrane pemphigoid, and retinal vasculitis. In these cases the rheumatoid arthritis approved dosing regimen is used: two 1000-mg intravenous infusions separated by 2 weeks (cycle 1) then every 24 weeks or based on clinical evaluation, but not sooner than every 16 weeks. Interferon alfa-2a is associated with flulike symptoms and depression, which may limit patient acceptance.

[1]Not FDA approved for this indication.

TABLE 4	Drug-Induced Uveitis*	
DRUG: NAME/CLASS	**ROUTE**	**TYPE OF UVEITIS**
Brimonidine (Alphagan, Lumify)	Topical	Granulomatous anterior uveitis
Metipranolol (OptiPranolol)[2]	Topical	Granulomatous anterior uveitis
Prostaglandin analogues	Topical	Anterior uveitis, cystoid macular edema
Vancomycin	Intravitreal	Retinal vasculitis
Triamcinolone acetate	Intravitreal	Sterile endophthalmitis
Antivascular endothelial growth factor agents	Intravitreal	Anterior uveitis
Cidofovir (Vistide)	Intravitreal/intravenous	Anterior uveitis/hypotony
Rifabutin (Mycobutin)	Oral	Hypopyon anterior uveitis
TNF-α inhibitors (most cases seen with etanercept)	Subcutaneous/intravenous	All forms of uveitis
Bisphosphonates	Oral/intravenous	Anterior uveitis/scleritis
Fluoroquinolones	Oral	Anterior uveitis/pigment dispersion/ocular hypertension
Sulfonamides	Oral	Anterior uveitis
Protein kinase inhibitors	Oral/intravenous	All forms of uveitis
Immune checkpoint inhibitors	Intravenous	Anterior uveitis
Vaccines (BCG, influenza, HBV, VZV, HPV, SARS-CoV-2)		Anterior uveitis (mostly)

*This is not an exhaustive list.
[2]Not available in the United States.
BCG, Bacillus Calmette-Guérin; *HBV*, hepatitis B virus; *HPV*, human papillomavirus; *TNF-α*, tumor necrosis factor-α; *VZV*, varicella-zoster virus.

Drug-Induced Uveitis

Uveitis has been causally linked to a variety of medications, ranging from ophthalmic topicals and injectables to systemically administered drugs taken orally and intravenously (Table 4). Although the incidence of drug-induced uveitis is low, the list of implicated medications is increasing. Few generalizations about pathogenesis are applicable, because both the types of medications known to cause uveitis and proposed pathways leading to intraocular inflammation are diverse. The mechanisms of drug-induced inflammation, however, can be placed into two broad categories: primary or direct injury to ocular tissue and secondary through systemic immune-mediated injury.

Establishing the diagnosis of drug-related uveitis is challenging. Critical findings including a temporal association between drug exposure and onset of uveitis symptoms and signs. The time interval might be relatively short (hours to days) if caused by primary injury to tissue or delayed in terms of weeks if mediated via a systemic immune response. The resolution of signs of uveitis after withdrawal or reduction in dose of medication offers further supporting evidence. Recurrence of ocular inflammation with rechallenge of the medication is often considered the standard for establishing causation. It is also a potentially hazardous method of achieving a definitive diagnosis because the clinical endpoint is harmful. Finally, alternative causes of uveitis need to be excluded. The confidence in making a diagnosis of drug-induced uveitis is always strengthened by finding similar cases reported in the literature.

Complications of Uveitis

Chronic uveitis gives rise to a variety of ocular complications such as secondary glaucoma; macular edema; corneal dysfunction; neovascularization of the iris, angle, and retina; retinal tears and detachments; cyclitic membrane formation; and uveal effusion, as well as other conditions. These ocular complications are typically approached by controlling or eliminating ocular inflammation and managing the structural/functional problems according to standards guidelines.

Disease-Specific Recommendations

Strength of recommendations for disease-specific noncorticosteroid immunomodulatory therapy is constrained by the relative lack of prospective clinical trials, drug-to-drug comparison trials, studies that have included patients with diverse forms of uveitis, and the small size of studies. Given these limitations, the strength of recommendations is tempered by a level of evidence for most drugs of 2B or lower on the Oxford Centre for Evidence-Based Medicine level of evidence scale. Mycophenolate preparations,[1] azathioprine[1], methotrexate[1], cyclophosphamide[1], cyclosporine[1], sirolimus (Rapamune)[1], infliximab[1], adalimumab, and etanercept[1] have demonstrated varying degrees of success in controlling inflammation, improving visual outcome, and reducing corticosteroid use in severe anterior, intermediate, and posterior uveitis and in panuveitis. Control of inflammation and improved visual acuity in Vogt-Koyanagi-Harada disease have been achieved with systemic methotrexate[1], azathioprine[1], mycophenolate preparations[1], infliximab[1], adalimumab[1], and interferon alfa-2a.[1] The uveitis of Behçet disease, juvenile idiopathic arthritis, pars planitis, and sympathetic ophthalmia responds to chlorambucil.[1] Mycophenolate preparations[1] have had success in various forms of anterior, intermediate, and posterior uveitis. The inflammation of Behçet disease has been controlled with azathioprine[1], infliximab[1], adalimumab[1], rituximab[1], and interferon alfa-2a.[1] Sarcoid uveitis has responded to infliximab[1] and adalimumab.[1] The systemic disease of juvenile idiopathic arthritis has been successfully managed with methotrexate, cyclosporine[1], mycophenolate mofetil[1], azathioprine[1], and TNF-α inhibitors adalimumab and infliximab.[1] Therapeutic vitrectomy and/or laser ablation has been used in different forms of noninfectious uveitis, but evidence of long-term effectiveness is sparse.

Systemic Drug Use in Pregnancy and in Children

Because the teratogenic potential of many immunosuppressive drugs is incompletely understood, it may be prudent to discuss

Uveitis

575

---

[1] Not FDA approved for this indication.

contraception when they are administered to women. The largely unknown teratogenic effects of immunosuppressive agents in men should also be considered. Although prednisone is well tolerated during pregnancy, its use should be carefully comanaged with an obstetrician.

The effects of immunosuppressive drugs are less well studied in children than in adults. Children on immunosuppressive agents should not receive live virus vaccine for 3 months after immuno-suppressive use has ended. This would include high-dose cortico-steroids. The impact of immunosuppressive drugs and systemic corticosteroids on growth and their collateral effects on social development are not inconsequential. Osteoporosis, adrenal sup-pression, and heightened susceptibility to infections related to cell-mediated immunity are among the side effects that require monitoring in children. Calcium supplements and vitamin D may be beneficial in some circumstances.

References

Agarwal M, Dutta Majumder P, Babu K, et al: Drug-induced uveitis: a review, *Indian J Ophthalmol* 68(9):1799–1807, 2020.
Dick AD, Rosenbaum JT, Al-Dhibi HA, et al: Guidance on noncorticosteroid systemic immunomodulatory therapy in noninfectious uveitis. Fundamentals of Care for UveitiS (FOCUS) Initiative, *Ophthalmology* 125:757–773, 2018.
Foster CS, Kothari S, Anesi SD, et al: The Ocular Immunology and Uveitis Foundation preferred practice patterns of uveitis management, *Surv Ophthalmol* 61:1–17, 2016.
Jabs DA, Nussenblatt RB, Rosenbaum JT, Standardization of Uveitis Nomenclature (SUN) Work Group: Standardization of uveitis nomenclature for reporting clinical data. results of the first international workshop, *Am J Ophthalmol* 140:509–516, 2005.
Jap A, Soon-Phaik C: Viral anterior uveitis. diagnosis and management, *Focal Points* 34(5):1–18, 2016. Available at https://store.aao.org/clinical-education/product-line/focal-points.html.
Kempen JH, Daniel E, Gangaputra S, Dreger K, et al: Methods for identifying long-term adverse effects of treatment in patients with eye diseases: the Systemic Immunosuppressive Therapy for Eye Diseases (SITE) Cohort Study, *Ophthalmic Epidemiol* 15(1):47–55, 2008.
Levy-Clarke G, Jabs DA, Read RW, et al: Expert panel recommendations for the use of anti-tumor necrosis factor biologic agents in patients with ocular inflammatory disorders, *Ophthalmology* 121:785–796, 2014.e783.
Lower CY, Lima BR: Pediatric uveitis, *Focal Points* 32(3):1–11, 2014. Available at https://store.aao.org/clinical-education/product-line/focal-points.html.
Schwartzman S: Advancements in the management of uveitis, *Best Prac Res Clin Rheumatol* 30:304–316, 2016.
Wakefield D, McCluskey P, Wildner G, et al: Inflammatory eye disease: pre-treatment assessment of patients prior to commencing immunosuppressive and biologic therapy: recommendations from an expert committee, *Autoimmun Rev* 16:213–222, 2017.
Yeh S, Suhler ER, Moorly RS, et al: Biologic response modifiers in uveitis, *Focal Points* 30(3):1–16, 2012. Available at https://store.aao.org/clinical-education/product-line/focal-points.html.

VISION REHABILITATION

Method of
August Colenbrander, MD; and Donald C. Fletcher, MD

CURRENT DIAGNOSIS

- The need for vision rehabilitation needs to be considered whenever patients indicate that they have difficulty performing visual tasks.
- Sometimes, however, patients do not recognize the visual causes of their complaints, therefore:
  - Vision rehabilitation needs to be considered whenever visual acuity is reported as 20/50 or less.
  - Vision rehabilitation also needs to be considered for all patients with reported visual disorders, such as visual field deficits or contrast vision deficits, who have not received this service yet,

CURRENT THERAPY

- Simple cases of reduced visual acuity can be addressed with a variety of magnifying devices, ranging from stronger glasses to electronic devices.
- Improved task lighting can often be helpful.
- Orientation and mobility training can be indicated for patients with visual field loss, even if their visual acuity is still adequate.
- As for any other specialized service, referral to a dedicated low vision service may be indicated.

Vision rehabilitation refers to the multidisciplinary effort of assisting those with various degrees of vision loss in coping with the *consequences* of that loss. To describe vision rehabilitation, the nature of vision itself must be understood. Vision is the major source of information about our environment. The eyes alone contribute as much information to the brain as all other organs combined. It is not surprising therefore that many people fear loss of vision almost as much as loss of life.

Most people will state that "we see with our eyes." On closer examination, this is not true. An isolated eyeball cannot produce any vision; our brain, however, can produce exquisite visual imagery in our dreams, without any input from the eyes.

The ultimate goal of vision is to facilitate interaction with the environment, not just to read letters on a letter chart. To achieve this goal, the visual process goes through three distinct stages. Each stage comes with its own specific problems.

- First is the *optical stage*, where the refractive media of the eye deliver an image to the retina. Familiar problems in this area include refractive errors and cataracts.
- Second is the *receptor stage*, where the optical image is translated into neural impulses. Age-related macular degeneration (AMD) is a significant problem of the receptor stage, which is becoming increasingly common as the population ages.
- Third are various stages of *neural processing*, initially in the inner retina (glaucoma), then in the visual cortex, and finally in higher cortical centers, where the visual input gives rise to visual perception and to visually guided behaviors, actions, and interactions.

The most common visual problems vary for different ages. Today, brain-damage-related vision problems (cerebral visual impairment [CVI]) are the single most prevalent cause of visual impairment in *infants and young children*. Given that vision is so important for normal development, vision loss in infants constitutes a developmental emergency and should be detected and addressed as early as possible. When a child does not smile back at the mother, the mother may be inclined to leave the baby in its crib, instead of holding him or her to provide extra tactile stimulation to compensate for missing visual stimulation.

At *school age* and later, visual health is critical because reading becomes important for academic development. For *adults*, vision is important for maintaining independence in activities of daily living (ADL) and development of vocational skills. For *seniors*, vision loss may exacerbate other age-related dysfunctions. Studies of the elderly have shown correlations between visual impairment and depression, falls, and reduced longevity. In all of these instances, early detection and early intervention are essential; the primary care physician plays a crucial role in this respect.

Four Aspects of Vision Loss

Vision is a complex phenomenon.

A convenient framework for discussing the various impacts of vision loss is to consider four aspects of visual functioning (Figure 1). At a basic level, we may consider how various external causes may result in *structural changes* to the eyes and the visual pathways. For this aspect, the focus is on the tissue;

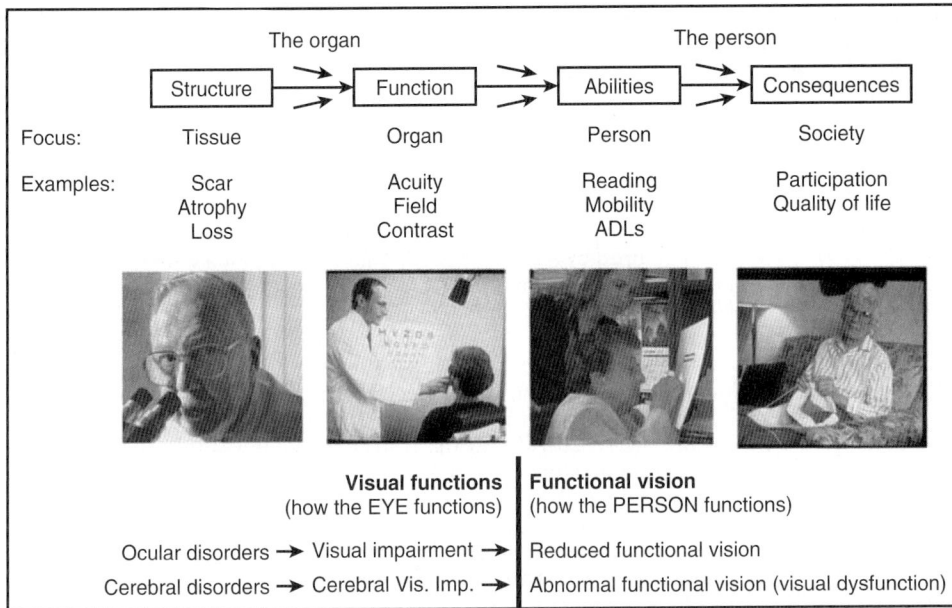

Figure 1 Aspects of vision loss.

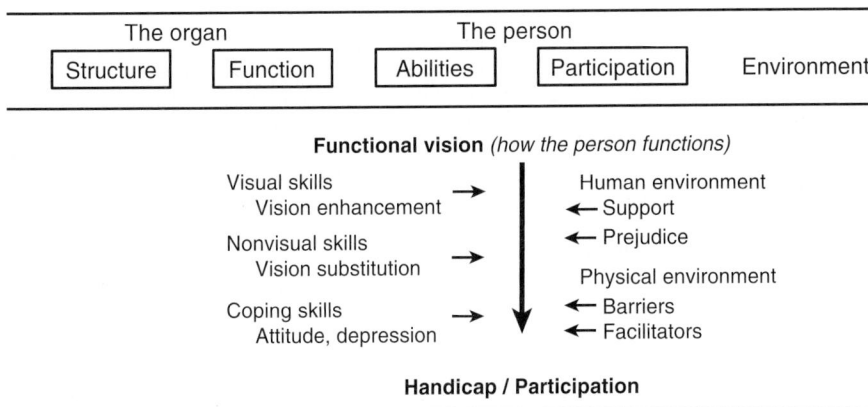

Figure 2 Comprehensive vision rehabilitation.

an ocular pathologist is needed to describe the pathologic condition. However, structural changes alone do not determine how well the eyes actually function. Clinicians need to measure various *organ functions*, such as visual acuity, visual field, and contrast sensitivity.

Yet even knowing how the eyes function does not tell us how the person functions. In other words, the *abilities* of the person to perform tasks, such as reading, mobility, face recognition, and ADL, must be considered. Occupational therapists (OTs) and other rehabilitation professionals work with patients to teach them how residual vision can be used most effectively. OTs also assess the person in a societal context. For example, do the visual changes have an impact on the person's *participation* in society, on his or her ability to perform necessary tasks, and on general satisfaction with one's quality of life? It is clear that to cover all aspects of vision rehabilitation, a team approach is necessary and that the patient must be part of that team.

A single ADL may cover several of the above aspects. When reading, the aspect of minimum print size falls under organ function (retinal resolution). Reading speed (words/minute) and reading endurance (hours/day) define abilities of the person; reading endurance may be poor, even if reading acuity is adequate. Reading enjoyment, finally, falls under the aspect of quality of life.

It is helpful to draw a line between the organ side of Figure 1 on the left and the person side on the right. On the left side of the diagram, we discuss *visual functions*, which describe how each eye functions. On the right side, we speak of *functional vision*, which describes how the person functions in vision-related activities. Medical specialists are well versed in dealing with the left side of the diagram. Yet the ultimate goal of all interventions is to improve the patient's quality of life. It is the function of vision rehabilitation to make sure that "eye" doctors become "people" doctors by extending their interest to the right side of the diagram as well.

Comprehensive Vision Rehabilitation

Considering all of these aspects, comprehensive vision rehabilitation involves much more than the patient's performance on a letter chart and requires teamwork by different professionals who specialize in different aspects of vision loss. All vision loss starts with some medical condition, so primary care physicians are well positioned to coordinate team activities. Primary care physicians need to be aware of what other team members can contribute and should know where to locate vision rehabilitation resources and to make appropriate referrals.

Figure 2 illustrates that comprehensive vision rehabilitation involves much more than the traditional optical low vision care offered in the past, and is still relevant today.

Low vision is a term used to describe individuals whose vision (with appropriate optical correction) is less than normal (low) but who are not blind (vision). Unfortunately, many people in this category do not yet receive the services they need. Such services should include adequate refractive, medical, and surgical care as well as rehabilitative care. The latter may include vision enhancement, vision substitution, and vision assistance as well as the honing of coping skills.

Vision enhancement, which is the traditional focus of low vision care, is primarily oriented at improving residual visual function through visual aids, including a wide range of magnification devices. Additionally, enhancement of contrast, illumination, and filters need to be explored.

Low vision is distinct from blindness (i.e., no vision). For blindness, the emphasis of rehabilitation is entirely on vision substitution. Patients with severe or profound low vision may combine the use of low vision rehabilitation skills with some blindness rehabilitation skills.

Vision substitution expands the options for rehabilitation by optimizing the use of other senses. This can range from using simple tactile markings to sense the position of a stove dial to devices such as talking books, a long cane for travel, and braille for reading. Vision enhancement and vision substitution are not mutually exclusive. A patient may use a magnifier to read price tags and may prefer talking books for recreational reading. A patient with retinitis pigmentosa, which causes reduced night vision, may have normal mobility in the daytime and need a cane at night. Digital audio books may have braille labels.

Vision assistance. A special form of vision substitution involves using the eyes of others or artificial intelligence (AI). Family members, caregivers, and office personnel should be familiar with *sighted guide* techniques to effectively assist visually impaired patients with minimal embarrassment. *Guide dogs* are also a possibility. Using a guide dog requires training of the patient as well as of the dog so that they can work as a team. Dog users must also demonstrate mastery of long cane travel skills. New glasses with built in cameras and speakers can utilize AI through Bluetooth connection to the patient's phone to describe their immediate environment. This new technology promises great utility in the future for the blind and visually impaired.

Coping skills. How different patients will accept visual aids may differ greatly. It is important to recognize that vision loss often causes a reactive depression. On the one hand, a depressed patient will be less receptive to rehabilitative suggestions. On the other hand, demonstration of rehabilitative success can be a powerful tool to lift a reactive depression and to motivate the patient for further success. It has been shown that the teaching of general problem-solving skills may improve the effectiveness of vision rehabilitation.

Many professionals may be involved in vision rehabilitation. Technicians may prescribe various magnifiers, rehabilitation workers may teach daily living skills, and psychologists may address depression. Acceptance of the work of these professionals will be improved if the trusted primary care physician is credited with making the referrals.

Beyond the factors that directly involve the patient, the environment must also be considered.

The *human environment* is important. As patients go through the stages of adaptation, a supportive home environment is essential. As patients are counseled, it is important to include spouses, children, or significant others to make sure that they understand the condition, know what can be expected, and know how to support the patient. Answering family and caregiver questions directly is often better than leaving this to the patient, who initially may not have absorbed everything that was said. An overprotective environment, which deprives patients of opportunities to do things for themselves, can be as detrimental as an overdemanding one that puts too much emphasis on the patient's shortcomings. The same holds true for the work or school environment and for social groups.

Initially, patients often feel isolated and believe that they are the only ones experiencing these problems. *Peer support groups* can be helpful; in these groups, patients can experience how others are dealing with similar problems.

Finally, the *physical environment* needs to be considered. An uncluttered environment, where things have a defined, fixed place is helpful because it reduces the need for searching. Good general illumination and task lighting often help, because at higher illumination levels retinal cells that are damaged but not

dead can still contribute to vision. Good contrast is important: Do not serve milk in a white Styrofoam cup; mark the edges of steps and stairs. The triangles and circles on men's and women's bathrooms are designed to be visible for those with very low vision; braille labels in elevators are useful for people who are totally blind.

How Blind Is Blind?

The most common visual function test is the letter chart, developed by Snellen in 1862. That test determines how large a letter, or other symbol, must be to be recognized by the patient. That size is then compared with the size recognized by a standard observer. If the magnification requirement is 2×, visual acuity is said to be 1/2; if it is 5×, visual acuity is said to be 1/5, etc. That fraction can be recorded in different ways; in the United States, it is customary to use 20 as the numerator (1/2 = 20/40, 1/5 = 20/100); in the British Commonwealth, 6 is used as the numerator (6/12, 6/30); in Europe, decimal fractions are common (0.5, 0.2).

Those calculations are simple; unfortunately, the terminology used to describe various ranges of vision loss is confusing. Figure 3 shows progressively degraded pictures with examples of the terminology used to describe different degrees of visual impairment. The visual acuity level represented by each picture can be determined from the number of lines that are readable on the low vision letter chart.

The first picture shows the visual acuity level that is labeled as "low vision" by the World Health Organization (WHO). Although the bottom lines of the letter chart cannot be read, the appearance of the room is near normal. The next picture shows what the US Social Security Administration considers "statutory blindness" for its programs. Although reading regular print is not possible without magnification devices, it is clear that this is far from actual blindness. Other US programs use a different definition for "legal blindness," and the WHO does not consider a person "blind" until he or she has reached the status of the last picture. At that level, reading even the special letter chart is not possible, but one can still navigate the room. Even this level of visual impairment does not constitute actual blindness.

The widespread use of the word "blindness" is unfortunate because it cannot be used with modifiers. One is either blind or sighted; one cannot be "a little bit blind." This black-and-white thinking has hampered the acceptance of vision rehabilitation. Terms such as *vision loss* or *visual impairment* are preferred because they can be used with modifiers, including mild, moderate, severe, profound, and total vision loss. Although "legal blindness" and "severe vision loss" (ICD-9-CM) have the same definition, there is a big difference between telling a patient "you *are* legally blind" and "you *have* a severe visual impairment." The first statement might be followed by "I am sorry, there is nothing more we can do for your eyes"; the second statement leads to the question, "What can we do to help you cope with this problem?"

Vision Rehabilitation Techniques and Devices

Having considered the general outlines of vision rehabilitation, some details of rehabilitative interventions can be discussed. Primary care physicians should know what vision rehabilitation techniques are available so that they can make appropriate referrals.

Optical Problems

The most commonly encountered visual problems are those involving the optical system of the eye.

Refractive errors are the easiest visual problems to deal with. Refractive errors can be corrected with glasses or contact lenses, and for those who hate glasses, by refractive surgery. Even if there are other causes of vision loss, determining the best refractive correction is still important.

Uncorrected refractive error accounts for about half of all visual impairment worldwide. In developed countries, the question may be why people do not avail themselves of the solutions that are available. In developing countries, availability and accessibility

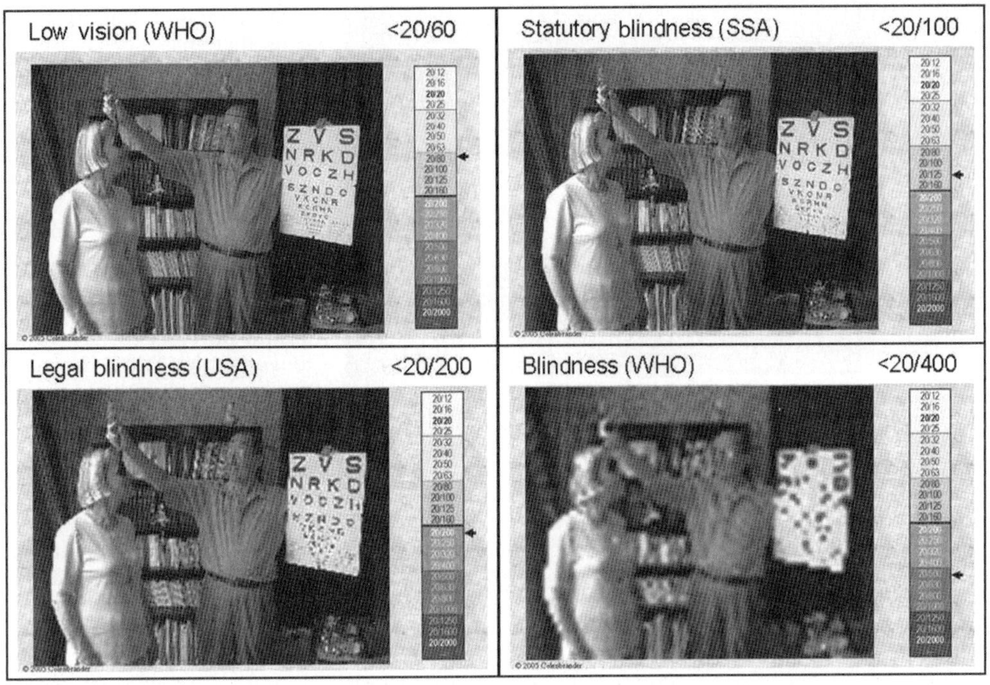

Figure 3 Ranges of vision loss.

of eye care and of the means for correcting refractive errors often do not exist. Providing these services is a matter of infrastructure, not of individual healthcare.

Opacities disrupt visual image formation. Cataracts are the most familiar opacity; they can be removed by surgery. Other opacities of a temporary or permanent nature may occur in the cornea, in the anterior chamber, or in the vitreous cavity. Corneal and conjunctival infections may cause corneal scarring, as is the case in trachoma, a condition that does not exist in the developed world anymore but is still a major cause of vision loss worldwide.

Letter chart acuity is a good way to measure optical problems. It should be understood, however, that letter chart acuity only measures the function of the retinal area where the letter read is projected. Even for a patient with 20/200 acuity, this area is less than 1 degree in diameter. For optical problems this does not matter because foveal defocus predicts equal defocus in all other areas of the retina. For retinal problems, however, visual acuity alone is not sufficient to characterize the visual status.

Magnification is the primary way to compensate for reduced acuity. One way to provide magnification is to bring print closer to the eye. For older adults, this requires reading glasses with extra power. Alternatively, large print may be helpful. Larger print on medicine labels, as required in several states, can reduce medication errors by older adults, who often take several medications. Handheld magnifiers are another option; today, many have built-in LED illumination to provide more light. Video-magnifiers with a table-mounted large screen are ideal for prolonged reading; they can also enhance contrast and brightness, while some devices can even read the text out loud. Tablets, smartphone apps, and dedicated devices can provide similar advantages in a portable form. Today, these electronic means of magnification are increasingly popular because they can provide not only magnification but also contrast enhancement. They also have a larger field of view and allow a more comfortable reading distance with binocular viewing.

Retinal Problems

While primitive forms of cataract surgery have existed for centuries, the study of retinal disorders has only been possible since the invention of the ophthalmoscope in 1851. The ability to effectively treat some retinal disorders is even more recent. Important retinal disorders include the following.

Age-related macular degeneration (AMD) is the most frequent diagnosis encountered in low vision rehabilitation services in the Western world. Because the condition is age-related, its frequency will increase in the future as our population ages. This has caused profound changes in the nature of low vision care. Until the mid-20th century, most low vision care was provided by special education teachers serving young students in schools for the blind. Today, the majority of low vision patients are seniors. This has resulted in a significant influx of OTs into the field with skills in addressing multiple geriatric impairments. Yet the needs of seniors to be served still outstrip the available services.

Given that macular degeneration affects central vision and the ability to read, most patients will ultimately seek rehabilitation help. However, if only one eye is affected, AMD may go unnoticed. The patient may only complain when the second eye starts to deteriorate; at that point, the damage in the first eye may be beyond repair. Therefore, it is useful to ask patients to periodically cover each eye to see whether there is any vision difference between the eyes. If there is, this is a reason for referral.

Glaucoma is another age-related condition. It causes loss of peripheral vision and affects central vision only in the late stages. Glaucoma often goes undetected because patients are not spontaneously aware of visual field loss, as little as they are spontaneously aware of an increased blood pressure. Therefore, glaucoma must be sought out, primarily by measuring the intraocular pressure.

Diabetic retinopathy is not limited to seniors. As the incidence of diabetes is rising worldwide, so is the incidence of diabetic retinopathy. Even if treated adequately, it will cause scattered blind spots throughout the visual field.

There are many other hereditary and nonhereditary retinal conditions that may cause vision loss, but they occur in smaller numbers. They all require the help of vision rehabilitation professionals to help patients cope effectively.

Scotomata. Whatever the cause, retinal conditions will generally cause localized blind spots (scotomata). Therefore, when retinal damage is suspected, visual acuity alone is no longer a sufficient descriptor of visual impairment because the retinal area where the letter chart symbol is projected does not predict anything about other retinal areas. In addition to letter chart acuity, the condition of the visual field and the presence of blind spots (scotomata) must be considered (Figure 4).

Figure 4 shows a retinal image, where a word is projected across a ring scotoma that leaves only a small central island of vision. This patient will be able to recognize the central letter but

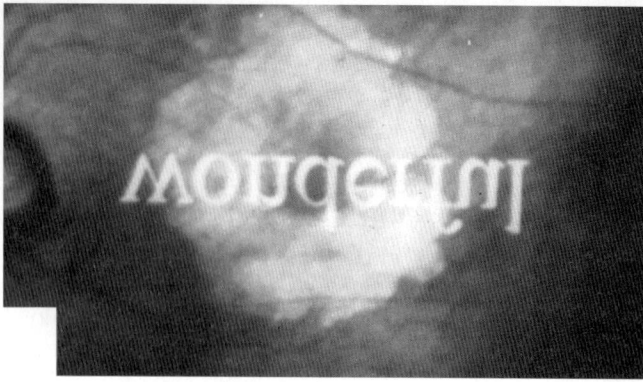

Figure 4 Ring scotoma.

will not be able to read the word. Clinicians must be careful when providing such patients with magnification because too much magnification will mean that fewer letters fit into the central area. This example also makes it clear that when retinal involvement is suspected, a reading test may be more informative than a letter chart test, given that reading requires a larger retinal area.

Neural Processing Problems

As stated earlier, the most important stages of the visual process take place after the retinal receptors have translated the optical image into neural impulses.

The first transformations take place in the *inner retina*. Here, the input from 100 M receptors in each eye is preprocessed and compressed for transmission through 1 M nerve fibers in each optic nerve. The optic nerve fibers do not simply transmit a pixel-by-pixel image, as does a digital camera. Different retinal ganglion cells probably transmit different aspects of the image, such as edges, movement, color, brightness, and so on. These separate "movies" are transmitted in parallel. At a later stage of neural processing, these different aspects of the image are merged again to contribute to a single visual perception.

At the first synaptic station in the lateral geniculate nucleus, only 20% of the incoming connections come from the optic nerves; the other 80% come from other cortical centers and probably contribute to filtering based on attention and other factors.

In the visual cortex, the visual information is analyzed for shapes and contours. In higher cortical centers, the visual information is further processed. Here, the flow of information is no longer strictly visual because it is combined with information from other senses. This results in identification and recognition of objects through comparison to stored concepts (through the ventral stream to the temporal lobe of the brain) and in spatial location of an object (through the dorsal stream to the parietal lobe of the brain), which then result in voluntary or involuntary visually guided action.

Our knowledge of these processes is still relatively new. It has been greatly helped by new modalities for neural and retinal imaging. Today, neural processing problems are increasingly recognized in all age groups.

In young children, CVI is now recognized as the most frequent cause of visual perceptual problems. CVI is often caused by perinatal ischemia, which may cause cortical as well as subcortical changes (periventricular leukomalacia). Because this ischemia is not localized, impairments are often not limited to the visual system. Schools for the blind have increasingly developed into schools for children with multiple disabilities.

In contact sports, the results of repeated subclinical injuries are now recognized.

In veterans, traumatic brain injuries may cause problems that may be hard to define. Often visual interpretation and decision making are impaired; oculomotor system problems are often found. Traffic accidents may cause similar damage.

In older adults, strokes may cause more localized problems and agnosias for specific tasks. In all of these cases, the term *visual impairment* may be used when visual acuity and/or visual field are impaired. The term *visual dysfunction* may be more appropriate when the visual input from the eyes to the brain is normal but the processing of this information in the brain is not.

Patient-Centered Functional Priorities

Vision problems affect all aspects of a patient's life. It is no longer sufficient for clinicians to determine that nothing more can be done about the *causes* of vision loss, because much more can be done about the *consequences* of vision impairment.

To determine the range of services that may be appropriate for an individual with vision impairment, the American Academy of Ophthalmology recommends consideration of the following functional priority areas:

- Reading—for many patients, this is their foremost concern.
- ADL—even though reading may be the most prominent complaint, most people spend the larger part of their day performing vision-dependent activities other than reading for self-care and home management.
- Safety—Patients with visual field loss must be made explicitly aware of this loss and the problems it may cause in navigating the environment. Are they at risk for falls? How do they cross the street? Do they drive?
- Community participation—can the individual still participate in community events, including religious gatherings?
- Physical, cognitive, and psychosocial well-being—because many patients with vision loss are older, this is an important aspect that should not be overlooked. If cognitive problems exist, it may affect the recommendations to be made.

Based on these considerations, patient-centered priorities can be set and specific rehabilitation goals formulated that reflect the patient's needs and desires. The primary care physician can then make appropriate referrals for rehabilitation.

References

Bourne RA, et al: Magnitude, temporal trends, and projections of the global prevalence of blindness and distance and near vision impairment: a systematic review and meta-analysis, et al. *Lancet Glob Health* 5(9):e888–e897, 2017.

Colenbrander A: Measuring vision and vision loss. In Tasman W, Jaeger EA, editors: *Duane's Ophthalmology*, Vol. 5. Philadelphia, 2013, Lippincott Williams & Wilkins.

Colenbrander A: Towards the development of a classification of vision-related functioning—a potential framework. In Dutton GH, Bax M, editors: *Visual Impairment in Children Due to Damage to the Brain*, London, 2010, Mac Keith Press.

Fletcher DC, Schuchard RA: Preferred retinal loci relationship to macular scotomas in a low-vision population, *Ophthalmology* 104:632–638, 1997.

Fletcher DC, Schuchard RA, Watson G: Relative locations of macular scotomas near the PRL: effect on low vision reading, *J Rehabil Res Dev* 36:356–364, 1999.

Schoessow KA: Shifting from compensation to participation: a model for occupational therapy in low vision, *Br J Occup Ther* 73:160–169, 2010.

Website Sources

The website of the American Academy of Ophthalmology (www.aao.org) contains much medical information. For rehabilitation related information, search for "low vision" and "rehabilitation".

The AFB website (www.AFB.org) has information for all age groups, including a section on aging.

The MDsupport website (www.MDsupport.org) specializes in support and documentation for AMD patients and care givers.

The Lighthouse Guild International in New York (www.lighthouseguild.org) offers extensive resources for all forms of vision loss.

These websites contain links to many more websites with additional information and often can provide information about local resources.

Infectious Diseases

AMEBIASIS

Method of
Koji Watanabe, MD, PhD

CURRENT DIAGNOSIS (SEE ALSO BOX 1)

- Amebiasis is transmitted by the ingestion of fecally contaminated water or food and by high-risk sexual behaviors (men who have sex with men [MSM] or oral–anal sexual contact).
- Although self-limiting mild to moderate colitis is the most common disease presentation, various severe illnesses (liver abscess, peritonitis, pleurisy, and pericarditis) can also occur.
- Diagnostic value of microscopic stool or abscess ova and parasite examination (O&P) is low. Antigen detection in stool shows high sensitivity for severely diarrheal and/or dysentery cases (amebic colitis), but shows relatively low sensitivity for mild colitis or asymptomatic cases. Serology shows high sensitivity but cannot distinguish current infection from past infection, and it is ideally used in conjunction with fecal antigen detection or polymerase chain reaction (PCR).

CURRENT THERAPY (SEE ALSO BOX 2)

- Infected individuals who are asymptomatic should be treated with a luminal agent (e.g., paromomycin), because they can be a source of new infection and can develop invasive amebiasis after long-term asymptomatic infection.
- Mild to severe colitis and extraintestinal disease require initial treatment with a tissue-active agent (e.g., metronidazole) followed by a luminal agent.
- Reinfection can occur frequently in endemic settings. The clinician should discuss methods to prevent re-exposure to *Entamoeba histolytica* with treated patients.

Epidemiology and Risk Factors for Acquisition

Amebiasis is transmitted by oral ingestion of the transmissible cyst form of *Entamoeba histolytica* in human stools. Transmission occurs by the ingestion of fecally contaminated food and water, mainly in developing countries. It also transmits directly from human to human by sexual contact or in institutions for the cognitively impaired. Food- or water-borne infection occurs in settings of poor sanitation. It is estimated to be the second most common cause of parasite infection–related mortality worldwide, accounting for 40,000 to 70,000 deaths annually. In developed countries, people who travel to or immigrate from developing countries are at higher risk for this parasitic disease. In the United States, amebiasis is the second most common cause of diarrhea in returning travelers. However, over the last two decades amebic infection has been increasingly reported as a sexually transmitted infection in East Asian developed countries and Australia. In one report from Taiwan, men who have sex with men (MSM) and people engaging in oral–anal sex were more likely to be seropositive for *E. histolytica*. While older studies from the United States have shown that amebiasis in MSM was due to nonpathogenic *Entamoeba dispar*, more recently MSM was shown to be an independent risk factor for amebiasis-related mortality. Also, *E. histolytica* infection has been reported as a common comorbidity among HIV-infected MSM or as a sexually transmitted infection in developed European countries. It is important for primary care physicians to take detailed histories of sexual behavior as well as travel whenever amebiasis is suspected.

Pathophysiology and Susceptible Host Factors to Invasive Diseases

E. histolytica has two different forms: the tissue-invasive "trophozoite form" and the infectious "cyst form," which is responsible for transmission. Cysts are notable for environmental stability, demonstrating considerable resistance to chlorination and desiccation, with several outbreaks resulting from the contamination of drinking water. Once cysts are ingested, excystation occurs at the terminal ileum or large intestine, forming motile trophozoites. Trophozoites bind to the mucous layer and the underlying intestinal epithelial cells via a parasite Gal/GalNAc lectin. Blockade of activity of the Gal/Gal lectin prevents contact-dependent cytolysis. Moreover, it has been shown that antilectin IgA in stool or breast milk has a protective effect against future acquisition of amebic infection in cohort studies. These results indicate that the Gal/GalNAc lectin plays a crucial role in amebic infection.

Host factors are also important for susceptibility to amebiasis. Amebiasis is more common in malnourished children, and the nutritional hormone leptin is protective, with a single nucleotide mutation of leptin receptor being the predominant genetic factor controlling amebiasis susceptibility in Bangladeshi children. Amebic liver abscess (ALA) is 10 times more common in men than in women and is uncommon in children.

Clinical Manifestations and Complications of Amebiasis

Asymptomatic self-limiting infection is the most common disease form of amebiasis. Up to 80% to 90% of people exposed to cysts have no or mild symptoms and clear the infection spontaneously. However, asymptomatic infection persists for a long time in some individuals who are reported as asymptomatic cyst passers or as fecal occult blood–positive, which is incidentally diagnosed by colonoscopy. These asymptomatically infected individuals can be a source of a new infection in the community. Also, some develop symptomatic invasive diseases after long-term latent infection.

Symptomatic intestinal amebiasis (amebic colitis) generally has a subacute onset. Usually it takes 1 to 3 weeks from disease onset to make a diagnosis. Abdominal symptoms range from mild diarrhea to severe dysentery with abdominal pain, diarrhea, and bloody stools. Weight loss and fever are common but not universal symptoms. Intestinal fistula or perforation of the large intestine, resulting in peritonitis, is a rare but life-threatening complication of intestinal amebiasis, which is called as "fulminant amebiasis." The very young or old, malnourished people, pregnant women, and patients using corticosteroids are at increased risk of fulminant amebiasis. Toxic megacolon also can be caused by amebiasis. Amebic colitis sometimes mimics acute appendicitis. In this situation, appendectomy without amebicidal treatment may result in severe postoperative complications, such as abdominal sepsis, gastrointestinal fistula, or hemorrhage. Periodic acid–Schiff (PAS) stain, or ideally, immunoperoxidase with anti-*E. histolytica* antibodies, in addition to routine hematoxylin and eosin (H&E) stain can help to identify the parasite by the histopathology. Thus, intestinal amebiasis sometimes presents as severe and complicated clinical illnesses.

E. histolytica infection also may have extraintestinal dissemination. Liver abscess is the most common form of extraintestinal amebiasis. Patients usually present with 1 to 2 weeks of fever with or without right upper quadrant abdominal pain. Other common symptoms may include cough, sweating, malaise, weight loss, anorexia, and hiccough. Two-thirds of patients lack intestinal symptoms. Physical examination reveals hepatomegaly and tenderness over the liver in approximately half of cases. Complications can occur by direct invasion of trophozoites or the indirect effect of inflammation. Up to10% of patients with ALA have accompanying thoracic amebiasis (pleuritic and pleural effusion). Pericarditis is the next most common form of extraintestinal amebiasis; it may result from rupture of a liver abscess in the left lobe or through extension of pleural amebiasis. Cerebral amebic abscesses are a rare form of extraintestinal amebiasis; they usually accompany other metastatic lesions, such as liver abscesses and thoracic amebiasis.

Thus, amebiasis can have various clinical presentations. The diagnosis can be very difficult to make in severe cases and in atypical clinical presentations because of secondary bacterial infection at the site of amebic invasion.

Diagnosis

Sensitivity of each diagnostic test is shown in Box 1. Although microscopic stool ova and parasite examination (O&P) is frequently used in many countries including the United States, it has low sensitivity; moreover, accuracy is highly dependent on the skill of the person who carries out. Identification of trophozoites by microscope in aspirated fluid from amebic abscess is more challenging because trophozoites are present only at the edge of the abscess. Moreover, microscopic examination cannot distinguish pathogenic *E. histolytica* from nonpathogenic *E. dispar* or *Entamoeba moshkovskii* by shape.

Currently, the combination of antigen detection in stool and/or sera and serologic testing is the best diagnostic pathway. Antigen detection in feces by the TechLab *E. histolytica* II enzyme-linked immunosorbent assay (ELISA), or the TechLab E. HISTOLYTICA QUIK CHEK membrane enzyme immunoassay, is rapid to perform (<2 hours, or <30 minutes) and can distinguish *E. histolytica* from *E. dispar* and *E. moshkovskii*. These antigen tests have highly sensitive diagnostic value for amebic colitis, that is, Bristol stool scale 6 or 7 (60% to 95%), whereas sensitivity is relatively low for asymptomatic carrier, that is, Bristol stool scale 5 or lower (20% to 50%). In one report, when used on patients' sera, ELISA showed high sensitivity in ALA cases but only before metronidazole treatment began. Real-time polymerase chain reaction (PCR) in stool is superior in sensitivity to stool antigen detection, but is still technically complex for diagnostic use in clinical settings. Serologic tests are sensitive (approximately 90% during the convalescent phase) and noninvasive diagnostic tools for amebiasis. Antibodies are detectable in 70% or more of patients within 5 to 7 days of acute infection and persist for years after treatment. Therefore, a negative serologic result is helpful for exclusion of disease, whereas a positive result cannot distinguish between present and previous infection. Multiplex PCR tests for intestinal pathogens are commercially available (e.g., FilmArray GI Panel from BIOMERIEUX) and show high sensitivity. Moreover, they can detect many intestinal pathogens, including protozoa. However, they are still expensive (about $100 USD per sample) for the routine diagnostic method in the clinical settings.

582

BOX 1 Sensitivity of Tests for Diagnosis of Amebiasis*

Test	Colitis	Liver Abscess
Microscopy (stool)	25%–60%	10%–40%
Stool antigen detection (e.g., E. histolytica II enzyme-linked immunosorbent assay (ELISA)	80%	40%
Serum antigen detection	65%	>95%
Microscopy (abscess fluid)	N/A	<20%
Real time polymerase chain reaction	>95%	>95%
Serologic testing (indirect hemagglutination)		
Acute	70%	70%–80%
Convalescent	>90%	>90%
Histopathology by biopsy	45%	N/A

*Before the initiation of therapy.
Modified from Mandell G, Bennett JE, Dolin R, et al. *Mandell, Douglas, and Bennett's Principles and Practice of Infectious Diseases*. 7th ed. Philadelphia: Elsevier Saunders; 2009.

BOX 2 Treatment Recommendations for Amebiasis in Adults

Asymptomatically Infected Individuals
Paromomycin (Humatin) 30 mg/kg/d PO tid × 5–10 days
or
Iodoquinol (Yodoxin)[2] 650 mg PO tid × 20 days

Mild to Severe Intestinal and Extraintestinal Disease
Metronidazole (Flagyl)* 750 mg PO tid × 10 days
or
Tinidazole (Tindamax) 2 g PO once daily × 5 days
Followed by
Paromomycin[1] 30 mg/kg/d PO tid × 5–10 days
or
Iodoquinol 650 mg PO tid × 20 days

*Use of intravenous form of metronidazole (500mg q8h) is limited to patients who cannot take oral medications.
[1]Not FDA approved for this indication.
[2]Not available in the United States
Modified from Mandell G, Bennett JE, Dolin R, Blaser MJ. *Mandell, Douglas, and Bennett's Principles and Practice of Infectious Diseases*. 7th ed. Philadelphia: Elsevier Saunders; 2009.

Histopathologic examination using biopsy or resected samples is sometimes useful for the diagnosis of intestinal amebiasis. As mentioned, PAS stain in addition to H&E can increase sensitivity in detection of *Entamoeba*. However, identification of *Entamoeba* in biopsy specimens is often challenging. About half of cases with gross ulcerative lesions in the large intestine, in which *E. histolytica* was proven by PCR, had a negative result on histopathology.

Therapy

Recommended treatment regimens are shown in Box 2. Therapy for invasive infection differs from therapy for noninvasive infection. Noninvasive infections (treatment for asymptomatically infected individuals) require treatment with luminal-active agents: paromomycin (Humatin) is currently recommended because of its high potency in asymptomatic cyst passers. Recently, it is increasingly reported that macroscopically visible colonic ulcers by *E. histolytica* are unexpectedly diagnosed from asymptomatic individuals. Treatment for asymptomatic patients with colonic ulcers is currently undetermined; however, tissue-active agents are commonly administered prior to luminal-active agents in reported cases.

For symptomatic patients, tissue-active agents should be administered before luminal-active agents. Most patients with mild to moderate colitis and uncomplicated liver abscess respond to treatment with tissue-active agents, such as metronidazole (Flagyl) and tinidazole (Tindamax). Tinidazole has the advantage of less frequent dosing than metronidazole. Treatment with tissue-active agents should be followed by luminal-active agents because parasites persist in the intestine in up to 40% to 60% of patients who receive tissue-active agents. Broad-spectrum antibiotics and/or surgical treatment should be added to tissue-active agents in patients with fulminant colitis in which perforation and peritonitis or bacteremia are suspected. Therapeutic needle aspiration or catheter drainage is not routinely required for uncomplicated liver abscesses. Those interventions in addition to medical treatment are recommended if there is clinical deterioration or lack of response to initial medical treatment, or if alternative diagnoses need to be excluded. Also, some reports suggest that clinicians should consider those interventions for patients with a high risk of abscess rupture, as defined by a cavity with a diameter of more than 5 cm or by the presence of lesions in the left lobe, although these criteria were not conclusive in case-control studies.

Symptoms (diarrhea, dysentery, fever, pain, and tenderness) and laboratory markers (white blood cell counts, red blood cell counts, and C-reactive protein) rapidly improve after effective treatment even in patients with extraintestinal lesions. In contrast, radiologic findings, such as abscess size, often remain unchanged for months after completion of treatment.

Monitoring After Treatment and Disease Prevention

Although routine monitoring after treating amebiasis is not recommended, it is well known that reinfection frequently occurs in endemic situations, including both water- or food-borne infections and sexually transmitted infections. In developed countries, in order to prevent reinfection, it is important for the primary physician to inform patients of behaviors that will place them at risk for acquisition of the cyst and how to avoid them, such as avoiding nonsterilized water or food in developing countries, unsafe homosexual contact, and oral–anal sexual contact. In developing countries, more than 1 billion people still have no access to safe food and water, resulting in the urgent need for an effective vaccine. Induction of acquired mucosal immunity is the current goal for vaccine development. Although there is currently no vaccine in human clinical trials, a vaccine containing the naïve or recombinant Gal/GalNAc lectin of E. histolytica has strong immunogenicity and protective effect against amebic colitis and liver abscess in animal models. Continuous effort will be needed to develop an effective vaccine to save the lives of affected people in endemic areas.

References

Barwick RS, Uzicanin A, Lareau S, et al: Outbreak of amebiasis in Tbilisi, Republic of Georgia 1998, *Am J Trop Med Hyg* 67:623–631, 2002.
Blessmann J, Tannich E: Treatment of asymptomatic intestinal *Entamoeba histolytica* infection, *N Engl J Med* 347:184, 2002.
Chavez-Tapia NC, Hernandez-Calleros J, Tellez-Avila FI, et al: Image-guided percutaneous procedure plus metronidazole versus metronidazole alone for uncomplicated amoebic liver abscess, *Cochrane Database Syst Rev* CD004886, 2009.
Gunther J, Shafir S, Bristow B, et al: Short report: amebiasis-related mortality among United States residents, 1990–2007, *Am J Trop Med Hyg* 85:1038–1040, 2011.
Haque R, Mollah NU, Ali IK, et al: Diagnosis of amebic liver abscess and intestinal infection with the TechLab *Entamoeba histolytica* II antigen detection and antibody tests, *J Clin Microbiol* 38:3235–3239, 2000.
Hung CC, Chang SY, Ji DD: Entamoeba histolytica infection in men who have sex with men, *Lancet Infect Dis* 12:729–736, 2012.
Hung CC, Wu PY, Chang SY, et al: Amebiasis among persons who sought voluntary counseling and testing for human immunodeficiency virus infection: a case-control study, *Am J Trop Med Hyg* 84:65–69, 2011.
Kobayashi T, Watanabe K, Yano H, et al: Underestimated Amoebic appendicitis among hiv-1-infected individuals in Japan, *J Clin Microbiol* 55:313–320, 2016.
Korpe PS, Liu Y, Siddique A, et al: Breast milk parasite-specific antibodies and protection from amebiasis and cryptosporidiosis in Bangladeshi infants: a prospective cohort study, *Clin Infect Dis* 56:988–992, 2013.
Leder K, Weller PF: Intestinal and extraintestinal *Entamoeba* histolytica amebiasis. UpToDate. Available at: http://www.uptodate.com/contents/search. [Accessed 09 February 2022].
Petri Jr WA, Haque R: *Entamoeba* species, including amebic colitis and liver abscess. In Bennett JE, Dolin R, Blaser MJ, editors: *Mandell, Douglas, and Bennett's principles and practice of infectious diseases*, ed 8th, Philadelphia, 2015, Elsevier Saunders, pp 3047–3058.
Saidin S, Othman N, Noordin R: Update on laboratory diagnosis of amoebiasis, *Eur J Clin Microbiol Infect Dis* 38:15–38, 2019.
Shirley DT, Watanabe K, Moonah S: Significance of amebiasis: 10 reasons why neglecting amebiasis might come back to bite us in the gut, *PLoS Negl Trop Dis* 13:e0007744, 2019.
Yanagawa Y, Shimogawara R, Endo T, et al: Utility of the rapid antigen detection test E. histolytica quik chek for the diagnosis of *Entamoeba histolytica* infection in nonendemic situations, *J Clin Microbiol* 58:e01991-20, 2020.

ANTHRAX

Method of
Shingo Chihara, MD

CURRENT DIAGNOSIS

Cutaneous Anthrax
- Incubation period of 1 to 7 days from exposure to cattle
- Painless or pruritic lesion progresses to ulcer and eschar
- Significant swelling
- Gram stain and culture of lesion

Gastrointestinal
- Incubation period of 1 to 6 days after consumption of raw or undercooked meat
- Nonspecific symptoms followed by abdominal pain, ascites
- Diarrhea uncommon
- Obtain blood culture and ascitic fluid for culture and Gram stain

Inhalational
- Incubation period of 1 to 7 days (up to 43 days)
- Biphasic: fever, malaise, myalgia followed by dyspnea
- Widened mediastinum seen on chest x-ray and computed tomography (CT) of chest
- Blood cultures turn positive in most

Injection
- Injection drug use
- Significant swelling seen; eschar rare

CURRENT THERAPY

Systemic Anthrax With Possible/Confirmed Meningitis
- Ciprofloxacin (Cipro) 400 mg IV every 8 hours or levofloxacin (Levaquin) 750 mg IV every 24 hours or moxifloxacin (Avelox)[1] 400 mg IV every 24 hours
  plus
- Meropenem (Merrem)[1] 2 g IV every 8 hours or imipenem/cilastatin (Primaxin)[1] 1 g IV every 6 hours or doripenem (Doribax)[1] 500 mg IV every 8 hours
- If penicillin-susceptible strains, then penicillin G 4 million units IV every 4 hours or ampicillin[1] 3 g IV every 6 hours could be an alternative to carbapenems
  plus
- Linezolid (Zyvox)[1] 600 mg IV every 12 hours or clindamycin (Cleocin) 900 mg IV every 8 hours or rifampin (Rifadin) 600 mg IV every 12 hours or chloramphenicol 1 g every 6 to 8 hours

Systemic Anthrax When Meningitis Has Been Excluded

- Ciprofloxacin 400 mg IV every 8 hours or levofloxacin 750 mg IV every 24 hours or moxifloxacin[1] 400 mg IV every 24 hours
  or
- Meropenem[1] 2 g IV every 8 hours or imipenem/cilastatin[1] 1 g IV every 6 hours or doripenem[1] 500 mg IV every 8 hours
  or
- Vancomycin (Vancocin)[1] 60 mg/kg/day IV divided every 8 hours (goal trough 15–20 μg/mL)
  or
- If penicillin-susceptible strains, then penicillin G 4 million units IV every 4 hours or ampicillin[1] 3 g IV every 6 hours
  plus
- Clindamycin[1] 900 mg IV every 8 hours or linezolid[1] 600 mg IV every 12 hours
  or
- Doxycycline 200 mg IV×1, then 100 mg IV every 12 hours, or rifampin[1] 600 mg IV every 12 hours

Oral Treatment for Cutaneous Anthrax Without Systemic Involvement

- One of the agents below for 7 to 10 days in naturally-acquired cases and for 60 days in bioterrorism-associated cases
- Ciprofloxacin 500 mg PO every 12 hours
- Doxycycline 100 mg PO every 12 hours
- Levofloxacin 750 mg PO daily
- Moxifloxacin[1] 400 mg PO daily
- Clindamycin[1] 600 mg PO every 8 hours
- If penicillin-susceptible strain
- Amoxicillin[1] 1 g PO every 8 hours
- Penicillin VK 500 mg PO every 6 hours

[1]Not FDA approved for this indication.

Anthrax has been described for centuries and the name is derived from Greek for "burnt coal" owing to eschar formation from cutaneous anthrax. Anthrax is rarely seen in developed countries, including the United States, but it is important to be aware of this condition because of its potential as a bioterrorism agent. When anthrax is suspected, the clinician needs to contact the local or state health department immediately. Anthrax has historical significance because it was the agent used in Koch's postulate during the 19th century when Koch proved that *Bacillus anthracis* is responsible for anthrax in cattle.

Background

B. anthracis is the bacterium responsible for anthrax. It forms spores that can survive in soil for years. It is hyperendemic in the Middle East and in sub-Saharan Africa. Systemic anthrax is primarily a disease of grazing animals. In naturally-acquired anthrax, humans are accidentally infected from exposure to the animal or its products.

Epidemiology

Since the mid-20th century, there has been a precipitous decline in anthrax owing to animal and human vaccines, improvement in factory hygiene, sterilization procedures for imported animal products, and increased use of alternatives to animal hides or hair. Cutaneous anthrax comprises over 95% of naturally-acquired human anthrax and there are an estimated 2000 cases annually. Between 1900 and 2001 there were 18 cases of inhalational anthrax in the United States, of which 16 were fatal. Over the last decade, there have been several cases of inhalational and cutaneous anthrax related to African drum makers. In late 2001, there were 22 cases of anthrax in the United States from spores delivered in the mail, of which five were fatal. In 1979, accidental release of dried anthrax spores from a biologic weapons facility in Sverdlovsk in the former Soviet Union resulted in 68 deaths from inhalation anthrax.

Pathophysiology

B. anthracis is a gram-positive, encapsulated, spore forming, nonhemolytic, nonmotile rod-shaped bacterium. Infection with anthrax requires three components: the edema factor, the lethal factor, and protective antigen. The edema factor combines with protective antigen and becomes edema toxin, which causes edema and impairment of the immune system. The lethal factor combines with protective antigen and becomes lethal toxin, which causes lysis of macrophages. For cutaneous anthrax, these exotoxins result in extensive edema and tissue necrosis locally. In inhalation anthrax, spores that reach the alveoli or alveolar ducts are phagocytized by the alveolar macrophage and transported to the mediastinal lymph nodes where they replicate and cause hemorrhagic mediastinitis. With gastrointestinal tract infection, *B. anthracis* is transported from the gastrointestinal tract to mesenteric lymph nodes where they multiply and cause mesenteric lymphadenitis, ascites, and sepsis.

Clinical Manifestations

There are four distinct clinical presentations: cutaneous, inhalation, gastrointestinal tract, and injection anthrax, depending on the site of entry. Meningitis is a devastating complication that could occur with any of the four infections.

Cutaneous Anthrax

Cutaneous anthrax is the most common form and seen in developing countries as a result of contact with infected animals or animal products such as wool, hair, or hides. Spores invade through either skin abrasions or hair follicles. Subsequently, they germinate and multiply. The incubation period is commonly 5 to 7 days with range of 1 to 19 days. The lesions appear in exposed areas such as head, neck, forearms, and hands and begin as a small, painless papule. They are pruritic at times and form blisters. Subsequently, they evolve into painless necrotic ulcers with a black, depressed eschar with extensive edema and lymphadenopathy.

Inhalation Anthrax

Inhalation anthrax occurs when spores are aerosolized while working with contaminated animal products or when they are released intentionally in bioterrorism. The incubation period is 1 to 7 days but could be as long as 43 days. The course of disease is usually biphasic. Initially, nonspecific symptoms such as fever, malaise, and myalgia are present, resembling influenza. These symptoms last for several days before the bacteremic phase starts. The manifestations include rapidly, fulminant progressive respiratory symptoms such as severe dyspnea, as well as hypoxemia and shock. Once in this phase, the patient dies within a few days despite support in the intensive care unit. Therefore it is important to suspect anthrax in the prodromal phase, which is difficult owing to its rarity and lack of specific symptoms. Widening of the mediastinum on a chest x-ray may be helpful in establishing the diagnosis. This finding was seen in 7 out of 10 cases of inhalation anthrax from 2001. Hilar abnormalities, pulmonary infiltrates, or consolidation and pleural effusion may be seen.

Gastrointestinal Tract Anthrax

Gastrointestinal tract anthrax occurs after ingestion of raw or undercooked meat from an animal infected with anthrax. Gastrointestinal infection is relatively common and has been reported from mouth to ascending colon. The incubation period is 1 to 6 days. Initially, nonspecific symptoms such as asthenia, headache, low-grade fever, facial flushing and conjunctival injection occur. They are followed by abdominal pain, abdominal distention from ascites, nausea, and vomiting. Diarrhea occurs less frequently. As the disease progresses, abdominal pain becomes severe and findings of hypotension and intravascular depletion are seen. When the infection occurs in the oropharynx, necrotic ulcers with pseudomembranes cause pain and edema.

Injection Anthrax

An outbreak of injection anthrax was described in 2009. It was reported in Scotland among injection heroin users. Among the 47 confirmed cases, typical eschar formation seen in cutaneous anthrax was not seen in all but one case. Prominent edema was seen in most patients and some developed compartment syndrome.

Meningitis

Meningitis is a complication seen with all forms of anthrax. About half of patients with inhalation anthrax develop hemorrhagic meningitis. Symptoms such as altered mental status, seizures, cranial nerve palsies, and myoclonus may be seen. When anthrax is suspected, lumbar puncture should be done on presentation unless there are contraindications.

Diagnosis

When diagnosis of anthrax is suspected, the provider must notify the local department of health and the clinical microbiology laboratory. There has been reported transmission of anthrax to laboratory personnel handling *B. anthracis* and specimen handling in biosafety level 3 facilities is recommended. Because the genus *Bacillus* is part of the normal skin flora, it is crucial for the microbiology laboratory to distinguish *B. anthracis* from other non-*anthracis* species of *Bacillus*. Conventional culture and staining are used for distinction. *B. anthracis* is nonmotile and nonhemolytic and those characteristics are used to distinguish it from non-*anthracis* species of *Bacillus*. Most microbiology laboratories have the ability to make a presumptive identification of an organism, and the identification is confirmed by a reference laboratory.

Specimen Collection

When collecting clinical specimens for suspected anthrax, proper personal protective equipment such as disposable gloves, disposable aprons, and boots, should be used. When there is any potential of aerosolization of spores, then face shields and respirators are recommended. Hand washing with soap and water will reduce the endospore contamination of the skin, but alcohol handrubs are not effective against these endospores. For cutaneous anthrax, the edge of the eschar should be lifted, and two specimens of vesicular fluid should be collected by rotating a swab. One swab will be used for culture and Gram stain while the other would be used for polymerase chain reaction (PCR). Punch biopsy of the cutaneous lesion is an alternative. When inhalational anthrax is suspected, blood cultures must be obtained prior to use of antibiotics. If pleural fluid is present, then thoracentesis should be performed for Gram stain, culture, and PCR. For alimentary tract anthrax, blood cultures must be obtained. If there are oral lesions, then specimens could be collected with swabs similar to a cutaneous lesion. If ascites is present, then paracentesis should be performed for Gram stain, culture and PCR. For meningitis, cerebrospinal fluid (CSF) should be collected for culture, Gram stain and PCR.

There are unique findings observed in routine laboratories with systemic anthrax. Marked hemoconcentration may be seen in the complete blood count, and the initial white blood cell count is frequently within normal limits. In chemistry, decreased sodium, increased blood urea nitrogen, mild transaminitis and hypoalbuminemia are seen. Inflammatory markers such as erythrocyte sedimentation rate and C-reactive protein are elevated in most cases except in cases of injection anthrax, when C-reactive protein is low.

Treatment

Supportive Care

Hospitalization is required for all patients with systemic infections. Only uncomplicated cutaneous anthrax could be treated on an outpatient basis. Close monitoring is warranted because the patient status may deteriorate rapidly. Hemodynamic support should be given, including fluids, vasopressors, blood products, and invasive hemodynamic monitoring. Mechanical ventilation may be needed because of respiratory distress, airway protection for altered mental status, or for airway edema. Adjunctive corticosteroids may be indicated in four situations:

patients with history of endocrine or corticosteroid therapy; edema of head or neck; anthrax meningitis; or vasopressor-resistant shock. Pleural fluid and ascites should be drained aggressively. Surgery is indicated in certain situations. Surgery for cutaneous anthrax has led to dissemination and poor outcome. Therefore, in cutaneous anthrax, indication for surgery is limited to tracheotomy for airway obstruction and surgery for compartment syndrome. In gastrointestinal anthrax, surgery might be considered for complications such as bowel ischemia or infarct and perforation. In injection anthrax, removal of necrotic nidus would help reduce the toxin and spore reservoir.

Antimicrobial Treatment for Systemic Disease with Possible Meningitis

At least three intravenous antibiotics with good penetration to the central nervous system are recommended. At least one drug should have bactericidal activity, and at least one drug should inhibit protein synthesis. These should be continued for at least 2 weeks or until clinically stable, whichever is longer. The fluoroquinolone class is bactericidal, has good penetration to the central nervous system, and has no reported resistance by *B. anthracis*. Intravenous ciprofloxacin (Cipro) is the primary bactericidal component in the treatment of systemic disease. Levofloxacin (Levaquin) and moxifloxacin (Avelox)[1] are considered to be alternatives. The carbapenem class has good central nervous system penetration, and meropenem (Merrem)[1] is the preferred second antibiotic in treatment of systemic disease with possible meningitis. Imipenem/cilastatin (Primaxin)[1] and doripenem (Doribax)[1] are considered alternatives. Penicillin G or ampicillin[1] could be used in place of carbapenems when the isolate is known to have a minimum inhibitory concentration (MIC) of less than 0.125 µg/mL. As for protein synthesis inhibitor, linezolid (Zyvox)[1] is preferred because it provides good central nervous system penetration. If there is contraindication to linezolid use such as drug–drug interaction or myelosuppression, then clindamycin (Cleocin)[1] is the alternative. When both linezolid and clindamycin cannot be used, rifampin (Rifadin)[1] could be used for synergistic effect in combination with the bactericidal drugs. Chloramphenicol is another antibiotic that is a protein synthesis inhibitor. It could be used if linezolid, clindamycin, and rifampin are unavailable. Doxycycline (Vibramycin) is an inhibitor of protein synthesis but does not adequately penetrate the central nervous system. Therefore doxycycline should not be used when meningitis is not ruled out. If the patient had been exposed to aerosolized spores, then the patient should be transitioned to oral antibiotics after completion of initial intravenous combination therapy to prevent relapse from spores.

Antimicrobial Treatment for Systemic Disease when Meningitis is Ruled Out

At least two antimicrobial agents are recommended for systemic anthrax without meningitis. At least one should be bactericidal and at least one should be a protein synthesis inhibitor. This combination should be administered intravenously for at least 2 weeks or until clinically stable, whichever is longer. For penicillin-susceptible strains, penicillin G is considered equivalent to ciprofloxacin. Vancomycin (Vancocin)[1] is an acceptable alternative bactericidal agent. Clindamycin[1] and linezolid[1] are equivalent first choices for protein synthesis inhibitors. Doxycycline is an alternative agent. If the patient had been exposed to aerosolized spores, then the patient should be transitioned to oral antibiotics after completion of initial intravenous combination therapy to prevent relapse from spores.

Treatment for Cutaneous Anthrax without Systemic Involvement

A single oral antibiotic is adequate to treat cutaneous anthrax without systemic involvement. Fluoroquinolones and doxycycline are considered first-line agents. Clindamycin[1] is a second-line agent when first-line agents are unavailable or contraindicated. Penicillin or amoxicillin[1] may be used if the isolate is found to be

---

[1]Not FDA approved for this indication.

sensitive in vitro. It is important to give an adequate dose because resistance may develop when underdosed.

Antitoxins

There are three antitoxins in the Centers for Disease Control and Prevention (CDC) Strategic National stockpile: raxibacumab, obiltoxaximab, and anthrax immune globulin intravenous (AIGIV). These agents are not readily available to the public. They inhibit binding of protective antigen to the anthrax toxin receptor and translocation of lethal factor and edema factor into cells. There are human and animal data from the pre-antibiotic era that suggest that there is lower mortality in those who received the antitoxin in cutaneous anthrax compared with those who did not. Whether this agent should be given for systemic anthrax is controversial owing to lack of data. Because the mortality rate with systemic anthrax is high whereas the complication of antitoxin treatment is low, the potential benefit from antitoxins outweighs the potential risk from the antitoxins in systemic anthrax. This agent should be given in addition to appropriate antibiotics when systemic anthrax is suspected.

Pregnancy

Overall management is similar to that in the nonpregnant patient. In pregnancy, ciprofloxacin is preferred over doxycycline for both treatment and prevention. Newer fluoroquinolones such as levofloxacin and moxifloxacin[1] are not preferred because embryo toxicity has been observed in animal studies. This was not seen with ciprofloxacin. Transplacental transmission of anthrax is known to occur. Ciprofloxacin, levofloxacin, meropenem,[1] ampicillin,[1] penicillin, clindamycin,[1] and rifampin[1] are known to have adequate concentration in the placenta and at least one agent should be used with treatment.

Prognosis

Uncomplicated cutaneous anthrax has a mortality rate of less than 2% with treatment. Injection anthrax has a mortality rate of 28%, and gastrointestinal anthrax has a mortality rate of 40%. Inhalational anthrax has mortality of 45% despite antibiotics and modern intensive care. Meningitis from anthrax is almost always fatal.

Prevention

Postexposure prophylaxis should be started as soon as possible after exposure. Sixty days of antibiotics for immediate protection and a three-dose series of Anthrax Vaccine Adsorbed (AVA, BioThrax) for long-term protection are recommended by the United States Advisory Committee on Immunization Practices. Ciprofloxacin and doxycycline are recommended as first-line antibiotic therapy for postexposure prophylaxis and are FDA-approved for this indication. Alternative agents include levofloxacin, moxifloxacin, amoxicillin, or penicillin VK (if sensitive); and clindamycin. AVA should be administered at diagnosis and at 2 and 4 weeks. AVA is not FDA-approved for postexposure prophylaxis. Raxibacumab and obiltoxaximab, which are two monoclonal antibodies held in the United States Strategic National Stockpile, have been approved for prevention of inhalation anthrax when alternative preventive therapies are not available or not appropriate.

---

[1]Not FDA approved for this indication.

References

Anthrax. Available at http://www.cdc.gov/anthrax/ [accessed 3.1.2025].

Hendricks KA, Wright ME, Shadomy SV, et al: Centers for disease control and prevention expert panel meetings on prevention and treatment of anthrax in adults, *Emerg Infect Dis* 20, 2014. https://doi.org/10.3201/eid2002.130687.

Knox D, Murray G, Millar M, et al: Subcutaneous anthrax in three intravenous drug users, *J Bone Joint Surg* 93:414–417, 2011.

Logan NA, Hoffmaster AR, Shadomy SV, Stauffer KE: In Versalovic J, editor: *Manual of clinical microbiology*, 10th ed., Washington DC, 2011, ASM Press, pp 381–402.

Meaney-Delman D, Zotti ME, Creanga AA, et al: Special considerations for prophylaxis for and treatment of anthrax in pregnant and postpartum women, *Emerg Infect Dis* 20, 2014. https://doi.org/10.3201/eid2002.130611.

Ruoff KL, Clarridge J, Bernard K: In Garcia LS, editor: *Clinical microbiology procedures handbook*, ed 3rd, Washington DC, 2010, ASM Press. 3.18.1.

Singh K: Laboratory-acquired infections, *Clin Infect Dis* 49:142–147, 2009.

BABESIOSIS

Method of
Cheston B. Cunha, MD; and Burke A. Cunha, MD

CURRENT DIAGNOSIS

- Suspect babesiosis in patients from Ixodes tick-endemic areas who present with a malaria-like illness (MLI) with fever, chills, headache, fatigue, and malaise.
- Clinically, babesiosis usually presents as an acute febrile illness with high fevers (>102 °F), relative bradycardia, and shaking chills accompanied by fatigue and myalgias.
- Myalgias may suggest an influenza-like illness (ILI).
- Severe headaches may suggest an alternate diagnosis (e.g., meningitis).
- Some patients with babesiosis may be short of breath and may go on to develop acute respiratory distress syndrome (ARDS).
- Consider babesiosis for unexplained fevers following blood transfusion.
- In prolonged fevers that meet the definition of fever of unknown origin (FUO), consider babesiosis in patients from endemic areas.
- With babesiosis, there are usually no localizing signs except for splenomegaly. Importantly, no rash is present. If rash is present, consider an alternate diagnosis.
- In babesiosis, nonspecific laboratory test results, considered together, are helpful in excluding or narrowing diagnostic possibilities.
- Common nonspecific laboratory findings of babesiosis include a normal/slightly decreased white blood cell count, relative lymphopenia, atypical lymphocytes, thrombocytopenia, elevated total bilirubin, and high lactate dehydrogenase levels. Sera are mildly elevated.
- The erythrocyte sedimentation rate is usually highly elevated (>90 mm/h) as are serum ferritin levels.
- Definitive babesiosis diagnosis is by peripheral blood smears (thick and thin); thick smears are best for the detection of babesia and thin smears are best to assess the degree of parasitemia.
- In normal hosts, the degree of parasitemia is usually low (1%–5%), but high in compromised hosts (>10%). Severe babesiosis may occur in asplenic individuals (Howell-Jolly bodies reflect the degree of splenic dysfunction), the immunosuppressed, the elderly, and those with coinfections (e.g., ehrlichiosis, Lyme disease).
- If present, babesiosis is diagnosed by peripheral stained blood smears demonstrating the characteristic (but uncommon) "Maltese cross" in tetrads (four merozoites).
- In nonmalarious areas, babesiosis may be diagnosed by demonstrating intraerythrocytic ring forms on the peripheral smear.
- Babesiosis, like malaria, has intracellular ring forms, but babesiosis, unlike malaria, has no intracellular pigment (hemozoin).
- Alternatively, *Babesia microti* serology in the Northeastern United States is diagnostic if IgM titers are highly elevated (>1:64).
- Polymerase chain reaction to detect Babesia is more sensitive than blood smear review. It is particularly useful in patients with a low level of parasitemia.

CURRENT THERAPY

- Preferred therapy is atovaquone (Mepron)[1] plus azithromycin (Zithromax).[1]
- Alternatively, clindamycin (Cleocin)[1] plus quinine[1] may be used.
- In addition to antibabesia therapy, exchange transfusion may be lifesaving in severe cases.

- For severe cases, continue therapy until degree of parasitemia is <5%.
- Recurrent or persistent babesiosis should be treated for >2 weeks after resolution of parasitemia.
- Doxycycline is not effective in babesiosis.
- Coinfection with other tick-borne pathogens is rare, but possible.

[1]Not FDA approved for this indication.

Epidemiology

Babesiosis is a tick-borne zoonosis that clinically presents as a malaria-like illness (MLI). There are many *Babesia* species, but only five are pathogenic in humans. The geographic distribution of babesiosis mimics that of hard-bodied *Ixodes dammini* (*I. scapularis*) ticks and their vertebrate hosts (e.g., dogs, cats, cattle, and rodents). The primary reservoir for babesiosis in the Northeastern United States is the white-footed mouse (*I. dammini* nymphs) and the white-tailed deer (*I. dammini* adults). Sporadic cases of babesiosis also occur in states with the tick vector/vertebrate hosts. Babesiosis may also be acquired by blood/blood product transfusions.

Clinical Features

In the Northeastern United States, babesiosis is usually *B. microti* and clinically manifests as an MLI. Babesiosis may be asymptomatic (IgG seropositive) or a mild, self-limited influenza-like illness (ILI). The incubation period for naturally acquired babesiosis is 1 to 6 weeks and 6 to 9 weeks for transfusion-acquired babesiosis. Clinical presentations in normal hosts are subacute with fever, fatigue, headache, malaise, and anorexia often mimicking Epstein-Barr virus infectious mononucleosis (with false-positive Monospot test results). Babesiosis presenting in patients with prolonged fevers of unknown origins (FUOs) and anorexia/weight loss may mimic a lymphoreticular malignancy. Presentation may be acute in those with impaired splenic function, those on immunosuppressives, or the elderly. Babesiosis may be viewed clinically as the "malaria of Long Island/Nantucket" as it presents with many malarial features, e.g., fever, chills, headache, sweats, myalgias. Excluding epidemiologic considerations, babesiosis differs in geographic distribution from malaria. Clinically, babesiosis differs from malaria in two important aspects. The clinical hallmarks of malaria are acute onset, intermittent fevers, and the classic "malaria paroxysm." Babesia reproduce by asynchronous asexual budding, which is clinically manifest as constant/nonintermittent fever. With malaria, fevers are intermittent with fever periodicity related to the *Plasmodium* species. Only *P. falciparum* has no fever periodicity and like babesiosis has no hepatic phase. Malaria and babesiosis both have extraerythrocytic ring forms, but babesiosis has two distinct morphologic features: extracellular merozoites (tetrads), known as "Maltese crosses," and no extraerythrocytic pigment, which malaria does have.

Unless the liver or spleen is enlarged, the physical features in babesiosis are limited to the fever. The fever curve of babesiosis is remittent without periodicity; fever is between 102 °F and 105 °F and accompanied by relative bradycardia. Rash is not a feature. When babesiosis is suspected, the presence of a rash is either indicative of coinfection, e.g., Lyme disease, or an alternative cause, e.g., viral or drug exanthem. Babesiosis should not be in the differential diagnosis of Rocky Mountain spotted fever with rash on the wrists/ankles. Babesiosis may clinically resemble ehrlichiosis. Peripheral blood smears are the best way to differentiate babesiosis from ehrlichiosis. Nonspecific laboratory abnormalities in babesiosis include normal/decreased white blood cell (WBC) count (leukopenia). Relative lymphopenia is usually present. Atypical lymphocytes are frequently present in the peripheral smear. Thrombocytopenia is a constant finding. The erythrocyte sedimentation rate (ESR) is highly elevated (usually >90 mm/h and often >100 mm/h) as is C-reactive protein (CRP). Since the pathophysiology of babesiosis is that of an acute hemolytic anemia, like malaria, intravascular hemolysis in babesiosis is manifested by increased lactate dehydrogenase (LDH)/total bilirubin. Increased LDH and total bilirubin are the most sensitive indicators of the

TABLE 1   Babesiosis

PREFERRED THERAPY	ALTERNATE THERAPY
Azithromycin (Zithromax)[1] 500 mg PO×1, then 250 mg PO q24h×7 days **plus** Atovaquone suspension (Mepron)[1] 750 mg PO q12h×7 days	Clindamycin (Cleocin)[1] 600 mg PO q8h×7 days **plus** Quinine[1] 650 mg PO q8h×7 days

From Cunha CB, Cunha, BA, editors: *Antibiotic Essentials*. 17th ed. New Delhi: Jaypee Brothers Medical Publishers; 2020, p. 271.
[1]Not FDA approved for this indication.

degree of intravascular hemolysis in babesiosis. The hemoglobin/hematocrit is decreased later in more severe cases. Ferritin levels are highly elevated and prolonged (higher/longer) than would occur with acute-phase ferritin elevations. Since babesiosis impairs T cell function, as in malaria, serum protein electrophoresis often shows polyclonal gammopathy reflecting compensatory B cell hyperactivity. Serum transaminases are mildly elevated, but alkaline phosphatase is unelevated. Cold agglutinins are not a feature of babesiosis. In patients with decreased/absent splenic function, Howell-Jolly bodies are present in the peripheral smear. The number of Howell-Jolly bodies present is inversely proportional to the degree of splenic dysfunction.

Diagnosis of babesiosis is microscopic or serologic. Like malaria, babesiosis may be diagnosed on Giemsa stained blood smears. If malaria is not a diagnostic consideration (geographic distribution, blood transfusion), the presence of intraerythrocytic ring forms is diagnostic. Less common, but more specific, are pathognomonic tetrads (Maltese crosses) of babesiosis in peripheral smears. Also, unlike malaria, there is no extraerythrocytic pigment in babesiosis. Alternatively, elevated IgM *Babesia* species titers are diagnostic.

Therapy

The preferred therapy of babesiosis consists of 7 days combination therapy of azithromycin (Zithromax)[1] plus atovaquone (Mepron).[1] Alternatively, clindamycin (Cleocin)[1] plus quinine[1] for 7 days may be used (Table 1).

Treatment failure may occur in those with impaired T cell function, e.g., patients with HIV or with decreased splenic function. In such cases, exchange transfusion may be lifesaving.

[1]Not FDA approved for this indication.

References

Bonoan JT, Johnson DH, Cunha BA: Life-threatening babesiosis in an asplenic patient treated with exchange transfusion, azithromycin and atovaquone, *Heart Lung* 27:424–428, 1998.

Cunha BA, Raza M, Schmidt A: Highly elevated serum ferritin levels are a diagnostic marker in babesiosis, *Clin Infect Dis* 60:827–829, 2015.

Cunha BA, Mickail N, Laguerre M: Babesiosis mimicking Epstein Barr Virus (EBV) infectious mononucleosis: another cause of false positive Monospot test, *J Infect* 62:531–532, 2012.

Cunha BA, Cohen YZ, McDermott B: Fever of unknown origin (FUO) due to babesiosis in an immunocompetent host, *Heart Lung* 37:481–484, 2008.

Cunha BA, Nausheen S, Szalsa D: Pulmonary complications of Babesiosis: case report and literature review, *Eur J Clin Microbiol Infect Dis* 26:505–508, 2007.

Cunha BA, Crean J, Rosenbaum G: Lipid abnormalities in babesiosis, *Am J Med* 15:758–759, 2000.

Cunha CB: Infectious diseases differential diagnosis. In Cunha BA, editor: *Antibiotic Essentials*, ed 12th, Sudbury, MA, 2013, Jones & Bartlett, pp 474–506.

Hildebrandt A, Gray JS, Hunfeld KP: Human babesiosis in Europe: what clinicians need to know, *Infection* 41:1057–1072, 2013.

Kim N, Rosenbaum GS, Cunha BA: Relative bradycardia and lymphopenia in patients with babesiosis, *Clin Infect Dis* 26:1218–1219, 1998.

Krause PJ, Daily J, Telford SR, et al: Shared features in the pathology of babesiosis and malaria, *Trends Parasitol* 23:605–610, 2007.

Larkin JM: Ticks and tick-related illness, *Med Health RI* 91:209–211, 2008.

Leiby DA: Transfusion-transmitted Babesia spp: bull's-eye on Babesia microti, *Clin Microbiol Rev* 24:14–28, 2011.

Merch K, Holmaas G, Frolander PS, et al: Severe human Babesia divergens infection in Norway, *Int J Infect Dis* 23:37–38, 2014.

Nathavitharana RR, Mitty JA: Diseases from North America: focus on tick-borne infections, *Clin Med* 15:74–77, 2015.

Panduranga V, Kumar A: Severe babesiosis presenting as acute respiratory distress syndrome in an immunocompetent patient, *Conn Med* 78:289–291, 2014.

Rosenbaum GS, Johnson DH, Cunha BA: Atypical lymphocytosis in babesiosis, *Clin Infect Dis* 20:203–204, 1995.

Sharon KP, Krause PJ: Babesiosis. In Cunha BA, editor: *Tickborne infectious diseases diagnosis and management*, New York, 2007, Information Healthcare, pp 111–120.

Usmani-Brown S, Halperin JJ, Krause PJ: Neurological manifestations of human babesiosis, *Handb Clin Neurol* 114:199–203, 2013.

Wudhikarn K, Perry EH, Kemperman M, et al: Transfusion-transmitted babesiosis in an immunocompromised patient: a case report and review, *Am J Med* 124:800–805, 2011.

BACTERIAL MENINGITIS

Method of
Martha Muller, MD

CURRENT DIAGNOSIS

Patient Age Often Determines Clinical Presentation:
- Neonates: nonspecific symptoms
- Classic features: Fever, headache, neck stiffness, altered mental status
- Cerebrospinal fluid (CSF) evaluation
- Elevated opening pressure
- Elevated white blood cell count
- Decreased glucose: CSF–to–blood glucose ratio less than 0.60
- Elevated protein

CURRENT THERAPY

Neonates Younger Than 2 Months
- Most common organisms: *Streptococcus agalactiae, Escherichia coli* or other gram-negative enteric organism, occasional *Listeria monocytogenes*
- Empiric therapy: ampicillin, cefotaxime, or ceftriaxone (should be discussed with a pharmacist to determine risk factors for use)

Infants and Children Older Than 2 Months
- Most common organisms: *Streptococcus pneumoniae, Neisseria meningitidis, Haemophilus influenzae* type B
- Empiric therapy: ceftriaxone and vancomycin (used for potential penicillin-resistant *S. pneumoniae*)

Adults
- Most common organisms: *S. pneumoniae, N. meningitidis*
- Empiric therapy: ceftriaxone and vancomycin

Adults Older Than 50 Years
- Most common organisms: *S. pneumoniae, N. meningitidis, L. monocytogenes*
- Empiric therapy: ceftriaxone, vancomycin, and ampicillin

Bacterial meningitis is a serious, life-threatening infection of the central nervous system. This inflammation of the meninges and subarachnoid space, including the cerebrospinal fluid (CSF), may potentially affect the brain cortex and parenchyma. Bacterial meningitis can occur via several pathophysiologic mechanisms (Table 1). In the neonatal period, most of the offending organisms have colonized mucosal surfaces after contact and aspiration of maternal intestinal and genital tract secretions during the delivery process. The most common mechanism noted outside of the neonatal period involves nasopharyngeal colonization, penetration of the nasopharyngeal mucous membrane barrier with entrance to the interstitial space, and entrance into the capillary

TABLE 1	Pathophysiologic Mechanisms Associated With the Development of Bacterial Meningitis
MECHANISM	**EXAMPLES**
Hematologic	Nasopharyngeal colonization with penetration
Traumatic	Skull fractures
Iatrogenic	Cochlear implantation; ventriculoperitoneal shunt placement
Congenital	Dermal sinus
Contiguous infection	Sinuses; middle ear

bloodstream with subsequent delivery to the meninges or choroid plexus. Once organisms penetrate the CSF, an advantage in their favor exists. In a usual physiologic state, there is essentially an absence of capsule-specific immunoglobulins, complement factors, polymorphonuclear lymphocytes, and other plasma cells within the CSF, making the environment conducive to bacterial proliferation. Available host defenses are apparently ineffectual against encapsulated organisms. The cerebral vasculature is the primary mark for inflammation. Inflammatory changes result in blood-brain barrier disruption, edema, vasospasm and potential arterial thrombosis, as well as cerebral vein occlusions.

Additionally, bacterial and neutrophil-associated inflammatory products may traverse the pial barrier, potentially resulting in neuronal necrosis or cranial nerve compression.

The majority of bacterial meningitis cases occur sporadically. Globally, reported cases of bacterial meningitis increased between 2006 and 2016, with poverty strongly correlated to incidence. Incidence reported in higher-resourced countries has decreased to 0.5 to 1.5 per 100,000 population. Africa continues to bear a significant burden of bacterial meningitis, with incidence reaching 1000 per 100,000 population. Worldwide, bacterial meningitis is linked with significant morbidity and mortality, evidenced by approximately 16 million reported cases in 2013, associated with 1.6 million years lived with disability annually. Although dependent on many factors, including etiologic agent, age, risk factors, and so on, case fatality rates for bacterial meningitis have been reported to be between 17% and 40%.

A disease formerly dominated by *Haemophilus influenzae* in infants has now transitioned to one caused by *Streptococcus pneumoniae*, largely affecting older adult patients. On the whole, *S. pneumoniae* meningitis causes meningitis in children older than 5 years of age and in adults older than 65 years of age. Contrastingly, *Neisseria meningitidis* tends to cause meningitis in older children and young adults. *Streptococcus agalactiae* dominates as the most common organism implicated in bacterial meningitis in neonates and young infants.

Many intrinsic and extrinsic factors increase the risk for developing bacterial meningitis and also affect the potential offending bacteria (Table 1). Additionally, general factors such as poor living conditions and crowded daycare centers influence the potential development of bacterial meningitis.

Diagnosis

The clinical presentation of bacterial meningitis is greatly influenced by patient age. Neonates and infants generally present with nonspecific signs and symptoms, including poor feeding, respiratory distress, fussiness, general weakness, and irritability. Although not universal in babies with bacterial meningitis, fever may also be present in less than 40% and seizures may be present in 15% to 34%. Similarly, hypothermia may be a presenting symptom. In general, patients with bacterial meningitis beyond the neonatal period present with more classic symptoms, including fever, neck stiffness, photophobia, significant headache, nausea, and vomiting. Those patients with associated systemic compromise have higher potential for poor disease outcome.

TABLE 2	Anticipated Cerebrospinal Fluid Findings in Bacterial Meningitis
CSF PARAMETER	**TYPICAL FINDINGS**
White blood cell count	>1000 cells/mm^3 (may be affected by immunosuppression, neutropenia, atypical pathogens)
Glucose	<40 mg/dL (CSF–to–blood glucose ratio <0.60)
Total protein	>100 mg/dL (increased above normal values for age)
Gram stain	Positivity depends on bacterial burden. Stains positive 97% of the time when cultures grow >10^5 CFU Specific yield of 70%–90% for *Streptococcus pneumoniae* Specific yield of 30%–90% for *Neisseria meningitidis* Sensitivity low for *Listeria monocytogenes* as few organisms are generally present in CSF
CSF opening pressure	>200 mm H$_2$O (may be >300 mm H$_2$O; continued elevation for first 24–48 hours before decrease)

CFU, Colony-forming units; *CSF*, cerebrospinal fluid.

Physical examination findings are also associated with age, generally displaying more characteristic findings with increasing age. Meningeal irritation may be demonstrated by neck stiffness, the Brudzinski sign (hips and knees flex reflexively when the neck is flexed), and the Kernig sign (flexion of the thigh with the hip and knee at 90-degree angles results in pain on knee extension), with reported sensitivity as low as 9% for Brudzinsky sign and 5% for Kernig sign. A high degree of suspicion for bacterial meningitis in the appropriate clinical setting should be maintained despite physical examination findings as they are not always indicative of the disease. An adult prospective study demonstrated that the classic signs of meningeal irritation demonstrated a sensitivity of only 5% to 30%. Adult patients older than 65 years may present without typical symptoms. Additionally, patients with bacterial meningitis in this population may frequently present with nonspecific confusion. These older adult patients may also have nuchal rigidity that is not associated with bacterial meningitis.

In general, lumbar puncture should be sought without delay, with few contraindications to suggest otherwise. Contraindications include shock, respiratory compromise, and coagulopathy. Indications for obtaining neuroimaging before conducting a lumbar puncture include the presence of focal neurologic findings in children and immunocompromised condition, previous history of central nervous system disease, new-onset seizure, and focal neurologic findings in adults. CSF examination is crucial to the diagnosis of bacterial meningitis. CSF obtained for suspected bacterial meningitis should routinely be evaluated for cell count (red blood cells; white blood cells, with differential as appropriate), glucose, protein, Gram stain, and culture (Table 2). CSF culture serves as the gold standard for diagnosis, with reported positivity in 50% to 90% of patients. CSF should be evaluated as soon as possible after obtaining it as white blood cells deteriorate within 30 minutes, and elevated white blood cell counts have the potential to metabolize CSF glucose. In general, characteristic CSF findings include elevated white blood cells, low glucose, and elevated protein values (Table 2). It is important to note that the CSF white blood cell count may infrequently be normal, especially very early in the course of illness. Blood cultures should also be obtained for patients with concerns for bacterial meningitis, with reported positivity in 50% to 80% of cases.

The receipt of antibiotics before CSF evaluation may lend to decreased organism recovery via culture. Effective antibiotic therapy can result in sterile cultures within 2 hours for *N.*

meningitidis and begin the sterilization process within 4 hours for *S. pneumoniae*. Additional factors that may adversely affect CSF diagnostic utility include the potential for 24 to 48 hours or longer before obtaining culture results, inadequate CSF specimen volumes, fastidious organisms requiring special growth parameters, and inappropriate specimen attainment and transportation to the laboratory. Although CSF glucose and protein values in children may rarely be affected (in general, irregular values tend to persist for many days despite appropriate therapy), a diagnosis of bacterial meningitis may often still be made based on the CSF analyses in the setting of antibiotic pretreatment. Polymerase chain reaction (PCR) is a promising tool in the arsenal for diagnosis of bacterial meningitis, especially in the setting of antibiotic pretreatment, and its evaluation and clinical use are expanding. Notably, the World Health Organization endorses the use of real-time PCR when considering *S. pneumoniae, N. meningitidis,* and *H. influenzae* type B for patients with potential meningitis. The diagnostic precision of PCR has been most widely evaluated for *S. pneumoniae, N. meningitidis,* and *H. influenzae* and has been reported to be as high as 95% to 100% in cases of culture-proven bacterial meningitis. A prospective study from Sweden reviewing CSF from repeat lumbar puncture demonstrated PCR positivity in 89% of samples taken on days 1 to 3; 70% of samples taken on days 4 to 6; and 33% of samples taken on days 7 to 10. In contrast, all CSF cultures taken from the same samples were negative. With its increasing utilization, PCR sensitivity has been reported as 61% to 100%, 88% to 94%, and 72% to 92% for *S. pneumoniae, N. meningitidis,* and *H. influenzae,* respectively. Additionally, false-negative PCR results are rare, occurring in approximately 5% of cases. Latex agglutination and coagglutination techniques, best for detection of bacteria that are actively proliferating and shedding polysaccharide, are infrequently used for the diagnosis of bacterial meningitis.

Complications of bacterial meningitis may occur any time during the course of the illness and include circulatory collapse, disseminated intravascular coagulation, gangrenous digits, focal neurologic findings, seizures, and subdural effusions.

The differential diagnosis of bacterial meningitis in infants and young children includes otitis media, pharyngitis, pneumonia, retropharyngeal abscess, and lymphadenopathy. Additional diagnoses include brain abscess, tuberculous meningitis, aseptic meningitis, meningitis caused by atypical organisms, and sinusitis.

Antibiotic Management

Successful treatment is characterized by a delicate balance between prompt antibiotic administration and host inflammatory response regulation. Underscored by an almost 100% mortality noted for untreated bacterial meningitis, prompt, appropriate antibiotic administration is paramount, generally increasing the chances of survival. This is particularly notable for infants and children in whom case fatality rates are decreased to less than 10% and less than 5%, respectively, for meningococcal meningitis in the setting of appropriate therapy.

Empiric antibiotic therapy should be chosen based on a variety of factors, including most likely bacterial etiology (local antibiograms and resistance patterns should be considered) (Tables 3 and 4), ability to penetrate the blood-brain barrier and achieve adequate CSF levels, and bactericidal mechanism of action. Beta-lactam antibiotics are frequently used to treat bacterial meningitis and are generally effective against the most commonly associated bacteria. CSF concentrations of these antibiotics, even in the setting of minimal meningeal inflammation, are generally adequate for the minimal inhibitory concentrations for susceptible bacteria. Bacterial resistance patterns also greatly influence empiric antibiotic therapy. Worldwide, penicillin resistance in *S. pneumoniae* has affected recommendations to use vancomycin as part of the empiric antibiotic regimen. Antibiotics should be provided parenterally at maximal clinically indicated doses (Table 5). Antibiotic therapy should not be delayed by the need to obtain neuroimaging. Once a specific organism is isolated, antibiotic therapy should be tailored to treat the organism, completing an appropriate duration of therapy (Table 6).

TABLE 3 Empiric Antibiotic Therapy Based on Contributing Factors*

CONTRIBUTING FACTOR	POTENTIAL ORGANISMS	ANTIBIOTIC THERAPY
Age		
<1 month	*Streptococcus agalactiae*, *Escherichia coli* (gram-negative enteric organisms), *Listeria monocytogenes*	Ampicillin and cefotaxime or ceftriaxone (discuss use in this population with pharmacist)
1–2 years	*Streptococcus pneumoniae*, *Neisseria meningitidis*, *Haemophilus influenzae* type B, *S. agalactiae*, *E. coli*	Ceftriaxone or cefotaxime and vancomycin[1]
2–50 years	*S. pneumoniae*, *N. meningitidis*	Ceftriaxone or cefotaxime and vancomycin[1]
>50 years	*S. pneumoniae*, *N. meningitidis*, *L. monocytogenes*	Ceftriaxone or cefotaxime, ampicillin and vancomycin[1]
Head trauma Penetrating trauma	*Staphylococcus aureus*, coagulase-negative staphylococci, aerobic gram-negative organisms (including *Pseudomonas aeruginosa*)	Vancomycin with either cefepime[1] or meropenem
Neurosurgery	*S. aureus*, coagulase-negative staphylococci, aerobic gram-negative organisms (including *P. aeruginosa*)	Vancomycin with either cefepime[1] or meropenem
CNS shunt placement	*S. aureus*, coagulase-negative staphylococci, aerobic gram-negative organisms (including *P. aeruginosa*)	Vancomycin with either cefepime[1] or meropenem

*Modified from Tunkel AR, Hartman BJ, Kaplan SL, et al: Practice guidelines for the management of bacterial meningitis, *Clin Infect Dis* 39:126–1284, 2004.
[1]Not FDA approved for this indication.

TABLE 4 Special Patient Characteristics Associated With Specific Organisms

BACTERIA	PATIENT CHARACTERISTICS
Streptococcus pneumoniae	Immunocompromised status
Neisseria meningitidis	Complement deficiencies, asplenia, smoking, antibody deficiency
Haemophilus influenzae type B	Native American children; Alaskan Native children
Listeria monocytogenes	Immunocompromised status
Staphylococcus aureus	Neurosurgical procedures, shunt device placement, trauma, underlying disease (e.g., diabetes mellitus), HIV, cardiovascular disease, intravenous drug use

TABLE 6 Duration of Antibiotic Therapy for Uncomplicated Infections Caused by Specific Organisms

PATHOGEN	DURATION OF THERAPY
Streptococcus agalactiae (group B streptococcus)	14 days
Escherichia coli (gram-negative enteric organisms)	21 days
Listeria monocytogenes	21 days
Streptococcus pneumoniae	10–14 days
Neisseria meningitidis	7 days
Haemophilus influenzae type B	7–10 days

TABLE 5 Antibiotics Commonly Used to Treat Bacterial Meningitis

ANTIBIOTIC	ADULT DOSING	PEDIATRIC DOSING
Ampicillin	2 g every 4 hours	300–400 mg/kg/day divided every 4–6 hours; maximum daily dose: 12 g/day
Cefotaxime[2]	2 g every 4–6 hours	225–300 mg/kg/day divided every 6–8 hours
Ceftriaxone	2 g every 12 hours	50 mg/kg/dose every 12 hours
Cefepime[1]	2 g every 8 hours	50 mg/kg/dose every 8 hours
Meropenem	2 g every 8 hours	40 mg/kg/dose every 8 hours
Vancomycin*[1]	15–20 mg/kg/dose every 8–12 hours	15 mg/kg/dose every 6 hours

*Appropriate loading and level monitoring should be performed by a pharmacist.
[1]Not FDA approved for this indication.
[2]Not available in the United States.

Adjunctive Therapy

With a goal of decreasing inflammation leading to neuronal death and brain damage, dexamethasone (Decadron)[1] administration is the cornerstone of adjunctive therapy for bacterial meningitis. Data from studies evaluating the effect of steroids on outcomes of infants and children with bacterial meningitis have demonstrated improved meningeal inflammatory indices and decreased audiologic and neurologic sequelae compared with those receiving placebo; this benefit is most notable for *H. influenzae* meningitis. The data for dexamethasone use to treat *S. pneumoniae* meningitis in children are less vigorous. Additionally, animal models of bacterial meningitis demonstrated decreased vancomycin concentrations and penetration rates in the CSF for those animals receiving dexamethasone. This is important given the potential need to use vancomycin in the treatment of penicillin-resistant *S. pneumoniae* bacterial meningitis.

The American Academy of Pediatrics Committee on Infectious Diseases does endorse the use of dexamethasone for *H. influenzae* type B meningitis. However, the committee does not make a recommendation for routine dexamethasone use in *S. pneumoniae* meningitis. They do provide a consideration of its use in children older than 6 weeks after risks and benefits have been reviewed. There are inadequate data to make a recommendation for dexamethasone use during the neonatal period. The available data demonstrating decreased unfavorable outcomes in adults when using dexamethasone have prompted the Infectious Diseases Society of America to routinely recommend dexamethasone for adults with suspected or proven pneumococcal meningitis. When given, dexamethasone should be provided at a dose of 0.15 mg/kg every

[1]Not FDA approved for this indication.

6 hours for 2 to 4 days. It should be given 10 to 20 minutes before or concurrent with the first dose of antibiotic therapy.

Vaccination Prevention

Between 1990 and 2013, global mortality caused by *S. pneumoniae*, *N. meningitis*, and *H. influenzae* type B decreased by 29%, 25%, and 45%, respectively. Conjugate vaccination strategies have played an important role in improving that landscape. The introduction of *H. influenzae* type B and *S. pneumoniae* conjugate vaccines during the 1990s and 2000s contributed to reports of a decrease in bacterial meningitis in both vaccinated and nonvaccinated populations. The additional benefit of whole-population herd immunity was also described with the introduction of pneumococcal conjugate vaccines. The introduction of conjugated *H. influenzae* type B vaccination programs provided a significant contribution to reducing bacterial meningitis, wherein bacterial meningitis caused by this organism has decreased by almost 100%. Interestingly, initiation of the 7-valent pneumococcal conjugate vaccine (Prevnar 7) in the United States was accompanied by a noted decrease in meningitis caused by vaccine serotypes, initially in children followed by a decrease in adults. However, a concurrent increase in nonvaccine serotypes was noted in response. Likewise, the introduction of the 13-valent pneumococcal conjugate vaccine (Prevnar 13) has also been met with an increased prevalence of nonvaccine serotypes causing bacterial meningitis. Since 2015 there has been a brisk increase in incidence of invasive pneumococcal disease, including meningitis, secondary to non-PCV13 serotypes. Despite the concerns regarding serotype replacement, receipt of several pneumococcal conjugate vaccines in the United States led to a 66% and 33% decrease in rates of pneumococcal meningitis for children younger than 2 years and adults older than 65 years, respectively. Vaccination against *N. meningitidis* has also resulted in a decrease in bacterial meningitis, demonstrating a rate decrease from 13.5 per 100,000 in 1968 to 1985 to 5.2 per 100,000 in 1989 to 2011. Many higher-resourced countries have seen a significant decrease in the incidence of serogroup-C meningitis related to vaccination. Serogroup-B meningitis rose with the decline of serogroup-C meningitis in higher-resourced countries. In 2015 the United Kingdom introduced serogroup-B vaccine 4CMenB (Bexsero), reporting an overall 75% decline in invasive disease.

Immunization against *H. influenzae* type B, *S. pneumoniae*, and *N. meningitidis* has been incorporated into the routine childhood vaccination schedule in the United States. The Advisory Committee on Immunization Practices provides specific vaccine recommendations.

Outcomes/Sequelae

The consideration of patient outcomes is multifactorial, including patient age; time to antibiotic administration, especially as it relates to symptom onset; host factors such as immune response to infection; and time to CSF sterilization. In general, the greatest morbidity and mortality are seen at the extremes of ages (i.e., neonates and older adults). Mortality associated with bacterial meningitis has been 20% to 25% for numerous decades. Pneumococcal meningitis is associated with the highest case fatality rates, reported as 20% to 37% in high-income countries and as high as 51% in low-income countries. This is in contrast with case fatality rates reported as 3% to 10% worldwide for meningococcal meningitis. A study reported that risk factors implicated in the development of neurologic complications in the pediatric population include age less than 12 months; bacterial etiology, especially *S. pneumoniae*; altered level of consciousness on presentation; delayed presentation; and delayed antibiotic administration.

An important immediate complication related to bacterial meningitis in pediatric patients is the development of subdural effusions. Subdural effusions are described in 20% to 39% of pediatric patients with bacterial meningitis and are notably more common in infants younger than 1 year compared with their older peers. Importantly, although there is the potential for infection, most subdural effusions in this clinical scenario are asymptomatic, demonstrating spontaneous resolution.

Neurologic difficulties have been reported in 20% to 30% of bacterial meningitis events. Similarly, long-standing neuropsychological sequelae have been reported in as many as 50% of those who survive bacterial meningitis. Compared with their well siblings who did not have bacterial meningitis, infants and children with bacterial meningitis are more likely to experience seizures, hearing loss, cognitive disturbances, and behavioral concerns. Similarly, there have been reports of disturbed executive functioning, memory, and intelligence in adults who have recovered from bacterial meningitis.

Seizures, hearing loss, and cognitive impairment are the most commonly reported disabilities after a diagnosis of bacterial meningitis. Seizures complicate bacterial meningitis and have an individual link to increased morbidity. In children, the development of long-standing neurologic complications is less concerning when associated seizures that occur early during the course of illness are easily controlled. In contrast, prolonged or difficult-to-control seizures and seizures developing 72 hours after admission are more likely to be associated with neurologic sequelae and are often indicative of a cerebrovascular event. Neurologic complications have been reported in as many as 50% of those who survive bacterial meningitis. Hearing loss is a common complication of bacterial meningitis. In fact, sensorineural hearing loss has been described as the most broadly reported neurologic sequelae of bacterial meningitis. Hearing loss has the potential to be transient or permanent and is often associated with *S. pneumoniae* meningitis. Sustained hearing loss is generally sensorineural, with incidence reported as 14% for mild hearing loss and 5% for severe hearing loss. The hearing loss typically occurs during the initial days of the infection and can be transient or permanent, underscoring the need for formal hearing evaluation to occur in all patients diagnosed with bacterial meningitis.

References

American Academy of Pediatrics: *Red book report of the committee on infectious diseases 2018-2021*, ed 31.

Brouwe MC, van de Beek D: Epidemiology of community-acquired bacterial meningitis, *Curr Opin Infect Dis* 31:78–84, 2018.

Bystritsky RJ, Chow FC: Infectious meningitis and encephalitis, *Neurol Clin* 40:77–91, 2022.

Costerus JM, et al: Community-acquired bacterial meningitis, *Curr Opin Infect Dis* 30:135–141, 2017.

Davis LE: Acute bacterial meningitis, *Continuum (Minneap Minn)* 24:1264–1283, 2018.

Diallo K, et al: Molecular diagnostic assays for the detection of common bacterial meningitis pathogens: a narrative review, *EBioMedicine* 65:103274103274, 2021.

Figueiredo AHA, et al: Acute community-acquired bacterial meningitis, *Neurol Clin* 809–820, 2018.

Hasbun R: Progress and challenges in bacterial meningitis, *JAMA* 328:2147–2154, 2022.

Kim KS: Acute bacterial meningitis in infants and children, *Lancet Infect Dis* 10:32–42, 2010.

Lexicomp Online: *Adult Lexi-Drugs Online*, Hudson, Ohio, 2021, UpToDate, Inc.

Lexicomp Online: *Pediatric and Neonatal Lexi-Drugs Online*, Hudson, Ohio, 2021, UpToDate, Inc.

Liechti FD, et al: Bacterial meningitis: insights into pathogenesis and evaluation of new treatment options: a perspective from experimental studies, *Future Microbiol* 10:1195–2213, 2015.

McGill F, et al: Acute bacterial meningitis in adults, *Lancet* 388:3036–3047, 2016.

Obaro S: Updating the diagnosis of bacterial meningitis, *Lancet Infect Dis* 19:1160–1161, 2019.

Oordts-Speets AM, et al: Global etiology of bacterial meningitis: a systematic review and meta-analysis, *PLOS One* 13, 2018. https://doi.org/10.1371/journal.pone.0198772. e0198772.

Pajor MJ, et al: High risk and low prevalence diseases: Adult bacterial meningitis, *Am J Emerg Med* 65:76–83, 2023.

Posadas E, et al: Pediatric bacterial meningitis: An update on early identification and management, *EB Medicine* 15:1–20, 2018.

Saez-Llorens X, McCracken GH Jr: Bacterial meningitis in children, *Lancet* 361:2139–2148, 2003.

Syrogiannopoulos GA, et al: Global epidemiology of vaccine-preventable bacterial meningitis, *PIDJ* 41:e525–e529, 2022.

Tunkel AR, et al: Practice guidelines for the management of bacterial meningitis, *CID* 39:1267–1284, 2004.

Van de beek D, et al: Community-acquired bacterial meningitis, *Lancet* 398:1171–1183, 2021.

van de Beek D, et al: Community-acquired bacterial meningitis, *Nat Rev Dis Primers* 2(1–20), 2016.

Wall EC, et al: Acute bacterial meningitis, *Curr Opin Neurol* 34:386–395, 2021.

Zainel A, Mitchell H, Sadarangani M: Bacterial meningitis in children: Neurological complications, associated risk factors, and prevention, *Microorganisms* 9:535, 2021.

Young S and Saguil A: Bacterial meningitis in children. *Am Fam Physician* 105(3):311-312.

BRUCELLOSIS

Method of
Patrick L. Allen, MD

CURRENT DIAGNOSIS

- Brucellosis presents with a variety of nonspecific clinical syndromes, most commonly an unusually persistent, undulating fever often accompanied by musculoskeletal pains. Rare complications include meningitis and endocarditis.
- The key to the diagnosis of brucellosis is maintaining a high degree of clinical suspicion in patients with a suggestive clinical history, such as travel to an endemic area, consumption of unpasteurized dairy products, close contact with potentially infected mammals, or inadvertent laboratory exposure.
- There is no gold standard for the diagnosis of *Brucella* infection. Multiple blood cultures should be drawn but have variable yield. Serologic tests may be helpful but require cautious interpretation, especially in endemic areas. Polymerase chain reaction (PCR) is promising but will require more standardization before widespread acceptance.

CURRENT THERAPY

- Combination therapy with multiple antibiotics is needed to successfully treat and to prevent recurrence.
- Doxycycline (Vibramycin) for 6 weeks plus either rifampin (Rifadin)[1] for 6 weeks or a parenteral aminoglycoside for 1 to 3 weeks are the most commonly recommended regimens.
- Longer therapy, often with three antibiotics in combination, is needed for localized and complicated disease.

[1]Not FDA approved for this indication.

TABLE 1	Characteristics of *Brucella* Species		
SPECIES	**PRIMARY HOST**	**OTHER HOSTS**	**ZOONOTIC SPREAD**
Brucella melitensis	Goats and sheep	Camels, cattle, yaks, alpacas, ibex	Yes
Brucella abortus	Cattle	Elk, bison, camels, moose	Yes
Brucella suis	Pigs, wild hogs	Hares, horses, reindeer, armadillo	Yes
Brucella canis	Dogs	Foxes, coyotes, cats, racoons	Less common
Brucella ovis	Sheep	Deer, goats, cattle	Not reported
Brucella ceti	Whales, dolphins, porpoises	Narwhals	Rare
Brucella pinnipediae	Seals	Whales, dolphins, porpoises	Rare
Brucella inopinata	Unknown		Rare
Brucella neotomae	Wood rats	Mice, guinea pigs	Rare
Brucella microti	Vole	Foxes	Not reported
Brucella papionis	Nonhuman primates		Not reported

History

Brucellosis, also called Malta fever, Mediterranean fever, and Undulant fever, has plagued humanity for millennia and was described by Sir David Bruce, a Scottish physician serving in the Royal Army Medical Corps. In 1887 he linked it with the causal pathogen, a bacteria later given the doubly eponymous name *Brucella melitensis* (from Malta). Later, additional species were identified, some of which also cause human disease.

As a public health interest, brucellosis is a disease reportable to the Centers for Disease Control (CDC). *Brucella* spp. can be easily cultured, grown, stored, and aerosolized in laboratories. This, together with the high infectivity of aerosolized specimens and a very low infectious dose, explains why brucellosis is recognized as a potential bioterrorism agent. Though its low case fatality rate (about 1%) and long incubation period make it an unlikely modern bioterrorism weapon (and is therefore listed by the CDC as a category B, "second highest priority," bioterrorism agent), the potential morbidity and economic ramifications of a widespread attack should not be underestimated. Fortunately, to date, *Brucella* has never successfully been used as a bioterrorism agent against humans.

Epidemiology

Brucellosis is now rare in the United States but is the world's most widespread zoonosis, found in animals as divergent as alpine ibex, African lions, and Antarctic seals. In humans it is noted as a top neglected disease by the World Health Organization (WHO). Though 500,000 human cases are reported worldwide each year, experts estimate the true incidence is substantially, perhaps 10-fold, higher. Much of the world

is endemic, particularly the Middle East and Mediterranean Europe. The control of brucellosis requires well-functioning veterinary and animal husbandry systems; thus it is not surprising that the highest incidence rates of brucellosis are often found in the least developed nations of the world or after times of political instability. For example, when the Syrian conflict starting in 2011 devastated local animal care infrastructure, human brucellosis cases surged in the following years. The United States successfully eradicated *Brucella melitensis* in the 1970s and has nearly eliminated other zoonotic species in livestock; however, *Brucella* continues to be identified in certain populations of bison and elk (in the greater Yellowstone area), as well as in some deer and boar populations. These wild animals do occasionally interact with and infect neighboring domestic animals. Table 1 lists a variety of species of brucellosis, their usual hosts and whether they are considered zoonotic.

In infected ruminants such as cattle and goats, spontaneous abortions are the hallmark clinical presentation, and consumption of infected aborted tissue is the primary means of transmission from animal to animal for *B. melitensis* (causing caprine brucellosis) and *B. abortus* (causing bovine brucellosis, also called contagious abortion). *B. suis* (causing swine brucellosis) also causes abortions and is sexually transmitted in pigs and wild swine. *B. canis,* primarily infecting domestic and wild dogs, is rarely transmitted to humans and requires substantial direct contact, such as assisting with birthing. Other species of *Brucella,* such as *B. ovis* (causing ovine brucellosis, infertility in male sheep), are not considered zoonotic, though rare cases of human transmission have been reported with some species (see Table 1).

The most common cause of human infection is the consumption of unpasteurized dairy products, because the bacteria concentrate in the mammary glands of cattle, goats, and camels. Of the approximately 100 cases of brucellosis diagnosed each year in the United States, most are owing to the consumption of illegally imported soft cheeses from Mexico. Other causes include direct contact with infected animals such as hunters who field-dress animals or meat industry workers who slaughter animals or clean animal products. Brucellosis is the most common laboratory-acquired infection, and this mode of transmission comprises 2% of all human brucellosis cases globally. Laboratory workers can be infected by inadvertent direct contact of infected specimens to mucosal or nonintact skin or through inhalation while sniffing open cultures. Fortunately, when humans are infected with *Brucella*, they are an accidental, dead-end host; human-to-human transmission is exceptionally rare.

Pathophysiology

Brucella spp. are gram-negative, aerobic, nonmotile, facultative intracellular coccobacilli of the family *Brucellaceae*. They are slow-growing, taking several hours to double. The three most virulent species (see Table 1) have a unique smooth lipopolysaccharide (LPS) that induces an unusually tame immune response in humans. After invading the host's mucosa, brucellae are ingested by macrophages and dendritic cells. There the bacteria employ a variety of sophisticated mechanisms to survive in specialized vacuoles and continue to replicate inside of the endoplasmic reticulum without affecting host-cell integrity. Programmed cell death is initially inhibited by the bacteria until sufficient replication has occurred. Brucellae then induce cell necrosis and release new pathogens, which travel through the bloodstream to regional lymph nodes and eventually to macrophage-rich tissues such as the liver, spleen, and bone marrow where chronic infection is established. Granuloma formation occurs in the lungs, liver, and other organs. Brucellae inhibit tumor necrosis factor-alpha, subsequently inhibiting macrophages and natural killer cells. Humoral immunity plays a limited role in controlling this mostly intracellular infection, though the production of antibrucellae antibodies are useful diagnostically. On the other hand, interferon-γ, causing the classic fevers associated with the disease, is a very important and effective host response against brucellae.

Clinical Manifestations

Brucellosis can affect any organ in the body. Its incubation period is usually 3 to 4 weeks but can be anywhere from 5 to 60 days. Asymptomatic and mild, self-limited infections do occur, but the rate remains unclear. In those with clinical brucellosis, fever is the invariable presentation, though it can be acute, relapsing, or prolonged over days to weeks. Other constitutional symptoms such as rigors, chills, sweats, generalized weakness, and fatigue are common. Skeletal complications such as arthralgias, peripheral arthritis, sacroiliitis, and lumbar spondylitis are the most common complications (40%) and are more difficult to treat, with three times the therapeutic failure rates of nonosteoarticular disease. Brucellosis can cause orchitis and epididymitis in men and spontaneous abortions in women. Other complications include hepatitis, liver granulomas, hepatosplenomegaly, lymphadenopathy, and pneumonia. Neurobrucellosis is rare (5%) and can consist of meningitis, meningoencephalitis, brain or epidural abscesses, and/or demyelination disorders. Endocarditis is also rare, occurring in about 2% of cases but responsible for about 80% of brucellosis deaths. Lab findings may include anemia, mild leukopenia, relative lymphocytosis, elevated transaminases, and elevated inflammatory markers. Children can be affected by brucellosis but are more likely than adults to have a mild course of illness.

Diagnosis

Any prolonged, recurrent, or unexplained fever should evoke a detailed clinical history. If that history reveals travel to an endemic area, consumption of any unpasteurized dairy product, close contact with a potentially infected animal, or potential accidental laboratory exposure, this should prompt a thorough diagnostic evaluation for brucellosis.

Unfortunately, there is no single reliable laboratory test as the gold standard for the diagnosis of brucellosis. The definitive diagnosis relies on isolation of the organism by culture. Blood cultures are of variable sensitivity (10%–90%), and yields improve with multiple blood draws over time, especially if drawn while febrile. Bacteremia is more persistent and therefore more easily diagnosed in early infection; with longer duration of illness, successful culture becomes increasingly elusive. Cerebrospinal fluid should be cultured in patients with any neurologic signs or symptoms, though this also has a low sensitivity (15%–30%). Bone marrow cultures have a higher sensitivity than blood cultures in many, but not all, studies and may slightly increase diagnostic yield. However, most recommend against routine bone marrow cultures, because blood cultures are much more easily obtained and may reveal brucellae, even in patients in whom the diagnosis is not initially being considered. In cases of suspected brucellosis, cultures should be incubated for 4 weeks owing to slow bacterial doubling time; the routine practice of discarding samples after 5 to 7 days increases the chances for a missed diagnosis.

Several techniques may be employed to improve the diagnostic yield of blood cultures. Lysis of white blood cells releases intracellular bacteria, and several experts recommend lysis-centrifugation as the method of choice for brucellae cultures. However, newer automated blood culture detection systems perform with even better sensitivity and faster time to detection of positive cultures. Laboratory personnel must be notified of any clinical suspicion for *Brucella* so that they can take appropriate protective precautions and avoid accidental exposure to the highly infectious bacteria.

In the absence of a positive culture, serologic tests are well established and indispensable diagnostic tools, though they do require cautious interpretation. Numerous serologic assays are available, each with its own unique limitations. Furthermore, individual immune responses to *Brucella* are highly variable, further complicating the interpretation of serologic assays. The standard agglutination test (SAT), developed in 1897, remains the most widely used diagnostic test worldwide, reliably detecting antibodies to the smooth LPS found in the three most common species infecting humans. If coupled with compatible symptoms of brucellosis, a titer of >1:160 (or 1:320 in endemic areas) confirms the diagnosis. A fourfold increase in titers over time is also diagnostic, though usually impractical. The prozone phenomenon, in which antibodies are so abundant that they interfere with expected agglutination, may cause false negative results. In that case, a true positive test will emerge with retesting after serial dilutions. False negatives can also be seen in long-standing chronic infection, as agglutinating antibodies wane over time and are replaced by nonagglutinating antibodies later in infection. False positives can occur owing to cross-reaction of antibodies with several other pathogens that share the smooth LPS, including *Francisella tularensis*, *Escherichia coli* O116 and O157, *Salmonella urbana*, *Yersinia enterocolitica* O:9, *Vibrio cholerae*, *Stenotrophomonas maltophilia*, and *Afipia clevelandensis*. Titers tend to decrease with successful treatment in most patients, but 3% to 5% have immunoglobulin M (IgM) persistence after 2 years, so following SAT titers after treatment is not recommended.

The 2-mercaptoethanol test (2-ME) is a microagglutination assay, similar to SAT but more specific to IgG; it does not react during early disease but can be used to monitor serologic response to treatment. Immunocapture agglutination tests such as Brucellacapt are useful for their sensitivity and single-step simplicity and can also be monitored to assess treatment success. Enzyme-linked immunosorbent assay testing has improved sensitivity over SAT and is recommended for suspected neurobrucellosis or when other serologic tests are negative in suspected brucellosis but is less specific than SAT. The serum dipstick assay offers rapid detection of IgM antibodies, most useful in recently acquired disease. The rose Bengal test (RBT) is a widely used buffered plate agglutination assay, using a suspension of *Brucella abortus* in an acid buffer. The RBT has several advantages over the SAT. It does not have the drawback of the prozone phenomenon. It is more sensitive in chronic infections, because it detects both agglutinating and nonagglutinating antibodies. The RBT is also technically simple, rapid, and cheap, making it an ideal screening test. However, test positivity tends to endure, limiting its usefulness in highly endemic areas where repeated exposure to *Brucella* is likely. A positive RBT should be followed up by a more specific agglutination test, especially in endemic areas. Another alternative is to perform serial dilution of a positive RBT serum specimen; persistent positivity at a >1:8 dilution is more suggestive of true clinical disease.

Nucleic acid amplification assays such as PCR offer striking sensitivity, rapid results, and early detection in as little as 10 days after exposure. First developed in 1990, various genomic targets have since been used to develop several assays. However, much of the developing world lacks the needed infrastructure to implement its use. Further, high interlaboratory variability and a lack of standardization have precluded widespread implementation efforts.

Treatment

Antibiotic therapy is indicated in all diagnosed cases of brucellosis and must be able to penetrate macrophages and act in the acidic intracellular environment. Monotherapy is associated with unacceptably high relapse rates, as are short treatment courses. Therefore WHO guidelines recommend 6 weeks of doxycycline (Vibramycin) plus either streptomycin for 2 to 3 weeks or rifampin (Rifadin)[1] for 6 weeks—both are popular worldwide. Seven days of gentamicin may be used as a substitute for streptomycin.[1] oxycycline plus an aminoglycoside is associated with lower relapse rates than doxycycline plus rifampin (5% vs 12%), but gentamicin requires parenteral, usually intramuscular, administration. Thus doxycycline plus rifampin is an easier and more popular choice, despite slightly higher relapse rates and a potential to increase rifampin resistance in areas coendemic with tuberculosis. In vitro resistance testing is often discrepant with in vivo activity and should not be a therapeutic consideration for brucellosis.

Localized disease is more difficult to treat in terms of likelihood of relapse; treatment often involves a combination of three antibiotics for an even more lengthy treatment course (Table 2). In addition to medical therapy, patients with endocarditis almost always benefit from valve replacement, because this has been shown to reduce mortality.

Monitoring

Patients should be expected to defervesce after an average of 4 to 5 days after initiation of appropriate therapy. Fevers lasting longer than 1 week should prompt consideration for treatment failure or an alternative diagnosis. Clinical relapse is defined as the reappearance of signs or symptoms of brucellosis and is ideally confirmed with positive blood cultures or increasing serology titers. Relapse with brucellosis may occur at a rate of around 5% to 10%, even with good adherence to recommended treatment regimens. Relapses typically present within 12 months after treatment and have a milder clinical course than the incident illness. Risk factors for relapse include male gender, bacteremia, duration of illness <10 days, and thrombocytopenia. Reinfection is also common in endemic areas. Relapses and reinfections are successfully treated with a repeated course of the previously mentioned combination treatment regimens.

Prevention

For individuals, the single most important measure to prevent *Brucella* infection is to avoid any consumption of unpasteurized dairy products, especially when sourced from endemic areas. Even in well-developed nations, brucellae persist in wild animal reservoirs

---

[1] Not FDA approved for this indication.

TABLE 2	Treatment of Brucellosis Syndromes
CLINICAL SYNDROME	**MANAGEMENT**
Nonlocalized disease	Doxycycline (Vibramycin) 100 mg po bid × 6 weeks + streptomycin 1 g IM daily × 2–3 weeks Doxycycline 100 mg po bid × 6 weeks +gentamicin[1] 5 mg/kg IV daily × 7 days Doxycycline 100 mg po bid × 6 weeks + rifampin (Rifadin)[1] 600–900 mg po daily × 6 weeks
Pregnancy (<36 weeks gestation)	Trimethoprim-sulfamethoxazole (Bactrim DS)[1] 5 mg/kg of TMP component po bid + rifampin[1] 600–900 mg po daily × 4 weeks
Localized disease:	
Osteoarticular (spondylitis, sacroileitis, peripheral arthritis)	Triple therapy: Doxycycline 100 mg po bid × 3 months + rifampin[1] 600–900 mg po daily × 3 months + aminoglycoside as above
Neurobrucellosis	Triple therapy: Doxycycline 100 mg IV or po bid + rifampin[1] 600–900 mg po daily + ceftriaxone[1] 2 g IV q12h until CSF studies normalize
Endocarditis	Surgical valve replacement + aminoglycoside × 4 weeks + doxycycline 100 mg po bid × 6 weeks to 6 months + trimethoprim-sulfamethoxazole[1] × 6 weeks to 6 months

[1] Not FDA approved for this indication.

and can easily pass into neighboring domestic animals. Unpasteurized products at risk include raw milk, soft cheeses, and ice cream. Fermented dairy products such as yogurt, hard cheeses, and sour milk may carry lower infectious risks but should still be avoided if unpasteurized. On a population level, the implementation of routine pasteurization has been shown to markedly reduce human brucellosis cases, and resources should be leveraged to improve consistent access to pasteurization worldwide. Unfortunately, many developing countries currently lack this infrastructure; in these areas, brucellae are found at alarming rates in dairy products.

Hunters and slaughterhouse workers should use rubber gloves while dressing animals and practice meticulous hand hygiene after any contact with killed animals or animal products. It should be noted that infected animals often appear healthy. Veterinarians and park rangers should take similar precautions.

Laboratories must be notified of specimens that have any suspicion for brucellosis. Labs must be meticulously compliant with established laboratory biosafety standards, such as avoiding splashes and aerosolizing procedures, and sniffing culture media. Adequate ventilation should be maintained, and protective barriers should be used where appropriate. In endemic areas, every positive blood culture vial should be initially processed in safety cabinets until brucellae is ruled out, because unanticipated infections are common.

Healthcare personnel caring for patients infected with *Brucella* should adhere to universal precautions, but no additional isolation measures or precautions are recommended, because human-to-human transmission is exceptionally rare. Currently there is no available vaccine to protect humans from brucellosis, though the WHO considers its development a high priority.

Ultimately, eradication among domesticated and wild animals is the only way to reliably prevent zoonotic disease. In domesticated animals, culling (selective slaughtering) of infected animals based on serologic screening is an important surveillance measure in developed countries but is not feasible in most developing nations. Vaccines are available for some animals, including cattle, sheep, goats, and camels. The most commonly used vaccines, S19 and RB-51, are live attenuated vaccines that can infect humans. Veterinarians can be exposed by accidental needle stick or by accidental spray onto mucosa while vaccinating animals. Humans potentially exposed to infectious vaccine products should take prophylactic antibiotics for 3 weeks (doxycycline and rifampin for S19 or doxycycline alone for RB-51) and should undergo serial diagnostic testing.

To add to the challenges of eliminating brucellosis from domesticated animals, we still have much to learn about the complete extent of *Brucella* in the wild. With animal reservoirs well established in so many species throughout the world, complete eradication of brucellosis is likely an unattainable goal.

References

Centers for Disease Control and Prevention: *Bioterrorism agents/diseases*. Available at https://emergency.cdc.gov/agent/agentlist-category.asp, 2018. Accessed 4.13.23.

Centers for Disease Control and Prevention: *Brucellosis*. Available at https://www.cdc.gov/brucellosis/clinicians/, 2021. Accessed 04.13.23.

Corbel MJ: *Brucellosis in humans and animals*, Geneva, 2006, World Health Organization.

"Etymologia: *Brucella* [broo-selʹə]." *Emerg Infect Dis* 14(8):1337, 2008. https://doi.org/10.3201/eid1408.089999.

Gilbert D, Brucella sp: *The sanford guide to antimicrobial therapy web edition*, Dallas, TX, 2019, Antimicrobial Therapy, Inc.. Available at https://webedition.sanfordguide.com/en/sanford-guide-online/disease-clinical-condition/brucella-sp. Accessed 4.13.23.

Gilbert D, Brucellosis: *The sanford guide to antimicrobial therapy web edition*, Dallas, TX, 2023, Antimicrobial Therapy, Inc. Available at https://webedition.sanfordguide.com/en/sanford-guide-online/disease-clinical-condition/brucellosis. Accessed 4.13.23.

Lalsiamthara J, Lee JH: Development and trial of vaccines against Brucella, *J Vet Sci* 18(S1):281–290, 2017.

Hull NC, Schumaker BA: Comparisons of brucellosis between human and veterinary medicine, *Infect Ecol Epidemiol* 8(1):1500846, 2018.

Pappas G, Akritidis N, Bosilkovski M, Tsianos E: Brucellosis, *N Eng J Med* 352:2325–2336, 2005.

Yagupsky P, Morata P, Colmenero JD: Laboratory diagnosis of human brucellosis, *Clin Microbiol Rev* 33(1):e00073-19, 2020.

CURRENT THERAPY

- If possible, the clinician should first consider discontinuing concurrent antibacterial therapy.
- Treatment should be initiated only after a positive test result for *C. difficile* toxin unless the patient is at high risk for *C. difficile* infection or is severely ill, in which case empirical therapy is justified.
- Treatment recommendations depend on the severity of the disease and whether the patient has a first-time diagnosis or recurrence.
- Clinical parameters that guide treatment include increasing age, leukocytosis, elevation of serum creatinine, and presence of hypotension, shock, ileus, or megacolon.
- Taken orally, fidaxomicin (Dificid) is preferred for initial therapy and recurrences, although it is much more costly than vancomycin, which remains an acceptable choice. Metronidazole (Flagyl)[1] oral, can be used for non-severe disease if these are not available.
- Intravenous metronidazole and or rectal vancomycin (enema)[1,6] can be added for severe disease.
- FMT (fecal microbiota therapy) is a safe and effective option for recurrent disease that does not respond to oral therapies, and has shown promise in studies of severe or fulminant *C. difficile* infection.
- Live biotherapeutic agents containing fecal microbiota (Rebyota) and bacterial spores (Vowst) have recently become available and may restore gut dysbiosis similar to FMT.
- Antimicrobial stewardship programs are a safe and cost-effective method of reducing the burden of *C. difficile* infections.

[1]Not FDA approved for this indication.
[6]May be compounded by pharmacists.

CLOSTRIDIOIDES DIFFICILE COLITIS

Method of
Jeffery D. Semel, MD

CURRENT DIAGNOSIS

- *Clostridium difficile* (renamed *Clostridioides difficile*) infection is diagnosed by a combination of clinical and laboratoryfindings.
- Diagnosis requires a positive test for the presence of *C. difficile* toxins.
- GDH, or glutamate dehydrogenase, produced by *C. difficile*, can be detected in stool. However, it is not specific and can be produced by non-toxigenic *C. difficile.*
- Enzyme immunoassay testing for toxin A and or B has a variable sensitivity and specificity and a turnaround time of about 24 hours and correlates well with disease activity.
- Nucleic acid amplification testing (NAAT) has a high sensitivity and specificity and a turnaround time of less than 4 hours; correlates less with disease activity, thus identifying patients with colonization as well as active infection. Increasingly, combination testing is being employed to imrove diagnostic accuracy.
- Laboratory testing for *C. difficile* toxins should only be performed on patients with ≥3 unformed stools per 24 hours, who are not on laxatives and is not useful as a test of cure.
- Pathologic findings can help to confirm diagnosis.
- NAAT followed by toxin A/B will distinguish between active infection and colonization in most cases.

Pseudomembranous colitis is an inflammatory disease of the colon that is almost always associated with the toxin-producing bacteria *Clostridioides difficile*. In very rare cases, other organisms can be responsible. In this article I discuss *C. difficile* as an important cause of pseudomembranous colitis.

Epidemiology and Risk Factors

C. difficile is the most common infectious cause of health care–associated diarrhea. Studies in US hospitals showed that mortality rates related to *C. difficile* infection nearly quadrupled from 1999 through 2004. An active population and laboratory based study done by the US Centers for Disease Control and Prevention in 2011 suggested that 453,000 new cases occur in the United States annually; with a 30-day mortality rate of 6.4%. Higher rates of infection were found in whites, females, and those > 65 years of age. A Canadian study in 2011 prospectively followed 5422 hospitalized patients and showed that 7.4% had asymptomatic colonization only (60% of these were positive at the time of admission); 2.8% developed *C. difficile* infection during hospitalization. A follow-up CDC study encompassing years 2011 to 2017 following determined efforts to control *C. difficile* infection revealed a decrease in health care-associated but not community-associated *C. difficile* infections. Progress in controlling *C. difficile* has continued; a 2023 CDC report showed a 13% decrease in hospital onset *C difficile* from the prior year.

Risk factors for the development of *C. difficile* infection include advanced age, antimicrobial or chemotherapeutic drug exposure, severe underlying illness, prior hospitalization (acute or long-term care), use of feeding tubes, recent gastrointestinal surgery, and gastric acid suppression. Exposure to antibiotics has been shown to lead to an alteration in the type and quantity of bacterial species found in the normal human intestinal microbiome. Most antibiotics have been associated with *C. difficile* infection.

Increased antimicrobial duration and dosage appear to be associated with higher risk of *C. difficile* infection.

Epidemic strains have been described by pulsed-field gel electrophoresis (e.g., PCR ribotype 027) that are associated with decreased regulatory gene function and increased toxin production. The risk and severity of infection are increased after exposure to the NAP1 strains. Failure of standard first-line therapy for *C. difficile* infection may increase to 10% to 35% during infection with Nap-like strains.

C. difficile infection occurs rarely without prior antibiotic exposure. Healthy peripartum women, children, and postsurgical patients rarely have *C. difficile* infection develop after a single dose of an antibiotic. Newborns have a higher rate of colonization but generally a low rate of *C. difficile* infection.

Microbiology and Pathophysiology

C. difficile is a gram-positive, spore-forming, anaerobic rod. *C. difficile* can exist as either a spore or vegetative form. The vegetative form is highly oxygen sensitive; slight exposure can kill the bacteria. The spore form is highly heat-stable and can survive harsh conditions such as the high acidity of the stomach. Spores have been shown to resist many commercial disinfectants. *C. difficile* reproduces in intestinal crypts and releases exotoxins A and B. Most invasive strains contain both toxins, but nontoxigenic strains exist and do not cause colitis. Collectively, toxins A and B disrupt cellular integrity, attract neutrophils, and activate inflammatory cytokines. Shallow ulcers are formed. Toxin production may fluctuate during active infection. Ulcer formation leads to the release of proteins, mucus, and inflammation manifesting as a pseudomembrane. A pseudomembrane is virtually pathognomonic for *C. difficile* infection.

Transmission occurs via the fecal–oral route, person to person, or via fomites. Following exposure to antibiotics, the normal gut flora is altered ("dysbiosis"), allowing *C. difficile* to become more dominant. Exposure to *C. difficile* spores may result in no acquisition, asymptomatic colonization, mild diarrhea, or infection. Evidence showing colonization occurring during hospitalization as opposed to prior to hospitalization poses an increased risk for *C. difficile* infection, suggests that colonization in some patients induces immunity, and that more virulent strains are present in the hospital. Colonization of asymptomatic hospitalized patients with *C. difficile* ranges from 0% to 22% and is higher in residents of long-term care facilities.

In addition, the host immune response to spore exposure is important in determining the clinical outcome. Approximately 60% of people have detectable levels of antibodies to toxin A and B. It is likely that prior exposure to *C. difficile* spores or related clostridial species and subsequent colonization stimulates antibody production and immunity. Deficient levels of antitoxin antibodies are a risk factor for *C difficile* infection. *C. difficile* has been found to be capable of creating a biofilm in vitro, which may impair the antibacterial activity of antibiotics such as metronidazole (Flagyl). Various studies are attempting to define the role of active or passive immunotherapy, including vaccination with nontoxigenic *C. difficile*, to prevent *C. difficile* infection. Another factor favoring *C. difficile* growth is the loss of gut microbiome members with bile metabolizing capacity leading to enrichment of primary conjugated bile acids, which can promote germination of *C. difficile* spores and decreased binding to toxins.

Clinical Features

C. difficile infection is diagnosed by a combination of clinical and laboratory findings. Diarrhea is defined as the passage of three or more unformed stools in a 24-hour period. Symptoms include fever, diarrhea, and cramplike abdominal pain. Patients can have nausea, vomiting, or hematochezia. In severe cases, abdominal tenderness and distention are present. Signs of septic shock can develop. The extent of leukocytosis frequently correlates with disease severity. Plain abdominal radiographs might show distended loops of bowel, ileus, or, in severe cases, toxic megacolon. Computed tomography (CT) image findings include colonic wall thickening and dilatation, mesenteric edema, and, rarely,

perforation. Endoscopy can reveal pseudomembranes. However, sigmoidoscopy or colonoscopy may be complicated by perforation in severely ill patients and should be performed with caution.

Differential Diagnosis

The differential diagnosis includes bacterial causes such as *Shigella*, *Salmonella*, or *Campylobacter* species, protozoan infections such as *Entamoeba histolytica* or *Strongyloides stercoralis* (immunosuppressed patients), inflammatory disorders such as ulcerative colitis or Crohn's disease, drug toxicity (e.g., chemotherapeutic agents), and vascular disorders such as ischemic bowel disease.

Diagnosis

Various tests have been developed for the diagnosis of *C. difficile* infection. Glutamate dehydrogenase (GDH) is a protein produced by *C. difficile* and can be detected in stool. It is very sensitive for *C. difficile* but can be produced by non-toxigenic *C. difficile* and thus is non-specific.

Enzyme immunoassays (EIA) for toxin A and or B detect toxin production. The sensitivity is 63%–94% and specificity is 75%–100%. GDH and toxin assays correlate well with clinical disease activity, but may not detect the presence of small amounts of toxin.

Molecular tests such as nucleic acid amplification testing (NAAT) can be performed in less than 4 hours. The sensitivity is approximately 93% and specificity is 97%. These tests target toxin genes and do not always correlate with clinical disease. Since the introduction of PCR, the number of cases diagnosed has increased further (though some may represent colonization). Increasingly, two-step testing using NAAT or GDH followed by toxin testing is being employed to distinguish between infection and colonization. When NAAT or GDH are positive but toxin testing is negative, active infection with very low toxin production, or asymptomatic colonization, is present; clinical judgment is necessary to guide therapy.

Treatment

If possible, the clinician should first consider discontinuing concurrent antibacterial therapy, unless there is a compelling clinical indication to continue. Antimotility agents should be avoided because decreased gut motility can increase the potential for tissue toxin exposure and toxic megacolon. Treatment for *C. difficile* infection should be initiated only after a positive *C. difficile* test result unless the patient is at high risk for *C. difficile* infection or is severely ill, in which case empirical therapy is reasonable even with negative test results.

Antibacterials used to treat *C. difficile* infection can be administered orally, intravenously, or rectally. Oral therapies are preferred. Oral vancomycin (Vancocin) is not absorbed in the gastrointestinal tract and is eliminated in the feces. Fidaxomicin (Dificid), a macrocyclic antibiotic, has been shown to have equal efficacy to vancomycin but with a potentially lower rate of *C. difficile* recurrence. Fidaxomicin is approved for patients 18 years or older. Oral metronidazole (Flagyl),[1] a nitroimidazole antibiotic, is eliminated primarily in the urine, although 6% to 15% is eliminated in the feces, but is less effective than fidaxomicin or vancomycin.

Recommendations for the treatment of *C. difficile* infection depend on the severity of the disease. Clinical parameters that correlate with severity include increasing age, leukocytosis, and elevation of the serum creatinine.

In addition to clinical findings, a white blood cell count of at least 15,000 cells/μL or a serum creatinine at least 1.5 times the premorbid level suggests the possibility of severe infection. The Society for Healthcare Epidemiology of America (SHEA) and the Infectious Diseases Society of America (IDSA) published treatment guidelines in 2018 and a "focused" update in 2021. Fidaxomicin 200 mg by mouth twice daily for 10 days is now considered the treatment of choice for an initial episode. The average retail price (USD, Singlecare.com, February 2022) of a 10-day course of fidaxomicin is $5262.00, compared with vancomycin, $491.00. In view of significant cost differences between fidaxomicin and vancomycin, the guidelines state that "implementation depends upon available resources and vancomycin remains an acceptable alternative". If these drugs are not available, metronidazole (Flagyl)[1] 500 mg three times daily by mouth can be used but should be avoided if the disease is severe.

Patients with an initial episode that is complicated by hypotension, shock, ileus, or megacolon should be treated fidaxomicin 200 mg, twice daily, PO, or via nasogastric tube, plus metronidazole[1] 500 mg IV every 8 hours. If the patient has a complete ileus, the clinician may consider adding a rectal instillation of van comycin[1,6] 500 mg every 6 hours. It is recommended that trained personnel administer the enema to decrease the chances of rectal perforation if the rectal route is chosen.

Monitoring

The response to therapy should be monitored clinically. Reversal of hemodynamic instability, decreasing stool frequency, and a declining white blood cell count are objective measures of response. Stool tests for *C. difficile* toxin are not valuable for monitoring disease elimination, because these tests can remain positive after improvement.

Complications and Recurrence

Another challenging problem in *C. difficile* infection is recurrence. Recurrence is defined as another episode that occurs within eight weeks following resolution of the initial episode. Recurrence occurs in approximately 20% to 30% of cases. Continued use of antibacterials (other than treating agents), increased age, female sex, use of proton pump inhibitors or corticosteroids, living in a nursing home, longer hospitalization, severe underlying disease, and inadequate antitoxin antibody response are risk factors for relapse.

The 2021 IDSA/SHEA guideline update now recommends fidaxomicin in one of two strategies, 200 mg oral twice daily for 10 days or 200 mg twice daily for 5 days followed by once every other day for 20 days as the treatment of choice for *C. difficile* recurrences. Alternatively, vancomycin can be prescribed in a tapered and pulsed regimen (vancomycin 125 mg PO 4 times per day for 2 weeks, followed by 125 mg PO 2 times per day for 1 week, followed by vancomycin 125 mg PO once daily for 1 week, followed by 125 mg PO once every 2 to 3 days for 2 to 8 weeks). Cost considerations apply as discussed in treatment of the initial episode. The updated guidelines also suggest that bezlotoxumab (Zinplava), a monoclonal antibody directed against *C. difficile*, given as a single intravenous infusion with standard of care antibiotics, be considered after a recurrence for high risk patients. Bezlotoxumab should be used with caution in patients with congestive heart failure.

Another option for recurrent *C. difficile* infection is fecal reconstitution or fecal microbiota therapy (FMT). The goal is to reverse dysbiosis and restore normal colonic flora. Healthy donor stool is infused via colonoscopy, intraduodenal, or by frozen capsule. Numerous studies have shown the efficacy of FMT, although the exact place, timing and mode of installation continue to be under evaluation. A second FMT installation may improve efficiency. Donor stool must be screened for infectious agents prior to installation. A randomized, double-blind study using live purified *Firmicutes* spores, taken by mouth in an attempt to reverse dysbiosis, showed good efficacy in patients with 3 or more recurrences and who remained positive for *C. difficile* toxin by EIA.

An emerging alternative to FMT for *C. difficile* recurrences may be live biotherapeutic products. Two have been recently approved by the FDA: fecal microbiota live-JSLM (Rebyota) and fecal macrobiota spores live-BRPK (Vowst). Fecal microbiota live is administered by rectal enema. Fecal microbiota spores are administered by oral capsules. Both products should not be used

for active treatment, have shown efficacy for prevention of further recurrence, and have moderate gastrointestinal side effects.

While FMT has an established role for recurrences, a systematic review of FMT for severe or fulminant *C. difficile* infection in 240 patients has recently shown promising results. Some patients required mutiple FMTs and or further adjunctive antimicrobials. Additionally, the effects of therapeutic antibiotics such as vancomycin have come under scrutiny. Oral vancomycin itself may cause a decrease in stool diversity and an increase in vancomycin-resistant enterococci while often not fully eradicating *C. difficile*. Despite the frequency of relapse, antimicrobial resistance of *C. difficile* to metronidazole and vancomycin has been low; however, some recent reports of resistance to vancomycin have emerged and continued vigilance has been advocated. Total colectomy is often considered as a last measure for patients who remain critically ill despite standard therapy. The exact indications for surgery are not clear, although refractory shock, signs of peritonitis, megacolon, and multiorgan failure are most often cited. As expected, the mortality rate after total colectomy is high, ranging from 35% to 80%.

There is insufficient evidence to support the evidence of probiotics[7] for prevention or treatment of *C. difficile* colitis or recurrences and are no longer recommended.

Prevention

Given the difficulties in controlling the spread of *C. difficile*, prevention is critical. *C. difficile* spores resist desiccation and can survive in the hospital environment for months. Environmental contamination is highest in and around the rooms of patients with *C. difficile* infection. The risk of hospital-associated *C. difficile* has been found to be increased for patients occupying the bed of a previous patient who received antibiotics. Items that have been found to harbor *C. difficile* spores include clothing, blood pressure cuffs, telephones, toilets, doorknobs, oral and rectal thermometers, and other medical equipment. In addition, the hands of health care workers have been found to be a vehicle of transmission.

Current recommendations for prevention of transmission of *C. difficile* include the following. Careful hand hygiene with soap and water is essential. Programs to monitor the compliance and technique of hand hygiene are recommended. Alcohol-based hand rubs, which are widely used, have been shown to be less effective at removing spores than conventional hand washing. Thus alcohol-based hand rubs should not be used for *C. difficile* isolation when *C. difficile* outbreaks are present. Barrier precautions with gowns and gloves should be used. Programs to ensure adequate and effective cleaning of health care facilities after use are recommended. Disposable electronic thermometers are recommended. Antimicrobial stewardship programs aimed at promoting the judicious use of antibacterial therapy have been found to be effective in reducing *C. difficile* infection rates and are encouraged. Finally, should continued antibiotic therapy be required in a high-risk patient with or without prior *C. difficile* infection, prophylaxis with vancomycin[1] 125 mg daily may decrease the risk of colitis.

---

[1]Not FDA approved for this indication.
[7]Available as a dietary supplement.

References

Centers for Disease Control and Prevention. 2023 National and State Healthcare-Associated Infections Progress Report. https://www.cdc.gov/healthcare-associated-infections/php/data/progress-report.html. November 2024.

DuPont HL, DuPont AW, Tillitson GS: Microbiota restoration therapies for recurrent Clostridioides difficile infection reach an important new milestone, *Ther Adv Gastroenterol* 17:1–11, 2024.

Fisbein SRS, Hink T, Reske KA, et al: Randomized controlled trial of oral vancomycin treatment in *Clostridioides difficile* colonized patients, *mSphere* 6: e00936–20, 2021.

Fischer M, Sipe B, Cheng Y, et al: Fecal microbiota transplant in severe and severe-complicated *Clostridium difficile*: A promising treatment approach, *Gut Microbes* 8(3):289–302, 2017.

---

[1]Not FDA approved for this indication.
[6]May be compounded by pharmacists.

Greentree DH, Rice LB, Donskey CJ: Houston, We have a problem: Reports of Clostridioides difficile isolates with reduced vancomycin susceptibility, *Clin Infect Dis* 75:1661–1664, 2022.

Jiang ZD, Ajami NJ, Petrosino JF, et al: Randomised clinical trial: faecal microbiota transplantation for recurrent Clostridum difficile infection - fresh, or frozen, or lyophilised microbiota from a small pool of healthy donors delivered by colonoscopy, *Aliment Pharmacol Ther* 45(7):899–908, 2017.

Johnson SW, Brown SV, Priest DH: Effectiveness of oral vancomycin for prevention of healthcare facility-onset *Clostridioides difficile* infection in targeted patients during systemic antibiotic exposure, *Clin Infect Dis* 27:ciz966, 2019, https://doi.org/10.1093/cid/ciz966. {epub ahead of print}.

Johnson S, Lavergne V, Skinner AM et al: Clinical practice guideline by the Infectious Diseases Society of America (IDSA) and Society for Healthcare Epidemiology of America (SHEA): 2021 focused update guidelines on management of *Clostridioides difficile* infection in adults, *Clin Infect Dis* 73(5):e1029–e1044, 2021.

Kyne L, Warny M, Qamar A, et al: Asymptomatic carriage of *Clostridium difficile* and serum levels of IGG antibody against toxin A, *N Engl J Med* 342:390–397, 2000.

Song YN, Yang DY, van Zanten SV, et al: Fecal microbiota transplantation for severe or fulminant Clostridioides difficile infection: systematic review and meta-analysis, *J Can Assoc Gastro* 5:e1–e11, 2022.

Oksi J, Aalto A, Sailla P, et al: Real-world efficacy of bezlotoxumab for prevention of recurrent *Clostridium difficile* infection: a retrospective study of 46 patients in five university hospitals in Finland, *Eur J Clin Microbiol Infect Dis* 38:1947–1952, 2019.

Shim JK, Johnson S, Samore MH, et al: Primary symptomless colonisation by *Clostridium difficile* and decreased risk of subsequent diarrhea, *Lancet* 351:633, 1998.

Song YN, Yang DY, van Zanten SV, et al: Fecal microbiota transplantation for severe or fulminant *Clostridioides difficile* infection: systematic review and meta-analysis, *J Can Assoc Gastro* 5:e1–e11, 2022.

Turner NA, Krishnan J, Nelson A, etal: Assessing the Impact of 2-step Clostridioides difficile testing at the healthcare facility level, *Clin Infect Dis* 77:1043–1049, 2023.

CAT SCRATCH DISEASE

Method of
Ronen M. Ben-Ami, MD

CURRENT DIAGNOSIS

- The combination of a compatible clinical syndrome of regional lymphadenopathy with a primary inoculation lesion and cat contact is highly suggestive of cat scratch disease.
- Results of *Bartonella henselae* serology are helpful in confirming the diagnosis; however, up to 20% of patients remain seronegative throughout their disease.
- Detection of *B. henselae* DNA by polymerase chain reaction from pus obtained by needle aspiration or lymph node biopsy is a highly sensitive diagnostic modality and may be particularly useful in seronegative patients.

CURRENT THERAPY

- Typical cat scratch disease is a self-limiting disease; therefore, systemic antimicrobials are not routinely indicated in immunocompetent patients with uncomplicated cat scratch disease.
- Indications for antimicrobial therapy include an immunocompromised host, endocarditis, retinitis, and other atypical syndromes.
- Treatment may also be considered for patients who have typical cat scratch disease and who have extensive or bulky lymphadenopathy and are highly symptomatic.
- Suppurative lymph nodes should be drained by large-bore needle aspiration.

Cat scratch disease is a worldwide zoonotic infection caused by *Bartonella henselae*, an intracellular, pleomorphic, gram-negative bacillus. Other *Bartonella* species have rarely been implicated. The disease typically manifests as benign regional lymphadenopathy, but atypical disease can involve almost any organ system and is associated with significant morbidity.

Epidemiology

B. henselae infection is widespread among domestic cats and other felids worldwide, and serologic studies indicate a higher prevalence in warm, humid climates. Transmission among cats occurs via an arthropod vector, the cat flea *Ctenocephalides felis*. *B. henselae* bacteremia is detected at higher rates in feral cats than in domesticated cats and in kittens compared with adult cats, explaining the higher infectivity of these animals. Cats infected with *B. henselae* are asymptomatic. Transmission to humans occurs via a scratch, bite, or lick; contamination of cat scratches by flea feces may enhance *Bartonella* transmission.

Cat scratch disease has been estimated to occur in the United States at a rate of 4.5 per 100,000 population with the highest incidence in southern regions (6.4 cases/100,000 population) and in children aged 5 to 9 years (9 cases/100,000 population). There is some seasonality, with incidence peaking between September and January. Although traditionally considered a disease of childhood, epidemiologic surveys have found a similar incidence of cat scratch disease in adults, and 6% of patients are 60 years of age or older. Cat contact is the most important risk factor: Almost all patients are cat owners or were otherwise exposed to cats, and about one-half can recall a recent bite or scratch, most commonly by a kitten.

Clinical Manifestations

Cat scratch disease is divided into two clinical syndromes. Typical cat scratch disease is a subacute, self-limiting regional lymphadenopathy and constitutes 80% to 90% of cases. Atypical cat scratch disease encompasses Parinaud oculoglandular syndrome and other clinical entities with systemic extranodal involvement. Bacillary angiomatosis and bacillary peliosis are manifestations of *B. henselae* infection in immunocompromised persons and are not discussed here.

Typical Cat Scratch Disease

A primary skin lesion, usually a papule or pustule, appears at the site of inoculation 3 to 10 days after cat contact and persists for 1 to 3 weeks. Regional lymphadenopathy develops within 1 to 7 weeks and resolves spontaneously after 2 to 4 months. The primary lesion is still present in about two-thirds of patients when they present for evaluation of lymphadenopathy. The most commonly involved lymph nodes are, in descending order of frequency, axillary and epitrochlear nodes, head and neck nodes, and femoral and inguinal nodes. One-third of patients develop lymphadenopathy at multiple sites. Lymph nodes are often painful and red; suppuration occurs in 10% of nodes. Mild constitutional symptoms, including low-grade fever and malaise, are noted in about one-half of the cases. Rash, night sweats, anorexia, and weight loss are uncommon. Infection results in lifelong immunity.

Atypical Cat Scratch Disease

Parinaud oculoglandular syndrome, the most common form of atypical cat scratch disease, is a specific type of regional lymphadenopathy that occurs after conjunctival inoculation of *B. henselae*. The syndrome includes granulomatous conjunctivitis and preauricular lymphadenopathy. Endocarditis and encephalitis represent severe forms of *B. henselae* infection and are more common in older adult patients. Encephalitis manifests with various degrees of altered mental status, agitation, headache, and seizures. Cerebrospinal fluid lymphocytic pleocytosis occurs in only one-third of cases, and brain imaging studies usually fail to show any abnormalities. Neuroretinitis manifests as sudden unilateral loss of visual acuity. The diagnosis is suspected on the basis of typical findings on fundoscopic examination: papilledema and macular exudates in a starlike configuration. However, these findings are not pathognomonic of cat scratch disease. Other ocular findings include uveitis, optic neuropathy, and retinal vessel occlusion. Infrequent manifestations are self-limiting granulomatous hepatitis and splenitis and osteoarticular disease. Prolonged fever of unknown origin has been described in children and adolescents, taking the form of relapsing fever in one-half of the cases.

TABLE 1	Antibiotic Treatment Regimens for Cat Scratch Disease			
CLINICAL SYNDROME	**FIRST CHOICE**	**SECOND CHOICE**	**COMMENTS**
Typical cat scratch disease	Not indicated*	Azithromycin (Zithromax)[1] 500 mg PO on day 1, then 250 mg PO × 4 days	Drain suppurative nodes using large-bore aspiration
Endocarditis	Gentamicin[1,†] 1 mg/kg IV q8h × >14 days plus doxycycline 100 mg IV/PO bid × 6 weeks	Doxycycline 100 mg PO bid plus rifampicin (Rifadin)[1] 300 mg PO bid × 6 weeks	Some experts recommend extending oral doxycycline treatment × 3–6 months Surgical valve excision may be required
Neuroretinitis	Doxycycline 100 mg PO bid plus rifampicin[1] 300 mg PO bid × 4–6 weeks	NA	Spontaneous resolution is the rule; the utility of treatment remains unproven
Other atypical cat scratch disease	As for neuroretinitis	NA	Treatment duration should be individualized

*Treatment may be considered for patients with bulky or extensive lymphadenopathy and for immunocompromised patients.
†A once-daily dose of 3 mg/kg may be associated with lower nephrotoxicity but was not assessed in clinical trials. Adjust dose to achieve peak serum concentration of 3 to 4 mcg/mL and trough concentrations of <1 mcg/mL.
[1]Not FDA approved for this indication.
NA, Not available.

Diagnosis

A compatible clinical syndrome in a person with a positive history of cat exposure suggests cat scratch disease. The diagnosis is most commonly confirmed with specific serologic assays. The immunofluorescence assay and the enzyme-linked immunosorbent assay are comparably sensitive, although cross-reactivity can occur with other organisms such as *Chlamydia* species, *Coxiella burnetii*, and non-*henselae Bartonella* species. A single elevated titer of immunoglobulin (Ig)M or IgG in the acute phase or a fourfold increase of IgG in convalescent serum supports the diagnosis.

Biopsy and histopathologic examination of lymph nodes are usually only performed when malignancy is suspected. Necrotizing granulomas are typically observed. The pleomorphic gram-negative bacilli are best visualized with the Warthin-Starry stain; however, the sensitivity of this method is too low to be clinically useful. Similarly, culture lacks sensitivity and requires prolonged incubation, making it impractical for routine use.

Polymerase chain reaction assays for the detection of *B. henselae* in pus aspirated from suppurative lymph nodes or primary skin lesions are highly sensitive and specific, and they can be performed with a rapid turnaround time. However, these assays are not widely available in most clinical microbiology laboratories.

Differential Diagnosis

Cat scratch disease should be differentiated from other infectious and noninfectious causes of regional lymphadenopathy. Importantly, lymphoma and solid tumors with metastases to lymph nodes may be confused with cat scratch disease. Malignancy should be suspected in patients who have marked constitutional symptoms, who are seronegative, or whose lymphadenopathy fails to resolve spontaneously after more than 6 months. Unlike cat scratch disease, pyogenic lymphadenitis manifests with rapid progression, high-grade fever, and a septic-appearing patient. Mycobacterial infection, syphilis, bubonic plague, tularemia, histoplasmosis, and sporotrichosis should be considered based on the presence of specific risk factors and endemic exposures. *Bartonella* endocarditis must be differentiated from other causes of culture-negative endocarditis, specifically Q fever and brucellosis.

Treatment

Because of the self-limiting course of typical cat scratch disease, patients usually only require observation and reassurance of its benign nature. The goals of therapy are alleviation of symptoms in patients with bulky lymphadenopathy and drainage of suppurating lymph nodes to prevent spontaneous formation of chronic sinus tracts. If drug treatment is initiated, azithromycin[1] is the agent of choice based on a small, randomized placebo-controlled study that

showed more rapid resolution of lymphadenopathy in the azithromycin arm as determined by ultrasonography. Suppurative nodes should be drained by large-bore needle aspiration. Incisional drainage is best avoided because it can promote sinus tract formation.

Atypical cat scratch disease syndromes usually require treatment, but there are scant data to support specific regimens, and treatment duration is not well defined. For patients with endocarditis, treatment with an aminoglycoside for at least 14 days is associated with a higher likelihood of recovery and survival. Uncontrolled data suggest that, for patients with neuroretinitis, treatment with antibiotics and corticosteroids is associated with better visual outcomes than treatment with antibiotics alone (Table 1).

Complications

Typical cat scratch disease usually resolves without sequelae, at a rate that varies according to antibiotic treatment. For untreated patients, lymph nodes return to normal size after up to 3 months, whereas for patients treated with azithromycin resolution occurs within 30 days. The overall prognosis of *B. henselae* neuroretinitis is favorable. However, moderate and severe loss of vision is present at follow-up in 14% and 6% of affected eyes, respectively. Neurologic deficits of patients with encephalitis are usually self-limited but may take weeks to months to fully resolve. Musculoskeletal complications, which affect about 10% of patients with cat scratch disease, are typically transient, but some patients may go on to develop chronic arthropathy.

Prevention

Flea control in domestic cats can reduce the likelihood of *Bartonella* bacteremia and transmission to humans. Bites and scratches should be promptly rinsed. HIV-infected patients and other immunocompromised persons should be cautioned about the risks of cat exposure because they are susceptible to disseminated visceral *B. henselae* infection, as well as other zoonotic infections such as toxoplasmosis.

References

Goaz S, Rasis M, Binsky Ehrenreich I, et al: Molecular diagnosis of cat scratch disease: a 25-year retrospective comparative analysis of various clinical specimens and different PCR assays, *Microbial Spectr* 10: e0259621, 2022.
Habot-Wilner Z, Trivizki O, Goldstein M, et al: Cat-scratch disease: ocular manifestations and treatment outcome, *Acta Ophthalmol* 96(4):e524–e532, 2018.
Landes M, Maor Y, Mercer D, et al: Cat scratch disease presenting as fever of unknown origin is a unique clinical syndrome, *Clin Infect Dis* 71:2818–2824, 2019.
Nelson CA, Saha S, Mead PS: Cat-Scratch Disease in the United States, 2005-2013, *Emerg Infect Dis* 22:1741–1746, 2016.
Raoult D, Fournier PE, Vandenesch F, et al: Outcome and treatment of *Bartonella* endocarditis, *Arch Intern Med* 163:226–230, 2003.
Rolain JM, Brouqui P, Koehler JE, et al: Recommendations for treatment of human infections caused by *Bartonella* species, *Antimicrob Agents Chemother* 48:1921–1933, 2004.

[1]Not FDA approved for this indication.

CHIKUNGUNYA

Method of
Scott Kellermann, MD, MPH; and Rick D. Kellerman, MD

CURRENT DIAGNOSIS

- Clinically, chikungunya is a diagnosis of exclusion, particularly when laboratory testing is not available. Accurate diagnosis depends on the patient's clinical symptoms and the epidemiology of endemic disease.
- Acute symptoms include incapacitating relapsing bilateral symmetric polyarthralgia accompanied by high fever, headache, backache, and fatigue. Some may have a pruritic maculopapular rash at onset.
- Chronic symptoms include episodic incapacitating symmetric polyarthralgia. Many have long-term asthenia and depression.
- For individuals presenting ≤8 days after onset of symptoms, chikungunya virus can be detected via real-time reverse-transcription polymerase chain reaction (RT-PCR).
- For individuals presenting ≥8 days after onset of symptoms, chikungunya virus serologic testing via enzyme-linked immunoassay (ELISA) or indirect fluorescent antibody (IFA) should be performed.
- Immunoglobulin (Ig)M anti–chikungunya virus antibodies are detectable starting about 5 days (range 1–12 days) and persist for several weeks to 3 months.
- IgM antibody levels peak 3 to 5 weeks after the onset of illness and persist for approximately 2 months.
- IgG antibodies begin to appear about 2 weeks after onset of symptoms and persist for years.
- A positive IgG antibody indicates prior chikungunya infection; it does not delineate whether arthritic symptoms are a consequence of prior infection.

CURRENT THERAPY

- Two chikungunya vaccines have been developed: a live-attenuated vaccine (IXCHIQ) and a virus-like particle vaccine (VIMKUNYA).
- On August 22, 2025, the U.S. Food and Drug Administration suspended the U.S. license for IXCHIQ.
- Medical treatment is primarily supportive.

The word *chikungunya* is a derivation of the Kimakonde (a Mozambique dialect) word *kungunyala*, meaning "to become desiccated or contorted." In the Democratic Republic of the Congo, it is called *buka-buka*, translated as "broken-broken," reflecting the incapacitating arthralgias that are common manifestations of chikungunya fever.

Epidemiology

It is believed that chikungunya virus originated in Africa and migrated to Asia 200 years ago. Evidence derived from molecular genetics suggests it evolved around 1700; the first recorded outbreak of this disease was probably in 1779.

Chikungunya was first diagnosed in Tanganyika in 1952 and is found in a large percentage of countries in Africa, Asia, and Southeast Asia and in India. Interestingly, some medical historians believe that a pandemic of chikungunya occurred in the Western Hemisphere in the 1800s but was diagnosed as dengue fever. The 21st-century researchers who have examined the accounts of this pandemic now speculate that it was caused by chikungunya because the cases exhibited severe joint arthritis, which is more indicative of chikungunya than dengue. The virus then disappeared from the Americas until it reemerged on Caribbean island of Saint Martin in 2013. Chikungunya virus often causes large outbreaks with high attack rates, affecting one-third to three-quarters of the population. Dense human populations and lack of herd immunity likely contribute to the volatile nature of chikungunya epidemics in many regions. In India during 2006, more than 1,250,000 cases of chikungunya were reported, with *Aedes aegypti* implicated as the vector. Between December 2013 and June 2023, 3,684,554 chikungunya cases (suspected and laboratory confirmed) were reported in 50 countries or territories in the Americas. Between 2014 and 2015, most countries in the Latin Caribbean with chikungunya outbreaks reported one or two annual epidemic waves followed by a period with lower incidence or no cases. Montserrat Island reported an explosive epidemic with a cumulative incidence of 85,493 cases per 100,000 inhabitants. Similarly, a serosurvey in Jamaica after the chikungunya epidemic in 2014 to 2015 showed a seroprevalence of 83.6%. A lifelong immunity and protection elicited by chikungunya infection suggests a limited potential for chikungunya recirculation in these locations in the near future.

After the outbreak in the Americas, there were more than 4000 cases reported in U.S. travelers from 2014 to 2017, 13 of which were locally acquired in the continental United States.

However, considering the large immunologically chikungunya-naïve population in North America, combined with the projected expansion of the ranges of *A. aegypti* and *A. albopictus* due to climate change, autochthonous chikungunya transmission in North America could substantially increase in the future.

In 2024 there were 199 travel-related cases of chikungunya in the United States; however, since 2019, no locally acquired chikungunya cases have been reported from U.S. states or territories.

Chikungunya epidemics appear suddenly and unpredictably and proceed explosively.

Risk Factors

Individuals at the highest risk of contracting chikungunya and experiencing more severe symptoms are those who have chronic arthritis, have underlying chronic medical conditions, are over the age of 65 years, or are pregnant. Travelers who spend extended periods of time in endemic areas are at greater risk of exposure, including missionaries, humanitarian aid workers, and those who frequently work outdoors.

Pathophysiology

Chikungunya is an arthropod-transmitted single-stranded RNA alphavirus of the family Togaviridae. Patients develop viremia within a few days of infection. The virus invades and replicates within the joints. Animal models of chikungunya virus pathogenesis suggest the virus directly infects the synovium, tenosynovium, and muscle, leading to production of proinflammatory cytokines and chemokines and recruitment of leukocytes. Typically, infectious virus is cleared from the circulation within days and from joints within a couple of weeks.

There is a wide range of frequency and severity of protracted disease, with chronic musculoskeletal symptomology occurring in 25% to 75% of patients. Why some patients develop chronic joint pain whereas others do not is not well understood. Three hypotheses have been proposed to explain chronic arthritis: persistent viral replication, persistent viral RNA driving an inflammatory response, and autoimmunity. Ongoing T cell activation has been reported in chronic arthritis due to chikungunya virus, but rheumatoid factor and anticyclic citrullinated peptide testing are typically negative.

As with dengue fever and yellow fever, chikungunya cycles from mosquito to human to mosquito. The mosquito *A. aegypti* is the usual vector for transmission of chikungunya. *A. aegypti* is well adapted to urban settings and is widely distributed in the tropics and subtropics worldwide. It prefers the human host. *A. aegypti* breeding sites are associated with elements of human habitation that are seemingly innocuous (e.g., flower vases, water storage vessels, tires, birdbaths). Eggs, which hatch when submerged, are laid on the walls of these artificial water containers. *A. aegypti* enters homes and will feed indoors and outdoors. A single *A. aegypti* mosquito can infect more than one human because this species may feed on another host if its blood meal is interrupted.

A. albopictus, the Asian tiger mosquito, is also a vector. Both species are found in the southeastern and eastern parts of the United States and limited parts of the southwest.

Both A. aegypti and A. albopictus struggle to survive at temperatures <10°C.

The risk of person-to-mosquito transmission is highest during the viremic first week of illness. Human and nonhuman primates are the main amplifying reservoirs for the virus. Transmission is possible through a needle stick, handling of blood, and aerosol laboratory exposure. No transfusion-related cases have been identified. Previous infection will convey permanent immunity.

Prevention

A virus-like particle vaccine (called VIMKUNYA) uses a molecule that resembles the virus closely enough to prompt an immune response to help prevent illness. This vaccine does not use a live or weakened form of the chikungunya virus. VIMKUNYA is manufactured by Bavarian Nordic. The vaccine was licensed by the U.S. Food and Drug Administration (FDA) in February 2025, and the Advisory Committee on Immunization Practices (ACIP) approved recommendations for use in U.S. travelers and laboratory workers in April 2025.

The ACIP recommends the virus-like particle vaccine for people age 12 years and older traveling to a country or territory where a chikungunya outbreak is occurring.

In addition, the vaccine may be considered for people age 12 years and older who are traveling or moving to a country or territory without an outbreak but with elevated risk for U.S. travelers if planning to stay for an extended period of time (e.g., 6 months or more).

On August 22, 2025, the U.S. Food and Drug Administration suspended the U.S. license for the live-attenuated IXCHIQ.

The best preventive measures are wearing permethrin-treated, bite-proof long sleeves and trousers and using a mosquito repellent such as 30% DEET, 20% oil of lemon eucalyptus, or 30% picaridin. Travelers to endemic areas should choose a hotel or lodging with air conditioning or with screens on windows and doors; however, this has only a limited effect because most contacts between the Aedes mosquitoes and humans occur outside. Travelers with underlying medical conditions and women late in their pregnancy (because their fetuses are at increased risk) might consider avoiding visiting areas with ongoing chikungunya outbreaks. The CDC's website has excellent information regarding preventive measures: https://www.cdc.gov/chikungunya/prevention/index.html. Customary blood handling procedures are recommended.

If a chikungunya epidemic were to occur in the United States, the standard public health measures of avoidance and mosquito control would be major lines of defense. To prevent local spread, the patient diagnosed with chikungunya should use mosquito repellent for 1 week after the onset of fever.

Clinical Manifestations

Chikungunya virus infection should be considered in patients with acute onset of fever and polyarthralgia, especially in travelers who have returned within 12 days from areas with endemic chikungunya. Joint pain may precede fever; in one outbreak in 2017 among more than 1300 patients in Dhaka, Bangladesh, joint pain preceded fever in 90% of cases.

The incubation period of the chikungunya virus ranges from 1 to 12 days, most typically 3 to 7 days. Chikungunya infection may be divided into an acute phase (<3 months) and chronic phase (>3 months). The acute phase may be further subdivided into viremic (1–3 weeks) and subacute postviremic (4–12 weeks) phases.

The viremic phase is characterized by sudden onset of high-grade fever (often >39°C); severe, incapacitating polyarthralgia/polyarthritis; myalgias; conjunctivitis; and exanthema. Polyarthralgia is reported in 87% to 98% of cases and represents the most characteristic symptom. The joint pain is mostly polyarticular, bilateral, and symmetric and occurs mainly in peripheral joints (wrists, ankles, and phalanges) and some large joints (shoulders, elbows, and knees). Joint swelling is less frequent, occurring in 25% to 42% of cases. Typically, the fever lasts for 2 days and then will defervesce abruptly.

Headache and an extreme degree of prostration may persist for a variable period, usually about 5 to 7 days. Symptoms typically resolve in 7 to 10 days. Rare complications include uveitis, retinitis, myocarditis, hepatitis, nephritis, hemorrhage, and neurologic problems such as myelitis, meningoencephalitis, Guillain-Barré syndrome, and cranial nerve palsies. In 40% to 50% of cases, skin involvement is present, consisting of a pruritic maculopapular rash, predominantly on the thorax, localized petechiae, and facial edema.

In the subacute phase, fever settles but articular symptoms and fatigue persist. Polyarthritis is usually symmetric and involves small and large joints. Tenosynovitis and bursitis can also occur, which are usually very painful. Patients who have concomitant comorbidities such as osteoarthritis, heart failure, respiratory disease, renal disease, and diabetes are likely to have more severe manifestations of acute infection. Chikungunya infection may also exacerbate underlying rheumatic diseases and relapses of autoimmune arthritis in patients who were in remission before infection.

The chronic phase of the disease may follow a pattern similar to rheumatoid arthritis, peripheral spondylarthritis, undifferentiated arthritis, and fibromyalgia. The ankles, knees, hips, wrists, elbows, and metacarpal-phalangeal joints are mainly involved. The joint disease may be relapsing or unremitting and incapacitating. Occasionally, the polyarthritis may meet the 2010 American College of Rheumatology diagnostic criteria for rheumatoid arthritis, and bone erosions may develop. Rehabilitation therapy must be initiated early to improve functionality. Factors such as age older than 45 years, high viral load ($\geq 10^9$ copies/mL) during the acute phase, and severe immunologic response in the postviremic phase are predictors of the development of chronic symptoms.

Approximately 20% of patients with chronic chikungunya infection may have chronic pain with neuropathic features including paresthesia, tingling, numbness, and itching.

A study of pregnant women conducted on the island of Réunion during the 2005–2006 epidemic showed that the mother-to-child (vertical) transmission rate was approximately 50% when chikungunya infection occurred in the intrapartum period, 2 days before or after delivery. Delivery by cesarean section did not prevent the transmission of virus. The babies were born healthy; however, they developed fever, weakness, and thrombocytopenia between 3 and 7 days. Neurocognitive outcome was poor in children with perinatal transmission from infected mothers. Although chikungunya virus RNA has been detected in breast milk, there have been no reported cases transmitted though breast milk. Even in endemic areas, women are encouraged to breastfeed.

In a study of 4000 patients with travel-acquired chikungunya in the United States, 18% were hospitalized, and 4 patients died. Hospitalization rates were highest among patients <10 years old (31%) and patients ≥70 years old (33%) and were higher among males than females.

Diagnosis

Chikungunya virus infection should be considered in patients presenting with an acute onset of fever and polyarthralgia and relevant epidemiologic exposure where mosquito-borne transmission of chikungunya virus infection has been reported. In humans, chikungunya viremia may exceed 10^9 RNA copies/mL; in addition, plasma viremia may be present before onset of symptoms. In the setting of symptomatic infection, viremia usually disappears after 6 to 7 days of illness; however, the virus has been isolated after 8 days, and chikungunya genomic products can be detected as late as day 17 of illness. Instructions for serum diagnostic testing are found on the CDC's website: https://www.cdc.gov/chikungunya/hcp/diagnosis-testing/index.html.

Chikungunya virus RNA can be detected by real-time reverse-transcription polymerase chain reaction (RT-PCR) during the first 5 days after onset of symptoms with excellent sensitivity and specificity (100% and 98%, respectively). For individuals presenting 8 or more days after onset of symptoms, chikungunya virus serologic testing via enzyme-linked immunoassay (ELISA) or indirect fluorescent antibody (IFA) should be performed. A positive result establishes a diagnosis of chikungunya virus infection.

Immunoglobulin (Ig)M anti–chikungunya virus antibodies (detected by direct ELISA) are present starting about 5 days (range 1–12 days) after onset of symptoms and persist for several weeks to 3 months. IgG antibodies begin to appear about 2 weeks after onset of symptoms and persist for years. A positive IgG antibody test result indicates prior chikungunya infection; it does not delineate whether arthritic symptoms are a consequence of prior infection. The time between possible exposure and clinical history should be evaluated carefully when making a diagnosis of chronic chikungunya viral arthritis in a patient with a positive IgG test. Chikungunya virus antibodies normally develop toward the end of the first week of illness; therefore to definitively rule out the diagnosis, convalescent-phase samples should be obtained from patients whose acute-phase samples test negative.

Viral culture is mainly a research tool and should be handled under biosafety level (BSL) 3 conditions.

A complete blood count may show lymphopenia and thrombocytopenia. Liver enzymes may elevate, and the serum creatinine might also increase. There are no pathognomonic radiologic findings, and biologic markers of inflammation are normal or modestly elevated.

In many parts of the world, chikungunya is a clinical diagnosis of exclusion, particularly when laboratory testing is not readily available. The probability of accurate clinical diagnosis is predicated on the epidemiology of endemic diseases and the patient's clinical symptoms.

Differential Diagnosis

Prominent arthralgia, high fever, diffuse rash, and absence of respiratory symptoms can help distinguish chikungunya from other illnesses. The differential diagnosis for chikungunya includes influenza, malaria, rickettsia, and a multitude of viruses. Zika, dengue, and chikungunya viruses are transmitted by the same mosquitoes, may have similar clinical features, and can occasionally coinfect the same individual. Typically, the signs and symptoms of Zika virus are mild, though Zika infection in pregnancy can result in serous congenital malformations. Clinically differentiating chikungunya from dengue may be difficult; however, in chikungunya, the onset of fever is typically more abrupt and shorter-lived, with severe arthralgia, rash, and lymphopenia more prevalent, whereas infection with dengue is more likely to present with neutropenia, thrombocytopenia, and the potential of hemorrhage, shock, and death. The accurate diagnosis of dengue virus infection is essential because proper clinical management of dengue can improve outcomes. Seasonally, chikungunya is more likely to be seen in the summer months when *Aedes* mosquitos proliferate. In regions where cocirculation of multiple arboviruses is present, a Trioplex RT-PCR assay can discern the presence of Zika, chikungunya, and dengue infection.

Treatment

Most chikungunya infections are self-limiting and will improve with supportive care, hydration, and analgesia. There is no specific antiviral therapy for acute chikungunya virus infection.

In the acute viremic phase (1–3 weeks), acetaminophen (up to 500–1000 mg three times daily) is useful. If acetaminophen is inadequate for symptom relief and once dengue is excluded, any nonsteroidal antiinflammatory drug (NSAID) may be used. During the acute infection, systemic glucocorticoids and other immunosuppressive medications should be avoided, as these agents may exacerbate the infection, especially during the viremic phase. Because of the risk of bleeding complications, avoid aspirin and other NSAIDs until dengue has been excluded.

In the subacute phase (4–12 weeks), if there is evidence of severe synovitis and joint swelling, prednisone 10 to 20 mg daily for 5 days tapered over 10 days can be efficacious. The lowest effective glucocorticoid dose possible with a short trial is usually sufficient; however, the individual response to therapy varies substantially. More severely affected patients may require higher doses (0.5 mg/kg daily), and some patients require up to 1 to 2 months of glucocorticoid therapy. Adding oral steroids to NSAIDs will aid in ameliorating symptomology. Weak opioids like codeine or tramadol may be also considered at the lowest dose for the shortest duration necessary.

In the chronic phase (>3 months) of chikungunya arthritis with ongoing synovitis or tenosynovitis, disease-modifying antirheumatic drugs (DMARDs) can be used. The most commonly used DMARD is methotrexate[1] as a single dose at 7.5 to 15 mg/week, along with folic acid[1] 1 mg/day. Renal function should be assessed. There is limited experience using sulfasalazine[1]. Methotrexate is recommended if there is severe persistent inflammatory polyarthralgia and arthritis affecting more than five joints. In patients with a complete response for at least 6 months, discontinuation of DMARD therapy should be attempted. In patients who are nonresponsive to methotrexate, a tumor necrosis factor (TNF)-α inhibitor[1] is an appropriate consideration.

Because of the rapidly changing situation in Africa and other areas with endemic chikungunya, clinicians should frequently check the CDC and World Health Organization websites for management guidelines.

Monitoring

Chikungunya is a nationally notifiable disease. Cases should be immediately reported to state or local health department officials to facilitate diagnosis and mitigate the risk of local transmission.

Complications

In a 2018 meta-analysis of studies in the Americas, 52% of chikungunya-infected patients in the American continent developed protracted articular symptoms. Because of its potential for chronicity, chikungunya is properly considered a major world health problem. Healthcare professionals should be prepared to address the physical, psychological, and social demands of the lingering sequelae of chikungunya.

Chikungunya is one of the agents researched as a potential biologic weapon.

---

[1] Not FDA approved for this indication.

References

Adams LE, Martin SW, Lindsey NP: Epidemiology of dengue, chikungunya, and Zika virus disease in the US states and territories, *Am J Trop Med Hyg* 101(4):884–890, 2017. 2019.

Amaral JK, Sutaria R, Schoen RT: Treatment of chronic chikungunya arthritis with methotrexate: a systematic review, *Arthritis Care Res (Hoboken)* 70(10):1501–1508, 2018.

August A, Attarwala H, Himansu S: A phase 1 trial of lipid-encapsulated mRNA encoding a monoclonal antibody with neutralizing activity against chikungunya virus, *Nat Med* 27(12):2224–2233, 2021.

CDC Yellow Book 2024: *Chikungunya.* Centers for Disease Control and Prevention. Available at: https://wwwnc.cdc.gov/travel/yellowbook/2024/infections-diseases/chikungunya

Cerny T, Schwarz M, Schwarz U: The range of neurological complications in chikungunya fever, *Neurocrit Care* 27:447–457, 2017.

de Souza W, Ribeiro G, de Lima S: Chikungunya: a decade of burden in the Americas, *The Lancet Regional Health Americas*, January 08, 2024.

Edington F, Varjão D, Melo P: Incidence of articular pain and arthritis after chikungunya fever in the Americas: a systematic review of the literature and meta-analysis, *Jt Bone Spine* 85:669, 2018.

Gérardin P, Sampériz S, Ramful D: Neurocognitive outcome of children exposed to perinatal mother-to-child chikungunya virus infection: the CHIMERE cohort study on Reunion Island, *PLoS Negl Trop Dis* 8(7):e2996, 2014.

Lindsey NP, Staples JE, Fischer M: Chikungunya virus disease among travelers-United States, 2014-2016, *Am J Trop Med Hyg* 98:192, 2018.

Ng W, Amaral K, Javelle E, Mahalingam S: Chronic chikungunya disease (CCD): clinical insights, immunopathogenesis and therapeutic perspectives, *QJM: Int J Med* 117(7), 2024.

O'Driscoll M, Salje H, Chang AY, Watson H: Arthralgia resolution rate following chikungunya virus infection, *Int J Infect Dis* 112(1–7), 2021.

Pathak H, Mohan MC, Ravindran V: Chikungunya arthritis, *Clin Med* 19(5):381–385, 2019.

Schilte C, Staikovsky F, Couderc T: Chikungunya virus-associated long-term arthralgia: a 36-month prospective longitudinal study, *PLoS Negl Trop Dis* 7(3):e2137, 2013.

Taksandel A, Vilhekar KY: Neonatal chikungunya infection, *J Prevent Infect Control* 1(8), 2015.

Zeller H, Van Bortel W, Sudre B: Chikungunya: its history in Africa and Asia and its spread to new regions in 2013–2014, *J Infect Dis* 214(suppl 5):S436–S444, 2016.

CHOLERA

Method of
Mark Pietroni, MD, MBA

Cholera affects about 3 million people per year and kills approximately 100,000. It can kill within hours of the onset of symptoms, and even today the impact of an outbreak of cholera can be catastrophic in locations in which the water and sanitation infrastructure is weak, especially in crisis or war situations. The 21st century has already seen large-scale cholera epidemics in Haiti, Zimbabwe, Pakistan and Yemen, as well as many smaller outbreaks in countries and areas in which cholera is endemic. When cholera is untreated, mortality can be as high as 60% to 70%, but even in epidemics, with appropriate management and well-run diarrhea treatment centers, mortality can be reduced to well below 1%.

Oral rehydration therapy (ORT) is now the mainstay of treatment (Table 1). Developed in the 1960s in Dhaka, Bangladesh, ORT was used to great effect during the Bangladesh Liberation War of 1971. Cholera broke out in the refugee camps outside Calcutta, and the medical services ran out of intravenous fluid. ORT was not accepted as routine therapy by the medical profession at that time. The courageous decision to treat people with ORT saved thousands of lives and convinced the world of the effectiveness of ORT in the management of cholera.

Pathophysiology

Cholera is caused by a gram-negative, comma-shaped bacterium called *Vibrio cholerae*. Clinical disease is caused by two serogroups: *V. cholerae* O1 (which has two biotypes: classical and El Tor) and *V. cholerae* O139. Humans are the only known natural host, and asymptomatic human carriage is rare. *V. cholerae* is rapidly killed by boiling water, but it can lie dormant for months in blue-green algae, crustaceans, and copepods in brackish water, especially in estuaries. The Ganges delta provides an ideal habitat and is believed to be the place cholera first emerged.

Human infection is caused by ingestion of contaminated food or drink or from poor hand hygiene in epidemic situations. Relative or absolute achlorhydria facilitates passage through the stomach. Proliferation occurs in the small intestine, where a number of toxins are released. This results in massive secretion of isotonic fluid into the gut. The fluid passes out of the anus full of vibrios to perpetuate the cycle of transmission. Killing the host does not appear to interrupt this cycle!

The cholera toxin is secreted only by the O1 and O139 serogroups. It has two subunits: A (active) and B (binding). Subunit B binds to receptors in the small intestine and subunit A activates adenylate cyclase. This causes the active secretion of a number of ions into the gut, which drags water by osmosis and also blocks the reabsorption of sodium from the gut. The net result is a massive loss of water, sodium chloride, and bicarbonate. This cannot be replaced by drinking a sodium solution because sodium reabsorption is blocked. However, the addition of glucose to a solution of sodium activates a sodium–glucose co-transporter; sodium is absorbed and water follows by osmosis. This is the basis of oral rehydration therapy for diarrhea today.

Clinical Presentation and Diagnosis

Cholera manifests as an acute watery diarrhea without blood in the stool or (usually) abdominal cramps. The majority of cases are clinically indistinguishable from other causes of watery diarrhea. About 10%-20% will develop dehydration but most require only oral rehydration fluid as treatment. However, some will progress to classic or severe cholera.

The classic picture is of the rapid onset of profuse watery diarrhea (rice-water stool) and vomiting, which is painless and can result in circulatory collapse within hours without effective treatment. The history is usually less than 24 hours, although it may be longer if the patient is taking oral rehydration solution. Abdominal cramps can occur. Fever is absent. Patients usually remain alert, but severe electrolyte abnormalities such as hypoglycemia and hyponatremia can cause a reduced level of consciousness or convulsions, especially in children. Acidosis is often severe and results in tachypnea, which is commonly misdiagnosed as pneumonia. Patients should be reassessed for the presence or absence of pneumonia 1 to 2 hours after adequate rehydration. The diagnosis of cholera can be confirmed by the presence of rapidly motile vibrios detected by dark-field microscopy or by stool or rectal swab culture. However, the classic history, appearance of the stool, and rapid presentation mean that the diagnosis is usually clinical.

Treatment

A clinical syndrome of acute watery diarrhea (three or more watery stools in the last 24 hours) of short duration (24–48 hours) with or without vomiting associated with dehydration in anyone older than 2 years in an endemic or epidemic situation should be treated as cholera. Children younger than 2 years may be managed in the same way, but other diagnoses such as rotavirus should be considered. The mainstay of management (whatever the causative organism) is appropriate early rehydration, and time should not be wasted worrying about investigations or which antibiotic to use (Figure 1).

TABLE 1	Composition (mEq/L) of Common Solutions Used for Rehydration						
SOLUTION	**NA+**	**K+**	**CL−**	**HCO3−**	**CITRATE**	**CA2+**	**GLUCOSE OR CARBOHYDRATE**
Intravenous Solution							
Normal saline	154	—	154	—	—	—	—
Ringer's lactate	130	4	109	28	—	3	—
Ringer's lactate + D5	130	4	109	28	—	3	278
Cholera saline (Dhaka solution)	133	13	98	48	—	—	140
Oral Solution							
Standard ORS	90	20	80	—	10	—	111
Hypo-osmolar ORS	75	20	65	—	10	—	75
ReSoMal*	45	40	76	—	7	—	125

Abbreviations: D_5 = 5% dextrose; ORS = oral rehydration solution; ReSoMal = reduced osmolarity ORS for malnourished children.
Reprinted with permission from Harris JB, Pietroni M: Approach to the child with acute diarrhea in developing countries. UpToDate. Available at http://www.uptodate.com/contents/approach-to-the-child-with-acute-diarrhea-in-developing-countries (accessed August 11, 2016).
*Also contains Mg 6 mmol/L, Zn 300 μmol/L, Cu 45 μmol/L.

Management of patients presenting with acute watery diarrhea

Patient with acute watery diarrhea

Look for other associated symptoms (history of bloody stools, signs of malnutrition, swelling of feet/legs, history of cough with rapid breathing, abnormal sleepiness, pallor, etc.)

Full medical assessment

Assessment for dehydration

Assess	Condition	Normal	Irritable/less active*	Lethargic/comatose*
	Eyes	Normal	Sunken	Sunken
	Tongue	Normal	Dry	Dry
	Thirst	Normal	Thirsty (drinks eagerly)	Unable to drink*
	Skin pinch	Normal	Goes back slowly*	Goes back very slowly*
	Radial pulse	Normal	Reduced*	Uncountable or absent*
Diagnosis		No sign of dehydration	If at least 2 signs, including one (*) sign, are present, diagnose *some dehydration*	If some dehydration plus one of the (*) signs are present, diagnose *severe dehydration*
Management		A	B	C

A. No sign of dehydration—ORS
• 50 mL ORS per kg body weight *plus* ongoing losses
• Send patient home with 4 packets of ORS
• Continue feeding, including breast milk for infants and young children

B. Some dehydration—ORS
• 80 mL ORS per kg body weight over 4–6 hours plus ongoing losses
• Observe patient for 6–12 hours
• Continue feeding, including breastmilk for infants and young children
• Reassess patient and dehydration status hourly.
• In case of frequent vomiting (>3 times in 1 hour): Treat with IV fluid

C. Severe dehydration—Start IV fluid immediately (100 mL/kg)

IV solution containing sodium, potassium, chloride and bicarbonate (e.g., Ringer's Lactate)

Children <1 year or malnourished
30 mL/kg in first 1 hour
70 mL/kg in next 5 hours

Adults and children >1 year
30 mL/kg in first 1/2 hour
70 mL/kg in next 2 1/2 hours

• Encourage the patient to take ORS as soon as he/she is able to drink
• Antibiotic, if needed, after rehydration
• Zinc[1] 20 mg/day for 10 days in children 6 months to 5 years old, 10 mg/day for 10 days in children under 6 months

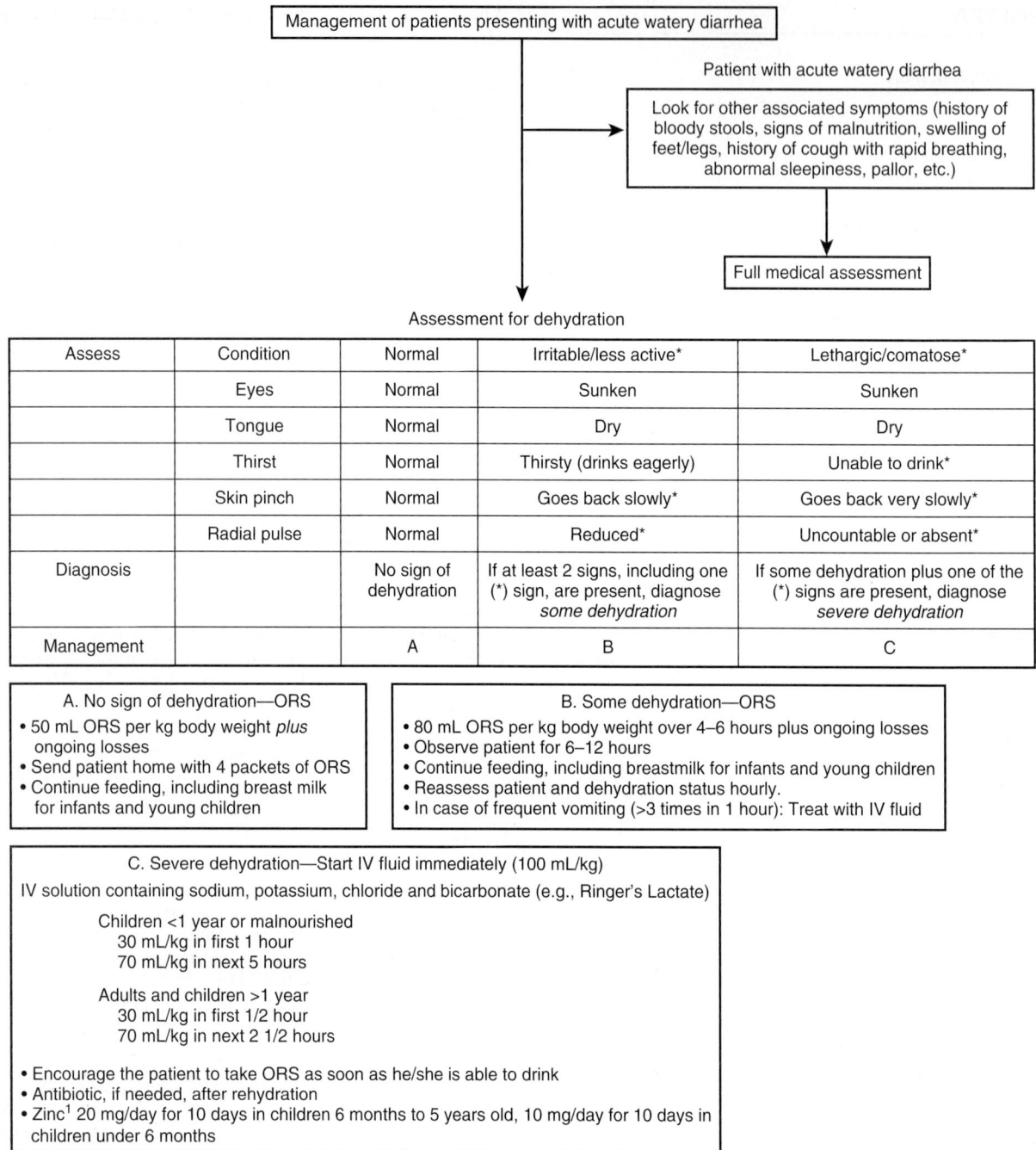

Figure 1 Quick identification of cholera cases can be made using a standard case definition. During an outbreak, cholera should be suspected in any patient who is older than 2 years, is attending a health facility, and has a history of acute watery diarrhea (passage of at least three stools in the last 24 hours) of a short duration (less than 24 hours), with or without vomiting, and with signs of dehydration. (Flow chart modified from International Centre for Diarrhoeal Disease Research, Bangladesh (ICDDR,B) internal treatment protocol.) *Abbreviation:* ORS = oral rehydration solution.

The initial assessment should be brief but must:
• Confirm the diagnosis of acute watery diarrhea
• Assess the level of dehydration
• Assess the presence or absence of malnutrition
• Recognize any other comorbidities

Accurate assessment and rapid, appropriate treatment of dehydration is critical to the management of cholera. A simple scoring system based on five clinical signs is sufficient and can accurately predict patients with 5% to 10% (some) dehydration and greater than 10% (severe) dehydration. Common mistakes include overreliance on individual clinical signs and giving too little intravenous fluid during the initial phase and too much during the recovery phase. Patients with less than 5% (no) dehydration and 5% to 10% (some) dehydration can be managed with oral rehydration alone (Box 1) unless there is a reduced level of consciousness or inability to take fluids by mouth. Those with 5% to 10% (some) dehydration must

be reassessed every 1 to 2 hours to make sure that hydration is improving.

Patients with severe dehydration require an immediate intravenous fluid bolus of 100 mL/kg given over 3 hours with one third in the first 30 minutes (double the duration in children who are younger than 1 year or have malnutrition). If possible, the intravenous fluid should contain sodium, potassium, and bicarbonate—Ringer's lactate or cholera saline—but normal saline with 5 to 10 mmol/L of potassium may also be used. Oral rehydration should start at the same time. Once the intravenous fluid bolus has finished, further intravenous fluids are usually not required.

Patients are best managed using a cholera cot, especially in an epidemic situation. The cholera cot is a bed (or sometimes a chair) covered with a nonabsorbent sheet with a hole that allows the passage of stool and urine directly to a bucket under the bed (Figure 2). The sheets and bucket should be replaced three times a day and between patients. They may be washed, sterilized, and

BOX 1 — Fluids for Patients without Signs of Dehydration

Acceptable
Oral rehydration solution (optimal for both repletion and maintenance)
Salted drinks (salted rice water or salted yogurt drink)
Broth or soup (salted vegetable or meat soup)
Water
Rice water
Coconut water (unsweetened)
Weak tea (unsweetened)
Fresh fruit juice (unsweetened)

Unacceptable
Carbonated beverages
Sweetened juices
Coffee
Medicinal teas or infusions

Fluids containing salt should be encouraged. Unacceptable fluids include carbonated beverages and sweetened juices; the sugar in these fluids may worsen diarrhea. Coffee and medicinal teas or infusions are also unacceptable since they can have diuretic and purgative effects.

Reprinted with permission from Harris JB, Pietroni M: Approach to the child with acute diarrhea in developing countries. UpToDate. Available at http://www.uptodate.com/contents/approach-to-the-child-with-acute-diarrhea-in-developing-countries (accessed August 11, 2016).

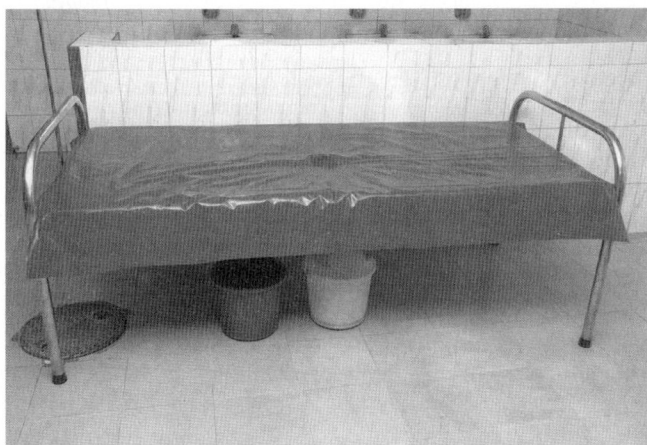

BOX 2 — Antibiotics in Cholera

Antibiotics should be given to all patients with severe dehydration. Choice of antibiotic depends on local sensitivity pattern. If ciprofloxacin is used a 3-day course is now needed due to rising MICs.

First-Line Drug (If Susceptibility Report Is Not Available)
Adults
Azithromycin (Zithromax)[1] 1 g (500 mg × 2) PO as a single dose after correcting severe dehydration

Children
Azithromycin[1] 20 mg/kg PO as a single dose after correction of dehydration and cessation of vomiting (if any)

Second-Line Drug (Not Recommended for Children < 5 Years or Pregnant Women)
Adults
Ciprofloxacin (Cipro)[1] 1 g (500 mg × 2) PO for 3 days after correction of severe dehydration

Children
Ciprofloxacin[1] 20 mg/kg PO for 3 days after correction of dehydration and cessation of vomiting (if any)

Third-Line Drugs
Doxycycline (Vibramycin) 300 mg as a single dose after food (not in children or pregnant women)

[1]Not FDA approved for this indication.

Figure 2 Cholera cot.

reused. Patients do not need to use a toilet (which can be several times an hour), linen is not soiled, and body fluids are prevented from running on the floor. This system enables adequate infection control to be maintained with limited resources.

After an initial assessment has been made and fluids started, a fuller clinical assessment can take place. Patients with significant comorbidities can require individually tailored treatment plans.

Antibiotics reduce the length of stay and fluid requirement in patients with severe dehydration due to cholera (Box 2). A single dose is sufficient, but this should be repeated if the dose is vomited back. The choice of antibiotic should be guided by local sensitivities where these are available. If not, a single dose of azithromycin (Zithromax)[1] 1 g in adults and 20 mg/day for 10 days in children 6 months to 5 years old, 10 mg/day for 10 days in children under 6 months. All children between 6 months and 5 years of age should receive zinc[1] 20 mg/day for 10 days because this reduces subsequent mortality and further episodes of diarrhea.

Recovery from cholera is rapid, and mortality is extremely low if the dehydration is treated appropriately. The Cholera Hospital run by the International Centre for Diarrhoeal Disease Research, Bangladesh (ICDDR,B), in Dhaka treats around 120,000 patients a year. The average length of stay is 16 hours, and the mortality rate is zero.

Prevention

Because the transmission of cholera is feco-oral, cholera can be prevented by good hand hygiene and by providing safe drinking water and appropriate sanitation. Standard food and hygiene precautions should be followed by people travelling in endemic areas (e.g., eat only boiled or fried foods; drink only boiled or bottled water). The FDA recently approved a single-dose live oral cholera vaccine, called Vaxchora in the United States. Vaxchora is indicated for adults 18–64 years old who are traveling to an area of active cholera. Two other oral inactivated cholera vaccines, Dukoral and ShanChol, are not available in the United States. These two cholera vaccines provide around 60% to 80% efficacy for 6 months. They are not recommended for the occasional traveler or tourist but may be given to people working in high-risk situations, such as aid workers in a cholera outbreak. The World Health Organization recommends the use of oral cholera vaccine in endemic areas as part of disease control programmes and maintains a global cholera vaccine stockpile for use in epidemic situations.

References

Ali M, Nelson AR, Lopez AL, Sack D: Updated global burden of cholera in endemic countries. *PLoS Negl Trop Dis* 9(6):e0003832, 2015. https://doi.org/10.1371/journal.pntd.0003832.
Alam NH, Ashraf H: Treatment of infectious diarrhea in children, *Paediatr Drugs* 5:151–165, 2003.
Harris JB, Pietroni MAC: Approach to the child with acute diarrhea in resource limited countries. In: UpToDate, Calderwood, S.B. & Bloom, A. (Eds), UpToDate, Waltham, MA, 2017.
Pietroni MAC: Case management of cholera, *Vaccine* 38(1):A105–A109, 2020.
Roy SK, Tomkins AM, Akramuzzaman SM, et al: Randomised controlled trial of zinc supplementation in malnourished Bangladeshi children with acute diarrhea, *Arch Dis Child* 77:196–200, 1997.
Saha D, Karim MM, Khan WA, et al: Single-dose azithromycin for the treatment of cholera in adults, *N Engl J Med* 354:2452–2462, 2006.
UNICEF Cholera Toolkit www.unicef.org/cholera_toolkit/ especially Chapter 8: Case management and infection control in health facilities and treatment sites pp 110–135. Accessed 10/3/2018.

[1]Not FDA approved for this indication.

COVID-19

Method of
Matthew Decker, MD, JD

CURRENT DIAGNOSIS

- The disease COVID-19 is caused by the SARS-CoV-2 virus.
- Symptoms include fever, chills, cough, sore throat, dyspnea, fatigue, nausea, vomiting, diarrhea, headache, and myalgia.
- Transmission occurs primarily via respiratory droplets.
- Diagnosis is made based upon polymerase chain reaction or antigen testing of a respiratory sample, usually via nasopharyngeal swab.
- Currently circulating variants are more infectious but generally cause milder illness.

CURRENT THERAPY

- Vaccination is the mainstay of prevention of both infection and progression to severe COVID-19.
- Previous regimens for pre- and postexposure prophylaxis are no longer effective against circulating variants.
- Antiviral medications are recommended for patients at high risk of progression to severe COVID-19 in both the inpatient and outpatient settings.
- Patients with moderate to severe disease warrant hospitalization.
- Corticosteroids are recommended for patients with a new or worsening oxygen requirement secondary to COVID-19.

Epidemiology

The COVID-19 pandemic, caused by the novel coronavirus SARS-CoV-2, emerged in late 2019 in Wuhan, China. By May 2023, it had spread globally, resulting in 774 million confirmed cases and over 7 million deaths worldwide. In the United States alone, nearly 7 million hospitalizations and around 1.2 million deaths occurred. Tragically, these impacts were particularly severe among racial and ethnic minorities and other marginalized communities, which faced higher risks of contracting SARS-CoV-2, hospitalization due to COVID-19, and mortality.

Pathophysiology

SARS-CoV-2, like other coronaviruses, is an enveloped positive-stranded RNA virus primarily spread through respiratory particles when infected individuals cough, sneeze, or talk. Transmission typically occurs within about 6 feet but can extend further in enclosed, poorly ventilated spaces. The risk of transmission depends on exposure type, duration, and preventive measures. Both asymptomatic and presymptomatic individuals can transmit the virus, with higher transmission risk from symptomatic cases.

The incubation period is usually up to 14 days but can be shorter with newer variants, even as early as 3 days. Peak infectiousness occurs within the first 10 days postinfection, aligning with high viral RNA levels in the upper respiratory tract. However, prolonged RNA detection does not necessarily indicate continued infectiousness, as polymerase chain reaction (PCR) tests can remain positive for up to 90 days. Factors affecting viral shedding duration include patient age, illness severity, and antiviral treatment.

SARS-CoV-2 evolves through random mutations, leading to various variants. The Omicron variant, dominant since November 2021, especially the JN.1 subvariant, constitutes a significant proportion of cases in the United States. Omicron shows increased transmissibility and immune evasion but is generally associated with milder illness.

COVID-19 manifests in two phases: a viral replication phase with typical upper respiratory symptoms and an inflammatory phase characterized by dysregulated immune responses, tissue damage, thrombosis, hypoxemia, and endothelial dysfunction. Early treatment with antivirals is crucial during the replication phase, whereas immunosuppressive, antiinflammatory, and antithrombotic therapies are more beneficial later in the disease course.

Prevention

SARS-CoV-2 primarily spreads through respiratory droplets, so reducing transmission risks involves practices like covering coughs and sneezes, wearing masks, isolating when symptomatic, and thorough handwashing. Healthcare workers should use proper personal protective equipment (PPE) when dealing with COVID-19 patients, following CDC guidelines on infection control and PPE use in healthcare settings.

Vaccination is the most effective way to prevent COVID-19, and all eligible individuals should be vaccinated per the latest CDC recommendations. This includes everyone aged 6 months and older, with vaccine type, dosage, and timing based on age and medical history. Pregnant, lactating individuals, and those trying to conceive are also encouraged to get vaccinated.

In the United States, there are mRNA vaccines (Pfizer-BioNTech, Moderna) and a recombinant spike protein with adjuvant vaccine (Novavax) available. The Comirnaty (Pfizer-BioNTech) and Spikevax (Moderna) vaccines are FDA approved for persons 12 years of age and older. Under the FDA emergency use authorization (EUA), the Pfizer-BioNTech and Moderna vaccines labeled "2024–2025 formula" are available for persons 6 months to younger than 12 years of age, while Novavax is available for those 12 years or older. The previously used adenovirus vector vaccine (Johnson & Johnson/Janssen) is no longer in use. Mild to moderate local and systemic reactions are common postvaccination but are typically short-lived. Rare adverse events like thrombosis with thrombocytopenia and mild myocarditis/pericarditis have been reported, but the risk is outweighed by the benefits of vaccination.

Monoclonal antibodies were previously used for preexposure prophylaxis but are no longer effective against the Omicron variant, losing FDA authorization for both pre- and postexposure prophylaxis. The CDC has updated isolation guidelines, recommending isolation until at least 24 hours after symptoms and fever resolve without the use of fever-reducing medications, followed by 5 days of enhanced precautions.

Clinical Manifestations

COVID-19 can manifest with various symptoms, including fever, chills, myalgia, cough, shortness of breath, headache, sore throat, congestion, runny nose, nausea, vomiting, diarrhea, or loss of taste/smell. Symptoms are typically milder in children compared with adults.

The severity of COVID-19 ranges from asymptomatic or mild cases to critical illness. Treatment decisions are based on the severity and risk of progression. The categories of illness severity are:

1. *Asymptomatic or presymptomatic infection:* Individuals who test positive for SARS-CoV-2 via PCR or antigen testing but have no symptoms consistent with COVID-19.
2. *Mild illness:* Individuals who have any of the various signs and symptoms of COVID-19 but do not have shortness of breath, dyspnea, or abnormal chest imaging.
3. *Moderate illness:* Individuals who show evidence of lower respiratory disease during clinical assessment or imaging and who have an oxygen saturation (SpO_2) $\geq 94\%$ on room air.
4. *Severe illness:* Individuals who have an $SpO_2 < 94\%$ on room air, a ratio of arterial partial pressure of oxygen to fraction of inspired oxygen <300 mm Hg, a respiratory rate >30 breaths/min, or lung infiltrates >50%.
5. *Critical illness:* Individuals who have respiratory failure, septic shock, or multiple organ dysfunction.

Pulse oximetry is vital for assessing COVID-19 severity but may underestimate hypoxemia in individuals with darker skin. Clinical context is crucial for accurate interpretation.

TABLE 1	Underlying Medical Conditions Associated With Higher Risk for Severe COVID-19

Asthma

Cancer

Cerebrovascular disease

Chronic kidney disease

Chronic lung diseases limited to:
Bronchiectasis
Chronic obstructive pulmonary disease
Interstitial lung disease
Pulmonary embolism
Pulmonary hypertension

Chronic liver diseases limited to:
Cirrhosis
Nonalcoholic fatty liver disease
Alcoholic liver disease
Autoimmune hepatitis

Cystic fibrosis

Diabetes mellitus type 1 and type 2

Down syndrome

Heart conditions
Heart failure
Coronary artery disease
Cardiomyopathies

HIV

Mental health conditions limited to:
Mood disorders, including depression
Schizophrenia spectrum disorders

Dementia

Obesity

Physical inactivity

Pregnancy and recent pregnancy

Primary immunodeficiency

Smoking, current and former

Solid organ or blood stem cell transplantation

Tuberculosis

Use of corticosteroids or other immunosuppressive medications

Risk factors for severe illness include age >50 (especially >65), immunosuppression, lack of vaccination, and certain underlying health conditions like asthma, cancer, chronic kidney/lung diseases, diabetes, heart conditions, obesity, and others (Table 1).

Co-infections are rare, and treatments are not routinely indicated without specific evidence (e.g., focal consolidation for bacterial pneumonia). Latent infections like hepatitis B, herpes zoster, and tuberculosis can occur, especially in patients on immunomodulators. Nosocomial infections remain a concern for hospitalized COVID-19 patients.

Diagnosis

Testing symptomatic individuals is crucial for diagnosing COVID-19, typically through PCR or antigen tests from upper respiratory tract specimens (nasal/nasopharyngeal). PCR is more sensitive and considered the gold standard, whereas antigen tests are faster but less sensitive.

A single negative PCR test rules out infection in symptomatic patients. Negative antigen tests should be repeated in 48 hours or followed by PCR. A positive PCR or antigen test confirms infection. Repeat PCR testing is unnecessary within 90 days of a positive result.

TABLE 2	Dosing Regimens for Nonhospitalized Adults
DRUG NAME	**DOSE**
Ritonavir-boosted nirmatrelvir (Paxlovid)	eGFR ≥ 60 mL/min Nirmatrelvir 300 mg with ritonavir 100 mg PO twice daily for 5 days eGFR ≥ 30 to < 60 mL/min Nirmatrelvir 150 mg with ritonavir 100 mg PO twice daily for 5 days
Remdesivir (Veklury)	200 mg IV on day 1 then 100 mg IV once daily on days 2 and 3
Molnupiravir (Lagevrio)[1]	800 mg PO every 12 hours for 5 days

[1]Not FDA approved for this indication.
eGFR, Estimated glomerular filtration rate.

Antibody testing does not diagnose current infection or assess immunity postvaccination. Chest radiography assesses infection severity and complications, whereas CT scans are reserved for clinical worsening or additional pathology evaluation.

Lab tests include complete blood count with differential, metabolic profile, and inflammatory markers (C-reactive protein, ferritin, D-dimer). COVID-19 may show lymphopenia, leukopenia/leukocytosis, thrombocytopenia, elevated liver enzymes, and inflammatory markers. Elevated D-dimer may indicate venous thromboembolism suspicion.

Treatment

Treatment recommendations for COVID-19 vary depending on whether the patient is hospitalized, the illness severity, and the need for supplemental oxygen.

Nonhospitalized Adults With Mild to Moderate COVID-19 Who Do Not Require Supplemental Oxygen

Patients at high risk of progressing to severe COVID-19 should receive antiviral treatment in addition to supportive care. Ritonavir-boosted nirmatrelvir (Paxlovid) is the preferred antiviral and should be administered within 5 days of symptom onset. However, caution is needed because of significant drug interactions, contraindications in patients with severe kidney or liver impairment, and other specific considerations.

If ritonavir-boosted nirmatrelvir is not feasible, a 3-day course of IV remdesivir (Veklury) is recommended within 7 days of symptom onset. Molnupiravir (Lagevrio)[1] is an alternative but is considered less effective and should be used cautiously, especially in pregnant patients. See Table 2 for more details.

Systemic corticosteroids like dexamethasone[1] should not be used solely for COVID-19 unless indicated for treating an underlying condition. Concerns about viral rebound or symptom recurrence should not deter appropriate antiviral therapy, as treated patients with ritonavir-boosted nirmatrelvir have not shown severe COVID-19 progression because of these reasons.

Adults Hospitalized for Reasons Other Than COVID-19

Patients with mild to moderate COVID-19 who are at high risk of progressing to severe illness should be managed similarly to nonhospitalized adults with mild to moderate COVID-19 who do not need supplemental oxygen. This includes supportive care measures and monitoring for symptom progression.

For thromboprophylaxis, therapeutic dose heparin[1] (low molecular weight or unfractionated) is recommended unless contraindicated. This helps prevent thromboembolic complications in high-risk patients.

[1] Not FDA approved for this indication.

TABLE 3 — Dosing Regimens for Hospitalized Adults

DRUG NAME	DOSE
Abatacept (Orencia)[1]	10 mg/kg actual body weight (up to 1000 mg) administered as a single IV dose
Baricitinib (Olumiant)	eGFR ≥ 60 mL/min 4 mg PO once daily eGFR 30 to < 60 mL/min 2 mg PO once daily eGFR 15 to < 30 mL/min 1 mg PO once daily eGFR < 15 mL/min Use not recommended Give for up to 14 days or until hospital discharge, whichever comes first
Dexamethasone[1]	6 mg PO or IV once daily for up to 10 days or until hospital discharge, whichever comes first
Heparin[1]	Therapeutic dose of SUBQ LMWH or IV UFH Prophylactic dose of SUBQ LMWH or UFH
Infliximab (Remicade)[1]	5 mg/kg actual body weight as single IV dose
Remdesivir (Veklury)	200 mg IV once, then 100 mg IV once daily for 4 days or until hospital discharge, whichever comes first
Tocilizumab (Actemra)	8 mg/kg actual body weight (up to 800 mg) as single IV dose

[1]Not FDA approved for this indication.
eGFR, Estimated glomerular filtration rate; *LMWH*, low-molecular-weight heparin; *SUBQ*, subcutaneous; *UFH*, unfractionated heparin.

Adults Hospitalized With COVID-19 But Do Not Require Supplemental Oxygen

Dexamethasone or other systemic corticosteroids should not be used. Patients at high risk of progressing to severe COVID-19 should be treated with a 5-day course of IV remdesivir. Remdesivir should be continued even if the patient progresses to a more severe illness. Therapeutic heparin[1] (low molecular weight or unfractionated) is also recommended unless contraindicated. For more detailed information, please refer to Table 3.

Adults Hospitalized With COVID-19 Requiring Conventional Oxygen

Patients who require minimal conventional oxygen may be treated with remdesivir monotherapy based on guidelines. However, for most patients in this category, a combination of dexamethasone[1] plus remdesivir is recommended.

A therapeutic dose of heparin should be utilized for all hospitalized patients with COVID-19, barring any contraindications to the same.

Patients receiving dexamethasone and experiencing rapidly increased oxygen needs along with systemic inflammation may benefit from additional immunomodulatory therapy. Preferred options include oral baricitinib (Olumiant) or IV tocilizumab (Actemra), with IV abatacept (Orencia)[1] and IV infliximab (Remicade)[1] being acceptable alternatives.

Adults Hospitalized With COVID-19 Requiring High-Flow Nasal Cannula Oxygen or Noninvasive Ventilation

All patients in this category should receive dexamethasone.[1] Remdesivir should be considered for these patients, especially if they are immunocompromised, within 10 days of symptom

[1]Not FDA approved for this indication.

onset, or have a positive antigen test. If an immunomodulator has not already been initiated, it should be started. Oral baricitinib is the preferred immunomodulator, with IV tocilizumab as the preferred alternative. Additional alternative immunomodulators include IV abatacept[1] and IV infliximab.[1]

Adults Hospitalized With COVID-19 and Requiring Mechanical Ventilation or Extracorporeal Membrane Oxygenation

All patients should be administered dexamethasone.[1] If the patient has not already received a second immunomodulator, either oral baricitinib or IV tocilizumab should be added. Remdesivir and anticoagulant therapy should be considered as with patients requiring high-flow nasal cannula oxygen or noninvasive ventilation.

Critically Ill Adults With COVID-19

In general, best practices for critically ill patients with COVID-19 mirror the care for other severe pulmonary diseases. Notable recommendations for COVID-19 include using norepinephrine as a first-choice vasopressor, considering low-dose corticosteroid therapy for patients with refractory septic shock who have completed a course of corticosteroids for COVID-19, and avoiding awake prone positioning to prevent the need for intubation. Prone ventilation is recommended for 12 to 16 hours per day for mechanically ventilated adults with refractory hypoxemia. Paradoxically, critically ill patients should receive prophylactic doses of heparin. Moreover, patients initially started on therapeutic heparin dosing outside the intensive care unit should be switched to prophylactic dosing.

Miscellaneous Therapies

Throughout the COVID-19 pandemic, various therapies have garnered attention as potential treatments or preventatives for COVID-19. However, many of these therapies were never proven effective, whereas others, initially effective or approved, have not stood the test of time. Therapies for which there is a recommendation against their use or insufficient evidence include hydroxychloroquine[1], anti–SARS-CoV-2 monoclonal antibodies, COVID-19 convalescent plasma, interferon[1], anakinra (Kineret)[1], inhaled corticosteroids, vilobelimab (Gohibic)[1], canakinumab (Ilaris)[1], antiplatelet therapy, fluvoxamine (Luvox)[1], IVIG[1], ivermectin (Stromectol)[1], metformin[1], vitamin C[7], vitamin D[7], and zinc.[7]

Furthermore, several common medications were initially believed to be either helpful or harmful during COVID-19 infection, including angiotensin-converting enzyme inhibitors, angiotensin receptor blockers, statins, NSAIDs, acid suppressive therapy, and systemic or inhaled corticosteroids. Patients should continue taking these medications for their underlying medical conditions unless advised otherwise by their healthcare provider based on their clinical condition.

Nonhospitalized Children With COVID-19

Supportive care is recommended for all nonhospitalized children with COVID-19. Additionally, children aged 12 years or older at high risk of severe COVID-19 can be treated with ritonavir-boosted nirmatrelvir within 5 days of symptom onset or remdesivir within 7 days of symptom onset. Molnupiravir[1] has not been authorized by the FDA for use in children. For children under the age of 12, no antiviral is approved or recommended for the prevention of severe COVID-19.

Children Hospitalized With COVID-19

Overall, children hospitalized with COVID-19 receive treatment almost identical to their adult counterparts. The primary difference lies in the administration of immunomodulators beyond dexamethasone. Whereas adults typically receive these

[1]Not FDA approved for this indication.
[7]Available as dietary supplement.

medications promptly, current recommendations for children suggest withholding immunomodulators unless patients do not show rapid improvement (i.e., within 24 hours) with dexamethasone.

Complications

Some patients experience new persistent or recurrent symptoms more than 4 weeks after SARS-CoV-2 infection. These syndromes have been termed "long COVID," "post-COVID conditions," and "post-COVID-19 syndrome," although the nomenclature is evolving. Symptoms can vary widely in terms of quality and severity, and they may persist even in patients whose initial illness was mild. Common symptoms include upper respiratory symptoms, brain fog, myalgia, gastrointestinal complaints, pain, menstrual irregularities, and sexual dysfunction. The prevalence of "long COVID" is estimated to range from 5% to 30% among patients infected with SARS-CoV-2. Evaluation and management recommendations are continually evolving, with a focus on addressing the specific symptoms of each patient.

Multisystem inflammatory syndromes in children and in adults are serious complications of COVID-19 infection. These conditions are characterized by severe inflammation and features similar to Kawasaki disease in the context of a current or recent SARS-CoV-2 infection. Patients typically present with fever, laboratory evidence of inflammation, and severe illness affecting multiple organ systems. Treatment involves the administration of intravenous immunoglobulin[1] and methylprednisolone[1], along with consideration of additional immunomodulators. Low-dose aspirin[1] is also recommended. In cases of significant cardiac involvement, therapeutic anticoagulation should be considered.

---

[1] Not FDA approved for this indication.

References

American Academy of Pediatrics. "Management Strategies in Children and Adolescents with Mild to Moderate COVID-19." Available at www.aap.org/en/pages/2019-novel-coronavirus-covid-19-infections/clinical-guidance/outpatient-covid-19-management-strategies-in-children-and-adolescents/. Accessed 30 Mar. 2024.

Bhimraj A, Morgan RL, Shumaker AH, Baden L, Cheng VC, Edwards KM, Gallagher JC, Gandhi RT, Muller WJ, Nakamura MM, O'Horo JC, Shafer RW, Shoham S, Murad MH, Mustafa RA, Sultan S, Falck-Ytter Y. Infectious Diseases Society of America Guidelines on the Treatment and Management of Patients with COVID-19. Infectious Diseases Society of America 2023; Version 11.0.0. Available at https://www.idsociety.org/practice-guideline/covid-19-guideline-treatment-and-management/. Accessed 30 Mar. 2024.

Centers for Disease Control and Prevention. "COVID Data Tracker." Centers for Disease Control and Prevention. Available at www.covid.cdc.gov/covid-data-tracker/#variant-proportions. Accessed 30 Mar. 2024.

Centers for Disease Control and Prevention. "Healthcare Workers." Centers for Disease Control and Prevention, Available at www.cdc.gov/coronavirus/2019-ncov/hcp/clinical-care/clinical-considerations-presentation.html. Accessed on 30 Mar. 2024.

Centers for Disease Control and Prevention. "Post-COVID Conditions: Information for Healthcare Providers." Available at www.cdc.gov/coronavirus/2019-ncov/hcp/clinical-care/post-covid-conditions.html. Accessed 30 Mar. 2024.

Centers for Disease Control and Prevention. "Preventing Respiratory Viruses | Respiratory Illnesses | CDC." Available at www.cdc.gov/respiratory-viruses/prevention/index.html. Accessed 30 Mar. 2024.

Centers for Disease Control and Prevention. "Underlying Medical Conditions Associated with High Risk for Severe COVID-19: Information for Healthcare Providers." Underlying Medical Conditions Associated with Higher Risk for Severe COVID-19: Information for Healthcare Professionals. www.cdc.gov/coronavirus/2019-ncov/hcp/clinical-care/underlyingconditions.html. Accessed 30 Mar. 2024.

COVID-19 Treatment Guidelines Panel. Coronavirus Disease 2019 (COVID-19) Treatment Guidelines. National Institutes of Health. Available at https://www.covid19treatmentguidelines.nih.gov/. Accessed 30 Mar. 2024.

Epidemic and Pandemic Preparedness and Prevention. COVID-19 Epidemiological Update – 15 March 2024. Available at www.who.int/publications/m/item/covid-19-epidemiological-update-15-march-2024. Accessed 30 Mar. 2024.

Siegal DM, Tseng EK, Schünemann HJ, et al.: ASH living guidelines on use of anticoagulation for thromboprophylaxis in patients with COVID-19: executive summary, *Blood Adv* (2025) 9(6):1247–1260, 2025.

World Health Organization. "Clinical Management of COVID-19: Living Guideline, 18 August 2023." Available at www.who.int/publications/i/item/WHO-2019-nCoV-clinical-2023.2. Accessed 30 Mar. 2024.

EBOLA VIRUS DISEASE

Method of
Uma Malhotra, MD

CURRENT DIAGNOSIS

- Detection of viral RNA in the blood by reverse transcriptase-polymerase chain reaction (RT-PCR) beginning 3 days after the onset of symptoms.
- Repeat testing may be necessary for patients with illness duration shorter than 3 days.
- Details on specimen collection and handling can be found on the Centers for Disease Control and Prevention (CDC) and World Health Organization (WHO) websites.

CURRENT THERAPY

- Intensive fluid management to correct volume losses and electrolyte abnormalities.
- Aggressive use of antiemetics, antidiarrheals, and rehydration solutions.
- Respiratory and hemodynamic support.
- Blood products for management of coagulopathy.
- Evaluate and treat any concomitant infections.
- Two monoclonal antibody therapies, REGN-EB3 (Inmazeb) and mAb114 (Ebanga), have been approved by the US Food and Drug Administration (FDA) for the treatment of adults and children with disease due to Ebola virus (*Orthoebolavirus zairense*).
- Strict infection control measures, with contact and droplet precautions, must be used.
- Personnel trained in the correct use of personal protective equipment (PPE) should care for the patients.
- The rVSV-ZEBOV Ebola vaccine (Ervebo), a replication-competent, live attenuated vaccine is now approved by the FDA for the prevention of disease caused by Ebola virus in adults aged ≥18 years at high risk for occupation exposure. A second two-component vaccine, Ad26.ZEBOV/MVA-BN-Filo (Zabdeno and Mvabea),[5] given in two doses 8 weeks apart, has been found to be safe and immunogenic when given to at-risk populations in regions where there is no active disease transmission and is expected to provide longer protection against Ebola virus.

---

[5] Investigational drug in the United States.

Filoviridae, derived from the Latin word "filum," meaning threadlike, is a family of viruses with a filamentous structure that can cause severe hemorrhagic fever and fulminant septic shock. The family includes the genera *Orthoebolavirus* and *Orthomarburgvirus*, with the former consisting of six viruses: Ebola virus (*Orthoebolavirus zairense*), Sudan virus (*Orthoebolavirus sudanense*), Bundibugyo virus (*Orthoebolavirus bundibugyoense*), Tai Forest virus (*Orthoebolavirus taiense*), Reston virus (*Orthoebolavirus restonense*), and Bombali virus (*Orthoebolavirus bombaliense*). Orthoebolaviruses cause Ebola disease, with three species known to cause large outbreaks in humans: Ebola virus causing Ebola virus disease (EVD), Sudan virus causing Sudan virus disease (SVD), and Bundibugyo virus causing Bundibugyo virus disease (BVD).

Epidemiology

Ebola virus, first recognized in Central Africa in 1976, has caused several outbreaks in the region, including the 2014 West African epidemic, with an initial estimated case fatality rate as high as 70%, although as the epidemic evolved, lower fatality rates in the range of 30% to 40% were observed. The 2014 epidemic resulted in over 28,000 cases and 11,000 deaths, with more than 800 infections occurring in healthcare workers. The virus has also caused multiple outbreaks in the Democratic Republic of the Congo (DRC), most recently in 2022.

Sudan virus, first recognized in Sudan in 1976, has been associated with a case-fatality rate of approximately 50%. It has been the causative agent for multiple outbreaks in Sudan, Uganda, DRC, with the most recent outbreak occurring in Uganda in January–February 2025. Bundibugyo virus, first seen in Uganda in 2007 and most recently in the DRC in 2012, has caused outbreaks with a case-fatality rate of approximately 30%. Tai Forest virus has been identified as the cause of illness in one person after exposure during a necropsy on a chimpanzee. Reston virus, discovered after an outbreak of lethal infection in macaques imported into the United States in 1989, is maintained in animal reservoirs in the Philippines. Bombali virus RNA has been found in African bats. Ebola virus outbreak updates can be found on the World Health Organization (WHO) website.

Risk Factors/Transmission

Outbreaks generally begin when an individual becomes infected through contact with the tissue or body fluids of an infected animal. The virus then spreads to others who come into contact with the infected individual's blood, skin, or other body fluids. Before the 2014 epidemic in West Africa, outbreaks occurred in remote regions with low population density and were controlled within short periods. However, this epidemic showed that movement of infected individuals facilitates the extensive and rapid spread of the virus.

Transmission occurs most commonly through direct contact of broken skin or mucous membranes with virus-containing body fluids from an infected person, the most infectious being blood, feces, and vomit. During the early phase of illness, the level of virus in the blood is typically quite low, but then increases rapidly to very high levels in advanced stages of the illness, when patients become highly infectious. In fact, corpses of persons who die of Ebola are highly infectious, and ritual washing of bodies at funerals has played a significant role in the spread of infection. The virus has also been detected in urine, semen, saliva, breast milk, tears, and sweat, and can persist in some of these fluids much longer than in blood. Ebola virus may also be transmitted through contact with contaminated surfaces, where the virus can remain infectious from hours to days.

Transmission to healthcare workers may occur when appropriate personal protective equipment (PPE) is not used, especially when caring for severely ill patients in advanced stages of illness. During the 2014 outbreak in West Africa, a large number of healthcare workers became infected. In Sierra Leone, the incidence of confirmed cases at the peak of the epidemic was about 100-fold higher in healthcare workers than in the general population. Several factors have contributed to the high rates of infections among health providers, including failure to recognize infection among patients and corpses, limited availability and training in the use of appropriate PPE, and inadequate management of contaminated waste and burial of corpses. Although there is no evidence of respiratory transmission, the virus is highly infectious when released in laboratory experiments as a small-particle aerosol; therefore healthcare workers may be at risk if exposed to aerosols generated during procedures.

Human infection can occur through contact with infected wild animals during hunting, butchering, and preparing meat, with several episodes having occurred after contact with infected gorillas or chimpanzees. To prevent infection, food products should be properly cooked to inactivate the virus, and basic hygiene measures should be followed. Direct transmission of virus infection from bats to wild primates or humans has not been proven, although Ebola RNA sequences and antibodies have been detected in bats in Central Africa. Bats likely form a major reservoir.

Pathophysiology

Ebola virus is a negative-sense, single-stranded RNA virus resembling rhabdoviruses and paramyxoviruses in its genome organization and replication mechanisms. The tubular virions contain the nucleocapsid surrounded by an outer envelope, which is derived from the host cell membrane and studded with viral glycoprotein spikes. The virions attach to host cell receptors through the spikes and are then endocytosed into vesicles. Initially, productive infection occurs primarily in dendritic cells, monocytes, and macrophages, resulting in impaired interferon production and release of proinflammatory cytokines, which have secondary effects on innate and adaptive immune responses, inflammation, and vascular integrity. Neutrophils are activated, with resultant degranulation, and lymphocytes undergo apoptosis. The virus then spreads to regional lymph nodes, resulting in further rounds of replication, followed by dissemination to the liver, spleen, thymus, and other lymphoid tissues.

When the virus infects cells, it hijacks the cell and forces it to become a virus-producing factory, churning out new copies of the virus, which results in a loss of cellular function and eventual cell death by apoptosis. As the disease progresses, there is extensive tissue necrosis accompanied by a systemic inflammatory response induced by the release of various cytokines, chemokines, and proinflammatory mediators, as well as a severe coagulopathy triggered by the release of tissue factors. This systemic inflammatory response may contribute to gastrointestinal dysfunction, and ultimately there is a multisystem failure caused by the damage to vascular and coagulation systems.

Clinical Manifestations and Laboratory Findings

Patients with EVD typically have an abrupt onset of symptoms at an average of 8 to 10 days after exposure, with a range of 2 to 21 days. The first phase of the illness is characterized by high fever, chills, headaches, myalgia, and malaise. The second phase is marked by gastrointestinal symptoms, which develop by days 3 to 5, and includes watery diarrhea, nausea, vomiting, and abdominal pain. Patients may also develop chest pain, hiccups, shortness of breath, conjunctival injection, and rash. The rash is usually diffuse erythematous, maculopapular, involving the face, neck, trunk, and arms. Respiratory symptoms such as cough are rare. Common neurologic symptoms include delirium, manifested by confusion, slowed cognition, or agitation, and less frequently, seizures.

The final phase, beginning in the second week, is marked by either progression to shock and death or gradual recovery. Fatal disease is characterized by development of multisystem failure usually as a consequence of massive fluid losses that lead to shock, loss of consciousness, and renal failure. Major bleeding, typically hemorrhage from the gastrointestinal tract, is infrequent and seen in less than 5% during the terminal phase of illness. Patients who survive begin to improve during the second week of illness, with a prolonged convalescence marked by weakness, fatigue, myalgias, headache, and memory loss. About half of the survivors are plagued by chronic debilitating joint pain, and a quarter experience eye problems. Other manifestations have included hearing loss, sloughing of skin, and hair loss, which may result from necrosis of dermal structures. The virus can persist in the eye for months, leading to uveitis, cataracts, and sometimes blindness. The prevalence of uveitis, unlike other causes, continues to increase until at least 2 years after symptom onset, with about 33% of the patients affected by that point.

During acute illness patients typically develop leukopenia, lymphopenia, thrombocytopenia, serum transaminase elevations, and proteinuria. They may develop renal insufficiency and electrolyte disturbances as a result of the gastrointestinal losses. Severe cases develop coagulation abnormalities with prolonged prothrombin and partial thromboplastin times, and elevated fibrin degradation products, consistent with disseminated intravascular coagulation.

Diagnosis

The approach to evaluating patients depends on whether or not appropriate signs and symptoms are evident, and if an exposure occurred within 21 days of the onset of symptoms. Infection control precautions must be used for all symptomatic patients with an identifiable risk for EVD. All symptomatic patients should be isolated in a single room with a private bathroom, and contact and droplet precautions should be implemented. Only essential personnel who are well trained in the use of PPE should interact with the patient. Phlebotomy and laboratory testing should be limited to essential tests. Both the Centers for Disease Control and Prevention (CDC) and the WHO have provided detailed recommendations for approach to the evaluation of persons who may have been exposed to the virus.

Rapid diagnostic tests are the most commonly used tests for diagnosis. Viral RNA is generally detectable by reverse transcriptase-polymerase chain reaction (RT-PCR) in the blood 3 days after the onset of symptoms. Repeat testing may be necessary for patients with illness duration shorter than 3 days. A negative RT-PCR test 72 hours or greater after the onset of symptoms rules out EVD. Details on specimen collection and handling can be found on the CDC website. For clinicians outside the United States, the WHO has issued guidance for the collection and shipment of specimens from patients with suspected disease.

Rapid immunoassays that detect virus antigen have also been developed. However, the tests are associated with both false positives and false negatives. Therefore they must be verified using RT-PCR test. The rapid immunoassays are mostly useful to make a provisional diagnosis in the appropriate clinical setting when RT-PCR is not readily available.

Differential Diagnosis

Acute onset of febrile illness in a person who lives or has recently been in West or Central Africa may be caused by a variety of local infectious diseases, which must be considered in the differential diagnosis. **Malaria** may have similar findings and might occur concurrently. Examination of blood smears and rapid antigen tests are typically used to diagnose malaria. **Typhoid** is characterized by fever and abdominal pain and is diagnosed by blood cultures.

Patients with **Lassa fever** may develop a severe clinical syndrome resembling EVD and progress to fatal shock. The illness is restricted to West Africa, where it is transmitted through exposure to the aerosolized excretions of rodents and diagnosed by RT-PCR testing and/or serology. Clinical manifestations of **Marburg virus disease** are similar to EVD, and cases have been identified in Central Africa. The diagnosis is made by RT-PCR. Patients with **influenza** may have a similar initial presentation, but respiratory signs and symptoms are prominent.

Therapy

Good supportive care can significantly improve the chances of recovery from EVD. Mortality rates have been as low as 18% among those cared for in the US and Europe, receiving careful fluid and electrolyte management, nutritional support, and critical care. Large volumes of intravenous fluids and electrolytes are often needed to correct dehydration and electrolyte abnormalities resulting from gastrointestinal losses. Supportive care is required for complications such as shock, hypoxia, hemorrhage, and multiorgan failure. Patients may develop secondary bacterial infections, which may require concurrent management with antimicrobials. Infection prevention and control measures are critical; all bodily fluids and tissues must be considered potentially infectious. The illness is associated with high rates of pregnancy-associated hemorrhage and fetal death. The CDC and the American College of Obstetrics and Gynecology have issued recommendations for the care of pregnant women with EVD. However, there are no definitive data to recommend cesarean delivery over vaginal delivery or the preferred timing for delivery. According to WHO guidelines from 2020, labor should not be induced. Additionally, procedures such as cesarean delivery, episiotomy, and vacuum extraction should only be performed for maternal indications, with the overall goal of reducing maternal morbidity and mortality.

Several monoclonal antibodies (mAbs) have been evaluated in animal studies and in clinical trials. Two products, mAb114 (ansuvimab-zykl [Ebanga]) and REGN-EB3 (atoltivimab/maftivimab/odesivimab [Inmazeb]) were approved for use by the FDA in 2020 and recommended for use by the WHO for EVD. The first product, mAb114, was isolated from a survivor of EVD and shown to protect 100% of macaques from lethal infection when administered up to 5 days after virus challenge. The second product, REGN-EB3, contains three mAbs (atoltivimab, maftivimab, odesivimab) that target the virus surface glycoprotein, providing potent virus neutralization. In rhesus macaques, a single infusion prevented death, even when administered after the onset of illness. The antibodies showed modest reductions in overall mortality in the range 14.6% to 17.8% compared with ZMapp[5], a three mAb combo, that had previously shown a small reduction in mortality compared with placebo (22% vs. 37%). Clinicians may contact the CDC's Emergency Operations Center for additional information on use of experimental therapeutics for treatment of EVD. Notably, no licensed therapeutics are currently available for the treatment of illness caused by Sudan virus or other Ebola virus species.

Long-Term Follow-Up

The WHO suggests close follow-up of patients after hospital discharge for the first year. A suggested schedule is first follow-up 2 weeks after discharge, then monthly for 6 months, and then every 3 months to complete 1 year. Survivors with ocular findings require follow-up to assess for cataracts. Semen testing should be done at follow-up visits until negative for Ebola virus RNA. If semen testing is unavailable, then WHO recommends that men practice safe sex for 12 months from onset of illness.

If patients develop fever, then they should be assessed for relapse while also being evaluated for other causes of infection. Development of uveitis and meningitis may suggest relapse. Spinal fluid analysis should be done when meningitis is suspected, even if the blood tests are negative for Ebola virus RNA.

Prevention

Two vaccines have shown promise in the prevention of EVD. The recombinant vesicular stomatitis virus–Zaire Ebola vaccine (rVSV-ZEBOV) has been found to have an efficacy of 97.5% when given as part of a ring vaccination strategy, where contacts of infected people are vaccinated, as are any subsequent contacts of those people. The greatest role for the vaccine may be in disease prevention when given promptly postexposure. The FDA-approved rVSV-ZEBOV (Ervebo) in December 2019. In the United States, the vaccine is recommended for preexposure prophylaxis in adults at risk for occupation exposure to the Ebola virus.

A second vaccine, Ad26.ZEBOV/MVA-BN-Filo (Zabdeno and Mvabea) was introduced in the DRC in November 2019 in response to the ongoing Ebola epidemic. Given in two doses, Zabdeno (first dose) and Mvabea (second dose 8 weeks later), this prime-boost vaccine has been found to be safe and immunogenic. In contrast to the rVSV-ZEBOV vaccine, which is being employed in a ring vaccination strategy for healthcare workers in the outbreak area, the Ad26.ZEBOV/MVA-BN-Filo vaccine will be given to at-risk populations in regions where there is no active disease transmission and is expected to provide longer protection. Several candidate vaccines against Sudan virus are in development.

Recommendations for travelers to an area affected by an Ebola outbreak or those residing in such an area are as follows:

[5] Investigational drug in the United States.

- Practice careful hand hygiene and avoid contact with an infected person's blood or body fluids, including personal items that may have come in contact with blood and body fluids.
- Avoid unprotected contact with the body of a deceased person who was infected with EVD.
- Avoid contact with bats and nonhuman primates, including blood, bodily fluids, and tissues from these animals.
- Monitor health for 21 days after return from an Ebola endemic region, and seek medical care immediately if any symptoms develop.

Healthcare workers at risk for exposure to Ebola must wear PPE and notify appropriate health officials at their institutions if they have unprotected contact with the blood or bodily fluids of a person infected with Ebola disease. Finally, institutions must have proper infection control and sterilization measures in place for handling of biohazardous materials. Clinicians may contact the CDC for additional information on use of experimental therapeutics and vaccines for prophylaxis after a high-risk occupational exposure to Ebola virus.

Monitoring

Local authorities may have specific regulations for management of asymptomatic individuals with Ebola virus exposure. This includes self-monitoring versus direct observation by a health official and the need for quarantine. In general, asymptomatic persons who have had an exposure should be monitored for 21 days after the last known exposure and should immediately report the development of fever or other clinical manifestations suggestive of EVD to the health authorities.

References

Biedenkopf N, Bukreyev A, Chandran K, et al.: Renaming of genera Ebolavirus and Marburgvirus to Orthoebolavirus and Orthomarburgvirus, respectively, and introduction of binomial species names within family Filoviridae, *Arch Virol* 168(8):220, 2023.
Center for Disease Control and Prevention: *Ebola, Health Care Providers.* https://www.cdc.gov/ebola/site.html#hcp. Accessed October 8, 2025.
Feldmann H, Sprecher A, Geisbert TW: Ebola, *N Engl J Med* 382(19):1832–1842, 2020.
Willet V, Dixit D, fisher D, et al.: Summary of WHO infection prevention and control guideline for Ebola and Marburg disease: a call for evidence based practice, *BMJ* 384:2811, 2024.
World Health Organization: *Ebola Virus Disease.* https://www.who.int/health-topics/ebola/#tab=tab_3. Accessed October 8, 2025.

FOODBORNE ILLNESSES

Method of
Anita Devi K. Ravindran, MD; and Viswanathan K. Neelakantan, MD

CURRENT DIAGNOSIS

- Infective foodborne illnesses are innumerable and are caused by various microorganisms. Some microorganisms are established agents, several others are emerging pathogens, and the pathogenicity of the remainder is still under speculation.
- Classification of these illnesses is best done according to their incubation periods, the symptoms they produce, or both.
- Nausea and vomiting predominate in illnesses with short incubation periods caused by preformed toxins, whereas diarrhea predominates in those with long incubation periods caused by toxins produced in the intestine.
- Undercooked charcuterie, meat, poultry, and seafood account for a majority of foodborne illness, but dairy products, salads, pastries, fruits, and vegetables can also cause illness.
- Contaminated water acts as a vehicle in almost all instances.

CURRENT THERAPY

- The majority of infective foodborne illnesses with symptoms confined to the gastrointestinal tract, although apparently alarming, are self-limiting and need only supportive measures including replacement of water and electrolytes.
- Antimicrobial agents are indicated only in certain patients, including those with systemic illnesses, extremes of age, immunocompromised and malnourished states, and severe life-threatening illness.
- Antitoxin is useful in botulism poisoning.
- Vaccines are available against *Vibrio cholerae, Salmonella typhi*, hepatitis A virus, and rotavirus, but their effectiveness and cost-effectiveness are debatable.

The Centers for Disease Control and Prevention (CDC) estimates that each year roughly one in six Americans (about 48 million people) gets sick from foodborne illnesses; 128,000 are hospitalized, and 3000 die. These figures are higher in developing nations, and many cases are not brought to light because they occur in remote villages. The 2011 estimates provide the most accurate picture of infective foodborne illnesses, of which bacteria, viruses, and parasites account for the majority. Processing of ready-to-eat foods increases the risk of acquiring foodborne illness because of increased food handling, leading to introduction and growth of pathogens. Increased international travel and migration have also resulted in a greater risk because travelers are at high risk for developing foodborne gastroenteritis caused by pathogens to which they have not been exposed at home.

Classification of Foodborne Illnesses

Agents causing foodborne diseases may be classified in several ways. The most common scheme is a taxonomic combined with a classification based on mode of action (Tables 1 to 3).

Bacteria

Aeromonas Species

Species of *Aeromonas* are ubiquitous and autochthonous in aquatic environments, more so after the tsunami that followed the Indonesian earthquake in December 2004. These aeromonads share many biochemical characteristics with members of the Enterobacteriaceae. The mesophilic species *Aeromonas caviae, Aeromonas hydrophila*, and *Aeromonas veronii* are principally associated with gastroenteritis; *A. caviae* particularly infects children younger than 3 years.

Transmission is documented as occurring from a contaminated piped water source, as seen in community-based outbreaks, especially among children. The probability of occurrence of *Aeromonas* infection increased significantly when the mean seasonal temperature exceeded 14°C (57°F), and this was exacerbated where the mean free chlorine concentration fell below 0.1 mg/L.

Aeromonas species are potential food-poisoning agents. *A. hydrophila* is psychrotrophic and has been associated with spoilage of refrigerated animal products including chicken, beef, pork, lamb, fish, oysters, crab, and milk.

The incubation period for *Aeromonas*-associated traveler's diarrhea is 1 to 2 days. It usually causes a sporadic illness. Usually a mild to moderate but self-limiting diarrhea occurs, but it can be severe enough in children to require hospitalization. *Aeromonas* gastroenteritis can occur as a nondescript enteritis, as a more-severe form accompanied by bloody stools, as the etiologic agent of a subacute or chronic intestinal syndrome, as an extremely rare cause of cholera-like disease, or in association with episodic traveler's diarrhea. By far the most common presentation of *Aeromonas* gastroenteritis is watery enteritis. The most serious

TABLE 1 Classification of Foodborne Illnesses

SIGNS AND SYMPTOMS OR MECHANISM	PATHOGENS
Based on Symptoms and Duration of Onset	
Nausea and vomiting within 6 h	*Staphylococcus aureus, Bacillus cereus*
Abdominal cramps and diarrhea within 8–16 h	*Clostridium perfringens, Bacillus cereus*
Fever, abdominal cramps, and diarrhea within 16–48 h	*Salmonella, Shigella, Vibrio parahemolyticus,* enteroinvasive *Escherichia coli, Campylobacter jejuni*
Abdominal cramps and watery diarrhea within 16–72 h	Enterotoxigenic *E. coli, Vibrio cholerae* O1, O139 Bengal, *Vibrio parahemolyticus,* NAG (nonagglutinable) vibrios, *Norovirus*
Fever and abdominal cramps within 16–48 h	*Yersinia enterocolitica*
Bloody diarrhea without fever within 72–120 h	Enterohemorrhagic *E. coli* O157:H7
Nausea, vomiting, diarrhea, and paralysis within 18–36 h	*Clostridium botulinum*
Based on Pathogenesis	
Food intoxications resulting from the ingestion of preformed bacterial toxins	*Staphylococcus aureus, Bacillus cereus, Clostridium botulinum, Clostridium perfringens*
Food intoxications caused by noninvasive bacteria that secrete toxins while adhering to the intestinal wall	Enterotoxigenic *E. coli, Vibrio cholerae, Campylobacter jejuni*
Food intoxications that follow an intracellular invasion of intestinal epithelial cells	*Shigella, Salmonella*
Diseases caused by bacteria that enter the bloodstream via the intestinal tract	*Salmonella typhi, Listeria monocytogenes*
Based on Toxin Production	
The organisms responsible produce two major types of toxins, or they may be invasive, with no toxin production.	
Secretory toxins are enterotoxins produced by microbes that colonize the intestines in large numbers by attaching to the mucosal epithelial cells without invasion of mucosa, and, hence, there is no fever or other systemic symptoms as a result of lack of inflammatory response. Massive quantities of fluid and electrolytes are lost into the large bowel as its reabsorbing capacity is exceeded by the hypersecretion of isotonic fluid produced by the enterotoxins.	*Vibrio cholerae,* enterotoxigenic *E. coli, Shigella dysenteriae, Salmonella typhimurium*
Cytotoxins are those that destroy the epithelial cells of the mucosa.	*Shigella dysenteriae* elaborating Shiga toxin, causing destructive colitis, enterohemorrhagic *E. coli,* producing a similar toxin causing hemorrhagic colitis and hemolytic uremic syndrome (HUS), and *Vibrio parahemolyticus)* *Clostridium perfringens,* which produces a secretory enterotoxin, also has a cytotoxic action.
Secretory toxins, cytotoxins, and/or neurotoxins that are preformed are ingested directly in food.	*Bacillus cereus, Staphylococcus aureus, Clostridium botulinum*
Certain invasive microbes produce systemic symptoms such as fever, headache, and myalgia, in addition to gastrointestinal symptoms.	Salmonellosis typhoid fever, shigellosis, and brucellosis

complication resulting from *Aeromonas* gastroenteritis is hemolytic uremic syndrome.

Pathogenesis
Mesophilic *Aeromonas* spp. can express a range of virulence factors, including attachment mechanisms and production of a number of toxins. Toxins include aerolysin (a pore-forming cytolysin that attaches to cell membrane, leading to leakage of cytoplasmic contents) and a cytotonic enterotoxin with activity similar to that of cholera toxin. Strains of *A. hydrophila* produce lectins and adhesins, which enable adherence to epithelial surfaces and gut mucosa.

Laboratory Diagnosis
Samples are best transported using Cary-Blair medium. *Aeromonas* forms a bull's-eye–like colony on the selective medium cefsulodin irgasan novobiocin (CIN) agar owing to fermentation of D-mannitol. Ampicillin blood agar has an advantage over CIN agar in that hemolytic colonies can readily be tested for oxidase. *Aeromonas* species produce hemolysis on sheep blood agar.

Treatment
In *Aeromonas* infections, ciprofloxacin (Cipro)[1] 500 mg PO or 400 mg IV twice daily is the antimicrobial treatment of choice. Piperacillin-tazobactam (Zosyn)[1] 4.5 g IV three times daily or ceftazidime (Fortaz)[1] 2 g IV daily may be added in severe infections. The organism is also susceptible to aminoglycosides and carbapenems. Resistance is now becoming a problem because *Aeromonas* can produce β-lactamases and carbapenemases. Therefore it is preferable to initiate therapy with a fluoroquinolone when the organism is isolated.

Bacillus cereus
Bacillus cereus is found abundantly in the environment and vegetation. It is known to produce two forms of food poisoning, emetic and diarrheal. The emetic (short-incubation) type of illness is associated with contaminated fried rice that is not refrigerated. The organism is present in uncooked rice, and the spores survive boiling. The illness is usually self-limiting, with recovery

---

[1]Not FDA approved for this indication.

TABLE 2 Common Organisms Implicated in Infective Foodborne Illness

ETIOLOGIC AGENT	USUAL INCUBA-TION PERIOD	SYMPTOMS	DURATION OF SYMPTOMS	COMMON VEHICLES
Upper Gastrointestinal Tract Symptoms (Nausea, Vomiting) Occur First or Predominate				
Staphylococcus aureus (preformed toxin)	1–6 h	Sudden onset of severe nausea and vomiting Abdominal cramps, diarrhea, and fever may be present	24–48 h	Unrefrigerated or improperly refrigerated meat, potato and egg salads, cream pastries
Bacillus cereus (preformed toxin)	1–6 h	Sudden onset of severe nausea and vomiting Diarrhea may be present	24 h	Improperly refrigerated cooked or fried rice, meat
Lower Gastrointestinal Tract Symptoms (Abdominal Cramps, Diarrhea) Occur First or Predominate				
Bacillus cereus (diarrheal toxin)	10–16 h	Abdominal cramps, watery diarrhea, nausea	24–48 h	Meat, stew, gravy, vanilla sauce
Clostridium perfringens (toxin)	8–16 h	Watery diarrhea, nausea, abdominal cramps; fever is rare	24–48 h	Meat, poultry, gravy, dried or precooked foods, time- and/or temperature-abused food
Vibrio cholerae	2 h to 5 d	Rice-water purging diarrhea leading to dehydration, shock, acidosis, renal failure, abdominal pain Cholera sicca is a severe form; patient dies before diarrhea is manifest; ileus and abdominal bloating result	2–7 d	Sewage-contaminated water Seafood: fish, shellfish, crabs, oysters, clams Contaminated rice, millet gruel, vegetables
Vibrio parahaemolyticus	12–24 h	Watery diarrhea, abdominal cramps, nausea, vomiting Neurologic symptoms can occur, as with *Clostridium botulinum* and *Trichinella spiralis*	2–5 d	Raw or undercooked seafood
Shigella	1–4 d	Abdominal cramps, fever, diarrhea Stool might contain blood and mucus	4–7 d	Food or water contaminated with fecal matter Ready-to-eat food touched by infected food worker
Salmonella (not *typhi*)	1–3 d	Diarrhea, fever, abdominal cramps, vomiting	4–7 d	Contaminated eggs, unpasteurized milk or juice, cheese, contaminated raw fruits and vegetables
Enterotoxigenic *Escherichia coli*	1–3 d	Watery diarrhea, abdominal cramps, some vomiting	3–7 d (or longer)	Food or water contaminated with human feces
Shiga toxin–producing *E. coli*, including *E. coli* O157:H7	2–6 d	Severe diarrhea that is often bloody; abdominal pain and vomiting Usually little or no fever	5–10 d	Undercooked beef, especially hamburger, unpasteurized milk and juice, raw fruit and vegetables (e.g., sprouts), salami (rarely), contaminated water
Campylobacter jejuni	2–5 d	Diarrhea, cramps, fever, vomiting Diarrhea may be bloody	2–10 d	Raw and undercooked poultry, unpasteurized milk, contaminated milk
Vibrio vulnificus	1–7 d	Vomiting, diarrhea, abdominal pain Fever, bleeding within the skin, ulcers requiring surgical removal Can be fatal to people with liver disease or weakened immune systems	2–8 d	Undercooked or raw seafood, especially oysters
Yersinia enterocolitica	3–7 d	Appendicitis-like symptoms: diarrhea, vomiting, fever, abdominal pain	Can remit and relapse over weeks to 1 mo	Drinking water, food contaminated with human fecal matter
Cyclospora	7–10 d	Diarrhea (usually watery), loss of appetite, weight loss, stomach cramps, nausea, vomiting, fatigue	Can remit and relapse over weeks to 1 mo	Fresh herbs and produce (e.g., raspberries, basil, lettuce)
Giardia lamblia (beaver fever)	7–10 d	Diarrhea (acute or chronic), stomach cramps, flatulence, weight loss, malabsorption, developmental delay	Days to weeks	Drinking water, food contaminated with human fecal matter

ETIOLOGIC AGENT	USUAL INCUBA-TION PERIOD	SYMPTOMS	DURATION OF SYMPTOMS	COMMON VEHICLES
Entamoeba histolytica	1–4 wk	Intestinal: diarrhea, fever, abdominal pain, dysentery, colitis, bowel perforation, ameboma Extraintestinal amebiasis: liver abscess with anchovy-sauce pus, spread to viscera, lungs, and brain	Days to weeks	Drinking water Food contaminated with human fecal matter
Both Upper and Lower Gastrointestinal Tract Symptoms				
Rotavirus	18–36 h	Acute onset of fever and vomiting followed 12–24 h later by frequent watery stools	3–7 d	Contaminated drinking water, food, fomites
Norovirus and other caliciviruses	12–48 h	Nausea, vomiting, cramping, diarrhea, fever, myalgia, some headache Diarrhea is more prevalent in adults; vomiting is more prevalent in children	12–60 h	Food (including shellfish) or water contaminated with human fecal matter Ready-to-eat food touched by an infected food worker
Generalized Symptoms				
Listeria monocytogenes	9–48 h or GI symptoms; 2–6 wk for invasive disease	Fever, muscle aches, nausea or diarrhea Pregnant women can have mild flulike illness, and infection can lead to premature delivery or stillbirth Elderly and immunocompromised patients can have bacteremia or meningitis	Variable	Fresh soft cheese, unpasteurized milk, ready-to-eat deli meat, hot dogs
Balatidium coli	4–5 d	Mostly asymptomatic Chronic diarrhea, occasional dysentery, nausea, foul breath, colitis, abdominal pain, weight loss, deep intestinal ulcerations, possible perforation of the intestine, pneumonia-like illness	Variable	Water contaminated with pig feces
Salmonella typhi	8–14 d	Fever, anorexia, lethargy, malaise, headache, rose spots, constipation or diarrhea, hepatosplenomegaly	4–6 wk	Contaminated water; contaminated food, mainly via food handlers; shellfish from polluted water
Ascoris lumbricoides	4–16 d	Nausea, abdominal pain, intestinal obstruction, malnutrition, Loeffler's syndrome (cough, pneumonitis, eosinophilia), biliary colic, colangitis, pancreatitis, appendicitis	Variable (chronic)	Soil-contaminated raw food, food handlers, water
Trichinella spiralis	1–2 wk	Asymptomatic or chronic diarrhea, abdominal pain Allergy leading to rash, periorbital edema, vasculitis, intramural thrombi Weakness of jaw, biceps, diaphragm, intercostals Eosinophilia, subconjunctival, splinter hemorrhages Muscle penetration: myalgia, orbital pain, diplopia Chronic phase: neurologic symptoms	Variable Acute phase: 1–3 wk	Raw or undercooked meat of pig, horse, wild boar, bush pig, warthog, bear
Infective cysticerci of *Taenia solium* (pork tape worm)	2 months on average	Seizures, vasculitis, focal neurologic deficits, intracranial hypertension, hydrocephalus, mental changes, encephalitis and Brun's syndrome (intermittent obstruction of cerebral aqueduct), myosists, vasculitis	Highly variable	Undercooked charcuterie (pork), contaminated raw vegetables, salads, water
Hepatitis A	15–50 d	Diarrhea, dark urine, jaundice, flulike symptoms, fever, headache, nausea, aversion to food, vomiting, abdominal pain; distaste for cigarettes	Variable: 2 wk to 3 mo	Food (including shellfish) or water contaminated with human fecal matter Inadequately cooked clams, oysters, mussels, cockles Contaminated lettuce, slush beverages, frozen strawberries and salad items Ready-to-eat foods touched by an infected food worker

Continued

Foodborne Illnesses

615

TABLE 2 Common Organisms Implicated in Infective Foodborne Illness—cont'd

ETIOLOGIC AGENT	USUAL INCUBATION PERIOD	SYMPTOMS	DURATION OF SYMPTOMS	COMMON VEHICLES
Brucella species	1–8 wk	Flulike illness; undulating fever, malaise, arthralgia, anorexia, hepatosplenomegaly, pleurisy, nausea, vomiting, diarrhea, new onset of increased desire to sleep after lunch	Variable	Unpasteurized dairy products, undercooked meat, bone marrow Contact with laboratory cultures and tissue samples Accidental injection of live brucellosis vaccine
Hepatitis E	3–8 wk	Prodrome: anorexia, nausea, vomiting, arthralgia, myalgia, weight loss, dehydration, abdominal pain Icteric phase: jaundice, pruritus, light-colored stool Urticaria, diarrhea, malaise	Variable (several weeks)	Fecally contaminated drinking water and food Raw and undercooked shellfish incriminated in sporadic outbreaks Possibly zoonotic spread
Microsporidium: *Encephalitozoon,* *Pleistophora,* *Nosema,* *Vittaforma,* *Trachipleistophora,* *Brachiola,* *Microsporidium,* *Enterocytozoon*	Unknown	Watery or bloody or unspecified diarrhea, abdominal discomfort, cramps, flatulence, weight loss, loss of appetite, wasting syndrome, subfebrile temperatures Extraintestinal: pneumonitis, myositis, keratoconjunctivitis, seizures, nephritis, cholangiopathy	Variable; self-limiting (1–2 wk) in immunocompetent patients	Contaminated water, food, or inhalation

Abbreviation: GI=gastrointestinal.

TABLE 3 Rare and Emerging Infections

ETIOLOGIC AGENT	USUAL INCUBATION PERIOD	SYMPTOMS	DURATION OF SYMPTOMS	COMMON VEHICLES
Bacillus subtilis	10 min to 14 h (average, 2.5 h)	Vomiting, diarrhea, abdominal cramps, nausea, headache, flushing, sweating	1.5–8 h	Sausage rolls, meat pasties, turkey stuffing, chicken stuffing, pizza, whole-grain bread, steak pie, pork sandwiches
Cyanobacteria: *Microcystic aeuroginosa,* *Anabaena circinalis,* *Anabaena flosaquae,* *Aphanizomenon flosaquae,* *Cylindrospermopsis racibarskii*	3–6 h	Diarrhea, vomiting, allergic reactions, breathing difficulty, dizziness, tingling and numbness, liver and kidney toxicity	8–16 h	Drinking water from untreated surface sources, inhaling aerosols from jet-skis and boats, consuming dietary supplements contaminated by microcystin
Anisakis	Few hours to days	Gastric: abdominal pain, nausea, vomiting Allergic: urticaria, anaphylaxis Intestinal: ileus, perforation, peritonitis, stenosis	2 wk	Raw, lightly pickled, or salted marine fish: Mackerel, squid, horse mackerel, salmon, bonito Squid, cuttlefish Sushi, sashimi
Astrovirus	1–4 d	Watery diarrhea (especially in children), vomiting, fever, anorexia, abdominal pain	3–4 d	Sewage-polluted water and food
Pleisomonas shigelloides	5 d	Diarrhea with blood and mucus, abdominal pain, headache, nausea, chills, fever, vomiting	1–7 d	Contaminated water used for drinking or rinsing foods to be eaten raw Contaminated raw shellfish, salted fish, crabs, oysters
Cyclospora	7 d	Frequent watery diarrhea, weight loss, abdominal pain, bloating, flatulence, vomiting, nausea, low-grade fever, fatigue, malabsorption, cholecystitis	1–4 wk Relapse is common	Fecally contaminated fresh raspberries, snow peas, mesclun

TABLE 3 Rare and Emerging Infections—cont'd

ETIOLOGIC AGENT	USUAL INCUBA-TION PERIOD	SYMPTOMS	DURATION OF SYMPTOMS	COMMON VEHICLES
Iosospora belli	8–11 d	Diarrhea, steatorrhea, headache, fever, malaise, abdominal pain, vomiting, dehydration, weight loss Mesenteric lymph node, liver, spleen involvement	Variable; runs a chronic course in immunocompromised patients	Contaminated food and water
Edwardisella tarda	Not defined	Nausea, vomiting, diarrhea, dysentery, colitis, wound infections, septicemia	Variable: 1–2 wk or longer	Fecal contamination of food, water, raw fish
Citrobacter species	Not defined	Diarrhea, hemolytic uremic syndrome, thrombocytopenic purpura		Meat and milk Parsley (in green butter) from organic gardens using pig manure
Arizona	Not defined	Diarrhea		Cream pie, chocolate eclairs, custard, eggs, chicken, turkey
Achromobacter xylosoxidans	Not defined	Abdominal pain, diarrhea, headache, vomiting		Raw milk, spoiled canned food, contaminated well water

in a day. It is mediated by a heat-stable, preformed enterotoxin resembling that of *Staphylococcus aureus*. The first major outbreak of *Bacillus cereus* food poisoning was in 1971 in England. The diarrheal (long-incubation) type of illness is produced by a heat-labile diarrheal enterotoxin formed in the intestine, which activates adenylate cyclase, causing intestinal fluid secretion, similar to *Escherichia coli* LT toxin and the toxin of *Clostridium perfringens*.

Pathogenesis
During the slow cooling of cooked rice, spores germinate and vegetative bacteria multiply; then they sporulate again. Sporulation is also associated with toxin production. The toxin is heat stable and can easily withstand the temperatures used to cook fried rice.

Laboratory Diagnosis
The disease is diagnosed by the isolation of *B. cereus* from the incriminated food (emetic type) or from stool and food (diarrheal type). Isolation from stools alone is not sufficient because gastrointestinal colonization with *B. cereus* occurs in many persons.

Treatment
B. cereus food poisoning may be symptomatically managed with replacement of fluids and electrolytes. Antimicrobials have no role in treatment. *B. cereus* is also known to produce a variety of ocular and systemic infections such as meningitis, osteomyelitis, pneumonia, and endocarditis. These are usually not foodborne, and it is in this situation that vancomycin (Vancocin)[1] becomes the drug of choice, with clindamycin (Cleocin)[1] and carbapenems being the alternative drugs, both being used along with aminoglycosides for synergistic action.

Campylobacter jejuni
Campylobacter jejuni are harbored in the reproductive and alimentary tracts of some animals. Other than gastrointestinal symptoms, the patient has malaise and headache. The organism may be shed in the patient's stool for up to 2 months. Bacteremia is observed in a small minority of cases. The disease is usually self-limiting. Guillain-Barré syndrome and Reiter's syndrome are recognized sequelae.

Pathogenesis
As few as 500 organisms can cause enteritis. The organism is invasive but generally less so than *Shigella*. *Campylobacter* produces adenylate cyclase–activating toxins resembling *E. coli* LT and cholera toxin.

Laboratory Diagnosis
The feces may be inoculated in enrichment medium or on selective media such as Campy-BAP or Skirrow's medium.

Treatment
Indications for antibiotic therapy in *C. jejuni* infections are prolonged fever, severe diarrhea, dysentery, and persistent symptoms for more than a week. Therapy of *Campylobacter* infection with ciprofloxacin (Cipro 500 mg orally twice daily for 7 days) early in the course of the illness shortens its duration. Unfortunately, this has led to the emergence of fluoroquinolone-resistant *Campylobacter* infections. Erythromycin eradicates carriage of susceptible *C. jejuni* and might shorten the duration of illness if given early in the disease. Erythromycin (Ery-Tab)[1] 250 mg PO four times daily is the drug of choice in *Campylobacter* enteritis. Azithromycin (Zithromax)[1] is also useful and has the advantage of shorter duration of therapy.

Gentamicin (Garamycin), carbapenems, amoxicillin-clavulanate (Augmentin),[1] and chloramphenicol[1] are useful in systemic infections. The usual duration of treatment is 2 weeks. The therapy is prolonged in immunocompromised persons and in patients with endovascular infections.

Clostridium botulinum
Clostridum botulinum is widely distributed in soil, in sediments of lakes and ponds, and in decaying vegetation. *C. botulinum* elaborates the most potent toxin known in humans. When the toxin is ingested, paralysis occurs, often requiring prolonged artificial ventilation. Common signs and symptoms include vomiting, thirst, dry mouth, constipation, ocular palsies, dysphagia, dysarthria, bulbar paralysis, and death due to respiratory paralysis. Coma or delirium occurs in some. Infants present with lethargy, poor feeding, loss of head control, and sometimes sudden infant death syndrome (SIDS).

The incriminated foods are corn syrup, home-canned or bottled meat, fruits, fish, vegetables, herb-infused oils, and cheese sauce. Infant botulism is associated with consumption of honey; honey should not be given to infants younger than 1 year.

Pathogenesis
Not all strains of *C. botulinum* produce botulinum toxin. Toxigenic types of the organism, designated A, B, C1, D, E, F, and G, produce immunologically distinct forms of botulinum toxin. Lysogenic phages encode toxin C and D serotypes.

---

[1]Not FDA approved for this indication.

[1]Not FDA approved for this indication.

Foodborne botulism is not an infection but an intoxication because it results from the ingestion of foods that contain the preformed clostridial toxin. If contaminated food has been insufficiently heated or canned improperly, the spores can germinate and produce botulinum toxin. The toxin is released only after cell lysis and death. The toxin resists digestion and is absorbed by the upper gastrointestinal tract and enters the blood. The toxin blocks release of acetylcholine by binding to receptors at synapses and neuromuscular junctions and causes flaccid paralysis.

Laboratory Diagnosis
Spoilage of food or swelling of cans or presence of bubbles inside the can indicate growth of *C. botulinum*. Food is homogenized in broth and inoculated in Robertson cooked meat medium and blood agar or egg-yolk agar, which is incubated anaerobically for 3 to 5 days at 37°C. The toxin can be demonstrated by injecting the extract of food or culture into mice or guinea pigs intraperitoneally.

Treatment
Hospitalization in an intensive care unit with immediate administration of botulinum antitoxin is vital in the management of botulism. The antitoxin neutralizes only toxin molecules unbound to nerve endings and does not reverse the paralysis. It should be given within 24 hours after the diagnosis is made. Penicillin is the antimicrobial of choice. Intubation and mechanical ventilation are needed for respiratory failure. If swallowing difficulty persists, intravenous fluids or alimentation should be given through a nasogastric tube.

Clostridium perfringens
C. perfringens is heat resistant and elaborates two toxins that can induce specific pathology in the human intestinal tract. It is the third leading cause of foodborne illnesses in United States, after norovirus and *B. cereus*. It is present abundantly in the environment, vegetation, sewage, and animal feces.

Human diseases caused by this organism are the more common *C. perfringens* type A food poisoning and the less common, but more serious, *C. perfringens* type C food poisoning producing necrotic enteritis. Necrotic enteritis is characterized by vomiting, severe abdominal pain, and bloody diarrhea. The incubation period is 2 to 5 days. Progression to necrosis of the jejunum and death occur.

Pathogenesis
Spores in food can survive cooking and then germinate when the food is improperly stored. When these vegetative cells form endospores in the intestine, they release enterotoxins. Food poisoning is mainly caused by type A strains, which produce alpha and theta toxins. The toxins result in excessive fluid accumulation in the intestinal lumen.

Laboratory Diagnosis
Because the bacterium is present normally in intestines, isolation from feces might not be sufficient to implicate it as the cause of the illness. Similarly, isolation from food, except in large numbers ($>10^9/g$), might not be significant. The homogenized food is diluted and plated on selective medium, as well as Robertson cooked meat medium, and subjected to anaerobic incubation. The isolated bacteria must be shown to produce enterotoxin.

Treatment
Food poisoning due to *Clostridium perfringens* is managed conservatively with hydration and replacement of electrolytes. *C. perfringens* is susceptible to benzylpenicillin (penicillin G), which may be useful in managing severe infections (1 mU IV every 4 hours). Vancomycin,[1] clindamycin,[1] cefoxitin (Mefoxin), and

metronidazole (Flagyl) are alternatives. *C. perfringens* type C toxoid vaccine[2] (two doses, 4 months apart) is preventive in pigbel.

Cronobacter sakazakii
Cronobacter sakazakii causes neonatal meningitis or necrotizing enterocolitis and bacteremia, which results in an alarming mortality rate. Surviving patients sometimes develop ventriculitis and cerebral abscess. *C. sakazakii* has been isolated from infant formulas.

Enterobacter species are generally resistant to the cephalosporins, except cefepime (Maxipime),[1] but are responsive to carbenicillin (Geocillin),[1] piperacillin (Pipracil),[1] ticarcillin (Ticar),[1] amikacin (Amikin),[1] and tigecycline (Tygacil).[1]

Enterohemorrhagic Escherichia coli
Many serogroups of *E. coli*, including O4, O26, O45, O91, O111, O145, and O157, are pathogenic, but the most common pathogenic serotype is O157:H7. Cattle are the main sources of infection; most cases are associated with the consumption of undercooked beef burgers and similar foods from restaurants and delicatessens. The latest outbreak of *E. coli* O157:H7 during the fall of 2019 and 2020 was linked to leafy greens (romaine salad greens). Several outbreaks of *E. coli* O157:H7 illnesses were identified as being caused by the REPEXH01 strain, which is classified as a "persistent" strain causing illness over many years.

Pathogenesis
Enterohemorrhagic *E. coli* (EHEC) strains can produce one or more types of cytotoxins, which are collectively referred to as Shiga-like toxins because they are antigenically and functionally similar to Shiga toxin produced by *Shigella dysenteriae*. (Shiga-like toxins were previously known as verotoxins.) The toxins provoke cell secretion and kill colonic epithelial cells, causing hemorrhagic colitis and hemolytic-uremic syndrome (HUS), leading occasionally to disseminated intravascular coagulation (DIC). A fibrin layer forms in the glomerular capillary bed, and acute renal failure occurs due to DIC. These are most likely to occur in children, elderly patients, and pregnant women. The young recover fully, but at times dialysis is warranted.

Laboratory Diagnosis
Laboratory diagnosis is performed by culturing the feces on McConkey's agar or sorbitol McConkey's agar. Strains can then be identified by serotyping using specific antisera. Shiga-like toxins can be detected by enzyme-linked immunosorbent assay (ELISA), and genes coding for them can be detected by DNA hybridization techniques.

Treatment
Hydration with electrolyte replacement is the mainstay of treatment in *E. coli* O157:H7 infection, and patients should be monitored closely and constantly for the development of HUS, which requires management in an intensive care setting with blood transfusion and dialysis. Although dysentery is self-limiting, the use of rifaximin (Xifaxan), a nonabsorbable agent, is recommended in those who are increasingly susceptible to infections. In the absence of dysentery, early institution of drugs like ciprofloxacin (Cipro) or azithromycin (Zithromax),[1] especially in traveler's diarrhea, decreases the duration of illness.

Enterotoxigenic Escherichia Coli
Enterotoxigenic *E. coli* (ETEC) is now ubiquitous in nature. Wild animals and cattle act as reservoirs of the organism. *E. coli* is carried normally in the intestine of humans and animals. Some specific serotypes harbor plasmids that code for toxin production.

---

[1]Not FDA approved for this indication.

[2]Not available in the United States.
[1]Not FDA approved for this indication.

This bacterium is responsible for a majority of traveler's diarrhea. The disease is self-limiting and resolves in a few days.

Pathogenesis

The bacteria colonize the gastrointestinal tract by means of fimbriae, attaching to specific receptors on enterocytes of the proximal small intestine. Enterotoxins produced by ETEC include the LT (heat-labile) toxin and the ST (heat-stable) toxins. LTs are similar to cholera toxin in structure and mode of action, consisting of A and B subunits. The B (binding) subunit of LTs binds to specific ganglioside receptors (GM1) on the epithelial cells of the small intestine and facilitates the entry of the A (activating) subunit, which activates adenylate cyclase. Stimulation of adenylate cyclase causes an increased production of cyclic adenosine monophosphate (cAMP), which leads to hypersecretion of water and electrolytes into the lumen and inhibition of sodium reabsorption.

Laboratory Diagnosis

The sample of feces is cultured on McConkey's agar. The ETEC stains are indistinguishable from the resident *E. coli* by biochemical tests. These strains are differentiated from nontoxigenic *E. coli* present in the bowel by a variety of in vitro immunochemical, tissue culture, or DNA hybridization tests designed to detect either the toxins or the genes that encode for these toxins. With the availability of a gene probe method, foods can be analyzed directly for the presence of ETEC in about 3 days. LTs can be detected by ligated rabbit ileal loop test and by observing morphologic changes in Chinese hamster ovary cells and Y1 adrenal cells. ELISA, immunodiffusion, and coagglutination are also used in diagnosis.

Listeria monocytogenes

Listeria monocytogenes is quite hardy and resists the deleterious effects of freezing, drying, and heat remarkably well for a bacterium that does not form spores. It is capable of growing at 3°C and multiplies in refrigerated foods. The latest implicated food in a February 2021 outbreak is queso fresco cheese.

Pathogenesis

L. monocytogenes invades the gastrointestinal epithelium. Once the bacterium enters the host's monocytes, macrophages, or neutrophils, it is bloodborne and can grow. Its presence in phagocytes also permits access to the brain and transplacental migration to the fetus in pregnant women. Granulomatosis infantisepticum is a feature of listeriosis. The pathogenesis of *L. monocytogenes* centers on its ability to survive and multiply in phagocytic host cells.

Laboratory Diagnosis

The diagnosis of listeriosis is most commonly made by isolation of *L. monocytogenes* from a normally sterile site. β-Hemolytic colonies, which test negative for catalase, hydrolyze hippurate, and have a positive cAMP reaction, form on blood agar. Serologic testing is not useful in diagnosing acute invasive disease, but it can be useful in detecting asymptomatic disease and gastroenteritis in an outbreak or in other epidemiologic investigations. Stool testing is not commercially available.

Treatment

Ampicillin[1] (2 g IV every 4 hours) is the drug of choice in *Listeria monocytogenes* infections. Aminoglycosides are added for synergistic effect. Trimethoprim-sulfamethoxazole (TMP-SMX)[1] (Bactrim, 20 mg of trimethoprim/day IV every 6 hours) is an alternative for patients allergic to penicillin. Ampicillin and TMP-SMX may be used in combination. Vancomycin (Vancocin),[1] linezolid (Zyvox),[1] carbapenems, macrolides, and tetracyclines are also effective. Cephalosporins are ineffective in the treatment of listeriosis and should not be used. The duration of therapy is highly

variable depending on the clinical situation and is 14 days for bacteremia, 21 days for meningitis, 42 days for endocarditis, and 56 days for neurologic infections. Patients whose disease is promptly diagnosed and treated recover fully, but permanent neurologic sequelae are common in patients with cerebral illnesses. Consuming only pasteurized dairy products and fully cooked meats, meticulously cleaning utensils, and thoroughly washing fresh vegetables before cooking will prevent foodborne listerial infections. Pregnant women and others at risk should avoid soft cheeses and thoroughly reheated ready-to-serve and charcuterie foods.

Nontyphoidal Salmonellosis

Nontyphoidal salmonellosis consists of several causative organisms classified under the family Enterobacteriaceae; one such organism is *Salmonella enteritidis*. It does not occur normally in humans, but several animals act as reservoirs.

The diarrhea may be watery, with greenish, foul-smelling stools. This may be preceded by headache and chills. Other findings include prostration, muscle weakness, and moderate fever. In August 2020, a multi-state outbreak of *Salmonella enteritidis* was linked to peaches packed or supplied by Prima Wawona packing company. An outbreak of *Salmonella stanley* infection was linked to wood ear mushrooms (dried mushrooms, also called kikurage/dried black fungus) imported to to the U.S. Yet another nontyphoidal Salmonella infection reported in July 2020 was caused by *Salmonella newport*. The likely source was identified as potentially contaminated red onions. A food-borne illness recently reported from Mexico was caused by *Salmonella poona* and linked to consumption of cucumbers. Newly reported include *Salmonella reading* and *Salmonella abony linked* to consumption of alfalfa sprouts.

Pathogenesis

The organism penetrates and passes through the epithelial cells lining the terminal ileum. Multiplication of bacteria in lamina propria produces inflammatory mediators, recruits neutrophils, and triggers inflammation. Release of lipopolysaccharides and prostaglandins causes fever and also loss of water and electrolytes into the lumen of the intestine, resulting in diarrhea.

Laboratory Diagnosis

Culture in selenite F broth and then subculture on deoxycholate citrate agar isolates the organisms. Plates are incubated at 37°C overnight, and growth is identified by biochemical and slide agglutination tests.

Treatment

The antibiotics recommended for gastroenteritis due to nontyphoidal salmonellosis are ciprofloxacin (Cipro)[1] 500 mg PO twice daily, and ceftriaxone (Rocephin) 2 g IV daily, for 3 to 7 days. Amoxicillin (Amoxil)[1] and TMP-SMX[1] are also effective. Therapy is prolonged in bacteremia, endocarditis, or meningitis.

Shigella Species

Shigella species belong to the family Enterobacteriaceae. Bacillary dysentery is caused by *Shigella flexneri*, *Shigella boydii*, *Shigella dysenteriae,* and *Shigella sonnei*. *S. flexneri* is most common in developing countries where hygiene is poor and clean drinking water is unavailable; *S. sonnei* is most common in developed countries. The watery diarrhea that is present initially becomes bloody after a day or two owing to spread of infection from the ileum to the colon. The illness is caused by exotoxin acting in the small bowel.

Extraintestinal manifestations are recognized, including HUS, Reiter's syndrome, meningitis, Ekiri syndrome (reported in Japanese children and consisting of a triad of encephalopathy due to cerebral edema, bizarre posturing, and fatty degeneration of liver), vaginitis, lung infections, and keratoconjunctivitis. Toxic megacolon, pneumatosis coli, perforation, and rectal prolapse are recognized complications.

Tossed salads, chicken, and shellfish are the commonly incriminated foods. Person-to-person spread by anal intercourse or oral

---

[1]Not FDA approved for this indication.

sex also occurs. Prepared food acts as a vehicle of transmission. Spread of infection is also linked to flies.

Children are at high risk during the weaning period, and increasing age is associated with decreased prevalence and severity. Children in daycare centers, persons in custodial institutions, migrant workers, and travelers to developing countries are also at high risk.

Pathogenesis

The virulence factor is a smooth lipopolysaccharide cell wall antigen, which is responsible for the invasive features, and the Shiga toxin, which is both cytotoxic and neurotoxic. Shigellae survive the gastric acidity and invade and multiply within the colonic epithelial cells, causing cell death and mucosal ulcers, and spread laterally to involve adjacent cells but rarely invade the bloodstream.

Laboratory Diagnosis

Shigellosis can be correctly diagnosed in most patients on the basis of fresh blood in stool. Neutrophils in fecal smears strongly suggest infection. Any clinical diagnosis should be confirmed by cultivation of the etiologic agent from stools. Cary-Blair medium is the transport medium of choice, and MacConkey agar or deoxycholate citrate agar (DCA) as well as a highly selective medium such as xylose-lysin deoxycholate (XLD), Hektoen enteric (HE), or Salmonella-Shigella (SS) agar are also used.

Treatment

Ciprofloxacin (Cipro, 500 mg PO twice daily for 3 days) is the antibiotic of choice for shigellosis. Alternative agents are pivmecillinam (Selexid),[2] ceftriaxone (Rocephin),[1] and azithromycin (Zithromax).[1]

Staphylococcus aureus

A notable incident of staphylococcal food poisoning occurred in February 1975 when 196 of 344 passengers and one flight attendant aboard a jet from Tokyo to Copenhagen via Anchorage contacted a gastrointestinal illness characterized by nausea, vomiting, and abdominal cramps. The flight attendant and 142 passengers were hospitalized. Symptoms developed shortly after a ham and omelet breakfast had been served. S. aureus was incriminated as the offending agent and ham as the vehicle of the outbreak. The source was traced to a cook with pustules on his fingers.

S. aureus is ubiquitous in the environment. Only strains that produce enterotoxin cause food poisoning. Food is usually contaminated by infected food handlers.

Pathogenesis

If food is stored for some time at room temperature, the organism can multiply in the food and produce enterotoxin. Most food poisonings are caused by enterotoxin A, and the isolates commonly belong to phage type III. These are heat stable, and ingestion of as little as 23 μg of enterotoxin can induce symptoms. The toxin acts on the receptors in the gut, and sensory stimulus is carried to the vomiting center in the brain by vagus and sympathetic nerves.

Because the ingested food contains preformed toxin, the incubation period is very short. In severe illness, profound hypotension occurs. Death is known to occur at extremes of age and in the malnourished.

Laboratory Diagnosis

The presence of a large number of S. aureus in food can indicate poor handling or sanitation; however, it is not sufficient evidence to incriminate the food as the cause of food poisoning.

Staphylococcal food poisoning can be diagnosed if staphylococci are isolated in large numbers from the food and their toxins are demonstrated in the food or if the isolated S. aureus is shown to produce enterotoxins. Dilutions of food may be plated on Baird-Parker agar or mannitol salt agar. Enterotoxin may be detected and identified by gel diffusion.

Treatment

Therapy is mainly supportive. Antibiotics have no role in the treatment because they are not antitoxins. Intravenous fluids and electrolyte replacement are imperative in the severely dehydrated patient.

Yersinia Species

The Yersinia species that cause food poisoning are commonly Yersinia enterocolitica and rarely Yersinia pseudotuberculosis. Pigs and other wild or domestic animals are the hosts, and humans are usually infected by the oral route. Serogroups that predominate in human illness are O:3, O:5, O:8, and O:9.

Yersiniosis is common in children and occurs most often in winter. Y. enterocolitica is associated with terminal ileitis and Y. pseudotuberculosis with mesenteric adenitis, but both organisms can cause mesenteric adenitis and symptoms that cause a clinical picture resembling appendicitis, resulting in surgical removal of a normal appendix. Rarer strains of Y. enterocolitica are likely to cause systemic infections, especially in patients with diabetes or in iron overload states. In Japan, a form of vasculitis, called Izumi fever, occurs, and in Russia a scarlet fever–like illness has been reported.

Pathogenesis

Yersinia organisms can survive and grow during refrigerated storage. Strains that cause human yersiniosis carry a plasmid that is associated with a number of virulence traits. Ingested bacteria adhere and invade M cells or epithelial cells.

Laboratory Diagnosis

Suspect food is homogenized in phosphate-buffered saline and inoculated into selenite F broth and held at 4°C for 6 weeks. The broth is subcultured at weekly intervals on deoxycholate citrate (DCA) or Yersinia-selective agar plates. This is termed cold-enrichment technique.

Treatment

Antibiotics are not recommended for gastroenteritis caused by Yersinia enterocolitica and the less-common Yersinia pseudotuberculosis, but bacteremia and extraintestinal infections require treatment with ciprofloxacin[1] (500 mg PO or 400 mg IV twice daily for 2 weeks). Third-generation cephalosporins (cefotaxime[1] [Claforan]), amoxicillin[1] (Amoxil), TMP-SMX[1] (Bactrim), amoxicillin-clavulanate[1] (Augmentin), carbapenems, and gentamicin (Garamycin) are also effective agents in therapy.

Viruses

Noroviruses

Noroviruses (formerly called Norwalk or Norwalk-like viruses and small round structured viruses [SRSV]) and sapoviruses belong to the family Caliciviridae and are the most common cause of gastroenteritis. They account for about 90% of epidemic nonbacterial outbreaks of gastroenteritis around the world. Norovirus infection often affects people during the winter months and is therefore sometimes called winter vomiting disease; however, people may be affected at any time of the year. After a norovirus infection, immunity lasts only for 14 weeks and is incomplete. Persons with blood group O are more susceptible to infection, whereas those with groups B and AB are partially protected. Norovirus infection outbreaks more commonly occur in closed or semiclosed communities, such as prisons, dormitories, cruise ships, schools, long-term

---

[1]Not FDA approved for this indication.
[2]Not available in the United States.

[1]Not FDA approved for this indication.

care facilities, and overnight camps—places where infection can spread rapidly from human to human or through tainted food and surfaces. Infection outbreaks can also result from food handled by an infected person.

Outbreaks have often been linked to consumption of cold foods, including salads, sandwiches, and bakery products. Salad dressing, cake icing, and oysters from contaminated waters have also been implicated in gastroenteritis outbreaks. Weight loss, lethargy, low-grade fever, headache, and (rarely) ageusia occur. Vomiting is more likely with infections caused by norovirus than sapovirus.

Pathogenesis

Norovirus strains that infect humans are found in genogroups I, II, and IV. GII.4 strains are more commonly associated with person-to-person transmission, and GI strains are identified more commonly in shellfish-associated outbreaks.

Noroviruses were shown to differentially bind to histo-blood group antigens, and the binding pattern correlates with susceptibility to infection and illness. A number of enzymes are important in the synthesis of histo-blood group antigens, including fucosyl transferase-2 (FUT-2, secretor enzyme), FUT-3 (Lewis enzyme), and the A and B enzymes. The glycan produced by FUT-2 H type 1, serves as a viral receptor for noroviruses.

Laboratory Diagnosis

The virus can be recovered from the infected person's stool and vomitus during illness for about 2 weeks. Electron microscopy and reverse-transcriptase polymerase chain reaction (RT-PCR) antigen-detection assays are performed on stool samples. Serologic assays are not available for clinical use. However, infection can be diagnosed by identifying a fourfold or greater increase in antibody titer between acute and convalescent sera using norovirus virus-like particles as antigen.

Treatment

There is no specific treatment for norovirus infection. Hydration is generally adequate for most patients. In developing countries, oral rehydration therapy is the treatment of choice. Effective hand washing, careful food processing, and education of food handlers along with chlorination of water are important preventive measures. A vaccine for norovirus is in clinical trials.

Rotavirus

Among the seven rotavirus species (A to G), rotavirus A, B, and C can cause disease in humans. Rotavirus A is the most common and is the major cause of waterborne outbreaks in humans. Infections are referred to as infantile diarrhea, winter diarrhea, or acute viral gastroenteritis. Children 6 months to 2 years of age, premature infants, the elderly, and the immunocompromised are particularly prone to more-severe symptoms caused by infection with group A rotavirus. Rotavirus can survive in water for days to weeks, depending on water quality and temperature. Waterborne outbreaks are most common, followed by spread by fomites. Rotaviruses infect intestinal enterocytes; diarrhea may be caused by malabsorption secondary to the destruction of enterocytes, villus ischemia and activation of the enteric nervous system, and intestinal secretion stimulated by the action of rotavirus nonstructural protein 4 (NSP4), a novel enterotoxin and secretory agonist with pleiotropic properties.

Outbreaks caused by group B rotavirus, also called adult diarrhea rotavirus, have also been reported in the elderly and adults. Such infections are rare and usually subclinical. Group C rotavirus has been associated with rare and sporadic cases of diarrhea in children in many countries. Subclinical infection to severe gastroenteritis leading to life-threatening dehydration can occur. The illness has an abrupt onset, with vomiting often preceding the onset of diarrhea. Up to one third of patients have fever of about 39°C. The stools are characteristically watery and only occasionally contain red or white cells. Symptoms generally resolve in a week.

Respiratory and neurologic features in children have been reported. Rotavirus infection has been associated with other clinical conditions including sudden infant death syndrome (SIDS), necrotizing enterocolitis, Kawasaki's disease, and type 1 diabetes.

Laboratory Diagnosis

Electron microscopy, direct antigen detection assays (ELISA, immunochromatography, latex agglutination), and nucleic acid detection (e.g., RT-PCR, polyacrylamide gel electrophoresis [PAGE]), are used mainly in epidemiologic studies during outbreaks.

Treatment

Dehydration due to group A rotavirus infection is treated with early institution of oral and intravenous fluids. The role of probiotics,[7] bismuth subsalicylate (Pepto Bismol),[1] inhibitors of enkephalinase, and nitazoxanide (Alinia)[1] are not clearly defined. Antimicrobials and antimotility agents should be avoided. A marked fall in deaths from childhood diarrhea following introduction of rotavirus vaccines (Rotarix, RotaTeq) has been reported from various parts of the world, and surveillance information has not revealed an association of any serious adverse reactions with the vaccine.

Other Pathogens

Cryptosporidium

Transmission of *Cryptosporidium* is usually by the fecal-oral route, often through food and water contaminated by livestock mammal feces. Persons most likely to be infected by *Cryptosporidium parvum* are infants and young children in daycare centers; those whose drinking water is unfiltered and untreated; those involved in farming practices such as lambing, calving, and muck-spreading; people engaging in anal sexual practices; patients in a hospital setting (from other infected patients or health care workers); veterinarians; and travelers.

Pathogenesis

Cryptosporidium spp. are believed to be noninvasive. Malabsorption resulting from the intestinal damage caused by prolonged protozoal infection can be fatal. Although host cells are damaged in cryptosporidiosis, the means by which the organism causes damage is not known. Mechanical destruction and the effects of toxins, enzymes, or immune-mediated mechanisms, working alone or together, may be instrumental. In the immunocompromised, the illness is much more debilitating, with cholera-like diarrhea.

Laboratory Diagnosis

Traditionally, cryptosporidiosis is diagnosed by microscopic observation of developmental stages of the organism in an intestinal biopsy specimen. Oocysts can be recovered from stool samples by formalin-concentration techniques, staining with a modified Ziehl-Neelsen acid-fast stain. Serologic tests (ELISA, immunofluorescence antibody, PCR) are of added value.

Treatment

Nitazoxanide (Alinia, 500 mg PO twice daily for 3 days) is recommended with antiretrovirals for HIV-positive patients. Fluid replacement and antidiarrheal agents are also given.

Trichinosis

Trichinosis is due to *Trichinella spiralis* infection, commonly as a result of consuming improperly cooked pork. Recent outbreaks

---

[1]Not FDA approved for this indication.
[7]Available as dietary supplement.

TABLE 4 Seafood Poisoning Caused by Neurotoxins Identified from Marine Dinoflagellate Species

TYPE OF POISONING	TOXINS	SOURCES OF TOXINS	PRIMARY VECTOR	ACTION TARGET
PSP	Saxitoxins and gonyautoxins	*Alexandrium* spp., *Gymnodinium* spp., *Pyrodinium* spp.	Shellfish	Voltage-gated sodium channel 1
NSP	Brevetoxins	*Kerenia brevis, Chatonella marina, C. antiqua, Fibrocapsa japonica, Heterosigma akashiwo*	Shellfish	Voltage-gated sodium channel 5
	Yessotoxins	*Protoceratium reticulatum, Lingulodinium polyedrum Gonyaulax spinifera*	Shellfish	Voltage-gated calcium/ sodium channel?
CFP	Ciguatoxins	*Gambierdiscus toxicus*	Coral reef fish	Voltage-gated sodium channel 5
CFP	Maitotoxins	*Gambierdiscus toxicus*	Coral reef fish	Voltage-gated calcium channel
AZP	Azaspiracids	*Protoperidinium crassipes*	Shellfish	Voltage-gated calcium channel
Palytoxin poisoning	Palytoxins	*Ostrepsis siamensis*	Shellfish	$Na_+K_+ATPase$

in North America have been attributed to consumption of bear meat rather than pork. The parasite lodges in the extraocular muscles, deltoid, biceps, intercostals, diaphragm, tongue, or masseter and produces severe weakness with pain, fever, and cough along with splinter hemorrhages and eosinophilia.

Moderate *T. spiralis* infection is treated with mebendazole (Vermox 200–400 mg PO three times daily for 3 days) or albendazole[1] (Albenza 400 mg PO twice daily for 7–14 days). For severe infections, prednisone is added in a dose of 1 mg/kg/day for 5 days.

Neurocysticercosis

Neurocysticercosis is caused by *Taenia saginata* infection, commonly as a result of consuming improperly cooked pork or contaminated raw vegetables and water. The parasite lodges in the central nervous system and skeletal muscle and presents as intracranial calcifications and ring-enhancing lesions on radioimaging studies. Other than leukocytosis, eosinophilia, and raised erythrocyte sedimentation rate, antibodies to species-specific antigens of *T. solium* can be detected by immunosorbent assay and complement fixation-tests. Treatment is aimed at controlling seizures and relief of hydrocephalus. Albendazole (15 mg/kg/day for 8–28 days) or praziquantel (50–100 mg/kg/day in three divided doses for a month) are given for parenchymal cysticerci with glucocorticoids to suppress the inflammatory response around the dying parasites. Surgery may be required to reduce intracranial pressure.

Dinoflagellate toxins

Dinoflagellates, a very large and diverse group of eukaryotic algae in the marine ecosystem, are the major group producing toxins that impact humans. Dinoflagellate toxins are structurally and functionally diverse, and many present unique biological activities. Five major seafood poisoning syndromes caused by toxins have been identified from the dinoflagellates (Table 4): paralytic shellfish poisoning (PSP), neurotoxic shellfish poisoning (NSP), amnesic shellfish poisoning (ASP), diarrheic shellfish poisoning (DSP) and ciguatera fish poisoning (CFP). Symptoms include allergic manifestations, neurologic including paresthesia of the extremities, headache, ataxia, vertigo, cranial nerve palsies,

and paralysis of respiratory muscles as well as gastrointestinal. Symptomatic treatment and antihistamines are the mainstay of treatment.

Tetrodotoxin poisoning

It is a neurotoxin concentrated in the skin and viscera of puffer fish, and other fishes of the order Tetraodontiformes and in some amphibian, octopus, and shellfish species. Human poisonings occur when the flesh or organs of the fish are improperly prepared and eaten. Tetrodotoxin acts by blocking the conduction of nerve impulses along nerve fibers and axons and interferes with the transmission of signals from nerves to muscles. Onset of symptoms usually is 30–40 minutes but may be as short as 10 minutes; it includes lethargy, paraesthesia, emesis, ataxia, weakness, and dysphagia; ascending paralysis occurs in severe cases with high mortality (1-2 mg is lethal). Management is symptomatic.

Group B Sreptococcus (GBS)

GBS bacteria is found in 15%–30% of adult human intestines and urinary tract. Rarely implicated in infections of skin, joints, heart and brain, a recent outbreak of food-borne illness caused by the Type III GBS ST283 strain was reported in Singapore during the period of January–July 2015. It is the largest of its kind and first association to food-borne transmission of GBS to people via consumption of "yusheng-style" raw fresh water fish. The primary case presented with giddiness and suffered bouts of vomiting and diarrhea. Further studies are ongoing to establish the link between increase in cases of Group B streptococcus (GBS) infection to consumption of raw fish. Treatment is symptomatic.

Newer Trends in Foodborne Illness

New or unusual pathogens and food hazards are identified in course of investigating outbreaks. In 2011, a novel outbreak of sprout-associated illness caused by a strain of *Escherichia coli* O104:H4 was reported from Germany and France. This enteroaggregative and Shiga toxin-producing strain caused severe illness leading to HUS and death. In 2008, an outbreak following consumption of chicken caused by *Arcobacter butzleri* (found in poultry) was reported from Wisconsin. The calcivirus Sapovirus is emerging as the likely cause of oyster-associated foodborne

---

[1]Not FDA approved for this indication.

Bagged spinach
Carrot juice
Peanut butter
Broccoli powder on a snack food
Dry dog food
Frozen potpies
Canned chilli sauce
Hot peppers
White and black pepper
Raw cookie dough (likely the flour)
Hazelnuts
Fenugreek sprouts
Papayas
Pine nuts
Raw scrapped tuna
Clover sprouts
Herbs
Avocado, guacamole

Reprinted from Braden C, Tauxe R: Emerging trends in foodborne diseases, *Inf Dis Clinics N Am* 27:517-533, 2013.

BOX 2	Miscellaneous Organisms Implicated in Foodborne and Waterborne Illnesses

Adenovirus 40, 41
Bacillus anthracis
Bacillus mycoides
Burkholderia cepacia
Burkholderia pseudomallei
Clostridium bifermentans
Corynebacterium diphtheriae
Coxiella burnetii
Dientamoeba fragilis
Enterococcus faecalis, E. faecium
Erysipelothrix rhusiopathiae
Francicella tularensis
Henipa virus
Klebsiella spp.
Leptospira spp.
Mycobacterium bovis
Parvovirus B
Pediococcus
Pestivirus
Picobirnavirus
Proteus spp.
Pseudomonas aeruginosa
Pseudomonas cocovenanans
Reovirus
Streptobacillus moniliformis
Taenia solium, T. saginata
Torovirus
Toxoplasma gondii

outbreaks in Japan. New and unsuspected food vehicles are also being identified that had not been previously recognized as problematic (Box 1).

Changing patterns of disease presentation have seen important foodborne challenges emerging. Chagas disease is emerging as a foodborne infection linked to fresh, unpasteurized acai and guava juice. Infected triatomid insects present in fruits are implicated. Outbreaks of Nipah virus encephalitis in Bangladesh and India have been linked to drinking of palm sap, toddy, and well water contaminated with urine of feeding giant fruit bats, the vector of Nipah virus.

More syndromes and other systemic disease presentations are being linked to foodborne infection. The feco-oral transmission of pathogens leading to other systemic manifestation include Campylobacter sp. (Guillain-Barre syndrome, irritable bowel syndrome), Toxoplasma gondii (behavior changes and neuropsychiatric manifestations) and *Salmonella choleraesuis* (aortitis). Foodborne outbreak of Group G streptococci (GGS) pharyngitis in a school dormitory in Japan (2016) presented with sore throat and fever in a majority; implicated food was a broccoli salad.

Miscellaneous

Many other organisms are implicated in foodborne and waterborne illnesses (Box 2). Some are discussed elsewhere in this book. Amebiasis, brucellosis, cholera, hepatitis A and E, giardiasis, typhoid fever, and other foodborne intestinal nematodes and cestodes are covered in the infectious diseases section of this text and are not covered in this section.

References

Abebe E, Gugsa G, Ahmed M: Review on major food-borne zoonotic bacterial pathogens, *J Trop Med*, 2020. 4674235, 202.

Almeria S, Chacin-Bonilla L, Maloney JG, Santin M: *Cyclospora cayetanensis*: a perspective (2020-2023) with emphasis on epidemiology and detection methods, *Microorganisms* 28;11(9):2171, 2023.

Bennett JE, Dolin R, Blaser MJ, editors: *Mandell, Douglas, and Bennett's Principles and Practice of Infectious Diseases*, 9th ed, Philadelphia, 2020, Elsevier.

Bintsis T: Review: foodborne pathogens, *AIMS Microbiol* 3(3):529–563, 2017.

Centers for Disease Control and Prevention: *A-Z Index For Foodborne Illness 2019*, 2019. Available at https://webarchive.library.unt.edu/web/20201221005535/ https://www.cdc.gov/foodsafety/diseases/index.html.

Chau ML, Chen SL, Yap M, et al: Group B streptococcus infections caused by improper sourcing and handling of fish for raw consumption, Singapore, 2015-2016, *Emerg Infect Dis* 23(12):2002–2010, 2017.

Fernández-Bravo A, Figueras MJ: An update on the genus *Aeromonas*: taxonomy, epidemiology, and pathogenicity, *Microorganisms* 8:129, 2020.

Gamarra RM: Food poisoning …drugs and diseases. *Medscape.* Updated June 19, 2018. Available at: https://emedicine.medscape.com/article/175569-overview?&icd=login_success_email_match_fpf

Khan Shahbaz M, Witola William H: Past, current, and potential treatments for cryptosporidiosis in humans and farm animals: a comprehensive review, *Front Cell Infect Microbiol* 13:1115522, 2023.

Katikou P, Gokbulut C, Kosker A, et al: An updated review of tetrodotoxin and its peculiarities, *Mar Drugs* 20(1):47, 2022.

LeClair CE, McConnell K: Rotavirus. *StatPearls.* Updated January 2, 2023. Available at: https://www.ncbi.nlm.nih.gov/books/NBK558951/

Lee H, Yoon Y: Etiological agents implicated in foodborne illness world wide, *Food Sci Anim Resour* 41(1):1–7, 2021.

Marcus EN, Danzl DF, Ganetsky M: Overview of shellfish, pufferfish, and other marine toxin poisoning, *UpToDate*, 2024. Available at: https://www.uptodate.com/contents/overview-of-shellfish-pufferfish-and-other-marine-toxin-poisoning, .

Pakbin B, Brück WM, Brück TB: Molecular mechanisms of *Shigella* pathogenesis; recent advances, *Int J Mol Sci* 24(3):2448, 2023.

Parak M, Asgari A, Nourian YH, Ghanei M: A review of poisoning with various types of biotoxins and its common clinical symptoms, *Toxicon* 240:107629, 2024.

Pavithra M, Chitra P, Karthik M, Ananthi P: Review in: toxic effects of cyanobacteria, *Int J Adv Res Biol Sci* 10(4):56–70, 2023.

Pires SM, Desta BN, Mughini-Gras L, et al: Burden of foodborne diseases: think global, act local, *Curr Opin Food Sci* 39:152–159, 2021.

Sekhi RJ: Diarrhea in children an infants caused by *E. coli*: a review article, *Eur J Res Devel Sustainabil* 3(2):89–92, 2022.

Versalovic J, Landry ML, Jorgensen JH, Warnock DW, Funke G, Carroll KC, eds: Section II: Bacteriology. In: *Manual of Clinical Microbiology*, 10th ed, Washington, DC, 2022, ASM Press..

Wiegand TJ: Tetrodotoxin. In: Wexler P, ed: *Encyclopedia of Toxicology*, 4th ed, vol 8, Philadelphia, 2024, Elsevier.

GIARDIASIS

Method of
Rodney D. Adam, MD

CURRENT DIAGNOSIS

- Giardiasis is the most common intestinal protozoan infection worldwide.
- Most cases result from exposure to contaminated drinking or recreational water.
- The clinical manifestations range from asymptomatic to chronic diarrhea with malabsorption and weight loss.
- The diagnosis can be established by stool microscopy or by immunoassays of fecal specimens.
- Occasionally, the trophozoites can be found in duodenal specimens when fecal assays are negative.
- Serologic testing plays no role in the diagnosis.
- Irritable bowel symptoms are very common after successful treatment of giardiasis.

CURRENT THERAPY

- The treatment of choice is metronidazole (Flagyl)[1] or tinidazole (Tindamax); tinidazole can be given as a single dose.
- Albendazole (Albenza)[1] and nitazoxanide (Alinia) are alternative agents.
- Paromomycin (Humatin),[1] a poorly absorbed aminoglycoside, is commonly recommended during early pregnancy when other agents are avoided.
- True drug resistance has not been documented, but refractory or recurrent cases can be treated by two drugs: a nitro-imidazole combined with quinacrine (Atabrine)[2] or albendazole.[1]

[1]Not FDA approved for this indication.
[2]Not available in the United States.

624

Giardia lamblia is the most common parasitic cause of diarrhea. It is found globally with manifestations that range from asymptomatic to chronic diarrhea with weight loss and malnutrition. Infection occurs when cysts are ingested, most commonly from contaminated water or more direct fecal oral transmission. Less commonly, infections are acquired from food or from zoonotic sources. The cysts excyst in the small intestine and replicate as trophozoites, which cause the disease associated with the organism. The diagnosis is made by the microscopic detection of cysts or trophozoites from fecal samples or by immunoassays of fecal samples. The treatment of choice for symptomatic patients is tinidazole (Tindamax) or metronidazole (Flagyl),[1] while treatment of asymptomatic people depends on the circumstances. Irritable bowel syndrome is common after symptomatic infection, so patients with persistent symptoms should only be treated when persistent infection is documented.

Background

Giardia lamblia (syn. *Giardia intestinalis, Giardia duodenalis*) was initially described by Leeuwenhoek in the 17th century while doing a microscopic examination of his own diarrheal feces. However, *G. lamblia* was not widely accepted as a human pathogen until the 1960s, when a number of outbreaks were reported in travelers to endemic areas. The presumed source of infection

[1]Not FDA approved for this indication.

in these cases was contaminated drinking water. Subsequently, *Giardia* has become the most commonly identified parasitic cause of diarrhea, and, along with *Cryptosporidium* species, is among the most commonly identified parasitic causes of water-borne diarrheal disease.

Organism

Giardia species are members of the diplomonad (two bodies) group of flagellated protozoans. The infectious form of the life cycle consists of the environmentally resistant cyst, which infects its host on ingestion. It is oval in shape, is about 8 μm × 12 μm in size and contains four nuclei. It excysts into pear-shaped trophozoites in the proximal small intestine that are about 10 to 12 μm by 5 × 7 μm in size. Two symmetrically placed nuclei are in the body of the trophozoites and four pairs of flagella aid with motility. A ventral concave disk uses primarily mechanical means to attach to the intestinal wall of the host. While still in the small intestine, some of the trophozoites then encyst into the cyst form, which is passed in the feces to continue the cycle of infection. The *Giardia* species are all parasitic and were initially assigned to species on the basis of host of origin. However, in 1952, they were divided into three species (*Giardia agilis,* amphibians; *Giardia muris,* rodents; *G. duodenalis* [*G. lamblia*], mammals and birds) that could easily be distinguished on the basis of morphologic appearance of the trophozoites. Subsequently, the *G. lamblia* morphologic group has been divided into additional species based on differences that can be seen at the ultrastructural or molecular level. Of the organisms that remain assigned to *G. lamblia,* all are found in mammals but are divided into eight genotypes or assemblages (A through H) on the basis of molecular differences with varying host specificities. Only genotypes A and B have been regularly found in humans. It is likely that at least some of these eight genotypes will eventually be assigned to separate species.

Epidemiology

Giardiasis is the most commonly diagnosed human protozoan infection and is one of the most commonly identified forms of gastroenteritis. Most cases occur from ingestion of contaminated water or by human-to-human transmission through the fecal–oral route. Thus the epidemiology of human infections can be understood by examining these mechanisms of transmission. In the United States most cases are sporadic and occur more often in the summer, probably reflecting infection from recreational water exposure. Infections were more commonly reported in children from ages 1 to 9 years, especially those younger than 4 years of age. In general, the incidence is higher in the northern states, perhaps because cysts survive longer in cool, moist environments.

Direct human-to-human transmission by the fecal oral route also occurs, leading to the higher prevalence found in children in daycare centers. The occasional reports of food-borne transmission most likely occurred because of food being contaminated by infected food handlers.

The greater incidence in children could reflect an increased use of recreational water facilities, daycare exposure, or increased susceptibility to symptomatic disease. The epidemiology of giardiasis in the United States is similar to that found in other developed countries located in temperate regions. However, in developing regions with inadequate availability of purified water, the epidemiology is very different. For example, in a shantytown near Lima, Peru, children were almost universally infected by the age of 2 years, and when treated, they were rapidly reinfected, but there were no symptoms that could clearly be correlated with their infections. Perhaps an outbreak at a ski resort town in the United States can explain these different epidemiologic patterns. In this water-borne outbreak, tourists were disproportionately affected despite drinking from the same water source as the local residents. The conclusion was that the local residents had repeatedly been exposed to water contaminated by *Giardia* cysts and were less susceptible to symptomatic disease.

The degree of zoonotic transmission of giardiasis remains controversial. Human acquisition of infection from dogs or cats has not been well documented, and usually the *Giardia* genotypes found in cats or dogs are distinct from those found in humans (A and B), even in regions where both are endemic. However, genotypes A and B have sometimes been identified in dogs or other animals, so the question is not totally resolved. On the other hand, beavers have been implicated as a source of contaminated water leading to human infections.

Risk Factors
People with hypogammaglobulinemia, and possibly those with IgA deficiency, are at increased risk for prolonged giardiasis. In animal models, deficiency in cell-mediated immunity (CMI) has been associated with increased risk, but in humans the increased risk has not been associated with defects in CMI.

Pathogenesis
Infection is initiated by the ingestion of as few as 10 cysts. After passage through the acidic environment of the stomach, each cyst excysts into two trophozoites in the proximal small intestine. However, gastric acidity is not required, and people with achlorhydria or who are treated with suppressors of gastric acid remain vulnerable to giardiasis. The trophozoites replicate in the proximal small intestine, where they attach to the intestinal mucosa by their ventral disks. The attachment appears to occur by mechanical means facilitated by the suction generated by the ventral disk and the four pairs of flagella as they provide motility. Although the trophozoites attach to the intestinal wall and leave imprints after separating from the wall, there is no well-documented evidence of invasion, either of the intestinal wall or at extraintestinal sites. Toxins have not been identified as causes of diarrhea. However, cysteine proteases, which are also involved in encystation, may be important contributors to the symptoms. The host parasite interaction leads to enterocyte apoptosis and epithelial barrier disruption. The host immune response is mediated through a TH17 response that includes IgA production. An inadequate immune response results in persistence of organisms and an excessive response may be responsibility for the prolonged diarrhea and malabsorption that is commonly found in symptomatic people. Irritable bowel syndrome as well as chronic fatigue are common after giardiasis with a rate over 30% in a large Norwegian outbreak in 2004. The trophozoites are coated with a cysteine-rich protein encoded by one of a family of related genes, and expression can be switched from one to another, perhaps contributing to the chronicity of the infection.

Prevention
The strategies for prevention should be determined by the most prevalent risk factors in specific situations. For travelers to endemic regions, the major risk is from the ingestion of contaminated water. Therefore drinking water should be purified by boiling for 1 minute or by filtration through a pore size of <1 μm. Halogenization with iodine or chlorine requires a prolonged contact time (hours) to inactivate cysts and is not recommended. In daycare centers and for food handlers, the best preventive measure is effective hand washing. In addition, children or workers who are infected should be treated.

Clinical Features
Most people with giardiasis are symptom-free, but the percentages range from rates of diarrhea no higher than background among children in some highly endemic regions to attack rates of nearly 100% in visitors to endemic regions. Symptomatic patients typically present for evaluation only after several days or even weeks of illness because of the subacute onset. The symptoms of giardiasis typically develop after an incubation period of 1 to 2 weeks and consist of diarrhea that is characterized by loose, foul-smelling stools and abdominal discomfort described as cramping or bloating (Table 1). Fatigue is very common, but fever is unusual and, when present, is mild and occurs only within the first few days. Malabsorption and weight loss are often present. The majority of cases resolve within several weeks, but occasionally the symptoms

TABLE 1	Symptoms of Giardiasis*
SYMPTOM	**AVERAGE (%)**
Diarrhea	95
Abdominal cramps	70
Weakness or malaise	70
Nausea	60
Weight loss	50
Anorexia (decreased appetite)	50
Abdominal distention (bloating/distension)	50
Flatulence	50
Vomiting	30
Fever	20

From Adam RD. Giardiasis. *Hunter's Tropical Medicine and Emerging Infectious Diseases,* Eds: Magill AJ, Ryan ET, Hill DR, Solomon T. Elsevier, 2019.
*The table includes the approximate frequency of the signs and symptoms reported in six studies of symptomatic giardiasis, but it is important to note that there is substantial variability of symptoms among studies.

will last for months in the absence of treatment. The prolonged symptoms are often due to postinfectious irritable bowel syndrome and/or chronic fatigue, especially if not accompanied by weight loss. Relapse is relatively uncommon after effective treatment.

Diagnosis
The gold standard of diagnosis has been the microscopic evaluation of three separate fecal samples, including concentrated specimens for cysts or, less commonly, trophozoites. The identification of trophozoites is typically associated with symptomatic infection, but cysts may be found in symptom-free persons. Because of the challenges in obtaining three fecal specimens and the interobserver variability in skill at identifying *Giardia* cysts, antigen detection tests have come into widespread use. The enzyme immunoassays are more commonly used and have high degrees of sensitivity and specificity. A direct fluorescent assay is slightly more sensitive than the enzyme immunoassays and can also detect *Cryptosporidium* species, but it requires the availability of fluorescent microscopy. Polymerase chain reaction (PCR) tests have also been described and are more sensitive but more expensive and not widely available. Some patients have negative workups of stool samples, but *Giardia* trophozoites can be detected in duodenal contents with the string test. The patient swallows a capsule on a string, which is left in situ for 4 hours to overnight. The string is then removed and examined microscopically for trophozoites. Alternatively, endoscopy with sampling of duodenal contents and duodenal biopsy can be used. Endoscopy has the added advantage of being able to detect other possible diagnoses, such as celiac disease or tropical sprue.

Differential Diagnosis
The diagnosis of giardiasis should be suspected in patients presenting with prolonged (>5–7 days) diarrhea without blood in the stools and no fever. In patients presenting relatively early in the course of illness, the major considerations in the differential diagnosis are other infectious etiologies of diarrhea, particularly *Campylobacter jejuni*, *Salmonella*, *Cryptosporidium*, and *Cyclospora cayetanensis*. Thus patients presenting with compatible symptoms should have stool samples submitted for culture and for microscopic examination for ova and parasites (O and P). Watery diarrhea is uncommon, and bloody stools are not seen with giardiasis; thus these findings should prompt the search for other etiologies.

For patients presenting with more prolonged symptoms, a number of noninfectious illnesses should be added to the differential diagnosis. Irritable bowel syndrome and lactose intolerance are among the more common etiologies and should be considered in patients

TABLE 2 Treatment of Giardiasis

DRUG	DOSE		FREQUENCY	DURATION	EFFICACY (%)
	ADULT	PEDIATRIC*			
Metronidazole[1] (Flagyl)	250 mg	5 mg/kg	tid	5–7 days	90–100
Tinidazole (Tindamax)	2 g	50 mg/kg	Single dose	Single dose	90–100
Secnidazole[1] (Solosec)	1.5 g	30 mg/kg[†]	Single dose	Single dose	90–100
Quinacrine[2] (Atabrine)	100 mg	2 mg/kg	tid	5–7 days	80–100
Furazolidone[2] (Furoxone)	100 mg	1.5 mg/kg	qid	10 days	80–94
Paromomycin[1] (Humatin)	500 mg	8–10 mg/kg	tid	10 days	55–90
Albendazole[1] (Albenza)	400 mg qd	15 mg/kg	Daily	5 days	90–100
Nitazoxanide (Alinia)	500 mg bid	7.5 mg/kg	bid	3 days	70–80

[†]Approved for adults and patients ≥12 years of age.
*The adult dose is the maximum pediatric dose.
[1]Not FDA approved for this indication.
[2]Not available in the United States.

presenting with diarrhea but no weight loss. Gluten enteropathy, tropical sprue, and, rarely, Whipple's disease are among the noninfectious etiologies of diarrhea accompanied by weight loss.

Treatment

Patients with symptomatic giardiasis should be treated. The criteria for treatment of patients with asymptomatic giardiasis are not well defined, but in general, patients in regions with low prevalence or linked with outbreaks should be treated. On the other hand, in settings where the prevalence is high and recurrence rates are high, there is probably no value to treating asymptomatic infection.

The most commonly used agents for treatment of giardiasis are the nitroimidazoles. Metronidazole (Flagyl),[1] tinidazole (Tindamax), and secnidazole (Solosec)[1] are available in the United States, while orinidazole (Tiberal)[2] is available in other countries (Table 2). These agents are completely absorbed from the gastrointestinal tract and are inactivated primarily by hepatic metabolism. Metronidazole has been available in the United States for decades and has generally been considered the drug of choice for treatment of giardiasis in most situations. More recently, tinidazole has become available and has a high degree of efficacy when given as a single dose. A meta-analysis of 60 randomized clinical trials for treatment of giardiasis concluded that tinidazole was more effective than metronidazole or albendazole. Metronidazole is mutagenic in bacterial assays and showed some carcinogenic activity in an animal model. However, carcinogenicity in humans has not been documented. Serious adverse reactions to the nitroimidazoles are rare, but nausea and a metallic taste are common and may decrease the compliance of patients with metronidazole. The problem with noncompliance can be addressed by the use of tinidazole or the other agents that can be given as a single dose.

Albendazole (Albenza)[1] is a tubulin inhibitor that was introduced as a broad-spectrum antihelminthic, but it also has good activity against *Giardia* trophozoites. It is generally well tolerated and in areas with endemic helminth infections has the added advantage of antihelminthic activity.

The first trimester of pregnancy poses a special problem because none of the agents have been adequately studied or approved for use during this time. Paromomycin (Humatin)[1] is a nonabsorbed aminoglycoside and is expected to be safe during pregnancy. Therefore it is usually the preferred choice in that setting; however, it is somewhat less effective than other agents. Specialty consultation should be considered for treatment of patients in their first trimester. Metronidazole is used

extensively during the second and third trimesters for other indications; thus it can be considered the drug of choice for those patients.[1] Albendazole is known to be teratogenic and should be avoided during pregnancy.

Nitazoxanide (Alinia) has been approved in the United States for treatment of giardiasis (and cryptosporidiosis) and is very well tolerated. However, the somewhat lower efficacy compared with nitroimidazoles and albendazole, along with the requirement for twice daily dosing, limits its role.

Treatment failures are not uncommon but may or may not be due to true drug resistance because in vitro cultures are not routinely performed, and in vitro testing is not standardized. When treatment failure occurs, the patient may respond to the same or an alternative drug. Treatment-refractory cases have been treated successfully with a combination of metronidazole[1] plus quinacrine[2] or albendazole.[1] The most common reason for persistence of symptoms after treatment is due to postgiardiasis irritable bowel syndrome, which can occur in over 30% of patients. Thus it is important to reevaluate stool specimens from patients with symptoms that persist after therapy.

Diet

Lactose intolerance is quite common while patients have giardiasis and potentially for months thereafter, so lactose ingestion should be moderated or eliminated as needed.

[1]Not FDA approved for this indication.
[2]Not available in the United States.

References

Adam RD: Giardia duodenalis: biology and pathogenesis, *Clin Microbiol Rev* 34(4):e0002419, 2021.

Coffey CM, Collier SA, Gleason ME, Yoder JS, Kirk MD, Richardson AM, Fullerton KE, Benedict KM: Evolving epidemiology of reported giardiasis cases in the United States, 1995–2016, *Clinical Infectious Diseases* 72:764–770, 2020.

Cooper MA, Sterling CR, Gilman RH, Cama V, Ortega Y, Adam RD: Molecular analysis of household transmission of *Giardia lamblia* in a region of high endemicity in Peru, *J Inf Dis* 202:1713–1721, 2010.

Hanevik K, Dizdar V, Langeland N, Hausken T: Development of functional gastrointestinal disorders after giardia lamblia infection, *BMC Gastroenterology* 9:27, 2009.

Lengerich EJ, Addiss DG, Juranek DD: Severe giardiasis in the United States, *Clin Infect Dis* 18:760–763, 1994.

Morrison HG, McArthur AG, Gillin FD, Aley SB, Adam RD, Olsen GJ, Best AA, Cande WZ, Chen F, Cipriano MJ, et al: Genomic minimalism in the early diverging intestinal parasite, *Giardia lamblia Science* 317:1921–1926, 2007.

Ordonez-Mena JM, McCarthy ND, Fanshawe TR: Comparative efficacy of drugs for treating giardiasis: a systematic update of the literature and network meta-analysis of randomized clinical trials, *Journal of Antimicrobial Chemotherapy* 73:596–606, 2018.

Singer SM, Fink MY, Angelova VV: Recent insights into innate and adaptive immune responses to *Giardia*, *Advances in Parasitology* 106:171–208, 2019.

HUMAN IMMUNODEFICIENCY VIRUS: TREATMENT AND PREVENTION

Method of
Allison Cormier, MD; and Tyler K. Liebenstein, PharmD

CURRENT DIAGNOSIS

- National guidelines recommend universal screening for human immunodeficiency virus (HIV) infection for all adult and adolescent patients in all healthcare settings after notification that testing will be done, unless the patient specifically declines testing (opt-out testing). Patients with behavioral risk factors, sexually transmitted diseases, or tuberculosis should be screened annually.
- Revised HIV testing algorithms reflect the increased sensitivity of newer diagnostic assays during early infection, such as fourth-generation HIV-1/2 antigen/antibody combination immunoassays.
- Acute HIV infection is recognized as a variable syndrome including fever, pharyngitis, rash, and arthralgias. As many as one-half of patients may be asymptomatic during seroconversion and early infection.

CURRENT THERAPY

- Combination antiretroviral therapy (ART) should be offered to all patients with HIV infection, regardless of CD4 helper T-lymphocyte (CD4 T-cell) count.
- Initial ART regimens preferred for most patients include a combination of two nucleoside analogue reverse transcriptase inhibitors (NRTIs) and an integrase strand transfer inhibitor (INSTIs), which are often coformulated into single-tablet preparations that can be administered once daily.
- Although ART decisions are often made by providers with specialized training, all providers who care for people living with HIV should be aware of the risk of antiretroviral drug interactions, particularly interactions involving the pharmacokinetic-enhancing agents ritonavir (Norvir) and cobicistat (Tybost).
- All sexually active adult and adolescent patients should receive information about HIV preexposure prophylaxis (PrEP) to reduce the risk of HIV acquisition. Both oral and injectable medication options are available for PrEP.

Introduction

Remarkable advances in therapeutics, leading to the development of antiretroviral therapy (ART), have transformed human immunodeficiency virus (HIV) infection from an almost universally fatal illness to a chronic disease that can be managed over decades with an enlarging repertoire of treatment options. Further developments in ART have also provided opportunities for preventing HIV infection in high-risk individuals. This chapter provides an overview of the current understanding of HIV pathogenesis and epidemiology and discusses guidelines for the initial evaluation and long-term management of HIV infection in adult patients.

Pathophysiology

HIV is an enveloped, single-stranded RNA virus belonging to the family Retroviridae. It was recognized as the causative agent of AIDS within 3 years after the initial description of the syndrome in 1981, and ongoing characterization of its molecular biology has provided the identification of multiple targets for drug development. Two types of human immunodeficiency viruses exist: HIV-1 and HIV-2. HIV-1 has worldwide distribution, accounts for most infections outside western Africa, and is the focus of this chapter.

HIV-2 infection is endemic in West Africa and has limited spread outside this area. It should be considered in infections in patients of West African origin or those who have had sexual contact or shared needles with people of West African origin. HIV-2 generally has a longer asymptomatic stage, lower plasma HIV-2 viral loads, and overall lower mortality rate. Approximately 25% to 30% of patients with HIV-2 who do not receive ART will have HIV-2 RNA levels below the rate of detection, and some will also have clinical progression and a decreased CD4 helper T-lymphocyte (CD4 T-cell) count. HIV-2 can progress to AIDS over time. HIV-1 and HIV-2 coinfection may occur and should be a consideration in patients from high prevalence HIV-2 areas. Patients diagnosed with HIV-2 infection should be managed by an HIV specialist.

Genetic heterogeneity of HIV-1 is reflected in categorization of the virus into three groups (M, O, and N) and several subtypes (B, C, D, AE, and CRF01_AE), some of which have overlapping geographic distribution around the world. Subtype C is prevalent in southern and eastern Africa, China, India, South Asia, and Brazil and accounts for 50% of HIV subtypes, whereas subtype B, the most common subtype in the United States, accounts for 12%.

The HIV viral genome is encoded in single-stranded RNA, packaged in core protein structures, and surrounded by a lipid bilayer envelope that is derived from the cell membrane of the host cell as the virus buds from the cell surface after replication.

This outer viral membrane contains HIV-specific glycoproteins, including gp120 and gp41, which facilitate attachment and entry into host cells through interaction with the cell surface receptor, CD4, and coreceptors CCR5 and CXCR4. CD4 T cells are the predominant host cell affected by HIV; this molecular tropism explains the immune system destruction manifested in chronic HIV infection and provides the rationale for clinical staging of HIV infection using CD4 T-cell counts. After host cell entry, the key enzyme responsible for viral replication is reverse transcriptase, an RNA-dependent DNA polymerase that is packaged within the virion core. This enzyme facilitates conversion of the HIV genome into a double-stranded DNA intermediate molecule. The second key enzymatic step is integration of this intermediate nucleic acid product into the host genome, which is facilitated by the viral protein integrase. Protein synthesis with packaging of new viral particles ensues, utilizing an HIV-specific protease. The integrase inhibitor class of drugs acts by blocking this step of integration.

Natural History

Within 1 to 4 weeks after the initial HIV infection, seroconversion may be accompanied by a nonspecific, self-limiting illness, often referred to as *acute retroviral syndrome*. This illness has variable manifestations but may include fever, malaise, myalgias, arthralgias, generalized lymphadenopathy, pharyngitis, and rash. The associated rash may be maculopapular, urticarial, or roseola-like. An illness resembling acute infectious mononucleosis syndrome, similar to that caused by Epstein-Barr virus (EBV) or cytomegalovirus (CMV), and aseptic meningitis has been described. Diagnosis of acute HIV infection requires a high index of suspicion, which does not commonly occur unless the patient reports a recent history of high-risk exposure.

During the acute phase of infection, high levels of viremia are present (often exceeding 10 million copies/mL) as HIV becomes widely disseminated throughout the body and the host defenses begin to counteract circulating virus through cell-mediated and humoral (antibody-mediated) immune mechanisms. Antibodies against HIV usually become detectable 2 to 4 months after infection. The initial, high-level viremia plateaus and then begins to decrease as neutralizing antibodies are established. Ongoing replication is partially controlled by the immune response, resulting in a steady-state level of viremia. This virologic level differs from patient to patient and is one of the determinants of the rate of disease progression. A small number of HIV-infected persons are able to control viral replication to levels below the limit of detection, and they tend to have a more benign course of disease. In these patients, designated *elite suppressors* by researchers, HIV replication continues to occur, and HIV RNA can be isolated from latently infected cells by means of specialized laboratory techniques.

After the establishment of HIV infection and seroconversion, a period of asymptomatic infection ensues, during which patients are free from evidence of immune suppression and opportunistic infections (OIs) are uncommon. This phase of clinical latency lasts a median of 8 to 10 years, based on observational studies from the pre-ART era. Ongoing viral replication leads to a gradual decrease in CD4 T-cell counts.

The symptomatic stage of HIV infection can begin at any time after infection, but clinical manifestations become more likely as the CD4 count decreases farther below the normal range of 800 to 1200 cells/mm^3. For example, *Pneumocystis jirovecii* (formerly *Pneumocystis carinii*) pneumonia (PJP) usually occurs in patients with a CD4 count less than 200 cells/mm^3 or a percentage less than 10%. CMV retinitis occurs almost exclusively in patients with a CD4 count less than 50 cells/mm^3 or a percentage less than 5%. Mucocutaneous candidiasis (oral thrush), herpes zoster, HIV-associated nephropathy, peripheral neuropathy, tuberculosis, and community-acquired bacterial pneumonia occur with increased frequency at earlier stages of infection and are less reliably predicted by CD4+ T-cell measurement.

Diagnosis

The current recommended testing algorithm incorporates a fourth-generation antigen/antibody combination HIV-1/2 immunoassay with a confirmatory HIV-1/HIV-2 antibody differentiation immunoassay. The fourth-generation assay detects both HIV-1 and HIV-2 antibodies and HIV p24 antigen. It has increased sensitivity because of its ability to diagnose acute/early infection, because HIV p24 antigen is detected before seroconversion has occurred. If the fourth-generation combination assay is positive, the HIV-1 and HIV-2 antibody differentiation immunoassay both confirms the positive result and determines if the patient is infected with HIV-1 or HIV-2. If the fourth-generation assay is positive but the confirmatory antibody differentiation immunoassay is indeterminate or negative, a plasma HIV RNA level should be obtained.

In facilities where fourth-generation testing is not available, a two-step approach is utilized via enzyme-linked immunosorbent assay (ELISA) to detect HIV antibodies with subsequent confirmation using an HIV-1/HIV-2 differentiation assay. An ELISA can detect HIV IgM and IgG antibodies as early as 3 weeks after virus exposure. This modality has excellent sensitivity and specificity for diagnosing chronic HIV infection; however, diagnosis may be missed in patients with early HIV infection who have not yet had seroconversion. If concern exists for acute/early HIV infection, plasma HIV RNA can be assessed.

False-negative and false-positive tests occur rarely. False-negative screening tests can occur with ELISA-only testing during acute/early HIV infection. This occurs less often using the fourth-generation antigen/antibody assay, which is more sensitive in detecting early HIV infection by identifying the p24 antigen. False-positive screening test results can occur for several non-HIV reasons, including cross-reaction from alloantibodies in pregnant women, autoantibodies from autoimmune diseases or malignancy, and the influenza vaccine. False-positive results in both screening and confirmatory testing are particularly uncommon.

Indeterminate test results occur when the initial screening test is positive and subsequent confirmatory testing is indeterminate or negative. In the event of a positive fourth-generation antigen/antibody test and negative HIV differentiation assay, the detection of p24 antigen would yield a positive result, but the differentiation assay would be negative, as no antibody is present. In all patients with indeterminate test results, a plasma HIV RNA should be obtained, as viremia is present before antibody seroconversion. A detectable plasma HIV RNA level is diagnostic of HIV infection. If HIV RNA is negative, the patient should be reassured that HIV infection is unlikely. A repeat screening test can be repeated after 3 months for further reassurance. If the patient had a recent high-risk exposure, another plasma HIV RNA can be performed in 1 to 2 weeks. All patients with indeterminate testing should be

counseled to avoid activities with potential to transmit HIV to others until evaluation is completed.

Consent

HIV screening should be voluntary and pursued only after discussion with the patient regarding testing. In the United States, written consent is no longer obligatory in any state, but individual states may have policies regarding documentation of the consent process and related counseling. Confidentiality, access to posttesting counseling, and services to support prompt linkage to HIV care for patients with positive results are important resources in HIV testing settings.

Screening

Early detection of HIV infection and subsequent initiation of ART can dramatically reduce morbidity and mortality of affected patients. A relatively normal life span is possible in patients in the United States who are diagnosed early in their infection and successfully treated. Such early treatment also can reduce the transmission of HIV. One-time testing is recommended for patients without high-risk factors for HIV exposure in patients 13 to 75 years of age. Pregnant women should be screened for HIV early in their pregnancy, even if they have been screened during prior pregnancies.

In patients with elevated risk of HIV exposure, more frequent testing is recommended. Men who have sex with men (MSM), along with patients who have sex with sexual partners who have HIV or with persons of unknown serostatus may benefit from HIV screening at least every 6 months. This is especially important in patients 13 to 24 years of age because this demographic group has experienced the highest rate of new infections in recent years. Other high-risk groups include patients who use injection drugs as well as sex workers.

Approach to the Patient with HIV Infection

HIV patient care is an ever-changing field, with routinely updated professional guidelines and new medications. The quality of care received by patients with HIV has been shown to correlate with the healthcare provider's experience and comfort in treating these patients. Referral to an HIV specialist is recommended for new HIV diagnoses, complications of HIV or antiretroviral drugs, and for treatment failure.

All patients with HIV should have a comprehensive history, physical examination, and laboratory evaluation when establishing care. This baseline evaluation can help establish and define the patient's goals and plan of care. In a patient who has already established treatment with ART and presents for initial evaluation with a new healthcare provider, it is important to document the complete antiretroviral history and drug resistance testing results, if available.

Patients with HIV are often faced with many medical, psychiatric, and social issues. These are best addressed through a patient-centered, multidisciplinary approach. In patients with a new diagnosis of HIV, it is important to counsel them regarding HIV infection and assess their understanding of the disease and its transmission. They should also be assessed for readiness to initiate ART, potential high-risk behaviors, mental illness, substance abuse, social support, medical comorbidities, and/or economic factors, because these are potential issues that may impair adherence to ART.

Antiretroviral Therapy

There are currently six major classes of antiretroviral medications used to treat patients with HIV. Although dozens of such medications are available, only a small selection of agents is currently preferred as initial treatment regimens (Table 1). For most patients, ART includes a combination of two NRTIs plus a third medication from a different class, although two-drug regimens are preferred for some patients.

When to Initiate Antiretroviral Therapy

Combination ART first became available in the mid-1990s and provided life-saving therapy for millions of patients suffering from HIV and AIDS. Although the early ART regimens were effective in helping patients with AIDS recover, they were also associated with many toxicities and side effects. In 2006, the U.S.

TABLE 1 Recommended Initial Regimens for Most People with HIV

GENERIC NAME (TRADE NAME) AND RECOMMENDED ADULT DOSING	SINGLE TABLET REGIMEN?	IMPORTANT POINTS
INSTI + 2 NRTIs		
Bictegravir/emtricitabine/tenofovir alafenamide (Biktarvy)* 50/200/25 mg—1 tablet by mouth once daily	Yes	Bictegravir has been shown to increase serum creatinine from baseline by a median 0.1 mg/dL as a result of inhibition of creatinine secretion, not a true reduction in GFR
Dolutegravir/abacavir/lamivudine (Triumeq) 50/600/300 mg—1 tablet by mouth once daily	Yes	Dolutegravir has been shown to increase serum creatinine from baseline by a mean of 0.15 mg/dL as a result of inhibition of creatinine secretion, not a true reduction in GFR Dolutegravir has a drug interaction with metformin (maximum daily metformin dose is 1000 mg) Must be confirmed HLA-B*5701 negative before starting treatment to avoid abacavir hypersensitivity reaction
Dolutegravir (Tivicay)† 50 mg—1 tablet by mouth once daily *PLUS* Tenofovir alafenamide/emtricitabine (Descovy) 25/200 mg—1 tablet by mouth once daily *OR* Tenofovir disoproxil fumarate/emtricitabine (Truvada) 300/200 mg—1 tablet by mouth once daily	No	Dolutegravir has been shown to increase serum creatinine from baseline by a mean of 0.15 mg/dL because of inhibition of creatinine secretion, not a true reduction in GFR Dolutegravir has a drug interaction with metformin (maximum daily metformin dose is 1000 mg) Descovy generally preferred over Truvada because of fewer bone and kidney toxicities
INSTI + 1 NRTI		
Dolutegravir/lamivudine (Dovato) 50/300 mg—1 tablet by mouth once daily	Yes	This two-drug regimen should not be used in those with HIV RNA >500,000 copies/mL, HBV coinfection, or in whom ART is to be started before the results of HIV genotypic resistance testing for reverse transcriptase or HBV testing are available Dolutegravir has been shown to increase serum creatinine from baseline by a mean of 0.15 mg/dL as a result of inhibition of creatinine secretion, not a true reduction in GFR Dolutegravir has a drug interaction with metformin (maximum daily metformin dose is 1000 mg)

*Biktarvy [package insert]. Foster City, CA: Gilead Sciences, Inc.; 2021.
†Tivicay [package insert]. Research Triangle Park, NC: ViiV Healthcare; 2021.
ART, Antiretroviral therapy; *GFR,* glomerular filtration rate; *HBV,* hepatitis B virus; *HIV,* human immunodeficiency virus; *HLA,* human leukocyte antigen; *INSTI,* integrase strand transfer inhibitor; *NRTI,* nucleoside analogue reverse transcriptase inhibitor.
Modified from Panel on Antiretroviral Guidelines for Adults and Adolescents. Guidelines for the Use of Antiretroviral Agents in Adults and Adolescents with HIV. Department of Health and Human Services. Available at: https://clinicalinfo.hiv.gov/sites/default/files/guidelines/documents/adult-adolescent-arv/guidelines-adult-adolescent-arv.pdf (Table 6).

Department of Health and Human Services, the International AIDS Society–USA, and the British HIV Society recommended CD4 counts of 200 cells/mm³ as the threshold for initiating ART treatment in asymptomatic patients. More recently, the paradigm has shifted toward earlier initiation of ART based on accumulating evidence for the beneficial effects of treatment initiation earlier in the course of infection. Antiretroviral therapies have advanced significantly since their conception, consisting of multiple drug classes, fewer toxicities, less pill burden, and overall improved tolerance. Failure to suppress viral loads on these medications is more likely to result from therapy nonadherence than medication failure.

HIV patients are now achieving normal life spans, and non–AIDS-defining illnesses are becoming more prominent. Cardiovascular, renal, and hepatic disease complications are lower in patients who started ART at higher CD4 thresholds (>350 cells/mm³). Earlier initiation of ART is also associated with reduced risk of transmission and improved immune restoration.

Current Recommendations for Antiretroviral Therapy

ART should be offered to all patients with HIV infection, regardless of CD4 T-cell count. The goal of ART is to prevent morbidity, mortality, and transmission associated with HIV. This is accomplished by maximally inhibiting HIV replication to achieve an undetectable HIV viral load. Based on guidelines from the U.S. Department of Health and Human Services, INSTI-based regimens are currently the first-line recommendation as initial therapy for most patients with HIV based on high rates of virologic suppression and tolerability demonstrated in large clinical trials. Nonnucleoside reverse transcriptase inhibitor (NNRTI) and protease inhibitor (PI) regimens are recommended in certain clinical situations (Table 2). Monotherapy with any antiretroviral drug is not recommended because of increased risk of drug resistance and therapy failure.

Selection of an Antiretroviral Regimen

ART regimens should be individualized based on a regimen's side-effect profile, pill burden, potential drug interactions, virologic

| TABLE 2 | Recommended Initial Regimens in Certain Clinical Situations |

GENERIC NAME (TRADE NAME) AND RECOMMENDED ADULT DOSING	SINGLE TABLET REGIMEN?	IMPORTANT POINTS
INSTI + 2 NRTIs		
Elvitegravir/cobicistat/tenofovir alafenamide/emtricitabine (Genvoya) 150/150/10/200 mg—1 tablet by mouth once daily *OR* Elvitegravir/cobicistat/tenofovir disoproxil fumarate/emtricitabine (Stribild) 150/150/300/200 mg—1 tablet by mouth once daily	Yes	Genvoya generally preferred over Stribild because of fewer bone and kidney toxicities Drug interactions with other medications are prevalent with both products because of cobicistat, a CYP3A4 inhibitor
Raltegravir (Isentress HD) 600 mg—2 tablets by mouth once daily *OR* Raltegravir (Isentress) 400 mg—1 tablet by mouth twice daily *PLUS* Tenofovir alafenamide/emtricitabine (Descovy) 25/200 mg—1 tablet by mouth once daily *OR* Tenofovir disoproxil fumarate/emtricitabine (Truvada) 300/200 mg—1 tablet by mouth once daily	No	Isentress HD generally preferred over Isentress because of once-daily dosing Descovy generally preferred over Truvada (Isentress HD) because of fewer bone and kidney toxicities
NNRTI + 2 NRTIs		
Rilpivirine/tenofovir alafenamide/emtricitabine (Odefsey) 25/25/200 mg—1 tablet by mouth once daily *OR* Rilpivirine/tenofovir disoproxil fumarate/emtricitabine (Complera) 25/300/200 mg—1 tablet by mouth once daily	Yes	Rilpivirine should only be used if HIV RNA <100,000 copies/mL and CD4 >200 cells/mm^3 Odefsey generally preferred over Complera because of fewer bone and kidney toxicities PPIs contraindicated with rilpivirine H2 blockers may be used once daily but must be spaced 12 hours apart from rilpivirine Should be taken with food
Doravirine/tenofovir disoproxil fumarate/lamivudine (Delstrigo) 100/300/300 mg—1 tablet by mouth once daily OR Doravirine (Pifeltro) 100 mg—1 tablet by mouth once daily PLUS Tenofovir alafenamide/emtricitabine (Descovy) 25/200 mg—1 tablet by mouth once daily	Yes, for Delstrigo	May be taken with or without food Doravirine does not have any restrictions with acid-suppressive medications
Efavirenz/tenofovir disoproxil fumarate/emtricitabine (Atripla) 600/300/200 mg—1 tablet by mouth once daily	Yes	High rates of neuropsychiatric adverse effects (e.g., vivid dreams, depression, suicidal ideation)
PK-enhanced PI + 2 NRTIs		
Darunavir/cobicistat/emtricitabine/tenofovir alafenamide (Symtuza) 800/150/200/10 mg—1 tablet by mouth once daily *OR* Darunavir/cobicistat (Prezcobix) 800/150 mg—1 tablet by mouth once daily *OR* Darunavir (Prezista) 800 mg—1 tablet by mouth once daily + Ritonavir (Norvir) 100 mg—1 tablet by mouth once daily *PLUS* Tenofovir alafenamide/emtricitabine (Descovy) 25/200 mg—1 tablet by mouth once daily *OR* Tenofovir disoproxil fumarate/emtricitabine (Truvada) 300/200 mg—1 tablet by mouth once daily *OR* Abacavir/lamivudine (Epzicom) 600/300 mg—1 tablet by mouth once daily	Yes, for Symtuza	Prezcobix generally preferred over the combination of Prezista and Norvir because of single tablet and potentially fewer GI side effects and drug interactions Drug interactions with other medications are prevalent with both cobicistat and ritonavir because of CYP3A4 inhibition Ritonavir also inhibits and induces several other CYP enzymes Careful attention should be given to manage drug interactions Descovy generally preferred over Truvada because of fewer bone and kidney toxicities If using Epzicom, must be confirmed HLA-B*5701 negative before starting therapy to avoid abacavir hypersensitivity reaction
Atazanavir/cobicistat (Evotaz) 300/150 mg—1 tablet by mouth once daily *OR* Atazanavir (Reyataz) 300 mg—1 tablet by mouth once daily + Ritonavir (Norvir) 100 mg—1 tablet by mouth once daily *PLUS* Tenofovir alafenamide/emtricitabine (Descovy) 25/200 mg—1 tablet by mouth once daily *OR* Tenofovir disoproxil fumarate/emtricitabine (Truvada) 300/200 mg—1 tablet by mouth once daily	No	Darunavir-containing regimens generally preferred over atazanavir-containing regimens Atazanavir is known to increase serum bilirubin. This generally does not require further workup if the patient is asymptomatic Evotaz generally preferred over the combination of Reyataz and Norvir because of single tablet and potentially fewer GI side effects and drug interactions Drug interactions with other medications are prevalent with both cobicistat and ritonavir because of CYP3A4 inhibition. Ritonavir also inhibits and induces several other CYP enzymes. Careful attention should be given to manage drug interactions Descovy generally preferred over Truvada because of fewer bone and kidney toxicities

CYP3A4, Cytochrome P450 3A4; *GI*, gastrointestinal; *H2*, histamine H$_2$ receptor; *HIV*, human immunodeficiency virus; *HLA*, human leukocyte antigen; *INSTI*, integrase strand transfer inhibitor; *NNRTI*, non-nucleoside reverse transcriptase inhibitor; *NRTI*, nucleoside reverse transcriptase inhibitor; *PI*, protease inhibitor; *PPI*, proton pump inhibitor.
Modified from Panel on Antiretroviral Guidelines for Adults and Adolescents. Guidelines for the Use of Antiretroviral Agents in Adults and Adolescents with HIV. Department of Health and Human Services. Available at: https://clinicalinfo.hiv.gov/sites/default/files/guidelines/documents/adult-adolescent-arv/guidelines-adult-adolescent-arv.pdf (Table 6).

efficacy, cost, and resistance testing results. Before starting ART in any patient with HIV, the following factors must be considered:

- Pretreatment HIV RNA level
- Pretreatment CD4 T-cell count
- HIV genotypic drug resistance testing results
- HLA-B*5701 status (if planning to use an abacavir-based ART regimen)
- Patient's individual preference
- Anticipated medication adherence

Other factors that are important to consider when choosing an initial regimen include the patient's medical comorbidities (cardiovascular, renal, psychiatric disease), pregnancy or the potential to become pregnant, and coinfections with tuberculosis, hepatitis C virus, and hepatitis B virus (HBV).

The currently recommended ART for most patients includes two NRTIs ("backbone"), abacavir/lamivudine (ABC/3TC [Epzicom]) or either tenofovir alafenamide/emtricitabine (TAF/FTC [Descovy]) or tenofovir disoproxil fumarate/emtricitabine (TDF/FTC [Truvada]), plus an INSTI (see Table 1). Single-tablet regimens coformulated with an INSTI and the NRTI backbone are available. INSTI-based regimens are well tolerated, have convenient dosing, and provide excellent virologic suppression. Regimens including NNRTI or PK-enhanced PIs remain effective but are now only recommended in certain clinical scenarios.

The NRTI combinations of ABC/3TC (Epzicom), TAF/FTC (Descovy), and TDF/FTC (Truvada) are available as fixed-dose combination tablets. The 3TC and FTC components have few adverse effects. The main differences among these combinations involve ABC, TAF, and TDF. The advantages of TAF and TDF include activity against HBV, and HLA-B*5701 testing is not required before use. TDF has some association with lower lipid levels compared with TAF, but also may cause decreased renal function and reduced bone mineral density. TAF is associated with less bone and kidney toxicity, and its use is preferred in patients with underlying bone and kidney disease or those at risk for these conditions. The advantage of ABC is that it has less bone mineral loss and less nephrotoxicity than TDF and does not require dose adjustment in patients with renal insufficiency. Potential drawbacks to ABC include an observed association with cardiovascular events in some studies and a hypersensitivity syndrome, necessitating screening for HLA-B*5701 before treatment initiation.

Once the combination NRTI backbone has been chosen, a third drug from another class must be added to the regimen. Current recommendations for most patients favor the INSTI class because of its high efficacy, fewer side effects, and no significant CYP3A4-associated drug interactions.

Darunavir (DRV [Prezista])–based regimens may still be preferred in certain patients with difficulty maintaining medication adherence, and a high genetic barrier to resistance is favored or in a situation when ART should be initiated before receiving resistance testing results. Darunavir boosted with ritonavir (Norvir) (DRV/r) or cobicistat (Tybost) (DRV/c [Prezcobix]) has a low rate of transmitted PI resistance, a high genetic barrier to resistance, and a low rate of treatment-emergent resistance. A dolutegravir (DTG [Tivicay])- or bictegravir (BIC)-containing regimen (BIC/TAF/FTC [Biktarvy]) is also a consideration for patients in whom it is necessary to initiate ART before receiving resistance testing results because of its high barrier of resistance.

NNRTI-based regimens include efavirenz (EFV [Sustiva]), rilpivirine (RPV [Edurant]), or doravirine (DOR [Pifeltro]) and may be appropriate choices in certain patients with good medication adherence. These medications have a low genetic barrier to resistance. EFV has minimal PK interactions with rifamycins, which makes it an excellent option in patients who require treatment for tuberculosis. EFV has a high rate of central nervous system–related side effects, which lowers its overall tolerability for some patients. RPV has fewer side effects than EFV, but its virologic efficacy is reduced in patients with high baseline HIV RNA and low CD4 T-cell counts. RPV also requires acid for absorption; it is contraindicated with proton pump inhibitors and must be spaced 12 hours apart from histamine 2 receptor antagonists.

More recently, two large, randomized controlled trials showed that a two-drug regimen of DTG plus lamivudine (DTG/3TC [Dovato]) was noninferior to DTG plus TDF/FTC. This two-drug regimen is another potential initial option for most people with HIV, except for patients with pretreatment HIV RNA greater than 500,000 copies/mL, who are known to have active HBV coinfection, or who will initiate ART before results of HIV genotype testing for reverse transcriptase or HBV testing are available.

Long-Acting Injectable Antiretroviral Therapy

In 2021, the first complete long-acting injectable ARV regimen, cabotegravir (CAB) and rilpivirine (RPV), Cabenuva, was approved as an option to replace the current ARV regimen in adults with HIV. Once-monthly or every-2-month CAB/RPV intramuscular (IM) injections can be used as an optimization strategy for people with HIV currently on oral ART with documented viral suppression (HIV-1 RNA less than 50 copies per mL) for at least 3 months. Candidates for CAB/RBV long-acting injections should have no baseline resistance to either medication, have no prior virologic failures, should not have HBV infection (unless also receiving an oral HBV active regimen), should not be pregnant or planning to become pregnant, and should not be receiving medications with significant drug interactions with CAB or RPV. Before initiation of the IM injection, patients should receive oral CAB (Vocabria) and oral RPV (Edurant) for approximately 1 month as an oral lead-in period to assess tolerance to these drugs. CAB/RPV (Cabenuva) injections should be administered by healthcare providers as gluteal IM injections. Administration variances of +/–7 days are allowed. The product is refrigerated and should be brought to room temperature before administration. Unopened vials may remain at room temperature for up to 6 hours. Medication drawn into a syringe may remain in the syringe for up to 2 hours.

Monitoring Response to Antiretroviral Therapy

HIV disease progression and response to ART can be monitored via CD4 T-cell count and HIV RNA (viral load). The CD4 T-cell count should be measured before initiation of ART and provides information regarding the patient's immune function and risk of OI. Recommendations for monitoring viral load and CD4 T-cell count are shown in Table 3.

CD4 T-cell counts can be highly variable, and significant change is only considered with 30% difference in absolute count or an increase or decrease in CD4 percentage by 3 percentage points. CD4 T-cell recovery is most rapid in the first 3 months after initiating ART, later followed by more gradual increases. For most patients on ART, adequate response is considered as an increase in CD4 count in the range of 50 to 150 cells/mm³ during the first year of treatment. Subsequent increases may average 50 to 100 cells/mm³ per year until a steady-state level is reached. Peripheral blood CD4 T-cell counts in most HIV patients will continue to increase over a decade as long as viral suppression is maintained. Most individuals will eventually recover CD4 counts within the normal range (>500 cells/mm³). For approximately 15% to 20% of patients, especially those who initiate ART at very low CD4 counts (<200 cells/mm³), low CD4 counts may persist, which is associated with increased morbidity and mortality. These patients should be evaluated for reversible causes of CD4-positive T-cell lymphopenia, including offending medications, untreated coinfections, and underlying malignancy. In patients with appropriate virologic suppression, the addition of more antiretroviral agents or transitioning to a different ART regimen has not been demonstrated to improve CD4 T-cell recovery.

CD4 T-cell counts should be repeated 3 months after ART initiation to monitor immune reconstitution and can be monitored in many patients at 3- to 6-month intervals for the first 2 years of ART. In virally suppressed patients with consistent CD4 counts between 300 and 500 cells/mm³ for at least 2 years, CD4 counts can be checked annually. Although ART is recommended for all patients with HIV, patients who remain untreated should have

TABLE 3 Recommendations on the Indications and Frequency of Viral Load and CD4 T-Cell Count Monitoring

CLINICAL SCENARIO	VIRAL LOAD MONITORING	CD4 T-CELL COUNT MONITORING
Before initiating ART	At entry into care If ART initiation is deferred, repeat before initiating ART In patients not initiating ART, repeat testing is optional	At entry into care If ART is deferred, every 3–6 months
After initiating ART	Preferably within 2–4 weeks (and no later than 8 weeks) after initiation of ART; thereafter, every 4–8 weeks until viral load is suppressed	3 months after initiation of ART
After modifying ART because of drug toxicities or for regimen simplification in a patient with viral suppression	4–8 weeks after modification of ART to confirm effectiveness of new regimen	Monitor according to prior CD4 count and duration on ART, as outlined below.
After modifying ART because of virologic failure	Preferably within 2–4 weeks (and no later than 8 weeks) after modification; thereafter, every 4–8 weeks until viral load is suppressed. If viral suppression is not possible, repeat viral load every 3 months or more frequently if indicated	Every 3–6 months
During the first 2 years of ART	Every 3–4 months	Every 3–6 months
After 2 years of ART (VL consistently suppressed, CD4 consistently 300–500 cells/mm³) After 2 years of ART (VL consistently suppressed, CD4 consistently >500 cells/mm³)	Can extend to every 6 months for patients with consistent viral suppression for greater than or equal to 2 years.	Every 12 months Optional
While on ART with detectable viremia (VL repeatedly >200 copies/mL)	Every 3 months or more frequently if clinically indicated	Every 3–6 months
Change in clinical status	Every 3 months	Perform CD4 count, and repeat as clinically indicated

ART, Antiretroviral therapy; *VL,* viral load.

Modified from Panel on Antiretroviral Guidelines for Adults and Adolescents. Guidelines for the Use of Antiretroviral Agents in Adults and Adolescents with HIV. Department of Health and Human Services. Available at: https://clinicalinfo.hiv.gov/sites/default/files/guidelines/documents/adult-adolescent-arv/guidelines-adult-adolescent-arv.pdf (Table 4).

CD4 counts monitored every 3 to 6 months to assess the need for OI prophylaxis.

Viral load functions as a marker for ART response and should be monitored at initiation of therapy and regularly thereafter. The pretreatment viral load can also provide useful information regarding selection of an initial ART. Commercially available HIV-1 RNA assays do not detect HIV-2 viral load. Decreases in viral load following ART initiation are associated with a reduction in risk of disease progression to AIDS or death. Optimal viral suppression is defined as a viral load persistently below the level of detection. Low-level viremia refers to a patient with confirmed detectable HIV RNA less than 200 copies/mL. This may be detected using real-time polymerase chain reaction (PCR) assays and may be predictive of developing viral rebound. Viral rebound, or virologic failure, is considered to occur when a patient with confirmed virologic suppression has HIV RNA greater than or equal to 1000 copies/mL. If virologic suppression occurs and the patient is found to have a single isolated detectable HIV RNA level with return to virologic suppression in subsequent tests, this is referred to as a *virologic blip*. This is not usually associated with virologic failure and does not require a change in ART. Acute illness, stress, and recent immunizations are a few potential causes of virologic blips. A repeat viral load can be rechecked in 3 months to confirm return to appropriate viral suppression.

If a patient has a very high HIV viral load at the time of ART initiation, it may take several weeks for a measurable virologic response to occur. Certain ART regimens may also have slower rates of virologic suppression than others. A patient who has received ART for at least 24 weeks and has not yet had documented virologic suppression should be evaluated for antiretroviral drug resistance.

The use of ART to prevent HIV transmission is called *treatment as prevention* (TasP), also known as *Undetectable = Untransmittable* (U = U). Maintaining HIV RNA levels less than 200 copies/mL with ART prevents HIV transmission to sexual partners. Patients who start ART should use another form of prevention with sexual partners for at least the first 6 months of treatment and until an HIV RNA level less than 200 copies/mL has been achieved. Patients who have HIV and who rely on ART for prevention require high ART adherence because transmission is possible during periods of poor compliance or treatment interruption.

Treatment Failure

Patients who are receiving ART and do not achieve HIV RNA levels below the lower limit of detection or are shown to have sustained virologic rebound are at risk for developing resistance mutations to their current ART regimen, especially at HIV RNA levels greater than 500 copies/mL. Virologic failure has a strong association with suboptimal medication adherence and drug intolerance/toxicity leading to self-discontinuation of ART.

Some factors that may increase the risk of ART nonadherence include active substance use, neurocognitive impairment, and mental illness. Unstable housing and other socioeconomic and psychosocial factors can make ART adherence particularly difficult. The patient's inability to afford the medication may lead to intermittent adherence or nonadherence. Some patients will stop taking ART as a result of adverse effects of their regimen. Others may not be able to adhere to a high pill burden or frequency of dosing.

Less common causes of treatment failure include existing or newly developed drug resistance. Patients with HIV-2 or HIV-1/HIV-2 coinfection can have innate resistance to certain ART regimens. Others may have adverse drug-drug interactions with other medications, suboptimal virologic potency, or error in their medication prescription.

If a patient is experiencing virologic failure, it is important to determine the cause because there is potential for choosing a subsequent therapy regimen that promotes better adherence. Management of a patient who is experiencing treatment failure is often complex; consultation with an HIV specialist can prove beneficial.

Drug Resistance and Resistance Testing

Two types of resistance assays exist to assess viral strains and direct treatment strategies: genotypic and phenotypic. These assays provide useful information in regard to resistance to NRTIs, NNRTIs, PIs, and INSTIs. In some settings, INSTI resistance tests must be ordered separately. In patients with newly diagnosed HIV infection, resistance testing can guide therapy selection to optimize virologic response. Genotypic assays detect drug resistance mutations by sequencing reverse transcriptase, protease, and integrase genes. Interpreting these test results requires knowledge of the mutations selected by different antivirals and the potential for cross-resistance to other drugs. Clinical trials have shown that consultation with HIV specialists regarding drug resistance interpretation improves virologic outcomes.

Adverse Drug Reactions and Drug-Drug Interactions

Adverse drug reactions to ART are common, especially when first initiating therapy. Generally, reactions such as nausea, fatigue, and headache often resolve within 1 to 2 weeks of starting ART. Severe or persistent adverse drug reactions should prompt consideration of change to a different agent. Each ART drug class has different characteristic adverse drug reactions. Additionally, each individual ART agent carries its own characteristic adverse drug reactions (Table 4). As drug therapies have evolved and new medications discovered, preferred agents have been updated to avoid those that

TABLE 4	Monitoring Recommendations for Antiretroviral Toxicity of Selected Drugs*	
DRUG	**TOXICITY**	**MONITORING**
NRTIs		
Abacavir (Ziagen)	Liver Abacavir hypersensitivity syndrome	LFTs Screening for HLA-B*5701 (should be confirmed negative before abacavir initiation) Symptoms of abacavir hypersensitivity may include fever, rash, nausea, vomiting, diarrhea, abdominal pain, malaise, fatigue, or respiratory symptoms such as sore throat, cough, or shortness of breath
Emtricitabine (Emtriva)	Minimal toxicity Liver Hyperpigmentation/skin discoloration	Serum creatinine LFTs HBV (before initiation of therapy) Severe acute exacerbation of hepatitis may occur in patients with HBV/HIV coinfection who discontinue emtricitabine. For patients in whom discontinuation of tenofovir is necessary, ensure that an agent active against HBV is administered
Lamivudine (Epivir)	Minimal toxicity Liver	Serum creatinine LFTs HBV (before initiation of therapy) Severe acute exacerbation of hepatitis may occur in patients with HBV/HIV coinfection who discontinue lamivudine. For patients in whom discontinuation of tenofovir is necessary, ensure that an agent active against HBV is administered
Tenofovir (disoproxil fumarate [Viread], alafenamide [Vemlidy])	Renal toxicity (tubulopathy) Decreased bone mineral density Liver	Serum creatinine Urine glucose and protein (before initiation of therapy and as clinically indicated during therapy) Serum phosphorus (in patients with chronic kidney disease) Bone mineral density testing (if history of bone fracture or risk factors for bone loss) LFTs HBV (before initiation of therapy) Tenofovir alafenamide (Vemlidy) is associated with lower rates of bone and kidney toxicity compared with tenofovir disoproxil fumarate Severe acute exacerbation of hepatitis may occur in patients with HBV/HIV coinfection who discontinue tenofovir. For patients in whom discontinuation of tenofovir is necessary, ensure that an agent active against HBV is administered
NNRTIs		
Efavirenz (Sustiva)	Rash Neuropsychiatric symptoms Hyperlipidemia Hepatotoxicity Prolonged QT interval	LFTs Lipid panel (before initiation of therapy and as clinically indicated during therapy) Signs and symptoms of neuropsychiatric effects (e.g., vivid dreams, depression, suicidal ideation)
Rilpivirine (Edurant)	Rash Depression, insomnia, headache Hepatotoxicity Prolonged QT interval	LFTs Lipid panel

Continued

DRUG	TOXICITY	MONITORING
Doravirine (Pifeltro)	Nausea Dizziness Abnormal dreams	No specific tests
PIs		
All	GI intolerance, nausea, vomiting, diarrhea Hyperglycemia Insulin resistance Hepatotoxicity Fat maldistribution Hyperlipidemia	Serum glucose LFTs (before initiation of therapy and as clinically indicated during therapy)
Atazanavir (Reyataz)	Indirect hyperbilirubinemia	Bilirubin
Darunavir (Prezista)	Skin rash	Darunavir contains a sulfonamide moiety; Stevens-Johnson syndrome, toxic epidermal necrolysis, acute generalized exanthematous pustulosis, and erythema have been reported Risk of cross-reactivity between darunavir and sulfonamide medications is very low. However, use caution in patients with severe sulfonamide allergies
INSTIs		
All	INSTIs typically well tolerated for most patients GI intolerance Insomnia Headache Depression and suicidal ideation (rare, usually in patients with preexisting psychiatric conditions) CPK elevation, muscle weakness, and rhabdomyolysis (primarily reported with raltegravir [Isentress]) Possible association with weight gain	LFTs Serum creatinine (dolutegravir [Tivicay] and bictegravir) CPK (if signs of muscle toxicity)

CPK, Creatinine phosphokinase; *GI*, gastrointestinal; *HBV*, hepatitis B virus; *HIV*, human immunodeficiency virus; *HLA*, human leukocyte antigen; *INSTI*, integrase strand transfer inhibitor; *LFT*, liver function test; *NRTI*, nucleoside reverse transcriptase inhibitor; *NNRTI*, non-nucleoside reverse transcriptase inhibitor; *PI*, protease inhibitor. Table is not all inclusive.
https://clinicalinfo.hiv.gov/sites/default/files/guidelines/documents/AdultandAdolescentGL.pdf. Section accessed March 9, 2021 [Appendix B, table 20].
Modified from Panel on Antiretroviral Guidelines for Adults and Adolescents. Guidelines for the Use of Antiretroviral Agents in Adults and Adolescents with HIV. Department of Health and Human Services. Available at: https://clinicalinfo.hiv.gov/sites/default/files/guidelines/documents/adult-adolescent-arv/guidelines-adult-adolescent-arv.pdf.

have tended to cause more frequent and severe adverse effects. For example, older agents in the NRTI class (e.g., stavudine [Zerit] and didanosine [Videx]) were commonly associated with hepatic steatosis, lipodystrophy, and insulin resistance. Newer-generation NRTIs, which have much lower rates of these serious adverse effects, have largely supplanted the use of these older drugs.

All providers who care for patients who receive ART should be aware of the possibility of adverse drug-drug interactions of antiretroviral drugs with other medications. The use of the pharmacokinetic-enhancing agents ritonavir (Norvir) and cobicistat (Tybost) in many combination ART regimens can pose serious risks to patients who receive other drugs metabolized through the cytochrome P450 pathway, including numerous anticoagulant drugs and synthetic glucocorticoids. When prescribing or altering one or more drugs in an ART regimen, the potential for drug interactions must be explored. It is critical to carefully review the patient's other medications for potential interactions. If multiple drugs with similar or conflicting metabolic pathways are prescribed, healthcare providers should carefully monitor for appropriate therapeutic efficacy and concentration-related toxicities. Consultation with a pharmacist to evaluate drug interactions is recommended.

Viral Hepatitis Coinfection
Approximately 5% to 10% of patients with HIV in the United States have coinfection with chronic HBV. Disease progression to cirrhosis, end-stage liver disease, and hepatocellular carcinoma is more rapid in these patients. Some antiretroviral toxicities and complications may be attributed to flares of HBV after initiation or discontinuation of ART.

FTC, 3TC, TDF, and TAF[1] are approved for treatment of HIV and are also active against HBV. Discontinuation of these drugs can potentially cause significant hepatic damage resulting from reactivation of HBV. The anti-HBV drug entecavir (Baraclude) has activity against HIV.[1] When entecavir is used to treat HBV in patients with HBV/HIV coinfection who are not taking ART, the drug can select for the *M184V* mutation, resulting in HIV resistance to 3TC and FTC. When 3TC is the only active drug used to treat HBV in coinfected patients, 3TC resistance develops in approximately 40% to 90% of patients after 2 to 4 years on 3TC monotherapy.

Before ART is initiated, all patients who test positive for HBV surface antigen (HBsAg) should also be tested for HBV DNA using a quantitative assay. This test should be repeated every 3 to 6 months to ensure effective HBV suppression. In patients with HBV/HIV coinfection, immune reconstitution following initiation of treatment for HIV, HBV, or both can be associated with elevated transaminases.

Complications
Diagnosis and Management of Opportunistic Infections
The widespread availability and use of ART have significantly reduced OI-related mortality in persons with HIV infection. OIs

---

[1] Not FDA approved for this indication.

continue to cause considerable morbidity and mortality, however, because of the increasing number of undiagnosed cases of HIV and patients who have known HIV infection but are not on ART or are unable to maintain adherence to ART.

PJP is an infection caused by a ubiquitous fungus, *P. jirovecii*. Most cases occur in patients with an advanced compromised immune system (CD4 count less than 100 cells/mm³). The most common manifestations are dyspnea, fever, nonproductive cough, and chest discomfort. Onset of symptoms is usually subacute and progressive over days to weeks. Patients with mild cases may present with normal pulmonary physical examination findings at rest but develop dyspnea, tachycardia, and rales with exertion. Hypoxemia is often present to varying severity. Laboratory findings are consistent with lactate dehydrogenase levels greater than 500 mg/dL and elevated serum 1,3 β-d-glucan. Chest radiography may show diffuse, bilateral, ground-glass interstitial infiltrates, but chest radiography can appear unremarkable in patients with early disease. In patients with normal chest plain films, computed tomography (CT) of the chest can show underlying abnormalities consistent with PJP. HIV-infected patients, including pregnant women and those on ART, should receive PJP chemoprophylaxis if they have CD4 counts less than 200 cells/mm³. Patients who receive pyrimethamine (Daraprim)-sulfadiazine for treatment or suppression of toxoplasmosis do not require additional prophylaxis for PJP. Trimethoprim-sulfamethoxazole (TMP-SMX [Bactrim]) is the first-line prophylactic agent at one double-strength tablet daily (which also confers prophylaxis against toxoplasmosis[1]) or three times weekly. In those who cannot tolerate TMP-SMX, alternative prophylactic options include atovaquone (Mepron), dapsone,[1] dapsone plus pyrimethamine (Daraprim)[1] plus leucovorin,[1] and aerosolized pentamidine (Nebupent).

Toxoplasma gondii is a protozoan infection and is associated with reactivation of latent tissue cysts. Patients at greatest risk have CD4 counts less than 50 cells/µL. Clinical disease is rare in patients with CD4 counts greater than 200 cells/µL. In patients with AIDS, the typical presentation of infection is focal encephalitis, including headache, confusion, focal motor weakness, and fever. In the absence of treatment, disease progression may lead to seizures, coma, and death. CT and magnetic resonance imaging (MRI) of the brain may show multiple contrast-enhancing lesions within the gray matter of the cortex or basal ganglia, often with associated edema. HIV-infected patients with toxoplasma encephalitis are usually seropositive for toxoplasma IgG antibodies. Definitive diagnosis requires the combination of clinical presentation, identification of one or more mass lesions via CT or MRI, and detection of the organism in a sample, with brain biopsy being the most preferred method. The therapy of choice includes pyrimethamine plus sulfadiazine plus leucovorin.[1]

Disseminated *Mycobacterium avium* complex (MAC) disease typically occurs in patients with CD4 counts less than 50 cells/mm³. Other factors associated with increased susceptibility to MAC disease include HIV RNA levels greater than 100,000 copies/mL, previous OIs, and previous colonization of the respiratory or gastrointestinal tract with MAC. In HIV-infected patients with AIDS who are not on ART, MAC disease usually presents as a disseminated, multiorgan infection. Symptoms may be minimal at first but may include fever, night sweats, weight loss, diarrhea, fatigue, and nonspecific abdominal pain. Laboratory abnormalities may include anemia out of proportion for that expected from HIV alone and an increase in liver alkaline phosphatase. Physical examination or imaging may note nonspecific hepatomegaly, lymphadenopathy, and/or splenomegaly. Diagnosis is based on a combination of clinical symptoms and the isolation of MAC from cultures obtained from blood, lymph nodes, bone marrow, or other sterile sites. Initial treatment should consist of at least two antimycobacterial medications in an effort to prevent the development of resistance.

Infectious disease specialists should be consulted regarding treatment. MAC isolates should be tested for susceptibility to clarithromycin (Biaxin) and azithromycin (Zithromax).

Cryptococcus neoformans meningitis occurs more commonly in patients with CD4 counts less than 100 cells/µL. It can present as a subacute or acute meningoencephalitis associated with fever, headache, and malaise. Classic meningeal symptoms may be absent. Disseminated disease is usually present when diagnosed in a patient with HIV infection and can involve virtually any organ. Diagnosis of meningitis via cerebrospinal fluid (CSF) often demonstrates elevated opening pressure, elevated protein, low-to-normal glucose, and lymphocytic pleocytosis. Numerous yeast forms may be visualized on Gram stain or India ink preparations of CSF. The CSF cryptococcal antigen (CrAg) is often positive. Serum CrAg may be positive in both meningeal and nonmeningeal involving infections, and its presence can be detected weeks to months before the onset of symptoms. A positive serum CrAg should proceed to lumbar puncture to rule out meningeal disease. Treatment of cryptococcosis occurs in three stages: induction, consolidation, and maintenance therapy.

CMV disease can cause disseminated and localized end-organ damage in HIV-infected patients with suppressed immune states with CD4 counts less than 50 cells/mm³. Clinical disease is usually the result of reactivation of latent infection. Risk factors include not receiving or failing to respond to ART, previous OIs, high level of CMV viremia, and high HIV viral load (>100,000 copies/mL). Retinitis is the most common clinical manifestation of CMV end-organ disease and is often unilateral, but it can progress to bilateral if therapy or immune recovery are not pursued. Retinitis may present with floaters, scotomata, or peripheral visual field defects. Colitis is another manifestation of CMV disease and may be associated with weight loss, abdominal pain, significant diarrhea, and malaise. Hemorrhage and bowel perforation can be life threatening. CMV viremia can be measured via PCR and is usually present in end-organ disease.

Mucocutaneous candidiasis of the oropharynx and esophagus occurs commonly in HIV-infected patients and is often an indication of underlying immune suppression (CD4 count <200 cells/mm³). Oropharyngeal candidiasis is usually painless and affects the oropharyngeal mucosa and tongue surface. Esophageal candidiasis may be associated with retrosternal discomfort and odynophagia. Oropharyngeal candidiasis is usually diagnosed clinically. Diagnosis of esophageal candidiasis is made based on symptoms, response to therapy, or visualization of mucosal lesions on examination.

Many treatment guidelines recommend initiating ART within 2 weeks for most diagnosed OI. In patients with cryptococcal meningitis and possible tuberculous meningitis, ART should be deferred because of the risks of serious immune reconstitution syndrome outweighing the benefits of ART. In patients with AIDS-associated OI for which no effective therapy exists (e.g., progressive multifocal leukoencephalopathy [PML], cryptosporidiosis, and microsporidiosis), improvement in immune function with ART can potentially improve disease outcomes.

Neurologic Complications

Both central nervous system disease and peripheral nerve abnormalities are common in advanced AIDS. HIV infection can directly cause distal sensory neuropathy, which may manifest as dysesthesia or hypersensitivity, decreased reflexes, and chronic neuropathic pain. Inflammatory demyelinating polyneuropathy (e.g., Guillain-Barré syndrome) has known associations with some enteric pathogens and causes ascending motor weakness, typically without sensory involvement. CMV infection may cause polyradiculopathy, transverse myelitis, and encephalitis/ventriculitis in patients with CD4 counts lower than 50 cells/mm³. CMV end-organ disease, including retinitis (a vision-threatening condition), requires prompt diagnosis and initiation of appropriate anti-CMV therapy.

Focal central nervous system lesions can arise from infectious and malignant conditions. Cerebral toxoplasmosis usually occurs in patients with prior exposure to *T. gondii* who develop

---

[1] Not FDA approved for this indication.

reactivation disease when the CD4 count is less than 100 cells/mm[3]. The main differential diagnosis for one or several enhancing brain lesions includes toxoplasmosis and primary central nervous system lymphoma (PCNSL). PCNSL is associated with EBV, and detection of nucleic acid for EBV in CSF carries a high specificity for this condition in the proper radiographic context. PML, a rare and potentially devastating demyelinating condition, is caused by reactivation of the JC virus and can manifest as focal neurologic deficit, seizures, or cognitive dysfunction. *C. neoformans* is a common cause of meningitis in AIDS patients and may manifest with central nervous system mass lesions, pulmonary disease, or gastrointestinal disease. Worldwide, tuberculosis accounts for a large proportion of HIV-associated meningitis cases; less commonly, it can manifest as single or multiple focal lesions (tuberculomas). Neurosyphilis should be considered in patients with unexplained neurologic disease and sexual risk factors.

Respiratory Complications

Respiratory illnesses are among the most common causes of morbidity in HIV-infected patients. Community-acquired bacterial pneumonia occurs at a significantly higher rate in HIV-infected patients compared with noninfected patients, regardless of CD4 T-cell count, and it is one of the most common reasons for hospitalization. *P. jirovecii* pneumonia (PJP) manifests with fever, cough, and dyspnea. Findings on physical examination and chest radiography can be variable, making the diagnosis difficult in the absence of high clinical suspicion. Elevated lactate dehydrogenase and oxygen desaturation with ambulation can be diagnostic clues. More than 90% of cases occur among patients with CD4 counts lower than 200 cells/mm[3]. The diagnosis is established by visualization of organisms in induced sputum (sensitivity, 50% to 90%) or in bronchoalveolar lavage specimens (sensitivity, 90% to 99%), most commonly with the use of immunofluorescent staining.

The risk of reactivation of latent TB is increased 100-fold in patients with HIV infection. Patients with HIV infection who are latently infected have a 10% annual risk of developing symptomatic tuberculosis, compared with a 10% lifetime risk among the general population. The risk of reactivation increases with decreasing CD4 T-cell count, and patients with counts lower than 350 cells/mm[3] are more likely to have atypical radiographic presentations, including middle- and lower-lobe infiltrates without cavitation. Patients with low CD4 T-cell counts are more likely to have extrapulmonary tuberculosis. Diagnostic approaches to tuberculosis in patients with HIV infection are similar to those in patients without HIV infection. Tuberculin skin testing can be used to diagnose latent tuberculosis infection, although the recommended cutoff for a positive test is 5 mm of induration. Treatment of coinfection with *Mycobacterium tuberculosis* and HIV requires consultation with experienced clinicians and pharmacists because of extensive drug-drug interactions among antiretroviral drugs and rifamycins.

Gastrointestinal Complications

Oropharyngeal candidiasis (thrush) commonly manifests as white plaques on the tongue, palate, or buccal mucosa that are painless and are easily scraped off. Although thrush is typically uncomplicated and easily treatable with topical preparations such as nystatin (Mycostatin) and clotrimazole (Mycelex troche), in the proper clinical setting it can alert the clinician to the presence of esophageal candidiasis. Esophageal involvement should be suspected in patients with dysphagia and odynophagia; retrosternal chest pain may also be present. Thrush is usually present but is not required for the diagnosis, which is often made on clinical grounds rather than being confirmed with endoscopy. Patients with esophageal candidiasis typically respond after several days of treatment, and 7 to 14 days of antifungal therapy is usually sufficient. For cases not responsive to empiric treatment for candidiasis, referral for endoscopy should be considered. Esophagitis caused by CMV or herpes simplex virus requires a histopathologic diagnosis.

Acute diarrhea, defined as three or more loose or watery stools per day for 3 to 10 days, is common among patients with HIV infection, and more than 1000 different enteric pathogens have been described. Data from a large cohort indicate that the most common pathogens isolated are *Clostridium difficile*, *Shigella* spp., *Campylobacter jejuni*, *Salmonella* spp., *Staphylococcus aureus*, and MAC. Culture of the stool can yield a microbiologic diagnosis in many cases, particularly for acute diarrheal illnesses caused by *Campylobacter*, *Yersinia*, *Salmonella*, and *Shigella* species. Infection with *C. difficile*, the most common bacterial enteric pathogen in the United States for both HIV-infected and HIV-uninfected persons, is diagnosed in most settings by detection of cytotoxin in the stool by enzyme immunoassay (EIA) or PCR, although the more laborious tissue culture is considered the gold standard. Enteric viruses are present in 15% to 30% of HIV-infected persons with acute diarrhea. Definitive diagnosis is not feasible in most clinical laboratories; viral enteritis should be suspected in the setting of community outbreaks because of the high transmissibility of viral pathogens. Treatment is supportive with fluid resuscitation and antimotility agents.

Chronic diarrhea (duration 30 days) was a common manifestation of advanced-stage AIDS in the pre-ART era. Most pathogens that cause acute gastroenteritis can also cause chronic symptoms. Pathogens that should be suspected in cases of chronic watery diarrhea include protozoa such as *Cryptosporidium parvum*, *Isospora belli*, and *Microsporidia* spp. These entities are self-limiting in the absence of severe immunosuppression. In advanced HIV infection, pathogen-specific antimicrobial therapy is infrequently effective, and symptoms commonly do not improve without immune reconstitution in response to ART. *Giardia lamblia* causes watery diarrhea, abdominal bloating, and occasionally malabsorption syndrome, and it can occur at any CD4 T-cell count. CMV infection can affect any segment of the gastrointestinal tract and is a common cause of chronic diarrhea. Diagnosis of gastrointestinal CMV disease is difficult without biopsy. Detection of CMV viremia with PCR does not correlate well with presence of CMV disease in HIV-infected patients, and CMV can be undetectable in serum in patients with extensive gastrointestinal disease.

Other Conditions

ART has dramatically increased the survival of individuals living with HIV, and the older adult population with HIV is expanding. There are few clinical trials or studies systematically focused on this cohort. Older adults with HIV may develop comorbidities that can complicate their HIV management. ART-related CD4 T-cell recovery in older patients has been observed to be slower and to be of lower magnitude than in younger patients. Hepatic and renal functions decrease as the body ages and may lead to impaired drug elimination and increased drug exposure in older adult patients.

Immune Reconstitution Inflammatory Syndrome

Immune reconstitution inflammatory syndrome (IRIS) is a collection of inflammatory disorders often associated with paradoxical worsening of preexisting infectious diseases after initiation of ART. IRIS is usually accompanied by an increase in CD4 T-cell count and can occur at any CD4 count. It usually occurs in the first 4 to 8 weeks after initiation of ART. Clinical features are often associated with the type and location of the preexisting OI and can be localized or systemic. Patients should continue ART and should receive treatment for the underlying OI as quickly as possible. If the patient's presentation involves paradoxical worsening of a previously diagnosed OI that is already receiving treatment, OI therapy should also be continued. Disseminated MAC accounts for up to one-third of cases of IRIS in the United States. Other important causes of IRIS are tuberculosis, CMV infection, viral hepatitis, and candida infections.

Management of Human Immunodeficiency Virus in Pregnancy and Women of Childbearing Potential

Human Immunodeficiency Virus in Pregnant Women

Every pregnant woman with HIV should be given ART regardless of her immunologic or virologic status in order to improve her health and prevent transmission of HIV to the fetus.

Increased perinatal transmission risk exists in pregnant women who experience early HIV infection and high-level viremia. Pregnant women with newly diagnosed HIV infection should start ART as soon as possible to prevent perinatal HIV transmission. The goal of ART is to achieve and sustain viral suppression throughout the pregnancy. Resistance testing should be performed before initiating ART, but therapy may be started before receiving resistance testing results. The ART regimen can be modified at a later date once resistance testing results are available.

Although there originally was a concern for increased risk of neural tube defects (NTDs) with DTG based on preliminary information from a study in Botswana in 2018, the most recent data from this study indicate that there is no longer a significant difference in NTDs with the use of DTG-based regimens compared with non–DTG-based regimens. Therefore, the U.S. Department of Health and Human Services guidelines on the use of antiretroviral drugs during pregnancy recommend DTG as a preferred agent in pregnant women with HIV.

In a patient already taking a regimen containing EFV [Sustiva] who presents for prenatal care during the first trimester and has virologic suppression, EFV can be continued. The risk of fetal NTDs is limited to the first 5 to 6 weeks of pregnancy, and pregnancy is often not recognized before weeks 4 to 6. Unnecessary changes to a patient's ART regimen during pregnancy may result in loss of viral suppression with increased risk of perinatal transmission.

In a pregnant patient with an HIV RNA viral load greater than or equal to 1000 copies/mL (or viral load is unknown) near delivery, IV infusion of zidovudine (Retrovir) during labor is recommended regardless of the patient's antepartum ART regimen or resistance profile. Maternal ART should be continued following delivery. Following delivery, patients should continue to follow up with their HIV healthcare provider as recommended for non-pregnant adults.

Maternal adherence to ART significantly reduces but does not completely eliminate the risk of transmission of HIV in breast milk. Postnatal HIV transmission can occur despite maternal ART adherence, and patients should be counseled to avoid breastfeeding. There have also been reports of mother-to-child transmission of HIV via mothers pre-masticating food and feeding it to their infants.

Preexposure Prophylaxis of Human Immunodeficiency Virus Infection

Globally, up to 2 million new HIV infections occur per year. It is estimated that up to 40,000 new HIV infections occur annually in the United States. The highest incidence of new HIV infections occur in MSM, especially among young African American males. For uninfected patients with a high risk of HIV acquisition, preexposure prophylaxis (PrEP) is an evidence-based method for preventing infections in those at risk. All sexually active adult and adolescent patients should receive information about PrEP and its role in preventing HIV acquisition. Clinicians should offer to prescribe PrEP to adults and adolescents whose sexual or injection behaviors and epidemiologic context place them at substantial risk of acquiring HIV infection. Available PrEP options include oral tenofovir disoproxil fumarate-emtricitabine (TDF/FTC [Truvada]), oral TAF/FTC (Descovy), and IM CAB (Apretude) (Tables 5 and 6). Efficacy is dependent on medication

637

TABLE 5	Guidance for Daily Oral Preexposure Prophylaxis Use	
	SEXUALLY ACTIVE ADULTS AND ADOLESCENTS	**PERSONS WHO INJECT DRUGS**
Identifying substantial risk of acquiring HIV infection	Anal or vaginal sex in the past 6 months *AND* any of the following: • HIV-positive sexual partner (especially if partner has an unknown or detectable viral load) • Bacterial STI in past 6 months • History of inconsistent or no condom use with sexual partner(s)	HIV-positive injection partner *OR* Sharing injection equipment
Clinically eligible	*All of the following conditions are met:* • Documented negative HIV test result within 1 week before initially prescribing PrEP • No signs/symptoms of acute HIV infection • Estimated creatinine clearance ≥30 mL/min • No contraindicated medications	
Dosage	• Daily, continuing, oral doses of FTC/TDF (Truvada), ≤90-day supply *OR* • For men and transgender women at risk for sexual acquisition of HIV; daily, continuing oral doses of FTC/TAF (Descovy), ≤90-day supply	
Follow-up care	*Follow-up visits at least every 3 months to provide the following:* • HIV Ag/Ab test and HIV-1 RNA assay, medication adherence and behavioral risk reduction support • Bacterial STI screening for MSM and transgender women who have sex with men • Access to clean needles/syringes and drug treatment services for PWID *Follow-up visits every 6 months to provide the following:* • Assess renal function for patients aged ≥50 years or who have an eCrCl <90 mL/min at PrEP initiation • Bacterial STI screening for all sexually active patients *Follow-up visits every 12 months to provide the following:* • Assess renal function for all patients • Chlamydia screening for heterosexually active women and men • For patients on FTC/TAF, assess weight, triglyceride and cholesterol levels	

eCrCl, Estimated creatinine clearance; *HIV,* human immunodeficiency virus; *MSM,* men who have sex with men; *PrEP,* preexposure prophylaxis; *PWID,* persons who inject drugs; *STI,* sexually transmitted infection.
Modified from Preexposure Prophylaxis for the Prevention of HIV Infection in the United States—2021 Update: A Clinical Practice Guideline. U.S. Public Health Service. Available at: https://www.cdc.gov/hiv/pdf/risk/prep/cdc-hiv-prep-guidelines-2021.pdf (Table 1a).

TABLE 6 Guidance for Cabotegravir Injection Preexposure Prophylaxis Use

	SEXUALLY ACTIVE ADULTS AND ADOLESCENTS	PERSONS WHO INJECT DRUGS
Identifying substantial risk of acquiring HIV infection	Anal or vaginal sex in the past 6 months *AND* any of the following: • HIV-positive sexual partner (especially if partner has an unknown or detectable viral load) • Bacterial STI in past 6 months • History of inconsistent or no condom use with sexual partner(s)	HIV-positive injection partner Sharing injection equipment
Clinically eligible	*All of the following conditions are met:* • Documented negative HIV test result within 1 week before initial CAB injection • No signs or symptoms of acute HIV infection • No contraindicated medications or conditions	
Dosage	• 600 mg CAB (one 3-mL injection in the gluteal muscle) • Initial dose • Second dose 4 weeks after first dose • Every 8 weeks thereafter	
Follow-up care	*At follow-up visit 1 month after first injection:* • HIV Ag/Ab test and HIV-1 RNA assay *At follow-up visits every 2 months (starting with third injection— month 3):* • HIV Ag/Ab test and HIV-1 RNA assay • Access to clean needles/syringes and drug treatment services for PWID *At follow-up visits every 4 months (starting with third injection— month 3):* • Bacterial STI screening for MSM and transgender women who have sex with men *At follow-up visits every 6 months (starting with fifth injection— month 7):* • Bacterial STI screening for all heterosexually active women and men *At follow-up visits every 12 months (after the first injection):* • Assess desire to continue injections for PrEP • Chlamydia screening for heterosexually active women and men *At follow-up visits when discontinuing CAB injections:* • Re-educate patients about the "tail" and the risks during declining CAB levels • Assess ongoing HIV risk and prevention plans • If PrEP is indicated, prescribe daily oral FTC/TDF or FTC/TAF beginning within 8 weeks after last injection • Continue follow-up visits with HIV testing quarterly for 12 months	

CAB, Cabotegravir; *HIV,* human immunodeficiency virus; *MSM,* men who have sex with men; *PrEP,* preexposure prophylaxis; *PWID,* persons who inject drugs; *STI,* sexually transmitted infection.
Modified from Preexposure Prophylaxis for the Prevention of HIV Infection in the United States—2021 Update: A Clinical Practice Guideline. U.S. Public Health Service. Available at: https://www.cdc.gov/hiv/pdf/risk/prep/cdc-hiv-prep-guidelines-2021.pdf. (Table 1b).

adherence; PrEP reduces the risk of acquiring HIV from sex by approximately 99% when taken as prescribed.

Before initiating PrEP, it is important to obtain a brief, targeted sexual and drug use history to identify patients likely to benefit from PrEP. The 2021 PrEP guidelines published by the U.S. Public Health Service recommend a dialogue around The "Five Ps": partners, practices, protection from sexually transmitted infections (STIs), past history of STIs, and pregnancy intention. It is important to determine sexual practices with a patient's main sexual partner, casual partners, or any anonymous partners. A drug history over the prior 6 months should be obtained and include injection drug use and sharing of needles. Clinicians should also briefly screen all patients for alcohol use disorder and the use of illicit non-injection drugs (e.g., amyl nitrite, stimulants) because use of these substances may affect sexual risk behavior. Clinicians should also consider the epidemiologic context of patient sexual practices as the risk of HIV acquisition is determined by both the frequency of specific sexual practices and the likelihood that a sex partner has HIV. Communities and populations that have higher HIV prevalence are more likely to lead to HIV exposure, indicating a greater need for risk-reduction methods (e.g., PrEP).

Patients screened for PrEP must be screened for common bacterial STIs, including serologic testing for syphilis and nucleic acid amplification tests for gonorrhea and chlamydia. This includes swabs of the oropharynx in patients who participate in oral sex and anal swabs for recipients of anal intercourse. Screening for trichomonas and bacterial vaginosis are not required before initiating PrEP because they lack strong correlation with HIV coinfection.

HIV testing with confirmed results within 1 week before initiating therapy is required to document that patients do not have HIV when they start taking PrEP medications. Plasma HIV testing with a fourth-generation antibody/antigen (Ab/Ag) test should be obtained to confirm that the patient does not have undiagnosed HIV infection. Additional HIV RNA testing should be performed in patients with signs or symptoms of acute HIV infection in the past 4 weeks, those with indeterminate antigen/antibody test results, and patients with high-risk HIV exposure in the preceding 4 weeks. Testing for both HIV Ab/Ag and HIV-1 RNA should be obtained at least every 3 months after oral PrEP initiation or every 2 months when CAB injections are given.

TDF/FTC (Truvada) is generally tolerated well by most patients; however, screening for persons at increased risk of adverse effects should be performed before PrEP initiation. TDF is associated with renal and bone toxicity in some patients; serum creatinine should be measured as TDF/FTC is not recommended for PrEP in patients with creatinine clearance less than 60 mL/min. In patients without reduced kidney function but who have risk factors for developing renal disease, urinalysis to document baseline proteinuria can be obtained for monitoring purposes. A different formulation of tenofovir, TAF (tenofovir alafenamide fumarate), has less association with renal and bone toxicity compared with TDF. In the United States, once-daily TAF/FTC (Descovy) can be prescribed for PrEP in high-risk MSM and transgender women, particularly those who have bone or renal contraindications to TDF, including those with a creatinine clearance as low as 30 mL/min. CAB (Apretude), administered IM every 2 months, is another option for PrEP in those at risk for renal toxicity because it may be administered irrespective of renal function.

Screening for undiagnosed HBV infection should be performed via hepatitis B surface antigen, hepatitis B core antibody, and hepatitis B surface antibody. If the patient's serology shows nonimmunity, vaccination against HBV should be pursued, as individuals engaging in high-risk sexual and drug-use behaviors have an increased risk of HBV infection. If the patient's serology reveals chronic HBV, it must be determined whether the patient requires HBV treatment. TDF (Viread) and TAF (Vemlidy) are first-line treatment choices for chronic HBV and can be used for PrEP[1] and treatment of chronic HBV. In those with chronic HBV who do not require HBV treatment, there is a low risk of HBV flare if TDF or TAF is discontinued.

TDF is also associated with decreased bone density; therefore patients considering PrEP should be screened for osteoporosis risk factors. The greatest amount of bone loss has been associated with the first 6 months of treatment. In patients with known osteopenia or osteoporosis, the risk of acquiring HIV versus further bone loss should be considered. Because of a lack of clear benefit, neither baseline nor serial dual-energy x-ray absorptiometry (DEXA) scans are recommended before initiation of PrEP or for PrEP monitoring. Because of lower rates of bone and renal toxicity, TAF or CAB should be considered over TDF in patients with significant risk for bone-related complications.

Providers should offer PrEP with TDF/FTC (Truvada) to women seeking to conceive and to pregnant or breastfeeding women whose sexual partner has HIV, especially when the partner's viral load is detectable or unknown. In patients who are pregnant, the risk of acquiring HIV must be considered against the risk of using antiretroviral medication during pregnancy. The 2021 PrEP guidelines published by the U.S. Public Health Service recommend that providers discuss the risks and benefits of all available alternatives for safer conception. Although each case should utilize shared decision making, generally the potential benefit of preventing HIV transmission to an infant during pregnancy outweighs theoretical risk to maternal or infant health.

Initiating Preexposure Prophylaxis
The combination tablet of TDF/FTC (Truvada) or TAF/FTC (Descovy) should be taken once daily for a duration of as long as the infection risk continues. It should be dispensed as a 90-day supply and renewed at each 3-month clinic follow-up. Condom use is encouraged while using PrEP. For patients who are not willing to use condoms consistently, the Centers for Disease Control and Prevention (CDC) recommends condom use to prevent acquisition of HIV (and other STIs) for the first 7 days after starting oral PrEP if engaging in receptive anal sex and 21 days if engaging in receptive vaginal sex. Common side effects of TDF/FTC and TAF/FTC include nausea and vomiting. These symptoms usually improve and resolve within the first 4 weeks of use.

CAB injections (Apretude) also be used for PrEP and may be especially appropriate for patients with significant renal disease, those who have difficulty with adherence to oral PrEP, and those who prefer injections every 2 months to an oral PrEP dosing schedule. CAB is administered as a 600 mg (3 mL) IM injection at baseline and at 1 month, followed by every 2 months thereafter. CAB injections should be administered in a healthcare setting; they should not be self-administered by patients. In studies, an oral CAB (Vocabria) lead-in phase was utilized before beginning IM injections, but this is not required before initiating CAB injections for PrEP unless patients are especially concerned about side effects with the first dose. Common side effects of CAB injections include

injection site reactions, such as pain, tenderness, and induration. Over-the-counter pain medication and/or warm compresses or heating pads can be used if needed to manage injection site pain.

Preexposure Prophylaxis Monitoring and Follow-Up
Patients on oral PrEP should have routine follow-up with their prescribing medical provider approximately every 3 months, although some clinicians may wish to schedule contact more frequently at the beginning of PrEP, either by phone or clinic visit. More frequent follow-up should occur for patients with exposures or symptoms of STIs or medication side effects. Patients prescribed CAB for PrEP should return for follow-up visits 1 month after the initial injection and then every 2 months. Recommendations for follow-up screening tests are provided in Tables 5 and 6.

Postexposure Prophylaxis of Human Immunodeficiency Virus Infection
The most effective means to prevent HIV infection include preventing exposure to the virus. In the event that an isolated occupational, sexual, or injection drug–related exposure occurs, postexposure prophylaxis (PEP) can be a second line of defense against HIV acquisition.

Occupational Exposure
Healthcare personnel include all paid and unpaid persons working in a healthcare setting with potential for exposure to infectious materials such as bodily fluids, contaminated medical supplies, or environmental surfaces. In the occupational setting, prevention of exposures to blood and bodily fluids from infected sources is the key to preventing occupationally acquired HIV infection. The overall risk of becoming infected with HIV after inadvertent exposure to body fluids from an HIV-infected patient is low. It is estimated that the average risk for HIV transmission following percutaneous exposure to HIV-infected blood is 0.3% and after mucous membrane exposure is 0.09%. The average risk of HIV transmission following nonintact skin exposure has not been defined; however, it is estimated to be lower than mucous membrane exposure. Healthcare personnel at the highest risk are those who received an accidental inoculation containing blood from a known HIV-infected source.

Initial Laboratory Evaluation
All patients initiating PEP after potential HIV exposure should be tested for HIV antigens and antibodies at baseline before PEP initiation. If baseline HIV testing indicates existing HIV infection, PEP should not be initiated. Repeat HIV testing should be performed at 4 to 6 weeks and 3 months following the exposure to determine if HIV infection has occurred. Administration of PEP should not be delayed while awaiting the results of HIV testing and can be discontinued if the source patient is found to not have HIV infection. PEP is most effective when taken as soon as possible following exposure.

Initiating Postexposure Prophylaxis/Choosing Appropriate Postexposure Prophylaxis Therapy
PEP is most effective when initiated as soon as possible following the exposure incident. If PEP is delayed, the effectiveness of therapy may be significantly reduced if initiated 72 hours or more following exposure. Initiating therapy after 72 hours might still be considered if the exposure is proven to be of an extremely high risk of transmission.

The current recommendation for PEP therapy is TDF/FTC (Truvada)[1] plus RAL (Isentress)[1] or DTG (Tivicay)[1] for 4 weeks. Overall, this regimen has acceptable tolerability, convenient dosing, and minimal drug interactions. In patients with significant underlying renal disease, an acceptable PEP alternative is zidovudine plus lamivudine (Combivir)[1] in addition to RAL or DTG.

---

[1] Not FDA approved for this indication.

[1] Not FDA approved for this indication.

PEP regimens include three (occasionally more) antiretroviral medications. Because of the potential for medication-related side effects, it is important to choose a PEP regimen with a lower toxicity profile to improve patient tolerance and encourage completion of PEP therapy.

HIV PEP should be offered to pregnant or breastfeeding healthcare providers based on the same criteria as any other provider with a similar exposure. Risk of HIV transmission from mother to child during acute HIV infection is increased during pregnancy and breastfeeding.

Additional resources regarding PEP are available (e.g., PEPline at https://nccc.ucsf.edu/clinician-consultation/pep-post-exposure-prophylaxis; 888-448-4911).

References

Baeten JM, Donnell D, Ndase P, et al: Antiretroviral prophylaxis for HIV prevention in heterosexual men and women, *N Engl J Med* 367(5):399–410, 2012.
Centers for Disease Control and Prevention: *HIV Surveillance Report*, vol.32. http://www.cdc.gov/hiv/library/reports/hiv-surveillance.html, 2019. Published May 2021.
Dominguez KL, Smith DK, Thomas V, et al: *Updated guidelines for antiretroviral postexposure prophylaxis after sexual, injection drug use, or other nonoccupational exposure to HIV-United States, centers for disease control and prevention*, U.S. Department of Health and Human Services, 2016.
Global UNAIDS: *AIDS Update*, 2021. https://www.unaids.org/sites/default/files/media_asset/2021-global-aids-update_en.pdf.
Grant RM, Lama JR, Anderson PL, et al: Preexposure chemoprophylaxis for HIV prevention in men who have sex with men, *N Engl J Med* 363(27):2587–2599, 2010.
Panel on Opportunistic Infections in Adults and Adolescents with HIV. Guidelines for the prevention and treatment of opportunistic infections in adults and adolescents with HIV: recommendations from the Centers for Disease Control and Prevention, the National Institutes of Health, and the HIV Medicine Association of the Infectious Diseases Society of America. Available at https://clinicalinfo.hiv.gov/sites/default/files/guidelines/documents/Adult_OI.pdf.
Kuhar DT, Henderson DK, Struble KA, et al: Updated US Public Health Service guidelines for the management of occupational exposures to human immuno- deficiency virus and recommendations for postexposure prophylaxis, *Infect Control Hosp Epidemiol* 34(9), 2013.
US Public Health Service: Preexposure prophylaxis for the prevention of HIV infection in the United States—2021. https://www.cdc.gov/hiv/pdf/risk/prep/cdc-hiv-prep-guidelines-2021.pdf.

INFECTIOUS MONONUCLEOSIS

Method of
Ben Z. Katz, MD

CURRENT DIAGNOSIS

- The classic triad of acute infectious mononucleosis consists of fever, lymphadenopathy, and pharyngitis.
- The diagnosis of infectious mononucleosis is usually based on the clinical picture, the presence of at least 10% atypical lymphocytes in the peripheral blood, and positive heterophil serology (monospot test).

CURRENT THERAPY

- In most patients, infectious mononucleosis is self-limited and requires only symptomatic treatment.
- Steroids and antiviral therapy have no place in the therapy of uncomplicated acute infectious mononucleosis in healthy persons.

Epidemiology and Risk Factors

One must distinguish between the epidemiology of Epstein-Barr virus (EBV) infection and that of infectious mononucleosis (IM), the most common symptomatic manifestation of primary EBV infection. Almost all adults have been infected with EBV. The symptomatology of primary EBV infection varies with the infected person's age at the time, with younger children usually having inapparent or mild infections. In developing countries and in lower socioeconomic groups in industrialized nations, up to 90% of children acquire primary EBV infection by 6 years of age, and IM almost never develops. In contrast, in higher socioeconomic groups, only 40% to 50% of adolescents have previously experienced EBV infection. From 10% to 20% of susceptible adolescents and adults contract EBV every year thereafter, with IM developing in about half of these patients.

Pathophysiology

Saliva is the main vehicle for transmission of EBV, a double-stranded DNA herpesvirus. Transmission usually requires direct and prolonged contact with infected oropharyngeal secretions, with salivary exchange being the main mode of transmission. The infection begins with viral replication in oropharyngeal epithelial cells and then spreads to local B lymphocytes, which then disseminate throughout the reticuloendothelial system and induce vigorous T- and NK-cell responses and neutralizing antibodies. The atypical lymphocytes that are produced are mainly suppressor T cells directed against EBV-infected B cells.

It is thought that most of the clinical manifestations of IM are due to these T- and NK-cell responses, which might explain why young children, whose immune responses are incompletely developed, are often asymptomatic with primary EBV infection. It is also possible that viral load determines symptomatology, and, because young adults likely spread more virus via salivary exchange than toddlers, young adults are more likely to be symptomatic. All EBV-seropositive persons shed virus in saliva intermittently throughout their lives. EBV may rarely be spread via blood transfusion or transplantation.

Clinical Manifestations

IM is usually an acute, self-limited, benign lymphoproliferative disease. EBV is responsible for nearly all heterophil-positive and most heterophil-negative cases. Other causes of heterophil-negative mononucleosis include cytomegalovirus, toxoplasmosis, hepatitis A and B, adenovirus, HIV, rubella, and human herpesvirus 6.

The classic triad of IM consists of fever, lymphadenopathy, and pharyngitis. Other typical findings include lymphocytosis with atypical lymphocytes and the presence of heterophil antibodies. After a 4- to 6-week incubation period, the illness begins with a 3- to 5-day prodrome of malaise, headache, and fatigue, typically followed in about half of the cases by onset of the triad. Additional symptoms can include anorexia, nausea, vomiting, periorbital or facial edema, and generalized lymphadenopathy, which is usually symmetrical. Splenomegaly occurs by the second or third week of illness in about half of all cases; rarely, splenic rupture can occur, which very rarely may be fatal. Hepatomegaly occurs in 10% to 15%, with clinical hepatitis occurring in about 5% of cases. Up to 20% of patients have a rash that may be erythematous, maculopapular, morbilliform, scarlatiniform, or urticarial, especially if ampicillin or one of its derivatives has been given to treat pharyngitis. Other symptoms can include arthritis and jaundice.

IM is a self-limited disease in nearly all patients. Median illness duration is 16 days.

Diagnosis

The diagnosis is usually based on the clinical picture, atypical lymphocytosis, and positive heterophil serology. Most adolescents and young adults with IM have most or all of these features, as well as an elevated white blood cell count with a relative lymphocytosis. Atypical lymphocytes generally represent more than 9% to 10% of the white blood cell count. Many infected persons also have mild thrombocytopenia and elevated hepatocellular enzymes. Heterophil antibody positivity is usually measured as a positive monospot test. If IM is suspected and heterophil antibodies are negative, specific titers for EBV, including viral capsid antigen (VCA) IgM and IgG, early antigen (EA), and Epstein–Barr nuclear antigen (EBNA), should be obtained, as well as serologic testing for cytomegalovirus

(CMV) and toxoplasmosis, the two most. common causes of heterophil-negative infectious mononucleosis. Acute EBV infection is characterized by the presence of IgM and IgG VCA antibodies and EA antibodies and the absence of EBNA antibodies.

Differential Diagnosis

If liver chemistry values are markedly elevated and antibodies against EBV, CMV, and toxoplasmosis are unrevealing, serology for hepatitis A, B, and C should be measured. If risk factors are present, HIV antibodies should be checked. A throat culture is indicated in patients with pharyngitis or tonsillitis because the tonsillitis of acute IM can be indistinguishable from that of group A streptococcal pharyngitis.

Treatment

In most patients, IM is self-limited and requires only symptomatic treatment, including bed rest, acetaminophen (Tylenol, 10–15 mg/kg every 4–6 hours), aspirin (10–15 mg/kg every 4–6 hours), or nonsteroidal antiinflammatory agents such as ibuprofen (Advil, 5–10 mg/kg every 6–8 hours). Saline gargles can be useful in treating a sore throat. In severe cases, meperidine (Demerol, 1–1.5 mg/kg every 3–4 hours) may be required.

Although a short, tapering course of corticosteroid therapy (e.g., a Medrol Dosepak[1]) is often prescribed, there is little evidence for its clinical efficacy, and caution is warranted. Infection is ultimately self-limited in nearly all cases, and rare reports of neurologic or septicemic complications after steroid use have appeared. Long-term immune responses following steroid use appear to be normal. Corticosteroid therapy should, however, be considered for the treatment of severe cases of IM associated with hemolysis, respiratory embarrassment, or thrombocytopenic purpura. The use of corticosteroids in atypical or antibody-negative cases is inappropriate because the diagnosis of lymphoma can then be confounded.

Parenteral administration of acyclovir[1] (Zovirax, 10–20 mg/kg IV every 8 hours) to patients with acute IM secondary to EBV reduces the level of oropharyngeal viral replication; however, replication returns to the previously high levels after cessation of treatment, and the drug has little or no effect on the clinical course. Acyclovir administered in high doses orally (20 mg/kg, maximum dose of 800 mg qid for 5 days) is also ineffective. Antiviral therapy is therefore not recommended for acute IM in a normal host.

In immunosuppressed or severely ill patients, however, specific therapy has a role in many cases. For example, etoposide (VePesid)[1], a drug that reduces macrophage activation, is often used in cases of infection-associated hemophagocytic syndrome. In posttransplant lymphoproliferative disorders, first-line therapy is often a reduction in immunosuppression; other options include rituximab[1] (Rituxan, 375 mg/m² IV weekly for 4 weeks). Oral leukoplakia in patients with AIDS responds to oral acyclovir[1] (20 mg/kg, maximum dose of 800 mg qid for 20 days), whereas a tapering course of steroids (as recommended earlier) may be used for lymphocytic interstitial pneumonitis (see below).

Monitoring

Quarantine is not indicated. Ampicillin and related drugs should be avoided when treating secondary bacterial complications because of their association with rash in persons with IM. Contact sports should be avoided as long as splenomegaly is still evident because of the rare possibility of splenic rupture, which usually occurs within 3 weeks of onset of IM but has been reported as late as 7 to 10 weeks into the illness.

Complications

Complications of acute IM can be neurologic (seizures, cranial nerve palsies, aseptic meningitis, encephalitis, optic neuritis, transverse myelitis, infectious polyneuritis [Guillain-Barré syndrome],

[1]Not FDA approved for this indication.

psychosis, Alice in Wonderland syndrome, or acute cerebellar ataxia), hematologic (hemolytic or aplastic anemia, thrombocytopenic purpura, agranulocytosis, or agammaglobulinemia), cardiac (pericarditis or myocarditis), pulmonary (cough or atypical pneumonia), renal (glomerulonephritis, acute kidney failure, or acute interstitial nephritis), or ophthalmologic (conjunctivitis) in nature. In about 10% of adolescents and young adults, fatigue can persist for 6 months or longer, and many of these patients meet the criteria for chronic fatigue syndrome. Young adults with more severe acute IM and certain predisposing gastrointestinal symptoms and laboratory findings are more likely to meet criteria for chronic fatigue syndrome 6 months later.

Rare patients have very high titers of EBV antibodies, and a chronic active EBV infection associated with unusual clinical manifestations such as uveitis or lymphoma can occur. EBV is also associated with lymphoproliferative disorders in persons with underlying abnormal immune systems. These include X-linked lymphoproliferative syndrome, in which affected males usually die of acute EBV infection, and the related infection-associated hemophagocytic syndrome, which is most commonly (about 75% of the time) triggered by EBV and seems to be due to an overly exuberant macrophage response to EBV-infected lymphocytes. Transplant recipients can acquire EBV-associated lymphoproliferative disease that can range from asymptomatic infection to fatal IM or lymphoma. Finally, although not seen much anymore due to combination antiretroviral therapy, patients with AIDS are susceptible to several serious complications of EBV infection, including lymphocytic interstitial pneumonitis, oral leukoplakia, leiomyosarcoma, and lymphoma.

References

Candy B, Hotopf M: Steroids for symptom control in infectious mononucleosis, *Cochrane Database Syst Rev*(3)CD004402, 2006.
Cohen JI, Jaffe ES, Dale JK, et al: Characterization and treatment of chronic active Epstein–Barr virus disease: A 28-year experience in the United States, *Blood* 117:5835–5849, 2011.
Jason LA, Cotler J, Islam MF, Sunnquist M, Katz BZ. Risks for developing ME/CFS in college students following infectious mononucleosis: a prospective cohort study. *Clin Infect Dis* 73:e3740-6, 2021.
Katz BZ: Commentary on "Steroids for symptom control in infectious mononucleosis (Review)" by B Candy and M Hotopf, *Evid Based Child Health* 7:447–449, 2012.
Katz BZ, Reuter C, Lupovitch Y, Gleason Y, McClellan D, Cotler J, Jason LA: A validated scale for assessing the severity of acute infectious mononucleosis, *J Pediatr* 209:130–133, 2019.
Odumade OA, Hogquist KA, Balfour Jr HH: Progress and problems in understanding and managing primary Epstein- Barr virus infections, *Clin Microbiol Rev* 24(1):193–209, 2011.
Rouphael N, Talati NJ, Vaughan C, et al: Infections associated with haemophagocytic syndrome, *Lancet Infect Dis* 7:814–822, 2007.
Soltys K, Green M: Posttransplant lymphoproliferative disease, *Pediatr Infect Dis J* 24:1107–1108, 2005.

INFLUENZA

Method of
Jeffrey A. Linder, MD, MPH

CURRENT DIAGNOSIS

- Influenza should be considered in any patient with respiratory symptoms between October and May in North America.
- The single most important piece of information when considering a diagnosis of influenza is the community prevalence of influenza.
- During influenza outbreaks, sudden onset of fever and cough has a positive predictive value of about 85%.
- Rapid testing should be done with molecular tests (e.g., reverse transcriptase polymerase chain reaction [RT-PCR]), which have a high sensitivity and specificity.

CURRENT THERAPY

- The influenza vaccine is the best means of preventing influenza. The inactivated influenza vaccine is recommended for all persons age 6 months and older.
- Influenza vaccination should be prioritized for essential workers and people at high-risk for influenza or COVID-19 complications.
- The antivirals zanamivir (Relenza) and oseltamivir (Tamiflu) can be used for prophylaxis of influenza in unimmunized patients, in close contacts of infected patients, and during institutional outbreaks of influenza.
- Early antiviral treatment should not be delayed and should be used for patients who are hospitalized; have severe, complicated, or progressive illness; or are at higher risk for complications.
- Antivirals may be prescribed within 48 hours of symptom onset for outpatients not at higher risk for influenza complications.

BOX 1   Influenza Vaccine Recommendations.

- All persons aged ≥6 months should be vaccinated annually
- Vaccination efforts should prioritize essential workers and people at higher risk of influenza and COVID-19 complications:
  - Age 6 months to 5 years
  - Age ≥50 years
  - Chronic pulmonary (including asthma), cardiovascular (except hypertension), renal, hepatic, neurologic, hematologic, or metabolic (including diabetes mellitus) disorders
  - Immunosuppressed
  - Pregnant during the influenza season
  - Age 6 months to 18 years old receiving long-term aspirin therapy and who therefore might be at risk for Reye syndrome
  - Residents of nursing homes and other long-term care facilities
  - American Indians/Alaska Natives
  - Morbidly obese (body mass index ≥40)
- Vaccination efforts should also prioritize those likely to transmit influenza to higher risk people:
  - Healthcare personnel
  - Household contacts and caregivers of children aged <5 years and adults aged ≥50 years, with particular emphasis on vaccinating contacts of children aged <6 months
  - Household contacts and caregivers of persons with medical conditions that put them at higher risk for severe complications from influenza

---

Influenza is a highly contagious viral infection that should be considered in any patient with respiratory symptoms between October and May in North America. Influenza infects 5% to 20% of the population of the United States in a typical year, sickens 3% to 11% of Americans, and is responsible for up to 810,000 hospitalizations and 61,000 deaths per year. Influenza can range in severity from mild illness to life-threatening disease. Those at highest risk of hospitalization, death, or complications from influenza are children younger than 2 years old, adults older than 65 years, people of any age who have underlying medical conditions or immune compromise, and pregnant women.

Information about influenza changes rapidly. Emergence of severe acute respiratory syndrome coronavirus 2 (SARS-CoV-2) and associated coronavirus disease 2019 (COVID-19) has complicated influenza diagnosis and management. To care optimally for patients with influenza-like illness during the influenza season, clinicians need to keep abreast of updated recommendations and the current prevalence of influenza and COVID-19 in their community. The influenza vaccine remains the best means of reducing the incidence, severity, and complications from influenza, but antiviral medications and symptomatic treatments have an important role in the prevention and treatment of influenza (Box 1).

Microbiology

There are two types of influenza viruses, A and B. Influenza A is separated into subtypes based on two surface antigens: hemagglutinin (H) and neuraminidase (N). The predominant circulating strains of influenza in recent decades have been influenza A (H1N1), influenza A (H3N2), and influenza B. Influenza A (H3N2) subtypes generally cause more severe influenza and are associated with higher mortality than other types. Influenza viruses undergo slight genetic changes from year to year, termed *antigenic drift*. Major changes in surface glycoproteins are termed *antigenic shift* and can result in severe pandemic influenza in a nonimmune population, which happened with an antigenically novel influenza A (H1N1) virus in 2009. Because of antigenic drift, and because immunity to a given type or subtype of influenza provides limited cross-immunity to other types and subtypes, the influenza vaccine needs to be reformulated and administered most years.

Patients contract influenza by being exposed to small- and large-sized respiratory droplets and aerosols from an infected person or contact with surfaces harboring influenza virus. Influenza has a latency of 1 to 4 days before the onset of symptoms. Adults are infectious from the day before symptom onset through approximately day 7 of illness, but immunosuppressed adults and children shed the virus for longer periods. Symptoms generally last from 7 to 14 days.

Beyond the emergence of SARS-CoV-2 in 2019, several other novel, highly pathogenic respiratory viruses—avian influenza A (H5N1), avian influenza A (H7N9), and Middle East respiratory syndrome coronavirus (MERS-CoV)—have case-fatality rates ranging from 35% to 53%. Collectively there have been more than 5000 human cases. These pathogens, if they acquire the ability to be highly transmissible between humans, have the potential to cause pandemic respiratory disease.

Prevention

Influenza vaccination is between 20% and 90% effective in preventing influenza or complications of influenza. Influenza vaccination is highly cost-effective and can even be cost-saving in high-risk groups. Influenza vaccination is less effective in younger children, in adults older than 65 years, in adults with comorbid conditions, and when there is a poor match between the influenza vaccine and circulating influenza. The Centers for Disease Control and Prevention (CDC) Advisory Committee on Immunization Practices puts out annual recommendations and supplementary updates on the prevention and treatment of influenza (www.cdc.gov/flu). The Advisory Committee on Immunization Practices recommends vaccinating all persons 6 months of age and older.

At present in the United States, there are three commonly administered, recommended types of influenza vaccine: quadrivalent inactivated influenza vaccine (IIV4), quadrivalent recombinant influenza vaccine (RIV4), and quadrivalent live attenuated influenza vaccine (LAIV4). The IIV4 (Afluria Quadrivalent, Fluarix Quadrivalent, FluLaval Quadrivalent, Fluzone Quadrivalent, Flucelvax Quadrivalent, Fluzone High-Dose, Fluad Quadrivalent), adjuvant IV3 (Fluad), and RIV4 (Flublok Quadrivalent) vaccines are administered as an intramuscular injection.

Different products are approved for administration in different lower age limits. A high-dose IIV4 (Fluzone High-Dose Quadrivalent) and an adjuvanted IIV4 (Fluad Quadrivalent) are available for patients aged 65 years or older, who are less likely to respond immunologically to standard inactivated influenza vaccine (IIV). The RIV4 (Flublok Quadrivalent) is only licensed for persons age 18 years or older. The main adverse effect of the IIV is soreness at the injection site. Patients often report a mild immune response of fever, malaise, myalgia, and headache that can last for 1 to 2 days, but rates of most of these symptoms are no different from those in patients who receive placebo injection.

Allergic reactions to egg proteins or other vaccine components (e.g., antibiotics and inactivating compounds) include hives, angioedema, asthma, and anaphylaxis. For patients with egg allergy who have only hives, any otherwise appropriate IIV or RIV can be administered. For patients with more severe reactions to egg or who received treatment for an allergic reaction can also receive any recommended IIV or RIV in an inpatient or outpatient medical setting and observed for at least 15 minutes by a clinician able to recognize and manage severe allergic reactions. The recombinant influenza vaccine (RIV4; FluBlok Quadrivalent) and cell culture derived quadrivalent (ccIIV4; Flucelvax, Quadrivalent) are considered egg free, but patients who had a severe allergic reaction to a previous dose of an egg-based vaccine should receive ccIIV4 or RIV4 in a supervised inpatient or outpatient setting. Patients who have had severe allergic reaction to influenza vaccine should not receive the vaccine.

Vaccination should be deferred in patients with confirmed or suspected COVID-19 or with any acute febrile illness, but patients with more moderate illness can be vaccinated. Guillain-Barré syndrome was associated with the 1976 swine flu vaccine, but there is no consistent evidence that modern influenza vaccines are associated with Guillain-Barré syndrome.

The LAIV4 (FluMist Quadrivalent) is administered as a nasal spray and is approved for patients ages 2 to 49 years. The LAIV4 is contraindicated in children aged 2 to 4 years with recurrent wheezing or asthma; children who are receiving aspirin or aspirin-containing products; patients with comorbid conditions or immunosuppression; pregnant women; family members or close contacts of severely immunosuppressed patients, who require a protected environment (e.g., hematopoietic stem cell transplant recipients); cerebrospinal leak or cochlear implants; and receipt of oseltamivir (Tamiflu) or zanamivir (Relenza) in the previous 48 hours, peramivir (Rapivab) in the previous 5 days, or baloxavir (Xofluza) in the previous 17 days. The LAIV4 should not be administered to those with severe nasal congestion. Adverse effects of the LAIV4 include runny nose, nasal congestion, headache, sore throat, chills, and tiredness, although these are only slightly more common than in patients receiving placebo. Those receiving the LAIV4 should avoid contact with severely immunosuppressed persons for 7 days.

Patients should be vaccinated in the fall when the seasonal vaccine becomes available, ideally before the end of October. In the event of vaccine shortages, higher-risk patients should receive priority (see Box 1). Patients should continue to be vaccinated until February and beyond because in the majority of recent influenza seasons the peak has been February or later. Children 6 months to 8 years of age who have not been previously immunized against influenza should be given two doses separated by at least 4 weeks.

Evaluation

Community Prevalence of Influenza

In caring for a patient with suspected influenza, the single most important piece of data is the community prevalence of influenza among patients with influenza-like illness. This ranges from near 0% during summer months to approximately 30% during a typical influenza seasonal peak. The prevalence may be higher during a particularly severe outbreak. In the United States clinicians can check the local prevalence of influenza and COVID-19 among patients with influenza-like illness through the CDC (www.cdc.gov/flu) and their state department of public health.

History and Physical Examination

Beyond the local prevalence of influenza, the diagnosis of influenza rests on the patient's history. All methods of diagnosing influenza—symptom complexes, clinician judgment, and testing—generally are highly specific but have poor sensitivity. Thus it is important to consider a diagnosis of influenza in any patient with respiratory symptoms during influenza season. Influenza is classically described as the very sudden onset of fever, headache, sore throat, myalgias, cough, and nasal symptoms. Children can also have otitis media, nausea, and vomiting. In differentiating influenza from nonspecific upper respiratory tract infections, it is most useful to consider the circulating prevalence of influenza, the abruptness of onset, and the severity of symptoms. Although COVID-19 and influenza symptoms overlap, COVID-19 may be more likely to include more profound shortness of breath, loss of taste or smell, nausea, vomiting, or diarrhea.

Certain symptom complexes have been shown in trials of antiviral treatment to strongly suggest influenza. For example, in an area with circulating influenza, prior to the emergence of SARS-CoV-2, the acute onset of cough and fever had a positive predictive value as high as 85%. Other studies have shown that clinician judgment performed as well as or better than hard-and-fast symptom complexes or rapid testing.

The physical examination in influenza primarily serves to identify the severity of influenza, complications, and worsening of underlying medical conditions. Clinicians should record vital signs and perform examinations of the ears, nose, sinuses, throat, neck, lungs, and heart for all patients suspected of having influenza.

Testing

Testing may not be required to make a diagnosis of influenza, but can help differentiate influenza from other respiratory viruses. Treatment for patients at high risk for influenza complications should not wait for test results. Testing may also help inform antiviral use, antibiotic prescribing, site-of-care decisions, and infection control measures. Specimens (nasopharyngeal swab, nasal swab, nasal wash, or nasal aspirate, depending on the particular test) should ideally be collected within 3 to 4 days of symptom onset.

Molecular assays such as reverse transcriptase polymerase chain reaction (RT-PCR) testing are highly sensitive (90% to 95%) and specific. Some can produce results in 15 to 45 minutes, and some can differentiate influenza types and subtypes. RT-PCR should be considered for hospitalized patients, institutional outbreaks, or other situations when clinicians are concerned about false-negative rapid test results. Other nucleic acid amplification tests, which can differentiate influenza from other respiratory pathogens, are becoming more available. The CDC recommends that all hospitalized patients with suspected influenza be tested with a high-sensitivity, high-specificity molecular assay.

Rapid influenza diagnostic tests (RIDTs) are much less sensitive (50% to 70%) and somewhat less specific (90%) than molecular tests. Negative results do not exclude the possibility of influenza, especially if the circulating prevalence of influenza is high (>30%). Some RIDTs can distinguish influenza A from influenza B and can provide a point-of-care result in less than 15 minutes.

In the event of a high prevalence of influenza or a high risk of complications from influenza, empiric antiviral treatment is indicated. Testing may be particularly helpful for hospitalized patients to rule out a need for antibiotics, but antiinfluenza treatment should not be withheld solely on the basis of a negative test result. Chest radiography, cultures, and blood tests are not routinely indicated, but they should be obtained for patients with suspected pneumonia or to identify other suspected complications.

Complications

Complications of influenza include primary complications, suppurative complications, and worsening of comorbid conditions. Primary complications of influenza include viral pneumonia, which is a

TABLE 1 Antiviral Agents for the Treatment and Prophylaxis of Influenza.

ANTIVIRAL AGENT	TREATMENT*		PROPHYLAXIS†		COMMENTS
	CHILDREN	ADULTS	CHILDREN	ADULTS	
Oseltamivir (Tamiflu)	Any age‡ Dose for 5 days bid: <1 year: 3 mg/kg per dose; ≤15 kg: 30 mg; 16–23 kg: 45 mg; 24–40 kg: 60 mg; >40 kg: 75 mg	75 mg PO bid for 5 days	3 months to 1 year: 3 mg/kg/day‡ Dose qd: ≤15 kg: 30 mg; 16–23 kg: 45 mg; 24–40 kg: 60 mg; >40 kg: 75 mg	75 mg PO qd	For patients with creatinine clearance < 30 mL/min, oseltamivir adult dosing should be reduced to 30 mg qd for treatment and to 30 mg qod for prophylaxis
Zanamivir (Relenza)	Approved for children ≥7 years; 10 mg (2 inhalations) bid for 5 days	10 mg (2 inhalations) bid for 5 days	Approved for children ≥5 years; 10 mg (2 inhalations) qd	10 mg (2 inhalations) qd	Avoid in patients with chronic lung disease (e.g., asthma, chronic obstructive pulmonary disease)
Peramivir (Rapivab)	≥6 months: One 12-mg/kg dose, up to 600 mg maximum IV over minimum 15 min	≥13 years: One 600-mg IV dose over a minimum of 15 min	NA	NA	For patients with creatinine clearance 30–49 mL/min, the dose should be reduced to 200 mg; For patients with creatinine clearance 10–29 mL/min, the dose should be reduced to 100 mg
Baloxavir (Xofluza)	≥12 years: <80 kg: one 40-mg dose; ≥80 kg: one 80-mg dose	<80 kg: one 40-mg dose; ≥80 kg: one 80-mg dose	≥12 years: <80 kg: one 40 mg dose ≥80 kg: one 80 mg dose	<80 kg: one 40-mg dose; ≥80 kg: one 80-mg dose	For patients within 2 days of illness onset. Avoid in pregnant women or breastfeeding mothers

*Suspected or confirmed influenza among persons with severe influenza or for persons at higher risk for influenza complications up to 5 days after symptom onset. For outpatients not at higher risk for influenza complications, treatment should be started within 48 hours of symptom onset.
†Prophylaxis should be given for 7 days after last known exposure and for institutional outbreaks for at least 2 weeks or until 1 week after the end of the outbreak.
‡Oseltamivir is approved by the US Food and Drug Administration for treatment in children 14 days and older and prophylaxis in children 1 year and older. Treatment in children <14 days old and prophylaxis in children <1 year old is recommended by the Centers for Disease Control and Prevention and the American Academy of Pediatrics.
IV, Intravenous; *NA*, not approved; *PO*, per os (orally).
Adapted from Centers for Disease Control and Prevention. Influenza Antiviral Medications: Summary for Clinicians. Available at https://www.cdc.gov/flu/professionals/antivirals/index.htm (accessed July 7, 2022).

VIII Infectious Diseases

644

feared complication and is likely a main cause of death in pandemic influenza. Other, less common primary complications of influenza include myositis and rhabdomyolysis, Reye syndrome, myocarditis, pericarditis, toxic shock syndrome, and central nervous system disease (e.g., encephalitis, transverse myelitis, and aseptic meningitis). Children can have a severe course with influenza, including signs and symptoms of sepsis along with febrile seizures. Suppurative complications of influenza include bacterial pneumonia, otitis media, and sinusitis. Influenza can cause worsening of comorbid conditions such as asthma, chronic obstructive pulmonary disease, congestive heart failure, and chronic kidney disease.

Chemoprophylaxis

Antiviral medications can be used to prevent influenza in patients who did not receive the influenza vaccine, cannot receive the influenza vaccine, received the vaccine in the prior 2 weeks (before reliable immunity develops), or in the event of poor matching between vaccine and circulating influenza strains (Table 1). Chemoprophylaxis should also be considered for close contacts of patients with confirmed influenza or for patients with immune deficiency who are unlikely to respond to the influenza vaccine but who are at high risk for having complications from influenza (see Box 1).

Amantadine (Symmetrel) and rimantadine (Flumadine) are not recommended for chemoprophylaxis or treatment because of a high prevalence of resistant influenza A strains. The neuraminidase inhibitors oseltamivir (Tamiflu), and zanamivir (Relenza) are approximately 80% effective in preventing influenza in household contacts of persons with influenza, and more than 90% effective

in preventing influenza in institutional settings. Chemoprophylaxis should be taken for 7 days after last known exposure. For hospital or long-term care facility outbreaks, chemoprophylaxis should be taken and for a minimum of 2 weeks or until 1 week after the end of the outbreak. For patients allergic to or unable to respond to the vaccine, chemoprophylaxis should be used for the duration of circulating influenza. The IIV can be given to patients receiving chemoprophylaxis. The LAIV should not be given from 2 days before to 14 days after taking an antiviral medication. Patients who receive the LAIV in this window should be revaccinated at a later date.

Treatment

The influenza vaccine is the best means of reducing influenza-related morbidity and mortality, but its limitations include production problems, low vaccination rates, and variable effectiveness. Given these limitations, there is an important role in management for influenza-specific antiviral medications (see Table 1). Antiviral medications reduce the duration of influenza symptoms by approximately 1 day, reduce complications requiring antibiotics by 30% to 50%, might decrease hospitalizations, decrease mortality among hospitalized patients, and are cost-effective. Early antiviral treatment, which should not wait for test results, starting up to 5 days after symptom onset can reduce complications for patients who are hospitalized; have severe, complicated, or progressive illness; or are at higher risk for complications (see Box 1). For outpatients not at higher risk for complications, antiviral treatment must be started within 48 hours of symptom onset.

Oseltamivir (Tamiflu) is taken as a capsule or oral suspension. The dose of oseltamivir should be reduced in patients with renal disease. Adverse effects of oseltamivir include nausea, vomiting, and perhaps behavioral changes. Oseltamivir, oral or enterically administered, is the drug of choice for hospitalized patients and those with severe illness. Zanamivir (Relenza) is taken as an oral inhaled powder and is not recommended for patients with underlying lung or heart disease. Adverse effects of zanamivir include worsening of underlying lung disease and allergic reactions. Amantadine and rimantadine are not recommended because of a high prevalence of resistant influenza A strains.

Peramivir (Rapivab), an intravenous neuraminidase inhibitor, was approved in the United State in December 2014 for patients within 48 hours of symptom onset. Peramivir has been associated with diarrhea, rashes including Stevens-Johnson syndrome, and neuropsychiatric changes.

Baloxavir (Xofluza), a cap-dependent endonuclease inhibitor, is active against both influenza A and B. Baloxavir has been associated with diarrhea. It has the advantage of requiring only one dose.

Antibiotics are generally not necessary, but they should be prescribed to treat suppurative complications of influenza. Antitussives such as guaifenesin with codeine (Robitussin AC) help coughing patients to sleep at night. β-Agonists, such as albuterol (Proventil)[1], can help patients with cough, especially if there is wheezing on examination. Analgesics and antipyretics such as acetaminophen (Tylenol) and ibuprofen (Motrin) reduce fever and generally help patients to feel better. Patients should be encouraged to rest and drink plenty of fluids.

Patients with suspected influenza should minimize contact with others to avoid spreading the infection. Use of face masks and hand hygiene can reduce the transmission of influenza.

---

[1]Not FDA approved for this indication.

References

Centers for Disease Control and Prevention: Influenza (Flu): information for health professionals, http://www.cdc.gov/flu/professionals/index.htm. Accessed 7 July 2022.

Ebell MH, Afonso AM, Gonzales R, et al: Development and validation of a clinical decision rule for the diagnosis of influenza, *J Am Board Fam Med* 25:55–62, 2012.

Falsey AR, Murata Y, Walsh EE: Impact of rapid diagnosis on management of adults hospitalized with influenza, *Arch Intern Med* 167:354–360, 2007.

Grohskopf LA, Alyanak E, Ferdinands JM, et al: Prevention and control of seasonal influenza with vaccines: Recommendations of the Advisory Committee on Immunization Practices — United States, 2021–22 Influenza Season, *MMWR Recomm Rep* 2021;70(No. RR-5):1–28. DOI: http://dx.doi.org/10.15585/mmwr.rr7005a1.

Tokars JI, Olsen SJ, Reed C: Seasonal incidence of symptomatic influenza in the United States, *Clin Infect Dis* 66:1511–1518, 2018.

LEISHMANIASIS

Method of
Carol Shetty, MD

CURRENT DIAGNOSIS

- Leishmaniasis is diagnosed through direct identification from tissue samples through Giemsa staining, culture, or detection of DNA through PCR.
- For cutaneous and mucocutaneous disease, tissue samples are obtained via scraping or biopsy; for visceral disease, aspirate or biopsy specimens are obtained from the spleen, bone marrow, liver, or enlarged lymph nodes.
- When definitive diagnosis cannot be made from tissue sampling, serologic studies can aid with diagnosis, but are frequently negative.

CURRENT THERAPY

- Simple cutaneous leishmaniasis can be monitored without treatment, or treated with local therapies, including heat therapy, cryotherapy with liquid nitrogen, topical ointments and creams containing paromomycin,[1] intralesional injection of pentavalent antimonial drugs, and laser treatments.
- Complex cutaneous and visceral leishmaniasis are treated with a limited number of highly toxic drugs:
  - Intravenous liposomal amphotericin B (AmBisome), which is highly effective and nontoxic, is the gold standard treatment for leishmaniasis, but its high cost precludes use in developing countries. It is the preferred treatment in pregnancy and does not have known teratogenic effects.
  - Amphotericin B deoxycholate (Fungizone) can be used to treat infections resistant to pentavalent antimonials,[1] but results in infusion-related side effects and delayed side effects.
  - The pentavalent antimonials, sodium stibogluconate (Pentostam)[10] and meglumine antimoniate (Glucantime),[2] are the most commonly used therapies because of availability. Pentavalent antimonials have a dose-dependent toxicity that includes anorexia, pancreatitis, and QT prolongation.
- Second line medications:
  - Pentamidine isethionate (Pentam 300)[1] is a highly toxic therapy used for treatment-resistant forms of cutaneous leishmaniasis.
  - Paromomycin sulfate[1] is an aminoglycoside that can be used as an alternative treatment of visceral leishmaniasis in the Indian subcontinent and resource-limited settings.
- Oral medications:
  - Miltefosine (Impavido) is the first recognized oral treatment for systemic leishmaniasis. It does not require hospitalization for administration and generally has mild side effects.
  - Azole medications have also been used, but evidence is insufficient to support their use alone in the treatment of leishmaniasis.

[1]Not FDA approved for this indication.
[2]Not available in the United States.
[10]Available in the United States from the Centers for Disease Control and Prevention.

Leishmaniasis comprises a spectrum of diseases caused by intracellular protozoan parasites from the genus *Leishmania* that infect humans and other mammals. In humans, *Leishmania* parasites cause three main clinical syndromes: visceral leishmaniasis (VL), also known as kala-azar; cutaneous leishmaniasis (CL), and mucosal leishmaniasis (MCL).

Epidemiology

Over 20 species of *Leishmania* cause disease in humans. *Leishmania* parasites are transmitted by the bite of the female phlebotomine sand fly, an important vector in a variety of transmissible diseases. *Leishmania* are found in 98 countries in a wide geographic distribution in Central and South America, Southern Europe, Africa, the Middle East, and Asia. Forms of CL and VL are endemic variably across this geographic distribution, with the Middle East, Mediterranean basin, Central and South America, and Central Asia accounting for 95% of CL cases, and most cases of VL occurring in Brazil, East Africa, and India.

The species responsible for causing VL are *Leishmania donovani* in South Asia and East Africa and *L. infantum* (*L. chagasi*) in the Mediterranean basin, Central Asia, and Latin America. CL and MCL are caused by several species of *Leishmania*, the most common being *L. major* and *L. tropica* in Europe, Africa, and Asia and *L. mexicana*, *L. braziliensis*, *L. amazonensis*, *L. panamensis*, *L. guyanensis*, and *L. peruviana* in the Americas.

Transmission of leishmaniasis can be zoonotic (transmission from animal to vector to human) or anthroponotic (transmission from human to vector to human).

Leishmaniasis has a growing global burden of disease with an estimated global annual incidence of approximately 657,000; growing prevalence of 4.6 million and disability-adjusted life-years burden of 697,000. It is considered one of the 20 neglected tropical disease by the World Health Organization (WHO), with current efforts to optimize treatment for children given a high burden of pediatric disease. The WHO South-East Asia region is the only region to have developed a regional strategic framework to eliminate VL between 2022 and 2026.

Risk Factors

Risk factors for leishmaniasis are primarily associated with human exposure within the geographic distribution of the phlebotomine sand flies and factors that aid in transmission. In Europe, Africa, and Asia, colonization and urbanization have been identified as the major risk factors for outbreaks of CL, with crowded and unsanitary housing conditions serving as a breeding ground for sand flies. In the Americas, activities that disturb sandfly habitats such as deforestation, mining, building of infrastructure such as roads, and tourism have led to human outbreaks of leishmaniasis with species previously affecting animals. Climate change has led to changes in temperature and rainfall that have increased the geographic range of phlebotomine sand flies, leading to increased global spread of leishmaniasis. Poverty and crowded living conditions are significant risk factors for leishmaniasis. Conflict and civil and political unrest are associated with increased incidence of leishmaniasis through displacement of populations and health system decline.

In most immunocompetent individuals, infection with VL typically does not lead to clinical symptoms. However, infants younger than 2 years and malnourished or severely immuno-compromised individuals are at risk for developing acute VL when exposed to the infection. People living with human immunodeficiency virus (HIV) who are coinfected with leishmaniasis are at high risk from developing severe infection with poor outcomes. Immunosuppressive medications, hematologic malignancies, and cirrhosis have also been noted to lead to poorer clinical outcomes.

Pathophysiology

There are two main forms of the *Leishmania* parasite. Within the phlebotomine sand fly, *Leishmania* exist as extracellular, flagellated promastigotes, and within mammalian host cells they are obligate intracellular nonflagellated amastigotes. *Leishmania* are inoculated to skin cells by the bite of the phlebotomine sand fly in their flagellated (promastigote) form (Figure 1). The promastigotes are then recognized by several types of receptors and ingested into resident macrophages, monocytes, neutrophils, and dendritic cells. The main factor in the virulence of *Leishmania* is an abundant surface of the glycoconjugate lipophosphoglycan. On entering the cell, the promastigotes transform into amastigotes, using hydrolases to acidify the pH and selectively inhibiting production of reactive oxygen species to promote their survival within the phagocyte of the cell. The host's immune response controls how the parasites multiply, infect new cells, and spread to other tissues. Most mammalian hosts are asymptomatic because of control of *Leishmaniasis* infection, which is characterized with a robust cellular immune response driven by production of interleukin-12 (IL-12). In contrast, manifestation of acute or chronic disease is associated with the absence of a robust cellular immune response and high levels of nonprotective serum antibodies, which is often characterized by high levels of IL-10 production. A balance between Th1 and Th2 cytokine secretion is important for controlling the infection, with exaggerated response of either helper T cell 1 (Th1) or Th2 leading to more severe disease.

Prevention

Despite promising work with leishmaniasis vaccines, there are currently no human vaccines available for the immune protection against leishmaniasis. There are three main vaccine candidates in clinical trials, two of which are in late preclinical trials (mRNA vaccine LEISH F2/F3 and live attenuated vaccine LmCen$^{-/-}$) and one of which is currently in phase II (therapeutic) trials (viral vector vaccine ChAd63-KH) (Figure 2). Therefore, prevention of contraction of leishmaniasis primarily consists of measures to prevent sand fly bites through the use of insect repellants, insecticide-impregnated bed nets and reservoir control within communities. Phlebotomine sand fly bites cannot penetrate through clothing, thus protective clothing is effective at prevention. Recent examples of interventions designed to reduce zoonotic transmission of leishmaniasis include extermination of rodent populations living near urban dwellings and interventions to reduce canine infections. Early diagnosis and treatment of leishmaniasis aids in epidemiologic control.

Clinical Manifestations

Visceral Leishmaniasis

VL, also known as kala-azar ("black fever" in Hindi), is the most severe form of leishmaniasis. When left untreated, symptomatic VL is 100% fatal. However, only a small fraction of those infected with parasites causing VL will show clinical manifestations (ratio ranging from 4:1 to 50:1 depending on parasite virulence and human living conditions). The classic manifestation of VL is known as kala-azar and manifests as slow progression of fever, malaise, weight loss, and hard splenomegaly (with hepatomegaly less common). The incubation period is typically 4 to 6 months but can range from a few weeks to several years. In VL, *Leishmania* parasites replicate within phagocytes of the reticuloendothelial system. Accumulation of parasites in the spleen, liver, and bone marrow result in severe anemia, hemolysis, and splenic sequestration. Laboratory manifestations include anemia and pancytopenia, renal impairment, hypergammaglobulinemia, and elevated liver enzymes and bilirubin later in the disease course. Advanced disease is marked by profound weight loss, hypoalbuminemia, edema, and hepatic dysfunction with resulting jaundice and ascites.

Post Kala-azar Dermal Leishmaniasis

Post–Kala-azar dermal leishmaniasis (PKDL) is a complication of VL on the skin that manifests years after treatment, especially in East Africa and South Asia. In East Africa, PKDL typically manifests as hypomelanotic macules, whereas in South Asia it manifests as polymorphic maculopapulonodular lesions (Figure 3).

Cutaneous Leishmaniasis

Leishmania parasites cause a spectrum of cutaneous manifestations. The most common clinical manifestation is localized CL, which results from multiplication of *Leishmania* within phagocytes of the skin cells. CL lesions classically appear as pink papules on exposed areas of skin that develop into nodules that ulcerate. The ulcers may be covered by hyperkeratotic eschar. The lesions heal spontaneously, often without treatment, over months to years into atrophic, depressed scars. The incubation period ranges from 1 week to several months. Some species have distinct manifestations; lesions caused by *L. major* and *L. mexicana* tend to evolve and resolve quickly, whereas those caused by *L. braziliensis, L. tropica*, can have longer periods of incubation and spontaneous healing.

CL can be classified as simple or complex. Simple CL has no mucosal involvement, a single or a few small (<1 cm) skin lesions, is amenable to local treatment, occurs in an immunocompetent host, and resolves without therapy. Complex CL may manifest with local subcutaneous nodules, regional adenopathy, multiple lesions (>4) of substantial size (>5 cm), are not amenable with local treatment, may involve the face, fingers, toes, joints, or

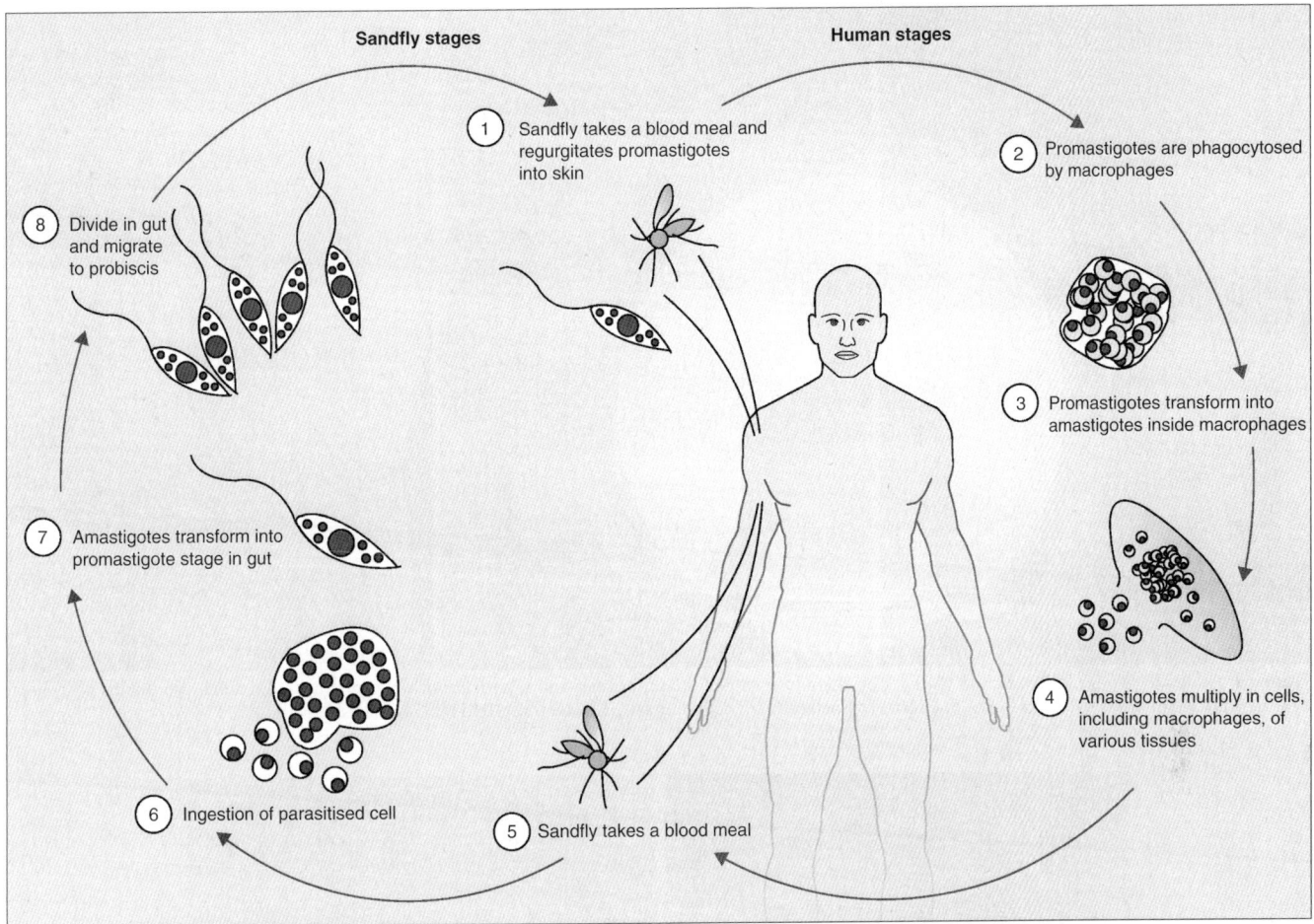

Figure 1 Leishmania life cycle. (From Burza S, Croft SL, Boelaert M: Leishmaniasis, *Lancet* 392[10151]:951–970, 2018)

Leishmaniasis Vaccine Pipeline

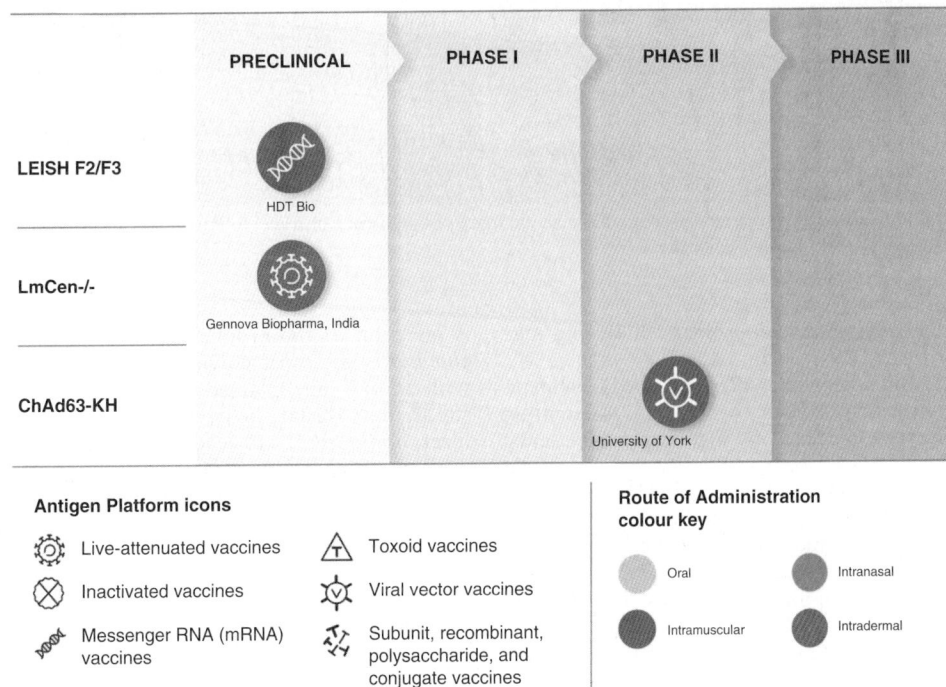

Figure 2 Overview of leishmaniasis vaccine candidates in clinical trials. (From Kaye PM, Matlashewski G, Mohan S, et al: Vaccine value profile for leishmaniasis, *Vaccine*, 41:S153–S175, 2023.)

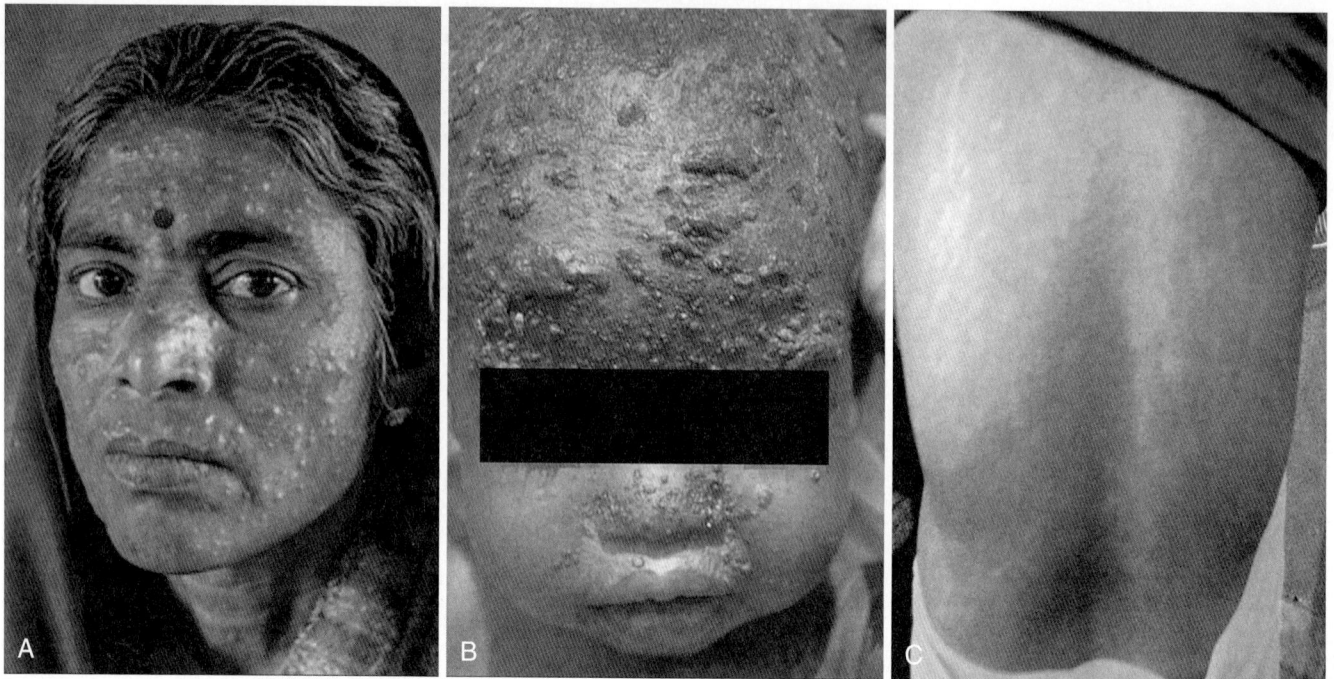

Figure 3 A female patient (A) and child (B) with erythematous maculopapular rash and a patient with hypopigmented macula (C) due to post–kala-azar dermal leishmaniasis. (From Burza S, Croft SL, Boelaert M: Leishmaniasis, *Lancet* 392[10151]:951–970, 2018)

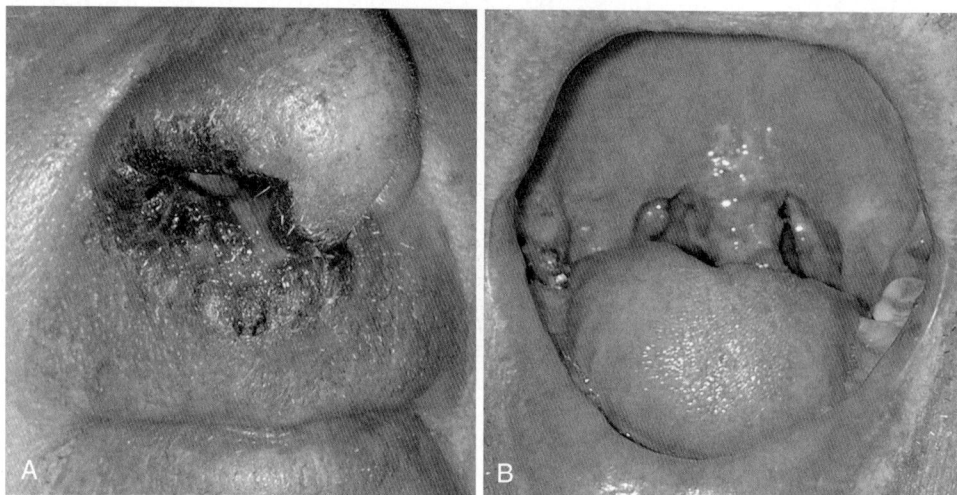

Figure 4 Severe oronasal mucocutaneous leishmaniasis in a 73-year-old man with a history of travel to Panama. (From Burza S, Croft SL, Boelaert M: Leishmaniasis, *Lancet* 392[10151]:951–970, 2018)

genitalia, may occur in an immunocompromised host, and may be associated with other clinical syndromes.

L. tropica can cause an uncommon syndrome called Leishmaniasis recidivans, in which new papules form around the margin of a healed primary lesion, mediated by a robust cell-mediated immune response.

A rare clinical manifestation is diffuse cutaneous leishmaniasis (DCL), in which soft nodules or plaques do not ulcerate, but spread to the face and extensors and gradually extend to the entire body. This is typically caused by *L. aethiopica, L. mexicana,* and *L. amazonensis* in immunocompromised patients. *L. infantum,* although most commonly associated with VL, can cause CL with slowly growing nodular lesions. It can be differentiated from leprosy by the preservation of sensation.

Mucosal Leishmaniasis

Progression of untreated or partially treated CL can result in parasite metastasis to the nasal mucosa leading to MCL, which is infection of the oropharynx and larynx (Figure 4). *L. braziliensis* is the most common cause of MCL. MCL manifests with chronic unexplained rhinorrhea or nasal congestion, epistaxis, sore throat, hoarseness, cough, mucosal bleeding, and ulcerations. MCL can lead to tissue necrosis and facial disfiguration with total or partial destruction of mucus membranes of the nose, mouth, and throat and life-threatening complications. It typically evolves slowly (over 3 years) and does not heal spontaneously.

Diagnosis

Leishmaniasis is diagnosed by direct visualization from tissue sampling. When concern exists for CL, care should be taken to remove debris, eschar, and exudate from the lesion, and a scraping or full-thickness skin biopsy can be collected. The standard for diagnosis is histopathologic visualization of *Leishmania* in a Giemsa-stained smear or parasite culture from the collected tissue sample. Polymerase chain reaction (PCR) detection of *Leishmania* DNA further increases the diagnostic sensitivity and can allow for species identification. In those who develop mucosal symptoms, tissue samples from the nasopharynx can be collected by an otolaryngologist. For evaluation of VL, aspirate or biopsy specimens are obtained from the spleen, bone marrow, liver, or enlarged lymph nodes. When tissue sampling has not been definitive of a diagnosis of VL, serologic tests can aid diagnosis; however, negative serology results are common in CL and MCL, as well as in VL when patients are immunosuppressed. Antibody detection by dipstick testing is a diagnostic tool that can help aid the decision for or against treatment.

Differential Diagnosis
Visceral Leishmaniasis
Local disease patterns influence the differential diagnosis of VL. Other infectious diseases such as malaria, disseminated histoplasmosis, hepatosplenic schistosomiasis, typhoid fever, brucellosis, tuberculosis, endocarditis, relapsing fever, African trypanosomiasis and syphilis are often on the differential diagnosis depending on the geographic location. Chronic diseases such as lymphoma and leukemia, sarcoidosis, malignant histiocytosis, and cirrhosis are also on the differential.

Cutaneous Leishmaniasis
Insect bites, furuncular myiasis, and bacterial tropical ulcers are in the differential for acute CL lesions. For chronic CL lesions, the differential includes leprosy, lupus vulgaris, discoid lupus erythematosus, and sarcoidosis.

Treatment
Local Therapies
In immunocompetent hosts, simple CL is typically observed for spontaneous healing. Simple CL may be treated with local therapies, including heat therapy, cryotherapy with liquid nitrogen, topical ointments and creams containing paromomycin,[1] intralesional injection of pentavalent antimonial drugs, and laser treatments.

Systemic Therapies
Complex CL (defined in "Clinical Manifestations"), MCL, and VL require systemic treatment. Treatment of systemic leishmaniasis consists of a limited number of established but relatively toxic drugs that require hospitalization.

Amphotericin B Drugs
The gold standard for treatment of VL is liposomal amphotericin B (AmBisome), because it is highly effective and nontoxic. Unfortunately, the high cost of the medication precludes its use in developing countries. Liposomal amphotericin B is delivered intravenously. For VL, the regimen approved by the US Food and Drug Administration (FDA) for immunocompetent individuals is 3 mg/kg/day on days 1 to 5, 14, and 21 for a total dose of 21 mg/kg. Immunosuppressed individuals should receive 4 mg/kg/day on days 1 to 5, 10, 17, 24, 31, and 38 for a total dose 40 mg/kg. Liposomal amphotericin B is the preferred treatment in pregnancy and does not have known teratogenic effects.

Amphotericin B deoxycholate (Fungizone) is an alternative for VL[1] and MCL resistant to pentavalent antimonials. For MCL, it is administered at the low dosage of 0.5 to 1 mg/kg/dose every other day for a cumulative total dose of 20 to 45 mg/kg. For VL, 1 mg/kg/dose daily or every other day is administered for a total of 15 to 20 doses. It is relatively toxic; doses exceeding 1 mg/kg/day frequently result in severe infusion-related side effects (fever, chills, and bone pain) and delayed side effects (renal toxicity).

Pentavalent Antimonials
Pentavalent antimonials (Sb) are the mainstay of treatment for all forms of leishmaniasis. Two essentially equivalent preparations are available. Sodium stibogluconate (Pentostam) is available in English-speaking countries; however, it is not FDA approved or commercially available and in the United States must be accessed through a protocol sponsored by the Centers for Disease Control and Prevention. Meglumine antimoniate (Glucantime)[2] is available in Southern Europe and Latin America. The recommended dosage of both preparations is for 20 mg/kg/day for 28 days, delivered intramuscularly or intravenously.

Sb-resistant VL (i.e., Bihar, India), treatment should be prolonged for 40 to 60 days. In cases of CL, pentavalent antimonials can be delivered intralesionally combined with cryotherapy. Sb has a dose-dependent toxicity that includes anorexia, pancreatitis, and QT prolongation.

Second-Line Drugs
Older drugs have limited current use. Pentamidine isethionate (Pentam 300)[1] is a highly toxic therapy used to treat Sb-resistant forms of CL that is given intramuscularly. CL is treated with 3 to 4 mg/kg every other day for 3 to 4 doses. MCL is treated with 2 to 4 mg/kg every other day for 15 doses. VL is treated with 4 mg/kg/dose every other day for 15 to 30 doses. Toxicity resulting from excess drug exposure manifests as myalgias, nausea, headache, and hypoglycemia.

Paromomycin sulfate[1] is an old aminoglycoside that has been reevaluated and can be the drug of choice for VL in the Indian subcontinent and resource-limited settings. It is given intramuscularly at the dose of 11 mg/kg/day for 21 days. Elevations of alanine aminotransferase (ALT) and aspartate aminotransferase (AST) liver enzymes are expected during therapy.

Oral Drugs for Leishmaniasis
Miltefosine (Impavido) is the first recognized oral treatment for VL, currently available in the United States. It is hexadecylphosphocholine that was originally developed as an anticancer agent and was initially available in Germany and India. The FDA-approved regimen is 50 mg twice daily (if 30–44 kg) or 50 mg thrice daily (if ≥45 kg) for 28 days. Miltefosine administration does not require the patient to be hospitalized for monitoring. Mild gastrointestinal toxicity may be common. Miltefosine is contraindicated in pregnancy.

Azole medications have also been used for treatment of leishmaniasis; however, evidence is insufficient to support their use alone in the treatment of leishmaniasis.

Monitoring
Monitoring parameters depend on the toxicity of treatment. Liposomal amphotericin B is typically well-tolerated, and patients should be monitored with baseline and once or twice weekly complete blood count (CBC) and serum chemistries for renal toxicity and electrolyte abnormalities (i.e., hypokalemia and hypomagnesemia). For patients taking amphotericin B deoxycholate, they should additionally be monitored for symptoms of infusion-related reaction such as headache, fever, nausea, vomiting, hypotension, and tachypnea. For patients taking pentavalent antimonials, baseline and weekly CBC; serum chemistries, including liver function tests, lipase/amylase; and electrocardiogram should be obtained. Patients should be monitored for side effects, including headache, fatigue, nausea, myalgias, and arthralgias. Patients on miltefosine should have baseline and weekly renal and hepatic function tests and CBC. They should be monitored for side effects, including nausea, vomiting and diarrhea, dizziness and motion sickness, and scrotal pain.

---

[1] Not FDA approved for this indication.

[2] Not available in the United States.
[1] Not FDA approved for this indication.

Monitoring Response to Treatment

In patients with VL who initiate treatment, fever improves by 3 to 5 days and fatigue improves during the first week. Anemia and pancytopenia begin to improve in the second week of therapy. Splenomegaly improves 1 to 2 months after completion of therapy but can take up to 1 year to regress completely. Test of cure is not typically conducted. Relapses can occur after apparent clinical cure from 2 to 8 months after treatment has been discontinued.

In patients with CL, lesions respond quickly to treatment; however, only one third of patients experience complete healing via reepithelization of lesions by the end of the treatment course.

Complications

Secondary bacterial infections can occur over CL lesions, leading to purulent drainage and localized cellulitis, which can be disabling especially in communities in which social stigma is high. Complications of CL, including MCL, or metastasis to the nasopharynx and oropharynx was described earlier.

When untreated, VL is 100% fatal. Complications of VL resulting from effects on the reticuloendothelial system include splenic rupture, uncontrolled bleeding, and disseminated intravascular coagulation (DIC). Hemophagocytic lymphohistiocytosis (HLH) is a rare complication of VL resulting from the uncontrolled activation of cytotoxic T-lymphocytes and natural killer (NK) cells. PKDL as a complication of VL was described earlier. Coinfection of VL and HIV increases the risk of developing VL, and VL also accelerates HIV disease progression.

When to Refer

When suspecting leishmaniasis, primary care physicians should feel empowered to initiate a workup, including biopsy of skin lesions. In the United States, given the rarity of leishmaniasis and barriers to accessing treatment, with a high index of suspicion or with confirmed diagnosis of leishmaniasis, patients generally should be referred to an infectious disease physician.

Note

Historically, the term "Old World" leishmaniasis has been used to describe disease occurring in Europe, Asia, and Africa, whereas "New World" leishmaniasis refers to disease occurring in Central and South America. For the purposes of this article, these terms have been replaced with the specific geographic locations.

Resources

Aronson N, Herwaldt BL, Libman M, et al: Diagnosis and treatment of leishmaniasis: clinical practice guidelines by the Infectious Diseases Society of America (IDSA) and the American Society of Tropical Medicine and Hygiene (ASTMH), *Clin Infect Dis* 63(12):1539–1557, 2016, https://doi.org/10.1093/cid/ciw742.

Berry I, Berrang-Ford L: Leishmaniasis, conflict, and political terror: A spatiotemporal analysis, *Soc Sci Med* 167:140–149, 2016, https://doi.org/10.1016/j.socscimed.2016.04.038.

Burza S, Croft SL, Boelaert M: Leishmaniasis, *The Lancet* 392(10151):951–970, 2018, https://doi.org/10.1016/S0140-6736(18)31204-2.

Institute For Health Metrics and Evaluation Global Burden of Disease: Leishmaniasis: level 3 cause. https://www.healthdata.org/research-analysis/diseases-injuries-risks/factsheets/2021-leishmaniasis-level-3-disease, 2019. [Accessed 8 December 2024].

Kaye PM, Matlashewski G, Mohan S, et al: Vaccine value profile for leishmaniasis, *Vaccine* 41:S153–S175, 2023, https://doi.org/10.1016/j.vaccine.2023.01.057.

Pace D: Leishmaniasis, *J Infect* 69:S10–S18, 2014, https://doi.org/10.1016/j.jinf.2014.07.016.

Regional Strategic Framework for Accelerating and Sustaining Elimination of Kala-Azar in the South-East Asia Region, 2022, World Health Organization, South-East Asian Region, 2022.

Scarpini S, Dondi A, Totaro C, et al: Visceral leishmaniasis: epidemiology, diagnosis, and treatment regimens in different geographical areas with a focus on pediatrics, *Microorganisms* 10(10):1887, 2022, https://doi.org/10.3390/microorganisms10101887.

World Health Organization. Leishmaniasis. https://www.who.int/news-room/factsheets/detail/leishmaniasis. [Accessed 2/1/24].

World Health Organization. Paediatric drug optimization for neglected tropical diseases Meeting report, September 2023. [Accessed 3/19/24].

LEPROSY

Method of
Carolina Talhari, MD, PhD; Maria Lucia Penna, MD, PhD; and Gerson O. Penna, MD, PhD

CURRENT DIAGNOSIS

- Contact of susceptible person with untreated leprosy cases; travel to or residence in a leprosy-endemic country
- Skin lesion(s) with altered sensation
- Thickened or enlarged peripheral nerve, with sensory loss and/or weakness in the muscles supplied by the nerve
- Presence of acid-fast bacilli in a slit-skin smear
- Skin biopsy with the presence of acid-fast bacilli or typical lesions, thereby aiding disease classification

CURRENT THERAPY*

Paucibacillary Leprosy (6 Months)
Adult (50–70 kg)
- Dapsone: 100 mg daily
- Rifampin (Rifadin)[1]: 600 mg once a month under supervision
- Clofazimine (Lamprene): 50 mg daily and 300 mg once a month under supervision

Child (<10 years)
- Dapsone: 1 mg/kg daily
- Rifampin[1]: 10 mg/kg once a month under supervision
- Clofazimine: 1 mg/kg/day

Multibacillary Leprosy (12 Months)
Adult (50–70 kg)
- Dapsone: 100 mg daily
- Rifampin (Rifadin)[1]: 600 mg once a month under supervision
- Clofazimine (Lamprene): 50 mg daily and 300 mg once a month under supervision

Child (<10 years)
- Dapsone: 1 mg/kg daily
- Rifampin[1]: 10 mg/kg once a month under supervision
- Clofazimine: 1 mg/kg/day

*As recommended by the World Health Organization (WHO).
[1]Not FDA approved for this indication.

Epidemiology

Leprosy is a chronic disease caused by *Mycobacterium leprae* that affects skin and nerves, often resulting in physical disabilities. The disease has been found around the world, showing that transmission occurs regardless of climate.

Disease transmission has ceased in nearly all developed nations, most likely because of better nutrition and socioeconomic development. Currently, new autochthonous cases are found in all tropical countries, with India, Brazil, and Indonesia having the highest number of cases annually. Some insular countries located in the Pacific and Indian Oceans have the highest rates of new case detection, indicating a high risk of transmission. In 2020 there was a reduction of 27.7% in the global leprosy registered prevalence and 37.1% in the new cases detection rate compared with 2019. According to the World Health Organization (WHO), this decrease is probably caused by less detection and reporting during the coronavirus disease 2019 (COVID-19) pandemic.

In the Gulf region of the United States, mostly in the states of Louisiana and Texas, native cases are still diagnosed. There are armadillos *(Dasypus novemcinctus)* in the area that have been infected with strains of *M. leprae* found also in autochthonous human cases. This suggests that leprosy might be a regional zoonosis, even though *M. leprae* was introduced into the Americas by Europeans and Africans. There are also records of *M. leprae* infection in armadillos in Central and South America. Furthermore, cases in African chimpanzees raise the possibility that these animals could be helping maintain leprosy transmission in Africa.

The mechanisms of leprosy transmission are not well known because there is no easy way to diagnose infection. It is presumed that in endemic areas, infection is much more frequent than actual disease onset. The incubation period can vary from a few months to more than 10 years, with an average of 2 to 5 years for paucibacillary (PB) leprosy and 5 to 10 years for multibacillary (MB) leprosy.

It is known that MB cases excrete large numbers of viable bacilli through nasal mucus, suggesting that transmission may be by the respiratory route; in fact, this is believed to be the main source of transmission. Because *M. leprae* can be eliminated from ulcerated skin lesions, breast milk, urine, and feces and it remains viable in the environment for many days, especially in humid climates, it is possible to theorize the existence of many different forms of transmission. The role of insects as vectors of bacilli is arguable.

Leprosy cases are not uniformly distributed in a community but tend to form clusters within different geographic regions, villages, or groups of domiciles. In most countries, cases are more common among men, and the 15- to 29-year-old age group tends to present the highest risk of disease. In areas where transmission is decreasing, the incidence tends to be higher among older adults, affecting those who lived during a period with a higher risk of infection.

Until 2008, *M. leprae* was the only agent responsible for leprosy. In that year, a new species called *Mycobacterium lepromatosis* sp. was described in Mexico as responsible for a diffuse form of the disease associated with increased morbidity and mortality. However, the clinical significance of this new entity, both in magnitude and in distribution, as well as particularities of the immune response to this pathogen, are not well known.

Risk Factors

In endemic areas, the main risk factors are a history of household contact with leprosy cases and low socioeconomic status. It is estimated that home contacts of patients with MB leprosy show a 5 to 10 times increased risk of becoming ill; PB leprosy case contacts present a 2 to 3 times increased risk compared with a group with no history of home exposure. In general, the increased risk between contacts reflects the proximity of these individuals, inside the house, with the potential source of infection. Also important is the sharing of other factors by household members, such as genetic markers, behavior, diet, intercurrent infections, and contextual aspects related to socioeconomic and environmental conditions.

An important fact in leprosy is that, even when living for a long time and in the same house with an untreated MB leprosy patient, most people do not get sick. It is estimated that 90% of the population have natural defenses against *M. leprae*. Today, there is evidence that susceptibility and resistance to *M. leprae* are genetically determined. The low frequency of genetically determined susceptibility may be the cause of the wide difference between infection and disease that is believed to exist.

Studies from the past decade confirmed the association between risk of incident leprosy and socioeconomic factors as demonstrated by the Norwegian study almost a century ago.

Prevention

Vaccination with bacille Calmette-Guerin (BCG)[1] reduces the risk of leprosy, with studies showing a variable efficacy of 20% to 80%. The revaccination of household contacts also provides protection, especially against the MB forms of the disease.

Chemoprophylaxis of contacts or high-risk groups with a single dose of rifampin (Rifadin)[1] has been shown to be effective for a period of 2 years. However, although the chemoprophylaxis trials reported a benefit, the relatively short duration of protection indicates functional limitations.

Combined strategies, including active community case-finding, the integration of rapid diagnostic tests to identify multibacillary leprosy among contacts, and potential immunization, are recommended as effective control measures with significant potential to reduce leprosy incidence.

Improving socioeconomic conditions in the general population in endemic areas is also a very effective strategy for disease control. This can be seen when comparing the current epidemiologic situation in the Hawaiian Islands with Micronesia or the Marshall Islands, where leprosy continues with a high incidence rate.

Pathophysiology

M. leprae is an intercellular microorganism with a specific tropism for skin and peripheral nerve cells. It cannot be cultivated in vitro but can be inoculated in mouse footpads and armadillos, although growth is quite slow. Active *M. leprae* infection is characterized by a wide clinical range, varying from a disease in which few bacilli are present in the body to one in which a high bacterial load is found in skin lesions.

Upon entering the organism, *M. leprae*, through its pathogen-associated molecular patterns (PAMPs), is recognized by pattern recognition receptors (PRRs) expressed in antigen-presenting cells (APCs), mainly dendritic cells (DCs), macrophages, monocytes, fibroblasts, and Schwann cells. Thus the innate immune response of the host is initiated, in which a local inflammatory response can eliminate the bacilli, avoiding the disease, or when this does not occur, the innate immunity can regulate the response of host adaptive immunity according to the pattern of cytokines produced by APCs.

In adaptive immunity, the bacilli multiply within macrophages, enter the lymph stream and bloodstream, reach the regional lymph nodes, and from there move on to the organs of the mononuclear phagocyte system. The mycobacterial antigens are then processed and presented by APCs that can be Langerhans cells, DCs, or others from the monocyte-macrophage system that induce the hapten-protein conjugates to link the HLA-DR class II molecules to the CD4 T lymphocytes. In patients in whom there is stimulation of the T-helper 1 cell response, these lymphocytes will produce interferon (IFN)-γ cytokines, tumor necrosis factor (TNF-α), interleukin-2 (IL-2), IL-17, IL1-β, and IL-12, which will promote the differentiation of macrophages in epithelioid cells that will undergo a fusion process resulting in giant cells. This inflammatory response will be sufficient to reduce *M. leprae* in the tuberculoid form of leprosy. In the presence of massive tissue infiltration by CD4 T lymphocytes, large production of these cytokines occurs along with the chemokine CXCL-10, leading to edema and tissue inflammation of the leprosy type 1 reaction. The production of TNF-α and IFN-γ by Schwann cells will lead to neural damage, which is also more significant in the type 1 reaction.

On the other hand, in the presence of stimulation of the TH2 subpopulation of T lymphocytes, these will produce the cytokines IL-4, IL-5, IL-6, IL-13, TNF-α, IL-10, and transforming growth factor (TGF)-β, the latter two produced by regulatory T lymphocytes (T-regs). TGF-β, IL-4, and IL-10 are suppressors of macrophage activation, leading to an insufficient immune cell response to combat the level of *M. leprae* proliferation within the macrophages. This characterizes the more infectious forms of the disease at the lepromatous end of the spectrum. The cytokines IL-4, IL-5, IL-6, and IL-13 activate plasma cells and B lymphocytes, which together with complement activation will form the immunocomplexes that will trigger leprosy type 2 reactions.

---

[1] Not FDA approved for this indication.

[1] Not FDA approved for this indication.

Clinical Manifestations

Because of the complexity of the parasite-host relation and the variable efficacy of the host's cellular immune response, the clinical manifestations of the disease cross a wide spectrum. This can vary from an isolated nerve lesion or a single skin patch to a systemic disease with the presence of nodules or tubercles, generally on the face. The disease can affect several organs beyond skin and nerves, including eyes, testicles, and kidneys. In 1966, Ridley and Jopling proposed a case classification system that takes into consideration clinical, bacteriologic, histopathologic, and immunologic parameters: tuberculoid leprosy (TL), borderline-tuberculoid leprosy (BTL), borderline-borderline leprosy (BBL), borderline-lepromatous leprosy (BLL), and lepromatous leprosy (LL). Indeterminate leprosy (IL) can be considered the first clinical manifestation of the disease. Indeterminate leprosy can resolve spontaneously or evolve into one of the other clinical forms.

Indeterminate Leprosy

This is characterized by one or more hypochromic macules with imprecise borders and reduced thermal sensitivity, although pain and tactile sensation may be preserved (Figure 1). These may occur as areas of sensory disturbance with no alteration in skin color, sweat glands, or hair growth. Any alteration in nerve function is preliminary, therefore there are no physical disabilities described with this classification. Slit-skin smear (SSS) test readings are negative.

Tuberculoid Leprosy

This type is characterized by erythematous or hypochromic skin lesions with clear, raised borders (Figure 2). These are limited in number with an asymmetric distribution and altered thermal sensation. Pain and tactile sensation may also be altered. Reduced perspiration and restricted partial or full alopecia may also be seen. Nerves can be affected intensively, but this usually only happens to a few. SSS results are negative.

Among children, TL lesions may have the appearance of nodules or tubercles, generally only one on the face, named nodular benign leprosy of childhood. Although these lesions tend to regress spontaneously, treatment should continue as per standard ethical practice.

Borderline-Tuberculoid Leprosy

This form is characterized by lesions similar to those seen at the TL end of the spectrum, although they are more numerous. In general, there are more than five lesions with a diameter of 10 cm or more, less clearly defined borders, and containing possible satellite lesions (Figure 3). These lesions tend to be more symmetric and several nerves may be affected. However, most patients with this disease type will still have a negative SSS test.

Borderline-Borderline Leprosy

This is a relatively rare variation, given that it commonly evolves quickly toward the lepromatous pole, often spurred on by reaction episodes. There are usually many foveal lesions (infiltrated plaques with expanding outer borders and well-defined inner borders with apparently normal skin in the middle) (Figure 4). Generally, nerves are intensively affected, and SSS tests are almost always positive.

Borderline-Lepromatous (Virchowian) Leprosy

A wide number of lesions are present with a range of possible clinical manifestations (infiltrations, papules, plaques, foveae, and nodules) that are common to the lepromatous form. However, with this type there is a tendency to see some delimitation between the lesions and areas of healthy skin. SSS test is positive with a high bacterial load.

Lepromatous (Virchowian) Leprosy

This form has the highest bacterial burden of human bacterial infections. Extensive lesions tend to be symmetric, erythematous,

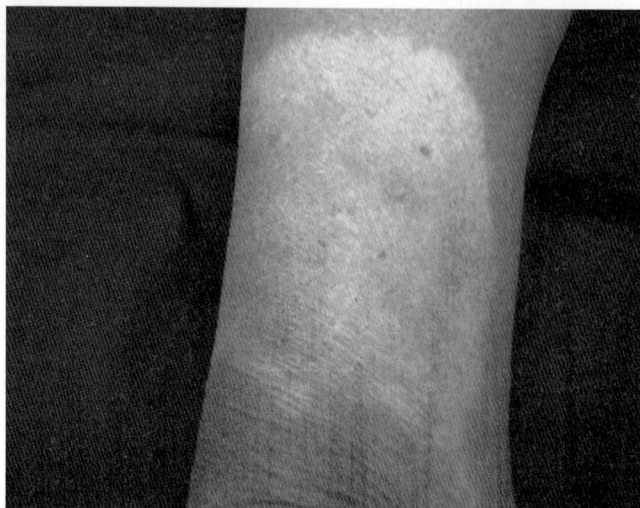

Figure 1 Indeterminate leprosy.

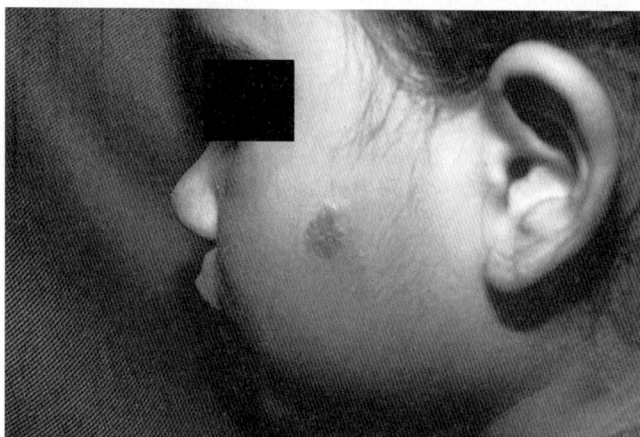

Figure 2 Tuberculoid leprosy in a child.

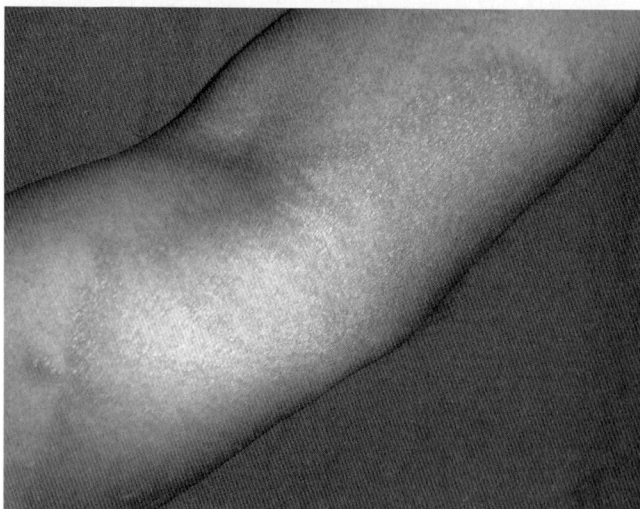

Figure 3 Borderline-tuberculoid leprosy.

infiltrated, and without clear delineation from normal skin areas. Simple lesions evolve to become papules, tubercles, and nodules that can eventually ulcerate and that are especially full of bacilli (Figure 5). There is diffuse infiltration of the face, with auricular appendages affected in the vast majority of cases and bilateral madarosis also common. Hands and feet may also be infiltrated or show signs of xerodermia. LL is a systemic disease that can affect the liver, spleen, adrenal glands, lymph nodes, eyes, and

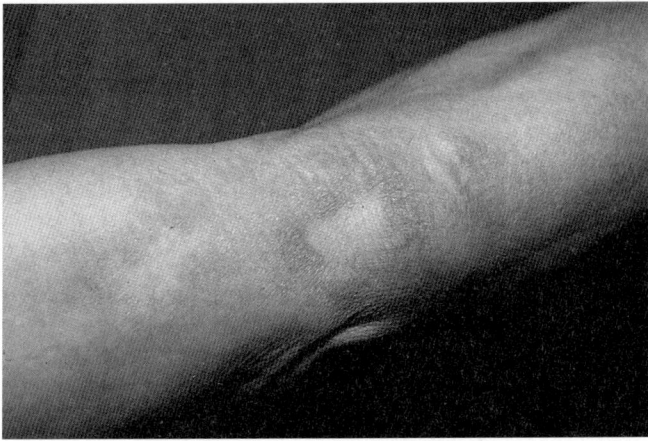

Figure 4 Borderline-borderline leprosy.

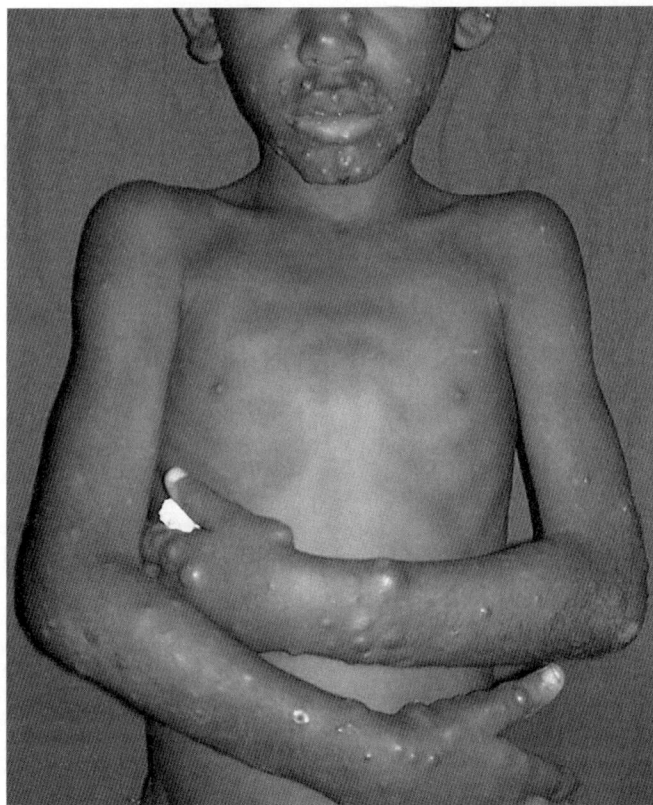

Figure 5 Lepromatous (Virchowian) leprosy.

nose when patients are not treated properly and opportunely. Nasal obstruction can be present with little or no response to vasoconstrictors. Often the nasal cavities will be affected, and the oropharynges will be full of nasal secretion highly abundant in bacilli. Subsequent nasal dryness can lead to secondary ulceration and infection with possible perforation and destruction of the nasal septum, resulting in what is commonly referred to as saddle nose. With olfactory bulb dysfunction, anosmia will often be the outcome. Lesions to the palate, lips, gum, and uvula can further compromise the pharynx, nasopharynx, and tonsils. The eyes may show erythema, dryness, dacryocystitis, lagophthalmos, and/or diminished sensation in the cornea. Likewise, iritis and iridocyclitis may be present, so proper intervention is necessary to ensure prevention of early onset of blindness. The testes may also be directly affected by bacilli, as witnessed by atrophy of the testicular parenchyma and diffuse fibrosis with

eventual sterility and alteration of sexual function. When secondary amyloidosis is present, renal insufficiency may result.

Variations of Lepromatous Leprosy
Histoid Lepromatous Leprosy (or Wade Lepromatous)
This form of leprosy is rare. Nodular lesions are present, well defined, and of varying sizes. These may be round or oval with a reddish or pink color. These lesions contain a large number of bacilli and are normally associated with sulfone resistance. Histiocytes with a spongy appearance are present under histologic analysis.

Diffuse Lepromatous Leprosy
Described by Lucio, Alvarado, and Latapi, this is a diffuse form of LL, also called *beautiful leprosy* because this form confers a pinkish and healthy appearance to the skin. It is more frequently seen in Mexico and is characterized by the diffuse infiltration of the skin, altered sensation that starts in the hands and feet, loss of eyebrows, and telangiectasias in the face and torso. A mycobacterium was isolated in cases of diffuse lepromatous leprosy (DLL) with Lucio phenomenon, whose DNA cannot be amplified using usual *M. leprae* primers. As a result, a new species has been proposed under the name *M. lepromatosis*.

Pure Neural Leprosy
This type presents only nerve lesions without any cutaneous patches. The most common nerves affected are the ulnar, tibial, and fibular nerves. The radial, median, facial, trigeminal, and auricular nerves, among others, may also be damaged.

Neuropathic pain is often present spontaneously or when the nerve is palpated, either with or without thickening of the nerve. This can evolve to sensory loss, paresthesia, or muscular atrophy in the corresponding area, in addition to autonomic dysfunction and nerve abscess.

Leprosy Diagnosis
The patient is examined to locate any possible skin lesions with diminished sensation and/or areas of sensory alteration that may be caused by compromised peripheral nerves. Lighting must be adequate, and it is important to observe the entire body surface moving from head to toe. Where there are possible signs of disease, thermal, pain, and tactile sensation testing should be done, also looking for areas of alopecia and/or anhidrosis. It must be noted if there is any type of physical disability.

The SSS test consists of collection and examination of skin smears taken from a suspected lesion, both earlobes, and both elbows, and helps classify a patient as PB with a negative examination result or MB when positive.

The SSS test results will generally be negative in IL, TL, and BTL, which are considered the PB group. Conversely, they tend to be positive in LL, BLL, and BBL, which are considered the MB group.

Ideally, the SSS test reading should be expressed quantitatively as a bacteriologic index (BI) so it is possible to monitor the patient's progress during treatment. In patients with a positive SSS test at the time of diagnosis, it is recommended to repeat it at the end of therapy. Smear microscopy is important for differential diagnoses between reactions and relapse.

The histologic examination of a skin biopsy also helps provide a more precise disease classification and can help confirm the diagnosis in cases that have a negative SSS test. In IL, there is a nonspecific inflammatory infiltrate, consisting of lymphocytes and sometimes histiocytes, around superficial and deep vessels that affects the cutaneous appendages, especially the neural fillets. The TL and BTL forms are characterized histologically by the presence of granulomas-histiocytes, which differentiate into epithelioid cells, giant cells, and lymphocytes, located around vessels, cutaneous appendages, and nervous fillets. Bacillus research is almost always negative. In BLL and LL forms, the inflammatory infiltrate is characterized by the predominance of foamy or

TABLE 1 Main Differential Diagnosis by Leprosy Forms

INDETERMINATE LEPROSY	TUBERCULOID AND BORDERLINE-TUBERCULOID LEPROSY	BORDERLINE-BORDERLINE, BORDERLINE-LEPROMATOUS, AND LEPROMATOUS LEPROSY
Pityriasis alba	Seborrheic dermatitis	Erythema nodosum
Seborrheic dermatitis	Dermatophytosis	Diffuse (anergic) cutaneous leishmaniasis
Localized scleroderma (morphea)	Granuloma annulare	Cutaneous and mucosal leishmaniasis
Residual hypochromia and achromia	Cutaneous leishmaniasis	Systemic lupus erythematous and other rheumatologic diseases
Pityriasis versicolor	Discoid lupus erythematous	Neurofibromatosis (von Recklinghausen disease)
Vitiligo	Pityriasis rosea Gibert	Pityriasis rosea Gibert
Hypochromic nevus	Psoriasis	Congenital syphilis, secondary syphilis, tertiary syphilis
	Sarcoidosis	Cutaneous lymphoma (Mycosis fungoides)
	Secondary syphilis	
	Cutaneous tuberculosis	

vacuolated histiocytes, with large numbers of bacilli that are isolated or grouped in structures called globias.

To establish an accurate diagnosis of leprosy, the primary care physician must conduct a comprehensive clinical assessment emphasizing the identification of characteristic skin lesions—hypopigmented or erythematous patches with sensory impairment—and palpation of peripheral nerves for thickening or tenderness. A detailed patient history should be obtained to evaluate lesion duration, progression, sensory alterations, and exposure risk factors. Sensory testing and nerve examination are essential to detect anesthesia and nerve involvement. Confirmatory investigations include SSS for acid-fast bacilli and, if necessary, histopathological examination of skin or nerve biopsies. In regions with limited access to laboratory resources, clinical diagnosis is sufficient to warrant the beginning of the standard leprosy treatment regimen, keeping in mind that this is the only dermatologic disease with altered sensation in lesions. The WHO suggests the classification of cases as either PB or MB based on the number of skin lesions, with MB cases having five or more such patches.

Available serologic testing does not show sufficient accuracy for disease diagnosis or infection. Studies published in the past decade confirmed the association between risk of incident leprosy and socioeconomic factors, as demonstrated by the Norwegian study almost a century ago.

Among serologic tests, the IgM anti–PGL-1 rapid test, such as the Fast ML Flow Hanseníase, has been integrated into the Brazilian public health system for surveillance and the diagnosis of leprosy contacts. This test detects anti–PGL-1 antibodies, which correlate with bacterial load, and has demonstrated higher seropositivity rates compared with ELISA and SSS tests, particularly in MB patients. However, it is important to emphasize that a negative result does not exclude leprosy in contacts, nor does a positive result confirm an active case of the disease.

Real-time polymerase chain reaction is available for leprosy and can act as a means of confirmation for diagnosis of PB leprosy cases.

Differential Diagnosis

Differential diagnoses of leprosy include a variety of skin conditions, given the wide range of clinical manifestations in leprosy. The sensory loss symptomatic of leprosy can also be difficult to determine in children and in other diseases that produce changes in the normal skin characteristics (Table 1).

Treatment

Leprosy treatment, like tuberculosis treatment, must deal with the resistance of *M. leprae* and its persistence. Single-drug therapy selects drug-resistant bacilli and should be avoided. Therapy duration has, as a target, the reduction of the number of persistent bacilli that could lead to relapses. Standard multidrug therapy (MDT) with dapsone, rifampin (Rifadin)[1], and clofazimine (Lamprene) for 12 months for MB cases and 6-month MDT with dapsone and rifampin for PB cases has dramatically changed the prognosis for leprosy patients. However, the especially regarding the necessary length of time for treatment, both in terms of the proportion of relapse cases and other outcomes, such as physical disability. The use of rifampin once a month was determined for financial reasons, and there is no study comparing this schedule with daily use. For this reason, research on new drugs and treatment regimens continues.

Shorter regimens were used but had shown high relapse rates: daily doses of rifampin[1] and ofloxacin (Floxin)[1] for 4 weeks; single-dose course of rifampin, ofloxacin, and minocycline (Minocin)[1] for single-lesion patients.

Fluoroquinolones (pefloxacin[2], ofloxacin[1], and moxifloxacin [Avelox][1]), macrolides (clarithromycin [Biaxin][1]), and tetracycline (minocycline)[1] are effective against *M. leprae*. Only rifampin, its derivative rifapentine (Priftin)[1], and moxifloxacin are bactericidal drugs; all others are bacteriostatic.

In cases of intolerance or resistance to dapsone, this can be removed from the drug regimen, and for PB leprosy patients, clofazimine is used instead. For MB leprosy patients, in these cases, minocycline[1] or ofloxacin[1] can be used instead of dapsone, without alteration in treatment duration. When similar intolerance or resistance is related to rifampin[1], this should be substituted with a daily dose of 400 mg of ofloxacin[1]. This alternate course lasts 6 months for PB leprosy cases and 24 months for MB leprosy cases.

For those who cannot take either dapsone or rifampin, PB leprosy patients can be treated with ofloxacin (400 mg/day)[1] or minocycline (100 mg/day)[1], and clofazimine (50 mg/day) in self-administered doses for 6 months. Similarly, MB patients can use ofloxacin[1] plus minocycline[1] plus clofazimine during the first 6 months of treatment (intensive phase), followed by 18 months with daily doses of ofloxacin or minocycline and clofazimine (maintenance phase).

In 2024 an open-label, proof-of-concept study showed complete clearance of *M. leprae* in nine MB patients with bedaquiline (Sirturo)[1] monotherapy for 8 weeks. After monotherapy, the patients started standard multidrug therapy for 12 months. The study shows promising results but has notable limitations, including a small sample size, potential biases, and reliance on the mouse footpad assay. Without a control group, it is unclear

---

[1] Not FDA approved for this indication.
[2] Not available in the United States.

whether bedaquiline alone is responsible for the observed effects. Furthermore, no monotherapy has been proven effective for leprosy or tuberculosis to date.

Perspectives on the Use of a Uniform Treatment for All Forms, Regardless of Clinical or Laboratory Classification

Despite the success of MDT, the complexity of operationalization of the scheme throughout the healthcare system, the prolonged treatment time, and the difficulty of patient adherence reinforce the need for shorter regimens that can be easily implemented in primary care. Since 2002, the WHO has recommended clinical studies to investigate the viability of uniform multidrug therapy (U-MDT) for all leprosy cases, regardless of classification, with 6 months' duration. The first randomized and controlled study on U-MDT, "Estudo independente para determinar efetividade do esquema Uniforme de MDT de seis doses (U-MDT) em pacientes de hanseníase (U-MDT-CT-BR)," was performed in Brazil and evaluated the efficacy of daily intake of dapsone plus clofazimine and monthly rifampicin[1] for 6 months for both PB and MB leprosy patients, regardless of classification criteria. Between 2012 and 2020, 15 scientific articles were published from U-MDT-CT-BR; these showed that reduction in the duration of treatment did not increase relapse rates, reaction frequency, or neural damage. The Brazilian study also demonstrated no statistical differences in BI decrease between regular MDT and U-MDT. Moreover, the same study showed that U-MDT reduced *M. leprae*–specific antibodies during and after treatment.

Together with the results from other four studies performed in China, India, and Bangladesh, U-MDT-CT-BR supports the premise that U-MDT is the best option and should be adopted in endemic countries to treat leprosy patients in the field worldwide. These studies led the WHO to recommend the addition of clofazimine to PB leprosy treatment in 2019.

Studies published between 2019 and 2020 confirmed the association between genetic susceptibility and recurrence, as well as the emergence of resistant strains of *M. leprae*. The authors showed that recurrence or reinfection is not related to time of treatment but rather to individual genetic susceptibility. Additionally, a population-based study for the search for *M. leprae* resistance reported the emergence and transmission of resistant strains in a former leprosy colony located in the Brazilian Amazon. Taken together, these studies demonstrated the need to save the unnecessary use of these drugs and strongly support the decision to adopt the shorter uniform treatment for leprosy.

Dapsone and rifampin resistance have been reported. Although reports of clofazimine-resistant isolates of *M. leprae* are rare, multidrug-resistant leprosy reports are increasing and should be regularly monitored.

Leprosy Reactions and Control

Over the course of this chronic disease, approximately 30% of patients develop acute inflammatory episodes called leprosy reactions. These reactions can occur before diagnosis, as well as during or after MDT treatment. They are commonly grouped into (1) type 1 (reversal) reactions (T1Rs) resulting from vigorous cell-mediated immune response and (2) type 2 reactions (T2Rs), the clinical manifestation of which is frequently erythematous nodosum leprosum (ENL) that comes about mainly from immunocomplex deposits. In patients with BBL and BLL, it is possible to have both reaction types simultaneously. There is also Lucio phenomenon, which is an immune system response with important clinical manifestations. Its physiopathology is not well understood, with abundant infection of *M. leprae* in endothelium, which can lead to thrombosis in the most superficial cases from immunocomplex deposits with hemorrhaging and cutaneous infarction.

In the literature, a robust association has been demonstrated between bacterial load and the frequency of leprosy reactions. A reaction can be set off by various factors, such as pregnancy, childbirth, vaccinations, puberty, intercurrent infections, stress (physical, psychological, or surgical), use of potassium iodate/iodide (SSKI), and immune reconstitution inflammatory syndrome (IRIS) linked to antiretroviral and/or immune-based therapies.

Those patients who experience leprosy reactions during MDT treatment should continue taking their regimen without modification while also beginning a specific and concurrent treatment for the appropriate reaction type.

Type 1 Reaction or Reversal Reaction

Clinically, lesions become more erythematous and infiltrated, and those with previously diminished sensation can become more sensitive to touch. Desquamation may occur, and some lesions may even ulcerate. New lesions can erupt along with edema in the hands, feet, and face, as well as general systemic symptoms. These reactions can last for years in some patients. It is important to begin an immediate intervention given that neuritis is the most common, serious, and potentially disabling clinical manifestation of T1R.

The drug of choice for T1R treatment is prednisone (or prednisolone [Millipred]) with a dosage of 1 to 2 mg/kg/day for at least 12 weeks, at which point it can be tapered off until discontinuing the medication around the 24th week.

Alternative drugs for a type 1 reaction include the following:
- Azathioprine (Imuran)[1]: 1 to 2 mg/kg/day, until reaction control
- Cyclosporine (Neoral, Sandimmune)[1]: 5 to 8 mg/kg/day, until reaction control
- Clofazimine: 300 mg to 30 days/200 mg to 30 days/100 mg to 30 days

Type 2 Reaction

This occurs in MB leprosy patients, and ENL is the most frequent clinical manifestation of T2Rs. Other variations of T2R are polymorphic erythema and vasculitis.

Clinically, ENL is a systemic condition with the eruption of painful and often symmetric erythematous nodules on the arms and legs. When deeper, these nodules are more easily palpated than the more visible ones but will often ulcerate. Neuritis is frequent, although it is less aggressive than seen in T1Rs. The systemic impact can produce edema, myalgia, fever, malaise, asthenia, weight loss, cephalalgia, iritis, episcleritis, iridocyclitis, glaucoma, epistaxis, arthralgia, and orchiepididymitis with testicular atrophy, glomerulonephritis, chronic renal insufficiency, hepatosplenomegaly, and amyloidosis.

The most common medication used for ENL is thalidomide (Thalomid) in variable dosage, from 100 to 400 mg/day, depending on the severity of the reaction. The distribution of thalidomide is restricted in some countries because of its teratogenic effects. For this reason, it should be given under strict supervision with proper medical, ethical, and legal measures in place.

For ENL associated with neuritis, iritis, orchitis, and/or hand-foot reactions or for women of childbearing age, a course of corticosteroids should be given (prednisone at 1–2 mg/kg/day).

In chronic cases and those that are nonresponsive to treatment, it is possible to administer clofazimine along with steroids at the initial dosage of 100 mg three times per day for a maximum of 12 weeks. This should be reduced to 100 mg twice daily for another 12 weeks and finally 100 mg/day for 12 to 24 weeks. Cyclosporine (Neoral, Sandimmune)[1] may also offer some benefit to the patient with serious ENL, as can the association of azathioprine (Imuran)[1], methotrexate[1], and corticosteroids.

Alternative drugs for a type 2 reaction include the following:
- Azathioprine[1]: 1 to 2 mg/kg/day, until reaction control
- Cyclosporine[1]: 5 to 8 mg/kg/day, until reaction control
- Methotrexate[1]: 15 mg (IM/SC or PO)/week, until reaction control
- Pentoxifylline (Trental)[1]: 1200 mg/day, until reaction control

---

[1] Not FDA approved for this indication.

TABLE 2	Differences Between Reaction Type 1 and Relapse
REVERSAL REACTION	**RELAPSE**
Generally occurs during course of multidrug therapy or within 6 months of treatment completion	Occurs at least 2 years after treatment completion
Sudden and unexpected onset	Slow and insidious onset
Can be accompanied by fever and malaise	In general, no systemic symptoms present
Old lesions become erythematous, shiny, and infiltrated	Old lesions may present erythematous edges
In general, many new lesions	Few new lesions
There may be ulceration of the reaction lesions	Ulceration may occur on arms and legs in addition to the lesions
Regression with desquamation	No desquamation present
Can quickly affect several nerve trunks, with presence of pain, sensory alteration, and decreased motor function	May affect a single nerve, and functional alterations often take place very slowly
Excellent response to corticosteroid therapy	Does not respond well to corticosteroid therapy
Bacteriologic index stable or decreases	Bacteriologic index increases

- Clofazimine: 300 mg to 30 days/200 mg to 30 days/100 mg to 30 days

Lucio Phenomenon
Lucio phenomenon can occur in LL patients. The skin lesions can be discrete and limited in number, pinkish or cyanotic, often very painful, and potentially necrotizing and ulcerative. This condition can lead to death. Treatment is based on a course of corticosteroid therapy appropriate for each patient.

Differential Diagnosis Between Relapse and Reaction
Relapse rates are very low, whereas reactions are quite frequent, even after completing treatment. Table 2 shows the main differences between reaction type 1 and type 2 relapse. Recently an *M. leprae* whole genome sequencing technique was used to discriminate between cases of relapse and reinfection.

Complications
Leprosy complications are the result of permanent nerve damage. Lesions to the large nerve trunks, such as the ulnar, median, and tibial, cause motor and sensory loss leading to disabilities such as claw hand and footdrop.

The absence of sensation in the hands, soles of the feet, and cornea leaves these areas predisposed to common wounds and pressure ulcers. This reality demands that patients take specific care to avoid ulcers and detect them as soon as possible to prevent secondary infection. In addition, corneal ulcers can result in blindness.

Acknowledgment
We thank Dr. Anna Maria Salles for the patient pictures.

References
Andrade KVF, Nery JS, Pescarini JM, et al: Geographic and socioeconomic factors associated with leprosy treatment default: an analysis from the 100 Million Brazilian Cohort, *PLoS Neglected Trop Dis* 13(9):e0007714, 2019.

Barreto J, Sammarco Rosa P, Adams L, et al: Bedaquiline monotherapy for multibacillary leprosy, *N Engl J Med* 391(23):2212–2218, 2024.
Butlin CR, Pahan D, Maug AKJ, et al: Outcome of 6 months MBMDT in MB patients in Bangladesh—preliminary results, *Lepr Rev* 87:171–182, 2016.
Cruz RCDS, Bührer-Sékula S, Penna GO, et al: Clinical trial for uniform multidrug therapy for leprosy patients in Brazil (U-MDT/CT-BR): adverse effects approach, *An Bras Dermatol* 93:377–384, 2018.
Gonçalves H de S, Pontes MA, Bührer-Sékula S, et al: Brazilian clinical trial of uniform multidrug therapy for leprosy patients: the correlation between clinical disease types and adverse effect, *Mem Inst Oswaldo Cruz* 107(Suppl 1):74–78, 2012.
Han XY, Sizer KC, Velarde-Félix JS, et al: The leprosy agents Mycobacterium lepromatosis and Mycobacterium leprae in Mexico, *Int J Dermatol* 51:952–959, 2012.
Hungria EM, Bührer-Sékula S, Oliveira RM, et al: Mycobacterium leprae-specific antibodies in multibacillary leprosy patients decrease during and after treatment with either the regular 12 doses multidrug therapy (MDT) or the uniform 6 doses MDT, *Front Immunol* 9:915, 2018.
Hungria EM, Oliveira RM, Penna GO, et al: Can baseline ML Flow test results predict leprosy reactions? An investigation in a cohort of patients enrolled in the uniform multidrug therapy clinical trial for leprosy patients in Brazil, *Infect Dis Poverty* 5(1):110–120, 2016.
International Federation of Anti-Leprosy Associations: Available at http://www.ilep.org.uk/about-ilep/. [Accessed July, 2022].
Kroger A, Pannikar V, Htoon MT, et al: International open trial of uniform multidrug therapy regimen for 6 months for all types of leprosy patients: rationale, design and preliminary results, *Trop Med Int Health* 13:594–602, 2008.
Moura RS, Penna GO, Cardoso LP, et al: Description of leprosy classification at baseline among patients enrolled at the uniform multidrug therapy clinical trial for leprosy patients in Brazil, *Am J Trop Med Hyg* 92(6):1280–1284, 2015.
Moura RS, Penna GO, Fujiwara T, et al: Evaluation of a rapid serological test for leprosy classification using human serum albumin as the antigen carrier, *J Immunol Methods* 412:35–41, 2014.
Nery JS, Pereira SM, Rasella D, et al: Effect of the Brazilian conditional cash transfer and primary health care programs on the new case detection rate of leprosy, *PLoS Neglected Trop Dis* 8(e3357):e3360, 2014.
Pedrosa VL, Dias LC, Galban E, et al: Leprosy among schoolchildren in the Amazon region: a cross-sectional study of active search and possible source of infection by contact tracing, *PLoS Neglected Trop Dis* 12:e0006261, 2018.
Penna GO, Bührer-Sékula S, Kerr LRS, et al: Uniform multidrug therapy for leprosy patients in Brazil (U-MDT/CT-BR): results of an open label, randomized and controlled clinical trial, among multibacillary patients, *PLoS Neglected Trop Dis* 11:e0005725, 2017.
Penna ML, Bührer-Sékula S, Pontes MA, et al: Results from the clinical trial of uniform multidrug therapy for leprosy patients in Brazil (U-MDT/CT-BR): decrease in bacteriological index, *Lepr Rev* 85(4):262–266, 2014.
Penna ML, Penna GO, Iglesias PC, et al: Anti-PGL-1 positivity as a risk marker for the development of leprosy among contacts of leprosy cases: systematic review and metaanalysis, *PLoS Neglected Trop Dis* 10:e0004703, 2016.
Pescarini JM, Strina A, Nery JS, et al: Socioeconomic risk markers of leprosy in high-burden countries: a systematic review and meta-analysis, *PLoS Neglected Trop Dis* 12(7), 2018:e0006622.
Rosa PS, D'Espindula HRS, Melo ACL, et al: Emergence and transmission of drug/multidrug-resistant Mycobacterium leprae in a former leprosy colony in the Brazilian Amazon, *Clin Infect Dis* 570, 2019.
Saavedra DP, Nobre ML, Guimarães RA, et al: A multicenter evaluation of leprosy rapid test fast ML Flow hanseníase in Brazil, *Eur J Clin Microbiol Infect Dis* 44(4):985–995, 2025.
Santos SD, Penna GO, Costa MCN, et al: Leprosy in children and adolescents under 15 years old in an urban center in Brazil, *Mem Inst Oswaldo Cruz* 111:359–364, 2016.
Shen J, Yan L, Yu M, et al: Six years' follow-up of multibacillary leprosy patients treated with uniform multi-drug therapy in China, *Int J Dermatol* 54:315–318, 2015.
Stefani MMA, Avanzi C, Bührer-Sékula S, et al: Whole genome sequencing distinguishes between relapse and reinfection in recurrent leprosy cases, *PLoS Neglected Trop Dis* 11(6):e0005598, 2017.
Talhari C, Mira MT, Massone C, et al: Leprosy and HIV coinfection: a clinical, pathological, immunological, and therapeutic study of a cohort from a Brazilian referral center for infectious diseases, *J Infect Dis* 202:345–354, 2010.
Talhari C, Talhari S, Penna GO: Clinical aspects of leprosy, *Clin Dermatol* 33:26–37, 2015.
Talhari S, Neves RG, Penna GO: Oliveira MLWR. In *Hanseníase, manaus, gráfica tropical*, 2006.
Uaska Sartori PV, Penna GO, Bührer-Sékula S, et al: Human genetic susceptibility of leprosy recurrence, *Sci Rep* 10:1284, 2020.
Vieira MCA, Nery JS, Paixão ES, Andrade KVF, Penna GO, Teixeira MG: Leprosy in children under 15 years of age in Brazil: a systematic review of the literature, *PLoS Neglected Trop Dis* 12(10):e0006788, 2018.
WHO Global leprosy (Hansen disease) update: 2020: impact of COVID-19 on global leprosy control, *WER* 36:421–444, 2021.

LYME DISEASE AND POST-TREATMENT LYME DISEASE SYNDROME

Method of
Emma Taylor-Salmon, MD; and Eugene D. Shapiro, MD

CURRENT DIAGNOSIS

- Lyme disease, caused by the spirochete *Borrelia burgdorferi*, is the most common vector-borne infection in both the United States and Europe.
- Early localized Lyme disease is a clinical diagnosis based on the presence of a single erythema migrans rash. The rash manifests as an expanding circular macule that is often uniformly erythematous but occasionally can have central clearing that gives it the appearance of a target lesion. Erythema migrans usually appears 7 to 14 days after a tick bite (although the bite often is not recognized). If untreated, it persists for about 2 to 4 weeks.
- Early disseminated Lyme disease can manifest as multiple erythema migrans, cranial nerve palsy, lymphocytic meningitis, radiculomyelitis (Bannwarth syndrome), or carditis.
- Arthritis is the primary manifestation of late Lyme disease. Typically it is an oligoarthritis that most often involves a single knee.
- Patients with no objective signs but only nonspecific symptoms (e.g., arthralgia, myalgia, fatigue, or perceived cognitive difficulties) are highly unlikely to have active Lyme disease as the cause regardless of the results of antibody tests.
- Antibody test results for Lyme disease are usually negative in patients with erythema migrans (single or multiple); therefore testing for antibody generally is only indicated for patients with noncutaneous manifestations of Lyme disease.
- The immunoglobulin G (IgG) antibody test has good sensitivity for patients with Lyme disease 4 weeks or more after initial infection.
- Tests for antibodies to *Borrelia burgdorferi* should use a two-tier procedure. Standard two-tier tests begin with a sensitive quantitative test, usually either a whole-cell or a C-6–based peptide enzyme-linked immunosorbent assay (ELISA); if that result is either positive or equivocal, a more specific test, the Western immunoblot, is done to confirm a positive test result. The presence of antibodies against at least either two (for IgM) or five (for IgG) proteins of *B. burgdorferi* is required for the immunoblot result to be considered positive. Modified two-tier antibody tests, which use a second (different) ELISA assay as the second-tier test, rather than an immunoblot, have been approved for use by the US Food and Drug Administration (FDA) and can replace the standard two-tier test.
- In patients with symptoms present for 4 to 6 weeks or longer, Lyme disease should not be diagnosed based on a positive IgM antibody result alone.
- Sensitivity of polymerase chain reaction assays of both blood and cerebral spinal fluid are poor because concentrations of *B. burgdorferi* in these fluids are low.
- Once serum antibodies to *B. burgdorferi* develop, both IgG and IgM antibodies may persist for decades despite adequate treatment; therefore elevated concentrations of antibodies in serum do not necessarily indicate active infection.

CURRENT THERAPY

- An oral course of doxycycline (Vibramycin)[1] for 10 days or of either amoxicillin (Amoxil)[1] or cefuroxime axetil (Ceftin) for 14 days is highly effective for treating erythema migrans (either localized or multiple).
- A 14- to 21-day course of the same antimicrobials also is highly effective in treating noncutaneous manifestations of early disseminated Lyme disease, although patients with Lyme meningitis or complete atrioventricular block should be treated either parenterally with ceftriaxone (Rocephin),[1] cefotaxime (Claforan),[1] or, in some instances, orally with doxycycline.[1]
- A 28-day course of an oral regimen is recommended for the treatment of Lyme arthritis.
- Doxycycline is contraindicated in women who are either pregnant or breast-feeding.
- The most effective preventive measure is avoidance of tick-infested areas. If exposure is unavoidable, visual inspection and prompt removal of embedded ticks, use of tick repellents with *N,N*-diethyl-3-methylbenzamide (DEET), and use of protective clothing have all been found to be modestly effective.
- An infected tick generally must be attached for 36 to 72 hours or longer for there to be a substantial risk of transmission of *Borrelia burgdorferi*. If a tick that has been embedded for at least 36 hours is removed, a single dose of doxycycline 8.8 mg/kg, maximum 200 mg,[1] given within 72 hours of removing the engorged tick, can be effective in preventing Lyme disease.
- Multiple or prolonged courses of antibiotics have not been shown to be effective and are not recommended for patients with only chronic, subjective symptoms after completing appropriate antibiotic treatment for Lyme disease.

[1]Not FDA approved for this indication.

Epidemiology and Ecology

Lyme arthritis was first described in 1977 when an unusual cluster of children with arthritis in Lyme, Connecticut, was reported. Soon after, Willy Burgdorfer identified the causative bacterial agent, a spirochete that was later named *Borrelia burgdorferi*, in *Ixodes scapularis*, the deer tick. Lyme disease, the most common vector-borne illness in both the United States and Europe, is transmitted by hard-bodied ticks of the *Ixodes* genus. In the United States, *I. scapularis* (in the East and upper Midwest) and *Ixodes pacificus*, the Western black-legged tick (on the Pacific coast), can be vectors of Lyme disease. More than 90% of all cases in the United States occur in nine states: Connecticut, Maryland, Massachusetts, Minnesota, New Jersey, New York, Pennsylvania, Rhode Island, and Wisconsin. In Europe and in Asia, *Ixodes ricinus* (the sheep tick) and *Ixodes persulcatus* (the taiga tick) can transmit *B. burgdorferi*. *Ixodes* ticks feed once in each of the three stages of their 2-year life cycle: larva, nymph, and adult. There are a number of genomospecies of *B. burgdorferi* sensu lato that cause Lyme disease. In the United States, Lyme disease is almost exclusively caused by *B. burgdorferi* sensu stricto, whereas in Europe and in Asia, *Borrelia afzelii* and *Borrelia garinii*, in addition to *B. burgdorferi* sensu stricto, are the major causes of Lyme disease.

Lyme disease is a zoonosis. The primary reservoir for *B. burgdorferi* is small mammals, such as mice and chipmunks, although birds and other mammals, such as foxes and coyotes, can also serve as reservoirs of the organism. Deer are not a competent reservoir for *B. burgdorferi*, but they are important for supporting the life cycle of the deer tick. Ticks are uninfected when they hatch. They can become infected after they feed on an infected animal. The bacteria live in the midgut of the tick, which must remain attached to a host for 36 to 48 hours or longer for the spirochete to travel to the salivary glands so it can be injected into the host. Although ticks may become infected at any stage of the life cycle, nymphs are more likely to transmit the organism. This is because their small size (<2 mm) makes them more difficult to detect than adult ticks. Consequently, nymphal ticks are less likely than are adult ticks to be removed before the organism can be transmitted. The most important risk factor for Lyme disease is exposure to ticks in an area in which the disease is endemic. Most cases of Lyme disease occur in the spring and summer, which correlates with peak activity of nymphal ticks and with frequent outdoor activity of humans.

Pathophysiology

The pathogenesis of Lyme disease is predominantly driven by the host immune response to the spirochete. During the first stage of infection, after transfer of the organism to the skin, inflammation ensues that leads to an erythematous lesion at the site of inoculation. The spirochete does not produce toxins; however, it can disseminate via the bloodstream or through the lymph vessels. After dissemination, the spirochete can adhere to distal tissues, and an immune-mediated inflammatory reaction at these sites leads to the characteristic clinical manifestations of Lyme disease.

Prevention

No vaccine is currently available to prevent Lyme disease in humans. The most effective preventive measure is avoidance of tick-infested areas. Tick repellents that contain N,N-diethyl-3-methylbenzamide (DEET) and the use of protective clothing (long sleeves and pants) have been found to be modestly effective at preventing Lyme disease. If exposure is unavoidable, frequent visual inspection with prompt removal of ticks is recommended. In endemic areas, if a nymphal or adult Ixodes tick is removed that is partially engorged (has been attached for at least 36 hours), a single dose of doxycycline[1] administered within 72 hours of removing the tick can be effective in preventing Lyme disease.

Clinical Manifestations

The clinical manifestations of Lyme disease can be divided into three stages: early localized disease, early disseminated disease, and late disease. About two-thirds of patients with Lyme disease in the United States have early localized disease, which is characterized by a single erythema migrans (EM) rash at the site of the tick bite (although the tick bite is recognized in only a minority of cases). The rash starts as an erythematous macule or papule and then expands as an annular macule that is often uniformly erythematous (about two-thirds of cases of EM in the United States), although it can have central clearing that gives it the appearance of a classic target lesion. EM usually appears 7 to 14 days (range 3–30 days) after the tick bite and, if untreated, may expand to an average of 15 cm in diameter before resolving after 2 to 4 weeks or longer. The rash may be asymptomatic or it may be accompanied by systemic symptoms such as fever, malaise, headache, stiff neck, myalgia, or arthralgia.

The second most common manifestation of Lyme disease is multiple EM, which accounts for 15% to 23% of the reported cases in the United States. Multiple EM, a manifestation of early disseminated Lyme disease, occurs when the spirochete disseminates via the bloodstream and appears as multiple erythematous round or ovoid macules that are usually smaller than most single EM lesions and are often accompanied by fever and other systemic symptoms. Other manifestations of early disseminated Lyme disease include cranial nerve palsy (especially facial palsy), lymphocytic meningitis, radiculomyelitis, and carditis. Cranial nerve palsies, especially facial nerve palsy, occur more commonly in children and account for approximately 3% to 5% of all cases of Lyme disease. In most cases, facial nerve palsy resolves within 4 to 8 weeks, usually leaving minor, if any, obvious residua. Lyme meningitis occurs less frequently (1%–2% of cases) and typically has a subacute presentation similar to, though often of longer duration than, that of enteroviral meningitis. There is a mononuclear pleocytosis in (CSF). Increased intracranial pressure with papilledema is not uncommon. Neurologic involvement in Lyme disease is more common in Europe and in Asia, presumably because local strains of the bacteria are more neurotropic. Carditis, which is found in fewer than 1% of cases, typically causes various degrees of heart block, which usually is asymptomatic and may be detected only with an electrocardiogram, but may manifest as syncope, dyspnea, or dizziness as a result of complete heart block. Sudden death due to Lyme carditis has been reported but is very rare.

Arthritis is the main manifestation of late Lyme disease and in North America accounts for approximately 6% to 8% of reported cases. Lyme arthritis typically is an oligoarthritis that involves a single knee about 90% of the time. Symptoms of arthritis develop 2 to 6 months after the tick bite and present with objective signs of inflammation of the joint. Arthritis typically resolves 2 to 6 weeks after appropriate treatment, although it may persist or recur in 10% to 20% of treated patients.

In Europe and in Asia, uncommon manifestations of Lyme disease include borrelial lymphocytoma, a painless nodule commonly located on the ear, breast, or scrotum; and acrodermatitis chronica atrophicans, a chronic fibrosing skin lesion, typically is found on the extensor surfaces of the extremities.

Diagnosis

Early localized Lyme disease is a clinical diagnosis based on a history of potential exposure to ticks in an endemic area and the presence of the characteristic EM rash. Antibodies to the organism typically appear 3 to 4 weeks after the initial infection. Consequently, serologic tests are not indicated in patients with EM because most will not have detectable antibodies. Although more patients with multiple EM may be seropositive at the time of presentation, a majority will still be seronegative early on. Moreover, detectable antibodies may never develop in patients who are treated early in their courses.

In patients with extracutaneous manifestations of Lyme disease, serologic testing is useful in making a diagnosis. Differential diagnosis for those with signs of meningitis include bacterial and viral meningitis. For those with cranial nerve palsies the differential diagnosis includes idiopathic (Bell's) palsy and lymphoma. For those with arthritis the differential diagnosis includes septic arthritis, rheumatologic disease such as lupus or juvenile idiopathic arthritis and leukemia.

Tests for antibodies to B. burgdorferi should use a two-tier procedure. In the standard two-tier test, a sensitive quantitative test, usually an enzyme-linked immunosorbent assay (ELISA) against either "whole cell" or C6 peptide–related antigens of the bacteria, is performed. If the result of the quantitative test is either positive or equivocal, a Western immunoblot is done to confirm the specificity of the result. Modified two-tier antibody tests, which use a second (different) ELISA assay as the second-tier test, have been approved for use by the FDA and can replace the standard two-tier test. As with most infections, once they develop, elevated concentrations of both IgM and IgG antibodies may persist for decades in symptom-free patients who have been cured of Lyme disease. A positive test result is evidence of prior exposure to the organism and is not evidence of active infection. In addition, false-positive antibody test results are common, especially in patients with a low prior probability of Lyme disease, such as those with chronic nonspecific symptoms such as arthralgia, myalgia, or fatigue, who do not have concomitant objective findings associated with Lyme disease. False-positive IgM test results are especially common. A diagnosis of Lyme disease should rarely be based on a positive IgM test result alone, especially in patients who have had symptoms for a month or longer.

Polymerase chain reaction (PCR) assays can detect the organism in skin biopsies, CSF, blood, or synovial fluid. However, because concentrations of the organism are low in both the blood and the CSF, sensitivity of PCR assays of these fluids is poor. Because the rash is so characteristic and because virtually all patients with Lyme arthritis will have a positive result for IgG antibodies to B. burgdorferi, such assays rarely are needed to make a diagnosis. The organism can be cultured using special media, but sensitivity generally is poor, and it takes weeks for the organism to grow.

Differential Diagnosis

The differential diagnosis of Lyme disease depends on the clinical stage of the illness. All of the symptoms associated with Lyme disease (e.g., myalgia, arthralgia, fever, fatigue) are so nonspecific that, if only these symptoms are present, they are not a sufficient indication to order a serologic test for Lyme disease (because the prior probability that Lyme disease is the cause of these symptoms is so low), unless these symptoms are accompanied by more specific signs of Lyme disease, such as frank arthritis, nuchal rigidity, or facial nerve palsy.

---

[1] Not FDA approved for this indication.

Single EM may be confused with ringworm, cellulitis, nummular eczema, granuloma annulare or insect bites. Southern tick-associated rash illness (STARI) manifests in a rash identical to EM. However, it occurs at the site of a bite from the Lone Star tick *(Amblyomma americanum)* and is most common in the south-central United States. The cause of STARI is unknown, but, unlike with Lyme disease, it is not associated with significant extracutaneous manifestations. Multiple EM may look very similar to erythema multiforme. Lymphocytic meningitis occurs with numerous viral infections, most commonly enterovirus. There are many other causes of carditis, including a number of viruses, as well as rheumatologic diseases such as lupus and rheumatic fever. Other causes of facial nerve palsy include idiopathic (Bell's) palsy and tumors (lymphoma, acoustic neuroma). There is substantial variation in how Lyme arthritis manifests. Most often it is a subacute arthritis that may mimic rheumatoid arthritis or other more chronic arthritides, with fewer than 50,000 white blood cells/mL in the synovial fluid. However, it can present acutely and may mimic acute bacterial arthritis (like that due to *Staphylococcus aureus*), with more than 100,000 white blood cells/mL in synovial fluid.

Relapse Versus Reinfection

Resistance of *B. burgdorferi* to recommended antimicrobials has not been reported. First-line antimicrobial therapy for Lyme disease is highly efficacious, and bacteriologic treatment failures are very rare. In a study of patients with two or more episodes of EM that occurred years apart, it was shown that the episodes were caused by different strains of bacteria, indicating that reinfection, rather than persistence of the original organism, was the cause of repeated episodes of EM. Reinfection rarely occurs in patients with late Lyme disease, indicating that most such patients are immune. On the other hand, patients with early Lyme disease who are treated may become reinfected from a new tick bite, presumably because the organism was killed before a protective immune response could occur. Persistent or recurrent arthritis does occur in 10% to 20% of patients with Lyme arthritis. So-called antibiotic-refractory arthritis occurs when frank arthritis persists despite two or more courses of antimicrobial treatment. This may be due to either an autoimmune process or slow clearance of antigens of dead organisms. There is no evidence that the cause is failure of the antibiotic to kill the organisms.

Post-Treatment Lyme Disease Syndrome and "Chronic" Lyme Disease

A small minority of patients with Lyme disease who have completed appropriate treatment may continue to have nonspecific symptoms, such as fatigue, arthralgia, myalgia, or perceived cognitive difficulties, for weeks or months after completing treatment. These have been termed *post-treatment Lyme disease symptoms* and, if they persist for 6 months or longer and are disabling, are referred to as *post-treatment Lyme disease syndrome* (PTLDS). It is not clear whether the frequency or the nature of these symptoms in patients with PTLDS is greater than that among the general population. In addition, several placebo-controlled, randomized clinical trials of prolonged courses (≥6) of intensive antimicrobial treatment (e.g., with ceftriaxone[1]) in patients with PTLDS have found there was virtually no benefit and substantial risk of adverse side effects of this treatment. Consequently, the Infectious Diseases Society of America, the American Academy of Pediatrics, the American Academy of Neurology, the American College of Rheumatology, and expert professional societies from many European countries do not recommend prolonged treatment with antimicrobials in patients with PTLDS. These patients are distinguished from patients with so-called chronic Lyme disease, who have complaints similar to those with PTLDS but who do not have evidence of ever having had Lyme disease. Of course, prolonged antimicrobial treatment is not indicated for these patients, who might better be described as having medically unexplained symptoms. Patients with either PTLDS or "chronic Lyme disease" are best managed by focusing on alleviating symptoms rather than with additional courses of antibiotic therapy. This is because long-term treatment with

antibiotics has not been shown to provide benefit and is associated with substantial risks. Managing these patients can be challenging. Ideally, management decisions should be directed by a clinician who can form a long-term therapeutic relationship with the patient and who has substantial experience managing medically unexplained symptoms. Clinicians need to be aware that while there is no scientific evidence to support the existence of "chronic" Lyme disease, many of these patients are suffering and, thus, are vulnerable to those who would offer inappropriate and potentially harmful therapies.

Prevention

The tick bite that transmits the infection is not recognized in most patients with Lyme disease. This is because most people who recognize that a tick is attached remove the tick before it can transmit the infection. It is worth trying to identify the species and degree of engorgement of a tick, because if it is not an *Ixodes* tick, it cannot transmit *B. burgdorferi,* and if it has not been feeding for at least 36 hours, then transmission is unlikely. Ticks that have been removed can be submitted to local public health authorities for identification. However, public health departments often also perform a PCR assay to test for the presence of *B. burgdorferi.* Although a negative result can be reassuring, a positive result may be misleading; because the assay is very sensitive, it could detect very small numbers of bacteria, and the predictive value of a positive result for risk of Lyme disease is unknown.

A single dose of doxycycline (8.8 mg/kg, maximum 200 mg)[1] taken within 72 hours of a deer tick bite was effective in preventing Lyme disease. However, because the risk of Lyme disease after a recognized tick bite is low, prophylaxis generally is not recommended routinely, but only for those at higher risk, such as someone in an endemic area who removes an engorged nymphal stage deer tick.

Treatment

Antimicrobial treatment of Lyme disease is highly effective and complications are rare (Table 1). The recommendations for treatment are summarized in the table. Antimicrobials that are highly effective and are considered first-line agents to treat Lyme disease orally (PO) include doxycycline,[1] amoxicillin (Amoxil),[1] and cefuroxime axetil (Ceftin). Amoxicillin is the preferred agent for women who are either pregnant or breastfeeding. Because the risk of teeth staining is low, use of doxycycline for 21 days or less of treatment in children younger than 8 years of age is now considered acceptable. Doxycycline is the preferred oral agent due to its good activity against other tick-borne illnesses such as human granulocytic anaplasmosis. Although macrolides such as azithromycin (Zithromax),[1] clarithromycin (Biaxin),[1] and erythromycin (EES)[1] are effective for treating early Lyme disease, they may not be as effective as the first-line agents. When parenteral treatment is indicated, ceftriaxone (Rocephin)[1] is the preferred agent because of once-daily administration. Alternative antimicrobials such as cefotaxime (Claforan)[1] and penicillin G (Pfizerpen-G)[1] also are highly effective, although penicillin G is rarely used because of need for frequent dosing due to its short half-life.

For patients with single EM or multiple EM, a 10-day course of doxycycline or a 14-day course of either amoxicillin or cefuroxime is recommended. For cranial nerve palsy (without apparent meningitis) or carditis that is asymptomatic and for which the patient is not hospitalized, a 14-day course of a first-line oral antimicrobial is recommended. For complicated carditis (complete heart block) and for meningitis, a 14-day course of a parental agent is recommended, although for patients who are not severely ill, 14 days of doxycycline[1] PO is an acceptable alternative for treating meningitis. Some experts complete a course of initial parenteral treatment with oral therapy after the patient has improved clinically. Patients with Lyme meningitis should be carefully evaluated for increased intracranial pressure which, if present, should be managed appropriately. There is no evidence that steroids are beneficial for patients with facial palsy due to Lyme disease. For treatment of Lyme arthritis, a 28-day course of an oral antimicrobial

---

[1] Not FDA approved for this indication.

[1] Not FDA approved for this indication.

TABLE 1	Antimicrobials Recommended to Treat Lyme Disease		
MANIFESTATION	**FIRST-LINE AGENTS**	**ALTERNATIVE AGENTS**	**DURATION**
Single or multiple erythema migrans, cranial nerve palsy, carditis that is asymptomatic or for which the patient is not hospitalized	Doxycycline (Vibramycin)[1] 4.4 mg/kg/day in 2 divided doses (maximum 100 mg/dose)	Azithromycin (Zithromax)[1] 10 mg/kg/day in 1 dose (maximum 500 mg/dose)	14 days; for single EM, 10-days of doxycycline or 7–10 days of azithromycin is effective
	Amoxicillin (Amoxil)[1] 50 mg/kg per day in 3 divided doses (maximum 500 mg/dose)	Clarithromycin (Biaxin)[1] 7.5 mg/kg in 2 divided doses (maximum 500 mg/dose)	
	Cefuroxime axetil (Ceftin) 30 mg/kg PO in 2 divided doses (maximum 500 mg/dose)	Erythromycin (EES)[1] 12.5 mg/kg in 4 divided doses (maximum 500 mg/dose)	
Severe carditis, meningitis,* radiculomyelitis	Ceftriaxone (Rocephin)[1] 50–75 mg/kg IV in 1 dose (maximum 2 g/dose)	Cefotaxime (Claforan)[1] 150–200 mg/kg/day IV in 3 divided doses (maximum 2 g/dose) Penicillin G (Pfizerpen)[1] 200,000–400,000 U/kg/day in 6 divided doses (maximum 4 million U/dose)	14 days; for severe carditis and for meningitis, an oral agent may be used to complete a course of treatment after substantial clinical improvement
Lyme arthritis†	Same oral agents used for EM	Same oral agents used EM	28 days

*Some experts treat Lyme meningitis with doxycycline (Vibramycin),[1] administered orally, 4.4 mg/kg/day in 2 divided doses (maximum 100 mg/dose), for 14 days.
†Patients with persistent or recurrent arthritis 4 weeks after completing treatment may receive either a second 4-week course of treatment orally or 2 weeks of treatment with a parenterally administered antimicrobial listed above.
[1]Not FDA approved for this indication.

is recommended. Nonsteroidal antiinflammatory drugs may be effective for treating the pain and inflammation associated with Lyme arthritis.

References

Centers for Disease Control. Lyme disease: Lyme disease. Available at [https://www.cdc.gov/lyme/index.html Accessed June 12, 2024].
Dersch R, Torbahn G, Rauer S: Treatment of post-treatment Lyme disease symptoms-a systematic review, *Eur J Neurol* 31, 2024:e16293, .
Lantos PM, Rumbaugh J, Bockenstedt LK, Falck-Ytter YT, et al: Clinical practice guidelines by the Infectious Diseases Society of America (IDSA), American Academy of Neurology (AAN), and American College of Rheumatology (ACR): 2020 guidelines for the prevention, diagnosis and treatment of Lyme disease, *Clin Infect Dis J* 23(72):1–8, 2021.
Steere AC, Strle F, Wormser GP, et al: Lyme borreliosis, *Nat Rev Dis Primers* 2:1–18, 2016.

MALARIA

Method of
Stephanie Spivack, MD

CURRENT DIAGNOSIS

- Malaria is an infection with protozoa of the genus *Plasmodium*. Five species are known to infect humans: *P. falciparum, P. vivax, P. ovale, P. malariae,* and *P. knowlesi*. Malaria is endemic in tropical regions of Africa, Asia, Latin America, the Caribbean, Oceania, and the Middle East.
- Malaria can range from mildly symptomatic to life threatening and is responsible for considerable morbidity and mortality worldwide. Children and pregnant women are especially vulnerable.
- Malaria should be suspected in people who are returning from endemic areas with fever. Other common symptoms include headache, myalgias, arthralgias, and malaise.
- The cornerstone of diagnosis is visualization of parasites on Giemsa-stained thick and thin blood smears. Rapid diagnostic tests (RDTs) can make a diagnosis quickly but cannot differentiate species of *Plasmodium* or quantify parasite burden, so should always be performed in conjunction with microscopy.

CURRENT THERAPY

- Treatment is based on disease severity, species of *Plasmodium* involved, expected drug susceptibility based on the area where the infection was acquired, and prior use of chemoprophylaxis. If chemoprophylaxis was used, a different medication should be selected for treatment.
- For uncomplicated malaria that is chloroquine sensitive, chloroquine or hydroxychloroquine (Plaquenil) can be used. Malaria that is presumed to be sensitive includes *P. falciparum* from certain areas of Central America, the Caribbean, and the Middle East; all *P. ovale, P. knowlesi[1], and P. malariae;* and *P. vivax,* unless acquired in Papua New Guinea or Indonesia.
- For uncomplicated *P. falciparum* malaria that is chloroquine resistant, options in the United States include artemether-lumefantrine (Coartem; preferred), atovaquone-proguanil (Malarone), or quinine sulfate (Qualaquin) in combination with doxycycline[1], tetracycline[1], or clindamycin[1].
- Intravenous (IV) artesunate is the first-line treatment for severe malaria. If this is unavailable, it should be acquired promptly, and an oral antimalarial option be used until it is available.
- Infections with *P. vivax* and *P. ovale[1]* should be treated with primaquine or tafenoquine (Krintafel) at the end of therapy to prevent relapse from hypnozoites (dormant liver forms); glucose-6-phosphate dehydrogenase (G6PD) levels should be tested before administering these medications.
- Travelers to endemic areas should use chemoprophylaxis in combination with mosquito avoidance to prevent infection; options include atovaquone-proguanil, doxycycline, mefloquine, chloroquine (if traveling to an area with chloroquine-sensitive malaria), primaquine[1] and tafenoquine (Arakoda).

[1]Not FDA approved for this indication.

Introduction

Malaria is a parasitic infection caused by protozoa of the genus *Plasmodium*. Malaria is transmitted by the bite of the female *Anopheles* mosquito.

Malaria is an enormous health problem globally and disproportionately affects impoverished populations in the tropics. In 2023 there were 263 million reported cases with 597,000 deaths in 83 countries. The World Health Organization (WHO) African Region carries the vast majority of the disease burden, with 94% of cases and 95% of deaths in 2023. Malaria can be particularly devastating for children and pregnant women. In the WHO African Region, children under 5 years old accounted for 76% of malaria deaths in 2023. Infections during pregnancy can result in premature delivery, low birth weight, and perinatal death. In addition to its burden on health, malaria also has a considerable economic impact. It is estimated that for each 10% reduction in malaria incidence, the gross domestic product (GDP) can increase up to 2% in high-burden low-income countries.

There has been significant global investment in efforts to control malaria with the eventual goal of elimination. This is a multipronged effort, including distribution of insecticide-treated bed nets, indoor residual spraying, improved access to testing and medication, targeted chemoprophylaxis, and development and implementation of vaccinations.

Risk Factors and Protective Factors

People who travel to or live in areas of malaria transmission are at risk of acquiring malaria. Each person's individual risk depends on a variety of factors, including their itinerary, sleeping and living accommodations, adherence to mosquito avoidance measures and chemoprophylaxis, time of year, local weather conditions, and density of local mosquito populations. Temperature and rainfall are major determinants for mosquito activity. Mosquitoes are most active when the temperature is above 20°C (68°F) and during the rainy or wet season. Because *Anopheles* bite between dusk and dawn, people who sleep without window screens, air conditioning, or bed nets are at higher risk. Notably, because of climate change, the range of mosquitoes is expanding toward the poles and toward higher altitudes as the temperature in these areas grows warmer, which will put new populations at risk for malaria. In subtropical climates, the mosquito biting season is also growing longer. Outbreaks of malaria have been associated with severe weather events like extreme rainfall and flooding; these events are expected to become more frequent as a result of climate change.

People who live in high-transmission areas during childhood develop partial acquired immunity from repeated infections and generally do not become severely ill from malaria. Acquired immunity increases with age, number of infections, and time spent in an endemic area. However, this immunity is quickly lost when people move to nonendemic areas. Therefore immigrants who return to visit friends and relatives (VFR) are a high-risk population because they may consider themselves immune and not take protective measures. Patients from this group may present to care with a self-diagnosis of malaria because they are highly familiar with this disease and its symptoms.

There are multiple genetic mutations in erythrocytes that are protective against malaria as well. For example, people who have erythrocytes lacking these Duffy antigen chemokine receptors (DARCs) are less likely to develop infection with *P. vivax*, which uses these receptors to enter cells. Mutations in hemoglobin are thought to inhibit parasite growth within erythrocytes. The most common of these is hemoglobin S heterozygosity (HbAS, or sickle cell trait), which has a prevalence of more than 25% in some malaria-endemic areas. Hemoglobin C (HbC) mutation, α-thalassemia, and other hemoglobinopathies are also protective. Neonates younger than 6 months rarely acquire malaria; this is thought to be from both maternal immunity and from the protective effects of fetal hemoglobin (HbF). People with glucose-6-phosphate dehydrogenase (G6PD) deficiency also have some protection; this is thought to be due to enhanced phagocytosis of infected G6PD-deficient erythrocytes. Many more examples of protective mutations exist; these are varied and still being fully elucidated.

Epidemiology

There are five species of *Plasmodia* associated with human disease: *P. falciparum*, *P. vivax*, *P. ovale*, *P. malariae*, and *P. knowlesi*. *P. falciparum* is the predominant species in sub-Saharan Africa and causes the majority of morbidity and mortality worldwide. *P. vivax* and *P. ovale* occupy different niches with some overlap, with *P. ovale* primarily in sub-Saharan Africa and *P. vivax* in the other areas. *P. malariae* is found worldwide but less frequently than *P. falciparum*. *P. knowlesi* is found primarily in Southeast Asia and is the only species with a zoonotic reservoir of macaques; it is unknown if it can be spread from human to human without the macaque as an intermediate host.

Malaria is transmitted from human to human (with the exception of *P. knowlesi*) by the bite of the female *Anopheles* mosquito. More than 30 types of *Anopheles* have been associated with malaria transmission worldwide. Infrequent cases of malaria transmission have been reported from mother to child, from blood transfusions, and from solid organ transplants. Rare cases of malaria have been reported around airports from mosquitoes that were unintentionally transported by airplane. Autochthonous (local) transmission can occur in nonendemic areas when a returning traveler with malaria is bitten by a mosquito before seeking treatment; this mosquito in turn can bite a resident and spread the parasite. There were 10 such cases of local transmission in the United States in 2023. "Imported" cases of malaria in travelers returning from endemic areas are much more common; the Centers for Disease Control and Prevention (CDC) reports approximately 2000 such cases in the United States annually.

Parasite Life Cycle

The life cycle of *Plasmodium* is completed in two hosts: the *Anopheles* mosquito and the human. First, an infected female mosquito introduces sporozoites (infective stage) into the human when taking a blood meal. These sporozoites travel through the blood to the liver, where they mature into schizonts, which then rupture to release merozoites (asexual blood stage) into the bloodstream. *P. vivax* and *P. ovale* have an additional hypnozoite (dormant) stage in the liver. These merozoites infect erythrocytes and develop into trophozoites (active stage). Some trophozoites will develop into schizonts, which release more merozoites, continuing the cycle in humans. Other trophozoites will differentiate into gametocytes (sexual stage), which are ingested by another *Anopheles* taking a blood meal. In the mosquito, the parasite will develop and eventually make its way back to the salivary gland of the mosquito, ready to continue its cycle with a new human host.

Clinical Manifestations

After an exposure, the typical incubation period is 8 to 14 days, but can vary widely based on the infecting species, the size of the exposure, and whether the host has prior immunity or took chemoprophylaxis. Incubation periods of up to 1 year have been reported.

Malaria classically presents with an acute febrile illness with paroxysms of chills and rigors, followed by fevers, then profuse sweating, and finally fatigue. The fever can rise above 40°C (104°F). The paroxysms can be accompanied by headaches, myalgias, arthralgias, malaise, and fatigue; less common symptoms include abdominal pain and diarrhea. The interval of fever paroxysms depends on the infecting species. In general, *P. knowlesi* causes fevers every 24 hours; *P. falciparum*, *P. vivax*, and *P. ovale* cause fevers every 48 hours (tertian fever); and *P. malariae* causes fevers every 72 hours (quartan fever). These paroxysms are caused by schizonts rupturing in the blood at regular intervals. Patients may be asymptomatic between paroxysms.

On physical examination, patients may have pallor, splenomegaly, and occasionally jaundice. Splenomegaly is caused by sequestration of both infected and noninfected erythrocytes in the spleen; splenic rupture has been associated with all species but most commonly with *P. vivax*. In asplenic patients, malaria can progress rapidly with high degrees of parasitemia.

The most common laboratory finding is anemia; this is typically normocytic but can be microcytic if there is an underlying nutritional deficiency or hemoglobinopathy. Additional nonspecific findings include leukocytosis or leukopenia, thrombocytopenia, elevated blood urea nitrogen (BUN) and creatinine, and elevated transaminases. There are no characteristic radiographic findings.

Nonfalciparum Malaria

Infections with *P. vivax* and *P. ovale* are less likely to cause severe malaria than *P. falciparum*. *P. falciparum* infects erythrocytes of all ages, while *P. vivax* and *P. ovale* infect only reticulocytes, resulting in lower parasite burdens. *P. falciparum* trophozoites and schizonts also sequester in microvasculature, where they can avoid detection and destruction while multiplying, leading to higher parasite burdens. However, *P. vivax* has been associated with severe cases in Papua New Guinea and Indonesia. *P. vivax* and *P. ovale* produce liver hypnozoites that may reactivate and cause relapses of malaria months or even years after the initial infection. *P. malariae* causes milder disease with an indolent course and can remain undetected for years. *P. knowlesi* presents similarly to *P. falciparum*. Because it replicates every 24 hours, it can cause daily fever spikes, high levels of parasitemia, and severe complications. Of note, mixed infections with more than one species can occur.

Severe Malaria

Severe malaria is diagnosed when patients have at least 1 of 12 clinical, laboratory, or radiographic findings: impaired consciousness, prostration, convulsions, acidosis, hypoglycemia, severe anemia, renal impairment, jaundice, pulmonary edema, bleeding, shock, and hyperparasitemia. The complete criteria are listed in Table 1.

The respiratory failure seen in severe malaria is caused by sequestration of infected erythrocytes in the pulmonary vasculature leading to a local inflammatory response and noncardiogenic pulmonary edema; this may require mechanical ventilation. Renal failure associated with severe malaria may require renal replacement therapy. Hypoglycemia is multifactorial, due to reduced hepatic gluconeogenesis, increased glucose consumption by tissues and parasites, excess insulin secretion by the pancreas, and poor oral intake. Lactic acidosis is a common finding in severe malaria, present in an estimated 85% of cases; hypovolemia, microvascular obstruction from sequestration, and anemia all contribute to reduced oxygen delivery to tissues. The anemia seen in malaria is multifactorial, due to hemolysis, phagocytosis of both infected and uninfected erythrocytes, and impaired erythropoiesis from inflammation.

Mortality from severe malaria approaches 100% if untreated but falls to 10% to 20% when treated promptly and effectively. Nonimmune individuals can progress to severe malaria quickly, so inpatient monitoring is recommended for all nonimmune patients with malaria until they are clinically improving.

Cerebral Malaria

Cerebral malaria occurs when infected erythrocytes become sequestered in the cerebral microvasculature. This can lead to altered or decreased level of consciousness, seizures, and can progress to coma. The diagnosis of cerebral malaria is made clinically when other causes of encephalopathy have been ruled out. The only way to confirm a diagnosis is by autopsy; there are reports of children who were diagnosed with cerebral malaria but were later found not to have consistent findings on autopsy. New biomarkers and imaging techniques are being studied to improve diagnostic accuracy. Children are more likely than adults to have persistent neurologic deficits after recovery; these can include hemiplegia, cerebellar ataxia, extrapyramidal rigidity, hearing impairment, and cognitive impairment.

Malaria During Pregnancy

Pregnant women are particularly vulnerable to poor outcomes from malaria, especially people who are nonimmune and in their

TABLE 1	Features of Severe Malaria
FINDING	**DESCRIPTION**
Impaired consciousness	Adults: Glasgow coma score <11 Children: Blantyre coma score <3
Prostration	Inability to sit, stand, or walk without assistance
Convulsions	More than 2 episodes in 24 hours
Acidosis	• A base deficit of >8 mEq/L, *or* • Plasma bicarbonate level of <15 mmol/L, *or* • Venous plasma lactate ≥5 mmol/L
Hypoglycemia	Blood or plasma glucose <2.2 mmol/L (<40 mg/dL)
Severe anemia	• Hemoglobin concentration ≤5 g/dL, *or* • Hematocrit of ≤15% in children <12 years, *or* • Hematocrit of <7 g/dL and <20% in those ≥12 years, *with* • Parasite count >10,000/µL
Renal impairment	• Plasma or serum creatinine >265 µmol/L (3 mg/dL), *or* • Blood urea nitrogen (BUN) >20 mmol/L
Jaundice	Plasma or serum bilirubin >50 µmol/L (3 mg/dL) *with*: • *Plasmodium falciparum* parasite count >2.5% parasitemia, *or* • *Plasmodium knowlesi* parasite count >20,000 parasites/µL
Pulmonary edema	• Consistent radiologic findings, *or* • Oxygen saturation <92% on room air, *plus* • Respiratory rate >30/min
Bleeding	• Recurrent or prolonged bleeding from the nose, gums, or venipuncture sites, *or* • Hematemesis, *or* • Melena
Shock	• Compensated shock (capillary refill ≥3 seconds, *or* temperature gradient on leg, but no hypotension) • Decompensated shock (systolic blood pressure <70 mm Hg in children or <80 mm Hg in adults, with evidence of impaired perfusion [cool extremities or prolonged capillary refill])
Hyperparasitemia	*Plasmodium falciparum:* • In nonimmune travelers: parasitemia ≥5% • All patients: parasitemia >10% *Plasmodium knowlesi:* • Parasite density >100,000 parasites/µL *Plasmodium vivax:* • No established thresholds

first pregnancy. Possible adverse outcomes in the fetus include premature delivery, intrauterine growth restriction, low birthweight, and perinatal mortality. Pregnant women can experience hypoglycemia and pulmonary edema. Parasites can infect the placenta, leading to congenital malaria in the neonate, or to recurrence of malaria in the mother.

Other Complications

Malaria can predispose to other infections; there is a well-documented association with bacteremia. Malaria may also increase the morbidity and mortality of other diseases by causing relative immunosuppression, dehydration, anemia, and malnutrition.

Laboratory Diagnosis

There are multiple methods available for confirming a diagnosis of malaria. The gold standard is visualization of parasites on

Giemsa-stained thick and thin blood smears. The thick smears allow for screening of a large amount of blood, and the thin smears allow for species identification based on morphology. Quantification of parasitemia can be performed on both thick and thin smears. On microscopic examination, *P. falciparum* will have classic ring-form trophozoites inside infected erythrocytes, sometimes with more than one trophozoite per erythrocyte, as well as banana-shaped gametocytes outside of erythrocytes; *P. vivax* and *P. ovale* cause enlargement of infected erythrocytes with Schüffner's dots in the cytoplasm, as well as the presence of schizonts in the peripheral blood (these are sequestered in infections with *P. falciparum*); *P. malariae* has characteristic band forms (thick trophozoites stretching across infected erythrocytes); and *P. knowlesi* is difficult to distinguish from *P. falciparum*. Parasitemia is quantified based on the number of infected erythrocytes; gametocytes do not cause disease and are not included in this calculation. Patients may have symptomatic malaria with a negative blood smear; this is more likely in individuals who are immunocompromised or those who have an infection with *P. vivax* or *P. ovale*. Smears should be repeated three times at intervals of 12 to 24 hours to increase sensitivity. Smears are also used to monitor treatment response; parasitemia should decrease with treatment. The major limitation of microscopy is that it requires a trained microscopist; because of the time-sensitive nature of malaria diagnosis, a microbiologist should always be available. The sensitivity and specificity approach 100% but can be operator dependent.

Rapid diagnostic tests (RDTs) are a valuable point-of-care tool. RDTs detect an antigen present in the malaria parasite; they can provide a result in 15 minutes or less and can use a fingerstick blood sample so do not require phlebotomy. There are multiple RDTs available with different targets: histidine-rich protein 2 (HRP2), *Plasmodium* lactate dehydrogenase (pLDH), and aldolase. HRP2 is produced only by *P. falciparum*, while pLDH and aldolase are produced by all species. The BinaxNOW test manufactured by Abbott Pharmaceuticals is commercially available in the United States and uses a combination of HRP2 and aldolase. According to the package insert, for patients with >5000 parasites/μL, the BinaxNOW test has a sensitivity of 99.7% and specificity of 94.2% for *P. falciparum*; it has a sensitivity of 93.5% and specificity of 99.8% for *P. vivax*.

All RDTs should be used in combination with microscopy. A positive RDT cannot determine the infecting species of *Plasmodia* or determine the degree of parasitemia. RDTs may remain positive for days or weeks even after malaria has been sufficiently treated, so they cannot be used to monitor treatment response. Therefore they are most useful for rapidly making a diagnosis and initiating treatment when a trained microbiologist is not immediately available.

Some *Plasmodia* have evolved to evade detection by RDTs. These parasites have a mutation that results in the absence of HRP2. Patients infected with these parasites may have a missed diagnosis of malaria resulting in delayed treatment, leading to further disease complications and further spread of these parasites. These mutated parasites have been reported 41 countries and now exceed 15% of all malaria reported in Brazil, Djibouti, Eritrea, Nicaragua, and Peru.

Polymerase chain reaction (PCR) tests have high sensitivity and specificity and can likely detect malaria even in cases with a low degree of parasitemia where a smear or RDT may be falsely negative. However, these tests have limited clinical utility because they are not readily available. Likewise, serology is generally not useful in the clinical setting because antibodies take days to weeks to develop.

Differential Diagnosis

The differential diagnosis of malaria is broad. There are multiple variables to consider, including the patient's age, health, and immune status; their specific travel and exposure history; their vaccine history; and their adherence to insect avoidance and chemoprophylaxis. Patients may present with more than one infection at once; testing and therapy should be guided by history and physical examination.

Some diseases to consider include hepatitis viruses; enteric illnesses including typhoid fever; arboviruses including dengue, chikungunya, Zika, and Oropouche; zoonotic infections including leptospirosis and hantavirus; and viral hemorrhagic fevers including Ebola and Marburg viruses. The trophozoites of malaria may be confused with babesia on blood smear, but the two can be differentiated by morphology and by the exposure history. In patients with prominent headaches, bacterial meningitis can be considered. Finally, respiratory viruses like influenza present very similarly to malaria. Ultimately, these are differentiated from malaria by diagnostic testing with microscopy and possibly RDTs.

Antimalarial Drugs
Treatment of Uncomplicated Malaria

The key to successful malaria treatment is early initiation of therapy. Malaria, particularly *P. falciparum* and *P. knowlesi*, can progress quickly if treatment is delayed. An infectious disease or tropical medicine specialist should be consulted if available. The CDC has a Malaria Hotline for expert consultation (available from 9 AM to 5 PM Eastern Standard Time at (770) 488-7788, or toll-free at (855) 856-4713; after hours, a malaria expert can be reached through the Emergency Operations Center at (770) 488-7100).

Four main factors should be considered when choosing a treatment course: the species of *Plasmodium* involved; the clinical status of the patient (uncomplicated vs. severe malaria); the expected drug susceptibility based on the area acquired; and the prior use of antimalarial treatment or chemoprophylaxis.

For uncomplicated *P. falciparum*, or if the species is unknown, that is acquired in an area where malaria is typically chloroquine sensitive (Central America west of the Panama Canal, Haiti, Dominican Republic, parts of the Middle East), oral chloroquine or hydroxychloroquine (Plaquenil) can be used. For *P. falciparum* acquired from all other areas, artemisinin-based combination therapies (ACTs) are the preferred treatment. Artemether-lumefantrine (Coartem) is preferred when available. Additional ACTs available outside the United States include artesunate-amodiaquine, artesunate-mefloquine, dihydroartemisinin-piperaquine, artesunate + sulfadoxine-pyrimethamine, and artesunate-pyronaridine. In the United States, if artemether-lumefantrine is not available, alternatives include atovaquone-proguanil (Malarone), mefloquine, or a combination of quinine sulfate with doxycycline[1], tetracycline (preferred)[1], or clindamycin[1]. Please see Table 2 for dosing details and side effects. Treatment doses of mefloquine carry a high risk of neuropsychiatric side effects, so this is generally not preferred unless there are no other options.

Infections with *P. vivax*, *P. ovale*, *P. malariae*, and *P. knowlesi* can be assumed to be chloroquine sensitive with the exception of *P. vivax* infections acquired in Papua New Guinea or Indonesia. These infections can be treated with chloroquine or hydroxychloroquine. ACTs, quinine combinations, and mefloquine will be effective as well. *P. vivax* and *P. ovale*[1] require additional antirelapse treatment to treat liver hypnozoites and prevent recurrence. This can be achieved with primaquine or tafenoquine (Krintafel). Of note, both medications can cause hemolytic anemia in patients who have G6PD deficiency; a G6PD level must be checked and return within normal range before these drugs are given. Additionally, tafenoquine (Krintafel) can only be used in patients who are aged 16 years or older, have no history of psychotic disorder, and received treatment with chloroquine for the acute phase.

During treatment, thick and thin blood smears should be checked every 12 to 24 hours. Once the patient is clinically improving and the parasitemia is improving, care can be transitioned to the outpatient setting.

---

[1] Not FDA approved for this indication.

TABLE 2 Medication Options for the Treatment of Malaria

Treatment for Uncomplicated Malaria

DRUG	INDICATION	ADULT DOSING	PEDIATRIC DOSING	SIDE EFFECTS	COMMENTS
Artemether-lumefantrine (Coartem)	*Plasmodium falciparum* that is chloroquine resistant (everywhere except part of Central America, Caribbean, Middle East) Alternative for chloroquine-sensitive *P. falciparum* Alternative for *P. vivax*[1], *P. ovale*[1], *P. malariae*[1], *P. knowlesi*[1]	1 tab = 20 mg artemether + 120 mg lumefantrine 1 dose = 4 tabs Day 1: 1 dose at 0 hours, 1 dose 8 hours later Days 2 and 3: 1 dose BID	Can be used if ≥5 kg 5 to <15 kg: 1 tab per dose 15 to <25 kg: 2 tabs per dose 25 to <35 kg: 3 tabs per dose ≥35 kg: 4 tabs per dose Day 1: 1 dose at 0 hours, 1 dose 8 hours later Days 2 and 3: 1 dose BID	Palpitations, headache, dizziness, fever, anorexia, nausea, vomiting, abdominal pain, sleep disorder, arthralgias, myalgias	Preferred for chloroquine-resistant *P. falciparum* Can be used in pregnancy
Atovaquone-proguanil (Malarone)	*P. falciparum* that is chloroquine resistant (everywhere except part of Central America, Caribbean, Middle East) Alternative for chloroquine-sensitive *P. falciparum* Alternative for *P. vivax*[1], *P. ovale*[1], *P. malariae*[1], *P. knowlesi*[1]	Adult tab = 250 mg atovaquone + 100 mg proguanil 4 tabs QD × 3 days	Can be used if ≥5 kg Pediatric (ped) tab = 62.5 mg atovaquone + 25 mg proguanil 5 to <8 kg: 2 ped tabs QD × 3 days 8 to <10 kg: 3 ped tabs QD × 3 days 10 to <20 kg: 1 adult tab QD × 3 days 20 to <30 kg: 2 adult tabs QD × 3 days 30 to <40 kg: 3 adult tabs QD × 3 days ≥40 kg: 4 adult tabs QD × 3 days	Abdominal pain, nausea, vomiting, headache, dizziness, elevated transaminases	Use with extreme caution in renal dysfunction with CrCl <30 mL/min after carefully weighing risks and benefits. Proguanil can accumulate and cause cytopenias in patients with renal dysfunction.
Quinine sulfate (Qualaquin) with doxycycline, tetracycline, or clindamycin	*P. falciparum* that is chloroquine resistant (everywhere except part of Central America, Caribbean, Middle East) Alternative for chloroquine-sensitive *P. falciparum* Alternative for *P. vivax*[1], *P. ovale*[1], *P. malariae*[1], *P. knowlesi*[1]	Quinine sulfate: 542 mg base (650 mg salt [2 capsules]) TID × 3 days Use quinine for 7 days for infections from Southeast Asia *Plus* one of the following: Doxycycline[1]: 100 mg BID × 7 days, *or* Tetracycline[1]: 250 mg QID × 7 days, *or* Clindamycin[1]: 20 mg/kg/day divided TID × 7 days. Do not exceed 1.8 g/day	Use doxycycline and tetracycline only if >8 years old Quinine sulfate: 8.3 mg base/kg (10 mg salt/kg) TID × 3 days Use quinine for 7 days for infections from Southeast Asia Doxycycline[1]: 2.2 mg/kg BID × 7 days Tetracycline[1]: 25 mg/kg/day divided QID × 7 days Clindamycin[1]: 20 mg/kg/day divided TID × 7 days	Quinine: dizziness, nausea, vomiting, tinnitus, QT prolongation, hypoglycemia Doxycycline: photosensitivity, esophagitis, GI upset Tetracycline: photosensitivity, GI upset Clindamycin: nausea, vomiting, diarrhea including from *Clostridioides difficile*, hypersensitivity reactions	Avoid doxycycline and tetracycline in pregnancy; quinine and clindamycin can be used Quinine is contraindicated with myasthenia gravis, optic neuritis, history of hypersensitivity reactions to mefloquine or quinidine (may be cross-reactive), prolonged QT interval Use quinine with caution in patients with atrial fibrillatoin or cardiac arrhythmias. Use with caution with mild to moderate hepatic impairment. Avoid in severe hepatic impairment Dose reduction of quinine recommended in renal impairment with GFR <50

TABLE 2 Medication Options for the Treatment of Malaria—cont'd

DRUG	INDICATION	ADULT DOSING	PEDIATRIC DOSING	SIDE EFFECTS	COMMENTS
Mefloquine	*P. falciparum* that is chloroquine resistant (everywhere except part of Central America, Caribbean, Middle East) Alternative for chloroquine-sensitive *P. falciparum* Alternative for *P. vivax, P. ovale*[1], *P. malariae*[1], *P. knowlesi*[1]	Dose 1: 750 mg Dose 2 at 6–12 hours: 500 mg	Dose 1: 15 mg/kg (max 750 mg/dose) Dose 2 at 6–12 hours: 10 mg/kg (max 500 mg/dose)	Vomiting, neuropsychiatric side effects (vivid dreams, insomnia, anxiety, depression, paranoia, hallucinations)	Safe in pregnancy Avoid with major psychiatric disorders
Chloroquine phosphate (Aralen)	Preferred for all chloroquine-sensitive malaria Chloroquine-sensitive *P. falciparum* (part of Central America, Caribbean, and Middle East) *P. vivax* except from Papua New Guinea and Indonesia *P. ovale, P. falciparum, P. malariae, P. knowlesi*[1]	Dose 1: 600 mg base (1000 mg salt) Doses 2, 3, and 4 at 6, 24, and 48 hours: 300 mg base (500 mg salt)	Dose 1: 10 mg/kg base (16.7 mg/kg salt) Doses 2, 3, and 4 at 6, 12, and 48 hours: 5 mg/kg base (8.3 mg/kg salt	QT prolongation, GI upset, headache, dizziness	Safe in pregnancy
Hydroxychloroquine (Plaquenil)	Chloroquine-sensitive *P. falciparum* (part of Central America, Caribbean, and Middle East) *P. vivax* except from Papua New Guinea and Indonesia *P. ovale, P. falciparum, P. malariae, P. knowlesi*[1]	Dose 1 = 620 mg base (800 mg salt) Doses 2, 3, and 4 at 6, 24, and 48 hours: 310 mg base (400 mg salt)	Dose 1 = 10 mg/kg base (12.9 mg/kg salt) Doses 2, 3, and 4 at 6, 24, and 48 hours: 5 mg/kg base (6.5 mg/kg salt)	QT prolongation, GI upset, headache	Safe in pregnancy For use only for if malaria is chloroquine sensitive

Treatment of Severe Malaria

DRUG	INDICATION	ADULT DOSING	PEDIATRIC DOSING	SIDE EFFECTS	COMMENTS
Artesunate	Severe malaria from any species of *Plasmodium*	2.4 mg/kg/dose IV Give at 0, 12, and 24 hours. Check smear 4 hours after 3rd dose If parasitemia >1%, give 1 dose daily until parasitemia <1% and patient able to take oral therapy, then transition to an oral regimen	2.4 mg/kg/dose IV* Give at 0, 12, and 24 hours. Check smear 4 hours after 3rd dose If parasitemia >1%, give 1 dose daily until parasitemia <1% and patient able to take oral therapy, then transition to an oral regimen		Monitor for posttreatment hemolysis with weekly labs (blood count, reticulocyte count, total bilirubin, and lactate dehydrogenase) × 4 weeks

Antirelapse Treatment

DRUG	INDICATION	ADULT DOSING	PEDIATRIC DOSING	SIDE EFFECTS	COMMENTS
Primaquine	Use in combination with a primary regimen for *P. vivax* and *P. ovale*[1] infections	30 mg base QD × 14 days[3] ≥70 kg: 30 mg QD until a total dose of 6 mg base/kg has been completed	<70 kg: 0.5 mg base/kg QD × 14 days (max 30 mg base/dose)	QT prolongation, GI upset	Check G6PD before use**

Continued

Malaria

TABLE 2 Medication Options for the Treatment of Malaria—cont'd

DRUG	INDICATION	ADULT DOSING	PEDIATRIC DOSING	SIDE EFFECTS	COMMENTS
Tafenoquine (Krintafel)	Use in combination with a primary regimen for *P. vivax* and *P. ovale*[1] infections	300 mg × 1 dose on day 1 or 2 of chloroquine or hydroxychloroquine therapy	Only for adolescents ≥16 years 300 mg single dose on day 1 or 2 of chloroquine or hydroxychloroquine therapy	Diarrhea, vomiting, headache, keratopathy (reversible), psychiatric symptoms (insomnia, anxiety, depression, abnormal dreams)	Can only be used if malaria was treated with chloroquine or hydroxychloroquine Check G6PD before use** Use in caution with history of psychiatric disease

*Some experts recommend using a higher dose of 3 mg/kg/dose in children <20 kg based on pharmacokinetic modeling. This dose is not approved by the FDA.

**In the case of intermediate G6PD deficiency, primaquine may be used at a dose of 45 mg weekly for 8 weeks with monitoring for hemolysis. In the case of G6PD deficiency, weekly chloroquine 300 mg (base) weekly can be used for 1 year.

[1]Not FDA approved for this indication.

[3]Exceeds dosage recommended by the manufacturer.

BID, Twice daily; *CrCl*, creatinine clearance; *GFR*, glomerular filtration rate; *GI*, gastrointestinal; *QD*, daily; *QID*, four times daily; *tab*, tablet; *TID*, three times daily.

Drug resistance remains a critical challenge for malaria treatment. Chloroquine was the main treatment option after its introduction in the 1980s, but resistance developed and spread rapidly. Resistance to cycloguanil (the active metabolite of proguanil) has been documented, and cases of atovaquone-proguanil (Malarone) failure have been reported. In Southeast Asia, there are regular cases of reduced quinine susceptibility and mefloquine resistance, with scattered cases in Africa and South America. Concerns about artemisinin resistance are now being investigated, with documented cases of slow parasite clearance and clinical failure of ACTs in Southeast Asia.

Treatment of Severe Malaria

If patients have any manifestation of severe malaria, IV artesunate should be initiated promptly. Artesunate lowers parasitemia more rapidly than any oral option. If artesunate is not in stock, efforts should be made to obtain it promptly; an oral antimalarial regimen can be initiated until it arrives. If nausea, vomiting, or lack of enteral access are barriers to oral medication, antiemetics and nasogastric tubes should be used as needed to deliver the drug; oral medications can be discontinued when artesunate is available. Artesunate is now manufactured by AMIVAS and available from major drug distributors. Pharmacists can call (855) 5AMIVAS ([855] 526-4827) to identify the closest distributor. Alternative options include obtaining the drug from a nearby hospital or transferring the patient to another hospital where artesunate is available. Guidance on obtaining artesunate can be found on the CDC's web page (https://www.cdc.gov/malaria/hcp /clinical-guidance/iv-artesunate-us.html).

Artesunate is administered at 0, 12, and 24 hours. A blood smear should be checked 4 hours after the third dose. If the parasitemia is still greater than 1%, artesunate should be continued daily for a maximum of 7 total days, with smears checked every 12 to 24 hours. When parasitemia is less than 1%, the patient can be transitioned to oral antimalarial treatment. Artesunate is only available in an IV formulation; an appropriate oral regimen can be chosen based on the factors detailed earlier. Patients should complete a full course of the oral regimen to prevent relapse.

Artesunate is generally well tolerated; the only contraindication to administering it is a known allergy. Postartemisinin hemolytic anemia has been reported, sometimes requiring transfusion. It is more likely to occur in cases with a high degree of parasitemia. After treatment with artesunate, blood work should be checked weekly, including hemoglobin, LDH, haptoglobin, bilirubin, and reticulocyte count. If any instances of postartemisinin hemolysis are detected, they should be reported to the Food and Drug Administration's (FDA) MedWatch program (https://www.fda.gov/safety/medwa tch-fda-safety-information-and-adverse-event-reporting-program).

Exchange transfusion, previously recommended to remove infected erythrocytes in patients with hyperparasitemia, is no longer recommended.

Antimalarial Drugs in Pregnancy

Chloroquine, hydroxychloroquine, artemether-lumefantrine (Coartem), mefloquine, or a combination of quinine sulfate and clindamycin[1] are options for treating uncomplicated malaria in pregnant women and can be used at all gestational ages. Atovaquone-proguanil (Malarone) is not recommended unless there are no alternative options because of a lack of evidence. Doxycycline and tetracycline are not recommended because of the risk for adverse tooth and bone development in the fetus.

Primaquine and tafenoquine (Krintafel) also cannot be given during pregnancy because they cross the placenta and can cause hemolytic anemia in G6PD-deficient fetuses. For patients with *P. vivax* or *P. ovale*, weekly chloroquine prophylaxis should be continued for the duration of the pregnancy, and primaquine or tafenoquine given after delivery. If the infant is being breastfed, it should be screened for G6PD deficiency before the administration of primaquine or tafenoquine in the mother. If primaquine and tafenoquine cannot be administered after delivery, chloroquine prophylaxis should be continued for 1 year. For pregnant women with severe malaria, aggressive treatment including IV artesunate should be used.

Treatment of Pediatric Patients

The treatment of malaria in pediatric patients depends on their age and weight. For children who weigh ≥5 kg, the treatment options for the acute phase are the same as those for adults, with the drug dose adjusted for patient weight; the pediatric dose should never exceed the recommended adult dose. For children under 8 years of age, doxycycline[1] and tetracycline[1] are generally not recommended due to the potential for tooth and bone malformation. For children who weigh <5 kg, mefloquine or a combination of quinine sulfate with clindamycin[1] are the only approved options. If these drugs are not available or not tolerated, artemether-lumefantrine or atovaquone-proguanil can be considered. In children with infection with *P. vivax* or *P. ovale*[1], primaquine or tafenoquine (Krintafel) should only be given after screening for G6PD deficiency is completed.

Prevention of Malaria

For travelers to areas with malaria transmission, a combination of insect avoidance and chemoprophylaxis is recommended; neither is 100% effective when used alone.

The *Anopheles* mosquito is a nocturnal feeder that bites between dusk and dawn; therefore maintaining safe living and sleeping conditions is important for preventing infection. This involves sleeping in an air-conditioned room or a room with window screens, sleeping under an insecticide-treated

---

[1]Not FDA approved for this indication.

mosquito net, using an insecticide spray or coils in living and sleeping areas, and wearing clothing that covers exposed parts of the body. In addition, a mosquito repellent should be applied to exposed skin when there is potential for mosquito bites. Repellents with diethyltoluamide (DEET) as the active ingredient are the most effective; ethyl butylacetylaminopropionate (IR3535) or picaridin are alternatives. Clothing and nets can be pretreated with permethrin for additional protection. Sunscreen should be applied before insect repellent if both are being used.

There are multiple options for chemoprophylaxis; the choice depends on the geographic area of travel. Options include atovaquone-proguanil (Malarone), doxycycline, chloroquine (in areas with chloroquine-sensitive malaria), mefloquine, and tafenoquine (Arakoda); primaquine has been used off-label. See Table 3 for details. In people with prolonged exposure to *P. vivax* or *P. ovale*, primaquine[1] or tafenoquine (Arakoda) should be given at the end of travel as terminal prophylaxis to kill liver hypnozoites. Detailed recommendations based on country can be found at the

CDC web page (https://wwwnc.cdc.gov/travel/yellowbook/2024 /preparing/yellow-fever-vaccine-malaria-prevention-by-country).

In infants, children, and adolescents, weight-based atovaquone-proguanil can be used for prophylaxis if the child weighs ≥5 kg. Chloroquine and mefloquine can be given to all infants and children. Doxycycline can be given to those older than 8 years. Primaquine[1] can be used in areas where *P. vivax* predominates, as long as G6PD levels are normal.

Pregnant women should be advised to avoid areas with malaria transmission until after delivery if possible. If this is not possible, chloroquine (if in an area with chloroquine-sensitive malaria) and mefloquine are the only safe options for prophylaxis during pregnancy. Doxycycline, primaquine, and tafenoquine are contraindicated. In those who are planning to become pregnant, conception does not need to be delayed after taking chemoprophylaxis due to the short half-life of these medications.

To prevent transmission of malaria to others, blood donation should be deferred after returning from an endemic area; the recommended interval to avoid donation ranges from 3 months to 3 years depending on the length of the exposure.

There have been expansive concerted efforts in endemic areas to reduce malaria transmission and move toward global malaria

---

[1] Not FDA approved for this indication.

TABLE 3 Options for Malaria Chemoprophylaxis

DRUG	ADULT DOSING	PEDIATRIC DOSING	SIDE EFFECTS	COMMENTS
Atovaquone-proguanil (Malarone)	1 adult tab = 250 mg atovaquone + 100 mg proguanil 1 adult tab QD Begin 1–2 days before arrival in endemic area, continue throughout stay and for 7 days after leaving area	1 pediatric tab = 62.5 mg atovaquone + 25 mg proguanil 5 to <8 kg: ½ ped tab QD 8 to <10 kg: ¾ ped tab QD 10 to <20 kg: 1 ped tab QD 20 to <30 kg: 2 ped tab QD 30 to <40: 3 ped tab QD ≥40 kg: 1 adult tab QD Begin 1–2 days before arrival in endemic area, continue throughout stay and for 7 days after leaving area	Minimal at prophylactic dose	Avoid in renal dysfunction when CrCl <30 mL/min Avoid in pregnancy and breastfeeding of infants under 5 kg
Doxycycline	100 mg QD Begin 1–2 days before arrival in endemic area, continue throughout stay and for 28 days after leaving area	Children ≥8 years old: 2.2 mg/kg QD (max 100 mg) Begin 1–2 days before arrival in endemic area, continue throughout stay and for 28 days after leaving area	Photosensitivity, esophagitis, GI upset	Avoid in pregnancy and in children <8 years old
Mefloquine	1 tablet = 228 mg base (250 mg salt) 1 tablet weekly Start 1–2 weeks before arrival in endemic area, continue throughout stay and for 4 weeks after leaving area	Weekly dose: ≤9 kg: 4.6 mg/kg base (5 mg/kg salt) per dose[6] >9–19 kg: ¼ tablet weekly >19–30 kg: ½ tablet >30–45 kg: ¾ tablet >45: 1 tablet Start 1–2 weeks before arrival, continue throughout stay and for 4 weeks after leaving area	Vomiting, neuropsychiatric side effects (vivid dreams, insomnia, anxiety, depression, paranoia, hallucinations)	Safe in pregnancy Avoid with major psychiatric disorders Some areas of Southeast Asia have mefloquine resistance**
Chloroquine	300 mg base (500 mg salt) per dose Take weekly Start 1–2 weeks before arrival in endemic area, continue weekly throughout stay, and for 4 weeks after leaving area	5 mg/kg base (8.3 mg/kg salt) per dose Do not exceed adult dose Take weekly Start 1–2 weeks before arrival in endemic area, continue weekly throughout stay, and for 4 weeks after leaving area	QT prolongation, GI upset, headache	Can be used in pregnancy Can only be used in areas with chloroquine-sensitive malaria*

Continued

TABLE 3 Options for Malaria Chemoprophylaxis—cont'd

DRUG	ADULT DOSING	PEDIATRIC DOSING	SIDE EFFECTS	COMMENTS
Primaquine***	2 tablets = 30 mg base (52.6 mg salt) Take daily Start 1–2 days before arrival in endemic area, daily throughout stay, and for 7 days after leaving area	0.5 mg/kg base (0.8 mg/kg salt) Take daily Start 1–2 days before arrival in endemic area, daily throughout stay, and for 7 days after leaving area	QT prolongation, GI upset	Recommended for areas where *P. vivax* predominates Check G6PD deficiency Cannot be used in pregnancy or breastfeeding unless infant is tested for G6PD deficiency
Tafenoquine (Arakoda)	200 mg per dose Start once daily for 3 days (loading dose) before arriving in endemic area, continue once weekly throughout stay, and for 1 week after leaving area	Not recommended	Headache, back pain, dizziness, nausea, and diarrhea	Prevents both *P. vivax* and *P. falciparum* Check for G6PD deficiency Cannot be used for children or during pregnancy or breastfeeding unless infant is tested for G6PD deficiency Not recommended with history of psychotic disorders

Terminal Prophylaxis After Prolonged Exposure to *P. vivax* or *P. ovale*

DRUG	ADULT DOSING	PEDIATRIC DOSING	SIDE EFFECTS	COMMENTS
Primaquine[1]	30 mg QD Take for 14 days after leaving malaria-endemic area Administer in addition to primary prophylaxis	0.5 mg base/kg/dose QD (max 30 mg) Take for 14 days after departure from malaria-endemic area Administer in addition to primary prophylaxis	QT prolongation, GI upset	Not needed if primaquine is used for primary chemoprophylaxis*** Check for G6PD deficiency Cannot be used in pregnancy or breastfeeding unless infant is tested for G6PD deficiency
Tafenoquine (Arakoda)	200 mg as a single dose, 7 days after the last dose of primary prophylaxis	Only approved for adults ≥18 years	Headache, back pain, dizziness, nausea, and diarrhea	Check for G6PD deficiency Cannot be used for children or during pregnancy or breastfeeding unless infant is tested for G6PD deficiency Not recommended with history of psychotic disorders

*This includes areas with chloroquine-sensitive *P. falciparum* (parts of Central America, the Caribbean, and the Middle East) and areas where *P. vivax* is predominant. The CDC web page has detailed information by country: https://wwwnc.cdc.gov/travel/yellowbook/2024/preparing/yellow-fever-vaccine-malaria-prevention-by-country.
**Mefloquine resistance has been reported on the borders of Thailand with Burma (Myanmar) and Cambodia, in the western provinces of Cambodia, in the eastern states of Burma on the border between Burma and China, along the borders of Burma and Laos, and in southern Vietnam.
***Primaquine is not FDA approved for primary chemoprophylaxis.
[6]May be compounded by pharmacists.
[1]Not FDA approved for this indication.
BID, Twice daily; *CrCl,* creatinine clearance; *GFR,* glomerular filtration rate; *GI,* gastrointestinal; *QD,* daily; *QID,* four times daily; *tab,* tablet; *TID,* three times daily.

elimination. The WHO estimates that 2.1 billion cases and 11.7 million deaths were averted from 2000 to 2022 because of these large-scale interventions. The mainstay of these interventions involves the distribution of insecticide-treated nets (ITNs) and administration of indoor residual spraying (IRS) of insecticides; these measures have been challenged in the past 2 decades by the evolution of mosquitoes that are resistant to pyrethroids, the insecticide used in most of these measures; nets and sprays that use alternatives or combinations of insecticides are being developed and implemented. Additional preventive measures include targeted chemoprophylaxis for pregnant women and seasonal chemoprophylaxis for children; better access to diagnostic tests; and improved access to ACTs. Urbanization, improvements to infrastructure, and socioeconomic advances also reduce transmission.

Finally, vaccines are emerging as an important component of malaria prevention. There are currently two vaccines available for use. The RTS,S/AS01 vaccine (Mosquirix)[2] was approved by the World Health Organization in 2021 and is administered at 0, 1, and 2 months, with a fourth dose 18 months after the third dose, to children aged 5 to 17 months; the R21/Matrix-M vaccine[2] is administered at 0, 1, and 2 months, with a fourth dose given 12 months after the third dose, for children aged 5 to 36 months and was approved in 2023. These vaccines have been introduced in eight countries with additional implementation planned. These vaccines target the circumsporozoite antigen in the preerythrocytic stage of the parasite life cycle. They reduce childhood morbidity and mortality but do not interrupt the transmission cycle. It is estimated that between 417 and 448 deaths are averted per every 100,000 children vaccinated. Notably, these vaccines are only effective against *P. falciparum;* they do not provide cross-protection

[2]Not available in the United States.

against the other species. There are efforts underway to develop vaccines with new targets that may prevent transmission, as well as use new technology like DNA- and mRNA-based vaccines and adjuvants. Finally, monoclonal antibodies to provide passive protection against malaria are being investigated.

References

CDC Yellow Book: *Malaria*. Available at https://wwwnc.cdc.gov/travel/yellowbook /2024/infections-diseases/malaria. Accessed April 4, 2025.

Centers for Disease Control and Prevention. *Clinical Guidance: Malaria Diagnosis & Treatment in the U.S.* Available at https://www.cdc.gov/malaria/hcp/clinical-guidance/index.html. Accessed April 4, 2025.

Centers for Disease Control and Prevention. *Locally Acquired Malaria Cases Identified in the United States.* Available at https://www.cdc.gov/han/2023/han00494.html. Accessed April 4, 2025.

Fairhurst RM, Wellens TE: Malaria *(Plasmodium species)*. Mandell, Douglas, and Bennett's principles and practice of infectious diseases—electronic, ed 9, Elsevier eBooks, 2019, pp 3299–3320.

Muppidi P, Wright E, Wassmer SC, Gupta H: Diagnosis of cerebral malaria: tools to reduce *Plasmodium falciparum* associated mortality, *Front Cell Infect Microbiol* 13:1090013, 2023. Available at https://doi.org/10.3389/fcimb.2023.1090013. Accessed 4 April 2025.

World Health Organization. Malaria vaccine: WHO position paper—May 2024. *Weekly Epidemiological Record No 19*, pp 225–248.

World Health Organization. *Malaria.* Available at https://www.who.int/news-room/fact-sheets/detail/malaria. Accessed April 4, 2025.

World Health Organization. *WHO guidelines for malaria.* Available at https://www.who.int/publications/i/item/guidelines-for-malaria. Accessed April 4, 2025.

World Health Organization. *World malaria report 2024.* Available at https://www.who.int/teams/global-malaria-programme/reports/world-malaria-report-2024. Accessed April 4, 2025.

Yadav A, Verma K, Singh K, et al: Analysis of diagnostic biomarkers for malaria: prospects on rapid diagnostic test (RDT) development, *Microb Pathog* 196:106978, 2024. Available at https://doi.org/10.1016/j.micpath.2024.106978. Accessed 4 April 2025.

MEASLES (RUBEOLA)

Method of
Jane A. Weida, MD, MS

CURRENT DIAGNOSIS

- Measles is a highly contagious but vaccine-preventable viral illness with a prodrome of high fever, cough, conjunctivitis, and coryza
- The incubation period is about 10 days to the onset of fever; the typical rash appears after about 14 days
- Measles produces a red maculopapular rash beginning on the face and then becoming generalized
- A pathognomonic enanthem, Koplik spots (small, clustered blue-white lesions on a bright-red base), may appear on buccal mucosa during the prodromal period
- Patients usually have a history of exposure, particularly of travel to an endemic area or of contact with carriers or non-immunized individuals

CURRENT THERAPY

- No specific antiviral therapy is available
- Adequate hydration
- Bed rest
- Antipyretics
- Antibiotics if needed for bacterial complications
- The American Academy of Pediatrics and World Health Organization recommend carefully dosed vitamin A for those diagnosed with measles, recognizing that high doses should be avoided due to toxicity
- Vaccination is the best way to prevent measles

Epidemiology

Before measles vaccines were introduced, measles caused millions of deaths worldwide each year. In the decade before the first measles vaccine was licensed in 1963, there were about 549,000 reported measles cases (although it is estimated that the actual incidence was much higher, possibly 3–4 million) and 495 deaths annually in the United States.

Measles was declared to have been eliminated from the United States in 2000, but outbreaks in increasing numbers have occurred since then. The number of cases was particularly high in 2025, with 1,491 confirmed cases as of September 16 2025, reflecting declining immunization rates and misleading or conflicting advice from federal health personnel. These numbers clearly surpass the 285 total cases in 2024. As of September 16, 2025, measles had been reported in 42 states with 803 cases reported in Texas, 100 in New Mexico and 90 in Kansas. The majority of the cases (92%) occurred in unvaccinated persons or those whose immunization status was unknown. Of the 1,491 cases, 12% were hospitalized. Those under the age of 5 years were more likely to be hospitalized. There had been three deaths: two in children in Texas and one adult in New Mexico. All three were unvaccinated.

In response to the measles outbreak in the United States, the Centers for Disease Control and Prevention (CDC) issued a Health Alert Network Health Advisory regarding guidance for the summer 2025 travel season. The advisory emphasized the important role that clinicians and public health officials play in preventing the spread of measles, including being vigilant for cases of febrile rash illnesses. It also emphasized that the measles-mumps-rubella (MMR) vaccination remains the most important tool for preventing measles.

From a historical perspective, there were 58 measles cases in 2023, 121 in 2022, 49 in 2021, and 13 in 2020. In 2019 there were 1282 cases in 31 states, the largest outbreak since 1992. The majority of the cases were in those who were not vaccinated.

Most measles cases in the United States are caused by exposure of unimmunized persons to those who contracted the illness after international travel to an endemic area or exposure when there is a local outbreak. Travelers with measles continue to bring the disease to the United States. Measles can spread when it reaches an area where groups of people are unvaccinated, especially areas where immunity dips below 95%.

Measles continues to be a major problem in many regions of the world. Worldwide, there were over 10 million cases of measles in 2023, with over 100,000 measles deaths that year. Although it is estimated that worldwide from 2000 to 2023, measles vaccination saved 60.3 million lives, millions of children across the world remain unvaccinated.

Being unvaccinated is the largest risk factor for measles in the United States. Infants who have lost maternal immunity but are too young to be immunized are at higher risk, as are individuals with vitamin A deficiency. Travel to international areas where measles is more common or to international/domestic areas where there is an outbreak also increases the risk of contracting the disease. If measles is suspected in a patient, a careful travel history should be obtained.

Pathophysiology

Measles is caused by an RNA respiratory virus of the family Paramyxoviridae and genus *Morbillivirus*. It is one of the most highly contagious communicable diseases. The virus spreads from person to person via respiratory droplets from coughing or sneezing or via direct contact. Measles is so infectious that when one person has it, up to 90% of the people close to them can contract it if they are nonimmune. The virus can stay in the air for up to 2 hours after an infected person has exited a room. Someone can get infected simply by walking through a room from which a person with measles has exited.

Patients are usually contagious from about 4 days before to about 4 days after the rash appears. The fact that the disease is contagious before the onset of symptoms makes quarantining particularly difficult. The incubation period is generally 10 days before the prodrome and 14 days before the onset of the rash, but it may vary from 6 to 21 days.

Unlike many other viruses that affect the respiratory or gastrointestinal systems, the major effect of the measles virus is on the immune system. The measles virus suppresses the immune response to other pathogens, which can make the individual susceptible to secondary infections. This immune suppression can last for a few weeks to a few months, but in some cases, it may last for 2 to 3 years. The immune response triggered by the measles virus may explain the serious long-term neurologic complications.

Once a measles infection has cleared, the affected person gains lifelong immunity, provided that they remain immunocompetent. Infants are protected by maternal antibodies for about 1 month in the case of an immunized mother and for about 4 months in the case of a mother who had a prior measles infection.

Prevention

The best way to prevent measles is with measles vaccination. The CDC recommends MMR vaccination at 12 to 15 months of age, with the second dose at 4 to 6 years of age. One dose is about 93% effective, while two doses are 97% effective at preventing measles.

The measles vaccine uses a live attenuated virus, most commonly administered as part of the MMR (measles-mumps-rubella) or MMRV (measles-mumps-rubella-varicella) combination vaccine. The "herd immunity" strategy attempts to protect individuals and the public with an overall population immunization rate of 95%.

The CDC defines evidence of immunity to measles as:
- Adults born before 1957, except healthcare personnel (see later)
- Documentation of receipt of MMR vaccine
- Laboratory evidence of immunity or disease

The diagnosis of disease without laboratory confirmation does not count as evidence of immunity.

Healthcare personnel with no evidence of immunity should complete a 2-dose series of MMR, at least 4 weeks apart, regardless of their year of birth. Adults born in 1957 or later without evidence of immunity should receive 1 to 2 doses of the vaccine. Students at postsecondary institutions, international travelers, and close contacts of immunocompromised persons who do not have evidence of immunity should complete a 2-dose series at least 4 weeks apart. The vaccine should not be given to pregnant women or severely immunocompromised individuals.

Individuals immunized between 1963 and 1967 may have received a relatively ineffective inactivated measles vaccine and should consider receiving the currently available live attenuated virus vaccine, especially if there is a local outbreak.

International travelers should be protected against measles. Infants 6 to 11 months of age who are traveling internationally should receive 1 dose of MMR vaccine. Children 12 months of age and older who are traveling abroad should have documentation of 2 doses of MMR vaccine at least 28 days apart.

Despite the importance of measles prevention, some parents refuse to vaccinate their children. A study published in the United Kingdom in 1998 claimed to find a link between autism and MMR vaccine. The study was later proven to be erroneous and fraudulent. Subsequent repeated studies have consistently shown that there is no link between vaccines and autism. Clinicians must educate parents about the crucial importance—which cannot be overstated—of MMR vaccination.

The MMR immunization should be avoided if a patient has had a previous life-threatening allergic reaction to the vaccine or if the patient has a severe primary or acquired immunodeficiency. Clinical judgment should direct immunization of patients with HIV illness or systemic immunosuppressive treatment, depending on the significance of their immunocompromise.

There are additional situations when vaccination with the measles virus should receive special consideration:

Tuberculosis: For patients with untreated tuberculosis, antituberculosis therapy should be started before immunizing. Because the MMR vaccination may temporarily suppress tuberculin skin test reactivity and may affect the interferon-γ release assay (IGRA), tuberculin skin or IGRA testing should be postponed for 4 to 6 weeks after MMR immunization.

Pregnancy: The MMR immunization should be avoided if a woman is pregnant or will become pregnant in the subsequent 28 days, primarily to avoid the rubella component of the MMR or MMRV vaccine.

Newborns and infants: Passive measles immunization from maternal antibodies fades within 1 to 2 months of age. If there is a local outbreak, infants may be vaccinated as early as 6 months of age. Measles vaccine administered before 9 months of age is not considered valid and the child should be reimmunized with a second and third dose, a minimum of 1 month apart, on or after the first birthday. The MMRV vaccine should not be administered to children under the age of 48 months due to the varicella component.

Postexposure prophylaxis: A susceptible individual exposed to measles has three options: administration of the measles vaccine, administration of immunoglobulin, or a combination of both. The measles vaccine, if administered within 72 hours of exposure, may provide some protection. Intramuscular immunoglobulin (0.25 mL/kg, maximum of 15 mL) may provide protection or modify the severity of the illness if administered within 6 days of exposure. Although the measles vaccine and immunoglobulin can be simultaneously administered, the vaccine is not considered valid in this situation because the immunoglobulin may attenuate the immunogenicity of the vaccine. Therefore the vaccine should be readministered 6 months later. Immunoglobulin may also be administered to severely immunocompromised individuals regardless of immunization status.

Office and Hospital Management Protocols

Physician office protocols: Physician offices should develop a protocol for management of patients with suspected measles. Because measles is so contagious, it is generally recommended that patients with suspected measles not be seen in the medical office. Rather, they should be seen in a specially designated area that is only accessible to caregivers who are immune, in a car in the office parking lot, or during a home visit. Office staff should be educated about the contagious nature of measles, and healthcare professionals should have proof of immunity.

Hospital protocols: Patients admitted to the hospital are preferably managed in negative-pressure isolation rooms using airborne precautions. Healthcare personnel should have proof of immunity.

Clinical Signs and Symptoms

Measles generally presents with a prodrome that includes high fever, malaise, anorexia, conjunctivitis, photophobia, coryza, and nonproductive croupy cough. Fever may reach over 40°C. Conjunctivitis may include redness, swelling, photophobia, and discharge. Koplik spots, which are small, clustered blue-white spots surrounded by a red ring that appear on the buccal mucosa, are pathognomonic but are not always present. A general rule is that if a patient has a rash without a fever, the diagnosis is not measles.

The measles rash is erythematous, maculopapular and blanching. It usually appears first on the face and behind the ears and then spreads to the trunk and extremities. The rash lasts 3 to 7 days. Patients are contagious 4 days before and 4 days after appearance of the rash. Recovery begins soon after the rash appears. As the rash fades, the skin desquamates.

Diagnosis

Measles is usually diagnosed clinically, based on the presenting signs, vaccination history, and travel exposure history. Clinical diagnosis can be difficult when the incidence of measles is low. The World Health Organization (WHO) clinical case definition for measles is a person with fever and maculopapular rash and at least one of the symptoms of cough, coryza, or conjunctivitis.

Laboratory findings include leukopenia, unless there is a secondary bacterial infection, as well as thrombocytopenia and proteinuria. Laboratory confirmation by real-time reverse transcriptase polymerase chain reaction (RT-PCR) testing, using a nasopharyngeal or throat swab, can help establish a diagnosis promptly. RT-PCR is available at many state public health laboratories. The most commonly used serologic test is virus-specific immunoglobulin M (IgM) in serum or oral fluid. IgM antibodies generally appear at the time of the rash, but they may not be detectable until 4 or more days after the rash appears. IgG antibodies appear a few days later. Viral cultures may be obtained, although measles is technically difficult to culture.

Measles is a reportable illness in the United States; therefore suspected cases must be reported to the local health department without delay. All cases of suspected measles should be reported even before laboratory confirmation. Clinicians can contact their local health department if there are questions as to which specimens to collect.

Differential Diagnosis

During the prodromal stage, measles can easily be mistaken for other viral upper respiratory illnesses. Although Koplik spots are pathognomonic, they are easy to overlook. Once the rash has appeared, measles can still be mistaken for other illnesses, including erythema infectiosum, infectious mononucleosis, enterovirus, Kawasaki disease, chikungunya, Rocky Mountain spotted fever, rubella, and scarlet fever.

Treatment

No specific antiviral treatment is available for measles. Treatment is supportive, including rest, adequate fluids, and antipyretics. Patients should be kept on bed rest until they are afebrile. Prompt recognition and treatment of secondary bacterial infections is essential.

The use of vitamin A in the treatment of measles has been confusing and controversial. Vitamin A does not provide protection from, does not stop the spread of, and is not a treatment for measles. The American Academy of Pediatrics recommends treatment with vitamin A[1], under direction of a healthcare professional, for those infected with measles regardless of hospitalization status. It is given immediately when the disease is diagnosed and then repeated the next day, usually in oral capsule or liquid form, in the following doses:
- Children 12 months or older: 200,000 IU (60,000 µg retinol activity equivalent [RAE])
- Infants 6 through 11 months of age: 100,000 IU (30,000 µg RAE)
- Infants younger than 6 months: 50,000 IU (15,000 µg RAE)
- An additional (i.e., a third) age-specific dose of vitamin A administered 2 through 6 weeks can be given to children with clinical signs and symptoms of vitamin A deficiency.

The WHO recommends that all children and adults with measles receive 2 doses of vitamin A[1] given 24 hours apart. This is especially important in undernourished children who are deficient in vitamin A, although the WHO notes that low vitamin A levels may also occur in well-nourished children. The WHO indicates that vitamin A can help prevent eye damage and blindness and may reduce the number of deaths from measles.

Excessive doses of vitamin A may result in toxicity manifested by anorexia, nausea, vomiting, diarrhea, dizziness, malaise, and skin changes (rash, itching, desquamation). In severe cases, vitamin A toxicity may result in increased intracranial pressure. Clinicians in Texas have reported cases of vitamin A toxicity.

Most patients with measles do not need hospitalization. For those who do, both standard and respiratory precautions should be initiated. Respiratory precautions should continue for 4 days after onset of rash for healthy children and for the duration of the illness for immunocompromised patients.

For those who have been exposed to measles and are not immune, MMR should be administered within 72 hours of exposure or immune globulin (GamaSTAN) administered within 6 days of exposure.

[1] Not FDA approved for this indication.

Complications

Complications of measles can occur in up to 40% of patients. Complications are highest in the very young, the very old, and those who are malnourished. Often the complications affect the respiratory tract, with pneumonia being the leading cause of death associated with measles. Pneumonia may be caused by a secondary bacterial or viral infection or by the measles virus itself. Otitis media is another common complication. Gastrointestinal complications include diarrhea and stomatitis. Measles keratoconjunctivitis is a common complication, especially in children with vitamin A deficiency. Measles causes about 1 to 2 deaths per 1000 as a result of respiratory or neurologic complications.

Measles can cause severe central nervous system complications. Some patients develop acute encephalitis. About 5% to 10% of these individuals may develop severe sensorineural hearing loss. About 0.05% to 0.1% of patients may develop measles postinfectious demyelinating encephalomyelitis. Adolescents tend to have a higher rate of this complication. Immunosuppressed patients may develop measles inclusion body encephalitis, which results in neurologic deterioration and death within months after the acute measles infections. This is a severe acute demyelinating disease, which usually starts several days after appearance of the rash. Seizures, fever, coma, and other neurologic signs may develop. Mortality is 10% to 20%. About one-third of survivors are left with neurologic deficits or respiratory problems, including bronchiectasis. Subacute sclerosing panencephalitis is a rare delayed neurologic complication of measles, occurring in about 2 in 10,000 patients. The rate may be higher in those younger than 15 months. This complication causes seizures and progressive intellectual and behavioral deterioration about 7 to 10 years, or even up to 15 years, after a measles infection. This complication is almost always fatal.

The complications of measles, as well as the disease itself, are best managed by prevention with immunization. Clinicians must continue to stress the vital importance of measles immunization to their patients. This has become even more crucial while measles cases continue to rise and while erroneous and misleading information is disseminated by some public officials. Vaccination remains the best defense against contracting measles.

References

American Academy of Pediatrics: *Measles Frequently Asked Questions*. https://www.aap.org/en/patient-care/measles/measles-frequently-asked-questions/?srsltid=AfmBOoqydIwpbzrc-rPN2Etlr2OliY8OURFm3uOMmJZdVQK-31FwKJ75J.

Center for Disease Control and Prevention: *Emergency Preparedness and Response Health Alert Network (HAN) - 00522 | Expanding Measles Outbreak in the United States and Guidance for the Upcoming Travel Season*. Available at: https://cdc.gov/han/2025/han00522.html.

Center for Disease Control and Prevention: *Measles Cases and Outbreaks*. Available at: https://cdc.gov/measles/data-research/index.html.

Center for Disease Control and Prevention: *Measles—Clinical Overview of Measles*. Available at: https://cdc.gov/measles/hcp/clinical-overview/index.html.

Center for Disease Control and Prevention: *Progress Toward Measles Elimination—Worldwide*, 2000- 2023. Available at: https://cdc.gov/mmwr/volumes/73/wr/mm7345a4.htm.

Center for Disease Control and Prevention: *Vaccines & Immunizations—Immunization Schedules*. Available at: https://cdc.gov/vaccines/hcp/imz-schedules/index.html.

Clark EH, Ashley P, Shandera WX: Viral and rickettsial infections: measles. In Papadakis MA, Rabow MW, McQuaid KR, Ghandi K, editors: *Current medical diagnosis and treatment 2025*, 64th ed, 2025, pp 1354–1357.

Kimberlin DW, Banergee R, Barnett ED, Lynfield R, Sawyer MH, editors: *Measles: in red book:2024-2027 Report of the Committee on infectious disease*, 33rd ed, Itasca, IL, 2024, American Academy of Pediatrics. Available at: https://publications.aap.org/redbook/book/755/chapter/14079321/Measles.

NMHealth: *Infectious disease epidemiology bureau: measles outbreak guidance*, 2025. Available at: https://www.nmhealth.org/about/erd/ideb/mog/.

Tesini BL: *Common viral infections in infants and children: measles in merck manual professional version*, 2023. Available at: https://www.merckmanuals.com/professional/pediatrics/common-viral-infections-in-infants-and-children/measles-#Symptoms-and-Signs_v1022950.

Texas Announces First Death in Measles Outbreak: *Texas Health And Human Services*. Available at: https://www.dshs.texas.gov/news-alerts/texas-announces-first-death-measles-outbreak.

World Health Organization: *Measles*, 2024. Available at: https://www.who.int/news-room/fact-sheets/detail/measles.

METHICILLIN-RESISTANT *STAPHYLOCOCCUS AUREUS*

Method of
Elissa Rennert-May, MD, MSc; and John M. Conly, MD, DSc

CURRENT DIAGNOSIS

- Healthcare-associated methicillin-resistant *Staphylococcus aureus* (HA-MRSA) is endemic in many hospital settings. The strains are polyclonal, resistant to many non–β-lactam antimicrobials, and typically cause pneumonia, line-related infection, surgical site infection, bacteremia, and infrequently skin and soft tissue infections.
- Strains of community-associated MRSA (CA-MRSA) have risen exponentially. The strains are clonal, sensitive to many non–β-lactam antimicrobials, harbour multiple virulence factors, and typically cause pyogenic skin and soft tissue infections and occasionally severe necrotizing pneumonia, fasciitis, and multifocal osteomyelitis.
- HA-MRSA infections typically affect patients with multiple co-morbidities in the healthcare setting, but CA-MRSA typically affects previously healthy persons.
- It can be difficult to differentiate infectious syndromes due to β-hemolytic streptococci versus CA-MRSA.

CURRENT THERAPY

- Methicillin-resistant *Staphylococcus aureus* (MRSA) strains harbor resistance to the β-lactam antimicrobials, including oxacillin, dicloxacillin, cloxacillin[2], nafcillin, methicillin[2], and first-, second-, and third-generation cephalosporins.
- Healthcare-associated MRSA (HA-MRSA) strains are typically resistant to macrolides, clindamycin (Cleocin), aminoglycosides, and quinolones (with the exception of delafloxacin [Baxdela]) and are variably resistant to tetracycline and trimethoprim-sulfamethoxazole (Bactrim). They are sensitive to vancomycin (Vancocin) and the lipoglycopeptides, fusidic acid[2], rifampin (Rifadin)[1], the oxazolidinones linezolid (Zyvox) and tedizolid (Sivextro), daptomycin (Cubicin), ceftaroline (Teflaro), and ceftobiprole (Zevtera).
- Community-associated MRSA (CA-MRSA) strains are resistant to macrolides and quinolones (with the exception of delafloxacin [Baxdela]) but usually are sensitive to aminoglycosides such as gentamicin (Garamycin), clindamycin, (Cleocin) and trimethoprim-sulfamethoxazole (Bactrim)[1], in addition to vancomycin (Vancocin), the lipoglycopeptides, fusidic acid[2], rifampin (Rifadin)[1], the oxazolidinones linezolid (Zyvox) and tedizolid (Sivextro), daptomycin (Cubicin), ceftaroline (Teflaro), and ceftobiprole (Zevtera).
- Empiric antimicrobial therapy should be guided by the clinical presentation, and when full sensitivities are available, the antimicrobials may be tailored accordingly.

[1]Not FDA approved for this indication.
[2]Not available in the United States.

Epidemiology

Staphylococcus aureus is one of the most frequently encountered bacteria causing human infections and may be considered as either methicillin-sensitive *S. aureus* (MSSA) or methicillin-resistant *S. aureus* (MRSA). MRSA was first described in 1961 and is resistant not only to the traditional antistaphylococcal β-lactam antibiotics (methicillin[2], nafcillin, oxacillin, cloxacillin[2], and dicloxacillin) but also other important β-lactam antibiotics, including the first- to fourth-generation cephalosporins and the carbapenem family, thus eliminating an important class of antibiotics from the clinician's armamentarium. The only β-lactams that have activity against MRSA are the advanced-generation cephalosporin agents ceftaroline (Teflaro) and ceftobiprole (Zevtera).

MRSA strains acquired in the hospital or other healthcare settings have traditionally been referred to as healthcare-associated MRSA (HA-MRSA), whereas community-associated MRSA (CA-MRSA) has referred to isolates acquired in the community setting and in the absence of traditional hospital or healthcare exposures for at least 1 year (overnight stays in an acute care or long-term care facility, surgery, dialysis, or presence of a central venous catheter). The term *community-onset HA-MRSA* has been used to describe the occurrence of MRSA infection in the setting of the presence of a healthcare exposure within the past year. MRSA has been recognized as a healthcare-associated pathogen since the 1970s and became endemic in hospitals in many countries, including the United States, United Kingdom, and many European countries, with exceptions being Denmark, the Netherlands, Scandinavia, and Canada. For several decades, MRSA was typically considered a hospital pathogen. Novel and virulent MRSA strains arising in the community and not associated with any traditional healthcare exposure risks were first encountered in the late 1990s in the United States, Australia, and some European countries and have since risen explosively on a global basis to become the predominant clone of *S. aureus* associated with community infections. Methicillin resistance among community isolates of *S. aureus* has been reported to be as high as 75% in some US communities. More recently livestock-associated MRSA (LA-MRSA) has been reported on a global basis, and transmission of these strains from swine, cattle, and horses has been implicated as a source of human infections, particularly in farmers, abattoir workers, and veterinarians. Recent work has demonstrated a role of φSa3 prophage in how human-adapted ST398 clones evolve and may play a role in virulence.

Specific genetic and molecular distinctions initially distinguished the HA- and CA-MRSA strains (Table 1) and have been used to characterize MRSA strains as likely of community versus healthcare origin. The HA-MRSA strains were found to harbor large staphylococcal cassette chromosome (SCC*mec*) types known as SCC*mec* types I, II, or III; to have multidrug resistance to non–β-lactam antimicrobials; to have the absence of specific virulence characteristics such as carriage of the Panton-Valentine Leukocidin *(PVL)* gene; and to have varying multilocus sequence types (ST5, ST239, ST 247, ST250). On the other hand, the CA-MRSA strains have been found to harbor SCC*mec* types IV, V, and more recently VI to XV have been described; to have paucidrug resistance to non–β-lactam antimicrobials; to have the presence of specific virulence characteristics such as carriage of the *PVL* gene, and to have multilocus sequence types ST1, ST8, and ST80. LA-MRSA strains often are nontypeable or harbor SCC*mec* V, have high rates of tetracycline resistance, carry multiple virulence factors, and are most often multilocus sequence types ST398 or ST9. However, over the past few years, healthcare-associated strains have moved into the community and likewise community strains have spread rapidly within hospitals, and the original distinctions between CA-MRSA and HA-MRSA from an epidemiologic perspective have become increasingly blurred. The point of transmission of MRSA is not always possible to identify with certainty, making the classification of CA and HA strains increasingly imprecise.

Risk Factors

The risk factors for HA-MRSA may be viewed from the perspective of the healthcare environment and patient-specific risk factors. A major risk factor for acquiring HA-MRSA is exposure to a healthcare setting and particularly in hospital or other institutional

[2]Not available in the United States.

TABLE 1 General Features Differentiating HA- and CA-MRSA*

CHARACTERISTIC	HA-MRSA	CA-MRSA
Drug resistance to non–β-lactams	Multiresistance	Pauciresistance
Pathogenicity islands	Few	Multiple
Age predilection	Older	Younger
Comorbidities	Multiple	None
Traditional risk factors	Healthcare contact, prolonged hospital stay, poor hand hygiene, contaminated equipment, invasive procedures, medical devices, recent antibiotic use	Crowded community environment, lack of cleanliness, loss of skin integrity, intravenous drug user, homelessness, incarceration, aboriginal, HIV+, contact sports, athletes, military, chronic skin disorder, veterinary worker

*Features are generalizations only given the appearance of community strains replacing traditional hospital strains in the health care setting and the appearance of typical HA strains in the community setting.
CA, Community-associated; HA, healthcare-associated; HIV, human immunodeficiency virus; MRSA, methicillin-resistant *Staphylococcus aureus*.

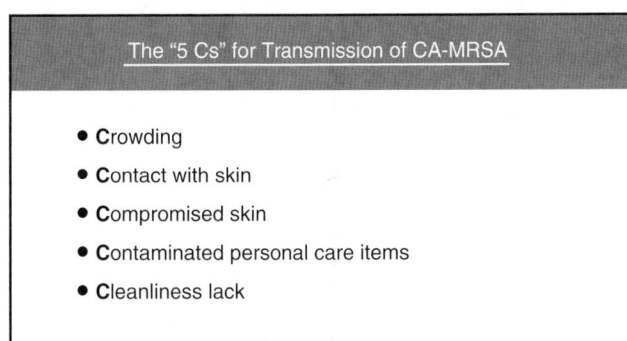

The "5 Cs" for Transmission of CA-MRSA

- **C**rowding
- **C**ontact with skin
- **C**ompromised skin
- **C**ontaminated personal care items
- **C**leanliness lack

Figure 1 The five Cs implicated in transmission of community-associated methicillin-resistant *S. aureus*. Adapted from the US Centers for Disease Control and Prevention.

settings where the prevalence of carriage of MRSA among patients is high. Additional risk factors in the healthcare environment include poor hand hygiene practices among hospital employees, contaminated bedside equipment and surfaces, overcrowding, and reduced healthcare worker-to-patient ratios. Patient risk factors (see Table 1) include aging, multiple comorbidities, receipt of antibiotics within the preceding 3 months, prolonged duration of hospital stay, admission to a long-term care facility or hospital in the previous year, invasive procedures, and the presence of indwelling catheters or other devices. In addition, the recent COVID-19 pandemic has led to some settings experiencing increased nosocomial rates of MRSA and with strains with increased numbers of virulence genes and may be considered an additional risk factor. Initial risk groups for CA-MRSA were injection drug users, homeless populations, incarcerated persons, and indigenous peoples. The Centers for Disease Control and Prevention have suggested the five Cs (Figure 1 and Table 2) as contributing factors implicated in the transmission among these groups. The initial risk groups have expanded (Table 3) to include men who have sex with men (MSM), athletes (especially those involved in team and contact sports), military personnel, those with a prior history of abscesses, individuals with chronic skin disorders, individuals with recent antibiotic receipt, underserved urban populations, individuals who have contact with colonized pets or livestock, and veterinary workers. In the drug-using and underserved urban populations, prevalence and social networking studies have identified hospices, shooting galleries, and crack houses as key sites in which CA-MRSA transmission may occur. Recent outbreaks have been reported in hospital nurseries, daycare settings, nursing home workers, schools, and college dormitories. Sexual transmission has been reported, but it may reflect close skin-to-skin genital contact rather than a true sexually transmitted pathogen. CA-MRSA has now become endemic in the general population in many communities, and the elderly and the very young seem to have a predilection for infection, especially if other risk factors

are present. Risk groups for LA-MRSA include farmers, their family members and farm hands who are engaged in livestock production (especially swine and cattle), abattoir workers, veterinarians, and veterinary assistants. There is concern about increasing threats to food safety and public health with the rise in strains of both LA-MRSA and LA-MSSA in livestock farms, especially in swine populations. Recent transmission of strains of LA-MRSA has been reported in the hospital setting as well.

Pathophysiology

The resistance to the antistaphylococcal β-lactam antibiotics in MRSA strains is imparted by the presence of an altered configuration for a specific penicillin-binding protein (PBP) known as PBP2a in the cell wall of staphylococci. Normally the PBPs would act as a site for the attachment of the active moieties of the β-lactam agent, which then would inhibit further cell wall assembly. The alteration in the configuration of PBP2a occurs as the result of the presence of the SCC*mec* gene in *S. aureus*, which confers resistance to the β-lactam antibiotics. The origins of the *mec* gene and its insertion into the SCC-*mec* element are not known with certainty. Once the MRSA strains acquired resistance to the antistaphylococcal β-lactam antibiotics in the healthcare setting, it is not difficult to appreciate how it emerged as a predominant pathogen in the hospital setting over the years, with increasing acuity of illness in the patient populations and increased use of broad-spectrum antimicrobials.

The appearance and rapid spread of CA-MRSA with the clinical impression of more virulent and lethal infections than what had been seen with traditional HA-MRSA strains may be explained by several factors. The SCC*mec* IV genetic element is very widely distributed among *S. aureus* isolates, which may explain its appearance in multiple settings globally, and these strains appear to have more rapid growth rates than typical HA-MRSA strains, larger numbers of virulence factors, pathogenicity islands, and higher levels of expression of the virulence factors produced. Recently α-type phenol-soluble modulins were described in strains of CA-MRSA, which are produced at very high levels and are potent lysins of neutrophils. High levels of α-toxin production by these strains, which act as pore-forming toxins for multiple cell types, may also contribute to their virulence. The vast majority of CA-MRSA strains also produce the genes for PVL and it functions as a dermonecrotic factor in skin lesions, a potent cell lysin in high concentrations, and a potent inflammatory mediator in lower concentrations. However, there is controversy about the role of PVL as a single predominant virulence factor, because strains of CA-MRSA that have this gene knocked out have demonstrated no difference in pathogenicity in both vertebrate and invertebrate animal models and in human settings when the PVL is not present.

TABLE 2 Risk Factor Associations Reported for CA-MRSA Infections

RISK CATEGORIES	FACTOR	DETAILS FROM REPORTS
High-risk populations	Younger and older age	Age distribution in CA-MRSA younger than HA-MRSA High rate of CA-MRSA in children under 2 years CA-MRSA more common in children compared to adults Outbreaks in hospital nurseries Outbreaks in nursing homes with elderly residents
	Indigenous populations: Native or Aboriginal or African American	Aboriginal communities in midwestern United States, Canada, and Australia Alaskan natives More common in African Americans
	Athletes (predominantly contact sports)	Outbreaks on football teams Outbreaks on wrestling team Other competitive sports
	Persons who inject drugs (PWIDs)	Reports of PWIDs with MRSA transmission Canadian report of USA300 strain outbreak
	Men who have sex with men (MSM)	CA-MRSA described in HIV+ population of MSM
	HIV+ individuals	Risk associated with overlapping social networks, intravenous drug use, hemodialysis, and CD4 counts <200 reported as independent risks
	Military personnel	3% of US Army soldiers colonized
	Inmates of correctional facilities	Reports of outbreaks in US prisons Two outbreaks (total 10 inmates) in Canada
	Students in elementary schools and college dormitories	Reports of outbreaks in schools and college dormitories
Previous positive MRSA cultures	MRSA carriage Past MRSA infection	Colonized soldiers more likely to get CA-MRSA disease Prior abscess risk factor for CA-MRSA
Medical history	Chronic skin disorder	Dermatologic condition most common underlying medical disorder for CA-MRSA infection Classroom contact of index CA-MRSA case had chronic dermatitis
	Recurrent or recent antibiotic use	Antibiotic use associated with CA-MRSA infection in rural Alaska
Environmental	Homelessness and living in shelters Overcrowding Contact with colonized pet Veterinary workers and family members	Medically underserved populations at higher risk of CA-MRSA Reports of USA300 strain outbreak involving individuals living in shelters or homeless Close contact implicated in jail outbreaks Neonatal intensive care unit transmission Family dog source of recurrent infection Veterinarians working with horses and livestock Family members of animal care workers Small animal veterinarians Swine farmers

CA, Community-associated; *HA,* healthcare-associated; *HIV,* human immunodeficiency virus; *MRSA,* methicillin-resistant *Staphylococcus aureus.*
Adapted from Barton-Forbes M, Hawkes M, Moore D, et al. Guidelines for the prevention and management of community associated methicillin resistant *Staphylococcus aureus* (CA-MRSA): a perspective for Canadian Health Care Practitioners. *Can J Infect Dis Med Microbiol.* 2006;17(suppl C):1B–24B.

TABLE 3 Principles of Empiric Treatment of Minor Skin and Soft Tissue Infections (Folliculitis, Furuncles, Small Abscesses Without Cellulitis, Impetigo, Secondarily Infected Lesions Such as Eczema, Ulcers, or Wounds) Where the Etiology Is Unknown But May Include MRSA as a Possibility

Recommendations

One or more of the following measures may be employed:
- Local therapy using hot soaks, elevation, and dressings as appropriate
- Incision and drainage of furuncles or small abscesses without antimicrobial therapy
- Topical 2% mupirocin ointment (Bactroban) or fusidic acid[2] for impetigo and secondarily infected lesions if local strains are likely sensitive
- Topical antiseptics may be considered
- Antimicrobial therapy is recommended in addition to local measures if one or more of the following is present: multiple sites of infection, evidence of progression, clinical evidence of systemic symptoms and signs, presence of comorbidities, extremes of age, immunosuppression, septic phlebitis, or difficult site for incision and drainage.
- In follow-up, routine screening for colonization of the nares or other body sites is not recommended.

[2]Not available in the United States.
MRSA, Methicillin-resistant *Staphylococcus aureus.*

Prevention

Controlling the spread of HA-, CA-, or LA-MRSA from an infected or colonized person to others in the hospital, family, or community is a key goal of prevention. In the hospital setting, strict adherence to hand hygiene, application of barrier precautions (gloves, gowns, and private rooms) for patients colonized or infected with MRSA, environmental and equipment cleaning, and antimicrobial stewardship are the key preventive strategies.

Active surveillance cultures to identify colonized patients and decolonization may be effective in selected settings, but its general application is controversial. In the community setting, practicing hygienic measures including good personal hygiene, consistent hand hygiene, ensuring all draining skin and soft tissue lesions have adequate dressings, not sharing potentially contaminated personal articles, and keeping the household environment hygienic are important. Public health organizations may also contribute to the prevention of CA-MRSA by instituting education programs targeting healthcare providers and individuals in high-risk groups in the community, and by promoting appropriate antimicrobial use. In sports settings, in addition to the basic hygienic measures mentioned previously, avoidance of sharing of towels and other personal items, showering after every practice or tournament, cleaning of communal showering and bathing areas, and cleaning or laundering of equipment after each use are also important.

Clinical Manifestations

The specific clinical infections associated with MRSA parallel those associated with MSSA. Almost any body site, organ, or appendage may be affected by infections due to *S. aureus*, but there are specific predilections associated with HA- and CA-MRSA. In the hospital or other healthcare setting, the most commonly encountered infections include pneumonia, line-related infection, surgical site infection, bacteremia, and less often skin and soft tissue infections. In the community setting, the most common sites (>80%) are skin and soft tissue infections (furuncles, cellulitis, and soft tissue abscesses) and less commonly severely invasive infections such as necrotizing pneumonia, necrotizing fasciitis, multifocal osteomyelitis/septic arthritis, epidural abscess, pelvic septic thrombophlebitis, and bacteremia with toxic shock syndrome. The skin and soft tissue infections often affect young previously healthy patients and are characteristically very painful and pyogenic with an initial black eschar that patients presume was a "spider bite" as the initiating process.

Diagnosis

The diagnosis of MRSA infections is based on the clinical presentation and the isolation of the causative organism from purulent discharge, sputum, or urine, or from specimens obtained from normally sterile body fluids (joint fluid, abscess or tissue aspirates, and blood). The organism appears on Gram stain as a gram-positive organism in clusters and is usually seen in association with neutrophils and may be either intracellular or extracellular. The organism is very hardy and grows readily on typical media in the microbiology laboratory within 24 to 48 hours. Some laboratories are using rapid agglutination tests to detect the PBP2a protein or polymerase chain reaction (PCR)-based techniques to provide same-day or next-day identification. In settings where no cultures have been obtained or in the setting of toxic shock syndrome where cultures are often negative, the diagnosis may be difficult and only suspected based on a typical clinical presentation.

Treatment

MRSA strains harbor resistance to the β-lactam antimicrobials, including oxacillin, dicloxacillin, cloxacillin[2], nafcillin,

methicillin[2], and first-, second-, and third-generation cephalosporins. The newer advanced-generation cephalosporin antimicrobials ceftaroline (Teflaro) and ceftobiprole (Zevtera) have activity against MRSA strains. The majority of HA-MRSA strains are resistant to macrolides, clindamycin (Cleocin), aminoglycosides, and quinolones (with the exception of delafloxacin [Baxdela]) and are variably resistant to tetracycline and trimethoprim-sulfamethoxazole (Bactrim)[1], depending on local epidemiologic patterns. They are sensitive to vancomycin (Vancocin) and the lipoglycopeptides such as dalbavancin (Dalvance), telavancin (Vibativ), and oritavancin (Orbactiv) and usually sensitive to fusidic acid[2], rifampin (Rifadin)[1], the oxazolidinones linezolid (Zyvox) and tedizolid (Sivextro), and daptomycin (Cubicin). For hospitalized patients where *S. aureus* is considered a possible etiology of any major infectious syndrome, it should be considered as methicillin-resistant until proven otherwise. Empiric choices of vancomycin or lipoglycopeptides such as dalbavancin (Dalvance), telavancin (Vibativ) or oritavancin (Orbitactiv), linezolid (Zyvox) or tedizolid (Sivextro), daptomycin (Cubicin) or advanced-generation cephalosproins such as ceftaroline (Teflaro) or ceftobiprole (Zevtera) should be considered as appropriate to the presenting syndrome. CA-MRSA strains are resistant to macrolides and often quinolones (with the exception of delafloxacin [Baxdela]) but usually are sensitive to aminoglycosides such as gentamicin (Garamycin), clindamycin, and trimethoprim-sulfamethoxazole (Bactrim)[1], but the resistance patterns vary depending on local resistance patterns. In addition, these strains are sensitive to vancomycin (Vancocin) and the lipoglycopeptides, fusidic acid[2], rifampin (Rifadin)[1], linezolid (Zyvox), daptomycin (Cubicin), ceftaroline (Teflaro), and ceftobiprole (Zevtera). LA-MRSA strains are almost always resistant to tetracyclines; often resistant to quinolones, macrolides, and clindamycin, and variably resistant to aminoglycosides and trimethoprim-sulfamethoxazole. In addition, these strains are sensitive to vancomycin (Vancocin) and the lipoglycopeptides, fusidic acid[2], rifampin (Rifadin)[1], the oxazolidinones linezolid (Zyvox) and tedizolid (Sivextro), daptomycin (Cubicin), ceftaroline (Teflaro) and ceftobiprole (Zevtera). Treatment guidelines for MRSA with a focus on the ambulatory setting have been published in Canada, the United Kingdom, and the United States, and provide both empiric choices for common infectious presentations of unknown etiology and definitive treatment once an etiology of MRSA is known. New guidelines for *S. aureus* bacteremia are currently under development by the Infectious Diseases Society of America. The treatment options for both empiric and definitive use where MRSA is considered or proven are presented in Tables 3 through 6 and represent a constellation of the various guidelines that have been published. A recent randomized controlled trial assessed the efficacy of combination therapy in patients with MRSA bacteremia (vancomycin or daptomycin with flucloxacillin[2]). They found that the number of patients with persistent bacteremia after 5 days was lower in the combination arm. However, due to increased nephrotoxicity in the combination arm the trial was stopped early. Further studies are required to determine the role and benefit of combination therapy for MRSA infections.

---

[2] Not available in the United States

[1] Not FDA approved for this indication.
[2] Not available in the United States

TABLE 4	Principles of Empiric Treatment of Non–Life-Threatening Skin and Soft Tissue Infections Other Than Minor Skin Infections Where the Etiology Is Unknown But May Include MRSA as a Possibility

Recommendations
- Antibiotic choice should be based on the severity of illness at presentation, clinical judgment, and regional susceptibility patterns of strains
- Empiric therapy for CA-MRSA and β-hemolytic streptococci is recommended*

*The IDSA guideline suggests to differentiate purulent and nonpurulent cellulitis and reserve empiric therapy for β-hemolytic streptococci only in nonpurulent cellulitis but acknowledges it is an area of controversy. The previous UK and Canadian guidelines explicitly recommend coverage for β-hemolytic streptococci and do not differentiate cellulitis into different types. Some of the guidelines that exist have not been updated and hence knowledge of local susceptibility patterns is important.
CA, Community-associated; *IDSA,* Infectious Diseases Society of America; *MRSA,* methicillin-resistant *Staphylococcus aureus.*

TABLE 5 Principles of Empiric Treatment of Life-Threatening Infections Where the Etiology Is Unknown But May Include MRSA as a Possibility

Recommendations
- Include MRSA coverage, regardless of prevalence rates of CA-MRSA in the community
- Include an agent effective against MSSA until susceptibility results become available

CA, Community-associated; *MRSA*, methicillin-resistant *Staphylococcus aureus*; *MSSA*, methicillin-sensitive *Staphylococcus aureus*.

TABLE 6 Guidelines for the Management of MRSA Infections

CLINICAL DISEASE	KEY FEATURES	MANAGEMENT PRINCIPLES	ANTIMICROBIAL CHOICES AND COMMENTS*
Skin and Soft Tissue Infection (SSTI)			
Localized lesion	Infected scratches and minor wounds Insect bites Furuncles Small abscesses Absence of systemic illness	Culture selectively† No antibiotic therapy recommended *Exceptions: multiple sites of infection, evidence of progression, systemic symptoms and signs, presence of comorbidities, extremes of age, immunosuppression, septic phlebitis, or difficult site for incision and drainage: antimicrobial therapy is recommended in addition to local measures* Cover draining lesions Emphasize personal hygiene Close follow-up Return if worsening	Generally not indicated, although some evidence exists for treatment with clindamycin PO or trimethoprim-sulfamethoxazole (Bactrim)[1] PO, in conjunction with incision and drainage for small simple abscesses Topical antibacterial (e.g., mupirocin [Bactroban] or fusidic ointment[2]) therapy may be considered Systemic antimicrobial therapy indicated if one or more of the following: multiple sites of infection, evidence of progression, systemic symptoms and signs, presence of comorbidities, extremes of age, immunosuppression, septic phlebitis, or difficult site for incision and drainage
Cellulitis (not extensive) or multiple abscesses with minimal or no associated systemic features for oral treatment consideration	Classic features of rubor, dolor, calor, and swelling suggesting cellulitis with or without associated drainage or exudate	Culture site (if purulent or drainage) Drainage of abscess or needle aspiration Oral therapy in older child and adult Appropriate infection control measures Imaging for extent and complications as appropriate Close follow-up Return if worsening	*Empiric:* Include coverage for β-hemolytic streptococci¶ Clindamycin (Cleocin) 300–450 mg tid-qid PO for adults and 30–40 mg/kg/day[3] ÷ q6–8h PO for children TMP-SMX (Bactrim)[1] 1–2 DS tab bid PO for adults and 8–12 mg/kg/day (of TMP) ÷ q12h PO for children PLUS coverage for β-hemolytic streptococci (e.g., amoxicillin, cephalexin [Keflex]) Doxycycline (Vibramycin) 100 mg bid PO for adults and 4.4 mg/kg/day mg/kg/day ÷ q12h PO for children** PLUS coverage for β-hemolytic streptococci (e.g., amoxicillin, cephalexin) Delafloxacin (Baxdela) 450 mg bid PO for adults *Comment:* Recently became the first fluoroquinolone approved by the FDA for MRSA SSTI Linezolid (Zyvox) 600 mg bid PO for adults and 30 mg/kg/day ÷ q8h PO for children, not to exceed 600 mg/dose; for children older than 12 years of age 600 mg bid PO *Comment:* Linezolid is more expensive than the other options and may not always be readily available depending on the setting *Comment:* If parenteral therapy considered, see choices for severe SSTI Tedizolid (Sivextro) 200 mg PO/IV once daily for 6 days; safety and efficacy have not been established for children *Proven MRSA:* As above, based on sensitivity testing If parenteral therapy necessary, see choices for SSTI with systemic features Lefamulin (Xenleta) was recently approved for community acquired pneumonia related to *S. aureus* and ABSSSI[1] in the United States. Ceftobiprole has been recently approved for three indications, including acute bacterial skin and skin structure infections (ABSSSI), community-acquired bacterial pneumonia (CABP), and *Staphylococcus aureus* bacteraemia *Comment:* Dose and frequency for SAB is 667 mg (ceftobiprole medocaril sodium: 667 mg equivalent to 500 mg of ceftobiprole) every 6 hours on days 1 to 8 and every 8 hours from day 9 onwards Dose and frequency for ABSSSI and CABP is 667 mg (=500 mg ceftobiprole) every 8 hours

TABLE 6 Guidelines for the Management of MRSA Infections—cont'd

CLINICAL DISEASE	KEY FEATURES	MANAGEMENT PRINCIPLES	ANTIMICROBIAL CHOICES AND COMMENTS*
Cellulitis (severe or rapidly spreading or extensive) or complicated SSTI (deep soft tissue infection, surgical or traumatic wound infection, large or multiple abscesses, or infected ulcers and burns) and/or associated systemic features for parenteral treatment consideration	Classic features of rubor, dolor, calor, and swelling suggesting cellulitis with or without associated drainage or exudate with systemic features of fever, chills, malaise, prostration	Culture (blood if febrile, site if purulent) Hospitalize as appropriate Drainage of abscess or needle aspiration Parenteral therapy Imaging for extent and complications as appropriate Appropriate infection control measures Consultation as indicated	*Empiric:* Include coverage for β-hemolytic streptococci¶ Vancomycin (Vancocin) 15–20 mg/kg/dose q8–12h IV for adults and 40–60³ mg/kg/day ÷ q6h IV for children *Proven MRSA:* Based on sensitivity testing Vancomycin 15–20 mg/kg/dose q8–12h IV for adults and 40–60³ mg/kg/day ÷ q6h IV for children Clindamycin 600–900 mg q8h IV/IM for adults and 30–40 mg/kg/day³ ÷ q6–8h IV for children Linezolid 600 mg q12h PO/IV for adults and 30 mg/kg/day ÷ q8h PO/IV for children, not to exceed 600 mg/dose; for children older than 12 years of age 600 mg bid PO/IV Tedizolid (Sivextro) 200 mg PO/IV once daily for 6 days; safety and efficacy have not been established for children Ceftaroline (Teflaro) 600 mg IV q12h for adults; safety and efficacy have not been established for children Daptomycin (Cubicin) 4 mg/kg/dose once daily IV for adults and under investigation in children Dalbavancin (Dalvance) 1000 mg IV followed by 500 mg IV 1 week later for adults; safety and efficacy not established in children Telavancin (Vibativ) 10 mg/kg/dose IV once daily Oritavancin (Orbactiv), given as a single 1200 mg 3-hour infusion; not approved for children Delafloxacin (Baxdela) 300 mg bid IV *Comment:* Linezolid, tedizolid, daptomycin, ceftaroline, ceftobiprole, dalbavancin, oritavancin and telavancin are more expensive than the other options and may not always be readily available depending on the setting
Necrotizing fasciitis (NF)	Clinically indistinguishable from group A streptococcus NF disease Extreme toxicity High complication rate	Cultures (blood, tissue) Imaging for extent and complications Surgical débridement Consultation as indicated Parenteral therapy Infection control measures	*Empiric:* Include coverage for β-hemolytic streptococci Vancomycin 15–20 mg/kg/dose q8–12h IV for adults and 40–60³ mg/kg/day ÷ q6h IV for children Clindamycin 600–900 mg q8h IV/IM for adults and 30–40 mg/kg/day³ ÷ q6–8h IV for children *Proven MRSA:* Based on sensitivity testing Vancomycin 15–20 mg/kg/dose q8–12h IV for adults and 40–60³ mg/kg/day ÷ q6h IV for children Clindamycin 600–900 mg q8h IV/IM for adults and 30–40 mg/kg/day³ ÷ q6–8h IV for children Linezolid 600 mg q12h PO/IV for adults and 30 mg/kg/day ÷ q8h PO/IV for children, not to exceed 600 mg/dose; for children older than 12 years of age 600 mg bid PO/IV TMP/SMX¹ 8–12 mg/kg/day (of TMP) ÷ q8–12h IV for adults and 8–12 mg/kg/day (of TMP) ÷ q6h IV for children *Comments:* Adjuncts such as IVIG (Gamunex)¹ may be considered in severe cases with septic shock Few data available for the use of TMP-SMX in this indication

Musculoskeletal Infection (MSI)

CLINICAL DISEASE	KEY FEATURES	MANAGEMENT PRINCIPLES	ANTIMICROBIAL CHOICES AND COMMENTS*
Osteomyelitis/septic arthritis	Preceding trauma Tendency for multifocal involvement Disease in adjacent muscle not uncommon Progression to chronic osteomyelitis possible May be complicated by deep venous thrombosis	Cultures (blood, bone, and tissue) Imaging for extent and complications Involve surgical team (early débridement and drainage) Consultation as indicated Parenteral therapy Consider combination therapy for severe cases or if slow to respond Infection control measures Look for other infected sites (imaging)	*Empiric:* Vancomycin 15–20 mg/kg/dose q8–12h IV for adults and 40–60³ mg/kg/day ÷ q6h IV for children Clindamycin 600–900 mg q8h IV/IM for adults and 30–40 mg/kg/day³ ÷ q6–8h IV for children Linezolid¹ 600 mg q12h PO/IV for adults and 30 mg/kg/day ÷ q8h PO/IV for children, not to exceed 600 mg/dose; for children older than 12 years of age 600 mg bid PO/IV Daptomycin¹ 6 mg/kg/dose once daily IV for adults and 6–10 mg/kg once daily for children TMP/SMX¹ 8–12 mg/kg/day (of TMP) ÷ q8–12h IV for adults and 8–12 mg/kg/day (of TMP) ÷ q6h IV for children *Comments:* Linezolid and daptomycin are more expensive than the other options and may not always be readily available depending on the setting Few data available for the use of TMP-SMX in these indications for children *Proven MRSA:* As above, based on sensitivity testing Addition of rifampin (Rifadin)¹ may be considered for osteomyelitis

Continued

Methicillin-Resistant Staphylococcus Aureus

677

TABLE 6	Guidelines for the Management of MRSA Infections—cont'd		
CLINICAL DISEASE	**KEY FEATURES**	**MANAGEMENT PRINCIPLES**	**ANTIMICROBIAL CHOICES AND COMMENTS***
Pyomyositis	May be extensive Tendency for multifocal involvement	Cultures (blood, tissue) Imaging for extent and complications Surgical drainage Consultation as indicated Parenteral therapy Infection control measures	

Respiratory Tract Infection (RTI)

Pneumonia	Influenza-like prodrome, hemoptysis, fever, shock, leukopenia, pneumatoceles, multifocal abscesses, consolidation, frequent empyema, respiratory failure, and high mortality	Cultures (blood, pleural fluid, sputum) Imaging for extent and complications Consultation as indicated Intensive care unit as appropriate Infection control measures Combination parenteral therapy Chest tube drainage for empyema	*Empiric:* Vancomycin 15–20 mg/kg/dose q8–12h IV for adults and 40–60[3] mg/kg/day ÷ q6h IV for children Linezolid 600 mg q12h PO/IV for adults and 30 mg/kg/day ÷ q8h PO/IV for children, not to exceed 600 mg/dose; for children older than 12 years of age 600 mg bid PO/IV Clindamycin 600–900 mg q8h IV/IM for adults and 30–40 mg/kg/day[3] ÷ q6–8h IV for children TMP/SMX[1] 8–12 mg/kg/day (of TMP) ÷ q8–12h IV for adults and 8–12 mg/kg/day (of TMP) ÷ q6h IV for children Telavancin (Vibativ) 10 mg/kg/dose IV once daily for adults for hospital or ventilator acquired pneumonia Ceftaroline (Teflaro) 600 mg IV q12h for adults with community-acquired pneumonia; safety and efficacy have not been established for children Ceftobiprole (Zevtera) has been recently approved for three indications, including acute bacterial skin and skin structure infections (ABSSSI),community-acquired bacterial pneumonia (CABP) and *Staphylococcus aureus* bacteraemia. Dose and frequency for SAB is 667 mg every 6 hours on days 1 to 8 and every 8 hours from day 9 onwards. Dose and frequency for ABSSSI and CABP is 667 mg (=500 mg ceftobiprole) every 8 hours safety and efficacy have not been established for children *Comment:* Daptomycin not indicated because it is inactivated by lung surfactant *Proven MRSA:* As above, based on sensitivity testing

Other

Sepsis syndrome Bacteremia Native valve endocarditis	Shock Multiple-organ failure May have purpura fulminans Associated SSTI, MSI, and RTI May be complicated by Waterhouse-Friedrichsen syndrome High mortality	Blood cultures Culture any pus or fluid collection Look for primary or secondary focus Imaging for identification of source including echocardiography Consultation as indicated ICU care Imaging: look for occult abscesses, bone infection, or endocarditis Involve surgery and other specialists as needed Infection control measures Parenteral, multidrug therapy Prolonged therapy for endovascular source infections	*Empiric:* Vancomycin 15–20 mg/kg/dose q8–12h IV for adults and 40–60[3] mg/kg/day ÷ q6h IV for children Daptomycin 6 mg/kg/dose once daily IV for adults and 4–10[3] mg/kg/dose once daily for children[1] *Comments:* Doses of daptomycin of up to 10 mg/kg/dose[3] once daily have been used in adults in this indication Some recommendations have included linezolid in this setting at the doses described above *Proven MRSA:* As above, based on sensitivity testing. *Comment:* New IDSA guidelines for the treatment of *S. aureus* bacteremia are in progress Ceftobiprole has been recently approved for three indications, including acute bacterial skin and skin structure infections (ABSSSI),community-acquired bacterial pneumonia (CABP) and *Staphylococcus aureus* bacteraemia, including right-sided infective endocarditis.

*Choice of antimicrobial therapy depends on local susceptibility patterns.

†Patients with risk factors, as a part of an outbreak investigation, patients with slowly responding or recurrent lesions.

¶The IDSA guideline suggests to differentiate purulent and nonpurulent cellulitis and reserve empiric therapy for β-hemolytic streptococci only in nonpurulent cellulitis but acknowledges it is an area of controversy. The UK and Canadian guidelines explicitly recommend empiric coverage for β-hemolytic streptococci and do not differentiate cellulitis into different types. A recent randomized controlled trial in the United States found no significant difference in efficacy between clindamycin and trimethoprim-sulfamethoxazole when used for treatment of uncomplicated skin and soft tissue infections, which were thought to be secondary to either β-hemolytic streptococci or *S. aureus*. Another recent placebo-controlled trial in the United States found that clindamycin or trimethoprim-sulfamethoxazole in conjunction with incision and drainage improved outcomes in patients with simple small abscesses (<5 cm) compared with incision and drainage alone.

[1]Not FDA approved for this indication. Dosing has varied in published reports and specific dosing guidelines are not available.

[2]Not available in the United States.

[3]Exceeds dosage recommended by the manufacturer.

**Not recommended for pediatric patients younger than 8 years of age or in pregnancy.

ICU, Intensive care unit; *IDSA,* Infectious Diseases Society of America; *IVIG,* intravenous immunoglobulin; *MRSA,* methicillin-resistant *Staphylococcus aureus*; *TMP-SMX,* trimethoprim-sulfamethoxazole.

References

Barton-Forbes M, Hawkes M, Moore D, et al: Guidelines for the prevention and management of community associated methicillin resistant *Staphylococcus aureus* (CA-MRSA): a perspective for Canadian Health Care Practitioners, *Can J Infect Dis Med Microbiol* 17(Suppl. C):1B–24B, 2006.

Brown NM, Brown EM: Guideline Development Group: Treatment of methicillin-resistant Staphylococcus aureus (MRSA): updated guidelines from the UK, *J Antimicrob Chemother* 76(6):1377–1378, 2021.

Brown NM, Goodman AL, Horner C, et al: Treatment of methicillin-resistant Staphylococcus aureus (MRSA): updated guidelines from the UK, *JAC Antimicrob Resist* 3(1):dlaa114, 2021, https://doi.org/10.1093/jacamr/dlaa114.

Chambers HF, Deleo FR: Waves of resistance: *Staphylococcus aureus* in the antibiotic era, *Nat Rev Microbiol* 7:629–641, 2009. https://doi.org/10.1038/nrmicro2200.

Daum RS, Miller LG, Immergluck L: A placebo-controlled trial of antibiotics for smaller skin abscesses, *N Engl J Med* 376(26):2545–2555, 2017.

David MZ, Daum RS: Community-associated methicillin resistant *Staphylococcus aureus*: epidemiology and clinical consequences of an emerging epidemic, *Clin Microbiol Rev* 23:616–687, 2010. https://doi.org/10.1128/CMR.00081-09.

File TM, Goldberg L, Das A, et al: Efficacy and safety of intravenous-to-oral lefamulin, a pleuromutilin antibiotic, for the treatment of community-acquired bacterial pneumonia: the phase III Lefamulin Evaluation Against Pneumonia (LEAP 1) trial, *Clin Infect Dis* 69:1856–1867, 2019.

Fluit AC: Livestock-associated *Staphylococcus aureus*, *Clin Microbiol Infect* 18:735–744, 2012. https://doi.org/10.1111/j.1469-0691.2012.03846.x.

Geriak M, Haddad F, Khulood R, et al: Clinical data on daptomycin plus ceftaroline versus standard of care monotherapy in the treatment of methicillin-resistant *Staphylococcus aureus* bacteremia, *Antimicrob Agents Chemother*, 2019. https://doi.org/10.1128/AAC.02483-18.

Gu J, Shen S, Xiong M, et al: ST7 Becomes One of the Most Common Staphylococcus aureus Clones After the COVID-19 Epidemic in the City of Wuhan, China, *Infect Drug Resist* 16:843–852, 2023.

Klevens RM, Morrison MA, Nadle J, et al: Invasive methicillin resistant *Staphylococcus aureus* infections in the United States, *JAMA* 298:1763–1771, 2007.

Kock R, Becker K, Cookson B, et al: Methicillin resistant *Staphylococcus aureus* (MRSA): burden of disease and control challenges in Europe, *Euro Surveill* 15:19688, 2010.

Lakhundi S, Zhang K: Methicillin-resistant *Staphylococcus aureus*: molecular characterization, evolution, and epidemiology, *Clin Microbiol Rev* 31, 2018. e00020-18. https://doi.org/10.1128/CMR.00020-18.

Lastinger LM, Alvarez CR, Kofman A, et al: Continued increases in the incidence of healthcare-associated infection (HAI) during the second year of the coronavirus disease 2019 (COVID-19) pandemic, *Infect Control Hosp Epidemiol* 20:1–5, 2022.

Lee SI, Lee GY, Park JH, Yang SJ: High prevalence of clonal complex 398 methicillin-susceptible and -resistant Staphylococcus aureus in pig farms: clonal lineages, multiple drug resistance, and occurrence of the staphylococcal cassette chromosome mec IX, *Foodborne Pathog Dis* 20(3):100–109, 2023.

Liu C, Bayer A, Cosgrove SE, et al: Clinical practice guidelines by the Infectious Diseases Society of America for the treatment of methicillin resistant *Staphylococcus aureus* infections in adults and children: executive summary, *Clin Infect Dis* 52:285–292, 2011. https://doi.org/10.1093/cid/cir034.

Miller LG, Daum RS, Creech CB, et al: Clindamycin versus trimethoprim-sulfamethoxazole for uncomplicated skin infections, *N Engl J Med* 372(12):1093–1103, 2015.

Popovich KJ, Aureden K, Ham DC, et al: SHEA/IDSA/APIC Practice Recommendation: Strategies to prevent methicillin-resistant Staphylococcus aureus transmission and infection in acute-care hospitals: 2022 Update, *Infect Control Hosp Epidemiol* 44(7):1039–1067, 2023, https://doi.org/10.1017/ice.2023.102.

Saei HD, McClure JA, Kashif A, etal: The Role of Prophage φSa3 in the Adaption of Staphylococcus aureus ST398 Sublineages from Human to Animal Hosts, *Antibiotics (Basel)* 13(2):112, 2024, https://doi.org/10.3390/antibiotics13020112.

Tong SYC, Lye DC, Yahav D, et al: Effect of vancomycin or daptomycin with vs without an antistaphylococcal β-lactam on mortality, bacteremia, relapse, or treatment failure in patients with MRSA bacteremia: a randomized clinical trial, *JAMA* 323(6):527–537, 2020.

Weidmann MD, Berry GJ, Zucker JE, et al: Bacterial pneumonia and respiratory culture utilization among hospitalized patients with and without COVID-19 in a New York City hospital, *J Clin Microbiol* 60(7):e0017422, 2022.

MPOX

Method of
Scott Kellermann, MD, MPH; and Rick D. Kellerman, MD

CURRENT DIAGNOSIS

- Clinical suspicion is based on history and symptoms, including suggestive skin lesions and high-risk epidemiologic characteristics.
- Clinical manifestations are usually mild but may become life threatening.
- Prodromal symptoms may include fatigue, headache, fever, chills, myalgias, and backache.
- A rash may develop at the site of inoculation, including the anogenital and perioral areas, and may or may not spread to the trunk and acral areas. Most commonly, there are 1 to 20 skin lesions. The lesions typically develop simultaneously, spread centrifugally, and evolve from macular to papular to vesicular (filled with clear fluid) to pustular (filled with opaque fluid) to pseudopustules (containing solid debris) and finally to scab formation. The lesions are deep seated, may be umbilicated, are pruritic, and are frequently painful.
- Clade Ib mpox is mainly transmitted heterosexually. At highest risk are those with multiple casual sexual partners, sex workers and their clients, and household contacts.
- Clade Ib mpox can cause a rash that may cover much of the body, including the face and torso.
- Children with clade Ib mpox are infected through contact with infected animals and/or infected household members and experience more severe disease than adults.
- Those at highest risk of clade IIb mpox include gay, bisexual, or other men who have sex with men with multiple sexual partners.
- The incubation period of mpox is usually from 5 to 13 days but can range from 4 to 21 days.
- People may be contagious 1 to 4 days before symptoms appear and remain infectious until all crusts have sloughed off and the lesions have reepithelialized.
- Diagnosis is confirmed by demonstration of the presence of monkeypox virus DNA by polymerase chain reaction testing or next-generation sequencing of a clinical specimen or isolation of monkeypox virus in culture from a clinical specimen.
- Histopathologic diagnosis is nonspecific.

CURRENT THERAPY

- The JYNNEOS vaccine is approved by the U.S. Food and Drug Administration (FDA) and preferred for prevention of clade IIb mpox. It is expected to be protective against monkeypox virus regardless of clade.
- Vaccination before exposure and postexposure prophylaxis protocols exist.
- Certain high-risk infected individuals should be considered for treatment with tecovirimat (Tpoxx)[1].

[1]Not FDA approved for this indication.

In November 2022, following the current best practice of not naming diseases after animals or geographic locations, the World Health Organization (WHO) changed the name of the disease previously referred to as *monkeypox* to *mpox*. Until the International Committee on the Taxonomy of Viruses decides on a different name, the virus will continue to be called monkeypox.

The monkeypox virus is an *Orthopoxvirus*, the same genus as smallpox (variola) and cowpox (vaccinia). Mpox is a contagious zoonotic disease and is endemic in certain parts of Africa. It was first isolated in 1958 in Copenhagen from a colony of laboratory monkeys sent from Singapore for polio virus research. In 1970 the first proven case of human mpox was diagnosed in the Democratic Republic of the Congo (DRC) (formerly the Republic of Zaire). Despite initially being named *monkeypox*, African rodents such as Gambian pouched rats, dormice, and African squirrels, rather than monkeys, are considered to be the most likely reservoirs of the virus.

There have been isolated cases and a few outbreaks of mpox in various countries, including the United Kingdom and the United States.

In 2003 the United States reported an outbreak of 71 probable cases (35 laboratory confirmed) that resulted from direct contact with prairie dogs sold as pets. The prairie dogs were found to have been infected when they were housed with Gambian pouched rats imported from Ghana. There were no reported deaths in the 2003 outbreak. Cases in a 2018 outbreak in the United Kingdom were eventually traced back to travelers who had visited Nigeria.

From January to May 2022, most suspected cases of mpox occurred in the DRC, with 1284 cases and 58 deaths reported. In May 2022, cases of clade IIb mpox were confirmed in the United Kingdom and traced to an individual who had traveled from Nigeria. On July 23, 2022, the WHO declared this outbreak of mpox a public health emergency of international concern (PHEIC). Worldwide, clade IIb mpox has spread to 123 countries resulting in 103,610 cases with 234 deaths. As of September 2, 2024, the United States has recorded 33,799 cases with 60 deaths. Clade IIb mpox is still circulating in the United States at low levels.

In September 2023 a new lineage of clade I monkeypox virus emerged in a previously largely unaffected region in South Kivu, DRC. Phylogenetically, this clade Ib lineage constitutes a cluster distinct from other clade I lineages that are now denoted clade Ia. The subsequent human-to-human spread of clade Ib resulted in 2672 confirmed mpox cases in South Kivu between January 1 and October 20, 2024. Since January 1, 2024, the DRC has reported more than 47,000 suspected mpox cases and more than 1000 suspected deaths. Of these, about 9000 cases have been confirmed through laboratory testing, with more than 40 confirmed deaths. From South Kivu, clade Ib spread to other provinces and to nearby countries including Burundi, the Central African Republic, Congo (Brazzaville), and Uganda. On August 14, 2024, for the second time in 2 years, the WHO declared another mpox outbreak a PHEIC. In the United States, clade Ib mpox has been diagnosed in travelers who recently visited areas with sustained clade Ib mpox transmission. Regarding the clade Ib mpox, the CDC has assigned a low risk to the general population within the United States. (https://www.cdc.gov/mpox/situation-summary/index.html).

Epidemiology

The eradication of smallpox in 1977 and the discontinuation of routine smallpox immunization paved the way for mpox to gain worldwide clinical relevance. This hypothesis was supported by a 2005 to 2007 study in the DRC that reported a 20-fold increase in mpox compared with the incidence in the 1980s. Those who were not immunized for smallpox had a fivefold higher risk of mpox infection compared with those who were vaccinated.

Transmission

A variety of animals, including nonhuman primates, and especially rodents, may contract mpox. Symptoms and severity of symptoms may differ among animals, varying from mild to febrile disease, upper respiratory symptoms, and a papular-pustular rash. Animal-to-animal transmission may occur through the fecal-oral route, respiratory droplets, contact with wounds, and eating infected meat.

As a zoonotic infection, animal-to-human transmission of mpox has been confirmed. Animal-to-human transmission can result from contact with infected papules, vesicles, pustules, or body fluids; by ingesting infected meat; or through bites and scratches.

Human-to-human transmission of monkeypox virus occurs primarily from transfer of infectious material through microabrasions in the skin and/or mucous membranes during sexual and/or close intimate contact. There is the potential for spread through large respiratory droplets during prolonged face-to-face contact (e.g., within a 6-foot radius for ≥3 hours in the absence of personal protective equipment [PPE]).

Fomites may present a transmission risk through resuspension of dried material from infected lesions (e.g., shaking contaminated linens).

Transmission may occur through an inadvertent needle-stick injury while collecting samples from a cutaneous lesion.

Vertical transmission of monkeypox virus from mother to child has been proven.

Although the virus has been found in semen and vaginal secretions, these seem to be minor drivers of infection, regardless of monkeypox viral load.

Emerging data suggest the possibility of monkeypox virus transmission 1 to 4 days before symptom onset.

Clades

Two distinct clades of mpox, clade I and clade II, exist in different geographic regions of Africa. Clade I is prevalent in Central Africa, whereas clade II is common in West Africa. The mortality risk associated with mpox varies with respect to the clade.

Clade II

Clade II consists of two subclades, clades IIa and IIb. Clade IIa is a West African zoonosis, having a low mortality.

Clade IIb is disproportionately spread among men who have sex with men, suggesting amplification of transmission through sexual networks. In a U.S. study of 7500 cases of mpox clade IIb from May 17 to July 22, 2022, 99% of the cases were male, and 94% reported recent male-to-male sexual or intimate conduct. Similar to data from other countries, 41% of these patients were HIV positive. It is unknown whether HIV infection increases a person's risk of acquiring mpox disease after exposure; however, the risk of progressing to severe mpox disease has been reported to be higher in those who are immunologically suppressed. During the outbreak that began in 2022, persons who experienced severe manifestations of mpox and who had HIV with CD4 counts <200 cells/mL presented significant treatment challenges.

Coinfections with sexually transmitted infections ranged from 16% to 29%, with gonorrhea, chlamydia, and syphilis the most commonly reported.

The global case fatality rate with clade IIb epidemics during the first mpox PHEIC in 2022 was approximately 0.03%. Outcomes from clade IIb infections in the United States are favorable. This may be a result of milder clade IIb infections, a healthier patient population, greater availability of supportive medical care, and because most older adults in the United States are vaccinated against smallpox.

Clade I

Clade I is subdivided into clade Ia and clade Ib.

Clade Ia is mainly a rodent-transmitted zoonotic infection and has shown little predilection for human-to-human spread. Most infected humans are children.

The current clade Ib outbreak, in densely populated regions of the DRC, is linked to sustained human-to-human transmission in previously unaffected individuals. The 2024 clade Ib outbreak in the DRC had a case fatality rate of 2.7% with substantially higher mortality rates in children.

In the current mpox clade Ib outbreak, transmission is primarily through heterosexual sexual transmission. Household transmission is not uncommon. In a report of 108 polymerase chain reaction (PCR)-confirmed cases, the median age of patients was 22 years, 52% were female, and 29% were sex workers. In adults, mpox clade Ib primarily affects the genitourinary system, indicative of sexual transmission, whereas children mostly manifest extragenital lesions. Available data indicate these cases are initially spread through intimate or sexual contact between adults and then spread through direct contact occurring within households, frequently involving children.

Risk Factors

Those at highest risk of exposure in the ongoing clade IIb outbreak are gay, bisexual, or men who have sex with men with multiple sexual partners.

For clade Ib, those at risk include individuals with multiple casual sexual partners, sex workers and their clients, and household contacts.

The risks for both clade Ib and clade IIb also include health workers who have the possibility of repeated exposure, laboratory personnel working with orthopoxviruses, clinical laboratory and healthcare personnel performing diagnostic testing for monkeypox virus, and outbreak response team members. People residing in the same household with those who have an mpox infection, especially children or close community contacts, are also at risk.

Pathophysiology

Monkeypox virus is a large, linear, double-stranded DNA virus with a genome size of around 190 kb. The virus replicates in the cytoplasm of vertebrate and invertebrate cells, although DNA viruses typically replicate and express their genomes in the nucleus. The virus invades the cell, replicates in the cytoplasm, and causes cell death.

After viral entry through skin or mucous membranes, the monkeypox virus replicates at the inoculation site and then spreads to local lymph nodes. This is followed by a viremia that leads to viral spread and seeding at other sites.

The large size of the monkeypox virus readily generates an immune response. Monkeypox virus infection stimulates an adaptive immune response comprising activated effector CD4+ and CD8+ T cells, neutralizing IgM and IgG antibodies and the production of Th1-inflammatory cytokines. Genomic analysis reveals that the virus may be actively mutating and adapting to human host immune responses.

Prevention

General safety measures, such as the use of PPE, should be employed by healthcare workers and laboratory researchers who may come in contact with the monkeypox virus. Hospitalized patients with confirmed or suspected mpox should be isolated. Lesions should be covered by gloves, a gown, or a sheet. Routine cleaning and disinfection procedures should be followed, and special attention should be paid to soiled laundry. Intubation, extubation, and any procedures likely to spread oral secretions should be performed in an airborne infection isolation room. Although there is no definitive epidemiologic evidence that mpox is spread by the airborne route, the use of an N95 respirator is suggested. To date, there have been no cases of mpox transmitted by blood transfusion, organ transplantation or implantation, infusion, or transfer of human cells, tissues, or cellular or tissue-based products. Patients and household members who are isolated at home should use well-fitting face masks and gloves. Lesions should be covered (e.g., long sleeves, long pants), and good hand hygiene should be routine. Laundering linens and towels with detergent and water should be sufficient.

Activities that could aerosolize dried material from lesions (e.g., use of portable fans, dry dusting, sweeping, vacuuming) should be avoided. If possible, use a separate bathroom if there are others living in the same household. Those infected with mpox should avoid contact with animals (specifically mammals), including pets.

It is recommended that condoms be used for 12 weeks after contracting the illness.

Vaccinations

Immunization against smallpox will confer cross-reactive protection against mpox.

Because of the antigenic similarities and therapeutic targets shared by all viruses in the orthopoxvirus genus, mpox vaccines are expected to be protective against monkeypox virus, regardless of clade.

There are two available vaccines that can reduce the risk of developing mpox: the modified vaccinia Ankara (MVA) vaccine (JYNNEOS in the United States, IMVANEX in the European Union, and IMVAMUNE in Canada) and the ACAM2000 vaccine.

JYNNEOS

The JYNNEOS vaccine is recommended as the primary vaccine to prevent mpox because it is associated with fewer side effects than the ACAM2000 vaccine. JYNNEOS is a live, nonreplicating modified vaccinia Ankara virus that was approved in 2019 by the U.S. Food and Drug Administration (FDA) for the prevention of mpox in high-risk adults 18 years of age and older. JYNNEOS is administered subcutaneously as a 2-dose series delivered 28 days apart. The standard regimen for JYNNEOS involves a subcutaneous (SC) route of administration with an injection volume of 0.5 mL. An alternative regimen involving intradermal (ID) administration with an injection volume of 0.1 mL may be used under an Emergency Use Authorization (EUA). Both the standard (0.5 mL SC) and the alternative (0.1 mL ID)[1] regimens have been found to be effective for mpox prevention.

There is an adequate supply of JYNNEOS vaccine; therefore clinicians can preferentially administer JYNNEOS via the subcutaneous route. The JYNNEOS vaccine is licensed as a series of 2 SC doses administered 28 days (4 weeks) apart. The CDC routinely recommends vaccination for people with sexual risk factors for mpox who have not been diagnosed with mpox during the ongoing outbreak or have not already received 2 doses of the JYNNEOS vaccine.

Peak immunity is expected to be reached 14 days after the second dose of JYNNEOS vaccine. Because JYNNEOS is based on a live, attenuated, nonreplicating orthopoxvirus, it may be administered without regard to timing of other vaccines.

Across 32 U.S. jurisdictions, among males aged 18 to 49 years eligible for JYNNEOS vaccination, mpox incidence was 14 times higher among unvaccinated males compared with those who had received a first vaccine dose ≥14 days earlier.

JYNNEOS dosing regimens can be found at https://www.cdc.gov/mpox/hcp/vaccine-considerations/index.html.

ACAM2000

The ACAM2000 vaccine is approved for immunization against smallpox and on August 29, 2024, the FDA approved an expanded indication for ACAM2000 for mpox prevention. In the United States, there is a large supply of ACAM2000, but this vaccine has more known side effects and contraindications. ACAM2000 was not used during the clade IIb mpox outbreak; therefore resources related to ACAM2000 for the mpox outbreak have been archived.

Vaccination Before Exposure

The WHO indicates that mass vaccination is not required or recommended for monkeypox virus at this time. Primary preventive (preexposure) vaccination is only recommended for individuals at high risk of exposure.

Postexposure Prophylaxis

The WHO recommends post-exposure preventive vaccination for contacts of cases, ideally within 4 days of first exposure (and up to 14 days in the absence of symptoms).

Pregnancy/Breastfeeding

Mpox can pose considerable hazards to the fetus. Miscarriages, stillbirth, preterm birth, and neonatal mpox have been reported when pregnant women contract mpox. Fetal ultrasound monitoring is recommended in cases of maternal monkeypox virus infection, and subsequent management should be based on the presence of ultrasound anomalies such as fetal hepatomegaly or hydrops. The sensitivity of molecular detection of monkeypox virus in the amniotic fluid is unknown, although by analogy with cytomegalovirus, toxoplasmosis, and Zika virus infections, it is likely that monkeypox virus is shed in the amniotic fluid when the fetal kidneys produce sufficient urine (i.e., after 18–21 weeks' gestation).

Though most nonpregnant adults with mpox experience mild illness, those with the infection who are pregnant, recently pregnant, or breastfeeding should be prioritized for treatment. These individuals may be at increased risk of severe disease and transmitting infection to the fetus or newborn. After consultation with the CDC, tecovirimat (Tpoxx)[1] should be considered for first-line treatment (see the "Treatment" section) (https://www.cdc.gov/mpox/hcp/clinical-care/pregnancy.html). Animal studies have suggested the risk of teratogenicity from brincidofovir (Tembexa)[1] and cidofovir[1].

JYNNEOS can be offered to pregnant or breastfeeding women who are otherwise eligible. The risks and benefits of JYNNEOS should be discussed with the patient using shared decision

---

[1] Not FDA approved for this indication.

making. There is limited information on the effects of mpox during pregnancy. Pregnant women appear to have similar signs and symptoms as those who are not pregnant.

Direct contact between a mother with mpox and her newborn is not advised. There is probable increased risk of severe infection in newborns.

Children

Treatment for mpox is based on clinical presentation and severity, regardless of clade. As with adults, children and adolescents with mpox should be closely monitored throughout their illness and likely will benefit from supportive care and pain control. Decisions about supportive treatment for children closely align with treatment plans for adults. Available and appropriate medical countermeasures (e.g., tecovirimat[1], cidofovir[1]) should be considered for those with severe disease or life-threatening complications. Additionally, treatment should be considered for those with severe immunodeficiency or who are immunocompromised, conditions affecting skin integrity (e.g., eczema), children <1 year of age, or adolescents who are pregnant or breastfeeding. These medications must be accessed through clinical trials or are available for compassionate use under the expanded access–investigational new drug protocol. For more information, visit https://www.cdc.gov/mpox/php/data-research/clade-i-mpox-in-children-in-africa-and-potential-impacts-on-children-in-the-united-states.html.

For the pediatric population, particular attention should be paid to keeping skin lesions covered and preventing children from scratching lesions or touching their eyes after touching lesions, which may result in autoinoculation and more severe illness.

Historically, children infected with monkeypox virus have been more likely to have severe disease. However, this was not the case in the global clade IIb outbreak. During the 2023 to 2024 clade Ib outbreak in the DRC, a substantially higher morbidity and mortality was seen in children under age 5 years. Although children younger than 15 years made up 34.2% of confirmed clade Ib cases in the DRC, a similar age-related proportion of mpox cases in the United States is not expected because, compared with the DRC, U.S. household sizes are smaller and there is availability of cleaning and disinfecting products, better access to medical care, and more robust patient information systems.

Clinical Manifestations

In patients with classic mpox, the incubation period from time of exposure to clinical illness is usually 5 to 13 days, but it may be up to 21 days. Emerging data suggest the possibility of monkeypox virus transmission 1 to 4 days before symptom onset.

The clinical manifestations of mpox are usually mild, and patients may have subclinical infection or be asymptomatic. In rare situations, patients may develop life-threatening illness. The duration of symptoms is usually 2 to 4 weeks. Most patients recover without specific treatment. Systemic symptoms are common and may occur during a prodromal stage, or shortly thereafter. In addition to rash, other symptoms may include conjunctivitis, cough, dyspnea, nausea, vomiting, dysphagia, sore throat, headache, fatigue and photophobia.

Prodromal symptoms may include fever, malaise, headache, sore throat, or cough, and (in many cases) swollen lymph nodes. Lymphadenopathy is a characteristic feature of mpox, and lymphatic swelling may occur in the submandibular, cervical, axillary, or inguinal nodes and may be bilateral. A person may be contagious during this period. In some clade Ib mpox cases, patients have presented with a rash without a recognized prodrome.

During the 2022 clade IIb outbreak, it was noted that patients frequently presented with lesions located on the anogenital and perioral areas alone, presumably at the site of inoculation, with some developing a small number of lesions on the trunk or acral areas of the body. The rash may or may not spread in a centrifugal pattern to the rest of the body. The total number of lesions may vary from a few to 100 but most commonly, there are 1 to 20 lesions. Over the ensuing 2 to 4 weeks, the lesions simultaneously evolve in 1- to 2-day increments from macular to papular, to vesicular (filled with clear fluid), to pustular (filled with opaque fluid),

to pseudopustules (containing solid debris), and to eventual scab formation. The lesions are deep seated, may be umbilicated, are pruritic, and are frequently painful. They may evolve in the same stage on the same area of the body or on different areas of the body. Occasionally there may be lesions at differing stages of development. Lesions remain in the pustular phase for 5 to 7 days before crusts begin to form. Healing lesions may itch. Crusts form and desquamate over the subsequent 7 to 14 days, and in most cases, the condition resolves around 3 to 4 weeks after symptom onset.

For both clade Ib and clade IIb monkeypox virus infection, lesions often occur in the genital and anorectal areas or in the mouth. The rash is not always disseminated across many sites on the body. It does not always appear on palms and soles. The rash may be confined to only a few lesions or only a single lesion. Rectal symptoms (e.g., purulent or bloody stools, rectal pain, or rectal bleeding) have been frequently reported with anogenital involvement.

Despite similarities in disease presentation between clades Ib and IIb, clade Ib infections in adults appear to be somewhat more severe, with higher total lesion counts and more frequent secondary bacterial infection, and urogenital and systemic complications. In the situation of transmission of clade Ib by sexual contact, lesions have appeared on the genital, oral, or anal areas, similar to those seen in patients with clade IIb in other regions of the world.

In children, the lesions of clade Ib are extragenital and symptoms more severe than with clade IIb.

Patients are no longer considered infectious after all crusts have sloughed off and the lesions have reepithelialized. An excellent monograph can be found at https://www.cdc.gov/mpox/hcp/clinical-signs/?CDC_AAref_Val=https://www.cdc.gov/poxvirus/mpox/clinicians/clinical-recognition.html.

Diagnosis

The diagnosis can be most easily confirmed by PCR testing of fluid from open lesions. Unlike the lesions seen in herpes simplex virus, which are usually filled with fluid and easily unroofed, mpox lesions may contain solid material, making them difficult to unroof with a swab. Two swabs from each of two to three lesions should be collected for testing. Using two sterile synthetic swabs (including, but not limited to, polyester, nylon, or Dacron with a plastic, wood, or thin aluminum shaft), swab the lesion vigorously to collect adequate DNA. Do not use cotton swabs. Unroofing or aspiration of lesions before swabbing is not necessary, nor is it recommended owing to the risk for sharps injury. All recommended PPE should be worn when collecting a specimen from a person with suspected or confirmed mpox.

Diagnosis may also be confirmed through the use of electron microscopy, culture, and immunohistochemical analysis. Genomic sequencing may be used in some situations. The use of serum IgM and IgG antibody testing may provide supportive information. Histopathologic diagnosis is nonspecific.

The CDC's standardized case definition and national notification for mpox infection can be found at https://www.cdc.gov/mpox/hcp/case-definitions/index.html (Table 1).

Differential Diagnosis

The differential diagnosis of mpox includes other poxviruses, particularly smallpox and chickenpox. Other conditions to be considered in the differential diagnosis include hand, foot, and mouth disease; herpes zoster; herpes simplex; measles; impetigo; scabies; candidiasis; dermatitis herpetiformis; orf; bullous disease; insect bites; contact dermatitis; molluscum contagiosum; and drug eruptions. Pharyngeal features of mpox may be mistaken for bacterial tonsillitis or primary syphilis. Papules, vesicles, and pustules may be present in the genital and perianal areas and can be confused with sexually transmitted illnesses such as herpes, syphilis, chancroid, or lymphogranuloma venereum. Distinguishing between varicella and mpox might be challenging; however, lymphadenopathy is a distinctive feature of mpox compared with varicella. Also, unlike varicella lesions, which are vesicular fluid filled lesions, mpox lesions are typically pseudopustules that simulate the appearance of pustules but contains solid debris.

TABLE 1 — Criteria for Mpox Diagnosis

Epidemiological Criteria

Within 21 days of illness onset:
- Reports having contact with a person or people with a similar appearing rash or who received a diagnosis of confirmed or probable mpox OR
- Had close or intimate in-person contact with individuals in a social network experiencing mpox activity; this includes men who have sex with men (MSM) who meet partners through an online website, digital application ("app"), or social event (e.g., a bar or party) OR
- Traveled outside the US to a country with confirmed cases of mpox or where MPXV is endemic OR
- Had contact with a dead or live wild animal or exotic pet that is an African endemic species or used a product derived from such animals (e.g., game meat, creams, lotions, powders, etc.)

Criteria to Distinguish a New Case from an Existing Case

For surveillance purposes, a new case of mpox virus infection meets the following criteria:
- Healthy tissue has replaced the site of all previous lesions after they have scabbed and fallen off; *and* new lesions are present that have tested positive for orthopoxvirus or mpox virus DNA by molecular methods or genomic sequencing

Case Classification

Suspect

Meets clinical criteria *and* epidemiologic criteria *and* there is no evidence of a negative test for either nonvariola orthopoxvirus or mpox virus

Probable

Meets presumptive laboratory criteria

Confirmed

Meets confirmatory laboratory criteria

The symptoms during the prodromal period may be similar to those of influenza, SARS-CoV-2, and other viral respiratory illnesses. Symptoms may be particularly variable in patients with HIV or other types of immunocompromise.

Treatment

Currently there is no treatment approved specifically for monkeypox virus infections. For most patients with mpox, who do not have severe disease or risk factors for severe disease, supportive care and pain control will assist recovery.

Because of the developing evidence base about these therapies and because treatment of mpox will evolve with time, before initiation of treatment, consultation is recommended with the state health department authorities and the CDC Emergency Operations Center (800-488-7100) or the CDC's Clinical Consultation Team (eocevent482@cdc.gov; 770-488-7100).

Updated information regarding indications for treatment of mpox can be found on the CDC website at https://www.cdc.gov/mpox/hcp/clinical-care/index.html.

Those at high risk include the following:
- Are severely immunocompromised patients (e.g., those with HIV with CD4 <200, or solid organ transplant recipients)
- Have atopic dermatitis and other conditions affecting skin integrity
- Are children
- Are pregnant or breastfeeding

In the United States, high-risk patients may meet the criteria to receive tecovirimat (Tpoxx, ST-246) under the CDC-held Expanded Access–Investigational New Drug (EA-IND) protocol.

Tecovirimat is a potent inhibitor of an orthopoxvirus protein required for the formation of infectious virus particles that are essential for dissemination within an infected host.

Tecovirimat was made available for treatment of certain patients with mpox during the global outbreak of mpox that began in 2022. During this outbreak, tecovirimat was the agent most commonly used and was well tolerated. The PALM007 trial was launched in October 2022 by the National Institute of Allergy and Infectious Diseases (NIAID) and the Democratic Republic of the Congo (DRC)'s National Institute for Biomedical Research. Initial analyses released in August 2024 indicated that tecovirimat did not reduce the duration of mpox lesions among children and adults with clade I mpox in the DRC. However, the study's 1.7% overall mortality was much lower than the mpox mortality of 3.6% or higher reported among cases analyzed together across all of the DRC, showing that better outcomes among people with mpox can be achieved when they are hospitalized and provided high-quality supportive care.

The STOMP trial was launched in September 2022 by NIH/NIAID. Initial analyses released in December 2024 indicated that tecovirimat did not reduce the time to resolution of mpox lesions or have an effect on pain among adults with mild to moderate clade II mpox and a low risk of developing severe disease.

The role of tecovirimat in treatment of mpox in patients with severe immunocompromise, including advanced HIV, has not been determined and requires additional clinical trials. Tecovirimat can be administered as an oral drug or an intravenous injection based on the weight of the patient. The duration of treatment is 14 days. Tecovirimat is well tolerated; the most common side effects are headache and nausea.

Brincidofovir (also known as CMX001 or Tembexa)[1] is made available for treatment of mpox to clinicians who request and obtain an FDA-authorized single-patient emergency use IND (e-IND). Eligibility criteria for brincidofovir among adult and pediatric patients (including neonates) with mpox include the following:
- Lab-confirmed mpox
- Have severe disease
- *OR* are at high risk for progression to severe disease
- *AND* meet any of the following: experience clinically significant disease progression while receiving tecovirimat or who develop recrudescence (initial improvement followed by worsening) of disease after an initial period of improvement on tecovirimat
- *OR* are otherwise ineligible or have a contraindication for oral or intravenous tecovirimat
- *OR* are severely immunodeficient (e.g., uncontrolled HIV infection with CD4 <200)

Severely immunodeficient patients without prior tecovirimat use can simultaneously initiate combination therapy with brincidofovir and tecovirimat.

Nearly all patients who receive brincidofovir are severely immunocompromised and receive brincidofovir concomitantly with tecovirimat[1] and/or vaccinia immune globulin intravenous[1].

Brincidofovir should not be used simultaneously with cidofovir[1]. Animal studies have suggested a risk of teratogenicity from brincidofovir; therefore it is not recommended to be used for the treatment of pregnant women and used only with caution in women of childbearing age.

Cidofovir (Vistide) is an antiviral medication that is approved by the FDA for the treatment of cytomegalovirus (CMV) retinitis in patients with acquired immunodeficiency syndrome and is commercially available in intravenous formulation. Data are not available on the effectiveness of cidofovir in treatment of mpox infection in humans. However, there is evidence of cidofovir efficacy against orthopoxviruses in in vitro and animal studies. It is unknown whether a person with severe mpox will benefit from treatment with cidofovir, although its use may be considered in such patients. Clinicians can switch patients between IV cidofovir and brincidofovir immediately without a drug holiday.

Vaccinia immune globulin: Data are not available on the effectiveness of vaccinia immune globulin intravenously (VIGIV [CNJ-016])[1] for treatment of mpox infection in humans. It is unknown whether a person with severe mpox will benefit from treatment

---

[1] Not FDA approved for this indication.

with VIGIV. As of July 23, 2025, the Administration for Strategic Preparedness and Response is no longer able to supply VIGIV from the Strategic National Stockpile for treatment of mpox due to limited supply, other than for infants less than 6 months of age. Typically, patients who receive VIGIV concomitantly receive tecovirimat and either brincidofovir or cidofovir[1].

Complications

Severe manifestations of mpox include ocular involvement (e.g., conjunctivitis, blepharitis, periocular cellulitis, keratitis, corneal ulceration, and loss of vision), neurologic complications (e.g., encephalitis/encephalomyelitis), myopericarditis and complications associated with mucosal lesions (oral, rectal, genital, and urethral).

Mpox may be life threatening in the severely immunocompromised and in young children. Secondary infections of the mpox lesions may occur. Mpox can be transmitted to the fetus during pregnancy, and newborns may contract it through close contact during and after birth. Miscarriages and stillbirth have been associated with mpox contracted during pregnancy.

The outbreak of clade Ib in the DRC, with its relatively high mortality rate and rapid spread to other previously mpox free African countries, is cause for international alarm.

References

Brosius I, Vakaniaki E, Mukari G: Epidemiological and clinical features of mpox during the clade Ib outbreak in South Kivu, Democratic Republic of the Congo: a prospective cohort study, *Lancet*, 2025.

Centers for Disease Control and Prevention: Mpox caused by human-to-human transmission of monkeypox virus with geographic spread in the Democratic Republic of the Congo. Available at https://emergency.cdc.gov/han/2023/han00501.asp.

Centers for Disease Control and Prevention. Monkeypox: Information for Health Care Professionals. Available at: https://www.cdc.gov/poxvirus/monkeypox/clinicians/index.html. Updated August 19, 2022.

Dashraath P, Nielsone-Saines K, Mattar C, et al: Guidelines for pregnant individuals with monkeypox exposure (correspondence), *Lancet*, 2022. https://doi.org/10.1016/S01406736(22)01063-7. Published online June 21.

DeWitt ME, Polk C, Williamson J, et al: Global monkeypox case hospitalization rates: a rapid systematic review and meta-analysis, *eClinicalMedicine* 54:101710-101710, 2022.

Huhn GD, Bauer AM, Yorita K, et al: Clinical characteristics of human monkeypox, and risk factors for severe disease, *Clin Infect Dis* 41:1742, 2005.

Kaler J, Hussain A, Flores G, et al: Monkeypox: a comprehensive review of transmission, pathogenesis, and manifestation, *Cureus* 14(7):e26531, 2022. https://doi.org/10.7759/cureus.26531.

Kwok KO, Wei WI, Tang A, et al: Estimation of local transmissibility in the early phase of monkeypox epidemic in 2022, *Clin Microbiol Infect* 28:1653.e1, 2022.

Levy V, Branzuela A, Hsieh K, et al: First clade Ib monkeypox virus infection reported in the Americas — California, November 2024, *MMWR (Morb Mortal Wkly Rep)*, 2025.

Masirika LM, Udahemuka JC, Schuele L, et al: Ongoing mpox outbreak in Kamituga, South Kivu province, associated with monkeypox virus of a novel clade I sublineage, Democratic Republic of the Congo, 2024, *Euro Surveill* 29:2400106, 2024.

Miller MJ, Cash-Goldwasser S, Marx GE et al Severe monkeypox in hospitalized patients — United States, august 10–October 10, 2022. *MMWR Morb Mortal Wkly Rep*. ePub: October 26, 2022.

Minhaj FS, Ogale YP, Whitehill F, et al: Monkeypox outbreak — nine states, May 2022, *MMWR Morb Mortal Wkly Rep* 71:764–769, 2022. https://doi.org/10.15585/mmwr.mm7123e1.

Ministere De La Sante Publique. Hygiene et Prevoyance Sociale Institut National De Sante Publique Centre des Operations D'urgences de Sante Publique Rapport journalier de l'épidémie de Mpox en RDC - Sitrep N°85 - Données du 13 Novembre 2024 (Semaine épidémiologique 46.

Mitjà O, Ogoina D, Titanji BK: Monkeypox, *Lancet* 401:60–74, 2023.

Moore MJ, Rathish B, Zahra F: Monkeypox[Updated 2022 Jul 16]. In *StatPearls [internet]*., treasure Island (FL), StatPearls Publishing, 2022. Available from: https://www.ncbi.nlm.nih.gov/books/NBK574519/.

National Institute of Health News Release. https://www.nih.gov/news-events/news-releases/nih-study-finds-tecovirimat-was-safe-did-not-improve-mpox-resolution-or-pain.

Nicaise N, Folayan M, Komakech A: Evolving epidemiology of mpox in Africa in 2024, *N Engl J Med*, 2025.

Philpott D, Hughes CM, Alroy KA, et al: Epidemiologic and clinical characteristics of monkeypox cases — United States, May 17–July 22, 2022, *MMWR Morb Mortal Wkly Rep* 71:1018–1022, 2022. https://doi.org/10.15585/mmwr.mm7132e3.

Rao AK, Petersen BW, Whitehill F, et al: Use of JYNNEOS (smallpox and monkeypox vaccine, live, nonreplicating) for preexposure vaccination of persons at risk for occupational exposure to orthopoxviruses: recommendations of the Advisory Committee on Immunization Practices — United States, 2022, *MMWR Morb Mortal Wkly Rep* 71:734–742, 2022. https://doi.org/10.15585/mmwr.mm7122e1.

Sherwat A, Brooks JT, Birnkrant D, Kim P: Tecovirimat and the treatment of monkeypox— past, present, and future considerations, *N Engl J Med* 387:579–581, 2022. https://doi.org/10.1056/NEJMp2210125.

Thornhill JP, Barkati S, Walmsley S, et al: For the SHARE-net Clinical Group. Monkeypox virus infection in humans across 16 countries—April–June 2022, *N Engl J Med* 387:1–14, 2022. https://doi.org/10.1056/NEJMoa2207323.

Vakaniaki EH, Kacita C, Kinganda-Lusamaki: Sustained human outbreak of a new MPXV clade I lineage in eastern Democratic Republic of the Congo, *Nat Med* 30:2791–2795, 2024.

Weaver JR, Isaacs SN: Monkeypox virus and insights into its immunomodulatory proteins, *Immunol Rev* 225:96–113, 2008. https://doi.org/10.1111/j.1600-065X.2008.00691.x. PMID: 18837778; PMCID: PMC2567051.

WHO 2022–24 mpox (monkeypox) outbreak: global trends. https://worldhealthorg.shinyapps.io/mpx_global/#43_Case_profile_(overall) Date accessed: September 24, 2024.

WHO Disease Outbreak News, *Mpox - Democratic Republic of the Congo*. Available at: https://www.who.int/emergencies/disease-outbreak-news/item/2024-DON522.

MUMPS

Method of
Kristen Rundell, MS, MD

CURRENT DIAGNOSIS

- Parotitis (swelling of the parotid salivary glands): unilateral or bilateral
- Fever
- Headache
- Malaise
- Myalgias
- Anorexia
- Increased serum amylase

CURRENT THERAPY

- Supportive care
- Warm or cold packs on the parotid
- Analgesics and/or antipyretics (such as acetaminophen [Tylenol] or ibuprofen [Motrin])
- IV fluids or hospitalization for cases of pancreatitis, meningitis, or severe orchitis

Epidemiology

Mumps is an extremely contagious, self-limiting virus that had disease rates of 99% until the vaccine was introduced in 1967. Since 2006, there have been several outbreaks in the United States. These usually present in young people, previously vaccinated. There is increased transmissibility on college campuses, in close knit communities, and large social gatherings. During 2020, there were significantly decreased number of cases, probably due to social distancing. For the United States and Finland, mumps is almost eradicated. For the rest of the world, mumps is still endemic as a result of a vaccination rate of only 61%.

Pathophysiology

Mumps is a single-stranded RNA virus and a member of the *Paramyxovirus* genus. It is transmitted through respiratory secretions, saliva, and contact with contaminated fomites.

Prevention

With the high rate of transmission and no antiviral therapy, prevention for mumps relies on community immunity as a result of high vaccine rates. There are two formulations of the mumps vaccine currently available in the United States: the measles-mumps-rubella vaccine (MMR) and the measles-mumps-rubella-varicella vaccine (MMRV, ProQuad). The dosing schedule for children calls for the first dose at age greater than 12 months to

15 months, and the second dose for children greater than 4 years to 6 years of age. For infants aged 6 through 11 months who are traveling internationally, a single MMR vaccine is recommended. These children should be revaccinated with 2 doses of MMR vaccine with the first dose at ages 12 months to 15 months and the second dose at ages 4 years to 6 years. During an epidemic, a single dose for adults born before 1957 is recommended and may be required by some health care professionals. The first dose gives approximately 80% immunity. Persons receiving both doses may still get the mumps virus if there is outbreak or if they travel to an endemic area. To avoid exposure or contraction of the disease during travel, it is suggested that travelers wash hands frequently and use alcohol-based sanitizers to decrease the contraction or spread of disease.

The vaccine is contraindicated for patients who are pregnant or planning to conceive in the 28 days after vaccination. Vaccine administration is also contraindicated for those who have a severe anaphylactic reaction to the vaccine or one of the components, and those individuals who are severely immunocompromised.

Clinical Manifestations

The incubation period for the mumps virus is 16 to 18 days. At the onset of the illness, patients may develop acute viral infection symptoms of fever, headache, and malaise. The parotitis, swelling of the parotid gland, is the diagnostic hallmark of the mumps virus. This is caused by the infection and inflammation of the parotid ductal epithelium. The swelling may last up to 10 days. Close to 30% of persons may not have this symptom and may be only mildly symptomatic.

Diagnosis

Diagnosis is made by the history and the constellation of symptoms and physical findings. It is difficult to use IgM to determine active infection, because the response may be short in duration, delayed, or even absent. PCR testing is available and requires early sampling.

Differential Diagnosis

Viral infections such as parainfluenza (also in the paramyxovirus genus) coxsackievirus, influenza A, Epstein-Barr, adenovirus, HIV, and cytomegalovirus may present with similar symptoms as mumps. There are also noninfectious etiologies of parotitis, which include salivary stones or tumors, sarcoid, Sjögren's syndrome, and thiazide diuretics.

Therapy (or Treatment)

Treatment for mumps virus is largely supportive. For complicated cases of pancreatitis, meningitis, encephalitis, and orchitis, patient may need to be hospitalized for additional care. The additional care usually includes fever reduction, analgesia, fluid resuscitation, and treatment of secondary bacterial infections.

Monitoring

For persons with active mumps, it is suggested that they be isolated from school or work for 5 days after the onset of symptoms. Shedding of virus usually occurs 4 days prior to the onset of symptoms. For this reason, it is difficult to slow down outbreaks of the disease. The last outbreak in the United States was in 2010.

Complications

Complications from mumps are rare. In children, pancreatitis and hearing loss are the sensorineural complications most often diagnosed. For adolescents and adults the complications are more common and usually more severe. These include aseptic meningitis; orchitis in males, which rarely leads to sterility; oophoritis in females; pancreatitis; and arthritis. Even more uncommon are Guillain–Barré/ascending polyradiculitis, transverse myelitis, facial palsy, interstitial nephritis, and myocardial involvement.

Mumps in pregnancy has been associated with increased fetal loss. There are no known teratogenic effects.

References

American Academy of Pediatrics: Mumps. In Pickering LK, Baker CJ, Kimberlin DW, Long SS, editors: *Red Book: 2009 Report of the committee on Infectious Diseases*, ed 28, Elk Gove Village IL, 2009, American Academy of Pediatrics, pp 468–472.
Centers for Disease Control and Prevention (CDC): Exposure to mumps during air travel—United States, April 2006, *MMWR Morb Mortal Wkly Rep* 55(401), 2006.
Centers for Disease Prevention and Control Website 4/28/24.
Dayan GH, Rubin S: Mumps outbreaks in vaccinated population: are available mumps vaccines effective enough to prevent an outbreak? *Clin Infect Dis* 47:1458, 2008.
Kleiman MB: Mumps virus. In Lenette EH, editor: *Laboratory Diagnosis of Viral Infections*, ed 2, New York, 1992, Marcel Dekker. p. 549.
Kutty PK, Barskey AE, Gallagher KM: *Mumps. Infectious diseases related to travel*, CDC Yellowbook, 2012(chapter 3).
Wharton M, Cochi SLK, William S: Measles, mumps and rubella vaccines, *Infect Dis Clin North Am* 4:47, 1990. www.cdc.gov/travel/yellowbook.

MYALGIC ENCEPHALOMYELITIS/CHRONIC FATIGUE SYNDROME

Method of
Stephen J. Gluckman, MD

CURRENT DIAGNOSIS

- Myalgic encephalomyelitis/chronic fatigue syndrome is defined as:
  - A substantial new-onset reduction in the ability to engage in preillness levels of occupational, educational, social, or personal activities
  - Accompanied by (often profound) fatigue that is not alleviated by rest
  - Associated with unrefreshing sleep
  - Worsened with physical or mental exertion
  - Persisting for more than 6 months
  - Frequently associated with cognitive impairment, orthostatic intolerance, joint and muscle pain, and depression.
- A typical story is a previously highly functioning individual who develops characteristic symptoms after an acute illness or significant stress.
- Should be differentiated from an isolated symptom of fatigue.
- The diagnosis is clinical, and individual patients may not completely fit the definition that was established for research purposes.
- There is no proven etiology and no specific diagnostic test or physical finding.

CURRENT THERAPY

- There is no proven cure or drug treatment.
- The physician should validate symptoms, provide education, offer support, and set reasonable expectations.
- Specific associated symptoms such as sleep disturbance, pain, and depression should be aggressively managed.
- Cognitive behavioral therapy and graded exercise therapy have been shown to be of possible benefit.
- Avoid excessive testing and unproven, sometimes costly, treatment with antimicrobials, corticosteroids, immunoglobulins, or other unproven drugs or alternative therapies.

Myalgic encephalomyelitis/chronic fatigue syndrome (ME/CFS) is an often misunderstood syndrome that should not be confused with malingering, hypochondriasis, or just fatigue. Patients with ME/CFS are truly suffering from their often disabling symptoms. The absence of an objective finding does not alter the validity of the patient's symptoms. It is impossible to successfully treat a patient with ME/CFS unless the clinician believes the patient is genuinely symptomatic. ME/CFS also should not be confused with the isolated symptoms of fatigue. Fatigue is a common patient complaint, whereas ME/CFS has a much lower prevalence.

Definition

ME/CFS is not a new disease; the syndrome has been described since at least the mid-1700s. However, since that time, it has been mistakenly ascribed to a number of incorrect pathologic and infectious causes. In the past, it has been called *febricula, neurasthenia, effort syndrome, Da Costa syndrome, chronic brucellosis, chronic Lyme disease, chronic Epstein-Barr syndrome, total allergy syndrome, chronic candidiasis,* and *multiple chemical sensitivity syndrome.* It has also been falsely attributed to infection with xenotropic murine leukemia virus–related virus (XMRV) and related retroviruses, such as murine leukemia virus (MLV). None of these possible causes has proved to be correct.

In 1988, in an attempt to be descriptive rather than to attribute an incorrect etiology to the disease, the term *chronic fatigue syndrome* was coined. Therefore the name is relatively new, but the syndrome is not. The disease is chronic, and fatigue is a cardinal feature, but it is more than being chronically tired. This working case definition was published by the Centers for Disease Control and Prevention and then modified in 1992 by the National Institute of Allergy and Infectious Diseases. In March 2015 the Institute of Medicine (IOM; now the National Academy of Medicine [NAM]) issued an extensive and thorough review of the topic. This comprehensive report has three major themes: (1) ME/CFS has acquired a great deal of negative connotation with associated misunderstanding and prejudice; (2) the criteria for diagnosis were greatly simplified, with emphasis on the major features (Box 1); and (3) by using the term *disease* and by supplying ample reference support in the document, the IOM unequivocally underscores the very real nature of this malady. The IOM report is by far the most thorough examination of the topic, and it unequivocally supports the validity of this disease.

One note of caution: This case definition is an epidemiologic and research tool and not a strict clinical tool. It is useful for studying the disease. However, some patients do not completely fit this definition. ME/CFS can nonetheless be diagnosed by a knowledgeable clinician who is willing to consider this diagnosis.

Because some immune abnormalities are often seen in these patients, some people have called this *chronic fatigue and immune dysregulation syndrome (CFIDS).* The immune abnormalities seen in patients with ME/CFS are mild and differ from patient to patient. Most significant, these patients are not immunosuppressed or at risk for opportunistic infections.

It has been noted that many of the symptoms of fibromyalgia overlap with ME/CFS, and some clinicians consider fibromyalgia and ME/CFS to be different aspects of the same disease because both often include pain and fatigue. These different names for the same syndrome can be confusing to patients and clinicians, and it is important to explain this when managing patients with ME/CFS.

A mention should be made in regard to long-haul COVID syndrome. In this entity, patients have persistent symptoms after recovering from acute COVID-19. There are a number of reasons for persistent symptoms, including lingering or permanent organ damage as the result of a severe episode of COVID-19 and/or posttraumatic stress disorder (PTSD) related to the trauma of being intubated in an intensive care setting. In addition, COVID-19 triggers typical ME/CFS in some persons.

BOX 1	Criteria for Myalgic Encephalomyelitis/Chronic Fatigue Syndrome

Diagnosis requires that the patient have the following three symptoms:
- A substantial reduction or impairment in the ability to engage in preillness levels of occupational, educational, social, or personal activities that persists for more than 6 months and is accompanied by fatigue, which is often profound, is of new or definite onset (not lifelong), is not the result of ongoing excessive exertion, and is not substantially alleviated by rest
- Postexertional malaise
- Unrefreshing sleep
  At least one of the two following manifestations is also required:
- Cognitive impairment
- Orthostatic intolerance

Epidemiology

Although chronic fatigue is an extremely common symptom, ME/CFS is not. The former has been noted to have a prevalence of 10% to 25% in a number of studies. However, the point prevalence of ME/CFS has been estimated to be in the range of 0.1%. ME/CFS is overrepresented in young and middle-aged women, but it has been described in both men and women and in all age groups.

Pathophysiology

The cause of ME/CFS is unknown. Much effort has gone into trying to discern an infectious, endocrine, immune, or psychiatric cause, but to date none has been proven. Research has suggested a number of possible abnormalities that may be associated with the pathogenesis of ME/CFS including immune system, endocrine/metabolic dysfunction, cardiovascular aberrations, and gut dysbiosis, but causality for any of these has not been established.

Studies have shown a link between ME/CFS and the presence of certain genes that mediate immune and stress responses. The findings suggest that difficulty managing stress may be linked to the development of ME/CFS. They also suggest that there may not be a single cause of ME/CFS but that there may be a number of stress-related triggers (physical or emotional) in those with a genetic predisposition. ME/CFS can be triggered by many infectious diseases in addition to COVID-19. This is consistent with the typical course, in which a previously healthy person develops an acute illness that resolves but initiates ME/CFS.

Clinical Features and Diagnosis

Although there is, as yet, no diagnostic test, the history, physical examination, and laboratory testing are generally very characteristic and allow a clinician to confidently make the diagnosis in most cases. The typical story is one of a previously highly functioning person who develops an acute illness or other stressor. The acute problem resolves; however, from that time on, symptoms of ME/CFS are triggered. Despite often profound symptoms, physical examination is persistently normal, as is laboratory testing. *In fact, if there are significant abnormalities on physical examination or testing, those abnormalities are not consistent with ME/CFS and should be further evaluated.* Symptoms are exacerbated by physical activity. The pre-ME/CFS medical history of the patient is not one of multiple medical problems. Affected patients are typically high-functioning persons who are "struck down" with this disease. Features to emphasize in addition to the case definition noted in Box 1 are included in Box 2.

In a patient with a typical history and examination, laboratory testing should be limited (Box 3). Testing for diseases with a low pretest likelihood runs the serious risk of false positive results.

| BOX 2 | Frequent Features of Chronic Fatigue Syndrome |

- Sudden onset of fatigue after a relatively common illness or other stressor
- Previously active and healthy person
- Symptoms very sensitive to exacerbation by physical activity
- Normal physical examination and laboratory testing
- Altered sleep
- "Foggy" thought processes
- Lack of progression to organ failure or any significant objective organ abnormality
- Joint and muscle aching without physical evidence of inflammation
- Feverish feeling (sustained elevated temperatures [>37.4°C] should prompt a search for an alternative diagnosis because the patient with chronic fatigue syndrome is not truly febrile)
- Diffuse aching that is not well localized to joints or muscles but without erythema, effusion, or limitation of motion
- Muscles that are easily fatigued (however, strength is normal, as are biopsies and electromyograms)
- Occasional mild cervical and/or axillary lymphadenitis (painful lymph nodes [lymphadenia] are a common complaint, but this is not a true lymphadenopathy)

| BOX 3 | Diagnostic Testing |

Tests to Perform
- Complete blood count
- Comprehensive chemistry screen
- Thyroid-stimulating hormone
- Perhaps: Cosyntropin (Cortrosyn) stimulation test, sleep study
- Additional testing *only* with specific clinical indications

Do Not Routinely Perform
- ANA testing
- Serology for cytomegalovirus, Epstein-Barr virus, *Bartonella*, *Babesia*, *Ehrlichia*, and *Anaplasma*
- MRI, SPECT, or PET scans
- Tilt-table testing

ANA, Antinuclear antibody; *MRI*, magnetic resonance imaging; *PET*, positron emission tomography; *SPECT*, single-photon emission computed tomography.

This can result in further testing, diagnostic confusion, and unnecessary treatments. Specifically, the signs and symptoms of ME/CFS are not those of systemic lupus, Lyme disease, cytomegalovirus, bartonellosis, ehrlichiosis, or babesiosis, among others. Serologic testing for these diagnoses is not helpful and can be harmful if the presence of antibodies results in the initiation of unwarranted medications. The presence of antibodies does not mean active disease. The analogy that patients can relate to is to remind them that they likely have antibodies to chickenpox but that they clearly do not have active chickenpox. For similar reasons, neuroimaging without objective clinical findings is not indicated. Although abnormalities can be found, they are nonspecific and of no clinical utility. Tilt-table testing is abnormal in many patients with ME/CFS; however, testing is expensive and uncomfortable, and abnormal results do not alter management. Of course, if history, physical examination, and initial laboratory testing do reveal abnormalities, as noted earlier, further laboratory evaluation should be undertaken to elucidate the cause of the aberration(s).

| BOX 4 | Therapy for Chronic Fatigue Syndrome |

- Educate the patient and their support system about the diagnosis of chronic fatigue syndrome. Emphasize the validity of the diagnosis and of the patient's symptoms. Make sure there is an understanding about expectations.
- Aggressively manage specific symptoms of sleep disturbance, pain, and depression.
- Consider cognitive behavioral therapy.
- Emphasize the need for gradual, graded exercise. Give the patient a specific "prescription" for this.
- Avoid the temptation to prescribe antimicrobials, corticosteroids, or other medications with no proven benefit and the potential to do harm.
- Discuss the pros and cons of using unstudied, expensive, or potentially dangerous "alternative therapies."

Treatment

There is no established cure for ME/CFS, but patients should be counseled that a number of things can be done to manage this often disabling illness (Box 4). These can be divided into things the clinician should do and things the patient should do.

Things the Clinician Should Do

To successfully manage ME/CFS, a clinician must believe that the patient is truly symptomatic. Patients with ME/CFS are not malingering. Because they often appear well and have consistently normal objective testing, they often become very defensive about their limitations. They are sensitive to the validity of their symptoms. Not only are they suffering but they are also blamed for it. Many patients with ME/CFS are partially or totally disabled. Their outward healthy appearance belies the internal sense of ill health. It is common for relatives and colleagues to believe they are malingering. A vicious cycle of frustration, anger, and depression commonly ensues.

As part of establishing the validity of the diagnosis, a clinician should review the history of ME/CFS, emphasizing that this is not a new disease but was originally described centuries ago.

For successful management, the clinician should give the patient enough time, specifically inquire about other diagnoses the patient is concerned about, and explain why they are not correct. The clinician should see the patient at regular intervals.

The clinician should also ensure that the patient has reasonable expectations. Most patients with ME/CFS have not had previous chronic illnesses or significant prolonged limitations. It is often necessary to review the information about ME/CFS with the patient's family and to emphasize that this disabling illness is not volitional.

Although it is generally wise to avoid a discussion about whether the origin of ME/CFS is psychiatric or organic, depression is an expected consequence of any chronic illness. Depression has specific treatments, and it should be aggressively diagnosed and treated. The patient should be told that successful management of depression will help them cope with ME/CFS.

If a sleep disturbance exists, it also should be aggressively managed, if necessary, by a sleep specialist. Sleep deprivation makes other symptoms more difficult to deal with.

Chronic pain is very enervating. If pain is prominent, that also should be aggressively managed, often by a pain specialist.

It is important for the clinician to be cautious about ascribing all of a patient's symptoms to ME/CFS. Such patients are, of course, not protected from getting additional, unrelated illnesses. Each symptom should be considered on its own before defaulting it to ME/CFS.

Complementary therapies must be discussed, or the patient might get the impression that the clinician is not comfortable in considering them; this can partially undermine the clinician-patient relationship. Although all are of unproved benefit and often undetermined risk, "complementary" therapies that are not dangerous (e.g., acupuncture) or expensive are reasonable to consider.

Things the Patient Should Do

Of the 350 studies that have looked at treatment options for ME/CFS, only cognitive-behavioral therapy and graded exercise therapy have been shown to be of possible benefit. In cognitive behavioral therapy, the patient undergoes a series of 1-hour sessions designed to alter beliefs and behaviors that might delay recovery. Although exercise can exacerbate symptoms, deconditioning will also do so. Limiting activity can worsen weakness and depression. The risk of exacerbating symptoms can be reduced by cautiously setting less ambitious activity/exercise goals. Because many patients with ME/CFS were particularly active before the onset of their illness and are impatient to get their former lives back, they often need strict guidelines to try to prevent overdoing exercise while at the same time getting a clear prescription to exercise. The exercise prescription should be individualized based on the degree of impairment, but it is wise to initially set goals on the low side to avoid exacerbating symptoms. It is important to acknowledge that both cognitive behavioral therapy and graded exercise are controversial, with several interest groups opposed to these modalities. As for cognitive behavioral therapy, it is safe and there is nothing to lose. As for exercise, the emphasis should be on very gradual to minimize the risk for exacerbation. Many patients have some time each day when they can perform some activities. They should be counseled to try use that time constructively with minimal-impact activities such as sewing, painting, or writing.

As part of the management of ME/CFS, patients, their families, and, when appropriate, their employers must reframe their expectations. Patients with ME/CFS have a chronic, disabling illness. Families and others must understand that patients cannot do all that they were able to do before the onset of ME/CFS and that patients cannot "will" the disease away any more than they could will away a more visible disability.

Things That Should Not Be Done

There are many suggested remedies for ME/CFS. Most are either unstudied or disproved. In particular, treatments that are expensive or potentially harmful should be avoided. There is no role for antimicrobial therapy. There is no role for antiviral therapy, including treatment for retroviruses. There is no role for intravenous immunoglobulin, corticosteroids, special diets, or vitamin treatments.

Prognosis

The likelihood of complete recovery from ME/CFS is only fair. The disease tends to wax and wane over time, but in only a minority of patients does it completely resolve. If sustained improvement occurs, it is generally over several years. Several features have been associated with a poorer prognosis, including age older than 38 years, more than eight symptoms, duration longer than 1.5 years, less than 16 years of formal education, a history of a dysthymic disorder, and a sustained belief that the disease results from a physical cause.

Monitoring

Despite the lack of very effective treatment, many patients benefit from regular monitoring of their condition. Knowing they have scheduled visits minimizes the number of crises and emergency visits and allows the patient to reconnect with a validating physician. Follow-up on a quarterly basis is a reasonable interval.

References

Bateman L, Bested AC, Bonilla HF, et al: Myalgic encephalomyelitis/chronic fatigue syndrome: essentials of diagnosis and management, *Mayo Clin Proc* 96:2861, 2021.

Bouquet J, Gardy JL, Brown S, et al: RNA-seq analysis of gene expression, viral pathogen, and B-cell/T-cell receptor signatures in complex chronic disease, *Clin Infect Dis* 64:476, 2017.

Clark MR, Katon W, Russo J, et al: Chronic fatigue: risk factors for symptom persistence in a 2 1/2-year follow-up study, *Am J Med* 98:187–195, 1995.

Fulcher KY, White PD: Randomised controlled trial of graded exercise in patients with the chronic fatigue syndrome, *BMJ* 314:1647–1652, 1997.

Goertzel BN, Pennachin C, de Souza Coelho L, et al: Combinations of single nucleotide polymorphisms in neuroendocrine effector and receptor genes predict chronic fatigue syndrome, *Pharmacogenomics* 7:475–483, 2006.

Goldenberg DL, Simms RW, Geiger A, et al: High frequency of fibromyalgia in patients with chronic fatigue seen in a primary care practice, *Arthritis Rheum* 33:381–387, 1990.

Grach SL, Seltzer J, Chon TY, Ganesh R: Diagnosis and management of myalgic encephalomyelitis/chronic fatigue syndrome, *Mayo Clin Proc* 98:1544, 2023.

Green CR, Cowan P, Elk R, et al: National Institutes of Health pathways to prevention workshop: advancing the research on myalgic encephalomyelitis/chronic fatigue syndrome, *Ann Intern Med* 162:860, 2015.

Haney E, Smith ME, McDonagh M, et al: Diagnostic methods for myalgic encephalomyelitis/chronic fatigue syndrome: a systematic review for a National Institutes of Health Pathways to Prevention Workshop, *Ann Intern Med* 162:834, 2015.

Hanson SW, Abbafati C, Aerts JC, et al: Global Burden of Disease Long COVID Collaborators: estimated global proportions of individuals with persistent fatigue, cognitive and respiratory symptom clusters following symptomatic COVID-19 in 2020 and 2021, *JAMA* 328:1604–1615, 2022.

IOM (Institute of Medicine): *Beyond Myalgic encephalomyelitis/chronic fatigue syndrome: redefining an illness*, Washington, DC, 2015, The National Academies Press. https://www.ncbi.nlm.nih.gov/25695122.

Komaroff AL, Lipkin WI: ME/CFS and Long COVID share similar symptoms and biological abnormalities: road map to the literature, *Front Med (Lausanne)* 10:1187163, 2023.

Lightfoot Jr RW, Luft BJ, Rahn DW, et al: Empiric parenteral antibiotic treatment of patients with fibromyalgia and fatigue and a positive serologic result for Lyme disease. A cost-effectiveness analysis, *Ann Intern Med* 119:503–509, 1993.

Lim EJ, Ahn YC, Jang ES, et al: Systematic review and meta-analysis of the prevalence of chronic fatigue syndrome/myalgic encephalomyelitis (CFS/ME), *J Transl Med* 18:100, 2020.

Myalgic Encephalomyelitis/Chronic Fatigue Syndrome. https://www.cdc.gov/me-cfs/management/index.html.

Paul BD, Lemle MD, Komaroff AL, Snyder SH: Redox imbalance links COVID-19 and myalgic encephalomyelitis/chronic fatigue syndrome, *Proc Natl Acad Sci U S A* 118, 2021.

Schwartz RB, Garada BM, Komaroff AL, et al: Detection of intracranial abnormalities in patients with chronic fatigue syndrome: comparison of MR imaging and SPECT, *Am J Roentgenol* 162:935–941, 1994.

Walitt B, Singh K, LaMunion SR, et al: Deep phenotyping of post-infectious myalgic encephalomyelitis/chronic fatigue syndrome, *Nat Commun* 15:907, 2024.

Wessely S, Chalder T, Hirsch S, et al: The prevalence and morbidity of chronic fatigue and chronic fatigue syndrome: a prospective primary care study, *Am J Public Health* 87:1449–1455, 1997.

White PD, Goldsmith KA, Johnson AL, et al: Comparison of adaptive pacing therapy, cognitive behaviour therapy, graded exercise therapy, and specialist medical care for chronic fatigue syndrome (PACE): a randomised trial, *Lancet* 377:823–836, 2011.

NECROTIZING SKIN AND SOFT-TISSUE INFECTIONS

Method of
Kalyanakrishnan Ramakrishnan, MD

CURRENT DIAGNOSIS

- Physical examination of the affected area may detect:
  - Exquisite pain and tenderness out of proportion to local signs of infection.
  - Cutaneous anesthesia, firm woody subcutaneous tissue, edema, and tenderness extending outside involved skin margins, hemorrhage or bullae of the overlying skin, and soft tissue crepitus.
  - Laboratory Risk Indicator for Necrotizing Fasciitis (LRINEC) score is useful in diagnosing necrotizing fasciitis. Imaging (computed tomography [CT] or magnetic resonance imaging [MRI] in adults; ultrasonography [US] in children) is usually confirmatory. Imaging should not delay surgery if indicated based on suspicion.

CURRENT TREATMENT

- Empiric high-dose intravenous polymicrobial antibiotics and surgical debridement remain the cornerstones of initial management of necrotizing skin and soft-tissue infections. Organism-specific antibiotics are continued until resolution of infection and debridement complete (usually 7–14 days).

Epidemiology

Necrotizing skin and soft tissue infections are rare with an estimated annual incidence of 1000 cases in the United States. These infections may be polymicrobial or monomicrobial. Polymicrobial infections are more common (70%–80%) and generally caused by synergistic activity of aerobes and anaerobes originating from the bowel or genitourinary tracts. They are more prevalent among older and immunocompromised patients, individuals with significant comorbidities, and those with underlying abdominal pathology. These infections typically involve the trunk and perineal regions, and follow penetrating abdominal injuries or surgery, genital or perianal sepsis, or decubitus ulcers. They have a more indolent course and thus are easier to diagnose. Monomicrobial infections (20%–30%) frequently follow minor trauma and are usually caused by group A streptococcus (GAS), occasionally by methicillin-resistant *Staphylococcus aureus* (MRSA), or by clostridia. They are more aggressive, involve the extremities and occur more often in younger healthy individuals. Type 3 infections follow exposure to contaminated fresh or warm seawater or ingestion of raw seafood; organisms responsible include *Aeromonas hydrophila, Vibrio vulnificus, Mycobacterium marinum, Pasteurella multocida, Haemophilus* and *Klebsiella* species. Type 4 (fungal) infections generally follow burns or major trauma. Both types 3 and 4 infections are rare, progress rapidly, and have a high mortality rate, especially in immune-suppressed patients.

Risk Factors

Cardiopulmonary disease, debility, diabetes mellitus, hepatorenal disease, immunocompromised states, obesity, arteriovenous/lymphatic insufficiency, and senescence all increase risk of skin and soft tissue infections by reducing tissue vascularity and oxygenation, increasing fluid stasis and risk of trauma, and decreasing ability to counter infections. Diabetes mellitus and hepatic cirrhosis favor polymicrobial infections due to staphylococcus and streptococcus species, anaerobes, and gram-negative bacilli. Neutropenia, intravenous drug use, and hot tub exposure promote pseudomonas infection. Human and animal bites cause infections with oral flora, staphylococci, *Pasteurella multocida*, and anaerobes. Poor sanitation and soil contamination propagate clostridial infections. Postoperative infections typically follow wound contamination with microorganisms from the patient during surgery.

Pathophysiology

Necrotizing skin and soft tissue infections advance rapidly, breaking down and traversing anatomic barriers, initiating extensive destruction of the subcutaneous tissue, fascia, and muscle and damaging the neurovascular bundle, thrombosing the subcutaneous vessels, and causing overlying skin necrosis. Most infections follow a rift in the protective cutaneous barrier due to trauma or increased tissue tension. Necrotizing fasciitis may also result from blunt injuries (bruise, muscle strain) and, occasionally vascular or lymphatic spread from a distant focus of infection. Various toxins expressed by the organisms (GAS and clostridia) display local and systemic effects (platelet aggregation and thrombosis, decreasing phagocytosis, neutrophil function and vascular tone, myocardial inhibition) triggering the systemic inflammatory response syndrome (SIRS) and multiple organ failure.

Prevention

Preserving cutaneous integrity prevents infection. Abrasions and lacerations should be washed with antibacterial solutions, foreign bodies should be removed, and dead/devitalized tissue excised to minimize infection risk. Preoperative skin cleansing with chlorhexidine/alcohol (Hibiclens) or povidone iodine diminishes rates of superficial and deep incisional infections. Intranasal 2% mupirocin ointment (Bactroban) twice daily with chlorhexidine total body wash daily for 5 days in nasal carriers of MRSA reduces hospital-acquired deep surgical–site infections, as does administering antibiotics (aminopenicillins, a second- or third-generation cephalosporin) 60 minutes before incision, sterile surgical technique, minimal tissue handling, and minimally invasive surgery.

Clinical Manifestations

Features of inflammation (redness, warmth, swelling, pain) and loss of function characterize necrotizing skin and soft tissue infections. Altered mental status, anorexia, diaphoresis, fatigue, fever, hypotension, nausea, and tachycardia suggest systemic spread of infection. The extremities, trunk, or anogenital regions are usually involved. Induration denotes cutaneous involvement. Patients with necrotizing fasciitis have severe pain disproportionate to the physical findings and rapid progression of infection. Examination reveals cutaneous anesthesia, firm and woody subcutaneous tissue, edema and tenderness extending beyond involved skin, hemorrhage or bullae of the overlying skin, and crepitus (indicates soft tissue gas; seen especially with gas-forming organisms such as clostridia). Tense edema and bullae have high specificity and positive predictive value for necrotizing fasciitis. Fournier gangrene is a form of polymicrobial necrotizing soft-tissue infection involving the loose groin and genital skin, where subcutaneous vessel thrombosis causes extensive tissue loss.

Diagnosis

Diagnosis is based on a strong clinical suspicion followed by confirmatory laboratory and imaging studies (if time permits), and surgery. Leukocytosis with a marked left shift, elevated C-reactive protein, elevated serum creatinine and creatine phosphokinase (denotes muscle injury), and low serum bicarbonate (suggests acidosis) signify severe infection. The LRINEC score (https://www.mdcalc.com/lrinec-score-necrotizing-soft-tissue-infection) uses six different laboratory parameters (hemoglobin, white blood cell count, C-reactive protein, glucose, creatinine, sodium) to predict risk of necrotizing fasciitis (score $\geq$ 6 suggestive, $\geq$ 8 strongly predictive). White blood cell count (< 15,000 mm^3) and serum sodium (> 135 mmol/L) levels alone are useful in ruling out necrotizing fasciitis (99% negative predictive value). Gram stains and cultures of aspirates or tissue biopsies, and blood cultures are valuable for detecting the infecting organisms and systemic spread; contamination may yield false-positive results. Biopsy or debridement typically demonstrates swollen gray soft tissue with undermining of the overlying skin, a brownish and odorous exudate and non-contractile muscle. Imaging (plain x-rays, ultrasonography [US], computed tomography [CT], magnetic resonance imaging [MRI]) may show edema or thickening, fluid collections or free air in the soft tissues. US, CT and MRI are highly sensitive (MRI highest) in detecting deep soft tissue involvement characteristic of necrotizing fasciitis; specificity is lower. US is sufficient in children, whose tissues are thin enough to allow adequate evaluation on imaging. Imaging should not delay debridement, if considered necessary.

Therapy

Patients with necrotizing skin and soft-tissue infections typically require in-hospital management, because many have underlying unstable comorbid illnesses, systemic sepsis, severe dehydration and acidosis, muscle breakdown, and organ dysfunction. Initial resuscitation may require airway and oxygen support, large-volume rehydration, and invasive monitoring. High-dose intravenous (IV) broad-spectrum antibiotics effective against the usually infecting polymicrobial spectrum of pathogens are commenced, followed by early and aggressive debridement of all necrotic tissue. IV antibiotics are maintained until the patient is afebrile for 48 to 72 hours and tolerates oral intake, debridement is completed and culture results are available. For polymicrobial necrotizing fasciitis acceptable antimicrobial choices include vancomycin plus piperacillin/tazobactam (Zosyn), a carbapenem (meropenem [Merrem], ertapenem [Invanz] or imipenem-cilastatin [Primaxin]), or cefotaxime (Claforan) with metronidazole (Flagyl) or clindamycin (Cleocin). Streptococcal and clostridial infections are treated with penicillin G and clindamycin. Antibiotic options in methicillin-susceptible *S. aureus* infections include nafcillin oxacillin or cefazolin. Options for methicillin-resistant *S. aureus* (MRSA) infections and in penicillin-allergic patients include vancomycin, daptomycin (Cubicin), or linezolid (Zyvox). Antibiotic doses are modified in children. Recommended duration is 7 to 14 days; longer as needed. Doxycycline combined with ciprofloxacin (Cipro) treats *Vibrio vulnificus* infection. Ceftriaxone (Rocephin) or cefotaxime combined with doxycycline is useful in aeromonos infections. Doxycycline is contraindicated in children (< 8 years), as is ciprofloxacin (< 17 years), unless the infection is considered life-threatening. Fungal infections respond well to fluconazole (Diflucan), voriconazole (Vfend) or amphotericin B; the antifungals usually continued for 2 weeks after resolution of symptoms. Debridement/drainage is repeated until all diseased tissue or collections are eliminated and healing begins. Wound vacuum dressings help remove drainage and encourage formation of healing granulation tissue. The tissue defect heals by secondary intention or may require skin grafting or flap closure. Hyperbaric oxygen (3–4 daily treatments at 2–3 atmosphere pressure for 30–90 minutes each) is useful, especially in clostridium-related synergistic infections. Adding intravenous immunoglobulin[1] 0.5–2 g/kg daily for 3 days has shown some success, and is an option in critically ill hemodynamically unstable patients not responding to conventional measures, especially in those with streptococcal toxic shock syndrome. Fournier gangrene is managed along the same principles as above.

Monitoring

Patients in shock or with acute respiratory distress syndrome, SIRS, or multi-organ failure are best managed in an intensive care unit and often require invasive monitoring, cardiorespiratory and renal support, and occasionally, endotracheal intubation.

Complications

Significant disfigurement, limb loss, respiratory and renal failure, and mortality (14%–50%) may eventuate despite timely and appropriate treatment; the mortality influenced by age, extent of infection, degree of biochemical/acid-base imbalance, presence of comorbidities, and treatment delay.

---

[1]Not FDA approved for this indication.

References

Kaafarani HMA, King DR: Necrotizing skin and soft tissue infections, *Surg Clin North Am* 94:155–163, 2014.

Hakkarainen TW, Kopari NM, Pham TN, Evans HL: Necrotizing soft tissue infections: review and current concepts in treatment, systems of care and outcomes, *Curr Probl Surg* 51:344–362, 2014.

Morgan MS: Diagnosis and management of necrotizing fasciitis: a multiparametric approach, *J Hosp Infect* 75:249–257, 2010.

Stevens DL, Bisno AL, Chambers HF, et al: Practice guidelines for the diagnosis and management of skin and soft tissue infections: 2014 update by the Infectious Diseases Society of America, *Clin Infect Dis* 59:e10–e52, 2014.

Ramakrishnan K, Salinas RC, Agudelo Higuita NI: Skin and soft tissue infections, *Am Fam Physician* 92:474–483, 2015.

OSTEOMYELITIS

Method of
Wissam El Atrouni, MD, MSc; John Sojka, MD; Mitchell C. Birt, MD; and Kim Templeton, MD

CURRENT DIAGNOSIS

- Osteomyelitis in adults typically occurs as a result of spread from adjacent soft tissues or direct inoculation of bone, such as after trauma or surgery. Hematogenous bacterial seeding leading to osteomyelitis is more common in children than in adults. When it occurs in adults, it is almost exclusively in the spine.
- Open fractures can lead to osteomyelitis due to contamination of bone at the time of injury; even small soft tissue wounds can indicate the presence of an open fracture. Because of the risk of infection, open fractures should be treated emergently.
- Infections around implanted hardware, especially joint arthroplasties or hardware in the spine, require urgent referral. These infections can occur at the time of hardware placement or later because of hematogenous seeding from distant infections. Patients with late arthroplasty infections usually demonstrate new pain in the area of a previously well-functioning joint.
- Diabetes mellitus is one of the more common chronic health conditions that increases the risk of developing osteomyelitis. Osteomyelitis in this population of patients usually occurs in the foot as a result of progressively deepening soft tissue ulcers and secondary infection. These infections are frequently polymicrobial.
- Initial evaluation of patients suspected of having osteomyelitis includes obtaining plain films. However, plain film findings are usually not specific for infection. Additional radiographic modalities, such as magnetic resonance imaging scan and/or a variety of nuclear medicine studies, can provide additional information regarding diagnosis and extent of involvement.

CURRENT THERAPY

- In the absence of sepsis, antibiotics for patients with suspected osteomyelitis are not started until adequate cultures can be obtained, through aspiration or biopsy of the bone, or during surgical debridement of the affected area.
- Antimicrobial therapy for osteomyelitis in adults typically lasts 4 to 6 weeks, whereas in children it may only be needed for 2 to 3 weeks, depending on the clinical picture.
- Surgical intervention for osteomyelitis of long bones is indicated for patients with chronic infections, infections adjacent to joint replacements, or to address bone abscesses. Surgery in these instances requires extensive debridement of infected and necrotic bone to remove all microabscesses and then irrigation to dilute any remaining bacterial load.
- Treatment of patients with diabetes-related foot infections and underlying osteomyelitis may require revascularization of the affected limb to decrease the need for amputation.

Introduction

Normal bone is typically highly resistant to infection. Infections in bone can arise when the host immune system is compromised or there is injury to the bone. Osteomyelitis occurs either due to hematogenous spread, extension from infections in adjacent soft tissues or joints, or as a result of direct inoculation of the bone due to trauma or surgery. Osteomyelitis can lead to devastating outcomes, including amputation or sepsis, if not addressed early, especially in patients with other health conditions.

Various classification systems have been developed to describe osteomyelitis. The Lew and Waldvogel classification described the etiology of the infection (in order of decreasing frequency: contiguous focus, vascular insufficiency, or hematogenous); however, this classification system does not guide or indicate the results from treatment. The Cierny-Mader system is based on the location (intramedullary) and extent (localized vs. diffuse) of the infection, as well as the degree of compromise of the patient. Unlike the Lew and Waldvogel classification, the Cierny-Mader (C-M) staging systems correlates with outcomes and can help guide treatment. Mandell et al. recommend considering C-M type 1 as early (intramedullary) hematogenous osteomyelitis, type 2 as early contiguous spread, and types 3 (localized) and 4 (diffuse) as more advanced disease. More recently, the BACH classification has been developed, incorporating variables of Bone involvement, Antimicrobial availability, soft tissue Coverage, and Host status. Each variable is further rated based on complexity and given a level of 1(lowest) to 3 (highest) complexity. The BACH classification has demonstrated good interobserver reliability across subspecialties, and current prospective studies are being completed to establish prognosis and outcomes based on initial BACH classification.

Osteomyelitis can be described as acute, usually being present for 2 weeks or less, subacute, and chronic. Chronic osteomyelitis can be more challenging to eradicate because of the development of avascular areas of bone (sequestra) and surrounding bone sclerosis (involucra) that help to wall off the sequestra, making it difficult to adequately address these areas with systemic antibiotics.

Epidemiology

The incidence of osteomyelitis appears to be increasing, especially among adults. This may be because of the availability of more sensitive evaluation and diagnostic measures or an actual increase incidence. If the latter, this may reflect the increased prevalence of comorbidities, such as diabetes mellitus, or the aging of the population, as the risk of developing osteomyelitis increases with age. The reported age- and sex-adjusted annual incidence has been reported to be approximately 24 cases per 100,000 person-years and is higher among men than women.

Although sex and gender have been found to impact all health conditions, the role of these factors are less clear in osteomyelitis. Whereas at least some differences in rates of infection, in general, between women and men are likely societal or gender related in terms of exposure to pathogens, sex-based differences in infection risk have also been identified related to levels of innate immunity, as females tend to have a more efficient immune response than do males. Immunity is controlled, in part, by both chromosomal and hormonal factors: estradiol appears to be protective against infection, in part by stimulating humoral immunity, whereas progesterone and testosterone suppress innate immune responses. However, the impact of gonadal hormones in modulating the immune system is clearer in animal models than in studies of humans. Current studies have identified sex-based differences in prevalence of respiratory, gastrointestinal, urinary tract, and genital tract infections. Additional research is needed to assess for similar differences in osteomyelitis.

Demographic differences have been noted in children and young adults with osteomyelitis. African American children have the highest rates of hospitalization related to osteomyelitis, whereas the lowest rates are among children of Asian or Hispanic descent. In addition, children who live in households with low median incomes or whose care is covered by private funds or Medicaid are more likely than children from other socioeconomic backgrounds to be hospitalized with acute osteomyelitis.

Pathogenesis

Osteomyelitis can occur via hematogenous seeding, direct extension from an adjacent area of infection, or because of inoculation of the bone as a result of trauma or surgery (Figure 1). *Staphylococcus aureus,* in particular, has receptors for fibronectin, laminin, collagen, and sialoglycoproteins that are present in the bone matrix, leading to seeding of the bone and consequent inflammatory reaction. Hematogenous osteomyelitis is more common among children than among adults. In adults, hematogenous osteomyelitis is almost exclusively seen in the spine, resulting from seeding of the disc space from a distant infected site (Figure 2). This can then involve the adjacent vertebral bodies and, with time, result in epidural extension. When hematogenous osteomyelitis occurs in the long bones of children and adolescents, it is almost always in the metaphysis. It is thought that this reflects the circulation in that area, with slowing of bone flow in the terminal capillaries along the area of the physis. In young children, there is connection between the metaphyseal and epiphyseal vessels that can allow infection of the epiphysis and eventually the adjacent joint. This is much less likely to occur in adults.

Bone infections due to trauma are typically related to presence of open fractures. Open fractures usually reflect significant levels of trauma to the bone and secondary soft tissue involvement. Infections can arise in these situations due to direct contamination of the soft tissues and bone with materials from the environment, including clothing, grass, and dirt, with contained bacteria. Open fractures are graded with the system described by Gustilo and Anderson and range from small puncture wounds over the fracture site to soft tissue stripping from the bone to open fractures with associated vascular injury. This classification system can help in determining the prognosis: patients with higher-grade injuries typically have a greater incidence of subsequent infection—up to 50% among patients with concomitant vascular injury. Although a small puncture wound over a fracture may seem inconsequential, these wounds usually indicate that bone was exposed at some point and was at risk for bacterial contamination. Open fractures are surgical emergencies, and patients with these injuries need immediate referral.

Bone infections can develop at sites of prior surgery, especially past surgical sites that include implantation of hardware. Many of these infections are thought to occur during the time of hardware placement. Although such infections can occur at the site of any hardware, it is most common among patients who have undergone joint arthroplasty and is one of the most devastating complications of these procedures. The rate of infection after primary joint arthroplasty ranges from 0.3% to 2.4% for total hip arthroplasties and 1.0% to 3.0% for total knee arthroplasties. Infection rates are higher among patients who undergo revision surgeries. Patients with infected arthroplasties may present in the first few weeks after surgery or may note onset of new pain in a previously well-functioning joint. The bacteria in these cases not only exist on the surface of the implant but also extend into adjacent bone and soft tissues (Figure 3). Patients with prior surgery of the spine, with or without the placement of hardware, are also at risk of developing late infections in the range of 0.2% to 9%. Suspected infections in areas of prior surgery, especially if implants are in place, require urgent referral.

Osteomyelitis is more likely to occur in patients with serious and/or chronic health conditions, including obesity, malignancy, immune compromise, substance abuse, and malnutrition. One of the most common of conditions increasing the risk for development of osteomyelitis is diabetes mellitus. An estimated 25% of diabetic patients will develop a foot ulcer at some point in their lifetime, with increased morbidity and mortality, compared with patients with diabetes without foot ulcers. Of these foot ulcers, 20% to almost 60% will harbor underlying osteomyelitis (Figure 4). Whereas men are more likely than women to develop diabetic foot ulcers and then present with ulcers that are deeper, there are no clear sex-based differences in prevalence of consequent osteomyelitis in this group of patients. Some of the differences identified between women and men with diabetes mellitus in developing foot ulcers may be more reflective of gender-based differences in self-care.

Infected foot ulcers are the most common risk factor for lower extremity amputations in this population. Diabetic foot ulcers

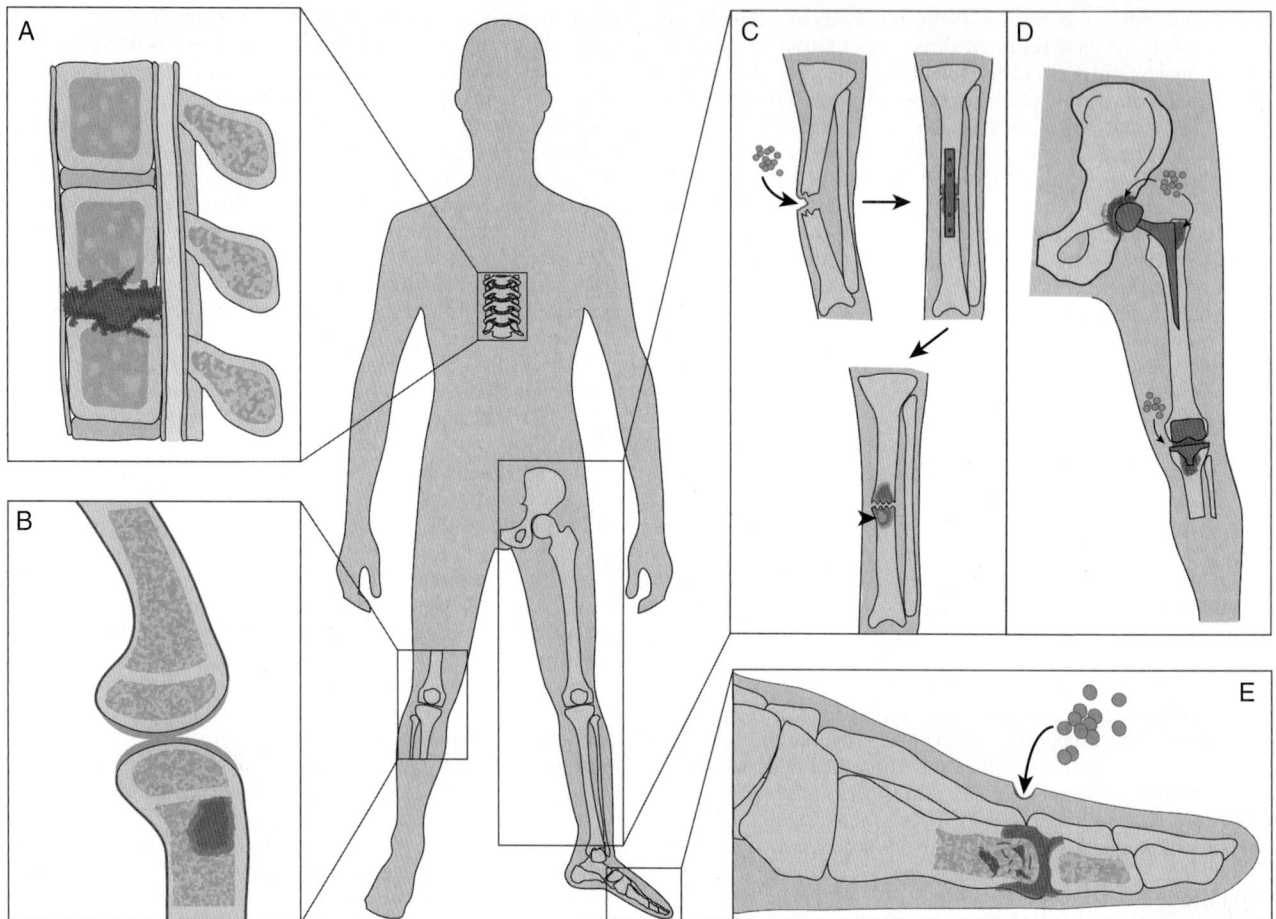

Figure 1 A diagram showing three categories of osteomyelitis. (A and B) Primary hematogenous (bloodborne) spread of bacteria mainly afflicts the vertebral bodies at all ages or the metaphysis of skeletally immature patients. (C and D) Contiguous bone infection is most commonly seen with direct contamination of bacteria in open fractures or joint replacement surgery with prosthetic implants. (E) Vascular or neurologic disease associated osteomyelitis most commonly affects the lower extremity. (From Birt MC, Anderson DW, Toby WB, Wang J: Osteomyelitis: recent advances in pathophysiology and therapeutic strategies *J Orthop* 14:45–52, 2017.)

usually start as superficial breaks in the skin or ulcers, which if they become chronic are at risk of infection. Infections of foot ulcers in the setting of diabetes are greater among patients with peripheral neuropathy or peripheral vascular disease; these comorbidities can also lead to masking of the signs and symptoms of inflammation, making a diagnosis of infection more challenging. Superficial infections in diabetic foot ulcers can eventually affect deeper tissues, in some patients progressing to osteomyelitis, increasing the risk of progression to amputation. Men have been found to be more likely than women to undergo amputations in this setting, whereas women are more likely to heal their ulcers without requiring amputation. This may be because of the severity of the presenting ulcers among men, who are also are more likely to have a history of lower extremity revascularization procedures.

Depth of the ulcer, especially in the presence of elevated inflammatory markers, can aid in the diagnosis of osteomyelitis. Involvement of bone can be confirmed with plain films; other imaging modalities, such as magnetic resonance imaging (MRI), white blood cell (WBC) scintigraphy, and 18F-fluorodeoxyglucose positron emission tomography/computed tomography (CT) may be useful in confirming the diagnosis but have variable reported sensitivities and specificities.

Treatment of these ulcers and associated infections is multidisciplinary: in addition to administration of antibiotics for culture-confirmed infections and potential surgical debridement of involved tissue, treatment includes local wound care (although evidence of type of wound care is mixed); evaluating and addressing, if needed or possible, peripheral vascular disease; off-loading

of the involved portion of the extremity; and appropriate glycemic control.

Microbiology

In children, most cases of acute hematogenous osteomyelitis are caused by a single organism, most commonly *S. aureus*. These cases typically involve the vascular metaphysis of long bones. Coagulase-negative staphylococci can also be an etiology in infants in intensive care with vascular catheters. Other gram-positive cocci include streptococci: *Streptococcus pneumoniae* in incompletely immunized children, or young children with underlying conditions and *Streptococcus pyogenes* (group A), especially after primary varicella-zoster and *Streptococcus agalactiae* (group B) in neonates. Culture-negative cases occur frequently, and these are usually presumed to be due to *S. aureus* and treated as such. In children 6 to 36 months old, *Kingella kingae*, a gram-negative component of the oral flora, is a major pathogen that causes non–long bone osteomyelitis. *Haemophilus influenzae* type b (Hib) is a rare cause of hematogenous osteomyelitis in young children after the wide implementation of Hib vaccination. Enteric gram-negative bacilli can cause osteomyelitis in infants and children with sickle cell disease. Those with hemoglobinopathies and HIV infection are also at risk for *Salmonella* osteomyelitis.

In adults, hematogenous osteomyelitis primarily presents as vertebral osteomyelitis and is caused by *S. aureus* in more than half of cases in case series in developed countries. The proportion of the cases of hematogenous osteomyelitis due to methicillin-resistant *S. aureus* (MRSA) depends on local epidemiology. Other

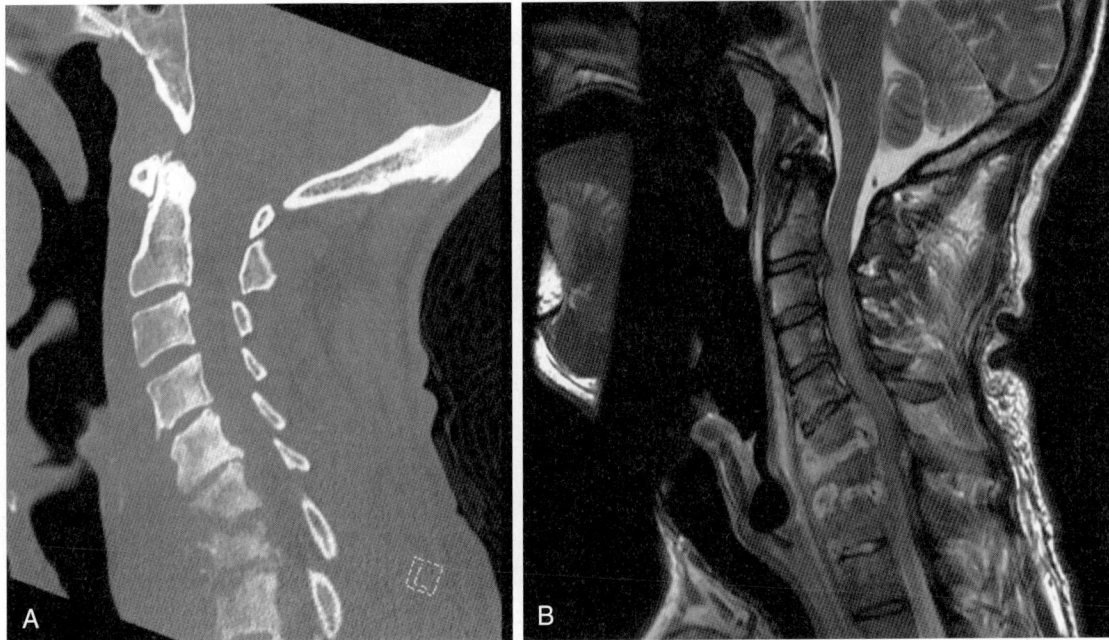

Figure 2 (A) Sagittal computed tomography scan demonstrating C6–8 spondylodiskitis. Note the cortical irregularity of the vertebral end plates. There is disc space narrowing and loss of the normal cervical spine curvature. Severe cortical destruction is present due to bacterial infection of the bone and intervertebral disc. (B) Sagittal T2 magnetic resonance imaging reveals diffuse T2 signal throughout the vertebral body and disc. Evident is loss of the normal cortical line of the endplates compared with adjacent levels and hyperintensity that extends posteriorly to the soft tissues.

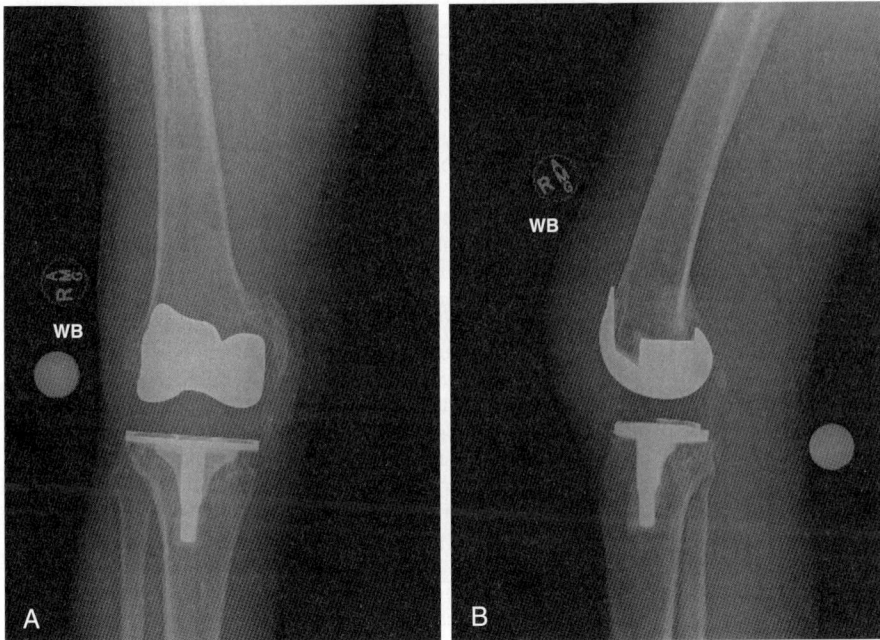

Figure 3 (A) Anteroposterior radiograph of an infected total knee arthroplasty. The radiograph shows resorption of the bone, especially the femur, adjacent to the implant. (B) Lateral radiograph of the knee demonstrating lucencies extending posterior along the femur and interface between the femur and implant.

etiologic organisms include aerobic gram-negative bacilli after genitourinary instrumentation, pyogenic streptococci including group B and C/G in diabetics, viridans and anginosus-group streptococci, enterococci, *Pseudomonas aeruginosa,* coagulase-negative staphylococci in patients with indwelling venous catheters, and injection drug users. In endemic areas, *Brucella* species and *Mycobacterium tuberculosis* should be considered. Disseminated *Mycobacterium avium* complex can involve the spine in patients with AIDS. Fungal vertebral osteomyelitis is rare but can occur in people at risk such as individuals who live in endemic areas for dimorphic fungi like *Histoplasma, Blastomyces,* and *Coccidioides;* intravenous drug users who can get *Candida* osteomyelitis; and immunocompromised hosts who can develop infections with *Aspergillus.*

Among adults with trauma or open fractures, diabetic and vascular insufficiency foot infections are more likely to develop polymicrobial osteomyelitis with staphylococci, streptococci, enterococci, gram-negative bacilli, and anaerobes (Table 1). After animal or human bites, *Pasteurella multocida, Eikenella corrodens,* and oral anaerobic gram-positive cocci are usually identified.

Clinical Manifestations

Patients with osteomyelitis typically present with pain and tenderness in areas with or without prior injury. They may experience pain with activity but also note pain at rest and that awakens them at night. Symptoms may be acute and localized or gradual onset and nonspecific; the latter may be subtle, making clinical

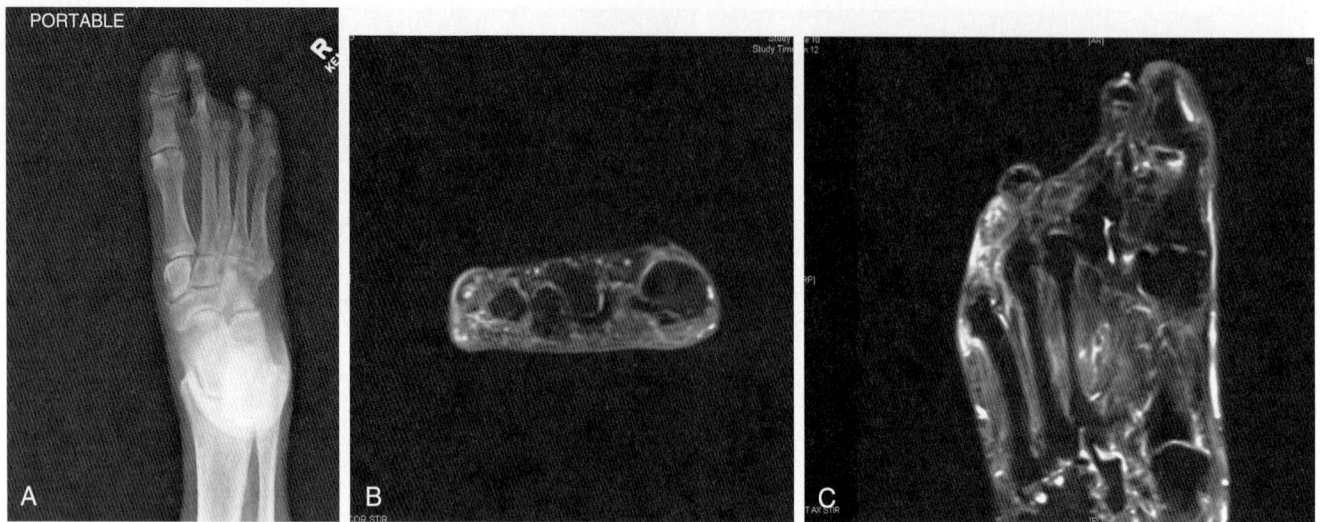

Figure 4 Osteomyelitis associated with diabetes/vascular insufficiency. (A) Anteroposterior radiograph revealing diffuse osteopenia within the fifth toe and subtle cortical disruption along lateral aspect of the proximal phalanx. Note previous amputation of third toe. Patients with loss of protective sensation and poor vascular supply have recurrent or multiple episodes of wound infections that can extend to involve adjacent bone. (B and C) Coronal and axial short tau inversion recovery (STIR) magnetic resonance images. Hyperintense STIR signal along the proximal phalanx and adjacent soft tissues of the fifth toe, consistent with infection and inflammation.

TABLE 1	Microbiology of Osteomyelitis

Common >50%	Rare <5%
• *Staphylococcus aureus* (MSSA, CA-MRSA)	• *Salmonella*
• Coagulase-negative staphylococci	• *Mycobacterium tuberculosis*
Occasional 25%–50%	• *Brucella*
• Streptococci	• *Coxiella*
• Enterococci	• Dimorphic fungi
• *Pseudomonas*	• *Mycobacterium avium* complex
• *Enterobacter*	• Atypical mycobacteria
• *Proteus*	• *Aspergillus*
• *Escherichia coli*	• *Mycoplasma*
• *Serratia*	• *Tropheryma*
• Anaerobes *(Finegoldia, Clostridium, Bacteroides)*	• *Actinomyces*
	• *Bartonella*
	• *Pasteurella*
	• *Eikenella*

CA, Community-associated; *MRSA,* methicillin-resistant *Staphylococcus aureus;* *MSSA,* methicillin-susceptible *S. aureus.*
Adapted from BennettJE, Dolin R, Blaser MJ: *Mandell, Douglas, and Bennett's principles and practice of infectious diseases,* ed 9. Philadelphia: Elsevier; 2020:1419–1429.

suspicion crucial. There may be noted warmth and erythema, especially in more superficial bones. Patients may also present with fever and other systemic signs of infection. Symptoms of pain at rest and constitutional signs may be interpreted as representing an underlying neoplasm, especially in children, in whom osteomyelitis and Ewing sarcoma often have nearly identical presentations. Patients whose bone infection has involved an adjacent native joint are reluctant to use that joint and have significant pain, even with limited attempts at range of motion. Patients with long bone infections, especially children, are reluctant to use that extremity, including bearing weight, if the infection involves a lower extremity. Patients with new onset pain in the setting of implanted hardware, especially joint arthroplasties, should be assumed to have an infection until proven otherwise. Patients with vertebral osteomyelitis, who are more commonly older men, usually present with unremitting back pain, fever, and occasionally leg pain.

The diagnosis of vertebral osteomyelitis can be difficult to make, because the symptoms may seem consistent with degenerative changes in the spine, especially in the typically older population affected by both conditions. In addition, initial plain radiographs may prove nondiagnostic. Concern about the presence of vertebral osteomyelitis requires urgent additional evaluation or referral. Continued infections in this area can lead to epidural extension and development of a spinal epidural abscess. Whereas these abscesses are more common among men, women are more likely to develop related neurologic deficits, potentially related to a relatively smaller spinal canal. Neurologic changes in this setting require rapid referral.

Diagnosis/Confirmation

The clinical diagnosis of osteomyelitis is confirmed by a combination of serum studies (WBC, erythrocyte sedimentation rate [ESR], C-reactive protein [CRP], procalcitonin), radiographic findings, microbiology or culture results, and pathology, if the patient undergoes surgery. Probe to bone test is a physical exam finding that can be helpful in evaluation diabetic foot ulcers. Plain radiographs are an inexpensive initial study; however, their sensitivity in diagnosing osteomyelitis is limited, as the findings of bone loss and periosteal reaction can be attributed to a number of aggressive bone conditions, including neoplasms. In addition, bone loss of approximately 30% to 40% is required before being noted on plain radiographs. MRI provides additional sensitivity and specificity in diagnosis, even in early osteomyelitis, especially if obtained with and without contrast. MRI findings include reduced T1- and heightened T2-weighted bone marrow signals, representing fatty marrow replaced by inflammation. Contrast enhancement patterns can also help to differentiate infection from neoplasia. CT is an alternative to MRI if the latter is not available or the patient is unable to tolerate the examination. CT findings can include gas along fascial planes, decreased density of infected bone, soft tissue masses, and abscesses, as well as identifying the course of overlying sinus tracts. Nuclear medicine imaging modalities are more expensive than other imaging options. Whereas in some reports nuclear medicine imaging modalities have been noted to be more sensitive in identifying osteomyelitis, they are less specific, with high false-positive rates. However, they can be useful in imaging areas in which hardware is present, because such metal can significantly limit the details seen on MRI or CT. Nuclear medicine imaging modalities include three-phase Tc99m MDP scan—ideal for bones not affected by underlying conditions, gallium 67 scan (usually performed as sequential bone then gallium scan for comparison), 111-indium radiolabeled WBC

TABLE 2 Medical Treatment of Osteomyelitis

ORGANISM	FIRST CHOICE	ALTERNATIVE
MSSA	Nafcillin, oxacillin, or cefazolin	Vancomycin; some add rifampin[1] to nafcillin/oxacillin
MRSA	Vancomycin or daptomycin (Cubicin)[1]	Linezolid (Zyvox)[1] or levofloxacin[1] + rifampin[1]
Penicillin-susceptible *Streptococci*	Penicillin G, ceftriaxone, or cefazolin	Vancomycin
Enterococci and Streptococci with penicillin MIC >0.5	Penicillin G, ampicillin with optional gentamicin	Vancomycin with addition of gentamicin
Enterobacteriaceae	Ceftriaxone or ertapenem (Invanz)[1]	Ciprofloxacin or levofloxacin[1]
Pseudomonas aeruginosa	Cefepime[1], meropenem[1], or imipenem	Ciprofloxacin or ceftazidime

[1]Not FDA approved for this indication.

MIC, Minimum inhibitory concentration; *MRSA*, methicillin-resistant *Staphylococcus aureus*; *MSSA*, methicillin-susceptible *S. aureus*.

Adapted from Bennett, J. E., Dolin, R., & Blaser, M. J. (2020). *Mandell, Douglas, and Bennett's principles and practice of infectious diseases* (9th ed., pp. 1418–1429).

scans, or Tc99m sulfur colloid bone marrow scans performed in sequence with WBC scans. These additional imaging modalities are usually used in complicated cases or cases in which the diagnosis is unclear based on other, less expensive tests.

The identification of the infecting organism is crucial to optimal medical management. In cases of presumed osteomyelitis, antibiotics should be withheld until material for culture is obtained, usually via needle aspiration of the area, assuming the patient is stable without sepsis or significant soft tissue infection or purulence. If the patient requires surgical debridement, tissue can be sent for culture and for pathologic evaluation. Pathology in these instances can help to rule out neoplasia and will demonstrate acute, chronic, or acute on chronic inflammatory cells. Swab cultures of draining sinuses demonstrate poor correlation with adjacent bone cultures, except for *S. aureus*. Material obtained for culture should be sent for both aerobic and anaerobic assessment.

Treatment
Medical Treatment

Vertebral osteomyelitis without associated neurologic deficit or nerve compression, and acute hematogenous osteomyelitis in children, are usually treated with systemic antimicrobials without the need for surgical debridement. Most other osteomyelitis syndromes in adults require a combination of medical and surgical treatments to eradicate infection and restore function. A cornerstone of medical therapy for osteomyelitis is identification of the causative organisms in culture. In the absence of associated active soft tissue infection or sepsis, antimicrobials are usually held until adequate cultures are obtained either by aspiration/biopsy or during surgical debridement of the affected bone. Vancomycin (Vancocin) and beta-lactams including cephalosporins have been used extensively for the treatment of osteomyelitis (Table 2). Although most experience is with intravenous antimicrobials, some data support the use of highly orally bioavailable antibiotics like trimethoprim-sulfamethoxazole (Bactrim)[1], rifampin[1], clindamycin, and quinolones. In the OVIVA trial, published in 2019 in the *New England Journal of Medicine*, investigators randomized 1054 participants with bone or joint infections at 26 UK centers, within 7 days of surgery or start of antibiotic treatment, to IV or oral antibiotics to finish 6 weeks. Definite treatment failure within 1 year of randomization occurred in 14.6% in the IV group and 13.2% in the oral group, meeting the noninferiority criteria of the oral therapy. Most commonly used oral antibiotics in the trial were ciprofloxacin, combination ciprofloxacin/rifampin[1], oral penicillins[1], clindamycin, and doxycycline.[1] Since this and other retrospective reports, oral antibiotic therapy for management of osteomyelitis has been used more, especially as an acceptable alternative to IV therapy.

Duration of antimicrobial treatment is generally 4 to 6 weeks based on experimental models and limited prospective studies. Parenteral antimicrobials can be continued outside the hospital using peripherally inserted central catheters. Dalbavancin (Dalvance)[1] is a novel, long-acting lipoglycopeptide with a half-life of 14.4 days and potent activity against most gram-positive pathogens causing osteomyelitis. In a small randomized clinical trial published in 2019, 80 participants with their first episode of osteomyelitis were randomized 7:1 to receive either two doses of dalbavancin[1] 1 week apart via a 30-minute IV infusion or standard of care therapy (oral or IV) per investigator judgment for 4 to 6 weeks. At 1 year follow-up, clinical response was similar between the two arms.

In children with hematogenous osteomyelitis, parenteral therapy can be changed to oral when the child is afebrile and able to tolerate oral medications, and duration of therapy as short as 2 to 3 weeks has been reported to be effective.

Fracture site infections after open fractures are treated with debridement, cultures, and organism-directed antimicrobial therapy. Considering that it is common to use or retain fracture fixation devices, long-term oral antimicrobial suppression after induction treatment for 6 weeks is used until fracture healing is documented on imaging. At that point, antimicrobial suppression can be stopped.

Vertebral osteomyelitis treatment might require drainage of associated paravertebral or psoas abscesses by interventional radiology. Duration of antimicrobial therapy might be longer than 6 weeks in patients with undrained abscesses, MRSA infections, or end-stage renal disease. Follow-up at the end of treatment includes assessment of resolution or improvement in pain and in level of inflammation markers such as ESR and CRP. A 25% or more reduction in these inflammation markers at the end of therapy is associated with treatment success. Repeat MRI is not routinely recommended and is reserved for patients with failure to improve or worsening symptoms. In 1 to 2 years after successful therapy, spontaneous fusion of the affected vertebral levels usually occurs.

In managing diabetic foot osteomyelitis, it is helpful to use the International Working Group on the Diabetic Foot/Infectious Diseases Society of America classification system of foot infection in people with diabetes (DFI). Infections are classified as mild, moderate, or severe. Infections are mild when at least two items are present (local swelling/induration, erythema up to 2 cm from the wound, local tenderness/pain, increased warmth, purulent discharge). Infection is moderate if erythema extends more than 2 cm from the wound or is deeper than the skin and subcutaneous tissue (tendon, muscle, joint, bone). Infection is severe if associated with the systemic inflammatory response syndrome (fever, tachycardia, tachypnea, leukocytosis). Management also requires evaluation of the vascular supply to the affected area, and revascularization is needed in patients with peripheral arterial disease to optimize surgical outcome and minimize need for amputation. Because most moderate and severe diabetic foot infections are polymicrobial, use of antimicrobials with anaerobic spectrum of activity is recommended (piperacillin-tazobactam [Zosyn], ampicillin-sulbactam [Unasyn], cephalosporins with metronidazole [Flagyl], carbapenems (ertapenem [Invanz]/imipenem [Primaxin][1]/meropenem [Merrem][1]), quinolones with metronidazole, or clindamycin). Targeting *P. aeruginosa* empirically in cases of DFI is usually not needed if a patient has not grown it on recent cultures, has not had recent antibiotic exposure, and lives in a temperate climate. In diabetic foot-related osteomyelitis treated with minor amputation and a positive bone margin culture or

Osteomyelitis

---

[1]Not FDA approved for this indication.

pathology, 3 weeks of antibiotics are generally recommended, whereas 6 weeks are usually recommended if no amputation or bone resection is done.

Surgical Treatment

Surgery is often performed in conjunction with antibiotic treatment in cases of osteomyelitis of long bones, especially in cases of chronic osteomyelitis or in the presence of bone abscesses, typically in cases of chronic osteomyelitis or in the presence of bone abscesses, especially in the presence of implanted hardware. Surgery for osteomyelitis of the spine is usually reserved for patients whose infection does not completely respond to antibiotic treatment or who develop neurologic deficits. Surgical treatment of osteomyelitis of long bones is primarily performed with wide excisional debridement and copious irrigation. The order in which the operations are performed is very important because a large bacterial load can be pushed further into surrounding bone and soft tissues by irrigating before debridement. The adage "the solution to pollution is dilution" accurately describes the intent of copious irrigation at a site of bone infection.

Bacteria identified within bone, either causing a biologic breakdown of the structure of the bone (infection) versus bacteria on or near bone (colonization), are two distinct clinical pictures. The structure of bone is similar to that of sponge; bacteria resulting in osteomyelitis can "hide" in the caverns and nooks of cancellous bone quite readily, leading to small local abscess communities in the bone, bone marrow, and surrounding soft tissues, making it difficult to eradicate them through the host inflammatory response or with systemic antibiotics. In addition, bacteria in these areas may not be exposed to antibiotic agents, WBCs, or irrigation solutions. Therefore, they can exist and multiply until the bone reacts and begins to break down at the site of the infection. Given this analogy, it is understandable that there is the need to irrigate a site of osteomyelitis thoroughly to dilute the bacterial load and then allow antibiotics the opportunity to work to eliminate the remaining pathogens from the infected bone.

To rid the bone of infection, surgeons typically debride bone that is obviously infected and/or necrotic, whereas healthy bone can and will be removed up to the margin of infected bone to improve the likelihood of healing in the absence of infection. This is critical to the success of the procedure but can lead to large defects. In addition, adjacent soft tissues should be sharply debrided back to healthy, bleeding tissue. As a result, WBCs can come into the area along with antibiotic agents delivered via the healthy, small blood vessels to complete the task of eliminating the bacteria. It is important that tissue removed during these procedures is sent for culture, as well as for pathologic examination.

Debridement involving infected bone with orthopedic implants adjacent to the site can be challenging. These implants and any surrounding necrotic tissue can be colonized by bacteria, often in the form of a surrounding glycocalyx or exopolysaccharide coating that envelops the bacteria. In some patients, this can necessitate the removal of rods, plates, screws, or the components of a joint replacement, as systemic antibiotics are unable to access bacteria housed in this biofilm. Removing the implant results in removal of the glycocalyx and reduces the bacterial load but frequently necessitates subsequent reconstructive surgeries.

Specific debridement techniques vary from surgeon to surgeon; however, the goal is to decrease the bacterial load at both the bone and the soft tissue levels. The techniques involve excisional debridement of the infected bone with irrigation of the bone that is left behind and presumed to be "healthy" tissue. In the case of long bone infections, reaming of the intramedullary canal can be performed as a debridement technique. Newer devices that have the capability to ream while simultaneously irrigating and aspirating the intramedullary content are on the market. These devices have demonstrated a unique and efficient method for debulking the infectious load at the site of the long bone infection. These devices are able to assist with effective debridement throughout

the entire length of the long bone without requiring a large soft tissue incision, therefore limiting the surgical insult to the surrounding soft tissues and preserving the blood supply necessary to deliver WBCs and antibiotics to the infected region.

Often, with obviously purulent infections, several surgical procedures are required to accomplish the task of bacterial elimination. The initial bacterial load can be so great that even after significant tissue (both bone and soft tissue) has been excised and irrigated, the surgeon cannot confidently close the wound for the completion of the case. Surgical decision making may include a second or third procedure to assess the site and determine the need for further tissue removal and irrigation versus wound closure. When multiple (staged) procedures are performed, wound coverage techniques can help to continue to minimize or eliminate bacteria during the patient's hospitalization.

A vacuum-assisted closure (VAC) device is one such coverage technique. These devices apply a vacuum or negative pressure environment to the wound with an evenly applied suction level to allow for continued bacterial debridement while keeping the wound covered during the time that the patient is out of the operating room. The VAC can be applied after the excisional debridement and irrigation procedure has been completed. VACs are typically used in anticipation of a return to the operating room for a second or third procedure.

A wound VAC device is applied to the bed of the wound using three key elements: (1) a sponge substrate (for even application of the suction), (2) a plastic tape to seal the wound edges, and (3) a suctioning device or pump to apply the negative pressure to the wound. Once applied, these devices can continue to promote healthy tissue growth and create a hostile environment for bacteria, thereby limiting bacterial proliferation.

Outcomes

Recovery after the diagnosis of osteomyelitis is widely variable, and it is difficult to provide concrete expectations for these patients as robust data are lacking. Limited studies provide objective outcome measures often reporting simply on clearance of infection, with failures of treatment considered recurrence of infection or the need for amputation. However, there has been an improvement in outcomes of these infections with a multidisciplinary approach to treatment and specialized care.

Advancements in materials and subsequent use of antimicrobial grafts has become commonplace in surgical management of osteomyelitis. Bone substitutes mixed with broad-spectrum antibiotics can provide stability and local high concentrations of antimicrobials. A recent prospective study from South Africa of 28 patients diagnosed with chronic osteomyelitis revealed promising surgical results. Eleven patients were treated surgically with 100% having remission, defined as no clinical signs of infection off antibiotics with a 12-month minimum follow-up. Surgical treatment included debridement with gentamycin lavage in intramedullary infections or antibiotic-impregnated bone cement with combined medullary and cortical infections. After clearance of infection with 6 weeks of oral antibiotic therapy, a second procedure was completed for bony stabilization or reconstruction. Surgical management of osteomyelitis remains variable, with many techniques and differing strategies, This, in addition to the variation in defining treatment outcomes, makes it difficult to compare results of surgical interventions. For the diagnosis of chronic osteomyelitis, surgical intervention is often necessary to remove the nidus of involved bone as the sequestrum and/or abscess will have poor penetration of systemic antibiotics. In a recent systematic review of surgical treatment of chronic osteomyelitis, authors found eradication in 92% of cases across 16 studies. The total amputation rate in this study was 7%. Hochen et al. reported on a prospective cohort of patients with long bone osteomyelitis. The authors concluded that patients with uncomplicated osteomyelitis can achieve functional outcomes similar to their matched cohort in the general population. Patients with complicated osteomyelitis scored worse on functional outcome measures, although they were significantly improved after successful treatment of lower extremity osteomyelitis.

The management of osteomyelitis surrounding a total joint arthroplasty can be complex, as this requires addressing infected bone and soft tissue while maintaining joint stability and function. Treatment in this setting requires surgical intervention, including debridement with component exchange in a one- or two-stage progression based on surgeon preference and host factors. Success rates range from 30% to over 90% based on many factors including infection chronicity, organism, and patient factors. Highest success rates are achieved with staged revision arthroplasty, which includes removing all implants using an antibiotic-filled temporary implant and systemic antibiotics for 6 weeks, followed by reimplantation of permanent implants.

Conclusion

Patient outcomes after treatment of osteomyelitis have improved over the years with development of new imaging technologies to improve diagnostic accuracy, development of new antibiotics and antibiotic delivery methods, and expanded surgical techniques. Most importantly, treatments, both medical and surgical, are based on a better understanding of the pathogenesis of this infection. However, given the continued increase in prevalence of osteomyelitis, we need additional research to better understand the contribution of various risk factors and patient comorbidities so that we can improve prevention efforts and continue to tailor multidisciplinary interventions.

References

Birt MC, Anderson DW, Toby EB, Wang J: Osteomyelitis: Recent advances in pathophysiology and therapeutic strategies, *J Orthop* 14:45–52, 2016.

Bouchoucha S, Gafsi K, Trifa M, et al: Intravenous antibiotic therapy for acute hematogenous osteomyelitis in children: a short versus long course, *Arch Pediatr* 20:464–469, 2013.

Camilleri-Brennan J, James S, McDaid C, et al: A scoping review of the outcome reporting following surgery for chronic osteomyelitis of the lower limb, *Bone Jt Open* 4(3):146–157, 2023.

Chong BSW, Brereton CJ, Gordon A, Davis JS: Epidemiology, microbiological diagnosis, and clinical outcomes in pyogenic vertebral osteomyelitis: a 10-year retrospective cohort study, *Open Forum Infect Dis* 5(3), 2018. Epub.

Cierny G, Mader JT, Penninck JJ: The Classic: A clinical staging system for adult osteomyelitis, *CORR* 414:7–24, 2003.

Crenshaw AH, ed: Campbell's Operative Orthopedics, 8 ed. edition

Dartnell J, Ramachadran M, Katchburian M: Haematogenous acute and subacute paediatric osteomyelitis: a systemic review of the literature, *J Bone Joint Surg Br* 94(5):584, 2012.

Dias SP, Brouwer MC, van de Beek D: Sex and Gender Differences in Bacterial Infections, *Infect Immun* 90(10), 2022:e0028322, .

Euba G, Murillo O, Fernadez-Sabe N, et al: Long-term follow up trial of oral rifampin-cotrimoxazole combination versus intravenous cloxacillin in treatment of chronic staphylococcal osteomyelitis, *Antimicrob Agents Chemother* 53:2672–2676, 2009.

Fan L, Wu X-J: Sex difference for the risk of amputation in diabetic patients: A systematic review and meta-analysis, *PLoS ONE* 16(3), 2021:e0243797, .

Ferguson J, Alexander M, Bruce S, O'Connell M, Beecroft S, McNally M: A retrospective cohort study comparing clinical outcomes and healthcare resource utilisation in patients undergoing surgery for osteomyelitis in England: a case for reorganising orthopaedic infection services, *J Bone Jt Infect* 6(5):151–163, 2021.

Gay L, Melenotte C, Lakbar I, Mezouar S, Devaux C, Raoult D, Bendiane M-K, Leone M, Mege J-L: Sexual Dimorphism and Gender in Infectious Diseases, *Front Immunol* 12, 2021:698121, .

Gehrke Alijanipour P, Parvizi J: The management of an infected total knee arthroplasty, *Bone Joint J* 97-B(10 Suppl A):20–29, 2015.

Gustilo RB, Mendoza RM, Williams DN: Problems in management of type III (severe) open fractures: a new classification of type III open fractures, *J Trauma* 24:742–746, 1984.

Hotchen AJ, Dudareva M, Ferguson JY, Sendi P, McNally MA: The BACH classification of long bone osteomyelitis, *Bone Joint Res* 8(10):459–468, 2019.

Hotchen AJ, Dudareva M, Corrigan RA, Ferguson JY, McNally MA: Can we predict outcome after treatment of long bone osteomyelitis? *Bone Joint J* 102-B(11):1587–1596, 2020.

Kim UJ, Bae JY, Kim S-E, et al: Comparison of pyogenic postoperative and native vertebral osteomyelitis, *Spine J* 19:880–887, 2019.

Kremers HM, Nwojo ME, Ransom JE, et al: Trends in the epidemiology of osteomyelitis: a population-based study, 1969 to 2009, *JBJS(A)* 97:837–845, 2015.

Lew DP, Waldvogel FA: Osteomyelitis, *Lancet* 364(9431):369–379, 2004.

Lew DP, Waldvogel FA: Current concepts: osteomyelitis, *NEJM* 336:999–1007, 1997.

Li H-K, Rombach I, Zambellas R, Walker AS, McNally MA, Atkins BL, Lipsky BA, for the OVIVA Trial Collaborators: Oral versus Intravenous Antibiotics for Bone and Joint Infection, *New England Journal of Medicine* 380(5):425–436, 2019.

Lindbloom BJ, James ER, McGarvey WC: Osteomyelitis of the foot and ankle: diagnosis, epidemiology, and treatment, *Foot Ankle Clin N Am* 19:569–588, 2014.

Lipsky BA, Senneville E, Abbas ZG, et al: Guidelines on the diagnosis and treatment of foot infection in persons with diabetes (IWGDF 2019 update), *Diabetes Metab Res Rev* 36(S1):e3280, 2020.

Mandell JC, Khurana B, Smith JT, et al: Osteomyelitis of the lower extremity: pathophysiology, imaging, and classification, with an emphasis on diabetic foot infection, *Emerg Radiol* 25:175–188, 2018.

Marais LC, Ferreira N, Aldous C, Le Roux TL: The outcome of treatment of chronic osteomyelitis according to an integrated approach, *Strategies Trauma Limb Reconstr* 2016 Aug;11(2):135–42.

Masters EA, Trombetta RP, de Mesy Bentley KL, et al: Evolving concepts in bone infection: redefining "biofilm", "acute vs. chronic osteomyelitis", "the immune proteome" and "local antibiotic therapy", *Bone Res* 7:20, 2019.

Mian HM, Lyons JG, Perrin J, et al: A review of current practices in periprosthetic joint infection debridement and revision arthroplasty, *Arthroplasty* 4(31), 2022.

Miller M, ed: Review of Orthopaedics, 3rd ed.

Okubo Y, Nochioka K, Testa M: Nationwide survey of pediatric acute osteomyelitis in the USA, *J Pediatric Ortho* 26:501–506, 2017.

Park KH, Cho OH, Lee JH, et al: Optimal duration of antibiotic therapy in patients with hematogenous vertebral osteomyelitis at low risk and high risk of recurrence, *Clin Infect Dis* 262:1262–1269, 2016.

Rappo U, Puttagunta S, Shevchenko V, et al: Dalbavancin for the Treatment of Osteomyelitis in Adult Patients: A Randomized Clinical Trial of Efficacy and Safety, *Open Forum Infectious Diseases* 6(1), January 2019.

Rodham P, Panteli M, Vun JSH, Harwood P, Giannoudis PV: Lower limb post-traumatic osteomyelitis: a systematic review of clinical outcomes, *Eur J Orthop Surg Traumatol* 2023 Jul;33(5):1863-1873.

Rossboth S, Lechleitner M, Oberaigner W: Risk factors for diabetic foot complications in type 2 diabetes-A systematic review, *Endocrinol Diabetes Metab* 2020 Aug 17;4(1):e00175.

Samara E, Spyropoulou V, Tabard-Fougère A, et al: Kingella kingae and osteoarticular infections, *Pediatrics* 144(6), 2019. Epub.

Schaper NC, van Netten JJ, Apelqvist J, Bus SA, Fitridge R, Game F, Monteiro-Soares M, Senneville E, Editorial Board IWGDF: Practical guidelines on the prevention and management of diabetes-related foot disease (IWGDF 2023 update), *Diabetes Metab Res Rev* 40(3):e3657, 2024.

Senneville E, Lipsky BA, Abbas ZG, et al: Diagnosis of infection in the foot in diabetes: a systematic review, *Diabetes Metab Res Rev* 36(S1):e3281, 2020.

Sircar K, Jung N, Kernich N, Zarghooni K, Eysel P, Yagdiran A, Herren C: Risk Factors for Neurologic Deficits in Patients With Spinal Epidural Abscess: An Analysis of One-Hundred-Forty Cases, *Global Spine J*, 2023:21925682231194467, .

Talha KM, Baddour LM, Ishaq H, Ramesh R, Arshad V, Tariq W, Fischer KM, Berbari EF, Sohail MR, Palraj R: Native Vertebral Osteomyelitis in Patients with Staphylococcus Aureus Bacteremia, *Am J Med Sci* 363(2):140–146, 2022.

Vanherwegen A-S, Lauwers P, Lavens A, Doggen K, Dirinck E: on behalf of the Initiative for Quality Improvement and Epidemiology in multidisciplinary Diabetic Foot Clinics (IQED-Foot) Study Group. Sex differences in diabetic foot ulcer severity and outcome in Belgium, *PLoS ONE* 18(2), 2023:e0281886, .

Zalavras CG, Marcus RE, Levin LS, Patzakis MJ: Management of open fractures and subsequent complications, *JBJS (A)* 4:884–895, 2007.

Zhang LX, Wang YT, Zhao J, Li Y, Chen HL: Sex Differences in Osteomyelitis of the Foot in Persons With Diabetes Mellitus: A Meta-Analysis, *Wound Manag Prev.* 67(5):19–25, 2021.

PLAGUE

Method of

Nelson Iván Agudelo Higuita, MD; Douglas A. Drevets, MD; and Brian Scott, DO

CURRENT DIAGNOSIS

- Plague should be suspected when a person develops abrupt onset of fever, lymphadenopathy, or sepsis and there is history of a flea bite or possible exposure to an infected animal or person.
- *Yersinia pestis* is an aerobic gram-negative coccobacilli that exhibits bipolar staining with Giemsa, Wright's, and Wayson stains.
- Automated diagnostic systems may misidentify *Y. pestis* as another organism.

CURRENT THERAPY

- Timely and appropriate management is imperative for a good outcome.
- Despite their toxicities, aminoglycosides are the treatment agents of choice.
- Respiratory droplet precautions should be instituted when pneumonic plague is suspected.
- Postexposure prophylaxis is indicated for close contacts.

Historical descriptions indicate that *Yersinia pestis* probably caused Justinian's Plague (AD 541), which led into the first plague pandemic. The second plague pandemic, also known as the Black Death, began in Central Asia in 1347 and then spread to Europe, Asia, and Africa. It killed an estimated 50 million people. The current (third) plague pandemic began in China and then spread worldwide along shipping routes in 1899–1900. *Y. pestis* is a gram-negative, nonmotile, facultatively anaerobic, non-spore-forming coccobacillus that is approximately 0.5 to 0.8 μm in diameter and 1 to 3 μm in length. Genomic sequencing shows that *Y. pestis* is a recently emerged clone of *Y. pseudotuberculosis*.

Epidemiology
Plague is a zoonosis for which urban and sylvatic rodents (e.g., rats, prairie dogs, and marmots) are the most important enzootic reservoirs. Additionally, domestic cats and dogs have been linked to human disease. Human plague occurs in North and South America, Asia, and Africa. Recent outbreaks reported to the World Health Organization (WHO) have occurred in the Democratic Republic of Congo (2005, 2006, 2020), China (2009), and Peru (2010). Plague is endemic in Madagascar, and between 2004 and 2009, 30% of all human cases worldwide were reported from this country. The largest epidemic in a quarter of a century was identified August 1, 2017, and was contained November 27, 2017. A total of 2417 cases (77% pneumonic) with a 9% case fatality ratio were reported. The last outbreak of plague occurred in August 2021 from two nonbordering regions in Madagascar, Itasy and Haute Matsiatra. Both are known endemic areas, with the Ambalavao district in Haute Matsiatra having served as the main epicenter during the 2017 epidemic. From 2000 to 2009, a total of 21,725 cases of plague with a 7.4% fatality rate were reported worldwide. The incidence of plague in most of the world is otherwise declining. In 2018, only 5 countries reported cases of plague. In North America, most human cases occur in New Mexico, Arizona, California, Colorado, and Texas. Between 1900 and 2012, 1006 confirmed or probable cases have occurred in the U.S. with over 80% of these attributable to bubonic plague. In the United States, an average of seven human cases have been reported annually. More information can be found on the WHO and Centers for Disease Control and Prevention websites.

Modes of Transmission
Most human infections are transmitted from rodent to humans via the bite of an infected flea. Infection also can be acquired by contact with body fluids from infected animals, such as during field dressing of game or by inhalation of respiratory droplets from animals, particularly cats, or humans with pneumonic plague.

Bioterrorism Threat
Plague was used as an agent of biowarfare by the Japanese in World War II and was a focus of intensive research and development in the former Soviet Union during the Cold War. Primary pneumonic plague is the most likely form of exposure because of biowarfare or bioterrorism. Recent increases in terrorism worldwide have increased the focus of public health management groups to develop comprehensive statements regarding plague as a biological weapon.

Pathogenesis and Clinical Syndromes
Transdermal inoculation of bacilli from the bite of an infected flea ultimately leads to infection of the regional lymph nodes in which massive replication of bacteria creates the bubo (derived from the Greek *bubon* or "groin"), a swollen, erythematous, and painful lymph node in the groin, axilla, or cervical region. Bacteremia and septicemia frequently develop and lead to secondary infection of other organs including the lungs, spleen, and central nervous system. Primary pneumonic plague is a rare natural occurrence and results from the inhalation of respiratory droplets containing *Y. pestis* bacilli from another case of pneumonic plague, usually in humans or in cats. Although plague in dogs is rare, human outbreaks have been traced to sick dogs with wildlife exposure. Secondary pneumonic plague results from seeding of the lungs by blood-borne bacteria in the setting of either bubonic or septicemic plague. Septicemic plague also begins with transdermal exposure but manifests as primary bacteremia/septicemia without the bubo. Less common manifestations include meningitis, pharyngitis, and gastroenteritis. In addition, inhalation of respiratory droplets produced by intense manipulation of human corpses or animal carcasses are another potential form of infection. Direct skin contact with infected blood from a corpse or carcass could also result in bubonic plague. Finally, transmission of antimicrobial resistant *Y. pestis* has been documented during outbreaks of pneumonic plague.

Bubonic plague is an acute febrile lymphadenitis that develops 2 to 8 days after inoculation. Inflamed lymph nodes are usually 1 to 6 cm in diameter and painful. Abrupt onset of fever is an almost universal finding and occurs simultaneously with, or up to 24 hours before, the appearance of the bubo. Headache, malaise, and chills are frequent, along with nausea, vomiting, and diarrhea. Most patients are tachycardic, hypotensive, and appear prostrate and lethargic with episodic restlessness. Leukocytosis with a left shift is typical. Complications include pneumonia, shock, disseminated intravascular coagulation, purpuric skin lesions, acral cyanosis, and gangrene. The differential diagnosis of bubonic plague includes tularemia and Group A β-hemolytic streptococcal adenitis with bacteremia.

Symptoms of septicemic plague are similar to those caused by other gram-negative bacteria, and are very similar to those of bubonic plague except that abdominal pain is more common in septicemic plague. Septicemic plague must be differentiated from fulminating septicemia caused by other gram-negative bacteria. Primary pneumonic plague has an abrupt onset of fever and influenza-like symptoms 1 to 5 days after inhalation exposure. Symptoms include shortness of breath, cough, chest pain, and bloody sputum with rapid progression to fulminating pneumonia and respiratory failure. Patients with secondary pneumonic infection show respiratory symptoms in addition to those attributed to the bubo or sepsis. Radiographic findings include patchy bronchopneumonia, multilobar consolidations, cavitations, and alveolar hemorrhage and are not pathognomonic of *Y. pestis*. Plague pneumonia must be differentiated from severe influenza, inhalation anthrax, and overwhelming community-acquired pneumonia.

Plague meningitis is rare but almost always universally fatal if untreated. This entity is most commonly seen as a complication of primary axillary bubonic plague. Plague meningitis can develop during appropriate treatment administration, particularly if treatment initiation was delayed or if the clinical course has been protracted.

Diagnosis
Plague is diagnosed by demonstrating *Y. pestis* in blood or body fluids such as a lymph node aspirate, sputum, or cerebrospinal fluid. A tentative diagnosis of bubonic plague can be made rapidly with fluid aspirated from a bubo showing gram-negative

coccobacilli with bipolar staining. It is important to remember that automated diagnostic systems might misidentify *Y. pestis*. In an outbreak in Colorado, the misidentification of *Y. pestis* as *Pseudomonas luteola* delayed the recognition of the outbreak. *Y. pestis* has also been misidentified as *Y. pseudotuberculosis* with matrix-assisted laser desorption/ionization time-of-flight mass spectometry (MALDI-TOF). Serology showing a fourfold rise in antibody titers to F1 antigen or a single titer of more than 1:128 is also diagnostic. Rapid tests using monoclonal antibodies to detect *Y. pestis* F1 antigen in bubo aspirates and sputum have been developed and field tested. The use of mass spectrometry as a more rapid and cost-effective diagnostic tool has also been studied.

Treatment

The aminoglycosides (gentamicin[1] and streptomycin), the fluoroquinolones (ciprofloxacin [Cipro] moxifloxacin [Avelox] and levofloxacin [Levaquin]) and doxycycline (Vibramycin) are considered first line therapy for all forms of plague with the exception of pneumonic and septicemic plague, in which doxycycline is considered an alternative agent. For plague meningitis, the first line therapy consists of levofloxacin or moxifloxacin with chloramphenicol. Typical minimal inhibitory concentrations for 90% (MIC_{90}) of tested strains for the fluoroquinolones are less than 0.03 to 0.25 μg/mL compared with less than 1.0 μg/mL and less than 1.0 μg/mL to 4.0 μg/mL for gentamicin and streptomycin, respectively, and less than 1.0 μg/mL for doxycycline. Streptomycin (15 mg/kg up to 1 g intramuscularly [IM] every 12 hours) and gentamicin (5 to 7 mg/kg/day intravenously [IV]/IM in one or two doses daily) are the drugs of choice for severe infection. For adults, standard fluoroquinolone dosing includes ciprofloxacin 400 mg IV every 8 hours or 750 mg orally every 12 hours; levofloxacin 750 mg IV/orally daily; and moxifloxacin 400 mg IV/orally daily. Doxycycline is administered starting with a 200 mg loading dose followed by 100 mg IV/orally every 12 hours. Chloramphenicol (25 mg/kg IV/orally every 6 hours) can be used in select circumstances. Antibiotic therapy should be continued for a total of 10 days; some experts will extend the duration of therapy to 14 days when a bacteriostatic agent like a tetracycline is used.

Prevention and Control

Standard infection control procedures should include a disposable surgical mask, latex gloves, devices to protect mucous membranes, and good hand washing. Hospitalized patients with known or suspected pneumonic plague should be isolated under respiratory droplet precautions for at least 48 hours after appropriate antibiotics are initiated. Patients without respiratory plague can be managed under standard precautions. Pre-exposure prophylaxis is not routinely recommended but can be considered under certain circumstances and for up to 48 hours after the last potential exposure. Postexposure prophylaxis should be given to individuals with close contact (less than 2 meters) with an infectious case or who have had a potential respiratory exposure. The recommended adult antibiotics for prophylaxis are doxycycline or ciprofloxacin in the same doses used for treatment. Postexposure prophylaxis can be given orally and should be continued for 7 days following exposure. Currently, there is no licensed plague vaccine. An encapsulated *Y. pseudotuberculosis*, strain V674pF1, is an efficient live oral vaccine against pneumonic plague in mice. Messenger RNA (mRNA)– lipid nanoparticle (LNP) vaccines may prove to be promising as well. An mRNA-LNP vaccine targeted against the F1 capsule antigen provided rapid and effective immunity in mice against *Y. pestis* after a single dose. With further research and development, this could be an important tool against future outbreaks. Recently, flea resistance to insecticides such as DDT and Deltamethrin in Madagascar has prompted an immediate need for alternative insecticides to prevent future plague outbreaks.

---

[1]Not FDA approved for this indication.

References

CDC. Maps and Statistics. http://www.cdc.gov/plague/maps/index.html.
Cooley KM, Fleck-Derderian S, McCormick DW, Nelson CA: Plague meningitis: a systematic review of clinical course, antimicrobial treatment, and outcomes, *Health Security* 21(1):22–33, 2023.
Jullien S, de Silva NL, Garner P: Plague transmission from corpses and carcasses, *Emerg Infect Dis* 27(8):2033–2041, 2021.
Kon E, Levy Y, Elia U, et al: A single-dose F1-based mRNA-LNP vaccine provides protection against the lethal plague bacterium, *Sci Adv* 10;9(10):eadg1036, 2023.
Nelson CA, Meaney-Delman D, Fleck-Derderian, et al: Antimicrobial treatment and prophylaxis of plague: recommendations for naturally acquired infections and bioterrorism response, *MMWR Recomm Rep* 70(3):1–27, 2021.
World Health Organization: Plague around the world in 2019, *Weekly Epidemiological Record* 94(25):289–292, 2019.

POST-ACUTE COVID SYNDROME

Method of
Victor S. Sierpina, MD; Justin Seashore, MD; Sagar Kamprath, MD; and Cathy Xie, DO

CURRENT DIAGNOSIS

- *Post-acute COVID syndrome* is defined as symptoms extending 3 weeks to 3 months after the acute disease occurs, and *long-haul COVID* is defined as symptoms persisting beyond 3 months after the infection has resolved.
- Predominant symptoms are new-onset shortness of breath, cough, palpitations, fatigue, and brain fog. Other common symptoms include gastrointestinal disturbances, headache, hair loss, new-onset nondescript pain, depression, anxiety, and posttraumatic stress disorder.
- Results of testing are not part of the current definition as many patients were not tested and are or were asymptomatic carriers.
- The broad spectrum of clinical manifestations of post-acute COVID syndrome should encourage clinicians and medical educators to include it in the differential diagnosis of any of a number of new or worsening complaints.

CURRENT TREATMENT

- Evidence for optimal management of long-haul COVID may be lacking at this time but is evolving, with best practices being described by multiple professional bodies.
- Multidisciplinary management and rehabilitation are essential to whole-person care.
- Organ- and system-specific care is appropriate and must be prioritized as to serious versus milder long-term problems.
- Self-management and peer support can plan important roles and must include shared decision making.
- Appropriate consultation and use of currently established disease-specific and organ-specific practice guidelines are foundational to optimal treatment planning.
- Quality-of-care principles for long-haul COVID include providing access to care, reducing the burden of illness, taking clinical responsibility, offering continuity of care, providing multidisciplinary rehabilitation, conducting evidence-based investigation and management, and continuing further research and development on appropriate and evidence-based clinical services.

Over the past 3 years, we have endured an ever-changing multimodal disease process, devastating millions of people not only with severe infection but also with mild or asymptomatic forms of the disease. Our understanding and definitions of the spectrum of conditions that encompasses post-acute COVID syndrome and long-haul COVID is an ongoing discovery. It is estimated that 10% to 30% of COVID-infected patients may be left with residual symptoms. With over 500,000 million worldwide known cases and many not reported, untested, or asymptomatic, post-acute COVID syndrome can be expected to affect a huge number of people.

Equally concerning is the puzzling discovery that those with even mild or asymptomatic COVID infections may develop post-acute COVID syndrome. Vaccination is largely protective of severe disease, though the syndrome may still occur in a small number of these patients. Children generally do not experience severe post-acute COVID syndrome, although psychological, mental health, and gastrointestinal symptoms are of increasing concern in this group and are often difficult to dissect from pre-existing conditions.

Some key ongoing questions include the following:
• What is the underlying biology of long-haul COVID?
• How many people become infected with long-haul COVID and who is most at risk?
• What is the relationship between long-haul COVID and other post-infection syndromes?

We endeavor to address these questions, though much further research is needed. We present here a holistic and methodical foundational program that uses minimally invasive procedures and management strategies. This approach will offer patients with post-acute COVID syndrome an improved quality of life with low-risk, cost-effective, common-sense healthcare approaches. The evidence base for this approach is grounded in current best practices but continues to evolve with new knowledge about the course of post-acute COVID syndrome. In parallel, we must guide patients away from high-risk, high-cost invasive therapies that have no proven benefit.

Healthcare professionals must be cognizant of the range of real physical long-term effects of COVID-19 and should address them with clinical discernment, understanding, and empathy. They should be careful not to label all such presentations as related to stress, anxiety, depression, or other psychological epiphenomena. The role of peer support is clearly important to those with post-acute COVID syndrome who may otherwise feel isolated and misunderstood.

Pathophysiology

COVID-19 is caused by the severe acute respiratory syndrome coronavirus 2 (SARS-CoV-2) and is genetically similar to the severe acute respiratory syndrome (SARS) and Middle East respiratory syndrome (MERS) coronaviruses that were responsible for the SARS outbreaks earlier in the century. SARS and MERS infections have been found to result in long-term postviral syndromes, some extending a decade a more after the initial disease. Coronaviruses that circulate among humans are usually benign and are responsible for about one-fourth of all common cold illnesses, with a total of seven human coronaviruses in known existence. However, it is likely that bats, a natural animal reservoir, facilitated mutation of the virus in China in late 2019. Another spillover possibility, escape of modified virus from a research laboratory in Wuhan, is still being debated. This novel coronavirus is composed of single-stranded RNA with its envelope surrounded by spike proteins resembling a crown, typically transmitted through respiratory droplets as well as fecal-oral transmission. The incubation period is about 5 days, though some variants such as the Delta variant have a shorter cycle and are potentially followed by 1 week of worsening symptoms that may lead to hospitalization in severe cases. Interferon is a key component that affects the mechanism of viral infection. Higher viral loads and delayed interferon responses are seen in severe infection, and it may be likely that patients most susceptible to severe disease cannot adequately mount an effective early antiviral response.

The virus attaches to cells via the ACE2 receptor, found in our tongue, nose, throat, stomach, small intestine, liver, brain, kidneys, and lungs. In the lungs, it binds to type 2 alveolar cells, where it replicates. The cells subsequently send a distress signal of cytokines and downregulate the ACE2 receptor, decreasing angiotensin 1 to 9 and angiotensin 1 to 7 (pro-vasodilation and antifibrotic). Angiotensin 1 receptors become more stimulated, which leads to a proinflammatory and profibrotic stage. COVID-19 also favors disordered endothelial function, which contributes to protein accumulation in the alveolar space seen in the "cytokine storm" directly related to capillary leak and the cases of ARDS seen in advanced states of the disease. Unfortunately, this is not only limited to the lungs, but predisposes the entire body system to a prothrombotic state, as seen in cases of stroke and other types of ischemic dysfunction. In this inflammatory state, vascular endothelial and smooth muscle cells produce large amounts of IL-6. This stimulates the acute-phase response, increasing fibrinogen production and favoring clot formation.

COVID-19 remains a complex disease process of the endothelium, and future treatments may focus on antiinflammatory therapies and promoting endothelial homeostasis. Obesity is one of the major risk factors for the cytokine storm as it induces a constant state of low-grade inflammation characterized by acute-phase reactants, reactive oxygen species, and proinflammatory cytokines. However, moderate exercise over time enhances the immune system, mobilizing NK and CD8+ T cells, and overall improves immunosurveillance and lowers inflammation.

Prevention

Conventional prevention includes the well-known guidelines from the Centers for Disease Control and Prevention (CDC) regarding masking, social distancing, hand washing/avoidance of touching the face, various isolation and quarantine measures, and vaccination. Large droplets are the primary mode of spread, which can be greatly mitigated with widespread mask wearing in addition to adequate ventilation.

Monoclonal antibodies may also be used in acute infection as they bind to the spike proteins of the coronavirus and can reduce the viral load, theoretically reducing the severity of the illness. Immunotherapy continues to evolve as certain formulations are more or less effective against emerging variants.

Given that over 99% of the recent cases in 2022 within the United States were caused by the omicron variant, bamlanivimab[5] and etesevimab[5] (administered together)[5] and REGEN-COV (casirivimab and imdevimab)[5] are not recommended because they have reduced activity against this variant. Paxlovid[5] (nirmatrelvir and ritonavir, approved for Emergency Use Authorization [EUA] by the U.S. Food and Drug Administration [FDA]), sotrovimab[5] (no longer has EUA), remdesivir (Veklury), molnupiravir[5] (Lagevrio, approved for EUA), and most recently bebtelovimab[5] (approved for EUA) are recommended for those with mild-to-moderate COVID-19 who are at risk for progression to severe disease. The monoclonal antibodies leronlimab[5] and tocilizumab (Actemra),[1] which have been efficacious in treating HIV, have been shown to reduce IL-6 levels in COVID-19 and are being further studied. Healthcare providers can consult with the National Institutes of Health's COVID-19 guidelines to decide whether these therapies are beneficial for individual patients as they are expected to evolve with new variants.

These measures may be used for patients with COVID-19 who are not sick enough to be hospitalized but are at risk for hospitalization because of medical comorbidities such as diabetes, immunosuppression, or obesity. Vaccination along with booster are still recommended for these patients. Access, cost, and administration hurdles impede the availability of immunotherapies worldwide.

The recent mRNA vaccines offer hope for prevention of infection and transmission, with current projections of 94.5% efficacy

---

[1] Not FDA approved for this indication.
[5] Investigational drug in the United States.

in reducing severe disease. Additionally, as new variants occur, these newly developed vaccines continue to protect up to 100% against severe COVID-19 infections. However, it is recommended to continue masking and engaging in social distancing even after vaccination. Some recent reports have indicated that patients suffering with post-acute COVID symptoms found that getting the COVID vaccine relieved these symptoms. The exact mechanism of this is unknown and bears further study but may have to do with clearing residual virus or reducing autoimmune and inflammatory processes.

Rates of anxiety and depression have increased during the pandemic, and this subsequently attenuates the immune system. Managing these appropriately and promptly can improve immunity as well as quality of life. Spending time outside and engaging in physical activity can also help strengthen the immune system and mitigate the cabin fever of COVID-19. Breathing techniques such as resonant breathing, singing, or 4-7-8 breathing can also help increase parasympathetic tone, increase heart rate variability, and decrease stress. At least 7 hours of sleep before vaccination provides a more robust antibody response from the immune system.

Other less proven but widely used methods include use of various supplements such as vitamin C,[1] vitamin D,[1] quercetin,[7] zinc,[1] probiotics,[7] luteolin,[7] melatonin,[7] and other supplements. None of these methods have been proven in prospective trials, but they are widely used, and there is some historical evidence for their utility and mechanisms of action in other coronavirus-like infections such as the common cold. An open discussion with patients regarding the limited evidence for them may be helpful while respecting patient autonomy and desire for agency in selecting self-care strategies in the presence of fear and uncertainty.

Vitamin C remains a potent antioxidant and anecdotally beneficial in several studies. The ongoing Lessening Organ Dysfunction With VITamin C—COVID-19 (LOVIT-COVID) clinical trial (NCT04401150) is assessing high-dose intravenous vitamin C for inpatients with COVID-19. For prevention, one may focus on increasing consumption of foods high in vitamin C such as citrus.

Vitamin D is an important regulator of human immune function and may stimulate the innate immune response to provide front-line protection against infectious agents. On the whole, people are spending less time outside in the sunlight, which hampers the production of the active form of vitamin D. Recently it was noted that higher vitamin D levels correlated with fewer COVID-19 cases and mortality. This could be a result of low vitamin D being a marker of a sedentary lifestyle and thus likely overall health risk. Whether or not one is COVID positive, taking vitamin D may be beneficial in a dose of around 4000 IU daily. There is also evidence that vitamin K_2[1] may be helpful in the absorption of vitamin D, but it should be avoided in patients on blood thinners.

Quercetin is a naturally occurring dietary flavonoid with antiviral properties and may disrupt the infectious mechanism of the coronavirus. It is an antioxidant found in many plant foods including capers, red onions, apples, leafy greens, dill, cilantro, fennel, berries, sweet potato, tomatoes, broccoli, and tea. Quercetin can also be purchased as a supplement. It is often combined with vitamin C to increase absorption and taken up to 500 mg twice a day.

Zinc impairs replication in RNA viruses and may enhance cytotoxicity when used with a zinc ionophore such as quercetin. Long-term zinc supplementation may result in copper deficiency, thus replacing copper is recommended.

N-acetylcysteine,[1] a glutathione precursor, at 600 mg orally twice per day, may help improve oxidative stress and inflammatory response in patients with upper respiratory tract infections.

N-acetylcysteine assists the liver in reducing glutathione, which in turn helps the liver in removing toxins. A case report has noted that glutathione supplementation has improved dyspnea in COVID-19 patients. These may represent a novel treatment approach in blocking nuclear factor kappa B (NF-κB) and attenuating the cytokine storm seen in COVID-19.

Several trials to assess various adaptogens, probiotics, and dietary supplements such as nicotinamide riboside[7] are currently underway as additional therapies for long-haul COVID. Hyperbaric oxygen therapy, montelukast (Singulair),[1] and deupirfenidone[5] are being evaluated to help with COVID-related respiratory complaints. Histamine-1 and histamine-2 antagonists show promise by inhibiting the virus from entering ACE-2–expressing cells. In addition, use of selective serotonin reuptake inhibitors (SSRIs) and serotonin-norepinephrine reuptake inhibitors (SNRIs) has been associated with reduced risk of intubation or death in COVID-19. As future trials ensue, we may have clearer direction in treating the long-term effects of COVID-19.

Clinical Manifestations

The multifaceted aspects of long-haul COVID are shown in Figure 1. According to the CDC, the most commonly reported long-term post-acute COVID symptoms are outlined in Box 1.

Diagnosis

The predominant symptoms leading patients to seek help are focused on new-onset shortness of breath, cough, palpitations, fatigue, and brain fog. Other common symptoms include gastrointestinal disturbances, headache, hair loss, new-onset nondescript pain, depression, anxiety, and posttraumatic stress disorder (PTSD).

Post-acute COVID syndrome is defined as symptoms extending 3 weeks to 3 months after the acute disease occurs, and *long-haul COVID* is defined as symptoms persisting beyond 3 months after the infection has resolved. Results of testing are not part of the current definition as many patients were not tested and are or were asymptomatic carriers. Even antibody testing is not entirely reliable as we are unsure of the durability of post-infection IgG results.

Persons with the following risks were two to three times more likely to develop long-haul COVID: persistent cough, hoarseness, headache, diarrhea, loss of appetite, and shortness of breath in the first week.

Persons with more than five symptoms in the first week of illness were four times more likely to develop long-haul COVID than those with fewer symptoms. The five most predictive symptoms of long-haul COVID in the first week of illness were fatigue, headache, shortness of breath, hoarse voice, and myalgia. Long-haul COVID was also more likely to occur in women, older adults, and those with obesity. An autoimmune component may explain the higher rate of post-acute COVID syndrome in women.

Indeed, post-acute COVID syndrome may comprise four or more syndromes rather than one distinct postviral entity, and it may include post–intensive care syndrome, post–viral fatigue syndrome, and long–haul COVID. Symptoms may fluctuate and present in nonlinear and nonsequentially unpredictable ways.

Such conditions have been seen in other post-infectious conditions, largely as a result of the persistence of the immune response, ongoing inflammation, and effects on blood coagulation.

After the Spanish flu of 1918, which killed an estimated 50 million people, late-occurring neurologic sequela included long-lasting brain damage in up to 1 million people. SARS and MERS as well as myalgic encephalomyelitis or chronic fatigue syndrome are other syndromes that share overlapping symptoms with post-acute COVID syndrome.

---

[1] Not FDA approved for this indication.

[5] Investigational drug in the United States.

[7] Available as dietary supplement.

Long-haul COVID is an evolving clinical problem that has important public health and long-term considerations as the pandemic continues and it becomes endemic.

Therapy

Once post-acute COVID syndrome or long-haul COVID is suspected or diagnosed, determining the patient's baseline status helps organize and systematize clinical interventions. Addressing evolving exacerbations and life-threatening manifestations must take priority. It is important to avoid unproven, high-cost, invasive experimental therapies outside of clinical trials. The general principles of management are described in a monograph by the National Institute for Health and Care Excellence (NICE) (Box 2).

For clinicians, a standardized approach to patients in the initial setting is important. Functional and behavioral assessments are of central importance as the rehabilitation of patients requires management of both. Multidisciplinary teams to direct care and address newly developing symptoms should be utilized when available.

To begin evaluation of the patient with post-acute COVID syndrome, the clinician should perform initial screening with standardized questionnaires including shortness-of-breath scales, such as the University of California, San Diego Shortness of Breath Questionnaire (SOBQ), and activity scales that assess activities of daily living (ADLs) and instrumental activities of daily living (iADLS). Nutritional evaluation (e.g., the subjective global assessment [SGA]), the Generalized Anxiety Disorder 7-Item

Questionnaire (GAD-7), the Patient Health Questionnaire-9 (PHQ-9), the International Education Standard-6 (IES-6), and the Impact of Event Scale-Revised (IES-R) are examples of behavioral assessments that can be used to evaluate anxiety, depression, and PTSD along with an ongoing symptoms evaluation. Use of these scales with each visit allow for individualized evaluations of improvement (Box 3).

Utilizing a multidisciplinary rehabilitation team including physicians, rehabilitation therapists, psychologists, nutritionists, and social workers to review these screenings allows the healthcare provider to develop a personalized, patient-centered approach to care.

Shared decision making with patients is key, given the vast number of symptoms patients may be experiencing. Discussing which are most troubling and limiting to the patient is of importance in goal setting. From this baseline, the healthcare provider can establish plans to address the most severe symptoms initially and determine those that can be readdressed in the future.

Acute COVID-19 presents with a broad range of symptoms, therefore patients recovering from this illness show heterogeneity that may be phenotypic. Some have few or no residual symptoms after the acute infection, while others show sustained symptoms at higher or lesser clinical penetrance.

Pulmonary

For many, respiratory symptoms may be the predominating indication, therefore a proper pulmonary examination is important.

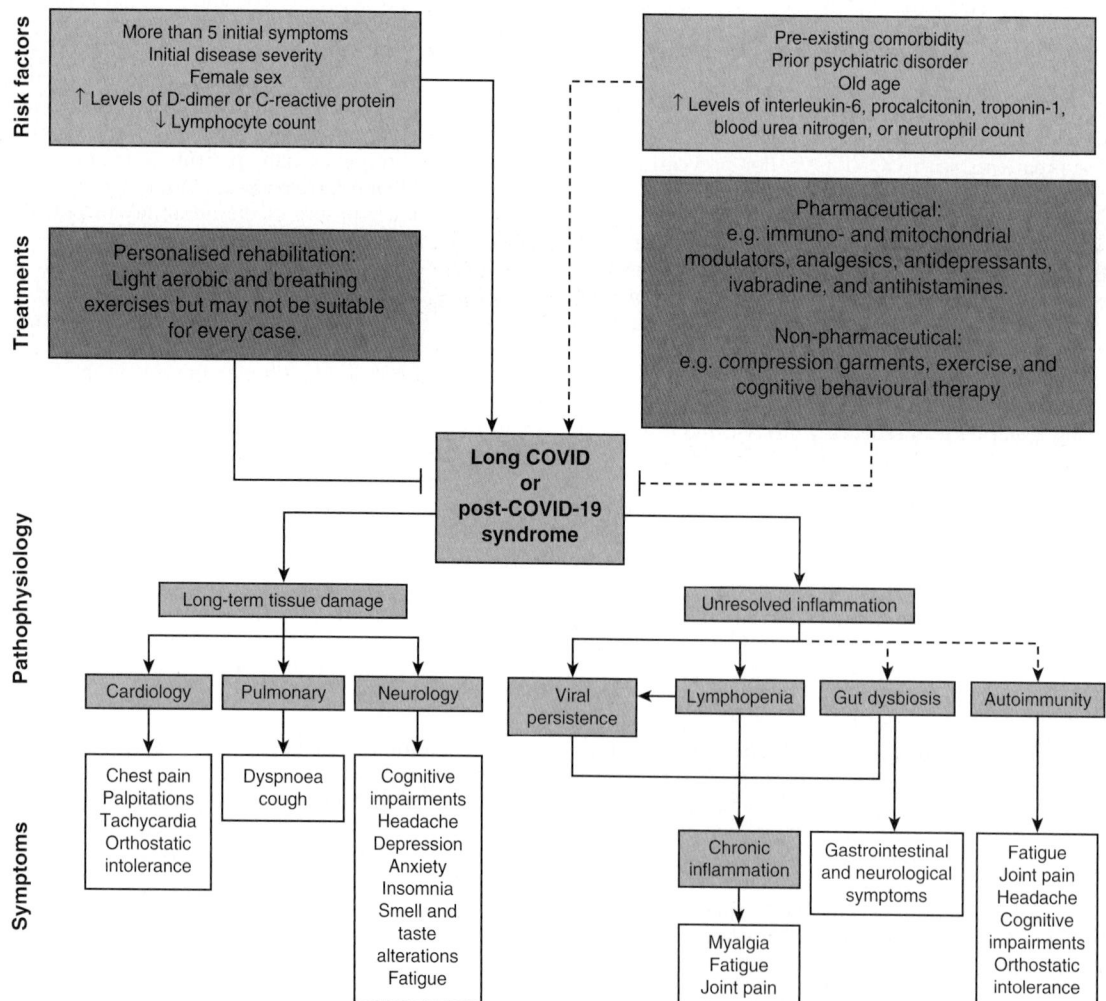

Figure 1 An overview of the symptoms, putative pathophysiology, associated risk factors, and potential treatments involved in long-haul COVID. *Dashed lines* represent areas where evidence is relatively lacking compared with the *solid lines*. (Modified from Yong SJ: Long COVID or post-COVID-19 syndrome: putative pathophysiology, risk factors, and treatments, *Infect Dis (Lond)* 53(10):737–754, 2021.)

BOX 1 — Symptoms Commonly Reported Among Patients with Post-Acute COVID Conditions

- Dyspnea or increased respiratory effort
- Fatigue
- Post-exertional malaise* and/or poor endurance
- "Brain fog," or cognitive impairment
- Cough
- Chest pain
- Headache
- Palpitations and/or tachycardia
- Arthralgia
- Myalgia
- Paresthesia
- Abdominal pain
- Diarrhea
- Insomnia and other sleep difficulties
- Fever
- Lightheadedness
- Impaired daily function and mobility
- Pain
- Rash (e.g., urticaria)
- Mood changes
- Anosmia or dysgeusia
- Menstrual cycle irregularities

*Post-exertional malaise (PEM) is the worsening of symptoms following even minor physical or mental exertion, with symptoms typically worsening 12 to 48 hours after activity and lasting for days or even weeks.

From Centers for Disease Control and Prevention: Clinical Care Information for COVID-19. Post-COVID Conditions: Overview for Healthcare Providers. Available at: https://www.cdc.gov/coronavirus/2019-ncov/hcp/clinical-care.html.

Pulse oximetry, pulmonary function testing, a 6-minute walk test, and chest x-ray are good starting points. Utilization of pulmonary rehabilitation will guide patients through this new sensation of shortness of breath and reduce symptom burden. This aspect of rehabilitation should not be limited to patients with only abnormal pulmonary function testing. Home monitoring with pulse oximetry is recommended. It is also important to eliminate other factors for dyspnea such as smoking, air pollutants, extremes in temperature, or excess exercise.

Several breathing techniques have been offered to help patients deal with breathlessness, improve diaphragmatic breathing, and help normalize lung function (Box 4).

The question of whether to use inhaled bronchodilators remains. A potential practice is to begin a trial with a short-acting agent to be used when symptomatic, and if the patient notes temporary benefit and the need to use it frequently, a long-acting beta agonist plus an inhaled corticosteroid can be considered. COVID-19 is known to induce an inflammatory response, and this may abate symptoms. Step-down therapy should be planned as one would do for asthma.

As pulmonary symptoms such as cough and shortness of breath have predominated presenting concerns in patients with post-acute COVID syndrome, a program at Yale called RECOVERY has been developed that could be a model for approaching pulmonary and other systems (Figure 2).

Cardiac

Another key organ affected by COVID-19 infection is the heart. Cardiotoxicity from the infection can cause inflammation of the heart (myocarditis), rhythm disturbances, and damage to the heart muscle (cardiomyopathy). Sudden cardiac death, heart attacks, and heart failure have all been observed, including

---

BOX 2 — Management of Post-Acute COVID Syndrome

These recommendations are for healthcare professionals who provide care for patients with ongoing symptomatic COVID-19 or post-acute COVID syndrome in primary care and community settings or in multidisciplinary assessment and rehabilitation services.

Self-Management and Supported Self-Management

- Give advice and information on self-management to people with ongoing symptomatic COVID-19 or post-acute COVID syndrome, starting from their initial assessment. This should include the following:
  - Ways to self-manage their symptoms, such as setting realistic goals
  - Who to contact if they are worried about their symptoms or if they need support with self-management
  - Sources of advice and support, including support groups, social prescribing, online forums, and apps
  - How to obtain support from other services, including social care, housing, and employment, and advice about financial support
- Information about new or continuing symptoms of COVID-19 that patients can share with their family, careers, and friends (see the section on common symptoms of ongoing symptomatic COVID-19 and post-acute COVID syndrome [https://www.nice.org.uk/guidance/NG188]).
- Explain that it is not known if over-the-counter vitamins and supplements are helpful, harmful, or have no effect in the treatment of new or ongoing symptoms of COVID-19.
- Support patients in discussions with their employer, school, or college about returning to work or education, for example by having a phased return. For advice on returning to work, follow national guidelines such as the NICE guideline on workplace health: long-term sickness absence and capability to work.

Multidisciplinary Rehabilitation

- Assess patients who have been referred to integrated multidisciplinary rehabilitation services to guide management. Include the physical, psychological, and psychiatric aspects of rehabilitation. Ensure that any symptoms that could affect the patient's ability to safely start rehabilitation have been investigated first (see recommendations for multidisciplinary rehabilitation teams [https://www.nice.org.uk/guidance/NG188]).
- Work with the patient to develop a personalized rehabilitation and management plan that is recorded in a rehabilitation prescription and includes the following:
  - Areas of rehabilitation and interventions based on their assessment
  - Helping the patient decide and work toward goals
  - Symptom management for all presenting symptoms, for example advice and education on managing breathlessness, fatigue and "brain fog."
- Encourage patients to keep a record or use a tracking app to monitor their goals, recovery, and any changes in their symptoms (see recommendations for follow-up and monitoring [https://www.nice.org.uk/guidance/NG188]).

Support for Older Adults and Children

- Consider additional support for older adults with ongoing symptomatic COVID-19 or post-acute COVID syndrome, for example short-term care packages, advance care planning and support with social isolation, loneliness, and bereavement, if relevant.
- Consider referral from 4 weeks for specialist advice for children with ongoing symptomatic COVID-19 or post-COVID-19 syndrome.

University of Texas Medical Branch Health (UTMB) Post COVID Recovery Clinic intake questionnaire
https://www.utmbhealth.com/post-covid-19-clinic
University of California, San Diego Shortness of Breath Questionnaire (SOBQ)
https://doi.org/10.1378/chest.113.3.619
Activities of Daily Living/Instrumental Activities of Daily Living
https://www.alz.org/careplanning/downloads/lawton-iadl.pdf
Subjective Global Assessment (SGA)
https://nutritioncareincanada.ca/sites/default/uploads/files/SGA%20Tool%20EN%20BKWT_2017.pdf
Generalized Anxiety Disorder 7-Item Questionnaire (GAD-7)
https://adaa.org/sites/default/files/GAD-7_Anxiety-updated_0.pdf
Patient Health Questionnaire-9 (PHQ-9)
https://www.apa.org/depression-guideline/patient-health-questionnaire.pdf
Impact of Event Scale-Revised (IES-R)
https://emdrfoundation.org/toolkit/ies-scoring.pdf

About 80% of the work of breathing is done by the diaphragm. After illness or general deconditioning, the breathing pattern may be altered, with reduced diaphragmatic movement and greater use of neck and shoulder accessory muscles. This results in shallow breathing, increasing fatigue and breathlessness, and higher energy expenditure. The "breathing control" technique is aimed at normalizing breathing patterns and increasing the efficiency of the respiratory muscles (including the diaphragm), resulting in less energy expenditure, less airway irritation, reduced fatigue, and improvement in breathlessness. The patient should sit in a supported position and breathe in and out slowly, preferably in through the nose and out through the mouth, while relaxing the chest and shoulders and allowing the tummy to rise. They should aim for an inspiration to expiration ratio of 1:2. This technique can be used frequently throughout the day, in 5–10 minute bursts (or longer if helpful).

Other breathing techniques—such as diaphragmatic breathing, slow deep breathing, pursed lip breathing, yoga techniques, Buteyko—are used in strategies to manage patients' breathing patterns and breathlessness but require specialist advice to identify which technique best suits each patient.

From Greenhalgh T, Knight M, A'Court C, Buxton M, Husain L. Management of post-acute covid-19 in primary care. BMJ. 2020;370:m3026.

Takotsubo heart syndrome. Beta blockers and immunotherapy may be indicated.

Cardiac symptoms such as palpitations or increased resting heart rate can be further evaluated with long-term ambulatory cardiac monitoring. A cardiopulmonary exercise test or echocardiogram can assist in delineating cardiac from pulmonary symptoms.

The appropriate type of testing and therapy for post-COVID cardiac syndrome will need to be determined. Electrocardiogram and rhythm monitoring, echocardiography, cardiac biomarkers, and close clinical observation with directed questions about cardiac function will be required for months and perhaps years. Cardiac biopsy may be needed in select cases as well as special imaging such as cardiac magnetic resonance imaging.

Long-term physiotherapy and ongoing cardiology consultation may be needed. Special consideration to cardiac rehabilitation must be given to patients with post-acute COVID syndrome, and modifying or suspending rehabilitation exercises is indicated for the following:

- Saturation <88% to 93%
- Heart rate <40 beats per minute or >120 beats per minute
- Systolic blood pressure <90 mm Hg or >180 mm Hg
- Body temperature fluctuations >37.2°C
- Respiratory symptoms and fatigue that worsen during exercise and do not alleviate after rest
- Symptoms such as chest tightness or pain, difficulty breathing, severe cough, dizziness, headache, unclear vision, palpitations, sweating, and instability

Fatigue

Prevention of deconditioning while considering the risks associated with overexertion can be a balancing act in the patient with post-acute COVID syndrome.

Exercise rehabilitation for athletes and others requires careful titration and personalization as excessive exercise can set back progress. This is also seen in treatment of fibromyalgia and chronic fatigue syndrome in which even slowly graded increases in exercise can cause worsening. It is likely that what we have learned from other conditions such as fibromyalgia and chronic fatigue syndrome, now called *myalgic encephalomyelitis/chronic fatigue syndrome* (ME/CFS), may be transferrable and helpful.

NICE guidelines for these conditions were revised in 2021 and may inform care for patients with post-acute COVID syndrome, but they are still controversial. It is important to consider safe approaches from complementary and integrative medicine, including mind-body therapies, yoga, tai chi, acupuncture,

personalized nutritional and fitness prescriptions, and carefully selected supplements, minerals, and vitamins.

A general rule of thumb for rehabilitation of patients with post-acute COVID syndrome is that if a patient feels excessively fatigued the day following exercise, so-called *postexercise malaise*, the program must be backed down to prevent overdoing. Controlled breathing exercises, careful pacing, goal setting, low intensity of exercise, and stress reduction are all critical.

Detailed guidelines on returning to sports activities are provided in the Stanford Hall consensus statement (see references). These guidelines can help address appropriate measures, timing, and rehabilitation of multiple systems (i.e., pulmonary, cardiac, neurologic, psychological, musculoskeletal) and overall exercise rehabilitation for returning to vigorous activities. The risk associated with post-acute COVID syndrome deconditioning is significant and must be considered on returning athletes to activity.

Dysautonomia

Providers should be familiar with syndromes such as chronic fatigue syndrome, postural orthostatic tachycardia syndrome, and mast cell activation syndrome. These syndromes are commonly brought up within the post-acute COVID syndrome community.

Dysautonomia may be particularly challenging as it presents with rapid heartbeat, anxiety, numbness, dizziness, low blood pressure, and extreme fatigue. Orthostatic intolerance, a postural orthostatic tachycardia (POT)-like syndrome, may be caused by viral or autoimmune damage to the autonomic nervous system. This condition is best managed with established measures such as patient education, maintaining volume and vascular tone, gradually adjusting positional changes, performing structured exercises including isometrics, wearing compression garments, and in some cases using pharmacologic agents to manage palpitations and to retain sodium and fluid. These pharmacologic agents include fludrocortisone (Florinef),[1] midodrine (Proamatine), and others affecting adrenergic surge such as beta blockers, methyldopa,[1] and clonidine (Catapres).[1]

---

[1] Not FDA approved for this indication.

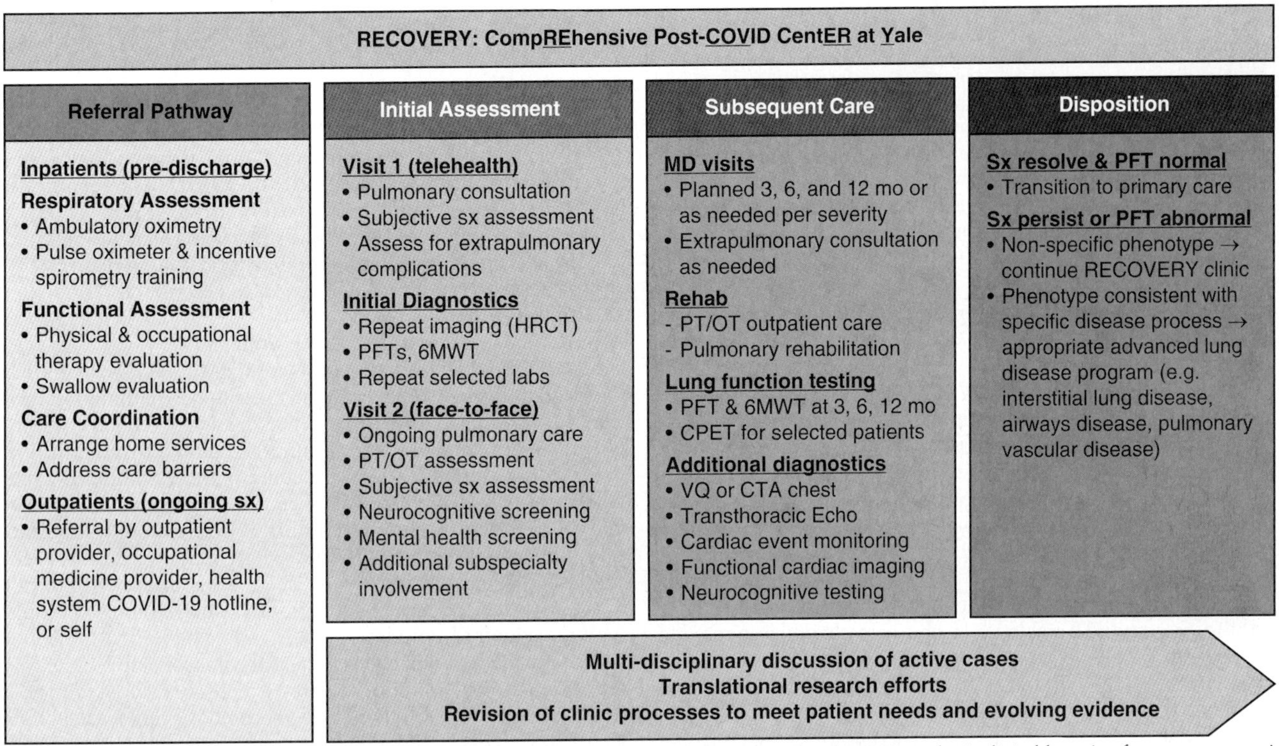

Figure 2 The RECOVERY Clinic Model. (From Lutchmansingh DD, Knauert MP, Antin-Ozerkis DE, et al.: A clinic blueprint for post-coronavirus disease 2019 RECOVERY: Learning from the past, looking to the future, *Chest* 159(3):949–958, 2021.

Neurologic

Patients with COVID-19 may suffer severe central nervous system insults resulting in strokes, severe brain inflammation (encephalomyelitis, a multiple sclerosis–like or Guillain-Barré type of demyelination), weakness, numbness, confusion, delirium, memory loss, headache, and psychosis. A complaint of enduring "brain fog" is common. Some of these problems occur early, and others occur late. They may be difficult to detect in patients in the intensive care unit who are very sick, hypoxemic, or sedated and when magnetic resonance imaging is difficult to obtain. The Mayo Clinic recommends that brain fog be managed like chemobrain including coping strategies and stress relief. Methylphenidate (Ritalin),[1] donepezil (Aricept),[1] modafinil (Provigil),[1] and memantine (Namenda)[1] have been suggested as options. Luteolin,[7] a flavonoid, has some promise of benefit.

Full neuropsychological testing and/or neurologic consultation should be considered in cases in which post-COVID cognitive changes persist. Occupational, physical, and speech/language therapy may play an important role.

Anosmia is another neurologic symptom of COVID and can be quite debilitating, though patients often recover with time. It can lead to loss of appetite, weight loss, and depression. Therapy for persistent anosmia can include olfactory training, which includes repeated sniffing of a set of odorants to speed recovery.

Mental Health

Mental health support for many will be of importance as patients cope with so many unknowns in their post-COVID world. Sorting out somatic from psychosomatic problems requires clinical acumen, patience, perseverance, and continuity of care. Psychiatric consequences may be severe and related to the immune response and/or from psychological stressors such as social isolation, worries about a potentially fatal illness, concerns about infecting others, stigma of disease, impact on employment, finances, and relationships in general.

The immune response to coronaviruses induces local and systemic production of cytokines, chemokines, and other inflammatory mediators, all of which combine to worsen the burden of preexisting depression, anxiety, PTSD, and other mental health disorders, particularly in female patients.

Mental health issues may end up being one of the most serious, enduring, yet largely hidden impacts seen in the post-COVID patient; thus management and monitoring must address this domain to maintain a holistic approach. Children and adolescents may be most affected.

Therapeutic trials of holistic, integrative, and functional medicine are appropriate given low harm and potential benefit. These may include antiinflammatory diets, acupuncture, meditation, and selected supplements such as fish oil,[1] magnesium,[1] SAMe,[7] valerian,[7] B vitamins,[1] and others.

Hematologic

Thrombotic sequelae and hypercoagulable states require monitoring and management, and prolonged anticoagulation may be required, especially in those with significant deep venous thromboses or pulmonary or cardiac emboli. Many patients will need transient anticoagulation, though some may require ongoing therapy if clotting abnormalities persist. Endothelial damage is now recognized as a perpetuating factor in post-acute COVID syndrome.

Gastrointestinal

If diarrhea and other gastrointestinal complaints continue, this likely reflects viral impact on the microbiota. Gastrointestinal symptoms are prominent in affected children. An antiinflammatory diet, Mediterranean-type diet, hypoallergenic elimination diet, or other personalized nutritional strategies should be considered. Optimizing nutritional support for vulnerable older adults and those with continued anosmia and dysgeusia is likewise vital. Though not yet well defined in terms of dosing and speciation, replacing microbiota with food-sourced or encapsulated prebiotics and probiotics is worth considering as a safe and potentially useful strategy in this population. Microbiome changes also affect

---

[7] Available as dietary supplement.

[1] Not FDA approved for this indication.
[7] Available as dietary supplement.

cognitive and mood function in the central nervous system via the gut-brain axis.

Renal

Acute kidney injury during the infectious stage may result in longer-term decreases in glomerular filtration rate and other renal parameters. This is likely to be worse in those already at risk with existing chronic kidney disease, diabetes, or hypertension. Nephrology consultation should be sought in appropriate cases.

Endocrine

Loss of control of diabetes and even diabetic ketoacidosis has been observed after resolution of acute COVID-19 symptoms, sometimes weeks or months later. New cases of prediabetes and diabetes types 1 and 2 have been reported. COVID-19 may also activate latent autoimmune thyroid disease, resulting in thyroiditis or thyrotoxicosis in the aftermath and resolution of respiratory disease. Risks for osteoporosis may also increase as a result of a multiplicity of factors such as immobilization, inflammation, steroid use, and other lifestyle or dietary factors. Weight gain and inactivity during lockdowns contributed to these conditions as well.

Being alert to the potential for the development or exacerbation of endocrinologic issues will enhance the healthcare provider's ability to respond quickly and appropriately when managing these patients.

Dermatologic

There is broad range of dermatologic presentations that include rash, chilblains, urticaria, and "COVID-toe," but they are usually self-limiting and not prolonged. They are treated with topical steroids, antihistamines, or oral steroids. Hair loss (telogen effluvium) is a particularly distressing problem from COVID and must be addressed for its emotional and cosmetic impact. It may be short-lived, but if prolonged it must be part of a holistic program of care including dermatologic consultation, particularly if there is an ongoing autoimmune or inflammatory etiology.

Monitoring

Supportive and rehabilitative care are still the mainstay of treatment for post-acute COVID syndrome. This includes adequate rest, nutrition, immune support, activity modification, mental and cognitive stimulation, stress management, and heart and lung rehabilitation, including supplemental oxygen for some patients. Utilizing standard and evidenced treatments for lung, heart, neurologic, and renal problems is a logical start. Given protracted and relapsing symptoms, it is important to reassure patients that most cases will recover with time and supportive symptomatic care. Registries and post-COVID clinics are needed to track and manage these serious sequelae of COVID-19. Our awareness is the first line of defense. The diffuse and protean manifestations of PCS should motivate our clinicians and medical educators to include it in the differential diagnosis of many other presenting complaints.

Multidisciplinary teams are key to long-term management but are not always easily accessible. Self-care, online, and other forms of support groups have sprung up widely for emotional, social support and peer-led practical advice in managing post-acute COVID syndrome. Much of the knowledge about this syndrome has been brought to public and professional awareness by such peer groups. Further research support in this area will be helpful.

Quality-of-care principles for long-haul COVID include providing access to care, reducing the burden of illness, taking clinical responsibility, offering continuity of care, providing multidisciplinary rehabilitation, conducting evidence-based investigation and management, and continuing further research and development on appropriate and evidence-based clinical services. Given the disproportionate impact of COVID on communities of color, additional attention must be given to social determinants of health, healthcare access, and enhanced research efforts regarding the genetic and racial differences in disease impact, both acute and long-term. Determining phenotypic differences in susceptibility to post-acute COVID syndrome and personalized rehabilitation are key future directions.

Complications

Understanding of COVID-19 and its potential long-term complications is evolving and offers many opportunities for clinicians and researchers to examine. As with COVID-19 infection itself, long-term complications may broadly affect multiple body systems. Addressing these symptoms starts with recognition.

One persistent neurologic complication that remains of concern is cognitive decline, which many describe as "brain fog." Additional symptoms of neuropathic pain and headaches may require further evaluation by a neurologist.

Myocardial inflammation seen in some COVID-19 infections may lead to future reduced cardiac function, arrhythmias, scarring, or cardiomyopathy. The prevalence currently remains unknown but is a major concern in our younger population and athletes.

Pulmonary complications are common in hospitalized patients who require ventilatory assistance. Our experience in the post-COVID population shows that fibrotic conversion, if it occurs, is rare, but reduction in diffusion capacity may persist. This reduction is a sign of parenchymal disease and should be monitored if patients develop future reductions in lung volumes compared with the standard population.

Hematologic complications such as thrombosis and long-term risk remain unknown, and further study is necessary. For example, it is unknown whether COVID-19 and a thrombosis can be safely considered a short-term event and managed as a provoked clot or if there is a prolonged inflammatory cascade that leaves a sustained risk.

The behavioral health component also remains of utmost importance because so much is not known, and the duration of symptoms is not clear. Management of PTSD, anxiety, and depression for patients with long-term complications should be included in strategies addressing the care of this new and ever-growing at-risk population.

Acknowledgment

We wish to thank Ms. Julie Trumble of the University of Texas Medical Branch Moody Medical Library for her incredibly diligent work on helping us assemble and keep updated on the literature on this evolving topic with weekly literature reviews in the past year.

References

Alwan NA: Surveillance is underestimating the burden of the COVID-19 pandemic, *Lancet* 396(10252):e24, 2020.

Barker-Davies RM, O'Sullivan O, Senaratne KPP, et al: The Stanford Hall consensus statement for post-COVID-19 rehabilitation, *Br J Sports Med* 54(16):949–959, 2020.

Calabrese M, Garofano M, Palumbo R, et al: Exercise training and cardiac rehabilitation in COVID-19 patients with cardiovascular complications: state of art, *Life (Basel)* 11(3):259, 2021.

Centers for Disease Control and Prevention. Post COVID Conditions. https://www.cdc.gov/coronavirus/2019-ncov/hcp/clinical-care/post-covid-conditions.html. Accessed 3/12/22.

COVID-19 rapid guideline: managing the long-term effects of COVID-19, London, 2020, National Institute for Health and Care Excellence (UK).

Crook H, Raza S, Nowell J, Young M, Edison P: Long covid—mechanisms, risk factors, and management—state of the art review, *BMJ* 374:n1648, 2021, https://doi.org/10.1136/bmj.n1648.

Dani M, Dirksen A, Taraborrelli P, et al: Autonomic dysfunction in 'long COVID': rationale, physiology and management strategies, *Clin Med (Lond)* 21(1):e63–e67.d, 2021.

Flottorp A, Brurber K, Fink P, Knoops H, Wyller V: New NICE guideline on chronic fatigue syndrome: more ideology than science? *Lancet* 399(Feb 12):611–613, 2022. https://www.thelancet.com/journals/lancet/article/PIIS0140-6736(22)00183-0/fulltext.

Greenhalgh T, Knight M, A'Court C, Buxton M, Husain L: Management of post-acute covid-19 in primary care, *BMJ* 370:m3026, 2020.

Logue JK, Franko NM, McCulloch DJ, et al: Sequelae in Adults at 6 Months after COVID-19 infection, *JAMA Netw Open* 4(2):e210830, 2021.

Mahase E: Long covid could be four different syndromes, review suggests, *BMJ* 371:m3981, 2020.

Mendelson M, Nel J, Blumberg L, et al: Long-COVID: an evolving problem with an extensive impact, *S Afr Med J* 111(1):10–12, 2020.

Nabavi N: Long covid: How to define it and how to manage it, *BMJ* 370:m3489, 2020.

Nalbandian A, Sehgal K, Gupta A, et al. Post-acute COVID-19 syndrome. *Nature Medicine*. Available at https://doi.org/10.1038/s41591-021-1283-z

NIHR Themed Review, Living with Covid19. 2020:1-29.

PSITTACOSIS

Method of
Stephanie Spivack, MD

CURRENT DIAGNOSIS

- Psittacosis is an infection with *Chlamydia psittaci,* a bacterium that is transmitted by infected birds, especially those in the parrot family.
- Psittacosis should be considered in patients with community-acquired pneumonia (CAP) who have been exposed to birds or those who are not improving on β-lactam antibiotics.
- Psittacosis causes 1% of CAP cases and typically presents with acute onset of fever, dry cough, and headache. It can also present as an influenza-like illness.
- Laboratory findings are nonspecific and include leukocytosis with elevated neutrophil count, as well as elevated inflammatory markers. Mild hepatic and renal impairment may be seen. Chest x-ray may reveal lobar or multilobar consolidations.
- There is no gold standard for diagnosis. Culture is not recommended because it is hazardous to laboratory personnel. Serology is the most widely available test; ideally, acute and convalescent samples should be collected. Polymerase chain reaction (PCR) is sensitive and specific but is only available through the Centers for Disease Control and Prevention (CDC) and specialty labs; it is not part of commercially available multiplex PCR tests.

CURRENT THERAPY

- When psittacosis is suspected, treatment should be initiated before receiving confirmatory results.
- The first-line treatment is with tetracyclines; for example, with 7 to 10 days of doxycycline 100 mg twice daily. Macrolides are an alternative for those who cannot take tetracyclines, including pregnant persons and children under 8 years of age. Azithromycin (Zithromax)[1] is preferred over erythromycin[1] and can be given for 5 days.
- Psittacosis is a reportable disease; cases are investigated by public and animal health authorities to prevent further spread of disease.

[1]Not FDA approved for this indication.

Psittacosis, also referred to as ornithosis (which more accurately represents the fact that infection can be acquired from all bird types) or occasionally "parrot fever," is an infection with the bacterium *Chlamydia psittaci* (also known as *Chlamydophila psittaci,* though this reclassification is not widely accepted), an intracellular gram-negative organism. The clinical syndrome was first described in the 1870s and the organism was isolated in the 1930s. It has been reported worldwide in people of all ages, though it is most commonly reported in those aged 40 to 64. Humans are infected through inhalation of secretions from infected birds. *C. psittaci* is responsible for approximately 1% of cases of community-acquired pneumonia (CAP) and is likely underdiagnosed due to testing limitations.

Risk Factors
The major risk factor for developing psittacosis is exposure to birds. *C. psittaci* has been isolated from over 460 species of birds but is found most frequently in psittacine (parrot-type) birds, including parrots, parakeets, macaws, cockatiels, lories, and budgerigars. *C. psittaci* has also been isolated from poultry (turkeys, chickens, ducks, geese), pigeons, doves, finches, sparrows, birds of

prey, and shorebirds. The strains from psittacine birds and turkeys are the most virulent in humans. There is a baseline prevalence of 5% to 8% in bird populations, but this can increase dramatically when birds are subject to the stress of breeding and shipping. Infected birds may appear sick but are often asymptomatic.

Most cases of psittacosis have been reported in people with close contact to birds, including pet owners and those who are exposed through their occupation (workers at pet shops, zoos, poultry farms, abattoirs, or through veterinary or wildlife work). The most common mode of transmission is through inhalation of dried secretions, including feces, urine, and respiratory secretions. However, mouth-to-beak transmission from kissing pet birds has been reported.

In approximately one-quarter of cases, there is no known bird contact. Other reported exposures include gardening and lawnmowing (presumably due to bird secretions in the environment) and exposure to the placental tissue of mammals including horses and sheep. Human-to-human transmission has been reported but is rare. Cases are generally sporadic, but outbreaks have been reported. Notably, ingestion of poultry products is not a known risk factor.

Clinical Manifestations
The typical incubation time after exposure is 5 to 14 days, though longer periods have been reported. The classic presentation is an acute onset of fevers, chills, nonproductive cough, and prominent headache, sometimes with photophobia, which can lead to a misdiagnosis of meningitis. Other nonspecific symptoms can include myalgias, fatigue, diarrhea, poor appetite, pharyngitis, rhinorrhea, and dyspnea. A pulse-temperature dissociation has been reported, with relative bradycardia in the setting of fever.

Typical laboratory findings include leukocytosis with elevated neutrophils and elevated inflammatory markers including erythrocyte sedimentation rate (ESR), C-reactive protein (CRP), and procalcitonin. Renal and hepatic dysfunction can be seen and are typically mild. Proteinuria and hyponatremia can accompany renal dysfunction.

A variety of findings can be seen on chest x-ray. Patients may have unilateral or bilateral, lobar or multilobar consolidations, or a normal chest x-ray. As with other atypical pneumonias, the imaging findings may appear to be more severe than the clinical presentation and examination might suggest. Pleural effusions occur in up to half of cases but are typically small. If bronchoscopy is performed, findings can include hyperemia and swelling of the mucosa.

Diagnosis
There is no gold standard of diagnosis; a suspected diagnosis can be confirmed with serology or PCR. There are multiple serologic methods available; the complement fixation (CF) test is widely used but cannot distinguish between *Chlamydia* species. The microimmunofluorescent antibody (MIF) test is more sensitive and specific. The diagnosis is confirmed if there is a fourfold rise in titers between acute and convalescent specimens collected at least 2 weeks apart, or a single high titer. Polymerase chain reaction (PCR) testing is sensitive and specific and can be performed on sputum, nasopharyngeal or oropharyngeal swabs, fluid from bronchoalveolar lavage (BAL), blood, or tissue. However, PCR for *C. psittaci* is not included on commercially available multiplex PCR tests; it must be requested through the CDC or specialty labs. Culture is not recommended because it is technically difficult and is a hazard to laboratory workers.

Differential Diagnosis
The differential diagnosis includes other organisms responsible for an atypical CAP, including *Chlamydia pneumoniae, Mycoplasma pneumoniae,* and *Legionella* species. The presentation can also be similar to that of respiratory viruses including influenza and COVID-19. Other organisms like *Coxiella, Coccidioides,* and *Histoplasma* can be considered.

Psittacosis

Therapy

Because testing is not widely available, treatment for psittacosis should be started empirically based on compatible clinical findings with relevant exposure history. Psittacosis can also be considered in a patient with CAP who is not responding to β-lactam therapy.

The first-line therapy is with tetracyclines, including doxycycline and minocycline (Minocin); for example, doxycycline 100 mg twice daily. A typical duration is 7 to 10 days. Macrolides are considered second-line therapy and are an alternative for patients who cannot take tetracyclines, for example, pregnant persons and children younger than 8 years old. When macrolides are used, azithromycin (Zithromax)[1] is preferred over erythromycin[1]; a typical duration is 5 days. In critically ill patients, the potential risk of using first-line tetracyclines must be weighed against the benefits.

Monitoring

Symptoms generally improve within 24 to 48 hours of starting therapy. Rare treatment failures and relapses have been reported; if this occurs, a different class of medication should be used. Patients who have recovered may develop a reinfection, even if they have serologic evidence of antibodies. Radiographic resolution occurs after an average of 6 weeks.

Complications

Cases may range from asymptomatic or very mild infections to severe pneumonia with multisystem organ failure. Complications involving nearly every organ system have been described. These include culture-negative endocarditis, myositis, and pericarditis; meningitis and encephalitis; cold agglutinins and hemophagocytic syndromes; and reactive arthritis. C. psittaci has also been associated with ocular adnexal lymphoma (OAL), but it is unclear what role it plays in disease pathogenesis. Additionally, adverse pregnancy outcomes have been reported in patients who develop psittacosis while pregnant. Mortality is low (1%) in the age of antibiotics.

Prevention

In hospitalized patients, standard infections prevention measures are sufficient. No prophylaxis is recommended for contacts of infected patients.

Psittacosis is a reportable disease, and confirmed cases are investigated by both public health agencies and animal health agencies to prevent the spread of disease to additional humans and animals. Infected birds should be quarantined and treated by veterinary professionals.

---

[1] Not FDA approved for this indication.

References

Balsamo G, Maxted AM, Midla JW, et al: Compendium of measures to Control Chlamydia psittaci infection among humans (psittacosis) and pet birds (avian chlamydiosis), J Avian Med Surg 31(3):262–282, 2017. Available at https://doi.org/10.1647/217-265. Accessed 31 March 2025.

Centers for Disease Control. Psittacosis. Available at https://www.cdc.gov/psittacosis/about/index.html [Accessed 03/31/2025].

Hogerwerf L, DeGier B, Baan B, Van Der Hoek W: Chlamydia psittaci (psittacosis) as a cause of community-acquired pneumonia: a systematic review and meta-analysis, Epidemiol Infect 145(15):3096–3105, 2017. Available at https://doi.org/10.1017/S0950268817002060. Accessed 31 March 2025.

Li X, Xiao T, Hu P, et al: Clinical, radiological and pathological characteristics of moderate to fulminant psittacosis pneumonia, PLoS One 17(7), 2022:e0270896. Available at https://doi.org/10.1371/journal.pone.0270896. Accessed 31 March 2025.

Nieuwenhuizen AA, Dijkstra F, Notermans DW, van der Hoek W: Laboratory methods for case finding in human psittacosis outbreaks: a systematic review, BMC Infect Dis 18(1):442, 2022. Available at https://doi.org/10.1186/s12879-018-3317-0. Accessed 31 March 2025.

Schlossberg D: Psittacosis (due to Chlamydia psittaci). Mandell, douglas, and bennett's principles and practice of infectious diseases—electronic, ed 9, Elsevier eBooks, 2019, pp 2320–2322.

Yung AP, Grayson ML: Psittacosis-a review of 135 cases, Med J Aust 148(5):228–233, 1988. Available at https://doi.org/10.5694/j.1326-5377.1988.tb99430.x. Accessed 31 March 2025.

Q FEVER

Method of
Sarah Kurz, MD

CURRENT DIAGNOSIS

- Indirect immunofluorescence antibody using the *Coxiella burnetii* antigen is the most commonly used diagnostic modality (immunoglobulin [Ig]G phase I, IgG phase II, IgM).
- Acute disease is diagnosed by either a fourfold rise in the titer between acute and convalescent plasma samples *or a* positive IgM *or* positive polymerase chain reaction (PCR).
- Persistent or chronic disease is diagnosed by evidence of a lesion in combination with an IgG phase I titer at least 1:800 *or* a positive biopsy *or* a positive PCR.
- Endocarditis is the most common manifestation of chronic disease and is typically confirmed serologically in the appropriate clinical context (compliment fixation titer of 1:200 or higher to phase I antigen); vegetation is only seen in half the cases.
- In persistent or chronic infection, the IgG phase I titer is typically much higher than the IgG phase II titer.
- With tissue samples, standard histopathologic stains are negative, although PCR assays can be run from blood, heart valves, and joint fluid.

CURRENT THERAPY

- Acute Q fever: 14 days of doxycycline or minocycline (Minocin)
- Endocarditis (native valve): doxycycline *plus* hydroxychloroquine (Plaquenil)[1] for 18 months
- Endocarditis (prosthetic valve): doxycycline *plus* hydroxychloroquine[1] for 2 years

[1] Not FDA approved for this indication.

Coxiella burnetii is the bacteria that causes the disease referred to as Q fever. It is a gram-negative coccobacillus that is an intracellular pathogen and has a spore stage that helps it withstand harsh environmental conditions. Acute infection leads to antibodies mostly against phase II antigens, whereas chronic infections more typically have IgG antibodies directed against phase I antigens.

Pathophysiology

Q fever is a zoonotic disease transmitted to humans from animals, but human-to-human transmission has also been documented. The organism is likely maintained in soft ticks and arthropods that then infect domestic and a variety of other small mammals. *C. burnetii* infections are most common in farm animals such as cows, sheep, and goats that are usually asymptomatic. The bacteria can be found in the urine, feces, milk, and birth products of these infected animals. At time of delivery, the placenta contaminates the environment and can persist in air samples for up to 2 weeks after delivery and in the soil for longer. There is also a large wildlife reservoir. Windborne spread from a contaminated environment can happen as far as 10 km away from the initial site. The bacteria are distributed worldwide except for New Zealand, Polynesia, and Antarctica. *C. burnetii* is highly pathogenic and even a single germ may be capable of producing infection. The larger the size of the inoculum, the higher the chance of developing significant disease.

Q fever can be transmitted to humans when people breathe in dust that has been contaminated with infected animal products. Another mode of transmission to humans that has been proposed is the consumption of contaminated, unpasteurized dairy products. *C. burnetii* can cause a range of diseases from asymptomatic infection to a flu-like illness, as well as endovascular infections. Transmission can also happen in laboratory settings. People who work as veterinarians, in dairy or livestock farms, or researchers at facilities with sheep, cows, or goats are at higher risk. It is also considered a potential bioterrorism agent.

The microorganisms replicate in the lungs and then invade the bloodstream. The vascular invasion typically corresponds to development of systemic symptoms including high fever, fatigue, myalgias, headache, chills, and diarrhea. There are a variety of possible clinical manifestations that have to do with the initial inoculum (dose of microorganisms inhaled) and the strain of *C. burnetii*. The development of endocarditis and more chronic infection with *C. burnetii* seems to be more related to host factors, and patients who have existing valve lesions, arterial aneurysms, or who are pregnant or have cancer are at higher risk. The incubation period averages 20 days.

Clinical Manifestations
Most commonly, disease in humans manifests as asymptomatic (as high as 60%) or mild, self-limited disease. Only around 5% of patients will go on to have the chronic form of the disease. Common clinical syndromes associated with *C. burnetii* include self-limited febrile illness, pneumonia, endocarditis, or hepatitis. Much less common clinical manifestations include meningitis, encephalitis, and osteomyelitis. Women infected during pregnancy might be at higher risk of preterm delivery, miscarriage, or stillbirth.

A self-limited febrile illness is the most common form of Q fever, and patients who are seropositive for *C. burnetii* often do not recall having pneumonia or other severe illness. Common laboratory abnormalities include mild thrombocytopenia and mildly elevated transaminases. In patients who develop pneumonia, less than 50% of them have a cough but all have fever; a severe headache is commonly present and can be a useful diagnostic clue. Radiographic findings can be variable, with pleural-based opacities seen commonly, as well as multiple rounded opacities, hilar lymphadenopathy, and pleural effusions.

Acute Q fever can also present as an isolated hepatitis. This is characterized by elevated liver enzymes (typically two to four times the upper limit of normal) associated with a fever, chills, and headache. It has a good prognosis. If a liver biopsy is performed, the typical pathologic finding is a "doughnut" granuloma. In terms of neurologic manifestations, severe headache is common in acute Q fever pneumonia, but there is no robust evidence of serious brain involvement. Aseptic meningitis and encephalitis have been reported but in a very small minority of cases.

A small percentage (5%) of those who get infected with *C. burnetii* can go on to develop chronic Q fever, which is usually an endovascular infection within the 2 years after primary infection but can be seen as early as 3 months. Endocarditis is the most common manifestation of chronic Q fever. Chronic Q fever has also been referred to as "persistent focalized infection" as there is no chronic manifestation of the disease without a focal lesion. Abnormal native valves or prosthetic valves predispose to the development of *C. burnetii* endocarditis. Any part of the vascular tree can be affected, and aortic aneurysms are also predisposed to infection. Patients may have fatigue, night sweats, weight loss, and symptoms of heart failure such as swelling of their lower extremities. People with valvular disease or vascular disease along with immunocompromised patients are more at risk for developing this more serious and chronic form of the disease.

Diagnosis
The diagnosis of Q fever is typically made serologically with indirect immunofluorescent antibody (IFA) using *C. burnetii* antigen and paired patient plasma samples to demonstrate a significant rise (fourfold or more) in the immunoglobulin (Ig)G IFA titer between acute and convalescent plasma samples. The first sample should be taken as early in the acute illness as possible, ideally during the first week of symptoms, and the second sample should be taken 3 to 6 weeks later. In most cases, the first IgG IFA will be low or normal and the second will show a fourfold or greater rise in titer. There are two distinct antigenic phases (phase I and phase II) of the disease to which humans develop an antibody response. In acute infection, the predominant response is to phase II antigen, and thus higher IgG IFA phase II antibody titers are seen compared with IgG IFA phase I. The reverse is true in chronic infection, where a rising IgG phase I titer is seen and may be higher than IgG phase II. In acute disease, a positive IgM or a positive polymerase chain reaction (PCR) are also diagnostic. IgM typically starts to rise by the end of the first week of illness and can remain elevated for months or longer, which does limit its diagnostic utility. IgM antibodies are less specific than IgG antibodies, and IgM titers should never be sent without concurrently sending IgG titers.

For persistent (chronic) localized infections such as endocarditis or osteomyelitis, the diagnosis is made by the presence of a lesion on imaging (such as a vegetation, nodular valvular thickening, or chordae rupture on echocardiogram or evidence of osteomyelitis radiographically) in the setting of an IgG phase I titer at least 1:800, a positive PCR from serum, or biopsy sample in the appropriate clinical setting.

The Duke Criteria are used to help rule in or out a diagnosis of endocarditis and either IgG phase I titer at least 1:800. A single blood culture positive for *C. burnetii* is considered a major Duke criterion for the diagnosis of endocarditis.

Therapy
It is important not to delay treatment when Q fever is suspected even while the diagnostic workup is ongoing. Efficacious treatment must be intracellularly active and effective at an acidic pH. The treatment of choice for acute Q fever in adults is 14 days of doxycycline 100 mg two times per day. If a patient is intolerant of doxycycline, then trimethoprim/sulfamethoxazole[1] (Bactrim) 160 mg/800 mg two times per day for 14 days or moxifloxacin (Avelox)[1] (less robust literature on dosing) are reasonable alternatives. For pregnant women, trimethoprim/sulfamethoxazole 160 mg/800 mg two times per day should be given throughout pregnancy up to 32 weeks' gestation.

For the treatment of endocarditis, two antibiotics are required for a much longer period of time. The current preferred regimen is doxycycline 100 mg two times per day *plus* hydroxychloroquine (Plaquenil)[1] 200 mg three times per day for 18 months for patients with native valve endocarditis and 2 years for patients with prosthetic valve endocarditis. For patients with prosthetic valve endocarditis, surgery is critical for cure of the infected prostheses.

Prevention
There is no vaccine available for Q fever in the United States. In the United States, the majority of occupationally related Q fever outbreaks occur at biomedical research facilities where workers are exposed to infected pregnant sheep. The CDC has put in place guidance for such facilities to create a medical surveillance and health education monitoring program along with engineering controls and use of personal protective equipment when appropriate. In the healthcare setting, the use of standard precautions by providers is sufficient to prevent Q fever transmission during routine care of patients with Q fever.

Monitoring
There is debate about the best way to follow and monitor patients, but there is consensus that all patients with acute Q fever should be monitored for the development of cardiovascular infections. Q fever endocarditis used to be considered almost universally fatal, and the changes in monitoring and treatment have transformed this clinical manifestation into a curable disease. Some advocate for early transthoracic echocardiogram during the acute phase of the disease to look both for acute endocarditis and valvular lesions, which predispose patients to the development of *C.*

[1] Not FDA approved for this indication.

Q Fever

709

burnetii endocarditis. Others argue that valvopathy is not significantly associated with the development of endocarditis and that universal transthoracic echocardiograms during the acute phase of the disease are an unnecessary cost.

Serology should be monitored every 3 months for up to 2 years after an episode of acute Q fever as rising serologic titers warrant additional evaluation for a focal lesion (cardiovascular, osteomyelitis) with transthoracic echocardiogram or radiology.

Patients being treated for *C. burnetii* endocarditis should be followed by an infectious diseases specialist and should have periodic monitoring for serologic response while on treatment with recommendations varying from monthly to every 3 to 6 months while on therapy and every 3 months for the first 2 years after therapy is complete. Successful treatment is accompanied by declining antibody titers and declining erythrocyte sedimentation rate, and correction of anemia. Hydroxychloroquine can cause retinal toxicity, so all patients should have a baseline ophthalmic exam and follow-up exams every 6 months while on therapy.

Complications

Up to 20% of patients can go on to develop extended significant fatigue after acute infection with Q fever. This has been termed "Q fever fatigue syndrome" (QFFS) and can include fatigue, headaches, seats, arthralgias, and myalgias, as well as large, painful lymph nodes. Studies looking at treatment of QFFS have concluded that patients should not be given extended courses of doxycycline.

References

Anderson A, Bijlmer H, Fournier PE, et al. (2013). Diagnosis and Management of Q Fever — United States, 2013: Recommendations from CDC and the Q Fever Working Group (Vol. 62, No. 3. Morbidity and Mortality Weekly Report. https://www.cdc.gov/mmwr/preview/mmwrhtml/rr6203a1.htm.

Bennett JE, Dolin R, Blaser MJ: *Principles and Practice of Infectious Diseases. Volume 2*, ed 9, Elsevier, 2020.

Eldin C, Melenotte C, Mediannikov O, et al: From Q fever to Coxiella burnetii infection: a paradigm change, *Clin Microbiol Rev* 30:115–190, 2017.

España PP, Uranga A, Cillóniz C, Torres A: Q Fever (Coxiella Burnetii), *Semin Respir Crit Care Med* 41(4):509–521, 2020.

Marin M, Raoult D: Q Fever, *CMR* 12:518–553, 1999.

Melenotte Cléa, Epelboin Loïc, Million Matthieu, et al: Acute Q Fever Endocarditis: A Paradigm Shift Following the Systematic Use of Transthoracic Echocardiography During Acute Q Fever, *Clinical Infectious Diseases* 69(11):1987–1995, 2019.

Million M, Raoult D: Recent advances in the study of Q fever epidemiology, diagnosis and management, *J Infect* 71:S2–S9, 2015.

Morroy G, Keijmel Sp, Delsing CE, et al: Fatigue following acute Q-fever: a systemic literature review, *PLoS ONE*, 2016. 11e0155884.

Redden P, Parker K, Henderson S, Fourie P, Agnew L, Stenos J, Graves S, Govan B, Norton R, Ketheesan N: Q fever - immune responses and novel vaccine strategies, *Future Microbiol* 18:1185–1196, 2023.

RABIES

Method of
Alan C. Jackson, MD

CURRENT DIAGNOSIS

- A history of animal bite or exposure is often absent in rabies acquired in North America.
- Pain, paresthesias, and pruritus are early neurologic symptoms of rabies, probably reflecting infection in local sensory ganglia.
- Autonomic features, hypersalivation, gooseflesh, cardiac arrhythmias, and priapism, are common.
- Hydrophobia is a highly specific feature of rabies.
- Paralytic features may be prominent, and the clinical presentation can resemble that of Guillain-Barré syndrome.
- Saliva samples for reverse transcription polymerase chain reaction (RT-PCR) and a skin biopsy should be obtained to detect rabies virus antigen or RNA to make a laboratory diagnosis of rabies.

CURRENT THERAPY

Rabies Prophylaxis
Details of an exposure determine whether postexposure rabies prophylaxis should be initiated.
- Wound cleansing is important after potential rabies exposure.
- Active immunization with a schedule of four doses of rabies vaccine (RabAvert or Imovax Rabies) at intervals is recommended. The four- dose series is a new Centers for Disease Control and Prevention (CDC) recommendation and is not yet reflected in the package insert, which calls for five doses.
- Passive immunization (if previously the patient was not immunized) consists of infiltrating human rabies immune globulin (HyperRAB, Imogam Rabies, or KamRAB) into the wound, with the remainder of the 20 IU/kg dosage given intramuscularly.

Rabies Cases
- There is no established effective therapy for rabies, but there is an increasing number of survivors who received supportive care in critical care units, particularly in India.
- Palliation is important for many fatal cases of rabies.

Rabies is an acute infection of the nervous system caused by rabies virus, which is a member of the family Rhabdoviridae in the genus *Lyssavirus*. Other lyssaviruses have only very rarely caused rabies in locations outside of the Americas.

Pathogenesis

Rabies virus is usually transmitted by bites from rabid animals. Transmission has rarely occurred through an aerosol route (in a laboratory accident or in a cave containing millions of bats) or by transplantation of infected organs or tissues (e.g., corneas). The virus is in the saliva of the rabid animal and is inoculated into subcutaneous tissues or muscles via a bite.

During most of the long incubation period (lasting 20–90 days or longer), the virus is close to the site of inoculation. The virus binds to the nicotinic acetylcholine receptor at the postsynaptic neuromuscular junction and travels toward the central nervous system (CNS) in peripheral nerves by retrograde fast axonal transport. There is rapid dissemination throughout the CNS by fast axonal transport. Under natural conditions, degenerative neuronal changes are not prominent, and it is thought that the rabies virus induces neuronal dysfunction by mechanisms that are not well understood. Oxidative stress due to mitochondrial dysfunction is thought to play an important role. In rabies vectors, the encephalitis is associated with behavioral changes that lead to transmission by biting. After the CNS infection is established, the virus spreads by autonomic and sensory nerves to multiple organs, including the salivary glands of rabies vectors in which the virus is secreted in saliva.

Clinical Features

In North America, where the bat is the most common rabies vector for human disease, a history of an animal bite is often absent, and there may be no known contact with animals. Many bats are small, and bat bites or scratches may not be recognized. The incubation period is usually between 20 and 90 days, and it rarely lasts 1 year or longer. Prodromal features are nonspecific and include malaise, headache, and fever, and patients can also have anxiety or agitation. Approximately half of patients experience pain, paresthesias, or pruritus at the site of the wound, which has often healed, and these symptoms likely reflect infection and inflammation involving local sensory ganglia. Approximately 80% of patients with rabies have encephalitic rabies; approximately 20% have paralytic rabies.

In encephalitic rabies, there are characteristic periods of generalized arousal or hyperexcitability separated by lucid periods. Autonomic dysfunction is common and includes hypersalivation, gooseflesh, cardiac arrhythmias, and priapism. Hydrophobia is the most characteristic feature of rabies and occurs in 50% to 80% of patients; contractions of the diaphragm and other inspiratory muscles occur on swallowing. This can become a conditioned reflex, and even the sight or thought of water can precipitate the muscle contractions. Hydrophobia is thought to be caused by inhibition of inspiratory neurons near the nucleus ambiguus.

In paralytic rabies, prominent muscle weakness usually begins in the bitten extremity and progresses to quadriparesis; typically there is sphincter involvement. Patients have a longer clinical course than in encephalitic rabies. Paralytic rabies is often misdiagnosed as Guillain-Barré syndrome.

Coma subsequently develops in both clinical forms. With aggressive medical therapy, a variety of medical complications develop, and multiple organ failure is common. Survival is very rare and has usually occurred in the context of incomplete postexposure rabies prophylaxis that included administration of one or more doses of rabies vaccine.

Epidemiology

Worldwide about 60,000 human deaths per year are attributed to rabies. The impact is particularly significant in terms of years of life lost because children are commonly the victims. Most human rabies cases occur through transmission from dogs in developing countries with endemic dog rabies, particularly in Asia and Africa. Travelers to endemic regions may develop rabies after they return home if they have not received effective postexposure rabies prophylaxis after an exposure. In the United States and Canada, transmission of rabies virus occurs most commonly in human cases from insect-eating bats, and often there is no known history of a bat bite or exposure to bats. A bat bite might not be recognized. The rabies virus variants responsible for most human cases are found in silver-haired bats and tricolored bats, and also in Brazilian (Mexican) free-tailed bats. These are small bats. Other rabies vectors in North American wildlife include skunks, raccoons, and foxes, but these species are rarely responsible for transmission to humans. This is likely because postexposure rabies prophylaxis is administered after recognized exposures.

Diagnosis

Most cases of rabies can be diagnosed clinically or the diagnosis will be strongly suspected, which is particularly important so that appropriate barrier nursing techniques can be initiated to prevent exposures of many health care workers. Some patients are potential candidates for an aggressive therapeutic approach. A serum-neutralizing titer can be useful for diagnosis in a previously unimmunized person, but a positive titer might not develop until the second week of clinical illness or later, and the result of the test might not be readily available. Detection of rabies virus antigen in a skin biopsy obtained from the nape of the neck using a fluorescent antibody technique is a useful diagnostic test. Detection of rabies virus ribonucleic acid (RNA) in saliva or in skin biopsies using RT-PCR amplification is an important recent advance for rapid rabies diagnosis. Rabies virus antigen can be detected in brain tissue obtained by brain biopsy or postmortem. Negative antemortem diagnostic laboratory tests do not exclude rabies and the tests may need to be repeated on subsequent samples.

Prevention

After a rabies exposure is recognized, rabies can be prevented with initiation of appropriate steps, including wound cleansing and active and passive immunization. After a human is bitten by a dog, cat, or ferret, the animal should be captured, confined, and observed for a period of at least 10 days; initiation of postexposure rabies prophylaxis is not necessary if the animal remains healthy. The animal should also be examined by a veterinarian prior to its release. If the animal is a stray, unwanted, shows signs of rabies, or develops signs of rabies during the observation

period, the animal should be killed immediately, and its head should be transported under refrigeration for a laboratory examination. The brain should be examined via an antigen-detection method using the fluorescent antibody technique and viral isolation using cell culture or mouse inoculation.

The incubation period for animals other than dogs, cats, and ferrets is uncertain; these animals should be killed immediately after an exposure, and the head should be submitted for examination. If the result is negative, one may safely conclude that the animal's saliva did not contain rabies virus; if immunization has been initiated, it should be discontinued. If an animal escapes after an exposure, it should be considered rabid unless information from public health officials indicates this is unlikely, and rabies prophylaxis should be initiated. The physical presence of a bat might warrant postexposure prophylaxis when a person (such as a small child or sleeping adult) is unable to reliably report contact that could have resulted in a bite.

Local wound care should be given as soon as possible after all exposures, even if immunization is delayed, pending the results of an observation period. All bite wounds and scratches should be washed thoroughly with soap and water. Devitalized tissues should be débrided.

Purified chick embryo cell culture vaccine (RabAvert) and human diploid cell vaccine (Imovax Rabies) are licensed rabies vaccines in the United States and Canada. Other vaccines grown in either primary cell lines (hamster or dog kidney) or continuous cell lines (Vero cells) are also satisfactory and available in other countries. A regimen of four 1-mL doses of rabies vaccine should be given IM in the deltoid area (anterolateral aspect of the thigh is also acceptable in children). The four-dose series is a CDC recommendation and is an update from the five doses recommended in the current package insert. Ideally, the first dose should be given as soon as possible after exposure, but failing that, it should be given regardless of the length of a delay. Three additional doses should be given on days 3, 7, and 14. Additional vaccine doses may be indicated for immunocompromised patients. Pregnancy is not a contraindication for immunization. Live vaccines should not be given for 1 month after rabies immunization. Preexposure rabies immunization is useful for people at high risk of a rabies exposure.

Local and mild systemic reactions are common. Systemic allergic reactions are uncommon, and anaphylactic reactions may be treated with epinephrine and antihistamines. Corticosteroids can interfere with the development of active immunity. Immunosuppressive medications should not be administered during postexposure therapy unless they are essential. The risk of developing rabies should be carefully considered before deciding to discontinue vaccination because of an adverse reaction. A serum-neutralizing antibody determination is necessary only after immunization of immunocompromised patients. Less-expensive vaccines derived from neural tissues are still used in some developing countries; these vaccines are associated with serious neuroparalytic complications.

Human rabies immune globulin (Imogam Rabies, HyperRAB, or KamRAB) should also be administered as passive immunization for protection before the development of immunity from the vaccine. It should be given at the same time as the first dose of vaccine and no later than 7 days after the first dose. Rabies vaccine and human rabies immune globulin should never be administered at the same site or in the same syringe. The recommended dose of human rabies immune globulin is 20 IU/kg; larger doses should not be given because they can suppress active immunity from the vaccine. After wounds are washed, they should be infiltrated with human rabies immune globulin (if anatomically feasible), and the remainder of the dose should be given IM in the gluteal area. Current updated recommendations by the World Health Organization do not recommend giving the remainder of the dose intramuscularly under certain circumstances. If the exposure involves a mucous membrane, the entire dose should be administered IM. With multiple or large wounds, the human rabies immune globulin might need to be diluted for adequate infiltration of all of the wounds. Adverse effects of human rabies immune globulin include local pain and low-grade fever.

After an exposure, a previously immunized patient should receive two 1-mL doses of rabies vaccine on days 0 and 3, but the patient should not receive human rabies immune globulin.

Management of Human Rabies

About 33 people have survived rabies, and there have been many recent survivors in India due to supportive critical care measures, and most have neurological sequelae (see Jackson, 2025a, b). The possibilities for an aggressive approach were reviewed (see Jackson et al., 2003). There was one survivor in Wisconsin in 2004 who did not receive rabies vaccine. It is now doubtful whether the therapy she received played a significant role in her favorable outcome because a similar approach has failed in many cases (see Jackson, 2013, 2025a, b), and there are concerns about its scientific rationale (see Zeiler and Jackson, 2016). There was a recent survivor with severe neurological sequelae in Mexico in 2022. This patient did not receive rabies vaccine until after the onset of disease. Palliation is an important alternative approach and may be appropriate for many patients in whom rabies develops (see Jackson, 2025b).

References

Fooks AR, Banyard AC, Horton DL, et al: Current status of rabies and prospects for elimination, *Lancet* 384:1389–1399, 2014.
Jackson AC, Fooks AR, editors: *Rabies: scientific basis of the disease and its management*, 5th ed., London, UK, 2025, Elsevier Academic Press (in press).
Jackson AC: Therapy of human rabies. In Jackson AC, Fooks AR, editors: *Rabies: scientific basis of the disease and its management*, 5th ed., London, UK, 2025a, Elsevier Academic Press (In press).
Jackson AC: Treatment of rabies. In: Hirsch MS, Edwards MS, Hall KK, editors. *UpToDate*. Waltham, MA: Wolters Kluwer, 2025b (in press).
Jackson AC: Pathogenesis. In Jackson AC, Fooks AR, editors: *Rabies: scientific basis of the disease and its management*, 5th ed., London, UK, 2025c, Elsevier Academic Press (in press).
Jackson AC: Demise of the Milwaukee protocol for rabies. *Clin Infect Dis*, 2025d (in press).
Jackson AC: Current and future approaches to the therapy of human rabies, *Antiviral Res* 99:61–67, 2013.
Jackson AC, Warrell MJ, Rupprecht CE, et al: Management of rabies in humans, *Clin Infect Dis* 36:60–63, 2003.
Manning SE, Rupprecht CE, Fishbein D, et al: Human rabies prevention—United States, 2008: Recommendations of the Advisory Committee on Immunization Practices, *MMWR Recomm Rep* 57(RR-3):1–28, 2008.
World Health Organization: *WHO expert consultation on rabies. Third report, WHO Technical Report Series 1012*, Geneva, 2018, WHO.
Zeiler FA, Jackson AC: Critical appraisal of the Milwaukee protocol for rabies: this failed approach should be abandoned, *Can J Neurol Sci* 43:44–51, 2016.

RAT-BITE FEVER

Method of
Jatin M. Vyas, MD, PhD

CURRENT DIAGNOSIS

- Exposure to rats is the major risk factor. Transmission can occur with simple contact with infected animals or excreta.
- A maculopapular rash and septic arthritis after initial symptoms of fever or sepsis should raise the suspicion of rat-bite fever.
- Clinicians must maintain a high index of suspicion for this diagnosis.
- Notify microbiology laboratory of clinical suspicion (slow growth, 5%–10% CO_2 microaerophilic conditions, 20% normal rabbit serum media supplementation, and avoidance of sodium polyanethol sulfonate when collecting blood cultures from the patient).

CURRENT THERAPY

Bite Site
- Clean and disinfect the bite site.
- Administer tetanus toxoid (tetanus-diphtheria toxoids, Td), if indicated.
- Postexposure rabies prophylaxis (Imovax Rabies) for animal bites should be considered in consultation with local public health authorities, though there are no reports of rat-to-human transmission of the rabies virus.

Established and Suspected Cases
- Give intravenous penicillin G at a dose of 1.2 million U/day for 5 to 7 days, followed by oral penicillin (PenVK)[1] or ampicillin (Omnipen)[1] 500 mg qid for an additional 7 days.
- For penicillin-allergic patients, consider doxycycline (Vibramycin)[1] 100 mg IV/PO twice daily or tetracycline (Achromycin)[1] 500 mg PO four times daily.
- *S. moniliformis* can be resistant to gentamicin (Garamycin),[1] tobramycin (Nebcin),[1] ciprofloxacin (Cipro),[1] and levofloxacin (Levaquin).[1]

[1]Not FDA approved for this indication.

Rat-bite fever (RBF) is a systemic, febrile disease caused by infection with *Streptobacillus moniliformis* or *Spirillum minus*. As the name implies, this infection is transmitted by a rat bite. However, the bacteria can also be transmitted by simple contact with infected rats or even through ingestion of food contaminated with rat excreta. Diagnosis can be difficult, and a high degree of suspicion is necessary to make a correct diagnosis. Recognition and early treatment are crucial, because case fatality is as high as 25% in untreated cases.

Epidemiology

S moniliformis is part of the normal respiratory flora of the rat. From 50% to 100% of healthy wild, laboratory, and pet rats harbor *S moniliformis* in the nasopharynx. *S moniliformis* is also excreted in the urine. *S minus* causes rat-bite fever mostly in Asia, but this organism is found worldwide. *S minus* has been demonstrated in rat conjunctival secretions and blood. Thus rat-bite fever can be transmitted not only from a bite but also through scratches, handling of dead rats, handling litter material, or by contamination of rat excreta.

Although the rat is the natural reservoir and major vector of the disease, *S moniliformis* has also been found in other rodents such as mice, squirrels, gerbils, and weasels. No precise data are available on the true incidence of rat-bite fever because it is not a reportable disease. It appears to be unusual in Western countries, a rarity that might reflect failed diagnosis, empiric treatment of infected bites and scratches caused by animals, or spontaneous recovery.

Risk Factors

The major risk factor is exposure to rats, either as an occupational hazard for persons such as laboratory workers, veterinarians, or pet shop employees, or for persons who have rats for pets or feed rats to snakes, especially children. Classically, homelessness and lower socioeconomic status were described as major factors, but most cases reported in the last few years have involved pet rats. Thirty percent of patients with rat-bite fever do not report any exposure to rats or other rodents. Therefore the lack of documented exposure does not exclude this diagnosis.

Pathophysiology

Very little is known about the pathophysiology of *S moniliformis* infections. Presumably, the failure of local control by dendritic cells, tissue macrophages, neutrophils, and other components of the innate immune system results in deeper infection, leading to bacteremia. Studies using histologic analysis have revealed intravascular thrombosis near the port of entry.

Prevention

The role of prophylactic antibiotics is unknown, but some authors recommend the use of oral penicillin V (PenVK)[1] after documented exposure to rats and a break in the skin. Penicillin V should be given for 3 days at a dose of 2 g per day for adults. Primary prevention should be encouraged for patients with occupational risk by using protective gloves to handle animals or cages.

Clinical Manifestations

Rat-bite fever is a systemic febrile disease. Classically, following a rat bite and a short incubation of 2 to 10 days, systemic dissemination of the organism is associated with an abrupt onset with intermittent relapsing fever, rigors, myalgias, arthralgias, headache, sore throat, malaise, and vomiting. These symptoms are followed within the first week by the development of a maculopapular rash in 75% of patients. The rash can be pustular, purpuric, or petechial, and it typically involves the extremities, in particular the palms and soles. The bite site typically heals promptly, with minimal inflammation and no significant regional lymphadenopathy.

Following the rash, approximately 50% of infected patients develop an asymmetric migrating polyarthritis, which appears to be exceedingly painful and affects large and middle-sized joints. Joint effusion appears more common in adults. Infection can occur in any tissue. Although most cases of rat-bite fever resolve spontaneously, there have been reports of complications. These include meningitis, endocarditis (including prosthetic valve endocarditis), myocarditis, pericarditis, pneumonia, brain abscess, septic arthritis, DIC (disseminated intravascular coagulation), and infarcts of the spleen and kidneys. The mortality rate in untreated cases is around 10% to 15%, and it rises to more than 50% in the rare cases with cardiac involvement.

Two closely related variants have been described. In Havervill fever, the organism is transmitted by ingestion of contaminated food. Havervill fever tends to occur in epidemics and also causes rashes and arthritis, but upper respiratory tract symptoms and vomiting appear more prominent. It is important to note that these patients do not provide a history of exposure to rodents. Sodoku is a rat-bite fever caused by *S minus*; it is common in Japan. The course is more subacute, arthritic symptoms are rare, and if the bite initially heals, it then ulcerates and is associated with regional lymphadenopathy and a distinctive rash. *S minus* cannot be grown using synthetic media, and thus microbiologic diagnosis rests on visualization of these organisms in infected tissues.

Diagnosis

Diagnosis is difficult and requires a high clinical index of suspicion. The initial symptoms of rat-bite fever are nonspecific, triggering a broad differential diagnosis. Additionally, the fastidious nature of this organism makes isolation from blood cultures difficult. Clinicians should ask about rodent exposure when compatible symptoms are seen in patients. Rat-bite fever should not be ruled out in the absence of bite history, because transmission can occur without a bite, and pet owners or laboratory workers can minimize the significance of the bite, especially in the absence of a local reaction.

No reliable serologic test is available, and the definitive diagnosis requires isolation of *S moniliformis* from the wound, blood, or synovial fluid in patients with septic arthritis. The microbiology

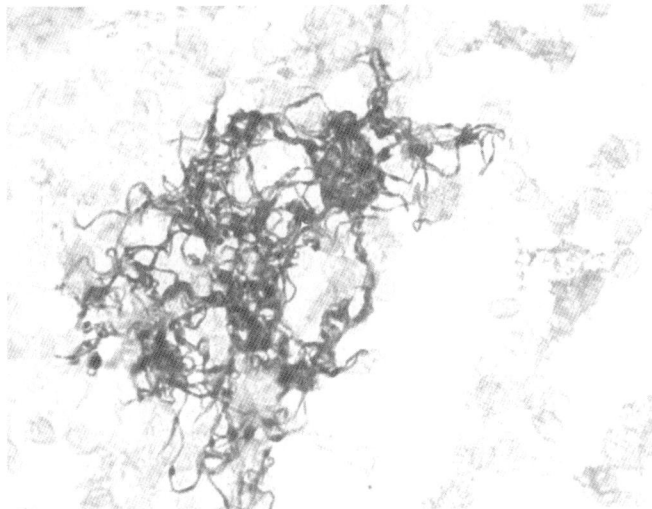

Figure 1 Gram stain of *Streptobacillus moniliformis*. Gram stain of growth from anaerobic bottle, ×100 magnification [microphotography]. Reprinted with permission from Partners' Infectious Disease Images; accessed on August 11, 2016, from http://www.idimages.org/images/detail/?imageid=373.

laboratory should be specifically notified of any clinical suspicion to enhance the chances of recovering the pathogen.

S moniliformis is a highly pleomorphic, nonencapsulated, nonmotile, gram-negative rod, which can stain positively on Gram stain (Figure 1). It is often dismissed as proteinaceous debris because of its numerous bulbous swellings with occasional clumping (*moniliformis*="necklace-like"). It grows slowly and requires a microaerophilic environment with 5% to 10% CO_2 or anaerobic conditions and media supplementation with 20% normal rabbit serum. Cultures can take up to 7 days to turn positive. Some experts recommend holding blood cultures for 21 days to permit sufficient time to grow this organism. *S moniliformis* is also inhibited by sodium polyanethol sulfonate, a common adjunct in most commercial blood culture media at a concentration as low as 0.0125%. *S moniliformis* has been identified using polymerase chain reaction amplification and 16S ribosomal ribonucleic acid (rRNA) sequencing, which shows great promise though it is available at reference laboratories. Fatty acid profiles obtained by gas-liquid chromatography can also be used for identification.

S minus, the other etiologic agent of rat-bite fever, is a short, thick, gram-negative, tightly coiled spiral rod that measures 0.2 to 0.5 μm and has two to six helical turns.

Differential Diagnosis

Differential diagnosis for fever, rash, and polyarthritis is broad. Malaria, typhoid fever, and neoplastic disease can cause relapsing fevers, and the presence of a rash and polyarthritis might suggest viral and rickettsial diseases including Rocky Mountain spotted fever. An asymmetric oligoarthritis suggests disseminated gonococcal and meningococcal diseases in the context of cutaneous lesions on the palms and soles. Lyme disease, leptospirosis, or secondary syphilis can have a similar clinical presentation. Finally, when classic infectious symptoms such as fever or rash are missing, any causes of polyarthritis, from crystal-induced arthropathies to rheumatoid arthritis, should be considered.

Treatment

All established cases of rat-bite fever should be treated with antibiotics because of the associated mortality and potential for complications. Intravenous penicillin G at a dose of 1.2 million units per day should be initiated as soon as the clinical diagnosis is

---

[1]Not FDA approved for this indication.

made. Empiric therapy is necessary and should not be delayed for laboratory confirmation of this bacterial infection. The intravenous treatment should continue for 5 to 7 days. After treatment with IV penicillin and suitable clinical response, therapy should be continued with oral penicillin (PenVK)[1] or ampicillin (Omnipen)[1] at a dose of 500 mg qid for an additional 7 days. For patients allergic to penicillin, intravenous doxycycline (Vibramycin)[1] at a dose of 100 mg every 12 hours or oral tetracycline (Achromycin)[1] at a dose of 500 mg four times a day can be used.

Streptomycin[1] and cephalosporins including cefotamxine (Claforan)[1] have been reported to be potentially useful. Other antibiotics including azithromycin (Zithromax),[1] erythromycin,[1] carbapenems,[1] aztreonam (Azactam),[1] clindamycin (Cleocin),[1] vancomycin (Vancocin),[1] and nitrofurantoin (Macrodantin)[1] have shown efficacy in vitro, but they lack good clinical correlation to recommend them for routine use. Erythromycin has been associated with treatment failures. Trimethoprim-sulfamethoxazole (Bactrim),[1] polymyxin B,[1] gentamicin (Garamycin),[1] tobramycin (Nebcin),[1] ciprofloxacin (Cipro),[1] and levofloxacin (Levaquin)[1] should not be used because in vitro resistance has been demonstrated.

Typically, the bite site heals promptly. It should be cleaned and disinfected, as is typical for management of other wounds. Tetanus prophylaxis (tetanus-diphtheria toxoids, Td) administration is indicated as required by the patient's immunization record. Rabies prophylaxis (Imovax Rabies) is usually not required for rodent bite, but consultation with local public health authorities is encouraged. There are no reports of transmission of the rabies virus from rats to humans.

---

[1]Not FDA approved for this indication.

References

Abusalameh M, Mahankali-Rao P, Earl S, et al: Discitis caused by rat bite fever in a rheumatoid arthritis patient on tocilizumab-first ever case, *Rheumatology (Oxford)* 57:1118–1120, 2018.

Adam JK, et al: Notes from the field: fatal rat-bite Fever in a child - San Diego County, California, 2013, *MMWR Morb Mortal Wkly Rep* 63(50):1210–1211, 2014.

Chen PL, Lee NY, Yan JJ, et al: Prosthetic valve endocarditis caused by *Streptobacillus moniliformis*: A case of rat bite fever, *J Clin Microbiol* 45:3125–3126, 2007.

Crews JD, Palazzi DL, Starke JR: A teenager with fever, rash, and arthralgia. *Streptobacillus moniliformis* infection, *JAMA Pediatr* 168(12):1165–1166, 2014.

Elliott SP: Rat bite fever and *Streptobacillus moniliformis*, *Clin Microbiol Rev* 20:13–22, 2007.

Fenn DW, et al: An unusual tale of rat-bite fever endocarditis, *BMJ Case Rep*. 2014, 2014.

Giorgiutti S, Lefebvre N: Rat bite fever, *N Engl J Med* 381(18):1762, 2019.

Graves MH, Janda JM: Rat-bite fever (*Streptobacillus moniliformis*): A potential emerging disease, *Int J Infect Dis* 5:151–155, 2001.

Hall CW, Al Hammadi A, Hasan, MR, Kapoor AK: Recognising rat-bite fever—a rare metastatic infection with *Streptobacillus moniliformis*, *Lancet Infect Dis* 24(1):e69, 2024.

Holroyd KJ, Reiner AP, Dick JD: *Streptobacillus moniliformis* polyarthritis mimicking rheumatoid arthritis: An urban case of rat bite fever, *Am J Med* 85:711–714, 1988.

King HY. Rat Bite Fever. UpToDate. http://www.uptodate.com/contents/rat-bitefever; [accessed April 21, 2018].

Lambe DW Jr, McPhedran AM, Mertz JA, Stewart P: *Streptobacillus moniliformis* isolated from a case of Haverhill fever: Biochemical characterization and inhibitory effect of sodium polyanethol sulfonate, *Am J Clin Pathol* 60:854–860, 1973.

Miura Y, Nei T, Saito R, Sato A, Sonobe K, Takahashi K: Streptobacillus moniliformis bacteremia in a rheumatoid arthritis patient without a rat bite: a case report, *BMC Res Notes* 8(1):694, 2005 Nov 19, https://doi.org/10.1186/s13104-015-1642-6.

Schachter ME, Wilcox L, Rau N, et al: Rat-bite fever, Canada, *Emerg Infect Dis* 12:1301–1302, 2006.

Stehle P, Dubuis O, So A, Dudler J: Rat bite fever without fever, *Ann Rheum Dis* 62:894–896, 2003.

Torres-Miranda D, Moshgriz M, Siegel M: Streptobacillus moniliformis mitral valve endocarditis and septic arthritis: the challenges of diagnosing rat-bite fever endocarditis, *Infect Dis Rep* 10(2):7731, 2018.

Washburn RG: Streptobacillus moniliformis (rat–bite fever). In Mandell GL, Bennett JE, Dolin R, editors: *Principles and Practice of Infectious Diseases, vol 2*, 6th ed, Philadelphia, 2005, Elsevier, pp 2708–2710.

RELAPSING FEVER

Method of
Diego Cadavid, MD

CURRENT DIAGNOSIS

- There are two forms of relapsing fever: epidemic and endemic.
- Epidemic relapsing fever is transmitted from person to person by the body louse *Pediculus humanus*.
- Endemic relapsing fever is transmitted from rodent reservoirs to humans exposed to endemic areas by soft-bodied ticks of the genus *Ornithodoros*.
- The hallmark of relapsing fever is two or more febrile episodes separated by periods of relative well-being.
- The diagnosis is confirmed by visualization of the etiologic spirochetes in thin peripheral blood smears prepared at times of febrile peaks by phase-contrast or darkfield microscopy or light microscopy after Wright or Giemsa staining.

CURRENT THERAPY

- The antibiotic of choice for treatment of relapsing fever is doxycycline except in children or pregnant women. In children <8 years of age, erythromycin[1] or oral penicillin is used instead of tetracycline (Table 3).
- Relapsing fever, if severe or complicated with neuroborreliosis, requires treatment with the intravenous antibiotics ceftriaxone or penicillin G (Table 3).
- The louse-borne epidemic form is treated with a single dose, whereas the endemic tick-borne form is treated with multiple doses for at least 1 week (Table 3).
- Antibiotic treatment of relapsing fever results in the Jarisch-Herxheimer reaction (JHR) in as many as 60% of cases, more often in the epidemic than in the endemic forms. It is characterized by the sudden onset of tachycardia, hypotension, chills, rigors, diaphoresis, and high fever. To reduce the risk of JHR, antibiotics should be started between but not at times of febrile peaks.

[1]Not FDA approved for this indication.

Relapsing fever is one of several diseases caused by spirochetes. Other human spirochetal diseases are syphilis, Lyme disease, and leptospirosis. Notable features of spirochetes are wavy and helical shapes, length-to-diameter ratios of as much as 100 to 1, and flagella that lie between the inner and outer cell membranes. The spirochetes that cause relapsing fever are in the genus *Borrelia*. Other *Borrelia* species cause Lyme disease, avian spirochetosis, and epidemic bovine abortion. Table 1 shows the main *Borrelia* species of relapsing fever, their vectors, and an estimate of their geographic ranges. In the United States, relapsing fever was considered a disease endemic only in the West. However, the recent finding of relapsing fever–like *Borrelia* in ticks and dogs in the eastern United States suggests that the risk of relapsing fever may extend into the East.

Epidemiology

There are two forms of relapsing fever: epidemic transmitted to humans by the body louse *Pediculus humanus* (louse-borne relapsing fever [LBRF]) and endemic transmitted to humans by soft-bodied ticks of the genus *Ornithodoros* (tick-borne relapsing

TABLE 1 | Relapsing Fever *Borrelia* Species Pathogenic to Humans

RELAPSING FEVER	*BORRELIA* SPECIES	ARTHROPOD VECTOR	DISTRIBUTION OF DISEASE
Endemic	*Borrelia hermsii*	*Ornithodoros hermsi*	Western North America
	Borrelia turicatae	*Ornithodoros turicata*	Southwestern North America and northern Mexico
	Borrelia venezuelensis	*Ornithodoros rudis*	Central America and northern South America
	Borrelia hispanica	*Ornithodoros marocanus*	Iberian peninsula and northwestern Africa
	Borrelia crocidurae	*Ornithodoros erraticus*	North and East Africa, Middle East, southern Europe
	Borrelia duttoni	*Ornithodoros moubata*	Sub-Saharan Africa
	Borrelia persica	*Ornithodoros tholozani*	Middle East, Greece, Central Asia
	Borrelia uzbekistan	*Ornithodoros pappilipes*	Tajikistan, Uzbekistan
	Borrelia miyamotoi	Ixodes spp.	Asia, Europe, North America
Epidemic	*Borrelia recurrentis*	*Pediculus humanus*	Worldwide (recently only in East Africa including immigrants to Europe)

TABLE 2 | Frequent Clinical Manifestations of Tick-Borne Relapsing Fever

SIGN OR SYMPTOM	FREQUENCY (%)
Headache	94
Myalgia	92
Chills	88
Nausea	76
Arthralgia	73
Vomiting	71
Abdominal pain	44
Confusion	38
Dry cough	27
Ocular pain	26
Diarrhea	25
Dizziness	25
Photophobia	25
Neck pain	24
Rash	18
Dysuria	13
Jaundice	10
Hepatomegaly	10
Splenomegaly	6

fever [TBRF]). In LBRF, itching caused by skin infestation with lice leads to scratching, which may result in crushing of lice and release of infected hemolymph into areas of skin abrasion. Louse infestation is associated with cold weather and a lack of hygiene. Migrant workers and soldiers at war are particularly susceptible to this infection. Historically, massive outbreaks of LBRF occurred in Eurasia, Africa, and Latin America, but currently the disease is found only in Ethiopia and neighboring countries. However, immigrants can spread LBRF to other parts of the world.

The main risk factor for TBRF is exposure to endemic areas (Table 1). The risk of infection increases with outdoor activities in areas where rodents nest, like entering caves or sleeping in rustic cabins. *Ornithodoros* ticks are soft-bodied and feed for short periods of time (minutes), usually at night. They can live many years between blood meals and may transmit spirochetes to their offspring transovarially. Infection is produced by regurgitation of infected tick saliva into the skin wound during tick feeding. There are several natural vertebrate reservoirs for TBRF, but most common are rodents (deer mice, chipmunks, squirrels, and rats). In contrast, the body louse *Pediculus humanus* is a strict human parasite, living and multiplying in clothing. Hard-tick-borne relapsing fever (HTBRF) is an emerging infectious disease throughout the temperate zone caused by *Borrelia miyamotoi*. *Borrelia miyamotoi* is a spirochete closely related to the bacteria that cause TBRF. It is more distantly related to the bacteria that cause Lyme disease. First identified in 1995 in ticks from Japan, *B miyamotoi* has since been detected in two species of North American ticks, the black-legged or "deer" tick (Ixodes scapularis) and the western black-legged tick (Ixodes pacificus). These ticks are already known to transmit Lyme disease, anaplasmosis, and babesiosis.

Clinical Diagnosis

Relapsing fever should be suspected in any patient presenting with two or more episodes of high fever and constitutional symptoms spaced by periods of relative well-being. The index of suspicion increases if the patient has been exposed to endemic areas for TBRF or to countries where LBRF still occurs (Table 1). Whereas LBRF is usually associated with a single febrile relapse, TBRF usually has multiple relapses (up to 13). Only about 10% of cases of HTBRF have febrile relapses. In LBRF the second episode of fever is typically milder than the first; in TBRF the multiple febrile periods are usually of equal severity. The febrile periods last from 1 to 3 days, and the intervals between fevers last from 3 to 10 days. During the febrile periods, numerous spirochetes are circulating in the blood. This is called *spirochetemia* and is sometimes unexpectedly detected during routine blood smear examinations. Between fevers, spirochetemia is not observed because the numbers are low. The fever pattern and recurrent spirochetemia are the consequences of antigenic variation of abundant outer membrane lipoproteins of relapsing fever *Borrelia* species that are the target for serotype-specific antibodies.

The mean latency between exposure to ticks in the endemic form or to lice in the epidemic form and onset of symptoms is 6 days (range, 3–18 days). Because *Ornithodoros* ticks feed briefly and painlessly at night, patients with TBRF may not be able to recall having been bitten by a tick. The clinical manifestations of TBRF and LBRF are similar, although some differences do exist. Table 2 lists the frequency of the most common manifestations of TBRF. The usual initial presentation is sudden onset of chills followed by high fever, tachycardia, severe headache, vomiting, myalgia and arthralgia, and often delirium. In the early stages, a reddish rash may be seen over the trunk, arms, or legs. The fever remains high for 3 to 5 days, and then it clears abruptly. After an asymptomatic period of 7 to 10 days, the fever and other constitutional symptoms can reappear suddenly. The febrile episodes gradually become less severe, and the person eventually recovers completely. As the disease progresses, fever, jaundice, hepatosplenomegaly, cardiac arrhythmias, and cardiac failure may occur, especially with LBRF. Jaundice is more common at times of relapses. Patients with LBRF are more likely to develop petechiae on the trunk, extremities, and mucous membranes; epistaxis; and blood-tinged sputum. Rupture of the spleen may rarely occur. Multiple neurologic complications can occur as a result of disseminated intravascular coagulation in LBRF and as a result of infection of the meninges and cranial and spinal nerve roots by spirochetes in TBRF. The most common neurologic complications of TBRF are aseptic meningitis and facial palsy. Relapsing fever in pregnant women can cause abortion, premature birth, and neonatal death. Sometimes patients can have nonfebrile relapses, consisting of periods of severe headache, backache, weakness, and other constitutional symptoms without fever that occur at the time of expected relapses. Delirium may persist for weeks after the fever resolves, and, rarely, symptoms may be protracted.

Relapsing fever may be confused with many diseases that are relapsing or cause high fevers. These include typhoid fever, yellow fever, dengue, African hemorrhagic fevers, African trypanosomiasis, brucellosis, malaria, leptospirosis, rat-bite fever, intermittent cholangitis, cat-scratch disease, and echovirus 9 infection, among others. Relapsing fever *Borrelia* spp. have antigens that are cross reactive with Lyme disease *Borrelia* spp. and inasmuch as the endemic areas of relapsing fever and Lyme disease overlap to some extent, confusion between the two infections can be expected. In fact, the same species of ticks can transmit HTBRF and Lyme disease, although erythema migrans rash is rare in the former and common in the latter.

Laboratory Diagnosis

Although the pattern of recurring fever is the clue to diagnosing relapsing fever, confirmation of the diagnosis requires demonstration of spirochetes in peripheral blood taken during an episode of fever. The comparatively large number of spirochetes in the blood during relapsing fever provides the opportunity for the simplest method for laboratory diagnosis of the infection, light microscopy of Wright- or Giemsa-stained thin blood smears or darkfield or phase-contrast microscopy of a wet mount of plasma. The blood should be obtained during or just before peaks of body temperature. Between fever peaks, spirochetes often can be demonstrated by inoculation of blood or cerebrospinal fluid (CSF) into special culture medium (BSK-H with 6% rabbit serum available from Sigma) or experimental animals. Enrichment for spirochetes is achieved by using the platelet-rich fraction of plasma or the buffy coat of sedimented blood. In the United States the most common causes of relapsing fever are *Borrelia hermsii* and *Borrelia turicatae*; both grow in BSK-H medium and in young mice or rats. Whereas direct visual detection of organisms in the blood is the most common method for laboratory confirmation of relapsing fever, immunoassays for antibodies are the most common means of laboratory confirmation for Lyme disease. Although serologic assays have been developed for the agents of relapsing fever, these are not widely available and of dubious utility. The antigenic variation displayed by the relapsing fever species means there are hundreds of different "serotypes." If a different serotype or species is used for preparing the antigen, only antibodies to conserved antigens may be detected. For this reason, a standardized enzyme-linked immunosorbent assay (ELISA) with Lyme disease *Borrelia* as antigen may be the best available serologic assay for relapsing fever. ELISA for *Borrelia burgdorferi* antibodies is routinely done across the United States and Europe. If a positive result for IgM or IgG antibodies is obtained, the Western blot for antibodies to *B burgdorferi* antigens would be expected to discriminate current

TABLE 3 Treatment Options for Tick-Borne Relapsing Fever*

Adults

Nonsevere forms

1. Doxycycline (Doryx oral), 100 mg PO bid for 1–2 wk[†]

2. Tetracycline (Sumycin), 500 mg PO qid for 1–2 wk

3. Erythromycin (Erythrocin),[1] 500 mg PO tid for 1–2 wk

Severe forms

1. Ceftriaxone (Rocephin),[1] 2 g IV qd for 1–2 wk

2. Penicillin G parenteral aqueous (Pfizerpen),[1] 4 million U IV q4h for 1–2 wk

Children (≤8 y)

Nonsevere forms

1. Erythromycin suspension oral (EryPed),[1] 30–50 mg/kg/d divided tid for 1–2 wk

2. Azithromycin oral suspension (Zithromax),[1] 20 mg/kg on the first day followed by 10 mg/kg/d for 4 more days

3. Penicillin V (Pen-Vee K),[1] 25–50 mg/kg/d divided qid for 1–2 wk

4. Amoxicillin (Amoxil),[1] 50 mg/kg/d divided tid for 1–2 wk

Severe forms

1. Ceftriaxone (Rocephin),[1] 75–100 mg/kg/d IV for 1–2 wk

2. Penicillin G parenteral aqueous (Pfizerpen),[1] 300,000 U/kg/d given IV in divided doses q4h for 1–2 wk

Abbreviations: IV = intravenous; PO = orally.
[1]Not FDA approved for this indication.
*The same oral agents are used for treatment of louse-borne (epidemic) relapsing fever but given as a single dose.
[†]In general, treatment for 1 wk is recommended in early/milder cases and for up to 2 wk for more severe cases.

or past Lyme disease from relapsing fever, as well as from syphilis, another cause of false-positive Lyme disease ELISA results. Other frequent laboratory abnormalities can occur in relapsing fever but are not diagnostic. These include elevated white blood cell count with increased neutrophils, thrombocytopenia, increased serum bilirubin, proteinuria, microhematuria, prolongation of the prothrombin time (PT) and partial thromboplastin time (PTT), and elevation of fibrin degradation products.

It may also be possible to confirm infection with relapsing fever borrelias, including *Borrelia miyamotoi*, by directly probing blood and/or CSF samples for fragments of the bacterium's genetic sequence, which few laboratories may be able to do.

Treatment

Relapsing fever *Borrelias* are very sensitive to several antibiotics, and antimicrobial resistance is rare. Table 3 summarizes the treatment options for adults and children younger than 8 years. Children older than 8 years can be treated with the same antibiotics as adults, but the doses should be adjusted by weight. Before antibiotics are given, the possibility of causing the Jarisch-Herxheimer reaction (JHR) should be considered (see later). The tetracycline antibiotics are most commonly used for treatment of LBRF and TBRF. The first antibiotic of choice in adults and children older than 8 years is doxycycline (Doryx). In general, shorter treatments are needed for LBRF than for TBRF. Single-dose therapy is usually recommended for LBRF. In contrast, in TBRF even multiple doses of tetracyclines for up to 10 days may fail to prevent relapses, and retreatment can be required. *B. miyamotoi* is susceptible in vitro to doxycycline, azithromycin, and ceftriaxone. Physicians have successfully treated patients infected with *B miyamotoi* with a 2 to 4-week course of doxycycline.

Alternative oral antibiotics to the tetracyclines are erythromycin (E-Mycin)[1], azithromycin (Zithromax)[1], amoxicillin (Amoxil)[1], penicillin[1], and chloramphenicol (Chloromycetin).[1] However, oral chloramphenicol is not available in the United States. Erythromycin, azithromycin, and penicillin do not appear as effective as the tetracyclines; however, they are recommended for children younger than 8 years and for pregnant women. Amoxicillin is another alternative for young children with early Lyme disease; however, it is ineffective for human granulocytic ehrlichiosis, which sometimes occurs as a co-infection with Lyme disease. *Borrelia miyamotoi* may be resistant to amoxacillin.

Although treatment with antibiotics is usually given orally, they may need to be given intravenously if severe vomiting makes swallowing impractical. If there are symptoms and signs of meningitis or encephalitis without clinical or radiologic signs of increased intracranial pressure, the CSF should be examined to rule out central nervous system (CNS) infection. The finding of elevation of CSF cells and protein demands the use of parenteral antibiotics, such as penicillin G[1] or ceftriaxone (Rocephin).[1] Optimally, antibiotic treatment should be started during afebrile periods when the spirochetemia is low. Starting therapy near the peak of a febrile period may induce JHR, in which high fever and a rise and subsequent fall in blood pressure, sometimes to dangerously low levels, may occur. Dehydration should be treated with fluids given intravenously. Severe headache can be treated with pain relievers such as codeine, and nausea or vomiting can be treated with prochlorperazine (Compazine).

Jarisch-Herxheimer Reaction

Antibiotic treatment of relapsing fever causes JHR in as many as 60% of cases. JHR is more common in LBRF than in TBRF. It can also occur in HTBRF. It is characterized by the sudden onset of tachycardia, hypotension, chills, rigors, diaphoresis, and high fever. Patients with JHR have said that they felt as if they were going to die. JHR is caused by the rapid killing of circulating spirochetes 1 to 4 hours after the first dose of antibiotic, which results in the release of large amounts of *Borrelia* lipoproteins in the circulation followed by massive release of tumor necrosis factor and other cytokines. If possible, patients with JHR should be transferred to an intensive care unit for close monitoring and treatment. Over several hours, the temperature declines and the patient feels better. Large amounts of intravenous fluids (0.9% sodium chloride solution) may be required to treat hypotension. Steroids and nonsteroidal antiinflammatory agents have no effect on the frequency or severity of the JHR. One study found that pretreatment with anti-TNF-alpha monoclonal antibody (Humira)[1] suppressed JHR after penicillin treatment for LBRF and reduced the associated increases in plasma cytokines. Death can occur as a result of JHR secondary to cardiovascular collapse in up to 5% of patients with treated LBRF and much less frequently in TBRF.

Outcome

Complete recovery occurs in 95% or more of adequately treated patients. The prognosis for untreated cases or if treatment is delayed varies. A mortality rate as high as 40% is reported in untreated epidemics of LBRF. Relapsing fever also has a high mortality rate in neonates. Some neurologic sequelae can occur in patients with TBRF complicated with neuroborreliosis.

Prevention

Prevention of TBRF involves avoidance of rodent- and tick-infested dwellings such as animal burrows, caves, and abandoned cabins. Wearing clothing that protects skin from tick access (e.g., long pants and long-sleeved shirts) is also helpful. Repellents and acaricides provide additional protection. Diethyltoluamide (DEET) repels ticks when applied to clothing or skin, but it must be used with caution. It loses its effectiveness within 1 to several hours when applied to skin and must be reapplied; it is absorbed through the skin and may cause CNS toxicity if used excessively. Picaridin (KBR 3023), which has been used as an insect repellent for years in Europe and Australia, is now available in the United States in 7% solution as Cutter

Advanced Repellent (Spectrum Brands). The US Centers for Disease Control and Prevention (CDC) is recommending it as an alternative to DEET. Permethrin Insect Repellent, an acaricide, is more effective than DEET but should not be applied directly to skin. When applied to clothing, it provides good protection for 1 day or more. In LBRF, prevention can be achieved by promoting personal hygiene and by dusting undergarments and the inside of clothing with malathion[1] powder[2] or lindane[1] powder[2] when available. Widespread antibiotic use may be necessary to control epidemics of LBRF, using one or two doses of 100 mg doxycycline[1] given within 1 week of exposure.

---

[2]Not available in the United States

References

Barbour AG, Hayes SF: Biology of *Borrelia* species, *Microbiol Rev* 50:381–400, 1986.
Bryceson AD, Parry EH, Perine PL, et al: Louse-borne relapsing fever, *Q J Med* 39:129–170, 1970.
Cadavid D, Barbour AG: Neuroborreliosis during relapsing fever: Review of the clinical manifestations, pathology, and treatment of infections in humans and experimental animals, *Clin Infect Dis* 26:151–164, 1998.
Fekade D, Knox K, Hussein K, et al: Prevention of Jarisch-Herxheimer reactions by treatment with antibodies against tumor necrosis factor alpha, *N Engl J Med* 335:311–315, 1996.
Kazragis RJ, Dever LL, Jorgensen JH, Barbour AG: In vivo activities of ceftriaxone and vancomycin against *Borrelia* spp. in the mouse brain and other sites, *Antimicrob Agents Chemother* 40:2632–2636, 1996.
Melkert PW: Fatal Jarisch-Herxheimer reaction in a case of relapsing fever misdiagnosed as lobar pneumonia, *Trop Geogr Med* 39:92–93, 1987.
Southern P, Sanford J: Relapsing fever, *Medicine* 48:129–149, 1969.
Taft W, Pike J: Relapsing fever. Report of a sporadic outbreak including treatment with penicillin, *JAMA* 129:1002–1005, 1945.

RUBELLA AND CONGENITAL RUBELLA

Method of
Dee Ann Bragg, MD

CURRENT DIAGNOSIS

- Given its clinical overlap with other viral syndromes, suspected rubella infection must be confirmed with laboratory testing.
- Rubella serology or viral polymerase chain reaction (PCR) testing are available options for confirming a suspected diagnosis.

CURRENT THERAPY

- Rubella infection is largely self-limited with no specific treatment indicated.
- Infection during pregnancy should prompt further evaluation and counseling regarding risks and potential outcomes.
- Treatment of children with congenital rubella syndrome requires a multidisciplinary effort based on individual manifestations.
- Vaccination is essential in reducing the risk of rubella and congenital rubella syndrome.

Rubella typically presents in children and adults as a mild viral illness, but is one of the TORCH infections (toxoplasmosis, other, rubella, cytomegalovirus, herpes) known to cause congenital anomalies. Although vaccination efforts have led to the successful eradication of rubella in the United States, it remains a significant cause of morbidity and death worldwide. Its name is derived from Latin and means "little red." Initially considered a variant

---

[1]Not FDA approved for this indication.

of measles or scarlet fever, rubella was first described as its own entity in the German medical literature in 1814. Thus it is still often referred to as "German measles" in common nomenclature.

Pathophysiology and Virology
Rubella virus, a single-stranded RNA virus and the only member of the Rubivirus genus, is part of the Togaviridae family and is the causative agent of rubella infection. There are 13 recognized genotypes of rubella, each with minor differences in nucleotide sequencing and gene expression. Rubella typically presents as a mild and self-limited illness. During pregnancy, however, it can infect the placenta and disrupt organogenesis by creating systemic inflammation and inhibiting actin assembly. Outcomes of antenatal infection are variable but can include miscarriage, fetal death, and congenital rubella syndrome (CRS).

Multiple factors are involved in the pathogenesis of CRS. Rubella infection can cause necrosis of the chorionic epithelial and endothelial cells. These cells then enter fetal circulation and can incite thrombotic or ischemic lesions in the eyes, ears, brain, and heart. The virus also appears to trigger an immune-modulated upregulation of interferon and cytokines, which can alter the normal development and differentiation of fetal cells.

Epidemiology
Although rubella is less contagious than other viruses such as influenza or measles, large epidemics are associated with significant morbidity from complications including encephalitis, fetal loss, deafness, and blindness. Norman Gregg, an Australian ophthalmologist, was the first to recognize the teratogenic potential of rubella when in 1941 he noted an unusually high incidence of congenital cataracts after an area outbreak.

Rubella was successfully eradicated from the United States in 2004 due to widespread vaccination efforts, and most sporadic cases since that time have been documented in foreign-born young adults. In endemic areas, annual springtime outbreaks are common. However, sporadic cases can occur year-round in temperate climates. Outbreaks typically affect early school–aged children, and the mean age for an infected host is 5 to 9 years. Because lifelong immunity develops after natural infection, large cyclical epidemics tend to occur every 3 to 8 years as population immunity wanes.

Humans are the only known host of rubella infection, and the virus is transmitted from person to person through respiratory droplets. After transmission, rubella virus replicates in the respiratory mucosa and cervical lymph nodes before entering systemic circulation and spreading to target organs.

Clinical Manifestations
Acquired Rubella
After an incubation period of about 14 days (range, 12–23), a variety of clinical symptoms can appear. These are generally mild, and about 50% of cases are asymptomatic. In children, a skin rash is typically the initial manifestation of rubella. The rash usually appears on the face and then progresses downward from the head to the feet. It lasts about 3 days and is characteristically maculopapular, presenting with small pink non-coalescing papules that are occasionally pruritic. Bathing or showering in hot water tends to make the rash more evident.

Adults more often have a prodromal period of low-grade fever, malaise, and adenopathy lasting 1 to 5 days before the onset of skin findings. Lymphadenopathy may begin up to a week before the rash and can last for several weeks. The postauricular nodes are particularly commonly involved, and posterior cervical or suboccipital nodes may also be affected.

Sequelae
Polyarthritis and polyarthralgia are the most common complications of rubella, particularly in adult women, in whom they are seen up to 70% of the time. They appear with such frequency that they are often considered intrinsic to the virus itself rather than complications. Joint symptoms typically present around the same time or just after the onset of the rash. They usually last 3 to 4 days but can remain for up to 1 month. The most commonly affected joints are fingers, wrists, and knees. Chronic arthritis is rarely observed.

Other complications are uncommon but can carry a high degree of morbidity and death. Hemorrhagic events are more likely in children than adults and occur in about 1 in 3000 cases. They manifest as a result of vascular damage or thrombocytopenia. Skin purpura is the most common presentation, but gastrointestinal, cerebral, or intrarenal hemorrhage can occur. Encephalitis occurs in about 1 in 6000 cases, more commonly in adults than children. Rare complications include orchitis, neuritis, progressive panencephalitis, and Guillain-Barré syndrome.

Congenital Rubella Syndrome (CRS)
CRS can present transiently with low birth weight, thrombocytopenic purpura, or hemolytic anemia. However, permanent defects are the hallmark of CRS because it classically involves a triad of cataracts, cardiac anomalies, and sensorineural deafness. Of these, hearing loss is the most common and sometimes the only complication observed. Cardiac abnormalities can include patent ductus arteriosus, ventricular septal defect, pulmonary artery hypoplasia, and coarctation of the aorta. Other ocular defects such as glaucoma, retinopathy, and microphthalmia can also occur. Additional manifestations can include microcephaly, intellectual disability, psychomotor retardation, and delayed speech.

Notably, it can take 2 to 4 years for certain neurologic, endocrine, or cardiac abnormalities associated with CRS to manifest. Diabetes mellitus, thyroid disease, autism, and progressive panencephalopathy can all occur as late effects of CRS.

The risk of CRS and its associated congenital defects is greatest when infection occurs in the first trimester. Up to 85% of infants born under these conditions are found to be affected, whereas defects are rare when infection occurs after 20 weeks' gestation.

Diagnosis
Given its nonspecific nature and similarity to other viral infections, clinical diagnosis of rubella is challenging and largely unreliable. Suspected infection should be confirmed by 1 of 3 diagnostic methods: (1) rubella immunoglobulin M (IgM) serology, (2) a demonstrated rise in rubella virus immunoglobulin G (IgG) between acute and convalescent phases, or (3) detection of rubella virus by PCR.

Among the existing options for laboratory diagnosis, rubella IgM is the most accessible and widely used. However, collection timing is important to consider. Rubella IgM will only be detectable in about 50% of cases on the day of rash appearance but will be present in nearly all cases by 7 to 10 days after the rash. It will then remain positive for 4 to 12 weeks. Importantly, serum IgM testing is most sensitive and specific in the setting of local outbreaks. False-positive results occur more frequently in sporadic cases, and in those instances, additional means of analysis should be performed to confirm diagnosis.

Rubella IgG testing can be used to diagnose acute rubella infection under two circumstances: either (1) a negative rubella IgG during acute infection followed by a positive IgG in the convalescent phase, or (2) a fourfold increase in IgG titer over 10 to 14 days. IgG avidity testing may also be useful. This measures the strength of antigen-antibody binding, which is typically weaker in acute infection and increases over time. Therefore a low avidity index would indicate a more recent infection.

Viral isolation of rubella by PCR is quite valuable for diagnostic confirmation and can be performed on samples obtained from throat or nasopharyngeal swabs. These tests are not as widely available in postvaccination settings and may need to be performed in conjunction with local health departments or national epidemiology centers.

Diagnosis of CRS in infants can similarly be confirmed by one of three methods: (1) rubella IgM detection in serum or cord blood, (2) persistence of rubella IgG >6 months of age (past the time frame of passive maternal immunity), or (3) PCR isolation of rubella virus from respiratory or urinary samples. Because both rubella virus and IgM remain positive for several months in patients with CRS, the time frame for testing is less crucial than in cases of postnatal infection.

Treatment

There is no specific treatment for rubella and, because acquired cases are generally mild and self-limiting, basic supportive care is recommended. Detection of rubella infection in pregnancies before 18 weeks' gestation should prompt further investigation including maternal-fetal medicine referral, detailed ultrasound examination, support for adverse outcomes including neonatal hospice services, and follow-up examination and screening of the newborn. Maternal infections after 18 weeks can be followed with routine ultrasound monitoring along with newborn evaluation and testing.

Prevention

Rubella Vaccine

The first rubella vaccines became available in 1969, and a number of strains have been developed since that time. Of these, the RA 27/3 vaccine has been the most enduring, and all other strains were discontinued at the time of its introduction in 1979. The RA 27/3 rubella vaccine is a live attenuated virus that is administered in conjunction with measles and mumps as MMR, or with measles, mumps, and varicella as MMRV (ProQuad). Single-antigen rubella vaccine is not available in the United States.

Vaccination against rubella is safe and effective. Adverse events such as fever and rash are mild and are generally attributable to the measles and mumps portions of the vaccines. After a single dose, more than 95% of those vaccinated have serologic confirmation of rubella immunity, with evidence of lifelong immunity in the vast majority of responders. MMR or MMRV is recommended for all children at 12 months of age, followed by a second dose between 4 and 6 years of age. The second dose is generally indicated to stimulate measles and mumps immunity in those who did not respond to the first vaccine. MMR and MMRV are contraindicated in immunosuppression, pregnancy, and in patients with a history of anaphylaxis to neomycin or other vaccine components.

Preconception Counseling and Prenatal Care

Rubella immunity, defined as serum rubella IgG of 10 IU/mL or greater, should be documented in all women attempting to conceive. MMR vaccine should be given in cases of nonimmunity, and although it is recommended at least 4 weeks before conception, inadvertent vaccination after that time is unlikely to be associated with adverse events. Rubella IgG should likewise be checked in all pregnant females as part of routine obstetric care, and MMR should be administered postpartum to nonimmune women.

Eradication and Future Goals

Despite widely available effective vaccines and evidence of sustained eradication in the Western Hemisphere, there are still approximately 100,000 cases of CRS annually worldwide. Although some African and Asian nations have introduced routine rubella vaccination, public health efforts have been inconsistent in many developing countries. Dedicated personnel and funding will likely be necessary to decrease rubella incidence and its complications on a global scale.

References

Baltimore RS, Nimkin K, Sparger K, et al: Case 4-2018: a newborn with thrombocytopenia, cataracts, and hepatosplenomegaly, *N Engl J Med* 378:564–572, 2018.
Bouthry E, Picone O, Hamdi G, et al: Rubella and pregnancy: diagnosis, management and outcomes, *Prenat Diagn* 34:1246–1253, 2014.
Centers for Disease Control and Prevention: *Epidemiology and Prevention of Vaccine-Preventable Diseases, 13th Edition*. Hamborsky J, Kroger A, Wolfe S, eds. Washington, DC: Public Health Foundation, pp 325–340, 2015.
Lambert N, Strebel P, Orenstein W, et al: *Rubella, Lancet* 385(9984):2297–2307, 2015.
Papania M, Wallace G, Rota P, et al: Elimination of endemic measles, rubella, and congenital rubella syndrome from the western hemisphere: the US experience, *JAMA Pediatr* 168:148–155, 2014.
Tipples G: Rubella diagnostic issues in Canada, *J Infect Dis* 204(Suppl 2):S659–S663, 2011.

SALMONELLOSIS

Method of
Tanya Rodgers, MD

CURRENT DIAGNOSIS

- Nontyphoidal salmonellosis should be suspected in individuals with gastroenteritis known to have high-risk exposures such as eating raw or contaminated eggs and poultry, or recent contact with reptiles.
- Testing is typically not necessary as most cases are self-limited and resolve in 3 to 7 days.
- Consider polymerase chain reaction or cultures (stool) in patients with fever, blood in stool, or in healthcare workers or food handlers who can transmit infection to others.
- Obtain blood cultures if bacteremia is suspected, as well as in those at risk for severe infection such as immunocompromised patients and those with vascular grafts, prosthetic valves, or joints.

CURRENT THERAPY

- Primary treatment is supportive care with oral hydration and electrolyte replacement as most salmonella infections cause self-limited gastroenteritis.
- Antidiarrheal agents are not recommended as they can prolong gastrointestinal transit time and lengthen course of illness.
- In uncomplicated infections, antibiotic treatment is not recommended as it does not shorten course of illness and can prolong bacterial shedding.
- Antibiotics are reserved for patients with bacteremia, those with suspected invasive disease as demonstrated by presence of severe diarrhea, fever and extraintestinal symptoms, and those at high risk for complications.

Salmonellosis is infection with the bacteria *Salmonella*. Nontyphoidal salmonellosis is one of the leading bacterial causes of diarrhea, causing approximately 150 million illness and 60,000 deaths globally each year.

Epidemiology

Salmonella is the most common cause of foodborne illness in the United States, causing more than 1.4 million cases, 25,000 hospitalizations, and 450 deaths each year—30% of all deaths associated with foodborne illness. *Salmonella* is the second most common bacterial isolate found in stool culture after *Campylobacter jejuni*. Most human cases (>95%) occur after the ingestion of contaminated food. The most common sources are poultry, eggs, and milk products, but infection has also been linked to meat, shellfish, nut butters, spices, flour, fruits and vegetables, and herbal supplements. New food sources are being identified continuously. The remaining cases of *Salmonella* infection are associated with ingestion of contaminated water; from handling reptiles (turtles and iguanas), live poultry, and household pets; and from person-to-person spread. Peak occurrence is during the summer months. *Salmonella* outbreaks can be widespread and span multiple states or even multiple countries, but the majority of infections (>80%) are sporadic.

Pathophysiology

Salmonella enterica is a motile, gram-negative facultative anaerobic rod-shaped bacillus in the Enterobacteriaceae family. There are more than 2500 serotypes that are categorized as either typhoidal or nontyphoidal. Typhoidal serotypes cause enteric fever (typhoid fever) and are adapted to human hosts, whereas nontyphoidal serotypes typically cause mild disease in humans and are adapted to many animal hosts. Serotypes are often designated by name, often from the location of first isolation, and sometimes designated by formula. The most frequently isolated serotypes associated with foodborne illness in the United States are *S.* Enteritidis, *S.* Newport, and *S.* Typhimurium.

Salmonella causes illness by attaching and invading the distal ilium and proximal colon. To do so, bacteria must survive the highly acidic gastric environment and avoid lysis by bile salts. This explains why patients with gastric hypoacidity are at increased risk for infection, including infants, patients with pernicious anemia, and those taking antacids. The initial host response to *Salmonella* infection involves neutrophil infiltration followed by lymphocytes and macrophages. This response is suppressed in immunocompromised individuals who are also at higher risk for severe infection. Once attachment invasion in established, *Salmonella* can spread beyond the gastrointestinal mucosa into draining mesenteric lymph nodes, then to liver, spleen, and the bloodstream.

Clinical Manifestations

The most common presentation of *Salmonella* infection is gastroenteritis with nausea, vomiting, and diarrhea occurring 6 to 48 hours after ingestion. Initial presentation is often associated with fever, chills, abdominal cramps, myalgias, and headaches. The incubation period and severity of illness are dependent on ingested dose of bacterium. Stool is typically nonbloody: if blood is present, *Shigella* or *Escherichia coli* infection is more likely. The course is usually self-limited and lasts 3 to 7 days; however, dehydration can be severe and leads to approximately 2.2 hospitalizations per 1 million people annually.

Approximately 5% of patients with *Salmonella* infection will develop bacteremia or invasive infections such as osteomyelitis, meningitis, endovascular infection, endocarditis, pneumonia, or septic arthritis. Rarely, intraabdominal infections can occur in the form of hepatic or splenic abscesses. The risk for invasive infection is higher among infants, older adults, people with atherosclerosis, hemoglobinopathies, cancer, and those who are immunocompromised. Vascular complications occur in 10% to 25% of adults with bacteremia, whereas localized infection occurs in 5% to 10%. If septic arthritis occurs, it is typically monoarticular, although reactive polyarthritis can occur and is thought to be a systemic immune response and not polyarticular infection.

Approximately 0.5% of people infected with *Salmonella* become chronic carriers, which is defined as having positive stool or urine culture at 12 months after acute infection. Infants, women, patients with gallstones and kidney stones, and people co-infected with *Schistosoma haematobium* are more likely to become chronic carriers.

Diagnosis

Infection with nontyphoidal salmonella should be suspected in patients with acute gastroenteritis, particularly if they are known to have ingested raw eggs, undercooked poultry, contaminated water, or have recently handled reptiles or live poultry. In most cases testing is not necessary as illness is self-limited. Testing is indicated when symptoms are severe, include bloody stool, or occur in high-risk patients or in healthcare providers or food handlers. Testing includes stool collection, and most labs now perform polymerase chain reaction (PCR) assay, which is both more sensitive and faster compared with stool culture. Reflex bacterial stool culture should be performed on the PCR-positive specimens to determine antimicrobial sensitivity to guide treatment. Rectal swabs and serologic antigen testing are less sensitive and are not recommended.

Blood cultures should be obtained when bacteremia is suspected due to clinical presentation, and in those patients at high risk for complications such as infants, patients with HIV infection or other immunocompromised hosts, patients with vascular grafts or prosthetic heart valves or joints, and those requiring hospitalization. If there is concern for endovascular infection further imaging should be considered, such as computed tomography or magnetic resonance imaging. Invasive infection is confirmed when *Salmonella* is isolated from either a blood culture or a tissue/fluid culture from the suspected site of infection.

Salmonella is a reportable infection, and most states mandate isolates or clinical material be submitted to local public state health laboratories.

Treatment

Acute gastroenteritis caused by nontyphoidal salmonella in an immunocompetent individual is typically self-limited and does not require antibiotic treatment. Care should focus on supportive measures including hydration and electrolyte replacement with reduced osmolarity oral rehydration solution for patients who can tolerate oral intake. For those who are experiencing severe dehydration, shock, altered mental status, or failure of oral hydration, isotonic IV hydration is recommended. Antiemetics such as prochlorperazine (Compazine) or promethazine (Phenergan) may be used as needed for 1 to 2 days to facilitate oral fluid repletion. Antidiarrheal medications are not recommended as they slow transit time and can lengthen the course of illness.

Antibiotic treatment is not recommended for use in immunocompetent individuals who are not at high risk for complication, as antibiotics do not shorten the course of nonsevere illness. In addition, antibiotics have been shown to prolong bacterial shedding, increase risk of relapse, and prolong the carrier state. This is thought to be due to suppressing endogenous flora in the gastrointestinal tract. If, however, patients exhibit severe symptoms, including diarrhea greater than nine times per day or signs of dehydration, antibiotics are recommended. Bloody diarrhea is not an indication for antibiotics, as it is more typically linked with *Shigella* or *E. coli*. The treatment of enterohemorrhagic *E. coli* with antibiotics has been linked to Shiga toxin–mediated hemolytic uremic syndrome.

Antibiotics are recommended for patients at increased risk for developing invasive *Salmonella* infection, including:

- Infants <3 months of age, at increased risk for salmonella meningitis
- Adults >50 years of age, at increased risk for endovascular infection
- Immunosuppressed individuals, at increased risk for bacteremia, including those with organ transplants, malignancies, hemoglobinopathies, and those receiving corticosteroids or other immunosuppressing medications
- Patients with vascular grafts or prosthetic joints, at increased risk for locally invasive infection

Antibiotics are also recommended when bacteremia is suspected due to high or persistent fever or extraintestinal symptoms. For patients with *Salmonella* bacteremia, antibiotics can speed recovery by 1 to 2 days. If endovascular infection is suspected, treating empirically with both a third-generation cephalosporin and a fluoroquinolone is recommended pending susceptibility data.

Antibiotic resistance of *Salmonella* isolates varies by serotype and geographic region and must be considered when choosing antibiotic regimens. Older antibiotics including chloramphenicol, ampicillin, and trimethoprim-sulfamethoxazole (Bactrim)[1] have very high resistance rates and should not be used as first-line treatment. Nalidixic acid[2] resistance, which has been shown to predict lack of response to fluoroquinolones, has been linked to worldwide use of fluoroquinolones in animals raised for human consumption. Stool isolates from *Salmonella*-infected travelers to Southeast Asia demonstrate up to 41% nalidixic acid resistance. In 2005, the FDA withdrew approval for fluoroquinolone use in livestock, and the National Antimicrobial Resistance Monitoring System continues to carry the most current information on

---

[1] Not FDA approved for this indication.
[2] Not available in the United States.

CLINICAL SYNDROME	PATIENT CHARACTERISTICS	ANTIBIOTICS	DURATION OF TREATMENT
Acute gastroenteritis	Immunocompetent patients >12 months to <50 years	Antibiotic treatment not recommended	3–7 days
	Infants <12 months	Azithromycin[†1] 10 mg/kg PO on day 1 (maximum 500 mg) followed by 5 mg/kg (maximum 250 mg) once daily for 4 additional days	
	Infants <3 months	Azithromycin as above Ceftriaxone[1] 50–75 mg/kg/d IV/IM q12h (maximum 2 g/d) Amoxicillin[1] 30 mg/kg/d PO divided q12h	
Severe gastroenteritis (fever, severe diarrhea >9×/day, hospitalization)	Adults	Ciprofloxacin[†1] 500 mg PO q12h or levofloxacin[1] 750 mg PO q24h Trimethoprim-sulfamethoxazole[1] 160 mg/800 mg PO q12h	3–7 days or until fever resolves
		Cefixime 400 mg PO daily divided q12h or q24h Azithromycin[1] 1 g PO on day 1, followed by 500 mg once daily	5–7 days
	Children	Azithromycin[†1] 10 mg/kg PO on day 1 (maximum 500 mg) followed by 5 mg/kg (maximum 250 mg) once daily for 4 additional days Ceftriaxone[‡1] 75–100 mg/kg IV or IM divided q12h or q24h (maximum 1 g per dose)	
At risk for invasive disease	Adults >50 years • Patients with atherosclerosis and endovascular grafts • Joint prosthesis • Immunocompromised including patients with HIV	Ceftriaxone[1] 1–2 g IV/IM q24h *plus* Ciprofloxacin[1] 500 mg q12h *or* Trimethoprim-sulfamethoxazole[1] PO 1 double-strength tablet q12h Amoxicillin[1] 500 mg PO q12h	7–14 days
Bacteremia and other extraintestinal infections	Adults	Ceftriaxone[1] 2 g IV q24h Cefotaxime[1] 1–2 g IV q8h Ciprofloxacin[1] 400 mg IV q12h or 500 mg PO q12h Levofloxacin[1] 500–750 mg IV q24h Trimethoprim-sulfamethoxazole[1] 8–10 mg/kg/d divided 3 times per day, or oral 1–2 double-strength tablets twice daily Ampicillin 2 g IV q24h Amoxicillin[1] 500 mg q8h, or 875 mg q12h Azithromycin[1] 500 mg IV q24h	7–14 days (At least 14 days in immunocompromised patient, and in patients with HIV with CD4 count <200 2–6 weeks)
	Children	Ceftriaxone[1] 50–75 mg/kg/d IV/IM divided q12h or q24h (maximum 2 g/d) Cefotaxime[1] 50–60 mg/kg IV/IM q8h (maximum 2 g/dose) Ciprofloxacin[§1] 10 mg/kg IV q8–12h (maximum 400 mg/dose) or oral 10–20 mg/kg q12h (maximum 1.5 g/day) Trimethoprim-sulfamethoxazole[1] 8–12 mg/kg IV divided q12h (maximum 160 mg of trimethoprim)	7–14 days
Chronic carriers	Adults	Ciprofloxacin[1] 750 mg PO q12h Trimethoprim-sulfamethoxazole[1] 1 double strength tablet q12h Amoxicillin[1] 1 g PO q8h	1 month 3 months 3 months

*Once culture and sensitivity data are available, adjust antibiotics accordingly.
[†]Preferred in the absence of contraindication.
[‡]Reserved for severe infection.
[§]Not routinely first line-use but justied in severe cases where alternatives are not available.
[1]Not FDA approved for this indication.

resistance reports on its website. Despite this, rates of *Salmonella* antibiotic resistance have been steadily increasing in the United States with 8.6% nalidixic acid resistance, 3.5% resistance to ceftriaxone[1], and 0.5% resistance to ciprofloxacin.[1] Multidrug resistance has long been noted to nontyphoid *Salmonella* isolates and has been linked to increased virulence and higher morbidity and mortality.

For nonpregnant adults and adolescents with severe illness who can tolerate oral therapy, fluoroquinolones (either ciprofloxacin[1]

500 mg twice daily or levofloxacin[1] 750 mg) are the recommended first-line treatment. If fluoroquinolones are contraindicated, alternatives include trimethoprim/sulfamethoxazole (Bactrim DS)[1] 160 mg/800 mg twice daily, cefixime (Suprax)[1] 400 mg divided every 12 or 24 hours, azithromycin (Zithromax)[1] 1 g followed by 500 mg once daily, or amoxicillin[1] 1 g three times per day. Depending on the medication, oral therapy duration is 3 to 7 days or until fever resolves (Table 1). For immunocompromised patients, those unable to tolerate oral therapy or those with bacteremia, IV

antibiotics are recommended for 7 to 14 days and 2 to 6 weeks in patients with HIV and CD4 counts less than 200. Initial treatment is ceftriaxone[1] 2 g every 24 hours plus ciprofloxacin[1] 400 mg IV every 12 hours, with plans to deescalate to targeted therapy once susceptibilities are available. If bacteremia is persistent, further investigation for endovascular or prosthetic complications is necessary, and if localized invasive infection is confirmed a 6-week course of antibiotics with IV ceftriaxone or ampicillin plus surgical management is recommended. Patients with endocarditis typically require valve replacement. If localized infection develops, surgical debridement in addition to antibiotics is needed.

For children requiring antibiotic treatment who can tolerate oral medication, first-line treatment is azithromycin[1] 10 mg/kg (maximum 500 mg) on day 1, followed by 50 mg/kg (maximum 250 mg) once daily for an additional 4 days pending culture results. If azithromycin is contraindicated, ciprofloxacin[1] or levofloxacin[1] can be considered while understanding the possible risk for cartilage damage. Amoxicillin[1] and trimethoprim-sulfamethoxazole[1] also can be considered, depending on local resistance patterns.

Monitoring

Asymptomatic shedding of *Salmonella* bacteria in stool can persist for a median of 5 weeks after acute infection. Routine follow-up stool cultures are not recommended for immunocompetent individuals; however, cultures may be useful for patients with persistent or relapsing symptoms. In addition, local health departments may recommend follow-up stool cultures for patients who are healthcare workers or food handlers. Stool samples should be taken at least 1 week after antibiotic treatment is completed and at least 1 month after acute illness onset. Testing should be performed on three separate stool samples taken at least 24 hours apart. Approximately 1% of patients will become chronic carriers of *Salmonella*, defined as shedding bacteria in their stool for more than 12 months after acute infection. Chronic carriers should be treated with amoxicillin[1] 1 g orally three times per day for 3 months. Alternative treatments include trimethoprim-sulfamethoxazole[1] twice daily for 3 months, or ciprofloxacin[1] 750 mg twice daily for 1 month. Ultimately, the antimicrobial selected should be dictated by sensitivities.

Prevention

Education is the cornerstone of prevention. Promoting both good hand hygiene and avoidance of cross-contamination are essential. All people should be encouraged to wash hands with soap and water after defecation and urination and before preparing and consuming food, with special attention to food handlers. Good hand hygiene should also follow contact with animals or their environments, in particular reptiles such as turtles and iguanas. The CDC recommends that children under 5 years of age and immunocompromised patients avoid contact with reptiles, live poultry such as chickens and ducks, and petting zoos and country farms. Risk can be decreased by immediate hand hygiene after contact.

Additional preventative measures include the following:
- Avoid ingestion of raw eggs.
- Thoroughly cook poultry to internal temperature of at least 160 degrees.
- Pasteurize eggs and dairy.
- Wash raw fruits and vegetables before consumption.
- Wash food preparation surfaces and utensils with soap and warm water before use.
- Avoid contaminating food that will not be cooked (such as salad) with food that will be cooked (such as raw chicken).

Patients with diarrhea should remain out of work until diarrhea resolves, should wash hands frequently, and should avoid preparing food for others. Do not offer empiric or preventative antibiotic therapy to asymptomatic contacts of patients with acute or persistent watery diarrhea, but instead follow appropriate infection prevention and control measures.

[1] Not FDA approved for this indication.

References

Acheson D, Hohmann EL: Nontyphoidal salmonellosis, *Clin Infect Dis* 32(2):263–269, 2001, https://doi.org/10.1086/318457.

Angulo FJ, Molbak K: Human health consequences of antimicrobial drug--resistant salmonella and other foodborne pathogens, *Clin Infect Dis* 41(11):1613–1620, 2005, https://doi.org/10.1086/497599.

Buchwald DS, Blaser MJ: A review of human salmonellosis: II. Duration of excretion following infection with nontyphi salmonella, *Clin Infect Dis* 6(3):345–356, 1984, https://doi.org/10.1093/clinids/6.3.345. [Accessed 12 October 2020].

Crowe SJ, et al: Vital signs: multistate foodborne outbreaks — United States, 2010–2014, *MMWR Morb Mortal Wkly Rep* 64(43):1221–1225, 2015, https://doi.org/10.15585/mmwr.mm6443a4. [Accessed 25 February 2021].

Cybulski J, et al: Clinical impact of a multiplex gastrointestinal polymerase chain reaction panel in patients with acute gastroenteritis, *Clin Infect Dis* 67(11), 2018https://doi.org/10.1093/cid/ciy357. [Accessed 11 April 2023].

Humphries RM, et al: In vitro susceptibility testing of fluoroquinolone activity against salmonella: recent changes to CLSI standards, *Clin Infect Dis* 55(8):1107–1113, 2012, https://doi.org/10.1093/cid/cis600. [Accessed 24 Sept. 2021].

Mead PS, et al: Food-related illness and death in the United States, *Emerg Infect Dis* 5(5):607–625, 1999, https://doi.org/10.3201/eid0505.990502. www.ncbi.nlm.nih.gov/pmc/articles/PMC2627714/.

Mulvey MR, et al: Emergence of multidrug-resistant salmonella enterica serotype 4,[5],12:I:- Involving human cases in Canada: results from the canadian integrated program on antimicrobial resistance surveillance (CIPARS), 2003-10, *J Antimicrob Chemother* 68(9):1982–1986, 2013, https://doi.org/10.1093/jac/dkt149. [Accessed 28 May 2022].

Nakaya H, et al: Life-threatening infantile diarrhea from fluoroquinolone-resistant salmonella enteric typhimurium with mutations in both GyrA and ParC, *Emerg Infect Dis* 9(2):255–257, 2003, https://doi.org/10.3201/eid0902.020185. www.ncbi.nlm.nih.gov/pmc/articles/PMC2901941/. [Accessed 16 October 2020].

Olsen SJ, et al: A nosocomial outbreak of fluoroquinolone-resistant salmonella infection, *N Engl J Med* 344(21):1572–1579, 2001, https://doi.org/10.1056/nejm200105243442102. [Accessed 29 April 2022].

Patà Z, et al: Nontyphoidal salmonella outbreaks associated with chocolate consumption: a systematic review, *Pediatr Infect Dis*, 2024https://doi.org/10.1097/inf.0000000000004252.

Smith K: *Outbreak of multidrug-resistant salmonella typhimurium associated with rodents purchased at retail pet stores --- United States, December 2003--October 2004*, Center for Disease Control, 2019. www.cdc.gov/mmwr/preview/mmwrhtml/mm5417a3.htm. [Accessed 6 December 2019].

Su L-H, et al: Antimicrobial resistance in nontyphoid salmonella serotypes: a global challenge, *Clin Infect Dis* 39(4):546–551, 2004, https://doi.org/10.1086/422726. academic.oup.com/cid/article/39/4/546/368085.

Voetsch AC, et al: FoodNet estimate of the burden of illness caused by nontyphoidal salmonella infections in the United States, *Clin Infect Dis* 38(s3):S127–S134, 2004, https://doi.org/10.1086/381578. [Accessed 7 August 2020].

SEPSIS

Method of
Hilary Faust, MD; Rabab Nasim, MD; and Jeannina Smith, MD

CURRENT DIAGNOSIS

Sepsis
- Life-threatening end organ dysfunction caused by dysregulated host inflammatory response to infection

Septic Shock
- A subset of sepsis in which particularly profound circulatory, cellular, and metabolic abnormalities are associated with a greater risk of mortality than with sepsis alone

Sequential Organ Failure Assessment Score
- Assessment of severity (not diagnosis) of sepsis (https://www.mdcalc.com/calc/691/sequential-organ-failure-assessment-sofa-score)
- Comprises measurements of respiratory, cardiovascular, central nervous system, renal, coagulation, and hepatic dysfunction
- Validated as a predictor of mortality and prolonged intensive care unit (ICU) stay
- May apply less favorably in certain populations, including African American patients

Quick Sequential Organ Failure Assessment Score

- Screening tool for organ dysfunction in adults (>18 years old) (https://www.mdcalc.com/calc/2654/qsofa-quick-sofa-score-sepsis)
- May apply less favorably to patients in ICU and emergency department settings
- A score ≥2 prompts for evaluation for sepsis and is used for screening, *not* diagnosis
  - Altered mental status (Glasgow Coma Scale score <15)
  - Respiratory rate ≥22/min
  - Systolic blood pressure ≤100 mm Hg

Laboratory Findings

- Lactic acidosis (≥2 mmol/L)
- Hypoxia (Pao_2:Fio_2 <400)
- Hyperbilirubinemia (≥1.2 mg/dL)
- Acute kidney injury (creatinine ≥1.2)
- Thrombocytopenia (<150,000/μL)
- Leukocytosis or leukopenia (white blood cell count <4000 or >12,000/μL)
- Elevated C-reactive protein or procalcitonin levels

Physical Findings

- Altered mental status (Glasgow Coma Scale score <15)
- Increased capillary refill (>2 seconds)
- Anuria and oliguria (urine output <500 mL/day)
- Tachypnea (respiratory rate >22/min)
- Tachycardia (heart rate >90 beats/min)
- Hypothermia or hyperthermia (temperature <36°C or >38°C)
- Hypotension (systolic blood pressure <90 mm Hg or mean arterial pressure <65 mm Hg)

CURRENT THERAPY

Initial 3 Hours of Triage (or Within 1 Hour of Presumptive Diagnosis)*

- Initiate adequate fluid resuscitation with balanced crystalloid solution at 30 mL/kg
- Obtain blood, urine, and other appropriate cultures (sputum, cerebrospinal fluid, abscess fluid, indwelling vascular catheters, tissues)
- Administer empiric antimicrobial therapy based on suspected source of infection
- Perform appropriate imaging studies as allowed by clinical circumstances
- Obtain source control with procedural or surgical intervention, as appropriate

Subsequent Interventions

- Add norepinephrine (Levophed) as first-line vasopressor for persistent hypotension (mean arterial pressure ≤65 mm Hg) after adequate fluid resuscitation
- Initiate therapy with dobutamine (Dobutrex) for inotropic support if there is suspicion of contributory cardiogenic shock
- Initiate therapy with hydrocortisone (Solu-Cortef)[1] plus fludrocortisone (Florinef)[1] for patients with continued hypotension after adequate fluid resuscitation and vasopressors
- Maintain glycemic control with a target blood glucose level <180 mg/dL
- Administer unfractionated or low-molecular-weight heparin for prophylaxis against deep vein thrombosis
- Administer proton pump inhibitors for stress ulcer prophylaxis

*Note: All interventions should be undertaken simultaneously and initiated within 1 hour after making a presumptive diagnosis of sepsis.
[1]Not FDA approved for this indication.

Definitions

Sepsis is defined as a life-threatening dysregulated inflammatory response of the body caused by infection resulting in end organ damage. Sepsis was typically fatal in the preantibiotic era, and morbidity and mortality remain substantial. The cardinal finding is organ dysfunction that is unrelated to the primary site of infection. Organ systems affected by sepsis most commonly include the cardiovascular system, respiratory system, renal system, and central nervous system. Endocrinologic, hematologic, and gastrointestinal/hepatic involvement is also common. Uncontrolled sepsis typically progresses to septic shock, implying a graver degree of illness with associated increased mortality. Septic shock is broadly defined as a subset of sepsis in which the underlying circulatory cellular/metabolic abnormalities are profound enough to substantially increase mortality; clinical markers of this degree of severity include persistent hypotension (mean arterial pressure [MAP] <65) requiring vasopressors and elevated serum lactate levels (>2 mmol/L or 18 mg/dL) despite adequate volume resuscitation.

Pathophysiology

Infection of the host by a microorganism leads to innate and adaptive immune activation. The functions of these innate and adaptive systems are to isolate the source of infection, deprive pathogens of the ability to replicate, and eliminate them. This process is highly regulated with many different cell types and mediators involved, striking a delicate balance between proinflammatory and antiinflammatory effects. When appropriately regulated, there is localized tissue injury or destruction mediated by the host immune system; this damage is subsequently repaired after resolution of the infection.

Sepsis is the failure of localization such that immune activation becomes generalized and leads to tissue injury or destruction remote from the site of infection. How the immune system enters this state of dysregulation remains poorly understood, though it likely represents interplay between the host's immune system and the pathogen itself. Some microbes promote generalized immune activation via the elaboration of specific pathogen-associated molecular patterns or the elaboration of exotoxin (typically by gram-positive bacteria) and endotoxin (gram-negative–derived lipopolysaccharide). Immune recognition of these mediators leads to generalized tissue destruction by means of ischemia, direct cytotoxicity, and accelerated programmed cell death. Damage-associated molecular patterns from cell death may further amplify the inflammatory response, leading to a cascading activation of the generalized immune response.

The host response is highly heterogenous, making it difficult to predict who will be at a higher risk of developing sepsis or progressing to septic shock. Genetic predisposition to sepsis and sepsis mortality has long been recognized, with specific genetic loci increasingly identified as risk factors. An enormous amount of research over the past four decades has elucidated many of the pathways and mediators involved. Tumor necrosis factor-alpha; platelet-activating factor; interleukin (IL)-1, IL-6, and IL-8; eicosanoids; complement pathway proteins; interferons; and nitric oxide are among the biologically active molecules characterized to date. As sequencing and analytic methods have grown more powerful over the last decade, studies utilizing integrated genomics have identified various genetic variants more likely to have pathogenic response to infections. Certain endotypes within sepsis reflecting differential gene expression such as sepsis response syndromes 1 and 2 and the Dutch molecular diagnosis and risk stratification of sepsis (MARS) 1 to 4 endotypes are noted to have differential mortality rates and treatment response. These studies provide a platform for future exploration of a "precision medicine approach" to targeted therapeutic intervention to improve sepsis outcomes, but they are not yet clinically relevant.

Microbiology

Sepsis may be caused by viral, bacterial, fungal, or parasitic infections, with bacterial infections being the most widely recognized and studied. The role of viruses in sepsis has been underappreciated historically, perhaps due to diagnostic challenges. The SARS-CoV-2 pandemic has demonstrated that viral sepsis can be highly morbid, though many other common viruses can cause sepsis, including influenza, respiratory syncytial virus, adenovirus, and parainfluenza, among others.

Bacterial infection is the most common cause of sepsis, and early empiric antimicrobial therapy is generally directed against bacterial organisms. Common causes of sepsis include gram-positive pathogens such as *Staphylococcus aureus* and *Streptococcus pneumoniae*. Among gram-negative pathogens, *Escherichia coli, Klebsiella* spp., and *Pseudomonas aeruginosa* are most often reported. The emergence of resistant organisms, particularly methicillin-resistant *S. aureus* and gram-negative bacteria harboring extended-spectrum β-lactamases, increases the risk of antibiotic failure and attendant mortality.

Fungal pathogens and parasites may cause sepsis as well. In recent years, non-*albicans Candida* species continue to increase in incidence, particularly among patients who are immunocompromised. *Candida* bloodstream infections caused increasing rates of sepsis from 2017 to 2021, with non-*Albicans* species comprising nearly two thirds of cases. Endemic fungi such as *Blastomyces, Histoplasma, Coccidioides,* and *Paracoccidioides* may cause highly morbid disease in certain regions. *Plasmodium* infection remains a leading cause of sepsis worldwide, with impacts from climate change threatening to expand the geographic distribution of these parasites and their insect vectors.

Epidemiology
Sepsis and septic shock are among the leading causes of death globally and often reported as the leading cause of death of hospitalized patients in the United States. The most recent World Health Organization reports of incidence and mortality estimate a rate of 189 cases per 100,000 person-years worldwide, with an overall mortality of 26.7%. Risk of mortality exists on a continuum, with more modest rates in early sepsis and much higher rates (exceeding 40%) in cases of septic shock. Although community-acquired sepsis is more common, hospital-acquired sepsis is associated with higher morbidity and mortality. Risk of mortality also increases at the extremes of age (i.e., elderly and infant patients), in the presence of preexisting immunocompromising conditions, and in cases arising from antimicrobial-resistant or nosocomial organisms. Disparities in mortality rates are observed across demographic groups, with higher mortality rates in the United States among non-Hispanic African American men and among rural populations.

Etiologies of sepsis depend on geographic location and reflect underlying patterns of infectious disease. Pneumonia is the leading cause of sepsis in the United States, followed by abdominal infections, bloodstream infections, and urinary tract infections. Worldwide, diarrheal illnesses are the most common cause, with pneumonia representing the leading cause of worldwide mortality. It is important to note that in nearly 50% of cases, an underlying pathogen is unable to be identified; culture negativity is an independent predictor of death in patients with sepsis, and the choice of antimicrobial therapy is often empirical based on clinical presentation, epidemiology, patient risk factors, and local patterns of antimicrobial resistance.

Clinical Manifestations
Because sepsis involves diffuse immune dysregulation and multiorgan dysfunction, no single symptom, physical finding, laboratory abnormality, or radiographic finding can be relied upon to make or exclude the diagnosis. Isolation of a particular microorganism in the setting of end organ dysfunction is highly suggestive, although not pathognomonic in all cases. Increasing numbers of physical findings and biomarkers associated with organ system dysfunction correlate with an increasing likelihood of the diagnosis of sepsis, and thus an adequate diagnostic workup entails a thorough clinical and laboratory evaluation.

Typical clinical findings include hypoxia and/or hypercarbia, oliguria, acute kidney injury (AKI), hypoperfusion, sepsis-induced cardiomyopathy, hyperglycemia or hypoglycemia, thrombocytopenia, anemia, coagulopathy, ileus, acute liver injury, hyperbilirubinemia, lactic acidosis, hyper/hypothermia, and hypotension. Due to sepsis-related endothelial dysfunction, septic shock typically manifests as a distributive shock with relatively warm extremities, a wide pulse pressure, and flushing of the skin, although such findings are not universally present. In advanced stages of septic shock, excessive sympathetic tone may lead to a relative imbalance in peripheral vasoconstriction, resulting in microcirculatory dysfunction that can be manifested by delayed capillary refill.

Diagnosis
The diagnosis of sepsis ultimately relies on the clinical suspicion of infection in the setting of end organ dysfunction. Due to the varied presentation and need for early intervention, early screening for sepsis during initial triage and clinical evaluation is essential. Estimated rates of missed or delayed diagnosis of sepsis are as high as 20%, with delays in diagnosis delaying proper management. Several screening tools are available for clinical use. The quick Sequential Organ Failure Assessment screening tool (https://www.mdcalc.com/calc/2654/qsofa-quick-sofa-score-sepsis) is one such tool that identifies organ dysfunction, distinguishing uncomplicated infection from sepsis, although its sensitivity has been shown to be low in some subsequent studies. Clinical deterioration scores such as the Modified Early Warning Score (MEWS), National Early Warning Score (NEWS), and others may be helpful in identifying patients at risk of decompensating, but are not designed to discriminate between septic and nonseptic patients. A constellation of other supportive evidence establishes a greater or lesser likelihood of the presence of sepsis (see the "Current Diagnosis" box). If clinical suspicion of an underlying infection warrants obtaining blood and/or fluid cultures, the diagnosis of sepsis can be presumed and justifies the initiation of empiric treatment. It is rare that specific microbiologic identification and antibiotic susceptibilities are available to guide initial therapy; therefore careful attention to clinical history, physical examination, laboratory findings, and a high index of suspicion are essential to making a timely clinical diagnosis.

Biomarkers in Sepsis
The need for a prompt diagnosis and treatment of sepsis has led to intense research into biomarkers for diagnosis and prognostication. Over 250 biomarkers have been identified in sepsis, although procalcitonin and C-reactive protein remain the principal biomarkers in wide clinical use. Procalcitonin is a precursor to calcitonin that is often upregulated in systemic inflammation (especially due to bacterial infection). Data shows that the use of procalcitonin is beneficial as a tool to deescalate antibiotics in patients who present with sepsis, particularly those with community-acquired pulmonary infections. A randomized trial has shown use of procalcitonin to guide discontinuation of antibiotic therapy to be associated with a reduction in 28-day mortality in patients with pneumonia, pyelonephritis, or primary bloodstream infections, suggesting that this may be a useful approach to antimicrobial deescalation even in cases of septic shock. In moderate-to-severe COVID-19 infection, elevated C-reactive protein markers are predictive of poor clinical outcomes and are used to guide immunomodulatory therapy. Identifying sepsis biomarkers with superior diagnostic performance to procalcitonin and C-reactive protein is an area of active study. Some promising examples include decoy receptor 3, group II phospholipase A2, sCD163, CD64, and heparin-binding protein, but they require further research and validation before they become available for widespread clinical use.

Treatment
Screening and Early Treatment
Sepsis and septic shock are medical emergencies, and it is recommended to begin treatment and resuscitation immediately (within the first 3 hours of triage or within 1 hour of presumed diagnosis, with expedited timelines in severe cases). Clinicians should

not wait for microbiological confirmation or evidence of worsening end organ dysfunction before initiating therapy. Current guidelines from the Surviving Sepsis Campaign, an international initiative to improve sepsis outcomes, emphasize the importance of early screening and initiation of treatment, with reliance on protocolized resuscitation and early treatment measures. These protocols, commonly referred to as *sepsis bundles* or *sepsis resuscitation bundles,* emphasize timely culture and laboratory collection, early supportive and resuscitative measures, timely initiation of broad-spectrum antimicrobial therapy, and reassessment of clinical status and response to interventions. Compliance with these protocols has been shown to decrease sepsis morbidity and mortality, and ongoing performance improvement programs focused around increasing the adequacy of sepsis bundles and adherence to them are important to improving health system outcomes.

For all patients with sepsis and septic shock, recommended early interventions include measuring serum lactate; obtaining laboratory data including markers of renal, hepatic, and cardiac function; obtaining blood cultures and cultures of suspected sources of infection; performing radiographic imaging of potential infectious sources; and administering broad-spectrum antibiotics. If serum lactate exceeds 2 mg/dL, it should be repeated within 6 hours of presentation.

Initial Resuscitation

For patients with evidence of hypoperfusion or hypotension on presentation (MAP <65 mm Hg, systolic blood pressure <90 mm Hg, diastolic blood pressure <60 mm Hg, lactate level >4 mg/dL, or clinical evidence of hypoperfusion) it is generally recommended to administer IV crystalloid solution as first-line therapy. The patient's volume status should be carefully assessed during and after resuscitation, with direction toward improving MAP above 65 mm Hg, maintaining urine output above 0.5 mL/kg, and decreasing lactate by 20%. While a volume of 30 mL/kg is often cited as a "standard" dose, appropriate fluid resuscitation is specific to the patient and clinical context. Normal saline (0.9%) has historically been a mainstay of IV resuscitation, although its use has been linked with hyperchloremic acidosis, AKI, and requirement for renal replacement therapy. Balanced crystalloid solutions like lactated Ringer solution (also known as Hartmann solution) or Plasma-Lyte A, which have electrolyte compositions more similar to plasma, have improved performance over normal saline solution and should be used when available.

Colloids like albumin are more effective at volume resuscitation compared with crystalloids in septic shock, although the translation of this finding to improved outcomes remains uncertain. The Saline versus Albumin Fluid Evaluation trial and the Albumin Italian Outcome Sepsis trial failed to demonstrate a mortality benefit when using albumin solution for fluid resuscitation compared with crystalloid solution, although post hoc analyses have suggested possible improved effects in cases of septic shock. The Surviving Sepsis Campaign has suggested the use of albumin in patients requiring large volumes of fluid resuscitation based on these data, and other populations (e.g., patients with cirrhosis, malnutrition) may also benefit from albumin resuscitation. Use of synthetic colloids such as pentastarch[2] or hydroxyethyl starch are associated with increased risk of mortality, AKI, and other serious adverse events. Both have no role and should be avoided in septic patients.

Antimicrobial Therapy

National and international guidelines recommend early empiric broad-spectrum antibiotics for all patients with suspected sepsis. Timely initiation (within 1 hour of suspected septic shock or known sepsis and within 3 hours of suspected sepsis without shock) of appropriate antimicrobials is critical because the risk of mortality increases with every hour antibiotic administration is

[2] Not available in the United States.

delayed. In circumstances where obtaining body fluid for culture may be significantly delayed (e.g., intraabdominal infection, CNS infection), antibiotic therapy should not be withheld in hopes of increasing the yield of culture data.

Empiric antibiotic regimens should be tailored to suspected sources of infection, local patterns of resistance, risk factors for nosocomial/resistant infection, and prior culture results (if available). Inadequate therapy is much more likely in patients infected with resistant pathogens including methicillin-resistant *S. aureus*, vancomycin-resistant enterococci, and resistant gram-negative bacteria, as well as in nosocomial sepsis. Attention to community and institutional resistance patterns and antibiogram data is vital in determining empiric regimens. The increasing availability of multiplex molecular assays can increase the sensitivity of culture data and rapidly guide appropriate antimicrobial therapy. Panels that use nucleic acid amplification testing capable of identifying a variety of common respiratory, enteric, and CNS pathogens are becoming more widely available and can decrease the time to identifying causative organisms and ensuring adequate treatment for patients with sepsis while facilitating appropriate antimicrobial deescalation.

Deescalation from early broad-spectrum antibiotic therapy, generally within 72 hours of initial treatment or within 24 hours of definitive culture results, has been shown to be safe in patients suffering from both sepsis and septic shock. Because a causative organism is often not isolated, decisions regarding antibiotic deescalation should be tailored to clinical circumstances, patient history, and clinical course. There is no definitive data that deescalation of broad-spectrum antibiotics increases the risk of cultivating antibiotic-resistant organisms.

Monitoring Treatment Response

After initial IV fluid resuscitation and the administration of empiric antimicrobial therapy, close ongoing monitoring of treatment response is essential in the treatment of sepsis. The decision to administer additional IV fluid resuscitation requires close attention to the clinical course after initial fluid resuscitation and the patient's ability to tolerate additional IV fluid, particularly in patients who have concomitant heart failure, limited respiratory reserve, and chronic kidney disease. Serial measurement of serum lactate levels (with a target of a 20% reduction) and serial assessment of capillary refill time (with a goal refill time <3 seconds) have been associated with lower overall IV fluid administration and possible improvements in 28-day mortality. Both methods are widely available and require no specialized monitoring or intensive operator training.

While in the past attention was paid to static parameters like central venous pressure and a central venous oxygenation ($Scvo_2$) to objectively guide fluid resuscitation, these parameters have fallen out of favor after failing to improve outcomes and possibly resulting in overresuscitation. Emphasis on dynamic parameters indicating fluid responsiveness, including pulse pressure variation, stroke volume variation, respirophasic variation of the inferior vena cava (IVC), and response to passive leg raise testing can be used to predict fluid responsiveness.

Pulse pressure variation is calculated as a difference in systolic and diastolic arterial blood pressure and for mechanically ventilated patients is a good indicator of volume responsiveness. A systematic review of 29 studies reported a higher area under the receiver operating characteristic curve for pulse pressure variation compared with central venous pressure (0.94 vs. 0.55) as an indicator of fluid responsiveness. Stroke volume variation greater than 10% measured by echocardiography is also associated with fluid responsiveness. According to one study, stroke volume variation showed a sensitivity and specificity of 94% each, and another meta-analysis reported that it resulted in shorter length of hospital stay. Use of point-of-care ultrasonography to assess respirophasic variation in the IVC, with a change in IVC diameter of greater than 20% during spontaneous unsupported respiration, has been associated with potential fluid responsiveness. In patients on invasive mechanical ventilation who are not making respiratory effort, variation of 12% to 18% has likewise been associated with volume responsiveness, though sensitivity and specificity are poor. IVC variation is subject to numerous confounding factors, and is not recommended as a sole means of determining fluid responsiveness. Other maneuvers, including the passive leg raising test, have demonstrated similar performance and may be employed in concert with each other to determine an individual patient's likelihood to respond to administration of IV fluid. Improved means of determining fluid responsiveness remains an active area of research.

Vasopressor Support

If there is persistent hypotension despite adequate fluid resuscitation, support of blood pressure with vasopressors is recommended. Blood pressure targets are generally based on MAP, with a goal of MAP above 65 mm Hg being appropriate for most patients. High MAP targets may improve renal function in patients with chronic hypertension but have been associated with increased rates of arrythmia. Likewise, lower MAP targets may be appropriate in certain chronic conditions like cirrhosis.

Timing of vasopressor administration remains an area of ongoing clinical investigation. Randomized controlled trials of early vasopressor initiation in early sepsis and patients in the intensive care unit (ICU) have not demonstrated a mortality benefit over protocolized fluid resuscitation in the CLOVERS and CLASSIC trials. CENSER found earlier resolution of shock and lower incidence of cardiogenic pulmonary edema and arrythmia, although this did not translate into reduced 28-day mortality. Choice of fluid resuscitation or early vasopressor initiation should therefore be tailored based on individual patient characteristics, such as history of clinical evidence of volume depletion, history of end-stage renal disease or congestive heart failure, or evidence of volume overload.

Norepinephrine is recommended as the first-line agent recommended for septic shock, and addition of vasopressin and epinephrine as potential second-line agents is recommended. Some clinical trials have suggested vasopressin may reduce the need for renal replacement therapy, though this finding has not been demonstrated consistently. Due to demonstrated increased risk from arrythmia compared with norepinephrine, use of dopamine for renal protection is no longer recommended unless norepinephrine is not available. Dobutamine or epinephrine is recommended if evidence of hypoperfusion persists and there is suspicion for contribution from cardiogenic shock (including stress-induced cardiomyopathy). Delays in obtaining central access should not preclude administration of vasopressor therapy when indicated, as risks of complication from extravasation are relatively low with careful monitoring. While the threshold for safe dosing of peripheral vasopressors remains an area of active study, maintenance of blood pressure with peripherally administered vasopressor therapy has a favorable risk/benefit profile pending the timely establishment of central access.

Source Control

A survey for potential sources of infection should be performed concomitantly with early resuscitation efforts. Elimination of the source of infection is critical to the treatment of sepsis and septic shock. Conditions that require emergent intervention, such as necrotizing fasciitis, cholangitis, and intestinal infarction should be ruled out within the first 6 hours after presentation. Potentially infected indwelling devices should be removed as soon as possible. Necrotic tissue should be debrided and abscesses drained if either condition is detected. Practitioners must consider the risks and benefits of the specific invasive procedures and the timing of such interventions for each patient individually. Imaging studies such as computed tomography of the head, chest, abdomen, and pelvis are commonly necessary to assess for potential sources or sequelae of infection. An exception to the mandate to drain or debride infected collections is the presence of infected pancreatic necrosis, in which case a step-up approach including endoscopic and/or percutaneous drainage, preferably delayed by at least 2 weeks, is preferred.

Steroid Use

Patients with critical illness can develop relative or, more rarely, absolute adrenal insufficiency. Administration of low-dose glucocorticoids, typically hydrocortisone[1] 200 to 300 mg in divided doses, has consistently been associated with faster reversal of septic shock and decreased vasopressor requirement. However, the data conflict as to whether there is a mortality benefit associated with steroid use. A large meta-analysis found that there was no overall association of glucocorticoid use with improved mortality but did find improved 28-day, ICU, and hospital mortality with combined administration of hydrocortisone and fludrocortisone[1]. Subsequent studies have found that response to steroids interacts may depend on underlying shock endotype, with benefit in the SRS1 endotype and possibly associated harm in the SRS2 endotype. Pending more definitive clinical data on shock endotypes and treatment outcomes, the benefits of glucocorticoid therapy (with coadministration of mineralocorticoid when feasible) likely outweigh potential harm, and should be considered in all critically ill sepsis patients. Steroids should be tapered as soon as vasopressor support is no longer required.

Nutrition in the Critically Ill Patient

Critically ill patients are in a state of catabolism, and studies have shown that early enteral nutrition (defined as within 48 hours of admission to the critical care unit) can decrease the risk of infection and mortality. Various guidelines recommend initiation of enteral nutrition within 24 to 72 hours of ICU admission for septic shock in patients without contraindication to enteral nutrition; patients who are requiring high levels of vasopressor support (>0.3 mcg/kg/min or equivalent), have escalating vasopressor requirements, or are suffering from intraabdominal infections should not receive enteral nutrition until their clinical condition stabilizes. There is theoretical risk of precipitating mesenteric ischemia or nonocclusive bowel necrosis with the introduction of enteral feeding when patients are on high doses of vasopressors, and secondary effects of enteral feeding (e.g., nausea/vomiting, aspiration) may pose additional risks to this patient population.

Randomized controlled trials investigating early parenteral nutrition in critically ill patients have failed to demonstrate mortality benefit or superiority over enteral feeding. While parenteral nutrition may reduce the risk of GI complications from enteral nutrition, its use is associated with increased length of ICU stay and increased systemic costs. In patients who are unable to receive enteral nutrition for a prolonged period (≥7 days), parenteral nutrition should be considered. Close attention to liver function, triglyceride levels, secondary infection, and intravascular volume status should be paid to patients on parenteral nutrition, with transition to enteral feeding when clinically feasible.

Glycemic Control

It is recommended to target blood glucose target between 140 and 180 mg/dL for critically ill patients rather than tighter control with intensive insulin therapy. Several studies have shown that tighter blood glucose control has no benefit and is associated with increased incidence of hypoglycemia and a higher risk of mortality. Clinical trial data from the 2021 CONTROLING study demonstrated that the use of individualized glucose targets based on pre-ICU glycated hemoglobin levels resulted in higher rates of severe hypoglycemia and increased mortality in nondiabetic patients; thus a goal of less than 180 mg/dL is appropriate for this population.

Summary

Sepsis remains a life-threatening medical emergency and a leading cause of death in the United States and worldwide. Early recognition and aggressive management are vital to improving outcomes, yet the diagnosis continues to require a high index of suspicion, timely evaluation, and robust clinical judgment. Major challenges include diagnostic uncertainty, low yield of current culture techniques, and antimicrobial overuse and resistance. Improvements in diagnostic and prognostic biomarkers, technologies to

---

[1] Not FDA approved for this indication.

identify responsible microbes, identification of biologically based endotypes, and precision therapies are promising areas for future inquiry and improvement in sepsis care.

References

Evans L, Rhodes A, Alhazzani W, et al: Surviving sepsis Campaign: international guidelines for management of sepsis and septic shock 2021, *Crit Care Med* 49(11):e1063–e1143, 2021.

Kyriazopoulou E, Liaskou-Antoniou L, Adamis G, et al: Procalcitonin to reduce long-term infection-associated adverse events in sepsis. a randomized trial, *Am J Respir Crit Care Med* 203(2):202–210, 2021.

Lyu QQ, Chen QH, Zheng RQ, Yu JQ, Gu XH: Effect of low-dose hydrocortisone therapy in adult patients with septic shock: a meta-analysis with trial sequential analysis of randomized controlled trials, *J Intensive Care Med* 35(10):971–983, 2020.

Meyhoff TS, Hjortrup PB, Wettersley J, CLASSIC Trial Group et al: Restriction of intravenous fluid in ICU patients with septic shock, *N Engl J Med* 386(26):2459–2470, 2022.

National Heart, Lung, and Blood Institute Prevention and Early Treatment of Acute Lung Injury Clinical Trials Network, Shapiro NI, Douglas IS, Brower RG, et al: Early restrictive or liberal fluid management for sepsis-induced hypotension, *N Engl J Med* 388(6):499–510, 2023.

Rudd KE, Johnson SC, Agesa KM, et al: Global, regional, and national sepsis incidence and mortality, 1990-2017: analysis for the global burden of disease Study, *Lancet* 395(10219):200–211, 2020.

SMALLPOX

Method of
Raul Davaro, MD

CURRENT DIAGNOSIS

- Human-to-human transmission of variola virus occurs by inhalation of large, virus-containing airborne droplets of saliva from an infected person.
- Before smallpox was eradicated, the disease had a secondary household or close contact attack rate of approximately 60% among unvaccinated individuals.
- There are four main clinical forms of smallpox, each with different characteristics.
- During the smallpox era, the case-fatality rate differed for the different clinical forms, but it was approximately 30% overall in unvaccinated individuals.

CURRENT THERAPY

- Tecovirimat (Tpoxx) and brincidofovir (Tembexa) have been approved for treatment of smallpox.
- Isolating patients in a negative-pressure room and ensuring vaccination is the main course of therapy.

Smallpox is caused by the variola virus (VARV) and is highly infectious by the respiratory route. Susceptible persons have up to a 90% chance of contracting the disease if they are exposed to someone who is infected, and the overall fatality rate is estimated at 30% among those who have not been vaccinated. The VARV is unique among the orthopoxviruses in that it is known to be a sole human pathogen.

The World Health Organization (WHO) declared smallpox eradicated in 1980 and today is the only human disease to be eliminated by the WHO. The eradication of smallpox through vaccination has not eliminated the risk of reintroduction of the infection by the accidental or intentional release of the VARV.

This viral infection, spread by respiratory droplets, continued to have worldwide distribution at the beginning of the 20th century. Because smallpox confers immunity in the survivors of an attack, its persistence depends on the contact of nonimmune persons with infected persons in the initial 2 weeks of acquiring the infection.

The WHO designed an Intensified Eradication Program based on a ring vaccination strategy that began in 1966 and eradicated smallpox from humans in an unprecedented effort in less than 10 years. The last natural case was documented in Somalia in 1977. Routine immunization against smallpox ceased in the United States in 1972 and worldwide in 1980. It was thought that without a human reservoir, the reemergence of this infection would not occur.

Smallpox virus stocks are still available in the United States at the Centers for Disease Control and Prevention in Atlanta, Georgia, and in Russia at the State Center for Virology and Biotechnology in Novosibirsk, Siberia. These stocks are maintained under strict biocontainment measures. In the aftermath of the terrorist attacks on September 11, 2001, and the deliberate distribution of *Bacillus anthracis* afterward, President Bush announced plans to immunize healthcare workers and first responders against smallpox by 2003. Although the plan fell short of its goals, 40,000 first responders and healthcare workers were vaccinated by the end of 2003.

The Agent

Smallpox is a single, linear, double-stranded DNA virus that belongs to the *Orthopoxvirus* genus, family Poxviridae. The poxviruses replicate in the cell cytoplasm. They are brick shaped and measure about 300 nm × 250 nm × 200 nm.

Epidemiology

The natural reservoir of smallpox is the patient suffering from the disease. Smallpox spreads from person to person through droplet nuclei or fine-particle aerosols released from the pharynx of an infected person. Smallpox can also be transmitted by fomites such as clothing and bedding. Smallpox patients are not infectious until the third day of the clinical disease, typically 1 day before the skin eruption. The secondary attack rate of smallpox is 37% to 88% among unvaccinated contacts, depending on many variables.

Clinical Presentation

Smallpox occurs as either variola major or variola minor (alastrim). Variola major had a mortality rate of 30% compared with 1% for variola minor.

After an incubation period of 10 to 14 days, the illness begins with intense prostration and high fever lasting 4 to 6 days (Figure 1). Headache, photophobia, and vomiting are noted. During the prodrome phase, most patients are bedridden. Around the fourth day, the fever breaks and the patient feels better.

The initial cutaneous lesions of smallpox appear as small, red spots on the face, in the mouth and pharynx, and on the forearms. Initially, smallpox lesions are small papules, but they change into vesicles and pustules within 1 to 2 days. The initial lesions are shotty and do not disappear with pressure. Most patients exhibit lesions on their soles and palms. A typical feature of variola is that the exanthem everywhere is in the same state of evolution, unlike the exanthem of chickenpox, in which lesions exhibit all stages of evolution. At the end of days 8 to 10, the skin rash crusts and dries; it takes 3 to 4 weeks from the onset of the disease for all the scabs to fall off. The period of contagiousness ends when the last scab falls off. Scarring and pitting of the skin are common sequelae.

Patients with the hemorrhagic disease develop severe prostration, high fever, abdominal pain, petechiae, and extensive cutaneous ecchymoses. In the malignant or flat form, the lesions fail to progress to the pustular stage. In the hemorrhagic and the malignant forms, death invariably occurs within 1 week.

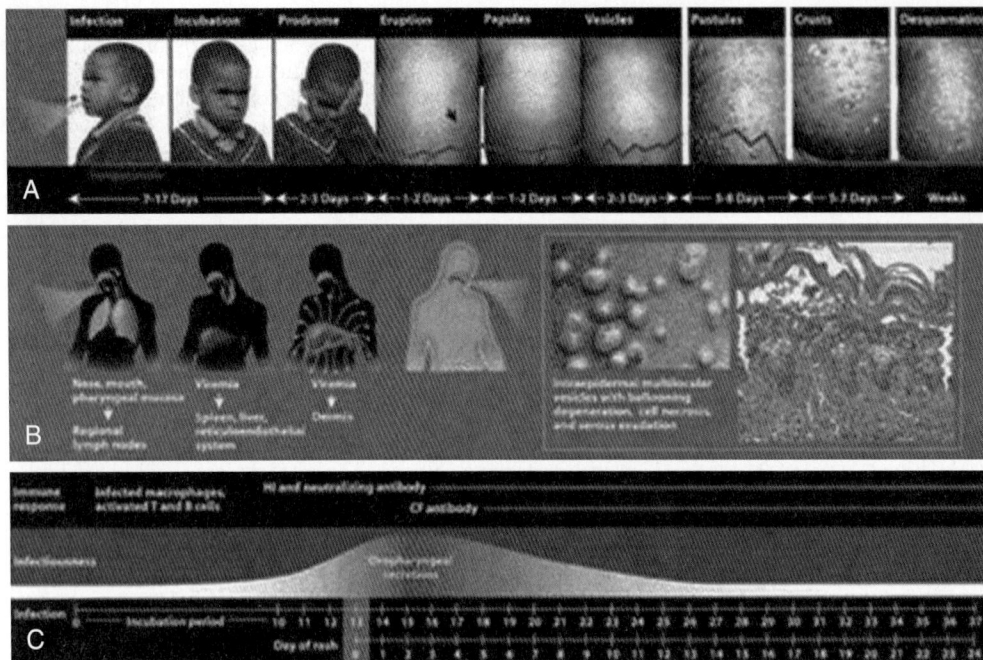

Figure 1 Clinical manifestations and pathogenesis of smallpox and the immune response. (A) The initial phases of infection and the clinical manifestations include temperature spikes and progressive skin lesions (photographs of lesions courtesy of Dr. David Heymann, World Health Organization). (B) The pathogenesis of the infection. The photographs on the *right* show the characteristic features of the vesicles caused by smallpox (H&E, ×90). (C) The immune response to smallpox and the period of infectiousness. *CF*, Complement fixation; *HI*, hemagglutination inhibition. (Reprinted with permission from Breman JG, Henderson, DA: Diagnosis and management of smallpox, *N Eng J Med* 346:1300–1308, 2002.)

Complications

Bacterial infections of the skin and other organs are common. Ocular involvement may result in blindness. Encephalitis (1 in 500 cases of variola major) is a devastating complication.

Differential Diagnosis (Figure 2)

Many rashes can be confused with smallpox, especially at the outset of the eruption when the rash is maculopapular. Monkeypox, herpes zoster, chickenpox, herpes simplex, impetigo, scabies, erythema multiforme, and syphilis are conditions that can be confused with smallpox (Box 1). When smallpox was endemic, chickenpox was the most common condition confused with smallpox. The most useful clinical points of smallpox are the following:

- Centrifugal distribution of the lesions
- All the lesions in the same stage of development
- Progression of the rash from the face to the arms, trunk, and legs
- A severe prodrome phase that lasts 4 days
- In an epidemic, known contact with an active case

Diagnosis

The identification of a suspected case of smallpox should be treated as an international health emergency. Clinical samples may be collected from vesicular or pustular fluid, blood, tonsillar swabs, and skin biopsy and must be transported to a biosafety level 4 facility for processing and testing with real-time polymerase chain reaction assays to detect virus DNA.

Lesions of varicella zoster virus (chickenpox, herpes zoster) demonstrate multinucleated giant cells on Tzanck smears; lesions of smallpox do not. Serology or electronic microscopy is not recommended for the diagnosis of smallpox because these modalities cannot distinguish among different orthopoxviruses.

Treatment

A suspected case of smallpox should be placed in a negative-pressure room with strict respiratory and contact isolation precautions. Ideally, to minimize the risk of contagion in healthcare personnel, patients with smallpox should be assisted by providers documented to have been immunized against this condition. Patients with smallpox require careful care of their eyes to avoid complications, and this is accomplished with daily eye rinsing. Patients must receive adequate nutrition and hydration. Skin and soft tissue infections must be treated with an antistaphylococcal β-lactam and, initially pending results of cultures, an antimicrobial with activity against methicillin-resistant *Staphylococcus aureus*. The US Food and Drug Administration (FDA) approved tecovirimat (Tpoxx) in 2018 for the treatment of smallpox. The safety of tecovirimat was demonstrated in 359 healthy human volunteers in whom the most frequently reported adverse effects included headache, nausea, and abdominal pain.

The recommended dosage of tecovirimat in adults weighing at least 40 kg is 600 mg (three 200-mg capsules) taken twice daily orally for 14 days. No adequate and well-controlled studies in pregnant women were conducted; therefore, there are no human data to establish the presence or absence of tecovirimat-associated risk. Common adverse reactions in healthy adult subjects (≥2%) were headache, nausea, abdominal pain, and vomiting.

In 2021 the FDA approved brincidofovir (Tembexa), a prodrug of cidofovir, for treatment of smallpox. It is indicated for treatment of human smallpox disease caused by VARV in adult and pediatric patients, including neonates. Brincidofovir dosage in adults weighing more than 48 kg is 200 mg by mouth weekly for 2 doses, given on days 1 and 8. In patients with a weight below 48 kg, the dosage is 4 mg/kg by mouth weekly for 2 doses, given on days 1 and 8.

The Strategic National Stockpile currently contains two smallpox therapeutics: tecovirimat and cidofovir.[1]

Vaccines and Vaccination

The current smallpox live vaccine, ACAM2000 (Sanofi Pasteur Biologics), is based on the traditional Jenner vaccine (using the related virus, vaccinia) and is administered in a single percutaneous dose. Vaccination after exposure—but before the rash is present—can abort or attenuate the clinical manifestations of the disease. This live vaccine is contraindicated for persons with

---

[1] Not FDA approved for this indication.

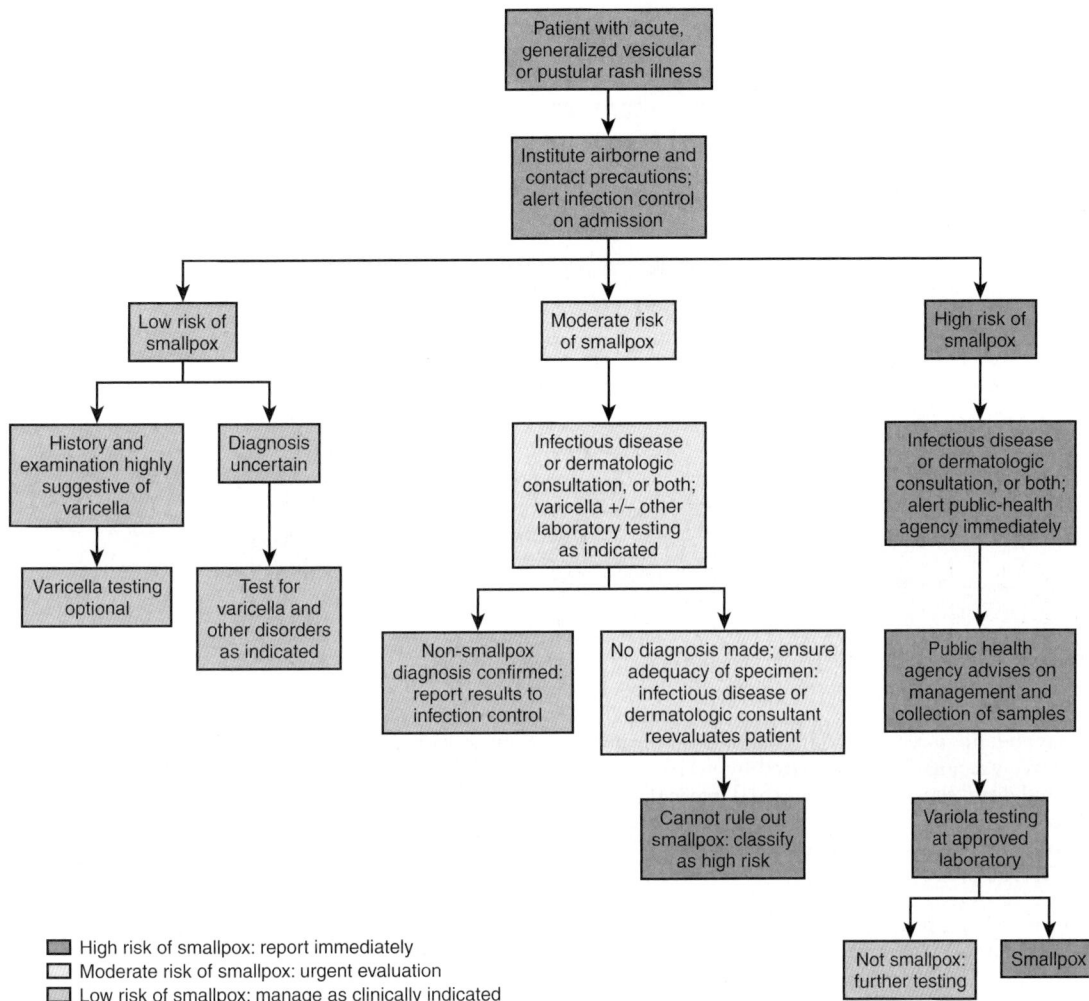

Figure 2 Algorithm for assessing patients for smallpox. (Reprinted with permission from Moore ZS, Seward JF, Lane JM: Smallpox, *Lancet*, 367:425–435, 2006.)

BOX 1	Conditions That Might Be Confused With Smallpox

Maculopapular Stage
- Measles
- Rubella
- Drug eruptions
- Secondary syphilis
- Erythema multiforme
- Scabies, insect bites
- Acne
- Scarlet fever

Vesicular/Pustular Stage
- Chickenpox
- Disseminated herpes zoster
- Disseminated herpes simplex virus
- Drug eruptions
- Contact dermatitis
- Erythema multiforme (including Stevens-Johnson syndrome)
- Enteroviral infections
- Secondary syphilis
- Acne
- Generalized vaccinia
- Monkeypox
- Impetigo
- Scabies, insect bites
- Disseminated molluscum contagiosum

severe immunosuppression, and newer-generation vaccinations have been developed for these populations. The virus begins growing at the injection site causing a localized infection or "pock" to form. A red, itchy sore spot at the site of the vaccination within 3 to 4 days is an indicator that the vaccination was successful; that is, there is "a take." A blister develops at the vaccination site and then dries up, forming a scab that falls off in the third week, leaving a small scar. If no evidence of vaccine take is apparent after 7 days, the person can be vaccinated again.

The vaccine causes local and systemic symptoms. There is an eruption at the injection site with redness and pain, systemic symptoms such as fever, and headaches. Swelling and tenderness of regional lymph nodes begin 3 to 10 days after vaccination and can last up to a month.

The Modified Vaccinia Ankara (MVA [JYNNEOS]) was compared with ACAM2000. The immune responses and attenuation of the major cutaneous reaction suggest that this MVA vaccine protected against variola infection.

The smallpox vaccine is the only known way to prevent smallpox in an exposed person. When given within 4 days of viral exposure, the vaccine can prevent or significantly lessen the severity of smallpox symptoms. Vaccination 4 to 7 days after exposure may offer some protection from the disease and may lessen its severity.

Complications

The vaccine (ACAM2000) is not without risk: it is estimated that pericarditis or myocarditis may develop in 5.7 per 1000 vaccinees. In addition, eczema vaccinatum, generalized vaccinia, progressive vaccinia, and vaccinia encephalitis can also occur (Table 1). The most common complication is inadvertent autoinoculation causing self-limited satellite lesions. Generalized vaccinia results from viremia and may be life-threatening in immunocompromised patients. Progressive vaccinia is characterized by necrosis at the inoculation site and distal sites such as bones and internal organs. Progressive vaccinia is often a fatal complication. Myopericarditis was observed with the use of adult vaccines in the United States in 2002 (see Table 1).

Contraindications to Vaccination

Persons who are immune compromised or who have severe eczema or who are pregnant should not receive postexposure vaccination against smallpox. However, in the event of exposure to a patient with smallpox, no absolute contraindication is applicable.

Use in Warfare

Because natural smallpox has been eradicated, the only possibility of a smallpox outbreak is the deliberate release of smallpox in a population by a nation or a terrorist group to inflict casualties in a civilian population. Preemptive vaccination of first responders and ring immunization of those exposed are the means available to avoid the massive propagation of smallpox. Smallpox stocks have been earmarked for destruction since the eradication of the disease in 1980. Yet, successive meetings of the World Health Assembly have postponed making a final recommendation while the threat of reemergence from elsewhere remains. At its last meeting in September 2018, the Advisory Committee on Variola Virus Research told WHO that live virus is still needed for the development of new antivirals, with split opinions on whether it is needed for diagnostics.

References

Adalja AA, Toner E, Inglesby TV: Clinical management of potential bioterrorism related conditions, N Engl J Med 372:954–962, 2015.
Breman JG, Henderson DA: Diagnosis and management of smallpox, N Engl J Med 346:1300–1308, 2002.
Breman JG: Smallpox, The Journal of Infectious Diseases 224(Suppl_4):S379–S386, 2021, https://doi.org/10.1093/infdis/jiaa588.
Centers for Disease Control and Prevention: Smallpox vaccination. Information for Health Care professionals. Available https://www.cdc.gov/smallpox/index.html [accessed 04.11.24].
Grosenbach DW, Honeychurch K, Rose EA, et al: Oral tecovirimat for the treatment of smallpox, N Engl J Med 379:44–53, 2018.
Pittman PR, Hahn M, Lee HeeChoon S, et al: Phase 3 efficacy trial of modified vaccinia ankara as a vaccine against smallpox, N Engl J Med 381:1897–1908, 2019.
World Health Organization. Smallpox. https://www.who.int/health-topics/smallpox [accessed 05/21/2024].

TETANUS

Method of
Bumsoo Park, MD, PhD

CURRENT DIAGNOSIS

- Tetanus is essentially a clinical diagnosis based on characteristic clinical manifestations.
- Characteristic clinical manifestations include trismus (or lockjaw; inability to open the mouth), risus sardonicus (sneering smile), neck stiffness, dysphagia, opisthotonus (hyperextension of the spine), and rigidity and spasms of upper and lower extremities.
- Anaerobic culture of *Clostridium tetani* from the wound can be confounded because it can be cultured from wounds with a low suspicion for tetanus.
- The immunoglobulin G (IgG)-based serologic antibody test can be confounded by previous immunization.
- Both IgM- and IgG-based point-of-care rapid test is under development and requires further investigation before becoming a mainstay diagnostic procedure.
- Given there is no reliable confirmatory test, differential diagnosis must be considered to prevent any delay in treatment of suspected tetanus and potential for resultant complications.

CURRENT TREATMENT

- The mainstay of tetanus treatment is acute, hospital-based, prompt intervention in both emergency and intensive care setting.
- Antitetanus immune globulin should be administered to rapidly neutralize tetanus toxin as soon as the diagnosis is made.
- Intramuscular human tetanus immune globulin (HyperTET) is widely available as the first-line choice. Intramuscular or intravenous equine tetanus antitoxin[1] (after an intradermal hypersensitivity testing) can be a reasonable alternative if this is the only available option.
- Clinicians may consider intrathecal administration[1] of the immune globulin in addition to intramuscular administration given potential additional benefits.

- Active immunization using tetanus toxoid is not only for prophylaxis but also for acute tetanus treatment because tetanus infection does not induce natural immunity.
- Antibiotics should be administered to inhibit local proliferation of *Clostridium tetani*. Clinicians may choose either penicillin (preferably intramuscular benzathine penicillin [Bicillin LA][1] given its benefit of single dose) or oral metronidazole (Flagyl)[1] depending on availability and preference.
- Benzodiazepines such as intravenous diazepam should be considered for proper sedation and control of muscle spasms as indicated.
- Intravenous magnesium sulfate[1] should be considered given its benefits, including control of muscle spasms, stabilizing autonomic dysfunction, reduced need for mechanical ventilation, and shorter hospital stays.
- Prompt airway management using either tracheostomy (preferred if there is laryngeal spasm) or endotracheal intubation is essential in cases of moderate-to-severe tetanus.
- To control autonomic instability, intravenous clonidine[1] can be administered to stabilize fluctuating blood pressure. Labetalol may be used to control tachycardia[1] and hypertension.
- Local wound care such as debridement and abscess drainage as well as minimization of risk of pressure ulcers is important.
- Optimization of nutrition should be considered given the catabolic state and resultant weight loss during the disease process.
- Other nursing measures that must be considered include upper airway suctioning, prophylaxis of deep vein thrombosis, nasogastric tube feeding, and/or urinary catheterization.

[1]Not FDA approved for this indication.

Tetanus is a toxin-mediated infectious disease caused by the bacterium *Clostridium tetani*. Since it was first discovered in the 1880s, tetanus remains an important public health entity with significant morbidity risk and potential for mortality with no specific measure for cure while being a vaccine-preventable condition.

Microbiology and Epidemiology

Clostridium tetani is a gram-positive, spore-forming, obligate anaerobic bacillus. It exists as spores ubiquitously in the environment, particularly in the soil, on rusty surfaces, in animal feces, and even in the human gastrointestinal tract. Spores remain dormant and viable for several months and are highly resistant to heat or usual antiseptics, yet they can be destroyed via autoclave at 121°C and 103 kPa (~1.01 atmospheric pressure) for 15 minutes. Tetanus is transmitted through open wounds or skin cuts as direct inoculation of the spores. Neonates can be infected via the umbilical cord if contaminated by cutting with unsterile instruments and the mother is unimmunized or inadequately immunized against tetanus. There is no risk of person-to-person transmission.

Since the tetanus toxoid-containing vaccine was developed in late 1940s, the incidence has markedly decreased. In the United States, approximately 20 to 25 cases of tetanus were reported yearly between 2020 and 2022 compared to annual 500 to 600 cases in the prevaccine era. This decline in incidence is similar in more economically developed area such as European countries. However, tetanus is still a major burden in less economically developed countries where immunization coverage is underestablished and access to hygienic umbilical cord care is limited. In 2019 a total of 56,903 cases of tetanus occurred in South Asia and Sub-Saharan Africa. Whereas most of the tetanus cases occur in elderly populations in high-income countries with approximately 11% case-fatality rate, neonates are widely affected in low-income countries, where the neonatal case-fatality rate even reaches 80% to 100%. The disease burden is significantly higher in males than females.

Risk Factors

Tetanus is a vaccine-preventable disease; thus, being unimmunized or inadequately immunized is a major risk factor for disease. Older people in high-income countries who were born before the vaccine program was established or whose antibody titer has waned from previous immunization are at increased risk. Neonates in less economically developed countries where vaccination coverage is underdeveloped are born with a risk of tetanus when their mothers are unimmunized. Additional risk factors include congenital or acquired immunosuppression, intravenous (IV) drug use, and diabetes mellitus.

In terms of local factors, the term "tetanus-prone wounds" is theoretically defined as wounds that are oxygen-deficient because *C. tetani* is obligate anaerobe, most often referred to the wounds that are severe, crushed, devitalized, or contaminated with dirt or rust. However, it has been reported that even minor skin disruptions such as scratches while gardening, unsterilized piercing, or animal bite may cause tetanus. Thus, any wounds except clean minor cuts should be regarded as tetanus-prone wounds.

Pathophysiology

When inoculated into the human system, the spores of *C. tetani* transform into motile bacilli that produce a potent exotoxin called tetanospasmin which is a zinc-dependent metalloproteinase that cleaves its target protein. The toxin is absorbed into the circulation and reaches lower motor neuron endings, where it inhibits the target protein synaptobrevin (a family of vesicle-associated membrane protein [VAMP]), which is essential for the release of neurotransmitters from presynaptic vesicles. Thus, the initial symptom of tetanus is flaccid paralysis. Then, the toxin is transported proximally in an extensive retrograde fashion along the axonal cytoplasm to reach motor nuclei in the brainstem and spinal cord. There, the toxin is taken up by GABAergic and/or glycinergic interneurons, where it inhibits the release of GABA and glycine, which are inhibitory neurotransmitters, resulting in motor rigidity, spasms, and autonomic hyperactivity.

Clinical Manifestations

The incubation period from the injury to the onset of symptoms can range from a few days to a few months (typically 3–21 days, average 7–10 days). Although the incubation period is not a determinant of disease severity, the period of onset (the interval between the first symptom and first proximal muscle spasm) is regarded as a predictor of disease severity, and early tracheal intubation and mechanical ventilation are usually required if the interval is less than 48 hours. The most widely used tetanus severity index is the Ablett Classification (Table 1), which clinicians should refer to for clinical decision making in directing treatment.

Non-neonatal Tetanus

Tetanus may manifest as localized tetanus (limited to an area of the entry point), cephalic tetanus (Figure 1; limited to head and neck area, including cranial nerve palsies), and generalized tetanus (where all muscle groups are affected). Localized tetanus can occur as a result of low toxin load with favorable prognosis or simply as an early manifestation of generalized tetanus, which is more common than localized cases. Because tetanospasmin reaches the motor nuclei of the shortest motor axons first, muscles innervated by motor cranial nerves are affected first, followed by trunk muscles, and finally the extremities. When it affects facial muscles, inability to open the mouth (trismus or lockjaw) and characteristic sneering smile (risus sardonicus) (Figure 2) are common initial symptoms. This may result in difficulty chewing and swallowing, pooled saliva from hypersalivation, and stiffness of neck muscles, which may potentially become lethal due to continued coughing spells and dysphagia followed by aspiration, laryngeal spasms, and airway obstruction. Rigidity of trunk and paraspinal muscles follows, and the hyperextension of the spine leads to characteristic opisthotonus (Figure 3). Abdominal rigidity may occur. When it eventually affects proximal limb muscles, exaggerated deep tendon reflexes and ankle clonus may commonly occur.

TABLE 1   Ablett Classification of the Severity of Tetanus

Grade 1: Mild

Mild-to-moderate trismus
General spasticity
No spasms
No dysphagia
No respiratory distress

Grade 2: Moderate

Moderate-to-severe trismus
Intermittent short spasms
Mild dysphagia
Mild tachypnea

Grade 3: Severe

Severe trismus and severe rigidity
Prolonged spasms
Severe dysphagia
Severe tachypnea
Anoxic spells
Tachycardia

Grade 4: Very Severe

Grade 3 plus following:
Violent autonomic disturbances with persistent or intermittent
    episodes of severe hypertension and tachycardia alternating with
    hypotension and bradycardia

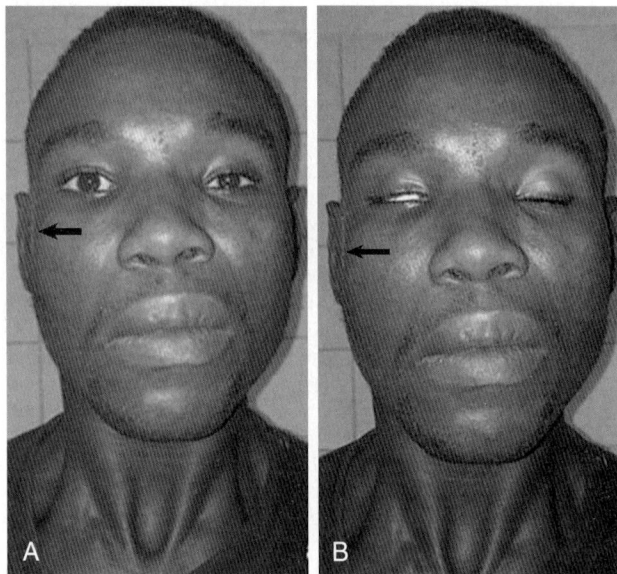

Figure 1 A case of cephalic tetanus. This is a 36-year-old man who presented with right facial nerve palsy followed by dysphagia. He had a physical assault with a gunstock on right zygomatic bone 7 days earlier and had a linear untreated right zygomatic wound that he did not seek medical attention for at the time. Note the linear wound *(arrow)* on right face with right facial droop and the inability of completely closing right eye.

Autonomic nervous system can be affected in very severe cases, and this may even occur during the early course of the disease. Hypertension and tachycardia are two common signs, but this can be complicated by fluctuating hypotension and bradycardia, which makes it difficult to manage. Other autonomic manifestations such as bowel and/or bladder dysfunction may occur. Increased respiratory secretion can result in fatal airway obstruction.

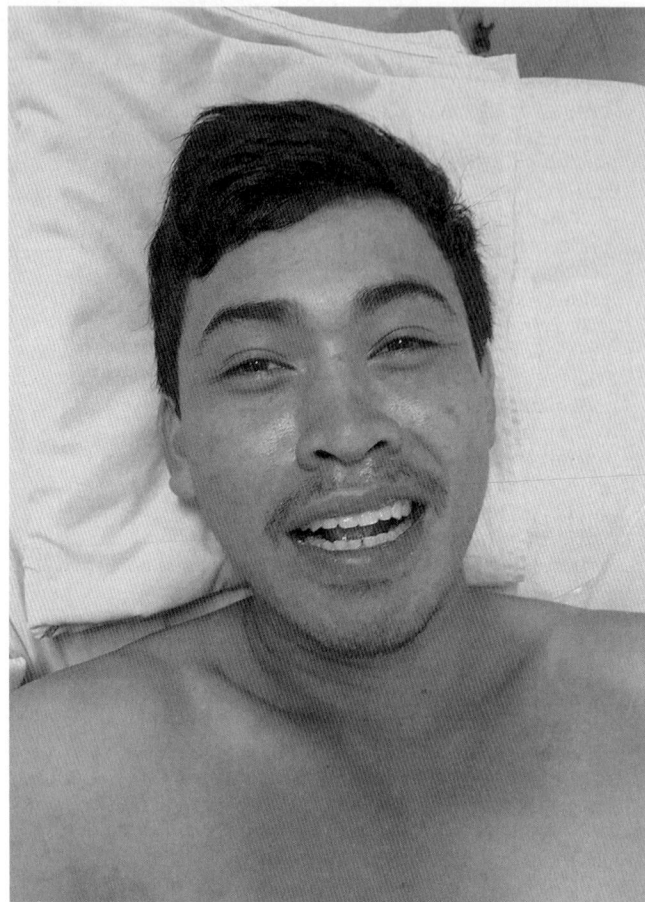

Figure 2 A typical appearance of risus sardonicus. Note the sneering smile of the face, wrinkled forehead, and "crow's feet" at the lateral palpebral margins from the tonic contraction of the muscles of facial expression.

Neonatal Tetanus

Most tetanus cases and deaths occur in low-income countries, where newborns are mostly affected; therefore, it is important for clinicians to promptly recognize symptoms in neonates for timely intervention. Even though it manifests similarly with non-neonatal tetanus, as described earlier, neonatal tetanus may initially manifest as more vague symptoms such as inability to feed, fever, neck stiffness, and respiratory distress. Low birth weight and age at onset within the first 7 days are associated with a higher risk of neonatal mortality.

Complications

Acute respiratory failure should be the most prioritized complication for clinicians to consider first, and this may occur secondary to laryngeal obstruction, prolonged respiratory muscle spasms, aspiration pneumonia, and sedative medications. Rarely, patients may develop acute respiratory distress syndrome (ARDS) due to either lung injury from mechanical ventilation or secondary bacterial sepsis. Cardiac involvement is possible, which includes arrhythmias (most frequently, isolated supraventricular and ventricular extrasystoles), sudden asystole due to autonomic dysfunction, and acute myocardial infarction in elderly patients with underlying coronary artery disease due to sympathetic hyperactivity. Severe muscle spasms may lead to tongue biting, compression fractures of midthoracic vertebrae, rhabdomyolysis, myoglobinuria, and renal failure. Long-term immobility may result in pressure ulcers and deep vein thrombosis. Mortality rate approximates 10% to 11% in high-income countries but reaches 80% to 100% in low-income countries.

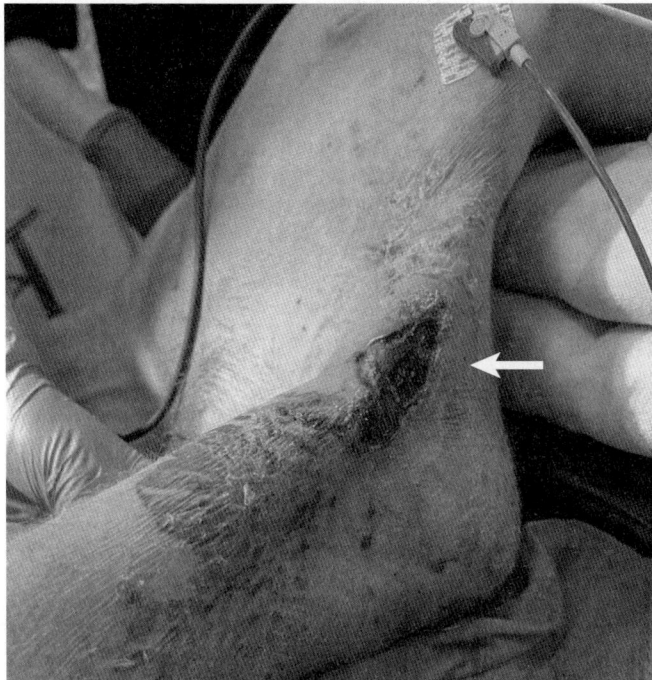

Figure 3 A typical appearance of opisthotonus. Note the hyperextended spine from the paraspinal muscle spasms.

TABLE 2	Conditions That Mimic Clinical Manifestations of Tetanus	
CLINICAL FEATURES	**DIFFERENTIAL DIAGNOSIS**
Trismus	Acute tonsillar abscess, temporomandibular joint disease, extrapyramidal reaction to drugs, dental pathology
Neck stiffness	Cervical spine disease; extrapyramidal reaction to drugs such as antipsychotics, antiemetics, or metoclopramide; meningitis; subarachnoid hemorrhage
Abdominal rigidity	Acute abdomen
Dysphagia	Myasthenia gravis, acute bulbar paralysis, rabies
Muscle spasms	Seizures, spasticity due to spinal cord disease, stiff man syndrome

Diagnosis

Tetanus is essentially a clinical diagnosis based on characteristic clinical manifestations. An anaerobic culture of *C. tetani* from a wound may be confounded because it can be cultured from wounds with a low suspicion for tetanus. There is no reliable serologic test for tetanus. Tetanus IgG antibody test via enzyme-linked immunosorbent assay may be considered, but it can be difficult to interpret the result because positive antibody can be confounded by previous immunization. Toxin bioassay from serum sample is available and may be useful in selective settings, but a negative assay cannot exclude the diagnosis. Both IgM- and IgG-based, point-of-care rapid tetanus test has been developed (SD BIOLINE Tetanus, Gentaur Europe BVBA, Kampenhout, Belgium), but it requires further investigation before licensed clinical use. One useful bedside examination tool is the spatula test, in which a spatula (tongue depressor) is inserted into the patient's mouth to gently touch the posterior pharynx. Normally, it creates a gag reflex, whereas the patient with tetanus bites the spatula, making it difficult to withdraw. Given there is no reliable confirmatory test, differential diagnosis must be considered to prevent any delay in treatment of suspected tetanus and potential for resultant complications (Table 2).

Treatment

The mainstay of tetanus treatment is acute, hospital-based, prompt intervention in both emergency and intensive care settings. It involves tetanus-specific intervention (toxin neutralization and antibiotics), control of muscle spasms, and supportive care.

Neutralization of Toxin

Tetanus toxin irreversibly binds to neurons, and the antitoxin (or tetanus immune globulin [TIG]) can only neutralize unbound toxins; therefore, the immune globulin should be administered as soon as tetanus diagnosis is made on clinical suspicion. Intramuscular human TIG, HyperTET (Grifols, Los Angeles, CA), is approved by the US Food and Drug Administration and available in the United States. The Centers for Disease Control and Prevention currently recommends a single dose of 500 units[3] for

both children and adults because it is as effective as high dose with causing less discomfort. Evidence from randomized controlled trials (RCTs) of intramuscular (IM) human TIG is scarce. A meta-analysis of 12 clinical trials showed mortality rate ranging from 16% to 83% in subjects receiving IM TIG. If human TIG is not available, IM or IV equine antitoxin (administered as 10,000–21,000 units depending on manufacturer directions) is a reasonable alternative (not licensed in the United States) if this is the only available format. An intradermal hypersensitivity testing (using 0.1 mL in a 1:10 dilution) is needed before equine antitoxin is given due to a risk of anaphylaxis. A recent RCT of 272 adults by a Vietnamese group showed no advantage of IM human TIG (3000 units) over IM equine antitoxin (21,000 units) in terms of duration of hospital/intensive care unit stay, duration of mechanical ventilation, in-hospital deaths, and adverse events. Intrathecal (IT) administration[1] of antitoxin has been controversial. The Vietnamese trial cited earlier showed that the IT approach is safe but did not provide overall benefit when added to IM administration. On the other hand, the meta-analysis of 942 patients in 12 clinical trials referenced previously found that the combined relative risk of mortality for IT over IM was 0.71 (95% confidence interval 0.62–0.81), suggesting benefits for tetanus treatment. Especially for neonatal tetanus, a comparative analysis showed that neonates who received IT human TIG in addition to equine antitoxin showed significant benefits in terms of hospital stay and mortality rate compared to the control group who received equine antitoxin only. Thus, clinicians may consider IT administration in addition to IM administration.

Active Immunization

Active immunization using tetanus toxoid is not only for prophylaxis but also for acute tetanus treatment because tetanus infection does not induce natural immunity. A tetanus toxoid should be given at a separate location of the TIG administration.

Use of Antibiotics

The theoretical background of using antibiotics is to inhibit local proliferation of *C. tetani*. Either penicillin or metronidazole has been used. Benzathine penicillin (Bicillin LA)[1] as a single IM dose of 1.2 million units or IV benzyl penicillin as 2 million units every 4 hours for 10 days can be given. Oral metronidazole (Flagyl)[1] is as effective as penicillins when it is given as 500 mg

---

[3] Exceeds dosage recommended by the manufacturer.

[1] Not FDA approved for this indication.

every 6 to 8 hours for 7 to 10 days. Theoretically, penicillin can inhibit GABA receptors, which may potentiate tetanospasmin activity, but evidence from an RCT showed no difference between penicillins and metronidazole in its outcome. Thus, clinicians may choose either penicillin (preferably benzathine penicillin, given its benefit of single dose) or metronidazole depending on availability and preference.

Control of Muscle Spasms

Another important modality in tetanus treatment is proper sedation and control of muscle spasms. Benzodiazepines are first-line therapy for this indication because they are GABA agonists that may potentially inhibit tetanospasmin activity and are readily available. Diazepam is most commonly used and well established given its wide availability and long half-life. It may be administered intravenously as 10 to 30 mg in 5-mg boluses every 5 minutes[3] or via a nasogastric tube as 10 to 40 mg every 1 to 2 hours[3] until severe spasms are controlled. Very little GABA is released in tetanus; thus, a large dose (up to 1000 mg/day)[3] of diazepam may be required to achieve adequate sedation and muscle relaxation. Midazolam (Versed)[1] may be considered because it is rapid-onset and short-acting, but there is little evidence of midazolam use in tetanus treatment and no direct comparative study between diazepam and midazolam. IV magnesium sulfate acts through calcium channel blockade and provides muscle relaxation and anticonvulsant effects. Per a recent systematic review, the use of magnesium sulfate[1] had no survival benefit but was found to be effective for reducing spasms along with diazepam, provided better autonomic control, reduced need for mechanical ventilation, and resulted in shorter hospital stays with very low magnesium toxicity reported. In terms of its dosage, most studies used an IV loading dose of 75 to 80 mg/kg followed by an infusion dose of 2 to 3 g per hour until muscle spasm control is achieved. IT baclofen (Lioresal)[1] may be considered because it can provide prompt muscle relaxation, but it has a potential risk of respiratory depression, cardiovascular instability, and central nervous system infection via cerebrospinal fluid contamination. Furthermore, there has been no RCT in its use, and most of the literature are case reports or series. Otherwise, several reports have been published for their successful use of dantrolene (Dantrium)[1] infusion, botulinum toxin A (Botox),[1] propofol (Diprivan),[1] and ketamine (Ketalar),[1] but these options would require further evidence before becoming mainstay of treatment.

Airway Management

Prompt airway management is essential in cases of moderate-to-severe tetanus. Access to mechanical ventilation is associated with improved outcome. Either tracheostomy or endotracheal intubation can be applied. If laryngeal spasm is present, tracheostomy is preferable to endotracheal intubation for both children and adults because it can lower the risk of tracheal stenosis after a prolonged mechanical ventilation compared to endotracheal intubation.

Control of Autonomic Disturbances

Autonomic dysfunction can be another major challenge for clinicians after respiratory failure is controlled. A retrospective study showed that autonomic dysfunction happened in one-third of the cases, and it can be a poor prognostic factor. IV clonidine[1] (α_2-adrenergic agonist) has been widely studied and was found to be effective for minimizing blood pressure fluctuations. The β-blocker labetalol was reported to successfully control hypertension and tachycardia.[1] Studies also showed that IV morphine[1] was able to counteract autonomic hyperactivity without needing sympathetic blockers but carries a risk of sedation at higher doses and with prolonged use.

Nursing and Other Supportive Measures

Proper local wound care with debridement and abscess drainage, as well as minimization of risk of pressure ulcers, is important. Optimization of nutrition should be a consideration because of a catabolic state secondary to continuous muscle hyperactivity, spasms, and multifactorial stress reactions, and patients may lose up to 15% of their body weight. Nasogastric tube feeding can be required in most cases because of trismus and dysphagia. Most patients also require urinary catheterization; urinary retention is common, and the bladder distention may provoke autonomic instability. Upper airway suctioning to prevent aspiration pneumonia and the prophylaxis of deep vein thrombosis are also warranted.

Prevention

Absorbed tetanus toxoid, a base of current tetanus vaccine, was developed by inactivating tetanus toxin with formaldehyde treatment in the 1920s. Clinical efficacy against tetanus after complete vaccine series reaches 100%. There are four available tetanus toxoid-based vaccines: DT, DTaP, Td, and Tdap. DT (pediatric diphtheria-tetanus toxoid) and DTaP (Daptacel, Infanrix) are pediatric vaccines that contain identical amounts of tetanus toxoid as adult vaccines but 3 to 4 times as much diphtheria toxoid. DTaP additionally contains acellular pertussis vaccine. On the other hand, Td (adult tetanus-diphtheria) and Tdap (Adacel, Boostrix) are adult vaccines with less diphtheria vaccine component. As with DTaP, Tdap additionally contains acellular pertussis vaccine.

Primary Immunization Series

In children younger than 7 years, primary series of four doses of DTaP is recommended at 2, 4, 6, and 15 to 18 months. A booster or fifth dose is recommended at 4 to 6 years of age. After age 7, an adult dose or Tdap is recommended as an adolescent booster at 11 to 12 years of age. DT can be of limited use when the pertussis component is contraindicated or a provider decides not to administer pertussis vaccine. For the adult population, if they did not receive Tdap at or after age 11 years, they should receive one dose of Tdap first, then Td or Tdap every 10 years. If they did receive Tdap at or after age 11, they may receive Td or Tdap every 10 years counting from the last Tdap.

Pregnancy Consideration

Tdap is recommended to be administered during each pregnancy between 27 and 36 weeks' gestation, regardless of the timing of previous tetanus immunization. Although this vaccination primarily targets pertussis, it should be understood as tetanus prevention, especially in areas where neonatal tetanus is common. A recent systematic review recognized that the key intervention to reduce neonatal mortality from neonatal tetanus was vaccination of pregnant women with tetanus toxoid.

Postexposure Prophylaxis

Proper prophylactic measures should be considered or initiated after open wound formation with any type of injury to prevent tetanus (Table 3). Regarding tetanus toxoid, DTaP is recommended for age younger than 7 years, while Tdap (preferred to Td) is a primary choice for individuals at 11 years or older. Td may be administered if the patient was previously vaccinated with Tdap. Neither tetanus toxoid nor TIG is required if a patient has already completed 3 or more doses of tetanus vaccine. However, for clean and minor wounds, tetanus toxoid–containing vaccine should still be given if it is 10 years or more since the last tetanus vaccine dose. For all other wounds, even after completing primary series, tetanus toxoid–containing vaccine should still be given if it is 5 years or more since the last tetanus vaccine dose.

---

[3] Exceeds dosage recommended by the manufacturer.
[1] Not FDA approved for this indication.

TABLE 3	Postexposure Prophylaxis for Tetanus in Wound Management		
PREVIOUS DOSES OF TETANUS TOXOID–CONTAINING VACCINES	**CLEAN, MINOR WOUNDS**	**ALL OTHER WOUNDS**	
Unknown or <3 doses	Tetanus toxoid	Tetanus toxoid + TIG	
≥3 doses	None (or tetanus toxoid only if ≥10 years since previous dose)	None (or tetanus toxoid only if ≥5 years since previous dose)	

TIG, Tetanus immune globulin.

References

Hao NV, Loan HT, Yen LM, et al: Human versus equine intramuscular antitoxin, with or without human intrathecal antitoxin, for the treatment of adults with tetanus: a 2 x 2 factorial randomised controlled trial, *Lancet Glob Health* 10:e862–e872, 2022.

Kumar AVG, Kothari VM, Krishnan A, Karnad DR: Benzathine penicillin, metronidazole and benzyl penicillin in the treatment of tetanus: a randomized, controlled trial, *Ann Trop Med Parasitol* 98:59–63, 2004.

Li J, Liu Z, Yu C, et al: Global epidemiology and burden of tetanus from 1990 to 2019: A systematic analysis for the Global Burden of Disease Study 2019, *Int J Infect Dis* 132:118–126, 2023.

Nepal G, Coghlan MA, Yadav JK, et al: Safety and efficacy of magnesium sulfate in the management of tetanus: a systematic review, *Trop Med Int Health* 26:1200–1209, 2021.

Recommended Adult Immunization Schedule for Ages 19 Years or Older, United States, 2024. Accessed: https://www.cdc.gov/vaccines/schedules/downloads/adult/adult-combined-schedule.pdf.

Recommended Child and Adolescent Immunization Schedule for Ages 18 Years or Younger, United States, 2024. Accessed: https://www.cdc.gov/vaccines/schedules/downloads/child/0-18yrs-child-combined-schedule.pdf.

Tiwari TSP, Moro PL, Acosta AM, Hall E, Wodi AP, Hamborsky J, editors: *Epidemiology and Prevention of Vaccine-Preventable Diseases,* ed 14, Washington, DC, 2021, Department of Health and Human Services, Centers for Disease Control and Prevention, pp 315–328.

Yen LM, Thwaites CL: Tetanus, *Lancet* 393:1658–1668, 2019.

TICKBORNE RICKETTSIAL DISEASES (ROCKY MOUNTAIN SPOTTED FEVER AND OTHER SPOTTED FEVER GROUP RICKETTSIOSES, EHRLICHIOSES, AND ANAPLASMOSIS)

Method of
Robert Wittler, MD

CURRENT DIAGNOSIS

- Early diagnosis of Rocky Mountain spotted fever (RMSF) and other tickborne rickettsial diseases is made clinically. RMSF should be considered in the setting of fever, headache, rash, and a history of possible tick exposure. The rash is not always present and typically occurs 2 to 4 days after the onset of fever.
- Diagnostic laboratory tests for rickettsial diseases, particularly RMSF, are usually not helpful in making a timely diagnosis during the initial states of illness.
- Tickborne rickettsial diseases can be confirmed by polymerase chain reaction (PCR) during the acute stage if readily available (whole blood for ehrlichiosis and anaplasmosis and skin biopsy or whole blood for RMSF) or at later stages by subsequently demonstrating a fourfold increase between acute and convalescent (ideally 2 to 4 weeks apart) serum immunoglobulin G (IgG) indirect immunofluorescence antibody titers. PCR of whole blood for RMSF has low sensitivity, although sensitivity increases in patients with severe disease.
- Typical findings of ehrlichiosis and anaplasmosis include fever, headache, malaise, leukopenia, thrombocytopenia, and elevated serum transaminases. Rash is often not present.

CURRENT THERAPY

- Treatment of choice for all tickborne rickettsial diseases in patients of all ages (including children less than 8 years of age) is doxycycline (Vibramycin).
- The dose for doxycycline is 100 mg twice daily (intravenously [IV] or orally depending on severity of illness) for adults. For children weighing <45 kg,[1] the recommended dose is 2.2 mg/kg/dose IV or orally twice daily.
- Delay in recognition and appropriate treatment is the most important factor associated with death from RMSF. Empiric treatment within 5 days of the onset of symptoms with doxycycline is the best way to prevent morbidity and death. Treatment decisions should never be delayed while awaiting laboratory confirmation, nor should treatment be discontinued solely on the basis of a negative test result with an acute-phase specimen.
- Although optimal duration of therapy has not been well studied, a common treatment course for RMSF and ehrlichiosis is at least 3 days after the patient defervesces (typically the minimum total course is 5–7 days) or longer for severe illness. Anaplasmosis should be treated for 10 days to provide appropriate therapy for possible coinfection with *Borrelia burgdorferi*.
- Historically chloramphenicol has been recommended for the treatment of RMSF during pregnancy based on adverse effects of older tetracycline drugs (but not specifically doxycycline). Although there is limited evidence, doxycycline has not been associated with teratogenicity or maternal hepatic toxicity during pregnancy, and doxycycline has been used successfully to treat tickborne rickettsial disease in several pregnant women without adverse effects.
- Chloramphenicol is not an alternative treatment for human monocytic ehrlichiosis (HME) or HGA. Chloramphenicol treatment of RMSF has been associated with a greater risk of death compared with doxycycline treatment.
- Limited case report data suggest that rifampin[1] can be used as an alternative to doxycycline for the treatment of confirmed (RMSF ruled out) mild anaplasmosis during pregnancy or with documented tetracycline allergy.

[1]Not FDA approved for this indication.

Tickborne rickettsial diseases in humans often share clinical features but are epidemiologically and etiologically distinct. In the United States included diseases are (1) Rocky Mountain spotted fever (RMSF) caused by *Rickettsia rickettsii*; (2) other spotted fever group (SFG) rickettsioses, caused by *Rickettsia parkeri* and *Rickettsia* species 364D; (3) *Ehrlichia chaffeensis* ehrlichiosis, also called human monocytic ehrlichiosis (HME); (4) other ehrlichioses, caused by *Ehrlichia ewingii* and *Ehrlichia muris*-like agent; and (5) anaplasmosis, caused by *Anaplasma phagocytophilum*, also called human granulocytic anaplasmosis (HGA). The reported incidence of tickborne rickettsial diseases has increased in the United States. Tickborne rickettsial diseases, especially RMSF, continue to cause severe illness and death in otherwise healthy adults and children, despite the availability of effective antibiotic therapy. SFG rickettsioses (including RMSF), ehrlichioses, and anaplasmosis are nationally notifiable diseases in the United States. Providers report potential cases to state or local health departments. In 2010, the reporting category of RMSF was changed to spotted fever rickettsiosis, as serology does not readily distinguish RMSF from other SFG rickettsioses.

Epidemiology

Tickborne rickettsial pathogens are maintained in natural cycles involving domestic or wild vertebrates and ticks. The epidemiology of each disease reflects the geographic distribution and seasonal activities of the tick vectors and the natural vertebrate hosts, as well as the human activities resulting in tick exposure. Although cases have been reported in every month, most cases occur during April to September, coincident with peak levels of tick host-seeking activity.

RMSF is the rickettsiosis in the United States that is associated with the highest rates of severe and fatal outcomes. The case-fatality rate in the preantibiotic era was ~25%. Current case-fatality rates are estimated at 5% to 10%. From 2008–2012, the estimated average annual incidence from passive surveillance of SFG rickettsioses was 8.9 cases per million persons. Reported annual incidence has increased during the past two decades. The highest incidence occurs in persons aged 60 to 69 years, and the highest case-fatality rate is among children aged <10 years. Additional epidemiologic risk factors for fatal RMSF include age ≥40 years, alcohol abuse, and glucose-6-phosphate dehydrogenase deficiency. From 2008 to 2012, 63% of reported SFG rickettsiosis cases came from Arkansas, Missouri, North Carolina, Oklahoma, and Tennessee. SFG rickettsiosis has been reported from all the contiguous 48 states and the District of Columbia.

In the United States, the tick species most frequently associated with transmission of *R rickettsii* is the American dog tick, *Dermacentor variabilis*, which is found primarily in the eastern, central, and Pacific Coast regions. The Rocky Mountain wood tick, *Dermacentor andersoni*, is associated with transmission in the western United States. Larval and nymphal stages of most *Dermacentor* spp ticks usually do not bite humans. Adult *D variabilis* and *D andersoni* ticks bite humans, but the principal hosts are deer, dogs, and livestock.

The brown dog tick, *Rhipicephalus sanguineus*, which is located throughout the United States, is an important vector in parts of Arizona and along the United States–Mexico border. All stages (larvae, nymphs, and adults) of *Rh sanguineus* bite humans and can transmit *R rickettsii*. Domestic dogs are the preferred host. On Arizona tribal lands, the warm climate and proximity of ticks to domiciles (tick-infested dogs) provide a suitable environment for *Rh sanguineus* to remain active year-round, resulting in cases of RMSF in Arizona every month of the year.

Rickettsia parkeri is transmitted by the Gulf Coast tick, *Amblyomma maculatum*. *R parkeri* rickettsiosis cases have not been documented in children, and no fatal cases have been reported. The first confirmed case of Rickettsia species 364D was in 2010 and likely transmitted by the Pacific Coast tick, *Dermacentor occidentalis*. All reported cases have been from California.

The average annual incidence of ehrlichiosis from 2008 to 2012 was 3.2 cases per million persons, with the most common cause being *E chaffeensis*. The highest incidence is in persons aged 60 to 69 years. The case fatality rate is ~3% and is highest among children aged <10 years, adults aged ≥70 years, and immunosuppressed persons. *E chaffeensis* is transmitted to humans by the lone star tick, *Amblyomma americanum*, which is the most commonly encountered tick in the southeastern United States, with a range that extends into areas of the Midwest and New England. Arkansas, Delaware, Missouri, Oklahoma, Tennessee, and Virginia have the highest reported incidence. The white-tailed deer is an important natural reservoir for *E chaffeensis*, and most cases occur during May to August.

The principal vector for *E ewingii* ehrlichiosis is also *A americanum*. Cases have primarily been reported from Missouri. No fatal cases of *E ewingii* ehrlichiosis have been reported. *Ehrlichia muris*–like agent (EML) has recently been recognized as a human pathogen. Reported cases have been from Minnesota and Wisconsin. The blacklegged tick, *Ixodes scapularis*, is an efficient vector for EML in experimental studies. EML agent DNA has been detected in *I scapularis* collected in Minnesota and Wisconsin but has not been detected in *I scapularis* from other states.

The incidence of human anaplasmosis during 2008–2012 was 6.3 cases per million persons. Incidence is highest in the northeastern and upper midwestern states, and the geographic range seems to be expanding. The case fatality rate is <1%. *I scapularis* is the vector for *Anaplasma phagocytophilum* in the northeastern and midwestern United States, whereas the western blacklegged tick, *Ixodes pacificus*, is the principal vector along the West Coast. The seasonality is bimodal, with the first peak June–July and a smaller peak in October, corresponding to the emergence of the adult stage of *I scapularis*. *I scapularis* also transits *Borrelia burgdorferi* (Lyme disease), *Babesia microti* (babesiosis), *Borrelia miyamotoi* (tickborne relapsing fever), and deer tick virus (a cause of tickborne encephalitis). Simultaneous infections with *A phagocytophilum* and *B burgdorferi* or *B microti* have occurred.

Pathophysiology

The agents causing RMSF, ehrlichiosis, and anaplasmosis are all obligate intracellular pathogens, but the target host cells they infect and subsequent pathology vary by organism.

R rickettsii is transmitted from the tick to humans via a painless bite, which often goes unrecognized. The organism resides in the salivary gland of the tick and is passed during acquisition of a blood meal. *R rickettsii* can be transmitted as early as 10 to 24 hours after tick attachment. When transmitted to a human host, *R rickettsia* localize and multiply in vascular endothelial cells, and, less commonly, underlying smooth muscle cells of small and medium vessels, resulting in vasculitis. The vasculitis is the underlying mechanism for most of the clinical features and laboratory abnormalities of RMSF. Injury to the vascular endothelium results in increased capillary permeability, microhemorrhage, and platelet consumption. Late-stage complications of pulmonary edema (acute respiratory distress syndrome) and cerebral edema are consequences of the microvascular leakage.

E chaffeensis predominantly infects monocytes and tissue macrophages and replicates in cytoplasmic vacuoles called morulae. Unlike RMSF, direct vasculitis and endothelial injury are rare in human monocytic ehrlichiosis. Frequent pathologic findings include granuloma formation, myeloid hyperplasia, and megakaryocytosis in the bone marrow. The severe pathology and multiorgan involvement in severe and fatal HME in immunocompetent patients is believed to be due to dysregulation of the host immune response that leads to tissue damage and eventually multiorgan failure. *E ewingii* has a predilection for neutrophils, and morulae can be observed in granulocytes of the blood, cerebrospinal fluid (CSF), and bone marrow.

A phagocytophilum is found predominantly in neutrophils in the peripheral blood and tissues from infected individuals. *A phagocytophilum* has the unique ability to selectively survive and multiply within cytoplasmic vacuoles (morulae) of polymorphonuclear cells by delaying their apoptosis. Infection with *A phagocytophilum* induces a systemic inflammatory response, which is believed to be the mechanism for tissue damage. Pathologic findings with human granulocytic anaplasmosis include normocellular or hypercellular bone marrow, erythrophagocytosis, hepatic apoptosis, focal splenic necrosis, and mild interstitial pneumonitis and pulmonary hemorrhage.

Clinical Manifestations

A detailed history should include information about known tick bites or activities that might be associated with tick exposure. Unrecognized tick bites are common. A history of a tick bite within 14 days of illness onset is reported in only 50% to 60% of RMSF cases and 68% of ehrlichiosis cases. Absence of a tick bite should never dissuade providers from considering tickborne rickettsial disease in the appropriate clinical context. Contact with pets, especially dogs, and a history of tick attachment or recent tick removal from pets can be useful in assessing human tick exposure.

Tickborne rickettsial diseases commonly have nonspecific clinical signs and symptoms early in the course of disease. Although there is overlap in the clinical presentations of tickborne rickettsial diseases, the frequency of certain associated signs and symptoms (e.g., rash and other cutaneous findings) and typical laboratory findings differ by pathogen and assist providers in developing a differential diagnosis, beginning appropriate antibacterial treatment, and ordering confirmatory diagnostic tests.

Symptoms of RMSF typically begin 3 to 12 days after the bite of an infected tick or 4 to 8 days after discovery of an attached tick. The incubation period is generally shorter (≤5 days) in patients who develop severe disease. Initial symptoms are often nonspecific and include the sudden onset of fever, chills, malaise, and myalgia. Clinical suspicion for RMSF should be maintained in cases of nonspecific febrile illness and sepsis of unclear cause, particularly during the spring and summer months.

The classic triad of fever, rash, and reported tick bite is present in only a minority of RMSF patients during the initial presentation to health care; therefore it is crucial not to wait for development of this triad before considering a diagnosis of RMSF and beginning treatment. A rash typically occurs 2 to 4 days after the onset of fever; however, many patients initially seek medical care before the rash. In one large series of patients with RMSF, 88% of patients had a rash, but only 49% had a rash in the first 3 days. Children more frequently have rash (97%) and develop the rash earlier. The rash typically begins as small, blanching macules on the ankles, wrists, or forearms that then spreads to the palms, soles, arms, legs, and trunk, usually sparing the face. The generalized petechial rash appears later (day 5 or 6) and is indicative of advanced disease. An inoculation eschar is rarely present with RMSF. In addition to rash, the most frequent clinical findings at any point in the illness are fever (99%), headache (91%), and myalgia (82%).

The total white blood cell count is typically normal or mildly increased with RMSF, and increased numbers of immature neutrophils are often present. Thrombocytopenia, slight elevations of AST or ALT, and hyponatremia might be present, particularly as the disease advances. Laboratory values cannot be relied on to guide early treatment decisions because they are often within or slightly deviated from normal reference values early in the course. When CSF is obtained, a lymphocytic (less commonly neutrophilic) pleocytosis can be present, along with a moderately elevated CSF protein. CSF glucose is generally normal.

R parkeri rickettsiosis is a milder illness compared with RMSF; no severe manifestations or death has been reported. Symptoms develop a median of 5 days (range, 2–10 days) after the bite of an infected tick. The first manifestation in nearly all patients is an inoculation eschar, which generally is nonpruritic, nontender or mildly tender, and surrounded by an indurated, erythematous halo and occasionally a few petechiae. Shortly after the onset of fever (0.5–4 days later), a nonpruritic maculopapular or vesicopustular rash develops in 90% of patients. The rash primarily involves the extremities and trunk and in ~half of patients involves the palms and soles. Headache (86%) and myalgia (76%) are common. Laboratory findings include modest elevation of hepatic transaminases (78%), mild leukopenia (50%), and thrombocytopenia (40%).

Few patients with *Rickettsia* species 364D have been reported, so the full clinical spectrum has yet to be described. It does appear to be relatively mild and characterized by an eschar or ulcerative skin lesion with regional lymphadenopathy. Fever, headache, and myalgia occur, but rash has not been a notable feature.

Symptoms of *E chaffeensis* ehrlichiosis typically occur a median of 9 days (range, 5–15 days) after an infected tick bite. Fever (96%), headache (72%), malaise (77%), and myalgia (58%) are common. Abdominal pain, vomiting, and diarrhea can occur, particularly in children. Rash (maculopapular, petechial, or diffuse erythema) occurs in approximately one-third of patients and is more frequent in children. The rash occurs a median of 5 days after illness onset and can involve the palms and soles. Neurologic manifestations are present in ~20% of patients. Characteristic laboratory findings in the first week include leukopenia, thrombocytopenia, and elevated levels of hepatic transaminases. *Ehrlichia ewingii* and *Ehrlichia muris*-like agent ehrlichiosis have similar clinical and laboratory features as *E chaffeensis* ehrlichiosis, although rash and gastrointestinal symptoms are less common.

Symptoms of human granulocytic anaplasmosis typically occur 5 to 14 days after an infected tick bite. Fever (92%–100%), headache (82%), malaise (97%), and myalgia (77%) are common.

Rash is present in <10% of patients, and central nervous system involvement is rare. Laboratory findings are similar to ehrlichiosis.

Diagnosis

Early diagnosis and initiation of treatment of tickborne rickettsial diseases is based on clinical and epidemiologic findings, as rapid confirmatory assays are often not available or reliable to guide treatment decisions early in the clinical course. Confirmatory diagnostic tests are serologic assays, nucleic acid detection, immunostaining of biopsy tissue, blood-smear microscopy, and culture.

Assays using paired acute and convalescent sera (ideally collected 2–4 weeks apart) are the standard for serologic confirmation. Assays are insensitive during the first week of rickettsial infection. After 7 days of illness, the sensitivity increases. Assays are highly sensitive 2 to 3 weeks after illness onset. Early therapy with doxycycline may diminish or delay the development of antibodies in RMSF.

A diagnosis of tickborne rickettsial diseases is confirmed with a ≥fourfold increase in antibody titer in patients with a clinically compatible acute illness. A single IgG antibody reciprocal titer ≥64 is supportive of, but not confirmatory for, the diagnosis. In the United States, R rickettsia–reactive IgG antibody reciprocal titers ≥64 can be found in 5% to 10% of the population who do not acutely have RMSF. Some laboratories also perform assays for IgM antibodies. However, because of the lower specificity of IgM compared with IgG assays, IgM titers should not be used as a stand-alone method for diagnosis.

PCR amplification of DNA from whole blood specimens collected during the acute stage of illness is particularly useful for confirming E chaffeensis, A phagocytophilum, E ewingii, and EML agent infections due to the tropism of those organisms for circulating cells. PCR detection of R rickettsia in whole blood is less sensitive, as low numbers of rickettsiae typically circulate in the blood in the absence of advanced disease. Tissue specimens such as a skin biopsy are a more useful source of SFG rickettsial DNA compared with blood samples. Doxycyline treatment decreases the sensitivity of PCR. Obtaining blood before treatment is recommended to decrease false-negative results.

Immunostaining of a skin punch biopsy is useful for diagnosing RMSF with 100% specificity and 70% sensitivity. Microscopic examination of blood smears or buffy-coat preparations during the first week of illness may reveal leukocyte morulae in patients infected with E chaffeensis or anaplasmosis, although it is relatively insensitive, and accuracy is dependent on having experienced microscopists. Culture is the reference standard for microbiologic diagnosis, but the agents that cause tickborne rickettsial diseases require cell culture techniques that are not widely available.

Differential Diagnosis

The differential diagnosis of fever and rash is broad, and during the early stages of illness tickborne rickettsial diseases can be indistinguishable from many viral exanthams, particularly in children. In addition to viral infections, conditions that should be considered include meningococcemia, Kawasaki disease, secondary syphilis, disseminated gonococcal infection, bacterial endocarditis, scarlet fever, leptospirosis, typhoid, drug eruptions, Stevens-Johnson syndrome, toxic shock syndrome, and thrombotic thrombocytopenic purpura.

Treatment

Doxycycline is the drug of choice for treatment of all tickborne rickettsial diseases in patients of all ages and should be initiated immediately in persons with signs and symptoms suggestive of rickettsial disease. Treatment decisions should never be delayed awaiting laboratory confirmation. Multiple studies have noted a delay in appropriate treatment of tickborne rickettsial diseases, particularly after the fifth day of illness for RMSF, to be a significant potentially preventable risk factor for severe disease, increased mortality rates, and long-term sequelae. Because of the nonspecific signs and symptoms of tickborne rickettsial diseases, concomitant empiric treatment for other conditions in the differential diagnosis should be administered (e.g., treatment with ceftriaxone for meningococcemia).

The recommended dose of doxycycline is 100 mg twice daily (IV or oral) for adults and 2.2 mg/kg twice daily (IV or oral) for children weighing <45 kg.[1] Oral therapy is appropriate for patients with early-stage disease who can be treated as outpatients. The recommended duration of therapy for RMSF and ehrlichiosis is at least 3 days after fever resolves and until evidence of clinical improvement is noted; typically, the minimum total course is 5 to 7 days. Severe or complicated disease could require a longer course. HGA should be treated for 10 days to provide appropriate therapy for possible coinfection with Lyme disease.

The use of doxycycline to treat children with suspected tickborne rickettsial disease should no longer be a subject of controversy. The American Academy of Pediatrics and CDC recommend doxycycline as the treatment of choice for children of all ages with suspected tickborne rickettsial disease. Doxycycline used at the recommended dose and duration for RMSF in children aged <8 years, even after multiple courses, has not resulted in tooth staining or enamel hypoplasia.

Chloramphenicol in the past was used as an alternative drug for treating RMSF. However, chloramphenicol has been associated with a higher risk of death compared to patients treated with a tetracycline; in vitro evidence indicates that chloramphenicol is not effective treatment for ehrlichiosis or anaplasmosis. Chloramphenicol is no longer available in the oral form in the United States, and the IV form is not readily available at all institutions.

Chloramphenicol has been recommended for the treatment of RMSF during pregnancy based on adverse effects of older tetracycline drugs (but not specifically doxycycline). Although there is limited evidence, doxycycline has not been associated with teratogenicity or maternal hepatic toxicity during pregnancy, and doxycycline has been used successfully to treat tickborne rickettsial diseases in several pregnant women without adverse effects.

Rifamycins demonstrate in vitro activity against *E chaffeensis* and *A phagocytophilum*. Case reports document favorable outcomes in small numbers of pregnant women treated with rifampin for anaplasmosis. Rifampin[1] could be an alternative for treatment of confirmed mild anaplasmosis (RMSF ruled out) during pregnancy or documented allergy to tetracycline-class drugs. Rifampin is not acceptable treatment for RMSF or potential coinfection with *B burgdorferi*.

Treatment of symptom-free persons seropositive for tickborne rickettsial disease is not recommended, regardless of past treatment, because antibodies can persist for months to years after infection.

Monitoring and Complications

Fever with tickborne rickettsial diseases typically subsides within 24 to 48 hours when treated with doxycycline in the first 4 to 5 days of illness. Lack of a clinical response within 48 hours of early treatment with doxycycline could indicate the illness is not a tickborne rickettsial disease, and alternative diagnoses or coinfection should be considered. Severely ill patients may require >48 hours of treatment before clinical improvement is noted. Patients with mild disease treated on an outpatient basis need close follow-up to ensure they are responding appropriately.

Patients with evidence of organ dysfunction, severe thrombocytopenia, mental status changes, or the need for supportive therapy should be hospitalized. Other considerations for hospitalization include the likelihood and ability to take oral medication and existing comorbid conditions, including the patient's immune status. Infection with RMSF and to a somewhat lesser extent HME are most likely to have a severe disease or death. Severe, late-stage manifestations of RMSF include meningoencephalitis, acute respiratory distress syndrome (ARDS), acute renal failure, arrhythmia, and seizures. Severe manifestations of HME include ARDS, shock-like syndromes, renal failure, hepatic failure, coagulopathies, and hemorrhagic complications.

Severe or life-threatening manifestations are less frequent with anaplasmosis than with RMSF or HME. Predictors of a more severe course of anaplasmosis include advanced age, immunosuppression, comorbid medical conditions, and delay in diagnosis and treatment. Confirmed *A phagocytophilum* coinfection has been reported in <10% of patients with Lyme disease. Response to treatment can provide clues to possible coinfection with Lyme disease or babesiosis. If the clinical response to treatment with doxycycline is delayed, coinfection or an alternate infection should be considered. Conversely, if Lyme disease is treated with a beta-lactam antibiotic in a patient with unrecognized *A phagocytophilum* infection symptoms could persist.

Prevention

The best prevention for all the tickborne rickettsial diseases is to avoid tick bites, perform regular tick checks on humans and pets, and promptly remove attached ticks. Longer periods of tick attachment increase the probability of transmission of tickborne diseases. Repellents and protective clothing can reduce the risk for tick bites. Products containing 20% to 30% N,N-Diethyl-meta-toluamide (DEET) effectively repel ticks and can be applied directly to the skin. DEET is not recommended for use on infants younger than 2 months. Permethrin-treated or -impregnated clothing can significantly reduce tick bites. Prophylactic treatment is not recommended in persons who have had recent tick bites and are well.

References

Biggs HM, Behravesh CB, Bradley KK, et al: Diagnosis and management of tickborne rickettsial diseases: Rocky Mountain spotted fever and other spotted fever group rickettsioses, ehrlichioses, and anaplasmosis—United States, *MMWR Recomm Rep* 65:1–44, 2016.

Buckingham SC, Marshall GS, Schutze GE, et al: Clinical and laboratory features, hospital course, and outcome of Rocky Mountain spotted fever in children, *J Pediatr* 150:180–184, 2007.

Cross R, Ling C, Day NPJ, McGready R, Paris DH: Revisiting doxycycline in pregnancy and early childhood—time to rebuild its reputation? *Expert Opin Drug Saf* 15:367–382, 2016.

Dahlgren FS, Holman RC, Paddock CD, Callinan LS, McQuiston JH: Fatal Rocky Mountain spotted fever in the United States, 1999–2007, *Am J Trop Med Hyg* 86:713–719, 2012.

Hamburg BJ, Storch GA, Micek ST, Kollef MH: The importance of early treatment with doxycycline in human ehrlichiosis, *Medicine (Baltimore)* 87:53–60, 2008.

Helmick CG, Bernard KW, D'Angelo LJ: Rocky Mountain spotted fever: clinical, laboratory, and epidemiological features of 262 cases, *J Infect Dis* 150:480–488, 1984.

Ismail N, McBride JW: Tick-borne emerging infections: ehrlichiosis and anaplasmosis, *Clin Lab Med* 37:317–340, 2017.

Kirkland KB, Wilkinson WE, Sexton DJ: Therapeutic delay and mortality in cases of Rocky Mountain spotted fever, *Clin Infect Dis* 20:1118–1121, 1995.

Kjemtrup AM, Padgett K, Paddock CD, et al: A forty-year review of Rocky Mountain spotted fever cases in California shows clinical and epidemiologic changes, *PLoS Negl Trop Dis* 16:1–18, 2022.

Marshall GS, Stout GG, Jacobs RF, et al: Antibodies reactive to Rickettsia rickettsii among children living in the southeast and south central regions of the United States, *Arch Pediatr Adoles Med* 157:443–448, 2003.

---

[1] Not FDA approved for this indication.

TOXIC SHOCK SYNDROME

Method of
Alwyn Rapose, MD

CURRENT DIAGNOSIS

- Clinical diagnosis: High index of suspicion when there is a combination of fever, rash—initially erythematous followed by desquamation, hypotension, and multiorgan injury.
- There needs to be a thorough search for a focus of infection like retained foreign body or tampon, deep-seated abscess or peritonitis, necrotizing fasciitis, or postoperative wound infection.
- Blood cultures and deep tissue cultures (from the site of the suspected infection) are recommended in all cases.

CURRENT THERAPY

- Aggressive fluid resuscitation.
- Broad antibiotic coverage initially, followed by deescalation to target the organism identified in cultures.
- Intravenous immunoglobulin[1] may help in patients who fail to respond to standard care.

[1]Not FDA approved for this indication.

Introduction

Toxic shock syndrome (TSS) is an acute illness, which as the name suggests is caused by a toxin, and the patient presents with hypotension (shock) and multiorgan involvement (syndrome). It was initially described in children with *Staphylococcus aureus* infection, but a similar syndrome is associated with *Streptococcus* infections as well as clostridial infections in children and adults. Different toxins—acting either directly or via different cytokine pathways—have been implicated in the pathogenesis of the disease. TSS carried a high mortality risk (40% to 60% in streptococcal TSS). However, early recognition and aggressive interventions have resulted in much improved outcomes in the era of modern medicine.

Historical Aspects

A review of the medical literature indicates this was first described in 1978 when J. Todd and colleagues reported a collection of seven cases in children. In the early years following its description, a majority of cases were seen in young menstruating women who used tampons, with the onset of illness within a few days of onset of their menstrual period. A large number of investigators evaluated tampons, contraceptive sponges, sanitary pads, and other medical and surgical materials and as the medical community became more familiar with this syndrome, there was a decrease in tampon-associated TSS and an increased incidence of nonmenstrual TSS associated with respiratory infections, necrotizing skin infections, deep-seated abscesses, and postoperative infections including gynecologic surgeries.

TSS is classically associated with *S. aureus* infection. The clinical features included fever, skin rash, hypotension, and multiorgan involvement with various combinations of respiratory, renal, and hepatic injury. Similar features following infection with *Streptococcus pyogenes* (group A *Streptococcus* [GAS] as well as other streptococci) resulted in a description of streptococcal toxic shock–like syndrome (TSLS). In patients with complications of medical or spontaneous abortions and infection with *Clostridium species* similar clinical features were seen along with very high mortality, and this condition was also included when describing TSS.

Pathogenesis

The *S. aureus* isolates from patients with menstruation-related TSS revealed a toxin that was first called toxic shock syndrome toxin 1 (TSST-1). Since then, however, multiple other toxins associated with *S. aureus* (enterotoxins B-F) have been described to be associated with TSS. Similarly, streptococcal exotoxins (A, B, and C)—superantigens—are potent activators of T lymphocytes and can also directly cause high fever (pyrotoxins) and shock, as well as tissue damage.

These bacterial toxins induce production of tumor necrosis factor (TNFα), interferons (IFNγ), interleukins (IL-1, IL-2), and other cytotoxins by human monocytes and lymphocytes that result in a cascade of proinflammatory cytokines (cytokine storm). These cytokines are responsible for fever, damage to vascular endothelium resulting in tissue injury, as well as the loss of intravascular volume and hypotension.

In contrast, clostridial infection is associated with direct tissue damage by secreted clostridial toxins.

Clinical Features

The surveillance case definition developed by the Centers for Disease Control and Prevention (CDC) included five clinical criteria: Fever, rash, hypotension, and involvement of three or more organ systems. The rash usually subsided with desquamation, which is the fifth clinical criterion. The patient may have prodromal symptoms like myalgia, arthralgia, and headache. Fever associated with a diffuse erythematous skin rash (sheets of erythema) involving the face trunk and extremities is rapidly followed by hypotension, decreased urine output, and features of septic shock (Figures 1 through 3). Detailed history taking and a thorough clinical examination is essential to determine the focus of infection—either menstrual tampon, retained foreign body, necrotizing infection in a closed space (fasciitis), postoperative wound infection, or, more recently described, peritonitis-associated TSS. Subtle differences between TSS and TSLS have been described. Clostridial infection following septic abortion or other gynecologic surgery is associated with severe abdominal and pelvic pain, uterine tenderness (endometritis), and a foul-smelling vaginal discharge. A delay in diagnosis and intervention results in a rapid progression of systemic involvement. A cytokine storm in the lungs can result in respiratory complications like acute respiratory distress syndrome (ARDS), and there can be acute renal injury secondary to hypotension or toxin-induced acute interstitial nephritis, shock liver, and in severe situations, altered mental status. In the recovery phase, the erythematous rash subsides with desquamation.

Management

Early diagnosis, rapid intervention with intravenous (IV) fluids, IV antibiotics as well as IV immunoglobulin (IVIG)[1] in some circumstances, along with supportive therapy like mechanical ventilation in patients with respiratory failure and dialysis for patients with severe renal injury, are key to survival in patients with TSS. Patients in circulatory shock are treated in an intensive care unit with ionotropic agents such as norepinephrine (Levophed), phenylephrine, and vasopressin (Pitressin) to provide pressor support. A multidisciplinary team, including intensivists, infectious disease specialists, pulmonologists, and nephrologists, is required for the management of these patients because they often develop respiratory failure and acute renal injury.

Removal of the focus of infection—be it an infected tampon, retained products of conception, surgical drainage of deep-seated abscess, aggressive debridement in patients with necrotizing fasciitis, or postoperative wound infection—is an essential component in the management of TSS.

Blood cultures should be obtained at presentation, and tissue cultures should be obtained at the time of surgery. Ascitic fluid cultures are essential in cases with suspected peritonitis.

[1]Not FDA approved for this indication.

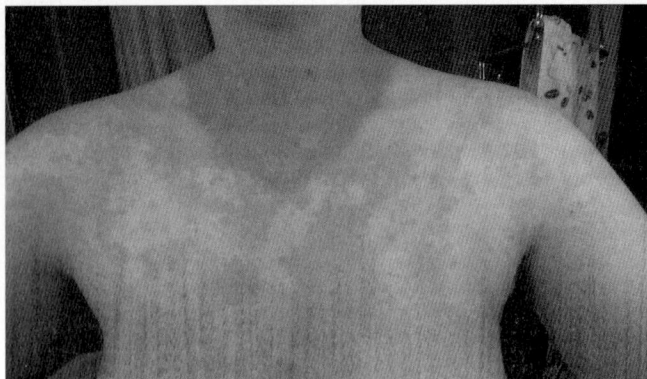

Figure 1 Diffuse erythematous rash on the trunk.

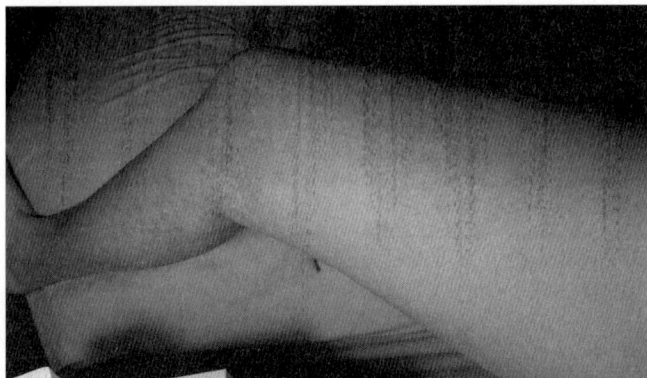

Figure 2 Diffuse erythematous rash on the lower extremity.

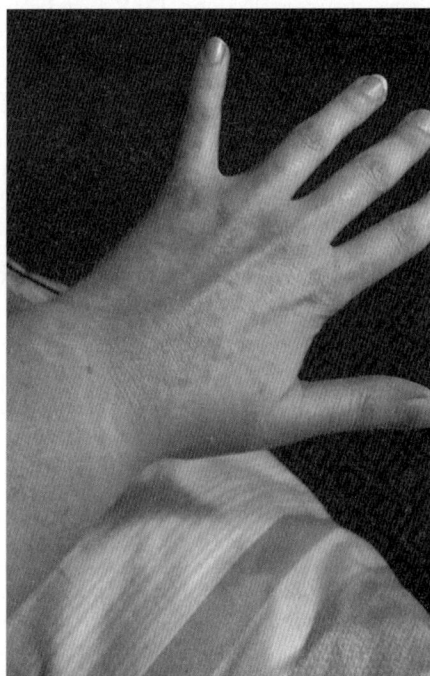

Figure 3 Diffuse erythematous rash on the upper extremity.

Patients should be initially treated with aggressive IV fluid resuscitation along with antibiotic combinations that will provide broad coverage against *Staphylococcus*, *Streptococcus*, and anaerobic organisms. Vancomycin (15 to 20 mg/kg every 12 hours) along with a carbapenem (meropenem [Merrem] 1 g every 8 hours, imipenem [Primaxin] 500 mg every 6 hours, or ertapenem [Invanz] 1 g every 24 hours), or vancomycin along with

piperacillin-tazobactam (Zosyn 4.5 g every 6 to 8 hours) (though there has been reported a higher risk of nephrotoxicity with this compared to the combination of vancomycin with carbapenem) is often the first choice for broad coverage. These antibiotics need dose adjustments based on a patient's renal function. In addition, antibiotics like clindamycin (600 to 900 mg every 8 hours) and linezolid (Zyvox 600 mg every 12 hours) are included because of their direct antitoxin effect (suppress toxin production and accelerate phagocytosis). These antibiotics do not need renal dose adjustments. When the patient is on vancomycin, there should be close monitoring of vancomycin troughs or vancomycin area under the curve, as well as creatinine, to optimize vancomycin dosage and reduce the risk of nephrotoxicity. If linezolid is used, vancomycin will not be required. Newer agents like ceftaroline (Teflaro 600 mg every 12 hours) also provide coverage against methicillin-resistant *S. aureus* (MRSA). The results of microbiology cultures help guide the final antibiotic choice (deescalation of antibiotics). If an infection is caused by a *Streptococcus* species, and no *S. aureus* is identified, vancomycin/ceftaroline can be discontinued and IV penicillin (12 to 24 million units per day as a continuous infusion or in six divided doses) combined with clindamycin is recommended. The duration of antibiotic therapy depends on the patient's clinical response. IVIG[1] has been used in patients who are failing standard therapy. It probably acts by providing antiinflammatory mediators and antibodies against some of the toxins and superantigens and has been shown to improve survival especially in TSLS.

New Research and Developments

Newer antibiotics recently approved for use in skin and skin structure infections, including dalbavancin (Dalvance), oritavancin (Orbactiv), delafloxacin (Baxdela), and omadacycline (Nuzyra), have great coverage against *S. aureus*, including MRSA and *Streptococcus*. However, these have not been approved for use in TSS.

There is ongoing research into the development of immunological agents (monoclonal antibodies and vaccines) that can target toxins and other superantigen-induced cytokine pathways. These nonantibiotic therapies have the potential to block the toxin-induced shock without the side effects commonly associated with antibiotic use.

---

[1]Not FDA approved for this indication.

References

Bonne SL Kadri SS: Evaluation and management of necrotizing soft tissue infections, *Infect Dis Clin N Am* 31(3):497–511, 2017.

Burnham JP, Kollef MH: Understanding toxic shock syndrome, *Intensive Care Med* 41(9):1707–1710, 2015.

Emgard J, Bergsten H, McCormick JK, et al: MAIT cells are major contributors to the cytokine response and group A streptococcal toxic shock syndrome, *Proc Natl Acad Sci USA* 116(51):25923–25931, 2019.

Jayouhey E, Bolze PA, Jamen C, et al: Similarities and differences between staphylococcal and streptococcal toxic shock syndromes in children: results from a 30-case cohort, *Front Pediatr* 6:360, 2018.

Krakauer T: FDA-approved immunosuppressants targeting staphylococcal super antigens: mechanisms and insights, *Immunotargets Ther* 6:17–29, 2017.

Krakauer T: Staphylococcal superantigens: pyrogenic toxins induced toxic shock, *Toxins (Basel)*. 11(3), 2019.

Linner A, Darenberg J, Sjolin J, et al: Clinical efficacy of poly-specific intravenous immunoglobulin therapy in patients with streptococcal toxic shock syndrome: a comparative observational study, *Clin Infect Dis* 59(6):851–857, 2014.

Reingold AL, Hargrett NT, Shands KN, et al: Toxic shock syndrome surveillance in the United States. 1980 to 1981, *Ann Intern Med* 96(6 Pt 2):875–880, 1982.

Shibl AM: Effect of antibiotics on production of enzymes and toxins by microorganisms, *Rev Infect Dis* 5(5):865–875, 1983.

Tierno Jr PM, Hanna BA: Ecology of toxic shock syndrome: amplification of toxic shock syndrome toxin 1 by materials of medical interest, *Rev Infect Dis* 11(Suppl 1):S182–S186, 1989.

Todd J, Fishaut M: Toxic-shock syndrome associated with phage-group-1 staphylococci, *Lancet* 2:1116–1118, 1978.

Wannamaker LW: Streptococcal toxins, *Rev Infect Dis* (5 Suppl 4)S723–S732, 1983.

Zumla A: Super antigens, T cells and microbes, *Clin infec Dis* 15(2):313–320, 1992.

TOXOPLASMOSIS

Method of
Jihoon Baang, MD

Introduction

Toxoplasma gondii, a widespread protozoan parasite, infects a significant portion of the global population. Its interaction with humans can result in a wide array of presentations, ranging from asymptomatic dormant forms and illnesses resembling acute mononucleosis to reactivation of the dormant organism, causing disease in various body parts, particularly the brain. In pregnant women, the parasite can infect the fetus, leading to substantial morbidity worldwide. Although most infections fortunately remain dormant, toxoplasmosis continues to be a major cause of morbidity, particularly in pregnant patients in resource-limited settings and among immunocompromised individuals.

Epidemiology and Risk Factors

Toxoplasmosis is a cosmopolitan zoonotic disease that has important implications for public health because it affects one-third of the world's population. The prevalence of *Toxoplasma gondii* varies widely depending on geographic area. For example, the United States has a prevalence of roughly 10% compared with other places such as Brazil and France, which has a prevalence of greater than 50%.

Toxoplasma gondii, a parasitic protozoan, relies on cats and their relatives as its sole definitive hosts, making them instrumental in the parasite's propagation. Three primary transmission routes contribute to the spread of toxoplasmosis. Firstly, foodborne transmission occurs when undercooked meat (particularly pork, lamb, and venison) from an infected animal is consumed. This mode of transmission is more prevalent in countries and cultures with a preference for undercooked meat. Secondly, cats, particularly kittens, can directly spread the parasite. An infected kitten may shed millions of oocysts for up to 3 weeks, contaminating soil, water, and its litter box. The third route involves congenital transmission from an infected mother to her unborn child, particularly when the infection is newly acquired. This can result in significant morbidity for the fetus. Though rare, additional transmission methods include organ transplantation from an infected donor, blood transfusions, and improper handling of infected tissue or blood within a laboratory setting.

Pathophysiology

T. gondii exists in three forms: the oocysts, tachyzoites and bradyzoites, and they all play a different role in the life cycle of this disease. The major route of infection for *T. gondii* is the gastrointestinal tract. The parasite gains access through the gastrointestinal tract, most commonly through oocysts (i.e., the egg stage) that can exist in contaminated soil, food, and water or through bradyzoites, which exist in tissue and can be transmitted through the ingestion of meat harboring *T. gondii*. Once the parasite enters the gastrointestinal tract, it transforms into tachyzoites which can rapidly multiply within the intestinal epithelium and spread throughout the body. Patients are often asymptomatic but can also develop a mononucleosis-like syndrome of fever, myalgias, and night sweats during this phase.

T. gondii tachyzoites can infect mammalian cells, but, in a normal host, the immune system can effectively reduce the burden of tachyzoites, leading to the elimination of the majority of tachyzoites in human tissue. Murine models suggest T cells, macrophages, and type 1 cytokines such as IFN-gamma and IL-12 play an important role in controlling *T. gondii*. Tachyzoites can change into bradyzoites and remain dormant in various tissues of the body, primarily the brain, skeleton, heart muscle and eye, without causing any symptoms for the remainder of a person's life. Bradyzoites can reactivate when a person who is harboring *T. gondii* becomes immunosuppressed and can lead to diseases in various parts of the body, mainly the brain, skeletal muscle, myocardium, and eye. The tissue cyst form will differentiate into tachyzoites, leading to uncontrolled proliferation that results in tissue destruction, most commonly in the brain and eye.

Clinical Presentation

When thinking about the diagnosis of *T. gondii* infection, there are a few clinical points that should be considered in the clinical reasoning process. The first is that the clinical presentation is influenced by the immune status of the host that it infects. The second is appreciation of the protean clinical manifestation of this cosmopolitan protozoan. The third is understanding the life cycle of this protozoan. And last, but not least, is understanding the limitations of various available diagnostic tests and how to interpret them in a certain clinical setting.

Clinical presentation will be categorized as presentation in a normal host, an immunocompromised host, and a pregnant patient for the convenience of this chapter. The genotype of *T. gondii* also influences the clinical presentation but it is seldom checked in clinical practice.

Clinical Presentation in the Normal Host

When a normal host encounters this protozoan, usually through soil and water contaminated with oocysts excreted from cats or the ingestion of undercooked meat harboring cyst bradyzoites, most of the time, they will have little to no symptoms. When they do have symptoms, they can develop flulike symptoms characterized by fevers, myalgias, and painless enlargement of cervical lymph nodes although rarely larger than 3 cm. Diffuse lymphadenopathy can be observed but is less common. It can mimic other "mononucleosis-like syndromes," such as acute HIV; viral hepatitis, such as hepatitis A virus; acute Epstein Barr virus (EBV); or acute cytomegalovirus (CMV) infection, and these should be considered in the differential diagnosis when considering acute toxoplasmosis. Symptoms can last for weeks and months but are almost always self-limiting. More severe presentations, such as hepatitis, pneumonitis, and myocarditis, have been reported but these are relatively rare manifestations in a normal host and other more common causes should be considered before considering acute toxoplasmosis. Not uncommonly, chorioretinitis can be the sole presentation of acute toxoplasmosis in a normal host and can manifest itself as visual disturbances or floaters. There have been epidemiologic and animal studies suggesting a link between psychiatric illnesses such as schizophrenia with toxoplasmosis, but a definitive link has not been established.

Clinical Presentation in the Immunocompromised Host

In marked contrast, toxoplasmosis has a much more morbid clinical course in the immunocompromised host, with a wider range of clinical presentations. The compromised immune system either cannot contain the infection when it happens, or the mechanism involved in keeping the infection dormant breaks down, leading to reactivation of the infection. Acute toxoplasmosis can lead to more severe disease in the immunocompromised host, sometimes leading to disseminated disease and ultimately death if left untreated. Dormant bradyzoites can reactivate and change to tachyzoites, the invasive form of *T. gondii*. This can lead to a wide range of clinical syndromes depending on the anatomic site it reactivates in. The protean clinical manifestation of toxoplasmosis is impressive and can involve any organ but most commonly involves the eye or the brain. Diagnosis can be challenging because it can often mimic other infections, routine culture data are unrevealing, and the diagnostic studies are often not as reliable in the immunocompromised host. A thorough exposure (e.g., adopted new kittens recently) history based on the life cycle of this protozoan can sometimes be helpful in the diagnostic reasoning process. A high index of clinical suspicion is needed in the early diagnosis of this disease.

The most common site of reactivation is the brain, in which reactivation leads to toxoplasma encephalitis (TE). It is the most common central nervous system (CNS) infection in patients with

HIV with a CD4 count less than 100 cells/mm³ who are not taking any prophylactic regimen. TE can present with a wide range of signs and symptoms depending on the anatomic lesion that it reactivates in the brain. It can present with mild headaches to various degrees of confusion and focal neurologic deficits including cranial nerve abnormalities. Symptoms often will progress over weeks and sometimes months. Patients can present acutely with seizures and cerebral hemorrhage. Sometimes they can present with neuropsychiatric symptoms with paranoid psychosis. In short, there are no pathognomonic clinical findings in TE, emphasizing the importance of maintaining an index of suspicion. It leads to a variety brain pathology, including ventriculitis and meningo-encephalomyelitis, rarely hydrocephalus, and, most commonly, focal areas of enhancing lesions in the brain. It often will present as ring enhancing lesions on brain imaging studies but can be difficult to differentiate between other diseases, such as CNS lymphoma, and other more indolent infections, such as tuberculosis and fungal infections.

T. gondii can involve the lungs and lead to pneumonia. The symptoms are nonspecific, and patients will often present with a worsening cough and shortness of breath that progresses over days to weeks. It is not uncommon to present without fevers. The clinical presentation and imaging findings can look nearly identical to *Pneumocystis jirovecii* pneumonia. The imaging findings can also resemble viral pneumonitis, pulmonary tuberculosis, and fungal pneumonias from histoplasmosis, coccidioidomycosis, and mycoplasma pneumonia.

The impressive range of manifestation is owing to the protozoan's ability to infect and remain dormant in any organ tissue in the form of bradyzoites. Because of this, although much less common, toxoplasmosis can present as myocarditis, pancreatitis, myositis, hepatitis and various ocular findings, most commonly chorioretinitis. We will discuss ocular toxoplasmosis separately because of the unique challenges it poses.

Toxoplasmosis of the Eye

Toxoplasmosis, a protozoal infection caused by *Toxoplasma gondii,* is a leading cause of posterior uveitis worldwide. The infection can occur following an episode of acute infection or reactivation of a dormant bradyzoite, and congenital transmission is also possible. Though some patients with ocular toxoplasmosis may be asymptomatic, others may experience eye pain, photophobia, blurry vision, and floaters. Early diagnosis and treatment of subclinical congenital toxoplasmosis is crucial because untreated chorioretinitis, the most common late manifestation of congenital toxoplasmosis, can result in blindness. In patients who are immunocompromised, larger retinal lesions with diffuse retinal necrosis may be present and may indicate a prodrome to the development of toxoplasma encephalitis.

Toxoplasmosis in Pregnancy

Congenital toxoplasmosis occurs when a pregnant mother with an acute infection transmits the disease to her fetus through the placenta. The incidence and severity of the disease depend on the gestational age at the time of maternal infection. The transmission risk is inconsistent throughout pregnancy. Congenital infection during early pregnancy is rare. However, when the primary maternal infection occurs in the latter half of pregnancy, congenital infection is more frequently observed. Most infected infants are born healthy, but around 22% may develop clinical disease by 3 years of age. Fetal outcomes associated with congenital toxoplasmosis can be severe, including miscarriage, stillbirth, or severe CNS sequelae. It is crucial to monitor and manage maternal infections during pregnancy to minimize the risk of congenital transmission and its associated complications.

Diagnosis

The diagnosis of toxoplasmosis is typically made through a combination of a clinical syndrome compatible with toxoplasmosis and positive serologic studies. In certain clinical scenarios, especially

in congenital infections in utero, the detection of *T. gondii* DNA in various body fluids and tissue can provide a definitive diagnosis. Histopathologic diagnosis through a biopsy of affected tissue is also possible but often pursued in a clinical scenario where other diagnoses need to be excluded. It is essential to consider a patient's immune status because the presentation of toxoplasmosis can vary depending on the host's immune response.

The detection of antibodies against *T. gondii* is the most common laboratory test used in the diagnosis of toxoplasmosis. Both immunoglobulin (Ig)M and IgG antibody tests should be performed initially, and the results should be combined with the patient's clinical presentation to establish a diagnosis. It is important to note that a single serologic test is rarely sufficient to confirm acute or chronic toxoplasmosis. Often, multiple tests at different time points are required. Accurately differentiating between acute and chronic infections is particularly crucial for pregnant patients because chronic infections pose minimal risk to the fetus and acute infections are more likely to result in congenital toxoplasmosis.

IgG and IgM antibodies against *T. gondii* can be easily detected in most laboratories using commercially available kits. If toxoplasmosis is suspected, *Toxoplasma*-specific IgG testing serves as a convenient initial step to determine the host's immune response to the organism. A positive IgG test signifies past exposure to *T. gondii* and the presence of the parasite in the host's body. A negative IgG test often implies no exposure to *T. gondii*, but it can also represent an early infection or, rarely, a false-negative test result, typically in individuals with compromised immune systems.

The IgM plays a role in differentiating between acute and chronic infections. A negative test result generally indicates a chronic infection, though a positive IgM test is less informative due to its lack of specificity. Because the IgM antibody can persist for over 18 months, it is less useful for determining the infection's timing. In pregnant patients, the timing of infection is crucial. One test that can be used is the IgG avidity test. This is based on the observation that the functional affinity of *T. gondii*–specific IgG antibodies is initially low after infection and increases over time, which can help ascertain the infection's age. A high avidity pattern reliably predicts an infection older than 4 months, whereas a low avidity pattern suggests an acute infection but is not as reliable. IgE antibodies can also be checked. These antibodies have shorter half-lives, which makes it more useful than IgM in determining whether someone has an acute infection. The IgA antibodies do not bring value in adults compared with the IgM as it can persist in recently infected patients for more than a year. However, IgA antibodies are more sensitive in detecting congenital toxoplasmosis and should be checked in fetuses and newborns with a high clinical suspicion for the condition. The avidity test, along with IgA and IgE antibodies, is not widely available in most labs; however, it can be performed at the Palo Alto Medical Foundation in the United States. None of the current commercial assays in the United States have been approved by the U.S. Food and Drug Administration for the use in infants, and all specimens from neonates should be sent to the Palo Alto Medical Foundation for testing. Table 1 summarizes the basic interpretation of serologic studies in individuals greater than a year old.

Polymerase chain reaction (PCR) amplification serves as an important tool for detecting *T. gondii* DNA in a variety of body fluids and tissues. This method has proven to be effective in diagnosing diverse forms of toxoplasmosis, including congenital, ocular, cerebral, and disseminated cases. The use of PCR on amniotic fluid has significantly transformed the diagnosis of fetal *T. gondii* infection by enabling early detection, thereby circumventing the need for more invasive procedures on the fetus. PCR allows for the precise identification of *T. gondii* DNA in numerous sample types, such as brain tissue, cerebrospinal fluid (CSF), vitreous and aqueous fluid, bronchoalveolar lavage (BAL) fluid, urine, amniotic fluid, and peripheral blood.

Histopathologic diagnosis of toxoplasmosis has become less common owing to the invasive techniques required for tissue

TABLE 1	Toxoplasmosis Laboratory Diagnosis	
IGG RESULT	**IGM RESULT**	**REPORT/INTERPRETATION FOR HUMANS***
Negative	Negative	There is no serologic evidence of infection with *Toxoplasma*.
Negative	Equivocal	This is a possible early acute infection or a false-positive IgM reaction. Obtain a new specimen for IgG and IgM testing. If results for the second specimen remain the same, the patient is probably not infected with *Toxoplasma*.
Negative	**Positive**	This is a possible acute infection or a false-positive IgM result. Obtain a new specimen for IgG and IgM testing. If results for the second specimen remain the same, the IgM reaction is probably a false-positive.
Equivocal	Negative	This is indeterminate. Obtain a new specimen for testing, or retest this specimen for IgG in a different assay.
Equivocal	Equivocal	This is indeterminate. Obtain a new specimen for both IgG and IgM testing.
Equivocal	**Positive**	This is a possible acute infection with *Toxoplasma*. Obtain a new specimen for IgG and IgM testing. If results for the second specimen remain the same or if the IgG becomes positive, both specimens should be sent to a reference laboratory with experience in diagnosis of toxoplasmosis for further testing.
Positive	Negative	This individual is infected with *Toxoplasma* for 6 months or more.
Positive	Equivocal	This individual is infected with *Toxoplasma* for probably more than 1 year, or this is a false-positive IgM reaction. Obtain a new specimen for IgM testing. If results with the second specimen remain the same, both specimens should be sent to a reference laboratory with experience in the diagnosis of toxoplasmosis for further testing.
Positive	**Positive**	This is a possible recent infection within the last 12 months or a false-positive IgM reaction. Send the specimen to a reference laboratory with experience in the diagnosis of toxoplasmosis for further testing.

*Except infants.
Source: NCCLS. Clinical Use and Interpretation of Serologic Tests for *Toxoplasma gondii*; Approved Guideline. NCCLS document M36-A [ISBN 1-56238-523-2]. NCCLS, 940 West Valley Road, Suite 1400, Wayne, PA 19087-1898 USA, 2004.

collection and the growing prevalence of PCR usage. Detecting tachyzoites in body fluids and tissue samples can confirm the presence of an acute infection, although this can be challenging to demonstrate. Meanwhile, the identification of bradyzoites may indicate either chronic infection or reactivation disease, depending on the host's condition.

Therapeutic response can serve as a diagnostic tool in certain cases. For patients presenting with ring-enhancing lesions in the brain who cannot undergo a brain biopsy and have inconclusive cerebrospinal fluid (CSF) results, a course of treatment for toxoplasma encephalitis should typically yield clinical and radiologic improvements within 14 days. If a clinical response is observed, it is generally considered sufficient for confirming the diagnosis of toxoplasma encephalitis.

Treatment

Treatment for *T. gondii* primarily targets the tachyzoite stage of the parasite but is unable to eliminate bradyzoites embedded within tissue, which can result in relapse in certain scenarios. In immunocompetent individuals, acute toxoplasmosis usually does not warrant treatment. However, if visceral involvement or severe symptoms are present, a 2- to 4-week course of therapy might be advantageous. On the other hand, treatment is typically necessary for acute toxoplasmosis and reactivation disease in immunocompromised hosts, ocular toxoplasmosis with visual disturbances, acute toxoplasmosis in pregnant patients, and cases of congenital toxoplasmosis.

The treatment regimen remains consistent across various clinical scenarios except for pregnant patients in their first trimester owing to the teratogenicity of pyrimethamine. Nevertheless, the dose and duration of treatment can vary depending on the specific situation and immune status of the host. The dose is typically higher and duration of treatment longer in patients who are immunocompromised.

Pyrimethamine (Daraprim) serves as the cornerstone of toxoplasmosis treatment and should be incorporated when possible. As a folic acid antagonist, it is associated with dose-dependent bone marrow suppression. This side effect can be mitigated through the coadministration of folinic acid (leucovorin).[1] Pyrimethamine monotherapy is not recommended owing to the high doses required for effective treatment. The addition of a second drug, such as sulfadiazine, adds synergy, allowing pyrimethamine to be used at substantially lower, nontoxic levels compared with when administered alone. Clindamycin,[1] atovaquone (Mepron),[1] and azithromycin (Zithromax)[1] can be used to replace sulfadiazine, if the patient is unable to tolerate sulfadiazine. Trimethoprim-sulfamethoxazole (Bactrim)[1] monotherapy has been shown in a small trial to be as effective as pyrimethamine combined with sulfamethoxazole and can be used if the patient is unable to tolerate pyrimethamine. For ocular toxoplasmosis, intravitreous injection of clindamycin[1] and dexamethasone[1] can be used, although a small, randomized trial did not show any difference in outcome compared with an oral regimen.

In pregnant patients, chronic *T. gondii* infection poses little risk to the fetus and does not need treatment. In acute or recent infection, treatment should be initiated. If a patient is in their first trimester (<14 weeks), spiramycin (Rovamycine)[2] should be started. In their second and third trimesters (>14 weeks), a pyrimethamine-sulfadiazine regimen can be used.

Because of the inability to eradicate bradyzoites embedded in tissue, secondary prophylaxis is recommended for immunocompromised patients to prevent relapse until immune reconstitution is achieved. For patients with HIV, this typically involves maintaining a CD4 count greater than 200/mm^3 for over 6 months. Transplant recipients, on the other hand, may require lifelong secondary prophylaxis to prevent the recurrence of infection.

Effective management of toxoplasmosis necessitates not only addressing the various side effects associated with treatment but also possessing the flexibility to switch to alternative regimens when a patient's tolerance to the initial therapy proves inadequate. This adaptability is crucial in optimizing patient outcomes

---

[1] Not FDA approved for this indication.
[2] Not available in the United States.

TABLE 2　Summary of Treatment Regimens for Toxoplasmosis

HOST	REGIMEN AND DURATION
Primary infection in immunocompetent host	No treatment in general but can treat with same regimen as below for 2–4 weeks in severe disease
Treatment of immunocompromised host/reactivation disease/ocular toxoplasmosis	Preferred: Pyrimethamine[1] (PO) 200 mg loading dose followed by 50 mg (<60 kg); 75 mg (≥60 kg) daily + sulfadiazine 1 g (<60 kg); 1.5 g (≥60 kg) + folinic acid (leucovorin)[1] 10–25 mg PO daily for 6 weeks or longer depending on clinical response and then secondary prophylaxis
	If unable to tolerate pyrimethamine: Trimethoprim/sulfamethoxazole[1] 10 mg/kg/day (trimethoprim component) divided in two to three doses for monotherapy for 6 weeks
	If unable to tolerate sulfadiazine: Can change to clindamycin[1] 600 mg IV/PO q8–q6h or atovaquone (Mepron)[1] 1500 mg PO q12h or azithromycin[1] 900–1200 mg PO daily with pyrimethamine 25–50 mg and leucovorin for 6 weeks or longer
Secondary prophylaxis	Sulfadiazine 500–1000 mg PO qid + primethamine[1] 25–50 mg PO daily + folinic acid[1] 10–25 mg PO daily until immune reconstitution
	Clindamycin[1] 300–450 mg PO q6-q8h +primethamine[1] 25–50 mg PO daily + folinic acid[1] 10–25 mg PO daily
	Atovaquone[1] 1500 mg PO daily with food
Pregnancy	First trimester: Spiramycin (Rovamycine)[2] 1 g q8h
	Second and 3rd trimester: Pyrimethamine (PO) 50 mg twice daily loading dose for 2 days then 50 mg daily + sulfadiazine 75 mg/kg/d in two divided doses for 2 days then 50 mg/kg twice daily + folinic acid[1] 10–20 mg PO daily until delivery
Fetal/congenital toxoplasmosis	Pyrimethamine + sulfadiazine + leucovorin[1]: expert consultation is recommended

[1]Not FDA approved for this indication.
[2]Not available in the United States.

and ensuring successful treatment. A summary of treatment for toxoplasmosis is provided in Table 2.

Prevention

Currently, no vaccines are available for the prevention of toxoplasmosis or for reducing the risk of reactivation. Preventative measures are crucial, particularly for seronegative pregnant women and individuals who are immunocompromised. Toxoplasmosis can occasionally be transmitted through donor organs, and routine screening is a standard practice in many transplant programs. Familiarity with the modes of transmission is the first step in mitigating the risk of acquiring toxoplasmosis. This includes avoiding areas potentially contaminated with cat feces or wearing gloves when exposure is unavoidable, such as when cleaning a kitten's litter box. Freezing meat to –20°C (–4°F) for at least 48 hours or cooking meat thoroughly is sufficient to eliminate bradyzoites that may be present within the meat. Washing fruits and vegetables under running water and consistently washing hands after outdoor activities are simple interventions that can minimize the risk of acquiring oocysts.

References

Bennett JE, Dolin R, Blaser MJ: Preface to the eighth edition. In Bennett JE, Dolin R, Blaser MJ, editors: *Mandell, douglas, and bennett's principles and practice of infectious diseases*, Eighth Edition, xxvii. Philadelphia, 2015, W.B. Saunders, pp 3355–3387.

CDC - DPDx Homepage, February 21, 2023. https://www.cdc.gov/dpdx/index.html, 2023. Accessed 03/01/2023.

Montoya JG, Liesenfeld O: Toxoplasmosis, *Lancet.* 363(9425):1965–1976, 2004.

NCCLS: *Clinical Use and interpretation of serologic tests for toxoplasma gondii; approved guideline. NCCLS document M36-A [ISBN 1-56238-523-2]*, 2004. NCCLS, 940 West Valley Road, Suite 1400, Wayne, PA 19087-1898 USA.

Panel on Guidelines for the Prevention and Treatment of Opportunistic Infections in Adults and Adolescents with HIV. Guidelines for the Prevention and Treatment of Opportunistic Infections in Adults and Adolescents with HIV. National Institutes of Health, Centers for Disease Control and Prevention, HIV Medicine Association, and Infectious Diseases Society of America. Year. Available at https://clinicalinfo.hiv.gov/en/guidelines/adult-and-adolescent-opportunistic-infection. Accessed 03/01/2023 [pp CC-1 – CC-15].

TYPHOID FEVER

Method of
Tamilarasu Kadhiravan, MD

CURRENT DIAGNOSIS

- Typhoid fever typically manifests as an undifferentiated acute febrile illness.
- Soft splenomegaly, normal or low white blood cell count, and elevated liver enzymes are subtle diagnostic pointers.
- Blood culture, drawn before antibiotic administration, is the most useful investigation.
- Consider presumptive treatment in appropriate epidemiologic settings.

CURRENT THERAPY

- Intermediate susceptibility and resistance to fluoroquinolones are widespread among *Salmonella enterica* Typhi.
- High-dose fluoroquinolones are suboptimal for treating such infections.
- Azithromycin (Zithromax)[1] is the preferred drug for uncomplicated typhoid fever.
- Ceftriaxone (Rocephin)[1] is preferred for treating hospitalized and seriously ill patients.
- Extensively drug-resistant (XDR) typhoid fever, which is resistant to ceftriaxone and fluoroquinolones, is an emerging threat.

[1]Not FDA approved for this indication.

Typhoid fever is a bacteremic infection caused by the gram-negative bacillus *Salmonella enterica* serovar Typhi. *S enterica*

Paratyphi also causes an illness clinically indistinguishable from typhoid fever. Humans are the only known host of *S enterica* Typhi, and it is transmitted by ingestion of contaminated food or water. Improvement in sanitation and hygiene led to the elimination of typhoid fever from the developed world long before the advent of antibiotics. On the other hand, in parts of the world lacking sanitation, it continues to be an important cause of febrile illness despite the availability of effective antibiotics.

Epidemiology

Typhoid fever is endemic in the developing world, especially the South and South East Asian countries of India, Nepal, Pakistan, Bangladesh, Vietnam, and Indonesia. Annual incidence in endemic settings is typically more than 100 cases per 100,000 population, and it predominantly affects children and young adults. Apart from sick persons with typhoid fever, convalescent carriers and asymptomatically infected food handlers (long-term carriers) are the sources of infection. Potential vehicles of infection include food or water consumed from roadside eateries, ice cubes and ice cream made from contaminated water, and raw vegetables and fruits. In contrast, most cases of typhoid fever in developed countries are imported by travel, especially to the Indian subcontinent.

Pathogenesis and Clinical Features

Following ingestion, the bacilli invade and multiply in the small-intestinal lymphoid tissue before entering the bloodstream. This primary bacteremia leads to widespread seeding of the reticuloendothelial system and intestinal lymphoid tissue, where the infection is amplified and spills over into the circulation. Onset of symptoms usually coincides with this secondary bacteremia. Interestingly, unlike other gram-negative bacteremic infections, septic shock develops relatively late in the course of illness, and the infection can be eminently cured by oral antibiotic therapy. Nonetheless, it should be emphasized that any delay in initiating antibiotic therapy increases the risk of complications (Box 1).

During the first week, temperature gradually increases in a stepladder fashion. Localizing symptoms are usually minimal. Anorexia, lassitude, and malaise are often marked. Headache and vomiting are common; however, a supple neck helps rule out meningitis. Abdominal symptoms such as constipation, loose stools, and abdominal pain are not infrequent, but they are nonspecific and often overlooked. Soft, tender enlargement of liver or spleen is seen in about half the patients. Rose spots and relative bradycardia, though classic, are rare. When the infection goes untreated, hypertrophied lymphoid tissue of the Peyer's patches can ulcerate toward the end of the second week, resulting in torrential gastrointestinal bleeding, small intestinal perforation, and secondary bacterial peritonitis. Patients with severe illness can present with a muttering delirium described as *coma vigil*. Untreated typhoid fever often resolves spontaneously in about 4 to 6 weeks. However, the risk of death is high (>10%), and relapses are frequent. Many patients excrete *S enterica* Typhi in feces and urine during convalescence (convalescent carriers), and some of them continue to excrete beyond 1 year (long-term carriers). Recovery from typhoid fever offers very little protection against disease following subsequent exposures.

Current Pattern of Antimicrobial Susceptibility

Since 1990, a sea change has occurred in the antimicrobial susceptibility of *S enterica* Typhi in endemic countries and elsewhere. Unregulated use of fluoroquinolones initially led to the emergence of *S enterica* Typhi strains with decreased susceptibility. These strains had a subthreshold increase in minimal inhibitory concentration (MIC) that was not detected by conventional disk-diffusion testing. Hence, resistance to nalidixic acid (NegGram)[2] (a quinolone) was often used as a surrogate marker for such strains. Currently, determination of MIC is recommended to identify fluoroquinolone susceptibility. Most infections in endemic countries are now caused by *S enterica* Typhi

---

| BOX 1 | Complications of Typhoid Fever |

Abdominal
Paralytic ileus
Intestinal hemorrhage
Intestinal perforation
Secondary peritonitis
Symptomatic liver dysfunction
Acalculous cholecystitis

Extra Abdominal
Encephalopathy
Cerebellar dysfunction
Myocarditis
Osteomyelitis and soft tissue abscesses
Multiorgan dysfunction syndrome
Hemophagocytic syndrome
Hemolysis
Glomerulonephritis

Long-term
Gallbladder cancer

---

with intermediate susceptibility or resistance to fluoroquinolones. Not surprisingly, this change is reflected in far-away geographic locales such as the United States and the United Kingdom. Of late, sporadic instances of resistance to azithromycin and third-generation cephalosporins have been reported. Notably, widespread emergence of extensively drug-resistant (XDR) *S. enterica* Typhi with extended-spectrum β-lactamase–mediated resistance to third-generation cephalosporins has been reported in the Sindh province of Pakistan. In 2019, two-thirds of *S. enterica* Typhi isolates from Karachi, Pakistan, were resistant to third-generation cephalosporins. Travel-associated XDR-typhoid cases have been reported from several countries in the Europe and North America.

Diagnosis

Clinical features are nonspecific, and laboratory testing is essential to confirm a diagnosis of typhoid fever. A soft splenomegaly, absence of leukocytosis, mild leukopenia, and modest elevation of transaminases are subtle pointers to a diagnosis of typhoid fever. Blood culture drawn early in the illness before initiation of antibiotics is often fruitful and is the gold standard for the diagnosis of typhoid fever. Clinical practice guidelines recommend against using serologic and nucleic acid amplification tests to diagnose typhoid fever. The time-honored Widal test, which detects agglutinating antibodies to somatic and flagellar antigens of *S enterica* Typhi, adds little to decision making. Initial enthusiasm about rapid serologic tests such as Typhidot and Tubex TF has not been confirmed in community-based studies. None of these tests are sensitive enough to rule out typhoid. In a patient who has nonlocalizing acute febrile illness lasting more than 5 to 7 days in a suggestive epidemiologic setting (residence in or travel to endemic area; outbreaks), it is prudent to treat presumptively for typhoid fever, after reasonably ruling out competing diagnoses such as malaria, dengue, leptospirosis, and rickettsial infection.

Treatment

Fluoroquinolones (ciprofloxacin [Cipro] or ofloxacin [Floxin][1] 7.5 mg/kg twice a day for 5–7 days) were unparalleled in efficacy for treating fully susceptible *S enterica* Typhi strains. However, their use was associated with frequent treatment failures, prolonged defervescence, and higher rates of complications in nalidixic acid-resistant *S. enterica* Typhi (NARST) infections. Given the high prevalence of reduced susceptibility, fluoroquinolones are no longer considered the drug of choice. Several alternatives have been evaluated in randomized, controlled trials for treating uncomplicated typhoid fever caused by NARST (Table 1). Ease of oral administration, proven

---

[2]Not available in the United States.

[1]Not FDA approved for this indication.

DRUG	DOSAGE	FEVER CLEARANCE TIME (MEDIAN OR MEAN)	RATE OF TREATMENT FAILURE	RELAPSE RATE	COMMENTS
High-dose ofloxacin (Floxin)[1]	10 mg/kg[3] bid × 7 d	8.2 d	36%	<1%; insufficient data	Not recommended
Gatifloxacin (Tequin)[2]	10 mg/kg qd × 7 d	4.4 d	9%	3%	Serious concerns about dysglycemia; resistance emerging in Nepal
Azithromycin (Zithromax)[1]	10–20[3] mg/kg qd × 7 d	4.4 d	9%	<1%; insufficient data	Effective in XDR-typhoid. Unproven in complicated typhoid fever
Cefixime (Suprax)[1]	10 mg/kg[3] bid × 7 d	5.8 d	27%	9%	High cost; not recommended
Ceftriaxone (Rocephin)[1]	60 mg/kg qd × 7 d	2.8 d	7%	7%	Experts suggest treatment for 10–14 d

Data from Arjyal A, Basnyat B, Nhan HT, et al: Gatifloxacin versus ceftriaxone for uncomplicated enteric fever in Nepal: an open-label, two-centre, randomised controlled trial. Lancet Infect Dis 2016;16:535. Dolecek C, Tran TP, Nguyen NR, et al: A multi-center randomised controlled trial of gatifloxacin versus azithromycin for the treatment of uncomplicated typhoid fever in children and adults in Vietnam. PLoS One 2008;3:e2188; Pandit A, Arjyal A, Day JN, et al: An open randomized comparison of gatifloxacin versus cefixime for the treatment of uncomplicated enteric fever. PLoS One 2007;2:e542; and Parry CM, Ho VA, Phuong le T, et al: Randomized controlled comparison of ofloxacin, azithromycin, and an ofloxacin-azithromycin combination for treatment of multidrug-resistant and nalidixic acid-resistant typhoid fever. Antimicrob Agents Chemother 2007;51:819.

[1]Not FDA approved for this indication.
[2]Not available in the United States.
[3]Exceeds dosage recommended by the manufacturer.

efficacy, and safety (under FDA review) make azithromycin (Zithromax)[1] a good first choice for uncomplicated typhoid fever. In hospitalized seriously ill patients and treatment failures, parenteral ceftriaxone (Rocephin)[1] is preferred. Usually, it takes about 4 to 7 days for defervescence after the initiation of antibiotics.

Recently, combining oral azithromycin (500 mg qd) with ceftriaxone (2 g qd) for inpatient or cefixime (Suprax)[1] (400 mg qd) for outpatient treatment was found to shorten the fever clearance time by about 7 hours, and fewer patients had persistent bacteremia on Day 3 (17% vs 4%). This clinical trial had certain limitations, and I do not recommend using a combination of antibiotics to treat typhoid fever. An ongoing multicountry clinical trial is expected to bring clarity to this issue. Nonetheless, practice guidelines recommend dual antibiotic treatment in certain special circumstances: (1) to cover for other pathogens such as rickettsia or suspected bacterial sepsis, (2) in patients with typhoid intestinal perforation, and (3) in seriously ill patients with suspected or confirmed XDR-typhoid. Despite in vitro susceptibility, aminoglycosides and first- and second-generation cephalosporins are not effective clinically for treating typhoid fever. Azithromycin (20 mg/kg qd for 7 days)[3] and meropenem (Merrem[1]; 20 mg/kg tid for 14 days) are the only options currently available for the treatment of XDR-typhoid. Antipyretics should be used for symptom relief; ibuprofen (Motrin; 10 mg/kg every 6 hours) is superior to acetaminophen (Tylenol; 12 mg/kg every 6 hours). However, ibuprofen should be avoided when dengue fever is a possibility. A soft, low-residue diet is traditionally advised to prevent intestinal perforation. Such a practice, however, is not founded on scientific evidence. Treatment of *S enterica* Paratyphi infection is identical to that of *S enterica* Typhi infection.

Prevention

Sustained improvement in sanitation and access to safe drinking water are essential to control typhoid fever in endemic areas. Avoiding potentially contaminated food and beverages and being vaccinated before travel decrease the risk of typhoid fever among travelers (see the article on travel medicine). Mass administration of the Vi polysaccharide vaccine (Typhim Vi, Typherix [outside United States]) has been found to confer herd immunity and is a potential tool for the control of typhoid fever in endemic settings. The typhoid conjugate vaccine (Typbar-TCV)[2] is being used to control XDR-typhoid outbreaks.

References

Chatham-Stephens K, Medalla F, et al: Emergence of extensively drug-resistant *Salmonella* Typhi infections among travelers to or from Pakistan - United States, 2016-2018, *MMWR Morb Mortal Wkly Rep* 68:11, 2019.

GRAM Typhoid Collaborators: Estimating the subnational prevalence of antimicrobial resistant *Salmonella enterica* serovars Typhi and Paratyphi A infections in 75 endemic countries, 1990-2019: a modelling study, *Lancet Glob Health* 12:e406, 2024.

Jin C, Gibani MM, Pennington SH, et al: Treatment responses to azithromycin and ciprofloxacin in uncomplicated *Salmonella* typhi infection: a comparison of clinical and microbiological data from a controlled human infection model, *PLoS Negl Trop Dis* 13:e0007955, 2019.

Meiring JE, Khanam F, Basnyat B, etal: Typhoid fever, *Nat Rev Dis Primers* 9:71, 2023.

Nabarro LE, McCann N, Herdman MT, etal: British Infection Association guidelines for the diagnosis and management of enteric fever in England, *J Infect* 84:469, 2022.

Qureshi S, Naveed AB, Yousafzai MT, et al: Response of extensively drug resistant *Salmonella* Typhi to treatment with meropenem and azithromycin, in Pakistan, *PLoS Negl Trop Dis* 14:e0008682, 2020.

Vinh H, Parry CM, Hanh VT, et al: Double blind comparison of ibuprofen and paracetamol for adjunctive treatment of uncomplicated typhoid fever, *Pediatr Infect Dis J* 23:226, 2004.

Wijedoru L, Mallett S, Parry CM: Rapid diagnostic tests for typhoid and paratyphoid (enteric) fever, *Cochrane Database Syst Rev*(5), 2017:CD008892.

Zmora N, Shrestha S, Neuberger A, et al: Open label comparative trial of mono versus dual antibiotic therapy for typhoid fever in adults, *PLoS Negl Trop Dis* 12:e0006380, 2018.

[1]Not FDA approved for this indication.
[2]Not available in the United States.
[3]Exceeds dosage recommended by the manufacturer.

VARICELLA (CHICKENPOX)

Method of
Martha Riese, MD

CURRENT DIAGNOSIS

- Historically, varicella has been diagnosed clinically. Symptoms include a pruritic vesicular rash, fever, malaise, abdominal pain, and anorexia.
- Polymerase chain reaction (PCR) testing is available for confirmation of the diagnosis. An open vesicular lesion is swabbed for specimen collection.

CURRENT THERAPY

- For immunocompetent individuals 1 to 12 years of age, treatment is supportive.
- Acyclovir (Zovirax) or valacyclovir (Valtrex) treatment is used to reduce the severity of symptoms and/or risk of complications in those who are younger than 1 year or older than 12 years of age, pregnant women, or for those who are immunocompromised.
- Postexposure prophylaxis with the varicella vaccine (Varivax)[1] is recommended for healthy patients exposed to the virus who do not have evidence of immunity or previous vaccination.
- Varicella zoster immunoglobin (Varizig) administration is recommended for high-risk individuals with exposure history.

[1]Not FDA approved for this indication.

Epidemiology

Varicella infection is caused by the varicella zoster virus (VZV) and is commonly known as chickenpox. This virus is highly contagious and spreads rapidly. Varicella exhibits a seasonality with infections being more common in the winter and spring. Individuals living in tropical climates are typically affected at an older average age than those living in more temperate climates. Historically, prior to the availability of vaccinations, greater than 90% of people were seropositive for varicella by adolescence in temperate areas and less than 5% of adults remained susceptible.

The economic and healthcare burden of varicella is significant. In 1995, the varicella virus vaccine (Varivax) became licensed and available in the United States, beginning an era of reduced morbidity and mortality from the virus. Since the addition of the varicella virus vaccine into the vaccination schedule in the United States in 1996, the overall incidence of the disease has decreased by approximately 92%, and varicella-related deaths have declined by 94%. However, even with the availability of the vaccine and its proven effectiveness at reducing the overall burden of disease, there are still many industrialized countries that have not incorporated it into their national vaccination programs.

Risk Factors

The only risk factor for infection with varicella is exposure to the virus. Adults, immunocompromised patients, infants, and pregnant women are at greatest risk for complications. Specifically, pregnant women, newborns, and the fetus are at high risk for complications.

Following the resolution of the primary infection, the virus remains dormant in the sensory nerve ganglia and can be reactivated at a later time, causing herpes zoster (shingles).

Pathophysiology

The VZV is a double-stranded DNA virus from the Herpesviridae family. The illness is spread by respiratory droplets or direct contact with open vesicular lesions. The virus enters through the respiratory system, mucosa, or conjunctiva. The incubation period is typically 10 to 21 days. The virus replicates in the regional lymph nodes of infected individuals and then is spread throughout the body.

Varicella infection typically confers lifelong immunity, but secondary infections in immunocompetent individuals have been documented on rare occasions. It is thought that subclinical reinfection is common.

Prevention

A live-attenuated varicella virus vaccine, Varivax, has been available since 1995. Currently, in the United States, a two-shot series is recommended for all children and adults who do not have evidence of immunity. The two-shot series of Varivax is more effective than a single dose of the vaccine at preventing infection and complications. A single dose of the vaccine has been shown to prevent infection and reduce the risk of complications, but to a lesser degree than when two shots are administered.

Evidence of immunity is defined as appropriately timed administration of the varicella vaccine, laboratory confirmation of disease, history of diagnosis of varicella or herpes zoster confirmed by a healthcare provider, or birth in the United States before 1980 (although birth prior to 1980 should not be considered sufficient evidence for healthcare workers, pregnant women, or the immunocompromised).

The United States follows the routine childhood vaccination schedule recommended by the Advisory Committee on Immunization Practices (ACIP). In keeping with that schedule, Varivax is recommended for initial administration to healthy children between the ages of 12 and 15 months. The second dose is recommended between ages 4 and 6 years. For children who receive the vaccine series between age 7 and 13 years, the minimum required interval between doses is 3 months. For adolescents over age 13 who have not been previously vaccinated, the first dose should be administered and the second dose should be given 4 to 8 weeks later. The second dose may still be given if more than 8 weeks have lapsed between doses without the need to repeat the series. The varicella vaccine can be safely administered with other vaccines during childhood.

A combination measles-mumps-rubella-varicella (MMRV) vaccine is available. The CDC recommends that the MMRV vaccine not be administered as a first dose to children under age 4 years due to a risk of febrile seizures. Rather, the MMR and varicella vaccines should be administered separately. The MMRV vaccine is preferred for the second scheduled dose after age 4 years through 12 years and for the first dose at age 48 months or older.

Varicella postexposure prophylaxis with Varivax[1] and/or the varicella zoster immune globulin (Varizig) is recommended to people exposed to active disease who do not have evidence of immunity. The varicella vaccine should optimally be administered to these individuals within 3 to 5 days of exposure to the virus. If the time from exposure exceeds 5 days, the vaccine is still recommended. These individuals should be encouraged to receive the second dose at the appropriate dosing interval.

For individuals without evidence of immunity who are at the highest risk of severe varicella infection and complications, varicella zoster immune globulin may be given following exposure to active disease. The immune globulin should be given within 10 days of exposure for high-risk patients. Patients given the varicella immune globulin should be evaluated for eligibility of future immunization with the varicella vaccine. If they are deemed eligible, an interval of 5 months should lapse prior to the administration of the varicella vaccine.

Varicella immunoglobulin can also be considered for those with contraindications to the varicella vaccine. Contraindications to the varicella vaccine include patients who are pregnant or might

[1]Not FDA approved for this indication.

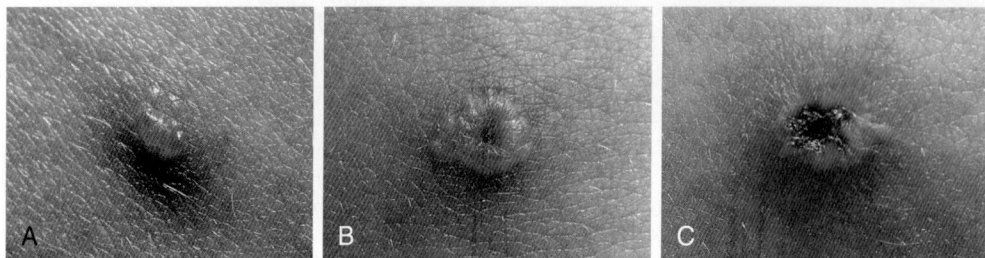

Figure 1 A, "Dewdrop on a rose petal"; a thick-walled vesicle with clear fluid forms on a red base. **B,** The vesicle becomes cloudy and depressed in the center (umbilicated); the border is irregular (scalloped). **C,** A crust forms in the center and eventually replaces the remaining portion of the vesicle at the periphery.

be pregnant, malignant neoplasms affecting the bone marrow or lymphatic system, those receiving prolonged immunosuppressive therapy (>2 weeks), moderate or severe concurrent illness, family history of congenital hereditary immunodeficiency, receipt of blood products within the past 3 to 11 months, or history of anaphylactic reaction to gelatin, neomycin, or other components of the vaccine.

Clinical Manifestations

Varicella infection is typically self-limited, with healthy children often having less severe disease than infected adults. Infections often start with a prodrome of fever, chills, malaise, abdominal pain, and pharyngitis that is followed by the appearance of the vesicular pruritic rash on an erythematous base. The lesions have been described as having a "dewdrop on a rose petal" appearance (Figure 1). The rash typically appears on the scalp, face, trunk, and extremities. Lesions may also appear on the mucous membrane of the cornea, conjunctiva, oropharynx, respiratory tract, and vagina. Following the initial prodrome, the first crop of lesions appears as erythematous macular lesions. The lesions commonly transition to papules, then to clear, fluid-filled vesicles, and the vesicles eventually crust over, usually in 1 to 2 days. New crops of lesions continue to appear throughout the course of the illness over approximately 4 to 5 days, ranging between 1 and 7 days. The presence of lesions in different stages is highly characteristic of varicella infection (Figure 2) and helps differentiate the clinical findings of chickenpox from smallpox. Individuals are infectious approximately 1 to 2 days before the onset of the rash until all lesions are crusted over and no new lesions are forming. The stage of the illness when the open vesicles are present is considered to be highly contagious.

Breakthrough infections in previously immunized patients have been documented. These are infections occurring at least 6 weeks following immunization and result from inadequate immunity to the virus. The course of the breakthrough infections in these patients is often shorter and milder with less than 50 lesions. Lesions may not progress to vesicles and or have the typical appearance, potentially making the diagnosis more challenging.

Diagnosis

Historically, the diagnosis of varicella has been based on typical clinical findings. When diagnosing varicella, the history and physical exam are of paramount importance. Noting the characteristics of the rash, including onset and evolution, are helpful in the diagnostic process. The disease is usually self-limiting. An atypical presentation or rash can make the diagnosis based on clinical symptoms difficult. The use of PCR testing is available for confirmation of the diagnosis. An open vesicular lesion is swabbed in order to collect the specimen to be tested. Other sources such as cerebrospinal fluid, blood, saliva, tissue biopsy, and throat swabs may also be used for PCR testing.

Differential Diagnosis

The differential diagnosis of a varicella infection can include hand, foot, and mouth disease; atopic dermatitis; eczema herpeticum; guttate psoriasis; impetigo; viral exanthem; allergic reactions; shingles; and smallpox. Herpes zoster typically presents unilaterally in a dermatomal pattern. Smallpox has been eradicated from natural transmission, but infection via bioterrorism or laboratory

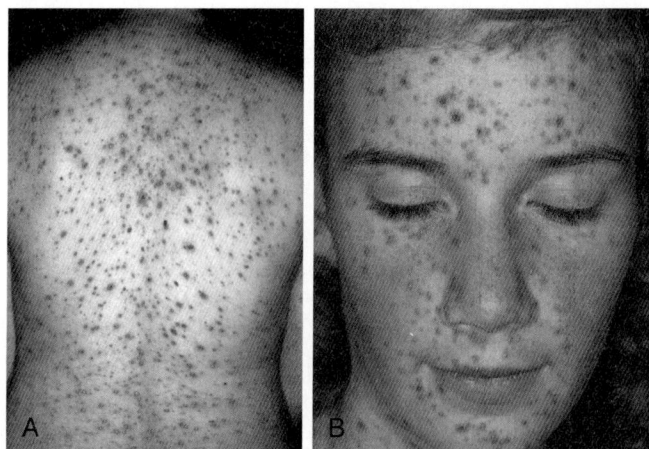

Figure 2 The disease starts with lesions on the trunk (A) and then spreads to the face (B) and extremities.

exposure must be considered if a suspicious rash is present. The rash seen with smallpox is typically more uniform in appearance and follows a more significant prodrome of symptoms.

Treatment

Treatment of varicella infection in healthy children older than 1 year and less than 12 years is symptomatic. Treating fever, malaise, and pharyngitis with ibuprofen or acetaminophen can improve patient comfort. Avoidance of salicylate use is important to reduce the risk of Reye syndrome.

Treatment of adults and children over the age of 12 years involves symptomatic care and antiviral medications such as acyclovir (Zovirax) and valacyclovir (Valtrex). Valacyclovir is more bioavailable and therefore recommended as the first-line treatment. Dosing for valacyclovir is 20 mg/kg up to a maximum of 1000 mg per dose, given three times daily for 5 days. Acyclovir can also be used as treatment, and the recommended dosing for individuals greater than 40 kg is 800 mg five times daily for 5 days. For children over 2 years of age and individuals less than 40 kg, liquid suspension acyclovir (200 mg/5 mL) is dosed 20 mg/kg every 6 hours for 5 days. The maximum dose of acyclovir is 3200 mg daily. If antiviral treatment is deemed necessary it should be started as soon as possible, ideally within 24 hours of rash onset.

For infants less than 12 months of age and immunocompromised individuals, IV antiviral medications are recommended. For adults, dosing of IV acyclovir is 10 to 15 mg/kg every 8 hours for 7 to 10 days. IV acyclovir for infants less than 12 months of age or immunocompromised children is 30 mg/kg/day divided every 8 hours for 7 to 10 days. Ideal body weight should be used to calculate the dosing regimen. With symptomatic improvement, absence of fever for 24 hours, and absence of new lesion development, switching to oral antiviral medication can be considered. For affected individuals with renal impairment, renal dose adjustments are recommended.

Pregnant women with any pulmonary involvement, including upper respiratory symptoms, should be treated with antivirals.

Complications

Approximately 1 in 1000 children with varicella infection will suffer from severe complications. Complications related to varicella infection include pneumonia, secondary bacterial skin or soft tissue infections due to *Staphylococcus aureus* or *Streptococcus pyogens*, encephalitis, cerebellitis, hepatitis, and even death. Severe complications occur more commonly in immunocompromised individuals, children younger than 1 year, those older than 12 years, adults, and newborns born to mothers that were infected with varicella. Neonates are most susceptible to a severe, even life-threatening disease if the mother develops varicella infection within 5 days prior to delivery or 2 days following birth.

Reye syndrome is another complication that has been associated with varicella infection. This illness presents with symptoms of nausea, vomiting, headaches, excitability, confusion, combativeness, and often progresses to a coma. An association with salicylate administration to febrile children was found to increase the risk of Reye syndrome. Children should not be given salicylates, including aspirin, due to this risk.

Congenital varicella can result in abnormalities of the brain, limbs, and eyes, as well as scarring of the skin and low birth weight. Children with mothers infected during the first and second trimesters have a greater risk of developing congenital varicella syndrome than those infected during the third trimester. Infections during the third trimester increase the risk of disseminated varicella. Infants born to mothers who were infected during pregnancy have an increased risk of developing herpes zoster (shingles) during the first few years of life.

Herpes Zoster

Vaccination

Herpes zoster infections are caused by a reactivation of the latent VZV that has been dormant in the sensory nerve ganglia of individuals who were previously infected with varicella. Patients over the age of 50 or those with a decreased amount of cell-mediated immunity appear to be most susceptible to herpes zoster. Herpes zoster infection typically only affects one side of the body and is distributed within a single dermatome. Disseminated zoster, or disseminated shingles, is characterized by a widespread rash that is not localized to a single dermatome.

There are two vaccines available to help prevent herpes zoster (shingles). Shingrix, a recombinant zoster vaccine, is the currently preferred vaccine and is recommended for individuals over the age of 50 years. Shingrix is given as a two-dose series with doses separated by 2 to 6 months apart. The second vaccine, Zostavax (zoster vaccine live), is a single-dose live-attenuated virus that has been available since 2006 and is approved to prevent shingles in patients ≥50 years of age. Currently, Zostavax has a recommendation from the Centers for Disease Control and Prevention (CDC) for administration to immunocompetent patients who are 60 years of age or older. Zostavax is safe for use in healthy individuals over the age of 60 who are allergic to Shingrix, who prefer Zostavax, or who do not have access to the Shingrix vaccine.

The Shingrix vaccine is preferred over Zostavax as it confers greater efficacy of herpes zoster prevention as well as fewer occurrences of postherpetic neuralgia (PHN)[1]. Shingrix provides a longer duration of protection. Patients who have had shingles in the past, have had Zostavax previously, or those who are uncertain if they have previously had varicella should still receive the Shingrix vaccine series if they otherwise meet the administration criteria.

---

[1]Not FDA approved for this indication.

Treatment

Treatment of acute herpes zoster with antiviral medication is recommended to aid in diminishing symptoms of the shingles rash, including severity and duration, as well as prevent new lesion formation and decrease viral shedding. Treatment is also thought to potentially decrease the risk of developing PHN.

Dosing regimens for immunocompetent adults include valacyclovir (Valtrex) 1000 mg three times daily for 7 days; famciclovir (Famvir) 500 mg three times daily for 7 days; or acyclovir (Zovirax) 800 mg five times daily for 7 days.

Children who are 11 years of age or younger or those who are immunocompromised with an acute herpes zoster infection should be treated with IV acyclovir 30 mg/kg/day divided every 8 hours for 7 to 10 days. Immunocompromised patients with disseminated herpes zoster should be treated with IV acyclovir therapy. Dosing is 10 mg/kg every 8 hours for 7 days. Ideal body weight should be used to calculate the dose for obese patients.

Treatment has been shown to be most effective if initiated within the first 72 hours of symptom onset. Initiating treatment past 72 hours in immunocompetent adults is recommended if new lesions are still appearing. There is limited evidence available on the efficacy in initiating treatment past 72 hours in immunocompetent patients if new lesions are no longer appearing. Immunocompromised adults should be treated with antiviral medication as soon as possible even if 72 hours have lapsed since the onset of the illness.

Pregnant women should also receive early initiation of treatment regardless of the number of lesions present. Acyclovir is preferred for use in pregnant women; recommended dosing is 800 mg five times daily for 7 days.

Postherpetic Neuralgia

PHN can occur following herpes zoster infection. Symptoms of PHN include severe pain in the area of previous zoster infection even after the rash has resolved. PHN can last for a few days or up to several years. Tricyclic antidepressants, pregabalin (Lyrica), and gabapentin (Neurontin) have the most research to support their use in the reduction of pain from PHN. Some evidence supports the use of topical capsaicin (Zostrix) and lidocaine patches (Lidoderm) in the treatment of herpes zoster. Acetaminophen and nonsteroidal antiinflammatory agents are commonly used, though studies of their effectiveness is limited.

References

Center for Disease Control and Prevention. Shingles Vaccine. Available at https://www.cdc.gov/vaccines/vpd/shingles/hcp/index.html. [Accessed on January 2, 2020].

Center for Disease Control and Prevention. Varicella. Available at https://www.cdc.gov/chickenpox/hcp/index.html. [Accessed on December 27, 2019].

Dooling KL, Guo A, Patel M, et al: Recommendations of the advisory committee on immunization practices for use of herpes zoster vaccines, *MMWR Morb Mortal Wkly Rep* 67:103–108, 2018.

Leung J, Marin M: Update on trends in varicella mortality during the varicella vaccine era—United States, 1990-2016, *Human Vaccines & Immunotherapeutics* 14(10):2460–2463, 2018.

Marin M, Guris D, Chaves S, et al: Prevention of varicella: recommendations of the Advisory Committee on Immunization Practices (ACIP), *MMWR Recomm Rep* 56:1–40, 2007.

Marin M, Leung J, Gershon AA: Transmission of vaccine-strain varicella-zoster virus: a systematic review, *Pediatrics* 144(3):20191305, 2019.

Marin M, Marti M, Kambhampati A, et al: Global varicella vaccine effectiveness: a meta-analysis, *Pediatrics* 137(3):e20153741, 2016.

Varicella and herpes zoster vaccines: WHO position paper, June 2014. Recommendations, *Vaccine* 2016(34):198–199, 2014.

World Health Organization. Immunization, vaccines and biologicals: varicella (2015). Available from http://www.who.int/immunization/diseases/varicella/en/ [Accessed on December 29, 2019].

Wutzler P, Bonanni P, Burgess M, et al: Varicella vaccination- the global experience, *Expert Review of Vaccines* 16(8):833–843, 2017.

VIRAL MENINGITIS

Method of
RosaMarie Maiorella, MD; and Carlos Anthony Casillas, MD, MPH

CURRENT DIAGNOSIS

- Typical presentation includes fever, headache, and neck stiffness or pain. Constitutional symptoms include mild lethargy, myalgias, nausea, and vomiting.
- Neonates often present with nonspecific signs and symptoms including temperature instability (fever or hypothermia), lethargy, irritability, and poor feeding.
- Cerebrospinal fluid (CSF) profile should be performed. Results show elevated white blood cell count (often but not always with mononuclear cell predominance), normal to slightly elevated protein, normal glucose, normal to slightly elevated opening pressure, and negative bacterial Gram stain and culture.
- Diagnostic polymerase chain reaction (PCR) and serologic studies can identify the etiologic agent.
- Consider neuroimaging before lumbar puncture if there is concern for increased intracranial pressure or if encephalitis is possible.

CURRENT THERAPY

- Symptomatic and supportive management includes analgesia, antipyretics, antiemetics, and intravenous fluids.
- Hospitalization is recommended for infants (younger than 1 year), elderly patients (older than 65 years), and immunocompromised patients, as well as for patients presenting with altered mental status, seizures, focal neurologic signs, or the absence of classic viral CSF findings.
- Few medications, with the exception of acyclovir (Zovirax) for HSV, effectively treat viral meningitis.

Epidemiology

The true epidemiology of viral meningitis is unknown because it is not a reportable disease. However, the Centers for Disease Control and Prevention (CDC) estimate 25,000 to 50,000 hospitalizations per year. There is also yearly variation in disease burden. Causes of viral meningitis vary by age group, immune status, season, and geography. There is increased incidence in summer and early fall owing to the high prevalence of enteroviruses and arthropod-borne viruses (arboviruses). Among children, incidence of hospitalization due to viral meningitis peaks immediately after birth and again at age 5. Common etiologic agents include enteroviruses, herpes simplex virus (HSV), arboviruses, lymphocytic choriomeningitis virus (LCMV), cytomegalovirus (CMV), varicella zoster virus (VZV), and Epstein–Barr virus (EBV). See Table 1 for features of the common and some less-common viral agents that cause meningitis.

Pathophysiology

Viral infection begins at the mucosal surface of the respiratory tract or gastrointestinal tract, with viral replication occurring in regional lymph nodes. A secondary viremia then occurs that provides access to the central nervous system (CNS). Symptoms of viral meningitis are due to either an immune response to the virus within the CNS (e.g., enterovirus) or direct viral invasion of neural tissue (e.g., HSV1/2).

Prevention

To prevent spread of viral agents responsible for meningitis, hand-washing and other infection-control measures are most important. The infection-control precautions necessary during patient contact depend on mode of transmission of the virus (see Table 1). Vaccines are available for some of the viruses that are known to cause meningitis, including polio (an enterovirus), mumps, measles, varicella, and influenza.

Clinical Manifestations

Viral meningitis can be difficult to distinguish from bacterial meningitis. Fever, headache, and neck stiffness and pain are the usual presenting complaints. Headache can be localized to the frontal or retro-orbital areas and may be associated with photophobia. Although neck stiffness and pain are usually present, neck rigidity (positive Kerning's sign or positive Brudzinski's sign) is not always present on examination. Constitutional symptoms can include lethargy, myalgias, and nausea or vomiting. There is often a history of concomitant viral respiratory or gastrointestinal illness at the time of presentation. Seizures can occur with viral causes of meningitis, especially HSV, but should prompt consideration of other diagnostic possibilities.

In contrast to children and adults, neonates often present with nonspecific findings such as temperature instability, lethargy, irritability, and poor feeding. See Table 1 for clinical manifestations associated with specific etiologic agents.

Viral meningitis can also manifest with signs of encephalitis, in which case the encompassing diagnosis is meningoencephalitis. Encephalitis or meningoencephalitis are likely if any of the following are present: altered mental status, seizures, focal neurologic deficits (including aphasia, anosmia, ataxia, cranial nerve deficits, motor weakness, or involuntary movements), or behavioral changes.

Diagnosis

Diagnosis of viral meningitis requires lumbar puncture for CSF studies including cell count, protein, glucose, Gram stain and culture, and specific viral studies. Although a lymphocytic pleocytosis is associated with viral infections, most viral CNS infections initially have a neutrophilic pleocytosis. However, neutrophilic pleocytosis is also associated with bacterial meningitis. In viral meningitis, though CSF protein is normal to slightly elevated, CSF glucose is normal, and no organisms are identified on CSF bacterial Gram stain or culture compared with elevated CSF protein, low CSF glucose, and positive CSF bacterial culture in bacterial meningitis.

Studies to identify a specific virus as the etiologic agent are recommended for patients with severe illness or a complicated course. Viral cultures of CSF are not generally useful given their poor sensitivity, and serologic viral studies require both acute and convalescent titers to demonstrate antibody response to the suspected viral antigen. CSF PCR studies that detect viral DNA or RNA are more sensitive than viral culture and provide more rapid results than serologic viral studies (see Table 1). Multiplex PCR techniques allow for testing of multiple viruses and bacteria with a single CSF sample and a single test. Where available, multiplex PCR may result in considerable savings in time and effort, while improving diagnostic capacity. In some cases, it is useful to perform viral PCR studies on blood (HSV, EBV, CMV, and human herpesvirus [HHV]6), urine (CMV), stool (enterovirus), and skin vesicles (HSV) to further support the diagnosis. However, a positive PCR study from blood, urine, stool, or skin does not provide direct evidence of CNS infection by the same virus. For example, enterovirus isolated from the stool can represent asymptomatic infection or prior infection but may also be isolated from the stool at the same time as concomitant enteroviral meningitis. Methods of diagnosis continue to be investigated, with Metagenomic Next Generation Sequency demonstrating promise as a method that can enhance pathogen identification in conjunction with CSF PCR testing.

Most other testing is not helpful, but further testing (including complete blood count, renal profile, liver function, pancreatic enzymes, and HIV studies) should be guided by the patient's presentation and clinical status.

Neuroimaging (computed tomography [CT] or magnetic resonance imaging [MRI]) should be obtained before lumbar puncture if there is concern for increased intracranial pressure. It is also recommended if symptoms of encephalitis are present (including altered consciousness, seizures, focal neurologic deficits, behavioral changes) to exclude other CNS disease.

TABLE 1 Clinical and Laboratory Characteristics of Viral Meningitis

VIRUS	TRANSMISSION	KEY CLINICAL FEATURES	DIAGNOSIS	COMMENTS
Enterovirus	Fecal-oral	May have rash on exam (e.g., Coxsackie, hand–foot–mouth) Patients with impaired humoral immunity or those <2 wk old can present with a sepsis-like syndrome with multiorgan dysfunction, DIC, cardiovascular collapse	CSF enterovirus PCR	More prevalent in summer and fall
Parechovirus	Fecal-oral and respiratory	Can cause sepsis-like illness in neonates <3 mo CSF will often have few to no WBCs	CSF parechovirus PCR	More prevalent in the summer and fall
Herpes simplex viruses 1 and 2	Vertical transmission during birth (HSV2), horizontal transmission via contact (HSV1 or HSV2)	10%–30% of adults have symptoms of meningitis with primary HSV2 infection; look for genital vesicular lesions on exam Mollarets meningitis: >3 episodes of fever and meningismus lasting 2–5 d, with spontaneous resolution; episodes may be months to years apart often due to chronic HSV2 CNS infection	CSF HSV1/HSV2 PCR	Meningitis is uncommon with nonprimary HSV2 infection
Arboviruses	Subcutaneous inoculation via mosquito or tick and rarely through ingestion of unpasteurized milk from infected livestock Prevention: Minimize tick and mosquito exposure with personal protection measures including insect repellents and covering exposed skin	Zika virus associated with Guillan-Barré syndrome and in newborn infants microcephaly; sexual transmission is possible	CSF arboviral PCR Zika RT-PCR (performed at CDC Arbovirus laboratory on CSF or serum within first 5–7 days of symptoms); Zika IgM cross reacts with other flaviviruses (e.g., Dengue)	More prevalent in summer and fall Geographic distribution within the U.S.: Eastern equine encephalitis: Eastern U.S. Western equine encephalitis: Western U.S. St. Louis encephalitis: Across the U.S. (majority of cases in Central and Eastern U.S.) West Nile virus: Across the U.S. California encephalitis (LaCrosse): Midwestern, mid-Atlantic, and Southeastern U.S. Zika virus: Small epidemics occurred in Southeastern U.S. and Gulf Coast states. Currently, there is no local transmission of zika virus in the continental U.S.
Lymphocytic choriomeningitis virus	Virus is present in rodent secretions, feces, and urine Ingestion of contaminated food, exposure of open wounds, or inhalation of aerosolized virus Lab workers, pet owners, and those living in impoverished conditions are highest risk for illness	Accompanied by a flulike illness	Serum LCMV titers (acute and convalescent) CSF findings: May have decreased glucose and WBC count >1000/mL	More prevalent in winter and spring
Cytomegalovirus	Exposure to infected body fluids (e.g., saliva, blood)		CSF CMV PCR	Reactivation of prior infection typically only occurs in the immunosuppressed

Continued

VIII Infectious Diseases

TABLE 1	Clinical and Laboratory Characteristics of Viral Meningitis—cont'd

VIRUS	TRANSMISSION	KEY CLINICAL FEATURES	DIAGNOSIS	COMMENTS
Epstein–Barr virus	Exposure to infected body fluids (e.g., saliva, blood)	Alice in Wonderland syndrome: altered body image and distortion of visual perception	CSF EBV PCR	Most common neurologic complication with primary infection
HIV	Exposure to contaminated blood or other body fluids (e.g., transfusion, sexual contact, percutaneous blood exposure)	During primary infection, a subset have meningitis or meningoencephalitis May expect thrush and cervical lymphadenopathy	HIV studies	Treatment with HAART
Human herpesvirus 6	Respiratory	Roseola: febrile illness followed by viral exanthem	CSF HHV6 PCR	HHV6 has been demonstrated in the CSF of asymptomatic persons Immunosuppressed persons at risk for symptomatic infection and reactivation
Varicella	Respiratory	Typical vesicular skin lesions of chickenpox on exam CSF pleocytosis has also been demonstrated with reactivation; can also occur in the absence of cutaneous findings of herpes zoster ("zoster sine herpete")	CSF VZV PCR	Rarely diagnosed during acute chickenpox infection; usually a postinfectious complication Other neurologic sequelae of varicella infection are more common than aseptic meningitis; most common is cerebellar ataxia
Mumps	Respiratory	Parotitis on exam is the most prominent sign of infection Aseptic meningitis can precede or follow clinical exam findings CSF profile can demonstrate an unusually high protein with a mild pleocytosis and normal glucose	Serum titers	More common in winter and spring
Measles	Respiratory	CSF pleocytosis in ≤30% of patients with measles; patients are usually without clinical meningitis	Serum titers	In the U.S., most cases are imported (e.g., occur in returning travelers), but in recent years there have been outbreaks of measles in the U.S. associated with pockets of unvaccinated people
Influenza	Respiratory	Aseptic meningitis is a less common neurologic complication of influenza infection (encephalopathy is more common)	CSF influenza PCR	More prevalent in winter Increased risk of neurologic complication in young patients and in those with pre-existing medical disease
COVID-19	Respiratory	CSF profile can demonstrate pleoyctosis and elevated protein	CSF SARS-CoV-2 RT PCR	Rare complication of COVID-19 infection

Abbreviations: CMV = cytomegalovirus; CNS = central nervous system; CSF = cerebrospinal fluid; DIC = disseminated intravascular coagulopathy; HHV = human herpesvirus; HSV = herpes simplex virus; LCMV = lymphocytic choriomeningitis virus; PCR = polymerase chain reaction; VZV = varicella zoster virus; WBC = white blood cell.

Differential Diagnosis

The major item on the differential diagnosis for viral meningitis is bacterial meningitis. The bacterial meningitis score, validated in children 29 days to 19 years, is a clinical prediction rule that identifies patients as at very low risk (0.1%) for bacterial meningitis if they lack all of the following: positive CSF Gram stain, CSF absolute neutrophil count (ANC) of at least 1000 cells/μL, CSF protein of at least 80 mg/dL, peripheral blood ANC of at least 10,000 cells/μL, and a history of seizure before or at the time of presentation. While C-reactive protein (CRP) is not generally useful because it can be high in viral meningitis and low in the initial stages of bacterial disease, elevated serum procalcitonin levels (>0.5 μg/mL in children and >0.2 μg/mL in adults) are more sensitive and specific for distinguishing viral from bacterial meningitis.

Other diagnoses to consider include parameningeal infections (i.e., subdural or epidural empyema, brain abscess), meningitis due to fungi, mycobacteria, rickettsia, mycoplasma, parasites, and other CNS infectious or inflammatory processes including malignancy, drug exposure, rheumatologic disease (e.g., systemic lupus erythematosus), or autoimmune (e.g., anti-NMDA receptor encephalitis).

Treatment

Symptomatic care remains the mainstay of therapy for viral meningitis. Therapy should be directed at pain and fever control (e.g., ibuprofen [Motrin], acetaminophen [Tylenol], ketorolac [Toradol]), management of nausea and vomiting (e.g., ondansetron [Zofran]), and intravenous fluids. Hospitalization is recommended for patients younger than 1 year, the elderly, and the immunocompromised. Patients who present with altered mental status, seizures, focal neurologic signs, or a CSF profile that does not have the classic viral profile should also be hospitalized for clinical management and for antibiotic treatment until bacterial meningitis can be excluded. Advanced care including management of respiratory failure, cardiovascular instability, seizures, disturbed fluid and electrolyte balance, and cerebral edema may be necessary.

Empiric antibiotic coverage may be considered while awaiting CSF culture results in the young, elderly, and immunocompromised, especially if there is suspicion of bacterial meningitis or partially treated bacterial meningitis.

Acyclovir (Zovirax) should be initiated in cases of suspected HSV while waiting PCR confirmation. Dosing of acyclovir is age and weight dependent: 20 mg/kg per dose IV every 8 hours for patients younger than 12 years; 10 mg/kg per dose IV every 8 hours for patients older than 12 years.

In the immunocompromised patient, HHV6 may be treated with foscarnet (Foscavir)[1] or ganciclovir (Cytovene)[1], and CMV may be treated with ganciclovir, valganciclovir (Valcyte), foscarnet, or cidofovir (Vistide). Case reports suggest benefit of such antiviral therapies in the immunocompromised, but no controlled trials have been performed.

Complications

The prognosis of viral meningitis depends on cause and severity of illness as well as age. Non-HSV viral meningitis has low mortality rates in adults and children alike. Mortality and morbidity are associated with other organ system involvement, including meningoencephalitis. Although up to 10% of infants hospitalized with non-HSV viral meningitis experience seizures, altered mental status, or increased intracranial pressure during the acute illness, studies have shown no evidence of long-term neurodevelopmental delay. Most adults recover fully within a week without long-term sequelae. Persistent neurologic sequelae (including headaches, incoordination, concentration difficulties, muscle weakness, and focal neurologic deficits) occur more often in patients with meningoencephalitis.

HSV is associated with high rates of morbidity and mortality. Neonatal isolated CNS HSV has a 4% mortality rate even with acyclovir treatment; mortality is 50% without acyclovir treatment. Unfortunately, acute treatment does not affect morbidity, as 70% of infants with neonatal CNS HSV infection will suffer from neurodevelopmental impairments. Improved outcomes have been shown with long-term oral acyclovir suppression therapy. Outside of the neonatal period, CNS HSV infection has a 28% mortality rate with antiviral treatment (70% mortality rate without treatment). Long-term neurologic sequelae occur in two-thirds of survivors who received antiviral therapy, compared with virtually all of those who did not receive treatment.

References

Centers for Disease Control and Prevention: Zika Virus. http://www.cdc.gov/zika/index.html. Accessed March 1, 2024.

Centers for Disease Control and Prevention. Recent reports of human *Parechovirus* (PeV) in the United States—2022. Available at: https://emergency.cdc.gov/han/2022/han00469.asp. Accessed 15 March, 2023.

Dubos F, Korczowski B, Aygun DA, et al: Serum procalcitonin level and other biological markers to distinguish between bacterial and aseptic meningitis in children: a European multicenter case cohort study, *Arch Pediatr Adolesc Med* 162:1157–1163, 2008.

Elbaz M, Gadoth A, Shepshelovich D, et al.: Systematic review and meta-analysis of foodborne tick-borne encephalitis, Europe, 1980-2021, *Emerg Infect Dis* 28(10):1945–1954, 2022.

Nigrovic LE, Fine AM, Monuteaux MC, et al: Trends in the management of viral meningitis at United States children's hospitals, *Pediatrics* 131:670–676, 2013, [PMID: 23530164].

Nigrovic LE, Kuppermann N, Macias CG, et al: Clinical prediction rule for identifying children with cerebrospinal fluid pleocytosis at very low risk of bacterial meningitis, *JAMA* 297:52–60, 2007.

Tao L, Humphries RM, Banerjee R, Gaston DC: Re-emergence of Parechovirus: 2017-2022 national trends of detection in cerebrospinal fluid, *Open Forum Infect Dis* 10(3):ofad112, 2023.

Xu H, Chen P, Guo S, et al: Progress in etiological diagnosis of viral meningitis, *Front Neurol* 14:1193834, 2023.

WHOOPING COUGH (PERTUSSIS)

Method of
Raul Davaro, MD

CURRENT DIAGNOSIS

- Pertussis, also known as whooping cough, is an acute respiratory tract infection that has increased in incidence in recent years.
- The diagnosis depends on clinical signs and laboratory testing. Both culture and polymerase chain reaction testing can be used to confirm the diagnosis; serologic testing is not standardized or routinely recommended.

CURRENT THERAPY

- Macrolide antibiotics such as azithromycin are first-line treatments to prevent transmission; trimethoprim/sulfamethoxazole is an alternative in cases of allergy or intolerance to macrolides.
- Current immunization recommendations in the United States consist of administering five doses of the diphtheria and tetanus toxoids and acellular pertussis (DTaP) vaccine to children before 7 years of age and administering a tetanus toxoid, reduced diphtheria toxoid, and acellular pertussis (Tdap) booster between 11 and 18 years of age.

Pertussis is a respiratory infection caused by *Bordetella pertussis*, a gram-negative, pleomorphic aerobic coccobacillus. Infection due to *B. pertussis* affects persons of all ages, with a clinical presentation ranging from a relatively mild-cough illness to a severe illness with pneumonia, seizures, encephalopathy, respiratory failure, and/or death.

Prior to the introduction of whole-cell pertussis vaccines in the United States during the 1940s, the annual number of reported cases often exceeded 200,000. The introduction of childhood pertussis vaccines dramatically altered the epidemiologic landscape of pertussis, with reported cases declining to a nadir of just over 1000 (0.47/100000 population) by the mid-1970s. However, despite substantial declines in disease since the prevaccine era, pertussis remains a significant health problem worldwide, with incidence increasing in several countries in recent years.

Epidemiology

Pertussis is highly contagious and is transmitted via aerosolized droplets through close contact during coughing or sneezing. Studies have identified household members as the source in 75% of cases in infants, mothers being the likely source in almost one-half of these cases. Pertussis shows no seasonality transmission.

During 2000–2016, 339,420 pertussis cases were reported. The majority were in white (88.2%) and non-Hispanic (81.3%) persons, 9.9% were hospitalized, and 0.1% were fatal; however, differences existed by age. Infants had the highest incidence (75.3/100,000 population), accounting for 88.8% of death.

---

[1]Not FDA approved for this indication.

The resurgence of pertussis, probably due to several reasons, including vaccine-driven selection, increased disease awareness and testing, improved diagnostics, and waning immunity.

Transmission

Pertussis is highly contagious and can spread rapidly from person-to-person through contact with airborne droplets. The human nasopharynx can be densely colonized with both commensal bacteria and pathogens, including *B. pertussis*. Infected individuals aerosolize pertussis-containing droplets by coughing or sneezing. Persons with pertussis are most infectious during the mucous producing stage and the first 2 weeks after cough onset.

Pertussis is considered far more contagious than polio, smallpox, rubella, mumps, and diphtheria. Studies showed that one infected person can transmit *B. pertussis* to as many as 12 to 17 other susceptible individuals, while polio and smallpox can be transmitted to 5 to 7, rubella 6 to 7, mumps 4 to 7, and diphtheria 6 to 7 susceptible individuals.

Microbiology and Pathophysiology

Bordetella are small gram-negative, aerobic, nonsporulating coccoid rods. *B. pertussis* infection and disease occur after four important steps: (1) attachment, (2) evasion of host defenses, (3) local damage, and (4) systemic manifestations.

Filamentous hemagglutinin (FHA) and fimbriae (FIM) are two major adhesins and virulence determinants for *B. pertussis*. They are required for tracheal colonization, are highly immunogenic, and are components of certain acellular pertussis vaccines. However, there is likely redundancy in the adhesion role of B. *pertussis* proteins, and it has been suggested that virulence factors such as pertactin (PRN) may mediate attachment in the absence of FHA. Pertussis toxin (PT) also acts as an adhesion and has specific recognition domains for human cilia. Evasion of host defenses occurs primarily through adenylate cyclase toxin (ACT) and PT. PT targets the innate immune system of the lung by inactivating or suppressing G protein–coupled signaling pathways. Through this mechanism of action, PT delays the recruitment of neutrophils to the respiratory tract and targets airway macrophages to promote *B. pertussis* infection.

Immunity

Immunity to pertussis, acquired either from natural infection or through vaccination, is not lifelong. It has been estimated that natural pertussis infection yields 3.5 to 30 years of protection, the estimated protection obtained from the whole-cell pertussis vaccine is 5 to 14 years, and that from the acellular vaccine is 4 to 7 years.

Clinical Symptoms

Pertussis symptoms begin 7 to 10 days after exposure. The disease is characterized by three stages: catarrhal stage, consisting of symptoms indistinguishable from a minor upper respiratory tract infection; paroxysmal stage, named for its characteristic cough consisting of intermittent, sudden bursts of cough, followed by whoop on inspiration and posttussive emesis (the paroxysms of cough are rapid and numerous, occurring up to 15 times in a 24-hour period); and convalescent stage, when paroxysms wane in number and severity. Patients are most contagious during the catarrhal stage. The paroxysmal stage usually lasts 1 to 6 weeks but can be as long as 10 weeks. Almost 80% of adults with confirmed pertussis have an illness involving a cough of at least 3 weeks' duration, and 27% still had a cough after 90 days.

Although symptoms can be prolonged, there is no evidence for chronic infection or long-term carriage of *B. pertussis*. Paroxysms can recur with subsequent respiratory illnesses months after initial illness and are not associated with recurrent isolation of *B. pertussis*. Adolescents and adults frequently have diseases that may not be recognized as pertussis. Whoop is uncommon, but paroxysms of cough and posttussive emesis are common manifestations. A study of adolescents and adults with prolonged cough illness found that 13% to 20% had infections with *B. pertussis*. Pertussis leads to the hospitalization in older children and adolescents in only about 1% to 7% of those affected. Among adults, people older than 65 years are at the highest risk of pertussis hospitalization. Complications also are uncommon in adults, occurring in about 5%, but can include syncope, rib fractures, pneumonia, and otitis media.

Among immunized patients, especially adolescents and adults, a prolonged cough may be the only manifestation of pertussis. A number of studies have documented that between 13% and 32% of adolescents and adults with an illness involving a cough of 6 days' duration or longer have serologic evidence of infection with *B. pertussis*.

Diagnosis

A positive culture of nasopharyngeal secretions (preferably an aspirate) on selective Regan–Lowe medium is the gold standard for the diagnosis of pertussis. PCR is a rapid test and has excellent sensitivity. However, PCR tests vary in specificity. It is recommended to obtain culture confirmation of pertussis for at least one suspicious case when there is suspicion of a pertussis outbreak. PCR may provide accurate results for up to 4 weeks. After the fourth week of cough, the amount of bacterial DNA in the nasopharynx rapidly diminishes, which increases the risk of obtaining false-negative results. PCR assay protocols that include multiple target sequences allow for speciation among *Bordetella* species.

Treatment

Antimicrobial therapy administered during the catarrhal stage may ameliorate the disease. Antimicrobial therapy is indicated before test confirmation if the clinical presentation is suggestive of pertussis or the patient is at high risk of severe or complicated disease (e.g., is an infant). The duration of treatment for pertussis and postexposure prophylaxis (PEP) is 5 days. After the paroxysmal cough is established, antimicrobial agents have no effect on the course of illness but are recommended to limit the spread of organisms to others. The resistance of *B. pertussis* to macrolide antimicrobial agents has been reported, but rarely. Penicillins and first- and second-generation cephalosporins are not effective against *B. pertussis*.

Trimethoprim-sulfamethoxazole (Bactrim)[1] is an alternative for patients older than 2 months who cannot tolerate macrolides or who are infected with a macrolide-resistant strain, but studies evaluating trimethoprim-sulfamethoxazole as treatment for pertussis are limited (Table 1).

Hospitalized young infants with pertussis should be managed in a setting/facility where these complications can be recognized and managed urgently. Exchange transfusions or leukapheresis have been reported to be life-saving in infants with progressive pulmonary hypertension and markedly elevated lymphocyte counts.

Prevention

In the United States, all vaccines available for preventing pertussis are acellular pertussis formulations combined with tetanus and diphtheria toxoids. Five doses of pertussis-containing vaccine (DTaP [Daptacel, Infanrix]) are recommended prior to entering school: four doses of DTaP before 2 years of age and one dose of DTaP before school entry. Adolescent and adult formulations, known as Tdap vaccines (Adacel, Boostrix), contain reduced quantities of diphtheria toxoid and some pertussis antigens compared with DTaP. A single dose is recommended universally for people 11 years and older, including adults of any age, in place of a decennial tetanus and diphtheria vaccine (Td). Booster doses of Tdap are not recommended for any group of people except pregnant women. The Centers for Disease Control and Prevention (CDC) recommends the use of PEP with antimicrobials in persons at high risk of developing severe pertussis and those who will have close contact with those at high risk of developing severe pertussis.

---

[1]Not FDA approved for this indication.

TABLE 1 Pertussis Treatment

ANTIBIOTIC	DOSING	COMMENTS
Azithromycin (Zithromax)	Children: 10 mg/kg/day for 3 days, or 10 mg/kg on day 1, then 5 mg/kg/day on days 2 through 5 Adults: 500 mg/day for 3 days, or 500 mg on day 1, then 250 mg/day on days 2 through 5	Preferred therapy due to ease of use and tolerability. Preferred agent for infants younger than 1 month Prolongation of the QT interval
Clarithromycin (Biaxin)	Children: 7.5 mg/kg twice daily for 7 days Adults: 500 mg twice daily for 7 days	Fewer adverse effects than erythromycin, but typically more than azithromycin Prolongation of the QT interval CYP3A4 inhibitor; use with caution with other CYP3A4 medications
Erythromycin, delayed release (Ery-Tab)	Children: 40 to 60 mg/kg/day in three or four divided doses for 7 to 14 days Adults: 666 mg three times per day for 7 to 14 days	Gastrointestinal adverse effects limit use Risk of hypertrophic pyloric stenosis in infants CYP3A4 inhibitor; use with caution with other CYP3A4 medications
Trimethoprim/ sulfamethoxazole	Children: 8/40 mg/kg/day divided into two doses for 14 days Adults: one double-strength tablet (160/800 mg) twice daily for 14 days	May be effective for those with intolerance to macrolide antibiotics Caution in pregnancy; contraindicated in infants younger than 2 months, or in mothers breastfeeding infants younger than 2 months

CYP, Cytochrome P450.
From Kline JM, Lewis WD, Smith EA, Tracy LR: Pertussis: A reemerging infection, *Am Fam Physician* 88:507–514, 2013.

References

American Academy of Pediatrics. Pertussis. In: Kimberly DW, Brady MT, Jackson MA, Long SS, eds. *Red Book: 2018 Report of the Committee on Infectious Diseases.* 31st ed. Itasca, IL: AAP.

Ebell MH, Marchello C, Callahan M: Clinical diagnosis of bordetella pertussis infection: A systematic review, *J Am Board Fam Med* 2017; 30:308–319.

Hewlett EL, Edwards KM: Pertussis—not just for kids, *N Engl J Med* 2005; 32:1215–1222.

Kilgore PE, Salim AM, Zervos MJ, Schmitt HJ: Pertussis: microbiology, disease, treatment and prevention, *Clin Microbiol Rev* 2016; 29:449–486.

Kline JM, Lewis WD, Smith EA, Tracy LR: Pertussis: A reemerging infection, *Am Fam Physician* 2013; 88:507–514.

Liang JL, Tiwari T, Moro P, et al: Prevention of pertussis, tetanus, and diphtheria with vaccines in the united states: recommendations of the Advisory Committee on Immunization Practices (ACIP), *MMWR Recomm Rep* 2018; 67(No. RR-2):1–44.

Skoff TH, Hadler S, Hariri S: The epidemiology of nationally reported pertussis in the United States, 2000-2016, *Clin InfecDis* 2019; 68:1634–1640.

YELLOW FEVER

Method of
Lucius M. Lampton, MD

CURRENT DIAGNOSIS

- Yellow fever is a historically important mosquito-borne Flavivirus with high morbidity and mortality.
- Travel to yellow fever–endemic areas in Sub-Saharan Africa and tropical Central and South America is the essential risk factor.
- Symptoms may include abrupt onset of fever, relative bradycardia, headache, and, if severe, jaundice, hemorrhage, and multiorgan failure.
- Diagnosis is with viral culture and serologic tests.
- Although infectious disease experts consider it improbable that yellow fever outbreaks will return to the continental United States, this reemerging disease is threatening to become more prevalent and deadly in tropical South America and Africa. Travel-related cases should be anticipated in the United States and its territories, as well as the possibility of brief episodes of local dissemination in areas bordering the Gulf of Mexico, where the vector, the *Aedes aegypti* mosquito, can be found.

CURRENT THERAPY

- Prevention is key and accomplished by vaccination and mosquito avoidance and control.
- Supportive care is the only treatment.

Epidemiology

Yellow fever is one of the great epidemic diseases of tropical Africa and the Americas. It receives its appellation "yellow" from the symptom of jaundice, which appears in severe disease, and it is caused by an RNA virus, specifically a Flavivirus (a family name derived from yellow fever, with *flavus* Latin for yellow), that is held in natural reservoirs by forest monkeys and spread to people via mosquitoes. The disease, termed an acute hemorrhagic fever, infects humans, all species of monkeys, and certain other small mammals and is transmitted among its hosts by several species of mosquitoes.

There are three types of yellow fever infection: urban, jungle, and intermediate. In urban or classical yellow fever, human-to-human spread occurs by the bite of the *A. aegypti* mosquito, which breeds in urban unpolluted water and bites principally in the daytime. Reinvasion of this mosquito in Central and South America has occurred beginning in the 1970s owing to increases in breeding sites resulting from urbanization and the collapse of vector control efforts. In jungle or sylvatic yellow fever, which was first recognized in 1933, the disease is perpetuated by enzootic infection of mammalians, usually monkeys, disseminated by several different mosquitoes: in South America via the *Haemagogus* and *Sabethes* spp.; in East Africa via *Ae. africanus*; and in West Africa via a variety of species of *Aedes*. Human infection arises by jungle exposure to these mosquitoes. In intermediate or savannah yellow fever, which commonly occurs in Africa, the virus disseminates from mosquitoes to humans residing or working in areas bordering jungles. This cycle also involves spread of the virus from monkey to human or from human to human via the bite of a mosquito.

Yellow fever, also termed Yellow Jack, the Saffron Scourge, fièvre jaune, Bronze John, and Black Vomit (the Spanish name is *vómito negro*), is the deadliest arthropod virus ever to emerge in the Americas. Both the molecular taxonomic research of viral strains and the annals of history reveal an African origin. Most authorities assert it was introduced to the new world by *A. aegypti*–infested slave ships voyaging from West Africa, with its first recognition in the Americas occurring in Yucatan, Mexico, in 1648 (although research suggests the disease was present in the Americas as early as 1498). Over the next two and a half centuries, yellow fever erupted with regularity in American and European port cities, with hundreds of thousands of deaths, earning the virus deserved recognition as one of the worst plagues the world had ever seen. Two of the most significant North American epidemics occurred in Philadelphia in 1793 and in the Mississippi Valley in 1878. American epidemics were the result of the introduction of the mosquito vector and infected humans along routes of trade, especially sea and river ports and rail lines, with particular virulence associated with the Gulf region where A. aegypti resided. Early attempts at control focused on quarantine and sanitary measures. The devastation associated with American epidemics was an important impetus in the nation's early public health and sanitation movements for the creation of city, state, and national boards of health.

Although two 19th-century physicians, Josiah Nott and Carlos Juan Finlay, suggested the mosquito was the infectious agent for yellow fever, it was not until 1900 that the work of the US Army Commission in Cuba under Major Walter Reed established that the vector of the urban form of this disease was the A. aegypti mosquito, with its viral cause not established until after 1928. Max Theiler developed an attenuated vaccine strain in 1937, which was recognized with a Nobel Prize. In what is acknowledged as one of the most successful campaigns in history against infectious disease, mosquito eradication efforts and this vaccine effectively controlled and eliminated urban yellow fever in the Americas and the West Indies, with the last large outbreak occurring in the continental United States in New Orleans in 1905. However, the disease persisted in its jungle form in forest areas in Africa and South America. Vaccine administration remains incomplete in endemic areas, and outbreaks periodically recur. As well, mosquito eradication efforts in both the Americas and Africa have recently slackened, with the resulting resurgence of A. aegypti into nearly all of the tropical American countries, placing this region at extraordinary risk for urban outbreaks. While only travel-related cases have been documented in Asia, theoretic anthroponotic dissemination could also take place there in the many areas where the urban vector resides.

Official statistics suggest the incidence of yellow fever fluctuates, with 90% of the 200,000 annual cases reported in Africa. However, authorities warn that these statistics considerably underestimate (owing to underreporting) the true magnitude of epidemics, which field studies estimate as 50 times greater. A frightening prospect associated with failing mosquito control in urban habitats is the potential reemergence of yellow fever similar to the recent rapid resurgence of dengue, which is also transmitted by the vector A. aegypti. Experts contend that one of the most profound mysteries of tropical medicine is that this dangerous virus has not emerged more frequently where a susceptible, unimmunized human population and the vector density coexist. However, since the 1980s, a resurgence of yellow fever has been seen across South America and Africa, which augurs potential risk for the United States. While yellow fever outbreaks remain unlikely in the Unites States, travel-related cases should be expected, as well as the possibility of brief urban cycle transmission in the American Southeast.

The 2015–2025 outbreaks in South America and Africa portend ominously that yellow fever appears to be moving from its typical rural setting toward urban areas. A large urban outbreak in Angola, which began in December 2015 and subsequently spread to the Democratic Republic of the Congo, resulted in 962 confirmed cases and 393 deaths and included multiple travel-related cases appearing in nonendemic areas internationally such as China. The outbreak in Brazil was first recognized in December 2016, with more than 2251 confirmed cases and 772 deaths noted as of June 1, 2019, including two dozen travel-related cases. This upsurge of human cases, which is the highest observed in the Americas for decades, reflects the spread into densely populated metropolitan areas, such as Rio de Janeiro and Sao Paulo, which in the past were not considered at risk for transmission.

In the current outbreak, all human cases have been linked only to Haemagogus and Sabethes mosquitoes. In late May 2025, the Pan American Health Organization (PAHO) reported a more than eight-fold increase in human yellow fever cases across South America compared with the previous year; there were more than 221 confirmed cases, including 89 deaths, compared with 61 confirmed cases and 30 deaths in the same period in 2024. These cases were located in Bolivia, Brazil, Colombia, Ecuador, and Peru. Almost all of these cases occurred in unvaccinated individuals. As of 2025, according to World Health Organization (WHO) data, 13 countries in South and Central America and 34 countries in Africa are endemic for, or have large areas that are endemic for, yellow fever.

In response to yellow fever's reemergence in Africa, the WHO launched the Yellow Fever Initiative in 2006, vaccinating in mass campaigns more than 105 million people in West Africa and attempting to secure a global vaccine supply. This campaign, which has primarily utilized fractional dosing, appears to be currently successful in holding the virus to lower numbers of cases. In 2017, the Eliminate Yellow Fever Epidemics (EYE) strategy was initiated with more than 50 partners supporting 40 at-risk countries in the Americas and Africa to prevent, detect, and contain global outbreaks. By 2026, it is projected that 1.38 billion people will be vaccinated against the disease. In March 2018, Brazil's health minister announced that all of the country's 78 million people will be targeted in a large-scale vaccination campaign.

Yellow fever remains the most dangerous arbovirus ever to inhabit the Western Hemisphere. Despite ongoing vaccination and mosquito control efforts in endemic areas, sylvatic and intermediate transmission cycles persist and appear to be expanding toward urban spread. Public health leaders encourage clinicians to utilize heightened suspicion and awareness for the virus, especially among travelers to tropical areas. Recent yellow fever outbreaks underscore boldly the potential threat this disease poses for the international community.

Risk Factors

Travel to yellow fever–endemic areas in Sub-Saharan Africa and tropical Central and South America, between the 15th parallel north and the 15th parallel south, is the essential risk factor.

Pathophysiology

Yellow fever virus has three types or cycles of transmission: urban, jungle (sylvatic), and intermediate (savannah). In urban yellow fever, the virus is spread by the bite of an A. aegypti mosquito infected about 2 weeks previously by feeding on a person with viremia. In jungle (sylvatic) yellow fever, the virus is transmitted by various forest canopy mosquitoes that acquire it from wild primates and then disseminate it to humans who are visiting or working in the jungle. Incidence of the disease is highest during months of peak temperature, rainfall, and humidity in South America and during the late rainy and early dry seasons in Africa. In the intermediate (savannah) cycle, which is most common in Africa, transmission of the virus to humans results from humans living or working in jungle border areas, with the virus spread from monkey to human or from human to human by mosquitoes. Humans infected with the virus are infectious to mosquitoes (what is termed being "viremic") shortly before the onset of illness and up to 5 days after onset. Yellow fever is not transmissible by contact, only via a vector's bite.

Prevention

Yellow fever is a mosquito-borne infection that can be prevented by mosquito avoidance and vaccination. Recovery from yellow fever imparts lifelong immunity against the virus.

Mosquito control is an essential component of any strategy to prevent the spread of yellow fever. Before the development of the vaccine and after the mosquito was proven as the vector, eliminating mosquito-breeding sites and decreasing exposure to A. aegypti mosquitoes proved successful in ending yellow fever outbreaks in North America and also in the building of the Panama Canal. Today, it remains critical not only to reduce the number of mosquitoes through larvicides and insecticides but also to limit mosquito bites through the use of house screening, mosquito netting, the wearing of protective attire, and the use of insect repellants such as diethyltoluamide (DEET). During jungle outbreaks, mosquito elimination is impractical and evacuation is essential until individuals are immunized and mosquitoes controlled. To prevent further mosquito transmission during outbreaks, infected patients should be isolated in well-screened rooms sprayed with insecticides.

Immunization is the most effective and reliable way to prevent yellow fever in areas in which it is endemic. Live attenuated yellow fever virus vaccine (17D strain) (YF-VAX) should be given (0.5 mL subcutaneously every 10 years) at least 10 days before travel to endemic areas in Africa and Central and South America. A single dose of vaccine gives greater than or equal to 99% protection and confers lifelong immunity. (Although required by some countries, a booster dose of the vaccine is not medically needed.) Although infection is uncommon in most of the endemic areas, vaccination is legally required for entry into many of these countries. The typically well-tolerated vaccine is contraindicated in pregnant women, in individuals with concurrent febrile illness or compromised immunity, and in infants younger than 6 months. If infants aged 6 to 8 months cannot avoid travel to a high-risk location, parents should discuss immunization with their physician, since the vaccine is usually not offered until the age of 9 months. In the United States, the vaccine is given only at US Public Health Service-authorized Yellow Fever Vaccination Centers. The International Certificate of Vaccination is valid for 10 years from 10 days after immunization or immediately after reimmunization.

After the 2016 outbreaks depleted global vaccine supplies, experts suggested as a dose-sparing strategy the utilization of a fractional dose of the vaccine among children 2 years of age or older and among nonpregnant adults.[3] In an observational study, a one-fifth dose of the vaccine induced seroconversion in 98% of recipients. Since 2018, mass vaccination campaigns in Africa and South America have utilized primarily fractional dosing. Recent studies indicate that fractional dosing is effective and non-inferior to standard doses at inducing seroconversion although there is concern about slower seroconversion and earlier antibody waning.

Clinical Manifestations

Yellow fever is characterized by the swift onset of fever, rigors, myalgias, headache, nausea, and vomiting. With an incubation period lasting 3 to 9 days, the illness is typically biphasic, with a two-stage course during which the pulse slows and kidney involvement occurs along with bleeding disorders. Between 5% and 50% of the cases are so mild they are inapparent. In those cases recognized, the pulse is usually rapid initially but by the second day becomes slow for the degree of fever (Faget sign). A tendency to bleed may be seen early in the disease. Often, the face is flushed, with facial edema and conjunctival injection. Restlessness, irritability, and leukopenia are also common. In most cases, this initial period of mild infection resolves after 1 to 3 days, occasionally longer, and the illness concludes with rapid recovery and no sequelae. However, approximately 15% of those infected progress further into the moderate to severe phases. In these cases, the falling fever and remission of symptoms 2 to 5 days after onset are only transitory, and a deadly phase soon begins with renewal of malignant symptoms. This stage of the illness, called intoxication, is marked by the fever returning, and although the pulse remains slow, the blood pressure drops, with resultant renal failure. The flushed face is replaced by a dusky pallor, with swollen, bleeding gums and a pronounced hemorrhagic tendency with telltale black vomit (one of the disease's monikers and classic symptoms) and melena. The skin and eyes may appear yellow (jaundice), the symptom that gave rise to the disease's popular name. (However, this jaundice is generally a symptom of convalescence more than acute disease.) Liver and renal failure (which may progress to acute tubular necrosis) and epigastric tenderness with hematemesis and gastrointestinal hemorrhage often occur. There may be oliguria, albuminuria, disseminated intravascular coagulopathy, backache, dizziness,

ecchymoses, myocarditis, agitated delirium, intractable hiccups, seizures, coma, and multiple organ failure. During recovery, bacterial superinfections, particularly pneumonia, may occur.

In terminal cases, death usually transpires within 7 days of onset and is rare beyond 10 days of illness. In patients with intoxication (malignant yellow fever), a 30% to 60% mortality may be seen, with survival depending on the quality of supportive management. At autopsy, the kidneys, liver, heart, and spleen appear to be the organs most impacted by the disease.

Diagnosis

Yellow fever is suspected in patients in endemic areas or returning from them if they develop classic clinical features such as sudden fever with relative bradycardia and jaundice. Mild infection often escapes recognition by the patient or clinician. Complete blood count, urinalysis, liver function tests, coagulation studies, viral blood cultures, and serologic tests should be done. Leukopenia with relative neutropenia is common, as are thrombocytopenia, prolonged clotting, and increased prothrombin time. Bilirubin and aminotransferase levels may be elevated acutely and for several months. Albuminuria, which occurs in 90% of patients, may reach 20 g/L. This finding helps differentiate yellow fever from viral hepatitis. In malignant yellow fever, hypoglycemia and hyperkalemia may occur terminally.

Diagnosis is confirmed by viral culture, serology, the identification of viral antigens and virus-specific immunoglobulin M (IgM) and neutralizing antibodies in serum by several rapid diagnostic methods, or detecting characteristic midzonal hepatocyte necrosis at autopsy. Suspected or confirmed cases must be quarantined and health departments notified. Needle biopsy of the liver during illness is contraindicated because of high risk of hemorrhage.

Differential Diagnosis

Mild yellow fever appears clinically like a broad expanse of other infections presenting with similar symptoms, including dengue, viral hepatitis, malaria, typhus, Q fever, typhoid, Rift Valley fever, leptospirosis, drug-induced syndromes, and toxic causes. Yellow fever may be distinguished from malaria by the findings of conjunctival suffusion or relative bradycardia. The other viral hemorrhagic fevers, which include dengue, Lassa fever, Marburg disease, Ebola, Crimean-Congo hemorrhagic fever, and Bolivian and Argentine hemorrhagic fevers, usually present without jaundice. As well, albuminuria is a reliable hallmark of yellow fever that allows its differentiation from other causes of viral hepatitis.

Treatment

Since no antiviral therapy is currently available, treatment is supportive, focused on aggressive symptom management designed to correct the acid-base imbalance and electrolyte abnormalities caused by emesis, heart failure, and renal derangements. Placement in an intensive care unit is recommended. Transfusions of blood, fresh-frozen plasma, and vitamin K[1] may be utilized with hemorrhagic symptoms. As well, a proton pump inhibitor, H2 blocker, and sucralfate (Carafate)[1] can be helpful as prophylaxis for gastrointestinal bleeding and should be considered in all hospitalized patients. Antipyretics, oxygen, vasopressors, and IV hydration may also be helpful. Avoidance of sedatives and drugs metabolized hepatically is prudent, and medication dosing should be adjusted in the face of declining renal function. Antibiotic therapy for secondary bacterial sepsis is often necessary during the recovery period. Owing to the increased risk of bleeding, avoidance of aspirin and other nonsteroidal antiinflammatory drugs, such as naproxen and ibuprofen, is recommended. Therapeutic use of monoclonal antibodies (mAbs) is being studied, and initial research reveals potential to neutralize yellow fever virus and prevent severe disease in animal models.

Complications

The majority of those infected with yellow fever will be asymptomatic or experience only mild disease with total recovery. The mortality rates in tropical America range from 45% to 75%, compared with less than 30% in Africa. This difference suggests genetic factors

---

[3] Exceeds dosage recommended by the manufacturer.

[1] Not FDA approved for this indication.

play a role in the course of the illness, as well as the viral strain. The convalescence of a yellow fever patient is usually prolonged and varies from patient to patient. Although uncommon, late death (weeks after the acute illness) can occur as a result of cardiac complications or renal failure. Profound asthenia and fatigue usually last for 1 to 2 weeks, but in some cases can last many months. Jaundice and the elevation of liver enzymes have been known to last an extended period (several months) during convalescence. Survival of an attack imparts lifelong immunity against subsequent infection.

References

A Global Strategy to Eliminate Yellow Fever Epidemics 2017–2026, Geneva: World Health Organization; 2018.

Centers for Disease Control and Prevention. Yellow fever. Available at: https://www.cdc.gov/yellowfever/index.html [accessed June 1, 2025].

Fauci AS, Paules CI: Yellow fever—once again on the radar screen in the Americas, *N Engl J Med* 376:1397–1399, 2017.

Fernandes EG, Gomes Porto VB, de Oliveira PMN, et al: Yellow fever vaccine–associated viscerotropic disease among siblings, São Paulo State, Brazil, *Emerg Infect Dis* 29(3):493–500, 2023.

Hamer DH, Angelo K, Caumes E, et al: Fatal yellow fever in travelers to Brazil, 2018, *MMWR Morb Mortal Wkly Rep* 67:340–341, 2018.

Juan-Giner A, Namulwana ML, Kimathi D: Immunogenicity and safety of fractional doses of 17D-213 yellow fever vaccine in children (YEFE): a randomised, double-blind, non-inferiority substudy of a phase 4 trial, *Lancet Infect Dis* S1473-3099(23)00131–7, 2023.

Moritz UG Kraemer, et al: Spread of yellow fever virus outbreak in Angola and the Democratic Republic of the Congo 2015–16: a modelling study, *The Lancet Infectious Diseases* 17(3):330–338, 2017.

National Notifiable Diseases Surveillance System (NNDSS): Yellow Fever Case Definition 2019. Available at: https://ndc.services.cdc.gov/case-definitions/yellow-fever-2019/ [accessed June 1, 2025].

Pan American Health Organization (PAHO). *Clinical management of yellow fever in the region of the Americas. Experiences and recommendations for health services.* Washington, DC: PAHO; 2023.

Pan American Health Organization/World Health Organization (PAHO/WHO): *Epidemiological update. Yellow fever in the region of the Americas.* 21 March 2024. Washington, DC: PAHO/WHO; 2024.

Ricciardi MJ, et al: Therapeutic neutralizing monoclonal antibody administration protects against lethal yellow fever virus infection, *Sci Transl Med* 15, eade5795(2023).

Roukens AH, Visser LG: Fractional dose yellow fever vaccination, coming of age, *Lancet Infect Dis* S1473-3099(23)00205-0, 2023.

Silva NIO, Sacchetto L, de Rezende IM, et al: Recent sylvatic yellow fever virus transmission in Brazil: the news from an old disease, *Virol J* 17(1):9, 2020.

Thongsripong P, et al: *Aedes aegypti* and *Aedes albopictus* (Diptera: Culicidae) oviposition activity and the associated socio-environmental factors in the New Orleans area, *J Med Entomol* 60(2):392–400, 2023.

Wilder-Smith A, Monath TP: Responding to the threat of urban yellow fever outbreaks, *The Lancet Infectious Diseases* 17(3):248–250, 2017.

World Health Organization. Yellow fever factsheet. Available at: https://www.who.int/news-room/fact-sheets/detail/yellow-fever [accessed June 1, 2025].

ZIKA VIRUS DISEASE

Method of
Scott Kellermann, MD, MPH; and Rick D. Kellerman, MD

CURRENT DIAGNOSIS

- Zika virus is a flavivirus transmitted by the *Aedes* mosquito.
- In many parts of the world, in a "pure" Zika epidemic, the diagnosis can be ascertained on clinical grounds. However, dengue and chikungunya have similar clinical presentations and may confound the clinical diagnosis.
- For individuals presenting ≤7 days after onset of symptoms, the diagnostic test of choice is a nucleic acid amplification test (NAAT) of serum (or whole blood) or urine.
- For individuals presenting >7 days after onset of symptoms, Zika virus immunoglobulin (Ig)M antibody testing is recommended. Because of the short period and low level of Zika virus RNA in serum, a negative NAAT does not exclude recent Zika infection. IgM generally is detectable >7 days post onset of symptoms and persists months to years. IgM testing is complicated by cross-reactive antibodies to other flaviviruses,

- The CDC has approved a single Trioplex real-time polymerase chain reaction (RT-PCR) assay to evaluate for the presence of Zika, chikungunya, and dengue infection. It is available through the CDC and other qualified laboratories.
- Zika virus is a neurotropic virus that particularly targets neural progenitor cells. The major complication of Zika virus disease is the potential risk of microcephaly as a result of vertical transmission.

CURRENT THERAPY

- At present, there is no treatment or vaccine for Zika virus disease.

Zika virus is a mosquito-borne flavivirus. In 1947, in a quest to solve the dilemma of yellow fever, researchers at the East African Research Institute in Uganda placed a caged rhesus macaque in the canopy of the nearby Zika Forest. The monkey developed a fever, and from its serum a transmissible agent was isolated that in 1952 was described as Zika virus. Initially, Zika virus, borne by arboreal mosquitoes such as *Aedes africanus*, infected wild primates and rarely infected humans, even in highly enzootic areas. Results of serologic and entomologic investigations suggest that Zika virus had an extensive geographic distribution in Africa and Asia earlier than 2007; however, fewer than 20 cases in humans were reported before 2007, and all had mild, self-limiting clinical manifestations. From 2007 to 2016, Zika went from a poorly known virus, causing sporadic human infections in Africa and Asia, to a nearly pandemic neurotropic virus with active circulation detected in 89 countries and territories. After its original identification, the first major Zika outbreak outside of Africa took place in 2007 on Yap Island, where an estimated 73% if the population age 3 years or older was infected with the Zika virus. In 2013 to 2014, an outbreak affecting an estimated 30,000 people occurred in French Polynesia. During this outbreak, 3% of donated blood samples tested positive for Zika virus by NAAT. Other isolated outbreaks followed. In 2015 to 2016, a major outbreak occurred in Brazil and other South American, Central American, and Caribbean countries. The first locally transmitted cases on the U.S. mainland were reported in 2016. As Zika virus migrated from Africa to Asia, the Asian lineage of the virus emerged. The results of sequence homology demonstrate that the strain responsible for outbreaks throughout the Americas was phylogenetically closest to the Asian lineage. The Zika virus appears to have mutated in character while expanding its geographic range, transforming from a localized endemic, mosquito-borne infection producing only a mild illness to a disease with explosive outbreaks linked with neurologic disorders including Guillain-Barré syndrome and microcephaly.

In November 2016, the World Health Organization declared, "The Zika virus and associated consequences remain a significant enduring public health challenge requiring intense action but no longer represent a public health emergency of international concern." The incidence in the Americas and the world has significantly waned after 2017. Since 2019 there have been no confirmed reports of mosquito transmission of Zika virus in the continental United States or its territories.

Epidemiology

Transmission is primarily through a bite of an infected mosquito; however, transmission through maternal-fetal exposure, sex (including vaginal, anal, and oral sex), blood product transfusion, organ transplantation, and laboratory contact has been documented.

Zika virus is most often transmitted by the daytime-active *Aedes* mosquitoes, such as *A. aegypti* and *A. albopictus* (Asian tiger mosquito). With the exception of West Nile virus, which is predominantly spread by *Culex* species mosquitoes, the arboviruses reaching the Western Hemisphere have all been transmitted by *Aedes* mosquitoes.

A. albopictus is a relatively new arrival to the United States, entering in the mid-1980s having been transported in used tires shipped from northern Asia. *A. aegypti*, on the other hand, likely arrived in the Americas in the 17th century aboard slave ships sailing from Africa. The distribution of *A. aegypti* is more widespread now than ever recorded, extending across all continents including North America. Although *A. aegypti* has likely maintained an intermittent presence in the United States for approximately 375 years, its distribution has been assumed to be limited by cold temperatures to boundaries roughly southward of the average 10°C winter isotherm. However, *A. aegypti* has been found in a Capitol Hill neighborhood of Washington, DC, and genetic evidence suggests that they survived at least four consecutive winters in the region. It is assumed that *A. aegypti* mosquitoes are capable of adapting for persistence in a northern climate.

Most significantly, pregnant mothers may vertically transmit the virus to the developing fetus, potentially resulting in microcephaly. Zika virus has been isolated in semen and vaginal secretions. Male-to-female and female-to-male sexual transmission of the Zika virus has been reported. Blood transfusions have been a source of transmission outside of the United States. The blood supply in the United States is tested for Zika virus.

The Zika pandemic is an example of a "perfect storm" in which a new American subclade emerged from the Asian lineage of the virus and was introduced into a uniformly susceptible population that had not been previously exposed to Zika virus.

Risk Factors

The risk of Zika virus infection for pregnant women is pronounced because of the potential link to microcephaly of the infant. The risk is greatest if the infection occurs early in pregnancy. There is no evidence that pregnant women are more susceptible to Zika virus infection or that the disease is more severe during pregnancy. The Centers for Disease Control and Prevention (CDC) reports that although Zika virus has been found in breast milk and possible Zika virus infections have been identified in breastfeeding babies, Zika virus transmission through breast milk has not been confirmed. Because current evidence suggests that the benefits of breastfeeding outweigh the risk of Zika virus spreading through breast milk, the CDC encourages mothers to breastfeed, even if they were infected or lived in or traveled to an area with risk of Zika.

Based on what is known about similar arbovirus infections, once a person has been infected and developed antibodies to Zika virus, they are likely to be protected from a future Zika virus infection. Once a woman has cleared the virus, she is not thought to be at risk for having a subsequent child with a Zika-related birth defect.

Pathophysiology

The Zika virus is a member of the Flaviviridae virus family, which includes dengue, yellow fever, West Nile, and Japanese encephalitis viruses. Zika is a single-stranded, positive-sense RNA virus that has been fully sequenced with a genome of approximately 11 kilobases. It is one of many arthropod-borne arboviruses. Monkeys are the common vertebrate host of the virus. Arboviruses oftentimes have complex natural transmission cycles involving mammals, birds, and blood-feeding arthropod vectors.

Arboviruses, particularly yellow fever and dengue, have been problematic in the Americas at least since the 16th century. However, since the year 2000, there has a dramatic resurgence of arboviruses, with unprecedented increases in dengue and the emergence of new viruses such as Zika and chikungunya.

Prevention

Population-based mosquito control measures are recommended to prevent the spread of Zika virus. Although yellow fever has historically been prevented entirely by aggressive mosquito control, in the modern era, vector control has been problematic because of the expense, logistics, public resistance, and the development of resistance to the pesticides used and their collateral adverse effects on the environment. Although a chemical war against the vector may provide short-term control, programs for improving urban infrastructure and environmental sanitation with a stable supply of potable water would offer more durable results. Among the best preventive measures against Zika virus are house screens, air conditioning, and removal of yard and household debris and containers that provide mosquito-breeding sites—luxuries often unavailable to impoverished residents of crowded urban locales where such epidemics take their greatest toll.

Releasing mosquitoes that are sterile or genetically modified to die before they can reproduce is being investigated, as are novel control strategies using *Wolbachia* to prevent mosquitoes from transmitting arboviruses.

Individuals who have contracted Zika virus should take precautions to avoid mosquito bites during the first week of illness (the likely window of viremia) to reduce the spread of infection to others.

Individuals who have traveled to an area with Zika virus transmission and return to an area with no Zika virus mosquito transmission should avoid mosquito bites for 3 weeks (the period during which they could become viremic).

Because of the association between Zika virus infection and microcephaly in fetuses, pregnant women or women considering pregnancy and who are contemplating international travel should consult their healthcare provider and the CDC's travel guidelines: https://www.cdc.gov/zika/geo/index.html.

A number of authorities have advised that pregnant women avoid or consider postponing travel to areas below 6500 feet (2000 meters) where exposure to Zika virus is a potential. Regions above 6500 feet (2000 meters) are deemed safe because the *Aedes* mosquitos are rare in these locations and the risk for exposure to Zika virus is minimal.

Anyone with Zika virus infection or exposure (via travel to or residence in mosquito transmission areas or unprotected sexual contact with an individual who has traveled to or resided in mosquito transmission areas) who has a pregnant partner should abstain from unprotected sex for the duration of the pregnancy. The CDC recommends that women who have had Zika virus exposure through travel or sexual contact and do not have ongoing risks for exposure should wait at least 8 weeks from date of diagnosis, symptom onset (if symptomatic), or last possible exposure before attempting to conceive. During this waiting period, either abstinence should be practiced or barrier contraception with condoms should be used. This 8-week waiting period may decrease the risk of maternal-fetal transmission of the Zika virus.

Zika virus typically remains in the semen for longer periods of time than other body fluids. Accordingly, the CDC recommends abstinence or barrier contraception be used for least 3 months from date of diagnosis, symptom onset (if symptomatic), or after the last possible exposure before attempting conception with their partner.

Zika virus RNA usually clears from semen after about 3 months but has been detected in semen up to 188 days after onset of illness. Between 2015 and July 2018, 52 cases of confirmed sexual transmission of Zika virus infection had been reported in the United States. The longest period from symptom onset in the index case to potential sexual transmission to a partner was between 32 and 41 days; most reports are of much shorter intervals. There is a lack of evidence that the risk of sexual transmission differs in symptomatic and asymptomatic men. Recommendations for men with possible Zika virus exposure whose partners are pregnant are advised to consistently and correctly use condoms during sex or abstain from sex for the duration of the pregnancy.

Zika virus RNA is usually detectable in the serum for about 2 weeks and clears from urine after about 6 weeks. In one description of shedding dynamics in adults, Zika virus RNA was

TABLE 1	Prevention of Mosquito Bites

- Remove yard debris (e.g., old tires) and containers that collect water and may provide mosquito breeding sites.
- Wear long-sleeved shirts, long pants, and socks. Tuck pants into socks.
- Apply permethrin to outer clothing.
- Use window screens.
- Use mosquito netting at night if sleeping quarters are not screened.
- Use mosquito netting when children younger than 2 months of age—before they can use mosquito repellents—must go outside.
- Apply mosquito repellents directly to exposed skin. When applying mosquito repellents to the face, spray it on the hands, then rub it in. Avoid the eyes and mouth.
- Do not allow young children to apply mosquito repellents themselves. Children who rub mosquito repellent into their own skin are prone to putting their hands into their mouths or touching their eyes.
- Adults should apply mosquito repellent on children by putting the repellent on their own hands and rubbing it into the child's skin.
- To limit the total amount of mosquito repellent that might be absorbed, do not apply to skin under clothing or on skin that is broken (i.e., cuts, rashes).
- Do not use mosquito repellents near food. Wash hands before eating or drinking.
- Wash off mosquito repellent from the skin when it is no longer needed.
- At the end of the day, wash treated skin with soap and water.

identified in the plasma (57%), urine (93%), and saliva (69%) of participants; estimated median times to clearance were 11.5, 24, and 14 days, respectively.

Documented reports of sexual transmission have primarily involved transmission from a man to a woman; however, transmission has also been documented from a man to another man and from a woman to a man.

Avoiding mosquito bites is important for disease control (Table 1). There are hundreds of insect repellents sold in the United States. Though research is limited, *A. aegypti* and *A. albopictus* mosquitoes seem to be most effectively repelled by products that contain at least 30% oil of lemon eucalyptus, 25% DEET (N,N-diethyl-m-toluamide), or 20% picaridin. Ten percent DEET provides protection for about 2 hours, and 30% DEET protects for about 5 hours. Anything over 50% DEET does not provide longer protection. The CDC recommends oil of eucalyptus not be used in children younger than 3 years. There are no age restrictions for DEET or picaridin. Products containing IR3535, 2-undecanone, and products made from natural plant oils such as citronella, lemongrass oil, cedar oil, rosemary oil, cinnamon oil, and geraniol seem to be ineffective against Zika-transmitting mosquitoes. Insect repellents can be used with sunscreen, but the sunscreen should be applied first.

Additional protection from mosquito bites can be achieved by treating outer clothing with permethrin. Permethrin, a derivative of *Chrysanthemum cinerariifolium,* is an insect repellent and insecticide. Though it is poorly absorbed and rapidly inactivated, permethrin should not be applied directly to the skin and should not be used on underclothing. The Environmental Protection Agency recommends that clothes treated with permethrin be washed separately from clothes that are not treated. If washed together, underclothing may absorb permethrin into the fabric, which may increase the risk of absorption through the skin. Permethrin-treated clothing will retain repellent activity through multiple washes. The Environmental Protection Agency indicates there is no evidence that exposure to permethrin results in adverse effects for pregnant or nursing mothers or adverse developmental effects in their children. Permethrin is listed as pregnancy category B. It can be used on the outer clothing of children older than 2 months of age.

At present, no Zika vaccines are available, although phase 1 and phase 2 studies are underway and several DNA and mRNA vaccine platforms appear promising.

Clinical Manifestations

The incubation period for Zika virus is estimated to be 3 to 12 days. A study after the Yap outbreak indicated that of those with serologic evidence of infection, 38% were symptomatic. Clinical manifestations of Zika virus infection include acute onset of low-grade fever (37.8–38.5°C); a pruritic macular or papular rash on the face, trunk, extremities, palms, and soles; arthralgia, notably in the small joints of the hands and feet; and nonpurulent conjunctivitis. Clinically, Zika virus disease is presumed if two or more of these symptoms are present. In more than 60 years of observation, severe disease requiring hospitalization is uncommon and case fatality is low.

Clinical manifestations in infants and children with postnatal infection are similar to the findings in adults. Arthralgia may be difficult to detect in infants and young children. It may present as irritability, pain on palpation or pain with passive movement of a limb, walking with a limp, or difficulty moving or refusing to move an extremity.

Diagnosis

In a "pure" Zika epidemic, a diagnosis can be ascertained on clinical grounds. However, dengue and chikungunya have similar clinical presentations and have been epidemic in the Americas, confounding the clinical diagnosis.

For individuals presenting ≤7 days after onset of symptoms, detection of Zika virus RNA is through a nucleic acid amplification test (NAAT) of serum (or whole blood) or urine. For all diagnostic testing processed on specimen types other than serum, it is necessary to also obtain a concurrent serum specimen for reflex IgM testing.

For individuals presenting >7 days after onset of symptoms, serologic testing for IgM antibodies to Zika virus should be performed. Plaque reduction neutralization tests (PRNT) may resolve false-positive IgM antibody results caused by nonspecific reactivity and help identify the infecting virus. However, due to cross-reactivity, PRNT might not discriminate between flaviviruses antibodies, especially after a secondary flavivirus infection.

For infant diagnosis, PRNT cannot distinguish between maternal and infant antibodies in specimens collected from infants at or near birth. Based on what is known about other congenital infections, maternal antibodies are expected to become undetectable by 18 months of age.

All serologic results should be interpreted with caution because there can be cross-reactivity with other flaviviruses (such as dengue virus). In regions where cocirculation of multiple arboviruses is present, a Trioplex RT-PCR assay can discern the presence of Zika, chikungunya, and dengue infection.

Cross-reactivity may also be observed in individuals who have been vaccinated against yellow fever or Japanese encephalitis.

The CDC website should be consulted for Zika virus testing recommendations for women who are symptomatic or asymptomatic during pregnancy. Instructions for testing can be found on Table 2.

There is no role for Zika virus testing in asymptomatic individuals who are not pregnant.

Instructions for monitoring infants with potential exposure to Zika virus can be found at https://www.cdc.gov/zika/hcp/clinical-pregnant/index.html.

Physicians who deliver an infant suspected of experiencing the effects of maternal Zika virus infection should consult the CDC to discuss blood, placental, and umbilical cord sampling. Clinicians should be alert to brain and eye defects in an infant, which might prompt suspicion of prenatal Zika virus infection. These findings might provide a signal to the reemergence of Zika virus, which is particularly important in geographic regions lacking ongoing comprehensive Zika virus surveillance.

Zika virus infection is a nationally notifiable disease.

Differential Diagnosis

Differential diagnosis encompasses a wide variety of other viral diseases such as dengue, chikungunya, Mayaro virus disease, Ross River fever, Barmah Forest disease, o'nyong-nyong disease,

TABLE 2	Testing Pregnant Women for Zika Virus*

Asymptomatic Pregnant Patient

Lived in or traveled to the United States and its territories during pregnancy:
- Because no confirmed cases of Zika virus disease have been detected in the United States and its territories since 2018, routine Zika virus testing is not recommended.

Traveled to an area with an active CDC Zika Travel Health Notice during pregnancy:
- NAAT testing may be considered up to 12 weeks after travel.

Traveled to an area with current or past Zika virus transmission outside the United States and its territories during pregnancy:
- Routine testing is not recommended.
- If the decision is made to test, NAAT testing can be done up to 12 weeks after travel.

Symptomatic Pregnant Patient

Lived in or traveled to an area with an active CDC Zika Travel Health Notice during pregnancy *or* had sex during pregnancy with someone living in or with recent travel to an area with an active CDC Zika Travel Health Notice:
- Specimens should be collected as soon as possible after onset of symptoms up to 12 weeks after symptom onset.
- Perform dengue and Zika virus NAAT and IgM testing on a serum specimen and Zika virus NAAT on a urine specimen.
- If Zika NAAT is positive and the Zika IgM is negative, repeat the NAAT test on newly extracted RNA from the same specimen to rule out false-positive results.
- If both dengue and Zika virus NAATs are negative but either IgM antibody test is positive, confirmatory PRNTs should be performed against dengue, Zika, and other flaviviruses endemic to the region where exposure occurred.

*Travel Resource: CDC: Countries and Territories at Risk for ZIKA (https://www.cdc.gov/zika/geo/index.html).
IgM, Immunoglobulin M; *NAAT*, nucleic acid amplification test; *PRNTs*, plaque reduction neutralization tests.

and Sindbis fever. In addition, the CDC lists group A streptococcus, leptospirosis, malaria, rickettsia, rubella, measles, parvovirus, enterovirus, and adenovirus in the differential diagnosis.

Dengue virus, chikungunya virus, and Zika virus infections have similar clinical manifestations and are transmitted by the same mosquito vector. However, chikungunya usually presents with high fever and intense joint pain affecting the hands, feet, knees, and back. Unlike Zika infection, conjunctivitis is far less common. Dengue infection usually manifests with high fever, severe muscle pain, and headache and may be associated with hemorrhage, and, similar to chikungunya, conjunctivitis is unusual. Coinfection with Zika, chikungunya, and dengue viruses has been described.

Treatment

At present, there is no treatment or vaccine for Zika virus disease. Because symptoms are usually absent or mild, most acutely infected patients do not access the medical system and treat themselves symptomatically. Antiviral medication is ineffective. The mainstays of management are bed rest and supportive care. When multiple arboviruses are cocirculating, testing for a specific viral diagnosis, if available, can be important in anticipating, preventing, and managing complications.

Although the Zika virus has not been associated with hemorrhagic fever, it is imperative to avoid aspirin and nonsteroidal antiinflammatory medications until dengue is excluded to reduce the risk of hemorrhage. The use of aspirin should be avoided in children because of the risk of Reye syndrome.

Because of the rapidly evolving knowledge about the Zika virus, clinicians are encouraged to freely consult the CDC and the World Health Organization (WHO) websites for clinical guidance.

Monitoring

For pregnant women with confirmed or possible Zika virus infection, serial fetal ultrasounds (every 3–4 weeks) should be

considered. Guidelines for monitoring pregnant females with a potential exposure to Zika virus can be found at https://www.cdc.gov/zika/hcp/clinical-pregnant/index.html.

Complications

The major complication of Zika virus disease is the potential risk of microcephaly as a result of vertical transmission. Amniocentesis has been used to detect the presence of Zika virus in amniotic fluid of women who had ultrasound confirmation of microcephalic fetuses. The virus has been isolated in the brains of newborns and miscarried fetuses. It is unclear whether there may be contributory factors to the development of microcephaly, such as nutritional and environmental factors or concomitant infection with other microorganisms.

Maternal infection with Zika virus may lead to placental infection and injury as the virus can be transmitted across the placenta to the fetal brain. Zika virus targets neuronal progenitor cells and neuronal cells at other stages of maturity. Neuronal growth and proliferation are disrupted, impairing normal brain development. The infant is particularly vulnerable in the first half of pregnancy, as this is the stage of peak neuronal proliferation and migration.

Zika-associated birth defects can occur whether or not the pregnant woman has had symptoms of the infection during pregnancy. The U.S. Zika Pregnancy and Infant Registry conducted a study of 6799 live-born infants from pregnancies with laboratory evidence of confirmed or possible Zika virus infection born between December 1, 2015, and March 31, 2018. In the U.S. states and territories, 5.3% of mothers with symptoms compatible with Zika virus infection during pregnancy delivered a baby with Zika-associated birth defects, compared with 4.2% of mothers infected with Zika virus who were asymptomatic. In this study, 8% of pregnant women with confirmed Zika virus infection in the first trimester delivered babies with Zika-associated birth defects. Approximately two-thirds of pregnant women in this cohort reported asymptomatic infections. Severity of maternal symptoms and signs, maternal virus load, and preexisting dengue antibodies do not appear to be predictors of infant outcome.

Among infants with any Zika-associated birth defect, one-third had more than one defect reported.

Infants may have a craniofacial disproportion and abnormal cranial shape. The fontanelles may be closed or very small and the sutures may be uneven or overlapping. A recognizable phenotype of microcephaly spectrum in congenital Zika syndrome has been identified. This includes anomalies of the shape of the skull and redundancy of the scalp consistent with fetal brain disruption sequence, which is present in 70% of infants but often is subtle. Additional features consistent with fetal immobility may be present, ranging from dimples (30.1%), distal hand/finger contractures (20.5%), and feet malposition (15.7%) to generalized arthrogryposis (9.6%). Neurologically, there may be changes in motor activity, severe muscle hypertonia, feeding difficulties, and excessive and inconsolable crying. Brain imaging may show calcifications, abnormal gyral patterns, enlarged ventricles, and marked decreases in the volume of gray and white matter. The corpus callosum may be thin or absent. The brainstem and cerebellum may be underdeveloped. Especially in infants between 3 and 6 months of age, seizures may arise, and children may exhibit visual problems, hearing loss, and impaired growth. Children exposed to Zika virus in utero who do not have overt signs of Zika virus–associated clinical manifestations or abnormal neuroimaging may have a higher risk of neurodevelopmental delay. The virus's strong affinity for neural cells might cause neurologic damage that only becomes apparent as children age. The full range of birth defects and disabilities associated with Zika virus disease remains to be fully delineated, and it is unclear whether infants and children who contract Zika in infancy or early childhood may develop neurologic complications.

Retrospective data from the French Polynesia Zika virus outbreak from October 2013 to April 2014 indicate a close association with Guillain-Barré syndrome. Of the 42 patients diagnosed with Guillain-Barré syndrome, 41 had anti–Zika virus IgM or

IgG (98%), and all had neutralizing antibodies against Zika virus (100%) compared with 54 of 98 in the control group (56%).

An escalating spectrum of neurologic complications associated with Zika virus infection is being established.

References

Gorshkov K, Shiryaev S, Fertel S: Zika virus: origins, pathological action, and treatment strategies front, *Microbiology* 9:3252, 2019.

Honein MA: Recognizing the global impact of Zika virus infection during pregnancy, *N Engl J Med* 378:1055–1056, 2018.

Mitchell P, Mier-y-Teran-Romero L, Biggerstaff B: Reassessing serosurvey-based estimates of the symptomatic proportion of Zika virus infections, *Am J Epidemiol* 188(1):206–213, 2019.

Musso D, Ko A, Baud D: Zika virus infection—after the pandemic, *N Engl J Med* 381:1444–1457, 2019.

Roth N, Reynolds M, Lewis E: Zika-associated birth defects reported in pregnancies with laboratory evidence of confirmed or possible Zika virus infection — U.S. Zika Pregnancy and Infant Registry, December 1, 2015–March 31, 2018, *MMWR Morb Mortal Wkly Rep* 71(3):73–79, 2022.

Wang Y, Ling L, Zhang Z: Current advances in Zika vaccine development, *Vaccines (Basel)* 10(11):1816, 2022.

World Health Organization: Zika virus. Available at https://www.who.int/newsroom/fact-sheets/detail/zika-virus.

ACUTE FACIAL PARALYSIS

Method of
Louito Edje, MD, MHPE

CURRENT DIAGNOSIS

- A thorough history, including timeline of onset and progression, is imperative.
- Neurologic examination of the head and neck with House-Brackmann baseline scoring is helpful in prognostication and communication with specialists.
- Facial palsy is rare in children, with the most common cause being borreliosis.
- 93.6% of children have complete improvement.
- 70% of adult patients fully recover in 6 to 9 months; the rest will have some degree of aberrant nerve regeneration resulting in post–facial paralysis synkinesis.
- For cases lasting longer than 3 weeks that are slowly progressive and accompanied by accessory symptoms such hyperacusis, tinnitus, or nystagmus, additional evaluation, including electrodiagnostic testing and magnetic resonance imaging with and without contrast, is needed.

CURRENT THERAPY

- Oral corticosteroids are first-line therapy for adults and children.
- Corticosteroids are most effective if administered within 72 hours of symptom onset.
- Combination oral steroids and antivirals should be used to decrease synkinesis.
- Antiviral therapy alone is not recommended.
- Early intervention with additional diagnostic testing is required if there is no improvement after the third week or complete paralysis is present at onset.
- Corneal care should include dexpanthenol (Panthoderm) ophthalmic ointment[2], artificial tears, and eye protection for full paralysis.
- Physical therapy is useful in severe paralysis at onset or persistent paralysis.

[2]Not available in the United States.

Epidemiology

The most common cause of peripheral facial paralysis (PFP) is Bell palsy, 60% to 75% of which is idiopathic. There is no association with sex, facial laterality, or seasonality. Bell palsy affects 7 to 40 cases per 100,000, most commonly in patients ages 30 to 45, with one in three resulting in permanent deficit of facial nerve function. The lifetime incidence is 1 in 60, with an 8% to 12% chance of recurrence. It is more common in patients with uncontrolled hypertension, obesity, and diabetes. A meta-analysis in 2022 found the incidence in 809 pregnant women to be 0.05%, with the incidence of pregnancy in all patients with PFP to be 6.62%. It is more common in the third trimester of pregnancy (68.82%).

Pathophysiology

The facial nerve passes through the petrous bone, exiting through the stylomastoid foramen giving off five branches to innervate the face, including the anterior two-thirds of the tongue, salivary glands, and the lacrimal glands (Figure 1).

Two main hypotheses for Bell palsy are viral reactivation and a cell-mediated autoimmune inflammatory response affecting the seventh cranial nerve. This nerve is responsible for lid closure, hearing, taste, salivary production, and tear formation. It is thought that inflammation leads to edema, subsequent epineural compression, and ischemia of the nerve. Edema can also activate collagen synthesis, which in turn causes fibrous compression. Elevated levels of herpes simplex type 1 DNA have been found in the geniculate ganglion and saliva of patients.

Risk Factors and Prevention

The majority of patients with Bell palsy fully recover. Risk factors for a protracted course or permanent deficits are House-Brackmann (HB) grade (more favorable recovery with HB III and IV than HB V and VI, 82.9% vs. 68.2%, $p < .001$), presence of hypertension at the time of diagnosis, personal or family history of Bell palsy, and extent of nerve denervation. Younger patients recover better than patients over age 60. Women recover better than men.

In one study, 65% of patients with less than 50% denervation had full recovery within 1 month; however, 90% of those with less than 75% denervation have full recovery in 2 months. Diabetes was found to be associated with an unfavorable outcome ($p = 0.07$). Pregnancy-induced hypertension and preeclampsia are also risk factors. Risk is higher in the third trimester, possibly because of edema and hypercoagulability. Prevention of Bell palsy can be done by avoiding alcohol consumption, exercising regularly, avoiding stress, and decreasing tobacco use.

Clinical Manifestations

Diagnosis

The diagnosis of Bell palsy is clinical; it manifests with sudden-onset unilateral facial paresis or paralysis. There may be facial asymmetry at rest or synkinesis of the forehead, eyelid, or mouth. This may manifest with a complaint of inability to close the lid, drooling, retroauricular pain, ipsilateral cheek paresthesia, or hyperacusis. A thorough neuroclinical examination of the head and neck (including otoscopy) may show facial asymmetry at rest or actively, brow ptosis, lagophthalmos, protective Bell phenomenon (superior rotation of the globe with attempted eye closure), increased tear film or epiphora, corneal hyperesthesia, flattened nasolabial fold, displacement of the nasal ala inferomedially, downturning of the oral commissure, salivary incompetence, and disturbance of taste. The constellation of facial findings on physical examination can be graded using the House-Brackmann grading system (Table 1).

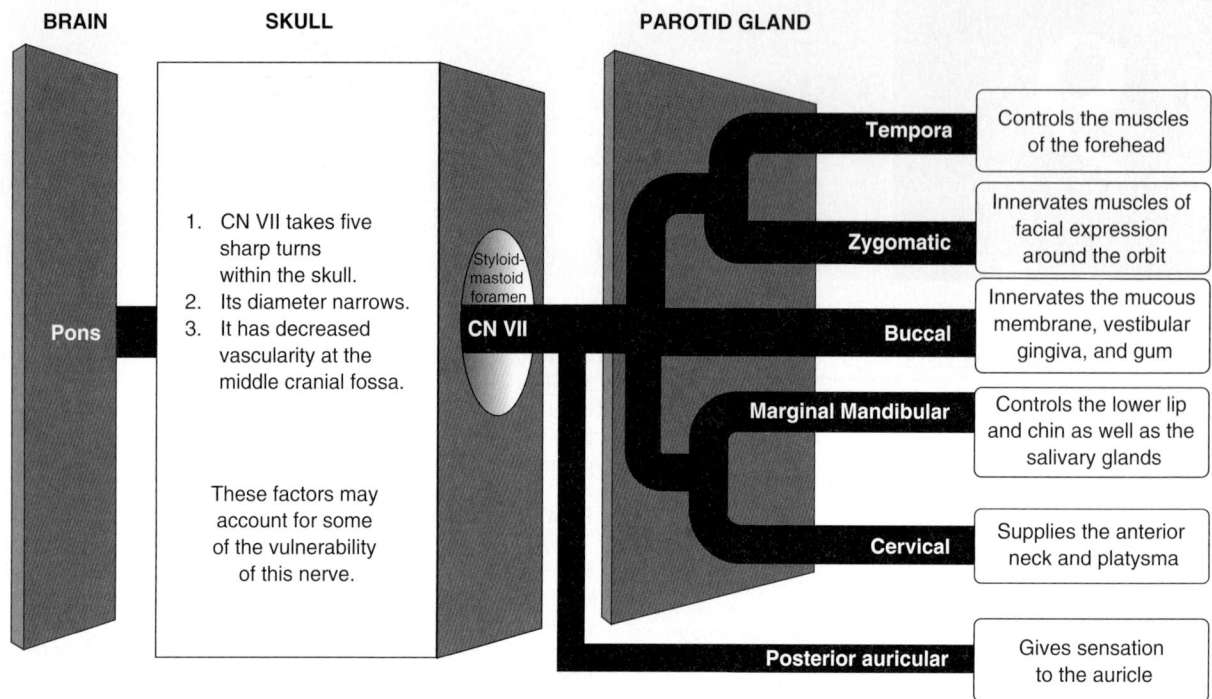

BRAIN **SKULL** **PAROTID GLAND**

Pons

Styloid-mastoid foramen

CN VII

1. CN VII takes five sharp turns within the skull.
2. Its diameter narrows.
3. It has decreased vascularity at the middle cranial fossa.

These factors may account for some of the vulnerability of this nerve.

Tempora — Controls the muscles of the forehead

Zygomatic — Innervates muscles of facial expression around the orbit

Buccal — Innervates the mucous membrane, vestibular gingiva, and gum

Marginal Mandibular — Controls the lower lip and chin as well as the salivary glands

Cervical — Supplies the anterior neck and platysma

Posterior auricular — Gives sensation to the auricle

Figure 1 Facial nerve schematic. Cranial nerve *(CN)* VII has a serpiginous path through the skull with narrowing to 0.68 mm and traversing a watershed area of decreased vascularity through the middle cranial fossa, all of which are considered contributory to its vulnerability.

Diagnostic testing is not routinely recommended except in severe HB grades and recurrent or bilateral facial palsy. In those cases, blood chemistries to consider include a complete blood count with differential, rheumatoid factor, and erythrocyte sedimentation rate. A 2020 meta-analysis found neutrophil-to-lymphocyte ratio to be a marker for inflammation and higher in Bell palsy than other causes. In children, a *Borrelia* serologic study should be performed because of its high incidence in that population (34%–56%). If a patient presents with complete facial paralysis, electrodiagnostic testing such as electroneurography, which tests for nerve conduction and axonal degeneration, and electromyography should be considered for prognostication. Cases lasting longer than 3 weeks that are slowly progressive, accompanied by accessory symptoms such as hyperacusis, tinnitus, or nystagmus, need additional evaluation, including magnetic resonance imaging of the head with and without contrast enhancement. If cerebrospinal fluid examination is required, consider head computed tomography before the procedure to prevent herniation.

When to Communicate With a Specialist

If corneal involvement is suspected, consult ophthalmology. With complete unilateral facial paralysis at onset, bilateral paralysis, change in hearing, or otic involvement with tympanic membrane abnormality, consider consulting otolaryngology. For symptoms persisting beyond 3 months, refer to neurology and physical therapy (PT).

Differential Diagnosis

Causes other than Bell palsy need to be considered with slowly progressive symptoms, focal neurologic deficits, and bilateral facial palsy. The differential includes Epstein-Barr virus, cytomegalovirus, Lyme disease, mumps virus, rubella virus, varicella zoster, herpes simplex 1, *Mycoplasma pneumoniae*, coxsackievirus, stroke, herpes zoster oticus (for those who present with otalgia or vesicles), systemic infection (human immunodeficiency virus, Miller Fisher variant of Guillain-Barré syndrome, neuroborreliosis), rickettsia, Sjögren syndrome, granulomatous disease (sarcoidosis, Melkersson-Rosenthal syndrome, in which alternating contralateral/ipsilateral facial palsy occurs with oral swelling and lingua plicata), trauma (petrous bone fractures), pontine infarct,

and benign or malignant tumors (masses of the cerebropontine angle, parotid tumors). Stroke can be differentiated from Bell palsy by involvement of the muscles of the forehead. With middle cerebral artery stroke, or other central cause, the frontalis muscle functions normally, whereas the mid and lower facial functions will be affected.

Therapy (or Treatment)
Medical

In children, weight-based dosing of oral prednisolone (Omnipred)[1], 1mg/kg/day (up to max 50 mg/day) given orally for 7–10 days without taper, is recommended. In adults, randomized controlled studies and meta-analyses provide strong evidence in support of use of glucocorticoids for management of Bell palsy. The most common dosing in the primary literature for adults is prednisone[1] 50 mg daily for 10 days or prednisone[1] 60 mg daily for 5 days, followed by a 5-day taper. These regimens are most effective if administered within 72 hours of symptom onset (odds ratio [OR] 2.36, $p < .05$).

A meta-analysis of high-quality randomized clinicals trials showed significantly better improvement with glucocorticoids and more rapid recovery of nerve function. A randomized controlled trial (RCT) of 496 patients in four treatment limbs showed benefit of prednisolone versus placebo alone, antiviral therapy alone, or combination therapy. This study also showed improved synkinesis and autonomic dysfunction. The number of people needed to be treated (NNT) with steroids to prevent one person from having facial paresis, synkinesis, or autonomic disturbance is 10.

One study found no difference in recovery of nerve function between patients treated with acyclovir (Zovirax)[1], steroids, and physiotherapy. In a Cochrane review of 10 studies, there was no consensus on the optimal antiviral dosing used for combination therapy (Figure 2).

For the reactivation of latent viral infection hypothesis, combination therapy with oral corticosteroids and antivirals leads to a lower rate of synkinesis (NNT = 12). In three trials in patients with severe facial nerve palsy (HB V and VI), there was no difference between combined treatment (steroids

[1] Not FDA approved for this indication.

TABLE 1 House-Brachmann Facial Palsy Grading

GRADE	RESTING SYMMETRY	FOREHEAD	EYE	MOUTH
I	Normal			
II (mild)	Normal	Good function	Complete closure, little effort	Slight asymmetry, little effort
III (moderate)	Normal	Slight function	Complete closure, maximum effort	Slight asymmetry, maximum effort
IV (moderate)	Normal	No function	Incomplete closure, maximum effort	Asymmetry, maximum effort
V (severe)	Asymmetry	No function	Incomplete closure, maximum effort	Slight function, maximum effort
VI (severe)	Total paralysis			

The House-Brackmann facial palsy grading is the most commonly used, in which HB I is normal movement and HB VI is complete loss of forehead, eye, and mouth movement. Other grading systems include the Sunnybrook scale and eFACE—a smartphone app with high test-retest reliability that provides real-time video examination of a patient's facial function. The patient-rated outcome measure Facial Disability Index Score and Stennert Index are also used.

Medication	Dosing	Renal	Liver	Adverse Effects
Valacyclovir (Valtrex)[1]	Adults & children >12 years: 1 g tid for 7 days	CrCl <10 mL/min 500 mg qd	None	GI upset, headache, dizziness, elevated LFTs, aplastic anemia
Prednisone[1]	Adults: 60 mg qd for 5 days, then 40 mg qd for 5 days Children: 2 mg/kg qd for 7–10 days		Undefined	Headache, jitters, edema, hyperglycemia, elevated BP

[1]Not FDA approved for this indication.

Figure 2 Standard therapy with precautions and adverse effects for adults and children. *BP*, Blood pressure; *GI*, gastrointestinal; *LFTs*, liver function tests.

and antivirals) and glucocorticoid monotherapy. If the cause is zoster oticus (Ramsay Hunt syndrome), treat urgently with acyclovir (Zovirax) 800 mg PO five times per day for 7 days, valacyclovir (Valtrex) 1000 mg three times a day for 7 days, or famciclovir (Famvir) 500 mg three times a day for 7 days. Antiviral monotherapy has limited effectiveness regardless of the HB grading.

Corneal care with dexpanthenol (Panthoderm) ophthalmic ointment[2] and artificial tears is useful, with nocturnal moisture-retaining eye protection for full paralysis. Pregnant patients should be treated as other patients, with early corticosteroids.

In one small 4-week pilot study (N = 7), injecting stem cells (extracellular vesicles containing messenger RNA [mRNA], micro-RNA, and other bioactive compounds decrease inflammation) into and around the affected facial nerve several times over 4-week periods in patients with recalcitrant disease showed a decrease in HB scores in all patients.

Nonmedical

PT should be offered to patients with severe facial paralysis or persistent symptoms beyond 3 to 4 months. An extended systemic review of RCTs found positive impact (improved facial function and patient-reported outcomes) of facial exercise therapy for facial nerve paralysis in four of seven high-quality trials. However, this varied in the level of effectiveness based on the onset of treatment after onset of the facial palsy and the severity of the palsy. PT is effective early in combination with other treatment. Mime therapy—self-massage, relaxation exercises, breathing exercises coordinated with facial movements, pronunciation of letters and words in 10 sessions of 45 minutes

over 4 weeks—also is of some benefit in patients with persistent symptoms.

Surgical

Surgical decompression is reserved for recalcitrant cases only, due to small study size and low certainty from RCTs on surgery for early management of Bell palsy. Even then, in severe cases, surgical decompression did not improve prognosis compared with conservative treatment alone.

Prognosis

Multivariable logistic regression analysis in one study found favorable outcomes were more likely to occur in patients under age 40, HB grading I or II, well-controlled blood pressure, absence of diabetes, and presence of good electrodiagnostic nerve function. According to the National Capital Nervous Facialis Study (NCNFS), 70% of adults recover in 6 to 9 months without therapy, whereas 4% have severe synkinesis from abnormal reinnervation. A study of data from 17 hospitals highlights the potential role of machine learning models in predicting the difference in outcomes between use of prednisolone, acyclovir, both, or neither.

Monitoring and Complications

HB grading should be used to monitor patient quality of life in persistent cases. Inability to fully close the lid can lead to corneal ulceration and permanent visual impairment. When damaged neurons regenerate, they do so making aberrant connections, for example, connecting to the lacrimal gland instead of the salivary gland, thus causing tearing while eating. These are called crocodile tears. Additionally, persistent abnormal facial motion or synkinesis is permanent in one in three patients. There is a 4% higher cumulated risk of nonhemorrhagic stroke in patients with Bell palsy over the general population (1.6%). Use of prednisolone can cause hyperglycemia and should be used judiciously while treating patients with type 2 diabetes.

References

Dalrymple SN, Row JH, Gazewood J: Bell palsy: rapid evidence review, *Am Fam Physician* 107(4):415–420, 2023.

Dreschnack PA, Belshaku I: Treatment of idiopathic facial paralysis (Bell's palsy) and secondary facial paralysis with extracellular vesicles: a pilot safety study, *BMC Neurol* 23(1):342, 2023. https://doi.org/10.1186/s12883-023-03400-6.

Ildiko G, Madhok VB, Daly F, Frank S: Antiviral treatment for Bell's palsy (idiopathic facial paralysis), *Cochrane Database Syst Rev* 9(9), 2019. https://doi.org/10.1002/14651858.CD001869.pub9.

Gupta KK, Balai E, Tang HT, Ahmed AA, Doshi JR: Comparing the use of high-dose to standard-dose corticosteroids for the treatment of Bell's palsy in adults-a systematic review and meta-analysis, *Otol Neurotol* 44(4):310–316, 2023. https://doi.org/10.1097/MAO.0000000000003823.

Heckmann JG, Urban PP, Pitz S, Guntinas-Lichius O, Gágyor I: The diagnosis and treatment of idiopathic facial paresis (Bell's palsy), *Dtsch Arztebl Int* 116(41):692–702, 2019. https://doi.org/10.3238/arztebl.2019.0692.

Khan AJ, Szczepura A, Palmer S, et al: Physical therapy for facial nerve paralysis (Bell's palsy): an updated and extended systematic review of the evidence for facial exercise therapy, *Clin Rehabil* 36(11):1424–1449, 2022. https://doi.org/10.1177/02692155221110727.

Luo JT, Hung YC, Chen GJ, Lin YS: Predicting early treatment effectiveness in bell's palsy using machine learning: a focus on corticosteroids and antivirals, *Int J Gen Med* 17:5163–5174, 2024. https://doi.org/10.2147/IJGM.S488418, PMID: 39539927; PMCID: PMC11559179.

Menchetti I, McAllister K, Walker D, Donnan PT: Surgical interventions for the early management of Bell's palsy, *Cochrane Database Syst Rev* 1(1), 2021. https://doi.org/10.1002/14651858.CD007468.pub4.

Neiderman NC, Narin N, Netanyahu Y, et al: Bell's palsy and pregnancy: incidence, comorbidities and complications. A meta-analysis and systematic review of the literature, *Clin Otolaryngol* 48(4):576–586, 2023. https://doi.org/10.1111/coa.14042.

Rajangam J, Lakshmanan AP, Rao KU, et al: Bell palsy: facts and current research perspectives, *CNS Neurol Disord: Drug Targets* 23(2):203–214, 2024. https://doi.org/10.2174/1871527322666230321120618.

Rim HS, Byun JY, Kim SH, Yeo SG: Optimal Bell's palsy treatment: steroids, antivirals, and a timely and personalized approach, *J Clin Med* 13(1):51, 2023. https://doi.org/10.3390/jcm13010051.

ALZHEIMER'S DISEASE

Method of
Katarzyna Wilamowska, MD, PhD; and Janice E. Knoefel, MD, MPH

CURRENT DIAGNOSIS

- There is insufficient evidence on benefits versus harms in screening for cognitive impairment in older adults (Category I).
- Cognitive screening tools can be useful along with an overall patient assessment (see Table 3).
- Rule out reversible causes of dementia with blood work and imaging (see "Diagnostic Evaluation" section)
- Diagnosis of Alzheimer's disease (AD) is clinical, but consider referral to dementia specialist if there are ambiguous findings.

CURRENT THERAPY

- There is no known cure.
- Acetylcholinesterase inhibitors and *N*-methyl-D-aspartic acid (NMDA) receptor antagonists temporarily improve day-to-day function but do not slow the progression of neuronal cell death.

- Since the early 2020s, disease-slowing treatment for mild AD has become available but carries a high burden of diagnostic testing, multiple IV infusions, need for intensive side effect monitoring and moderate risks of hemorrhage, stroke, and death.
- Behavioral symptoms of AD are best treated with psychosocial interventions; use pharmacology as a last resort.
- Caregiver training and support is extremely important; it will impact the health of patient and caregiver alike.
- High caregiver burden can result in early institutionalization and poor patient outcomes.

Alzheimer's disease (AD) is considered the most common (60%–80%) individual cause of major neurocognitive disorders (NCDs), previously known as dementia. As of 2021, more than one in nine (11.3%) Americans aged 65 or older are living with AD. By 2050, the number of Americans living with AD will double to a projected 12.7 million.

AD is not a result of normal aging (Table 1). There is no cure and, after a prolonged debilitating disease process, AD is fatal. Although we continue to learn more about the pathophysiology of AD, it is known to have indolent asymptomatic deposition of abnormally folded extracellular amyloid-β (Aβ) and clumping tau proteins in the brain that may precede symptoms by more than 20 years. As the disease progresses, amyloid plaques, neurofibrillary tangles, and brain inflammation develop, culminating in neuronal cell death. Research is not yet able to accurately predict the appearance of cognitive symptoms based on these processes.

As with many disorders listed in the *Diagnostic and Statistical Manual*, Fifth Edition (DSM-5), dementia carries with it a stigma that may lead patients, family, and friends to avoid or reject the diagnosis. Conversely, a patient with AD, due to the cognitive impact of the disease, may not be aware of their deficits. Diagnosis of AD is often delayed (especially in unbefriended older adults) until the inability for independent living and self-care, usually seen as reduction in instrumental activities of daily living (IADLs), brings the patient to the attention of medical professionals.

Screening

Screening for cognitive impairment in older adults continues to be controversial. The US Department of Veterans Affairs, the Canadian Task Force on Preventive Health Care (CTFPHC), the National Institute for Health Care and Excellence (NICE), and the Royal Australian College of General Practitioners (RACGP) recommend against screening for cognitive impairment of asymptomatic older adults. The European Federation of Neurological Societies (EFNS) has no recommendations for asymptomatic individuals, and the US Preventive Services Task Force (USPSTF) states that the current evidence is insufficient to assess the balance of benefits and harms of screening for cognitive impairment in older adults. However, all these organizations encourage screening, workup, and referrals for cognitive impairment in patients where memory or other cognitive concerns are detected by the patient, knowledgeable informant, or medical practitioner.

On the other hand, the International Association of Gerontology and Geriatrics (IAGG) recommends screening for cognitive impairment of patients with known risk factors for dementia. The Gerontological Society of America (GSA) and the Alzheimer's Association recommend regular screening for cognitive impairment through the Medicare Annual Wellness Visit with coverage for "detection of cognitive impairment" approved by Medicare since 2011.

Risk Factors and Prevention

The strongest risk factors for AD are unmodifiable: age and genetics.

AD is not a normal part of aging, and aging alone does not cause AD. The percentage of Americans with AD increases with age, with the prevalence of AD in those aged 65 to 74 at 5.3%, 75 to 84 at 13.8%, and 85 or older at 34.6%.

TABLE 1 — Examples of Changes With Normal Aging Versus Alzheimer's Disease

COGNITIVE DOMAIN AFFECTED	NORMAL AGING	ALZHEIMER'S DISEASE
Learning and Memory	Sometimes forgetting names or appointments but remembering them later	Forgetting important dates or events Asking for the same information over and over
Executive Function	Occasional error in balancing a checkbook, omission of a recipe ingredient, taking the wrong turn while driving, making a bad decision once in a while	Difficulty completing daily tasks, trouble driving to a familiar location, managing a budget, or remembering rules to a favorite game Poor judgment when dealing with money; victim of financial fraud Less attention to personal grooming
Complex Attention	Misplacing things occasionally but able to find them by retracing their steps	Putting items in unusual places, losing things, unable to retrace steps to find them, may accuse others of stealing
Language	Sometimes having trouble finding the right word	Trouble following or joining a conversation May struggle with vocabulary: word finding, calling things by the wrong name
Perceptual-motor	Vision changes related to cataracts, glaucoma, age-related macular degeneration	Difficulty reading, judging distances, determining color/contrast No longer knows how to use daily household objects (e.g., hairbrush, TV remote, phone)
Social Cognition	Sometimes feeling weary of work, family, and social obligations Developing very specific ways of doing things and getting upset at change in routine	Decreased participation in hobbies, social activities, work projects, or sports Changes in mood and personality; confused, suspicious, depressed, fearful, or anxious Easily upset

Several identified genes increase the risk of AD, and people with a first-degree relative (parent or sibling) with AD have a 2.5 times lifetime risk of developing AD compared with the general population. AD with mendelian family history is rare and is more likely in early-onset Alzheimer's disease (EOAD, symptom onset before age 65). Of families with EOAD, 86% have a mutation in one of three causative genes: PSEN1 (chromosome 14; most frequent), APP (chromosome 21; important in trisomy 21 populations), and PSEN2 (chromosome 1; extremely rare). An estimated 5% to 10% of all AD cases are EOAD.

In late-onset AD, homozygote APOE4 gene has the strongest impact on risk, but by no means is it a guarantee of disease development. In fact, since the early 2010s, there has been credible evidence that lifestyle modifications can decrease the impact of this vulnerability gene marker. Of note, studies of racial or ethnic backgrounds on AD development are inconclusive and, at best, illustrate nonbiologic determinants of health.

Modifiable risk factors include optimizing cardiovascular health, preventing brain cell injuries, decreasing harmful substance exposure, and promoting protective behaviors.

Optimizing cardiovascular health involves controlling hypertension while monitoring for and correcting adverse effects such as cerebral hypoperfusion, and stroke, controlling hyperlipidemia and diabetes with appropriate treatment, encouraging smoking cessation, and recognizing and treating insomnia and obstructive sleep apnea. These are generally considered to be "vascular risks."

Preventing brain cell injury starts in early life with consistent helmet use, avoidance of sports-related concussions, and with counseling and treatment of substance-use disorders. Recognition and treatment of obstructive sleep apnea can prevent injury to brain cells.

The lifetime dose of over-the-counter (OTC) and prescribed medications with potent anticholinergic action have been shown to increase risk for dementia. Reduction and/or cessation in the use of these medications must be encouraged. Frequently implicated are first-generation antihistamines, overactive bladder antimuscarinics, muscle relaxants, and tricyclic antidepressants. Many persons unwittingly use first-generation antihistamines for years in sleep-inducing OTC medications, unaware of the risk to cognitive function.

Protection includes ameliorating sensory impairment (vision and hearing loss), treating mood disorders, encouraging a healthy diet and exercise, and enhancing brain plasticity in cognitive and social functions. All these behaviors have a transient effect that diminishes once the intervention is abandoned.

Diagnosis

Diagnostic Criteria

Diagnosis of dementia involves meeting the diagnostic criteria for an all-cause major neurocognitive disorder, which necessitates the following:

- Evidence of cognitive decline from previous functional and performance baseline in a **minimum of two cognitive domains** (complex attention, executive function, learning and memory, language, perceptual motor, or social cognition)
- Cognitive deficits interfere with patient's ability to function independently
- Deficits cannot be better explained by delirium, affective disturbances, or other disorders

AD diagnosis is clinically classified as **probable** AD or **possible** AD dementia. Core clinical criteria for probable AD dementia are the following:

- Insidious onset
- Clear-cut history of worsening cognition
- Initial and most prominent cognitive deficits in one of the categories:
  - **Amnestic presentation:** Most common. Presents with impairment in learning and recall of recently learned information. Deficits in other cognitive domains could be present.
  - **Nonamnestic presentation:**
    - **Language presentation:** Deficits in word finding and verbal communication dominate, but deficits in other cognitive domains should be present.
    - **Visuospatial presentation:** Deficits are in spatial cognition, including object agnosia, impaired face recognition, simultanagnosia, alexia and path-finding. Deficits in other cognitive domains should be present.
    - **Executive dysfunction:** The most prominent deficits are impaired reasoning, judgment, and problem solving. Deficits in other cognitive domains should be present.

The diagnosis of probable AD dementia should *not* be applied when there is evidence of other major NCDs such as vascular dementia (VaD), Lewy body dementia (LBD), frontotemporal dementia, primary progressive aphasia, or other active neurologic disease (e.g., Parkinson disease), nonneurologic comorbidity, or medication use causing substantial cognitive effect (see "Differential Diagnoses" section).

Possible AD dementia diagnosis is applied in circumstances of atypical disease course that fulfills the aforementioned core diagnostic criteria or in an etiologically mixed presentation.

Differential Diagnoses

The diagnosis of AD must be differentiated from other states of altered cognition (Table 2). Furthermore, in older adults, the presence of delirium, postoperative cognitive dysfunction, post–COVID-19 "brain fog," mild cognitive impairment, or new onset anxiety or mood disorder may be a first sign of future development of major neurocognitive disorder and should trigger closer follow-up.

- Delirium: Develops over a short period of time (hours or days), with change from baseline involving fluctuating levels of attention and awareness throughout the day. Level of activity may range from hyperactive to hypoactive (often underdiagnosed), or mixed. Delirium may be incited by acute infection, change in medical condition, injury, substance intoxication or withdrawal (e.g., drug abuse, OTC or prescribed medications), toxin exposure, or multiple etiologies. Resolution may be acute with correction of underlying cause, but symptoms may persist for weeks or months.
- Postoperative cognitive dysfunction: Develops after receiving anesthesia. Although multifactorial in origin, it is thought to be triggered by the immune/inflammatory response to surgery. Typically affects cognitive domains of learning and memory, and executive function. Resolution is typical within 6 months.
- Post–COVID-19 "brain fog": Develops after COVID-19 infection of any severity, including asymptomatic positive tests. Current presumed etiologies include multifactorial delirium, viral-induced immune and inflammatory response, SARS-CoV-2–induced coagulopathy, and direct viral invasion of the central nervous system (CNS). Some cases resolve within days or weeks; others have been persistent and may indicate a new cognitive baseline for the patient. There is some emerging evidence of hypometabolic lesions of the brain that can be visualized with positron emission tomography (PET) scanning.
- Mild cognitive impairment (MCI): Insidious onset of symptoms of **minor** neurocognitive disorder where cognitive impairment **does not** interfere with ability to function independently. May affect any cognitive domain and presage development of major neurocognitive disorder. Symptoms may not progress and do not resolve unless substance/medication induced.
- Anxiety or mood disorder: Onset is often insidious but may be acute. If new onset of anxiety or depression occurs, it may be the first symptom of a major neurocognitive disorder. Rather than a new onset of mental disorder, such as bipolar disorder or attention-deficit/hyperactivity disorder (ADHD), consider chronic undiagnosed cognitive disorder with atypical presentation or "new" presentation due to loss of compensatory mechanisms. Resolution depends on appropriate recognition and cognitive/pharmacologic treatment.
- Substance use disorder: Onset may be acute or progressive. Etiology is typically from chronic use but may be brought to medical attention due to discontinuation or overdose. Substances typically indicated are alcohol, stimulants, marijuana, and opioids. Impact is primarily to executive function, memory, and learning domains. Complete resolution of symptoms can occur with prolonged abstinence from substance and correction of nutritional deficiencies, but masked VaD may be present as sequelae of chronic substance use. Cannot exclude that the presence of neurocognitive changes incited substance use disorder or its escalation.

- Major NCDs that are not AD: All are progressive and do not resolve. Treatment varies with category and can, in fact, worsen cognitive and behavioral outcomes if misdiagnosed. For brevity, only the most common major NCDs are listed in full detail.
  - VaD: Presentation may affect any cognitive domain, although executive function domain deficits tend to be favored, while memory may be initially preserved. Onset of impairment appears to be abrupt, especially in patients with cardiovascular risk factors. Physical examination findings are focal in nature (but may be subtle) and often include motor function difficulties, especially slow gait or poor balance. Five percent to 10% of all dementias are of vascular etiology alone.
  - LBD: An umbrella term for NCDs due to misfolded α-synuclein deposition including dementia with Lewy bodies (DLB) and Parkinson disease dementia (PDD). Presentation characteristic of rapid eye movement (REM) sleep disturbances (acting out dreams), visual hallucinations, and marked visuospatial impairment. Parkinsonian motor symptoms may or may not be present at time of diagnosis (see Chapter 173 on Parkinson disease). Patients in this group are often exquisitely sensitive to neuroleptic medications precipitating marked confusion or delirium, and rapidly deteriorating balance and gait. Five percent of all patients with dementia are of DLB etiology alone.
  - Frontotemporal lobar degeneration (FTLD): Group of disorders that includes behavioral variant FTLD, primary progressive aphasia, Pick disease, corticobasal degeneration, and progressive supranuclear palsy. Pathologic changes involve intracellular tau and TDP-43 protein inclusions preferentially in frontal and temporal lobes leading to marked atrophy. Presentation encompasses marked changes in personality and behavior and/or difficulty producing or comprehending language. Symptoms may worsen when treated with anti-Alzheimer's medications.
  - Mixed: Presents as a combination of component NCDs with AD, VaD, and, to a lesser degree, LBD. Increases in likelihood with age, with highest occurrence in the 85 years and older age group. Over 50% of people with dementia have evidence of more than one type of pathology on postmortem examination.
- Other diagnoses to consider include traumatic brain injury, chronic traumatic encephalopathy syndrome, prion disease, Huntington disease, human immunodeficiency virus (HIV) infection, neurosyphilis, cryptococcosis, brain tumor, subdural hematoma, normal-pressure hydrocephalus, hypoxia secondary to heart failure, hypothyroidism, hypercalcemia, hypoglycemia, temporal arteritis, systemic lupus erythematosus, hepatic or renal failure, metabolic conditions, epilepsy, multiple sclerosis, and severe vitamin B_{12} deficiency.

Diagnostic Evaluation

History

Focused history is needed from the patient and at least one knowledgeable informant. Current cognitive and functional difficulties should be discussed, as well as fluctuation of symptoms. Behavior linked to stress, fatigue, or being away from a patient's normal surroundings should also be understood and may clue the clinician into diagnosis and treatment needs.

A thorough medication review should be performed with focus on adverse medication effects, goals of care, and deprescribing where possible. Supplements, OTC medications, and herbal remedies need to be evaluated in a nonjudgmental fashion. Reviewing current and past substance use at the same time may reveal more information than if asked separately.

Timeline of the start of functional decline generally precedes presentation to provider by several years. This may be elicited by asking about anecdotes that may have seemed funny or odd at the time (e.g., "Remember when Mom was making her specialty dish and forgot part of the recipe?" or "Remember when Dad took a long time to drive home, even though he was 5 minutes away?").

COGNITIVE DISORDER	ONSET	ETIOLOGY	CHARACTERISTICS SPECIFIC TO DISORDER	TIME TO RESOLUTION
Delirium	Acute	Multifactorial	Fluctuating levels of attention and awareness	Days, weeks, months
Postoperative cognitive dysfunction	Immediately after anesthesia	Multifactorial Immune/inflammatory response to surgery	Memory and executive function domains most affected	Typically within 6 months
Post–COVID-19 "brain fog"	Positive COVID-19 infection	Multifactorial Viral-induced inflammation Viral-induced coagulopathy Viral invasion of CNS	May affect any cognitive domain	Weeks, months, or persistent
Mild cognitive impairment (MCI)	Insidious	Multifactorial May be reversible if due to substance or medication intoxication Amnestic most common	May affect any cognitive domains; not severe enough to interfere with independent function	Resolves after substance/ medication cessation, or persistent
Anxiety or mood disorder	Chronic or new onset	If new onset, consider prodromal neurocognitive disorder or atypical presentation of previously undiagnosed anxiety/ mood disorder	Depression: "pseudodementia" may appear to affect multiple cognitive domains, but upon closer evaluation cognition changes are due to depression Anxiety: suspiciousness, restlessness, insomnia, fearfulness	May improve with combination of cognitive therapy and appropriate medications; recalcitrant disorders may benefit from ECT
Substance use disorder	Progressive due to use, or acute due to overdose or cessation of substance	Alcohol-related brain damage Chronic stimulant use disorder Chronic marijuana use disorder Chronic opioid use disorder	Memory and learning Executive function domains most commonly affected May have VaD component	May improve with cessation of substance and/or repleting nutritional deficiencies, or persistent

Major Neurocognitive Disorders

COGNITIVE DISORDER	ONSET	ETIOLOGY	CHARACTERISTICS SPECIFIC TO DISORDER	TIME TO RESOLUTION
Alzheimer's disease (AD)	Insidious, most common individual cause of dementia	Misfolded amyloid-β and tau protein deposition leading to neuronal death	Short-term memory loss, language, visuospatial, or executive function most impacted	Progressive
Lewy body dementia (LBD): umbrella term for dementia with Lewy bodies and Parkinson disease dementia	Insidious or pseudoacute in the setting of sleep deprivation	Misfolded α-synuclein (Lewy bodies) deposition in substantia nigra and cortex leading to degradation of dopaminergic neurons	Visual hallucinations, REM sleep disorders; may have bradykinesia, rigidity, or gait changes (see Chapter 173 on Parkinson disease) Very sensitive to neuroleptic medications	Progressive
Frontotemporal lobar degeneration (FTLD)	Insidious, symptoms develop earlier in life than AD	Tau and TDP-43 protein inclusions in frontal and temporal lobes Most common cause of dementia in people younger than 60	Behavioral, personality, language changes; memory typically preserved in early disease May have worsening symptoms when treated with cholinesterase inhibitors or NMDA antagonists	Progressive
Vascular dementia (VaD)	Stepwise progression	Cardiovascular risk factors, strokes, infarcts	May affect any cognitive domains; focal findings or gait/balance changes on examination	Progressive
Mixed dementia	Insidious, increases with age	Commonly a combination AD and VaD but can have LBD components	Mixed characteristics of component disorders	Progressive

CNS, Central nervous system; *ECT,* electroconvulsive therapy; *NMDA,* N-methyl-ᴅ-aspartic acid; *REM,* rapid eye movement.

TABLE 3 Brief List of Self-Administered and Office Screening Tools for Evaluation of Suspected Major Neurocognitive Disorders and Caregiver Burden

TOOL	PREVISIT OR TIME TO ADMINISTER IN OFFICE	PREFERRED PERSON TO ANSWER	COGNITIVE DOMAINS EVALUATED	DESCRIPTION
IADL	Previsit / <5 min	Patient	Executive function, apraxia, agnosia	Instrumental activities of daily living
ADL	Previsit / <5 min	Patient	Executive function, apraxia, agnosia	Activities of daily living
AD8	Previsit / <5 min	Informant	Memory, executive function, apraxia, agnosia	Good at eliciting early cognitive changes in a variety of dementias; asks informant about judgment, less interest in hobbies, repeats things, trouble using tools, forgets month or year, finances, trouble remembering appointments or daily things
GPCOG	Previsit / <5 min	Patient and Informant	Memory, executive function, aphasia	Recall, orientation, recent news recall; patient questionnaire is paired with an informant questionnaire that asks about memory, finances, wordfinding, ADLs
Short (16 questions) or full (26 questions) IQCODE	Previsit / >10 min	Informant	Memory, executive function, apraxia, agnosia	Asks informant about changes in cognitive function, physical function, patient personality, and behavior
Mini-Cog	<5 min	Patient	Memory, executive function, apraxia	Three-item recall plus clock drawing
MIS	<5 min	Patient	Memory	Four-item recall
SLUMS	6–10 min	Patient	Memory, executive function, aphasia, apraxia, agnosia	Orientation, five-item recall, math, animals, attention, clock, figures, story
MOCA: may require extra training and licensing	6–10 min	Patient	Memory, executive function, aphasia, apraxia, agnosia	Small trails B, copy figure, clock, naming, verbal fluency, five-word recall, similarities, orientation, attention
Trail making tests (TMT)	<5 min	Patient	Executive function	Older patients with a TMT-A $\geq$ 54 seconds or a TMT-B $\geq$ 150 seconds have a threefold (95% confidence interval, 1.3–7.0) increased risk of performing poorly during driving
Zarit Burden Interview	Previsit / 22 questions	Caregiver	Measures perceived social, physical, financial, and emotional burden	Higher scores indicate greater caregiver burden
Revised Memory and Behavior Problems Checklist	Previsit / 24 questions	Caregiver	Focused and caregiver reactions to problematic behaviors in patients with dementia	Higher scores indicate greater caregiver burden

AD8, Ascertain Dementia 8-Item Informant Questionnaire; *ADL*, activities of daily living; *GPCOG*, General Practitioner Assessment of Cognition; *IADL*, instrumental activities of daily living; *IQCODE*, Informant Questionnaire on Cognitive Decline in the Elderly; *MIS*, Memory Impairment Screen; *MoCA*, Montreal Cognitive Assessment; *SLUMS*, Saint Louis University Mental Status Examination.

Any medical illnesses or conditions that may have triggered the decline should be elucidated (e.g., "Mom has never been the same since that infection last year" or "Dad woke up one morning and couldn't see out of his right eye, but he didn't mention it until a few weeks later as it didn't bother him").

NCDs expose the affected individual to multiple safety concerns, and these must be discussed to detect current problems, to avoid future adverse events, and to plan for the future. Triggers for further evaluation include "close calls" for motor vehicle accidents, falls, getting lost or locked out, or falling victim to scams.

Cognitive Status Examination

Although qualitative impressions of cognitive status are helpful in raising suspicions, quantitative evaluation of cognitive status is needed for diagnosis and for tracking decline. No single screening tool evaluates all cognitive domains: learning and memory, executive function, complex attention, language, perceptual-motor/visuospatial skills, and social cognition. With the limited time of a primary care visit, one is compelled to leverage previsit and office waiting times for completion of clinical questionnaires by patient and informant before the appointment, as well as some in-clinic screening tools that may be administered by a medical assistant, nurse, or medical provider (Table 3). These screening tools may aid in the clinical decision making of the provider but need to be interpreted with caution. For example, there may be cases where the patient passes a cognitive screen but fails an entire cognitive domain within the screen, warranting further evaluation.

Physical Examination

The neurologic examination should attempt to rule out Alzheimer's dementia with findings indicative of other major neurocognitive etiologies. Asymmetry in sensation/motor/strength/reflexes is suggestive of VaD. Tremor and bradykinesia hint at Parkinson disease syndromes. Abnormalities of eye movement in vertical gaze may signify progressive supranuclear palsy. Peripheral neuropathy, although most likely secondary to diabetes, may indicate B_{12} deficiency, hypothyroidism, alcoholism, or neurosyphilis.

Laboratory Testing
Reversible or treatable causes of neurocognitive impairment may be revealed by checking complete blood count (CBC); electrolytes including blood glucose, renal, liver and thyroid function; syphilis; HIV; and vitamins B_{12} (cobalamin), B_9 (folate), B_1 (thiamine), and D (calciferol).

If EOAD is suspected based on family history and early age of symptom presentation, consider genetic counseling before testing for PSEN1, PSEN2, or APP. There is currently no clinical diagnostic benefit to testing for the APOE4 gene; however, this should be tested if antiamyloid infusion therapy is considered.

Neuroimaging
Although neuroimaging research continues to move forward on describing brain imaging changes and correlation to the development of major NCDs, this does not promise a diagnosis from structural neuroimaging alone. At present, there is some controversy as to whether clinical neuroimaging is needed in routine cognitive workups, but we recommend routine brain magnetic resonance imaging (MRI) to screen for and rule out stroke, tumors, hematomas, or normal pressure hydrocephalus, and perhaps suggest FTLD with focal cortical atrophy.

Of note: There can be significant crossover in presentation between FTLD and AD. As such, Medicare provides conditional reimbursement for PET for brain amyloid.

When to Refer
Ultimately, the diagnosis of AD in the primary care setting is done clinically after ruling out the aforementioned differential diagnoses, with more ambiguous cases referred to dementia specialists including geriatricians, geriatric psychiatrists, neurologists, or neuropsychologists. If finding a specialist nearby proves difficult, consider directing your efforts to the closest Alzheimer's Disease Research Center (ADRC).

Treatment
Counseling
AD is a life-altering diagnosis. Although many patients have heard of AD, they may not know of the progressive nature and likely debilitation ahead of them. While the patient is decisional, planning for future decisions may be reassuring to both patient and families. It is essential to discuss protection of themselves, their assets, and their wishes pertaining to current and future management of financial, legal, and healthcare concerns.

Caregiver Support
On average, a person diagnosed with AD survives 3 to 11 years after diagnosis; some may live 20 years or more. The progressive dependence of patients with AD brings to focus the importance of their caregivers. More than 11 million family members, friends, and neighbors provide care for people with dementia. They provide emotional support, ensure a safe care environment, assist in household tasks and personal care, provide health and medical care at home, navigate healthcare systems, serve as surrogate decision makers, arrange services of community-based organizations, and provide needed information during patient medical and nursing visits.

Eighty-three percent of caregivers are family, friends, and unpaid caregivers, often undertaking this role on the foundation of love or obligation to the care recipient. Most begin this role without adequate training or support. This is not without cost: caregivers report physical, emotional, and financial strain, with one in four finding it difficult to take care of their own health. Increased caregiver burden correlates with decreases in care

recipient quality of life, hastens placement, and increases risk of hospitalization and mortality. (See Table 3 for tools to evaluate caregiver burden.)

Management of Cognitive Symptoms
Until June 2021, Food and Drug Administration (FDA)-approved medications for treatment of AD would only ameliorate symptoms, not alter the progression of the disease. There are two classes of these medications: acetylcholinesterase inhibitors (AChEIs) and N-methyl-D-aspartic acid (NMDA)-receptor antagonists (Table 4).

AChEIs increase the available acetylcholine between neuronal synapses, enhancing neurotransmission. These medications are most effective in mild to moderate AD. Donepezil (Aricept), rivastigmine (Exelon), and galantamine (Razadyne) are AChEIs currently approved by the FDA. Historically, the first FDA-approved medication for treating AD was tacrine, but this was withdrawn later due to hepatotoxicity and the advent of safer AChEIs.

NMDA-receptor antagonists function by inhibiting the excitation of NMDA receptors by the neurotransmitter glutamate, preventing influx of Ca^{2+}. This inhibition has the effect of both decreasing excitotoxicity of the neurons involved (reducing symptoms) and restoring the amyloid-β induced Ca^{2+} imbalance (potential neuroprotective role).

A new class of medications, distinct from the symptomatic therapies discussed previously, became available to select patients in 2021: monoclonal antibodies directed against amyloid. As the accumulation of amyloid beta plaques in the brain is part of the AD disease pathologic process, there is hope that this new class of drug can provide clinical benefit. This class of infusible medications in meant to be time limited and not indefinite. As more research and real-world use data is collected, guidelines may change.

The first of this class was aducanumab (Aduhelm), a recombinant human immunoglobulin gamma 1 (IgG1) monoclonal antibody directed against aggregated soluble and insoluble forms of amyloid beta. This medication was withdrawn from the market by its manufacturer in 2024 as other medications in this class entered the marketplace. A second drug in this class, lecanemab (Leqembi) was traditionally FDA approved in July 2023 for the treatment of AD initiated in early AD (mild cognitive impairment due to AD or mild AD dementia). The third antiamyloid monoclonal antibody therapy is donanemab (Kinsula), which was approved in July 2024. Approval of these medications remain controversial because the amyloid hypothesis of AD is only part of the complex physiology of this condition. Medications in this class require monthly or twice-monthly infusions/injections and have very significant symptom and MRI monitoring guidelines for use. Treatments are approved for 9 months (twice monthly for lecanemab) or for 6, 12, and 18 months once monthly (donanemab) dependent on appearance of amyloid on follow-up amyloid scan.

Numerous vitamins and supplements have been studied in prevention and treatment of cognitive behaviors in AD; however, the evidence of benefit is inconclusive and not subject to FDA scrutiny.

Multiple studies have shown aerobic exercise has a positive overall effect on cognitive function and may even slow the progression of AD. Cognitive stimulation (engagement in a range of activities aimed at general enhancement of cognitive and social functioning) has also been shown to have beneficial effects on cognitive function, while music-based therapies and psychological treatment can improve symptoms of anxiety, depression, and quality of life in those with AD. Cognitive training (guided practice of standard tasks designed to engage particular cognitive functions with a range of difficulty levels to suit the individual's level of ability) has been shown to provide a few months of benefit to cognitive function.

Management of Behavioral Symptoms
Behavioral symptoms in AD are common reasons for acute care appointments, emergency department visits, or psychiatric admissions in persons with major NCDs. Although more difficult to implement, the most effective treatment is nonpharmacologic.

TABLE 4 FDA-Approved Medications for Treating Cognitive Symptoms of Alzheimer's Disease*

	DONEPEZIL (ARICEPT)		RIVASTIGMINE (EXELON)		GALANTAMINE (RAZADYNE)	MEMANTINE (NAMENDA)	COMBINED MEMANTINE-DONEPEZIL (NAMZARIC)
Stage of AD	Mild to moderate	Moderate to severe	Mild to moderate	Mild to moderate	Mild to moderate	Moderate to severe	Moderate to severe
Mechanism	AChEI					NMDA receptor antagonist	Shared characteristics of component medications
Route of administration	Tablet ODT	Tablet	Oral capsule Oral solution	Patch	Tablet XR tablet Oral solution	Tablet Oral solution	XR tablet
Doses	5 mg, 10 mg ODT: 5 mg, 10 mg Transdermal weekly patch (Adlarity): 5 mg/day, 10 mg/day	10 mg, 23 mg	1.5 mg, 3 mg, 4.5 mg, or 6 mg Oral sol: 2 mg/mL	Patch 4.6 mg/24 hr (9 mg rivastigmine) Patch 9.5 mg/24 hr (18 mg rivastigmine)	4 mg, 8 mg, 12 mg Oral sol: 4 mg/mL XR: 8 mg, 16 mg, 24 mg	5 mg, 10 mg Oral sol: 2 mg/mL XR: 7 mg, 14 mg, 21 mg, 28 mg	XR: 7 mg–10 mg, 14 mg–10 mg, 21 mg–10 mg, 28 mg–10 mg
Target daily dose	10 mg	23 mg	6 mg BID	9.5 mg/24 hours once daily	Tabs: 12 mg BID XR: 24 mg QD	10 mg XR: 28 mg	28 mg–10 mg
Renal impairment	No dose adjustment	No dose adjustment	May be able to tolerate lower doses	No dose adjustment	Do not exceed 16 mg/day; none if CrCl < 9 mL/min	5 mg BID XR: 14 mg	14 mg–10 mg
Hepatic impairment	Use with caution	Use with caution	May be able to tolerate lower doses	No dose adjustment	Do not exceed 16 mg/day	Use with caution	Use with caution
Frequency	Once daily	Once daily	BID	Daily	Varies	Once daily in evening	Once daily in evening
Minimum interval between dose increases	4–6 weeks between 5 mg and 10 mg	At least 3 months at 10 mg before increasing to 23 mg	2 weeks	4 weeks	4 weeks	1 week	1 week
Administration cautions		23 mg tablet should not be split, crushed, or chewed because this may increase its rate of absorption	Should be taken with meals	The patch should be replaced with a new one every 24 hr The same site should not be used within 14 days	Should be taken with meals	XR: do not divide, crush, or chew	Do not divide, crush or chew
Most common adverse effects	Nausea, diarrhea, insomnia, vomiting, muscle cramps, fatigue, and anorexia May cause bladder outflow obstructions		Nausea, vomiting, anorexia, dyspepsia, and asthenia	Nausea, vomiting and diarrhea	Nausea, vomiting, diarrhea, dizziness, headache, decreased appetite, and weight decreased May cause bladder outflow obstructions	Dizziness, headache, confusion, and constipation	Headache, diarrhea, dizziness May cause bladder outflow obstructions

*See chapter text for aducanumab commentary.
AChEI, Acetylcholinesterase inhibitor; AD, Alzheimer's disease; BID, twice daily; CrCl, creatinine clearance; NMDA, N-methyl-D-aspartic acid; ODT, orally disintegrating tablet.

TABLE 5	Initial Treatment of Common Behavioral Symptoms in Alzheimer's Disease			
BEHAVIORAL SYMPTOM	**CONSIDERATIONS**	**TREATMENT**	**FOLLOW-UP**	**CAUTION**
Agitation	Change in patient's environment (most common cause)	If possible, remove the new trigger. If not, caution 3–4 week adjustment period	1–2 weeks	Reassure caregiver and allow for more frequent contact
	Lack of caregiver training/ knowledge	Provide in office training on redirection, reassurance, de-escalation Alzheimer's Association offers free online classes on living with Alzheimer's disease for caregivers	1–2 weeks	Evaluate for caregiver strain as this will have lasting impact on both caregiver and patient health and may lead to early institutionalization of patient
	Unreported pain	Acetaminophen 500 mg daily Can slowly scale up to 1000 mg BID Use the lowest effective dose	3–4 weeks	Medication review of other APAP-containing medications; contraindicated in concurrent hepatic illness
	Infection	Determine source and treat appropriately	After treatment	Many common antibiotics can trigger behavioral issues; review Beers criteria and use with caution
	Drug reaction	Review medications with Beers criteria	1–2 weeks	Due to lower renal and hepatic clearances, drug effect may last longer than expected
Anxiety	Start at half of recommended adult dose, and taper slowly	Cognitive behavioral therapy, anxiolytics	3–4 weeks	Avoid benzodiazepines or sedative-hypnotics
Depression	Start at half of recommended adult dose, and taper slowly	Cognitive behavioral therapy, antidepressants	3–4 weeks	
Restlessness/ pacing	Ensure proper use of assistive devices or walking buddy	Create an environment that encourages safe walking or other forms of exercise If patient no longer mobilizes, consider fidget blanket	At next visit	
Anorexia/ cachexia	Due to AD progression: may have lost cognitive domains to prepare food, remember mealtimes, execute coordinated chew/ swallow control	Optimize social supports, deprescribe medications that interfere with eating, provide appealing food and feeding assistance	At next visit	Avoid appetite stimulants or high-calorie supplements Do not recommend percutaneous feeding
Insomnia	Wake-sleep cycle inversions are common in AD; patients have good sleep, just not at hours expected by caregiver	May be corrected with cognitive behavioral therapy, bright-light exposure during waking hours, increasing daytime activity, replacing caffeine with decaf, trial of melatonin[7]	At next visit	Avoid benzodiazepines or sedative-hypnotics
Aggression	See all preceding agitation sections	Apply all nonpharmacologic interventions possible As last resort consider AChEI, then antipsychotics/ anticonvulsants	1–2 weeks	Avoid benzodiazepines

[7]Available as dietary supplement.

AD, Alzheimer's disease; *AChEI*, acetylcholinesterase inhibitor; *APAP*, acetaminophen; *BID*, twice daily.

Some behavior disturbances are induced by brain changes due to AD. In early stages of the disease, these are repetition, wandering, and refusing assistance. In moderate AD, pacing, agitation, antisocial or oversexualized behavior, resistance to care, and aggression can be common. In late AD, resistance to care, physical aggression, and repetitive vocalizations such as moaning or screaming may appear. The disease process notwithstanding, the most common cause of new behavioral symptoms is an environmental trigger, either internal (e.g., infection, pain) or external (e.g., new housing, change in caregivers or daily routine). To manage the behavior, the trigger must be identified.

Patient-centered and adaptive dementia communications skills are key to solving most behavioral symptoms of AD: making eye contact before speaking, using simple language, speaking slowly and clearly, communicating empathy through actions (smiling), asking only one question at a time, and allowing adequate time for the patient to respond (Table 5).

Although it is appropriate to consider anxiolytics and antidepressants in the treatment of anxiety and depression associated with AD, the treatment of agitation and aggression is more nuanced. It is in these cases that we should strive for excellent individualized psychosocial care. Unfortunately, there are times when the patient's agitation and aggression can be disruptive to care and distressing to the caregiver, resulting in a request for medication to the medical provider. If this is the case for your patient, consider an AChEI as the initial prescription because this medication has been shown to have benefits for apathy, delusions, and purposeless motor behaviors. If a patient has been on maximal dose AChEI for some time and now has new behavioral symptoms, deprescribing should be considered as the AChEI action may have outlived its usefulness. At this time, and at all times in the care of persons with dementia, one very important consideration is the length and quality of restorative night-time sleep. This should be one the first and foremost symptoms for management at all stages of these illnesses.

If AChEIs are unsuccessful, antipsychotics (in order of trial: quetiapine [Seroquel][1], risperidone [Risperdal][1], olanzapine [Zyprexa][1]) or anticonvulsants (given in order of trial: carbamazepine [Tegretol][1], valproate [Depakene][1]) should be carefully considered, starting at half the adult dose and titrating slowly to effect or lack of tolerance to adverse reactions. Thorough documentation of behavioral issues triggering prescription and deprescription trials should be maintained for these medications. Note there is a strong national movement to decrease use of antipsychotics in dementia care, especially in nursing homes.

Monitoring

AD is a progressively debilitating neurocognitive disorder with the patient slowly losing the ability to accurately report symptoms or concerns and being increasingly dependent on the care of others. The Reisberg Functional Assessment Staging (FAST) scale was designed to reflect the progressive activity limitations of AD and has been well validated since its initial publication in 1988. Key points of the FAST scale are (1) it progresses through all steps in sequence, therefore out-of-sequence changes should trigger workup for non-AD causes; and (2) when a patient reaches stage 7, the patient is considered eligible for hospice benefits.

In addition to monitoring the patient's health and well-being, special attention must be paid to the caregiver's needs, signs of caregiver burnout, and, despite all best efforts of the caregiver, if the patient requires a higher level of care than can be provided in the current home care setting.

---

[1] Not FDA approved for this indication.

References

Bruijnen CJWH, Dijkstra BAG, Walvoort SJW, et al: Prevalence of cognitive impairment in patients with substance use disorder, *Drug Alcohol Rev* 38(4):435–442, 2019. https://doi.org/10.1111/dar.12922.

By the 2023 American Geriatrics Society Beers Criteria® Update Expert Panel: American Geriatrics Society 2023 updated AGS Beers Criteria® for potentially inappropriate medication use in older adults, *J Am Geriatr Soc* 71(7):2052–2081, 2023. https://doi.org/10.1111/jgs.18372.

Cummings J, Zhou Y, Lee G, Zhong K, Fonseca J, Cheng F: Alzheimer's disease drug development pipeline: 2024, *A& D Transl Res & Clin Interv* 10(2), 2024. https://doi.org/10.1002/trc2.12465.

McKhann GM, Knopman DS, Chertkow H, et al: The diagnosis of dementia due to Alzheimer's disease: recommendations from the National Institute on Aging–Alzheimer's Association workgroups on diagnostic guidelines for Alzheimer's disease, *Alzheimer's & Dementia* 7(3):263–269, 2011. https://doi.org/10.1016/j.jalz.2011.03.005.

Nakamura ZM, Nash RP, Laughon SL, Rosenstein DL: Neuropsychiatric complications of COVID-19, *Curr Psychiatry Rep* 23(5):25, 2021. https://doi.org/10.1007/s11920-021-01237-9.

Patnode CD, Perdue LA, Rossom RC, et al: *Screening for cognitive impairment in older adults: an evidence update for the U.S. Preventive services task Force*, Agency for Healthcare Research and Quality (US), 2020. http://www.ncbi.nlm.nih.gov/books/NBK554654/. Accessed 8 August 2025.

Vaucher P, Herzig D, Cardoso I, Herzog MH, Mangin P, Favrat B: The trail making test as a screening instrument for driving performance in older drivers; a translational research, *BMC Geriatr* 14(1):123, 2014. https://doi.org/10.1186/1471-2318-14-123.

CENTRAL NERVOUS SYSTEM NEOPLASMS

Method of
Mark Kraemer, MD; and Mahua Dey, MD

CURRENT DIAGNOSIS

- Neuroimaging (preference for magnetic resonance imaging [MRI] with and without contrast) should be obtained in patients with concerning headaches, new onset seizures, and/or new neurologic deficits.
- Urgent consultation with neurosurgery and neurooncology is recommended for newly discovered brain masses. Newly discovered pituitary masses should also prompt consultation with endocrinology.
- Tissue should be obtained for pathological diagnosis of both primary and metastatic central nervous system (CNS) tumors. CNS tissue sampling should be reserved for tumors without another identifiable source. Meningiomas may be diagnosed on MRI alone.

CURRENT THERAPY

- High-dose corticosteroids are often first employed for symptom relief of symptomatic central nervous system (CNS) tumors. In general, corticosteroids should be used with caution only in the setting of symptomatic lesions with associated edema. Steroids should not be given if a diagnosis of primary CNS lymphoma is considered.
- Surgical resection is typically pursued for most primary brain tumors and large symptomatic metastatic tumors. Small asymptomatic meningiomas often do not require surgical resection but should be followed closely with surveillance magnetic resonance imaging.
- Radiotherapy is used as primary treatment for small metastatic tumors, or as adjuvant therapy in many primary CNS tumors.
- Owing to the blood-brain barrier, chemotherapy has limited survival benefit in many CNS tumors. New immunotherapies are being developed as a way to improve therapeutic options.

Introduction

Brain tumors are a diverse group of neoplasms that are broadly divided into primary and metastatic. Patients generally present with progressive neurologic deficits over a variable time course depending on tumor location, size, and growth rate. Interestingly, small lesions may produce obvious deficits if there is disruption of eloquent brain regions (e.g., motor/sensory cortex, Broca/Wernicke areas, visual apparatus). On the contrary, large, slow-growing lesions in clinically silent brain regions may present with only subtle deficits over long periods of time. For example, large frontal lobe meningiomas may be discovered after multiple years of slow progressive loss of executive function, even leading to significant disruption in family, social, and work life before clinical identification. New-onset seizures should also raise suspicion for a new brain neoplasm.

Yet, the most common presenting symptom among patients with new brain tumors is nonspecific headaches. This provides a diagnostic dilemma for clinicians, who frequently encounter patients presenting with headaches. Various guidelines have been developed for identifying high-risk headaches, which include onset, duration and frequency, character, associated clinical signs, past medical history, and other factors, including head

TABLE 1 Concerning Headache Features, Adapted From the National Institutes of Health

Headache Features

Sudden, severe headache that may be accompanied by a stiff neck	Headache and loss of sensation or weakness in any part of the body
Severe headache accompanied by fever, nausea, and/or vomiting unrelated to another illness	Headache associated with convulsions and/or shortness of breath
First or worst headache, often accompanied by confusion, weakness, double vision, or loss of consciousness	Two or more headaches a week
Headache that worsens over days or weeks	Persistent headache in someone who has been previously headache-free, particularly >50 years of age
Recurring headache in children	New headaches in someone with a history of cancer or HIV/AIDS
Headache after a head injury	

National Institutes of Health. *Headache.* Last reviewed March 8, 2023. Accessed August 29, 2023. https://www.ninds.nih.gov/health-information/disorders/headache

injury. The National Institutes of Health compiled a list of concerning headache features that should drive additional clinical workup (Table 1).

Neuroimaging with high-quality magnetic resonance imaging (MRI) is the gateway to treatment for neoplasms in the central nervous system (CNS). In high-acuity situations and/or low-resource environments, MRI may not be feasible and thus noncontrast computed tomography (CT) of the brain may be performed. CT images of brain tumors, even with iodine-based contrast, provide poor resolution of most brain neoplasms. Yet, CT does provide high sensitivity for acute hemorrhage, which can be helpful. However, among patients with subacute symptom onset, urgent high-quality (1- to 2-mm slice thickness) MRI with and without gadolinium contrast is the critical first step in diagnosis. Tumor features on MRI help guide treatment and further workup. For example, multifocal enhancing lesions centered along the gray–white matter junction raise suspicion for metastatic disease. Solitary lesions with imaging findings suggestive of significant necrosis and edema raise suspicion for a high-grade glioma. Urgent consultation with neuroradiology and neurosurgery is recommended for further patient triage and management after a new lesion is identified.

Treatment for most brain tumors involves biopsy and/or surgical resection. Adjuvant therapy including radiation, chemotherapy, and immunotherapy is dependent on tumor pathologic diagnosis and patient clinical factors. Primary tumors are graded 1 to 4 based upon risk of recurrence according to the World Health Organization (WHO) Classification of Tumors. The WHO regularly updates tumor grading and classification based on currently available high-quality research. Historically, brain tumors were categorized based primarily on histologic features, including cell morphology/tissue architecture, evidence of necrosis, and level of mitoses. Today, molecular and genomic studies and techniques play a larger role in the categorization of CNS tumors (Table 2). Currently, genomic testing of neoplasms is regularly performed for both classification and guiding individualized adjuvant therapy. With rapidly evolving diagnostic and therapeutic tools available, patients with CNS neoplasms are surviving longer than ever before. Local control of CNS disease, whether primary or metastatic, is chief among treatment objectives for patient quality of life and to preserve functional status.

TABLE 2 Glioma Types and Molecular Pathology

TUMOR TYPE	GENES/MOLECULAR PROFILES CHARACTERISTICALLY ALTERED
Astrocytoma, IDH mutant	*IDH1, IDH2, ATRX, TP53, CDKN2A/B*
Oligodendroglioma, IDH mutant, and 1p/19q-codeleted	*IDH1, IDH2, 1p/19q, TERT* promoter, *CIC, FUBP1, NOTCH1*
Glioblastoma, IDH wildtype	IDH-wildtype, *TERT* promoter, chromosomes 7/10, *EGFR*

IDH, Isocitrate dehydrogenase.

Metastatic Tumors

Metastatic tumors are the most common neoplastic lesions identified in the brain. Tumors are primarily spread through hematogenous mechanisms and may be deposited anywhere within the brain. Classically, however, metastatic tumors are identified at the junction of the superficial gray and deep white matter, likely a reflection of the longer relative mean transit time of blood and tumor cells through the small vascular networks found in these locations (Figure 1). Metastatic cells cross the blood-brain barrier (BBB) where they may further disseminate along the perivascular spaces, leptomeninges and even spread through cerebrospinal fluid (CSF) into distant regions of the CNS. The most common pathologies in order of incidence include lung, breast, melanoma, and renal cell carcinoma. Both the lung and liver serve as a hematogenous filter for many other cancers, which provides the brain relative protection from cancers of the abdomen and genitourinary tract. Yet, occasionally prostate, colon, and other cancers may metastasize to the brain.

Clinical suspicion for metastatic disease should prompt whole-body imaging. Diagnosis may occur through several pathways, ideally with input from a multidisciplinary team including radiologists, oncologists, neurosurgeons, and pathologists. Generally, tissue diagnosis should be performed with biopsy of safe target tissues, for example a peripheral lung mass. However, in patients with large symptomatic brain tumors, initial tissue diagnosis may be obtained with craniotomy and tumor debulking. Local control of CNS disease drives prognosis and adjuvant treatment in patients with metastatic cancer, and thus removal of large symptomatic lesions may be the first and most obvious step regardless of the pathologic diagnosis. Even among radio- and chemotherapy-sensitive tumors, debulking and relief of local mass effect is a critical initial step in management to avoid imminent patient deterioration. However, for smaller lesions with mild or moderate mass effect, we typically recommend tissue diagnosis through biopsy of non-CNS tissues, which is generally lower risk.

Treatment of CNS metastatic disease depends upon tumor pathology, lesion location and size, clinical performance status, and systemic disease burden. Treatment tools including surgery, radiotherapy, chemotherapy, and immunotherapy must be weighed against potential toxicities and associated risks. Generally, surgery is reserved for larger (>2 to 3 cm), radio-resistant tumors in patients with good functional status. As most metastatic tumors arise at the gray-white junction near the surface of the brain, many tumors may be microsurgically resected with high success and tolerable risk. Neurosurgeons typically admit patients into the intensive care unit postoperatively for at least 12 to 24 hours for close neuromonitoring before transitioning to general care status. Tight blood pressure control and normal coagulation status are key concerns perioperatively. In the absence of prior epilepsy, patients with supratentorial tumors should be placed on antiepileptic prophylaxis (levetiracetam [Keppra][1] 500 mg twice

---

[1] Not FDA approved for this indication.

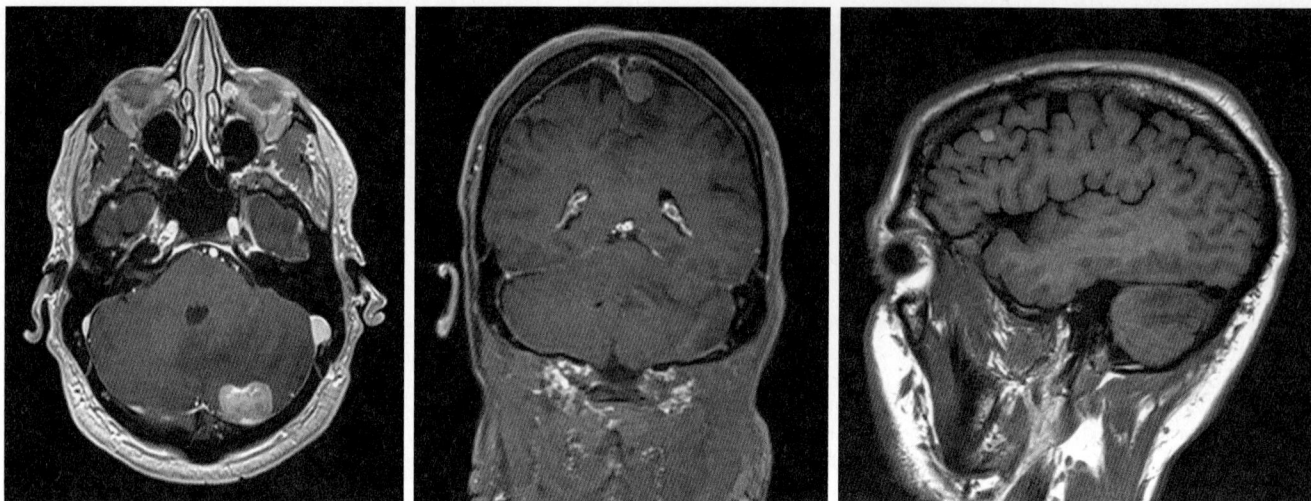

Figure 1 Metastatic tumors often arise at the gray-white junction and avidly enhance after contrast administration. This patient with a history of melanoma presented with multiple metastatic lesions, including a large right cerebellar tumor (*left image*, MRI T1 axial with contrast), a small tumor near the falx (*middle image*, MRI T1 coronal with contrast), and a left middle temporal gyrus tumor (*right image*, MRI sagittal T1 FLAIR).

daily) for at least 3 months postoperatively. Infratentorial tumors typically do not require seizure prophylaxis. Patients with prior epilepsy should continue their current therapy or may require dose escalation. High-dose corticosteroids (typically intravenous dexamethasone [Decadron]) are used both pre- and postoperatively and tapered based upon the severity of edema. Of note, patients with neuroimaging characteristics concerning for lymphoma should not be given corticosteroids until a tissue specimen is obtained. Repeat MRI with and without contrast is obtained within 48 hours after surgery to evaluate the extent of resection and survey for perioperative complications, including hemorrhage, stroke, and hydrocephalus.

Most CNS metastatic tumors are radioresistant. Small cell lung cancer is a notable exception; it is highly sensitive to chemoradiation and there is little role for surgery even in large metastases. Randomized studies have shown benefit in patient survival and local recurrence rates for patients undergoing postoperative radiotherapy. At most centers, radiotherapy is delivered with a linear accelerator, which precisely delivers ionizing radiation to target tissues. Gamma Knife and CyberKnife, two separate technologies, may also be used. Brain radiotherapy may be performed on the entire brain (whole-brain radiotherapy, WBRT) or more precisely targeted. Modern techniques for WBRT include hippocampal sparing protocols, which have been shown to have lower incidence of memory decline (a well-known complication of WBRT). WBRT has the benefit of treating micrometastases not yet visible on imaging. Targeted radiotherapy is usually preferred for one or few metastatic lesions (typically lesions <2 cm in circumference and five or fewer total lesions; this is institution/clinician dependent), which may be performed in either fractionated or single high-dose regimens. In patients with one or more small, nonoperative tumors, stereotactic radiosurgery (SRS) is standard of care. In SRS, a single fraction of high-dose radiation (typically 21 Gy) is precisely administered to the tumor with a 1-mm margin. Such treatments require the expertise of a comprehensive team including radiation oncologists, neurosurgeons, and medical physicists. When administered in this fashion, all cells in the target region are obliterated in one treatment with 70% to 90% local control rates at 1 year. Alternatively, fractionated radiotherapy may be preferred in patients who have already undergone surgical resection, because it is less toxic on nearby nontargeted healing tissues (e.g., incision sites) and performed no earlier than 2 weeks postoperatively. Currently investigators are exploring the role of preoperative SRS in larger CNS metastasis. Traditionally, radiosurgery is not performed in larger lesions (>3 cm) due to significant brain edema

and necrosis. However, SRS performed immediately before surgery (~1 to 2 days) has the potential benefit of sterilizing the tumor bed and expediting systemic therapy.

Radionecrosis is a well-known toxicity of radiosurgery and manifests as fibrinoid necrosis of the blood vessel walls and necrosis of the surrounding brain tissue. Radiographically, radionecrosis may occur as early as 3 months or delayed up to 3 years after radiation. Its appearance is often similar to tumor recurrence on MRI. Radionecrosis is more likely to occur when treating larger tumors, and may be influenced by other adjuvant treatments and/or specific tumor pathologies. Recently, laser interstitial thermal therapy (LITT) has been used for treatment of post–SRS-treated lesions concerning for recurrence versus radionecrosis. LITT is a minimally invasive procedure performed by neurosurgeons in which a laser probe is stereotactically placed to ablate the region of concern. LITT is not currently standard of care, but multiple centers are currently evaluating its utility with promising outcome.

Patients with metastatic CNS disease require ongoing close follow-up with an interdisciplinary oncology team. Control of CNS disease is paramount for patient quality of life and function, and thus treatment of new metastatic brain tumors is often addressed before other systemic disease. Recently, there has been an explosion of new cancer-specific targeted agents approved by the U.S. Food and Drug Administration (FDA) or currently in clinical trials. It is now common to see patients with metastatic cancer survive multiple years after initial diagnosis. This paradigm shift means that patients are often treated for multiple new metastatic brain lesions over the course of their disease.

Primary Tumors
Meningioma

Tumors arising from the arachnoid cap cells along the surface (and rarely the ventricles) of the brain are the most common primary brain neoplasms. Meningiomas are often discovered incidentally during brain imaging performed for other reasons. Atypical of most CNS neoplasms, which cannot be reliably diagnosed with imaging alone, meningiomas have a classic appearance on MRI. Tumors arise from the extraaxial dural surfaces with homogenous enhancement and a classic dural tail (Figure 2). Asymptomatic patients with small tumors and without concerning radiographic features (e.g., surrounding T2 signal in adjacent parenchyma to suggest brain invasion, proximity to eloquent regions) are often observed with serial MRI. However, meningiomas have variable growth rates, and it is difficult to determine the clinical characteristics of the tumor at

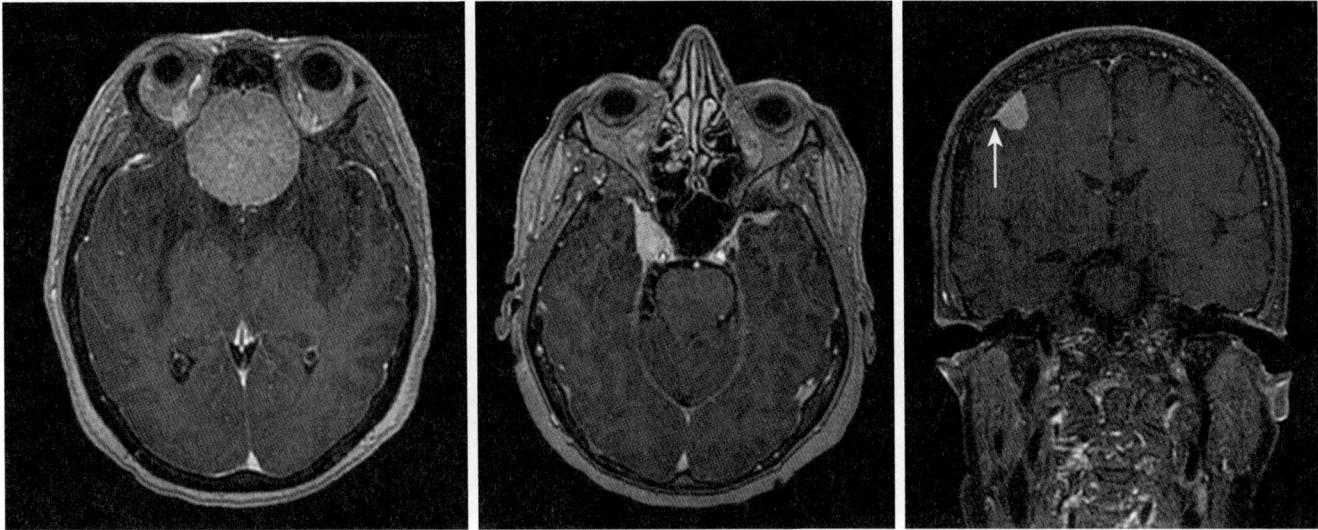

Figure 2 Meningiomas are heterogeneously enhancing tumors found along the dura mater, often demonstrating a tail *(arrow)*. *Left image* shows an axial magnetic resonance imaging (MRI) T1 with contrast image of a large olfactory groove meningioma in a patient presenting with slow progressive executive function decline over the course of years. *Middle image* shows a much smaller meningioma in a patient with neurofibromatosis I causing compression of the right optic nerve. The *right image* shows an axial T1 MRI image of a small asymptomatic convexity meningioma, which may be followed conservatively in the absence of clinical symptoms or interval growth.

the time of identification. For example, small tumors with minimal or negligible growth may never cause clinical symptoms throughout the patient's life span. Tumors causing clinical symptoms and/or demonstrating significant growth on imaging require treatment. Surgical resection of meningiomas may be complicated by lesion location, blood supply, and proximity/ encasement of eloquent tissues (e.g., cerebral arteries and/or nerves). Goals of surgery include maximal safe resection with a margin of normal surrounding dura mater. Meningiomas are graded I to III by the WHO, with the vast majority (>90%) being grade I at the time of pathologic diagnosis. Grade II and III meningiomas are likely to recur and usually qualify for adjuvant radiotherapy. At the time of publication, there are no FDA-approved targeted therapies, although investigators are keen to develop new drugs.

Gliomas

Multiple tumors arise from the glial cells, or nonneuronal "helper" cells of the brain. In order of incidence, the three major categories include astrocytoma (WHO grades I–IV), oligodendroglioma (WHO grades II–III) and ependymoma (WHO grades II–III). Most of these tumors occur sporadically, although several familial syndromes are also implicated including neurofibromatosis type I, Li-Fraumeni, and Lynch syndrome. Other well-known risk factors include male gender, non-Hispanic White ethnicity, advanced age, and exposure to ionizing radiation. Gliomas are generally categorized into high-grade (WHO grades III and IV) and low-grade (WHO grade I and II) categories based on recurrence risk and aggression. Primary brain tumors require tissue for pathologic and molecular diagnosis, which is obtained through either stereotactic biopsy or craniotomy for tumor resection.

Unlike metastatic tumors, which are typically well circumscribed, gliomas present unique surgical challenges due to their nondistinct borders. Detailed anatomical knowledge and high magnification with surgical microscopes are critical tools for neurosurgeons. New tools including the orally administered prodrug 5-aminolevulinic acid (5-ALA [Gleolan]) have been developed to improve resection of gliomas. 5-ALA allows photodynamic detection of tumor cells during surgery when illuminated with blue light from a microscope. Additionally, when tumors involve eloquent brain areas (motor cortex, Broca/Wernicke regions, insular lobe), neurosurgeons may elect to perform surgery with the patient awake. Gliomas may invade such regions without completely impairing function, therefore complete tumor resection is

not possible without creating permanent deficits. Because adjuvant therapies depend in part on performance status, all efforts are taken to avoid creating new deficits during surgery. Awake craniotomy with cortical mapping improves safety in tumor resection in eloquent brain regions. Specialized MRI sequences including diffusion-tensor imaging may also be used to evaluate nearby white-matter tracts for surgical planning and to improve safety of resection. Lastly, intraoperative MRI may also be used to guide maximally safe surgical resection by providing real-time feedback during surgery.

High-Grade Glioma

Among adults, high-grade gliomas are most common. In particular, glioblastoma (astrocytoma, WHO grade IV) is the most common type of glioma, which represents more than half of new primary malignant brain tumors and 59% of all gliomas. Despite significant research efforts over the course of decades, these tumors continue to have very poor prognosis with only 6.9% of patients surviving 5 years after diagnosis. Owing to their rapid growth, patients with high-grade gliomas often present with signs and symptoms of elevated intracranial pressure, including headaches, vision changes/papilledema, nausea, and vomiting. Imaging characteristics of high-grade gliomas include heterogeneously enhancing intraaxial masses with extensive surrounding vasogenic edema (Figure 3). Tumors may be quite large at the time of diagnosis with areas of necrosis centrally, suggesting growth that has outmatched blood supply. Gross total resection of the tumor likely provides a relative survival benefit; however, due to their diffuse borders, recurrence is the natural history of the disease.

After surgical resection, high-grade gliomas are treated with a combination of fractionated radiotherapy and chemotherapy (Table 3). At most centers, the oral drug temozolomide (Temodar), an alkylating chemotherapy, remains the standard of care, which is administered concurrently with local radiotherapy. Temozolomide confers a survival advantage compared with patients with glioblastoma undergoing radiotherapy alone, and the addition of tumor treating fields (TTFields), a helmet-like device that emits low-intensity, intermediate-frequency alternating electric fields, has been shown to have added survival benefit. Various molecular markers have been shown to modulate prognosis, including methylation of the promoter of O6-methylguanine-DNA methyltransferase (MGMT) and mutation of isocitrate dehydrogenase (IDH). Both IDH mutations and MGMT methylation confer improved prognosis based upon response to available chemotherapies.

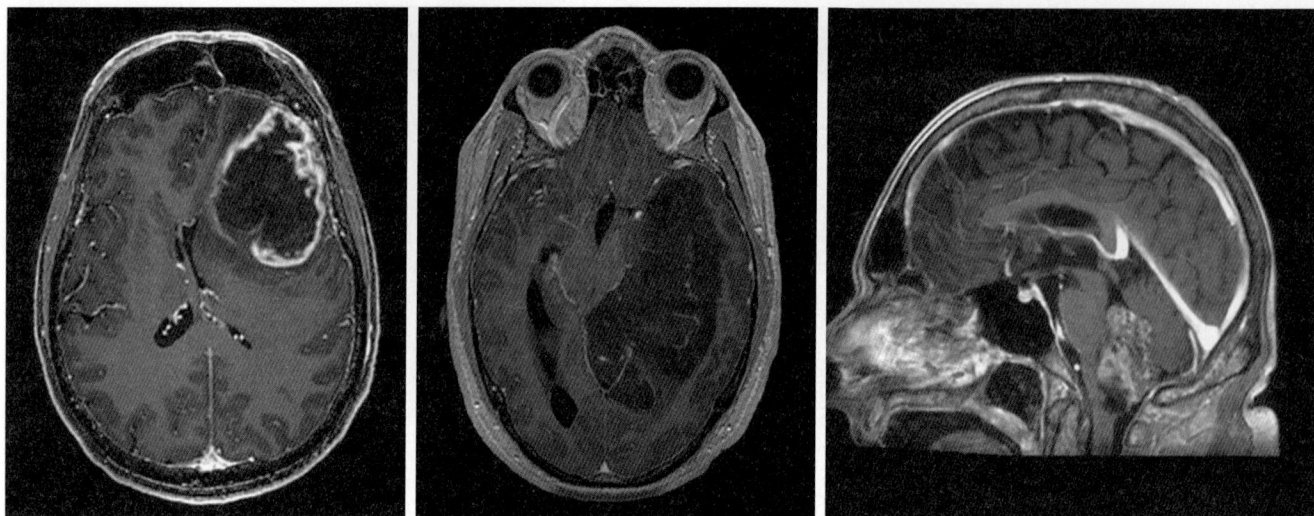

Figure 3 High-grade gliomas including glioblastoma, or grade IV astrocytoma (*left image,* axial T1 magnetic resonance imaging [MRI] with contrast), demonstrate heterogenous enhancement and often significant mass effect and central necrosis due to aggressive growth. Low-grade gliomas (*middle image,* grade II astrocytoma, axial T1 MRI with contrast) grow more slowly and often do not enhance or demonstrate necrosis; however, they also infiltrate normal surrounding brain structures. The *right image* (sagittal T1 MRI with contrast) shows a patient with a heterogeneously enhancing tumor in the fourth ventricle, which turned out to be a grade II ependymoma. Given their location within the ventricles, ependymomas are highly susceptible to distal seeding of the neural axis.

Patients with high-grade gliomas should be followed closely by an interdisciplinary oncology team with routine MRI surveillance. Tumor recurrence is expected but may be difficult to distinguish from radiotherapy treatment effects (pseudoprogression). Depending on the patient's performance status, additional treatment options may include additional surgery and/or salvage chemotherapy and radiation. Both lomustine (Gleostine, an alkylating agent) and bevacizumab (Avastin, an inhibitor of neovascularization) are FDA approved for progressive glioblastoma. Despite radiographic and symptomatic improvement with these drugs, there appears to be no significant overall survival benefit. Glioma treatment is an active area of research with multiple new potential emerging technologies including immunotherapy and tumor vaccines.

Low-Grade Glioma

Low-grade gliomas (WHO grades I–II) have improved prognosis; however, their clinical course is rarely benign. Grade I astrocytoma (pilocytic astrocytoma) is a rare exception, which may be cured with gross total resection alone because of its distinct border. Yet, this tumor is found more often in the pediatric population and rarely in adults. The clinical behavior of low-grade gliomas is variable and depends on pathologic diagnosis. Unlike high-grade tumors, low-grade gliomas are slower growing and less likely to present with signs and symptoms of elevated intracranial pressure. Rather, patients more often present with seizures. Imaging often demonstrates a nonenhancing mass, with variable amounts of surrounding edema (Figure 3). Nearly all low-grade gliomas have mutations in IDH, which confers a prognostic advantage over IDH wild-type gliomas. The natural history of many low-grade gliomas unfortunately involves progression to high-grade subtypes. After surgical resection and/or biopsy, most patients with low-grade gliomas will undergo both radiation and chemotherapy, which confers a survival benefit.

Ependymomas

Ependymomas (WHO grades II–III) are also tumors that arise from glial origin; however, they account for 5% or less of all adult primary tumors. On imaging, ependymomas typically demonstrate heterogenous enhancement and may have cystic components (Figure 3). Unlike other gliomas, ependymomas form from cells along the ventricles and therefore may spread through the CSF. Both cranial and spinal imaging are often ordered to evaluate for seeding of distant locations within the thecal canal.

Treatment is primarily surgical, with known survival benefit from gross total resection. Depending on success of the operation and histological grading, patients may undergo postoperative fractionated radiotherapy to the tumor site and/or additional targeted radiotherapy to distant tumor sites. Likely owing to their rarity, no chemotherapy regimen has been thoroughly investigated.

Primary CNS Lymphoma

Primary CNS lymphoma (PCNSL) is a rare aggressive non-Hodgkin lymphoma affecting the brain, spinal cord, and CSF. This tumor is most seen in elderly and immunocompromised patients, but it also affecting immunocompetent individuals. Imaging typically reveals a homogenously enhancing solitary tumor with a nonuniform, fluffy-appearing periphery. Importantly, if PCNSL is a diagnostic consideration, corticosteroids should not be administered until a tissue diagnosis has been made. Corticosteroids are cytotoxic and may decrease diagnostic accuracy during tissue examination. Diagnosis is typically confirmed with stereotactic brain biopsy. There is no role for surgical resection, even in large tumors, because of its exquisite sensitivity to chemoradiation. Because of the CNS BBB, early experience with traditional therapy regimens for diffuse large B-cell lymphoma was ineffective in PCNSL. However, in high doses methotrexate effectively traverses the BBB and continues to be the backbone of current chemotherapy regimens. Although radiotherapy (specifically WBRT) has fallen out of favor because of cognitive impairment, this remains an active area of study with several ongoing trials. Despite maximal therapy, disease recurrence is common with 5-year survival between 30% and 40%.

Pituitary Adenomas

Tumors of the pituitary are a diverse group of tumors and account for a growing number (17.2%) of newly discovered CNS tumors. Patients often present with endocrinopathies and/or vision changes, which occurs because of the proximity of the dorsum sellae and the nearby optic chiasm. Tumors less than 1 cm are considered microadenomas, whereas growth greater than 1 cm defines a macroadenoma. When tumors grow large enough to displace the optic chiasm, patients classically present with bitemporal peripheral vision loss. Initial workup includes a full endocrine workup. Tumors are classified by their secretory activity (functional tumors), or lack thereof (nonfunctional tumors). Table 4 shows the typical laboratory findings among the most common subtypes. Small asymptomatic (nonfunctional)

TABLE 3	Adjuvant Treatment for Gliomas	
	TUMOR TYPE	**ADJUVANT TREATMENT**
Low grade	Diffuse astrocytoma (WHO grade II)	Radiotherapy (RT)
	Oligodendroglioma, IDH mutant, 1p19q codeleted (WHO grade II)	Standard RT + adjuvant PCV or Standard RT + adjuvant TMZ or Standard RT + concurrent and adjuvant TMZ or Observation (in very selective low-risk cases)
	IDH-mutant astrocytoma (WHO grade II)	Standard RT + adjuvant TMZ or Standard RT + concurrent and adjuvant TMZ or Standard RT + adjuvant PCV or Observation (in highly selected low-risk patients)
	Ependymoma (WHO grade II)	Standard RT
High grade	IDH-mutant astrocytoma (WHO grade III)	Standard RT with adjuvant TMZ (preferred) or Standard RT with concurrent and adjuvant TMZ
	IDH-mutant astrocytoma (WHO grade IV)	Standard RT with concurrent and adjuvant TMZ or Standard RT with adjuvant TMZ or Standard RT alone or Standard RT with concurrent and adjuvant TMZ + alternating electric field therapy
	Oligodendroglioma, IDH mutant, 1p19q codeleted (WHO grade III)	Standard RT and neoadjuvant or adjuvant PCV or Standard RT with concurrent and adjuvant TMZ or Standard RT and adjuvant TMZ
	Anaplastic ependymoma (WHO grade III)	RT
	Glioblastoma IDH wild-type (WHO grade IV)	Hypofractionated RT + concurrent and adjuvant TMZ or Standard RT + concurrent TMZ and adjuvant TMZ + alternating electric field therapy or Standard RT + concurrent TMZ and adjuvant TMZ or Hypofractionated RT alone

PCV, Procarbazine, CCNU or lomustine, and vincristine; *TMZ,* temozolomide.

TABLE 4	Pituitary Adenomas, Frequency, Secretion Profile, and Clinical Manifestations		
ADENOMA SUBTYPE	**FREQUENCY**	**SECRETION PROFILE**	**CLINICAL SYMPTOMS**
Prolactinoma	27%	Prolactin	Amenorrhea-galactorrhea
Somatotroph adenoma	15%–18%	Growth hormone	Acromegaly
Corticotroph adenoma	10%	ACTH	Cushing disease
Gonadotroph adenoma	10%	FSH, LH	Nonfunctional
Thyrotroph adenoma	1%	TSH	Hyperthyroidism, hypothyroidism, or silent
Other	30%–40%	–	Nonfunctional

ACTH, Adrenocorticotropic hormone; *FSH,* follicle-stimulating hormone; *LH,* luteinizing hormone; *TSH,* thyroid-stimulating hormone.
Mete O, Lopes MB. Overview of the 2017 WHO Classification of Pituitary Tumors. *Endocr Pathol.* 2017;28:228-243.

microadenomas may be managed conservatively with routine surveillance. However, treatment for most symptomatic pituitary adenomas is surgical. Prolactinomas are an exception, due to highly efficacious medical therapy with dopaminergic agonists (cabergoline [Dostinex] and bromocriptine [Parlodel]). Yet, all large pituitary adenomas causing significant mass effect should be urgently referred for surgery to preserve vision. Surgery is often performed transnasally using endoscopes with high success. However, very large tumors may require craniotomy for successful resection. Similar to other CNS tumors, patients with pituitary adenomas require close follow-up with a multidisciplinary team involving both neurosurgery and endocrine.

References

Bang A, Schoenfeld JD: Immunotherapy and radiotherapy for metastatic cancers, *Ann Palliat Med* 8:312–325, 2019.

Brown PD, et al: Postoperative stereotactic radiosurgery compared with whole brain radiotherapy for resected metastatic brain disease (NCCTG N107C/CEC.3): a multicentre, randomised, controlled, phase 3 trial, *Lancet Oncol* 18:1049–1060, 2017.

Baumert BG, et al: Temozolomide chemotherapy versus radiotherapy in high-risk low-grade glioma (EORTC 22033-26033): a randomised, open-label, phase 3 intergroup study, *Lancet Oncol* 17:1521–1532, 2016.

Buckner JC, et al: Radiation plus procarbazine, CCNU, and vincristine in low-grade glioma, *N Engl J Med* 374:1344–1355, 2016.

Fabian D, et al: Treatment of glioblastoma (GBM) with the addition of tumor-treating fields (TTF): a review, *Cancers* 11, 2019.

Garzon-Muvdi T, Bailey DD, Pernik MN, Pan E: Basis for immunotherapy for treatment of meningiomas, *Front Neurol* 11:945, 2020.

Grabowski MM, et al: Combination laser interstitial thermal therapy plus stereotactic radiotherapy increases time to progression for biopsy-proven recurrent brain metastases, *Neurooncol Adv* 4:vdac086, 2022.

Mete O, Lopes MB: Overview of the 2017 WHO classification of pituitary tumors, *Endocr Pathol* 28:228–243, 2017.

Mitchell DK, et al: Brain metastases: an update on the multi-disciplinary approach of clinical management, *Neurochirurgie* 68:69–85, 2022.

Mittal S, et al: Alternating electric tumor treating fields for treatment of glioblastoma: rationale, preclinical, and clinical studies, *J Neurosurg* 128:414–421, 2018.

Nieder C, Grosu AL, Gaspar LE: Stereotactic radiosurgery (SRS) for brain metastases: a systematic review, *Radiat Oncol* 9:155, 2014.

Ostrom QT, et al: CBTRUS statistical report: primary brain and other central nervous system tumors diagnosed in the United States in 2015-2019, *Neuro Oncol* 24:v1–v95, 2022.

Patchell RA, et al: A randomized trial of surgery in the treatment of single metastases to the brain, *N Engl J Med* 322:494–500, 1990.

Putora PM, et al: Treatment of brain metastases in small cell lung cancer: decision-making amongst a multidisciplinary panel of European experts, *Radiother Oncol* 149:84–88, 2020.

Schaff LR, Grommes C: Primary central nervous system lymphoma, *Blood* 140:971–979, 2022.

Stupp R, et al: Radiotherapy plus concomitant and adjuvant temozolomide for glioblastoma, *N Engl J Med* 352:987–996, 2005.

Stupp R, et al: Effect of tumor-treating fields plus maintenance temozolomide vs maintenance temozolomide alone on survival in patients with glioblastoma: a randomized clinical trial, *JAMA* 318:2306–2316, 2017.

Wick W, et al: Lomustine and bevacizumab in progressive glioblastoma, *N Engl J Med* 377:1954–1963, 2017.

GILLES DE LA TOURETTE SYNDROME

Method of
Alonso G. Zea Vera, MD

CURRENT DIAGNOSIS

- Multiple motor tics and one or more phonic tics have been present for some time during the illness, although not necessarily concurrently.
- The tics may wax and wane in frequency but have persisted for more than 1 year since the first tic onset.
- Onset occurs before 18 years of age.
- The disturbance is not caused by the direct physiologic effects of a substance or a general medical condition.

CURRENT THERAPY

- Educate the patient and family about tics, their waxing and waning course, and its natural history. Long-term reductions in tics may occur in the late teens, irrespective of pharmacologic therapy.
- If necessary, provide information to educate teachers and classmates to reduce social impairment.
- Assess for the presence of comorbidities including attention-deficit/hyperactivity disorder (ADHD), obsessive-compulsive disorder (OCD), anxiety, mood problems, learning problems, and behavior problems.

- Consider nonpharmacologic and pharmacologic treatment for the most impairing symptoms first. Tics do not always need to be treated, and other comorbidities may be more impairing.
- Treatment of ADHD, OCD, anxiety, mood problems, learning problems, and behavior problems should follow evidence-based guidelines and may require specialty evaluation (neurology, psychiatry, and psychology). Stimulants are not contraindicated in patients with Tourette syndrome.
- Comprehensive Behavioral Intervention for Tics could be considered in motivated families and can be offered even if tics are not impairing. Families should be counseled about the time and effort required and the scarcity of trained providers in some areas. Patients who are very young or have severe untreated comorbidities may not be able to participate in this therapy.
- Alpha-agonists are the most common first-line medications used in the treatment of tics and are particularly beneficial for patients with comorbid ADHD. Commonly used second-line medications include topiramate (Topamax)[1] or baclofen (Lioresal).[1] Dopamine receptor antagonists are usually restricted to severe and refractory cases.
- Monitor the benefits and side effects at regular intervals. Counsel parents that tics fluctuate and that brief worsening of symptoms is common. Brief exacerbations do not necessarily require a change in therapy.
- Do not begin treatment with more than one central nervous system drug simultaneously, and avoid changing medication regimens too fast. Start one medication, wait 2 to 4 weeks, and then reassess all symptoms before starting the next medication.
- Maintain stable dosing during the school year; consider tapering medications in the summer.
- Consider weaning tic-suppressing medications in the middle to late teen years if tics are well controlled.

[1]Not FDA approved for this indication. Tourette syndrome (TS) is a neuropsychiatric illness characterized by multiple motor tics and phonic tics that persist for longer than 1 year (see the Current Diagnosis box). Transient tics have been reported in up to ~25% of children from kindergarten to sixth grade. However, the prevalence of TS is closer to 0.3% to 1.5% of the population, and boys are three to four times more likely to be affected than girls. The prevalence of tic disorders is even higher in children with intellectual disabilities.

Clinical Manifestations

Tics are sudden, recurrent, nonrhythmic, patterned movements (i.e., motor tics) or vocalizations (i.e., phonic tics; also called *vocal tics*). Tics are fragments of normal behavior that present out of context and are not goal-directed. What separates tics from normal actions is their exaggerated character in intensity, frequency, and repetition. Tics usually follow a somatotopic distribution, with tics being more frequent in the eyes, face, neck, phonic muscles (i.e., phonic tics), and shoulders compared with the trunk and extremities.

Tics can be divided into simple or complex tics. Simple tics are brief and involve a single muscle or small group of muscles. Common simple motor tics include eye blinking, facial grimace, head jerk, and shoulder shrug. Common simple phonic tics include throat clearing, sniffing, and coughing. Complex tics can be a series of simple tics or a seemingly purposeful coordinated sequence of actions or sounds. Examples of complex motor tics include jumping, touching, or copropraxia (i.e., performing obscene gestures). Examples of complex phonic tics include echolalia (i.e., repeating others' words), palilalia (i.e., repeating their own words), or coprolalia (i.e., utterance of foul language). Simple tics are more frequent than complex tics.

The possibility of developing coprolalia or copropraxia often causes significant distress in patients and families. These phenomena are commonly considered a core symptom of TS by the general population leading to names like *the cursing disease*. This perception has been fueled by inaccurate and exaggerated portrayals of people with TS in the media. Coprophenomena is only present in 10% to 20% of patients.

Tics have a characteristic waxing and waning pattern. Patients frequently report the resolution of old tics (although they may recur later) and the appearance of new tics. Tics tend to be exacerbated by stress, anxiety, excitement, anger, fatigue, and acute illnesses. Parents often notice more tics when the child is bored or unoccupied with an activity. On the contrary, tics are often diminished during focused mental or physical activities, and they usually do not affect activities of daily living, occupational activities, or recreational activities. Although tics are commonly reported to be absent during sleep, studies using polysomnography have shown that they may persist during it.

Patients with tics often describe an uncomfortable sensation preceding the tics, known as a premonitory urge, that remits once the tic is performed. This urge can be described as a physical sensation (i.e., itch or pressure) in a specific body area or a general ill-defined feeling. The majority of older children and adults report premonitory urges associated with at least one of their tics. However, younger children are less likely to report it. It is unclear if this is caused by the absence of an urge or the lack of awareness of the urge. Some young children that deny urges may report that their tics are "painful," even with mild tics. Further questioning may reveal that the pain appears shortly before the tic and disappears after the tic, suggesting a premonitory urge.

Tics can often be suppressed, although only momentarily, leading to the misinterpretation that tics are voluntary actions. The ability to suppress tics improves with age. Patients frequently report that the premonitory urge worsens when suppressing their tics and that the release of the tic brings relief. Some patients report a "rebound effect" with many tics occurring after a prolonged period of tic suppression. For example, some children who suppress their tics in school report an increased frequency of tics when they get home.

A natural course has been described in TS. The onset of tics is usually between 4 and 8 years of age. Children often present with motor tics first, followed by the development of phonic tics. Tic severity usually increases in the later elementary school years and early adolescence and decreases by late adolescence and early adulthood. Most TS patients have minimal tics or may "outgrow" their tics when they become adults. However, a minority of patients may continue to have bothersome tics throughout life.

Comorbidities

About 85% of patients with Tourette syndrome have at least one psychiatric comorbidity and ~60% have 2 or more. The most common comorbidities are obsessive-compulsive disorder (~65%; OCD) and attention deficit and hyperactivity disorder (~55%; ADHD). Anxiety, mood disorders, and sleep problems are also common. ADHD symptoms frequently are present before tic onset, but OCD symptoms are more likely to appear after the onset of tics. TS patients should be screened for these conditions regularly.

Diagnosis

TS is a primary tic disorder diagnosed based on clinical criteria (see Current Diagnosis box) listed in the *Diagnostic and Statistical Manual of Mental Disorders,* fifth edition (DSM-5). Other primary tic disorders include *provisional tic disorder, persistent (chronic) motor* or *vocal tic disorder, other specified tic disorder,* and *unspecified tic disorder.* The diagnosis depends on correctly recognizing that the abnormal movements are tics through a careful history and physical examination. Laboratory and imaging studies can be used to rule out other conditions but are rarely needed. Sometimes tics are interpreted as a symptom of a different condition. Coughing or sniffing tics may be attributed to asthma, chronic cough, or allergies. Blinking tics could lead to the diagnosis of poor vision or dry eyes.

Secondary tics, those caused by an underlying condition, are rare. Causes of secondary tics include drug-induced movement disorders, structural lesions (i.e., trauma, tumors), and a variety of neurodevelopmental and neurodegenerative disorders. Complex or atypical cases with multiple comorbidities or multiple abnormalities identified on a general or neurologic examination should be referred for specialist consultation.

Tics may resemble other movement disorders, such as stereotypy, chorea, ballism, dystonia, and myoclonus. Stereotypies are repetitive, simple movements that start before 3 years of age, are suppressible, and usually occur when a child is excited. Chorea consists of a sequence of random, continual, involuntary, nonpurposeful, nonrhythmic movements. Choreic movements often flow from one body part to another. Ballism is a large-amplitude choreic movement affecting the proximal limb. Myoclonus is an involuntary, sudden, shocklike movement. Chorea, ballism, and myoclonus cannot be volitionally suppressed. Dystonia is produced by overflow of motor contractions, leading to abnormal postures, and its twisting movements typically are slower than tics.

An important mimic of TS is *functional tic-like behavior.* This is a subtype of functional movement disorder characterized by ticlike behaviors. Although previously considered uncommon, a large increase of this phenotype was reported during the coronavirus 2019 (COVID-19) pandemic. In contrast with TS, it more commonly presents with an abrupt onset of ticlike behaviors in adolescents and young adults, with a preponderance in female patients. Onset of ticlike movements after 12 years of age is highly suggestive of functional tic-like behavior disorder. Functional ticlike behaviors involve the arms or trunk more than the face, interfere more with voluntary actions, are less suppressible, and are more suggestible. Other functional neurologic symptoms can be present. The diagnosis of functional ticlike disorder is challenging because it can also present in patients with TS, and the characteristics of these two conditions may overlap. Evaluation by a specialist is recommended in these cases.

A controversial diagnosis that includes tics as a core symptom is pediatric autoimmune neuropsychiatric disorders associated with streptococcal infections (PANDAS). PANDAS criteria include an abrupt onset or exacerbation of tics or obsessive-compulsive symptoms in prepubertal children after documented group A β-hemolytic streptococcal (GABHS) infections. PANDAS criteria imply an immunologic etiology for tics triggered by GABHS infections, similar to Sydenham chorea. However, PANDAS is not associated with arthritis, carditis, or nephritis and is not thought to be a rheumatic disease.

Several factors have contributed to the controversy in PANDAS. Both tics and GABHS infections are common in childhood, therefore separating a causal from an incidental relationship is challenging. The definition of *abrupt* exacerbation is also unclear because TS is characterized by a waxing and waning pattern, and exacerbations can present after infectious and non-infectious triggers. An elevated GABHS serologic titer (i.e., anti-streptolysin O, and anti-DNase B) are commonly used to prove the temporal association of tic exacerbation and a recent GABHS infection. However, prospective studies have shown that these titers can remain elevated for many months without evidence of an acute infection, making them unreliable markers of recent infections.

Large prospective studies, using serial throat cultures and serologic testing, compared patients with TS or OCD and patients meeting the PANDAS criteria. These studies found similar frequencies of exacerbations and exacerbations associated with GABHS infections in both groups. Most exacerbations in both groups were not related to GABHS infections. More recent studies evaluating the association between GABHS infections with onset and exacerbations of tics in patients with chronic tic disorders also failed to show a relationship. As a result, it has been suggested that patients meeting the PANDAS criteria represent a subgroup of patients with TS or OCD, and the proposed immunologic link between GABHS infections and tics has been questioned. Testing patients with tics for GABHS in the absence of symptoms of an acute infection is not recommended. The American Academy of Pediatrics has published a clinical report on the diagnosis and management of patients with suspected PANDAS.

Treatment

The first step in treating TS is educating the patient, parents, and other adult caregivers. Parents, teachers, and other adult caregivers are discouraged from telling the child to stop ticcing because this produces emotional anxiety that may worsen the tics. Educational materials for teachers aim to promote a conducive environment for the child at school. The patient is encouraged to openly

TABLE 1	Therapy for Tics in Tourette Syndrome		
MEDICATION	STARTING DOSE	TITRATION	GOAL DOSE
Clonidine (Kapvay)[1]	0.05 mg qhs	0.05 mg every 3–7 d	0.05–0.1 mg tid
Clonidine patch (Catapres-TTS)[1]	Catapres TTS-1 weekly*	Weekly as needed	Catapres TTS-1, TTS-2, or TTS-3 weekly*
Guanfacine (Intuniv)[1]	0.5 mg qhs	0.5 mg every 3–7 d	1–4 mg divided bid
Baclofen (Lioresal)[1]	10 mg qhs	10 mg every 3–7 d	40–90 mg/d divided bid/tid
Clonazepam (Klonopin)[1]	0.5 mg qhs	0.5 mg every wk	1–2 mg bid
Topiramate (Topamax)[1]	25 mg qhs	25–50 mg weekly	50–100 mg bid
Pimozide (Orap)	1 mg qhs	1 mg every 3–5 d	1–4 mg/d divided daily or bid
Haloperidol (Haldol)	0.25–0.5 mg qhs	0.25–0.5 mg every 5–7 d	1–4 mg/d divided daily or bid
Fluphenazine (Prolixin)[1]	0.5 mg qhs	0.5 mg every 3–5 d	1–4 mg/d divided daily or bid
Risperidone (Risperdal)[1]	0.5 mg qhs	0.5 mg every 3–5 d	1–4 mg/d divided daily or bid
Ziprasidone (Geodon)[1]	20 mg qhs	20 mg every wk	20–80 mg/d divided daily or bid
Aripiprazole (Abilify)	1 mg qhs	1 mg every wk	1–20 mg daily or divided bid
Botulinum toxin type A (Botox)[1]	Not applicable	Not applicable	30–300 units in one or more focal sites, injected once every 3 mo

*The system areas are 3.5 cm² (Catapres TTS-1), 7.0 cm² (Catapres TTS-2), and 10.5 cm² (Catapres TTS-3), and the amount of drug released is directly proportional to the area.
[1]Not FDA approved for this indication.

talk about his or her tics to classmates to promote understanding and minimize bullying. However, if bullying is present, it should be addressed with the school. Comorbidities should be considered early in the treatment of TS. Although tics are often the most noticeable symptom, other symptoms like inattentiveness, hyperactivity, obsessive or compulsive behaviors, depression, and anxiety may be more impairing to the patient. Untreated comorbidities can also worsen the severity of tics and hamper its treatment.

Not all patients with tics need tic-suppressing treatment. The decision to start treatment depends on the level of impairment caused by tics, which may not correlate with objective markers of tic frequency or severity. Younger children are usually less bothered by their tics, even if they are frequent. However, adolescents may find tics more disruptive, even if infrequent. Treatment should be considered when there is functional interference, social interference, pain, or classroom or occupational disruption. Occasionally, parents request treatment preemptively (i.e., even if tics are not causing impairment) because of fear that the tics may worsen or result in bullying in the future. Preemptive treatment is generally not recommended for TS. Finally, it is important to keep in mind that tic-suppressing treatment rarely stops tics completely. The goal of treatment is to decrease tics to a level that is not impairing.

Initial treatment of tics consists of pharmacotherapy, psychotherapy, or a combination of both. Clinical trials enrolling patients with TS are usually small and show small effect sizes. A recent systematic review found that comprehensive behavioral intervention for tics (CBIT) had the highest level of confidence in the evidence with an effect size similar to medications. In CBIT, patients learn to increase self-awareness of tics and premonitory urges and to perform antagonistic movements. CBIT effects can persist months to years after concluding therapy, and it has been recommended in highly motivated families given the lack of side effects, even if tics are not impairing. However, CBIT is limited by the amount of effort and time required as well as the scarce availability of trained providers in some areas. Very young patients or patients with severe untreated comorbidities may be unable to complete the program.

Because TS is a chronic, nonfatal disorder, it is prudent to start pharmacotherapy with medications that carry the least side effects. The most commonly used tic-suppressing medications belong to two classes: α_2-adrenergic agonists and dopamine receptor blocking agents (Table 1). Because of their favorable side-effect profile,

α_2-adrenergic agonists are usually the first-line treatment. Clonidine (Catapres; Kapvay)[1] and guanfacine (Tenex; Intuniv)[1] have shown benefits in both tics and ADHD symptoms, making them an excellent choice in patients with comorbid ADHD. The main side effects are sedation and lightheadedness caused by mild hypotension. Sedation is more common with clonidine. The clonidine patch (Catapres-TTS)[1] may produce less peak sedation, but it commonly produces local skin irritation.

Among tic-suppressing medications, dopamine receptor blocking agents have the higher effect size and confidence in the evidence. However, they are associated with severe side effects including acute akathisia, dystonic reactions, tardive dyskinesia, cognitive blunting, acute anxiety with somatizations and school refusal, sedation, weight gain, metabolic syndrome, hyperprolactinemia, and QT prolongation. Some experts recommend baseline electrocardiograms, weight, blood pressure, fasting glucose, prolactin level, and lipid profile with follow-up monitoring every 3 months to detect drug-induced metabolic syndrome. Diet modification, routine exercise, or pharmacologic therapy may be needed. Dopamine receptor antagonists are usually restricted to the most severe cases and managed in specialty clinics.

Other medications used for tics with limited evidence include topiramate (Topamax)[1] and baclofen (Lioresal).[1] These can be used as second-line agents. The decision to use these medications can also be guided by comorbidities (i.e., using topiramate in patients with comorbid migraines). Medications used for refractory patients include botulinum toxin type A (Botox)[1] and tetrabenazine (Xenazine).[1] Finally, deep brain stimulation has emerged as a potential therapy for medically refractory patients.

The importance of effectively treating comorbid conditions cannot be overstated. The frequently held concern that ADHD stimulant therapy may worsen tics may lead families to avoid these medications, even if indicated. The landmark Treatment of ADHD in Children with Tics study and subsequent meta-analyses showed that children treated with methylphenidate (Ritalin) had, on average, reduced tic severity, contrary to the belief that stimulants exacerbate tics. The presence of tics is not an absolute contraindication to the use of stimulants in ADHD. However, if symptoms of OCD, anxiety, or autism spectrum disorder are present, ticcing or compulsions may escalate on stimulants. If a patient has done well for months to

[1]Not FDA approved for this indication.

years on stimulants for ADHD before an exacerbation of tics, it usually is not necessary to discontinue stimulants.

Complications

Patients with TS have a poorer quality of life, more suicidal thoughts, and more difficulties with school and work. TS patients also have a higher frequency of self-injurious behaviors, which can be tic-related or not. Most patients with TS (~60%) report pain associated with one of their tics during their lifetime. A recent study also found a higher frequency of cervical spine disorders in adult patients with TS. Although rare, in severe cases tics have resulted in serious complications such as vertebral artery dissection or spinal compression.

Summary

TS is a complex neuropsychiatric illness that may need pharmacologic and nonpharmacologic therapies. Cooperation among the primary care physician, neurologist, psychiatrist, and psychologist is imperative for the comprehensive care of severely affected patients. If a patient has mild tics and few or no comorbid symptoms, pharmacologic therapy may not be needed. However, if the tics are severe in the presence of many neuropsychiatric symptoms, it is reasonable to refer patients to specialists.

References

Board of Directors. Pediatric acute-onset neuropsychiatric syndrome (PANS): clinical report, *Pediatrics* 155(3):e2024070334, 2025.
Martino D, Hedderly T: Tics and stereotypies: a comparative clinical review, *Park Relat Disord* 59:117–124, 2019.
Ricketts EJ, Wolicki SB, Danielson ML, et al: Academic, interpersonal, recreational, and family impairment in children with Tourette syndrome and attention-deficit/hyperactivity disorder, *Child Psychiatry Hum Dev* 53(1):3–15, 2022.
Isung J, Isomura K, Larsson H, et al: Association of Tourette Syndrome and Chronic Tic Disorder With Cervical Spine Disorders and Related Neurological Complications, *JAMA Neurology* 78(10):1205–1211, 2021.
Pringsheim T, Okun MS, Muller-Vahl K, et al: Practice guideline recommendations summary: treatment of tics in people with Tourette syndrome and chronic tic disorders, *Neurology* 92(19):896–906, 2019.
Espil FM, Woods DW, Specht MW, et al: Long-term Outcomes of Behavior Therapy for Youth With Tourette Disorder, *J Am Acad Child Adolesc Psychiatry* 61(6):764–771, 2022.
Pringsheim T, Ganos C, McGuire JF, et al: Rapid Onset Functional Tic–Like Behaviors in Young Females During the COVID–19 Pandemic, *Mov Disord* 36(12):2707–2713, 2021.

INTRACEREBRAL HEMORRHAGE

Method of
Mohamed AlShamrani, MD; and Ronda Lun, MD

CURRENT DIAGNOSIS

- Intracerebral hemorrhage is a medical emergency: immediate imaging must be obtained in anyone with acute onset focal neurologic deficits
- Noncontrast CT is the gold standard; CT angiography can be helpful for prognostic factors and to rule out underlying vascular malformations
- Obtain magnetic resonance imaging +/− magnetic resonance venogram (MRV) if etiology of bleed is unclear

CURRENT THERAPY

- Ensure the airway is protected because level of consciousness could deteriorate rapidly
- Medical treatment:
  - Achieve hemostasis by correcting coagulopathies
  - Blood pressure lowering

- Immediate treatment of elevated blood glucose and elevated body temperature
- Surgical treatment:
  - Posterior fossa decompression for cerebellar hemorrhages
  - Extraventricular drainage for hydrocephalus
  - Evacuation of hematoma may be necessary as a lifesaving measure
  - Minimally invasive surgery could be indicated in select patients

Introduction

Intracranial hemorrhage (ICH) refers to bleeding within the skull, in any intracranial compartment (i.e., subdural, subarachnoid, epidural, or intraparenchymal) (see Figure 1). However, the term is commonly used for intraparenchymal hemorrhages specifically, which will be the focus of this chapter. ICH can be further categorized as "spontaneous" or "secondary," with the latter inferring that there is an underlying lesion (i.e., vascular malformation, tumor) or alternative explanation (i.e., trauma) for the bleed (Table 1). Spontaneous ICH is synonymous with hemorrhagic stroke, referring to spontaneous intraparenchymal bleeding in the absence of identifiable secondary causes. It represents 10% to 15% of all strokes and is the second most common subtype after ischemic strokes. Although the absolute incidence of ICH has increased over the past three decades due to population growth, aging, and increased use of antithrombotic medications, the long-term prognosis remains poor, with approximately 50% mortality at 1 year and loss of functional independence in nearly 75% of survivors.

Pathophysiology

ICH occurs when an arterial intracranial blood vessel bursts and a hematoma is formed due to accumulation of extravasated blood. The hematoma then causes mass effect with compression of adjacent healthy brain tissue, causing neuronal dysfunction and cell death from cytotoxic edema. Hematoma expansion (HE) occurs in up to one-third of patients with ICH in the first 6 hours and is a potentially targetable surrogate outcome for improving survival and preventing disability. The risk for HE is greatest at within 3 hours after symptom onset and the predicted probability of HE is inversely associated with time, although delayed expansion after 24 hours can rarely be encountered. Concurrent with the cessation of active bleeding, vasogenic edema will develop and peak over the next 2 to 7 days. Extension of the blood into the ventricular system may cause acute hydrocephalus due to obstruction of venous outflow. Even small volumes of HE are

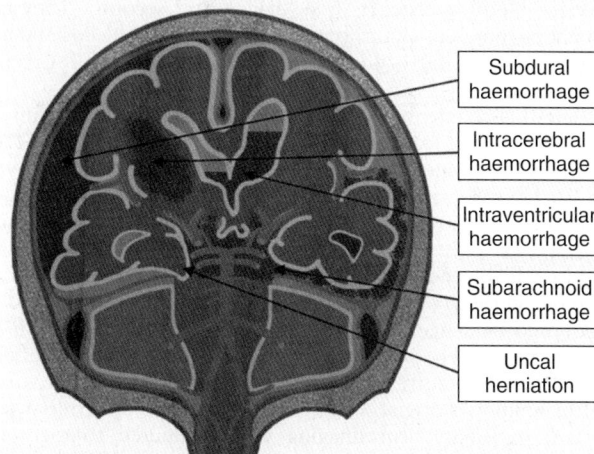

Figure 1 Intracranial compartments. (From https://www.sciencedirect.com/science/article/pii/S0263933915001088.)

TABLE 1	Spontaneous Versus Secondary Causes of Intracerebral Hemorrhage	
SPONTANEOUS ICH	**SECONDARY ICH**	
Hypertensive vasculopathy	Vascular malformations (dural arteriovenous fistula, arteriovenous malformation, cavernous malformation, capillary telangiectasias)	
Cerebral small vessel disease	Cerebral venous thrombosis	
Cerebral amyloid angiopathy	Hemorrhagic conversion of ischemic infarct	
	Moyamoya disease	
	Septic emboli/mycotic aneurysm	
	Brain tumors	
	Vasculitis (infectious, systemic autoimmune disease, primary CNS)	
	Reversible cerebral vasoconstriction syndrome	
	Drugs/toxins (cocaine, amphetamines)	

CNS, Central nervous system; ICH, intracerebral hemorrhage.

TABLE 2	Glasgow Coma Scale	
RESPONSE	**SCALE**	**SCORE**
Eye opening response	Eyes open spontaneously	4 points
	Eyes open to verbal command	3 points
	Eyes open to pain	2 points
	No eye opening	1 point
Verbal response	Oriented	5 points
	Confused conversation, but able to answer questions	4 points
	Inappropriate responses, words discernible	3 points
	Incomprehensible sounds or speech	2 points
	No verbal response	1 point
Motor response	Obeys verbal command for movement	6 points
	Purposeful movement to painful stimulus	5 points
	Withdraws from pain	4 points
	Flexion response, decorticate posture	3 points
	Extensor response, decerebrate posture	2 points
	No motor response	1 point
Total Possible Points		15 points

associated with an increased risk for adverse outcomes: the development of a teaspoon of new parenchymal hemorrhage is associated with quadruple the odds of mortality, and the development of even 1 mL of new ventricular hemorrhage has been shown to be associated with increased risk of disability and death. Ultimately, increased intracranial pressure (ICP) from the mass effect may cause supratentorial herniation, midline shift, and secondary brain injury.

Location of ICH is a helpful predictor in determining the underlying pathogenesis of the ICH. Chronic hypertension is the most common risk factor responsible for subcortical and infratentorial hemorrhages, such as those in the basal ganglia, thalamus, brainstem, and cerebellum. The pathogenesis of hypertensive hemorrhages is attributed to chronic exposure to high pressures in the branching arterioles from major intracranial vessels, resulting in lipohyalinosis of the small arterioles. These relatively fragile vessel walls may then rupture and result in ICH. On the contrary, lobar hemorrhages and convexity subarachnoid hemorrhages in adult patients over the age of 55 are often attributed to cerebral amyloid angiopathy (CAA). This disease process is characterized by the deposition of abnormal amyloid beta proteins in the small to medium-sized vessels of the brain, resulting in weakened vascular integrity over time, which increases the risk for arterial rupture. Amyloid-related hemorrhages typically spare the deep gray matter and brainstem, reflecting the distribution of amyloid deposits, most of which are detected only on MRI sequences sensitive for blood byproducts (see "Diagnosis" section). They are thought to represent clinically silent cerebral microbleeds and are an important risk factor to recognize for increased risk for recurrent ICH.

While this chapter focuses on arterial ICH, it is important to recognize that bleeding from a ruptured venous blood vessel may occur rarely, and that venous hemorrhages are not considered a subtype of ICH. However, it needs to be ruled out as a potential secondary etiology for parenchymal hemorrhage, as the treatment and prognosis are drastically different. Counterintuitively, the mechanism by which venous hemorrhages occur is due to formation of thrombus in the venous drainage of the brain, leading to buildup of ICP and blockage of cerebrospinal fluid (CSF)/blood outflow from the brain. The backlog of pressure leads to venous infarction, petechial hemorrhage, and ICH. In any patient with a lobar ICH of unknown origin or ICH that crosses typical arterial territories, immediate neuroimaging with computed tomography venogram (CTV) or magnetic resonance venogram (MRV) should be pursued to rule out underlying cerebral venous sinus thrombosis (CVST) as the ultimate culprit. This is especially true of lobar hemorrhages in patients who are younger than 55 years of age.

Clinical Manifestations

Neurologic deficits due to ICH are sudden in onset but unlike its ischemic stroke counterpart—where stroke deficits are maximal at onset—neurologic signs and symptoms attributed to ICH tend to worsen with time. As the hematoma expands, patients can deteriorate rapidly, resulting in decreased level of consciousness and requiring intubation. Initial clinical manifestations vary depending on hemorrhage location. The most frequent location for ICH related to chronic hypertension is within the basal ganglia—more specifically the internal capsule/thalamus/putamen/pons. Thus the most common symptomatology includes hemiplegia, hemi-body sensory loss, dysarthria, ataxia, and visual field loss. Cortical bleeds are most frequently associated with CAA and may clinically manifest with aphasia, apraxia, and hemianopia, in addition to the symptomatology mentioned previously. Epileptic seizures may be seen either at the onset of disease or later, as a manifestation of cortical irritation from blood/scar tissue. Headaches, nausea, vomiting, and decreased level of consciousness are common in the context of increased ICP but may also result from other mechanisms such as brainstem compression, development of hydrocephalus, or herniation.

Diagnosis

ICH is a medical emergency: the development of acute neurologic deficits should immediately raise concern for stroke, thus rapid assessment and management are crucial. Initial assessment should prioritize the ABCs of resuscitation (airway, breathing, and circulation) before proceeding with assessment for neurologic deficits. The most commonly used rapid stroke assessment scale is the National Institute of Health Stroke Severity scale (NIHSS). However, another frequently used clinical assessment tool is the Glasgow Coma Scale (GCS) (Table 2), which is often used to assess indications for intubation in the context of decreased level of consciousness. A threshold of GCS 8 or less is used as an indication for intubation. Immediate neuroimaging should be obtained to confirm the diagnosis and rule out other diseases that may

NONCONTRAST CT MARKER	DEFINITION	ILLUSTRATION
Density Markers		
Swirl sign	Area of hypodensity within the hematoma that may be completely encapsulated within the hematoma or may be connected to the wall of the hematoma	
Hypodensity sign	Area of hypodensity within the hematoma that is not connected to the wall of the hematoma	
Blend sign	Area of hypodensity adjacent to an area of hyperdensity within the hematoma with a well-defined margin and a density difference of >18 Hounsfield units	
Shape Markers		
Island sign	At least 3 satellite hematomas adjacent but separate to the main hematoma or 4 small hematomas that are connected to the main hematoma	

Original artwork by Lubna Allabboudy (allabboudylubna@gmail.com).

present in a similar manner, including ischemic stroke and subarachnoid hemorrhage. The noncontrast CT scan is the gold standard for emergent assessment of ICH. Noncontrast CT scans can be used to differentiate ischemic strokes from ICH and to assess ICH size and mass effect on surrounding brain tissue. The initial noncontrast CT scan can also help in assessing certain morphologic markers within the hematoma that have been associated with a higher chance of expansion and potentially worse outcomes. Definitions and visual illustrations of some of these noncontrast CT markers of HE can be found in Table 3. Administration of CT iodinated contrast to facilitate CT angiography may be pursued to look for active contrast extravasation (known as the *spot sign*), which can also be helpful in identifying hemorrhages at a high risk of expansion. CT angiography can also investigate for underlying lesions such as tumor or vascular malformations. Emergent MRI may be used as the initial imaging modality in select centers, although more commonly MRI is obtained in a delayed fashion to investigate the etiology of the bleed. Useful MRI sequences include T2* susceptibility-weighted images (SWI) or gradient-echo (GRE) sequences, which are sensitive for the detection of deoxyhemoglobin, a byproduct of blood. Additional pursuit of imaging such as CTV or MRV should be considered when there is clinical or radiologic suspicion for CVST. Catheter angiography may be pursued when diagnostic suspicion for underlying vascular malformation is high particularly when other more common etiologies are ruled out such as hypertension, CAA, and CVST. The hematoma might obscure an underlying lesion in the acute phase. If the suspicion for an underlying lesion (e.g., malignancy, vascular malformation) is high, repeating an MRI and/or catheter angiography after the resolution of the hematoma can be considered.

Therapy

Treatment of ICH comprises a combination of medical and surgical approaches and generally follows two important principles. During the acute period, stabilizing the hematoma and decreasing the risk for HE is crucial and may be achieved through hemostasis and blood pressure (BP) control. Second, addressing mass effect and its downstream complications may be done through surgery and osmolar therapies.

Emergency Medical Treatment

The two mainstays of medical treatment in ICH are hemostasis and BP control.

Hemostatic abnormalities may not only cause ICH but potentially worsen outcomes if not corrected. Patients with known coagulation factor deficiency or platelet disorders should have replacement of the appropriate factor(s). Patients with significant thrombocytopenia should be considered for platelet transfusion. Those taking vitamin K antagonists (i.e., warfarin) with elevated international normalized ratio (INR) should have their INR corrected rapidly. Either fresh frozen plasma (FFP) or prothrombin complex concentrates (PCC) (50 units/kg, maximum dose 3000 units) may be used, although PCC may be superior in achieving a faster INR normalization rate than FFP and is the preferred agent. Vitamin K (phytonadione 10 mg IV) needs to be given concurrently due to the short half-life of PCC; the onset of action of vitamin K starts approximately 2 hours after administration and will continue to peak over the next 12 to 14 hours. Other hemostatic factors such as rFVIIa (recombinant factor VIIa [NovoSeven RT])[1] are not currently recommended, although there are ongoing clinical trials evaluating its efficacy in patients presenting in an early time window from symptom onset. Patients taking direct oral anticoagulants (DOACs) may be eligible for specific reversal agents, such as idarucizumab ([Praxbind] 2.5 g IV boluses twice, no more than 15 minutes apart) for dabigatran (Pradaxa), and andexanet alfa (Andexxa, Ondexxya) for factor Xa inhibitors (such as rivaroxaban [Xarelto], edoxaban [Savaysa, Lixiana][1], or apixaban [Eliquis]). If andexanet alfa is not available, some clinicians may choose to use PCC to reverse factor Xa inhibitors if there is biochemical evidence of activity at time of presentation or confirmed recent ingestion. Patients taking antiplatelet agents before development of their ICH should not routinely receive platelet transfusion if their platelet count is normal, as it has been found to be harmful rather than beneficial. Protamine sulfate can be considered in patients on low-molecular-weight heparin[1] or heparin infusion.

Elevated BP is frequently encountered in acute ICH due to a variety of physiologic responses. However, high BP is a major risk factor for developing HE and thereby worse outcomes after ICH. The INTERACT-3 clinical trial demonstrated improved outcomes at 3 months after implementing a care bundle within 6 hours of presentation, which included intensive lowering of systolic BP to <140 mm Hg, strict glucose control, antipyretic treatment, and rapid reversal of warfarin-related anticoagulation. However, excessive BP lowering may be associated with increased risk for renal insufficiency. For those presenting with severely elevated SBP (>220 mm Hg), lowering to 140 mm Hg is practically challenging and may be harmful, thus many clinicians may choose to target a BP that is 25% lower than the patient's initial SBP instead.

As per INTERACT-3, the acute care of intracerebral hemorrhage should also include strict glucose control (target 6.1–7.8 mmol/L in those without diabetes and 7.8–10.0 mmol/L in those with diabetes), treatment of elevated body temperatures (target body temperature ≤37.5°C), and rapid reversal of vitamin K antagonist–related anticoagulation (target international normalized ratio [INR] <1.5) within 1 hour of treatment.

Surgical Management

There are multiple scenarios where surgical management of ICH should be considered immediately.

1. Cerebellar hemorrhages: Due to the limitations in space for expansion in the posterior fossa, it is generally accepted that any cerebellar hemorrhage with brainstem compression and/or hydrocephalus and/or neurologic deterioration should have immediate surgical decompression.
2. Intraventricular extension and hydrocephalus: insertion of an extraventricular drainage (EVD) device should be considered for ICH with intraventricular hemorrhage (IVH) extension causing impaired consciousness or hydrocephalus.
3. Supratentorial, medium-sized (i.e., volumes of 30–80 mL) ICH: minimally invasive surgery may be indicated if it can be performed within 24 hours of symptom onset, particularly if the hemorrhage is lobar in location.

Surgical decompression is often indicated for cerebellar hemorrhages, intraventricular extension, and hydrocephalus. Due to the limitations in space for expansion in the posterior fossa, it is generally accepted that any cerebellar hemorrhage with brainstem compression and/or hydrocephalus and/or neurologic deterioration should have immediate surgical decompression. Hematoma evacuation with decompressive craniectomy for deep basal ganglia hemorrhages may be considered as a lifesaving measure in deteriorating patients; however, its efficacy for prevention of functional disability is not well established. In patients with IVH causing hydrocephalus or deteriorating level of consciousness, EVD should be considered. There is limited evidence for irrigation of extraventricular drains with alteplase (Activase)[1], and its use is not routinely recommended based on the current level of evidence. A summary of therapeutic options for ICH is outlined in Table 4.

Inpatient Medical Treatment

Medical treatment of ICH should be continued beyond the emergency setting to prevent further complications during hospitalization. Maintenance of normoglycemia and normothermia should be the standard of care, as hyperglycemia and hypothermia have both been associated with poorer long-term outcomes. Universal dysphagia screening before initiation of an oral diet should be implemented to reduce the risk of aspiration pneumonia—a common complication during the first weeks of hospitalization. To mitigate the risk for urinary tract infections, indwelling foleys should not be inserted without appropriate clinical indication and, if needed in the acute phase, should be removed as soon as deemed possible. All patients should have intermittent pneumatic compression devices for prevention of venous thromboembolism (VTE) beginning the day of hospital admission. Once the patient has been deemed clinically and radiologically stable, they may be transitioned to a pharmacologic agent for VTE prophylaxis. A common practice is repeating brain imaging after 24 to 48 hours from onset to prove hematoma stability before the initiation of pharmacologic VTE prophylaxis. Osmolar therapies such as hypertonic saline and mannitol should be considered in patients who are at risk of increased ICP and subsequent complications such as brain herniation, but these are considered temporizing measures until definitive surgical intervention. Prophylactic use of antiseizure medications is not recommended as a routine practice in ICH.

---

[1] Not FDA approved for this indication.

---

[1] Not FDA approved for this indication.

TABLE 4 Summary of Therapies in the Treatment of Intracerebral Hemorrhage

MEDICAL TREATMENT OPTIONS

Hemostasis	Known coagulation factor deficiency: replacement of appropriate factors
	Vitamin K antagonist–related ICH: • Target INR of <1.5 • FFP or prothrombin complex concentrates • Vitamin K
	DOAC-related ICH: • Idarucizumab (Praxbind) for dabigatran (Pradaxa) • Andexanet alfa (Andexxa) for rivaroxaban (Xarelto), edoxaban (Savaysa, Lixiana)[1], or apixaban (Eliquis) • Consider using FFP if andexanet alfa is not available
	Antiplatelet-related ICH: • Do not give platelet transfusion
	Heparin infusion or LMWH-related ICH: • Consider protamine sulfate
	Ongoing trials for rFVIIa (NovoSeven RT)[1]—not currently recommended
Blood pressure control	SBP between 150 and 220 mm Hg: • Lowering SBP to 140 mm Hg is safe and improves functional outcomes • Avoid drastic lowering of SBP to 120 mm Hg or less to avoid compromising systemic perfusion pressures to other organs (i.e., kidneys)
	SBP >220 mm Hg: • Lowering SBP is still indicated, although practically challenging to 140 mm Hg. Consider lowering SBP by at least 25% reduction

Surgical Treatment Options

Decompressive surgery	Posterior fossa/cerebellar hemorrhages: • Surgery is indicated for any cerebellar hemorrhage with brainstem compression and/or hydrocephalus and/or neurologic deterioration • Threshold of 3 cm in hematoma diameter for surgical intervention
	Supratentorial/deep hemorrhages: • Surgery may be considered a lifesaving measure in deteriorating patients but does not improve functional outcomes
Minimally invasive surgery	Supratentorial (lobar) hemorrhages between 30 and 80 mL • Rapid access (i.e., performed within 24 hours of symptom onset) was associated with improved 6-month functional outcomes
Extraventricular drainage	Indicated for patients with hydrocephalus and decreased level of consciousness
	Irrigation with alteplase (Activase)[1] is not currently indicated

Prevention of Secondary Injury and Complications

Monitoring	Dedicated stroke unit or intensive care unit with neuroscience expertise • Frequent vital sign checks (including blood pressure), neurologic assessments, and continuous cardiopulmonary monitoring if on continuous IV antihypertensives • EEG should be considered for decreased level of consciousness • Continuous intracranial pressure monitoring may be considered for transtentorial herniation, significant IVH, hydrocephalus, or decreased level of consciousness
Glucose	Strict glucose control (target 6.1–7.8 mmol/L in those without diabetes and 7.8–10.0 mmol/L in those with diabetes)
Temperature	Antipyretic treatment targeting body temperature <37.5°C
Seizure control	Antiepileptics should be considered in those with clinical seizures. It is not routinely recommended as prophylaxis
Dysphagia	Dysphagia assessment needs to be performed before initiation of oral diet to prevent aspiration pneumonia
Urinary tract infection	Foley catheters should not be routinely used
Venous thromboembolism	Intermittent pneumatic compression devices are indicated on first day of hospitalization. Pharmacologic prophylaxis may be considered upon proving radiologic hematoma stability

[1]Not FDA approved for this indication.

DOAC, direct oral anticoagulant; *EEG*, electroencephalogram; *FFP*, fresh frozen plasma; *ICH*, intracerebral hemorrhage; *INR*, international normalized ratio; *IVH*, intraventricular hemorrhage; *LMWH*, low-molecular-weight heparin; *SBP*, systolic blood pressure.

Intracerebral Hemorrhage

787

TABLE 5 Components of ICH Score and FUNC Score and Their Associations With Outcomes

	ICH SCORE	FUNC SCORE
Scoring	Glasgow Coma Scale: 3–4: 2 points 5–12: 1 point 13–15: 0 points	Glasgow Coma Scale: ≥9: 2 points ≤8: 0 points
	ICH volume (cm^3): ≥30: 1 point <30: 0 points	ICH volume (cm^3): <30: 4 points 30–60: 2 points >60: 0 points
	Intraventricular hemorrhage: Yes: 1 point No: 0 points	Pre-ICH cognitive impairment: No: 1 point Yes: 0 points
	ICH location: Infratentorial: 1 point Not infratentorial: 0 points	ICH location: Lobar: 2 points Deep: 1 point Infratentorial: 0 points
	Age (years): ≥80: 1 point <80: 0 points	Age (years): <70: 2 points 70–79: 1 point ≥80: 0 points
	Total: 0–6 (higher score suggests worse prognosis)	Total: 0–11 (lower score suggests worse prognosis)
Association with outcomes in original publication	*Association with 30-day mortality:* 0: 0% mortality 1: 13% mortality 2: 26% mortality 3: 72% mortality 4: 97% mortality >5: 100% mortality	*Association with 90-day functional independence:* 0–4: 0% independent 5–7: 13% independent 8: 42% independent 9–10: 66% independent 11: 75% independent

Prognostication and decisions around withdrawal of care should not be made for at least 48 hours.
ICH, Intracerebral hemorrhage.

Monitoring

ICH patients should be cared for in a dedicated stroke or intensive care unit wherever possible, as this has been shown to be associated with better outcomes. Frequent vital sign checks, neurologic assessments with validated scales such as GCS and NIHSS, and continuous cardiopulmonary monitoring should be part of the standard treatment plan. BP monitoring is especially crucial because it is the only therapy that has the potential to improve functional outcomes, thus hypertensive patients should have repeat BP checks every 15 minutes until the desired BP target is achieved and maintained for 24 hours. Electroencephalography (EEG) monitoring should be considered in any patient who has persistent unexplained decreased level of consciousness (LOC), due to frequent subclinical seizures in ICH patients. Continuous monitoring of ICP is not universally indicated but may be considered in patients with evidence of transtentorial herniation, significant IVH, hydrocephalus, or decreased level of consciousness (i.e., GCS ≤8).

Complications

Prognostication

ICH patients typically present very severely (i.e., decreased LOC, debilitating deficits), and recovery in ICH tends to be much slower than its ischemic stroke counterpart. It is a devastating disease with limited treatment options, and a vital role for the clinician is providing accurate prognostication to family members/patients. The most widely used prognostication tool is the ICH score, which was initially developed to predict 30-day mortality but has since been validated to predict long-term mortality up to 1 year (Table 5). Other prediction scores include the FUNC score, which was originally developed to predict the chances of meaningful functional recovery (see Table 5), although its use is less widely implemented. It is generally recommended that prognostication should be deferred to at least 48 to 72 hours after time of presentation to optimally assess the patient's clinical trajectory and allow time for radiographic stability to ensue.

Acute Neurologic Deterioration

Acute neurologic deterioration is associated with increased risk for long-term disability and mortality, and may result from HE, seizures, increasing mass effect, development of ventricular hemorrhage, and cerebral herniation. Approximately one-fifth of patients will experience early neurologic deterioration. Antiepileptic medications should not be initiated unless a clinical seizure is witnessed or suspected and confirmed with EEG.

Long-Term Complications

The long-term sequelae of ICH include physical disability, cognitive impairment, mood disorders, localization-related epilepsy, and increased risk for recurrent ICH. There may be an increased risk for ischemic stroke in patients with a history of ICH due to avoidance of antithrombotic medications. Important predictors for recurrent ICH include microhemorrhages detected on MRI, uncontrolled hypertension, prior lacunar stroke, older age, and ongoing anticoagulation therapy, although it is still an ongoing, active area of research. Patients with ICH who require long-term anticoagulation (i.e., atrial fibrillation, mechanical heart valves, hypercoagulable disorders) should be assessed by a neurologist or thrombosis specialist to optimize risk factor control, and the risk for future ICH should be weighed against the need for antithrombotic therapy. Data from the ENRICH trial suggest that minimally invasive surgery when performed within 24 hours of symptom onset for a patient with supratentorial, medium-sized ICH may improve functional outcomes at 6 months. In patients with ICH due to CAA that have concurrent atrial fibrillation, nonpharmacologic methods of reducing the risk of cardioembolic ischemic stroke may be considered, such as left appendage closure to reduce the risk of ICH recurrence.

TABLE 6 · Ongoing Clinical Trials in Intracerebral Hemorrhage

CLINICAL TRIAL NAME	PRIMARY COUNTRY	INTERVENTION ASSESSED	STATUS
Surgical Trials			
Early Minimally Invasive Image Guided Endoscopic Evacuation of Intracerebral Hemorrhage (EMINENT-ICH)	Switzerland	Early minimally invasive image-guided hematoma evacuation with the best medical treatment compared with best medical treatment alone	Recruiting
Ultra-Early, Minimally inVAsive intraCerebral Hemorrhage evacUATion Versus Standard trEatment (EVACUATE)	Australia	Ultra-early, minimally invasive hematoma evacuation vs. standard care within 8 hours of ICH	Recruiting
Efficacy and Safety of NeuroEndoscopic Surgery for IntraCerebral Hemorrhage (NESICH)	China	Neuroendoscopic hematoma removal vs. standard conservative in patients with spontaneous supratentorial deep ICH	Recruiting
A Prospective, Multicenter Study of Artemis, a Minimally Invasive Neuro Evacuation Device, in the Removal of Intracerebral Hemorrhage (MIND)	United States	Artemis device plus medical management vs. medical management alone in supratentorial ICH	Active, not recruiting
Dutch Intracerebral Hemorrhage Surgery Trial (DIST)	Netherlands	Minimally invasive endoscopic-guided surgery vs. standard medical management for spontaneous supratentorial ICH	Recruiting
Acute Medical Therapy			
Recombinant Factor VIIa (rFVIIa) for Hemorrhagic Stroke Trial (FASTEST)	United States	Recombinant factor VIIa (NovoSeven RT)[1] plus best standard therapy vs. placebo plus best standard therapy within 2 hours of symptom onset	Recruiting
Fingolimod as a Treatment of Cerebral Edema After Intracerebral Hemorrhage (FITCH)	United States	Single dose of fingolimod (Gilenya)[1] vs. placebo in patients with primary spontaneous ICH	Completed, pending results
Stopping Hemorrhage With Tranexamic Acid for Hyperacute Onset Presentation Including Mobile Stroke Units (STOP-MSU)	Australia	Tranexamic acid (Cyklokapron)[1] vs. normal saline given within 2 hours of symptom onset in mobile stroke units	Completed, pending results
Rehabilitation/Prevention			
Avoiding Anticoagulation After IntraCerebral Hemorrhage (A3ICH)	France	Anticoagulation with apixaban (Eliquis)[1] vs. no anticoagulation with left atrial appendage closure vs. usual care	Recruiting
Anticoagulation in ICH Survivors for Stroke Prevention and Recovery (ASPIRE)	United States	Apixaban[1] vs. aspirin in patients with ICH and nonvalvular atrial fibrillation	Recruiting
EdoxabaN foR IntraCranial Hemorrhage Survivors With Atrial Fibrillation (ENRICH-AF)	Canada	Edoxaban (Savaysa, Lixiana)[1] vs. no antithrombotic therapy or antiplatelet monotherapy in high-risk atrial fibrillation patients after ICH	Recruiting
Prevention of Stroke by Left Atrial Appendage Closure in Atrial Fibrillation Patients After Intracerebral Hemorrhage	Sweden	Left atrial appendage occlusion vs. medical therapy in patients with nonvalvular atrial fibrillation after ICH	Recruiting
Prevention of Hypertensive Injury to the Brain by Intensive Treatment in IntraCerebral Hemorrhage (PROHIBIT-ICH)	United Kingdom	Intensive BP treatment (target <120/80 mm Hg) guided by telemetric home monitoring vs. standard primary care (target 130/80 mm Hg) in survivors of hypertension-related ICH	Recruiting
Statins In Intracerebral Hemorrhage (SATURN)	United States	Continuation vs. discontinuation of statin drugs after spontaneous lobar ICH	Recruiting
MOBILE Health Intervention in Intracerebral Hemorrhage Survivors	Hong Kong	Mobile stroke app vs. standard care for management of hypertension in ICH survivors	Recruiting
Triple Therapy Prevention of Recurrent Intracerebral Disease EveNts Trial (TRIDENT)	Australia	Telmisartan (Micardis)[1], amlodipine (Norvasc)[1], and indapamide[1] vs. placebo for prevention of recurrent stroke in ICH survivors	Recruiting
Study of Antithrombotic Treatment After IntraCerebral Hemorrhage (STATICH)	Denmark	Anticoagulation vs. no anticoagulation in ICH survivors with atrial fibrillation	Recruiting
Colchicine for the Prevention of Vascular Events After an Acute Intracerebral Hemorrhage (CoVasc-ICH)	Canada	Colchicine[1] for the prevention of vascular events after an acute ICH	Completed, pending results

[1]Not FDA approved for this indication.
BP, Blood pressure; *ICH*, intracerebral hemorrhage.

Prevention

Primary Prevention

Hypertension is the major modifiable risk factor for hemorrhagic strokes. Uncontrolled hypertension accounts for approximately 74% of ICH worldwide, and treatment of hypertension is effective as both primary and secondary prevention. Use of antithrombotic medication is another modifiable risk factor for ICH. For patients who require long-term anticoagulation for atrial fibrillation or VTE, DOACs carry a much lower risk for ICH than warfarin and should be first-line therapy unless patients have a specific indication otherwise (i.e., valvular atrial fibrillation, mechanical valve, antiphospholipid syndrome). Patients should not be on antiplatelet agents without appropriate clinical indication, as chronic antiplatelet therapy is a known risk factor for ICH.

Secondary Prevention

Hypertension is not only an important risk factor for ICH but is also implicated in other cardiovascular diseases. Treatment of hypertension is effective for attenuating the risk for recurrent hemorrhagic strokes and prevention of ischemic strokes. For patients at a high risk of cardiovascular events who previously experienced an ICH, the RESTART trial has shown that antiplatelet therapy may be resumed without an increased risk of recurrent ICH. The decision to start anticoagulants after an ICH, however, is not as clear-cut and will depend on the balance of risk for ICH occurrence and clinical indications for requiring anticoagulation. Important factors to consider include the suspected etiology of ICH, control of risk factors before the last ICH, age/comorbidities, and patient preference. Finally, statin therapy is not currently indicated for primary or secondary prevention of intracerebral hemorrhage. Lower levels of low-density lipoprotein (LDL) may be associated with increased risk for ICH, but research is ongoing to better understand this relationship.

Ongoing Research

There are multiple ongoing clinical trials in the intracerebral hemorrhage field that have the potential to change the way we treat the disease. These are summarized in Table 6 and broken down in terms of acute surgical trials, acute medical trials, and those evaluating optimal management of comorbidities after ICH.

References

Primary and secondary prevention of ischemic stroke and cerebral hemorrhage: JACC focus seminar, *J Am Coll Cardiol* 75(15):1804–1818, 2020. https://doi.org/10.1016/j.jacc.2019.12.072.

Shoamanesh (Co-chair) A, Patrice Lindsay M, Castellucci LA, et al. Canadian stroke best practice recommendations: management of spontaneous intracerebral hemorrhage, 7th edition update 2020. *Int J Stroke*. Published online November 11, 1747493020968424, 2020. https://doi.org/10.1177/1747493020968424.

O'Donnell MJ, Xavier D, Liu L, et al: Risk factors for ischaemic and intracerebral haemorrhagic stroke in 22 countries (the INTERSTROKE study): a case-control study, *Lancet Lond Engl* 376(9735):112–123, 2010. https://doi.org/10.1016/S0140-6736(10)60834-3.

Salman RAS, Frantzias J, Lee RJ, et al: Absolute risk and predictors of the growth of acute spontaneous intracerebral haemorrhage: a systematic review and meta-analysis of individual patient data, *Lancet Neurol* 17(10):885–894, 2018. https://doi.org/10.1016/S1474-4422(18)30253-9.

Ma L, Hu X, Song L, et al: The third intensive care bundle with blood pressure reduction in acute cerebral haemorrhage trial (INTERACT3): an international, stepped wedge cluster randomised controlled trial, *Lancet* 402(10395):27–40. 2023. https://doi.org/10.1016/S0140-6736(23)00806-1.

Greenberg SM, Ziai WC, Cordonnier C, et al: 2022 Guideline for the management of patients with spontaneous intracerebral hemorrhage: a guideline from the American heart association/American stroke association, *Stroke* 53(7):e282–e361, 2022. https://doi.org/10.1161/STR.0000000000000407.

Hemphill JC, Bonovich DC, Besmertis L, Manley GT, Johnston SC: The ICH score: a simple, reliable grading scale for intracerebral hemorrhage, *Stroke* 32(4):891–897, 2001. https://doi.org/10.1161/01.str.32.4.891.

Rost NS, Smith EE, Chang Y, et al: Prediction of functional outcome in patients with primary intracerebral hemorrhage: the FUNC score, *Stroke* 39(8):2304–2309, 2008. https://doi.org/10.1161/STROKEAHA.107.512202.

Shoamanesh A: Anticoagulation in patients with cerebral amyloid angiopathy, *Lancet* 402(10411):1418–1419, 2023. https://doi.org/10.1016/s0140-6736(23)02025-1.

Morotti A, Boulouis G, Dowlatshahi D, Li Q, Barras CD, Delcourt C, et al: Standards for detecting, interpreting, and reporting noncontrast computed tomographic markers of intracerebral hemorrhage expansion, *Ann Neurol* 86(4):480–492, 2019. https://doi.org/10.1002/ana.25563.

ISCHEMIC CEREBROVASCULAR DISEASE

Method of
Alvaro Cervera Alvarez, MD, PhD; and Geoffrey A. Donnan, MD

CURRENT DIAGNOSIS

- Early recognition of stroke is crucial to transport patients to hospitals with dedicated stroke units.
- Advanced neuroimaging allows the use of reperfusion therapies with a prolonged time window.

CURRENT THERAPY

- Most strokes are preventable and, therefore, risk factor management and stroke education are crucial.
- Admission to a stroke unit is the most effective and widely available resource for the majority of patients.
- Thrombolysis and thrombectomy have revolutionized the management of acute stroke, greatly improving the outcome.

Treatment of ischemic stroke has improved significantly in the past few years, and mortality and disability rates owing to this condition have decreased. The management of patients in stroke units and the demonstration of the efficacy of thrombolysis and thrombectomy have been crucial in this achievement. Control of vascular risk factors has decreased the number and severity of events. However, recent studies have found an increased incidence of ischemic stroke in the young. Improved management has included high-quality rehabilitation, which has to start early to improve the recovery (i.e., functional independence) of stroke survivors. The multidisciplinary management of stroke can be improved with specific educational programs aimed at increasing awareness of stroke in the general population and among professionals. The concept of "Time is Brain" has great value in emphasizing that stroke is an emergency. Because the window for the available time-dependent treatments is very narrow, avoiding delay is the major goal in the prehospital phase of acute stroke care. Therefore it is important to transport all stroke patients as soon as possible to the closest hospital with a stroke unit. In rural or remote areas with no stroke unit facilities, telemedicine has proven to be a valid alternative.

Prevention

Lifestyle modification can be a major contributor to reducing the risk of ischemic stroke. Strategies to achieve this protection include avoiding smoking and excessive alcohol consumption, keeping a low/normal body mass index, practicing regular exercise, and having a diet low in salt and saturated fat, high in fruits and vegetables, and rich in fiber. In addition, a Mediterranean diet supplemented with nuts is associated with a decreased risk of vascular events. There is no need to add vitamin supplements to the diet because they do not affect stroke prevention.

Regular assessment of vascular risk factors (e.g., hypertension, diabetes, hypercholesterolemia) is important because their control can significantly reduce the incidence of vascular events. In the case of blood pressure, this can be done with diet and pharmacologic therapy, aiming at normal levels of 120/80 mm Hg. After an ischemic stroke, blood pressure should be lowered even in patients with normal blood pressure. Diabetes should be managed with lifestyle modification and pharmacologic therapy as required, and blood pressure needs to be more tightly controlled in these patients (<130/80 mm Hg). The best antihypertensive treatments for diabetics are angiotensin-converting enzyme inhibitors or angiotensin receptor antagonists. Hypercholesterolemia

TABLE 1	Prevention of Stroke in Patients With Atrial Fibrillation

CHA2DS2-VASc SCALE

RISK FACTOR	SCORE
Congestive heart failure	1
Hypertension	1
Age ≥75	2
Age 65–74	1
Diabetes mellitus	1
Stroke or transient ischemic attack	2
Vascular disease	1
Female sex	1

should be managed with lifestyle modification and a statin. After a noncardioembolic ischemic stroke, high-dose statins are beneficial in all patients for secondary prevention.

Postmenopausal hormone replacement therapy should be avoided for the primary or secondary prevention of stroke because it can increase the risk of new vascular events. Other strategies to prevent stroke include the treatment of obstructive sleep apnea with continuous positive airway pressure breathing.

Antithrombotic Therapy

Low-dose aspirin[1] can be used for the primary prevention of stroke in women or of myocardial infarction in men. Nevertheless, its effect is very small, and it cannot be recommended on a population-wide basis. Aspirin is beneficial for the prevention of stroke in patients with asymptomatic carotid stenosis.

In patients with atrial fibrillation, the CHA2DS2-VASc scale (Table 1) is used to decide whether to use anticoagulation. If the score (https://www.mdcalc.com/chads2-score-atrial-fibrillation-stroke-ris) is 2 or more, treatment with oral anticoagulants is indicated. With a score of 1, the decision should be made according to the presence of risk factors, risk of bleeding, and patient choice. If the score is 0, there is no need to start antithrombotic treatment, neither antiplatelets nor anticoagulants. All patients with stroke or transient ischemic attack (TIA) should be anticoagulated, unless strictly contraindicated. Patients with valvular atrial fibrillation require anticoagulation with warfarin, aiming at an international normalized ratio (INR) of 2.0 to 3.0. Patients with prosthetic heart valves should also receive warfarin, and the target INR depends on the prosthesis type. In nonvalvular atrial fibrillation, the treatment options include warfarin (INR 2.0 to 3.0) or a direct oral anticoagulant (dabigatran [Pradaxa], apixaban [Eliquis], rivaroxaban [Xarelto], and edoxaban [Savaysa]). The direct oral anticoagulants are associated with a decreased risk of intracranial hemorrhage compared with warfarin. Dabigatran (150 mg, twice daily) and apixaban (5 mg, twice daily) have shown to be superior to warfarin in stroke prevention. The dose of the direct oral anticoagulants needs to be adjusted depending on age, renal function, and/or weight.

After an ischemic stroke, all patients should receive antithrombotic therapy. Antiplatelet agents are the first choice unless anticoagulation is required. The most effective regimen is clopidogrel (Plavix) or aspirin plus dipyridamole (Aggrenox). However, low-dose aspirin is a reasonable alternative. During the first 3 weeks after a minor stroke or TIA, the combination of aspirin plus clopidogrel or aspirin and ticagrelor (Brilinta) can be more effective in reducing ischemic events than clopidogrel alone, although the evidence is scarce. However, dual antiplatelet treatment is not recommended in the long term, except if there is an association with

[1] Not FDA approved for this indication.

unstable angina or non–Q wave myocardial infarction, or if there has been a recent stenting. Anticoagulation is usually indicated for secondary prevention if the stroke cause is cardioembolic and in specific situations, such as aortic arch atheroma or fusiform aneurysms of the basilar artery. However, level 1 evidence is lacking for these approaches.

Management of Carotid Stenosis

In patients with asymptomatic carotid stenosis (≥60%), surgery is indicated only if the risk of stroke is high. Endarterectomy is the treatment of choice if the stenosis is symptomatic (i.e., has been associated with an ipsilateral stroke or TIA), and severe (70% to 99%). Surgery should be performed in centers with a perioperative complication rate of less than 6% and as soon as possible after the last ischemic event.

Endarterectomy may be indicated for certain patients with moderate stenosis (50%–69%), although it should be performed only in centers with a perioperative complication rate of less than 3% to be effective. In cases of symptomatic carotid lesions, angioplasty plus stenting is a reasonable alternative, mainly in patients younger than 70 years. If stenting is performed, a combination of clopidogrel and aspirin is required immediately before the procedure and for at least 1 month after to prevent stent thrombosis.

In patients with intracranial atheromatosis and stroke recurrences, intensive medical treatment is the preferred option. Angioplasty and stenting are not recommended.

Management of Patent Foramen Ovale

The presence of a patent foramen ovale (PFO) is associated with cryptogenic stroke in the young. There is evidence that in selected patients with stroke or TIA (<60 years of age, nonlacunar stroke, and exclusion of other causes of stroke) the percutaneous transcatheter closure of the PFO is associated with a significant reduction of new vascular events, although with more frequent atrial fibrillation postprocedure, usually transient. Otherwise, there is no evidence indicating that anticoagulation is more effective than antiplatelets for stroke prevention in patients with PFO.

Management of Acute Ischemic Stroke

All stroke patients should be treated in a stroke unit, because this is associated with a reduction of death, dependency, and the need for institutional care. This effect is present in all stroke patients, irrespective of gender, age, stroke subtype, and stroke severity. Patients with stroke should have a careful clinical assessment, including a neurologic examination. The use of a stroke rating scale, such as the National Institutes of Health Stroke Scale, provides important information about the severity of stroke.

Urgent cranial computed tomography (CT) is mandatory after an ischemic stroke before starting any therapy. Alternatively, magnetic resonance imaging (MRI) or CT perfusion (CTP) can be performed, providing additional information about the selection of patients for mechanical thrombectomy within 6 to 24 hours from symptom onset. However, there is not enough evidence to recommend its routine use in the acute stroke setting.

For the detection and early management of the medical complications of stroke, neurologic status, pulse, blood pressure, temperature, and oxygen saturation should be monitored. Similarly, serum glucose levels need to be monitored and hyperglycemia needs to be treated with insulin accordingly. Normal saline is recommended for fluid replacement during the first 24 hours after stroke. If the patient has a fever, treatment with acetaminophen (paracetamol) may be used while sources of infection are being sought. Reducing blood pressure is recommended only in patients with extremely high blood pressure or when indicated by other medical conditions. Blood pressure should be lowered gradually, avoiding abrupt changes.

Thrombolysis

All patients suffering an ischemic stroke within 4.5 hours of onset should receive thrombolytic treatment, with intravenous tissue plasminogen activator (tPA [Activase] or tenecteplase [TNKase]) unless contraindicated, because it is effective in improving stroke

BOX 1 | Treatment of Acute Ischemic Stroke With Intravenous Thrombolysis

- Infuse 0.9 mg/kg (maximum dose 90 mg) of tPA (Activase) over 60 minutes, with 10% of the dose given as a bolus over 1 minute or tenecteplase (TNKase) in a single bolus (0.25 mg/kg, max 25 mg).
- Admit the patient to a stroke unit for monitoring. Perform neurologic assessment and blood pressure measurement every 15 minutes during the infusion, every 30 minutes thereafter for the next 6 hours, and then hourly until 24 hours after treatment. Administer antihypertensive medications to maintain systolic blood pressure ≤180 mm Hg and diastolic ≤105 mm Hg.
- If intracranial hemorrhage is suspected, discontinue the infusion and obtain an emergency CT scan.
- Obtain a follow-up CT scan at 24 hours before starting anticoagulants or antiplatelet agents.

CT, Computed tomography; *tPA,* tissue plasminogen activator.

BOX 2 | Reperfusion Therapies in Acute Ischemic Stroke

Symptom onset between 0 and 4.5 hours:
- No contraindications for thrombolysis.
  - Perform CT scan.
  - Administer IV tPA (Activase) or tenecteplase (TNKase).
  - Perform multimodal imaging (this could be done beforehand if it does not delay treatment with IV tPA).
  - MT: if occlusion of intracranial internal carotid artery or middle cerebral artery (segment 1, M1), NIHSS score ≥ 6, no premorbid disability (mRS 0–1), and ASPECTS ≥ 6. Groin puncture within 6 hours of symptom onset.

Contraindications for thrombolysis:
- Perform multimodal imaging.
  - Proceed to MT: if occlusion of intracranial internal carotid artery or middle cerebral artery (M1), NIHSS score ≥ 6, no premorbid disability (mRS 0–1), and ASPECTS ≥ 6. Groin puncture within 6 hours of symptom onset.

Symptom onset between 4.5 and 9 hours or wake-up stroke:
- Perform multimodal imaging.
  - If no contraindications for thrombolysis, administer IV tPA (Activase) or tenecteplase if significant penumbra according to EXTEND or WAKE-UP trials.
  - Proceed to MT if significant penumbra according to DAWN or DEFUSE 3 trials (this varies depending on age, NIHSS, and size of infarct core).
  - Standard medical management if no criteria for thrombolysis or MT.

Symptom onset between 9 and 24 hours:
- Perform multimodal imaging.
  - If occlusion of the intracranial internal carotid artery, middle cerebral artery (M1), or both.
  - Proceed to MT if significant penumbra according to DAWN or DEFUSE 3 trials (this varies depending on age, NIHSS, and size of infarct core).
  - Otherwise, standard medical management.

Other circumstances:
1. MT could be a reasonable option in selected cases with distal occlusion of the middle cerebral artery (M2 or M3).
   - MT is a reasonable therapeutic option for selected patients with occlusion of the anterior cerebral arteries, vertebral arteries, basilar artery, or posterior cerebral arteries.
   - Selected patients could benefit from MT even with premorbid conditions (mRS > 1), ASPECTS < 6, or NIHSS score < 6.
2. Patients with large ischemic cores can also benefit from MT, although there is a higher risk of vascular complications.

ASPECTS, Alberta stroke program early CT score; *CT,* computed tomography; *IV,* intravenous; *mRS,* modified Rankin Scale; *MT,* mechanical thrombectomy; *NIHSS,* National Institutes of Health Stroke Scale; *tPA,* tissue plasminogen activator.

outcome (Box 1). It is very important to start treatment as soon as possible, because pooled analysis has demonstrated that earlier treatment results in a better outcome. Thrombolysis with tPA is effective in all different population subgroups, including the very elderly, even with significant comorbidities. The therapeutic window can be extended up to 9 hours from onset when using advance imaging, such as perfusion-diffusion MRI or CTP. This approach has also been shown to be effective in wake-up strokes. Tenecteplase (TNKase)[1] is an alternative to tPA. Due to its easier administration and association with better outcome, it is recommended as the first line agent in many guidelines.

Endovascular Thrombectomy

Mechanical thrombectomy using stent retrievers, in addition to thrombolysis, is more effective in improving outcomes than thrombolysis alone in anterior circulation strokes and a large artery occlusion, with a time window of up to 6 hours. This treatment is also effective when there are contraindications for intravenous thrombolysis. In a recent metaanalysis of five major trials (MR CLEAN, ESCAPE, REVASCAT, SWIFT PRIME, and EXTEND IA), endovascular thrombectomy led to significantly reduced disability at 90 days compared with control (odds ratio 2.49), with a number needed to treat of 2.6. All subgroups of patients benefit from this effect. Therefore health authorities have to implement access to thrombectomy within a reasonable time frame in a network, including stroke centers. Recent evidence shows that similar results are obtained when treating basilar artery occlusion.

There is recently published evidence indicating that the therapeutic window could be extended significantly when using multimodal imaging to select patients who have marked penumbra. Thus the DAWN trial showed that patients with ischemic penumbra could benefit from thrombectomy up to 24 hours since symptom onset, in comparison with standard care. This result was replicated by the DEFUSE 3 trial, although it included patients up to 16 hours from onset. Also, recent studies showed that thrombectomy can be beneficial in patients with a large ischemic core, although there is a higher risk of vascular complications. In Box 2, there is a simplified algorithm for the use of reperfusion therapies in acute ischemic stroke.

In large urban areas, mobile stroke units can significantly improve the management of acute stroke patients. These specialized units are ambulances equipped with CT scans and staff expert in acute stroke care. The use of mobile stroke units is associated with a faster thrombolytic treatment and a better functional outcome in comparison with the standard of care (transferring patients to emergency services). Also, these mobile units could facilitate a faster access to endovascular thrombectomy.

Antithrombotic Drugs

All ischemic stroke patients should receive a low dose of aspirin daily. This can be started as soon as possible in patients who have not received reperfusion therapies, but always within 48 hours after onset. However, in patients who received thrombolysis, aspirin should be delayed for 24 hours. The use of other antiplatelet agents during the acute phase of stroke cannot be recommended based on available evidence. Similarly, early administration of unfractionated heparin, low-molecular-weight heparin, or heparinoids is not indicated in patients with acute ischemic stroke.

Treatment of Stroke Complications

Brain edema develops between the second and fifth day after stroke onset and is the cause of early deterioration and death. In

---

[1] Not FDA approved for this indication.

the case of a malignant infarction of the middle cerebral artery, the mortality rate is 80%. In patients younger than 60 years, with this pattern of cerebral infarction, hemicraniectomy has been effective in reducing mortality and severe disability, as shown in the pooled analysis of the DECIMAL, DESTINY, and HAMLET trials. Decompressive hemicraniectomy is also effective in reducing mortality in patients older than 60 years, although the rates of severe disability are very high. Surgery needs to be performed within 48 hours after symptom onset. Surgical decompression is also indicated in the case of large cerebellar infarctions that compress the brainstem.

Stroke-associated infections require appropriate antibiotics, but prophylactic administration is discouraged. Venous thromboembolism is a frequent complication after stroke, but its incidence can be reduced with appropriate hydration and graded compression stockings. If the risk of deep venous thrombosis or pulmonary embolism is high, the use of subcutaneous heparin or low-molecular-weight heparin is beneficial. Early mobilization is an effective way of preventing complications, such as aspiration pneumonia or pressure ulcers. Anticonvulsants are administered only to prevent recurrent seizures but are not used prophylactically.

In the case of urinary incontinence, specialist assessment and management are recommended. Dysphagia is common after stroke and is associated with a higher incidence of medical complications and increased mortality. Malnutrition also predicts a poor functional outcome and increased mortality, and it is important to assess the swallowing capacity and the nutritional status of the patient.

Rehabilitation should be started after admission to the stroke unit. The optimal timing of first mobilization is unclear, but mobilization within the first few days appears to be well tolerated. However, very early mobilization can be associated with a worse outcome, as shown in the AVERT trial. An early, lower-dose, out-of-bed activity regimen is preferable to very early, frequent, higher-dose intervention. It is important to assess cognitive deficits and depression during the patient's hospital stay, because this may require specific intervention, although evidence about the type is lacking.

References

Albers GW, Marks MP, Kemp S, et al: DEFUSE 3 Investigators. Thrombectomy for stroke at 6 to 16 hours with selection by perfusion imaging, *N Engl J Med* 378(8):708–718, 2018.

AVERT Trial Collaboration Group, Bernhardt J, Langhorne P, et al: Efficacy and safety of very early mobilisation within 24h of stroke onset (AVERT): a randomised controlled trial, *Lancet* 386(9988):46–55, 2015.

Campbell BCV, Ma H, Ringleb PA, et al: EXTEND, ECASS-4, and EPITHET Investigators. Extending thrombolysis to 4·5-9 h and wake-up stroke using perfusion imaging: a systematic review and meta-analysis of individual patient data, *Lancet* 394(10193):139–147, 2019.

Campbell BCV, Mitchell PJ, Churilov L, et al: Tenecteplase versus alteplase before thrombectomy for ischemic stroke, *N Engl J Med* 378(17):1573–1582, 2018.

Goyal M, Menon BK, van Zwam WH, et al: Endovascular thrombectomy after large-vessel ischaemic stroke: a meta-analysis of individual patient data from five randomised trials, *Lancet* 387(10029):1723–1731, 2016.

Jovin TG, Li C, Wu L, et al: Trial of thrombectomy 6 to 24 hours after stroke due to basilar-artery occlusion, *N Engl J Med* 387(15):1373–1384, 2022.

Nogueira RG, Jadhav AP, Haussen DC, et al: DAWN Trial Investigators. Thrombectomy 6 to 24 hours after stroke with a mismatch between deficit and infarct, *N Engl J Med* 378(1):11–21, 2018.

Palaiodimou L, Katsanos AH, Turc G, Asimakopoulos A-G, et al.: Tenecteplase vs alteplase in acute ischemic stroke within 4.5 hours: a systematic review and meta-analysis of randomized trials, *Neurology* 103(9):e209903, 2024.

Powers WJ, Rabinstein AA, Ackerson T, et al: American Heart Association stroke council. 2018 guidelines for the early management of patients with acute ischemic stroke: a guideline for healthcare professionals from the American Heart Association/American Stroke Association, *Stroke* 49(3):e46–e110, 2018.

Sarraj A, Hassan AE, Abraham MG, et al: SELECT2 investigators. Trial of endovascular thrombectomy for large ischemic strokes, *N Engl J Med* 388(14):1259–1271, 2023, https://doi.org/10.1056/NEJMoa2214403. Epub 2023 Feb 10. PMID: 36762865.

Stroke Foundation: *Clinical guidelines for stroke management*, 2022. Melbourne Australia.

Turc G, Hadziahmetovic M, Walter S, et al: Comparison of mobile stroke unit with usual care for acute ischemic stroke management: a systematic review and meta-analysis, *JAMA Neurol* 79(3):281–290, 2022.

Vahedi K, Hofmeijer J, Juettler E, et al: Early decompressive surgery in malignant infarction of the middle cerebral artery: a pooled analysis of three randomised controlled trials, *Lancet Neurol* 6:215–222, 2007.

▦ MIGRAINE

Method of
Natalia Murinova, MD

◉ CURRENT DIAGNOSIS

- Migraine is a prominent primary headache disorder characterized by intense unilateral pain, typically accompanied by nausea, vomiting, and sensitivity to light and sound.
- It is a significant global health concern, affecting over one billion individuals and ranking as the second leading cause of disability due to its incapacitating nature.
- The post–COVID-19 era has introduced additional complexities in managing migraine, compounding the challenges faced by those suffering from this condition.

◉ CURRENT THERAPY

- Acute treatment of migraine
  - Nonspecific
    - Acetaminophen; nonsteroidal antiinflammatory drugs (NSAIDs); antiemetics
  - Specific migraine medication classes
  - U.S. Food and Drug Administration–approved for acute treatment of migraine with or without aura in adults
    - Triptans, serotonin (5-HT1B, 5-HT1D, 5-HT1F) receptor agonists
    - Ditans, oral serotonin (5-HT1F) receptor agonists
    - Gepants, oral calcitonin gene-related peptide (CGRP) receptor antagonists
- Preventive treatment of migraine
  - Nonspecific therapies
    - Beta-blockers; tricyclics; antiepileptics; N-methyl-D-aspartate (NMDA)
  - Specific therapies
    - Anti-CGRP medications
    - OnabotulinumtoxinA (Botox) injections

Definition

Migraine is a primary headache disorder not caused by any known structural cause. International Headache Society (IHS) criteria define migraine and explain clinical variability seen in patients.

The headache episode in migraine as defined by the IHS has at least two of four defining features (one-sided, pulsating, moderate-to-severe, and aggravated by movement) and at least one of two associated features (nausea and/or vomiting, light and sound sensitivity). In its most common form, migraine is an episodic, recurrent headache lasting 4 hours or longer per episode if left untreated. The frequency varies from rare episodes to everyday headache.

In its more malignant forms, migraine is chronic, daily, nonstop pain with rare or no pain-free time. There is significant clinical variability: unilateral location and pulsating pain is present in around 50% of migraine sufferers. Most patients are disabled from pain; environmental oversensitivity to light, sound, and smell; inability to function; and often transient cognitive dysfunction such as difficulty with concentration. There is a subset of migraine with aura, most commonly the visual symptoms associated with fully reversible visual changes that can mimic transient ischemic attack or stroke.

Many medical providers fail to recognize migraine because they default to the most classic migraine presentation with visual aura with unilateral, pulsating pain with nausea and vomiting. Because migraine can manifest in many different ways, this makes diagnosis challenging. If a patient presents to a medical provider with recurrent moderate-to-severe headaches, migraine diagnosis should be considered. In general, most migraine experts consider a headache migraine unless there is a warning sign or some atypical feature. However, there are a number of neurologic disorders that mimic migraine. For example, stroke can present with migraine-like headache. The majority of people with "sinus headache" can also suffer from migraine. For patients' safety, other causes of headache and other neurologic disorders need to be ruled out. The clinical presentation differs from person to person, and we should consider migraine diagnosis as a possibility in anyone with recurring, disabling headaches and impaired function.

Epidemiology

Migraine affects more than 1 billion people worldwide. Based on the most recent data available, the prevalence of migraine in the United States shows that it affects approximately 15.9% of adults, with a higher incidence in women, reported at 21%, and men at 10.7%. Onset can occur as early as age 5 years and prevalence peaks in young people, but it can occur at any age. Though migraine can be transient, migraine affects people during their most productive years of life. The Global Burden of Disease Study 2016 measured how disabling various disorders are across the world and assessed how disorders affect disability-adjusted life years. In Global Burden of Disease 2016, migraine was the second-most disabling disorder, after low back pain. In one study, 88% of patients diagnosed with sinus headache had migraine.

Risk Factors

Migraine is most commonly seen in young women with a family history of migraine. There are many risk factors that can be cumulative for a given individual who presents with migraine. Lifestyle factors that lead to migraine include high-stress work, nutrition (high carbohydrate diet), physical inactivity, and chronic stress. Therefore a young person with genetic susceptibility to migraine with stress at work, physical inactivity, poor nutrition, and sleep deprivation has increased risk for developing migraine. It is estimated that in 1 year, up to 3% of episodic migraine cases become chronic. Risk factors for migraine chronification are obesity, acute medication overuse, caffeine overuse, stressful life events, depression, and sleep disorders. Comorbid conditions often seen in migraine include anxiety, depression, and insomnia, and these conditions have bidirectional effect.

Pathophysiology

Although migraine was once considered exclusively a disorder of the blood vessels, compelling evidence has led to the realization that a migraine represents a highly choreographed interaction between major inputs from both peripheral and central nervous systems, with the trigeminovascular system and the cerebral cortex among the main players. Migraine was initially thought to be a purely vascular disorder, but it is understood that migraine involves the neuropeptide calcitonin gene-related peptide (CGRP). During a migraine attack, there seems to be increased release of CGRP in the dura mater, which results in vasodilation and inflammation. Studies have shown that if CGRP is given intravenously to people with migraine, most will have a migraine episode in the next few hours.

Diagnosis and Workup

The main questions are whether the patient presents with headache that meets migraine criteria and whether they need neuroimaging (Table 1). We diagnose migraine using IHS criteria (https://ichd-3.org/1-migraine/). Migraine is divided into two major subtypes. Migraine without aura is the most common, characterized by a headache with severe unilateral pain, photophobia, phonophobia, and functional impairment. Migraine with

TABLE 1	Precision Questions Helpful in Migraine Diagnosis
1. Is this a new kind of headache?	New headache needs further history; make sure this is not a migraine mimic.
2. Use "red flag" questions, such as do you have any other condition such as cancer?	"Red flag" questions are used to exclude secondary headache.
3. How many total headache days do you have per month? Lump all headache days.	Total headache days >15 days per month are suggestive of chronic migraine.
4. How long do your headaches last with no treatment?	Duration of headache without therapy should be more than 4 hours for migraine diagnosis. With shorter duration, consider other diagnosis, such as trigeminal autonomic cephalgia.
5. What associated symptoms do you have?	For migraine, look for associated nausea and light and sound sensitivity.
6. How many days per month do you use an acute therapy for any pain?	Medication overuse headache is commonly seen with chronic migraine, and any medication used for any pain can cause this.

aura is most commonly characterized by reversible visual changes that precede and sometimes accompany the migraine pain. The success of migraine treatment depends on making the correct diagnosis. This requires careful headache history, because many patients diagnose themselves with sinus headache or tension-type headache or other type of headache. Identifying classic symptoms has a high probability of accurate diagnosis. The headache pattern should distinguish migraine from other primary headaches (tension or cluster headache) while realizing that most patient with migraine-type headaches can also have coexisting tension-type headaches. Chronic migraine is defined as having more than 15 days of headaches per month of combination of migraine and tension-type headaches. The clinical history and neurologic examination target need to exclude secondary headache that can manifest as migraine-type headaches. Patients with secondary headaches can also have a primary headache like migraine. In most patients the diagnosis is made using their history and IHS criteria. Diagnostic imaging is not indicated in otherwise healthy patients with migraine with normal neurologic examination. Patients with "red flags" such as abnormalities during the neurologic examination, fever, unintentional weight loss, history of cancer, transplant, or immunodeficiency need further workup with neuroimaging. Which kind of neuroimaging should be performed is a common question: Magnetic resonance imaging of the brain with and without contrast is the preferred imaging modality.

Treatment

The pharmacologic treatment addresses acute treatment, used for management of acute headache episodes, and preventive treatments that have shown efficacy in decreasing migraine attacks in the long term. In an effort to lessen both the frequency and severity of migraine episodes, patients previously had to commit to long-term daily preventive medication regimens, often stretching over many months or even years. The pharmaceutical landscape, however, has evolved with the advent of innovative treatments such as anti-CGRP monoclonal antibodies. These newer options, which are typically administered via subcutaneous injections just once a month, have not only simplified migraine prevention but also boast higher patient adherence rates, likely owing to their convenience and well-tolerated side effect profiles. This breakthrough in migraine therapy marks a

TABLE 2 Migraine Treatment by Severity and Phenotype

	CLINICAL MIGRAINE PHENOTYPE	STRATEGY	MEDICATION
Increasing migraine severity	Mild to moderate	Acetaminophen NSAID	Acetaminophen (Tylenol)[1] 1000 mg Naproxen sodium (Aleve)[1] 220–660 mg Ibuprofen (Motrin) 800 mg
	Moderate to severe	NSAID + triptan + antinausea	Naproxen (Aleve) 440 mg + ondansetron (Zofran)[1] 8 mg ODT + triptan later for rescue if necessary
		Triptan (5HT1B agonist 5HT1D agonist) Ditan (5HT1F agonist) Gepant (CGRP antagonist)	Sumatriptan (Imitrex) (6 mg SQ injection; 20 mg nasal solution; 25, 50, and 100 mg oral tablet) Zolmitriptan (Zomig) (2.5, 5 mg nasal solution; oral tablet; ODT) Rizatriptan (Maxalt) (5 mg, 10 mg oral tablet; ODT) Naratriptan (Amerge) (1, 2.5 mg PO tablet) Eletriptan (Relpax) (20, 40 mg PO tablet) Almotriptan (Axert) (6.25, 12.5 mg PO tablet) Frovatriptan (Frova) (2.5 mg PO tablet) Lasmiditan (Reyvow) 50, 100, 200 mg PO tablet Ubrogepant (Ubrelvy) 50, 100 mg PO tablet Rimegepant (Nurtec ODT) 75 mg ODT
	Severe attack difficult to treat and refractory migraine		Triptan + NSAID + antinausea drug Gepant + NSAID + antinausea drug Ditan + NSAID + antinausea drug Ketorolac (Toradol)[1] IM 60 mg Indomethacin[1] oral or rectal Prochlorperazine (Compazine)[1] 5, 10 mg Dexamethasone[1] or prednisone[1]

[1]Not FDA approved for this indication.
ODT, Oral disintegrating tablet.
From Pringsheim T, Davenport W, Mackie G, et al: Canadian Headache Society guideline for migraine prophylaxis, *Can J Neurol Sci* 39(Suppl 2):S1–59, 2012.

BOX 1 First-Line Acute Therapy of Migraine

- Naproxen (Aleve)[1] 440 mg + ondansetron (Zofran)[1] 8 mg ODT + triptan later for rescue if necessary

Triptans
- Sumatriptan (Imitrex) 6 mg SQ injection; 20 mg nasal solution; 25, 50, and 100 mg oral tablet
- Zolmitriptan (Zomig) 2.5, 5 mg oral tablet; ODT; nasal spray
- Rizatriptan (Maxalt) 5, 10 mg oral tablet; ODT
- Naratriptan (Amerge) 1, 2.5 mg oral tablet
- Eletriptan (Relpax) 20, 40 mg oral tablet
- Almotriptan (Axert) 6.25, 12.5 mg oral tablet
- Frovatriptan (Frova) 2.5 mg oral tablet

Ditans
- Lasmiditan (Reyvow) 50, 100, 200 mg oral tablet

Gepants
- Ubrogepant (Ubrelvy) 50, 100 mg oral tablet
- Rimegepant (Nurtec ODT) 75 mg oral disintegrating tablet
- Zavegepant (Zavzpret) 10 mg nasal spray

[1] Not FDA approved for this indication.

BOX 2 Steps for Acute Treatment for Migraine Headache

Step 1: Choose options that are not known to lead to MOH.
- Antiemetics: Ondansetron (Zofram)[1] (tablet, dispersible tablet), prochlorperazine (Compazine)[1] (tablet, suppository), promethazine (Phenergan)[1] (tablet, suppository), metoclopramide (Reglan)[1]
- Natural supplements/herbs: Feverfew tea,[7] Boswellia,[7] magnesium[7]
- Anesthetic: Lidocaine nasal spray[1]
- Gepants: Ubrogepant (Ubrelvy), rimegepant (Nurtec ODT), and zavegepant (Zavzpret nasal spray)
- Neuromodulation: Cefaly (supraorbital stimulation), Gammacore (vagal nerve stimulation), SpringTMS (transcranial magnetic stimulation), Relivion (external combined occipital and trigeminal neurostimulation), Nerivio (remote electrical neuromodulation)
- Nonmedication options: Rest, ice, meditation, biofeedback, distraction, essential oils[7]

Step 2: NSAIDs, longer acting are generally considered less likely to lead to MOH.
- Diclofenac (tablet,[1] capsule,[1] powder), ketorolac,[1] naproxen,[1] ibuprofen
- Step 3: Limit any acute medications such as triptans to 1–2 days per week to avoid MOH.
- Triptans: Sumatriptan (Imitrex) (tablet, nasal spray, injection), rizatriptan (Maxalt) (tablet, dispersible tablet), eletriptan (Relpax), zolmitriptan (Zomig) (tablet, dispersible tablet, nasal spray), almotriptan (Axert), frovatriptan (Frova), naratriptan (Amerge)
- Ergotamines: dihydroergotamine DHE 45 injection, Migranal nasal spray

MOH, Medication overuse headache.
[1] Not FDA approved for this indication.
[7] Available as a dietary supplement.

substantial leap forward, offering patients a more user-friendly approach to managing their condition. Many patients who previously found little relief from conventional oral treatments are now experiencing a substantial reduction in the frequency and severity of migraines, thanks to the latest therapeutic advancements. This improvement has been a significant stride forward in migraine management.

The treatment strategy for migraines has shifted from using mostly nonspecific pain medications such as aspirin and acetaminophen to migraine-specific therapies such as triptans, ditans, and gepants and other treatments such as neuromodulation (Table 2; Boxes 1–3).

Level A Therapies, Established as Effective and FDA Approved for EM

- AEDs: Topiramate (Topamax) (caution if low weight or history of kidney stones), divalproex sodium (Depakote) (caution of weight gain), sodium valproate (Depakene)
- Beta-blockers: Propranolol (Inderal), timolol (Blocadren), metoprolol (Lopressor) (the only Level A medication that is not FDA approved)

Specific Preventive Migraine Therapies FDA Approved for EM and CM

- Anti-CGRP monoclonal antibodies: erenumab-aooe (Aimovig), fremanezumab-vfrm (Ajovy), galcanezumab-gnlm (Emgality)
- Gepants: Rimegepant (Nurtec ODT) and atogepant (Qulipta)
- Neuromodulation devices: Cefaly (supraorbital stimulation), Gammacore (vagal nerve stimulation)

Level B Therapies, Probably Effective for EM, not FDA Approved for EM

- Antidepressants: Amitriptyline, venlafaxine (Effexor XR)
- Beta-blockers: Atenolol (Tenormin), nadolol (Corgard)

Level C Therapies, Possibly Effective for EM, not FDA Approved

- Calcium channel blockers and angiotensin-converting-enzyme inhibitors: Verapamil (Calan), lisinopril (Prinivil)
- AEDs: Carbamazepine (Tegretol)
- Beta-blockers: Pindolol (Visken)
- Antihistamines: Cyproheptadine (Periactin)
- Angiotensin-receptor blockers: candesartan (Atacand), clonidine (Catapres)

AED, Automated external defibrillator; *CGRP*, calcitonin gene-related peptide; *CM*, chronic migraine; *EM*, episodic migraine; *FDA*, US Food and Drug Administration.

Acute Treatment

Mechanism of Acute Migraine Medications

Migraine pain is considered to be caused by dura mater release of CGRP, with subsequent vasodilation and neurogenic inflammation. Triptans and ergots are agonists of serotonin 5-HT1B and 5-HT1D receptors, and their activation prevents CGRP release. Activation of 5-HT1B (serotonin) receptors by triptans may lead to constricted blood vessels, which raise concerns for individuals with a risk of ischemic events. Ditans are selective oral serotonin (5-HT1F) receptor agonists, which is thought to stop plasma protein release by action of the trigeminal ganglion. 5-HT1F receptors are not present in vessels, and because of this there is no concern of vasoconstriction making them a safe options for patient with history of cardiovascular disease. Gepants such as ubrogepant (Ubrelvy), rimegepant (Nurtec ODT), and atogepant (Qulipta) are oral CGRP receptor antagonists. There is a new gepant, zavegepant (Zavzpret), that is an intranasal treatment.

The American Headache Society guideline for acute treatment in 2015 summarized evidence-based assessment of acute treatments for migraine: "The specific medications—triptans and dihydroergotamine (nasal spray [Migranal, Trudhesa], inhaler[5]) are effective (level A)," whereas "effective nonspecific medications include acetaminophen, NSAIDs (nonsteroidal antiinflammatory drugs), opioids (butorphanol nasal spray)[1] (not recommended), sumatriptan/naproxen (Treximet), and the combination of acetaminophen/aspirin/caffeine (e.g., Excedrin Migraine)" also have level A evidence. "Ergotamine tartrate (Ergomar) and other forms of dihydroergotamine, ketoprofen

(Orudis),[1] intravenous and intramuscular ketorolac (Toradol),[1] flurbiprofen (Ansaid),[1] intravenous (IV) magnesium (in migraine with aura),[1] and the combination of isometheptene compounds, codeine/acetaminophen,[1] tramadol/acetaminophen (Ultracet),[1] prochlorperazine (Compazine),[1] droperidol (Inapsine),[1] chlorpromazine (Thorazine),[1] and metoclopramide (Reglan)[1] are probably effective (level B)."

It is important to educate patients on appropriate use of acute therapy, because medication overuse headache (MOH) can develop. This is defined as the presence of more than 15 headache days per month while taking any acute medications for any pain, even if not headache related, more than 15 days per month and 10 days per month for migraine-specific treatments such as triptans. MOH is often difficult to treat and may be medication and procedure refractory. We strongly recommend keeping an electronic headache diary with emphasis on monitoring days per month of acute medication use and setting a limit on maximum monthly use (most headache clinics recommend 1 to 2 days per week maximum). An electronic headache diary app, such as https://migrainebuddy.com/, can be very helpful in documenting headache days and medication use. The novel class of medications known as gepants is not associated with MOHs and may be a suitable treatment option for patients experiencing MOH due to triptan use.

An oral nonopioid analgesic, such as naproxen (Aleve),[1] is often adequate for acute treatment of mild-to-moderate migraine without nausea or vomiting. Migraine-specific agents should be considered when migraine episodes are moderate to severe. The acute migraine-specific pharmacotherapies include triptans, ergotamines, ditans, and gepants.

Many acute therapies are effective only for some patients and can cause significant side effects. Patients who do not respond to one triptan may respond to another triptan or a different mode of administration of the same triptan. Note that triptans are contraindicated in patients with vascular risk factors. Patients are advised to test the effectiveness of triptan medications across at least four headache episodes, documenting any relief in symptoms and noting the occurrence of any adverse effects.

- Sumatriptan (Imitrex) (6 mg subcutaneous [SQ] injections; 20 mg nasal solution; 25, 50, and 100 mg oral tablet)
- Zolmitriptan (Zomig) (2.5, 5 mg nasal solution; oral tablet or oral disintegrating tablet)
- Rizatriptan (Maxalt) (5, 10 mg oral tablet; oral disintegrating tablet)
- Naratriptan (Amerge) (1, 2.5 mg oral tablet)
- Eletriptan (Relpax) 20, 40 mg oral tablet
- Almotriptan (Axert) (6.25, 12.5 mg oral tablet)
- Frovatriptan (Frova) (2.5 mg oral tablet)
- Dihydroergotamine (D.H.E. 45, Migranal, Trudhesa) should be considered in patients who are refractory to triptans, although they have the same vascular disease contraindication.
- Dihydroergotamine (D.H.E. 45, 1 mg SQ or IV; Migranal 0.5 mg/spray into each nostril; Trudhesa 0.725 mg/spray into each nostril)

A number of new agents became available in 2020.

New Acute Migraine Treatment: Ditans and Gepants

The one approved ditan is lasmiditan (Reyvow), which is an oral serotonin (5HT1F) receptor agonist. The gepants approved for acute migraine treatment are ubrogepant (Ubrelvy) and rimegepant (Nurtec ODT), which are oral CGRP receptor agonists. These drugs were approved by the US Food and Drug Administration (FDA) in 2020 for acute migraine treatment with and without aura in adults.

Ditans for Acute Migraine Treatment

Ditans are the only group of medications known to selectively bind serotonin 1F receptor (5-HT1F) on the trigeminal neurons. Ditans do not cause vasoconstriction via the serotonin 1B receptor on blood vessels as triptans do and therefore are not contraindicated in patients with known vascular risk factors. A majority of patients in clinical studies had at least one cardiovascular risk

---

[1] Not FDA approved for this indication.
[5] Investigational drug in the United States.

factor, only a few of the subjects had ischemic heart disease, and none had ischemic events attributed to lasmiditan during the trial within 48 hours. To date, no clinical trials are available that have compared lasmiditan to other acute headache treatments. The most common side effects in clinical trials were dizziness, paresthesias, and sedation. Cognitive changes and confusion were also reported. Lasmiditan can cause impaired driving ability, and there is a drug warning against driving and operating machinery for at least 8 hours after taking this drug. It is important to mention this to the patient. Because of the central nervous system (CNS) action, other concomitant CNS depressants should be avoided. Caution is also advised with heart rate–lowering medications. It is not known whether ditans can cause serotonin syndrome.

There is no available evidence that supports limiting the use of ditans with selective serotonin reuptake inhibitors or serotonin-norepinephrine reuptake inhibitors because of concerns for serotonin syndrome. However, given the seriousness of serotonin syndrome, caution is warranted, especially in a patient taking other medications and supplements. No data for pregnancy and breastfeeding are available at this time.

It is important to note that lasmiditan is classified as a controlled substance. It may be considered as an alternative treatment for patients who cannot use triptans, for instance, in urgent care scenarios. However, to minimize the risk of MOHs, its use should be restricted to 1 or 2 days per week.
- Lasmiditan (Reyvow 50, 100, or 200 mg PO as a single dose; maximum: one dose in 24 hours)

Gepants for Acute Migraine Treatment
Gepants are the only group of oral medications known to selectively bind and antagonize CGRP receptors. Gepants do not cause vasoconstriction, because they do not bind to serotonin 1B receptor on blood vessels as triptans do and therefore are not contraindicated in patients with known vascular risk factors. CGRP levels tend to increase with migraine, and patients with migraine injected with CGRP develop migraine within a few hours. No clinical trials are available that have compared gepants to other acute headache treatments. Gepants are well tolerated, and the most commonly reported side effect compared with placebo is nausea in ubrogepant trials. Because gepants are metabolized via CYP3A4 via the liver, coadministration with strong inhibitors of CYP3A4 such as ketoconazole and CYP3A4 inducers such as rifampin should be avoided. No data for pregnancy and breastfeeding are available at this time.
- Ubrogepant (Ubrelvy 50–100 mg PO as a single dose; may repeat once based on response and tolerability after ≥2 hours)
- Rimegepant (Nurtec 75 mg PO as a single dose; maximum: 75 mg/24 hours)
- Zavegepant (Zavzpret [10 mg/spray] intranasally one spray in one nostril /dose/24 hours) is the first intranasal gepant.

Neuromodulation Therapies for Migraine
There are currently several FDA-approved neuromodulation devices for use in migraine, all of which use noninvasive stimulation to modulate brain function. All are considered to have nonsignificant risks and are generally well tolerated by patients. Neuromodulation can be used for acute treatment of migraine. These devices generally require patient payment, although they are generally free of charge for veterans or military active duty personnel.
- Remote electrical neuromodulation device (Nerivio)
- External trigeminal neurostimulation device (Cefaly)
- Single-pulse transcranial magnetic stimulation device (Savi Dual)
- External vagal nerve stimulation device (GammaCore)
- External combined occipital and trigeminal neurostimulation device (Relivion)

Preventive Treatment
There is emphasis on prevention of migraine attacks for many patients, because acute therapy is often less effective in more severe cases. Consider preventive treatments for patients who have more than 4 migraine days per month, are disabled by migraine, who are missing work, who are using the emergency room for headache treatment, or who are prone to overusing acute medications. Preventive treatments should also be considered for patients with serious medical problems, such as heart disease or stroke.

Medical providers should consult the American Academy of Neurology/American Headache Society guidelines. All guidelines were consistent in their recommendations of treatments for first-line use. All rated topiramate, divalproex/sodium valproate, propranolol, and metoprolol as having the highest level of evidence.

Level A: Effective
- Divalproex (Depakote ER)/sodium valproate (Stavzor) 500 to 1000 mg/day
- Metoprolol (Lopressor)[1] 25 to 200 mg/day
- Petasites (butterbur)[7] 50 to 75 mg bid
- Propranolol (Inderal) 40 to 240 mg/day
- Timolol (Blocadren) 10 to 15 mg bid
- Topiramate (Topamax) 25 to 200 mg/day

Level B: Probably Effective; should be considered for patients requiring migraine prophylaxis
- Amitriptyline (Elavil)[1] 10 to 150 mg/day
- Fenoprofen (Nalfon)[1] 200 to 600 mg three times per day[a]
- Feverfew[7] 50 to 150 mg bid; 2.08 to 18.75 mg three times per day for MIG-99 preparation
- Ibuprofen (Advil, Motrin)[1] 200 mg twice a day[a]
- Ketoprofen (Orudis)[1] 50 mg three times per day[a]
- Magnesium[1] 600 mg per day
- Naproxen (Naprosyn)[1]/naproxen sodium (Anaprox DS)[1] 500 to 1100 mg/day or naproxen sodium 550 mg twice a day[a]
- Riboflavin (vitamin B_2)[7] 400 mg/day
- Venlafaxine (Effexor ER)[1] 150 mg extended release/day
- Atenolol (Tenormin)[1] 25 to 100 mg/day

Anti–Calcitonin Gene-Related Peptide Monoclonal Antibodies for Preventive Treatment
Since 2018, CGRP receptor antagonist monoclonal antibodies have been FDA approved for preventive treatment of both episodic and chronic migraine: erenumab-aooe (Aimovig), galcanezumab-gnlm (Emgality), fremanezumab-vfrm (Ajovy), and eptinezumab-jjmr (Vyepti). The first three are intended for self-injection at home. Before covering, most medical insurances require trial of at least two to three classes of preventive therapies with highest level of evidence including beta-blockers (propranolol or timolol), antiseizure medications (divalproex sodium or topiramate), and tricyclics or SNRIs (duloxetine [Cymbalta][1]). They are effective in about one-third of patients with migraine with super-responders, have low side effect profile, and do not interact with any medications. They are not indicated during pregnancy or breast-feeding owing to lack of evidence. When prescribing erenumab-aooe (Aimovig), a newer side effect to be aware of is hypertension; monitoring blood pressure is advisable because of the potential, albeit rare, occurrence of elevated levels. Additionally, Aimovig may lead to gastrointestinal side effects, particularly constipation. It is crucial to discuss any preexisting constipation or gastrointestinal conditions with patients before initiating this medication.
- Erenumab-aooe (Aimovig) 70 to 40 mg SQ once a month self-administered by patient
- Fremanezumab-vfrm (Ajovy) 225 mg SQ monthly or 675 mg every 3 months (quarterly), which is administered as three consecutive subcutaneous injections of 225 mg each
- Galcanezumab-gnlm (Emgality) 240 mg (two consecutive subcutaneous injections of 120 mg each) once as a loading dose, followed by monthly doses of 120 mg injected subcutaneously

---

[1] Not FDA approved for this indication.
[7] Available as dietary supplement.
[a] Used for 1 month or less.

Gepant Anti–Calcitonin Gene-Related Peptide Receptor Antagonists for Migraine Prevention

Atogepant (Qulipta) was approved in 2021 for prevention of migraine at doses from 10 mg to 60 mg a day. Rimegepant (Nurtec ODT) received additional FDA approval for migraine prevention in 2021 at the dose of 75 mg every other day.

Chronic Migraine Treatment

Patients with chronic forms of migraine can be especially difficult to treat. Many patients are prone to developing MOH. Overuse is defined as taking acute medication 10 or more days per month for triptans, ergotamines, opioids, and combination analgesics and 15 or more days per month for nonopioid analgesics (including aspirin, NSAIDs, and acetaminophen). People can develop MOH at much lower levels of regular medication use for any pain. Medical providers should ensure that patients are aware of the risk of MOH and limit medication use well below these levels. We recommend not using acute medication more than 1 to 2 days per week on average, and this includes all acute treatment options apart from gepants, lidocaine, and neuromodulation devices. Neuromodulation is a great option for management of acute exacerbation in patients with chronic migraine because daily use does not lead to rebound and worsening headaches. Always consider preventive medications and lifestyle changes in patients with chronic migraines, because acute medications cause MOH when used 15 or more days per month.

MOH often leads to clinically refractory migraine. Taking acute medications to abort migraine attacks more than 10 days per month can lead to increased neuronal excitability, depletion of central serotonin production, and increased release of CGRP. Clinical observation suggests that both preventive and acute treatment for the primary headache usually fail unless the offending medication or medications that caused MOH are stopped. Recent research suggests that the most effective approach to treating medication-overuse headaches (MOHs) is to discontinue the overused acute medications and simultaneously implement a preventive treatment strategy.

Treatments for chronic migraine include:

- Topiramate (Topamax)[1] 25 to 200 mg/day
- OnabotulinumtoxinA (Botox)[1] 155 units injections by medical providers every 3 months
- Erenumab-aooe (Aimovig)[1] 70, 140 mg SQ once a month self-administered by patient
- Fremanezumab-vfrm (Ajovy)[1] 225 mg SQ monthly, or 675 mg every 3 months (quarterly), which is administered as three consecutive subcutaneous injections of 225 mg each.
- Galcanezumab-gnlm (Emgality)[1] 240 mg (two consecutive subcutaneous injections of 120 mg each) once as a loading dose, followed by monthly doses of 120 mg injected subcutaneously
- Atogepant (Qulipta)[1] 10 to 60 mg daily orally

Monitoring

Primary care providers should consider regular follow-up of their patients every few months or more frequently until patients are stable and have gained therapeutic success. We recommend adding multimodal therapy at each visit, and this can include exercise, sleep therapy, nutrition therapy, stress reductions, and supplements in addition to pharmacotherapy reevaluation. We use the visits to address migraine comorbidities, especially anxiety and sleep. With regular monitoring, medication dose can be optimized for maximum efficacy and the least possible side effects. Acute pharmacotherapy escalation in patients who are not optimally controlled can backfire and lead to development of MOH. When a patient experiences significantly worsening headache on 15 or more days per month and has history of migraine, acute medication frequency of use needs to be assessed. MOH may resolve after the acute medication is stopped; however, in many patients with comorbid anxiety and insomnia, more treatment should be considered. In patients with MOH we should consider preventive therapy and neuromodulation therapy. Compliance with medication therapy can be improved by education offered by caring providers and establishing therapeutic alliance with patients by using motivational interviewing skills.

References and Further Recommended Reading

Chou DE, Shnayderman Yugrakh M, Winegarner D: Acute migraine therapy with external trigeminal neurostimulation (ACME): a randomized controlled trial, *Cephalalgia* 39:3–14, 2019.

Chun-Pai Yang, Liang Chih-Sung, Chang Ching-Mao, et al: Comparison of new pharmacologic agents with triptans for treatment of migraine: a systematic review and meta-analysis, *JAMA Netw Open* 4(10):e2128544–e2128544, 2021.

Dodick DW, Lipton RB, Ailani J, et al: Ubrogepant for the treatment of migraine, *N Engl J Med* 381:2230–2241, 2019.

Goadsby PJ, Wietecha LA, Dennehy EB, et al: Phase 3 randomized, placebo-controlled, double-blind study of lasmiditan for acute treatment of migraine, *Brain* 142:1894–1904, 2019.

Halker Singh RB, Ailani J, Robbins MS: Neuromodulation for the acute and preventive therapy of migraine and cluster headache, *Headache* 59(Suppl 2):33–49, 2019.

Headache Classification Committee of the International Headache Society: The international classification of headache disorders, 3rd edition (beta version), *Cephalalgia* 33(9):629–808, 2013.

Kuca B, Silberstein SD, Wietecha L, Berg PH, Dozier G, Lipton RB: Lasmiditan is an effective acute treatment for migraine: a phase 3 randomized study, *Neurology* 91:e2222–e2232, 2018.

Lipton RB, Croop R, Stock EG, et al: Rimegepant, an oral calcitonin gene-related peptide receptor antagonist, for migraine, *N Engl J Med* 381:142–149, 2019.

Lipton RB, Dodick DW, Silberstein SD, et al: Single pulse transcranial magnetic stimulation for acute treatment of migraine with aura: a randomised, double-blind, parallel-group, sham-controlled trial, *Lancet Neurol* 9:373–380, 2010.

Marmura MJ, Silberstein SD, Schwedt TJ: The acute treatment of migraine in adults: the American headache society evidence assessment of migraine pharmacotherapies, *Headache* 55:3–20, 2015.

Misra UK, Kalita J, Bhoi SK: High-rate repetitive transcranial magnetic stimulation in migraine prophylaxis: a randomized, placebo-controlled study, *J Neurol* 1–9, 2013.

Ornello R, Andreou AP, De Matteis E, Jürgens TP, Minen MT, Sacco S: Resistant and refractory migraine: Clinical presentation, pathophysiology, and management, *EBioMedicine* 99, 2024.

Puledda F, Silva EM, Suwanlaong K, Goadsby PJ: Migraine: from pathophysiology to treatment, *J Neurol* 270(7):3654–3666, 2023.

Russo AF, Hay DL: CGRP physiology, pharmacology, and therapeutic targets: migraine and beyond, *Physiol Rev* 103(2):1565–1644, 2023.

Steiner Timothy J, Stovner Lars Jacob: Global epidemiology of migraine and its implications for public health and health policy, *Nat Rev Neurol* 19(2):109–117, 2023.

Stovner LJ, Nichols E, Steiner TJ, et al: Global, regional, and national burden of migraine and tension-type headache, 1990–2016: a systematic analysis for the Global Burden of Disease Study 2016, *Lancet Neurol* 17(11):954–976, 2018.

Stovner LJ, Nichols E, Steiner TJ, Vos T: Headache in the Global Burden of Disease (GBD) studies. In *Societal impact of headache*, New York, NY, 2019, Springer, Cham, pp 105–125.

Sussman M, Benner J, Neumann P, Menzin J: Cost effectiveness analysis of erenumab for the preventive treatment of episodic and chronic migraine: results from the US societal and payer perspectives, *Cephalalgia* 38:1644–1657, 2018.

Szperka CL, et al: Migraine care in the era of COVID–19: clinical pearls and plea to insurers, *Headache* 2020.

Tassorelli C, Grazzi L, de Tommaso M, et al: Noninvasive vagus nerve stimulation as acute therapy for migraine: the randomized PRESTO study, *Neurology* 91:e364–e373, 2018.

Vollbracht S, Rapoport AM: The pipeline in headache therapy, *CNS Drugs* 1–13, 2013.

Yarnitsky D, Dodick DW, Grosberg BM, et al: Remote electrical neuromodulation (REN) relieves acute migraine: a randomized, double-blind, placebo-controlled, multicenter trial, *Headache* 59:1240–1252, 2019.

MULTIPLE SCLEROSIS

Method of
Caitlin Jackson-Tarlton, MD

CURRENT DIAGNOSIS

- Multiple sclerosis (MS) is an immune-mediated demyelinating disease of the central nervous system (CNS).
- The McDonald criteria, the most widely used diagnostic criteria, incorporate a patient's symptoms, physical examination, magnetic resonance imaging (MRI) findings, and, when applicable, cerebrospinal fluid (CSF) analysis and other ancillary tests.

---

[1] Not FDA approved for this indication.

- The core MS phenotypes are relapsing and progressive MS. Diagnosis of relapsing-remitting multiple sclerosis (RRMS) requires recurrent episodes of acute CNS demyelinating attacks (also referred to as *relapses* or *flares*). Clinically isolated syndrome (CIS), a single demyelinating episode and often first attack of MS, may meet McDonald criteria for RRMS based on MRI and CSF results.
- Primary progressive multiple sclerosis (PPMS) is heralded by progressive neurologic impairment from disease onset in the absence of any preceding attacks. Secondary progressive multiple sclerosis (SPMS) is progressive neurologic disease after a history of relapsing MS.
- Radiologically isolated syndrome (RIS) is the presence of CNS demyelinating lesions on MRI in a patient lacking symptoms and physical examination findings typical of demyelination. RIS and CIS not meeting McDonald criteria may later develop into clinically definite MS requiring clinical and radiologic monitoring.

CURRENT THERAPY

- Acute attacks of MS are treated with high-dose corticosteroids and, in severe cases, plasma exchange. These therapies facilitate time to recovery but do not prevent future relapses.
- Disease-modifying therapies (DMTs) reduce the number of new attacks and new MRI lesions. To date, there are no curative treatments.
- There are many distinct and effective DMT choices approved for CIS, RRMS, and SPMS with activity (ongoing clinical attacks and/or new MRI lesions).
- The single approved therapy for PPMS is ocrelizumab (Ocrevus). Treatment for RIS remains uncertain with trials ongoing.
- Medications vary in their mechanism of action, efficacy, side effect profile, and mode of delivery. DMT choice should be individualized considering the patient's age, severity of MS, presence of comorbidities, family planning, and patient preference. Insurance coverage often plays a role given the substantial cost of these medications.
- Novel MS medications, including further oral medications, and infusion-based monoclonal antibodies are currently under scientific evaluation.

Multiple sclerosis (MS) is an immune-mediated inflammatory demyelinating disease of the central nervous system (CNS) that affects approximately 1 million people in the United States alone.

Risk Factors

Women are at least twice as likely as men to develop of MS. Other known risk factors for development of MS include ethnicity, genetic background, and socioeconomic and environmental exposures. White individuals, particularly those born and reared in extreme northern or southern latitudes, are particularly susceptible to MS, although recent data suggest that African Americans may have a more severe clinical course. Genetic susceptibility is associated with the *HLA-DRB1* major histocompatibility allele, as well as interleukin-2 and interleukin-7 receptors. Obesity, particularly during adolescence, and low serum vitamin D levels are both associated with an increased risk of development of MS and may influence the severity of its clinical course. The association between MS and infection with Epstein-Barr virus (infectious mononucleosis) has been studied extensively. A recent large longitudinal study of U.S. military recruits strengthened this association by demonstrating that Epstein-Barr infection preceded the development of MS in

those who were subsequently diagnosed with MS. Further, the risk of developing MS was increased 32-fold after Epstein-Barr infection but was not increased by other viruses such as cytomegalovirus. Given that Epstein-Barr infection is very common and MS quite uncommon, this suggests that exposure to the virus may be necessary but insufficient for developing MS. Comorbid chronic vascular diseases and mood disorders complicate and worsen the MS disease course. Cigarette smoking is associated with an increased risk for development of MS and likely is associated with an increased severity and clinical course.

Pathophysiology

The etiology and pathophysiology of MS as a whole remains uncertain. However, most evidence supports an inflammatory autoimmune demyelinating disease induced by environmental factors in a genetically susceptible host. Animal models including experimental allergic encephalomyelitis and Theiler murine encephalomyelitis virus also point to an autoimmune inflammatory demyelinating etiology, most likely associated with viral infection. Studies that suggested chronic cerebrospinal vascular insufficiency has an important association with MS have been refuted.

Pathophysiology likely varies among individual patients with MS. Four distinct pathologies in active demyelinating MS lesions have been described. Pattern 1 displays marked macrophage infiltration without humoral abnormalities. Pattern 2 shows distinct humoral abnormalities with complement activation and immunoglobulin (Ig) deposition. Pattern 3 involves primary oligodendrocyte degeneration and early loss of myelin-associated glycoprotein. Pattern 4 reveals oligodendrocyte dystrophy in periplaque white matter. Early studies suggest that there could be a therapeutic advantage with different therapies for different types of demyelinating disease.

Prevention

Currently, there is no known way to definitively prevent the development of MS. Patients with a single clinical attack of demyelination and abnormal magnetic resonance imaging (MRI) ("high-risk" clinically isolated syndrome) have a delayed onset to MS diagnosis with immunomodulatory therapy. Two recent small randomized, double-blinded, placebo-controlled trials of individuals with radiologically isolated syndrome (RIS) showed treatment with dimethyl fumarate (Tecfidera)[1] and teriflunomide (Aubagio)[1] substantially reduced the risk of clinical demyelinating attacks. Additional studies on the treatment of RIS are ongoing but currently no agent has a U.S. Food and Drug Administration (FDA)-approved indication for RIS.

Clinical Manifestations

The clinical course of MS is varied. Approximately 85% of patients present with a relapsing-remitting course. This entails an acute impairment within the CNS, with symptoms depending on the area of inflammation. An acute demyelinating cause of a focal neurologic symptom is suggested by an onset over hours to days, with a plateau of impairment over a few weeks. Symptoms then improve either spontaneously or with the use of corticosteroids over a number of days to weeks or longer. However, symptoms might not completely resolve, leaving an individual with permanent neurologic disability. Inflammation within the optic nerve (optic neuritis) is heralded by painful, unilateral, and monocular visual deficit (often a central scotoma). Symptoms of brainstem dysfunction include binocular diplopia, sensory deficits unilaterally on the face and contralaterally on the arm and leg, significant dysarthria, and vertigo. Cerebellar dysfunction is seen with ataxia that is typically unilateral. Spinal cord inflammation is indicated by a distinctive, usually gradually rising sensory level of deficit that commonly is accompanied by bowel and bladder impairment and paraparesis or quadriparesis, depending on a thoracic versus cervical level of the lesion.

---

[1]Not FDA approved for this indication.

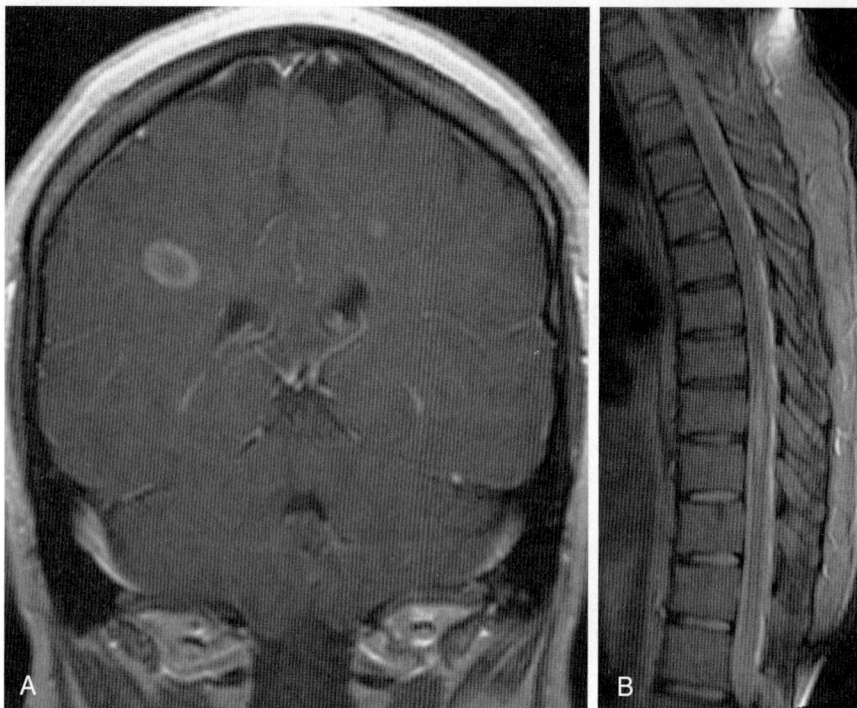

Figure 1 Magnetic resonance image showing brain T_1 gadolinium-enhancing lesions (A) and T_2 thoracic spine (B) typical of multiple sclerosis.

Progressive forms of MS include secondary progressive multiple sclerosis (SPMS) and primary progressive multiple sclerosis (PPMS). These are heralded by a slow (months to years) but steady and insidious, progressive neurologic deficit. Most commonly, progressive MS presents with a progressive myelopathy consisting of an upper motor neuron gait disorder often with progressive weakness, spasticity, and neurogenic bladder and bowel impairment. Occasionally, patients with progressive MS have insidious sensory loss, cerebellar ataxia, or dementia, in isolation or in association with the myelopathy. SPMS is diagnosed when a patient has had a prior history of at least one clinical attack (relapse) followed by more than 1 year of progressive neurologic disease. PPMS is diagnosed with progressive CNS disease consistent with MS and typical MRI brain or spinal lesions from onset without any prior relapse, often with cerebrospinal fluid (CSF) abnormalities that support the diagnosis.

Diagnosis

The diagnosis of MS is formalized by the continually revised McDonald criteria. Criteria must only be applied to individuals presenting with a syndrome typical for demyelination, and alternative diagnoses must be considered and excluded. A diagnosis of relapsing-remitting multiple sclerosis (RRMS) entails having two or more clinical attacks (relapses) in the accompaniment of objective clinical evidence of two or more lesions. The 2017 McDonald criteria allow some patients with a single clinical attack, clinically isolated syndrome (CIS), who meet additional criteria through MRI and/or CSF analysis, so-called dissemination in time and space, to be diagnosed with relapsing remitting multiple sclerosis.

Progressive MS is diagnosed when there is progressive CNS disease characteristic of MS for at least 1 year and at least two of the following: (1) one or more demyelinating MRI brain lesions typical for MS, (2) two or more demyelinating spinal cord lesions typical for MS, or (3) the presence of CSF-specific oligoclonal bands (Figure 1).

Occasionally, visual-evoked potentials and somatosensory-evoked potentials are used to further document dissemination of MS within the CNS. Serologic investigations are done primarily to rule out MS mimickers depending on and directed by any accompanying systemic symptoms and the clinical setting in individual patients. These may include antineuronal antibodies (aquaporin-4-IgG and myelin oligodendrocyte glycoprotein-IgG), antinuclear antibodies, erythrocyte sedimentation rate, anticardiolipin antibodies, vitamin B12, Lyme serology, and/or body imaging for sarcoidosis.

Differential Diagnosis

Referral to a neurologist is recommended when a diagnosis of MS is suspected. Other CNS diseases can mimic relapsing or progressive MS. Neuromyelitis optica is an autoimmune disease with severe acute attacks that are typically restricted to the optic nerves and spinal cord. However, other brainstem and deep cerebral structures, such as the area postrema, cerebral white matter, and diencephalon, can also be involved. Brain MRI findings are usually not consistent with MS, at least early on in the disease, and a specific water channel autoantibody (aquaporin-4-IgG) is found in serum in most cases.

Clinical syndromes of CNS demyelination with myelitis, optic neuritis, and acute disseminated encephalomyelitis (ADEM) with serologic presence of antibodies to myelin oligodendrocyte glycoprotein (MOG) are increasingly recognized and are now referred to as myelin oligodendrocyte glycoprotein antibody-associated disease (MOGAD). ADEM is an acute, typically monophasic, and postinfectious CNS inflammatory demyelinating presentation that is more common in children and may or may not be associated with anti-MOG antibodies.

Optic neuritis may be further mimicked by acute ischemic optic neuropathy. This condition is typically painless, occurs suddenly, and occurs in patients with advanced age and preexisting vascular risk factors.

Progressive myelopathies that mimic PPMS or SPMS include a compressive myelopathy (e.g., cervical spondylosis, disc disease, or neoplastic infiltration), nutritional deficiencies (e.g., vitamin B12 or copper deficiency), infectious causes (e.g., HTLV1), genetic causes (e.g., adrenoleukodystrophy), paraneoplastic disease (e.g., CRMP-5 auto-antibodies), systemic disorders (e.g., sarcoidosis), or a progressive vascular cause (e.g., dural arteriovenous fistula).

Treatment

Acute demyelinating MS attacks (relapses) may be treated with high doses of corticosteroids. These may be given orally or intravenously; however, high doses of corticosteroids are necessary and are superior to low doses. For example, a typical regimen is intravenous methylprednisolone (Solu-Medrol) 1000 mg once daily for 3 to 5 days without oral corticosteroid tapering doses. The oral equivalent to this intravenous regimen is prednisone 1000 to 1250 mg orally once daily for 3 to 5 days with no oral corticosteroid taper afterward. Gastrointestinal intolerance occurs in some patients, and concomitant use of stomach-protecting agents such as proton pump inhibitors may be recommended. Typical acute corticosteroid side effects include insomnia, irritability, and increased appetite. There are rare but well-known associations with avascular necrosis of the hip and acute psychosis. Chronic corticosteroid side effects such as diabetes mellitus, cataracts, osteoporosis, adrenal suppression, weight gain, and cushingoid habitus are more associated with chronic corticosteroid use and not short courses of steroids.

Generally, only MS attacks that are associated with functional impairment (vision loss, diplopia, motor weakness, and ataxia) are treated because clinical recovery is hastened, but final clinical recovery is not found to be altered by this therapy. Occasionally, patients have very severe acute attacks of MS or other demyelinating disease that does not improve with use of high-dose corticosteroids. In these patients, the use of plasma exchange (typically seven exchanges over approximately 14 days) is recommended. Approximately 45% of patients experience functional recovery within 1 month after plasma exchange. Side effects of plasma exchange therapy include paresthesias related to hypocalcemia, anemia, thrombocytopenia, or complications of central venous access that is required for many patients. Intravenous immunoglobulin (Gammagard)[1] has not yet been shown to improve severe clinical attacks of demyelinating disease.

Disease-modifying therapies (DMTs) are chronic immunomodulatory treatments used to reduce the number of clinical attacks of MS (somewhere between 30% and 70%, depending on the agent) and to reduce new inflammatory MRI lesions (somewhere between 40% and 95%, depending on the agent). The traditional approach to choosing a DMT is to start most patients on an agent that is relatively safe but of lower efficacy and only "escalating" if the disease is not controlled. This strategy is referred to as an "escalation approach." Newer therapies are more efficacious but have the potential for more side effects and have less evident long-term risks. Starting with higher efficacy DMTs to minimize breakthrough disease that may leave permanent neurologic disability is known as an "induction approach" and is increasingly used by some MS experts. Trials are ongoing to compare long-term MS outcomes of these two treatment strategies. Either way, patients and healthcare professionals should realize that the medications are specifically for reduction in relapse-related disease and do not provide a cure or any symptomatic benefit.

Chronic parenteral therapy for RRMS includes the use of type 1 β interferons, glatiramer acetate (Copaxone), natalizumab (Tysabri), alemtuzumab (Lemtrada), ocrelizumab (Ocrevus), ofatumumab (Kesimpta), and ublituximab (Briumvi) (Table 1). Alternatively, oral therapies can be used and include teriflunomide, sphingosine-1-phosphate (S1P) receptor modulators, and the fumarates. The S1P receptor modulators include fingolimod (Gilenya), siponimod (Mayzent), ozanimod (Zeposia), and ponesimod (Ponvory). Dimethyl fumarate was the first fumarate available. More recently, diroximel fumarate (Vumerity) and monomethyl fumarate (Bafiertam) have been approved. Cladribine (Mavenclad) is an oral medication for treatment-resistant disease as a second-line therapy. The FDA product labels for most of these parenteral and oral therapies have recently been updated to specifically include CIS and SPMS with activity (ongoing relapses and/or new MRI lesions co-occurring with progressive disease) as approved indications for their use. Cladribine is not recommended for CIS because of its side effect profile. Ocrelizumab is approved for treatment of all clinical courses of CNS demyelinating disease, including CIS, RRMS, SPMS with activity, and PPMS course.

The side effect profile is well known for traditional injectable agents such as interferons and glatiramer acetate (see Table 1), and they have been safely used for many years. The safety profile for oral therapies seems satisfactory, but their long-term

side effect profile is still being assessed. For fingolimod, first-dose monitoring for 6 hours is required to assess heart rate and rhythm, and an eye exam is needed to screen for macular edema before initiating the medication and after several months. Serious infections including progressive multifocal leukoencephalopathy (PML) and disseminated varicella-zoster have been reported. Additional S1P receptor modulators have been developed with similar but distinct receptor binding in an effort to improve the side effect profile. One such agent, siponimod, was studied and approved for use in individuals with secondary progressive MS with ongoing disease activity. As a result of more selective binding, siponimod has fewer cardiac side effects, requiring first-dose cardiac monitoring only in select circumstances. It does, however, require CYP genotyping before initiation because of genetic differences in drug metabolism. Ponesimod requires first-dose cardiac monitoring in some individuals but does not require genetic testing. Ozanimod does not require genetic screening or cardiac monitoring, although there is a theoretical risk of serotonin syndrome, and the concurrent use of monoamine oxidase inhibitors is not recommended.

Teriflunomide may be associated with liver disease, reactivation of tuberculosis, and teratogenicity. Dimethyl fumarate is associated with flushing and gastrointestinal discomfort, and rare patients have developed PML when taking this medication. Diroximel fumarate, a structurally similar drug, showed improved gastrointestinal tolerability compared with dimethyl fumarate in a clinical trial. Monomethyl fumarate, the active metabolite of dimethyl fumarate and diroximel fumarate, was not studied in a trial specific to patients with MS but was approved based on mechanism of action and safety data when studied in healthy individuals.

Highly effective MS therapy may be indicated with natalizumab, alemtuzumab, or anti-CD20 agents (ocrelizumab, ofatumumab, and ublituximab) if first-line medications are intolerable, if therapeutic response is suboptimal (continued MS attacks or marked ongoing and new inflammatory disease on MRI despite therapy), or when a concerning clinical onset (severe attack, incomplete recovery, and/or high lesion burden) occurs.

Natalizumab is clearly associated with the development of PML, a severely impairing and often fatal opportunistic brain infection caused by reactivation of the dormant JC virus. In North America, natalizumab is only available through the Tysabri Outreach: Unified Commitment to Health prescribing program. Risk factors for PML in natalizumab-treated patients include the presence and index value of JC virus serum antibody (JCV-Ab), duration of therapy of at least 2 years, and history of prior immunosuppressive medication therapy (e.g., methotrexate, azathioprine). Seropositivity of patients with MS for JC virus antibody is over 55%. The seroconversion rate from JC virus Ab negativity to positivity is approximately 2% to 5% per year, and false-negative results are rare (<3%). Currently, no cases of PML have been found in patients persistently seronegative for JCV-Abs. Risk prevalence estimation after 2 years of treatment in JCV Ab–positive patients ranges from 1:250 for those without a history of immunosuppression to 1:90 in those with a history of prior immunosuppressive therapy. Evidence is emerging for extending the dosing interval to every 6 to 8 weeks in select individuals as a strategy to lower the risk of PML but maintain drug efficacy.

Ocrelizumab (anti-CD20 B cells; humanized form), an every-6-month infusion, is approved for relapsing MS and is the only therapy approved for PPMS. Initial clinical trials of ocrelizumab showed an increased rate of breast cancer in patients treated with ocrelizumab compared with those on placebo or interferons. As such, the FDA approval label recommends advising patients regarding a potential increased malignancy rate and that patients follow standard breast cancer screening guidelines. More recently, long-term follow-up safety data from several clinical trials, including open-label extension periods, were published and showed no increased risk of malignancy, including breast cancer, compared with matched reference MS and general populations. Ofatumumab is another anti-CD20 B-cell–depleting monoclonal

---

[1]Not FDA approved for this indication.

TABLE 1 Approved Immunomodulatory Therapy for Multiple Sclerosis

MEDICATION	DOSING	SIDE EFFECTS	MONITORING	ADDITIONAL INFORMATION
Interferon β1a (Avonex)	30 μg IM injection every week	Flulike symptoms (fever, chills, arthralgias, myalgias, and headaches), elevated LFTs, anemia, leukopenia, thrombocytopenia, depression, localized injection site rejections	CBC with differential, AST, ALT, ALP, and total bilirubin level at baseline, at 3 months, at 6 months × 2 years, and then annually Thyroid function cascade on initiation of therapy	Premedication with acetaminophen can ameliorate postinjection flulike symptoms
Interferon β1a (Rebif)	22-μg or 44-μg SC injection three times per week	Flulike symptoms (fever, chills, arthralgias, myalgias, headaches), elevated LFTs, anemia, leukopenia, thrombocytopenia, depression, localized injection site rejections	CBC with differential, AST, ALT, ALP, and total bilirubin level at baseline, at 3 months, at 6 months × 2 years, and then annually Thyroid function cascade on initiation of therapy	Premedication with acetaminophen can ameliorate postinjection flulike symptoms
Peginterferon β1a (Plegridy)	125 μg SC every 2 weeks	Flulike symptoms (fever, chills, arthralgias, myalgias, headaches), elevated LFTs, anemia, leukopenia, thrombocytopenia, depression, localized injection site rejections	CBC with differential, AST, ALT, ALP, and total bilirubin level at baseline, at 3 months, at 6 months × 2 years, and then annually Thyroid function cascade on initiation of therapy	Premedication with acetaminophen may ameliorate postinjection flulike symptoms
Interferon β1b (Betaseron, Extavia)	250-μg SC injection every other day	Flulike symptoms (fever, chills, arthralgias, myalgias, headaches), elevated LFTs, anemia, leukopenia, thrombocytopenia, depression, localized injection site rejections	CBC with differential, AST, ALT, ALP, and total bilirubin level at baseline, at 3 months, at 6 months × 2 years, and then annually Thyroid function cascade on initiation of therapy	Premedication with acetaminophen can ameliorate postinjection flulike symptoms
Glatiramer acetate (Copaxone)	20-mg SC injection daily or 40-mg SC injection three times per week	Injection site reactions (erythema, edema, pruritus, pain), transient chest pain, palpitations, facial flushing, anxiety, shortness of breath	None	
Fingolimod hydrochloride (Gilenya)	0.5 mg PO once daily	Headache, flulike symptoms, diarrhea, back pain, liver enzyme elevations, cough, hypertension, macular edema, and infections (disseminated varicella and herpes, rare cases of PML, opportunistic bacterial and fungal infections), increased risk of skin cancer; may cause a decrease in pulmonary function New FDA labeling required, investigating unexplained deaths occurring during treatment with fingolimod	CBC with differential, AST, ALT, and bilirubin at baseline and periodically thereafter Serology for VZV-IgG to determine immunity; if negative, vaccinate; if live-attenuated vaccine, give at least 4 weeks before initiation Latent infection screening (HIV, hepatitis, TB) in those at high risk Fundus examination at baseline and in 3–4 months for macular edema, repeated annually in those with diabetes mellitus or uveitis or if visual symptoms develop ECG, HR, and BP before first dose; first dose must be monitored for 6 hours for HR reduction and BP changes; 6-hour monitoring after oral dose must be repeated for patients who discontinue therapy for ≥2 weeks Periodic skin examinations	Should not be used in patients with recent MI, unstable angina, stroke, TIA, second- or third-degree AV block, CHF, SSS without cardiac pacing, or QTc > 500 ms, or with class Ia or III antiarrhythmic drugs Overnight continuous ECG monitoring recommended for those with preexisting cardiac or cerebrovascular disease; recurrent syncope; severe, untreated OSA; use of β-blockers; or prolonged QTc Caution for redemonstration of severe inflammatory disease on discontinuation

Drug	Dosing	Adverse effects	Monitoring	Additional considerations
Siponimod (Mayzent)	Requires oral titration; the recommended maintenance dosage for most is 2 mg PO once daily The recommended maintenance dosage in patients with a CYP2C9*1/*3 or CYP2C9*2/*3 genotype is 1 mg PO once daily Contraindicated in CYP2C9*3/*3 genotype	Herpes infection, upper respiratory infection, fungal skin infection, hypertension, macular edema; may cause a decrease in pulmonary function	CYP2C9 genotype determination CBC with differential, AST, ALT, and bilirubin at baseline and then periodically Serology for VZV-IgG to determine immunity; if negative, vaccinate; if live-attenuated vaccine, give at least 4 weeks before initiation Latent infection screening (HIV, hepatitis, TB) in those at high risk Fundus evaluation (OCT) at baseline and then annually for those with diabetes and uveitis or if visual symptoms develop Recent ECG (within past 6 months) and baseline BP	Concomitant use of moderate or strong CYP3A4 inducers (e.g., modafinil, efavirenz [Sustiva]) is not recommended for patients with CYP2C9*1/*3 and CYP2C9*2/*3 genotype Should not be used in patients with MI, unstable angina, stroke, TIA, or class III/IV CHF in the past 6 months or in patients with second- or third-degree AV block or in those with SSS unless the patient has a pacemaker First-dose monitoring is recommended for patients with certain preexisting cardiac conditions; initial monitoring procedures must be repeated for interruption of treatment of ≥4 consecutive doses Unknown whether rebound disease occurs with discontinuation, as seen in fingolimod
Ponesimod (Ponvory)	Requires oral titration; maintenance dose is 20 mg PO once daily	Herpes infection, upper respiratory infection, fungal skin infection, hypertension, macular edema, increased rate of cutaneous malignancies; may cause a decrease in pulmonary function	CBC with differential, AST, ALT, and bilirubin at baseline and then periodically Serology for VZV-IgG to determine immunity; if negative, vaccinate; if live-attenuated vaccine, give at least 4 weeks before initiation Latent infection screening (HIV, hepatitis, TB) in those at high risk Fundus evaluation (OCT) at baseline and then annually for those with diabetes and uveitis or if visual symptoms develop Recent ECG (i.e., within past 6 months) and baseline BP Periodic skin examinations	Should not be used in patients with MI, unstable angina, stroke, TIA, or class III/IV CHF in the past 6 months or in patients with second- or third-degree AV block or those with SSS unless the patient has a pacemaker First-dose monitoring is recommended for patients with certain preexisting cardiac conditions; initial monitoring procedures must be repeated for interruption of treatment of ≥4 consecutive doses Unknown whether rebound disease occurs with discontinuation, as seen in fingolimod
Ozanimod (Zeposia)	Requires oral titration; maintenance dose is 0.92 mg PO once daily	Herpes infection, upper respiratory infection, fungal skin infection, hypertension, macular edema; may cause a decrease in pulmonary function	CBC with differential, AST, ALT, and bilirubin at baseline and periodically thereafter Serology for VZV-IgG to determine immunity; if negative, vaccinate; if live-attenuated vaccine, give at least 4 weeks before initiation Latent infection screening (HIV, hepatitis, TB) in those at high risk Fundus evaluation (OCT) at baseline and then annually for those with diabetes and uveitis or if visual symptoms develop Recent ECG (within past 6 months) and baseline BP	Should not be used in patients with MI, unstable angina, stroke, TIA, or class III/IV CHF in the past 6 months or in patients with second- or third-degree AV block or those with SSS unless the patient has a pacemaker Do not use in severe untreated OSA or with concomitant use of an MAOI Cardiac monitoring and genetic testing not needed Unknown whether rebound disease occurs with discontinuation, as seen in fingolimod
Teriflunomide (Aubagio)	7 mg or 14 mg PO once daily	Diarrhea, abnormal LFTs, nausea, alopecia, hepatotoxicity, may cause significant birth defects if used during pregnancy, hypertension, TB reactivation, peripheral neuropathy, can worsen psoriasis, hypophosphatemia, transient acute renal failure, hyperkalemia	CBC at baseline, 6 months, and then annually AST, ALP, and bilirubin monthly for 6 months and then annually Latent infection screening (HIV and hepatitis) in those at high risk Tuberculin skin test and pregnancy test (women of childbearing potential) at baseline BP at baseline and then periodically	Do not use in severe hepatotoxicity, pregnancy, or with concomitant leflunomide use Prolonged half-life: recommend removal by activated charcoal or cholestyramine when required Pregnancy: teratogenic, accelerated washout recommended before conception

Continued

TABLE 1 Approved Immunomodulatory Therapy for Multiple Sclerosis—cont'd

MEDICATION	DOSING	SIDE EFFECTS	MONITORING	ADDITIONAL INFORMATION
Dimethyl fumarate (Tecfidera)	120 mg PO twice daily for 1 week, then 240 mg PO twice daily	Flushing, abdominal pain, nausea, diarrhea, infection (rare cases of PML, disseminated herpes), lymphopenia, hepatotoxicity	CBC with differential at baseline and then every 6–12 months; if lymphopenia occurs, monitor more frequently; may need to discontinue AST, ALT, ALP, and bilirubin at baseline Latent infection screening (HIV, hepatitis, TB) in those at high risk	Discontinue in sustained lymphopenia (<0.5 × 10⁹/L) because increases risk of infections including PML or LFT elevation (>20× upper limit of normal or jaundice)
Monomethyl fumarate (Bafiertam)	95 mg PO twice daily for 1 week, then increase to 190 mg PO twice daily	Flushing, infection, lymphopenia, abdominal symptoms but generally less than dimethyl fumarate, hepatotoxicity	CBC with differential at baseline, at 6 months, and then annually AST, ALT, ALP, and bilirubin at baseline Latent infection screening (HIV, hepatitis, TB) in those at high risk	
Diroximel fumarate (Vumerity)	231 mg PO twice daily for 1 week, then increase to 462 mg PO twice daily	Flushing, infection, lymphopenia, abdominal symptoms but generally less than dimethyl fumarate	CBC with differential at baseline, at 6 months, and then every 6–12 months AST, ALT, ALP, and bilirubin at baseline Latent infection screening (HIV, hepatitis, TB) in those at high risk	Improved gastrointestinal intolerance
Ocrelizumab (Ocrevus)	300 mg IV once followed by a 300 mg dose 2 weeks later, then 600 mg IV every 24 weeks	Infusion reactions, respiratory tract infections, herpes infections, neutropenia, reduced immunoglobulins Possible increased risk of cancer including breast cancer; follow standard cancer screening	Rule out active hepatitis and latent TB before first dose; consult liver specialist if history of hepatitis before first dose Immunoglobulins at baseline and then annually	Do not administer if signs of infection; delay until infection resolves If IgG <150 mg/dL or 150–500 mg/dL with recurrent infections, consider IVIg replacement Administer vaccines >6 weeks before ocrelizumab infusions; live and live-attenuated vaccines not recommended until B cell counts recover after discontinuation
Ofatumumab (Kesimpta)	Initial dosing: 20 mg SC injection at weeks 0, 1, and 2 Subsequent dosing: 20 mg SC injection every 4 weeks starting at week 4	Injection reactions most common within 24 hours of the first injection Respiratory tract infections, herpes infections, neutropenia, reduced immunoglobulins	Rule out active hepatitis and latent TB before first dose Immunoglobulins at baseline and then annually	Do not administer if signs of infection; delay until infection resolves If IgG <150 mg/dL or 150–500 mg/dL with recurrent infections, consider IVIg replacement Administer live and live-attenuated vaccines >4 weeks and inactivated vaccines >2 weeks before initiation; live and live-attenuated vaccines not recommended until B cell counts recover after discontinuation
Ublituximab (Briumvi)	150 mg IV once followed by a 450-mg IV dose 2 weeks later, then 450 mg IV every 24 weeks	Infusion reactions possible, recommend patient monitoring for 1 hour after the first two infusions Respiratory tract infections, urinary tract infections, neutropenia, reduced immunoglobulins	Rule out active hepatitis before first dose Immunoglobulins at baseline and then annually	Do not administer if signs of infection; delay until infection resolves. If IgG <150 mg/dL or 150–500 mg/dL with recurrent infections, consider IVIg replacement Administer live and live-attenuated vaccines >4 weeks and inactivated vaccines >2 weeks before initiation; live and live-attenuated vaccines not recommended until B cell counts recover after discontinuation

Drug	Dosing	Adverse effects	Monitoring/Recommendations
Natalizumab (Tysabri)	300 mg IV once every 4 weeks	Urticaria and anaphylaxis, headache, arthralgias, nausea, depression, infections (urinary tract, pneumonia, herpes simplex or reactivation) Rare hypersensitivity reactions can occur and are often associated with antibodies against natalizumab; if occurs, DMT switch is required	Baseline JCV Ab serologic study every 6 months while JCV negative; if JCV seropositive, consider another DMT If conversion occurs while on drug, strong consideration should be given to switching DMT with interim close monitoring; extended dosing interval of 6–8 weeks can be considered, but long-term a switch is recommended If PML is suspected, discontinue immediately, PLEX to remove the drug, MRI head with and without gadolinium with diffusion-weighted imaging; CSF for JCV PCR Risk of PML may be greater in patients with prolonged therapy and those previously treated with immunosuppressive medications; prescribing professional requires TOUCH enrollment Caution for redemonstration of severe inflammatory disease on discontinuation
Alemtuzumab (Lemtrada)	IV infusion over 4 h × two treatment courses First course: 12 mg/day on 5 consecutive days Second course: 12 mg/day on 3 consecutive days 12 months after the first treatment course	Infusion reactions with anaphylaxis; rarely MI, stroke, cervicocephalic artery dissections Autoimmune thyroid disorders, immune thrombocytopenia, antiglomerular basement membrane disease Malignancies including thyroid cancer, melanoma, lymphoproliferative disorders Opportunistic infections (PML, herpes, varicella, and other viral, bacterial, and fungal infections)	CBC with differential; serum creatinine; urinalysis with urine cell counts at baseline, then monthly; and TSH at baseline and then every 3 months until 48 months after last dose ALT, AST, bilirubin at baseline and then periodically until 48 months after last dose Serology for VZV-IgG to determine immunity; if negative, vaccinate; if live-attenuated vaccine, give at least 6 weeks before initiation Ensure no infections (HIV, hepatitis, TB) before treatment Baseline and yearly skin and cervical examinations Contraindicated if HIV positive Premedicate with high-dose corticosteroids, and give herpetic prophylaxis at time of first dose, continuing for at least 2 months or until CD4+ lymphocyte count is >200 cells/μL, whichever occurs later Complete all necessary immunizations at least 6 weeks before initiation No live virus vaccines after a course of alemtuzumab until lymphocyte counts normalize
Cladribine (Mavenclad)	Two treatment courses (1.75 mg/kg per treatment course); one course per year for a total of 2 years Treatment course is divided into 2 treatment weeks separated by 4 weeks: each treatment week consists of 4–5 days on which a patient receives a single daily dose (dose depending on body weight)	Anemia, thrombocytopenia, lymphopenia, upper respiratory tract infection, headache, hypersensitivity reaction, may increase risk of malignancies	CBC 2 and 6 months after the start of each treatment course and then annually thereafter Ensure no infections (HIV, hepatitis, TB) before treatment Serology for VZV-IgG to determine immunity; if negative, vaccinate, if live-attenuated vaccine, give at least 4–6 weeks before initiation If lymphocyte count at month 2 is <200 cells/mL, hold cladribine, monitor monthly until month 6, and then administer herpes prophylaxis Follow standard cancer screening guidelines Contraindicated in infections (HIV, active hepatitis, TB), current malignancy, pregnant women, and women and men of reproductive potential who do not plan to use contraception during dosing and for 6 months after the last dose in each treatment course Administer live-attenuated or live vaccines at least 4–6 weeks before starting; avoid vaccination with live-attenuated or live vaccines during and after treatment

Ab, Antibody; *ALP,* alkaline phosphatase; *ALT,* alanine aminotransferase; *AST,* aspartate aminotransferase; *AV,* arrioventricular; *BP,* blood pressure; *CBC,* complete blood count; *CHF,* congestive heart failure; *ECG,* electrocardiogram; *HIV,* human immunodeficiency virus; *HR,* heart rate; *IgG,* immunoglobulin G; *IV,* intravenous; *IVIg,* intravenous immunoglobulin G; *JCV,* JC virus; *LFT,* liver function test; *MAOI,* monoamine oxidase inhibitor; *MI,* myocardial infarction; *OCT,* optical coherence tomography; *OSA,* obstructive sleep apnea; *PCR,* polymerase chain reaction; *PLEX,* plasma exchange; *PML,* progressive multifocal leukoencephalopathy; *PO,* by mouth; *SC,* subcutaneously; *SSS,* sick sinus syndrome; *TB,* tuberculosis; *TIA,* transient ischemic attack; *TOUCH,* Tysabri Outreach: Unified Commitment to Health; *TSH,* thyroid-stimulating hormone; *VZV-IgG,* varicella zoster virus immunoglobulin G.

antibody that has a similar risk profile to ocrelizumab but is given monthly through an autoinjector. The most recently FDA-approved anti-CD20 B-cell–depleting agent, ublituximab, is given every 6 months as an intravenous infusion and again shares a similar side effect profile.

Alemtuzumab is a monoclonal antibody (anti-CD52; T and B cells) for RRMS with major safety precautions that include potential for malignancy and the development of autoimmune thyroid disease, immune thrombocytopenia, and, rarely, antiglomerular basement membrane disease. More recently, serious and life-threatening infusion reactions including strokes and arterial dissections have been reported with alemtuzumab.

Mitoxantrone is a chemotherapy agent that is approved for SPMS, but given its severe side effect profile (acute and delayed cardiotoxicity, acute myelogenous leukemia), it is rarely used today. Daclizumab (Zinbryta) (anti-CD25, interleukin [IL]-2 receptor) was withdrawn voluntarily from the market because of case reports of an association with presumably immune-mediated encephalitis.

Available, although limited, evidence suggests that autologous bone marrow transplantation with stem cell delivery is a promising therapy for select patients with MS. It appears that individuals most likely to benefit are young, are ambulatory, have recent disease onset, and have ongoing disease activity despite having tried first- and second-line agents. Risks are "front-loaded" and include the adverse effects resulting from cytotoxic agents (nausea, mucositis, and alopecia) and myelosuppression (infection and hemorrhage). Late toxicity includes engraftment syndrome, infertility, infection, myelodysplastic syndromes, and secondary autoimmune disorders. Several large randomized controlled trials are ongoing to supplement existing evidence.

The mechanism of action of most DMTs is to modulate the immune system. This can have important implications on timing of vaccine delivery (see Table 1) and vaccine response. Immunization status should be discussed early, and generally patients should be encouraged to update their vaccines as per public health guidelines. Administration of non–live vaccines is considered safe in patients with MS, including those taking a DMT, although response may be diminished with specific DMTs such as anti-CD20 B-cell–depleting agents and S1P receptor modulators. If a patient is experiencing an acute MS relapse, vaccination should be deferred until after symptoms resolve or plateau. If a patient has recently received a course of steroids, it is recommended to wait 4 to 6 weeks before vaccinating if possible. The inactivated seasonal influenza vaccine and non–live coronavirus disease 2019 (COVID-19) vaccines are recommended in all patients with MS. Guidelines regarding the number and timing of COVID-19 vaccinations are continuously changing as the understanding and epidemiology of COVID-19 evolve. Currently, consideration should be given to vaccination against COVID-19 before initiation of anti-CD20 B-cell–depleting agents and S1P receptor modulators because both have been shown to impair vaccine response. The Centers for Disease Control and Prevention recently recommended Shingrix, a recombinant non–live vaccine against herpes zoster, to individuals older than 18 years of age who are immunocompromised, such as those with MS on immunosuppressing DMTs. Live and live-attenuated vaccines should be avoided in persons with MS if possible. When needed, administration should be done before initiation of DMT, with timing dependent on the specific agent used (see Table 1). For instance, immunity against varicella-zoster should be confirmed before initiating an S1P receptor modulator given reports of disseminated varicella on fingolimod. This requires a live vaccination series to be completed at least 1 month before beginning the S1P modulator to allow time for the vaccine to take effect.

Pregnancy and Lactation

Given the demographics of people diagnosed with multiple sclerosis, the use of DMTs around pregnancy and lactation is a commonly encountered scenario. Generally, DMTs are avoided during pregnancy because this is a time when new attacks and new lesions are less likely to occur, although an increase is often seen postpartum. No agent has FDA approval for use in pregnancy. Pregnancy registries show no clear or major safety risks regarding the use of interferons and glatiramer acetate during pregnancy, and these agents are occasionally continued on a case-by-case basis. Natalizumab has risk for severe MS rebound disease when stopped, and pregnancy does not appear to be protective against this. Therefore some clinicians will continue natalizumab off-label until 30 to 34 weeks of gestation with extended interval dosing (every 6–8 weeks) and then resume 1 to 2 weeks postpartum with screening of the newborn for hematologic abnormalities. FDA labels recommend a 6-month washout from last dose to time of conception for anti-CD20s, although based on pharmacokinetics, some clinicians will allow a shorter washout after discussion with the patient. It is recommended that the patient avoid becoming pregnant for at least 4 months after the last alemtuzumab infusion.

Oral agents are contraindicated during pregnancy. It is recommended that conception only be attempted 6 months after the last cladribine dose for both men and women. A 2-month washout is recommended for fingolimod but risk for rebound of MS disease activity exists, so a switch to another agent is often entertained in advance of pregnancy planning. Teriflunomide is teratogenic and requires an accelerated washout or 24-month waiting period. Dimethyl fumarate can be stopped at the time of conception planning.

With respect to lactation, oral agents should again be avoided because they are small molecules and can pass into breast milk. Injectables and infusion-based monoclonal antibodies are sometimes used off-label on a case-by-case basis by MS experts because breast milk transfer of these large molecules appears to be minimal and risk of exposure to the newborn is low.

Monitoring

Most, if not all, patients with MS should be followed by a neurologist at least occasionally. Recommendations for clinical assessment range from 6 to 18 months, depending on clinical activity of relapses and disability. The ideal scheduling of repeat brain MRI scans is controversial and varies depending on MS clinical activity and whether medications are initiated, changed, or discontinued, but general recommendations are every 1 to 2 years in stable patients.

Complications

MS is one of the main causes for neurologic impairment at a young age. Often patients need gait assistance when impairment becomes more severe. This includes the use of a single gait aid, such as a cane or walking stick, or an ankle-foot orthosis for symptomatic foot drop. Dalfampridine (Ampyra) is a potassium channel blocker that has been shown to improve walking speed. Contraindications include a history of seizures and moderate to severe renal impairment.

Spasticity associated with upper motor neuron weakness in the lower extremities may be treated with an active daily exercise program directed by physical therapists and physiatrists. Judicious use of baclofen (Lioresal) is helpful (typically starting at 5 mg three times daily, with no more than a maximum of 80 mg per day). Baclofen side effects include drowsiness and liver enzyme elevations. Some patients with significant lower extremity weakness are assisted in their gait by the leg support provided by spasticity, and if spasticity is reduced pharmacologically, this can in fact worsen their gait. Alternatives to baclofen include tizanidine (Zanaflex) and clonidine (Catapres).[1] For focal spasticity, botulinum toxin (Botox) injection can be used. Gabapentin (Neurontin)[1] can be helpful as an adjuvant therapy, particularly in those with neuropathic pain or for monotherapy in those who failed first-line agents. Oral cannabinoids (tetrahydrocannabinol and cannabidiol [Sativex][2]) have favorable evidence for

---

[1] Not FDA approved for this indication.
[2] Not available in the United States.

patient-reported symptoms of spasticity, spasms, and central pain but may have cognitive side effects. Benzodiazepines have antispasticity properties but are not typically first line because of side effects and potential for dependency. Dantrolene (Dantrium) has been shown to be effective but is rarely used because of hepatoxicity.

Patients often experience symptoms of neurogenic bladder dysfunction. This includes symptoms of urinary urgency and urge-related incontinence. Bladder stimulants such as caffeine may aggravate urinary symptoms. Patients with neurogenic bladder should be investigated for completeness of bladder emptying. If there is severe impairment in bladder emptying, urinary catheterization often is recommended. If bladder emptying is complete or only mildly impaired (<100 mL postvoid residual), use of medications such as oxybutynin (Ditropan), solifenacin (Vesicare), and tolterodine (Detrol) may be recommended for urge-related symptoms. These anticholinergic medications can cause confusion and should be used with caution in older adults or those with cognitive dysfunction. Mirabegron (Myrbetriq) may be preferable in such situations as it selectively acts as a beta-3 adrenergic receptor agonist to relax the detrusor smooth muscle but requires monitoring for hypertension. Regardless of drug choice, ongoing monitoring of bladder emptying is recommended. Some patients require formal urodynamic evaluation for complex bladder symptoms.

Constipation is a common symptom that may exacerbate neurogenic bladder symptoms. Treatment includes physical exercise, dietary fiber supplementation, and hydration. Stool softeners, promotility agents, bulking agents, or enemas may be required. Sexual dysfunction can occur in men and women, including reduced libido either with or without difficulty achieving erection and/or orgasm. Management may include nonpharmacologic and pharmacologic strategies similar to those used in non–MS-related sexual dysfunction.

Fatigue is a common MS-related symptom. A complete sleep history to ensure appropriate sleep hygiene is imperative. This includes initiating sleep promptly, maintaining sleep throughout the night, and awakening feeling refreshed. Encouragement of a formal exercise program to facilitate restful sleep and daytime vigor is important. Obstructive sleep apnea, restless leg syndrome, and other parasomnias must be ruled out as additional contributing factors to fatigue. If sleep hygiene is entirely normal and late afternoon fatigue remains a problem, pharmacologic therapy for MS-related fatigue can be considered. Medications that have been used for debilitating MS fatigue that does not respond to nonpharmacologic management include amantadine hydrochloride (Symmetrel)[1], modafinil (Provigil)[1], armodafinil (Nuvigil)[1], amphetamines (including methylphenidate [Ritalin][1]), and fluoxetine (Prozac).[1] None of these medications has FDA approval specific to MS fatigue. A recent randomized, double-blind, crossover trial determined amantadine, modafinil, and methylphenidate were not superior compared with placebo and their use is often limited by their side effect profile.

Neuropathic pain and other uncomfortable sensations can occur in MS. Neuropathic pain agents such as gabapentin[1], pregabalin (Lyrica)[1], duloxetine (Cymbalta)[1], and tricyclic antidepressants are frequently used. Paroxysmal attacks of sensory (Lhermitte phenomenon and trigeminal neuralgia) and motor (painful tonic spasms) symptoms can cause discomfort and interfere with function. Both sensory and motor symptoms are typically very sensitive to low-dose carbamazepine (Tegretol).[1]

Mood disorders such as anxiety and depression are prevalent in MS. Treatment includes nonpharmacologic management such as cognitive-behavioral therapy, and medications may be warranted in some patients. Pseudobulbar affect, uncontrollable episodes of laughter or crying, may occur. If this symptom is bothersome to the patient, dextromethorphan/quinidine (Nuedexta) is approved for this indication. Selective serotonin reuptake inhibitors, serotonin-norepinephrine reuptake inhibitors, and tricyclic antidepressants have been used off-label for pseudobulbar affect.

MS is a common CNS inflammatory demyelinating disease with heterogenous presentation and prognosis. CIS, RRMS, and active SPMS are treated with corticosteroids to hasten resolution of acute relapses and chronic immunomodulatory medications to reduce the number of future clinical attacks and new MRI lesions. Ocrelizumab is the only medication approved for PPMS. Symptomatic care is important in these patients, including the treatment of gait disorder, spasticity, neurogenic sphincter dysfunction, fatigue, paroxysmal symptoms, neuropathic pain, and mood disorders.

References

Hittle M, Culpepper WJ, Langer-Gould A, et al: Population-Based Estimates for the Prevalence of Multiple Sclerosis in the United States by Race, Ethnicity, Age, Sex, and Geographic Region, *JAMA Neurol* 80(7):693–701, 2023.

Kjetil B, et al: Longitudinal analysis reveals high prevalence of Epstein-Barr virus associated with multiple sclerosis, *Science* 375(6578):296–301, 2022.

Nourbakhsh B, Revirajan N, Morris B, et al: Safety and efficacy of amantadine, modafinil, and methylphenidate for fatigue in multiple sclerosis: a randomised, placebo-controlled, crossover, double-blind trial, *Lancet Neurol* 20(1):38–48, 2021.

Reich DS, Lucchinetti CF, Calabresi PA: Multiple sclerosis, *N Engl J Med* 378:169–180, 2018.

Thompson AJ, Banwell BL, Barkhof F, et al: Diagnosis of multiple sclerosis: 2017 revisions of the McDonald criteria, *Lancet Neurol* 17(2):162–173, 2018.

Wallin MT, Culpepper WJ, Campbell JD, et al: The prevalence of MS in the United States: a population-based estimate using health claims data, *Neurol* 92(10):e1029–e1040, 2019.

MYASTHENIA GRAVIS

Method of
Taylor B. Harrison, MD; and William P. Roche, MD

CURRENT DIAGNOSIS

- Myasthenia gravis (MG) is an autoimmune disorder that affects the neuromuscular junction, resulting in fatigable skeletal muscle weakness.
- Diagnosis may be based on clinical history and exam in combination with identification of autoantibodies (e.g., Ach-R Abs) or abnormalities on electrodiagnostic testing.
- Myasthenic crisis, defined by respiratory failure, can stem from respiratory or oropharyngeal weakness. It may develop abruptly and typically occurs in the setting of illness, change in medications, or early in the disease course.

CURRENT THERAPY

- Mild symptoms can respond well to anticholinesterase inhibitors such as pyridostigmine (Mestinon).
- A wide range of medications may be used to treat MG, including steroids, nonsteroidal immunosuppressants, as well as intravenous immunoglobulin (IVIG)[1] and plasmapheresis. Thymectomy may be considered in patients with acetylcholine receptor antibodies.
- It is important to recognize that certain medications may worsen MG.
- Myasthenic crisis is a medical emergency, and patients should be treated in the intensive care unit with close respiratory monitoring and possibly intubation. IVIG[1] and plasmapheresis are treatment options for myasthenic crisis.

[1]Not FDA approved for this indication.

[1]Not FDA approved for this indication.

Epidemiology

Myasthenia gravis (MG) is the most common acquired disorder of neuromuscular transmission, with an incidence of 8 to 30 per million annually. The prevalence is a mean of 175 per million, reflecting the disease's low mortality rate in the era of current therapies. An estimated 700,000 people are living with MG worldwide, with between 36,000 to 125,000 living in the United States.

There exists a bimodal age distribution with two peaks of incidence: the first peak in the second to third decades of life, and a second peak in the seventh to eighth decades. Women predominate in early-onset MG (defined by onset <50 years of age), whereas men predominate with late-onset disease (>50 years of age).

Risk Factors

MG is associated with thymoma: approximately one-third of patients with thymoma will develop myasthenia, and 10% of myasthenic patients have a thymoma. Certain human leukocyte antigen (HLA) subtypes, which are known to predispose to autoimmune disorders in general, also increase the risk of MG. Other autoimmune disorders are present in about 15% of myasthenic patients, most commonly thyroiditis, followed by systemic lupus erythematosus and rheumatoid arthritis. A small percentage of patients may have a myasthenia-myositis overlap syndrome.

Pathophysiology

To understand the pathophysiology, a review of normal physiology is needed. In normal muscle contraction, an action potential (AP) travels down a motor nerve to the presynaptic axon terminal. At the axon terminal, the AP triggers voltage-gated calcium channels to open, causing calcium influx. Calcium influx causes synaptic vesicles containing acetylcholine to fuse with the cell membrane, resulting in exocytosis of acetylcholine into the synaptic cleft. Acetylcholine diffuses across the synaptic cleft and binds with nicotinic acetylcholine receptors (AChRs) on the cell membrane of the muscle fiber. The AChRs are ligand-gated ion channels that, once opened, allow cation influx, generating an end plate potential (EPP). When the EPP reaches a threshold value, it triggers voltage-gated sodium channels in the postsynaptic membrane to open, resulting in further cation influx and membrane depolarization, resulting in a muscle fiber AP and muscle fiber contraction. Excess acetylcholine is then broken down by the enzyme acetylcholinesterase (AchE) in the synaptic cleft.

The safety factor is an important concept in understanding the muscle fatigability of MG. The safety factor is the ratio of postsynaptic EPP generated by a quantity of acetylcholine to the threshold required to generate an all-or-none muscle fiber AP and thus muscle fiber contraction. In the healthy state, more acetylcholine is released than is needed to generate a muscle fiber AP. In myasthenia the safety factor is lower, and sufficient acetylcholine may not be released to generate successive APs with repeated contractions. Exercise will result in insufficient neuromuscular transmission over time because of this reduction in safety factor, and as muscle fibers fail to reach threshold to generate an AP, fatigable weakness ensues.

MG is caused by antibodies targeting antigens of the postsynaptic membrane of the neuromuscular junction. In MG, the normal action of acetylcholine at the postsynaptic muscle cell membrane is disrupted by one of several antibody-mediated mechanisms. Most commonly, antibodies are formed against the AChR itself. These AChR antibodies interrupt normal transmission by cross-linking the receptors causing increased turnover or complement-mediated degradation or by inducing conformational changes in the channel, keeping acetylcholine from activating the channel. Other antibodies have been found to cause MG, including antibodies against muscle-specific kinase (MUSK), lipoprotein-related protein 4 (LRP4), or agrin. The postsynaptic cell membrane is folded into secondary synaptic folds, increasing the surface area of the cell membrane, and AChRs are organized in clusters at the peaks of these folds (adjacent to the nerve axon terminal).

TABLE 1	Medications That May Exacerbate or Precipitate Myasthenia Gravis

Black Box Warnings

Telithromycin (Ketek)[2]

Fluoroquinolones (ciprofloxacin [Cipro], moxifloxacin [Avelox], levofloxacin [Levaquin])

Drugs to Avoid

D-penicillamine (Cuprimine)

Checkpoint inhibitors (ipilimumab [Yervoy], pembrolizumab [Keytruda], nivolumab [Opdivo])

Quinine

IV magnesium

Use Only With Caution

Macrolides (erythromycin, azithromycin [Zithromax], clarithromycin [Biaxin])

Aminoglycosides (gentamycin [Garamycin], neomycin, tobramycin)

Procainamide (Pronestyl)

Desferrioxamine (Desferal)

Beta blockers (propranolol, metoprolol [Lopressor], carvedilol [Coreg])

Statins (atorvastatin [Lipitor], pravastatin [Pravachol], rosuvastatin [Crestor], simvastatin [Zocor])

[2]Not available in the United States.

MUSK, LRP4, and agrin are proteins that participate in AChR clustering on these peaks. Antibody-mediated disruption of the function of these proteins causes reduced AChR concentration on the postsynaptic membrane with reduced safety factor, resulting in a myasthenia phenotype.

Some patients do not have antibodies that are detectable by current serologic testing. These patients are presumed to have antibodies against components of the postsynaptic membrane that have not yet been identified.

Prevention

Although there is no recognized prevention for developing myasthenia, exacerbations (myasthenic crises) are preventable by avoiding certain drugs. In particular, beta blockers, some antibiotics (aminoglycosides, fluoroquinolones, and macrolides), and chelating agents (penicillamine [Cuprimine]) should be avoided in myasthenic patients (Table 1). Statins should be used cautiously and only at the lowest effective dose.

Clinical Manifestations

Patients with MG will present with weakness of the extraocular, bulbar, axial, or limb muscles. The most characteristic feature of the weakness seen in myasthenia is fatigability; that is, the tendency of a muscle to get weaker with repeated use. Thus when thinking about weakness from MG, it is important to get a sense of whether the patient's symptoms are exacerbated by exercise or demonstrate a diurnal fluctuation (with the most typical pattern being weakness that is worse at the end of the day).

Ocular symptoms (ptosis and diplopia) are the first symptoms of myasthenia in approximately 60% of patients, and in 15% to 20% of all myasthenic patients, weakness remains limited to the eye muscles (so-called ocular myasthenia). Patients will complain of a drooping eyelid or binocular double vision (which improves with closing one eye) that frequently fluctuates throughout the day or with activity. On physical examination, these patients have ptosis or limitations in extraocular movements that are triggered or exaggerated by sustained upgaze for 60 seconds (so-called upgaze paresis). The extraocular manifestations are rarely symmetric, and the ptosis is very often more significant on one side.

Weakness of the limbs tends to be symmetric and usually affects proximal more than distal muscles. Patients will frequently complain of reduced ability to perform repetitive actions of the proximal muscles, such as lifting an arm to comb hair or climbing stairs. On physical examination, fatigability can be demonstrated by having the patient activate the deltoids (arm abduction) or iliopsoas (hip flexion) either against gravity for 2 minutes or against examiner resistance for 5 repetitions of 5 seconds each. Typically, myasthenic patients with weakness of these muscle groups will have a significant decrement in strength between the first repetition and the last. Similar maneuvers can be performed using whichever muscle groups are affected, according to the patient's complaints.

Bulbar weakness manifests as difficulty with speech (dysarthria) or swallowing (dysphagia). These symptoms may also be fatigable; for example, patients may notice more difficulty enunciating toward the end of the day or at the end of a speech, or more trouble swallowing toward the end of a meal or when eating chewy foods such as steak. If shortness of breath is present, it typically improves moving from a supine to sitting position, which helps with diaphragm excursion. Strength of sniff and cough can be easily assessed at the bedside, and weakness of neck flexion may indicate risk for diaphragmatic weakness.

Sensation is not affected in MG. If a patient has sensory loss, static weakness that does not fluctuate with exercise, or other neurologic symptoms aside from weakness, this should prompt the examiner to consider an alternate diagnosis. Deep tendon reflexes are normal in MG.

Diagnosis

It is important to understand the proper diagnostic algorithm for MG, which is based on the combination of clinical history, examination findings, presence of autoantibodies, and results of electrodiagnostic testing. In the setting of a good clinical history and positive examination findings, the presence of pathologic autoantibodies is likely sufficient to confirm the diagnosis. When the clinical history or examination is suggestive but autoantibodies are not present, electrodiagnostic testing is important to confirm a suspected diagnosis, particularly if immunosuppressive or interventional therapies are considered.

Bedside tests to support a diagnosis include the ice pack test and edrophonium. Placement of ice over a ptotic eyelid may lead to clinical improvement, as cool temperature slows down the breakdown of Ach in the synapse due to slowed action of AchE. This effectively increases the amount of available acetylcholine to the neuromuscular junction and can thus improve muscle weakness.

Laboratory evaluation of autoantibodies is standard of care in patients with suspected MG. In generalized MG, AChR Abs are generally present in up to 85% of affected individuals with generalized MG. AChR Abs may include blocking, binding, and modulating antibodies. Of those patients with generalized MG who are seronegative for AChR Ab, approximately 30% to 40% are seropositive for MUSK antibodies. In ocular MG, where symptoms are limited to ptosis or binocular diplopia, only about 15% are seropositive for autoantibodies, and if present, those autoantibodies are AChR Ab. The low density lipoprotein 4 antibodies (LPR4) can be present in up to 5% of patients. In the otherwise seronegative patient for AChR and MUSK antibodies, an estimated 18% of patients may have LPR4 antibodies, but there is significant variation among study populations. The vast majority are seronegative and require further evaluation for confirmation of the diagnosis.

Electrodiagnostic testing for a disorder of neuromuscular transmission includes slow repetitive nerve stimulation (RNS). A stimulator is used to depolarize a motor nerve (resulting in an all-or-none nerve AP) and generate a muscle twitch recorded as a compound motor action potential (CMAP). A train of stimuli (between 4 and 6) are performed at a rate of 3 to 5 per second. In MG the dysfunction at the postsynaptic muscle membrane results in some muscle fibers not achieving depolarization sufficient to cause an all-or-none muscle fiber AP, and the size of the overall CMAP (from multiple muscle fibers) is reduced. The threshold for abnormality is a CMAP decrement of >10%, generally between the first and fourth stimuli. If a baseline study at rest is normal, the patient is asked to exercise the muscle for 1 minute, and the study is repeated at 1-minute intervals to assess for the development of decrement. It should be noted that the sensitivity of RNS is increased with the presence of fatigable weakness on examination, because the clinical correlate of a decrement is weakness. Aside from distal hand muscles, trapezius or facial muscles such as nasalis can be studied.

Single-fiber electromyography looks for "jitter" or loss of synchronization of individual muscle fibers innervated by a single anterior horn cell in the spinal cord. This is the most sensitive electrodiagnostic test for MG.

Differential Diagnosis

The differential diagnosis for diplopia and ptosis includes cranial nerve palsies: oculomotor (cranial nerve III), trochlear (cranial nerve IV), and abducens (cranial nerve VI). Horner's syndrome may also cause ptosis due to weakness in Mueller's muscle, although other signs such as anisocoria (unequal pupils) that is worsened in the dark is present. Thyroid eye disease may cause any of these symptoms as well. The differential diagnosis for appendicular weakness without sensory loss includes myopathy, pure motor neuropathy, anterior horn cell disease, or a central nervous system pathology involving the motor pathways. These causes of weakness result in static rather than fluctuating weakness.

The main differential diagnosis for fatigable weakness as seen in MG is the Lambert-Eaton myasthenic syndrome (LEMS). LEMS is caused by antibodies against voltage-gated calcium channels on the presynaptic neuromuscular junction and may be paraneoplastic (small cell carcinoma of the lung) or autoimmune. MG and LEMS can be differentiated by the presence of postexercise facilitation of reflexes (after 10 seconds of sustained exercise), as well as antibody and electrodiagnostic testing.

Therapy

Overall, the treatment goal is to achieve freedom from symptoms or functional limitations, recognizing that patients may still have some weakness of some muscles (this is known as minimal manifestation status). Mainstays of treatment include anticholinesterase inhibitors, as well as oral steroids, and a variety of immunosuppressants, as well as intravenous immunoglobulin (IVIG)[1], and plasmapheresis may be used. Broadly, medical therapy can be classified as symptomatic or disease-modifying, the latter with an immunomodulatory effect targeting the underlying disease pathophysiology.

It should be noted that there exists wide variation in therapeutic approaches, and there are limited head-to-head data comparing individual medications. Current treatments, as well as advances in clinical care, have significantly improved the mortality rate of MG and outcomes of myasthenic crisis.

Symptomatic Therapy

Pyridostigmine (Mestinon) is an AchE inhibitor that increases the amount of acetylcholine in the synaptic cleft by slowing its breakdown by AchE and should be considered as initial therapy. Onset of action is typically within 30 minutes, with benefit generally lasting 3 to 4 hours. It is initially dosed 60 mg 3 times daily by mouth and may be increased to 120 mg every 3 to 4 hours while awake, with the total dose typically not exceeding 480 mg/d. It does not penetrate the central nervous

---

[1] Not FDA approved for this indication.

system, and most side effects are gastrointestinal. Side effects may include nausea, vomiting, abdominal cramping, diarrhea, sweating, blurred vision, or muscle twitching and cramps. Anticholinergic agents such as glycopyrrolate (Robinul) 1 mg or hyoscyamine sulfate (Levsin)[1] 0.125 mg with each pyridostigmine dose can usually treat these muscarinic side effects effectively. Data suggest that MUSK Ab–positive patients may have a lesser response to acetylcholinesterase therapy compared with AChR–seropositive patients. In the setting of ocular myasthenia, there appears to be more of response in ptosis compared with diplopia.

Corticosteroids

Corticosteroids, typically prednisone[1], are a mainstay of immunotherapy and used when pyridostigmine alone does not achieve an adequate treatment response. Two general approaches exist, using either a low-dose or high-dose regimen. Decisions may be dictated by the severity of weakness, presence of significant bulbar dysfunction, or comorbid conditions (such as diabetes). A "low-dose" approach is used with milder disease and includes initiation of 10 to 20 mg daily, and increasing by 5 mg orally weekly to a lower target dose (generally 40–60 mg/d). Oral high-dose (1 mg/kg/d) steroid therapy may be used with moderate-severe weakness and generally has a latency of 2 to 4 weeks before onset of benefit with maximal benefit in 5 to 6 months. It is important to recognize that early clinical deterioration is possible (reported up to 50%) approximately 7 to 10 days after treatment initiation, generally when steroids are dosed at 1 mg/kg/d or higher. In those patients for whom high-dose therapy is introduced, concomitant treatment with either IVIG or plasma exchange (PLEX), discussed herein, may provide protection against early clinical deterioration.

For a patient who has achieved the treatment goal of minimal manifestation on a particular dose of steroids, it is important to consider weaning the dose to reduce side effects. A common approach is a slow taper decreasing 5 mg/d per month on alternate days, with a slower taper once a total dose of 10 mg daily is achieved. Many patients can be maintained on low doses of steroids.

Some patients have an inadequate response to steroids or intolerable side effects or are unable to taper because of recurrence of symptoms. These patients are typically treated with alternative, steroid-sparing, immunomodulatory therapies. Some patients with comorbidities that limit steroid dosing are started on steroids and nonsteroidal immunosuppressant medications concurrently.

Thymectomy

Thymectomy is considered standard of care for those with thymoma, which is present in approximately 15% of patients with generalized MG. A randomized controlled trial supports thymectomy in AChR Ab–positive patients with at least moderately severe disease. Thymectomy patients demonstrated improved outcomes compared with placebo, required less steroids, fewer required steroid-sparing immunosuppressants, and experienced fewer hospitalizations. Thymectomy is controversial for mild symptoms, purely ocular disease, older age (>60 years), and there exist various surgical approaches. It is considered standard of care to pretreat with IVIG or PLEX before surgery if patients are symptomatic before surgery.

Other Immunomodulatory Therapies

Azathioprine (Imuran)[1] is a purine analog that inhibits nucleic acid synthesis, as well as T- and B-cell proliferation. It is a commonly used steroid-sparing immunosuppressant that is considered first line and has shown efficacy in a randomized clinical trial. Azathioprine allows reduced steroid dose, reduces relapse rate, and prolongs duration of remission. Treatment is generally started at 50 mg daily, increasing by 50 mg every 1 to 2 weeks to approximately 150 to 200 daily (2–3 mg/kg/d), generally in split doses. Onset of action is estimated at 4 to 8 months, and therapy requires regular blood count and liver function monitoring. Side effects include a flulike illness at initiation (reported in up to 10%–20%, requires cessation), leukopenia, and transaminitis. Thiopurine methyltransferase enzyme testing can be performed, if available, before starting to identify patients at high risk of bone marrow suppression (although monitoring of blood counts is favored by many practitioners).

Intravenous immunoglobulin (IVIG, Gammagard)[1] has been shown to improve weakness in MG. Its mechanism of action is unclear but is presumed to stem from neutralizing circulating pathogenic autoantibodies. A dose of 2 g/kg spread over 5 days is a common algorithm for initial treatment, although in patients who previously tolerated it, IVIG could be given as 1 g/kg/d over 2 days. Onset of action is typically within the first week, and benefit may be sustained for 3 to 4 weeks after treatment. Side effects include headache (sometimes severe and related to aseptic meningitis), thrombosis because of increased serum viscosity, and renal failure. Avoidance of sucrose-containing products may decrease risk of renal failure. Slowed infusion rates may help avoid decompensation of heart failure. Patients on maintenance dosing may receive IVIG 1 g/kg every 3 to 4 weeks.

Mycophenolate mofetil (CellCept)[1] inhibits guanosine nucleotide synthesis that is needed for B and T lymphocytes. Although there have been two negative randomized clinical trials, there are several retrospective reports supporting efficacy, and consensus expert opinion is that it remains a treatment option. It is started at 500 mg twice daily and titrated to 1000 to 1500 mg twice daily. Side effects include nausea, vomiting, diarrhea, and leukopenia. It has teratogenic potential and should not be used in pregnancy.

Cyclosporine (Sandimmune)[1] is a calcineurin inhibitor that has suppressed inflammatory cytokines and has multiple effects on T-cell function. It is initiated at approximately 3 mg/kg daily as a twice-daily split dose and may be titrated up to 5 mg/kg/d with a target trough level <300 ng/mL. Onset of action is approximately 2 to 3 months. Side effects include hirsutism, hypertension, clinically significant nephrotoxicity, and increased cancer risk (including dermatologic cancers). Cyclosporine level may be affected by multiple drug interactions, and concomitant medications should be reviewed.

Methotrexate (Trexall)[1] is a folate antimetabolite that may be dosed orally or subcutaneously. A typical oral dose is initiated at 10 mg weekly and titrated to 15 to 25 mg orally once a week. It is recommended that the patient take folate[1] supplementation of approximately at least 1 mg daily. Side effects include stomatitis (folate supplementation may help prevent this), bone marrow suppression, and interstitial lung disease (rare). It is important to note that methotrexate is a known teratogen and should be avoided in women of childbearing potential.

Plasmapheresis or PLEX removes plasma from the circulation and replaces it, typically with albumin, with the net effect of removing pathologic autoantibodies and inflammatory cytokines. Typically, five exchanges are performed over a period of 1 to 2 weeks, and benefit is typically observed by the third exchange. PLEX requires placement of a vas cath or (if to be used as a maintenance therapy) a permacath. When used as a maintenance therapy, 1 to 2 exchanges are typically performed, at variable intervals, as frequently as weekly. There is a risk of deep venous thrombosis or line infection. Hypotension may occur because of citrate-induced hypovolemia, and it may be associated with hypocalcemia. Angiotensin-converting enzyme (ACE) inhibitors need to be held 24 hours because of bradykinin-related vasodilation.

Rituximab (Rituxan)[1] is a CD20 antibody that has been evaluated in a randomized controlled trials. Data support efficacy, particularly in MUSK Ab patients and modest evidence for treatment-refractory AChR Ab myasthenia and for double-seronegative myasthenia. It is dosed 325 mg/m² weekly for 4

---

[1] Not FDA approved for this indication.

weeks, although it can also be dosed 1 g/m² with a second dose 2 weeks later. Dosing may be repeated at 6-month intervals. Side effects include infusion-related symptoms including pruritus, headache, hypotension, nausea, and chills. Rituximab may additionally result in leukopenia, anemia, or thrombocytopenia. Infusion-related symptoms can be pretreated with acetaminophen and diphenhydramine.

Eculizumab (Soliris) is a complement inhibitor that was FDA approved for AChR Ab–generalized MG in 2017. It is dosed at 900 mg weekly for 4 weeks, followed by 1200 mg for the fifth week and thereafter 1200 mg every 2 weeks. Generally, only mild infusion reactions are reported, typically managed by pretreatment acetaminophen and diphenhydramine, although there is risk for severe meningococcal infection. Meningococcal immunization is recommended before treatment initiation.

Cyclophosphamide (Cytoxan)[1] is typically reserved for treatment-refractory patients. It may be administered orally with a daily dose ranging from 1.5 to 5 mg daily. Potential side effects of oral cyclophosphamide include cystitis and bladder cancer, leading many treating physicians to use IV pulse dosing. A common approach for pulse dosing is 1 gm/m² monthly for 6 months (less toxic). Onset of action with pulse dosing is relatively quick, generally about 1 month.

Efgartigimod (Vyvgart) is a neonatal Fc receptor (FcRn) blocker, which was FDA approved for AChR Ab generalized MG in 2022. It has a novel mechanism of action that effectively reduces IgG levels, including levels of pathogenic autoantibodies. As such, efgartigimod has been likened to "plasma exchange in a bottle." It is administered intravenously at a dose of 10 mg/kg weekly for a total of four treatments (a treatment cycle) and, depending on response, repeat cycles may be given after 8 weeks. Side effects include infusion reaction, headache, and respiratory and urinary tract infections. If a patient has an active infection at the time of a cycle, it is recommended that the treatment cycle be delayed.

Rozanolixizumab (Rystiggo) is a humanized IgG4 monoclonal antibody that blocks the neonatal Fc receptor, thus reducing the amount of circulating IgG. This new medication was FDA approved for both AChR Ab and MUSK Ab–positive MG in 2023, the first approved treatment for both AChR and MUSK Ab MG. It is administered (via weight-based dosing) by subcutaneous infusion once weekly for 6 weeks with subsequent treatment cycle timing contingent upon clinical status (though not to occur before 9 weeks after the first dose of the last infusion cycle). Side effects include headache, diarrhea, urinary tract infection, and herpes simplex infection. If a patient has an active infection at the time of a cycle, it is recommended that the treatment cycle be delayed.

Zilucoplan (Zilbrysq) is a small peptide that functions as a complement inhibitor that was FDA approved for AChR Ab MG in 2023. It is dosed at 0.3 mg/kg via subcutaneous injection daily and constitutes the first self-administered injectable drug for treatment of AChR Ab MG. As it is not a monoclonal antibody, there is no need for supplemental dosing if a patient requires IVIG or plasma exchange for additional treatment of symptoms. Common side effects include injection site bruising, headache, and diarrhea.

Nipocalimab (IMAAVY) is an FcRn-blocking monoclonal antibody that was FDA approved in 2025 for patients with AChR and MUSK Ab MG 12 years and older. As with other drugs that share this mechanism, it decreases circulating levels of IgG. It is infused intravenously with a loading dose of 30 mg/kg followed by 15 mg/kg every 2 weeks. The most common adverse events included respiratory tract infections, peripheral edema, and muscle spasms. If a patient has an active infection at the time of a cycle, it is recommended that the treatment cycle be delayed.

Treatment Considerations in Pregnancy

Pregnancy and postpartum status have been reported to be triggers for worsening of myasthenia. Ideally, prepregnancy planning allows for optimization of clinical status to improve pregnancy outcomes. These patients require expert multidisciplinary care through the postpartum period. In pregnancy the treatment of choice is pyridostigmine, with steroids being the immunosuppressant of choice. Azathioprine[1] and cyclosporine[1] are relatively safe in expectant mothers who are not satisfactorily controlled or cannot tolerate corticosteroids. IVIG[1] and PLEX may also be treatment options. The newer FDA-approved medications have limited safety data in pregnancy.

Transient neonatal myasthenia may affect the newborn infant. This is difficult to predict and requires close attention for signs after delivery. Neonatal critical care support should be readily available for these infants.

Monitoring

After a diagnosis of MG is confirmed, additional testing or monitoring is indicated. The frequency of clinical assessment should be dictated by the severity and nature of the patient's symptoms, as well as the impact of the disease on function. Patients with MG should be managed in concert with a neurologist. Refractory MG is defined by symptoms that affect function and are unchanged or worse after corticosteroids and at least two other immunosuppressive agents used in adequate doses for adequate duration. Patients meeting criteria for refractory MG should be referred to a physician or medical center with expertise in MG.

Computed tomography of the chest should be performed to screen for thymoma. Assessment of thyroid function is important. If immunomodulatory medications are used for disease control, TB screening should be performed.

Pulmonary and swallowing dysfunction may be encountered. Pulmonary function testing should be performed for patients with symptomatic generalized MG, particularly if there are complaints of dyspnea. Speech therapy referral for a swallow evaluation should be performed if there is concern for dysphagia.

Periodic laboratory monitoring is required with use of immunomodulatory medications, which may vary depending on the specific medication used. Suggested tests and monitoring algorithms are detailed in Table 2.

Complications

The most severe complication of MG is myasthenic crisis, which is defined by worsening of weakness requiring intubation or noninvasive ventilation. Myasthenic crisis may be seen in up to 20% of patients at some point in disease course. Myasthenic crisis is most commonly encountered in the setting of concomitant illness, change in medications, or early in the disease course because maximum weakness occurs in the first year of the disease in 66% of patients. Respiratory failure can result from respiratory muscle weakness, oropharyngeal weakness, or a combination of both. It is important to recognize that new respiratory or swallowing complaints can quickly escalate, and patients with these complaints should be quickly assessed. One can assess diaphragm strength by the force of a strong sniff or cough; patients should be able to count to 20 after a deep breath. Staccato speech or dyspnea that precludes speaking in full sentences is of high concern for myasthenic crisis. Spirometry with forced vital capacity <2 L or negative inspiratory force of <40 cm H_2O should be sent to the hospital for further evaluation. Assessment of swallowing function by speech therapy and possible modified barium swallow should be considered in the context of dysphagia for solids and liquids.

IVIG and PLEX have comparable outcomes for the treatment of patients with moderate-to-severe weakness. The response to PLEX may be more predictable than IVIG in severe MG

---

[1] Not FDA approved for this indication.

[1] Not FDA approved for this indication.

TABLE 2	Suggested Medication Monitoring
MEDICATION	**SUGGESTED MONITORING**
Azathioprine (Imuran)	CBC, LFTs weekly for the first month then monthly to every 3 months
Cyclosporine (Sandimmune)	Monthly CBC, LFTs, renal function monthly for 3 months then quarterly Periodic trough level Blood pressure checks
Cyclophosphamide (Cytoxan)	CBC (attention to neutrophil count), electrolytes and renal function, LFTs, UA every 2–4 weeks
Eculizumab (Soliris)	CBC, renal function, LFTs
IVIG (Gammagard)	Renal function monthly, with repeated dosing maybe every 3 months
Methotrexate (Trexall)	CBC, LFTs monthly initially, then at stable dose at least every 3 months
Mycophenolate mofetil	CBC every 2 weeks for first month, then monthly to quarterly
Plasma exchange	Blood pressure and serum calcium
Prednisone	Weight and blood pressure Periodic potassium and HbA1c Bone density test Periodic eye exam
Rituximab (Rituxan)	CD20 counts may be considered but varies among providers
Efgartigimod (Vyvgart)	Evaluate the need to administer age-appropriate immunizations (live attenuated or live vaccines) according to immunization guidelines before initiation of a new treatment cycle
Rozanolixizumab (Rystiggo)	Avoid live and live-attenuated vaccines during treatment Delay treatment cycle in the setting of active infection
Zilucoplan (Zilbrysq)	Ensure meningococcal vaccination at least 2 weeks before starting treatment Appropriate vaccinations for encapsulated bacteria (e.g., *Streptococcus pneumoniae*) as per immunization guidelines
Nipocalimab (IMAAVY)	Avoid live and live-attenuated vaccines during treatment Delay treatment cycle in the setting of active infection

CBC, Complete blood count; *HbA1c*, hemoglobin A1c; *IVIG*, intravenous immunoglobulin; *LFTs*, liver function tests; *UA*, urinalysis.

exacerbations, and retrospective data suggests PLEX may be more effective than IVIG in myasthenic crisis. PLEX, however, may be associated with more complications, as well as longer hospital stay and associated hospital costs.

References

Farmakidis C, Pasnoor M, Dimachkie M, Baron R: Treatment of myasthenia gravis, *Neurol Clin* 36:311–337, 2018.
Gilhus NE: myasthenia gravis, *N Engl J Med* 375:2570–2581, 2016.
Myasthenia Gravis Foundation of America. Myasthenia Gravis:. Available at http://myasthenia.org/. Accessed March 21, 2025.
Narayanaswami P, Sanders DB, Wolfe G, et al: International consensus guidance for management of myasthenia gravis:2020 update, *Neurology* 96(3):114–122, 2020.
Tannemaat MR, Huijbers MG, Verschuuren JJ: Myasthenia gravis—pathophysiology, diagnosis, and treatment, *Handb Clin Neurol* 200:283–305, 2024.
Wilfe GI, Kaminski HJ, Aban IN, et al: Randomized trial of thymectomy in myasthenia gravis, *N Engl J Med* 375:511–522, 2016.

NEUROFIBROMATOSIS (TYPE 1)

Method of
Jason E. Marker, MD, MPA

CURRENT DIAGNOSIS

- Neurofibromatosis type 1 (NF1) can be diagnosed by physicians based on well-defined diagnostic criteria that can be met with a careful history and physical exam.
- Additional testing may be needed in some cases (including genetic testing) to confirm the diagnosis or to provide information that will be important for both short- and long-term management.
- NF1 has important genetic underpinnings, can have extremely variable expression within families, and will evolve in its need for medical intervention throughout the lifetime of the patient.

CURRENT THERAPY

- There is no treatment for NF1. However, there are many therapies for both the common and uncommon manifestations and complications of the condition.
- Many therapies are similar to those used for non-NF1 patients with the same symptoms. However, there are some manifestations where unique therapies are needed, and physicians need to know the difference between these.
- Proper monitoring of the patient aids in the identification of treatable symptoms and allows opportunities for anticipatory guidance and counseling.
- There are several emerging therapies related to the heritability of NF1 that are important for patients of childbearing age to be aware of.

Introduction and Epidemiology

Neurofibromatosis encompasses three distinct genetic entities: NF1, NF2-related schwannomatosis (formerly neurofibromatosis type 2 and hereafter referred to as NF2), and schwannomatosis related to genetic variants other than NF2 (hereafter referred to as schwannomatosis.) Because NF1 is so much more common (incidence of 1:1900 to 1:3000 livebirths) than NF2 (incidence of 1:25,000 to 1:33,000 livebirths) and schwannomatosis (incidence of 1:40,000 to 1:1.7M livebirths), when the word *neurofibromatosis* is used (or the older name, Von Recklinghausen disease), it is generally referring to NF1. NF1 is the primary topic of this chapter.

NF1 is an autosomal dominant genetic disorder and is progressive in that its clinical manifestations evolve over the lifespan. About half of the cases of NF1 are familial and the remainder are the result of new, spontaneous mutations. Life expectancy is reduced by 5 to 15 years and is related to the severity of the clinical manifestations, higher rates of malignant tumors (both disease-specific and others not directly tied to NF1), and excess hypertensive and vascular disease risk. There is no predilection based on ethnic origin or country of birth.

Risk Factors

NF1 is an autosomal dominant condition and affects 50% of the offspring of parents where one parent is affected, making family history the primary predictable risk factor. Advanced paternal age increases the likelihood of a de novo mutation.

Eighty percent of newly occurring mutations are believed to come from the paternally derived chromosome. Parental mosaicism can confound risk stratification and must be considered in pre-conception counseling.

Pathophysiology

NF1 is the result of mutations in the *NF1* gene (chromosome 17q11.2) that codes for the protein neurofibromin. Neurofibromin is a protein in the GTPase-activating family that stimulates the RAS pathway for tumor suppression. Loss of neurofibromin results in "de-suppression" of tumor growth within susceptible tissues. Although genetic penetrance in NF1 is complete, NF1 is highly variable in its expression (even within families). This is because germline mutations must be coupled with somatic mutations in order for symptoms to manifest clinically.

Several thousand distinct *NF1* mutations have been identified. Many small mutations have demonstrated no genotype-phenotype correlation, while some individuals (1% to 5% of NF1 patients) will have complete loss of the 1.4 to 1.5 Mb of the *NF1* gene and are severely affected. Due to the large size of this gene, mutations in the *NF1* gene occur more often than in any other human gene.

Somatic and germline (rare) mosaicism occurs and can result in phenotypically unaffected offspring who could later transmit the mutated gene to their own children. Also, some individuals with neurocognitive symptoms have been found to have haploinsufficiency (heterozygous for a pathogenic variant with an intact second allele).

Prevention

There is no specific prevention for any of the clinical manifestations of NF1. Due to its variable expression, some individuals will simply be more or less affected. To the extent that having a diagnosis of NF1 *could* cause academic challenges, interpersonal hardships, and social isolation, robust anticipatory guidance throughout the lifespan can help these individuals develop proper support systems and personal resilience, preventing some of the morbidity of the disease.

Affected individuals of child-bearing age now have the option of genetic testing of fertilized eggs to select unaffected eggs for implantation. This is an emerging prevention strategy.

Clinical Manifestations

There are a number of clinical manifestations of NF1. Because of the variability of expression of the *NF1* gene, these manifestations may be variably present in any affected individual. The following section on diagnosis will discuss how these clinical manifestations fit into the diagnostic criteria for NF1.

Café-au-lait spots are flat, irregularly shaped, uniformly hyperpigmented macules that appear during the first year of life and then increase in number through childhood. These macules are present in 95% of adults with NF1 but tend to fade and become more indistinct later in life. Among the general population of individuals who do not have NF1, 15% will have one to three café-au-lait macules.

Freckling (primarily in areas of skin apposition like the axillae and inguinal folds) is distinct from café-au-lait macules as the freckles are smaller, more clustered, and generally appear later in childhood than the café-au-lait macules.

Lisch nodules are tan-colored hamartomas of the iris. Lisch nodules do not affect vision and may be seen with simple ophthalmoscopy (although the use of a slit lamp will help identify small nodules and distinguish them from iris nevi). These nodules are seen in up to 90% of adults with NF1, but fewer than 10% of children under 6 years old.

Neurofibromas present as several types of lesions with variable characteristics, risk of pathology, and symptomatology. Cutaneous peripheral neurofibromas are benign peripheral nerve sheath tumors that are generally soft, mobile, and fleshy.

They may be dermal or epidermal on a broad or pedunculated base. These neurofibromas are nontender, are usually more common on the trunk, and can number from a few to thousands. Cutaneous peripheral neurofibromas do not degenerate into malignant peripheral nerve sheath tumors (MPNSTs). Plexiform neurofibromas can be superficial or deep inside the body. They tend to be more diffuse and involve plaques and tangles of abnormal tissues that can grow into a complex mass. On whole-body scanning, 50% of patients with NF1 will have at least one plexiform neurofibroma. Large plexiform neurofibromas can create symptoms by compressing nearby structures and, unlike cutaneous neurofibromas, they have the capacity to degenerate into MPNSTs. Nodular neurofibromas are firm and rubbery. Unlike the cutaneous neurofibromas, they are sometimes tender, often deeper and usually less mobile. They are not as invasive as the plexiform neurofibromas but can undergo degeneration into MPNSTs.

Optic pathway gliomas (OPGs) occur in 15% of children younger than 6 (but rarely in older individuals) and can grow anywhere along the optic tracts. Most individuals are asymptomatic, but advanced tumors can affect vision or even upset the normal function of the hypothalamus with growth rate variations and premature or delayed puberty.

Orthopedic abnormalities are primarily long-bone dysplasias and pseudoarthroses. Anterolateral bowing of the tibia (usually unilateral) in infants and young children can easily go undetected until a pathologic fracture develops at the onset of ambulation. One half of fractures occur during the toddler years. Long-bone pseudoarthrosis has a male predisposition (1.7:1) and NF1 accounts for 50% to 70% of all long-bone pseudoarthroses. Other orthopedic findings in NF1 patients may include short stature (13% have a height less than 2 standard deviations below the mean), scoliosis (10% to 15% of NF1 patients are affected), sphenoid wing dysplasia (leading to facial asymmetry), osteoporosis, and macrocephaly.

Neurologic abnormalities encompass cognitive defects and learning disabilities as well as the risk of seizures. Although profound intellectual disability is rare (the likelihood of having an IQ <70 is similar to the general population), 81% of NF patients will have some impairment in one or more areas of cognitive functioning. While less than half of NF1 patients have a specific learning disability, more than half will have some amount of neuropsychological impairment, including speech articulation problems, ADD, or impairment of executive functioning. Seizures occur twice as often in patients with NF1 (prevalence 4% to 6%) as in the general population and can be of any type and occur at any age.

Other manifestations of concern: Rarely, other central nervous system (CNS) neoplasms develop. CNS astrocytomas usually arise during childhood and, when not an incidental finding on a scan being done for another purpose, may present with symptoms of increased intracranial pressure. Rare brainstem gliomas are usually symptomatic at presentation. Malignant peripheral nerve sheath tumors are highly malignant tumors that can arise from a preexisting plexiform or nodular neurofibromas. The lifetime risk of developing an MPNST in a patient with NF1 is 5% to 13% and most commonly occurs in teenagers and young adults. MPNSTs are usually diagnosed when a plexiform or nodular neurofibroma goes through a period of pain, change in consistency, and rapid growth. Hypertension, including hypertension as early as childhood, is common among NF1 patients. Although rare, renal neurovascular lesions can be the cause, and NF1 patients with hypertension should be evaluated for renal artery stenosis. Macrocephaly, congenital heart disease (primarily pulmonic stenosis and mitral valve defects), cerebrovascular dysplasia, and increased incidence of irritable bowel syndrome and constipation have been observed, more commonly in individuals with NF1, though not fully studied.

Diagnosis

The diagnosis of NF1 can be made reliably by a primary care team, but a multidisciplinary team of subspecialists is often involved in the long-term care of these individuals, including during the diagnostic phase. A comprehensive history (including a detailed family history) and examination should be undertaken. Additional testing or referral, as indicated by the initial evaluation, should be pursued to clarify the diagnosis, seek findings amenable to treatment, and facilitate proper anticipatory guidance and patient/family education.

The US National Institutes of Health (NIH) Consensus Conference in 1997 (with minor revisions in 2021) set forth the following diagnostic criteria for NF1:

At least two of the following clinical features must be present to make the diagnosis of NF1:

- Six or more café-au-lait macules greater than 5 mm (prepubertal) or greater than 15 mm (postpubertal) in longest diameter
- Two or more neurofibromas of any type (or a single plexiform neurofibroma)
- Freckling in the axillary or inguinal regions
- Optic pathway glioma
- Two or more Lisch nodules or two or more choroidal abnormalities (see below)
- A distinctive bony lesion (sphenoid dysplasia or a long-bone dysplasia with or without pseudoarthrosis)
- A heterozygous pathogenic NF1 variant allele fraction of 50% in apparently normal tissue (like WBCs)

A child with ONE of the above clinical findings AND a first-degree relative with NF1 based on these criteria meets diagnostic criteria for NF1.

These criteria are both sensitive and specific, and are met by 97% of NF1 patients by the age of 8 years (100% by the age of 20 years). Nearly half of individuals with a new sporadic mutation fail to meet these criteria by the age of 1 year. Therefore, in an infant with one clinical feature, close observation is needed to determine if other criteria will be met. If, by the age of 4 years, only one criterion is met, referral for a genetic diagnosis may be warranted if not already obtained.

Other specific testing may be needed to make the diagnosis, to determine the extent of involvement of the disorder, or to decide on treatment. These include the following:

- Dermatologic evaluation: If the identification of café-au-lait spots, whether café-au-lait spots meet diagnostic criteria, or the identification of criteria-meeting freckling is in question, referral to Dermatology may be needed. Likewise, the spectrum of neurofibromas is broad and a dermatologist may be needed to properly identify these lesions.
- Lisch nodules: Although occasionally seen with the naked eye or through an office ophthalmoscope, formal ophthalmologic consultation is recommended to look for small Lisch nodules and to assess for optic disk findings suggestive of OPGs or increased intracranial pressure. Choroidal abnormalities seen on optical coherence tomography/near infrared imaging (OCT/NIR) fall into this same diagnostic category.
- Optic pathway gliomas: Ophthalmologic evaluation is recommended as noted earlier. Brain MRI imaging is not recommended for asymptomatic patients with normal ophthalmologic evaluations.
- Orthopedic abnormalities: Plain radiographs of long bones or CT imaging of craniofacial bones may be needed to identify the diagnostic findings in these areas.
- Neurologic abnormalities: Because new focal seizures or change in previous seizure frequency or type could be the result of a new intracranial neoplasm, neuroimaging is warranted with any new seizure activity.
- Other manifestations of concern: MPNSTs are best differentiated from benign plexiform or nodular neurofibromas by positron emission tomography (PET) scan. Evaluating for renal artery stenosis in individuals with new onset hypertension (including children) is indicated.
- Genetic counseling and testing: Genetic testing is usually reserved for cases where the diagnosis remains in question following a thorough history, examination, and nongenetic

testing. Additionally, genetic testing may be indicated for family members of the affected individual. Knowing that expression is extremely variable, preconception, embryonic preimplantation, or prenatal (amniocentesis or chorionic villi sampling) testing for individuals in families with NF1 should be considered.

Differential Diagnosis

Because of the well-established diagnostic criteria and availability of genetic testing, the differential diagnosis of NF1 is limited. As noted at the outset, NF2 and schwannomatosis are lumped together with NF1 under the general diagnosis of neurofibromatosis. Schwannomatosis is a complex regional pain syndrome with some common underlying pathophysiology but no overlapping symptoms and unrelated genetics. NF2 will be discussed briefly in the discussion to come.

Legius syndrome includes café-au-lait macules, axillary freckling, and macrocephaly. It does *not* include neurofibromas or CNS tumors, however. Like NF1, Legius syndrome is an autosomal dominant disorder for loss of a tumor suppressor protein, but it affects an entirely different gene.

Constitutional mismatch repair-deficiency syndrome (CMMR-D) is a rare autosomal recessive condition that results in café-au-lait macules (and occasionally axillary freckling and Lisch nodules). Unlike in NF1, individuals with CMMR-D are at risk for hematologic malignancies in infancy and childhood, brain tumors (primarily glioblastomas) in mid-childhood, and colorectal cancer in adolescence and young adulthood. Rhabdomyosarcomas and optic pathway gliomas may occur rarely in CMMR-D.

NF2 is caused by the *NF2* gene on chromosome 22, which encodes for the tumor suppressor protein merlin (or schwannomin), which is a functionally different protein than that produced by *NF1*. Key differences between NF1 and NF2 include the following points about NF2:

- Few or nonexistent café-au-lait macules
- No Lisch nodules
- No risk of MPNSTs
- Spinal root tumors are schwannomas in NF2 (neurofibromas in NF1)
- No cognitive impairment
- High prevalence of bilateral acoustic schwannomas and resulting hearing loss in 90% to 95% of patients by the age of 30 years
- 60% to 80% have cataracts
- Presence of meningiomas

Noonan syndrome is characterized by short stature and may include café-au-lait macules that may meet the size and number criteria for NF1. Sometimes, the facial features of Noonan syndrome can overlap with the appearance of NF1. However, the webbed neck of Noonan syndrome and the association with pulmonic stenosis are not part of NF1. Although the RAS signaling pathway is involved in Noonan syndrome, the underlying genetics are entirely different.

Surveillance and Therapy

In 2020, the FDA approved oral selumetinib (Koselugo), an oral selective mitagen-activated protein kinase (MEK) inhibitor, for pediatric patients 2 years of age and older with NF1 who have symptomatic, inoperable plexiform neurofibromas. The research that led to this approval showed statistically and clinically significant decreases in the size of these neurofibromas, as well as the pain and disability that often accompanies them. It remains unclear whether selumetinib treatment decreases the likelihood of malignant transformation of plexiform neurofibromas into MPNSTs. Similar medications are currently under study at this time, including MEK inhibitors for adults with MPNSTs.

The following areas of surveillance should be undertaken. Where research or expert opinion suggests a proper frequency, it is listed, although shared decision making with the patient/family as well as communication with your medical colleagues will be required to develop appropriate timelines. Therapeutic options are listed here for many of the common issues NF1 patients face, while the management of less common complications is outlined in the next section.

- Yearly examination of the skin for new neurofibromas and any signs of change within an existing neurofibroma should be done. Especially when nodular or plexiform neurofibromas exist (those at risk of malignant transformation), any history of rapid change or new pain should be evaluated thoroughly. A PET scan can distinguish between benign and malignant lesions. Referral to surgical and/or dermatologic colleagues should be made regarding these nodular or plexiform neurofibromas (for biopsy and management decisions) and should be strongly considered for all but the most clear and superficial cutaneous neurofibromas.
- Cutaneous neurofibromas that develop pruritus are often not responsive to antihistamines, although the itching is often improved by the use of gabapentin (Neurontin)[1].
- Yearly blood pressure measurement, even in children and young adults, should be done. Once the diagnosis of essential hypertension is made following testing that excludes the diagnosis of renal artery stenosis, blood pressure should be controlled following standard blood pressure goals and treatment algorithms. Hypertension that becomes hard to control may prompt an evaluation for pheochromocytoma, a rare finding in NF1.
- Growth tracking of weight, height, and head circumference should be done through childhood and adolescence in the usual manner. Additionally, any signs of premature or delayed puberty should be evaluated further. Growth and pubertal abnormalities should prompt an age-appropriate endocrinology referral for additional testing (serum, urine, and/or neuroimaging) and treatments based on these results.
- Neurodevelopmental and academic assessment should be undertaken, involving family members and school personnel when appropriate. Individuals who develop neuropsychiatric and academic problems should undergo formal neurodiagnostic testing, and any identified diagnoses should be treated. These treatments are no different than those used for non-NF1 individuals who carry the same neuropsychiatric diagnosis. Neuroimaging is not indicated in the evaluation of neuropsychiatric conditions unless neurologic deficits exist.
- NF1 patients who develop seizures are treated with the usual seizure management algorithms following neuroimaging to look for new intracranial pathologies. An electroencephalogram (EEG) is not indicated for asymptomatic individuals.
- Evaluation for skeletal changes including scoliosis, facial asymmetry, or long bone abnormalities should be performed yearly during childhood and adolescence, and then at the typical wellness visits into young adulthood (with prompting in these older ages to report any changes that are noticed between visits). Any abnormalities that are encountered should prompt additional imaging and referral to subspecialty care.
- Women with NF1 develop osteoporosis at an earlier age than their non-NF1 peers and should undergo earlier screening in accordance with this fact and with other standard risk factors they may have. When diagnosed, this osteoporosis is treated like it would be for any other patient.
- For unclear reasons, women with NF1 have an increased risk of HER2(+) breast cancer, especially women under the age of 40 (at the age of 70, the risk approximates that of the general population). These are usually invasive ductal carcinomas (the most common type overall) and are managed in the usual way. These patients need both earlier education about, and screening for, breast cancer (often starting at age 30). NF1 patients with breast cancer have poorer 5-year survival rates.
- Formal ophthalmologic evaluation for visual screening, slit lamp and intraocular examination should take place yearly at least through adolescence, usually in the context of a comprehensive examination. Lisch nodules are nonpatho-

logic and no treatment is needed, but any signs of elevated intracranial pressure or optic disc pathology warrant further testing and management. The optimal frequency of MRI surveillance of an optic pathway glioma is unknown but should be based on symptomatology, size, and rate of progression.
- Brain MRI is not recommended as a routine screening test. It may be a part of the initial diagnostic workup but should not need to be repeated for asymptomatic patients who are otherwise receiving comprehensive surveillance. Of note, "NF-associated bright spots" may be seen on MRI imaging, and the data are inconclusive on the relationship between these spots and any pathologic process. These spots often resolve spontaneously by late childhood. Increased brain volume may be observed but is not definitively tied to any NF1 symptoms.
- Whole body MRI screening or MRI of nonbrain areas of potential concern (such as visible but stable and asymptomatic plexiform or nodular neurofibromas) is not recommended by most authorities. Likewise, screening PET scanning is not recommended.

Management of Complications

The previous section outlines the surveillance of and treatment for most of the common concerns for patients with NF1. Rarely, more significant complications present themselves. These are listed here along with their management plan.

- Symptomatic cutaneous neurofibromas that are cosmetically unacceptable, painful, itchy, or disfiguring will sometimes need to be managed. Once it is clear that the lesions in question are truly simple cutaneous neurofibromas, they may be removed in any manner, including by excision, cryotherapy, laser, or electrodessication.
- Symptomatic plexiform neurofibromas that have not degenerated into MPNSTs that are deemed in need of management or removal should be managed by a multidisciplinary team of surgeons and oncologists who are familiar with this type of tumor. These invasive tumors require nonstandard operative approaches and consideration of emerging chemotherapeutic agents.
- MPNSTs are often due to a co-mutated SUZ12 gene (which lies contiguous to NF1). Individuals with large or complete deletions of the NF1 gene (those who are generally more severely affected) are at an increased risk of this complication. MPNSTs are usually managed by surgeons and oncologists familiar with NF1 and often involve surgical excision with adjunctive radiation and possibly emerging chemotherapeutic agents.
- Optic pathway gliomas are most commonly found to be low-grade pilocystic astrocytomas. As such, they are often sensitive to the standard oncologic treatments for that type of tumor—but when to observe and when to proceed to treatment is controversial.
- Because the bony architecture of pathologic skeletal lesions is inherently abnormal in these patients, the risk of complications from corrective treatments is higher than in non-NF1 patients. Your local orthopedic colleagues need to be aware of this and obtain tertiary care backup when needed. Amputation is often the best long-term plan for long bone lesions.
- Refractory hypertension in the absence of renal artery stenosis that is ultimately found to be the result of pheochromocytoma should be managed by a multidisciplinary team experienced in the management of this diagnosis. It is managed in the same manner as non-NF1 patients with a pheochromocytoma.
- Short stature is often correctible with growth hormone therapy. However, this treatment is not often used because it compounds the inherent protumorgenic nature of NF1. In extreme cases of short stature when growth hormone is used, clinicians need to be alert to the evolution and potential malignant degeneration of new or existing tumors.

---

[1] Not FDA approved for this indication.

- NF1 patients are at a high risk of psychosocial issues arising from the symptoms they may experience from their NF1, its lack of treatability, and its genetic underpinnings. These symptoms may affect relationship building and reproductive decisions. Extra professional support may be needed, particularly during adolescence.

Although pregnancy is not a "complication" of NF1, its management can certainly be complicated by the diagnosis. Pregnant NF1 patients have increased morbidity (but not mortality) due to hypertensive and vascular complications. These complications should be anticipated and managed by an appropriately trained medical team. Genetic counseling should be recommended, ideally prior to conception, and steps taken to ensure proper evaluation and surveillance for the newborn.

References

Defendi GL: Genetics of neurofibromatosis type 1 and type 2. Available at https://emedicine.medscape.com/article/950151-overview. Accessed 15 November 2018.

Evans DG: Neurofibromatosis type 2. Available at https://www.uptodate.com/contents/neurofibromatosis-type-2. Accessed 15 November 2018.

Food and Drug Administration Package Insert for selumetinib (Koselugo). Available at: https://www.accessdata.fda/gov/drugsatfda-docs/label/2020/213756s000lbl.pdf. Accessed 15 November 2018.

Ferner RE, Huson SM, et al: Guidelines for the diagnosis and management of individuals with neurofibromatosis 1, *J Med Genet* 44:81–88, 2007.

Hart L: Primary care of patients with neurofibromatosis 1, *The Nurse Practitioner* 30(6), 2005.

Hersh JH: Committee on Genetics of the American Academy of Pediatrics: Health Supervision of Children with Neurofibromatosis, *Pediatrics* 121:633–645, 2008.

Human Genetics Society of Australia: *Choosing Wisely Australia: 5 Things Clinicians and Consumers Should Question*, October 2016. Available at http://www.choosingwisely.org.au/getmedia/bbc1ca07-7340-49ca-9e85-ad4c1a7bc197/GESA_Choosing_Wisely_Recommendations.pdf.aspx. Accessed 15 November 2018.

Korf BR: Neurofibromatosis type 1 (NF1): Management and prognosis. Available at https://www.uptodate.com/contents/neurofibromatosis-type-1-nf1-management-and-prognosis. Accessed 29 January 2022.

Korf BR: Neurofibromatosis type 1 (NF1): Pathogenesis, clinical features, and diagnosis. Available at https://www.uptodate.com/contents/neurofibromatosis-type-1-nf1-pathogenesis-clinical-features-and-diagnosis. Accessed 29 January 2022.

Legius E, Messiaen L, Wolkenstein P, et al. Revised diagnostic criteria for neurofibromatosis type 1 and Legius syndrome: an international consensus recommendation, *Genet Med* 23(8):1506–1513, 2021.

Selumetinib PPI Dec 2021: https://den8dhaj6zs0e.cloudfront.net/50fd68b9-106b-4550-b5d0-12b045f8b184/22c94947-0a99-4b03-9d06-866a301712bc/22c94947-0a99-4b03-9d06-866a301712bc_viewable_rendition__v.pdf.

Selumetinib PPI April 2020: https://www.accessdata.fda.gov/drugsatfda_docs/label/2020/213756s000lbl.pdf.

Stewart DR, Korf BR, et al: Care of adults with neurofibromatosis type 1: a clinical practice resource of the American College of Medical Genetics and Genomics (ACMG), *Genet Med* 20(7):671–682, 2018 Jul.

Tonsgard JH: Clinical manifestations and management of neurofibromatosis type 1, *Sem Pediatr Neurol*, Elsevier 13:2–7, 2006.

Williams VC, Lucas J, et al: Neurofibromatosis type 1 revisited, *Pediatrics* 123:124–133, 2009.

NONMIGRAINE HEADACHE

Method of
Stephen Ross, MD

PEARLS

- Most important for headache evaluation is the history and physical examination, particularly the neurological examination.
- If headache is a symptom of a secondary disease or condition, the causative process must be treated at the same time symptomatic headache treatment is administered.
- Symptomatic headache treatment is selected based on the headache characteristics/phenotype regardless of the underlying contributing conditions.

CURRENT DIAGNOSIS

- Characteristics that should lead to evaluation for secondary disease contributions to headache include worst experienced headache, significant change in headache pattern, new onset headache in context of recent trauma, immunocompromised state, or new active constitutional symptoms such as fever, stiff neck, or hypertension.
- A more extensive diagnostic evaluation should be considered for any patient with headache who also has "red flags" (see Table 2).

CURRENT THERAPY

- Specific therapy for secondary cause of headache should be initiated when identified. Examples include the following:
  - Antihypertensive treatment for hypertension
  - Antibiotics for bacterial meningitis
  - Immunosuppressant for central nervous system sarcoidosis
- Symptomatic therapy for headache should be selected based on the headache phenotype.
- Four principal phenotypes of headache include the following:
  - Migrainous (unilateral, throbbing, photophobia, nausea, with/without aura)
  - Musculoskeletal (bilateral, nonthrobbing, absence of photophobia and nausea)
  - Trigeminal autonomic cephalgia (unilateral, severe, brief, associated with ipsilateral autonomic features and/or restlessness)
  - Neuralgia (very brief, recurrent, electric shock/burning, and/or jolt pain)

Evaluation and Diagnosis

Gathering of a thorough history and physical examination (Table 1) allows creation of the differential diagnosis.

- Determine the need for diagnostic studies to evaluate for potential secondary contributors. Based on the presence/newness/intensity/evolution of "red flags" (Table 2), you must consider performing diagnostic studies. Depending on the differential diagnosis, evaluation may include brain and/or cervical spine imaging, spinal tap, and blood studies. Specific treatment can be initiated for some identified secondary contributors. Examples include decompression surgery for cervical spinal stenosis, antibiotics for bacterial meningitis, and sodium replacement for hyponatremia.
- Discern the dominant headache phenotype (Figure 1) to guide symptomatic treatment. The two forms of secondary headache therapy are (1) the specific treatment, which addresses underlying etiology, and (2) the symptomatic treatment, which is selected based on the dominant headache phenotype. Often headache phenotypes can be segregated into one or more of the following themes: migraine (covered in the chapter Migraine), tension-type headaches, trigeminal autonomic cephalalgias (TACs), and cranial neuralgias. The symptomatic treatment mirrors that used for the parallel primary headache disorders (see the following). For example, you may use ubrogepant for treatment of migrainous headache secondary to closed-head trauma in the same way you use ubrogepant for the diagnosis of primary migraine without aura.

Headache Type and Therapy

The first step in evaluation of the patient with a suspected nonmigraine headache via history and physical is to discern potential primary and/or secondary contributors to the pain.

TABLE 1 Headache Characteristics

Is there more than one type?	What is the location/radiation?	Is there any positional component?	Is there anything that triggers it?	Is there any pattern to occurrence (e.g., always 1 hour after going to bed, every spring)?
When was the onset?	What does it feel like (e.g., throbbing, pressure, burning)?	Are there any associated features (e.g., nausea, photophobia, ptosis, lacrimation)?	Is there anything that relieves it?	What treatments have been tried so far? What is the response to these?
What is the duration?	What is the frequency?	What is the intensity, along with ramp?	Is there any family history of this?	Is there any change with Valsalva?

TABLE 2 Headache Red Flags

Onset after age 50 years	"Thunderclap" onset of pain	Positional exacerbation	Onset with recent malignancy, nontrivial head trauma, or seizures	Persistent or unexplained vomiting
Worst headache of life	Marked change in pain pattern	Precipitated by Valsalva maneuvers	Unexplained fever	Meningeal signs
First headache of life	Unusual associated features (blindness, diplopia, confusion, weakness)	Lack of response to abortive medications	Significant blood pressure elevation	Abnormal neurologic examination

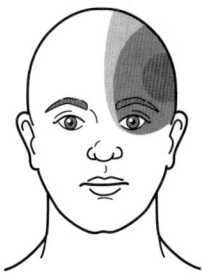

Migraine
Throbbing
Unilateral
Mod-severe
Nausea
Photophobia
Phonophobia
Aura

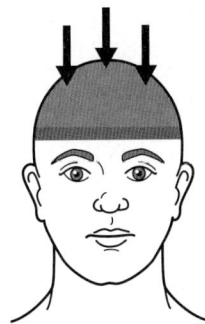

Tension-type Headache
Pressing
Bilateral
Mild-moderate

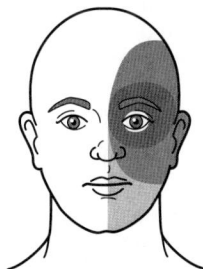

Trigeminal Autonomic Cephalalgia
Unilateral
Orbital/temple
Severe
Ptosis, lacrimation, rhinorrhea, nasal congestion
Restlessness

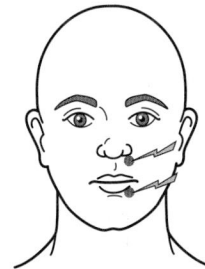

Cranial Neuralgia
Electric/stabbing
Unilateral
Severe
Triggered by innocuous stimuli

Figure 1 Headache phenotypes.

- *Primary contributor* implies the headache is caused by a primary headache disorder. Examples include migraine, tension-type headache, and cluster headache.
- *Secondary contributor* implies the headache is a symptom of an alternate disease process/condition. Examples include headache secondary to severe hypertension, headache secondary to subarachnoid hemorrhage, and headache secondary to meningitis.

Symptomatic treatment is similar for primary and secondary etiologies but varies according to the pain phenotype (Table 3).

General principles are to start low-dose pharmacotherapy and then titrate upward as needed to control pain, with the understanding that often it can take 3 to 4 weeks before benefit of preventive treatments is experienced. If the pain is not adequately controlled despite maximum dose or if treatment is not tolerated, then a second-line treatment should be considered. If there has been some, but not enough, improvement with the first treatment, then a second treatment can be added. If there has been no improvement with the first treatment, taper off the first while adding the second treatment.

An example of a first-line treatment for migraine would be topiramate (Topamax). An example of a second-line treatment for migraine would be amitriptyline (Elavil).

Migraine
Please see the chapter on Migraine.

Tension-Type Headache
Tension-type headache is experienced by almost everyone at some point in their lives. Most do not seek medical evaluation but rather self-manage, typically with over-the-counter simple analgesics or topical modalities such as heat. Diagnostic criteria are listed in Table 4.

The presence or absence of "emotional tension" does not define this condition. Many individuals experience tension-type headache who are not stressed and do not have anxiety or depression. If a person is experiencing stress or is anxious, this can act as a trigger for tension-type headache, as well as the other primary headache conditions. Tension-type headache has both episodic and chronic forms. Chronic is defined as having symptoms at least 15 days/month for greater than 3 months.

TABLE 3 Symptomatic Headache Treatment

MIGRAINOUS	TENSION-TYPE	CLUSTER-LIKE	NEURALGIFORM
Covered in Migraine chapter	Heat, massage, analgesic cream	Sumatriptan, zolmitriptan[1], oxygen	Carbamazepine, oxcarbazepine[1]
	Acetaminophen, NSAID	gammaCore	Topiramate[1], gabapentin, baclofen[1]
	Physical modalities	Verapamil[1]	Gamma-knife surgery
	Relaxation techniques	Galcanezumab	Microvascular decompression surgery
	Amitriptyline[1]	Topiramate[1], lithium[1]	
	Venlafaxine[1], tizanidine[1], baclofen[1]	For select types—indomethacin[1]	

[1]Not FDA approved for this indication.
NSAID, Nonsteroidal antiinflammatory drug.

TABLE 4 International Headache Society Criteria for Tension-Type Headache

AT LEAST TWO OF THESE FOUR CHARACTERISTICS	BOTH OF THE FOLLOWING
Bilateral location	No nausea or vomiting
Pressing or tightening (nonpulsating) quality	No more than one of photophobia or phonophobia
Mild or moderate intensity	
Not aggravated by routine physical activity, such as walking or climbing stairs	

BOX 1 International Headache Society Criteria for Cluster Headache

At least five attacks
Severe unilateral orbital, supraorbital, and/or temporal pain lasting 15–180 min
Either or both of the following:
- At least one of the following symptoms or signs, ipsilateral to the headache:
  - Conjunctival injection and/or lacrimation
  - Nasal congestion and/or rhinorrhea
  - Eyelid edema
  - Forehead and facial sweating
  - Miosis and/or ptosis
- A sense of restlessness or agitation
Occurring with a frequency between one every other day and eight per day
Not better accounted for by another diagnosis

Treatment principles for tension-type headache generally start with physical modalities/relaxation techniques (e.g., local heat, massage, analgesic cream) and/or as needed acetaminophen 325 mg or nonsteroidal antiinflammatory drugs (e.g., ibuprofen 200 mg, aspirin 325 mg, naproxen 220 mg, diclofenac 50 mg). If this is inadequate, titrate the dose (e.g., acetaminophen 325 mg up to 1000 mg, ibuprofen 200 mg up to 800 mg) and/or refer for additional physical/cognitive modalities (e.g., physical therapy, myofascial release therapy, biofeedback therapy, cognitive-behavioral therapy). FDA-approved preventive treatments are lacking. If preventive treatment is needed, consider a tricyclic antidepressant (e.g., amitriptyline[1] starting with 10 mg or 25 mg at bedtime, titrating up to 150 mg if needed/tolerated). Allow 3 to 4 weeks to assess efficacy before titration to the next dose. It is recommended to prescreen the patient with an electrocardiogram (ECG) and monitor for side effects. Once you reach 100 mg, check amitriptyline blood level and repeat ECG. Alternatives could include venlafaxine (Effexor)[1], starting at 37.5 mg or 75 mg (two to three times per day or once per day if using the long-acting form) and titrating if needed to 225 mg; tizanidine (Zanaflex)[1] starting with 4 mg one-half pill two to three times per day titrating if needed to two pills three times per day; baclofen (Lioresal)[1] starting with 5 mg or 10 mg three times a day, titrating if needed up to 20 mg four times a day; or mirtazapine (Remeron)[1], starting with 7.5 mg or 15 mg every day at bedtime, titrating if needed up to 45 mg.

Trigeminal Autonomic Cephalalgias

TACs are syndromes characterized by intense pain and autonomic symptoms in a trigeminal distribution most commonly in the ophthalmic (V1) distribution. Common features of TACs include (1) unilateral, side-locked location (i.e., pain stays on one side of the head), typically in the V1 distribution, and (2) associated ipsilateral autonomic features including conjunctival injection, lacrimation, nasal congestion/rhinorrhea, eyelid edema, miosis and/or ptosis, and facial sweating. These disorders can be differentiated based on attack duration/frequency.

The most common TAC type is a cluster headache, which occurs 100 times less frequently than migraine headache. Diagnostic criteria include (1) duration lasting 15 to 180 minutes, (2) more likely to have associated ipsilateral autonomic features, and (3) more likely to have agitation/activation during the attack (Box 1).

Triptans or high-flow oxygen are first-line abortive treatments. Preference is given to faster acting agents (e.g., sumatriptan [Imitrex] 6 mg subcutaneous [SC] injection or 20 mg nasal[1], or zolmitriptan [Zomig][1] 5 mg nasal; these may be repeated again in 1 to 2 hours if needed but have a maximum of two doses in a 24-hour period). Oxygen is best administered by nonrebreather face mask at 6 to 12 L/min for 7 to 15 minutes. An alternate abortive treatment is gammaCore, a noninvasive vagus nerve stimulator that may be administered to the anterior neck as a set of three 2-minute stimulations. Other options include intranasal or intramuscular dihydroergotamine (DHE 45) or 1 mL of 4% intranasal lidocaine.[1] Short-term preventives can include oral steroids or occipital nerve blocks.

First-line preventive treatment is short-acting verapamil[1] starting at 40 to 80 mg oral three times a day, titrating if needed to 480 mg (total daily dose, although there are studies taking the dose up to 720 mg three times a day). An effective alternative is

[1]Not FDA approved for this indication.

[1]Not FDA approved for this indication.

galcanezumab (Emgality) given as three consecutive 100-mg SC shots (300 mg) each month while cluster headache is active. This is a monthly self-injection that blocks one of the neurotransmitters (calcitonin gene-related peptide) that propagates messages along the pain pathways. GammaCore may also be used for prevention therapy. Third-line considerations are topiramate[1] or lithium.[1]

A second type of TAC is episodic paroxysmal hemicrania. This has the same diagnostic criteria as cluster headache with one exception, duration. These patients present with severe, frequent, and brief (<30 minutes) attacks associated with ipsilateral autonomic symptoms and/or restlessness. This condition is diagnosed and treated with indomethacin (Indocin).[1] Give 25 mg orally three times a day with meals; if no improvement after 1 week, titrate to 50 mg three times a day; if no improvement is seen in 1 week, can further titrate to 75 mg three times a day; if no improvement is seen in 1 week after titration up, consider an alternate etiology.

A third type of TAC patients may experience is hemicrania continua. This is a unilateral, daily constant pain with exacerbations of pain intensity associated with autonomic/activation features similar to cluster headache. Diagnosis is mainly with indomethacin trial as previously mentioned, which often results in complete symptomatic relief. Sometimes patients continue the medication after a diagnostic trial and need to be weaned off very slowly.

A fourth type of TAC patients may experience is a short-lasting, unilateral, neuralgiform headache attack. The differentiating feature from other TAC types is very brief attacks (5 to 240 seconds) of stabbing orbital and temporal pain. Treatment is mainly done with lamotrigine (Lamictal).[1] Second-line treatments for this type of headache include topiramate[1] or gabapentin (Neurontin).[1]

Cranial Neuralgias

Most headache disorders are secondary to pathophysiology in the brain; however, individual nerves can be irritated in the peripheral nervous system that can lead to pain in the face and head. Common types include trigeminal neuralgia, glossopharyngeal neuralgia, and occipital neuralgia.

Trigeminal neuralgia presents as short paroxysmal attacks of severe unilateral shock-like pain mostly in the V2 (maxillary)/V3 (mandibular) distribution of the trigeminal nerve. Triggers include eating, drinking, brushing teeth, touching the face, and even talking. First-line symptomatic treatment for trigeminal neuralgia includes carbamazepine (Tegretol) 100 mg two times a day titrating up to 1200 mg/day (monitoring level and metabolic panel) or oxcarbazepine (Trileptal)[1] 150 to 300 mg two times a day titrating up to 2400 mg/day. Second-line agents can include baclofen[1], pregabalin (Lyrica)[1], gabapentin[1], topiramate[1], and lamotrigine.[1] For refractory cases, consider referral for Gasserian ganglion percutaneous techniques, which are deep face injections typically performed by pain management specialists (e.g., neurology, anesthesiology). Other treatment options include gamma-knife treatment or microvascular decompression performed by neurosurgeons.

Glossopharyngeal neuralgia presents as stabbing pain in the ear, angle of jaw, tongue base, and tonsillar region. Triggers include chewing, swallowing, coughing, yawning, and talking. There is a lack of evidence-based treatment; thus symptomatic treatment is similar to trigeminal neuralgia as detailed earlier.

Occipital neuralgia presents as a paroxysmal stabbing pain in the greater, lesser, and third occipital nerve distribution. Examination can reveal local tenderness in the territory of the affected nerve. Treatment includes occipital nerve block using anesthetic along with glucocorticoid, targeting tender points palpated in the near greater and lesser divisions of the occipital nerve. Alternative treatment options include gabapentin[1], pregabalin[1], and amitriptyline.[1]

---

[1]Not FDA approved for this indication.

References

Bendtsen L, Zakrzewska JM, Abbott J, et al: European Academy of Neurology guideline on trigeminal neuralgia, *Eur J Neurol* 26(6):831–849, 2019.

Do TP, et al: Red and orange flags for secondary headaches in clinical practice: SNNOOP10 list, *Neurology* 92(3):134–144, 2019.

Gronseth G, Cruccu G, Alksne J, et al: Practice parameter: the diagnostic evaluation and treatment of trigeminal neuralgia (an evidence-based review): report of the quality standards subcommittee of the American Academy of Neurology and the European Federation of Neurological Societies, *Neurology* 71(15):1183–1190, 2008.

Headache Classification Committee of the International Headache Society (IHS): The international classification of headache disorders, 3rd edition, *Cephalalgia* 38(1):1–211, 2018.

Jensen RH: Tension-type headache - the normal and most prevalent headache, *Headache* 58(2):339–345, 2018.

Kahriman A, Zhu S: Migraine and tension-type headache, *Semin Neurol* 38(6):608–618, 2018.

Robbins MS, Starling AJ, Pringsheim TM: Treatment of cluster headache: the American Headache Society evidence-based guidelines, *Headache* 56(7):1093–1106, 2016.

OPTIC NEURITIS

Method of
Tanyatuth Padungkiatsagul, MD

CURRENT DIAGNOSIS

- Vision is impaired, including visual acuity, visual field, and/or color perception.
- Patients typically have eye pain that is worse with eye movement.
- Relative afferent pupillary defect (RAPD) can be observed if one eye is affected or both eyes are asymmetrically affected.
- The anterior optic nerve has a normal appearance in two-thirds of affected patients.

CURRENT THERAPY

- Consider IV methylprednisolone (Solu-Medrol, 1 g/day IV for 3 days) followed by oral steroids (1 mg/kg per day for 11 days).
- Avoid low-dose oral steroid monotherapy, as this is associated with a higher relapse rate.
- If brain MRI or blood testing suggest a high-risk, clinically isolated syndrome, consider disease-modifying therapy to delay progression to Multiple Sclerosis (MS) or Neuro-myelitis optica (NMO).
- If clinical features suggest acute optic neuritis associated with NMO spectrum disorder (NMOSD) or myelin oligodendrocyte glycoprotien antibody–associated disease (MOGAD), intravenous methyprednisolone should be started promptly and consider plasma exchange therapy in patient responding suboptimally..
- If the patient's history and testing suggest MS, NMOSD, or recurrent MOGAD, consider specific maintenance treatment for these conditions.

Epidemiology

The incidence of optic neuritis is approximately 1 to 5 in 100,000. Though it typically affects women in their fourth decade of life, 1 in 4 patients are male, and patients have been reported ranging from the first to seventh decades of life. Optic neuritis occurs worldwide in persons of various ethnicities.

Optic neuritis can be classified as a clinically isolated syndrome or in association with a disease such as multiple sclerosis

(MS) or neuromyelitis optica spectrum disorder (NMOSD). NMOSD is clinically distinguished by more frequent involvement of the optic nerves and spinal cord and less involvement of the brain than MS and by distinct pathophysiology. A recently identified distinct classification is myelin oligodendrocyte glycoprotien antibody–associated disease (MOGAD) optic neuritis. Approximately half of patients with optic neuritis as a clinically isolated syndrome develop MS. A small percentage develop NMOSD.

Risk Factors

A diagnosis of a disease associated with optic neuritis, such as MS or NMOSD, increases the risk of developing optic neuritis. In one study, more than 70% of patients with MS and 100% of patients with neuromyelitis optica (NMO) had unilateral optic neuritis at some point. Patients with recurrent MOGAD flares or persistent elevated serum MOG-IgG may be at risk for recurrent optic neuritis.

Pathophysiology

Most optic neuritis occurs as a result of inflammation causing demyelination of the ganglion cell axons that compose the optic nerve. This is thought to be an immune-mediated process.

Prevention

Disease-modifying therapies have been shown to reduce risk of neurologic relapses in patients with MS or NMOSD. These therapies presumably also decrease the risk of MS-, NMOSD-, or recurrent MOGAD optic neuritis because optic neuritis is a common relapse syndrome in these conditions.

Clinical Manifestations

A typical optic neuritis patient experiences acute or subacute loss of vision characterized by decreased visual acuity, visual field loss, and/or color vision loss, accompanied or preceded by pain in the affected eye that is worse with eye movements. However, 8% of patients do not have pain. Other symptoms include positive visual phenomena in 30% of patients. Other signs include a relative afferent papillary defect in cases where one eye is affected or both eyes are asymmetrically affected and a mildly swollen optic nerve head in approximately one-third of patients. Optic neuritis in NMOSD is more likely to have bilateral involvement and severe visual impairment. The spectrum of MOGAD optic neuritis is being defined with initial case series describing a higher prevalence of and more severe optic nerve head swelling than MS- or NMOSD-associated optic neuritis.

The natural history of clinically isolated optic neuritis includes resolution of pain 3 to 5 days after onset and nadir of vision 7 to 14 days after onset. Spontaneous improvement in vision is typically evident within 3 weeks, and almost 70% of affected patients recover 20/20 visual acuity even in the absence of treatment. MOGAD optic neuritis also usually has a favorable final visual outcome. Optic neuritis associated with NMOSD tends to have less spontaneous recovery of vision and early recognition is important due to benefits of early treatment.

Diagnosis

The diagnosis is based on the clinical presentation. Where there is uncertainty, magnetic resonance imaging (MRI) of the orbits, including fat-saturated sequences (T2 and T1 with and without gadolinium contrast), can help visualize inflammation in the retrobulbar optic nerve. Changes on MRI involving the chiasm or more than 50% of the optic nerve are suggestive of NMOSD optic neuritis. MOGAD optic neuritis also has distinct imaging features, including perioptic nerve sheath enhancement.

Optic neuritis is often associated with other demyelinating syndromes, most commonly MS. Therefore it is important to screen for historical and current neurologic impairment through history and examination. MRI and/or and cerebrospinal fluid analysis documenting evidence of dissemination in time and space is diagnostic of MS in patients with clinically isolated optic neuritis. In addition, for patients not meeting criteria for MS at time of presentation with clinically isolated optic neuritis, MRI of the brain has been shown to be an important prognostic indicator for development of MS. MRI of the brain showing 0, 1, or more than 3 lesions typical for MS is associated, respectively, with a 25%, 60%, and 78% risk of progression to clinically definite MS.

Less commonly, optic neuritis is associated with other demyelinating syndromes such as NMOSD. This should be considered in patients with severe vision loss, bilateral involvement, or history of prior optic neuritis, transverse myelitis, or area postrema syndrome. A serum antibody, aquaporin-4 (AQP-4)-IgG, has been identified as a pathologic agent in this disorder. Testing for this is commercially available with a published sensitivity and specificity of 63% and 99%, respectively. Positive testing for AQP4-IgG in a patient with optic neuritis is diagnostic of NMOSD per published consensus criteria. A serum MOG-IgG is commercially available and aids in the identification of MOGAD optic neuritis.

Differential Diagnosis

Atypical features for optic neuritis such as systemic symptoms, history of cancer, pain that persists beyond 2 weeks, progressive vision loss beyond 14 days, no spontaneous improvement in vision, retinal hemorrhages, cotton-wool spots, or macular exudates should prompt diagnostic evaluation for etiologies other than optic neuritis. Diagnostic considerations for other optic neuropathies should cover a broad range of etiologies such as vascular (e.g., anterior ischemic optic neuropathy), compressive (e.g., optic nerve sheath meningioma, glioma), inflammatory (e.g., lupus, vasculitis sarcoidosis), infectious (e.g., syphilis, tuberculosis, Lyme disease), and infiltrative optic neuropathies (e.g., lymphoma, metastasis). Investigations may be tailor to each patient depending on the patient's clinical presentation and risk factors.

Treatment and Monitoring

The Optic Neuritis Treatment Trial (ONTT) was a randomized trial comparing placebo, oral prednisone, and IV methylprednisolone (1 g/day IV for 3 days) followed by oral prednisone (1 mg/kg per day for 11 days) for acute optic neuritis. IV steroids hastened recovery of vision without affecting final visual outcome compared with placebo treatment. Treatment with low-dose oral prednisone alone (1 mg/kg/day for 14 days) was associated with no improvement in vision and increased risk of relapse compared with placebo treatment. The 15-year follow-up results, published in 2008, demonstrated persistence of visual recovery. Studies have demonstrated non-inferiority of high-dose oral steroids (1250 mg prednisone/day for 3 days) to IV methylprednisolone with regards to vision recover following acute optic neuritis.

Many clinicians offer IV or high-dose oral steroid treatment to hasten visual recovery. Monotherapy with low-dose oral prednisone should be avoided. Regardless of the decision to treat or not with steroids, all patients should be monitored closely. Continued progression of vision loss, failure to spontaneously recover vision, or persistent pain should prompt additional diagnostic workup as well as consideration for additional IV steroid therapy for atypical optic neuritis. If this is not effective, plasma exchange has been reported as an effective acute therapy for atypical optic neuritis including NMOSD and MOGAD optic neuritis.

In patients with acute optic neuritis and NMOSD or acute optic neuritis on the NMO-spectrum, treatment with plasma exchange or rituxamab (Rituxan)[1] should be considered to improve functional visual outcome.

---

[1] Not FDA approved for this indication.

In patients with a clinically isolated syndrome, consideration should be given to institution of disease-modifying therapy for MS based on the type and number of lesions on brain MRI and oligoclonal bands in cerebrospinal fluid. Several clinical trials have shown an association between early treatment with MS therapies and decreased incidence of progression to clinically definite MS in patients with a recent clinically isolated syndrome and clinically silent lesions on brain MRI.

In patients who meet diagnostic criteria for either MS or NMOSD, consideration should be given to treating the underlying disease. Eculizumab (Soliris), inebilizumab (Uplizna), and satralizumab (Enspryng) have shown to reduced risk of relapse and increased remission rate in AQP-4-IgG-positive NMOSD. Decisions regarding chronic therapy following MOGAD optic neuritis are currently based on recurrence and persistently elevated serum antibody titers.

Complications

Though more than 70% of patients with optic neuritis recover objectively normal visual acuity, many have residual subjective visual disturbances. These often worsen or recur in heat, which is known as Uhtoff's phenomenon.

Complications of steroid therapy include insomnia, agitation, and stomach irritation. Long-term side effects of steroid treatment for this condition are rare owing to the brief period of treatment. Complications of disease-modifying therapies for MS, NMOSD, and MOGAD are reviewed elsewhere.

References

Cree BAC, Bennett JL, Kim HJ, et al. Inebilizumab for the treatment of neuromyelitis optica spectrum disorder (N-MOmentum): a double-blind, randomised placebo-controlled phase 2/3 trial, *Lancet* 394:1352–1363, 2019.

Chen JJ, Flanagan EP, Jitprapaikulsan J, et al: Myelin oligodendrocyte glycoprotein antibody-positive optic neuritis: clinical characteristics, radiologic clues, and outcome, *Am J Ophthalmol* 195:8–15, 2018.

Morrow SA, Fraser JA, Day C: Effect of treating acute optic neuritis with bioequivalent oral vs intravenous corticosteroids: a randomized clinical trial, *JAMA Neurol* 75(6):690-6, 2018.

Moss HE: Visual consequence of medications for multiple sclerosis: the good, the bad, the ugly and the unknown, *Eye Brain*. 29:13–21, 2017.

Optic Neuritis Study Group: Visual function 15 years after optic neuritis, *Ophthalmology* 115:1079–1082, 2008.

Pittock SJ, Berthele A, Fujihara K, et al: Eculizumab in aquaporin-4-positive neuromyelitis optica spectrum disorder, *N Engl J Med* 381:614–625, 2019.

Thompson AJ, Banwell BL, Carroll WM, et al: Diagnosis of multiple sclerosis: 2017 revisions of the McDonald criteria, *Lancet Neurol*. 17:162–173, 2018.

Winferchuk DM, Banwell B, Bennett JL, et al: International consensus diagnostic criteria for neuromyelitis optica spectrum disorders, *Neurology* 85:177–189, 2015.

Yamamura T, Kleiter I, Fujihara K, et al.: Trial of Satralizumab in neuromyelitis optica spectrum disorder, *N Engl J Med* 381:2114–2124, 2019.

PARKINSON DISEASE

Method of
Brian James Nagle, MD, MPH

CURRENT DIAGNOSIS

- The cardinal features of Parkinson disease are "TRAP":
  - Tremor at rest
  - Rigidity
  - Akinesia or bradykinesia
  - Postural instability
- It is responsive to levodopa and has unilateral onset and a progressive course.
- Consider alternative diagnosis for rapid gait impairment or frequent falls at onset, cerebellar signs, symptoms symmetric or restricted to legs at onset, lack of progression in 5 years, early bulbar or respiratory dysfunction, severe autonomic failure, or lack of development of typical nonmotor symptoms.

CURRENT THERAPY

- There is no benefit to starting medication early given no evidence of disease-modifying benefits, but exercise may be neuroprotective.
- In early disease, levodopa, dopamine agonists (DAs), and monoamine oxidase-B (MAO-B) inhibitors are all efficacious.
  - Levodopa is superior for treating motor symptoms but carries risk of dyskinesias.
  - Avoid DAs and anticholinergics in those over 70 years because of side effect profile.
  - MAO-B inhibitors as monotherapy are beneficial for 2 to 3 years before additional medication is needed.
  - For patients under 60 years, anticholinergics (for tremor-predominant Parkinson disease) or amantadine (Symmetrel) can be considered.
- For motor fluctuations, MAO-B inhibitors, DAs, catechol-O-methyltransferase inhibitors, amantadine, and istradefylline (Nourianz) can be useful adjunctives.
- Deep brain stimulation (DBS) is useful for treating levodopa-resistant tremor; reserve focused lesioning for nonsurgical candidates with limited life expectancy.
- DBS and continuous levodopa-carbidopa intestinal gel (Duopa enteral suspension) have the best efficacy for reducing motor fluctuations, but novel delivery options are now available, including continuous subcutaneous pumps for both foslevodopa-foscarbidopa (Vyalev) and apomorphine (Vyalev).

Epidemiology

Parkinson disease (PD) is the second most common neurodegenerative disease, affecting about 1 million individuals in the United States, and is expected to increase to 1.2 million by the year 2030. Individuals with PD account for about 0.3% of the general population over the age of 40 years. Annual incidence is about 90,000 cases of PD each year. Males tend to be affected more than females, with lifetime risk of 2% and 1.3%, respectively, in those 40 years and older.

Pathophysiology

PD is a progressive neurodegenerative disease that results from loss of the dopaminergic neurons in the substantia nigra pars compacta (SNpc) of the midbrain, leading to an imbalance of motor pathways in the basal ganglia. The hallmark pathologic feature of PD is the presence of cytotoxic intracellular inclusions called Lewy bodies, which result from the misfolding and subsequent aggregation of the alpha-synuclein protein. The trigger of this misfolding is unknown, but most theories involve an environmental trigger in genetically susceptible individuals. Lewy bodies are also found outside of the SNpc with a preference for particular neuronal populations both centrally and peripherally, which correspond with symptoms seen at varying stages of PD, including the premotor stage. One theory suggests that misfolded proteins are transferred between these neuronal cell populations and induce alpha-synuclein misfolding in adjacent cells in a prion-like fashion. Current research is looking to uncover the pathologic mechanism for potential pharmacologic targets.

Risk Factors

Although age is the greatest risk factor with a mean age of onset of 60 years, 5% to 10% of cases occur before the age of 50 years. The majority of cases are sporadic or idiopathic. Having one first-degree relative increases the risk of PD by two to three times, and a pathogenic variant with known significance can be found in 10% to 15% of PD cases. Although genetic testing is not routinely done, there are commercially available panels that typically include the seven most common genes and can be considered with genetic counseling when there is a strong family history. One such pathogenic variant is a mutation in *GBA1*, which also causes Gaucher disease. Seen predominantly in those of Ashkenazi Jewish descent, its role in PD is likely related to the decreased activity of glucocerebrosidase, leading to lysosomal dysfunction that promotes accumulation of alpha-synuclein. Another common pathogenic variant involves mutations to leucine-rich repeat kinase 2 (*LRRK2*), which likely represents a distinct subset given it has been shown to have distinct pathologic findings and phenotype with slower progression and fewer nonmotor features. Inherited cases tend to have an earlier age of onset than idiopathic cases, and ongoing studies are looking for novel genetic and epigenetic variants because disease-modifying targets may vary for different genetic variants. Environmental factors that are associated with PD risk include pesticides, well water, heavy metals, traumatic brain injury, and some industrial chemicals. Conversely, caffeine, smoking, physical activity, and nonsteroidal antiinflammatory medications have been associated with decreased risk of PD.

Clinical Manifestations

Symptoms of PD can be divided into those that are either motor or nonmotor. Motor symptoms include the four cardinal symptoms: tremor at rest, rigidity, akinesia or bradykinesia, and postural instability. Tremor (an oscillating, rhythmic movement) is often the presenting symptom, though there are people who never develop tremor. The PD tremor typically occurs unilaterally at onset in one of the upper extremities but can also involve the legs and jaw. It is slower in frequency (4 to 6 Hz) and larger in amplitude than essential tremor and enhanced physiologic tremor, though early on amplitude may be small. It typically occurs at rest, though can occur after a few seconds with prolonged posture, known as a reemergent tremor. Although the tremor usually disappears or reduces during action, it can persist, though it should be more pronounced at rest. It often increases with stress and distraction, which can be observed during conversation or while distracted performing a motor task in another extremity or stating the days of the week backward. Another phenomenon patients may describe is an internal tremor or buzzing when no observable external tremor can be seen.

Bradykinesia (slowness of movements) is often seen with akinesia or hypokinesia (decreased amplitude of movements), and patients will describe difficulty with dexterity, changes in handwriting (micrographia), and slowing of reaction time. Additional signs are reduced arm swing during gait, decreased blink rate, and hypomimia (masked facies). Hypophonia (low or soft volume) is another common feature that may be noticed initially by the family. To test for bradykinesia, use rapid-alternating movements (RAMs) with emphasis on making big and fast movements, such as opening and closing the hand, finger tapping, supinating and pronating the hand, and tapping of toes and heels. When observing RAMs, it is important to note speed, amplitude, and rhythm, as patients may inadvertently gradually decrease the amplitude to maintain speed (decrement) or have brief pauses in the rhythm (hesitation). Gait changes due to bradykinesia are often noted by the family because of slowing with a quick, shortened stride often described as shuffling. It is important to listen to the patient's gait as scuffing of the soles on the floor can often be heard. Hesitation during gait is often referred to as "freezing of gait," occurring particularly at doorways and corners.

Rigidity is the resistance to passive movement that is independent of velocity ("lead pipe rigidity"), as opposed to spasticity, which is velocity dependent with resistance felt during rapid passive movements and absent when slow. The classic "cogwheel rigidity" is simply a tremor superimposed over the rigidity. Patients may describe stiffness with movements. Rigidity can be tested in the neck and all extremities with passive movements. Subtle rigidity can be enhanced via distraction such as contralateral activation by asking the patient to perform a RAM in the contralateral limb. This is distinct from dystonia, an abnormal sustained contraction of muscles that can lead to abnormal posturing, which can also be seen in PD. If dystonia occurs in the extremities they may describe cramping of muscles or gait difficulty due to curling of their toes or inversion of their foot. Cervical dystonia often causes neck stiffness and/or pain that limits activities like driving. Dystonia can also occur in the eyelids with difficulty opening the eyes (blepharospasm).

Postural instability is the lack of corrective movements to maintain balance and often presents as gait instability or imbalance. Patients will often develop stooped posture due to dysfunction of both motor and sensory pathways, including increased tone in axial flexors and paraspinal muscle weakness. This abnormal posturing can progress to camptocormia, but some may also lean to one side (Pisa syndrome). The abnormal axial posturing often does not persist in the supine position. Postural instability can be tested with the pull test, where patients are warned that the examiner will pull their shoulders from behind and instructed to protect themselves from falling by resisting the pull or taking a step backward. An abnormal response is when the examiner, who is standing close behind, needs to catch the patient because of lack of a protective response. This is best performed with the examiner standing in front of a wall to avoid falling backward with the patient. It is not necessary to test this in a patient who requires an assistive device to walk, as it can be implied that they are unable to stand unassisted.

Nonmotor symptoms can affect many other organ systems and may require multiple specialists for management. These can be broadly divided into those that are neuropsychiatric, autonomic, sleep, and sensory. Common nonmotor symptoms include depression and/or anxiety, constipation, rapid eye movement sleep behavior disorder, anosmia, orthostatic hypotension, and urinary urgency and frequency.

Diagnosis

The gold standard for diagnosis remains the histologic features noted above at autopsy. In 2015 the International Parkinson and Movement Disorder Society (MDS) published updated MDS Clinical Diagnostic Criteria for Parkinson Disease (MDS-PD Criteria), which first requires presence of clinical parkinsonism, defined as bradykinesia (both slowness *and* decrement in speed or amplitude) plus tremor and/or rigidity. Postural instability was not included as this is typically seen later in the disease course, and early onset of postural instability should indicate an alternative diagnosis. If parkinsonism is present, established PD diagnosis can be made with at least two supportive criteria, including clear and dramatic response to dopaminergic therapy (levodopa or dopamine agonist), levodopa-induced dyskinesias (involuntary writhing movements), marked motor fluctuations with end-of-dose wearing off, rest tremor of an extremity, anosmia, or evidence of cardiac sympathetic denervation with metaiodobenzylguanidine scintigraphy. Red flags that should warrant considering alternative diagnoses include rapid gait impairment or frequent falls, bilateral and symmetric symptoms at onset, lack of progression in 5 years, early bulbar or respiratory dysfunction, severe autonomic failure, or lack of development of typical nonmotor symptoms. The MDS-PD Criteria also define absolute exclusion criteria, which if present rule out PD, such as cerebellar signs, downward vertical gaze palsy, frontotemporal dementia, or parkinsonism restricted to the lower extremities. A thorough review of medication history is also important to evaluate for history of dopamine-blocking neuroleptics and time course that would suggest drug-induced parkinsonism. The most common associated drug classes are antipsychotics and antiemetics.

Ancillary testing can include magnetic resonance imaging of the brain to rule out vascular or other structural cause of secondary parkinsonism. Although dopamine transporter (DAT) positron emission tomography or single-photon emission computed tomography with reduced tracer uptake in the striatum can demonstrate nigrostriatal degeneration, making it suitable for distinguishing between neurodegenerative and nondegenerative etiologies (essential tremor, vascular, or drug-induced), it cannot distinguish PD from other neurodegenerative forms of parkinsonism, such as Lewy body dementia or multiple system atrophy (MSA).

Seeding amplification assay technologies that amplify minute amounts of misfolded alpha-synuclein to detect its presence in cerebrospinal fluid and tissue are under investigation and show promise as a future ancillary test, though this may not differentiate PD from other alpha-synucleinopathies. Skin biopsies with immunohistochemical staining for phosphorylated alpha-synuclein are another ancillary test undergoing investigation and have even been shown to differentiate PD from MSA.

The Unified Parkinson's Disease Rating Scale (UPDRS) was designed to rate severity of disease and should not be used to diagnose PD. Part III (Motor Examination) of the UPDRS is frequently used for tracking a patient's response to treatment and progression of disease. The Hoehn and Yahr Staging Scale is used to categorically stage progression (Table 1).

Current Therapy

The most recent guidelines for treatment were published in 2021 by the American Academy of Neurology for treatment in early PD. The MDS published more extensive guidelines in 2018 for both early and advanced PD.

Currently there are no disease-modifying therapies to slow or stop progression of PD, thus treatments are considered to be symptomatic for both motor and nonmotor symptoms. Nonpharmacologic therapies include physical, occupational, and speech therapies. In particular, the Lee Silverman Voice Treatment (LSVT) LOUD program focuses on voice projection to counter hypophonia, and the LSVT BIG program focuses on improving balance, posture, and gait. Studies using dietary supplements (e.g., coenzyme Q10 and creatine) to prevent or delay progression are either still investigational or have been shown not to be useful. Exercise is associated with decreased risk, but with regard to slowing progression, evidence is still insufficient and under investigation. There are also several PD-focused exercise programs, such as dance, tai chi, and boxing. There is no particular PD diet, but the Mediterranean diet is recommended as some studies have shown benefits in nonmotor symptoms.

In patients presenting with early stages of PD, that is mild symptoms that are either minimally or nondisabling, it is important to consider the impact of symptoms on their life, as physically nondisabling symptoms may still cause anxiety in social situations or interfere with their job. Other factors to consider are age, comorbidities, and the efficacy and side effect profiles of available treatments. For those that are nondisabling and do not affect the patient's life, it is reasonable to monitor symptoms clinically, as early initiation of treatment has not been shown to slow progression.

Pharmacologic treatments in early disease (Table 2) fall into two categories of medications: dopaminergic (levodopa, dopamine agonists [DAs], and monoamine oxidase-B [MAO-B] inhibitors) and nondopaminergic (anticholinergics and amantadine). There are benefits and risks with all three dopaminergic classes. Although levodopa is the most effective treatment for motor symptoms, it does carry a risk of developing dyskinesias. This typically occurs with daily doses greater than 400 mg, so it is important to use the lowest effective dose (150 to 300 mg/day). Patients at higher risk of developing dyskinesias tend to be younger at onset, female, low weight, and have increased severity of disease. It is also important to note that there can be both short-term and long-term effects, so titration should be

TABLE 1	Hoehn and Yahr Staging Scale
STAGE	**DESCRIPTION**
1	Symptoms are unilateral only; minimal to no disability
2	Symptoms are bilateral, balance is intact; minimal disability
3	Mild to moderate bilateral symptoms, impaired balance; physically independent
4	Severe disability; able to walk and stand unassisted
5	Wheelchair or bedridden if unassisted

TABLE 2	Treatment of Motor Symptoms in Early Parkinson Disease			
DRUG CLASS	**DRUG NAMES**	**DOSING**	**SIDE EFFECTS**	**COMMENTS**
Levodopa	Carbidopa-levodopa IR (Sinemet)	25 mg/100 mg; 0.5–2 tabs TID	Dyskinesia, orthostatic hypotension, drowsiness, nausea, hallucinations	Titrating too quickly avoided, can take 2–3 months for benefit Higher risk of dyskinesia when levodopa >400 mg/day
Dopamine agonists (nonergot)	Pramipexole (Mirapex)	IR: 0.125–1.5 mg TID ER: 0.375–4.5 mg daily	Impulse control disorder, hallucinations, orthostatic hypotension TD: Skin irritation	Avoided in elderly because of increased risk of side effects Slow taper when discontinuing
	Ropinirole (Requip)	IR: 0.25–8 mg TID XL: 2–24 mg daily		
	Rotigotine patch (Neupro)	TD: 2–8 mg/24 hr		
MAO-B inhibitors	Rasagiline (Azilect)	0.5–1 mg daily	Nausea, orthostatic hypotension, dyskinesia Serotonin syndrome with SSRI, rare in PD	Will likely need additional medication after 2–3 years of monotherapy
	Selegiline (Eldepryl)	5 mg daily or BID		
Anticholinergics	Benztropine (Cogentin)	0.5–6 mg daily total; divided 2–4 doses	Nausea, dry mouth, blurred vision, constipation, urinary retention, confusion	Can reduce tremor in tremor-predominant PD Avoided in elderly
	Trihexyphenidyl (Artane)	1–15 mg daily total; divided 3–4 doses		
NMDA antagonist	Amantadine IR (Symmetrel)	50–100 mg BID or TID	Confusion, hallucinations, myoclonus, livedo reticularis, leg edema, insomnia, dry mouth	Discontinuation requires gradual taper Also used as adjunct to reduce dyskinesias

BID, Twice daily; *ER*, extended-release; *IR*, immediate-release; *MAO-B*, monoamine oxidase-B; *NMDA*, N-methyl-D-aspartate receptor; *PD*, Parkinson disease; *SSRI*, selective serotonin reuptake inhibitor; *TD*, transdermal; *TID*, three times daily; *XL*, extended-release.

TABLE 3 Comparison of Carbidopa-Levodopa Formulations in Advanced Parkinson Disease

FORMULATION	DRUG NAMES	DOSAGE FORMS & IR EQUIVALENT*	LEVODOPA PHARMACOKINETICS	COMMENTS
C/L IR	Sinemet† C/L IR ODT (Parcopa)† C/L IR (Dhivy)†	Sinemet/Parcopa: 25 mg/100 mg tab (most common) 10 mg/100 mg tab 25 mg/250 mg tab Dhivy: 25 mg/100 mg tab (scored for ¼-tab dose increments)	Peak: 30–60 mins Half-life: 1.5–2 hr Frequency: every 2–3 hr, 4–8 times daily	Carbidopa prevents peripheral conversion, reducing side effects and increasing levodopa distribution in CNS Crush or chew for more rapid onset ODT useful with dysphagia
C/L CR	Sinemet CR	25 mg/100 mg ≈ 1 tab IR 50 mg/200 mg ≈ 2 tabs IR	Peak: 1.5–2 hr Half-life: 1.6 hr Frequency: every 4–8 hr (25–100 mg); every 6–8 hr (50–200 mg)	Wax matrix lowers bioavailability; variable, unpredictable response limits daytime use; primarily used overnight
C/L/entacapone	Stalevo	12.5 mg/50 mg/200 mg ≈ 0.5 tab IR 18.75 mg/75 mg/200 mg ≈ 0.75 tab IR 25 mg/100 mg/200 mg ≈ 1 tab IR 31.25 mg/125 mg/200 mg ≈ 1.25 tabs IR 37.5 mg/150 mg/200 mg ≈ 1.5 tabs IR 50 mg/200 mg/200 mg ≈ 2 tabs IR	Peak: 1–2 hr Half-life: 1.1–3.2 hr Frequency: every 2–8 hr, 3–8 times daily	Can combine dose with IR to increase C/L without increasing entacapone Can cause diarrhea and turn body fluids orange Increased risk of dyskinesias
C/L ER	Rytary	23.75 mg/95 mg ≈ 0.5 tab IR 36.25 mg/145 mg ≈ 0.75 tab IR 48.75 mg/195 mg ≈ 1 tab IR 61.25 mg/245 mg ≈ 1.25 tab IR	Peak: 1–4.5 hr Half-life: 1.9 hr Frequency: every 4–8 hr, 3–5 times daily	Can cause headaches Granule ratio: 1 IR:2 ER Sprinkle capsule contents into applesauce for more rapid onset
C/L intestinal gel	Duopa enteral suspension	Levodopa dose: Morning bolus: 100–200 mg over 10–30 min Daily maintenance: 20–120 mg/hr (max 2 g daily) Bolus: 10–40 mg every 1–2 hr as needed	Peak: 2.5–3 hr; therapeutic plasma levels 10–30 min after bolus Half-life: similar to IR Frequency: administered over 16 hr daily	Requires GJ-tube Some patients may need routine nighttime oral C/L after daily infusion
Foscarbidopa-foslevodopa SC injection	Vyalev subcutaneous infusion	12 mg/240 mg per mL Continuous infusion rate (mL/hr): based on total levodopa daily (TLD) oral dosing in mg, [(TLD × 1.3)/240]/[number of hours patient is typically awake (e.g., 16 hr)] Optional loading dose: 0.5–1.1 mL Optional on-demand dose: 0.10, 0.15, 0.20, 0.25, or 0.30 mL	Peak: 2 hr Half-life: similar to IR Frequency: continuous over 24 hr	Infusion site reactions include erythema, nodules, pain
Levodopa oral inhalation	Inbrija†	INH: 84 mg per dose	Peak: 15–30 min Half-life: 1–2 hr Frequency: 1 dose per off-period, ≤5 doses daily	Used as needed for early wearing off

*Equivalent reference is carbidopa-levodopa IR 25 mg/100 mg tablet.
†Can be used as on-demand therapy.
C/L, Carbidopa-levodopa; *CNS,* central nervous system; *CR,* controlled-release; *ER,* extended-release; *GJ-tube,* gastrojejunostomy tube; *INH,* inhaled; *IR,* immediate-release; *ODT,* oral dissolving tablet.

gradual with interval changes around every 3 to 4 months based on response to treatment, as rapid titration can lead to unnecessarily higher total daily doses that increase the risk of dyskinesias. Studies comparing immediate release (IR) formulation with controlled-release (CR) formulation have not shown a difference in early disease, and no studies have compared extended-release (ER) formulation with IR in early disease. It is important to note that protein competes with levodopa in the gut for absorption. Early in the disease course, patients may be less affected clinically by taking levodopa too close to meals; to get the greatest bioavailability, it should be recommended to take levodopa 30 minutes before or after eating. It is also important to note that tremor can be resistant to levodopa in some patients, which is important to keep in mind when assessing response to treatment.

Levodopa-sparing dopaminergic therapy for early disease includes the use of either DAs or MOA-B inhibitors, which can be considered for patients who are at higher risk of developing dyskinesias. Treatment with DA monotherapy can show improvement up to 5 years without needing the addition of levodopa. DAs should only be considered in patients under 60 years given the increased risk of side effects in the elderly. DAs should also be avoided in patients who have a history of impulse control disorder, cognitive impairment, hallucinations, or excessive daytime sleepiness. Patients should be warned about side effects and asked to involve a family member or caregiver in monitoring. Transdermal or ER formulations of DAs may also reduce the risk or severity of side effects. No specific DA has been shown to be superior, though the nonergot DAs (ropinirole, rotigotine, and

TABLE 4 Adjunct Treatments of Motor Symptoms in Advanced Parkinson Disease

DRUG CLASS	DRUG NAMES	DOSING	SIDE EFFECTS	COMMENTS
Dopamine agonists*	Apomorphine (Apokyn)[†]	SC: 2–6 mg (0.2–0.6 mL), ≤5 doses daily	Nausea, orthostatic hypotension	Requires in-office or nurse-monitored titration
	Apomorphine (Onapgo)	SC infusion pump: 2–6 mg/hr, continuous infusion over 16 hr	Nausea, orthostatic hypotension, infusion site nodules, somnolence, insomnia, headaches, dyskinesia	Helps to reduce total levodopa daily dose
MAO-B inhibitors*	Safinamide (Xadago)	50–100 mg daily	Nausea, orthostatic hypotension, dyskinesia	
	Zonisamide (Zonegran)[1]	25–100 mg daily	Serotonin syndrome with SSRI; rare in PD	
COMT inhibitors	Entacapone (Comtan)	200 mg with dose of C/L, up to 8 times daily	Potentiates levodopa; may worsen dyskinesias, hallucinations, hypotension, hyperhidrosis	Orange body secretions (urine, sweat, etc.)
	Tolcapone (Tasmar)	100–200 mg TID		Generally avoided because of hepatotoxicity, requiring monitoring
	Opicapone (Ongentys)	25–50 mg nightly		
NMDA antagonist*	Amantadine ER (Gocovri)	68.5–274 mg nightly	Confusion, hallucinations, myoclonus, livedo reticularis, leg edema, insomnia, dry mouth	Reduces dyskinesias; can also reduce off time
	Amantadine ER (Osmolex ER)	129–322 mg nightly		Gradual taper if discontinued
Adenosine A2A antagonist	Istradefylline (Nourianz)	20–40 mg daily	Dyskinesia	Reduces off time

[1]Not FDA approved for this indication.
*Refer to Table 2 for additional medications; dopamine agonists, MAO-B inhibitors, and amantadine used for early PD are also used as adjunct to levodopa.
[†]Used for on-demand therapy.
COMT, Catechol-O-methyltransferase; *ER*, extended-release; *MAO-B*, monoamine oxidase-B; *NMDA*, N-methyl-D-aspartate receptor; *PD*, Parkinson disease; *SC*, subcutaneous; *SL*, sublingual; *SSRI*, selective serotonin reuptake inhibitor; *TID*, three times daily.

pramipexole) are preferred over ergot DAs (bromocriptine [Parlodel], pergolide[2], cabergoline[1]) given the increased risk of cardiac fibrosis with the latter. Selection of DA should take cost and ease of use into consideration, and initiation should start with the lowest dose with a slow increase to the lowest dose of clinical efficacy. If side effects are seen, a slow, staged taper should be used to avoid DA withdrawal syndrome. MAO-B inhibitors rasagiline (Azilect) and selegiline (Eldepryl, Zelapar) have been shown to provide some benefit in early PD, though the response is not as robust as levodopa or DAs, and most patients require another medication in 2 to 3 years. Concomitant use of MAO-B inhibitors and serotonin reuptake inhibitors carries a risk of serotonin syndrome, though they do not need to be avoided altogether as this is rarely seen in PD.

Nondopaminergic therapy for early PD with anticholinergics (benztropine [Cogentin] and trihexyphenidyl [Artane]) can be considered in young patients with tremor-predominant PD but should be avoided in the elderly because of risks of cognitive impairments and association with increased dementia risk. Amantadine IR (Symmetrel) can also be used as monotherapy in early disease with young patients.

As the disease progresses, most patients will need some formulation of levodopa (Table 3), and many will also require use of adjunct therapy (Table 4). In advanced PD, nigrostriatal dopaminergic presynaptic neurons are no longer able to store and release dopamine, which makes patients more susceptible to the pulsatile nature of oral medications, resulting in "wearing off," the reemergence of PD motor and nonmotor symptoms. This can take many forms and in some can be predominantly nonmotor, so asking patients if they feel *any* symptoms that indicate it is time for their next dose or if they miss a dose can be helpful to bring this to light. Dyskinesias can occur when levodopa peaks, and some may

also experience them when wearing off (diphasic dyskinesia). It is important to distinguish whether the dyskinesias are bothersome, as most nonbothersome dyskinesias do not need to be treated. As mentioned previously, high-protein meals can affect absorption, as can constipation. It is also important to ask about dietary supplements, such as the bean *Mucuna pruriens* which contains naturally occurring levodopa, as supplements are not regulated, and the amount of levodopa has been shown to vary drastically and rarely corresponds with the label. Strategies to reduce motor fluctuations include switching carbidopa-levodopa from an IR formulation (Sinemet) to ER (Rytary) to minimize the pulsatility, or adding a catechol-O-methyltransferase inhibitor, MAO-B inhibitor, DA, or adenosine-A2A antagonist. When wearing off is unpredictable or sudden, use of on-demand therapies (levodopa or apomorphine [Apokyn]) can help reverse or lessen the symptoms (Tables 3 and 4). When dyskinesias are bothersome, amantadine is commonly used. Clozapine (Clozaril)[1] can be used to treat dyskinesia and psychosis but is seldom used first-line because of the risk of agranulocytosis and need for frequent lab monitoring.

The most effective treatments currently for motor fluctuations and dyskinesias are deep brain stimulation (DBS) and continuous levodopa-carbidopa intestinal gel (CLIG; Duopa enteral suspension), which is delivered via a percutaneous gastrojejunostomy tube with a small battery-powered pump. DBS modulates pathways in the brain that reduce symptoms and allow reduction of dopaminergic therapy. CLIG reduces pulsatility with its continuous infusion. A continuous subcutaneous apomorphine infusion pump (Onapgo) that can help reduce daily carbidopa-levodopa doses was recently approved by the FDA in 2025. Another continuous subcutaneous pump that delivers phosphorylated carbidopa-levodopa (Vyaley) received FDA approval in 2024. Focused lesioning can be done in a variety of ways, resulting in permanent destruction of a specific target in the brain to reduce

[1]Not FDA approved for this indication.
[2]Not available in the United States.

[1]Not FDA approved for this indication.

TABLE 5 Treatment of Nonmotor Symptoms in Parkinson Disease

SYMPTOMS	MANAGEMENT	CONSIDERATIONS
Constipation*	Physical activity and hydration Stopping offending medications Nutrition: bran/wheat germ cereal, applesauce, and prune juice blended, 2 tablespoons 1–2 times daily Fiber: methylcellulose (Citrucel) daily Stool softener: docusate (Colace) Osmotic laxative: PEG (Miralax), milk of magnesia, or lactulose (Kristalose) Stimulant laxative: senna (Senokot) or bisacodyl (Dulcolax, oral or suppository) Enema	Avoid psyllium husk fiber supplements (Metamucil), which can worsen constipation with dehydration. Counsel on importance of prevention. Constipation often requires multiple agents with combination daily treatments for prevention and more aggressive, as needed, treatments. Constipation can decrease absorption and efficacy of oral medications.
Gastroparesis*	Diet modification (smaller frequent low-fat meals), H2 blockers, domperidone[2] For nausea, can consider ondansetron (Zofran)[1]	Avoid prochlorperazine (Compazine), promethazine (Phenergan), and metoclopramide (Reglan), which can worsen PD motor symptoms. Avoid PPIs, which may further slow gastric emptying.
Orthostatic hypotension*	Increased hydration, liberal salt intake, compression stockings +/− abdominal binders Droxidopa (Northera), fludrocortisone (Florinef)[1], or midodrine (Proamatine); can cause or worsen supine hypertension Pyridostigmine (Mestinon)[1]; does not cause supine hypertension	Degree of neurogenic orthostatic hypotension can be assessed with tilt table testing. If supine hypertension is present, instruct patient to sleep with head elevated 30 degrees; shorter-acting antihypertensive can be considered at bedtime. Orthostatic hypotension often requires comanagement with cardiology.
Pedal edema*	Compression stockings or elastic bandage wrap Lymphedema management clinic	Avoid diuretics, which can cause or worsen orthostatic hypotension.
Neurogenic bladder* (urinary retention, urgency, and frequency)	May be on-off fluctuations (especially if occurring primarily at night), optimize PD meds Mirabegron (Myrbetriq), vibegron (Gemtesa) Clean technique intermittent catheterization Referral to urologist or urogynecologist	Avoid anticholinergics given increased risk of confusion. BPH is frequent in older men, so urology referral can help rule out structural etiology.
Psychosis (hallucinations/ delusions)	Pimavanserin (Nuplazid) only FDA-approved treatment Quetiapine (Seroquel)[1] and clozapine (Clozaril),[1] lowest risk of worsening PD	Clozapine requires prescriber to be on registry and frequent CBC monitoring.
REM sleep behavior disorder (RBD)	Melatonin[7] Low-dose clonazepam (Klonopin)[1] if OSA ruled out or treated	Patients typically report vivid dreams; if no sleep partner, you can ask about falling out of bed, dramatic changes in position in bed, or noticing items knocked off nightstand upon waking.
Insomnia	Assessing timing of arousal; may be akathisia from wearing off; can use C/L CR or ER dose before bed or middle of night	Sleep study can be helpful as poor sleep quality or excessive daytime sleepiness may be due to OSA.
Restless legs syndrome	May be akathisia from wearing off, optimize meds If no response to dopaminergic changes, gabapentin (Neurontin)[1] or pregabalin (Lyrica)[1] can help In younger patients, can consider low-dose nonergot DA	
Mood disorders (anxiety, depression)	Episodic: likely on-off fluctuations, optimize PD meds Static: initiating antidepressant (SSRI, SNRI, bupropion [Wellbutrin], TCA); talk therapy, psychotherapy, transcranial magnetic stimulation	Bupropion (Wellbutrin) is least likely to worsen RBD.
Cognitive dysfunction	If due to on-off fluctuation, optimize meds Adding AChE inhibitor; rivastigmine patch (Exelon) preferred; if not tolerated, can use donepezil (Aricept)[1], galantamine (Razadyne)[1], or memantine (Namenda)[1]	Fluctuations in cognition are common. Transdermal patch is preferred over oral formulation because of fewer side effects; for skin irritation with patch, spray area with fluticasone (Flonase),[1] and dry it before applying patch.
Impulse control disorder	Reviewing medications Slow taper of DA, if taking	Impulse control disorder can manifest as gambling, excessive shopping or cleaning, hypersexuality, overeating, or excessive time and focus on a hobby.
Drooling	Hard, sour candy/lozenges RimabotulinumtoxinB (Myobloc) or incobotulinumtoxinA (Xeomin) injections in parotid +/− submandibular salivary glands	Complaints of dysphagia can be due to sialorrhea.
Dysphagia	Episodic: represents wearing off, consider on-demand therapy Speech-language pathology referral, modified barium swallow study, diet modification If severe, may require percutaneous gastrostomy tube	Dysphagia increases risk of aspiration pneumonia. C/L ODT (Parcopa) can be very useful when dysphagia occurs.
Weight loss	Monitoring, supplemental shakes, referral to nutritionist or dietician	Weight loss has a poorer prognosis; earlier dementia and death are possible.

Continued

TABLE 5	Treatment of Nonmotor Symptoms in Parkinson Disease—cont'd	
SYMPTOMS	**MANAGEMENT**	**CONSIDERATIONS**
Pain	Determining pain type For musculoskeletal, PT for stretching; if dystonia, stretching and botulinum toxin injections For neuropathic pain, gabapentin (Neurontin)[1], pregabalin (Lyrica)[1], or TCA For radicular pain, PT for core strengthening and treating for neuropathic pain; if severe, considering imaging and referral to surgeon	

*Symptom of dysautonomia.
[1]Not FDA approved for this indication.
[2]Not available in the United States.
[7]Available as dietary supplement.
AChE, Acetylcholinesterase; *BPH*, benign prostatic hypertrophy; *CBC*, complete blood count; *C/L*, carbidopa-levodopa; *CR*, controlled-release; *DA*, dopamine agonist; *ER*, extended-release; *H2*, histamine H2-receptor; *ODT*, oral dissolving tablet; *OSA*, obstructive sleep apnea; *PD*, Parkinson disease; *PEG*, polyethylene glycol; *PPI*, proton pump inhibitor; *PT*, physical therapy; *RBD*, REM sleep behavior disorder; *REM*, rapid eye movement; *SNRI*, serotonin and norepinephrine reuptake inhibitor; *SSRI*, selective serotonin reuptake inhibitor; *TCA*, tricyclic antidepressant.

tremor but does not reduce motor fluctuations or other PD features. Whereas prior lesioning techniques required surgery or radiation, focused ultrasound lesioning can be done nonsurgically, though it should be reserved for those who are not candidates for DBS and those with a limited life expectancy given the lack of long-term data.

Monitoring

PD is a neurologic disease that affects multiple systems in the body, thus a comprehensive review of systems at each visit should be completed. Table 5 highlights common nonmotor symptoms and management strategies. Management often requires a multidisciplinary approach.

Patients should undergo cognitive screening annually. The Montreal Cognitive Assessment is more sensitive than the Mini-Mental State Examination for identifying mild cognitive impairment. Cognitive decline can be treated with rivastigmine transdermal patch (Exelon), which is better tolerated than the oral formulation and is the only acetylcholinesterase inhibitor shown to improve cognition in PD. It was also shown to reduce falls. If rivastigmine is not tolerated, donepezil (Aricept),[1] galantamine (Razadyne),[1] or memantine (Namenda)[1] can be trialed.

Complications

When a patient is admitted to the hospital, great care should be taken to ensure they receive their PD medications in a timely fashion. Many formulations are not available in hospitals and require patients to bring their own medications, particularly in advanced disease. Patients should not have carbidopa-levodopa or DAs stopped acutely because of risk of dopamine withdrawal.

Psychosis occurs in about half of patients and presents as visual illusions (misinterpretation of visual stimuli), hallucinations (visual or presence), and/or delusions. Visual hallucinations are generally well-formed and recurrent. Auditory hallucinations are less common and occur with visual hallucinations, rarely in isolation. When delusions are present, they are often paranoid in character with common themes of abandonment and spousal infidelity. PD psychosis diagnosis can be made when at least one of these occurs after the onset of PD and is recurrent or continuous for at least 1 month. The only FDA-approved treatment is pimavanserin (Nuplazid), a selective inverse agonist of serotonin receptor 2A, and evidence suggests it has a lower mortality than other antipsychotics. Clozapine (Clozaril)[1] is effective, though as noted earlier, requires frequent lab monitoring, so it is often reserved for refractory cases. Quetiapine (Seroquel)[1] is frequently used, though clinical studies have not shown benefit (Table 5).

Although PD clinical course is very heterogenous with varying rates of progression and symptomology, it generally follows a gradual and steady progression. When acute changes are seen, infections and metabolic derangements should be ruled out. Death is generally from another cause, complications from a fall, or related to failure to thrive or aspiration pneumonia in the setting of dysphagia.

References
Bisaglia M: Mediterranean diet and Parkinson's disease, *Int J Mol Sci* 24(1):42, 2022.
Brücke T, Brücke C: Dopamine transporter (DAT) imaging in Parkinson's disease and related disorders, *J Neural Transm (Vienna)* 129(5–6):581–594, 2022.
Calabresi P, Mechelli A, Natale G, et al: Alpha-synuclein in Parkinson's disease and other synucleinopathies: from overt neurodegeneration back to early synaptic dysfunction, *Cell Death Dis* 14(3):176, 2023.
Fox SH, Katzenschlager R, Lim SY, et al: International Parkinson and movement disorder society evidence-based medicine review: update on treatments for the motor symptoms of Parkinson's disease, *Mov Disord* 33(8):1248–1266, 2018.
Jan A, Gonçalves NP, Vaegter CB, et al: The prion-like spreading of alpha-synuclein in Parkinson's disease: update on models and hypotheses, *Int J Mol Sci* 22(15):8338, 2021.
Postuma RB, Berg D, Stern M, et al: MDS clinical diagnostic criteria for Parkinson's disease, *Mov Disord* 30(12):1591–1601, 2015.
Pringsheim T, Day GS, Smith DB, et al: Dopaminergic therapy for motor symptoms in early Parkinson disease practice guideline summary: a report of the AAN guideline subcommittee, *Neurology* 97(20):942–957, 2021.
Skrahina V, Gaber H, Vollstedt EJ, ROPAD Study Group, et al: The Rostock International Parkinson's Disease (ROPAD) study: protocol and initial findings, *Mov Disord* 36(4):1005–1010, 2021.
Thaler A, Alcalay RN: Diagnosis and medical management of Parkinson disease, *Continuum (Minneap Minn)* 28(5):1281–1300, 2022.
Yoo D, Bang JI, Ahn C, et al: Diagnostic value of α-synuclein seeding amplification assays in α-synucleinopathies: a systematic review and meta-analysis, *Parkinsonism Relat Disord* 104:99–109, 2022.

REHABILITATION OF THE STROKE PATIENT

Method of
Natalie Blonien, DPT; and Deanna Jewell, DO

CURRENT DIAGNOSIS

- The diagnosis of stroke will have been made before rehabilitation.

CURRENT THERAPY

- Individualized rehabilitation services in acute and postacute settings supplied by a multidisciplinary team provides the best outcome for stroke patients.
- Rehabilitation programs that are intensive, repetitive, and salient task-specific interventions performed in enriched environments promote neuroplasticity and functional recovery.
- Evidence-based interventions that are individualized for a patient and address specific needs are critical

---

[1]Not FDA approved for this indication.

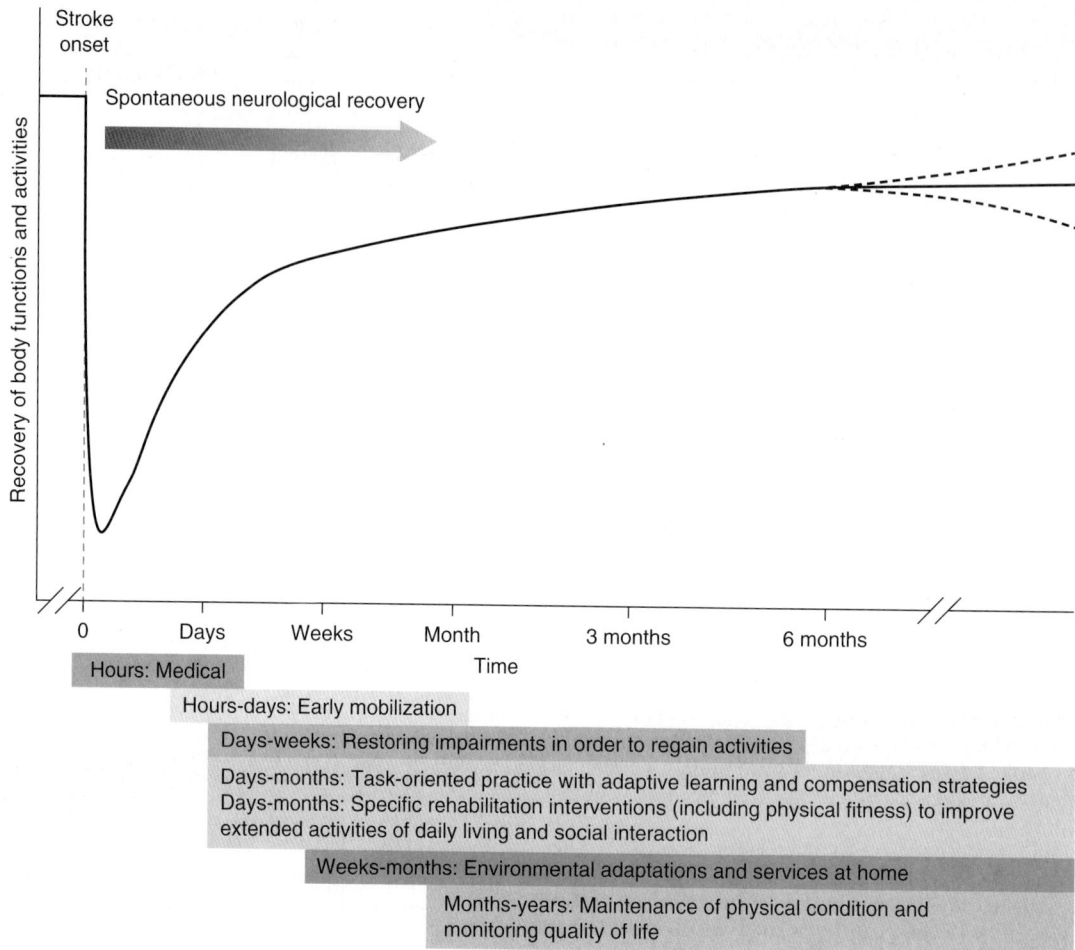

Figure 1 Framework for neurologic recovery of function after stroke. (Langhorne P, Bernhardt J, Kwakkel G: Stroke rehabilitation, *Lancet* 377(9778):1693–1702, 2011.)

Globally, one in four people will have a stroke. The mortality from stroke has decreased with advances in prevention, recognition, and delivery of care, but it remains a leading cause of long-term disability. Stroke is a cerebrovascular accident (CVA), which can be either ischemic or hemorrhagic. Ischemic CVA is more common, accounting for 90% of all strokes. There is wide diversity in stroke patients and stroke severity. Of those admitted to a hospital, about 65% of survivors receive rehabilitation services and more than 30% have persistent deficits in autonomy, engagement, and participation in society. CVA reduces mobility in more than half of stroke survivors aged 65 and older.

The current guidelines for adult stroke rehabilitation include both medical and rehabilitation involvement. This includes prevention, medical management of comorbidities, and an individualized rehabilitation program that includes appropriate assessments and treatments based on the international classification of functioning, disability, and health. The goal of rehabilitation is to enable stroke survivors to reach and maintain their optimal functional levels by providing the skills and tools needed to attain independence and self-determination. The current treatment approach is based on cortical reorganization after an injury, known as neuroplasticity, which can be influenced by rehabilitation. Best practice and research strongly support intensive, repetitive, and salient task-specific interventions to promote neuroplasticity and functional recovery.

Stroke rehabilitation programs have demonstrated reduction in mortality and improved functional outcomes and consist of an interdisciplinary team of healthcare providers involved at different points in the continuum of care. There is strong evidence that organized, interprofessional stroke care can reduce mortality rates, long-term disability, and institutional care. It can also enhance recovery and increase independence in activities of daily living (ADLs). Physical medicine and rehabilitation physicians (physiatrists) or neurologists

with specialized training/board certification in rehabilitation medicine direct the healthcare team with the support of rehabilitation nurses, as well as physical therapists (PTs), occupational therapists (OTs), and speech and language pathologists (SLPs). Other essential providers include neuropsychologists, psychiatrists, pharmacists, social workers, case managers, vocational counselors.

Rehabilitation services for patients who have had a stroke can be provided throughout the continuum of care. The average acute care admission is 4 days in the United States and involves acute stroke treatments and prophylactic care. Rehabilitation therapies are initiated in this phase, but medical management is the priority. After the patient is medically stable, their severity of deficits and medical needs determines the level of postacute care recommended. Options for postacute care in the United States include inpatient rehabilitation facility (IRF), skilled nursing facility (SNF), nursing home, or long-term acute care hospital (LTACH). Those with milder deficits can discharge home with outpatient rehabilitation services or home health. The first 3 months after a stroke is the greatest phase of neurologic recovery, in which rehabilitation plays a fundamental role (Figure 1).

Medical management involved during the acute care admission and postacute setting is focused on subsequent stroke prevention, including management of hypertension, dyslipidemia, diabetes, weight loss, physical activity, nutrition, and smoking cessation. Medical complications can occur after a stroke that negatively affect recovery, including skin breakdown, joint contractures, deep venous thrombosis and pulmonary embolism, bowel and bladder dysfunction, pain, falls, seizures, depression, and pneumonia.

IRFs provide the highest level of intensity of rehabilitation care under direct supervision of a physiatrist. This consists of 3 hours of therapy (PT, OT, SLP) 5 days a week or 15 hours per week

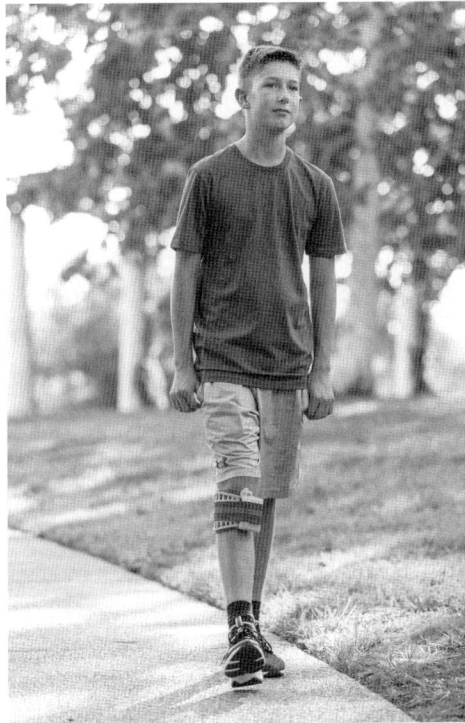

Figure 2 Functional electrical stimulation (FES) used in gait. (Lazaro RT, Reina-Guerra SG, Quiben M, ed:. *Umphred's Neurological Rehabilitation,* 7th ed. Philadelphia: Elsevier; 2019. Fig. 32.5.)

equivalent. All members on the rehabilitation team are expected to have specialized stroke expertise. An IRF is appropriate for the patient who requires close physician medical management of acute and chronic medical conditions, skilled nursing, and multiple therapy services. The outcomes for IRF demonstrate greater functional recovery and return to community. SNFs provide daily nursing care and rehabilitation services. In contrast to IRFs, the intensity of therapies is less, and there is physician oversight but not necessarily direct daily supervision. The recommendation for IRF versus SNF requires collaborative decision-making involving the entire rehabilitation team to maximize the functional outcome of the patient while considering individual factors.

After postacute care, the rehabilitation team, the patient, and their support system determine the least restrictive environment for discharge. The goal is to return home with appropriate support services within the home or outpatient services. Assessment of patient goals and the home environment is critical. If discharge to the community is not feasible, a transition to a long-term residential facility may be necessary.

With any level of stroke rehabilitation care, limitations in access to medical and therapy resources can be barriers to optimal functional recovery. Prestroke health status, length of time needed for recovery, and systemic inequities in the healthcare system, such as adequate insurance coverage and availability of skilled providers, can affect outcomes.

Hemiplegia

Hemiplegia is weakness of the unilateral arm and leg, which is commonly seen after stroke. Rehabilitation of motor function involves physical and occupational therapies. Electrical stimulation, such as functional electrical stimulation (FES) and neuromuscular electrical stimulation (NMES), delivers a current using transcutaneous electrodes applied to a muscle group to elicit a muscle contraction. NMES is an effective intervention for patients who have had a stroke and have limited volitional control. FES and NMES are essentially the same, but FES is the term used when electrical stimulation is being used within a functional task. For example, FES is used as an orthotic to assist with drop foot during gait and to improve function (Figure 2). As a modality

or as an orthotic, evidence supports that patients who have had a stroke show improvement in muscle activation of the muscles stimulated even when not wearing the device, thus promoting the recovery. In upper limb recovery, there is a statistically significant benefit from FES when applied within 2 months of stroke on ADL participation. NMES can be applied to the shoulder joint in the prevention or correction of shoulder subluxation or the wrist and hand during task-specific training.

Lack of bimanual upper extremity use significantly limits ADLs and participation in occupations. The intervention of constraint-induced movement therapy (CIMT) involves casting or immobilizing the uninvolved upper extremity to force the use of the hemiparetic side when it demonstrates a baseline ability to have volitional control of finger and wrist extension. The protocol varies between 3 and 6 hours per day for 5 days a week for 2 weeks or modified dosing of 1 hour per day for 3 days a week for 10 weeks. CIMT in the chronic phase of recovery demonstrates improvement in upper extremity participation in ADLs, motor function, and strength

Mirror therapy is a form of visual imagery. A mirror is placed in midline and a patient regards the image of the nonparetic limb as if it were the affected side while performing movement. Mirror therapy has been found effective in improving neglect and motor impairments in patients with moderate-to-severe involvement. It is recommended as an adjunct to therapy in the clinic and is easily performed in the home with basic equipment and training.

Virtual reality is a promising intervention but has yet to be adapted to widespread clinical practice. Virtual reality is used to assist with both upper and lower limb recovery with evidence to support a correlation between neuroplasticity changes and functional recovery; however, the underlying mechanism is unclear.

Patients who demonstrate limited motor return can use equipment to compensate for hemiplegia. This can include adaptive equipment, orthotics, and mobility devices. OTs are primarily involved in the evaluation process for upper extremity orthotics and equipment related to adaptations for ADLs. This can include upper extremity slings, shower benches, dressing aids, and adaptive utensils (Figure 3). PTs are primarily involved in the evaluation of orthotics, assistive devices, and wheelchairs. Careful consideration and expertise are needed when recommending equipment to maximize function and minimize waste.

Joint Contracture

Development of a joint contracture on the hemiparetic side within the first year after stroke typically occurs at elbow flexors, wrist flexors, and plantarflexors due to loss of range of motion and is more likely with the presence of spasticity. Contractures can cause pain and difficulty with performing ADLs. PTs and OTs commonly prescribe individualized daily stretching. Static positioning of the shoulder in maximal external shoulder rotation for 30 minutes a day in early stroke rehabilitation is effective in preventing shoulder contracture. Orthotics are commonly prescribed for both the upper and lower extremity joints at risk for developing contractures. Wrist hand orthoses are often fabricated by OTs, and evidence supports bracing in conjunction with early spasticity treatments to minimize contracture development. PTs will recommend the use of ankle foot orthoses (AFOs) to be worn for gait to remediate or prevent the development of ankle plantarflexion contractures and assist with foot positioning during the swing phase. In nonambulatory patients, resting ankle splints that position the foot at 90 degrees help minimize the development of plantarflexion contractures to improve sitting posture and participation in transfers.

Gait and Balance Impairment

Impairment related to gait and balance contributes to falls. Multiple factors can contribute to falls, including low balance confidence, motor or sensory impairment, cognition, and visual and perceptual issues. PTs are primarily involved in the assessment of gait, balance, and risk of falls.

There are many different approaches to physical rehabilitation. Successful treatments are based on individualized interventions to specifically address the patient's impairments and functional

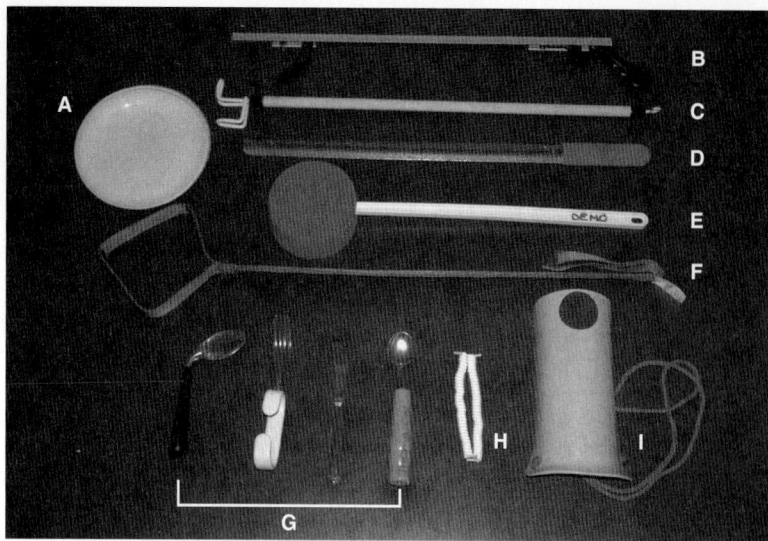

Figure 3 Adaptive equipment to assist with activities of daily living. (Gonzalez-Fernandez M, Feldman D: Rehabilitation of the stroke patient. In: Kellerman RD, Rakel DP, eds: *Conn's Current Therapy 2023*. Philadelphia: Elsevier; 2023:780-784.)

limitations. The use of intensive and repetitive functional task training to facilitate restoration of gait and gait-related activities is well supported in the literature. Compensations strategies, such as the use of an AFO with an assistive device, can improve balance and gait. Evidence suggests that lower extremity resistance training can improve functional mobility, but evidence is limited for carryover into improvement in gait. Treadmill training with or without body weight support is commonly used in research and clinical settings. There is promising evidence for the use of robotic assistive walking, which appears to be more beneficial than a treadmill for patients after acute stroke who are unable to walk even with the assistance of body weight support. Limitations in the clinical use of robotic devices include the cost of the equipment and availability in the clinic.

Spasticity

Spasticity is velocity dependent increase in muscle tone with passive range of motion and is caused by an upper motor neuron injury. Complications of spasticity include pain, decreased range of motion, impaired gait, impaired ADLs, impaired functional mobility balance and stability, compensatory gait patterns, and interference with transfers.

Spasticity is commonly seen after CVA and usually develops within weeks. There are nonpharmacologic, pharmacologic, and surgical options to manage tone. Pharmacologic treatment includes oral medications and focal treatment. Oral medications used to treat spasticity include baclofen (Lioresal), dantrolene (Dantrium), and tizanidine (Zanaflex). Baclofen can also be administered via an intrathecal baclofen pump to treat severe spasticity. Focal treatment consists of chemodenervation with botulinum toxin injections. Botulinum toxin A (Botox, Dysport, or Xeomin) and botulinum toxin B (Myobloc)[1] block the release of acetylcholine from the neuromuscular junction, causing denervation of the muscle and reduced muscle activity. The benefits from botulinum toxin injections typically last for 3 months. Nonpharmacologic considerations include orthotics, stretching, transcutaneous electrical stimulation, and hydrotherapy. Other modalities used in conjunction with therapy and pharmacologic treatments include NMES and vibration therapy. NMES was discussed in the section on hemiplegia and is used over the spastic muscles. Vibration therapy applies localized muscle vibration to either the spastic muscles or the antagonist muscle. Both NMES and vibration therapy are found to improve short-term management of spasticity in conjunction with conventional therapy but with limited long-term effect.

Pain

Several subtypes of pain may manifest after stroke, including neuropathic pain, hemiparetic shoulder pain, thalamic/ central-poststroke pain, complex regional pain syndrome (CRPS) and spasticity related pain. Central-poststroke pain is due to stroke in the lower brainstem, thalamus, or subthalamic region involving the spinothalamic tract. Treatment includes psychosocial support, along with trial of anticonvulsants (gabapentin [Neurontin][1] or pregabalin [Lyrica]), tricyclic antidepressants (amitriptyline),[1] or serotonin-norepinephrine reuptake inhibitor (duloxetine [Cymbalta]). Poststroke shoulder pain is multifactorial, and the differential includes CRPS, spasticity, glenohumeral subluxation, bicipital tendonitis, and impingement. The most common pattern of spasticity in the shoulder after CVA is an adducted internally rotated shoulder, which can become painful. Another potential cause of post-CVA shoulder pain is glenohumeral subluxation. The glenohumeral joint is stabilized by the rotator cuff. Due to flaccid paralysis initially after a CVA, the rotator cuff is unable support the weight of the humeral head in the glenoid fossa, resulting in inferior subluxation. Shoulder pain results in functional impairments of the upper limb and negatively affects rehabilitation, leading to depression and poor health-related quality of life. Noninvasive standard of care provided by PTs and OTs includes posture and positioning of the limb, restoring scapular and humeral alignment, stretching within a pain-free range, strengthening the scapular and shoulder muscles, taping, and thermal modalities such as ice or heat treatments. NMES may be helpful to reduce pain. Botulinum toxin injections to the subscapularis and pectoralis major have been shown to be effective in treating spasticity related pain and improve range of motion. Patients suspected to have subacromial injury or inflammation may benefit from subacromial corticosteroid injection. Acupuncture may also be beneficial for improving pain. Medical interventions should be used in conjunction with conventional therapy to improve outcomes.

Depression

Depression is reported in up to 23% to 40% of patients who have had a stroke and is associated with a history of depression, severe disability, cognitive impairment, history of previous stroke, and female sex. It is imperative to screen for and address symptoms of depression early in recovery because it can negatively affect participation in rehabilitation.

No drug class has been found to be superior in treating poststroke depression. Decision on type of antidepressant will typically be made based on side effect profile. Medications commonly used and studied in treating depression in poststroke patients include selective serotonin reuptake inhibitors (escitalopram [Lexapro] or

---

[1] Not FDA approved for this indication.

citalopram [Celexa]) and tricyclic antidepressants (nortriptyline). Medications commonly used and studied in treating depression in poststroke patients include selective serotonin reuptake inhibitors and selective-norepinephrine reuptake inhibitors.

Exercise for depression has been well studied in the general population with positive results. There seems to be a transient positive impact of exercise on depression symptoms after a stroke in patients who performed 1 month of exercise, but it does not appear this effect lasts beyond the termination of the exercise program.

Dysphagia

Dysphagia is difficulty swallowing due to impaired oropharyngeal coordination. It affects up to 65% of patients and places them at risk of dehydration, malnutrition, aspiration, and pneumonia. Screening for dysphagia is conducted at an acute care hospital because patients should refrain from eating or drinking until evaluated by a trained team member, preferably an SLP. All patients with concern for pharyngeal dysphagia should undergo fiberoptic endoscopic examination or videofluoroscopy swallow study. On diagnosis of dysphagia, an effective treatment plan can be administered based on diagnostic results. This can include enteral feedings, swallow therapy with compensatory strategies, and diet modifications. Common evidence-based swallow therapy interventions include swallowing exercises, environmental modifications that include proper body positioning, and safe swallow advice.

Communication

Communication impairment can consist of aphasia, dysarthria, or apraxia of speech and is primarily evaluated and treated by SLPs. Damage to the language-dominant hemisphere typically causes aphasia, which is impaired ability to use language. The type of aphasia is predictive based on the location of the lesion, with characteristic features including fluency, comprehension, and repetition. Dysarthria is a group of motor speech disorders resulting from weakness or lack of coordination that affects articulation. Apraxia of speech is a disorder of motor planning and movement despite having normal strength. This presents decreased rate of speech, sound errors, increased sounds and duration between sounds, and abnormal sound intonation and rhythm. Communication disorders can negatively affect social participation and quality of life and can contribute to depression. A variety of evidence-based treatment approaches for aphasia are available, and no treatment is the most effective. Support is provided for early daily aphasia therapy in the acute setting, with overall improved long-term communication outcomes. Skilled interventions provided in the chronic phase of rehabilitation continue to prove effective. There is support for bouts of intensive speech and language therapy delivery, but dosing and timing are inconclusive.

Dysarthria and apraxia of speech are considered disorders that affect the motor control or motor planning of speech. Behavioral treatments include focus on supporting the physiology of respiration and sound production, strategies to address articulation, and rate of speech generation. Apraxia of speech management includes strategy training and gesture training. They should be individually tailored to meet the patient's strengths and goals. Evidence indicates that patients may benefit from using augmentative communication devices to supplement speech, such as a simple communication board or a computerized device.

Cognitive Dysfunction

Cognitive dysfunction is associated with mortality, increased disability, and increased SNF placement. Deficits in cognitive domains can include attention, memory, executive functioning, and perceptual and visuospatial abilities. Cognitive screening with a validated screening tool is recommended for all patients who have had a stroke. The Montreal Cognitive Assessment and Mini Mental Status Examination are commonly used assessments to screen for cognitive impairment after a stroke. Formal neuropsychological examination may be useful after a screening tool is administered.

Nonpharmacologic cognitive rehabilitation is performed by OTs and SLPs. The standard of practice recommends that interventions should be actively applied to improve everyday function. Promoting recovery of cognitive impairment is positively correlated with time spent in enriched environments while participating in tasks that increase cognitive engagement. This can include books, games, virtual reality, and music. Frequently, compensatory strategies are recommended to support cognitive deficits, such as memory. This includes electronic and nonelectronic memory aids. Poststroke patients with mild memory impairments can benefit from internalized strategies, such as visual imagery, along with external memory aids. The more severe a memory impairment, the less likely internal strategies are effective. Overall, cognitive rehabilitation has been found to improve attention, memory, visual neglect, and executive functioning.

Physical activity and exercise have a small positive effect on cognition, and studies suggest that exercise has a protective effect on cognitive decline in older adults without cognitive impairment. It is recommended as an adjunctive therapy to improve cognition and memory. Pharmacologic considerations are primarily based on evidence for individuals with vascular dementia and includes N-methyl-D-aspartate receptor agonist (memantine [Namenda][1]) or cholinesterase inhibitors (donepezil [Aricept],[1] rivastigmine [Exelon],[1] and galantamine [Razadyne][1]).

Visual and Perceptual Impairment

Visual impairments after a stroke can involve impaired eye movements, visual field loss, or deficits related to perceptual or visuospatial capabilities; these can affect mobility and ADLs. Assessments of visual impairments can be clinically performed primarily by neurologists, physiatrists, neuroophthalmologists, and OTs. A thorough evaluation to determine the type and severity of visual impairment is necessary to implement appropriate treatments. Studies suggest that training in visual scanning strategies can improve perceptual impairments caused by neglect. Also, increasing the sensory information during scanning tasks to include audio with visual input can enhance these effects. Targeted strengthening eye exercises for convergence insufficiency are recommended for the treatment of impaired eye muscle strength and coordination. Support is conflicting for the use of prism glasses to compensate for visual field loss. Computer-assisted training interventions may be considered to improve visual perception related to neglect.

Bladder and Bowel Dysfunction

Potential issues include overactive bladder, urinary retention, urinary incontinence, fecal incontinence, and constipation. Urinary incontinence is correlated with poor outcomes, including slow recovery, prolonged hospitalization, and the need for nursing home care. Many factors contribute to urinary incontinence, including damaged neuormicturition pathways, impaired cognition, difficulty with mobility, and communication impairment. Premorbid urologic history should be obtained. Removal of a Foley catheter within 24 hours of IRF admission or 48 hours of acute admission is recommended, followed by random and postvoid residual bladder scans to assess for urinary retention and intermittent catheterization as needed. Communication and cognitive awareness of need to void should be assessed so strategies can be provided. Bowel management includes assessment of bowel habits, medications, and fluid and fiber intake. Treatment of both bowel and bladder dysfunction should be based on the contributing factors and can include the use of toileting schedules, pharmacologic intervention, pelvic floor muscle training, communication skills, and addressing functional mobility.

---

[1] Not FDA approved for this indication.

Conclusions

Stroke rehabilitation requires a well-coordinated interdisciplinary team approach that systematically evaluates a stroke patient to identify impairments that affect activities and participation in daily life. Evidence-based interventions that are individualized for a patient and address specific needs are critical. Research demonstrates that coordination within an interdisciplinary team is important to optimize functional outcomes. Advocacy for appropriate acute rehabilitation care to optimize functional recovery and for continued rehabilitation services beyond acute stroke management is vital.

References

Avvantaggiato C, Casale R, Cinone N, et al: Localized muscle vibration in the treatment of motor impairment and spasticity in post-stroke patients: a systematic review, *Eur J Phys Rehabil Med* 57(1):44–60, 2021.

Bath PM, Lee HS, Everton LF: Swallowing therapy for dysphagia in acute and subacute stroke, *Cochrane Database Syst Rev* (10), 2018.

Brady MC, Kelly H, Godwin J, et al: Speech and language therapy for aphasia following stroke, *Cochrane Database Syst Rev* (6), 2016.

Bruni MF, Melegari C, De Cola MC, et al: What does best evidence tell us about robotic gait rehabilitation in stroke patients: a systematic review and meta-analysis, *J Clin Neurosci* 48:11–17, 2018.

Centers for Disease Control and Prevention. Stroke. Available at. https://www.cdc.gov/stroke/facts.htm. Accessed 05/15/24.

Cicerone KD, Goldin Y, Ganci K, et al: Evidence-based cognitive rehabilitation: systematic review of literature from 2009 through 2014, *Arch Phys Med Rehabil* 100(8):1515–1533, 2019.

De Sire A, Moggio L, Demeco A, et al: Efficacy of rehabilitative techniques in reducing hemiplegic shoulder pain in stroke: systematic review and meta-analysis, *Ann Phys Rehabil* 65(5):101602, 2022.

Eraifej J, Clark W, France B, et al: Effectiveness of upper limb functional electrical stimulation after stroke for the improvement of activities of daily living and motor function: a systematic review and meta-analysis, *Syst Rev* 6(1):40, 2017.

Johnston TE, Keller S, Denzer-Weiler C, et al: A clinical practice guideline for the use of ankle-foot orthoses and functional electrical stimulation post-stroke, *J Neuro Phys Ther* 45(2):112–196, 2021.

Lazaro Rolando T, et al: *Umphred's neurological rehabilitation*, ed 7, Elsevier Health Sciences (US), 2020.

Teasell R, Salbach NM, Foley N, et al: Canadian stroke best practice recommendations: rehabilitation, recovery, and community participation following stroke. part one: rehabilitation and recovery following stroke; 6th Edition Update 2019, *Int J Stroke* 15(7):763–788, 2020.

Thieme H, Morkisch N, Mehrholz J, et al: Mirror therapy for improving motor function after stroke, *Cochrane Database Syst Rev* (7), 2018.

Todhunter-Brown A, Sellers CE, Baer GD, et al.: Physical rehabilitation approaches for the recovery of function and mobility following stroke, *Cochrane Database Syst Rev* 2(2):CD001920, 2025.

Winstein CW, Stein J, Arena R, et al: Guidelines for adult stroke rehabilitation and recovery, *Stroke* 47:98–169, 2016.

SEIZURES AND EPILEPSY IN ADOLESCENTS AND ADULTS

Method of
Jose A. Padin-Rosado, MD

CURRENT DIAGNOSIS

- Obtain a thorough clinical history, including a detailed description of the paroxysmal events from the patient and from witness accounts.
- Perform a complete physical and neurologic examination.
- Perform laboratory tests including electrolytes, blood glucose, liver function, and toxicology.
- Obtain a lumbar puncture if signs of infection are present.
- Neuroimaging is strongly recommended. Magnetic resonance imaging (MRI) is the preferred test because of its higher resolution. Head computed tomography (CT) is acceptable in the acute setting to rule out hemorrhage.
- Routine electroencephalography (EEG) with sleep deprivation and activation procedures should be performed as close to the time of occurrence of the paroxysmal event to increase the diagnostic yield.

CURRENT THERAPY

- Choose the right medication for the type of epilepsy and epilepsy syndrome.
- Consider the side-effect profile, cost, and drug dosing schedule, and adapt to the unique patient characteristics taking into consideration the patient's comorbidities.
- Aim for monotherapy whenever possible.
- Start low and increase slowly when initiating antiseizure drug (ASD) therapy to minimize side effects and increase compliance.
- An adequate ASD trial with titration of the medication until clinical effectiveness or side effects occur is recommended.
- When switching from one drug to another, consider overlapping medications to provide protection until the first drug is discontinued.
- If the patient fails two antiseizure drug trials either in monotherapy or polytherapy, refer the patient to an epilepsy center for evaluation.
- If the patient is seizure free after 2 years of treatment, consider withdrawing ASDs for epilepsies of unknown etiology or epilepsy syndromes known to resolve.

Epilepsy is a disease characterized by an enduring predisposition to generate seizures and by the neurobiologic, cognitive, psychological, and social consequences of this condition. Epilepsy is commonly defined as having two or more unprovoked seizures greater than 24 hours apart. However, as per the classification proposed by the International League Against Epilepsy (ILAE) in 2014, a single seizure can be classified as epilepsy if risk of seizure recurrence is high (see the "Classification" section later in this chapter).

A seizure is defined as transient signs or symptoms caused by abnormal excessive synchronous activity of brain neurons. Seizures can be classified as either acute symptomatic (provoked) or unprovoked. Acute symptomatic seizures are associated with a transient systemic or brain insult and will usually not require treatment with antiepileptic drugs because of the transient nature of the precipitant and the associated low risk for development of epilepsy. Unprovoked seizures, on the other hand, may represent the beginning of epilepsy.

Epidemiology

Epilepsy is one of the most common neurologic conditions, affecting more than 50 million people worldwide. The prevalence of epilepsy (number of people with active epilepsy) is approximately 1% in the United States, with 3.4 million people (3 million adults and 470,000 children) suffering from the disease. The incidence of epilepsy (number of new cases) is around 150,000 each year or 55 per 100,000 population. The incidence is higher in patients younger than 2 years of age and in those older than 65 years of age. The risk of developing epilepsy is slightly higher in men than in women. African Americans and disadvantaged populations are affected at a higher rate than Caucasians. The lifetime risk of developing a seizure is around 9% to 10%.

Classification

Definition of Epilepsy

In 2014, the ILAE published a practical definition of epilepsy. This definition classifies epilepsy as a disease of the brain characterized by any of the following criteria: at least two unprovoked or reflex seizures occurring more than 24 hours apart; one unprovoked or reflex seizure and a probability of recurrent seizures similar to the general recurrence risk (60%) after two unprovoked seizures, occurring over the next 10 years; or diagnosis of an epilepsy syndrome.

In 2017, the ILAE released a major revision of both the classification of the epilepsies and epilepsy syndromes and the classification of seizure types. The classification of the epilepsies and epilepsy syndromes has three levels: (1) classification of the seizure type, (2) classification of the epilepsy type, and (3) diagnosis

ILAE 2017 Classification of Seizure Types Expanded Version[1]

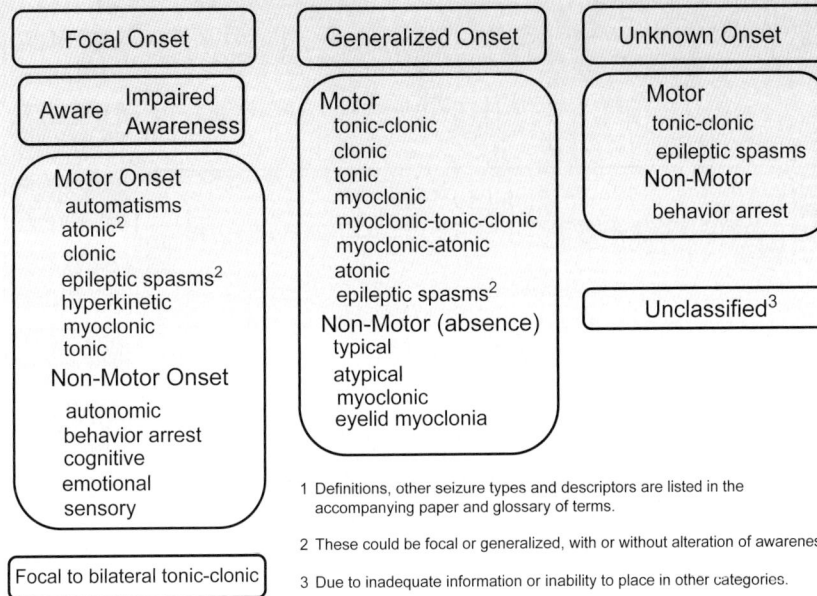

Figure 1 Classification of seizure types. From Fisher RS, Cross JH, French JA, et al.: Operational classification of seizure types by the International League Against Epilepsy: Position Paper of the ILAE Commission for Classification and Terminology, *Epilepsia* 58(4):522–530, 2017.

Seizures and Epilepsy in Adolescents and Adults

833

of an epilepsy syndrome whenever possible. The cause and associated comorbidities are considered at each diagnostic step because these carry treatment implications.

The first step is to classify the type of seizure (Figure 1 and Box 1). It assumes that the patient has been diagnosed with an epileptic seizure and then organizes the seizures by where they originate in the brain into either a *focal-onset seizure*, formerly known as *partial-onset seizure* (emanating from networks in one lobe or hemisphere), *generalized-onset seizure* (engaging bilateral neural networks), and *unknown-onset seizures*. The term *secondary generalized seizure* is replaced by *focal to bilateral tonic-clonic seizure*, and it is placed in a special category. Then focal-onset seizures can be optionally classified into seizures with preserved awareness as *focal aware seizures* (formerly known as *simple partial seizures*) and seizures with impaired awareness as *focal impaired awareness seizures* (formerly known as *complex partial seizures*). Focal-onset seizures, generalized-onset seizures, and unknown-onset seizures can be optionally and further subdivided into whether they have associated motor symptoms or other nonmotor symptoms. In some settings, classification into seizure type will be the only attainable level possible for diagnosis because there may be no access to EEG, video, and imaging studies or too little information available to make a higher level of diagnosis.

The second step is to classify the type of epilepsy (Figure 2). This step in the classification assumes that the patient fulfills the diagnosis of epilepsy (according to the ILAE 2014 definition of epilepsy discussed earlier) and classifies the epilepsies into *focal* (focal clinical features and EEG with focal epileptiform abnormalities), *generalized* (bilateral clinical features and EEG with generalized epileptiform abnormalities), *combined generalized and focal* (features of both on clinical evaluation and on EEG), and *unknown* type (either no clinical information available and normal or no EEG available).

The third step is the diagnosis of an epilepsy syndrome whenever possible. A *syndrome* refers to a cluster of features such as seizure type, EEG findings, and imaging features that tend to occur together and may provide information regarding treatment implications and prognosis. Within the generalized

---

BOX 1 | Changes in Seizure Type Classification from 1981 to 2017

- Change of "partial" to "focal"
- Certain seizures types can be either of focal, generalized, or unknown onset.
- Seizures of unknown onset may have features that can still be classified.
- Awareness is used as a classifier of focal onset seizures.
- The terms *dyscognitive, simple partial, complex partial, psychic,* and *secondary generalized* were eliminated.
- New focal seizure types include automatisms, autonomic, behavioral arrest, cognitive, emotional, hyperkinetic, sensory, and focal to bilateral-tonic-clonic seizures. Atonic, clonic, epileptic spasms, myoclonic, and tonic seizures can be either focal or generalized.
- New generalized seizure types include absence with eyelid myoclonia, myoclonic absence, myoclonic-tonic-clonic, myoclonic atonic, and epileptic spasms.

From Fisher RS, Cross JH, French JA, et al.: Operational classification of seizure types by the International League Against Epilepsy: Position Paper of the ILAE Commission for Classification and Terminology, *Epilepsia* 58(4):522–530, 2017.

---

epilepsies, a well-known subgroup, known as the *idiopathic primary generalized epilepsies*, exists and includes four distinct syndromes: *childhood absence epilepsy, juvenile absence epilepsy, juvenile myoclonic epilepsy,* and *generalized-tonic-clonic seizures*.

From the moment the patient is diagnosed with having an epileptic seizure, a cause should be sought. Etiologies include structural etiology (structural abnormality seen on brain MRI that is strongly associated with the development of seizures), such as temporal lobe seizures from mesiotemporal sclerosis; genetic etiology (epilepsies with a presumed genetic mutation), such as benign familial neonatal epilepsy with mutation in *KNCQ2* or *KNCQ3* (potassium channels); infectious

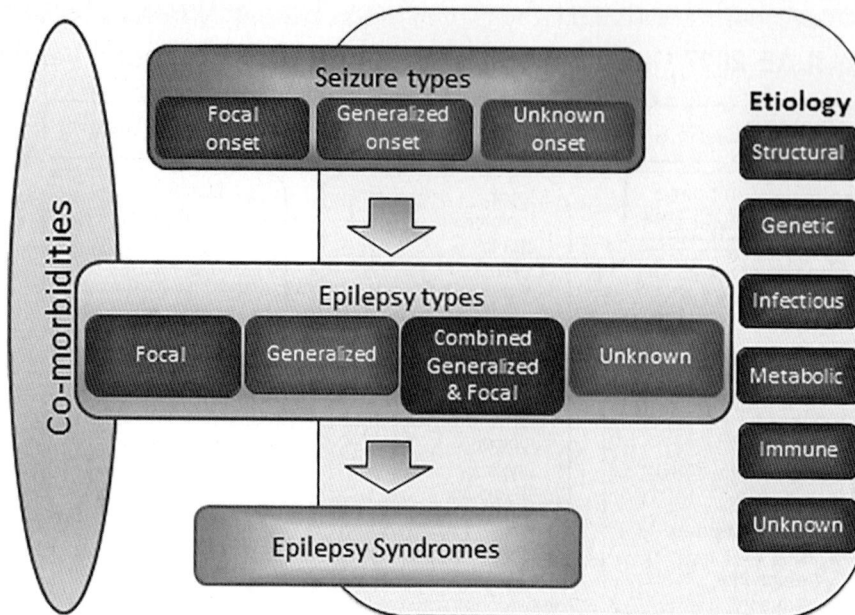

Figure 2 Classification of the epilepsies. From Scheffer IE, Berkovic S, Capovilla G, et al.: ILAE classification of the epilepsies: Position paper of the ILAE Commission for Classification and Terminology, *Epilepsia* 58(4):512–521, 2017.

etiology, such as neurocysticercosis; metabolic etiology, such as porphyria and pyridoxine-dependent seizures; immune etiology, such as anti-NMDA receptor encephalitis and anti-LG1 encephalitis; and unknown etiology.

Comorbidities should be considered for every patient with epilepsy at each stage of classification, just like etiology. Comorbidities include learning, psychological, and behavioral problems. The term *benign* is replaced by *self-limiting* (likely spontaneous resolution of a syndrome) and *pharmacoresponsive* (the epilepsy syndrome will be controlled with appropriate ASD treatment). This classification is aimed at providing tools for improved diagnosis and understanding of etiology and targeted therapies to the patient's disease.

Diagnosis

The diagnosis of a seizure and epilepsy is largely a clinical one and is highly dependent on the history and physical examination. The clinical history should be obtained from the patient and from a witness. After the aforementioned is obtained, the information is analyzed to determine whether indeed the paroxysmal event in question represents a true seizure or a seizure mimicker. If the event of concern represents a seizure, then it is further classified into *focal* or *generalized* and into *acute symptomatic*, a transient phenomena with lower seizure recurrence, or *unprovoked*, which confers a higher risk for seizure recurrence and development of epilepsy.

The clinical history is aimed at obtaining a clear description of the prodromal or premonitory state, the pre-ictal state, the ictal state, and the post-ictal state. The prodromal state occurs hours to days before the ictus and is most commonly seen in generalized seizures (but may also occur in focal onset seizures) and consists of behavioral changes, mood swings, fatigue, and changes in sleep patterns. Regarding the pre-ictal period, the patient should be questioned about the presence of warning signs immediately before the seizure onset, also known as *auras*. An aura is a simple partial seizure or a seizure without impaired awareness. An aura points to a focal seizure onset, and we can potentially determine the lobe of onset according to the description of the aura. For example, a rising gastric sensation and a sensation of déjà vu points to seizure onset in the temporal lobe, and visual hallucinations point to the occipital lobe.

The clinician then asks the patient what happened during the event (ictal period). Issues to consider include the level of awareness, the presence of ability to speak, the presence of automatisms (lip-smacking, ipsilateral hand automatisms, and contralateral dystonia points to ipsilateral temporal lobe seizures), other behavior, and the duration of the event (true seizures usually last less than 2 minutes, whereas nonepileptic events are usually of longer duration).

The next questions focus on what happened after the event (post-ictal period). These include whether there is any confusion or fatigue, how long it takes the patient to come back to baseline, the presence of tongue bites and muscle aches, and the presence of urinary incontinence (commonly seen with true seizures). The clinician also asks about triggers including sleep deprivation, stress, drug intake, and alcohol withdrawal.

Other information to obtain includes the presence of diurnal variations—for example, frontal lobe seizures usually occur at nighttime and generalized tonic-clonic and myoclonic seizures occur mostly during the morning. If more than one seizure occurs, the clinician then asks the patient about the maximum seizure-free period; seizure frequency to assess for disease severity and response to treatment; number of visits to the hospital or emergency department to assess for seizure severity; and the presence of falls or injuries during seizures to assess for risks and degree of seizure control.

Medical history should include questions regarding the patient's prenatal history and development to assess for remote symptomatic causes of seizures; history of febrile seizures; history of central nervous system (CNS) lesions (tumors, stroke) and infections; history of brain trauma, specifically with associated penetrating injuries with intraparenchymal blood, skull fractures, and prolonged loss of consciousness; and family history of epilepsy.

Social history should include questions about level of education and employment. Patients with a higher level of education usually will have a better understanding of their diagnosis and prognosis. Employment is important because patients at higher risk for development of subsequent seizures after a first seizure have a higher risk of injury if they work in a high-risk job (e.g., in construction handling heavy machinery). Patients with altered awareness during a seizure should not drive. Clinicians should be familiar with the specific state laws regarding driving in patients with seizures and epilepsy. Use of drugs and alcohol are risk factors for the development of a first provoked seizure, and some illegal drugs may exacerbate or cause seizures. Patients should be discouraged from using illegal drugs and from excessive intake of alcohol. Review of current medications or newly started medications should be performed to determine whether any can precipitate seizures (e.g., tramadol, bupropion).

After the medical history is obtained, a thorough physical and neurologic examination should be performed. The clinician should look for skin abnormalities such as neurocutaneous manifestations of diseases (tuberous sclerosis and neurofibromatosis). It is also important to test for muscle strength to rule out subtle weakness or post-ictal Todd paralysis; look for lateral tongue/cheek bites, which are commonly seen in true epileptic seizures; also look for bruises, scrapes from falls, burns, and muscle and back pain commonly seen in compression fractures caused by convulsive seizures.

The evaluation of a new-onset seizure should be aimed at determining whether the seizure represents an acute symptomatic seizure, usually a transient phenomenon or an unprovoked seizure.

If the history and physical examination points to a probable acute symptomatic seizure, then life-threatening conditions should be ruled out (e.g., hemorrhage, CNS infection, neoplasms) as soon as possible. Basic laboratory tests should be ordered including complete blood count, electrolytes (sodium), blood glucose, liver function tests, and toxicology to rule out drug use. If signs of CNS infection are present (fever, nuchal rigidity), consider performing a lumbar puncture. Emergency neuroimaging (usually head CT in an acute setting) should also be performed. If the patient continues to be altered or confused or to have focal deficits not explained by neuroimaging or is not at baseline 30 to 60 minutes after a seizure, emergency EEG or continuous video EEG monitoring should be performed to look for subclinical seizures. If there is evidence of provoking factors (sleep deprivation, alcohol or drug use), normal neuroimaging, and the patient is back to baseline, then the EEG can be delayed and performed in the outpatient setting. The EEG is important because some patients with symptomatic seizures can also have epileptiform abnormalities that may require ASD treatment, such as an alcohol withdrawal seizure with focal interictal epileptiform discharges (IEDs) originating from an area of encephalomalacia caused by a fall.

Unprovoked seizures are classified into seizures of unknown etiology and seizures with a preexistent brain lesion (remote symptomatic). If the initial workup points to a probable unprovoked seizure, an MRI with epilepsy protocol (3 Tesla MRI with 1- to 3-mm slices and coronal fluid–attenuated inversion recovery sequences) interpreted by a neuroradiologist should be performed to rule out subtle lesions such as cortical dysplasias and mesiotemporal sclerosis, which confer a higher risk for development of epilepsy. Also, the EEG is of paramount importance to stratify patients at risk for recurrent seizures. The EEG should be performed with sleep deprivation and with activating procedures and as close as possible to the seizure (within 24 hours) to increase the yield of detecting interictal epileptiform abnormalities. There is a 51% chance of recording epileptiform abnormalities if the EEG is performed 24 hours after a seizure.

Differential Diagnosis

The diagnosis of a seizure or epilepsy can be challenging. There are many paroxysmal conditions, both psychiatric and organic, that may mimic seizures. Of all the seizure mimickers, psychogenic nonepileptic attacks (also known as *psychogenic nonepileptic seizures*) are the condition most commonly misdiagnosed as epilepsy. The estimated prevalence of psychogenic nonepileptic attacks is 2 to 33 per 100,000, and most patients are younger females. The clinical history and physical examination usually points to the diagnosis of psychogenic nonepileptic attacks. Red flags include poor control on multiple ASDs with a series of normal EEGs, psychiatric history, unusual triggers such as pain and

getting upset, diagnosis of chronic pain syndrome and fibromyalgia, seizures in outpatient clinics or at doctor visits (presence of an audience), and a never-ending list of symptoms on review of systems. Some of these patients also have a history of sexual, emotional, or physical abuse. The physical examination may reveal give-way weakness and histrionic behavior. The "gold standard" for the diagnosis of psychogenic nonepileptic events is continuous video EEG monitoring. The combination of atypical semiology and lack of EEG findings during the paroxysmal event allows for a definitive diagnosis. Common behaviors seen during a nonepileptic paroxysmal event include position of convenience, ictal eye closure, retained awareness with bilateral motor features resembling a convulsive event, opisthotonic posturing (arched back), pelvic thrusting, crying/weeping, ictal stuttering, baby talk, side-to-side head movements, pseudo-sleep, irregular out-of-phase motor activity (like a fish out of water), gradual onset and termination, prolonged attacks, and stop-and-go phenomena.

Syncope is the second most common paroxysmal event misdiagnosed as seizures. Syncope represents a transient lack of blood flow to the brain. Some features are helpful in differentiating syncope from true seizures, and these include prodromal symptoms of general malaise, sweating, dizziness, nausea, palpitations and chest pain, and loss of consciousness with rapid recovery after hitting the ground as a result of rapid brain reperfusion. The challenging part is the fact that many syncopal events show "convulsive-like" behavior such as clonic phenomena, making the diagnosis more challenging. Syncopal events are usually shorter than typical convulsive seizures, and recovery is faster with no post-ictal state and usually no tongue-bites or urinary incontinence, a feature commonly seen in true convulsive seizures. The most common type of syncope is vasovagal and is precipitated by some situations such as pain and sight of blood. The other type is reflex syncope caused by micturition, cough, the Valsalva maneuver, and defecation. The EEG shows a typical progression of generalized slowing followed by suppression without any associated ictal features. Cardiac mechanisms should be explored because some could be life-threatening (e.g., Brugada syndrome or other arrhythmias) and require immediate intervention.

Migraines, especially complicated migraines, and migraine auras cause positive focal symptoms such as visual auras, sensorimotor phenomena, and weakness, which could potentially mimic partial seizures. However, the course of migraines is in the range of minutes, and the course of seizures is in the range of seconds. A complicated migraine may be misdiagnosed as Todd paralysis. Patients with migraines do have a history of headaches and retained awareness during the attack; these two features favor the diagnosis of migraine headaches.

Transient ischemic attacks (TIAs) should not be misdiagnosed as seizures because this entity has marked focal negative phenomena (weakness, numbness, aphasia), whereas seizures present mostly positive phenomena (movement, automatisms, jerking). Positive symptoms rarely occur during TIAs (limbshaking TIA).

Other conditions that may mimic seizures include hypoglycemia, panic attacks, paroxysmal movement disorders, nonepileptic myoclonus, sleep disorders, parasomnias, cataplexia, and hypnic jerks. It is important therefore to obtain a detailed history, followed by continuous video-EEG monitoring to try to capture these events for final diagnostic purposes, because it is not uncommon to misdiagnose and mislabel these conditions as epilepsy.

Treatment

Treatment should be initiated only if the potential benefit from treatment exceeds the potential for harm. In general, if the patient has an acute symptomatic seizure, treatment with an antiseizure drug is usually not necessary because these seizures are caused by a transient and reversible precipitating factor. In these cases, it is best to treat the provoking factor (discontinue the offending drug or treat the electrolyte abnormality) or allow sufficient time for the acute provoking etiology to resolve.

If an acute symptomatic cause cannot be found, then it is possible that the patient's seizure represents the first unprovoked seizure of an underlying epileptic disorder. About 150,000 adults will have an unprovoked first seizure. Unprovoked seizures are classified into *remote symptomatic seizures* (preexistent brain lesion) or *seizures of unknown etiology*. The rate of seizure recurrence after an unprovoked single seizure ranges from 31% to 56% over 2 to 5 years, and most patients will experience a recurrence in the first year. Seizure recurrence rates are significantly higher if there is a prior brain insult (twofold increase), if the EEG shows epileptiform abnormalities, if there is an abnormality on neuroimaging, and if the seizure occurs out of sleep (nocturnal seizure). If any of the aforementioned factors are present, then ASD treatment may be warranted. If ASD treatment is recommended, then patients should be advised that the risk of side effects will range from 7% to 31%, and they are mild and reversible. Patients should be informed that immediate ASD therapy will reduce the risk of seizure recurrence in the first 2 years after the seizure but will not improve the long-term (>3 years) chance of attaining seizure remission. Also, a single seizure can potentially be treated if the consequences of a recurrent seizure will significantly affect quality of life such as driving, work, or general safety. If two or more unprovoked seizures separated by 24 hours occur or if seizure recurrence risk is equal to 60% or more after a single event, then epilepsy is diagnosed, and treatment with an ASD is strongly recommended.

The goal of therapy is complete seizure freedom with no side effects. Around 50% to 60% of patients become seizure free on a single drug. Unfortunately, this is not possible in 30% to 40% of patients, necessitating referral to epilepsy centers for evaluation to rule out seizure imitators, evaluate for the presence of possible surgically remediable syndromes, and to try other options including diets and/or devices (vagal nerve stimulator, responsive nerve stimulator).

When starting ASD treatment, it is important to choose the medication that is effective for the seizure type or epilepsy syndrome. Of all available ASDs, five have a "broad spectrum" of action (work for both focal and generalized seizures): valproate (Depakote), lamotrigine (Lamictal), levetiracetam (Keppra), topiramate (Topamax), and zonisamide (Zonegran).[1] Consider a broad-spectrum ASD if the type of seizure is unknown. All of the available ASDs are effective against focal seizures except ethosuximide (Zarontin); this medication is only effective for treatment of typical absence epilepsy.

Next, consider the side-effect profile, cost, and drug dosing schedule, and adapt to the unique patient characteristics taking into consideration the patient comorbidities (Tables 1 and 2). For example, drugs with a once-a-day dosing schedule are optimal for patients with a history of prior poor compliance and for older adults; in patients taking multiple drugs for other comorbidities, administration of liver enzyme inducers (phenytoin) should be avoided. If the patient suffers from obesity, topiramate should be considered. In patients with migraine, either valproate or topiramate should be considered because these drugs are also effective for migraine prophylaxis.

Aim for monotherapy whenever possible to decrease side effects and drug interactions. Begin titration with a low dose, and increase slowly to maximize compliance and decrease side effects. If mild side effects occur, reassure the patient because most are usually transient.

Increase the ASD dose until seizure freedom is achieved or until side effects occur. If side effects occur, decrease the dose to the maximum tolerated dose. When switching from one ASD to another, always overlap the medications. For example, if a new medication is added, consider titrating to the effective dose before decreasing the failed medication. This approach provides some protection against breakthrough seizures during medication transitions.

If polytherapy is needed, consider ASDs with different mechanisms of action (rational polytherapy) such as a sodium channel blocker with a GABA enhancer or synergistic mechanisms (e.g., valproate and lamotrigine). Consider medications with parenteral formulations and a rapid time to therapeutic onset for rapid control of seizures if you are planning to discharge the patient from the emergency department with an adequate therapeutic dose. Drug levels should be obtained when compliance is an issue. Medication drug levels are a guide and not a goal. Always follow the patient's clinical response to ASDs.

In general it is reasonable to consider ASD discontinuation in patients who have been seizure free for 2 years. The reported relapse rate after discontinuing ASDs is around 41% or less. Factors associated with higher relapse include symptomatic epilepsy, age of onset between 10 and 12 years, cognitive delay, abnormal neurologic examination, juvenile myoclonic epilepsy, symptomatic partial epilepsy, abnormal EEG, family history of seizures or epilepsy, poor initial response to a drug, and more than one drug before discontinuation. If epileptiform abnormalities are seen and there is worsening of the EEG (increased EEG abnormalities) during discontinuation, then relapse rates are higher. Therefore consider performing an EEG before and after AED discontinuation.

Characteristics of Specific Antiseizure Drugs

Phenytoin

Phenytoin (Dilantin) is one of the most used antiseizure medications. It is effective for treatment of focal seizures and generalized seizures, prophylaxis after neurosurgical procedures,[1] and status epilepticus that does not respond to benzodiazepines. It can exacerbate absence seizures and myoclonus. Phenytoin exerts its antiepileptic effect by blocking sodium channels, thereby preventing post-tetanic potentiation. It is metabolized by the cytochrome P450 enzyme system in the liver and follows zero-order or nonlinear kinetics, therefore very steep elevations in blood levels can occur with minimal drug increases when the blood level is close to 20 μg/mL. Idiosyncratic reactions include blood dyscrasias and hepatitis, but these are rare. Common cumulative side effects include gum hyperplasia, coarsening of facial features, hirsutism, ataxia caused by cerebellar degeneration, nystagmus, drowsiness, lethargy, rash, headaches, nausea, vomiting, bone marrow hypoplasia, vitamin K and folate deficiency, and osteoporosis. Phenytoin is a strong inducer of hepatic enzymes, and it alters the metabolism of other drugs.

Fosphenytoin sodium (Cerebyx) is a prodrug, with phenytoin as its active metabolite. This medication is intended for parenteral administration; it is better tolerated than parenteral phenytoin because it is an aqueous solution with a neutral pH and can be administered three times as fast as phenytoin (150 mg/min vs. 50 mg/min). It has fewer cardiovascular side effects, including less hypotension, because, unlike phenytoin, it is not mixed with polyethylene glycol and will not cause vein irritation or purple glove syndrome because of its neutral pH.

Carbamazepine

Carbamazepine (Tegretol) is one of the most used ASDs in the world. It has been used in the United States since 1974 for

---

[1] Not FDA approved for this indication.

[1] Not FDA approved for this indication.

DRUG	HALF-LIFE	INITIAL DOSAGE	MAINTENANCE DOSAGE	INCREMENT	DOSING SCHEDULE	ADVERSE EFFECTS
Carbamazepine (Tegretol)	12–17 h	200 mg BID	600–1800[3] mg	200 mg q wk	TID–QID	Hyponatremia, leukopenia, rare aplastic anemia and hepatitis
Gabapentin (Neurontin)	5–7 h	300 mg QD	1200–3600 mg	300 mg q3–7 d	TID	60% removed by hemodialysis, prolonged half-life to 51 h with hemodialysis. Dosed 300 mg after hemodialysis
Lacosamide (Vimpat)	13 h	50mg QD	300–600 mg[3]	100 mg q wk	BID	Extra 50% of dose after each hemodialysis. Can prolong PR interval at high doses
Lamotrigine (Lamictal)	25 h alone 60 h with VPA	6.25–12.5 mg QD to QOD	400 mg alone 100 mg with VPA	12.5–25 mg	BID q2wk	Life-threatening rash, especially with rapid titration and VPA. Titration and maintenance doses vary based on other AEDs
Levetiracetam (Keppra)	7 h	500 mg QD	2000–4000[3] mg	500 mg q wk	BID	Decrease dose in chronic renal insufficiency, severe hepatic disease
Oxcarbazepine (Trileptal)	9–11 h	300 mg QD	900–2400 mg	300 mg q wk	BID	Hyponatremia. Fewer side effects than carbamazepine
Phenobarbital	80–100 h	30–60 mg QD	60–120 mg	30 mg q1–2 wk	QD–BID	Sedation, Dupuytren contractures, rebound seizures with rapid tapering
Phenytoin (Dilantin)	22 h	200 mg QD	200–300 mg	100 mg q wk	QD–BID	Gum hypertrophy, hirsutism, cerebellar ataxia or atrophy, peripheral neuropathy, rare hypersensitivity, hepatitis
Pregabalin (Lyrica)	6 h	50 mg QD	150–600 mg	50 mg q3–7d	BID–TID	Weight gain
Topiramate (Topamax)	21 h	25 mg QD	200–400 mg	25 mg q1–2wk	BID	Cognitive impairment at >400 mg/day, rare kidney stones, glaucoma, oligohidrosis
Valproic acid (Depakene)	9–16 h	250 mg QD	750–3000 mg	250 mg q3–7 d	TID–QID	Tremor, weight gain, alopecia, thrombocytopenia. Rare hepatitis and pancreatitis. Risk of teratogenesis and neural tube defects
Zonisamide (Zonegran)	63 h	100 mg QD	200–400 mg	100 mg q2wk	BID	Kidney stones, oligohidrosis, rare blood dyscrasias

ASD, Antiseizure drug; *BID*, two times daily; *d*, day; *h*, hour; *q*, every; *QD*, every day; *QID*, four times daily; *QOD*, every other day; *TID*, three times daily; *VPA*, valproic acid; *wk*, week.

[3]Exceeds dosage recommended by the manufacturer.

TABLE 2 Choice of Antiseizure Drug in Special Situations

SPECIAL SITUATION	DRUG OF CHOICE	COMMENTS
Partial seizures	Carbamazepine, lamotrigine, levetiracetam, oxcarbazepine, topiramate, gabapentin	
Refractory partial seizures	Lacosamide, pregabalin, zonisamide	Second-line treatment
Generalized epilepsies	Lamotrigine, topiramate, valproic acid,[1] zonisamide[1]	Avoid valproic acid in women
Absence seizures	Ethosuximide, lamotrigine,[1] valproic acid, topiramate[1]	Ethosuximide is the choice for only pure absence seizures and is insufficient in other associated generalized tonic-clonic or myoclonic seizures
Juvenile myoclonic epilepsy	Valproic acid,[1] topiramate,[1] lamotrigine,[1] zonisamide,[1] levetiracetam	Avoid valproic acid in women
Myoclonic seizures	Clonazepam, valproic acid,[1] levetiracetam	Lamotrigine occasionally exacerbates myoclonic seizures
Women of childbearing potential	Lamotrigine, topiramate, levetiracetam, oxcarbazepine	Avoid enzyme-inducing agents that alter steroid hormones and OCP levels; use OCPs with ≥50 μg of estrogen; OCPs increase the elimination of lamotrigine. Significant increased risk of teratogenicity with valproic acid
Older adult patients	Lamotrigine, gabapentin, levetiracetam, topiramate	Avoid polypharmacy and highly protein-bound ASDs and ASDs with high drug-drug interactions
Depression	Lamotrigine,[1] topiramate[1]	
Bipolar disorder	Valproic acid,[1] carbamazepine, lamotrigine, topiramate[1]	
Migraine	Valproic acid, topiramate	Consider the choice according to sex, side-effect profile, and seizure type
Chronic pain	Pregabalin,[1] gabapentin[1]	
Neuropathic pain	Carbamazepine,[1] gabapentin,[1] pregabalin	

ASD, Antiseizure drug; *OCP,* oral contraceptive pill.
[1]Not FDA approved for this indication.

treatment of focal epilepsies and generalized tonic-clonic seizures. It is highly effective and usually well tolerated. Carbamazepine, like phenytoin, blocks sodium channels. This medication is metabolized in the liver, and the major metabolic pathway is epoxidation to CBZ 10-11-epoxide. This epoxide confers most of the toxicity associated with this drug. It undergoes autoinduction and therefore induces its own metabolism in the first 3 to 5 weeks, and it takes longer to reach steady-state blood levels. Usually the extended-release formulations (Carbatrol and Tegretol XR) are better tolerated than the immediate-release formulations. Idiosyncratic side effects are rare and include aplastic anemia, agranulocytosis, hyponatremia, thrombocytopenia, hepatitis, and Stevens-Johnson syndrome. White blood cell counts may decrease mildly and do not require intervention unless the level decreases below 3000/mm^3. Dose-related side effects include diplopia, dizziness, nausea, and ataxia.

Phenobarbital

Phenobarbital (Luminal) was the most commonly used ASD of the 20th century. It is inexpensive and long acting, but it has fallen out of favor for newer ASDs because of its poor side-effect profile. It is used for treatment of focal-onset, generalized seizures and neonatal seizures.[1] It is a barbiturate and acts on the GABA-A barbiturate binding site and therefore prolongs the duration of calcium channel opening, stabilizing neuronal membranes. It has a very long half-life (70 to 120 hours) in adults and therefore is suitable for once-a-day administration. It is a powerful inducer of microsomal liver enzymes. Side effects include cognitive problems, sedation, psychomotor slowing, depression, coarsening of facial features, osteopenia, folic acid deficiency, Dupuytren contractures, megaloblastic anemia, and hepatitis (autoimmune reaction). Withdrawal of this medication should be performed very slowly because of the high risk of withdrawal seizures.

Primidone (Mysoline) is metabolized to phenobarbital (main active metabolite) and phenylethylmalonamide. It is a second-line agent used for treatment of focal seizures and secondary generalized seizures, and the side-effect profile is similar to phenobarbital.

Valproic Acid

Valproic acid (Depakene) and its sodium salt divalproex (Depakote) are broad-spectrum medications and the drugs of choice for treatment of primary generalized epilepsies such as juvenile myoclonic epilepsy, absence epilepsy, photosensitive epilepsy, and Lennox-Gastaut syndrome (LGS); they are a second-line choice for epileptic spasms. They are also approved for treatment of focal-onset epilepsies, although higher doses are needed to treat focal epilepsy. A parenteral form (Depacon) is available for treatment of status epilepticus. It works by enhancing GABA function; it may increase GABA by stimulation of glutamate decarboxylase

(GAD) and by selective modulation of voltage-gated sodium channels. Divalproex sodium (Depakote) is a powerful inhibitor of both oxidation and glucuronidation. Common side effects include dyspepsia, thinning and curling of hair, weight gain, tremor, rashes, bone marrow suppression, polycystic ovarian syndrome, amenorrhea with anovulatory cycles, thrombocytopenia, hepatitis and pancreatitis that could be life threatening, hyperammonemia, and sedation. Valproic acid should not be given to women of childbearing potential because of the high risk of fetal defects (10%), specifically neural tube defects. Decreased IQ scores have been noted in children whose mothers were treated with valproate during pregnancy.

Ethosuximide

The mechanism of action of ethosuximide (Zarontin) is blockade of T-type calcium channels, and it is indicated for treatment of typical absence epilepsy. This medication will not work to control any other seizure types. Common side effects are minimal and include dyspepsia, nausea, loss of appetite, and tiredness.

Felbamate

Felbamate (Felbatol) is effective for treatment of multiple seizure types, but it was briefly withdrawn from the U.S. market in 1994 because of the occurrence of aplastic anemia and hepatic failure. It is now available only for patients with intractable seizures in whom other medications have failed and when the benefits outweigh the risks. Its mechanism of action is blockade of NMDA receptors, modulation of sodium channels, and blockade of calcium channels. The risk for hepatic failure is 14 in 110,000 patients and increases with polytherapy.

Gabapentin

Gabapentin (Neurontin) is similar to the structure of GABA but has no effect on the GABA receptor. It enhances GAD, thereby increasing levels of GABA. This medication has no drug interactions. It is excreted entirely unchanged in the kidneys. Gabapentin is used for treatment of focal seizures with or without secondary generalization. It is ineffective in myoclonus and primary generalized seizures, and it is ineffective at lower doses. The dose should be adjusted in patients with renal disease according to creatinine clearance.

Pregabalin

Pregabalin (Lyrica) is an analogue of GABA, but like gabapentin (Neurontin), it has no effect on the GABA receptor. It has no drug interactions, and it is usually well tolerated. It must be dose-adjusted in patients with renal failure, and it is 50% removed after hemodialysis. It is used as an adjunct in adult patients with focal epilepsies. Common side effects include dizziness, drowsiness, weight gain, dry mouth, and edema.

Lamotrigine

Lamotrigine (Lamictal) works by sodium channel blockade and inhibits release of glutamate. It is broad spectrum, and it is used for adjunctive treatment of focal-onset seizures with or without secondary generalization, for crossover to monotherapy, and in LGS. It is also effective for treatment of atypical absence seizures,[1] tonic/atonic seizures, and myoclonic seizures, although it may cause exacerbations in some patients with juvenile myoclonic epilepsy. It is one of the preferred drugs to treat older adult patients and pregnant women because of its favorable safety and pharmacokinetic profile. Lamotrigine levels should be closely watched and will increase significantly with coadministration of valproate; these two medications cause a synergistic therapeutic effect but could also increase adverse reactions (rash). It could cause a rash (5%) if the drug is titrated too quickly; this rash could progress into a life-threatening condition

[1] Not FDA approved for this indication.

(Stevens-Johnson syndrome; 0.1%) and is more common in children with concomitant valproate use. If rash occurs, the medication should be discontinued immediately. Other common side effects include tremor, insomnia, headaches, ataxia, and somnolence. Pregnancy increases lamotrigine clearance by 50%, necessitating dose adjustments; therefore lamotrigine levels should be monitored before, during, and after pregnancy, and doses should be adjusted accordingly.

Levetiracetam

Levetiracetam (Keppra) is one of the most widely used ASDs because of its good pharmacokinetics, favorable side-effect profile, and multiple formulations, including parenteral and liquid (ease of administration). It is a broad-spectrum drug. It has a unique mechanism of action (binds to synaptic vesicle protein 2A-SV2A). It does not induce liver enzymes and therefore does not affect the metabolism of other drugs and does not bind to proteins in plasma. This medication must be dose-adjusted in patients with renal disease and after hemodialysis (add an extra 500 mg). It is one of the only ASDs that decreases the interictal epileptic burden (the other one is Depakote). It is approved for adjunctive treatment of primary generalized tonic-clonic seizures in adults and children 6 years of age and older with idiopathic generalized epilepsy, adjunctive treatment of focal onset seizures in adults and children 4 years of age and older, and adjunctive treatment of myoclonic seizures in adults and adolescents 12 years of age and older with juvenile myoclonic epilepsy. It is also used off-label for prophylaxis in patients after traumatic brain injury and in status epilepticus. Common adverse effects include behavioral changes (avoid in patients with psychiatric conditions), somnolence, asthenia, headache, dizziness, and flulike symptoms. It does not have any serious idiosyncratic reactions and is safe for older adults and probably safe to take during pregnancy. Consider obtaining levels during pregnancy because clearance is increased during pregnancy, necessitating dose adjustments.

Brivaracetam

Brivaracetem (Briviact) is a chemical analogue of levetiracetam with a similar mechanism of action but a higher affinity (20-fold) for the SV2A receptor. Like levetiracetam, it exhibits linear kinetics with a favorable side-effect profile. It is indicated for adjunctive treatment of focal-onset seizures with or without secondary generalization in adults and children 16 years of age and older. It does not have added therapeutic benefit if coadministered with levetiracetam. It may increase serum concentrations of carbamazepine epoxide and phenytoin.

Oxcarbazepine

Oxcarbazepine (Trileptal) is an analogue of carbamazepine but without the toxic epoxide. Thus it is better tolerated than carbamazepine (Tegretol). It is metabolized to the 10 monohydroxy metabolite, which confers its pharmacologic effect. It is used as monotherapy or adjunctive therapy for focal epilepsies in adults, as monotherapy for focal epilepsies in children 4 years of age and older, and as adjunctive therapy in children 2 years of age and older. It may exacerbate myoclonic seizures and absence seizures. It interacts with oral contraceptives, thereby reducing its efficacy. Hyponatremia is rare in children but may be higher in older adult populations. Other side effects include dizziness, fatigue, and headache, and these are dose dependent. Patients who develop rash with carbamazepine (Tegretol) may develop rash if treated with oxcarbazepine (Trileptal) because of cross-reactivity.

Tiagabine

Tiagabine (Gabitril) works by reversible inhibition of the GABA-transporter-1, thereby increasing the availability of

GABA in the synaptic cleft. It is approved as an adjunctive medication for treatment of refractory focal-onset seizures. It can worsen absence seizures and cause status epilepticus in patients with primary generalized epilepsy. Common side effects include tremor, nervousness, dizziness, abdominal pain, diarrhea, and emotional lability.

Topiramate

Topiramate (Topamax) is a broad-spectrum ASD with multiple mechanisms of action. It works by inhibiting sodium conductance and weakly inhibiting carbonic anhydrase, blocks the AMPA glutamate receptor, and enhances GABA. It is approved for adjunctive treatment of focal-onset seizures or primary generalized epilepsy and for treatment of LGS. Enzyme inducers (e.g., phenytoin) decrease topiramate levels by 50%. This medication will need dose adjustments in patients with renal failure. Topiramate (Topamax) reduces the levels of oral contraceptives, thereby decreasing its effectiveness. Common side effects include word-finding difficulties, weight loss (decreased appetite), paresthesias in the fingers and mouth, kidney stones, anhidrosis caused by the drug's carbonic-anhydrase effect, acute myopia in closed-angle glaucoma, ataxia, and tiredness. Usually doses >400 mg are poorly tolerated.

Zonisamide

Zonisamide (Zonegran) is a broad-spectrum ASD used for treatment of focal epilepsy with or without secondary generalization. It is also effective for treatment of myoclonus (juvenile myoclonic epilepsy)[1] and absence seizures (T-type calcium channel blockade). This ASD has a structure similar to the sulfonamides; therefore it is contraindicated in patients with allergies to these antibiotics. It has a long-half life (>60 hours); therefore it can be taken once a day, which increases compliance. The major mechanism of action is the blockade of sodium channels; it also works on T-type calcium channels and weak inhibition of carbonic anhydrase. Enzyme inducers and valproate (Depakote) decrease half-life. The most common adverse reactions include anorexia with associated weight loss, headache, mental slowing, confusion, ataxia, dizziness, kidney stones (1%), oligohidrosis, and paresthesias (carbonic anhydrase inhibition).

Vigabatrin

Vigabatrin (Sabril) is a structural analogue of GABA and binds irreversibly to the GABA-T (GABA transaminase), thereby increasing GABA concentrations in the brain. It is indicated for treatment of epileptic spasms in tuberous sclerosis and in refractory focal-onset epilepsies. It may exacerbate absence seizures and myoclonic seizures and, like tiagabine, may cause generalized spike-and-wave status epilepticus in patients with absence seizures or primary generalized epilepsy. This ASD causes visual field defects (nasal constriction and concentric constriction with preserved central vision), and these may be irreversible. Other side effects include fatigue, dizziness, headache, tremor, and double vision.

Rufinamide

Rufinamide's (Banzel) mechanism of action is probable modulation of sodium channels (prolongation of inactive state of the channel). It is indicated as adjunctive treatment of seizures associated with LGS in both children and adults.

Lacosamide

Lacosamide (Vimpat) has a novel mechanism of action by enhancing the slow inactivation of voltage-gated sodium channels. It is approved for the adjunctive treatment and conversion

to monotherapy and monotherapy treatment of focal onset epilepsies. It is also used off label for treatment of status epilepticus in the intensive care unit because of availability of an IV formulation. This medication does not have significant drug interactions.

Clobazam

Clobazam (Onfi) is a benzodiazepine with a 1,5 substitution instead of the common 1,4 substitution; therefore it has less anxiolytic and sedative effects. It works by binding to the GABA-A receptor. It is approved for the adjunctive treatment of LGS. It may also be effective for treatment of primary or focal seizures with secondary generalized seizures[1] as well as catamenial epilepsy.[1] It has no significant clinical interactions. Side effects include sedation, dizziness, ataxia, and weakness. No idiosyncratic reactions have been identified.

Perampanel

Perampanel (Fycompa) is a noncompetitive AMPA receptor antagonist and is indicated in the adjunctive treatment of focal-onset seizures with or without secondary generalization and in primary generalized seizures in adults and adolescents 12 years of age and over. The recommended dose is 8 to 12 mg/day for focal seizures and 8 mg/day for primary generalized seizures. This medication has a black box warning because it can cause severe psychiatric and behavioral reactions (aggressiveness, suicidality, homicidal threats and ideation, and irritability). Common adverse effects include somnolence, headache, dizziness, and fatigue.

Eslicarbazepine

Eslicarbazepine (Aptiom) is a prodrug of S-licarbazepine with a mechanism of action similar to oxcarbazepine (Trileptal) sodium channel blockade. It is approved as monotherapy or adjunct therapy for treatment of focal-onset seizures. Common adverse effects include dizziness, nausea, diplopia, and headache.

Cannabidiol

Cannabidiol (EPIDIOLEX) is the first prescription pharmaceutical formulation of purified CBD oil approved by the FDA (in June 2018) for the treatment of seizures associated with LGS and Dravet syndrome in patients 1 year of age and older.

The most common side effects of this drug include increase in liver enzymes, especially when used in conjunction with valproate or valproate and clobazam, decreased appetite, diarrhea, rash, tiredness, sleepiness, and infections.

Fenfluramine

Fenfluramine (Fintepla) is a phenethylamine that is structurally similar to serotonin and exerts its antiepileptic effect by increasing the release of serotonin, which stimulates multiple 5-HT receptor subtypes, and by acting as a positive modulator of sigma receptors. This medication was approved by the FDA in June 2020 for treatment of seizures in Dravet syndrome and LGS in patients 2 years of age and older. The most common side effects include decreased appetite, weight loss, diarrhea, fatigue, lethargy, and pyrexia. It has few relative drug-drug interactions.

Everolimus

Everolimus (Afinitor) is a rapamycin derivative that inhibits mTOR (mammalian target of rapamycin). mTOR overactivation has been linked to the pathogenesis of tuberous sclerosis complex (TSC), therefore it can target the etiology of the disease. It was approved by the FDA as adjunctive treatment for TSC with partial onset seizures in patients 2 years of age and older. The most common adverse effects are stomatitis, pyrexia, pneumonia, diarrhea, and hypercholesterolemia.

---

[1] Not FDA approved for this indication.

Special Populations

Women

Epilepsy is one of the most common conditions occurring in women of reproductive age (1.1 million). Women of reproductive age who are taking ASDs for epilepsy should be counseled on the possibility of teratogenicity from ASD therapy and the potential interaction with contraception. Some ASDs (enzyme inducers) affect oral contraceptives (OCPs), leading to decreased effectiveness and unwanted pregnancies. These ASDs are phenobarbital, phenytoin, carbamazepine, oxcarbazepine, eslicarbazepine, felbamate, topiramate (doses >200 mg/day), lamotrigine (doses >300 mg/day), primidone, rufinamide, and clobazam. OCPs can reduce the levels of lamotrigine, leading to breakthrough seizures. In patients taking these ASDs, a second barrier method versus changing to a non–enzyme-inducing ASD is recommended. Seizures during pregnancy will remain the same or decrease, but around 15% to 30% will have an increase in seizure frequency. Most women (84% to 92%) with epilepsy who were seizure free 9 months before the pregnancy will remain free from seizures during the pregnancy. Blood levels of lamotrigine, phenytoin, carbamazepine (to a lesser extent), and possibly levetiracetam and the active oxcarbazepine metabolite, will decrease during pregnancy because of increased clearance; therefore these ASD levels should be monitored and medication dosages adjusted as needed. The risk to the fetus from seizures (especially convulsive seizures) is higher than the risk to the fetus from ASDs. More than 90% of female patients with epilepsy will deliver a normal baby. The rates of congenital malformations in women with epilepsy taking ASDs is around 4% to 6% (double that of the general population) but remain low. The risk of malformations increases with polytherapy and with higher dose of ASDs. Valproate/valproic acid is the ASD that carries the highest teratogenicity (6% to 10%), mostly associated with neural tube defects. It also produces long-term cognitive problems, with a reduction in children's IQs when mothers take valproate (Depakote) during pregnancy. Therefore valproic acid is contraindicated and should not be used as a first-line treatment in women of childbearing potential. Women of childbearing potential who have epilepsy should be supplemented with folic acid at a dose of 0.4 mg/day to decrease the risk of congenital malformations if they become pregnant. Breast-feeding is an important concern in the postpartum period in women taking ASDs. Even though some ASDs (e.g., primidone and levetiracetam) transfer into breast milk, breast-feeding is encouraged. The infant should be monitored for increased sedation if mothers are on those two ASDs.

Older Adults

The current world population is aging, and the risk for epilepsy increases dramatically after 65 years of age. The recognition of seizures in this group may be more complicated because the presentation may be atypical. Also, many other conditions may mimic seizures in older adults, making diagnosis a challenging proposition. The most common seizure type in older adults is complex partial seizures, which present with confusion, staring, change in mental status, and unresponsiveness. The most common cause of epilepsy in this group is cerebrovascular disease. Other conditions that may cause epilepsy include neurodegenerative conditions (Alzheimer disease), head trauma, and brain tumors. When treating older adult patients, the pharmacokinetic and pharmacodynamic properties of medications should be considered. Older adults have reductions in protein binding, renal elimination, and hepatic metabolism, thereby conferring a higher risk for idiosyncratic reactions and altered kinetics. Gabapentin, lamotrigine, levetiracetam, pregabalin, and oxcarbazepine are usually well tolerated and recommended as first-line treatment in this patient population. AEDs with hepatic enzyme–inducing mechanisms are not recommended in older adult patients because of the potential for interactions with other drugs. Fortunately, seizures in this population are easy to control, and monotherapy is usually effective.

Drug-Resistant Epilepsy

Drug-resistant or intractable epilepsy is defined as the failure of adequate trials of two tolerated, appropriately chosen and used ASDs used in monotherapy or polytherapy to achieve sustained seizure freedom. Drug-resistant epilepsy affects one-third of patients living with epilepsy.

These patients should be referred to an epilepsy center for further management, including evaluation by an epileptologist who will perform a detailed clinical and physical examination and order further diagnostic tests including video EEG monitoring to record the patient's events for final diagnostic purposes and to evaluate for possible epilepsy surgery. Surgical resection of the epilepsy focus is the only available treatment to cure epilepsy. Seizure freedom rates after temporal lobectomy are 70% to 90% for mesiotemporal sclerosis and 40% to 70% for neocortical resections. In patients who are not suitable candidates for epilepsy surgery, dietary treatment or neuromodulation is recommended. Dietary options include the ketogenic diet, the modified Atkins diet, and the low glycemic index diet.

These diets can be used as adjunctive therapy in combination with ASDs and devices, such as the vagus nerve stimulator (VNS), responsive neurostimulation system (RNS), and deep brain stimulator (DBS). These diets have similar seizure reduction rates (around 50%) in one-half of patients. The low glycemic index diet is better tolerated and less restrictive than the modified Atkins diet and the classic ketogenic diet.

The VNS, RNS, and DBS are approved for treatment of pharmacoresistant epilepsy in the United States. The VNS works by delivering an intermittent mild current to the left vagus nerve. The mechanism of action is unknown but believed to include alterations in the reticular activating system, the central autonomic network, the limbic system, and the diffuse noradrenergic projection system. With long-term use, this device provides >50% seizure reduction in about 50% to 60% of patients, with around 8% becoming seizure free after 2 years. The new SenTiva generator (LivaNova, London, UK) combines traditional VNS therapy with seizure detection technology via changes in cardiac rhythms.

RNS therapy (Neuropace, Mountain View, CA) was approved by the FDA in 2013 for treatment of refractory focal-onset seizures. This device continuously monitors and detects abnormal electrical activity that can lead to a seizure and then delivers electrical stimulation to the area of seizure generation to try to abort the seizure. It has two leads, and either subdural or depth electrodes or a combination of both can be used and placed close to or over the epileptogenic zone. These leads are connected to the generator that seats on the skull. Treatment with the RNS system is recommended in patients who are not amenable to surgery and have multifocal epilepsy with no more than two discrete seizure onset zones. The median seizure reduction at 5 years was >65%, with 15% of patients achieving seizure freedom.

The FDA approved DBS in 2018 for adjunctive treatment of patients with drug-resistant focal onset epilepsy who are 18 years of age of older. This device is particularly useful if the seizure focus is difficult to localize to one or two brain regions. Leads are placed in the anterior nucleus of the thalamus for delivery of electrical stimulation. According to the Stimulation of the Anterior Nuclei of the Thalamus for Epilepsy (SANTE) trial with 110 patients randomized to receive active stimulation versus sham stimulation, a median reduction in seizures of 69% from baseline was observed at the end of 5 years, and seizure severity and quality of life improved significantly.

References

Ahmed NS, Spencer SS: An approach to the evaluation of a patient for seizures and epilepsy, *Wisc Med J* 103(1):49–55, 2004.

Benbadis S: The differential diagnosis of epilepsy: a critical review, *Epilepsy Behav* 15:15–21, 2009.

Britton JW: Antiepileptic drug therapy: when to start, when to stop, *Continuum Lifelong Learning Neurol* 16:105–120, 2010.

Fisher RS, Cross JH, French JA, et al: Operational classification of seizure types by the International League Against Epilepsy: Position Paper of the ILAE Commission for Classification and Terminology, *Epilepsia* 58:522–530, 2017.

Fisher RS, Acevedo C, Arzimanaglou, et al: ILAE official report: a practical clinical definition of epilepsy, *Epilepsia* 55:475–482, 2014.

Gavvala JR, Schuele SU: New-onset seizure in adults and adolescent: a review, *JAMA* 36:2657–2668, 2016.

Harden CL, Meador KJ, Pennell PB, et al: Management issues for women with epilepsy—focus on pregnancy (an evidence- based review): II. Teratogenesis and perinatal outcomes: Report of the Quality Standards Subcommittee and Therapeutics and Technology Subcommittee of the American Academy of Neurology and the American Epilepsy Society, *Epilepsia* 50:1237–1246, 2009.

Harden CL, Pennell PB, Koppel BS, et al: Management issues for women with epilepsy—focus on pregnancy (an evidence- based review): III. Vitamin K, folic acid, blood levels, and breast-feeding: Report of the Quality Standards Subcommittee and Therapeutics and Technology Assessment Subcommittee of the American Academy of Neurology and the American Epilepsy Society, *Epilepsia* 50:1247–1255, 2009.

Hesdorffer DC, Logroscino G, Benn EKT, et al: Estimating risk for developing epilepsy: a population-based study in Rochester, Minnesota, *Neurology* 76:23–27, 2011.

Krumholz A, Wiebe S, Gronseth G, et al: Practice parameter: evaluating an apparent unprovoked first seizure in adults (an evidence-based review): Report of the Quality Standards Subcommittee of the American Academy of Neurology and the American Epilepsy Society, *Neurology* 69:1996–2007, 2007.

Kwan P, Brodie MJ: Effectiveness of first antiepileptic drug, *Epilepsia* 42(10):1255–1260, 2001.

Kwan P, Brodie MJ: Early identification of refractory epilepsy, *N Engl J Med* 342(5):314–319, 2000.

Kwan P, Arzimanoglou A, Berg AT, et al: Definition of drug resistant epilepsy: consensus proposal by the ad hoc Task Force of the ILAE Commission of Therapeutic Strategies, *Epilepsia* 51(6):1069–1077, 2010.

Ochoa JG: Antiepileptic Drugs. Available at https://emedicine.medscape.com/article/1187334-overview. (Accessed March 22, 2018).

Perucca E: The pharmacological treatment of epilepsy: recent advances and future perspectives, *Perucca Acta Epileptologica* 3:22, 2021.

Riva A, Golda A, Balagura G, et al: New Trends and Most Promising Therapeutic Strategies for Epilepsy Treatment, *Frontiers in Neurology* 1-13, 2021.

Salanova V, et al: Long-term efficacy and safety of thalamic stimulation for drug resistant partial epilepsy, *Neurology* 84(10):1017–1025, 2015.

Scheffer IE, Berkovic S, Capovilla G, et al: ILAE classification of the epilepsies: Position Paper of the ILAE Commission for Classification and Terminology, *Epilepsia* 58:512–521, 2017.

SLEEP DISORDERS

Method of
**Meghna P. Mansukhani, MD; Bhanu Prakash Kolla, MD; and
Erik Kent St. Louis, MD, MS**

Sleep is a universal biological imperative for all mammals. Sleep deprivation and sleep disorders are frequent and underappreciated determinants of health status. Sleep is essential for survival, and sleep loss and sleep disorders are associated with major health problems, including cardiovascular, metabolic, neuropsychiatric, and neoplastic disorders, as well as neurobehavioral-associated accidents and risks. Healthy sleep must be regarded along with nutrition and exercise as key pillars for good health.

Recent evidence has suggested that a chief purpose of sleep may be to maintain cerebral metabolic homeostasis, clearing waste products that accumulate during wakefulness such as beta-amyloid, a protein known to abnormally accumulate in Alzheimer's disease. Insufficient sleep quantity appears to be associated with a variety of health problems and may contribute to mortality and dementia risk. Total sleep deprivation, as well as selective deprivation of nonrapid eye movement (NREM) or rapid eye movement (REM) sleep, may be lethal in laboratory animals. Adequate sleep quality is similarly necessary to ensure optimal daytime functioning because basic vigilance, attention and cognitive performance, and overall quality of life are each substantially eroded by disordered sleep, and insufficient sleep

and sleep-disordered breathing (SDB) pose significant health hazards. Unfortunately, insufficient sleep quantity and quality is a widespread public health crisis in children and adults worldwide in the developed world, and primary sleep disorders are a highly prevalent cause of morbidity, an important contributor to mortality, and a public health hazard that raises risk for motor vehicle collisions and catastrophic occupational injuries and accidents.

The clinical specialty of sleep medicine initially emerged during the 1970s and 1980s, surrounding growing clinical application of diagnostic polysomnography (PSG). While the main diagnostic use remains evaluation and initial treatment for SDB, PSG and related techniques have tremendous utility for the evaluation of selected patients with nocturnal events, periodic limb movement disorder (PLMD), narcolepsy and related primary central nervous system (CNS) hypersomnias.

In this chapter, we review the classification of common sleep disorders, a practical bedside approach toward interviewing and examining patients with sleep problems, advantages and limitations of diagnostic implements within the sleep laboratory, and summarize diagnostic and therapeutic approaches to common sleep disorders.

The International Classification of Sleep Disorders

The International Classification of Sleep Disorders (ICSD) provides a common nomenclature and taxonomy for disorders of sleep for clinicians and researchers alike. The most current ICSD, ICSD-3, divides sleep disorders into six distinct categories. The ICSD-3 nomenclature is shown in Box 1, and the most common sleep complaints and disorders are presented and discussed in detail throughout this chapter.

Clinical Approach to the Sleep Medicine Patient: The Interview and Examination

The three most common clinical presenting sleep-related complaints are hypersomnia, insomnia, and unusual behaviors or events at night (parasomnias). Hypersomnia, which is excessive sleepiness during waking hours, is often multifactorial and may be related to insufficient sleep quantity, quality, or timing; SDB; sedating medications; or certain medical, psychiatric, or neurologic conditions. Insomnia may be regarded as a problem in initiating or maintaining sleep under conditions that are normally conducive to sleep. Parasomnias are unusual behaviors that are often dangerous to the patient or bed partner during sleep.

Insomnia is a subjective complaint. To some patients it is not at all bothersome to require 20 to 30 minutes to fall asleep, while to others it seems very wrong. While insomnia is fundamentally a subjective symptom, the manifestations follow common patterns. Sleep latency, the time taken to fall asleep, varies significantly, but initial sleep latency longer than 30 minutes may be considered prolonged, once proper sleep-conductive conditions have been established (lights off, dark and quiet sleep environment without distracting stimuli). There is also significant variation in what degree of subjective sleep disruption reflects sleep-maintenance insomnia, as normal individuals may briefly awaken as often as 10 to 15 times each hour, with most such arousals being below the threshold of conscious awareness. Multiple nocturnal awakenings that are disturbing to the patient, especially when there is difficulty reinitiating sleep and prolonged wake after sleep-onset time, may be regarded as sleep-maintenance insomnia. Patients admitting to insomnia should be asked to estimate what amount of their problem is ascribable to an active mind or worries, restless legs, or body pain. Disturbing influences in the sleep environment such as the ambient light, temperature, and noise conditions in the bedroom should be sought. A precise diagnosis is not possible without detailed knowledge of sleep and wake behavior over the entire circadian cycle during a more protracted time, such as 1 to 2 weeks. A sleep diary can be very helpful in gaining needed insights for diagnosis. Increasingly, helpful information about

Insomnia
- Chronic insomnia disorder
- Short-term insomnia disorder
- Other insomnia disorder
  Isolated symptoms and normal variants
- Excessive time in bed
- Short sleeper

Sleep-Related Breathing Disorders
The continuum of obstructive sleep-disordered breathing: snoring, Upper-airway resistance syndrome, and obstructive sleep apnea (OSA)

Obstructive sleep apnea (OSA) disorders
- OSA, adult
- OSA, pediatric

Central sleep apnea syndromes
- Central sleep apnea with Cheyne-Stokes breathing
- Central apnea due to medical disorder without Cheyne-Stokes breathing
- Central sleep apnea due to high altitude periodic breathing
- Central sleep apnea due to a medication or substance
- Primary central sleep apnea
- Primary central sleep apnea of infancy
- Primary central sleep apnea of prematurity
- Treatment-emergent central sleep apnea

Sleep-related hypoventilation disorders
- Obesity hypoventilation syndrome
- Congenital central alveolar hypoventilation syndrome
- Late-onset central hypoventilation with hypothalamic dysfunction
- Idiopathic central alveolar hypoventilation
- Sleep-related hypoventilation due to a medication or substance
- Sleep-related hypoventilation due to a medical disorder
- Sleep-related hypoxemia disorder
  Isolated symptoms and normal variants
- Snoring
- Catathrenia

Central Disorders of Hypersomnolence
- Narcolepsy Type I
- Narcolepsy Type II
- Idiopathic hypersomnia
- Kleine-Levin syndrome
- Hypersomnia due to a medical disorder
- Hypersomnia due to a medication or substance
- Hypersomnia associated with a psychiatric disorder
- Insufficient sleep syndrome
  Isolated symptoms and normal variants
- Long sleeper

Circadian Rhythm Sleep-Wake Disorders
- Delayed sleep-wake phase disorder

- Advanced sleep-wake phase disorder
- Irregular sleep-wake rhythm disorder
- Non-24-hour sleep-wake rhythm disorder
- Shift work disorder
- Jet lag disorder
- Circadian rhythm sleep-wake disorder not otherwise specified

Parasomnias
NREM-related parasomnias
- Disorders of arousal (from NREM sleep)
- Confusional arousals
- Sleepwalking
- Sleep terrors
- Sleep-related eating disorder

REM-related parasomnias
- REM sleep behavior disorder
- Recurrent isolated sleep paralysis
- Nightmare disorder

Other parasomnias
- Exploding head syndrome
- Sleep-related hallucinations
- Sleep enuresis
- Parasomnia due to a medical disorder
- Parasomnia due to a medication or substance
- Parasomnia, unspecified
  Isolated symptoms and normal variants
- Sleep talking

Sleep-Related Movement Disorders
- Restless legs syndrome
- Periodic limb movement disorder
- Sleep-related leg cramps
- Sleep-related bruxism
- Sleep-related rhythmic movement disorder
- Benign sleep myoclonus of infancy
- Propriospinal myoclonus at sleep onset
- Sleep-related movement disorder due to a medical disorder
- Sleep-related movement disorder due to a medication or substance
- Sleep-related movement disorder, unspecified

Isolated symptoms and normal variants
- Excessive fragmentary myoclonus
- Hypnagogic foot tremor and alternating leg muscle activation
- Sleep starts (hypnic jerks)

Other Sleep Disorders
- Fatal familial insomnia
- Sleep-related epilepsy
- Sleep-related headaches
- Sleep-related laryngospasm
- Sleep-related gastroesophageal reflux
- Sleep-related myocardial ischemia

Abbreviations: CNS = central nervous system; NREM = non–rapid eye movement [sleep]; REM = rapid eye movement [sleep].

Sleep Disorders

843

timing and duration of sleep may be logged in applications for personal mobile computing devices.

The patient and physician may at times have difficulty differentiating between hypersomnia and complaints of fatigue (a sense of lacking enough energy to carry out usual daily activities, without the tendency toward dozing or nodding off inadvertently). A quick, incisive bedside test that helps distinguish between hypersomnia and fatigue is the Epworth Sleepiness Scale (ESS), a short questionnaire asking the patient his or her likelihood of dozing inadvertently during usual permissive daytime sedentary settings including reading, watching television, or traveling in a car. An online version is available at http://www.stanford.edu/~dement/epworth.html. Scores over 10 are considered abnormal and indicative of a possible underlying primary sleep disorder and suggest the need for further evaluation. Complaints of hypersomnia must be placed into the context of the sleep history with particular emphasis on the quantity, timing, and quality of sleep.

Patients may also present with complaints of disturbing or unusual activities during sleep (parasomnias). Key diagnostic points in determining the diagnosis for parasomnias include their onset, duration, frequency, time of night, stereotypy, injuries sustained, and whether there is any further behavioral change following the parasomnia episode.

Collateral history obtained from a bed partner may be particularly instructive. Patients should be asked whether they are reported to snore, whether the snoring is intermittent or constant, and if the snoring volume is related to sleeping in a supine position. Disruptive snoring loud enough to be heard outside a closed bedroom door, or witnessed stop-breathing episodes indicating apneas or self-awareness of arousals related to a snort or gasp, are particularly suggestive symptoms of obstructive sleep apnea (OSA). Symptoms such as morning dry mouth and sore throat, frequent morning headaches, or heartburn may indicate a higher likelihood of significant SDB. Patients should be asked about awareness of restless legs symptoms or movements during sleep, and whether they have been told of peculiar sleep-related behaviors or evidence of acting out their dreams, yelling or thrashing in sleep, or exhibiting sleep walking or other amnestic behaviors during sleep.

In addition to a detailed sleep history, taking a thorough general medical history is important because sleep disorders are frequently tightly linked to other diseases. OSA is closely associated with hypertension, coronary artery disease, cerebrovascular disease, atrial fibrillation, obesity, and the metabolic syndrome. Congestive heart failure, even when well compensated, is frequently associated with central sleep apnea syndrome. Restless legs syndrome and periodic limb movements in sleep (PLMS) are more common in patients with systemic iron deficiency or renal impairment, or in those with spinal cord or peripheral nerve pathologies. Hypoventilation is more prevalent in patients with neuromuscular disease; advanced obstructive lung disease; kyphosis; and in traumatic, vascular, neoplastic, or degenerative disorders that affect the medullary centers of the brain. Various genetic syndromes such as trisomy-21 produce craniofacial abnormalities predisposing to OSA due to anatomic narrowing of the upper airway.

Physical examination in sleep medicine focuses on signs indicating predisposition or associated sequelae of SDB. Careful inspection of the oropharynx and nares is particularly important because significant oropharyngeal narrowing is the chief anatomic substrate for obstructive SDB, while nasal septal deviation or other nasal obstruction, in addition to a thickened neck and overweight body habitus, may also contribute toward sleep apnea. Careful inspection for signs of neuromuscular disease, such as weakness of cervical flexor or extensor muscles, fasciculations or thoracoabdominal paradox, may help detect the underlying cause for sleep-related hypoventilation. Elevated blood pressure, a cardiac gallop, wet rales, and peripheral edema may be present as signs of systemic hypertension, heart failure, or cor pulmonale associated with untreated SDB.

Diagnostic Tools in the Sleep Laboratory
Polysomnography
Laboratory polysomnography (PSG) is the "gold standard" for formal assessment of suspected SDB, hypersomnia, or parasomnias. PSG is a diagnostic test most often performed in a sleep laboratory; attended by trained technicians; and combining evaluation of sleep, breathing, and movement. During PSG, several polygraphic physiologic variables are analyzed, including electroencephalography (EEG) as well as chin electromyography (EMG) to allow determination of sleep staging, limb EMG leads to analyze periodic leg movements that may disrupt sleep, oronasal airflow measured by a thermistor and nasal pressure sensors, electrocardiography, and respiratory effort measured by inductance plethysmography or piezocrystal monitors. Body position is also analyzed to delineate effects of sleeping position on breathing.

Each 30-second epoch of the PSG is subsequently scored by a sleep technologist as either wake, NREM sleep (N1 or N2

light NREM, or N3 slow wave sleep), or REM sleep according to well-defined guidelines. Sleep architecture, or the composition of sleep by different stages, varies greatly by age, but in middle-aged adults is approximately 60% to 75% N1-N2, 10% to 20% N3, and 15% to 25% REM sleep. Children usually have higher, and elderly individuals have lower, percentages of N3 and REM. Arousals from sleep and their mechanisms, whether due to breathing, movement, or spontaneous causes, are determined. Accordingly, a precise determination of the duration of a patient's total sleep time, sleep efficiency (total time spent asleep divided by time in bed), and disrupting influences on sleep, such as abnormal respiration or movement, may be determined. The effects of confounding medications and medical disorders on sleep architecture, such as selective-serotonin reuptake inhibitors (SSRI) that suppress and delay REM sleep, or benzodiazepines that reduce the N3 and REM amounts and increase sleep stage shifting leading to heightened light NREM N1 and N2, must also be considered.

Attended PSG is advantageous because it allows precise measurement of sleep and relevant cardiorespiratory and neurologic behaviors and allows intervention with therapeutic positive airway pressure (PAP) trials if indicated. Disadvantages of PSG include patient inconvenience, a foreign sleep environment, and expenses due to highly trained personnel and technology. For those patients whose disease severity is difficult to predict, or who may have other complicating medical illnesses that would render interpretation of an out-of-center cardiopulmonary sleep test inaccurate (such as those with significant cardiopulmonary or neurologic diseases), or those who may require noncontinuous PAP modalities, or for those with parasomnia symptoms, attended PSG and treatment design is needed. Split-night PSG remains a cost-effective strategy for many patients.

PSG is currently the only way to actually measure sleep; although the sleep state is currently defined by the variables measured in PSG (EEG, EMG, and EOG), the science of sleep medicine may develop other ways of characterizing the sleep state that are more convenient, precise, and correlate even better with health and disease.

Home Sleep Apnea Testing
PSG is comprehensive, but for patients with characteristic clinical presentations for OSA syndrome, it is often possible to arrive at a diagnosis using a significantly reduced number of recording channels that may be conducted in the home setting. A recent systematic review concluded that many commercially available home monitoring devices do not perform well in sensitivity or specificity. The best out-of-center testing devices use similar measures as PSG but exclude EEG, EMG, or EOG channels needed to score sleep. Thus, these devices typically measure at a minimum airflow using thermistors and nasal pressure transducers, breathing effort using respiratory impedance plethysmography, oxygen saturation using pulse oximetry, and snoring. Using these signals, the frequency of apneas and hypopneas per hour of recording, called the respiratory event index (REI), may be determined. Some testing devices add markers for sleep, such as actigraphy (see below), position sensors, or pattern recognition of pulse or autonomic variability to estimate sleep time (called peripheral arterial tonometry). Home sleep apnea testing (HSAT) devices are thus far only considered for evaluation of OSA syndrome and are not suitable for diagnostic evaluation of other sleep disorders. Because of limited sensitivity, they are best employed when there is a high pretest probability that the patient has at least moderately severe OSA syndrome. Patients appropriate for HSAT would be those who satisfy three criteria: have a high likelihood of having at least moderately severe OSA, will be good candidates for either autotitrating continuous PAP (CPAP) or an oral appliance, and do not have underlying diseases that either will obscure HSAT or who may have other disorders

that require PSG for diagnosis. Because of the poor sensitivity of HSAT, a negative result should be cause for PSG: the patient should have had a high pretest probability for having at least moderately severe OSA.

For medically uncomplicated patients fitting the above criteria, using HSAT followed by APAP most often leads to similar results as attended PSG with CPAP therapy based upon in-lab titration of pressure. This strategy is increasingly being used, largely owing to reduced costs. These good results depend, however, upon expert PAP mask fitting and follow-up. It is best to remember that treatment is chronic and requires ongoing follow-up. More is written about this in the section on OSA below.

Multiple Sleep Latency and Maintenance of Wakefulness Testing

The multiple sleep-latency test (MSLT) provides an objective measure of sleepiness compared with normal individuals lacking primary sleep disorders. The chief clinical indication for MSLT is for evaluation of narcolepsy and related primary CNS hypersomnias such as idiopathic hypersomnia and Kleine-Levin syndrome. A MSLT is carried out during the daytime in a sleep laboratory following nocturnal PSG, with four or five nap opportunities at standard times and intervals, usually at 9:00 and 11:00 AM and 1:00, 3:00, and 5:00 PM. Careful inspection of each nap is subsequently performed to determine the timing of sleep onset relative to commencement of each nap, and whether REM sleep occurs during each nap. A mean sleep latency is then calculated from the average initial sleep latency from each nap. Mean sleep latencies shorter than 8 minutes are considered abnormal and indicative of pathologic excessive daytime sleepiness. Whether or not a sleep-onset REM period (a SOREM, i.e., reaching REM sleep within 15 minutes of sleep onset during a nap) is captured is also considered and tabulated. More than one SOREM is abnormal and is consistent with the diagnosis of narcolepsy.

There are several considerations prior to performing and interpreting a valid MSLT. Patients should be instructed to sleep well for at least 2 weeks preceding the study, to allow at least 6 to 7 hours per night (and when possible, extending time in bed to 8-9 hours), and many sleep specialists document the quantity of sleep before the test with actigraphy monitoring or a sleep diary to ensure adherence to this recommendation and exclude the contaminating influence of insufficient sleep quantity. If it is safe and practically possible to do so, patients should be instructed to taper or discontinue sedative, stimulant, or REM suppressant medications (i.e., opiate analgesics, antidepressants, or other psychotropic or CNS active drugs) with the oversight and permission of other relevant treating primary care, psychiatry, and pain physicians at least 2 weeks prior to MSLT, and certain psychotropic drugs such as fluoxetine (Prozac) with a long elimination half-life should be discontinued for at least a month prior to MSLT to avoid decrease in MSLT sensitivity for delay of REM latency. Patients should undergo a full-night diagnostic PSG the night before a MSLT study to ensure that there is not another primary sleep disorder, such as SDB or PLMD, that could provide an alternative reason for significant sleepiness and to ensure that sufficient sleep quantity of 6 hours or more is obtained.

While the MSLT is designed to assess sleepiness, the maintenance of wakefulness test (MWT) is used to assess the ability to remain awake. The MWT is most useful when an objective measure of the effectiveness of treatment for disorders causing hypersomnolence is needed. The patient is seated in a dim room in a comfortable, semi-reclined position and asked to remain alert but passive for four 40-minute periods that are 2 hours apart. EEG, EOG, and chin EMG are measured, and the signals are analyzed to detect any epochs of unequivocal sleep during each 40-minute period. Normal patients have a mean time to epochs of unequivocal sleep of 30.4 minutes; however, the data is not normally distributed, and 42% of all patients remain awake for the entire 40 minutes on all four opportunities. Since simulated and actual driving performance is compromised with sleep times of 19 minutes or less on MWT, this is a reasonable threshold for the distinction of clinically significant daytime sleepiness, and driving or other safety sensitive tasks should be curtailed when sleep latencies are 19 minutes or shorter.

Actigraphy Monitoring

Wrist actigraphy monitoring is utilized to provide a rigorous estimation of sleep quantity and its circadian pattern. The actigraphy monitor may be worn like a wristwatch and contains an accelerometer that detects movements, which are recorded over time periods lasting up to weeks. The magnitude and pattern of movements may be analyzed and modeled to infer the sleep-wake pattern and provides a graphic representation of the patient's sleep schedule. The test is used in the evaluation of suspected circadian rhythm disorders, to assess response to treatment of insomnia, and for investigating patients with hypersomnia prior to PSG and MSLT to more accurately document the adequacy of sleep prior to the assessment for sleepiness. Recent applications utilizing the accelerometer in smartphones and wrist-worn fitness devices show promise, but most have not been validated as diagnostic tools.

Diagnostic and Therapeutic Approach to Common Sleep Disorders
Insomnia

The insomnia disorders all share three basic components: repeated complaints of insomnia, which may involve difficulties falling asleep, staying asleep, poor sleep quality, or waking undesirably early; an adequate time and opportunity for sleep; and a complaint of resultant daytime impairment. Insomnia is the most common of sleep complaints: nearly 45% of people were affected intermittently within the past year in some large studies, and up to 15% suffer chronic insomnia disorders. Risks for insomnia include female sex, older age, and a psychiatric or medical comorbidity. Chronic insomnia should be distinguished from short-term insomnia, which may occur in anyone occasionally (e.g., the night before an important job interview, or during increased stress). Per the ICSD-3, the sleep disturbance and associated daytime symptoms have to occur at least three times a week for at least three months to meet criteria for chronic insomnia disorder (see Box 1). Insomnia may begin in childhood, continue throughout a patient's lifetime, and appear as a manifestation of neurologic hyperarousal, with demonstrable increases in cerebral metabolism via functional MRI and increases in beta and theta EEG activity as well as generalized increased metabolism and stress hormone production compared with normals in either wake or sleep states. To a lesser extent, these same markers for hyperarousability are seen in other causes of primary insomnia (see Box 1).

In the past, insomnia was classified into primary and secondary, with secondary insomnia being far more common. Secondary insomnia was thought to be a result or accompaniment of an underlying illness. This may be incorrect. For example, it has previously been thought that treatment of secondary insomnia ought to focus on treatment of the underlying disorder. Newer evidence indicates that this approach may be suboptimal for the following reasons: secondary insomnia does not reliably improve when the underlying disorder does; secondary insomnia in general responds to treatment directed at insomnia; and in some cases, the underlying disorder, such as depression, responds better to treatment when the insomnia is addressed directly and concurrently. Furthermore, in several illnesses, such as depression, insomnia may predate the depression by months, and insomnia is a risk factor for future development of many psychiatric illnesses. In addition, primary insomnia was further divided into subtypes of idiopathic insomnia, psychophysiologic (learned) insomnia and paradoxical insomnia (sleep state misperception). Secondary insomnia was also divided into various subtypes such as inadequate sleep hygiene, insomnia due to medical condition, mental disorder, drug or substance. However, it is rare to encounter patients who fit under one of these subtypes exclusively. Most patients with insomnia, primary and secondary, tend to have some diagnostic criteria listed under many of these subtypes. Thus, in the current ICSD-3 insomnia is no longer classified into primary and secondary insomnia and no distinction is made between various etiologic subtypes of primary and secondary insomnia.

Chronic insomnia may be preceded in predisposed individuals by precipitating factors such as illness or stress and may be propagated by behavioral or maladaptive cognitive factors. Some individuals do not appear to require precipitating or propagating factors to develop chronic insomnia and have underlying redisposition toward insomnia. They are prototypic for an underlying predisposition toward insomnia. These individuals manifest insomnia from infancy and persist despite optimization of sleep hygiene and habit. However, in most cases of insomnia, precipitating and/or propagating influences may be found through careful interview and help establish a secure diagnosis.

In these individuals, identifiable precipitating causes that may be traumatic, stressful periods or struggles, medical illness, drugs, or toxins. However, even when the cause is removed, a conditioned response built upon associated and at times maladaptive sleep-related behaviors ensues. Instead of beginning to relax for sleep under permissive circumstances, the affected patient experiences paradoxical arousal as they approach their sleep conditions. The patient under the influence of the precipitating cause may have spent many hours worrying, uncomfortable, clock-watching, or otherwise raising their anxiety levels. Propagating factors include these same behaviors that help maintain sleeplessness once it has begun and may additionally include irregular sleep schedules and the use of drugs. Abuse of alcohol may contribute or be secondary to the sleep disturbance.

Effective treatment strategies for insomnia focus on removing any residual precipitating influences and mitigating or eliminating propagating influences. The main therapies for insomnia are sleep hygiene, behavioral therapies, cognitive therapies, and pharmacologic therapies. Patients often respond best to combined modalities. There is high-level evidence that combined cognitive/behavior therapies (CBT) are at least as effective as pharmacologic therapy for most patients with insomnia. CBT also appears to have enhanced rates of insomnia remission, so these approaches ought generally to be employed first. The addition of hypnotics to CBT has resulted in more rapid remission in some, but not all, studies. Growing recognition of the adverse effect profile of sedative-hypnotic drugs, particularly zolpidem (Ambien), which has been associated with heightened risks of falls and sleep walking, sleep eating, and related amnestic behaviors, has also encouraged a shift toward an earlier application of behavioral approaches to coping with insomnia.

In childhood, the most common causes of insomnia are behavioral. Insomnia may occur when parents fail to establish and enforce an appropriate nightly bedtime, so that their child may subsequently stall and refuse to go to bed in a timely fashion. In other cases, insomnia may occur when a child cannot fall asleep until a usual condition is present, such as being held, rocked, or fed. Appropriate advice and treatments include strict limit-setting for bedtime resistance; maintaining regular sleep schedules with avoidance of napping during the daytimes; and curtailing disrupting influences, such as television watching, gaming, and computer use. Suggesting a nightly cell phone or personal device (i.e., iPod, iPad, or Wii U) check-in procedure is especially helpful in teenage children, and caffeinated soda and excessively stimulating activities should be avoided during the evenings. Selected

children benefit from incentives such as a patient-parent contract that offers privileges for slightly later bedtimes on weekends after the child adheres regularly to a specified sleep schedule during school nights.

Four considerations for restoring normal sleep hygiene to discuss with all insomnia patients in the office include these three central concepts:

- Maintain a regular sleep schedule. Go to bed and arise at the same time each day. Ideally, the schedule should match the patient's biologic clock, with nocturnal sleep and bedtime/rise time matching their tendency for sleepiness and alertness (sleep education/hygiene).
- Avoid lying sleepless in bed. After 20 to 30 sleepless minutes spent trying to fall asleep, the patient should be instructed to leave the bedroom to pursue a quietly distracting activity, such as reading mundane material or watching a boring television program, and waiting until he or she feels sleepy enough to return to bed. Patients should explicitly avoid reading in bed, listening to the radio in bed, or watching television in bed if they are having difficulty initiating or maintaining sleep. This is a practical form of stimulus control (Table 1).
- Avoidance of clock-watching behavior. Patients should be instructed to remove clocks from their bedrooms or hide the clock face so as to make the insomnia period timeless and of uncertain duration. Falling asleep should not be a race against time, and repetitive checking of the time only serves to reinforce anxiety and further activate the mind (see stimulus control, Table 1). For the same reason, when watching television, discourage patients from watching news shows with scrolling tickertape newsflashes with clock time shown.
- Schedule thinking time earlier in the evening, well in advance of the sleep period. Patients who worry, plan, or think out their problems in bed should be encouraged to schedule a time earlier in the evening, well in advance of their normal bedtime, to attempt to work out these concerns prior to carrying them into bed. This "constructive worry" or "worry time" represents a practical form of cognitive and stimulus control therapy.

There are numerous other associated issues and behaviors that may be useful for application in selected patients, such as cutting down overall time in bed (sleep restriction), establishing a regular and relaxing bedtime routine (such as by taking a relaxing bath, listening to soothing music, or having a light snack before bed), avoiding daytime naps, avoiding caffeinated beverages after noontime, and establishing a regular morning exercise routine and avoiding evening exercise. It is important for the physician to avoid overloading the patient with too many considerations and tasks at once, however, as the burden of implementing these suggestions then becomes tantamount to too many obtrusive "swing thoughts" during a golf swing. One or two concepts to start with are sufficient, and once mastered and implemented, the patient can gradually phase in other ideas over time. Relaxation training and cognitive behavioral therapy can be very helpful in selected receptive patients who have failed the above typical self-help measures, and as a last resort, periodic or even scheduled chronic pharmacotherapy can also be implemented.

There are now several highly effective and tolerable hypnotic medications available for short-term, intermittent, and chronic use. The class of nonbenzodiazepine receptor agonists (the so-called "Z" drugs, or zolpidem [Ambien], zaleplon [Sonata], and eszopiclone [Lunesta]) are preferred by most sleep specialists but some of them remain costlier than the older generation choices, including the benzodiazepines—which have adverse effects on sleep architecture—as well as diphenhydramine (Benadryl) and trazodone (Desyrel),[1] which each have less specific

---

[1] Not FDA approved for this indication.

TABLE 1	Therapeutic Tools for Treating Insomnia	
THERAPY TYPE	**SPECIFIC THERAPIES/COMPONENTS**	**GOALS**
Education/sleep hygiene	Improve knowledge about behaviors that foster or hinder healthy sleep	Improve opportunity and environment for sleep
Behavioral therapies	Stimulus control • Unmodified extinction • Graduated extinction • Positive routines/faded bedtime with response cost • Scheduled awakenings • Sleep restriction	Dissociate anxiety or conditioned autonomic response from the process or location of going to sleep
	Relaxation training • Progressive muscle relaxation • Passive relaxation • Autogenic training-biofeedback • Imagery training • Meditation • Hypnosis • Paradoxical intention	Increase pressure for sleep by decreasing the time allotted for sleep, increasing the probability of successful sleep attempts Reduce physiologic and/or cognitive arousal that hinders or disrupts sleep Reduce performance anxiety that confounds ability to successfully go to sleep
Cognitive therapies	Cognitive restructuring Decatastrophizing Reappraisal Attention shifting	Decrease unrealistic expectations about sleep, misconceptions, or misattributions regarding causes of insomnia, consequences of insomnia, ability to control sleep; produce a more appropriate and adaptive mind-set
Pharmacologic therapies	Hypnotics Sedating antidepressants Herbal supplements	Enhance sleepiness at appropriate times or to enhance convenience of sleep time and/or duration

sleep-promoting effects and more adverse effects and potential for drug-drug interactions, especially in elderly patients. Zolpidem is now available in sublingual (Edluar) and mist (Zolpimist) formulations, as well. Intermediate- (Intermezzo) and long-acting preparations of zolpidem (Ambien CR) are also available that can be taken at bedtime to help with sleep onset and maintenance insomnia; the intermediate-acting preparation can be taken during a middle of the night awakening, provided there is at least 4 hours of sleep time remaining. The clinical pharmacology of the most commonly prescribed and most useful hypnotic medications are summarized in Table 2. A concern with each of these may be the potential for habituation of efficacy; fall risk; and the potential to cause sleepwalking, sleep eating, or other amnestic behaviors during sleep. If these adverse effects result, the hypnotic drug should be promptly discontinued with a shift toward the use of cognitive behavioral therapy strategies. In women, zolpidem should be used with particular caution given the slower metabolism of the drug, thereby promoting vulnerabilities to carryover sedation and unpleasant "hangover" type feelings or driving safety risks during the commute the next morning. Pharmacologic therapy of insomnia may be bolstered by the advent of suvorexant (Belsomra), a novel hypocretin antagonist that has a wake-suppressing rather than sleep-promoting mechanism of action. However, it should be noted that the higher doses that were primarily studied were determined as overly sedating and unsafe by the FDA and only the lower doses were approved. Further clinical experience will likely be necessary to establish the role of this medication as a treatment for insomnia.

Sleep-Disordered Breathing

Breathing during sleep is carefully regulated to maintain homeostasis of oxygen, carbon dioxide, and blood pH. The mechanisms and homeostatic set points for ventilation vary systematically between wake, non-REM sleep, and REM sleep. In wake, the resulting ventilatory pattern is governed by careful integration of classic feedback systems designed to keep blood pH at approximately 7.40, arterial $PaCO_2$ at approximately 38 to 45 mm Hg, and PaO_2 greater than approximately 60 mm Hg with cortical influences that govern functions such as speaking, laughing, eating, singing, and other voluntary activities. During non-REM sleep, ventilation is considerably more rhythmic and is governed almost exclusively by the chemoresponsive feedback systems indicated above; during REM sleep, the chemoresponsive feedback system is further influenced by additional input from REM-influenced neurons, resulting in a less rhythmic and less-carefully regulated metabolic milieu.

Significant deviation from these norms is termed "sleep-disordered breathing" (SDB), and is marked by several distinct event types. Apneas are total or near-total cessations of airflow. Hypopneas are significant declines in tidal volume sufficient to result in significant reduction in oxygenation. Excess effort for breathing may result in arousals from and disturbance of sleep, and are termed respiratory effort-related arousals (RERAs). These types of events are often related as a rate, either as the apnea-hypopnea index (AHI; apneas+hypopneas per hour of sleep), the respiratory disturbance index (apneas+hypopneas+RERAs per hour of sleep), or the REI (apneas+hypopneas per hour of recording when sleep is not measured directly). In addition to these types of SDB, the general baseline minute ventilation may fall to the point where sustained hypoventilation takes place during sleep, termed sleep-related alveolar hypoventilation.

Obstructive SDB: Snoring and OSA

The dynamic upper-airway obstruction, which occurs as a result of sleep in some persons, leads to a continuum of SDB varying from mild snoring to hypopneas to obstructive apneas. The likelihood and extent of upper-airway collapse is determined by the neural input into the dilating upper-airway muscles, influence of sleep state, and upper-airway anatomy. Obstructive events are

TABLE 2 Clinical Pharmacology of Hypnotic Medications

	MECHANISM OF ACTION	DOSAGE (MG)	DURATION OF ACTION ($T^{1/2}$)	TYPICAL ADVERSE EFFECTS	INTERACTIONS
Diphenhydramine (Benadryl)	H1	25–50	Intermediate (2.4–9.3 h)	Dry mouth, constipation, urinary retention	Nonsignificant
Trazodone (Desyrel)[1]	SRI	50–150	Short (3–6 h)	Dry mouth, dizziness, rash	CYP substrate; several others
Triazolam (Halcion)	BRA	0.125–0.5	Short (1.5–5.5 h)	Tolerance	CYP induction
Temazepam (Restoril)	BRA	7.5–30	Intermediate (8–18 h)	Tolerance	Nonsignificant
Melatonin[2]	MT1–MT2	1–3	Ultra-short (35–50 min)	Hangover type effect	None
Zolpidem (Ambien)	NBRA	5, 10	Short (2–2.6 h)	Amnestic behavior	Numerous
Zaleplon (Sonata)	NBRA	5, 10	Short (1 h)	Headache, amnestic behavior	Several
Eszopiclone (Lunesta)	NBRA	1–3	Intermediate (6 h)	Headache, amnestic behavior, rash possible	Nonsignificant
Ramelteon (Rozerem)	MT1-MT2	8, 16[3]	Short (1–2.6 h)	Hyperprolacti nemia	Ketoconazole (Nizoral), rifampin
Doxepin (Silenor)	H1	3,6	Intermediate (12-15 h)	Dizziness, tachycardia	Nonsignificant
Suvorexant (Belsomra)	Orexin antagonist	10-20	Intermediate (12 h)	Headache, dizziness, abnormal dreams	CYP3A4 inducer
Lemborexant (Dayvigo)	Orexin antagonist	5-10	Intermediate (≤7 h)	Drowsiness, fatigue, headache	CYP3A4 substrate
Daridorexant (Quviviq)	Orexin antagonist	25–50	Intermediate (8 h)	Drowsiness, fatigue	CYP3A4 substrate

Abbreviations: $t^{1/2}$=half-life of drug; h=hours; H1=antihistaminergic H1 receptor blocker; SRI=serotonin reuptake inhibitor; BRA=benzodiazepine receptor agonist; CYP substrate=metabolized by cytochrome metabolism, susceptible to enzyme inhibition and elevated serum levels by multiple drugs; CYP induction=cytochrome enzyme inducer, may cause multiple potential drug-drug interactions via this mechanism; NBRA=nonbenzodiazepine benzodiazepine receptor agonist; MT1/MT2=melatonin type 1 and type 2 receptor agonist.

[1]Not FDA approved for this indication.
[2]Available as dietary supplement.
[3]Exceeds dosage recommended by the manufacturer.

more likely to occur in REM sleep when muscle tone is lowest, during transitions from lighter non-REM sleep to deep non-REM sleep when sleep is unstable, or when muscle tone is decreased by substances such as alcohol or drugs. The single biggest risk factor for snoring or OSA is obesity, wherein fatty deposition reduces upper-airway dimension, humoral factors reduce net dilating forces of the muscles, and the mechanical effects of obesity reduce lung volumes and the stabilizing effect of tracheal traction on the upper airway. Beyond obesity, many but not all patients have a predisposing anatomy of a narrowed oropharynx, such as a low-lying palate or redundant soft palate tissue, a thickened tongue base, or a narrow hypopharynx, although nasal anatomy with septal deviation or chronic congestion may also aggravate the problem.

Snoring without other symptoms, signs, or polysomnographic evidence of upper-airway obstructions such as hypersomnia, frequent associated arousals, or significant airflow limitation is termed primary snoring. While snoring may be a socially objectionable symptom or disruptive to the patient's sleep partner, snoring in isolation is otherwise not considered to be abnormal and such patients may be reassured if their bed partners are not bothered by their snoring. If treatment is desired, options include relieving nasal obstruction if present, commercially available lubricant throat sprays, mandibular positioning devices, and nasal or upper-airway surgical approaches such as nasal septal repair or uvulopalatopharyngoplasty (UPPP, or UP3 procedure). An otorhinolaryngology consultation may be helpful in determining which surgical approaches may be most beneficial for the individual.

OSA is an extremely common public health problem present in at least 2% to 4% of the general population and has been linked to development of hypertension and is a risk factor for incidental development of stroke, coronary artery disease, congestive heart failure, and atrial fibrillation. OSA has been shown to be associated with a wide variety of endothelial and metabolic abnormalities that favor vascular disease, and when patients with moderate to severe OSA are compared to normals or treated OSA patients, they appear to have a higher mortality and cardiovascular event frequency. Thus, the two main reasons to detect and treat OSA are to improve symptoms and to decrease cardiovascular risks. There are good data to show that treatment of OSA improves symptoms and quality of life. Data regarding the reversal of cardiovascular risk are not as firm, but most experts agree that at least moderate and severe OSA ought to be treated, regardless of symptom severity.

OSA severity is rated by the polysomnographic AHI, the hourly rate of apneas and hypopneas averaged over the total sleep time, or, in the case of HSAT, by the REI. An AHI of 4 per hour or less is considered normal. Mild OSA is diagnosed with an AHI of 5 to 14 per hour, moderate OSA with AHI of 15 to 29 per hour, and severe OSA with AHI being 30 per hour or higher. In most laboratories, correlation of the AHI with specific sleep stages and body positions is usually performed to determine whether positional therapy may be offered, as many patients have OSA only during the supine sleep position (position-dependent OSA), and some manifest OSA only during REM sleep in the supine position.

A form of OSA called the upper-airway resistance syndrome is defined by a clinical complaint of hypersomnia, often accompanied by snoring but without an abnormally high frequency of overt apneas or hypopneas resulting in significant decline in oxygen saturation. PSG confirms repetitive arousals related to the increased respiratory effort (respiratory effort-related arousals, or RERAs, during PSG) required to overcome upper-airway obstruction. Because of the similar pathogenesis and treatment response to relieve upper-airway obstruction, this is considered a variant of OSA.

Therapeutic options for snoring and sleep apnea include reducing nasal congestion or obstruction, positional therapy, nasal continuous positive airway pressure, oral appliances, the nasal expiratory positive airway pressure device, oral pressure therapy (OPT), or surgical management (Table 3). Patients with OSA have higher morbidity from vascular events and higher motor vehicle accident rates. Assessment and appropriate counseling for weight loss, cardiovascular risk factors, and driving while untreated (or extreme caution) should be part of a treatment plan.

Weight loss. Weight loss may reduce soft tissue in the neck, making the oropharynx less compressible. The improvement in lung volumes accompanied by weight loss also favor enhancement of longitudinal traction on the upper airway, the so-called "tracheal tug." About 30% to 40% of patients who are able to achieve substantial weight loss may become cured of their OSA. Careful follow-up is needed because many remissions are not permanent. Alcohol and other substances that reduce upper-airway tone or cause sedation or reduced responsiveness worsen OSA and should be prudently avoided.

Positional therapy. Among the lifestyle or behavioral changes, positional therapy involves employing one or more simple strategies to enforce sleep only in nonsupine body positions, usually on the side. One method is the "tennis ball in T-shirt" approach. The patient wears a snug-fitting T-shirt with a pocket sewn onto the back between the shoulder blades with two or three tennis or wiffle balls inserted into it to discourage the patient from turning onto the back during sleep. Other options include similar commercially marketed shirts or vests (the FDA-approved ZZoma sleep apnea pillow, the "snoring backpack," and similar strategies) and body pillows propped or wedged behind the patient or hugged by the patient. A correctional device for positional sleep apnea is also approved in the European Union. Unfortunately, shoulder or hip pain often limits the application of positional therapy, especially in elderly persons, and long-term adherence or compliance remains poor, with only about one-third of patients able to perpetuate positional therapy strategies in long-term follow-up. Patients with position-dependent OSA should be counseled to be cautious for development of severe OSA problems during any future anticipated prolonged periods of supine sleep, such as postoperative recovery periods following surgery or following a major injury.

Positive airway pressure. The mainstay of treatment for OSA for the majority of patients remains positive airway therapy (PAP). The main components of PAP appliances are the blower unit, which delivers calibrated pressures to hold open the airway; tubing to conduct the pressurized air to the patient; an interface such as a nasal or oronasal mask; and a harness to hold the mask firmly to the patient's face during use. Of the PAP therapies, continuous positive airway pressure (CPAP), which delivers a continuous set pressure between 5 and 20 cm H_2O, is usually first tried in the setting of PSG; in many sleep centers, the practice of performing split-night PSG (an initial diagnostic phase followed by a treatment phase of CPAP titration toward an optimal pressure for the individual patient) allows diagnosis and treatment

prescription to occur in an efficient manner. If an optimal pressure cannot be determined by laboratory titration or data is not available to guide prescription of a specific pressure for a patient, application of an autotitrating PAP device may be considered, offering flexibility for delivering a relatively wide range of self-adjusting treatment pressures as the patient changes sleep position and enters different sleep stages through the night with accordingly varying apnea severity. Autotitrating PAP has been found to be efficacious in most patients diagnosed with OSA by HSAT. However, close clinical follow-up is needed in all patients who have recently started PAP.

PAP is typically delivered through an interface chosen as most comfortable by the patient, either a nasal mask, nasal pillows, or an oronasal. Nasal pillows, a type of cannula that provides a tight seal within the nares, and a newer tube-like frame that sits in front of and not within the nares are most effective at lower treatment pressures; they may be favored by many patients with claustrophobia but may dislodge at higher pressures or with frequent nocturnal movement. Nasal masks of various types are used in many patients, but if mouth breathing and consequent leak are a problem, a chin strap may be added, or an oronasal face mask may be substituted. Many newer PAP machines offer the feature of pressure relief during exhalation, which may enhance patient tolerability at higher level PAP pressures by "giving way" as the patient expires. Bilevel positive airway pressure (BPAP) may also be employed at higher treatment pressures if CPAP is not well tolerated. Setting a pressure delta ≥4 cm between the inspired and expired pressure may also add a degree of positive pressure ventilation for patients with concurrent sleep-related hypoventilation from an intrinsic pulmonary disease or neuromuscular respiratory muscle weakness.

The FDA recently approved the use of tirzepatide (Zepbound), a gluucaon-like-peptide-1 agonist, for the treatment of moderate to severe OSA in adults with obesity, to be used in conjunction with dietary and physical activity measures for weight loss.

Oral appliances. Oral appliances may be fitted by a dental sleep specialist. They provide a means of advancing the mandible that pull the tongue base forward slightly, opening the oropharyngeal airway to some degree and obviating some apnea and hypopnea events. The device is most effective for mild to moderate severity and supine position-dependent OSA and generally less predictably effective for most cases of severe OSA. However, the use of oral appliances is increasing due to greater availability of competent dental professionals working with the devices, awareness that for some patients adherence is better with OAs than PAP, and improvements in appliance design that allow enhanced efficacy in some instances. Because oral appliances are less reliably effective in controlling SDB, repeat testing—either with out-of-center sleep testing or PSG after maximal adjustment—is needed to confirm efficacy.

Nasal valve appliances. An expiratory nasal resistance valve appliance (Provent) was approved by the FDA for treatment of OSA. The device may be an alternative for some patients with OSA who fail to tolerate CPAP therapy. The device is a small, disposable oval appliance that is affixed over each of the patient's nares by self-adhesive with an airflow port that offers resistance to expiratory airflow, thereby producing expiratory positive airway pressure and preserving nasal and oropharyngeal airway patency with minimal impedance to inspiratory airflow. The device was proven to significantly reduce polysomnographic AHI and subjective sleepiness on the ESS in a sham-controlled randomized trial. Because they are disposable, a new device must be affixed each night. Appropriate patient characteristics and long-term results are not yet clear, but these may be considered in patients who do not prefer CPAP or oral appliances and are agreeable to follow-up to ensure efficacy.

Oral pressure therapy. A newer option for treatment of mild to moderate OSA is OPT (Winx), which combines an oral appliance with negative intraoral pressure to help keep the tongue and soft palate in a more anterior position, enlarging the retrolingual

| TABLE 3 | Treatment of Sleep-Related Breathing Disorders |

SLEEP-RELATED BREATHING DISORDER	TREATMENT MODALITY		GOAL
OSA syndrome	Lifestyle/behavior modification	• Weight loss	Reduced weight may result in improvement airway patency
		• Alcohol avoidance	Alcohol worsens OSA; avoidance of exacerbating factor is encouraged
	Positive airway pressure	• Positional therapy	Enhance airway patency by nonsupine sleeping
		• Continuous positive airway pressure (CPAP)	Counteract collapsing forces in upper airway; "stent" open the upper airway
		• Bilevel positive airway pressure (BPAP)	End expiratory pressure stents open airway; inspiratory pressure enhances minute ventilation or decreases hypopneas
	Upper airway stimulation	Inspire™	Stimulation to upper airway muscles during sleep resulting in increased airway patency
		• Autotitrating positive airway pressure (APAP)	Uses feedback algorithms to adjust pressure in response to airway conditions in order to provide airway patency with minimal mean pressure
	Oral appliances	• Mandibular positioning devices • Tongue retention devices	Enhance airway patency by stabilizing lateral pharyngeal walls and enhancing AP airway dimensions at the velopharyngeal level
	Surgical modification of the upper airway	• Palatal surgeries (uvulopalatopharyngo plasty, others)	Enhance airway patency by reconfiguring soft tissues and/or skeletal structures
		• Maxillo-mandibular advancement	Enhance airway patency by reconfiguring soft tissues and skeletal structures
Central sleep apnea syndromes	Correct underlying disorders (treat heart failure, etc.)	• Various	Reduce stimuli to ventilatory hyperresponsiveness
	Gases	• Oxygen	Reduce responsiveness to variation in CO_2
	Positive airway pressure	• CPAP	Reduce stimulation to ventilate by decreasing lung water, improving V/Q matching, reducing airway resistance
	Transvenous phrenic nerve stimulation (Remede)	• Noninvasive positive pressure ventilation (NIPPV), also referred to as BPAP-ST (Avoid in heart failure patients with ejection fraction<45%)	Provide ventilatory assistance in order to avoid hypercapnia/hypoxemia associated with central apneas or hypopneas, thus reducing hyperventilatory feedback
		• Adaptive servoventilation (Avoid in heart failure patients with ejection fraction<45%)	Provide ventilatory assistance in proportion to needs, reducing or eliminating variability in ventilation and ventilatory drive; avoid hypercapnia/hypoxemia associated with central apneas or hypopneas, thus reducing hyperventilatory feedback.
			Cause diaphragmatic contraction, creating a negative intrathoracic pressure mimicking a normal breathing pattern and augmenting airflow to decrease central apnea.
Hypoventilation syndromes	Positive airway pressure	• Noninvasive positive pressure ventilation (NIPPV), also referred to as BPAP-ST	Provide ventilatory assistance in order to avoid hypercapnia/hypoxemia associated with central apneas or hypopneas
		• Tracheostomy with mechanical ventilation	Provide ventilatory assistance in order to avoid hypercapnia/hypoxemia associated with central apneas or hypopneas, protect or control airway

and retropalatal space. There is as yet limited experience with the device; however, this may be an option for some patients who are averse to or intolerant of other therapies.

Surgery. Surgical modifications of the upper airway are principally of two basic approaches, palatal approaches, tongue-based procedures (genioglossus advancement, hyoid myotomy and suspension, lingualplasty), or maxillomandibular advancement (MMA). Palatal approaches such as UPPP, or "UP3" performed by otorhinolaryngologists are effective for relief of snoring but mostly ineffective for treatment of OSA, especially if severity is

moderate or greater in degree. MMA appears to be quite effective in mild to moderate OSA and can even be applied with good effect even in selected severe OSA cases; however, morbidity from perioperative pain is considerable and long-term outcomes remain unclear. A hypoglossal nerve stimulation implant (Inspire) is a novel surgical treatment for PAP-intolerant patients. A randomized controlled trial published in 2014 demonstrated efficacy and reasonable tolerability; because this device was only recently FDA approved, there is limited clinical experience with it. This treatment is indicated for patients with moderate to severe OSA

(AHI 15-65/hour), with an inability to tolerate PAP, less than 25% central disordered breathing events, and lack of concentric collapse on drug-induced sedated endoscopy. It is more effective in patients with a BMI less than 32, but those with a BMI 32 to 35 kg/m² may be eligible. The reduction in AHI is about two-thirds, and one in three patients who are deemed to be candidates do not respond to the treatment. Follow-up PSGs are generally required to titrate stimulation settings. Side effects may include tongue discomfort and headache.

Central Sleep Apnea Syndrome

Central sleep apnea syndrome results from an unstable ventilatory drive during sleep, resulting in periods of insufficient ventilation and compromise of gas exchange despite a patent oropharyngeal airway. Clinically, patients may share similar symptoms with those with OSA, including snoring, except patients with central sleep apnea more frequently complain of insomnia than hypersomnia. Central sleep apnea has a heterogeneous pathophysiology and may be idiopathic or due to high-altitude-induced periodic breathing, due to Cheyne-Stokes breathing, or narcotic-induced. Neurologic causes—such as brainstem infarction or neurodegenerative disorders, including multiple system atrophy—may also cause central apnea. In heart failure, the presence of central sleep apnea syndrome or Cheyne-Stokes breathing imparts a poor prognosis. A high-quality clinical trial showed that on average, CPAP did not reduce mortality. However, central sleep apnea is often at least partially resistant to treatment with conventional nasal CPAP therapy, and while CPAP may effect improved mean oxygenation, frequent arousals that fragment sleep often continue. However, a recent large multicenter randomized control trial, the SERVE-HF study, showed elevated all-cause and cardiovascular mortality risk in patients with central sleep apnea and symptomatic heart failure with an estimated ejection fraction of ≤45% who were randomized to ASV. Therefore, use of ASV in this patient population is not advised at the current time. Remede, a phrenic nerve stimulator, has recently been approved by the FDA as a treatment option in selected cases with central sleep apnea.

Treatment-Emergent Central Sleep Apnea Syndrome

Treatment-emergent central sleep apnea syndrome is a subtype of central sleep apnea wherein patients have significant obstructive/anatomical problems with ventilation, but also have unstable ventilatory patterns noted in patients with central sleep apnea syndromes. These patients have a clinical and PSG presentation of OSA, but once the upper airway is opened with CPAP, they experience frequent central apneic events that may or may not later resolve with continued exposure to PAP in the home setting. Some patients clearly continue to manifest frequent central sleep apneic events more than five times per hour, leading to the suboptimal outcomes of persisting clinical complaints of hypersomnia and medical risk. Treatment-emergent central sleep apnea syndrome may occur in as many as 4% to 15% of those with OSA. There is emerging evidence that alternative modes of PAP—particularly ASV—may be superior to conventional CPAP for treatment of treatment-emergent central sleep apnea syndrome. A randomized controlled trial recently showed that ASV more reliably relieves SDB, while CPAP fails to control SDB in up to one-third of cases. However, there is also evidence to suggest that treatment-emergent central sleep apnea resolves over time in a substantial number of patients who continue to remain on CPAP therapy.

Sleep-Related Hypoventilation

The causes of hypoventilation during sleep include primary pulmonary parenchymal disorders, neuromuscular conditions affecting bellows musculature, or restrictive physiology of the chest wall accompanying kyphoscoliotic disorders or morbid obesity. While each of these disorders may also ultimately cause daytime hypoventilation, sleep recumbency, especially supine sleep positioning, and REM sleep stage (which leads to relative paralysis of the chest wall and sole dependency on diaphragmatic excursion to drive respiratory effort) often lead to exclusive or initial sleep-related hypoventilation with subsequent medical risk consequent to suboptimal nocturnal oxygenation. Failure to treat significant nocturnal hypoventilation may result in the development of sequelae of hypoxemia such as polycythemia, pulmonary hypertension, and right heart failure, or of hypercapnic respiratory failure. Treatment most often involves use of NIPPV (see Table 4). A newer modality of positive pressure ventilation, volume-assured pressure support ventilation (AVAPS™), consists of a short delivery of a provider-set tidal volume, which, when coupled with a set backup respiratory rate, assures delivery of a minimum minute ventilation, even when changes in the patient's muscular strength or ventilatory load change. These therapies are best titrated in the context of a supervised overnight laboratory polysomnogram under the direction of a sleep or pulmonary medicine specialist. One must be careful not to resort to the potentially dangerous solution of added oxygen therapy alone in severe COPD or neuromuscular etiologies of sleep-related hypoventilation, because as ventilation fails and hypercapnea results, the hypoxic drive to breathe may become the chief factor leading to continued ventilatory effort and oxygen in this context may precipitate acute respiratory failure in some individuals. A morning arterial blood gas on room air following PSG is indicated to assess for potential hypercapnia and assess the impact of ventilatory support. In the context of severe hypercapnia (i.e., Pco_2 of 55 or greater), serial arterial blood gases to monitor the effects of ventilatory support, oxygenation, and accumulating hypercapnia may help determine whether nocturnal mechanical ventilatory support is indicated.

Narcolepsy and Central Disorders of Hypersomnolence

Narcolepsy is the prototypical central disorder of hypersomnolence. Narcolepsy is categorized further as Narcolepsy Type I (previously called narcolepsy with cataplexy) and Narcolepsy Type II (previously called narcolepsy without cataplexy). Cataplexy is a distinctive and highly specific symptom characterized by emotionally provoked muscle atonia intruding into wakefulness that is seen in a minority of patients overall and may precede but more often follows onset of the main symptom of hypersomnia. In the absence of cataplexy, a diagnosis of Narcolepsy Type I may also be made if cerebrospinal fluid (CSF) hypocretin-1 concentration, measured by immunoreactivity, is <110 pg/mL or <1/3 of mean values obtained in normal subjects with the same standardized assay. In Narcolepsy Type II, there is no cataplexy, and the CSF hypocretin level does not meet the above criteria or has not been measured. In addition to sleepiness and cataplexy, the full clinical pentad of narcolepsy also includes symptoms of sleep paralysis (the inability to move the body upon awakening), hypnogogic hallucinations (the intrusion of dream imagery and mentation into conscious awareness following awakening), and sleep-maintenance insomnia (with frequent nocturnal arousals and difficulty maintaining sleep). However, narcolepsy is most frequently monosymptomatic, with the sole symptom being pervasive, enduring sleepiness and decreased vigilance with a tendency toward dozing off inadvertently in permissive settings and the overwhelming desire to nap during the daytime, especially in the afternoons. Naps are most often highly refreshing; scheduled naps can be utilized to therapeutic advantage or indeed, in rare patients, as the sole treatment for those bent on avoiding stimulant pharmacotherapy. Narcolepsy is relatively uncommon, affecting approximately 1:2000 of the general population. While the etiology of narcolepsy remains unknown, most experts continue to favor a long hypothesized autoimmune cause. Major advances in the understanding of the neurobiology of narcolepsy over the past two decades have included the clear linkage of the HLA DQB1*0602 haplotype in up to 90% patients having narcolepsy with cataplexy, discovery of wake-promoting hypocretin/

TABLE 4	Clinical Pharmacology of Stimulant and Wake-Promoting Medications				
	MECHANISM OF ACTION	DOSAGE (MG)	DURATION OF ACTION ($T\frac{1}{2}$)	TYPICAL ADVERSE EFFECTS	INTERACTIONS
Modafinil (Provigil)	Unknown	100–600[3]	Intermediate (15 h)	Tremor, jitteriness, palpitations, hypertension	Oral contraceptives
Armodafinil (Nuvigil)	Unknown	150–450[3]	Intermediate (15 h)	Tremor, jitteriness, palpitations, hypertension	Oral contraceptives
Pitolisant (Wakix)	Histamine-3 receptor inverse agonist/ antagonist	8.9-35.6 mg	Long (8-24 h)	Headache, nausea, insomnia	Antihistamines, oral contraceptives, CYP2D6 inhibitors, CYP3A4 inducers, mirtazapine, TCAs and other QT-prolonging agents
Solriamfetol (Sunosi)	DNRI	75-150 mg	Intermediate (7 h)	Headache, nausea, anxiety, insomnia	Dopamine agonists, CNS stimulants, sympathomimetics, esketamine, MAOIs, SNRIs, bupropion
Methylphenidate (Ritalin)	DNRI	15–100[3]	Short (2–4 h)	Tremor, jitteriness, palpitations, hypertension	Nonsignificant
Methylphenidate SR (Concerta)[1]	DNRI	18–72	Intermediate (3.5 h)	Tremor, jitteriness, palpitations, hypertension	Nonsignificant
Amphetamine/ dextroamphetamine (Adderall)	DNRI	15–100[3]	Intermediate (10–13 h)	Tremor, jitteriness, palpitations, hypertension, QTc prolongation	Beware MAOIs, SSRIs, SNRIs, TCAs, bupropion (Wellbutrin)
Dextroamphetamine (Dexedrine)	DNRI	15–100[3]	Long (10–28 h)	Tremor, jitteriness, palpitations, hypertension, QTc prolongation	Beware MAOIs, SSRIs, SNRIs, TCAs, bupropion
Lisdexamfetamine (Vyvanse)[1]	DNRI	20–100[3]	Short (<1 h as prodrug) (10–28 h as dextroamphetamine)	Tremor, jitteriness, palpitations, hypertension, QTc prolongation	Beware MAOIs, SSRIs, SNRIs, TCAs, bupropion
Methamphetamine (Desoxyn)[1]	DNRI	15–100[3]	Intermediate (9–15 h)	Tremor, jitteriness, palpitations, hypertension, QTc prolongation	Beware MAOIs, SSRIs, SNRIs, TCAs, bupropion

[1]Not FDA approved for this indication.
[3]Exceeds dosage recommended by the manufacturer.
Abbreviations: $t\frac{1}{2}$=half-life of drug; h=hours; DNRI=dopamine and norepinephrine monoamine reuptake inhibitor; QTc=corrected QT interval; MAOI=monoamine oxidase inhibitor; SSRI=serotonin selective reuptake inhibitor; SNRI=selective norepinephrine reuptake inhibitor; TCA=tricyclic antidepressant (the potential interaction with all these agents is largely theoretical concern for potentiation of serotonin syndrome).

orexin peptides produced by the perifornical posterolateral hypothalamus, and low to unmeasurable CSF hypocretin in nearly 90% of narcolepsy with cataplexy patients. Within the last few years, epidemic narcolepsy-cataplexy following H1N1 vaccination in Europe and Asia also provided further support for the autoimmune hypothesis of narcolepsy. Unfortunately, these tantalizing discoveries have not yet yielded clear insight into pathogenic mechanisms nor more specific therapies for patients, and the mainstay of treatment for the condition remains the use of older stimulant and wake-promoting medications, or prescribed therapeutic napping, as naps are most often highly refreshing and restorative in narcolepsy patients. Supportive laboratory evidence for narcolepsy includes a relatively normal polysomnogram to exclude other causes of hypersomnia such as OSA or PLMD, followed by a confirmatory MSLT, which demonstrates mean sleep latency shorter than 8 minutes and two or more sleep-onset REM periods during four or five nap opportunities.

Idiopathic hypersomnia is a closely related condition often difficult to distinguish from narcolepsy without cataplexy, although a few nuanced clinical features tend to distinguish it from narcolepsy, chiefly a characteristically reported unrefreshing nocturnal sleep and nap quality. Idiopathic hypersomnia has previously been further subclassified as variants with or without prolonged sleep period, although these phenotypes are overlapping and current diagnostic standards have eliminated this distinction. Other similar enigmatic and poorly understood primary CNS hypersomnias include posttraumatic hypersomnia when there is a history of temporally related antecedent substantial head injury, and recurrent hypersomnia, also known as the Kleine-Levin syndrome, which in addition to hypersomnia includes other neuropsychiatric sequelae such as cognitive and behavioral changes like hypersexuality and hyperphagia. Hypersomnia is also commonly associated with as many as 50% of those with myotonic dystrophy type 1.

The mainstay of treatment for each of these conditions is stimulant and wake-promoting agent therapy, with the goal of improved vigilance and psychomotor functioning. Stimulants and wake-promoting agents range in intensity from lower to higher intensity and efficacy/tolerability options, from modafinil (Provigil) and armodafinil (Nuvigil) on the milder end of the spectrum—although selected narcolepsy patients respond quite well to these drugs—to methylphenidate (Ritalin), and to the amphetamine/dextroamphetamine (Adderall). Relevant clinical pharmacology of the stimulant medications commonly used in clinical practice are summarized in Table 4. Patients with uncontrolled hypersomnias should be cautioned against driving, operating dangerous machinery, or engaging in other similarly dangerous activities or hobbies while they are drowsy, as they may be prone to sudden and unpredictable sleep attacks. Sodium oxybate (gamma hydroxy butyrate) is an FDA approved tightly controlled substance for the treatment of sleepiness and cataplexy in patients with narcolepsy. Sodium oxybate (Xyrem) is usually given in two divided doses, before bedtime and in the middle of the night; it can be dangerous in the setting of uncontrolled OSA or respiratory conditions and central nervous system depressants. An extended-release preparation, Lumryz, is now available as an extended-release sodium oxybate preparation taken once nightly at bedtime, starting at 4.5 g and increased by 1.5 g at weekly intervals as needed to a maximum of 9 g. Another oxybate salts product (Xywav) was recently FDA approved for the treatment of idiopathic hypersomnia and narcolepsy. For idiopathic hypersomnia, it can be taken once (≤3 g at bedtime) or twice nightly (≤2.25 g at bedtime and then 4 hours later) and gradually increased in increments of ≤1.5 g per night weekly up to a maximum of 6 g nightly. For narcolepsy, it is dosed twice nightly (≤2.25 g at bedtime and repeated 4 hours later) and can be increased 1.5 g/night per week up to a maximum of 9 g nightly based on efficacy and tolerability. Other REM suppressing medications such as tricyclic antidepressants, SSRIs and SNRIs are also used in the treatment of cataplexy.

Circadian Rhythm Sleep Wake Disorders

Circadian rhythm sleep disorders result in misalignment of the timing of the sleep period relative to the desired bed and rise times, resulting in concurrent insomnia and hypersomnia symptoms despite normal total sleep time. The most common circadian rhythm disturbances are actually exogenous influences on the patient and his/her circadian axis, which in these cases is functioning normally but is unable to adjust rapidly enough to the required new temporal milieu. These exogenous disorders include jet lag disorder and shift work disorder, resulting either from imposed transmeridian travel or alternating work shifts, respectively, that disturb the patient's environmental entraining cues and homeostatic drives for sleep and wakefulness, thereby resulting in misalignment of the patient's endogenous biological sleep drive and typical sleep schedule to the clock time and environment to which they must rapidly adapt.

Jet lag disorder results when an individual crosses across several transmeridian time zones in a single day. Crossing one or two time zones is usually not too difficult for the traveler to accommodate, but crossing three time zones typically causes symptoms of jet lag. Flying eastward is generally much more difficult than flying westward, as patients more easily accommodate phase delay then phase advancing, or "loss" of time. Treatments for jet lag syndrome usually involve efforts to rapidly reentrain the patient to the new environment, and protocols for advance prepartion including setting back (for eastward travel) or setting ahead (for planned westward travel) one's daily routine 2 to 3 weeks prior to the trip so that the traveler is already partially reset in his or her circadian routine before departing. Also critical is attempting to rapidly adapt to the

new time zone, such as by seeking regular sunlight exposure during the daytime and avoiding light exposure in the evening. Brief use of a hypnotic medication and regular daily doses of melatonin[7] 0.5 to 5.0 mg at bedtime for the first few nights after arrival can help reset the sleep schedule in the new time zone.

Shift-work sleep disorder results from workers who must constantly and regularly alter or rotate their work schedules between different shifts (so-called "swing shifts") or workers who must accommodate a regularly scheduled second or third shift (i.e., shifts other than a day shift). Shift workers often have difficulty adapting and shifting their sleep-wake schedules and develop symptoms of insomnia or hypersomnia. Shift workers must be educated to prioritize regularly obtaining a sufficient quantity of sleep, regardless of their work circumstances. Swing shift workers should also be counseled to avoid working more than five night shifts in a row, as night shift work frequently leads to a greater degree of sleep deprivation over time. Shift workers should also be counseled to avoid rotating swing shifts whenever possible, to strictly avoid scheduling overtime duty, and to avoid long commutes (and to exercise special caution to avoid drowsy driving). Judicious use of caffeinated beverages, or prescribed stimulant therapy with modafinil may be helpful for enhancing vigilance in some patients, but should be used with caution as they might interfere with sleep initiation.

The two most common endogenous circadian disorders are delayed sleep-wake phase disorder (DSWPD) and advanced sleep-wake phase disorder (ASWPD), disorders that are most prevalent in opposite extremes of life. DSWPD is seen most often in adolescents and young adults who are biological night owls in their circadian preference, preferring a delayed bedtime and rise time (i.e., bedtimes well past midnight and subsequent arising times in the late morning or early afternoon). DSWPD patients have an extreme and enduring form of this tendency, however, resulting in persisting misalignment of the patient to societal norms. Adolescent and young adult patients present with profound intractable initial insomnia due to their inability to fall asleep at a conventional bedtime as required for school or most daytime occupations, and profound daytime hypersomnia due to their inability to arise and function in the morning hours. Diagnosis is easily recognized by clinical history and sleep diaries, with or without adjunctive actigraphy to objectively verify the pattern of consistent delayed sleep-phase periods. Contrarily, ASWPD is more common in elderly individuals who are biological larks (i.e., preferring an early bedtime and early rise time by nature). However, the ASWPD elderly are unable to stay awake for desired evening activities (often even unable to go out to dinner with friends), and awaken undesirably early in the morning with a consequent inability to fall back asleep in early morning hours. The presentation can mimic depression, whose hallmark biological sign is often noted to be an early morning awakening; care should be taken to carefully distinguish between these two diagnoses. Treatment of each is difficult; options include specifically timed bright light therapy, with or without light restriction, and timed administration of low dose melatonin. The time of administration differs for the two disorders, and is determined by the patient's own endogenous dim light melatonin onset and arise time, and the phase response curve for light and melatonin administration. Bright light therapy is administered at approximately 2500 lx intensity for at least 30 minutes. The timing of bright light administration is first thing in the morning after arising in DSWPD, where a phase-advancing influence is desired; for ASWPD patients, bright light is prescribed in the late afternoon and early evening hours where it will have a phase-delaying effect. Weeks to a few months of regular therapy are necessary to achieve effect. Adherence is difficult and compliance unable to be verified. Specifically timed melatonin usually given at very low doses for this indication (contrary to its use in higher supraphysiologic doses as a hypnotic agent by many patients in other contexts of

---

[7]Available as a dietary supplement.

insomnia, or its high-dose use in REM sleep behavior disorder [RBD]) may also be administered, but its dose and timing are complicated; it must be given in accordance with the circadian phase response curve to have optimal effects and to avoid complicating the problem. For most patients with DSWPD, immediate release melatonin 0.5 mg should be administered at approximately 1 hour before desired bedtime; in ASWPD, melatonin would instead be given prior to the time point of 8 hours following the patient's usual rise time (so as to have a phase-delaying effect). Adjunctive light restriction is recommended in the late afternoon and evenings for DSWPD to avoid precipitating additional phase delays—such as the avoidance of working with luminescent computer screens or viewing video media from close distance in the late evenings—and some experts advocate the use of commercially available blue light restricting glasses as biologically reasonable, as blue light stimuli in evening hours may exacerbate phase delay and confound other recommended treatment effects. However, the efficacy of blue light restriction currently lacks explicit evidence from large clinical trials. As a last resort, the measure of chronotherapy, a progressive delay of bedtime every few days, is prescribed, with the bed and rise times being progressively and successively delayed until the desired bed and rise times are achieved. Attempts to then entrain the patient on this schedule with the aforementioned measures are again attempted with scheduled bright light and prescribed timed melatonin dosing. This is a lengthier process for DSWPD patients and necessitates work restriction during the approximate 2-week time frame necessary to achieve a turnaround of the desired patient's sleep/wake schedule.

Parasomnias and Other Nocturnal Events

Parasomnias are nocturnal events that disrupt sleep but usually do not appreciably disturb sleep quality. As such, nocturnal events do not typically present with symptoms of insomnia or hypersomnia unless there are other comorbid primary sleep disorders such as OSA, which is a frequent comorbidity presenting along with the parasomnias, especially in adult patients.

Parasomnias may arise from either NREM or REM sleep. The NREM parasomnias are essentially all variations on the theme of disorders of arousal, where the behavioral sleep state lingers into awakening, leaving arousal from sleep incomplete. Consequent clinical manifestations are surprisingly heterogeneous and often age related, with specific syndromes such as sleep terrors (also called night terrors) in children, sleep walking and confusional arousals seen in children and adults, and sleep-related eating behavior seen almost exclusively in adults, especially those receiving zolpidem or other newer prescribed hypnotics. NREM disorders of arousal are especially common in children in the first decade of life and are regarded as a relatively normal variant (and perhaps in some cases simply representing an exaggerated manifestation of the physiological difficulty in arousing from the characteristically deeper N3 NREM sleep inherent in the developing brain). As such, pediatric parasomnias are frequently outgrown; however, in some patients, they do endure throughout life. In adult patients who present with newly evolved nocturnal events proven to be NREM disorders of arousal, one should be highly suspicious of comorbid primary sleep disorders that provoke arousing events, such as SDB or PLMD.

REM parasomnias include nightmares and RBD. Nightmares are undesirable, disturbing dreams that lead to sudden arousal from sleep with heightened autonomic sequelae of sweating, hypervigilance, tachycardia, and tachypnea. Nightmares and vivid dreaming are present in between 10% and 50% of normal young children and in about 50% of adults, but become abnormally disturbing in content or frequency much less frequently, and the true prevalence of nightmare disorder remains unknown. Patients who present with a chief complaint of frequent nightmares should be reassured as to their biological nature and receive a detailed physical and neurologic history and examination to exclude potential provoking comorbid causes such as a recent medication change in type or dosage, mood

or anxiety disorder, or primary sleep disorder such as SDB. If no certain readily reversible triggering cause may be identified, referral for consideration of hypnosis, behavior treatment in the form of imagery rehearsal therapy, or pharmacotherapy with clonazepam (Klonopin)[1] may be helpful in some cases. Nightmares that involve flashbacks of previous traumatic events, most often also with similar daytime flashbacks, suggest the alternative diagnosis of posttraumatic stress disorder (PTSD) and the need for psychiatric evaluation. Recent evidence has suggested that alpha-blocking medications such as prazosin (Minipress)[1] or terazosin (Hytrin)[1] may be helpful in suppressing nightmares associated with PTSD.

RBD is characterized by potentially injurious dream enactment behaviors that mirror frightening dream content (characteristically involving fighting off attackers or defending oneself against assailants). In RBD, bed partners will describe objective witnessed dream enactment manifested by violent limb thrashing movements such as punching or kicking and screaming or shouting vocalization during sleep. While RBD patients rarely leave the bed and sleepwalk, falls or other injurious behavior to self or the bed partner are frequent. Importantly, RBD is strongly associated with future development of neurodegenerative disorders. Elderly patients newly diagnosed with RBD harbor up to an 91.9% risk of developing Parkinsonism within 15–25 years of symptom onset, with a shorter-term risk of 30% to 50%, so that all patients with RBD require serial neurologic examinations and follow-up. RBD in young adults may, however, be caused by antidepressant medications, especially the SSRIs, and removal of the offending drug may lead to resolution of dream enactment in some cases. Diagnosis of RBD is by clinical history as well as confirmatory evidence for increased REM sleep muscle tone evident on polysomnographic electromyogram (EMG) leads in the chin and limbs (known as REM sleep without atonia). Treatment options include melatonin,[7] initially at doses of 3 to 6 mg and gradually titrating toward 12 mg nightly as needed to suppress witnessed injurious behaviors, or clonazepam (Klonopin)[1] 0.5 to 1.0 mg increased to 2 to 3 mg nightly. Great care should be taken to first exclude comorbid OSA prior to use of clonazepam, a potential respiratory and upper-airway suppressant.

Nocturnal epilepsies or psychogenic nonepileptic spells may also arise from sleep or apparent sleep and are additional diagnostic considerations in the differential diagnosis of parasomnias. A high degree of stereotypy (one attack being essentially identical to the next) with multiple attacks within a single night are features suggestive of organic partial extratemporal (frontal lobe) epilepsy, even in the absence of EEG changes between or during an episode. In children, benign rolandic epilepsy may lead to stereotyped episodes of facial twitching and drooling, with or without secondary generalized tonic clonic seizures. Children or adults with autosomal dominant nocturnal frontal lobe epilepsy (ADNFLE) may present with bizarre brief motor behavior (typically of 10- to 60-second duration) without postictal sleepiness. ADNFLE has recently been mapped in several kindreds as a channelopathy, producing a defect of the neuronal nicotinic acetylcholine receptor. Psychogenic nonepileptic spells are instead characterized by nonstereotypic and often prolonged attacks that arise from a behavior state of apparent sleep that is instead confirmed during video-EEG PSG to represent normal waking EEG background. Distinguishing features for the differential diagnosis of nocturnal events are shown in Table 5.

Sleep-Related Movement Disorders

Sleep-related movement disorders include restless legs syndrome (RLS), periodic limb movement disorder (PLMD), leg cramps, bruxism, rhythmic movement disorder, and others.

[1]Not FDA approved for this indication.
[7]Available as dietary supplement.

TABLE 5 Distinguishing Features of Nocturnal Events

	PREMONITORY SYMPTOMS	BEHAVIORAL CHARACTERISTICS	DURATION	FREQUENCY	EEG/PSG FINDINGS
NREM Parasomnias					
Night terrors	None	Inconsolable screaming	Minutes	1 or less nightly	Arousal from N2-N3
Confusional arousals	None	Confused, amnestic	Seconds to minutes	1 or less nightly	Arousal from N3>N2
Sleepwalking	None	Ambulation, amnesia	Minutes	1 or less nightly	Arousal from N3 » N2
REM Parasomnias					
Nightmares	Dream recall	Arousal, frightened, palpitations	Seconds	Generally 1/nightly	Arousal from REM
RBD	Variable dream recall	Thrashing, complex motor behavior	Seconds to minutes	>1/night, second>first half	REM sleep without atonia
Epilepsies					
BECTS	Facial twitching, hypersalivation	Focal motor or GTC, postictal	Seconds to minutes	>1/night	Arousal from NREM, IEDs EEG pattern
ADNFLE	Bizarre stereotyped motor behavior	Focal motor, bizarre motor	Seconds, < 1 min	1 or multiple attacks/night	Arousal from N2
TLE	Aura variable	CPS, postictal	1–2 min	1 or multiple attacks/night	Arousal from N2
Psychogenic spells	Variable	Variable	often>5 min	1 or multiple attacks/night	Normal awake EEG

Abbreviations: NREM=nonrapid eye movement sleep; N2=stage 2 NREM sleep; N3=stage 3 NREM sleep; REM=rapid eye movement sleep; IEDs=interictal epileptiform discharges; EEG=electroencephalogram; PSG=polysomnogram; BECTs=benign epilepsy of childhood with centro-temporal spikes; ADNFLE=autosomal dominant nocturnal frontal lobe epilepsy; TLE=temporal lobe epilepsy; RBD=REM sleep behavior disorder.

RLS and PLMS

Diagnosis of RLS is based completely on a clinical history and typically requires four central elements of the described symptoms: an uncomfortable urge to move the legs, with or without uncomfortable leg sensations; temporary relief by movement; symptoms occurring solely or predominantly at rest; and nocturnal worsening of symptoms. About 50% of patients with RLS will carry a positive family history of the disorder, but positive family history is not necessary for the diagnosis. The nature of the symptoms as described by the patient may be quite variable with regard to the symptom quality, location or distribution, temporal occurrence, frequency, and severity. RLS symptoms are usually described as uncomfortable, although not really painful, with a sense of a creepy-crawly or prickling discomfort, often below the knees and centered about the shins or calves, but sometimes more proximally in the thighs, or even isolated to the feet and ankles. Symptoms may occur in the arms as well, especially proximally near the shoulders. Augmentation is common, occurring in about 50% of patients treated with dopaminergic drugs and involves a worsening of the symptoms: symptom onset occurs earlier during the day, becomes more intense, and spreads up to the arms. RLS has been linked to deficient iron stores and dopaminergic neurotransmission in the brain and is more common in patients with parkinsonism, multiple sclerosis, epilepsy, and in those with chronic renal insufficiency.

While periodic limb movements of sleep (PLMS) are seen in 80% to 90% of RLS patients, PLMS are not necessary for the diagnosis of RLS. Furthermore, PLMS are also extremely frequent in the general population, seen in 5% to 15% of younger adults and as many as 45% of elderly individuals. PLMD is diagnosed when PLMS is thought to cause daytime hypersomnia in the absence of other sleep disorders.

Nonpharmacologic treatments including warm or cool baths, massage, stretching, or even the application of spontaneous compression devices have been reported to be effective anecdotally and in small case series, but an evidence base for these measures remains poor, and most patients seeking medical care for the symptom have severe enough symptoms to merit pharmacologic treatment.

Iron and pharmacologic treatments for RLS are outlined in Table 6. Iron deficiency, or even low normal body iron stores, may worsen or precipitate symptoms. Measuring a serum ferritin should be considered early in all RLS patients, with iron replacement therapy begun if serum ferritin values are less than 50 mcg/L. Iron therapy can be constipating or cause GI distress, and the formulation of iron with added vitamin C (Ferrex 150 Plus, Vitelle Irospan) is often better tolerated by those who cannot stomach ferrous sulfate.

Carbidopa-levedopa (Sinemet)[1] may be used for patients with only intermittently disturbing symptoms, but chronic nightly use of carbidopa-levodopa, especially above a dosage of 200 mg daily, may raise the risk of augmentation. For nightly use, the newer dopaminergic agonist medications pramipexole (Mirapex) or ropinirole (Requip) remain a mainstay of treatment. Pramipexole may be initiated at 0.125 to 0.25 mg nightly and titrated every few days to the 0.375 to 0.50 mg range or beyond if needed for symptom control. Doses beyond 1.0 mg are typically not additionally effective and appear to raise augmentation risk. Ropinirole may be initiated at 0.5 to 1.0 mg with gradual upward titration to the 4 to 6 mg[3] range as needed and tolerated. Generally, dosing 1 hour prior to bedtime is sufficient, but if earlier evening or late afternoon symptoms emerge, cautious application of divided doses may be utilized, and some experts advice at least a low morning dosage administered daily to achieve a more chronic steady state of dopamine administration since this may be a sensible strategy to minimize augmentation risk. For either initial first-line therapy, or particularly when patients are beginning to

[1] Not FDA approved for this indication.
[3] Exceeds dosage recommended by the manufacturer.

Sleep Disorders

TABLE 6 Clinical Pharmacology of Treatments for Restless Leg Syndrome

	MECHANISM OF ACTION	DOSAGE	TYPICAL ADVERSE EFFECTS	INTERACTIONS
Iron Replacement				
Ferrous sulfate[1]	Fe	324 mg, 1 tab every alternate day	Nausea, constipation	None
Ferrous fumarate+vit C[1]	Fe	200/125 mg, 1 tab every alternate day	Nausea, constipation	None
Carbidopa-Levodopa (Sinemet)[1]	DA	25/100 1–2 prn	Nausea, dizziness, ICD	None
Pramipexole (Mirapex)	DA	0.125–1.0 mg[2] qhs	Nausea, dizziness, ICD	None
Ropinirole (Requip)	DA	1–6 mg[2] qhs	Nausea, dizziness, ICD	None
Rotigotine (Neupro Transdermal Patch)	DA	1–3 mg qam	Nausea, dizziness, ICD	None
Gabapentin (Neurontin)[1]	Unknown	300–1200[2] mg qhs	Nausea, dizziness, pedal edema, weight gain	None
Gabapentin Enacarbil (Horizant)	Unknown	600 mg	Nausea, dizziness, pedal edema, weight gain	None
Pregabalin (Lyrica)[1]	Unknown	100–600 mg qhs	Nausea, dizziness, pedal edema, weight gain	None
Tramadol (Ultram)[1] Codeine	MRA MRA[1]	50 mg 400 mg qhs 30–60 mg	Nausea, dizziness Nausea, dizziness	None None
Oxycodone[1]	MRA	5–15 mg	Nausea, dizziness	None

[1]Not FDA approved for this indication.
[2]Exceeds dosage recommended by the manufacturer.
Abbreviations: mg=milligrams; Fe=iron replacement; DA=dopamine agonist; MOR=mu opiate receptor agonist.

experience earlier symptom onset during the day and may have failed the other short-acting dopaminergic drugs pramipexole and ropinirole, a rotigotine (Neupro) patch has been an advent in RLS management and often may be substituted for those other agents to provide more day-long symptom relief and reduce a growing augmentation tendency. Rotigotine offers several other advantages, as its transdermal delivery system provides continuous day-long release of medication that may minimize peak/trough serum concentration variation and minimize the occurrence of other potential adverse effects. Rotigotine also appears to result in augmentation less frequently than other dopaminergic drugs. All patients receiving dopaminergic agents should be counseled upfront about the approximate 15% idiosyncratic risk of impulse control disorder symptoms (such as pathologic gambling, shopping, or hoarding/punding behaviors), and be forewarned that should such problems result, the medication must be withdrawn and another nondopaminergic drug substituted for symptom control. Typical dose-related adverse effects are also described further in Table 6.

Gabapentin (Neurontin)[1] is increasingly becoming an alternative first-line medication for RLS, dosed 300 to 1200[3] mg every night at bedtime as needed and tolerated. Gabapentin may be the agent of choice in patients with comorbid anxiety, pain and insomnia or in patients who are intolerant, resistant to, or have developed augmentation with dopamine agonist medications. On the other hand a dopamine agonist is still generally the first choice for pharmacologic treatment of RLS in severe cases and may be preferred over gabapentin in patients with comorbid depression, obesity, metabolic syndrome, OSA and history of falls. Gabapentin enacarbil (Horizant) is a prodrug of gabapentin that is better absorbed and carries an indication for RLS, but generic gabapentin is also frequently effective and well tolerated, and there has been no head-to-head trial showing superiority of the more expensive prodrug gabapentin encarbil over that of gabapentin. Other alternatives include clonazepam[1] and tramadol (Ultram).[1] For patients unresponsive to these measures, opiate treatment with oxycodone (Roxicodone)[1] 5 to 15 mg at bedtime, hydromorphone (Dilaudid),[1] or methadone (Dolophine)[1] are often effective. A large randomized trial showed that the combination oxycodone-naloxone (Targiniq ER)[1] resulted in substantial improvements in RLS symptoms in patients who had previously shown inadequate response to dopamine agonists. Small case series suggest other alternatives for refractory RLS such as carbamazepine (Tegretol),[1] oxcarbazepine (Trileptal),[1] and lamotrigine (Lamictal).[1] The impact of comorbid OSA should also be considered, as optimization of treatment for SDB may improve both subjective RLS symptoms as well as PLMD frequency in many patients. A novel TOMAC (tonic motor activation) device was recently approved by the FDA for RLS based on a promising multicenter trial showing safety, efficacy, and tolerability in 133 patients with medication-refractory RLS.

Sleep-Related Leg Cramps

Sleep-related leg cramps are a common and enigmatic problem affecting 7% to 10% of children and up to 70% of elderly adults. Unfortunately, despite their extremely common occurrence and impact on the quality of life of cramp sufferers, little is known about the pathophysiology or treatment of this condition. Cramps are painful, involuntary sustained muscle contractions, lasting 2 to 10 minutes and affecting the unilateral or bilateral calves, thighs, or feet, with residual tenderness of the affected muscle lasting up to an hour or longer. The clinical approach to sleep-related leg cramps is to first determine whether they are also present during daytime in addition to sleep. If daytime cramping is prominent, exclusion of a precipitating neuromuscular disorder is paramount, including amyotrophic lateral sclerosis, peripheral neuropathy, myositis, or cramp-fasciculation syndrome. In elderly men, peripheral vascular disease and other systemic medical comorbidities are also common. (The reader is referred to the chapter on neuromuscular disorders for further advice on the diagnosis of these conditions.) A neurologic examination should be conducted on all cramp sufferers, and those having sensorimotor findings, fasciculations, or pathologic reflex findings should be referred for EMG, serum creatinine kinase, or additional blood and urine tests for exclusion of symptomatic causes of neuropathy as appropriate. While additional testing for electrolyte abnormalities such as hypomagnesemia, hypocalcemia, hyponatremia, and hypokalemia can be considered, they are of extremely low yield. When examination findings are normal and cramps are isolated to the sleep state, further diagnostic work-up can usually be avoided. Symptomatic treatment measures for sleep-related leg cramps include tonic water with lemon and advising adequate hydration and nightly stretching of the calves and thighs. Prescription quinine (Qualaquin)[1] carries a FDA black box warning for leg cramp treatment and is essentially no longer used for this indication. For refractory frequent cramp sufferers, a sodium-channel blocking anticonvulsant such as carbamazepine[1], oxcarbazepine[1], or lamotrigine[1] may also be considered.

Sleep-Related Bruxism

Sleep-related bruxism, rhythmic grinding of the teeth during sleep, may lead to significant tooth wear and dental or jaw pain. The condition is usually idiopathic, although it may be associated with psychiatric conditions such as mood or anxiety disorders, especially if it is also present during daytime. Treatment usually involves dental referral for consideration of a fitted mouth guard, although in extreme cases pharmacotherapy with clonazepam[1] or consideration of botulinum toxin (Botox)[1] may be necessary.

Other Sleep-Related Movement Disorders

Sleep-related rhythmic movement disorder usually occurs in patients with psychomotor maldevelopment and involves repetitive head and neck or axial body movements. This behavior is not strictly voluntary and often persists during PSG into deep drowsiness or light NREM sleep, so behavioral treatments alone are often ineffective. Head banging behavior, sometimes into the headboard of the bed, can be injurious at times: a protective helmet or treatment with clonazepam[1] is advisable in some cases. Most other movement disorders, such as organic tremors, myoclonus, or dyskinesias generated by the basal ganglia, are suppressed during sleep but may reemerge during drowsiness or nocturnal awakenings.

Propriospinal myoclonus at sleep onset is characterized by myoclonic jerks having their primary and earliest onset in abdominal and axial muscles prior to spreading to the limbs and may be associated with thoracic spinal cord pathology. Spinal imaging with MRI is advised. Treatment with clonazepam[1] is usual for this uncommon diagnosis, although it is unfortunately often ineffective, and many cases of propriospinal myoclonus are instead found to represent a functional movement disorder.

Isolated Symptoms and Normal Variants

These conditions are felt largely to represent either normal variants or otherwise largely benign disorders. The definition of long and short sleepers are somewhat arbitrary, but may be considered as greater than 10 hours or shorter than 5 hours of habitual sleep. Short or long sleep time are each assumed to be variants of normal behavior in the absence of hypersomnia or nighttime symptoms of insomnia.

Sleep talking, or somniloquy, in isolation is rarely of concern. History is often lifelong in such patients. When sleep talking is newly evolved in an elderly individual or a younger patient receiving antidepressant therapy, RBD should be considered in the differential diagnosis, and the patient should be questioned about other potential evidence for dream enactment behavior. A careful medication history and neurologic examination alone will usually dictate whether further evaluation with PSG may be indicated, but in most cases isolated sleep talking is not a cause for concern.

Sleep starts, hypnic jerks or physiologic myoclonus are near universal in their occurrence and often associated with recent excessive caffeine intake or emotional or physical stress. A history of occurrence of jerks limited to the arms, legs, or axial musculature causing arousal within the first 5 to 10 minutes of sleep, and lacking later recurrence during the night, is typical. Reassurance and avoidance of precipitating factors is advised; however, if hypnic jerks are excessive or recur later in the night, PSG is occasionally necessary to distinguish this benign diagnosis from PLMD or propriospinal myoclonus. Propriospinal myoclonus at sleep onset is characterized by myoclonic jerks having their primary and earliest onset in abdominal and axial muscles prior to spreading to the limbs and may be associated with thoracic spinal cord pathology. Spinal imaging with MRI is advised. Treatment with clonazepam[1] is usual for this uncommon diagnosis.

Other Sleep Disorders

Undesirable influences in the patient's sleep environment can serve to regularly distract or disturb him or her from initiating or maintaining sleep. Typical influences include a bed partner who snores loudly or who causes bed motion due to restless or disturbed sleep; pets who sleep in bed with the patient and cause awakening; environmental noise from neighborhood dogs, car alarms, or neighboring freeway or train way; too much outdoor ambient light; or undesirable household ambient temperature. There is considerable overlap in this category of environmental sleep disturbance with inadequate sleep hygiene, as activating stimuli in the environment may lead the patient toward chronic insomnia and adapting undesirable sleep-related behaviors that serve to further disrupt restful sleep.

Sleep-Related Medical and Neurologic Disorders

Fatal familial insomnia is an exceedingly rare, autosomal dominant variant form of familial Creutzfeldt-Jakob disease, a prion disorder that leads to progressive insomnia and progressive cognitive impairment, with death inevitably occurring within 3 years of onset. Aggregate prion protein accumulates in the thalamus and other brain regions, and relentlessly progressive insomnia, panic disorder, hallucinosis, and dementia ensue. Unfortunately, no treatments are currently known for this rare disorder.

Conclusions

Sleep disorders are common and result in significant patient morbidity, daytime dysfunction, and impaired quality of life. Untreated sleep disordered breathing (SDB) may also raise the risk for hypertension, vascular events, and mortality. The most common presenting symptoms of sleep disorders include insomnia, characterized by difficulty initiating and maintaining sleep with poor sleep quality, and hypersomnia, the symptom of excessive daytime sleepiness. Evaluation begins with a detailed history and physical examination, which in select cases may require support and clarification by polysomnography and multiple sleep-latency testing. Fortunately, effective therapies are available for the majority of sleep disorders. Insomnia typically requires behavioral or pharmacologic interventions, while SDB may be effectively treated in most cases with positive airway pressure (PAP) therapy. Primary CNS hypersomnias including narcolepsy require stimulant management in most cases, while most parasomnias benefit from clonazepam.[1] Circadian sleep disorders may require timed light and melatonin therapies. Patients having

---

[1]Not FDA approved for this indication.

[1]Not FDA approved for this indication.

RLS and PLMD should be evaluated for iron deficiency and may enjoy symptom control through dopaminergic or other alternative symptomatic treatments. The majority of patients with sleep disorders benefit from a careful clinical evaluation and appropriately selected therapies.

References

American Academy of Sleep Medicine: *International Classification of Sleep Disorders: Diagnostic and Coding Manual*, ed 3-TR, Darien, IL, 2024, American Academy of Sleep Medicine. 2024.

Costanzo MR, Ponikowski P, Javaheri S, et al: Sustained 12 month benefit of phrenic nerve stimulation for central sleep apnea, *Am J Cardiol* 121(11):1400–1408, 2018.

Kapur VK, Auckley DH, Chowdhuri S, et al: Practice guideline for diagnostic testing for adult obstructive sleep apnea: an American Academy of Sleep Medicine clinical practice guideline, *J Clin Sleep Med* 13(3):479–504, 2017.

Kent D, Stanley J, Aurora RN, et al: Referral of adults with obstructive sleep apnea for surgical consultation: an American Academy of Sleep Medicine clinical practice guideline, *J Clin Sleep Med* 17(12):2507–2531, 2021.

Patil SP, Ayappa I, Caples SM, et al: Treatment of adult obstructive sleep apnea with positive airway pressure: an American Academy of Sleep Medicine clinical practice guideline, *J Clin Sleep Med* 15(2):335–343, 2019.

Sateia MJ, Buysse DJ, Krystal AD, et al: Clinical practice guideline for the pharmacologic treatment of chronic insomnia in adults: an American Academy of Sleep Medicine clinical practice guideline, *J Clin Sleep Med* 13(2):307–349, 2017.

Suurna MV, Klasner M: Neurostimulation for obstructive sleep apnea, *Otolaryngol Clin North Am* 57(3):457–465, 2024.

SPORTS-RELATED HEAD INJURIES

Method of
Brandon Hockenberry, MD; Margaret Pusateri, MD; and Christopher McGrew, MD

CURRENT DIAGNOSIS

- Initial evaluation of any sports-related head injury should follow standard emergency medicine procedures.
- Presence of any "red flag" symptoms is concerning for a more serious head injury (skull fracture and intracranial hemorrhage) and requires emergency evaluation.
- If "red flag" symptoms are present and advanced imaging is indicated, a noncontrast computed tomography (CT) scan of the head is the initial study of choice.
- If no "red flag" symptoms are present, one of several validated neuropsychological tests should be administered to evaluate cognitive function (e.g., Sports Concussion Assessment Tool, version 5 [SCAT 5]; https://bjsm.bmj.com/content/bjsports/early/2017/04/26/bjsports-2017-097506SCAT5.full.pdf).
- Ultimately, concussion is still a clinical diagnosis.
- Advanced neuroimaging, fluid biomarkers, genetic testing, helmet sensors, and video surveillance have all been purported as possible prognostic indicators but require further validation.

CURRENT THERAPY

- Blood pressure control is critical for patients with intracranial hemorrhage.
- Small intracranial hemorrhages without midline shift or significant symptoms may be monitored, but surgical decompression is otherwise required.
- For patients requiring sedation, propofol (Diprivan)[1] is often preferred due to its short half-life, which makes it easier to monitor neurologic status.
- Mannitol can also be used to help lower intracranial pressure.
- For posttraumatic seizures, phenytoin (Dilantin)[1] is the preferred medication.

- If there is any concern for concussion, the athlete should immediately be removed from play.
- An athlete should never be allowed to return to play on the same day as the injury.
- After an initial rest period of 24–48 hours, an athlete should begin progressing through return-to-play and return-to-learn protocols (https://www.cdc.gov/headsup/providers/return_to_activities.html).
- In the first 24 hours after injury, acetaminophen is the treatment of choice for associated headaches; nonsteroidal antiinflammatory drugs (NSAIDs) and aspirin can worsen an undiagnosed intracranial hemorrhage.
- If headaches persist longer than 3–5 days, medications that do not pose a risk for rebound headaches (e.g., tricyclic antidepressants) can be used.
- Good sleep hygiene is important for recovery. If insomnia persists for more than 2–3 days after injury, medications can be considered.
- Typical recovery time is up to 2 weeks in adults and 4 weeks in children.
- Access to a multidisciplinary team including physical therapists, neurologists, and psychiatric providers is beneficial for athletes with complicated or prolonged recoveries.
- If an athlete has a history of a learning disability, depression, anxiety, or chronic headaches, recovery can be complicated by an exacerbation of the underlying disease.

[1]Not FDA approved for this indication.

Introduction and Epidemiology

Sports-related head injuries include a heterogenous group of insults to the brain caused by either a direct impact to the head or an impact to the body associated with energy transfer into the head.

In the United States, sports are among the leading causes of head injuries. Specifically between the ages of 15 and 24 years, athletic activities are the second leading cause of head injuries; only motor vehicle accidents have a higher incidence. Athletic and recreational activities vary widely in terms of biomechanics and kinetics, resulting in a wide range of associated risks. Many sports are limited by the speed at which an athlete can run (e.g., rugby or soccer), but others allow athletes to compete at much higher speeds, some nearly equivalent to those of motor vehicles (e.g., cycling or skiing). These sports potentially put athletes at a higher risk for more severe head injuries.

Sports- and recreation-related traumatic brain injuries (SRR-TBIs) are monitored by the National Electronic Injury Surveillance System—All Injury Program (NEISS-AIP). According to this program, there were more than 3.4 million visits to emergency departments (EDs) across the United States for SRR-TBIs between 2001 and 2012, or approximately 340,000 per year.

Concussion is by far the most common head injury associated with athletic activity. It is estimated that 1.7 to 3.0 million concussions per year are related to sports and recreational activities. The overall rate is 2.5 concussions per 10,000 athletic events, and concussions make up 5% to 18% of reported injuries in the National Collegiate Athletic Association. It is estimated that 50% of concussions go unreported or undiagnosed. The most common severe head injury is a subdural hematoma, which accounts for greater than 90% of all sport-related catastrophic head injuries. These are most often seen in American football, cheerleading, and skiing/snowboarding and occur in less than 1 per 100,000 athletic events. Fatalities from sports-related head injuries are very rare; however, subdural hematoma is a serious injury. In one study, it was reported that American football players with subdural hematoma had a fatality rate of 8.5% and a 48% rate of suffering permanent neurologic deficits.

Risk Factors

Every athlete is potentially at some risk for a head injury during activity. Many factors contribute to relative risk, with the type of activity being the largest contributing factor. In their younger years, males sustain the most head injuries playing football or wrestling, whereas bicycling and basketball take over top spots after the high school and college years. In females, bicycling and horseback riding contribute the most head injuries. It should be noted that some activities have higher incidence rates of head injuries than the aforementioned activities (e.g., men's/women's ice hockey) but are not as commonly played and therefore do not contribute to the sheer volume of injuries that other activities do. With respect to concussion specifically, men's ice hockey and football have the highest incidence rates (5.5 to 6.5 concussions per 10,000 athletic events) in the high school and college populations. On the women's side, soccer and lacrosse have the highest rates (3 to 3.5 concussions per 10,000 athletic events).

Children and teens are at increased risk for head injuries because they are developmentally immature and more frequently participate in activities that have a higher risk for head trauma. Overall, 70% of all SRR-TBIs are in the age group of 0 to 19 years. In the young athlete, a larger head-to-neck ratio, smaller amount of neck/shoulder musculature, and thinner cranial bones all contribute to an increased chance that a blow to the head will cause a head injury. The active elderly have better balance, fewer falls, and fewer TBIs than their more chronically ill counterparts. Therefore increased age is not an independent risk factor for SRR-TBIs.

At the high school and college levels, males have more concussions than do women in sheer numbers but a lower incidence rate overall. Females may have greater risk because of decreased neck musculature compared with males. Female sex has been associated more commonly with abnormal imaging, surgical intervention, complication, and death. A history of previous concussion increases risk for future concussions compared with nonconcussed athletes, and the greatest risk for repeat concussion is during the 10-day period after the most recent concussion.

Pathophysiology

The pathophysiology of SRR-TBIs and sports-related concussion (SRC) is multifactorial. Several mechanisms have been identified. Biomechanically, a combination of acceleration, deceleration, and rotational/translational forces directly applied or transmitted to the head affect change at the level of individual cells. Metabolic derangements, neurotransmitter dysfunction, changes in cerebral blood flood, neuroinflammation, microstructural damage, and diffuse axonal injury have all been implicated as potential pathways. Helmet-based measurement studies have attempted to quantify head impacts, providing information on force, frequency, and location. However, results vary widely among athletes diagnosed with concussions. In addition, the accuracy of the data detected by helmet sensors and video surveillance systems has been called into question; it does not necessarily reflect the impact on the brain itself, and there is no evidence to support the use of such systems to attempt to diagnose SRC.

Assessment and Diagnosis of Sports-Related Head Injury

The initial assessment of any sports-related head injury should follow standard emergency medicine procedures. Assessment of the "ABCs" (airway, breathing, and circulation) and evaluation for concomitant cervical spine injury should be the first steps in management. The presence of any red flag symptoms (Box 1) should raise concerns for a serious head injury, such as an intracranial hemorrhage or skull fracture, and requires immediate evaluation in the ED, likely advanced head or neck imaging, and possible specialist consultation. The appropriate emergency action plan should be initiated and the athlete stabilized and transported to the designated medical facility.

Once in the ED, the decision whether to obtain images needs to be made. Some assessment tools have been developed, such as the Pediatric Emergency Care Applied Research Network (PECARN; https://www.mdcalc.com/pecarn-pediatric-head-injury-trauma-

algorithm) and Canadian CT Head Injury algorithms. A Glasgow Coma Scale score below 14, palpable skull fracture, or presence of red flag symptoms would all be reasons to image acutely. The initial imaging test of choice after head injury is a noncontrast head CT, which will show fractures, intracranial hemorrhage, midline shifts, and signs of edema. CT with angiography will show decreased blood flow into cerebral vessels because of increased intracranial pressure. However, if increased intracranial pressure due to malignant brain edema or an expanding hematoma is suspected, more invasive intracranial pressure monitoring is a more accurate measure and will be more useful to management (see Box 1).

If no red flag symptoms are present and the athlete does not require emergency medical treatment, he or she should be removed from the field of play if there is any suspicion for possible SRC. Several brief neuropsychological tests have been developed to evaluate cognitive function. Examples of practical and validated tests include the SCAT 5 and the Standardized Assessment of Concussion (SAC). The SCAT 5 is broken down into six steps: immediate or on-field assessment, symptom evaluation, cognitive screening, neurologic screening, delayed recall, and decision. In addition to an assessment of the aforementioned red flag symptoms, the immediate or on-field assessment section of the SCAT 5 also includes a review of observable signs (e.g., lying motionless on the playing field, facial injury after head trauma, and blank or vacant look), a memory assessment using the Maddocks Questions (Box 2), a measure of the Glasgow Coma Scale (Table 1), and a cervical spine assessment. It has been found that standard orientation questions (name, location, and year) are not reliable in the immediate assessment of SRC. The Maddocks questions, which focus on sport-specific memory assessment, provide better information to help the examiner determine whether there is a concern for an SRC. Once the initial assessment is complete, if there is any concern for an SRC, the athlete should be removed from the sporting environment and not allowed to return to play on the day of injury.

Diagnosis of SRC remains a clinical diagnosis. Over the past two decades, multiple investigations have focused on the use of advanced neuroimaging (e.g., functional magnetic resonance imaging [f-MRI] and electroencephalogram [EEG]) and

---

BOX 1	**Red Flag Symptoms**

Persistent vomiting
Seizure
Severe "worst headache of my life"
Focal neurologic deficit
Blurred vision
Slurred speech
Significant drowsiness/poor awakening
Poor orientation to person/place/time
Declining mental status

The presence of any of these symptoms should prompt consideration of emergency department evaluation and head imaging. If no red flags are present, the clinician may be able to send the athlete home safely and follow up in the office the next day.

BOX 2	**Memory Assessment: Maddocks Questions**

What venue are we at today?
What half is it now?
Who scored last in the game?
What team did you play last week?
Did your team win the last game?

Note: Can be adapted to specific sports as necessary.
These questions help make diagnosis of concussion. No official score cutoff is diagnostic; however, inability to answer them all correctly should raise suspicion for concussion or more severe head injury. Questions can be changed slightly if they are not relevant to a sport, such as swimming.

TABLE 1   Glasgow Coma Scale

BEST EYE RESPONSE (E)	BEST VERBAL RESPONSE (V)	BEST MOTOR RESPONSE (M)
Eye opening spontaneously: 4	Oriented: 5	Obeys commands: 6
Eye opening to voice: 3	Confused: 4	Localizes to pain: 5
Eye opening to pain: 2	Inappropriate words: 3	Flexion/withdrawal from pain: 4
No eye opening: 1	Incomprehensible sounds: 2	Abnormal flexion to pain: 3
	No verbal response: 1	Abnormal extension to pain: 2
		No motor response: 1

Used to rate the severity of head injury. Scores in each category are added for a total of 15 points. Athletes with concussion typically have a Glasgow Coma Scale score of 14 (losing 1 point in the verbal response category) or 15. Scores less than 14 should prompt a visit to the emergency department for head imaging.

body fluid analysis (blood, saliva, and cerebrospinal fluid) as potential tools to aid in the diagnosis of SRCs. (In addition, these modalities have been explored as potential prognostic indicators, attempting to predict clinical recovery or assess the cumulative risk of repetitive trauma.) At this time, advanced neuroimaging, fluid biomarkers, and genetic testing are important research tools but require further validation to determine their ultimate clinical utility in the evaluation and diagnosis of SRC.

Clinical Manifestations

Clinical manifestations after an SRR-TBI and SRC can be varied. The brain itself is a complex organ. Depending on which area is injured, different symptoms may present. With regard to the more serious diseases, such as intracranial hemorrhages or diffuse axonal injury, the athlete is often critically injured, again demonstrating red flag symptoms and signs of increased intracranial pressure. However, SRC is an evolving injury within the acute phase and can often have an initially subtle presentation. Signs and symptoms rapidly change, especially over the first 24 to 48 hours. Classically, symptoms fall into one of four categories: physical (headache, nausea, and dizziness), cognitive (difficulty concentrating and slowed reaction times), emotional (anxiety and irritability), and sleep disturbances (insomnia and hypersomnia). As part of the SCAT 5 and other concussion assessment tools, an in-depth symptom checklist is used to evaluate SRCs both initially and during follow-up. For example, Table 2 outlines the SCAT 5 symptom checklist. It is important to note that there are no specific scoring guidelines that are diagnostic of concussion. The scores are most commonly used to monitor an athlete's recovery, tracking improvement or decline over time. Of note, higher scores at the time of initial injury are associated with longer recoveries.

Treatment

Presence of red flag symptoms listed in Box 1 or a Glasgow Coma Scale score of less than 14 should raise suspicion for a more severe SSR-TBI, such as a skull fracture or intracranial hemorrhage, rather than a typical concussion. If an athlete sustains an SSR-TBI other than concussion, he or she should be evaluated in the ED. In the event of an intracranial hemorrhage of any kind, the largest concern is increasing intracranial pressure. Strict blood pressure control is incredibly important, because an increased blood pressure will increase the pressure in the bleeding vessel and thus the rate and severity of the bleed. Intracranial hemorrhages may be monitored if the bleed is small and not causing a midline shift or significant symptoms. However, definitive treatment with surgical decompression is preferred for subdural and epidural hemorrhages. Most patients will require intubation, sedation, and intracranial pressure monitoring. For sedation, propofol (Diprivan)[1] is the preferred agent at many institutions

[1] Not FDA approved for this indication.

TABLE 2   SCAT 5 Symptoms Checklist

SYMPTOM	SEVERITY
Headache	0 1 2 3 4 5 6
"Pressure in head"	0 1 2 3 4 5 6
Neck pain	0 1 2 3 4 5 6
Nausea and/or vomiting	0 1 2 3 4 5 6
Dizziness	0 1 2 3 4 5 6
Blurred vision	0 1 2 3 4 5 6
Balance problems	0 1 2 3 4 5 6
Sensitivity to light	0 1 2 3 4 5 6
Sensitivity to noise	0 1 2 3 4 5 6
Feeling slowed down	0 1 2 3 4 5 6
Feeling like "in a fog"	0 1 2 3 4 5 6
"Don't feel right"	0 1 2 3 4 5 6
Difficulty concentrating	0 1 2 3 4 5 6
Difficulty remembering	0 1 2 3 4 5 6
Fatigue or low energy	0 1 2 3 4 5 6
Confusion	0 1 2 3 4 5 6
Drowsiness	0 1 2 3 4 5 6
More emotional	0 1 2 3 4 5 6
Irritability	0 1 2 3 4 5 6
Sadness	0 1 2 3 4 5 6
Nervous or anxious	0 1 2 3 4 5 6
Trouble falling asleep (if applicable)	0 1 2 3 4 5 6
Total number of symptoms	Of 22
Symptom severity score	Of 132

There is no score cutoff that is diagnostic of concussion; it is simply used to monitor a patient's improvement or decline over time. Higher scores at time of injury are associated with longer recovery times.
SCAT 5, Sports Concussion Assessment Tool version 5.

because it has a short half-life, making it easier to monitor the patient's neurologic status. In the presence of malignant brain edema, mannitol (Osmitrol) can be added to decrease intracranial pressure when strict blood pressure and pain control has failed. For a TBI causing posttraumatic seizure, phenytoin (Dilantin)[1] remains the preferred medication, although many institutions will use older antiepileptic drugs such as valproate (Depakote)[1] or carbamazepine (Tegretol)[1] as treatments of choice.

TABLE 3 Graduated Return-to-Play Protocol as Outlined by the Consensus Statement on Concussion in Sport

STAGE	AIM	ACTIVITY	GOAL OF EACH STEP
1	Symptom-limited activity	Daily activities that do not provoke symptoms	Gradual reintroduction of work/school activities
2	Light aerobic exercise	Walking or stationary cycling at slow to medium pace; no resistance training	Increase heart rate
3	Sport-specific exercise	Running or skating drills; no head impact activities	Add movement
4	Noncontact training drills	Harder training drills (e.g., passing drills); may start progressive resistance training	Exercise, coordination, and improved thinking
5	Full-contact practice	After medical clearance, participate in normal training activities	Restore confidence and assess functional skills by coaching staff
6	Return to sport	Normal game play	

Start step 1 after initial 24- to 48-hour period of rest. Each step should take a minimum 24 hours to progress through.

TABLE 4 Example of a Graduated Return-to-Learn Protocol as Outlined by the Consensus Statement on Concussion in Sport

STAGE	AIM	ACTIVITY	GOAL OF EACH STEP
1	Daily activities that do not give the child symptoms	Typical activities of the child during the day as long as he or she does not increase symptoms (e.g., reading, texting, screen time). Start with 5–15 min at a time and build up	Gradual return to typical activities
2	School activities	Homework, reading, or other cognitive activities outside of the classroom	Increase tolerance to cognitive work
3	Return to school part time	Gradual introduction of schoolwork. May need to start with a partial school day or increased breaks during the day	Increase academic activities
4	Return to school full time	Gradually progress school activities until a full day can be tolerated	Return to full academic activities and catch up on missed work

Unlike the return-to-sport protocol, there is no minimum required time for each stage. Some children may be able to tolerate a full school day immediately after injury without difficulty, depending on symptom severity.

The current recommendation for the management of SRC is to remove the athlete from play and not allow a return on the same day. The athlete should avoid physical exertion and mental activities that make symptoms worse. After an initial rest period of 24 to 48 hours, the patient should begin progressing to both physical (noncontact) and mental activities. The athlete should return to normal activities of daily living as much as is tolerated without symptom exacerbation. The newest consensus statement on concussion in sport outlines not only a return-to-play protocol but also a return-to-learn protocol. These are outlined in Tables 3 and 4. Children and adolescents should not return to sport until they have fully returned to school. It is important to note that there is no evidence to suggest that any medications or nutritional supplements will improve rate of recovery from concussion. Medications in concussion treatment are primarily used for symptomatic relief.

Monitoring Concussions

After concussion diagnosis, the clinically stable athlete can be sent home if a responsible adult is available to accompany him or her. Sleep is encouraged, and the athlete need not be awakened for evaluation. The athlete should be followed up in a qualified healthcare provider's office within 24 to 48 hours for reevaluation. Follow-up examination should include a symptom severity checklist (see Table 2), history, and neurologic examination at a minimum. Completing a full SCAT 5 evaluation is unnecessary if the athlete had one done at time of injury and still has symptoms. Advanced neuroimaging with MRI is not needed to monitor a concussion and by definition should be normal.

As the athlete returns to play, close supervision under a qualified healthcare provider such as a certified athletic trainer or physical therapist is ideal but not always possible. When an athlete has progressed through the return-to-play protocol (see Table 3), follow-up with an appropriate qualified healthcare provider should be arranged to obtain full medical clearance to return to full contact activity.

Management of Concussion Complications

Headaches are among the most common symptoms of a concussion and often the symptom that bothers the athlete the most. In the acute period after injury, medications have some potential to mask important symptoms. For the first 1 to 2 hours after the injury, it is important to be able to accurately monitor the patient for a changing clinical picture, which could suggest that the head injury is not a concussion but rather an evolving epidural or subdural hematoma. For the first 24 hours, NSAIDs and aspirin should be avoided because they can thin the blood and potentially make an undiagnosed hematoma become a more significant bleed. Acetaminophen (Tylenol) is the preferred medication for headache in the first 24 hours. After the first day, it is safe to switch to ibuprofen (Motrin), which may have more benefit. If headaches are not improving after 3 to 5 days, it is advisable to switch to another medication that does not pose the risk of creating rebound headaches. Tricyclic antidepressants are a good choice and work very well. Nortriptyline (Pamelor)[1] at a low dose (25 mg/d) is generally well tolerated in children as well as adults and may be stopped abruptly without withdrawal

---

[1] Not FDA approved for this indication.

symptoms once the athlete is feeling well and ready to progress back to activities.

Sleep disturbances in athletes with concussion are also very common. Many will not sleep well the first night after injury and want to nap during the day. Other athletes may sleep much more than usual after initial injury. Although there are no clear studies proving the optimal amount of sleep, current trends are to try to return the athlete to normal sleep cycles and daily living as much as possible. An emphasis on sleep hygiene over the first few days is standard. If insomnia persists after 2 to 3 days, medications may be considered. Melatonin[7] is available over the counter, has very few side effects, and is generally well tolerated. The next step would be amitriptyline (Elavil)[1] at a low dose (10– 25 mg/d). This can be especially effective if the athlete has both headaches and poor sleep because it is more sedating than nortriptyline.

A concussion is expected to last no more than 14 days in an adult and less than 4 weeks in the pediatric population. Each individual physician will have a different comfort level treating concussion; however, it is reasonable to consider a referral to a specialty physician once an athlete has passed the normal expected recovery time and is not categorized as a "prolonged concussion." Each city or region will have a different culture about who takes care of the prolonged concussions. Neurologists, sports medicine physicians, and physical medicine and rehabilitation physicians are all well equipped to take care of these athletes. Physical therapists, particularly those who specialize in vestibular rehabilitation, can be very helpful to patients with continued balance problems, concentration difficulties, and other visual symptoms. Last, neuropsychologists can be extremely helpful in difficult cases. Some athletes have complicated clinical histories prior to the injury. Attention-deficit/hyperactivity disorder, depression, anxiety, and chronic headaches can all make the clinical picture very confusing when the athlete is having symptoms such as concentration difficulties, mood swings, insomnia, or headaches that are not improving as expected. It is important to remember that many athletes would not rate their symptom severity score as all zeros at baseline, so expecting them to achieve this goal after injury is impractical. When this scenario is suspected, referral for neuropsychiatric testing can help to divide out which symptoms may be concussion related and which could be more chronic in nature.

Prevention

Helmets have been shown to reduce sports-related skull fractures and intracranial hemorrhages but have not been shown to decrease rates of concussion. Mouth guard use decreases the rate of dental injuries and lip lacerations but has not been definitively proven to decrease the rate of concussion or other brain injuries. Sport-specific rule changes have resulted in reduced rates of head injury. The most prominent and well-studied example is that of youth ice hockey. Introduction of the 2013 Canadian national body checking policy change disallowing body checking in Pee Wee hockey players below the age of 13 years resulted in a 50% relative reduction in injury rate and a 64% reduction in concussion rate in 11-year-old and 12-year-old hockey players in Alberta. Reduction of contact practices in certain team sports such as American football reduces exposure to head injury as well. Finally, epidemiologic evidence has demonstrated that the most likely period for repeat SRC is in the first 10 days after the most recent concussion, so disallowing contact activity during this interval has potential to reduce repeat concussions.

---

[1]Not FDA approved for this indication.
[7]Available as a dietary supplement.

References

Black AM, Hagel BE, Palacios-Derflingher L, et al: The risk of injury associated with body checking among Pee Wee ice hockey players: an evaluation of Hockey Canada's national body checking policy change, *Br J Sports Med* 51:1767–1772, 2017.

Coronado VG, Haileyesus T, Cheng TA, et al: Trends in sports-and recreation-related traumatic brain injuries treated in US emergency departments: The National Electronic Injury Surveillance System—All Injury Program (NEISS-AIP), 2001– 2012, *J Head Trauma Rehabil* 30:185–197, 2015.

Gessel LM, Fields SK, Collins CL, et al: Concussions among United States high school and collegiate athletes, *J Athl Train* 42:495–503, 2007.

Harmon KG, Clugston JR, Dec K, et al: American Medical Society for Sports Medicine position statement on concussion in sport, *Br J Sports Med* 53:213–225, 2019.

Kerr ZY, Roos KG, Djoko A, et al: Epidemiologic measures for quantifying the incidence of concussion in national collegiate athletic association sports, *J Athl Train* 52:167–174, 2017.

Leddy J, Haider M, Ellis M, et al: Early subthreshold aerobic exercise for sports related concussion: a randomized clinical trial. *JAMA Pediatr,* 173(4):319–325, 2019.

McCrory P, Meeuwisse W, Dvorak J, et al: Consensus statement on concussion in sport—the 5th international conference on concussion in sport held in Berlin, October 2016, *Br J Sports Med* 51:838–847, 2017.

Munivenkatappa A, Agrawal A, Shukla DP, et al: Traumatic brain injury: Does gender influence outcomes? *Int J Crit Illn Inj Sci* 6(2):70–73, 2016.

Nagahiro S, Mizobuchi Y: Current topics in sports-related head injuries: a review, *Neurol Med Chir (Tokyo)* 54:878–886, 2014.

Patricios JS, Schneider KJ, Dvorak J: Consensus statement on concussion in sport: the 6th International Conference on Concussion in Sport-Amsterdam, October 2022, *Br J Sports Med* 57(11):695–711, 2023.

Sarmiento K, Thomas K, Daugherty J, et al: Emergency department visits for sports and recreation-related traumatic brain injuries among children—United States, 2010-2016, *MMWR* 68:237–242, 2019; number 10.

Steenerson K, Starling AJ: Pathophysiology of sports-related concussion, *Neurol Clin* 35:403–408, 2017.

TARGETED TEMPERATURE MANAGEMENT (THERAPEUTIC HYPOTHERMIA)

Scott Leikin, DO; Jennifer Wang, DO; and Adel Bassily-Marcus, MD

CURRENT THERAPY

- Targeted temperature management (therapeutic hypothermia) should be considered following resuscitation from cardiac arrest to reduce the risk of anoxic brain injury.
- There does not appear to be a benefit to cooling to a temperature of 33°C when compared to cooling to a temperature of 36°C (97°F).
- There is a paradigm shift of therapeutic hypothermia to preventing fever and instituting a targeted temperature.
- Cooling pads are the most commonly used method to induce hypothermia.

Introduction

Inducing patients to a targeted temperature to reduce anoxic brain injury post cardiac arrest has now become the standard of care at medical institutions around the world. Although the theory has multiple applications for multiple conditions, post cardiac arrest is the most common and studied indication and the focus of this chapter. Although each institution has their own protocol, there are common tenets that are included in each institution's protocols. Current nomenclature is Targeted Temperature Management (TTM) as the theories on ideal temperature for the post cardiac arrest patient have evolved from therapeutic hypothermia. The evolution of TTM is important to understand, as the current theory is fever prevention is where the benefit is and fever is what is associated with poor neurologic outcomes in the post cardiac arrest time period.

The first multicenter, randomized control study on post cardiac arrest care was conducted in Europe and published in the New England Journal of Medicine (NEJM) in 2002. A total of 3551 patients were deemed eligible, but only 275 were included. In the study, 137 were assigned to hypothermia (32 to 34°C as measured by bladder temperature for 24 hours) and 138 to normothermia. To qualify in the study, subjects must have had a witnessed cardiac arrest, with an initial rhythm of ventricular fibrillation (VF) with return of spontaneous circulation (ROSC). The results showed a favorable neurologic outcome in 75/136 patients (55%) in the hypothermia group compared to 54/137 patients (39%) in the normothermia group at 6 months as measured by the Pittsburgh cerebral-performance category. The mortality difference at 6 months was 41% in the hypothermia group and 55% in the normothermia group. This validated the utilization of mild therapeutic hypothermia to improve neurologic outcomes and decrease mortality for witnessed VF cardiac arrest.

In 2002, a NEJM study described survival with good neurologic outcome to hospital discharge in patients who were unconscious after ROSC in out-of-hospital cardiac arrest. In the study, 77 patients were assigned to normothermia or moderate hypothermia (core body temperature of 33°C within 2 hours of ROSC for 12 total hours). Usually, out-of-hospital cardiac arrests have survival rates of only 5% to 35%. The investigators found 21/43 (49%) patients in the hypothermia group survived and had a favorable neurologic outcome compared to 9/34 (26%) in the normothermia group with (P = .046). The authors concluded that moderate hypothermia improved outcomes in patients with coma after ROSC in out-of-hospital cardiac arrest patients.

In 2010, the American Heart Association (AHA) released a class I recommendation for post VF/VT TTM. Pulseless electrical activity/asystole was given a IIb recommendation. TTM is generally defined as a core temperature of 33 to 36°C. Since this recommendation, TTM has been adopted as common practice post cardiac arrest in comatose adult patients.

In May 2011, the Society of Critical Care Medicine published "Targeted temperature management in critical care: A report and recommendations from five professional societies" and determined that TTM with a core body temperature goal of 32 to 34°C be used for post out-of-hospital VF/VT arrest.

In December 2013, the NEJM published a study titled "Targeted Temperature Management at 33°C versus 36°C after Cardiac Arrest." This international multicenter study aimed to determine the optimal temperature associated with improved neurologic outcomes for out-of-hospital cardiac arrest patients. They found no significant 180-day neurologic outcome or mortality difference between the patients in the 33°C arm and the patients in the 36°C arm. There were no adverse effects or benefits to patients cooled to 33°C. The authors concluded that in patients who were unconscious after ROSC was obtained in out-of-hospital cardiac arrest, a temperature of 33°C did not confer a benefit compared to a temperature of 36°C. This shifted the paradigm of therapeutic hypothermia to preventing fever and instituting a targeted temperature.

The International Liaison Committee on Resuscitation and the AHA Emergency Cardiovascular Care Committee and the Council on Cardiopulmonary, Critical Care and Perioperative and Resuscitation reviewed 5045 studies, of which 6 were RCTs and 5 were observational. They recommended: target core temperatures between 32 and 36°C for at least 24 hours and against using pre-hospital cooling with cooled intravenous fluids.

The theoretical benefits of TTM are that it can reduce brain oxygen usage by 6% for every 1°C reduction while also preventing inflammation and cerebral edema. TTM is currently being studied for encephalopathy, bacterial meningitis, cardiogenic shock, traumatic brain injury, and organ donation.

Initiation

With few absolute contraindications, TTM should be considered in all patients who achieved ROSC post cardiac arrest regardless of the underlying rhythm during the cardiac arrest. Many post cardiac arrest patients with ROSC will go to the cardiac catheterization lab for an angiogram and this should not delay the initiation of TTM. Determining the etiology for the cardiac arrest is still extremely important and should not have a bearing on the initiation of TTM. The patient populations in whom TTM is considered a relative contraindication include intracranial hemorrhage, exsanguination, hypotension refractory to multiple vasopressors, severe sepsis, and pregnancy. At our tertiary care academic medical center, the only absolute contraindications are cryoglobulinemia, traumatic injury leading to cardiac arrest, and family refusal or advanced directives that preclude the use of TTM.

Eligibility requires a comatose patient; the patient should not be able to follow commands or respond to noxious stimuli. This is equivalent to a Richmond Agitation Sedation Score of –4 or –5 or Glasgow Coma Scale <8. The patient must have a sustained cardiac rhythm that results in adequate brain perfusion.

The most studied rhythms in cardiac arrest which benefited from TTM were VT or VF. It is uncertain whether pulseless electrical activity and a "nonshockable rhythm" would benefit from TTM but we would advocate that any patient regardless of the underlying rhythm have TTM utilized if ROSC is obtained. This is in line with the 2015 AHA guidelines on post cardiac arrest care and emergency cardiovascular care. The guideline committee came to this conclusion because cohorts who did not receive TTM had such significant neurologic morbidity that the benefits were considered to outweigh the risks. Significant head trauma should be ruled out in patients who present to an emergency department with a noncontrast head computed tomography (CT) scan. Ideally, TTM should be initiated as soon as ROSC is obtained but it is acceptable to initiate it within the first 6 hours, and even up to 12 hours post arrest. We strongly advocate initiating the process as soon as feasible. We would also recommend that pacer pads be applied to the patient's skin and kept in place. The target core temperature should be maintained at the desired temperature for 24 hours. Based on a review of the literature, initiating a core temperature between 32 and 36°C for these patients with external cooling pads is the target.

The most commonly used method to induce hypothermia is with external cooling pads. Once the process is started, the time to target temperature should be within 2 hours. Other less commonly used options include ice bags at the groin, chest, axilla, and neck, and infusing cold saline. Cooled intravenous saline will reduce core temperature by 1°C every 30 minutes. The 2015 AHA guidelines recommend against cooling patients in the prehospital setting with intravenous cooled saline, as survival and neurologic recovery were not shown to be improved in various trials. Urinary catheters with temperature probes are often used to measure core temperature. Other acceptable methods of temperature measurement include esophageal, rectal, central, tympanic, or nasal probes. Axillary and oral temperature measurements are not reliable in measuring core temperature. Potential complications of cooling include electrolyte abnormalities, hyperglycemia, coagulopathy, and arrhythmias.

Maintenance

In TTM, the targeted core temperature should be maintained within 0.5°C for 24 hours. Shivering should be avoided as it creates heat, thereby increasing oxygen demand. Bedside Shivering Assessment Scale (BSAS) should be utilized to help guide therapy for shivering. For sedation purposes, our recommended first-line treatment is propofol (Diprivan) 15 to 20 µg/kg/min. Midazolam (Versed) 1 to 2 mg/h is an alternative. Fentanyl 25 µg/h infusion can be used if adequate sedation is not achieved.

The BSAS treatment algorithm should be utilized to eliminate shivering. In the BSAS, neuromuscular blockade with an agent such as cisatracurium (Nimbex) 0.15 mg/kg IV bolus followed by an infusion of 1 μg/kg/min can be used, although this protocol may mask seizures. The lowest dose that eliminates shivering using agents with a short half life is recommended because hypothermia slows medication metabolism and elimination.

TTM may worsen or cause hemodynamic derangements and arrhythmias, such as hypotension and bradycardia, that are common post cardiac arrest. Maintenance of a mean arterial pressure (MAP) at or above 65 mm Hg will help ensure adequate brain perfusion.

TTM patients are mechanically ventilated, and some institutions use esophageal probes to track body temperature, although this is less common, as it is invasive. Oxygen saturation should be maintained at 94% to 96% to avoid hypoxia or hyperoxygenation. Hyperglycemia is common with TTM, so serum glucose should be checked at set intervals, with a goal <180 mg/dL. If serum glucose is persistently >200 mg/dL despite treatment, an insulin drip should be considered. Electrolyte abnormalities, especially hypokalemia, are common during TTM. Therefore, the serum potassium level should be checked every 4 to 6 hours and replenished if lower than 3.5 meq/L. Rewarming may increase potassium levels.

It has been reported in the literature that up to 66% of TTM patients will develop an infection. Fever and leukocytosis may be present in the absence of infection and are not reliable indicators of infection. A comprehensive plan needs to be developed for every patient when signs of infection are potentially present. Even if a high percentage of patients develop an infection, this has not been shown to affect mortality.

Rewarming
Rewarming should occur 24 hours after achieving the targeted temperature. Rewarming should not occur at a rate that is faster than 0.2°C/h until the patient reaches 37°C; this will likely take between 6 to 12 hours. Once at 37°C, this temperature should be maintained for 48 to 72 hours, as rebound hyperthermia is associated with poor neurologic outcomes. Electrolyte abnormalities such as hyperkalemia, hypoglycemia, and hypotension may occur. Blood pressure should be carefully monitored during the rewarming period.

Post-Therapeutic Hypothermia/Prognosis
The AHA recommends 72 hours before prognosticating neurologic recovery. Presence of at least two of the following: incomplete brain stem reflexes, presence of myoclonus, unreactive electroencephalography (EEG), and absent cortical somatosensory-evoked potentials suggest poor neurologic outcome. A full neurologic examination should be done daily. Involving neurology or neurocritical care is advised to help prognosticate neurologic recovery in post cardiac arrest TTM patients.

References
Badjatia N, Strongilis E, Gordon E: Metabolic impact of shivering during therapeutic temperature modulation the bedside shivering assessment scale, *Stroke* 39(12):3242–3247, 2008, https://doi.org/10.1161/STROKEAHA.108.523654.

Bernard, Gray, Buist: Treatment of comatose survivors of out-of-hospital cardiac arrest with induced hypothermia. *New England Journal of Medicine*, 346:557–563, 2002, https://doi.org/10.1056/NEJMoa003289.

Callaway Clifton W, et al: American heart association guidelines update for cardiopulmonary resuscitation and emergency cardiovascular care, *Circulation* 132(18):S315–S367, 2015, https://doi.org/10.1161/CIR.0000000000000252, 3 Nov. 2015.

Donnino MW, Anderson LW, Berg KM, Reynolds JC: Temperature management after cardiac arrest an advisory statement by the advanced life support task force of the international liaison committee on resuscitation and the american heart association emergency cardiovascular care committee and the council on cardiopulmonary, critical care, perioperative and resuscitation, *Circulation* 132(25):2448–2456, 2015. https://doi.org/10.1161/CIR.0000000000000313.

Friedman OA: *Critical care: targeted temperature management after cardiac arrest,* In JM Orpopello, V Kvetan, SM Pastores. Eds. New York, NY: McGraw Hill, Lange, 2017.

Moler MD, Silverstein FS, Hulubkov R, et al: Therapeutic hypothermia after out-of-hospital cardiac arrest in children, *New Eng Journal of Medicine*, 372:1898–1908, 2015, Available at: https://doi.org/10.1056/NEJMoa1411480.

Nielson MD, PhD,Wetterslev N, MD, PhD, J, & Cronberg, MD, PhD, T: Targeted temperature management at 33°c versus 36°c after cardiac arrest. *New England Journal of Medicine* 369:2197–2206, 2013, Available at: https://doi.org/10.1056/NEJMoa1310519.

Nunnally M, Jaeschke R, Bellingan G: Targeted temperature management in critical care: a report and recommendations from five professional societies, *Critical Care Medicine* 39(5):1113–1125, 2011, https://doi.org/10.1097/CCM.0b013e318206bab2.

T.: Mild therapeutic hypothermia to improve the neurologic outcome after cardiac arrest, *New England Journal of Medicine* 346:549–556, 2002, https://doi.org/10.1056/NEJMoa012689.

Scirica BM: Therapeutic hypothermia after cardiac arrest, *Circulation, Clinician update* 127(2):244–250, 2013, https://doi.org/10.1161/CIRCULATIONAHA.111.076851.

Yunen JR, Tolentino R: *Critical care: chapter: controversies in therapeutic hypothermia,* In JM Oropello, V. Kvetan, SM Pastores. Eds.). New York, NY: McGraw Hill Lange, 2017.

TRIGEMINAL NEURALGIA

Method of
Karlynn Sievers, MD; and Hugh Silk, MD, MPH

CURRENT DIAGNOSIS

The International Headache Society Diagnostic criteria (classic) are as follows:
- Recurrent paroxysms of unilateral facial pain in the distribution(s) of one or more divisions of the trigeminal nerve, with no radiation beyond, and fulfilling criteria B and C
- Characteristics of pain:
  - Last from a fraction of a second to 2 min
  - Severe intensity
  - Electric shock-like, shooting, stabbing, or sharp in quality
  - Precipitated by innocuous stimuli to the affected trigeminal distribution
- Demonstration on magnetic resonance imaging (MRI) or during surgery of neurovascular compression (not simply contact), with morphologic changes in the trigeminal nerve root
- Not better accounted for by another diagnosis
- International Headache Society Diagnostic criteria (secondary)
- Same as previous except
  - Secondary trigeminal neuralgia secondary to another disease process

CURRENT THERAPY

- Medications
  - Carbamazepine: start 100 mg twice daily and increase by 200 mg/day to a maximum of 1200 mg/day (number needed to treat = 2)
  - Alternative treatments are available but have not been proven to be as effective (Table 1).
- For some patients with refractory or severe symptoms, surgical treatment (e.g., microvascular decompression, radiosurgery, alternative invasive procedures) can be helpful.

Epidemiology
The incidence of trigeminal neuralgia is estimated to be 5.9/100,000 women and 3.4/100,000 men. The peak incidence is in patients aged 60 to 70 years. It has also been called "tic

TABLE 1 Treatment Options for Trigeminal Neuralgia With Evidence of Effectiveness

TREATMENT TYPE	EVIDENCE OF EFFECTIVENESS
Medical therapy	
Carbamazepine (Tegretol)	Likely to be beneficial (gold standard)
Oxcarbazepine (Trileptal)[1]	Likely to be beneficial*
Baclofen (Lioresal)[1]	Likely to be beneficial,* particularly in patients with TN caused by MS
Gabapentin (Neurontin)[1]	Unknown effectiveness
Lamotrigine (Lamictal)[1]	Unknown effectiveness
Surgical therapy	
Microvascular decompression	Trade-off between benefits and harms*
Stereotactic radiosurgery	Trade-off between benefits and harms*
Percutaneous destructive radiosurgical techniques	Trade-off between benefits and harms*

*Based on observational studies and/or consensus.
[1]Not FDA approved for this indication.
MS, Multiple sclerosis; *TN,* trigeminal neuralgia.

douloureux" because of facial spasms that often accompany the disorder.

Risk Factors

Increasing age is a risk factor. Trigeminal neuralgia is rarely diagnosed in patients below 40 years of age. Other risk factors include multiple sclerosis (the incidence of trigeminal neuralgia in this population is 2% to 5%), stroke, and hypertension (especially in women). There is no racial predominance.

Pathophysiology

It is currently hypothesized that trigeminal neuralgia results from demyelination of the fifth cranial nerve, leading to electrical transmission of nerve impulses that are not mediated by neurotransmitters and that generate pain. Demyelination is most commonly caused by aberrant or tortuous blood vessels that cause nerve compression but can also be attributed to sources such as multiple sclerosis or amyloid deposition.

The most used classification system for trigeminal neuralgia has three categories: classical, secondary, and idiopathic. With classical trigeminal neuralgia, there is no underlying cause for the demyelination other than vascular compression, as described previously. With secondary trigeminal neuralgia, an alternate cause such as multiple sclerosis or tumor is responsible for the demyelination. A third category would include idiopathic trigeminal neuralgia, where there are no radiologic findings that account for the patient's symptoms.

Prevention

There is no known method for the prevention of trigeminal neuralgia.

Clinical Manifestations

Trigeminal neuralgia is a clinical diagnosis made based on recurrent attacks of unilateral facial pain. The pain is intense and is usually described as sharp, shock-like, or stabbing. Any of the branches of the trigeminal nerve can be affected, but the maxillary branch is the most common and the ophthalmic branch the least common. The pain lasts for seconds, and most patients are asymptomatic between attacks (though some will have a mild, dull, persistent ache around the affected nerve). Attacks can recur infrequently or hundreds of times per day.

Often, patients have trigger zones that will set off paroxysms of pain with minimal stimulation. Activities such as chewing, teeth brushing, or touching a trigger area can set off attacks; sometimes even minimal stimulation such as a light breeze can trigger an episode. Not all patients have trigger zones; however, the presence of these is nearly pathognomonic for trigeminal neuralgia.

Diagnosis

The diagnosis is clinical, based on the commonly described symptoms listed earlier. Diagnosis of trigeminal neuralgia should be considered in all patients who describe unilateral intense paroxysmal facial pain on three or more occasions. Careful examination of the head and neck and thorough neurologic examination should be performed in all patients. Exam findings are typically normal in patients with trigeminal neuralgia; therefore exam abnormalities should prompt reconsideration of the diagnosis. Sensory abnormalities (including vision or hearing loss), facial muscle weakness, or loss of the corneal reflex are not associated with trigeminal neuralgia and warrant further workup.

Laboratory studies are typically not helpful in making the diagnosis. Temporal mandibular joint or dental radiographs may be helpful to rule out other pathology for those who present with mid or lower face symptoms. Magnetic resonance imaging ([MRI] with and without contrast) of the brain can be helpful in distinguishing between classic and symptomatic trigeminal neuralgia and should be considered in all patients with new onset of symptoms. There is some early evidence that structural MRI techniques can help identify changes associated with trigeminal neuralgia and to predict those patients who will respond well to surgical intervention, but more research is needed in this area.

Differential Diagnosis

The differential diagnosis includes other types of headaches (migraine, cluster headache, paroxysmal hemicrania), dental sources (cracked teeth, caries, dental abscess), infectious causes (sinusitis, otitis media, postherpetic neuralgia), nervous system pathology (intracranial tumors, multiple sclerosis), temporomandibular joint syndrome, and giant cell arteritis. Many of these other diagnoses will have specific examination findings.

Treatment

Medical treatment should be initiated for all new cases of trigeminal neuralgia. Carbamazepine (Tegretol) has been shown in multiple randomized controlled trials to reduce pain in trigeminal neuralgia and is considered the gold standard for medical treatment. The number needed to treat is 2. Dosing starts at 100 mg twice daily and increases gradually in increments of 200 mg/day to a maximum of 1200 mg/day. Carbamazepine can have side effects such as drowsiness, dizziness, hepatotoxicity, pancreatitis, blood dyscrasias, and ataxia. Consensus opinion is that it has a greater than 50% failure rate for long-term (5–10 years) pain control. Oxcarbazepine (Trileptal)[1] can also be used, though the data are not as robust as for carbamazepine (level B for oxcarbazepine vs level A for carbamazepine). Medication should start at 600 mg/day in two divided doses and then be increased to 300 mg every third day to a maximum of 1800 mg. For both medications, testing for the HLA-B*15:02 allele should be considered in at-risk patients (e.g., those of Asian ancestry) to avoid Stevens-Johnson syndrome. Pimozide (Orap)[1] has been promoted as equal to carbamazepine; however, the studies are of low quality with no adverse effect comparison, and pimozide has many potentially serious side effects. Tizanidine (Zanaflex)[1] has been shown to be as effective as carbamazepine but also with low-quality studies. Lamotrigine (Lamictal)[1] can be used in patients who do not tolerate carbamazepine or as an adjunct to those without full benefit from carbamazepine, but the dose must be titrated slowly; therefore it is not as effective for acute pain control. Baclofen (Lioresal)[1] and gabapentin (Neurontin)[1] may be useful in patients with multiple sclerosis who also have trigeminal neuralgia, but evidence is lacking regarding their effectiveness in classical trigeminal neuralgia. Topical lidocaine has been used intraorally for those with significant oral pain from trigeminal neuralgia;

---

[1]Not FDA approved for this indication.

however, again, there are no well-designed studies of its efficacy. A new sodium channel blocker (Vixotrigine)[5] with affinity for the Na_v 1.7 sodium channel is being investigated with some promising evidence of effectiveness, but it is still in clinical trials and not yet available for prescription. Eslicarbazepine (Aptiom)[1] is a third-generation antiepileptic that is being investigated as well; 88.9% of patients had good pain relief, but there was a high rate of side effects (71%). Sumatriptan (Imitrex) has been used extensively for migraine headache and is now being tried for refractory trigeminal neuralgia symptoms.[1] Dosing is 3 mg subcutaneously or 50 mg twice daily orally. With this dosing, baseline pain scores decreased after 15 minutes, and these effects persisted after discontinuation of treatment for 1 week. Primary side effects with sumatriptan included dizziness and rebound headaches.

Recent studies have shown some weak data that botulinum toxin A (Botox)[1] can be an effective treatment in reducing both the intensity of pain and frequency of paroxysms in trigeminal neuralgia; adverse events include facial asymmetry and edema or hematoma at the injection site. Alcohol injections[1] and cryotherapy have also been used to treat the pain of trigeminal neuralgia.

For some patients with refractory or severe symptoms, surgical treatment can be helpful. Microvascular decompression and radiosurgery are both common techniques for the treatment of trigeminal neuralgia, with microvascular decompression generally considered to be first-line surgical intervention. Other surgical techniques can include radiofrequency thermocoagulation, glycerol rhizolysis, stereotactic radiosurgery, balloon compression, peripheral nerve section, partial sensory root section, and gamma-knife radiosurgery. Studies have noted sensory side effects, and most evidence for neurosurgical approaches comes from observational studies.

Neuromodulation is an alternative for patients with symptoms refractory to pharmacotherapy who do not want to pursue surgical treatment. Both central and peripheral neuromodulation have been studied, but evidence of effectiveness is very limited. Other newer treatments as an alternative to surgery include ozone injection around the Gasserian ganglion, nerve combing, cryotherapy, low level laser therapy, and carbon dioxide laser therapy. Though these therapies have shown some signs of

reduction in pain, they are newer and are still undergoing trials to determine efficacy.

Treatment for secondary trigeminal neuralgia typically includes treating the underlying cause.

Monitoring

Although there is no standard protocol for monitoring patients with trigeminal neuralgia, the condition is extremely painful, and there have been incidents reported of patients accidently overdosing on medications or taking their own lives. Therefore it is recommended that patients be monitored at regular intervals to make sure that their pain is controlled and to monitor for side effects from treatment.

Management of Complications

The disease can have relapses and remissions. Medications or alternative treatments should be reinstituted as needed. Tests should be run as needed based on side effect symptoms, and treatments should be stopped and others considered based on efficacy and patient tolerance.

References

Burman K, Khandelwal A, Chaturvedi A: Recent advances in trigeminal neuralgia and its Management: a Narrative Review, *J Neuroanesthesia Crit Care* 8(2):112–117, 2021. 2021.

Cruccu G, Stefano G, Truini A: Trigeminal neuralgia, *N Engl J Med* 383:754–762, 2020, https://doi.org/10.1056/NEJMra1914484.

Gubian A, Rosahl SK: Meta-analysis on safety and efficacy of microsurgical and radiosurgical treatment of trigeminal neuralgia, *World Neurosurg* 103:757–767, 2017.

International Headache Society: International Classification of Headache Disorders (3rd edition – beta version). Available at http://www.ihs-headache.org/ichd-guidelines/ihs-guidelines. Accessed March 15, 2022.

Khan M, Nishi SE, Hassan SN, et al: Trigeminal neuralgia, glossopharyngeal neuralgia, and mysfascial pain dysfunction syndrome: an update, *Pain Res Manag* 7438326, 2017, https://doi.org/10.1155/2017/7438326. Epub 2017 Jul 30. Accessed March 7, 2021.

Lambru G, Zakrzewska J, Matharu M: Trigeminal neuralgia: a practical guide, *Practical Neurol* 21:392–402, 2021.

Obermann, M. Recent advances in understanding/managing trigeminal neuralgia. *F1000Res2019 – Review*. PMID 31069052.

Wiffen PJ, Derry S, Moore RA, et al: Carbamazepine for acute and chronic pain. In *The cochrane library*, Chichester, UK, 2013, John Wiley & Sons, Ltd. (Search date 2010).

Zhang J, Yang M, Zhou M: Non-antiepileptic drugs for trigeminal neuralgia, *Cochrane Database Syst Rev* 12, 2013.

---

[5] Investigational drug in the United States.
[1] Not FDA approved for this indication.

ALCOHOL USE DISORDER

Method of
David A. Frenz, MD

CURRENT DIAGNOSIS

- Unhealthy alcohol use (UAU) represents a continuum of alcohol use associated with negative health consequences, including addiction.
  - *Hazardous use* increases the risk of health consequences.
  - *Harmful use* has caused health consequences but does not meet the threshold for addiction.
  - *Alcohol use disorder* (AUD) represents addiction as defined by the *Diagnostic and Statistical Manual of Mental Disorders,* fifth edition, text revision *(DSM-5-TR).*
- A single-question screener (SQS) is a clinically efficient means to assess for UAU.
  - When negative, UAU has been reliably excluded.
  - When positive, the Alcohol Use Disorders Identification Test (AUDIT) should be administered.
- The AUDIT stratifies patients into four groups.
  - A score <8 points is a negative screen; UAU has been excluded unless there is clear evidence of malingering or deception.
  - A score of 8 to 15 points is consistent with hazardous use.
  - A score of 16 to 19 points is consistent with harmful use.
  - A score >19 points is worrisome for addiction and requires further assessment.
- Checklists based on the *DSM-5-TR* can be used to assess for addiction.

CURRENT THERAPY

- Some patients with AUD are physiologically dependent on alcohol and require medically managed withdrawal (detoxification) to prevent severe and complicated withdrawal syndromes.
  - Carefully selected patients can be withdrawn on an ambulatory basis using the Short Alcohol Withdrawal Scale (SAWS) and lorazepam.
- All patients with UAU should receive counseling.
  - The goal is to reduce alcohol-related risks and harms, not achieve abstinence.
  - Counseling can take the form of simple advice, motivational interviewing (MI), chain analysis, and cognitive-behavioral therapy (CBT).
- Simple advice involves educating patients about drink sizes, daily and weekly drinking limits, pacing and spacing, and avoiding and managing triggers.
  - The National Institute on Alcohol Abuse and Alcoholism (NIAAA) offers a variety of free patient materials to facilitate these discussions and serve as behavioral prescriptions.

- MI helps patients recognize that their current choices and behaviors are ultimately not consistent with their stated goals and values.
  - Patients seemingly discover this "on their own" through skillful conversations involving open questions, reflective listening, and other communication techniques.
  - Recognition and felt discrepancy provide the psychic energy or motivation for patients to change.
- Chain analysis helps patients recognize the many intermediate steps between a stimulus to drink alcohol and eventually consuming it.
  - Patients can "break the chain" by developing and following action plans for each link in chain.
- CBT helps patient recognize how their distorted (irrational) beliefs drive alcohol use.
  - Numbing, avoiding, and chemical coping are often the result of rigid demands, awfulizing, frustration intolerance, and depreciation beliefs.
  - Clinicians help patients transform their irrational beliefs into rational, flexible preferences; this tends to reduce alcohol use.
- Addiction pharmacotherapy should be considered for all patients with AUD.
  - Acamprosate (Campral) and naltrexone (ReVia, Vivitrol) reduce drinking and have favorable side-effect profiles.
  - Medication selection is based on patient preference, factors such as medication compliance, and end-organ function.

Classification

UAU represents a continuum of alcohol use associated with negative health consequences, including addiction. This conceptualization has been adopted by the United States Preventive Services Task Force (USPSTF) and is the basis for screening, brief intervention, and referral to treatment (SBIRT), the contemporary graded approach to management described in this chapter.

UAU consists of three mutually exclusive categories (Box 1). *Hazardous use* increases the future risk of negative health consequences; *harmful use* has already caused adverse health consequences but does not meet the criteria for addiction; and *alcohol use disorder* (AUD), or *addiction,* is defined by the *DSM-5-TR.*

Hazardous use is anchored in binge drinking and weekly consumption limits. A binge is alcohol consumption that results in legal intoxication (blood alcohol concentration [BAC] ≥0.08 gram percent). For healthy adults, this is typically >3 drinks for women and men ≥65 years of age, and >4 drinks for men <65 years of age, where one U.S. standard drink contains 14 grams of ethanol (Table 1). Alcohol intoxication is strongly associated with immediate risks including injuries, suicide, and violence.

Over longer timescales, alcohol is associated with a broad range of conditions including infectious diseases, many cancers, cardiovascular diseases, gastrointestinal diseases, mood disorders, and epilepsy. Consuming >7 drinks per week increases all-cause mortality in a linear manner, regardless of gender. AUD is defined in the *DSM-5-TR* as "a problematic pattern of alcohol use leading to clinically significant impairment or distress, as manifested by

BOX 1   The Alcohol-Use Continuum

Low Risk Use, Including No Use
Consumption of alcohol below amounts identified as hazardous; and use in circumstances not defined as hazardous (context)
Example: One glass of wine with dinner several days per week

Hazardous Use
Alcohol use that increases the risk for health consequences

Hazardous Consumption
Females; males ≥65 years of age: >3 drinks/day and/or >7 drinks/week
Males <65 years of age: >4 drinks/day and/or >7 drinks/week

Hazardous Context
Example: Alcohol use during pregnancy

Harmful Use
Alcohol use with health consequences in the absence of addiction
Example: College student who sustains a forehead laceration secondary to falling down while intoxicated

Alcohol Use Disorder
Addiction to alcohol per the *Diagnostic and Statistical Manual of Mental Disorders (DSM-5-TR)*
• Mild: 2–3 criteria
• Moderate: 4–5 criteria
• Severe: ≥6 criteria

The shaded portion represents unhealthy alcohol use (UAU).

BOX 2   Two-Step Process for Screening for Unhealthy Alcohol Use (UAU) and Associated Management

Step 1: Single-Question Screener (SQS)
How many times in the past year have you had X or more drinks in a day?
where X = 4 for females and males ≥65 years of age; and X = 5 for males <65 years of age

Management
0 times: None/done (negative screen)
≥1 times: Proceed to Step 2

Step 2: Alcohol Use Disorders Identification Test (AUDIT)
Administer full-scale AUDIT (10 items)
(https://auditscreen.org/check-your-drinking)

Management
<8 points: None/done (negative screen)
8–15 points: Brief intervention
16–19 points: Brief intervention and continued monitoring
>19 points: Assess for Alcohol Use Disorder (AUD), initiate treatment if present

TABLE 1   U.S. Standard Drinks: By Definition, One Standard Drink Contains 14 Grams of Ethonol

BEVERAGE	ALCOHOL BY VOLUME	DRINK SIZE
Beer (regular)	5%	12 fl oz
Wine	12%	5 fl oz
Distilled spirits*	40%†	1.5 fl oz

*Examples include vodka, gin, whiskey, rum, and tequila
†80 proof
Data from U.S. Department of Agriculture and U.S. Department of Health and Human Services. Dietary Guidelines for Americans, 2020–2025 (9th ed). Washington, DC: U.S. Department of Agriculture, 2020, p. 49

at least two [criteria], occurring within a 12-month period." The *DSM-5-TR* outlines 11 criteria such as "alcohol is often taken in larger amounts or over a longer period than was intended" and "recurrent alcohol use resulting in a failure to fulfill major role obligations at work, school, or home." Consumption (frequency and quantity), the defining features of hazardous use, has never been part of the construct.

Harmful use exists when alcohol-related harm has occurred but the "problematic pattern" and/or criterion threshold for AUD have not been satisfied.

Epidemiology
Large, population-based surveys have found that 17.1% to 24.4% of Americans binge drink, with considerable regional variability. This translates into healthcare settings. For example, a cross-sectional study of 2.7 million primary care patients determined that 6.1% exceeded recommended daily consumption limits (male: 8.7%; female: 3.8%).

A similar pattern exists for AUD. The third wave of the National Epidemiologic Survey on Alcohol and Related Conditions (NESARC-III), a cross-sectional survey of American adults, found that 13.9% and 29.1% of the population met criteria for AUD in the preceding year and on a lifetime basis, respectively. Coincidentally, the corresponding prevalence is 13.9% in primary care settings.

Diagnosis
In light of its prevalence and considerable harms, the USPSTF recommends "screening for UAU in primary care settings in adults 18 years or older, including pregnant women, and providing persons engaged in risky or hazardous drinking with brief behavioral counseling interventions to reduce unhealthy alcohol use."

Various screening instruments exist. The author prefers a two-step process beginning with a single-question screener (SQS)[a] to reduce the testing burden for both patients and clinicians (Box 2). Positive screens are then clarified with the AUDIT (https://auditscreen.org/check-your-drinking). Both instruments are in the public domain and may be used without formal permission or licensing.

Although patients with UAU can engage in malingering and deception, the reported sensitivity of the SQS ranges from 0.73 to 0.88. Its negative predictive value (NPV), which depends on prevalence, is 0.94 to 0.98 when 5% to 15% of those screened have UAU. Said differently, this corresponds to a 2% to 6% false-negative classification ("miss rate") at typical base rates in primary care.

Patients with significantly elevated AUDIT scores (>19 points) require careful assessment for AUD. This can be accomplished through structured clinical interviews ("checklists" based on *DSM-5-TR* criteria) or referral to a mental health professional for diagnostic assessment. Suggested checklists include the Structured Clinical Interview for DSM-5 Disorders (SCID-5-CV; Module E) and the Mini International Neuropsychiatric Interview (MINI; Module I).

Treatment
Management of UAU depends on patient classification (see Box 1). Most patients, including those with AUD, are appropriate for initial treatment in primary care settings.

Some patients with AUD are physiologically dependent on alcohol and require medically managed withdrawal (detoxification) to prevent severe and complicated withdrawal syndromes. The latter includes withdrawal seizure and withdrawal delirium (delirium tremens).

---

[a]Also known as the NIAAA single-item question or one of the AUDIT-C (consumption) questions.

BOX 3   Ambulatory Withdrawal Management

Step 1: Administer the Prediction of Alcohol Withdrawal Severity Scale (PAWSS)

Score < 4: Proceed to Step 2

Score ≥ 4: Consider consultation with an addiction medicine physician

https://www.mdcalc.com/calc/10102/prediction-alcohol-withdrawal-severity-scale

Step 2. Assess for additional risk factors*

Absent: Proceed to Step 3

Present: Consider consultation with an addiction medicine physician

Step 3. Administer the Revised Clinical Institute Withdrawal Assessment for Alcohol (CIWA–Ar)

Score < 10: Proceed to Step 4

Score ≥ 10: Consider consultation with an addiction medicine physician

https://www.mdcalc.com/calc/1736/ciwa-ar-alcohol-withdrawal

Step 4. Administer the Short Alcohol Withdrawal Scale (SAWS)

Score < 12: Proceed to Step 5

Score ≥ 12: Consider consultation with an addiction medicine physician

https://z.umn.edu/adle

Step 5. Initial home treatment plan

- Thiamine 100 mg by mouth per day for 5 days
- Patient to measure SAWS at least 4 times per day
- Lorazepam 1 mg by mouth ×1 when SAWS ≥ 12 for the first time. Contact physician right away for additional instructions

Step 6. Updated home treatment plan

- Patient should check in with physician daily for 5 days
- Goal is to keep SAWS < 12
- Suggested lorazepam taper
  - Day 1: 1 mg by mouth every 6 hours
  - Day 2: 1 mg by mouth every 8 hours
  - Day 3: 1 mg by mouth every 12 hours
  - Day 4: 1 mg by mouth
- Consider consultation with an addiction medicine physician if SAWS ≥ 12 despite suggested taper
- Decrease lorazepam frequency if patient reports sedation or mental clouding
- Maintain a low threshold for recalling the patient to clinic for an in-person examination

*Withdrawing from other substances; physiologic dependence on opioids; opioid use disorder; consuming > 8 standard drinks per day; previously tried/failed ambulatory withdrawal management; pregnancy; older age; epilepsy; history of non-alcohol related seizure; clinically significant laboratory abnormalities; active psychiatric symptoms; cognitive impairment; absence of a reliable caregiver; communication barriers; inability to check in with provider daily or return to clinic, if needed.

Adapted from the American Society of Addiction Medicine's Clinical Practice Guideline on Alcohol Withdrawal Management

Primary care clinicians can attempt ambulatory withdrawal management if withdrawal scores are low/mild and risk factors for severe and complicated withdrawal are absent (Box 3).

Goals

Total abstinence from alcohol has traditionally been the treatment goal; however, this disease-oriented outcome is difficult to achieve and maintain in both clinical trials and "real-world" settings. The author prefers pragmatic, patient-oriented treatment goals ("progress not perfection") that are consistent with the trend toward non-abstinent recovery.[b] This is analogous to other chronic diseases in which improvement is celebrated (e.g., reduction in hemoglobin A_{1c}), even if the ideal state has not been achieved.

For patients who meet *DSM-5-TR* criteria for AUD, a reduction in severity represents clinical progress, for example, when a patient who fulfilled seven criteria ("severe") at baseline now fulfills three criteria ("mild"). Remission is achieved when no criteria for AUD have been satisfied for at least 3 months, except for the criterion for craving. As noted previously, consumption is not part of the *DSM-5-TR* construct: abstinence is not required for remission.

Relapse is a nonclinical term that generally means that drinking has interrupted a period of continuous abstinence. The author suggests using more clinically accurate categories in the UAU spectrum.

Counseling

The USPSTF recommends behavioral counseling interventions for patients with UAU. This generally begins with simple advice about drink sizes, daily and weekly drinking limits, pacing and spacing, and avoiding and managing triggers. The NIAAA offers a variety of free patient materials to facilitate these discussions and serve as behavioral prescriptions (https://bit.ly/3Jb6mHh).

MI is a person-centered style of counseling that is used to address ambivalence about changing one's behaviors. Systematic reviews have consistently demonstrated its effectiveness for various alcohol-related outcomes, although a recent meta-analysis questioned its efficacy in maintaining abstinence in primary care settings. The method involves open questions, reflective listening, and other communication techniques (Box 4). The goal is to lead patients to recognize that their current choices and behaviors are ultimately inconsistent with their stated goals and values. This discrepancy, when recognized and felt, provides the psychic energy or motivation for the patient to change. Self-help books can provide structure and cadence for office visits and can serve as out-of-session "homework" between visits (https://amzn.to/3usxUD0).

Chain analysis helps patients recognize the many intermediate steps between a stimulus to drink alcohol and eventually consuming it. Patients can "break the chain" by developing and following action plans for each link in the chain. Patient worksheets can be used to analyze their behaviors and serve as tools that they can use in the community (https://cls.unc.edu/wp-content/uploads/sites/3019/2016/06/Chain-Analysis-Worksheet.pdf).

CBT helps patients recognize how their distorted (irrational) beliefs cause unhealthy negative emotions and behaviors, including drinking. Irrational beliefs take four general forms:
- Rigid demands: Must, should, ought
- Awfulizing: "It's awful ... Terrible ... End of the world"
- Frustration intolerance: "I can't stand it"
- Depreciation beliefs: "I'm no good," "She's no good," "It's no good"

For example, a patient may experience family conflicts or financial adversities. Frustration intolerance may lead them to use alcohol to numb, avoid, or chemically cope with the situation.

CBT helps patients transform their irrational beliefs into flexible preferences (e.g., "My financial situation is challenging, but I've had money problems before and can tolerate it). These new rational beliefs tend to reduce alcohol use. Patient worksheets (https://web.archive.org/web/20210512220141/http://www.oxfordclinicalpsych.com/view/10.1093/med:psych/9780199743049.001.0001/med-9780199743049-interactive-pdf-005.pdf) and inexpensive self-help books (https://www.amazon.com/REBT-Pocket-Companion-Clients-2nd/dp/1914938194) can support these efforts.

---

[b] Sometimes referred to as "harm reduction." The author considers the term confusing as all of medicine is ultimately harm reduction. Of greater concern, the term is potentially pejorative and can interfere with the therapeutic alliance.

BOX 4 Motivational Interviewing

The patient completed the SQS (positive) and AUDIT (score = 17) as part of a well-adult examination. This exchange demonstrates Open questions, Affirming, Reflecting and Summarizing (OARS), which support the first fundamental task of motivational interviewing: engaging.

Provider: Thanks for filling out that paperwork before our visit. [A]
Patient: No problem.

Provider: Would it be okay to discuss some of your answers?
Patient: Sure.

Provider: It looks like you're drinking alcohol on most days. [S]
Patient: Yeah, I have a few glasses of wine with dinner.

Provider: Seems like that might be a change from last year. [O]
Patient: Probably. Work has been stressful.

Provider: Say more. [O]
Patient: We're short-staffed, so I've been working a ton of hours. And customers have been tough to deal with—they want everything yesterday.

Provider: How do you think that's connected to wine? [O]
Patient: I'm pretty wound up after work. I guess wine helps me relax and chill out.

Provider: What else? [O]
Patient: Well, work is always on my mind. Wine takes that down a few notches. It also helps me sleep.

Provider: Work has been stressful, and alcohol helps you with tension and worry. [S]
Patient: Yeah; it calms me down.

Provider: And getting good sleep is important to you. [R]
Patient: Totally—I need energy and have to be mentally sharp for my job.

Provider: You're stuck in a vicious cycle at work, and alcohol helps you cope with that—so it's helpful from that standpoint. [R]
Patient: [Nods in agreement]

The patient's AUDIT score suggests alcohol-related problems. The provider might segue to problem items in the following way.

Provider: But it seems like alcohol might have some downsides, too. [S]
Patient: Maybe.

Medications

Addiction pharmacotherapy, sometimes described as *medication-assisted treatment* (MAT),[c] is generally reserved for patients with AUD (Box 5). Disulfiram (Antabuse), which was approved by the U.S. Food and Drug Administration in 1951, has generally fallen into disuse secondary to lack of efficacy, medication interactions, and potential for various harms.

Naltrexone (ReVia [oral], Vivitrol [IM]) and acamprosate (Campral) both improve drinking outcomes, although with various nuances depending on trial design and type of data analysis. In placebo-controlled trials, acamprosate but not naltrexone increased abstinence, while naltrexone but not acamprosate reduced heavy drinking. Head-to-head trials found differences between the

medications; however, they were ultimately equivalent when these data were subject to meta-analysis. Overall, the author selects one medication over the other based on patient preference and factors such as medication compliance and end-organ function.

The literature continues to evolve on the off-label use of medications including baclofen (Lioresal), gabapentin (Neurontin), and topiramate (Topamax). In the author's opinion, these should generally be prescribed in consultation with an addiction medicine specialist after patients have tried and failed adequate therapeutic trials of acamprosate and naltrexone despite robust psychosocial treatments.

Comorbidities

Other mental disorders frequently co-occur[d] with AUD and often precede its onset. In this context, AUD may represent a maladaptive coping mechanism for affective and anxious symptoms and for psychological trauma. Nascent evidence is mixed on treatment priorities and modalities. In the absence of firm guidance, management is empiric and should likely occur in consultation with local mental health experts.

Similarly, medical conditions such as chronic pain syndromes often co-occur with AUD and portend poorer drinking outcomes. Here, too, the literature is incipient, and management should occur in consultation with local experts (e.g., addiction medicine, pain medicine).

Uncertainties and Controversies

Alcoholic Anonymous (AA) formed in the 1930s and continues to play a central role in the recovery community. Its effectiveness has long been debated secondary to defects in trial design such as standardization of interventions, selection bias, blinding, and patient attrition. A recent systematic review focused primarily on manualized Twelve-Step Facilitation (TSF), a standardized, professionally delivered treatment that facilitates involvement in AA. It found that TSF improved complete abstinence compared with MI and CBT, and it was equivalent for six remaining outcomes such as drinking intensity and alcohol-related consequences. The certainty of evidence was variable and ranged from very low to high, depending on the outcome. None of the studies included a true control condition (e.g., wait list control) or compared TSF to addiction pharmacotherapy. The author takes a "might help, can't hurt" posture but does not consider community-based (peer-led) AA a substitute for treatments for which there is stronger evidence.

ASAM maintains a comprehensive guideline *(The ASAM Criteria)* for assessing patients and matching them to the most appropriate level of care (e.g., outpatient vs. residential treatment) based on their clinical characteristics (https://www.asam.org.asam-criteria/asam-criteria-4th-edition). It first appeared in 1991 and is widely used by treatment providers and funders (health plans, government agencies). The framework represents expert opinion for which outcome data are sparse. Some have more bluntly noted that matching patients to treatment options based on expert opinion is little better than assigning patients by chance. The author considers *The ASAM Criteria* a helpful rule of thumb but gives considerable weight to patient preferences in terms of treatment setting. A carefully supervised trial of office-based addiction treatment is reasonable if a patient is unwilling or unable to pursue a higher level of care, provided imminent danger[e] is absent.

---

[c]The author prefers to describe addiction pharmacotherapy as *disease-modifying therapy* (DMT) because medications are often the primary or sole treatment for addiction, especially for other substance use disorders such as opioid addiction.

[d]There is an old, ungrammatical saw in addiction medicine: "Which came first and which came worse?" Did generalized anxiety disorder (GAD), for example, develop first and then chemical coping and AUD followed? Or, did AUD develop first and then anxious symptoms instead represent a substance-induced anxiety disorder? This is often difficult to establish by history and only becomes evident on a post hoc basis.

[e]ASAM's doctrine of imminent danger consists of three components: (1) a strong probability that certain behaviors will occur; (2) the likelihood that such behaviors will present a significant risk of serious adverse consequences to the individual and/or others; and (3) the likelihood that such adverse events will occur in the very near future, within hours and days, rather than weeks or months.

BOX 4 | Addiction Pharmacotherapy

Acamprosate

Brand name: Campral

Usual maintenance dosing: 666 mg by mouth three times per day

Mechanism of action: Postulated to be a gamma-amino butyric acid (GABA) agonist, glutamate antagonist, or both

Elimination: Excreted unchanged in urine

Adverse effects: Principally gastrointestinal, especially diarrhea

Prescribing pearls:
- Obtain baseline renal function test. Moderate impairment does not preclude therapy but requires monitoring. Do not use if eGFR <30 mL/min
- Initiate therapy at usual maintenance dose. Reduce dose to 666 mg two times per day for patients <60 kg. Reduce dose to 333 mg three times per day for eGFR 30–60 mL/min
- Gastrointestinal symptoms, if they develop, generally occur with initiation of treatment and are dose-related and transient. Consider temporary dose reduction (e.g., 333 mg three times per day for 7 days) for severe symptoms that threaten ongoing therapy
- Can be safely used with benzodiazepines and alcohol. May be started during medically managed withdrawal. Patients who resume drinking should be encouraged to continue taking acamprosate

Naltrexone

Brand names: ReVia (oral), Vivitrol (injectable)

Usual maintenance dosing: ReVia 50 mg by mouth daily; Vivitrol 380 mg intramuscularly every 4 weeks

Mechanism of action: Opioid antagonist

Elimination: Extensively metabolized by the liver, primarily excreted in urine

Adverse reactions: Opioid withdrawal syndrome, including precipitated withdrawal if opioid tolerant; hepatotoxicity; injection site reactions

Prescribing pearls:
- Patient must be opioid-free for ≥7 days before initiating therapy. Consider urine toxicology if abstinence cannot be reliably established by history
- Obtain baseline liver function tests. Alcohol-related transaminase elevations are common at baseline and should improve as alcohol consumption decreases. Do not use if transaminases are >5 times normal
- Obtain baseline renal function test. Moderate impairment does not preclude therapy but requires monitoring. Do not use if eGFR <30 mL/min
- Initiate oral therapy at 25 mg per day, titrating to usual maintenance dose over 7–14 days
- Mild opioid withdrawal symptoms, if they develop, generally occur with initiation of treatment, are dose-related and transient (they are likely caused by antagonism of endogenous opioids, e.g., endorphins). Consider temporary oral dose reduction (e.g., 12.5 mg per day for 7 days) for severe symptoms that threaten ongoing therapy
- Repeat liver function tests at 1 month and periodically thereafter
- Can be safely used with benzodiazepines and alcohol. May be started during medically managed withdrawal. Patients who resume drinking should be encouraged to continue taking naltrexone
- Always establish tolerability with the oral formulation before switching to injectable

Data from Center for Substance Abuse Treatment. Incorporating alcohol pharmacotherapies into medical practice. Treatment Improvement Protocol (TIP) Series 49. HHS Publication No. (SMA) 09-4380. Rockville, MD: Substance Abuse and Mental Health Services Administration, 2009.

References

The ASAM Clinical Practice Guideline on Alcohol Withdrawal Management, *J Addict Med* 14(3S Suppl 1):1–72, 2020. PMID: 32511109.

American Psychiatric Association: *Diagnostic and statistical manual of mental disorders*, ed 5, text revision, Arlington, VA, 2022, American Psychiatric Association, p 553ff.

Bahji A, Bach P, Danilewitz M, et al.: Comparative efficacy and safety of pharmacotherapies for alcohol withdrawal: a systematic review and network meta-analysis, *Addiction* 117(10):2591–2601, 2002.

Hall K, Gibbie T, Lubman DI: Motivational interviewing techniques—facilitating behaviour change in the general practice setting, *Aust Fam Physician* 41(9):660–667, 2012. PMID: 22962639.

Miller WR, Rollnick S: *Motivational interviewing*, ed 4, New York, 2023, Guilford Press, pp 49–140.

Saitz R: Unhealthy alcohol use, *N Engl J Med* 352(6):596–607, 2005. PMID: 15703424.

Saitz R, Miller SC, Fiellin DA, Rosenthal RN: Recommended use of terminology in addiction medicine, *J Addict Med* 15(1):3–7, 2021. PMID: 32482955.

Searight HR: Counseling patients in primary care: evidence-based strategies, *Am Fam Physician* 98(12):719–728, 2018. PMID: 30525356.

Sim MG, Wain T, Khong E: Influencing behaviour change in general practice. Part 1—brief intervention and motivational interviewing, *Aust Fam Physician* 38(11):885–888, 2009. PMID: 19893835.

Sim MG, Wain T, Khong E: Influencing behaviour change in general practice. Part 2—motivational interviewing approaches, *Aust Fam Physician* 38(12):986–989, 2009. PMID: 20369152.

Spithoff S, Kahan M: Primary care management of alcohol use disorder and at-risk drinking. Part 1: screening and assessment, *Can Fam Physician* 61(6):509–514, 2015. PMID: 26071154.

Spithoff S, Kahan M: Primary care management of alcohol use disorder and at-risk drinking. Part 2: counsel, prescribe, connect, *Can Fam Physician* 61(6):515–521, 2015. PMID: 26071155.

Stuart MR, Lieberman JA: *The fifteen minute hour: efficient and effective patient-centered consultation skills*, ed 6, Boca Raton, FL, 2019, CRC Press.

Tiglao SM, Meisenheimer ES, Oh RC: Alcohol withdrawal syndrome: outpatient management, *Am Fam Physician* 104(3):253–262, 2021. PMID: 34523874.

US Preventive Services Task Force: Screening and behavioral counseling interventions to reduce unhealthy alcohol use in adolescents and adults: US Preventive Services Task Force recommendation statement, *J Am Med Assoc* 320(18):1899–1909, 2018. PMID: 30422199.

AUTISM SPECTRUM DISORDER

Method of
Meelie Bordoloi, MD

CURRENT DIAGNOSIS

- The diagnosis of autism spectrum disorder (ASD) relies on diagnostic criteria listed in the *Diagnostic and Statistical Manual of Mental Disorders* (DSM-5) with core features present from the early childhood developmental period.
- Key features of autism spectrum disorder include:
  - Impairment of functions of daily living.
  - Deficits in social-emotional reciprocity, nonverbal communication, and developing/maintaining relationships.
  - Presence of repetitive behaviors like repeated movements or speech, cognitive rigidity, intense focus on specific interests or unusual reactions to sensory experiences.
  - Presence of diverse range of symptoms and abilities, with severity determined by the level of support required in daily life.
  - Presence or absence of intellectual development and/or impairment or absence of functional language.
  - Presence of comorbid psychiatric conditions such as anxiety, depression, attention-deficit/hyperactivity disorder being common.

871

CURRENT THERAPY

- The goal of treatment is to enhance functioning in different settings, independence, and improved quality of life.
- The objectives of early intervention and individualized approaches to treatment is to lead to significant long-term improvements.
- Applied Behavior Analysis (ABA), a behavioral intervention focusing on positive reinforcement, remains the cornerstone of evidence-based treatment of autism spectrum disorder.
- Comprehensive programs providing social skills training, speech-language therapy, occupational therapy, and educational interventions are crucial supports to improve functioning.
- There is no single pharmacologic agent to treat autism. Aripiprazole (Abilify) and risperidone (Risperdal) are approved by the US Food and Drug Administration for the treatment of symptoms of aggression in autism.
- Comorbid psychiatric conditions such as attention-deficit/hyperactivity disorder, anxiety, depression should be treated with pharmacological agents based on severity. Comorbid medical and genetic conditions should be treated accordingly.
- Continued medical/psychiatric care and family support are crucial.
- Ongoing research explores new therapies, including technology-based interventions and pharmacologic treatments.

TABLE 1 Risk Factors for Autism

RISK FACTORS	CONDITIONS
Genetic	Highest risk in identical twins followed by nonidentical twins and close relatives
	Genetic mutations and copy number variations polygenic
Environmental	
Perinatal factors	Exposure to air pollution
	Exposure to pesticides such as organochlorines, organophosphates, and pyrethroids
	Exposure to heavy metals (lead, mercury, arsenic)
	Increased parental age
	Maternal infections such cytomegalovirus and rubella
	Medication use like valproate in pregnancy
	Maternal immune activation
	Birth complications like prematurity, low birth weight and conditions leading to hypoxia
	Maternal obesity and diabetes (lower risk)
Neurobiologic	Abnormal brain development and connectivity
	Imbalance between neurotransmitter systems (glutamate/GABA)
	Abnormalities in synaptic function and plasticity

Epidemiology

Autism spectrum disorder (ASD) prevalence is on the rise globally. The World Health Organization reports that 1 in 100 children has autism. According to the Centers for Disease Control and Prevention (CDC) 2022 data, an estimated 1 in 31 children in the United States (3.2%) are diagnosed with ASD by age 8, with boys being three times more likely to be diagnosed than girls. Reasons for the increase are multifactorial and are due to a combination of changes in definition (change in diagnostic criteria of ASD from DSM-4 to DSM-5), improved diagnostic tools and increased awareness. Siblings of individuals with ASD have a significantly higher risk, with a reported prevalence of 18.5%. Around 33% to 45% of individuals with ASD also have intellectual disability, up to 50% have attention-deficit/hyperactivity disorder (ADHD), and up to 30 % experience epilepsy. Most common psychiatric comorbidities include ADHD (~50%), anxiety disorders (up to 40%), and depression (up to 40%). The presence of intellectual disability or global developmental delay increases the likelihood of having a genetic condition related to ASD. Most common genetic conditions associated with autism include tuberous sclerosis complex, fragile X syndrome, neurofibromatosis type 1 and 22q11.2 deletion syndrome.

Pathophysiology

ASD arises from a complex interplay of genetic, environmental, and neurobiologic factors (Table 1).

A robust genetic influence is evidenced by a strong concordance rate in identical twins (60%–90% in monozygotic twins) with indications of a mix of genetic and environmental factors evidenced by a concordance rate of up to 20% in dizygotic twins. Other proof of genetic contributions includes uneven sex distribution, higher prevalence among siblings (3%–6%), and greater ASD risk with closer genetic relationships. ASD is considered a polygenic disorder characterized by incomplete penetrance and variable expressivity. Structural changes in chromosomes like microdeletions or microduplications in regions like 16p11.2 and 22q11.2 have been associated with autism. De novo mutations, combinations of single-nucleotide polymorphism, and copy number variations (CNVs) in certain chromosomes are also commonly seen. Sometimes, ASD can be inherited as part of single-gene disorders such as fragile X syndrome, Rett syndrome, and tuberous sclerosis, but it is important to remember that these conditions are rare in the population. Overall, genetic conditions play a role in 20% to 25% of cases.

Environmental factors include prenatal, perinatal, and postnatal influences. Increased parental age, both for mothers and fathers, has been associated with a higher risk of having a child diagnosed with ASD. Studies show that mothers aged 30 or older and fathers aged 40 or older tend to have a greater risk compared to younger parents. Certain infections during pregnancy, such as rubella or cytomegalovirus, have been linked to an increased risk of ASD. Notably, any condition causing immune activation during pregnancy also carries a risk. Among medications, the use of valproate during pregnancy was associated with an absolute risk ranging from 2.5% to 4.42%. Birth complications such as low birth weight, prematurity, fetal distress, or any condition leading to a state of hypoxia in the baby can increase the risk of ASD. Environmental factors such as exposure to air pollution preconception, during pregnancy, and in early infancy, particularly at levels typically found in large cities, have been associated with an increased risk of autism. Gestational exposure to pesticides, for example, organochlorines, organophosphates, and pyrethroids, have been linked to ASD. Heavy metal (mercury, lead, arsenic) exposure during pregnancy and the early developmental period have been associated with ASD.

During infancy, children diagnosed with ASD may experience a more rapid increase in head circumference and exhibit greater overall brain volume compared to typically developing peers. Neurobiologic changes occur in individuals with ASD. They often exhibit atypical brain structure and connectivity patterns, including reduced gray matter volume in specific regions and abnormal white matter tracts linking various brain areas. Studies also indicate a potential disruption in the delicate balance between excitatory (glutamate primarily) and inhibitory (γ-aminobutyric acid [GABA] primarily) neurotransmission. Irregularities in the regulation of these neurotransmitter systems could potentially underlie certain characteristics of ASD. Other important neurobiologic changes include abnormalities in synaptic function and plasticity.

Although a recent systematic review study by Prada et al. (2025) has suggested a potential association between prenatal acetaminophen exposure and neurodevelopmental outcomes, extensive large

TABLE 2	Clinical Signs and Symptoms of Autism in Children Up to 2 Years of Age
DEFICITS	**SIGNS**
Social communication problems	Limited eye contact Difficulty following gaze Indifference to caregivers Does not respond to their name Speech delays
Nonverbal communication issues	Echolalia Scripted language Challenges with nonverbal cues such as facial expressions, eye contact Using gestures to communicate needs
Repetitive activities and fixated interests	Difficulty with transitions Stereotyped movements like rocking, hand flapping, tiptoe walking Intense focus on certain activities or objects such as dinosaurs, trucks, trains
Other signs	Unusual sensory sensitivities Delayed motor skills Loss of previously acquired skills

TABLE 3	Clinical Signs and Symptoms of Autism More Evident in the Later Childhood Developmental Period After Age 2 Years of Age
Impaired joint attention	Difficulty focusing on the same object or activity with another person while communicating about it
Nonverbal communication difficulties	Challenges understanding or using facial expressions, gestures, and body language
Pragmatic language deficits	Difficulty using language appropriately in different situations, taking turns, or adjusting communication style
Trouble understanding nonverbal communication	Misinterpreting emotions, sarcasm, humor, or other subtle meanings in language
Difficulty inferring intentions or beliefs of others	Cannot understand others point of view or beliefs
Lack of interest in social interaction	Preferring solitary play or using others as tools
Delayed development of attachment	Difficulty forming close bonds with caregivers
Limited social interaction with peers	Few friendships or difficulty maintaining them
Perseverative questioning	Repetitive questioning about a preferred topic
Scripted play	Acting out scenes or dialog verbatim from movies, TV shows, or other media
Difficulty shifting attention	Difficulty moving attention to nonpreferred activities
Sensory	Hypersensitivity and hyposensitivity

scale cohort studies and meta-analyses, along with epidemiological studies, have not demonstrated a causal relationship between acetaminophen and ASD. This consensus is consistently reinforced by the World Health Organization and leading U.S. medical organizations.

Theories of the pathogenesis of ASD that have been debunked include the refrigerator mother theory, vaccination theory, and chelation therapy.

Clinical Manifestations

ASD manifests as a diverse neurodevelopmental condition characterized by a wide array of clinical features, including abnormalities in social communication, interpersonal skills and interactions, and repetitive behaviors, interests, and activities. Early indicators of this disorder are often present before 18 months of age and are brought to the pediatrician's attention by caregiver concerns. Clinical signs and symptoms of children younger than age 2 years with ASD are listed in Table 2. Presentation in the first 2 years of life is characterized by reduced gaze to faces or shared smiles, lack of orientation to name by 12 months, lack of pointing or gesturing by 14 months or lack of pretend play by 18 months. Key determinants in the early developmental period include absent or limited interest in playing with children, including siblings, inability to maintain relationships because of difficulty with use of pragmatic language, lack of recognition of social cues (especially nonverbal), and inability to take turns, leading to conflicts with peers at school or other settings. Table 3 lists signs and symptoms of children with ASD who are in the later childhood developmental period. Children with ASD often exhibit theory of mind deficits. In other words, they have trouble inferring the emotions, thoughts, and ideas of others. This inability to comprehend the mental and emotional states of other individuals compounds the patient's challenges with social interactions and back-and-forth conversations.

Repetitive behaviors, the other core symptom of ASD with a reported incidence of 37% to 95% includes stereotypical movements involving parts of or the whole body like hand flapping, rocking, swaying, and walking on tiptoes (among others).

Cognitive rigidity and fixated interests are also hallmark symptoms of ASD. Atypical responses to sensory stimuli (noise, textures, odors, and more) are also commonly seen. Intellectual and language impairment are specifier conditions for ASD (per DSM-5), and symptoms from both are prevalent and can coexist. Interestingly, children with ASD may have learning difficulties without intellectual impairment and should be

encouraged to request academic support through a referral for an Individualized Education Plan (IEP), which could result in obtaining special services to improve academic and scholastic performance.

Of note, the presence of comorbid neurodevelopmental disorders makes ancillary symptomatology wide and diverse. Symptoms of anxiety, ADHD, depression, tics, auditory and visual hallucinations, aggression from impaired impulse control, and disruptive behaviors are frequently observed. Other general clinical features include sleep problems (e.g., bedtime resistance, initial and maintenance insomnia), feeding problems (because of inflexibility with certain tastes and textures), leading to atypical food intake and, subsequently, development of gastrointestinal (GI) problems such as weight abnormalities, nutritional deficiencies, diarrhea, and constipation. Symptoms of coexistent medical comorbidities, for example, epilepsy, are also widely prevalent. Finally, it is important to be aware of "special skills" that children with ASD may have in memory, mathematics, calendar calculation (among various others), and appreciate neurodiversity in all spheres.

Diagnosis

An individual is diagnosed with ASD based on direct observation and clinical assessment per criteria mentioned in DSM-5 defining difficulties in two areas: social communication and interactions and restricted, repetitive patterns of behaviors, activities, or interests. These difficulties cause significant impairment in daily functioning and cannot be better explained by intellectual disability and global developmental delay. Specifiers include the presence/absence of intellectual impairment, language impairment, catatonia and other neurodevelopmental disorders or behavioral problems. A comprehensive evaluation based on a detailed psychiatric and medical history obtained from the patient (as applicable), parents, caregivers, teachers, therapists, and any other important person or in other settings in their lives is the reference standard. Gathering a developmental history, a three-generation family history (when applicable) of ASD and other neurodevelopmental disorders, for example, intellectual disability, language delay, ADHD, and seizures, are crucial in the process. A thorough psychosocial assessment to obtain a history of trauma and other adverse childhood experiences is important to differentiate autism from other conditions. Standard diagnostic tools are used to support clinical assessment. The *Autism Diagnostic Observation Schedule*, second edition (ADOS- 2), is the reference standard. It can be applied from the age of 12 months to adulthood. Other tools with varying levels of accuracy and reliability in use are available, as well. Accompanying testing to support the diagnosis and assess areas of need, impairment, and problem severity include testing for speech, language, intelligence, and adaptive functioning. A physical examination should be performed whenever appropriate to determine the presence of other medical conditions.

Screening and Surveillance

Global consensus emphasizes the importance of early identification of autism. The American Academy of Pediatrics recommends initial screening at 18 months and again at 24 months. The Modified Checklist for Autism in Toddlers, Revised with Follow-Up (MCHAT-RF) is a first-tier standardized screening tool used for children 16 to 30 months. The MCHAT-RF has a specificity of 85% and specificity of 95%. A first-tier screen's purpose is to detect ASD in a general population. Second-tier screens like the Screening Tool for Autism in Toddlers and Young Children (STAT) for children aged 24 to 36 months are used to distinguish ASD from other neurodevelopmental disorders. A positive screening test should be followed by a referral for a comprehensive evaluation for ASD, which may include a psychiatric assessment by a child psychiatrist, medical evaluation by a developmental pediatrician, a standardized testing such as ADOS conducted by a psychologist, and speech and occupational therapy evaluation by a qualified clinician. A detailed medical examination should include a family history of genetic conditions commonly associated with autism along with a physical examination to determine head circumference (early acceleration of head growth), weight (reduced or increased as a result of specific dietary preferences), dysmorphic features (clinical syndromes), muscle tone and reflexes (mild hypotonia). Testing for hearing is often recommended and a Wood's lamp examination may be done if there is suspicion for tuberous sclerosis. A lead level is commonly indicated along with other routine blood tests. Currently, genetic counseling is frequently conducted, particularly considering the demand for precision medicine. Chromosomal microarray (CMA) is a widely used first-line test that analyzes an individual's entire genome for chromosomal abnormalities, including deletions or duplications of genetic material. Although CMA can detect CNVs associated with ASD, its yield is limited, identifying a genetic cause in only 5% to 14% of individuals. Another commonly used genetic test is whole-exome sequencing (WES). WES, which focuses on the exome, can identify mutations in individual genes potentially contributing to ASD. WES offers a broader scope than CMA, with a detection rate of 8% to 20%. Newer technologies such as whole-genome sequencing (WGS) and next-generation sequencing (NGS) panels are promising tools. A groundbreaking tool in this area is CRISPR-Cas9 technology (clustered regularly interspaced short palindrome repeats) which explores the gene with advanced precision and compares findings with genomes of typical individuals. Just as importantly, electroencephalography to rule out seizure disorders and magnetic resonance imaging of the brain to detect any underlying disorder may be warranted.

Management

The goal of management of this condition is to have improved social communication, better adaptive skills, academic success,

TABLE 4	Autism Treatment Strategies
Behavioral approaches	Applied Behavior Analysis (ABA)
Developmental approaches	Speech and language therapy, occupational therapy, social skills training, play-based programs such as Early Start Denver Model
Education therapies at school	Treatment and Education of Autistic and Related Communication-Handicapped Children (TEACCH) program
Family therapies	Family-based interventions help improve communication, coping strategies, and understanding of ASD
Academic support	Through Individualized Educational Plan (IEP)
Pharmacotherapy	Use of medications for comorbid medical and psychiatric problems
Complementary and alternative therapies	Limited evidence supports dietary interventions, nutritional supplements, and sensory-based interventions

ASD, Autism spectrum disorder.

and an overall improved state of functioning. Table 4 lists a variety of treatment strategies for ASD.

Referral to early childhood intervention programs is the key to successful outcomes and can be done before confirmation of the diagnosis. State-run early intervention programs funded by PART C of Individuals with Disabilities Education Act (IDEA) cater to children from birth to 3 years old diagnosed with developmental delay. These programs offer comprehensive services. For children 3 and older, eligibility for social services is conducted by the public school system and referral to an early prevention program such as Head Start can be made. If indicated, the child may be provided speech therapy, language and social skills therapy occupational therapy and behavioral interventions. Another evidence-based intervention program is the Early Start Denver Model (ESDM), which is a play-based intervention fostering social communication, emotional regulation, and play skills through naturalistic interactions. It can be beneficial for children as early as 12 and 48 months. Parent training and an individualized approach are the additional key components of this program. Applied Behavioral Analysis, often called the gold standard in the management of autism is based on the principles of learning theory and boasts of an individualized approach with a focus on skill development. Educational interventions at school through an IEP are crucial supports. Once the child is close to adulthood, transition-related skills should be taught and may include driving and vocational lessons. For children with severe intellectual disability, concerns about guardianship should be brought up and discussed with the parent/caregiver. Throughout all this, a crucial factor is the presence and unconditional support from family and teachers.

As ASD can result in sleep problems and nutritional deficiencies as mentioned previously, regular visits with their psychiatrist or primary care physician are recommended. Referral to specialists may also be warranted. It is necessary to treat comorbid psychiatric conditions such as ADHD, anxiety, depression, and aggression along with medical symptoms that crop up due to associated medical or genetic conditions.

Pharmacotherapy

There is no single pharmaceutical agent indicated in autism. Pharmacotherapy is used for treatment of co-occurring symptoms (Table 5). Atypical antipsychotics aripiprazole (Abilify) and risperidone (Risperdal) are FDA approved for treatment of aggression in children. Treatment of coexistent depression, anxiety, and obsessive, compulsive behaviors are achieved by using selective

TABLE 5 Pharmacotherapy

CATEGORY	TYPES	INDICATIONS	SIDE EFFECTS (NOT EXHAUSTIVE)
Atypical antipsychotics	Aripiprazole (Abilify), risperidone (Risperdal)	Aggression	Extrapyramidal symptoms, metabolic syndrome, hypotension, seizures
Selective serotonin reuptake inhibitors	Fluoxetine (Prozac), sertraline (Zoloft), escitalopram (Lexapro), citalopram (Celexa) fluvoxamine (Luvox)	Anxiety, depression, irritability,[1] obsessive-compulsive disorder	Nausea, diarrhea, headaches, low libido, black box warning for suicidal ideations in individuals <24 years of age
Serotonin-norepinephrine reuptake inhibitors	Atomoxetine (Strattera), venlafaxine (Effexor),[1] duloxetine (Cymbalta)[1]	Attention-deficit/hyperactivity disorder (ADHD), anxiety, depression	Nausea, diarrhea, headaches, low libido, black box warning for suicidality <24 years of age
Stimulant	Methylphenidate and amphetamines	ADHD	Tachycardia, insomnia, lack of appetite, growth lag, seizures
α_2-Agonists	Clonidine (Kapvay), guanfacine (Intuniv)	ADHD, sleep,[1] impulse control[1]	Dry mouth, hypotension, somnolence, headache
Melatonin[7]		Sleep	Abdominal cramps, daytime fatigue, alertness decreased

[1]Not FDA approved for this indication.
[7]Available as a dietary supplement.

serotonin reuptake inhibitors. Comorbid ADHD is often treated with stimulants, though nonstimulants like atomoxetine (Strattera) have good evidence to support their use in this population. α2-agonists such as clonidine (Kapvay) and guanfacine (Intuniv) are commonly used for impulse control, as well, especially in poor responders to stimulants. Sleep is commonly treated with clonidine[1] or melatonin.[7] N-acetylcysteine (NAC)[1] can improve the hypothesized excitation: inhibition imbalance in ASD. GI issues like constipation are also commonly treated. Seizures are often treated with antiepileptics.

Alternative treatments for ASD vary widely, encompassing biologically derived approaches, for example, dietary supplements and specialized diets, alongside more intrusive interventions such as hyperbaric oxygen therapy, chelation, and injectable medications. However, the medical literature regarding numerous alternative therapies for ASD remains sparse.

Newer Approaches

Emerging therapies show promise; however, they require cautious interpretation of the evidence because of inconsistent outcomes. Oxytocin (Pitocin)[1] is a neuropeptide produced in the hypothalamus and has shown some promise in improvement in social functioning and repetitive behaviors. Bumetanide (Bumex)[1] has been proposed as a potential treatment for autism because of its chloride-related antagonist effects, which are associated with GABAergic inhibition. Balovaptan[5] is a potent, selective vasopressin 1a receptor antagonist that can improve social interaction and help recognize emotions in faces. Suramin,[1] an antiparasitic drug, reverse-transcriptase inhibitor has shown promise in improvement in language and social skills and in reducing repetitive behaviors. Nirsevimab (Beyfortus),[1] a recombinant IgG1-κ monoclonal antibody has been shown to improve social communication, cognitive skills, and repetitive behaviors in trials. CM-AT, a pancreatic enzyme therapy, seems to enhance language and social interaction in children. Transcranial magnetic stimulation has been noted to improve communication skills in young children. Topical CBD (cannabinoid),[5] called Zyn002, is also being studied in children currently High-dose Leucovorin (folinic acid) can improve core symptoms of verbal communication and social reciprocity with medium-to-large effect sizes in children with folate receptor autoantibodies or specific folate metabolism gene polymorphisms.

[1]Not FDA approved for this indication.
[7]Available as dietary supplement.
[5]Investigational drug in the United States.

References

Aishworiya R, Valica T, Hagerman R, Restrepo B: An Update on Psychopharmacological Treatment of Autism Spectrum Disorder, *Neurotherapeutics* 19(1):248–262, 2022.
Breakthroughs in treatment of Autism. Available at https://www.abtaba.com/blog/autism-treatment-breakthrough
Lai MC, Kassee C, Besney R, Bonato S, Hull L, Mandy W, et al: Prevalence of co-occurring mental health diagnoses in the autism population: a systematic review and meta-analysis, *Lancet Psychiatry* 6(10):819–829, 2019.
Laura Weissman. Autism spectrum disorder in children and adolescents: Surveillance and screening in primary care UpToDate, Connor RF (Ed), Wolters Kluwer.
Marilyn Augustyn. Autism spectrum disorder (ASD) in children and adolescents: Terminology, epidemiology, and pathogenesis UpToDate, Connor RF (Ed), Wolters Kluwer.
Marilyn Augustyn, L Erik von Hahn Autism spectrum disorder in children and adolescents: Clinical features UpToDate, Connor RF (Ed), Wolters Kluwer.
Marilyn Augustyn, L Erik von Hahn Autism spectrum disorder in children and adolescents: Evaluation and Diagnosis UpToDate, Connor RF (Ed), Wolters Kluwer.
Prada D, Ritz B, Bauer AZ, Baccarelli AA: Evaluation of the evidence on acetaminophen use and neurodevelopmental disorders using the Navigation Guide methodology, *Environ Health* 14;24(1):56, 2025.
Rosen Tamara E, Mazefsky Carla A, Vasa Roma A, Lerner Matthew D: Co-occurring psychiatric conditions in autism spectrum disorder, *Int Rev Psychiatry* 30(1):40–61, 2018.
Shaw KA, Williams S, Patrick ME, et al: Prevalence and early identification of autism spectrum disorder among children aged 4 and 8 years— Autism and Developmental Disabilities Monitoring Network, 16 sites, United States, 2022, *MMWR Surveill Summ* 74(2):1–22, 2025.
Wang L, Wang B, Wu C, Wang J, Sun M: Autism Spectrum Disorder: Neurodevelopmental Risk Factors, Biological Mechanism, and Precision Therapy, *Int J Mol Sci* 24(3):1819, 2023, https://doi.org/10.3390/ijms24031819. PMID: 36768153; PMCID: PMC9915249.
World Health organization. Autism. https://www.who.int/news-room/questions-and-answers/item/autism-spectrum-disorders-(asd).

DELIRIUM

Method of
Tessa E. Rohrberg, MD

CURRENT DIAGNOSIS

- Delirium is a syndrome characterized by the acute onset of cerebral dysfunction with a change or fluctuation in baseline mental status, inattention, and either disorganized thinking or an altered level of consciousness.
- The *Diagnostic and Statistical Manual of Mental Disorders, Fifth Edition*, offers diagnostic criteria for delirium.

- Hyperactive delirium is the most easily recognized subtype and includes symptoms of irritability, restlessness, agitation, or uncooperativeness.
- Hypoactive delirium has been associated with a higher mortality and includes behaviors such as reduced motor activity, apathy, lack of awareness, or lethargy.
- Delirium usually lasts 1–2 weeks, but complications may persist beyond hospitalization.

CURRENT THERAPY

- Prevention is the most effective approach to treatment.
- Antipsychotic medication should not be used prophylactically to prevent delirium.
- Nonpharmacologic therapies are key in management.
- Pharmacologic therapies should be used when nonpharmacologic strategies are not effective or when patients present with a potential for harm to themselves or others.
- Caregivers should be included in a multidisciplinary treatment plan.

Epidemiology

Delirium can be seen in persons of all ages across many clinical settings. Prevalence is affected by patient age, underlying medical diseases, severity of acute insult, and baseline mental status. Although up to 29% of adults may experience delirium during non–intensive care unit (ICU) hospitalization, prevalence is as high as 82% in patients in the ICU with mechanical ventilation and 60% in patients following orthopedic surgery. In addition, up to 88% of patients may experience delirium at the end of life. Delirium may be missed in more than half of the cases. Patients with delirium may have increased length of hospital stay, long-term cognitive impairment, and higher mortality. National costs of delirium and associated complications have been reported up to $152 billion annually.

Pathophysiology

Although the exact etiology of delirium is unclear, it is often multifactorial and complex. Delirium is a syndrome that results from an acute insult causing cerebral dysfunction. Mechanisms contributing to delirium may include neurotransmitter imbalances and anatomic deficits. Neurotransmitter alterations—including serotonin imbalance, acetylcholine deficiency, dopamine excess, and/or melatonin deficiency—are thought to contribute. These alterations may lead to increased cytokine levels and an inflammatory response that changes the blood-brain barrier and cerebral oxidative metabolism. Higher cortical areas of the brain, such as the prefrontal and nondominant posterior parietal regions, have been implicated by brain imaging in patients with delirium. Other regions thought to be involved include the anterior thalamus, basal ganglia, and temporo-occipital cortex. More research is needed to fully elucidate the stress response and effect of risk factors.

Risk Factors

Many risk factors for developing delirium have been identified; they can be divided into predisposing and precipitating factors. See Table 1 for differentiation of these risk factors. A patient with many predisposing risk factors may experience delirium with only a minor precipitating event, whereas a patient with few predisposing risk factors may require multiple precipitating factors to develop delirium. Medications present a great risk for developing delirium. Those posing a higher risk comprise anticholinergics (including antihistamines, muscle relaxants, and urinary incontinence agents like oxybutynin [Ditropan]), benzodiazepines, dopamine agonists, and meperidine (Demerol); those that pose a moderate-to-low risk include antibiotics,

TABLE 1	Risk Factors for Delirium	
PREDISPOSING FACTORS	PRECIPITATING FACTORS
Male sex	Dehydration
Age >65 years	Trauma
Previous diagnosis of delirium	Hypoxia
Chronic pain	Infection
Medical comorbidities	Ischemia
Alcohol abuse	Shock
Terminal illness	Recent surgery/anesthesia
Dementia	Urinary or stool retention
Depression	Uncontrolled pain
Elder abuse	ICU environment
Recurrent falls	Sleep deprivation
Malnutrition	Physical restraints or immobility
Polypharmacy	Mechanical ventilation
Sensory impairment	Foley catheter
Pressure ulcers	Coma
Urinary or fecal incontinence	Medications

ICU, Intensive care unit.

anticonvulsants, antiemetics (metoclopramide [Reglan]), antidizziness agents, antihypertensives, antivirals, corticosteroids, opiates, nonsteroidal antiinflammatory drugs, sedatives, and tricyclic antidepressants.

Data have revealed not only the high incidence of delirium in patients with acute COVID-19 infection but also the concerning long-term cognitive effects that may persist beyond the acute phase of infection. While factors such as elevated viral load, viral persistence, direct central nervous system involvement of SARS-CoV-2, the subsequent inflammatory cascade, and prolonged hospitalization contribute to the risk of acute delirium, the lasting impact on cognitive function is becoming increasingly evident. Delirium is also associated with worse hospital outcomes and increased mortality in patients with COVID-19 infection. Lasting cognitive impairment appears to be one of the most prevalent neurologic manifestations following the acute phase of COVID-19, underscoring the need for extended follow-up studies to better understand the implications. Addressing these long-term effects requires a comprehensive, multidisciplinary approach to both prevention and management, alongside continued support for patients and caregivers.

Clinical Manifestations

The three subtypes of delirium are hyperactive, hypoactive, and mixed. Hyperactive delirium is more commonly recognized in the clinical setting. It typically includes irritability, agitation, restlessness, and uncooperative behaviors. Patients may also have fast or loud speech, combativeness, fast motor responses, nightmares, tangentiality, or persistent thoughts. This subtype is seen in patients experiencing withdrawal from substances of abuse, including drugs or alcohol. Hypoactive delirium may be more difficult to distinguish and thus is associated with more severe complications, including a higher mortality. Hypoactive delirium is frequently found in the elderly and includes sluggishness, apathy, lethargy approaching stupor, lack of awareness, slowed movements, sparse or slow speech, and staring. Metabolic dysfunction—such as hepatic encephalopathy or hypercapnic respiratory failure—may make it more difficult to identify hypoactive symptoms. Delirium may also present with a mixed level of activity and may fluctuate rapidly between hyperactivity and hypoactivity

TABLE 2	Differential Diagnosis of Delirium		
	DELIRIUM	**DEMENTIA**	**DEPRESSION**
Features	Confusion and inattention	Memory loss	Sadness, anhedonia
Onset	Acute	Insidious	Slow
Course	Fluctuating, worse at night	Chronic, progressive, stable over course of a day	Single episode or recurrent
Duration	Hours to months	Months to years	—
Consciousness	Altered	Normal	Normal
Attention	Impaired	Normal, except in late stages	May be impaired
Orientation	Fluctuates	Poor	Normal
Speech	Incoherent	Mild errors	Normal or slow
Thought	Disorganized	Impoverished	Normal
Illusions	Common (visual hallucinations)	Rare, except in late stages	Not usually
Psychomotor changes	Yes	No	Yes
Reversible	Usually	Rarely	Possibly

or between normal and disturbed psychomotor activity. Mixed delirium may be misdiagnosed as sundown syndrome.

Diagnosis

The diagnosis of delirium may be missed due to its multifactorial etiology, atypical symptoms of hypoactive delirium, and resemblance to other comorbidities. Diagnosis is dependent on early recognition through routine monitoring. The *Diagnostic and Statistical Manual of Mental Disorders*, Fifth Edition, text revision, includes diagnostic criteria for delirium that includes the following:

1. A disruption in attention, including inability to maintain concentration and awareness of the environment.
2. An alteration in cognitive processes of memory, orientation, language or development of a perceptual disturbance.
3. The disruption from baseline occurs acutely, usually within hours to days, and fluctuates over time.
4. The history, examination, and clinical data indicate that the disruption results from another medical condition, substance abuse or withdrawal, adverse medication reaction, or exposure to toxins. The disruption cannot be related to dementia and cannot happen in a state of unconsciousness or coma.

The diagnosis of delirium can be further specified as acute (lasting a few hours or days) or persistent (lasting weeks to months), and a hyperactive, hypoactive, or mixed level of activity. Evaluation for the diagnosis of delirium should be done for underlying causes and can be individualized for each patient. Laboratory and radiologic testing usually consists of a complete blood count, comprehensive metabolic panel, urinalysis with microscopy, blood cultures, electrocardiography, and chest radiography. Additional testing might include an arterial blood gas, urine drug screen, serum ammonia, blood alcohol level, computed tomographic (CT) imaging of the head, and cardiac biomarkers. It is important to screen for drug or alcohol withdrawal, as this can present with delirium.

Differential Diagnosis

Many other diseases may closely resemble delirium. Cognitive impairment and mood disorders may be confused with delirium, including dementia or depression. See Table 2 for a comparison of characteristics of these diseases. In the elderly and those with postoperative side effects, it is important to consider urinary and fecal retention. The Critical Illness, Brain Dysfunction and Survivorship (CIBS) Center website (http://www.icudelirium.org) has many mnemonics that can be useful when one is considering other circumstances that mimic delirium. One such mnemonic is "I WATCH DEATH."

Infection	Sepsis, urinary tract infection, pneumonia, HIV, SARS-CoV-2
Withdrawal	Alcohol, barbiturates, sedative-hypnotics, opiates
Acute metabolic	Acidosis, alkalosis, electrolyte disturbance, renal or hepatic failure
Trauma	Head injury, heat stroke, postoperative, burns
Cenral nervous system pathology	Abscess, hemorrhage, subdural hematoma, seizures, encephalitis, meningitis, stroke, tumors, hydrocephalus, syphilis
Hypoxia	Anemia, hypotension, respiratory failure, congestive heart failure, carbon monoxide poisoning
Deficiencies	Vitamin B12, folate, thiamine, niacin
Endocrinopathies	Hypo/hyperthyroid, hypo/hyperglycemia, hyperparathyroidism, adrenal disease
Acute vascular	Hypertensive emergency, pulmonary embolism, arrythmia, myocardial infarction
Toxins/drugs	Anticholinergics, benzodiazepines, alcohol, illicit drugs, pesticides, solvents
Heavy metals	Lead, mercury, manganese

Monitoring

Although many assessment tools exist, the Confusion Assessment Method (CAM) is the most effective screening tool, with a sensitivity of 94% to 100% and a specificity of 90% to 95%. Screening should be performed by a trained health professional and done at least once per shift in patients at moderate to high risk. One should routinely monitor for precipitating factors, including changes in medications, laboratory values, clinical symptoms, and physical examination findings.

Prevention

Prevention is the key to decreasing delirium incidence, hospital costs, and complications. Delirium may be preventable up to 40% of the time. Efforts should involve a multidisciplinary and multicomponent approach. This includes early mobilization, cognitive reorientation activities using calendars and clocks, promotion of normal sleep-wake cycles using protocols that control light and noise stimuli, clustering of patient activities, and improving access to sensory equipment like glasses or hearing aids. Other key interventions include nutrition and fluid replacement, adequate pain management, and the prevention of constipation. Although antipsychotic medications should not be used for the prevention of delirium, home psychiatric medications should be restarted when possible so as to lower the risk for delirium.

TABLE 3 Prevention and Treatment of Delirium

NONPHARMACOLOGIC	PHARMACOLOGIC
Identify underlying etiology	**Typical Antipsychotics**
Medication review	Haloperidol (Haldol)[1] 0.5–1.0 mg
Early mobilization	PO q4h or IM/IV q30–60min prn;
Cognitive reorientation	maximum dose 30 mg q24h
Sensory enhancement	**Atypical Antipsychotics**
Pain management	Risperidone (Risperdal)[1] 0.25–2 mg PO
Cluster activities	qd–bid; maximum dose 6 mg q24h
Sleep-wake cycle	Quetiapine (Seroquel)[1] 12.5–200 mg
enhancement	PO bid; maximum dose 400 mg
Family and caregiver support	q24h
Nutritional and fluid	Olanzapine (Zyprexa)[1] 2.5–10 mg
replacement	PO qd or 5-10 mg IM
Prevention of constipation	q2-4h prn; max 30 mg q24h
Restart home psychiatric	Ziprasidone (Geodon)[1] 20–40 mg PO
medications	bid or 10 mg IM daily; maximum
Routine use of the Confusion	80 mg PO q24h or 40 mg IM q24h
Assessment Method	Aripiprazole (Abilify)[1] 10–30 mg PO
	qd; maximum dose 30 mg q24h
	Benzodiazepines
	Lorazepam (Ativan)[1] 0.5–2 mg PO/
	IM/IV q4h prn; maximum dose 10
	mg q24h

[1]Not FDA approved for this indication.

Treatment

Treatment of delirium includes the identification and management of the underlying etiologies, assessment of risk factors, and review of the medication list. Delays to initiation of treatment may result in the prolongation of symptoms, the possibility of long-term cognitive impairment, and higher mortality. Treatment is primarily aimed at prevention utilizing the nonpharmacologic measures described earlier. The Hospital Elder Life Program (HELP) is a widely used evidence-based model that uses this approach and involves physicians, nurses, caregivers, family members, and patients. Research has shown that support of family and caregiver involvement can further increase the effectiveness of this model and can contribute to shorter length of hospitalization, reduced healthcare costs, and a decreased incidence of delirium. Pharmacologic therapies are used when nonpharmacologic strategies are not effective. There are currently no antipsychotic medications that are approved by the US Food and Drug Administration for the treatment of delirium. Antipsychotics should be reserved for patients in whom behavioral interventions have failed or are not possible or in those who have a potential for harm to themselves or others. Antipsychotic medications should be used at the lowest effective dose for the shortest possible duration. Haloperidol (Haldol)[1] is the antipsychotic medication used most often for delirium management; however, atypical antipsychotic medications have been shown to be as effective. Haloperidol, risperidone (Risperdal)[1], and quetiapine (Seroquel)[1] are considered the safest when used for delirium. Quetiapine (Seroquel)[1] is the preferred agent for those with Lewy body dementia or Parkinson disease due to fewer extrapyramidal effects. Benzodiazepines should not be used for delirium unrelated to alcohol or benzodiazepine withdrawal. Nonopiate medications should be used initially to treat pain in patients diagnosed with delirium. If sedation is required in ICU patients with delirium, studies suggest the use of dexmedetomidine (Precedex) rather than benzodiazepines. See Table 3 for delirium prevention and treatment strategies.

Complications

Delirium is associated with significant long-term complications. Although cognitive impairment following a diagnosis of delirium may improve with time, lasting effects are possible.

[1]Not FDA approved for this indication.

A longer duration of delirium in critically ill patients has been associated with worse long-term executive function and global cognition. The severity of lasting cognitive impairment has been compared to mild Alzheimer disease or moderate traumatic brain injury. Other complications include the development of mood disorders, loss of function in activities of daily living (ADLs), hospital readmission, longer duration of mechanical ventilation, and increased lengths of stay in the ICU and in hospital. Family members and caregivers may also experience stress in caring for their loved ones with cognitive impairment. Adverse effects of medications used in the treatment of delirium are also impactful and can include extrapyramidal symptoms, QT interval prolongation, insulin resistance, sedation, increased risk of falls, and hypotension. Mortality in patients suffering from delirium is as high as 39% during hospitalization, with a 10% increased risk of death per hospital day. Patients diagnosed with delirium are also up to three times more likely to die at 6 months after discharge. Mortality is greater in those with hypoactive delirium.

References

American Geriatric Society Abstracted Clinical Practice Guideline for Postoperative Delirium in Older Adults. *J Am Geriatr Soc* 63:142-150, 2015.

Critical Illness, Brain Dysfunction, and Survivorship (CIBS) Center. Available at http://www.icudelirium.org. Accessed January 22, 2020.

Delirium. In: American Psychiatric Association: *Diagnostic and Statistical Manual of Mental Disorders*, 5th ed, text revision, Arlington, VA, 2022.

Downing LJ, Caprio TV, Lyness JM: Geriatric Psychiatry Review: Differential Diagnosis and Treatment of the 3 D's - Delirium, Dementia, and Depression, *Curr Psychiatry Rep* 15:365, 2013, Available at: https://doi.org/10.1007/s11920-013-0365-4, Accessed 27 April 2020.

Giussani G, Westenberg E, Garcia-Azorin D, et al: Prevalence and trajectories of post-COVID-19 neurological manifestations: A systematic-review and meta-analysis. *Neuroepidemiology.* Published online January 25, 2024. Available at https://doi-org.kumc.idm.oclc.org/10.1159/000536352, Accessed 18 March 2024.

Hospital Elder Life Program (HELP) for Prevention of Delirium. Available at http://www.hospitalelderlifeprogram.org. Accessed January 29, 2020.

Jaqua EE, Nguyen VTN, Chin E: Delirium in Older Persons: Prevention, Evaluation, and Management, *Am Fam Physician* 108(3):278–287, 2023.

Pandharipande PP, Girard TD, Jackson JC, et al: Long-term cognitive impairment after critical illness, *New Engl J Med* 369(14):1306–1316, 2013.

Salluh JIF, Wang H, Schneider EB, et al: Outcome of delirium in critically ill patients: systematic review and meta-analysis, *BMJ* 350:h2538, 2015, Available at: https://doi.org/10.1136/bmj.h2538, Accessed 29 January 2020.

Wang YY, Yu JR, Xie DM, et al: Effect of the tailored, family-involved hospital elder life program on postoperative delirium and function in older adults, *JAMA Internal Medicine* 180(1):17–25, 2019.

DRUG USE DISORDERS

Method of
William M. Greene, MD; and Mark S. Gold, MD

CURRENT DIAGNOSIS

- Screen for substance use in all primary care and emergency settings.
- The clinical interview remains the mainstay of diagnosis.
- Clinicians should have a low threshold for ordering a urine drug test.
- Collateral information should be obtained from family or other sources.
- DSM-5 offers current diagnostic criteria for substance use disorders (Box 1).

CURRENT THERAPY

- Effective pharmacologic and psychosocial treatments exist.
- Formal detoxification is indicated for dangerous withdrawal states or in patients with serious medical comorbidity.

- Pharmacologic relapse prevention options are substance specific, and particularly useful options exist for nicotine and opioids.
- Psychosocial treatments remain a mainstay of substance treatment and range along a continuum of intensity from outpatient counseling to long-term residential treatment.
- Patients should be referred to mutual aid meetings (e.g., Narcotics Anonymous, SMART Recovery) to complement other therapies.
- Indefinite remission is an attainable goal for many—a relapse does not constitute total failure but provides an opportunity to reevaluate the treatment approach.

Epidemiology

Widespread pathologic use of intoxicating substances, both legal and illegal, remains one of the greatest public health concerns facing our nation. According to the 2022 National Survey on Drug Use and Health, among Americans aged 12 years and older, 70.3 million (24.9% of the population) used an illicit drug within the preceding year. By order of frequency, these drugs included cannabis, hallucinogens, prescription pain reliever misuse, cocaine, prescription sedative/tranquilizer misuse, prescription stimulant misuse, methamphetamine, inhalants, and heroin. In addition, 50.9 million Americans (18.1%) aged 12 years and older used tobacco within the previous month, mostly in the form of cigarettes; another 23.5 million (8.3%) vaped nicotine. Each year in the United States, approximately 480,000 people die from an illness attributable to cigarette smoking, making this the foremost cause of preventable death. Overdose deaths have remained a matter of pressing national concern in the United States; opioids were involved in 75.4% of the estimated 107,000 overdose deaths in 2021. Per CDC data, synthetic opioids such as fentanyl accounted for approximately 3000 deaths in 2013; by 2018, they accounted for over 30,000; as of 2021, synthetic opioid deaths have skyrocketed to 71,000. U.S. life expectancy increases ended in 2010 and started falling in 2014, with fatal overdoses playing a key role in this shift. Fatal drug overdoses in the United States have more than quadrupled between 1999 and 2020. Overall, the estimated annual economic cost of tobacco, alcohol, and illicit drugs in the United States is more than $740 billion, including costs related to crime, lost work productivity, and health care.

From 1997 to 2019, the rate of past-month cigarette use among 12- to 17-year-olds steadily dropped from 28.3% to 3.7%. The 2022 Monitoring the Future survey data confirm that cigarette smoking has continued to fall to the lowest rate in the survey's history (i.e., past month use among 12th graders is now at only 4.0%, compared with 36.5% in 1997). Encouraging though these trends may be, they are counterbalanced by explosive growth of nicotine vaping. Among 12- to 17-year-olds, past-month vaping of nicotine increased from 7.5% in 2017 to 18.1% in 2019. Similarly, past-month vaping of cannabis among 12- to 17-year-olds increased from 3.6% in 2017 to 10.1% in 2019. Concurrent with pandemic-related disruptions, the number of 12th graders who reported any lifetime illicit drug use dropped significantly, from historical norms of 47% to 50% to only 41% in 2022. Despite advances in our understanding and treatment of substance use disorders, drug use remains an epidemic, especially in the areas of drugged driving and drug use (including tobacco) during pregnancy.

Diagnosis

The fifth edition of the *Diagnostic and Statistical Manual of Mental Disorders* (DSM-5), published in 2013, eliminated the diagnostic categories of substance abuse and substance dependence. In the interest of consistency and clarity and based on large-population data, they were replaced by a new diagnostic entity: "substance use disorder" (see Box 1). Those familiar with DSM-IV terminology found the new criteria quite familiar, as they essentially represent a combination of the old abuse and dependence criteria.

BOX 1 DSM-5 Diagnostic Criteria for "Substance Use Disorder"

A problematic pattern of use leading to clinically significant impairment or distress as manifested by two or more of the following in a 12-month period:
- Often taken in larger amounts or longer period than intended
- Persistent desire or unsuccessful efforts to cut down or control use
- Great deal of time spent in activities necessary to obtain, use, or recover from effects
- Craving, or strong desire or urge to use
- Recurrent use resulting in failure to fulfill major role obligations at work, school, or home
- Continued use despite having persistent/recurrent social or interpersonal problems caused or exacerbated by the substance
- Important social, occupational, or recreational activities are given up or reduced because of use
- Recurrent use in situations in which use is physically hazardous
- Continued use despite knowledge of having a persistent/recurrent physical or psychological problem likely to have been caused or exacerbated by the substance
- Tolerance (needing increased amounts for desired effect, or diminished effect with same amount)
- Withdrawal (manifested by characteristic syndrome or taking more to relieve/avoid withdrawal)

Specify current severity:
- Mild: Two to three criteria are met
- Moderate: Four to five criteria are met
- Severe: Six or more criteria are met

When diagnosing a substance use disorder, the specific substance for which criteria are met must be listed. In addition, it is also important to document the severity of the disorder based on the number of symptoms present. Examples of specific diagnoses using current nomenclature would be "cannabis use disorder, moderate" or "opioid use disorder, severe." This simpler evidence-based diagnostic schema eliminated some of the confusion previously surrounding the term "dependence," which was often mistaken to be synonymous with "physiological dependence." It has long been understood, in the context of certain prescribed drugs, that the presence of tolerance and withdrawal is not pathologic in nature; rather, these represent an expected state of neuroadaptation. This fact is reflected in the current substance use disorder criteria for opioids, stimulants, and sedatives. For these three categories, the tolerance and withdrawal criteria are not considered to be met if present when the substance is taken solely under appropriate medical supervision. It should be noted this exception does not apply to cannabis, even if it is "prescribed."

Despite the importance and usefulness of the DSM-5, many patients (and clinicians) may still be left wondering if the problem at hand would appropriately be characterized as "addiction." Though not definitive, moderate to severe substance use disorders are generally synonymous with the concept of addiction. In a 2011 public policy statement, the American Society of Addiction Medicine offered the following short definition of addiction, which has been well received:

Addiction is a primary, chronic disease of brain reward, motivation, memory and related circuitry. Dysfunction in these circuits leads to characteristic biological, psychological, social and spiritual manifestations. This is reflected in an individual pathologically pursuing reward and/or relief by substance use and other behaviors. Addiction is characterized by inability to consistently abstain, impairment in

TABLE 1 Pharmacotherapy for Nicotine Dependence

DRUG	MECHANISM OF ACTION	DOSAGE	INSTRUCTIONS	COMMENTS
Nicotine patch (Nicoderm CQ)	NRT	7 mg, 14 mg, 21 mg	1 patch daily	Tapering of doses recommended to discontinue
Nicotine gum (Nicorette)	NRT	2 mg, 4 mg	Chew slightly then "park" on oral mucosa	Tapering of doses recommended to discontinue
Nicotine lozenge (Commit)	NRT	2 mg, 4 mg	Absorbed through oral mucosa; minimize swallowing	Tapering of doses recommended to discontinue
Nicotine inhaler (Nicotrol inhaler)[2]	NRT	4 mg/cartridge	6–16 cartridges/day	By prescription only; tedious administration
Nicotine nasal spray (Nicotrol NS)	NRT	0.5-mg/spray	1–2 sprays in each nostril q1h; max 80 sprays/day	By prescription only
Bupropion HCl (Wellbutrin[1], Zyban)	Inhibits reuptake of NE and DA	150-mg SR tab, 300-mg XL tab	300 mg PO (divided qd [XL tab]-bid [SR tab]) daily for 7–12 weeks	Helps with comorbid depression; can help prevent weight gain
Varenicline (Chantix)	Partial agonist at $\alpha_4\beta_2$ nicotinic acetylcholine receptor	0.5 mg, 1 mg	0.5 mg PO qd for 3 days, then 0.5 mg PO bid for 4 days, then 1 mg PO bid for 11 weeks	May smoke during first week; may continue for an additional 12 weeks

[1]Not FDA approved for this indication.
[2]Not available in the United States.
DA, Dopamine; *max*, maximum; NE, norepinephrine; NRT, nicotine replacement therapy; SR, sustained release; XL, extended release.

behavioral control, craving, diminished recognition of significant problems with one's behaviors and interpersonal relationships, and a dysfunctional emotional response. Like other chronic diseases, addiction often involves cycles of relapse and remission. Without treatment or engagement in recovery activities, addiction is progressive and can result in disability or premature death.

Tobacco and Nicotine

Nicotine is the main addictive component in tobacco. It is administered via smoking (e.g., cigarettes, cigars, pipes, hookah) or in smokeless formulations (e.g., dip, chew, snuff, snus) and now also via vaporization (e.g., electronic cigarettes, vaping devices). Adverse health effects are not equivalent among the different routes of administration; cigarette smoking is recognized as the most harmful mode of administration. Beyond standard nicotine pharmacodynamics, smoking in particular reduces brain monoamine oxidase (MAO) activity, resulting in higher levels of synaptic dopamine and norepinephrine thus enhancing nicotine's addictive effects.

After administration, nicotine rapidly binds to nicotinic acetylcholine receptors in the central nervous system (CNS), where it acts as a mild psychostimulant and mood modulator in a non-impairing, yet profoundly addictive, manner. When the user is tired, smoking has a stimulating effect. When the user is anxious or stressed, smoking exerts a calming effect. Given the rapidity of CNS effects, smoking is akin to injection of a drug, but without the needle. Given its short half-life, repeated self-administration serves to effectively relieve unpleasant withdrawal symptoms from the nicotine itself. Repeated use quickly leads to both physiologic and psychological dependence.

As with other misused drugs, cue-induced cravings play an important role in maintaining tobacco addiction. For example, the smell of the smoke, the sound of the lighter, and the feel of the cigarette on the lips all contribute to an overall process addiction beyond just addiction to the nicotine itself. Further complicating matters, tobacco use is also strongly associated with alcohol use, with which it has synergistic toxic effects.

Toxicities from tobacco use are well described and include severe pulmonary disease, cardiovascular disease, and carcinomas of the upper aerodigestive tract and of the bladder. Even secondhand smoke, previously considered harmless, is now correctly regarded as a serious health risk to the nonsmoker and a "drug" itself. Cigarette smoke contains much more than nicotine—over 7000 separate chemical components have been identified, at least 250 of which are known to be harmful, and at least 69 of which are known carcinogens. Additionally, secondhand tobacco exposure in utero can cause serious adverse health effects in the developing fetus.

Although cessation may prove difficult for even the most motivated tobacco users, effective treatments for tobacco use disorder now exist. Clinical trials indicate that a combination of counseling and medications offers the best chance for success and should be offered to patients willing to make a quit attempt. A wide range of FDA-approved nicotine replacement therapies are readily available and have similar rates of efficacy (Table 1). Patches (Nicoderm CQ), gums (Nicorette), and lozenges (Commit) are available over the counter, but the nasal spray (Nicotrol NS) and inhaler (Nicotrol Inhaler[2]) are available by prescription only. Recently electronic cigarettes and vaping devices have gained popularity, but unlike other nicotine products, they are not regulated as drugs by the FDA.

Nonnicotine prescription medications with proven efficacy are available. Bupropion HCl (Wellbutrin, Zyban) is an antidepressant that was serendipitously noted to dramatically reduce nicotine cravings in some patients; it is now widely used for this purpose (as Zyban). Varenicline (Chantix) was specifically developed to treat tobacco use disorder and represents a considerable advancement, with improved smoking cessation rates. It acts as a partial agonist at the nicotine receptor and effectively serves to satisfy cravings while simultaneously blocking the effects of exogenously administered nicotine. Although probably the most effective agent, varenicline carries some risk of psychiatric side effects, but this should not deter use. Previous attempts to develop a "nicotine vaccine" (e.g., NicVAX)[5] have not come to fruition, though ongoing efforts in the immunopharmacotherapy arena remain ongoing.

Nicotine replacement, bupropion, and varenicline are all considered first-line pharmacotherapy. Bupropion but not varenicline may also be used in combination with nicotine replacement therapies. All pharmacotherapy options are enhanced with the coadministration of counseling or behavioral therapies.

---

[2]Not available in the United States.
[5]Investigational drug in the United States.

Helpful resources for patients interested in quitting include www.smokefree.gov (a government website dedicated to helping people quit smoking), 1-800-QUIT-NOW (a free phone-based service with coaches and educational materials), and a variety of resources available through the American Cancer Society and American Heart Association.

Cannabis

Cannabis (marijuana, pot, weed, grass, ganja, bud, reefer) remains the most used illicit drug in the world. As of 2022, 61.9 million Americans aged 12 or older (22% of the U.S. population) reported using marijuana during the preceding year. Cannabis is readily harvested from *Cannabis sativa* or *Cannabis indica*; it is typically smoked, though it may be ingested or vaporized. Despite a recent trend wherein states have legalized cannabis for medicinal and/or recreational purposes, it is still listed as a Schedule I drug by the Drug Enforcement Agency (DEA), which implies a high potential for abuse and no currently accepted medical use. Delta-9-tetrahydrocannabinol (THC) is the active ingredient, which exerts its desired psychoactive effects at CB_1 receptors diffusely throughout the CNS. Average THC concentration of commercial cannabis plants has been steadily increasing due to selective breeding: annual analysis of the DEA's record of seizures indicates that the average THC concentration increased from approximately 1% in 1975, to approximately 10% in 2008, to approximately 15% in 2021. Growing evidence strongly suggests that higher THC concentrations are associated with increased harm (e.g., adverse neurocognitive and psychiatric effects, development of cannabis use disorder). Additionally, various high potency cannabis concentrates have been developed including hashish, hash oil/butane hash oil, "wax," "shatter," and vape oil. Some of these preparations may contain THC concentrations ranging from 20% to 80% or even higher.

Acute psychoactive effects of cannabis include euphoria, relaxation, heightened sensations, increased appetite, distorted sense of time, slowed reaction time, illusions and hallucinations, paranoia, and anxiety. Acute somatic effects include conjunctival injection, xerostomia, increased heart rate and blood pressure, muscle relaxation, and reduced intraocular pressure. There is no known risk of dangerous overdose. Withdrawal symptoms are generally mild and may include irritability, cravings, diminished appetite, and insomnia. Cannabis is now recognized as unequivocally addictive. Users of this drug commonly develop tolerance and demonstrate loss of control and continued use despite negative consequences—the hallmarks of addiction. Among Americans aged 12 or older in 2022, it is estimated that 6.7% (or 19 million people) had a cannabis use disorder within the past year.

Not surprisingly, with hundreds of chemicals identified in its smoke, chronic cannabis use poses significant health risks. Chronic cannabis use is associated with respiratory symptoms, bronchitis, myocardial infarction, stroke, impaired immunity, persistent disruption of memory and attention, various psychiatric disorders (e.g., anxiety, depression, mania, psychosis), and low birth weight when used during pregnancy.

Currently, treatment of cannabis use disorder remains psychosocial, with various forms of individual and group therapy demonstrating benefit. To date, insufficient evidence supports use of pharmacotherapy targeted at cannabis use disorder. Various existing drugs (including fluoxetine [Prozac][1], lithium[1], and buspirone[1]) have been investigated. However, well-controlled clinical trials to support their use are lacking. Preliminary data suggest that dronabinol (Marinol)[1] may be of some utility in relieving cravings and withdrawal symptoms without causing intoxication.

Cocaine, Methamphetamine, and Other Stimulants

As a class, cocaine and other stimulants work primarily by enhancing dopamine transmission in a dose-dependent fashion, either directly (amphetamines) or by blocking reuptake (cocaine). Cocaine and a variety of amphetamines (e.g., amphetamine/dextroamphetamine

[Adderall], dextroamphetamine [Dexedrine], methamphetamine [Desoxyn], methylphenidate [Methylin, Ritalin]) are available for legitimate medical use as Schedule II drugs. Cocaine (in 4% solution) is still used as a topical anesthetic, and amphetamine derivatives are used to treat attention-deficit/hyperactivity disorder (ADHD), narcolepsy, obesity, and binge-eating disorder (only lisdexamfetamine [Vyvanse] is FDA approved for this indication). Any of these agents may be misused, and all have significant addictive potential. Even newer safer agents such as modafinil (Provigil) and armodafinil (Nuvigil) are associated with use disorders, albeit less commonly than the traditional stimulants.

Prescription stimulant misuse may involve the ingestion of excessive doses to achieve a euphoric high or nonmedical use or diversion of prescriptions (e.g., students sharing medication to facilitate studying). When taken at prescribed doses for an appropriate condition, even methamphetamine is generally safe and effective. In contrast, when it is synthesized in clandestine laboratories and smoked or injected in high doses, methamphetamine (crystal meth, ice, crank, speed) is alarmingly dangerous. No other commonly abused drug is so strongly associated with permanent brain damage, resembling that seen in victims of traumatic brain injury. As ADHD becomes more widely recognized and treated, physicians must be aware of the potential for misuse of their well-intentioned prescriptions. To this end, several recent pharmacologic developments have resulted in improved treatment options. Extended-release formulations of methylphenidate (e.g., Concerta) and amphetamine/dextroamphetamine (Adderall XR) are considered to have less misuse potential than their short-acting counterparts. Better still, the formulation of lisdexamfetamine includes the amino acid lysine coupled with the amphetamine molecule, consequently acting as a prodrug with the lowest misuse potential of all stimulants approved for ADHD.

Cocaine and other stimulants induce sympathomimetic effects including tachycardia, hypertension, mydriasis, and diaphoresis. When taken at the doses typically used to achieve euphoria, these drugs are commonly associated with seizures, myocardial infarction, hemorrhagic stroke, dyskinesia/dystonia, and psychosis. Withdrawal is generally experienced as a crash and includes fatigue, depressed mood, increased appetite, and intense cravings. Considered nonaddictive until about 1980, cocaine is now widely recognized as one of the most addictive drugs, particularly in the base form (crack or freebase). MDMA (methylenedioxymethamphetamine), also known as ecstasy or molly, shares the pharmacodynamic properties of the stimulants combined with serotoninergic effects of the hallucinogens.

Currently no medication has demonstrated efficacy in treating cocaine or stimulant use disorders. Pharmacologic treatment remains symptomatic during the acute withdrawal phase. Stimulant-induced psychosis and mania respond well to traditional psychotropics when warranted; however, to date, no medications have reliably demonstrated efficacy in preventing relapse. In the arena of immunopharmacotherapy, efforts to date to develop a safe and effective "cocaine vaccine" have not yet come to fruition but may hold future promise. In the meantime, traditional psychosocial treatments remain the mainstay of clinical care.

Opioids

Opioids are categorized as (1) endogenous (endorphins, enkephalins, dynorphins), (2) opium alkaloids (morphine, codeine), (3) semisynthetic (heroin, oxycodone [Roxicodone, OxyContin]), or (4) synthetic (methadone [Dolophine], fentanyl [Sublimaze, Duragesic]). The last three categories have a wide range of clinical uses including analgesia, anesthesia, antidiarrhea, cough suppression, acute withdrawal management, and maintenance therapy.

Opioids exert their clinical effect at mu, delta, and kappa opioid receptors. The effect on mu receptors is considered the most important, with its activation directly linked to both analgesic and euphoric effects. Most humans subjectively experience therapeutic opioid doses with a neutral to mildly aversive response. However, when used in sufficient quantities by genetically vulnerable persons, some users experience energy, relief of emotional

---

[1] Not FDA approved for this indication.

TABLE 2 Useful Medications in Treating Opioid Use Disorders

DRUG	UTILITY	FORMS	ADMINISTRATION	NOTES
Naloxone (Narcan)	Overdose; additive to prevent abuse[1]	SC, IM, IV	0.4–2 mg q2–3 min prn	$T_{1/2}$ = 1 h; wears off quickly
Naltrexone (ReVia, Vivitrol)	Prevention of relapse	PO, IM	ReVia: 50–100 mg PO daily Vivitrol: 380 mg IM q4wk	Potential for hepatotoxicity; precipitates withdrawal; useful for ETOH as well
Clonidine (Catapres, Catapres-TTS patch)[1]	Withdrawal	PO, transdermal	0.1–0.2 mg PO tid prn; 0.1–0.3 mg q24h transdermal via weekly patch	Monitor for hypotension
Lofexidine (Lucemyra)	Withdrawal	PO	0.18 mg tabs, 3 tabs PO Q5-6h prn	Monitor for hypotension
Methadone (Dolophine)	Withdrawal; maintenance	PO	Start 20–30 mg PO qd Target 80–120 mg PO qd	Restricted to methadone clinics
Buprenorphine (Subutex[2], Suboxone [with naloxone], Buprenex injection[1])	Withdrawal; maintenance	SL, IM, IV	Start 2–4 mg SL qd-bid Target 4–24 mg SL daily divided qd-tid	No longer requires special DEA certification
Buprenorphine (Sublocade, Brixadi)	Maintenance	SQ	Monthly or weekly SQ injections, as directed	Long-acting injectable agents for patients already stabilized on transmucosal agent

[1]Not FDA approved for this indication.
[2]Not available in the United States.
DEA, Drug Enforcement Administration; ETOH, ethanol.

pain, and a profound euphoria. Intoxication manifests with miosis, impaired consciousness, slurred speech, bradycardia, and depressed respiration. Overdose is potentially fatal via respiratory depression, but it is quite amenable to treatment with repeated doses of naloxone (Narcan). The withdrawal syndrome is characterized by a constellation of miserable but not life-threatening symptoms including mydriasis, piloerection, muscle cramps, diaphoresis, vomiting, lacrimation, rhinorrhea, chills, insomnia, cravings, and autonomic hyperactivity.

Since pain was recognized as "the fifth vital sign" in the 1990s, concurrent with heavy marketing campaigns from pharmaceutical companies, the United States experienced a veritable explosion of widespread opioid prescribing for nonmalignant pain. An industry of pain management developed, with the unfortunate side effect of having a sizable proportion of its output being used nonmedically. It is important for prescribers to recognize the addictive potential of prescription opioids matches—or in some cases even exceeds—that of heroin. As prescribing patterns returned to sanity, the second wave of the opioid epidemic began in 2010 with the rapid rise in heroin-related overdose deaths. As drug cartels quickly began to substitute heroin with fentanyl, the third wave began in 2013, characterized by an even more dramatic rise in overdose deaths involving fentanyl. In 2024, some have noted the development of what appears to be a fourth wave, characterized by widespread use of stimulants (primarily methamphetamine) concurrent with fentanyl.

The most common method of prescription opioid misuse involves simply taking more than prescribed, usually by the appropriate route of administration. Alternatively, individuals with opioid use disorders commonly take their medications via nasal insufflation or inject them intravenously. The extended-release property of certain medications, such as oxycodone (OxyContin), can easily be circumvented by crushing the pills, which greatly enhances the euphoric effect. Even transdermal fentanyl patches (Duragesic) can be misused by any number of methods, such as applying heat to a worn patch, employing complex extraction techniques described online, or simply sucking on the patch itself. If the prescription is used up before its renewal date, the user must either supplement the supply or face the unpleasant effects of withdrawal.

There is no shortage of methods to obtain opioids illicitly. These include seeing multiple prescribers (doctor shopping), purchasing online at foreign "pharmacies" or on the "dark web," general trade

or purchase on the black market, or diversion from hospitals and pharmacies by healthcare professionals. As of 2023, all states have implemented controlled substance databases (i.e., prescription drug monitoring programs [PDMPs]) aimed at curbing the problem of use disorders involving opioids and other prescription drugs.

Acute opioid withdrawal management is achieved by one of two basic strategies: (1) symptomatic treatment with unrelated medications, or (2) substitution with a cross-tolerant (opioid) drug with less potential for misuse (Table 2). The first strategy commonly employs the use of clonidine (Catapres)[1], an α_2-adrenergic agonist, to help with the autonomic component of withdrawal. Since 2018, lofexidine (Lucemyra) has been FDA approved for this purpose and offers similar benefits with improved side effect profile. These α_2 agents are typically used in combination with other symptomatic treatments on an as-needed basis, using agents such as diazepam (Valium) for anxiety, loperamide (Imodium) for diarrhea, and promethazine (Phenergan)[1] or ondansetron (Zofran)[1] for nausea.

The second strategy typically involves either methadone or buprenorphine (with naloxone [Suboxone, Zubsolv]). Methadone, a pure mu agonist with a half-life of approximately 36 hours, is usually started in the 20- to 30-mg range and titrated cautiously by 10 mg every 4 to 7 days. Induction and maintenance therapy with methadone occurs only in the setting of a highly regulated and federally approved methadone clinic. Buprenorphine, a mu partial agonist (and kappa antagonist), is usually administered sublingually and has a half-life similar to that of methadone. It was approved in 2002 for office-based treatment of opioid addiction, making pharmacotherapy much more widely available. Caution should be used to avoid administering buprenorphine too soon (before the onset of withdrawal syndrome); otherwise acute withdrawal can actually be precipitated. Buprenorphine is available either alone (in a generic sublingual monotherapy product) or in combination with naloxone (Suboxone, Zubsolv). Here, the role of naloxone is primarily to deter intravenous use, because naloxone has negligible bioavailability when taken sublingually as prescribed. The FDA has recently approved longer-acting injectable formulations of buprenorphine, including a monthly subcutaneous injection (Sublocade) and more recently a weekly or monthly subcutaneous injection (Brixadi). These newer formulations have

---

[1]Not FDA approved for this indication.

been a welcome addition to the armamentarium used to fight the opioid epidemic; they improve compliance and largely eliminate diversion issues but do pose additional logistical hurdles with respect to insurance approval and administration.

Buprenorphine and methadone are useful in managing acute withdrawal as well as in long-term maintenance therapy for preventing relapse to heroin or the opioid of choice. As maintenance therapy, these agents serve to block euphoria, satisfy cravings, and reduce illicit use, with consequent verifiable harm reduction. Buprenorphine, with a built-in ceiling effect because of its unique pharmacology, is much safer than methadone, which is often fatal in overdose. Increasing evidence supports the benefit of continuing long-term maintenance therapy indefinitely, as discontinuation is often associated with relapse and other adverse outcomes. Buprenorphine is increasingly being initiated in emergency department settings, and this trend is associated with improved patient outcomes. Increasingly, buprenorphine is being used as an analgesic as well (Butrans transdermal patch, Belbuca buccal strip), and it may be the ideal choice in patients with comorbid pain and addiction who have demonstrated an inability to use other opioids safely. Effective December 29, 2022, the requirement for a special DEA license (or "X-waiver") to prescribe buprenorphine has been eliminated; now any physician with a DEA number may prescribe buprenorphine, even to treat opioid use disorder.

Also approved for safe and effective opioid relapse prevention is naltrexone, an opioid antagonist, which is available in both oral (ReVia, generic) and intramuscular depot formulations (Vivitrol).

Sedative-Hypnotics

This class of drugs includes a wide array of compounds (benzodiazepines, barbiturates, and various related compounds) (Table 3), most of which have at least some addictive potential. Overall these medications do much more good than harm and are useful in treating anxiety disorders, insomnia, seizures, and muscle spasms. They are also important in managing withdrawal states and useful as a component of surgical anesthesia. These drugs act as CNS depressants, and their primary mechanism of action is to enhance inhibitory GABA neurotransmission. The risk of toxicity is by respiratory depression, which is magnified by concomitant use of opioids or other CNS depressants, such as alcohol.

Sedative-hypnotic intoxication and withdrawal states closely resemble those of alcohol except for the more protracted time course of withdrawal. Anxiety, restlessness, insomnia, tremor, nystagmus, tachycardia, and hypertension usually appear 2 to 12 hours after the last dose, and symptoms gradually resolve over 1 to 2 weeks. Withdrawal seizures, psychosis, and delirium are fairly common. Detoxification is best accomplished on an inpatient basis and typically involves tapering doses of a long-acting benzodiazepine (e.g., clonazepam [Klonopin], diazepam, clorazepate [Tranxene]) at a rate of about 10% of the initial daily requirement per day. Acute sedative overdose is managed primarily with supportive care and airway management. Flumazenil (Romazicon) 0.2 to 0.5 mg/min IV may be used for acute benzodiazepine overdose, but only with caution because it can precipitate severe acute withdrawal symptoms.

Since their introduction in the 1960s, benzodiazepines, given their enhanced safety profile, have largely replaced barbiturates. However, barbiturates still in common use include phenobarbital and butalbital. Phenobarbital, used mainly for treating seizures, is considered to have a relatively low potential for misuse. Butalbital, compounded with caffeine plus acetaminophen or aspirin (Fioricet, Fiorinal), has moderate misuse potential, typically in combination with other drugs. Carisoprodol (Soma), though not a barbiturate, is metabolized into meprobamate, a barbiturate-like drug. Commonly taken in combination with opioids and other sedatives, carisoprodol is highly misused.

Alprazolam (Xanax) stands out among its peers as the single most misused, most addictive, and yet currently most prescribed sedative-hypnotic. Its rapid onset (T_{max} 1 to 2 hours) and relatively short half-life (6 to 14 hours) contribute to its abuse liability and

TABLE 3	Common Sedative-Hypnotics, Equivalent Dose Conversions	
GENERIC NAME	**TRADE NAME**	**DOSE (MG)**
Benzodiazepines		
Diazepam	Valium	10
Alprazolam	Xanax, Niravam	0.5–1
Lorazepam	Ativan	2
Clonazepam	Klonopin	1–2
Chlordiazepoxide	Librium	25
Clorazepate	Tranxene	7.5
Oxazepam	Serax	10–15
Temazepam	Restoril	15
Triazolam	Halcion	0.25
Flurazepam	Dalmane	15
Barbiturates		
Phenobarbital	N/A	30
Pentobarbital	Nembutal	100
Secobarbital	Seconal	100
Butalbital (with caffeine and aspirin or acetaminophen)	Fiorinal, Fioricet	100
Amobarbital	Amytal	100
Related Compounds		
Carisoprodol	Soma	700
Meprobamate	Miltown, Equanil	1200
Chloral hydrate	Noctec	500
Methaqualone[2]	Quaalude	300
Ethchlorvynol[2]	Placidyl	500
Zolpidem	Ambien	20
Zaleplon	Sonata	20
Eszopiclone	Lunesta	3

[2]Not available in the United States.
N/A, Not applicable.

propensity for withdrawal seizures. Diazepam, historically the most prescribed sedative, also has a relatively rapid onset and significant addictive potential, but its long half-life makes it an ideal agent for use in treating withdrawal from other sedatives. Flunitrazepam (Rohypnol, "roofies") is a benzodiazepine that causes anterograde amnesia, outlawed in the United States because of its use in drug-facilitated sexual assaults.

γ-Hydroxybutyric acid (GHB) and baclofen (Lioresal) also act as GABAergic CNS depressants, with intoxication and withdrawal states consistent with the class. Oddly, GHB is considered a Schedule I drug with high abuse potential and no accepted medical use, but when marketed as sodium oxybate (Xyrem), GHB is available as a Schedule III drug (with special restrictions) for use in treating narcolepsy. Baclofen, on the other hand, appears to have rather low addictive potential and may actually play a role in the treatment of alcoholism.[1]

Relatively newer sedatives—such as zolpidem (Ambien), zaleplon (Sonata), and eszopiclone (Lunesta)—are benzodiazepine-like drugs with CNS depressant activity, collectively known as the "Z drugs"; they are approved for the short-term treatment of

[1] Not FDA approved for this indication.

insomnia and have at least some potential for misuse and dependence. Clonazepam (Klonopin) is generally considered to have the lowest potential for euphoria and addiction and is thus the agent of choice if a benzodiazepine must be given to patients with a relative contraindication, such as a history of any drug use disorder.

Conclusion

Despite intensive supply-reduction strategies, improved primary prevention efforts, and the many recent pharmacotherapy advances, drug use disorders remain largely unchanged in their overall scale with the notable exceptions of the increased use of more dangerous opioids (fentanyl) and increased vaping of both nicotine and cannabis. Another notable exception is the significant reduction in tobacco use since the turn of the century. It is estimated that 25% of patients seen in office settings and 50% of those seen in emergency departments have active problems related to substance use. All patients in primary care settings should be screened for tobacco, alcohol, and illicit drug use. Patients should be asked directly about substance use at the initial point of contact (e.g., emergency departments, primary care offices), and clinicians should maintain a healthy degree of skepticism toward patients' responses, remembering that many patients minimize substance use. When any suspicion exists, urine drug screens should be readily used without hesitation or fear of communicating mistrust. A variety of affordable quick screen kits are available, which can be sent out for laboratory confirmation of positive results if necessary.

Physicians and other health care professionals are in a unique position to intervene with drug use disorders at the individual level because these disorders are commonly encountered in clinical practice. The problem must first be identified and, depending on the skill set of the primary provider, patients should be treated or referred appropriately. All clinicians are encouraged to incorporate formal SBIRT (screening, brief intervention, and referral to treatment) into routine clinical practice. Current procedural terminology (CPT) codes and a reimbursement schedule for screening and brief intervention may be located online at https://www.samhsa.gov/sbirt/coding-reimbursement. Screening may involve written or verbal assessments of substance use to determine whether or not the patient exhibits a problematic level of use. The brief intervention aspect of SBIRT targets those with milder substance use disorders and provides effective strategies for intervention before the need for more extensive or specialized treatment arises. Referral to specialized treatment is generally recommended for patients with moderate-to-severe substance use disorders. Data suggest this approach can be successful in modifying problematic substance use behavior. In addition to formal treatment, physician referral to local mutual aid meetings (Narcotics Anonymous, Alcoholics Anonymous, SMART Recovery, Celebrate Recovery) has proved beneficial. Ample scientific evidence supports the effectiveness of these programs. Local chapters will readily provide physicians with the names and telephone numbers of members willing to welcome newcomers (www.aa.org; www.na.org).

Physicians are usually well equipped to treat the sequelae of drug use disorders, but they often forget that addiction itself is a treatable disease entity. Treatment ranges in intensity along a continuum that includes medically managed inpatient detoxification, partial hospitalization, intensive outpatient treatment, and outpatient care. The American Society of Addiction Medicine provides patient placement criteria that dictate the appropriate level of treatment based on a multidimensional assessment. Healthcare professionals should be familiar with the treatment centers in their area; these can place the patient in the appropriate level of care.

It is important to remember that relapse is a characteristic of addiction and does not equate to treatment failure but rather indicates a need for an adjustment in the level of treatment or monitoring. Other chronic diseases, such as diabetes and hypertension, necessitate ongoing monitoring and adjustment of treatment interventions as needed, and the same is true of substance use disorders. Data on the treatment and monitoring of recovering physicians (a subgroup of individuals with addiction that boasts a 5-year success rate >78%) teach us the lesson that adequate initial treatment coupled with ongoing monitoring is critical. Sustained recovery from a substance use disorder is readily attainable and is characterized by voluntary sobriety, improved personal health, and improved citizenship.

References

American Psychiatric Association: *Diagnostic and statistical manual of mental disorders*, ed 5, Washington, DC, 2013, American Psychiatric Publishing.

American Society of Addiction Medicine: *Public policy statement: definition of addiction*. Available at http://www.asam.org/docs/publicy-policy-statements/1definition_of_addiction_long_4-11.pdf, 2011.

Bailey JA, Hurley RW, Gold MS: Crossroads of pain and addiction, *Pain Med* 11:1803–1818, 2010.

DuPont RL, McLellan AT, White WL, et al: Setting the standard for recovery: physicians health programs, *J Subst Abuse Treat* 36:159–171, 2009.

Gold MS, Kobeissy FH, Wang KK, et al: Methamphetamine- and trauma-induced brain injuries: comparative cellular and molecular neurobiological substrates, *Biol Psychiatry* 66:118–127, 2009.

Kelly JF, Humphreys K, Ferri M: Alcoholics Anonymous and other 12–step programs for alcohol use disorder, *Cochrane Database Syst Rev* (3), 2020. https://doi.org/10.1002/14651858.CD012880.pub2.

Miech RA, Johnston LD, Patrick ME, O'Malley PM, Bachman JG, Schulenberg JE: *Monitoring the future national survey results on drug use, 1975–2022: secondary school students. Monitoring the future monograph series*, Ann Arbor, MI, 2023, Institute for Social Research, University of Michigan. Available at https://monitoringthefuture.org/results/publications/monographs/.

Office of National Drug Control Policy: *The economic costs of drug abuse in the United States: 1992–2002*, Washington, DC, 2004, Executive Office of the President. [Publication No. 207303].

Pardo B, Taylor J, Caulkins JP, et al: *The future of fentanyl and other synthetic opioids*, Santa Monica, CA, 2019, RAND Corporation. Also available in print form https://www.rand.org/pubs/research_reports/RR3117.html.

Scholl L, Seth P, Kariisa M, et al: Drug and opioid-involved overdose deaths — United States, 2013–2017, *MMWR Morb Mortal Wkly Rep* 67:1419–1427, 2019.

Substance Abuse and Mental Health Services Administration: *Key substance use and mental health indicators in the United States: results from the 2022 National Survey on Drug Use and Health (HHS Publication No. PEP23-07-01-006, NSDUH Series H-58)*, Center for Behavioral Health Statistics and Quality, Substance Abuse and Mental Health Services Administration, 2023. https://www.samhsa.gov/data/report/2022-nsduh-annual-national-report.

EATING DISORDERS

Method of
Nandini Datta, PhD

Bulimia Nervosa

CURRENT DIAGNOSIS

- Binge-eating episodes occur at least once per week for 3 months (eating objectively large quantities of food in a discrete period of time accompanied by a loss of control while eating).
- Compensatory purging episodes occur at least once per week for a period of 3 months (e.g., self-induced vomiting, laxatives, diuretics, excessive and compulsive exercise, enemas) to prevent weight gain.
- Shape and weight are overvalued and impact self-worth and self-esteem.
- Weight is at or above expected range given age, height, and historical growth curves.

CURRENT TREATMENT

- Cognitive behavioral therapy (CBT) is the most evidence-based treatment for bulimia nervosa (BN).
- Interpersonal psychotherapy (IPT) is an appropriate alternative.

- Family-based treatment (FBT) is useful for adolescents with BN.
- Antidepressant treatment (selective serotonin reuptake inhibitors [SSRIs]) may be useful in augmenting psychotherapy or as an alternative in the event that psychotherapy is not effective, refused, or unavailable. It is not as effective as CBT and thus not a front-line approach.

Diagnosis

To diagnose bulimia nervosa (BN), an individual must engage in recurrent binge episodes with compensatory behaviors (e.g., self-induced vomiting, diuretic or laxative use, excessive and compulsive exercise). A binge is a discrete episode of eating a quantity of food that is more than the average person would eat in the same setting, accompanied by a loss of control or feeling as though one cannot stop eating. Nonpurging forms of bulimia occur when an individual uses extreme dietary restriction/fasting and/or exercise as a means of compensating for binge episodes. A disproportionate emphasis on weight and shape in one's self-evaluation is also required in diagnosing BN. DSM-5 criteria require that these episodes occur at a minimum of once weekly for 3 months. Unlike individuals with anorexia nervosa (AN), who may binge and purge, individuals with BN are within range of or above the median body mass index (BMI).

Significant health consequences may accompany BN. Laboratory studies often reveal electrolyte abnormalities, which can lead to cardiac arrhythmias and cardiac arrest in severe cases. Physical examination may detect enamel decay and parotid gland enlargement as a consequence of recurrent vomiting. When ipecac[1] is used to induce vomiting, severe cardiac and skeletal myopathies may develop. Laxative abuse is associated with metabolic acidosis and elevated serum amylase levels. BN has an elevated risk for mortality (crude mortality of 3.9%–6% in an inpatient sample), with many dying by suicide. Most common comorbid psychiatric diagnoses are mood, anxiety, personality disorders (specifically borderline personality disorder), and substance use disorders.

Epidemiology

BN behaviors typically first occur in middle adolescence (ages 14–16), with onset of full syndrome BN in later adolescence and early adulthood (ages 17–24). The lifetime prevalence estimate of DSM-5 BN ranges from 4% to 6.7%, and while less is known about males, at minimum they are estimated to account for between 10% to 25% of all cases. Symptoms may persist for a number of years, with intermittent periods of remission. A review of existing treatment studies suggests that approximately 45% of patients fully recover, with 27% improving considerably and the remaining 23% exhibiting a chronic course.

Etiology

BN can be explained by a confluence of biologic, sociocultural, psychological, and familial factors. From a biologic standpoint, BN aggregates in families; in twin studies, about half of the variance in heritability can be explained by genetic factors. Serotonin levels may be reduced, and imaging studies show abnormal serotonergic circuitry in the orbital-frontal cortex. Internalization of cultural ideals of beauty may present as a focus on thinness for women, where for males there is often pressure to be muscular with low body fat. Participation in sports where weight and appearance are tied to performance (e.g., gymnastics, wrestling) may increase risk. Early puberty and childhood obesity are common precipitants, as are experiences with peer weight-related teasing. Personality characteristics of individuals with BN may include perfectionism, impulsivity, and instability in interpersonal relationships. Childhood sexual and physical abuse increases the risk for BN.

Treatment

Given the significant physical, social, and emotional consequences associated with BN, effective treatment requires

---

[1] Not FDA approved for this indication.

addressing wide-ranging difficulties. Over 70 randomized controlled treatment trials (RCTs) exist for adults with BN, yet only four focus on adolescents. Most studies have examined behavioral therapies, medications, or a combination thereof. CBT is established as the treatment of choice for adults with BN and has been subjected to a large number of RCTs. The underlying assumption of CBT is that bulimic behaviors are maintained by dysfunctional attitudes about shape, weight, and physical appearance, which thereby lead to an overemphasis of these aspects in self-evaluation. Excessive dieting typically ensues, resulting in physiologic and psychological deprivation that increases vulnerability to binge eating. Feelings of guilt and fear about weight gain are mitigated through engaging in purging behaviors. CBT targets this cycle through the use of self-monitoring to increase an awareness of patterns in behaviors, thoughts, and emotions that maintain BN symptoms.

CBT is found to be more effective than no treatment, pill placebo, nondirective supportive psychotherapy, nutritional counseling, stress management, and antidepressant medication therapy. Response to CBT is good, with approximately 50% recovered and 20% with significant reductions in symptoms at the end of treatment. CBT is acceptable and feasible with adolescents; however, a more recent RCT had a 20% rate of abstinence, compared with previous rates of 56% in a case series and 36% in a guided self-help (GSH) version at the end of treatment. Compared with an alternative intervention, interpersonal psychotherapy (IPT), CBT demonstrates a greater probability of remission and reduction in symptoms at the end of treatment. However, these initial differences appear to diminish at a 1-year follow-up, suggesting that, while less efficient, IPT is a viable alternative. IPT was adapted for BN to target interpersonal factors thought to contribute to the development and maintenance of the disorder. IPT has yet to be studied with adolescents.

More recently, CBT has been expanded to address other maintaining features of eating disorders broadly (e.g., interpersonal difficulties, clinical perfectionism, low self-esteem, and mood intolerance). Enhanced CBT (CBT-E) addresses these features and is delivered in a focused or broad (addressing aforementioned maintaining features) format. For individuals with more complex psychopathology, the broad version may be more effective. Further, a novel treatment, integrative cognitive affective therapy for BN (ICAT-BN), may be preferable to CBT-E for individuals with greater affective lability and stimulus seeking behaviors.

Other interventions show promise in the treatment of BN and require further examination. For adolescents, FBT may be helpful, demonstrating higher rates of binge/purge abstinence (40%) than supportive psychotherapy in one study, and higher than CBT (FBT: 39% vs. CBT: 20%) in another. Derived from FBT for AN, parents are supported to directly change dysfunctional eating behaviors. For adults, dialectical behavior therapy (DBT) has been shown to significantly decrease binge/purge episodes when delivered in an individual format. Similar effects were found when an appetite-awareness component was added to standard DBT.

Antidepressants (SSRIs) are the most studied medication treatment for BN. Fluoxetine (Prozac) demonstrates greater reductions in binge eating, purging, and eating-related cognitions than placebo when prescribed at higher doses (60 mg/day). A small pilot study of fluoxetine with adolescents suggests it is acceptable and may decrease BN symptoms. Antidepressants alone are not as effective as when combined with CBT, or as CBT alone.

Binge-Eating Disorder

CURRENT DIAGNOSIS

- Recurrent episodes of binge eating, defined as eating an objectively large amount of food in a discrete period of time with a sense of lack of control during the episode.

- Binge eating is associated with at least three of the following: eating more rapidly than normal; eating until uncomfortably full; eating outside of physical hunger; eating alone because of embarrassment; and subsequent feelings of self-disgust, depression, or guilt.
- There is marked distress associated during a binge eating episode.
- These episodes occur at least once per week over 3 months.
- There is no associated compensatory behavior (e.g., purging), and bingeing does not occur in the context of another eating disorder diagnosis (anorexia or BN).

CURRENT TREATMENT

- CBT and IPT have good evidence of efficacy among adults.
- GSH CBT may be effective for those with less psychopathology.
- DBT requires further study to determine whether good outcomes are sustained over time.
- There is no evidence-based treatment for young patients with binge eating disorder (BED).
- Pharmacologic treatments should be considered as an adjunct to psychotherapy.

Diagnosis

Binge episodes are typically characterized by eating quantities that are larger than others would eat in a similar setting and are accompanied by a feeling of being out of control. Individuals with BED do not engage in compensatory behaviors (e.g., self-induced vomiting, excessive exercise) as in BN. The ICD-11 also recognizes subjective binge episodes, when smaller amounts of food are consumed with loss of control. DSM-5 criteria require that the episodes occur at a minimum frequency of once per week over a 3-month period. Binge eating (BE) is commonly associated with feelings of guilt and embarrassment and may result in attempts to hide eating. Furthermore, during binge episodes, eating is often rapid and results in feeling uncomfortably full. Most individuals with BED have at least one comorbid psychiatric diagnosis (79% of respondents in one study).

Epidemiology

Lifetime prevalence of BE among adult females was 3% and 3.6% in two separate studies, and 2.1% in males. It occurs at equal rates across ethnic and racial groups. BE most typically onsets in later adolescence or early adulthood, although it does occur in children and is often associated with overweight and obesity, as well as psychological symptoms. Among adolescents with obesity, an estimated 1% meet the criteria for BED, and up to 26% experience BE/loss of control eating. In BED, obesity often predates dieting and subsequent BE, with women having an earlier onset of both dieting and BE. Remission rates in BED are higher than in other eating disorders, although duration and severity is similar to BN.

Etiology

The etiology of BED is unknown. Restrictive dieting, body image dissatisfaction, pressure to be thin, low self-esteem, depressive symptoms, and limited social support increase the risk for the onset of adolescent BE. Increased rates of BE in families suggests there may be a genetic link. Heritability estimates range between .39 and .45. Potential medical causes for BE include CNS tumors, Kleine-Levin syndrome, Kluver-Bucy syndrome, Prader-Willi syndrome, and gastrointestinal pathology, and these causes should be ruled out during assessment. Comorbid psychiatric disorders are common among adults with BED, including mood disorders, anxiety disorders, and, at lesser frequency, substance use disorders and personality disorders. There are high rates of obesity among individuals with BED; however, psychiatric symptoms are linked to the severity of BE rather than obese status.

Treatment

Treatment for adults with BED has received considerable attention in RCTs compared with other eating disorder diagnoses. Most treatments target reduction in BE, psychological symptoms, and weight loss for those who are overweight, as determined by BMI categories. CBT has been applied in multiple formats (group, GSH, CD-ROM delivered, and in combination with medication) and appears to have the highest rates of abstinence. Individual CBT outperformed group CBT in one trial, and a GSH version was more effective in reducing BE than behavioral weight-loss (BWL). CBT targets underlying dysfunctional attitudes and behaviors that maintain BE. An alternative treatment, interpersonal psychotherapy (IPT), is a time-limited psychodynamic therapy targeting interpersonal difficulties that underlie the disorder. IPT is helpful in reducing the frequency of BE. IPT, CBT, and motivational interviewing (MI) all lead to improvements in cognitive restraint, disinhibition, and shape and weight concerns thought to maintain BE.

DBT is another treatment adapted for BED with the aim of targeting affected regulation difficulties formulated to be a maintaining mechanism of BE. Women in a small trial comparing group DBT to a waitlisted group had significantly greater decreases in BE and related eating disorder thoughts and behaviors, with over half abstinent from BE at follow-up. However, compared with supportive psychotherapy, the rate of abstinence, while achieved more quickly in the DBT group, did not differ between the groups at follow-up. Pilot data suggest comprehensive DBT (individual, group, and skills coaching) may be effective.

Pharmacologic treatments targeting BE and weight loss have been tested alone and in combination with psychotherapy. There may be improvement in weight loss with addition of pharmacotherapy. The combination of CBT with topiramate (Topamax)[1] resulted in greater weight loss and better psychosocial outcomes than CBT with fluoxetine.[1] A high dose of the SSRI escitalopram (Lexapro)[1], anticonvulsants topiramate and zonisamide (Zonegran)[1], lisdexamfetamine (Vyvanse) at a dose of 50 mg or 70 mg, and the selective norepinephrine reuptake inhibitor atomoxetine (Strattera)[1] were each associated with significantly decreased binge eating and weight in separate placebo-controlled trials.

Anorexia Nervosa

CURRENT DIAGNOSIS

- Persistent restriction of energy (caloric) intake relative to requirements, leading to significantly low weight (e.g., accounting for age, sex, developmental trajectory, and physical health).
- Ongoing behavior interfering with weight gain driven by a fear of becoming fat.
- Disturbance in the perception of shape, weight, overvaluation of weight, and shape in self-evaluation, or lack of acknowledgment of seriousness of low weight.
- Either meets criteria for restricting type, with absence of binge or purge behaviors, or binge eating/purging type.

CURRENT TREATMENT

- FBT for adolescents with AN has the most evidence supporting its efficacy to date.
- AFT may be a helpful alternative.
- There are no first-line treatments for adults with AN.
- CBT may prevent relapse in weight-restored individuals.

---

[1]Not FDA approved for this indication.

Diagnosis

AN is characterized by dietary restriction that is severe enough to lead to seriously low weight, fear of weight gain, and difficulty or inability to accurately perceive shape or weight. Secondary amenorrhea is no longer required for a diagnosis of AN in the DSM-5. Individuals may be classified as AN-restricting subtype or AN-binge/purge subtype. The definition of low weight is less than "minimally normal" among adults or "minimally expected" among children and adolescents. Growth charts normed by age and gender are necessary to calculate expected BMI for individuals under 18 and growth curves may help detect deviations from an individual's growth trajectory. A BMI at or below the 10th percentile is a benchmark reflecting malnourishment associated with AN, and BMI below 18.5 kg/m^2 may be used as guidelines. When an individual meets all criteria for AN, but despite significant weight loss weighs within or above the median BMI range, atypical AN (AAN) may be diagnosed. Otherwise, AAN is associated with the same psychological and physical features of AN.

A wide variety of medical and psychiatric symptoms accompany AN. Potentially life-threatening medical conditions may develop as a result of semistarvation. Vital sign abnormalities (e.g., bradycardia, orthostasis, hypothermia) and amenorrhea are common consequences of malnutrition. Bone loss resulting in osteopenia and, in more severe cases, osteoporosis may occur. Abnormal laboratory findings may occur in some patients with AN who use laxatives, diuretics, and diet pills and who engage in self-induced vomiting.

The lifetime rate of comorbid psychiatric diagnoses among adolescents with AN is approximately 55%. Most commonly, these comorbidities include anxiety disorders (social anxiety, separation anxiety, generalized anxiety and obsessive compulsive disorder [OCD]), depression, and substance abuse. There is significant overlap in OCD symptoms and AN, thus careful consideration must be given to the content of obsessions and compulsions in diagnosis. In AN, obsessional preoccupations are related to eating, food, weight, and shape, and compulsions may appear as calorie counting, excessive exercise routines, and mealtime rituals. Depressive symptoms such as dysphoric thought, low energy, difficulty concentrating, and low self-esteem also manifest in AN and may not indicate a separate depressive disorder.

Epidemiology

Peak age of onset for AN is between 14 and 18 years. Lifetime prevalence of females with a DSM-5 diagnosis of AN in the United States is estimated to be between .8% and 3.6%, based on method of data collection. The incidence of AN among males is less studied, but recent estimates suggest that 1 out of every 4 cases are male. Little is known about the prevalence of AN across racial and ethnic groups. A recent study did not reflect significantly higher rates of AN among non-Hispanic white adolescents compared with Hispanic and non-Hispanic black peers; however, other evidence suggests that it is less common among persons of African origin.

AN has the highest mortality rate of any psychiatric illness, with reports as high as 5% per decade. Rates of chronicity obtained from long-term adult follow-up studies (AN diagnosis persisting greater than 5 years) are estimated between 7% and 15%. Death occurs most commonly secondary to medical complications of starvation or suicide. Prognosis for adolescents with short duration of illness (less than 3 years) is better than adults.

Etiology

The causal mechanisms of AN are multiply determined through the interface of biologic/genetic, psychological, and sociocultural factors. Heritability estimates from twin studies range from 48% to 74%, and family aggregation studies report that AN occurs at about five times the expected rate in affected families. The interactional effect between genes and developmental processes is reflected in studies demonstrating greater heritability among 17-year-old twins compared with 11-year-old twins. Hormonal changes during adolescence could mediate gene expression during puberty, explaining this difference.

Perfectionistic and avoidant personality features are associated with AN and are likely heritable. Neurocognitive features including cognitive rigidity and an overly detailed style of information processing are common and may represent an endophenotype as those who are recovered, as well as unaffected siblings who demonstrate similar cognitive styles. Common developmental challenges associated with adolescence may also precipitate or emerge as a consequence of AN. These include navigating issues of autonomy, self-efficacy, and intimacy. Sociocultural factors including exposure to a Westernized "thin ideal" of beauty for females and an overly muscular ideal for males may be internalized, thereby triggering extreme dieting or exercise. Furthermore, activities where weight or appearance is intertwined with performance may also elevate risk (e.g., gymnastics, ballet, wrestling, figure skating).

Treatment

Given the severity of psychological, social, and health consequences of AN, both close medical monitoring and psychotherapy are the standard of care. In severe cases, inpatient medical monitoring may be required, and standard criteria for hospitalization are available for physicians to treat common consequences of starvation like bradycardia, hypotension, and orthostatic vital sign abnormalities. Findings from RCTs among adults are inconclusive because of dropout rates as high as 50%. Medication trials of antidepressants (serotonin reuptake inhibitors and tricyclics) have high dropout rates and show little to no improvement of weight or eating disorder behaviors. Therefore these should not be used independent of psychotherapy. A recent trial demonstrated an average of 1 lb per month greater weight gain for those taking olanzapine (Zyprexa)[1] than not; however, potential risks, including tardive dyskinesia and metabolic side effects, need be considered. CBT may help prevent relapse for individuals who are already weight-restored. For underweight individuals, findings are mixed, and nonspecific therapies such as nonspecific supportive clinical management (NSCM) showed better outcomes compared with IPT and CBT at end of treatment. However, improvements in NSCM appear to decline over time, and IPT may catch up to CBT.

Recent treatment studies have focused on improving retention. For example, an enhanced version of outpatient CBT (CBT-E), which employs motivational enhancement strategies, retained 64% of the original sample, improving on previous trends in attrition. Individuals completing treatment had clinically significant improvements in weight and eating disorder psychopathology. When CBT-E was compared with focal psychodynamic therapy and treatment as usual (TAU) in the community, weight gain and improvements in eating disorder symptoms were more rapid. However, focal psychodynamic treatment had the highest rates of recovery at follow-up (35%), though these were only significantly higher than the TAU group.

FBT, otherwise known as *Maudsley family therapy*, has been studied in seven RCTs with superior outcome to other individual therapies. This outpatient treatment empowers parents to disrupt self-starvation and other behaviors that maintain AN. In the initial phase of treatment, parents take full control over managing eating-related behaviors. FBT demonstrates rates of remission ranging from 49% (full remission in weight and eating disorder thoughts and behaviors) to 89% for partial remission. Rates of relapse are about 10% and there is minimal dropout, suggesting it is acceptable to families. FBT delivered in a parent-focused format may be just as effective and preferable to conjoint FBT for families with high levels of expressed criticism.

AFT may be an alternative approach for individuals whose family members are unable to participate. The focus in AFT is on helping an adolescent move toward healthy individuation and increased self-efficacy. AN is conceptualized as an ineffective strategy that the adolescent has adopted in managing common

---

[1]Not FDA approved for this indication.

developmental challenges. In AFT, adolescents learn new skills to support eating and weight gain and parents are involved in separated collateral sessions. CBT has also been studied in adolescents; compared with TAU and hospitalization, it appeared to be the most cost-effective approach.

Avoidant-Restrictive Food Intake Disorder

CURRENT DIAGNOSIS

- Disturbance in eating/feeding resulting in persistent failure to meet nutritional and/or energy (caloric) needs.
- The disorder must result in one of the following consequences: significant weight loss or faltering growth; significant nutritional deficiency; dependence on nutritional supplements or enteral feeding; and interference with psychosocial functioning.
- The eating/feeding disturbance is not better explained by another medical or psychiatric condition or by cultural or religious practices.

CURRENT TREATMENT

- There are no established treatments for this new diagnosis, though clinical trials are currently underway.
- CBT or family interventions that employ behavioral strategies are being explored as potential treatment options.

Diagnosis

Avoidant-restrictive food intake disorder (ARFID) is a new diagnosis included in the DSM-5, which reflects the recognition of "food neophobia" or extreme picky eating as challenges. Individuals with ARFID can be of any age and exhibit clinically significant feeding/eating difficulties, which result in failure to meet energy (caloric) or nutritional needs. In response, individuals have low weight or failure to meet expectations for growth, significant nutritional deficiency, a need for enteral feeding or oral nutritional supplementation, and/or impairment in psychosocial functioning. Although there may be failure to thrive or to make expected weight gain/weight loss, ARFID is distinguished from AN by the absence of body image disturbance driving restrictive eating symptoms. Low weight can be determined through clinical judgment and examination of developmental trajectory using growth charts. Nutritional deficiency may be assessed through dietary history, as well as physical examination. Related medical consequences may follow those seen in malnourished individuals with AN (e.g., bradycardia, anemia, hypothermia) and can be life threatening. Individuals with ARFID treated in an inpatient setting are more likely to require nasogastric feeding than those with AN. If limited food intake is better explained by cultural or religious practice, an eating disorder in which there is disturbance in experience of shape/weight, or current physiologic or psychiatric conditions that explain the symptoms, ARFID is not diagnosed. Further, in the event of a coexisting medical diagnosis, food refusal is serious enough to warrant separate clinical attention. Thorough assessment should include examination of feeding, and eating history, psychiatric symptoms, development, and underlying medical causes must be ruled out before making a diagnosis.

Individuals with ARFID often exhibit selective eating, food neophobia, and hypersensitivity to sensory features of food (texture, taste, temperature, appearance). Similar clinical presentations may have varying etiology, requiring individualized treatment plans. In some, development of food avoidance can be traced to a specific aversive event, trauma, or related gastrointestinal problem, or may arise out of a choking, swallowing, or vomiting phobia. Individuals may also have a lack of drive or interest in eating or heightened textural sensitivity, which is also common in autism spectrum disorders.

Epidemiology

No data exist on prevalence, course, and outcome of this disorder. Surveillance studies are underway in the United Kingdom and Canada for related "food avoidance emotional disorder," with overlap in clinical features. In a school-age sample (ages 8–13), prevalence of ARFID was 3.2%. In pediatric inpatient ED programs, rates of ARFID are reported to be between 5% and 14% comprised of a higher proportion of males than other ED diagnoses and tend to be younger. ARFID appears to arise most commonly in infancy and early childhood but can occur at any age and last into adulthood. Preliminary data suggest ARFID occurs at equal rates in males and females. There is no evidence to guide for whom clinical intervention is warranted versus those whose symptoms resolve over time.

In one study, 53% of individuals ages 9 to 22 had at least one co-occurring lifetime psychiatric diagnosis, the most common being an anxiety disorder. Severity of symptoms among those with a sensory sensitivity profile of ARFID was related to increased risk for current and lifetime conduct, neurodevelopmental and disruptive disorders. Increased severity in the fear of aversive consequences profile was associated with increased risk for current and lifetime anxiety, obsessive-compulsive, and trauma-related disorders.

Treatment

There are no systematically studied treatments to date for ARFID; however, behavioral interventions with contingency management have been successfully used among children who have food neophobia in the context of a developmental disability. Given limited data, individualized treatment plans are best derived through assessment of medical history, temperament, psychiatric symptoms, and development. Food avoidance may be treated through use of behavioral strategies (e.g., shaping, chaining, contingency management, extinction) that systematically desensitize individuals to a wider range of foods. Related anxiety management techniques (relaxation training, visualization for mastery) and cognitive strategies derived from CBT may address maintaining psychiatric features. CBT was successfully applied in a case study of young adults with food neophobia, and a transdiagnostic CBT model with family involvement proved useful in a case study of a pediatric patient. Mirtazapine has been used with pediatric patients in two case studies with demonstrated increases in rate of weight gain, improvements in anxiety and eating. In most severe cases of malnutrition, hospitalization for medical stabilization purposes may be needed before outpatient therapy.

References

Bulik CM, Berkman ND, Brownley KA, et al: Anorexia nervosa treatment: a systematic review of randomized controlled trials, *Int J Eat Disord* 40:310–320, 2007.

Call C, Walsh B, Attia E: From DSM-IV to DSM-5: changes to eating disorder diagnoses, *Curr Opin Psychiatry* 26:532–536, 2013.

Couturier J, Isserlin L, Norris M, et al: Canadian practice guidelines for the treatment of children and adolescents with eating disorders, *J Eat Disord* 8(4):1–80, 2020.

Hay P: Current approach to eating disorders: a clinical update: 2020, *Intern Med J* 50:24–29, 2020.

Keery H, et al: Attributes of children and adolescents with avoidant/restrictive food intake disorder, *J Eat Disord* 7:31, 2020.

Kreipe R, Palomski A: Beyond picky eating: avoidant/restrictive food intake disorder, *Curr Psychiatry Rep* 14:421–431, 2012.

Le Grange D, Lock J, editors: *Eating disorders in children and adolescents: a clinical Handbook*, New York, 2011, The Guilford Press.

Peat C, Brownley K, Berkman N, et al: Binge eating disorder: evidence-based treatments, *Curr Psychiatry* 11:32–39, 2013.

Shapiro J, Berkman N, Brownley K, et al: Bulimia nervosa treatment: a systematic review of randomized controlled trials, *Int J Eat Disord* 40:321–336, 2007.

Smink F, van Hoeken D, Hoek H: Epidemiology of eating disorders: incidence, prevalence and mortality rates, *Curr Psychiatry Rep* 14:406–414, 2012.

Steinhausen H, Weber S: The outcome of bulimia nervosa: findings from one-quarter century of research, *Am J Psychiatry* 166:1331–1341, 2009.

Stice E, Marti CN, Rohde P: Prevalence, incidence, impairment and course of the proposed DSM-5 eating disorder diagnoses in an 8-year prospective community study of young women, *J Abnorm Psychol* 122(2):445–457, 2013.

GENERALIZED ANXIETY DISORDER

Method of
Natalie C. Dattilo, PhD; and Andrew W. Goddard, MD

CURRENT DIAGNOSIS

- Generalized anxiety disorder (GAD) is the most common psychiatric disorder seen in the primary care setting.
- GAD is characterized by feelings of dread, negative anticipation, and worry that are difficult to control and may include hypervigilance, excessive reassurance seeking, and behavioral avoidance of anxiety-provoking situations.
- Symptoms of GAD most often include agitation, irritability, restlessness, muscle aches or tension, dizziness, fatigue, racing heart, dry mouth, nausea, decreased sexual desire, sleep or appetite disturbances, and an inability to relax.
- A thorough medical examination and laboratory work may be indicated to rule out underlying physiologic causes, adverse reaction to medication, caffeine or substance use, and drug or alcohol withdrawal.
- Symptoms that are persistent, disruptive, or distressing warrant treatment.
- The Generalized Anxiety Disorder – 7 (GAD-7) is a screening instrument used to assess symptoms of GAD in primary care settings. Scores of 5, 10, and 15 are taken as the cut-off points for mild, moderate, and severe anxiety, respectively. When used as a screening tool, further evaluation is recommended when the score is 10 or greater.

CURRENT THERAPY

- Effective treatments for GAD include serotonergic antidepressants, certain forms of psychotherapy, or a combination of both.
- Educate the patient and family members about treatment options as well as realistic treatment expectations.
- Depending on the patient's preference, treatment may include a selective serotonin reuptake inhibitor (SSRI) or a serotonin norepinephrine reuptake inhibitor (SNRI), starting at low doses with careful titration so as not to exacerbate anxiety symptoms.
- Treatment may also include a trial of cognitive-behavioral therapy (CBT) monotherapy or in combination with medication management.
- Refer to or consult with a psychiatrist for patients with severe or particularly complex cases or for patients with a less-than-expected response to treatment.
- Refer to a CBT specialist for patients with a preference for behavioral, skills-based, or nonmedication therapy or for whom pharmacotherapy may be contraindicated.

Epidemiology

Anxiety disorders are among the most prevalent psychiatric disorders in the world. In the United States, it is estimated that an anxiety disorder is diagnosed in approximately 16 million adults each year and approximately 30 million meet criteria for an anxiety disorder over the course of their lifetimes. Second to depression, anxiety disorders are the most common mental health problem seen by physicians in the general medical setting. In fact, patients with anxiety are more likely to present initially to a generalist physician office than to a mental health care provider.

Anxiety disorders tend to be chronic and disabling and impose a high individual and societal burden. It has been estimated that the United States spends approximately $40 billion to $60 billion per year for costs associated with anxiety disorders. These include not only direct costs associated with treatment but also indirect costs associated with lost productivity. Thus early detection and treatment is critically important.

Risk Factors

Risk factors associated with anxiety disorders include personal or family history of anxiety; recent increase in stressful life events; lack or perceived lack of social support; ineffective emotional coping strategies; being female; experiencing childhood adversity, including trauma or witnessing a traumatic event; having a chronic health condition or serious illness; having an acute or chronic pain condition; and substance abuse. Having a genetic predisposition to developing an anxiety disorder is likely, although environmental stressors clearly play a role. Research has also shown that patients suffering from anxiety are generally more sensitive to physiologic changes than nonanxious patients. This heightened sensitivity leads to diminished autonomic flexibility, which may be the result of faulty central information processing in anxiety-prone persons.

Pathophysiology

Current evidence suggests that anxiety symptoms are likely caused by dysregulation in the central nervous system fear circuit. Physical and emotional manifestations of this dysregulation can result in a state of hyperarousal. Several neurotransmitter systems have been implicated in the development of this state.

The most commonly considered are the serotoninergic and noradrenergic neurotransmitter systems. Very simply, it is believed that an underactivation of the serotoninergic system and an overactivation of the noradrenergic system are involved, resulting in dysregulation of physiologic arousal and the emotional experience of this arousal. Disruption of the γ-aminobutyric acid (GABA) system has also been implicated because of the response of many of the anxiety-spectrum disorders to treatment with benzodiazepines.

There has also been some interest in the role of corticosteroid regulation and its relation to symptoms of fear and anxiety. Corticosteroids might increase or decrease the activity of certain neural pathways, affecting not only behavior under stress but also the brain's processing of fear-inducing stimuli. The stress response is hardwired into the brain and is most often triggered when survival of the organism is threatened. The stress response, however, can be triggered not only by a physical challenge or threat but also by the mere anticipation (or fear) of threat. As a result, when humans chronically and erroneously believe that a threatening event is about to occur, they begin to experience the physical and psychological symptoms of anxiety and panic.

Finally, a subcortical neural structure, the amygdala, serves an important role in coordinating the cognitive, affective, neuroendocrine, cardiovascular, respiratory, and musculoskeletal components of fear and anxiety responses (fear expression). It is central to registering the emotional significance of stressful stimuli and creating emotional memories. The amygdala receives input from neurons in the sensory cortex. When activated, the amygdala stimulates regions of the midbrain and brainstem, causing autonomic hyperactivity, which can be correlated with the physical symptoms of anxiety.

Prevention

No biological markers are specific enough yet to detect anxiety early, and there is no available evidence to suggest that current medications prove efficacious in preventing these disorders. Therefore, it is important to screen for specific risk factors, such as family history and substance abuse. If a person is anxiety prone, he or she should first be encouraged to adopt healthy lifestyle habits. Exercise has been shown to relieve tension, anxiety, and stress. Patients should avoid stimulants such as caffeine and nicotine, which can exacerbate symptoms. Reducing alcohol intake should be encouraged as well. Educating patients on healthy sleep habits can prevent conditioned (or secondary) insomnia issues. It is also recommended that anxiety-prone persons reduce subjective levels of stress by practicing effective methods of relaxation and other stress management activities, like meditation, yoga, social connection, gratitude journaling, and pleasant event scheduling.

Clinical Manifestations

GAD is characterized by subjective feelings of worry, dread, or anticipation of negative events and can include hypervigilance and avoidance of anxiety-producing situations. Physical symptoms can include jitteriness or shakiness, trembling, muscle aches and tension, sweating, cold or clammy hands, dizziness, or vertigo; fatigue; racing or pounding heart; hyperventilation; sensation of a lump in the throat, choking sensation, or dry mouth; numbness and tingling in the hands, feet, or other body parts; upset stomach, nausea, vomiting, or diarrhea; decreased sexual desire; and sleep and appetite disturbances.

Psychological symptoms include, most predominantly, unrealistic or excessive worry and apprehension, hypervigilance or an inability to relax, distractibility, indecisiveness, and insecurity. Patients often express feelings of impatience, agitation, irritability, and fear. They may ask multiple questions repeatedly in an attempt to quell the anxiety through excessive information or reassurance seeking. In GAD, the worries a patient may express tend to be nonspecific and all-encompassing. They tend to be "worst-case scenario" and "what if?" thinkers. Some patients also exhibit specific phobias such as fear of being far from home or fear of social contact. Patients with GAD may report difficulty falling asleep because they "can't turn their mind off" at night. If a patient reports these symptoms or displays one of several behavioral manifestations of GAD leading to significant distress and/or impairment of function, the condition is unlikely to remit on its own and treatment is warranted.

Diagnosis

A diagnosis of GAD is made when a patient meets the specific diagnostic criteria outlined in the *Diagnostic and Statistical Manual of Mental Disorders, Fifth Edition* (DSM-5). Persons with GAD experience uncontrollable, excessive anxiety and worry involving several areas of functioning on most days for at least 6 months. The anxiety must be associated with at least three of the following symptoms: restlessness, fatigue, impaired concentration, irritability, muscle tension, or sleep problems. Patients tend to express chronic excessive nervousness, exaggerated worry, tension, and irritability that appear to have no cause or are more intense than the situation warrants. Physical signs such as headaches, trembling, twitching, or sweating often develop, which lead to further worries. GAD symptoms tend to wax and wane over time, with short-term exacerbations of acute anxiety in response to stress. Symptoms show substantial overlap with those of other medical and psychological disorders, particularly major depressive disorder, substance abuse disorders, and other anxiety disorders, which tends to complicate diagnosis.

Differential Diagnosis

It is important to perform a thorough medical workup when initially assessing the patient with anxiety symptoms. The differential diagnosis can include several organic causes, such as endocrine dysfunction, intoxication or withdrawal, hypoxia, metabolic abnormalities, and neurologic disorders. It is also important to rule out other comorbid psychiatric disorders. Severe depression, bipolar disorder, prodromal schizophrenia, delusional disorder, and adjustment disorder can often be accompanied by severe anxiety. Many organic causes can be ruled out by a thorough history and basic laboratory work, including thyroid-stimulating hormone, urine toxicology, electrocardiogram, complete blood count, and metabolic panel. The most common medical conditions associated with anxiety are presented in Box 1.

The list of drugs suspected of causing anxiety is extensive. Drugs commonly associated with anxiety include stimulants such as amphetamine, cocaine, methamphetamine, and caffeine. Drugs such as lysergic acid diethylamide (LSD) and 3,4-methylenedioxymethamphetamine (MDMA, or "ecstasy") can also cause acute

---

BOX 1 — Medical Conditions Often Associated With Anxiety Symptoms

Cardiopulmonary
Angina
Mitral valve prolapse
Pulmonary embolism
Chronic obstructive pulmonary disease (COPD)
Asthma

Endocrine
Hyperthyroidism
Pheochromocytoma
Cushing syndrome
Menopause

Gastrointestinal
Gastroesophageal reflux
Irritable bowel syndrome (IBS)
Gastritis

Neurologic
Dementia
Substance intoxication or withdrawal
Seizure disorder
Migraine

---

and chronic anxiety. Prescription medications to consider include sympathomimetics, antihypertensives, and nonsteroidal antiinflammatory drugs (NSAIDs).

Treatment and Monitoring

Current practice guidelines indicate that the treatment of an anxiety disorder begins with education. Many people are confused, scared, or frustrated by the symptoms and behavior and are reassured to know they are not alone and that there are effective interventions. The patient should receive an appropriate medical workup, such as a physical examination, and studies (e.g., electrocardiogram, thyroid-stimulating hormone) when indicated. After ruling out a medical condition, developing a good working alliance with the patient provides a basis for ongoing disease management and prevents unnecessary utilization or overutilization of the medical system, as well as potential exacerbation of symptoms.

A combination of psychotherapy and medication management is recommended as first-line treatment for GAD. CBT has the strongest empirical support to date for the treatment of anxiety. Mindfulness-based stress reduction (MBSR) has an emerging evidence base as an effective alternative or complementary behavioral treatment program for anxiety. Both offer a skills-based approach to treatment. In CBT, the therapist and patient work collaboratively and in an active and problem-solving manner. It is structured and generally short term with an emphasis on reducing symptoms and preventing "flare-ups" by monitoring and changing unhelpful or inaccurate thinking patterns that result in feelings of anxiety and worry. Another critical component of CBT for GAD is learning and applying behavioral relaxation techniques (e.g., diaphragmatic breathing, guided imagery, progressive muscle relaxation) and distress tolerance skills (e.g., mindfulness, acceptance). Volumes of evidence support the efficacy of CBT interventions for GAD, but success requires commitment to treatment on the part of the patient. Its efficacy is also contingent upon the ability of the therapist and the length of time in treatment. Studies show that when compared with patients undergoing monotherapy, patients treated with a combination of CBT and medication experience nearly twice the remission rate.

SSRIs have been shown to be the best-tolerated class of medication, and response rates are significantly higher than

TABLE 1	Pharmacotherapy for the Treatment of Generalized Anxiety Disorder	
DRUG	**STARTING DOSE**	**TARGET DOSE**
Selective Serotonin Reuptake Inhibitors		
Paroxetine (Paxil)*	10 mg qd	10–60 mg qd
Escitalopram (Lexapro)*	5–10 mg qd	10–20 mg qd
Sertraline (Zoloft)	12.5–25 mg qd	50–200 mg qd
Fluoxetine (Prozac)	10 mg qd	20–40 mg qd
Serotonin-Norepinephrine Reuptake Inhibitors		
Venlafaxine (Effexor XR)*	37.5 mg qAM	150–300 mg qAM[†]
Duloxetine (Cymbalta)*	30 mg qd	60–90 mg qd
Other		
Buspirone (BuSpar)	5 mg bid–tid	10 mg tid

*U.S. Food and Drug Administration indication for generalized anxiety disorder.
[†]Exceeds dosage recommended by the manufacturer.

placebo for GAD. SSRI medications includes fluoxetine (Prozac),[1] fluvoxamine (Luvox),[1] citalopram (Celexa),[1] escitalopram (Lexapro), paroxetine (Paxil), and sertraline (Zoloft).[1] Some improvement in symptoms should be noted within 3 or 4 weeks, and the dose should be increased if no improvement is seen. In treating any anxiety disorder, SSRIs should be started at low doses and gradually titrated up to therapeutic levels to avoid an initial exacerbation of anxiety. Pharmacotherapy options for the treatment of GAD are presented in Table 1.

Benzodiazepines, which have been commonly used in the past to treat anxiety disorders, are not recommended except in cases of extreme impairment of function and only for very short-term use. The tolerability and lack of addiction potential make the SSRIs more desirable for long-term management, but the delay in response makes short-term symptom relief with a benzodiazepine desirable for those with the greatest impairment. Because of the risk for rebound anxiety when withdrawing from benzodiazepines with short half-lives, such as alprazolam (Xanax), many prefer the longer-acting benzodiazepines, such as clonazepam (Klonopin).[1] However, the addiction potential and the potential for abuse with either drug make this the treatment option of last resort.

If the patient does not respond to the combination of CBT and medication, a reevaluation of symptoms might reveal a comorbid disorder missed on the first examination. Comorbid psychiatric disorders significantly lower the likelihood of recovery from anxiety and increase recurrence rates. Some clinicians try switching to a different SSRI before considering the next step in treatment; however, a referral to a psychiatrist or integrated care consultant for further evaluation and management may be necessary. Treatment-refractory anxiety can be extremely frustrating for the patient, the patient's family, and the treating physician. If benzodiazepine treatment was initiated, this frustration can and does often lead to an increased dependence on the medication and a requirement of increasingly higher doses to achieve the same effect. For long-term gains, therapy in addition to medication treatment should be recommended.

Education is critical to reassure the patient that effective treatment is available, but that patience may be necessary until the right combination of modalities is found. Although all anxiety disorders display a significant amount of chronicity,

most patients have an improved outcome with appropriate treatment. Response rates improve when comorbidity is low. Patients with an earlier onset of symptoms (childhood or adolescence) can generally expect a more chronic course and their anxiety symptoms may be more difficult to treat. Patients rarely have a spontaneous remission of symptoms, but most can continue to function despite the symptoms. Nevertheless, time to resolution of symptoms is shortened and overall functioning typically improves with treatment.

Pharmacotherapy often helps to prevent relapse, and rates are improved when effective treatment is continued for 12 months. When considering termination of pharmacologic treatment, the risk for relapse in GAD should be discussed with the patient. When discontinuing the SSRIs, a slow taper is recommended, with close monitoring for withdrawal symptoms (e.g., headache, gastrointestinal upset, restlessness, and other flulike symptoms). Also monitor for rebound anxiety symptoms. If relapse occurs, reinstituting treatment is indicated, and many patients opt for indefinite treatment to maintain remission of symptoms. Lifelong management with pharmacotherapy or psychotherapy, or both, is not unusual for many patients. For many, a maximum reduction of symptoms, rather than a full remission, is an acceptable outcome.

Complications
Untreated anxiety disorders can lead to, or worsen, other mental and physical health conditions, including bruxism (teeth grinding), cognitive impairment, depression, gastrointestinal disorders, headache, insomnia, heart disease, substance abuse, and significantly impaired quality of life.

Conclusion
Anxiety disorders are highly prevalent in the United States. GAD is one of the most common psychiatric conditions seen in primary care, second only to major depression. This condition can be disabling and costly to the patient and to the health care system. Despite the prevalence of anxiety disorders, patients often remain undiagnosed and untreated, and patients with unrecognized anxiety disorders tend to be higher utilizers of general medical care. Patients with anxiety disorders can present with multiple somatic complaints and comorbid disorders, causing great effort and expense in identifying the cause of unexplained symptoms. Once an anxiety disorder is identified, patients may be treated using well-tested and efficacious pharmacologic and psychotherapeutic treatments. Helpful resources for patients and families are listed in Table 2.

TABLE 2	Helpful Resources for Family Members and Patients With Anxiety Disorders
ORGANIZATION	**WEBSITE**
American Family Physician	www.familydoctor.org/condition/generalized-anxiety-disorder
American Psychiatric Association	www.psychiatry.org/patients-families/anxiety-disorders
American Psychological Association	www.apa.org/topics/anxiety
Anxiety Disorders Association of America	www.adaa.org
Association for Behavioral and Cognitive Therapies	www.abct.org
Mental Health America	www.mentalhealthamerica.net/conditions/anxiety-disorders
National Institute of Mental Health	www.nimh.nih.gov/index.shtml

[1]Not US Food and Drug Administration (FDA) approved for this indication.
[1]Not FDA approved for this indication.

References

American Psychiatric Association: *Diagnostic and Statistical Manual of Mental Disorders*, ed 5, Washington, DC, 2013, American Psychiatric Association.

American Psychiatric Association: *Practice Guideline for the Treatment of Patients with Panic Disorder*, ed 2, Washington, DC, 2009, American Psychiatric Association.

Campbell-Sills L, Stein MB: *Guideline Watch: Practice Guidelines for the Treatment of Patients With Panic Disorder*, Arlington, VA, 2006, American Psychiatric Association.

Davidson JRT, Feltner DE, Dugar A: Management of generalized anxiety disorder in primary care: Identifying the challenges and unmet needs, *Prim Care Companion J Clin Psychiatry* 12:2010.

Gabbard GO: *Gabbard's Treatment of Psychiatric Disorders*. ed 3, Washington, DC, 2001, American Psychiatric Publishing.

Goddard AW, Coplan JD, Shekhar A, et al: Principles of the pharmacotherapy of anxiety disorders. In Charney DS, Nestler EJ, editors: *The Neurobiology of Mental Illness*, ed 2nd, New York, 2004, Oxford University Press, pp 661–682.

Kessler RC, Berglund P, Demler O, et al: Lifetime prevalence and age-of-onset distributions of DSM-IV disorders in the National Comorbidity Survey Replication, *Arch Gen Psychiatry* 62:593–602, 2005.

Kroenke K, Spitzer RL, Williams JBW, et al: Anxiety disorders in primary care: Prevalence, impairment, comorbidity, and detection, *Ann Intern Med* 146:317–325, 2007.

Lépine JP: The epidemiology of anxiety disorders: Prevalence and societal costs, *J Clin Psychiatry* 63(Suppl. 14):4–8, 2002.

Sadock BJ, Sadock VA: *Kaplan and Sadock's Synopsis of Psychiatry: Behavioral Sciences/Clinical Psychiatry*, ed 10, Philadelphia, 2007, Lippincott Williams & Wilkins.

Spitzer RL, Kroenke K, Williams JBW, Lowe B: A brief measure for assessing generalized anxiety disorder, *Arch Intern Med* 166:1092–1097, 2006.

Stein MB: Attending to anxiety disorders in primary care, *J Clin Psychiatry* 64(Suppl. 15):35–39, 2003.

MAJOR DEPRESSIVE, BIPOLAR AND RELATED MOOD DISORDERS

Method of
Ila Durkin, MD; Muaid Ithman, MD; and Matthew Macaluso, DO

CURRENT DIAGNOSIS

- Screen for depression in all primary care settings.
  - The Patient Health Questionnaire 9-Item (PHQ-9) is patient-rated, free, and easily implemented in the outpatient setting.
  - The Edinburgh Postnatal Depression Scale (EDPS) is a 10-item patient-rated free scale used for peripartum depression.
- Screen for bipolar disorder before prescribing antidepressants for depression; on average bipolar II disorder (BDII) goes misdiagnosed as major depressive disorder (MDD) for 10 years. Consider BDII if there is a family history of bipolar, if there have been multiple failed trials of antidepressants, or if psychosis has been present during depressive episodes. The Mood Disorders Questionnaire (MDQ) is a brief, patient self-report, screening that can be used in clinic to assist with screening for bipolar disorder.
- In addition to the core symptom of depressed mood, the SIGE-CAPS mnemonic is a useful tool in medical education to teach the diagnostic criteria for MDD: sleep, interest, guilt, energy, concentration, appetite, psychomotor, and suicide (see Table 1).
- In addition to the core symptoms of euphoric or agitated mood and increased energy, the DIGFAST mnemonic is another mnemonic used in medical education to teach students the symptoms of mania and hypomania used to diagnose bipolar I and II disorders: distractibility, impulsivity, grandiosity, flight of ideas, activity, sleep, and talkativeness (see Table 2).

CURRENT THERAPY

- Psychotherapy and lifestyle changes, without pharmacotherapy, is a reasonable first-line treatment for mild or uncomplicated major depressive disorder (MDD).

- First-line pharmacotherapy for MDD includes oral antidepressants such as selective serotonin reuptake inhibitors (SSRIs) and serotonin-norepinephrine reuptake inhibitors (SNRIs). Second-line treatment strategies include switching antidepressants or adding a medication, procedural intervention such as repetitive transcranial magnetic stimulation, or psychotherapy for augmentation (see Table 4).
- Antidepressants must be given an adequate trial (therapeutic dose for 6 wk) before deeming the medication ineffective.
- First-line pharmacotherapy of mania, hypomania or depression in bipolar disorders is a mood stabilizer monotherapy or a mood stabilizer and second-generation antipsychotic combination (see Table 5).
- Antidepressant monotherapy should be avoided to treat bipolar depression because of the risk of manic switch or a mixed episode. Parenthetically, a prior edition of the American Psychiatric Association Practice Guidelines suggested that oral antidepressant monotherapy (e.g., SSRIs) could be used to treat depressive episodes associated with bipolar II disorder. However, using traditional oral antidepressants such as SSRIs and SNRIs to treat bipolar depression can be associated with manic switching and is off-label, with the exception of the combination of fluoxetine and olanzapine (Symbyax), which has unique properties thought to be safe and effective.
- Treatment-resistant MDD, mania, hypomania, or bipolar depression should be referred to a psychiatrist. Treatment resistance is generally defined as the failure of two or more adequate medication trials. It's important to remember that, as Dr. Sheldon Preskorn states, "patients don't fail medications. Medications fail patients."

Pathophysiology

Biopsychosocial factors play a role in the development of mood disorders such as major depressive disorder (MDD), bipolar I disorder (BDI), and bipolar II disorder (BDII). Dysregulation of monoamine neurotransmitters such as norepinephrine, serotonin, and dopamine form the building blocks of most biologic theories. Heritability is approximately 40% for MDD and up to 90% for bipolar disorder; thus there is a strong genetic predisposition to mood disorders. Psychosocial factors should be taken into consideration and might include stressful or life-changing events (e.g., moving cities, the death of a loved one, or childbirth), sleep disruptions, adverse childhood experiences, poverty, racism or discrimination, chronic medical conditions, or substance use (e.g., cannabis associated with an exacerbation of mania). There is not typically one identifiable triggering event for an acute depressive or manic episode but rather a culmination of biopsychosocial factors leading to a disruption of intricate neuroregulatory mechanisms and neural circuits.

MDD has a 12-month prevalence of approximately 7% in the United States. The prevalence varies greatly with age and sex such that the prevalence in youth is three times that in adults over 60, and the prevalence for females is twice that of males. The 12-month prevalence of BDI is 1.5% in the United States, with an almost equal distribution between males and females. The peak age of onset for a manic episode is 20 to 30 years, but onset occurs throughout the lifecycle. BDII has a slightly lower 12-month prevalence of 0.8% in the United States; however, this is difficult to estimate because BDII diagnosis from symptom onset typically lags by 10 years. For this reason, age of onset is not a reliable factor to use in distinguishing between BDI and BDII disorders. This is particularly problematic in clinical practice, because the more mood episodes a patient with bipolar disorder experiences, the more frequent and severe the episodes become in the future (i.e., kindling).

Prevention

One way to prevent worsening or untreated mood disorders is to screen for them regularly. The US Preventive Services Task Force (USPSTF) recommends screening for depression in adults, especially older adults and pregnant or postpartum women. The Patient Health Questionnaire 9-item (PHQ-9) is a patient-rated scale commonly used in the primary care setting to screen for MDD and for suicide risk in any adult. The Edinburgh Postnatal Depression Scale (EDPS) is a 10-item patient-rated scale that is more a more sensitive screen for depression in the peripartum period. The Mood Disorder Questionnaire (MDQ) is a 17-item patient-rated scale that can be used in the primary care setting to assess for bipolar disorders. Because each of these screening tools are free in the public domain and patient-rated, they are straightforward to use in the outpatient primary care setting.

In addition to screening for MDD and bipolar disorders, practicing trauma-informed care can help prevent worsening of mood disorders. In 1998 a landmark study, The Adverse Childhood Experiences (ACE) Study, found that ACEs directly affect long-term mental and physical health of adults, even when controlling for other common lifestyle risk factors. This study also highlighted the prevalence of ACEs as more than half of study participants reported a history of at least one ACE. Trauma-informed care in its essence is recognizing the prevalence of trauma and its effects on health and behavior. Free resources are available to learn about trauma-informed care and how to implement this into your practice; one such online resource is https://www.aces aware.org.

Diagnosis

MDD is diagnosed when a patient has five or more depressive symptoms for 2 weeks or longer as defined by the *Diagnostic and Statistical Manual of Mental Disorders*, Fifth Edition, Text Revision; at least one of the depressive symptoms must be depressed mood or anhedonia (loss of interest or pleasure). As shown in Table 1, the mnemonic SIGECAPS can be used to recall the depressive symptoms used for diagnosis. These symptoms must cause clinically significant distress or impairment in functioning; milder symptoms may be more difficult to detect or observe because of efforts by the patient to maintain some or all prior functioning. Symptoms cannot be attributable to the effects of a substance (e.g., illicit substances or in some cases prescribed drugs) or of a medical condition because this would indicate a different depressive disorder (substance/medication-induced depressive disorder or depressive disorder due to another medical condition, respectively). It is imperative to screen for previous manic or hypomanic episodes because this would indicate a diagnosis of bipolar disorder, which has a different treatment strategy than MDD, including the use of different classes of medication than commonly used in MDD. Responses to a significant stressor, including bereavement, may share some of the same symptoms as MDD, and in these instances it is important to consider the cultural context of the patient's response to the stressor. Also, it is important to take into consideration the history of a previous major depressive episode, because a stressor may trigger a recurrence of MDD.

BDI is diagnosed when a patient has at least one manic episode; the manic episode may have been preceded by or may be followed by hypomanic or major depressive episodes. A manic episode is defined as at least 7 days of abnormally and persistently elevated, expansive or irritable mood, and increased energy, accompanied by three additional symptoms (four if the mood is only irritable). As shown in Table 2, the mnemonic DIGFAST can be used to recall the additional symptoms used to diagnose a manic episode. To be considered a manic episode, the symptoms must cause marked impairment in functioning, lead to hospitalization, or be accompanied by psychosis (delusions or hallucinations). If mania occurs as a result of antidepressant treatment and continues to meet diagnostic criteria for a manic episode beyond the physiologic effects of that treatment, this is sufficient to diagnose a manic episode and therefore a BDI diagnosis.

BPII is diagnosed when a patient has both hypomanic and major depressive episodes. A hypomanic episode is defined similarly to a manic episode with several key differences. Hypomanic

TABLE 1	SIGECAPS Mnemonic for Diagnosis of a Major Depressive Episode*	
S	Sleep	Insomnia or hypersomnia, nearly every day.
I	Interest	Markedly diminished interest or pleasure in all, or almost all, activities most of the day, nearly every day; by subjective account or observed by others.
G	Guilt	Feelings of worthlessness or excessive or inappropriate guilt (which may be delusional) nearly every day.
E	Energy	Fatigue or loss of energy nearly every day.
C	Concentration	Diminished ability to think or concentrate, or indecisiveness, nearly every day; subjective account or observed by others.
A	Appetite	Significant weight loss without dieting or weight gain or decrease or increase in appetite nearly every day. In children, this may be failure to make expected weight gain.
P	Psychomotor	Psychomotor agitation or retardation nearly every day; observed by others, not merely subjective.
S	Suicide	Recurrent thoughts of death, recurrent suicidal ideation with or without a specific plan, or a suicide attempt.

*Also included in the diagnostic criteria is depressed mood most of the day, nearly every day; subjective account or observed by others. In children and adolescents this may be irritable mood. Lasts at least 2 weeks.

TABLE 2	DIGFAST Mnemonic Used to Diagnose a Manic or Hypomanic Episode*	
D	Distractibility	Distractibility, as reported or observed
I	Impulsivity	Excessive involvement in activities that have a high potential for painful consequences
G	Grandiosity	Inflated self-esteem or grandiosity
F	Flight of ideas	Flight of ideas or subjective experience that thoughts are racing
A	Activity	Increase in goal-directed activity or psychomotor agitation
S	Sleep	Decreased need for sleep
T	Talkativeness	More talkative than usual or pressure to keep talking

*Also included in the diagnostic criteria is abnormally and persistently elevated, expansive, or irritable mood, and abnormally and persistently increased activity or energy, lasting at least 1 week for mania or 4 days for hypomania and present most of the day, nearly every day.

episodes last at least 4 days instead of 7 as with mania, are not severe enough to cause marked impairment in functioning, nor can they be severe enough to require hospitalization, and are not accompanied by psychosis. Although hypomanic episodes do not cause marked impairment in functioning, they do cause an unequivocal change in functioning or behavior, which is uncharacteristic for the patient and observable by others. Examples of this would be patients who are still going to work but are unable to perform at a level that is typical for them. A history of major depressive episode is necessary to make a BDII diagnosis. A major depressive episode in the context of BDI or BDII disorder uses the same diagnostic criteria as a depressive episode occurring as part of a MDD (see Table 1). If manic or hypomanic symptoms

TABLE 3	Mood Episodes That Must or Must Not Be Present When Diagnosing Mood Disorders		
	MDD	**BDI**	**BDII**
Major depressive episode	Yes	Maybe	Yes
Manic episode	Never	Yes	Never
Hypomanic episode	Never	Maybe	Yes

BDI, Bipolar I disorder; *BDII*, bipolar II disorder; *MDD*, major depressive disorder.

are attributable to the effects of a substance (e.g., illicit substance or potentially a prescribed drug) or of a medical condition, the diagnosis would instead be either substance/medication-induced bipolar and related disorder or bipolar and related disorder due to another medical condition.

As displayed in Table 3, the overlap of diagnostic criteria and mood episodes for MDD, BDI, and BDII can make it difficult to distinguish between these mood disorders. BDII is often misdiagnosed as MDD for multiple reasons; patients typically present to their providers for treatment of their major depressive episodes but not for their hypomanic episodes, or patients might also misremember or minimize the significance of past hypomanic episodes. Clinicians might also miss the subtleties of hypomania in their haste to screen for mania. If a patient has a history of recurrent MDD starting in adolescence and characterized by multiple failed antidepressant trials, a diagnosis of BDII should be considered, especially if the family history is positive for bipolar disorder or if the depressive episodes include psychotic symptoms. Mood lability, decreased need for sleep, and increased energy or activity are symptoms that have a higher predictive accuracy when assessing for hypomanic episodes. The Mood Disorders Questionnaire (MDQ) is a brief, patient self-report, screening that can be used in clinic to assist with screening for bipolar disorder.

Treatment

Major Depressive Disorder

For mild and uncomplicated MDD it is reasonable to consider starting with lifestyle changes and referral to a psychotherapist for psychotherapy. This is provided a thorough medical workup has been completed to rule out other conditions manifesting with symptoms of depression (e.g., anemia or hypothyroidism). The descriptors *mild* and *uncomplicated* mean there are few symptoms in excess of those required to make the diagnosis, symptoms are minimally distressing but manageable, symptoms result in only minor/minimal impairment in functioning, there is no psychosis, and the current episode is the first episode of depression. Lifestyle modification includes regular exercise, practicing good sleep hygiene (see Healthy Sleep Habits at the American Academy of Sleep Medicine's https://sleepeducation.org), management of any poorly controlled and/or chronic medical problems (e.g., diabetes, obstructive sleep apnea) and addressing substance use disorders, including substance misuse, whether prescription, over the counter, or illicit. Psychotherapy interventions include acceptance and commitment therapy, behavioral activation therapy, cognitive-behavioral therapy, interpersonal psychotherapy, mindfulness-based cognitive therapy, problem-solving therapy, and short-term psychodynamic psychotherapy. If depression is moderate to severe, if it has not responded to nonpharmacologic interventions, or if the patient has had success previously with antidepressant medication, then pharmacotherapy should be considered in addition to psychotherapy and lifestyle changes, if appropriate. Patient motivation and ability to access the treatment in question is important.

First-line pharmacotherapy is monotherapy with a selective serotonin reuptake inhibitor (SSRI), serotonin-norepinephrine reuptake inhibitor (SNRI), or "other" reuptake inhibitors including bupropion, mirtazapine, trazodone, vilazodone (Viibryd), or vortioxetine (Trintellix) (Table 4). It is important to remember

that antidepressants can take 6 weeks or more to achieve full effect. Therefore setting realistic expectations for the treatment team and patients is important, as is ensuring an adequate trial of an antidepressant, usually defined as between 6 and 12 weeks of at least a midrange dose. Second-line pharmacotherapy options for partial responders or nonresponders to first-line treatment include switching to another antidepressant or augmentation with a second antidepressant or nonantidepressant medication, as listed in Table 4. Tricyclic antidepressants (TCAs) and monoamine oxidase inhibitors (MAOI) are older antidepressants but considered third-line agents because of their side effect profiles (e.g., TCAs can be lethal in overdose, and MAOIs have dietary restrictions relative to tyramine-containing foods and drinks). Please see references listed at the end of this chapter for more information on TCAs or MAOIs.

If a patient has tried and failed two adequate trials of antidepressants (an adequate dose for 6 weeks), referral to a psychiatrist should be considered for treatment-resistant depression (TRD). Treatment options for TRD include electroconvulsive therapy (ECT), repetitive transcranial magnetic stimulation, intranasal esketamine (Spravato), or vagal nerve stimulation (VNS).

ECT uses an electric current to induce a seizure while the patient is anesthetized, two to three times a week for a total of 12 treatment sessions. ECT is one of the most effective treatments for TRD and can be considered a life-saving treatment because it works for severely ill patients, patients at risk, and patients who do not respond to other treatments. Transcranial magnetic stimulation uses magnets to induce an electric current that is focused on the dorsolateral prefrontal cortex. This can be performed in a clinic setting, 5 days per week for 6 weeks of treatment. Intranasal esketamine is an N-methyl-D-aspartate receptor antagonist and is administered in the clinic setting under direct supervision of a licensed healthcare provider with monitoring for at least 2 hours afterward for resolution of adverse effects, which include blood pressure elevation, sedation, a feeling of intoxication or drunkenness, nauseas and vomiting, dissociation, and psychotomimetic symptoms. Invasive VNS is a surgically implanted device that delivers electrical impulses to the brain via the vagus nerve. External, noninvasive VNS devices are available commercially but are not currently approved by the US Food and Drug Administration (FDA) for TRD, although the devices have been FDA approved for use in cluster headaches and migraines.

Some alternative treatments for MDD can be beneficial additions for some patients in addition to traditional treatment and carry minimal or different risks. One such treatment is bright light therapy which uses 10,000-lux white light (with an ultraviolet filter) for 30 minutes in the morning (and also sometimes at mid-day); the patient must be facing but not staring into the light box and remove all eyeglasses, corrective lenses, contact lenses, etc. Adverse effects can include manic switching in at risk patients, eye strain, headache, floaters, etc. When in doubt about safety, consult with an ophthalmologist. Supplements such as omega 3 fatty acids, vitamin B9 (folate) or vitamin D have little evidence to support their efficacy in mood disorders, but also have limited risk for adverse effects. St. John's wort[7] has been shown to be superior to placebo in treating MDD. However, it is a potent inducer of CYP3A4 and interacts with medications such as digoxin, warfarin, and oral contraceptives; combined with other serotonergic antidepressants this can contribute to serotonin syndrome.

For MDD, 40% of patients will achieve symptomatic remission within 3 months and 80% within 1 year. The antidepressant used, at the dose at which remission was achieved, should be continued for at least 6 months to minimize the risk of symptomatic relapse. Each successive major depressive episode increases the risk of recurrence (80%–90% increase in risk after the second episode). Therefore it is generally recommended to

---

[7] Available as a dietary supplement.

TABLE 4	Antidepressants and Medications for Augmentation			
CLASS	MEDICATION	MINIMUM EFFECTIVE DOSE (MG/DAY)	THERAPEUTIC DOSE RANGE (MG/DAY)*	PRESCRIBING TIPS
SSRI	citalopram (Celexa)	20	10–40	Maximum dose 20 mg/day if >60 years
	escitalopram (Lexapro)	10	10–20	Max dose 10 mg/day if >60 years. Very well tolerated.
	fluoxetine (Prozac)	20	10–80	Dose in the morning because this can be activating. Long half-life, so no discontinuation syndrome.
	fluvoxamine (Luvox)[1]	50	50–300	Works well for OCD. Has a lot of drug-drug interactions.
	paroxetine (Paxil)	20	10–60[3]	More likely to cause discontinuation syndrome. Not recommended during pregnancy.
	sertraline (Zoloft)	50	50–200	More likely to cause GI upset.
SNRI	desvenlafaxine (Pristiq)	50	50–100	Active metabolite of venlafaxine, better tolerated than venlafaxine.
	duloxetine (Cymbalta)	60	60–120	Helpful for chronic pain at higher doses.
	levomilnacipran (Fetzima)	40	20–120	Helpful for chronic pain, but not available as generic yet.
	venlafaxine (Effexor)	75	75–375[3]	More likely to cause discontinuation syndrome. Works well for anxiety.
NDRI	bupropion SR (Wellbutrin SR)	150	150–300	Activating; can cause weight loss. Least likely to have sexual side effects. Lowers seizure threshold.
NaSSA	mirtazapine (Remeron)	30	15–60[3]	Dose at bedtime, helps with insomnia and anorexia.
SARI	nefazodone (Serzone)	400	100–600	Contraindicated in patients with known hepatic impairment.
	trazodone (Desyrel)	150	150–600	Usually used as adjunct for insomnia, 25–100 mg at bedtime.
SPARI	vilazodone (Viibryd)	20	10–40	Must be taken with food. Less likely to cause sexual side effects or weight gain.
SMS	vortioxetine (Trintellix)	10	5–20	Less likely to cause sexual side effects or weight gain.
Medications used for augmentation	aripiprazole (Abilify)	2	2–20	Can be activating, dose in the morning.
	brexpiprazole (Rexulti)	2	0.5–3	Might be better tolerated than aripiprazole.
	buspirone (BuSpar)[1]	15	15–60	Works well for anxiety and can help mitigate sexual side effects of antidepressants.
	lithium[1]	600–900	†	Has antisuicidal properties.
	modafinil (Provigil)[1]	100	100–400	Non–habit-forming stimulant, useful for low energy.

[1]Not FDA approved for this indication.
[3]Exceeds dosage recommended by the manufacturer.
*Does not include dose adjustments for hepatic or renal impairment.
†Target plasma level 0.4–0.8 mmol/L is suggested.
GI, Gastrointestinal; hs, at bedtime; NaSSA, noradrenergic/specific serotonergic agent; NDRI, norepinephrine dopamine reuptake inhibitor; OCD, obsessive-compulsive disorder; SARI, serotonin-2 antagonists/serotonin reuptake inhibitor; SMS, serotonin modulator and stimulator; SNRI, selective serotonin-norepinephrine reuptake inhibitor; SPARI, serotonin-1A partial agonist/serotonin reuptake inhibitor; SRI, selective serotonin reuptake inhibitor.

continue antidepressant treatments indefinitely after two major depressive episodes to prevent recurrent episodes.

Bipolar I Disorder and Bipolar II Disorder

As shown in Table 5, the mainstay of bipolar treatment is with mood stabilizers. Mood stabilizers include lithium, some anticonvulsants, and most second-generation antipsychotics (SGA). Lithium has antisuicidal and neuroprotective properties, is efficacious in mania and depression and is the best prophylactic agent. It can be a lifesaving medication for patients but also intimidating for physicians to manage; for this reason,

the authors think it prudent to discuss lithium management in more detail. The controlled-release tablets (Lithobid) given once daily at bedtime are better tolerated, with a starting dose of 300 mg in the elderly or 600 to 900 mg in non-elderly patients. Trough lithium levels should be obtained 5 days after starting the medication or after dose adjustments; draw laboratory samples in the morning before taking morning medications. It is essential that these levels be *measured at trough*, or about 12 hours after the last dose was administered; otherwise the levels are not accurate. Lithium has a narrow therapeutic range of 0.8 to 1.2 mmol/L for acute mania

TABLE 5 Mood Stabilizers

CLASS	MEDICATION	MANIA OR HYPOMANIA INDICATION	BIPOLAR DEPRESSION INDICATION	THERAPEUTIC DOSE RANGE (MG/DAY)*	PRESCRIBING TIPS
Lithium salt	lithium	First line as mono or combo therapy	First line	600–1800†	Up to fourfold increase in levels when used with ACEIs, thiazide diuretics or NSAIDs.
Anticonvulsant	carbamazepine (Tegretol)	Second line as combo therapy	Third line	300–1600†	Teratogenic, avoid use in women of childbearing age. Multiple drug interactions.
	lamotrigine (Lamictal)	–	First line	100–500	Strict titration schedule to decrease risk of SJS.
	oxcarbazepine (Trileptal)[1]	Third line as combo therapy	–	600–1200	Lower potential for side effects or drug interactions as compared to carbamazepine.
	valproic acid (Depakote)	First line as mono or combo therapy	Second line	750–3000†	Teratogenic, avoid use in women of childbearing age. Helpful in mixed episodes (manic or hypomanic and depressive symptoms).
SGA	aripiprazole (Abilify)	First line as mono or combo therapy	–	15–30	Compared to other SGAs, less risk for sedation, metabolic effects, and EPS. Available as a LAI.
	asenapine (Saphris)	First line as mono or combo therapy	–	10–20	Available in sublingual film or transdermal patch.
	brexpiprazole (Rexulti)[1]	–	–	2–4	Compared to other SGAs, less risk for sedation, metabolic effects and EPS.
	cariprazine (Vraylar)	First line as mono or combo therapy	–	3–12[3]	Compared to other SGAs, less risk for sedation, metabolic effects, and EPS.
	clozapine (Clozaril)[1]	Third line	–	350–700†,[3]	Requires weekly or monthly laboratory studies with REMS due to agranulocytosis.
	lurasidone (Latuda)	–	First line	20–120	Lower risk of weight gain, must be taken with a meal.
	olanzapine (Zyprexa)	First line as mono or combo therapy	First line in combo with fluoxetine	10–20	High risk of weight gain and metabolic syndrome, consider starting metformin.
	paliperidone (Invega)[1]	–	–	6–12	Available as an LAI. No dose adjustment needed for hepatic impairment.
	quetiapine (Seroquel)	First line as mono or combo therapy	First line	100–800	Sedating, which can be helpful during acute mania. Can cause hypotension so titrate slowly.
	risperidone (Risperdal)	First line as mono or combo therapy	–	2–6	Available as a LAI. Can cause hyperprolactinemia.
	ziprasidone (Geodon)	First line as mono or combo therapy	–	80–160	Lower risk of weight gain, must be taken with a meal.

[1]Not FDA approved for this indication
[3]Exceeds dosage recommended by the manufacturer.
*Does not include dose adjustments for hepatic or renal impairment.
†Monitor using trough blood levels.
ACEIs, Angiotensin-converting enzyme inhibitors; *EPS*, extrapyramidal symptoms; *LAI*, long-acting injectable; *NSAIDs*, nonsteroidal antiinflammatory drugs; *REMS*, risk evaluation and mitigation strategy; *SGA*, second-generation antipsychotic; *SJS*, Stevens-Johnson syndrome.

in nonelderly adults, 0.6 to 1.0 mmol/L for maintenance in nonelderly adults and 0.4 to 0.8 mmol/L for elderly patients. Trough levels above 1.4 mmol/L are toxic, ranging in severity from mild to severe toxicity. Mild lithium toxicity symptoms are tremor, nausea, diarrhea, vomiting, abdominal pain, weakness and sedation, whereas moderate-to-severe toxicity can lead to delirium, coma, and renal failure. As shown in Table 6, medications can affect lithium levels; nonsteroidal antiinflammatory drugs (NSAIDs) and thiazide diuretics have the greatest potential to increase lithium concentrations. Lithium is excreted primarily through the kidneys; thus conditions

such as diarrhea, vomiting, or heavy sweating can also affect lithium levels, leading to toxicity. Patients and their families should be educated on the signs of lithium toxicity and encouraged to contact their provider during acute illnesses or medication changes to ensure their lithium is managed appropriately.

For acute mania, the treatment setting is generally inpatient because these patients often lack insight into their illness or into their need for treatment while also exhibiting impulsive involvement in activities that have a high potential for painful consequences (sexual indiscretions, substance use, driving recklessly). Medications contributing to mania or hypomania, such as

TABLE 6	Medication Effects on Lithium Levels
Medications That Increase Lithium Levels	
Thiazide diuretics	hydrochlorothiazide
	chlorthalidone
ACEIs	lisinopril
	enalapril
	ramipril
	benazepril
ARBs	losartan
	irbesartan
	olmesartan
	valsartan
NSAIDs	ibuprofen
	naproxen
	diclofenac
	indomethacin
	etodolac
	ketorolac
	fenoprofen
	ketoprofen
	nabumetone
	oxaprozin
	piroxicam
	meclofenamate
COX-2 inhibitor	celecoxib
Tetracyclines	doxycycline
	minocycline
	tetracycline
	demeclocycline
Antimicrobial	demeclocycline
Medications That Decrease Lithium Levels	
Methylxanthines	caffeine
	theophylline
Osmotic diuretics	mannitol
Carbonic anhydrase inhibitors	acetazolamide
	topiramate
	zonisamide
Diuretics, Antihypertensives, and Analgesics That Do Not Affect Lithium Levels	
Loop diuretics	furosemide
	bumetanide
Potassium-sparing diuretics	spironolactone
	amiloride
	triamterene
Calcium channel blockers	amlodipine
	diltiazem
	verapamil
	nifedipine
Central alpha agonists	clonidine
	guanfacine
Beta blockers	metoprolol
	atenolol
	propranolol
	labetalol
	nebivolol
	bisoprolol
	nadolol
Vasodilators	hydralazine
	isosorbide
	mononitrate
NSAIDs	sulindac
	aspirin
Other analgesics	acetaminophen
	tramadol
	opioids

ACEIs, Angiotensin-converting enzyme inhibitors; *ARBs,* angiotensin II receptor blockers; *COX-2,* cyclooxygenase-2; *NSAIDs,* nonsteroidal anti-inflammatory drugs.

antidepressants or stimulants, must be tapered and discontinued. Substance use should be addressed, including cannabis, which can cause or worsen psychosis. First-line treatment for mania or hypomania is lithium monotherapy or lithium combined with an SGA, valproic acid monotherapy or valproic acid combined with an SGA, or SGA monotherapy (see Table 5). Combination therapy is preferable if the patient has severe mania or psychosis, with *severe* being defined as requiring almost continual supervision to prevent harm to self or others. If the patient is already on a mood stabilizer, first optimize the dose before switching or adding medications. If symptoms are not controlled with first-line treatment, add another first-line medication such as lithium or valproic acid or add an SGA if not already prescribed. Other options for second-line treatment include change from one SGA to another or adding carbamazepine. A good indicator for treatment efficacy is total sleep time overnight, but measured objectively because the patient may feel subjectively that his or her sleep is adequate. Sleep aids can be helpful for severe mania but might not be necessary otherwise because mood stabilizers have sedating effects. For treatment-resistant mania or severe mania during pregnancy refer to a psychiatrist; ECT should be considered in these cases.

Bipolar depression is treated very differently than MDD in that antidepressant monotherapy should never be used, because of the risk of inducing a manic episode of mixed episode with both manic or hypomanic and depressive symptoms. It is especially more difficult to treat mixed episodes, and these patients are at an increased risk for suicide. Substance use should be addressed, including cannabis, which can cause or worsen psychosis. Just like in mania or hypomania, the first-line treatment is a mood stabilizer; if a patient is already on a mood stabilizer, it is important to optimize the dose before switching or adding other medications. There are fewer designated first-line options for bipolar depression, as seen in Table 5, and second-line treatment is very similar to that of mania or hypomania in that combination therapy with an SGA can be trialed. Sleep issues should be addressed more like sleep issues of MDD rather than that of mania or hypomania, with emphasis on sleep hygiene as opposed to prescription sleep aides. If a patient historically has only ever had mild intermittent manic symptoms and their mood stabilizer has been optimized, then an antidepressant can be trialed if necessary. Signs of manic switching should be observed closely; if switching is present, the antidepressant should be stopped immediately. For treatment-resistant bipolar depression, refer to a psychiatrist, who might then recommend ECT.

Bipolar disorders are highly recurrent; 90% of patients who experience a manic episode will go on to have recurrent mood episodes, and 50% of BDII patients will have a recurrent mood episode within the first year of their first mood episode. It is recommended that the medication regimen that achieved remission be continued. If a patient is on an antipsychotic as combination therapy with another mood stabilizer, decreasing or tapering off the antipsychotic can be considered after 6 months of remission.

Monitoring

Long-term antidepressant use is relatively safe and does not require regular monitoring of laboratory values unless adverse side effects (ASEs) are suspected. Some antidepressants are more or less prone to certain ASEs, as shown in Table 4, and these nuances might help guide your treatment decisions. The most common side effects (insomnia, lethargy, nausea, vomiting, diarrhea) improve with time and, if tolerable, patients should be asked to wait it out rather than switching medications. If stopped suddenly, tapered off too rapidly, or, for antidepressants with a very short half-life, if a single dose is skipped, patients may experience discontinuation syndrome with flulike symptoms, shocklike sensations, dizziness or vertigo, insomnia, irritability, crying spells, poor concentration, and vivid dreaming. When coprescribing or increasing the dose of serotonergic medications there is a risk of serotonin syndrome. SSRIs have an antiplatelet effect and therefore increased risk of bleeding. SSRIs and SNRIs have a risk of hyponatremia that is not dose related, and older patients are at an increased risk. Most antidepressants, with a few exceptions as described in Table 4, can have sexual adverse effects; however, SSRIs have the highest rates.

At initiation of lithium, laboratory studies to monitor include complete blood count (CBC) with differential, thyroid studies, kidney function, calcium, electrolytes, urinalysis, pregnancy test, weight, and fasting glucose. Thyroid studies, kidney function, calcium, and electrolytes should be monitored 3 months after initiation and then annually. Trough lithium levels should be obtained 5 days after initiation or any dose change and annually thereafter. Lithium's ASE are generally dose related and most commonly include GI upset, tremor (propranolol[1] can be helpful), polyuria, and polydipsia (or nephrogenic diabetes insipidus). Using the controlled-release formulation once daily at bedtime and using the lowest therapeutic dose can help with ASE. Long-term lithium use increases the risk of hypothyroidism.

When initiating valproic acid, baseline laboratory values include CBC, liver function tests (LFTs), and weight; these should be repeated after 6 months. Pregnancy status should also be considered because valproic acid can be teratogenic. Females of childbearing potential who take valproic acid should consider taking folic acid[1] supplementation. Trough valproic acid levels should be obtained 5 days after initiation or any dose change. Patients receiving ongoing valproic acid treatment should have at least annual (more often if clinically indicated) therapeutic drug monitoring and repeat of the baseline screening laboratory tests. The ASEs are also generally dose related and include GI upset, weight gain, tremor, hair loss, lethargy, hyperandrogenism in women, thrombocytopenia, and pancreatitis. Once-daily dosing of the controlled-release formulation is often better tolerated in clinical practice. Very rarely, valproic acid can cause fulminant hepatic failure.

When initiating carbamazepine, baseline laboratory tests include urea, electrolytes, CBC, LFTs and weight; these should be repeated after 6 months. Trough carbamazepine levels should be obtained 5 days and 1 month after initiation or any dose change; carbamazepine is a hepatic enzyme inducer that induces its own metabolism, as well as that of other medications reliant on CYP 3A4 for their metabolism. Patients receiving ongoing carbamazepine treatment should have at least annual (more often if clinically indicated) therapeutic drug monitoring and repeat of the baseline screening laboratory tests. The most common ASEs include dizziness, diplopia, drowsiness, ataxia, nausea, and headaches; starting at a low dose, increasing slowly and using a controlled-release formulation can be helpful. Dry mouth, edema, hyponatremia, sexual dysfunction, rash, neutropenia and raised alkaline phosphatase and γ-glutamyl transferase are also ASEs of carbamazepine, although less common than those ASEs listed earlier. When prescribing carbamazepine to individuals of Asian ancestry (those descending from the Han dynasty), human leukocyte antigen genetic testing should be completed before starting carbamazepine and to decrease the risk of serious skin reactions.

Baseline laboratory values for antipsychotic therapy are fasting blood glucose and fasting lipid profile; these should be repeated at 4 months and annually thereafter. Other baseline laboratory values, which can be repeated as clinically indicated, include CBC, LFTs, and an electrocardiogram (ECG). At the baseline assessment and at least once annually thereafter, patients should be screened for symptoms of hyperprolactinemia, which include decreased libido, galactorrhea, erectile dysfunction, or menstrual changes; in men this can lead to irreversible gynecomastia. SGAs commonly cause weight gain and metabolic syndrome, with a few exceptions as shown in Table 5. Generally, weight gain and metabolic syndrome can be mitigated with adjunctive metformin.[1] Although SGAs have a lower incidence of extrapyramidal symptoms (EPS) when compared with first-generation antipsychotics, these movement disorders should be screened for at baseline and annually thereafter (twice annually in adults over the age of 65). EPS

include acute dystonic reaction, parkinsonism, akathisia (subjective and objective restlessness), and tardive dyskinesia (involuntary athetoid or choreiform movements). Other ASEs of SGAs include sedation, orthostatic hypotension, and anticholinergic symptoms.

Complications

According to the Centers for Disease Control and Prevention and to the National Institute of Mental Health, suicide is a major public health concern and a leading cause of death in the United States. Suicide rates have been steadily climbing over the past several decades, with firearms used in more than half of suicides. Patients with MDD, BDI, or BDII are at increased risk of suicide. It is recommended to screen universally for suicide risk using the PHQ-9, as well as decrease access to lethal means (e.g., weapons, stockpiles of medication, etc.): for example, encouraging patients to keep firearms locked and separate from ammunition. Risk factors for suicide include prior suicide attempts, current psychiatric symptoms, substance use, recent biopsychosocial stressors, history of ACEs, and access to lethal means. Research shows that nearly half of patients who attempted suicide had also consumed alcohol at the time of the attempt. It can be helpful to ask patients what their protective factors are against suicide or what do they have to live for; this might be family, friends, pets, or religious beliefs. Individuals experiencing suicidal ideation or other mental health crisis can call or text the 988 Suicide and Crisis Lifeline, which is available 24 hours a day. The Lifeline provides confidential free support to anyone in suicidal crisis or emotional distress. All health systems and clinics should have emergency processes and contract procedures in place for patients to use, which can include presenting to the emergency department when in crisis.

References

American Psychiatric Association. Clinical Practice Guidelines. Available at https://www.psychiatry.org/guidelines. Accessed February 18, 2024.
Cafer J: *Cafer's psychopharmacology: visualize to memorize 270 medication mascots*, ed 1, CaferMed LLC, 2020.
Diagnostic and statistical manual of mental disorders, ed 5, Text Revision. Washington, DC, 2022, American Psychiatric Association, pp 139–214.
Macaluso M, Johnston C, editors: *Handbook of practical psychopharmacology*, ed 1, Washington, DC, 2024, American Psychiatric Association.
Macaluso M, Preskorn SH, editors: *Antidepressants: from biogenic amines to new mechanisms of action, first edition, volume 250 of handbook of experimental pharmacology*, Switzerland, 2019, Springer Nature Switzerland AG.
Malhi GS, Bell E, Bassett D, Boyce P, Bryant R, Hazell P, et al: The 2020 Royal Australian and New Zealand College of Psychiatrists clinical practice guidelines for mood disorders. *Aust N Z J Psychiatry*, 55(1), 7–117. Available at: https://doi.org/10.1177/0004867420979353.
Rush AJ, Fava M, Wisniewski SR, et al: Sequenced treatment alternatives to relieve depression (STAR*D): rationale and design, *Control Clin Trials* 25(1):119–142, 2004, https://doi.org/10.1016/s0197-2456(03)00112-0.
U.S. Department of Veterans Affairs: VA/DoD Clinical Practice Guidelines. Management of Bipolar Disorders (BD). Available at https://www.healthquality.va.gov/guidelines/mh/bd/index.asp, 2023. Accessed 18 February 2024.
U.S. Department of Veterans Affairs: VA/DoD Clinical Practice Guidelines, *Management of Major Depressive Disorder (MDD)*, 2022. Available at https://www.healthquality.va.gov/guidelines/MH/mdd/. Accessed 18 February 2024.
U.S. Department of Veterans Affairs: VA/DoD Clinical Practice Guidelines. Assessment and Management of Patients at Risk for Suicide. Available at https://www.healthquality.va.gov/guidelines/mh/srb/index.asp, 2019. Accessed 18 February 2024.

OBSESSIVE-COMPULSIVE DISORDER

Method of
Matthew Macaluso, DO; and Matthew Boyte, MD

CURRENT DIAGNOSIS

- Obsessive-compulsive disorder (OCD) is characterized by the presence of obsessions (intrusive, persistent, and unwanted thoughts or images) and/or compulsions (repeated acts that may or may not be performed to reduce the subjective distress that is typically caused by obsessions).

[1] Not FDA approved for this indication.
[1] Not FDA approved for this indication.

- The disorder may present with only obsessions or compulsions alone, but they are most often seen together.
- The diagnosis is made based on clinical presentation, and rating scales such as the Yale-Brown Obsessive Compulsive Scale (Y-BOCS) may be used to aid in diagnosis and monitor response to treatment.
- Comorbidity with other psychiatric disorders is common among patients with OCD, and the diagnosis of OCD is often missed.

CURRENT THERAPY

- Selective serotonin reuptake inhibitors (SSRIs) and psychotherapy are considered first-line treatments for obsessive-compulsive disorder (OCD). Other strongly serotonergic drugs have been studied as well.
- Much of the response to treatment may be seen within the first 6 weeks, although optimized treatment may need to be continued for more than 6 months to appreciate the full therapeutic benefit.
- Clomipramine (Anafranil) may be considered for patients who do not respond to first-line treatments.
- Augmentation with second-generation antipsychotics may be a good option for patients who have an incomplete response to first-line treatments. Evidence also suggests augmentation with first-generation antipsychotics may be useful for treatment of tics associated with OCD.

Epidemiology

Obsessive-compulsive disorder (OCD) is a mental disorder that the World Health Organization recognizes as being 1 of the 10 most disabling illnesses by measures of lost income and decreased quality of life. The disorder affects approximately 1% of the population worldwide each year and has a lifetime prevalence of 2% to 3%. Males and females are equally affected in adulthood, although boys are affected at a higher rate than girls during childhood. Onset occurs most frequently in either late childhood or early adulthood. Often the disorder is unrecognized or misdiagnosed. Treatment is, consequently, estimated to be delayed after nearly 8 years untreated on average. Furthermore, access to evidence-based psychotherapies for the disorder are limited.

Etiology

Genetic factors have been determined to contribute approximately one-half of the risk of the development of OCD. There are also brain regions or circuits that are clearly affected in patients with the disorder. Hyperactivity in the caudate, thalamus, anterior cingulate cortex, and orbitofrontal cortex have all been demonstrated. Activity in the brain circuit involving these and other associated areas is referred to as the cortico-striato-thalamo-cortical loop.

Although pharmacological treatments target neurotransmitter systems, the role of neurotransmitter dysregulation or brain chemistry balance in OCD development is unclear. The hypothesis that decreased serotonergic activity is responsible for OCD symptoms is purely based on response to serotonin reuptake inhibitors rather than clear evidence of decreased serotonergic activity as having a causal relationship. The roles of glutamate and other neurotransmitters are being investigated but likewise require further research to establish their specific contributions to the disorder.

There does seem to be an association between immune dysregulation and OCD, although it is unclear whether this is causative or has clinical relevance. The temporal relationship between immune response and the sometimes rapid development of OCD symptoms has primarily been described in the childhood disorders *pediatric acute onset neuropsychiatric syndrome* (PANS) and *pediatric autoimmune neuropsychiatric disorder associated with* Streptococcus (PANDAS). A similar association in adult populations has not been as widely accepted.

Presentation and Diagnosis

OCD is characterized by obsessions and/or compulsions that are time-consuming and cause significant impairment. Although the disorder may present with either obsessions or compulsions alone, they are most often seen together. Obsessions are intrusive, persistent, and unwanted thoughts or images that are distressing for patients to experience. They are considered egodystonic, meaning they do not align with the patient's values and self-image. Compulsions are repeated acts that are performed to reduce the subjective distress that is typically caused by obsessions. The rituals patients perform may be in the form of behaviors that can be witnessed by others, such as cleaning or ordering. Alternatively, they may occur as mental acts, such as counting or praying. Patients may also avoid situations that worsen their distress. Some of the more common obsessions and compulsions encountered in clinical practice are presented in Table 1.

The diagnosis is made on the basis of criteria presented in the *Diagnostic and Statistical Manual of Mental Disorders* (DSM-5-TR). In addition to the aforementioned presence of obsessions, compulsions, or both, which are time-consuming and impairing, the criteria stipulate the symptoms must not be caused by the effects of a substance of abuse or another medical condition. Further, the symptoms must not be better explained solely by another mental disorder. Despite the well-established role of genetic contributions in the development of OCD, there is not currently a role for genetic testing in establishing the diagnosis. This is the case for most other psychiatric disorders as well. There have not been any clearly identified genetic markers, and the risk of developing OCD is likely multifactorial.

The level of insight patients have into their illness is variable, and it should be specified. Patients with minimal or absent insight have a poorer prognosis. Similarly, the presence or absence of tics should be specified as it may help guide treatment. Specifically, tics may improve with adjunctive antipsychotic medications as discussed in more detail later.

The differential diagnosis for OCD may include mood disorders, anxiety disorders, personality disorders, and psychotic disorders. Patients often do not recognize their obsessive thoughts to be consistent with those seen in OCD. As a result, many will report depression or anxiety rather than obsessions. For this reason, it is important to consider some features that can be useful in distinguishing OCD from other disorders. Obsessions are usually more irrational than depressive ruminations or anxious thoughts. Patients with OCD also tend to maintain more insight

TABLE 1	Examples of Obsessions and Compulsions	
OBSESSIONS	**COMPULSIONS**
Contamination (most common)	Washing/cleaning
Sexual (inappropriateness or deviance)	Asking for reassurance or avoidance
Religious (eternal damnation)	Praying or asking for forgiveness
Aggression (intrusive violent images or fear of harming others)	Asking for reassurance
Pathologic doubt (uncertainty about performing tasks correctly)	Checking repeatedly
Superstition (overvaluing numbers or other qualities)	Avoiding unlucky values or counting behaviors
Symmetry/order	Ordering or arranging

Grant JE: Obsessive-compulsive disorder, *N Engl J Med* 371(7):646–653, 2014; Hirschtritt ME, Bloch MH, Mathews CA: Obsessive-compulsive disorder, *JAMA* 317(13):1358–1367, 2017.

and be more aware of the irrational quality of their thoughts than those with psychotic disorders. OCD may be differentiated from obsessive-compulsive personality disorder (OCPD), in part, by the nature of the patient's obsessive thought content. Those with OCPD often fixate on topics they find to be consistent with their own values and of particular interest to them. On the other hand, patients with OCD find their obsessive thoughts to be distressing and not aligned with their desires or beliefs. Comorbidity is common among patients with OCD, and they should be screened for other disorders including major depressive disorder (MDD), anxiety disorders, and attention-deficit/hyperactivity disorder.

Monitoring

OCD symptom severity, progression, or improvement may be measured by using one of several validated scales. The Yale-Brown Obsessive Compulsive Scale (Y-BOCS) is one of the most commonly used scales and is clinician administered. The Dimensional Obsessive-Compulsive Scale (DOCS) and Obsessive-Compulsive Inventory–Revised (OCI-R) are self-report scales that may also be helpful in identifying symptoms. Measurement-based care is important when treating any psychiatric disorder.

Treatment

First-line treatment for OCD includes selective serotonin reuptake inhibitors (SSRIs) and psychotherapy. Patients who do not respond fully to these interventions may benefit from either switching to the tricyclic antidepressant (TCA) clomipramine or augmenting with antipsychotics. The American Psychiatric Association guidelines suggest that two or more trials of different SSRIs may be considered before a clomipramine trial. Interventional treatments may also be considered for treatment-resistant cases. These strategies are discussed in more detail later.

Selective Serotonin Reuptake Inhibitors

Because of their efficacy and an adverse effect profile that is better than that of TCAs, SSRIs are considered the first-line medications for the treatment of OCD. Although fluoxetine (Prozac), fluvoxamine (Luvox), paroxetine (Paxil), and sertraline (Zoloft) are the FDA-approved SSRIs for OCD treatment, citalopram (Celexa) and escitalopram (Lexapro) appear to have similar efficacy based on clinical experience and limited data from randomized controlled trials. It should be noted that the risk of arrhythmia associated with citalopram and, to a lesser extent, escitalopram limits the use of higher doses, particularly in the elderly population or individuals who are CYP2C19 poor metabolizers. Suggested starting doses and target doses for treating OCD with SSRIs are presented in Table 2. The serotonin and norepinephrine reuptake inhibitors (SNRIs) duloxetine (Cymbalta) and venlafaxine (Effexor) have similarly shown good efficacy, albeit with a less robust evidence base.

Optimizing treatment at high doses of medication taken over a period of 6 to 12 months may be necessary for treatment response, although some studies suggest that most of the benefit will be seen after 6 weeks. In other words, OCD patients require higher doses of SSRIs and other serotonergic drugs than MDD patients. With optimized treatment, 60% to 70% of patients respond to monotherapy with SSRIs, and a minority of patients achieve full remission of symptoms. These outcomes are less than ideal for patients, in the opinion of the authors. Among patients who do respond, treatment should be continued for a minimum of 1 to 2 years before considering a gradual taper of the medication. The risks and benefits of a proposed taper must be discussed with the patient.

Clomipramine

The TCA clomipramine may have a larger effect size for treatment of OCD than SSRIs, but this has not been demonstrated in head-to-head trials. The higher adverse effect burden of clomipramine, including xerostomia, headache, constipation, and sexual adverse effects, in addition to the necessity of serum

TABLE 2 Dosing Recommendations

MEDICATION	STARTING DOSE (MG/DAY)	TARGET DOSE (MG/DAY)
Fluoxetine (Prozac)	20	40–80
Fluvoxamine (Luvox)	50	200–300
Sertraline (Zoloft)	50	100–200
Paroxetine (Paxil)	20	40–60
Citalopram (Celexa)	20	40
Escitalopram (Lexapro)	10	20–40
Clomipramine (Anafranil)	25	150–250

Data from Del Casale A, Sorice S, Padovano A, et al: Psychopharmacological treatment of obsessive-compulsive disorder (OCD), *Curr Neuropharmacol* 17(8):710–736, 2019; Grant JE: Obsessive-compulsive disorder, *N Engl J Med* 371(7):646–653, 2014.

level monitoring in the higher dose range, are among the reasons SSRIs are preferred. Even so, patients who do not respond to SSRIs may reasonably be considered for a trial of clomipramine (see Table 2 for dosing recommendations).

Antipsychotics

Patients who have incomplete response to monotherapy from an SSRI may benefit from augmentation with a second-generation antipsychotic. The evidence for augmentation with either risperidone or aripiprazole is the strongest, although other antipsychotics may also be effective. First-generation antipsychotics, such as haloperidol, have evidence supporting use in Tourette disorder as well. This strategy may be particularly helpful for patients who have tics, and higher-potency dopamine D2 receptor antagonists should be considered for this subset of patients. Of note, antipsychotics are associated with a higher adverse effect burden, including long-term risks of metabolic syndrome and tardive dyskinesia. For this reason, psychotherapy should be considered as an addition to first-line medications before augmenting with antipsychotics.

Benzodiazepines

Benzodiazepines have limited efficacy for the treatment of OCD symptoms and carry the risk of dependence in addition to significant adverse effects. Benzodiazepines can also cause disinhibition in some patients. For these reasons, it is recommended that benzodiazepine use be time-limited for patients experiencing high levels of distress associated with their OCD symptoms. Patients should be counseled on the risks and recommendation for a short duration of treatment when benzodiazepines are prescribed.

Psychotherapy

Psychotherapy should be considered for all patients who are diagnosed with OCD. Exposure and response prevention (ERP) and cognitive therapy are two types of cognitive-behavioral therapy (CBT) that are the primary evidence-based psychotherapies for OCD. ERP consists of repeated exposures to stimuli that cause distress related to the patient's obsessions. The patient is asked not to engage in the compulsive behaviors associated with the obsessions or not to focus on obsessive thoughts. Over time, the patient should see that the stimuli are not as threatening as they initially perceived. Cognitive therapy involves challenging cognitive distortions. Examples of cognitive distortions often seen in OCD patients include overimportance of thoughts, overestimation of threat, overestimation of responsibility, intolerance of uncertainty, and perfectionism. Access to therapists who provide these manualized and evidence-based therapies is often insufficient, and computer-based therapy sessions may be considered as a way to improve access to patients who are unable to participate in person.

Other Treatments

Interventional treatment strategies may be considered in patients for whom first- and second-line treatments are ineffective. Deep brain stimulation (DBS), transcranial magnetic stimulation (TMS), and ablative surgery have all been shown to have efficacy in reducing symptom burden. DBS and ablative surgeries target structures in the cortico-striato-thalamo-cortical loop and should only be considered in severe cases because of their invasive nature. DBS requires the placement of electrodes into brain structures associated in OCD, whereas TMS uses a magnetic field to influence neuronal activity in these regions. These treatments require referral to specialized centers led by experts.

References

American Psychiatric Association: *DSM-5 task force: diagnostic and statistical manual of mental disorders: DSM-5*, ed 5, Washington, DC, 2013, American Psychiatric Association.

Bandelow Borwin, et al: World Federation of Societies of Biological Psychiatry (WFSBP) guidelines for treatment of anxiety, obsessive-compulsive and posttraumatic stress disorders – version 3. part I: anxiety disorders, *World J Biol Psychiatry* 24(2):79–117, 2022, https://doi.org/10.1080/15622975.2022.2086295.

Del Casale Antonio, et al: Psychopharmacological treatment of obsessive-compulsive disorder (OCD), *Curr Neuropharmacol* 17(8):710–736, 2019, https://doi.org/10.2174/1570159x16666180813155017.

Grant Jon E: Obsessive–compulsive disorder, *N Engl J Med* 371(7):646–653, 2014, https://doi.org/10.1056/nejmcp1402176.

Hirschtritt Matthew E, et al: Obsessive-compulsive disorder, *JAMA* 317(13):1358–1367, 2017, https://doi.org/10.1001/jama.2017.2200.

Katzman Martin A, et al: Canadian clinical practice guidelines for the management of anxiety, posttraumatic stress and obsessive-compulsive disorders, *BMC Psychiatry* 14(Suppl 1), 2014, https://doi.org/10.1186/1471-244x-14-s1-s1.

Pittenger Christopher, et al: Specialty knowledge and competency standards for pharmacotherapy for adult obsessive-compulsive disorder, *Psychiatry Res* 300:113853, 2021, https://doi.org/10.1016/j.psychres.2021.113853.

PANIC DISORDER

Method of
Cheryl Wehler, MD

CURRENT DIAGNOSIS

- Panic disorder (PD) is characterized by the presence of multiple untriggered panic attacks.
- These unexpected panic attacks are associated with significant anticipatory anxiety and/or changes in behavior to minimize the consequences or avoid another panic attack.
  - Patients worry about being negatively judged due to visible panic symptoms.
  - Patients worry about dying or "going crazy."
- The panic attacks are not attributable to another medical condition or to the effects of a substance (medication or drug of abuse).
- The panic attacks are not better explained by another mental disorder.
- Patients frequently present with concern about somatic symptoms (e.g., fear of heart attack because of shortness of breath and chest discomfort).
- Assess patients for suicidality, as suicide risk increases with panic attacks or recent diagnosis of panic disorder.

CURRENT THERAPY

- Pharmacology and psychotherapy are effective treatments for PD.
- Selective serotonin reuptake inhibitors (SSRIs), serotonin norepinephrine reuptake inhibitors (SNRIs), tricyclic antidepressants (TCAs), and benzodiazepines have demonstrated efficacy for the treatment of PD.

- The favorable safety profile of SSRIs and SNRIs make them first-line monotherapy agents.
- Although TCAs are effective, their side effects and greater toxicity in overdose limit their clinical utility.
- Monoamine oxidase inhibitors (MAOIs) also appear effective but are reserved for patients who are nonresponders to multiple first-line treatments because of their safety profile limitations.
- Benzodiazepines are not first-line monotherapy but are useful adjuncts to antidepressants if residual anxiety requires additional treatment.
- Although the more rapid response of benzodiazepines (compared with SSRIs/SNRIs) make them attractive, the inevitable physiological dependence make them less so.
- Patients with PD can be sensitive to medication side effects; therefore the adage "start low and go slow" is applicable to dosing.
- Cognitive behavioral therapy (CBT) or CBT with medications are first-line treatments for children and adults with PD.

Epidemiology

The 12-month prevalence estimate for panic disorder (PD) in the general population of the United States and Europe is approximately 2% to 3% in adults and adolescents. Non-Latino Caucasians and Native Americans have significantly higher rates than Latinos, African Americans, and Asian Americans. Adolescent and adult females are approximately twice as likely as males to be affected (although the clinical features of PD do not differ between males and females). The prevalence is highest in adult females. Prevalence rates decline in older individuals. The overall prevalence of PD is low in children (<14 years). PD is associated with the highest number of medical visits among all anxiety disorders.

Risk Factors

Risks factors for PD include a disposition to negativity, experience of childhood physical and sexual abuse, and family history, indicating genetic vulnerability. Respiratory disorders such as asthma are associated with panic disorder. Smoking is a risk factor for panic attacks and PD. PD is associated with social and occupational/physical disability and high economic cost. PD may be comorbid with a variety of other psychiatric diagnoses, such as depression, bipolar affective disorder, and other anxiety disorders.

Diagnosis

PD is defined by the *Diagnostic and Statistical Manual of Mental Disorders*, fifth edition (DSM-V) as recurrent unexpected panic attacks followed by at least 1 month of anticipatory anxiety about having another attack, and a significant change in behavior to avoid another panic attack. A panic attack, the core feature of panic disorder, is an abrupt surge of intense fear/anxiety with concurrent physical and cognitive symptoms (Box 1). To be diagnosed as having PD, a patient must have more than one panic attack that is not the result of an obvious trigger or cue. The best example might be a nocturnal panic attack in which the individual is waking from sleep, with no external cues, in a state of intense fear (panic) and experiencing physical and cognitive symptoms. Expected panic attacks, that is, those for which there is an obvious cue or trigger, also occur in patients with PD. In the United States and Europe, approximately half of individuals with PD experience expected panic attacks as well as unexpected panic attacks. The presence of expected panic attacks does not rule out the diagnosis but is insufficient to make the diagnosis of this disorder.

A thorough diagnostic evaluation, including a complete history and thorough physical examination, is necessary to rule out medical or substance-induced panic attacks and establish the diagnosis of PD. Atypical symptoms or features of a panic attack may be suggestive of a medical illness or pharmacologic substance as the precipitant. A workup that includes laboratory

BOX 1 DSM-5 Criteria for Panic Disorder

- Recurrent unexpected panic attacks. A panic attack is an abrupt surge of intense fear or intense discomfort that reaches a peak within minutes, and during which time four (or more) of the following symptoms occur:
  Note: The abrupt surge can occur from a calm state or an anxious state.
  - Palpitations, pounding heart, or accelerated heart rate
  - Sweating
  - Trembling or shaking
  - Sensations of shortness of breath or smothering
  - Feelings of choking
  - Chest pain or discomfort
  - Nausea or abdominal distress
  - Feeling dizzy, light-headed, faint, or unsteady
  - Chills or heat sensations
  - Parenthesis (numbness or tingling sensations)
  - Depersonalization (being detached from oneself) or derealization (feelings of unreality)
  - Fear of "going crazy" or losing control
  - Fear of dying
  Note: Culture-specific symptoms (e.g., tinnitus, neck soreness, headache, uncontrollable screaming or crying) may be seen. Such symptoms should not count as one of the four required symptoms [to diagnose PD].
- At least one of the attacks has been followed by 1 month (or more) of one or both of the following:
  - Persistent concern or worry about additional panic attacks or their consequences (e.g., losing control, having a heart attack, "going crazy")
  - A significant maladaptive change in behavior related to the attacks (e.g., behaviors designed to avoid having panic attacks, such as avoidance of exercise or unfamiliar situations)
- The disturbance is not attributable to the physiological effects of a substance (e.g., a drug of abuse, a medication) or another medical condition (e.g., hyperthyroidism, cardiopulmonary disorders)
- The disturbance is not better explained by another mental disorder (e.g., the panic attacks do not occur only in response to feared social situations, as in social anxiety disorder; in response to circumscribed phobic objects or situations, as in specific phobia; in response to obsessions, as in obsessive-compulsive disorder; in response to reminders of traumatic events, as in posttraumatic stress disorder; or in response to separation from attachment figures, as in separation anxiety disorder)

tests such as complete blood cell count, complete chemistry panel (including calcium level), thyroid-stimulating hormone (TSH) level, and urine drug screen may be helpful in determining a medical or substance-related cause. These tests may be followed by a chest radiograph, an electrocardiogram, and cardiac enzymes, as warranted. If the clinical examination or history is suggestive, a Holter monitor, EEG, CT scan, or urine catecholamine assay may be performed.

Clinical Manifestations

In the United States, the median age of onset for PD is 20 to 24 years. PD is rare in childhood but occurs in adolescents; their symptoms are similar to those in adults. Onset after age 45 is unusual. If untreated, the usual course is chronic, and attacks may wax and wane. Some individuals have a chronic course complicated by frequent attacks whereas others have rare episodic symptoms. A minority of individuals have full remission. Caffeine and several other substances can provoke a panic attack.

The severity and frequency of panic attacks vary widely. Individuals who have infrequent panic attacks resemble individuals with more frequent panic attacks with regard to symptoms, demographics, and family history. To be diagnosed with PD, an individual must have more than one full-symptom attack with more than four of the symptoms listed in Box 1. Individuals may, however, have limited-symptom attacks with fewer than four symptoms.

There are three symptomatic facets of PD: acute panic, anticipatory anxiety, and phobic avoidance. Phobic avoidance often includes restricting daily activities to minimize or avoid panic attacks. Panic disorder is associated with other psychopathology, such as other anxiety disorders, particularly agoraphobia.

Although medical illness can precipitate a panic attack, individuals with anxiety, particularly PD, may be hypervigilant and misinterpret mild physical symptoms as harbingers of a catastrophic or fatal illness. Individuals with PD often report feelings of anxiety that are associated with health or mental health concerns.

Panic attacks often contribute to the presentation of other psychiatric illnesses, such as other anxiety disorders and major depression. A thorough history that documents the onset of symptoms, possible triggers, and context of symptoms is critical to establishing the diagnosis of PD. In addition to the history of the present illness and current symptoms, a psychiatric review of symptoms, past psychiatric history, general medical history and current medications, substance use history, family history, and mental status exam are valuable in constructing a psychiatric differential diagnosis and then a final working diagnosis. For instance, an individual with a history of a past trauma presenting with flashbacks, nightmares, and triggered panic attacks may have posttraumatic stress disorder (versus panic disorder).

Suicidal behavior in individuals with anxiety disorders has long been attributed to co-occurring risk factors, such as depression. New research suggests that an anxiety disorder is associated with suicidal ideation and suicide attempts beyond the effects of co-occurring mental disorders. Panic attacks and a recent diagnosis of PD are associated with a higher rate of suicide attempts and suicidal ideation.

Differential Diagnosis

The differential diagnosis of PD is wide ranging (Table 1). PD is not diagnosed if panic attacks are the direct physiological consequence of another medical condition or substance. Medical conditions that can cause panic attacks include cardiopulmonary conditions such as arrhythmias and asthma or chronic obstructive pulmonary disease (COPD). Endocrine and neurologic disorders such as hyperthyroidism, pheochromocytoma, vestibular dysfunction, and seizures may also cause panic attacks. In addition, central nervous system (CNS) stimulants and withdrawal from CNS depressants may precipitate a panic attack. On the other hand, a panic attack may mimic a wide variety of medical disorders.

Treatment

PD is a common mental disorder. It is associated with social and occupational/physical disability and high economic cost. When symptoms cause significant distress or interfere with functioning, treatment is warranted. Regardless of the modality chosen, the goal of treatment is a reduction in the frequency and severity of panic attacks as well as the resultant anticipatory anxiety and avoidance behaviors.

Research has confirmed the efficacy of multiple psychosocial and pharmacologic interventions in treating PD. Choice of treatment depends on multiple factors, including patient preference; risks and benefits for an individual patient; cost; past treatment history; and co-occurring medical, psychiatric, or substance abuse issues.

Selective serotonin reuptake inhibitors (SSRIs), serotonin norepinephrine reuptake inhibitors (SNRIs), tricyclic antidepressants (TCAs), and benzodiazepines have demonstrated efficacy for the treatment of PD. The favorable safety profile of SSRIs and SNRIs makes them first-line monotherapy agents. Although TCAs are effective, their side effects and toxicity in overdose limit their clinical utility. Monoamine oxidase

TABLE 1	Differential Diagnosis of Panic Attacks
SYSTEM	**POSSIBLE DIAGNOSES**
Psychiatric	Mood disorder (panic attacks associated with depression or bipolar disorder)
	Anxiety disorders (panic attacks associated with social anxiety, specific phobia, posttraumatic stress disorder, generalized anxiety disorder, obsessive compulsive disorder)
	Agoraphobia
	Psychotic disorder (panic attacks associated with psychosis)
	Somatoform disorder
	Factitious disorder
Cardiac	Myocardial infarction
	Angina
	SVT or other arrhythmia
	Mitral valve prolapse
	Labile hypertension
Respiratory	Asthma
	COPD
	Pulmonary embolus
Neurologic	Seizure disorder
	Vestibular dysfunction
Endocrine	Thyroid disorder
	Hypoglycemia
	Adrenal dysfunction
	Hyperparathyroidism
	Pheochromocytoma
Substance	Excess caffeine
Use	Psychostimulants
Substance	Caffeine
Withdrawal	Nicotine
	Alcohol or sedative
	Opioid

TABLE 2	Pharmacologic Treatments of Panic Disorder		
MEDICATION (TRADE NAME)	**INITIAL DOSE (MG/DAY)**	**DOSE RANGE (MG/DAY)**	
SSRIs			
Citalopram (Celexa)[1]	10–20	20–40	
Escitalopram (Lexapro)[1]	5–10	10–20	
Fluoxetine (Prozac)	10–20	20–80	
Fluvoxamine (Luvox)[1]	50	100–300[†]	
Fluvoxamine CR (Luvox CR)[1]	100	100–300	
Paroxetine (Paxil)	10–20	20–60	
Paroxetine CR (Paxil CR)	12.5–25	25–75	
Sertraline (Zoloft)	25	50–200	
SNRIs			
Duloxetine (Cymbalta)[1]	30	60–120	
Venlafaxine (Effexor)[1]	25–50	150–225	
Venlafaxine ER (Effexor ER)	37.5	75–225	
TCAs			
Desipramine (Norpramin)	25–50	100–200	
Clomipramine (Anafranil)[1]	25	50–150	
Imipramine (Tofranil)[1]	25	50–150	
Nortriptyline (Pamelor)[1]	10–25	75–150	
MAOIs			
Phenelzine* (Nardil)[1]	45[†]	45-75[§]	
Benzodiazepines			
Alprazolam (Xanax)	0.25–0.5 tid	5–6	
Alprazolam XR (Xanax XR)	0.5–1	3–6	
Lorazepam (Ativan)[1]	0.25 tid	2–8[‡]	
Clonazepam (Klonopin)	0.25 bid	0.5–2[†]	

[1]Not FDA approved for this indication.
*Dietary restrictions required (low-tyramine diet); 2-week washout required before initiation and after termination of monoamine oxidase inhibitor (MAOI) trial.
[†]Divided doses may be given.
[‡]Total daily dosage divided across 2–4 doses/day.
[§]Usually administered tid.

inhibitors (MAOIs) also appear effective but are reserved for patients who are nonresponders to multiple first-line treatments because of their safety profile. Benzodiazepines are not first-line monotherapy but are useful adjuncts to antidepressants if residual anxiety requires additional treatment (Table 2).

An important consideration when using psychopharmacologic treatments in PD is the side-effect profile of a particular agent. Because patients with PD can be acutely sensitive to medication side effects, it is prudent to start medications at low doses and gradually increase them to therapeutic doses as tolerated. An effective dose is patient dependent—the goal is to prevent (versus respond to) panic attacks. If a decision is made to discontinue a SSRI, SNRI, or TCA, the medication should be gradually tapered when feasible.

Cognitive behavioral therapy (CBT) and CBT with medications are first-line treatments for children and adults with PD. CBT presents the most evidence of efficacy from random control trials. CBT for panic disorder generally includes psychoeducation, episode monitoring and response, self-awareness of anxious automatic thoughts and beliefs, controlled exposure to fear cues, modification of anxiety-reducing behaviors, and prevention of relapse. Psychosocial interventions, such as CBT, may enhance long-term outcomes by reducing the likelihood of relapse.

References

American Psychiatric Association: *Diagnostic and Statistical Manual of Mental Disorders*, ed 5, Arlington, VA, 2013, American Psychiatric Association.
American Psychiatric Association: *Practice Guideline for the Treatment of Patients with Panic Disorder*, ed 2, Arlington, VA, 2010, American Psychiatric Association.
Craske MG, Kircanski K, Epstein A, et al: Panic disorder: A review of DSM-IV panic disorder and proposals for DSM-V, *Depress Anxiety* 27:93–112, 2010.
Thibodeau MA, Welch PG, Sareen J, Asmundson GJG: Anxiety disorders are independently associated with suicide ideation and attempts: Propensity score matching in two epidemiological samples, *Depress Anxiety* 30:947–954, 2013.
Locke AB, Kirst N, Shultz CG: Diagnosis and management of generalized anxiety disorder and panic disorder in adults, *Am Fam Physician* 91(9):617–624, 2015.
Marchesi C: Pharmacological management of panic disorder, *Neuropsychiatr Dis Treat* 4:93–106, 2008.
Milrod B, Chambless DL, Gallop R, et al: Psychotherapies for panic disorder: a tale of two sites, *J Clin Psychiatry* 9, 2015, Jun (Epub ahead of print).
Stahl SM: *Stahl's Essential Psychopharmacology: The Prescriber's Guide*, ed 5, New York, 2014, Cambridge University Press.
Andrisano C, Chiesa A, Serretti A: Newer antidepressants and panic disorder: A meta-analysis, *Int Clin Psychopharmacol* 28:33–45, 2013.

POSTTRAUMATIC STRESS DISORDER

Method of
Natalie C. Dattilo, PhD

CURRENT DIAGNOSIS

- Posttraumatic stress disorder (PTSD) is quickly becoming one of the most common psychiatric disorders seen in the primary care setting.
- PTSD is diagnosed after a person experiences symptoms for at least 1 month following a traumatic event. However, symptoms may not appear until several months or even years later and can persist as a chronic condition.
- The disorder is characterized by three main types of symptoms: (1) reexperiencing the trauma through distressing recollections, (2) emotional numbness and behavioral avoidance, and (3) increased arousal such as feeling jumpy and easily angered.
- A thorough medical examination and laboratory workup may be indicated to rule out contributing physiologic factors and comorbidities, substance use or misuse, and drug or alcohol withdrawal.
- Symptoms that are persistent, disruptive, or distressing warrant treatment.
- The PTSD Checklist-5 (PCL-5) is a 20-item self-report measure that assesses the 20 *Diagnostic and Statistical Manual of Mental Disorders,* Fifth Edition (DSM-5) symptoms of PTSD. The gold standard for diagnosing PTSD is a structured clinical interview such as the Clinician-Administered PTSD Scale (CAPS-5). When necessary, the PCL-5 can be scored to provide a provisional PTSD diagnosis.

CURRENT THERAPY

- Effective treatments for PTSD include serotonergic antidepressants, certain forms of trauma-based psychotherapy, or a combination of both.
- Educating the patient and family members about treatment options and setting realistic treatment expectations are critical.
- Depending on the patient's preference, treatment may include a selective serotonin reuptake inhibitor (SSRI) starting at low doses with careful titration so as not to exacerbate anxiety or agitation.
- Treatment may also include a trial of cognitive-behavioral therapy, cognitive processing therapy, or prolonged exposure therapy to boost response rates and prevent relapse.
- Refer to or consult with a psychiatrist for patients with severe or particularly complex cases or for patients with a less-than-expected response to treatment.
- Refer to a cognitive-behavioral therapy specialist for patients with a preference for behavioral, skills-based, or nonmedication therapy or for whom pharmacotherapy may be contraindicated.

Epidemiology

In the United States, it is estimated that PTSD is diagnosed in approximately 10.5 million adults (3.5%) each year, and approximately 20.4 million (6.8%) will meet criteria over the course of their lifetimes. The lifetime prevalence of PTSD among men is 3.6% and among women is 9.7%. The 12-month prevalence is 1.8% among men and 5.2% among women. As with depression and anxiety disorders, patients with PTSD are more likely to present initially to a general practitioner's office than to a mental health care provider.

Owing, in part, to increased public awareness, PTSD is quickly becoming one of the most frequently seen clinical problems in primary care. Symptoms frequently overlap with other complaints, such as insomnia, irritability, or pain. Most behavioral symptoms of PTSD are a result of anxiety and hypervigilance, and the clinical presentation shares many phenotypic similarities with other anxiety disorders, such as panic disorder (PD) and generalized anxiety disorder (GAD).

Risk Factors

Risk factors associated with PTSD include exposure to trauma, being female, having lower levels of education and income, being divorced or widowed, having a history of behavioral or psychological problems, family history of behavioral or psychological problems including substance abuse, recent increase in stressful life events, lack or perceived lack of social support, ineffective emotional coping strategies, experiencing childhood adversity or trauma, having a chronic health condition or serious illness, having an acute or chronic pain condition, and substance abuse. Although a genetic predisposition to developing PTSD is likely, environmental stress and early trauma clearly play a role.

Pathophysiology

Our current understanding of PTSD is incomplete; however, several neurobiologic systems have been implicated in the pathophysiology and vulnerability toward developing PTSD after trauma exposure. As in other anxiety disorders, PTSD symptoms are believed to be due to dysregulation of neuronal activity within the central nervous system (CNS), in particular the fear circuit. This dysregulation causes a state of hyperarousal, which gives rise to the physical and emotional manifestations of the condition. Several neurotransmitter systems have been implicated in the genesis of this hyperaroused state. Overstimulation of the CNS and the autonomic sympathetic activity it generates affect the prefrontal cortex and the limbic system (e.g., amygdala, hypothalamus), both of which play an important role in our ability to discern stimuli as aversive or threatening and regulate our stress response.

The two most commonly implicated neurotransmitter systems to date include the serotoninergic and noradrenergic neurotransmitter systems. Very simply, it is believed that an underactivation of the serotoninergic system and an overactivation of the noradrenergic system are involved. These systems interact with other neuronal circuits in various regions of the brain, including the locus ceruleus (LC) and the limbic structures, resulting in a dysregulation of physiologic arousal and the emotional interpretation of this arousal, respectively. Disruption of the γ-aminobutyric acid (GABA) system has also been implicated because of the response of many of the anxiety-spectrum disorders to treatment with benzodiazepines.

There has also been some interest in the role of corticosteroid regulation and its relation to symptoms of fear and anxiety. Corticosteroids might increase or decrease the activity of certain neural pathways, affecting not only an individual's behavior under stress but also how the brain perceives and processes threatening stimuli. The stress response is hardwired into the brain and is most often triggered when survival of the organism is threatened. The stress response, however, can be triggered not only by a physical challenge or threat but also by the mere anticipation (or fear) of threat. As a result, when humans chronically and erroneously believe that a threatening event is about to occur, they begin to experience the physical and psychological symptoms of anxiety and panic.

The hypothalamic–pituitary–adrenal (HPA) axis is another neurocircuit implicated in the initiation of a stress response. The HPA axis assists with the adaptation to stress and the maintenance of homeostasis after challenge. It connects the CNS and the endocrine system, and a dysfunctional HPA axis is associated with numerous psychosomatic and psychiatric disorders. Corticotropin-releasing factor (CRF) is a molecule produced by cells in the hypothalamus in response to physical or psychological stress. Increased levels of CRF in the hypothalamus in response to stress results in the activation of the HPA axis and increased release of cortisol. It is believed that high CRF levels at the time of trauma may facilitate encoding of traumatic memory and enduring anxiety effects. Patients with PTSD exhibit increased cerebrospinal fluid levels of CRF and other abnormalities in the HPA axis system.

Finally, a subcortical neural structure, the amygdala, serves an important role in coordinating the cognitive, affective, neuroendocrine, cardiovascular, respiratory, and musculoskeletal components of fear and anxiety responses. It is central to registering the emotional significance of stressful stimuli and creating emotional memories. The amygdala receives input from neurons in the sensory cortex. When activated, the amygdala stimulates regions of the midbrain and brainstem, causing autonomic hyperactivity, which can be correlated with the physical symptoms of anxiety.

Prevention

No biological markers are specific enough yet to detect which individuals are more likely to develop PTSD after experiencing a trauma, and there is no available evidence to suggest that current medications prove efficacious in preventing this disorder. Therefore it is important to screen for specific risk factors, such as exposure to trauma (either recent or remote), family history of mental health issues, recent increase in stressful life events, or substance abuse. If a person is found to be at risk, but not symptomatic, he or she should first be encouraged to adopt healthy lifestyle habits. Aerobic exercise and other forms of physical activity have been shown to relieve stress and anxiety and improve mood relatively quickly. These patients should also be encouraged to avoid stimulants such as caffeine and nicotine, which can exacerbate symptoms and contribute to insomnia. It is also highly recommended that anxiety-prone persons manage stress by learning effective methods of behavioral relaxation, applied meditation, and other healthy stress reduction techniques.

Clinical Manifestations

PTSD can manifest in many ways. Behavioral signs may include increased alcohol consumption, change in communication, change in sexual functioning, emotional outbursts, inability to rest or relax, change in appetite, pacing, suspiciousness, self-destructive behavior, or social isolation. Cognitive signs may include changes in alertness, confusion, hypervigilance, memory problems, poor attention and concentration, poor decision making or problem solving, and suicidal ideation. Emotional signs may include agitation, anxiety, apprehension, depression, fear, feeling overwhelmed, grief, guilt, irritability, and loss of emotional control. Sleep is also affected for individuals suffering from PTSD, and they will often report insomnia or nightmares. Other common features include a sense of emotional detachment from others and unwanted or intrusive thoughts; however, these can be difficult for clinicians to identify and patients rarely self-report. Physical symptoms can include chills, difficulty breathing, dizziness, elevated blood pressure, fainting, fatigue, grinding teeth, headaches, muscle tremors, nausea, pain, profuse sweating, rapid heart rate, twitches, and weakness. These symptoms cause significant distress and impairment of function.

Diagnosis

A diagnosis of PTSD is made when the patient meets specific diagnostic criteria as outlined in the DSM-5. In previous versions of the DSM, PTSD was categorized as an anxiety disorder. The diagnosis of PTSD now falls under its own category of mental disorders, called "Trauma and Stressor-Related Disorders," owing to the myriad ways it can present clinically.

PTSD may develop after a person experiences, witnesses, or confronts a physically or psychologically traumatic event. The event may involve actual or threatened death, serious or life-threatening injury or threat of severe injury, or sexual violence or threat of sexual violence. An individual may directly experience the traumatic event; witness, in person, the traumatic event; or learn that the traumatic event occurred to a close family member or close friend. An individual may also develop PTSD after experiencing repeated or extreme exposure to aversive details of the traumatic events. Examples may be first responders collecting human remains or police officers repeatedly exposed to details of child abuse. Note: This does not apply to exposure through electronic media, television, movies, or pictures, unless exposure is work related.

The disorder is characterized by three main types of symptoms: (1) reexperiencing the trauma through distressing recollections, (2) emotional numbness and behavioral avoidance, and (3) increased arousal such as feeling jumpy and easily angered.

A diagnosis of PTSD can be made in adults, adolescents, and children over the age of 6 when one or more of the following reexperiencing symptoms are present:

- Spontaneous or cued recurrent, involuntary, and intrusive distressing memories of the traumatic events (Note: In children repetitive play may occur in which themes or aspects of the traumatic events are expressed.)
- Recurrent distressing dreams in which the content or affect (i.e., feeling) of the dream is related to the events (Note: In children there may be frightening dreams without recognizable content.)
- Flashbacks or other dissociative reactions in which the individual feels or acts as if the traumatic event is recurring (Note: In children trauma-specific reenactment may occur in play.)
- Intense or prolonged psychological distress at exposure to internal or external cues that symbolize or resemble an aspect of the traumatic events
- Physiologic reactions to reminders of the traumatic events

A diagnosis of PTSD can be made in adults, adolescents, and children over the age of 6 when two or more of the following emotional numbness or behavioral avoidance symptoms are also present:

- Inability to remember an important aspect of the traumatic events (not due to head injury, alcohol, or drugs)
- Persistent and exaggerated negative beliefs or expectations about oneself, others, or the world (e.g., "I am bad," "No one can be trusted," "The world is completely dangerous")
- Persistent, distorted blame of self or others about the cause or consequences of the traumatic events
- Persistent fear, horror, anger, guilt, or shame
- Markedly diminished interest or participation in significant activities
- Feelings of detachment or estrangement from others
- Persistent inability to experience positive emotions

In addition to reexperiencing and avoidance, a diagnosis of PTSD can be made in adults, adolescents, and children over the age of 6 when two or more of the following marked changes in arousal and reactivity are also present:

- Irritable or aggressive behavior
- Reckless or self-destructive behavior
- Hypervigilance
- Exaggerated startle response
- Problems with concentration
- Difficulty falling or staying asleep or restless sleep

Finally, the diagnosis is made if the symptoms have been present for at least 1 month and cause clinically significant distress or impairment in functioning.

Differential Diagnosis

It is important to perform a thorough medical workup when initially assessing the patient with PTSD symptoms. Differential diagnoses can include several organic causes, such as endocrine dysfunction, intoxication or withdrawal, hypoxia, metabolic abnormalities, and neurologic disorders. It is also important to consider and rule out any cooccurring psychiatric disorders. Major depression with or without suicidality, bipolar disorder, panic disorder, delusional disorder, polysubstance dependence, and adjustment disorder can often accompany PTSD, in addition to relationship problems and difficulty at work or in social situations.

It is not uncommon for patients with PTSD to report chronic pain or present with "ill defined" or "medically unexplained" somatic symptoms such as headaches, dizziness, tinnitus, and blurry vision or medical issues including diabetes, obesity, and cardiovascular, respiratory, musculoskeletal, neurologic, or gastrointestinal problems. Frequently reported medical comorbidities with PTSD across various studies include cardiovascular disease, especially hypertension, and immune-mediated disorders. Because PTSD is associated with limbic dysfunction and alterations in the HPA axis, neuroendocrine and immune function can be significantly disrupted, and because of its impact on the CNS, pseudo-neurologic symptoms and disorders of sleep–wake regulation are also common.

It is also not uncommon for patients with PTSD to "self-medicate" or cope with their symptoms by drinking alcohol, smoking cigarettes, or using drugs, including cannabis and prescription pain medications or anxiolytics. Studies show that people with PTSD have more issues with drugs and alcohol both before and after being diagnosed with PTSD. In addition, having PTSD increases the risk that one will develop a drinking or drug problem, even in the absence of any prior drug or alcohol use.

Treatment and Monitoring

Current practice guidelines for the treatment of PTSD begin with education. Many people are confused, scared, or frustrated by the symptoms and behavior and are reassured to know they are not alone and that there are effective interventions. The patient should receive an appropriate medical workup, including a physical examination and studies (e.g., electrocardiogram, thyroid-stimulating hormone) when indicated. In addition to treating any cooccurring or underlying medical conditions, developing a good working alliance with the patient and family provides a basis for ongoing disease management and prevents unnecessary utilization or overutilization of the medical system, as well as potential exacerbation of symptoms.

A combination of psychotherapy and medication management is recommended as first-line treatment for PTSD. Psychological treatments with the most robust empirical support include trauma-focused psychotherapies utilizing exposure techniques, cognitive restructuring, relaxation/stress modulation training, and psychoeducation.

Cognitive-behavioral therapy (CBT) is the most effective non-medication treatment for PTSD. The two types of CBT recommended for PTSD are cognitive processing therapy (CPT) and prolonged exposure (PE). In CPT one examines what he or she is thinking and telling him- or herself about the trauma and decides whether those thoughts are accurate or inaccurate. It can be done individually or in a group. PE works through repeated exposure to thoughts, feelings, and situations the person has been avoiding and helps him or her learn that reminders of the trauma do not have to be avoided. PE is done individually with a therapist. Both CPT and PE offer a skills-based approach to treatment. The therapist and patient work collaboratively and in an active and problem-solving manner. The work structured and generally short term with an emphasis on reducing symptoms. Volumes of evidence support the efficacy of CBT interventions for PTSD, but success requires commitment to treatment on the part of the patient. Its efficacy is also contingent upon the ability of the therapist and the length of time in treatment. Studies show that when compared with patients undergoing monotherapy, patients treated with a combination of CBT and medication experience nearly twice the remission rate.

If combination therapy is initiated owing to symptom severity or patient preference, the SSRIs have been shown to be the best-tolerated class of medications, and response rates are significantly higher than placebo. This class of medication includes fluoxetine

TABLE 1A — Pharmacotherapy for the Treatment of Posttraumatic Stress Disorder

DRUG	STARTING DOSE	TARGET DOSE
Selective Serotonin Reuptake Inhibitors		
Paroxetine (Paxil)	10 mg qd	10–60 mg qd
Escitalopram (Lexapro)*	5–10 mg qd	10–20 mg qd
Sertraline (Zoloft)	12.5–25 mg qd	50–200 mg qd
Fluoxetine (Prozac)*	10 mg qd	20–40 mg qd

*Not US Food and Drug Administration approved for this indication.

TABLE 1B — Evidence-Based Psychotherapy for the Treatment of Posttraumatic Stress Disorder

PSYCHOTHERAPY	DESCRIPTION	FORMAT
Trauma-Focused Cognitive-Behavioral Therapy (TF-CBT)		
Cognitive processing therapy (CPT)	Teaches you to reframe negative thoughts about trauma	Weekly individual or group meetings
Prolonged exposure (PE)	Teaches you to gain control by facing your fears	Weekly individual meetings

(Prozac),[1] fluvoxamine (Luvox), citalopram (Celexa), escitalopram (Lexapro), paroxetine (Paxil), and sertraline (Zoloft). Some improvement should be noted within 3 or 4 weeks, and the dose should be increased if no improvement is seen. In all cases, SSRIs should be started at low doses and gradually titrated up to therapeutic levels to avoid an initial exacerbation of anxiety or agitation. Pharmacotherapy and psychotherapy options for the treatment of PTSD are presented in Tables 1A and 1B.

Benzodiazepines, which have been commonly used in the past to treat anxiety symptoms, are not recommended except in cases of extreme impairment of function, for short-term use only, and only after a thorough substance abuse history has been obtained. The tolerability and lack of addiction potential make the SSRIs more desirable for long-term management, but the delay in response makes short-term symptom relief with a benzodiazepine desirable for those with the greatest impairment. Because of the risk for rebound anxiety when withdrawing from benzodiazepines with short half-lives, such as alprazolam (Xanax), many prefer the longer-acting benzodiazepines, such as clonazepam (Klonopin).[1] However, the addiction potential and the potential for abuse with either drug make this the treatment option of last resort.

If the patient does not respond to the combination of CBT and medication, a reevaluation of symptoms might reveal a comorbid disorder missed on first examination. Comorbid psychiatric disorders significantly lower the likelihood of recovery from PTSD and increase recurrence rates. Many clinicians try switching between SSRIs before considering the next step in treatment, but a referral to a psychiatrist for further evaluation and management may be necessary if this strategy does not work. Treatment-refractory anxiety can be extremely frustrating for both the patient and clinician. This can lead to increased dependence on benzodiazepines and an escalation of doses required for the same effect.

When approaching the start of therapy, the clinician should reassure the patient that effective treatment is available but that patience may be necessary until the right combination of modalities is found. Although PTSD, like all anxiety disorders, displays a significant amount of chronicity, most patients have an

[1]Not FDA approved for this indication.

Gabbard GO: Treatment of Psychiatric Disorders, vols. 1–2. 3rd ed, Washington, DC, 2001, American Psychiatric Publishing.

Goddard AW, Coplan JD, Shekhar A, et al: Principles of the pharmacotherapy of anxiety disorders. In Charney DS, Nestler EJ, editors: *The Neurobiology of Mental Illness*, ed 2nd, New York, 2004, Oxford University Press, pp 661–682.

Gupta M: Review of somatic symptoms in post-traumatic stress disorder, *Int Rev Psychiatry* 25:86–99, 2013.

Kessler RC, Berglund P, Demler O, et al: Lifetime prevalence and age-of-onset distributions of DSM-IV disorders in the National Comorbidity Survey Replication, *Arch Gen Psychiatry* 62:593–602, 2005.

Kroenke K, Spitzer RL, Williams JBW, et al: Anxiety disorders in primary care: Prevalence, impairment, comorbidity, and detection, *Ann Intern Med* 146:317–325, 2007.

Lepine JP: The epidemiology of anxiety disorders: Prevalence and societal costs, *J Clin Psychiatry* 63(Suppl. 14):4–8, 2002.

National Comorbidity Survey: NCS-R appendix tables: Table 1. Lifetime prevalence of DSM-IV/WMH-CIDI disorders by sex and cohort. Table 2. Twelve-month prevalence of DSM-IV/WMH-CIDI disorders by sex and cohort. 2005, Available at: http://www.hcp.med.harvard.edu/ncs/publications.php.

Sadock B, Sadock V: *Kaplan and Sadock's Synopsis of Psychiatry: Behavioral Sciences/Clinical Psychiatry*, ed 10, Philadelphia, 2007, Lippincott Williams & Wilkins.

Stein M: Attending to anxiety disorders in primary care, *J Clin Psychiatry* 64:35–39, 2003.

TABLE 2 Helpful Resources for Patients with Posttraumatic Stress Disorder

ORGANIZATION	WEBSITE
US Department of Veteran Affairs National Center for PTSD	https://www.ptsd.va.gov/index.asp
Anxiety and Depression Association of America (ADAA)	https://www.adaa.org/understanding-anxiety/posttraumatic-stress-disorder-ptsd
National Institute of Mental Health (NIMH)	https://www.nimh.nih.gov/health/topics/post-traumatic-stress-disorder-ptsd/index.shtml
American Academy of Family Physicians (AAFP)	http://www.aafp.org/afp/2000/0901/p1046.html

improved outcome with appropriate treatment. Response rates improve when comorbidity is low. Patients with an earlier onset of symptoms (childhood or adolescence) can generally expect a more chronic course and may be more difficult to treat. Occasionally, patients can have a spontaneous remission of symptoms and many can continue to function despite their symptoms. However, time to resolution of symptoms is shortened and overall functioning can improve with treatment.

Pharmacotherapy often helps to prevent relapse, and rates are improved when effective treatment is continued for 12 months. When considering termination of pharmacologic treatment, the risk for relapse in all the disorders should be discussed with the patient. When discontinuing the SSRIs, a slow taper is recommended, with close monitoring for withdrawal symptoms (e.g., headache, gastrointestinal upset, restlessness, and other flu-like symptoms). Also monitor for rebound anxiety symptoms. If relapse occurs, reinstituting treatment is indicated, and many patients opt for indefinite treatment to maintain remission of symptoms. Lifelong management with pharmacotherapy or psychotherapy, or both, is not unusual for many patients. For many, a maximum reduction of symptoms, rather than a full remission, is an acceptable outcome.

Complications

Untreated anxiety disorders can lead to, or worsen, other mental and physical health conditions, including bruxism (teeth grinding), cognitive impairment, depression, gastrointestinal disorders, headache, insomnia, heart disease, substance abuse, and significantly impaired quality of life.

Conclusion

PTSD is a highly prevalent psychiatric condition that can be disabling and costly to the patient and to the health care system. Despite the prevalence of PTSD and other mental health disorders, a high percentage of patients often remain undiagnosed and untreated. These untreated patients also tend to be higher utilizers of general medical care. Patients with PTSD often present with multiple somatic complaints and comorbid disorders, causing great effort and expense in identifying the cause of unexplained symptoms. Once PTSD is identified, patients may be treated using well-tested and efficacious pharmacologic and psychotherapeutic treatments. Helpful resources for patients and families are listed in Table 2.

References

American Psychiatric Association: *Diagnostic and Statistical Manual of Mental Disorders*, ed 5, Washington, DC, 2013, American Psychiatric Association.

American Psychological Association: *Clinical Practice Guideline for the Treatment of Posttraumatic Stress Disorder (PTSD) in Adults*, Washington, DC, 2017, American Psychological Association.

Bailey C, Cordell E, Sobin S, Neumeister A: Recent progress in understanding the pathophysiology of posttraumatic stress disorder: Implications for targeted pharmacological treatment, *CNS Drugs* 27:221–232, 2013.

SCHIZOPHRENIA

Method of
Brian J. Miller, MD, PhD, MPH

CURRENT DIAGNOSIS

- There are three primary symptom domains in schizophrenia:
  - Positive symptoms (i.e., hallucinations, delusions, disorganized thought, and abnormal psychomotor behavior)
  - Negative symptoms (i.e., restricted affect or avolition/asociality)
  - Cognitive symptoms (i.e., attention, language, memory, and processing speed)
- Symptoms last ≥ 1 month and there are continuous signs of illness for ≥ 6 months.
- There is significant impairment one or more major areas of functioning (work, interpersonal relations, or self-care).
- Rule out that psychosis is not due to a primary mood disorder, schizoaffective disorder, substance intoxication or withdrawal, or a general medical condition.

CURRENT THERAPY

- Antipsychotic medication, with monitoring for medication adherence and side effects.
- Adjunctive medications as needed, including antidepressants, mood stabilizers, benzodiazepines, beta-blockers, and anticholinergics.
- Aggressive monitoring for and management of medical comorbidities, substance use disorders, and suicidality, including collaboration with primary care physician.
- Psychosocial interventions.
- Involvement of family/support system in care.
- Long-term treatment, including outpatient medication management and therapy, with inpatient care for acute crisis intervention/illness exacerbation.

Schizophrenia is a complex, chronic, and often severe psychiatric disorder that is a leading cause of disability worldwide. Although the literal translation of the word schizophrenia is "split mind," patients with this disorder do not have a "split personality" or "multiple personality disorder" (known as dissociative identity disorder). Rather, schizophrenia is a psychotic disorder that interferes with a person's thinking, mood, behavior, and/or interpersonal relations. Schizophrenia often has devastating, lifelong consequences for affected individuals and their families and is associated with an increased risk of premature mortality, including deaths from suicide and cardiovascular disease. In this chapter, the epidemiology and diagnosis of schizophrenia are reviewed. We then discuss pharmacologic and psychosocial treatments for schizophrenia in the context of a chronic disease model. The risks of medical and substance use comorbidity and suicidality are also highlighted.

Epidemiology and Risk Factors

The etiology of schizophrenia is not known, but it is thought to involve interactions between genetic (or epigenetic) and environmental factors, including developmental problems that occur during gestation. The lifetime prevalence of schizophrenia is approximately 1% and is equal in men and women. The usual age of onset is in the late teens or early 20s to late 30s, although schizophrenia can have onset before age 10 (early onset) or after age 45 (late onset). The age of onset is usually younger for men than women.

Several lines of evidence support a genetic contribution to the risk of schizophrenia. There is a 40% lifetime risk of schizophrenia in a child of two parents with schizophrenia. Twin-twin concordance is 50% in monozygotic twins, and 12% in dizygotic twins. A recent genome-wide association study and meta-analysis found that schizophrenia is significantly associated with single nucleotide polymorphisms in the major histocompatibility complex region on chromosome 6p22.1 (which includes several immunity-related genes, particularly complement C4), although numerous other genes have been implicated. There are likely multiple candidate genes that increase the risk of schizophrenia, each with small effect size.

Replicated environmental risk factors for schizophrenia include season of birth (winter), advanced paternal age, prenatal stress throughout gestation (famine and acute maternal stress in the first trimester, prenatal infections with a myriad of different agents, loss of the father in the second or third trimester), obstetric complications (including gestational diabetes, low birth weight, asphyxia), severe childhood abuse, and cannabis use. It remains unclear whether some of these risk factors are causal to schizophrenia or represent early manifestations of disease.

Diagnosis

There are three primary symptom domains in schizophrenia: positive, negative, and cognitive symptoms. Positive symptoms are abnormalities of thought content, including hallucinations (abnormal sensory perceptions in the absence of external stimuli) and delusions (fixed, false beliefs), formal thought disorder (also called disorganized thinking), and abnormal psychomotor behavior (such as catatonia). Hallucinations are most commonly auditory but can occur in any sensory modality. Negative symptoms include impairments in emotional expression (blunted affect), motivation (avolition), social behavior (asociality), speech (alogia), and the ability to experience pleasure (anhedonia). Cognitive symptoms include impairments in attention, language, memory, processing speed, and executive function.

The most commonly used diagnostic criteria for schizophrenia are derived from the *Diagnostic and Statistical Manual of Mental Disorders*, Fifth Edition (DSM-5). These criteria include the presence of two or more characteristic symptoms—delusions, hallucinations, disorganized speech, grossly abnormal psychomotor behavior (such as catatonia), or negative symptoms (i.e., restricted affect or avolition/asociality)—for a significant portion of time during a 1-month period (or less if successfully treated), with continuous signs of the disturbance persisting for at least 6 months. At least one of these two characteristic symptoms should include delusions, hallucinations, or disorganized speech. During this period, there is significant impairment in one or more major areas of functioning, including work, interpersonal relations, or self-care. It must also be established that the disorder is not better accounted for by a primary mood disorder, schizoaffective disorder, substance intoxication or withdrawal, or other general medical condition. From these criteria, it is important to note that

delusions and hallucinations, although common, are not required for the diagnosis. Furthermore, although cognitive symptoms are also not required for the diagnosis, they are a tremendous cause of illness-related disability. A diagnosis of schizophrenia is most definitively made by interviewing the patient, obtaining collateral history from family and/or friends, and completing a medical workup (physical examination, routine blood and urine tests). According to DSM-5 (released May 2013), the diagnostic criteria no longer identify subtypes of schizophrenia, primarily because of a lack of utility for clinicians. Also of note, the Psychoses Workgroup for DSM-5 considered the addition of "attenuated psychosis syndrome" (i.e., prodromal or high-risk psychosis) as a diagnostic category. Ultimately, attenuated psychosis syndrome is listed in DSM-5 among conditions that require further research before consideration as a formal disorder. Nevertheless, the early identification of individuals with prodromal or high-risk psychosis, investigation of risk factors and biomarkers that might predict conversion to fulminant psychotic disorder, and early interventions for individuals with prodromal or high-risk psychosis are areas receiving significant attention and effort in the field. In keeping with a growing emphasis on early intervention to avert or minimize the chronicity of schizophrenia, we are seeing more dedicated "first-episode psychosis" and/or "early intervention" programs being established in outpatient settings

Treatment

At present there is no cure for schizophrenia. Although there is significant clinical heterogeneity within the disorder, schizophrenia is usually a chronic condition that requires long-term treatment. Comprehensive treatment involves outpatient medication management and psychotherapy, psychosocial interventions, involvement of the family/support system, inpatient care for acute crisis intervention/illness exacerbation, and collaboration with primary care physicians. Currently, there is a vigorous research effort for diagnostic, prognostic and theranostic biomarkers in schizophrenia, toward a more "personalized medicine" approach for patients.

Antipsychotic medications play an important role in the pharmacologic management of schizophrenia. So-called first-generation antipsychotics (FGAs) have been in clinical use since the introduction of chlorpromazine (Thorazine) in the 1950s. These agents block the dopamine D2 receptor, and common side effects include extrapyramidal side effects (EPS) (e.g., Parkinsonism, dystonia). The newer or "second-generation antipsychotics" (SGAs), in addition to D2 receptor blockade, are also serotonin 5-HT2 receptor antagonists. While the risk of EPS is lower for SGAs than FGAs, SGAs are associated with a heightened risk of weight gain and the metabolic syndrome. In 2024, the FDA approved the first non-D2 receptor antagonist for schizophrenia, Cobenfy (a combination of xanomeline and trospium chloride). Xanomeline is an M1 and M4 muscarinic acetylcholine receptor agonist. Trospium chloride is a peripheral (but not central) muscarinic receptor antagonist. Table 1 provides a more detailed description of antipsychotic medications. The Texas Medication Algorithm Project (TMAP) currently recommends a trial of a single (non-clozapine) SGA for newly diagnosed patients with schizophrenia, or patients never before treated with an SGA. However, neither the TMAP nor the American Psychiatric Association (APA) guidelines for the treatment of schizophrenia preferentially endorse a particular antipsychotic. Clozapine (Clozaril) is primarily used for "treatment-refractory" schizophrenia, usually defined as a lack of/partial response to an adequate trial of monotherapy with two or three different antipsychotics.

Adjunctive medications may also play an important role in the pharmacologic treatment of some patients with schizophrenia. These include antidepressants for depression and anxiety, mood stabilizers for depression or mood elevation, benzodiazepines for anxiety or agitation, beta-blockers for akathisia, and anticholinergics for EPS.

Medication nonadherence is a major treatment issue in patients with schizophrenia at all phases of the illness. Reasons for nonadherence are complex and multifaceted but may include medication side effects, impaired insight into illness, psychopathology in

	TABLE 1	Antipsychotic Medications			
AGENT	**MECHANISM OF ACTION***	**TYPICAL DOSING**	**SIDE EFFECTS†**	**SIDE EFFECTS†**	**NOTES**
First Generation					
Haloperidol (Haldol)	D₂-antagonist	1.5–15 mg/day	EPS/TD Akathisia	NMS Hyperprolactinemia	PO, IM, IV, and long-acting injection formulations
Loxapine (Adasuve)	D₂-antagonist	10 mg/day	Dysgeusia Sedation	Throat irritation	INH formulation; for treatment of acute agitation
Second Generation					
Aripiprazole (Abilify)	Partial D₂-agonist and 5-HT2A antagonist	10–30 mg/day	Weight gain (+) Dyslipidemia (+) Glucose dysregulation (+)	Headache EPS/TD Akathisia	PO, rapid-dissolving PO, IM, transdermal patch, and long-acting injection formulations
Asenapine (Saphris)	D₂-antagonist/5-HT₂ antagonist	10–20 mg/day	Weight gain (+) Dyslipidemia (+) Glucose dysregulation (+)	Sedation EPS/TD Akathisia	Rapid-dissolving PO formulation
Clozapine (Clozaril)	D₂-antagonist/5-HT₂ antagonist	300–900 mg/day	Weight gain (+++) Dyslipidemia (+++) Glucose dysregulation (++) Agranulocytosis Sedation	Orthostatic hypotension Seizures Myocarditis EPS/TD	PO and rapid-dissolving PO formulations
Iloperidone (Fanapt)	D₂-antagonist/5-HT₂ antagonist	12–24 mg/day	Weight gain (++) Dyslipidemia (+) Glucose dysregulation (+)	Dizziness Tachycardia Sedation EPS/TD	PO formulation
Lurasidone (Latuda)	D₂-antagonist/5-HT₂ antagonist	40–80 mg/day	Weight gain (+) Dyslipidemia (+) Glucose dysregulation (+)	Sedation Akathisia Nausea EPS/TD	PO formulation
Olanzapine (Zyprexa)	D₂-antagonist/5-HT₂ antagonist	5–30 mg/day	Weight gain (+++) Dyslipidemia (+++) Glucose dysregulation (++)	Sedation Dizziness Hyperprolactinemia EPS/TD	PO, rapid-dissolving PO, IM, and long-acting injection formulations
Paliperidone (Invega)	D₂-antagonist/5-HT₂ antagonist	6–12 mg/day	Weight gain (+) Dyslipidemia (+) Glucose dysregulation (+)	Tachycardia Headache EPS/TD	PO and long-acting injection formulations Active metabolite of Risperidone (Risperdal)
Quetiapine (Seroquel)	D₂-antagonist/5-HT₂ antagonist	200–800 mg/day	Weight gain (++) Dyslipidemia (+) Glucose dysregulation (+)	Sedation Headache Orthostatic hypotension EPS/TD	PO and extended-release PO formulations
Risperidone (Risperdal)	D₂-antagonist/5-HT₂ antagonist	2–6 mg/day	Weight gain (++) Dyslipidemia (+) Glucose dysregulation (+)	Sedation Hyperprolactinemia EPS/TD	PO, PO liquid, rapid-dissolving PO, and long-acting injection formulations
Ziprasidone (Geodon)	D₂-antagonist/5-HT₂ antagonist	80–160 mg/day	Weight gain (+) Dyslipidemia (+) Glucose dysregulation (+)	Sedation QTc prolongation EPS/TD	PO and IM formulations
Aripiprazole lauroxil (Aristada)	Partial D₂ agonist and 5-HT2A antagonist	441 mg/month or 882 mg/4–6 weeks	Weight gain (+) Dyslipidemia (+) Glucose dysregulation (+)	Headache EPS/TD Akathisia	Long-acting injection formulation
Aripiprazole (Abilify Asimtufii)	Partial D2 agonist and 5-HT2A antagonist	960 mg/2 mo	Weight gain (+)	Headache	Extended-release injection for IM use
Brexpiprazole (Rexulti)	Partial D2 and 5-HT1A agonist and 5-HT2 antagonist	1–4 mg/day	Weight gain (+) Dyslipidemia (+) Glucose dysregulation (+)	Increased triglycerides EPS/TD Akathisia	PO formulation

Continued

TABLE 1 Antipsychotic Medications—cont'd

AGENT	MECHANISM OF ACTION*	TYPICAL DOSING	SIDE EFFECTS†	SIDE EFFECTS†	NOTES
Cariprazine (Vraylar)	Partial D2 and D3 agonist	1.5–6 mg/day	Weight gain (+) Dyslipidemia (+) Glucose dysregulation (+)	Headache EPS/TD Akathisia	PO formulation
Lumateperone (Caplyta)	5-HT2A antagonist, partial D2 agonist, D1 receptor–dependent glutamate modulator, serotonin reuptake inhibitor	42 mg/day	Weight gain (+/-) Dyslipidemia (+/-) Glucose dysregulation (+/-)	Headache Somnolence Sedation	PO formulation
Olanzapine/ samidorphan (Lybalvi)	D2-antagonist/5HT2 antagonist (olanzapine), mu-opioid antagonist (samidorphan)	5 mg/10 mg to 20 mg/10 mg qd	Weight gain (++) Dyslipidemia (++) Glucose dysregulation (+)	Sedation Dizziness Hyperprolactinemia EPS/TD	PO formulation
Risperidone (Perseris)	D2-antagonist/5HT2 antagonist	90–120 mg/month	Weight gain (++) Dyslipidemia (+) Glucose dysregulation (+)	Sedation Hyperprolactinemia EPS/TD	Subcutaneous long-acting injection formulation
Risperidone (Uzedy)	D2-antagonist/5HT2 antagonist	50-125 mg/mo, or 100-250 mg/2 mo	Weight gain (++) Dyslipidemia (+) Glucose dysregulation (+)	Sedation Hyperprolactinemia EPS/TD	Extended-release injection for subcutaneous use

Other Antipsychotics

AGENT	MECHANISM OF ACTION*	TYPICAL DOSING	SIDE EFFECTS†	SIDE EFFECTS†	NOTES
Xanomeline/ trospium chloride (Cobenfy)	M1/M4 agonist (xanomeline) and peripheral M1/M4 antagonist (trospium)	100/40 mg to 250/60 mg/day in bid dosing	Weight gain (+/-) Dyslipidemia (+/-) Glucose dysregulation (+/-)	Hypertension Constipation Dyspepsia Nausea/vomiting	PO formulation

Abbreviations: D_2 = dopamine D_2 receptor; +++, severe risk; EPS = extrapyramidal side effects; $5\text{-}HT_2$ = serotonin $5\text{-}HT_2$ receptor; ++ = moderate risk; TD = tardive dyskinesia; + = mild or low risk; NMS = neuroleptic malignant syndrome.

*All first-generation and second-generation antipsychotics have an FDA black box warning for an "association with an increased risk of mortality in elderly patients treated for dementia-related psychosis." All second-generation agents are D_2 and $5\text{-}HT_2$ antagonists; however, many act on multiple receptors, including alpha-adrenergic, beta-adrenergic, histaminergic, muscarinic cholinergic, and D_1, and $5\text{-}HT_1$ receptors.

†EPS and TD are possible side effects with all antipsychotics, but they occur less frequently with second-generation than first-generation drugs.

all three symptom domains, lack of efficacy, and comorbid substance use. Over 70% of patients in the Clinical Antipsychotic Trials of Intervention Effectiveness (CATIE) Schizophrenia Trial discontinued medication within the first 18 months of treatment. Medication nonadherence leads to dramatically increased risk of illness relapse, hospitalization, and suicidal behavior and should be routinely assessed in clinical visits. The use of rapid-dissolving oral or long-acting injectable medications may improve adherence in some patients.

Psychosocial interventions are also a cornerstone of the comprehensive treatment of patients with schizophrenia, and when utilized in combination with medication, are more effective than antipsychotics alone. Psychotherapy, including cognitive-behavioral therapy, supportive therapy, and group therapy, promotes improved illness management and medication adherence. Involvement of the patient's family/support system in care, including family-based therapies and psychoeducation, has been shown to increase medication adherence and decrease illness relapse rates. Psychosocial rehabilitation, which may include assertive community treatment, social skills training, vocational rehabilitation, and cognitive remediation, can help maximize patients' psychosocial functioning. There is growing evidence that cognitive remediation therapy in combination with other psychosocial interventions, particularly vocational rehabilitation, can improve real-world functioning for patients with schizophrenia in a relatively short time period.

Although there is no "typical" patient with schizophrenia, the clinical course is often characterized by acute relapses of the illness with the inter-episode absence or attenuation of symptoms. Multiple factors increase a patient's risk of illness relapse, including

medication nonadherence, psychosocial stressors, substance use, medical illnesses such as infections, and the natural history of the disorder itself. Hospitalization may be required for acute exacerbations of psychotic symptoms, including hallucinations, delusions, and impaired self-care. Hospitalization may also be required if a patient represents an acute danger to self or others.

The concept of the recovery model and recovery-oriented care is a movement that is currently transforming the delivery of mental health services. Integral to the recovery model are certified peer specialists (CPS). A CPS is a licensed professional who has progressed in their own recovery from mental illness and works to assist patients with schizophrenia and other mental illness in regaining control over their own lives and over their own recovery process. CPSs provide peer support services, serve as consumer advocates, are resources for psychoeducation, and offer the unique perspectives based on their individual experiences.

Comorbidity

Schizophrenia is associated with an increased risk of premature mortality, and cardiovascular disease is a leading cause of death in this patient population. Multiple factors contribute to this risk, including a high prevalence of smoking, poor health habits, poor health care, medication side effects, and (perhaps) the pathophysiology of the disorder itself. SGAs as a class are associated with weight gain and an increased risk of metabolic syndrome. Over 40% of the 1460 patients in the CATIE Schizophrenia Trial met the criteria for metabolic syndrome at baseline. Recommendations for monitoring of patients on SGAs, based on a consensus statement from the American Diabetes Association and the APA, are described in Table 2. Primary care physicians play an important

TABLE 2 | Monitoring Second-Generation Antipsychotic (Excluding Clozapine)

	BASE-LINE	4 WEEKS	8 WEEKS	12 WEEKS	QUARTERLY	ANNUALLY	IF SYMP-TOMS ARISE	EVERY 5 YEARS	OTHER
Personal/family history*	X					X			
Pregnancy test†	X						X		
Weight/BMI	X	X	X	X	X				
Waist circumference	X					X			
Blood pressure	X			X		X			
Fasting glucose/HgbA1C	X			X		X			
Fasting lipid panel	X			X				X	
EKG‡	X						X		
Prolactin	X						X		
CBC with differential§									X

More frequent assessments may be warranted based on clinical status.
*Including obesity, diabetes, hypertension, and dyslipidemia.
†In all women of childbearing age.
‡For patients taking Ziprasidone (Geodon), which may prolong the QTc interval, and Clozapine (Clozaril).
§For patients taking Clozapine (Clozaril). CBC with differential required at baseline, then weekly for 6 months, then every other week for 6 months, then monthly thereafter. Baseline absolute neutrophil count (ANC) must be ≥ 1500/mm^3 (or ≥1000/mm^3 in patients with benign ethnic neutropenia) due to risk of agranulocytosis.

collaborative role with psychiatrists in the detection and management of metabolic disturbances in patients with schizophrenia, in order to minimize the cardiovascular risks associated with these comorbidities.

Patients with schizophrenia are also at an increased risk of suicide, which is also a leading cause of premature mortality. The prevalence of completed suicide in patients with schizophrenia is about 10%, and suicide attempts occur with even greater frequency. Clinicians should routine assess patients for suicidal ideation and, if present, explore risk factors for completed suicide, which include a suicidal plan and intent, previous suicide attempts, a family history of suicide, age, sex, access to lethal means, social isolation, and comorbid substance use. Medications, psychotherapy, and/or hospitalization may be required.

Comorbid substance use disorders predominate in patients with schizophrenia, with an estimated prevalence of 40% to 50%. Common substances of abuse include alcohol, marijuana, and cocaine. Patients with schizophrenia and comorbid substance use are at increased risk of medication nonadherence, illness relapse, hospitalization, suicidal and violent behavior, and an overall poor response to treatment. Furthermore, up to 70% to 90% of patients with schizophrenia are tobacco users, which contribute to the increased risk of medical comorbidity. Clinicians are encouraged to routinely screen for and address substance use in their treatment plans.

Conclusions

Schizophrenia is a complex, heterogeneous, and chronic psychiatric disorder. Comprehensive treatment usually involves long-term medication management and therapy, education for patients and their families, and psychosocial interventions. Primary care physicians play an important collaborative role in the detection and management of medical comorbidities, substance use disorders, and suicidality. Physicians, patients, and families are encouraged to become involved in the National Alliance on Mental Illness (NAMI; www.nami.org), which is a tremendous resource for help, support, education, and advocacy for patients with schizophrenia and other mental illness.

References

American Diabetes Association, American Psychiatric Association, American Association of Clinical Endocrinologists, et al: Consensus development conference on antipsychotic drugs and obesity and diabetes, J Clin Psychiatry 65:267, 2020.

American Psychiatric Association: Practice guideline for the treatment of patients with schizophrenia, ed 3, Am J Psychiatry 177:868, 2020.

Buchanan RW, Carpenter WT: Schizophrenia and other psychotic disorders. In Sadock BJ, Sadock VA, editors: Kaplan and Sadock's Comprehensive Textbook of Psychiatry, ed 8, Philadelphia, 2005, Lippincott Williams and Wilkins, pp 1329–1345.

Buckley PF, Miller BJ, Lehrer DS, et al: Psychiatric comorbidities and schizophrenia, Schizophr Bull 35:383, 2009.

Fusar-Poli P, Tantardini M, De Simone S, et al: Deconstructing vulnerability for psychosis: meta-analysis of environmental risk factors for psychosis in subjects at ultra high-risk, Eur Psychiatry 40:65–75, 2017.

Laursen TM, Munk-Olsen T, Vestergaard M: Life expectancy and cardiovascular mortality in persons with schizophrenia, Curr Opin Psychiatry 25:83, 2012.

Leucht S, Corves C, Arbter D, et al: Second-generation versus first-generation antipsychotic drugs for schizophrenia: a meta-analysis, Lancet 373:31, 2009.

Lieberman JA, Stroup TS, McEvoy JP, et al: Effectiveness of antipsychotic drugs in patients with chronic schizophrenia, N Engl J Med 353:1209, 2005.

McEvoy JP, Meyer JP, Goff DC, et al: Prevalence of the metabolic syndrome in patients with schizophrenia: baseline results from the Clinical Antipsychotic Trials of Intervention Effectiveness (CATIE), Schizophr Res 80:19, 2005.

Messias EL, Chen CY, Eaton WW: Epidemiology of schizophrenia: review of findings and myths, Psychiatr Clin North Am 30:323, 2007.

Nelson B, Amminger GP, Yuen HP, et al: Staged treatment in early psychosis: a sequential multiple assignment randomised trial of interventions for ultra high risk of psychosis patients, Early Interv Psychiatry 12:292, 2018.

Rodrigues-Amorim D, Rivera-Baltanás T, López M, et al: Schizophrenia: a review of potential biomarkers, J Psychiatr Res 93:37–49, 2017.

Shi J, Levinson DF, Duan J, et al: Common variants on chromosome 6p22.1 are associated with schizophrenia, Nature 460:753, 2009.

Torrey EF: Surviving Schizophrenia, ed 7, New York, 2019, Harper Perennial.

11 Respiratory System

ACUTE BRONCHITIS AND OTHER VIRAL RESPIRATORY INFECTIONS

Method of
Tomoko Sairenji, MD, MS

CURRENT DIAGNOSIS

- Most cases of acute bronchitis are caused by viruses, and it is diagnosed clinically.
- The predominant symptom of acute bronchitis is acute cough, with or without sputum.
- Other diseases such as asthma, pneumonia, chronic obstructive pulmonary disease exacerbation, and heart failure should be ruled out.

CURRENT THERAPY

- Antibiotics are not recommended for most cases of acute bronchitis.
- Dextromethorphan, guaifenesin, and honey may be considered to relieve cough symptoms.
- Patient education: Cough can last 3 weeks or more.

Etiology

Acute bronchitis is a common reason for ambulatory care visits. It is characterized by an acute cough and is most commonly caused by viruses such as rhinovirus, enterovirus, influenza A and B, parainfluenza, coronavirus, coxsackie, and respiratory syncytial virus (RSV). Bacterial causes such as *Mycoplasma pneumoniae*, *Chlamydia pneumoniae*, and *Bordetella pertussis* are much less common.

Pathophysiology

Acute bronchitis is caused by an acute inflammatory process in the mucosa of the trachea and bronchi with resultant injury to epithelium of the mucosa.

Clinical Manifestations

Cough is the primary symptom of acute bronchitis, but it can cause other symptoms such as nasal congestion, wheezing, dyspnea, fever, and nonspecific constitutional symptoms.

Diagnosis

Acute bronchitis is diagnosed clinically, characterized by an acute cough with or without sputum production. It is often a diagnosis of exclusion, in which other diseases such as asthma, pneumonia, chronic obstructive pulmonary disease exacerbation, and heart failure are ruled out. Initially, manifestations of acute bronchitis can be identical to the common cold and difficult to distinguish. Patients may have a mildly ill appearance, but fever is less common in bronchitis after the first few days. On auscultation, there may be wheezing or rhonchi that improve with coughing. A patient with a high temperature, otherwise abnormal vital signs, and a more toxic appearance should raise concern for pneumonia or influenza.

Laboratory testing is usually not necessary for the typical patient in the outpatient setting, but it can be done for influenza and pertussis when there is greater suspicion for these diseases.

Imaging such as chest x-rays are not necessary in most cases for patients who have normal vital signs, no bloody sputum, and a normal lung examination. However, it is recommended in those older than 75 years of age, because pneumonia does not always mount a fever or cause tachycardia in the elderly.

Differential Diagnosis

Common Cold/Upper Respiratory Infections

The common cold can be difficult to differentiate from acute bronchitis. On average, adults have 2 to 4, and young children as many as 6 to 10 episodes annually. It is most commonly caused by rhinoviruses but can also be caused by other respiratory viruses such as coronavirus, influenza, and RSV and parainfluenza viruses. The symptomatic trajectory of the common cold is sore throat, malaise, and low-grade fever for 1 to 2 days, followed by nasal congestion, rhinorrhea, and cough. Cough can occur in 30% to 40% of cases, and fluid can accumulate in the middle ear or sinus cavities. Common cold/upper respiratory infection (URI) symptoms are generally the worst on days 3 and 4 and start to improve by day 7. Symptoms that would warrant consideration for more serious disease are respiratory distress, difficulty swallowing, altered mental status, signs suggesting dehydration, stiff neck, rash, or sore throat for more than 5 days. Influenza (high fever with general myalgias), acute bacterial sinusitis (symptoms for more than 10 days without improvement, severe symptoms including fever ≥39°C, and purulent nasal discharge lasting more than 3 consecutive days), streptococcal pharyngitis (absence of cough with tender lymphadenopathy and tonsillar exudates), asthma exacerbations triggered by URI, and infectious mononucleosis (fatigue, fever, sore throat, and adenopathy more severe than typical URI) are other conditions on the differential. Testing is not warranted for the diagnosis of a common cold unless one of these diseases is suspected and needs to be ruled out.

Similar to acute bronchitis, antibiotics are strongly discouraged for the common cold because they provide no benefit in terms of reducing symptom severity or duration. If symptoms are severe, treatment focuses mostly on symptomatic management, of which most can be done using over-the-counter therapies. Rest and adequate hydration and nutrition are encouraged but have not been studied in trials. Acetaminophen and nonsteroidal antiinflammatory drugs can help with fever and discomfort. The combination of antihistamines and decongestants may be more beneficial than either component alone for nasal symptoms. When needed, dextromethorphan may provide symptom relief with cough suppression. Intranasal or inhaled cromolyn sodium[1] may help with rhinorrhea, throat pain, or cough. Various formulations of intranasal cromolyn sodium (NasalCrom) are available over the counter, and oral inhaled cromolyn sodium (Intal) is available by a

913

---

[1] Not FDA approved for this indication.

prescription. Regular use of vitamin C supplements[7] (1 to 2 g/d) may decrease duration of cold symptoms, but they are not effective if started after cold symptoms start. Oral zinc sulfate[1,7] may decrease URI symptom duration and severity, but it is not routinely recommended because of adverse effects (bad taste, nausea, and abdominal cramping).

Croup

Croup affects children with a peak incidence between 6 and 36 months of age, annually affecting 3% of those in this age range. Parainfluenza virus types 1 to 3 constitute 75% of all cases, but infection with many different viruses can produce this illness. Although some cases of croup can be caused by bacteria, it does not change how it is managed.

Croup is diagnosed clinically. Initially, patients experience cold-like symptoms: low-grade fevers and coryza. Inspiratory stridor, hoarseness, and a barking cough are typical findings that follow, peaking between 24 to 48 hours after onset. These symptoms are caused by mucosal inflammatory swelling of the larynx, trachea, and bronchi. Symptoms are often worse at night and can be exacerbated by emotional distress. Most (85%) cases are considered mild, but nasal flaring and retractions, increased respiratory rate, hypoxia, and tachycardia are indicators of more severe croup. Routine radiologic imaging is not encouraged, because the steeple sign that is often associated with croup is nonspecific and can be seen in other causes of glottic and subglottic narrowing such as epiglottitis and bacterial tracheitis.

Management of croup is dependent on the severity of the disease. Administration of corticosteroids (single dose of dexamethasone [Decadron][1] 0.6 mg/kg) are recommended for croup of any severity because it reduces return visits and hospitalization rates. Oxygen should be given to children with hypoxia or respiratory distress. Nebulized epinephrine[1] (0.5 mg/kg (max 5 mg) of 1:1000 L-epinephrine (adrenaline) diluted in 2–5 mL normal saline) is recommended for moderate or severe croup. It takes effect by vasoconstriction of the upper airway mucosa, leading to decreased edema. It has a quick onset of action, but efficacy wanes after 1 to 2 hours, so monitoring patients beyond 2 hours is recommended.

Humidified air has been commonly used for croup, but it has not been shown to be effective in decreasing croup symptoms or hospital admissions in moderate croup.

Pertussis

Pertussis should be suspected when patients have more than 2 weeks of a characteristic paroxysmal, whooping cough and posttussive emesis, or recent pertussis exposure. Most pertussis is caused by the bacteria *B. pertussis*. The number of outbreaks and pertussis incidence has been rising since the 1980s, with the most recent peak in 2024 (35,435 cases). In the early catarrhal stage (1–2 weeks), it is difficult to discern from a common cold. The cough becomes more frequent, and severe bouts characterize the ensuing paroxysmal stage (1–6 weeks, maximum of 10 weeks). Paroxysms of cough can be debilitating and cause posttussive emesis, weight loss, and other conditions related to severe cough, but there are few symptoms otherwise. After this stage, the cough gradually improves over the course of a few weeks.

Atypical presentations are not uncommon, because those who have acquired immunity can present with a lesser degree of paroxysm. Thus pertussis should be suspected if cough symptoms last more than 3 weeks. Infants may also have atypical presentation of cough without paroxysmal whooping.

Diagnosis can be confirmed with either culture, polymerase chain reaction (both better for early stages), or serology (accurate in later stage). Efficacy of antibiotics is questionable because treatment does not improve symptoms. However, antibiotics (Azithromycin [Zithromax][1] is first line; children, 10 mg/kg on day 1, then 5 mg/kg daily on days 2–5; adults, 500 mg on day 1, then 250 mg daily on days 2–5) are still recommended to decrease transmission. Immunization is critical to prevent further outbreaks of pertussis.

Bronchiolitis

Bronchiolitis is the most common cause for infant hospitalization of infants. RSV is the most common cause of bronchiolitis. Bronchioles become plugged with detached epithelium and inflammatory cells. Onset of upper respiratory symptoms is often soon followed by rapid development of wheezing and labored breathing. Infants with bronchiolitis typically do not have a marked response to asthma treatment with bronchodilators and corticosteroids, despite similar presenting symptoms. Treatment primarily consists of maintaining oxygenation and adequate hydration. Palivizumab (Synagis) is used to prevent hospitalization rate for highest-risk infants, such as those with premature birth, chronic lung disease, and hemodynamically significant congenital heart disease.

Therapy

Decreasing Antibiotic Use

Antibiotic use in the treatment of bronchitis is strongly discouraged in all major guidelines, but they are often prescribed. The strongest predictor of whether a patient will receive antibiotics is whether the clinician perceives the patient desires them. Patient education such as setting the expectation that cough from acute bronchitis can last 3 weeks, that antibiotics would not effectively aid in shortening the duration of symptoms, and explaining consequences of inappropriate antibiotic use such as antibiotic resistance and adverse effects is important. One in five patients treated with antibiotics will experience side effects such as headache, nausea, skin rash, diarrhea, and vaginitis. Patients are more likely to respond to this sort of education if they feel their concerns have been heard and addressed. In some cases, using a delayed prescription strategy wherein patients would need to call for a prescription or agree to pick up antibiotics after a certain number of days may be effective in decreasing antibiotic use. Providing methods for symptomatic management is also important for patients who desire treatment.

Recommended Cough Treatment

Dextromethorphan, guaifenesin, and honey may be considered to relieve cough symptoms. Dextromethorphan (12 years and older: 30 mg orally every 6–8 hours max 120 mg/day. Dextromethorphan immediate release dose for children: ages 6–12 years, 15 mg every 6–8 hours, max 60 mg/day; ages 4–6 years 7.5 mg every 6–8 hours max 30 mg/day. NOT recommended for children under 4 years) is a central-acting antitussive that reduces the cough reflex. In placebo-controlled studies, it was shown to decrease coughs by 19% to 36% (8–10 fewer coughs per 30 minutes) compared with placebo. Guaifenesin (12 years and older: [immediate-release] 200–400 mg orally every 4 hours, max 2400 mg/day; children 6–12 years: 100–200 mg every 4 hours, max 1200 mg/day; 2–6 years: 50–100 mg every 4 hours, max 600 mg/day; NOT recommended for children under 2 years) is an expectorant that increases respiratory tract secretions, hence decreasing mucus thickness. Study results vary, but it has been shown to decrease cough frequency and severity compared with placebo. Honey (5–10 mL [1–2 teaspoons once or twice daily]) has been compared with dextromethorphan, diphenhydramine, and no treatment in children. It was found to be better than no treatment in its effectiveness in decreasing cough severity and frequency and improving sleep quality. Honey is only an option for children older than 1 year, because of the risk of botulism.

Cough Treatments That Are Not Recommended

There is no evidence that centrally acting antitussive codeine[1] has any effect to decrease cough symptoms, and benzonatate (Tessalon Perles), a peripherally acting antitussive, has only been shown to be effective in conjunction with guaifenesin. Unfortunately, many over-the-counter therapies do not significantly impact acute bronchitis symptoms. Clinical trials have shown that ibuprofen

---

[7] Available as dietary supplement.
[1] Not FDA approved for this indication.

(Motrin)[1] and antihistamines are not effective in reducing symptoms of cough. The FDA warns against using cough medications that have antihistamines and antitussives in children younger than 4 years of age because of the high risk for potential harm. Use of beta-agonists is also not recommended, unless the patient presents with wheezing at the time of presentation.

References

Altunaiji S, Kukuruzovic R, Curtis N, et al: Antibiotics for whooping cough (pertussis), *Cochrane Database Syst Rev*(3):CD004404, 2007.

Barnett ML, Linder JA: Antibiotic prescribing for adults with acute bronchitis in the United States, 1996-2010, *JAMA* 311:2020–2022, 2014.

Ebell MH, Lundgren J, Youngpairoj S: How long does a cough last? Comparing patients' expectations with data from a systematic review of the literature, *Ann Fam Med* 11:5–13, 2013.

Kinkade S, Long N: Acute bronchitis, *Am Fam Physician* 94:560–565, 2016.

Oduwole O, Meremikwu MM, Oyo-Ita A, et al: Honey for acute cough in children, *Cochrane Database Syst Rev*(12):CD007094, 2014.

Petrocheilou A, Tanou K, Kalampouka E, et al: Viral croup: diagnosis and a treatment algorithm, *Pediatr Pulmonol* 49:421–429, 2014.

Russell KF, Liang Y, O'Gorman K, et al: Glucocorticoids for croup, *Cochrane Database Syst Rev*(1):CD001955, 2011.

Smith D, McDermott A, Sullivan J: Croup: diagnosis and management, *Am Fam Physician* 97:575–580, 2018.

Smith SM, Fahey T, Smucny J, et al: Antibiotics for acute bronchitis, *Cochrane Database Syst Rev*(3):CD000245, 2014.

Smith SM, Schroeder K, Fahey T: Over-The-Counter (OTC) medications for acute cough in children and adults in community settings, *Cochrane Database Syst Rev*(11):CD001831, 2014.

---

[1] Not FDA approved for this indication.

ACUTE RESPIRATORY FAILURE

Method of
Anthony J. Faugno III, MD; and Scott K. Epstein, MD

CURRENT DIAGNOSIS

- History and physical examination can give insight into the etiology of hypoxic and hypercapneic respiratory failure but may be insufficient to make a definitive diagnosis and guide therapy.
- An arterial blood gas is mandatory to define severity and whether hypoxic or hypercapneic (or both) respiratory failure is present.
- Additional diagnostic modalities, including chest radiograph, electrocardiogram, cardiac laboratory tests (troponin, brain natriuretic peptide), echocardiography, and selected use of a pulmonary artery catheter, can help identify a specific etiology.

CURRENT THERAPY

- Treatment of acute respiratory failure often begins with non-specific approaches such as oxygen and mechanical ventilation (noninvasive or invasive).
- The goal of mechanical ventilation is to improve gas exchange and rest the respiratory muscles while waiting for the beneficial effects of specific therapy aimed at the underlying cause (e.g., bronchodilators, antibiotics, and corticosteroids in acute exacerbations of chronic obstructive pulmonary disease [COPD]).
- Noninvasive ventilation avoids many complications associated with invasive ventilation and improves outcomes for patients with acute cardiogenic pulmonary edema and acute exacerbations of COPD.
- High-flow nasal cannula is emerging as the preferred therapy for hypoxic respiratory failure in patients with non-cardiogenic pulmonary edema who do not require urgent intubation.

- Invasive mechanical ventilation can be lifesaving but can cause clinical deterioration if not properly administered.
- Using low tidal volumes (6 mL/kg ideal body weight) can help avoid dangerous dynamic hyperinflation in acute exacerbations of COPD and further lung injury in acute lung injury (e.g., volutrauma, barotrauma).
- Once signs of improvement are evident, focus rapidly shifts to liberating the patient from the ventilator using spontaneous breathing trials to assess the need for ventilatory support followed by airway assessment to determine readiness for extubation.

The respiratory system serves many complex physiologic functions, the most important of which is gas exchange. Using the interface between the alveolar space and capillaries, O_2 is taken up and CO_2 is eliminated. Acute respiratory failure, a life-threatening entity, is present when this system fails, over the course of minutes to hours, resulting in hypoxemia (type I) or hypercapnia (type II), or both. Most patients with acute respiratory failure present with dyspnea, although the correlation with disease severity is poor. Indeed, dyspnea might seem mild in those with baseline chronic respiratory failure, and it might be absent in those with an underlying neurologic process (e.g., drug overdose). Other symptoms and signs such as cough, chest pain, orthopnea, fever, tachypnea, rales, and wheezing are insensitive and nonspecific.

This chapter outlines the general pathophysiology and therapeutic approach to acute respiratory failure by using the examples of three common entities: acute respiratory distress syndrome (ARDS), cardiogenic pulmonary edema (congestive heart failure [CHF]), and acute exacerbation of chronic obstructive pulmonary disease (AECOPD).

Definitions and Pathophysiology

Acute Hypoxic Respiratory Failure

Hypoxic respiratory failure is conventionally defined as an arterial oxygen tension (PaO_2) of less than 60 mm Hg. Because this definition ignores the inspired fraction of oxygen (FiO_2), some favor a PaO_2/FiO_2 ratio of less than 300. To account for the arterial CO_2 tension ($PaCO_2$), others favor an alveolar–arterial (A–a) O_2 gradient greater than 250 mm Hg, using the equation

$$A\text{--}a\ O_2\ gradient = PAO_2 - PaO_2$$
$$= (713 \times FiO_2) - (PaO_2 + PaCO_2/0.8)$$

where 713 is the barometric pressure (760) minus the water vapor pressure. A normal A–a O_2 is less than 10 mm Hg, but this threshold value increases with age. The determination of PaO_2 requires an invasive test, an arterial blood gas. Oxygenation can be continuously monitored noninvasively by pulse oximetry, which provides an estimate of arterial oxygen saturation (SaO_2). In general, an SaO_2 of 0.90 corresponds to a PaO_2 of 60 mm Hg, but the relation depends on temperature, pH, $PaCO_2$, and 2,3-diphosphoglycerate (2,3-DPG). Accuracy is adversely affected by low perfusion states, dark skin pigmentation, nail polish, dyshemoglobins (e.g., carboxyhemoglobin, methemoglobin), intravascular dyes, motion, and ambient light.

Clinicians tend to focus on PaO_2 and SaO_2, but the real parameter of interest is O_2 delivery (DO_2) to organs and tissues. DO_2 depends on cardiac output and O_2 carrying capacity of arterialized blood (CaO_2):

$$DO_2 = CO \times CaO_2$$

where

$$CaO_2 = k(Hb \times SaO_2) + 0.003\ PaO_2$$

where k is a constant. DO_2 decreases when cardiac output or hemoglobin is reduced despite a normal PaO_2 and SaO_2. The peripheral response to reduced DO_2 is an increased O_2 extraction ratio (O_2ER), allowing oxygen uptake $\dot{V}CO_2$, an indicator

TABLE 1 Pathophysiologic Mechanisms of Acute Hypoxic Respiratory Failure

MECHANISM	A–A O2 GRADIENT	PACO2	RESPONSE TO 100% O2	CAUSE
Diffusion abnormality	↑	↑ Normal	↑↑	Severe interstitial lung disease ARDS, pneumonia
Hypoventilation	Normal	↑	↑↑↑	Narcotic overdose, obesity hypoventilation syndrome, respiratory muscle weakness
↓ FiO2	Normal	Usually ↓	↑↑↑	High altitude, smoke inhalation
↓ MvO2	↑	Usually ↓	↑	ARDS, shock, CHF, PE
Shunt	↑	Usually ↓	None or ↑	ARDS, pneumonia, CHF, atelectasis, PE
$\dot{V}/\dot{Q}$ mismatch	↑	↑, Normal, ↓	↑↑↑	AECOPD, asthma, PE, ARDS, pneumonia

↑, Increased; ↓, decreased; *A–a O2*, alveolar–arterial O_2; *AECOPD*, acute exacerbation of chronic obstructive pulmonary disease; *ARDS*, acute respiratory distress syndrome; *CHF*, cardiogenic pulmonary edema; *FiO2*, fraction of inspired oxygen; *MvO2*, mixed venous oxygen saturation; *PaCO2*, partial pressure of arterial CO_2; *PE*, pulmonary embolism; $\dot{V}/\dot{Q}$, ventilation–perfusion ratio.

of metabolic demand, to remain constant. Cellular and organ dysfunction occurs when DO_2 and O_2ER are outstripped by metabolic demand. The balance between DO_2 and demand can be estimated by examining the mixed venous O_2 saturation (MvO_2) using the rearranged Fick equation:

$$MvO_2 = SaO_2 - \left(\dot{V}O_2/CO \times Hb\right)$$

When MvO_2 falls below 65% to 75%, imbalance is present. When cellular injury is present, extraction capabilities are limited and cellular hypoxia occurs despite "adequate" DO_2. Under these circumstances, the MvO_2 can be paradoxically normal. These parameters can be determined using a pulmonary artery catheter. The data obtained may be useful in individual patients, but randomized, controlled trials show no benefit when the pulmonary artery catheter is used routinely to guide therapy.

The pathophysiologic mechanisms of type I respiratory failure are listed in Table 1. The most common mechanism is ventilation–perfusion $\dot{V}/\dot{Q}$ mismatch, characterized by a widened A–a O_2 gradient, a dramatic increase in PaO_2 in response to supplemental O_2, and a variable $PaCO_2$. When areas of low $\dot{V}/\dot{Q}$ predominate (e.g., reduced ventilation with normal perfusion), the $PaCO_2$ may be low as the patient hyperventilates in an effort (only partially effective) to increase the PaO_2. When areas of high $\dot{V}/\dot{Q}$ predominate, much ventilation is wasted, and hypercapnia is also present. Areas of lung that are perfused but not ventilated characterize shunt. The resulting fall in PaO_2 depends on the percentage of cardiac output circulating through the shunt and the O_2 content of that blood. Supplemental O_2 has minimal or small effect on PaO_2 because the shunted blood is not exposed to the increased FiO_2. Therefore, treatment is aimed at decreasing shunt by improving ventilation to the affected area or reducing perfusion to that area. When shunt results from a unilateral process (e.g., pneumonia, atelectasis), placing the good lung in the dependent position decreases shunt perfusion, and oxygenation improves.

Acute Hypercapneic Respiratory Failure

Hypercapneic respiratory failure is defined as a $PaCO_2$ greater than 45 mm Hg. The equation used to determine $PaCO_2$ provides insight into the three basic mechanisms underlying hypercapnia:

$$PaCO_2 = k\left(\dot{V}CO_2\right)/V_E\left(1 - V_D/V_T\right)$$

where k is a constant, V_E is total minute ventilation (respiratory rate times tidal volume), and V_D/V_T is the dead space. Therefore, hypercapnia can result from increased CO_2 production $\dot{V}CO_2$, increased physiologic dead space (V_D/V_T), and decreased minute ventilation (Box 1). Increased VCO_2 alone is usually insufficient to cause hypercapnia because the respiratory system responds by increasing minute ventilation to keep $PaCO_2$ normal (37 to 43 mm Hg). Conversely, with abnormalities of respiratory muscle function or respiratory drive, or with increased dead space (and

BOX 1 Pathophysiologic Mechanisms of Hypercapnia

Increased Carbon Dioxide Production $\left(\dot{V}CO_2\right)$
Fever
Overfeeding
Seizure
Sepsis
Thyrotoxicosis

Decreased Ventilation (V_E)
Depressed respiratory drive
Phrenic nerve injury
Respiratory muscle weakness

Increased Dead Space (V_D/V_T)
Acute exacerbation of chronic obstructive pulmonary disease
Interstitial lung disease (e.g., pneumonia, interstitial fibrosis, etc.)
Pulmonary vascular disease

diminished reserve), the respiratory response to increased $\dot{V}CO_2$ may be insufficient, and hypercapnia results.

Treatment

Treatment of acute hypoxemic and hypercapneic respiratory failure combines nonspecific (e.g., supplemental O_2, mechanical ventilation) and specific therapy (Boxes 2 and 3).

Oxygen Therapy

In the hospital, 100% O_2 is supplied from a wall source with a regulator determining flow rate in liters per minute. The final delivered oxygen concentration (FiO_2) depends on this flow rate and the amount of room air breathed by the patient. The O_2 flow rate is almost never sufficient to meet all of the patient's ventilatory demands, so varying amounts of room air are entrained to meet these needs. The final inspired oxygen concentration depends on the relative fraction of each gas, total minute ventilation, and the pattern of breathing (including the inspiratory-to-expiratory ratio). O_2 may be administered using nasal prongs, a facial mask, or high-flow devices designed to deliver higher FiO_2 (Table 2). High-flow nasal cannula (HFNC) devices are more capable of meeting the inspiratory flow demands during respiratory distress (in excess of 40 L/min) and more reliably deliver the set FiO_2 because they can overcome the entrainment phenomenon. Other reported benefits of HFNC include reduction in respiratory rate and work of breathing and increased end expiratory lung volume. A modest amount of positive end expiratory pressure, approximately 0 to 5 cm H_2O, is supplied by HFNC when breathing with a closed mouth.

Regardless of oxygenation strategy it is important to titrate oxygen support to physiologic endpoints, generally a $SaO_2 > 92\%$. Recent clinical data suggest evidence of potential harm

BOX 2 Causes of and Treatments for Acute Hypoxemic Respiratory Failure

Acute Exacerbation of Chronic Obstructive Pulmonary Disease
Antibiotics
Bronchodilators
Systemic steroids

Acute Respiratory Distress Syndrome
Efforts to decrease lung water
Lung-protective mechanical ventilation
Treatment of specific etiology or removal of injurious trigger

Congestive Heart Failure
Afterload reduction
Diuretics
Inotropes

Lobar Collapse or Atelectasis
Bronchoscopy
Pulmonary toilet (airway suctioning to improve clearance of secretions)

Pneumonia
Antibiotics
Chest physiotherapy

Pneumothorax
Tube thoracostomy to drain pleural air and facilitate lung re-expansion

Pulmonary Embolism
Anticoagulation
Thrombolytic therapy

Status Asthmaticus
Bronchodilators
Systemic steroids

BOX 3 Causes of and Treatments for Acute Hypercapneic Respiratory Failure

Acute Exacerbation of Chronic Obstructive Pulmonary Disease
Antibiotics
Bronchodilators
Systemic steroids

Acute Respiratory Muscle Weakness (e.g., myasthenic crisis)
Acetylcholinesterase therapy

Drug Overdose
Flumazenil (Romazicon)
Naloxone (Narcan)
Other antidotes

Guillain-Barré Syndrome[1]
Immunoglobulin[1]
Plasmapheresis

Spinal Cord Injury
Intravenous methylprednisolone[1]

Status Asthmaticus
Bronchodilators
Systemic steroids

Toxin (e.g., botulinum toxin)
Antitoxin

[1]Not FDA approved for this indication.

for supraphysiologic blood oxygen tensions, and that an upper limit of supplemental oxygenation should be observed in all patients. The goal here is likely a PaO_2 between 70 and 120 mm Hg with an upper threshold of 98% SaO_2, though this requires further prospective evaluation. In hypercapneic patients (e.g., with AECOPD), high-flow O_2 can lead to worsening hypercapnia and acute respiratory acidosis. The mechanisms are multifactorial: worsening V/Q matching (increased dead space), decreased intracellular binding of CO_2, and minute ventilation inadequate for the amount of CO_2 produced. Therefore, the goal in these patients is to achieve a PaO_2 of 55 to 60 mm Hg (SaO_2 88% to 90%) with low-flow oxygen (~24% to 28% O_2). If this (often delicate) balance between maintaining tissue oxygenation and avoiding significant respiratory acidosis cannot be achieved, short-term mechanical ventilation may be required.

Mechanical Ventilation

Mechanical ventilation can be delivered noninvasively through a tight-fitting face mask or invasively via an endotracheal tube. The goals of mechanical ventilation are to correct severe arterial blood gas abnormalities, provide respiratory support while specific therapy is used, and unload and rest the respiratory muscles. The ventilator should be set to optimize patient–ventilator interaction and avoid dynamic hyperinflation and intrinsic positive end-expiratory pressure (PEEPi). PEEPi can worsen gas exchange, predispose to barotrauma, and cause hypotension.

Noninvasive Ventilation

Noninvasive ventilation is most commonly applied as continuous positive airway pressure (CPAP), when airway pressure is kept constant throughout the respiratory cycle, or by bilevel positive airway pressure (BiPAP), when inspiratory pressure support actively assists each inspiration. Noninvasive ventilation offers numerous advantages over invasive ventilation, including increased comfort; maintenance of normal swallowing, speech, and cough; less need for sedation; and avoiding the trauma of intubation.

The effective application of noninvasive ventilation starts with carefully explaining the procedure to the patient, followed by selection of a proper-fitting face mask. The mask is placed close to the face to acclimate the patient to high inspiratory flow. The mask is then secured using straps (but not too tightly), and ventilator settings are adjusted to minimize leaks and ensure comfort. The patient is reassessed frequently. Failure to improve within 2 to 4 hours (e.g., reduction in dyspnea, respiratory rate, accessory muscle use, and hypercapnia) signals noninvasive ventilation failure and need for intubation.

Noninvasive ventilation improves outcome (avoids intubation, decreases length of stay, improves survival) in a number of conditions (Table 3). Although randomized, controlled trials show dramatic benefit in AECOPD, other studies show no or uncertain benefit in community-acquired pneumonia, ARDS, pulmonary fibrosis, and routinely after planned extubation. One mechanism for improved outcome is the reduction in infection (pneumonia, sepsis) seen with noninvasive ventilation compared with intubated patients. Noninvasive ventilation should not be used in the presence of respiratory arrest, shock, excessive secretions, inability to protect the airway, an agitated or uncooperative patient, and facial abnormalities that preclude proper application of the mask. Comparison of noninvasive ventilation to high-flow nasal cannula in ARDS suggests evidence of harm in patients with more severe hypoxemia. This phenomenon is hypothesized to be related to ventilator-induced lung injury where tidal volumes are less strictly regulated in noninvasive as compared to invasive ventilation.

Invasive Ventilation

Invasive mechanical ventilation is delivered via an endotracheal tube. The set parameters include FiO_2 and positive end-expiratory pressure (PEEP). For volume-assist control, the clinician chooses respiratory rate and tidal volume. For pressure support, the clinician chooses the inspiratory pressure level above PEEP, and the patient determines respiratory rate. The

TABLE 2	Short-Term Oxygen Delivery Systems			
DELIVERY SYSTEM	**O$_2$ FLOW RATE (L/MIN)**	**FIO$_2$ RANGE**		**COMMENTS**
Basic Systems				
Nasal cannula (prongs)	1–6	0.22–0.40		Comfortable
				Facilitates communication and oral intake
				Humidification required at high flow rates
Simple masks	5–6	0.30–0.50		Mask acts as reservoir to increase FiO$_2$
				High flow combats CO$_2$ rebreathing
				Less comfortable
				Must be removed to facilitate communication and oral intake
				Easily displaced with movement
Reservoir Masks				
Nonrebreathing	4–10	0.60–1.00		One-way valve between the mask and the reservoir bag
				Inspired O$_2$ from wall source and reservoir bag
Partial rebreathing	5–10	0.35–0.90		Lacks one-way valve
Venturi masks	4–10	0.24–0.40		Uses Bernoulli principle (fixed amount of entrained room air added to O$_2$)
				Maximum delivered FiO$_2$ can be controlled
				Often used in COPD to avoid excessive FiO$_2$ and risk for hypercapnia
High-flow nasal cannula	10–60	0.21–1		Can overcome room air entrainment, set FiO$_2$ more accurate
				Generates modest amount of positive end expiratory pressure
				Reduces CO$_2$ rebreathing by anatomic dead space washout
				Reduction in work of breathing in select patients

COPD, Chronic obstructive pulmonary disease; *FiO$_2$,* fraction of inspired oxygen.

resulting tidal volume depends on inspiratory pressure level and patient factors including respiratory muscle strength and respiratory system mechanics. Initially the ventilator is set to meet most of the patient's minute ventilation, allowing respiratory muscle rest. Such full support should not be prolonged because diaphragmatic dysfunction can result. Most patients require sedation, but excessive sedation levels are associated with worse outcomes. Therefore, strategies to minimize continuous intravenous sedation using a sedation protocol or once-daily interruption of sedation are recommended.

Invasive mechanical ventilation, especially when prolonged, is associated with numerous complications including ventilator-associated pneumonia, sinusitis, airway injury, thromboembolism, and gastrointestinal bleeding. Therefore, once significant clinical improvement occurs, efforts should focus on rapidly removing the patient from the ventilator. This is achieved by daily screening for readiness (Box 4) followed by a 30- to 120-minute spontaneous breathing trial on minimal or no ventilator support. Patients tolerating the spontaneous breathing trial are extubated if they have a good cough, manageable respiratory secretions, and an adequate mental status to protect the airway. Approximately 25% of patients do not tolerate the spontaneous breathing trial; they should be returned to full ventilator support for 24 hours and undergo careful evaluation for reversible causes. The clinician should consider a more gradual approach to weaning these patients.

Specific Causes of Acute Respiratory Failure
Acute Exacerbation of Chronic Obstructive Pulmonary Disease
Patients with COPD can experience two or three exacerbations per year, especially if they are actively smoking. The best predictor of future exacerbations is a history of previous exacerbations. Other risk factors for exacerbation include serum eosinophilia, pulmonary hypertension and gastric reflux. Hospital mortality ranges from 2% to 11%, rising to 25% for those requiring critical care.

AECOPD is defined by increased sputum volume, purulence, and dyspnea. Physical examination is notable for tachypnea, use of accessory respiratory muscles, diminished breath sounds, prolonged expiratory phase with wheezing, thoraco-abdominal paradox (inward inspiratory abdominal motion), and Hoover sign (inward inspiratory motion of the lower rib cage). The latter two physical signs indicate the presence of dynamic hyperinflation and diaphragmatic dysfunction. AECOPD is further characterized by hypoxemia (resulting from V̇/Q̇ mismatch) and hypercapnia. Patients with more severe underlying disease might demonstrate evidence of acute and chronic respiratory acidosis.

Etiology and Diagnosis
Approximately 50% of AECOPDs result from bacterial infection (e.g., *Pneumococcus* species, *Haemophilus influenzae*, *Moraxella catarrhalis*, and *Pseudomonas* species). The remainder result from viral infection and air pollution. In many cases a cause cannot be identified, although there is increasing appreciation that acute myocardial infarction and pulmonary embolism may be present in up to 25%. Pulmonary embolism may be suggested by a PaCO$_2$ lower than baseline and the need for a higher than expected FiO$_2$ to maintain the SaO$_2$ at greater than 90%. Computed tomographic pulmonary arteriogram is recommended to make the diagnosis, because V̇/Q̇ scanning is nondiagnostic in nearly half of COPD patients, and false-positive high-probability scans occur.

Treatment
Treatment for AECOPD is based on high-quality evidence consisting of numerous randomized, controlled trials and well-performed meta-analyses. Bronchodilator therapy is essential. Nebulized combination therapy (albuterol and ipratropium [DuoNeb]) is effective, but it is not demonstrably superior to single-agent therapy delivered via a metered-dose inhaler. Theophylline should generally be avoided because toxicity outweighs benefits. Antibiotics improve outcome, especially in the

TABLE 3 — Efficacy of Noninvasive Ventilation in Various Conditions

CONDITION	QUALITY OF EVIDENCE	COMMENT
AECOPD	Strong	↓ Need for intubation
		↓ Nosocomial pneumonia
		↑ Survival
Acute cardiogenic pulmonary edema	Strong	↓ Need for intubation
		↑ Survival
Facilitating weaning in select patients	Strong	↓ Duration of intubation
		Most effective in AECOPD
High risk for extubation failure	Strong	↓ Need for reintubation
Extubation failure in heterogeneous patient population	Moderate	Not effective, two RCTs
Routinely after extubation	Moderate	Not effective, single RCT
Extubation failure in AECOPD	Moderate	Single case-control study
Type I RF, diffuse infiltrates, not ICH	Moderate	↓ Need for intubation
		May ↓ survival, requires close monitoring
Hypoxemic respiratory in ICH with diffuse pulmonary infiltrates	Moderate	↓ Need for intubation
		↑ Survival
Postoperative respiratory failure	Moderate	↓ Need for intubation
		↓ Nosocomial pneumonia
		↑ Survival
Asthma	Weak	Uncertain effect on mortality
		Uncertain effect on intubation
		Benefit may be in ACOS
Obesity hypoventilation	No RCTs	Probably effective in ↓ need for intubation
Do not intubate patients	Observational studies	Most effective with CHF, COPD
Pulmonary fibrosis	Observational studies	Not effective

ACOS, Asthma COPD Overlap Syndrome; *AECOPD*, acute exacerbation of chronic obstructive pulmonary disease; *CHF*, cardiogenic pulmonary edema; *COPD*, chronic obstructive pulmonary disease; *FiO₂*, fraction of inspired oxygen; *ICH*, immunocompromised host; *RCT*, randomized, controlled trial; *RF*, respiratory failure.

BOX 4 — Screening Criteria to Assess Readiness to Undergo a Trial of Spontaneous Breathing

Required Criteria
$PaO_2/FiO_2 \geq 150$ or $SaO_2 \geq 90\%$ or $FiO_2 \leq 40\%$ and PEEP ≤5 cm H_2O
Absence of hypotension

Additional Criteria (optional criteria)
Weaning parameters*
- Negative inspiratory force <–20 to –25 cm H_2O
- Respiratory rate (f) ≤35 breaths/min
- Spontaneous tidal volume (V_T) >5 mL/kg
- f/V_T <105 breaths/L per min

Absence of significant anemia (e.g., Hb ≥8–10 mg/dL)
Absence of fever (e.g., core temperature ≤38.5°C)
Adequate mental status: patient awake and alert or easily aroused.

---

* Recent studies indicate that these parameters are often unnecessary in deciding whether to initiate trials of spontaneous breathing.
Hb, Hemoglobin; *PEEP*, positive end-expiratory pressure.

---

presence of fever and increased sputum purulence and volume. Older agents, such as amoxicillin and tetracycline, appear to be less effective than newer macrolides and fluoroquinolones though local resistance patterns should drive antibiotic selection.

Corticosteroids enhance β-agonist activity and counteract the inflammatory state seen in AECOPD. Oral prednisone at a dose of 30 to 40 mg is recommended with a duration of 5 days being noninferior to longer courses. Intravenous therapy (methylprednisolone [Solu-Medrol] 125 mg every 6 hours for 72 hours followed by oral prednisone) should be used in the critically ill patient or when response to oral therapy is suboptimal. There is no role for mucolytic agents or chest physiotherapy during acute exacerbation. Continuation of beta blockers, previously thought to contribute to bronchoconstriction, may in fact be associated with decreased mortality and exacerbations because of impact on COPD comorbidities such as coronary artery disease.

Admission to the intensive care unit (ICU) is indicated for patients with hemodynamic instability, confusion, lethargy and coma, severe dyspnea unresponsive to emergency management, or severely abnormal gas exchange despite initial therapy (PaO_2 <40 mm Hg, $PaCO_2$ >60 mm Hg, pH <7.25). Randomized, controlled trials demonstrate that noninvasive ventilation decreases the risk for intubation and improves survival in AECOPD when there is severe dyspnea, hypoxemia, tachypnea, and significant respiratory acidosis ($PaCO_2$ >45 mm Hg and pH <7.35). Patients who fail noninvasive ventilation or who are not candidates require intubation and mechanical ventilation.

A major risk is the development of dynamic hyperinflation (PEEPi), which occurs when expiratory time is not sufficient to reach functional residual capacity. The resulting air trapping within the thorax can worsen gas exchange, predispose to barotrauma (e.g., pneumothorax), and cause hypotension. PEEPi is minimized by keeping delivered minute ventilation at 5 L/min or less; achieved by lowering tidal volume (e.g., 6 mL/kg ideal body weight) or respiratory rate (8 to 10 breaths/min), or by increasing inspiratory flow rate, allowing more time for expiration. PEEPi is suggested by an elevated plateau pressure or persistent expiratory flow at the time of the next ventilator breath. PEEPi can also increase work of breathing by increasing the patient's inspiratory effort to trigger the ventilator. When extrinsic PEEP is at or just below the PEEPi level, the patient triggers more easily and work of breathing is reduced. The approach to weaning and extubation in AECOPD is similar to that for other conditions, although the risk of failing a spontaneous breathing trial is increased.

Acute Respiratory Distress Syndrome
Etiology and Diagnosis
ARDS is the result of an acute process and is characterized by hypoxemia (PaO_2/FiO_2 <300) with bilateral diffuse alveolar infiltrates, and no evidence of cardiac etiology. Lung injury in this syndrome can result from both pulmonary and extrapulmonary etiologies. Pulmonary causes include pneumonia, gastric aspiration, near drowning, toxic gas inhalation, medication side effects, and lung contusion. Extrapulmonary causes include sepsis, pancreatitis, fat embolism, drug overdose, nonthoracic trauma, and massive transfusion. Conditions that can mimic the clinical findings of ARDS include CHF, diffuse alveolar hemorrhage (DAH), acute cryptogenic organizing pneumonia (COP), and acute eosinophilic pneumonia (AEP). These latter three entities can be diagnosed by bronchoscopy (DAH, AEP) or by open lung biopsy (COP), all of which are treated with high doses of corticosteroids.

Differentiating cardiogenic pulmonary edema from ARDS can be challenging, especially because these conditions can coexist. Physical findings of jugular venous distention and a positive third heart sound, abnormal electrocardiogram (ECG), elevated brain natriuretic peptide (BNP), and positive cardiac enzymes (troponin) point to a cardiac etiology. A chest radiograph showing cardiomegaly, vascular redistribution, widened vascular pedicle, perihilar alveolar infiltrates, and pleural effusions also suggests a cardiac cause. Bedside echocardiography can demonstrate reduced left ventricular function. A pulmonary artery catheter provides definitive evidence of an elevated pulmonary capillary wedge pressure and reduced cardiac output. That said, recent randomized, controlled trials demonstrate no improvement in survival with routine use of the pulmonary artery catheter in ARDS.

Treatment
The first principle of ARDS management is to prevent further lung injury by employing a lung protective ventilation strategy limiting the transpulmonary pressure, using the plateau pressure as a surrogate. In general this is accomplished by titrating the set tidal volume to 6 to 8 mL/kg of ideal body weight. Once this is achieved the tidal volume is titrated down to achieve a plateau pressure of 30 cm H_2O or less, with lower pressures being more protective. This plateau pressure is measured on the ventilator with an inspiratory hold, and approximates the alveolar pressure. Failing to accomplish this places the lungs at risk for further injury by creating significant shear stress with repeated opening of atelectatic areas (atelectrauma) and overdistending less affected areas (volutrauma, barotrauma). Using small tidal volumes often results in significant hypercapnia, which can have an independent protective effect (permissive hypercapnia). The application of PEEP recruits and opens atelectatic lung, thereby reducing harmful shear forces. The optimal level of PEEP remains uncertain; individual studies have tended to show no mortality benefit of a high PEEP versus a low PEEP ventilatory strategy, however trends in mortality reduction and decreased salvage therapy are seen with a higher PEEP strategy in meta-analysis.

The severity of ARDS is generally subdivided by PaO_2/FiO_2 ratios indicating mild (300 to 200), moderate (200 to 100), and severe (<100) disease; these thresholds correspond to rising risk of mortality. A PaO_2/FiO_2 ratio of less than 150 suggests a higher mortality ARDS phenotype where therapy in addition to lung protective ventilation may provide benefit. Placing the patient in the prone position appears to reduce mortality. The routine use of neuromuscular blockade is controversial with the most recent trial indicating no mortality benefit. Inhaled pulmonary vasodilators, used to optimize V/Q matching, do improve oxygenation but have no impact on mortality. The benefit of extracorporeal membrane oxygenation is yet unclear and is reserved for very severe, high-mortality disease to be used in expert centers. The use of corticosteroids lacked an evidence basis for many years; recent data is suggestive of benefit in a mixed population of ARDS with early use. The clearest benefit of steroids has been seen with treatment of ARDS related to SARs-CoV2 infection, where multiple randomized trials have confirmed a significant mortality benefit.

Cardiogenic Pulmonary Edema
Cardiogenic pulmonary edema occurs in patients with cardiomyopathy or acutely when ischemia is present. Diagnosis is suggested by jugular venous distension, a third heart sound, diffuse rales, abnormal ECG, and a chest radiograph showing cardiomegaly, diffuse alveolar infiltrates, and bilateral pleural effusion. A markedly elevated BNP or pro-BNP further suggests a cardiac etiology.

Therapy consists of oxygen, nitrates, diuretics, afterload reduction, and anti-ischemic therapy if the history or ECG is suggestive. Mechanical ventilation produces positive intrathoracic pressure, which improves cardiac function by decreasing both left ventricular preload and afterload, reversing hypoxemia, and decreasing work of breathing. In hemodynamically stable patients without active ischemia, CPAP at levels of 8 to 12 cm H_2O should be used. A meta-analysis of 15 randomized, controlled trials showed that noninvasive ventilation decreased the need for intubation and improved survival. CPAP and BiPAP appear to be equivalent, although many prefer BiPAP when hypercapnia is present.

Because cardiogenic pulmonary edema is rapidly reversible, intubated patients can often be extubated within 24 hours. That said, the transition from positive pressure ventilation to negative ventilation (e.g., T-piece or extubation) can precipitate pulmonary edema. These patients may benefit from lower peri-extubation respiratory support to anticipate postextubation pulmonary edema.

References
Acute Respiratory Distress Syndrome: The Berlin Definition, *JAMA* 307(23), 2012.

Acute Respiratory Distress Syndrome Network: Ventilation with lower tidal volumes as compared with traditional tidal volumes for acute lung injury and the acute respiratory distress syndrome, *N Engl J Med* 342:1301–1308, 2000.

Briel M, Meade M, Mercat A, et al: Higher vs lower positive end-expiratory pressure in patients with acute lung injury and acute respiratory distress syndrome: Systematic review and meta-analysis, *JAMA* 303(9):865, 2010.

Ely EW, Baker AM, Dunagan DP, et al: Effect on the duration of mechanical ventilation of identifying patients capable of breathing spontaneously, *N Engl J Med* 335:1864–1869, 1996.

Epstein SK: Complications in ventilator supported patients. In Tobin M, editor: *Principles and Practice of Mechanical Ventilation*, New York, 2006, McGraw Hill, pp 877–902.

Frat J-P, Thille AW, Mercat A, et al: High-flow oxygen through nasal cannula in acute hypoxemic respiratory failure, *N Engl J Med* 372(23):2185–2196, 2015.

Girardis M, Busani S, Damiani E, et al: Effect of conservative vs conventional oxygen therapy on mortality among patients in an intensive care unit: the oxygen-icu randomized clinical trial, *JAMA* 316(15):1583, 2016.

Kress JP, Pohlman AS, O'Connor MF, et al: Daily interruption of sedative infusions in critically ill patients undergoing mechanical ventilation, *N Engl J Med* 342:1471–1477, 2000.

Masip J, Peacock WF, Price S, et al: Indications and practical approach to noninvasive ventilation in acute heart failure, *European Heart Journal* 39(1):17–25, 2018.

Ouellette DR, Patel S, Girard TD, et al: Liberation from mechanical ventilation in critically ill adults: An official American College of Chest Physicians/American Thoracic Society Clinical Practice Guideline, *Chest* 151(1):166–180, 2017.

Rochwerg B, Brochard L, Elliott MW, et al: Official ERS/ATS clinical practice guidelines: noninvasive ventilation for acute respiratory failure, *Eur Respir J* 50(2):1602426, 2017.

Vogelmeier CF, Criner GJ, Martinez FJ, et al: Global strategy for the diagnosis, management, and prevention of chronic obstructive lung disease 2017 report. GOLD Executive Summary, *Am J Respir Crit Care Med* 195(5):557–582, 2017.

ASTHMA IN ADOLESCENTS AND ADULTS

Method of
Matthew A. Rank, MD; and Michael Schatz, MD, MS

CURRENT DIAGNOSIS

- Confirm the diagnosis by demonstrating an increase in forced expiratory volume in 1 second (FEV_1) or the forced vital capacity (FVC) by 10% or more after asthma therapy.
- Assess past severity by a history of exacerbations requiring oral corticosteroids, emergency department visits, hospitalization, or intubation.
- Identify environmental exposures, allergic sensitization, and comorbidities that may be aggravating asthma.
- Assess asthma based on symptom frequency, nocturnal awakenings, rescue therapy use, activity limitation, spirometry, and recent exacerbation history.

CURRENT THERAPY

- Nonpharmacologic therapy includes asthma education (especially regarding inhaler technique, self-monitoring, self-management, and importance of adherence to medication), reduction in environmental triggers, addressing any relevant psychosocial issues, and allergen immunotherapy for select patients.
- Preferred step therapy for long-term asthma management is low-dose inhaled corticosteroids, either scheduled or as needed, for mild asthma; low- or medium-dose inhaled corticosteroids combined with formoterol[1] scheduled and as needed for moderate asthma; and medium- or high-dose inhaled corticosteroids plus long-acting β agonists for severe asthma, plus additional consideration for other add-on therapies (long-acting muscarinic antagonist macrolide antibiotics, biologics, and oral prednisone).
- Asthma exacerbations should be treated with high-dose inhaled β agonists and early use of systemic corticosteroids.

[1]Not FDA approved for this indication.

Asthma is an extremely common chronic medical condition that causes substantial morbidity among its sufferers. In addition to discomfort, asthma can cause sleep disruption, missed school and work, limitations of recreational activities, and acute episodes requiring emergency hospital care. Although the past 40 years have seen the introduction of increasingly effective and convenient medications, recent surveys continue to suggest that asthma remains suboptimally controlled in a substantial proportion of patients. The purpose of this chapter is to describe an approach to assessment and therapy that leads to optimal asthma control. It is based on the Global Strategy for Asthma Management and Prevention (Global Initiative for Asthma [GINA] 2024) update and the 2020 Focused Updates to the Asthma Management Guidelines from the National Heart, Lung, and Blood Institute, but it includes recommendations from multiple sources.

Diagnosis

The first step in evaluating a patient with asthma is to confirm the diagnosis. This is particularly important in patients with atypical symptoms or a poor response to asthma therapy. Asthma is confirmed by demonstration of reversible airways obstruction, which most commonly is an increase in FEV_1 or FVC by 10% or greater for adults and adolescents. For some patients, 2 to 4 weeks of chronic inhaled asthma therapy or 2 weeks of oral corticosteroid therapy are necessary to demonstrate reversibility. The latter is particularly important in adults with a history of smoking in whom chronic obstructive pulmonary disease (COPD) is a diagnostic consideration. In patients with normal pulmonary function, asthma can also be confirmed by means of methacholine (Provocholine) or exercise challenge, which are two forms of a provocation challenge, along with before and after pulmonary function tests. In addition, an elevated fractional exhaled nitric oxide (FENO >50 ppb) can be suggestive of a diagnosis of asthma.

Particularly important masqueraders of asthma include vocal cord dysfunction, panic attacks, hyperventilation, deconditioning, and cough caused by postnasal drip, reflux, or angiotensin-converting enzyme (ACE) inhibitor therapy. All of these can also coexist with asthma, so their presence does not exclude asthma. Even when these conditions coexist with asthma, their diagnosis and appropriate therapy usually reduce the patient's respiratory symptoms. Other diagnostic considerations include syndromes of which asthma represents one part: allergic bronchopulmonary aspergillosis, eosinophilic granulomatosis with polyangiitis, and aspirin-exacerbated respiratory disease.

Assessment
Assessment of patients with asthma involves gathering details of past severity, identifying aggravating factors, and defining current asthma control status.

Current Status
Assessment of the current therapy the patient is actually taking is necessary for understanding the asthma's severity and to appropriately initiate or change therapy. It is particularly important to determine whether the patient is taking long-term control medications, such as inhaled corticosteroids, long-acting β agonists, leukotriene modifiers, long-acting muscarinic antagonists, oral corticosteroids, macrolides, or biologics. Both asthma control and risk factors for future exacerbations should be considered. Patients with at least three of the following symptoms in the past 4 weeks are defined as *uncontrolled* in the GINA 2024 guidelines: daytime asthma symptoms more than twice a week, night waking caused by asthma, rescue treatments more than twice a week other than use as pretreatment for exercise, and any activity limitation caused by asthma. Other tools to assess asthma control, such as the Asthma Control Test or the Asthma Control Questionnaire, can also be used to determine asthma control (Table 1).

Asthma can be a mild, infrequent illness or a severe daily one. Certain severity markers identify patients who are more likely to experience severe exacerbations or to have symptoms that are more difficult to control and who thus require more careful surveillance. These include a history of asthma hospitalization, especially requiring intensive care or intubation, past requirement for oral corticosteroids, and specific comorbid conditions (Table 2). In patients with prior severe exacerbations, the rapidity of the onset of the exacerbation should be ascertained. Some patients may have minimal day-to-day asthma symptoms but still have a high risk for asthma exacerbations.

Aggravating Factors
Factors that appear to trigger asthma symptoms should be assessed because they may be targets for avoidance therapy. Certain aspects of the patient's environment that can contribute to asthma triggering should be specifically ascertained, including occupational exposures, age of the home, pets, carpeting, visible mold, active or passive smoke, rodent, and cockroach exposure. Patients with persistent asthma should have in vitro or skin tests to identify allergic sensitization to pollens, house dust mites, mold spores, animal dander, and cockroaches that can contribute to the maintenance of asthma inflammation or can trigger episodes. The presence of comorbidities that can aggravate asthma, including obesity, rhinitis, sinusitis, gastroesophageal reflux, obstructive sleep apnea, and COPD, should be identified and treated. Finally, psychosocial factors to assess include a history or symptoms of anxiety or depression, attitudes toward asthma and asthma therapy, adherence to therapy, and social

TABLE 1 Determining Asthma Control in Patients 12 Years of Age and Older*

IN THE PAST 4 WEEKS, HAS THE PATIENT HAD	WELL CONTROLLED	PARTLY CONTROLLED	UNCONTROLLED
Daytime asthma symptoms more than two times per week?	None of these	1 to 2 of these	3 to 4 of these
Any night waking caused by asthma?			
Rescue needed more than two times per week other than for pretreatment for exercise?			
Any activity limitation caused by asthma?			

*Modified from Global Initiative for Asthma (GINA) 2023 guideline. Can consider using the Asthma Control Test or Asthma Control Questionnaire as other ways to assess asthma symptom control.

TABLE 2 Risk Factors for Future Asthma Exacerbations in Patients 12 Years of Age and Older*

Ever intubated or in the intensive care unit for asthma

Had one or more severe exacerbations in the past year

Frequent use of rescue inhaler (more than 200 puffs of rescue inhaler per month) or ≥3 rescue inhalers per year

Not adherent to ICS with good technique

Comorbid conditions: obesity, chronic rhinosinusitis, GERD, confirmed food allergy, pregnancy

Psychological or socioeconomic challenges

Low lung function: FEV_1 % predicted <60%, high bronchodilator reversibility

Exposures: Smoking, e-cigarettes, allergen exposure if sensitized, and air pollution

High blood eosinophils and high fractional exhaled nitric oxide

*Any of these risk factors increases the risk for exacerbations, even if the patient has few day-to-day asthma symptoms.
FEV_1, Forced expiratory volume in 1 second; GERD, gastroesophageal reflux disease; ICS, inhaled corticosteroid.
Modified from Global Initiative for Asthma (GINA) 2023 guideline.

support. These may be targets for therapy or may be helpful when creating an effective therapeutic plan and therapeutic alliance.

Long-Term Management
Nonpharmacologic Therapy
The first tenet of nonpharmacologic therapy in the long-term management of asthma is education. Patients must understand the inflammatory pathophysiology of asthma and the relationships among airway inflammation, bronchospasm, and symptoms. Patients should be informed that the cause of asthma is unknown and that there is no cure, but triggers can be identified and asthma can be controlled. They should receive education regarding self-assessment, either based on symptoms or peak flow monitoring, and regarding the recognition of early signs of an impending exacerbation.

The next step is to discuss and agree on the goals of therapy. Long-term goals of asthma management include the following:
- Achieve good control of symptoms.
- Maintain optimal pulmonary function.
- Maintain normal activity, including work, school, leisure activity, sleep, and exercise.
- Prevent recurrent exacerbations, especially those requiring urgent medical visits.
- Provide pharmacotherapy with minimal or no adverse effects.
- Achieve patient and family satisfaction with asthma care.

The healthcare provider should let the patient know that these are the expectations of optimal management and confirm that they are the patient's goals as well.

A very important component of nonpharmacologic therapy is the reduction of relevant environmental triggers. Information should be given regarding environmental control of pollen, mites, mold, animal dander, and cockroach antigens (Box 1) that appear to be relevant based on the history and results of skin or in vitro specific IgE tests. A multifaceted environmental mitigation plan is favored over single interventions. Inhalant allergen immunotherapy should be considered for patients who have persistent asthma when there is clear evidence of a relationship between symptoms and exposure to an allergen to which the patient is sensitive.

Pulmonary rehabilitation may be considered for people with shortness of breath and significant airflow obstruction.

Vaccination to reduce risks associated with respiratory infections is recommended and includes annual vaccines for influenza, updated vaccines for COVID-19, pertussis vaccination every 10 years, respiratory syncytial virus for people older than 60 years, and pneumococcal vaccine (PSV-20) for people with asthma older than 19 years.

Finally, psychosocial issues should be considered and addressed. For many patients, the education and therapeutic alliance described earlier adequately addresses psychosocial concerns. For other patients, poor past adherence requires identifying the barriers to adherence and finding solutions together. Resources for patients with poor social support should be identified. Clinically significant anxiety or depression that can make asthma harder to control should be treated.

Pharmacologic Step Therapy
The main principle of asthma pharmacologic step therapy is to add therapy in steps until control is achieved (step up) and decrease therapy in reverse steps (step down) to establish the lowest effective dose necessary to maintain control.

There are two types of asthma medications: quick-relief medications (Table 3) and long-term control medications (Table 4). Systemic corticosteroids can be used either short term to treat an exacerbation (see Table 3) or as long-term maintenance therapy for patients with severe disease (see Table 4). The generally recommended steps of pharmacologic therapy are shown in Table 5. Definitions of low-, medium-, and high-dose inhaled corticosteroids for each of the available preparations are given in Table 6. At each therapeutic step level, the GINA guideline has indicated preferred medications, which generally identify medications with the best balance of efficacy and safety in clinical trials for patients at that level of severity. However, these recommendations are based on population data and must be tailored to individual patient needs, circumstances, and responsiveness to therapy.

All patients with asthma should have an action plan that describes their pharmacologic self-management. Aspects of pharmacologic self-management include maintenance of the medication schedule, rescue therapy doses for increased symptoms, when and how to increase controller medication therapy, when and how to use prednisone, how to recognize a severe exacerbation, and when and how to seek urgent or emergency care. Controller medications may be increased with an upper respiratory infection or with symptoms requiring more than two doses of rescue therapy in 12 hours. Although doubling the dose of inhaled corticosteroids does not appear to generally be sufficient to provide a clinical benefit under these circumstances, quadrupling or

BOX 1 Measures to Control Environmental Factors That Can Worsen Asthma

Allergens

An approach that considers multiple relevant triggers is most likely to be successful.

Animal Dander

Remove the animal from the house, or, at a minimum, keep the animal out of the patient's bedroom, keep the bedroom door closed, and consider using a high-efficiency particulate air filter.

Dust Mites

Recommended

Encase mattress in a special dustproof cover.

Encase pillow in a special dustproof cover, or wash it weekly in hot water.

Wash sheets and blankets on the patient's bed in hot water weekly. Water must be hotter than 130°F to kill the mites. Cooler water used with detergent and bleach can also be effective.

Desirable

Reduce indoor humidity to 60% or less.

Remove carpets from the bedroom.

Avoid sleeping or lying on cloth-covered cushions or furniture.

Remove carpets that are laid on concrete.

Cockroaches

Keep all food out of the bedroom.

Keep food and garbage in closed containers.

Use poison baits, powders, gels, or paste (e.g., boric acid). Traps can also be used.

If a spray is used to kill cockroaches, stay out of the room until the odor goes away.

Pollens (from Trees, Grass, or Weeds) and Outdoor Molds

Try to keep windows closed.

If possible, stay indoors, with windows closed, during periods of peak pollen exposure, which are usually during the midday and afternoon.

Indoor Mold

Fix all leaks, and eliminate water sources associated with mold growth.

Clean moldy surfaces.

Dehumidify basements if possible.

Tobacco Smoke

Advise patients and others in the home who smoke to stop smoking or to smoke outside the home.

Discuss ways to reduce exposure to other sources of tobacco smoke, such as from daycare providers and the workplace.

Indoor and Outdoor Pollutants and Irritants

If possible, do not use a wood-burning stove, kerosene heater, fireplace, unvented gas stove, or heater.

Try to stay away from strong odors and sprays, such as perfume, talcum powder, hair spray, paints, new carpet, or particle board.

---

quintupling the dose may be helpful. Prednisone is usually needed for patients with incomplete or temporary responses to adequate doses of β agonists (2 to 6 puffs with a spacer, waiting at least 1 minute between puffs), substantial interference with sleep every night, requirement for 12 or more puffs of β agonist in a 24-hour period, or a peak flow less than 60% predicted. Home treatment of exacerbation is further discussed later in this chapter.

Persistent asthma is most effectively controlled with daily long-term control medications, specifically antiinflammatory therapy. For patients receiving long-term control medications, identify their current step of therapy, based on what they are actually taking (see Table 5), and their level of control (see Table 1). Data suggest that the use of antiinflammatory therapy for patients who were previously defined as having mild and intermittent asthma leads to reduced exacerbation risk and can be used as scheduled or intermittent therapy to reduce exacerbations. In general, step up one step for patients whose asthma is not well controlled. For patients with very poorly controlled asthma, consider increasing by two steps, a course of oral corticosteroids, or both. Before increasing pharmacologic therapy, consider adverse environmental exposures, poor adherence, poor inhaler technique, or comorbidities as targets for intervention. For patients with troublesome or debilitating side effects from asthma therapy, explore a change in therapy.

There are six biologic medications approved for severe asthma not controlled by standard therapy (see Table 4). These biologic medications can be considered for patients with frequent and/or severe asthma exacerbations, poor asthma control, or frequent and/or chronic use of systemic corticosteroids in spite of maximal standard therapy. It is at this point in asthma management—when considering biologics—that results from peripheral blood eosinophil counts, total serum IgE, fractional exhaled nitric oxide, and environmental skin tests can help inform biologic choice.

Follow-Up

Patients whose asthma is not controlled should be seen every 2 to 6 weeks (depending on their initial level of severity or control) until control is achieved. Once control is achieved, follow-up contact at 1- to 6-month intervals is recommended. These checkups should ensure continued control, identify other changes in the patient's status, and update the patient's action plan.

When well-controlled asthma has been maintained for at least 3 months, a step down in therapy can be considered to determine the minimum amount of medication required to maintain control or reduce the risk for side effects. Reduction in therapy should be gradual because asthma can deteriorate at a highly variable rate and intensity. Doses of inhaled corticosteroids may be reduced by about 25% to 50% every 3 months to the lowest dose possible to maintain control. Using a strategy that includes as-needed ICS can be effective for stepping down overall ICS dose. Many patients with persistent asthma relapse if inhaled corticosteroids are totally discontinued.

Patients should be encouraged to contact their asthma healthcare provider for signs of loss of asthma control, such as nocturnal symptoms, increasing β-agonist use, or activity limitation. Consultation with an asthma specialist is recommended if the patient has difficulties achieving or maintaining control of asthma, immunotherapy or an asthma biologic is being considered, the patient requires step 4 care or higher, or the patient has had an exacerbation requiring hospitalization.

Treatment of Exacerbations

Asthma exacerbations are acute or subacute episodes of progressively worsening shortness of breath, cough, wheezing, or chest tightness associated with decreases in expiratory airflow.

Home Management

Patients' action plans should direct their home therapy of asthma exacerbations according to the following recommendations.

Initial therapy can be with inhaled short-acting β agonists (2 to 6 puffs by metered-dose inhaler [MDI] or nebulizer). This may be repeated in 20 minutes. Formoterol, a rapid and long-acting β agonist, in combination with inhaled corticosteroids, can also be used for rescue treatments at home as part of a single maintenance and reliever treatment strategy, with the total number of puffs permitted varying by age and medication type (see Table 5, steps 1 to 4).[1] In 2022 Reddel et al. published an example of an action plan using SMART (see *J Allergy Clin Immunol* 1S:S31–S38, 2022). With a favorable response (minimal or no symptoms and peak expiratory

---

[1]Not FDA approved for this indication.

TABLE 3 Usual Dosages for Quick-Relief Medications for Patients 12 Years of Age and Older

MEDICATION	DOSAGE FORM	ADULT DOSE	COMMENTS
Inhaled Short-Acting β₂ Agonists (SABAs)			**Not recommended for long-term daily treatment**
Metered-Dose Inhaler		Applies to All Three SABAs	
Albuterol HFA (Proventil, Ventolin, ProAir)	90 μg/puff, 200 puffs/canister	2 puffs 5 min before exercise	An increasing use or lack of expected effect indicates diminished control of asthma.
Albuterol Breath Activated (ProAir RespiClick, ProAir Digihaler with eModule)	90 μg/puff, 200 puffs/canister	2 puffs q4–6h prn	Regular use exceeding 2 days/week for symptom control (not prevention of EIB) indicates the need for additional long-term control therapy. The Digihaler option allows for careful tracking of medicine use.
Levalbuterol HFA (Xopenex)	45 μg/puff, 200 puffs/canister	2 puffs q4–6h prn	Differences in potencies exist, but all products are essentially comparable on a per-puff basis. May double the usual dose for mild exacerbations. For levalbuterol, the patient should prime the inhaler by releasing 4 actuations before use. For HFA, periodically clean the HFA activator as the drug may block/plug the orifice. Nonselective agents (epinephrine [Primatene Mist], metaproterenol [Alupent]) are not recommended because of their potential for excessive cardiac stimulation, especially in high doses.
Nebulizer Solutions			
Albuterol (AccuNeb, Proventil)	0.63 mg/3 mL 1.25 mg/3 mL 2.5 mg/3 mL 5 mg/mL (0.5%)	1.25–5 mg in 3 mL saline q4–8h prn	May mix with budesonide (Pulmicort) inhalant suspension, cromolyn (Intal), or ipratropium (Atrovent)[1] nebulizer solutions. May double the dose for severe exacerbation.
Levalbuterol (R-albuterol) (Xopenex)	0.31 mg/3 mL 0.63 mg/3 mL 1.25 mg/0.5 mL 1.25 mg/3 mL	0.63 mg–1.25 mg q8h prn	Compatible with budesonide (Pulmicort) inhalant suspension. The product is a sterile-filled, preservative-free, unit-dose vial.
Inhaled SABA Combined With Inhaled Corticosteroid			
Albuterol/budesonide (Airsupra)	90 mcg albuterol/80 mcg budesonide	2 inhalations as needed, up to 12 puffs in a 24 hour period	Approved for people 18 years old and older
Anticholinergics			
Metered-Dose Inhalers			
Ipratropium HFA (Atrovent)[1]	17 μg/puff, 200 puffs/canister	2–3 puffs q6h	Multiple doses in the emergency department (not hospital) setting provide additive benefits to short-acting β agonists. It is the treatment of choice for bronchospasm caused by a β blocker. Does not block EIB. Reverses only cholinergically mediated bronchospasm; does not modify reaction to antigen. May be an alternative for patients who do not tolerate short-acting β agonists. Evidence is lacking for ipratropium producing added benefit to β₂ agonists for long-term control in asthma therapy.
Ipratropium with albuterol (Combivent Respimat)[1]	20 μg/puff of ipratropium bromide and 100 μg/puff of albuterol, 200 puffs/canister	2–3 puffs q6h	
Nebulizer Solutions			
Ipratropium bromide[1]	0.2 mg/mL (0.02%)	0.5 mg q6h	
Ipratropium bromide with albuterol (DuoNeb)[1]	0.5 mg/3 mL ipratropium bromide and 2.5 mg/3 mL albuterol	3 mL q4–6h	Contains EDTA to prevent discoloration of the solution. This additive does not induce bronchospasm.
Systemic Corticosteroid			
Methylprednisolone (Medrol) Prednisolone (Delta-Cortef, Prelone) Prednisone (Deltasone, Orasone)	2-, 4-, 6-, 8-, 16-, 32-mg tab 5-mg tabs; 5 mg/5 mL, 15 mg/5 mL 1-, 2.5-, 5-, 10-, 20-, 50-mg tabs; 5 mg/mL, 5 mg/5 mL	Short course (burst): 40–60 mg/day as a single dose or two divided doses for 3–10 days	Short courses (bursts) are effective for establishing control when initiating therapy or during a period of gradual deterioration. Action may begin within 1 hour. The burst should be continued until symptoms resolve. This usually requires 3–10 days but can require longer. There is no evidence that tapering the dose following improvement prevents relapse in asthma exacerbations.

TABLE 3 — Usual Dosages for Quick-Relief Medications for Patients 12 Years of Age and Older—cont'd

MEDICATION	DOSAGE FORM	ADULT DOSE	COMMENTS
Dexamethasone (Decadron)	0.5-, 0.75-, 1-, 1.5-, 2-, 4-, and 6-mg tablets and 0.5 mg/5 mL and 1 mg/5 mL	0.6 mg/kg as a single dose	Can be considered as an alternative for children presenting to the emergency department with asthma.
Steroid Injection			
Methylprednisolone acetate (Depo-Medrol)	40 mg/mL 80 mg/mL	240 mg[3]* IM once	May be used in place of a short burst of oral steroids in patients who are vomiting or if adherence is a problem.

*80 to 120 mg per package insert.
[1]Not FDA approved for this indication.
[3]Exceeds dosage recommended by the manufacturer.
EDTA, Edetic acid; *EIB*, exercise-induced bronchospasm; *HFA*, hydrofluoroalkane; *PEF*, peak expiratory flow; *tab*, tablet.

TABLE 4 — Usual Dosages for Long-Term Control Medications for Patients 12 Years of Age and Older

MEDICATION	DOSAGE FORM*	ADULT DOSE	COMMENTS
Systemic Corticosteroids			
Methylprednisolone (Medrol)	2-, 4-, 8-, 16-, 32-mg tab	7.5–60 mg qd in a single dose in AM or qod as needed for control	For long-term treatment of severe persistent asthma, administer a single dose in AM either daily or on alternate days. (Alternate-day therapy may produce less adrenal suppression.)
Prednisolone (Delta-Cortef, Prelone)	5-mg tab 5 mg/5 mL, 15 mg/5 mL	Short-course (burst) to achieve control, 40–60 mg/day as a single dose or two divided doses for 3–10 days	Short courses (bursts) are effective for establishing control when initiating therapy or during a period of gradual deterioration. There is no evidence that tapering the dose following improvement in symptom control and pulmonary function prevents relapse.
Prednisone (Deltasone, Orasone)	1-, 2.5-, 5-, 10-, 20-, 50-mg tab 5 mg/mL, 5 mg/5 mL	Short-course (burst) to achieve control, 40–60 mg/day as a single dose or two divided doses for 3–10 days	
Inhaled Combined Medications*			
Fluticasone and salmeterol (Advair Diskus, Wixela Inhub, Advair HFA and generic)	DPI: 100 μg/50 μg, 250 μg/50 μg, 500 μg/50 μg HFA: 45 μg/21 μg, 115 μg/21 μg, 230 μg/21 μg	1 inhalation bid[†] 2 puffs bid[†]	100/50 DPI or 45/21 HFA for patients not controlled on low- to medium- dose ICS 250/50 DPI or 115/21 HFA for patients not controlled on medium- to high- dose ICS
Fluticasone and salmeterol (AirDuo RespiClick, AirDuo Digihaler with eModule)	55 μg/14 μg, 113 μg/14 μg, 232 μg/14 μg	1 inhalation bid	
Budesonide and formoterol (Symbicort, Breyna, and generic)	HFA MDI: 80 μg/4.5 μg, 160 μg/4.5 μg	2 inhalations bid[†]	80/4.5 for patients not controlled on low- to medium-dose ICS 160/4.5 for patients not controlled on medium- to high- dose ICS
Mometasone and formoterol (Dulera)	50 μg/5 μg, 100 μg/5 μg, 200 μg/5 μg	2 inhalations bid[†]	100/5 for patients not controlled on low- to medium-dose ICS 200/5 for patients not controlled on medium- to high-dose ICS
Fluticasone furoate/vilanterol trifenatate (Breo Ellipta)	100 μg/25 μg 200 μg/25 μg	1 inhalation daily	200/25 for patients not controlled on 100/25
Fluticasone furoate/umeclidinium/vilanterol (Trelegy Ellipta)	100 μg/62.5 μg/25 μg 200 μg/62.5 μg/25 μg	1 inhalation daily	For patients not controlled on ICS/LABA
Inhaled Long-Acting Anticholinergic			
Tiotropium (Spiriva Respimat)	1.25 μg or 2.5 μg/actuation	2 puffs daily	Possibly more side effects compared with LABA as add-on therapy to ICS; more effective than placebo when added to ICS; effective when added to ICS/LABA

Continued

TABLE 4 Usual Dosages for Long-Term Control Medications for Patients 12 Years of Age and Older—cont'd

MEDICATION	DOSAGE FORM*	ADULT DOSE	COMMENTS
Long-Acting β₂ Agonists			
Inhaled Long-Acting β₂ agonists			Should not be used for relief of acute symptoms or exacerbations. Use only with ICS.
Salmeterol (Serevent Diskus)	DPI 50 μg/inhalation	1 inhalation q12h	Decreased duration of protection against EIB may occur with regular use.
Leukotriene Modifiers			
Leukotriene Receptor Antagonists			
Montelukast (Singulair, generic)	4-mg, or 5-mg chewable tab 10-mg tab	10 mg qhs for ≥15 yr old; 5 mg qhs for 6–14 yr old	Montelukast exhibits a flat dose-response curve. Doses >10 mg do not produce a greater response in adults. Black box warning for risk of serious neuropsychiatric events.
Zafirlukast (Accolate, generic)	10- or 20-mg tab	40 mg/day (20-mg tab bid)	For zafirlukast: Administration with meals decreases bioavailability; take at least 1 h before or 2 h after meals. Zafirlukast is a microsomal p450 enzyme inhibitor that can inhibit the metabolism of warfarin. Doses of this drug should be monitored accordingly. Monitor for signs and symptoms of hepatic dysfunction.
5-Lipoxygenase Inhibitor			
Zileuton (Zyflo)	600-mg tab, immediate-release or extended-release tab	2400 mg daily (600 mg qid for immediate release or 1200 mg bid for extended release)	Monitor hepatic enzymes (ALT). Zileuton is a microsomal p450 enzyme inhibitor that can inhibit the metabolism of warfarin and theophylline. Doses of these drugs should be monitored accordingly.
Methylxanthines			
Theophylline (Slo-Phyllin, Theobid, Theo-Dur)	Liquids, sustained-release tab, cap	Starting dose 10 mg/kg/day up to 300 mg max Usual max 800 mg/day	Adjust dosage to achieve serum concentration of 5 to 15 μg/mL at steady-state (≥48 h on same dosage). Because of wide interpatient variability in theophylline metabolic clearance, routine serum theophylline level monitoring is essential. Patients should be told to discontinue if they experience symptoms of toxicity. Various factors (diet, food, febrile illness, age, smoking, and other medications) can affect serum concentration.
Asthma Biologics			
Omalizumab (Xolair)	Subcutaneous (SQ) injection 150 mg/1.2 mL following reconstitution with 1.4 mL sterile water for injection Autoinjector 150 mg/mL and 75 mg/0.5 mL	150–375 mg SQ every 2–4 weeks, depending on body weight and pretreatment serum IgE level	For children 6 years of age and older with moderate to severe allergic asthma not controlled by inhaled corticosteroids. Monitor patient following injections; be prepared and equipped to identify and treat anaphylaxis that may occur. Do not administer more than 150 mg per injection site. Higher doses (up to 600 mg every 2 weeks) can be used for patients with comorbid nasal polyps. The dosing of omalizumab for nasal polyps is based on weight and IgE levels that is different from the dosing for asthma.

TABLE 4 Usual Dosages for Long-Term Control Medications for Patients 12 Years of Age and Older—cont'd

MEDICATION	DOSAGE FORM*	ADULT DOSE	COMMENTS
Benralizumab (Fasenra)	30 mg/mL single-dose prefilled syringe, 30 mg/mL autoinjector	30 mg SQ every 4 weeks for first 3 doses, then once every 8 weeks	For patients 12 years of age and older with severe eosinophilic asthma
Mepolizumab (Nucala)	100 mg/mL prefilled syringe, 100 mg/mL autoinjector	100 mg SQ every 4 weeks	For patients 12 years of age and older with severe eosinophilic asthma: 100 mg SQ every 4 wks. For patients with comorbid nasal polyps, the dose is the same as for asthma. For patients with eosinophilic granulomatosis with polyangiitis and hypereosinophilic syndrome, the dose of mepolizumab is 300 mg SQ every 4 weeks, with 3 separate 100-mg SQ injections given at least 5 cm apart on the upper arm, thigh, or abdomen. For children 6 to 11 years of age with severe eosinophilic asthma: 40 mg SQ every 4 weeks
Reslizumab (Cinqair)	Intravenous solution 10 mg/1 mL (10 mL)	3 mg/kg IV over 20 to 50 minutes every 4 weeks	For adults with severe eosinophilic asthma
Dupilumab (Dupixent)	Subcutaneous solution in prefilled syringe: 300 mg/2 mL and 200 mg/1.14 mL; Pen-injector: 300 mg/2 mL	400 mg SQ loading followed by 200 mg every other week OR 600 mg SQ loading followed by 300 mg every other week	For patients 12 years of age and older with moderate to severe eosinophilic or corticosteroid-dependent asthma. Consider using the 300-mg maintenance dose for patients with oral corticosteroid–dependent asthma, moderate-to-severe atopic dermatitis, or nasal polyps. For children 5 to 11 years of age, the dosing should be adjusted by weight: For 15 to 30 kg, use 100 mg every 2 weeks or 300 mg every 4 weeks; for >30 kg, use 200 mg every 2 weeks. For children 5 to 11 years of age who also have moderate-to-severe atopic dermatitis, use the atopic dermatitis dosing guidelines.
Tezepelumab-ekko (Tezspire)	Subcutaneous solution 210 mg/1.91 mL Pen 201 mg/1.91 mL	210 mg SQ every 4 weeks	For severe asthma in patients 12 years of age and older

*See Table 6 for estimated comparative daily dosages for inhaled corticosteroids.
†Dose depends on level of severity or control.
ALT, Alanine aminotransferase; *amp,* ampule; *cap,* capsule; *DPI,* dry powder inhaler; *EIB,* exercise-induced bronchospasm; *HFA,* hydrofluoroalkane; *ICS,* inhaled corticosteroid; *LABA,* long-acting β$_2$ agonist; *max,* maximum; *MDI,* metered-dose inhaler; *SABA,* short-acting β$_2$ agonist; *tab,* tablet.

flow [PEF] ≥80% predicted or personal best), the patient may continue β agonists every 3 to 4 hours for 24 to 48 hours. If repeated β agonists are needed, a short course of oral corticosteroids should be considered.

With an incomplete response to initial therapy (persistent wheezing and dyspnea and PEF 50% to 79% predicted or personal best), oral corticosteroids should be added, β agonists should be repeated, and the patient should contact the clinician that day.

With a poor response (marked wheezing and dyspnea at rest, PEF <50% predicted or personal best), oral corticosteroids should be added, the β agonist should be repeated immediately, and the patient should contact the clinician and usually proceed to the emergency department. For signs of severe distress (e.g., difficulty talking in full sentences, diaphoresis, drowsiness, confusion, or cyanosis), 911 should be called.

Emergency Department and Hospital Management

Assessment should rapidly determine the severity of the exacerbation based on the intensity of symptoms, signs (heart rate, respiratory rate, use of accessory muscles, chest auscultation), peak flow (unless the patient is too dyspneic to perform), and pulse oximetry. Treatment should begin immediately following recognition of an exacerbation severe enough to cause dyspnea at rest, peak flow less than 70% predicted or personal best, or pulse oximetry oxygen saturation less than 95%. While treatment is being given, a brief, focused history and a physical examination pertinent to the exacerbation can be obtained.

TABLE 5 Stepwise Approach for Managing Asthma in Patients 12 Years of Age and Older*

STEP	PREFERRED THERAPY	ALTERNATIVE THERAPY
1	As needed SABA or as needed low-dose ICS-formoterol[1]	
2	Low-dose ICS daily plus SABA or low-dose ICS taken whenever short-acting β agonist is taken or as needed low-dose ICS-formoterol[1]	
3	Scheduled and as needed low-dose ICS-formoterol[1] Limit to 12 puffs total per day or less	Medium-dose ICS plus as-needed SABA, low-dose ICS plus LABA *or* LTRA *or* tiotropium and as-needed SABA
4	Scheduled and as needed medium-dose ICS-formoterol[1] Limit to 12 puffs total per day or less	Medium-dose ICS plus LABA *or* LTRA *or* tiotropium and as-needed SABA
5	Medium-to-high dose ICS/formoterol plus as needed low-dose ICS/formoterol or as needed ICS/SABA OR High dose ICS/LABA plus as needed SABA or as needed ICS/SABA	Consider add-on therapy with macrolide antibiotics, tiotropium, LTRA, and/or biologics (anti-IgE, anti-IL5/5R, anti-IL4R, anti-TSLP). Oral corticosteroids as last resort.

*The stepwise approach is meant to assist, not replace, the clinical decision making required to meet individual patient needs.
[1]Not FDA approved for this indication.
ICS, Inhaled corticosteroid; *LABA,* long-acting β agonist; *LTRA,* leukotriene receptor antagonist; *SABA,* short-acting β agonist.
Modified from Global Initiative for Asthma (GINA) 2024 guideline; Expert Panel Working Group of the National Heart, Lung, and Blood Institute (NHLBI) administered and coordinated National Asthma Education and Prevention Program Coordinating Committee (NAEPPCC), Cloutier MM, Baptist AP, et al. 2020 Focused Updates to the Asthma Management Guidelines: A Report from the National Asthma Education and Prevention Program Coordinating Committee Expert Panel Working Group, *J Allergy Clin Immunol* 146(6):1217–1270, 2020.

TABLE 6 Estimated Comparative Daily Dosages for Inhaled Corticosteroids for Patients 12 Years of Age and Older

DRUG	DOSAGE FORM	DAILY DOSE		
		LOW (µg)	MEDIUM (µg)	HIGH (µg)
Beclomethasone (QVAR RediHaler)	40 or 80 µg/puff	100–200	>200–400	>400
Budesonide DPI (Pulmicort Flexhaler)	90 or 180 µg/inhalation	200–400	>400–800	>800
Budesonide/formoterol (Symbicort) pMDI	80 µg and 160 µg			
Ciclesonide (Alvesco)	80 or 160 µg/actuation	80–160	>160–320	>320
Fluticasone-HFA	MDI: 44, 110, 220 µg/puff	100–250	>250–500	>500
Fluticasone DPI (Flovent Diskus, ArmonAir RespiClick,[2] ArmonAir Digihaler,[2] Arnuity Ellipta), fluticasone-salmeterol DPI (Advair)	DPI: 50, 100, and 250 µg/inhalation (Flovent Diskus); 55, 113, and 232 µg/inhalation (ArmonAir RespiClick,[2] ArmonAir Digihaler); 50, 100, and 200 µg/inhalation	100–250	>250–500	>500
Fluticasone furoate (Arnuity Ellipta) and fluticasone furoate/vilanterol (Breo Ellipta)		100	100	≥200
Mometasone DPI (Asmanex)	110 or 220 µg/actuation	110–220	>220–440	>440
Mometasone HFA (Asmanex and Dulera)		200	200	≥400

[2]Not available in the United States.
DPI, Dry powder inhaler; *HFA,* hydrofluoroalkane; *MDI,* metered-dose inhaler.
Adapted from Global Initiative for Asthma. Global Strategy for Asthma Management and Prevention. 2024. Available at: https://ginasthma.org/2024-report/.

In patients with mild to moderate exacerbations (PEF >40% predicted), initial therapy includes oxygen to achieve oxygen saturation greater than 93% and an inhaled short-acting β agonist by nebulizer or MDI (4 to 8 puffs) with a holding chamber, which may be repeated up to three times in the first hour. Oral corticosteroids (prednisone 40 to 80 mg) are recommended if there is no immediate response to therapy or if the patient was recently treated with oral corticosteroids.

In patients with severe exacerbations (PEF <40% predicted), initial therapy includes oxygen as mentioned earlier, an inhaled high-dose short-acting β agonist (e.g., albuterol 5 mg) and ipratropium (Atrovent 0.5 mg)[1] by nebulizer, and oral or intravenous corticosteroids (prednisone or methylprednisolone [Solu-Medrol] 80 mg). The albuterol may be repeated every 20 minutes or used continuously for 1 hour.

Repeated assessments of symptoms, signs, PEF, and oxygen saturation determine the responsiveness of the exacerbation to therapy. Such assessments should be made in patients presenting with severe exacerbations after the initial bronchodilator treatment and in all patients after three doses of bronchodilator therapy (60 to 90 minutes after initial treatment). In patients who are improving, short-acting β agonists may be repeated every hour until a favorable response is achieved (no distress, PEF >70%). When this response is sustained for at least 60 minutes after the last treatment, the patient may usually be discharged on a course of oral corticosteroids (generally prednisone 40 to 60 mg for 5 to 10 days), initiation or continuation of medium-dose inhaled corticosteroids, and arrangement for outpatient follow-up.

In patients who are not improving with the aforementioned therapy, adjunctive therapy, such as with intravenous magnesium sulfate[1] (2 g IV over 15 to 30 minutes) or heliox, may be considered. Noninvasive ventilation or intubation and mechanical ventilation may be required for patients with respiratory failure in spite of treatment.

Summary

Asthma is a very common problem with the potential to cause substantial interference with quality of life. Although there is no cure for asthma, asthma can be well controlled in the majority of patients with proper management and an effective patient-clinician relationship. We hope that the method described herein for assessing and managing asthma will assist healthcare providers in helping their patients achieve well-controlled asthma.

---

[1]Not FDA approved for this indication.

References

2020 Focused Updates to the Asthma Management Guidelines: A Report from the National Asthma Education and Prevention Program Coordinating Committee Expert Panel Working Group. Available at: https://www.nhlbi.nih.gov/health-topics/asthma-management-guidelines-2020-updates.
Global Initiative for Asthma. Global Strategy for Asthma Management and Prevention. 2024. Available at: https://ginasthma.org/2024-report/.

ATELECTASIS

Method of
Alykhan S. Nagji, MD; Joshua S. Jolissaint, MD; and Christine L. Lau, MD

CURRENT DIAGNOSIS

- Hypoxia
- Tachypnea
- Diminished breath sounds
- Wheezing
- Radiologic signs of atelectasis

CURRENT THERAPY

- Chest percussion or vibration
- Nasotracheal or bronchoscopic suctioning
- Incentive spirometry
- Positive-pressure ventilation
- Ambulation
- Postoperative pain control

Atelectasis refers to the collapse of alveoli that affects segmental or lobar regions of the lung or the entire lung and results in hypoventilation. However, recent studies have suggested that the alveoli are not collapsed but are filled with fluid and foam. These hypotheses are not mutually exclusive; collapsed alveoli and fluid- and foam-filled alveoli may be present concurrently in an atelectatic lung. Although atelectasis is considered a benign condition, early treatment, reversal, and prevention are essential to an overall improved outcome.

Etiology

Compression Atelectasis

Compression atelectasis occurs when the transmural pressure distending the alveolus is reduced to a level that allows the alveolus to collapse. To best illustrate this mechanism, consider the patient who has undergone induction of anesthesia. The diaphragm is relaxed and is displaced cephalad. In the supine position, the pleural pressures increase to the greatest extent in the dependent lung regions and can compress the adjacent lung tissue.

Surfactant Impairment

Surfactant serves to reduce the alveolar surface tension, thereby stabilizing the alveoli and preventing collapse. Reduction in surfactant occurs with certain types of anesthesia. Studies have shown that hyperinflation by means of increased tidal volume, sequential air inflations to the total lung capacity, or even a single cycle of increased tidal volume can increase the release of surfactant, aiding in recruitment and stabilization of alveoli.

Gas Resorption

One mechanism by which gas resorption results in atelectasis involves the patent airway. In regions of the lung with increased ventilation compared to perfusion, which produces a ventilation/perfusion (V/Q) mismatch, there is low alveolar oxygen tension. Increasing the fraction of inspired oxygen (FIO_2) initiates a cascade of events that increases alveolar oxygen tension (PAO_2) and decreases alveolar nitrogen tension (PAN_2), which results in loss of alveolar volume secondary to increased absorption of oxygen.

Another mechanism by which gas resorption leads to atelectasis occurs after complete airway occlusion. In such cases, gas is trapped distal to the obstruction. Gas uptake by the proximal blood flow continues without additional gas inflow. This causes the alveoli to collapse.

Pathophysiology

The trapping of air and hyperinflation of the alveoli are produced from the aforementioned mechanisms. The gases that are trapped are absorbed by the blood perfusing through that region of the lung, which eventually causes collapse of the alveoli. The atelectasis produces alveolar hypoxia and pulmonary vasoconstriction to prevent V/Q mismatching and to minimize arterial hypoxia. This vascular response is effective only if a large part of the lung is not collapsed; otherwise, intrapulmonary shunting occurs.

Clinical Presentation

The signs and symptoms of atelectasis are often nonspecific. The natural course of atelectasis may lead to fever, cough, tachypnea, wheezing, rhonchi, and chest pain. On physical examination, atelectasis may manifest as an area of localized reduced breath sounds with constant wheeze or reduced chest wall expansion or both.

Diagnosis

Chest radiographs aid in the diagnosis of atelectasis. They provide both direct and indirect signs that may indicate an atelectatic etiology for the patient's symptoms.
Direct signs include:
- Displaced pulmonary vessels
- Air bronchograms
- Displacement of intralobar fissures (most reliable sign)
Indirect signs include:
- Pulmonary opacification
- Diaphragmatic elevation
- Hyperexpansion of unaffected lung
- Tracheal, heart, and mediastinal shift toward atelectatic side

- Shift of the hilum toward the collapsed lobe
- Segmental ipsilateral rib approximation

Treatment

Treatment of atelectasis is geared toward the underlying cause. It is important to recognize respiratory distress and to intubate the patient if appropriate.

If the etiology is that of an obstructive atelectasis, chest percussion or vibration and nasotracheal or bronchoscopic suctioning may help in the clearing of secretions. With regard to lung re-expansion, incentive spirometry, continuous or intermittent positive-pressure ventilation, and early ambulation may be used.

Those patients who have a nonobstructive atelectasis caused by a pneumothorax or pleural effusion benefit from tube thoracostomy or thoracentesis. Additionally, appropriate pain management in the postoperative setting allows for proper ventilation.

References

Duggan M, Kavanagh BP: Pulmonary atelectasis: A pathogenic perioperative entity, *Anesthesiology* 102:838–854, 2005.

Duggan M, Kavanagh BP: Atelectasis in the perioperative patient, *Curr Opin Anaesthesiol* 20:37–42, 2007.

Hubmayr RD: Perspective on lung injury and recruitment: A skeptical look at the opening and collapse story, *Am J Respir Crit Care Med* 165:1647–1653, 2002.

Peroni DG, Boner AL: Atelectasis: Mechanisms, diagnosis and management, *Paediatr Respir Rev* 1:274–278, 2000.

Wagner PD, Laravuso RB, Uhl RR, West JB: Continuous distributions of ventilation-perfusion ratios in normal subjects breathing air and 100 per cent O_2, *J Clin Invest* 54:54–68, 1974.

BACTERIAL PNEUMONIA

Method of
Arjun Muthusubramanian, MD, MPH; Alison N. Huffstetler, MD; and Katharine C. DeGeorge, MD, MS

CURRENT DIAGNOSIS

- The clinical diagnosis of pneumonia is aided by patient symptoms of fever, cough, shortness of breath, purulent sputum, or chest pain, and by chest radiography which may demonstrate lobar consolidation, pleural effusion, or cavitary lesions.
- When determining the appropriate treatment setting, use a validated scoring system such as the pneumonia severity index (PSI) or CURB-65 to predict disease severity and risk of death.
- Hospital-acquired pneumonia may be diagnosed in a hospitalized patient who develops a pulmonary infection greater than 48 hours after admission.

CURRENT THERAPY

- Treat outpatients with uncomplicated bacterial pneumonia empirically with high-dose amoxicillin or doxycycline. Only use a macrolide as monotherapy if local pneumococcal resistance is less than 25%.
- Use broad-spectrum antibiotics for empiric treatment of patients with hospital-acquired pneumonia and narrow therapy as soon as possible, based on culture results and sensitivities.
- If a patient has prior respiratory isolation of MRSA or *Pseudomonas aeruginosa*, then presumptive treatment should be initiated and cultures obtained to help guide, and potentially narrow therapy.

Pneumonia (PNA) is a leading cause of death in the United States and accounts for more than 400,000 emergency department (ED) visits annually. PNA often presents with shortness of breath, fever, productive cough, with leukocytosis, and radiographic findings of lobar infiltrate. Diagnosis and treatment should be based on underlying characteristics of the patient and their risk factors. The most common cause of community-acquired pneumonia (CAP) is *Streptococcus pneumoniae*, while hospital-acquired pneumonia (HAP) is more frequently caused by gram-negative bacteria and places patients at a risk for multi-drug resistant (MDR) organisms. Treatment of a non-severe case of PNA in an individual without comorbidities in an outpatient should be empiric and include high-dose amoxicillin or doxycycline; a macrolide should only be used if local pneumococcal resistance is less than 25%. Therapy for inpatients may rely on sputum and blood cultures with targeted antibiotic regimens to reduce cost and complications of therapy. Common treatment regimens for CAP requiring hospitalization include a respiratory fluoroquinolone (such as moxifloxacin [Avelox]) or a beta-lactam (ceftriaxone [Rocephin]) plus a macrolide. Empiric treatment regimens for HAP should be broad and based on local antibiograms, with consideration for coverage for *Pseudomonas aeruginosa* and/or methicillin-resistant *Staphylococcus aureus* (MRSA). Prevention of PNA is essential and pneumococcal vaccines should be routinely provided according to recommended schedules to children and to adults 65 and over.

This chapter discusses diagnosis and treatment of CAP and HAP in adults. While previous guidelines approached healthcare-associated pneumonia (HCAP) and HAP separately, these are now diagnosed and treated as a single disease process (HAP).

Epidemiology

CAP affects approximately 5 to 6 people per 1000 persons per year, with seasonal variance resulting in higher incidence during winter. The associated morbidity and mortality rates are high; in 2015, 16.1 deaths per 100,000 people in the US population were attributed to PNA. Treating these patients comes at a cost of $10.6 to $17 billion in the United States annually. Men are affected more frequently than women, and African Americans more frequently than Caucasians. The very young and elderly (aged ≥65 years) are affected more often than younger adults. Despite our best efforts, advances in medical therapies have not significantly decreased the mortality rate associated with PNA since the advent of penicillin in 1928.

The incidence of HAP is approximately 1.6 to 3.6 cases per 1000 hospital admissions. HAP is a leading cause of hospital-acquired infections (HAIs) and 22% of HAIs are accounted for by HAP. HAP most frequently occurs in patients outside of the intensive care unit (ICU); however, those in the ICU and on mechanical ventilation are at high risk of ventilator-associated pneumonia (VAP). HAP is associated with complications including respiratory compromise, septic shock, acute renal failure, and empyema.

Aspiration PNA is not a separate entity, but rather a subsect that describes the etiology of the particular infection. Microaspiration (aspiration of small amounts of oropharyngeal secretions) is expected in healthy adults during sleep; however, aspiration PNA refers, rather, to large-volume entry of oropharyngeal or upper gastrointestinal contents into the lower respiratory tract (macroaspiration). While 5% to 15% of CAP can be attributed to aspiration PNA, there is no solid data on the contribution of aspiration PNA to HAP.

Etiology

Risk Factors

Predisposing factors for development of PNA include several prescription medications (angiotensin converting enzyme [ACE] inhibitors, antipsychotic medications, glucocorticoids, H-2 blockers, proton pump inhibitors, and sedatives), tobacco use, alcohol use, malnutrition, use of dentures at night, bronchial obstruction due to foreign body, altered mental status due to reversible causes, and pulmonary edema. Nonmodifiable risk factors include immotile cilia, cystic fibrosis, chronic obstructive pulmonary disease

(COPD), Kartagener's syndrome, human immunodeficiency virus (HIV), lung cancer, and Young's syndrome.

Community-Acquired Pneumonia Pathogens

Worldwide, *S. pneumoniae* is the leading cause of PNA. In the United States, however, rates of streptococcal PNA have declined following implementation of the pneumococcal vaccine in both adults and children. "Typical" organisms that cause PNA in the United States include *Haemophilus influenza* (although less common following development of the *H. influenza* vaccine in 1987), *S. aureus*, group A streptococcus, *Moraxella catarrhalis*, anaerobes, and aerobic gram-negative bacteria. "Atypical" organisms include *Mycoplasma pneumoniae*, *Legionella* spp., *Chlamydia pneumoniae*, and *Chlamydia psittaci*.

Existing pulmonary infection with influenza, respiratory syncytial virus, human metapneumovirus, adenovirus, and rhinovirus increase the risk of developing a secondary bacterial PNA. Patients admitted to the ICU requiring invasive diagnostic testing frequently become infected with *S. pneumoniae*, but have disproportionate incidence of *Legionella*, *S. aureus*, *H. influenza*, and enteric gram-negative bacilli (*Klebsiella pneumoniae*, *P. aeruginosa*, *Acinetobacter* spp, *M. catarrhalis*). Identification of the organism responsible for CAP is only established in approximately 40% of cases.

Specific patient risk factors, including failure of outpatient therapy, should be considered to identify involved pathogens in CAP. Consider local trends and outbreaks for diagnosis of *Legionella*, *M. pneumoniae*, and *C. pneumoniae*. Alcoholism is frequently linked to anaerobic bacterial PNA, *K. pneumoniae*, *Mycobacterium tuberculosis*, and *S. pneumoniae*. Patients with high risk of aspiration also have higher rates of anaerobic oral flora underlying PNA. Patients with COPD frequently have PNA caused by *C. pneumoniae*, *H. influenza*, *Legionella* species, *M. catarrhalis*, *P. aeruginosa*, and *S. pneumoniae*. Exposure to animals such as bats, birds, or farm animals increases risk of *Histoplasma capsulatum* and *Coxiella burnetii* infections. HIV is a risk factor for *H. influenza*, *M. tuberculosis*, and *S. pneumoniae* in the early stages and a risk factor for *Pneumocystis jiroveci* in late stages with decreased CD4 count. Travel increases risk for *Blastomyces dermatitidis* and *Coccidioides* species. Severe infections that do not respond to initial therapy should raise concern for possible MRSA infection. When clinical management would be altered by confirmed diagnosis of microbial infection or aforementioned risk factors for particular causative organisms exist, effort should be made for more extensive diagnostic testing.

Hospital-Acquired Pneumonia

Acutely ill, hospitalized patients have a higher risk of aspirating, which accounts for many of the differences in involved pathogens in HAP as compared to CAP. Oropharyngeal colonization with microorganisms that are commonly found in hospitals may occur within 48 hours of admission. Aerobic gram-negative bacilli such as *Escherichia coli*, *K. pneumoniae*, *Enterobacter* spp., and *P. aeruginosa* are more commonly identified in patients with HAP, but gram-positive cocci are also identified. HAP, distinct from CAP, places patients at higher risk for MDR pathogens. Prior intravenous (IV) antibiotic use is a strong risk factor for MDR HAP. MRSA is also more common in patients with HAP, primarily due to prior IV antibiotic use as well. MDR *P. aeruginosa* is identified most frequently in patients who have received IV antibiotics, previously on mechanical ventilation, and with a history of COPD, cystic fibrosis, and bronchiectasis.

Diagnosis

Symptoms of PNA most often include fever, cough, shortness of breath, purulent sputum, and chest pain. Physical exam may demonstrate bronchial breath sounds and crackles, although breath sounds may also be entirely normal, especially in the elderly. Oxygen saturation is often reduced, and chest radiography may demonstrate lobar consolidation, pleural effusion, and/or cavitary lesions. Depending on the severity of illness, patients may be treated in the outpatient or inpatient acute care settings, or may require intensive care for ventilatory or vasopressor support.

TABLE 1	2007 Infectious Diseases Society of America/American Thoracic Society Criteria for Defining Severe Community-Acquired Pneumonia

Minor Criteria

Respiratory rate ≥30 breaths/min

PaO_2/FiO_2 ratio ≤250

Multilobar infiltrates

Confusion/disorientation

Uremia (BUN ≥20 mg/dL)

Leukopenia only due to infection (white blood cell [WBC] count <4000 cells/μL)

Thrombocytopenia (platelet count <100,000/μL)

Hypothermia (core temperature <36°C)

Hypotension requiring aggressive fluid resuscitation

Major Criteria

Septic shock with need for vasopressors

Respiratory failure requiring mechanical ventilation

BUN, Blood urea nitrogen.

Community-Acquired Pneumonia

Diagnosis of CAP requires the presence of symptoms (fever, cough, purulent sputum, pleuritis, and/or shortness of breath) plus chest radiographic findings consistent with PNA such as lobar consolidation, pleural effusion, and/or cavitary lesions. Blood oxygen saturation is frequently low and white blood cell counts may be elevated, often with a neutrophilic predominance. Presentation in the elderly may be more subtle, with atypical or absent symptoms, blunted febrile response, and lack of leukocytosis. A patient meets the criteria for severe CAP, as defined by Infectious Diseases Society of America/American Thoracic Society CAP severity criteria, when meeting either one major criterion or three or more minor criteria (Table 1). Chest radiography (CXR) is not indicated if clinical symptoms are met. For patients requiring hospitalization, 2022 evidence suggests point of care ultrasound may be more sensitive for pneumonia than CXR.

Patients diagnosed with bacterial PNA treated in the outpatient setting do not require specific microbial identification; neither noninvasive nor invasive testing is recommended for this population (including blood cultures, endotracheal aspirates, and urine antigen testing).

Expectorated sputum samples for gram stain and culture are not routinely recommended for outpatients. Sputum samples for gram stain and culture should be collected, ideally before initiation of treatment, from those who are hospitalized and who meet one of the following: (1) classified as having severe CAP, (2) being empirically treated for MRSA or *P. aeruginosa*, (3) having prior infection with MRSA or *P. aeruginosa*, or (4) having been hospitalized and have received parenteral antibiotics in the past 90 days. Early gram stain can direct initial empiric therapy, especially with findings of less common pathogens. Sputum samples become lower yield as the time between treatment initiation and collection of the sample increases. Inadequate samples (<10 inflammatory cells per epithelial cell) should not be sent for gram stain or culture. Nebulized hypertonic saline may be used to induce sputum sample when necessary.

Obtaining blood cultures are recommended for the same population of patients for whom sputum culture collection is indicated. In the general population of patients hospitalized with PNA, false positive blood cultures are common and can increase the duration of hospital stay and potentially misinform treatment decisions. Additionally, false positive blood cultures frequently lead to use of broad-spectrum antibiotics, increasing microbial resistance patterns.

Pneumococcal urinary antigen testing should only be obtained for those with severe CAP. Legionella urinary antigen testing routinely should be performed for those with severe CAP or when indicated by epidemiologic factors.

During times of community circulation of influenza, those with CAP should be tested for influenza virus, preferably via nucleic acid amplification. Although biomarkers such as procalcitonin (PCT) can be used to monitor response to therapy, PCT, soluble triggering receptor expressed by myeloid cells 1 (sTREM-1), and C-reactive protein should not be used to guide the diagnosis of bacterial PNA.

Hospital-Acquired Pneumonia

The diagnosis of HAP can be made in hospitalized patients who develop pulmonary infection ≥48 hours after hospital admission. Criteria for HAP require new or progressive findings on chest radiography, fever, leukopenia or leukocytosis, or altered mental status (for patients aged ≥70 years), and new or worsening clinical symptoms or signs consistent with bacterial PNA in the absence of mechanical ventilation.

Similar to the management of CAP, sputum and blood cultures should be obtained only when clinically indicated and biomarkers for diagnostic purposes are not routinely recommended. Low dose computed tomography for diagnosis of HAP may assist in diagnosis.

Treatment Setting

Determination of appropriate treatment setting is important for both patient outcomes and healthcare costs. Inpatient care of PNA can be 25 times as costly as outpatient management and also increases risk of thromboembolic events and superinfection with drug-resistant or virulent organisms. However, inappropriate outpatient management of patients at higher risk of death can lead to potentially avoidable morbidity and mortality.

Several scoring systems have been developed to help predict short-term mortality and need for hospital or ICU admission in patients with bacterial PNA. The following clinical decision aids are the most commonly used:

- *Pneumonia Severity Index (PSI):* Commonly used, well-validated scoring system that evaluates 20 items with emphasis on the age of the patient. Higher PSI scores indicate higher risk of requiring ICU level care or short-term mortality. See Table 2 for details of PSI scoring. Patients classified as risk classes I and II should be managed as outpatients; those with risk class III should be treated in an observation unit or with short-stay hospitalization; risk classes IV and V should be admitted to the hospital.
- *CURB-65:* Severity-of-illness score which incorporates confusion, uremia, respiratory rate, low blood pressure, and age ≥ 65 years into a prognostic model to determine a patient's candidacy for outpatient therapy. A CURB-65 score of ≥2 is indicative of likely need for hospitalization, with consideration for ICU care for those with of scores 3 or greater. This shorter scoring system may be less cumbersome in a busy setting, but the effect on hospital admission rates and patient outcomes have been studied less extensively than the PSI score.
- *SMART-COP:* Assists the physician in determining whether the patient requires ICU level care. The algorithm takes into account systolic blood pressure, multilobar chest x-ray findings of infiltrate, albumin, respiratory rate, tachycardia, confusion, oxygenation, and pH and stratifies patients into risk groups that estimate risk of requiring intensive respiratory or vasopressor support.

In addition to clinical judgment, PSI is preferred over CURB-65 in helping guide determination of the need for inpatient management of adults with CAP.

Patients with septic shock requiring vasopressor therapy in the setting of CAP should be admitted to the ICU. If there is clinical concern for impending airway compromise, the patient should be intubated and admitted to the ICU. In several clinical studies, patients who were critically ill and were not initially admitted to the ICU had higher rates of morbidity and mortality.

Treatment

General recommendations for empiric treatment of both CAP and HAP are detailed in Table 4. Antibiotics and supportive care (oxygen, IV fluids, and ventilatory or vasopressor support when necessary) is

TABLE 2	Pneumonia Severity Index	
RISK FACTORS		**POINTS**
Demographics		
Age, men		Age in years
Age, women		Age in years–10
Nursing home resident		+10
Comorbid Conditions		
Active Neoplasm		+30
Liver disease		+20
History of CVA		+10
Chronic heart failure		+10
Chronic renal failure		+10
Physical Exam		
Altered mental status		+20
Respiratory rate elevated >30		+20
Hypotension, SBP <90 mm Hg		+20
Temperature <95°C or >40°C		+15
Tachycardia, pulse >125 bmp		+10
Laboratory and Imaging Findings		
Acidosis, arterial pH <7.35		+30
Hyponatremia, Na <130 mmol/L		+20
BUN ≥30 mg/dL		+20
Glucose ≥250 mg/dL		+10
Hematocrit <30%		+10
PaO$_2$ <60 mm Hg		+10
Pleural effusion		+10
Total points		

Total points less than 51 indicates low incidence of death from CAP. Patients with increased total points have higher risk of death; the greatest risk for those greater than 130 total points with rate of death for adults diagnosed with CAP of 24.9%.
BUN, Blood urea nitrogen; *CAP*, community-acquired pneumonia; *CVA*, cerebrovascular disease; *SBP*, systolic blood pressure; *Na*, sodium; *PaO$_2$*, partial pressure of arterial oxygen.

TABLE 3	Risk Factors for Multi-drug Resistant Pathogens in Hospital-Acquired Pneumonia

Risk Factors for MDR Pathogens in Ventilator-Associated Pneumonia (VAP)

Prior intravenous antibiotic use within 90 days

Septic shock at time of VAP
ARDS preceding VAP
Hospitalization greater than or equal to 5 days prior to VAP
Acute renal replacement therapy prior to VAP

Risk Factors for MDR Pathogens in HAP, MRSA in VAP/HAP, and *Pseudomonas* in VAP/HAP

Prior Intravenous antibiotic use within 90 days

ARDS, Acute respiratory distress syndrome; *MDR*, Multi-drug resistant; *MRSA*, methicillin-resistant *Staphylococcus aureus*.

the mainstay of treatment for both community and hospital-acquired bacterial PNA. Antibiotic selection is guided by several factors:
- Age
- Severity of illness

TABLE 4 Empiric Antibiotic Therapy for Pneumonia for Adults

TYPE OF PNEUMONIA	SETTING	ANTIMICROBIAL THERAPY
Community-Acquired Pneumonia	Outpatient, patient without co-morbidities and without risk-factors for MRSA or *Pseudomonas aeruginosa*[1]	Amoxicillin 1 g 3 times daily OR Doxycycline 100 mg 2 times daily OR Macrolide (only if local pneumococcal resistance is <25%), such as azithromycin (Zithromax) 500 mg on day 1 followed by 250 mg daily or clarithromycin (Biaxin) 500 mg 2 times daily
	Outpatient, patient with co-morbidities[2]	Respiratory fluoroquinolone[3] OR β-lactam[4] PLUS macrolide or doxycycline
	Inpatient, non-severe	Respiratory fluoroquinolone[3] (levofloxacin or moxifloxacin) OR Select β-lactam (ampicillin+sulbactam [Unasyn],* cefotaxime [Claforan], ceftriaxone [Rocephin], or ceftaroline [Teflaro]) PLUS macrolide (azithromycin or clarithromycin)
	Inpatient, severe	Select β-lactam (ampicillin+sulbactam,* cefotaxime, ceftriaxone, ceftaroline) PLUS macrolide OR Select β-lactam PLUS respiratory fluoroquinolone[3] (levofloxacin or moxifloxacin)
	Prior respiratory isolation of *P. aeruginosa*	ADD piperacillin-tazobactam (Zosyn), cefepime (Maxipime), ceftazidime (Fortaz), imipenem (Primaxin), meropenem (Merrem),* or aztreonam (Azactam) to inpatient regimen
	Prior respiratory isolation of MRSA	ADD vancomycin or linezolid (Zyvox) to inpatient regimen
Aspiration Pneumonia	Outpatient	Amoxicillin/clavulanate (Augmentin) OR clindamycin OR levofloxacin OR moxifloxacin
	Inpatient	β-lactam/β-lactamase inhibitor (ampicillin/sulbactam,* piperacillin/tazobactam) OR carbapenem OR respiratory fluoroquinolone[3] OR 3rd or 4th generation cephalosporin (ceftriaxone, cefepime)
	Inpatient, risk of predominantly anaerobic infection[5]	ADD clindamycin to regimen
	Prior respiratory isolation of MRSA	ADD vancomycin or linezolid to inpatient regimen
Hospital-Acquired Pneumonia	Not at high risk of mortality[6] AND no risk factors for MRSA	Piperacillin/tazobactam OR cefepime OR levofloxacin OR carbapenem (imipenem, meropenem*) OR ceftolozane/tazobactam (Zerbaxa)
	Not at high risk of mortality AND risk factors for MRSA	Select β-lactam (cefepime, ceftazidime, imipenem, meropenem, or piperacillin/tazobactam) OR fluoroquinolone (levofloxacin, ciprofloxacin) OR aztreonam PLUS vancomycin or linezolid
	High risk of mortality, administration of intravenous antibiotics in past 90 days, VAP	Two of select β-lactam (cefepime, ceftazidime, imipenem, meropenem,* or piperacillin/tazobactam) OR fluoroquinolone (levofloxacin, ciprofloxacin) OR aminoglycoside (amikacin, gentamicin, tobramycin) OR aztreonam PLUS vancomycin or linezolid

[1]Risk-factors include prior respiratory isolation of MRSA or *P. aeruginosa* OR recent hospitalization and administration of intravenous antibiotics in the last 90 days.
[2]Presence of comorbid conditions (chronic heart, lung, liver, or renal disease; diabetes mellitus; alcoholism; malignancies, asplenia, immunosuppression [iatrogenic or pathologic]), Use of antimicrobials within the past 3 months, High-rate (>25%) of macrolide-resistant *S. pneumonia*.
[3]Respiratory fluoroquinolones include levofloxacin (Levaquin) 750 mg daily, moxifloxacin (Avelox) 400 mg daily, or gemifloxacin (Factive) 320 mg daily.
[4]Amoxicillin/clavulanate (Augmentin) 500 mg/125 mg 3 times daily, amoxicillin/clavulanate 875 mg/125 mg 2 times daily, cefuroxime (Ceftin) 500 mg 2 times daily, cefpodoxime (Vantin) 200 mg 2 times daily.
[5]Risk factors for predominantly anaerobic infection include patients with severe periodontal disease and necrotizing pneumonia or lung abscess.
[6]Risk factors for mortality include need for ventilatory support and septic shock.
*Not FDA approved for this indication.
MRSA, Methicillin-resistant *Staphylococcus aureus*; VAP, ventilator associated pneumonia.

- Risk of infection by MDR pathogen (Table 3 for risk factors)
- Setting (both timing and location) of PNA onset

Initiation of initial treatment should also be guided by geographic antibiograms, which should be available through local hospitals. The CDC Antibiotic Resistance Patient Safety Atlas provides similar information for the aggregate of hospital-acquired infections. Antibiotic therapy should be narrowed as soon as possible based on culture and subsequent sensitivity results, if culture was obtained.

PCT may be used as an indicator of response to therapy after diagnosis of CAP and HAP based on recent trial data. If PCT measurements decrease to less than 0.1 µg/L, a provider may consider discontinuation of antibiotics. For patients with COVID-19 and a superimposed bacterial PNA, consider use of PCT to identify utility of antibiotics.

In addition to antimicrobial therapy for those who require hospitalization, care should be taken to maintain appropriate oral hygiene and to maintain head of bed at 30 to 45 degrees in efforts to minimize risk of aspiration. Serum glucose goal should be less than 180 mg/dL. A few additional considerations exist for patients with severe PNA during hospitalization. These individuals should all receive dual antibiotic therapy, as noted in Table 4. For those who remain hypotensive despite adequate fluid resuscitation, consider screening for occult adrenal insufficiency within 24 hours of admission. Those with hypoxemia or respiratory distress may receive a closely monitored trial of non-invasive ventilation followed by intubation as indicated. Low-tidal volume ventilation (6 mL/kg of ideal body weight) should be utilized.

TABLE 5 Recommended Vaccinations for the Prevention of Pneumonia

VACCINE	POPULATION	RECOMMENDATIONS
Influenza	All persons older than 6 months	Annually If first lifetime dose of influenza vaccine (infants ≥6 months and children ≤9 years), 2nd dose should be given 4 weeks after 1st dose
Pneumococcal	Adults ≥50 years	Should receive 1 dose of pneumococcal conjugate vaccine (PCV15, PCV20, or PCV21) at age ≥50 years if patient is PCV-naïve or has unknown vaccination history, 1 dose of PCV20 or PCV21 ≥1 year after last PCV13 dose, 1 dose of PCV15, PCV20 or PCV21 ≥1 year after last PPSV23 dose, 1 dose of PCV20 or PCV21 ≥5 years since both PCV13 and PPSV23. If PCV20 or PCV21 is used, there is no indication for follow up with PPSV23.
	Adults 19–49 years who smoke tobacco or who have chronic heart disease (excluding hypertension), chronic lung disease, chronic liver disease, alcoholism, or diabetes mellitus	1 dose of either 15-valent or 20-valent or 21-valent pneumococcal conjugate vaccine (PCV15 or PCV20 or PCV21) if PCV-naïve or PCV7 at any age, 1 dose of PCV20 or PCV21 ≥1 year after last PCV13 dose, 1 dose of PCV15, PCV20 or PCV21 ≥1 year after last PPSV23 dose. If PCV20 or PCV21 is used, no additional PPSV23 is needed. If PCV15 is used, PPSV 23 is indicated 1 year after PCV15.
	All immunocompetent adults 65 years and older	Engage in shared clinical decision-making to see if 1 dose of pneumococcal conjugate vaccine PCV 15 (Vaxneuvance) or PCV 20 (Prevnar 20) or PCV 21 (Capvaxive) would be appropriate. Eligible adults may receive either PCV 15 in series with PPSV23 or PCV 20 or PCV21 alone. If PCV 15 is used, it should be administered first, followed by PPSV23 at least 1 year later. If they received dose of PPSV23 prior to age 65, dose of PCV 15 should be given at least 1 year after 1st dose of PPSV23 and dose of PPSV23 should be given at least 5 years after 1st dose of PPSV23.
	Adults 19 and older with immunocompromising conditions*	Eligible adults may receive either PCV 15 in series with PPSV23, PCV20, or PCV21 alone. If PCV 15 is used, administer 1 dose of PCV 15 first and then dose of PPSV23 at least 8 weeks after dose of PCV 15 and a second dose of PPSV23 5 years after 1st dose of PPSV23. At age 65 and older, administer one final dose of PPSV23 at least 5 years after previous dose of PPSV23 and at least 8 weeks after dose of PCV 15. Only 1 dose of PPSV23 is recommended after age 65 years.
	Adults 19 and older with cerebrospinal fluid leak or cochlear implant	Eligible adults may receive either PCV 15 in series with PPSV23 or PCV 20 alone or PCV21 alone. If PCV 15 is used, administer 1 dose of PCV 15 first and then dose of PPSV23 at least 8 weeks after the dose of PCV 13. At age 65 and older, administer one final dose of PPSV23 at least 5 years after previous dose of PPSV23. Only 1 dose of PPSV23 is recommended after age 65 years.
Haemophilus influenza type B (HiB)	All children younger than 5 years old, unvaccinated older children and adults with certain medical conditions,* people who receive bone marrow transplant	Administer 1 dose of HiB at age 2, 4, 6 (per product) and 12–15 months with minimum of age 6 weeks. Children with one dose at age >15 months need no further doses. For high-risk conditions, children age 12–59 months who previously received 1 or no doses should receive two additional doses of HiB, 8 weeks apart. For children who received two doses before 12 months of age should receive one additional dose. Hib may be given to high-risk adults.

*B- or T- lymphocyte deficiency, complement deficiencies, phagocytic disorders (excluding chronic granulomatous disease), HIV infection, chronic renal failure, nephrotic syndrome, leukemia, lymphoma, Hodgkin disease, generalized malignancy, multiple myeloma, solid organ transplant, iatrogenic immunosuppression, anatomical or functional asplenia.

Community-Acquired Pneumonia

Patients with suspected CAP should first be risk stratified using one of the PNA severity scoring indices discussed above and in Table 2. If being admitted to the hospital, the first dose of empiric antibiotic (see Table 4) should be administered in the ED as soon as the diagnosis of PNA is made. In addition to the established antibiotics noted in Table 4, the two antibiotics omadacycline (Nuzyra) and lefamulin (Xenleta) were approved in 2018 and 2019, respectively, for the treatment of CAP. Ceftolozane/tazobactam (Zerbaxa) was approved in 2019 for treatment of HAP and VAP. Both are available in IV and oral formulations and were shown to be non-inferior to treatment with moxifloxacin (Avelox) in the management of CAP. Patients may be transitioned from IV to oral antibiotics when they are hemodynamically stable, able to tolerate oral medications, and are able to absorb these medications enterally. When possible, an oral antibiotic should be chosen from the same or similar antibiotic class as the IV antibiotic used. Observation of inpatients after transition to oral antibiotics is not necessary as long as the patient is clinically stable and has a safe disposition plan. The recommended duration of antibiotic therapy is at least 3 days for beta lactams and 5 days for other antibiotics, with discontinuation only after the patient has been afebrile for at least 48 to 72 hours and remains clinically stable. Concern for a coexisting extrapulmonary infection may affect antibiotic selection and extend duration of therapy.

If a patient has prior respiratory isolation of MRSA or *P. aeruginosa*, then presumptive treatment should be initiated and cultures obtained to help guide, and potentially narrow therapy. If the patient was recently hospitalized, had IV antibiotics in the past 90 days, and locally validated risk factors for MRSA or *P. aeruginosa*, cultures should be obtained. If managing non-severe PNA, only initiate appropriate coverage if cultures return positive or if rapid nasal polymerase chain reaction is positive for MRSA. If PNA is characterized as severe, then initiate empiric coverage, while awaiting culture results to help guide de-escalation of or continuation of therapy. Oral fluoroquinolones and macrolides are more likely to have a clinical improvement as compared with amoxicillin. Treatment with probiotics[7] may improve the clinical course of CAP.

---

[7]Available as dietary supplement.

Hospital-Acquired Pneumonia

All patients with suspected HAP should be treated with broad spectrum antibiotics (see Table 4). Antibiotic choice should be governed by local antibiograms. The recommendations for further diagnostic testing, including cultures and PCR testing, were described in more detail in the diagnosis section. As described in Table 4, if the patient has risk factors for mortality or for MDR pathogens, then therapy with multiple agents is indicated. However, in selecting antimicrobial coverage, clinicians must weigh the benefit of initiating adequate coverage as soon as possible against the harms of uniform broad-spectrum coverage, such as increased resistance rates, risk of *Clostridium difficile* infection, and adverse drug effects. Whenever MRSA is suspected, treatment with vancomycin or linezolid (Zyvox) should be initiated; daptomycin (Cubicin) should not be used to treat pulmonary MRSA infection.

Prevention

Immunization against influenza, *S. pneumoniae*, and *H. influenza* is the best protection against bacterial PNA in adults and children. Recommended vaccine schedules are described in Table 5. In general, everyone should receive an annual influenza vaccine and individuals should receive *H. influenza* and pneumococcal immunization on a schedule based on age and risk factors. The pneumococcal vaccines have a 44% to 75% efficacy against invasive disease from *S. pneumoniae* for persons 65 and older and have been shown to be cost effective in populations aged 50 years and older. A systematic review demonstrated that the influenza vaccine effectively reduces PNA, hospital admission, and death. Annual influenza immunization is recommended as neuraminidase and hemagglutinin evolve rapidly, and new formulations targeting predicted strains are needed.

References

Centers for Disease Control and Prevention. FastStats - Pneumonia. https://www.cdc.gov/nchs/fastats/pneumonia.htm. Published 2017. Accessed March 10, 2018.

Kalil AC, Metersky ML, Klompas M, et al: Management of adults with hospital-acquired and ventilator-associated pneumonia: 2016 clinical practice guidelines by the infectious disease society of america and the american thoracic society, *Clin Infect Dis* 63(5):61–111, 2016, https://doi.org/10.1093/cid/ciw353.

Kaysin A, Viera AJ: Community- acquired pneumonia in adults: diagnosis and management, *Am Fam Physician* 94(9):698–706, 2016. http://www.aafp.org/afp/2016/1101/p698.html.

Kurotschka PK, Bentivegna M, Hulme C, Ebell MH: Identifying the best initial oral antibiotics for adults with community-acquired pneumonia: a network meta-analysis, *J Gen Intern Med* 39(7):1214–1226, 2024.

Jones RN: Microbial etiologies of hospital–acquired bacterial pneumonia and ventilator–associated bacterial pneumonia, *Clin Infect Dis* 51(S1):S81–S87, 2010, https://doi.org/10.1086/653053.

Mandell LA, Niederman MS: Aspiration pneumonia, *N Engl J Med* 380(7):651–663, 2019, https://doi.org/10.1056/NEJMra1714562.

Mandell LA, Wunderink RG, Anzueto A, et al: Thoracic society consensus guidelines on the management of community-acquired pneumonia in adults, *Clin Infect Dis* 44:S27–S72, 2007, https://doi.org/10.1086/511159.

Metlay JP, Waterer GW, et al: Diagnosis and treatment of adults with community-acquired pneumonia: an officialK clinical practice guideline of the american thoracic society and infectious diseases society of america, *Am J Respir Crit Care Med* 200(7):e45–e67, 2019. https://doi.org/10.1164/rccm.201908-1581ST.

Musher DM, Thorner AR: Community-acquired pneumonia, *N Engl J Med* 371(17):1619–1628, 2014. https://doi.org/10.1056/NEJMra1312885.

Wilson JW, Estes LL: *Mayo Clinic Antimicrobial Therapy: Quick Guide*, 2nd ed., 2012.

Centers for Disease Control and Prevention: *Immunization Schedules*, 2020. https://www.cdc.gov/vaccines/schedules/index.html.

BLASTOMYCOSIS

Method of
John M. Embil, MD; and Donald C. Vinh, MD

CURRENT DIAGNOSIS

- Blastomycosis is most commonly caused by the thermally dimorphic fungi *Blastomyces dermatitidis* and *gilchristii*, which together constitute the *B. dermatitidis* complex.

- *Blastomyces* spp. are endemic to the United States (southeastern and south central states bordering Mississippi and Ohio Rivers; upper Midwestern states bordering the Great Lakes) and to Canada (Manitoba and Ontario bordering the Great Lakes; Quebec adjacent to St. Lawrence River).
- Blastomycosis should be suspected in the appropriate clinical context in patients who have resided or traveled to an endemic area.
- Blastomycosis has a broad range of manifestations, mimicking other infectious (e.g., bacteria, mycobacteria) and neoplastic processes.
- Blastomycosis may be asymptomatic, or it can manifest with disease involving the lung, skin, bone and joints, genitourinary system, or central nervous system.
- Diagnosis requires microscopic examination and/or culture of clinical specimens. *Blastomyces* antigen detection is also useful. Serology has no diagnostic value.

CURRENT THERAPY

- Treatment varies with the severity of disease.
- Long-term suppressive therapy may be required for those who are immunosuppressed.

The *Blastomyces dermatitidis* complex are the thermally dimorphic fungi that most commonly cause blastomycosis. Although novel *Blastomyces* species have been identified, they appear to be much less common than the *B. dermatitidis* complex; these new species have distinct mycological features and may produce atypical presentation of disease. *Blastomyces* spp. exist in mycelial form in the environment but grow as yeast forms at body temperature. Although the *B. dermatitidis* complex is endemic to certain specific regions within North America, numerous cases have been reported from areas where it is not considered endemic. It is presumed that those patients acquired infection in the endemic areas and subsequently presented outside of these geographic locations. However, it is also possible that the natural reservoirs of the fungus are evolving. The clinical manifestations of blastomycosis can be diverse, and therefore this infection should be suspected within the appropriate clinical context in persons with a history of residence or travel to such endemic areas.

Epidemiology

Our knowledge of the exact geographic distribution of *B. dermatitidis* complex is limited by the fact that the fungus cannot be readily recovered from nature; thus identification of the endemic area has been largely derived from outbreak investigations and small case series. Most epidemiologic studies have depended upon recovery of *B. dermatitidis* in culture from clinical specimens or histologic visualization to establish the diagnosis. In addition, the incidence and prevalence of blastomycosis has been difficult to establish because suitable serologic or skin-prick assays (demonstrating acceptable sensitivity and/or specificity) to confirm infection are lacking. The geographic niche of *Blastomyces* spp. may therefore be greater than is currently believed.

The currently known areas of endemicity for *B. dermatitidis/gilchristii* are the south central and upper midwestern United States, including areas surrounding the Great Lakes. *B. dermatitidis* is also endemic in Wisconsin (1.3 cases per 100,000 population) and Mississippi (1.4 cases per 100,000 population), as well as parts of Missouri, Kentucky, Tennessee, Arkansas, and Alabama. In Canada, the major areas of endemicity include the province of Manitoba (0.62 cases per 100,000 population), the southern region of Quebec (0.46–0.79 cases per 100,000 population), and the Kenora region of the province of Ontario (7.11 cases per 100,000 population). Although most cases of blastomycosis are

BOX 1 Clinical Manifestations of Blastomycosis

Lung

Acute Pneumonia

Acute pneumonia is clinically indistinguishable from bacterial pneumonia.

Patients may present with fevers, chills, dyspnea, and cough, which initially might not be productive but, with time, may be accompanied by sputum production.

Radiographic findings can also be difficult to discern from those due to a bacterial pneumonia.

The radiographic pattern of pulmonary blastomycosis includes the following:

- Lobar infiltrates that mimic bacterial pneumonias
- Cavitary lung lesions and miliary patterns, which can mimic tuberculosis
- Mass lesions that may be mistaken for neoplasms
- Cystic lesions that resemble abscesses

There is no definitive plain radiograph or computed tomographic scan findings characteristic of pulmonary blastomycosis.

The spectrum of clinical pulmonary disease ranges from spontaneous resolution to pneumonia, with or without the acute respiratory distress syndrome; the latter is accompanied by high (50%–89%) mortality rates.

Chronic Pneumonia

A nonresolving pneumonia is one of the hallmarks of pulmonary blastomycosis.

Chronic pneumonia may be associated with fever, chills, weight loss, sputum-producing cough, and hemoptysis.

There is no characteristic radiographic appearance to help establish the diagnosis.

Skin

Cutaneous lesions are the most common extrapulmonary manifestations of blastomycosis. Lesions usually result from dissemination of a primary pulmonary lesion or rarely from direct inoculation.

Lesions can have a number of different appearances, with verrucae (wartlike lesions) and ulcers being the most common manifestations. The verrucous lesions have a heaped-up appearance with a raw excoriated center. These lesions can mimic squamous cell carcinomas. Cutaneous abscesses may be associated with these lesions.

Ulcerative lesions initially manifest as pustules that eventually erode, producing a bed of granulation tissue that is friable and bleeds when traumatized. Other skin lesions include subcutaneous nodules and isolated abscesses.

Bone and Joint

The most common manifestation of extrapulmonary blastomycosis, after cutaneous disease, is involvement of bones and joints.

Any bone may be involved, although the long bones and axial skeleton are the most commonly affected.

The radiographic findings are indistinguishable from bacterial osteomyelitis and arthritis.

Genitourinary Tract

In the genitourinary tract, the prostate has been reported to be commonly affected by blastomycosis.

Symptoms can mimic prostatitis, and patients can present with obstructive uropathy.

Central Nervous System

The central nervous system (CNS) is infrequently affected by B. dermatitidis. Infection may occur in isolation or with concomitant non-CNS infection.

CNS blastomycosis can occur in immunocompromised patients (e.g., HIV, solid organ transplant), as well as in patients with little/no risk factors (e.g., diabetes mellitus alone; persons with no underlying comorbidities).

Clinical manifestations depend on the area of involvement and range from focal neurologic findings (e.g., due to mass lesions in the brain parenchyma) to symptoms of meningitis due to involvement of the meninges.

Radiographically, the findings may be indistinguishable from bacterial processes. Other sites of involvement have been described but are infrequent compared with those summarized previously.

---

concentrated in these regions, it should be remembered that persons can acquire infection with *Blastomyces* spp. in these areas but present at a later time to healthcare providers in locations where blastomycosis is not usually observed. Inquiring about residence or travel to these areas is important to help establish the diagnosis.

Risk factors for acquiring blastomycosis have been defined by case reports, case series, and a small number of case-control studies and have not been conclusively established. Exposure while in endemic regions to soil, decaying wood, or to dust clouds generated by soil disruption is important; however, specific outdoor occupations or activities have not been confirmed. The fungus may also be associated with exposure to river waterways.

Ethnic ancestry may be a contributing factor to disease. In one study from Mississippi, African American ancestry and prior history of pneumonia were independent risk factors for blastomycosis; however, neither environmental nor socioeconomic risk factors were detected. These findings were in contrast to previously noted studies where race and gender were not identified as specific risk factors for acquisition of blastomycosis. One study in Canada noted an increased incidence among the Indigenous population of Manitoba. Thus it remains unclear if certain ethnic groups are at increased risk for disease or simply reflect differences in exposure.

Immunosuppression may also be an important risk factor, particularly for the tendency to develop severe disease. Blastomycosis has been reported in pregnant women, persons with diabetes mellitus, organ transplant recipients, and persons infected with HIV.

Dogs and humans are the species most commonly affected by *B. dermatitidis* complex. Anecdotally, dogs can serve as a sentinel marker for human disease (i.e., dogs present with systemic infection before their owners), leading to early suspicion of human infections by astute veterinarians. In such cases, it is speculated that humans and their pet dogs have a simultaneous exposure to the same source of fungus and therefore develop synchronous infection. This hypothesis, however, remains to be confirmed, and in a 2008 study, canine blastomycosis was not deemed to predict human disease among the human owners. Additional studies are required to establish the relationship between blastomycosis in humans and disease in their pet dogs.

The most common mode of transmission is presumed to be by inhalation of aerosolized conidia from the environment. There are, however, reports of cutaneous blastomycosis occurring after accidental cutaneous inoculation, for example in the laboratory setting during autopsy or after dog bites. The median incubation period, established by reviewing the results of point-source outbreaks, ranges from 30 to 45 days.

Pathophysiology

After inhalation of conidia into the lungs, the fungus is phagocytosed by alveolar macrophages. The human body temperature allows the fungus to transform to the yeast phase. It is speculated that a process similar to infection with *Mycobacterium tuberculosis* then occurs. The fungus might spread to other organs via the bloodstream and lymphatics. The primary defense against *B. dermatitidis* is through a suppurative response initially with

BOX 2 | Establishing the Diagnosis of Blastomycosis

Direct Examination

A wet preparation of respiratory secretions or a touch preparation of tissues examined under high magnification by light microscopy can reveal the characteristic thick-walled, broad-based budding yeast form. However, this method has a low diagnostic yield: 36% for a single specimen and 46% for multiple specimens.

Calcofluor white stains can help in identifying the pathogen but require fluorescence microscopy.

Histopathologic Examination

The fungus may be difficult to identify with hematoxylin and eosin stain.

If there is a high index of suspicion, the Gomori methenamine-silver stain should be used to optimize detection of thick-walled, broad-based budding yeast forms compatible with *Blastomyces dermatitidis*.

Culture

Diagnostic yield ranges from approximately 86% from sputum to 92% from specimens obtained by bronchoscopy.

Culture is the gold standard for diagnosis. However, the fungus can take several weeks to be isolated in culture.

Confirmation of identity traditionally requires demonstration of thermal dimorphism (mycelial-to-yeast conversion), which can further delay diagnosis. Commercially available nucleic acid probe assays can more rapidly provide definitive identification without the need to demonstrate thermal dimorphism.

Isolation of *B. dermatitidis* should not be considered a contaminant.

Serology

Current serologic assays are neither sensitive nor specific, and they should not be used to establish or refute a diagnosis or in therapeutic decision making.

Nucleic Acid Detection

This method permits genetic-based identification of *B. dermatitidis* from culture of clinical specimens, rather than relying on thermal dimorphism to confirm identity of the fungus, thus reducing the time required for its identification.

Antigen Detection

The only currently available antigen detection assay has its greatest sensitivity in urine, although antigens can be detected in serum and other body fluids.

Cross reaction with antigens from other fungi (e.g., *Histoplasma* spp.) can occur.

The greatest benefit of the antigen detection assay may be to follow efficacy of treatment in patients with established disease (antigen levels decrease with successful treatment or rise with recurrence).

Skin Testing

A commercially available standardized reagent for skin testing is not available.

Modified from Chapman SW, Bradsher RW, Campbell GD, et al: Practice guidelines for the management of patients with blastomycosis, *Clin Infect Dis* 30:679–683, 2000; and Martynowicz MA, Prakash UBS: Pulmonary blastomycosis: An appraisal of diagnostic techniques, *Chest* 121:768–773, 2002.

neutrophils, followed by influx of monocytes with establishment of cell-mediated immunity, resulting in noncaseating granuloma. The patient with intact immunologic responses can contain the process without progression to clinical disease. Alternatively, the patient can develop a symptomatic pneumonia and then mount a suitable immunologic response and recover. Impaired immunity favors the development of progressive pulmonary disease

with or without extrapulmonary manifestations. It has also been suggested that reactivation of disease can occur at pulmonary or extrapulmonary sites. The pathophysiology of *B. gilchristii* is thought to be similar to that of *B. dermatitidis*. A vaccine that protects humans against infection with *Blastomyces* spp. is unavailable.

Clinical Manifestations

After inhalation of the conidia, an initial infection can occur. Most primary infections (at least 50%) are asymptomatic or mild and usually go unrecognized, resolving spontaneously. In others, a symptomatic pneumonia can develop; recovery can occur either spontaneously or with therapy, without further progression. Some persons develop progressive pneumonia or extrapulmonary manifestations. The type of clinical manifestations (localized, extrapulmonary, or disseminated disease) can have a seasonal variation: persons with manifestations occurring early after exposure (1–6 months) developed localized pneumonia, whereas those who presented later after exposure (4–9 months) tended to have isolated extrapulmonary or disseminated disease. Blastomycosis has been termed "the great mimic," because its clinical manifestations are nonspecific and can be similar to those of many different clinical entities. The most common organ systems involved in blastomycosis, in descending order of frequency, include lung, skin, bone, genitourinary, and central nervous systems (CNS). Box 1 summarizes the key clinical manifestations of blastomycosis.

Blastomycosis in Special Populations

Children account for a small percentage of the cases of blastomycosis, ranging from 2% to 11%. Children demonstrate a similar spectrum of manifestations as in adults (excluding prostatic disease). The most common symptoms include cough, headache, chest pain, weight loss, fever, abdominal pain, and night sweats. It is postulated that children experience disseminated infection more frequently than do adults.

Although there are few published reports of blastomycosis in pregnancy, disease has been observed in pregnant women, with presumed subsequent intrauterine and perinatal transmission.

Blastomycosis has been reported in persons with advanced HIV and among those who have undergone solid organ transplants. In immunocompromised hosts, it appears that a significant percentage developed rapidly progressive pulmonary disease, leading to respiratory failure and death. For those who are immunocompromised, the reported mortality rate range is 30% to 40%, with death occurring within the first few weeks of disease onset.

Diagnosis

The most reliable technique for confirming the diagnosis of blastomycosis is recovery of the fungus in culture. Alternatively, direct observation of the pathogen by light microscopy or with calcofluor white stain or in histopathologic examination of tissue establishes a presumptive diagnosis. *Blastomyces* spp. are characteristically observed as a thick-walled, broad-based budding yeast. Because colonization does not occur, identification of *B. dermatitidis/gilchristii* should never be considered a contaminant. Serologic assays are extremely variable in their sensitivity and specificity and do not play a role in confirming or excluding the diagnosis, thus limiting their value in therapeutic decision making. A reliable skin test is unavailable, but a fungal cell wall antigen detection assay exists that can be performed on urine, serum, or cerebrospinal fluid and may aid in diagnosis; moreover, it may be of benefit to follow the efficacy of treatment in established infections. Box 2 summarizes techniques for establishing the diagnosis of blastomycosis.

Treatment

The treatment recommendations for blastomycosis from the Infectious Diseases Society of America (IDSA) are summarized in Table 1. Amphotericin B deoxycholate (Fungizone) is the agent with which there is the greatest experience, particularly for the treatment of patients with severe blastomycosis or for those who

| **TABLE 1** | Treatment Suggestions for Infections Caused by *Blastomycosis dermatitidis* |

TREATMENT RECOMMENDATIONS

MANIFESTATION	PRIMARY RECOMMENDATION	ALTERNATIVE RECOMMENDATION	COMMENTS
Pulmonary Infection			
Mild to moderate	Itraconazole (Sporanox) 200 mg PO tid × 3 days, then qd or bid × 6–12 mo	Fluconazole (Diflucan)[1] 400–800[3] mg/day or ketoconazole (Nizoral) 400–800 mg/kg × 6–12 mo	For itraconazole, measure serum levels after at least 2 wk, to ensure adequate drug exposure. Target level: >1.0 µg/mL and <10.0 µg/mL
Moderate to severe	Lipid formulation of amphotericin B (AmBisome[1], Abelcet, Amphotec[2]) 3–5 mg/kg/day OR Amphotericin B deoxycholate (Fungizone) 0.7–1 mg/kg/d for 1–2 wk or until improvement, followed by itraconazole 200 mg PO tid × 3 days then 200 mg PO bid × 6–12 mo		Amphotericin B toxicity can be attenuated by minimizing the duration of therapy and switching to oral therapy when the patient is stable For itraconazole, measure serum levels after at least 2 wk, to ensure adequate drug exposure. Target level: >1.0 µg/mL and <10.0 µg/mL
Disseminated Infection Not Involving the Central Nervous System			
Mild to moderate	Itraconazole 200 mg PO tid × 3 days then qd or bid × 6–12 mo		
Moderate to severe	Lipid formulation of amphotericin B 3–5 mg/kg/d OR Amphotericin B deoxycholate 0.7–1 mg/kg/d for 1–2 wk or until improvement, followed by itraconazole 200 mg PO tid × 3 days then 200 mg PO bid to complete at least 12 mo		To minimize toxicity, switching to oral therapy once the patient is stable should be considered Bone and joint infections are usually treated for at least 12 mo with itraconazole For itraconazole, measure serum levels after at least 2 wk, to ensure adequate drug exposure. Target level: >1.0 µg/mL and <10.0 µg/mL
Central Nervous System Involvement (with or without other manifestations)			
	Lipid preparations of amphotericin B[1] 5 mg/kg/d × 4–6 wk followed by an oral azole for ≥12 mo		It has been suggested that liposomal amphotericin B achieves higher CNS levels than other lipid formulations When switching to oral azole, options include fluconazole[1] 800 mg PO qd[3], itraconazole 200 mg PO bid or tid[3], or voriconazole (Vfend)[1] 200–400[3] mg PO bid Longer durations of therapy may be necessary in the immunocompromised host
Special Populations			
Immunocompromised	Lipid formulation of amphotericin B 3–5 mg/kg/d OR Amphotericin B deoxycholate 0.7–1 mg/kg/d for 1–2 wk or until improvement, followed by itraconazole 200 mg PO tid × 3 days then 200 mg PO bid to complete at least 12 mo		Lifelong suppression with itraconazole 200 mg PO qd may be required for those in whom immunosuppression cannot be reversed
Pregnant patients	Lipid formulation of amphotericin B 3–5 mg/kg/d		No duration of lipid formulation amphotericin B treatment provided; continue until clinical cure During pregnancy, azoles should be avoided because of potential teratogenicity If the placenta or newborn demonstrates evidence of infection, give amphotericin B deoxycholate 1.0 mg/kg/d
Children: mild to moderate	Itraconazole[1] 10 mg/kg/d for 6–12 mo		Maximum dose of itraconazole should be 400 mg/d
Children: moderate to severe	Amphotericin B deoxycholate 0.7–10.0 mg/kg/d OR Lipid formulation amphotericin B 3–5 mg/kg/d × 1–2 wk followed by itraconazole 10 mg/kg/d × 12 mo		

[1]Not FDA approved for this indication.
[3]Exceeds dosage recommended by the manufacturer.
[2]Not available in the United States.
bid, Twice daily; *CNS,* central nervous system; *PO,* orally; *qd,* daily; *tid,* three times daily.
Modified from Chapman SW, Bradsher RW, Campbell GD, et al: Practice guidelines for the management of patients with blastomycosis, *Clin Infect Dis* 30:679, 2000; and Chapman SW, Dismukes WE, Proia LA, et al: Clinical practice guidelines for the management of blastomycosis: 2008 update by the Infectious Diseases Society of America, *Clin Infect Dis* 46:1801–1812, 2008.

have CNS involvement. Lipid preparations of amphotericin B (Abelcet, AmBisome[1], Amphotec[2]) have been shown to be effective in animal models, although clinical trial data are unavailable for these agents in humans. Clinical experience suggests that the lipid formulations may be as effective but less toxic than the deoxycholate preparation.

It is generally accepted that in patients with severe disease or CNS involvement, amphotericin B–based products should be used to initiate therapy until the patient is stable, followed by stepdown to an azole, specifically itraconazole (Sporanox), to complete the total duration of therapy. Patients on itraconazole should have serum levels of the antifungal drug measured after at least 2 weeks of therapy, targeting a level >1.0 µg/mL and <10.0 µg/mL. Ketoconazole (Nizoral), although once recommended as the agent of choice, is less effective and more toxic than itraconazole. Experience with fluconazole (Diflucan)[1] for the treatment of blastomycosis is limited, although in vitro studies have demonstrated that fluconazole is effective against *B. dermatitidis*. Fluconazole does, however, have excellent penetration into the CNS; therefore fluconazole may be considered as an alternative treatment of CNS blastomycosis[1]. There are also an increasing number of reports of voriconazole (Vfend)[1] being used for the successful treatment of CNS blastomycosis, as well as in persons with refractory blastomycosis. A case series of patients with CNS blastomycosis suggested that voriconazole may be the most desirable azole for the management of CNS disease. Voriconazole therapeutic drug monitoring is necessary to ensure appropriate serum concentrations are attained while avoiding dose-related adverse effects (e.g., hepatic toxicities). Similarly, there are reports on the successful use of posaconazole (Noxafil)[1] and isavuconazole (Cresemba)[1] for blastomycosis. The echinocandins (caspofungin [Cancidas][1], micafungin [Mycamine][1], and anidulafungin [Eraxis][1]) have limited activity against *B. dermatitidis* and are not considered appropriate choices.

Table 1 summarizes the therapeutic options for treatment of various types of blastomycosis. Amphotericin B–based therapy is usually the treatment option of choice in persons who have severe disease. Whenever the patient is clinically stable, it is desirable to switch from the potentially toxic amphotericin B to a less toxic agent (usually an azole). It is important to note that amphotericin B in cumulative doses of 1.5 to 2.5 g for persons with disseminated blastomycosis, with life-threatening disease, or in those who are immunocompromised or pregnant, can lead to cure without relapses.

In patients with overwhelming pulmonary disease, amphotericin B–based products are the therapeutic agents of choice. Although acute respiratory distress syndrome (ARDS) can complicate the management of these patients, data on the beneficial role of corticosteroids in the management of patients with overwhelming pulmonary disease or ARDS are limited to few case reports. For patients with less severe pulmonary disease, an alternative to amphotericin B is a 6- to 12-month course of oral itraconazole. A similarly prolonged course of oral itraconazole is also appropriate for persons with bone and joint disease. The precise duration of therapy, however, is unknown and should be individualized. The same is true for cutaneous blastomycosis. For persons with CNS blastomycosis, an initial treatment course of 4 to 6 weeks with intravenous lipid formulation of amphotericin B should be followed with an oral azole to complete at least 12 months of therapy. For those who are immunocompromised, prolonged therapy is also necessary. Patients who are immunosuppressed and in whom the immunosuppression cannot be reversed can require lifelong suppressive itraconazole therapy at 200 mg per day. Additional details for the management of the various stages of blastomycosis should be sought from the most current version of the IDSA guidelines.

---

[1] Not FDA approved for this indication.
[2] Not available in the United States.

References

Bariola JR, Perry P, Pappas PG, et al: Blastomycosis of the central nervous system: a multicenter review of diagnosis and treatment in the modern era, *Clin Infect Dis* 50:797–804, 2010.

Bush JW, Wuerz T, Embil JM, Del Bigio MR, McDonald PJ, Krawitz S: Outcomes of persons with blastomycosis involving the central nervous system, *Diagn Microbiol Infect Dis* 76(2):175–181, 2013.

Chapman SW, Lin AC, Hendricks KA, et al: Endemic blastomycosis in Mississippi: epidemiological and clinical studies, *Semin Respir Infect* 12:219–228, 1997.

Chapman SW, Dismukes WE, Proia LA, et al: Clinical practice guidelines for the management of blastomycosis: 2008 update by the Infectious Diseases Society of America, *Clin Infect Dis* 46:1801–1812, 2008.

Chapman SW, Sullivan DC: Blastomyces dermatitidis. In Mandell GL, Bennett JE, Dolin R, editors: *Mandell, douglas, and bennett's principles and practice of infectious diseases*, 7th ed., Philadelphia, 2010, Elsevier, pp 3319–3332.

Choptiany M, Wiebe L, Limerick B, et al: Risk factors for acquisition of endemic blastomycosis, *Can J Infect Dis Med Microbiol* 20:117–121, 2009.

Crampton TL, Light RB, Berg GM, et al: Epidemiology and clinical spectrum of blastomycosis diagnosed at Manitoba hospitals, *Clin Infect Dis* 34:1310–1316, 2002.

Litvinov IV, St-Germain G, Pelletier R, Paradis M, Sheppard DC: Endemic human blastomycosis in Quebec, Canada, 1988–2011, *Epidemiol Infect* 141(6):1143–1147, 2013.

Martynowicz MA, Prakash UBS: Pulmonary blastomycosis: an appraisal of diagnostic techniques, *Chest* 121:768–773, 2002.

Meyer KC, McManus EJ, Maki DG: Overwhelming pulmonary blastomycosis associated with the adult respiratory distress syndrome, *N Engl J Med* 329:1231–1236, 1993.

Oppenheimer M, Cheang M, Trepman E, et al: Orthopedic manifestations of blastomycosis, *South Med J* 100:570–578, 2007.

Pappas PG: Blastomycosis in the immunocompromised patient, *Semin Respir Infect* 12:243–251, 1997.

Ward BA, Parent AD, Raila F: Indications for the surgical management of central nervous system blastomycosis, *Surg Neurol* 43:379–388, 1995.

CHRONIC OBSTRUCTIVE PULMONARY DISEASE

Method of
Alexis Waters, PA

CURRENT DIAGNOSIS

- Chronic obstructive pulmonary disease (COPD) is a condition of adults over age 40.
- The prevalence of COPD in the United States is 5.6%, representing about 18 million Americans.
- Further research is needed into the gender, racial, and ethnic disparities in who is diagnosed with and dies from COPD.
- COPD is the result of chronic inflammation caused by external irritants, most commonly tobacco smoke in high-income countries and household air pollution in low- and middle- income countries.
- Rare causes of COPD include α-1 antitrypsin deficiency, abnormal lung development, and infections, especially human immunodeficiency virus and tuberculosis.
- Chronic inflammation in COPD leads to reduced elasticity of the airways, increased mucus production, destruction of the alveoli, and changes to pulmonary vasculature.
- The three primary symptoms of COPD are dyspnea, chronic cough, and sputum production.
- Classification of COPD patients into group A, B, or E based on COPD Assessment Test (CAT) and Modified Medical Research Council Dyspnea Scale (mMRC) scores in addition to exacerbation history.
- COPD is a progressive disease that is characterized by periods of stability and episodes of exacerbation.
- The diagnosis and severity of COPD are determined through spirometry.

- Smoking cessation is the cornerstone of COPD management. Counseling and pharmacotherapy improve quit rates.
- Patients with COPD should receive both the pneumococcal, influenza, respiratory syncytial virus (RSV), and COVID-19 vaccines.
- Pulmonary rehabilitation improves activity capacity and quality of life and decreases dyspnea and hospitalization.
- Proper inhaler technique is necessary for maximal benefit from inhaled medications.
- Short-acting β-agonists are appropriate for mild, intermittent symptoms.
- A long-acting β-agonist (LABA), a long-acting antimuscarinic (LAMA), or both may be added in patients with more frequent or severe dyspnea. Inhaled corticosteroid (ICS) is considered in patients with eosinophilia.
- Attention should be paid to management of retained secretions.
- Noninvasive ventilation can decrease hypercapnia and dyspnea in patients with chronic hypercapnic respiratory failure.
- A selected group of patients with severe disease may benefit from surgical interventions, such as lung volume reduction surgery or lung transplantation.
- Exacerbations of COPD in outpatients may be managed with increased frequency of short-acting bronchodilators, systemic corticosteroids, and antibiotics.
- Palliative care is appropriate for patients with severe, refractory symptoms.

Epidemiology

Chronic obstructive pulmonary disease (COPD) is a condition that mostly impacts adults over age 40. In 2019 COPD caused approximately 3.23 million deaths worldwide and over 150,000 deaths in the United States. Before the coronavirus epidemic, COPD was the third leading cause of death and the seventh leading cause of poor health in the world and was the fourth leading cause of death in the United States. In the postpandemic landscape, COPD dropped to the fourth leading cause of death globally and the sixth leading cause of death in the United States. In the United States the prevalence of COPD in 2020 ranged from 3.2% (Hawaii) to 11.9% (West Virginia), with an average overall age-adjusted prevalence of 5.6%. This represents about 18.5 million people, one-third of whom may not yet be diagnosed or know that they have the condition. There are gender, racial, and ethnic differences in who is impacted by COPD in the United States. Women have consistently higher prevalence rates than men (5.9% vs. 5.2% in 2020), although men are more likely to die of the disease. Reported rates of COPD among Black or African Americans are often lower than for Hispanic or White Americans; however, data suggest that Black or African Americans are more likely to go undiagnosed. A study on Mexican Americans showed that this group developed COPD at much lower tobacco smoke exposure than European Americans. Further research is indicated to elucidate differences in risk factors for and pathogenesis of COPD among Americans from different racial, ethnic, and socioeconomic backgrounds.

Pathophysiology

COPD is an inflammatory disease of the lungs characterized by airflow obstruction. Chronic inflammation of and subsequent pathologic changes to the airways (the conducting portions of the lung), lung parenchyma (the portions of the lung involved in gas exchange), and pulmonary vasculature all contribute to the development of COPD. In most cases of COPD, an external irritant (such as tobacco or air pollution) causes an inflammatory response within the airways. The exact mechanism of inflammation is unknown but is thought to involve oxidative stress, an excess of proteases, and inflammatory cells including neutrophils and macrophages. A rare cause of COPD is α-1 antitrypsin deficiency, in which increased protease activity is the major pathologic factor. COPD can also develop in patients who have abnormal lung development and/or infections, especially human immunodeficiency virus and tuberculosis.

Regardless of the etiology, the end result of the inflammation is reduced elasticity of the airways, increased mucus production, and destruction of the alveoli. Reduced elasticity impacts the ability of the lung to exhale fully and causes airway collapse, ultimately causing air trapping, reduced carbon dioxide release, and hyperinflation. Increased mucus production physically inhibits air flow and gas exchange, while alveoli destruction reduces the area available for gas exchange. Pulmonary vasculature changes occur with the prolonged hypoxia caused by COPD, which causes vessels to constrict in response to the limited available oxygen. There is increasing evidence that direct damage to pulmonary vessel endothelium by external irritants also contributes to COPD pathology by leading to excessive arterial remodeling. Pulmonary hypertension is thus a common sequela of COPD and is associated with poor outcomes.

Prevention

Depending on its primary cause, prevention of COPD is aimed at reducing the relevant external irritant (tobacco or air pollution); in high-income countries, tobacco use is the major irritant, while in low- and middle-income countries, the primary cause is household air pollution. In the United States public health efforts at reducing cigarette smoking over the past few decades have led to a significant decrease in the number of Americans who use tobacco. In 1965 over 42% of American adults smoked, compared with fewer than 14% in 2018.

Clinical Manifestations

COPD is a treatable, though not curable, condition. It is characterized by periods of stability and episodes of exacerbation and is generally a progressive disease, particularly for patients who are continuously exposed to external irritants (tobacco smoke and/or air pollution). There are three primary symptoms of COPD: dyspnea, chronic cough, and sputum production. Other symptoms include wheezing, chest tightness, fatigue, and activity limitation. Patients do not need to have all three cardinal symptoms to have COPD. Many patients report variability in symptom severity, with multiple studies reporting that patients find symptoms most bothersome in the morning, when they frequently inhibit personal care activities necessary to prepare for the day. Shortness of breath and cough are the most common and most troublesome symptoms. Around 30% to 40% of people with COPD report that the disease impacts their ability to work, ability to sleep, familial relationships, and social lives.

According to the National Heart, Lung, and Blood Institute (NHLBI) and the World Health Organization (WHO), COPD exacerbations are characterized by increased dyspnea, worsening cough, and/or an increase or change in sputum that worsens over a time period of less than 14 days. Tachypnea and tachycardia may also be present. Patients with more severe COPD frequently experience more exacerbations, with around 10% to 20% of patients requiring at least one hospitalization each year. Most COPD exacerbations are thought to be caused by viral illnesses; bacterial infections are far less likely and are probably even more rare than exacerbations caused by air pollution or pulmonary embolism.

Diagnosis

A diagnosis of COPD should be considered in adults who have typical symptoms (shortness of breath, cough, sputum) and an appropriate exposure history (tobacco smoke and/or other environmental exposure). Spirometry, or pulmonary function tests (PFTs), are needed to definitively diagnose the airflow obstruction seen in COPD. PFTs consistent with COPD show that

TABLE 1	GOLD Criteria for Severity of Airflow Obstruction in COPD		
FEV$_1$/FVC < 0.70	GRADE	SPIROMETRY RESULT	OBSTRUCTION SEVERITY
	GOLD 1	FEV$_1$ ≥ 80% predicted	Mild
	GOLD 2	50% ≤ FEV$_1$ ≤ 80% predicted	Moderate
	GOLD 3	30% ≤ FEV$_1$ < 50% predicted	Severe
	GOLD 4	FEV$_1$ < 30% predicted	Very severe

FEV$_1$, Forced expiratory volume in 1 second; *FVC*, forced vital capacity; *GOLD*, Global Institute for Chronic Obstructive Lung Disease.

TABLE 2	Modified Medical Research Council Dyspnea Scale
mMRC Grade 0	I only get breathless with strenuous exercise.
mMRC Grade 1	I get short of breath when hurrying on the level or walking up the hill.
mMRC Grade 2	I walk slower than people of the same age on the level because of breathlessness, or I have to stop for breath when walking on my own pace on the level.
mMRC Grade 3	I stop for breath after walking about 100 m or after a few minutes on the level.
mMRC Grade 4	I am too breathless to leave the house, or I am breathless when dressing or undressing.

mMRC, Modified Medical Research Council.

TABLE 3	Chronic Obstructive Pulmonary Disease Assessment Test

In the ranges below, circle the number that best indicates how you feel:

I never cough.	0 1 2 3 4 5	I cough all the time.
I have no phlegm (mucus) in my chest at all.	0 1 2 3 4 5	My chest is completely full of phlegm (mucus).
My chest does not feel tight at all.	0 1 2 3 4 5	My chest feels very tight.
When I walk up a hill or one flight of stairs, I am not breathless.	0 1 2 3 4 5	When I walk up a hill or one flight of stairs, I am very breathless.
I am not limited doing any activities at home.	0 1 2 3 4 5	I am very limited doing activities at home.
I am confident leaving my home despite my lung condition.	0 1 2 3 4 5	I am not at all confident leaving my home because of my lung condition.
I sleep soundly.	0 1 2 3 4 5	I don't sleep soundly because of my lung condition.
I have lots of energy.	0 1 2 3 4 5	I have no energy at all.

the ratio of the forced expiratory volume in 1 second to the forced vital capacity (FEV$_1$/FVC) is ≤0.70 after bronchodilator use. These diagnostic criteria, along with further characterization of severity of airflow obstruction (Table 1), are established by the Global Institute for Chronic Obstructive Lung Disease (GOLD), a joint effort of the NHLBI and WHO. Importantly, severity of airflow obstruction may not correspond to severity of symptoms. To assess severity of symptoms, validated symptom assessments should be used; these include the Modified Medical Research Council Dyspnea Scale (mMRC, Table 2) and the COPD Assessment Test (CAT, Table 3). Results of these subjective tests can be used to guide treatment and assess response to treatment.

In addition to spirometry and symptom assessment, all patients diagnosed with COPD should be screened for α-1 antitrypsin deficiency. Imaging, either with chest radiograph or computed tomography (CT) scan, is not needed. However, in certain patients, CT may be useful; these patients include those with frequent exacerbations, those with subjective symptoms that are significantly out of proportion to spirometry results, and those with FEV$_1$ <45% of predicted. COPD patients who qualify should also undergo lung cancer screening with CT as recommended by the U.S. Preventive Services Task Force.

The most easily confused differential diagnosis for COPD is asthma; however, these conditions can be distinguished by the lack of response to bronchodilator therapy in COPD compared with an improvement in FEV$_1$ or FVC (sometimes to normal) in patients with asthma. Other possible diagnoses to consider in patients with symptoms consistent with COPD include heart failure, bronchiectasis (etiologies include infection, autoimmune disorders, and cystic fibrosis, among others), and other causes of airway obstruction (malignancy). Less common COPD mimics include tuberculosis, chronic bronchitis without airflow obstruction on COPD, obliterative bronchiolitis (often after hematopoietic stem cell transplant), and diffuse panbronchiolitis (seen in male nonsmokers of East Asian descent with chronic sinusitis).

Treatment of Stable COPD

Treatment of stable COPD is focused on improving patient quality of life, decreasing symptoms of dyspnea and shortness of breath, increasing activity capacity, preventing and treatment of complications and exacerbations, and prolonging life.

Smoking Cessation

Tobacco use is one of the leading contributors to the development of COPD. The only two interventions that have shown a direct impact on prolonging life in patients with COPD are management of chronic hypoxemic respiratory failure with long-term oxygen use, in addition to smoking cessation. Long-term tobacco cessation is difficult to achieve, and overall patient rates for long-term cessation are ~25%. It is important to target therapy with nicotine replacement and patient counseling, in addition to consideration of pharmacologic therapy. Of note, counseling provided by

healthcare providers of even 3 minutes' duration has been shown to significantly increase the quit rate. Nicotine replacement therapy (NRT) in the form of gum, lozenge, or patch has been very well tolerated. NRT is contraindicated in patients who have recently suffered myocardial ischemia or stroke. The literature disagrees at what point with these patients' resumption is considered safe, but on average greater than 2 weeks after an ischemic event is considered reasonable. Current safety data for e-cigarettes is largely absent in regards to the use of e-cigarettes; their use is not recommended with current therapy guidelines. Pharmacologic therapy in the form of varenicline (Chantix), bupropion (Zyban), or nortriptyline (Pamelor)[1] have been shown successful in augmenting smoking cessation rates (Table 4). However, literature supports that the largest success rates were seen in patients who had received counseling and NRT in addition to pharmacologic therapy.

---

[1] Not FDA approved for this indication.

TABLE 4 Smoking Cessation Medications*

MEDICATION	DOSAGE AND ADMINISTRATION
Nicotine transdermal (NicoDerm CQ)	21 mg/24 hr, 14 mg/24 hr, 7 mg/24 hr If >10 cigarettes/day, then use 21 mg/day for 6 wk, then 14 mg/day for 2 wk, then 7 mg/day for 2 wk If ≤10 cigarettes/day, then use 14 mg/day for 6 wk, then 7 mg/day for 2 wk
Nicotine lozenges (Nicorette)	4 mg, 2 mg Weeks 1–6, 1 lozenge every 1–2 hr Weeks 7–9, 1 lozenge every 2–4 hr Weeks 10–12, 1 lozenge every 4–8 hr
Nicotine gum (Nicorelief, Thrive)	4 mg, 2 mg Weeks 1–6, 1 gum every 1–2 hr Weeks 7–9, 1 gum every 2–4 hr Weeks 10–12, 1 gum every 4–8 hr
Nicotine nasal spray (Nicotrol NS)	10 mg/mL, 1 dose = 1 spray in each nostril Start with 1–2 doses/hr and adjust as needed Do not use more than 5 doses/hr Do not use for more than 3 mo
Bupropion hydrochloride SR (Zyban)	100 mg, 150 mg, 200 mg Days 1–3, 150 mg/day Then increase to 150 mg bid
Varenicline (Chantix)	0.5 mg, 1 mg Days 1–3, 0.5 mg/day Then increase to 0.5 mg bid Patients who quit at 12 wk may be treated an additional 12 wk

*The doses listed in this table assume normal renal and hepatic function.
bid, Twice daily.

Pulmonary Rehabilitation

Pulmonary rehabilitation programs are typically structured with both an exercise component in addition to an educational program. These are supervised by respiratory therapists and groups typically meet two to three times a week, for a 6- to 8-week duration. Educational material includes focuses on smoking cessation, energy conservation techniques in the setting of ADL (activities of daily living) and IADL (instrumental activities of daily living) performance, pursed lip breathing, nutrition, and management of acute exacerbation symptoms. The exercise element is formatted to patient activity tolerance level and includes activities such as strength and resistance training to assist with improvement of muscle mass; cardiovascular training with treadmill, walking, or stationary bike; and stretching exercises. Pulmonary rehabilitation has been shown to have significantly positive impact on measures of quality of life, reduction of dyspnea and shortness of breath, in addition to increased exercise capacity and tolerance. Early rehabilitation for patients discharged from the acute care setting with COPD exacerbations has been demonstrated to decrease mortality risk and hospital readmission. Pulmonary rehabilitation referrals within 1 year of posthospital discharge is only accessed by 2.7% of patients, and nearly 40% of the U.S. patient population has poor or difficult access to pulmonary rehab services. This represents the increasing need to consider pulmonary rehabilitation referrals, especially at the time of discharge, to improve patient outcomes. Creation of telehealth programs for pulmonary rehabilitation should be developed to increase patient access. Telehealth pulmonary rehabilitation programs appear to have similar outcomes compared with office-based programs and result in increased patient compliance and access to services.

Vaccinations

Influenza, COVID-19, and pneumococcal vaccinations are recommended for all patients with COPD. Influenza vaccination has demonstrated nearly a 38% reduction in influenza-related hospitalization in COPD patients with similar efficacy seen with either live attenuated or inactivated vaccine. A reduction in COPD exacerbations has also been seen in vaccinated COPD patients. COVID-19 vaccination is recommended in patients with COPD due to their higher risk of complications given their underlying pulmonary disease. Pneumococcal polysaccharide vaccine (PPSV23 [Pneumovax 23]) and pneumococcal conjugate vaccines (PCV15 [Vaxneuvance], PCV20 [Prevar 20], PCV21 [Capvaxive]) are recommended for patients with COPD less than 65 years of age and with FEV_1 less than 40% or other significant comorbidities, and for all patients 65 years of age or older. Pneumococcal vaccination has shown similar efficacy in decreased rates of community-acquired pneumonia, immunogenicity, and pneumococcal invasive disease. The CDC also recommends the new respiratory syncytial virus (RSV) vaccination (Abrysvo or Arexvy) for patients 60 years or older and/or with underlying chronic lung or heart disease. However, despite this data, overall vaccination rates remain low and should remain a key focus of patient education.

Medications

Medications used in the treatment of COPD are currently based on the recommendations in the GOLD guidelines. Medication recommendations are based on classification of symptoms, disease severity, and exacerbation history.

COPD medications are categorized predominantly by rescue medications versus maintenance therapy medications (Table 5). Commonly used medications for rescue therapy include short-acting β-agonists (SABAs), which stimulate the β-2 receptors that trigger bronchodilation and relaxation of smooth muscle of the airway. These are used as "rescue" or "as needed" medications because of their rapid onset of action (within minutes); however, their relatively short duration of action is about 4 to 6 hours. The long-acting β-agonists (LABAs) similarly have a rapid onset of action; however, their duration of action is longer than the short-acting agents of 12 to 24 hours. Side effect considerations include tachycardia, headache, hypokalemia, and tremor.

Additional medications that also impact bronchodilation include short-acting and long-acting antimuscarinics (SAMAs and LAMAs). Muscarinic antagonists function by inhibiting acetylcholine release, which minimizes smooth muscle constriction. Both SAMA and SABA therapy have been found to provide equivalent symptomatic relief in addition to improvement of FEV_1 in all COPD stages. However, when used in combination, they perform superiorly in symptom reduction and FEV_1 improvement compared with use in isolation. Side effects of muscarinic antagonists include urinary retention, tachycardia, and dry mouth.

Both LABA and LAMA therapy have been shown to decrease symptom reporting and reduce acute exacerbations, in addition to improvement seen in FEV_1. There is some preliminary data that exist suggesting that tiotropium (a LAMA) may perform superiorly over LABA therapy when compared as single agents. However, when used in combination LABA/LAMA therapy they have an even greater efficacy in symptom relief, reducing exacerbations, and improvement in pulmonary function compared with the individual agents alone.

Inhaled corticosteroids (ICS) improve lung function, decrease exacerbation frequency, and decrease airway inflammation. They have not been shown to be effective when used as monotherapy in COPD. Their benefit has best been demonstrated when used as part of combination therapy. Of note, ICS therapy does increase risk of pneumonia, particularly in those with severe disease. Triple therapy with ICS/LABA/LAMA is more efficacious than ICS/LABA, ICS/LAMA, and ICS alone; however, triple therapy should be reserved for those who are experiencing frequent exacerbations, not solely on classification of disease severity.

In the GOLD guidelines, medication recommendations are directed by a classification system based on symptom score from the CAT and the mMRC questionnaire and exacerbation history

TABLE 5	Commonly Used Inhaled Medications for Stable COPD
MEDICATION	**DOSAGE**
SABA	
Albuterol (multiple brands)	2 puffs every 4–6 hours, as needed
Levalbuterol (Xopenex)	1–2 puffs every 4–6 hours, as needed
SAMA	
Ipratropium (Atrovent)	2 inhalations 4 times a day
LABA	
Salmeterol (Serevent Diskus)	1 inhalation twice daily
Indacaterol (Arcapta Neohaler)	Inhale contents of 1 capsule every day
Olodaterol (Striverdi Respimat)	2 puffs once a day, same time of day
Arformoterol (Brovana)	2 mL nebulized twice daily
Formoterol (Perforomist)	2 mL nebulized twice daily
LAMA	
Tiotropium (Spiriva HandiHaler)	2 inhalations of the powder contents of 1 capsule once daily
Tiotropium (Spiriva Respimat)	2 inhalations once daily
Aclidinium (Tudorza Pressair)	1 inhalation twice daily
Umeclidinium (Incruse Ellipta)	1 inhalation daily
Glycopyrronium bromide inhalation powder (Seebri Neohaler)	1 capsule inhaled twice daily using a neohaler device
Glycopyrrolate inhalation solution (Lonhala Magnair)	1 vial inhaled twice daily
Revefenacin (Yupelri)	1 vial nebulized once daily
Combination Medications	
SABA/SAMA	
Albuterol/ipratropium (Combivent Respimat)	1 inhalation 4 times a day
LABA/LAMA	
Umeclidinium/vilanterol (Anoro Ellipta 62.5/25)	1 inhalation once daily
Olodaterol/tiotropium (Stiolto Respimat 2.5/2.5)	2 inhalations once daily
Formoterol/glycopyrrolate (Bevespi Aerosphere 4.8/9)	2 inhalations twice daily
Aclidinium/formoterol (Duaklir Pressair 400/12)	1 inhalation twice daily
ICS/LABA	
Budesonide/formoterol (Symbicort 160/4.5, 80/4.5)	2 inhalations twice daily
Fluticasone/salmeterol (multiple brands)	1–2 inhalations twice daily, depending on brand
Mometasone/formoterol (Dulera 100/5, 200/5)1	2 inhalations twice daily
Fluticasone/vilanterol (Breo Ellipta 100/25, 200/25)	1 inhalation once daily
LABA/LAMA/ICS	
Fluticasone/umeclidinium/vilanterol (Trelegy Ellipta 200/62.5/25, 100/62.5/25)	1 inhalation once daily
Budesonide/glycopyrrolate/formoterol (Breztri Aerosphere 160/9/4.8)	2 inhalations twice daily

ICS, Inhaled corticosteroids; *LABA*, long-acting β-2 agonist; *LAMA*, long-acting antimuscarinic agent; *SABA*, short-acting β-2 agonist.

(Figure 1). Exacerbation history is quantified as either 0 or 1 episode or 2 or more episodes (with at least one requiring hospitalization). On the CAT questionnaire, it entails a series of eight questions as they pertain to ability to perform daily tasks and overall symptoms throughout their day. The mMRC serves as a simple tool to measure breathlessness. The sum of these scores helps classify patients on the GOLD grid.

Patients who meet GOLD classification in group A have been deemed to benefit from initiation of bronchodilator therapy. The treatment is continued if the patient is noted to have benefited from therapy. Group B patients should be initiated on a long-acting bronchodilator in the form of a LABA or LAMA. If a patient continues to have significant symptom reports despite LAMA or LABA therapy, their treatment should be adjusted to a combination LAMA/LABA therapy. If patients in group B present with severe dyspnea, it is appropriate to initiate combination LAMA/LABA therapy rather than start with one agent in isolation. In new GOLD 2025 guidelines, groups C and D have been combined to group E "exacerbations" for classification. For patients in group E, the initial treatment choice is LAMA + LABA. If LABA therapy is cost prohibitive, adding ICS would be second-line treatment. For patients who have more asthmatic consistent symptoms, LABA/ICS would be first line rather than LABA/LAMA therapy in these patients. Patients who continue

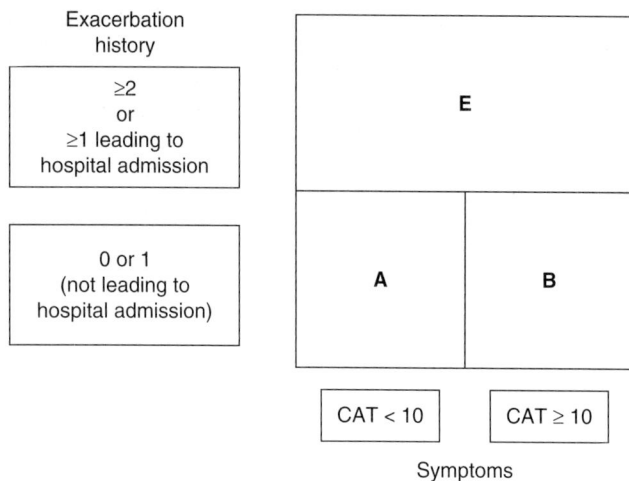

Figure 1 Exacerbation history. *CAT*, COPD Assessment Test.

to have persistent exacerbations despite dual therapy should be transitioned to triple therapy with LABA/LAMA/ICS combination medication. Providers should also consider adding LAMA/LABA/ICS as first line in group E if blood eosinophils are >300. If the patient had already been using LAMA/LABA in group E and continues to experience exacerbations, providers should consider ICS addition if blood eosinophils >100.

It is important to follow GOLD classification guidelines early and ensure patients are on an appropriate treatment-compliant regimen. This slows disease progression to group E and less likelihood of treatment discontinuation due to the patient's lack of perceived benefit of therapy.

In patients with persisting exacerbations on this treatment, the phosphodiesterase-4 inhibitor roflumilast (Daliresp) 500 mcg/day or prophylactic azithromycin (Zithromax)[1] 250 mg/day or 500 mg three times a week for 1 year is prescribed. These agents have shown to decrease exacerbation frequency compared with standard of care. Risks with therapy include increase in macrolide-associated antibiotic resistance, increased risk of hearing impairment, and QT prolongation. The PDE4 inhibitors do have increased side effect profiles compared with inhaler regimens. Patients may experience GI upset, headache, and abdominal discomfort. These are typically noted earlier in treatment courses and lessen as the patient continues therapy.

Difficulty with secretion management can lead to increased dyspnea, shortness of breath, and hypoxia. Medical management of secretions include use of guaifenesin[1] in addition to positive expiratory devices (PEP) such as an Aerobika or Acapella. For patients who have a poor cough reflex and would not tolerate PEP devices, home suctioning equipment could be considered to assist with secretion management.

Patient education remains a large component of COPD treatment. Incorrect inhaler technique is a significant factor in treatment failure. It is important to continue to review technique and disease understanding throughout their disease course, particularly before changing treatment regimen. Providers should keep in mind patient preference for inhaler delivery devices and that in-office spirometry may not be entirely reflective of resistance/effort patterns with home inhalers. To assist with appropriate medication delivery, patients should receive education on inhaler administration with spacer to ensure adequate aerosolization of the medication.

Noninvasive Ventilation

Noninvasive ventilation serves an important role in the management of chronic hypercapnic respiratory failure. Home bilevel positive airway pressure (BiPAP) qualification based on current

Medicare guidelines for patients with COPD can be pursued if treatment or consideration of obstructive sleep apnea (OSA) and use of continuous positive airway pressure (CPAP) have been ruled out. An arterial blood gas measurement is performed while the patient is awake and requires hypercapnia noted ($PaCO_2$ > 51) and nocturnal oximetry monitoring for a >2-hour recording time with SpO_2 noted <89% for at least 5 consecutive minutes during sleep. Inspiratory positive airway pressure (IPAP) and expiratory positive airway pressure (EPAP) are often frequently adjusted in the early stages to best mitigate hypercapnia and as best tolerated for patient comfort.

Surgical Remedies

Lung volume reduction (LVR) surgery is a special consideration for those patients with advanced disease who may not meet criteria for lung transplant. LVR performance has demonstrated improvement in pulmonary function, quality of life measurements, and activity tolerance. It has also helped improve patient function and overall nutritional status to optimize patients before consideration for transplant. Patients are evaluated under selection criteria outlined by the National Emphysema Therapy Trial (NETT). Inclusion criteria are based on age (75 years or less), no active smoking, and less than 20 mg daily of prednisone. LVR has been most effective in patients with upper lobe predominant emphysema visualized on CT, FEV_1 ≤45% predicted, and the ability to ambulate at least 140 m when evaluated with the 6-minute walk test. Patients are excluded from consideration if morbidly obese, FEV_1 <20% predicted and DLCO <20% predicted, concern for prior chest wall surgery or adhesions, and heterogeneous emphysema or interstitial disease on imaging.

Lung transplantation could be considered in patients with COPD who are younger than 65 years old for a single-lung transplant versus 60 years or younger for a double-lung transplant. Other criteria include FEV_1 20% to 25% or less, presence of pulmonary hypertension, requirement of chronic supplemental oxygen therapy, and $PaCO_2$ greater than 55 mm Hg. The most used prognostic model for patients being considered for lung transplantation is the BODE Index, which evaluates BMI, airflow limitation, dyspnea, and 6-minute walk distance. Patients who have additional significant organ dysfunction, are HIV positive, have active hepatitis B or C, or have recent/current underlying malignancy are excluded from consideration.

Endobronchial therapy with a Zephyr valve is a promising new intervention for COPD. With increasing evidence as provided by the LIBERATE trial, this has demonstrated clinically significant impact with use of the Zephyr valve. Within this procedure, one-way valves are placed within certain parts of the airway resulting in nonsurgical reduction of lung volume. This has improved patient reports on impact of quality of life, dyspnea, increased FEV_1, and notable increase in exercise capacity and tolerance.

Supplemental Oxygen

Long-term supplemental oxygen therapy (LTOT) is one of only two measures (other than smoking cessation) that has been shown to significantly decrease mortality risk in COPD patients. Patients qualify for home oxygen therapy if SpO_2 <88% either at rest or with exertion. LTOT for those who did not meet appropriate criteria for initiation (exertional, rest, or nocturnal need) did not demonstrate a decrease in frequency of exacerbations or an impact on mortality. There was a notable increase in healthcare costs to the patient. Home oxygen therapy is the second highest cost expenditure after hospitalizations in industrialized countries for COPD patients. Therefore LTOT is a meaningful intervention when used in the appropriate patient population but is not beneficial for all patients with COPD.

Opiate Therapy in Patients With COPD

Patients with underlying COPD may also be on concurrent opiate therapy whether for chronic pain or palliative management of end-stage COPD. Literature from 2021 has noted a correlation between opioid drug use in COPD patients and adverse outcomes.

---

[1] Not FDA approved for this indication.

This is partly associated with the understanding that opiates can contribute to suppression of respiratory drive. However, there appears to be risk associated regardless of short-acting versus long-acting formulations and dose when reviewing respiratory-related mortality events. There were decreased adverse events seen in patients who used combination opioid/nonopioid formulations versus opioid-only therapy. Opioid use was associated with nearly double the risk of mortality due to COPD- or pneumonia-related causes. It is difficult to delineate the significance of this because the studies are observational and do not currently identify indications for receipt of opiates (whether for non–COPD-related reasons vs. palliative treatment). It is important to counsel patients on risks associated with concurrent opiate therapy.

Treatment of Exacerbations of COPD

COPD exacerbations are defined by a worsening or "flare" of respiratory symptoms such as dyspnea, sputum production, and sputum purulence. These episodes can be mild (requiring only as-needed bronchodilator therapy), moderate (managed outpatient with antibiotics and/or corticosteroid therapy), or severe (requiring hospital admission or emergency department management). Indications for hospital admission include altered mental status, severe/worsening hypercapnia, tachypnea or respiratory distress, failure of response to outpatient treatment, or worsening hypoxic respiratory failure. Triggers for an acute exacerbation include environmental (smoking, allergens, pollen) or viral/bacterial infections. It should be noted that ~30% of exacerbations could be attributed to a bacterial cause.

If initial bronchodilator therapy is unsuccessful in exacerbation management, corticosteroid therapy is considered. Treatment courses have been shown to have similar outcomes of success with a 5-day course of prednisone (40 mg once a day) versus a 10- to 14-day course of prednisone therapy. The addition of antibiotic therapy should be considered for those patients who meet two of the three following criteria: (1) increased sputum volume, (2) increased sputum purulence, and (3) increased dyspnea. In selection of antibiotic therapy, it is important to consider prior sputum culture data and the presence of underlying pseudomonas or resistant pathogens. When antibiotic therapy is indicated, this can reduce risk of treatment failure, decrease hospitalization duration, and shorten overall recovery time. The initial agent of choice should be selected based on local area bacterial resistance patterns. Based on the antibiograms available, amoxicillin/clavulanate (Augmentin)[1], azithromycin (Zithromax), or doxycycline[1] would be appropriate choices. Treatment courses should be no longer than 5 to 7 days.

In the setting of a COPD exacerbation with acute hypercapnic respiratory failure, noninvasive ventilatory support is part of mainstay therapy. BiPAP is the initial treatment of choice with acute hypercapnic respiratory failure for improvement in tachypnea, respiratory distress, and $Paco_2$ levels. However, as some 2022 studies have shown patients with milder respiratory acidosis pH in the 7.20 to 7.35 range, it may be beneficial to treat with high-flow nasal cannula (HFNC). HFNC resulted in significant reduction in $Paco_2$ and respiratory rate. This is an important consideration in patients who are BiPAP intolerant, but further research is required to determine whether this is an appropriate first-line therapy in patients with mild respiratory acidosis.

[1] Not FDA approved for this indication.

References

Agrawal R, Moghtader S, Ayyala U, Bandi V, Sharafkhaneh A: Update on management of stable chronic obstructive pulmonary disease, *J Thorac Dis* 11(suppl 14):S1800–S1809, 2019. https://doi.org/10.21037/jtd.2019.06.12.

Celi A, Latorre M, Paggiaro P, Pistelli R: Chronic obstructive pulmonary disease: moving from symptom relief to mortality reduction, *Ther Adv Chronic Dis* 14:20406223211014028, 2021. https://doi.org/10.1177/20406223211014028. Published 2021 May 13.

Fiorentino G, Esquinas AM, Annunziata A: Exercise and chronic obstructive pulmonary disease (COPD), *Adv Exp Med Biol* 1228:355–368, 2020. https://doi.org/10.1007/978-981-15-1792-1_24.

Global Initiative for Chronic Obstructive Lung Disease: Global strategy for the diagnosis, management, and prevention of chronic obstructive pulmonary disease (2024 Report). https://goldcopd.org/2024-gold-report-2/.

Leard LE, Holm AM, Valapour M, et al: Consensus document for the selection of lung transplant candidates: an update from the International Society for Heart and Lung Transplantation, *J Heart Lung Transplant* 40(11):1349–1379, 2021. https://doi.org/10.1016/j.healun.2021.07.005.

Lee M, Mora Carpio AL: Lung volume reduction surgery. In *StatPearls.*, treasure Island (FL), StatPearls Publishing, 2022.

Plotnikow GA, Accoce M, Fredes S, et al: High-flow oxygen therapy application in chronic obstructive pulmonary disease patients with acute hypercapnic respiratory failure: a multicenter study [published correction appears in Crit Care Explor. 2021 Mar 19;3(3):e0376], *Crit Care Explor* 3(2):e0337, 2021. https://doi.org/10.1097/CCE.0000000000000337. Published 2021 Feb 12.

Quint J, Montonen J, Singh D, et al: New insights into the optimal management of COPD: extracts from CHEST 2021 annual meeting (October 17-20, 2021), *Expert Rev Respir Med* 16(4):485–493, 2022. https://doi.org/10.1080/17476348.2022.2056022.

Stellefson M, Wang M-Q, Kinder C: Racial disparities in health risk indicators reported by Alabamians diagnosed with COPD, *Int J Environ Res Public Health* 18(18):9662, 2021. https://doi.org/10.3390/ijerph18189662.

van der Leest S, Duiverman ML: High-intensity non-invasive ventilation in stable hypercapnic COPD: evidence of efficacy and practical advice, *Respirology* 24(4):318–328, 2019. https://doi.org/10.1111/resp.13450.

Vigneswaran J, Krantz S, Howington J: Economic considerations of lung volume reduction surgery and bronchoscopic Valves, *Thorac Surg Clin* 31(2):211–219, 2021. https://doi.org/10.1016/j.thorsurg.2021.02.006.

Walters JA, Tan DJ, White CJ, Wood-Baker R: Different durations of corticosteroid therapy for exacerbations of chronic obstructive pulmonary disease, *Cochrane Database Syst Rev* 3(3):CD006897, 2018. https://doi.org/10.1002/14651858.CD006897.pub4. Published 2018 Mar 19.

COCCIDIOIDOMYCOSIS

Method of
Divya Chandramohan, MD; and Gregory Anstead, MD, PhD

CURRENT DIAGNOSIS

- Maintain a high index of suspicion in patients from endemic areas and travelers
- Diagnostic tests include:
  - Serologic detection of immunoglobulin M and immunoglobulin G antibodies by immunodiffusion, complement fixation, and enzyme immunoassay (EIA)
  - Culture of sputum, exudates, cerebrospinal fluid, and tissue
  - Direct observation of *Coccidioides* spherules in histopathologic and cytologic specimens
  - Urine antigen EIA

CURRENT THERAPY

Pulmonary Infection
- No risk factors for dissemination; not severe disease; observe
- Risk factors; prolonged symptoms: fluconazole (Diflucan)[1] 400 mg/day or itraconazole (Sporanox)[1] 200 mg twice a day for 3 to 6 months
- Diffuse or severe pneumonia: amphotericin B (Fungizone) 1 mg/kg/day or lipid formulation of amphotericin (Abelcet, AmBisome)[1] 5 mg/kg/day; after improvement, switch to azole; treat for 1 year
- Chronic fibrocavitary disease: azole therapy for at least 1 year; resection in selected cases

Disseminated Disease
- Nonmeningeal, severe disease: amphotericin B 1 mg/kg/day or lipid formulation of amphotericin[1] 5 mg/kg/day; after improvement, switch to azole for 1 to 2 years; consider posaconazole (Noxafil)[1] suspension 200 mg four times daily or tablets 300 mg daily or voriconazole (Vfend)[1] 400 to 600 mg/day daily in refractory cases

- Nonmeningeal, slowly progressive: azole therapy for 1 to 2 years; itraconazole[1] preferred for bony involvement; consider posaconazole[1] or voriconazole[1] (as above) in refractory cases.
- Meningeal, central nervous system involvement: fluconazole[1] 800 to 2000 mg/day[2]; intrathecal amphotericin B[1] or voriconazole (Vfend)[1] 200 mg twice daily in refractory cases[1]; shunting for hydrocephalus; consider corticosteroids if vasculitis is present.

[1]Not FDA approved for this indication.
[2]Exceeds dosage recommended by the manufacturer.

Coccidioidomycosis (CM) is caused by soil fungi of the genus *Coccidioides*, divided genetically into *Coccidioides immitis* (California isolates) and *Coccidioides posadasii* (isolates outside California). There are no distinct differences in the disease caused by the two species. *Coccidioides* occurs only in the Western Hemisphere. In the United States, the Centers for Disease Control and Prevention reports that the range includes 12 states (AZ, CA, CO, ID, NM, NV, OK, OR, TX, UT, WA, and WY). The major endemic areas are characterized by arid to semiarid climates, hot summers, low altitude, alkaline soil, and sparse vegetation. Hyperendemic areas include the San Joaquin Valley of California and Pima, Pinal, and Maricopa Counties in Arizona. *Coccidioides* is also found in parts of Latin America (Mexico, Guatemala, Honduras, Nicaragua, Brazil, Bolivia, Argentina, Paraguay, Venezuela, and Colombia). Cases may be observed in nonendemic areas because of travel or reactivation of prior infection. In the United States an estimated 150,000 cases of CM occur annually, with the clinical presentation ranging from a self-limited respiratory infection to devastating disseminated disease. The incidence of CM is increasing in the United States because of rising populations and the resulting construction in the endemic areas. Risk factors for increased severity of CM include receiving immunosuppressive medications (corticosteroids, transplant drugs, and tumor necrosis factor–α antagonists); pregnancy (esp. the third trimester); genetic factors (i.e., defects in the interleukin-12/interferon-γ axis and STAT3 pathways, certain ABO blood group and human leukocyte antigen types); and specific races/ethnicities (African Americans, Asian–Pacific Islanders, and Native Americans). Outbreaks may occur after dust storms, earthquakes, droughts, and activities causing soil disruption, such as construction and archeological digs. Persons with occupations involving exposure to soil are also at risk for acquiring CM.

Coccidioides is dimorphic; in the soil, the organism exists in its mycelial form, which produces barrel-shaped arthroconidia. The usual means of infection is the inhalation of arthroconidia; uncommon routes include direct cutaneous inoculation and organ transplantation. Arthroconidia germinate to produce spherules filled with endospores, the characteristic tissue phase. Spherules rupture to release endospores, which form additional spherules (Figure 1). The spherules become surrounded by neutrophils and macrophages, which leads to granuloma formation. Both B and T lymphocytes are essential for host defense against this pathogen.

Clinical Manifestations

CM is asymptomatic in 60% of infected individuals. In the remaining 40% a self-limited, flu-like illness with dry cough, pleuritic chest pain, myalgias, arthralgia, fever, sweats, anorexia, and weakness develops 1 to 3 weeks after exposure. Primary infection may be accompanied by immune complex–mediated complications including an erythematous macular rash, erythema multiforme, and erythema nodosum. Acute infection usually resolves without therapy, although symptoms may persist for weeks. In 5% of these patients, asymptomatic pulmonary residua persist, including pulmonary nodules and cavitation. Immunocompromised patients may develop chronic progressive

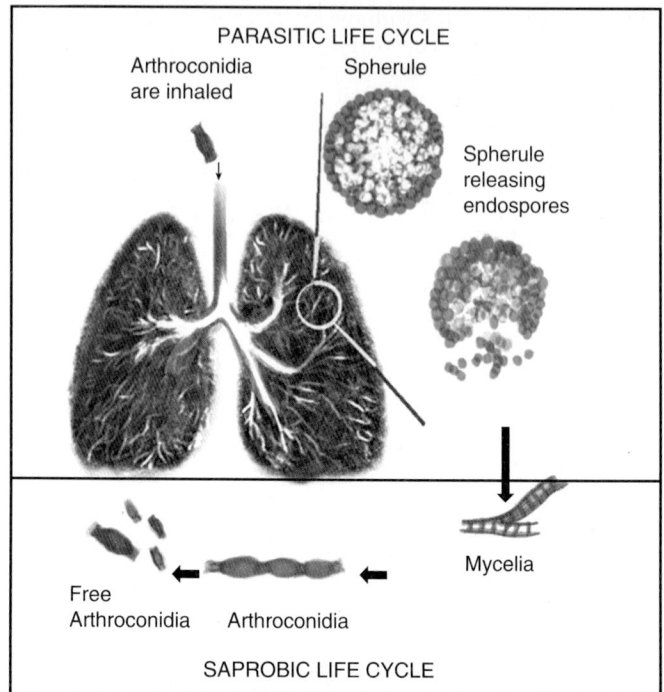

Figure 1 Life cycle of *Coccidioides* sp. indicating parasitic phase in the host and the saprobic phase present in environment.

pulmonary infection, with the evolution of thin-walled cavities that may rupture, leading to bronchopleural fistula and empyema formation.

Extrapulmonary disease develops in 1 of every 200 patients and can involve the skin, soft tissues, bones, joints, and meninges. The most common cutaneous lesions are verrucous papules, ulcers, or plaques. The spine is the most frequent site of osseous dissemination, although the typical lytic lesions may also occur in the skull, hands, feet, and tibia. Joint involvement is usually monoarticular and most commonly involves the ankle or knee. Fungemia may occur in immunocompromised patients and carries a poor prognosis.

In coccidioidal meningitis, the basilar meninges are usually affected. Cerebrospinal fluid findings include lymphocytic pleocytosis (often with eosinophilia), hypoglycorrhachia, and elevated protein levels. The mortality rate is greater than 90% at 1 year without therapy, and chronic infection is the rule. Hydrocephalus or hydrocephalus coexisting with brain infarction is associated with a higher mortality rate. CM is a great imitator and has many diverse clinical presentations, including immune thrombocytopenia, ocular involvement, massive cervical lymphadenopathy, laryngeal and retropharyngeal abscesses, endocarditis, pericarditis, peritonitis, hepatitis, and lesions of the male and female genitals and urogenital tracts.

Diagnosis

CM may be diagnosed by direct observation of spherules in tissues or in wet mounts of sputa or exudates. The growth of *Coccidioides* in culture usually occurs in 3 to 5 days, with sporulation after 5 to 10 days. Definitive identification is made by DNA probe or exoantigen testing. Laboratory personnel should exercise extreme caution when handling cultures of *Coccidioides*.

Serologic methods are useful in establishing the diagnosis and for monitoring the course of CM. Immunoglobulin M (IgM) antibodies are present soon after infection or relapse but then wane; quantification does not correlate with disease severity. The immunoglobulin G (IgG) antibody appears later and remains positive for months. Rising titers of IgG are associated with progressive disease, and declining titers are associated with resolution. The IgG antibodies can fix complement when combined with coccidioidal antigen and can be detected by immunodiffusion

(immunodiffusion complement fixation [IDCF]); titers of 1:16 or greater suggest disseminated disease. In the cerebrospinal fluid, a positive IDCF of any titer is considered diagnostic of meningitis and is much more sensitive than culture in making the diagnosis. An enzyme immunoassay (EIA) is also available for the detection of IgM and IgG antibodies, but it is less specific. The sensitivity and specificity of serologic testing is high for pleuropulmonary disease. Polymerase chain reaction testing on pleural fluid is not as sensitive and is comparable to pleural fluid culture. Adenosine deaminase levels in pleural fluid are inconsistently elevated. According to Infectious Diseases Society of America guidelines, an indeterminate EIA IgM and IgG test result should be considered nonreactive. If only the EIA IgM assay is reactive, this could be a false-positive result, and IgM/IgG testing should be repeated at a later time. A specific urinary antigen test is also available for the diagnosis of CM; this assay has a sensitivity of 71% in moderate to severe disease, compared with 84% for culture, 29% for histopathologic examination, and 75% for serologic testing. The majority of cases with disseminated or meningeal CM have elevated serum 1,3-β-D-glucan levels. However, 1,3-β-D-glucan values correlate poorly with coccidioidal complement fixation antibody titers.

Treatment

In most patients, primary pulmonary infection resolves spontaneously without treatment. However, all patients require observation for at least 2 years to document resolution of infection and to identify any complications as soon as possible. For patients who have risk factors for disseminated disease (listed earlier), treatment is necessary. Other indications for treatment are severe disease (infiltrates involving both lungs or more than half of one lung; significant hilar or mediastinal lymphadenopathy; complement fixation titers >1:16) and highly symptomatic disease (weight loss >10%; night sweats present for >3 weeks; symptoms present for >2 months).

For diffuse or severe pneumonia, therapy with amphotericin B deoxycholate (Fungizone) 0.5 to 1.5 mg/kg/day or a lipid formulation of amphotericin B (Abelcet or AmBisome)[1] 2 to 5 mg/kg/day should be given for several weeks, followed by an oral azole, such as itraconazole (Sporanox)[1] 200 mg twice daily or fluconazole (Diflucan)[1] 400 to 800 mg/day. The total duration of therapy should be at least 1 year; for immunosuppressed patients, oral azole therapy should be maintained as secondary prophylaxis. In HIV patients with CD4-positive T-cell counts greater than 250 cells/mm[3] who had focal pneumonias that responded to azoles, antifungals may be discontinued. Azole therapy may be used initially for less severe disease. During pregnancy, amphotericin B is the preferred drug, because of the teratogenicity of azoles.

An asymptomatic patient with a solitary nodule or pulmonary cavitation due to *Coccidioides* does not require specific antifungal therapy or resection. However, the development of complications from the cavitation, such as hemoptysis or bacterial or fungal superinfection, necessitates initiation of azole therapy. Resection of the cavities is an alternative to antifungal therapy. Rupture of a cavity into the pleural space requires surgical intervention with closure by lobectomy with decortication, in addition to antifungal therapy. For chronic pneumonia, the initial treatment should be an oral azole for at least 1 year. If the disease persists, one may switch to another oral azole, increase the dose if fluconazole was initially selected, or switch to amphotericin B. Resection should be performed for patients with refractory focal lesions or severe hemoptysis.

The treatment of disseminated infection without central nervous system involvement is based on oral azole therapy, such as itraconazole[1] or fluconazole[1] (400 mg/day, or higher in case of fluconazole). If there is little or no improvement or if there is vertebral involvement, treatment with amphotericin B is recommended (dosage as for diffuse pneumonia). Concomitant surgical débridement or stabilization is also recommended. In patients with refractory CM that has failed to respond to fluconazole,

itraconazole, and amphotericin B and its lipid formulations, treatment with posaconazole (Noxafil)[1] suspension 200 mg four times daily with a fatty meal or voriconazole (Vfend)[1], at doses of 400 to 600 mg/day, has been successful. A posaconazole tablet with improved oral bioavailability and an intravenous preparation are now available, and likely these new forms of posaconazole are more efficacious. The posaconazole tablet has been dosed at 300 mg/day[2]. Clinical experience with voriconazole is limited.

For coccidioidal meningitis, lifetime treatment with azoles is indicated. Fluconazole[1] at doses of 800 mg/day or higher[2] is recommended. There have been several reports of successful treatment of coccidioidal meningitis with voriconazole (Vfend)[1] 200 mg orally twice daily after a loading dose. Itraconazole is not recommended because of its irregular oral absorption. Limited studies exist for the use of isavuconazole (Cresemba)[1] in the treatment of CM, including coccidioidal meningitis. For patients with increased intracranial pressure at the time of meningitis diagnosis, repeated lumbar punctures are recommended. Obstructive hydrocephalus requires shunting. Intrathecal amphotericin B[1] is now strictly reserved for meningitis refractory to high-dose azoles or coccidioidal meningitis in the first trimester of pregnancy. In patients with CNS vasculitis with cerebrovascular accident due to CM, those that received corticosteroids were less likely to develop additional infarcts compared with those who did not. Reduction of immunosuppression is an important adjunct to antifungal therapy, including the initiation of antiretroviral therapy if the patient has HIV infection. In patients with AIDS and nonmeningeal coccidioidomycosis, antifungal therapy can be discontinued when the CD4 count exceeds 250 cells/mm[3].

---

[1] Not FDA approved for this indication.
[2] Exceeds dosage recommended by the manufacturer.

References

Ampel NM: Coccidioidomycosis: changing concepts and knowledge gaps, *J Fungi (Basel)* 6:354, 2020.

Bays DJ, Thompson 3rd GR: Coccidioidomycosis, *Infect Dis Clin North Am* 35:453–469, 2021.

Bays DJ, Thompson GR, Reef S, et al: Natural history of disseminated coccidioidomycosis: examination of the VA-armed forces database, *Clin Infect Dis* 73:e3814–e3819, 2020.

Diep AL, Hoyer KK: Host response to *Coccidioides* infection: fungal immunity, *Front Cell Infect Microbio* 10:581101, 2020.

Donovan FM, Zangeneh TT, Malo J, Galgiani JN: Top questions in the diagnosis and treatment of coccidioidomycosis, *Open Forum Infect Dis* 4:ofx197, 2017.

Gabe LM, Malo J, Knox KS: Diagnosis and management of coccidioidomycosis, *Clin Chest Med* 38:417–433, 2017.

Galgiani JN, Ampel NM, Blair JE, et al: Infectious Diseases Society of America (IDSA) clinical practice guideline for the treatment of coccidioidomycosis, *Clin Infect Dis* 63:e112–e146, 2016.

Gorris ME, Ardon-Dryer K, Campuzano A, et al: Advocating for coccidioidomycosis to be a reportable disease nationwide in the United States and encouraging disease surveillance across North and South America, *J Fungi (Basel)* 9:83, 2023.

Hartmann CA, Aye WT, Blair JE: Treatment considerations in pulmonary coccidioidomycosis, *Expert Rev Respir Med* 10:1079–1091, 2016.

Heidari A, Quinlan M, Benjamin DJ, et al: Isavuconazole in the treatment of coccidioidal meningitis, *Antimicrob Agents Chemother* 63:e02232-18, 2019.

Kassis C, Durkin M, Holbrook E, et al: Advances in diagnosis of progressive pulmonary and disseminated coccidioidomycosis, *Clin Infect Dis* 72:968–975, 2021.

Kim MM, Vikram HR, Kusne S, Seville MT, Blair JE: Treatment of refractory coccidioidomycosis with voriconazole or posaconazole, *Clin Infect Dis* 53:1060–1066, 2011.

McCotter OZ, Benedict K, Engelthaler DM, et al: Update on the epidemiology of coccidioidomycosis in the United States, *Med Mycol* 57(Suppl 1):S30–S40, 2019.

Odio CD, Marciano BE, Galgiani JN, Holland SM: Risk factors for disseminated coccidioidomycosis, United States, *Emerg Infect Dis* 23:308–311, 2017.

Stockamp NW, Thompson 3rd GR: Coccidioidomycosis, *Infect Dis Clin North Am* 30:229–246, 2016.

Thompson 3rd GR, Blair JE, Wang S, et al: Adjunctive corticosteroid therapy in the treatment of coccidioidal meningitis, *Clin Infect Dis* 65:338–341, 2017.

Thompson 3rd GR, Lewis 2nd JS, Nix DE, Patterson TF: Current concepts and future directions in the pharmacology and treatment of coccidioidomycosis, *Med Mycol* 157(Suppl 1):S76–S84, 2019.

Thompson 3rd GR, Sharma S, Bays DJ, et al: Coccidioidomycosis, *Chest* 143(3):776–781, 2013, https://doi.org/10.1378/chest.12-1312.

Van Dyke MCC, Thompson GR, Galgiani JN, Barker BM: The rise of *Coccidioides*: forces against the dust devil unleashed, *Front Immunol* 10:2188, 2019.

CYSTIC FIBROSIS

Method of
Hanna Phan, PharmD; and Cori L. Daines, MD

CURRENT DIAGNOSIS

- Cystic fibrosis (CF) is an autosomal recessive genetic disorder that causes dysfunction of the cystic fibrosis transmembrane conductance regulator (CFTR) on the apical surface of epithelial cells, leading to the inability to move adequate ions, specifically chloride, out of the cell.
- This defect leads to thick, dehydrated mucus in the respiratory tract that manifests as chronic cough and recurrent infections.
- Thickened secretions lead to disease manifestations in organs other than the lungs.
- Diagnosis is made via a sweat chloride test using quantitative pilocarpine iontophoresis.
- Close to 2000 *CFTR* mutations are known, leading to a multitude of clinical phenotypes and disease severity.

CURRENT THERAPY

- A given patient's overall treatment regimen is often based on various factors, including age, clinical presentation, organ systems involved, disease progression/severity, *CFTR* genotype, and comorbidities.
- Primary treatment includes augmented airway clearance with bronchodilators, mucolytics, or mucus hydrators along with mechanical airway vibration.
- For the vast majority of patients, secondary treatment includes use of a CFTR modulator.
- Nutritional therapy consists of enzymes and vitamin replacement for those who are pancreatic insufficient.

Epidemiology

Cystic fibrosis (CF) is an autosomal recessive, inherited multisystem disease caused by mutations of the *CFTR* gene on chromosome 7. There are currently close to 2000 known *CFTR* mutations. Carriage of the gene is highest in individuals of Northern European descent, leading to an incidence of 1 in 3000 non-Hispanic White people in the United States. The incidence is lower in Hispanic White people and those of African descent. There are more than 33,000 individuals with CF in the United States, more than 100,000 individuals worldwide, and approximately 1000 new diagnoses each year. The average life expectancy is increasing with new therapies but still varies among countries. In the United States and Canada, the median life expectancy is currently 61 years in babies born between 2019 and 2023.

Pathophysiology
Cystic Fibrosis Transmembrane Regulator
Genotypes and Phenotypes
The cystic fibrosis transmembrane conductance regulator (CFTR) is a protein in the adenosine triphosphate–binding cassette transporter family that has two transmembrane domains, two nucleotide-binding domains, and a regulatory domain. It shares structural elements with other membrane pumps. Mutations in the gene coding the CFTR fall broadly into six categories. The first category includes premature truncation mutations, leading to no full-length protein. The second category includes the *Phe508del* (i.e., *F508del*) mutation, which is the most common mutation and accounts for 75% of all mutations in the United

States. Class II mutations result in the cell degrading the CFTR before full maturation and function. Class III mutations result in a chloride channel at the cell surface that does not function (also called a *gating mutation*). Class IV mutations result in a chloride channel embedded at the cell surface that has decreased and ineffective chloride movement function, and class V mutations are promoter or splicing abnormalities that result in a reduced number of functional chloride channels at the cell surface. Class VI mutations result in a chloride channel that is not stable on the cell surface and, like class V mutations, insufficient quantities of chloride channel at the cell surface.

Understanding the genetics of any given individual with CF is vital in understanding the pathophysiology. Disease manifestation is directly related to the amount of chloride moved at the cell surface. Class I, II, and III mutations result in minimal chloride movement, less than 5% of normal, and "classic" or severe disease phenotype. The presence of one mutation in the class IV, V, or VI category results in greater chloride movement at the surface, typically 10% or more, and a "mild" or "nonclassic" phenotype. Approximately 15% of individuals with CF fall into this latter category and have some preserved chloride channel activity and milder disease phenotype.

Mechanism
CF affects all organs with epithelial cells expressing CFTR, which typically means the cells lining a ductal system and the fluid outside that system are affected. In the lungs, the respiratory epithelium is lined with cells that express CFTR. When CFTR does not move appropriate amounts of chloride, the chloride is trapped inside the cell, which leads to the epithelial sodium channel pumping additional sodium into the cell to balance. The resulting salt inside the cell creates an osmotic gradient across the cell surface, and water enters the cell. The water first comes from the periciliary fluid layer, dehydrating the fluid around the cilia, making it difficult for them to beat. Next, the water is removed from the outer mucus layer, also dehydrating it, making it thick and viscous. In the sinopulmonary tract, this inspissation of the mucus limits natural mucociliary clearance and leads to inflammation and an advantageous environment for bacterial colonization. Damage to the airways becomes irreversible and leads to a loss of lung function.

A similar process occurs in other organs with any epithelial cell lining a ductal system. In the pancreas, for instance, epithelial cells line the ducts of the exocrine pancreas. The cells pull water from the normal pancreatic excretion, dehydrating it and clogging the ducts. The enzymes then autodigest the exocrine pancreas, rendering it nonfunctional. The same is true in the biliary ducts of the liver. In the sweat glands, salt and water are trapped in the ducts, making the sweat very salty and leading to the diagnostic result of the sweat chloride test.

Clinical Manifestations
Pulmonary
The tracheobronchial tree in CF has poor mucociliary clearance, as noted previously. Patients with CF have excessive cough, make mucus, and might wheeze. They have periodic episodes of exacerbation in which excessive mucus builds up and bacterial infection occurs. The thick mucus becomes a source of persistent infection with bacteria that are unable to be cleared. Often, the infections are caused by bacteria that are not present in the normal undamaged airway, especially *Staphylococcus aureus* and *Pseudomonas aeruginosa*. When the bacteria become active and the patient experiences an exacerbation, the cough and sputum production will worsen. Exacerbations in children are often triggered by viruses and typical childhood illnesses, and in adults, exacerbations may also be triggered by other environmental factors. With exacerbation, there may be shortness of breath, chest pain, wheezing, dyspnea on exertion or at rest, and fatigue. Other symptoms of a pulmonary exacerbation include weight loss, poor appetite, and fever. Over time, there is progressive loss of lung function resulting from infections, mucus, and inflammation.

Symptoms become more persistent and bothersome over time, and exacerbations become more common. Additionally, more than 30% of individuals with CF also have asthma.

Sinuses

The sinuses in CF have the same mucostasis that occurs in the lungs. The mucus impaction leads to chronic sinus congestion and obstruction, persistent infections, and persistent inflammation. More than 50% of adults with CF have chronic sinusitis. Patients with CF are more likely to develop polyps as well. Symptoms include nasal congestion or drainage, sinus headache, and inability to smell.

Pancreas

Poor growth can occur because of insufficient nutrient breakdown and absorption, resulting in malabsorptive, greasy stools. Fat-soluble vitamins in the diet are also poorly absorbed because of the malabsorption of fat. Individuals with CF can develop significant deficiencies in vitamins A, D, E, and K. In general, the endocrine pancreas that makes insulin is not initially affected in CF. Over time, individuals with CF often develop CF-related diabetes (CFRD) caused by global inflammation of the pancreas. More than 40% of adults with CF will eventually develop CFRD.

Liver

In the liver, there is inspissation of the bile in the bile duct caused by excessive reabsorption of water from the bile. The resulting blockage of the bile ducts leads to hepatic inflammation. In general, this is asymptomatic for the patient with CF and is found by checking laboratory levels of liver function tests. Occasionally, this bile blockage is severe and leads to chronic inflammation and biliary cirrhosis of the liver. A small percentage of individuals with CF, typically less than 5%, have cirrhosis with portal hypertension, esophageal varices, and splenomegaly and would need a liver transplant.

Intestines

Excessive reabsorption of fluid in the gut can lead to constipation and even small bowel obstruction. This can also occur when stools are malabsorptive. Some people with CF will have rectal prolapse caused by straining, with either malabsorptive or constipated stools. Other manifestations of CF in the intestines can be a result of medication side effects.

Sweat Glands

Excessive salt is trapped in the sweat, leading to excessive salt loss in the sweat and possible electrolyte imbalance and dehydration.

Genitourinary

Men with CF generally all have congenital absence of the vas deferens, rendering them naturally infertile. Men still produce sperm but do not have the other structures.

Other

CF causes clubbing of the fingers, which is usually more prominent as lung disease progresses. CF-related arthropathies occur in a small percentage of individuals with CF, usually caused by inflammatory markers in circulation that deposit in the joints. Mental health issues, such as depression and anxiety, are common in teenagers and adults with CF, with an incidence of approximately 30%. Medications taken by people with CF may also contribute to mental health challenges.

Diagnosis

Because CF is an insidiously progressive disease, it is important to make an early diagnosis and begin therapies as soon as possible. In the United States the majority of diagnoses are made via newborn screening. Depending on the state, testing involves immunoreactive trypsinogen levels with possible genetic panels of mutations. When the state reports a positive newborn screen, the care provider must order/obtain a sweat chloride test on the infant. Diagnoses are then based on the results of the screens. The Cystic Fibrosis Foundation guidelines state that a positive sweat diagnosis of CF is greater than 30 mmol/L chloride, with 30 to 60 mmol/L chloride being the intermediate zone. Consensus remains that if a child has two mutations, symptoms, and an abnormal sweat chloride (30–60 mmol/L), this is consistent with a diagnosis of CF. Children with symptoms and a sweat chloride greater than 60 mmol/L have CF as well. A secondary diagnosis of CFTR-related metabolic syndrome (CRMS) designates those individuals whose diagnoses are unclear. Those with one mutation and an intermediate sweat (30–60 mmol/L) or those with two mutations and a negative sweat (<30 mmol/L) are followed prospectively for the development of symptoms and should have yearly sweat tests and periodic evaluations for the evolution of symptoms at a certified CF center, where the testing methodology is certified by the national Cystic Fibrosis Foundation.

As newborn screening has only been widely available for the past 15 to 25 years, teenagers and adults who did not receive newborn screening are still being diagnosed the traditional way, which is the presence of symptoms and a positive sweat test. Here again, a positive sweat means a value of 60 mmol/L, whereas a value of 30 mmol/L or greater deserves further investigation, such as genetic testing. Sweat tests should be done at a certified CF center. Traditional symptomatology per the Cystic Fibrosis Foundation is represented in the following:

- Very salty-tasting skin
- Persistent coughing, at times with phlegm
- Frequent lung infections, such as pneumonia or bronchitis
- Wheezing or shortness of breath
- Poor growth or poor weight gain in spite of a good appetite
- Frequent greasy, bulky stools, or difficulty with bowel movements
- Nasal polyps
- Chronic sinus infections
- Clubbing or enlargement of the fingertips and toes
- Rectal prolapse
- Male infertility

If a diagnosis of CF is suspected because of symptomatology, a sweat test for a definitive diagnosis should be performed regardless of the patient's age or newborn screening status.

Treatment
Pulmonary Treatment
Nonpharmacologic Therapy

Because of the increased viscosity of airway secretions and the subsequent obstruction and even mucus plugging in CF, there is a fundamental need for airway clearance or chest physiotherapy as part of chronic care. As a core component of therapy in the pulmonary management of CF, airway clearance or chest physiotherapy helps loosen this mucus, and help with expectoration should be done routinely two times per day as part of chronic management for patients of all ages; increased frequency may be necessary during periods of pulmonary exacerbation. Manual physiotherapy or percussion and postural drainage is often the first technique introduced into care. Other airway clearance techniques can be used, depending on age and access to devices. These techniques include the use of autogenic drainage, the active cycle of breathing technique, high-frequency chest compression (e.g., vest), the use of oscillatory positive expiratory pressure (e.g., MetaNeb) devices, and exercise.

Chronic Pharmacologic Therapy

The selection of medications used in the pulmonary management of chronic CF is currently based on age and clinical need. This is based on current guidelines, U.S. Food and Drug Administration (FDA)-approved indications for newer agents (e.g., CFTR modulators), and current evidence in cases of off-label medication use. Such pharmacotherapy consists of various medication classes, including bronchodilators, mucolytics, inhaled antibiotics, anti-inflammatory agents, and CFTR modulators.

Inhaled medications are used in conjunction with chest physiotherapy to facilitate airway clearance, helping loosen mucus and expectoration, and suppress bacterial growth of pathogens in the airways. The use of a short-acting β-agonist, such as albuterol (Proventil, Ventolin)[1], in either metered-dose inhaler or aerosolized or nebulizer form, facilitates mucociliary clearance through bronchodilation and decreases occurrence of bronchospasm from subsequent inhaled therapies such as mucolytics (e.g., hypertonic saline [sodium chloride 7% (HyperSal, PulmoSal)][1]), dornase alfa (Pulmozyme), mannitol inhalation powder (Bronchitol), and antibiotics. Mucolytics are also fundamental in mucociliary clearance. Nebulized hypertonic saline, most commonly sodium chloride 7% and administered twice a day, increases hydration of sputum through osmotic action, thinning sputum for airway clearance. Dornase alfa breaks down extracellular DNA in sputum, thereby decreasing its viscosity. This nebulized mucolytic is most commonly administered daily, usually after the use of nebulized hypertonic saline in sequence. The use of hypertonic saline and dornase alfa is recommended to help improve lung function and reduce exacerbations. Approved in 2020 as a possible add-on maintenance therapy for persons with CF ages 18 years and older, mannitol inhalation powder (Bronchitol) is a dry powder formulation and thus does not require use of a nebulizer for administration and is dosed twice daily. Because of its acute bronchospasm risk, it should only be used in those who have passed the Bronchitol Tolerance Test, which is administered and performed under supervision. Inhaled corticosteroids with or without a long-acting β-agonist are not used to treat CF itself but are appropriate in cases of concurrent asthma.

Some patients with CF may require the use of an inhaled antibiotic to help suppress bacterial burden in the airways and improve patient outcomes, such as lung function and exacerbation frequency. Currently, the only FDA-approved inhaled antibiotics are tobramycin inhalation solution (Bethkis, Kitabis, Tobi), tobramycin inhalation powder (Tobi Podhaler), and aztreonam inhalation solution (Cayston) for patients with CF with *P. aeruginosa*. For patients who newly acquire *P. aeruginosa*, it is recommended to treat with an inhaled antibiotic for 28 days, with the preferred agent being tobramycin-inhaled solution, in an attempt to eradicate the pathogen. The use of an inhaled antibiotic to prevent acquisition of *P. aeruginosa* is not recommended. For patients with CF with the persistent presence of *P. aeruginosa* from respiratory cultures, the chronic use of inhaled antibiotics, such as tobramycin or aztreonam, is recommended to improve lung function and reduce exacerbations. For chronic use, cycling (e.g., on 28 days, off 28 days) of an inhaled antibiotic is common. The use of continuous inhaled antibiotic therapy in which two different inhaled antibiotics (e.g., tobramycin and aztreonam) are used rotationally is not routine but has been used by specialists in cases of multidrug-resistant pathogens, advanced or severe lung disease, or frequent acute exacerbations.

Antiinflammatory agents—specifically oral azithromycin and/or high-dose ibuprofen—are also noted in the current guidelines. Azithromycin (Zithromax), a macrolide antibiotic, is not used in chronic CF for its antiinfective properties but for its antiinflammatory and immunomodulatory properties. For patients with CF with the persistent presence of *P. aeruginosa* from respiratory cultures, the use of chronic azithromycin[1] is recommended to improve lung function and reduce exacerbations. Use in patients with CF who lack the persistent presence of *P. aeruginosa* can be considered to help reduce the frequency of exacerbations. Monitoring for the presence of nontuberculosis mycobacterium in respiratory cultures and the potential for drug interactions with azithromycin (e.g., medications that may prolong the QT interval) is recommended with the use of chronic azithromycin. A less commonly used antiinflammatory agent used among certified CF centers is high-dose ibuprofen.[1] The therapeutic benefit of slowing the loss of lung function is greatest in children 6 to 17 years

of age. This therapy requires therapeutic drug monitoring (i.e., pharmacokinetic assessment of serum ibuprofen levels) and dose adjustment. Subtherapeutic levels can have negative effects on lung function because of an increase in inflammatory mediators, and supratherapeutic levels increase the risk for toxicities (e.g., bleeding, nephrotoxicity). This therapy is less commonly used because of its potential for adverse effects, the need for laboratory monitoring, and the need for pharmacokinetic-based dosing. Routine, chronic use of systemic steroids such as prednisone is not recommended in the chronic management of CF.

CFTR modulators target the underlying defect in the CFTR protein; thus they are indicated for patients with CF with certain CF genotypes. The initial consideration for use and dosing of CFTR modulators is based on age, CF genotype, weight, concurrent therapy, ability to swallow tablets or capsules, and available dosage forms. There are three main types: potentiators, correctors, and amplifiers; however, the latter type is not currently available and is being developed and studied. Ivacaftor (Kalydeco) is a potentiator, increasing chloride movement through the CFTR protein channel. Ivacaftor is currently approved for patients aged 1 month or older who have at least one responsive mutation, based on clinical and/or in vitro assay data, such as various gating and conducting mutations. Lumacaftor is a corrector, facilitating correct formation and stabilization of the CFTR protein. Lumacaftor is combined with ivacaftor as Orkambi for the treatment of CF and is currently approved for patients aged 1 year or older whose genotype is homozygous *Phe508del*. Tezacaftor is also a corrector but is longer acting and has some differences compared with lumacaftor with regard to drug interactions and side effects. Like lumacaftor, tezacaftor is a corrector combined with ivacaftor as Symdeko for chronic treatment of CF. Symdeko is currently approved for patients aged 6 years or older whose genotype is homozygous *Phe508del*, as well as a number of mutations responsive to this combination based on in vitro data and/or clinical evidence. Elexacaftor and vanzacaftor are also correctors. Each binds to a different site on the CFTR protein than tezacaftor, providing an additive effect in improving cellular processing and trafficking of CFTR, resulting in improved outcomes, including lung function, symptoms (cough, sputum production), exacerbation rate, and nutritional status. Elexacaftor is combined with tezacaftor and ivacaftor as Trikafta and is currently approved for patients aged 2 years or older who have at least one *Phe508del* mutation or other responsive genotypes, based on in vitro data. Until early 2025, available CFTR modulators' standard dosing was twice a day. However, the approval of combination agent, vanzacaftor-tezacaftor-deutivacaftor (Alyftrek), established a once-daily dosing option for ages 6 years and older who have at least one *Phe508del* mutation or other responsive genotypes, based on in vitro data. Deutivacaftor is a deuterated ivacaftor, a potentiator with a longer half-life, resulting in once-daily dosing of vanzacaftor/tezacaftor/deutivacaftor (Alyftrek). Patients on lumacaftor-ivacaftor (Orkambi) or tezacaftor-ivacaftor (Symdeko) should be considered for transition to elexacaftor-tezacaftor-ivacaftor (Trikafta) or vanzacaftor-tezacaftor-deutivacaftor (Alyftrek) when of appropriate age. Ivacaftor (Kalydeco) is available as oral granule packets and tablets. Tezacaftor-ivacaftor (Symdeko) and elexacaftor-tezacaftor-ivacaftor (Trikafta) are available as oral granule packets and tablet blister packs with combination tablets (morning doses) and ivacaftor (evening doses). Vanzacaftor/tezacaftor/deutivacaftor (Alyftrek) is available as tablet blister packs with combination tablets. It is important to make patients/caregivers aware of the different-appearing packaging, prescribed dosing, and administration. A study published in 2023 demonstrated that "stepping down" certain chronic therapies (i.e., discontinuing inhaled mucolytic therapy such as hypertonic saline and/or dornase alfa) may be safe to consider among some adolescents and adults with CF taking elexacaftor-tezacaftor-ivacaftor (Trikafta). Studies to determine whether such approaches are appropriate for younger patients, if other chronic therapies can be considered as part of "stepping down" regimens, and if the approach can be applied

---

[1] Not FDA approved for this indication.

to patients on newer agents (e.g., vanzacaftor/tezacaftor/deutivacaftor [Alyftrek]) are ongoing.

CFTR modulators have variable monitoring considerations. Liver function tests for aspartate aminotransferase (AST), alanine aminotransferase (ALT), and total bilirubin should be done before starting therapy, followed by every month for the first 6 months for vanzacaftor-tezacaftor-deutivacaftor (Alyftrek) and elexacaftor-tezacaftor-ivacaftor (Trikafta), then every 3 months for the subsequent 12 months, and annually thereafter. For ivacaftor (Kalydeco), lumacaftor-ivacaftor (Orkambi), and tezacaftor-ivacaftor (Symdeko), AST and ALT should be followed every 3 months for the first year of therapy and annually thereafter. More frequent monitoring may be indicated if AST and/or ALT elevations are identified. More frequent (e.g., every 3–6 months) monitoring of fat-soluble vitamin serum levels (e.g., vitamins D, A, and E) during the first year of highly effective modulator therapy (e.g., elexacaftor-tezacaftor-ivacaftor [Trikafta]) could be also considered. As noncongenital lens opacities or cataracts have been reported in pediatric patients with ivacaftor, a baseline ophthalmologic examination (e.g., slit-lamp exam) is also recommended in patients who are younger than 18 years of age. Follow-up ophthalmologic examinations are recommended, but the frequency is not well defined by the manufacturer; however, in practice, follow-up is often at least annually. Doses should be taken with a fatty meal and with pancreatic enzymes (for those who require the use of pancreatic enzymes as part of CF management). All of the listed CFTR modulators are substrates and/or inducers of CYP3A4, as well as other CYP450 isoenzymes (e.g., CYP2C9), so screening for and managing drug interactions are essential. In addition, dosing modifications or discontinuation may be necessary for moderate or severe hepatic dysfunction. FDA-approved age and CF genotype indications for each of the CFTR modulators may be updated with ongoing clinical trials in young ages and other CF genotypes; thus it is recommended to check the latest FDA-approved indications when considering use.

Acute Pharmacologic Therapy

Many patients with CF, despite the use of chronic therapies, experience pulmonary exacerbations requiring treatment. In addition to increased frequency of airway clearance or chest physiotherapy, acute pulmonary exacerbations may require the use of systemic antimicrobials. Whenever possible, the selection of systemic antimicrobial agents should be guided by a patient-specific history of respiratory cultures and patient clinical response to past regimens.

When a systemic antimicrobial is required for outpatient management, an oral antibiotic is commonly used, with the duration of most agents being 10 to 14 days. For example, if a given patient has a history of P. aeruginosa, use of oral ciprofloxacin (Cipro)[1] or levofloxacin (Levaquin)[1] is typically 14 days, with few patients who may require up to 21 days of therapy based on exacerbation severity or clinical response. Patients who have inhaled antibiotics as part of their chronic regimen may continue treatment cycles during outpatient treatment for acute pulmonary exacerbation. Some CF centers may use home infusion services for intravenous (IV) antimicrobials; however, this requires additional logistic considerations, including nursing support, infusion equipment, and laboratory monitoring. In addition, factors related to adherence to airway clearance, social support system at home, and appropriateness of home IV access should be considered.

For inpatient management, the use of IV antibiotics is more common, and the use of oral antibiotic(s) may also be part of the regimen. P. aeruginosa is often "double covered" when possible, specifically when hospitalized and/or requiring IV antimicrobials, but the possibility of single coverage instead is currently being studied in a clinical trial. Double coverage involves the use of two agents active against P. aeruginosa from two different antibiotic classes (e.g., β-lactam and aminoglycoside). The use of inhaled and systemic (e.g., IV) antibiotics of the same class

---

[1] Not FDA approved for this indication.

(e.g., aminoglycosides) simultaneously is not common. Another approach is starting IV antimicrobials in the inpatient setting, with transition and completion of the therapy course with home infusion services.

There are special instances in which longer courses of medications such as antibiotics or antifungal therapy may be necessary. For example, in the treatment of nontuberculosis mycobacterium (e.g., Mycobacterium abscessus), multiple types of antibiotics (e.g., inhaled, IV, and/or oral) may be used for extended durations (e.g., months). In the treatment of allergic bronchopulmonary aspergillosis, antifungal therapy may be used in addition to systemic corticosteroids (e.g., prednisone) for extensive periods (e.g., weeks or months). These more complex antimicrobial treatment courses are often managed by specialists (e.g., pulmonary and/or infectious disease specialists).

Nutritional/Gastrointestinal Treatment
Nonpharmacologic Therapy
Persons with CF often have greater dietary energy intake needs. Consistent, high-calorie dietary intake can be a challenge because of several physiologic factors, including loss of taste or smell caused by chronic sinusitis and chronic gastroesophageal reflux. Behavioral factors may affect nutritional intake, necessitating behavioral intervention by dietitians and/or psychologists. For patients of all ages with continued suboptimal growth, the use of enteral feeding modes may also be necessary. For patients who have chronic constipation or a history of distal intestinal obstructive syndrome (DIOS), appropriate hydration and increased fiber content in the diet are recommended.

Infant formulas and breast milk do not provide adequate sodium for infants with CF. Because of excessive sodium loss through insensible loss, infants are at risk for developing hyponatremic hypochloremia dehydration. It is recommended that one-eighth teaspoon of table salt be provided from birth and increased to one-fourth teaspoon at 6 months through 1 year of age, divided throughout the day by feedings. Additional supplementation may be necessary for children and adults living in high-temperature climates and/or involved in considerable physical activities (e.g., sports).

Chronic Pharmacologic Therapy
For patients with pancreatic insufficiency, the use of pancreatic enzyme replacement therapy (PERT) is needed. There are various brands of PERT that contain various amounts of lipase, protease, and amylase. Pancreatic enzymes should be taken at mealtimes and snack times and in coordination with enteral feeds (when applicable). The dosing of PERT is based on the lipase component. Typical pancreatic enzyme initial dosing ranges from 500 to 1500 units of lipase per kilogram of body weight per meal, with a common maximum of 2500 units of lipase per kilogram per meal or, less commonly applied, 10,000 units of lipase per kilogram per day. Enzyme preparations come in a range of concentrations to accommodate all patient needs and minimize the number of capsules required. Given the number of medications a person with CF may require for chronic management, clinicians should be mindful about how many capsules are required per meal or snack when selecting a brand and strength of pancreatic enzyme. When maximal PERT dosing is reached and the patient continues to present with symptoms of malabsorption (e.g., steatorrhea), other etiologies should be investigated. Some clinicians may add an acid suppression agent (e.g., a proton pump inhibitor or H2 receptor antagonist) to help enhance the activity of pancreatic enzymes through decreasing duodenal acidity; however, the potential risks of long-term acid suppression (e.g., small intestinal bacterial overgrowth [SIBO]) should be considered. A proton pump inhibitor or H2 receptor antagonist may also be used to treat concurrent gastroesophageal reflux disease.

In pancreatic insufficiency, supplementation of fat-soluble vitamins (i.e., A, D, E, K) should be provided via specially formulated multivitamins, available in various dosage forms with dosing based on age. Monitoring of vitamin levels is often done at least annually, with adjustments in supplementation of individual vitamins (e.g., vitamin D, cholecalciferol) based on adherence to current treatment, age, and level of deficiency.

For those with chronic constipation or history of DIOS, chronic use of an osmotic laxative such as over-the-counter polyethylene glycol 3350 (MiraLAX)[1] may be helpful. Oral *N*-acetylcysteine (Mucomyst)[1] has also been used for the prevention of mucus accumulation in the gastrointestinal (GI) tract of some individuals with DIOS.

Acute Pharmacologic Therapy
Patients presenting with DIOS often require more aggressive treatment than that for chronic constipation related to CF. Treatment of DIOS may include laxatives at higher doses or the use of electrolyte intestinal lavage solution (e.g., GoLYTELY)[1] or hyperosmolar enemas. Oral and/or rectal administration[1] of *N*-acetylcysteine solution has also been used for the treatment of mucus accumulation in the GI tract of some individuals with DIOS.

Monitoring
Monitoring of pulmonary symptoms should be done at each encounter. Spirometry to assess lung function is recommended as part of CF clinic visits to assess changes in forced expiratory volume in 1 second (FEV_1) relative to baseline. In addition, routine respiratory cultures including screening for acid-fast bacilli and fungi to monitor for pathogens and susceptibilities are recommended. Nutritional status (e.g., weight, height, weight for length, body mass index) should also be monitored regularly. Annual routine laboratory testing is also done through CF centers and screenings for complications (e.g., CFRD). Recommended monitoring for the various chronic therapies is discussed in the previous section.

Management of Other Complications
In addition to the general manifestation of CF (e.g., pulmonary, growth, and nutrition), complications may appear with age and disease progression. The following are examples and general management approaches. Referral to other specialists, such as endocrinology, gastroenterology, otorhinolaryngology, or transplant (when appropriate for advanced disease), may be necessary.

Sinusitis
Treatment of the acute exacerbations of sinusitis can include systemic (e.g., oral) antibiotics, which are also used in pulmonary exacerbations. The use of intranasal irrigations of antimicrobials (e.g., gentamicin)[1] may also be considered, although guidelines defining and comparing intranasal irrigation agent selection, formulation, dosing, and monitoring are currently lacking.

Small Intestinal Bacterial Overgrowth
Treatment of SIBO in persons with CF is similar to treatment of those without CF, including the use of oral antibiotics (e.g., rifaximin [Xifaxan][1]). Nonpharmacologic treatment may include dietary manipulation, such as reducing carbohydrate consumption, resulting in a high-fat, low-carbohydrate diet.

Cystic Fibrosis–Related Diabetes
In addition to dietary modifications, when pharmacologic treatment is needed, insulin therapy includes a regimen consisting of long-acting insulin paired with carbohydrate counting and coverage with rapid-acting insulin. Insulin is the most appropriate therapeutic choice because there is a loss of β cell function. Acute pulmonary exacerbation or illness may complicate glucose control, especially if systemic corticosteroids are used as part of the management of severe, acute pulmonary exacerbations.

Hepatobiliary Disease
In addition to nutritional support, treatment with oral ursodeoxycholic acid or ursodiol (Actigall)[1] could be considered, though its use has become less common and is no longer recommended per recent guidelines due to lack of supportive data. Newer guidelines published in 2023 suggest ultrasound and other imaging should be done to guide therapy for hepatobiliary disease.

References
Farrell PM, White TB, Ren CL, et al: Diagnosis of cystic fibrosis: consensus guidelines from the Cystic Fibrosis Foundation, *J Pediatr* 181S, 2017. https://doi.org/10.1016/j.jpeds.2016.09.064.

Goetz DM, Brown RF, Filigno SS, et al: Cystic fibrosis foundation position paper: Redefining the CF care model, *J Cyst Fibros* 23(6):1055–1065, 2024. https://doi.org/10.1016/j.jcf.2024.08.007.

Kapnadak SG, Dimango E, Hadjiliadis D, et al: Cystic Fibrosis Foundation Consensus Guidelines for the care of individuals with advanced cystic fibrosis lung disease, *J Cys Fibr*, 2020. https://doi.org/10.1016/j.jcf.2020.02.015.

Lahiri T, Hempstead SE, Brady C, et al: Clinical practice guidelines from the Cystic Fibrosis Foundation for preschoolers with cystic fibrosis, *Pediatrics* 137(4), 2016.

Mayer-Hamblett N, Ratjen F, Russell R, et al; SIMPLIFY Study Group: Discontinuation versus continuation of hypertonic saline or dornase alfa in modulator treated people with cystic fibrosis (SIMPLIFY): results from two parallel, multicentre, open-label, randomised, controlled, non-inferiority trials, *Lancet Respir Med* 11(4):329–340, 2023.

Mogayzel Jr PJ, Naureckas ET, Robinson KA, et al: Cystic fibrosis pulmonary guidelines. Chronic medications for maintenance of lung health, *Am J Respir Crit Care Med* 187(7):680–689, 2013.

Mogayzel Jr PJ, Naureckas ET, Robinson KA, et al: Cystic Fibrosis Foundation pulmonary guideline. Pharmacologic approaches to prevention and eradication of initial Pseudomonas aeruginosa infection, *Ann Am Thorac Soc* 11(10):1640–1650, 2014.

Sellers ZM, Assis DN, Paranjape SM, et al: Cystic fibrosis screening, evaluation, and management of hepatobiliary disease consensus recommendations. *Hepatology* 79(5):1220–1238, 2024.

▌HISTOPLASMOSIS

Method of
Jihoon Baang, MD

CURRENT DIAGNOSIS

- For diagnosing histoplasmosis, one must consider signs, symptoms, imaging indicative of fungal processes, and non-invasive antigen and serologic tests. However, these tests are not always highly sensitive and should not deter you away from the diagnosis if clinical suspicion is high.
- Histopathology is the diagnostic gold standard though it may not always be necessary or feasible. If the diagnosis is uncertain, a biopsy of a suspicious lesion is advised if risks are acceptable. Importantly, a detailed skin (including mucosa) examination for lesions or ulcers should be done. While non-invasive fungal tests can pose challenges in identifying histoplasmosis, occasionally a straightforward skin punch biopsy can lead to the diagnosis histoplasmosis.
- Always take a good exposure history as it can be an important clue when diagnosing histoplasmosis.

CURRENT THERAPY

- Most patients with acute histoplasmosis recover spontaneously without treatment.
- Itraconazole is the mainstay of treatment with the most clinical experience, but if it cannot be used, posaconazole, isavuconazole, and voriconazole are reasonable alternative regimens.
- Severe cases and CNS infections may need IV amphotericin formulations.

---

[1] Not FDA approved for this indication.

Introduction

Histoplasmosis is a systemic mycosis caused by the dimorphic fungus *Histoplasma capsulatum*. This pathogen can lead to a variety of clinical manifestations, making diagnosis challenging. The infection primarily affects the lungs and commonly manifests as acute or chronic pulmonary disease, as well as disseminated disease in immunocompromised individuals. This chapter will cover the epidemiology, clinical features, diagnosis, and management of histoplasmosis, with a focus on the latest evidence-based guidelines and best practices for physicians.

Epidemiology

Histoplasmosis stands as the leading cause of infection among the endemic mycoses in humans. Though its prevalence is highest in North and Latin America, cases have been reported globally. Regions with the greatest concentration of histoplasmosis include southern Illinois, Indiana, western Ohio, Missouri, Kentucky, Tennessee, Mississippi, and Arkansas in the United States, as well as Rio de Janeiro State in Brazil. Emerging research indicates that the geographic distribution of histoplasmosis may be more extensive than previously recognized.

H. capsulatum flourishes in soil enriched by bird or bat guano, often in substantial amounts near bird roosts, chicken coops, rodent-infested abandoned buildings, and bat-inhabited caves where the soil is abundant in animal excretions rich in organic nitrogen. Because *H. capsulatum* can enter a state of latency and reactivate years later, cases have been reported in patients with a distant history of residing in or traveling to endemic regions.

Mycology and Pathogenesis

Histoplasma capsulatum var. *capsulatum* and *H. capsulatum* var. *duboisii* are the two varieties of *H. capsulatum* responsible for human histoplasmosis. *H. capsulatum* var. *duboisii* causes African histoplasmosis, which is predominantly observed in West Africa and Madagascar. This form is characterized by involvement of the skin, bone, lymph nodes, and subcutaneous tissue (also known as "triple tropism"). However, this chapter focuses exclusively on the manifestations and treatment of *H. capsulatum* var. *capsulatum*, hereafter referred to as *H. capsulatum*.

H. capsulatum is a thermally dimorphic fungal pathogen that predominantly grows as a mold in the environment and converts to yeast at 37°C during infection. Consequently, the organism exists in the yeast form when causing human disease but can be isolated as a mold in cultured clinical specimens. In tissues, *H. capsulatum* appears as small, 2- to 4-μm oval yeast forms with narrow-based budding, often in groups and clustering within macrophages. The size, budding pattern, and intracellular presence can aid in the histopathological diagnosis of histoplasmosis.

Disruption of soil containing *H. capsulatum* leads to the aerosolization of microconidia, which serve as the infectious particles. Upon inhalation, these microconidia are phagocytized but can survive and convert to the yeast phase within pulmonary macrophages. The subsequent dissemination through the reticuloendothelial system is typically contained rapidly in healthy hosts but can result in severe disease in the absence of normal immunity. Microconidia can be transported for several miles by air currents, meaning that individuals not in the direct vicinity of the disrupted soil are also at risk for developing histoplasmosis.

Clinical Manifestations

The majority of *H. capsulatum* infections remain asymptomatic, with less than 5% resulting in clinical symptoms. The presence and severity of clinical manifestations are influenced by factors such as the host's immune status, the infectious inoculum size, and the virulence of the infecting strain. Acute pulmonary histoplasmosis is the most frequently observed clinical presentation; however, a range of other symptomatic histoplasmosis syndromes have been documented, highlighting the diverse clinical manifestations of the fungus in humans. In some instances, the initial infection only becomes evident years later as an old, calcified granuloma incidentally found on a chest imaging study.

Acute Pulmonary Histoplasmosis

Acute pulmonary histoplasmosis typically manifests as a self-limited illness resembling infectious mononucleosis. Symptoms are nonspecific and may include fever, chills, malaise, nonproductive cough, and chest pain. Chest radiographs often reveal diffuse infiltrates in one or more lobes, frequently accompanied by enlarged hilar and mediastinal lymph nodes, providing a helpful diagnostic clue. In fewer than 10% of cases, it can also present with a persistently enlarged lymph node that can compress local structures and sometimes be mistaken for lymphoma. The nonspecific symptoms often mimic various upper respiratory infections, leading to a broad differential diagnosis. This includes common viral infections such as acute Epstein Barr virus and HIV infection, bacterial pneumonias, atypical pneumonias such as *Mycoplasma pneumonia* and *Legionella pneumonia*, as well as less common infections such as acute pulmonary blastomycosis. Nonetheless, more severe cases may arise, particularly in immunocompromised individuals. A history of substantial fungal spore exposure (e.g., cleaning a chicken coop) can often aid the diagnostic reasoning process in these cases. Severe respiratory distress, persistent symptoms, and even fatalities may occur in the absence of appropriate treatment. This underscores the importance of prompt diagnosis and timely intervention when warranted.

Chronic Pulmonary Histoplasmosis

A subset of patients with acute pulmonary histoplasmosis fails to clear their infection and progresses to develop chronic pulmonary infection. A portion of these patients may exhibit chronic cavitary disease. Chronic pulmonary histoplasmosis may be arbitrarily defined when the duration of symptoms from pulmonary histoplasmosis exceeds 6 weeks. Patients typically have structural lung disease, such as chronic obstructive pulmonary disease (COPD), and a history of smoking and often reside in areas where histoplasmosis is endemic, although this is not always the case. A combination of systemic and pulmonary signs and symptoms is typically observed in chronic pulmonary histoplasmosis. Common systemic symptoms include fevers, night sweats, weight loss, lack of appetite, subjective loss of energy, and malaise. Pulmonary symptoms consist of cough, occasional minimal hemoptysis, dyspnea, and sputum production. In patients with preexisting lung disease, distinguishing these symptoms from baseline symptomatology may be challenging. Radiologic studies typically reveal cavitary disease without hilar lymphadenopathy. Notably, patients can develop a "marching cavity," in which ongoing necrosis enlarges the cavity, potentially consuming the entire lobe. Mediastinal and hilar lymphadenopathy is less common in this form of histoplasmosis. Pleural effusions are rare, and their presence renders histoplasmosis a less likely cause of a patient's pulmonary process.

Other chronic pulmonary processes resembling chronic pulmonary histoplasmosis include tuberculosis, nontuberculous mycobacterial infections such as *Mycobacterium avium* complex, endemic fungal infections like blastomycosis and coccidioidomycosis, as well as immune-mediated processes such as granulomatosis with polyangiitis, sarcoidosis, and malignancy. A meticulous history and physical examination, along with serologic and histopathological studies, can be instrumental in differentiating between these disease processes.

Untreated, this form of histoplasmosis can lead to death due to progressive pulmonary insufficiency. With treatment, prognosis depends on coexisting pulmonary disease and degree of lung tissue damage but is generally favorable with regard to microbiological cure. However, relapses occur in up to 20% of cases even after prolonged treatment.

Disseminated Histoplasmosis

Most, if not all, episodes of histoplasmosis have a period of dissemination, during which infected macrophages spread throughout the body via the reticuloendothelial system. In most cases, this is a self-limited event, quickly contained upon immune system activation. However, about 1 in 2000 infections result in progressive disseminated disease. Almost invariably, these cases occur in immunocompromised hosts. Patients at risk for progressive disseminated disease include those with advanced HIV infection, solid organ transplant recipients, patients with hematologic malignancies, and those treated with immunomodulating agents, most notably corticosteroids or tumor necrosis factor α (TNF-α) inhibitors. Infants are also at risk.

Recognition of disseminated histoplasmosis can be challenging. Symptoms include fevers, malaise, anorexia, respiratory symptoms, and weight loss. Laboratory investigations often reveal elevated acute phase reactants, abnormal liver function tests, and pancytopenia. Hepatosplenomegaly and lymphadenopathy are common. Severe cases can be clinically indistinguishable from bacterial sepsis, and patients present with hypotension and multiorgan failure. A potential diagnostic clue is the presence of mucosal ulcerations, which are generally painful and can occur anywhere in the oral, pharyngeal, or laryngeal mucosa. Various morphologies may be seen, ranging from superficial to verrucous. Adrenal involvement resulting in adrenal insufficiency can occur. These patients present with enlarged adrenals on imaging and clinical symptoms of Addison's disease. Although survival without antifungal therapy has been described, disseminated histoplasmosis is generally fatal if left untreated.

Mediastinal Manifestations of Histoplasmosis

Mediastinal involvement in histoplasmosis can present as mediastinal fibrosis or granulomatous mediastinitis. Mediastinal fibrosis, also known as fibrosing mediastinitis, is a very rare complication of pulmonary histoplasmosis, where extensive fibrotic tissue forms in the mediastinum in response to infection. Males aged 20 to 40 years have the highest risk for this complication. The fibrosis, composed of mature collagen rather than granulomatous tissue, encases the mediastinal structures and can progress, ultimately leading to death. Prognosis relies on the extent of mediastinal structure involvement, with bilateral disease involving pulmonary veins particularly associated with poor outcomes. Currently, no satisfactory treatment exists.

Conversely, granulomatous mediastinitis, or mediastinal granuloma, is characterized by a caseous inflammatory mass within mediastinal lymph nodes. The majority of patients remain asymptomatic, and cases are frequently identified only through incidental imaging findings. Symptoms, when present, are related to the structures involved. The prognosis for this condition is more favorable, as the process typically resolves, and the affected lymph nodes calcify. The necessity for treatment in such cases remains uncertain.

Central Nervous System Histoplasmosis

Central nervous system (CNS) involvement in *H. capsulatum* infection is relatively rare. It may occur as part of progressive disseminated histoplasmosis in about 5% to 10% of cases, or it may present as isolated cases without other signs of dissemination. CNS histoplasmosis typically causes chronic lymphocytic meningitis, although parenchymal lesions can also occur. Symptoms resemble those of other chronic infectious meningitides, often involving a combination of systemic symptoms such as fever, weight loss, and night sweats, along with localizing symptoms like headaches, focal neurologic deficits, or behavioral changes. Treatment failures and relapses are common, and prognosis depends on the extent and reversibility of immunosuppression with appropriate treatment.

Other Manifestations of Histoplasmosis

H. capsulatum can affect all organ systems, either in the context of clinical disseminated histoplasmosis or as an isolated extrapulmonary infection. It is a known cause of endovascular and cardiac infections, including endocarditis involving both native and prosthetic valves. Pericarditis occurs in around 5% of patients with pulmonary histoplasmosis and is thought to be an immunologic reaction, often resolving with nonsteroidal antiinflammatory drugs (NSAIDs)

or corticosteroids. Bone, joint, and skin infections may also arise, presenting diagnostic challenges. Though urogenital involvement is frequently documented in autopsy series, it seldom causes clinical symptoms. However, there have been reported cases of *H. capsulatum* causing symptomatic prostatitis, nephritis, epididymitis, vaginal and penile ulcers, and ovarian involvement. Similarly, gastrointestinal involvement is found in up to 70% to 90% of disseminated histoplasmosis cases during autopsy, but specific symptoms are less common. Gastrointestinal histoplasmosis can lead to diarrhea, gastrointestinal bleeding, bowel perforation, or bowel obstruction. It should be considered in patients with refractory inflammatory bowel disease, particularly if they reside in endemic areas.

Diagnosis

Identifying histoplasmosis can be challenging because of the diverse clinical manifestations associated with this widespread fungus and the limitations of existing diagnostic tools. When suspecting histoplasmosis, it is typically advisable to employ a combination of diagnostic methods to increase the likelihood of accurate detection. Time frames for test results can differ, and in situations involving severe or disseminated infections, initiating empiric therapy could be crucial. When possible, acquiring tissue samples is key for establishing a definitive pathologic diagnosis and, in some cases, may be the only test that confirms the presence of histoplasmosis.

Histopathology is one of the most valuable techniques for diagnosing histoplasmosis. Necrotizing or nonnecrotizing granulomas are often observed. A skilled pathologist can identify the characteristic pattern of yeast forms, predominantly within macrophages but also outside of them. Yeast forms are best visualized using a methenamine silver stain, such as Gomori-Grocott methenamine silver stain (GMS). As an alternative, periodic acid–Schiff (PAS) staining can be employed. Differentiating histoplasmosis from other pathogens like small variants of Blastomyces dermatitidis, capsule-deficient *Cryptococcus* spp, endospores of *Coccidioides* spp, and *Candida glabrata*, or staining artifacts can be challenging, and seeking expert consultation is recommended in such instances. A thorough skin examination should be conducted because a simple skin biopsy can sometimes reveal the organism, particularly in cases of disseminated histoplasmosis.

Culture confirmation of histoplasmosis is desirable, but the yield of cultures can be limited, and results may take several weeks. In disseminated histoplasmosis, cultures are typically positive from multiple sites, such as blood and bone marrow. In acute pulmonary histoplasmosis, the yield of respiratory cultures ranges between 9% and 40%, depending on the extent of lung involvement. Mild to moderate cases often result in negative cultures. In chronic cavitary lung disease, the culture yield improves owing to the increased fungal burden, with *H. capsulatum* detected in up to 85% of cases. *H. capsulatum* growth can be observed in two distinct phases. In mold phase the fungus grows like mold on fungal medium, such as Sabouraud dextrose agar, at a temperature range of 25°C to 30°C. It may take up to 6 weeks to grow. On microscopy, tuberculate macroconidia with thick walls and surface projections (8–15 μm in diameter), which is considered diagnostic, and smooth-surfaced microconidia (2–4 μm in diameter) are observed. In the yeast phase, the fungus grows in tissues and on fungal medium at 37°C. Oval cells measuring 2 to 4 μm in diameter can be seen, best observed using methenamine silver or periodic acid-Schiff stains. The yeast may appear clustered within macrophages. Blood cultures have low sensitivity in detecting *H. capsulatum*. Fungal blood cultures can increase the sensitivity of histoplasmosis detection, but the lysis centrifugation method may offer further improvement. A positive fungal culture with microscopic features indicative of *H. capsulatum* should be confirmed through specific testing, typically using DNA probing.

Antibody testing for *H. capsulatum* can be helpful in diagnosing chronic forms of histoplasmosis, but it is important to interpret the results in conjunction with the patient's clinical presentation and other specific tests. This is because antibodies generally take 2 to 6 weeks to appear, limiting their utility in acute cases. The complement fixation (CF) test uses yeast and mycelial antigens, with a fourfold increase in titers considered diagnostic. A single titer of ≥1:32 is also indicative of infection. However, in the right clinical context, a lower titer (e.g., ≥1:8) should not be disregarded. CF seropositivity may persist at low levels for years after infection resolution, and cross-reactions can occur with other fungal infections, tuberculosis, lymphoma, and sarcoidosis. The immunodiffusion (ID) assay is more specific than the CF test, detecting the presence of M and H bands. The M band appears earlier and lasts longer, whereas the H band is less common and associated with disseminated disease and severe pulmonary infections. Any positive titer should prompt further investigation because many patients with confirmed histoplasmosis have antibody titers in the low positive range. In immunosuppressed patients, the sensitivity of serology tests is reduced, but positive serologies can still be detected in up to 50% of disseminated histoplasmosis cases. In summary, antibody testing can be a useful tool for diagnosing chronic histoplasmosis, but it should always be considered alongside the clinical scenario and additional testing methods.

The commercial assay for detecting polysaccharide antigens shed by *H. capsulatum* is a valuable diagnostic tool for histoplasmosis, particularly in immunocompromised patients. These assays can be performed on various body fluids, including urine, serum, cerebrospinal fluid (CSF), and bronchoalveolar lavage (BAL) fluid. Though earlier generations of the test demonstrated better performance in urine samples, recent advancements have resulted in equivalent accuracy for urine and serum assays. Detection of antigens in BAL fluid can complement the findings from urine and serum assays, potentially increasing overall sensitivity. Antigen detection assays are highly recommended for suspected histoplasmosis cases because they directly measure shedding, which is not affected by a patient's immune status. This makes the assay especially useful for immunocompromised patients with disseminated or chronic pulmonary histoplasmosis, as well as for monitoring disease activity. In patients with HIV, the urine test has a sensitivity of 95%, whereas the serum test has a sensitivity of 85%. However, in cases of limited disease with minimal fungal burden, antigen detection may be less successful. It is important to note that false positives can occur in patients with blastomycosis. Overall, antigen detection assays are a crucial adjunct to diagnosing histoplasmosis and should be considered in all suspected cases.

Treatment

The treatment of histoplasmosis varies based on clinical syndrome and severity of illness. A summary of current treatment is provided in Table 1. The Infectious Diseases Society of America (IDSA) emphasizes that its guidelines cannot always account for individual variation among patients and are not intended to

TABLE 1	Treatment Summary of Histoplasmosis		
CLINICAL SITUATION	**TREATMENT (FOOTNOTE FOR DOSING)**	**DURATION**	**ADDITIONAL INFORMATION**
Pulmonary Histoplasmosis			
Mild-moderate infection	Treatment typically unnecessary but can treat with itraconazole (Sporanox) for 6–12 weeks if symptoms persist >4 weeks		Check itraconazole blood levels after 7–10 days Final duration should be individualized Posaconazole (Noxafil)[1] is a reasonable alternative azole, although clinical data are limited
Acute and severe	Liposomal amphotericin B (AmBisome)[1] for 1–2 wks andhen itraconazole on average for 12 weeks		Check itraconazole blood levels after 7–10 days Final Duration should be individualized
Less severe	Itraconazole for 6–12 weeks		
Adjunctive treatment in patients with hypoxemia	Methylprednisolone[1]/prednisone[1] 0.5–1.0 mg/kg/day for 1–2 weeks		Can switch to oral prednisone 60mg and taper over 1–2 weeks
Chronic cavitary	Itraconazole for more than 1 year		Final duration should be individualized
Pulmonary nodule	None		
Extrapulmonary Histoplasmosis			
Pericarditis and rheumatologic syndromes	NSAIDS. If no response, may try methylprednisolone[1]/prednisone[1] 0.5–1.0 mg/kg/day for 1–2 weeks and itraconazole for 6–12 weeks		Prednisone 0.5 mg/kg/d with a taper over 1–2 weeks for severe cases
Mediastinal lymphadenitis	No treatment needed. If symptoms persist, may try prednisone[1] for 1–2 weeks and itraconazole for 6–12 weeks		
Mediastinal granulomatous	No treatment needed by if symptoms persist, may try itraconazole for 6–12 weeks		
Mediastinal fibrosis	Antifungal treatment is generally not effective. intravascular stent(s) may be needed if the process leads to vascular stenosis.		
CNS histoplasmosis	Liposomal amphotericin B[1] for 4–6 weeks and then itraconazole for more than 12 months May use fluconazole (Diflucan)[1] 800 mg as an alternative azole (better CNS penetration)		Until resolution of all CSF abnormalities, including clearance of Histoplasma antigen
Disseminated			
Severe	Liposomal amphotericin B[1] for 4–6 weeks and then itraconazole for more than 12 months		If persistently immunosuppressed may need lifelong suppression
Moderate	Itraconazole for more than 12 months		If feasible, reduction of immunosuppression is recommended

[1]Not FDA approved for this indication.
Liposomal amphotericin B 3 to 5 mg/kg/d; itraconazole 200 mg po three times a day for 3 days (loading dose), followed by 200 mg po twice daily; posaconazole DR 300 mg po twice daily for 2 doses (loading dose), followed by 300 mg po daily.

replace physician judgment with respect to specific patients or unique clinical situations. This is an important point because many of the treatment recommendations for histoplasmosis listed are not based on high-quality randomized trials.

For acute pulmonary histoplasmosis, no clinical trial evidence is available to guide treatment decisions, leading the IDSA guidelines to be relatively conservative. They reserve treatment only for "moderately severe to severe" cases, although no explicit definition of severity is provided. Additionally, treatment is not recommended for mild to moderate symptoms persisting for less than 4 weeks. In these cases, careful clinical judgment is essential. Although poor long-term outcomes are uncommon in patients with mild to moderate symptoms, symptom resolution upon antifungal treatment is typical. As a result, some experts choose to treat even mild to moderate acute pulmonary disease with a symptom duration of fewer than 4 weeks, contrary to IDSA guideline recommendations.

In most cases of acute pulmonary histoplasmosis, itraconazole (Sporanox) can be used. Fluconazolebe (Diflucan)[1] should be avoided because it has been shown to be inferior to itraconazole. Clinical data on voriconazole (Vefend),[1] posaconazole (Noxafil),[1] and isavuconazole (Cresemba)[1] are not as robust as those for itraconazole, but these drugs exhibit good in vitro activity and can be used if a patient cannot tolerate itraconazole. If a patient is hypoxic and requires mechanical ventilation, a lipid formulation of amphotericin B (AmBisome)[1] (3-5 mg/kg IV daily) should be used until clinical improvement. Once the patient is able to tolerate an oral regimen, a transition to itraconazole should be made. Adjunctive methylprednisolone[1] 0.5 to 1.0 mg/kg/day for 1 to 2 weeks should also be considered in cases of severe acute pulmonary histoplasmosis, although there are limited data on this approach. Treatment should be continued for 6 to 12 weeks. The treatment regimen for chronic pulmonary histoplasmosis is identical but will require at least 1 year of treatment with close follow-up for relapse once treatment is stopped.

There are limited data to guide the best approach for managing mediastinal complications related to histoplasmosis, which include mediastinal lymphadenitis, mediastinal granuloma, and mediastinal fibrosis. Many experts agree that in most of these scenarios, antifungal treatment is not required. Treatment may be considered if symptoms are severe or persist for longer than 1 month because it has been shown to help with faster resolution of symptoms. Adjunctive steroids may be used if the enlarged lymph nodes begin encroaching upon critical structures in the mediastinum. Patients with mediastinal fibrosis can develop progressive sclerosis of their mediastinal tissue, necessitating surgical removal of fibrotic areas and placement of intravascular stents. The role of steroids or antifungals in these situations remains unclear.

In disseminated histoplasmosis with moderately severe to severe symptoms, induction treatment with liposomal amphotericin B (AmBisome)[1] (3-5 mg/kg IV daily) is recommended for the first 1 to 2 weeks, followed by oral itraconazole for at least 1 year. For patients with acute progressive histoplasmosis, prompt initiation of treatment can be life-saving and should be initiated based on clinical suspicion because serologic studies can take days to weeks to result. For mild to moderate symptoms, the induction phase can be skipped, and treatment with oral itraconazole for 1 year should suffice. Lifelong suppression may be needed in patients who are immunosuppressed. If antifungals are stopped, close monitoring for relapse should be done.

CNS histoplasmosis should be aggressively treated with liposomal amphotericin B[1] (5 mg/kg daily intravenously) for 4 to 6 weeks, followed by oral itraconazole for at least 1 year. Repeat lumbar punctures should be performed every 1 to 2 weeks to assess CSF histoplasmosis antigen levels.

Patients can develop rheumatologic complications related to their histoplasmosis, including pericarditis and arthralgia. In most cases, these can be managed with NSAIDs. If symptoms

are severe and persistent, a 1- to 2-week trial of prednisone, combined with itraconazole for 6 to 12 weeks can be considered.

Prevention

Currently, there are no vaccines for histoplasmosis, although efforts to develop such vaccines continue. For immunosuppressed patients, including those with HIV who have a CD4 count of less than 150/µL and live in endemic areas, itraconazole[1] 200 mg daily can be used for chemoprophylaxis. Educational efforts targeting individuals at high risk of developing severe disease and those involved in high-risk activities can be helpful. Spraying 3% formalin on guano deposits should be considered before undertaking cleaning activities. Additionally, wearing an N95 mask during these high-risk activities, if feasible, should be considered.

Reference

Kauffman CA: "Histoplasmosis: a clinical and laboratory update." *Clin Microbiol Rev* 20(1):115–132, 2007.
Wheat LJ, Alison GF, Martin BK., et al: "Clinical practice guidelines for the management of patients with histoplasmosis: 2007 update by the infectious diseases society of America." Clin Infect Dis 45, no. 7 (October 1, 2007): 807–25.
Bennett JE, Raphael D, Martin JB: "Preface to the eighth edition." In Mandell, douglas, and bennett's principles and practice of infectious diseases (Eighth Edition), page edited by J.E. Bennett, R. Dolin, and M.J. Blaser, xxvii. Philadelphia: W.B. Saunders, 2015. pp 3162-3176
Guarner J, Brandt ME: Histopathologic diagnosis of fungal infections in the 21st century, *Clin Microbiol Rev* 24(2):247–280, 2011.
Hage CA, Ribes JA, Wengenack NL, et al: A multicenter evaluation of tests for diagnosis of histoplasmosis, *Clin Infect Dis* 53(5):448–454, 2011.

HYPERSENSITIVITY PNEUMONITIS

Method of
David I. Bernstein, MD; and Haejin Kim, MD

CURRENT DIAGNOSIS

- History of inhalational exposure to an identifiable environmental antigen associated with development of compatible clinical features.
- Objective evidence of acute inflammatory pneumonitis or chronic pneumonitis with fibrosis based on physical examination, lung function testing, radiographic features, and lung biopsy findings.
- In the acute form, clinical improvement in symptoms, lung function, and radiographic abnormalities with avoidance of the causative antigen(s).

CURRENT THERAPY

- Avoidance of contact with the offending antigen is essential and is often curative if performed early in the course of the disease.
- Although systemic corticosteroids are often required during the acute phase of hypersensitivity pneumonitis, their impact on disease progression and prognosis has not been determined.

Hypersensitivity pneumonitis (HP), also known as extrinsic allergic alveolitis, is an inflammatory disorder of the lungs mediated by immunologic hypersensitivity to a specific antigen, usually organic in nature. Although more than 200 causative antigens have been implicated, only a small number of individuals develop HP in response to exposure. Table 1 lists common causative agents in HP. Comprehensive lists of causative agents are available.

---

[1] Not FDA approved for this indication.

TABLE 1 Hypersensitivity Pneumonitis: Representative Sources and Causative Agents

CONDITION OR PERSONS AT RISK	SOURCE	CAUSATIVE ANTIGENS
Dairy farmers	Hay, grains, silage	Thermophilic actinomycetes
Bird fancier's or pigeon breeder's disease	Avian droppings or feathers	Avian proteins
Humidifier lung	Contaminated water	Thermophilic actinomycetes or other microorganisms
Chemical workers	Polyurethane foam, varnishes, lacquers	Isocyanates
Machine workers	Metalworking fluid	*Pseudomonas fluorescens, Aspergillus niger, Staphylococcus capitis, Rhodococcus* spp., *Bacillus pumilus*
Familial hypersensitivity pneumonitis	Contaminated wood dust in walls	*Bacillus subtilis*
Hot tub lung	Mold on ceiling	*Cladosporium* spp., *Mycobacterium avium*

Modified from Richerson HB, Bernstein IL, Fink JN, et al: Guidelines for the clinical evaluation of hypersensitivity pneumonitis: report of the subcommittee on hypersensitivity pneumonitis, *J Allergy Clin Immunol* 84:839–844, 1989.

TABLE 2 Clinical Features of Hypersensitivity Pneumonitis

FEATURE	ACUTE (INFLAMMATORY)	CHRONIC (FIBROTIC)
Identification of Source of Exposure to Causative Antigens		
Symptoms	Influenza-like illness ± cough/dyspnea within hours after antigenic exposure	Insidious progression with cough, exertional dyspnea, fatigue, and weight loss
Physical findings	Fever; normal chest examination or bibasilar crackles	Cyanosis; right-sided heart failure; lungs normal or bibasilar crackles
High-resolution computed tomography	Diffuse ground-glass infiltrates	Honeycombing, mosaic attenuation, reticular opacities, peribronchiolar interstitial thickening reflecting irreversible pulmonary fibrosis
Pulmonary function testing	↓ FEV_1 and FVC (restrictive pattern); ↓ TLC; ↓ PaO_2 on exercise challenge; ↓ D_{LCO}	
Other findings supportive of a diagnosis of HP	<ul><li>Improvement with avoidance of environmental exposure to suspect causative antigens (acute HP only)</li><li>Precipitating antibodies to HP antigens cultured directly from the environment may help identify specific causative microorganisms</li><li>BAL lymphocytosis with reduced CD4/CD8 ratio <1</li><li>Surgical lung biopsy: peribronchial interstitial lymphocytic and plasma cell infiltrates and/or noncaseating granulomas; pulmonary fibrosis in advanced cases of chronic HP</li></ul>	

BAL, Bronchoalveolar lavage; *D_{LCO},* carbon monoxide diffusion in the lungs; *FEV_1,* forced expiratory volume in 1 second; *FVC,* forced vital capacity; *HP,* hypersensitivity pneumonitis; *PaO_2,* arterial partial pressure of oxygen; *TLC,* total lung capacity.

Pathophysiology

HP is thought to involve primarily delayed type IV (cell-mediated) hypersensitivity and is not mediated by immunoglobulin E (IgE) antibodies. Bronchoalveolar fluid obtained from patients with HP may show a predominant CD8+ lymphocytosis supporting T cell–mediated disease. Viruses are thought to play a role in the development of HP through upregulation of costimulatory molecules on alveolar macrophages and dendritic cells, leading to increased activation of type 1 helper T cells. Adoptive transfer models in animals have shown that CD4+ T cells and cytotoxic T cells are the most important effector cells in experimental HP, rather than cytokines, antibodies, or complement alone.

Clinical Presentation and Diagnosis

The main clinical features for HP are listed in Table 2. Acute inflammatory HP is diagnosed if the history, physical findings, high-resolution chest CT, and pulmonary function tests indicate infiltrative and restrictive lung disease; exposure is documented to a recognized or new causative agent; and there is significant improvement in symptoms, lung function, and radiographic findings with avoidance of the offending cause. IgG antibody to the offending antigen (serum preciptins) may be demonstrated but is not required for diagnosis. Immediate skin test reactivity is not indicated. The clinician can differentiate acute from chronic fibrotic HP based on chest CT and lung biopsy findings (see Table 2). A careful home, environmental, and occupational history is essential to identify one or more causative antigens.

Treatment

The primary treatment is cessation of exposure to the sources of offending antigens at home or in the workplace. Effective environmental control measures may include modification of work habits, improvement in ventilation, or change in manufacturing procedures. Systemic corticosteroids are often required and aid in recovery during the acute phase, but there are no long-term studies of their impact on disease progression or survival rates. Referral to a specialist in hypersensitivity lung diseases is recommended for proper diagnosis and identification of the sources of causative antigens. Individuals with advanced lung disease who have undergone lung transplantation for HP have survival rates comparable to individuals with interstitial lung disease. Nintedanib (Ofev), a tyrosine kinase inhibitor, is approved for chronic progressive interstitial lung disease and can be considered in such patients with HP.[1]

---

[1]Not FDA approved for this indication.

References

Bernstein D, Lummus Z, Santilli G, et al: Machine operator's lung: A hypersensitivity pneumonitis disorder associated with exposure to metalworking fluid aerosols, *Chest* 108:636–641, 2006.

Girard M, Lacasse Y, Cormier Y: Hypersensitivity pneumonitis, *Allergy* 65:322–334, 2009.

Hamblin M, Prosch H, Vašáková M: Diagnosis, course and management of hypersensitivity pneumonitis, *Eur Respir Rev* 31(163):210169, 2022.

Hanak V, Golbin JM, Hartman TE, et al: High-resolution CT findings of parenchymal fibrosis correlate with prognosis in hypersensitivity pneumonitis, *Chest* 134:133–138, 2008.

Jacobs RL, Andrews CP, Coalson JJ: Hypersensitivity pneumonitis: Beyond classic occupation disease: Changing concepts of diagnosis and management, *Ann Allergy Asthma Immunol* 95:115–128, 2005.

Kern RM, Singer JP, Koth L, Mooney J, et al: Lung transplantation for hypersensitivity pneumonitis, *Chest* 147:1558–1565, 2015.

Lacasse Y, Assayag E, Cormier Y: Myths and controversies in hypersensitivity pneumonitis, *Semin Respir Crit Care Med* 29:631–642, 2008.

Morisset J, Johannson KA, Jones KD: Identification of diagnostic criteria for chronic hypersensitivity pneumonitis: an international modified delphi survey, *Am J Respir Crit Care Med* 197:1036–1044, 2018.

Nogueira R, Melo N, Novais E, et al: Hypersensitivity pneumonitis: Antigen diversity and disease implications, *Pulmonology* 25:97–108, 2019.

Schuyler M, Gott K, French V: The role of MIP-1alpha in experimental hypersensitivity pneumonitis, *Lung* 182:135–149, 2004.

LEGIONELLOSIS (LEGIONNAIRE'S DISEASE AND PONTIAC FEVER)

Method of
Shiwei Zhou, MD

Microbiology

Organisms of the Legionellaceae family are aerobic gram-negative, facultative intracellular bacteria with environmental reservoirs in water and soil. Among *Legionella* bacteria, *L. pneumophila* is the most common cause of human disease, with at least 16 serotypes. *L. micdadei* and *L. longbeachae* can also cause human disease.

Epidemiology

The incidence of legionellosis is six times as high as 2 decades ago, likely due to improved diagnostic modalities and an aging population. Patient risk factors for *Legionella* pneumonia include male sex, age >50, cigarette smoking, immunocompromise, and neuromuscular disease. Environmental risk factors include exposures to engineered water systems, such as cooling towers, hot tubs, and decorative fountains where there is stagnation of water with biofilm formation. Healthcare acquisition accounts for about 20% of reported cases of Legionnaire's disease in the United States.

Patients likely become infected by inhaling aerosols or through microaspiration of water contaminated with *Legionella*. Though *Legionella* infections are associated with outbreaks, they are not transmitted person-to-person. The incubation period is typically 2 to 10 days.

Clinical Features

The spectrum of illness caused by *Legionella* ranges from asymptomatic infection, nonspecific febrile illness (Pontiac fever), pneumonia (Legionnaire's disease), to extrapulmonary infection involving spleen, liver, kidneys, and heart.

Patients with Pontiac fever present with an acute, self-limited, flu-like illness with malaise, fatigue, myalgias, headache. They do not develop pneumonia, and symptoms usually resolve without treatment in a few days.

Legionnaire's disease presents as a pneumonia with high fever (can be as high as >40°C or 104°F) and relatively nonproductive cough. This can be difficult to distinguish from other bacterial pneumonia. Concomitant symptoms include watery diarrhea with nausea/vomiting and central nervous system complaints, such as headache or mental status changes. Laboratory findings such as hyponatremia, liver injury in a hepatocellular pattern, and elevation in creatine phosphokinase levels are also frequently reported.

Diagnosis

Legionella grows poorly on routine culture media. Diagnosis has typically relied on the *Legionella* urinary antigen; however, this only detects *L. pneumophila* serogroup 1, so a negative urinary antigen does not rule out legionellosis. Polymerase chain reaction testing on a respiratory specimen is able to detect all clinically relevant serogroups and has become an increasingly preferred diagnostic method.

On imaging, most patients will have a pulmonary infiltrate. On chest computed tomography (CT), immunosuppressed patients may demonstrate nodular, mass-like lesions with possible halo sign or even cavitation.

Treatment

Legionella is an intracellular pathogen, and effective antibiotics in the treatment of Legionnaire's disease must attain high levels within cells. Drug regimens, dosages, and common adverse effects are listed in Table 1.

TABLE 1	Antibiotic therapy for *Legionella* infection	
ANTIMICROBIAL AGENT	**DOSAGE**	**ADVERSE EFFECTS/COMMENTS**
Macrolides		
Azithromycin (Zithromax)*	500 mg PO or IV daily	A/E: GI side effects, QTc prolongation
Clarithromycin (Biaxin)[1]	500 mg PO or IV Q12h	A/E: More GI side effects than azithromycin, QTc prolongation
Fluoroquinolones		
Levofloxacin (Levaquin)*	750 mg PO or IV daily	A/E: Prolonged QTc, tendinopathy, photosensitivity, *C. difficile*, CNS reactions
Moxifloxacin (Avelox)[1]	400 mg PO or IV daily	A/E: Prolonged QTc, tendinopathy, photosensitivity, *C. difficile*
Tetracyclines		
Doxycycline[1,*]	100 mg PO or IV Q12h	A/E: GI upset, esophagitis, photosensitivity. Only for mild infection. Tetracyclines are not effective against *L. longbeachae*
Minocycline[1]	100 mg PO or IV Q12h	A/E: GI upset, esophagitis, photosensitivity, dizziness and vertigo, occasional blue coloring of tissues. Only for mild infection. Tetracyclines are not effective against *L. longbeachae*

*Drugs also used in treatment of community-acquired pneumonia.
[1]Not FDA approved for this indication.
A/E, Adverse effect; *CNS,* central nervous system; *GI,* gastrointestinal.

A macrolide (especially azithromycin [Zithromax]) or a respiratory fluoroquinolone (e.g., levofloxacin [Levaquin], moxifloxacin [Avelox][1]) is the treatment of choice. A 2021 meta-analysis of previous cohort studies found similar rates of mortality and clinical cure between macrolides and fluoroquinolones in the treatment of *Legionella* pneumonia. Alternative agents include tetracyclines (e.g., doxycycline,[1] minocycline [Minocin][1]) though they are not active against *L. longbeachae*. Of note, beta-lactams, monobactams, and aminoglycoside antibiotics are not effective against *Legionella*.

Among patients treated for community-acquired pneumonia, 1% to 10% may have legionellosis. An empiric regimen that includes azithromycin,[1] or a respiratory fluoroquinolone would provide coverage for most *Legionella* species. In patients with microbiologically confirmed legionellosis, copathogens are less common, so treatment can be narrowed to agents active against *Legionella* alone.

For hospitalized patients or those with severe disease, intravenous therapy is preferred. Patients can be transitioned to oral antibiotics when they are clinically improving, hemodynamically stable, and able to tolerate oral medications.

The duration of therapy of *Legionella* pneumonia for immunocompetent patients who responded to therapy and defervesce within 72 hours is 7 to 10 days. Patients with delayed response may need longer therapy. Radiographic changes will lag behind clinical improvement and may take months to clear completely.

For patients with immunocompromise who are at high risk of relapse, 2 to 3 weeks of treatment is reasonable based on clinical response. Combination therapy of both a macrolide and a fluoroquinolone has been used in patients with severe illness, but so far, data have not shown improved clinical outcomes.

---

[1] Not FDA approved for this indication.

References

Agarwal S, Abell V, File Jr TM: Nosocomial (Health Care-Associated) Legionnaire's Disease, *Infect Dis Clin North Am* 31(1):155–165, 2017, https://doi.org/10.1016/j.idc.2016.10.011.

Albin O, Mills JP, Saint S, Swanson M, Deng JC: A "fluid" diagnosis, *N Engl J Med* 385(23):2180–2185, 2021, https://doi.org/10.1056/NEJMcps2108991.

Jasper AS, Musuuza JS, Tischendorf JS, et al: Are fluoroquinolones or macrolides better for treating legionella pneumonia? A systematic review and meta-analysis, *Clin Infect Dis* 72(11):1979–1989, 2021, https://doi.org/10.1093/cid/ciaa441.

Sivagnanam S, Podczervinski S, Butler-Wu SM, et al: Legionnaires' disease in transplant recipients: A 15-year retrospective study in a tertiary referral center, *Transpl Infect Dis* 19(5):10.1111/tid.12745., 2017. https://doi.org/10.1111/tid.12745.

Torres A, Cillóniz C: Are macrolides as effective as fluoroquinolones in legionella pneumonia? Yes, but…, *Clin Infect Dis* 72(11):1990–1991, 2021, https://doi.org/10.1093/cid/ciaa442.

LUNG ABSCESS

Method of
Michael Persinger Jr., MD; and Morteza Khodaee, MD, MPH

CURRENT DIAGNOSIS

- Lung abscess is often a sequela of aspiration in patients with risk factors such as periodontal disease, alcoholism, or neurologic impairment.
- Sputum culture and Gram stain should be obtained before starting broad-spectrum antibiotics, if possible. Conventional culture methods often underdetect anaerobic or facultative anaerobic organisms.
- While chest radiography should be performed initially, it may fail to detect lesions in cases of extensive lobar consolidation or opacification. Computed tomography (CT) is the preferred diagnostic modality.

CURRENT THERAPY

- First-line therapy is systemic intravenous antibiotics with β-lactam/β-lactamase inhibitors (e.g., ampicillin-sulbactam [Unasyn][1]). Alternative intravenous (IV) options include carbapenems (e.g., meropenem[1]) or clindamycin (Cleocin) for penicillin-allergic patients. Third-generation cephalosporins (e.g., ceftriaxone [Rocephin][1]) with IV metronidazole (Flagyl) may also be used.
- Anaerobic coverage is essential. If methicillin-resistant *Staphylococcus aureus* (MRSA) is a concern, add vancomycin (Vancocin) or linezolid (Zyvox).
- Procedural interventions, including percutaneous thoracic tube drainage (PTTD) and endoscopic catheter drainage (ECD), were historically reserved for nonresponders, but more recent studies, including a narrative review from 2023, support earlier use to collect samples for culture, shorten hospitalization, and hasten recovery.
- Surgical resection is a last-line option, typically reserved for cases refractory to antibiotics and drainage. It carries an elevated mortality risk (~11%).

---

[1] Not FDA approved for this indication.

Definition and Classification

A lung abscess is a localized collection of necrotic pulmonary tissue and pus resulting from liquefactive necrosis, most commonly occurring in the setting of an active pulmonary infection. The process typically results in the formation of a walled-off cavity containing necrotic debris and purulent material, with or without an air-fluid level. These air-fluid levels develop when the abscess communicates with the bronchial tree, allowing partial drainage of fluid.

Lung abscesses are broadly categorized as either primary or secondary. A primary lung abscess, which accounts for the majority of cases, arises due to aspiration of oropharyngeal contents. This leads to the development of aspiration pneumonitis, which may progress to pneumonia and subsequent abscess formation. In contrast, secondary lung abscesses occur due to an underlying condition that predisposes to infection or impaired drainage. Such conditions include bronchial obstruction from malignancy, lymphadenopathy, tumors, or foreign bodies; hematogenous spread from infections such as right-sided endocarditis; contiguous spread from nearby structures such as subphrenic abscesses or empyema; and immunosuppressive states. Lung abscesses can also be classified by chronicity, with abscesses lasting more than 6 weeks considered chronic.

Epidemiology

While exact incidence rates are unknown, antibiotics have drastically reduced the incidence of lung abscesses. In addition to antimicrobial therapy, further advances in dental medicine and increased knowledge and management of periodontal disease have further decreased the incidence of lung abscesses. Typically, middle age to older adult males are more commonly affected than women of similar ages. Anatomically, the right lung is more commonly affected due to the wider and more vertically oriented right main bronchus. Within the right lung, the posterior segment of the upper lobe is most commonly affected. The superior segments of the lower lobes bilaterally are frequently involved, with the right being more common than the left.

Risk Factors

The most identified risk factors for lung abscess include alcoholism and periodontal disease, particularly gingivitis. Periodontal disease is associated with an increased oral bacterial burden, which can lead to infection if aspirated. Alcoholism increases the likelihood of overt aspiration due to impaired consciousness, although microaspiration events have also been documented in otherwise healthy individuals during sleep or while supine, potentially explaining the development of lung abscess in patients without obvious risk factors.

Additional predisposing factors include any condition that increases aspiration risk, such as neurologic dysfunction, gastro-esophageal reflux, dysphagia, impaired cough or gag reflex, seizure disorders, stroke, or the use of sedative medications (either therapeutic or recreational). Immunocompromised individuals—including those with malnutrition, HIV infection, malignancy, or those on chronic corticosteroids or other immunosuppressive therapies—are also at increased risk. In these cases, infections tend to be more severe, often involving aerobic gram-negative bacilli and complex or multiloculated abscesses.

In pediatric populations, important risk factors include foreign body aspiration, cystic fibrosis, congenital immunodeficiencies, and other pediatric lung parenchymal diseases. Among adults, underlying structural lung diseases such as chronic obstructive pulmonary disease (COPD) are important to consider. Up to 40% of patients presenting with lung abscess have some degree of COPD, which increases the risk of bronchial obstruction. It is also important to evaluate for potential underlying malignancy in any adult patient with a nonresolving lung abscess despite appropriate antibiotic therapy.

Pathophysiology

The most common mechanism of lung abscess formation is the aspiration of oropharyngeal secretions containing mixed aerobic and anaerobic flora. This event initiates an inflammatory response, resulting in aspiration pneumonitis. The inflammation impairs mucociliary clearance by damaging ciliated epithelial cells, which hinders the removal of mucus and pathogens from the lower respiratory tract. The localized pneumonitis activates the inflammatory cascade and leads to the release of cytokines such as tumor necrosis factor-α (TNF-α), interleukin (IL)-6, and IL-1. These mediators promote parenchymal tissue necrosis and cavitation.

As the inflammatory process progresses, the necrotic tissue becomes encapsulated, with increasing fibrosis and sharper demarcation of the abscess wall. If the abscess involves the bronchioles, partial drainage of pus may occur, resulting in an air-fluid level on imaging. Peripheral abscesses can eventually communicate with the pleural space. In turn, this can cause the development of a pleural effusion, typically exudative by Light's Criteria, with potential progression to empyema.

Clinical Manifestations

Lung abscess often presents as an indolent illness. Fever is the most commonly reported symptom, present in approximately 80% of cases. Other systemic symptoms include chills, fatigue, night sweats, and unintentional weight loss. Pulmonary symptoms may include cough—often productive of foul-smelling sputum—dyspnea, pleuritic chest pain, and hemoptysis. Given the variability in clinical presentation, a thorough physical examination and diagnostic workup are essential.

Diagnosis

On physical examination, findings may include decreased breath sounds and signs of focal consolidation such as rales or egophony. However, some patients may have a normal lung examination. Other supportive findings include digital clubbing, which is nonspecific and may reflect chronic pulmonary disease and malignancy; poor dentition or gingival inflammation; and neurologic signs such as impaired gag reflex or swallowing dysfunction.

Chest radiography may be diagnostic if it reveals a cavitary lesion with an air-fluid level (Figure 1A). Early in the disease course, before significant fibrosis has developed, radiographs may show nonspecific consolidation with or without cavitation. If the chest radiograph is inconclusive, contrast-enhanced computed tomography (CT) is recommended and remains the diagnostic gold standard (Figure 1B and C). CT is particularly valuable in assessing lesion architecture, identifying potential bronchial obstruction or malignancy, and guiding procedural interventions. Point-of-care lung ultrasound may be used, particularly in emergency or intensive care settings, but its utility depends on abscess location and

depth. Deep, multiloculated, or segmental lesions may be difficult to visualize sonographically. However, if the abscess is superficial in an anatomically favorable position (e.g., empyema), ultrasound may be used for needle guidance during aspiration.

Microbiologic diagnosis includes obtaining sputum for Gram stain and culture before the initiation of antibiotics, if possible. However, conventional techniques have limited sensitivity for detecting anaerobes, which are only identified in about 40% of cases. Emerging methods such as metagenomic next-generation sequencing may improve anaerobic pathogen detection in the future. If sputum cannot be obtained, bronchoscopy should be considered—particularly in critically ill or immunocompromised patients, or when obstruction is suspected. Image-guided needle aspiration or biopsy may also be considered if the clinical response to empiric antibiotics is suboptimal. If the abscess is superficial and easily accessible, it is reasonable to attempt to obtain an ultrasound-guided aspiration for antimicrobial sensitivities.

Blood cultures should be obtained from two separate venous sites to identify potential hematogenous spread. Laboratory evaluation typically includes a complete blood count, which may reveal leukocytosis, and inflammatory markers such as C-reactive protein, erythrocyte sedimentation rate, procalcitonin, and lactate. Tuberculosis should be excluded through sputum acid-fast bacillus (AFB) testing and interferon-γ release assay or tuberculin skin testing.

Differential Diagnosis

Several conditions may mimic lung abscess radiographically. Tuberculosis is a key differential diagnosis due to its potential to cause cavitary lesions. Other infectious mimics include hydatid cysts from echinococcosis and fungal infections such as aspergillosis, which may produce aspergillomas. Noninfectious causes include pulmonary neoplasms, which may either mimic or cause lung abscesses via bronchial obstruction. Pulmonary infarctions, such as those caused by embolism, and systemic vasculitides like granulomatosis with polyangiitis may also present with cavitary pulmonary lesions.

Microbiology

Lung abscesses are often polymicrobial, comprising both anaerobic and aerobic bacteria. Common anaerobes include species of *Bacteroides*, *Prevotella*, *Peptostreptococcus*, and *Fusobacterium*. Monomicrobial abscesses may be caused by *Streptococcus* species, *Staphylococcus aureus* (including methicillin-resistant *S. aureus* [MRSA]), *Klebsiella pneumoniae*, *Streptococcus pyogenes*, *Burkholderia pseudomallei*, *Nocardia*, or *Actinomyces*.

Treatment

Empiric antibiotic therapy is the cornerstone of lung abscess management. Initial treatment usually includes β-lactam/β-lactamase inhibitor combinations. First-line options include intravenous (IV) ampicillin-sulbactam (Unasyn[1]) 3 g every 6 hours or piperacillin-tazobactam (Zosyn) 3.375 g every 6 hours. If a nosocomial infection or MRSA is suspected, vancomycin (Vancocin) or linezolid (Zyvox) should be added.

An alternative regimen involves third-generation cephalosporins such as ceftriaxone (Rocephin[1]) 1 to 2 g daily in combination with agents targeting anaerobes, such as metronidazole (Flagyl) 500 mg IV every 6 to 8 hours or clindamycin (Cleocin) 600 to 900 mg IV every 6 to 8 hours. While clindamycin monotherapy was once standard, increasing resistance has limited its current use. In cases of treatment failure, broad-spectrum agents such as meropenem (Merrem)[1] 1 g IV every 8 hours may be considered. Antibiotic therapy should be tailored based on speciation and sensitivity from collected culture data.

The duration of intravenous therapy is variable, ranging from 5 days to 3 to 4 weeks, depending on clinical response. Once significant improvement is noted both clinically and radiographically, a transition to oral therapy can be made. Oral options include amoxicillin-clavulanate (Augmentin) 875/125 mg every 12 hours or clindamycin (Cleocin) 150 to 450 mg every 6 hours. Total

---

[1]Not FDA approved for this indication.

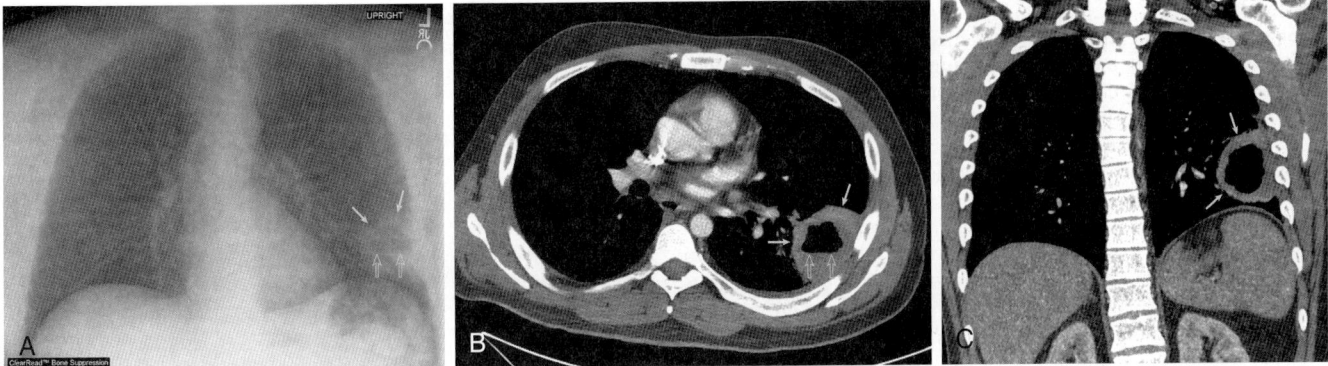

Figure 1 ClearRead Bone Suppression anteroposterior chest radiograph (A) with large left lower lobe thick-walled, cavitary lesion *(solid arrows)* with air-fluid level *(open arrows)*. Transverse (B) and coronal (C) chest computed tomography with large left lower lobe cavitary lesion *(solid arrows)* with air-fluid level *(open arrows)*.

antibiotic duration typically ranges from 3 to 8 weeks, depending on resolution. Shorter antibiotic courses have been associated with poorer outcomes or recurrence of the abscess. Therapy may be discontinued once imaging confirms complete resolution or stabilization of the abscess cavity with scar tissue development.

Procedural intervention may be necessary in cases of poor clinical response, to guide microbiologic diagnosis, to evaluate for obstruction, or for abscesses larger than 6 cm. Two primary drainage methods are used: percutaneous thoracic tube drainage (PTTD), typically guided by imaging and used for peripheral abscesses; and endoscopic catheter drainage (ECD), usually performed via bronchoscopy and preferred for more central lesions or when evaluating for obstructive etiology. ECD carries a lower complication risk and has demonstrated better success rates, while PTTD carries a higher risk of bronchopleural fistula. Both techniques also carry risks of bacteremia, pneumothorax, empyema, parenchymal seeding, and septic shock.

Surgical resection (via lobectomy or segmentectomy) is reserved as a last resort for cases unresponsive to medical and potential procedural management. Indications include chronic abscesses, contraindications to drainage, or complications such as rupture with pyopneumothorax or empyema. Surgical treatment is associated with higher mortality and should be pursued by a multidisciplinary team involving pulmonology, infectious disease, and interventional radiology.

Prognosis

Approximately 90% of patients respond to antibiotic therapy, with clinical improvement generally seen within 2 to 4 weeks. Radiographic resolution lags behind clinical recovery, and serial imaging should be used to confirm resolution. Poor prognostic indicators include large abscess size (>6 cm), immunocompromised status, presence of sepsis, advanced age, and underlying malignancy. Mortality ranges from 5% to 15%, with primary lung abscesses generally associated with better outcomes.

References

Hadid W, Stella GM, Maskey AP, Bechara RI, Islam S: Lung abscess: the non-conservative management: a narrative review, *J Thoac Dis* 16(5):3431–3440, 2024. https://doi.org/10.21037/jtd-23-1561.

Lee JH, Hong H, Tamburrini M, Park CM: Percutaneous transthoracic catheter drainage for lung abscess: a systematic review and meta-analysis, *Eur Radiol* 32(2):1184–1194, 2022, https://doi.org/10.1007/s00330-021-08149-5.

Nelson JK, Parsonnet J: Bacterial lung abscess. In Mandell D, Bennett's, editors: *Principles and practice of infectious diseases*, 9th Ed, Elsevier, Inc, 2020, pp 926–931.

Neuman M, Mahdavi R, Khoadee M: 37-year-old man • cough • increasing shortness of breath • pleuritic chest pain • Dx? *J Fam Pract* 70(3):143–149, 2021, https://doi.org/10.12788/jfp.0171.

Ramirez JA, File Jr TM: Pulmonary infections in adults: lung abscess and pleural effusion, *FP Essent* 550:30–36, 2025. PMID: 40094493.

Sabbula BR, Rammohan G, Sharma S, Akella J: Lung abscess. 2024 jun 8. In *StatPearls [Internet]*, Treasure Island (FL), 2025, StatPearls Publishing. (PMID: 32310380.

Sperling S, Dahl VN, Fløe A: Lung abscess: an update on the current knowledge and call for future investigations, *Curr Opin Pulm Med* 30(3):229–234, 2024, https://doi.org/10.1097/MCP.0000000000001058.

Umamoto K, Horiba M: Lung abscess as a secondary infection of COVID-19: a case report and literature review, *J Infect Chemother* 29(7):700–702, 2023, https://doi.org/10.1016/j.jiac.2023.02.005.

Vaarst JK, Sperling S, Dahl VN, Fløe A, Laursen CB, Gissel TN, Gjoerup PH, Bendstrup F: Lung abscess: clinical characteristics of 222 Danish patients diagnosed from 2016 to 2021, *Respir Med* 216:107305, 2023. https://doi.org/10.1016/j.rmed.2023.107305.

Zhang R, Yu J, Shang X, Wang Z, Li H, Cao B: Heterogeneity in clinical patterns of adult lung abscess patients: an 8-year retrospective study in a tertiary hospital, *BMC Pulm Med* 25(1):101, 2025, https://doi.org/10.1186/s12890-025-03487-2.

LUNG CANCER

Method of
Erin A. Gillaspie, MD, MPH; and Amanda S. Cass, PharmD

CURRENT DIAGNOSIS

- An improvement in lung cancer outcomes is achievable with use of low-dose computed tomography (LDCT) for lung cancer screening.
- The accurate staging of lung cancer is crucial to help guide treatment recommendations.
- Tissue diagnosis can be achieved through image-guided endobronchial and surgical biopsies.

CURRENT THERAPY

- All smokers should be counseled on smoking cessation.
- Treatment recommendations are based on stage of cancer and patient fitness to tolerate surgery.
- Surgically resectable non–small cell lung cancer (NSCLC) is more commonly approached in a minimally invasive fashion.
- Early-stage NSCLC is most often treated with definitive surgery with or without systemic therapy.
- Locally advanced NSCLC requires a multimodal treatment regimen often using a combination of radiation therapy, surgery, and systemic therapy.
- Recent approvals for immunotherapy and targeted therapy in earlier line setting necessitate earlier molecular and programmed death-ligand 1 (PD-L1) testing for some patients.
- Forty percent of patients will have an advanced stage of disease at diagnosis, and systemic therapy is the mainstay of treatment.
- All patients with stage IV disease should have molecular and PD-L1 testing to help guide therapy.
- Small cell lung cancer (SCLC) is aggressive, and the mainstay of treatment is systemic therapy combined with radiation therapy in early-stage disease or immunotherapy in advanced disease.

Epidemiology

Lung cancer is the leading cause of cancer-related mortality in the United States among both men and women. The overall incidence rate is decreasing, more rapidly among men, largely as a result of the declining use of tobacco. Despite this, men are still more likely to develop lung cancer in their lifetime (approximately 1 in 16 compared with about 1 in 17 for women). Lung cancer incidence by race and ethnicity has been studied. The highest incidence is among Black men and White females. Although Hispanic populations have a lower incidence and mortality rate overall, Cuban males have higher age-adjusted incidence rates. Lung cancer is predominantly a disease of older individuals, 65 to 84 years of age, with average age at diagnosis of 70 years.

Most cases are diagnosed at locally advanced or advanced stages of disease (76%), which accounts for the relatively poor overall survival. The 5-year overall survival is 22% overall and 26% for non–small cell lung cancer (NSCLC) and only 7% for small cell lung cancer (SCLC).

Epithelial lung cancers are divided into four major cell types: SCLC, adenocarcinoma, squamous cell carcinoma, and large cell carcinoma; the latter three types are collectively known as NSCLCs. All histologic types of lung cancer can develop in current or former smokers, although squamous and small cell carcinomas are most commonly associated with heavy tobacco use. It is essential to distinguish histologically between SCLC and NSCLC because these subtypes have different natural histories and therapeutic approaches. In addition, the molecular subtype of NSCLC has become an important part of treatment planning because some chemotherapeutic agents perform quite differently in squamous cell cancers versus adenocarcinoma. Further, patients with adenocarcinoma are more likely to harbor tumor mutations, making them candidates for targeted therapy.

Risk Factors

Tobacco use (cigarettes, cigars, and pipes) is by far the greatest risk factor for lung cancer, accounting for approximately 80% of lung cancer deaths. Risk increases as a function of both quantity and duration of tobacco exposure. Environmental tobacco smoke or secondhand smoke is also an established cause of lung cancer.

Radon gas is the second most common risk factor. Prolonged exposure to low-level radon in homes might impart a risk of lung cancer equal to or greater than that of environmental tobacco smoke.

Additional risk factors include asbestos, radiation, agent orange, chromium, cadmium, and arsenic. Individuals with occupations in rubber manufacturing, roofing, paving, and chimney sweeping are also felt to be at an increased risk for developing lung cancer. Finally, family history of lung cancer is a risk factor, but the exact genetic driver remains unclear. Notably, the incidence of lung cancer in never-smokers is increasing for reasons that are also unclear.

Prevention

Smoking cessation is the cornerstone of lung cancer prevention. Stopping tobacco use before middle age avoids more than 90% of the lung cancer risk attributable to tobacco. Moreover, smoking cessation in individuals with an established diagnosis of lung cancer is associated with improved survival and decreased toxicities from therapy.

The combination of smoking cessation counseling with medications leads to a higher likelihood of successful quit attempts. Medications that are approved by the U.S. Food and Drug Administration (FDA) include nicotine replacement therapy (nicotine patches [NicoDerm CQ], lozenges [Nicorette], gum [Nicorelief, Nicorette], spray [Nicotrol NS]), varenicline (Chantix), and bupropion (Zyban). Nicotine patches, which provide longer periods of nicotine replacement, should be used in combination with gum or lozenges to treat short-term cravings. The results of a multicenter, double-blind, randomized controlled trial, the Evaluating Adverse Events in a Global Smoking Cessation Study, compared varenicline, bupropion, nicotine patch, and placebo in

TABLE 1	The 5 As of Smoking-Cessation Counseling
Ask	Ask and record smoking status
Advise	Advise smokers on benefit of stopping in a personalized, appropriate manner
Assess	Assess motivation to quit
Assist	Assist in smokers' quit attempt
Arrange	Arrange follow-up with cessation services

more than 8000 smokers and found that the efficacy of each medication was higher than that of placebo. The results of this trial also demonstrated that there was no increase in neuropsychiatric symptoms in smokers exposed to varenicline, leading the FDA to remove the black box warning.

Patients must want to stop smoking and must be willing to work hard to achieve the goal of smoking abstinence to achieve success. Counseling using the 5 As (ask, advise, assess, assist, arrange) remains the recommended five major steps in intervention (Table 1). A shortened version, the 3 As, is an alternative for busy clinicians and involves asking and recording smoking status, advising the patient of health benefits, and acting on the patient's response.

Early Detection

Clinicians have an important opportunity to improve lung cancer outcomes through early detection. Increasing evidence demonstrates a mortality benefit when screening high-risk patients with low-dose computed tomography (LDCT). The U.S. Preventive Services Task Force recommends lung cancer screening with LDCT for individuals 50 to 80 years of age, current or former smokers who have quit within the past 15 years, and smokers who have at least a 20 pack-year history of smoking. Medicare covers LDCT screening for a similar group of high-risk individuals, differing only in the upper age limit (50–77 years of age). These policy decisions were made following the results of the National Lung Screening Trial (NLST).

The NLST was a large multicenter, randomized controlled trial performed in the United States that compared annual chest x-ray (CXR) with LDCT in 53,454 patients who were considered high risk for development of lung cancer. This trial was terminated early when it met its primary endpoint of achieving a 20% relative reduction in lung cancer mortality favoring the LDCT arm. Nearly twice as many early-stage cancers were detected in the LDCT group compared with the CXR group (40% vs. 21%). The overall rates of lung cancer death were 247 and 309 deaths per 100,000 person-years in the LDCT and CXR groups, respectively. Compared with the CXR group, the rate of death in the LDCT group from any cause was reduced by 6.7% (95% confidence interval, 1.2–13.6; $P = .02$). A common critique of the NLST is the high false-positive rate. However, across three rounds of screening in the LDCT arm, only 24.2% of screening examinations were positive and went on to require additional imaging or biopsy. The interpretation of screening LDCT continues to improve through the use of the American College of Radiology's structured reporting system, Lung-RADs, which has further decreased the false-positive rate.

Similarly, the Danish-Belgium Lung Cancer Screening Trial (NELSON) found a 26% relative reduction in lung cancer mortality when screening high-risk individuals with LDCT compared with no screening, further supporting the role for annual LDCT scans in high-risk individuals as part of health maintenance.

Clinical Manifestations

The tumor size, location, and manifestation of paraneoplastic syndromes determine the clinical presentation of most patients with lung cancer. Most patients with early-stage disease are

TABLE 2

TUMOR LOCAL EFFECT	DISTANT METASTASIS EFFECTS	PARANEOPLASTIC SYNDROME
Cough	Bone pain	Hypercalcemia
Dyspnea	Headache	SIADH
Hemoptysis	Nausea and vomiting	Lambert-Eaton syndrome
Chest pain	Seizure	Cerebellar ataxia
Hoarseness	Weight loss	Encephalitis
SVC syndrome	Fatigue	Cachexia/anorexia
Postobstructive pneumonia	Abdominal pain	Cushing syndrome
Pleural effusion	Spinal cord compression	
Pericardial effusion	Pathologic fracture	

TABLE 2 Clinical Signs and Symptoms of Lung Cancer

asymptomatic, and their cancer is discovered incidentally on CXR or LDCT scans (Table 2).

Peripheral tumors may invade the chest wall and can present with pain. Centrally located tumors may cause symptoms from direct invasion or compression of mediastinal structures. Symptoms may include cough, hemoptysis, wheezing, stridor, and postobstructive pneumonia. Patients may present with diaphragmatic paralysis caused by phrenic nerve invasion, superior vena cava (SVC) syndrome with facial edema, bluish discoloration of the upper chest, and shortness of breath. They may even have dysphagia from esophageal compression. Mediastinal lymph node involvement can cause disruption of the recurrent laryngeal nerve, leading to hoarseness. Tumors arising in the superior sulcus, so-called Pancoast tumors, can result in lower brachial plexopathy and Horner syndrome. Pleural effusion may also be the presenting sign for lung cancer and can cause pain, dyspnea, or cough (see Table 2).

Symptoms from metastatic disease may be the first sign of malignancy. Frequent sites of metastasis include supraclavicular and cervical lymph nodes, bone, brain, liver, and adrenal glands. Brain metastases occur in 10% to 30% of patients, and symptoms may include seizures, nausea and vomiting, headache, or focal neurologic dysfunction. Bony metastases commonly present with pain, pathologic fracture, or spinal cord compression. Liver metastases can cause biliary obstruction and jaundice; however, this is not particularly common. Constitutional symptoms include anorexia, weight loss, weakness, fever, and night sweats.

Some lung cancers are notable for ectopic production of hormones leading to paraneoplastic syndromes. These are most commonly described in SCLC; however, they can occur in rare cases of NSCLC. The most common paraneoplastic syndromes in NSCLC are tumor cachexia and hypercalcemia. The causes of tumor cachexia are not well characterized. Hypercalcemia is mediated by the production of parathyroid hormone–related peptide. The peptide stimulates the release of calcium from bones, resulting in an elevation in calcium in the blood and osteopenia. This syndrome is treated effectively with bisphosphonate therapy. Hypertrophic pulmonary arthropathy can occur with NSCLC or SCLC and is characterized by digital clubbing and periostitis of the long bones that are demonstrable on plain x-rays.

Paraneoplastic syndromes unique to SCLC include Lambert-Eaton myasthenic syndrome, syndrome of inappropriate antidiuretic hormone (SIADH), and Cushing syndrome. A patient presenting with Lambert-Eaton myasthenic syndrome should always be ruled out for malignancy; 50% of patients who present with this syndrome have cancer, and in 95% of those cases it is SCLC. Another paraneoplastic syndrome related to SCLC is SIADH. SIADH generally resolves within 1 to 4 weeks of initiating chemotherapy. During this period, serum sodium can usually be managed and maintained above 128 mEq/L via fluid restriction. Demeclocycline (Declomycin)[1] can be a useful adjunctive measure when fluid restriction alone is insufficient. Vasopressin receptor antagonists also have been used in the management of SIADH but are costly and have increased unique toxicities such as liver injury.

Cushing syndrome caused by ectopic production of adrenocorticotropic hormone by SCLC and pulmonary carcinoids results in electrolyte disturbances rather than the classic changes in body habitus. Treatment with standard medications such as metyrapone (metopirone)[1] and ketoconazole (Nizoral)[1] is largely ineffective.

Cerebellar degeneration may be associated with anti-Hu, anti-Yo, or P/Q channel autoantibodies. Cutaneous manifestations such as dermatomyositis are rare. Thrombosis including Trousseaus syndrome, marantic endocarditis, and coagulopathies is also uncommon and is usually associated with a poorer prognosis.

Diagnostic Techniques

Once lung cancer is suspected, tissue biopsy is required to make a definitive diagnosis. In patients with suspected metastatic disease, a biopsy of a distant site of disease is preferred for tissue confirmation because it provides diagnosis and staging information.

Several methods can be considered for biopsy, and the technique selected should be tailored to the location of the primary tumor and the presence of mediastinal nodal involvement or metastatic disease.

For peripheral lesions, a computed tomography (CT)-guided needle biopsy may be considered. This route of biopsy is associated with a risk of pneumothorax that requires intervention in approximately 5.6% of cases.

The advent of navigational bronchoscopy has allowed interventional pulmonologists to sample nodules both centrally and in the periphery of the lungs with very high yield. This may be coupled with endobronchial ultrasonography (EBUS) to allow for mediastinal staging in the same setting.

Mediastinal nodal involvement or direct extension into the mediastinum may be evaluated by bronchoscopy paired with endoscopic ultrasonography or surgically by mediastinoscopy.

Surgical biopsies using a minimally invasive approach (video-assisted thoracoscopic surgery [VATS] or robot-assisted thoracoscopic surgery) may be used as both diagnostic and therapeutic options. For patients presenting with a pleural or pericardial effusion, cytologic examination of the fluid may establish the diagnosis.

The tenets of biopsy are the same no matter which method is chosen: there should be adequate tissue for diagnosis, histologic subtyping, and molecular testing. If sufficient tissue is not obtained to further classify the subtype of lung cancer, additional procedures to obtain sufficient tissue are often warranted, particularly in patients with advanced-stage disease.

Staging

The accurate staging of lung cancer is crucial in guiding treatment recommendations (Tables 3 and 4). Staging makes use of imaging modalities combined with biopsy to help determine the size, location, and histology of a lesion. A complete history and physical examination along with an assessment of performance status is important in evaluating a patient's ability to tolerate therapy (Figure 1).

Imaging

CT scanning is a standard part of the workup for lung cancer and determining the candidacy for resection. Although excellent in

[1] Not FDA approved for this indication.

delineating the extent of the primary lesion disease and some sites of metastatic disease, it is the least sensitive and specific modality for the identification of lymph node involvement or distant metastatic disease. CT scan of the chest should always be obtained with extension through the adrenal glands, a common site of metastatic disease.

Positron emission tomography (PET) plays an important role in both nodal and extrathoracic staging. PET attempts to identify sites of malignancy based on glucose metabolism by measuring the uptake of ^{18}F-fluorodeoxyglucose (FDG). Rapidly dividing cells will preferentially take up ^{18}F-FDG and appear as a "hot spot." Combined ^{18}F-FDG PET-CT imaging has been shown to improve the accuracy of staging in NSCLC compared with visual correlation of PET and CT on either study alone. A standardized uptake value of >2.5 on PET is considered highly suspicious for malignancy. False negatives can be seen in diabetes, in lesions <8 mm, and in slow-growing tumors (e.g., carcinoid tumors or well-differentiated adenocarcinoma). Confirmation of PET scan abnormalities with tissue diagnosis remains important because this modality of imaging also carries the risk of false-positive upstaging, particularly in regions where histoplasmosis is prevalent.

Mediastinoscopy was once considered the gold standard diagnostic technique for the assessment of mediastinal lymph nodes. Mediastinoscopy can evaluate lymph node stations 2R, 4R, 2L, 4L, and 7, and it can uniquely resect whole lymph nodes to submit for analysis. This has been replaced in many centers by EBUS, which is less invasive and offers the ability to ultrasonographically evaluate each lymph node and to sample N1, N2, and N3 nodes. A review of available publications reveals a median sensitivity of 89% for EBUS and a very low risk of complications. In addition, cytologic rapid on-site evaluation confirms the adequacy of samplings at the time of procedure to enhance overall yield.

Brain magnetic resonance imaging (MRI) with contrast is mandatory in all patients with SCLC. An MRI of the brain should also be performed in all patients with NSCLC if the tumor is larger than 4 cm, lymph nodes are involved, or the patient has neurologic symptoms.

Assessing Treatment Candidacy

After establishing the stage of cancer, a meticulous evaluation should be performed before recommending therapy (see Figure 1). Workup should include history and physical examination, labs

TABLE 3	TNM Staging				
PRIMARY TUMOR (T)		**LYMPH NODES (N)**		**DISTANT METASTASIS (M)**	
T0	No evidence of primary tumor	N0	No regional lymph nodes involved	M0	No distant metastases
Tis	Carcinoma in situ	N1	Ipsilateral lymph node peribronchial and/or ipsilateral hilar or intrapulmonary lymph nodes involved	M1	Distant metastases present
T1	Tumor ≤3 cm, surrounded by lung or visceral pleura without bronchoscopic evidence of invasion more proximal than lobar bronchus	N2	Ipsilateral mediastinal or subcarinal lymph nodes involved	M1a	Separate tumor nodule(s) in contralateral lobe; pleural or pericardial nodule(s) or malignant pleural or pericardial effusion
T1a	Tumor ≤1 cm	N3	Contralateral mediastinal or hilar lymph nodes or ipsilateral or contralateral scalene or supraclavicular lymph nodes involved	M1b	Single extrathoracic metastasis
T1b	Tumor >1 cm but ≤2 cm			M1c	Multiple extrathoracic metastases in one or more organs
T1c	Tumor >2 cm but ≤3 cm				
T2	Tumor >3 cm but ≤5 cm or with any of the following: involves main bronchus but does not involve carina, invades visceral pleura, associated with atelectasis or obstructive pneumonitis				
T2a	Tumor >3 cm but ≤4 cm				
T2b	Tumor >4 cm but ≤5 cm				
T3	Tumor >5 cm but ≤7 cm or with any of the following: separate tumor nodule(s) in same lobe as primary or directly invades				
T4	Tumors >7 cm in greatest dimension or any tumor that invades the mediastinum, diaphragm, heart, great vessels, recurrent laryngeal nerve, carina, trachea, esophagus, or spine or a separate tumor in a different lobe of the ipsilateral lung				

TABLE 4	Staging Groups		
STAGE	**T**	**N**	**M**
Stage 0	Tis	N0	M0
Stage IA1	T1a	N0	M0
Stage IA2	T1b	N0	M0
Stage IA3	T1c	N0	M0
Stage IB	T2a	N0	M0
Stage IIA	T2b	N0	M0
Stage IIB	T1a to c	N1	M0
	T2a	N1	M0
	T2b	N1	M0
	T3	N0	M0
Stage IIIA	T1a to c	N2	M0
	T2a to b	N2	M0
	T3	N1	M0
	T4	N0	M0
	T4	N1	M0
Stage IIIB	T1a to c	N3	M0
	T2 a to b	N3	M0
	T3	N2	M0
	T4	N2	M0
Stage IVA	Any	Any	M1a
	Any	Any	M1b
Stage IVB	Any	Any	M1c

including a complete blood count, a comprehensive metabolic panel, nutritional assessment, pulmonary function testing and cardiac assessment—this generally includes at minimum an electrocardiogram and may require more comprehensive evaluation depending on history. Assessment of a patient's performance status has important prognostic and therapeutic implications and should be noted in all patients.

In patients who are being considered for surgery, smokers should be counseled to stop immediately. In addition to helping reduce the risk of perioperative pulmonary complications and death, it will help reduce the long-term consequences related to tobacco use.

Assessment of Cardiovascular Risk

Major cardiac-related adverse events occur in approximately 2% to 3% of patients after pulmonary resection. The Thoracic Revised Cardiac Risk Index is a validated tool that can be used to help guide which patients should be sent for additional preoperative consultation. Patients who score more than 1.5 on the cardiac risk index or those who describe limited exercise capacity or recent diagnosis of active heart disease all warrant evaluation by a cardiologist.

Assessment of Pulmonary Function

Patients undergoing pulmonary resection commonly have several coexisting conditions and exposures that can affect pulmonary function. It is therefore essential to ensure adequate pulmonary reserve before proceeding with resection. Spirometry and measurement of diffusing capacity of the lung for carbon monoxide (DLCO) should be obtained for all patients undergoing pulmonary resection. These are calculated as a percentage of the predicted value. The forced expiratory volume in 1 second, measured during spirometry, determines the mechanical function of the lung; that is, the airflow limitations of medium to large airways. The DLCO value provides a gross estimate of the function at the alveolar-capillary membrane. The DLCO (the actual and predicted postoperative percentage) has been shown in various studies to be the most important predictor of perioperative complications and mortality.

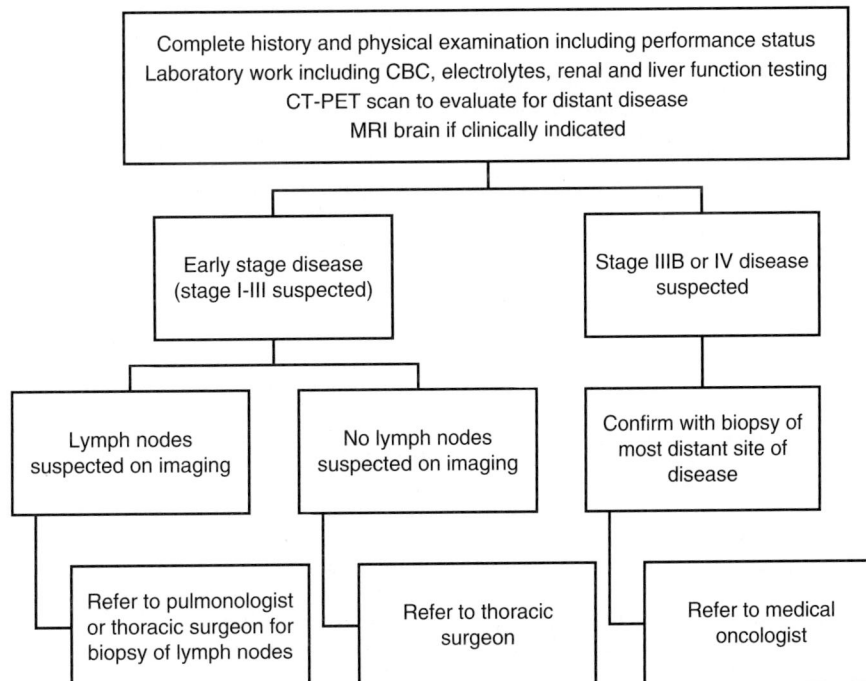

Figure 1 Approach to diagnosis. *CBC*, Complete blood count.

A postoperative predicted forced expiratory volume in 1 second or DLCO of less than 60% should prompt additional testing such as a shuttle walk test or stair-climbing exercise. If the postoperative predicted DLCO is less than 30% to 40%, this denotes an increased risk and warrants a formal cardiopulmonary exercise test with measurement of maximal oxygen consumption. This quantitative assessment has established thresholds associated with surgical risk. A ventilation-perfusion scan may also be helpful in patients with heterogeneous underlying lung disease.

Surgical Approach to Lung Cancer

The approach to surgery and extent of pulmonary resection are determined by the size and location of the tumor and the experience of the surgeon.

Open Lobectomy

Many pulmonary resections continue to be performed in open fashion via thoracotomy with division of muscle and removal of a small segment of rib to allow for rib spreading.

Surgery is performed with a special endotracheal tube (a double-lumen tube) that allows the operative lung to be collapsed while maintaining ventilation to the contralateral lung. After thoracotomy, the chest is inspected to rule out metastatic disease and confirm that the tumor is resectable.

Surgery begins with the removal of N1 and N2 lymph nodes, which are sent to pathology. A lobectomy is performed by isolating the arteries, vein, and bronchus associated with the lobe and dividing each along with the fissure that connects the upper, middle (right), and lower lobes. Once the lobectomy is completed, the remaining lung is reinflated to fill the pleural space, and chest tubes are positioned to help drain fluid and air while the patient recovers.

Lung resections carry a significant risk of perioperative morbidity, with 37% of patients experiencing some form of postoperative complication. Atrial arrhythmia and prolonged air leak are the most common complications. Other complications include infection, bleeding, hypoxia, and death.

Video-Assisted Lobectomy

Technologic advancements including VATS and robot-assisted thoracoscopic surgery have allowed most medical centers to transition to a minimally invasive approach for most pulmonary resections.

VATS for lobectomy is conducted in a similar fashion to an open lobectomy but uses two to three small ports in the chest, each measuring approximately 1 cm, and a slightly larger utility incision measuring 3 cm through which the specimen is removed. VATS differs from open surgery in both the length of incisions as well as minimal disruption or division of muscle fibers, and there is no rib spreading. A camera and special instruments have been designed to make the surgery possible.

Comparison of outcomes shows that both open surgery and VATS provide equal cancer-specific outcomes. Both VATS and open surgery have similar patterns of postoperative complications, although at a lesser rate for minimally invasive approaches. Additional benefits of VATS include earlier recovery, earlier discharge, less pain, less effect on pulmonary function, better quality of life, and increased delivery of adjuvant therapy.

Robot-Assisted Lobectomy

Robot-assisted lobectomies were first performed in 2003, and the use of this technology has continued to increase with time. Much like VATS, a robotic lobectomy is performed through small incisions.

This newer technology has several advantages over traditional thoracoscopic surgery in that it provides a three-dimensional, high-definition visualization compared with only a two-dimensional view in thoracoscopic surgery. In addition, the instruments have nine degrees of freedom and include the ability to staple and seal

vessels. Robotic surgery also boasts the same patient benefits as VATS.

Extent of Resection: Lobar Versus Sublobar Resection

Lobectomy has long been considered the standard of care and the optimal oncologic procedure for management of resectable lung cancer. More limited resections (including segmentectomy or wedge resection) were thought to be associated with a higher risk of recurrence and historically were reserved for patients with limited cardiopulmonary reserve.

The advent of CT screening for lung cancer and improvements in imaging technology have led to the identification of earlier-stage cancers (<2 cm), partially solid lesions, and completely ground glass lesions. This has prompted a renewed interest in the possibility of more limited resection that preserves more pulmonary function and thereby a patient's ability to undergo subsequent resections if required.

The CALB140503 trial published in 2023 randomized patients to lobar versus sublobar resection (wedge or segmentectomy) for node-negative tumors ≤2 cm. The oncologic outcomes for sublobar resection were noninferior, with similar patterns of postoperative morbidity and length of hospitalization. More surgeons have begun adopting a selective approach to sublobar resections in early-stage lung cancers that satisfy the above criteria and have a favorable biology—semisolid lesions without visceral pleural invasion.

Treatment: Non–Small Cell Lung Cancer
Stage I and II Lung Cancers

Surgery is recommended as part of the treatment regimen for stage I, stage II, and some stage IIIA NSCLCs. Stages I and II, based on the American Joint Committee on Cancer eighth edition staging system, include tumors that are node negative and up to 7 cm in size, tumors that involve the chest wall, and pericardium or satellite nodules in the same lobe. Surgery can also be considered for tumors involving the main bronchus and ipsilateral hilar nodes. There remains a great deal of debate on the optimal therapy for patients with N2 disease, in particular multistation or bulky disease. This will be discussed in further detail later in the chapter.

Comprehensive pathologic staging is just as important at the time of surgery as it is included in the workup. Lymph nodes should be sampled from N2 stations (on the right side, stations 4R, 7, and 9R; on the left side, stations 5, 6, 7, and 9L) and N1 stations (stations 10 to 14) at the time of surgery. There is notably a 6% to 8% rate of occult N2 disease discovered at the time of final pathology for patients with T1 tumors and negative preoperative assessments.

The Commission on Cancer 2020 Operative Standards were recently updated to reflect the new recommendations for extent of lymphadenectomy at the time of lung cancer resection. Each patient should have at least one separately submitted N1 or hilar lymph node as well as three distinct mediastinal lymph node (N2) stations submitted for pathologic assessment.

Patients with a primary tumor >4 cm or nodal involvement should be considered for neoadjuvant and/or adjuvant therapy. Studies have demonstrated that surgery can be performed safely with equivalent perioperative morbidity and mortality after neoadjuvant therapies.

Neoadjuvant Therapy

The movement of immunotherapy and targeted therapies into earlier stage treatment of lung cancer has dramatically increased in the last few years. There remains a great deal of debate as to the optimal timing and duration of therapy. There have been several FDA approvals in both neoadjuvant and adjuvant therapy in the last few years, with more anticipated in upcoming months.

Before initiating any neoadjuvant or adjuvant therapy, testing for PD-L1 status, EGFR mutations, and ALK mutations should be preformed. Immunotherapy has been shown to have less benefit in patients with EGFR or ALK mutations, and some of the

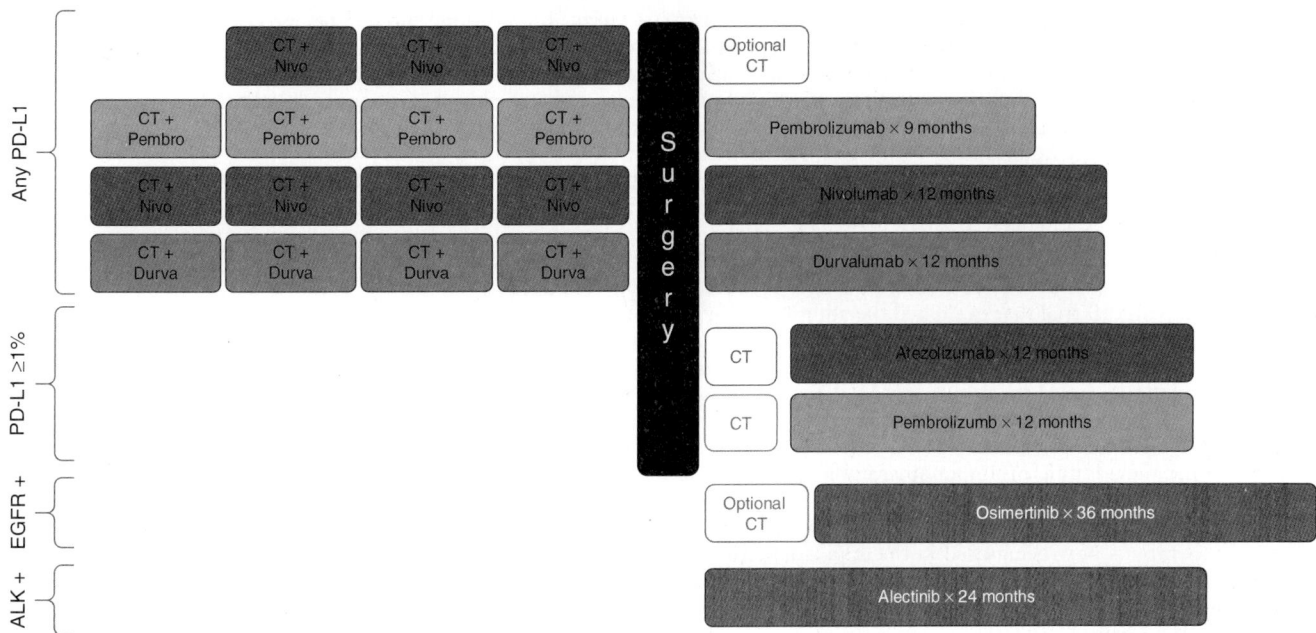

Figure 2 General treatment algorithm for lung cancer. *CT*, Chemotherapy.

neoadjuvant trials excluded these patients. Additionally, there are adjuvant targeted therapy options for patients with EGFR and ALK mutations. These results can be incorporated with other factors to determine which patients may benefit most from particular neoadjuvant or adjuvant treatment options (Figure 2).

In 2022, the PD-L1 inhibitor nivolumab (OPDIVO) was approved by the FDA in combination with platinum doublet chemotherapy for the neoadjuvant treatment of patients with resectable stage IB to IIIA NSCLC based on the phase III Check-Mate-816 trial. Patients were treated in the neoadjuvant setting with nivolumab (OPDIVO) in addition to chemotherapy or with chemotherapy alone, which resulted in event-free survival of 31.6 months and 20.8 months, respectively. This resulted in a 37% reduction in the risk of disease recurrence, disease progression, or death by 37% in this patient population. Surgery was performed safely with no increased perioperative morbidity or mortality. The pathologic complete response rate was 24% for patients receiving chemotherapy and immunotherapy versus 2.2% in the chemotherapy-only arm. The CheckMate-816 protocol left adjuvant therapy to the discretion of the treating physician, leading to a great deal of therapeutic variability.

There have also been several peri-adjuvant trials in this setting. The Aegean trial randomized 802 resectable Stage II–III patients to neoadjuvant chemotherapy with durvalumab (Imfinzi) versus chemotherapy alone for four cycles. Patients underwent surgery followed by additional durvalumab of placebo. Although data continue to mature, after a median follow-up of 11.7 months, the durvalumab arm showed a 32% reduction in the risk of disease progression and death. Likewise, the Keynote 671 trial randomized 797 patients with resectable stage II–III cancers to receive neoadjuvant chemotherapy and pembrolizumab (Keytruda) versus chemotherapy alone for four cycles. Patients went on to have surgery followed by additional pembrolizumab or placebo. The event-free survival at 24 months was 62.4% for the pembrolizumab arm versus 40.6% for the placebo arm. A pathologic complete response was achieved in 18.1% of patients in the pembrolizumab arm versus 4% in the placebo arm. Overall survival is not statistically different between the two groups.

Lastly, the CheckMate 77T randomized 461 patients with stage IIA to III NSCLC to receive four cycles of chemotherapy plus nivolumab (Opdivo) or placebo before surgery. Following surgery, patients received nivolumab or placebo monthly. The 18-month event-free survival was 70.2% in the nivolumab group

and 50.0% in the placebo group. A pathologic complete response occurred in 25.3% of patients in the nivolumab group and in 4.7% of patients in the placebo group. Overall survival data is not yet mature.

For patients who do not receive neoadjuvant therapy and have tumors that are determined on final pathology to be >4 cm or in patients with lymph node involvement, adjuvant therapy is recommended.

The benefit of adjuvant chemotherapy was firmly established in 2008 by a landmark meta-analysis (the Lung Adjuvant Cisplatin Evaluation Study) that demonstrated a 5.4% improvement in 5-year survival for patients treated with surgery followed by adjuvant chemotherapy compared with surgery alone. The benefit was primarily confined to patients with stage II or IIIA disease, with only a modest benefit in patients with tumors <4 cm. In 2011 the NSCLC Collaborative Group compiled a postoperative chemotherapy meta-analysis and reported a similar survival benefit in patients with stage II disease. There is no role for adjuvant chemotherapy in patients with stage IA NSCLC.

The optimal platinum-based chemotherapy regimen remains a topic of debate. Although the aforementioned trials employed different platinum doublets, cisplatin (Platinol)[1] and vinorelbine (Navelbine) was one of the most commonly used regimens. The E1505 trial assessed the addition of bevacizumab (Avastin) to cisplatin-based chemotherapy. Although this trial demonstrated no benefit in overall survival, a post hoc analysis compared the different platinum doublet regimens (pemetrexed [Alimta], gemcitabine [Gemzar], docetaxel [Taxotere], and vinorelbine) and found no difference in either overall survival or disease-free survival but noted that cisplatin plus pemetrexed was associated with improved tolerance and was preferred among physicians for patients with nonsquamous NSCLC.

If a decision is made to proceed with adjuvant chemotherapy, treatment should be started within 6 to 12 weeks after surgery, assuming that the patient has fully recovered, and should be administered for no more than four cycles. Although cisplatin-based chemotherapy is the preferred treatment regimen, carboplatin (Paraplatin)[1] can be substituted for cisplatin in patients who are unlikely to tolerate cisplatin for reasons such as reduced renal function, presence of neuropathy, or hearing impairment.

---

[1] Not FDA approved for this indication.

The use of PD-L1 inhibitors in the adjuvant setting has also been studied recently, and atezolizumab (Tecentriq) and pembrolizumab (Keytruda) both have FDA approval for this indication in patients who have resected NSCLC with PD-L1 ≥1% following platinum-based chemotherapy. The IMpower010 was a phase III trial that evaluated the addition of atezolizumab (Tecentriq) treatment for 1 year compared with basic supportive care in patients with stage IB to IIIA NSCLC following resection and platinum-based chemotherapy. Median disease-free survival was not reached in the atezolizumab (Tecentriq) arm compared with 35.3 months in the basic supportive care arm. The KEYNOTE-091 trial was a phase III trial that evaluated the addition of pembrolizumab (Keytruda) treatment for 1 year compared with basic supportive care in patients with stage IB to IIIA NSCLC following resection and platinum-based chemotherapy. Median disease-free survival was 58.7 months in the pembrolizumab (Keytruda) arm compared with 34.9 months in the placebo arm. However, it is unclear whether the addition of immunotherapy in the adjuvant setting is safer or more effective than when used in the neoadjuvant setting.

Targeted therapy is now being used in the adjuvant setting in select patient populations. Patients with stage IB to IIIA NSCLC who have undergone resection and whose tumors harbor an *EGFR* mutation can now receive osimertinib (Tagrisso) in the adjuvant setting. In a phase III trial, patients received adjuvant osimertinib (Tagrisso) for up to 3 years or placebo, with the primary outcome of disease-free survival in patients with stage II to IIIA NSCLC postresection. Of note, in this study, patients could receive adjuvant chemotherapy but were not required to. At 24 months, 90% of patients in the osimertinib (Tagrisso) arm were alive and disease free compared with 44% in the placebo group. The difference in overall survival was statistically significant, with a median overall survival of 38.6 months in the osimertinib (Tagrisso) group and 31.8 months in the placebo group.

Additionally, patients with stage IB to IIIA, completely resected, ALK positive NSCLC can receive adjuvant alectinib (Alecensa). In the phase III ALINA trial, patients received either alectinib for 2 years or 4 cycles of platinum chemotherapy. At 2 years, 93.8% of patients in the alectinib group and 63% of patients in the chemotherapy group were alive and disease free. Overall survival data is not yet mature. The results for both of these studies reinforces the importance of testing for EGFR or ALK mutations prior to initiation of any neoadjuvant or adjuvant therapy.

Postoperative radiation is usually reserved for patients in whom there is a concern for residual disease (e.g., patients with positive margins on final pathology). In patients with stage I and II disease who either refuse or are not suitable candidates for surgery, stereotactic body radiation therapy is a treatment option for patients with tumors that are ≤5 cm. Treatment is typically administered in three to five fractions delivered over 1 to 2 weeks and is associated with a disease control rate of approximately 90% and 5-year survival rates of up to 60%. Cryoablation is another technique occasionally used to treat small, isolated tumors (i.e., ≤3 cm). However, very little data exist on long-term outcomes with this technique.

Locally Advanced Lung Cancer

The treatment of locally advanced lung cancer is complex and requires a multidisciplinary approach. More treatment regimens are incorporating immune checkpoint inhibitors and targeted therapies to enhance progression-free and overall survival.

T3N1 Tumors

T3N1 is a relatively infrequent stage of lung cancer, but surgery has a well-defined role as the primary treatment for these tumors. T3 lung cancers range in size from 5 to 7 cm or invade structures that can be routinely taken en bloc with the lung: the chest wall, pericardium, or a single phrenic nerve. Often, hilar nodal involvement is discovered at the time of resection. The surgical goal is an en bloc resection with microscopically negative margins.

Surgical resection should be preceded with neoadjuvant therapy or followed by adjuvant systemic therapy as described previously. If a complete resection is not technically feasible, concurrent chemoradiotherapy is recommended as described in the following section.

Stage IIIA Tumors

This is a heterogenous group that comprises patients with (1) small tumors (T1 to T2) with ipsilateral mediastinal lymph node involvement (N2), (2) large tumors (T3 to T4) with ipsilateral lymph node involvement (N1), and (3) large tumors (T4) without lymph node involvement (N0). In the following sections, we will discuss some of the nuances in the subcategories of this complex group of tumors: N2 disease, T4 tumors, and superior sulcus tumors.

N2 Disease

The optimal management of N2 disease is perhaps the most challenging and controversial area in thoracic oncology. Tumor characteristics and nodal burden of disease as well as performance status play an important role in determining who should be considered for surgery. Patients with clinical stage I or II disease who are discovered to have N2-positive nodes at the time of resection should undergo lobectomy with mediastinal lymphadenectomy and then be referred for adjuvant chemotherapy as described previously. In most cases, pathologic involvement of mediastinal lymph nodes is documented preoperatively, and a multimodal approach is recommended because these patients are at high risk for local and distance recurrence.

The Intergroup 0139 study sought to help define the roles of therapy for N2 disease. The trial found no definitive survival benefit with surgery after neoadjuvant chemoradiotherapy compared with definitive chemoradiotherapy alone. The study outcomes were confounded by a very high mortality rate in patients undergoing pneumonectomy, which likely affected this outcome. Subgroup analysis did show a trend toward survival benefit in patients undergoing lobectomy as a part of trimodal treatment. In the aftermath of this trial, a more conservative surgical approach was adopted in many institutions offering resections to patients with single-site micrometastatic disease and who could undergo lobectomy rather than pneumonectomy.

More contemporary studies have demonstrated significantly higher median survival and freedom from recurrence compared with the INT0139 trial with the use of multimodal therapies, including immunotherapy and targeted therapies, leading to a more aggressive surgical approach for local control.

Patients who are deemed nonoperative should be considered for the PACIFIC regimen. The randomized, placebo-controlled, phase III trial demonstrated a significant improvement in progression-free survival and overall survival in patients treated with concurrent chemoradiotherapy followed by 1 year of therapy with the immune checkpoint inhibitor durvalumab (Imfinzi) compared with placebo. This trial has established this as a new standard of care for patients with locally advanced, unresectable disease.

While radiation was used in some cases postoperatively for patients with occult N2 disease identified at the time of surgery, the recent Lung ART trial evaluated the benefit of conformal radiation in completely resected patients with N2 disease. The trial found that postoperative radiation was not associated with an increased disease-free survival compared with no radiation. Thus postoperative radiation is not recommended as the standard of care for stage IIIA N2 NSCLC.

Esophagitis and pneumonitis are the two most common toxicities associated with concurrent chemoradiotherapy.

T4 Tumors

T4 tumors are locally aggressive with invasion of critical mediastinal structures such as the pulmonary artery, heart, aorta, SVC, trachea, esophagus, spine, or diaphragm. Surgery can be

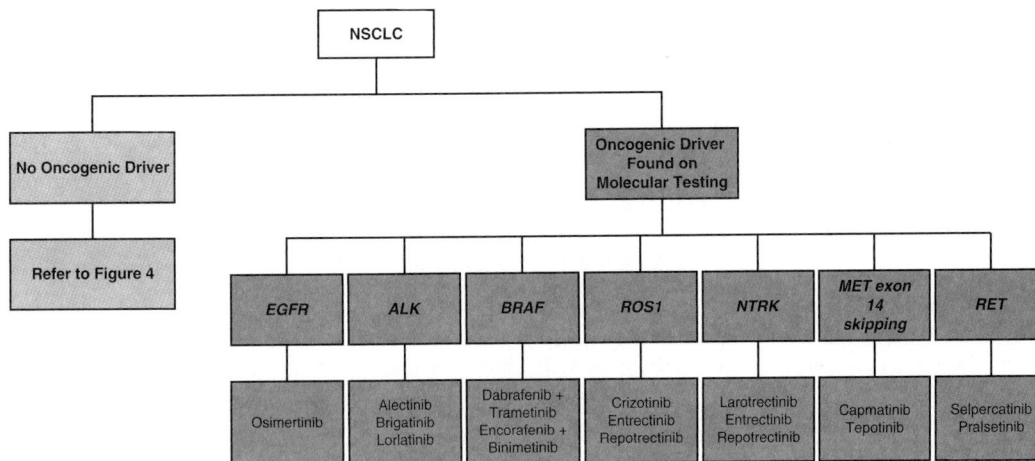

Figure 3 Treatment algorithm for metastatic non–small cell lung cancer.

considered as part of a multimodal therapy plan in high-volume centers with dedicated thoracic surgeons. Meticulous preoperative planning and, in some cases, a multidisciplinary surgical approach are necessary to ensure complete resection.

Superior Sulcus Tumors

Superior sulcus tumors, also known as *Pancoast tumors,* arise from the apical segment of the right upper or left upper lobe. These tumors may invade any of the structures in the apex of the chest: brachial plexus, subclavian artery, subclavian vein, musculature, ribs, paravertebral sympathetic chain, or spinal nerve roots. Patients may present with shoulder pain, Horner syndrome, or neurologic complications of the upper extremity.

As with other locally advanced tumors, a multidisciplinary approach is the mainstay of management of superior sulcus tumors. Complete staging is important to help determine resectability. MRI is often used in conjunction with other imaging modalities to better assess chest wall invasion and neurologic involvement.

Treatment with neoadjuvant chemoradiotherapy followed by surgery results in superior survival for patients with N0 or N1 disease. Surgery is generally completed 3 to 5 weeks after completion of chemoradiotherapy and involves en bloc resection of the tumor, chest wall, and any other involved structures with subsequent reconstruction.

Patients with unresectable disease (medical inoperability, positive mediastinal nodes) should be offered concurrent chemoradiotherapy followed by durvalumab consolidation as described previously.

Stage IIIB

Stage IIIB includes any tumors with contralateral mediastinal nodal involvement or large tumors (>5 cm) with ipsilateral mediastinal nodal involvement. These tumors are considered inoperable because surgery has not been shown to confer any survival benefit. These patients should be treated with concurrent chemotherapy and radiation followed by consolidation therapy with either durvalumab (Imfinzi) or osimertinib (Tagrisso) in patients with EGFR mutations. Durvalumab for 1 year was compared with placebo in the phase III PACIFIC trial and showed improved overall survival in stage IIIB NSCLC patients who did not progress following concurrent chemotherapy and radiation. The phase III LAURA trial compared osimertinib until disease progression versus placebo in patients with stage III EGFR positive NSCLC who did not progress during or after concurrent chemotherapy and radiation. Median progression-free survival was 39.1 months in the osimertinib arm and 5.6 months in the placebo arm. Overall survival data is not yet mature.

Stage IV

Approximately 40% of patients present with stage IV disease at the time of diagnosis. Moreover, a significant proportion of

patients who present with early-stage NSCLC will relapse despite initial curative-intent therapy. Systemic therapy depends on a patient's performance status, histology, and PD-L1 and molecular status. Of note, the early application of palliative care in conjunction with chemotherapy is associated with improved survival and a better quality of life.

Chemotherapy

Chemotherapy has been an important therapeutic option for decades in the treatment of patients with stage IV NSCLC. A landmark meta-analysis in 1995 established cisplatin-based regimens as the standard of care and conferred a survival benefit in patients with stage IV disease.

Treatment recommendations have continued to evolve over the years. Histology of the NSCLC has come to be very important in treatment consideration; phase III trials have demonstrated cisplatin[1] and pemetrexed to be superior to cisplatin[1] and gemcitabine (Gemzar) in patients with nonsquamous NSCLC, whereas cisplatin and gemcitabine was superior in patients with squamous cell histology. This survival difference is thought to be related to the differential expression of thymidylate synthase, one of the targets of pemetrexed, among tumor subtypes. Importantly, bevacizumab (Avastin), a monoclonal antibody that targets vascular endothelial growth factor (VEGF), was also established as unsafe to administer in patients with squamous NSCLC and is FDA approved in combination with carboplatin and paclitaxel as a first-line option only in patients with nonsquamous NSCLC.

In addition to histology, PD-L1 status and presence of oncogenic drivers guide treatment selections. The majority of patients with oncogenic drivers should be treated with targeted therapies regardless of PD-L1 status (Figure 3).

Immunotherapy

Immune checkpoint inhibitors have increasingly become part of the first-line treatment paradigm in patients with metastatic NSCLC and no driver mutations. Checkpoint inhibitors exert antitumor effects by inhibiting negative T-cell regulators. Regardless of histology, all patients with advanced-stage lung cancer should undergo programmed death-ligand 1 (PD-L1) testing as this will drive treatment decisions in the absence of an oncogenic driver (Figure 4). A phase III trial demonstrated a superior response rate and progression-free and overall survival rates when pembrolizumab (Keytruda) was compared with platinum-based chemotherapy in patients with tumors that were PD-L1 ≥50% and EGFR and ALK wild type. Cemiplimab (Libtayo) and atezolizumab (Tecentriq) have also been FDA approved as monotherapy in patients with NSCLC and PD-L1 of ≥50% and EGFR and ALK wild type. Similar results were also seen in a phase III

---

[1] Not FDA approved for this indication.

Lung Cancer

trial comparing nivolumab (OPDIVO) plus ipilimumab (Yervoy) with platinum-based chemotherapy. More recently, combination therapy with platinum-pemetrexed (Alimta) and pembrolizumab in nonsquamous NSCLC and platinum-taxane (paclitaxel [Taxol] or nab-paclitaxel [Abraxane]) and pembrolizumab in squamous cell lung cancer was found to be superior to chemotherapy alone regardless of the patient's PD-L1 status. Likewise, this was also seen with combination therapy including nivolumab (OPDIVO) plus ipilimumab (Yervoy) plus histology-appropriate platinum-based doublet chemotherapy, as well as cemiplimab (Libtayo) combined with histology-appropriate platinum chemotherapy. However, the additive benefit of chemotherapy to patients with tumors that are PD-L1 ≥50% to immunotherapy alone remains unclear beyond a small subset of analyses from the aforementioned trials. Combination chemotherapy with carboplatin (Paraplatin),[1]

paclitaxel, bevacizumab (Avastin), and atezolizumab (Tecentriq) has also been shown to be superior to carboplatin, paclitaxel, and bevacizumab in patients regardless of PD-L1 status and is also FDA approved as a first-line treatment option for nonsquamous NSCLC. For patients with PD-L1 of 1% to 49% or patients who are PD-L1 negative, chemotherapy plus immunotherapy combinations are preferred. However, for those patients who are not candidates for chemotherapy, there are two immunotherapy only options available for treatment. These patients can be treated with pembrolizumab (Keytruda) monotherapy or combination nivolumab (OPDIVO) and ipilimumab (Yervoy). In patients who are PD-L1 negative and not a candidate for chemotherapy, the only nonchemotherapy option that exists is nivolumab (Opdivo) and ipilimumab (Yervoy) combination therapy. Numerous other trials are currently ongoing to evaluate the use of immunotherapy in NSCLC, both alone and in combination with other immunologic agents, chemotherapy, targeted therapy, and radiotherapy.

Targeted Therapy

Driver mutations have been detected in 50% of nonsquamous NSCLCs, including *KRAS, EGFR, ALK, BRAF, HER2, ROS1, RET, PIK3CA, MET, NRAS, MEK1, AKT1, FGFR1, DDR2,* and *NTRK.* Targeted therapy has FDA approval for patients with *EGFR* mutations, *ALK* rearrangements, *ROS1* rearrangements, *NTRK1* rearrangements, *BRAF* mutations, *KRAS* mutations, *RET* rearrangements, and *MET* exon 14 skipping mutations (Figure 5). In patients who harbor a mutation and are also strongly PD-L1 positive, the presence of the mutation should drive selection of therapy (see Figure 3).

EGFR mutations have been reported in approximately 15% of North American patients with metastatic nonsquamous NSCLC, of which 90% are exon 19 deletions or exon 21 *L858R* point mutations. First- and second-generation *EGFR* tyrosine kinase inhibitors (TKIs) erlotinib (Tarceva), gefitinib (Iressa), and afatinib (Gilotrif) are approved as first-line therapy based on clinical trials demonstrating superior response rates, progression-free survival, and overall survival compared with chemotherapy in treatment-naive patients with *EGFR* mutation–positive NSCLC. Despite the observed survival benefits, most patients eventually develop therapeutic resistance. Furthermore, approximately 50% of patients who develop acquired resistance to *EGFR* TKI

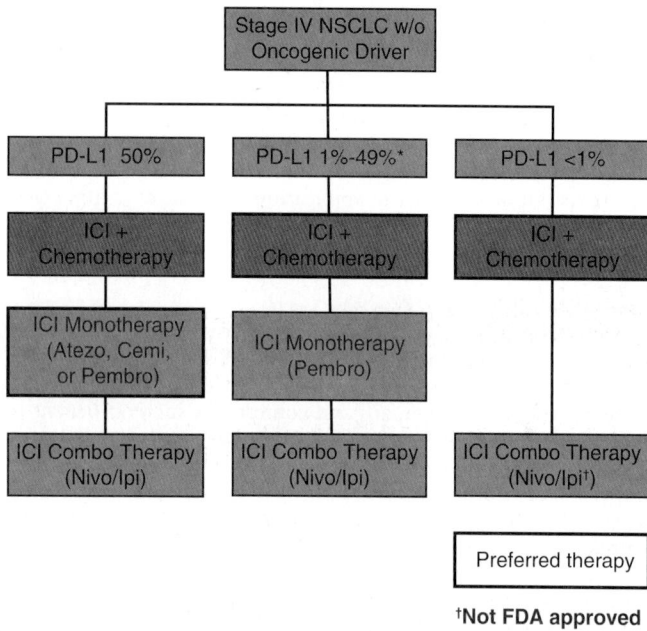

Figure 4 Algorithm for programmed death-ligand 1 *(PD-L1)* testing. *ICI,* Immune checkpoint inhibitor; *NSCLC,* non–small cell lung cancer.

[1]Not FDA approved for this indication.

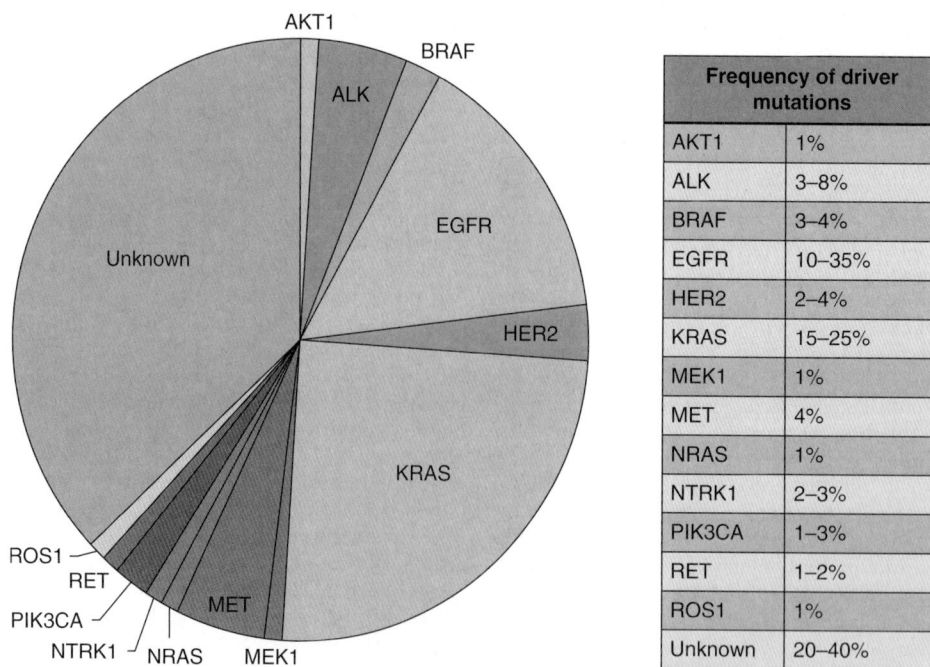

Frequency of driver mutations	
AKT1	1%
ALK	3–8%
BRAF	3–4%
EGFR	10–35%
HER2	2–4%
KRAS	15–25%
MEK1	1%
MET	4%
NRAS	1%
NTRK1	2–3%
PIK3CA	1–3%
RET	1–2%
ROS1	1%
Unknown	20–40%

Figure 5 Molecular mutations in nonsquamous, non–small cell lung cancer.

therapy acquire a second site mutation occurring within exon 20 (i.e., *T790M*). Consequently, osimertinib (Tagrisso), a third-generation mutant-specific *EGFR* inhibitor that irreversibly binds to the kinase domain of *EGFR*, was recently approved for patients with *T790M* mutations who have acquired resistance to first- and second-generation *EGFR* inhibitors. Osimertinib was also demonstrated in the FLAURA trial to have improved progression-free survival compared with the first-generation inhibitors erlotinib and gefitinib in patients with treatment-naive *EGFR* mutation–positive NSCLC, establishing osimertinib as the preferred first-line option for this cohort of patients.

Osimertinib (Tagrisso) in combination with chemotherapy has also been studied in the first-line treatment for EGFR-positive NSCLC compared with osimertinib alone. At 24 months, 57% of patients in the chemotherapy plus osimertinib compared with 41% of patients in the osimertinib group were alive and progression free. However, adverse events were much higher in the chemotherapy plus osimertinib group versus the osimertinib alone group, with grade 3 or higher adverse events occurring in 32% and 9% of patients, respectively. Overall survival data is immature, and osimertinib monotherapy remains the preferred treatment in these patients.

Another option for patients who have traditional EGFR mutations is lazertinib (Lazcluze) plus amivantamab (Rybrevant). This combination was studied in the MARIPOSA trial against osimertinib (Tagrisso), which showed an improvement in overall survival. At 36 months 60% of patients were alive in the lazertinib plus amivantamab group compared to 51% in the osimertinib group. It is important to note that the lazertinib plus amivantimab regimen is cumbersome on the patients. They have to come in every 2 weeks for the infusion, as well as take a large amount of supportive care medications to prevent EGFR skin toxicities and VTEs. In the lazertinib plus amivantamab group, 10% of patients discontinued treatment due to adverse effects compared to 3% in the osimertinib group.

Traditionally, patients with EGFR exon 20 insertion mutations have not had an option for targeted therapy because of the inherent resistance of EGFR exon 20 insertion mutations to traditional EGFR inhibitors. Amivantamab (Rybrevant) is a bispecific EGFR-MET antibody that engages both EGFR and MET pathways. This is approved in patients with EGFR exon 20 insertion mutations in the first-line setting based on a phase III PAPILLON trial that showed a progression-free survival of 31% of patients in the amivantamab plus chemotherapy arm and 3% of patients in the chemotherapy alone group at 18 months. Amivantamab was well tolerated, with the most common adverse events being infusion-related reactions and paronychia. Incidence of infusion-related reactions decreased after the first dose of amivantamab. Amivantamab is also approved in the second-line or later setting as monotherapy in patients with EGFR exon 20 insertion–positive NSCLC who have not previously received in the first-line setting.

ALK-positive NSCLC accounts for approximately 3% to 7% of patients diagnosed with NSCLC. Crizotinib (Xalkori) was the initial *ALK* TKI to gain accelerated approval by the FDA in 2011 after two open-label, randomized phase III trials demonstrated improved progression-free survival with crizotinib compared with chemotherapy in both first- and second-line settings. Ceritinib (Zykadia) is also approved as a first-line therapy option, demonstrating superior progression-free survival compared with chemotherapy in patients with *ALK*-positive NSCLC. More recently, alectinib (Alecensa), brigatinib (Alunbrig), and lorlatinib (Lorbrena) have demonstrated superior progression-free survival and central nervous system control when compared with crizotinib (Xalkori) and are all preferred first-line treatment options for first-line therapy for *ALK* positive NSCLC. Lorlatinib (Lorbrena) is also approved in patients who have progressed on a prior *ALK* inhibitor and is particularly effective in patients who develop a G1202R mutation as a mechanism of resistance to *ALK* inhibitor therapy.

ROS1 rearrangements occur in approximately 1% to 2% of NSCLC. Crizotinib (Xalkori), entrectinib (Rozlytrek), and repotrectinib (Augtyro) are the preferred first-line therapy for patients with *ROS1*-positive NSCLC. Ceritinib (Zykadia)[1] and lorlatinib (Lorbrena)[1] have also been shown to be active in this cohort of patients.

BRAF mutations occur in approximately 2% to 3% of patients with NSCLC, and more than 50% of these are *BRAF* V600E mutations. Dabrafenib (Tafinlar) and vemurafenib (Zelboraf)[1] have demonstrated promising results in phase II trials. However, impressive phase II trial results with BRAF inhibitor dabrafenib in combination with the MEK inhibitor trametinib (Mekinist) and BRAF inhibitor encorafenib (Braftovi) plus MEK inhibitor binimetinib (Mektovi) established this combination treatment as the preferred treatment options for patients with BRAF V600E–positive NSCLC.

NTRK rearrangements have been reported in 1% of patients with NSCLC. Larotrectinib (Vitrakvi), entrectinib (Rozlytrek), and repotrectinib (Augtyro) are the preferred treatment options in patients with NTRK-positive stage IV NSCLC.

Around 4% of patients with NSCLC have tumors that harbor a *MET* exon 14 skipping mutation. Tepotinib (Tepmetko) and capmatinib (Tabrecta) both received FDA approval based on phase II studies showing response rates of over 40% in these patients. Peripheral edema was the most common adverse event for both agents. Crizotinib (Xalkori)[1] has also shown benefit in this patient population; however, it does not have central nervous system (CNS) penetration compared with the newer MET inhibitors.

Two agents, selpercatinib (Retevmo) and pralsetinib (Gavreto), have received FDA approval for patients with NSCLC with *RET* translocations. *RET* translocations occur in up to 2% of patients with NSCLC. Approval for these agents was based on phase I/II trials that showed response rates of over 60%. The most common adverse events in both trials were hypertension and myelosuppression. Although interstitial lung disease can occur with both agents, there is a greater risk with pralsetinib (Gavreto) compared with selpercatinib (Retevmo). Of note, these agents also target VEGF and can cause delayed wound healing, so they should be held in patients undergoing surgical procedures.

Second-Line Therapy and Beyond

Second-line therapy for advanced NSCLC was almost never recommended until a seminal study in 2000 showed that docetaxel (Taxotere) improved survival compared with supportive care alone. Over a decade later, docetaxel and ramucirumab (Cyramza) received FDA approval after a phase III trial found the combination to impart a modest improvement in response rate, overall survival, and progression-free survival compared with docetaxel alone. More recently, nivolumab (OPDIVO) and atezolizumab (Tecentriq) received FDA approval in patients who progress on platinum-based chemotherapy, and pembrolizumab (Keytruda) is also approved in patients with tumors that are PD-L1 ≥1%. It should be noted that patients who progress on a first-line TKI or pembrolizumab should be considered for a platinum-based doublet as their second-line therapy, not single-agent docetaxel or docetaxel plus ramucirumab.

The *KRAS* mutation, which occurs in 15% to 25% of patients, has long been an undruggable target in NSCLC. However, sotorasib (Lumakras) is a GTPase inhibitor that is now approved in patients with NSCLC with *KRAS* G12C mutations who have progressed on platinum-based therapy. Approval was based on a phase II trial showing benefit in these patients. Treatment was well tolerated, and the most common adverse events were nausea, fatigue, and increased liver enzymes. Sotorasib (Lumakras) cannot be used in patients with other *KRAS* mutations. Studies of other *KRAS* inhibitors are ongoing for patients with non-G12C mutations. A second KRAS G12C inhibitor, adagrasib (Krazati), has also been FDA approved based on a phase II trial for patient with KRAS G12C mutated NSCLC in the second-line setting. Similar to sotorasib (Lumakras), the most common adverse events

---

[1] Not FDA approved for this indication.

with adagrasib (Krazati) were nausea, diarrhea, and increased liver enzymes. The role of sotorasib (Lumakras) and adagrasib (Krazati) in patients with NSCLC with *KRAS* G12C mutations in the first-line setting is currently unknown.

HER2 mutations occur in 2% to 4% of NSCLC patients. Fam-trastuzumab deruxtecan (Enhertu) is an antibody drug conjugate that is approved in the second-line or later setting in NSCLC patients with HER2 mutations based on phase II trials.

Oligometastatic Disease

The concept of oligometastatic disease (single-site metastatic disease) was first proposed in 1995. Studies at this time described patients with disease in the adrenal gland or brain as actually having a relatively favorable prognosis. For these lesions, the standard of care includes surgical resection of both the primary tumor and the metastasis if they present synchronously or resection of the recurrence. Generally, when the primary tumor and metastatic disease are identified at the same time, the metastatic site is treated first. If this cannot be successfully addressed, there is no benefit to resecting the primary tumor.

Treatment for Small Cell Lung Cancer

SCLC, which accounts for 15% to 20% of new lung cancer cases, is an aggressive disease characterized by rapid growth and early widespread metastasis. The primary etiologic agent responsible for SCLC is tobacco smoke. The aggressive nature of SCLC is underscored by its high mutational burden, including loss of expression of the tumor suppressor genes *p53* in 70% to 80% and retinoblastoma in almost 100% of tumors. Although there is a shift in recommendations for the staging of SCLC, most patients are still diagnosed using the traditional staging system of limited-stage disease (LD) and extensive-stage disease (ED). At the time of diagnosis, approximately 30% of patients have *limited-stage disease* (LD-SCLC), defined as tumors confined to the hemithorax that can be encompassed in a tolerable radiation port, whereas about 70% of patients have *extensive-stage disease* (ED-SCLC), defined as the presence of overt metastatic disease by imaging or physical examination. Regardless of stage at diagnosis, most patients relapse and develop chemotherapy-resistant disease, with a median survival of 12 to 20 months for patients with LD and 7 to 11 months for patients with ED; only 6% to 12% of patients with LD-SCLC and 2% of patients with ED-SCLC live beyond 5 years.

In patients with LD-SCLC, treatment with concurrent chemotherapy and radiation, followed by 2 years of durvalumab (Imfinzi) is the preferred treatment based on the phase III ADRI-ATIC trial, which showed improved progression-free survival and overall survival compared with chemotherapy alone. For decades, first-line therapy for ED-SCLC consisted of four to six cycles of platinum-based chemotherapy with either cisplatin[1] or carboplatin (Paraplatin)[1] plus either etoposide (Toposar) or irinotecan (Camptosar)[1] followed by observation. A recent phase III trial in patients with advanced-stage disease demonstrated superior survival when atezolizumab (Tecentriq) was combined with carboplatin and etoposide for four cycles followed by maintenance atezolizumab compared with carboplatin and etoposide alone, making combination chemotherapy with a checkpoint inhibitor a new treatment option for patients with this disease. Similar results were seen with durvalumab (Imfinzi) in combination with a platinum agent and etoposide and is another option for patients in the first-line setting.

Although up to 80% of patients will respond to first-line chemotherapy, most will eventually relapse. Topotecan (Hycamtin), lurbinectedin (Zepzelca), and tarlatamab (Imdelltra) are the only agents approved for second-line therapy. Additionally, patients who relapse >6 months after first-line therapy can repeat their original platinum-based treatment. Nivolumab (Opdivo)[1] or pembrolizumab (Keytruda)[1] can be used in the third-line setting but only in patients who have not received an immune checkpoint inhibitor in the first-line setting.

Radiation therapy is also an important component in the therapeutic armamentarium for patients with SCLC. Patients with LD are generally treated with concurrent chemoradiotherapy with four cycles of chemotherapy and radiation added to either cycle one or cycle two of therapy. For patients who are not candidates for concurrent chemoradiotherapy, sequential therapy can be considered with radiation after chemotherapy. Prophylactic cranial irradiation (PCI) should be considered in patients who have responded well to initial therapy. In patients with ED, thoracic radiation can be considered, although it has not been shown to improve overall survival. Similarly, a large phase III trial in patients without brain metastases following chemotherapy demonstrated no improvement in overall survival for patients treated with PCI compared with observation. Long-term toxicities, including deficits in cognition, have been reported after PCI, and for many patients observation with an MRI every 3 months has been adopted as the standard of care.

Surgery has for many decades played a very limited role in the treatment of SCLC because of its propensity to metastasize. The pendulum is beginning to shift for early-stage, node-negative SCLC. More contemporary studies have demonstrated that surgery may play a beneficial role in a select group of patients.

Invasive mediastinal staging should be performed for patients without evidence of metastatic disease. In node-negative patients with T1 and T2 tumors, a lobectomy followed by adjuvant chemotherapy should be offered to medically fit patients. The 5-year survival rate in this group of patients is 40% to 50%.

Monitoring

Routine disease monitoring is important both after curative treatment and during treatment for incurable disease.

Non–Small Cell Lung Cancer

The National Comprehensive Cancer Network guidelines have clear recommendations for the follow-up of NSCLC and SCLC divided by stage, and these are summarized here.

After completion of curative therapy for stages I and II, a history and physical examination along with a chest CT (+/–) with contrast every 6 months for the first 2 to 3 years should be performed. If after 2 to 3 years there are no findings that would require alternative monitoring, the patient can be transitioned to annual history, physical examination, and noncontrast LDCT scan of the chest.

Patients with stages I and II who were treated with radiation rather than surgery should be followed by a slightly more aggressive regimen. Patients should have a history and physical examination along with a chest CT (+/–) with contrast every 3 to 6 months for the first 3 years and then every 6 months for the next 2 years. At that time, if there are no findings that would require alternative monitoring, the patient can be transitioned to annual history, physical examination, and a noncontrast LDCT scan of the chest.

Patients with stages III and IV oligometastatic disease should likewise be followed with a history and physical examination along with a chest CT (+/–) with contrast every 3 to 6 months for the first 3 years and then every 6 months for the next 2 years. If there are no findings that would require alternative monitoring, the patient can be transitioned to annual history, physical examination, and a noncontrast LDCT scan of the chest.

Any residual or new radiographic abnormalities will require consideration of more frequent imaging. Please note that PET-CT and brain MRI are not routinely indicated as part of surveillance; however, they should be tailored to each patient and their primary sites of disease.

Symptoms of shortness of breath, cough, wheezing, new bone pain, headache, or constitutional symptoms should prompt immediate evaluation with imaging to rule out disease recurrence, and the patient's primary oncologist should be contacted.

---

[1] Not FDA approved for this indication.

While patients are being treated with palliative systemic therapy, scans are routinely obtained every 6 to 8 weeks while on chemotherapy or every 8 to 9 weeks while on immunotherapy.

Small Cell Lung Cancer

SCLC has a distinct follow-up recommendation. Patients who were diagnosed and treated for limited-stage disease should have follow-up with a history and physical examination along with CT scan of the chest/abdomen every 3 months for the first year and every 6 months for the subsequent 2 years. At that time, patients may transition to annual examinations and imaging. MRI scans of the brain are essential as well and are recommended every 3 to 4 months for the first year and every 6 months for the second year.

Patients with extensive-stage disease will require more frequent follow-up examinations. A history and physical examination with CT scans of the chest/abdomen should occur every 2 months for the first year, every 3 to 4 months for the second and third years, every 6 months for the fourth and fifth years, and then annually. Monitoring of the brain is the same as for limited-stage disease, with MRI of the brain recommended every 3 to 4 months for the first year and every 6 months for the second year.

Any patient, regardless of type of cancer, should have a survivorship plan created as part of their follow-up. These plans apply to survivors across the continuum of care. This comprehensive, individualized plan includes the aforementioned cancer-specific follow-up but also highlights important nutritional considerations, physical activity, and immunizations. Patients should be encouraged to continue routine screening for other malignancies and routine health maintenance. Ongoing smoking cessation should be encouraged.

Summary

The treatment of cancers is rapidly changing with the advent of immunotherapy, targeted therapy, localized radiation treatments, and minimally invasive surgical approaches. The intricacies of treatment, now more than ever before, demand a multidisciplinary approach to ensure that patients are provided with the best possible care to optimize both their quantity and quality of life.

References

Antonia SJ, Villegas A, Daniel D, et al: Durvalumab after chemoradiotherapy in stage III non-small-cell lung cancer, *N Engl J Med* 377(20):1919–1929, 2017.

Altorki N, Wang X, Kozono D, Watt C, et al: Lobar or sublobar resection for peripheral stage IA non-small-cell lung cancer, *N Engl J Med* 388(6):489–498, 2023.

Altorki NK, wang X, Wigle D, Gu L, et al: Perioperative mortality and morbidity after sublobar versus lobar resection for early-stage non-small-cell lung cancer: post-hoc analysis of an international, randomised, phase 3 trial (CALGB/Alliance 140503), *Lancet Respir Med* 6(12):915–924, 2018.

Deutsch M, Crawford J, Leopold K, et al: Phase II study of neoadjuvant chemotherapy and radiation therapy with thoracotomy in the treatment of clinically staged IIIA non-small cell lung cancer, *Cancer* 74:1243–1252, 1994.

Gaissert HA, Ferenandez FG, Crabtree T, et al: The Society of Thoracic Surgeons general thoracic surgery database: 2017 update on research, *Ann Thorac Surg* 104(5):1450–1455, 2017.

Gandhi L, Rodrigues Abreu D, Gadgeel S, et al: (Keynote-189). Pembrolizubman plus chemotherapy in metastatic non-small cell lung cancer, *NEJM* 327:2078–2092, 2018.

Horn L, Mansfield AS, Szczęsna A, et al: IMpower133 Study Group: first-line atezolizumab plus chemotherapy in extensive-stage small-cell lung cancer, *N Engl J Med* 379(23):2220–2229, 2018.

Paz-Ares L, Luft A, Vincente D, et al: (Keynote-407). Pembrolizumab plus chemotherapy for squamous non-small cell lung cancer, *NEJM* 379:2040–2051, 2018.

Peters S, Camidge RC, Shaw AT, et al: Alectinib versus crizotinib in untreated alk-positive non–small-cell lung cancer, *N Engl J Med* 377:829–838, 2017.

Reck M, Rodriguez-Abreu D, Robinson AG, et al: Pembrolizumab versus chemotherapy for PD-L1-positive non-small-cell lung cancer, *N Engl J Med* 375(19):1823–1833, 2016.

Soria JC, Ohe Y, Vansteenkiste J, et al: Osimertinib in untreated EGFR-mutated advanced non-small-cell lung cancer, *N Engl J Med* 378:113–125, 2018.

Spyratos D, Zaragoulidis P, Porpodis K, et al: Preoperative evaluation for lung cancer resection, *J Thorac Dis* 6(Supp1):S162–S166, 2014.

The National Lung Screening Trial Research Team: Reduced lung-cancer mortality with low-dose computed tomographic screening, *NEJM* 365:395–409, 2011.

Vyfhuis MAL, Bhooshan N, Burrows WM, et al: Oncological outcomes from trimodality therapy receiving definitive doses of neoadjuvant chemoradiation (≥60 Gy) and factors influencing consideration for surgery in stage III non-small cell lung cancer, *Adv Radiat Oncol* 2(3):259–269, 2017.

OBSTRUCTIVE SLEEP APNEA

Method of
Daniel Gorelik, MD; and Masayoshi Takashima, MD

CURRENT DIAGNOSIS

Symptoms
- Excessive daytime fatigue and somnolence
- Morning headaches
- Loud snoring and gasping for air
- Witnessed apneic episodes following loud snoring
- Frequent nocturia with no other underlying etiology
- Hypertension

Clinical Signs and Risk Factors
- Central obesity with body mass index (BMI) >30 kg/m^2
- Large neck circumference (>17 inches in men; >16 inches in women)
- Being male or a postmenopausal female
- Use of sedatives or alcohol before going to bed
- Family history of sleep apnea
- Craniofacial abnormalities: retrognathia, micrognathia, congenital malformations

CURRENT THERAPY

- Gold standard for treatment is positive airway pressure
- Weight loss, smoking cessation, avoidance of sedatives
- Improvement of sleep hygiene and sleep schedule
- Minimally invasive procedures (i.e., oral appliances, palatal stents, radiofrequency turbinate reductions) may be beneficial for a select patient population
- Surgical therapy is usually reserved for patients not tolerating or unable to use CPAP or BiPAP
- Implants for muscle stimulation
- Initial procedures are focused on decreasing upper airway resistance to improve compliance with CPAP or BiPAP
- Identification of anatomic sites of obstruction is critical to successful surgical outcomes

BiPAP, Bilevel positive airway pressure; *CPAP,* continuous positive airway pressure.

Sleep-disordered breathing encompasses the spectrum from upper airway resistance syndrome to obstructive sleep apnea (OSA). OSA is characterized by episodes of partial or complete upper airway collapse leading to cessation or reduction of airflow. Such events lead to oxygen desaturation and sleep fragmentation, causing excessive daytime sleepiness, morning headaches, depression, memory loss, impaired alertness, decreased libido, and reduced cognitive function. Nighttime symptoms are often more telling, and obtaining a sleep history from a bed partner is exceptionally helpful. The most common symptoms include loud snoring, restless sleep, choking or gasping episodes, and frequent awakening from sleep. Nocturnal perspiration, nocturia, and symptoms of nocturnal gastroesophageal reflux are also commonly associated with severe OSA.

As the severity of OSA typically increases with age, nightly hypoventilation and activation of the sympathetic nervous system lead to pathophysiologic derangements, such as hypertension, ischemic heart disease, myocardial infarction, stroke, arrhythmia, and premature death. An apnea-hypopnea index (AHI) of greater than 5 has been shown to be associated with increased risk of cerebrovascular accident. An AHI greater than 20 is associated with increased mortality. Patients with oxygen desaturation below 90% have an elevated incidence of cardiac arrhythmia.

BOX 1 Definitions of Sleep Medicine Terms

Apnea-hypopnea index (AHI): Sum of apneas and hypopneas per hour of sleep.

Obstructive apnea: Cessation of airflow for ≥10 s associated with ongoing ventilatory effort.

Obstructive hypopnea: (1) Decreased airflow by ≥30% which is ≥10 s and a ≥3% oxygen desaturation and/or associated with an arousal. (2) Decreased airflow ≥30% which is ≥10 s which is associated with a ≥4% oxygen desaturation

Obstructive sleep apnea (OSA): AHI >5 events per hour of sleep, often associated with oxygen desaturation <90%. Mild OSA is defined by an AHI of 5–15. Moderate OSA is an AHI 15–30, and severe OSA is an AHI >30.

Obstructive sleep apnea syndrome: OSA in association with daytime symptoms of excessive sleepiness or other neurobehavioral symptoms.

Primary snoring: Snoring with an AHI <5 and no complaints of excessive daytime sleepiness.

Respiratory effort–related arousals: Sleep fragmentation that is caused by arousals from increasing respiratory effort but that does not meet criteria for an apnea or hypopnea. The event lasts longer than 10 s.

Respiratory disturbance index: Sum of apneas, hypopneas, and respiratory effort–related arousals per hour of sleep.

Upper airway resistance syndrome (UARS): Snoring in association with AHI <5, frequent arousals, and abnormally negative midesophageal pressure (<−10 cm H_2O) or increased diaphragmatic electromyogram activity.

These potentially severe consequences, along with a patient's decreased quality of life, substantiate the need for early recognition and treatment.

Definitions of terms related to sleep apnea are listed in Box 1.

Epidemiology

On the basis of available population-based studies, the prevalence of OSA among adults between 30 and 60 years of age is estimated to be 6% for women and 13% for men. This represents relative increases over the last two decades of 14% to 55% among subgroups divided by age, gender, and body mass index (BMI). OSA remains undiagnosed in 70% to 80% of patients because their symptoms are often vague, and OSA must be diagnosed with polysomnography.

Risk Factors

When controlling for gender and BMI, patients over age 50 have an increased prevalence of OSA secondary to decreased muscle tone.

Obesity (BMI >30 kg/m^2) is a risk factor for OSA. A 10% increase in weight is associated with a sixfold increase in risk for development of OSA, and a 10% weight loss is associated with a 26% decrease in AHI. Patients undergoing bariatric surgery on average have postsurgical reductions in AHI of 29 events per hour. There is evidence of a potential link between OSA and insulin resistance.

Approximately 30% of hypertensive persons have OSA and up to 50% of OSA patients have hypertension. Resistant hypertension, which is defined as blood pressure greater than 140/90 mmHg despite therapy with at least three different antihypertensive classes, is especially prevalent in the OSA population. It is estimated that 90% of male patients and 77% of female patients with resistant hypertension have OSA. A dose-effect relationship between OSA severity and severity of hypertension has been established. Mechanisms for hypertension center around hypoxemia and hypercapnia leading to increased oxidative stress, decreased nitric oxide secretion, and increased catecholamine, angiotensin II, aldosterone, renin, and endothelin-1 secretion.

Male patients are nearly twice as likely to have OSA as female patients. Estrogen and progesterone might play a protective role because population-based studies have demonstrated that postmenopausal women have a two- to threefold increased risk of OSA compared to premenopausal women.

African Americans and Asians are at greater risk for OSA than Caucasians. Being African American is an independent risk factor for severe sleep-disordered breathing, with an odds ratio of 2.55 compared with Caucasians. Asians have a narrower cranial base, a higher Mallampati score, smaller thyromental distance, and steeper thyromental plane than Caucasians, which might account for their increased risk.

Pathophysiology

Airway obstruction leading to OSA can occur anywhere along the pathway from the nostrils, soft palate, base of tongue, hypopharynx, and the epiglottis. The airway lacks skeletal structure and is vulnerable to influences, such as muscle tone, fat deposition, and tissue redundancy.

Prevention

Lifestyle modification can prevent OSA. Patients should adopt a healthy and athletic lifestyle to develop good muscle tone and weight loss, avoid sedatives and alcohol at bedtime, establish regular sleeping patterns, avoid the supine sleeping position, and elevate the head when sleeping.

Diagnosis

Definitive diagnosis of OSA is made by polysomnography. Mild OSA is defined as an AHI of 5 to 15 per hour; moderate OSA is an AHI of 15 to 30 per hour; and severe OSA is an AHI greater than 30 per hour. There are several types of polysomnograms patients can obtain, ranging from Level 1 to 3. Level 1 sleep studies are performed in a sleep laboratory with a technician in attendance. It assesses at least seven channels of data (but usually 16+), including respiratory, cardiovascular, and neurological parameters. Level 1 sleep studies have long been the gold standard of diagnoses of sleep-disordered breathing and other sleep disorders. Patients spend the night in a sleep laboratory during which multiple physiologic variables are continuously monitored. These include electroencephalogram (EEG), electrooculogram (EOG), electromyogram (EMG), oronasal airflow, chest wall effort, body position, snore volume, electrocardiogram (ECG), and oxyhemoglobin saturation. Laboratory testing also includes a complete accounting of sleep variables, monitoring of cardiac rhythm, and assessment of possible restless legs syndrome (RLS) or periodic limb movements (PLMs) during sleep. This information enables the clinician to determine the severity of the condition and identifies potentially relevant comorbidities.

Level 2 sleep studies use the same equipment as Level 1 but do not have a technician in attendance. These are rarely offered or ordered. In recent years, Level 3 sleep studies have grown in popularity. These tests use portable monitors that allow sleep studies to be performed in a patient's home. Level 3 studies only measure three channels of data: oximetry, airflow, and respiratory effort. A thorough diagnostic study requires at least 6 hours of sleep, allowing assessment of variability related to sleep stages.

If there are sufficient apneas or hypopneas during the first half of the study (ideally 4 hours of diagnostic testing, with a minimum of 2 hours if an AHI >40 is confirmed), a split-night study may be performed, in which the second half of the night (minimum of 3 hours of sleep) is devoted to titration of continuous positive airway pressure (CPAP) therapy. If the criteria for a split-night sleep study are not achieved during the night, a second night for titration study is ordered. The split-night protocol is a cost-effective use of laboratory resources that is particularly well suited for patients with severe OSA.

A meta-analysis comparing Level 1 and 3 studies showed that Level 3 portable sleep studies displayed good diagnostic performance compared to Level 1 in-lab sleep studies in adult patients with high pre-test probability of moderate or severe OSA, and no unstable comorbidities. For patients suspected to have other types of sleep disorders, a Level 1 sleep study remains the gold standard.

According to the Institute for Clinical Systems Improvement (ICSI), polysomnography should be performed in patients with symptoms of OSA and one or more of the following: cardiovascular disease, hypertension, coronary artery disease, obesity, sleep complaints, type 2 diabetes mellitus, recurrent atrial fibrillation, and large neck circumference.

Treatment

Initially, patients should be counseled to avoid practices that can potentially worsen the severity of OSA. CNS depressants taken before sleep (alcohol, sleep medications, pain medications) can worsen upper airway collapse during sleep and should be discouraged. Weight loss and maintenance should always play a role in the treatment of these patients. Bariatric surgery may be an option for patients with obesity and comorbid OSA. Systematic reviews have shown a reduction of AHI and subjective improvement in these patients; however, it is important to note that OSA usually does not resolve following bariatric surgery. Myofunctional therapy, which is a series of isometric and isotonic exercises of the oral cavity and pharyngeal muscles, is designed to increase upper airway tone. Oral pressure therapy uses a mouthpiece to generate negative pressure to gently pull the palate forward, opening the retropalatal airway. End positive airway pressure (EPAP) therapy uses nasal appliances to increase expiratory resistance and prevent pharyngeal collapse.

In patients with positional OSA, defined as greater than a two-fold difference in AHI between supine and nonsupine positions, avoiding the supine position during sleep may suffice to normalize ventilation during sleep. There are several commercial devices worn around the neck or back that gently vibrate when a patient is supine. Nightly compliance rates are 75% to 96%.

Continuous Positive Airway Pressure Therapy

CPAP remains the therapeutic mainstay for primary treatment of OSA. It serves as a pneumatic stent for the upper airway and is effective in reducing the physiologic abnormalities measured on polysomnography. Additionally, CPAP is thought to augment lung volumes and elicit a reflex that increases tone in the upper airway musculature. Overall, it has been shown to reduce AHI, improve quality of life, and reduce cardiovascular risk.

There are many manufacturers of CPAP devices and many interfaces that help maximize comfort with treatment. Expiratory pressure release (EPR) is available through several CPAP manufacturers. EPR does not seem to compromise the effectiveness of CPAP therapy and improves the patient's sense of comfort with therapy, but it does not seem to systematically improve the level of adherence. Automatically adjusting positive airway pressure (APAP) is similar to CPAP, but instead of delivering a constant pressure, APAP adjusts delivered pressure breath to breath.

Bilevel respiratory-assist devices deliver alternating levels of positive airway pressure and may be considered an alternative therapeutic option when standard CPAP is not tolerated or when oxygen saturation is not raised sufficiently with standard CPAP. In some cases of severe OSA (in particular among patients with underlying pulmonary conditions), supplemental oxygen can be used in conjunction with CPAP therapy.

The main disadvantage with positive airway pressure treatment is poor compliance. CPAP adherence rates—defined as at least 4 hours per night—70% of nights are between only 39% and 50% overall CPAP compliance. Treatment is effective as long as the patient uses the device for the entire night, every night. APAP, CPAP desensitization, and the use of integrated heated humidifiers helped improve adherence to therapy. Improving nasal resistance with allergy management or nasal surgery has also shown to decrease CPAP pressures and improve CPAP compliance.

Oral Appliances

Oral appliances worn in the mouth during sleep can help maintain a patent airway, especially in patients with significant positional sleep apnea who sleep supine and experience airway collapse secondary to the tongue falling posteriorly. In general, there are two types of appliances, mandibular-advancement appliances and tongue-retaining devices. The mandibular-advancement appliances are currently used more often and have been more widely studied. They require viable dentition for retention and they are fitted to the maxillary and mandibular dentition to enable the protrusion of the mandible, therefore increasing oropharyngeal patency. The most common side effect is drooling. Temporomandibular joint pain might limit the viability of this therapy, and chronic use of the appliance can result in a change of the dental occlusion. A dentist with expertise in sleep medicine should ideally implement and monitor this type of treatment.

Surgical Procedures

If patients are not tolerating CPAP and a significant upper airway anatomic obstruction is identified, surgery should be considered. A variety of procedures help stabilize the retropalatal region, and others are intended to stabilize the retrolingual airway (Box 2). Sleep surgery has been shown to be most effective when addressing multiple levels of obstruction. Procedures are often combined for maximum effectiveness, such as septoplasty, turbinate reduction, tonsillectomy, uvulopalatopharyngoplasty, and genial tubercle advancement. With the advent of transoral robotic surgery (TORS), surgeons are now able to access the posterior oropharynx, base of tongue, and hypopharynx more easily, and procedures to address these areas are more common.

It is challenging to predict which patients are likely to have a successful surgical outcome. Much of this difficulty is associated with accurately identifying the site(s) of obstruction. The current gold standard is drug-induced sleep endoscopy (DISE), a procedure that examines the upper airway while the patient is in a drug-induced (propofol [Diprivan][1] or dexmedetomidine [Precedex]), sleep-resembling state. As the patient snores and obstructs, a flexible fiberoptic scope is passed through the nose to evaluate the upper airway for the site of obstruction. The advantage of a DISE in comparison to assessing the airway while awake is it can more naturally evaluate sites of obstruction during sleep. DISE has shown to alter surgical treatment plans in

---

| **BOX 2** | Treatments for Obstructive Sleep Apnea |

Nasal Obstruction
Septoplasty
Rhinoplasty or nasal valve surgery
Turbinate reduction
Adenoidectomy

Retropalatal Obstruction
Tonsillectomy
Uvulopalatopharyngoplasty
Z-palatoplasty
Lateral pharyngoplasty
Palatal stents
Radiofrequency soft palate surgery

Retrolingual Obstruction
Transoral robotic-assisted base of tongue reduction
Lingual tonsillectomy
Genioglossus advancement
Hyoid suspension
Tongue base suspension
Upper airway stimulation device (hypoglossal nerve stimulator)
Maxillomandibular advancement

50% of OSA patients. The VOTE system is the most commonly used scoring system that evaluates the four major anatomical areas for potential obstruction, including the velum (palate), oropharyngeal walls (lateral), tongue, and epiglottis. Both the extent and configuration of collapse are noted. Although there is no clear consensus that DISE improves surgical outcomes for sleep surgery, there are retrospective studies that have shown benefit. Patients with anterior-posterior palatal collapse on DISE compared to concentric collapse had better outcomes following UPPP. Another study found DISE helped identify patients with significant oropharyngeal lateral wall collapse and complete base of tongue obstruction. These features were inversely correlated with surgical success.

In recent years, the development of new implantable devices that allow for upper airway stimulation has offered a new solution for patients with specific anterior-posterior collapse of the upper airway. The upper airway stimulation device monitors respiratory patterns and stimulates primarily tongue muscles to protrude during inspiration, relieving OSA.

A substantially more invasive procedure, the maxillomandibular advancement, has been shown to be very effective in a number of case series. However, the only definitive surgical cure is tracheostomy, which completely bypasses the upper airway but is not without its comorbidities.

Monitoring

The patient's response to therapy needs to be monitored. In the case of CPAP therapy, monitoring of CPAP adherence is critical, because subjective reports are inaccurate. Resolution of excessive sleepiness is the desired outcome for patients who are symptomatic at baseline. If excessive sleepiness remains problematic despite documentation of desirable CPAP adherence, treatment with modafinil (Provigil) 100 to 400 mg in the morning might be considered. Other potential conditions affecting sleep need to be monitored and, if necessary, treated. Often, other conditions, such as poor sleep hygiene, RLS, PLMs, or psychophysiologic insomnia, interfere with adequate response to therapy.

For patients who undergo surgery, retesting is indicated. The interval at which retesting should be done depends on the type of surgery that was performed. Retesting 3 months following the surgical intervention is adequate in most cases.

References

Al Lawati NM, Patel SR, Ayas NT: Epidemiology, risk factors, and consequences of obstructive sleep apnea and short sleep duration, *Prog Cardiovasc Dis* 51:285–293, 2009.

Ancoli-Israel S, Klauber MR, Stepnowsky C, et al: Sleep-disordered breathing in African-American elderly, *Am J Respir Crit Care Med* 52:1946–1949, 1995.

Ashrafian H, Toma T, Rowland SP, et al: Bariatric surgery or non-surgical weight loss for obstructive sleep apnoea? A systematic review and comparison of meta-analysis, *Obes Surg* 25(7):1239–1250, 2015.

Cai A, Wang L, Zhou Y: Hypertension and obstructive sleep apnea, *Hypertens Res* 39:391–395, 2016.

Caples SM, Rowley JA, Prinsell JR, et al: Surgical modifications of the upper airway for obstructive sleep apnea in adults: a systematic review and meta-analysis, *Sleep* 33(10):1396–1407, 2010.

Chang JL, Goldberg AN, Alt JA, et al: International consensus statement on obstructive sleep apnea, *Int Forum Allergy Rhinol* 2023;13(7):1061–1482.

Dedhia RC, Strollo PJ, Soose RJ: Upper airway stimulation for obstructive sleep apnea: Past, present, and future, *Sleep* 38:899–906, 2015.

El Shayeb M, Topfer LA, Stafinski T: Diagnostic accuracy of level 3 portable sleep tests versus level 1 polysomnography for sleep-disordered breathing: a systematic review and meta-analysis, *CMAJ* 186(1):E25–E51, 2014. https://doi.org/10.1503/cmaj.130952.

Fujita S, Conway W, Zorick F, Roth T: Surgical correction of anatomic abnormalities in obstructive sleep apnea syndrome; Uvulopalatopharyngoplasty, *Otolaryngol Head Neck Surg* 89(6):923–934, 1981.

Heiser C, Steffen A, Boon M, et al: Post-approval upper airway stimulation predictors of treatment effectiveness in the ADHERE registry, *Eur Respir J* 53, 2019.

Hsin-Ching L, Friedman M, Hsueh-Wen C, et al: The efficacy of multilevel surgery of the upper airway in adults with obstructive sleep apnea/hypopnea syndrome, *The Laryngoscope* 118:902–908, 2008.

Institute for Clinical Systems Improvement (ICSI): *Diagnosis and Treatment of Obstructive Sleep Apnea in Adults*, Bloomington, MN, 2008, Institute for Clinical Systems Improvement.

Levendowski DJ, Seagraves S, Popovic D, Westbrook PR: Assessment of a neck-based treatment and monitoring device for positional obstructive sleep apnea, *J Clin Sleep Med* 10:863–871, 2014.

Li KK, Powell NB, Kushida C, et al: A comparison of Asian and white patients with obstructive sleep apnea syndrome, *Laryngoscope* 109:1937–1940, 1999.

Peppard PE, Young T, Palta M, et al: Longitudinal study of moderate weight change and sleep-disordered breathing, *JAMA* 284:3015–3021, 2000.

Peppard PE, Young T, Palta M, et al: Prospective study of the association between sleep-disordered breathing and hypertension, *N Engl J Med* 342:1378–1384, 2000.

Punjabi NM: The epidemiology of adult obstructive sleep apnea, *Proc Am Thorac Soc* 5:136–143, 2008.

Quan SF, Howard BV, Iber C, et al: The Sleep Heart Health Study: Design, rationale, and methods, *Sleep* 20:1077–1085, 1997.

Sher AE, Schechtman KB, Piccirillo JF: The efficacy of surgical modifications of the upper airway in adults with obstructive sleep apnea syndrome, *Sleep* 19(2):156–177, 1996.

Soares D, Sinawe H, Folbe AJ, et al: Lateral oropharyngeal wall and supraglottic airway collapse associated with failure in sleep apnea surgery, *Laryngoscope* 122:473–479, 2012.

Strollo PJ, Soose RJ, Maurer JT, et al: Upper-airway stimulation for obstructive sleep apnea., *N Engl J Med* 370:139–149, 2014.

Vilaseca I, Morello A, Montserrat JM, et al: Usefulness of uvulopalatopharyngoplasty with genioglossus and hyoid advancement in the treatment of obstructive sleep apnea, *Arch Otolaryngol Head Neck Surg* 128:435–440, 2002.

Wang Y, Sun C, Cui X, et al: The role of drug-induced sleep endoscopy: predicting and guiding upper airway surgery for adult OSA patients, *Sleep Breath* 22:478–482, 2018.

PLEURAL EFFUSION AND EMPYEMA

Method of
Marie Claire O'Dwyer, MBBCh, BAO, MPH; and Juana Nicoll Capizzano, MD

CURRENT DIAGNOSIS

- Asymmetric chest expansion and dullness to percussion have been reported to be the most accurate physical signs of a pleural effusion.
- Ultrasound (US) has higher diagnostic accuracy than chest radiograph (CXR) for diagnosis of pleural effusion and empyema.
- US is recommended to be performed routinely in addition to conventional CXR in the evaluation of pleural space infection, both for diagnostic purposes and for guidance of pleural space interventions.
- Point-of-care ultrasound (POCUS)-guided thoracentesis is the standard of care and improves safety and efficacy.
- Chest computed tomography (CT) should be obtained when pleural space infection is suspected.

CURRENT THERAPY

- Identify and treat the underlying causes of pleural effusion and empyema.
- Consider large-volume thoracentesis to assess symptomatic response and to determine potential benefit of definitive procedure.
- When a definitive procedure is needed to manage a malignant pleural effusion, decisions on whether an indwelling pleural catheter or a talc pleurodesis is preferred should take into account whether an effusion is loculated, whether the lung is fully expandable, and patient preferences.
- In cases of empyema chest tube placement, antibiotics with or without antifibrinolytics reduce the need for surgical drainage.

Pleural Anatomy

The pleura consists of two serous contiguous membranes: the visceral pleura, which covers the lungs and neurovascular structures, and the parietal pleura, which covers the chest wall. The visceral pleura is innervated by the autonomic nervous system and has no sensory innervation. The parietal pleura is innervated by sensory branches of the intercostal and phrenic nerves, hence irritation of the parietal pleura can cause pain. The space between the visceral and parietal pleura is known as the pleural cavity. In normal health the pleural cavity contains a small amount of serous fluid that plays an important role in lubrication and generates surface tension for optimal respiration. Alterations in health, either from acute illness (e.g., pneumonia, pulmonary embolism) or chronic conditions (e.g., heart failure, cirrhosis, nephrotic syndrome), can cause aberrations in pleural fluid homeostasis that lead to accumulation of fluid in the pleural space, known as a pleural effusion. Fluid is most likely to accumulate in areas or "recesses" where the lungs do not completely fill the pleural cavity. The costodiaphragmatic recess, where the costal and diaphragmatic parietal pleura meet, is the most common site of pleural effusion.

Clinical Presentation

There are many clinical presentations of pleural effusion. It may be an incidental finding on imaging performed for other reasons (e.g., a patient having a lung cancer screening with computed tomography [CT]). The size of the effusion does not always correlate with symptoms, and patients can be asymptomatic even with the presence of large pleural effusions. Symptomatic pleural effusions encompass a spectrum of mild to severe symptoms and may include shortness of breath at rest or on exertion, cough, pleuritic chest pain, and easy fatigability. A thorough history may also provide clues as to the underlying etiology of the effusion (e.g., symptoms of heart failure, chronic liver disease, pneumonia, or underlying malignancy).

Common clinical signs of a pleural effusion include reduced breath sounds, dullness to percussion, asymmetric chest expansion, reduced vocal resonance/tactile fremitus and egophony (an audible E to A change), and a pleural rub. Bronchial breath sounds may be auscultated above the level of the pleural effusion. Large pleural effusions may cause midline shift with the trachea deviated away from the side of the pleural effusion. The sensitivity and specificity of physical examination for detecting pleural effusions is limited. Asymmetric chest expansion and dullness to percussion have been reported to be the most accurate physical signs of a pleural effusion.

Imaging

Although traditionally chest radiograph has been the imaging of choice for diagnosis, ultrasound (US) has higher diagnostic accuracy for detecting pleural effusion. Bedside or *point-of-care ultrasound* (POCUS) is increasingly being incorporated into clinical practice. Importantly, the accuracy of POCUS for detecting pleural effusion is still high even when performed by physicians with limited POCUS training. Where available, POCUS can be considered first-line imaging rather than chest radiograph in the diagnosis of pleural effusion. *(See Image)*

Currently, chest x-ray is still performed as first-line imaging in the evaluation of respiratory symptoms in most centers, with POCUS being reserved for guiding thoracentesis. CT of the chest is typically also performed as part of the evaluation, unless the cause of the effusion is readily apparent clinically.

Etiology

Pleural effusion should be considered as a clinical presentation and not as a specific diagnosis. Just as there are many varied clinical presentations of pleural effusions, there are many varied underlying causes of pleural effusions. The most common four causes of pleural effusions in practice are pneumonia, cirrhosis, heart failure, and malignancy (Table 1).

Diagnosis

Management of a pleural effusion should be directed at treating the underlying cause of the effusion. A thorough history, physical examination, and directed workup (consider blood count and differential, electrolytes, hepatic function panel, lactate dehydrogenase [LDH], serum protein, cholesterol, and brain natriuretic peptide [BNP]) are recommended to assess for the underlying

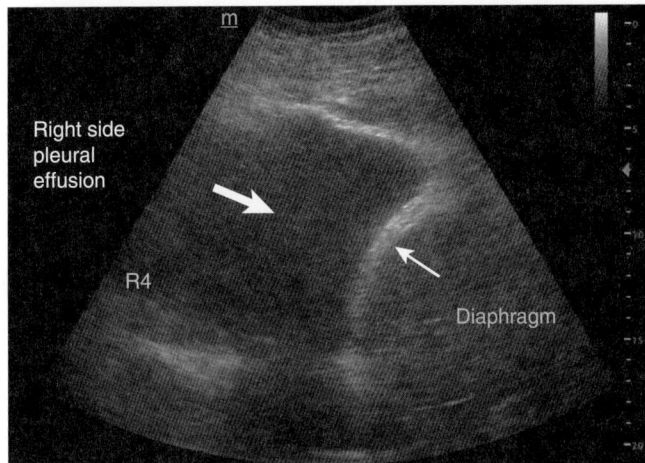

Figure 1 Ultrasound image of the lung shows moderate pleural effusion on the base of the right side. The *thin arrow* shows the diaphragm, and the *thick arrow* shows the anechoic area consistent with the effusion.

etiology of the effusion. In occasional cases where the clinical cause of the pleural effusion is readily apparent (e.g., post–coronary artery bypass graft [CABG] pleural effusion), a clinician may choose not to sample the pleural fluid. However, in most cases of pleural effusion, pleural fluid sampling is vital to determine the etiology and direct treatment.

Pleural Fluid Sampling

Pleural fluid sampling or thoracentesis is the diagnostic procedure of choice in the evaluation of a pleural effusion, performed using sterile procedural technique. US with sterile probe covers has dramatically improved the safety and success of thoracentesis and where available should be used to guide thoracentesis, particularly in the case of loculated effusions. Small-volume thoracentesis can be used for diagnostic purposes, whereas large-volume thoracentesis can provide additional symptom relief.

Examination of the pleural fluid includes inspecting the color, odor, and viscosity of the fluid at the bedside. The pleural fluid is then sent for laboratory analysis including biochemical (protein, LDH, pH, glucose), microbiologic (Gram stain and aerobic/anaerobic culture), and cytologic testing. It is of vital importance that the pleural fluid be handled correctly as deficiencies in this process can result in unreliable and inaccurate results. Ideally samples should be processed in the laboratory within 2 hours or refrigerated for no more than 48 hours. Cytologic analysis of pleural fluid for malignancy has a sensitivity of close to 60% for one sampling and rising to almost 75% after a second thoracentesis. In cases where two thoracentesis studies have yielded nondiagnostic results, guidelines recommend pursuing more invasive diagnostic testing, typically video-assisted thoracoscopic surgery (VATS) for pleural biopsies.

Pleural Manometry

Pleural fluid manometry is performed in some centers to measure pleural pressure, typically using a digital manometer attached to the thoracentesis needle. Although pleural manometry is not routine practice, it has potential utility in (1) detection of nonexpandable lung, (2) determination of likelihood of success of pleurodesis, and (3) minimizing risks of re-expansion pulmonary edema by stopping aspiration if pleural pressure drops by 15 mm Hg.

Light's Criteria

A seminal 1972 paper from Light and colleagues described an approach to interpreting pleural fluid analysis by classifying effusions as either transudates or exudates that is still relevant today. Using Light's criteria, an effusion is defined as exudative if any one or more of three criteria are met: a pleural fluid protein to serum protein ratio of greater than 0.5, a pleural fluid LDH to serum LDH ratio of greater than 0.6, and a pleural fluid LDH greater than two-thirds the upper limit of normal serum LDH concentration (see

TABLE 1	Light's Criteria		
CRITERIA		**EXUDATE**	**TRANSUDATE**
Pleural fluid protein to serum protein ratio		>0.5	≤0.5
Pleural fluid LDH to serum LDH ratio		>0.6	≤0.6
Pleural fluid LDH		Greater than two-thirds the upper limit of normal serum LDH	Less than or equal to two-thirds the upper limit of normal serum LDH

LDH, Lactate dehydrogenase.
Note exceptions do occur; for example, a patient with congestive heart failure on diuretics may have an exudative effusion.

TABLE 2	Causes of Pleural Effusions		
		EXUDATE	**TRANSUDATE**
Very common		Pneumonia	Congestive heart failure
Common		Malignancy Pulmonary embolism	Cirrhosis/hepatic hydrothorax
Uncommon		Post-CABG surgery Pancreatitis Viral pleuritis Drug-induced pleuritis Tuberculosis (varies by region)	Nephrotic syndrome Acute atelectasis Peritoneal dialysis Hypoalbuminemia
Rare		Esophageal rupture Chylothorax Systemic lupus erythematosus Rheumatoid pleuritis	Superior vena cava obstruction Constrictive pericarditis Myxedema

CABG, Coronary artery bypass graft.
Adapted from Karkhanis VS, Joshi JM: Pleural effusion: diagnosis, treatment, and management. *Open Access Emerg Me* 4:31–52, 2012.

Table 2). Light's criteria are 98% sensitive for identifying exudates and approximately 75% specific, so it is important to always consider the clinical context and results of additional workup to determine the etiology of the pleural effusion.

Treatment

After determining the etiology, treatment is directed at the underlying cause and preventing reaccumulation of pleural fluid. Malignant pleural effusion and infected pleural fluid (empyema) are two specific effusions that require specific, directed treatment as described next.

Malignant Pleural Effusions

Malignant pleural effusion affects almost one in six patients with cancer. It is a poor prognostic indicator that often suggests a limited life expectancy (median survival ranges generally <12 months and often significantly shorter). Management of malignant pleural effusion is individualized and guided by the patient's symptoms.

For asymptomatic patients, the harms of pleural interventions outweigh potential clinical benefits and thus should be avoided. For symptomatic patients, first-line management is large-volume thoracentesis via image guidance (POCUS or CT) where available. The goals of this approach are to assess magnitude of symptomatic benefit for the patient and to assess for expandable lung when coupled with pleural manometry. The use of pleural manometry has not been shown to reduce complications of thoracentesis, but it can be helpful to differentiate between fully expandable lung, entrapped lung, and trapped lung. This is important as treatment options for patients with malignant pleural effusions and nonexpandable lung are more limited.

More than 50% of patients with malignant pleural effusion experience relatively rapid fluid accumulation (within short weeks) and should be considered for a definitive pleural procedure. Individualized treatment plans that consider patient preferences, symptom burden, life expectancy, and risks of the procedure can help guide choice of definitive pleural procedure versus symptom palliation with noninvasive strategies (e.g., opioid pharmacotherapy).

Definitive pleural procedures can reduce the total number of interventions need, relieve symptoms, and improve overall quality of life. First-line treatment strategies include chemical pleurodesis or indwelling pleural catheters (IPCs).

IPCs are preferred in the presence of loculated effusions. They can be inserted as an outpatient procedure and have a low risk of treatment failure. Infections such as cellulitis or pleural space infection are the most common complications and can be treated with antibiotic therapy without the need for catheter removal. Spontaneous pleurodesis, which obliterates the pleural space preventing fluid reaccumulation, has been reported as occurring in 16% to 65% of cases where an IPC is placed. For patients with malignant pleural effusions, expandable lung, and good performance status who prefer not to have a long-term catheter, daily drainage or outpatient talc slurry pleurodesis through the IPC are strategies that can result in higher pleurodesis rates.

An IPC can be used regardless of whether fully expandable lung is present. In contrast, chemical pleurodesis for management of malignant pleural effusion should only be used in the presence of fully expandable lung. Graded talc is the most effective and safest chemical pleurodesis agent. This can be administered via a poudrage (sprayed directly on the pleura during thoracoscopy) or via a slurry through an indwelling catheter as mentioned. Both techniques have similar failure rates (22% vs. 24%).

About 30% of patients with malignant pleural effusions have nonexpandable lung (defined as a condition where the lung is unable to expand to the volume of the chest cavity, such as an endobronchial lesion causing lobar collapse), so treatment options are more limited. Generally an IPC is recommended. Intrapleural fibrinolytics introduced via IPC may be considered as they have been shown to help improve symptoms and promote drainage, although they are associated with bleeding complications and costs may be prohibitive.

Pleural Infection

There are approximately 1 million patients hospitalized in the United States each year with pneumonia. Of those hospitalized, 20% to 40% have a parapneumonic effusion. Parapneumonic pleural effusions can be classified as uncomplicated parapneumonic effusions that are free-flowing, sterile reactive effusions that often will not reaccumulate postdrainage, and some small effusions may resolve with antibiotics alone.

Complicated parapneumonic effusions arise from bacterial introduction into the pleural cavity. The glucose is decreased, the pleural fluid pH is less than 7.2, and cultures are negative. Loculations may be present in the effusion. Complete drainage of all loculations is required to prevent progression to empyema or organized effusion, and a chest drain (image-guided percutaneous catheter or thoracostomy tube) should be left behind in all cases. Early surgical intervention with thoracoscopic adhesiolysis may be considered if loculations are present. Alternatively, combination therapy with intrapleural tissue plasminogen activator (t-PA [Activase][1]) and deoxyribonuclease (DNase [Pulmozyme][1]) improves fluid drainage and may reduce the need for surgical intervention.

Delays in recognizing a complicated parapneumonic effusion, delays in antibiotic treatment, or incomplete drainage may contribute to the development of an empyema, or frank pus in the pleural space. From 5% to 10% of parapneumonic effusions progress to empyema, 30% require surgical drainage of the pleural space, and approximately 15% of these patients die. Twenty-five percent of patients will be hospitalized for a month with median duration of stay of 12 to 15 days. Standard therapy consists of antibiotics and tube drainage of the infected pleural fluid. Anaerobic pleural space infections may present more insidiously with loss of appetite and substantial weight loss and are more likely in patients who have poor dental hygiene and are at risk for aspiration.

In addition to IV antibiotics, chest tube thoracostomy is first-line management with a low threshold for surgical intervention if there is incomplete drainage, sepsis, or poor clinical improvement. Intrapleural administration of fibrinolytics may be of benefit in reducing frequency of failed drainage by cleaving intrapleural fibrous septations and may be of benefit in patients who are medically unable to tolerate surgery.

Failure to completely evacuate the empyema can lead to chronic infection. The presence of a bronchopleural fistula, either arising from a lung abscess or due to surgical complication, significantly increases this risk. In these situations, surgical interventions such as long-term drainage with an open thoracostomy, Eloesser flap, or rotational muscle flap may be required.

If the pleural space is incompletely drained but adequately sterilized with antibiotics, the effusion may progress to the organizational stage. This is characterized by heavy fibrin deposit with the formation of a thick peel throughout the pleura with loculations and trapping of the lung, preventing reexpansion. Patients may report significant dyspnea, and pulmonary function tests will show a restrictive pattern. Classic CT findings include thickened pleura with multiple loculations. Decortication, either via VATS or thoracotomy, is required to completely remove the peel from the parietal and visceral pleura.

---

[1] Not FDA approved for this indication.

References

Bhatnagar R, Piotrowska HEG, Laskawiec-Szkonter M, et al: Effect of thoracoscopic talc poudrage vs talc slurry via chest tube on pleurodesis failure rate among patients with malignant pleural effusions: a randomized clinical trial, *JAMA* 323(1):60–69, 2020, https://doi.org/10.1001/jama.2019.19997.

Garrison GW, Cho JL, Deng JC, et al: ATS core curriculum 2021. Adult pulmonary medicine: thoracic oncology, *ATS Sch* 2(3):468–483, 2021, https://doi.org/10.34197/ats-scholar.2021-0032RE. PMID: 34667994; PMCID: PMC8518653.

Hu K, Chopra A, Huggins JT, Nanchal R: Pleural manometry: techniques, applications, and pitfalls, *J Thorac Dis* 12(5):2759–2770, 2020, https://doi.org/10.21037/jtd.2020.04.04. PMID: 32642184; PMCID: PMC7330282.

Porcel José M: Identifying transudates misclassified by Light's criteria, *Curr Opin Pulm Med* 19(4):362–367, 2013, https://doi.org/10.1097/MCP.0b013e32836022dc.

Porcel JM, Light RW: Pleural fluid analysis: are Light's criteria still relevant after half a century?, *Clin Chest Med* 42(4):599–609, 2021, https://doi.org/10.1016/j.ccm.2021.07.003. PMID: 34774168.

Zaki HA, Albaroudi B, Shaban EE, et al: Advancement in pleura effusion diagnosis: a systematic review and meta-analysis of point-of-care ultrasound versus radiographic thoracic imaging, *Ultrasound J* 16(1):3, 2024, https://doi.org/10.1186/s13089-023-00356-z. PMID: 38261109; PMCID: PMC10805747.

PNEUMOCONIOSIS: ASBESTOSIS AND SILICOSIS

Method of
David N. Weissman, MD

CURRENT DIAGNOSIS

- For presentation in an adult of suggestive symptoms (e.g., dyspnea, cough), ask about jobs associated with inhaling mineral or metal dust.
- If pneumoconiosis is suspected, perform chest imaging. High-resolution chest computed tomography without contrast is more sensitive than chest x-ray and provides more detailed information about pattern of pulmonary involvement and related thoracic findings (e.g., adenopathy).
- Evaluate degree of impairment and whether a restrictive or mixed obstructive-restrictive disorder is present with spirometry, lung volumes, and diffusing capacity of the lung for carbon monoxide.
- Exclude alternative causes of interstitial lung disease (e.g., connective tissue disease, hypersensitivity pneumonitis, sarcoidosis).
- Lung biopsy is not usually needed but may be necessary if clinical findings are uncertain or atypical for pneumoconiosis.

CURRENT THERAPY

- Treatment is symptomatic and similar to that for other patients with chronic lung disease
- Give recommended vaccinations for respiratory pathogens.
- Provide empiric treatment with short- and long-acting inhaled bronchodilators and inhaled corticosteroids when they are found to provide symptomatic relief.
- Give supplemental oxygen therapy if pulmonary hypertension is present or to prevent pulmonary hypertension if O_2 saturation is less than 88% at rest, with exercise, or with sleep.
- Consider lung transplantation in the setting of end-stage lung disease.

The pneumoconioses are a group of interstitial fibrotic lung diseases predominantly associated with occupational exposures. They are caused by inhalation of mineral or metallic dust particles small enough to penetrate into the deep lung (respirable size range) (Table 1). These agents interact with pulmonary target cells, including alveolar macrophages and alveolar epithelial cells, to activate a cascade of inflammatory mediators including growth factors. Although exposure to these dusts can induce other types of respiratory disease as well, the final common pathway leading to pneumoconiosis is alveolar epithelial cell damage and interstitial fibrosis. This chapter focuses on silicosis and asbestosis, two common forms of pneumoconiosis.

Asbestosis

Asbestos is composed of strong, heat-resistant fibers of hydrated magnesium silicate classified morphologically as serpentine (chrysotile) or amphibole (crocidolite [riebeckite asbestos], amosite [cummingtonite-grunerite asbestos], anthophyllite asbestos, actinolite asbestos, and tremolite asbestos). In addition, certain asbestiform fibers (winchite, richterite, erionite) can cause adverse health effects identical to those of asbestos. Fiber dimensions and persistence in tissues are key determinants of toxicity. There is a dose–response effect between the quantity of asbestos inhaled and the severity of fibrotic lung disease. Asbestos is also a carcinogen, and increasing exposure is associated with increased risk for lung cancer, mesothelioma, ovarian cancer, and laryngeal cancer.

TABLE 1	Representative Pneumoconioses		
SOURCE	**MAIN CLINICAL FEATURES**	**OCCUPATION**	**DUST**
Crystalline silica	Silicosis, COPD, increased susceptibility to TB, lung cancer, autoimmune diseases	Mining, stone cutting, pottery, foundry work, artificial stone countertop work	Free crystalline silica (SiO_2)
Asbestiform fibers	Asbestosis, bronchogenic carcinoma, mesothelioma, various forms of benign pleural disease	Insulation, shipbuilding, construction, some mining (e.g., vermiculite mining in Libby, MT)	Various asbestiform fibers
Coal	Coal workers' pneumoconiosis, COPD	Coal mining	Coal mine dust
Hard metal	Hard metal lung disease (cobalt lung), asthma	Machinists, metal workers	Hard metal, composed primarily of tungsten carbide and cobalt

COPD, chronic obstructive pulmonary disease; *TB*, tuberculosis.

Asbestos is no longer mined in the United States, and almost all importation was banned in 2024. However, exposures continue to occur, especially in construction and renovation (due to reservoirs of asbestos that are still present in many older buildings), the heating trades (where asbestos is often encountered), and with exposure to older or recently imported asbestos-containing automotive friction products such as brake linings and clutch facings. Workers exposed to asbestos can carry it home on their clothing, resulting in exposure of family members. Living near geological formations prone to asbestos formation in California has been implicated as a risk factor for mesothelioma.

The Occupational Safety and Health Administration (OSHA) permissible exposure limit (PEL) for asbestos is 0.1 fiber per cc air. This limit was based in part on the limits of the analytical methodology used in exposure assessment. Exposure to the PEL every day over a 45-year working lifetime has been estimated to be associated with an increased risk of cancer (lung, mesothelioma, and gastrointestinal) of 336 cases per 100,000 exposed persons and an increased risk of asbestosis of 250 cases per 100,000 exposed persons.

Asbestosis causes symptoms of dyspnea and cough. Latency between initial exposure and disease onset is related to exposure intensity. In the United States, this period is generally about two or more decades. The disease can lead to chronic respiratory failure. Effects of smoking add to the severity of the disease and can cause obstructive findings in addition to the expected decreased lung volume and diffusion capacity associated with fibrotic lung diseases. Bibasilar inspiratory crackles on auscultation, finger clubbing, and bibasilar small, irregular parenchymal opacities on chest x-ray with extension to mid- and upper-zones with advancing disease are characteristic.

The International Labour Organization (ILO) has established a system for classification (grading) of radiographs for the presence of radiographic abnormalities in lung parenchyma and pleura that are associated with pneumoconiosis, as well as their severity. The ILO classification system is widely used in epidemiology, surveillance, administrative, and legal settings. The small opacity profusion grades of 0/1 and 1/0 are often considered as defining the boundary between normal and abnormal lung parenchyma.

High-resolution computed tomography (CT) is the most sensitive imaging method for suspected asbestosis. Findings associated with asbestos exposure include lower lobe or diffuse irregular opacities, bronchial wall thickening, rounded atelectasis, and pleural abnormalities such as pleural plaques and diffuse pleural thickening. The presence of pleural plaques on radiography (particularly bilateral calcified pleural plaques); or uncoated asbestos fibers or fibers coated with an iron-rich proteinaceous material (asbestos bodies) in sputum, bronchoalveolar lavage, or lung biopsy help differentiate asbestosis from idiopathic pulmonary fibrosis.

Criteria for Diagnosis

Diagnosis is supported by radiographic chest imaging or lung biopsy findings of interstitial lung disease compatible with asbestosis; documentation of exposure to asbestos by history, the presence of pleural plaques (bilateral pleural plaques are essentially pathognomonic for asbestos exposure), or the presence of asbestos bodies or an excessive burden of uncoated asbestos fibers in lung biopsy tissue or possibly via bronchoalveolar lavage or sputum; and no other likely explanation for the diffuse fibrotic lung disease.

Asbestos-Related Benign Pleural Disease

Pleural plaques are characteristic forms of localized parietal pleural thickening that are usually bilateral and asymmetrical, involve the lower lung fields or the diaphragm, and spare the costophrenic angles and apices. Pleural plaques are a marker for exposure to asbestos and are often associated with other asbestos-related conditions. Pleural plaques generally result in minimal reductions in forced vital capacity and do not degenerate into malignant lesions.

In contrast, diffuse visceral pleural thickening can result in adhesions between the visceral and parietal pleura with major decreases in forced vital capacity and respiratory insufficiency sufficient for considerathon of decortication.

Benign pleural effusions can occur in the first decade after asbestos exposure and contain erythrocytes and a mixed inflammatory cell infiltrate of lymphocytes, neutrophils, and eosinophils. The thickened visceral pleura and adjacent atelectatic lung tissue can result in a pleural-based area of rounded atelectasis, simulating a lung mass on chest radiography. CT can reveal the comet sign, a pleural band connecting the apparent mass to an area of thickened pleura.

Lung Cancer and Malignant Mesothelioma

Exposure to all forms of asbestos increases the risk of lung cancer. The peak risk occurs at about 30 to 35 years after the onset of exposure. Tobacco smoking increases this risk in a supra-additive fashion, increasing risk to a level greater than for asbestos or smoking alone. In contrast, smoking does not further increase the asbestos-associated risk for malignant mesothelioma. Asbestos-associated malignant mesothelioma can also affect the peritoneum (and sometimes the pericardium), but when it affects the pleura, this disease manifests with dyspnea, chest pain, and bloody pleural effusion (most often unilateral). A latency period of 30 years or longer after initial exposure is common. Biopsy and specialized immunohistochemical stains are typically required to distinguish malignant mesothelioma from benign mesothelial proliferations and various carcinomas such as adenocarcinomas. It is currently unclear when to screen asbestos-exposed individuals at increased risk for lung cancer with low-dose chest computed tomography.

Treatment

Treatment of asbestosis is primarily symptomatic and similar to that for other patients with chronic lung disease (Box 1). Lung transplantation should be considered in the setting of end-stage lung disease. Treatment of benign pleural disease is also symptomatic; as already noted, decortication is an option for managing severe cases of diffuse visceral pleural thickening. Depending on extent of disease, mesothelioma may be treated with surgery, radiation, chemotherapy, or some combination of these. In general, prognosis is poor. Mesothelioma-associated malignant pleural effusion can require palliation through procedures such as pleurodesis, pleurectomy, and decortication. Asbestos-associated lung cancer is managed in the same fashion as lung cancer occurring without a history of exposure to asbestos.

Nintedanib and Inhaled Treprostinil

Advanced asbestosis and silicosis cases can progress to pulmonary fibrosis and/or pulmonary hypertension. Nintedanib (Ofev) is approved for chronic progressive pulmonary fibrosis, hence it may be used in appropriately progressive asbestosis and silicosis cases.[1] Similarly, inhaled treprostinil (Tyvaso) is approved for interstitial lung disease (ILD) with pulmonary hypertension, and it may be used in appropriate cases of asbestosis and silicosis.[1] However, there are insufficient data to understand safety and effectiveness of either treatment, specifically in asbestosis or silicosis, since most patients studied have had other kinds of ILDs.

Silicosis

Silicosis is a fibrosing interstitial lung disease resulting from the inhalation of crystalline silicon dioxide (silica) in dust of respirable size. The commonest form of crystalline silica is quartz, which is the main component of sand and is present in most rocks. Noncrystalline (amorphous) silica, like that in diatomaceous earth or glass, does not cause silicosis. However,

heating amorphous silica, as occurs in foundries when molten metal is poured into clay castings, can convert amorphous silica into cristobalite, a hazardous form of crystalline silica. Mining, stone cutting, sandblasting, and foundry work are all examples of trades associated with exposure to respirable dust containing crystalline silica. The International Agency for Research on Cancer (IARC) has designated crystalline silica as a Group 1 human lung carcinogen.

In 2016, OSHA established a new PEL for respirable crystalline silica of 0.05 mg/m^3. It also established requirements for engineering and administrative controls, personal protective equipment, and medical surveillance including periodic chest radiography and spirometry obtained at least every 3 years. Reporting of silicosis cases to public health authorities is required in some states.

Radiographic Patterns of Silicosis

Three main radiographic patterns of silicosis have been described. Two are nodular interstitial patterns and one is an alveolar-filling pattern. The *simple* pattern is associated with nodules that are smaller than 10 mm and that are predominantly rounded and in the upper lung zones. *Progressive massive fibrosis* (PMF) is found in more advanced interstitial disease. It is associated with multiple coalescent larger nodules, upper lobe fibrosis, upward retraction of the hila, and compensatory hyperinflation of the lower lobes. The large upper-zone opacities can cavitate, sometimes in the setting of superimposed mycobacterial infection. Hilar adenopathy can occur in association with either pattern, sometimes with an egg-shell pattern of hilar node calcification. A third radiographic pattern is an alveolar-filling process. Overwhelming silica exposure over a short period can cause a pathologic response called *silicoproteinosis*, in which alveoli become flooded with proteinaceous fluid. The condition resembles idiopathic pulmonary alveolar proteinosis. The radiographic alveolar filling pattern favors the lower lung zones and is not necessarily associated with the changes of simple silicosis or PMF.

Silicosis Syndromes

Three syndromes of silicosis can be defined based on clinical course and radiographic pattern. Chronic silicosis develops slowly, usually 10 to 30 years after first exposure. It most often has the simple radiographic pattern, but it can be associated with PMF.

Accelerated silicosis develops more rapidly, within 10 years after first exposure. It is associated with higher intensity exposures and can be associated with either the simple or PMF radiographic patterns. Accelerated silicosis is differentiated from chronic silicosis by its more rapid course. Patients with accelerated courses are at greater risk for developing PMF. The clinical presentations of chronic and accelerated silicosis are variable but include cough, dyspnea, and a variety of chest findings ranging from a normal chest examination to crackles, rhonchi, or wheezing. PMF is associated with more severe symptoms and respiratory impairment. Findings compatible with both restrictive and obstructive lung disease (decreased forced vital capacity [FVC], forced expiratory volume at 1 sec [FEV$_1$], FEV$_1$/FVC, diffusion capacity) can occur, potentially leading to cor pulmonale and respiratory failure.

Acute silicosis is associated with very intense exposures to silica, leading to symptoms within a few weeks to a few years after exposure. Intense exposure results in lung injury caused by flooding of alveoli with proteinaceous material, or silicoproteinosis. As already noted, the radiographic appearance is that of an alveolar-filling pattern favoring the lower lung zones. Patients present weeks to a few years after exposure with cough, weight loss, fatigue, and occasional pleuritic chest pain, crackles on auscultation, and progression to respiratory failure often complicated by mycobacterial infection.

Criteria for Diagnosis

The diagnosis of silicosis is predicated on a history of exposure to respirable crystalline silica, typical chest x-ray findings, and

---

[1] Not FDA approved for this indication.

the lack of a more likely diagnosis. High-resolution CT detects changes of silicosis with greater sensitivity than chest radiography. Lung biopsy is seldom required for diagnosis in the setting of a good exposure history and typical findings on chest imaging.

Treatment

Treatment is primarily symptomatic and similar to that for other patients with chronic lung disease (see Box 1). Experimental therapies such as oral corticosteroid therapy and whole-lung lavage have been reported, but clinical benefit is unclear. As noted earlier for asbestosis, the role of treating progressive silicosis with the antifibrotic drug nintedanib or silicosis with pulmonary hypertension with inhaled treprostinil is also currently unclear. Lung transplantation should be considered for patients with end-stage lung disease.

All forms of silicosis, as well as substantial exposure to crystalline silica in the absence of silicosis, are associated with an increased risk of pulmonary tuberculosis and fungal infections. Patients should be evaluated for latent tuberculosis infection by tuberculin skin testing or with an interferon gamma release assay. A positive tuberculin skin test in a patient with a history of substantial silica exposure of at least 10 mm of induration should be considered evidence of tuberculosis infection, regardless of previous immunization with bacille Calmette-Guérin. If testing for latent tuberculosis infection is positive, an evaluation for active tuberculosis should be performed and active disease treated. As in other settings, treatment for active or latent infection should be provided using one of the drug treatment protocols recommended by the Centers for Disease Control and Prevention. Vaccination for respiratory pathogens such as influenza, respiratory syncytial virus, severe acute respiratory syndrome coronavirus-2, and pneumococci should be provided according to curent Centers for Disease Control and Prevention recommendations.

Disclaimer

The findings and conclusions in this report are those of the authors and do not necessarily represent the views of the National Institute for Occupational Safety and Health or the Centers for Disease Control and Prevention.

REFERENCE

Centers for Disease Control and Prevention: 2024. Adult immunization schedule by age. Available at: https://www.cdc.gov/vaccines/schedules/hcp/imz/adult.html, accessed 4/26/2024.
Krefft S, Wolff J, Rose C: Silicosis: an update and guide for clinicians, *Clin Chest Med* 41(4):709–722, 2020.
Maher TM: Interstitial lung disease: a review, *JAMA* 331(19):1655–1665, 2024.
Musk AW, de Klerk N, et al: Asbestos-related diseases, *Int J Tuberc Lung Dis* 24(6):562–567, 2020.
Spagnolo P, Ryerson CJ, et al: Occupational interstitial lung diseases, *J Intern Med* 294(6):798–815, 2023.

PULMONARY HYPERTENSION

Method of
Patrick Kicker, DO; Maria Theresa Opina, MD; and Dan Schuller, MD

CURRENT DIAGNOSIS

- Pulmonary arterial hypertension (PAH) is a type of pulmonary hypertension (PH) based on restricted flow because of vascular wall remodeling and increased pulmonary vascular resistance. PH does not equal PAH.
- The clinical presentation of PAH is subtle and nonspecific with dyspnea, fatigue, and exercise limitation. A high index of suspicion is required.

- Echocardiography is the recommended initial screening test but is not sufficient to provide a definitive diagnosis.
- Right heart catheterization is the gold standard for diagnosing PAH, based on a mean pulmonary artery pressure of ≥20 mm Hg.
- Multimodality risk stratification with combination of functional class assessment, echocardiography, exercise testing (6-minute walk test), B-type natriuretic peptide, and hemodynamic parameters are required at the time of initial diagnosis and for longitudinal monitoring.

CURRENT THERAPY

- Early referral to a PAH expert center is recommended for appropriate evaluation and treatment.
- General measures and supportive care include avoiding pregnancy and high-altitude travel, influenza, coronavirus disease 2019 (COVID-19), respiratory syncytial virus (RSV), and pneumococcal immunizations; supplemental oxygen for hypoxemia; diuretics and electrolyte replacement when needed; correction of anemia; and optimal evaluation and management of associated comorbidities.
- With a few exceptions, patients with PAH at low or intermediate risk should be treated with upfront combination therapy with endothelin receptor antagonists (ERAs) and phosphodiesterase-5 inhibitors (PDE5i).
- In high-risk patients with PAH, combination therapy including intravenous prostanoid and referral for lung transplantation is recommended.
- Sotatercept (Winrevair) is a novel activin signaling inhibitor approved therapy that regulates the vascular cell proliferation in PAH and will impact the therapeutic landscape.
- PAH requires a multidimensional approach to care that includes rehabilitation, psychosocial and spiritual support, and palliative care.

Definition and Classification

Pulmonary hypertension (PH) is defined by a mean pulmonary arterial pressure (mPAP) greater than 20 mm Hg at rest. The definition of pulmonary arterial hypertension (PAH) also implies a pulmonary vascular resistance (PVR) >2 Wood units and pulmonary capillary wedge pressure (PCWP) ≤15 mm Hg. Based on Ohm's law, resistance is directly proportional to a pressure gradient and inversely proportional to flow. Thus, the PVR is calculated by dividing the pressure gradient (mPAP minus PCWP) by the cardiac flow rate using the cardiac output or CO:

$$PVR = (mPAP - PCWP)/CO$$

Rearranging the equation to calculate the mPAP yields mPAP = (PVR × CO) + PCWP. From this simple equation, different hemodynamic profiles leading to PH can be distinguished (Figure 1). PH can occur because there is an increase in PVR (or precapillary PH), an increase in PCWP (or postcapillary PH), an increase in flow (high cardiac output state), or any combination of these. Isolated precapillary PH occurs when the mPAP is greater than 20 mm Hg to define the PH state, and the PVR is elevated (>2 Woods units) while the PCWP is normal (≤15 mm Hg). Likewise, isolated postcapillary PH occurs when the mPAP is greater than 20 mm Hg and the PCWP is greater than 15 mm Hg while the PVR is normal at less than 2 Woods units. Commonly, one finds combined pre- and postcapillary PH with all values abnormally elevated.

Understanding these equations permits appropriate classification, which has therapeutic implications, and insight into sudden clinical worsening with progression of the natural history of

HEMODYNAMIC PROFILES IN PULMONARY HYPERTENSION

Pulmonary Arterial Pressure = (Pulmonary Vascular Resistance)
(Cardiac Output) + Wedge Pressure

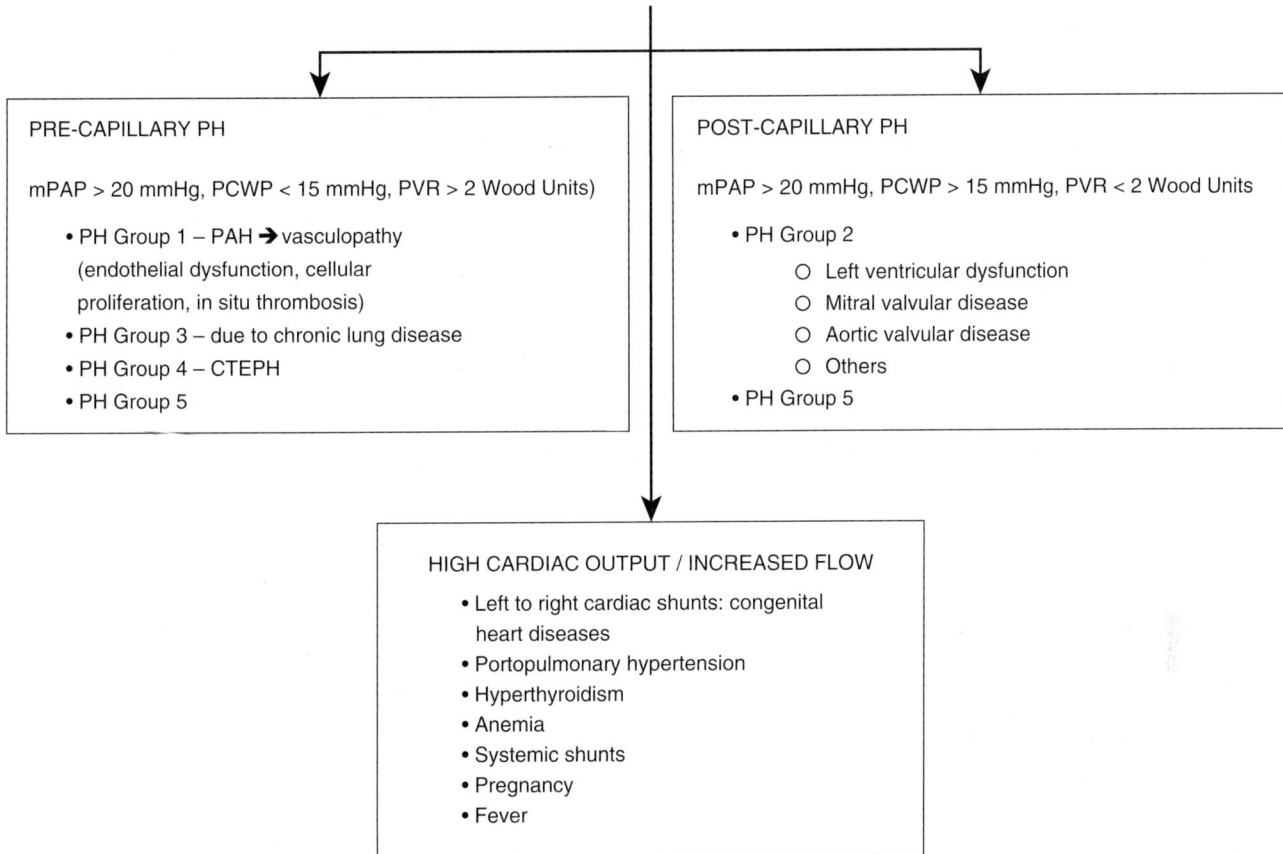

PRE-CAPILLARY PH

mPAP > 20 mmHg, PCWP < 15 mmHg, PVR > 2 Wood Units)

- PH Group 1 – PAH ➜ vasculopathy
  (endothelial dysfunction, cellular
  proliferation, in situ thrombosis)
- PH Group 3 – due to chronic lung disease
- PH Group 4 – CTEPH
- PH Group 5

POST-CAPILLARY PH

mPAP > 20 mmHg, PCWP > 15 mmHg, PVR < 2 Wood Units

- PH Group 2
  - ○ Left ventricular dysfunction
  - ○ Mitral valvular disease
  - ○ Aortic valvular disease
  - ○ Others
- PH Group 5

HIGH CARDIAC OUTPUT / INCREASED FLOW

- Left to right cardiac shunts: congenital
  heart diseases
- Portopulmonary hypertension
- Hyperthyroidism
- Anemia
- Systemic shunts
- Pregnancy
- Fever

Figure 1 Hemodynamic profiles in pulmonary hypertension.

the underlying conditions. For instance, a patient with idiopathic PAH can have an increase in pulmonary pressures caused by progression of the disease (precapillary) or from interval development of a high output state such as fever, anemia, or pregnancy, or from interval development of fluid overload or left ventricular dysfunction (postcapillary).

PH has a prevalence of 1% globally and is classified into five groups (Box 1) based on common underlying mechanisms or pathophysiology. Only PH group 1 is designated as PAH with restricted flow caused by vascular wall remodeling and increased PVR. PH group 2 is caused by left heart disease, a common condition that elevates pulmonary venous pressures; this group represents the highest proportion of patients with PH in the United States. PH group 3 is caused by chronic intrinsic lung diseases with chronic hypoxia and/or hypercapnia as a common mechanism; in patients with mild to moderate chronic obstructive pulmonary disease, the prevalence of PH is about 20% and increases to 50% in more advanced cases of the disease. PH group 4 is predominantly caused by chronic thromboembolic disease, which causes obliteration of the pulmonary vascular bed by chronic organized thrombus leading to increased PVR. PH group 5 consists of heterogeneous conditions with multifactorial mechanisms that affect PH.

PAH is a rare, progressive, incurable disease of the small pulmonary arteries characterized by precapillary PH, vascular cell proliferation, aberrant remodeling, and thrombosis in situ (Figure 2). This group is amenable to specific PAH therapies. PAH is further subdivided into categories because of various etiologies and risk factors linked to a common pathogenesis but with significant variability in presentation, natural history, and response to treatment.

Recent registry data from economically developed countries indicate a PAH incidence and prevalence of ~6 and 48 to 55 cases/million adults, respectively. In the United States, almost half of the cases of PAH are idiopathic, whereas approximately 25% are associated with connective tissue disease (predominantly scleroderma), nearly 10% with congenital heart disease, 5% with liver disease (porto-pulmonary hypertension), and 5% with drugs or toxins (e.g., methamphetamine [Desoxyn], dasatinib [Sprycel], or appetite suppressants). Schistosomiasis is a rare parasitic infection in the United States, but it is endemic in 74 countries. Worldwide, 85% of persons infected with schistosomiasis are in sub-Saharan Africa, and the disease represents the most common cause of PAH worldwide.

Heritable PAH has been associated with several genetic mutations (predominantly the bone morphogenetic protein receptor type 2 [*BMPR2*] gene, activin receptor-like kinase type 1 [*ALK1*], and endoglin) and accounts for almost 3% of cases in the United States. It is transmitted as an autosomal dominant trait, with incomplete penetrance estimated to be approximately 10% to 20%. Genetic anticipation, distinguished by decreasing age of disease onset, has been reported in families affected with heritable PAH.

Clinical Manifestations

The initial symptoms of PAH are often subtle and nonspecific; mean time between symptom onset and PAH diagnosis is approximately 2 years. Patients often report progressive or exertional breathlessness, fatigue, and exercise limitation. With progression, patients may present with near syncope or syncope, palpitations, or anginal chest pain. Early detection requires a high index of

BOX 1   Clinical Classification of Pulmonary Hypertension

Group 1: Pulmonary Arterial Hypertension
Idiopathic PAH
  Nonresponders at vasoreactivity testing
  Acute responders at vasoreactivity testing
Heritable PAH
Associated with drugs and toxins
PAH associated with:
  Connective tissue disease
  HIV infection
  Portal hypertension
  Congenital heart disease
Schistosomiasis
PAH with overt features of venous/capillaries pulmonary veno-
  occlusive disease/pulmonary capillary hemangiomatosis
  involvement
Persistent PH of the newborn

Group 2: Pulmonary Hypertension Associated with Left Heart Disease
Heart failure
  with preserved left ventricular ejection fraction
  with reduced or mildly reduced ejection fraction
Valvular heart disease
Congenital/acquired cardiovascular conditions leading to
  postcapillary PH

Group 3: Pulmonary Hypertension Associated with Lung Diseases and/or Hypoxia
Obstructive lung disease
Restrictive lung disease
Lung disease with mixed restrictive/obstructive pattern
Hypoventilation syndromes
Hypoxia without lung disease (e.g., high altitude)
Developmental lung disorders

Group 4: Pulmonary Hypertension Associated with Pulmonary Artery Obstructions
Chronic thromboembolic PH
Other pulmonary artery obstruction

Group 5: Pulmonary Hypertension with Unclear and/or Multifactorial Mechanism
Hematologic disorders (including chronic hemolysis and
  myeloproliferative disorders)
Systemic disorders (including sarcoidosis)
Metabolic disorders
Chronic renal failure with or without hemodialysis
Pulmonary tumor thrombotic microangiopathy
Fibrosing mediastinitis

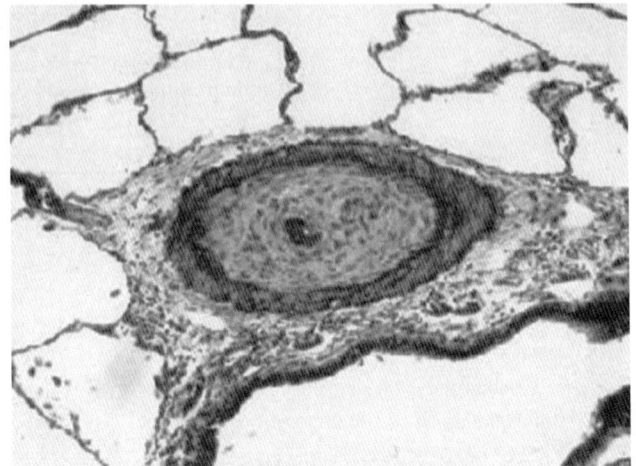

Figure 2 Typical advanced pulmonary arteriopathy in idiopathic pulmonary arterial hypertension. Note the proliferative changes in all three vessel layers, including intimal hyperplasia, medial hypertrophy, and adventitial fibrosis. (From Broaddus VC, Mason RJ, Ernst JD, et al, eds: *Murray & Nadel's Textbook of Respiratory Medicine*, 6th ed. Philadelphia: Elsevier; 2016.)

connective tissue diseases; evidence of liver cirrhosis or portal hypertension; venous insufficiency or varicosities suggestive of possible thromboembolic disease; and obvious signs of underlying cardiac or respiratory diseases, including obstructive sleep apnea. Suggestive electrocardiographic findings include right axis deviation greater than 110 degrees, which has a positive predictive value between 72% and 93% and a negative predictive value between 26% and 65%. Other associated findings include right atrial enlargement and right ventricular hypertrophy.

Diagnosis

The diagnostic evaluation is aimed at screening high-risk individuals, excluding secondary causes of PH, and evaluating possible associated conditions. In addition, various elements of the comprehensive examination are useful for subsequent risk stratification, which is required to select the best therapeutic option and assess prognosis. PAH is always a diagnosis of exclusion.

After reviewing pertinent previous medical records and performing a complete history and physical examination, the pivotal test in the diagnostic algorithm by the primary care provider or non-PH expert center is a transthoracic echocardiogram (TTE) to assess the probability of PH. An echocardiogram has an intermediate or high risk for PH based on a peak tricuspid regurgitation velocity 2.8 m/s or greater or right ventricular systolic pressure ≥35 mm Hg. In one series, TTE had a sensitivity of 87% (95% confidence interval, 84.8%, 90.0%) and specificity of 66% (95% confidence interval, 60.7%, 71.6%). After a positive screen, a decision must be made as to whether to fast track the referral of the patient to a PH expert center or locally advance the diagnostic evaluation with additional testing aimed at diagnosing common causes of PH and ruling out chronic thromboembolic PH (CTEPH). A comprehensive evaluation may include chest film, electrocardiogram, TTE, ventilation-perfusion lung scan, pulmonary function testing, 6-minute walk test, serologic evaluation (human immunodeficiency virus [HIV], antinuclear antibodies, brain natriuretic peptide [BNP or NT-pro BNP], and others), and right-side cardiac catheterization for hemodynamic assessment and vasoreactivity testing. Depending on the results, additional, contingent tests may include a transesophageal echocardiogram, stress echocardiogram, "bubble" echocardiogram, computed tomography (CT) scan of the chest with or without pulmonary angiogram, coagulopathy profile, blood gases, overnight oximetry, polysomnography, or cardiac magnetic resonance imaging (MRI). During cardiac catheterization, additional interventions, such as exercise or fluid challenges, pharmacologic interventions with vasoactive agents, and/or a left-side cardiac catheterization, may be useful to

suspicion because attribution to conditions such as asthma or "being out of shape" is a common error that can contribute to delay in diagnosis. Failure to respond to typical treatments for heart failure or asthma may be an important clue. Dysphonia or hoarseness caused by compression of the recurrent laryngeal nerve (Ortner's syndrome), which is caused by an enlarged pulmonary artery, occurs in less than 1% of patients. Early physical findings of PH may be nonspecific and include an accentuated pulmonary component of the second heart sound (P2) and a midsystolic ejection murmur. Physical findings in more advanced cases that involve right ventricular failure include a right parasternal lift, right ventricular gallop, diastolic murmur of pulmonary regurgitation, jugular venous distention, lower extremity edema, ascites, and signs of low cardiac output, including cool extremities. A murmur of tricuspid regurgitation may be audible, and this murmur intensifies with inspiration, unlike that of mitral regurgitation. Patients with suspected PH may also exhibit signs of associated conditions, such as telangiectasias, Raynaud's phenomenon, sclerodactyly, calcinosis, or malar erythema in

Low-risk criteria associated with a good prognosis include WHO functional class I–II, 6-minute walk test distance greater than 440 m, right atrial pressure (RAP) less than 8 mm Hg, and Cardiac Index ≥ 2.5 L/min/m^2.

Adverse PAH prognostic factors include PAH associated with connective tissue disease, HIV, heritable or porto-pulmonary hypertension; men greater than 60 years; renal insufficiency with estimated glomerular filtration rate (eGFR) less than 60 mL/min/1.73 m^2; WHO functional class III or IV; systolic blood pressure less than 110 mm Hg; heart rate greater than 96; all-cause hospitalization within 6 months; 6-minute walk test distance less than 165 m; BNP test greater than 800 pg/mL or NT-proBNP ≥ 1100 pg/mL; pericardial effusion; diffusion capacity <40% of predicted; and RAP >20 mm Hg.

Treatment

General supportive measures for patients with PH are listed in Box 2. The overall goals of therapy are to prevent clinical worsening; decrease hospital admissions; improve quality of life (decreased symptoms), WHO functional class (increased activity level), hemodynamics, 6-minute walk results; and optimize survival. For PH diagnostic groups 2 to 3, early and correct identification of the underlying conditions is paramount to prevent misclassification and provide optimal treatment, such as effective diuresis of heart failure, correction of hypoxemia for chronic obstructive pulmonary disease, use of continuous positive airway pressure for obstructive sleep apnea, and so forth. Cases consistent with mixed PH where the PVR is increased and believed to be out of proportion for the underlying PH group 2 or 3 disorder usually require referral to a PH expert center. PAH-specific therapies are not FDA approved for these patients and may lead to the development of pulmonary edema in patients with PH group 2 or worsening gas exchange in patients with PH group 3.

Patients with CTEPH–PH group 4 require therapeutic anticoagulation and consideration for pulmonary thromboendarterectomy or balloon pulmonary angioplasty at a center of expertise. Screening for antiphospholipid syndrome should be performed at CTEPH diagnosis and, if positive, lifelong anticoagulation with vitamin K antagonist is recommended over direct oral anticoagulants. Riociguat (Adempas), an activator of nitric oxide causing vasodilation, is indicated and FDA approved for patients with inoperable or persistent/recurrent CTEPH.

Specific PAH therapy is usually started for symptomatic patients in WHO functional class II, III, or IV if they show no acute vasoreactivity or if they do not maintain an acceptable sustained response to calcium channel blockers. Nonresponders to acute vasoreactivity testing who are at low or intermediate risk should be treated with initial oral combination therapy with an endothelin receptor antagonist (ERA) and a phosphodiesterase-5 inhibitor (PDE5i).

Currently available therapeutic choices include ERAs such as ambrisentan (Letairis), bosentan (Tracleer), or macitentan (Opsumit); PDE-5is such as sildenafil (Revatio) or tadalafil (Adcirca); combined macitentan and tadalafil (Opsynvi); soluble guanylate cyclase stimulator, riociguat (Adempas); prostacycline analog agents such as intravenous epoprostenol (Flolan, Veletri), intravenous or subcutaneous treprostinil (Remodulin), inhaled treprostinil (Tyvaso nebulized or Tyvaso-DPI), oral treprostinil (Orenitram); oral selective prostacycline receptor agonist selexipag (Uptravi) or inhaled iloprost (Ventavis); and subcutaneous activin signaling inhibitor sotatercept (Winrevair). Use of these medications should be done under the auspices of or at an expert referral center.

Based on the global experience over the last 3 decades and more than 40 randomized controlled trials performed on nearly 10,000 patients, we have learned the following: (a) In treatment-naïve patients with PAH, any monotherapy is better than placebo and associated with an improvement in exercise capacity and outcome; (b) in treatment-naïve and newly diagnosed (incident) patients with PAH, initial combination therapy improves symptoms, exercise capacity, and outcomes compared with monotherapy; and (c) in already treated (prevalent) patients with PAH, sequential combination therapy improves exercise capacity,

secure a definitive diagnosis, assess potential mixed etiologies, and determine the hemodynamic profile for risk stratification.

Vasoreactivity testing in patients with PAH can be accomplished with the use of inhaled nitric oxide,[1] intravenous epoprostenol sodium (Flolan),[1] or intravenous adenosine (Adenocard).[1] A positive vasodilator response is defined as greater than 10% decrease in mPAP to an absolute value of less than 40 mm Hg with no decrease in cardiac output. Patients who show acute vasoreactivity should be considered for a high-dose calcium channel blocker titration challenge under hemodynamic monitoring in an intensive care setting. For the minority of patients who demonstrate a favorable response to either oral diltiazem (Cardizem)[1] or nifedipine (Procardia),[1] the selection of drug and dosing will depend on the cumulative dose of the acute challenge, their heart rate, and hemodynamic tolerance.

Novel diagnostic tools that are being investigated for PAH but are not universally available yet include V/Q single-photon emission CT and dual-energy CT, three-dimensional dynamic contrast-enhanced MRI, parametric MRI mapping, intravascular ultrasound, and optical coherence tomography.

Risk Stratification

In addition to the etiologic classification of PAH, the World Health Organization (WHO) uses a functional classification for patients with PH, modeled after the New York Heart Association classification for heart failure. Patients with PAH are classified by severity of dyspnea and limitation of physical activity:

- Class I includes patients with no limitation on physical activity. Routine physical activities do not cause increased dyspnea, chest pain, fatigue, or presyncope.
- Class II includes patients with mild limitation of physical activities. These patients are comfortable at rest, but routine physical activities result in increased dyspnea, chest pain, fatigue, or syncope.
- Class III includes patients with marked limitation of physical activities. They are comfortable at rest, but activities that are less than ordinary result in dyspnea, chest pain, fatigue, or palpitations.
- Class IV includes patients unable to perform any physical activity without symptoms. Dyspnea or fatigue may be present at rest, and discomfort increases with any activity.

[1] Not FDA approved for this indication.

hemodynamics, and outcomes compared with patients who continue on background therapy.

In therapy-naïve (incident) patients with PAH, initial combination therapy with ambrisentan and tadalafil was associated with a significant lower risk of clinical failure events, defined as the first occurrence of a composite of death, hospitalization for worsening PAH, disease progression, or unsatisfactory long-term clinical response. On the other hand, bosentan added to sildenafil therapy in patients with PAH was not superior to sildenafil monotherapy in delaying the time to the first morbidity/mortality event. This discrepancy observed between two different drug combinations within the same categories of drugs may be explained by the known drug-drug interaction where bosentan significantly decreases the plasma concentration of sildenafil, but sildenafil increases the plasma concentrations of bosentan.

In a long-term, event-driven trial of predominantly prevalent patients with symptomatic PAH, macitentan monotherapy or added to background therapy significantly reduced morbidity and mortality.

In a randomized, double-blind trial, riociguat significantly improved exercise capacity and secondary efficacy endpoints including PVR, NT-proBNP, WHO functional class, time to clinical worsening, and dyspnea scores.

Among patients with PAH who remained symptomatic on monotherapy with bosentan or sildenafil, inhaled treprostinil improved exercise capacity and quality of life and was usually well tolerated.

In a large, event-driven trial of predominantly prevalent patients with PAH on background therapy, the oral selective prostacyclin receptor agonist selexipag reduced the risk of death or complications from PAH. In nonvasoactive and treatment-naïve patients at high risk, initial combination therapy including IV prostacycline analog agents is recommended. Intravenous epoprostenol receives the strongest recommendation for high-risk patients because it has reduced the 3-month rate of mortality, even as monotherapy. Referral for lung transplantation should also be considered.

In 2024, the U.S. Food and Drug Administration (FDA) approved the first-in-class activin signaling inhibitor sotatercept (Winrevair) for the treatment of adults with PAH to increase exercise capacity, improve WHO functional class and reduce the risk of clinical worsening events. Sotatercept, a novel fusion protein, binds activins and growth differentiation factors to restore balance between growth-promoting and growth-inhibiting signaling pathways. In a phase 2 clinical trial, treatment with sotatercept reduced pulmonary vascular resistance in WHO Class II and III patients with PAH receiving stable background therapy. Improvement from baseline in 6-minute walk distance and NT-proBNP levels were also noted. In a phase 3 clinical trial, treatment with sotatercept resulted in an improved 6-minute walk distance at 24 weeks when compared with placebo in WHO Class II and III patients with PAH receiving stable background therapy. Improvements were also reported in pulmonary vascular resistance, NT-proBNP level, WHO functional class, and time to death or clinical worsening. Sotatercept injection may be administered subcutaneously every 3 weeks by patients or caregivers with guidance, training and close monitoring.

The decision regarding initial therapy must be individualized and incorporates many factors and determinants of risk, including WHO functional class, progression of symptoms, hemodynamic assessment, 6-minute walk test, biomarkers of severity, comorbidities, access to emergent care, and psychosocial support.

Surgical options for advanced cases of PAH, including balloon graded atrial septostomy and lung transplantation, are beyond the scope of this chapter but remain important treatment options for patients with refractory disease.

Monitoring

Goal-directed therapy has been described, calling for periodic assessment every 3 to 6 months and possible escalation of therapy.

This approach has been associated with improved survival, with specific goals that include clinical stability, WHO functional class II, a 6-minute walk distance of greater than 400 m, and near-normal RAP and cardiac output.

Risk stratification using validated risk assessment tools such as REVEAL 2.0, REVEAL Lite 2 or COMPERA 2.0 should be used at the time of initial evaluation and regular follow-up.

Health coaching, goal setting, and periodic evaluation of advanced directives should always be incorporated in the longitudinal monitoring of patients with PAH.

The optimal management of patients with PH requires a holistic, multidimensional approach that incorporates shared decision making integrating medical care, rehabilitation, psychosocial support, spiritual support, palliative care, education, and participation in support groups.

Special Situations

Pregnancy and Birth Control

The effect of PH on pregnancy, although substantial, has been altered by recent treatments. Current guidelines recommend counseling of pregnant women and their partners on the outcomes associated with PH with discussion of possible termination of the pregnancy and the need for vigilant avoidance of pregnancy using contraceptive practices. However, some recent studies suggest that current treatment modalities are having some impact on better outcomes. The ROPAC study by Silwa et al. demonstrated that maternal and neonatal mortality was substantially lower than previously reported (4.6% and 2.7%, respectively). No maternal deaths occurred during gestation, and most occurred at least 1 week after delivery. Most of the maternal deaths occurred in those with more severe PAH. In a more recent meta-analysis of 19 studies published in 2020, a maternal mortality rate of 11.5 per 100 pregnancies was reported, with 81.6% occurring in the early postpartum period.

Physicians caring for pregnant patients with PH should consult an obstetrician, maternal fetal medicine specialist, pulmonologist, and geneticist if first-trimester termination is not an option.

Women with PH of childbearing potential should be provided with clear contraceptive advice because many of the PAH therapies are teratogenic, and the implications of contraception failure can be devastating.

Surgical Procedures

Perioperative mortality increased in patients with PH and was reported to be as high as 15% for emergency procedures in the PAH population. The decision to perform surgery should be individualized considering the potential risks and benefits. Multidisciplinary discussion with a PH physician, anesthesiologist and surgery should be considered and preoperative optimization of PAH therapy performed whenever possible.

Travel and Altitude

Travel for patients with PAH requires planning and coordination. Air travel may induce arterial hypoxemia and pulmonary vasoconstriction and increase right ventricular afterload. In-flight oxygen administration is advised for patients with PaO_2 <60 mm Hg and those already requiring supplemental oxygen at rest. Patients with PAH should be advised to travel preferably with company and bring a current list of their medications, extra doses, supplies, PH physician contact information, and information regarding local PH centers near their travel destination. In general, it is recommended to avoid altitudes >1500 m without additional supplemental oxygen.

COVID-19

Most of the major initial healthcare disruptions in the care for PAH caused by the coronavirus disease 2019 (COVID-19) pandemic have essentially resolved, and the evaluation, management, and follow-up of PAH have returned to prepandemic standards.

Many PAH-specific drugs (e.g., ERAs and PDE5i) have significant drug-drug interactions with nirmatrelvir/ritonavir (Paxlovid) and are contraindicated. Stopping the drug will not mitigate the interaction, and coadministration risks serious toxicity.

COVID-19 vaccination continues to be strongly recommended for patients with PH because they represent a high-risk population group.

References

Aryal SR, Moussa H, Sinkey R, et al: Management of reproductive health in patients with pulmonary hypertension, *Am J Obstet Gynecol MFM* 2:100087, 2020.

Benza RL, Gomberg-Maitand M, Elliot G, et al: Predicting survival in patients with pulmonary arterial hypertension. The reveal risk score calculator 2.0 and comparison with ESC/ERS- based risk assessment strategies, *Chest* 156(2):323–333, 2019.

Galiè N, Barberà JA, Frost AE, et al: Initial use of ambrisentan plus tadalafil in pulmonary arterial hypertension, *N Engl J Med* 373(9):834–844, 2015.

Hoeper MM, Badesch DB, Ghofrani HA, et al: STELLAR Trial Investigators: Phase 3 Trial of Sotatercept for Treatment of Pulmonary Arterial Hypertension, *N Engl J Med* 388(16):1478–1490, 2023.

Humbert M, Kovacs G, Hoeper MM, et al: 2022 ESC/ERS Guidelines for the diagnosis and treatment of pulmonary hypertension, *Eur Heart J* 43:3618–3731, 2022.

Jha N, Jha AK, Mishra SK, Sagili H: Pulmonary hypertension and pregnancy outcomes: systemic review and meta-analysis, *Eur J Obstet Gynecol Reprod Biol* 253:108–116, 2020.

McGoon MD, Ferrari P, Armstrong I, et al: The importance of patient perspectives in pulmonary hypertension, *Eur Respir J* 53(1):1801919, 2019.

Ryan JJ, Melendres-Groves L, Zamanian RT, et al: Care of patients with pulmonary arterial hypertension during the coronavirus (COVID19) pandemic, *Pulm Circ* 10(2):1–7, 2020.

Sahay S, Farber HW: Management of hospitalized patients with pulmonary arterial hypertension and COVID-19 infection, *Pulm Circ* 10(3):1–5, 2020.

SARCOIDOSIS

Method of
W. Ennis James, MD; and Brady Otten, MD

CURRENT DIAGNOSIS

- The diagnosis of sarcoidosis is one of exclusion.
- Tissue biopsy, confirming noncaseating granulomatous inflammation, is required in most cases.
- Initial evaluation should include screening for dangerous organ involvement.

CURRENT THERAPY

- Many cases of sarcoidosis do not require treatment.
- Treatment is typically indicated when sarcoidosis results in impaired quality of life or involves potentially dangerous organs.
- Corticosteroids are the most commonly used initial therapy but are associated with significant side effects.

Sarcoidosis is a multisystem granulomatous disease of unknown cause. The lung is most commonly affected, but any organ may be involved. The natural course of sarcoidosis is variable, ranging from an asymptomatic state to a progressive disease causing significant organ dysfunction that may be life-threatening. This variability in organ involvement and disease presentation often makes the diagnosis of sarcoidosis problematic.

Epidemiology

Sarcoidosis occurs worldwide and affects all races and ages. The disease is most common between ages 20 and 40, although analyses from large databases have revealed that the incidence and prevalence of the disease is bimodal, with a second peak between ages 45 and 65. Onset of disease tends to occur at an earlier age in Black people and males. A large analysis from an American national healthcare database found an incidence of 17.8 per 100,000 in African Americans and 8.1 per 100,000 in American White people, and a prevalence of 141 per 100,000 in African Americans and 50 per 100,000 in American White people. Incidence and prevalence rates were lower in Hispanic Americans than in White people and lower still in Asian Americans. The highest prevalence of sarcoidosis is found in White people in Scandinavia and in Black Americans. Sarcoidosis appears to affect more women than men across all racial/ethnic groups. In the United States, Black women have the highest prevalence of sarcoidosis, almost twice that of Black American men. The relative risk for having sarcoidosis increases significantly if a family member has it as well. In the United States nearly 20% of African Americans with sarcoidosis have an affected first-degree relative, compared with 5% in White people.

The clinical presentation and severity of sarcoidosis vary among racial and ethnic groups. The disease tends to be more severe in African Americans, whereas White people are more likely to be asymptomatic at report. Extrathoracic manifestations are more common in certain populations, such as ocular and cardiac sarcoidosis in Japanese populations, chronic uveitis and lupus pernio in African Americans, and erythema nodosum in Europeans. There is increasing evidence that genetic polymorphisms affect the risks and manifestations of the disease. This is consistent with the current theory that sarcoidosis does not have a single cause but is the result of an abnormal granulomatous host response to one of many potential antigens in a genetically susceptible person.

Immunopathogenesis

The exact immunopathogenesis of sarcoidosis is unknown, but it is thought to be similar to that of other granulomatous diseases. That is, antigen-presenting cells (APCs), usually either macrophages or dendritic cells, process and present an antigen via a human leukocyte antigen (HLA) class II molecule to T lymphocytes and their receptors. These T lymphocytes are usually of the CD4 T-helper 1 (T_H1) class. The antigen involved in this reaction is unknown, and there may be many antigens that are each associated with a specific HLA class II molecule and T-cell receptor. This could explain the inability to determine one specific cause of sarcoidosis and the varied phenotypic expressions of the disease.

The interaction of APCs and T lymphocytes activates the APCs to produce tumor necrosis factor α (TNF-α) and other cytokines. A proliferation of CD4 T_H1 lymphocytes also ensues, which results in the secretion of interferon-γ, interleukin (IL)-2, IL-12, and other cytokines. These cytokines activate and recruit monocytes and macrophages and transform them into giant cells, which are important building blocks of the granuloma. Additional factors may also lead to this series of immunologic events, such as the persistence of antigens like soluble AA amyloid fibrils that prevent antigen degradation.

The typical sarcoidosis lesion is a noncaseating (nonnecrotic) granuloma. The sarcoid granuloma consists of a compact core of macrophage-derived epithelioid and multinucleated giant cells surrounded by a perimeter of monocytes, lymphocytes, and fibroblasts. Granulomas can resolve spontaneously or with therapy; however, they can also persist and lead to persistent hyalinization and fibrosis. The development of such fibrosis can cause permanent organ dysfunction and in large part determines the prognosis.

Clinical Features and Clinical Course
Pulmonary Sarcoidosis

Between 30% and 60% of patients with pulmonary sarcoidosis are asymptomatic, and the disease is detected incidentally on chest x-ray. Some patients report with nonspecific pulmonary symptoms, such as dyspnea, cough, wheezing, and chest pain. Respiratory failure from sarcoidosis is extremely rare at report. Unlike in many other interstitial lung diseases, crackles

TABLE 1	Chest Radiograph Stages of Sarcoidosis		
RADIOGRAPHIC STAGE	**BILATERAL HILAR LYMPH NODE ENLARGEMENT**	**PARENCHYMAL DISEASE**	
I	Yes	No	
II	Yes	Nonfibrotic	
III	No	Nonfibrotic	
IV	No or yes	Fibrotic	

Adapted from Judson MA, Baughman RP. Sarcoidosis. In: Baughman RP, du Bois RM, Lynch JP, Wells AU, eds. *Diffuse Lung Disease: A Practical Approach.* Arnold; 2004:109-129.

BOX 1 Factors Associated With a Poor Prognosis in Sarcoidosis

- Symptomatic at report
- African American race
- Extrathoracic disease
- Stage II to III versus stage I on chest x-ray
- Age greater than 40 years
- Splenic involvement
- Lupus pernio
- Disease duration greater than 2 years
- Forced vital capacity less than 1.5 L
- Stage IV chest x-ray or aspergilloma
- Pulmonary hypertension

Data from Judson MA, Baughman RP. Sarcoidosis. In: Baughman RP, du Bois RM, Lynch JP, Wells AU, eds. *Diffuse Lung Disease: A Practical Approach.* Arnold; 2004:109-129.

---

are rarely heard on chest auscultation. Abnormalities on the chest radiograph occur in more than 90% of patients with pulmonary sarcoidosis. Bilateral hilar adenopathy occurs in 50% to 85% at disease report, and 25% to 50% have parenchymal infiltrates. On computed tomography, small nodules from granulomatous inflammation most commonly occur in the mid- and upper-lung zones and have a predilection for the bronchovascular bundles, subpleural locations, intralobular septa, and the airways.

A radiographic staging system was developed several decades ago (Table 1). Groups of patients with higher radiographic stages have more severe pulmonary dysfunction, lower remission rates, and greater mortality. However, there is significant overlap among these groups, and stages are highly inaccurate predictors of outcomes for individual patients.

Advanced pulmonary stage IV (fibrocystic) sarcoidosis displays destruction of the lung architecture, with upward traction of the hila, lung distortion, upper-lobe volume loss, fibrocystic disease, honeycombed cysts, and decreased lung volumes. Aspergillomas can develop in these large cystic lesions and may be associated with life-threatening hemoptysis. Bronchiectasis from airway distortion also can occur and is an additional potential cause of hemoptysis.

The cause of dyspnea in pulmonary sarcoidosis is multifactorial. It may be the result of abnormalities of gas exchange, lung mechanics, weakness of the respiratory muscles, obesity from corticosteroid therapy, pulmonary hypertension, or sarcoidosis involvement of the heart. Pulmonary function and the chest radiographic findings are often discordant and often do not correlate with symptom severity. In patients with pulmonary sarcoidosis with a normal lung parenchyma (stage I), the vital capacity, diffusing capacity, partial pressure of arterial oxygen (PaO_2) at rest, PaO_2 with exercise, and lung compliance are abnormal in 20% to 40% of cases. The majority of patients with pulmonary sarcoidosis have a vital capacity of greater than 70% of that predicted at diagnosis; however, those with abnormal lung parenchyma have abnormal pulmonary function tests 50% to 70% of the time.

Patients with stage IV fibrocystic sarcoidosis tend to have the most severe pulmonary dysfunction and often have a restrictive ventilatory defect found on spirometry. It is underappreciated, however, that endobronchial involvement and airway distortion from fibrosis may cause airflow obstruction to be the major abnormality found on pulmonary function testing. Wheezing may be the prominent reporting symptom of sarcoidosis, and many cases of sarcoidosis are misdiagnosed as asthma.

Only 3% to 5% of patients die of sarcoidosis. In the United States 75% of these deaths are the result of complications of advanced pulmonary fibrosis, including pulmonary hypertension, infection, and life-threatening hemoptysis, which may result from the development of aspergillomas. Despite these potential complications, the overall prognosis is favorable in patients with stage IV sarcoidosis, with a 10-year survival of over 80%. Staging systems, including one that incorporates the lung function, pulmonary artery to ascending aorta diameter ratio greater than 1, and the presence of greater than 20% fibrosis on imaging, can be useful predictors of mortality. Other organs that result in fatalities from sarcoidosis are the heart and the central nervous system

(CNS). In Japan, death from sarcoidosis is more commonly caused by cardiac than pulmonary involvement.

Patients who report with Löfgren syndrome (described in the next section) or with asymptomatic bilateral hilar adenopathy on chest radiograph have a good prognosis. African Americans tend to have a lower forced vital capacity and worse prognosis compared with White people and are more likely to develop new organ involvement within 2 years of diagnosis. Box 1 lists risk factors associated with a poor prognosis.

Extrapulmonary Sarcoidosis

The extrapulmonary manifestations of sarcoidosis are present in up to 67% of patients, can be the presenting manifestation of systemic sarcoidosis, and can affect the prognosis and treatment options for sarcoidosis.

The eyes and skin are the most common extrapulmonary organs involved with sarcoidosis. Ocular manifestations occur in 25% to 50% of patients; anterior uveitis is the most common manifestation. Symptoms of anterior uveitis may include red eyes, painful eyes, and photophobia. However, one-third of patients with anterior uveitis from sarcoidosis have no ocular symptoms. In addition, an intermediate or posterior uveitis can cause vision problems or can be asymptomatic. For these reasons, all patients with sarcoidosis should undergo an eye examination by an ophthalmologist. Other ocular manifestations of sarcoidosis include conjunctivitis, keratoconjunctivitis sicca (dry eyes), scleritis, and optic neuritis.

Skin lesions in sarcoidosis can be classified into two categories: specific lesions that demonstrate noncaseating granulomas on biopsy and nonspecific lesions that do not (Figure 1). The specific skin lesions are often papular and commonly occur around the nose, eyes, and nape of the neck. They also have a predilection for areas of previous scars and tattoos, which is often referred to as "scar sarcoidosis" and is highly specific to sarcoidosis. Lupus pernio is a type of specific skin lesion causing disfiguring lesions on the face, often with erythema and significant induration. These lesions have a tendency to appear on the nose, cheeks, medial and lateral sides of the eyes, and lateral sides of the mouth. Lupus pernio lesions are relatively recalcitrant to therapy and often respond only partially to corticosteroids. The most common nonspecific skin lesion is erythema nodosum, which is often seen with an acute sarcoidosis presentation of fever, arthritis (especially in the ankles), pulmonary symptoms, and bilateral hilar adenopathy on chest radiograph. This syndrome is known as *Löfgren syndrome* and tends to have a good long-term prognosis.

Cardiac and neurologic sarcoidosis can be life-threatening and is therefore important to recognize. Cardiac involvement is detected clinically in 5% to 10% of patients with sarcoidosis during life but has been found in up to 25% at autopsy. Cardiac sarcoidosis can cause left ventricular dysfunction, cardiac arrhythmias, and sudden cardiac death. All patients with sarcoidosis should be screened for cardiac sarcoidosis, which,

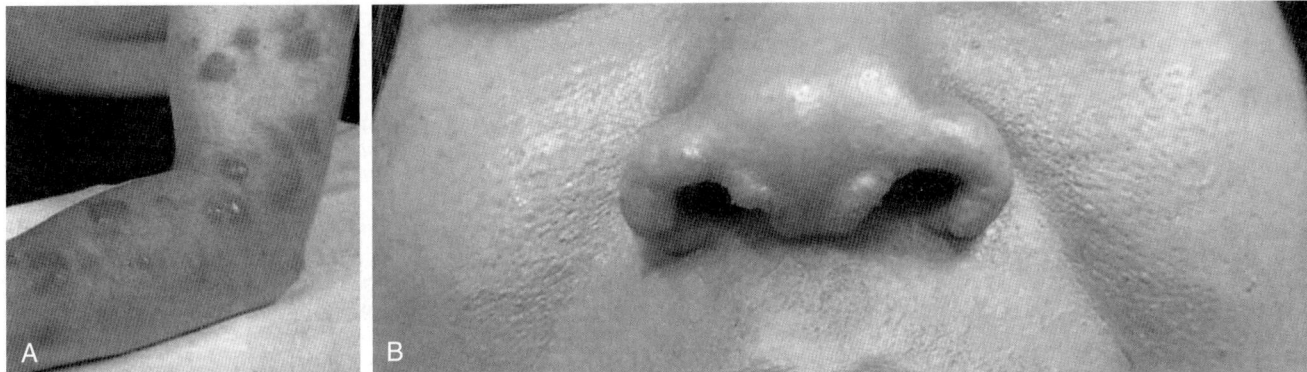

Figure 1 Skin lesions of sarcoidosis. (A) Sarcoid lesions may occur at any site, and they may take nodular, papular, or plaque forms. Biopsy is often necessary for diagnosis. (B) *Lupus pernio* is the term used to describe a dusky-purple infiltration of the skin of the nose, cheeks, or ears in chronic sarcoidosis. (Figure A from Forbes CD, Jackson WF. *Color Atlas and Text of Clinical Medicine*. 3rd ed. Mosby; 2003, with permission.)

at a minimum, should include an electrocardiogram (ECG), as well as eliciting symptoms of left ventricular dysfunction (e.g., orthopnea, peripheral edema) and cardiac arrhythmias (e.g., palpitations, sensation of skipped heartbeats, syncope). Transthoracic echocardiography (TTE) and Holter monitoring have been recommended by some as appropriate additional screening tests. Patients with either significant symptoms or abnormal ECG or TTE should undergo more definitive testing for the diagnosis of cardiac sarcoidosis. Cardiac magnetic resonance imaging (MRI) provides both diagnostic and prognostic data and is recommended over cardiac positron emission tomography (PET) as the initial test of choice; however, this may vary depending on local expertise and availability. The diagnosis of cardiac sarcoidosis is typically made noninvasively, based on a combination of a typical clinical presentation coupled with the detection of characteristic findings on advanced imaging after other possible etiologies have been excluded. Because myocardial involvement is patchy, endomyocardial biopsy is diagnostic in less than 25% and is not commonly performed to make the diagnosis of cardiac sarcoidosis.

Clinically apparent neurosarcoidosis occurs in less than 10% of patients with sarcoidosis. Palsy of the seventh cranial nerve is the most common manifestation of neurosarcoidosis, and it often predates the diagnosis of the disease. Sarcoidosis can affect any part of the peripheral nervous system and CNS and can cause a cranial nerve palsy, mononeuropathy or polyneuropathy, aseptic meningitis, seizures, mass lesions in the brain and spinal cord, hydrocephalus, and encephalopathy. Brain and spinal cord MRI with contrast is the imaging test of choice to evaluate for potential CNS sarcoidosis in patients with a compatible clinical presentation.

Sarcoidosis causes clinically apparent extrathoracic lymphadenopathy in more than 10% of patients. The spleen may be involved in up to 50% of patients, but it is usually asymptomatic and rarely causes hypersplenism. Histologic evidence of hepatic sarcoidosis is present in 50% to 80% of patients with sarcoidosis, although most of these patients are asymptomatic and have normal liver function tests. Hepatomegaly, abdominal pain, and pruritus are the most common symptoms associated with hepatic sarcoidosis but are present only in 15% to 25% of patients with hepatic involvement. Elevation of the serum alkaline phosphatase is the most common liver function test abnormality. Sarcoidosis rarely involves the thyroid, kidney, breast, genitourinary tract, and gastrointestinal tract.

Bone involvement is occasional, usually occurring as small cysts or cortical defects found in the small bones of the hands and feet, but can also be found incidentally on imaging of the long bones and axial skeleton. An acute sarcoid arthritis often is present at disease onset and has a good prognosis. This is commonly found in the ankles of patients who report with Löfgren syndrome. Chronic sarcoid arthritis is rare. It is usually a nondestructive arthropathy of the shoulders, wrists, knees, ankles, and small joints of the hands and feet.

Sarcoidosis of the upper respiratory tract is underappreciated and can occur in the nasopharynx, hypopharynx, larynx, or any of the sinuses. Sarcoidosis of the upper respiratory tract is often relatively recalcitrant to therapy, and sinus involvement is more common in those with lupus pernio.

Hypercalcemia or hypercalciuria leading to nephrolithiasis can occur with sarcoidosis and may result in renal dysfunction. These phenomena are the result of the enzyme 1α-hydroxylase in activated macrophages that convert 25-hydroxyvitamin D to 1,25-dihydroxyvitamin D, the active form of the vitamin, which results in increased gut absorption and increased renal excretion of calcium that can cause nephrolithiasis. Patients with sarcoidosis-associated hypercalcemia typically have low 25-hydroxyvitamin D levels with 1,25-dihydroxyvitamin D levels that are elevated or at the upper limits of normal in combination with a low or low-normal parathyroid hormone.

Patients can have constitutional symptoms such as fever, night sweats, weight loss, malaise, and fatigue at report. These symptoms may be associated with hepatic sarcoid involvement but also may be a sign of the systemic nature of the disease, presumably from cytokine release, rather than specific organ involvement. A small fiber neuropathy may occur with sarcoidosis and cause pain or autonomic dysfunction.

Diagnosis and Initial Workup

The diagnosis of sarcoidosis requires a compatible clinical picture, histologic demonstration of noncaseating granulomas, and exclusion of other diseases capable of producing a similar histologic and clinical picture. It is prudent to bear a healthy degree of skepticism in the diagnosis, and patients should be evaluated closely for additional clues supporting an alternative diagnosis. Mycobacterial and fungal diseases must always be considered as alternative causes of granulomatous inflammation. Therefore stains and cultures of tissue specimens for mycobacteria and fungi should always be obtained when the diagnosis of sarcoidosis is considered. Hypersensitivity pneumonitis, a granulomatous lung disease from inhalation of bioaerosols, may also mimic sarcoidosis. Bioaerosols from hot tubs and birds are the most common causes of hypersensitivity pneumonitis, and clinicians should specifically inquire about these two exposures in individuals who are being evaluated for sarcoidosis. Sarcoidosis is a systemic disease, so signs or symptoms of extrathoracic disease should be sought. All patients should be evaluated for "dangerous" extrapulmonary manifestations, including cardiac, CNS, renal, and ocular involvement, as well as sarcoidosis-associated hypercalcemia.

It is prudent to select a biopsy site associated with less morbidity, such as the skin, if a lesion is present. Transthoracic needle aspiration of mediastinal lymph nodes under ultrasound guidance (EBUS-TBNA) via bronchoscopy has a high yield for the diagnosis of pulmonary sarcoidosis and was recommended over mediastinoscopy on recently published guidelines. Transbronchial lung biopsy has a diagnostic yield of 40% to more than

Clinical or Laboratory Findings That Strongly Support a Diagnosis of Sarcoidosis Without a Tissue Biopsy

- Löfgren syndrome
- Heerfordt syndrome (uveoparotid fever)
- Asymptomatic bilateral hilar adenopathy on chest x-ray
- Lupus pernio

90% in pulmonary sarcoidosis. Endobronchial biopsy has a 40% to 60% sensitivity and adds to the yield of transbronchial biopsy.

Bronchoalveolar lavage (BAL) with examination of lymphocyte populations has been used in the evaluation of possible pulmonary sarcoidosis. In sarcoidosis, there is an increased number of BAL lymphocytes, and these are predominantly CD4⁺. It has been proposed that an increase in BAL lymphocytes and a BAL CD4/CD8 ratio greater than 3.5 makes the diagnosis of sarcoidosis highly likely.

Although serum angiotensin-converting enzyme (ACE) often is elevated in active sarcoidosis, the specificity and sensitivity of this test are inadequate for it to be used diagnostically. Serum ACE may be used as supportive evidence for the diagnosis, and it also may be used in some instances to follow disease activity.

Gallium-67 (^{67}Ga) scanning is cumbersome because it takes several days to complete and is infrequently used as a diagnostic test. However, bilateral hilar uptake and right paratracheal uptake (lambda sign) coupled with lacrimal and parotid uptake (panda sign) with ^{67}Ga strongly suggest a diagnosis of sarcoidosis. Fluorodeoxyglucose PET scanning (outside the CNS) and MRI studies using contrast (CNS and cardiac) have essentially replaced ^{67}Ga scanning for detecting sarcoidosis activity.

Ideally, the diagnosis of sarcoidosis requires a demonstration of noncaseating granulomas in at least one organ. However, according to recently published guidelines, certain clinical presentations are so specific for the diagnosis of sarcoidosis that biopsy may not be necessary. Extreme caution must be used in these situations to ensure that there is no clinical information that would suggest an alternative diagnosis that should prompt a tissue biopsy. Clinical or laboratory findings that strongly support the diagnosis of sarcoidosis without a tissue biopsy are listed in Box 2.

In addition to screening for neurologic (symptoms) and cardiac (symptoms, ECG) involvement, all patients should undergo evaluation by an ophthalmologist (even in the absence of ocular symptoms). Laboratory testing to evaluate for other organ involvement at the time of diagnosis should include serum calcium, creatinine, alkaline phosphatase, and a complete blood count with differential.

Treatment

Therapy is often not mandatory for sarcoidosis because the disease can remit spontaneously. Systemic antisarcoidosis therapy is indicated for dangerous organ involvement and for disease causing significant quality-of-life impairment. Potentially dangerous disease includes neurosarcoidosis, cardiac sarcoidosis, renal sarcoidosis, hypercalcemia that does not respond to dietary measures, and ocular sarcoidosis that does not respond to topical (eye drop) therapy. Therapy should also be considered when the disease is progressive and at risk of resulting in long-term morbidity. In general, treatment is discouraged for asymptomatic stage I pulmonary sarcoidosis, elevations of serum liver function tests, or specific levels of ACE.

The decision to treat sarcoidosis can be problematic because the disease has a variable prognosis that must be weighed against the potential side effects of therapy. It is often most prudent to monitor patients without therapy if they are asymptomatic or have only mild organ dysfunction. For pulmonary sarcoidosis, patients who are asymptomatic and those with mild disease that might spontaneously remit usually are not treated. For patients with clinical findings that predict spontaneous remission (e.g., erythema nodosum), the benefits of treatment often are offset by

the toxicity of therapy. Often these patients can be managed with supportive therapy such as nonsteroidal antiinflammatory drugs for arthralgias and fever or bronchodilators and inhaled corticosteroids for wheezing and cough.

It is recommended that patients with mild to moderate pulmonary sarcoidosis be observed for 2 to 6 months, if possible. Patients who improve will have avoided the toxicity of corticosteroids, and patients who deteriorate over this period should be considered for treatment. Patients with pulmonary dysfunction who neither improve nor deteriorate during the observation period may be given a corticosteroid trial, or they may be observed further. Patients with severe pulmonary dysfunction or pulmonary symptoms causing significant impairment should be treated.

Corticosteroids are considered first-line therapy for the treatment of sarcoidosis, but the dose, duration of therapy, and methods by which one can assess effectiveness have not been standardized. Topical corticosteroid therapy should be used whenever possible in an attempt to minimize systemic complications. This includes corticosteroid eye drops for anterior sarcoid uveitis and corticosteroid creams and injections for localized skin lesions. Prolonged use of topical steroids for ocular and cutaneous sarcoidosis is associated with an increased risk of side effects (glaucoma, cataracts, skin discoloration and thinning). Recent guidelines published by the European Respiratory Society provide some guidance to the dosing of oral steroid regimens. Pulmonary sarcoidosis usually is treated initially with 20 mg/day of prednisone or its equivalent. Higher doses may be required for neurosarcoidosis and cardiac sarcoidosis. Some advocate for doses as high as 1 mg/kg/day for cardiac and neurologic involvement, although this should not be considered standard practice for all presentations because studies have not consistently shown a clear benefit. Regardless of the starting dose, the patient should be evaluated within 2 to 12 weeks for a response, with the goal of tapering corticosteroids down to the lowest effective dose (ideally <10 mg/day) as quickly as possible. This dose is usually continued for at least 6 months. Patients failing to respond to therapy within 3 months are unlikely to respond to a more protracted course of therapy or a higher dose.

The relapse rate after corticosteroid therapy is withdrawn may be as high as 70%, and therefore patients need to be followed closely as the corticosteroid dose is tapered and discontinued. In some patients, there may be recurrent relapses requiring long-term, low-dose therapy. On occasion, the chronic prednisone dose needed to prevent relapse is less than 5 mg/day. Patients who relapse after corticosteroids have been withdrawn can be retreated with corticosteroids. However, corticosteroid-sparing agents should be considered in patients who are unable to taper the corticosteroids to less than 10 mg/day to control the disease.

Methotrexate (Trexall)[1] is the most studied alternative sarcoidosis medication and is usually used as a corticosteroid-sparing agent but at times can be used as replacement therapy. Methotrexate is most useful for pulmonary, skin, joint, and eye sarcoidosis. The goal weekly dose is 10 to 15 mg. Hydroxychloroquine (Plaquenil)[1] given once or twice daily may be used for sarcoidosis of the skin, joints, nerves, and for hypercalcemia from sarcoidosis, but it has not been shown to be beneficial for pulmonary sarcoidosis. Because of the risk of retinal toxicity, most patients should not receive a daily dose greater than 5 mg/kg/day or greater than 400 mg, whichever is lower. Azathioprine (Imuran)[1] is also useful as a second-line therapy for sarcoidosis. The initial dose is typically 50 mg once a day, which can be increased by 50 mg every 2 to 4 weeks as tolerated to a maximum dose of 2 mg/kg once daily. Leflunomide (Arava)[1] has also been shown to be useful in the treatment of pulmonary and extrapulmonary sarcoidosis. Monoclonal antibodies against TNF-α, such as infliximab (Remicade)[1] and adalimumab (Humira)[1], are useful agents in patients with

---

[1]Not FDA approved for this indication.

severe sarcoidosis and/or who fail to respond to the aforementioned treatments. Patients treated with these second-line and third-line medications should undergo regular drug-specific toxicity monitoring and may require modifications in therapy to avoid adverse effects. Minocycline (Minocin)[1] and doxycycline (Vibramycin)[1] (100 mg twice daily) may be useful for skin sarcoidosis. Cyclosporine is ineffective for pulmonary sarcoidosis. To date, the efficacy of antifibrotic medications in sarcoidosis remains unclear and its role (if any) in the treatment of fibrotic sarcoidosis requires further investigation. Therapy should also be considered for the nongranulomatous aspects of the disease. Sarcoidosis-associated small fiber neuropathy may respond to medications for neuropathic pain, monoclonal antibodies against TNF-α, or intravenous immunoglobulin[1]. Sarcoidosis-associated fatigue may benefit from a physical training program, neurostimulants, or monoclonal antibodies against TNF-α.

References

Baughman RP, Culver DA, Judson MA: A concise review of pulmonary sarcoidosis, *Am J Respir Crit Care Med* 183:573–589, 2011.

Baughman RP, Field S, Costabel U: Sarcoidosis in America: analysis based on health care use, *Ann Am Thorac Soc* 13:244–252, 2016.

Baughman RP, Nunes H, Sweiss NJ, et al: Established and experimental medical therapy of pulmonary sarcoidosis, *Eur Respir J* 41(6):1424–1438, 2013.

Baughman RP, Teirstein AS, Judson MA, et al: Clinical characteristics of patients in a case control study of sarcoidosis, *Am J Respir Crit Care Med* 164:1885–1889, 2001.

Baughman RP, Valeyre D, Korsten P, et al: ERS clinical practice guidelines on treatment of sarcoidosis, *Eur Respir J* 58(6):2004079, 2021. 16.

Belperio JA, Shaikh F, Abtin FG, et al: Diagnosis and treatment of pulmonary sarcoidosis: a review, *JAMA* 327(9):856–867, 2022.

Birnie DH, Sauer WH, Bogun F, et al: HRS expert consensus statement on the diagnosis and management of arrythmias associated with cardiac sarcoidosis, *Heart Rhythm* 11:1304–1323, 2014.

Chen ES, Song Z, Willett MH, et al: Serum amyloid A regulates granulomatous inflammation in sarcoidosis through Toll-like receptor-2, *Am J Respir Crit Care Med* 181:360–373, 2010.

Elliot CD, Maier LA, Wilson KC, et al: Diagnosis and detection of sarcoidosis: an official American Thoracic Society clinical practice guideline, *Am J Respir Crit Care Med* 201(8):e26–e51, 2020.

Hamzeh N, Steckman D, Sauer W, Judson MA: Pathophysiology and clinical management of cardiac sarcoidosis, *Nat Rev Cardiol* 12:278–288, 2015.

Judson MA: The clinical features of sarcoidosis: a comprehensive review, *Clinic Rev Allerg Immunol* 49:63–78, 2015.

Judson MA: The diagnosis of sarcoidosis, *Clin Chest Med* 29:415–427, 2008.

Judson MA, Costabel U, Drent M, et al: The WASOG sarcoidosis organ assessment Investigators. The WASOG sarcoidosis organ assessment instrument: an update of a previous clinical tool, *Sarcoidosis Vasc Diff Lung Dis* 31:19–27, 2014.

Lower EE, Baughman RP: Prolonged use of methotrexate in refractory sarcoidosis, *Arch Intern Med* 155:846–851, 1995.

Nardi A, Brillet P, Letoumelin P, et al: Stage IV sarcoidosis: comparison of survival with the general population and cause of death, *Eur Respir J* 38:1368–1373, 2011.

Tavee JO, Karwa K, Ahmed Z, et al: Sarcoidosis-associated small fiber neuropathy in a large cohort: clinical aspects and response to IVIG and anti-TNF alpha treatment, *Respir Med* 126:135–138, 2017.

Thillai M, Atkins CP, Crawshaw A, et al: BTS clinical statement on pulmonary sarcoidosis, *Thorax* 76(1):4–20, 2021.

TUBERCULOSIS AND OTHER MYCOBACTERIAL DISEASES

Method of
Lizbeth Cahuayme-Zuniga, MD

CURRENT DIAGNOSIS

- Latent tuberculosis infection (LTBI) is diagnosed in an asymptomatic individual who has been previously exposed to tuberculosis (TB) and has a positive blood interferon-gamma release assay (IGRA) or a tuberculin skin test (TST).
- A positive IGRA or TST does not distinguish LTBI from active TB disease.

- Active TB is diagnosed based on clinical manifestations, microbiological evidence, and radiographic evidence of disease.
- Culture is the gold standard microbiologic test for diagnosing TB disease. Microscopy (acid-fast bacilli [AFB] smear) and molecular nucleic acid amplification test (NAAT) are also useful for diagnosis.
- All patients with LTBI or TB disease should undergo human immunodeficiency virus (HIV) testing.

CURRENT THERAPY

- LTBI: the three preferred regimens are rifamycin-based regimens for 3 to 4 months.
- Treatment of TB disease should be done in conjunction with the local public health department.
- Drug-susceptible pulmonary TB disease: standard regimen: isoniazid (INH) + rifampin (RFP) + pyrazinamide (PZA) + ethambutol (EMB) for 2 months, followed by 4 months of INH + RFP. New shortened regimen: INH + Rifapentine (RPT) + Moxifloxacin (MOX) + PZA for 2 months, followed by 2 months of INH + RPT + MOX.
- Drug-susceptible extrapulmonary TB disease is typically treated as per pulmonary TB disease, but treatment and duration vary based on the anatomic site(s) involved.
- Treatment of drug-resistant TB disease should be done in consultation with a TB expert.

Tuberculosis

Epidemiology

Tuberculosis (TB) disease remains one of the significant causes of morbidity and mortality in the world. About one-fourth of the global population is estimated to have been infected with TB at some point. According to the World Health Organization (WHO), approximately 7.5 million individuals received a new TB diagnosis in 2022. *M. tuberculosis* was the second leading cause of death from an infectious agent, following COVID-19, and caused almost double the number of fatalities seen from human immunodeficiency virus (HIV). In this context, drug-resistant TB remains a deadly communicable disease in several parts of the world and poses a serious global health threat. The WHO estimated that 410,000 people developed multidrug-resistant (MDR) TB around the globe in 2022. Resistant strains contribute to 15% to 20% of global TB mortality.

Microbiology

TB is caused by one of the species from the *Mycobacterium tuberculosis* complex, which comprises at least nine species in the genus *Mycobacterium*. The species *Mycobacterium tuberculosis* sensu stricto causes most of the human TB worldwide, followed by *Mycobacterium africanum*, which causes human TB in West Africa, where it accounts for up to 50% of cases. Other Mycobacterium species that have been reported to cause TB disease in humans include *Mycobacterium bovis*, *Mycobacterium microti*, *Mycobacterium caprae*, *Mycobacterium canetti*, and *Mycobacterium pinnipedii*. *M. tuberculosis* is an aerobic, slow-growing, non–spore-forming, nonmotile bacillus. Its complex cell envelope is rich in high-molecular-weight lipids, which make it acid-fast (resist decolorization by acid solutions during staining procedures). It grows slowly and takes 3 to 8 weeks to be seen on solid media.

Transmissibility

In most cases, *M. tuberculosis* spreads from person to person via the airborne route. When a person with pulmonary TB disease coughs, sneezes, talks, or sings, they produce aerosolized particles (droplet nuclei) containing the tubercle bacilli that can remain suspended in the air for prolonged periods; when inhaled by another individual, they can reach the terminal air passages. Prolonged exposure and multiple aerosol inocula are usually required to establish infection. The probability of transmitting *M. tuberculosis* depends on several factors: (1) infectiousness of the patient with TB disease, especially when the sputum smear is positive for acid-fast bacilli (AFB) or if there is evidence of cavitary pulmonary TB because cavities carry a high bacterial load making patients highly contagious; (2) host susceptibility (i.e., immunosuppression due to use of steroids); (3) length of exposure to the individual with TB disease; (4) the environment in which the exposure takes place (highest risk in small and poor ventilated spaces); and (5) characteristics of the *M. tuberculosis* strain. Other less common modes of transmission include skin inoculation, aerosolization from a nonpulmonary source (i.e., irrigation of infected wounds), donor-derived transmitted infection, ingestion of unpasteurized contaminated milk (in the case of *Mycobacterium bovis*), and rarely venereal transmission.

Pathophysiology
Primary Initial Infection
After inhalation, the droplet nucleus carrying the tubercle bacilli is transported through the upper airways and arrives in the alveolar space of the middle or lower lung lobes. The immune response to *M. tuberculosis* is primarily cell-mediated. The tubercle bacilli are engulfed by alveolar macrophages, which may successfully kill the mycobacteria. Alternatively, a primary infection occurs when the mycobacteria release virulence factors that allow them to survive within the macrophage phagosomes, where they can replicate and eventually destroy the macrophages. Inflammatory cells are released, and focal pneumonitis occurs.

Latent Tuberculosis Infection
Following the primary infection, *M. tuberculosis* replicates in the initial focus of infection. It spreads via the lymphatics to the hilar lymph nodes and then through the bloodstream to more distant anatomic sites. The development of cellular immunity is delayed, and it takes approximately 4 to 8 weeks to contain the infection. The pathologic features of TB will depend on the degree of hypersensitivity and the local concentration of antigen. The formation of granulomas with caseous necrosis could be seen where the tubercle bacilli may remain in a state of latency for years. People with latent TB infection (LTBI) have no clinical evidence of TB disease and are not contagious to others, although they are at risk of developing active TB disease. In a small number of cases, people may develop a significant reaction in the initial pulmonary focus (the Ghon focus) and the draining regional lymph nodes (the Ranke complex), resulting in radiographically visible calcification. Among individuals infected with *M. tuberculosis* who develop a cellular CD4+ T-cell response, 90% to 95% will be able to contain the infection, avoiding the progression to active TB diseases. The tuberculin skin test (TST) and interferon-gamma release blood assays (IGRA) turn positive during this latency period. The onset of tuberculin hypersensitivity may be associated with erythema nodosum or phlyctenular keratoconjunctivitis (a severe unilateral inflammation of the eye).

Active Tuberculosis Disease
Once *M. tuberculosis* establishes an infection, its progression from LTBI to active TB disease will depend on host factors (most notably the immune system state) and microbial virulence. In certain people, such as children, patients of advanced age, or individuals living with HIV, the primary focus of infection may progress to pneumonia (known as progressive primary disease), and it may cavitate and spread. On average, 5% to 10% of those infected will develop active TB disease throughout their lifetime, usually within the first five years after initial infection. The greatest risk of progression is during the first 2 years following exposure. Host characteristics associated with progression from infection to TB disease include young children (<4 years old), silicosis, diabetes mellitus, diseases associated with immunosuppression such as HIV and immunosuppressive drugs such as corticosteroids, tumor necrosis factor (TNF) inhibitors, among others. TB disease occurs most often in the lung apices, but any part of the body can be affected. Those metastatic foci with the initial infection may become new nidus of infection and reactivate, causing TB disease. Common extrapulmonary sites include lymph nodes, pleura, pericardium, vertebra, gastrointestinal and genitourinary tract, eye, and meninges.

Prevention
Preventing the transmission of TB disease involves multiple measures. Some essential components include (1) early screening and detection of patients infected with *M. tuberculosis*, preventing them from progressing from LTBI to TB disease; (2) rapid identification and prompt airborne isolation of patients with suspected or confirmed TB disease; (3) early and adequate treatment of patients with TB disease; and (4) implementation of infection prevention and control measures (critical in situations where the risk of TB transmission is high, such as healthcare facilities, congregate settings, and households affected by TB).

Immunization
The bacille Calmette-Guérin (BCG) vaccine is a live-attenuated vaccine derived from *Mycobacterium bovis*. It is used in countries with high TB prevalence. It has been shown to prevent progression to severe forms of TB disease and dissemination, predominantly in young children. The BCG vaccine can alter TST results, and its effects depend on the vaccination age and the immunization interval before testing (it can give false-positive results due to cross-reactivity with BCG components). The BCG vaccine doesn't affect IGRA's results and is the test of choice for those individuals with prior vaccination. There is currently no licensed vaccine that is effective in preventing TB disease in adults; however, an investigational TB vaccine candidate (M72/AS01E) showed promising results in a Phase IIb trial in HIV-negative adults with evidence of LTBI when it demonstrated 50% efficacy (90% CI, 12-71) over approximately 3 years of follow-up. The development of TB vaccines is a priority, and until mid-2023, WHO reported 16 vaccine candidates in clinical trials.

Clinical Manifestations
Primary infection is usually asymptomatic. Patients with LTBI have no symptoms and no clinical evidence of disease. A person with active TB disease may be initially asymptomatic, but as the bacilli multiplies and the disease progresses, symptoms will appear according to the organ involvement. Patients with pulmonary TB classically present with a chronic cough, sputum production, and non-specific constitutional symptoms such as fever, chills, night sweats, and weight loss. Hemoptysis can occur, and it indicates advanced disease. Extrapulmonary TB can affect almost any organ in the body and can present with a wide range of manifestations depending on the anatomic site affected. TB lymphadenitis, or scrofula, is the most common form of extrapulmonary TB. Cervical adenopathy is the most common presentation. Over time, the lymph nodes can progress to abscess with sinus tract formation. Pleural TB is characterized by symptoms of unilateral pleural effusion, often accompanied by acute illness, cough, chest pain, fever, and dyspnea. Skeletal TB most often involves the spine. Spinal TB is known as Pott's disease, and it most often affects the thoracic spine; patients present with local pain, constitutional symptoms, or paraplegia secondary to cord compression. Central nervous system (CNS) TB's most common presentation is meningitis. Patients present initially with malaise, headache, fever, or personality change followed by protracted headache, meningismus, vomiting, confusion, and focal neurologic findings. If untreated, it can lead to seizures, stupor, and coma.

Diagnosis
Latent Tuberculosis

The first and most crucial step in diagnosing LTBI is ensuring that the person has no clinical, microbiological, or radiographic evidence of active TB disease. This is accomplished through a comprehensive medical history and detailed physical exam, assessing the patient's risk factors for primary infection and progression to TB disease, inquiring about any epidemiological exposures and prior BCG vaccination, addressing any symptomatology in conjunction with obtaining a chest radiograph looking for any radiographic signs suspicious of active TB as lung cavities, pleural effusions, airspace opacities or new lung lesions on serial examinations. The American Thoracic Society (ATS), Infectious Diseases Society of America (IDSA), and the Centers for Disease Control (CDC) recommend screening for LTBI based on the likelihood of infection (such as recent immigrants or closed TB contacts), the possibility of increased risk of progression to TB disease, and in cases where preventing therapy is beneficial for the patient. Initial testing is recommended in individuals whose activities put them at risk of infection, such as healthcare or correctional facility employees.

The U.S. Food and Drug Administration (FDA) has approved two methods of immunologic testing for M. tuberculosis infection: the blood IGRAs and the TST. These tests measure the TB-specific immune response as an indirect assessment of infection. However, they do not distinguish infection from disease and poorly predict TB progression. The TST detects cell-mediated immunity to M. tuberculosis through a delayed-type hypersensitivity reaction using a protein precipitate of heat-inactivated tubercle bacilli (purified protein derivative [PPD]–tuberculin). The TST (Tubersol) is administered by the intradermal injection of 0.1 mL of PPD into the volar surface of the forearm (Mantoux method) to produce a transient wheal. Based on risk stratification for different populations, the induration reaction is interpreted at 48 to 72 hours following established cut points. A reaction of 5 mm or greater is considered positive for close contacts of TB cases, immunosuppressed persons (including HIV, organ transplant recipients, patients taking the equivalent of ≥15 mg/day of prednisone for 1 month or longer, and TNF blockers users), and persons with fibrotic changes on chest radiograph consistent with old TB. A reaction of ≥10 mm is considered positive in people from countries where TB is endemic, injection drug users, residents, and employees of high-risk congregate settings (e.g., correctional facilities, nursing homes, homeless shelters, hospitals, and other healthcare facilities), mycobacteriology laboratory personnel, and children under 4 years of age. A reaction of 15 mm or greater is considered positive for all other people. TST contains antigenic compounds that cross-react with BCG and non-tuberculous mycobacteria, potentially causing false-positive reactions. False-negative reactions can occur in a few instances: in infants and young children, in immunocompromised hosts due to medical conditions or as a result of immunosuppressive drugs (e.g., high-dose steroids, TNF-inhibitor), during the first weeks following primary infection, in persons receiving vaccination with live virus, in patients with severe or disseminated disease, and following recent viral and bacterial infections.

IGRAs are in vitro, T-cell-based assays that measure interferon-gamma (IFN-γ) release by sensitized T-cells in response to highly specific M. tuberculosis antigens. It is the preferred test in persons who have received BCG (either as a vaccine or for cancer therapy) and in those who are unlikely to return for a TST reading. Currently, there are two commercially available IGRA platforms: the QuantiFERON TB Gold In Tube (QFT-GIT; Cellestis Limited, Carnegie, Victoria, Australia) and the T-SPOT TB test (T-SPOT, manufactured by Oxford Immunotec Ltd, Abingdon, United Kingdom). The QFT-GIT measures IFN-γ plasma concentration using an enzyme-linked immunosorbent assay (ELISA), while the T-SPOT assay enumerates T cells releasing IFN-γ using an enzyme-linked immunospot (ELISPOT) assay. False-positive IGRA results can be seen with infections due to *Mycobacterium marinum*, *Mycobacterium kansasii*, *Mycobacterium gordonae*, and *Mycobacterium szulgai*.

Active Tuberculosis

Active TB is diagnosed based on clinical manifestations, microbiological evidence, and radiographic evidence of disease. Four diagnostic modalities exist to help with the diagnosis, including image techniques, microscopy (AFB smear), culture-based methods, and molecular nucleic acid amplification test (NAAT).

In pulmonary TB, it is recommended that three sputum specimens be obtained for AFB smears, AFB cultures, and NAAT (when available). The NAAT assay confirms that the infecting mycobacteria are from the M. tuberculosis complex. Appropriate NAATs include the Hologic Amplified Mycobacteria Tuberculosis Direct and the Cepheid Xpert MTB/Rif test. The latter provides a real-time (polymerase chain reaction) PCR to detect M. tuberculosis and rifampicin (Rifadin, Rimactane) resistance in a single automated cartridge. Culture is the gold standard for detecting mycobacteria in clinical specimens and performing drug susceptibility testing and genotyping. Visible growth on solid media can take up to 8 weeks; liquid media growth results can be faster, 2 to 3 weeks. Induced sputum with hypertonic saline is recommended for patients unable to expectorate sputum. Flexible bronchoscopy can be pursued to obtain respiratory specimens when sputum smears are negative. If an AFB smear from respiratory specimens is positive but the NAAT is negative, then it is unlikely that the positive smear is due to active TB disease. If a patient suspected to have TB disease has a negative AFB smear but positive NAAT for a respiratory specimen, then a presumptive diagnosis of TB disease can be given. However, a negative NAAT is not enough to rule out pulmonary TB disease.

If there is a suspicion of active extrapulmonary disease, the fluid or tissue potentially affected should be sampled for testing, including AFB smear microscopy, AFB culture, NAAT, and histopathology. Adenosine deaminase levels can be measured in pleural, cerebral spinal fluid, ascitic, and pericardial fluids.

Treatment
Latent Tuberculosis Infection

The aim of treating LTBI is to prevent individuals at high risk of TB infection from progressing to TB disease. Without treatment, approximately 5% to 10% of immunocompetent persons with LTBI develop active TB disease in their lifetime. After confirming that active TB is not present, LTBI treatment can begin. The National Tuberculosis Controllers Association (NTCA) and the CDC updated guidelines in 2020 for treating LTBI for persons living in the United States. Three preferred and two alternative regimens are recommended for treating LTBI (Table 1). The preferred regimens are rifamycin-based, including 3 months of once-weekly isoniazid (Nydrazid) (INH) plus rifapentine (Priftin) (RPT), 4 months of daily rifampin (Rifadin, Rimactane) (RFP), and 3 months of daily INH plus RFP. These regimens are preferred due to their effectiveness, safety, and high completion rates. For those who are at risk of drug interactions or experiencing adverse effects with the preferred regimens, INH for either 6 or 9 months is an alternative. Six months of daily INH is strongly recommended as an alternative for HIV-negative adults and children of all ages. INH may cause or worsen peripheral neuropathy. To prevent this, vitamin B6, known as pyridoxine[1] (25–50 mg), should be administered with INH to patients at risk of peripheral neuropathy. A dose of 100 mg is recommended for those with established neuropathy. It is advisable to seek consultation from a TB expert if the patient has been in contact with someone who has known drug-resistant TB.

Active Tuberculosis Disease

Treatment should be started promptly after collecting specimens for a patient suspected of having active TB disease. Treatment should not be delayed while waiting for confirmation by culture or drug-susceptibility molecular test results. Before beginning

---

[1] Not FDA approved for this indication.

PREFERED REGIMENS	DURATION OF THERAPY	DOSAGES	FREQUENCY OF ADMINISTRATION
INH* + RPT	3 months	Adults and children aged >12 years: INH: 15 mg/kg; 900 mg maximum dose RPT: 10–14 kg: 300 mg; 14–25 kg: 450 mg; 25–32 kg: 600 mg; 32–49.9 kg: 750 mg; ≥50 kg: 900 mg maximum dose	Once weekly
RFP	4 months	Adults: 10 mg/kg, maximum dose 600 mg	Daily
INH* + RFP	3 months	Adults: INH: 5 mg/kg, maximum dose 300 mg RFP: 10 mg/kg, maximum dose 600 mg	Daily

*Vitamin B6 (pyridoxine)[1] is given in conjunction with INH.
[1]Not FDA approved for this indication.
INH, Isoniazid (Nydrazid); *RFP*, rifampin (Rifadin, Rimactane); *RPT*, rifapentine (Priftin).
Adapted from Sterling TR, Njie G, Zenner D, et al: Guidelines for the treatment of latent tuberculosis infection: Recommendations from the National Tuberculosis Controllers Association and CDC, *MMWR Recomm Rep* 69(No. RR-1), 2020.

therapy, a complete medical evaluation, including history and physical evaluation, baseline complete blood count, blood chemistries (including assessment of kidney and liver function tests), HIV screening, and pertinent imaging should be performed. Viral hepatitis screening for hepatitis B and C should be obtained if risk factors or if an abnormal liver function test at baseline. The treatment regimen for active TB disease relies on using multiple antibiotics to which the bacterial isolate is either presumed or known to be susceptible. TB regimens vary in duration, types of anti-TB drugs prescribed, and the dose and frequency of the drugs.

Drug Susceptible Pulmonary Tuberculosis. The standard 6-month regimen for treatment of drug-susceptible pulmonary disease in the United States (Table 2) consists of a 2-month intensive phase of four drugs: INH, RFP, pyrazinamide (Zinamide) (PZA), and ethambutol (Myambutol) (EMB), taken daily, followed by a continuation phase of INH and RFP for 4 months. If drug susceptibilities are available before starting treatment, EMB doesn't need to be included in the regimen. Once susceptibility to INH and RFP is confirmed, EMB can be discontinued. The CDC recommends continuous daily dosing of the above agents rather than intermittent dosing for the intensive and continuation phases of treatment. As discussed previously, pyridoxine (vitamin B6)[1] should be given throughout INH administration. Under certain conditions, the continuation phase may be extended beyond 4 months. In 2022, the CDC recommended a new 4-month regimen as a treatment option for drug-susceptible pulmonary TB (Table 3). This shortened regimen involves taking INH, high-dose RPT, PZA, and moxifloxacin (Avelox) (MOX)[1] daily for 2 months, followed by a 2-month continuation phase that consists of INH, high-dose RPT, and MOX. This new regimen is available to patients aged 12 and older. However, it should not be used during pregnancy or breastfeeding. Patients with HIV infection who are receiving efavirenz (Sustiva) (EFV)-based regimen for HIV treatment may use this medication. CDC recommends extending the continuation phase to 7 months in people with (1) cavitary pulmonary TB and whose sputum culture remained positive at completion of 2 months of therapy; (2) in people whose intensive phase didn't include PZA; (3) in patients with HIV who are not on antiretroviral therapy (ARV) during TB treatment; and (4) in the rare circumstance that patient was treated with once-weekly INH and RFP and whose sputum cultures remains positive at completion of the intensive phase.

Extrapulmonary Tuberculosis. The treatment regimens for extrapulmonary disease will depend on the anatomic site involved. Treatment for cutaneous, genitourinary, gastrointestinal, lymphatic, pleural, and pericardial TB is the same as for pulmonary

[1]Not FDA approved for this indication.

TABLE 2	Preferred Regimen for Drug Susceptible Pulmonary Tuberculosis	
INTENSIVE PHASE	**DURATION**	**ADULT DOSAGE FOR DAILY ADMINISTRATION**
INH* RFP PZA EMB	7 days per week for 8 weeks OR 5 days per week for 8 weeks	INH: 5 mg/kg (typically 300 mg) RFP: 10 mg/kg (typically 600 mg) PZA: 30–40 mg/kg EMB: 15–25 mg/kg
CONTINUATION PHASE	**DURATION**	**ADULT DOSAGE FOR DAILY ADMINISTRATION**
INH* RFP	7 days per week for 18 weeks OR 5 days a week for 18 weeks	INH: 5 mg/kg (typically 300 mg) RFP: 10 mg/kg (typically 600 mg)

*Vitamin B6 (pyridoxine)[1] is given in conjunction with INH.
[1]Not FDA approved for this indication.
EMB, Ethambutol (Myambutol); *INH*, isoniazid (Nydrazid); *PZA*, pyrazinamide (Zinamide); *RFP*, rifampin (Rifadin, Rimactane).

disease. In pericardial TB, the use of corticosteroids is not routinely recommended unless the patient is at a higher risk of complications (i.e., large pericardial effusions, high levels of inflammatory cells or markers in pericardial fluid, or early signs of constriction). In CNS TB, treatment is prolonged; the standard intensive phase regimen is the same as for pulmonary TB disease, but the continuation phase lasts 7 to 10 months. INH, RFP, and PZA penetrate the blood–brain barrier efficiently. EMB and injectable agents penetrate only when the meninges are inflamed. Adjunctive corticosteroids have been shown to improve survival in individuals with severe CNS TB and may reduce neurologic morbidity as well. Corticosteroids are only given if the patient is on anti-TB therapy.

Monitoring

During the treatment of LTBI or suspected/confirmed TB disease, patients are closely monitored to ensure they respond well to the therapy, adhere to the prescribed treatment, and do not experience any adverse reactions. Studies have found that the primary reason for relapse, treatment failure, or drug resistance is nonadherence to medication. Therefore, to ensure that patients take their medication as directed, directly observed therapy (DOT) is recommended as the standard of care for TB treatment. This approach involves observing patients swallowing their TB medication. Video DOT uses video-enabled devices to facilitate remote interactions and is recommended by the CDC as an alternative to in-person DOT. All patients diagnosed with LTBI or TB disease must undergo baseline HIV testing. In addition, if the patient has

TABLE 3	Four-Month Regimen for Drug Susceptible Pulmonary Tuberculosis			
MEDICATION	ADULT DOSAGE FOR DAILY ADMINISTRATION	INTENSIVE PHASE	CONTINUATION PHASE	
RPT	≥40 kg: 1200 mg	7 days/wk for 56 doses (8 wks)	7 days/wk for 63 doses (9 wks)	
MOX[1]	≥40 kg: 400 mg			
INH*	≥40 kg: 300 mg			
PZA	40–<55 kg: 1000 mg; ≥55–75: 1500 mg; >75 kg: 2000 mg		N/A	

*Vitamin B6 (pyridoxine)[1] is given in conjunction with INH.
[1]Not FDA approved for this indication.
INH, Isoniazid (Nydrazid); *MOX,* moxifloxacin (Avelox); *PZA,* pyrazinamide (Zinamide); *RFP,* rifampin (Rifadin, Rimactane); *RPT,* rifapentine (Priftin).

TABLE 4	Major Adverse Effects of First-Line Medications for the Treatment of Tuberculosis Disease
FIRST LINE MEDICATIONS	MOST COMMON ADVERSE EFFECTS
INH	Hepatotoxicity Dermatitis (Rash) Drug-induced lupus Peripheral neuropathy
Rifamycins (RFP, RPT, RFB)	Hepatotoxicity Dermatitis (Rash) GI upset Thrombocytopenia Hypersensitivity reactions
PZA	Hepatotoxicity Dermatitis (Rash) GI upset Gout
EMB	Optic neuritis Dermatitis (Rash)

EMB, Ethambutol (Myambutol); *INH,* isoniazid (Nydrazid); *PZA,* pyrazinamide (Zinamide); *RFB,* rifabutin (Mycobutin); *RFP,* rifampin (Rifadin, Rimactane); *RPT,* rifapentine (Priftin).

risk factors for hepatitis B and/or C, baseline serologies should also be checked.

Latent TB

Patients receiving LTBI treatment should be evaluated monthly for adherence, adverse effects, and signs or symptoms of TB disease. Baseline laboratory testing is not routinely indicated for all patients starting LTBI treatment. It is recommended that patients who are at risk for liver disease or who regularly use alcohol, inject drugs, have HIV, or are pregnant or less than 3 months postpartum undergo baseline liver function testing. For individuals who are at high risk of developing TB disease or have concerns about medication adherence, DOT for LTBI treatment should be considered. After baseline testing, routine periodic retesting (e.g., monthly) is recommended for persons with abnormal initial results and others at risk for hepatic disease. Patients who experience symptoms suggestive of hepatitis (e.g., fatigue, weakness, malaise, anorexia, nausea, vomiting, abdominal pain, pale stools, brown urine, chills) or who have jaundice should undergo laboratory testing.

Active TB

When treating TB disease, a monitoring plan specific to the patient should be developed in collaboration with the local Department of Health. As previously mentioned, all patients should have baseline HIV testing and, if indicated, viral hepatitis screening. All patients should have a baseline laboratory, including a complete blood count, metabolic chemistry panel, and liver function test. Patients should be evaluated monthly for medication response and adverse effects during therapy (Table 4). Periodic laboratory testing is recommended if there are abnormalities at baseline or if the patient experiences adverse drug effects. In cases of pulmonary TB, monthly sputum or other respiratory specimens should be obtained to evaluate the bacteriological response. If the patient remains culture-positive after at least 2 months of treatment, repeat drug susceptibility testing must be performed to exclude a resistant strain. Repeat chest radiographs can be pursued if clinically indicated (e.g., symptoms fail to improve). Treatment failure may occur due to medication nonadherence, drug resistance, malabsorption, or drug interactions.

Complications

Anti-TB medications can cause various adverse reactions such as nausea, vision loss, fatigue, dermatitis (rash), and hepatitis. The occurrence of these reactions is influenced by both the specific medication and the individual medical conditions. If there is an adverse reaction that cannot be attributed to a specific anti-TB medication, all anti-TB medications should be stopped. They should then be gradually reintroduced to identify the cause of the adverse reaction. Among the common side effects, it is

important to remark that all first-line agents can cause dermatitis (most commonly from PZA). A more severe form of dermatitis associated with fever and mucus membrane involvement suggests Steven-Johnson syndrome or toxic epidermal necrolysis and warrants prompt discontinuation of all medications and a dermatology evaluation. Drug-induced hepatitis is one of the major complications in the treatment of patients with TB. Two patterns of liver function test abnormalities may be seen: hepatocellular and cholestatic (usually caused by INH or PZA) and a cholestatic pattern (caused by RFP). EMB rarely causes hepatitis. It is generally recommended that medication be withheld if a patient's transaminase level exceeds three times the upper limit of normal or if it is associated with symptoms or five times the upper limit of normal if the patient is asymptomatic. INH, as discussed previously, may cause peripheral neuropathy, especially in individuals with a predisposing cause, such as alcoholism, diabetes, HIV, or malnutrition. Pyridoxine (vitamin B6)[1] should be used with INH to prevent INH-induced neuropathy. It is important to know that INH (rarely, RFP) can induce active systemic lupus erythematosus, especially in patients with sub-clinical disease. PZA impairs renal excretion of uric acid, increasing its level. Therefore, patients with a history of gout are at increased risk for PZA-related gout attacks. Patients taking ETB should undergo baseline and routine vision screenings (visual acuity and color vision) due to the risk of optic neuritis.

Special Situations

Tuberculosis and Tumor Necrosis Factor Inhibitors

TNF plays a significant role in the initial and long-term control of *M. tuberculosis* through various mechanisms. As a result, patients who receive TNF inhibitors are at higher risk of reactivation and severe disease. Therefore, before starting anti-TNF blockers, all patients should undergo a complete clinical evaluation, including a test for IGRA and radiographic imaging to screen for TB. If IGRA is not available, then a TST can be used instead. This screening process should continue annually after that. If LTBI is detected, all patients should receive appropriate treatment and initiation of TNF blocker should be delayed for at least a month.

Tuberculosis and HIV Coinfection

Individuals who have HIV are at a high risk of developing TB disease, even if their CD4+ T cell count is normal. Worldwide,

---

[1] Not FDA approved for this indication.

HIV-positive people account for about 12% of all new cases of active TB disease and 25% of all TB-related deaths. The level of immunodeficiency influences the severity of TB disease. In HIV-positive patients with CD4+ T counts above 200 cells/mm^3, the presentation of TB disease is similar to that of people who do not have HIV. However, in those with CD4 counts below 200 cells/mm^3, pulmonary cavity formation is less common, sputum bacillary load decreases, and it often affects the lower lobes. Initiation of TB treatment in patients with HIV is complex and requires the expertise of a healthcare physician who specializes in treating both conditions. In general, it must address potential drug interactions, optimal timing for initiating ART in ART-naive patients, and potential for the immune reconstitution inflammatory syndrome (a paradoxical worsening of signs and symptoms of infection after ART initiation). There are many drug interactions between rifamycin medications and various classes of ART. When TB occurs in patients already on ART, treatment for TB should be started immediately and ART modified according to any potential interactions and to maintain virologic suppression. For ART-naive patients, ART should be started within 2 weeks after TB treatment initiation in those with CD4+ T counts less than 50 cells/mm^3 when TB meningitis is not suspected and within 8 weeks of starting anti-TB treatment in those with higher CD4 cell counts. The optimal approach for initiation of ART in TB meningitis remains uncertain. The CDC/ATS/IDSA guidelines suggest delaying ART initiation until the completion of 8 weeks of TB treatment for TB meningitis patients, irrespective of their CD4 count.

Tuberculosis and Transplantation

TB is one of the most significant opportunistic infections that may affect solid-organ transplant (SOT) recipients and hematopoietic stem cell transplant (HSCT) recipients. In most cases, the infection is caused by the reactivation of LTBI in the recipient, mainly during the first few months after transplantation. Ideally, LTBI treatment should be started before transplantation. Pulmonary TB is the most common clinical presentation. However, indolent, severe, or disseminated forms are seen more frequently than in the general population. Treatment for TB in transplant patients is similar to that of nontransplant, but it is essential to consider interactions between rifamycins with immunosuppressive drugs such as calcineurin inhibitors and mTOR inhibitors.

Drug-resistant Tuberculosis

Drug-resistant TB continues to be a public health threat. Resistance to antituberculous agents can be either primary, meaning it has been present before the initiation of therapy and is due to transmission of a drug-resistant strain, or secondary, indicating the emergence of resistance after antituberculosis therapy. The most important risk factor for drug-resistant TB is prior antituberculosis treatment, especially in cases of incomplete medication adherence, inadequate drug absorption or dosing, and single-drug treatment. Other risk factors include infection acquired in regions where resistance is prevalent and known contact with a drug-resistant case. The WHO uses five categories to classify cases of drug-resistant TB: INH-resistant TB; RFP-resistant TB and MDR-TB (TB resistant to RFP and INH); extensively drug-resistant TB (XDR TB); and pre-XDR-TB. Pre-XDR-TB is XDR-TB resistant to RFP, plus any fluoroquinolone, plus at least one of either bedaquiline (Sirturo) (BDQ) or linezolid (Zyvox) (LZD)[1]. Detection of drug resistance requires bacteriological confirmation of TB and testing for drug resistance using rapid molecular diagnostic tests, culture methods, or sequencing technologies. Resistance to RFP, the most effective first-line drug, is of most significant concern. Both MDR-TB and RFP-resistant TB (RR-TB) require treatment with second-line drugs. Consultation with a TB expert is advised if MDR or XDR

---

[1] Not FDA approved for this indication.

TABLE 5	ATS/IDSA Criteria for Diagnosis of NTM Pulmonary Disease
CATEGORY	**CRITERIA**
Microbiologic	• At least two separate positive cultures from sputum samples or • At least one positive culture from a bronchoalveolar wash/lavage or biopsy or • Biopsy with mycobacterial histopathologic features and at least one positive culture from sputum or bronchial wash
Radiographic	• Nodular or cavitary opacities or • Multifocal bronchiectasis with small nodules
Clinical	• Pulmonary symptoms

ATS, American Thoracic Society; *IDSA,* Infectious Diseases Society of America; *NTM,* nontuberculous mycobacteria.

TB is suspected or confirmed. In the United States during 2021, INH-resistance at initial diagnosis was reported for 536 (8.9%), including 5.8% of cases among U.S.-born persons and 10.0% among non-U.S.–born persons. Globally, the estimated annual number of people who developed MDR-TB or RR-TB in 2022 was 3.3% among new cases and 17% among those previously treated. Three countries accounted for 42% of the estimated global number of people who developed MDR/RR-TB in 2022: India (27%), the Philippines (7.5%), and the Russian Federation (7.5%).

Nontuberculous Mycobacteria

Overview

Nontuberculous mycobacteria (NTM) are pathogens that can affect both immunocompetent and immunocompromised individuals and are found worldwide in the environment. The development of new molecular methods and advances in culture techniques have allowed the characterization of new NTM species. There are more than 170 species of NTM, of which more than half are considered pathogens. NTM are species other than the *Mycobacterium tuberculosis* complex and *Mycobacterium leprae*. The most clinically relevant species in the United States are the *Mycobacterium avium* complex (MAC) and *Mycobacterium abscessus* species. NTM causes six major clinical disease syndromes, of which NTM lung disease accounts for the majority of cases, and its incidence and prevalence are increasing globally and in the United States. Common extrapulmonary sites include lymph nodes, skin, and soft tissues. To be diagnosed with NTM lung disease, patients should meet all clinical, radiological, and microbiologic criteria; however, the decision to start treatment is complex, requiring careful analysis of risks and benefits on an individual basis. Treatment varies depending on the species and susceptibility patterns and typically involves a multidrug regimen to prevent the development of drug resistance. These complex infections should be managed in collaboration with an expert in NTM infections.

Pathogenesis

NTM are ubiquitous in the environment and can be found mostly in water (both natural and treated water sources) but also in soil, dust particles, and aerosols. NTM can produce different morphotypes and robust biofilms and are quite resistant to commonly used water disinfectants, making exposure extremely common. Unlike pulmonary TB, person-to-person transmission is unlikely, although *M. abscessus* transmission has been reported among patients with cystic fibrosis (CF). Mycobacteria are initially phagocytosed by macrophages, which produce IL-12, which upregulates IFN-γ, a critical pathway in the control of mycobacterial infections. When interrupted or altered by iatrogenic or genetic factors, it can lead to disseminated NTM disease. In patients infected with human immunodeficiency virus (HIV), disseminated NTM infections typically occurred when the CD4+ T-lymphocyte number had fallen below 50/μl. NTM pulmonary disease occurs frequently in patients with pre-existing structural lung disorders, such as chronic obstructive pulmonary disease (COPD), bronchiectasis, CF, pneumoconiosis, prior TB, pulmonary alveolar proteinosis, and esophageal motility disorders or as a manifestation of complex genetic disorders and environmental exposures. There is also an association between bronchiectasis, nodular pulmonary NTM infections, and a particular body habitus, predominantly in postmenopausal women.

Prevention
Patients with pre-existing lung conditions and immunosuppression are at a higher risk of developing NTM disease. Thus, they should be advised to avoid activities that could expose them to NTM infections, such as using hot tubs, saunas, steam rooms, taking prolonged showers, and cleaning swimming pools and fish tanks. Patients who are already colonized by NTM, if possible, should avoid medications that may predispose them to develop disease and increase the risk of dissemination (e.g., TNF antagonists and steroids). Healthcare-associated NTM infections are well-known, and their prevention requires that surgical wounds, injection sites, and intravenous catheters should not come into contact with tap water or tap water-derived fluids. Endoscopes should not be cleaned in tap water either.

Clinical Manifestations
Chronic pulmonary disease is the most common clinical manifestation of NTM. MAC, *M. kansasii*, and *M. abscessus* are the most common pulmonary pathogens in the United States. The symptoms of NTM pulmonary disease are variable and nonspecific and can be confused with other chronic pulmonary conditions. Commonly, patients have chronic or recurring coughs. Other symptoms vary and include sputum production, fatigue, malaise, dyspnea, fever, hemoptysis, chest pain, and weight loss. Constitutional symptoms are progressively more prevalent with advancing NTM lung disease.

NTM can also impact other parts of the body. When it affects the lymph nodes, it causes localized cervical lymphadenitis, the most common NTM disease in children. The lymph nodes, typically unilateral and painless, can enlarge and cause fistulous drainage to the skin. NTM can affect the skin and soft tissue, usually from direct inoculation after traumatic wounds, injections, and cosmetic procedures. It is mainly caused by the rapidly growing mycobacteria (RGM) species *M. abscessus*, *M. fortuitum*, and *M. chelonae*. Lesions can manifest in various forms, such as ulcers, papules, nodules, eschars, and sporotrichoid lesions. NTM can affect tendon sheaths, bursae, bones, and joints, usually from direct inoculation of the pathogen through accidental trauma, surgical incisions, puncture wounds, or injections. Clinical manifestations include pain, swelling, erythema, purulent drainage of the joint involved, and pathologic fractures, with or without systemic symptoms. Catheter-related infection is the most common healthcare-associated NTM infection. It is most often seen with long-term central IV catheters, mainly due to RGM. The patient presents with fever and signs of catheter site infection, such as erythema, local tenderness, and drainage. Disseminated infections occur exclusively in severely immunocompromised patients, such as those with advanced HIV infection/AIDS, hematologic malignancy, or receiving immunosuppressive drugs, including therapy with TNF inhibitors and high-dose steroids. Patients with AIDS and disseminated MAC generally present with high fever, weight loss, night sweats, abdominal pain, and chronic diarrhea and are found to have lymphadenopathy, hepato-splenomegaly, and involvement of the bone marrow.

Diagnosis
Diagnosing NTM lung disease requires clinical, radiographic, and microbiologic criteria and appropriate exclusion of other diagnoses (Table 1). Healthcare providers should have a high index of suspicion, particularly as the symptoms, such as chronic cough, sputum, fatigue, hemoptysis, malaise, and weight loss, are often nonspecific and may also reflect underlying lung disease. Two main radiographic manifestations exist: the nodular bronchiectatic form and the cavitary lung disease. The significance of NTM isolated from the sputum of individuals who meet the clinical and radiographic criteria must be interpreted in the context of the number of positive cultures and specific species isolated. It is important to note that NTM species can be isolated from respiratory specimens due to environmental contamination. The microbiological criteria require positive culture results from at least two sputum specimens or one positive culture from a bronchial wash, lavage, or lung tissue with granulomatous inflammation. Patients who do not meet all criteria require close monitoring as NTM pulmonary disease may develop over time.

Because treatments and outcomes differ depending on the NTM species, accurate identification of NTM species is critical. Acid-fast bacillus (AFB) staining cannot differentiate between *M. tuberculosis* and NTM. AFB cultures from the site of infection are needed to identify a causative NTM agent, but it may take several weeks for a laboratory to grow NTM. Molecular methods have replaced traditional biochemical tests or high-performance liquid chromatography for NTM identification. NAATs can classify NTM or complexes. NTM lymphadenitis is best diagnosed by excisional lymph node biopsy for AFB culture and histopathology. Tissue biopsies of affected areas may demonstrate noncaseating granulomatous changes on histopathology. Disseminated MAC is diagnosed by isolating the mycobacteria in AFB blood culture or the hematopoietic system, such as bone marrow, liver, or spleen. Drug susceptibility testing on isolated mycobacterial species is necessary to help guide treatment decisions.

Treatment
Treatment of NTM depends on several factors, including the specific organ affected, the species of NTM, drug susceptibility, comorbid conditions, and the patient's immune status, including any immunosuppressive medications they may be taking. NTM has intrinsic resistance to many antibiotics and can develop resistance to therapy. Therefore, treatment typically requires two to three antimicrobial agents for a prolonged period. It should be noted that not all cases of NTM pulmonary disease require treatment, and the decision to initiate treatment should be based on a careful evaluation of the potential risks and benefits of long-term use of many drugs. Antibiotic susceptibility testing can be performed at appropriate reference laboratories. However, because drug susceptibilities of the NTM agent may not be readily available, the selection of antibiotics is often empirically chosen based on the CDC/ATS/IDSA guidelines. Surgical or wound care management may be required in cases of extrapulmonary disease. NTM treatment requires consultation with an infectious diseases or NTM expert.

Mycobacterium Leprae Complex
Overview
Leprosy, or Hansen's disease, is a rare and often overlooked condition. There are fewer than 200 cases each year in the United States, most of which are imported from countries where the disease is more common. Leprosy is caused by the *Mycobacterium leprae* complex. It primarily affects the skin and nerves. Contrary to past beliefs, leprosy is not highly contagious and can be easily cured, but if left untreated, it can cause serious complications such as irreversible neuropathy, which can severely impair the quality of life.

Transmission
Prolonged contact with someone with untreated Hansen's disease over many months is needed to become infected. Approximately 95% of people are naturally immune and don't get infected. The

primary mode of transmission is thought to be by the respiratory route from either respiratory droplets or nasal secretions. Vertical transmission of leprosy from a mother with lepromatous leprosy is possible but extremely unlikely if she has been treated. Leprosy lesions have been reported in the area of a tattoo, suggesting inoculation of the mycobacteria from unsterilized needles. In the southeastern United States, exposure to infected armadillos is a risk factor for contracting leprosy.

Pathophysiology

Hansen's disease is a granulomatous infection caused by *Mycobacterium leprae* complex, which is comprised of *M. leprae* and *M. lepromatosis*. These organisms are gram-positive AFB that cannot be grown in culture. They replicate slowly, and the incubation period of the disease is, on average, approximately 5 years. The development of leprosy depends on many factors, including immune function and genetic predisposition. Th1 immune response is strong and associated with lower bacterial counts and limited disease, whereas Th2 response is weak and results in higher bacterial counts and more severe disease. *M. leprae* complex has an affinity for peripheral nerve cells, preferentially attacking Schwann cells, causing nerve demyelination and loss of axonal conductance, which presents clinically as numbness and neuropathy.

Prevention

Early diagnosis is imperative so that treatment can be initiated promptly to decrease leprosy complications and potential transmission. There is no FDA vaccine available specifically to prevent leprosy. However, the BCG vaccine[1] may provide some protection against it. Additionally, in household contact with infected patients, BCG vaccination decreases the likelihood of developing multibacillary disease.

Clinical Manifestations

There are varying degrees of severity in the presentation of this disease, and it largely depends on the immune response to the *M. leprosy* strain. Clinical manifestations will be associated with the involvement of the skin, nerves, and mucous membranes. A thorough skin examination should be completed to assess macules, papules, plaques, subcutaneous nodules, and infiltrative skin changes. *M. leprosy* has a predilection for the cooler part of the body, including the skin, cutaneous nerves, ears, nose, eyes, larynx, and testes. The earliest sensory change in leprosy skin lesions is a compromised perception of the difference between warm and cold temperatures. Peripheral nerves should be assessed for enlargement and tenderness to palpation. In advanced disease, a person may have loss of lateral eyebrows (superciliary madarosis) or eyelashes (ciliary madarosis), or both. Thickening and nodularity of skin on the face can lead to a "leonine facies" appearance. There may be deformities of the nose (so-called saddle nose) or perforation of the nasal septum. Claw hand, foot drop, or paralysis of an extremity can be seen. *M. lepromatosis* is associated with necrotizing vasculitis, also known as the Lucio phenomenon, a potentially fatal complication of leprosy.

Diagnosis

The disease caused by the *M. leprae* complex can present itself in a range of clinical and histopathologic forms. A high index of suspicion is essential in those at risk for leprosy in the United States, including patients from countries where leprosy is common, any contact with armadillos, and family history of leprosy. A skin biopsy for histopathology is most helpful to make a diagnosis. In endemic countries, leprosy is diagnosed by finding at least one of the following cardinal signs: (1) definite loss of sensation in a pale (hypopigmented) or reddish skin patch; (2) thickened or enlarged peripheral nerve, with loss of sensation and/or weakness of the muscles supplied by that nerve; or (3) microscopic detection of bacilli in a slit-skin smear. The WHO

developed a classification based on the number of lesions: the paucibacillary form, in cases where five or fewer skin lesions are present without any bacilli evident on skin smears, and the multibacillary form, when more than five lesions are present or with nerve involvement, or with the demonstrated presence of bacilli, irrespective of the number of the skin lesions. The Ridley-Jopling classification of leprosy is usually used in the United States. This schema classifies the disease depending on the degree of the host's cell-mediated immune response and includes five types. Disease types range from the polar tuberculoid form (TT) with a robust immune response, including well-formed granulomas, few bacilli, and more classic clinical manifestations, to the polar lepromatous type (LL) with minimal cell-mediated immune response, foamy macrophages without granulomas, and many bacilli seen on histopathology. Borderline tuberculoid (BT), midborderline (BB), and borderline lepromatous (BL) types have varying degrees of both cell-mediated and humoral responses. There are no serologic or skin tests. PCR can be used to detect *M. leprae* and *M. lepromatosis* DNA in tissue.

Treatment

Leprosy can be cured with multidrug therapy, making early recognition and treatment essential to prevent disability and mortality. As with other mycobacteria, multidrug therapy decreases the chances of drug resistance. In the United States, treatment consensus and consultation by the National Hansen's Disease Program (NHDP) are recommended. The U.S. NHDP offers a variety of resources to patients and healthcare providers. These resources include the opportunity to review histopathology specimens, consultation regarding molecular diagnosis of *M. leprae* complex, free antimicrobial therapy for patients, and educational materials for physicians and patients to understand the disease better and prevent injury and disability. Additionally, NHDP provides resources for surgical care and rehabilitation of patients referred for digit or limb-threatening wounds. NHDP contact information can be found at https://www.hrsa.gov/hansens-disease/index.html. The antibiotics routinely used in leprosy are dapsone (DAP), rifampin (Rifadin, Rimactane) (RFP),[1] and clofazimine (Lamprene) (CFZ). Alternative regimens include clarithromycin (Biaxin),[1] minocycline (Dynacin, Minocin, Myrac, Solodyn, Ximino),[1] and certain fluoroquinolones.

Monitoring

Once patients start treatment, they should be educated about the potential side effects of the medications. Close monitoring is recommended, with a detailed skin evaluation and whether new lesions have appeared. DAP can induce induced methemoglobinemia in people with glucose-6-phosphate dehydrogenase (G6PD) deficiency. Therefore, it is important to perform G6PD testing at the initiation of therapy. RFP can cause rash, gastrointestinal intolerance, and hepatitis and may turn body fluids to an orange-red color; in addition, it is important to note the significant interactions with other drugs. CFZ commonly causes red and dark skin pigmentation of varying intensity. Complications of Hansen's disease arise from injuries to the areas with reduced sensation, mainly the hands and feet. These injuries can lead to peripheral neuropathy complications, such as claw hand and foot drop. In such cases, patients may require evaluation and management by occupational and physical therapists.

---

[1] Not FDA approved for this indication.

References

Bennett J, Dolin R, Blaser M: Mycobacterium leprae (leprosy). In Bennett J, Dolin R, Blaser M, editors: *Mandell, Douglas, and Bennett's Principles and practice of infectious diseases*, ed 9, Elsevier, 2020, pp 3022–3034.

Bennett J, Dolin R, Blaser M: Infections caused by nontuberculous mycobacteria other than Mycobacterium avium complex. In Bennett J, Dolin R, Blaser M, editors: *Mandell, Douglas, and Bennett's Principles and practice of infectious diseases*, ed 9, Elsevier, 2020, pp 3049–3058.

---

[1] Not FDA approved for this indication.

Bennett J, Dolin R, Blaser M: Mycobacterium avium complex. In Bennett J, Dolin R, Blaser M, editors: *Mandell, Douglas, and Bennett's Principles and practice of infectious diseases*, ed 9, Elsevier, 2020, pp 3035–3048.

Bennett J, Dolin R, Blaser M: Mycobacterium tuberculosis. In Bennett J, Dolin R, Blaser M, editors: *Mandell, Douglas, and Bennett's Principles and practice of infectious diseases*, ed 9, Elsevier, 2020, pp 2985–3021.

Daley CL, Iaccarino JM, Lange C, et al: Treatment of nontuberculous mycobacterial pulmonary disease: an Official ATS/ERS/ESCMID/IDSA clinical practice guideline, *Clin Infect Dis* 71(4):e1–e36, 2020.

Nahid P, Dorman SE, Alipanah N, et al: Official American Thoracic Society/Centers for Disease Control and Prevention/Infectious Diseases Society of America clinical practice guidelines: treatment of drug-susceptible tuberculosis, *Clin Infect Dis* 63(7):e147–e195, 2016.

Office of AIDS Research Advisory Council, Centers for Disease Control and Prevention, National Institute of Health, HIV Medicine Association (HIVMA) of the Infectious Diseases Society of America (IDSA). Guidelines for the Prevention and Treatment of Opportunistic Infections in Adults and Adolescents with HIV. Available at: https://clinicalinfo.hiv.gov/en/guidelines/adult-and-adolescent-opportunistic-infection/whats-new-guidelines.

Sterling TR, Njie G, Zenner D, et al: Guidelines for the treatment of latent tuberculosis infection, *MMWR Recomm Rep* 69(1):1–11, 2020.

Tait DR, Hatherill M, Van Der Meeren O, Ginsberg AM, et al: Final Analysis of a Trial of M72/AS01E Vaccine to Prevent Tuberculosis, *N Engl J Med* 381(25):2429–2439, 2019, https://doi.org/10.1056/NEJMoa1909953. Epub 2019 Oct 29.

WHO: *Global Tuberculosis Report*, World Health Organization, 2023. https://www.who.int/teams/global-tuberculosis-programme/tb-reports/global-tuberculosis-report-2023 (2023).

Williams PM, Pratt RH, Walker WL, Price SF, Stewart RJ, Feng PI: Tuberculosis – United States, 2023, *MMWR Morb Mortal Wkly Rep* 73:265–270, 2024.

VENOUS THROMBOEMBOLISM

Method of
Moniba Nazeef, MD; and John P. Sheehan, MD

CURRENT DIAGNOSIS

- A comprehensive history is the most important diagnostic tool to assess risk factors including recent surgery, bedridden state, trauma, orthopedic procedure, or active cancer.
- Moderately high–sensitivity D-dimer assays (>85% sensitivity) can be used to exclude venous thromboembolism if there is low clinical probability but should be combined with imaging in all other cases.
- Venous compression ultrasonography is a noninvasive, affordable, and widely available test for the diagnosis of deep venous thrombosis. Computed tomography pulmonary angiography is the current gold standard for the diagnosis of pulmonary embolism.

CURRENT THERAPY

- The choice of initial therapy is frequently guided by the clinical scenario. Initial therapy includes unfractionated heparin, low-molecular-weight heparin, fondaparinux (Arixtra), or the direct oral anticoagulants—rivaroxaban (Xarelto) or apixaban (Eliquis).
- The traditional heparin-warfarin regimen has been increasingly supplanted by the use of direct oral anticoagulants.
- Standard treatment for a new episode of deep venous thrombosis or pulmonary embolism is 3 to 6 months of therapeutic anticoagulation. The recommended duration of anticoagulation for venous thromboembolism requires individualized analysis of the clinical presentation and patient specific factors that weigh both recurrence and bleeding risk.

Venous thromboembolism (VTE) is a significant health problem, with surveillance data suggesting that 60,000 to 100,000 people die of VTE each year in the United States. Approximately 50% to 60% of this disease burden is associated with a recent hospitalization, underscoring the importance of VTE prophylaxis. VTE comprises superficial vein thrombosis (SVT), deep venous thrombosis (DVT), and pulmonary embolism (PE). DVT typically starts in the deep veins of the lower extremities and progresses proximally. If untreated, a clot can break off and travel to the lungs where it is trapped in the pulmonary circulation, resulting in PE. DVT confined to the deep veins of the calf is termed *isolated distal DVT,* whereas involvement of the popliteal or more proximal veins is termed *proximal DVT.* SVT represents thrombosis in the superficial veins of the legs or arms and rarely progresses to DVT. The focus of this chapter is to understand the risk factors, diagnosis, treatment, and prevention of DVT and PE.

Pathophysiology/Risk Factors

Venous blood flow is maintained by a delicate homeostatic balance of prothrombotic and antithrombotic factors. Virchow's triad describes the major factors leading to VTE from a pathophysiologic standpoint: (1) intrinsic hypercoagulability, (2) endothelial damage, and (3) venous stasis. Most often, a combination of these factors leads to the development of VTE. Based on the presence or absence of typical clinical risk factors, VTE occurrences can be considered either provoked (e.g., postsurgical) or unprovoked (spontaneous). Furthermore, provoking risk factors may be transient/reversible (e.g., estrogen use) or nontransient/irreversible (e.g., lower extremity paresis), which has implications for decisions regarding duration of anticoagulant therapy (Table 1).

Acquired Risk Factors

Certain clinical conditions shift the balance between procoagulant and anticoagulant factors to promote thrombosis. These conditions include surgery, pregnancy and puerperium, inflammation, active cancer, major trauma, specific medications, and a variety of conditions that lead to immobility. A more comprehensive list is provided in Table 1. Many of these clinical conditions cause multiple changes relevant to VTE risk. For example, surgical interventions may induce endothelial damage, immobilization leading to venous stasis, platelet activation, and trigger inflammatory responses that increase fibrinogen, factor VIII, and von Willebrand factor levels. Orthopedic procedures involving the lower limbs and abdominopelvic surgeries in cancer patients are especially high risk from a VTE standpoint. Active cancer is associated with 20% of all VTE and involves a variety of mechanisms leading to hypercoagulability, including increased tissue factor expression, venous obstruction, indwelling catheters, reduced mobility, and chemotherapy.

Pregnancy and the puerperium, oral contraceptives (OC), and hormone replacement therapy (HRT) are important VTE risk factors in women. OC and HRT are associated with a number of changes in hemostatic protein levels and platelet function that appear globally prothrombotic. Higher estrogen content is associated with increased thrombotic risk and is modulated by a combination with specific progestins. Additionally, there is a higher risk of VTE in OC users with a positive family history, suggesting an underlying genetic predisposition.

A variety of conditions that involve prolonged immobilization enhance VTE risk. Cast immobilization of the lower extremity, paresis after neurologic events, multiple trauma, orthopedic surgeries, travel-associated immobility (>4 to 6 hours), or a bedridden state due to a variety of medical or surgical conditions result in stasis that promotes venous thrombosis. Many of these clinical situations are also associated with an inflammatory state that concomitantly increases intrinsic hypercoagulability of the blood. Venous wall injury may occur via a variety of mechanisms, including surgical interventions, indwelling intravenous catheters, trauma, and vasculitis.

Genetics of Venous Thromboembolism

Although acquired clinical risk factors are critical to assessing risk, the genetic contribution to VTE is also substantial, with heritability of VTE estimated at 40% to 47%. Like many

TABLE 1 Risk Factors for Venous Thromboembolism

Transient/Reversible

Surgery (esp. lower limb orthopedic surgery)
General anesthesia > 30 min
Immobility due to surgical or medical condition
Oral contraceptives/hormone replacement therapy
Pregnancy, puerperium
Major trauma
Acute inflammation
Indwelling venous catheters
Heparin-induced thrombocytopenia
May-Thurner syndrome
Travel-associated thrombosis
Medications including tamoxifen, L-asparaginase,
   immunomodulatory agents (lenalidomide [Revlimid]),
   erythropoietin

Permanent/Nonreversible

Active cancer
Antiphospholipid syndrome
Myeloproliferative neoplasms
Paroxysmal nocturnal hemoglobinuria
Lower extremity paresis from neurologic disease
Sickle cell disease
Nephrotic syndrome
Active autoimmune conditions (SLE, IBD, ITP, TTP)
Chronic infection/inflammation
Morbid obesity (BMI > 40)

BMI, Body mass index; *IBD,* inflammatory bowel disease; *ITP,* immune thrombocytopenic purpura; *SLE,* systemic lupus erythematosus; *TTP,* thrombotic thrombocytopenic purpura.

complex phenotypes, VTE has a multigenic basis in which most individual alleles make relatively small contributions to overall risk. Factor V Leiden and the prothrombin G20210A polymorphism are examples of such alleles (two- to fourfold relative risk). At least 17 genes have been identified that harbor VTE-associated variants. Importantly, family history remains an independent risk factor even after excluding known gene variants associated with thrombophilia, suggesting that unidentified genes also contribute to VTE risk. Deficiencies of the coagulation inhibitors antithrombin, protein C, and protein S are rare conditions with a more substantial effect on the relative risk of VTE (10- to 20-fold increase) but tend to be diagnosed erroneously in the setting of acute thrombosis. The multigenic basis of VTE has implications for thrombophilia testing that include: (1) identification of minor alleles (e.g., factor V Leiden) is not helpful for prediction of VTE recurrence risk, (2) a careful family history is generally more valuable than a thrombophilia evaluation, and (3) the *absolute* risk for carriers of thrombophilic alleles is generally quite small and does not justify indefinite anticoagulation. A robust estimate of individual genetic risk requires systematic screening of all known VTE risk genes or whole genome/exome sequencing approaches that are not routinely available. Thus current thrombophilia testing rarely contributes to clinical decision making in patients with VTE. Testing should never be pursued for provoked events and is best limited to selected situations such as presentations at a young age (<30 years) or known thrombophilic traits occurring in the context of a family history of VTE. A thorough personal and family history is generally sufficient to determine the likelihood of an underlying inherited hypercoagulable state.

Epidemiology and Natural History

The exact incidence of VTE is unknown, but it is estimated that about 300,000 to 600,000 Americans are affected by VTE each year. VTE incidence appears approximately 30% higher in African Americans and approximately 70% lower in Asian and Native American populations relative to Whites. Importantly, the incidence of VTE increases with age, particularly after age 50.

Whereas overall VTE is slightly more common in men, women have an increased incidence before age 40 based on the influence of pregnancy and contraceptives. In older age groups, the frequency of PE is increased relative to DVT. Finally, the incidence of VTE has been increasing steadily since the mid-1980s, which may, in large part, represent the increased use and enhanced sensitivity of computed tomography (CT) scans and magnetic resonance (MR) imaging.

The natural history of VTE is affected by the underlying clinical risk factors, provoked versus unprovoked nature of the event, reversibility of risk factors, and location/nature of the thrombotic event. In general, untreated thrombi tend to extend proximally, break off, and embolize to the pulmonary circulation, where they may result in infarction and pulmonary hypertension. The risk of PE is increased for proximal versus distal involvement with DVT. More than 75% of VTE starts in the calf veins, and 20% to 30% of these cases progress to involve proximal veins in the leg or pelvis. Approximately 50% of patients with untreated symptomatic proximal DVT develop symptomatic PE, whereas the incidence of asymptomatic PE is even higher. Importantly, 10% of symptomatic PE is rapidly fatal, and 30% of patients with untreated symptomatic nonfatal PE will have a fatal recurrence. Thus recognition of PE is of the utmost clinical importance. Anticoagulant therapy inhibits thrombus growth and largely prevents interval recurrence, whereas endogenous thrombolysis may result in partial or complete resolution of the thrombus. Uncommonly, progressive thrombosis in the presence of anticoagulation may occur in high-risk situations such as metastatic malignancy or the antiphospholipid syndrome.

The risk of VTE recurrence after stopping anticoagulation varies significantly based on clinical presentation. About 20% to 40% of VTE episodes are unprovoked in nature, which is associated with a substantially higher recurrence rate. For unprovoked clots, recurrence rate is estimated to be approximately 10% in 1 year, approximately 30% in 5 years, and approaches approximately 40% in 10 years. In contrast, the recurrence risk of VTE associated with surgery (a transient risk factor) is less than 3% per year. Recurrences tend to occur in a similar site to the initial event, which is particularly important in the case of PE, as 25% of PE presents as sudden death. In contrast, the risk of recurrent VTE is much smaller in isolated distal (calf) DVT compared with proximal DVT and PE.

Long-Term Complications of Venous Thromboembolism
Postthrombotic Syndrome

About 20% to 50% patients with DVT develop some degree of postthrombotic syndrome (PTS) within the subsequent 1 to 2 years. Chronic venous obstruction, inflammation, endofibrosis, and valvular dysfunction contribute to the chronic venous insufficiency of PTS. Risk factors for PTS include persistent DVT symptoms after 1 month, extensive or recurrent DVT, inadequate anticoagulation, and advanced age. Manifestations include chronic leg edema, pain, heaviness, erythema, and venous ulcers that may result in significant disability. PTS is largely nonreversible, emphasizing the importance of DVT prevention. Graduated compression stockings provide symptomatic relief by preventing pooling of blood in the lower extremities but do not prevent PTS. In the 5% to 10% of patients with severe PTS, active supportive care and consultation with vascular surgery, dermatology, or vein specialists should be sought early to avoid development of debilitating venous ulcers.

Chronic Thromboembolic Pulmonary Hypertension

Chronic thromboembolic pulmonary hypertension (CTEPH) is a long-term complication of PE affecting 3% to 4% patients despite adequate anticoagulation. CTEPH is characterized by progressive pulmonary hypertension and right-side heart failure due to remodeling of pulmonary vasculature by thrombotic material. Patients with large central or extensive pulmonary emboli, hemodynamic compromise, and right heart dysfunction at diagnosis are at highest risk. Chronic progressive dyspnea with exertion is the most common symptom, and the clinician must have a high clinical suspicion based on the patient's history of PE. An echocardiogram revealing elevated pulmonary arterial hypertension should trigger evaluation with a ventilation/perfusion (V/Q) scan. The presence of chronic mismatched segmental perfusion defects on the V/Q scan is diagnostic of CTEPH. If anatomically feasible, treatment of choice is pulmonary endarterectomy, which can reverse the hemodynamic and functional abnormalities. Early recognition and referral to a specialized surgical treatment center are critical to patient outcomes. Lifelong anticoagulation is recommended for all patients with CTEPH.

Diagnosis of Deep Venous Thrombosis

The diagnosis of DVT proceeds via determination of clinical probability, D-dimer screening, and confirmatory imaging.

Clinical Features

Diagnosis begins with evaluation of the clinical scenario for VTE risk factors and suspicious physical exam findings. Suggestive features in the patient's recent history include recent surgery or bedridden state, trauma or orthopedic procedure, active cancer, and other typical risk factors (Table 1). Classic symptoms of DVT include limb swelling, pain, and erythema. On exam, unilateral calf swelling, pitting edema, dilated veins, and tenderness on palpation can be seen. The clinical probability becomes stronger when more of these findings are present. Risk stratification systems such as the Wells model (Table 2) use these clinical features to rapidly classify patients as high (~60% thrombosis), moderate (~25%), or low (~5%) risk for DVT. Differential diagnosis of DVT includes trauma, cellulitis, osteomyelitis, chronic venous insufficiency, arterial ischemia, ruptured Baker cyst, hematoma, and superficial thrombophlebitis. Because neither history nor physical examination findings are specific for DVT, D-dimer screening and objective imaging must be pursued if sufficient clinical suspicion exists. A simplified algorithm for diagnosis of DVT is provided (Figure 1).

D-dimer Screening

D-dimer is a specific fibrin degradation product generated by plasmin cleavage of cross-linked fibrin clot, formed by thrombin and factor XIII activity. D-dimer represents a useful screening tool based on excellent sensitivity and a high negative predictive value for VTE. However, D-dimer lacks specificity, as it is increased in a variety of conditions, including acute inflammation, recent surgery or trauma, pregnancy, disseminated intravascular coagulation, advanced age, or cancer. The level of clinical suspicion also impacts interpretation of D-dimer results. Specific D-dimer assays vary in sensitivity and specificity, although qualitative testing has largely been replaced by enzyme-linked immunosorbent assay–based quantitative assays. More recently, highly sensitive assays (>95% sensitivity) using latex-enhanced immunoturbidimetric immunoassays provide rapid quantitation for use in the diagnosis of VTE. Point-of-care testing with specified cutoff values are also available. Thus the clinician should be familiar with the type of D-dimer testing available locally. Highly sensitive assays have a good negative predictive value to rule out VTE without further testing. Moderately high–sensitivity assays (>85% sensitivity) can be used to exclude VTE if there is low clinical probability but should be combined with imaging in all other cases. Qualitative or semiquantitative assays are generally not reliable for excluding thrombosis. Finally, if clinical suspicion for DVT or PE is high, a negative D-dimer should not be used to rule out VTE, and appropriate imaging should be pursued to confirm the diagnosis.

TABLE 2	Wells Model for Predicting Pretest Probability of Deep Vein Thrombosis	
CLINICAL VARIABLE		**POINTS**
Active cancer (treatment ongoing or within previous 6 months or palliative)		1
Recently bedridden >3 days or major surgery within 4 weeks		1
Pitting edema confined to the symptomatic leg		1
Dilated superficial veins (nonvaricose)		1
Previous documented DVT		1
Paralysis, paresis, or recent plaster immobilization of the lower extremities		1
Localized tenderness along the distribution of the deep venous system		1
Calf swelling 3 cm greater than asymptomatic side measured 10 cm below tibial tuberosity		1
Alternative diagnosis at least as likely as DVT		−2

Clinical probability by interpretation of total score: >2, high; 1 or 2, moderate; <1, low.
DVT, Deep venous thrombosis.

Imaging

Ultrasonography

Venous compression ultrasonography (CUS) is a noninvasive, affordable, and widely available test for the diagnosis of DVT. The

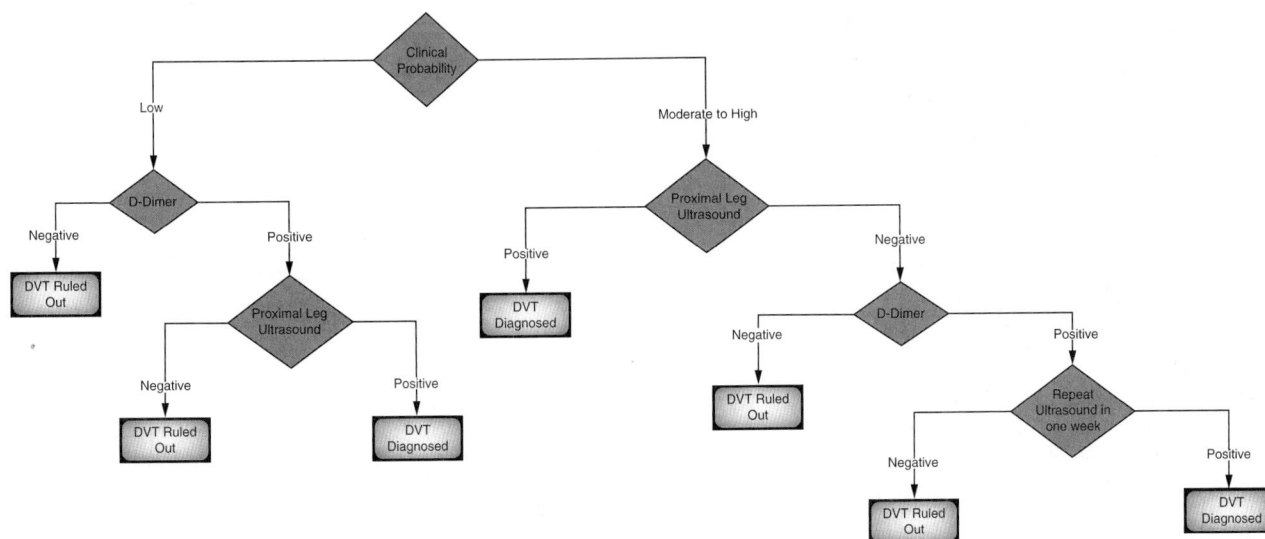

Figure 1 Suggested diagnostic algorithm for diagnosis of deep venous thrombosis *(DVT).*

deep veins are assessed by use of a compression probe with lack of compressibility in a venous segment indicative of thrombus. Duplex technology or color-coded Doppler scanning visualizes blood flow to allow accurate identification of deep veins. Lack of flow plus noncompressibility increases diagnostic accuracy and also facilitates diagnosis in veins that cannot be compressed (e.g., pelvic and subclavian veins). Venous ultrasonography has an excellent sensitivity and specificity (~94%) for diagnosis of proximal limb DVT. The common femoral, femoral, and trifurcation of calf veins are readily visualized. In most cases, a negative test is sufficient to rule out proximal VTE. Currently two methods for CUS are used: (1) the two-point compression technique, which only evaluates the proximal veins in the groin and popliteal fossa; and (2) whole-leg ultrasound scanning evaluating both proximal and distal veins. The sensitivity and specificity of CUS for calf vein DVT is significantly lower and highly operator dependent. Therefore many centers only perform the proximal vein assessment, which is reliable, reproducible, and efficient. If clinical suspicion remains high after a negative proximal vein ultrasound scan, repeat ultrasound scanning should be performed in about a week to assess for proximal extension in the deep venous system. If negative, no further testing is needed. A negative whole-leg CUS test result essentially rules out DVT and does not need follow-up testing. However, this approach is time-consuming and may lead to increased diagnosis of calf vein thromboses and potential overtreatment. The 3-month incidence of symptomatic proximal venous thrombosis in patients with a normal initial test are comparable at approximately 1% for both approaches. For upper extremities, compression ultrasonography is about 86% sensitive and specific.

Contrast Venography

Once the gold standard for diagnosis of DVT, contrast venography is rarely used because it is invasive and requires contrast exposure. CT and MR venography have a sensitivity and specificity of greater than 90% for DVT in lower extremities. However, these studies are also not widely used for diagnosis because of increased cost, radiation, and contrast exposure. CT and MR venography are useful to define anatomy in patients with multiple recurrent DVT (evaluation by CUS is problematic), an indeterminate abnormality on ultrasound scanning, or a thrombus diagnosed in the setting of very low clinical suspicion.

Diagnosis of Pulmonary Embolism

Similar to DVT, the diagnosis of PE requires determination of clinical probability, consideration of D-dimer testing, and confirmatory imaging.

Clinical Features

A patient presenting with risk factors for VTE and antecedent history of DVT should raise the suspicion for PE. The most common symptoms of PE are shortness of breath and chest pain. Pleuritic chest pain is typical, but PE may also present with substernal pressure or be confused with musculoskeletal pain. Other symptoms may include cough and hemoptysis. Clinical signs include tachypnea, tachycardia, and hypoxia. The findings of DVT in the lower extremities increase the probability of PE. The Wells model for PE provides a useful framework to estimate the pretest probability using these variables (Table 3).

Chest X-ray, Electrocardiography, and Troponin

Chest x-ray should be performed in all suspected cases. The classic Hampton hump or peripheral wedge-shaped opacity corresponding to a large pulmonary infarct is seldom appreciated and not very sensitive or specific. However, a chest x-ray is useful in assessing for other conditions such as pneumonia, pneumothorax, and pulmonary edema that can present in similar fashion. Electrocardiography (ECG) should be performed in anyone presenting with chest pain to rule out myocardial infarction. Evidence of right heart strain on ECG has predictive and prognostic value in assessment of PE. Similarly, a troponin level is usually obtained in evaluation for myocardial ischemia. An elevated troponin level

TABLE 3	Wells Model for Predicting Pretest Probability of Pulmonary Embolism	
CLINICAL VARIABLE		**POINTS**
Clinical signs and symptoms of DVT (minimum leg swelling and pain with palpation of the deep veins)		3
An alternative diagnosis is less likely than PE		3
Heart rate > 100 beats/min		1.5
Immobilization or surgery in the previous 4 weeks		1.5
Previous DVT/PE		1.5
Hemoptysis		1
Active cancer (treatment ongoing or within previous 6 months or palliative)		1

Clinical probability by interpretation of total score: >6, high; 4–6, moderate; <4, low.
DVT, Deep venous thrombosis; *PE*, pulmonary embolism.

in the absence of ECG evidence of ischemia can be suggestive of myocardial injury in the setting of massive or submassive PE.

Ventilation/Perfusion Scanning

V/Q scans have largely been replaced by computed tomography pulmonary angiography (CTPA). However, V/Q scans remain useful in selected patients with significant renal insufficiency (to avoid contrast dye) and young or pregnant females (to avoid radiation exposure). This technique uses inhaled and intravenous radioisotopes to evaluate ventilation and circulation in the pulmonary parenchyma and vasculature, respectively. A normal perfusion scan in the setting of a normal chest x-ray excludes PE. The addition of a ventilation scan increases specificity by accounting for other pulmonary disorders. A normal chest x-ray and ventilation scan in areas with multiple large perfusion defects that involve greater than 75% of a segment (V/Q mismatch) is associated with greater than 80% probability of PE and considered a high-probability V/Q scan. An intermediate-probability scan usually requires further diagnostic evaluation because it is considered nondiagnostic in most situations. Three-dimensional single-photon emission CT (SPECT) is now used by many centers in place of planar V/Q scans. SPECT may be more accurate than planar V/Q scanning, resulting in fewer nondiagnostic studies.

Computed Tomography Pulmonary Angiography

CTPA is the modality of choice for diagnosis of PE. It is a relatively noninvasive procedure that can provide prompt diagnosis of PE. With recent advancements, the availability of thin-slice scans provides a detailed analysis of pulmonary vasculature that increases the sensitivity for detecting thrombi at the subsegmental and peripheral arterial level. In contrast to V/Q scanning, CTPA provides detailed visualization of the lung parenchyma, which can detect peripheral pulmonary infarctions and alternative diagnoses. When required, the CTPA examination can be extended to include the iliac veins, providing a detailed view with a single contrast exposure. CTPA has excellent sensitivity and specificity for diagnosis of lobar and segmental PE. Diagnostic accuracy is lower at the subsegmental level, and results should be interpreted in the context of clinical probability, proximal lower extremity ultrasound results, and D-dimer level. A simplified algorithmic approach to diagnosis of PE is provided (Figure 2). CTPA use is limited by costs, exposure to potentially nephrotoxic contrast dye, and chest radiation. It should be avoided in younger women because of the associated increased risk of breast cancer.

Pulmonary Angiography

Once the gold standard for the diagnosis of PE, pulmonary angiography is an invasive procedure that has been replaced by CTPA and is now very rarely performed.

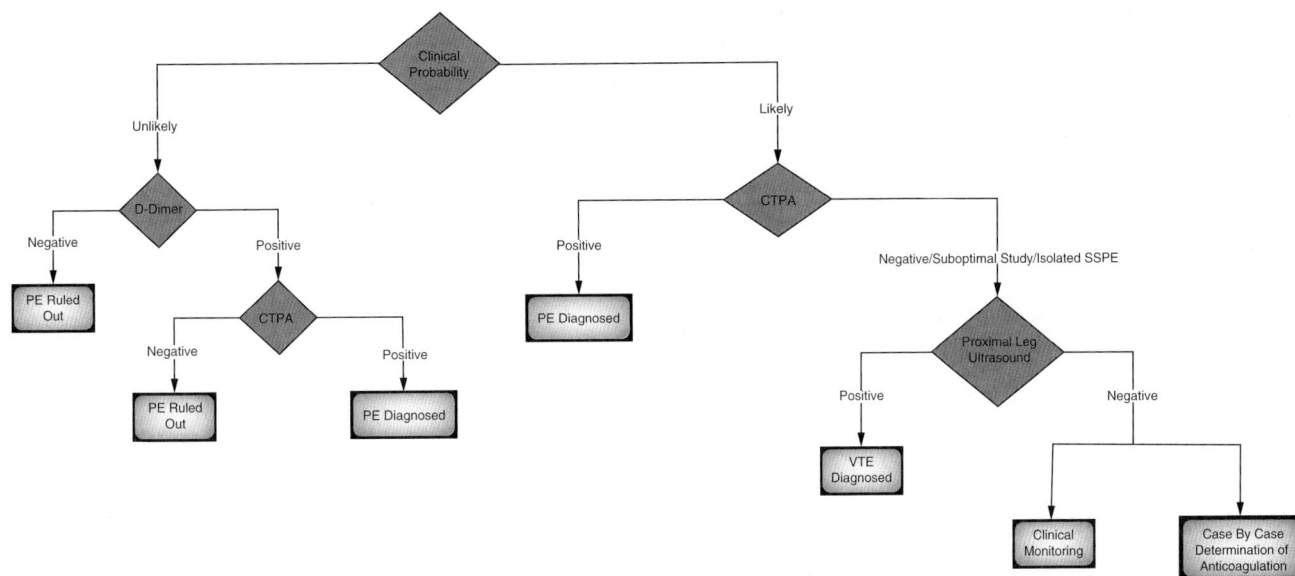

Figure 2 Suggested diagnostic algorithm for diagnosis of pulmonary embolism *(PE)*. *CTPA,* Computed tomography pulmonary angiography; *SSPE,* subsegmental pulmonary embolism.

Magnetic Resonance Angiography

Pulmonary contrast-enhanced magnetic resonance angiography (CE-MRA) is emerging as a useful alternative to CTPA in select patients such as younger females and those with severe iodinated contrast allergy. Currently, CE-MRA has limited availability and usefulness that is dependent on the expertise and experience of the available radiologist.

Diagnosis of Recurrent Deep Vein Thrombosis

The diagnosis of recurrent DVT can be challenging because signs and symptoms of PTS in the affected extremity can obscure the diagnosis. Clinical assessment of the probability for recurrent DVT is less well standardized than initial episodes; however, many predictive factors are expected to be shared. The clinician should assess for the presence of ongoing clinical risk factors, attempt to discern between chronic and acute signs and symptoms, and consider D-dimer testing. A negative D-dimer test can be used to exclude recurrent DVT, although the accuracy of this approach has not been well studied. If D-dimer testing is positive or has not been done, CUS is performed. The finding of noncompressibility of an ipsilateral femoral or popliteal vein segment, which was previously unaffected, can be considered diagnostic. For diagnosing recurrent DVT in a previously affected vein segment, an increase in thrombus diameter of at least 4 mm on serial CUS in combination with a D-dimer measurement can serve as helpful criteria. This diagnosis requires the expertise of an experienced radiologist with the previous ultrasound available for comparison. In practice, comparison with previous CUS is difficult, given the operator-dependent characteristics of the test. If comparison with the previous examination is equivocal or unavailable, CT or MR venography may be considered. An intraluminal filling defect suggests acute rather than remote thrombosis. Alternatively, a patient with initially equivocal CUS findings can undergo serial repeat examinations to detect DVT extension.

Treatment of Venous Thromboembolism

Anticoagulation Therapy for Venous Thromboembolism

Patients with newly diagnosed VTE should be promptly initiated on therapeutic anticoagulation. In the absence of a severely symptomatic lower extremity, high thrombus burden PE with right ventricular dysfunction or significant cardiovascular comorbidity, management is predominantly outpatient. In the presence of PE, a simplified PE severity index (sPESI; https://www.mdcalc.com/calc/1247/simplified-pesi-pulmonary-embolism-severity-index) is often used to assess appropriateness for outpatient therapy.

The sPESI score includes the following factors (1 point each): age greater than 80 years, history of cancer, chronic cardiopulmonary disease, pulse greater than 110 beats/min, systolic blood pressure less than 100 mm Hg, and arterial oxygen saturation less than 90%. Patients with a sPESI score greater than or equal to 1 are considered high risk and should be considered for initial inpatient management.

Choice of Initial Anticoagulant Therapy

The choice of initial therapy is frequently guided by the clinical scenario. Initial therapy includes unfractionated heparin (UFH), low-molecular-weight heparin (LWMH), fondaparinux (Arixtra), or the direct oral anticoagulants—rivaroxaban (Xarelto) or apixaban (Eliquis) (Table 4). Therapeutic UFH is administered intravenously (IV) and demonstrates complex pharmacokinetics (both hepatic and renal clearance) that requires laboratory monitoring of drug effect (activated partial thromboplastin time [aPTT] or anti–factor Xa activity). Thus UFH therapy requires hospital admission and has largely been replaced by other options. UFH may still be appropriate for patients experiencing inpatient VTE events, especially if a need for invasive procedures is anticipated (half-life, 1 to 2 hours). The therapeutic target range for UFH is a 1.5- to 2.5-fold increase over the baseline aPTT or 0.3 to 0.7 U/mL anti–factor Xa activity. In contrast, LMWH is administered subcutaneously and primarily cleared by the kidneys, resulting in predictable pharmacokinetics. Subcutaneous administration facilitates outpatient treatment, and predictable pharmacokinetics allow weight-based dosing without laboratory monitoring. Fondaparinux, a synthetic pentasaccharide, is exclusively cleared by the kidneys with a long half-life (17 to 21 hours) that allows for once-daily, weight-adjusted subcutaneous dosing. Fondaparinux similarly does not require routine laboratory monitoring, but caution is warranted in patients with mild renal insufficiency where drug accumulation may increase bleeding risk. Heparin therapy (UFH, LWMH, or fondaparinux) for VTE is administered for a *minimum* of 5 days followed by transition to longer-term oral anticoagulation with an oral vitamin K antagonist (VKA) or a direct oral anticoagulant (DOAC). Alternatively, rivaroxaban or apixaban can be initiated immediately after VTE diagnosis and bypass the need for heparin therapy (see later).

Historically, VKAs are the primary oral anticoagulants for the long-term treatment of VTE. Warfarin (Coumadin) is the VKA used almost exclusively in the United States. Warfarin and other VKAs inhibit vitamin K-dependent γ-carboxylation of the coagulation zymogens (proenzymes). This posttranslational

TABLE 4 Drugs for the Treatment of Venous Thromboembolism

DRUG	DOSING	ELIMINATION	HALF-LIFE	MONITORING
UFH	80 units/kg IV bolus, then 18 U/kg/hour initial infusion rate	Complex, hepatic/renal metabolism	1–2 hours	aPTT Anti–factor Xa activity
LMWH	Dalteparin (Fragmin): 200 U/kg SQ QD Enoxaparin (Lovenox): 1 mg/kg SQ BID	Predominantly renal	3–5 hours	None required*
Fondaparinux (Arixtra)	5.0 mg SQ QD (<50 kg) 7.5 mg SQ QD (50–100 kg) 10 mg SQ QD (>100 kg)	Renal	17–21 hours	None required*
Warfarin (VKA) (Coumadin)	Initially 5 mg PO QD, broad range (2.5–10 mg)	Extensive hepatic metabolism Renal excretion for metabolites	Pharmacokinetics: 20–60 hours, variable Pharmacodynamics: 42–72 hours†	PT/INR (2.0–3.0)
Dabigatran (Pradaxa)	Parenteral anticoagulant × 5–10 days, then dabigatran 150 mg PO BID	>80% renal, 20% biliary Prodrug	12–17 hours 14–17 hours (elderly)	None required
Rivaroxaban (Xarelto)	15 mg PO BID × 21 days; then 20 mg PO QD	66% renal, 33% biliary CYP450 substrate	5–9 hours 9–12 hours (elderly)	None required
Apixaban (Eliquis)	10 mg PO BID × 7 days, then 5 mg PO BID	25% renal, 75% biliary CYP450 substrate	8–15 hours	None required
Edoxaban (Savaysa)	Parenteral anticoagulant × 5–10 days, then edoxaban 60 mg PO QD (30 mg QD for ≤60 kg)	35% renal, 60% biliary	10–14 hours	None required

*Anti–factor Xa activity can be used in selected circumstances such as extremes of body weight (<45 kg or >100 kg).
†Pharmacodynamics of coagulation protein recovery most relevant to in vivo effect of VKA.
aPTT, Activated partial thromboplastin time; *BID*, twice daily; *INR*, international normalized ratio; *IV*, intravenous; *LMWH*, low-molecular-weight heparin; *PO*, orally; *PT*, prothrombin time; *QD*, once daily; *SQ*, subcutaneous; *UFH*, unfractionated heparin; *VKA*, vitamin K antagonist.

modification is required for both efficient protein secretion and function (membrane binding) of coagulation factors VII, IX, X, and II. Vitamin K is oxidized during γ-carboxylation of these coagulation factors, and warfarin inhibits enzymatic regeneration of the reduced form of vitamin K, creating a functional deficiency. This mechanism of action is the basis for (1) the reversibility of the warfarin by administration of the reduced form of vitamin K, (2) the reduction in warfarin effect by dietary vitamin K, and (3) the enhancement of the warfarin effect by many antibiotics, as bacterial flora are a major source of vitamin K. Warfarin also undergoes extensive metabolism by the liver, which provides multiple opportunities for drug interactions. Thus genetic variation in liver metabolism, variable dietary vitamin K intake, and numerous potential drug interactions generate substantial individual variation in warfarin dose requirements.

Warfarin (2.5- to 10-mg initial dose) is usually started the same day as heparin, overlapped with parenteral heparin therapy for a *minimum* of 5 days and discontinued once a therapeutic warfarin level is obtained on two consecutive days. The warfarin effect is monitored by the international normalized ratio (INR), which represents a prothrombin time that has been corrected for specific reagent sensitivity. The target INR for VTE treatment is 2.0 to 3.0. The pharmacodynamic effects of warfarin on the INR are primarily determined by the in vivo half-lives of the relevant coagulation factors. Thus the full effect of a warfarin dose change on the INR is usually not seen for 48 to 72 hours, correlating with the half-life of factors IX, X, and prothrombin (factor II). This delayed effect necessitates overlap with heparin therapy for at least 5 days, or longer if further warfarin dose titration is required to reach a therapeutic INR. Initial warfarin dosing should be conservative (2.5 mg daily) if enhanced sensitivity is expected, including patients that are elderly (>65 years old), low body weight (<45 kg), hypoalbuminemic (<2 g/dL), on antibiotic therapy, or have poor oral intake.

The traditional heparin-warfarin regimen has been increasingly supplanted by the use of DOACs. DOACs are orally available, low-molecular-weight compounds that directly inhibit the active site of either factor Xa (rivaroxaban, apixaban, edoxaban [Savaysa]), or thrombin (dabigatran [Pradaxa]). In general, these drugs possess predictable pharmacokinetics and relatively short half-lives, allowing fixed once- or twice-daily oral dosing without routine monitoring. Both rivaroxaban and apixaban are approved for initial use after the VTE diagnosis with a more intensive dose regimen that tapers to the standard maintenance dose after 21 days for rivaroxaban or 7 days for apixaban (Table 4). Edoxaban and dabigatran are approved for continued treatment of VTE at their standard maintenance dose after 5 to 10 days of a parenteral anticoagulant (usually LWMH). Differences in clearance mechanisms have implications for clinical usage. For instance, dabigatran is heavily dependent on renal clearance and can accumulate with increased bleeding risk in patients with significant renal insufficiency (CrCl < 30 mL/min). In contrast, apixaban dosing is less affected by renal insufficiency but should not be used in patients with significant liver dysfunction or biliary stasis.

Comparison of Warfarin Versus DOACs

DOACs demonstrate equivalent efficacy to the traditional combination of LMWH and warfarin in the treatment of VTE. Advantages of the DOACs include rapid onset of action, predictable dose response, no monitoring requirement, elimination of parenteral therapy (rivaroxaban and apixaban), no significant diet interactions, limited drug interactions, and an overall safety signal equivalent to or better than warfarin. Metaanalyses of DOAC trials demonstrate that fatal bleeding, intracranial hemorrhage (ICH), and clinically relevant, nonmajor bleeding are reduced with DOACs compared with warfarin. The rate of gastrointestinal (GI) bleeding was similar. Given the potentially life-changing nature of ICH, the lower rate with DOACs is particularly significant. Disadvantages of DOACs include cost, inability to monitor compliance with routine coagulation testing, the effect of renal function on drug clearance, and lack of widely available reversal

TABLE 5 Reversal Agents

DRUG	REVERSAL AGENT	DOSING	COMMENTS
Heparin	Protamine*	1–1.5 mg/100 U UFH IV	Hypersensitivity reactions, less effective vs. LMWH
Warfarin	Four-factor PCC (Kcentra) FFP Vitamin K	25–50 U/kg IV 2–4 L 1–10 mg PO or IV	Dose depends on INR, PCC favored over FFP Volume overload, transfusion reaction Reversal takes 6–24 hours
Dabigatran	Idarucizumab (Praxbind)	2.5 g IV for 2 doses (within 15 min)	Drug specific monoclonal Fab fragment
Rivaroxaban Apixaban Edoxaban	Andexanet alfa (Andexxa) (approved for reversal of rivaroxaban or apixaban only) Four-factor PCC†	800 mg IV bolus at 30 mg/min, then 960 mg infusion at 8 mg/min 50 U/kg IV	Reverses factor Xa active site inhibitors

*FDA approved for treatment of heparin overdose. Off-label uses: heparin neutralization (adults); intracranial hemorrhage associated with heparin or LMWH; LMWH overdose (adults).

†Evidence for reversal of factor Xa inhibitors by PCC is low quality.

Fab, Fragment antigen-binding; *FDA*, U.S. Food and Drug Administration; *FFP*, fresh frozen plasma; *INR*, international normalized ratio; *IV*, intravenous; *LMWH*, low-molecular-weight heparin; *PCC*, prothrombin complex concentrate; *PO*, orally; *UFH*, unfractionated heparin.

agents. The relatively short half-lives of DOACs and recent development of reversal agents (Table 5) partially overcome the reversibility advantage for warfarin. Largely based on safety profile and ease of use, recent guidelines provide a weak recommendation for DOACs over warfarin in patients without cancer.

Cancer-Associated Thrombosis

VTE associated with cancer accounts for approximately 20% of all cases and clearly is a heterogeneous patient population. Treatment of cancer-associated thrombosis is problematic in that patients are at increased risk for both VTE recurrence and bleeding complications. In addition to the multiple drug interactions that complicate VKA use in cancer patients, LMWH demonstrates significantly lower rates of recurrent VTE relative to VKA therapy. Thus LMWH for the first 6 months after the event has been the standard recommendation. The role of DOACs in cancer-associated thrombosis continues to evolve. Metaanalysis of subgroups from the large DOAC VTE trials demonstrates no difference in VTE recurrence or major bleeding compared with LMWH for primarily low-risk cancer patients. Subsequent comparison of edoxaban[1] and dalteparin (Fragmin) (Hokusai trial) in a broader population of active cancer patients demonstrated a lower rate of VTE recurrence but higher rate of major bleeding. A randomized study comparing rivaroxaban[1] to dalteparin (SELECT-D) demonstrated similar findings with reduced VTE rate and increased nonmajor bleeding in the DOAC arm. The increased bleeding was primarily observed in patients with upper GI or urothelial cancers in both studies. Ongoing studies will further address the role of DOACs in this setting. Duration of therapy is generally at least 6 months but may be modified based on disease response, bleeding risk, and prognosis.

Special Considerations in the Acute Management of Venous Thromboembolism

Although the vast majority of patients diagnosed with VTE should be promptly initiated on therapeutic anticoagulation, a limited number of acute presentations may require a modified approach as described in the following sections.

Massive Pulmonary Embolism With Hemodynamic Instability

Patients presenting with hemodynamically unstable PE (systolic blood pressure < 90 mm Hg for 15 minutes, requiring vasopressors or overt shock) are at high risk for right heart failure and death. The focus for these patients should be resuscitation (IV fluids, pressors, oxygenation, and airway control) and rapid confirmation of diagnosis (perfusion scan or CTPA). If highly unstable, then bedside echocardiogram may be used for a presumptive diagnosis based on right ventricular findings. Prompt thrombolytic therapy (tPA [Activase][1] 100 mg IV) or consideration of emergency endovascular therapy should be pursued, with the former being more readily available.

Patients who present with worsening right heart failure, preresuscitation cardiopulmonary arrest, free-floating thrombus, or high thrombus burden in the absence of systemic hypotension may also be considered for thrombolytic therapy. Many institutions have a PE response team to facilitate decision making and institution of therapy. However, for the majority of patients presenting with evidence of right ventricular dysfunction (by echocardiogram or CT) without systemic hypotension (i.e., submassive or intermediate risk PE), the use of thrombolytic therapy remains controversial. This controversy stems from both heterogeneity in patient selection for these trials and the inability to demonstrate long-term benefits over anticoagulation alone.

Broader use of thrombolytic therapy is primarily limited by the increased risk of major bleeding (9.2%) versus anticoagulation (3.4%), which includes a 1.5% incidence of intracranial bleeding. Contraindications include previous ICH, known intracranial vascular lesion or malignancy, ischemic stroke within 3 months, suspected aortic dissection, active bleeding or bleeding diathesis, and closed head/facial trauma within 3 months. Relative contraindications include poorly controlled hypertension, recent surgery (14 days), and pregnancy. The use of combined modalities (catheter-based fibrinolysis, pharmaco-mechanical clot dissolution) and lower doses of tissue plasminogen activator (tPA[1] 50 mg IV) may modulate the bleeding risk, but currently, broader application of thrombolytic therapy remains controversial.

Extensive Proximal Vein Lower Extremity Thrombosis

Proximal iliac vein thrombosis is often highly symptomatic and may result in severe PTS. Rarely, compromise of the arterial supply may occur, as described for phlegmasia alba dolens ("milk leg") and phlegmasia cerulea dolens. The former describes a swollen, white extremity with early compromise of arterial flow secondary to extensive DVT. The latter is an advanced stage characterized by severe swelling, cyanosis, and blue discoloration of the extremity—a precursor of venous gangrene. These entities are emergencies that require prompt anticoagulation, elevation, and consideration of endovascular intervention. The presence of bilateral proximal iliac vein thrombosis should prompt evaluation for inferior vena cava (IVC) thrombus or agenesis, particularly in

---

[1] Not FDA approved for this indication.

[1] Not FDA approved for this indication.

younger patients. Catheter-directed thrombolysis and endovascular approaches have been pursued in proximal iliofemoral venous thrombosis in an attempt to reduce the risk of severe PTS. Recent studies have been unable to demonstrate that the desired benefit in PTS reduction outweighs the increased risk of bleeding. Thus the routine use of thrombolytic therapy for proximal iliofemoral venous thrombosis cannot be recommended, and patient selection for this approach remains controversial.

Spontaneous Proximal Upper Extremity Thrombosis

The majority of upper extremity DVT is related to intravenous catheters, malignancy, or thrombophilia. Spontaneous upper extremity DVT in the absence of provocation is rare. This entity (Paget-Schroetter syndrome) tends to occur in a younger, often adolescent population with a recent history of exercise or strenuous activity usually involving the dominant upper extremity. This presentation in the absence of usual VTE risk factors should prompt an evaluation for venous thoracic outlet syndrome (TOS). Because of the younger age of these patients and significant disability associated with PTS in the upper extremity (particularly the dominant hand), the initial approach has included thrombolysis (within 14 days), anticoagulation, and evaluation for venous TOS. However, no rigorous comparison of these approaches or combinations of approaches has been undertaken. If evidence for venous TOS is demonstrated, first rib resection on the affected side is often recommended. In the absence of a predisposing anatomic abnormality, an underlying thrombophilic state or occult malignancy should be considered.

Venous Thromboembolism Presenting With Paradoxical Embolism

The occurrence of arterial embolism, most commonly cryptogenic stroke, in the presence of DVT and a right-to-left shunt (i.e., patent foramen ovale [PFO]) suggests the diagnosis of paradoxical embolus. Standard anticoagulation for VTE is recommended, followed by PFO closure when complete. If indefinite anticoagulation is planned, the additional benefit of PFO closure is unclear.

DOACs in End-Stage Renal Disease

Warfarin has been the mainstay for treatment of VTE in patients with end-stage renal disease (ESRD). Most DOACs cannot be used in patients with creatinine clearance less than 30 mL/min because of the lack of randomized trial data in this population. However, apixaban is FDA approved for use even in patients with ESRD without dose adjustment based on its predominantly hepatic clearance and pharmacokinetic data.

Apixaban has been increasingly used in these patients because of its convenient dosing and lack of UFH bridging that typically requires hospitalization. Several small-center studies and a large retrospective study of patients with ESRD and newly diagnosed VTE who received either apixaban or warfarin suggest apixaban is associated with lower incidence of major bleeding with comparable incidence of recurrent VTE and all-cause mortality. It must be borne in mind that bleeding rates in ESRD patients on anticoagulation are overall higher than the general population. At this time, an individualized approach is recommended based on patient risk factors for bleeding and recurrent thrombosis, as well as treatment duration and cost, in determining appropriateness of apixaban in such cases.

DOACs in Obesity

There is a lack of consensus regarding direct oral anticoagulant dosing for the management of VTE in obese patients, particularly morbidly obese patients, given the relative scarcity of randomized clinical trial data in patients with a body mass index greater than 40 kg/m² or weight greater than 120 kg. This stems from concern that fixed dosing in obese patients might lead to decreased drug exposure and lower efficacy.

Retrospective and prospective studies, as well as metaanalyses comparing DOAC with VKA in VTE, have shown similar efficacy and bleeding signal in obese patients. As a result, in patients with BMI greater than 40 kg/m² or weight greater than 120 kg,

the 2021 International Society on Thrombosis and Hemostasis (ISTH) guidelines suggest that standard doses of apixaban or rivaroxaban and weight-based LMWH are appropriate for the treatment of VTE and VTE prophylaxis. Data on other DOACs are not sufficient at this time.

Moreover, ISTH no longer recommends regularly monitoring peak or trough drug-specific DOAC levels because there are insufficient data to influence management decisions. It is therefore reasonable to consider using standard doses of apixaban or rivaroxaban in obese patients after weighing the risks and benefits.

In obese patients receiving LMWH for acute VTE, the initial LMWH dose is recommended according to *actual body weight* rather than a fixed maximum daily dose by American Society of Hematology guidelines. Routine monitoring of LMWH is no longer recommended because of the unclear effect of anti–factor Xa levels with bleeding and lack of standardization.

Acute Venous Thromboembolism With Contraindication to Anticoagulation

Occasionally patients diagnosed with acute VTE will have an absolute contraindication to anticoagulation. Placement of a temporary IVC filter may be considered in these patients to provide short-term protection from PE. However, the vast majority of contraindications to anticoagulation are temporary, and definitive anticoagulation therapy should be instituted as soon as feasible. IVC filter use is associated with increased risk of lower extremity DVT. Evaluation for IVC filter removal should be planned within 3 to 6 months, depending on the clinical scenario.

Isolated Subsegmental Pulmonary Embolism and Incidental Venous Thromboembolism

The enhanced sensitivity of current CT scanners and extensive use of CT angiography has led to an increased diagnosis of isolated subsegmental PE. Treatment of isolated subsegmental PE (where proximal DVT has been excluded) is controversial as the natural history and benefit of anticoagulation is unclear. If an isolated subsegmental defect occurs in a clinical context that is high risk for recurrent VTE (e.g., malignancy), therapeutic anticoagulation is preferred. Alternatively, for an isolated subsegmental PE occurring in a patient that is otherwise low risk for VTE recurrence, clinical surveillance is preferred. Based on the frequency of diagnostic and staging CT scans in cancer patients, an incidental diagnosis of VTE is not an uncommon finding. Although outcome data are limited in this setting, incidental VTE appears to have similar effects on mortality and risk of VTE recurrence. Because the outcomes for incidental and symptomatic VTE in cancer patients appear similar, most cases of incidental VTE should be treated similar to symptomatic VTE.

Special Circumstances for Anticoagulant Monitoring

The predictable dose responses for LMWH, fondaparinux, and the DOACs allow use without monitoring. However, select circumstances exist where monitoring may be desirable. LMWH is the preferred anticoagulant in pregnancy, but weight-based dosing may not be as accurate during pregnancy. Periodic confirmation of therapeutic target levels (0.5 to 1.2 U/mL anti–factor Xa activity) 4 hours after subcutaneous injection is often recommended. Likewise, the accuracy of weight-based LMWH dosing with a body weight less than 45 kg or greater than 100 kg is not extensively validated. Confirmation of therapeutic peak levels in these individuals is recommended. Similarly, a need for DOAC drug levels may arise when assessing compliance, bleeding with potential drug overdose, or for an emergent procedure. DOACs directed against factor Xa (rivaroxaban, apixaban, and edoxaban) are monitored with an anti–factor Xa activity assay using a drug-specific standard curve. Significant dabigatran drug effect is excluded with a normal thrombin time. Alternatively, dabigatran drug effect can be detected by prolongation of the aPTT or more specialized coagulation tests. The INR is not sensitive to dabigatran.

Reversal Agents

Acute reversal of anticoagulation may be required for drug overdose with clinically significant bleeding or emergent procedures. If the situation is nonemergent, holding warfarin (4 to 5 days depending on INR) or DOACs (2 to 3 days depending on renal function) is preferable. If urgent reversal is required, specific agents exist for UFH, warfarin, and, more recently, DOACs (Table 5). Although UFH overdose may be reversed with dose-adjusted protamine, the short half-life of UFH and potential toxicity of protamine often mitigate against use. Protamine is most commonly used to reverse high-dose UFH after cardiopulmonary bypass. LMWH overdose may also be treated with protamine,[1] but significantly less effectively. Warfarin is fully reversed by administration of four-factor prothrombin complex concentrate (PCC) or fresh frozen plasma (FFP). The four-factor PCC dose is modified based on the INR and favored over FFP, which may be complicated by volume overload and transfusion reactions. Immediate reversal with PCC or FFP should be followed with 5 to 10 mg vitamin K by the oral or IV route. Vitamin K takes 6 to 24 hours to act but is critical to maintaining anticoagulant reversal because the PCC or FFP effect will wane based on plasma half-life of the coagulation factors. Notably, high doses of vitamin K can result in relative warfarin resistance for the ensuing 1 to 2 weeks. Lower doses of vitamin K (1 to 2 mg) may be appropriate for less serious bleeding where early reinitiation of warfarin is anticipated. Highly specific agents for the reversal of DOACs are now available. Dabigatran is rapidly reversed by administration of idarucizumab (Praxbind), a humanized monoclonal fragment antigen-binding (Fab) fragment that neutralizes the parent drug and major metabolites. DOACs targeting factor Xa (rivaroxaban, apixaban, edoxaban) may be rapidly reversed with andexanet alfa (Andexxa), a truncated, inactive form of recombinant factor Xa that acts as a decoy for small molecules targeting the factor Xa active site. Andexanet alfa was approved for life-threatening bleeding in patients treated with rivaroxaban and apixaban based on an open-label, single-group study (ANNEXA-4). Given the relatively short half-lives of the DOACs, high cost, and association with increased risk of thromboembolic events for andexanet alfa, it should be reserved for truly emergent procedures or life-threatening anticoagulant-related bleeding. Use of andexanet alfa in patients treated with edoxaban or betrixaban is off-label.

[1] Not FDA approved for this indication.

Duration of Anticoagulation

Standard treatment for a new episode of DVT or PE has traditionally been 3 to 6 months of therapeutic anticoagulation. The recommended duration of anticoagulation for VTE requires individualized analysis of the clinical presentation and patient-specific factors that weigh both recurrence and bleeding risk (Figure 3).

Clinical Presentation

Recurrence risk varies widely based on clinical presentation (see Epidemiology and Natural History). The key distinction is between events that occur in the absence (unprovoked) versus the presence (provoked) of established VTE risk factors (Table 1). The majority of cases with clinical risk factors present may be categorized as transient/reversible (e.g., surgery, estrogen) or permanent/nonreversible (e.g., dense hemiplegia secondary to stroke). Surgery is a major transient risk factor for VTE with a low recurrence risk (3% at 5 years). Three months of anticoagulation is sufficient for this population, whereas shorter durations are associated with increased risk of recurrence. Estrogen-related events have a similarly low risk of recurrence if reexposure is avoided. A second category of VTE events occurs in association with a nonsurgical transient risk factor (leg injury, significant medical illness, travel association) and demonstrates an intermediate recurrence risk (15% at 5 years). This subgroup is substantially more heterogeneous than the surgical group, with a variety of triggering factors and broader recurrence risk estimates. VTE events associated with nonreversible clinical risk factors may require extended anticoagulation with periodic reassessment of risks and benefits. Unprovoked VTE demonstrates a high risk of recurrence (30% at 5 years) and, in many respects, behaves as a chronic disease. Finally, patients with an underlying malignancy represent approximately 20% of VTE cases but are usually excluded from natural history studies. Cancer-associated thrombosis demonstrates a 15% annualized recurrence risk with longer-term risk more difficult to estimate based on competing mortality from the underlying cancer. These patients have concomitant increased bleeding risk, complicating the risk-benefit analysis for anticoagulation.

Thrombus Site

Thrombus location significantly influences recurrence risk, with more proximal events demonstrating higher rates of recurrence. Patients with isolated distal or calf vein DVT are half as likely to have recurrent events compared with proximal DVT or PE. Patients presenting with proximal DVT have similar recurrence risk to patients with PE. However, patients initially

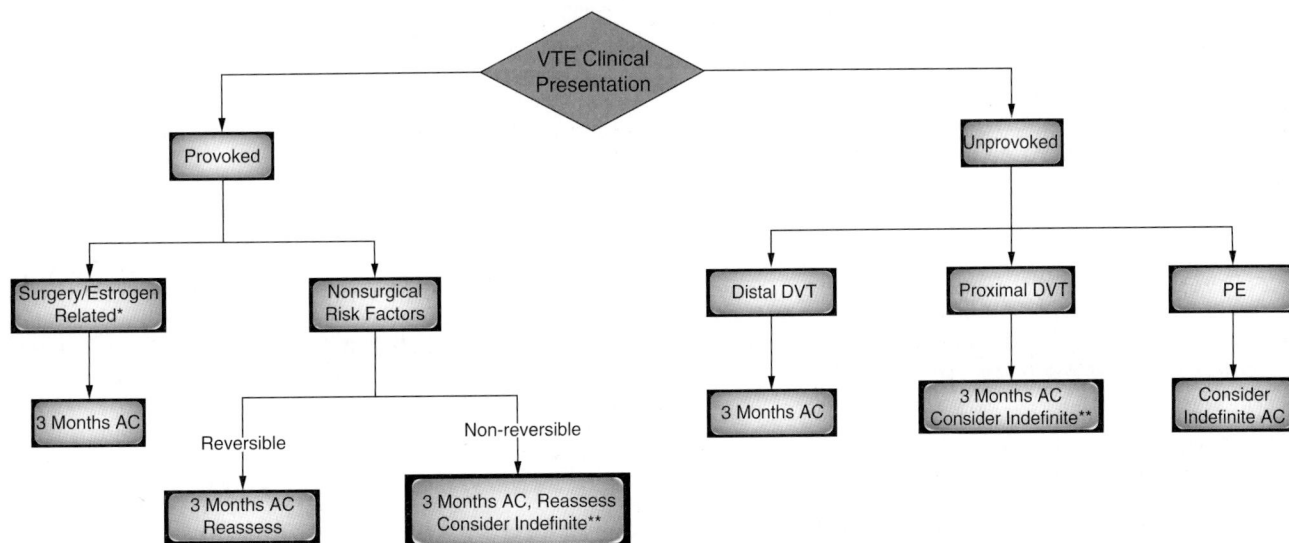

Figure 3 Suggested algorithm for treatment of venous thromboembolism *(VTE)*. *Estrogen-related includes oral contraceptives, hormone replacement therapy, pregnancy, and puerperium. **Indefinite anticoagulation *(AC)* includes reduced-dose direct oral anticoagulant options after initial 3 months therapeutic AC. *DVT,* Deep venous thrombosis; *PE,* pulmonary embolism.

presenting with PE are substantially more likely to have a PE recurrence relative to patients presenting with DVT only. This finding takes on particular importance when one considers the cause-specific mortality rate associated with PE is greater than 10%. Thus patients presenting with unprovoked PE deserve particular attention with regard to consideration of indefinite anticoagulation.

Standard Versus Indefinite Anticoagulation

Clinical presentation categorizes patients with regard to recurrence risk, which is critical to the decision between standard (3 months) and indefinite anticoagulation (Figure 3). This decision is also influenced by bleeding risk and requires clinical judgment. As mentioned earlier, VTE associated with surgical or estrogen-related provoking factors and distal DVT (provoked or unprovoked) should be treated with therapeutic anticoagulation for 3 months. Conversely, most patients with unprovoked proximal DVT or PE should be considered for indefinite therapy based on their substantial recurrence risk unless they also have high bleeding risk. There is little rationale for arbitrary extended periods of anticoagulation beyond the standard 3 to 6 months, unless awaiting resolution of a risk factor (e.g., extended immobilization). Prolongation of anticoagulation beyond 6 months in patients with unprovoked VTE delays but clearly does not prevent recurrence. A number of strategies, including postanticoagulation D-dimer testing (3 to 5 weeks) and risk stratification models, have attempted to identify patients with unprovoked VTE for which anticoagulation may be safely stopped. Postanticoagulation D-dimer testing is the most established strategy, further stratifying these patients into high (8.8%) and low (3.0%) first-year recurrence rates. Conversely, the presence of persistent or multiple antiphospholipid antibodies increases recurrence risk (1.8- to 4.5-fold) for patients presenting with unprovoked VTE. Alternative approaches to risk reduction in unprovoked VTE include indefinite anticoagulation with reduced-intensity DOACs or daily acetylsalicylic acid (ASA). ASA reduces recurrence risk by approximately one-third in unprovoked VTE but is inferior to reduced-dose rivaroxaban and apixaban (EINSTEIN CHOICE, AMPLIFY-EXT).

VTE associated with nonsurgical risk factors is more problematic with regard to definitive assessment of recurrence risk. Patients who suffer VTE with minor provocations may have a recurrence rate that approaches unprovoked VTE. These patients should be treated for at least 3 months and reassessed. Clinical factors that may impact a decision for indefinite anticoagulation include underlying cardiopulmonary disease (decreased ability to tolerate recurrence), ongoing inflammation (inflammatory bowel disease, autoimmune disease, chronic infections), prolonged immobilization (stroke), and male sex. For patients with a prolonged but ultimately reversible risk factor (i.e., stroke immobility improving with physical therapy), prolongation of anticoagulation until resolution of the underlying risk factor is reasonable. Similarly, travel-associated thrombosis may be a recurring risk that requires an intermittent prophylaxis plan. Bleeding risk assessment is important to decisions regarding recommended duration of therapy. Major risk factors for bleeding on anticoagulation include advanced age, previous bleeding history, cancer, renal or liver failure, previous stroke, diabetes mellitus, nonsteroidal inflammatory drugs or antiplatelet therapy, comorbidity and reduced functional capacity, recent surgery, frequent falls, and alcohol (Table 6). Additional risk assessment tools (e.g., HAS-BLED score) exist, primarily validated for warfarin therapy.

Clinical Decision Making

Particularly for clinical situations with modest evidence, shared decision making between physician and patient is desirable in determining the duration of anticoagulant therapy. Medical comorbidities affecting bleeding or fall risk in the elderly, patient anxiety about recurrent VTE events, and occupational/lifestyle risks for trauma may substantially affect anticoagulation

decisions. Family history should be obtained with particular attention to first-degree relatives affected by VTE, including unprovoked events and age of presentation. Questions regarding the underlying cause for a VTE event often drive requests for thrombophilia evaluations. These requests generally fail to acknowledge the complex, multigenic basis for VTE and rarely contribute to clinical decision making (see Genetics of Venous Thromboembolism). The clinical presentation and family history are substantially more useful than identification of minor thrombophilia traits, which are poor predictors of VTE recurrence. Finally, when a decision is made to pursue indefinite anticoagulation, periodic reassessment of this decision is important. The risk-to-benefit ratio of anticoagulation may change as the patient's medical history evolves. The hematology consultant serves an important role in facilitating difficult anticoagulation decisions.

TABLE 6 Risk Factors for Bleeding With Anticoagulant Therapy and Estimated Risk of Major Bleeding in Low-, Moderate-, and High-Risk Categories

Risk Factors

Age > 65 y

Previous bleeding

Cancer

Metastatic cancer

Renal failure

Liver failure

Thrombocytopenia

Previous stroke

Diabetes

Anemia

Antiplatelet therapy

Poor anticoagulant control

Comorbidity and reduced functional capacity

Recent surgery

Frequent falls

Alcohol abuse

Nonsteroidal antiinflammatory drug

Categorization of Risk of Bleeding

	ESTIMATED ABSOLUTE RISK OF MAJOR BLEEDING		
	LOW RISK (0 RISK FACTORS)	MODERATE RISK (1 RISK FACTOR)	HIGH RISK (≥2 RISK FACTORS)
Anticoagulation 0–3 mo			
Baseline risk (%)	0.6	1.2	4.8
Increased risk (%)	1.0	2.0	8.0
Total risk (%)	1.6	3.2	12.8
Anticoagulation after first 3 mo			
Baseline risk (%/y)	0.3	0.6	≥2.5
Increased risk (%/y)	0.5	1.0	≥4.0
Total risk (%/y)	0.8	1.6	≥6.5

Data from the Ninth Edition of the Antithrombotic Guideline (AT9).

TABLE 7 Risk Factor Stratification and Prophylaxis Options

RISK STRATIFICATION	RECOMMENDED PROPHYLAXIS	DURATION
Low Risk		
Same-day surgery Medical illness in a fully mobile patient	Early mobilization	–
Moderate Risk		
Most general surgery procedures	LMWH UFH IPC/GCS with or without pharmacologic prophylaxis as appropriate	5–14 days

Most acute medical illnesses	LMWH
	UFH
	Betrixaban*[2]
		Duration of inpatient stay
		Extended duration beyond hospitalization may
		    be appropriate for very high-risk patients in
		    whom bleeding risk is low

High Risk		
Hip or knee replacement surgery	LMWH UFH Fondaparinux Rivaroxaban Apixaban Dabigatran[†] Adjusted dose warfarin	At least 10–14 days Extended duration up to 4 weeks preferred ASA[1] may be used subsequently for extended duration of therapy
General surgery with active cancer, previous VTE	LMWH[‡] UFH Adjusted dose warfarin	Extended duration (4 weeks) for abdominopelvic surgeries in cancer patients
Major trauma, spinal cord injury	IPC with or without GCS, use pharmacologic prophylaxis when appropriate	

*FDA approved for patients hospitalized for acute medical illness at high risk of VTE.
[†]FDA approved for VTE prevention after hip replacement surgery.
[‡]Off-label use in cancer patients.
[1]Not FDA approved for this indication.
[2]Not available in the United States.
ASA, Acetylsalicylic acid; *DVT*, deep venous thrombosis; *FDA*, U.S. Food and Drug Administration; *GCS*, graduated compression stockings; *IPC*, intermittent pneumatic compression; *LMWH*, low-molecular-weight heparin; *UFH*, unfractionated heparin; *VTE*, venous thromboembolism.

Prevention of Venous Thromboembolism

About 60% of VTE events are associated with recent hospitalization or surgery, and up to 70% of these cases are preventable. However, less than half of hospitalized patients receive appropriate prophylactic measures. Given the significant morbidity and mortality associated with VTE, primary prophylaxis strategies in high-risk situations are of great medical importance and may provide a cost savings. Risk stratification of patients based on surgery or medical illness, patient characteristics (e.g., previous VTE, active cancer, duration of immobility), and bleeding risk impact recommendations for pharmacologic and mechanical prophylaxis. Pharmacologic agents include LMWH, fondaparinux, low-dose UFH, VKA, and DOACs. The focus in this section is primarily on heparin and DOACs given the available evidence. Mechanical prophylaxis includes graduated compression stockings (GCS) that are greater than 15 mm Hg at the ankle or intermittent pneumatic compression devices (IPCs). IPCs enhance lower extremity deep vein blood flow and may increase fibrinolytic activity. These modalities can be used alone or in combination for patients with high bleeding risk who cannot use pharmacologic prophylaxis. IPCs are considered more effective than GCS alone, particularly after orthopedic surgery.

General Surgery

For general surgery patients, well-established risk assessment tools such as the Caprini or Rogers scores stratify patients by VTE risk to identify those who would benefit from pharmacologic prophylaxis. In general, if the risk of VTE is moderate to high and bleeding risk is low, pharmacologic prophylaxis with LMWH or low-dose UFH should be given. If the bleeding risk is high, intermittent pneumatic compression with or without GCS should be used. Ideally, the minimal duration of prophylaxis is 5 to 10 days but varies widely based on duration of bed rest, inpatient stay, and comorbid conditions. In patients with active cancer undergoing abdominopelvic surgery, prophylaxis should be extended to 4 weeks after surgery.

Orthopedic Surgery

Orthopedic procedures are associated with high risk of VTE, especially those involving the lower extremities and pelvic region. For patients undergoing total hip or total knee arthroplasty, pharmacologic prophylaxis using LMWH, UFH, DOACs, or adjusted-dose warfarin should be used if no contraindication exists. LMWH is quite effective and safe with the benefit of long-term experience with these agents. Low-dose DOACs have shown comparable efficacy to enoxaparin in this population with a similar low absolute risk of bleeding. Low-dose apixaban (2.5 mg twice daily), rivaroxaban (10 mg daily), and dabigatran (220 mg daily) appear safer than higher doses. Prophylaxis should continue at least 10 to 14 days, and prolongation up to a month should be considered for major orthopedic surgery. Low-dose aspirin[1] has been shown to be effective for extended prophylaxis after initial acute phase of therapy (~5 days) with standard anticoagulants in patients undergoing total hip or knee arthroplasty; however, anticoagulants are generally favored for high-risk patients. IPCs should be used during the inpatient stay in addition to pharmacologic prophylaxis. If bleeding risk is high, IPCs should be used until pharmacologic agents can be safely

[1]Not FDA approved for this indication.

administered. For arthroscopic procedures of the knee and other low-risk procedures, prophylaxis is generally not indicated unless other risk factors exist. A summary of available agents and recommendations for prophylaxis is provided (Table 7).

Acute Medical Illness

For hospitalized patients with medical illnesses, the risk of VTE is approximately eightfold higher than the general population. Patients expected to be hospitalized with reduced mobility for more than 3 days, a previous history of VTE, active infection or malignancy, recent surgery or trauma, heart failure, or respiratory failure should be considered for prophylaxis. The Padua score is a prospectively validated risk assessment model that stratifies patients into groups with high (~11%) or low (0.3%) incidence of VTE. Current prophylaxis options for medical patients include LMWH, low-dose UFH, and fondaparinux.[1] When bleeding risk is considered moderate to high, mechanical prophylaxis using IPCs or GCS should be used until it is safe to add anticoagulants. For low-risk patients admitted for short duration or remaining ambulatory, withholding prophylaxis may be appropriate. Clinical context and bleeding risk assessment should also impact these decisions.

Although pharmacologic prophylaxis is typically limited to the acute illness during the inpatient stay, analysis of population-based data suggests that approximately 75% of VTE events occur well after discharge, at a median of almost 3 weeks. Furthermore, increased compliance with inpatient prophylaxis over time has not resulted in the expected decrease in the rate of VTE. The effect of extended DOAC prophylaxis (35 to 42 days) has been examined in medical patients for apixaban[1] and rivaroxaban. Reduced-dose apixaban and rivaroxaban demonstrated similar VTE prevention to standard enoxaparin prophylaxis but increased bleeding events. Extended prophylaxis is an area of ongoing investigation with unresolved issues that include appropriate patient selection and discerning the effects of specific anticoagulants versus prophylaxis duration on outcomes.

---

[1] Not FDA approved for this indication.

References

Chatterjee S, Chakraborty A, Weinberg I, et al: Thrombolysis for pulmonary embolism and risk of all-cause mortality, major bleeding, and intracranial hemorrhage: a meta-analysis, *JAMA* 311(23):2414–2421, 2014.

Connors JM: Thrombophilia testing and venous thrombosis, *N Engl J Med* 377:1177–1187, 2017.

Ellenbogen MI, Ardeshirrouhanifard S, Segal JB, Streiff MB, Deitelzweig SB, Brotman DJ: Safety and effectiveness of apixaban versus warfarin for acute venous thromboembolism in patients with end-stage kidney disease: a national cohort study, *J Hosp Med* 17:809–818, 2022, https://doi.org/10.1002/jhm.12926.

Heit JA, Crusan DJ, Ashrani AA, Petterson TM, Bailey KR: Effect of a near-universal hospitalization-based prophylaxis regimen on annual number of venous thromboembolism events in the US, *Blood* 130:109–114, 2017.

Kearon C, Akl EA, Ornelas J, et al: Antithrombotic therapy for VTE disease: CHEST guideline and expert panel report, *Chest* 149:315–352, 2016.

Kearon C, Parpia S, Spencer FA, et al: Antiphospholipid antibodies and recurrent thrombosis after a first unprovoked venous thromboembolism, *Blood* 131:2151–2160, 2018.

Konstantinides SV, Vicaut E, Danays T, et al: Impact of thrombolytic therapy on the long-term outcome of intermediate-risk pulmonary embolism, *J Am Coll Cardiol* 69:1536–1544, 2017.

Martin KA, Beyer-Westendorf J, Davidson BL, Huisman MV, Sandset PM, Moll S: Use of direct oral anticoagulants in patients with obesity for treatment and prevention of venous thrombo- embolism: updated communication from the ISTH SSC Sub- committee on Control of Anticoagulation, *J Thromb Haemost* 19(8):1874–1882, 2021.

Raskob GE, van Es N, Verhamme P, et al: Edoxaban for the treatment of cancer-associated venous thromboembolism, *N Engl J Med* 378:615–624, 2018.

Ortel TL: American Society of Hematology 2020 guidelines for management of venous thromboembolism: treatment of deep vein thrombosis and pulmonary embolism, *Blood Adv* 4(19):4693–4738, 2020.

Vedantham S, Goldhaber SZ, Julian JA, et al: Pharmacomechanical catheter-directed thrombolysis for deep-vein thrombosis, *N Engl J Med* 377:2240–2252, 2017.

Weitz JI, Lensing AWA, Prins MH, et al: Rivaroxaban or aspirin for extended treatment of venous thromboembolism, *N Engl J Med* 376:1211–1222, 2017.

Zoller B, Ohlsson H, Sundquist J, Sundquist K: A sibling based design to quantify genetic and shared environmental effects of venous thromboembolism in Sweden, *Thromb Res* 149:82–87, 2017.

VIRAL AND MYCOPLASMAL PNEUMONIAS

Method of
Cheston B. Cunha, MD; and Burke A. Cunha, MD

CURRENT DIAGNOSIS

Influenza (human, avian, swine)

- Mild influenza A or B presents acutely with headache, fever, sore throat, plus/minus rhinorrhea.
- Severe influenza A presents with an acute onset (patients often able to name the hour the influenza began) and rapidly become bed bound.
- Headache, myalgias, and prostration may be severe.
- With swine influenza, gastrointestinal symptoms (e.g., nausea/vomiting or diarrhea) may be prominent.
- Auscultation of the lungs is quiet, disproportionate to the degree of respiratory distress. Influenza is an interstitial process and not alveolar, which explains the absence of rales.
- With severe influenza, patients rapidly become hypoxemic. Hypoxemia is accompanied by an A-a gradient >35, which indicates a interstitial oxygen diffusing defect.
- Severe tracheobronchitis is common and manifested by hemoptysis.
- Relative lymphopenia with monocytosis occurs early followed by thrombocytopenia and later leukopenia. Low titer elevations of cold agglutinins are not infrequent (≥1:18).
- Patients may have chest pain exacerbated by breathing mimicking pleuritic chest pain. This is the result of direct intracostal muscle involvement with the influenza virus, which results in myositis and pain on inspiration.
- The chest radiograph in early influenza in mild to moderate cases is normal or near normal, with minimal, if any, increase in interstitial markings. The chest radiograph in fulminant cases shows symmetrical bilateral patchy infiltrates without pleural effusion in 48 hours.
- Severe influenza A is accompanied by severe hypoxemia cyanosis, and may be followed by an early fatal outcome.
- Influenza pneumonia most often presents alone without bacterial superinfection, but bacterial infection may accompany (e.g., MSSA/CA-MRSA) or follow influenza (e.g., *S. pneumoniae* or *H. influenzae*).
- Purulent sputum with influenza indicates concurrent bacterial pneumonia usually caused by *S. aureus* (methicillin-susceptible *Staphylococcus aureus* [MSSA]/methicillin-resistant *Staphylococcus aureus* [MRSA]). Bacterial pneumonia following influenza (after 1–2 weeks), is suggested by leukocytosis, focal or segmental pulmonary infiltrates, and purulent sputum; the pathogens are not *S. aureus,* but most commonly are *S. pneumoniae, H. influenzae,* and rarely Group A streptococcus.
- A laboratory diagnosis may be made by multiplex polymerase chain reaction (PCR) of respiratory secretions.

COVID-19

- COVID-19 is caused by a novel β-coronavirus (different than the novel β-coronaviruses causing severe acute respiratory syndrome [SARS] and Middle East respiratory syndrome [MERS]) identified as SARS-CoV-2.
- Common nonspecific laboratory abnormalities include leukopenia, relative lymphopenia, thrombocytopenia, and mildly elevated serum transaminases.
- Chest x-ray (CXR) early resembles that of influenza pneumonia (i.e., essentially unremarkable, without definite/discreet infiltrates).
- As COVID-19 pneumonia progresses, the CXR shows bilateral interstitial fuzzy/fluffy peripheral infiltrates.

- Chest computed tomography (CT) scans may show bilateral peripheral infiltrates with or without consolidation.
- Diagnosis of COVID-19 is by reverse transcription PCR (RT-PCR) of respiratory tract specimens or antigen testing. RT-PCR usually becomes positive early in the disease course (days).

Mycoplasma pneumoniae
- In a patient with community-acquired pneumonia (CAP) who has a dry, nonproductive cough without severe headache or myalgias, the most likely diagnosis is *M. pneumoniae*. *M. pneumoniae* CAP is commonly accompanied by nonexudative pharyngitis and/or loose stools or watery diarrhea.
- The temperature is usually less than 102°F (38.9°C) and is not accompanied by frank rigors or pleuritic chest pain.
- Relative bradycardia and elevations in the serum transaminases are not features of *M. pneumoniae* CAP.
- Respiratory viruses are often associated with mild elevations of cold agglutinins (≤1:16) but *M. pneumoniae* is the only pathogen causing CAP associated with highly elevated cold agglutinin titers (≥1:64). Elevated cold agglutinin titers occur in up to 75% of patients with *M. pneumoniae*, and occur early and transiently.
- In a patient with CAP, elevated cold agglutinin titers (>1:8) effectively rule out the typical pathogens, as well as *Legionella* species and *C. pneumoniae*.
- In the absence of an antecedent respiratory tract infection (e.g., nonexudative pharyngitis, otitis, etc., in the preceding 3 months), the presence of an increased *M. pneumoniae* ELISA IgM titer is diagnostic of acute infection.

CURRENT THERAPY

Viral Influenza
- The aim of therapy is to inhibit the influenza virus and prevent its attachment/spread to uninfected respiratory epithelial cells.
- The neuramidase inhibitors (oseltamivir and zanamivir) shorten the course of influenza by 1 to 2 days and have antiviral activity. These agents are active against both influenza A and B.
- Most strains of human and avian flu, but not swine flu, are resistant to amantadine (Symmetrel) or rimantadine (Flumadine).
- Oseltamivir (Tamiflu) is recommended for treatment of influenza within 2 days of illness onset (see Table 3).
- Amantadine and rimantadine may have an important therapeutic effect in severe influenza A by increasing distal airway dilation and increasing oxygen action.
- Peramivir (Rapivab) may be useful in those unable to take oral neuraminase inhibitors.

COVID-19
- Oral agents are now available to treat COVID-19 patients: Nirmatrelvir/ritonavir (Paxlovid) is more effective than molnupiravir (Lagevrio, approved for Emergency Use Authorization by the FDA) in preventing disease progression.
- Effective therapy for hospitalized patients with COVID-19 pneumonia is with remdesivir (Veklury) 200 mg (IV) for the first dose, then 100 mg (IV) q24h for 5 to 10 days.
- Dexamethasone[1] 6 mg IV/ PO daily for 10 days should be considered in patients who are hospitalized and require supplemental oxygen.

Mycoplasma pneumoniae
- The agents active against *M. pneumoniae* are macrolides, tetracyclines, quinolones, and ketolides. β-Lactam antibiotics are not active against *M. pneumoniae* because it does not contain a bacterial cell wall.

- Goals of therapy of *M. pneumoniae* CAP are to eradicate the infection, decrease the shedding of *M. pneumoniae* in respiratory secretions posttherapy, and to prevent post-treatment asthma.
- Therapy is equally efficacious with macrolides, doxycycline (Vibramycin), or a respiratory quinolone intravenously, orally, or in combination for 1 to 2 weeks.
- The mode of administration is determined by the severity of the CAP and the setting. Outpatients are usually treated orally. Patients hospitalized with severe CAP are initially treated intravenously and then changed to an oral agent.
- Macrolide resistance to *M. pneumoniae* has been described in children and reported in adults.

---

[1]Not FDA approved for this indication.

Influenza pneumonia is the most important cause of viral pneumonia in adults. Influenza A is the predominant type of influenza found in adults, and influenza B is more common in children. Influenza A has the potential for severe disease, occurs seasonally, and is the predominant type involved in influenza pandemics. *M. pneumoniae* CAP was first recognized decades ago as distinctive from bacterial and viral pneumonias. It was originally described by Eaton as "Eaton agent" pneumonia caused by a pleuropneumonia-like organism (PPLO), later shown to be caused by *M. pneumoniae*. *M. pneumoniae* is a common cause of pneumonia in all age groups, but the peak incidence of *M. pneumoniae* CAP is in young adults. *M. pneumoniae* CAP is a common cause of ambulatory CAP.

The term *atypical pneumonia* was first applied to viral pneumonias because the clinical laboratory and radiologic findings were different from those caused by typical bacterial pulmonary pathogens. In influenza pneumonia, the clinical findings are confined to the trachea, bronchi, lung parenchyma, and central nervous system. *M. pneumoniae* CAP is a systemic infection with a pulmonary component. Over the years, atypical pneumonia has come to refer to pneumonia caused by systemic nonviral/nonbacterial pathogen agents that have a pulmonary component. Viral pneumonias are no longer considered atypical pneumonias. Atypical pneumonias may be divided into nonzoonotic and zoonotic atypical CAPs. Nonzoonotic CAPs are most commonly caused by *M. pneumoniae*, *Chlamydia pneumoniae*, or *Legionella* species, whereas the three most common zoonotic atypical pneumonias are caused by *Chlamydia psittaci* (psittacosis), *Francisella tularensis* (tularemia), or *Coxiella burnetii* (Q fever). All of the atypical pneumonias are distinct clinical entities that may be differentiated on the basis of their characteristic pattern of extrapulmonary organ involvement. Although some viruses may occasionally have extrapulmonary manifestations (i.e., influenza, adenovirus with viral pneumonias), the primary clinical features are confined to the lungs. *M. pneumoniae* is a critical cause of nonzoonotic atypical CAP, particularly in the ambulatory setting. *M. pneumoniae* CAP may be severe in patients with impaired host defenses or those with severe, preexisting cardiopulmonary disease.

Influenza (Human, Avian, and Swine)
Viral influenza pneumonia affects children and adults. Influenza B is the primary cause of mild influenza in children and adults. Influenza A is primarily an infection of adults that may be mild to severe. Influenza A has the potential for pandemic spread (e.g., swine influenza [H_1N_1]).

Influenza occurs during the winter months, usually peaking in February. Influenza is spread by aerosolized droplet infection from person to person and via fomites. Influenza A is classified into subtypes based on hemagglutinin (H) and neuramidase (N) surface proteins. An important characteristic of the influenza A virus is antigenic drift, which refers to minor changes in surface protein shift in the neuramidase or hemagglutinin receptors. With influenza A, these surface receptor proteins are important in cellular adherence of the influenza virus and spread of influenza from respiratory epithelial cells. The vaccine for the flu season most often includes the influenza hemagglutinin and neuramidase types seen at the end of the preceding year's season. Prevention of attachment and spread of the virus is helpful in controlling the spread of influenza; vaccine protection conferred by specific antibody response to influenza A is highly protective (approximately 80% in noncompromised hosts).

During the years when influenza B has been prevalent, vaccines for the subsequent year contain an influenza B component.

Clinical manifestations of influenza A in adults varies considerably from mild to fatal infection. Mild infection is usually manifested as an acute febrile illness characterized by headache and myalgias with dry, unproductive cough and rhinorrhea. Mild influenza may be caused by influenza A or B and usually resolves in a few days without complications in normal hosts who have good cardiopulmonary function.

Severe influenza A (human, avian, swine) occurs in normal healthy adults and may be fatal. The onset of severe influenza A (human, avian, swine) is sudden, and the patient often recalls the exact hour of onset. The patient is febrile, with early/extreme prostration rendering the patient bedridden. Fever rapidly rises and may be accompanied by chills. Neck soreness, severe headache, and myalgias are typical. Sore throat, eye pain, conjunctival injection, and hemoptysis are frequently present. Chest pain worsened by deep inspiration is not truly pleuritic but rather reflects influenza A myositis of the intracostal muscles. Shortness of breath is related to the degree of hypoxemia. Severe influenza A causes an oxygen diffusion defect as manifested by an increased A-a gradient (>35). Profound hypoxemia may be accompanied by cyanosis. Hypotension caused by hypoxemia and vascular collapse may follow. The course of fulminant viral influenza A is of short duration.

Physical findings are few in viral influenza (i.e., conjunctival suffusion). Auscultation reveals absolutely quiet lungs because the infectious process is interstitial and not alveolar. Routine blood tests are usually unremarkable except for leukopenia, relative lymphopenia, and thrombocytopenia. Atypical lymphocytes are not present, but low titers of cold agglutinins may be present. Cold agglutinins (if present) have titers less than or equal to 1:18. In fatal cases, a pale blue hue of the skin may be noted, and there may be bleeding from multiple orifices before death. The chest radiograph in uncomplicated influenza A is unremarkable, with minimal perihilar bilateral increased prominence of interstitial markings possible. In severe influenza A pneumonia, the chest radiograph shows bilateral symmetrical perihilar infiltrates without pleural effusions in <48 hours.

Patients may die from severe influenza A without superimposed bacterial pneumonia. Most deaths during the 1918–1919 pandemic were young military recruits who died of influenza A pneumonia without bacterial pneumonia. Influenza may be complicated by bacterial pneumonia. Bacterial pneumonias complicating influenza may occur concurrently at presentation or may occur after an interval of improvement 1 to 2 weeks after the presentation of influenza. Influenza A presenting concurrently with bacterial pneumonia is caused by *Staphylococcus aureus*. In contrast to influenza alone, MSSA/CA-MRSA is manifested by an increase in fever, shaking chills, leukocytosis, purulent sputum, localized rales on auscultation, bacteremia, and focal/segmental infiltrates on chest radiograph that rapidly cavitate in less than 72 hours. Alternatively, patients with influenza A may develop a secondary bacterial infection 1 to 2 weeks later. Secondary bacterial pneumonia is less severe and is usually caused by *Streptococcus pneumoniae* or *Haemophilus influenzae*.

Viral influenza-like illnesses (ILIs) most often present during the winter months or influenza season. For clinical and therapeutic purposes, it is important to differentiate influenza A from viral ILIs in hospitalized adults. Some clinical features may point to a specific ILI viral etiology, but a specific viral diagnosis can be made by viral respiratory PCR of nasopharyngeal swab specimens. The only viral ILI likely to mimic influenza A presenting with a fulminant severe viral CAP is MERS. The mimics of ILIs are presented (Table 1). The main nonviral mimic of influenza A in hospitalized adults is Legionnaire's disease (LD). LD may be differentiated from influenza A and other viral ILIs by CXR findings and characteristic nonspecific laboratory tests. With LD CAP, the CXR shows one or more nonfocal infiltrates. Fever, usually greater than 102° F, is accompanied by relative bradycardia. With LD, the ESR is highly elevated (>90 mm/h), the ferritin is highly elevated (>2 times normal), and the serum phosphorus is decreased early, as is serum sodium. Although an elevated CPK and mild transaminitis often accompany LD, these findings are not uncommon in influenza A and some viral ILIs. There are few infections that may mimic the dry, productive cough of *M. pneumoniae* CAP. Pertussis is most likely to mimic mycoplasma. Pertussis, unlike mycoplasma, is not accompanied by watery diarrhea. The distinguishing laboratory feature of *M. pneumoniae* CAP is elevated cold agglutinins not found with pertussis. The key non-specific laboratory finding in pertussis is marked lymphocytosis (Table 2).

COVID-19 emerged from Wuhan, China in 2019 and spread worldwide early in 2020, resulting in a pandemic. COVID-19 is caused by a novel β-coronavirus (different than the novel β-coronaviruses causing SARS and MERS) identified as SARS-CoV-2. SARS-CoV-2 is thought to have been contracted from wild animals in food markets. COVID-19 spreads rapidly via airborne transmission, and may be spread from asymptomatic individuals.

Patients most commonly present with fever, headache, sore throat, dry cough, shortness of breath, and diarrhea (in some).

Clinically, the spectrum of COVID-19 ranges from asymptomatic cases to symptomatic cases. Symptomatic COVID-19 most often presents as a mild ILI; in more severe cases, it presents as a viral pneumonia (not unlike influenza pneumonia). Severe COVID-19 pneumonias have severe hypoxemia caused by an oxygen diffusion defect (high A-a gradient). Fatal cases are due to ARDS and/or myocarditis. Common nonspecific laboratory abnormalities include leukopenia, relative lymphopenia, thrombocytopenia, and mildly elevated serum transaminases. Serum LDH or CPK are often elevated. Elevated D-dimers also present frequently and may herald a subsequent coagulopathy.

Early CXR resembles that of influenza pneumonia (i.e., essentially unremarkable without definite/discrete infiltrates). As COVID-19 pneumonia progresses, the CXR shows bilateral Interstitial peripheral infiltrates. CXR demonstrates no/small bibasilar effusions. Chest CT scans may show bilateral nodular infiltrates with or without consolidation. Cavitation is not a feature of COVID-19 pneumonia. Co-infection or superinfection is a rare occurrence in COVID-19.

Diagnosis of COVID-19 is by RT-PCR of respiratory tract specimens. A positive RT-PCR result may be present early in the disease course, although it may not become positive for a few days. If clinical suspicion is high, serial testing may reveal RT-PCR + after 2 to 3 repeat tests. The RT-PCR should not be used as a test of cure. RT-PCR + may persist for 1 to 2 weeks after clinical recovery, although transmission should not occur during this time period. Antibody testing may become positive after several weeks.

COVID-19 seems to preferentially affect adults, with relative sparing of young children. Elderly patients with advanced lung/cardiac disease are particularly predisposed to severe disease/complications.

Anti-Influenza Therapy

Therapy of viral influenza is directed at inhibiting viral replication and preventing further infection of respiratory epithelial cells. The neuramidase inhibitors zanamivir (Relenza), oseltamivir (Tamiflu), and peramivir (Rapivab) have anti-influenza A and B activity. Neuramidase inhibitors decrease the severity and duration of influenza symptoms by 1 to 2 days. Current flu strains are resistant to amantadine and rimantadine, but these drugs may still be useful to increase peripheral airway dilation and oxygenation, which may be of critical importance in severe influenza A with severe hypoxemia. Mild influenza A/B may be

INFLUENZA-LIKE ILLNESSES (ILIS)	CHEST FILM FEATURES	CLINICAL CLUES
MERS	Ill-defined infiltrates (early) Bilateral dense interstitial nodular infiltrates (late) Severe cases often develop ARDS	Recent travel to Middle East or contact with MERS case Dry cough and sore throat Hemoptysis (in some) Diarrhea (common) WBC count normal, thrombocytopenia Elevated LDH
COVID-19	CXR: Ill-defined infiltrates (early) Bilateral, peripheral dense interstitial infiltrates Severe cases often develop ARDS	Fever and dry cough Diarrhea (common) Myocarditis (late, in some) ARDS (in some) Leukopenia Relative lymphopenia Thrombocytopenia Mildly elevated serum Transaminases (early) Elevated CPK (in some) Elevated D-dimer may herald coagulopathy
RSV	Clear CXR (early) Bilateral ill-defined infiltrates on CXR (late) Chest CT: GGO (non-specific)	Antecedent/concurrent rhinorrhea Hoarseness Lymphocyte/monocyte ratio >2
HPIV-3	Clear CXR (early) Bilateral ill-defined infiltrates on CXR (late)	Hoarseness Prolonged lymphocyte/monocyte ratio <2 Monocytosis
EV-D86	Clear CXR (early) Bilateral ill-defined infiltrates on CXR (late)	Diarrhea (common) Flaccid paralysis
Legionnaire's disease	Rapidly progressive, asymmetric, ill-defined infiltrates on CXR Consolidation and small pleural effusions (common) Cavitation (rare)	High fevers (>102 °F) Highly elevated ESR (>90 mm/h) Ferritin (>2 xn) Leukocytosis with relative lymphopenia Elevated CPK (in some) Mild transient elevated transaminases common (early) Microscopic hematuria (early)

Abbreviations: MERS = Middle East respiratory syndrome; COVID-19: Coronavirus disease; RSV = respiratory syncytial virus; HPIV = human parainfluenza virus; EV = enterovirus; GGO = ground gloss opacity; CXR = chest x-ray; ARDS = acute respiratory distress syndrome.

TABLE 2 Mimics of Mycoplasma pneumoniae in Community Acquired Pneumonia (CAP) Hospitalized Adults

MYCOPLASMA CAP MIMICS	CHEST FILM FEATURES	CLINICAL CLUES
C. pneumoniae	Ill-defined lower lobe infiltrates (often ovoid) No consolidation, cavitation or effusion	No seasonal predisposition Hoarseness Protracted dry cough Mycoplasma-like illness that doesn't respond to erythromycin Wheezing (in some) No diarrhea No cold agglutinins Rhinorrhea proceeds dry cough (1–2 weeks)
Pertussis	Perihilar illdefined infiltrates ("shaggy heart" sign) No consolidation, cavitation or effusions	Protracted dry cough Persistent cough (without typical "whoop" of children) Afebrile or minimal fevers Marked lymphocytes (> 60%) No cold agglutinins

treated with neuramidase inhibitors. Mild cases of influenza A should be treated at the onset of the illness. For severe influenza A, neuramidase inhibitors provide optimal anti-influenza therapy (Table 3). For human and avian influenza (H_5N_1), these antiviral drugs may be ineffective, but are effective against swine influenza.

COVID-19 Therapy

At the time of writing, optimal therapy of COVID-19 continues to evolve. Effective therapy for hospitalized patients with COVID-19 pneumonia who require oxygen is remdesivir (Veklury) 200 mg (IV) for the first does, then 100 mg (IV) q24h for 5 to 10 days. A 3-day course of IV remdesivir can be considered for high risk patients with mild disease. This can be administered as an outpatient treatment if an infusion center is able to offer this therapy. Oral therapy for COVID-19 is now available for high-risk patients. Nirmatrelvir with ritonavir (Paxlovid, approved by the FDA) is currently the most effective PO agent available. Due to the ritonavir component, drug-drug interactions need to be considered when prescribing this medication. Molnupiravir (Lagevrio,

TABLE 3 — Adult Anti-Influenza Antivirals

ANTIVIRAL	TREATMENT DOSE	PROPHYLACTIC DOSE
Mild Influenza A/B		
Zanamivir (Relenza)*	2 inhalations (5 mg per inhalation) q12h × 5 d	2 inhalations (5 mg per inhalation) q24h × 5 d
Influenza		
Baloxavir (Xofluza)	80 mg (PO) × 1 dose	80 mg (PO) × 1 dose
Oseltamivir (Tamiflu)*	75 mg (PO) q12h × 5 d†	75 mg (PO) q24h × 7 d
Peramivir (Rapivab)‡	600 mg (IV) over 30 min × 1 d	None

*Currently most human and avian influenza strains are resistant.
†For avian (H5N1) influenza, 150 mg (PO) q12h may be effective.
‡In general, begin influenza treatment within 2 days of illness onset. Peramivir may be initiated any time after symptom onset.

approved for Emergency Use Authorization by the FDA) is an alternate PO option but has lower efficacy than Paxlovid in preventing serious disease in high risk patients. Monoclonal antibodies are no longer recommended due to lack of activity against current circulating variants. Dexamethasone[1] has a role in limiting mortality in patients admitted with COVID-19 who require supplemental oxygen. Interlukin inhibitors (IL-6 in particular) have a role in select patients with COVID-19. Vaccines play a critical role in prevention of COVID-19, although the increasing number of genetic variants may blunt the effectiveness of existing vaccines.

Mycoplasma Pneumoniae

M. pneumoniae is a common cause of ambulatory CAP. It affects all age groups, and in normal hosts with intact cardiopulmonary function, *M. pneumoniae* CAP is usually a mild, self-limiting infection. However, *M. pneumoniae* derives its importance from difficulty in diagnosis, the necessity for non–β-lactam therapy, and because of its effect on peripheral airways.

M. pneumoniae CAP is one of the nonzoonotic causes of CAP (the others being *Legionella* and *Chlamydia pneumoniae*). *M. pneumoniae* is an atypical pneumonia that is a systemic infectious disease with a pulmonary component. It may be distinguished from other atypical pneumonias by its characteristic pattern of extrapulmonary organ involvement. *M. pneumoniae* CAP most closely resembles *C. pneumoniae* CAP clinically, but is very different from LD in terms of its epidemiology, age distribution, pattern of extrapulmonary organ involvement, and severity.

Clinically, *M. pneumoniae* presents as a subacute febrile illness. Temperatures rarely exceed 102°F (38.9°C). Rigors are not a feature of *M. pneumoniae* CAP, but patients may complain of chilly sensations. Mild headache and/or myalgias are not uncommon. The most common presenting symptom in *M. pneumoniae* CAP is the prolonged, nonproductive, dry cough. Patients with *M. pneumoniae* CAP often complain of or have mild nonexudative pharyngitis. Rhinorrhea and conjunctivitis are not features of *M. pneumoniae* CAP. Watery diarrhea is commonly present in *M. pneumoniae* CAP, but abdominal pain is not a clinical finding. Other extrapulmonary manifestations are uncommon or rare (e.g., meningoencephalitis, pericarditis, hemolytic anemia, glomerular nephritis, Guillain-Barré syndrome, erythema multiforme). *M. pneumoniae* has a distinctive pattern of extrapulmonary organ involvement that does not include cardiac involvement (relative bradycardia) or hepatic involvement, including normal serum glutamate-oxaloacetate transaminase

(SGOT) or serum glutamate-pyruvate transaminase (SGPT). The distinguishing laboratory feature of *M. pneumoniae* CAP is elevated cold agglutinin titers. Although a variety of infectious and noninfectious diseases are associated with cold agglutinin elevations, they are usually of low titer (i.e., <1:16). There are no pulmonary infections presenting as CAP that are associated with high elevations of cold agglutinin titers (i.e., ≥1:64). Although elevated cold agglutinins occur early in up to 75% of patients with *M. pneumoniae* CAP, they are still diagnostically important when present. In a patient with CAP and a cold agglutinin titer greater than or equal to 1:64, the diagnosis of *M. pneumoniae* CAP is very likely.

M. pneumoniae may be differentiated from the typical bacterial pneumonias because of the presence of extrapulmonary findings, including nonexudative pharyngitis, loose stools or watery diarrhea, erythema multiforme, and high cold agglutinin. Patients with typical bacterial CAP usually have a more acute onset of presentation, a productive cough, and temperatures that may exceed 102°F (38.9°C), often accompanied by chills. Patients with typical pneumonia often have pleuritic chest pain, which is not a feature of *M. pneumoniae* CAP. Among the atypical pneumonias, the zoonotic pneumonias (i.e., tularemia, psittacosis, Q fever) may be eliminated from consideration if there is a recent zoonotic contact history with the appropriate vector.

C. pneumoniae CAP resembles closely *M. pneumoniae* CAP. *C. pneumoniae* may be distinguished by the absence of cold agglutinins and the presence of hoarseness, which is a feature of *C. pneumoniae* CAP but not *M. pneumoniae* CAP. Loose stools or watery diarrhea are not usual features of *C. pneumoniae* CAP. The most common clinical problem is differentiating *Legionella* from *Mycoplasma* CAP; this may be done by appreciating the differences in the pattern of extrapulmonary organ involvement with each of these pathogens. *Legionella* may be clinically differentiated from *Mycoplasma* by acuteness of onset or severity, the presence of relative bradycardia, temperatures greater than 102°F (38.9°C), and the presence of abdominal pain. From a laboratory standpoint, highly elevated cold agglutinin titers argue strongly against the diagnosis of *Legionella* and point to *M. pneumoniae*. Nonspecific laboratory tests in a patient with CAP that suggest *Legionella* and argue against *M. pneumoniae* include otherwise unexplained hypophosphatemia, hyponatremia, microscopic hematuria, and increased creatinine. *Legionella* does not affect the upper respiratory tract as does *Mycoplasma* (e.g., nonexudative pharyngitis). Ear findings are not a feature of Legionnaires' disease but are common in *M. pneumoniae* CAP. The finding most likely to cause confusion between *M. pneumoniae* and *Legionella pneumophila* is the presence of loose stools or watery diarrhea, which is found in both.

M. pneumoniae may be cultured from the throat in viral culture media, but the diagnosis is usually made serologically. An elevated enzyme-linked immunosorbent assay (ELISA) or enzyme immuno-assay (EIA) IgM titer suggests acute or recent infection, but an elevated IgG titer indicates past exposure but not acute infection. Elevated IgG titers regardless of degree of elevation are not diagnostic of current infection with *M. pneumoniae* and only indicate previous antigenic exposure. *M. pneumoniae* ELISA IgM levels may take up to 3 months to decrease. Therefore, clinicians should take into account recent antecedent respiratory illness to properly interpret elevated IgM titers, including patients with nonexudative pharyngitis within 3 months prior to the presentation of CAP. The combination of an increased *M. pneumoniae* IgM titer and highly elevated cold agglutinin titers is virtually diagnostic of acute infection. Cold agglutinin titers are elevated transiently early and rapidly fall; the simultaneously elevated cold agglutinins and IgM titers of *M. pneumoniae* indicate active or current infection. In patients with CAP caused by another organism (e.g., *S. pneumoniae*), the presence of elevated *Mycoplasma* IgG titers does not indicate co-infection but only preexisting serologic exposure to *M. pneumoniae*.

---

[1] Not FDA approved for this indication.

TABLE 4	Antibiotics Effective Against *M. pneumoniae*
ANTIBIOTIC	**DOSE (ADULT)**
Mild/Moderate CAP	
Doxycycline	100 mg (IV/PO) q12h
Erythromycin	500 mg (base, estolate, stearate) (PO) q6h
Erythromycin lactobionate	1 g (IV) q6h
Clarithromycin (Biaxin)	500 mg (PO) q12h
Azithromycin (Zithromax)	500 mg (IV) q24h x 2 doses, followed by 500 mg (PO) q24h
Severe CAP	
Levofloxacin (Levaquin)	500 mg (IV/PO) q24h, or 750 mg IV/PO q24h (may allow for shorter duration of therapy)
Moxifloxacin (Avelox)	400 mg (IV/PO) q24h

CAP, Community-acquired pneumonia.

M. pneumoniae Therapy

M. pneumoniae has a predilection for the respiratory epithelial cells and resides on their surface. Mycoplasmas have no definite cell wall like the typical pathogens causing CAP. Their position on the surface of the respiratory epithelium and their absence of a cell wall necessitates the therapeutic approach, which includes non–β-lactam antibiotics with the capacity to penetrate into the *Mycoplasma* organisms. Traditionally, macrolides and tetracyclines have been used successfully to treat *M. pneumoniae*. Both tetracyclines and macrolides are effective against *Mycoplasma* because they interfere with intracellular protein synthesis at the ribosomal level. Tetracyclines penetrate intracellularly better than macrolides, with the exception of penetration into the alveolar macrophage, which is relevant in *Legionella* but not *M. pneumoniae* infections. Macrolides and tetracyclines are both active against *Mycoplasma*. Patients treated with macrolides or tetracyclines defervesce rapidly over 24 to 48 hours. Clinical defervescence manifests by an increased feeling of well-being and a decrease in fever. The dry cough persists during and after therapy regardless of the anti-*Mycoplasma* antimicrobial used.

There are important differences in the shedding rates of *Mycoplasma* from respiratory epithelial cells posttherapy when using tetracyclines instead of macrolides. Tetracycline therapy is associated with a more rapid decrease in shedding. Tetracyclines with better ability to penetrate intracellularly, such as doxycycline (Vibramycin), are the most rapid at decreasing *Mycoplasma* shedding, which is an important public health consideration. Mycoplasmas are transmitted by aerosolized droplet infection. Because patients with *Mycoplasma* have a prolonged cough, organisms not eliminated from respiratory epithelial cells may be aerosolized during coughing for weeks following the acute infection, spreading the infection to susceptible individuals via aerosolized droplets. The aim of therapy is to rapidly treat the patient's pneumonia and extrapulmonary sites of involvement. The secondary goal is to rapidly decrease shedding and aerosolization to prevent the spread of *Mycoplasma* to other individuals. An additional therapeutic goal is to decrease the incidence of post-*Mycoplasma* asthma seen in some patients. *M. pneumoniae* CAP may exacerbate preexisting asthma, but may also cause permanent post-CAP asthma in some individuals.

Until recently, doxycycline was the most active antimicrobial to use against *M. pneumoniae*. Currently, the "respiratory quinolones," levofloxacin (Levaquin) and moxifloxacin (Avelox), are highly active anti–*M. pneumoniae* antimicrobials. The respiratory quinolones and doxycycline penetrate cells efficiently and interfere with intracellular enzymes or protein synthesis of intracellular organisms. Respiratory quinolones and doxycycline are highly effective anti-*Mycoplasma* agents and rapidly decrease shedding of *M. pneumoniae* in respiratory secretions.

Therapy for *M. pneumoniae* is ordinarily 1 to 2 weeks. Patients who have impaired cardiopulmonary disease or are immunocompromised may require 2 full weeks of therapy. In patients with borderline cardiopulmonary function, *M. pneumoniae* as with other relatively low virulence pathogens may present as severe CAP. Antimicrobial therapy for typical or atypical CAP should be directed against the presumed pathogen and not based on co-morbidities. Normal healthy hosts are treated with the same antimicrobial as patients hospitalized with severe CAP. Patients hospitalized with compromised cardiopulmonary function caused by severe *M. pneumoniae* CAP are most often initially treated intravenously with doxycycline (Vibramycin), a macrolide, or a respiratory quinolone. Most patients with *M. pneumoniae* CAP present in the ambulatory setting, which permits therapy with oral doxycycline, a macrolide, or a respiratory quinolone (Table 4).

References

Cunha CB, Cunha, BA: *Antibiotic Essentials*, ed 17. New Delhi, 2020, Jaypee Medical Publishers.

Foster CB, Friedman N, Carl J, Piedimonte G: Enterovirus D68: a clinically important respiratory enterovirus, *Cleve Clin J Med* 82:26–31, 2015.

Gottlieb RL, Vaca CE, Paredes R, et al: GS-US-540-9012 (PINETREE) Investigators. Early remdesivir to prevent progression to severe Covid-19 in outpatients, *N Engl J Med* 2022 27;386(4):305–315.

Qu J, Yang C, Bao F, et al: Epidemiological characterization of respiratory tract infections caused by *Mycoplasma pneumoniae* during epidemic and post-epidemic periods in North China, from 2011 to 2016, *BMC Infect Dis* 17;18(1):335, 2018.

Uyeki TM, Bernstein HH, Bradley JS: Clinical practice guidelines by the Infectious Diseases Society of America: 2018 update on diagnosis, treatment, chemoprophylaxis, and institutional outbreak management of seasonal influenzae, *Clin Infect Dis* 5;68(6):895–902, 2019.

VIRAL RESPIRATORY INFECTIONS

Method of
Robert C. Welliver Sr., MD

CURRENT DIAGNOSIS

- Rapid diagnostic kits, preferably one of the numerous commercially available polymerase chain reaction (PCR) assays, are available for many common respiratory viruses. These tests are used increasingly to establish that antibiotic therapy is not necessary in many patients with febrile respiratory illnesses or with lower respiratory tract infections such as pneumonia and wheezing.
- The presence of wheezing on physical examination virtually excludes bacterial infection from consideration in subjects with lower respiratory disease (as previously defined).

CURRENT THERAPY

- The management of most viral respiratory infections consists of rest, adequate caloric and fluid intake, and management of fever and malaise, preferably with acetaminophen, or else with nonsteroidal antiinflammatory drugs (NSAIDs).
- Corticosteroids are essential, evidence-based, first-line therapy in the management of croup. With the exception of late-phase COVID-19 infections and virus-induced wheezing, they are of minimal benefit in other viral infections.
- Specific antiviral therapy is available only for influenza virus infection and coronavirus (SARS-CoV-2) infection. Beneficial effects of antiinfluenza antivirals have been more readily achieved for influenza infections in prevention rather than treatment.

Viral infections of the upper and lower respiratory tract are among the most common infections in humans, and they account for significant morbidity at all ages. Infants and young children can sustain six to eight such infections annually, and adults have an average of nearly two such infections per year. Rhinoviruses are the most commonly identified agents and cause illness year-round. Other common causative agents during winter months include influenza viruses and respiratory syncytial virus (RSV), while enteroviruses predominate in summer months. The parainfluenza viruses also commonly cause respiratory infection, particularly in autumn (type 1) and late spring or summer (type 3). SARS-CoV-2, the causative agent of COVID-19 disease, is now commonly recovered year-round, while other coronaviruses, metapneumoviruses, adenoviruses, and less virulent viral agents are identified less often.

Although each of these agents can cause a common cold, some viral infections are associated with characteristic patterns of respiratory disease. Most of these viruses can also exacerbate asthma, cystic fibrosis, and chronic obstructive pulmonary disease (COPD).

Common Colds

The "common cold" is the most prevalent of the viral respiratory illnesses. Pharyngitis or rhinitis is usually the earliest sign of a cold, beginning a few days after infection has taken place. Nasal congestion and clear or slightly cloudy rhinorrhea usually follow within 24 to 48 hours. Cough occurs in approximately 30% to 40% of those infected, and fluid can accumulate in the middle ear or sinus cavities if they become blocked as a result of mucosal swelling. Ear and sinus cavity infections occur when this fluid is trapped for a week or more. As many as 40% of subjects treated with either antibiotics or a placebo report beneficial effects, with equal frequency between groups.

Cough can be one of the most irritating symptoms during colds. Cough during colds is principally caused by secretions entering the upper airway (postnasal drainage) and not by inflammation of the airway itself. Therefore it is not surprising that cough suppressants, especially codeine, have little effect on cough induced by colds. Antihistamines have also been found to be ineffective in relief of cough during colds, and side effects occur frequently, principally sedation and dry mouth. The true benefit of antihistamines in the management of colds probably is that of inducing sleep.

Influenza-Like Illness

The influenza syndrome is defined as the abrupt onset of fever, headache, and striking degrees of malaise and prostration, often with intense myalgia. Respiratory symptoms can occur concurrently, but they may not always be prominent features. The principal causes of this syndrome are the influenza virus types A and B. The illness is generally self-limited, and most symptoms resolve over 4 or 5 days. Lassitude can persist for up to 2 weeks.

Influenza virus infection and influenza-like illness are best treated symptomatically, relying on rest, adequate intake of fluids and calories, and appropriate analgesic therapy. M2 proton channel inhibitors such as amantadine (Symmetrel) and rimantadine (Flumadine) have been approved for therapy. Positive outcomes from therapy with these agents have been observed only when therapy was instituted within 48 hours after the onset of symptoms, and symptomatic benefits are variable. Side effects, primarily agitation, are often distressing. Since 2016, resistance to M2 inhibitors has been commonly observed among circulating epidemic strains of influenza virus, and their use currently is generally not recommended.

More recently, inhibitors of the activity of influenza viral neuraminidase have been used in treatment and prevention of influenza virus infection in adults and children. The first such compound released, zanamivir (Relenza), was administered by inhalation but was unpopular because of its irritating effects on the airway. An oral compound, oseltamivir (Tamiflu), has been used to prevent and to treat influenza virus infection. As with M2 inhibitors, treatment should be started within the first 48 hours of symptoms, and prophylaxis should be instituted

within 48 hours of exposure. Treatment with oseltamivir shortens the duration of subsequent illness by only about 24 hours. Treatment can prevent some of the complications of influenza infection, including pneumonia. The drug may be more effective as a preventive agent, because it may be up to 90% effective in preventing culture-positive symptomatic influenza illness. The recommended dose for adults is 75 mg orally every 12 hours for 5 days. In children, the appropriate dose based on body weight is 30 mg twice daily for children weighing less than 15 kg, 45 mg twice daily for children weighing 15 to 23 kg, 60 mg twice daily for children weighing 23 to 40 kg, and 75 mg twice daily for children weighing more than 40 kg. The principal side effect is nausea, which can be reduced by taking the drug with food.

A new type of antiviral (baloxavir marboxil [Xofluza]) was released for treatment of influenza infections in 2018. This drug acts by a different mechanism than previous antivirals used to treat influenza infections. The advantages are that it is given as a single dose for the entire course of treatment and reduces the duration of influenza illness by approximately 24 hours. It does not seem more effective than oseltamivir in reducing influenza-related symptoms. Baloxavir is approved for use in adults and children 12 years of age or older. The dosing recommendation is one single dose of 40 mg for patients less than 80 kg (<176 lb) and 80 mg for patients of at least 80 kg (≥176 lb).

In 2009, a novel H1N1 strain of influenza caused a worldwide pandemic. This epidemic H1N1 strain currently circulates in a much more limited fashion, and symptoms are markedly less severe. Seasonal influenza A/H3N2 and type B strains continue to circulate in the world. The considerable majority of these epidemic and seasonal strains continue to show sensitivity to oseltamivir, whereas most are resistant to M2 inhibitors. All strains continue to show sensitivity to zanamivir.

Moreover, strains of avian influenza viruses, bearing antigenic types not included in the usual influenza vaccines, have become isolated from humans more frequently in the US. These avian influenza strains have traditionally only infected birds but, since 2024, they have been recovered from a variety of animals, particularly from cattle. Illness caused by these avian strains is generally milder than that caused by historically influenza strains, but a limited number of hospitalizations and one death due to avian influenza infections have recently occurred in the US, most strikingly among dairy farm workers. Transmission to humans has most often occurred after prolonged, direct exposure to cattle, but the virus is excreted in milk and remains infectious in unpasteurized, raw milk. Pasteurization is highly effective in inactivating avian influenza strains. These avian strains have uniformly proved susceptible to oseltamivir at the dosages suggested above.

Croup

Croup is defined as the occurrence of a triad of hoarseness or laryngitis; a deep, brassy, or barking cough; and inspiratory stridor. Airway obstruction in croup is caused by constriction in the subglottic area, often noted on radiographs by a steeple-shaped narrowing of the air column in this region. Affected children are usually afebrile and nontoxic in appearance.

Parainfluenza virus type 1 is the primary cause of croup, although infection with many different viruses can produce this illness. Influenza virus can cause a particularly severe form of croup. Bacterial secondary infection occurs uncommonly in croup, but it can result in fever and severe obstruction of the airway. Administration of dexamethasone (Decadron)[1] at 0.6 mg/kg either orally or intramuscularly (IM) markedly reduces the rate of hospitalization, admission to the intensive care unit (ICU), and intubation for croup.

Bronchiolitis

Bronchiolitis represents the most common cause for hospitalization of infants in developed countries. Infants present with a

---

[1] Not FDA approved for this indication.

TABLE 1 | Efficacy of Respiratory Syncytial Virus Vaccines

VACCINE AND AGE GROUP STUDIED	COMPONENT	DOSE, ROUTE	EFFICACY VS. LRTD	EFFICACY VS. SEVERE* LRTD	DURATION OF PROTECTION
Arexvy	Prefusion RSV F protein	120 mcg in 0.5 mL, IM			
Adults age 50–59 years with comorbidity or ≥60 years, well			83% reduction	94% reduction	67% reduction in LRTD over 2 years postvaccination
Abrysvo	Prefusion RSV, subtypes A and B	120 mcg in 0.5 mL, IM			
Adults ≥60 years			67% vs. LRTD with ≥2 LRT symptoms	86% vs. LRTD with ≥3 LRT symptoms	
Infant of mother vaccinated any time during pregnancy			51%–57% vs. any LRTD	69%–82% vs. severe LRTD	
Infant of mother vaccinated at 32–36 weeks' gestation			35%–57% vs. any LRTD	77%–91% vs. severe LRTD	
mRESVIA	mRNA for the RSV F protein	50 mcg† in 0.5 mL, IM			
Adults ≥60 years			80% vs. LRTD with ≥2 LRT symptoms		63% against LRTD at 6 months postvaccination

*Severe = marked tachypnea or hypoxia, or mechanical ventilation.
†Prefilled syringe contains 96 mcg, but 50 mcg is delivered during injection.
IM, Intramuscular; *LRT,* lower respiratory tract; *LRTD,* lower respiratory tract disease.
https://www.cdc.gov/rsv/hcp/vaccine-clinical-guidance/older-adults.html.

history of several days of upper respiratory symptoms, followed by the onset of wheezing and labored breathing. RSV is the most common cause of bronchiolitis and is the agent found in the most severe cases that result in respiratory failure. Contrasting with asthma, obstruction of the airway in bronchiolitis is a result of plugging of bronchioles with detached epithelium and inflammatory cells. Mucus plugging and constriction of smooth muscle are not prominent. Also in contrast with asthma is the absence of a sustained response to bronchodilators and corticosteroids among infants with bronchiolitis.

Therapy of bronchiolitis primarily consists of administration of supplemental oxygen and replacement of fluid deficits as needed. Ribavirin (Virazole)[1] is a compound with antiviral activity against RSV, but controlled studies have not demonstrated meaningful differences in outcomes between treated and untreated subjects. The compound is quite expensive and must be delivered orally or via a special aerosol generator. Ribavirin is now used almost exclusively in older, immunocompromised individuals with RSV infection. Even there, its effectiveness is controversial.

Palivizumab (Synagis), a monoclonal antibody against the fusion protein of RSV, has proved to be effective in reducing the rate of hospitalization for RSV infection by approximately 50% when given to high-risk infants. Infants who may be considered candidates for therapy include those with chronic lung disease, those born prematurely, and those with hemodynamically significant congenital heart disease. Doses of palivizumab (15 mg/kg) have been given on a monthly basis throughout the local RSV season, usually November through March. However, a newer monoclonal antibody named nirsevimab (Beyfortus) with an extended half-life has been approved for prevention of RSV infection in infants born prematurely or at term and should eventually replace palivizumab. Results of clinical trials and subsequent real-world experience indicate that the use of nirsevimab will reduce not only the rate of RSV hospitalizations but

also that of RSV lower respiratory infections severe enough to cause visits to acute care centers and emergency departments. Nirsevimab is given only once to infants born during or entering their first RSV season, starting from birth. The correct dose of nirsevimab is 50 mg IM for infants weighing less than 5 kg and 100 mg IM for those weighing 5 kg or more. Infants at risk born outside of the RSV season should receive nirsevimab at the start of the ensuing RSV season. Nirsevimab is approved for use in infants up to 24 months of age if they remain at risk for severe RSV infection in their second RSV season. The recommended dose is a total of 200 mg, administered as two 100-mg doses IM at one time. A similar compound, clesrovimab (Enflonsia), produced by a second company, has become available for the prevention of RSV lower respiratory illness and hospitalization in neonates and infants who are born during or entering their first RSV season. Clesrovimab is also a monoclonal antibody against the RSV fusion (F) protein, although it binds at a somewhat different site. The correct dose is 105 mg as a single IM injection regardless of the infant weight.

Although no licensed RSV vaccines (as opposed to monoclonal antibody preparations) are currently available for administration to infants, beginning in 2022, the Food and Drug Administration (FDA) has given approval for the use of RSV vaccines (Arexvy [GlaxoSmithKline], Abrysvo [Pfizer], and mRESVIA [Moderna]). A summary of these vaccines is presented in Table 1. These vaccines (all administered in 0.5 mL IM) are approved for prevention of RSV infection in adults 60 years of age or older. All three vaccines reduced the incidence of severe RSV lower respiratory tract disease (LRTD) by approximately 80%. Of note is the low frequency of RSV LRTD in control groups, ranging from 5.5 to 6.5 cases per 1000 patient-years in the year after placebo vaccination. In addition to adult vaccination, Abrysvo (but not Arexvy or mRESVIA) is also approved for use in pregnant women from 32 to 36 weeks' gestation during the RSV season to prevent RSV infection in their infants. Infants of mothers who received Abrysvo at any time during pregnancy had an 81% reduction in the development of RSV lower respiratory infection within 3 months after birth and a 69% reduction within 6 months after birth. Given that transplacental transfer of antibody may be reduced during the third trimester of pregnancy, it was subsequently demonstrated that maternal vaccination with Abrysvo from 32 through 36 weeks' gestational age reduced the rate of RSV lower respiratory infection RSV in infants by 34.7% and the risk of severe lower respiratory tract infection by 91.1% by 90 days of age (Table 1).

The CDC recommends a single dose of any FDA-licensed RSV vaccine for all adults aged 75 and older, and adults aged 60 to 74 who are at increased risk of severe RSV disease. While this is likely to change, RSV vaccines for adults are not currently considered annual vaccines, and there is no recommendation to administer them more than once. There are currently no RSV vaccine formulations approved for use in infants. A very low incidence of Guillain-Barré syndrome (GBS, an unusual form of neuropathy, usually ascending in distribution) has followed the use of Arexvy and Abrysvo, but not mRESVIA. The incidence during 1 to 42 days after vaccination was approximately twice that observed from 43 to 90 days after vaccination.

The GlaxoSmithKline RSV vaccine had a statistically significant association with GBS, while the Pfizer RSV vaccine had a similar, but not statistically significant, association. In the analysis, fewer doses of Pfizer RSV vaccine were administered compared with the GlaxoSmithKline RSV vaccine. For both vaccines, FDA estimated the risk of GBS to be on the order of 10 excess cases per 1 million vaccinated adults 60 or older.

Severe Acute Respiratory Syndrome Coronavirus–2 (COVID-19 or SARS-CoV-2)

The appearance of SARS-CoV-2 has profoundly affected healthcare worldwide. Although symptoms are generally milder in children, respiratory illness can at times be severe or even fatal. Symptoms are not readily distinguishable from other respiratory viral infections early on but may become severe as the illness progresses. Numerous antivirals and antibody formulations have been developed, but the use of antibodies has essentially been eliminated as variants of the parent virus have become resistant to antibody preparations, including convalescent plasma. A summary of the use of currently FDA-recommended preparations that can be used in adults and children is presented in Table 2.

Corticosteroids

The use of dexamethasone[1] is now recommended in patients hospitalized and with oxygen saturation values of 94% or less, as well as in subjects with critical illnesses (ICU admission, use of mechanically assisted ventilation or extracorporeal membrane oxygenation [ECMO]). In these patients, the appropriate dexamethasone dose is 6 mg intravenously (IV) or orally, for 10 days, or until the patient is discharged home. In children, the dose for dexamethasone is 0.15 mg/kg IV or IM every day for a maximum of 10 days. If dexamethasone is unavailable, the equivalent dose for adults of methylprednisone[1] is 32 mg IV or orally, and the equivalent dose of prednisone[1] is 40 mg IV or orally. The use of corticosteroids, particularly dexamethasone, is not supported by the Infectious Diseases Society of America (IDSA) for outpatients and those inpatients with no need for supplemental oxygen. The use of corticosteroids, particularly dexamethasone, is not supported by the IDSA for outpatients and those inpatients with no need for supplemental oxygen.

Tocilizumab

Tocilizumab (Actemra), an inhibitor of the proinflammatory cytokine interleukin-6, is suggested, in addition to standard therapy (i.e., corticosteroids) for progressive, severe, or critical disease if there is an elevation of inflammatory markers (e.g., C-reactive protein >75 mg/L). The recommended dosages for hospitalized adult and pediatric patients aged 2 years and older are: 12 mg/kg for patients weighing less than 30 kg and 8 mg/kg for patients 30 kg or more (maximum 800 mg/dose). The drug is administered by a 60-min infusion. Tocilizumab should not be used in patients already doing well on corticosteroids. If tocilizumab is unavailable, sarilumab (Kevzara)[1], at 200 mg every 2 weeks, may be substituted.

Convalescent Plasma

Among immunocompetent patients hospitalized with COVID-19, the IDSA guideline panel recommends against COVID-19

[1] Not FDA approved for this indication.

1018

TABLE 2 Recommended Antiviral Therapy for Severe Acute Respiratory Syndrome COVID-19 (SARS-CoV-2)

DRUG	PROPHYLAXIS	AMBULATORY, MILD-TO-MODERATE DISEASE	HOSPITALIZED, MILD-TO-MODERATE DISEASE, NO OXYGEN REQUIREMENT	HOSPITALIZED, MORE SEVERE DISEASE, SpO₂ ≤94%	HOSPITALIZED, CRITICAL ILLNESS (ICU, MECHANICAL VENTILATION, ECMO, SEPTIC SHOCK)
Remdesivir (Veklury)*	No recommendation	**Adults:** 200 mg on day 1, 100 mg on days 2 and 3 **Pediatrics:** 5 mg/kg on day 1, 2.5 mg/kg days 2 and 3	**Adults:** 200 mg on day 1, 100 mg on days 2 and 3 **Pediatrics:** 5 mg/kg on day 1, 2.5 mg/kg days 2 and 3	5 days recommended (10 days optional)	Suggest against use
Nirmatrelvir/ ritonavir (Paxlovid)†	No recommendation	**Adults:** Recommended for use within 5 days of disease onset, if patients have high risk of progression to severe disease **Children:** ≥12 years and at least 40 kg body mass	**Adults:** Recommended for use within 5 days of disease onset, if patients have high risk of progression to severe disease **Children:** ≥12 years and at least 40 kg body mass	No recommendation	No recommendation
Dexamethasone	No recommendation			Suggested	Recommended

*Remdesivir should not be used if patient ALT is >10 times the upper limit of normal.
†Paxlovid Therapy Pack contains 150 mg nirmatrelvir and 100 mg ritonavir tablets. The recommended dose for adults and children ≥12 years and at least 40 kg body mass is two nirmatrelvir tablets (300 mg) and one ritonavir tablet (100 mg) taken together every 12 hours for 5 days.
ALT, Alanine transaminase; *ECMO,* extracorporeal membrane oxygenation; *GFR,* glomerular filtration rate; *ICU,* intensive care unit; *SpO₂,* oxygen saturation.

convalescent plasma. Among immunocompromised patients hospitalized with COVID-19, the IDSA guideline panel suggests against the routine use of COVID-19 convalescent plasma. Among ambulatory patients with mild-to-moderate COVID-19 at high risk for progression to severe disease who have no other treatment options, the IDSA guideline panel suggests FDA-qualified high-titer COVID-19 convalescent plasma within 8 days of symptom onset rather than no high-titer COVID-19 convalescent plasma. Patients, particularly those who do not qualify for other treatments and place a higher value on the uncertain mortality reduction and a lower value on the potential adverse effects of convalescent plasma, would reasonably select convalescent plasma.

Neutralizing Antibody Preparations

Pemivibart (Pemgarda) is a monoclonal antibody against the COVID-19 spike protein, which was authorized for emergency use only for preexposure prevention of COVID-19 in immune compromised individuals 12 years or older, weighing at least 40 kg. The FDA has not approved pemivibart for routine therapeutic use or for postexposure prophylaxis. Pemivibart should only be used when there is a compelling need for prevention, when circulating COVID-19 strains are generally susceptible, and when no other effective formulations are available. The recommended first dose is 4500 mg, but subsequent doses (at an interval of 3 months) should be reduced. Anaphylaxis occurred with 4 of 243 (0.6%) infusions in one report.

Vilobelimab (Gohibic) is an antibody against the complement fragment C′5a, to reduce the hyperinflammation that can follow COVID-19 infection. It is currently available only in clinical trials or used off-label (under EUA) for treatment of COVID-19 in patients on mechanically assisted ventilation or ECMO. The dose used is 800 mg administered intravenously.

Janus Kinase Inhibitors

These compounds inhibit signaling among inflammatory cells using the nuclear factor kappa B pathway. One compound, baricitinib (Olumiant), has been used in addition to standard therapy (such as corticosteroids) to reduce the massive inflammation observed in severe COVID-19 infection. Baricitinib, 4 mg/kg PO once daily for up to 14 days, has been used in patients with severe COVID-19 receiving high-flow nasal cannula (HFNC) oxygenation but is not indicated for patients requiring mechanically assisted ventilation or ECMO. The dose must be halved in subjects with GFR values 30 to <60 mL/minute, and should not be used with GFR values of <30 mL/minute. Tofacitinib (Xeljanz)[1] may be used as an alternative to Baricitinib, using 10 mg/kg every 12 hours orally for up to 14 days.

Antivirals

Paxlovid (nirmatrelvir 300 mg/ritonavir 100 mg) is an antiviral protease inhibitor suggested for use in outpatients ≥12 years of age and weighing ≥40 kg with mild to moderate COVID-19 who are at high risk for progression to severe disease. Paxlovid should be initiated within 5 days of the onset of respiratory symptoms. Paxlovid dosing must be adjusted for renal insufficiency. If the glomerular filtration rate (GFR) is >30 to <60 mL/min, the dose should be reduced to one nirmatrelvir tablet (150 mg) and one ritonavir tablet (100 mg) every 12 hours. The drug should not be administered if the GFR is <30 mL/min.

Paxlovid has numerous interactions with other compounds, which may seriously affect the activity of the other drugs, as well as of nirmatrelvir/ritonavir itself. For important information about drug interactions, check https://www.fda.gov/media/1550 50/download.

Remdesivir (Veklury) is suggested for patients (ambulatory or inpatient), within 7 days of the onset of respiratory symptoms, who have mild-to-moderate COVID-19 and who are at high risk for progression to severe disease. Remdesivir may be administered for 5 days to hospitalized patients with SpO_2 values of ≤94% in room air. Remdesivir use is not supported for inpatients requiring mechanical ventilation or ECMO. Adults should receive a loading dose on day 1 of 200 mg, followed by 100 mg on days 2 and 3. For children (3–40 kg), the loading dose is 5 mg/kg, followed by 2.5 mg/kg on days 2 and 3.

Molnupiravir may be used for ambulatory patients or inpatients 18 years of age or older who have a mild-to-moderate risk of disease progression and no other treatment options. The drug has mutagenic potential and reproductive concerns, and thus should not be used during pregnancy. Molnupiravir (Lagevrio)[1] has not been approved, but has been authorized for emergency use by the FDA under an Emergency Use Authorization for the treatment of COVID-19. If used, administration of 800 mg orally every 12 hours should begin within 5 days of onset of illness and be continued for 5 days, but should not be used for initial therapy or for pre- or postexposure prophylaxis. Molnupiravir causes disorders of bone and cartilage growth in animals; therefore it should not be used in children <18 years of age.

Compounds not recommended in adults for use in COVID-19 include anakinra (Kineret)[1], chloroquine[1] and hydroxychloroquine (Plaquenil)[1], ivermectin (Stromectol)[1], colchicine[1], fluvoxamine[1] (except in clinical trials), lopinavir/ritonavir (Kaletra)[1], and inhaled steroids (except for other conditions, such as asthma). Bacterial secondary infection occurs with an estimated frequency of ≤4% in COVID-19, so antibiotics are not generally recommended. In children, Remdesivir (Veklury) has been used successfully, but there are no data to support the use of Janus kinase inhibitors, Paxlovid, or antibiotics. Molnupiravir use is contraindicated in children because of possible adverse effects on bone and cartilage.

---

[1]Not FDA approved for this indication.

References

Bhirmaj A, Morgan RL, Hirsch Shumaker A, et al: IDSA guidelines on the treatment and management of patients with COVID-19, *Infect Dis Society Am*, 2023. www.idsociety.org/practice-guideline/covid-19-guideline-treatment-and-management/.

Buckingham SC, Jafri HS, Bush AN, et al: A randomized, double-blind, placebo-controlled trial of dexamethasone in severe respiratory syncytial virus (RSV) infection: effects on RSV quantity and clinical outcome, *J Infect Dis* 185:1222–1228, 2002.

Flores G, Horwitz RI: Efficacy of β2-agonists in bronchiolitis: a reappraisal and meta-analysis, *Pediatrics* 100:233–239, 1997. https://www.cdc.gov/rsv/vaccines/older-adults.html.

IDSA Guidelines on the Treatment and Management of Patients with COVID-19 Available at: https://www.idsociety.org/practice-guideline/covid-19-guideline-treatment-and-management.

Muether PS, Gwaltney Jr JM: Variant effect of first- and second-generation antihistamines as clues to their mechanism of action on the sneeze reflex in the common cold, *Clin Infect Dis* 33:1483–1488, 2001.

Tavorner D, Danz C, Economos D: The effects of oral pseudoephedrine on nasal patency in the common cold: a double-blind single-dose placebo-controlled trial, *Clin Otolaryngol* 24:47–51, 1999.

Treanor JJ, Hayden FG, Vrooman PS, et al: Efficacy and safety of the oral neuraminidase inhibitor oseltamivir in treating acute influenza: a randomized controlled trial. US Oral Neuraminidase Study Group, *JAMA* 283:1016–1024, 2000.

AXIAL SPONDYLOARTHRITIS

Method of
Atul A. Deodhar, MD, MRCP; and Sonam R. Kiwalkar, MD, MEHP

CURRENT DIAGNOSIS

- *Axial spondyloarthritis* (axSpA) is an umbrella term that includes ankylosing spondylitis (AS, also called radiographic axSpA, or r-axSpA) and nonradiographic axial spondyloarthritis (nr-axSpA). The presence or absence of definitive sacroiliitis on radiographs differentiates r-axSpA from nr-axSpA. The latter is a condition with the same clinical features and similar disease burden, except that definitive radiographic features of sacroiliitis are lacking.
- In the absence of diagnostic criteria, the diagnosis of r-axSpA is made by the presence of definitive sacroiliitis on sacro-iliac (SI) joint radiographic imaging plus either chronic (>3 months) inflammatory back pain or restriction in spinal movements or chest expansion (Modified New York Criteria for Classification of AS).
- Because definitive sacroiliitis may take up to 10 years to appear on a radiograph from the start of chronic inflammatory back pain (the most common first symptom), early or mild disease can be missed.
- When axSpA is suspected with features of inflammatory back pain (usually starting before 45 years of age) along with other clinical features of spondyloarthritis—such as uveitis, psoriasis, enthesitis, asymmetric peripheral inflammatory arthritis, family history of spondyloarthritis, high C-reactive protein, inflammatory bowel disease, favorable response to nonsteroidal antiinflammatory drugs—but a radiograph of the SI joints is negative or uncertain for definitive sacroiliitis, magnetic resonance imaging) of the SI joints, and/or human leukocyte antigen-B27 typing may help in making the diagnosis.

CURRENT THERAPY

- Nonpharmacologic interventions include active physical therapy, self-directed physical exercise, patient education, and smoking cessation.
- Nonsteroidal antiinflammatory drugs (NSAIDs) are the first line of pharmacologic treatment.
- In patients who do not respond adequately to NSAIDs, treatment with a tumor necrosis factor-α inhibitor (TNFi), interleukin-17 inhibitor, or Janus kinase inhibitor (JAKi) is recommended.
- Retrospective analysis in cohorts of patients with r-axSpA using long-term TNFi therapy has shown a reduced rate of new bone formation in the spine, although no pharmaceutical agents have shown disease-modifying ability in placebo-controlled prospective studies to date.
- Conventional synthetic antirheumatic drugs such as sulfasala-zine (Azulfidine)[1] or methotrexate[1] can be used to treat peripheral arthritis in axSpA patients, but they do not have efficacy in axial disease.

[1]Not FDA approved for this indication.

Definition and Spectrum of the Disease

Axial spondyloarthritis (axSpA) is an umbrella term that includes ankylosing spondylitis (AS, also called radiographic axSpA, or r-axSpA) and nonradiographic axial spondyloarthritis (nr-axSpA). The presence or absence of definitive sacroiliitis on radiographic imaging differentiates *r-axSpA* from nr-axSpA.

axSpA is a chronic, immune-mediated inflammatory disorder involving the sacroiliac (SI) joints, the spine, and the peripheral joints and entheses. In some, spinal bony fusion develops gradually over several years and may lead to reduced spine and neck flexibility. The axial skeleton is always involved, and involvement of the peripheral joints and enthesitis occurs in approximately 30% of patients. Extramusculoskeletal manifestations (EMMs) include psoriasis, acute anterior uveitis, and inflammatory bowel disease (IBD) (i.e., Crohn disease or ulcerative colitis).

Epidemiology

Based on the 2009 to 2010 National Health and Nutritional Examination Survey (NHANES), the estimated prevalence of axSpA in the US population is about 1.0%, of which 0.5% of patients are reported to have AS. The prevalence of nr-axSpA is thus assumed to be the other 0.5%, because pelvic radiographs and SI magnetic resonance imaging (MRI) examinations were not carried out in this population-based study. Based on 2006 to 2014 data from the US Medicare Fee-for-Service and IBM MarketScan databases, a retrospective observational cohort study showed an increase in the diagnostic prevalence of AS and axSpA, which could possibly be attributed to increased disease awareness.

The prevalence of axSpA varies with geographic region and, in general, depends on the prevalence of human leukocyte antigen (HLA)-B27. Prevalence of HLA-B27 is less than 1% in Japan, 3% in African Americans, and more than 20% in some native populations of Eastern Siberia and Alaska; it is 8% in Western Europe and 10% to 16% in Scandinavian countries. Thus axSpA is rare in Japanese and African American populations. The prevalence of axSpA is about 0.5% in persons of European descent and 1.4% in those of Scandinavian ancestry, whereas it increases to 2% to 3% in natives of eastern Siberia and Alaska. The risk of axSpA is increased among those with an affected first-degree relative. The male-to-female ratio is 2:1 for the diagnosis of r-axSpA. In contrast, there is no difference in the prevalence of nr-axSpA among males and females, suggesting that male sex is a prognostic indicator for progression from nonradiographic to radiographic axSpA.

Pathogenesis

Genetics plays a major role in the pathogenesis of spondyloarthritis, and the *HLA-B27* gene has a major association with r-axSpA. *HLA-B27* is present in about 70% to 90% of patients with r-axSpA in most ethnic groups. The risk of disease in family members of patients with r-axSpA is 63% in monozygotic twins, 20% in dizygotic twins, 8.2% in first-degree relatives, 1% in second-degree relatives, and 0.7% in third-degree relatives. The overall contribution to r-axSpA heritability by *HLA-B27* is estimated to be approximately 20%. Some other genes associated with r-axSpA—such as endoplasmic reticulum aminopeptidases (ERAP-1 and ERAP-2) and interleukin-23 receptor (IL-23R)—have been implicated to play a role in the pathogenesis.

The following hypotheses have been put forth to explain the role of *HLA-B27* in the pathogenesis of axSpA:

- *Arthritogenic peptide presentation:* Certain antimicrobial peptides have molecular mimicry to self-peptides found in the joints, and it is hypothesized that *HLA-B27* presents these to cytotoxic T cells. The activated T-cell lymphocytes then lead to autoreactivity, arthritis, and spondylitis.
- *HLA-B27 heavy chain homodimer:* The heavy chains of the HLA-B27 molecule can form homodimers when they are expressed on the cell surface, resulting in their recognition by natural killer cell receptors. This can enhance the survival and proliferation of CD-4 T cells and increase the production of IL-17 in vivo.
- *HLA-B27 misfolding and unfolded protein response:* HLA-B27 assembly takes place in the endoplasmic reticulum (ER) before it is expressed on the cell surface. The misfolded HLA-B27 molecules accumulate in the ER, leading to cellular stress secondary to the unfolded protein response. This then activates the IL-23/IL-17 pathway of inflammation.
- *HLA-B27 shaping of the human gut microbiome:* The human body contains a large community of commensals and symbiotic bacteria, fungi, and viruses called *microbiota*. The term *microbiome* refers to the genomes of these microorganisms. The composition of the gut microbiome is influenced by genes and other environmental factors. It is postulated that HLA-B27 predisposes to AS by influencing the gut microbiome. Studies have shown that the microbiota composition of patients with AS differs from that of rheumatoid arthritis patients, as well as healthy controls. Further, *HLA-B27*–positive healthy individuals have a microbiome that differs from that of *HLA-B27*–negative subjects.

In animal models of spondyloarthritis, *HLA-B27* transgenic rats and mice did not develop spondyloarthritis when raised in a germ-free environment, but they developed spondyloarthritis-like disease when they were housed in a typical laboratory environment, suggesting a role for microbes in the pathogenesis of spondyloarthritis. More than 60% of patients with AS have subclinical acute or chronic intestinal inflammation. This loss of architectural and functional integrity in the intestinal epithelium enables the passage of microbial products into the submucosa and then into the systemic circulation. Innate and adaptive immune cells recognize these microbial products and produce proinflammatory cytokines. These microbial products and the immune cells travel from the gut to distant sites, such as peripheral joints and entheses, causing inflammation.

Clinical Manifestations

The most common manifestations of axSpA include chronic inflammatory low back, hip, and/or buttock pain. The typical characteristics of inflammatory back pain include age of onset before 40 years, insidious onset without any identifiable cause, improvement with exercise or activity and no improvement with rest, and pain in the second half of the night. Neck pain is rarely the presenting feature because of involvement of the cervical spine; when this is present, it is more commonly seen in women.

The limitation of spinal motion is initially the result of axial inflammation and later is secondary to the ossification of ligamentous structures, bony fusion of apophyseal joints, and outer fibers of the annulus fibrosus of the intervertebral disks, leading to the development of syndesmophytes.

Hip involvement is seen in up to 40% of patients. The typical symptoms are pain in the groin or radiation of pain to the medial thigh or the knee. Hip involvement is associated with significant functional impairment. Other peripheral joints—such as the ankles, knees, shoulders, and, to a lesser extent, the sternoclavicular joint, the temporomandibular joint, and small joints of the hands and feet—may also be involved.

Enthesitis is a classic feature of axSpA. Enthesitis manifests as pain, stiffness, and tenderness at the sites of insertions of ligaments, muscles, or tendons to a bone. Typical areas of enthesitis include the Achilles tendon, plantar fascia attachment to the calcaneum, costochondral junctions, and the paraspinal muscle attachment to the pelvic rim. Diffuse swelling of the toes or fingers, called *dactylitis* ("sausage digits"), is rarely seen in axSpA.

EMMs associated with axSpA include psoriasis, IBD, and uveitis. A large epidemiologic study found that 42% of axSpA patients had one or more EMMs; uveitis was present in 27%, IBD in 10%, and psoriasis in 11%. Uveitis seen in association with axSpA manifests as eye discomfort during the prodromal phase followed by an acute onset of eye redness, pain, photophobia, and miosis. The usual characteristics of uveitis associated with axSpA are acute in onset, unilateral, and involve the anterior part of the uvea. Even though overt IBD is seen in only 10% of axSpA patients, more than 60% have subclinical mucosal inflammation in the gut.

Diagnosis

There is a significant delay of 6 to 8 years in the diagnosis of axSpA from symptom onset. Diagnostic delay has the potential to lead to disease progression and structural damage to the spine, due to delayed treatment. There are many reasons for this, including the commonality of back pain in the general population and the rarity of axSpA as a cause of back pain. There are no specific physical findings or laboratory tests to diagnose axSpA; the diagnosis is based on pattern recognition and clinical reasoning. Patients with back pain are generally seen by nonrheumatologists who may not be familiar with features of inflammatory back pain and may not suspect axSpA. In an attempt to decrease this delay in diagnosis, the Spondyloarthritis Research and Treatment Network (SPARTAN) developed draft recommendations for the referral of adults with chronic back pain starting before the age of 45 years to a rheumatologist for evaluation of axSpA (Figure 1).

In the optimal clinical setting with a patient complaining of onset of chronic (>3 months) inflammatory back pain starting before 45 years of age, the presence of other features of spondyloarthritis (as described earlier), a positive *HLA-B27* test, and a plain radiograph of the SI joint showing definitive sacroiliitis, the diagnosis of r-axSpA would be straightforward. Radiographic findings such as sclerosis; joint erosions; or widening, narrowing, or ankylosis of the SI joint suggest sacroiliitis. However, the grading of sacroiliitis has poor reproducibility even in expert hands.

During this early stage of the disease (also known as *nr-axSpA*), MRI (without contrast) of the SI joints may show evidence of active inflammation and may also show structural changes such as sclerosis, fatty metaplasia, or erosions that aid in making the diagnosis. The required sequence of MRI and the features that suggest a diagnosis of nr-axSpA include the following:

- T1-weighted sequence, semicoronal and axial. Structural changes such as erosions and ankylosis can be seen. Fat metaplasia appears hyperintense.
- Fat-suppressed T2-weighted (short-TI inversion recovery [STIR]) sequence, semicoronal. Osteitis, representing active inflammation and reported as bone marrow edema; appears hyperintense.
- Erosion sensitive sequence, semicoronal (e.g., T1-weighted fat suppressed).

Refer adults who have chronic (>3 months) back/hip/buttock pain before age 45 and a score of 3 or more	Points
X-ray or MRI sacroiliitis	3
Elevated ESR or CRP	2
HLA-B27+	2
Uveitis	2
Inflammatory bowel disease	1
Psoriasis	1
Back pain has a good response to NSAIDs	1
Back pain improvement with exercise and not with rest	1
Alternating buttock pain	1
Family history of axial spondyloarthritis, uveitis, psoriasis or inflammatory bowel disease	1
Total	**Refer if score of 3 or more**

Figure 1 Draft referral recommendation for adults with chronic (>3 months) back/hip/buttocks pain with onset before age 45 years and a score of 3 or more.

When the clinical suspicion of axSpA is high but radiographic imaging of the SI joints is negative or inconclusive for sacroiliitis, the presence of the features previously noted on MRI of the SI joints may help in confirming a diagnosis of nr-axSpA.

The changes of inflammation on STIR imaging (i.e., "osteitis") can be seen in professional athletes, military recruits, and even in normal individuals because of mechanical stress ("false-positive MRI"). It is therefore important to emphasize that ruling out common causes of back pain, pattern recognition, and clinical reasoning is the key to a diagnosis of axSpA.

Plain radiographs of the spine may show characteristic changes in r-axSpA. Romanus lesions or the *shiny corner sign* and squaring of the vertebral body are seen as a result of erosions at the attachments of the spinal ligaments at the vertebral corners in early disease. This is followed by ossification of the outer layer of annulus fibrosus, leading to syndesmophyte formation on plain radiographs. In the late stages, ankylosis of the spine, also known as *bamboo spine*, may be seen in a small percentage of patients with r-axSpA. The role of low-dose computed tomography (CT) in the diagnosis of axSpA is currently being researched.

An elevated erythrocyte sedimentation rate (ESR) or C-reactive protein (CRP) is seen in only 30% to 40% of patients with active r-axSpA.

Differential Diagnosis

Chronic nonspecific back pain is common in the general population (19% according to the NHANES study); thus mechanical causes of back pain should be considered first.

Diffuse idiopathic skeletal hyperostosis (DISH) is sometimes mistaken for "bamboo spine of AS." DISH is a noninflammatory condition affecting the spine. It is more commonly seen in obese, diabetic males, often older than 50 years of age. Radiographically, DISH is characterized by calcification of the anterior longitudinal ligament involving at least four contiguous vertebral bodies, sometimes referred to as *flowing osteophytes*. The flowing osteophytes are bulky and typically appear on the right side of the spine. SI joints are not involved in patients with DISH.

Osteitis condensans ilii (OCI) can be mistaken for sacroiliitis but is usually an asymptomatic benign disorder of multiparous women. OCI is characterized by radiographic findings of a triangular area of dense sclerosis on the lower and inferior part of iliac side of the SI joint. OCI is not associated with erosions or ankylosis of the SI joints.

Inflammatory back pain with sclerotic changes on SI joint radiographs can also be seen in conditions such as (1) postpartum insufficiency fracture of the sacrum; (2) septic sacroiliitis from tuberculosis, brucellosis, fungi, and other infectious agents; and (3) rarely malignancies such as acute lymphoblastic leukemia.

Treatment

The goals of treatment of axSpA are to reduce symptoms, improve and maintain spinal flexibility and normal posture, reduce functional limitations, and prevent complications of the disease. The mainstay of treatment has been NSAIDs, exercise and physical therapy, biologics such as tumor necrosis factor-α inhibitors (TNFi) and interleukin-17 inhibitors (IL-17i), and small-molecule drugs such as Janus kinase inhibitors (JAKi).

Treatment of axSpA can be divided into nonpharmacologic, pharmacologic, and surgical interventions.

Nonpharmacologic Interventions

Nonpharmacologic interventions include active physical therapy (on land or aquatic), self-directed physical exercise, patient education, and smoking cessation. These are recommended during all stages of the disease.

Pharmacologic Interventions

Box 1 outlines pharmacologic interventions for the treatment of axSpA.

The use of biologics and small molecules has been associated with an increased risk of serious infections. While bacterial infections are seen in both classes of drugs, herpes zoster is seen mostly with JAKi and reactivation of latent tuberculosis is mostly seen with TNFi. Therefore screening for latent tuberculosis should be performed before these therapies are initiated.

Some of the side effects of TNFi and IL-17 therapy include injection-site reactions with subcutaneous preparations or infusion reactions with infliximab (Remicade) or golimumab (Simponi) or secukinumab (Cosentyx). Some of the other adverse effects of TNFi are the development of demyelinating disease, worsening of heart failure, recurrence of lymphoma or malignant melanoma, and paradoxical development of psoriasis-like skin lesions. Adverse events associated with IL-17i therapy include leukopenia, candidiasis, and the development or worsening of IBD. The ORAL Surveillance Study, a postmarketing safety trial in rheumatoid arthritis patients ordered by the FDA, showed a higher risk of major adverse cardiac events (fatal and nonfatal myocardial infarctions and nonfatal strokes) and a higher risk of cancers (excluding nonmelanoma skin cancers) in those on JAKi therapy compared with those on TNFi therapy. As a result, the FDA added a black box warning

Pharmacologic Interventions for the Treatment of Axial Spondyloarthritis

- NSAIDs are used in full doses either continuously or on an as-needed basis, depending on the severity of symptoms, comorbidities, and patient preferences. No particular NSAID is preferred over any other.
- If patients continue to have symptoms despite a 4-week trial of full-dose NSAIDs, therapy is escalated to either TNFi or IL-17i.
- Although certolizumab (Cimzia) is the only TNFi approved for nr-axSpA, all five TNFi agents are FDA approved for the treatment of AS.
  - Soluble receptor of TNF—Etanercept (Enbrel) 50 mg, SC injection once weekly.
  - TNFi monoclonal antibodies:
    - Adalimumab (Humira) 40 mg SQ every 2 weeks
    - Golimumab (Simponi) 50 mg SQ once a month or (Simponi Aria) 2 mg/kg IV at weeks 0, 4, and then every 8 weeks thereafter
    - Certolizumab pegol (Cimzia) 200 mg SQ twice a month or 400 mg SQ once a month
    - Infliximab (Remicade) 5 mg/kg IV infusion every 6 weeks
      - No TNFi is preferred over any other, except in patients with concomitant uveitis or IBD, in whom monoclonal antibodies are preferred over soluble receptor TNFi therapy.
      - In case of primary failure of TNFi, treatment can be switched to IL-17i or JAKi. In case of secondary failure of TNFi therapy (failing after initial benefit), either an alternative TNFi or IL-17i or JAKi can be used.
- IL-17Ai, secukinumab (Cosentyx) is given as 150 mg SQ at weeks 0, 1, 2, 3, and 4, followed by 150 mg or 300 mg SQ every 4 weeks. Ixekizumab (Taltz), another IL-17Ai, can also be used. It is given as 160 mg SQ once, followed by 80 mg SQ every 4 weeks. Bimekizumab (Bimzelx), a new agent that blocks IL-17A and IL-17F, has shown efficacy and safety similar to that of other anti–IL-17A agents. It is given as 160 mg SQ every 4 weeks. All are approved for the treatment of AS and nr-axSpA. In case of primary failure of IL-17i, treatment can be switched to TNFi or JAKi. In case of secondary failure of IL-17i therapy (failing after initial benefit), either an alternative IL-17i or TNFi or JAKi can be used.
- While both JAKi (tofacitinib [Xeljanz] 5 mg PO two times a day and upadacitinib [Rinvoq] 15 mg PO once a day) are approved for the treatment of AS, only upadacitinib is approved for nr-axSpA.
- Conventional synthetic DMARDs such as sulfasalazine (Azulfidine)[1], up to 3 g/day, and methotrexate[1], up to 25 mg/week, are effective in the treatment of peripheral joint involvement, but not of axial disease in axSpA.
- Local glucocorticoid injections for enthesitis or intraarticular injections for active peripheral arthritis can provide relief for flareups. However, injection of inflamed weight-bearing tendons such as the Achilles tendon is not recommended because of the risk of rupture.
- Systemic glucocorticoids do not have any benefit in axSpA and should be avoided.

[1]Not FDA approved for this indication.

axSpA, Axial spondyloarthritis; *DMARDs,* disease-modifying antirheumatic drugs; *FDA,* US Food and Drug Administration; *IL,* interleukin; *IV,* intravenously; *JAKi,* Janus kinase inhibitor; *nr-axSpA,* nonradiographic axial spondyloarthritis; *NSAIDs,* nonsteroidal antiinflammatory drugs; *SQ,* subcutaneously; *TNFi,* tumor necrosis factor inhibitor.

on tofacitinib (Xeljanz) and extended the warning to upadacitinib (Rinvoq) because it is in the same class of drugs.

Surgical Interventions

Total hip arthroplasty should be considered in patients with refractory hip pain or functional decline in the presence of radiographic evidence of structural damage. Spinal corrective osteotomies are occasionally necessary for fixed kyphotic deformities seen in advanced AS but should be undertaken only in centers of expertise.

Monitoring

Patients should be monitored regularly for disease activity, functional impairment, and medication safety. The frequency of monitoring is individualized. Assessment of disease activity can be performed by the following methods:

- Use of the Bath Ankylosing Spondylitis Disease Activity Index (BASDAI): This is a patient-administered questionnaire with six questions answered on a visual analog scale of 0 to 10. A BASDAI score of 4 or greater is indicative of active disease. Clinically significant improvement is defined as an absolute change of 2 or greater.
- Use of the Ankylosing Spondylitis Disease Activity Score (AS-DAS): This incorporates three questions used in the BASDAI, a patient global assessment of disease activity, and CRP. An AS-DAS score below 1.3 is defined as inactive disease; a score of 1.3 to 2.1 is low disease activity; 2.1 to 3.5 is high disease activity, and greater than 3.5 is very high disease activity. A reduction of 1.1 or greater in ASDAS is considered a significant improvement.

Structural damage resulting from axSpA can be measured using the modified Stoke Ankylosing Spondylitis Spine Score. This score correlates with disease activity as measured with the ASDAS.

Functional impairment can be measured by the Bath Ankylosing Spondylitis Functional Index. This is a patient-administered questionnaire that includes 10 activities of daily living. The Bath Ankylosing Spondylitis Metrology Index is an index of spinal and hip mobility in patients with AS. It includes lateral lumbar flexion, tragus-to-wall distance, modified Schober test, maximal intermalleolar distance, and cervical rotation.

The ESR and CRP may be useful in monitoring disease activity. MRI of the SI joints or spine is expensive and is not indicated to monitor disease activity of AS. Spine radiographs are not used for monitoring purposes in daily practice, although they may be used to counsel patients about lifestyle changes (such as stopping smoking) or to start biologic therapy.

Complications

A 2020 systematic review and meta-analysis identified hypertension (23%), cardiovascular disease (12%), and depression (11%) as the most common comorbidities in patients with axial spondyloarthritis. Cardiovascular disease is being recognized as a common comorbidity in patients with AS and is linked to chronic inflammation. All patients with AS should be counseled about the traditional risk factors for cardiovascular disease, and appropriate treatment should be instituted if necessary.

The prevalence of osteoporosis is approximately 25% after 10 years of axSpA. Vertebral fractures are seen in about 10% of patients with AS. The lower cervical spine is the most commonly involved area, where there is often also neurologic compromise. One should consider vertebral fractures in patients with neck and back pain that has changed in intensity or character from baseline. Another rare complication is the cauda equine syndrome from long-standing AS resulting from inflammation of the lumbosacral nerve roots caused by arachnoiditis. Cardiac manifestations include aortic valve insufficiency and conduction abnormalities. Pulmonary manifestations are rare and include chest expansion restriction from ossification of costovertebral joints and upper lobe–predominant interstitial lung disease. Patients with AS can have immunoglobulin A (IgA) nephropathy or, in late stages, renal amyloidosis if the disease is left untreated.

References

Baraliakos X, Østergaard M, Poddubnyy D, et al: Effect of secukinumab versus adalimumab biosimilar on radiographic progression in patients with radiographic axial spondyloarthritis: results from a head-to-head randomized phase IIIb study, *Arthritis Rheumatol* 76(8):1278–1287, 2024. https://doi.org/10.1002/art.42852.82.

Bennett AN, McGonagle D, O'Connor P, et al: Severity of baseline magnetic resonance imaging-evident sacroiliitis and HLA-B27 status in early inflammatory back pain predict radiographically evident ankylosing spondylitis at eight years, *Arthritis Rheum* 58(11):3413–3418, 2008.

Bittar M, Deodhar A: Axial spondyloarthritis: a review, *JAMA* 333(5):408–420, 2025. https://doi.org/10.1001/jama.2024.20917.

Brophy S, MacKay K, Al-Saidi A: The natural history of ankylosing spondylitis as defined by radiological progression, *J Rheumatol* 29(6):1236–1243, 2002.

Curtis JR, Winthrop K, Bohn RL, et al: The annual diagnostic prevalence of ankylosing spondylitis and axial spondyloarthritis in the United States using Medicare and MarketScan databases, *ACR open rheumatol* 3(11):743–752, 2021.

de Winter JJ, van Mens LJ, van der Heijde D: Prevalence of peripheral and extra-articular disease in ankylosing spondylitis versus non-radiographic axial spondyloarthritis: a meta-analysis, *Arthritis Res Ther* 18(1):196, 2016.

Deodhar A, Mease PJ, Reveille JD, et al: Frequency of axial spondyloarthritis diagnosis among patients seen by US rheumatologists for evaluation of chronic back pain, *Arthritis Rheum* 68(7):1669–1676, 2016.

Ramiro S, Nikiphorou E, Sepriano A, et al: ASAS-EULAR recommendations for the management of axial spondyloarthritis: 2022 update, *Ann Rheum Dis* 82:19–34, 2023.

Reveille JD: Genetics of spondyloarthritis - beyond the MHC, *Nat Rev Rheumatol* 8(5):296–304, 2012.

Reveille JD, Witter JP, Weisman MH: Prevalence of axial spondylarthritis in the United States: estimates from a cross-sectional Survey, *Arthritis Care Res* 64(6):905–910, 2012.

Rudwaleit M, Khan MA, Sieper J, et al: Commentary: the challenge of diagnosis and classification in early ankylosing spondylitis: do we need new criteria? *Arthritis Rheum* 52(4):1000–1008, 2005.

Ward MM, Deodhar A, Gensler LS, et al: Update of the American College of Rheumatology/Spondylitis Association of America/Spondyloarthritis Research and Treatment Network recommendations for the treatment of ankylosing spondylitis and nonradiographic axial spondyloarthritis, *Arthritis Care Res* 71(10):1285–1299, 2019. https://doi.org/10.1002/acr.24025.

Ytterberg SR, Bhatt DL, Mikuls TR, et al: ORAL Surveillance Investigators: cardiovascular and cancer risk with tofacitinib in rheumatoid arthritis, *N Engl J Med* 386(4):316–326, 2022.

COMMON SPORTS INJURIES

Method of
Andrew S.T. Porter, DO

CURRENT DIAGNOSIS

- Lateral Ankle Sprain—Pain over lateral ankle ligament(s) with localized swelling. Often associated with laxity and pain with anterior drawer and/or talar tilt test. Obtain x-rays based on the Ottawa ankle and foot rules.
- Medial Ankle Sprain—Less common than lateral ankle sprain. Pain in the deltoid ligament with localized swelling. Obtain x-rays based on Ottawa ankle and foot rules.
- High Ankle Sprain—Syndesmotic injury. Pain with squeeze test and/or dorsiflexion with external rotation.
- Osteochondral Ankle Injuries—Most commonly seen in the talar dome. Associated with an ankle inversion injury and ankle pain. Often have a joint effusion and soft tissue swelling and can have mechanical symptoms (catching, locking, crepitus, and a feeling of giving way). Obtain x-rays initially and then magnetic resonance imaging (MRI) to grade degree of injury.
- Anterior Cruciate Ligament (ACL) Injuries—Most common after noncontact injuries. Physical examination reveals a diffuse knee effusion, positive Lachman, and/or anterior drawer test. Obtain x-rays then MRI for further evaluation.
- Posterior Cruciate Ligament (PCL) Injuries—Occur with varus/valgus stress with the knee in full extension. Physical examination reveals a positive posterior drawer and sag sign. Obtain x-rays then MRI for further evaluation.
- Medial Collateral Ligament (MCL) Injuries—Occur with valgus stress or twisting with or without contact. Physical examination reveals localized effusion and a positive valgus stress testing and tenderness to palpation along the MCL. Graded 1 to 3.
- Osteochondral Knee Injuries—Most commonly seen in the femoral condyle. Associated with a knee injury. Knee pain and, often, mechanical symptoms of the knee. Palpation of the femoral condyles with the knee in flexion reproduces pain. Obtain x-rays initially and then MRI to grade degree of injury.
- Mallet Finger—Disruption of the extensor mechanism insertion into the distal phalanx.
- Jersey Finger—Occurs after avulsion of the flexor digitorum profundus tendon from its insertion on the distal phalanx.
- Proximal Interphalangeal (PIP) Joint Dorsal Dislocation—Injury to the volar plate with or without an avulsion fracture.
- Scaphoid Fracture—Pain over the scaphoid with or without a fall on an outstretched hand injury is a scaphoid fracture until proven otherwise. Obtain wrist x-rays with a scaphoid view.
- Tendinosis—Repetitive chronic tendon injuries result in scarring, disorganization of fibers, degeneration, and are without an inflammatory component.
- Stress Fractures—Most often seen in active patients as a result of excessive stress on normal bone from overactivity or normal stress on a bone that is deficient (osteoporotic, poor nutrition, or in female athlete triad). History is positive for bone pain, and physical examination reveals tenderness to palpation in the affected bone and often a positive tuning fork test, hop test, and fulcrum test. Obtain x-rays first, then MRI or bone scan if needed.
- Spondylolysis/Spondylolisthesis—Most often seen in young athletes with insidious onset low back pain and history of repetitive extension. Positive stork test. X-rays initially, and if negative, may proceed with limited CT and SPECT scan or MRI.

CURRENT THERAPY

- Lateral Ankle Sprain—Treat with RICE (rest, ice, compression, elevation) and early rehab. Return to play (RTP) is generally 1 to 4 weeks and is based on functional progression. RTP with ankle brace.
- Medial Ankle Sprain—Treat with RICE and early rehab. RTP with ankle brace.
- High Ankle Sprain—Treat with RICE and boot for 1 to 3 weeks and then rehab. RTP takes a longer time compared with lateral ankle sprain.
- Osteochondral Ankle Injuries—Degree of injury is graded via MRI, and this guides treatment and RTP.
- ACL Injuries—ACL tears often need reconstruction that is individualized in active patients who require knee stability.
- PCL Injuries—Isolated PCL injuries often heal conservatively with protected weight bearing in an extension brace and knee rehab.
- MCL Injuries—Often heal conservatively with bilateral hinged knee brace and knee rehab. Generally, RTP in 2 to 6 weeks.
- Osteochondral Knee Injuries—Degree of injury is graded via MRI, and this guides treatment and RTP.
- Mallet Finger—Treat with continuous full-extension stack splinting of the distal interphalangeal joint for 6 weeks and then nighttime splinting and activity splinting for 6 weeks.
- Jersey Finger—Treatment is referral to orthopedic surgeon for surgical intervention.

- PIP joint dorsal dislocation—Reduce dislocation and obtain x-rays. Treat with progressive extension blocking splint with 30° to 40° of flexion and decrease by 10° per week.
- Scaphoid Fracture—If x-rays with scaphoid view are negative, place in a short-arm thumb spica cast and follow up in 2 weeks. If x-rays remain negative but pain persists, obtain a CT or MRI. Treat nondisplaced scaphoid fractures with short-arm thumb spica cast: proximal-third fractures 12 to 20 weeks, middle-third fractures 10 to 12 weeks, and distal-third fractures 4 to 6 weeks.
- Tendinosis—Treat by creating inflammation to facilitate healing.
- Stress Fractures—Treat with general treatment for stress fractures plus specific treatment based on stress fracture site.
- Spondylolysis/Spondylolisthesis—Treat with extension blocking brace, rest, rehabilitation with core strengthening and lower extremity flexibility, and gradual RTP.

| BOX 1 | Ottawa Ankle and Foot Rules |

- An ankle x-ray series is indicated if there is pain in the malleolar zone and any of these findings are made:
  - Tenderness over the lateral malleolus
  - Tenderness over the medial malleolus
  - Inability to bear weight four steps immediately after the injury or in the emergency department or physician's office
- A foot x-ray series is indicated if there is pain in the midfoot zone and any of these findings are made:
  - Tenderness over the base of fifth metatarsal
  - Tenderness over the navicular bone
  - Inability to bear weight four steps immediately after the injury and in the emergency department or physician's office

*X-rays are indicated if any of these criteria are met.
Data from Bachmann and colleagues (2003) and Tiemstra (2012).

Ankle Injuries

The ankle is the most common joint injured in athletes. Ankle sprains are common, as they represent 25% of all sports-related injuries. The Ottawa ankle and foot rules help in the decision to obtain x-rays (Box 1). In general, treatment will consist of RICE (rest, ice, compression, elevation), early mobilization, and rehab. Prevention of ankle injuries is important and consists of ankle braces, ankle taping, neuromuscular training program, and regular sport-specific warm-up exercises.

Lateral Ankle Sprain

The most common ankle sprain is a lateral inversion sprain that results from landing on an inverted foot with or without plantarflexion. The lateral ankle ligaments are the anterior talofibular ligament (ATFL), calcaneofibular ligament, and the posterior talofibular ligament. The ATFL is the most commonly sprained ligament. Lateral ankle sprains are most commonly treated with RICE initially, then early ambulation, range of motion, progression into strengthening, and then proprioception rehabilitation. Proprioception rehabilitation includes balancing on one leg and performing balancing exercises on a wobble board. For example, patients can balance on one leg when brushing their teeth. Athletes should return to play (RTP) with a lace-up/velcro ankle brace after injury with or without taping. This added stability will help prevent future ankle injuries and also decrease the severity of ankle injuries. Most athletes will RTP in a few days to 4 weeks; this return is based on pain, obtaining full active range of motion and full strength, and functional stability.

Medial Ankle Sprain

Medial ankle ligament sprains are rare, account for < 10% of ankle injuries, and are often accompanied with a lateral malleolar fracture or syndesmotic injury. The medial ankle ligament is the deltoid ligament and is injured via external rotation or eversion. These ankle sprains are treated similarly to lateral ankle sprains.

High Ankle Sprain

High ankle sprains, also known as syndesmotic ankle sprains, occur through forced external rotation of a dorsiflexed foot most commonly but also occur by forced internal rotation of a fixed plantar flexed foot. The syndesmotic ligaments connect and stabilize the distal tibia to the distal fibula. The syndesmotic ligaments are the anterior tibiofibular ligament, posterior tibiofibular ligament, transverse tibiofibular ligament, interosseous ligament, and the interosseous membrane. Palpate the fibular head for pain. Pain on palpation of the fibular head might indicate a maisonneuve fracture, a fracture of the proximal third of the fibula associated with syndesmotic disruption. A high ankle sprain has a longer healing time compared to a lateral ankle sprain. Often these need immobilization with a boot or cast for 1 to 4 weeks to help with healing before beginning rehab. RTP after a high ankle sprain depends on pain, achieving a full active range of motion, full strength, and functional stability. Incomplete healing of a high ankle sprain can result in distal tibia and fibula instability.

Osteochondral Ankle Injuries

Osteochondral injuries are injuries to the articular surface of a joint. These injuries range from small undisplaced depressions and cracks in the osteochondral surface to small pieces of articular cartilage and bone that break off of the articular surface and float within the joint. Osteochondral injuries occur most commonly on weight-bearing articular surfaces. In osteochondral injuries, osteonecrosis of subchondral bone occurs, resulting in separation of cartilage and subchondral bone from underlying, well-vascularized bone. The term *osteochondral lesion* (OCL) is favored over the previously used term *osteochondritis dessicans* because there might not be an inflammatory component of the injury. OCLs are often associated with repeated trauma or overuse in athletes. OCLs typically present with pain in the affected joint and can develop with a specific injury or over several months in highly active athletes. OCLs are more common in younger patients with open physes (growth plates) and are referred to as juvenile OCLs. Adult OCLs describe this condition in skeletally mature patients.

Osteochondral injuries are a cause for pain in up to 25% of ankle injuries and need to be considered when a patient presents with ankle pain. Acute osteochondral injuries in the ankle most commonly affect the talar dome (Figures 1–3) but can also be found in the distal tibia (Figure 4). OCLs are first evaluated by x-rays (see Figures 1 and 2) and then graded by magnetic resonance imaging (MRI) (Table 1). CT scan (see Figure 3) is sometimes utilized as well. Grade 1 to 3 juvenile OCLs and grade 1 to 2 adult OCLs are treated conservatively. Conservative treatment consists of no weight bearing (NWB) in a cast or boot for 6 to 10 weeks followed by partial weight bearing (PWB) to full weight bearing (FWB) over 2 to 6 months, followed with an ankle brace for 3 months, and ensuring adequate calcium and vitamin D intake to facilitate healing. Nonsteroidal antiinflammatory drugs (NSAIDs) should be avoided because they can slow bone healing, and OCLs are probably not an inflammatory process. For grade 4 juvenile OCLs, grade 3 and 4 adult OCLs, and those that have not clinically healed with conservative care operative treatment is required. Operative treatment options depend on OCL size and type and include removal of the OCL followed by transchondral drilling and microfracture to stimulate fibrocartilage formation, fixation of the OCL with an osteochondral allograft, osteochondral autograft transfer, and autologous chondrocyte implantation.

Knee injuries—The knee joint lacks intrinsic bone stability, so most stability is from the major knee ligaments.

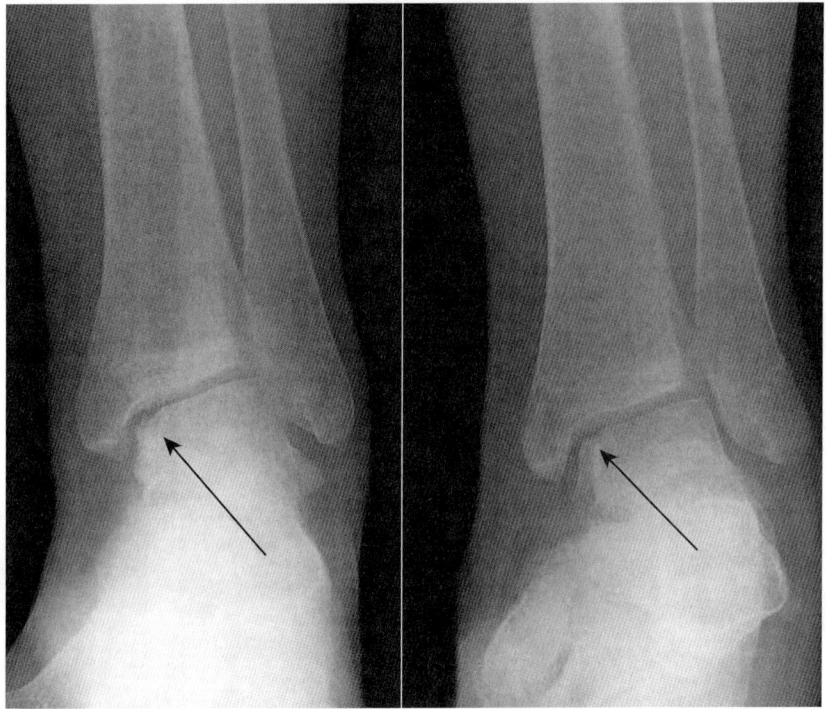

Figure 1 X-rays of the left ankle, AP and mortise views, which demonstrate a grade 2 osteochondral lesion (OCL) along the medial talar dome.

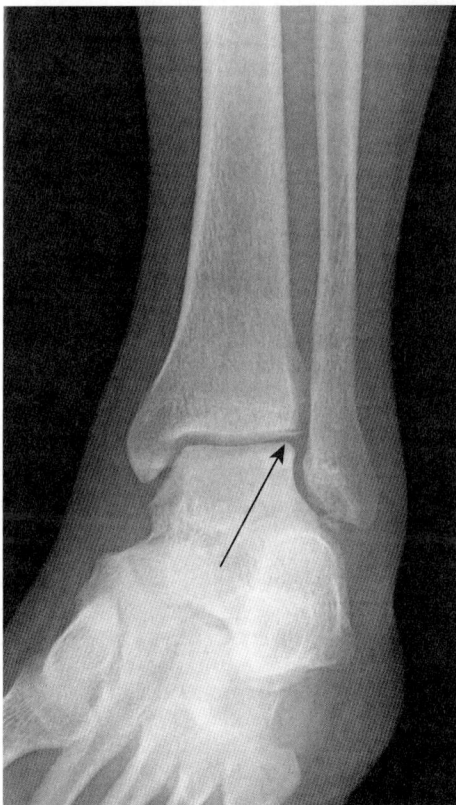

Figure 3 CT scan without contrast. Sagittal image of ankle, which demonstrates a grade 4 OCL of the talar dome.

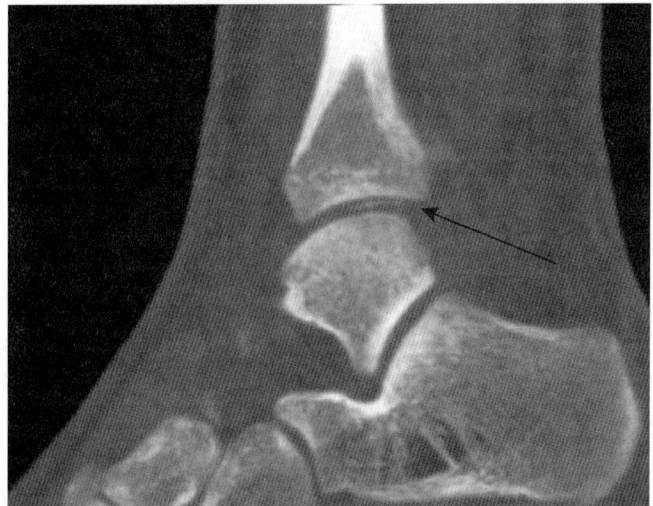

Figure 2 X-ray of the left ankle, mortise view, which demonstrates a grade 4 OCL along the lateral talar dome.

Anterior Cruciate Ligament Injuries

The anterior cruciate ligament (ACL) is the key stabilizer of the knee and is one of two major intraarticular knee ligaments, the other being the posterior cruciate ligament (PCL). Most ACL tears occur from noncontact injuries. Women experience ACL tears up to nine times more often than men do. The main function of the ACL is to prevent excessive anterior tibial translation relative to the femur. Patients who sustain an injury to their ACL often describe hearing a pop, feeling instability in their knee, experiencing pain immediately after the injury, and develop an associated knee effusion. On-the-field evaluation is ideal in an ACL injury, as the hamstrings will often start to tighten up shortly after the injury, preventing anterior tibial translation. This will prevent an isolated test of the ACL and give the false impression that an ACL endpoint is present when in fact the ACL is completely torn. The anterior drawer (Figure 5) and Lachman test (Figure 6) are the main physical examination tests to evaluate the ACL. Obtain x-rays and then MRI if an ACL tear is suspected. The blood supply to the ACL is poor and is provided by the middle geniculate artery off of the popliteal artery. Because of the poor blood supply, ACL tears often need reconstruction if athletes want to return to a high level of activity and knee stability is needed. ACL reconstruction timing is important and often will occur 3 to 4 weeks after injury to allow for swelling to decrease, ROM and strength to improve,

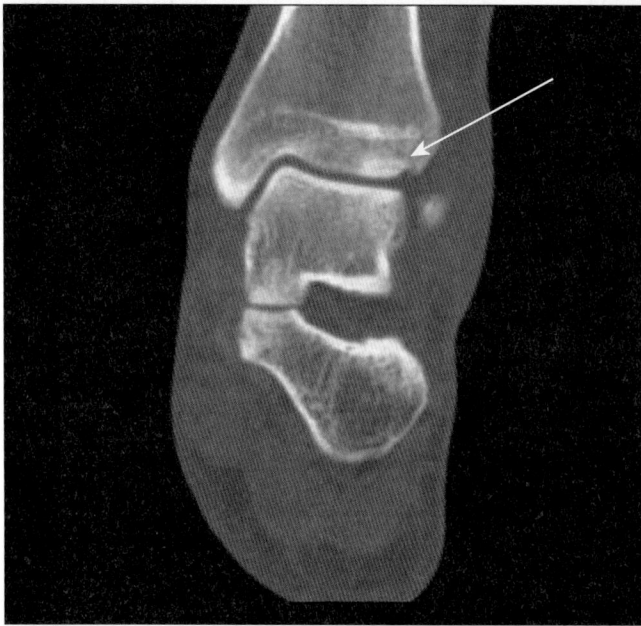

Figure 4 CT scan without contrast. Coronal image of ankle, which demonstrates a grade 1 OCL of the distal lateral tibia.

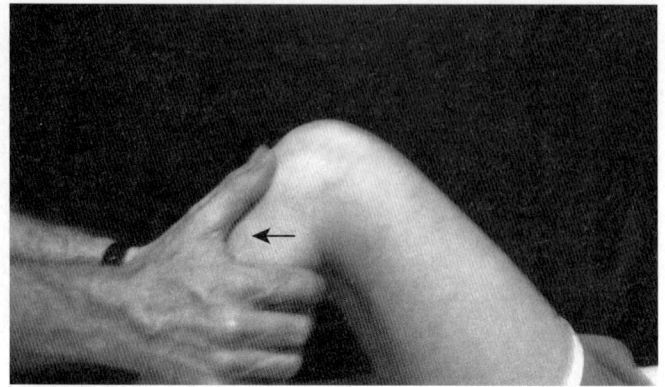

Figure 5 Anterior drawer test for ACL laxity. Patient's knee is flexed 90°. Examiner applies anterior force to the tibia in relation to the patient's femur to evaluate for laxity.

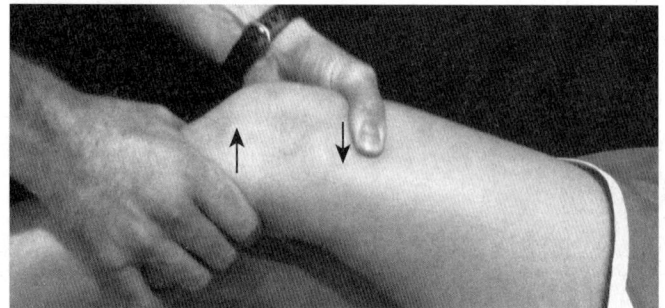

Figure 6 Lachman test for ACL laxity. Patient's knee is flexed 20°–30°. Examiner grasps the distal femur and proximal tibia and applies anterior force to the tibia and posterior force to the femur to evaluate for ACL laxity.

TABLE 1	Classification of Osteochondral Lesions	
STAGE	**PLAIN X-RAY FINDINGS**	**MRI FINDINGS**
1	Depressed osteochondral fragment	Articular cartilage thickening and low signal changes in subchondral bone
2	Osteochondral fragment attached by bone	Articular cartilage breached, no synovial fluid around fragment
3	Detached nondisplaced fragment	Articular cartilage breached, synovial fluid around fragment
4	Displaced fragment	Loose foreign body

and inflammation to decrease. Also during this presurgical time, it is important to have patients perform pre-hab (presurgical rehabilitation), focusing on AROM and knee strengthening. A knee effusion will cause the quadriceps muscles to weaken and atrophy. Hamstring tendon autograft, patella tendon autograft, quadriceps tendon autograft, and allograft are all used for ACL reconstruction. Each graft has advantages and disadvantages and should be discussed with the orthopaedic surgeon before reconstruction and individualized for each patient. Continuing to participate in high-level activity after an ACL tear if undiagnosed can lead to a knee dislocation and further intraarticular knee injury.

PCL Injuries
The PCL is the other major intraarticular knee ligament. Isolated PCL injuries are much less common than ACL injuries and make up only 3.5% of ligamentous knee injuries in sports, with the remaining 96.5% of PCL injuries associated with multiligamentous knee injuries. PCL injuries, unlike ACL injuries, are the result of external forces (e.g., a soccer player sliding into the goal post and tearing his or her PCL). The main function of the PCL is to resist posterior tibial translation. Posterior drawer testing (Figure 7) and a sag sign test (Figure 8) are the physical examination tests used to evaluate the PCL. Obtain x-rays then MRI if a PCL tear is suspected. The blood supply to the PCL is better than the blood supply to the ACL. Isolated PCL injuries (grades 1 and

2) are treated conservatively because surgical reconstruction has not been shown to be helpful. Conservative treatment consists of protected weight bearing in an extension brace followed by quadriceps rehabilitation and ROM exercises. RTP is generally 4 to 6 weeks after a PCL injury. Surgical intervention is recommended for associated injuries to the ACL, medial collateral ligament (MCL), and posterior lateral corner (grade 3 PCL injury).

MCL Injuries
The MCL is an extraarticular ligament that resists knee valgus forces. An MCL sprain results from a valgus stress to a partially flexed knee. Athletes will present with localized pain and swelling along the medial aspect of the knee. Most MCL injuries are isolated ligament injuries, but more severe MCL injuries can involve tears of the medial meniscus and ACL, commonly referred to as the "terrible triad." The MCL is examined by palpation and valgus stress testing at 0° and 30° of knee flexion. MCL injuries are graded 1, 2, or 3 depending on severity of injury. A patient with a grade 1 MCL sprain has pain in the MCL but no valgus stress testing laxity. A grade 2 MCL sprain has valgus stress testing laxity but a solid endpoint. A grade 3 MCL sprain has no endpoint with valgus stress testing. Thankfully, the MCL has a rich vascular supply and can often heal conservatively. Treatment consists of RICE for the first 1 to 2 weeks and a bilateral hinged knee brace to facilitate healing. Weight bearing and ROM and strengthening exercises are started when they are tolerable. RTP after an MCL injury depends on the grade and generally takes 2 to 6 weeks.

Osteochondral Knee Injuries
Osteochondral injuries occur in the knee as well as in the ankle. Osteochondral injuries of the knee most commonly affect the lateral aspect of the medial femoral condyle but can be found anywhere along the medial or lateral femoral condyle, patella, or trochlea. History is significant for knee pain, with or without swelling and mechanical symptoms (catching, locking, crepitus, and feeling of

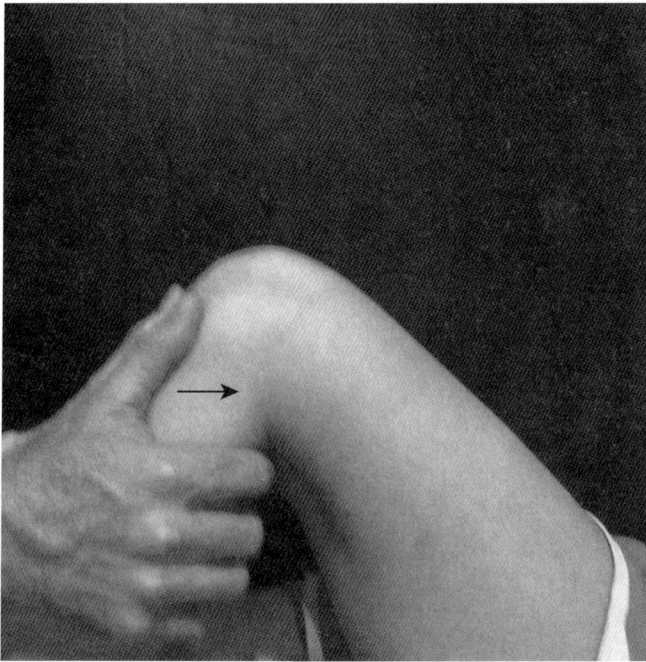

Figure 7 Posterior drawer test for PCL laxity. Patient's knee is flexed 90°. Examiner applies posterior force to the tibia in relation to the patient's femur to evaluate for laxity.

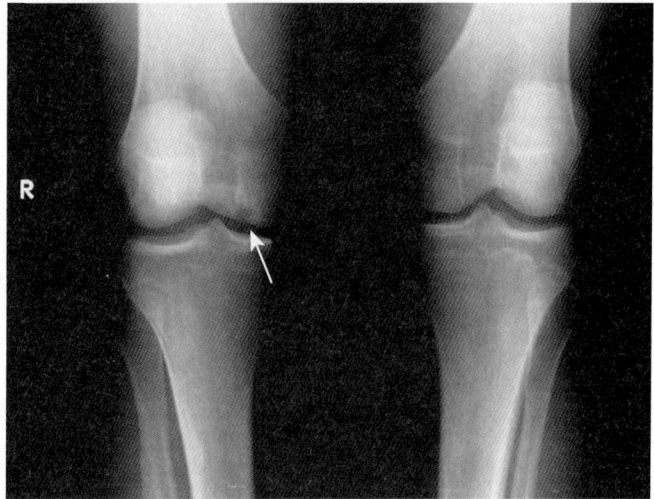

Figure 8 Sag sign test for PCL laxity. Examiner views the tibia condyles from the lateral side to evaluate for a posterior sag (displacement) in the appearance that would indicate a PCL injury.

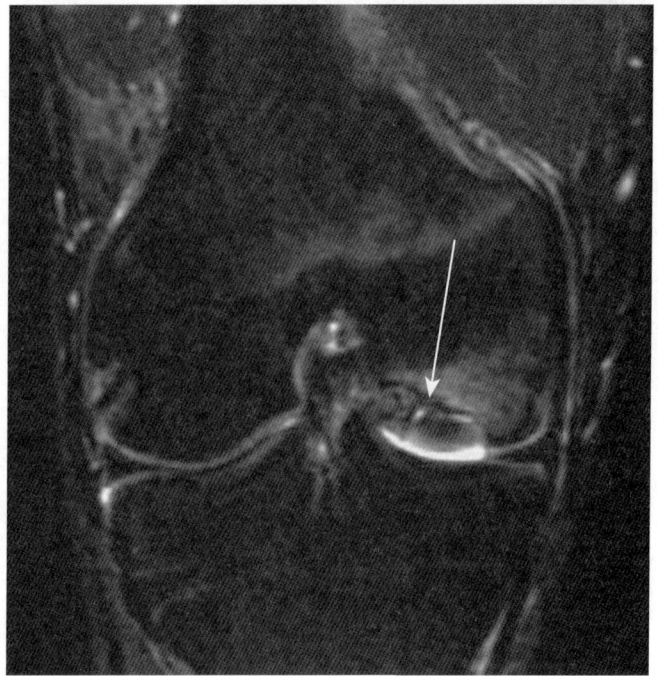

Figure 9 X-ray of the bilateral knees, AP view, which demonstrates a grade 1 OCL along the right knee medial femoral condyle.

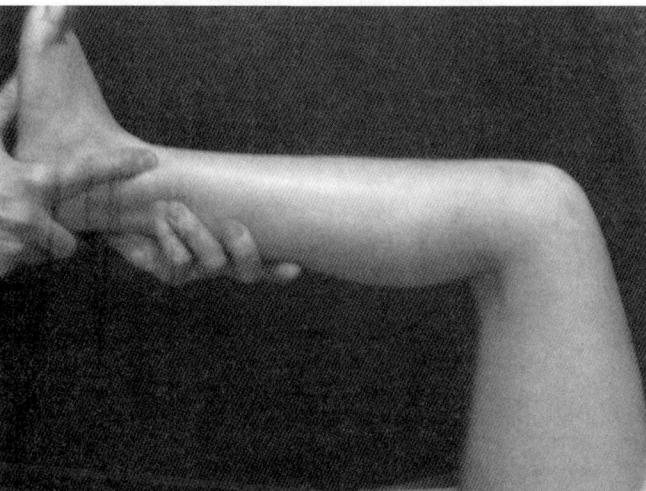

Figure 10 Magnetic resonance imaging (MRI) of the right knee, without contrast. Coronal T2 fat saturation image, which demonstrates a grade 4 OCL of the medial femoral condyle.

giving way). On palpation, patients can have pain in the affected area with knee flexion with or without crepitus. Obtain x-rays initially (Figure 9) and then grade the OCL severity by MRI (Figure 10). CT scans are also utilized sometimes. Grade 1 to 3 juvenile knee OCLs and grade 1 to 2 adult knee OCLs are treated conservatively. Grade 4 juvenile OCLs, grade 3 to 4 adult OCLs and all OCLs that have failed conservative care are treated operatively.

Hand Injuries

Mallet Finger

A mallet finger occurs after forced flexion of an actively extended distal interphalangeal (DIP) joint, resulting in disruption of the extensor mechanism insertion into the distal phalanx. Patients with a mallet finger are unable to actively extend the DIP joint. This injury can be associated with an avulsion fracture (Figure 11). For acute injuries, general treatment consists of continuous extension splinting of the DIP joint (0° to 10° of hyperextension) for at least 6 weeks. The 6-week clock starts over if the DIP joint

is allowed to flex at all during the initial 6 weeks of treatment or if, at the end of the 6 weeks, the mallet finger is not completely healed. After the initial 6 weeks, it is recommended to continue with nighttime splinting and activity splinting for another 6 weeks to ensure adequate healing and avoidance of surgery. To perform this splinting, a stack splint is well tolerated and is protective (Figure 12). Orthopaedic referral is indicated if the patient is unable to obtain full passive extension of the DIP joint or if the avulsion fracture involves over 30% of the joint space.

Jersey Finger

A jersey finger results from the avulsion of the flexor digitorum profundus tendon from its insertion on the distal phalanx. This commonly occurs in football and rugby players when the tip of their flexed finger is caught in a jersey and the DIP joint of the finger is then forcefully extended. After this injury occurs, the patient is unable to actively flex the DIP joint. Treatment is urgent referral to an orthopaedic surgeon for surgical intervention.

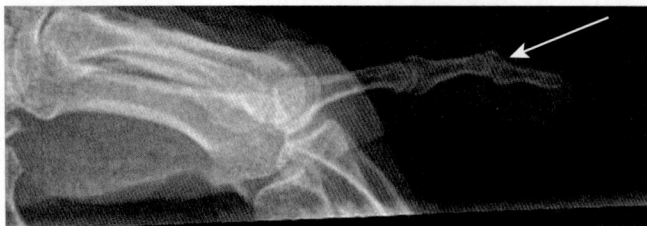

Figure 11 X-ray of the left hand, lateral view, which demonstrates a mallet finger of the fifth finger. Note the flexion of the DIP joint and avulsion fracture of the distal phalanx that involves about 30% of the joint space.

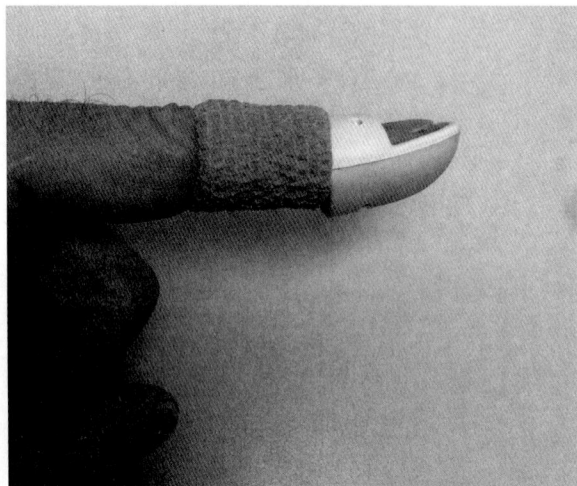

Figure 12 Stack splint with Coban wrap added for stability that immobilizes the DIP joint at neutral to 5° of hyperextension.

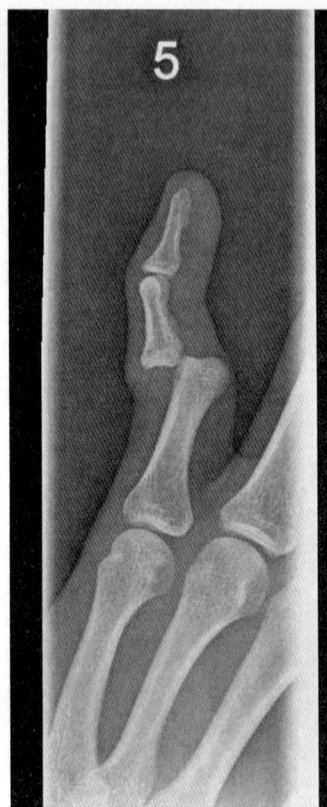

Figure 13 X-ray of the left hand, oblique view, which demonstrates a proximal interphalangeal (PIP) joint dorsal and lateral dislocation.

Proximal Interphalangeal Joint Dorsal Dislocation

Proximal interphalangeal (PIP) joint injuries are the most common joint injuries in sports. Most PIP dislocations are dorsal and result from hyperextension with an axial load. Dislocations are described by the position of the distal fragment in relation to the proximal fragment. PIP dorsal dislocations cause injury to the volar plate with or without avulsion fracture. Pre-reduction x-rays are preferred if they can be obtained promptly (Figure 13). X-rays of the finger with at least one view being a true lateral view should be obtained to rule out fracture. However, many PIP dorsal dislocations occur on the playing field and it is reasonable to reduce these dislocations, buddy tape the affected finger, and allow the patient to RTP with x-rays obtained after the athletic competition. Reduction is usually uncomplicated and is performed urgently via hyperextending the joint, applying traction in plane with the finger, then flexing the joint. Post reduction films are a necessity (Figure 14). Stability testing of the collateral ligaments should be performed after the reduction. Full flexion and extension of the PIP joint will be possible if the joint is stable. A stable joint without a large avulsion fragment should be treated with a progressive extension blocking splint (Figures 15 and 16). Start with 30° to 40° of flexion and decrease by 10° per week over 3 to 4 weeks, then buddy tape the injured finger with activity PRN (8). Some PIP dorsal dislocations have a lateral component to them and these are treated similar to pure dorsal dislocations (see Figure 13). Orthopaedic surgeon referral is indicated if there is a large avulsion fracture or the joint is unstable.

Scaphoid Fracture

The scaphoid bone is the most common carpal bone that is fractured and is a common injury that is encountered in primary care. Interestingly, scaphoid fractures occur most commonly in young men. Scaphoid fractures occur less commonly in young children and the elderly because of the relative weakness of the distal radius compared with the scaphoid in these age groups. Often a scaphoid fracture is caused by a FOOSH (fall on an outstretched hand)

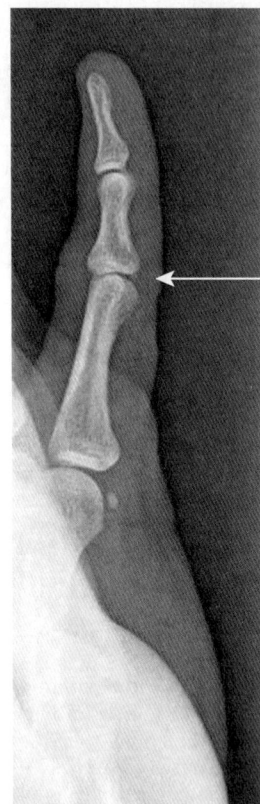

Figure 14 X-ray of the left hand, lateral status postreduction view, which demonstrates a relocated proximal interphalangeal (PIP) joint. Note the avulsion fracture of the middle phalanx.

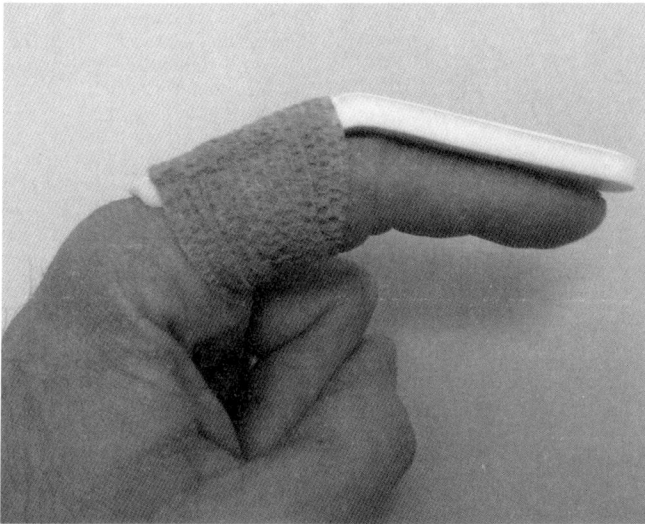

Figure 15 Dorsal extension blocking splint at 30°–40° of flexion at the PIP joint. Note that there is no pressure over the PIP joint volar plate and that flexion and extension at the DIP joint is possible.

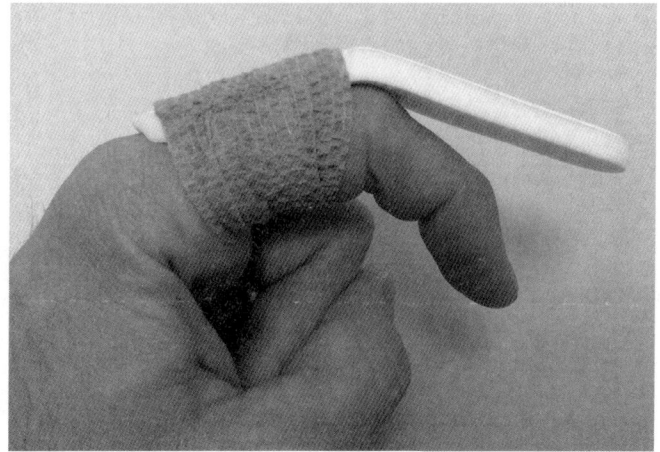

Figure 16 Dorsal extension blocking splint at 30°–40° of flexion at the PIP joint. This figure illustrates the freedom of motion that is possible at the PIP joint (full flexion and limited extension) and the DIP joint (full flexion and extension).

injury. On physical examination, if the patient has pain over the scaphoid tubercle or in the anatomical snuffbox with or without a history of a FOOSH injury, the clinician needs to have a high index of suspicion for a scaphoid fracture when evaluating the wrist x-rays. Obtain the standard wrist x-rays (AP, lateral, and oblique views) plus a dedicated scaphoid view (AP with ulnar deviation) and be aware that early imaging with x-rays is often unrevealing for a scaphoid fracture (Figure 17). If a fracture is not seen on x-rays, the clinician needs to have a high index of suspicion for a scaphoid fracture, place the patient in a short-arm thumb spica cast, and have the patient follow up in 2 weeks. If repeat x-rays remain negative and the patient continues to have scaphoid pain, proceed with an MRI of the wrist with T2 fat saturation views or a CT scan. If a scaphoid fracture is noted on imaging, the location of the scaphoid fracture will guide treatment. Because the blood supply to the scaphoid is distal to proximal, scaphoid fractures are harder to heal than other carpal fractures. Nondisplaced middle-third or proximal-third scaphoid fractures are treated with a long- or short-arm thumb spica cast with the wrist at 20° to 30° of extension and the thumb in slight extension and abduction for 10 to 20 weeks. Middle-third fractures should be immobilized for 10 to 12 weeks. Proximal-third fractures should be immobilized from 12 to 20 weeks. It is much easier to regain flexion in the wrist after casting than it is to regain extension. If the elbow is incorporated in the cast, it should be casted at 90° of flexion. A long-arm cast may decrease healing time, but it does not improve nonunion rates. A nondisplaced distal-third fracture should be treated in a short-arm thumb spica cast for 4 to 6 weeks. For displaced fractures or non-healing fractures, a referral to an orthopedic surgeon is recommended. Use acetaminophen for pain control and avoid nonsteroidal antiinflammatory drugs (NSAIDs) because NSAIDs can impair bone healing. Ensure adequate energy availability via diet and adequate calcium and vitamin D intake, and avoid tobacco exposure to help heal the fracture. Bone health and bone nutrition are a part of the big picture in fracture healing.

Overuse Injuries

Tendinosis

The paradigm and management of tendon overuse injuries is changing. The term *tendinitis* is generally used to refer to painful overuse tendon conditions and implies that inflammation is present. However, the most common pathology in chronic painful tendons is tendinosis. Tendinosis occurs after repetitive injuries to a tendon results in intertendinous scarring, disorganization of tendon fibers, and degeneration. Tendinosis does not have an inflammatory component. Early on in a tendon injury, there

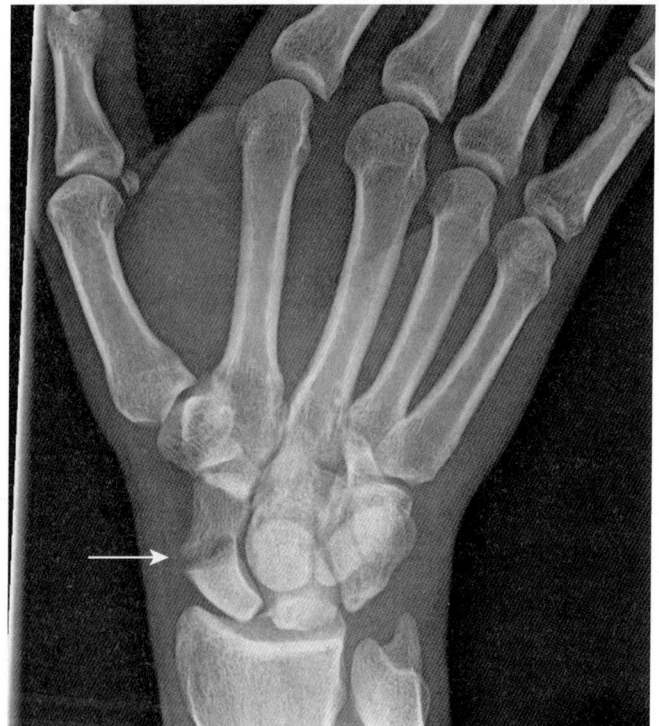

Figure 17 Scaphoid view x-ray (AP view with ulnar deviation) is important to obtain in addition to your standard wrist views (AP, lateral, and oblique) when scaphoid fracture is suspected. This scaphoid fracture was not seen on the x-rays on the day of the injury. Patient continued to have wrist pain and then presented 10 weeks later, and x-rays were obtained demonstrating the scaphoid fracture.

is inflammation resulting in tendinitis, but after about 6 weeks this generally evolves into tendinosis. Early activity modification and treatment of tendinitis with NSAIDs and rehabilitation may prevent the development of tendinosis. Tendinosis is a problematic condition that affects many active people, young and old. To address these more chronic tendon injuries, healing is facilitated by creating an inflammatory response. To create inflammation, treatments such as eccentric strengthening (Figure 18), deep soft tissue massage with tools (e.g., gua sha or Graston, or ASTYM) (Figure 19), nitroglycerin patches (Nitro-Dur),[1] and musculoskeletal ultrasound-guided percutaneous needle tenotomy (with or

---

[1] Not FDA approved for this indication.

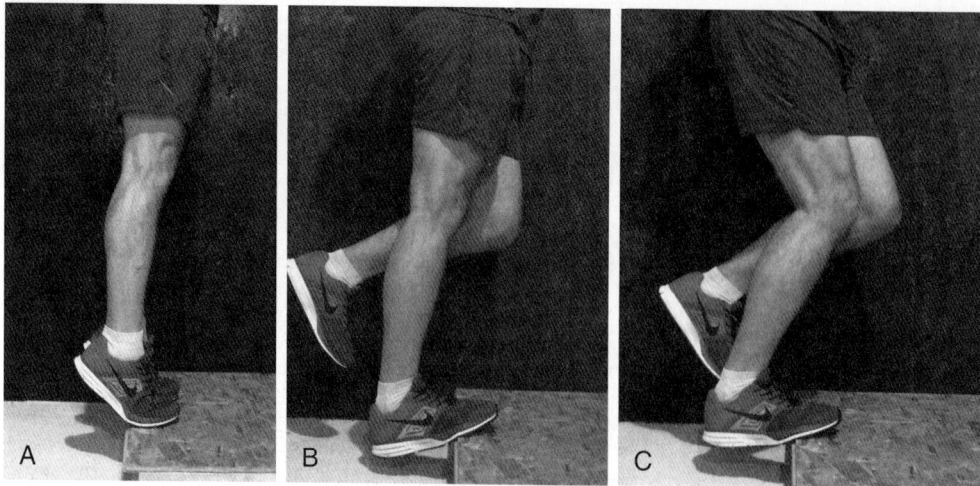

Figure 18 Eccentric exercises for Achilles tendinosis. (**A**) Patient begins with the injured leg straight and the ankle in flexion. The assistance of the uninjured leg was utilized to get in this starting position. (**B**) The ankle of the injured leg (right leg, in this case) is slowly lowered in a controlled fashion to full dorsiflexion to eccentrically strengthen (while lengthening the calf muscles) the right Achilles tendon. The left leg is then brought back down, and full plantarflexion in both ankles is performed, recruiting the uninjured leg to assist with getting back to position (**A**). (**C**) The eccentric exercise from (**B**) is repeated with the knee bent at 45°.

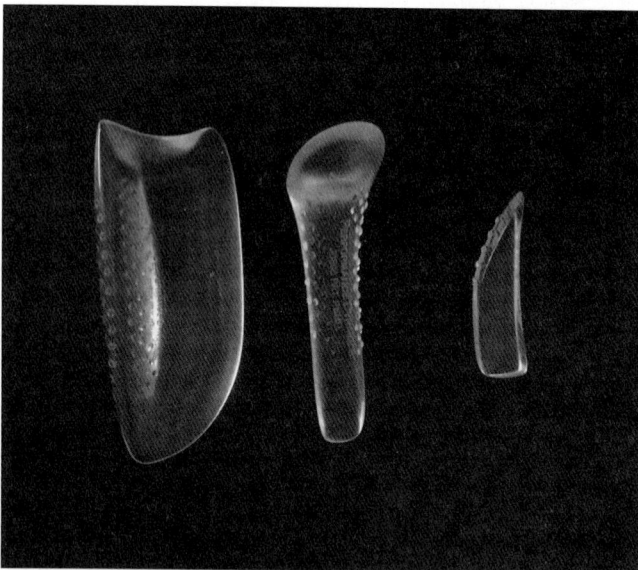

Figure 19 ASTYM® tools.

TABLE 2 Treatment of Tendinosis

TREATMENT MODALITY	DESCRIPTION
Deep soft tissue massage with tools (gua sha, Graston, ASTYM) (Figure 19)	One to three times per week for 4–6 wk; most common with athletic trainer certified or physical therapist
Nitroglycerin patches (Nitro-Dur)[1]	0.1 mg/h patch, apply Q24 h to a different location on tendon for at least 6 wk
Eccentric strengthening (Figure 18)	3 sets of 15 exercises, twice daily, for 12 wk
Musculoskeletal ultrasound-guided percutaneous needle tenotomy with or without autologous blood injection, prolotherapy, or platelet-rich plasma	Referral to primary care sports medicine physician

[1]Not FDA approved for this indication.

without injection of autologous blood, prolotherapy, or platelet-rich plasma) have all been utilized and have been shown to be effective (Table 2). It is important to avoid NSAIDs when trying to create inflammation because NSAIDs will prevent the inflammatory response. This concept of tendinosis diagnosis and treatment

TABLE 3 Stress Fracture Physical Exam Tests

PHYSICAL EXAM TEST	POSITIVE TEST
Palpation	Pain over affected bone with palpation
Stork test (Figure 22)	Back extension with rotation while standing on one leg increases pain in the pars interarticularis region
Fulcrum test	Pain in fracture site while applying a bending force (e.g., over the exam table) to distal extremity while proximal extremity is kept relatively immobilized
Hop test	Hopping 10 times on affected leg reproduces pain at fracture site
Tuning fork test	Vibrating tuning fork over fracture site results in pain at site

can be utilized for tendons throughout the body and is most commonly applied to the Achilles tendon, patella tendon, iliotibial (IT) band, piriformis, gluteus medius, hamstrings, biceps, common elbow flexor tendon, and common elbow extensor tendon.

Stress Fractures

Stress fractures occur when osteoclastic activity overwhelms osteoblastic activity. Bone injury unfolds over a continuum of time, starting with normal bone that progresses to stress reaction, then stress fracture, and finally fracture if the bone continues to be injured. This can occur as a result of excessive stress on normal bone from overactivity or normal stress on a bone that is deficient (osteoporotic, poor nutrition, or in female athlete triad). Stress fractures are common injuries in athletes and occur most often in the lower extremities. Running sports account for 69% of stress fractures. Stress fractures should be considered in someone who is active, presents with bone pain, and who performs repetitive activities with limited rest or with a recent increase in activity. Physical examination tests to perform in the area of interest are palpation, the tuning fork test, the fulcrum test, and the hop test (Table 3). If a stress fracture is suspected, x-rays should be obtained, keeping in mind that it takes 2 to 3 weeks for signs of stress fracture (i.e., periosteal reaction, callus formation, fracture line) to show up on an x-ray, and often stress fractures do not show up on x-rays. If x-rays are negative and a diagnosis is needed to help guide care and RTP, a bone scan or MRI with T2 fat saturation views (Figures 20 and 21) should be obtained. The bone scan and MRI are equally sensitive, but an MRI is more specific and avoids patient radiation exposure. An MRI is more expensive. Because a bone scan can stay positive for up to 18 months, clinical progress should not be monitored with a bone scan.

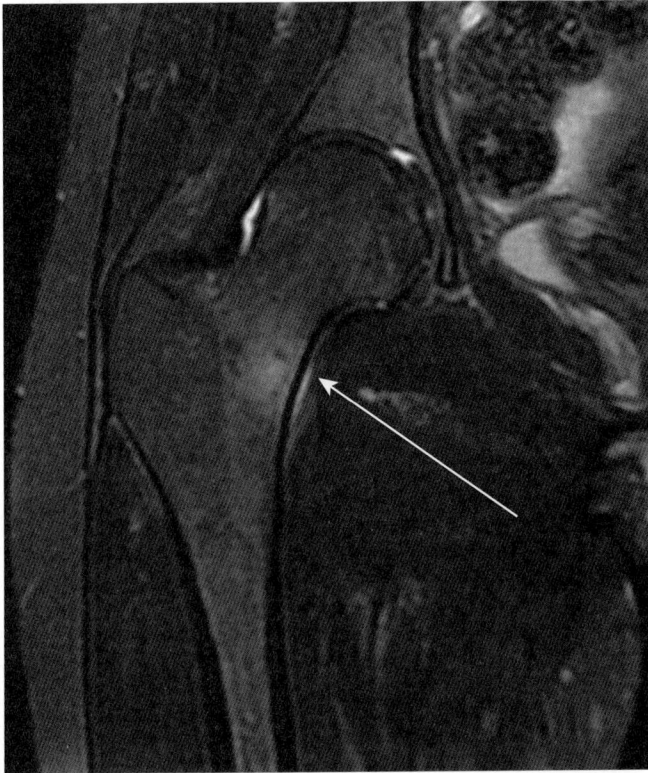

Figure 20 MRI of the right hip without contrast. Coronal T2 fat saturation image demonstrates a compression-sided femoral neck stress fracture (note surrounding bone edema in white).

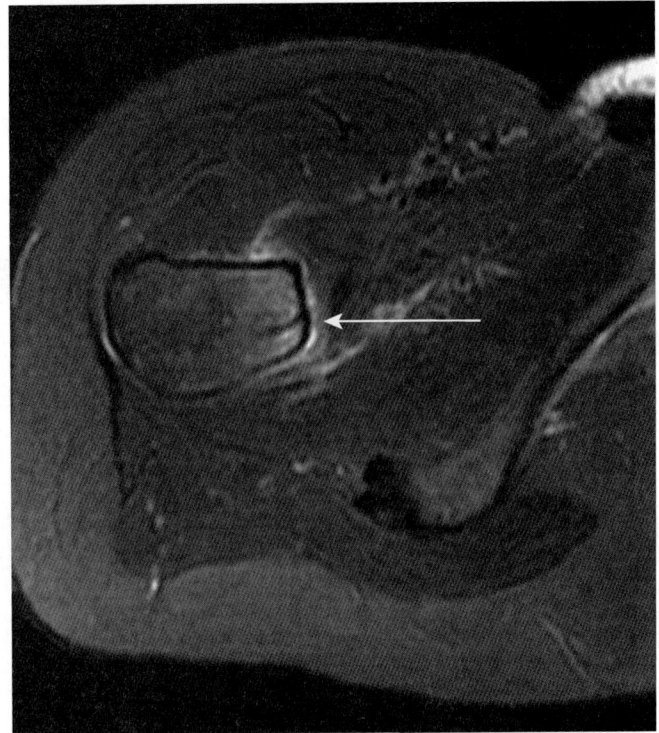

Figure 21 MRI of the right hip without contrast. Axial T2 fat saturation image that demonstrates a compression sided femoral neck stress fracture (note edema in white and probable fracture line in black that measures up to 11 mm).

To prevent stress fractures, athletes should distribute loading forces on the bone with cross training and biomechanical adjustments (i.e., orthotics, proper shoes, stretches, strengthening, running mechanics), consume sufficient calories to maintain adequate energy availability, and ensure appropriate intake of calcium and vitamin D. A study by Lappe of female Navy recruits showed reductions in stress fractures in those consuming 2000 mg of calcium[1] and 800 IU vitamin D[1] daily, either as a supplement or through consumption of dairy products. Tobacco should be avoided. Additionally, women of child bearing age should try to maintain regular menses by consuming adequate calories and avoiding a negative energy balance.

General treatment for stress fractures can be grouped into nutrition, medication, and biomechanical recommendations. Nutrition recommendations include optimizing energy availability in the diet, ensuring adequate calcium and vitamin D intake, and avoidance of tobacco exposure. Medication recommendations include using acetaminophen as needed for pain control and avoidance of NSAIDs. Biomechanical recommendations are to offload the affected bone and reduce activity to pain-free functioning and pain-free cross-training. Crutches may be needed to offload the injured area even more than a walking boot/cast or steal shank. The patient may require complete non-weight bearing (NWB) with the overall goal being to obtain pain-free ambulation during the initial treatment. Tables 4 and 5 outline recommended guidelines for protected weight bearing for specific stress fracture sites. Additional recommendations are to begin a rehabilitation program when tolerated and to stretch and strengthen supporting structures. Start a gradual increase in activity when the patient is pain-free.

Because of their propensity for delayed healing and nonunion, certain stress fractures are considered high risk, necessitate prompt treatment, and may ultimately require surgical fixation. Low-risk stress fractures have a lower incidence of delayed

TABLE 4	High-Risk Stress Fracture Initial Treatment
HIGH-RISK STRESS FRACTURE	**INITIAL TREATMENT (IF STABLE AND NONDISPLACED)**
Femoral neck (compression side) (Figures 20 and 21)	NWB for 6–8 wk then PWB to FWB over next 6–8 wk
Anterior tibia (tension side)	NWB for 6–8 wk then PWB to FWB over next 6–12 wk
Medial malleolus	Pneumatic lower leg boot for 6–8 wk
Navicular	NWB cast/boot for 6 wk then 6-wk RTP progression
Base of fifth metatarsal (Jones)	NWB cast/boot 6–8 wk
May consider surgery for quicker RTP	
Sesamoids	NWB cast/boot 6 wk

Abbreviations: NWB = non-weight bearing; PWB = partial weight bearing; FWB = full weight bearing.

TABLE 5	Low-Risk Stress Fracture Initial Treatment
LOW-RISK STRESS FRACTURE	**INITIAL TREATMENT**
Sacrum/pelvis	WBAT 7–12 wk
Femoral shaft	WBAT 6–8 wk
Posterior medial tibia (compression side)	WBAT boot 2–12 wk (longer time with cortical break) then transition to pneumatic tibial brace
Fibula	WBAT 1–4 wk
Metatarsal (2nd–5th)	Steel shank/walking boot 3–6 wk

Abbreviations: WBAT = weight bearing as tolerated.

[1] Not FDA approved for this indication.

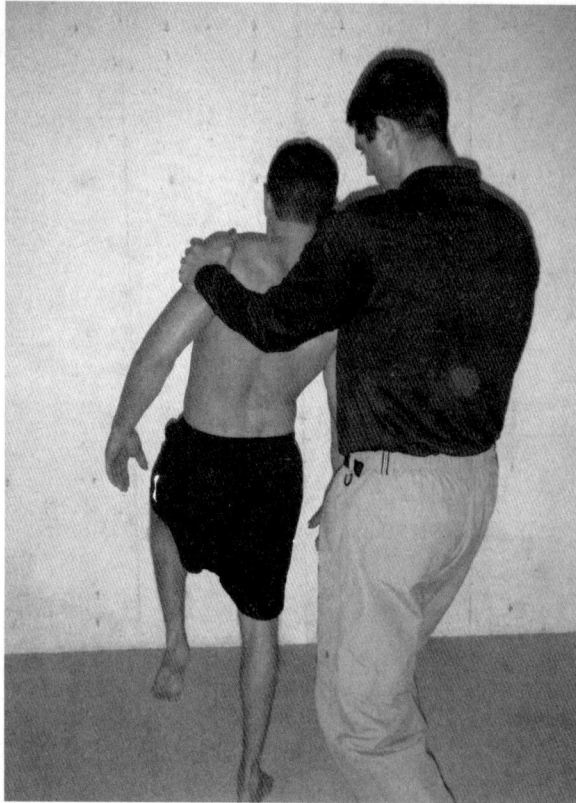

Figure 22 Stork test: To assess localized spondylolysis pain, a single leg hyperextension rotation test (stork test) is performed. The patient stands on one leg and hyperextends and rotates the spine. Reproduction of the patient's pain is suggestive of a spondylolysis.

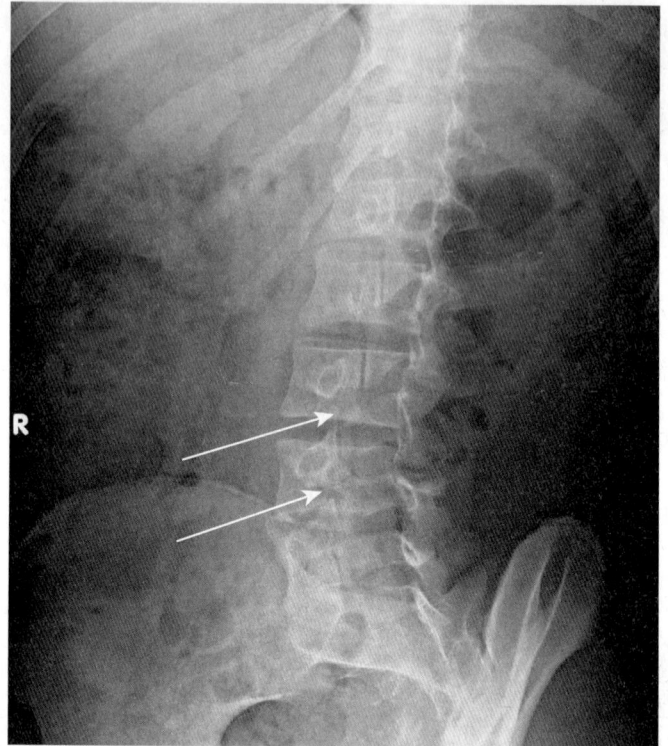

Figure 23 Oblique view x-ray of the lumbar spine, which demonstrates a L3 and L4 spondylolysis.

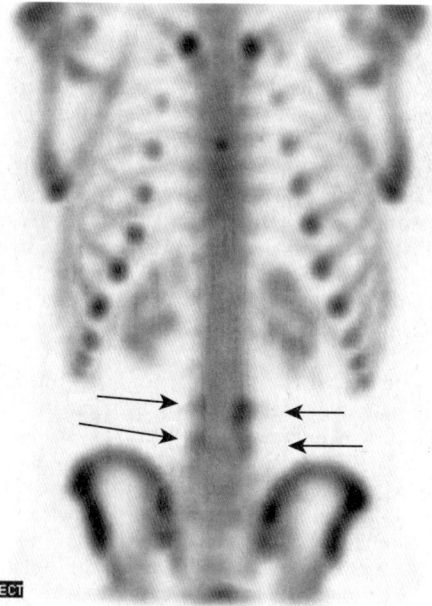

Figure 24 SPECT scan lumbar spine, PA view, which demonstrates an acute bilateral L3 and L4 spondylolysis.

healing and nonunion. High-risk stress fractures that appear stable and nondisplaced can be treated nonoperatively with close follow-up. Consider referral to an orthopaedic surgeon for failed conservative treatment. Biomechanical forces along the bone with activity are used to classify tibia and femur stress fractures. For example, during running, the tibia and femur have different forces exerted on different parts of the bone. The tibia compresses posteriorly, so there is more compression along the posterior tibia and more tension along the anterior aspect of the tibia. The femoral neck compresses inferiorly and medially with running, so there is more compression along the inferior medial aspect of the femoral neck and more tension along the superior lateral aspect of the femoral neck. These variable forces on different parts of the bone affect the potential for delayed healing and nonunion.

Spondylolysis and Spondylolisthesis

Spondylolysis is a nondisplaced stress fracture of the pars interarticularis. Spondylolisthesis occurs when there is bilateral spondylolysis with listhesis (slippage) of the vertebral body. Spondylolisthesis is graded 1 to 4 depending on how much slippage is present with each grade, accounting for 25% (i.e., grade 1 = 0–25%).

When a young athlete presents with low back pain, spondylolysis needs to be considered: this can be the cause of their pain up to 47% of the time. Spondylolysis is an overuse injury caused by repetitive hyperextension and/or rotation and has increased incidence in ballet dancers, gymnasts, divers, soccer players, and football linemen. L5 is the most common level for a spondylolysis. The history is significant for insidious onset of deep pain in the low back exacerbated by extension. Physical examination shows a positive Stork test (see Table 3), often with reproduction of pain on the side of weight bearing (Figure 22). If history and physical exam are suggestive of a pars interarticularis injury, x-rays of the lumbar spine, including oblique views, should be obtained. Oblique view x-rays provide the best view to identify a spondylolysis even though they only demonstrate spondylolysis about 30% of the time when it is present (Figure 23). If x-rays are negative, proceed with MRI or with SPECT scan. If the SPECT scan is positive (Figure 24), then proceed with limited CT scan (Figures 25 and 26). If radiation exposure is a concern, or if high-definition MRI is readily accessible, thinly sliced stacked axial cuts with T2 fat saturation views in all planes using a high-definition MRI is the test of choice (Figure 27). A spectrum of recommended treatments and conservative approaches that allow for a prompt and safe RTP

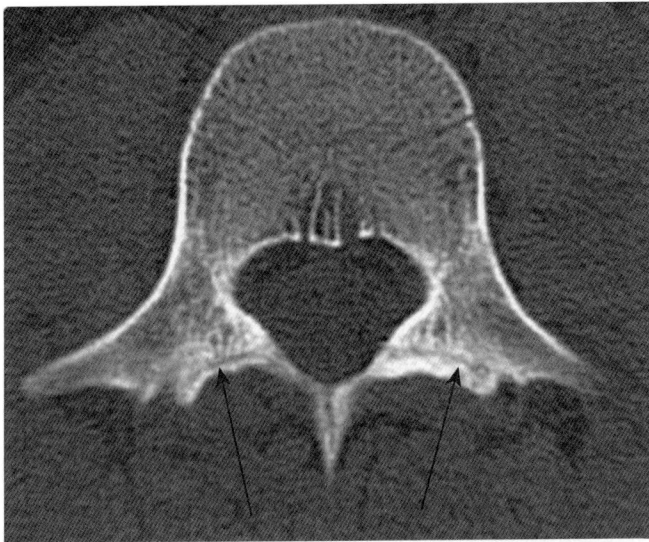

Figure 25 CT scan without contrast. Axial image at L3 shows bilateral pars interarticularis fractures that appear acute with jagged and nonsclerotic fracture edges.

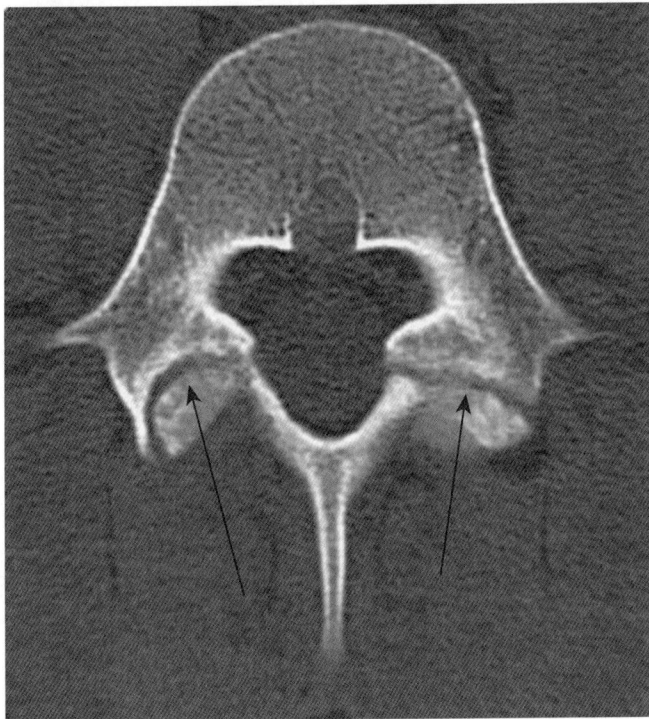

Figure 27 MRI lumbar spine without contrast. Axial T2 fat saturation image at L5 that demonstrates a right L5 spondylolysis signified by right pars interarticularis bone edema in white at L5.

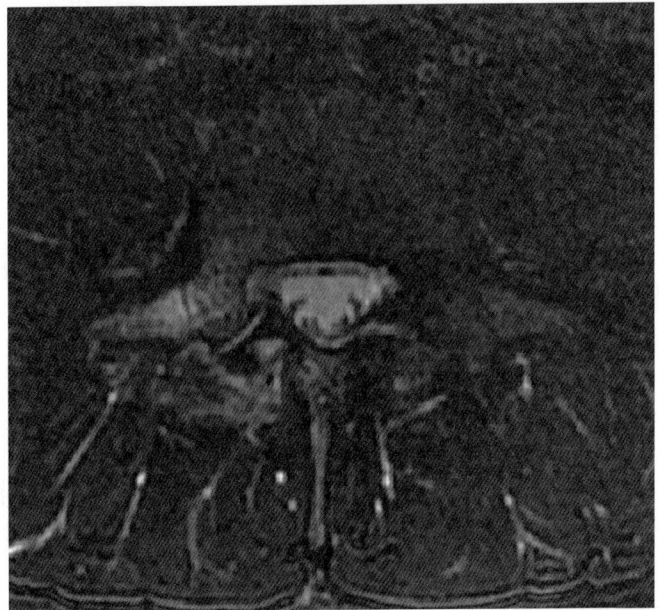

Figure 26 CT scan without contrast. Axial image at L4 shows bilateral pars interarticularis fractures. Right L4 pars fracture appears more chronic in appearance, with sclerotic fracture edges on the lateral aspect. Left L4 pars fracture appears more acute, with more jagged-appearing edges.

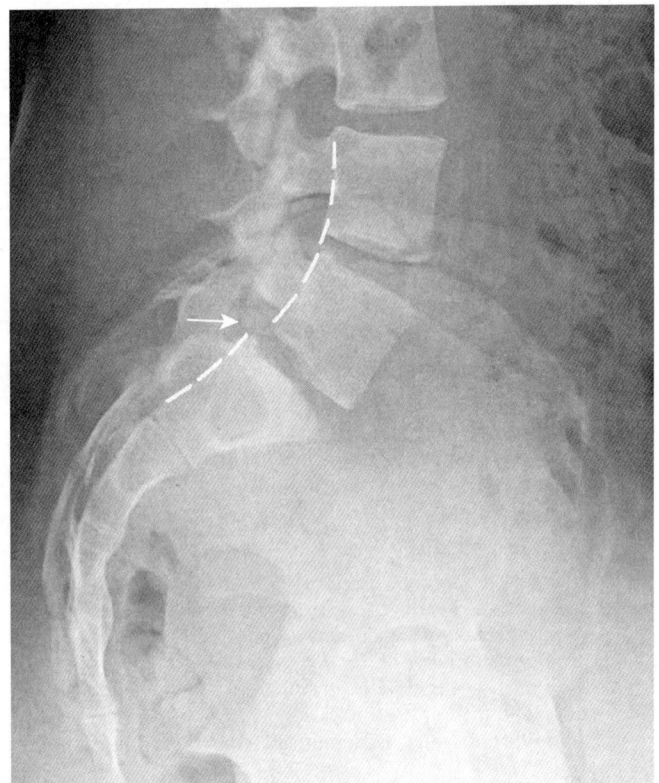

Figure 28 Lateral view x-ray of the lumbar spine, which demonstrates a grade 1 L5 spondylolisthesis.

are reasonable. For acute spondylolysis, the recommended treatment consists of a warm and form-extension-blocking back brace worn all day except for showering and bathing (23–24 hours per day) for the first month of treatment in conjunction with rest from activity. During the second month, use of the brace during the day with rehabilitation is suggested. Rehabilitation consists of core strengthening and lower extremity flexibility. The third month consists of a gradual return to activity, continuing core strengthening and flexibility, and wearing the brace with activity. When treating spondylolysis, a healed pars interarticularis injury is defined as pain-free activity that may include bony union of the pars interarticularis stress fracture or fibrous nonbony union.

Generally, the patient should wear the brace for at least 1 year with activity and sometimes longer depending on the severity of injury. Utilize acetaminophen for pain, avoid NSAIDs, ensure adequate energy availability, maximize calcium and vitamin D intake, and avoid tobacco exposure to facilitate bone healing.

The general goal for spondylolisthesis treatment is to prevent further slippage; treatment is similar to that for spondylolysis. Surgical referral is indicated for grade 2, 3, or 4 spondylolisthesis (Figure 28).

References

Almekinders LC: Anti-inflammatory treatment of muscular injuries in sports, *Sports Med* 15:139–145, 1993.

Bachmann LM, Kolb E, Koller M, et al: Accuracy of Ottawa ankle rules to exclude fractures of the ankle and mid-foot: systematic review, *Br Med J* 326:417–424, 2003.

Beynnon BD, Johnson RJ, Brown L: Knee. In DeLee JC, Drez D, Miller MD, editors: *DeLee & Drez's Orthopaedic Sports Medicine Principles & Practice*, 3rd ed., Philadelphia, 2009, Elsevier, pp 1579–1847.

Gellman H, Caputo RJ, Carter V, et al: Comparison of short and long thumb-spica casts for non-displaced fractures of the carpal scaphoid, *J Bone Joint Surg Am* 71:354–357, 1989.

Haskell A, Mann RA: Foot and ankle. In DeLee JC, Drez D, Miller MD, editors: *DeLee & Drez's Orthopaedic Sports Medicine Principles & Practice*, 3rd ed., Philadelphia, 2009, Elsevier, pp 1865–2205.

Kaeding C, Best TM: Tendinosis: Pathophysiology and nonoperative treatment, *Sports Health* 1:284–292, 2009.

Lappe J, Cullen D, Haynatzki G, et al: Calcium and vitamin D supplementation decreases incidence of stress fractures in female navy recruits, *J Bone Miner Res* 23:741–749, 2008.

Leggit JG, Meko CJ: Acute finger injuries: part I. Tendons and ligaments, *Am Fam Physician* 73:810–816, 2006.

Liem BC, Truswell HJ, Harrast MA: Rehabilitation and return to running after lower limb stress fractures, *Curr Sports Med Rep* 12:200–207, 2013.

Purcell L, Micheli L: Low back pain in young athletes, *Sports Health* 1:212–222, 2009.

Simon AM, Manigrasso MB, O'Connor JP: Cyclo-oxygenase 2 function is essential for bone fracture healing, *J Bone Miner Res* 17:963, 2002.

Tiemstra JD: Update on acute ankle sprains, *Am Fam Physician* 85:1170–1176, 2012.

CONNECTIVE TISSUE DISORDERS

Method of
Molly A. Hinshaw, MD; and Susan Lawrence-Hylland, MD

CURRENT DIAGNOSIS

Lupus Erythematosus
- The erythematous-violaceous and variably pruritic, tender, or scaly eruption is photosensitive.
- Mild to moderate systemic involvement may include arthritis and pleurisy.
- Severe systemic involvement may include nephritis, cerebritis, vasculitis, and severe cytopenias.
- Associated findings include antiphospholipid antibodies associated with thromboembolism or stroke, Raynaud%92 s phenomenon, and sicca symptoms.

Dermatomyositis and Polymyositis
- Photosensitive, violaceous-erythematous, poikilodermatous, and variably scaly patches occur around eyes, on extensor extremities (especially over joints), upper back, scalp, and dystrophic nail folds with prominent telangiectasias.
- Patients may have or develop myositis or pulmonary involvement.
- Age-appropriate cancer screening is required for adults.

Scleroderma
- Patients have firm, variably pruritic, and indurated plaques.
- Localized scleroderma (i.e., morphea or asymmetric sclerotic plaques) may be seen.
- Limited systemic sclerosis is characterized by symmetric sclerosis of distal extremities, and patients may have systemic disease.
- Diffuse systemic sclerosis is characterized by symmetric sclerosis of the trunk and proximal extremities, and patients may have systemic disease.
- Sclerodactyly (i.e., thickening of skin of digits) may occur in patients with systemic sclerosis.
- Pulmonary, cardiac, and gastrointestinal screening should be done for patients with systemic sclerosis.

- Patients with systemic sclerosis should be evaluated and monitored for renal crisis.
- Raynaud%92 s phenomenon may develop in patients with systemic sclerosis.

CURRENT THERAPY

Lupus Erythematosus
- Patients should be counseled on photoprotection measures.
- Localized cutaneous disease is treated with medium- to high-potency topical corticosteroids, and intralesional triamcinolone acetonide 10 mg/mL (Kenalog-10) is added if needed.
- Mild to moderate systemic involvement is treated with low- to medium-potency prednisone 5 to 20 mg/day and with antimalarials.
- Severe disease is treated with prednisone 1 mg/kg/day with a taper based on clinical response. Steroid-sparing agents include azathioprine (Imuran),[1] mycophenolate mofetil (CellCept),[1] methotrexate (Rheumatrex),[1] and cyclophosphamide (Cytoxan).[1]
- Thromboembolism or stroke is treated by anticoagulation with warfarin (Coumadin), aspirin, or heparin.
- Sicca syndrome is treated with frequent water intake, saliva replacement, artificial tears, routine dental care, and pilocarpine (Salagen).

Dermatomyositis and Polymyositis
- Patients should be counseled on photoprotection measures.
- Medium-potency topical corticosteroids and calcineurin inhibitors are used for cutaneous disease.
- Prednisone 1 mg/kg/day is first-line therapy for muscle or pulmonary disease.
- Methotrexate[1] 10 to 25 mg/week is a steroid-sparing agent used for muscle involvement.
- Hydroxychloroquine (Plaquenil)[1] 200 mg/day is used for persistent skin involvement.

Scleroderma
- For localized scleroderma, UVA[1] 20 to 60 J/cm² or psoralen plus UVA (PUVA) is used to resolve established lesions; high-potency corticosteroids and calcipotriene (Dovonex)[1] may help to reduce pruritus and inflammation in new lesions; and systemic prednisone[1] or methotrexate[1] may be used for rapidly progressive new lesions.
- Treatment of systemic sclerosis is primarily aimed at limiting complications.
- Physical therapy is used for contractures.
- Systemic sclerosis is treated with cyclophosphamide (Cytoxan),[1] mycophenolate mofetil (CellCept),[1] methotrexate[1] 10 to 25 mg/week, and photopheresis.
- Renal crisis is treated with captopril (Capoten)[1] 6.25 mg three to six times/day and titrated to effect.
- Raynaud's is treated with warming techniques, calcium channel blockers, antiadrenergic agents, antiplatelet drugs, and topical vasodilators.

[1]Not FDA approved for this indication.

Lupus Erythematosus

Lupus erythematosus is an autoimmune connective tissue disease that may localize to the skin or involve several organ systems. A complete review of systems with evaluation of positive findings is necessary to thoroughly assess patients for signs of systemic lupus as defined by the American Rheumatism Association. Cutaneous lupus erythematosus manifests in chronic, subacute, and acute forms. A punch biopsy from within an erythematous lupus lesion is useful for confirming the diagnosis.

Clinical Features

Discoid lupus and tumid lupus are the two forms of chronic cutaneous lupus erythematosus. Discoid lupus lesions are tender or pruritic, erythematous to violaceous, scaly plaques that typically occur on sun-exposed skin. The lesions resolve with scarring, and when the lesions affect the scalp, they cause scarring alopecia. Tumid lupus manifests as pruritic, erythematous to violaceous, nonscaly plaques that typically preferentially affect the face and trunk.

The lesions of subacute cutaneous lupus erythematosus occur as erythematous to violaceous, scaly macules and as annular or polycyclic patches. These lesions are commonly located on sun-exposed skin and heal without scarring.

Acute cutaneous lupus erythematosus is exemplified by malar erythema (i.e., butterfly rash) and by poikiloderma (i.e., hyperpigmentation, telangiectasias, and epidermal atrophy). It is a manifestation of systemic lupus erythematosus (SLE). Cutaneous lesions may be widespread. In addition to the American Rheumatism Association criteria, patients with SLE may also develop Raynaud's phenomenon, hypercoagulability, and overlap syndromes with Sjögren's disease, dermatomyositis, and other conditions.

Hydrochlorothiazide (HydroDIURIL), terbinafine (Lamisil), minocycline (Minocin), procainamide (Pronestyl), hydralazine (Apresoline), and isoniazid (Nydrazid) are a few of the pharmaceutical agents that cause drug-induced lupus. This disease manifests with synovitis, photosensitivity, and positive serology results, and it may have cutaneous lesions that do not necessarily abate with cessation of the medication.

Management

Prevention

All patients with lupus erythematosus should be counseled on photoprotection, including protecting skin from sunlight and avoiding sun exposure during peak hours (i.e., between 10 AM and 2 PM). Ultraviolet A and B wavelengths may cause lupus to flare. Broad-spectrum sunscreen with an SPF of 30 or higher and that contains titanium, zinc, Mexoryl (L'Oreal), or Helioplex (Neutrogena) should be used whenever patients are outdoors. Photoprotective clothing, available from multiple vendors, is useful for limiting sun exposure.

Patients with lupus are relatively immunosuppressed by their disease. Vaccinations should be kept up to date, although there is a debate about the necessity and safety of vaccination against meningococcal disease (*Neisseria meningitidis*) (Menactra, Menomune), varicella-zoster virus (Zostavax), and *Streptococcus* (Pneumovax).

Treatment of Cutaneous Lupus Erythematosus

Medium-potency topical corticosteroids should be used for lupus localized to the skin, and they are used as adjunct treatment for patients with systemic lupus. Use of triamcinolone 0.1% cream (Flutex) for lesions on the head and neck until symptoms subside or up to 2 weeks continuously is an appropriate starting strength. Ointment-based vehicles are useful for lesions on the trunk and extremities. They are also the vehicles of choice on the scalp of patients of African American descent. Foam or liquid- or lotion-based corticosteroids work well in the scalp of other ethnic groups and can be used on the trunk and extremities. If lesions persist, the corticosteroid can be occluded, or intralesional injections with triamcinolone can be repeated monthly as needed. Intralesional triamcinolone acetonide at concentrations of 5 mg/mL (Kenalog) can be injected into lesions on the face or neck and doses of 10 to 20 mg/mL (Kenalog-10, Kenalog) into lesions on the trunk or extremities. Intralesional corticosteroids may cause mild discomfort, atrophy of the skin or subcutis, or stretch marks. Topical calcineurin inhibitors such as pimecrolimus (Elidel)[1] or tacrolimus (Protopic)[1] may be used for maintenance treatment but are not recommended for new or active lesions because they do not work quickly. Recurrent or refractory cutaneous lesions require systemic treatment.

Treatment of Systemic Lupus Erythematosus

Antimalarials, including hydroxychloroquine (Plaquenil),[1] are disease-modifying agents that limit the progression of lupus. Hydroxychloroquine, chloroquine (Aralen),[1] and quinacrine[2] (at compounding pharmacies) raise the pH of inflammatory cells, inhibiting inflammatory pathways that cause end-organ damage in patients with SLE.

Hydroxychloroquine is typically used first at 200 mg daily for 2 weeks and then increased to 400 mg daily. Patients need laboratory monitoring and a baseline and then yearly eye examination because the medication may be deposited in the retina over time. Hydroxychloroquine exerts its effects within 2 to 3 months of beginning treatment. Its effects are diminished in smokers.

Depending on end-organ involvement in SLE, immunosuppression with systemic corticosteroids such as prednisone at doses of 1 mg/kg/day is appropriate. Steroid-sparing drugs such as methotrexate (Rheumatrex),[1] acitretin (Soriatane),[1] or mycophenolate mofetil (CellCept)[1] are added. After signs of inflammation subside, prednisone is tapered.

Treatment of Musculoskeletal Manifestations

Arthralgia is a common complaint that can usually be managed with acetaminophen or nonsteroidal antiinflammatory drugs (NSAIDs). For true arthritis unresponsive to the previously described measures, hydroxychloroquine[1] 200 mg twice daily can be added. After that, treatments similar to those used for rheumatoid arthritis can be added, although the antitumor necrosis factor agents usually are avoided in lupus. Methotrexate[1] 7.5 to 25 mg PO once weekly may be used along with folic acid[1] 1 mg daily to help limit side effects. Routine toxicity monitoring includes frequent complete blood cell counts and liver tests. Azathioprine (Imuran)[1] 0.5 to 2 mg/kg can be used with frequent monitoring of complete blood cell counts and liver tests. A sample for testing the thiopurine methyltransferase activity level should be drawn before initiating therapy because a genetic deficiency can lead to severe pancytopenia. Leflunomide (Arava)[1] 10 to 20 mg PO once daily can be used with frequent blood cell counts and liver tests. Low-dose glucocorticoids (prednisone 5–10 mg/day) may be used as a bridge to steroid-sparing therapy and to treat intermittent flares.

Treatment of Hematologic Manifestations

Autoimmune cytopenias are common and are often a defining feature of SLE. Lymphopenia (absolute lymphocyte count <1500 cells/microliter) does not require therapy. Hemolytic anemia in SLE is the result of antierythrocyte antibodies that activate complement, and it is treated with prednisone at a dose based on clinical severity. Typically, 1 mg/kg/day, or approximately 60 mg, is used for 4 to 6 weeks, with gradual tapering as long as the response is maintained. For severe hemolytic anemia, pulse methylprednisolone (Solu-Medrol) 1 g IV for 3 consecutive days can be tried, followed by the previously described standard dosing. For patients who do not respond to glucocorticoids or are unable to taper prednisone to low doses, other treatments can be used. They may include azathioprine[1] 1.5 to 2.5 mg/kg/day, mycophenolate mofetil[1] 1000 to 2000 mg/day in divided doses, danazol (Danocrine)[1] 300 to 600 mg/day in divided doses, intravenous immunoglobulin,[1] or rituximab (Rituxan)[1] 375 mg/m² weekly for four doses.

Immune thrombocytopenia results from antiplatelet antibodies that identify platelets for early destruction. Treatment is indicated when patients have signs or symptoms of spontaneous bleeding or when the platelet count drops below 50,000/mL. The initial treatment approach with glucocorticoids is similar to that used for hemolytic anemia. For patients with chronic thrombocytopenia or for those who cannot achieve an acceptable long-term dose of prednisone, steroid-sparing agents, including azathioprine,[1] mycophenolate mofetil,[1] danazol,[1] rituximab,[1] and intravenous

---

[1] Not FDA approved for this indication.

[2] Not available in the United States.

immunoglobulin[1] can be used in doses similar to those used for hemolytic anemia. Dapsone,[1] cyclosporine (Sandimmune, Neoral),[1] and cyclophosphamide (Cytoxan)[1] have also been used.

Thrombotic thrombocytopenia purpura may occur in SLE, and it must be differentiated from immune thrombocytopenia because treatment requires emergent plasmapheresis. Manifestations of thrombotic thrombocytopenia purpura include fever, microangiopathic hemolysis, and central nervous system and renal abnormalities.

Antiphospholipid antibodies include the lupus anticoagulant, anticardiolipin antibodies, and β_2-glycoprotein. They are associated with coagulopathy, thrombocytopenia, late-trimester miscarriage, and heart valve abnormalities. Antiphospholipid antibodies that can be determined with blood testing but are not associated with thromboembolism do not require treatment. Low-dose aspirin[1] may be considered but has not been shown to prevent future thrombosis. Hydroxychloroquine[1] 200 mg twice daily has been shown to reduce the risk. Patients with antiphospholipid antibodies who develop thromboembolism need lifelong treatment with warfarin (Coumadin). A goal international normalized ratio (INR) remains controversial because different studies advocate for high-intensity warfarin (INR >3) or low-intensity therapy (INR >2). For women who have suffered a miscarriage determined to be related to antiphospholipid antibodies, low-dose aspirin and heparin 5000 units SQ twice daily may increase the likelihood of a successful pregnancy.

Treatment of Renal Manifestations

Many patients with SLE have mild to severe renal involvement. Diagnosis by renal biopsy is important to establish the type of kidney involvement. Lupus nephritis is considered one of the more severe manifestations of the disease, and treatment is aimed at preventing renal failure. Treatment should be coordinated with a rheumatologist or nephrologist.

Class I disease requires no specific therapy. The class IIb pattern with more than 1 g of proteinuria can be treated with moderate-dose prednisone (20 mg/day for 6 weeks to 3 months), followed by tapering. Class III and IV patterns of disease have the same prognosis and are treated similarly with high-dose prednisone (1 mg/kg/day) for at least 6 weeks before tapering, based on clinical response, by 10 mg a week to a maintenance of 10 to 15 mg/day. In addition to prednisone, cytotoxic therapy is initiated with cyclophosphamide[1] 0.5 to 1 g/m^2 of body surface area monthly for 6 months and tapered to every 3 months, based on clinical response, for a total of 2 to 3 years. Cyclophosphamide has serious toxicities, including hemorrhagic cystitis, bone marrow suppression, infertility, teratogenicity, and increased risk of malignancy. 2-Mercaptoethane sulfonate sodium (Mesna)[1] can be given with each infusion to minimize bladder toxicity. Class V disease can be treated with prednisone alone, similar to class IIb disease, unless there are coexisting features of class III or IV disease, for which treatments outlined previously should be implemented.

An acceptable alternative to cyclophosphamide for class III and IV disease is mycophenolate mofetil[1] 2 to 3 g/day in divided doses combined with corticosteroids (dosing outlined earlier). This appears to be an effective therapy with fewer side effects than traditional therapy.

Treatment of Nervous System Manifestations

Neuropsychiatric involvement is common in patients with lupus. Symptoms can range from mild to severe and include headache, aseptic meningitis, neuropathy, myelopathy, cognitive dysfunction, seizures, cerebritis, and stroke. A thorough evaluation is necessary to define the cause of nervous system dysfunction and differentiate it from a medication side effect. For seizures, antiepileptic therapy is used, preferably in coordination with a neurologist. Lupus cerebritis and transverse myelitis are two of the more serious manifestations that need to be treated emergently with aggressive immunosuppression in coordination with a rheumatologist or neurologist. Treatment includes high-dose corticosteroids and cyclophosphamide,[1] similar to treatment for lupus nephritis.

Dermatomyositis and Polymyositis
Clinical Features

Dermatomyositis may affect skin and muscle. Cutaneous dermatomyositis manifests with violaceous erythema of characteristic areas, including the periorbital skin (i.e., heliotrope rash), upper back (i.e., shawl sign), dorsal hands (i.e., Gottron's papules), scalp, lateral thighs (i.e., Holster sign), and periungual skin, where dilated capillary loops and erythema are observed. Patients may report muscle weakness. As in lupus, a punch biopsy of an actively inflamed cutaneous lesion shows characteristic features.

Evaluation of patients with cutaneous dermatomyositis is not complete without assessment for systemic involvement. Serum aldolase is the most specific marker for myositis, and it can be used as a measure of response to treatment. Creatinine kinase and alanine aminotransferase levels may be elevated but are not specific indicators. An electromyogram shows dampening of signals, and a muscle biopsy shows a characteristic pattern of myositis. Inflammatory lung disease, diagnosed by the characteristic pattern on chest computed tomography, bronchoalveolar lavage, or biopsy, may be life limiting and therefore should be treated aggressively, similar to lung disease in scleroderma. Adult patients should have age-appropriate cancer screening because dermatomyositis is a paraneoplastic phenomenon in 10% to 50% of patients.

Some patients present with characteristic cutaneous dermatomyositis but no systemic involvement (i.e., dermatomyositis sine myositis). The risk of concurrent or subsequent cancer development is thought to be increased. These patients require monitoring for systemic involvement that may develop over time.

Treatment

Patients with dermatomyositis need photoprotection similar to patients with lupus. Periodic evaluation by clinical examination and review of systems allows for early intervention for developing visceral or muscle involvement.

Cutaneous dermatomyositis is treated the same as lupus (see earlier). Dermatomyositis with systemic involvement is initially treated with immunosuppression using prednisone at doses of 1 mg/kg/day. Steroid-sparing agents are incorporated early in the disease and include antimalarials (methotrexate,[1] azathioprine,[1] and mycophenolate mofetil[1]) at doses that are used in treating lupus.

Scleroderma
Clinical Features

Scleroderma is a sclerosing condition of skin or viscera, or both. The cause is unknown, but transforming growth factor-β plays a role. Type I and III collagens are excessively produced, as are other substances, including glycosaminoglycans, tenascin, and fibronectin.

Cutaneous scleroderma without Raynaud's phenomenon or clinically relevant systemic involvement is also known as *morphea*. Morphea has different distribution patterns, including guttate, linear, segmental, or diffuse distribution, but it is always characterized by indurated plaques that are inflammatory initially, have an advancing inflammatory ("lilac") border as they progress, and then become hyperpigmented. The cutaneous lesions may restrict movement of joints and can cause restricted growth of underlying structures, particularly when they develop in childhood.

Systemic sclerosis may affect the respiratory, renal, cardiovascular, genitourinary, and gastrointestinal systems and vascular structures. Raynaud's phenomenon may be the first presenting symptom of systemic sclerosis, and it can be severe, leading to digital ulcerations and autoamputation. The American College of Rheumatology has defined criteria for the diagnosis.

Tests for antinuclear antibodies are positive in approximately 95% of patients, who typically present with a homogeneous or

---

[1] Not FDA approved for this indication.
[1] Not FDA approved for this indication.

---

[1] Not FDA approved for this indication.

speckled pattern. A nucleolar pattern is more specific for systemic sclerosis. Anticentromere antibodies are present in 60% to 90% of patients with limited disease but are rare in diffuse disease. Topoisomerase I (Scl-70) antibodies are positive in 30% of patients with diffuse disease and are associated with pulmonary fibrosis. Anti-PM-Scl antibodies are present in overlap syndromes and are associated with myositis and renal involvement.

Treatment

Treatment of Limited Scleroderma

For limited scleroderma, treatment with topical medium-potency corticosteroids such as triamcinolone 0.1% ointment (Kenalog) plus calcipotriene (Dovonex)[1] 0.005% cream or intralesional triamcinalone[1] 20 mg/mL may slow progression of active lesions or improve the pruritus and cutaneous stiffness that typify cutaneous scleroderma. For rapidly evolving disease, prednisone[1] 1 mg/kg/day and methotrexate[1] 15 to 20 mg/week may help slow progression of disease. UVA[1] given over 36 treatments at doses of 30 to 60 mJ/cm^2 or PUVA (oral methoxsalen [8-MOP] 10 mg taken 2 hours before treatment with UVA light) can soften the existing plaques of morphea.

Treatment of Systemic Sclerosis: Raynaud's Phenomenon

First-line treatment for Raynaud's phenomenon is preventive, with cold avoidance and the use of warming techniques. If pharmacotherapy is required, extended-release calcium channel blockers such as nifedipine (Procardia XL)[1] starting at 30 mg/day or amlodipine (Norvasc)[1] starting at 5 mg/day may be useful. If this is not helpful, the α-blocker prazosin (Minipress)[1] 1 mg three times daily or the angiotensin receptor blocker losartan (Cozaar)[1] 50 mg daily may be helpful. Antiplatelet therapy with low-dose aspirin[1] (81 mg/day) or dipyridamole (Persantine)[1] 50 to 100 mg three or four times daily may be useful. Topical vasodilators such as nitroglycerin ointment (Nitro-Bid)[1] applied to the base of the affected finger three times daily can be helpful in refractory disease. Digit-threatening ischemia may be treated with an intravenous prostaglandin such as alprostadil (Prostin VR)[1] or iloprost (Ilomedine),[5] which require peripheral or central access. Patients with severe recurrent digital ischemia may ultimately benefit from surgical sympathectomy.

Treatment of Gastrointestinal Manifestations

The most common gastrointestinal manifestation is esophageal reflux caused by esophageal dysmotility. Proton pump inhibitors such as omeprazole (Prilosec)[1] 20 mg twice daily should be used and may prevent the development of esophageal strictures. Prokinetic drugs such as metoclopramide (Reglan)[1] 10 mg four times daily can be helpful. Erythromycin[1] 500 mg three or four times daily can help esophageal and gastric hypomotility. Small bowel hypomotility can lead to bacterial overgrowth, resulting in malabsorption and diarrhea. Rotating antibiotics that include metronidazole (Flagyl),[1] ciprofloxacin (Cipro),[1] and amoxicillin/clavulanate (Augmentin)[1] can be used.

Treatment of Pulmonary Manifestations

Inflammatory lung disease occurs commonly in patients with scleroderma and can be life limiting. Cyclophosphamide[1] at doses of up to 2 mg/kg/day for up to 2 years may slow progression of pulmonary disease. Pulmonary hypertension occurs more commonly in limited systemic sclerosis than in diffuse disease. Symptomatic patients may receive treatment with prostacyclin analogues, which require continuous infusions. The endothelin receptor antagonist bosentan (Tracleer)[1] can be given orally starting at 62.5 mg twice daily. Liver tests should be monitored frequently. At this point, care is typically coordinated with a cardiologist to monitor disease progression and treatment response. Anticoagulation for pulmonary hypertension may improve survival because of the frequent occurrence of pulmonary arterial thrombosis.

---

[1] Not FDA approved for this indication.
[5] Investigational drug in the United States.

Treatment of Renal Manifestations

Angiotensin-converting enzyme (ACE) inhibitors (e.g., captopril [Capoten[1]] beginning at 6.25 mg three to six times daily and titrated for blood pressure control) have dramatically reduced the incidence of renal failure and death due to renal crisis. Avoidance of prednisone at doses greater than 15 mg/day is also important in reducing the risk of renal crisis.

---

[1] Not FDA approved for this indication.

References

Atzeni F, Bendtzen K, Bobbio-Pallavicini F, et al: Infections and treatment of patients with rheumatic diseases, *Clin Exp Rheumatol* 26(Suppl. 48):S67–73, 2008.

Dziadzio M, Denton CP, Smith R: Losartan therapy for Raynaud's phenomenon and scleroderma, *Arthritis Rheum* 42(12):2646–2655, 1999.

Ginzler EM, Dooley MA, Aranow C, et al: Mycophenolate mofetil or intravenous cyclophosphamide for lupus nephritis, *N Engl J Med* 353(21):2219–2228, 2005.

Iorizzo LJ, Jorizzo JL: The treatment and prognosis of dermatomyositis: An updated review, *J Am Acad Dermatol* 59:99–112, 2008.

Matucci-Cerinic M, Steen VD, Furst DE, et al: Clinical trials in systemic sclerosis: Lessons learned and outcomes, *Arthritis Res Ther* 9(Suppl. 2):S7, 2007.

Nihtyanova SI, Denton CP: Current approaches to the management of early active diffuse scleroderma skin disease, *Rheum Dis Clin North Am* 34:161–179, 2008.

Pisoni CN, Sanchez FJ, Karim Y, et al: Mycophenolate mofetil in systemic lupus erythematosus: Efficacy and tolerability in 86 patients, *J Rheumatol* 32:1047–1052, 2005.

Steen VD: The many faces of scleroderma, *Rheum Dis Clin North Am* 34:1–15, 2008.

Subcommittee for Scleroderma Criteria of the American Rheumatism Association Diagnostic and Therapeutic Criteria Committee: Preliminary criteria for the classification of systemic sclerosis (scleroderma), *Arthritis Rheum* 23:581–590, 1980.

Tan EM, Cohen AS, Fries JF, et al: The 1982 revised criteria for the classification of lupus erythematosus, *Arthritis Rheum* 25:1271–1272, 1982.

Wallace DD: *Lupus Erythematosus*, ed 7, Philadelphia, 2006, Lippincott Williams & Wilkins2006.

FIBROMYALGIA

Method of
Lora Black, PhD; Timothy Sowder, MD; and Andrea L. Chadwick, MD, MSc

CURRENT DIAGNOSIS

- Fibromyalgia (FM) is a common condition, seen in 2% to 8% of the population, depending on the diagnostic criteria used.
- Hallmark symptoms of FM typically include widespread body pain, cognitive difficulties ("fibro fog"), poor sleep, and fatigue. Other associated symptoms may also include headaches, abdominal or pelvic pain, and symptoms of depression or anxiety.
- FM may occur independently of any other medical conditions but is also known to associate with other painful conditions such as osteoarthritis and autoimmune disorders such as lupus and rheumatoid arthritis.
- No blood tests or imaging modalities are useful for diagnosing FM; however, tender point examination and questionnaires are available for aiding in diagnosis.

CURRENT THERAPY

- Treatment should be multidisciplinary and focus on symptom management, lifestyle modifications, and psychological interventions.
- A variety of on-label and off-label medications are available to mechanistically address the altered pain processing underlying FM.

- Physical therapy, exercise, and psychological treatments such as cognitive-behavioral therapy are of the utmost importance in adequate management of FM symptoms.
- Seeing patients frequently to monitor medications, address side effects, and provide motivational interviewing and care is important to providing optimal patient pain relief and minimizing poor outcomes.

Epidemiology

The global prevalence of fibromyalgia (FM) has been estimated to be 2.7% (4.2% female, 1.4% male), but studies have produced varying results. Historically, studies have been conducted using the 1990 American College of Rheumatology (ACR) diagnostic criteria, which required pain to be present on palpation of at least 11/18 tender points to confirm a diagnosis of FM. Using these criteria, prevalence estimates range from 0.4% to 8.8% with 2.0% in the United States (3.4% of females and 0.5% of males, ratio ~7:1). The problems with these criteria include difficulty reproducing tender points, significantly higher rates in women (possibly because of the increased number of tender points in women or a higher pressure pain threshold in males), and a strong correlation with various measures of distress and negative affect. In 2010 the ACR released updated criteria that do not require a tender point assessment. These new criteria have yielded prevalence estimates of 7.7% in women and 4.9% in men for a ratio of 1.6:1, which is similar to that seen in other chronic pain conditions. The prevalence is similar in different countries, cultures, and ethnic groups; there is no evidence that FM has a higher prevalence in industrialized countries and cultures. There are also concerns about underdiagnosis of FM with only 12% to 28% of subjects identified during population-based surveys as fulfilling the ACR 1990 criteria having ever been diagnosed with FM.

Risk Factors

There are both genetic and environmental risk factors associated with the development of FM. FM has been thought to affect mostly women with initial studies predicting that women were up to seven times more likely to develop FM. More recent studies using updated criteria have found less of a discrepancy but still indicate an increased risk with women being 1.5 to 2 times more likely to be affected than men. FM can affect people of all ages, including children. Many patients are diagnosed when they are young or middle aged, but studies show that prevalence rises with age, peaking in people greater than 60 years old. It is postulated that perhaps widespread chronic pain in older patients is more likely to be attributed to osteoarthritis or other degenerative conditions instead of FM; however, the two conditions are known to coexist. Patients diagnosed with certain conditions like rheumatoid arthritis and lupus have been noted to be more likely to develop FM than others. Obesity, poor sleep, low physical activity levels, and decreased job or life satisfaction are potentially modifiable risk factors. There are many other conditions associated with FM, though the degree of contribution to actual disease development has yet to be determined. Individuals with FM are more likely have psychiatric disorders, including depression, anxiety, obsessive-compulsive disorder, and posttraumatic stress disorder. A history of childhood, adolescent, or adulthood abuse or traumatic events have also been linked with the development of FM and other centralized pain syndromes. Maladaptive cognitive features are poor prognostic factors for FM and can include catastrophizing and fear-avoidance of movement and activity. Lower education and other indicators of lower social status have been thought to place patients at an increased risk for FM, though other studies did not find a significant difference in developed and wealthy areas versus rural and poor areas.

Pathophysiology

FM can be thought of as a centralized pain state, where "centralized" refers to amplification of pain emanating from the central nervous system. Evidence suggests that dysfunction in central nervous system pain processing mechanisms underlie this condition and include central amplification of pain and nonpainful stimuli (including auditory, visual, and olfactory). Typical manifestations of central amplification include allodynia (pain resulting from a nonnoxious stimulus) and hyperalgesia (increased sensitivity to a painful stimulus), and temporal summation (progressive increase in the pain response to repetitive painful stimulus). This term "centralized pain" does not exclude that an individual's peripheral nervous system and its nociceptive input may be contributing to the patient's overall pain symptoms, but rather that they feel greater levels of pain than would be normally expected based on the degree of peripheral nociceptive input. However, it must be noted that many patients with FM do not have any identifiable structural or functional abnormalities in the periphery that would explain their widespread pain and associated symptoms. The concept of central amplification helps describe the heterogenous clinical features of FM as many of the same neurotransmitters that control sensory sensitivity and pain also control mood, memory, fatigue, and sleep. A variety of quantitative research methods have been employed to establish that central amplification is involved in the pathophysiology of FM, including quantitative sensory testing and functional, chemical, and structural brain neuroimaging. Functional magnetic resonance imaging has corroborated that nonnoxious stimuli such as mild pressure activates brain regions involved in pain processing compared with healthy controls. It has also been found that endogenous pain inhibitory pathways do not effectively operate in patients with FM. This defective inhibition is postulated to exist because of the altered homeostasis of inhibitory and excitatory neurotransmitters.

Clinical Manifestations

The patient with FM can experience a wide variety of symptoms, including pain, fatigue, sleep disturbance, cognitive dysfunction, and mood alterations. These patients typically present with chronic widespread pain for at least 3 months that is not fully explained by injury or inflammation. This pain is typically identified as being "all over," but drawings by patients show various localized areas of pain, which may migrate in intensity from time to time. Somatic pain is typically the dominant feature; however, visceral pain (including abdominal and pelvic pain) and headaches are also commonly seen. Most frequently, the affected areas include the shoulders, arms, lower back, buttocks, and thighs. Widespread pain in the joints is also common. The patients most generally experience pain that is throbbing, achy, and tender. This pain is often accompanied by generalized hypersensitivity, allodynia, and hyperalgesia, which is indicative of the underlying central amplification. Other symptoms can include numbness, tingling, burning, cramps, and sensitivity to light and sound. Exacerbating factors for these patients' pain include emotional distress, weather changes, sleeping problems, and strenuous activity. A total of 70% to 90% of patients with FM sleep fewer hours, have more frequent waking, and report nonrestorative sleep. They also suffer from significant fatigue, weakness, and stiffness that are worse in the morning and improve as the day progresses. A total of 76% of patients report mental confusion, forgetfulness, and concentration difficulties. This cognitive dysfunction is frequently described as being more bothersome than their widespread pain. These symptoms are so pervasive and disruptive that they are commonly referred to as "fibro fog." In addition, there is an affective component to the cognitive dysfunction that is usually described by patients as feeling fatigued and exhausted all the time, irrespective of how much sleep they get. Depression, anxiety, and posttraumatic stress disorder are comorbidities with high prevalence in this patient population, and their various symptoms can also be present in the patient with FM.

Diagnosis

FM is a condition with distinctive clinical characteristics that allow for it to be diagnosed in the primary care setting. Although many practitioners may have concern that the diagnosis of FM is controversial or that it may label patients in a negative manner, studies suggest that the opposite is true. Establishing the diagnosis of FM can actually provide substantial validity and relief for patients for their previously unexplained symptoms. Prompt diagnosis is a vital component of effective FM management and is linked with patients having greater satisfaction in health, which in turn leads to decreased healthcare use and its associated costs.

In the clinical setting, FM should be considered as a diagnosis in any patient presenting with chronic widespread or multifocal pain. It is commonly comorbid in patients with other chronic pain syndromes, those with thyroid dysfunction, and patients with rheumatic diseases. There exists other co-occurring pain syndromes that have been linked to the same pathophysiology as FM that may also spark a clinicians' suspicion for FM such as irritable bowel syndrome, interstitial cystitis, migraine headache, temporomandibular disorder, and chronic pelvic or genitourinary pain (e.g., interstitial cystitis, vulvodynia). It is very important to note that FM should *not* be considered a diagnosis of exclusion.

A thorough history including asking about pain during childhood and adolescence, other comorbid pain symptoms, a history of childhood or adulthood abuse, or other traumatic events will help elucidate whether FM should be considered in the differential diagnosis. An excellent physical exam including musculoskeletal, neurologic, assessment of tenderness or significant pain to palpation, and allodynia should always be performed. Laboratory tests are not necessary or useful to establish the diagnosis of FM, besides possibly helping sort through the differential diagnoses. Basic laboratory evaluation may include vitamin D levels, thyroid panels, erythrocyte sedimentation rate, C-reactive protein, and blood count or blood chemistries to guide an assessment of potentially treatable causes of diffuse musculoskeletal pain. Detailed serologic studies are not necessary unless the patient has other signs and symptoms of other potential comorbid diseases. No imaging studies are specific in diagnosing FM, and one must be careful in performing radiographs or other imaging studies, as these can have findings that are associated with the degenerative aging process but may not be the actual cause of the patient's ongoing pain symptoms.

The 1990 ACR tender point exam has been historically used to "diagnose" FM; however, it was originally developed to be used for research and was never intended to be used in clinical practice. Revised versions of diagnostic criteria were published in 2010 and again in 2016. These revised criteria do not require a tender point exam to elucidate a diagnosis and may be ascertained with a self-report questionnaire (Table 1). These criteria rapidly assess widespread pain symptoms and associated symptoms of poor sleep, cognitive difficulties, fatigue, and mood problems. Once diagnosed, treatment for FM can be initiated immediately, even if further tests or referrals to specialists are pending.

Differential Diagnosis

Although the diagnosis of FM can be difficult and time-consuming, providing the patient with an answer to their issues can decrease healthcare costs by decreasing biological testing and imaging, decreasing the number of visits, and decreasing the number and dosage of drugs prescribed. With such a wide variety of possible symptomatic expressions of FM, it is important to address the differential diagnoses in a systematic way. Arthralgias are commonly seen in osteoarthritis and spondyloarthritis but are also seen in rheumatic diseases like rheumatoid arthritis, Sjögren syndrome, systemic lupus erythematous, and polymyalgia rheumatica. Inflammatory, metabolic, and drug-induced myopathies and myalgias should also be ruled out. Myofascial pain syndrome, tendonitis, and bursitis are common pathologies that cause pain in localized areas. Neurologic disorders such as multiple sclerosis and myasthenia gravis should be considered in addition to radiculopathies and both peripheral and compressive neuropathies that could complicate the picture. Viral infections and Lyme disease should be considered as potential infectious causes. Endocrinopathies like hypothyroidism, Cushing syndrome, and hyperparathyroidism can cause weakness, but are unlikely to cause the

| TABLE 1 | American College of Rheumatology 2016 Revised Fibromyalgia Criteria |

A patient satisfies the modified 2016 fibromyalgia criteria if the following three conditions are met:
- Widespread pain index (WPI) ≥7 and symptom severity scale (SSS) score ≥5 *or* WPI of 4–6 and SSS score ≥9.
- Generalized pain, defined as pain in at least four of five regions, must be present. Jaw, chest, and abdominal pain are not included in generalized pain definition.
- Symptoms have been generally present for at least 3 months.

Ascertainment

WPI

Note the number of areas in which the patient has had pain over the last week. In how many areas has the patient had pain? Score will be between 0 and 19.
Left upper region (Region 1)
  Jaw, left
  Shoulder girdle, left
  Upper arm, left
  Lower arm, left
Right upper region (Region 2)
  Jaw, right
  Shoulder girdle, right
  Upper arm, right
  Lower arm, right
Left lower region (Region 3)
  Hip (buttock, trochanter), left
  Upper leg, left
  Lower leg, left
Right lower region (Region 4)
  Hip (buttock, trochanter), right
  Upper leg, right
  Lower leg, right
Axial region (Region 5)
  Neck
  Upper back
  Lower back
  Chest
  Abdomen

SSS Score

Fatigue
Waking unrefreshed
Cognitive symptoms
For the each of the three symptoms above, indicate the level of severity over the past week using the following scale:
  0 = No problem
  1 = Slight or mild problems, generally mild or intermittent
  2 = Moderate, considerable problems, often present and/or at a moderate level
  3 = Severe: pervasive, continuous, life-disturbing problems
The SSS score is the sum of the severity scores of the three symptoms (fatigue, waking unrefreshed, and cognitive symptoms) (0–9) plus the sum (0–3) of the number of the following symptoms the patient has been bothered by that occurred during the previous 6 months:
(1) Headaches (0–1)
(2) Pain or cramps in lower abdomen (0–1)
(3) Depression (0–1)
The final symptom severity score is between 0 and 12.

The fibromyalgia severity (FS) scale is the sum of the WPI and SSS.

A diagnosis of fibromyalgia is valid irrespective of other diagnoses and does not exclude the presence of other clinically important illnesses.

significant widespread pain seen in FM. There are other disorders that frequently overlap or co-occur with FM that should be optimally treated in conjunction. These include depression, anxiety, obsessive-compulsive disorder, posttraumatic stress disorder, tension headaches, migraines, temporomandibular disorder, chronic fatigue syndrome, irritable bowel syndrome, interstitial cystitis (painful bladder syndrome), chronic prostatitis, and vulvodynia. It is important for any clinician to distinguish that the patient's symptoms are not explained by another pathology or systemic disorder because treatment of these entities can vary greatly. However, the 2016 Revised Fibromyalgia Criteria does not exclude the diagnosis of FM if other conditions are present. Each of these problems should be considered as variables and optimally treated when attempting to diagnose this complex syndrome.

Treatment

FM is best approached by using an integrated, multidisciplinary approach where pharmacologic and nonpharmacologic treatments are provided in parallel. Engaging and motivating the patient toward their treatment goals as an active participant in their care is vital for success. As stated before, FM can be diagnosed and treated in the primary care setting. Referral to specialists should only be necessary when pain is refractory to therapy (e.g., comprehensive pain management clinic), those in whom the diagnosis is uncertain (e.g., to a rheumatologist or neurologist depending on symptoms), or those with significant comorbid mood or psychiatric disturbances. Forming treatment teams can be very useful and should include clinicians with expertise in exercise/physical activity (e.g., physical therapists), patient education, and pain psychology.

Most comprehensive guidelines on treatment of FM generally recommend that all patients should receive education on their condition, the importance of being an active participant in their care, and setting reasonable and attainable goals and expectations for treatment. Patients need to be informed that instead of searching for treatments to cure the condition, management of the condition should focus on pain reduction (not complete pain relief), increased physical functioning, and improved quality of life. This management should rely heavily on stress reduction, exercise and physical activity, adequate sleep, and improving function through cognitive restructuring (e.g., reducing catastrophizing, increasing self-efficacy). Pharmacologic treatments can be effective in alleviating some of the symptoms of FM, but rarely will patients achieve significant improvements without embracing these essential self-management strategies.

In the United States, there are three drugs currently approved by the U.S. Food and Drug Association (FDA) for the treatment of FM: (1) pregabalin (Lyrica), (2) milnacipran (Savella), and (3) duloxetine (Cymbalta). These drugs mechanistically treat FM through either increasing the activity of inhibitory neurotransmitters (milnacipran and duloxetine) or to decrease the activity of excitatory neurotransmitters (pregabalin). Table 2 highlights the FDA-approved medications in the pharmacologic treatment of FM. Careful initiation and titration are recommended to improve patient compliance and response, given the incidence of side effects or drug-drug interactions. There are a variety of commonly used drugs other than those listed previously, although none of them has FDA approval for the FM indication. These other medications have been shown in a variety of research studies to provide pain and symptom relief in FM and include gabapentin (Neurontin), tricyclic antidepressants (e.g., nortriptyline [Pamelor], amitriptyline [Elavil]), cyclobenzaprine (Flexeril), and venlafaxine (Effexor). Basic analgesics such as acetaminophen and nonsteroidal antiinflammatory drugs have little evidence supporting effectiveness for FM. Therapies such as low-dose naltrexone have been shown to be effective for improving pain symptoms in FM; however, this compound is not commercially available and must be compounded. The literature has reported that low doses from 0.5 to 9 mg daily of naltrexone can be used for FM, with randomized-controlled trials using doses of 4.5 mg daily. There exists no evidence that mu-opioid agonists are helpful in the long-term treatment of FM and ultimately increase central amplification over time, thereby increasing the potential for worsening pain and functioning whilst placing the patient at risk for dependence and addiction. Clinicians and patients should recognize that in many cases, treatment with pharmacologic agents may be ineffective. The choice of drug should always be discussed with the patient and should focus on targeting the most bothersome symptoms. Oftentimes multiple types of drugs/drug combinations are needed. If a drug is trialed and does not lead to clinically meaningful relief after 4 weeks at the full recommended dose, it should be tapered or stopped, and an alternative drug trialed.

Nonpharmacologic treatment for FM consists of educational and psychological interventions, in addition to physical modalities and should be an integral part of a comprehensive FM treatment plan. Education should be a foundational intervention applied immediately with diagnosis or early in the patient's treatment plan and should consist of information on the underlying pain mechanisms causing clinical pain and associated symptoms

| TABLE 2 | Comparison of FDA-Approved Pharmacologic Therapies for Fibromyalgia |

DRUG	DATE OF FDA APPROVAL	MECHANISM OF ACTION	AVAILABLE STRENGTHS	DOSING	COMMON SIDE EFFECTS
Duloxetine (Cymbalta)	June 16, 2008	Serotonin norepinephrine reuptake inhibition	20 mg; 30 mg; 60 mg	• 60 mg/day recommended total dose (doses >60 mg rarely helpful for pain) • Start 30 mg/day for 1 week or longer and then may increase to 60 mg/day	Dry mouth, somnolence, nausea, constipation, decreased appetite, hyperhidrosis
Milnacipran (Savella)	January 14, 2009	Serotonin norepinephrine reuptake inhibition	12.5 mg; 25 mg; 50 mg; 100 mg; convenience starter pack	• Convenience starter pack dosing: Start 12.5 mg daily × 1 day, then 12.5 mg bid × 2 days, then 25 mg bid × 4 days, then 50 mg bid • Max dose 100 mg bid (200 mg/day)	Nausea, constipation, hot flush, hyperhidrosis, vomiting, palpitations, increased heart rate, dry mouth, hypertension
Pregabalin (Lyrica)	June 21, 2007	Nonselective alpha-2-delta calcium channel blocker	25 mg; 50 mg; 75 mg; 100 mg; 150 mg; 200 mg; 225 mg; 300 mg	• Start at 75 mg bid (can start much lower in sensitive or older patient population) • May increase to 150 mg bid within 1 week • Max dose 225 mg bid (450 mg/day)	Dizziness, somnolence, dry mouth, peripheral edema, blurred vision, weight gain, abnormal thinking/cognitive difficulties

bid, Two times per day.

(e.g., central nervous system pain and sensory amplification) and information on the nature of the condition (e.g., nonprogressive, chronic, and lifelong with episodic flares, risk of other comorbid conditions). This will provide a strong foundation to then add psychological therapies, which are typically behavioral based and focused on acceptance theories.

Psychological treatments for managing chronic pain have been recognized as an important component of comprehensive care for fibromyalgia. A main tenet of these treatments is the focus on the biopsychosocial model, which emphasizes the connections between biological, psychological, and social factors in the experience of chronic pain. Although some patients with FM may benefit from addressing comorbid psychiatric conditions (e.g., anxiety, depression), there is evidence for the effectiveness of pain-focused psychological treatments, such as self-regulatory techniques, cognitive-behavioral therapy (CBT), and acceptance and mindfulness-based therapy, on pain-specific outcomes.

Two main types of psychological interventions are commonly used in FM: CBT and acceptance and commitment therapy (ACT). Cognitive-behavioral therapy for chronic pain (CBT-CP) aims to educate patients about the associations between psychological factors and the experience of pain, with a focus on the bidirectional relationships between thoughts, feelings, behaviors, and physical sensations. CBT-CP teaches a variety of pain-coping skills to increase patient's sense of control and autonomy. Cognitive strategies, such as cognitive restructuring, can be used to identify maladaptive thought patterns, reframe them, and increase the likelihood of using self-management skills. CBT-CP also emphasizes behavior-focused coping skills, such as activity pacing and sleep hygiene, to help patients implement behavior changes that are more effective for the self-management of fibromyalgia. CBT-CP has a strong evidence base and is considered the gold standard psychological treatment for many chronic pain conditions, including fibromyalgia. Numerous reviews and meta-analyses have shown CBT-CP to improve disability ratings, catastrophizing, pain ratings, and mood compared with treatment as usual.

ACT differs from CBT in its emphasis of context over content. Rather than challenging pain-related thoughts, as in CBT-CP, ACT-CP encourages patients to exercise psychological flexibility to accept their pain, pain-related thoughts, and physical limitations while still pursuing values-based actions. Similarly, ACT-CP can target the emotions that result from unhelpful thoughts rather than exclusively focusing on the thoughts themselves. Noticing the present moment is another critical component to ACT-CP and can be specifically used in FM to change the way in which they associate with the pain (e.g., describing aspects of the pain rather than judging it as bad or how it will negatively impact their life). Research has shown that ACT-CP is effective in the treatment of chronic pain conditions. A 2016 meta-analysis showed positive effects for anxiety, depression, functioning, pain intensity, and quality of life for these therapies compared with treatment as usual.

Self-regulatory techniques teach patients to monitor both physical and psychological cues and use specific skills to help regulate these cues as needed. Deep breathing, visual imagery, progressive muscle relaxation, mindfulness meditation, and biofeedback are skills often taught as part of relaxation/self-regulation training for management of fibromyalgia. Deep breathing, with an emphasis on diaphragmatic breathing, has been shown to improve pain thresholds and increase function among FM patients. Guided visual imagery is another relaxation technique that guides patients through visual images and cues in an effort to increase feelings of relaxation and can be helpful for self-management of pain. Progressive muscle relaxation comprises systematically tensing and relaxing muscle groups in an effort to decrease overall muscle tension that may contribute to pain levels. Mindfulness is based on Eastern meditation practices and emphasizes focusing on the present moment with acceptance, openness, and curiosity. Biofeedback is based on the learning principle that immediate feedback enhances learning and aims to extend voluntary control to pathophysiologic functioning. During biofeedback, specialized equipment is used to monitor physiologic functioning associated with stress (e.g., skin temperature, muscle tension, heart rate) and is brought to the attention of the patient in an effort to cue the use of self-regulation skills. Although self-regulation techniques have shown some utility as standalone treatments for chronic pain conditions, they appear to be most efficacious when used as part of other psychological or multidisciplinary treatments for fibromyalgia.

Physical activity, including active and passive modalities, is perhaps the most important nonpharmacologic treatment for FM. Physical therapy, including warm-water aquatherapy, can be used initially to help patients improve their conditioning and obtain education on how to incorporate movement and activity into their daily lives. Among different exercise interventions, aerobic exercise has been shown to be the most beneficial. Patients should start with low-to-moderate intensity activities (e.g., walking, stationary cycling, or swimming). Over time, patients can increase their intensity and duration over time to a goal of at least 20 min/day at least two to three times weekly. It is important to counsel patients on pacing themselves and that initially they may have more soreness or pain as they gradually build their physical conditioning and strength. Continuation of the exercise regimen is of paramount value as ongoing exercise has been associated with maintenance of improvements in FM. Passive forms of physical activity such as balneotherapy (heated spa treatments), manipulation, massage, transcutaneous electrical stimulation, and ultrasound have only weak evidence to support their use. Complementary and alternative medicine options that may be considered include acupuncture, yoga, tai chi, and qi gong meditation, but there are few high-quality evidence studies to support their use as first-line therapy.

Monitoring

No laboratory or imaging monitoring is required in the treatment of FM. Regular/frequent outpatient engagement with patients is recommended—to discuss the comprehensive care plan and focus on patient goals for treatment, as increased outpatient engagement has been shown to reduce morbidity and mortality (including risk of suicide) in patients with FM.

References

Arnold LM, Gebke KB, Choi EHS: Fibromyalgia: management strategies for primary care providers, *Int J Clin Pract* 70(2):99–112, 2016.

Bernardy K, Fuber N, Kollner V, Hauser W: Efficacy of cognitive-behavioral therapies in fibromyalgia syndrome - a systematic review and metaanalysis of randomized controlled trials, *J Rheumatol* 37(10):1991–2005, 2010.

Borchers AT, Gershwin ME: Fibromyalgia: a critical and comprehensive review, *Clinic Rev Allerg Immunol* 49:100–151, 2015.

Clauw DJ: Fibromyalgia: a clinical review, *JAMA* 311(15):1547–1555, 2014.

Glombiewski JA, Sawyer AT, Gutermann J, Koenig K, Rief W, Hofmann SG: Psychological treatments for fibromyalgia: a meta-analysis, *Pain* 151(2):280–295, 2010.

Hassett AL, Gevirtz RN: Nonpharmacologic treatment for fibromyalgia: patient education, cognitive-behavioral therapy, relaxation techniques, and complementary and alternative medicine, *Rheum Dis Clin North Am* 35(2):393–407, 2009.

Lami MJ, Martinez MP, Sanchez AI: Systematic review of psychological treatment in fibromyalgia, *Curr Pain Headache Rep* 17(7):345, 2013.

McCracken LM, Vowles KE: Acceptance and commitment therapy and mindfulness for chronic pain: model, process, and progress, *Am Psychol* 69(2):178–187, 2014.

Perrot S: Fibromyalgia: a misconnection in a multi-connected world?, *Eur J Pain*, 2019.https://doi.org/10.1002/ejp.1367. Available at: [Epub ahead of print].

Rahman A, Underwood M, Carnes D: Fibromyalgia. *BMJ* 348:g1224, 2014.

Rupp A, Young E, Chadwick AL: Low dose naltrexone's utility for non-cancer centralized pain conditions - a scoping review, *Pain Medicine* 24(11):1270–1281, 2023 Nov 2.

Talotta R, Bazzichi L, Di Franco M, et al: One year in review 2017: fibromyalgia, *Clin Exp Rheumatol* 35(Suppl. 105):S6–S12, 2017.

Thieme K, Mathys M, Turk DC: Evidenced-Based guidelines on the treatment of fibromyalgia patients: are they consistent and if not, why not? have effective psychological treatments been overlooked? *J Pain* 18(7):747–756, 2017.

Veehof MM, Trompetter HR, Bohlmeijer ET, Schreurs KM: Acceptance- and mindfulness-based interventions for the treatment of chronic pain: a meta-analytic review, *Cogn Behav Ther* 45(1):5–31, 2016.

Wolfe F, Clauw DJ, Fitzcharles M, et al: 2016 Revisions to the 2010/2011 fibromyalgia diagnostic criteria, *Semin Arthritis Rheum* 46(3):319–329, 2016.

JUVENILE IDIOPATHIC ARTHRITIS

Method of
Ashley Cooper, MD; and Michael J. Holland, MD

CURRENT DIAGNOSIS

- Juvenile idiopathic arthritis (JIA) is a clinical diagnosis. JIA is diagnosed when objective signs of arthritis persist in a child, with onset under 16 years of age, for at least 6 weeks in the absence of another identifiable cause.
- Children who present with musculoskeletal pain without accompanying objective signs of joint inflammation (swelling or painful, limited range of motion) are unlikely to have arthritis. In many children with JIA, swelling and joint limitation are more prominent than pain.
- Laboratory testing has limited value in diagnosing JIA. In some cases, no laboratory tests are needed to make the diagnosis. When clinically indicated, laboratory tests are used to exclude other causes of arthritis such as infection (including Lyme disease in endemic areas), malignancy, or underlying systemic autoimmune disease.
- The antinuclear antibody (ANA), rheumatoid factor (RF), and anti–cyclic citrullinated peptide (anti-CCP) have prognostic but *not* diagnostic value in JIA. These tests should not be drawn to evaluate musculoskeletal pain in children in the absence of objective signs of arthritis.

CURRENT THERAPY

- Medical therapy is individualized for each child based on severity and number of affected joints and comorbidities. The goal of treatment is to completely control joint inflammation to minimize symptoms and prevent damage.
- Many rheumatologists use a step-up treatment approach, titrating medication until inactive disease is achieved. In children with severe arthritis, early combination therapy is sometimes used. With appropriate use of currently available medications, most children with JIA can achieve clinically inactive disease.
- Current treatment options include scheduled nonsteroidal antiinflammatory drugs (NSAIDs), intraarticular corticosteroid injections, disease-modifying antirheumatic drugs (DMARDs, most commonly methotrexate), and biologic response modifiers (e.g., antitumor necrosis factor alpha, antiinterleukin-1, or antiinterleukin-6 therapy).
- With the currently available medications, most children with JIA do not require systemic corticosteroids. Steroids should *not* be prescribed to a child presenting with joint pain or swelling of unclear etiology.
- Optimal timing and approach to medication discontinuation in patients who have achieved inactive disease are unclear. Relapse rates are high after medication discontinuation in most JIA subtypes.
- A partnership between the child's rheumatologist and primary care provider is key to safe use of immune-modulating medications. Optimal management includes the following:
  - Medication toxicity monitoring with periodic laboratory studies
  - Prompt evaluation of infectious symptoms in immunosuppressed patients
  - Administration of age-appropriate vaccines (with avoidance of live virus vaccines in patients on immunosuppression)
  - Counseling of adolescents to avoid alcohol while on methotrexate and pregnancy while on teratogenic medications

- Children with JIA should remain physically active and be allowed to continue participating in sports and leisure activities as tolerated. Physical and/or occupational therapy is indicated for patients with limited mobility, deconditioning, or compromised activities of daily living.
- Regular screening for uveitis is an essential part of JIA management to allow prompt treatment of this sight-threatening complication.

Juvenile idiopathic arthritis (JIA) is an umbrella term that encom-passes multiple forms of chronic, immune-mediated arthritis that begin in childhood. The classification system currently used for JIA was established in 1995 by the International League of Associations for Rheumatology (ILAR). By replacing the term *juvenile rheumatoid arthritis* with *juvenile idiopathic arthritis* and defining additional subtypes, the ILAR criteria better reflect the clinical heterogeneity among children with arthritis. Absence of the term *rheumatoid* from the current nomenclature appropriately highlights that most cases of juvenile arthritis are not simply early-onset rheumatoid arthritis (RA), as only 5% of all children with JIA have rheumatoid factor (RF)-positive polyarticular disease.

The subtypes of JIA are summarized in Table 1 and include oligoarticular, polyarticular (RF negative and RF positive), enthesitis-related (a childhood-onset spondyloarthropathy closely related to ankylosing spondylitis), psoriatic, and systemic arthritis.

Although each of these conditions has a distinct phenotype, the presence of chronic inflammatory arthritis (and synovitis in particular) is the unifying feature and sine qua non of JIA. A careful history and physical exam are the most important tools in diagnosis. A complete exam of all joints should be performed in children with possible JIA as the pattern of affected joints impacts disease classification. Additional affected joints are often identified on exam that have not been apparent to patients and parents. Common pitfalls in diagnosis of arthritis in children include the following:

- *Diagnosing JIA in the absence of objective clinical signs of arthritis (joint inflammation).* Most children who present to the primary care office with joint pain (even chronic pain) do not have JIA. Isolated pain in the absence of objective findings of arthritis such as swelling predicts against JIA or other chronic rheumatic disease.
- *Attempting to rule in JIA with laboratory studies.* ANA tests can be positive in up to 30% of healthy children, and positive RF may also be seen in viral infection, bacterial infection, or malignant conditions. Due to the high frequency of positive results in children without rheumatic disease, these tests should not be drawn to evaluate for arthritis in the setting of normal exam findings.
- *Attempting to rule out JIA with laboratory studies.* Arthritis is a clinical diagnosis. If a child presents with chronic joint swelling, limited range of motion or contractures, one should not be falsely reassured by normal labs. Many children with arthritis have completely normal inflammatory markers and a negative ANA, and 95% of children with JIA are RF negative.

Risk Factors/Prevention

All JIA subtypes are generally thought to result from an aberrant immune response to an environmental trigger in a genetically predisposed person. A monozygotic twin concordance of 25% to 40% and increased autoimmunity in family members of children with JIA suggest a significant genetic contribution to disease development. Genome-wide association studies in the 2010s revealed susceptibility loci for JIA, though differences in genetic factors exist between clinical JIA subtypes. Strong genetic associations are rare for most JIA subtypes and many identified risk loci are associated with multiple autoimmune diseases. The exception is that 80% to 90% of children with enthesitis-related arthritis

(ERA) are human leukocyte antigen (HLA)-B27 positive. Testing for specific HLA alleles currently has no diagnostic utility in JIA. For the interested reader, Hersh and Prahalad reviewed the genetics of JIA, and Yasin and Schulert published a detailed review of the genetics and pathophysiology of systemic JIA (SJIA).

There is no known prevention for JIA.

Pathophysiology

Synovitis in JIA is characterized by synovial hypertrophy, edema, and hypervascularity. A mixed inflammatory infiltrate of T and B lymphocytes, plasma cells, macrophages, and dendritic cells is found in the synovial lining of affected joints. Infiltrating mononuclear cells produce proinflammatory cytokines and chemokines that contribute to bone and cartilage erosion and perpetuate recruitment of inflammatory cells.

SJIA is uniquely characterized by significant innate immune activation, including increased production of the proinflammatory cytokines interleukin-1 (IL-1) and 6 (IL-6). Some experts suggest that SJIA may therefore be better classified as an autoinflammatory disease.

Given their unique clinical phenotypes, the epidemiology, clinical manifestations, diagnosis, and management of the JIA sub-types will each be discussed separately. Some general principles of diagnosis and management reviewed in the "Current Diagnosis" and "Current therapy" sections earlier and introduced next under "Oligoarticular Juvenile Idiopathic Arthritis" are applicable to all JIA subtypes.

Oligoarticular Juvenile Idiopathic Arthritis

Epidemiology

Oligoarticular JIA is the most common JIA subtype, accounting for 40% to 50% of all cases, with an incidence of approximately 1 in 10,000 children per year. Peak age of onset is 1 to 4 years, with a female predominance. It is most commonly seen in children of Northern European descent.

Clinical Manifestations

Children with oligoarticular JIA present with arthritis in one to four joints, without spread to more than four joints in the first 6 months of disease. Oligoarthritis typically affects large joints in an asymmetric pattern. The most common presentation is arthritis of a single knee. Swelling is the predominant symptom, often with little or no apparent pain early in the disease course. Affected joints may have limited range of motion or contractures. A relatively painless limp is common, and is sometimes the first symptom apparent to parents. Stiffness is worse in the morning or after inactivity, though may be difficult for children to describe. Children with oligoarthritis may experience a persistent oligoarticular course (limited to four or fewer affected joints throughout the child's life) or an extended articular course (spread to five or more joints after the first 6 months of disease).

Diagnosis

A careful history and exam are key to diagnosis. Persistent joint swelling for more than 6 weeks, joint contracture, and/or gait disturbance are the most common presenting symptoms of oligoarticular JIA. Physical exam reveals joint effusion or thickened synovium indicating joint inflammation. Some children may also have warmth, decreased range of motion, contracture, or pain with range of motion on exam. Atrophy of adjacent muscles can be seen in chronic arthritis. Children with oligoarticular JIA are otherwise well appearing. Severe pain (especially with nighttime waking), extremely red or hot joints, *migratory* swelling, fevers, rash, pallor, or a generally ill-appearing child suggest an alternative diagnosis.

All forms of nonsystemic JIA are diagnosed on the basis of objective signs of arthritis, a history of at least 6 weeks of persistent symptoms, **the patient's clinical picture.** As there is no single test that can confirm the diagnosis of JIA, the value of lab testing is limited to excluding other diagnoses and for prognostic purposes in confirmed cases of JIA (see "Complications"). Radiographs have limited diagnostic value with the exception of detecting other conditions such as malignancy, though the presence of erosion(s) may be useful prognostically. MRI or musculoskeletal ultrasound can be useful in cases of equivocal or challenging physical exam (such as in obese patients).

Differential Diagnosis

In some patients with a classic clinical picture, no specific workup for other diagnoses is needed. Prompt evaluation by a pediatric rheumatologist is key to confirming the presence of arthritis, determining an appropriate individualized workup, and rapidly initiating treatment if a diagnosis of JIA is established.

Features that suggest the need to evaluate for alternative diagnoses include the following:

- Atypical demographics (age, ethnicity)—may suggest a different JIA subtype, such as ERA in older children (see "Enthesitis-Related Arthritis").
- Travel history—may suggest the need to evaluate for Lyme arthritis or tuberculosis in patients residing in or traveling to endemic areas.
- Atypical clinical features—severe pain, constitutional symptoms such as weight loss, fevers, fatigue, or an ill appearance should prompt consideration of infection, malignancy, inflammatory bowel disease, or a systemic collagen vascular disease such as lupus in a child with arthritis. Acute, subacute, or migratory arthritis suggests an infectious or postinfectious cause (including rheumatic fever). Episodic joint swelling, especially after trauma, may suggest a bleeding disorder or intraarticular vascular malformation.

Treatment

Treatment of JIA aims to completely control joint inflammation to control symptoms and mitigate the risk of joint damage. In oligoarticular JIA, either scheduled nonsteroidal antiinflammatory drugs (NSAIDs) or intraarticular corticosteroid injections are used as first-line therapy. NSAIDs must be administered at antiinflammatory doses on a scheduled basis to control inflammation, and may take 6 to 8 weeks to be effective. Naproxen (Naprosyn) is often preferred due to twice-daily dosing and available liquid formulation. Steroid joint injections can control inflammation rapidly and are often used for patients with contractures or severe arthritis to more rapidly restore physical function. Intraarticular steroid injections should not be repeated more frequently than every 3 to 6 months. In patients with arthritis refractory to NSAIDs or steroid injections, traditional or biologic disease-modifying antirheumatic drugs (DMARDs), such as methotrexate (Trexall) and tumor necrosis factor (TNF) inhibitors, can be used (some off-label) in a step-wise fashion until disease control is achieved. DMARDs should be prescribed and monitored by a rheumatologist.

Monitoring

JIA disease control is monitored by a rheumatologist on the basis of history and physical exam. The frequency of follow-up visits varies depending on the patient's disease course and medications. Assessments of functional status should be performed to identify patients who would benefit from physical and occupational therapy services or school accommodations. Eye screening for uveitis is a critical part of JIA monitoring (see "Complications"). Medication toxicity monitoring depends on the medication used:

- Daily NSAIDs: complete blood count (CBC), comprehensive metabolic panel (CMP), and urinalysis every 6 to 12 months.
- Methotrexate: CBC and CMP at baseline, 1 month after starting or dose escalation, and then every 3 months on stable doses. Urine pregnancy screening should be considered in girls of reproductive age.
- Biologic DMARDS: Similar lab screening to methotrexate, with some variation depending on the specific medication. Testing for tuberculosis should be performed before starting biologic medications.

Patients on immunosuppressive medications should be evaluated promptly for symptoms of infection. They should avoid live virus vaccines, but **should** receive all other age-appropriate vaccinations including an annual flu vaccine.

Complications

Articular complications include joint limitation, cartilage loss, bony erosion, contracture, and muscle atrophy, leading to chronic disability and pain, though these complications are less common with currently available treatments. A complication of arthritis unique to the growing child is local growth disturbance, most commonly seen as leg length discrepancy as a result of knee arthritis. Inflammation near the open growth plate can cause overgrowth of the affected limb in young children or premature growth plate closure leading to a shorter limb in adolescents.

Chronic anterior uveitis is a common complication of JIA, particularly oligoarticular and RF-negative polyarticular JIA. Chronic uveitis is treatable but carries a high risk of morbidity including cataract, glaucoma, synechiae (adhesions leading to an irregular pupil), band keratopathy (corneal calcium deposits), and blindness. Chronic uveitis is often completely asymptomatic until damage has occurred. Because it can only be detected by slit lamp exam performed by an eye doctor, regular screening is critical to early detection, treatment, and prevention of permanent damage. Uveitis is more likely to occur early in the course of disease, in patients who are ANA positive, and who have an early age of arthritis onset. Well-established screening recommendations guide the frequency of eye exams, ranging from every 3 to 12 months, depending on risk factors. Risk stratification for uveitis is the only use of ANA testing in patients with JIA. Uveitis may occur independent of active arthritis, so eye screening is a critical part of health maintenance for people with JIA throughout their lives. All children diagnosed with uveitis should see an ophthalmologist with experience treating uveitis. Topical corticosteroids are first-line therapy for anterior uveitis, though long-term use is not advisable given the risk of cataracts and glaucoma. Methotrexate[1] and the TNF inhibitors adalimumab (Humira) and infliximab (Remicade)[1] are used widely in children with refractory uveitis. Some patients require more aggressive treatment for uveitis than for arthritis.

Polyarticular Juvenile Idiopathic Arthritis

Epidemiology

Polyarticular arthritis has two subtypes. RF-negative polyarthritis has two peaks of onset (at 1–4 years and in adolescence) and accounts for 20% of all JIA. It is more common in girls and occurs in all ethnicities. RF-positive polyarthritis makes up only 5% of JIA, has a peak onset of 9 to 11 years, and is more common in girls and in non-White individuals.

Clinical Manifestations

Children with polyarthritis present with evidence of arthritis (swelling, morning stiffness, pain, limited range of motion) in five of more joints. Young children may present with gait disturbance or loss of milestones, while older children may present with prolonged morning stiffness or difficulty with activities of daily living and fine motor tasks. Large and small joints in the extremities are affected (often symmetrically). Long-standing disease can produce bony overgrowth of the small joints in the hands or joint deformities including wrist subluxation and boutonniere deformities of the fingers. Arthritis of the cervical spine (presenting with limited extension) and temporomandibular joint (TMJ; presenting with decreased mouth opening, jaw deviation, or retro/micrognathia) are common and cause significant morbidity. Mild to moderate systemic symptoms, including fatigue and weight loss, may be present; however, high-grade fevers should not occur.

Diagnosis

Diagnosis hinges on the presence of arthritis in five or more joints on physical exam (typically with some degree of wrist and hand involvement), at least 6 weeks of symptoms, and exclusion of other causes. There are no confirmatory tests; however, in patients with polyarticular JIA diagnosed clinically, the RF and anti–cyclic citrullinated peptide (anti-CCP) have prognostic value.

RF and anti-CCP positivity are associated with a more severe, erosive course. Some children with polyarticular JIA have normal inflammatory markers, while others have a moderately elevated erythrocyte sedimentation rate (ESR) and anemia of chronic disease. These findings are more useful for assessing overall health and monitoring response to therapy than in establishing an initial diagnosis, as they are nonspecific.

Differential Diagnosis

Reactive arthritis may present with polyarticular joint swelling but is typically acute in onset and characterized by more pain than is seen in JIA. The arthritis of acute rheumatic fever is typically exquisitely painful, has a unique migratory pattern, and is usually exquisitely responsive to NSAID therapy. While patients with polyarticular JIA may experience an *additive* arthritis pattern early in the disease course, *migratory* arthritis (i.e., swelling resolving completely in one joint and moving to another) is not seen in JIA. In patients with extreme pain, bone pain, pallor, or severe fatigue, malignancy such as leukemia or neuroblastoma should be considered. Polyarthritis can occur as a manifestation of other underlying autoimmune diseases, including systemic lupus erythematosus, mixed connective tissue disease, or inflammatory bowel disease. The best approach to evaluating for these conditions is a thorough history and physical exam. Oral ulcers, Raynaud phenomenon, or malar or discoid rashes raise concern for lupus. Because ANA tests are nonspecific and have a high positive rate in both the healthy and JIA populations, an ANA test in isolation is not helpful in evaluating for lupus unless it is negative (which essentially excludes lupus). In cases in which the history or physical raises concern for lupus, using a combination of several laboratory studies is more helpful. A reasonable initial workup for lupus when clinical suspicion is high includes an ANA, specific lupus antibodies (Smith, double-stranded DNA), ESR, C3 and C4 levels, CBC with differential to evaluate for cytopenias, a urinalysis, creatinine, and blood pressure measurement. Inflammatory bowel disease can present with inflammatory arthritis. Inflammatory bowel disease (IBD) should be considered in patients with significant oral ulcers, chronic abdominal pain and/or diarrhea, weight loss, significantly elevated ESR, or anemia.

Treatment

The goals of treatment are the same as for oligoarticular disease, although children with polyarticular JIA often require more aggressive medical therapy to attain inactive disease. Scheduled NSAIDs are often started first line or in conjunction with other medications for pain relief, but they are rarely effective as monotherapy. Intraarticular steroid injections may be used in combination with systemic therapy for severely affected or critical joints, but monotherapy with steroid injections is not a viable approach to treating this disease. Most children with polyarticular JIA require treatment with DMARDs for disease control. There are two general approaches to initiation of medications: step-up therapy and early aggressive (combination) therapy. The choice of approach may be driven by provider and/or patient preference or severity of disease. In a step-up approach, methotrexate is most commonly used as the first DMARD. Methotrexate (10–15 mg/m^2 or 0.5–1 mg/kg, maximum of 25 mg) once weekly is administered orally or subcutaneously, with sub-cutaneous dosing preferred by many pediatric rheumatologists on the basis of possible improved absorption and mitigation of side effects. Biologic medications shown to be effective in JIA refractory to methotrexate include TNF inhibitors (etanercept [Enbrel], adalimumab [Humira], golimumab [Simponi], and infliximab [Remicade][1]), the IL-6 inhibitor tocilizumab (Actemra), the T cell costimulation inhibitor abatacept (Orencia), and some Janus kinase inhibitors including tofacitinib (Xeljanz) and upadacitinib (Rinvoq). Selection of an initial biologic medication can be driven by a variety of factors including patient/parent preference, logistics of administration,

---

[1] Not FDA approved for this indication.

[1] Not FDA approved for this indication.

side effects, comorbid medical conditions, and (in our current health system) insurance restrictions. The anti-CD20 medication rituximab (Rituxan)[1] is sometimes used in patients with RF-positive disease, usually after failure of other medications.

An early aggressive approach, such as first-line combination therapy with methotrexate and a TNF inhibitor with or without adjunctive NSAIDs, intraarticular steroid injections, or a short oral steroid bridge, is sometimes used. With earlier aggressive use of DMARDs, treatment with systemic corticosteroids can now be avoided altogether in most children and limited to short bridging courses in the rarer cases they are needed. While systemic steroids can produce rapid improvements in pain, symptoms return quickly after discontinuation and their side effect profile makes long-term use unacceptable. Systemic steroids should **never** be initiated in a child presenting with musculoskeletal pain of unknown etiology, given the dangers of corticosteroids in undiagnosed infection or malignancy.

Monitoring

Monitoring of clinical disease and medications (NSAIDs, methotrexate, TNF inhibitors) is the same as described for oligoarthritis. Other biologic medications have similar monitoring requirements, including testing for latent tuberculosis (TB) before initiation. Some biologics have additional recommended laboratory monitoring parameters. Given the expertise needed to safely prescribe and monitor DMARDs, these medications should only be prescribed to children with JIA by a rheumatologist. In patients with systemic inflammation or anemia at presentation, these labs should be followed as adjunctive markers of disease activity, but normalization should not falsely reassure that arthritis is well controlled if the joint exam indicates otherwise. Children with polyarticular JIA who develop fever while on immunosuppression should be assessed promptly for infection.

Complications

Articular complications in polyarticular JIA include joint contractures, deformities, growth disturbances, and progressive, erosive disease. Cervical spine, TMJ, hip, and wrist involvement are associated with higher morbidity. Fortunately, with earlier aggressive treatment, severe joint destruction and severe physical disability are now less common. Surgical interventions are sometimes required for patients with severe micrognathia (mandibular distraction or reconstruction techniques), joint destruction (joint replacements), or severe growth disturbances (limb inequality procedures). Children with polyarticular JIA can also develop chronic uveitis. Similar to oligoarticular JIA, age of onset, duration of disease, and ANA status are risk factors for development of uveitis and direct frequency of eye screening. The exception is that uveitis is rare in RF-positive polyarticular JIA; thus eye screening is needed only once yearly in this subtype.

Enthesitis-Related Arthritis

Epidemiology

ERA is the only JIA subtype more common in boys, makes up 9% to 19% of all JIA, and has a peak age of onset of 10 to 13 years.

Clinical Manifestations

ERA is a childhood form of spondyloarthropathy and closely related to ankylosing spondylitis. Spondyloarthropathies are characterized by axial arthritis, although in children peripheral arthritis precedes axial disease, sometimes by years. Peripheral arthritis in ERA preferentially affects the lower extremities, often asymmetrically. Arthritis of the hips and sacroiliac joints, tenosynovitis (inflammation of tendon sheaths), and *enthesitis* (inflammation at the bony insertions of tendons, ligaments, or fascia) are common findings. *Tarsitis,* diffuse swelling of the dorsum of the foot, is relatively unique to ERA. Pain is more prominent in ERA than other JIA subtypes. Axial arthritis develops in some patients in late adolescence or adulthood. Uveitis in ERA is acute and symptomatic (with a red, photophobic eye), distinct from uveitis in other forms of JIA.

Diagnosis

ERA usually presents as monoarthritis or oligoarthritis in the lower extremities (hips, knees, ankles). Diagnosis is made on the basis of arthritis on exam with a history supporting a chronic course. HLA-B27 positivity can support the diagnosis, though the HLA-B27 is not a diagnostic test (as some ERA patients are B27 negative and many B27-positive individuals are healthy). Though most children do not have sacroiliitis or spinal arthritis at presentation, findings of inflammatory sacroiliac or spinal arthritis on radiographs or magnetic resonance imaging (MRI) strongly suggest this diagnosis.

Differential Diagnosis

School-aged children with ERA often present with arthritis of a single knee or ankle. In addition to the diagnostic considerations outlined earlier for oligoarthritis, ERA must be distinguished from oligoarticular JIA itself. Clues to diagnosis in this clinical scenario are older age (recall that the peak age of onset of oligoarticular JIA is 1–4 years), male gender, and supporting clinical features if present (tenosynovitis, enthesitis, acute symptomatic uveitis). In children presenting with hip symptoms, infectious and orthopedic conditions (including slipped capital femoral epiphysis or Perthes) should be considered. Rarely, older adolescents present with sacroiliitis. Low back stiffness, worse in the morning, helps distinguish from infectious and orthopedic conditions, though imaging is usually required to make this distinction with confidence. The vast majority of children with chronic low back pain have mechanical rather than inflammatory pain.

Treatment

The general approach to treatment of ERA is similar to polyarticular JIA, though for patients with sacroiliitis or spinal arthritis, TNF inhibition should be considered early in the disease course. The IL-17 inhibitor secukinumab (Cosentyx) is also approved for use in ERA, as well as juvenile psoriatic arthritis (see "Juvenile Psoriatic Arthritis").

Monitoring

Monitoring is very similar to polyarticular JIA with a few exceptions:
1. Children with ERA should be monitored closely for development of axial arthritis. This may include a combination of the following approaches: querying symptoms of inflammatory back pain, eliciting sacroiliac pain on exam, measuring spine mobility (with a modified Schober test), and/or imaging sacroiliac joints with x-ray or MRI.
2. Eye exams are only required once yearly and as indicated based on symptoms as uveitis in ERA is usually symptomatic.

Complications

Acute uveitis occurs in some patients with ERA and often responds to topical corticosteroids. Patients who develop a red or photophobic eye should be evaluated promptly by an eye doctor. Arthritis of the spine, sacroiliac joints, and hips can be difficult to control, sometimes leading to joint destruction, even in the setting of prompt and aggressive therapy. In adulthood, these patients are at risk for progressive, ascending ankylosis of the spine.

Juvenile Psoriatic Arthritis

Epidemiology

Juvenile psoriatic arthritis accounts for approximately 10% of JIA, is more common in girls, and has two peaks of onset: preschool and late childhood.

Clinical Manifestations

Psoriatic arthritis usually presents with peripheral joint involvement and can occur in a monoarticular, oligoarticular, or polyarticular pattern. Both small and large joints can be affected, often in an asymmetric pattern. *Dactylitis,* or a "sausage digit," is a unique feature of psoriatic arthritis not seen in other forms of JIA. Dactylitic fingers and toes exhibit diffuse swelling that extends beyond individual joints. Arthritis of the distal interphalangeal (DIP) joints is also unique to psoriatic arthritis among children with JIA. There is some clinical overlap between psoriatic arthritis and ERA. Enthesitis and tenosynovitis are prevalent features, and sacroiliitis can occur in up to 30% of adolescents. Nail changes, including pitting, horizontal ridges, and onycholysis, are common, and overt psoriasis occurs in about half of children. Both chronic uveitis (with risk factors similar to patients with oligo- and polyarticular JIA) and acute uveitis (in HLA-B27–posi-tive patients) can occur.

Diagnosis

Unlike adults, children with psoriatic arthritis often present with arthritis before skin disease. In patients with chronic arthritis and psoriasis, the diagnosis is relatively straightforward. In those with chronic arthritis without psoriasis, clinical clues to diagnosis include dactylitis, psoriatic nail changes (pitting or onycholysis), DIP involvement, or a first-degree relative with psoriasis.

Differential Diagnosis

Depending on the pattern of joint involvement, differential diagnosis includes other forms of JIA (oligoarticular, polyarticular, ERA) and other conditions listed previously in the differential of these JIA subtypes. Small joint involvement or dactylitis help distinguish psoriatic from oligoarticular JIA in young children with fewer than five affected joints.

Treatment

The treatment approach is similar to polyarticular JIA, though for patients with sacroiliitis, enthesitis, or dactylitis, TNF inhibition has the most well-established efficacy. There are also at least two groups of biologic DMARDs that are specifically indicated for use in psoriatic JIA (and in the case of secukinumab, for ERA), including IL-12/23 (ustekinumab [Stelara]) and IL-17 (secukinumab [Cosentyx]) inhibitors.

Monitoring

Monitoring is similar to other forms of JIA, including eye screening for chronic uveitis, as described for oligo- and polyarthritis, and monitoring for axial arthritis, as described for ERA. In addition, patients who have not developed skin manifestations should be monitored for development of psoriasis.

Complications

Articular and ocular complications are similar to other JIA subtypes, though children with psoriatic arthritis often have poorer functional outcomes and lower rates of remission off medication than those with oligo- or polyarticular JIA.

Systemic Juvenile Idiopathic Arthritis

Epidemiology

SJIA occurs in children of all ages and into adulthood (known as Still disease in adults). It is the only form of JIA that affects boys and girls equally. SJIA makes up 10% to 20% of JIA. It occurs in all ethnicities, with increased prevalence in some Asian countries including Japan.

Clinical Manifestations

SJIA is characterized by fever, rash, and arthritis. Fevers in SJIA are high grade, typically spiking once (quotidian) or twice (double quotidian) daily with return to normal temperature between fevers. The rash seen in SJIA is salmon-colored or erythematous, macular or urticarial, sometimes with associated Koebner phenomenon. A unique feature of the SJIA rash is its *evanescent* nature: it appears with fever and resolves or fades during afebrile periods. The arthritis in SJIA can affect any number of joints, in any pattern, and is not always present at disease onset. In some patients, the latent period between onset of systemic features and arthritis is weeks or months. Many patients exhibit nonspecific symptoms, including fatigue, irritability, and myalgia during fevers. Children with SJIA have significant systemic inflammation during periods of disease activity. Profoundly elevated white blood count, platelet count, ESR, CRP, ferritin, and anemia are common. SJIA is

truly a systemic disease, with some patients exhibiting lymphadenopathy, hepatosplenomegaly, and serositis (pleural or pericardial effusions). The most feared complication of SJIA is macrophage activation syndrome (MAS; see "Complications").

Diagnosis

SJIA is diagnosed based on the presence of quotidian fevers, evanescent Still rash, arthritis, and systemic inflammation, with exclusion of similar conditions. SJIA often leads to inpatient evaluation, given patients' high-grade fevers and ill appearance. Children who lack arthritis at the time of presentation are challenging to diagnose. In practice, SJIA is often presumptively diagnosed before arthritis has been present for 6 weeks (and sometimes in the absence of arthritis), as the severity of this disease can necessitate urgent treatment.

Differential Diagnosis

SJIA has a broad differential diagnosis that includes infectious (viral, bacterial, rickettsial), oncologic (leukemia, neuroblastoma), and inflammatory conditions (Kawasaki, polyarteritis nodosa, inflammatory bowel disease, among others). Involvement of infectious disease and oncology consultants can help exclude these mimics, particularly if treatment with corticosteroids is being considered. Additional workup, including infectious studies and bone marrow biopsy, is appropriate in cases of diagnostic uncertainty.

Treatment

The treatment paradigms have evolved more for SJIA than any other JIA subtype since the late 2000s. Traditionally, children with SJIA were treated with systemic corticosteroids, resulting in the full spectrum of anticipated morbidities (e.g., growth delay, infections, osteoporosis). Traditional DMARDs and TNF inhibitors are significantly less effective than for other JIA subtypes. Targeted therapy with inhibition of IL-1 (with anakinra [Kineret][1] or canakinumab [Ilaris]) or IL-6 (with tocilizumab [Actemra]) is the emerging standard of care, though optimal timing of these medications is unclear. Many pediatric rheumatologists are now using IL-1 or IL-6 blockade first line or after a failed NSAID trial to avoid or minimize corticosteroids. Since the 2010s, JAK inhibitors, including tofacitinib (Xeljanz)[1] have been used with some success in treatment-refractory cases. Systemic corticosteroids continue to have a role in severe disease or MAS. Other treatments for MAS include cyclosporine (Neoral)[1], etoposide (Toposar)[1], and emapalumab (Gamifant).

Monitoring

Monitoring is similar to polyarticular JIA, with a few exceptions. As uveitis is rare in SJIA, eye exams are needed only annually. Laboratory markers of systemic inflammation (including ferritin) are useful in monitoring disease activity and evaluating for impending MAS, which can develop even when disease otherwise appears well controlled. Given the serious and life-threatening nature of this disease, all children with SJIA should be followed closely by a pediatric rheumatologist or an adult rheumatologist with experience managing SJIA.

Complications

Articular complications of SJIA are similar to polyarticular JIA, though the arthritis of SJIA is often aggressive and destructive. There is emerging evidence that earlier treatment with targeted biologics may prevent progression to chronic polyarthritis. MAS is a serious complication of SJIA, characterized by unregulated production of proinflammatory cytokines, macrophage proliferation, and hemophagocytic activity in the bone marrow and other organs. MAS is a potentially fatal rheumatologic emergency. It is often suspected on the basis of rapidly worsening clinical status and the development of continuous fever. Laboratory findings include a profoundly elevated ferritin, elevated lactate dehydroge-nase and transaminases, falling blood cell counts, and paradoxi-cally low or falling ESR and fibrinogen in the setting of other signs of systemic inflammation. MAS is currently considered a secondary

---

[1] Not FDA approved for this indication.

form of hemophagocytic lymphohistiocytosis (HLH). Since at least 2013, interstitial lung disease has been recognized, more often in younger patients with predominant systemic symptoms and a history of MAS. This complication may be associated with markedly elevated levels of IL-18 and with the HLA-DRB*15 haplotype. A potential association between some cases of ILD in SJIA and exposure to IL-1 or IL-6 inhibitor drugs is currently being investigated.

References

Aeschlimann FA, Chong S, Lyons TW, et al: Risk of serious infections associated with biologic agents in juvenile idiopathic arthritis: a systematic review and meta-analyses, *J Pediatr* 204:162–171, 2019.

Clarke SLN, Sen ES, Ramanan AV: Juvenile Idiopathic arthritis-associated uveitis, *Pediatric Rheumatol Online J* 14:27, 2016.

Crayne CB, Beukelman T: Juvenile idiopathic arthritis: oligoarthritis and polyarthritis, *Pediatr Clin N Am* 65:657–674, 2018.

Hersh AO, Prahalad S: Genetics of juvenile idiopathic arthritis, *Rheum Dis Clin N Am* 43:435–448, 2017.

Lee JJL, Schneider R: Systemic juvenile idiopathic arthritis, *Pediatr Clin N Am* 65:691–709, 2018.

Petty RE, Southwood TR, Manners P, et al: International League of Associations for Rheumatology classification of juvenile idiopathic arthritis: second revision, Edmonton, 2001, *J Rheumatol* 31(2):390–392, 2004.

Shoop-Worrall SJW, Kearlsey-Fleet L, Thomson W, Verstappen SMM, Hyrich KL: How common is remission in juvenile idiopathic arthritis: a systematic review, *Semin Arthritis Rheum* 47:331–337, 2017.

Towe C, Grom AA, Schulert GS: Diagnosis and management of the systemic juvenile idiopathic arthritis patient with emerging lung disease, *Paediatr Drugs* 25(6):649–658, 2023.

Wong KO, Bond K, Homik J, Ellsworth JE, Karkhaneh M, Ha C, Dryden DM: *Antinuclear antibody, rheumatoid factor, and cyclic-citrullinated peptide tests for evaluating musculoskeletal complaints in children: Comparative Effective-ness Review No. 50*, Agency for Healthcare Research and Quality, 2012. Avail-able at https://effectivehealthcare.ahrq.gov/sites/default/files/pdf/musculoskeletal-complaints-tests-children_research.pdf. Accessed 1 January 2019.

Yasin S, Schulert GS: Systemic juvenile idiopathic arthritis and macrophage activation syndrome: update on pathogenesis and treatment, *Curr Opin Rheumatol* 30:514–520, 2018.

OSTEOARTHRITIS

Method of
Rachel Chamberlain, MD; Jacob Christensen, DO; and Christopher Bossart, MD

CURRENT DIAGNOSIS

- Risk factors for osteoarthritis (OA) include age, gender, genetics, and anatomic factors, which are nonmodifiable; modifiable risk factors include body mass index (BMI), tobacco use, trauma, physical activity, and muscle strength.
- OA is diagnosed using both clinical and radiologic information.
- Clinical signs and symptoms include joint pain, crepitus, mild swelling, and joint line tenderness to palpation. Symptoms wax and wane and may be related to activity but can be present at varying times of day.
- The Kellgren-Lawrence Classification system can help determine the grade of OA, but the ultimate determination of the severity is based on clinical factors.

CURRENT THERAPY

- First-line therapy for OA includes exercise, physical therapy, and weight loss (if the patient is overweight or obese).
- Nonsteroidal antiinflammatory drugs (NSAIDs) are the best studied pharmacologic treatment for OA pain. Their use must be balanced by their side effects and the patient's comorbid conditions.

- Injections of corticosteroids may be used for OA pain management, but their pain relief effects are not long term.
- Hyaluronic acid injections can be considered in patients with mild to moderate OA of the knee, but this is an expensive therapy and evidence of effectiveness is mixed.
- No current treatment either in systemic medications or injections alters the course of OA. Research in the long-term benefits of biologic agents is ongoing.
- Total joint replacement is an expensive but definitive treatment for many patients with OA. The referring clinician should consider the patient's overall health and help optimize the patient's health for a successful outcome when referring for a total joint replacement.

Osteoarthritis (OA), also known as degenerative joint disease, is the most common form of arthritis worldwide. OA is a significant cause of morbidity, disability, and decreased quality of life. It is one of the leading contributors to global years lived with disability (YLDs) by Global Disease Burden studies. It is the leading cause of lower extremity disability. OA affects about one in eight people in the United States, or 27 to 31 million, and about 250 million people worldwide, with the most commonly affected joints being the knees, hips, hands, feet, and spine. As the age of the population and the rates of obesity increase, the economic impact of OA also increases. It is estimated that OA costs 1% to 2.5% of GDP in developed countries, with the majority of cost for treatment (85%) coming from joint replacement surgeries.

OA has been previously characterized pathologically by varying levels of cartilage involvement. One may find fissures and microfibrillations in mild or early disease, and erosive destruction of the joint surfaces may be seen in more advanced disease. However, it is recognized that the effects of OA can be seen throughout the entire joint including the bone, synovium, menisci, and ligaments.

Pathogenesis

The pathogenesis of OA remains unclear. For decades, the traditional belief was that OA was a "wear and tear" condition associated with the cumulative stress of aging. This theory has not been shown to be true, or at least it is not an accurate depiction of "the whole story." Research investigating other possible mechanisms is gaining traction. More recent research areas of focus include what role inflammatory mediators, genetics, metabolic factors, proteases, and biomarkers may play in the development of OA.

Risk Factors

Despite the pathogenesis of OA being unclear, a number of factors have been identified to be associated with increased risk. These risk factors include age, gender, body mass index (BMI), genetics, tobacco smoking, trauma, chronic overuse, anatomic factors, and muscle strength.

Age—There is a clear correlation between aging and development of OA. It is also clear that the aging of joint tissues and the development of OA are separate and distinct processes. There are a number of aging changes within the joint that may contribute to development of OA including: thinning of articular cartilage, reduced hydration, accumulation of advanced glycation end-products (AGEs), and abnormal calcification ("chondrocalcinosis"). Based on population based radiographic surveys from the Framingham study, the prevalence of knee OA in patients aged 63 to 94 was 33%, and symptomatic knee OA was 9.5%.

Gender—OA is more common in women than men. Some have postulated that the correlation between age and OA explains the why OA is more common in the postmenopausal years; however, there is some evidence to suggest decreased estrogen exposure in women could also be a contributing factor.

BMI—Being overweight or obese has been well documented as a strong risk factor for development of OA. This is likely both related to increased mechanical forces and metabolic changes associated with obesity. Weight loss has also been shown to reduce the risk of developing knee OA.

Genetics—Twin studies have shown a genetic contribution of about 40% to 70% depending on the site of OA. There exists substantial heterogeneity depending on the site of involvement, and there is also racial variation, which makes studying this genetic component more difficult.

Trauma and chronic overuse—Trauma, which includes both major injuries and surgery, increases the risk of OA. For example, history of anterior cruciate ligament (ACL) tear in the knee is associated with increased risk of OA development regardless of whether surgical reconstruction is done. The mechanism for this is not completely understood. Chronic overuse as is seen in some occupations carries an increased risk of development of OA. For example, professional soccer players have an increased risk of developing knee OA, and professional baseball pitchers have a higher risk of developing elbow OA.

Biomechanical factors—Joint structural abnormalities may increase the risk of developing OA. The understanding of the role of muscle strength in OA is expanding. It is known that patients with knee and hip OA have reduced muscle strength in the surrounding muscles. However, it has been thought previously that this was a consequence of the symptoms of OA causing decreased activity, muscle atrophy, and subsequent weakness. There is more recent evidence to suggest that muscle weakness may actually predate the onset of knee OA.

Clinical Features

OA is characterized clinically by insidious onset, usage-related joint pain, which can be accompanied by mild stiffness. Pain can be present at varying times of day. Mild swelling may be present in OA; however, large effusion and history of trauma or injury should prompt further workup. Patients may complain of limitation in range of motion, as well as a sensation of giving way or buckling (particularly in knee OA). Tenderness to palpation along the joint lines is a common physical exam finding. Joint deformity is a sign of advanced disease. Symptoms are typically slowly progressive as is the disease course.

OA severity can be graded based on radiographic criteria or a combination of radiographic criteria and symptom severity. Perhaps the most commonly used radiographic criteria is the Kellgren-Lawrence method, classifying OA severity into grades 0 to 4 based on presence of joint space narrowing, osteophyte formation, and sclerosis of subchondral bone (Table 1). This method is certainly useful, though it should be mentioned that there are limitations to this method—namely, that there is somewhat poor correlation between radiographic findings and symptoms. It is estimated that up to 50% of people with radiographic findings of OA do not have any symptoms.

TABLE 1	Kellgren Lawrence Radiographic Classification of Osteoarthritis of the Knee
Grade 1	Doubtful joint space narrowing, possible osteophytic lipping
Grade 2	Definite osteophytes, possible joint space narrowing
Grade 3	Moderate osteophytes, definite joint space narrowing, some sclerosis, possible bone-end deformity
Grade 4	Large osteophytes, marked joint space narrowing, severe sclerosis, definite bone ends deformity

Data from Kellgren JH, Lawrence JS. Radiological assessment of osteo-arthrosis. *Ann Rheum Dis.* 1957;16:494–502.

Current Therapy

Treatment for OA is individualized based on patient symptoms, values, needs, goals, and response to therapies. There is no single treatment for OA, which reliably and consistently manages symptoms on its own. Therefore, a combination of therapeutic approaches is used in order to optimize function, minimize pain, and in some cases modify the process of damage to the joint. In general, safer treatments should be considered first before trying other treatments with higher risk profiles. Treatments can be placed into four categories: nonpharmacologic, pharmacologic, nonsurgical, and surgical interventions.

Nonpharmacologic Therapies

Nonpharmacologic therapies represent the mainstay of treatment for OA initially. These therapies include education, exercise, weight management, braces, assistive devices, psychologic therapies, manual medicine, and alternative therapies.

Education—It is important to inform patients about their diagnosis, the modifiable risk factors for their specific case, and their expected prognosis. Information should be provided regarding the various treatment options including their risks, benefits, costs, and alternatives. Doing this helps encourage active shared decision making and combat some of the common misconceptions about OA management. Patient involvement in setting goals and self-managing their condition improves adherence and can make a significant difference in patients' view of their disease.

Exercise—The goal of exercise therapy is reduction in pain and improvement in joint function. Various forms of exercise exist, and physical activity in general should be encouraged, providing it is done with patient symptoms as a guide. The forms of exercise with the best evidence for improvement, particularly in knee OA, are aerobic exercise and resistance strength training. Perhaps the most readily available form of aerobic exercise is walking, and formal walking programs have been shown to significantly improve OA symptoms, as well as quadriceps strength. Aquatic exercise has also been shown to be beneficial, and has the added benefit of decreased weight-bearing stress on joints.

Weight loss—In overweight and obese patients (BMI > 25), a reduction of 10% of baseline body weight has been shown to decrease OA-related joint pain. This is true of patients with knee and hip OA, but may also be beneficial in patients with OA of the hands in light of evidence that increased BMI is a risk factor for development of hand OA. Again, this may be partially related to metabolic changes.

Braces and assistive devices—Walking aids, such as a walking stick or cane, as well as knee braces for patients with joint malalignment, may be helpful, and should be considered as an adjunct treatment in appropriate patients. OA of the thumb is particularly amenable to splinting to improve pain.

Psychologic therapies—Chronic pain from OA can have significant effects on a patient's ability to function. Often as patients feel less able to perform the activities they enjoy, their mood is adversely affected, which in turn negatively affects their pain symptoms. There is some evidence that psychological interventions, such as cognitive behavioral therapy, are helpful in this regard.

Manual medicine—Manual techniques, whether performed by a physical therapist, doctor of osteopathic medicine (DO), massage therapist, or chiropractor, typically focus on improvement/maintenance of range of motion as well as joint mobility. There is some limited evidence to suggest manual manipulation may improve pain scores, particularly when combined with exercise therapy. However, more research in this area is needed.

Alternative therapies—There is currently insufficient evidence to recommend the use of acupuncture, therapeutic ultrasound, and neuromuscular electrical stimulation for treatment of OA.

Pharmacotherapy

Despite the fact that nonpharmacologic agents are first line, many patients with OA require drug therapy. Although no available medications predictably reverse or halt the inexorable progression of the disease, some medications do reduce pain and inflammation, enhancing the patient's quality of life.

Analgesics—The most common nonnarcotic analgesic agent currently used for OA is acetaminophen (Tylenol). The recommended dose for OA is 1 g administered every 8 hours or three to four times daily (not to exceed 4 g/day). However, even at a high dose, studies are mixed if acetaminophen is effective for OA pain. Adverse effects are rare, but caution must be exercised in patients who have preexisting renal or liver conditions. Duloxetine (Cymbalta) 60 mg daily is approved by the US Food and Drug Administration (FDA) for mild to moderate pain resulting from OA. In a double-blind, randomized, placebo-controlled study of patients with chronic pain due to OA of the knees, there was significant improvement with duloxetine versus the placebo. In treating OA, the regular use of opioids is not recommended or supported. Tramadol (Ultram) is commonly used, particularly in patients who have contraindications to nonsteroidal antiinflammatory drugs (NSAIDs), but we suggest caution in prescribing even this medication given potential for tolerance. While for years it has been suggested that opioids improve quality of life and function in patients with chronic pain from OA, there is no evidence to support this in OA. Opioids may be needed occasionally for intense pain, but the benefits are limited compared to the risks of tolerance, opioid misuse, addiction, overdose, and death.

Nonsteroidal antiinflammatory drugs—Pain in OA patients is often not adequately controlled with pure analgesics, whereas NSAIDs in adequate dosage can provide significant clinical improvement. The 2013 AAOS Guidelines on nonsurgical management of knee OA recommend NSAIDs with a strong strength of recommendation. If simple analgesics fail to provide adequate relief, one of the many currently available NSAIDs may be tried. Clinical trials with naproxen (Anaprox), diclofenac (Voltaren), and sulindac (Clinoril) showed significantly greater improvement when compared with high-dose acetaminophen. The chief limiting factor in the use of NSAIDs is the possible induced gastric pathologic changes, disturbed renal function, and potential increased cardiac events. In addition, many patients with OA may be on other platelet inhibiting medications and interactions should be taken into consideration. For patients ages 75 and above, topical NSAIDs are advised over oral given less toxicity and adverse effects. Cost and compliance also must be given consideration. Many of the NSAIDs are now available in dosage forms that can be given once or twice daily, which helps overcome the issue of noncompliance.

Cyclooxygenase 2 inhibitors—COX-2 inhibitors block prostaglandin synthesis and inflammatory mediators without the COX-1 effect of inhibiting gastric mucosal protection. In the United States, the COX-2–specific inhibiting NSAID that is FDA approved is celecoxib (Celebrex). It is equivalent to the older nonselective NSAIDs with regard to therapeutic effectiveness, but the risk of gastrointestinal injury and adverse effects on platelet aggregation is lessened. The risk of renal side effects is probably comparable with that of the conventional NSAIDs. A trial assessing the effect of celecoxib on cardiovascular events found a slightly higher risk of cardiovascular events, but primarily only at higher doses (400 mg/day or greater). In addition, celecoxib can be used with low-dose aspirin (81 mg) daily and anticoagulants, including warfarin. It is important to take into consideration that the cost of Celebrex is several times that of traditional NSAIDs.

Glucosamine and chondroitin sulfate—Glucosamine and chondroitin sulfate are over-the-counter dietary supplements that have gained moderate press touting their possible symptom-modifying effects. However, there is no significant evidence demonstrating that either of these used alone or in combination prevents or reduces arthritis in the knee. A Cochrane review shows mild improvement in pain scores at short-term follow-up with glucosamine compared with placebo, however only with certain preparations of the product. At this point, multiple organizations including the American College of Rheumatology and American Academy of Orthopedic Surgeons cannot recommend their use in treating OA.

Turmeric—Turmeric[7] has been used for treatment of many inflammatory disease processes, including OA, with modest improvement in pain. Curcumin[7] is the primary constituent within turmeric, and there is thought that regular intake can protect joints in individuals with OA. The studies to date are small and limited in number, but they do show modest reduction in pain among those with OA. Larger studies would be needed in order for a definitive recommendation to be made but given its low side effect profile and risk of adverse effects it seems to be a reasonable addition to treatment. However, turmeric may interact with other antiplatelet therapies, and this should be considered individually for each patient.

Disease-modifying drugs—To date, there are no known medications that reliably slow or stop the disease process of OA, and disease modifying antirheumatic drugs (DMARDs) are not recommended in the treatment of OA.

Intra-articular Injections

Corticosteroid injections (CSI)—Early in symptomatic OA it is preferable to attempt to control symptoms by nonpharmacologic therapy and with oral therapy, rather than by local injection. CSI are commonly used for OA. Steroids are strong antiinflammatory medications, and there is reasonable evidence that CSI decreases pain in the short term. There remain concerns that CSI may damage cartilage and therefore hasten the advancement of OA. Clinical trials remain mixed. However, when noninvasive therapies are not controlling OA pain or a patient has an OA flair, CSI can provide relief. CSI is thought to be relatively safe to be given three to four times per year, although this is an expert opinion and not based in sound evidence. The remote risk of introducing infection from the procedure is minimized by adhering to a meticulous aseptic technique. CSI is thought to be less problematic than systemic steroids when it comes to side effects such as raising blood sugar, but caution should be used in patients with diabetes, particularly uncontrolled DM. While arthrocentesis of a painful arthritic joint is commonly done, there is little evidence that this is an effective therapy, particularly after the short term.

Hyaluronic acid—Intra-articular hyaluronic acid (HA) injections have been approved by the FDA since 1997 as a medical device for OA of the knee. The clinical use of intra-articular HA in painful OA of the knee was introduced in Europe in the 1990s. The mechanism of action of HA is not completely understood, but it is thought to restore normal viscoelastic properties to the pathologically altered synovial fluid. Other possible beneficial effects include protection of the chondrocytes, antiinflammatory effects, and possible improvement of the mechanics of joint motion. Unfortunately, in non-industry-funded studies, head-to-head comparisons often fail to show superiority over cortisone and placebo injections. In addition, HA does not change the course of OA. Numerous preparations of FDA-approved HA products are in wide use in the United States. Initially, all HA products were extracted from rooster combs; however, that is no longer the case. In approximately 2% to 8% of patients injected with avian derived product, a subsequent pseudoseptic reaction can occur, mimicking an infected joint. Newer HA products are not animal-derived preparations but rather are developed from biological fermentation of streptococcal bacteria. In the United States, these products are only approved for knee OA. Drawbacks of intra-articular HA products include mixed evidence, cost, and less efficacy in patients with morbid obesity or severe (Kellrgan Lawrence Grade 4) OA.

Platelet rich plasma (PRP)—PRP injections have become popular in recent years, and evidence continues to grow supporting the use of PRP in knee osteoarthritis. PRP is not FDA approved for osteoarthritis at this time and therefore is not covered by insurance. PRP formulations and research methods vary widely, confounding study results and making FDA approval difficult. Thus the cost of PRP remains prohibitive for many patients. There are several systemic reviews showing improvement in knee OA pain and function from PRP injections compared with HA and CSI,

---

[7] Available as dietary supplement.

but the level of evidence remains weak and many studies have a high risk of bias. Though the research continues to have flaws, intra-articular PRP is gaining popularity, especially in knee OA, and may become a common treatment in the future.

Stem cells—Stem cell injections have become an intriguing area of research. The thought that intra-articular injections of stem cells can help improve/restart chondrogenesis, and regeneration of damaged cartilage is actively being researched. However, a recent systematic review of the literature shows only a low level of evidence for its use, all of which were studies deemed to be at high risk for bias. At this time, it is not considered a mainstay treatment for OA in the United States.

Surgical Management of Osteoarthritis

Surgical management of arthritis varies by which joint is affected, with knee arthritis being most common, followed by hip. Knee arthroscopy should not be used to manage knee OA and/or degenerative meniscus tears in the setting of OA, as there is little to no improvement compared with exercise. Additionally, arthroscopic partial menisectomy for degenerative meniscus tears may increase risk of developing OA. Hemiarthroplasty can be considered in patients with unicompartmental knee arthritis, and may carry less risks than total knee arthroplasty (TKA). In addition, a valgus-producing proximal tibial osteotomy may be beneficial in patients with symptomatic medial compartment knee OA. Total joint arthroplasty is an expensive surgery, though often well covered by insurance companies. The surgeries carry significant risks, including cardiovascular events, deep vein thrombosis, and prosthesis infection, which can lead to long hospitalizations for intravenous antibiotics and repeat surgeries. Not all patients have the pain relief and function improvement expected from total joint arthroplasty (TJA).

When referring a patient to orthopedic surgery for consideration of a total hip or knee arthroplasty, the clinician may be able to help prepare the patient to optimize their surgical outcome. This includes, but is not limited to, helping a patient with smoking cessation, weight loss, and diabetes control. Ideally, a patient would be tobacco/nicotine free for at least 8 weeks prior to surgery, would have a BMI less than 40, and would have a hemoglobin A1C ≤7.0. In addition, the referring clinician should take into consideration that patients with chronic pain and/or opioid use, depression and anxiety, liver cirrhosis/hepatitis C, and other chronic conditions may not have optimal outcomes from total joint replacement. It is acceptable to delay total knee arthroplasty up to 8 months to improve these modifiable risk factors without decreasing the patient's benefit from total joint arthroplasty. Arthroplasty procedures are also performed for arthritis of the shoulder, elbow, wrist, thumb, and ankle with varying degrees of evidence for pain and quality of life improvement. Surgical techniques and prostheses are undergoing advancements and improving patient outcomes for the less commonly done arthroplasty surgeries, and clinicians can expect this technology to continue to advance in the future.

Conclusions

OA remains a very common source of pain and disability throughout the world and also carries a significant financial burden. The pathophysiology of OA is more complex than previously believed, and is not fully understood. OA has both modifiable and nonmodifiable risk factors. Nonmodifiable risk factors include age, gender, and genetic risk/family history. Modifiable risk factors include weight loss in patients who are overweight or obese, eliminating tobacco exposure, trauma and overuse, and control of metabolic syndrome.

Nonpharmacologic therapy for OA is first-line treatment and includes education and management of patient expectations, weight loss, exercise, and physical therapy. Braces and assistive devices, cognitive behavioral therapy, manual therapy, and alternative therapy may also be considered but have less definitive evidence.

Pharmacologic therapy is usually required for OA, with acetaminophen being first line. Clinicians should educate patients on high dose acetaminophen and safe amounts to take to achieve therapeutic effect without danger to liver. NSAIDs are often more effective at controlling pain from OA, but do carry a higher risk profile for gastrointestinal bleeding, renal dysfunction, and cardiovascular events. Herbal medications such as glucosamine chondroitin and turmeric may also be beneficial but studies are mixed. Opioids should be avoided in management of OA pain, as there is no evidence that they improve function and quality of life (as previously proposed) but do carry very serious side effects.

Nonsurgical interventions such as intra-articular injections can be beneficial in managing pain from OA. It is important to counsel patients that none of the current injection therapies have data that they change the course of the disease process; they only help control pain and improve function. Corticosteroid injections often give the patient good pain relief but are often not long lasting. HA injections may also be beneficial, but many studies show equivocal pain improvement compared with cortisone and the cost is much greater. Studies are still ongoing at biologic agent injections such as PRP and stem cell therapies, and data is mixed. It is unclear if these expensive, non-FDA-approved therapies are beneficial at this time.

Total joint arthroplasty is the definitive treatment for OA, with the best data in hip followed by knee arthroplasty. These surgeries carry significant risks, especially in the older population that OA most commonly affects. In addition, surgery is very expensive and associated with significant time loss from work. Patients' chronic medical conditions should be well controlled prior to a total joint arthroplasty, to minimize risks of poor outcomes or adverse effects.

References

American Academy of Orthopedic Surgeons: Management of Osteoarthritis of the Hip Evidence-Based Clinical Practice Guideline, Available at: https://www.aaos.org/uploadedFiles/PreProduction/Quality/Guidelines_and_Reviews/OA%20Hip%20CPG_3.13.17.pdf. Accessed 15 March 2019.

Bartels EM, Juhl CB, Christensen R, et al: Aquatic exercise for the treatment of knee and hip osteoarthritis, *Cochrane Database of Systematic Reviews*, 2016. Available at: https://doi.org/10.1002/cca.1312.

Belk JW, Kraeutler MJ, Houck DA, et al: Platelet-rich plasma versus hyaluronic acid for knee osteoarthritis: a systematic review and meta-analysis of randomized controlled trials, *Am J Sports Med* 49:1,249–260, 2020.

Brown GA: AAOS Clinical Practice Guideline: Treatment of osteoarthritis of the knee: evidence-based guideline, *Journal of the American Academy of Orthopaedic Surgeons* 21(9):577–579, 2013, Available at: https://doi.org/10.5435/jaaos-21-09-577.

Conaghan, P. I56. DMARDs in Osteoarthritis: What is the evidence? *Rheumatology*, 53(suppl_1):i12–i13, 2014, Available at: https://doi.org/10.1093/rheumatology/keu061.003.

Dadabo J, Fram J, Jayabalan P: Noninterventional therapies for the management of knee osteoarthritis, *The Journal of Knee Surgery* 32(01):046–054, 2018, Available at: https://doi.org/10.1055/s-0038-1676107.

Dai WL, et al: Efficacy of platelet-rich plasma in the treatment of knee osteoarthritis: a meta-analysis of randomized controlled trials, *Arthroscopy* 33(3):659–670.e1, 2017 Mar, Available at: https://doi.org/10.1016/j.arthro.2016.09.024. Epub 2016 Dec 22. Review PubMed PMID: 28012636.

Fransen M, Mcconnell S, Harmer AR, Esch MV, Simic M, Bennell KL: Exercise for osteoarthritis of the knee, *Cochrane Database of Systematic Reviews*, 2015, Available at: https://doi.org/10.1002/14651858.cd004376.pub3.

Henrotin Yves, et al: Curcumin: a new paradigm and therapeutic opportunity for the treatment of osteoarthritis: curcumin for osteoarthritis management, *SpringerPlus* 2(1), 2013, Available at: https://doi.org/10.1186/2193-1801-2-56.

Hochberg MC, Altman RD, April KT, et al: American College of Rheumatology 2012 recommendations for the use of nonpharmacologic and pharmacologic therapies in osteoarthritis of the hand, hip, and knee, *Arthritis Care & Research* 64(4):465–474, 2012, Available at: https://doi.org/10.1002/acr.21596.

Idres FA, Samaan M. Intra-articular platelet-rich plasma vs. corticosteroid injections efficacy in knee osteoarthritis treatment: a systematic review, *Ann Med Surg (Lond)*, 6;85(2):102–110, 2023. https://doi.org/10.1097/MS9.0000000000000106.

Kohn MD, Sassoon AA, Fernando ND: Classifications in Brief: Kellgren-Lawrence Classification of Osteoarthritis, *Clin Orthop Relat Res* 474(8):1886–1893, 2016, Available at: https://doi.org/10.1007/s11999-016-4732-4.

Lin KY, et al: Intra-articular injection of platelet-rich plasma is superior to hyaluronic acid or saline solution in the treatment of mild to moderate knee osteoarthritis: a randomized, double-blind, triple-parallel, placebo-controlled clinical trial, *Arthroscopy* 35(1):106–117, 2019 Jan, Available at: https://doi.org/10.1016/j.arthro.2018.06.035. PubMed PMID: 30611335.

Laudy ABM, Bakker EWP, Rekers M, et al: Efficacy of platelet-rich plasma injections in osteoarthritis of the knee: a systematic review and meta-analysis, *Br J Sports Med*, 49:657–672, 2015.

McGrory B, Weber K, Jevsevar D, Sevarino K: Surgical management of osteoarthritis of the knee, *Journal of the American Academy of Orthopaedic Surgeons* 24(8), 2016, Available at: https://doi.org/10.5435/JAAOS-D-16-00159.

Migliorini F, Driessen A, Quack V, et al: Comparison between intra-articular infiltrations of placebo, steroids, hyaluronic and PRP for knee osteoarthritis: a Bayesian network meta-analysis, *Arch Orthop Trauma Surg*, https://doi.org/10.1007/s00402-020-03551-y.

Moyer RF, Birmingham TB, Bryant DM, et al: Valgus bracing for knee osteoarthritis: a meta-analysis of randomized trials, *Arthritis Care & Research* 67(4):493–501, 2015, Available at: https://doi.org/10.1002/acr.22472.

Nakagawa Yasuaki, et al: Short-term effects of highly-bioavailable curcumin for treating knee osteoarthritis: a randomized, double-blind, placebo-controlled prospective study, *Journal of Orthopaedic Science* 19(6):933–939, 2014, Available at: https://doi.org/10.1007/s00776-014-0633-0.

Oneill TW, Mccabe PS, Mcbeth J: Update on the epidemiology, risk factors and disease outcomes of osteoarthritis, *Best Practice & Research Clinical Rheumatology* 32(2):312–326, 2018, Available at: https://doi.org/10.1016/j.berh.2018.10.007.

Pas HI, Winters M, Haisma HJ, et al: Stem cell injections in knee osteoarthritis: a systematic review of the literature, *Br J Sports Med* 51(15):1125–1133, 2017 Aug, Available at: https://doi.org/10.1136/bjsports-2016-096793. Epub 2017 Mar 3. Review PubMed PMID: 28258177.

Sanders TL, Pareek A, Kremers HM: Long-term follow-up of isolated ACL tears treated without ligament reconstruction, *Knee Surgery, Sports Traumatology, Arthroscopy* 25(2):493–500, 2016, Available at: https://doi.org/10.1007/s00167-016-4172-4.

Siemieniuk RAC, Harris IA, Agoritsas T, et al: Arthroscopic surgery for degenerative knee arthritis and meniscal tears: a clinical practice guideline, *BMJ* 357, 2017https://doi.org/10.1136/bmj.j1982.

Sihvonen R, Paavola M, Malmivaara A, et al: *Br J Sports Med* 54:1332–1339, 2020.

Smithers CJ, Young AA, Walch G: Reverse shoulder arthroplasty, *Curr Rev Musculoskelet Med* 4(4):183–190, 2011, Available at: https://doi.org/10.1007/s12178-011-9097-4.

Towheed TE, Maxwell L, Anastassiades TP, et al: Glucosamine therapy for treating osteoarthritis, *Cochrane Database Syst Rev* (2)CD002946, 2005 Apr 18. Review PubMed PMID: 15846645.

Tsoukas D, Fotopoulos V, Basdekis G, Makridis KG: No difference in osteoarthritis after surgical and non-surgical treatment of ACL-injured knees after 10 years, *Knee Surgery, Sports Traumatology, Arthroscopy* 24(9):2953–2959, 2015, Available at: https://doi.org/10.1007/s00167-015-3593-9.

OSTEOPOROSIS

Method of
Alexei O. DeCastro, MD; Scott Bragg, PharmD; and Peter Carek, MD, MS

CURRENT DIAGNOSIS

- Screen for osteoporosis with bone mineral density (BMD) testing in females aged 65 years and older or in postmenopausal females younger than 65 at increased risk of osteoporosis.
- Current evidence is insufficient to recommend screening for osteoporosis in males.
- The radiographic definition of osteoporosis in postmenopausal females and males over 50 is a T-score ≤–2.5 at the femoral neck, total hip, or lumbar spine.
- Clinical osteoporosis can be diagnosed after a fragility fracture (i.e., low-trauma fracture to the vertebrae, proximal femur, distal radius, humerus, pelvis, proximal tibia, ribs).
- Consider decision support tools like the fracture risk assessment tool from the World Health Organization to assist in screening and treatment decisions.
- In patients with a fragility fracture, BMD testing is recommended to determine the severity of the disorder and guide treatment decisions.
- Consider workup of secondary causes of osteoporosis and risk factors for falls.
- Current evidence is insufficient to recommend routine vertebral fracture assessment and trabecular bone scores, although they may improve fracture risk assessment.

CURRENT THERAPY

- Recommend aspects of a healthy lifestyle including adequate intake of calcium and vitamin D, regular physical activity, adequate sleep, fall prevention strategies, and other lifestyle modifications (e.g., stop smoking, alcohol consumption in moderation).

- Mixed evidence exists on the benefit of taking calcium and vitamin D for primary prevention of osteoporotic fracture in adults over age 50. For secondary prevention, at least 1200 mg/day of calcium and 800 to 1000 IU/day of vitamin D are recommended. Dietary sources are preferred, but supplements may be necessary to meet goals.
- Mind-body, resistance, and aerobic exercise may reduce the risk of falls and fractures.
- Drug treatment for osteoporosis should prioritize evidence-based treatments that reduce vertebral, nonvertebral, and hip fracture. Therapies with better patient-oriented evidence include alendronate (Fosamax), risedronate (Actonel), zoledronic acid (Reclast), denosumab (Prolia), teriparatide (Forteo), abaloparatide (Tymlos), or romosozumab (Evenity).
- Pharmacologic treatment should be considered in patients with a fragility fracture, radiographic evidence of osteoporosis, and those with low bone mass and high 10-year fracture risk (i.e., 10-year hip fracture probability ≥3%, 10-year major osteoporosis-related fracture ≥20%).
- Treatment of premenopausal females, males younger than 50 years old, and adolescents with osteoporosis is controversial due to a lack of long-term safety and efficacy studies. A Z-score ≤–2.0 indicates osteoporosis, but treatment is often reserved for patients at very high fracture risk or patients with multiple fragility fractures.

Osteoporosis is a metabolic bone disease characterized by low bone mass and structural deterioration of bone tissue, which is associated with decreased bone strength and increased susceptibility to fractures. Its clinical relevance is increasing because of population growth of older adults and high morbidity and mortality associated with the disease. Osteoporosis is asymptomatic until a patient has a fracture, so identifying patients at high fracture risk is important. Once a vertebral fracture is present, patients may develop back pain, height loss, and/or thoracic kyphosis. Hip fractures can cause thigh or groin pain, typically limit a patient's mobility, and are associated with high rates of morbidity and mortality. Primary or secondary prevention of fractures in patients with osteoporosis is a challenge because screening on a population level is difficult, screening recommendations differ between organizations, and osteoporosis treatments have many risks.

The World Health Organization (WHO) defines radiographic osteoporosis as a bone mineral density (BMD) that is 2.5 or more standard deviations below the mean for a young, healthy person (*T*-score ≤–2.5). The BMD is assessed by dual-energy x-ray absorptiometry (DEXA) at the lumbar spine, total hip, and femoral neck. A clinical diagnosis of osteoporosis may be made if a patient has a fragility fracture, defined as a low-trauma fracture to the vertebrae, proximal femur, distal radius, humerus, pelvis, proximal tibia, or ribs. Low bone mass, previously known as osteopenia, is a milder degree of bone loss (*T*-score of –1.0 to –2.4). Although the risk of fracture increases significantly with decreasing BMD, large observational studies have demonstrated that osteoporotic fractures can occur across a wide spectrum of BMDs. Osteoporotic fractures may occur secondary to low bone quantity and/or poor bone quality that is not measured by DEXA scans. Qualitative determinants of bone strength are rarely assessed in practice but include trabecular bone scores, microcracks, mineralization defects, bone geometry, cell death, changes in bone size, and changes in bone turnover.

Epidemiology

Osteoporosis is the most common metabolic disorder of the skeleton. Based on 2018 data in the United States of adults over age 50, the prevalence of osteoporosis in females was 35.6% and in males it was 10.7%. Worldwide, the prevalence of osteoporosis and osteopenia was estimated at 19.7% and 40.4% of older adults based on a 2022 meta-analysis. For patients with osteoporosis, the lifetime risk of a fragility fracture is estimated to be 65% in females and 42% in males. Hip fractures are the most feared fragility fracture because they cause a mortality rate of 10% to 20% at 12 months, and up to 25% of those with hip fractures require long-term nursing care.

Despite screening recommendations and the ability to make a clinical diagnosis, many females with osteoporosis go unrecognized and untreated. In one study from an insurance claims database, less than 50% of females with a fragility fracture had an osteoporosis diagnosis within 1 year of the fracture, and less than 30% were treated with pharmacologic therapy.

Screening

Universal DEXA screening in all females older than 65 years and postmenopausal females at high fracture risk is important. Nonmodifiable risk factors include genetic background, advancing age, female sex, personal history of fracture, and family history of fracture in a first-degree relative. Modifiable risk factors include low body weight, hormonal deficiencies, smoking, alcohol misuse, an inactive lifestyle, and a diet low in calcium and vitamin D. In addition, certain medications affect calcium absorption or skeletal homeostasis, thereby increasing fracture risk. Routine assessment and minimizing high-risk medications (e.g., glucocorticoids, aromatase inhibitors, antiandrogen therapy, calcineurin inhibitors, enzyme-inducing anticonvulsants, proton pump inhibitors, antidepressants), when possible, can lower fracture risk. Other comorbid illnesses (e.g., chronic kidney disease, endocrine disorders, chronic inflammatory conditions) increase the risk of secondary osteoporosis, but better control of the underlying condition may reduce this risk.

Several decision support tools are available to identify patients at high risk for fracture. The most common risk assessment is the Fracture Risk Assessment Tool (FRAX), which incorporates easy-to-identify risk factors, helps determine the appropriateness of a DEXA, and provides a 10-year absolute fracture risk. Factors considered by FRAX include BMD of the femoral neck, previous fracture history, family history of fracture, age, sex, race/ethnicity, glucocorticoid use, alcohol misuse, current smoking status, and secondary osteoporosis causes. Though FRAX incorporates DEXA results, it does not require this information to estimate fracture risk. Inclusion of race/ethnicity in FRAX is controversial and may perpetuate inequities in care because people of color may have an underestimated risk and not be considered for antiresorptive treatment.

Other fracture risk assessment tools include the Simple Calculated Osteoporosis Risk Estimation (SCORE), the Osteoporosis Self-Assessment Tool (OST), and the Osteoporosis Risk Assessment Instrument (ORAI). These tools may be reasonable alternatives to FRAX because they can assess the need for a DEXA, rely on fewer factors than FRAX, and have comparable sensitivities for fracture assessment.

Screening recommendations vary across major practice guidelines. The U.S. Preventive Services Task Force (USPSTF) recommends screening for osteoporosis in females older than 65 years old (grade B recommendation) and in postmenopausal females younger than 65 who are at equal or greater risk of osteoporosis compared with an average 65-year-old female (grade B recommendation). It is important to note that if the 10-year fracture risk with FRAX is ≥9.3% in a patient less than 65 years old, then pursuing a DEXA scan is valuable to improve risk prediction and treatment decisions. Currently, the USPSTF guidelines state that insufficient evidence is available to support screening for osteoporosis in males. The Bone Health and Osteoporosis Foundation (BHOF) and the International Society for Clinical Densitometry recommend similar screening recommendations in females. They differ from USPSTF, though, by recommending screening in all males 70 years and older and males 50 to 69 years of age with elevated risk.

Other screening risk assessments, such as vertebral imaging and trabecular bone scores, may be considered in addition to DEXA scans to help identify asymptomatic vertebral fractures

or to quantify bone microarchitecture. These techniques may help better characterize 10-year fracture risk or guide pharmacologic treatment decisions, although neither vertebral imaging nor trabecular bone scores are discussed in the USPSTF guidelines because of limited data with these screening modalities relevant to improving patient-oriented outcomes.

The optimal rescreening interval remains unclear after an initial DEXA scan. Most guidelines recommend retesting after 2 to 3 years of antiresorptive therapy or in high-risk individuals not treated on medications. In patients receiving bisphosphonate therapy, a baseline DEXA and a repeat at 3 years may be a cost-effective strategy to minimize the number of DEXA scans if a patient improves as expected and is then able to begin a drug holiday. Data from Gourlay and colleagues suggests that waiting for 15 years to rescreen is a reasonable strategy in low-risk individuals with a normal T-score at baseline. Based on the same data, a rescreening period of 5 years is sensible in patients with low bone mass. Shared decision making should be used to determine when to stop screening because patient risk factors and life expectancy vary significantly.

Pathophysiology

A patient's BMD correlates strongly with subsequent fracture, which makes it an important screening and assessment tool, but other factors also influence risk. Several factors that lead to decreased bone strength include small bone size, increased length of the femoral neck, cortical porosity, and decreased viability of osteocytes.

Peak bone mass typically occurs in an individual's third decade of life. Differences in the peak bone mass may be secondary to genetic, hormonal, and environmental variables. Increases in body size and skeletal load play a role in determining peak bone mass. Physical activity during childhood enhances bone mass, whereas chronic diseases during childhood may decrease BMD. The contribution of single-gene polymorphisms to osteoporosis risk is unclear because osteoporosis is a polygenic disease and genetic variants seem to have small effect on BMD and fracture risk.

Bone resorption begins to overtake bone formation with advancing age. Hormonal deficiency causes bone loss because testosterone and estrogen help determine bone homeostasis (i.e., osteoclast-induced bone resorption vs. osteoblast-supported bone formation). In females, rapid estrogen loss after menopause initially affects trabecular bone density. After a few years, bone loss continues to occur more slowly and primarily affects cortical sites. During this phase, fewer osteoblasts are active, which reduces bone formation. Males are less likely to develop bone loss because of greater bone mass during puberty and no sudden loss of sex hormone production. Increasing age is an independent risk factor for bone loss. Another contributing factor is loss of muscle strength and coordination, which increases the risk for falls and fragility fractures.

Clinical Manifestations

There are typically no clinical manifestations of osteoporosis until a patient has a fracture. Patients may have height loss, back pain, and thoracic kyphosis after experiencing a vertebral fracture. Manifestations stemming from thoracic kyphosis could include dyspnea or constipation. Hip fractures typically result from a fall and are associated with pain, swelling, bruising, skeletal deformities, and a limited range of motion. Significant pain is often seen with both vertebral and hip fractures, although some patients may present with asymptomatic vertebral fractures that can be clinically inconspicuous. Functional disability is common after a fracture and may require rehabilitation to improve long-term functional status.

Diagnosis

Osteoporosis can be diagnosed radiographically or after a fragility fracture (i.e., low-trauma fracture to the vertebrae, proximal femur, distal radius, humerus, pelvis, proximal tibia, ribs).

Low-trauma fractures occur when falling from standing height or lower. The initial evaluation after a fragility fracture should include a personal and family history, pain assessment, evaluation for secondary osteoporosis causes, a physical examination, labs, and imaging tests. Most cases of osteoporosis are diagnosed by a screening DEXA of the total hip, femoral neck, or lumbar spine. Bone mass measurements by DEXA must be interpreted in relation to the patient's age, fracture history, family history, previous medication use, timing of menopause (only for females), and other concomitant disorders. Vertebral fracture assessment is another imaging modality that may augment risk assessment decisions when performed during a DEXA. A vertebral fracture assessment involves a spine radiograph and may identify asymptomatic vertebral fractures, which strongly correlate with future symptomatic vertebral fractures.

DEXA results are expressed as a *T*-score or a *Z*-score. The WHO established the *T*-score as the standard deviation (SD) difference between an individual's BMD compared with a sex- and race/ethnicity-matched young adult reference population. The *T*-score should be used for males aged 50 and older and postmenopausal females. A *T*-score that is –2.5 SD or more above the mean is diagnostic of osteoporosis, whereas a *T*-score that is between –1.0 and –2.4 SD below the mean is defined as low bone mass. Severe osteoporosis is defined as having a *T*-score of –2.5 SD or below plus a fragility fracture. Bone density measurements may be different across various bone sites in the same patient. These discrepancies may be related to differences in skeletal compartments (trabecular vs. cortical) at distinct sites. To classify the degree of osteoporosis, use the lowest *T*-score from the lumbar spine, total hip, or femoral neck.

The *Z*-score is the SD difference between a patient's BMD compared with a reference population matched for age, sex, and race/ethnicity. A low *Z*-score of –2.0 SD or below indicates osteoporosis and can identify patients in need of further workup or even osteoporosis treatment. *Z*-scores should be used in the evaluation of adult males younger than age 50, premenopausal females, and adolescents. Less evidence exists for characterizing the severity of disease and need for osteoporosis treatment in these populations, making patient care decisions difficult. Further research is needed to identify younger patients in need of screening with *Z*-scores and whether osteoporosis treatment for these patients changes long-term patient-oriented outcomes.

Prevention

Prevention of osteoporosis is important because bone loss with aging is difficult to treat. Lower peak bone mass established in early adulthood may determine bone strength and fracture risk decades later. Therefore prevention starts with good nutrition, maintenance of a healthy body weight, and weight-bearing exercise to optimize bone mass during adolescence and early adulthood. All patients should be counseled on avoiding smoking or reducing use if patients are unwilling to fully quit. Alcohol consumption should be limited to ≤2 drinks per day in males and ≤1 drink per day in females to lower fracture risk. Complete abstinence from alcohol remains a topic of debate, with the WHO recommending that no level of alcohol consumption should be considered safe when considering cancer and other risks. Interestingly, a 2022 meta-analysis showed that moderate alcohol intake (i.e., 1–2 drinks in males, 1 drink in females) is associated with higher BMD compared with higher intake or abstinence.

To inform treatment decisions, identifying secondary causes of osteoporosis is important. Examples of conditions causing secondary osteoporosis include rheumatoid arthritis, chronic kidney disease, multiple myeloma, hyperthyroidism, and hypogonadism. Better control of a comorbid condition causing secondary osteoporosis may reduce the risk of fracture. Medications that are harmful to bone health should be monitored and reevaluated when possible. Stopping medications associated with osteoporosis is reasonable after having a shared decision-making discussion with a patient to identify their preferences, the magnitude of benefits and risks from the drug, and whether treatment alternatives exist.

Primary prevention with bisphosphonates in postmenopausal patients with normal BMD or low bone mass can be considered as treatment may increase BMD and reduce subsequent fractures. Consult dosing guides if using a bisphosphonate for prevention versus treatment because lower doses or less frequent dosing intervals may be recommended. An interesting new study on zoledronic acid (Reclast) with doses at baseline and a repeat dose in 5 years[1] showed significant reductions in fragility fractures, any fractures, and major osteoporotic fractures.

Conversely, a 2022 systematic review commissioned by the USPSTF on hormone therapy for primary prevention of chronic conditions notably found more risk than benefit in postmenopausal patients with or without a hysterectomy (grade D recommendation). As a result, hormone therapy should be avoided if being used for osteoporosis primary prevention alone but may be considered if treating other conditions like vasomotor symptoms of menopause.

Calcium and vitamin D are both physiologically vital in bone formation. Studies are conflicting on the benefits of calcium and vitamin D_1 for primary prevention of fracture in older adults. Several studies with higher potential for bias have shown increases in BMD and reduction of fracture risk in high-risk adult patients given both calcium and vitamin D. As a result, the BHOF recommends 1200 mg of elemental calcium and 800 to 1000 IU of vitamin D_1 daily for postmenopausal females[1]. However, recent studies with lower potential for bias do not support calcium or vitamin D to reduce the risk of fractures or to increase BMD in older adults when used in primary prevention. Concerns about renal adverse events, particularly nephrolithiasis, exist with calcium consumption. Several studies have also raised concern that calcium supplements may increase coronary artery calcification, but evidence of harm on long-term patient-oriented outcomes remains unclear.

Treatment

Nonpharmacologic Therapy

Nondrug therapy for preventing fractures in patients with osteoporosis includes addressing fall risk factors. Common but preventable causes of falls may include vision deficits, gait abnormalities, dizziness, and balance problems. Referral to a physical therapist may help address both balance and gait issues while improving muscle strength. Performing a formal home safety evaluation and modifying a patient's living environment may reduce fall risk by improving lighting, using assistive devices, and removing home hazards. Frequent medication assessments are also important and may reduce the risk of falls if stopping ineffective or potentially inappropriate medications like those outlined by the American Geriatric Society Beers Criteria.

Regular physical activity with mind-body, aerobic, and resistance exercises are effective in increasing spine BMD. Patients should exercise at least 30 minutes three times per week incorporating a balance of moderate-intensity aerobic and resistance activity. Some evidence exists that high-intensity resistance and impact training in a closely supervised setting can provide greater benefit on BMD improvement than low impact exercise at home. In individuals experiencing a fragility fracture, acute or subacute rehab remains an important intervention to reduce long-term morbidity.

A balanced diet may reduce fall risk by preventing dehydration and ensuring that micronutrients support improved balance, muscle strength, and bone health. Although benefits with calcium and vitamin D on primary prevention remain unclear, adequate calcium and vitamin D consumption should be encouraged when used with antiresorptive therapies (e.g., bisphosphonates, denosumab) to reduce the risk of hypocalcemia and to ensure optimal effectiveness. Because optimal doses are not established, a daily intake of at least 1200 mg of calcium and 800 to 1000 IU of vitamin D_1 is recommended for all females over age 50 and all males

---

[1] Not FDA approved for this indication.

over age 70 by the BHOF. Calcium and vitamin D supplements are often used because of low dietary consumption and reduced vitamin D creation with decreased sun exposure in older adults. Both calcium carbonate and calcium citrate can be used, but caution should be used because of constipation and gastrointestinal disturbances.

Goal vitamin D levels and the optimal dosing strategy remain unclear, with mixed evidence on different goal values and replacement strategies. Some studies suggest that a serum 25-hydroxyvitamin D level of at least 30 ng/mL is needed to reduce falls and to improve physical function in the elderly. However, many experts advocate for treating only severely low 25-hydroxyvitamin D values <20 ng/mL because there is a lack of high-quality studies showing better patient-oriented outcomes with a treatment goal of ≥30 ng/mL. In patients with confirmed vitamin D insufficiency, administration of 50,000 IU of oral ergocalciferol (vitamin D$_2$ [Drisdol])[1] once weekly for 8 to 12 weeks was thought to be safe and effective. However, studies from 2015 to 2020 have shown that high-dose vitamin D may increase the risk of falls. Administration of vitamin D 1000 to 2000 IU per day with titration to 4000 IU per day remains a reasonable alternative. After starting vitamin D, a repeat serum 25-hydroxyvitamin D value can be obtained, but a goal value remains unclear.

Pharmacologic Treatment

All drugs approved by the U.S. Food and Drug Administration for treating osteoporosis reduce vertebral fracture risk. The antifracture effects of these medications are thought to be related to an increase in BMD and an improvement in qualitative measures of bone strength. For a summary of drug treatment dosing and prevention evidence on different types of fracture, see Table 1.

Bisphosphonates are often considered first-line medications because they work to reduce all types of osteoporotic fracture, are reasonably safe, can be taken orally, and are relatively inexpensive. The bisphosphonates reduce osteoclast resorption through the inhibition of farnesyl diphosphate synthase, a key enzyme that supports osteoclast activity. Alendronate (Fosamax) and risedronate (Actonel) are the preferred oral bisphosphonates based on their evidence of benefit. These drugs should be taken weekly to improve effectiveness and minimize adverse effects. Ibandronate (Boniva) is an alternative bisphosphonate that comes orally or in an intravenous (IV) formulation, but its antifracture data is weaker considering there is no evidence that it prevents against hip fractures. Zoledronic acid (Reclast) is the preferred IV bisphosphonate and is given as a once-yearly infusion. Zoledronic acid is the only osteoporosis therapy shown to reduce all-cause mortality and may be a preferred treatment in those who cannot tolerate or are nonadherent to oral bisphosphonates.

Treatment with a bisphosphonate after fracture historically has been delayed with theoretical concerns that treatment soon after surgery could disrupt bone remodeling and fracture healing. Current evidence shows that early administration of bisphosphonates does not impair fracture healing and in fact lowers the risk of subsequent fractures compared with delayed administration. A patient's life expectancy should be considered when contemplating treatment because bisphosphonates need to be used for 12 to 18 months before having antifracture benefit.

Side effects of oral bisphosphonates include esophageal and gastric irritation, musculoskeletal pain, nephrotoxicity, and hypocalcemia. Oral bisphosphonates must be taken with a full glass of plain tap water, and a 30- to 60-minute wait is required before eating or reclining to improve drug absorption and reduce gastrointestinal adverse effects. Intravenous zoledronic acid is associated with infusion reactions, nephrotoxicity, hypocalcemia, and atrial fibrillation. Patients with stage 4 or 5 chronic kidney disease should avoid all bisphosphonates with the concern for nephrotoxicity.

Atypical femur fractures and osteonecrosis of the jaw are rare but serious concerns with bisphosphonate therapy. Atypical femur fractures with bisphosphonates appear are seen more frequently in cohort studies when having higher cumulative doses and extended treatment durations. Young females are particularly prone to these fractures, which often require surgical intervention. Prodromal symptoms that have been linked to this syndrome include proximal femur pain, evidence of previous stress fracture, or cortical thickening on x-ray. Osteonecrosis of the jaw is another exceedingly rare complication with bisphosphonate use that also occurs with higher cumulative doses and extended treatment durations. While these complications are rare, concern for these events may prevent patients from starting a bisphosphonate.

The ideal duration of bisphosphonate therapy is unknown. Low-risk patients may consider discontinuing therapy after 3 to 5 years once the risks and benefits are weighed. Low-risk patients are defined as those that have a T-score that improves into a low bone mass range or normal range and have not had recent fragility fractures. In low-risk individuals, benefits from the initial bisphosphonate course may last for another 5 years or longer. High-risk patients (e.g., patients with a T-score still below −2.5, having recent fragility fractures) could have continued benefit of reducing vertebral fractures with bisphosphonates up to 10 years, but other types of fractures do not seem to be reduced, and the risk of complications (e.g., atypical fractures, osteonecrosis of the jaw, atrial fibrillation with zoledronic acid, esophageal irritation with oral bisphosphonates) may increase.

Denosumab (Prolia) is a monoclonal antibody that works similarly to estrogen by stopping osteoclast formation through inhibition of the receptor activator of nuclear factor κB ligand (RANKL) system. It is approved for treatment of males and postmenopausal females with osteoporosis who are at high risk for fracture and is given as a subcutaneous injection every 6 months. Like the preferred bisphosphonates, denosumab may significantly reduce the risk of vertebral, nonvertebral, and hip fractures compared with placebo. Unlike bisphosphonates, denosumab could be considered in patients with advanced chronic kidney disease with close monitoring for hypocalcemia.

Common side effects of denosumab include skin rash, upper respiratory tract infections, arthralgias, back pain, diarrhea, and hypocalcemia. The risk of severe hypocalcemia is high in patients with advanced kidney disease on dialysis, which prompted the FDA to issue a boxed warning in January 2024. Long-term risks of atypical fractures and osteonecrosis of the jaw have been reported with denosumab-like bisphosphonates, so it is recommended to reevaluate the need for continued treatment after 3 to 5 years. Starting sequential therapy with another osteoporosis treatment after stopping denosumab is recommended to avoid posttreatment decline in BMD, which starts around 9 to 10 months after the last dose.

Estrogen (e.g., conjugated equine estrogen [Premarin]), selective estrogen receptor modulators (e.g., raloxifene [Evista]), and mixed agents (e.g., bazedoxifene/conjugated equine estrogen [Duavee]) remain a niche treatment option with evidence of benefit but also many risks. These agents inhibit osteoclast apoptosis and secretion of osteoprotegerin on osteoblasts, which reduces osteoclast production. Conjugated equine estrogen is effective at reducing all types of fractures but is not recommended by USPSTF in primary prevention because of potential serious consequences. Complications associated with estrogen include thromboembolism, stroke, myocardial infarction, and some types of cancer. Raloxifene, on the other hand, improves BMD and reduces the risk of vertebral fractures but not nonvertebral or hip fractures. Unfortunately, raloxifene can exacerbate vasomotor symptoms (e.g., hot flashes, sweating) and increase the risk of thromboembolic events. Raloxifene may be considered in postmenopausal patients with osteoporosis who cannot tolerate other treatments or in postmenopausal females at high breast cancer risk. The combination of bazedoxifene and conjugated equine estrogens is approved for prevention of postmenopausal osteoporosis, but its use is not recommended by USPSTF for primary prevention of osteoporosis secondary to complications seen with estrogen therapy.

MEDICATION	ROUTE	DOSE/FREQUENCY	CLINICAL EVIDENCE OF EFFICACY		
			VERTEBRAL	HIP	NONVERTEBRAL
Alendronate (Fosamax)	Oral	Treatment: 70 mg weekly Prevention: 35 mg weekly	+	+	+
Risedronate (Actonel)	Oral	Prevention or treatment: 35 mg weekly or 150 mg monthly	+	+	+
Zoledronic acid (Reclast)	IV	Treatment: 5 mg yearly Prevention: 5 mg every 2 years or 5 mg once	+	+	+
Ibandronate (Boniva)	Oral	Prevention or treatment: 150 mg monthly	+	−	+
	IV	Treatment: 3 mg every 3 months	+	−	+
Denosumab (Prolia) Denosumab-bbdz (Jubbonti)	SubQ	Treatment: 60 mg every 6 months	+	+	+
Abaloparatide (Tymlos)	SubQ	Treatment: 80 µg daily	+	−	+
Teriparatide (Forteo, Bonsity)	SubQ	Treatment: 20 µg daily	+	−	+
Romosozumab (Evenity)	SubQ	Treatment: 210 mg monthly	+	+	+
Raloxifene (Evista)	Oral	Prevention or treatment: 60 mg daily	+	−	−
Bazedoxifene/ conjugated equine estrogen (Duavee)[1]	Oral	Prevention: 20/0.45 mg daily	+	−	+
Conjugated equine estrogen (Premarin)[1]	Oral	Prevention: 0.3–1.25 mg daily	+	+	+
Calcitonin (Miacalcin)	Nasal	200 IU (1 spray in one nostril) daily	+	−	−
	IM or SubQ	100 IU daily	+	−	−

[1]Not FDA approved for this indication.
IM, Intramuscular; *IU*, international units; *IV*, intravenous; *SubQ*, subcutaneous.

Calcitonin (Miacalcin) remains a short-term treatment option after vertebral fractures to reduce pain, but weak osteoporosis evidence and long-term concerns should limit use. Calcitonin works through a different mechanism by inhibiting osteoclast activity through the calcitonin receptor, but unfortunately only has benefit on reducing the risk of vertebral fractures. There are also concerns that long-term use is associated with a higher risk for malignancy.

Parathyroid hormones (i.e., teriparatide [Forteo], abaloparatide [Tymlos]) have recognized antifracture effects on both vertebral and nonvertebral sites compared with active bisphosphonate treatment, but these are typically reserved for patients with more severe osteoporosis. Unfortunately, there is mixed data on whether they reduce the risk of hip fracture compared with bisphosphonates. Parathyroid hormones stimulate osteoblast bone formation and increase serum calcium absorption in the gastrointestinal tract and reabsorption through the renal tubules. Adverse effects may include orthostatic hypotension, hypercalcemia, nausea, arthralgia, risk of renal stones, and leg cramps. Maintaining adequate calcium and vitamin D is recommended while taking parathyroid hormones, but caution should be exercised to avoid hypercalcemia.

Currently, parathyroid hormone analogs should be limited to 2 years and reserved for patients with very high fracture risk (e.g., severe osteoporosis, *T*-score <−3) or refractory to other agents. Parathyroid hormones can only be used for 2 years based on concerns for osteosarcoma, which has only been seen in laboratory animals exposed to high doses. Consequently, parathyroid hormones are contraindicated in patients with risk of osteosarcoma, such as those with Paget disease of the bone, previous skeletal radiation, or unexplained elevations of alkaline phosphatase. No evidence exists for combining parathyroid hormones with other osteoporosis treatments at the same time. However, it is recommended that after stopping a parathyroid hormone, sequential therapy with an antiresorptive should be started to avoid post-treatment bone loss.

Romosozumab (Evenity) is a monoclonal antibody often reserved for patients with severe osteoporosis secondary to safety concerns. Romosozumab works by binding and inhibiting sclerostin, which is a glycoprotein that inhibits osteoblast bone formation and, to a lesser degree, increases osteoclast bone resorption. There is robust evidence showing better effectiveness at reducing hip, vertebral, and nonvertebral fractures compared head to head with alendronate over 24 months. Preliminary studies on romosozumab raised concern for a higher risk of myocardial infarction and stroke, but these risks were not seen in all trials and long-term safety monitoring is ongoing. Romosozumab should be reserved for patients at very high fracture risk (e.g., severe osteoporosis, *T*-score <−3) or refractory to other antiresorptives because of safety concerns and high costs. When romosozumab is used, it is given as two consecutive subcutaneous injections (total dose of 210 mg) once every month for up to 1 year. Like other treatments, except bisphosphonates, sequential therapy with another antiresorptive medication is recommended to avoid bone loss after stopping treatment.

References

American Geriatrics Society Beers Criteria® Update Expert Panel: American Geriatrics Society 2023 updated AGS Beers Criteria® for potentially inappropriate medication use in older adults, *J Am Geriatr Soc* 71(7):2052–2081, 2023.

Barrionuevo P, Kapoor E, Noor A, et al: Efficacy of pharmacological therapies for the prevention of fractures in postmenopausal women: a network meta-analysis, *J Clin Endocrinol Metab* 104(5):1623–1630, 2019.

Bischoff-Ferrari HA, Dawson-Hughes B, Orav EJ, et al: Monthly high-dose vitamin D treatment for the prevention of functional decline: a randomized clinical trial, *JAMA Intern Med* 176(2):175–183, 2016.

Bolland MJ, Leung W, Tai V, et al: Calcium intake and risk of fracture: systematic review, *BMJ* 351, 2015:h4580.

Bolland MJ, Nisa Z, Mellar A, et al: Fracture prevention with infrequent zoledronate in women 50 to 60 years of age, *N Engl J Med* 392(3):239–248, 2025.

Chen SJ, Chen YJ, Cheng CH, et al: Comparisons of different screening tools for identifying fracture/osteoporosis risk among community-dwelling older people, *Medicine (Baltim)* 95(20):e3415, 2016.

Chen Y, Liu R, Hettinghouse A, et al: Clinical application of teriparatide in fracture prevention: a systematic review, *JBJS Rev* 7(1):e10, 2019.

Final Recommendation Statement: *Osteoporosis to prevent fractures: screening*, U.S. Preventive Services Task Force, 2025. https://www.uspreventiveservicestaskforce.org/uspstf/recommendation/osteoporosis-screening. .

Fink HA, MacDonald R, Forte ML, et al: Long-term drug therapy and drug holidays for osteoporosis fracture prevention: a systematic review. In *Comparative effectiveness review No. 218. (Prepared by the Minnesota evidence-based practice center under contract No. 290-2015-00008-I) AHRQ publication No. 19-EHC016-EF*, Rockville, MD, 2019, Agency for Healthcare Research and Quality.

Godos J, Giampieri F, Chisari E, et al: Alcohol consumption, bone mineral density, and risk of osteoporotic fractures: a dose-response meta-analysis, *Int J Environ Res Public Health* 19(3):1515, 2022.

Gourlay ML, Fine JP, Preisser JS, et al: Bone-density testing interval and transition to osteoporosis in older women, *N Engl J Med* 366(3):225–233, 2012.

Guirguis-Blake JM, Perdue LA, Coppola EL, et al: *Interventions to prevent falls in older adults: an evidence update for the U.S. Preventive Services Task Force. Evidence Synthesis No. 236, AHRQ Publication No. 23-05309-EF-1*, Rockville, MD, 2024, Agency for Healthcare Research and Quality.

Jeremiah MP, Unwin BK, Greenawald MH, Casiano VE: Diagnosis and management of osteoporosis, *Am Fam Physician* 92(4):261–268, 2015.

Khalid S, Calderon-Larranaga S, Sami A, et al: Comparative risk of acute myocardial infarction for anti-osteoporosis drugs in primary care: a meta-analysis of propensity-matched cohort findings from the UK Clinical Practice Research Database and the Catalan SIDIAP Database, *Osteoporos Int* 33(7):1579–1589, 2022.

LeBoff MS, Greenspan SL, Insogna KL, et al: The clinician's guide to prevention and treatment of osteoporosis, *Osteoporos Int* 33(10):2049–2102, 2022.

Lyles KW, Colon-Emeric CS, Magaziner JS, et al: Zoledronic acid and clinical fractures and mortality after hip fracture, *N Engl J Med* 357(18):1799–1809, 2007.

Naso CM, Lin S, Song G, et al: Time trend analysis of osteoporosis prevalence among adults 50 years of age and older in the USA, 2005–2018, *Osteoporos Int* 36(3):547–554, 2025.

Qaseem A, Hicks LA, Etxeandia-Ikobaltzeta I, et al: Pharmacologic treatment of primary osteoporosis or low bone mass to prevent fractures in adults: a living clinical guideline from the American College of Physicians, *Ann Intern Med* 176(2):224–238, 2023.

Reid HW, Selvan B, Batch BC, Lee RH: The break in FRAX: equity concerns in estimating fracture risk in racial and ethnic minorities, *J Am Geriatr Soc* 69:2692–2695, 2021.

Saag K, Petersen J, Brandi ML, et al: Romosozumab or alendronate for fracture prevention in women with osteoporosis, *N Engl J Med* 377(15):1417–1427, 2017.

U.S. Preventive Services Task Force, Grossman DC, Curry SJ, et al: Vitamin D, calcium, or combined supplementation for the primary prevention of fractures in community-dwelling adults: U.S Preventive Services Task Force recommendation statement, *JAMA* 219(15):1592–1599, 2018.

U.S. Preventive Services Task Force, Mangione CM, Barry MJ, et al: Hormone therapy for the primary prevention of chronic conditions in postmenopausal persons: U.S. Preventive Services Task Force recommendation statement, *JAMA* 328(17):1740–1746, 2022.

Walker MD, Shane E: Postmenopausal osteoporosis, *N Engl J Med* 389(21):1979–1991, 2023.

Watson SL, Weeks BK, Weis LJ, et al: High-intensity resistance and impact training improves bone mineral density and physical function in postmenopausal women with osteopenia and osteoporosis: the LIFTMOR randomized controlled trial, *J Bone Miner Res* 33(2):211–220, 2018.

Weaver J, Sajjan S, Lewiecki EM, Harris ST: Diagnosis and treatment of osteoporosis before and after fracture: a side-by-side analysis of commercially insured and medicare advantage osteoporosis patients, *J Manag Care Spec Pharm* 23(7):735–744, 2017.

Wells GA, Cranney A, Peterson J, et al: Alendronate for the primary and secondary prevention of osteoporotic fractures in postmenopausal women, *Cochrane Database Syst Rev* 1:CD001155, 2008.

Xiao PL, Cui AY, Hsu CJ, et al: Global, regional prevalence, and risk factors of osteoporosis according to the World Health Organization diagnostic criteria: a systematic review and meta-analysis, *Osteoporos Int* 33(10):2137–2153, 2022.

Zhang S, Huang X, Zhao X, et al: Effect of exercise on bone mineral density among patients with osteoporosis and osteopenia: a systematic review and network meta-analysis, *J Clin Nurs* 00:1–12, 2021.

Zhao J, Zeng X, Wang J, Liu L: Association between calcium or vitamin D supplementation and fracture incidence in community-dwelling older adults, *J Am Med Assoc* 318(24):2466–2482, 2017.

PAGET'S DISEASE OF BONE

Method of
Ian R. Reid, MD

CURRENT DIAGNOSIS

- Suspect the presence of Paget's disease in those patients with bone pain, bone deformity, isolated elevation of alkaline phosphatase, or lytic/sclerotic lesions on radiographs.
- Paget's disease is usually diagnosed from plain radiographs.
- Bone scintigraphy identifies the affected bones and allows some assessment of disease activity.
- Biochemical markers of bone turnover allow more precise assessment of turnover and response to therapy.
- Serum total alkaline phosphatase activity is the most cost-effective marker, although bone-specific alkaline phosphatase and procollagen type I N-terminal propeptide (PINP) are marginally more sensitive.

CURRENT THERAPY

- Zoledronate (zoledronic acid, Reclast) 5 mg given as a single infusion over 15 minutes; retreatment is seldom required within 5 years.
- Alendronate (Fosamax) 40 mg/day for 6 months; retreatment may be required between 2 and 6 years.
- Risedronate (Actonel) 30 mg/day for 2 months; retreatment may be required between 1 and 5 years.

Paget's disease is a focal skeletal condition in which one or more bones has a clearly circumscribed area of increased turnover (Figure 1A). Either osteoblasts or osteoclasts may predominate at a given time, resulting in sclerosis or lysis, respectively. Areas that are initially lytic often become sclerotic later, and it is common to see both changes within the same bone (see Figure 1B). Unaffected areas of the skeleton are completely normal, in marked contrast to some rare congenital conditions which are sometimes (inappropriately) referred to as early-onset or juvenile Paget's disease. Such conditions (e.g., familial expansile osteolysis, idiopathic hyperphosphatasia) have different etiologies, clinical presentations, and responses to treatment when compared to Paget's disease.

Etiology

Within pagetic bone, there is a loss of the usual tight control of bone cell function, and the bone-resorbing cells (osteoclasts) and bone-forming cells (osteoblasts) both exhibit overactivity. In the case of osteoclasts, this leads to local areas of bone loss, which can result in deformity or fracture. Osteoblast overactivity leads to the random laying down of new bone, which is disorganized in its structure, mechanically inadequate, and prone to deformity. Osteoblast overactivity can also lead to bone expansion, resulting in bone pain, premature arthritis (if it affects articular surfaces), and nerve compression (e.g., in the spine or skull). Figure 1B shows the effects of osteoblast and osteoclast overactivity on the structure of an affected tibia. The disease progresses along a long bone at a rate of about 1 cm per year, so most patients have had active disease for 1 or more decades before presentation. Typically, the disease progresses until the entire bone is involved. However, Paget's disease does not spread from one bone to another, so the number of affected bones remains constant throughout the disease course.

Paget's disease sometimes runs in families, and about 10% of patients are reported to have an affected relative. This observation has led to much work seeking genetic associations of the condition. It is now apparent that mutations of the gene for sequestosome 1

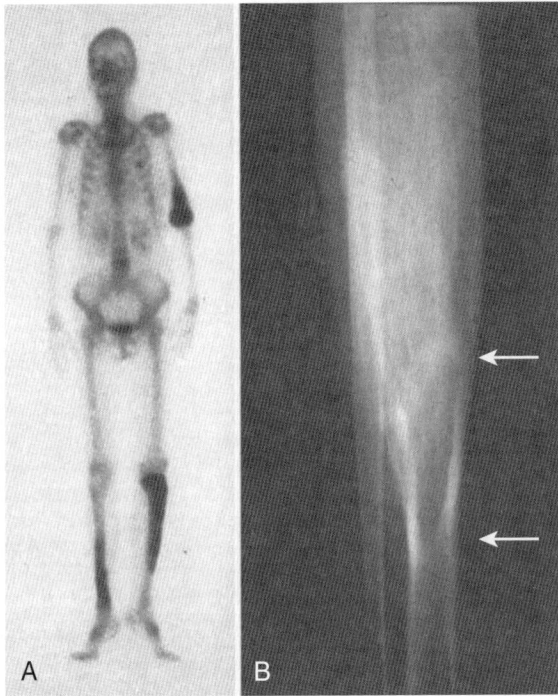

Figure 1 A, Bone scintigram in a patient with Paget's disease, demonstrating the multifocal nature of the condition and the presence of normal bone at other sites. B, Tibia affected by Paget's disease. The upper tibia is of increased density and width as a result of osteoblast overactivity, whereas the lower part of the affected bone shows a lytic region (*between arrows*) resulting from osteoclastic bone resorption. Below this, the bone is normal. Copyright I. R. Reid, used with permission.

are associated with Paget's disease in some families. Other research has focused on possible environmental causes, and a slow viral infection has been suggested. Evidence that the prevalence of Paget's disease has decreased dramatically in recent decades is consistent with altered exposure to an environmental agent. However, both the genetic and environmental hypotheses fail to account for the (multi-) focal nature of the condition, which resembles benign neoplasms resulting from an early single episode of hematogenous spread.

Altered gene expression in osteoblasts and bone marrow stromal cells from pagetic bone has been demonstrated, including increased levels of dickkopf-1, interleukin-1, and interleukin-6. These changes are likely to result in stimulation of osteoclast proliferation and inhibition of osteoblast growth, leading to development of the characteristic lytic bone lesions. This work suggests that the key abnormality may reside in the osteoblast, rather than the osteoclast, as was assumed in the past. Uncertainties remain regarding the primary abnormality giving rise to this condition.

Epidemiology

Paget's disease is classically a condition of older adults, most patients being older than 60 years of age at diagnosis. There is a male preponderance in some studies. It is overwhelmingly a condition of individuals with European forebears, particularly from the United Kingdom and Western Europe (excluding Scandinavia), where about 6% to 7% of the older population were once affected. Among older white Americans, the prevalence was about 2%. Prevalence and disease severity have decreased substantially, possibly reflecting change in an environmental etiologic factor. It is extremely uncommon in individuals with predominantly Asian or Polynesian ancestry, although it is observed in some black populations.

Clinical Presentation

The most common symptoms attributable to Paget's disease are bone and joint pain. The bone pain is typically worse at rest and may trouble patients particularly at night. With skull involvement, pounding

headaches can result. If Paget's disease leads to deformity of joint surfaces, premature arthritis occurs. This is particularly common at the hips. Deformity in long bones can occur, and involvement of the radius or weight-bearing bones of the lower limb often manifests in this way. Microfractures, which can be very painful, sometimes occur over the convexity of a deformed, weight-bearing bone. These can progress to complete fractures. Fractures can also occur through an area of active lytic disease in a weight-bearing bone.

Deafness is a common manifestation of Paget's disease and is caused by involvement of the bones of the middle ear or compromise of the eighth cranial nerve. More rarely, other neurologic syndromes can arise from nerve entrapment, including paraplegia as a result of spinal cord involvement.

Some pagetic patients are asymptomatic and are diagnosed because of an incidental finding of elevated circulating levels of alkaline phosphatase. The diagnosis may also result from an incidental radiographic finding, such as in studies of the urinary tract. Commonly, only one or two bones are involved, although disease may be more widespread. The pelvis, vertebral bodies, long bones, and skull are the most common sites, but almost any bone can be involved.

Diagnosis

Serum alkaline phosphatase, the most widely available marker of osteoblast activity, is usually elevated; however, if only one bone is involved, this test can be normal. In any patient with an elevation of alkaline phosphatase, it is important to determine whether this is coming from liver or bone. This question is usually addressed by other liver function tests, although assays of bone-specific alkaline phosphatase and of other osteoblast-specific markers (e.g., procollagen type I N-terminal propeptide [PINP]) are available. If the elevation of alkaline phosphatase is bony in origin, it is important to rule out other bone conditions such as metastatic cancers (e.g., breast, prostate). This is usually done by identifying the sites of skeletal abnormality on a bone scintigram and then obtaining plain radiographs of the abnormal areas.

Paget's disease has a characteristic appearance on plain radiographs, showing either bony rarefaction or sclerosis (depending on whether the osteoclastic or osteoblastic phase is predominating), disorganization of trabecular architecture, and the other abnormalities already discussed (e.g., deformity). Bone biopsy is not usually necessary to confirm the diagnosis.

Other biochemical markers of osteoblast or osteoclast activity, such as breakdown products of bone collagen, have been used in Paget's disease. Total alkaline phosphatase, bone alkaline phosphatase, PINP or N-terminal telopeptide of type I collagen (NTX) identified more than 95% of pagetic subjects in one cohort of pagetic subjects, although the poorer precision of NTX reduced its utility in monitoring the effects of treatment. Osteocalcin, C-telopeptide of type I collagen, and urinary free deoxypyridinoline are less useful for assessment of baseline activity and monitoring response to therapy. Total alkaline phosphatase remains the most widely used test because of its low cost and wide availability.

Treatment

Treatment of Paget's disease almost always relies on the potent bisphosphonates, primarily zoledronate (Reclast). These compounds have a very high affinity for the bone surface, where they remain for years. They are ingested by osteoclasts when bone is resorbed and inhibit a key enzyme in the mevalonate pathway, farnesyl pyrophosphate synthase. This results in disruption of the osteoclast cytoskeleton and cell death. Bisphosphonates are preferentially taken up at sites of high bone turnover, which accounts for their utility as bone scintigraphy agents, and therefore target active pagetic bone.

The preferred treatment is the potent intravenous bisphosphonate zoledronate (Reclast, generic), which is administered in a single dose of 5 mg over 15 minutes. It has been compared with the standard 2-month course of risedronate (Actonel) in two randomized, controlled trials. At 6 months, 96% of patients receiving zoledronate had a therapeutic response, compared with 74% of those randomized to risedronate ($P < 0.001$). Alkaline phosphatase levels normalized in 89% of patients in the zoledronate group and in 58% of those in the risedronate group ($P < 0.001$). Zoledronate showed a more rapid onset of action and superior effects on quality-of-life measures. Perhaps the most impressive data with zoledronate have been those from the open follow-up of responders in these studies. Six years after drug administration, relapse had occurred in 0.7% of those receiving zoledronate but in 20% of risedronate-treated patients. Therefore, zoledronate produces much more sustained responses to therapy than have hitherto been possible.

The first administration of an intravenous bisphosphonate may be accompanied by flu-like symptoms, which settle over 24 to 48 hours and usually do not recur. Their resolution can be hastened by the use of paracetamol (acetaminophen, Tylenol) or nonsteroidal anti-inflammatory agents. Dexamethasone[1] 4 mg daily for 3 doses, starting just before the infusion, is an effective prophylaxis. Intravenous bisphosphonates require a creatinine clearance of at least 35 mL/min. Potent oral bisphosphonates such as alendronate (Fosamax, generic) and risedronate (Actonel, generic) have been widely used, but are usually less effective than zoledronate. These are administered daily over periods of 2 to 6 months and produce good disease control. The duration of treatment chosen in the pivotal clinical trials was arbitrary to some extent, and individual patients may require longer or shorter initial courses to achieve remission. Oral bisphosphonates have a very low bioavailability. Therefore, they must be taken in a fasting state, with a glass of water, and at least 30 minutes before consumption of food or other fluids. Positively charged ions (including calcium supplements, antacids, and mineral supplements) bind avidly to bisphosphonates and impair their absorption, so they must be taken at a different time of day. Potent bisphosphonates can cause irritation to the upper gastrointestinal tract and should not be prescribed to patients with inflammation or ulceration in that region. Patients should remain upright for 30 minutes after taking oral bisphosphonates to minimize the risk of reflux and associated esophagitis or ulceration.

The injectable bisphosphonate pamidronate (Aredia, generic) has been used in the past for treatment of Paget's disease. It is typically given as a series of infusions of 60 to 90 mg, each administered over a period of 1 to 2 hours. Pamidronate produces partial or complete remissions of disease activity that last for up to several years.

Potent bisphosphonates can cause mild hypocalcemia, which is usually asymptomatic and not a cause for concern. However, in patients with marked vitamin D deficiency, hypocalcemia can be more severe and sustained. Therefore, it is important to ensure that patients are vitamin D sufficient before receiving these drugs—a serum 25-hydroxyvitamin-D level greater than 40 nmol/L is more than adequate. Some physicians prescribe calcium to patients receiving bisphosphonate therapy (given in the evening if the oral bisphosphonate is given in the morning) as a further protection against hypocalcemia.

In the past, the weak bisphosphonate etidronate (Didronel) was used to treat Paget's disease. This is much less effective than the agents discussed earlier. If used in high doses or for more than a few months, it carries the risk of producing osteomalacia, which can lead to bone pain and fractures. Therefore, it no longer has a place in the treatment of Paget's disease. Calcitonin (Miacalcin Injection) has also been relegated to an historical role only, because its efficacy is much less than that of the potent bisphosphonates and its effects are rapidly reversed after cessation of therapy. Denosumab (Prolia)[1] has some efficacy is inferior to zoledronate and is rapidly reversed after cessation.

There are several philosophical approaches to Paget's disease management, none of which is strictly evidence based. There is general agreement that patients with symptoms attributable to Paget's disease should receive treatment. This is clear-cut in patients who have bone pain at the site of a pagetic lesion, but it is a common observation that antipagetic drugs can produce variable degrees of improvement in pain from joints adjacent to pagetic bone. Patients with neurologic complications from spinal cord or other nerve entrapments also improve with antipagetic therapy.

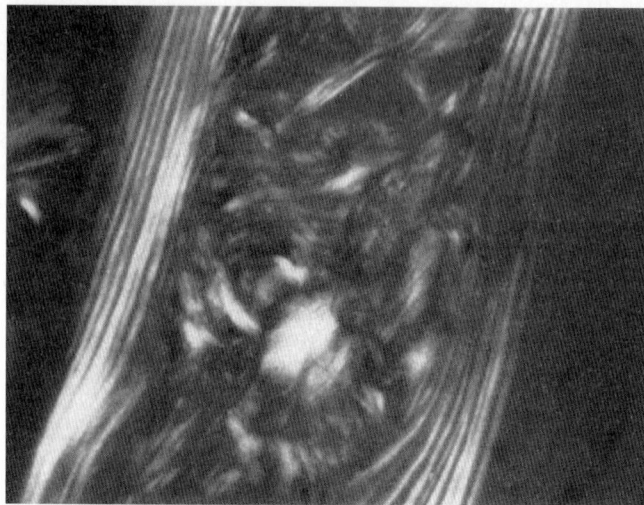

Figure 2 Section of a bone trabecula affected by Paget's disease, viewed under polarized light to show orientation of lamellae. In the center of the trabecula, the collagen fibers are chaotically laid down (woven bone), consistent with active Paget's disease. Over the outer surfaces, collagen is organized in parallel lamellae, indicating the restoration of normal bone microarchitecture after treatment with alendronate. Reprinted with permission from: Reid IR, Nicholson GC, Weinstein RS, et al: Biochemical and radiologic improvement in Paget's disease of bone treated with alendronate: A randomized, placebo-controlled trial. Am J Med 1996;101:341–48.

Treatment aimed at preventing complications of Paget's disease is variably endorsed, because there is no clinical trial evidence that treatment prevents the progression of deformity, the development of pagetic symptoms, or fracture. However, it is clear that treatment leads to a restoration of normal bone histology (Figure 2) and radiographic healing of lytic lesions and that, in the absence of such intervention, both bone lysis and deformity progress. It seems unreasonable to withhold safe therapies that are able to halt histologic and radiologic disease progression. Therefore, many experienced physicians endorse the provision of antipagetic therapy for individuals with lytic lesions in long bones; lesions at sites that are likely to lead to neurologic complications, arthritis, or deformity; or involvement of the skull that could compromise hearing. Expert opinion also supports the use of antipagetic therapy before elective surgery on pagetic bone, because this approach reduces the vascularity of pagetic bone and results in less perioperative blood loss. On the other hand, Paget's disease in asymptomatic patients whose future risk of complications is thought to be low (e.g., with involvement of the ilium) is commonly managed without specific pharmaceutical intervention, although the availability of a safe, single-dose treatment with zoledronate is increasing the inclination to treat.

When providing treatment targeted at these goals, it is important to consider how adequacy of therapy can be judged. In the case of patients with pain, maximal relief of pain is an important endpoint. Lytic lesions should be treated and monitored with sequential radiographs until healing is apparent. Activity at other sites can be assessed indirectly with biochemical markers of bone turnover, although these are much less sensitive in patients with monostotic disease. In this context, there can be considerable residual activity at a single affected site without the markers being abnormal. Bone scintigrams provide the most sensitive method of assessing local disease activity.

In the past, Paget's disease caused substantial morbidity in the elderly population. However, it is now possible to achieve adequate and sustained disease control with use of intravenous zoledronate. Prompt use of these agents, when indicated, can be expected to halt disease progression and to effectively prevent the development of significant complications from this condition.

---

[1] Not FDA approved for this indication.

References

Kanis JA: *Pathophysiology and Treatment of Paget's Disease of Bone*, London, 1991, Martin Dunitz.

Miller PD, Brown JP, Siris ES, et al: A randomized, double-blind comparison of risedronate and etidronate in the treatment of Paget's disease of bone, *Am J Med* 106:513–520, 1999.

Ralston SH, Langston AL, Reid IR: Pathogenesis and management of Paget's disease of bone, *Lancet* 372:155–163, 2008.

Reid IR, Davidson JS, Wattie D, et al: Comparative responses of bone turnover markers to bisphosphonate therapy in Paget's disease of bone, *Bone* 35:224–230, 2004.

Reid IR, Lyles K, Su GQ, et al: A single infusion of zoledronic acid produces sustained remissions in Paget disease: data to 6.5 years, *J Bone Miner Res* 26(9), 2011. 2261–70.

Reid IR, Miller P, Lyles K, et al: Comparison of a single infusion of zoledronic acid with risedronate for Paget's disease, *N Engl J Med* 353:898–908, 2005.

Reid IR, Nicholson GC, Weinstein RS, et al: Biochemical and radiologic improvement in Paget's disease of bone treated with alendronate: A randomized, placebo-controlled trial, *Am J Med* 101:341–348, 1996.

Singer FR, Bone III HG, Hosking DJ, et al: Paget's disease of bone: an Endocrine Society Clinical Practice Guideline, *J Clin Endocrinol Metab* 99(12):4408–22, 2014.

POLYMYALGIA RHEUMATICA AND GIANT CELL ARTERITIS

Method of
Mark A. Matza, MD, MBA; and Sebastian H. Unizony, MD

CURRENT DIAGNOSIS

Primary Polymyalgia Rheumatica

- Age is greater than 50 years.
- Symptoms include pain and stiffness involving the shoulder and hip girdles, and sometimes the neck and lower back. Symptoms are worse after immobilization (e.g., morning) and improve with activities.
- Constitutional symptoms such as fever, fatigue, and weight loss can be present. Peripheral arthralgias or arthritis (e.g., wrists) occasionally occur.
- Only 15%–20% of patients with primary or isolated polymyalgia rheumatica (PMR) develop giant cell arteritis (GCA).
- Upon disease onset, acute-phase reactants (erythrocyte sedimentation rate and C-reactive protein concentration) are typically elevated but can rarely be normal.
- Ultrasound can be used to assess for synovitis, tenosynovitis, or bursitis in the shoulders and hips.

Giant Cell Arteritis

- Age is greater than 50 years.
- Acute-phase reactants (erythrocyte sedimentation rate and C-reactive protein concentration) are elevated in approximately 95% of the cases before treatment with glucocorticoids is initiated.
- Symptoms include new-onset headaches (often temporal), scalp tenderness, jaw or tongue claudication, and vision impairment such as diplopia, amaurosis fugax, episodic blurry vision, and/or blindness.
- Approximately 50% of patients with GCA also have PMR symptoms.
- Constitutional symptoms such as fever, fatigue, and weight loss are often present. In addition, about 10% of GCA cases present only with fever and without other cranial or PMR manifestations.
- Temporal arteries may be prominent, beaded, or tender on examination, but they may also be normal. Vascular bruits and decreased pulses can be auscultated in the presence of large-vessel disease.
- Temporal artery biopsy is the diagnostic test of choice for patients presenting with cranial symptoms, but false-negative results may occur.

- Ultrasound can also be diagnostic in the appropriate clinical scenario when hypoechoic circumferential mural thickening (i.e., halo sign) is identified in the temporal arteries.
- Noninvasive cross-sectional imaging, including computed tomography angiography, magnetic resonance angiography, or positron emission tomography, can be used to evaluate for large-vessel involvement (e.g., aorta, subclavian arteries, axillary arteries.

CURRENT THERAPY

Primary Polymyalgia Rheumatica

- Prednisone at a dose of 15–20 mg/day (or equivalent glucocorticoid) is used initially. The starting dose should be continued for 1 full month to suppress the disease effectively and then tapered to 10 mg by the end of month 2 of treatment. Prednisone can then be tapered off at the rate of 1 mg/month for a total prednisone duration of approximately 1 year.
- Should symptoms recur with tapering, the glucocorticoid dose should be increased temporarily, followed by a new tapering attempt.
- Sarilumab (Kevzara), methotrexate[1] and tocilizumab (Actemra)[1] can be considered for relapsing patients or patients at high risk for glucocorticoid toxicity (e.g., poorly controlled diabetes mellitus). Sarilumab is now approved for the treatment of primary polymyalgia rheumatica patients who have persistent disease despite glucocorticoid use or who cannot tolerate glucocorticoids.

Giant Cell Arteritis

- Treatment should not be delayed while awaiting confirmatory testing (e.g., temporal artery biopsy), given the risk of blindness (15%–20%) in untreated patients.
- Prednisone[1] at a dose of 1 mg/kg or approximately 60 mg (or equivalent glucocorticoid) should be started immediately if the diagnosis is suspected.
- Pulse dose methylprednisolone[1] (1 g daily for 3 days) should be considered if vision changes occur (e.g., amaurosis fugax, monocular permanent vision loss).
- Tocilizumab (Actemra) is an effective drug for remission maintenance and glucocorticoid-sparing in GCA patients both with new-onset and relapsing disease.
- Once the disease activity is controlled, glucocorticoids are tapered off gradually.
- In patients receiving only glucocorticoids, tapers usually last 12 to 24 months, but relapses are common (up to 70% of cases), requiring dose adjustments and prolongation of glucocorticoid therapy.
- In patients receiving tocilizumab, glucocorticoid tapers are typically shorter (e.g., 6 months), and disease relapses are seen in only approximately 30% of the patients within 1 year.
- Approximately 40% of GCA patients in remission after treatment with tocilizumab (162 mg weekly) for 1 year may be able to discontinue tocilizumab and remain in remission for at least 2 more years.
- The use of low doses of aspirin[1] to prevent ischemic complications of GCA is controversial.
- Prophylaxis for glucocorticoid-induced osteoporosis with bisphosphonates, calcium, and vitamin D should be considered in all patients receiving glucocorticoids.
- Immunizations according to the national guidelines (influenza and pneumococcus) should be administered to all GCA patients, especially when they receive glucocorticoids and tocilizumab.

[1]Not FDA approved for this indication.

Primary polymyalgia rheumatica (PMR) and giant cell arteritis (GCA) are related and often overlapping systemic inflammatory disorders that typically affect patients older than 50 years of age. Women are more commonly affected than men, and Caucasians more so than African Americans, Asians, and Hispanics. Symptoms range from proximal muscle aching in primary PMR to blindness in GCA. Both conditions are characterized by elevated serum inflammatory markers (erythrocyte sedimentation rate [ESR] and C-reactive protein [CRP]). Most patients quickly respond to glucocorticoids (e.g., prednisone), but many of them fail to maintain long-term disease control during or after glucocorticoid tapers. Interleukin (IL)-6 receptor blockade with tocilizumab (Actemra) in combination with up to 6 months of prednisone has demonstrated efficacy for remission maintenance, glucocorticoid sparing, and quality-of-life improvement in GCA randomized clinical trials. Preliminary evidence suggests that tocilizumab[1] might also be beneficial in some patients with primary PMR.

Primary Polymyalgia Rheumatica

Clinical Presentation

Primary or isolated PMR is characterized by symmetric proximal joint pain and stiffness (i.e., shoulders and hips). The lifetime risks for primary PMR in women and men older than 50 years of age are 2.4% and 1%, respectively. Disease onset can be acute or subacute, but patients sometimes delay seeking medical attention for days to weeks. Symptoms are classically worse early in the morning and after periods of immobilization (e.g., a "long commute"). Morning stiffness is generally prolonged greater than 45 minutes. Involvement of the peripheral joints (e.g., wrists, knees, and ankles) is rare. Weight loss, fatigue, anorexia, and low-grade fever can be seen. Physical examination is usually unrevealing. However, some patients may demonstrate tenderness and limited active range of motion of the shoulder and hip girdles, but synovitis (e.g., joint swelling, effusion, or erythema) is absent. Range of motion with passive limb movements is typically better.

Apart from occurring in isolation (i.e., primary PMR), PMR symptoms can be seen in nearly 50% of patients with GCA (as discussed later).

Diagnosis

Diagnosis is made based on the clinical presentation and the exclusion of other conditions (e.g., rheumatoid arthritis, GCA, and regional noninflammatory rheumatisms [such as rotator cuff tendinopathy]). Almost all patients demonstrate increased serum ESR and/or CPR at disease onset before treatment is started. Patients have negative rheumatoid factor and anti-CCP antibodies. The response to glucocorticoids (e.g., prednisone) is also often a telling indication of PMR: most patients experience dramatic clinical improvements within 24 to 48 hours. Ultrasound can be used to detect synovitis, tenosynovitis, or bursitis in the shoulders and hips. GCA occurs in approximately 15% to 20% of patients with primary PMR. Therefore, these patients should be queried closely to detect any symptoms that suggest GCA—namely headaches, scalp tenderness, jaw claudication, and visual disturbances.

A minority of patients with presentations of PMR eventually declare their true underlying disorder to be rheumatoid arthritis. Such patients can convert from seronegative to seropositive (i.e., positive rheumatoid factor or anti-CCP antibodies) at some point during follow-up. The presence of distal joint symptoms (e.g., small joints of the hands) might help predict the evolution to rheumatoid arthritis (RA), but the development of RA cannot be predicted if seronegative at baseline. Rarely, late-onset spondyloarthritis initially can be confused with PMR.

Treatment

Patients with primary PMR are treated with glucocorticoids. Prednisone at a dose of 15 to 20 mg is often used to induce disease remission. Symptoms should dramatically improve within 1 to 2 days. Infrequently, patients require higher doses (e.g., 25 to 30 mg) over a longer period (e.g., 5 to 7 days) to achieve clear responses. However, in cases that do not demonstrate classic responses to glucocorticoids, ruling out other conditions (e.g., GCA) is mandatory. The initial glucocorticoid dose is maintained for about 4 weeks to ensure clear sustained resolution of the clinical manifestations and normalization of the inflammatory marker values. A gradual glucocorticoid taper is then begun to maintain the disease in remission. Patients usually taper the daily prednisone dose by 2.5 to 5 mg every 2 to 4 weeks until the dose of 10 mg is achieved. Subsequently, the taper progresses at a rate of 1 to 2.5 mg every 2 to 4 weeks until glucocorticoid discontinuation. The total duration of the treatment in the absence of a disease flare is about 12 to 18 months. Unfortunately, many patients relapse and require an increased prednisone dose and renewed tapering attempt once the disease is again controlled.

Most patients can eventually taper off prednisone completely; however, in some, a low dose of prednisone may be required to prevent the recurrence of symptoms. For patients with primary PMR who require excessive prednisone exposure to maintain disease control, methotrexate[1] or IL-6 blockade therapy with sarilumab (Kevzara) or tocilizumab (Actemra)[1] should be considered. Sarilumab is now approved for the treatment of PMR patients who have had an inadequate response to glucocorticoids or who cannot tolerate a glucocorticoid taper. Sarilumab is given at a dose of 200 mg by subcutaneous injection every 2 weeks and can be used in combination with a short glucocorticoid taper over approximately 14 weeks.

Giant Cell Arteritis

Clinical Presentation

GCA is the most frequent form of primary vasculitis in adults. The disease causes granulomatous inflammation in the large arteries, including the aorta and its primary branches—particularly the vessels of the head and neck. The epidemiology of GCA is identical to the one of primary PMR, with the exception that GCA is three times less frequent. The lifetime risks for GCA in women and men older than 50 years are 1% and 0.5%, respectively. The incidence of GCA increases with each decade and peaks around 73 years of age.

The onset of GCA is often subacute or acute. The most frequent clinical manifestations of this condition can be divided into four not mutually exclusive categories: cranial manifestations, PMR symptoms, constitutional symptoms, and signs and symptoms of large artery involvement.

The cranial manifestations of GCA include headache, jaw claudication, scalp tenderness, temporal artery abnormalities (e.g., prominent arteries, palpable beading, decreased pulsation, or tenderness), and visual symptoms (e.g., diplopia, amaurosis fugax, transient blurred vision, and blindness). The most frequent cranial manifestation is headache (60% to 70% of cases), which may involve not only the temporal region but also other cranial locations. The only unique feature of the GCA-related headache is that it is new for the patient. Jaw claudication, which is reported by 30% to 50% of patients, is very specific of GCA. Typically, patients with jaw claudication notice pain when eating foods that require vigorous chewing, such as meats. Jaw pain is exertional and resolves with mandibular rest. Less frequently, patients may report tongue or pharyngeal pain during mastication and swallowing.

About one-third of patients with GCA have visual manifestations, including diplopia, blurred vision, amaurosis fugax, and the most serious GCA complication—permanent vision loss or blindness. Unlike the slowly progressive blurred vision seen in elderly patients with cataracts, the blurred vision reported by GCA patients is usually monocular (although it

---

[1] Not FDA approved for this indication.

[1] Not FDA approved for this indication.

can be bilateral), acute, and short lived (e.g., minutes to hours). Blindness, which develops in 8% to 20% of patients, occurs in greater than 90% of the cases before GCA is suspected and treatment with glucocorticoids is initiated. This complication can develop abruptly but, more often, is preceded by episodes of blurred vision or amaurosis fugax. By the time blindness occurs, most patients have increased inflammatory markers in serum and also report other clinical manifestations (headaches, jaw claudication, PMR symptoms, etc.). The mechanism of vision loss in GCA is in the great majority of the cases ischemia of the head of the optic nerve (so-called anterior ischemic optic neuropathy). Unfortunately, blindness is generally irreversible.

Approximately 50% of patients with GCA also have PMR symptoms. In addition, most patients with GCA and primary PMR report nonspecific manifestations such as fever, malaise, fatigue, anorexia, or weight loss. At times, fever is the only presenting symptom of GCA, and high clinical suspicion is required to order confirmatory tests to make the diagnosis (e.g., temporal artery biopsy). Finally, despite the fact that nearly all patients have some degree of large-vessel involvement at least histologically, only about 30% of patients develop clinical manifestations related to it. Vascular inflammation can cause structural damage of the walls of elastic arteries, leading to dilation and dissection, as well as narrowing of the lumens of muscular arteries resulting in stenosis, occlusion, and distal ischemia. The most frequently affected vessels include the thoracic and abdominal aorta, and the vertebral, carotid, subclavian, axillary, and brachial arteries. Signs and symptoms related to the involvement of limb arteries may include extremity claudication, decreased peripheral pulses, blood pressure asymmetries, and vascular bruits. Involvement of the vertebral and, less often, the carotid circulation may cause transient ischemic attack and stroke. Aortic disease may lead to aortic aneurysm (mainly in the thoracic aorta) and less frequently aortic dissection. In most patients, however, large artery inflammation and subsequent arterial damage are clinically silent and only detected by vascular imaging.

Diagnosis

GCA is diagnosed based on a combination of clinical presentation, laboratories, imaging, and biopsy. The temporal arteries may be bulging, irregular, or tender on examination; however, they may also be normal, even if temporal artery biopsy subsequently confirms the presence of GCA. The laboratory hallmark of GCA is the elevation of the inflammatory markers ESR and CRP, which is seen in ~95% of untreated patients with new-onset disease. Although elevation of the inflammatory markers is highly sensitive for the diagnosis of GCA, the specificity of these tests is low (~30%).

A characteristic pattern of inflammation in a temporal artery, with granulomatous infiltrates composed of lymphocytes, macrophages, and giant cells, is the most specific test for the diagnosis of GCA. Because skipped lesions (i.e., diseased segments alternating with normal-appearing tissue) are common, multiple sections of biopsies of at least 1 to 2 cm should be examined to increase the diagnostic yield. In addition, simultaneous or sequential bilateral temporal artery biopsies may decrease the false-negative biopsy rate in up to 13% of cases.

Vascular imaging (i.e., ultrasound, MRA, CTA, and PET) has been increasingly incorporated into the care of patients with GCA. Changes suggestive of vasculitis can be found in the arterial walls and/or lumens. Characteristic mural lesions may include circumferential wall thickening or edema, contrast enhancement, and [18]fluorine-2-deoxy-D-glucose (FDG) uptake. Luminal lesions may include stenosis, occlusion, and aneurysmal dilatation. Temporal artery ultrasound scanning may reveal a characteristic "halo sign," caused by edema within and around the blood vessel wall. Several studies and meta-analyses have estimated the sensitivity (55% to 100%) and specificity (75% to 100%) of the halo sign for the diagnosis of GCA compared with clinical diagnosis as the gold standard.

Treatment

Treatment with high-dose glucocorticoids should not be delayed to obtain a temporal artery biopsy or ultrasound. A dose of prednisone[1] 1 mg/kg or approximately 60 mg (or prednisone equivalent) should be initiated promptly when a diagnosis of GCA is considered. Lower doses (e.g., 40 mg/day) can be used for individuals who are frail and elderly. If visual involvement has occurred, pulse dose methylprednisolone[1] 1000 mg daily for 3 days can be initiated, followed by high-dose oral glucocorticoids. The optimal duration of a prednisone taper in GCA is not certain. In one randomized clinical trial, the percentage of patients achieving sustained disease remission at 1 year was essentially the same regardless of whether patients received a 6-month or 12-month prednisone taper. Sustained remissions were achieved in only 14% and 18% of patients, respectively. Thus, although high-dose glucocorticoids are effective at controlling GCA and inducing remission in most patients, the great majority of patients experience disease flares whenever prednisone is tapered to a lower dose (e.g., <15 mg/day) or discontinued.

The interleukin-6 receptor blocker tocilizumab (Actemra) is now approved worldwide for the treatment of GCA in combination with glucocorticoids. The addition of tocilizumab leads to substantial improvement in the rate of glucocorticoid-free remissions at 1 year and a reduction in the cumulative prednisone dose by approximately 50%. Tocilizumab can be administered either intravenously (8 mg/kg each month)[1] or subcutaneously (165 mg each week). The high rate of treatment failure with regimens involving prednisone alone suggests that all patients without contraindications to tocilizumab (e.g., history of diverticulitis) should be treated with the combination of tocilizumab and prednisone initially, followed by an aggressive prednisone taper designed to discontinue prednisone within 4 to 6 months. In a trial of the interleukin-6 receptor blocker tocilizumab, 42% of patients who completed 1 year of weekly tocilizumab in disease remission were able to discontinue treatment and maintain treatment-free remissions for at least 2 more years. Some patients, on the other hand, may require ongoing tocilizumab or even tocilizumab plus prednisone to maintain disease control. Patients who are not able to discontinue prednisone entirely can usually be controlled well with the combination of tocilizumab and low-dose prednisone.

Aspirin[1] (81 mg/day), which has been shown in some retrospective studies and a meta-analysis to reduce the incidence of vision loss, should be considered in all patients without contraindications. Prophylaxis for glucocorticoid-induced osteoporosis with bisphosphonates, calcium, and vitamin D should be implemented, particularly since GCA tends to afflict elderly individuals, many of whom have significant comorbidities at baseline, including osteoporosis. Prophylaxis for *Pneumocystis jiroveci* pneumonia may also be considered in appropriate clinical circumstances, particularly when prolonged or recurrent courses of high-dose glucocorticoids are required in patients with underlying chronic pulmonary conditions (e.g., emphysema).

References

Akiyama M, Kaneko Y, Takeuchi T: Tocilizumab in isolated polymyalgia rheumatica: A systematic literature review, *Semin Arthritis Rheum*, 2020.

Buttgereit F, Dejaco C, Matteson EL, Dasgupta B: Polymyalgia rheumatica and giant cell arteritis: a systematic review, *JAMA* 315(22):2442–2458, 2016.

Dasgupta B, Cimmino MA, Maradit-Kremers H, et al: 2012 provisional classification criteria for polymyalgia rheumatica: a European league against rheumatism/American College of Rheumatology collaborative initiative, *Ann Rheum Dis* 71(4):484–492, 2012.

Hoffman GS: Giant cell arteritis, *Ann Intern Med* 165(9):ITC65–ITC80, 2016.

Kermani TA, Schmidt J, Crowson CS, et al: Utility of erythrocyte sedimentation rate and C-reactive protein for the diagnosis of giant cell arteritis, *Semin Arthritis Rheum* 41(6):866–871, 2012.

---

[1] Not FDA approved for this indication.

Koster MJ, Matteson EL, Warrington KJ: Large-vessel giant cell arteritis: diagnosis, monitoring and management, *Rheumatology (Oxford)* 57(suppl 2):ii32–ii42, 2018.

Lally L, Forbess L, Hatzis C, Spiera R: Brief report: a prospective open-label phase IIa trial of tocilizumab in the treatment of polymyalgia rheumatica, *Arthritis Rheumatol* 68(10):2550–2554, 2016.

Ruediger C, Nguyen L, Black R, et al: Efficacy of methotrexate in polymyalgia rheumatica in routine rheumatology clinical care, *Intern Med J*, 2020.

Soriano A, Muratore F, Pipitone N, et al: Visual loss and other cranial ischaemic complications in giant cell arteritis, *Nat Rev Rheumatol* 13(8):476–484, 2017.

Spiera RF, Unizony S, Warrington KJ, et al; SAPHYR Investigators: Sarilumab for relapse of polymyalgia rheumatica during glucocorticoid taper, *N Engl J Med* 389(14):1263–1272, 2023.

Stone JH, Tuckwell K, Dimonaco S, et al: Trial of tocilizumab in giant-cell arteritis, *N Engl J Med* 377(4):317–328, 2017.

PSORIATIC ARTHRITIS

Method of
William Tillett, MBChB, PhD; and Laura C. Coates, MBChB, PhD

CURRENT DIAGNOSIS

- Psoriatic arthritis (PsA) is a form of inflammatory arthritis genetically associated with the spondylarthritides (SpA) (e.g., ankylosing spondylitis, reactive arthritis, inflammatory bowel disease [IBD], arthritis).
- It is usually diagnosed in the presence of psoriasis (personal or family history), negative rheumatoid factor, and other typical features such as dactylitis and nail involvement.
- Presentation is highly heterogeneous with potential involvement in multiple domains (arthritis, enthesitis, dactylitis and axial disease, skin plaques, and nail dystrophy), as well as SpA-related extraarticular manifestations (IBD and uveitis).

CURRENT THERAPY

- Therapy for PsA aims to control musculoskeletal inflammation (arthritis, enthesitis, dactylitis, and axial disease) and cutaneous manifestations (skin plaques and nail dystrophy).
- Treatment usually follows a step-up approach with non-steroidal antiinflammatory drugs (NSAIDs), topical therapies (for skin plaques), conventional synthetic disease-modifying antirheumatic drugs (DMARDs; e.g., methotrexate [Trexall][1], leflunomide [Arava][1]) and biologics (tumor necrosis factor [TNF], interleukin [IL]-12/23, IL-17, and IL-23 inhibitors), and targeted synthetic DMARDs (apremilast [Otezla] and Janus kinase [JAK] inhibitors).
- PsA is commonly associated with comorbidities such as depression and increased cardiovascular risk with elements of the metabolic syndrome, which may affect therapeutic choice.

[1]Not FDA approved for this indication.

Epidemiology

Psoriatic arthritis (PsA) is a destructive inflammatory arthritis occurring in up to 20% of people with psoriasis. Psoriasis affects approximately 2% to 3% of the U.S. population. The exact prevalence of PsA among the general population has been difficult to estimate because of the heterogeneous nature of the disease and variety of different classification criteria. The lowest prevalence estimates come from Japan (0.001%), and the highest come from Italy (0.42%). Data from recent studies have been more consistent with prevalence estimates of 0.16% in North America and 0.19% in the United Kingdom. PsA affects men and women equally and can develop at any age, but it typically occurs in the 10 to 15 years after the diagnosis of psoriasis, usually between 30 and 50 years of age. The incidence of developing PsA among people with psoriasis is approximately 2% per year. In a recent prospective study of patients with psoriasis, 51 of 464 patients developed PsA over an 8-year follow-up period.

Risk Factors

A number of risk factors have been identified that appear to increase the risk of developing PsA. The presence of HLA-B27 is an established genetic risk factor. Increased rates of PsA are seen among those with more severe psoriasis (relative risk [RR] 5.4, $P = 0.006$). The site of psoriasis may also be important, and some reports suggest that intergluteal and scalp psoriasis confer an increased risk of developing PsA. Nail psoriasis (pitting, onycholysis, subungual hyperkeratosis, and oil drop discoloration) is also associated with an increased likelihood of developing PsA. Nail dystrophy occurs in 80% of patients with PsA but only 20% of patients with psoriasis alone. Obesity is a well-documented risk factor for developing both psoriasis and PsA. The higher the body mass index (BMI), the higher the risk of developing arthritis. Alcohol is a potentially modifiable risk factor with associated increased rates of both psoriasis and arthritis. Data relating to smoking as a risk factor are mixed, with reports suggesting both increased risk and a potentially protective effect.

Pathophysiology
Genetics

The exact etiology of PsA remains uncertain. Genetics are known to play a central role. However, the number of genes identified does not account for the strong heritability seen clinically. Approximately 40% of people with PsA will have a first-degree relative with the condition. PsA appears to have a stronger association with *HLA-B* and *HLA-C* alleles, whereas psoriasis is associated with the *HLA-C* allele. The *HLA-Cw6, B57, DR7,* and *B17* alleles are all associated with early-onset psoriasis. The *HLA-B7, HLA-B27, DR4, B*38,* and *DR7* alleles are associated with PsA. The *HLA-B39, B27,* and *DR7* alleles are associated with more progressive/destructive disease, whereas the *HLA-B22* allele appears to be protective.

Immunopathology

Tissue-specific autoantibodies have not yet been identified. The inflammatory arthritis is characterized by hypervascularity, hypertrophy/tissue proliferation, and inflammatory cell infiltrate. Lymphocytes (particularly T helper [Th]17 cells) and dendritic cells are known to play an important role. The cytokine profile for PsA shows a predominance of tumor necrosis factor [TNF]-α, IL-1, and IL-10.

Infection and Trauma

The temporal link between infections and the development of PsA raises the possibility of a pathologic role of bacteria or viruses. There are higher rates of both psoriasis and PsA in HIV-endemic areas, and psoriasis is often more extensive among patients with HIV. The gut microbiome is an area of current interest in which disturbance of the normal microbiota is being investigated as a possible immunologic trigger. Finally, a small number of epidemiologic studies have made the association with trauma and the subsequent development of PsA, but reports are inconclusive.

Prevention

There are no proven strategies to prevent the development of PsA, but observational studies have suggested that biologic use may delay or prevent the onset of arthritis, and ongoing research is focusing on this question. Current preventive strategies focus on early diagnosis and prevention of damage accumulation, loss of function, and disability. The treatment of comorbid conditions, pre–drug treatment screening, and drug dose optimization to minimize drug exposure are important prevention strategies.

Early diagnosis and treatment strategies focus on the prevention of damage and subsequent disability. Untreated inflammation results in damage to the articular surface and surrounding tissues with subsequent loss of movement, pain, limitation of function, and reduced quality of life. Erosion of the surface of the bone, narrowing of the joint space, and new bone formation (osteoproliferation) cause pain, reduced movement, and physical dysfunction. Observational studies have suggested that delay of diagnosis by as little as 6 months results in more damage and poorer physical function.

In the United Kingdom, annual screening of patients with psoriasis for arthritis is recommended using the Psoriasis Epidemiology Screening Tool (PEST) questionnaire. The questionnaire asks patients with psoriasis whether they have ever had pain in their joints, whether a doctor has ever told them they have arthritis, whether they have had nail pitting, whether they have had pain in their heel, and whether they have ever had a completely sausage-like swelling of a finger or toe without reason. A score of 3 or more is positive.

Clinical Manifestations
PsA is classified with the seronegative spondyloarthropathies that include axial spondyloarthritis (axSpA), reactive arthritis (ReA), and inflammatory bowel disease (IBD) arthritis. The seronegative spondyloarthropathies share many of the clinical and genetic features, such as HLA-B27 association, enthesopathy (inflammation at the tendon and ligament insertion to the bone), association with uveitis, spondyloarthritis, and asymmetric peripheral arthritis.

The following are classical patterns of PsA, although there is often overlap among these groups:

- Polyarthritis (five or more joints)
- Oligoarthritis (four or fewer joints)
- Monoarthritis (one joint)
- Spondyloarthritis (axial disease)
- PsA mutilans (digital shortening/telescoping caused by onycholysis)

Polyarthritis is the most common form, occurring in approximately 60% cases, whereas mutilans only occurs in 5% cases.

The signs of PsA are heterogeneous and include psoriasis, nail dystrophy, joint disease, enthesitis, dactylitis, and spondyloarthritis. These are discussed in the following sections.

Psoriasis
In its most common plaque form, the skin lesions of psoriasis are characterized by scaly plaques on the extensor surfaces. Psoriasis can be hidden in the scalp, ear, natal cleft, and umbilicus. Most patients develop psoriasis before developing arthritis, but a small proportion, approximately 10%, will develop psoriasis after the arthritis. A proportion of patients present with musculoskeletal symptoms but are unaware that they have skin psoriasis, which can be subtle in sites such as the hairline, intergluteal region, behind the ear, or umbilicus. Other patterns of psoriasis include guttate (small spots that can be widespread), palmar-plantar (palms and soles), and inverse (affecting the flexural creases).

Nail Dystrophy
Pitting (fine pits), onycholysis (lifting of the distal nail plate), hyperkeratosis (thickening of the nail plate), and oil drop discoloration (salmon-colored spots) are the most common nail manifestations of psoriasis. Other features include leukonychia, Beau lines, and longitudinal ridging. Nail pitting can be a clinically subtle but helpful sign to distinguish PsA from other types of arthritis. Nail dystrophy itself is associated with an increased risk of developing arthritis and can be the only manifestation of psoriasis.

Joint Disease
Inflammatory arthritis is the hallmark of PsA. The joints appear swollen and hot and are stiff and painful. The recognized patterns of joint involvement are inflammatory polyarthritis (five or more joints involved, which may be symmetric or asymmetric in distribution), oligoarticular (fewer than five joints), monoarticular (one joint), axial (spondyloarthritis), and mutilans (digital shortening caused by onycholysis).

Enthesitis
Inflammation at the insertion of the tendon or ligament to the bone (rather than the midportion of the tendon, which is more likely to be an overuse tendinopathy) may be a sign. Many sites can be affected by enthesitis. However, the most readily assessable are the Achilles insertion to the calcaneus, the lateral epicondyle of the elbow, and the medical condyle of the femur. Enthesitis is not commonly seen in rheumatoid arthritis and can be a useful distinguishing sign. The assessment of enthesitis can be challenging because many entheseal insertions correlate anatomically with myofascial tender points seen in fibromyalgia. Ultrasonography can be helpful to examine for sonographic features of enthesitis, such as insertional hypervascularity, osteoproliferation, and erosion.

Dactylitis
Also known as sausage finger, dactylitis is the swelling of an entire digit. Dactylitis occurs in 50% of patients with PsA at some point in their disease. The inflammation is at the joint, tendon, and extracapsular tissues.

Spondyloarthritis
Spondyloarthritis affects up to 50% of patients with PsA, but cohort studies have suggested that only one-half of these patients have symptoms of inflammatory back pain. Inflammatory back pain typically occurs before 40 years of age and will wake people in the second half of the night; they are characteristically stiff in the morning and feel better with exercise and nonsteroidal anti-inflammatory drugs (NSAIDs). The radiographic features are of sacroiliitis (sclerosis, erosions, and fusion), which can be asymmetric, and syndesmophytes (bone formation that can be fine or chunky), which can flow between vertebrae, causing fusion.

Other manifestations include uveitis (approximately 30% of patients; RR 3.5 compared with the general population), metabolic syndrome (elevated BMI, hypertension, and dyslipidemia), IBD (Crohn disease; RR 2.9 compared with the general population), and depression.

Diagnosis
In the absence of specific antibodies, the diagnosis of PsA remains clinical. The Classification Criteria for Psoriatic Arthritis (CASPAR) criteria were developed for use in clinical trials to ensure a consistent trial population and were also shown to apply in the clinical setting as diagnostic criteria (Box 1).

Differential Diagnosis
The other seronegative spondyloarthropathies are in the primary differential diagnosis. The absence of an infectious trigger or concurrent IBD discounts ReA and IBD arthritis. The presence or history of psoriasis (or a first-degree relative with psoriasis) is the most useful distinguishing feature in differentiating from axial spondyloarthritis.

Osteoarthritis is a common and clinically challenging differential, particularly in the hands. Young age of onset, the presence of nail psoriasis at the affected ray, and radiographic features of PsA are the most useful distinguishing features.

Gout is an important differential for two reasons. First, a history of a swollen toe is often mistaken as gout (or podagra). Second, uric acid is commonly mildly elevated in patients with PsA. A careful history and examination for other clinical features of PsA can be helpful, such as history of psoriasis, nail dystrophy at the affected toe, enthesitis, or axial symptoms. Ultrasonography to examine for sonographic features of crystal deposition or aspiration to examine for crystals may be required. Concurrent gout and PsA are rare but recognized.

BOX 1 | Classification Criteria for Psoriatic Arthritis

Confirmed inflammatory articular disease (joint, spine, or entheseal) with at least three points from the following features:
1. Current psoriasis (2 points)
2. Past personal history or family history of a first- or second-degree relative with psoriasis (1 point each)
3. Dactylitis (1 point)
4. Juxtaarticular new bone formation (ill-defined ossification near joint margins—excluding osteophyte formation—on plain hand and feet radiographs; 1 point)
5. Rheumatoid factor negativity (1 point)
6. Psoriatic nail dystrophy (onycholysis, pitting, and hyperkeratosis observed on current physical examination; 1 point)

Investigations to support the diagnosis include the following:
- Rheumatoid factor (RhF) and anticyclic citrullinated peptide (ACPA or Anti-CCP) are usually negative.
- Inflammatory markers such as C-reactive protein (CRP), plasma viscosity (PV), and erythrocyte sedimentation rate (ESR) can often be normal and do not exclude inflammatory joint disease.
- Plain radiographs can be helpful to distinguish PsA from rheumatoid arthritis (RA) or osteoarthritis (OA). The plain radiographic features of PsA are erosions, joint space narrowing, osteoproliferation (bone formation), ankyloses (fusion), and, in the mutilans form of the disease, osteolysis (bone resorption).
- Magnetic resonance imaging (MRI) and ultrasonography are both frequently used to assess for spondyloarthritis and articular and entheseal inflammation, respectively.

Therapy (or Treatment)

The treatment of PsA aims to control inflammation related to the disease to improve symptoms, maximize function, and prevent long-term complications. Different therapies may be chosen depending on the domains of disease (arthritis, skin, nails, enthesitis, dactylitis, axial disease) that are active in any one individual patient. In general, treatment of PsA follows a step-up approach with treatment escalated in case of nonresponse to the previous therapy. Ideally, treatment should follow a treat-to-target approach in which a treatment target, such as minimal disease activity (MDA), is reassessed at each visit, and therapy is assessed if the target is not met. This approach has been shown to improve disease control in the Tight Control of Inflammation in Early Psoriatic Arthritis (TICOPA) trial.

NSAIDs are used frequently to help manage pain and stiffness but do not seem to have a significant effect on the disease course. Particularly in the early stages of disease or in the case of disease flares, parenteral steroids (intraarticular or intramuscular) are used to control inflammation quickly, although there can be a risk of psoriasis flare on withdrawal of systemic steroids. The mainstay of therapy in PsA are disease-modifying antirheumatic drugs (DMARDs), which are grouped into three categories:
1. Conventional synthetic DMARDs (methotrexate[1], sulfasalazine [Azulfidine][1], leflunomide [Arava][1])
2. Biologic DMARDs (TNF inhibitors, interleukin [IL]-12/23, IL-17, or IL-23 inhibitors)
3. Targeted synthetic DMARDs (phosphodiesterase 4 [PDE4] and Janus kinase [JAK] inhibitors)

Conventional synthetic DMARDs (csDMARDs) are commonly used to treat skin psoriasis and peripheral arthritis. The use of these drugs is based on their efficacy in psoriasis and in rheumatoid arthritis, although the data supporting their efficacy in PsA are relatively lacking. The most commonly used csDMARD is methotrexate[1], although the placebo-controlled Methotrexate In PsA (MIPA) trial did not show a significant effect of methotrexate over placebo. Many rheumatologists discounted these data because of flaws in the study design (low target dose used, poor completion rate). Interestingly, in the supplementary data from the study, it seemed that patients with polyarticular disease responded much better to methotrexate than those with oligoarthritis. This may be caused by a differential response in different forms of arthritis, but it most likely relates to the sensitivity of the outcome measures used. The Study of Etanercept and Methotrexate in Combination or as Monotherapy in Subjects with Psoriatic Arthritis (SEAM-PsA) study compared first-line etanercept (Enbrel) versus methotrexate and showed superiority for etanercept but with 23% achieving MDA on methotrexate alone. Given that there is proven efficacy for the use of methotrexate in psoriasis, this drug is useful to manage patients with both peripheral arthritis and active psoriasis. Sulfasalazine[1] is also commonly used, and a number of studies support its efficacy. However, a Cochrane review in 2000 summarized the results of these studies and concluded that although it was effective, the effect size was relatively small. Leflunomide[1] is the conventional DMARD with the strongest trial data. The Treatment of Psoriatic Arthritis Study (TOPAS) in 2004 confirmed the efficacy of leflunomide versus placebo but came shortly before breakthrough trials with biologic therapies with superior results. Unlike RA, for which combination csDMARD is common, there is less evidence in PsA. A randomized controlled trial comparing methotrexate monotherapy with methotrexate plus leflunomide combination therapy (COMPLETE-PsA) found superior response in the combination arm but increased side effects, including liver test abnormalities and fatigue.

Despite the mixed data on the csDMARDs and their effect on clinical measures of disease activity, none of them has any proven effect on disease progression in the form of radiographic damage. Observational studies have suggested that early use of therapies and higher dosages used in more recent years may be associated with less radiographic damage, but this has not been formally tested. Recent studies have compared conventional and biologic drugs in early PsA. The Comparison Between Adalimumab Introduction and Methotrexate Dose Escalation in Patients with Inadequately Controlled Psoriatic Arthritis (CONTROL) study took patients with active disease despite moderate (15-mg) doses of methotrexate and compared methotrexate dose escalation with addition of adalimumab (Humira).[1] This showed superiority in MDA responses for adalimumab at week 16. There are very limited data in treating other domains of PsA, such as enthesitis and dactylitis, for which only small open-label studies are available. In axial PsA, as in other axial spondylarthritides, there is no evidence of efficacy of conventional drugs, and treatment algorithms rely on biologic therapies.

A number of biologic DMARDs (bDMARDS) have proven efficacy in PsA, and four have been licensed for use in this condition. There are five different TNF inhibitors (adalimumab, certolizumab pegol [Cimzia], etanercept, infliximab [Remicade], and golimumab [Simponi]), which have all shown efficacy across the key domains of PsA, including arthritis, enthesitis, dactylitis, skin disease, and nail disease. They have all shown long-term efficacy and retardation of radiographic damage, confirming their effect on structural progression. In most of the studies, around 50% of patients were also receiving a concomitant csDMARD (usually methotrexate). However, in PsA, in contrast with rheumatoid arthritis, there was no significant difference in efficacy seen with combination treatment over monotherapy biologics. A randomized trial recently addressed this point, comparing methotrexate monotherapy, etanercept monotherapy, and the combination

---

[1] Not FDA approved for this indication.

in a placebo-controlled trial. This study confirmed superiority of both etanercept arms over methotrexate monotherapy but did not find a difference in effect with concomitant use of csDMARDs.

As a secondary outcome in the PsA studies, there has been a significant difference seen in enthesitis and dactylitis using clinical measures. In the PsA studies and in specific psoriasis studies, the efficacy of TNF inhibitors has been proven for both skin and nail disease. As yet, there are no specific studies in axial PsA, but data in axial spondyloarthritis and/or ankylosing spondylitis have confirmed the efficacy of TNF inhibitors for spinal symptoms.

A number of interleukin inhibitors have been licensed for the treatment of PsA. Ustekinumab (Stelara), a p40 antibody that blocks the action of IL-12 and IL-23, is particularly effective for psoriasis, with proven superiority over TNF inhibitors. It also has evidence of efficacy for peripheral arthritis, enthesitis, and dactylitis. Surprisingly, however, despite a small positive open-label study, a randomized trial in axial spondyloarthritis was halted early, with no evidence of efficacy over placebo. Thus the phenotype of disease must be considered when choosing a therapy.

IL-17A inhibitors (secukinumab [Cosentyx] and ixekizumab [Taltz]) and the IL-17A and IL17F inhibitor bimekizumab (Bimzelx)[1] are now licensed and can be used for PsA and axial spondylarthritis, providing an alternative biologic option for those with PsA. A specific study in axial PsA has also shown efficacy of secukinumab. These drugs showed even higher responses in skin psoriasis, with head-to-head studies confirming superiority over ustekinumab and TNF inhibitors. Brodalumab (Siliq)[1], a human antibody against the IL-17 receptor, also blocks different forms of IL-17. It is licensed for the treatment of plaque psoriasis and has positive phase III data in PsA.

A number of specific IL-23 inhibitors have been approved for treatment of PsA, including guselkumab (Tremfya) and risankizumab (Skyrizi), which are also licensed for plaque psoriasis. These bind to the p19 subunit, providing specific blockade of IL-23 only, and have been shown to have impressive efficacy in skin psoriasis. Phase III trial data are available in PsA, with evidence of efficacy in peripheral arthritis, but again studies in ankylosing spondylitis and axial spondyloarthritis have been halted because of lack of efficacy in the spinal domain. Further studies will investigate the efficacy of these drugs, specifically in axial PsA.

In recent years, a third class of drugs, the targeted synthetic DMARDs (tsDMARDs), have also become available for the treatment of PsA. Apremilast is a phosphodiesterase 4 inhibitor with proven modest efficacy in the treatment of peripheral arthritis, psoriasis, enthesitis, and dactylitis but not in axial SpA. Although responses seem lower than with the biologic drugs, apremilast has a very reassuring safety profile with no requirement for regular blood monitoring. The other group of tsDMARDs in development focus on targeting the JAK pathway. Tofacitinib (Xeljanz) and upadacitinib (Rinvoq) are licensed for treatment of peripheral arthritis and showed improvements in arthritis, enthesitis, and dactylitis outcomes that were comparable with adalimumab, which was included in both studies as either an internal control or a head-to-head comparison. Tofacitinib showed modest efficacy on skin psoriasis, with seemingly higher responses seen in the upadacitinib PsA trial, although they are not specifically licensed for psoriasis. Studies in axial spondyloarthritis have confirmed that JAK inhibitors are also efficacious for axial disease with a license for tofacitinib in AS. Other JAK and tyronsine kinase inhibitors (TYK) inhibitors, with different selectivity for JAK pathways, are in phase II and III studies. A recent study identified safety concerns with tofacitinib compared with a TNF inhibitor, showing an increased risk of malignancy, cardiovascular disease, and venous thromboembolism, particularly in patients older than 65 years of age or those with preexisting cardiovascular risk factors. Caution is advised with JAK inhibitors, particularly in this population.

In all cases, the aim of treatment should be to minimize disease activity. The choice of therapy can be difficult because there are few head-to-head comparison studies, and many of the newer bDMARDs and tsDMARDs appear to have similar efficacy in arthritis. In cases with significant psoriasis, an argument could be made for IL-12/23, IL-17, or IL-23 inhibitors, for which superior efficacy has been shown in psoriasis and PsA trials. For those with axial disease, proven efficacy is limited to TNF, IL-17, and JAK inhibitors. In other cases, the choice of medication often depends on comorbidities, and therapies may be contraindicated (IL-17 inhibitors worsening active IBD) or helpful (TNF inhibitors).

Monitoring

Monitoring of PsA may include assessment of clinical disease activity measures, patient-reported outcomes, laboratory testing, and imaging. The majority of day-to-day disease monitoring consists of clinical outcome measures, often combined with patient-reported outcomes.

Ideally, all domains of the disease should be assessed to allow optimal choice of therapy. To assess arthritis, a full 68/66 joint count is required, rather than the reduced joint counts used in rheumatoid arthritis. Dactylitis is usually evident when joints are examined. Enthesitis can be assessed clinically, looking for tenderness and swelling at the site of key tendon attachments. In cases of doubt, ultrasound imaging can be helpful to look for inflammation and increased blood flow. Although rheumatologists are focused on musculoskeletal signs, when treating patients with PsA, they should also assess skin and nail manifestations. This can be a relatively brief assessment, such as looking at body surface area of skin psoriasis affected; it is important not to underestimate the effect of skin involvement on a patient's quality of life.

Multiple patient-reported outcomes are available to measure the patient's perspective in PsA, including questionnaires assessing pain, function, work disability, and other effects. The majority of these are research tools, and they are often combined with physician-assessed clinical measures to form composite scores. In clinical practice, some questionnaires may be used to assess the patient's perspective and encourage dialogue with patients.

As mentioned previously, treatment recommendations now state that a treat-to-target approach should be implemented in routine care of PsA. Recommendations state that the treatment target should ideally be remission, with the alternative target of low disease activity if remission is not feasible. Additional recommendations on treat-to-target have highlighted that the target of therapy should include both musculoskeletal and skin manifestations of disease. Thus the MDA criteria have been recommended for the target of treatment because these include measures of arthritis, psoriasis, enthesitis, and patient-reported pain, global activity, and functional ability.

Management of Complications

PsA is associated with a number of comorbidities. It is part of the spectrum of spondyloarthritis and has associated extraarticular manifestations (EAMs), including potential overlap with IBD and uveitis. The involvement of these other systems is important to recognize to aid diagnosis and then comanage patients to optimize outcome. Often therapies for PsA are also licensed for treatment of EAMs, allowing treatment of the disease as a whole.

Other comorbidities, not directly related to the disease complex, are also prominent in patients with psoriasis and PsA. Depression and anxiety are prevalent in up to one-half of the population and are important to address to maximize quality of life and to aid with adherence to therapy. Patients with psoriasis and PsA also have a much higher risk of metabolic syndrome and associated cardiovascular comorbidity. There

---

[1] Not FDA approved for this indication.

are higher rates of obesity, diabetes, hypertension, hyperlipidemia, and associated complications such as nonalcoholic fatty liver disease and cardiovascular events. The cardiovascular risk seems to be higher in those with severe active disease and provides another argument for effective control of inflammation. Beyond controlling disease, patients need support and interventions to manage their other risk factors such as weight, smoking, blood pressure, and lipid control.

References

Baraliakos X, Gossec L, Pournara E, et al: Secukinumab in patients with psoriatic arthritis and axial manifestations: results from the double-blind, randomised, phase 3 MAXIMISE trial, *Ann Rheum Dis* 80(5):582–590, 2021.

Charlton R, Green A, Shaddick G: On behalf of the PROMPT study group: Risk of uveitis and inflammatory bowel disease in people with psoriatic arthritis: a population-based cohort study, *Ann Rheum Dis* 77:277–280, 2018.

Coates LC, Soriano ER, Corp N, et al: Group for Research and Assessment of Psoriasis and Psoriatic Arthritis (GRAPPA): updated treatment recommendations for psoriatic arthritis 2021, *Nat Rev Rheumatol* 18:465–479, 2022, https://doi.org/10.1038/s41584-022-00798-0.

Coates LC, Moverley AR, McParland L et al, et al: Effect of tight control of inflammation in early psoriatic arthritis (TICOPA): a UK multicentre, open-label, randomised controlled trial, *Lancet* 386(10012):2489–2498, 2015.

Coates LC, Tillett W, D'Agostino MA, et al: Comparison between adalimumab introduction and methotrexate dose escalation in patients with inadequately controlled psoriatic arthritis (CONTROL): a randomised, open-label, two-part, phase 4 study, *Lancet Rheumatol* 4(4):e262–e273, 2022.

Deodhar A, Helliwell PS, Boehncke WH, et al: Guselkumab in patients with active psoriatic arthritis who were biologic-naive or had previously received TNFα inhibitor treatment (DISCOVER-1): a double-blind, randomised, placebo-controlled phase 3 trial, *Lancet* 395(10230):1115–1125, 2020.

Kristensen LE, Keiserman M, Papp K, et al: Efficacy and safety of risankizumab for active psoriatic arthritis: 24-week results from the randomised, double-blind, phase 3 KEEPsAKE 1 trial, *Ann Rheum Dis* 81(2):225–231, 2022.

Mease PJ, Gladman DD, Collier DH, et al: Etanercept and methotrexate as monotherapy or in combination for psoriatic arthritis: primary results from a randomized, controlled phase III trial, *Arthritis Rheumatol* 71(7):1112–1124, 2019.

Mease PJ, Helliwell PS, Hjuler KF, et al: Brodalumab in psoriatic arthritis: results from the randomized phase III AMVISION-1 and AMVISION-2 trials, *Ann Rheum Dis* 80(2):185–193, 2021.

Mease PJ, Rahman P, Gottlieb AB, et al: Guselkumab in biologic-naive patients with active psoriatic arthritis (DISCOVER-2): a double-blind, randomised, placebo-controlled phase 3 trial, *Lancet* 395(10230):1126–1136, 2020.

Ogdie A, Weiss P: The epidemiology of psoriatic arthritis, *Rheum Dis Clin North Am* 41(4):545–568, 2015.

Östör A, Van den Bosch P, Papp K, et al: Efficacy and safety of risankizumab for active psoriatic arthritis: 24-week results from the randomised, double-blind, phase 3 KEEPsAKE 2 trial, *Ann Rheum Dis* 81(3):351–358, 2022.

Taylor W, Gladman D, Helliwell P: Classification criteria for psoriatic arthritis: Development of new criteria from a large international study, *Arthritis Rheum* 54:2665–2673, 2006.

Tillett W, Charlton R, Nightingale A, et al: Interval between onset of psoriasis and psoriatic arthritis comparing the UK Clinical Practice Research Datalink with a hospital-based cohort, *Rheumatology* 56(12):2109–2113, 2017.

Van den Bosch F, Coates L: Clinical management of psoriatic arthritis, *Lancet* 391(10136):2285–2294, 2018.

Veale DJ, Fearon U: The pathogenesis of psoriatic arthritis, *Lancet* 391:2273–2284, 2018.

RHEUMATOID ARTHRITIS

Method of
Megan Krause, MD

CURRENT DIAGNOSIS

- Clinical diagnosis based on combination of history, examination, and supporting laboratory studies.
- Presentation is typically chronic symmetric polyarticular inflammatory arthritis.
- While not required for diagnosis, supporting laboratory studies include positive rheumatoid factor (RF), positive anticitrullinated protein antibodies (ACPA), elevated C-reactive protein (CRP), and elevated sedimentation rate (ESR).
- Radiographs can be normal at diagnosis. Findings of periarticular osteopenia and erosions are supportive of diagnosis of rheumatoid arthritis (RA).

CURRENT THERAPY

- Methotrexate (Otrexup, Rasuvo, Rheumatrex) initial dose typically 10 to 15 mg weekly with an increase based on disease activity up to 25 mg weekly orally or subcutaneously in conjunction with daily folic acid[1] 1 mg orally daily.
- Hydroxychloroquine (Plaquenil) 5 mg/kg orally per day with maximum of 400 mg daily.
- Sulfasalazine (Azulfidine-EN) initially dose typically 500 mg orally once daily or 500 mg twice daily, increasing up to goal dose of 1000 to 1500 mg twice daily.
- Leflunomide (Arava) 10 to 20 mg orally once daily.
- Azathioprine (Imuran) initial 1 mg/kg/day orally with increasing dose based on response to maximum of 2.5 mg/kg/day.
- Janus kinase inhibitors
  - Tofacitinib (Xeljanz) immediate release 5 mg orally twice daily or extended release 11 mg orally once daily.
  - Baricitinib (Olumiant) 2 mg orally once daily.
  - Upadacitinib (Rinvoq) 15 mg orally once daily.
- Tumor necrosis factor (TNF) inhibitors
  - Adalimumab (Humira, biosimilars) 40 mg subcutaneous every other week.
  - Certolizumab (Cimzia) 400 mg subcutaneous at week 0, 2, and 4, then 200 mg every other week or 400 mg every 4 weeks.
  - Etanercept (Enbrel, biosimilars) 50 mg subcutaneous every week.
  - Golimumab (Simponi, Simponi Aria)
    - Simponi: 50 mg subcutaneous every 4 weeks
    - Simponi Aria: 2 mg/kg intravenous at week 0, 4, and then every 8 weeks
  - Infliximab (Remicade, biosimilars) 3 mg/kg intravenous at week 0, 2, and 6 and then every 8 weeks but, if persistent disease activity, dose can be adjusted between 3 and 10 mg/kg every 4 to 8 weeks.
- Interleukin 6 (IL6) receptor inhibitors
  - Tocilizumab (Actemra, biosimilars)
    - Subcutaneous: if less than 100 kg: 162 mg every other week, increase to weekly if persistent disease activity; if more than 100 kg: 162 mg every week.
    - Intravenous: 4 mg/kg every 4 weeks, can be increased to 8 mg/kg every 4 weeks if persistent disease activity.
  - Sarilumab (Kevzara) 200 mg subcutaneous every 2 weeks.
- T cell co-stimulation inhibitors
  - Abatacept (Orencia)
    - Subcutaneous: 125 mg once weekly (with or without IV loading dose).
    - Intravenous: if less than 60 kg: 500 mg; if 60 to 100 kg: 750 mg; if more than 100 kg: 1000 mg with initial dosing at week 0, 2, and 4, and then every 4 weeks.
- B cell inhibitor
  - Rituximab (Rituxan, biosimilars) 1000 mg IV day 1 and 15, subsequent doses can be repeated at 24 weeks.
- Interleukin 1 receptor inhibitor
  - Anakinra (Kineret) 100 mg subcutaneous every day.

[1]Not FDA approved for this indication.

Epidemiology

Individuals can develop rheumatoid arthritis (RA) at any age, but a peak incidence is between 50 and 75 years. Women are affected at a frequency of two to three times greater than men. It is estimated that the prevalence is approximately 1% in the United States.

Risk Factors

The exact pathogenesis of RA is not completely understood. It is likely the consequence of the interplay of multiple factors, including genetic predisposition and epigenetic factors, along with environmental exposures that result in the systemic inflammatory process. The environmental factors are diverse and are likely not the same in all individuals. Cigarette smoking has been identified as a significant risk factor. Periodontal disease also is associated with development of RA. Silica is an example of an associated occupational exposure.

Multiple genetic risk factors have been identified. The shared epitope, referring to a specific sequence at the HLA-DRB1 locus, which is involved with antigen presentation, has been one of the most studied. Other genetic factors have been identified but individually contribute a small increase in risk.

Pathophysiology

The combination of genetics, epigenetic factors, and environmental exposures lead to downstream consequences of loss of tolerance to self. Both the innate and adaptive immune systems are activated in this process. Diverse immune cells including T cells, B cells, macrophages, and dendritic cells are involved in the pathogenesis. The production of cytokines contributes to the wide variety of downstream tissue targets that lead to the diverse clinical manifestations of RA. While RA frequently is diagnosed based on presentation of inflammatory arthritis, the production of cytokines and interplay of multiple cell types leads to the multiorgan dysfunction.

Prevention

It is not understood how to prevent the development of RA. Limiting known risk factors such as smoking and maintaining periodontal health would be reasonable recommendations.

Clinical Manifestations

Articular Manifestations

Classically, individuals will present with symmetric inflammatory polyarthritis (affecting five or more joints) frequently affecting the wrists, metacarpophalangeal joints (MCPs), proximal interphalangeal joints (PIPs), and metatarsophalangeal joints (MTPs). Both small and large joints can be affected. The distal interphalangeal joints (DIPs) and lumbar spine are spared.

On examination, the joints can be warm, erythematous, swollen, and tender. Range of motion of joints is frequently limited. The synovitis on exam can be described as boggy in contrast to bony hypertrophic changes of osteoarthritis.

Extraarticular Manifestations

One of the consequences of the systemic nature of RA is that the symptoms are not limited to the joints. The extraarticular manifestations can have significant impact both in terms of morbidity and mortality. High clinical suspicion is required, and evaluation is necessary to differentiate toxicity of medications versus a manifestation of RA. More data are required to understand how the advances in therapy will impact extraarticular manifestations.

Individuals with RA can develop subcutaneous nodules, which sometimes can be independent of disease activity. Rarely, individuals can develop a paradoxical increase in rheumatoid nodules with methotrexate.

Individuals can present with significant dryness of the mouth consistent with secondary Sjögren syndrome. Some of these individuals will have positive autoantibodies, such as SSA/Ro and SSB/La.

Pulmonary manifestations can be quite varied and have important implications for treatment. Pleural disease can be seen and can include pleural effusions and pleurisy. Pulmonary nodules can also be present. Interstitial lung disease can present in wide ranging patterns, including usual interstitial pneumonia (UIP), nonspecific interstitial pneumonia (NSIP), organizing pneumonia, and constrictive bronchiolitis.

Cardiac manifestations can include accelerated coronary artery disease. If the joint symptoms preclude significant exertion, patients may not present with classic angina. Pericardial disease can range from pericarditis, pericardial effusion, and constrictive pericarditis. Depending on the location, rheumatoid nodules affecting the heart can be associated with valve dysfunction and conduction abnormalities.

Episcleritis and scleritis can be associated with RA. A dreaded ocular complication of RA is peripheral ulcerative keratitis and corneal melt; this requires emergent ophthalmologic evaluation.

Frequently hematologic abnormalities can be associated with RA. Anemia of chronic disease, leukocytosis, and thrombocytosis can be frequently seen. A minority of individuals will develop Felty syndrome, which includes clinical manifestations of splenomegaly, leukopenia (frequently neutropenia), and frequent infections.

Entrapment syndromes such as carpal tunnel syndrome can be a presenting symptom of RA or develop over the course of the disease. In the case of carpal tunnel syndrome, it is the result of compression of the median nerve due to swelling of the flexor tendons.

RA can affect the cervical spine. The atlantoaxial joint can be prone to subluxation, which can result in myelopathy. A high clinical suspicion is required, as individuals may not present with neck pain and joint damage can obscure examination findings such as reflexes.

An increasingly rare manifestation is vasculitis secondary to RA. This can have multiple manifestations but can include cutaneous ulcers and mononeuritis multiplex.

Diagnosis

Rheumatoid arthritis is a clinical diagnosis based on the pattern of clinical and laboratory findings. Rarely at presentation, individuals can present with monoarticular (one joint) or oligoarticular (two to four joints) involvement, but typically when observed over time, individuals will have polyarticular involvement.

Tests to aid diagnosis include the RF, which refers to an immunoglobuin M (IgM) directed against immunoglobulin G (IgG). It is a nonspecific test and can be elevated related to age, as well other diseases that can mimic RA, such as hepatitis C. ACPA have the advantage of being more specific than RF with specificity as high as 95%. Individuals are considered to have seropositive RA when either RF or ACPA is positive; this occurs in approximately 70% to 80% of individuals. Acute phase reactants including CRP and ESR, when elevated, are supportive of the diagnosis but not required for the diagnosis. Anemia of chronic disease, thrombocytosis, and leukocytosis can also be supportive of the diagnosis but are nonspecific.

The American College of Rheumatology (ACR) and European League Against Rheumatism (EULAR) have developed classification criteria. Domains included the pattern of joint involvement, serology status (RF and ACPA), acute phase reactants (CRP and ESR), and duration of symptoms (cutoff of 6 weeks).

At presentation, x-rays can be normal. The earliest abnormality in RA on x-ray evaluation of the joints includes soft tissue swelling and periarticular osteopenia. Additional changes on x-rays include symmetric joint space narrowing and marginal erosions. If erosions are present at diagnosis, this is associated with a worse prognosis.

Differential Diagnosis

The differential diagnosis is broad for RA. Multiple infections can cause polyarticular joint pain. Viral etiologies can include hepatitis B, hepatitis C, and HIV. Parvovirus B19 can also be a mimic of RA; joint pain can be a prominent feature in adults in contrast to children who rarely have joint involvement. Typically the arthritis of parvovirus B19 will resolve spontaneously over a few weeks. Travel history is also an important element of the history; for example, Chikungunya and Dengue can present with arthritis symptoms. Rubella, both the illness and vaccine, can be associated. Bacterial infection such as endocarditis and Lyme disease can present with oligoarticular/polyarticular joint pain. Rheumatic fever is also in the differential and can present with migratory joint pain.

Inflammatory arthritis can be a manifestation of other systemic rheumatologic conditions including seronegative spondyloarthritis (psoriatic arthritis, arthritis secondary to inflammatory bowel disease, reactive arthritis, and ankylosing spondylitis/axial spondyloarthritis). The pattern of involvement can be helpful, as seronegative spondyloarthritis frequently presents in an asymmetric, large joint predominant, and lower extremity predominant fashion. Inflammatory arthritis can develop secondary to connective tissue disease such as systemic lupus erythematosus and systemic sclerosis. ANCA-associated vasculitis can also present with arthritis. Paraneoplastic syndromes can present with joint pain including hypertrophic osteoarthropathy.

Treatment

The goals of treatment of RA are to address both the short term and long term complications of RA. The overarching principle is "treat to target." The goal of therapy should be to achieve clinical remission or low disease activity. The treatment approach must be individualized and consider the comorbidities of the patient. The significant cost of the medications must also be considered in therapy decisions.

Analgesics and Nonsteroidal Antiinflammatory Drugs

Analgesics and nonsteroidal antiinflammatory agents can be utilized to help address breakthrough pain. However, these agents should not be the foundation of treatment. Their role can be used to help control symptoms while a maintenance strategy with conventional disease-modifying antirheumatic drugs (DMARDs) and/or biologics is being established, as there is delay to the full clinical benefit of these medications. Since these medications do not alter the natural history of the disease, they should not be used in isolation.

In patients with extensive damage related to RA, these medications can have a role in helping address pain. DMARDs and biologics are unable to address pain related to damage.

Glucocorticoids

Glucocorticoids are frequently used due to their rapid onset of action, which distinguishes them from DMARDs and biologics. These are frequently utilized at initial diagnosis or with flares of established disease. However, the side effects of corticosteroids limit their use. Corticosteroids should not be utilized in isolation to treat RA. Corticosteroids can be given in multiple administration forms, including oral, intramuscular, and intraarticular. The choice of which to use is dependent on the individual patient's scenario.

Conventional Disease Modifying Antirheumatic Drugs

Conventional DMARDs are immunosuppressants with the goal of inducing and maintaining remission of patients with RA.

Methotrexate

Methotrexate (Otrexup, Rasuvo, Rheumatrex), in the absence of contraindications, is typically the first-line medication utilized for RA. The exact mechanism specifically for RA is incompletely understood. Methotrexate inhibits dihydrofolate reductase which results in reduction of DNA synthesis and, as a result, cell replication. However, this is not the role in isolation as daily folic acid[1] is prescribed to help counter the side effects and does not reverse the therapeutic benefit. Methotrexate also increases the release of adenosine which leads to reduction of inflammation.

Methotrexate can be given in both oral and subcutaneous administration forms. Typically, the starting dose is 10 to 15 mg weekly with titration depending on clinical response, up to 25 mg weekly. At higher doses, gastrointestinal absorption can be limited, and this can be a situation to prefer the subcutaneous form.

Common side effects can include oral ulcers, nausea, fatigue, increased infection risk, cytopenias, and hepatotoxicity. Methotrexate requires routine blood monitoring specifically for cytopenia and hepatotoxicity. The toxicity of methotrexate is increased in the setting of renal dysfunction, and in this setting there should be consideration of dose reduction versus choosing an alternative agent.

[1] Not FDA approved for this indication.

Methotrexate is a teratogen. The recommendation is to wait 3 months from stopping methotrexate before trying to conceive.

Hydroxychloroquine

Hydroxychloroquine (Plaquenil) has multiple mechanisms of action including inhibition of antigen presentation via interference of toll-like receptors and acidification of lysosomes.

It is an oral medication with the dose range of 200 to 400 mg daily. It is a weight-based regimen, and when using real body weight, the dose is 5 mg/kg with the maximum of 400 mg daily.

Side effects can include photosensitive rash, hypoglycemia, hearing loss, and retinal toxicity. Hydroxychloroquine can deposit in the retina which can ultimately lead to vision loss if not identified. Individuals are recommended to have routine eye examinations so changes related to hydroxychloroquine, including bull's eye maculopathy, can be identified and hydroxychloroquine can then be discontinued if necessary. Eye comorbidities, such as macular degeneration, may complicate the ability to monitor for hydroxychloroquine toxicity and would need to be discussed with patient's eye provider.

Sulfasalazine

The exact mechanism of action of sulfasalazine (Azulfidine-EN) in RA is not currently well understood.

It is an oral medication that is utilized twice daily. The dose is typically started at 500 mg once or twice daily with titration of dose to 1000 to 1500 mg twice daily.

Side effects include rash, gastrointestinal side effects, cytopenias, and hepatoxicity. Laboratory monitoring is required to monitor for cytopenia and hepatotoxicity.

Leflunomide

Leflunomide (Arava) inhibits dihydroorotate dehydrogenase, which results in the reduction of pyrimidine synthesis and ultimately reduction of cellular replication.

It comes in an oral form. A loading dose is not required and frequently not used, as it can result in a side effect of diarrhea. Leflunomide has a very long half-life due to its entrance in the enterohepatocyte circulation.

Side effects include diarrhea, cytopenias, hepatoxicity, and increased infection risk. It requires routine laboratory monitoring for cytopenia and hepatotoxicity. It is contraindicated in pregnancy.

A cholestyramine (Questran)[1] washout procedure can be utilized to eliminate leflunomide when needed for a time sensitive scenario, such as a woman wanting to pursue pregnancy.

Azathioprine

Azathioprine (Imuran) is an inhibitor of purine synthesis and as a result of cellular replication.

It is an oral medication and the dosing is weight based. Azathioprine is typically started at 1 mg/kg/day and can be escalated up to a maximum of 2.5 mg/kg/day.

Side effects can include cytopenias, rash, nausea, diarrhea, and pancreatitis. Azathioprine requires routine monitoring for cytopenias and hepatotoxicity. A thiopurine methyltransferase (TPMT) level can be checked prior to initiation for assessment of the metabolism of azathioprine. If there are reduced levels of TPMT activity, then one would need to consider using a reduced dose or an alternative agent.

Azathioprine has been less commonly used as other agents have become available. Interstitial lung disease secondary to RA is one scenario in which it is still utilized.

Synthetic Disease Modifying Antirheumatic Drugs
Janus Kinase (JAK) Inhibitors

Tofacitinib (Xeljanz), baricitinib (Olumiant), and upadacitinib (Rinvoq) are targeted small molecules that inhibit Janus kinases (JAKs). Inhibition blocks intracellular signaling of cytokine receptors and results in decreased gene activation.

The JAK inhibitors are oral medications. Side effects can include cytopenia, hepatotoxicity, and cholesterol elevation. The U.S. Food and Drug Administration (FDA) updated warnings in 2021 regarding serious heart-related events, cancer including lymphoma and lung cancer, and thrombosis. Individual patient risk factors should be given attention. Routine lab monitoring is required to monitor for these complications. There are rare reports of bowel perforation, and currently there is a recommendation to avoid in the setting of diverticulitis.

Biologics
"Biologics" refers to medical therapies that are derived from living organisms such as humans, animals, or microorganisms in contrast to traditional nonbiological drugs that are chemically synthesized in a laboratory without the use of living organisms. Biologics may be produced by cutting-edge biotechnology methods such as gene-based and cellular technologies. Biologics can be used in combination with conventional DMARDs. "Biosimilar" drugs have a chemical structure and biochemical function that is similar to biologics. While not identical to their corresponding biologic, biosimilars are becoming increasingly available.

TNF Inhibitors
TNF inhibitors inhibit the effect of TNF alpha, a proinflammatory cytokine. There are five different TNF inhibitors: etanercept (Enbrel), adalimumab (Humira), certolizumab (Cimzia), golimumab (Simponi), and infliximab (Remicade). Etanercept has a component of the TNF receptor, allowing it to bind TNF alpha, and prevents it from binding to TNF receptors. The remaining are monoclonal antibodies targeting TNF alpha. Etanercept, adalimumab, certolizumab, and golimumab come in a subcutaneous form. Golimumab and infliximab are available as an infusion.

Side effects include injection site/infusion reactions. Patients must be counseled on infection risk to wide-ranging organisms, ranging from bacterial, viral, fungal, and mycobacterial. Individuals must undergo tuberculosis testing prior to initiation of therapies. There were initial concerns regarding lymphoma in the setting of TNF inhibitor use, but also underlying RA plays a role in the risk. TNF inhibitors can be associated with exacerbations of congestive heart failure. Multiple sclerosis would be a contraindication to TNF inhibitors.

Interleukin 6 Receptor Inhibitor (Tocilizumab and Sarilumab)
Tocilizumab (Actemra) and sarilumab (Kevzara) are both interleukin 6 (IL6) receptor inhibitors, which prevents activation of the receptors of IL6. This prevents the downstream activation of targets of IL6, a proinflammatory cytokine.

Tocilizumab comes as both infusion and subcutaneous versions. Sarilumab comes as a subcutaneous version.

Side effects include cytopenia, particularly neutropenia and thrombocytopenia, hepatotoxicity, and elevated cholesterol. Routine monitoring is necessary. Injection site/infusion reactions are also a risk. The infection concerns are similar to TNF inhibitors, with the risk pertaining to diverse organisms. Due to rare reports of bowel perforations, it is recommended to be avoided in the setting of diverticulitis.

T Cell Coactivation Inhibition
Abatacept (Orencia) prevents T cell coactivation by binding the costimulating signal (CD80/86) on antigen presenting cells and preventing it from binding T cells. Administration forms include subcutaneous injection and intravenous infusions. Side effects include injection/infusion site reactions. Infection risk is also a concern with abatacept.

B Cell Inhibition
Rituximab (Rituxan) depletes B cells by targeting CD20, which is present on B cells.

It is an intravenous medication. The timing of subsequent doses is typically every 6 months.

The risks of rituximab include infusion reactions. Infection risk is a concern with rituximab, particularly considering the long timeframe of effect. Careful attention must be given to prevent hepatitis B reactivation. Even patients with evidence of natural immunity via cleared infection would be a candidate for hepatitis B reactivation prophylaxis. Progressive multifocal leukoencephalopathy (PML) related to JC virus has been reported in patients receiving rituximab for the indication of RA. The risk is very low, and in multiple reports, patients were also on additional immunosuppressants such as chemotherapy.

Interleukin 1 Inhibition
Anakinra (Kineret) is an inhibitor of the IL1 receptor preventing the downstream activation of IL1, a proinflammatory cytokine. Risks are similar to other biologics in terms of infection, injection site reaction, cytopenia, and nausea. It is a daily subcutaneous injection.

Combination Therapy
Combination therapy is frequently utilized for treatment of RA. An indication to proceed with combination therapy is when disease activity is persistent despite therapeutic dosing with a single agent. A frequently used combination therapy is termed "triple therapy." This refers to the combination of methotrexate, sulfasalazine, and hydroxychloroquine. A single biologic can be utilized in combination with conventional DMARDs, most frequently methotrexate. Two biologics are not recommended to be utilized together, due to concern with increased infection risk.

Choice of Therapy
Multiple factors must be weighed in terms of the choice of therapy for RA. If there are no contraindications, methotrexate is typically used as the first choice. If there is an insufficient response to a maximized dose of methotrexate, including use of subcutaneous methotrexate, then combination therapy is frequently utilized. If methotrexate is unable to be tolerated, then leflunomide could be considered in its place. The combination therapy to be utilized with methotrexate could include triple therapy versus methotrexate in combination with a biologic or synthetic DMARD (JAK inhibitors). Triple therapy has been compared with methotrexate plus biologic therapy in multiple studies and overall thought to be equivalent in terms of achieving clinical response. The choice between the two is dependent on discussion with the patient. Consideration for the forms of administration would need to be taken into account. Comorbidities of the patient can restrict choices. Another consideration is cost and insurance coverage for different medications.

When patients have consistently achieved clinical remission, there can be consideration for reduction in treatment. There is increased risk of flare of disease when reducing medications. Patients would need to be counseled regarding this risk and monitored closely.

Special Scenarios
Pregnancy
As RA can affect women of childbearing age, the goals in terms of pregnancy must be understood for patients with RA. Methotrexate and leflunomide would be contraindicated in the setting of pregnancy. Methotrexate is associated with known congenital abnormalities. The recommendation would be to stop methotrexate 3 months prior to contraception. Leflunomide has a much longer half-life and the level could be checked and, if elevated, then could use cholestyramine[1] washout. If there is a possibility of pregnancy, then hydroxychloroquine or sulfasalazine are frequently used options in this setting. TNF inhibitors have been utilized in pregnancy. The recommendations would be to stop TNF inhibitors over the course of pregnancy with the specific TNF inhibitors having different recommendations; certolizumab is not thought to cross the placenta due to its chemical structure, and

---

[1]Not FDA approved for this indication.

in some individuals, this is continued throughout the pregnancy. Less information is available about the safety of other biologics in pregnancy and, if possible, would be avoided until further information is known.

Patients can have improvement in their clinical symptoms during pregnancy, which emphasizes the importance of an individualized approach during pregnancy. Patients should be counseled on the risk for flare in the postpartum setting.

Breastfeeding

Data is limited regarding the effects of medications for RA and breastfeeding. The potential benefits of breastfeeding would need to be weighed with potential risk. Methotrexate and leflunomide are avoided during breastfeeding. An individualized approach is necessary in conjunction with the patient and obstetrician.

Malignancy

Data is limited regarding the ideal choice of therapy in the setting of a history of malignancy. DMARDs are frequently preferred over biologics in the setting of prior malignancy. Specifically in the setting of lymphoproliferative disorders, if a biologic is indicated due to disease activity, rituximab is preferred over other biologic choices. Individualized decisions must be made in conjunction with the patient and their hematologist/oncologist.

Preoperative Management

Due to the risk of atlantoaxial instability in RA, particularly in long-standing disease, patients prior to surgery should be screened for this complication. Cervical spine x-rays with flexion and extension views would be recommended. The results should be reviewed with an anesthesiologist to assist with planning for positioning during surgery.

Management of immunosuppressant medications must be reviewed with the surgeon and take into account the nature of surgery as well as the pharmacokinetics of the immunosuppressants. Data are limited on the ideal management of immunosuppressants in this setting. Guidelines have been published in the setting of total hip and knee arthroplasty.

Monitoring

There are two components of monitoring for patients with RA. The first is to assess for disease activity both from the standpoint of the joints as well as extraarticular manifestations. From the joint perspective, there are multiple disease activity scores that can be utilized. Some rely solely on patient reported outcomes. Others are a combination of patient reported outcomes, exam findings, and provider global assessment. Swollen joint counts and tender joint counts are frequently utilized. Specifically for laboratory monitoring of disease activity, ESR and CRP can be utilized but do not trend with disease activity in all patients. ACPA and RF do not trend with disease activity and thus the values do not need to be repeated if positive.

Separately, drug toxicity must be assessed including clinical symptoms and laboratory monitoring. In addition, monitoring for development of infection is also necessary.

Management of Complications

If drug toxicity develops, depending on the nature of toxicity, the medication dose should either be reduced or discontinued. If the side effect likely reflects a class effect, consider an agent in a different drug class. If infection occurs while on immunosuppressant therapy, these medications should be held at least until the infection has resolved. Restarting would be dependent on the clinical scenario, including the nature of the infection and the specific treatment for RA.

References

Aletaha D, Neogi T, Silman AJ, et al: 2010 Rheumatoid Arthritis Classification Criteria: an American College of Rheumatology/European League Against Rheumatism Collaborative Initiative, *Arthritis Rheum* 62:2569–2581, 2010.
Aletaha D, Smolen JS: Diagnosis and management of rheumatoid arthritis: a review, *JAMA* 320:1360–1372, 2018.
Anderson J, Caplan L, Yazdany J, et al: Rheumatoid arthritis disease activity measures: American College of Rheumatology recommendations for use in clinical practice, *Arthritis Care Res (Hoboken)* 64:640–647, 2012.
Goodman SM, Springer B, Guyatt G, et al: 2017 American College of Rheumatology/American Association of Hip and Knee Surgeons guideline for the perioperative management of antirheumatic medication in patients with rheumatic diseases undergoing elective total hip or total knee arthroplasty, *Arthritis Care Res* 69:1111–1124, 2017.
Fraenkel L, Bathon JM, England BR, et al: 2021 American College of Rheumatology guideline for the treatment of rheumatoid arthritis, *Arthritis Care Res (Hoboken)* 72:924–939, 2021.
Hochberg M: *Rheumatology*, Seventh edition, Philadelphia, PA, 2019, Elsevier. 2019.
Smolen JS, Landewe R, Bijlsma J, et al: EULAR recommendations for the management of rheumatoid arthritis with synthetic and biologic disease-modifying antirheumatic drugs: 2016 update, *Ann Rheum Dis* 76:960–977, 2017.

TENDINOPATHY AND BURSITIS

Method of
Kyle Goerl, MD

CURRENT DIAGNOSIS

Tendinopathy
- Tendinitis is an inflammatory condition only present within the first weeks of a tendon injury.
- Tendinosis is a degenerative condition usually developing weeks after the initial injury.
- The diagnosis of tendinopathy is typically made clinically with a thorough history and physical examination.
- Most tendinopathies occur secondary to overuse and can be acute from trauma, chronic, or recurrent.
- Tendinopathies are usually characterized by pain, possible swelling, and dysfunction of the affected tendon.
- If the diagnosis is in question, magnetic resonance imaging and ultrasound are helpful diagnostic aides.

Bursitis
- Bursitis is an inflammatory reaction of a bursa.
- Bursitis is typically the result of overuse or trauma, but systemic illnesses can also cause bursitis.
- The olecranon, prepatellar, and trochanteric bursa are particularly susceptible to traumatic bursitis due to their location directly under the skin with minimal subcutaneous fat for protection.
- Bursitis rarely occurs alone, so a search should be conducted for an associated condition such as tendinopathy or a tendon tear.
- Imaging studies demonstrate that lateral hip pain is usually tendinopathy, not "trochanteric bursitis," a term that should be reserved for image-proven bursitis.
- Septic bursitis usually only affects the olecranon and prepatellar bursa, and care must be taken to distinguish it from aseptic bursitis.
- Common pathogens in septic bursitis include *Staphylococcus aureus* and β-hemolytic *Streptococcus*.
- If the diagnosis of septic bursitis is in question, aspiration should be performed and the aspirate sent for gram stain, cell count and differential, culture, and crystal analysis, and blood should be sent for culture, complete blood count, C-reactive protein, and erythrocyte sedimentation rate.

CURRENT THERAPY

Tendinopathy
- Given that tendonitis is an inflammatory condition, scheduled NSAIDs should be considered. Ice, bracing, activity modification, and rest are also effective.

- Tendinosis is not an inflammatory condition, so NSAIDs are not usually a part of the treatment regimen aside for pain control.
- Tendinosis responds well to physical therapy (PT) and, in particular, eccentric exercises. Deep tissue massage with tools is also an effective treatment modality.
- Steroid injections can be effective for short-term pain relief, but not for long-term healing, and should not be a routine part of the treatment plan. Steroid injections can be considered if the patient is in too much pain to perform PT, for disturbed sleep, or to help perform activities of daily living.
- Injections of blood products such as whole blood and platelet-rich plasma, prolotherapy, and sclerotherapy have varying levels of evidence supporting their effectiveness but are reasonable alternatives to surgery.
- When conservative measures fail, more invasive procedures such as tenotomy, tendon scraping, and open debridement should be considered, though rarely needed.

Bursitis

- Early treatment should include NSAIDs, ice, activity modification, and rest.
- If an associated condition like tendinopathy is discovered, appropriate treatment should target that condition as well and typically involves PT.
- In the event of septic bursitis, antibiotic treatment should be initiated. Parenteral medication should be seriously considered given the high failure rate of oral antibiotics.
- Surgery is rarely needed for bursitis.

TABLE 1	Differentiation Between Tendonitis and Tendinosis	
	TENDONITIS	**TENDINOSIS**
Pathology	Inflammatory	Degenerative
Timing	Days to weeks	Weeks to years
Imaging	Typically unnecessary	Radiographs initially Ultrasound or magnetic resonance imaging for persistent symptoms

TABLE 2	Common Tendinopathy Sites

Upper Extremity

1. Rotator cuff (especially supraspinatus)
2. Medial epicondyle
3. Lateral epicondyle (especially extensor carpi radialis brevis)
4. First dorsal compartment of the wrist (De Quervain)

Lower Extremity

1. Gluteus medius and gluteus minimus
2. Iliopsoas
3. Patellar
4. Achilles

Tendinopathy

Background

Tendon is a connective tissue used to attach muscle to bone. Normal tendon tissue is dense and has a highly regular and fibrillar pattern. Tendinopathy is the term used to describe a clinical syndrome typically resulting from overuse of a tendon. Traditionally, the term tendonitis has been used to describe all tendon injuries, but the suffix "–is" indicates the presence of inflammation, which is only present early in the tendinopathy disease process. Inflammation may have resolved and inflammatory cells may no longer be present, but the patient may still have pain. At that point, the disease process has changed from one of inflammation to a degenerative problem more appropriately termed tendinosis (Table 1).

Tendinopathies are characterized by pain, swelling, and impairment of functional activities of the affected region. They can be acute, chronic, or recurrent. The diagnosis is usually clinical based on history and physical examination. Typically, there is a history of repetitive motion, which can be anything from painting a wall to playing a sport such as tennis. If this historical information is lacking, then a systemic medical condition should be considered.

With repetitive activities and inadequate recovery time, tenocytes will begin producing inflammatory substances and the load-bearing matrix of the tendon will begin to break down and become fibrotic. The collagen matrix becomes disorganized with fibers separating and healing in an erratic, disorganized manner. There is an increase in mucoid ground substance, hypercellularity, and pathologic vessel and sensory afferent nerve formation. The abnormal nerve formation likely contributes to the sensation of pain. This histopathological degenerative process is more appropriately called tendinosis. The degenerative mechanism appears to be multifactorial, with contributions from:

1. Classic inflammatory mediators like interleukins, prostaglandins, and substance P
2. Altered load bearing on a tendon, as in shoulder impingement
3. Systemic influences such as aging

Tendinopathy is occurring at higher rates in the developed world secondary to an increase in recreational sport participation. Lower extremity tendons, like the Achilles and patellar tendons, bear a large amount of tensile force (Table 2). Thirty

percent of runners will suffer Achilles tendinopathy in their lifetime, with an odds ratio of 31:2 when compared to age-matched controls. Repetitive exposure is a risk factor. That said, 1 in 3 patients with Achilles tendinopathy do not participate in sports. With respect to patellar tendinopathy, jumping sports like volleyball and basketball are risk factors. Historically, most lateral hip pain was labeled "trochanteric bursitis." Research using imaging techniques, including magnetic resonance imaging (MRI) and ultrasound (US), has concluded that lateral hip pain around the greater trochanter is more likely due to tendon tears or tendinopathy of the gluteus medius and gluteus minimus muscle-tendon complex than inflammation of the trochanteric bursa. Rarely is there an actual bursitis present, so the diagnosis "trochanteric bursitis" should no longer be used regularly unless there is documented bursitis on an imaging study. This is important because the patient is more likely to benefit long-term from physical therapy (PT) as opposed to NSAIDs or steroid injections, due to the underlying pathology being more likely tendon-related than bursa-related. Without an imaging study, the better term for lateral hip pain, at this time, is Greater Trochanteric Pain Syndrome (GTPS).

Many upper extremity tendons, like those of the wrist, are adapted to gliding through synovial sheaths. The most commonly affected tendons in the upper extremity are the rotator cuff, specifically the supraspinatus tendon, and the common extensor tendon (more precisely, the extensor carpi radialis brevis) involved in lateral epicondylopathy, commonly known as *tennis elbow*. Despite names like tennis elbow and golfer's elbow, upper extremity tendinopathies (Table 2) are more likely due to repetitive motion from work- or hobby-related activities. When sports are a cause of upper extremity tendinopathy, they are typically those requiring overhead motion like baseball, volleyball, and tennis. Up to 35% to 50% of adult tennis players will develop an elbow tendinopathy during their lifetime. A common cause of tendinopathy in the wrist is De Quervain's tenosynovitis. De Quervain's tenosynovitis affects the first dorsal compartment of the wrist containing the abductor pollicis longus and extensor pollicis brevis tendons. As the term "tenosynovitis" suggests, this condition results in irritation and swelling of not only the tendons themselves, but of the synovial sheath encapsulating those tendons as well.

Some patients will develop tendinopathies without repetitive activity. Diseases of glucose metabolism and atherosclerosis are associated with a higher incidence of tendinopathy. Some common medications are also associated with tendinopathy including statins, fluoroquinolone antibiotics, and steroids, especially when steroids are injected intratendinously, which should be avoided.

Evaluation

On physical examination, the affected tendon will sometimes appear swollen, and it is typically tender to palpation. The affected tendon-muscle complex may exhibit restricted flexibility, and stretching it or activating it against resistance may reproduce the patient's pain.

When the diagnosis of a tendinopathy is in question, imaging can be helpful. Radiographs of the affected area should be considered to look for abnormalities, such as large calcifications within tendons. When the diagnosis is in question or the patient has failed a course of PT, advanced imaging should be considered. This is usually accomplished by either US or MRI. US can reveal thickening or structural changes within the tendon consistent with degeneration and other abnormalities like calcification. As tendinopathies are commonly associated with bursitis, bursal thickening consistent with bursitis may also be seen. Similar findings may be demonstrated on MRI.

Determining which imaging modality to use can be challenging. MRI is considered the gold standard for diagnosing tendinopathies and has the advantage of demonstrating an anatomic overview of the affected area, as well as providing soft tissue contrast. However, in trained hands, the advantages of US include ease of use, point-of-care examination, dynamic evaluation of the tendon and muscles, better resolution than MRI, and guidance for injections and procedures.

Prevention

Prevention is always the best option. Tendons do not respond well to acute changes in routine or long periods of rest. This should be kept in mind by athletes during the offseason, someone taking on a new labor job on an assembly line, or an administrative assistant with a new work space. These "potential patients" should be eased into their new routines, as all of these scenarios are classic setups for the development of a tendinopathy. Maintaining activity during the offseason and preparing one's self for changes in the workplace will help to mitigate the risk of tendinopathy development.

Treatment

Medications are rarely employed in the treatment of tendinosis, as the patient usually does not present to the clinician's office until long after the disease process has begun. If the patient is caught early enough, for example, within a week or two of the offending event (e.g., lateral epicondylitis a week after painting a house), then the disease process is still likely an inflammatory one and appropriately termed a tendonitis. In this case, scheduled NSAIDs (so long as the patient does not have medical contraindications to their use) are appropriate to try and stop the inflammatory process and ultimately prevent it from progressing to a degenerative process. Other effective treatments for tendonitis include activity modification, bracing, rest, and ice. However, if the patient has had pain for months, the process has likely progressed to tendinosis. The use of NSAIDs has been shown to negatively affect the repair mechanism involved in tendinosis, thus they should be used cautiously in this situation.

Expectations about healing tendinosis should be addressed early. To begin with, tendon healing takes significant time and effort on the part of the patient. Additionally, many of the treatment modalities used to heal tendons will produce a reasonable amount of pain in and of themselves. This is actually a good thing, as it indicates the patient is working hard enough to heal and that the healing process is occurring. It is not uncommon to have minor setbacks during the rehabilitation process. There should be

an overall trend from a state of disease to health, but the path to recovery is not typically linear. The initial management of tendinopathy should be rehabilitation through PT. The patient should be informed that the "work" of PT is not done at the therapist's office, but it is done at home on their own. Failing to adhere to the treatment program will almost ensure a lack of recovery.

The exercises performed in PT aim to reorganize the degenerative matrix, reduce tenocyte activity, improve tendon compliance, and provide analgesia. Specifically, eccentric exercises have proven to be an effective treatment. An eccentric exercise is one that strengthens the muscle-tendon complex while lengthening the complex. For example, if a patient is being treated for lateral epicondylosis, the eccentric exercise would be to move the wrist from extension to flexion against resistance, lengthening the common extensor tendon. Strengthening exercises also work to hypertrophy the muscle, which is commonly atrophied after long periods of abnormal use from compensatory movement by the patient to try and reduce pain. The time needed for the exercises to work well is 3 months, which correlates with the time needed to form new fibroblasts, the presumed mechanism by which eccentric exercises work.

PT exercises should be done bilaterally, as there is proven crossover effect for tendinopathies, whereby exercising the non-affected side actually improves the affected side. Adding static stretching to eccentric exercises has been shown to improve outcomes over eccentric exercises alone in patellar tendinopathy and should be included in an effective rehabilitation program. Before releasing an athlete back to sports activity, the final components of an optimal rehabilitation program include explosive concentric movements (i.e., weightlifting or box jumps), higher eccentric loading exercises (i.e., jumping from an elevated surface like a box and landing on the ground), and sports-specific movements like sprinting and cutting.

The other treatment modality commonly employed by a physical therapist in tendinosis is deep soft tissue massage with tools. These tools are used to scrape along the pathologic tendon, which promotes blood flow and inflammation leading to the breakdown of the degenerative tissue and ultimately healing of that tissue.

When these conservative measures fail, more aggressive treatment methods should be considered. It is important to point out that the following treatment options are supported by limited high quality evidence but are nonetheless reasonable alternatives to a surgical procedure. Less invasive methods include extracorporeal shockwave therapy and low-intensity pulsed US. Glyceryl trinitrate patches are sometimes used to promote blood flow and have been shown to provide some pain relief. Injections are common treatment modalities in tendinopathies. Steroid injections are commonly used, but usually provide short-term pain relief at best. There is evidence for long-term negative effects of steroids, so they should be used judiciously. A reasonable time to try a steroid injection is if the patient is experiencing so much pain that they are unable to perform therapy or activities of daily living, or they cannot sleep. US guidance in the hands of a trained physician can help ensure that the injection is placed properly and specifically, not intratendinously. Other treatment options requiring a more trained physician, such as a sports medicine specialist, include prolotherapy, sclerotherapy, and biological blood product injections. Prolotherapy, the injection of hypertonic glucose, is thought to work by inducing a local inflammation-repair mechanism. In sclerotherapy, a sclerotic agent, typically polidocanol (Asclera),[1] is injected to degrade the tendinopathy pain generators, namely the abnormal vessels and sensory nerves within the tendinopathic tissue. Blood products, including whole blood and platelet-rich plasma, are used with the intent to deliver a high concentration of growth factors to the tendinopathic tissue where blood flow is typically low.

If the tendinopathy does not respond to these treatment options, then more invasive measures are typically considered.

---

[1] Not FDA approved for this indication.

A tenotomy procedure uses a sharp object, typically a large bore needle or mechanized oscillating needle, to repetitively fenestrate the degenerated portion of tendon tissue, as noted on US guidance, to cause bleeding and stimulate tissue healing. There is a newer technique, whereby the outside of tendon is scraped with a needle or scalpel. The procedure is guided by increased color Doppler signal on US indicating high vascularity and presumed nerve formation. The recovery from these techniques is usually a minimum of 6 weeks, so they should be reserved for recalcitrant cases. Finally, an open procedure can be performed to remove macroscopically abnormal tissue through an incision in the tendon; unfortunately, the recovery for this sort of a procedure is the in the timeframe of 4 to 12 months.

Bursitis

Background

Bursas are fluid-filled sacs designed to reduce friction between various tissues including bones, skin, tendons, and muscles. Typically, there is little fluid within a bursa, but with irritation from overuse or trauma, the bursa may swell with fluid leading to pain and dysfunction. This is referred to as bursitis due to the inflammatory nature of the condition.

There are multiple locations in the body where bursitis more commonly occurs including the shoulder, elbow, hip, and knee. Bursitis usually develops from either trauma or overuse, but systemic illnesses like rheumatoid arthritis, diabetes mellitus, gout or pseudogout, and immunosuppression may also lead to bursitis. Bursas that are more susceptible to traumatic bursitis include the prepatellar, olecranon, and trochanteric bursas. They are closer to the skin and have little subcutaneous fat over them, thus they are more likely to sustain a direct impact. Both the olecranon and prepatellar bursa are at risk for chronic irritation and trauma as well. Olecranon bursitis is seen in patients who frequently rest on their elbows, as in desk workers and truck drivers. Prepatellar bursitis is seen in patients who kneel for work like carpet layers and house cleaners.

Septic bursitis is rare, and it most commonly affects the olecranon and prepatellar bursa. This occurs via direct inoculation from the traumatic event. The most common organisms isolated are *Staphylococcus aureus* followed by β-hemolytic *Streptococcus*, with about 10% being polymicrobial infections.

The other bursas in the body are more susceptible to overuse injuries. The bursas around the shoulder most commonly affected include the subacromial-subdeltoid bursa and the scapulothoracic bursa. Athletes who perform overhead movements in sports such as baseball, softball, tennis, volleyball, and swimming are at greater risk for irritating these bursas. Of course, athletes are not the only people at risk for bursitis. Manual laborers working with their arms, especially when flexed or abducted regularly, can also develop bursitis around the shoulder.

The hip and pelvis have multiple bursas, but the more commonly affected include the bursas around the greater trochanter and iliopsoas. As stated in the tendinopathy section, lateral hip pain is rarely caused by "trochanteric bursitis," but there are bursa present under the gluteus maximus, gluteus medius, and gluteus minimus muscle-tendon complexes. Bursitis in this region is rarely found without an associated problem like gluteal tendinopathy or iliotibial (IT) band syndrome. In fact, it is likely that one of these underlying problems led to the bursitis. There is also a bursa under the iliopsoas muscle as it crosses the iliopectineal eminence and anterior hip joint.

Rare causes of knee bursitis include irritation of the suprapatellar bursa, deep infrapatellar bursa, pes anserine bursa, semimembranosus bursa, and medial collateral ligament bursa (Voshell's bursa). Bursitis at these locations is almost always from chronic overuse. In the ankle, the retrocalcaneal bursa may also be irritated from overuse.

Evaluation

Evaluation of a patient with suspected bursitis should always begin with a thorough history. Usually the clinician will discover a history of either trauma or overuse, but the patient should be questioned about the presence of systemic illness as well. Physical exam of the affected region should include inspection for erythema and swelling. Warmth may be noted on palpation. Range of motion may be limited, but is not a consistent finding. Strength is rarely affected. The appearance of decreased strength may only reflect pain, not true weakness. True weakness would suggest an associated concern like tendinopathy or a tendon tear.

Patients presenting with shoulder pain should be evaluated for rotator cuff tendinopathy and scapulothoracic dysfunction and winging, which predispose the athlete to impingement and bursitis. For patients complaining of hip pain, another symptom they may complain of is snapping. The patient should be questioned if the snap is reliably reproducible. If so, then have the patient demonstrate the snap. Snapping laterally is typically the gluteus maximus muscle or iliotibial band snapping over the greater trochanter, and this is a risk factor for bursitis. If the snapping is anterior in the hip, it is likely the iliopsoas tendon snapping over the iliopectineal eminence or anterior femoral head, which can lead to iliopsoas bursitis. Unpredictable snapping or snapping on examination of the anterior hip and groin that is difficult to reliably reproduce should prompt an investigation for an intra-articular source.

For the olecranon and prepatellar bursas, special attention must be given to the fact that they are more likely to develop into a septic bursitis from a bacterial infection. If there is evidence of an abrasion in these particular areas, the physician needs to ensure there is not an associated infection. Erythema, progressive swelling, and painful range of motion may point toward the presence of an infection, but these symptoms are often present in aseptic bursitis as well, making the diagnosis difficult. Fever may be present, but its absence does not rule out infection. If there is any concern for infection, the bursa needs to be aspirated and fluid sent for cell count and differential, crystal analysis, Gram stain, and culture before starting antibiotics. Blood should also be sent for a complete blood count, C-reactive protein, erythrocyte sedimentation rate, and cultures.

Imaging is not always necessary to diagnose bursitis. Swelling and erythema over a known bursa may be enough to make a diagnosis, but if the diagnosis is in question, then imaging typically begins with radiographs. Radiographs can evaluate for bony abnormalities that may suggest an underlying reason for bursitis. For example, spurring on the undersurface of the acromion can be a risk factor for subacromial-subdeltoid bursitis. Radiographs can also be used to rule out fracture or evaluate for a foreign body, especially in the setting of olecranon or prepatellar bursitis.

Further evaluation is typically done with either MRI or US. MRI offers the advantage of global assessment of the affected region, as well as allowing enhancement of soft tissues. In skilled hands, US is an effective tool to demonstrate bursitis throughout the body (see Figure 3). US also has the distinct advantage of real-time imaging during a dynamic examination of the affected tissue. If aspiration or injection is needed, US can help guide the procedure. Both MRI and US modalities are useful in assessing for associated diagnoses like tendinopathy as well.

Treatment

Bursitis treatment usually begins with conservative measures like rest or activity modification, NSAIDs, compression, padded splinting, and ice. If the bursitis is acute, it is typically responsive to these basic treatments. As stated previously in this chapter, it is common to find associated problems with the bursitis. These include rotator cuff tendinopathy, gluteal tendinopathy, and iliotibial band syndrome. It is imperative that these issues be treated as well or the bursitis will likely reoccur. This typically requires a home exercise plan usually best directed by a physical therapist.

If these problems fail to respond to this conservative approach, including rehabilitation, then a steroid injection can be considered. There is reasonable evidence that doing the injection under US guidance will lead to better outcomes, especially for the subacromial-subdeltoid bursa, but blind injections are certainly reasonable if US is not available. Research reveals that steroid injections for GTPS demonstrate clinically relevant relief at 3 months post-injection when compared to usual care, but that difference disappears by 12 months. This is a common finding with steroid injections. Thus, it is reasonable to consider a steroid injection for pain relief, especially if the patient is unable to participate in PT, but it is unlikely to "fix" the patient's problem long-term.

For olecranon and prepatellar bursitis, the clinician must first differentiate between septic and aseptic bursitis. If the bursa is infected, following aspiration and lab collection, antibiotics must be initiated. The decision about whether to use oral versus parenteral antibiotics and whether admission is warranted depends upon the severity of the infection and the reliability of the patient. Oral therapy should be used cautiously, as treatment failure has been seen in up to 39% to 50% of patients. The duration of antibiotic treatment is usually 10 to 14 days. Surgical intervention is rarely necessary but should be considered in patients who fail to respond to incision, drainage, and appropriate antibiotics; if there is suspicion of a foreign body; or there is an inability to adequately drain the bursa.

With aseptic bursitis of the prepatellar and olecranon bursas, the clinician should resist the urge to aspirate and inject with steroids. Aspiration and injection is a possible treatment option but should only follow a failed conservative approach. This is due to the fact that, once drained, the bursa is likely to quickly fill with fluid again, and there is a risk for an iatrogenic infection. Steroids are also known to cause skin atrophy. A 6- to 8-week trial of the conservative approach is reasonable.

References

Ackermann PW, Renstrom P: Tendinopathy in Sport, *Sports Health* 4(3):193–201, 2012.

Chang A, Miller TT: Imaging of tendons, *Sports Health* 1(4):293–300, 2009.

Long SS, Surrey DE, Nazarian LN: Sonography of greater trochanteric pain syndrome and the rarity of primary bursitis, *Am. J. Roentgenol* 201(5):1083–1086, 2013.

Reilly D, Kamineni S: Olecranon bursitis, *J Shoulder Elbow Surg* 25(1):158–167, 2016.

Scott A, Docking S, Vicenzino B, et al: Sports and exercise-related tendinopathies: a review of selected topical issues by participants of the second International Scientific Tendinopathy Symposium (ISTS) Vancouver 2012, *Br J Sports Med* 47(9):536–544, 2013.

Seroyer ST, Nho SJ, Bach BR, Bush-Joseph CA, Nicholson GP, Romeo AA: Shoulder Pain in the Overhead Throwing Athlete, *Sports Health* 1(2):108–120, 2009.

Williams BS, Cohen SP: Greater trochanteric pain syndrome: a review of anatomy, diagnosis and treatment, *Anesth Analg* 108(5):1662–1670, 2009.

Wu T, Song HX, Dong Y, Li JH: Ultrasound-guided versus blind subacromial-subdeltoid bursa injection in adults with shoulder pain: A systematic review and meta-analysis, *Semin Arthritis Rheum* 45(3):374–378, 2015.

CHLAMYDIA TRACHOMATIS

Method of
Tracy L. Williams, MD

CURRENT DIAGNOSIS

- Screen all sexually active women less than 25 years of age for *Chlamydia trachomatis* annually regardless of symptoms per Centers for Disease Control and Prevention (CDC) recommendations.
- Symptomatic patients should be tested regardless of gender.
- Reinfection with *C. trachomatis* is common.
  - Retest all patients who have a history of *C. trachomatis* or *Neisseria gonorrhoeae* at 3 months after treatment, regardless of whether their partner(s) were treated.
  - If the patient does not follow up at 3 months, then retest upon presentation for medical care within the first 12 months posttreatment.
- Patients who screen positive for *C. trachomatis* need to be screened for gonorrhea, syphilis, and human immunodeficiency virus (HIV).
- Screen all pregnant women for chlamydia, gonorrhea, syphilis, and HIV at their first prenatal visit and again in the third trimester if they are at high risk for sexually transmitted infections (STIs).
- Perform a test of cure on pregnant patients at 4 weeks posttreatment and repeat in 3 months, preferably in the third trimester if the pregnant woman was diagnosed during the first trimester.

CURRENT THERAPY

- Doxycycline (Vibramycin) 100 mg orally twice a day for 7 days is the recommended regimen for nonpregnant patients and for presumptive treatment for *C. trachomatis.*
- Azithromycin (Zithromax) 1 g orally in a single dose is the recommended regimen for pregnant patients with *C. trachomatis.*
- All of the patient's recent sexual partners need referral and treatment.
  - The patient's last sexual contact should be referred and treated if it has been more than 60 days since the patient had a sexual partner.
  - The partner needs to be treated for *C. trachomatis* even if their personal STI results are negative.
- Counsel patients and their partners to abstain from sexual contact until 7 days after one-dose therapy or after the final dose of the 7-day regimen.
- The CDC recommends patients who test positive for *N. gonorrhoeae* only be treated for *C. trachomatis* when coinfection is not excluded.
- Doxycycline postexposure prophylaxis (doxy PEP)[1] is used as a prevention strategy for men having sex with men (MSM) and transgender women with a history of a bacterial STI in the past 12 months, taken as a single of 200-mg dose once within 72 hours of unprotected sex.

[1]Not FDA approved for this indication.

Epidemiology

Chlamydia trachomatis is the most common notifiable sexually transmitted infection (STI) in the United States, with an incidence of 1.65 million cases per year according to the Centers for Disease Control and Prevention (CDC) in 2023. Women ages 15 to 19 years are the most commonly affected, followed by women ages 20 to 24. The incidence of *C. trachomatis* has steadily climbed yearly since it became a federally mandated notifiable disease except during the COVID-19 era, which may be a reflection of a reduction of usual screening practices.

C. trachomatis costs an estimated $2.4 billion annually. Cost-benefit analyses have consistently shown prioritizing screening efforts in asymptomatic women to be cost-effective.

Risk Factors

The risk of contracting *C. trachomatis* increases with multiple sexual partners; unprotected sex including vaginal, oral, and anal intercourse; anal-receptive intercourse; and men having sex with men (MSM). The risk increases in the presence of other coinfections including human immunodeficiency virus (HIV) or herpes simplex virus (HSV). African Americans have a fourfold higher incidence compared with their White counterparts (13% vs. 2.4%, respectively).

Pathophysiology

C. trachomatis is an obligate intracellular parasite. It is found only in human cells but can live on fomites for up to 30 hours. Previous infections do not yield protection against future infections with *C. trachomatis*. *C. trachomatis* does not infect the squamous epithelium of the vaginal vault but can infect the urethra, the squamocolumnar junction of the cervix, the rectal mucosa, and the oropharynx.

Prevention

Prevention depends on screening of asymptomatic patients, who make up a large portion of the infected population. The US Preventive Services Task Force (USPSTF) recommends annual screening of all sexually active women younger than 25 years of age and for older women at increased risk. The CDC and the USPSTF found insufficient evidence to recommend routine screening of men based on cost-effectiveness, efficacy, and practicality. Screening is recommended for symptomatic men or men in areas with high prevalence of *C. trachomatis*, including MSM, men in correctional facilities, and men visiting STI clinics. Overall, screening of men is recommended as long as it does not divert resources from the screening of women. Symptomatic patients should be tested regardless of gender.

MSM are at high risk for bacterial and viral STI. The CDC recommends the following annual STI screening in this group:

- Urethral screening for *C. trachomatis* and *N. gonorrhoeae*. The preferred methodology is testing the urine using nucleic acid amplification technique (NAAT)
- Anal screening for both *C. trachomatis* and *N. gonorrhoeae* for men who participate in receptive anal intercourse
- Pharyngeal screening for *N. gonorrhoeae* but not *C. trachomatis* for men who have oral receptive sex

In 2024, the CDC added a prevention strategy targeting MSM and transgender women with a history of at least one bacterial STI (specifically, syphilis, chlamydia or gonorrhea) during the past 12 months. Clinicians are advised to counsel about the benefits and harms of using doxycycline (any formulation) 200 mg once within 72 hours (not to exceed 200 mg per 24 hours) of oral, vaginal, or anal sex. The approach, known as doxycycline post-exposure prophylaxis (doxy PEP)[1], should be offered through shared decision making. Necessity for continued use of doxy PEP should be reevaluated every 3 to 6 months.

Patients who screen positive for *C. trachomatis* need to be screened for other STIs, including gonorrhea, syphilis, and HIV.

Abstinence and monogamous relationships are ideal to help prevent the transmission of *C. trachomatis*. Safer sex practices to limit the spread of *C. trachomatis* include the consistent use of condoms. Epidemiologic studies show that people often base their decision to use condoms on their perception of their partner's risk. Given the high prevalence of asymptomatic *C. trachomatis* infections in certain American populations, selective condom use is not an effective strategy.

Clinical Manifestations

Most infections are asymptomatic. However, some women will report vaginal discharge, postcoital or intermenstrual bleeding, or lower abdominal pain. Men are more commonly symptomatic than women and may report dysuria or urethral discharge.

Untreated *C. trachomatis* in women has significant health sequelae. Approximately 40% of women with untreated *Chlamydia* go on to develop pelvic inflammatory disease (PID). Women with PID may become infertile (20%), develop debilitating chronic pelvic pain (18%), or suffer ectopic pregnancy (9%).

Men do not tend to experience as severe sequelae from *C. trachomatis*. The most common illness is urethritis, but men may also experience epididymitis, proctitis, and conjunctivitis. Reactive arthritis is also more common in men.

Diagnosis

Tests used for detection of *C. trachomatis* can be divided into molecular (NAAT, DNA probing, and hybrid capture), antigen detection (direct immunofluorescence and enzyme immunoassay), and cell culture.

The most reliable method of testing for *C. trachomatis* is NAAT. It is FDA approved for use on vaginal/endocervical secretions, male intraurethral swabs, and first-catch urine. It is not FDA approved for rectal or oropharyngeal use but is used off-label in laboratories as described earlier. The primary benefit of NAAT is the lack of a need for viable organisms to induce a positive test result; this increases its sensitivity to more than 95% because of the ability to detect *C. trachomatis* even if only one copy of the targeted RNA or DNA is present. Its specificity is also desirable at 99%.

C. trachomatis cell culture is used as the reference standard for all testing but has many limitations, including expense, long turnaround time (72 hours), and transport and specimen storage requirements. Its sensitivity is 80% to 85%. It is not readily available.

Limiting barriers to screening is important. If testing in the clinic is difficult to arrange, self-collected vaginal swab specimens perform at least as well as other approved specimens using NAAT. First-catch urine NAAT testing is also more acceptable to many patients, particularly asymptomatic men and women who do not otherwise need a pelvic examination.

Differential Diagnosis

Infection with *Chlamydia* is often asymptomatic but is included in the differential diagnosis of various organ system complaints. It should be ruled out in any sexually active patient presenting with urethritis, mucopurulent cervicitis, epididymitis, and proctitis. There is significant overlap in the symptoms caused by *C. trachomatis* with *N. gonorrhoeae*, so testing for both bacteria with NAAT is preferred. Other agents that are included in the differential diagnosis after *C. trachomatis* and *N. gonorrhoeae* have been ruled out include *Trichomonas vaginalis,* HSV, adenovirus,

---

[1] Not FDA approved for this indication.

BOX 1 Recommended Treatments for *Chlamydia trachomatis* by Clinical Syndrome

Nonpregnant Adolescents and Adults With Chlamydial Infection
Recommended regimen
- Doxycycline (Vibramycin) 100 mg orally twice daily for 7 days
Alternative regimens
- Azithromycin (Zithromax) 1 g orally in a single dose
- Levofloxacin (Levaquin)[1] 500 mg orally once daily for 7 days

Pregnant Patients With Chlamydial Infections
Recommended regimen
- Azithromycin 1 g orally in a single dose
Alternative regimen
- Amoxicillin[1] 500 mg orally three times/day for 7 days

Neonates With Chlamydial Infection
Recommended regimen
- Erythromycin base or ethyl succinate 50 mg/kg body weight/day orally divided into four doses daily for 14 days*

Infants and Children Who Weigh <45 kg With Chlamydial Infection
Recommended regimen
- Erythromycin base or ethylsuccinate 50 mg/kg/day orally divided into 4 doses daily for 14 days*
Alternative regimen
- Azithromycin suspension 20 mg/kg/day orally, one dose daily for 3 days**

Children Who Weigh ≥45 kg but Who Are <8 Years Old
Recommended regimen
- Azithromycin 1 g orally in a single dose

Children Aged ≥8 Years
Recommended regimens
- Azithromycin 1 g orally in a single dose
or
- Doxycycline 100 mg orally twice a day for 7 days

Inpatient and Outpatient PID
- Please refer to PID chapter for treatment regimens

---

[1] Not FDA approved for this indication.
* Infants <6 weeks of age who are treated with erythromycin should be followed for signs and symptoms of infantile hypertrophic pyloric stenosis.
** There are limited data about the effectiveness and optimal dosing of azithromycin for treating chlamydial infection among infants and children weighing <45 kg.
Providers should consult the Centers for Disease Control and Prevention's website at https://www.cdc.gov/sti/hcp/clinical-guidance/ for up-to-date treatment recommendations.
PID, Pelvic inflammatory disease.

Mycoplasma species, and *Ureaplasma*. More specifically, persistent urethritis after treatment with doxycycline can be caused by infection with *T. vaginalis* or doxycycline-resistant *Urea urealyticum* or *Mycoplasma genitalium*.

C. trachomatis should be ruled out in newborn infants with conjunctivitis in the first 30 days of life or pneumonia at 1 to 3 months of life, especially if they were born to mothers with untreated chlamydial infections.

Treatment

Recommendations for treatment regimens are summarized in Box 1. Doxycycline (Vibramycin) has become the preferred antibiotic for *C. trachomatis* in nonpregnant patients. It has demonstrated effectiveness not only for urogenital infection but also for rectal and oropharyngeal infection. Azithromycin (Zithromax) is the treatment of choice for pregnant patients and has shown efficacy for urogenital infection. It can also be considered as a suitable alternative if nonadherence to doxycycline arises. Presumptive treatment for *C. trachomatis* should be considered for high-risk patients with cervicitis. High-risk patients include women up to 25 years old; those with new or multiple sexual partners; those who engage in unprotected sex, especially if follow-up cannot be ensured; and those for whom a relatively insensitive diagnostic test is used in place of NAAT.

The CDC only recommends presumptive treatment for *C. trachomatis* for patients being treated for *N. gonorrhoeae* when coinfection is not excluded. Coinfection is common, as illustrated in a study that found 20% of men with *N. gonorrhoeae* and 42% of women with *N. gonorrhoeae* were also infected with *C. trachomatis*. Cotreatment is also recommended in the hope that it will impede the development of antimicrobial-resistant *N. gonorrhoeae*.

C. trachomatis is a reportable infectious disease. The patient is instructed to refer all of their sexual partners for testing and treatment if they have had sexual contact during the previous 60 days. If the patient has not been sexually active for the last 60 days, then the patient is to refer their most recent sexual contact for treatment. The patient's recent sexual partners should be treated empirically even if their personal STI evaluation returns negative results. The patient and their sexual partners should be counseled to abstain from sexual activity until after the final dose of the 7-day regimen or for 7 days posttreatment after a one-dose therapy. Reinfection, rather than recurrence, is the more common etiology of repeat *C. trachomatis* infection.

Expedited partner therapy is an option in certain cases. This entails the patient delivering the antibiotic to their partner(s) without a physician first seeing the patient. Patients are to give their partners written materials on the importance of following up with a physician if any signs of complications occur (e.g., pelvic pain in women or testicular pain in men). It can be used effectively in certain situations but is not routinely recommended in MSM because of the high risk for coexisting infections, especially undiagnosed HIV infection, in their partners. Please refer to the CDC website (https://www.cdc.gov/sti/hcp/clinical-guidance/expedited-partner-therapy.html) to check on legality in individual states. In general, using the traditional patient-physician model is preferred.

Infants born to women with untreated *C. trachomatis* infection are at increased risk for vertical transmission. Prophylactic treatment with oral erythromycin for *C. trachomatis* is not recommended. The state-mandated standard erythromycin eye ointment that all newborns receive is still indicated but is not adequate treatment if the infant ultimately develops conjunctivitis. Overall, infants born to infected mothers need to be closely monitored for any signs and symptoms of infection and treated appropriately.

Intrauterine devices (IUDs) have regained popularity in the United States after they were implicated in causing PID in the 1970s. The IUD has evolved, and now the risk of PID appears increased only in the first 3 weeks postinsertion. If *C. trachomatis* or PID is contracted with an IUD in place, practitioners must decide whether the IUD should be removed. Research has found insufficient evidence to mandate removal, but close follow-up is mandatory.

Monitoring

Repeat testing is recommended for all patients, including pregnant women, treated for *C. trachomatis* at 3 months regardless of the treatment status of the patient's partner(s) because reinfection is so common. If the patient does not follow up at 3 months, they should be retested upon presentation for medical care within the first 12 months posttreatment.

Test of cure, which is testing at 4 weeks posttreatment, is recommended only for pregnant patients. Testing for cure earlier than 3 to 4 weeks increases the rate of false positive results. Pregnant women who are at high risk for STIs include those who were treated for *C. trachomatis* during the pregnancy; these women also qualify to be rescreened in the third trimester for *N. gonorrhoeae*, HIV, and syphilis in addition to *C. trachomatis*.

Complications

C. trachomatis is a major public health concern because it results in serious health complications and sequelae. In women it can cause PID, endometritis, ectopic pregnancy, infertility, salpingitis, and perihepatitis (Fitz-Hugh–Curtis syndrome). In men it is associated with postgonococcal or nongonococcal urethritis and epididymitis. Reactive arthritis can occur in both men and women.

C. trachomatis is especially problematic in pregnancy because it is associated with an increased risk of preterm labor and preterm premature rupture of membranes. Infants born to women infected with *C. trachomatis* risk experiencing pneumonia and conjunctivitis.

C. trachomatis pneumonia can present as an afebrile pneumonia often with a staccato cough without wheezing between 1 and 3 months of life. *C. trachomatis* conjunctivitis, also known as ophthalmia neonatorum, is uncommon in the United States, but worldwide it is the number one cause of blindness. It usually presents within the 5th and 12th days of life but can present at up to 1 month of age. State-mandated prophylactic eye ointment given to babies at birth mainly helps prevent gonococcal ophthalmia; it does not prevent perinatal transmission of *C. trachomatis* from mother to infant. Therefore the screening of pregnant women and ultimate treatment of their *C. trachomatis* during pregnancy is the best method of preventing complications in newborn infants.

References

Bachmann LH, Barbee LA, Chan P, et al: CDC clinical guidelines on the Use of doxycycline postexposure prophylaxis for bacterial sexually transmitted infection prevention, United States, 2024, *MMWR Recomm Rep* 73(RR-2):1–8, 2024. https://doi.org/10.15585/mmwr.rr7302a1.

Bebear C, de Barbeyrac B: Genital *Chlamydia trachomatis* infections, *Clin Microbiol Infect* 15:4–10, 2009.

Blas MM, Canchihuaman FA, Alva IE, et al: Pregnancy outcomes in women infected with *Chlamydia trachomatis*: a population-based cohort study in Washington State, *Sex Transm Infect* 83:314–318, 2007.

Centers for Disease Control and Prevention (CDC). *Sexually Transmitted Infections Surveillance 2023.* Available at: https://www.cdc.gov/sti-statistics/annual/index.html. Accessed 3/26/2025.

Centers for Disease Control and Prevention (CDC): Sexually transmitted infections treatment guidelines, 2021, *MMWR Recomm Rep (Morb Mortal Wkly Rep)* 70(No.4):65–82, 2021.

Honey E, Augood C, Templeton A, et al: Cost effectiveness of screening for *Chlamydia trachomatis*: a review of published studies, *Sex Transm Infect* 78:406–412, 2002.

Johnson RE, Newhall WJ, Papp JR, et al: Screening tests to detect *Chlamydia trachomatis* and *Neisseria gonorrhoeae* infections—2002, *MMWR Recomm Rep (Morb Mortal Wkly Rep)* 51(RR-15):1–38, 2002.

Kramer A, Schewebke I, Kampf G: How long do nosocomial pathogens persist on inanimate surfaces? A systematic review, *BMC Infect Dis* 6:130, 2006.

LeFevre ML: U.S. Preventive Services Task Force: Screening for chlamydia and gonorrhea: U.S. Preventive services Task Force recommendation statement, *Ann Intern Med* 161(12):902–910, 2014.

Lyss SB, Kamb ML, Peterman TA, et al: *Chlamydia trachomatis* among patients infected with and treated for *Neisseria gonorrhoeae* in sexually transmitted clinics in the United States, *Ann Intern Med* 139:178–185, 2003.

CONDYLOMATA ACUMINATA

Method of
M. Chantel Long, MD

CURRENT DIAGNOSIS

- Condylomata acuminata are usually flesh-colored, brown, or gray and can be flat, plaquelike, or exophytic papules, giving them the classic "cauliflower" appearance.
- The lesions may be single or multiple and can range in size from minute to several centimeters in diameter.
- When the appearance of the lesion is typical, confirmatory tests are usually unnecessary.
- Suspicious lesions or uncertain diagnoses warrant biopsy to rule out malignancy.

Epidemiology

Condylomata acuminata, commonly known as genital warts, is a sexually transmitted disease caused by the human papilloma virus (HPV). It is estimated that 43 million people are infected with HPV in the United States, with the highest prevalence in adolescents and young adults. Lifetime incidence of HPV infection is greater than 50% and appears to be increasing, making it the most common sexually transmitted disease.

Risk Factors

Risk factors associated with HPV infection include sex with an infected partner, early age at first sexual intercourse, multiple sexual partners, history of sexually transmitted infections, cigarette smoking, and lack of condom use. The majority of patients whose sexual partner has condyloma will themselves develop condyloma within 3 months. An even larger percentage of people are believed to develop subclinical infection.

Pathophysiology

About 90% of warts are caused by HPV types 6 and 11; condyloma can be coinfected with types 16, 18, 31, 33, 35, and 45, which have oncogenic potential, especially in patients with HIV infection. Genital skin appears to be less susceptible to the oncogenic potential of HPV compared to the transformation zones of the cervix and anal canal.

The virus is easily transmitted via sexual contact. Vertical transmission and autoinoculation are possible. The average incubation period between infection and appearance of condyloma ranges from 3 months to several years. Condyloma can persist or recur after therapy, undergo malignant transformation, or spontaneously regress.

Prevention

Prevention options include HPV vaccination, abstinence, routine condom use, and limiting sexual partners. Once patients have condyloma, they should be encouraged to use condoms consistently. Educate patients that condoms can decrease transmission but might not completely prevent infection.

One HPV vaccine series is currently available in the United States. Gardasil 9 is a 9-valent HPV vaccine indicated for male and female patients aged 9 to 26 years for prevention of cervical cancer and genital warts. It may also be given to patients age 27 to 45 years based on shared clinical decision-making between the patient and clinician.

Clinical Manifestations

Most genital warts are asymptomatic on presentation, although patients can present with complaints of a "bump." Localized irritation, pruritus, pain, or bleeding can occur, and symptoms may vary based on the location and size of the lesions. Usually, the warts appear flesh-colored, brown, or gray and can be flat, plaquelike, or exophytic papules, giving them the classic "cauliflower" appearance. The lesions may be single or multiple and range in size from minute to several centimeters in diameter. Flat HPV lesions might not be grossly visible.

The majority of HPV infections are either subclinical or unrecognized. Clinically apparent disease might represent only a small portion of the actual infected area.

TABLE 1	Differential Diagnosis
LESION	**APPEARANCE**
Verruca vulgaris	Occurs anywhere Tends to be thicker, drier, and hyperkeratotic
Molluscum contagiosum	Occurs anywhere Smooth, round papules with central umbilication
Seborrheic keratoses	Occurs anywhere Multiple waxy, rough, hyperpigmented papules
Condyloma latum	Moist, rounded, white papules of syphilis
Pearly penile papules	Smooth, uniform, small, 1–2mm at corona, benign
Vestibular papillae	Both sides of vulva, female equivalent of pearly penile papules
Lichen planus	Purplish, pruritic rash or flat-topped polygonal papules
Nonpigmented nevi	Occurs anywhere Flat or raised, reddish or flesh colored

Diagnosis

When the clinical appearance of the lesion is typical, confirmatory tests are usually unnecessary. The entire anogenital tract should be examined because of the widespread nature of HPV. A magnifying glass and anoscopy may be helpful for thorough detection and examination. Application of dilute 3% to 5% acetic acid solution to the skin surface can help detect subtle HPV lesions by producing an acetowhitening of the condyloma; however, this is not a specific test and is not routinely recommended. Pap smears or tissue biopsy can provide histopathologic confirmation of the diagnosis. Biopsy is recommended to rule out malignancy in any suspicious lesions, such as large or rapidly growing condyloma; pigmented, atypical, friable, bleeding, or ulcerated lesions; sites of previous treatment failure; areas of recurrence; acetowhite lesions; or lesions in immunocompromised patients. Although costly and not recommended, HPV identification via DNA testing can be performed.

Differential Diagnosis

Table 1 outlines the differential diagnosis for condylomata acuminata.

Treatment

In the absence of dysplasia, the Centers for Disease Control and Prevention recommends no treatment of subclinical HPV infection. The goal of treatment is to eliminate symptoms, namely clinically apparent warts, rather than address the underlying HPV infection. Current treatments do not eradicate the virus.

Ideally, treatment of condyloma should continue until all warts are gone. A repeated course of therapy is often required to achieve a wart-free state. Recurrence may be due to latent HPV in the surrounding normal tissue, HPV reinfection, or improper selection or use of a therapy modality. Nearly all treatment regimens have similar efficacy and rates of intolerance and toxicity. All are known to cause local pain and irritation. Any given treatment has a 40% to 80% rate of wart clearance and up to a 50% recurrence rate. It is unknown whether eliminating warts will decrease infectivity of current or future sexual partners.

The factors to consider when deciding on treatment include location and size of the warts, the patient's tolerance and preference, cost, convenience, and the clinician's preference. Patient-applied options allow the patient greater control; however, this requires good compliance, and the warts must be accessible by the patient or caregiver. Provider-applied treatments are good choices for large treatment areas. Data regarding the efficacy of using more than one modality at a time are lacking. It is common practice for health care providers to combine treatment

TABLE 2 Treatment Regimens

DRUG	USE ON	ADVANTAGES	DISADVANTAGES	INSTRUCTIONS
Patient Applied				
Podofilox 0.5% gel or solution (Condylox)	Moist warts	Relatively inexpensive	Avoid in pregnancy Avoid on mucous membranes Do not exceed 10cm^2 area Do not exceed 0.5mL daily; can have systemic side effects	Apply bid × 3d, then 4d off Repeat weekly May use for 4–6 cycles[3]
Imiquimod 5% cream (Aldara)	Dry or moist warts		Avoid with large warts >10cm^2 Requires compliance Hypo- or hyperpigmentation of treated skin can occur Local inflammatory skin reaction	Apply nightly, 3 times per week Use up to 16 weeks Wash off after 6–10h
Sinecatechins 15% ointment (Veregen)	Dry warts		Avoid in pregnancy and genital herpes Avoid in immunocompromised patients	Apply tid Use up to 16wk Do not wash off
Provider Applied				
Trichloroacetic acid (TCA) (Tri-Chlor) or bichloroacetic acid (BCA)[2] 80%–90% solution	Small, few Moist warts	May use on vagina, cervix May use on anal warts May use in pregnancy	Avoid with dry and large warts	Apply sparingly with cotton tip Air dry Repeat weekly to every other week Do not allow to "run" on normal skin Neutralize with soap or sodium bicarbonate
Cryotherapy	Small, few, flat Dry or moist	May use in pregnancy May use liquid nitrogen in vagina, meatus, anus	Avoid with large warts Avoid cryoprobe use in vagina or anus	Freeze q1–2wk Freeze 1–2mm border May offer/need local anesthesia
Surgery	Small or large Dry or moist	May use on anal warts Use on large warts and large treatment areas	Avoid in patients with bleeding disorder	Scissors, shave biopsy, punch excision, curettage, cautery, laser
Interferon-α-2b injections (Intron A)	Refractory warts		Expensive Flulike side effects	Multiple intralesional injections Several times a week Often requires specialty referral
Laser vaporization	Refractory warts	May use on intraurethral and large warts as well as large treatment areas	Expensive	Requires specialty referral

[2]Not available in the United States.
[3]Exceeds dosage recommended by the manufacturer.

modalities. Table 2 outlines current therapy regimens. Podophyllin resin (Podocon-25) is no longer recommended. Failure to respond after four treatments or failure to clear within 3 months warrants a change in therapy modality and possible reevaluation of the diagnosis.

Advise patients to abstain from sexual activity while undergoing treatment for genital warts.

Monitoring
Counseling of patients regarding prevention and recognition of condyloma as well as screening and treatment of sexual partners should be part of the comprehensive management plan. One should consider testing for other sexually transmitted diseases because they often coexist with HPV. Encourage patients to discuss their HPV diagnosis with sexual partners. Asymptomatic partners likely harbor a subclinical infection, and examination for genital warts is appropriate if lesions are suspected. Discuss the need for smoking cessation and regular physician examinations, including Pap smears, as ways to prevent early HPV-related neoplasm.

Complications
Anogenital HPV infection with high-risk genotypes is associated with squamous cell carcinoma of the cervix, vagina, vulva, penis, and anus. Persistent HPV infection is the most important risk factor for development of cervical intraepithelial neoplasia and cancer.

References
American Academy of Pediatrics. Human papillomavirus. In: Pickering LK, Baker CJ, Kimberlin DW, Long SS, editors. Red Book: 2009 Report of the Committee on Infectious Diseases. 28th ed. Elk Grove Village, IL: American Academy of Pediatrics; 2009. p. 477–483.

Centers for Disease Control and Prevention: *Epidemiology and Prevention of Vaccine-Preventable Diseases. The Pink Book*, ed 12, Washington, DC, 2011, Public Health Foundation.

Centers for Disease Control and Prevention: 2010 Sexually transmitted diseases treatment guidelines, *MMWR* 59:1–5, 2010. 69–78.

Centers for Disease Control and Prevention. Anogenital warts and human papillomavirus (HPV) infection HPV information for clinicians. Available at www.cdc.gov/std/treatment-guiedlines/toc.htm [accessed December 28, 2021].

Gilbert SM, Lambert SM, Weiner D: Extensive condylomata acuminata of the penis: Medical and surgical management, *Infect Urol* 16:65–76, 2003.

Kodner CM, Nasrat S: Management of genital warts, *Am Fam Physician* 70:2335–2342, 2004.

GENITAL ULCER DISEASE: CHANCROID, GRANULOMA INGUINALE, AND LYMPHOGRANULOMA

Method of
Todd Stephens, MD

Chancroid, granuloma inguinale, and lymphogranuloma venereum (LGV) are important genital ulcer diseases that should be included in the differential diagnosis of patients presenting with anal or genital ulcers with or without inguinal adenopathy. Syphilis and herpes simplex virus testing should be considered on all such patients because of similarities in clinical presentation. Testing or treatment for other potential sexually transmitted infections (STIs), including HIV, should be considered given the high risk for concomitant infection.

Chancroid

History

Chancroid, also called soft sore, was first distinguished from the hard chancre of syphilis by Ricord in 1838. Ducrey, in Naples, demonstrated that inoculation of material from the chancroid ulcer into the skin of the forearm could reproduce the ulcer, and he went on to identify the causative organism, which bears his name.

Epidemiology

Chancroid is an important cause of genital ulceration in most countries of the developing world, accounting for about 10 million cases annually. Chancroid was diagnosed in 60% of patients who had genital ulcers and who presented to STI clinics in Africa before the HIV epidemic. Now, herpes simplex lesions represent a higher percentage. The prevalence of this disease is highest among commercial sex workers, and the presence of chancroid lesions significantly increases the risk of transmission of HIV. Although generally rare in industrialized countries, there have been several well-documented outbreaks in urban centers of North America, particularly among men who have sex with men.

Etiology

Chancroid is caused by *Haemophilus ducreyi*, a small anaerobic Gram-negative bacillus that forms streptobacillary chains on Gram stain and grows only on enriched media.

Clinical Features

After an incubation of 3 to 7 days, a papule appears that soon ulcerates, leaving a soft ulcer with an undermined edge and a purulent base. Vesicles are not seen. About half of patients develop unilateral inguinal adenopathy (Figure 1). Both the adenopathy and the lesions are very painful. Lesions can be single or multiple, and atypical presentations occur. Kissing lesions often occur on adjacent cutaneous surfaces. Not infrequently, a giant ulcer develops with several smaller satellite ulcers around the periphery, which can mimic the ulcerative phase of herpes simplex. More than half of the lesions occur on the prepuce, particularly in uncircumcised men. In women, the majority of lesions are on the fourchette, labia, and perianal area. Adenopathy can progress to bubo formation with tender, overlying erythema. These buboes can rupture and produce inguinal abscesses.

Diagnosis

Gram stain of smears obtained from the ulcer base has been advocated in the past for diagnosis, but this lacks both sensitivity and specificity. The preferred diagnostic modality is swabs for culture from the ulcer base or undermined edge. These are plated directly on enriched media (GC agar and Mueller-Hinton agar base) and incubated for 72 hours in an atmosphere of 5% carbon dioxide at 33°C. Polymerase chain reaction (PCR) and immunochromatography tests are also available.

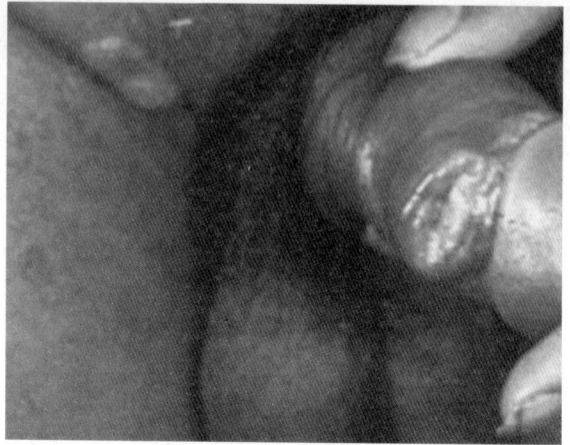

Figure 1 Chancroid. This photo shows an early chancroid ulcer on the penis along with accompanying regional inguinal adenopathy. (Courtesy of Dr. Pirozzi, Centers for Disease Control and Prevention.)

However, clinically, a probable diagnosis of chancroid can be made if all of the following four criteria are met: (1) the patient has one or more painful genital ulcers; (2) the clinical presentation, appearance of genital ulcers and, if present, regional lymphadenopathy are typical for chancroid; (3) the patient has no evidence of T. pallidum infection by darkfield examination or NAAT (i.e., ulcer exudate or serous fluid) or by serologic tests for syphilis performed at least 7–14 days after onset of ulcers; and (4) HSV-1 or HSV-2 NAAT or HSV culture performed on the ulcer exudate or fluid are negative.

Treatment

The Centers for Disease Control and Prevention (CDC) recommend a syndromal management approach in which a positive diagnosis is suggested if the patient has one or more painful ulcers and no evidence of syphilis or herpes simplex virus. Ulcers with painful adenopathy are pathognomonic (Table 1 lists antimicrobial treatment). The safety and efficacy of azithromycin (Zithromax) for pregnant and lactating women have not been established. Ciprofloxacin (Cipro)[1] is contraindicated during pregnancy and lactation. No adverse effects of chancroid on pregnancy outcome have been reported. Serologic testing for syphilis, HIV, and other appropriate STIs should be performed. Chancroidal ulcers should be kept clean with regular washing in soapy water and kept dry. Fluctuant buboes might require incision and drainage, which is preferable over needle aspiration. Treatment of all sexual partners within 60 days should be pursued, and treatment is similar to that for the source patient. Patients should not engage in sexual activity until the ulcers are healed.

Granuloma Inguinale (Donovanosis)

History

Granuloma inguinale was first recognized in India, where Donovan observed, in an oral lesion of the disease, the bodies that bear his name. There is considerable confusion about terminology between this disease and LGV, because various similar synonyms have been used inconsistently. Adding to the confusion, Donovan's name is associated with two tropical diseases that he discovered: leishmaniasis, with the discovery of intracellular protozoan inclusions that bear his name (Leishman-Donovan bodies), and granuloma inguinale (whose intracellular inclusions were believed to be caused by protozoa but are now known to be caused by bacteria).

---

[1]Not FDA approved for this indication.

FEATURES AND TREATMENT	CHANCROID	GRANULOMA INGUINALE	LYMPHOGRANULOMA VENEREUM
Clinical Features			
Incubation period	3–7 days	3–40 days	1–28 days
Primary lesion	Papule	Papule	Papule or vesicle
Ulcerative lesion painful	Yes	No	No
Lymphadenopathy	Yes (unilateral)	No	Yes (unilateral or bilateral)
Base	Purulent	Raised, easily bleeds	Nonvascular
Border	Round, raised, undermined edges	Irregular, expansion along skin folds	Irregular, ragged
Treatment			
Treatment of choice (any of the options listed)	Azithromycin (Zithromycin) 1g Ciprofloxacin (Cipro)[1] 500mg bid × 3d Ceftriaxone (Rocephin)[1] 250mg IM once	Azithromycin[1] 1g PO once a week or 500 mg qd for >3 weeks until all lesions have completely healed Doxycycline (Vibramycin) 100mg bid × 3 wks	Azithromycin[1] 1g weekly × 3wk Doxycycline 100mg bid × 3wk
Alternative treatment (any of the options listed)	Erythromycin (Ery-Tab)[1] 500mg qid × 7d	Azithromycin[1] 1g PO qwk × 3 wk Erythromycin[1] 500mg qid × 3 wk Ciprofloxacin[1] 750mg bid × 3 wk Ceftriaxone[1] 1 gm IM daily for at least 3 weeks and until all lesions have completely healed.	Erythromycin[1] 500mg qid × 3wk

[1]Not FDA approved for this indication.

Epidemiology

Endemic areas are localized to a few specific areas of the tropics, particularly India, Papua New Guinea, Brazil, and the eastern part of South Africa, particularly Durban. Commercial sex workers and men are primarily involved.

Etiology

The disease is caused by an encapsulated Gram-negative coccobacillus *Klebsiella granulomatis* (previously known as *Calymmatobacterium* or *Donovania granulomatis*).

Clinical Features

A firm, painless papule or nodule is the presenting sign of granuloma inguinale. The incubation period is variable from 3 to 40 days from inoculation. This nodule quickly ulcerates, and the base is highly vascular, is beefy red, and bleeds easily. Lymphadenopathy is not part of the clinical presentation of this disease, distinguishing granuloma inguinale from chancroid and LGV. However, the ulcer can be easily confused with chancroid, condyloma lata, ulcerated verrucous warts, and squamous carcinoma. Untreated, the ulcers slowly expand, particularly along skin folds toward the inguinal region or anus (Figure 2). The ulcers are flat and raised and have slightly hypertrophic margins, but the bases are typically free of pus and necrotic debris. Less-common presentations include extragenital lesions involving the neck and mouth; cervical lesions that resemble carcinoma; and involvement of the uterus, tubes, and ovaries, producing hard masses, abscesses, or frozen pelvis.

Diagnosis

Diagnosis requires the demonstration of intracellular Donovan bodies from Giemsa or Wright staining of smears taken from a swab of the ulcer base or from biopsy material.

Treatment

See Table 1 for antimicrobial treatment. Treatment should be continued until lesions are resolved and, if possible, a little longer to reduce the risk of relapse.

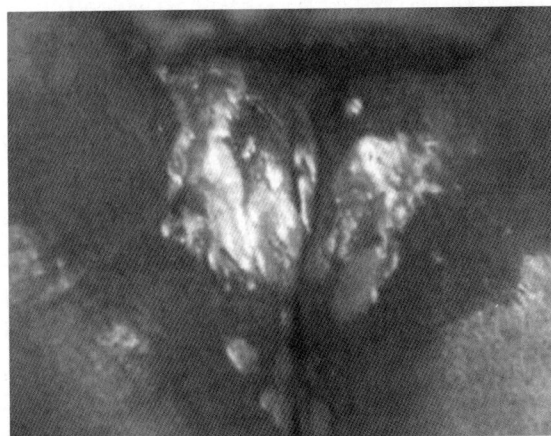

Figure 2 Granuloma inguinale. (Source: NEHC http://www.nhec.med.navy.mil/hp/sharp/std_pictures.htm)

Lymphogranuloma Venereum

History

LGV was first differentiated from syphilis in 1906 by Wasserman, though the first full description of the disease was given by Durand, Nicolas, and Favre in 1913. In 1925, Frei developed an intradermal skin test that gave positive responses in most LGV patients. The term "tropical bubo" was associated with the disease later.

Epidemiology

LGV is largely confined to the tropics and is not a common STI. The global overall incidence is in a decline. It is seen more commonly in men, but since 2004, there has been a resurgence manifesting as proctitis in North America and Europe among HIV-positive men who have sex with men.

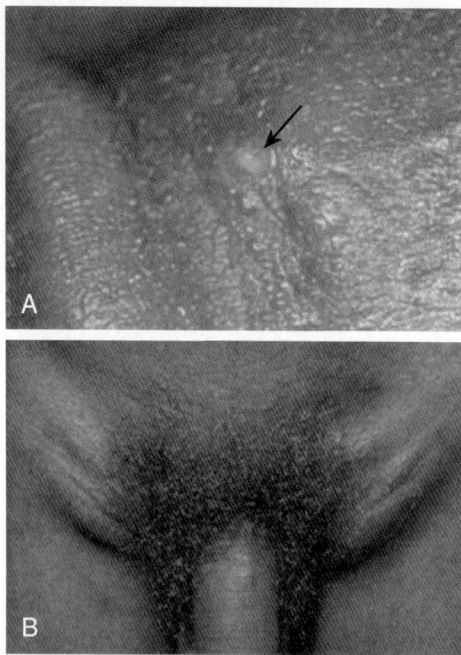

Figure 3 Lymphogranuloma venereum. **A,** Small ulcerative lesion near corona of penis *(arrow).* **B,** Bilateral inguinal adenopathy, with developing groove sign as adenopathy expands above and below the inguinal ligament. (**A** courtesy Ronald Ballard, Reproduced with permission from The Diagnosis and Management of Sexually Transmitted Infections in South Africa, 3rd ed., Johannesburg, South African Institute for Medical Research, 2000. **B** courtesy Connexions (http://cnx.org/content/m14883/latest/Case_10-pres1-1.jpg).)

Etiology

LGV is a chlamydial infection caused by the invasive L1, L2, and L3 serovars of *Chlamydia trachomatis,* an intracellular gram-negative bacterium.

Clinical Features

LGV is essentially a systemic disease whose natural course is divided into three distinct phases. The initial phase of LGV is normally an inconspicuous genital lesion beginning as a typically small, painless papule or vesicle occurring 1 to 28 days after inoculation. This papule or vesicle quickly ulcerates and heals without a scar, and it often goes unrecognized by the patient (Figure 3). However, the second phase of LGV is the development of increasingly painful lymphadenopathy, often with fever and malaise. The lymphadenopathy progresses to bubo formation over 1 to 2 weeks. When a sexually active adult patient presents with an inguinal bubo not associated with genital ulcers, LGV is an important diagnosis to consider. The infected nodes are usually unilateral (bilateral in a third of cases) and often coalesce into a matted mass that can project outwards above or below the inguinal ligament, producing the pathognomonic groove sign present in 20% of patients with LGV. The buboes are likely to rupture, forming multiple sinuses. Untreated, LGV can cause extensive lymphatic damage, resulting in elephantiasis of the genitalia. Anal involvement, likewise, can lead to perirectal abscesses, fistulas, and rectal strictures. These complications represent the late phase of LGV.

Diagnosis

The diagnosis of LGV can only be confirmed using PCR methods of smears, scrapings, or aspirated material. Alternatively, the ability to perform micro-immunofluorescence serology testing using a fluorescein-conjugated monoclonal antibody and viewing the slide with a fluorescence microscope can demonstrate the inclusion bodies within the cytoplasm of macrophages. Gram staining by itself lacks appropriate sensitivity or specificity. Additional laboratory findings include leukocytosis, elevated erythrocyte sedimentation rate, and increases in immunoglobulin G and cryoglobulins.

Treatment

Antimicrobial treatment is summarized in Table 1. Needle aspiration or incision and drainage of fluctuant buboes may be required for symptomatic relief but are not routinely recommended for treatment because drainage can delay healing. Fistula openings should receive sterile dressings. One of the primary goals of treatment of LGV is to prevent long-term complications such as anogenital strictures or fistulas. Plastic surgical operations may be of benefit in cases with extensive rectal strictures or elephantiasis of the genitalia. However, these surgical interventions should only be performed after a prolonged course of antibiotics. Scars should be monitored to detect malignant change.

Management of Sex Partners

Any person having had sexual contact with a patient with LGV within 60 days before the onset of the patient's symptoms should be examined and presumptively treated with azithromycin[1] 1gram orally as a single dose or doxycycline 100mg orally twice a day for seven days. Symptomatic patients should be treated with longer treatment regimens.

---

[1]Not FDA approved for this indication.

References

Centers for Disease Control and Prevention: Sexually Transmitted Diseases Treatment Guidelines, 2021, Granuloma Inguinale (Donovanosis). Available at https://www.cdc.gov/std/treatment-guidelines/donovanosis.htm.

Centers for Disease Control and Prevention: Sexually Transmitted Diseases Treatment Guidelines, 2015, *MMWR Recomm Rep* 64(No. RR-3):1–137, 2015. Available at http://www.cdc.gov/std/tg2015/toc.htm.

Habif T: In *Clinical Dermatology,* Philadelphia, 2004, Mosby, pp 325–329.

Leppard B: In *An Atlas of African Dermatology,* Oxon, UK, 2002, Radcliffe Medical Press, p 69, 151, 237.

Ndinya-Achola JO, Kihara AN, Fisher LD, et al: Presumptive specific clinical diagnosis of genital ulcer disease (GUD) in a primary health care setting in Nairobi, *Int J STD AIDS* 7(3):201–205, 1996.

O'Farrell N: Granuloma Inguinale. In Ryan E, Hill D, Solomon T, editors: *Hunter's Tropical Medicine and Emerging Infectious Diseases,* ed 10, Canada, 2020, Elsevier, pp 531–533.

Richens J, Mabey DC: Sexually transmitted infections (excluding HIV). In Cook GC, Zumla AI, editors: *Manson's Tropical Diseases,* ed 22, London, 2009, Saunders, pp 403–434.

Ronald A: Chancroid. In Hunter GW, Strickland GT, Magill AJ, editors: *Hunter's Tropical Medicine and Emerging Infectious Diseases,* ed 8, Philadelphia, 2000, WB Saunders, pp 367–369.

GONORRHEA

Method of
John Brill, MD, MPH

CURRENT DIAGNOSIS

- Gonorrhea (GC) is caused by the gram-negative diplococcus *Neisseria gonorrhoeae.*
- Asymptomatic gonococcal infections are common in men and women, particularly in extragenital locations.
- Molecular tests are more sensitive than culture for diagnosis, particularly in extragenital locations.
- All patients diagnosed with GC should be tested for other sexually transmitted infections, including human immunodeficiency virus (HIV).
- Annual screening for *N. gonorrhoeae* infection is recommended for all sexually active women aged less than 25 years and for older women at increased risk for infection.

CURRENT THERAPY

- Ceftriaxone (Rocephin) 500 mg IM is the first-line treatment for GC, with the addition of doxycycline (100 mg orally twice daily [BID] × 7 days) if concomitant chlamydia has not been ruled out. Persons weighing over 150 kg should be given a dose of ceftriaxone 1 g IM.
- The higher dosing of ceftriaxone compared with prior recommendations reflects a small increase in resistance. Doxycycline is now preferred over azithromycin due to a sevenfold increase in azithromycin resistance from 2014 to 2018.
- Only immunoglobulin E–mediated allergic reaction to penicillin (PCN) or cephalosporins (anaphylaxis, Stevens-Johnson syndrome, or toxic epidermal necrolysis) should contraindicate the use of ceftriaxone. Due to limited options, infectious disease consultation is recommended in this situation.

Epidemiology

Gonorrhea (GC) is the second most common reportable human infection in the United States, with 601,319 cases reported in 2023. After a historic low in 2009, rates had progressively increased in all US regions before seeing a decline in both 2022 and 2023 (Figure 1). Rates are significantly higher for men (228/100,000) than women (131/100,000). Rates are highest for persons in the 20- to 24-year-old age group, with a younger median age profile in women than men (Figure 2). The highest statewide rate is seen in Alaska (311 cases per 100,000), with the southeastern US having the highest regional rates (Figure 3). The greatest disparity by race or ethnicity is observed among non-Hispanic Black men and women, with rates eight times those of Whites (Figure 4).

Risk Factors

Risk factors for infection include unprotected intercourse, adolescent and young adult age, new/multiple sexual partners, and exchanging sex for money or drugs. Gonococcal infection is strongly associated with other sexually transmitted infections (STIs). In fact, at a county population level, the human immunodeficiency virus (HIV) infection rate carries the highest association with GC rates, superseding all other socioeconomic and demographic risk factors. Additional risk factors for GC include inconsistent condom use among persons who are not in mutually monogamous relationships, previous or coexisting STIs, and exchanging sex for money or drugs. Military recruits, incarcerated persons, and persons receiving care at public STI clinics are also at high risk.

Pathophysiology

Neisseria gonorrhoeae infects noncornified epithelial cells such as the urethra, endocervix, rectum, oropharynx, and conjunctiva. The bacteria divide by binary fission every 20 to 30 minutes, thus the rapid emergence of symptoms. *N. gonorrhoeae* attaches to different types of mucus-secreting epithelial cells via a number of alterable structures located on the surface of gonococci and additionally uses several mechanisms to counter the immune system. *N. gonorrhoeae* is primarily spread by infected secretions (oral, urethral) coming into contact with mucosal surfaces. Mother-to-child transmission is well established, hence the recommendation to treat all newborns prophylactically with erythromycin (Ilotycin) 0.5% ophthalmic ointment.

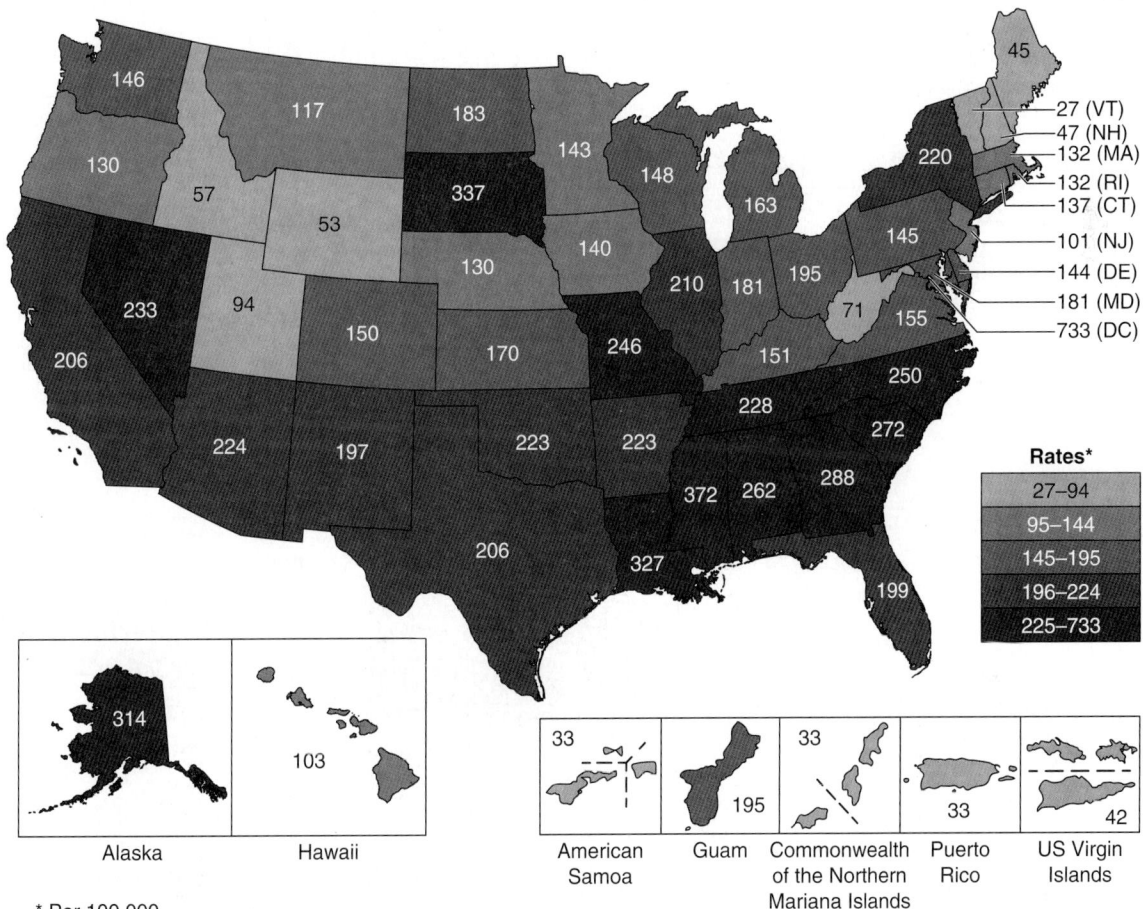

* Per 100,000.

NOTE: See Section A1.11 in the Appendix for more information on interpreting reported rates in US territories.

Figure 1 Gonorrhea—Rates of reported cases by Jurisdiction, United States and Territories, 2022. From CDC: Sexually Transmitted Disease Surveillance 2022. https://www.cdc.gov/std/statistics/2022/figures.htm. Accessed March 18, 2023.

Screening and Prevention

The US Preventive Services Task Force (USPSTF) recommends annual screening for *N. gonorrhoeae* infection in all sexually active women aged less than 25 years and in older women at increased risk for infection (e.g., those who have a new sex partner, more than one sex partner, a sex partner with concurrent partners, or a sex partner who has an STI)—a "B" recommendation. The USPSTF concludes that the current evidence is insufficient to assess the balance of benefits and harms of screening for GC in men—an "I" recommendation.

Men who have sex with men (MSM) without consistent condom use are at high risk for GC infection; the Centers for Disease Control and Prevention (CDC) recommends that sexually active MSM be screened at least annually at anatomic sites of exposure, with testing every 3 to 5 months for those at high risk. Mucosa that is infected by GC is more susceptible to HIV, even in asymptomatic states, raising the impetus for screening and treatment. Because the bacterium is an obligate human pathogen with adult transmission only via sexual contact, avoidance of intimate contact with an infected person is the ultimate mode of prevention. Male latex condoms, used correctly and consistently, are highly effective at preventing GC transmission; polyurethane male and female condoms are effective when intact but have higher breakage rates.

Clinical Manifestations

The most common symptom of genital GC infection is a mucopurulent urethritis or cervicitis. In men, genital GC typically manifests with urethral discharge and dysuria 2 to 5 days after exposure; however, approximately 30% of urethral infections are asymptomatic. About half of genitally infected women will show symptoms, most commonly vaginal discharge, dysuria, and itching, generally 5 to 10 days after exposure. The great majority of rectal and pharyngeal infections are asymptomatic. GC can also present as ocular and disseminated infection. Except for neonatal infections, believed to arise from perinatal transmission, diagnosis of gonococcal infection in infants and children should trigger a sexual abuse investigation, including multisite testing.

Diagnosis

Laboratory diagnosis of GC can be made by Gram staining of urethral secretions in symptomatic men, by culture of endocervical or urethral specimens, or by nucleic acid amplification testing (NAAT) of urine or the target location. Gram staining of urethral discharge showing leukocytes with intracellular gram-negative diplococci is extremely specific and sensitive. Gram staining is not sensitive enough to rule out infection in symptom-free men or in extraurethral locations. NAAT has largely replaced culture and appears to be more than twice as sensitive as culture in extragenital locations. The increased sensitivity of NAATs is due to their ability to produce a positive test result from as little as a single copy of the target DNA. False-positive test results can occur with

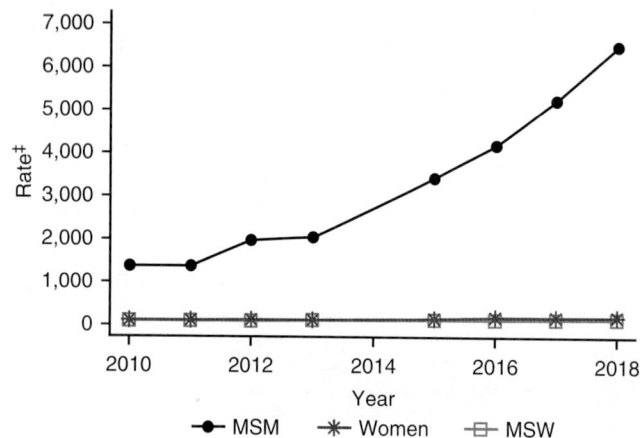

Figure 2 Gonorrhea—Estimated rates of reported gonorrhea cases by MSM, MSW, and women. STD Surveillance Network (SSuN), 2010 to 2018. From CDC: Sexually Transmitted Disease Surveillance 2018. https://www.cdc.gov/std/stats18/gonorrhea.htm. Accessed March 21, 2021.

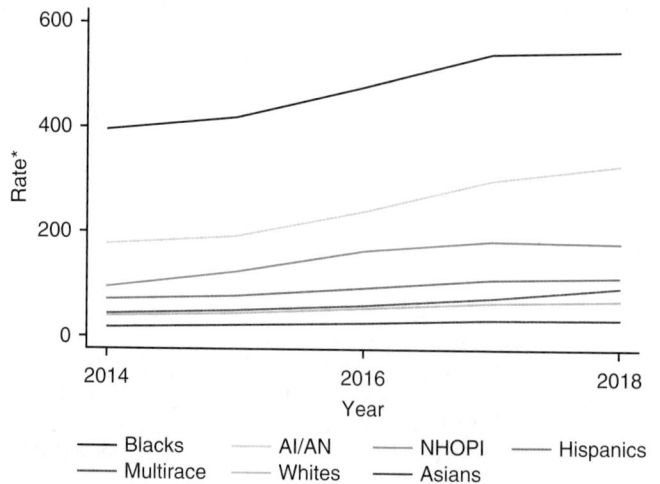

* Per 100,000.

Figure 4 Gonorrhea—Rates of reported cases by race/ethnicity, United States, 2014 to 2018. From CDC: Sexually Transmitted Disease Surveillance 2018. https://www.cdc.gov/std/stats18/gonorrhea.htm. Accessed March 21, 2021.

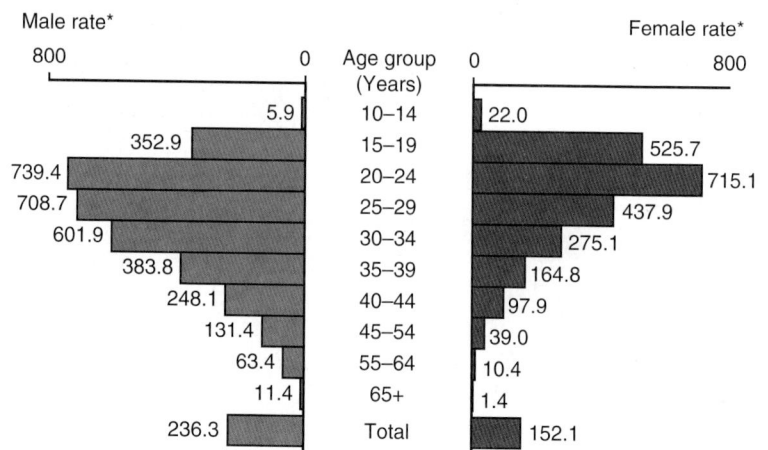

Male rate*	Age group (Years)	Female rate*
5.9	10–14	22.0
352.9	15–19	525.7
739.4	20–24	715.1
708.7	25–29	437.9
601.9	30–34	275.1
383.8	35–39	164.8
248.1	40–44	97.9
131.4	45–54	39.0
63.4	55–64	10.4
11.4	65+	1.4
236.3	Total	152.1

Figure 3 Rates of reported gonorrhea cases by age group and sex, United 2022. From CDC: Sexually Transmitted Disease Surveillance 2022. https://www.cdc.gov/std/statistics/2022/figures.htm. Accessed March 18, 2022.

* Per 100,000.

NOTE: Total includes cases of all ages, including those with unknown age.

NAAT, especially if NAAT has not been cleared by the US Food and Drug Administration (FDA) for use with these specimens or if it is ordered too soon after treatment because NAATs do not require viable organisms. Although this higher sensitivity has allowed the use of less invasively collected specimens, such as first-catch urine, specific site testing (pharyngeal or rectal specimens) will detect up to 80% more infections than urine screening alone, highlighting the importance of a careful exposure history and consideration of multiple-site screening in high-risk populations. Since the early 2010s, literature has also demonstrated that approved self-collection vaginal swabs are accurate and highly acceptable to patients.

Differential Diagnosis

Differential diagnosis of gonorrheal genital infections includes *Chlamydia trachomatis* (CT), *Mycoplasma genitalium*, *Trichomonas vaginalis*, and herpes simplex infection. In women, yeast vaginitis and bacterial vaginosis should be considered. Coinfection is common and cannot be ruled out on clinical grounds; therefore cotesting for CT and *Trichomonas* should be done in all patients, and all patients should be offered testing for HIV, syphilis, and hepatitis.

Gonococcal conjunctivitis is typically purulent and unilateral, but again, it cannot be distinguished clinically from other bacterial infections. Because gonococcal eye infections in adults generally result from autoinoculation, this diagnosis should prompt testing at other exposure sites.

Therapy

The 2024 CDC guidelines recommend a single intramuscular dose of ceftriaxone (Rocephin) 500 mg for the treatment of uncomplicated GC in persons weighing less than 150 kg, with the addition of oral doxycycline (100 mg twice daily [BID] for 7 days) if concomitant chlamydial infection has not been excluded. For persons weighing over 150 kg, a single 1-g IM dose of ceftriaxone should be used. If administration of IM ceftriaxone is not available, a single 800-mg oral dose of cefixime (Suprax) is an alternative regimen.

The risk for penicillin cross-reactivity is markedly lower with third-generation cephalosporins such as ceftriaxone (<1%) than first-generation cephalosporins. Only immunoglobulin E–mediated allergic reaction to penicillin (PCN) or cephalosporins (anaphylaxis, Stevens-Johnson syndrome, or toxic epidermal necrolysis) should contraindicate the use of ceftriaxone. Gentamicin[1] 240 mg IM × 1 *plus* azithromycin 2 g orally × 1 is an alternative regimen.

Expedited partner therapy (EPT) is a strategy of treating sex partners of patients with GC or chlamydia without examining the partner. EPT is advocated by the CDC to decrease reinfection rates, particularly where the likely alternative is no care. EPT is less efficacious for MSM, and shared decision making or in-person evaluation is recommended. A challenge for EPT with GC is the need for parental administration of the preferred therapy, ceftriaxone. If oral therapy seems to be the only option for a partner to be treated, cefixime[1] 800 mg (Suprax, two 400-mg single-dose tablets) should be used, again in conjunction with doxycycline 100 mg BID × 7 days if chlamydial infection has not been excluded.

Monitoring

The 2021 CDC monitoring guidelines contained several changes from prior recommendations:

- Because reinfection is common, occurring in 7% to 12% of patients, men and women with GC should be retested 3 months after treatment of the initial infection, regardless of

whether they believe that their sex partners were successfully treated.
- If the 3-month retesting does not occur, clinicians should retest whenever the individual next presents for care within 1 year of initial treatment.
- A test of cure is needed 7 to 14 days after treatment for people who are treated for a throat infection, as ceftriaxone levels are more variable in the pharynx.
- Pregnant women treated early in pregnancy should have a test of cure, as well as a retest in the third trimester.
- Those with persistent symptoms 3 weeks or more after treatment should have a test of cure.

Testing with NAAT in a shorter interval after treatment may result in false-positive test results because of the presence of DNA fragments. In this situation, testing should be repeated for CT and *Trichomonas* to reduce the potential for false-negative initial test results. For continued symptomatic genital infections despite appropriate therapy, culture with sensitivity testing is recommended.

Management of Complications

In men younger than 40, GC causes about 30% of cases of epididymitis, marked by unilateral testicular pain and swelling. Uncommon male complications of *N. gonorrhoeae* include inguinal lymphadenitis, penile edema, periurethral abscess or fistula, accessory gland infection (Tyson glands), balanitis, urethral stricture, and perhaps prostatitis. Female complications of GC are more frequent and burdensome; they include pelvic inflammatory disease, potentially leading to infertility or ectopic pregnancy. Disseminated gonococcal infections may occur in up to 2% of untreated patients. Certain gonococcal strains are more likely to cause disseminated gonococcal infections. Although patients are bacteremic, many appear nontoxic. Symptoms and signs may include fevers, myalgias, arthralgias, asymmetric polyarthritis, and a characteristic dermatitis consisting of a small number (<30) of skin lesions on the distal extremities that begin as papules and progress to pustules and ulcerations. Rarely, meningitis and endocarditis may occur. Hospitalization and consultation with an infectious disease specialist are recommended.

Prevention of Recurrent Infections

Doxycycline postexposure prophylaxis (Doxy PEP), the use of doxycycline to prevent bacterial STIs, was recommended by a 2024 CDC task force for certain high-risk individuals. The CDC recommends that providers should counsel gay, bisexual, and other MSM and transgender women (TGW) with a history of at least one bacterial STI (syphilis, chlamydia, or GC) during the past 12 months about the benefits and harms of using doxy PEP; other risk groups may be considered in a shared decision-making manner. The treatment consists of doxycycline[1] 200 mg, taken as soon as possible within 72 hours after having oral, vaginal, or anal sex, with a maximum dose of 200 mg every 24 hours. In clinical trials, serious adverse effects were rare and primarily gastrointestinal. A full discussion of the risk, benefits, and considerations may be found on the CDC website.

References

CDC: Sexually transmitted Infections Treatment Guidelines, 2021. Downloaded from https://www.cdc.gov/std/treatment-guidelines/gonorrhea.htm 2.25.25.

CDC: Clinical treatment of gonorrhea, 2024. Downloaded from https://www.cdc.gov/gonorrhea/hcp/clinical-care/index.html 2.25.25.

CDC Clinical Guidelines on the Use of Doxycycline Postexposure Prophylaxis for Bacterial Sexually Transmitted Infection Prevention, United States, 2024. Downloaded from https://www.cdc.gov/mmwr/volumes/73/rr/rr7302a1.htm 3.31.25.

United States Preventive Services Task Force: Final Recommendation Statement: Chlamydia and Gonorrhea Screenings. Available at www.uspreventiveservicestaskforce.org/Page/Document/RecommendationStatementFinal/chlamydia- and-gonorrhea-screening. Accessed Mar 21, 2021.

---

[1] Not FDA approved for this indication.

[1] Not FDA approved for this indication.

NONGONOCOCCAL URETHRITIS

Method of
Shannon Dowler, MD

CURRENT DIAGNOSIS

- The gold standard for rapid diagnosis of nongonococcal urethritis (NGU) in a clinic setting is a Gram stain of urethral discharge positive for greater than 2 WBC/hpf and negative for gram-negative diplococci (diagnostic for *Neisseria gonorrhea*). Microscopic diagnosis of this nature is often immediately available only in dedicated sexual health clinics.
- The majority of patients with NGU present to primary or urgent care, so clinical presentation in a male with symptoms of penile discharge and/or dysuria, with a positive sexual history, is adequate for a presumptive diagnosis while awaiting confirmatory testing.
- A urine sample (the first portion of the urine stream results in the highest yield) should be sent for nucleic acid amplification testing (NAAT).
- It is important to take a thorough sexual history and test exposed extragenital sites for infection, such as the throat and anus.
- In adolescents and young adults, a test of reinfection is recommended 12 weeks after treatment. In select patients where there is concern for nonadherence, or in pregnant patients with positive NAAT, test of reinfection/cure (TOR/C) is recommended in 4 weeks. All patients with a positive NAAT should have TOR/C in 3 to 4 months.
- Patients with recurrent infection or persistent symptoms should be evaluated for reinfection, drug resistance, or causes of NGU other than *Chlamydia*, such as *Trichomonas vaginalis* or *Mycoplasma genitalium*.
- New guidelines for the testing and management of *M. genitalium* should be reviewed.

CURRENT THERAPY

- If immediate test results are not available, empiric treatment to cover both *Chlamydia trachomatis* and *Neisseria gonorrhea* is recommended with ceftriaxone (Rocephin) 500 mg IM × 1 (1 g for patients ≥150 kg) and doxycycline 100 mg BID × 7 days. An alternate regimen in place of doxycycline is azithromycin (Zithromax) 1 g PO × 1 if patient nonadherence a concern.
- Stocking medications for the immediate treatment of *C. trachomatis*, *N. gonorrhea*, and *T. vaginalis* in the clinic is best practice and strongly recommended.
- Expedited partner therapy (EPT) is recommended, though state law should dictate this practice. The Guttmacher Institute maintains an active database of EPT rules by state.

Epidemiology

There are several etiologies of nongonococcal urethritis (NGU) in the United States, the most common being *Chlamydia trachomatis*. In 2021 the Centers for Disease Control and Prevention estimated that in the United States there were 1.6 million *C. trachomatis* infections reported—a slight decrease from 2019 likely tied to the lack of testing as a result of the COVID-19 pandemic. The second most common cause, in as much as 29% of cases, is *Mycoplasma genitalium*. With the first U.S. Food and Drug Administration-approved test for *M. genitalium* available in 2019, guidelines for management are rapidly evolving. Men who have sex with women are at higher risk for *Trichomonas vaginalis* than men who have sex with men, and the prevalence varies geographically. Historically, poor testing options for men have made it difficult to quantify the prevalence of NGU due to *T. vaginalis*, though with the advent of nucleic acid amplification testing (NAAT) testing, it is estimated to be the cause of up to 8% of cases. Other less common causes include *Ureaplasma urea lyticum*, herpes simplex virus (HSV), Mpox, and adenovirus.

Risk Factors

The risk factors for NGU include sexual activity without using barrier method protection, younger age (<25 years), high-risk sexual partners, multiple sex partners, and a history of sexually transmitted infection (STI). Other contributing factors include low socioeconomic status and racial and ethnic minority status.

Pathophysiology

NGU as a broad term describes the inflammation of the male urethra caused by infection other than *Neisseria gonorrhea*. Inflammation as a result of the infection causes a penile discharge that ranges in consistency from mucoid to mucopurulent and a range of dysuric symptoms from none to marked burning. Though the cause of NGU is most often bacterial (e.g., *C. trachomatis* and *M. genitalium*), it can also be caused by protozoa, *T. vaginalis*, viral etiologies (HSV), and other etiologies.

Prevention

The mainstay of public health primary prevention efforts includes the education of adolescents and young adults about the inherent risks of unprotected sex, multiple partners, and high-risk sexual partners. Efforts at "abstinence-only" education have resulted in poor outcomes. Encouraging the use of barrier methods of contraceptions, limiting the number of sexual partners, and avoiding high-risk partners are primary prevention strategies. Secondary prevention is geared toward making sexual health clinics widely available and affordable for all people, regardless of insurance status, and ensuring primary care and urgent care practices are equipped for screening, treatment of, and education on signs and symptoms of infection. Emergency departments also play a role in thoroughly screening at-risk patients who present for care.

In 2024, the first guidelines were released for the use of doxycycline for postexposure prophylaxis (DoxyPEP) for specific populations, including men who have sex with men and transgender women with a history of an STI in the prior year. Early studies reveal strong evidence to support DoxyPEP for the prevention of chlamydia, syphilis, and gonorrhea infections in select patient populations. Studies are underway to understand the potential impacts to the microbiome and antimicrobial resistance, but early utilization reveals significant reductions in infections in at risk populations.

Clinical Manifestations

Most men with NGU present with symptoms of dysuria and urethral discharge. Dysuria can range from intermittent and episodic discomfort to persistent pain. Discharge ranges from clear to mucoid to mucopurulent. Frankly purulent and abundant discharge should alert the clinician to strongly consider *N. gonorrhea*. Many men may not be aware of discharge, so asking questions about "crusting" on the penis or underwear can be helpful. The clinical examination is critical. "Milking" the penis can allow for urethral discharge to manifest at the tip of the penis. At times, the urethral meatus can be inflamed and red. In men with *T. vaginalis*, the symptoms are often more mild and vague, such as "a tingling feeling" or "itching inside the penis" with urination; discharge is less common. Clinicians should pay attention to the presence of significant findings such as enlarged lymph nodes, penile ulcers, warts, rashes, and scrotal/testicular pain. Patients may present with more than one infection.

Diagnosis

Though Gram stain of the urethral discharge is the gold standard for immediate diagnosis, this modality is rarely available in standard clinical practice. If Gram stain is available, the absence of gram-negative diplococci and the presence of greater than 2 WBC/hpf suggest a diagnosis of NGU. For all patients, further testing by NAAT should be undertaken. Based on patient risk, history, and exam, a clinician may opt to treat empirically even in the absence of WBCs.

A urine sample (ideally limited to the "first" portion of the stream) should be collected after physical examination. NAAT has high specificity and sensitivity, and results are often available within hours or within a day for many labs. There is not an indication for culture of any causes of NGU. In men who have sex with women, *T. vaginalis* should be strongly considered as an etiology. NAAT for *T. vaginalis*, *N. gonorrhea*, and *C. trachomatis* is available in the majority of labs. Alternatively, a urine sample can be spun for microscopy, and in experienced labs, *T. vaginalis* can be diagnosed with microscopy. Wet prep testing is not a reliable test for *T. vaginalis* in men. In January 2019, the first FDA-approved NAAT for *M. genitalium* was introduced to the U.S. market. Current CDC guidelines do not routinely recommend screening for *M. genitalium*. For patients who have refractory or recurrent symptoms, or those with negative NAAT for other pathogens, the diagnosis of *M. genitalium* should be strongly considered. Management of *M. genitalium* is addressed later in this section. Increasingly, nongenital sites of asymptomatic infection are being identified, particularly in the throat and anus. A thorough sexual history should include anatomic sites of sexual contact, and screening should be performed at those sites when a patient presents with symptoms or risk for sexually transmitted infections. Routine screening should also include sampling from extragenital sites. Numerous studies have confirmed that many patients with negative urine NAATs will have asymptomatic or minimally symptomatic *C. trachomatis* or *N. gonorrhea* infections in other sites of sexual contact.

Therapy/Treatment

Patients with characteristic symptoms who have a Gram stain performed that rules out *N. gonorrhea* should be treated for NGU empirically with doxycycline 100 mg BID × 7 days. This guidance in the 2021 CDC STI guidelines reflects a significant change. Alternatively, azithromycin (Zithromax) 1 g by mouth in one dose can be given; unfortunately, owing to emerging drug resistance, this should be reserved for patients where the likelihood of treatment nonadherence is very high. In the absence of Gram stain testing availability, empiric treatment coverage with both azithromycin and ceftriaxone (Rocephin) should be considered in patients with a history of recent infection, high-risk contacts, or symptoms of urethritis. All clinical locations that test and treat for sexually transmitted infections should maintain a supply of oral azithromycin and metronidazole (Flagyl), as well as intramuscular ceftriaxone to provide immediate treatment and reduce barriers to care such as transportation to a pharmacy, pharmaceutical insurance coverage, cost, and concerns about confidentiality, particularly in younger patients.

If trichomonas is suspected, new guidelines recommend men receive a one-time 2 g dose of metronidazole but women receive 500 mg BID × 7 days, a marked change from prior guidelines. Of note, the new guidelines also disabuse the historical potential for the interaction between alcohol and metronidazole and no longer list this as a contraindication. Additional regimens are available at the free-of-charge STD treatment guidelines page on the CDC website (cdc.gov). The STD treatment guideline app is an excellent public source tool for treatment guidelines.

If a patient presents with persistent symptoms despite appropriate treatment, the clinician must consider reinfection or drug resistance. If the patient had negative tests for *N. gonorrhea* and *C. trachomatis,* the clinician should consider empiric treatment for *T. vaginalis* with metronidazole 2 g PO ×1 or tinidazole (Tindamax) 2 g PO ×1 if the patient is a male who has sex with females. The possibility of *M. genitalium* should be considered in patients with NGU, particularly those with recurrent or persistent symptoms. *M. genitalium* has developed rapid drug resistance, with more than a third of infections now resistant to azithromycin. Monotherapy cure rates are less than 50%. Performing NAAT testing for recurrent or persistent symptoms in the absence of a confirmatory *C. trachomatis* or *N. gonorrhea* result should be undertaken. The guidelines for treatment recommend two step therapy beginning with doxycycline 100 mg BID × 7 days followed by moxifloxacin (Avelox)[1] 400 mg daily for 7 days. The CDC recommends testing partners of patients with symptomatic *M. genitalium* and treating if positive; alternatively, if testing is not an option for partners of positive cases, the same drug regimen can be used unless the partner is pregnant. For guidance on treatment in pregnancy, contact: https://www.stdccn.org/render/Public

All patients treated for NGU should be advised to abstain from sex for 1 week following completion of treatment to allow for clearance of infection. Known sexual partners should be treated with expedited partner therapy when allowed by state law. The patient should not resume sexual activity until the partner is adequately treated. Coordinating partner treatment and 1 week of posttreatment abstinence can be challenging to manage owing to patient nonadherence to recommendations. If uncertain how to manage patients not following guidelines, consider partnering with your local health department STD clinic. Positive tests should be reported to the health authority as indicated by state law. Suspected or confirmed drug resistance should be reported to the CDC at https://www.stdccn.org/render/Public

Monitoring

Partner treatment is recommended for all confirmed causes of NGU. Test of reinfection soon after treatment (4 weeks) is recommended in high-risk patients and test of reinfection in 12 weeks (3 months) for all patients with a positive NAAT for *C. trachomatis*, *N. gonorrhea*, or *T. vaginalis*. Because testing can remain positive in men following clinical cure, test of cure and test for reinfection for *M. genitalium* in the absence of symptoms is NOT recommended at this time.

Complications

Untreated *C. trachomatis* infection in men can cause epididymitis, prostatitis, and reactive arthritis. Autoinoculation to the eyes is a potential complication in untreated urethral infections and requires immediate treatment. Untreated infection in men can result in both genital and extragenital infections in partners; in women this has the potential to lead to chronic pelvic pain, infertility, and surgical complications of infection. Additionally, the presence of genital infection can serve as a cofactor in the acquisition or transmission of HIV.

---

[1] Not FDA approved for this indication.

References

BASHH guidelines. https://www.bashhguidelines.org/current-guidelines/urethritis-and-cervicitis/mycoplasma-genitalium-2018/ (Accessed April 18, 2020).

Centers for Disease Control and Infection: *Emerging infectious diseases: increasing macrolide and fluoroquinolone resistance in* Mycoplasma genitalium. wwwnc.cdc.gov/eid/article/23/5/16-1745_article, 2017 (Accessed April 28. 2020).

Centers for Disease Control and Prevention. Chlamydia. July 30, 2019. gov/std/stats18/chlamydia.htm (accessed April 18, 2020).

Guttmacher Institute. Partner treatment of STIs. Guttmacher.org/state policy/explore/partner-treatment-stis (accessed April 18, 2020)

US Food and Drug Administration: FDA permits marketing of first test to aid in the diagnosis of a sexually transmitted infection known as *Mycoplasma genitalium, January* 23, 2019. https://www.fda.gov/news-events/press-announcements/fda-permits-marketing-first-test-aid-diagnosis-sexually transmitted-infection-known mycoplasma. (accessed April 28, 2020).

SYPHILIS

Method of
Jennifer Frank, MD

CURRENT DIAGNOSIS

- Serologic testing includes both nontreponemal-specific testing (VDRL and RPR) and treponemal-specific testing (FTA-Abs [fluorescent treponemal antibody absorption] and TP-PA [*Treponema pallidum* particle agglutination]).
- Cerebrospinal fluid testing (VDRL [Venereal Disease Research Laboratory], protein, cell count) is performed to diagnose neurosyphilis.

CURRENT THERAPY

- Penicillin is first-line therapy for all types and stages of syphilis.
- Penicillin is the only recommended treatment for pregnant women and for congenital syphilis. Penicillin-allergic patients should undergo desensitization.

Epidemiology

The rate of primary and secondary syphilis reached a low point (2.1/100,000) in 2000 and has increased since that time, with the most recent data indicating a continued increase of 1% from 2022 to 2023 for all cases of syphilis. However, there was a 10.2% decrease from 2022 to 2023 for primary and secondary cases, the first significant decrease since 2001. Rates of primary and secondary syphilis are decreasing among men, women, most age groups, and all races. Forty-one states have shown decreased rates. Men who have sex with men (MSM) continue to have the highest rates of syphilis, accounting for approximately one-third of cases, although rates are decreasing. Congenital syphilis cases continued to increase by 3% from 2022 to 2023 with a total of 3882 cases.

Risk Factors

MSM and HIV-positive persons are at highest risk for primary and secondary syphilis. Approximately half of those diagnosed with primary and secondary syphilis are 15 to 24 years of age. Other risk factors include living in certain geographic areas in the United States or an urban area and being born to a mother infected with syphilis. Risk factors can reflect disparities such as access to sexual health care rather than solely sexual health behavior.

Pathophysiology

Syphilis is caused by infection with the spirochete *Treponema pallidum* subspecies *pallidum* (Figure 1). The average incubation period is 21 days (range 3–90 days). Primary infection manifests with signs and symptoms at the site of infection; secondary and tertiary syphilis manifest with systemic signs and symptoms. Syphilis is primarily sexually transmitted but may be transmitted perinatally or through nonsexual cutaneous transmission. Previous infection does not confer long- term immunity.

Prevention

Prevention includes both avoiding initial infection and preventing disease progression through early detection and treatment. Transmission of syphilis can be reduced (although not eliminated) by using condoms. Screening for syphilis in pregnancy combined with treatment of infected women reduces perinatal transmission. The two most common missed opportunities in prevention

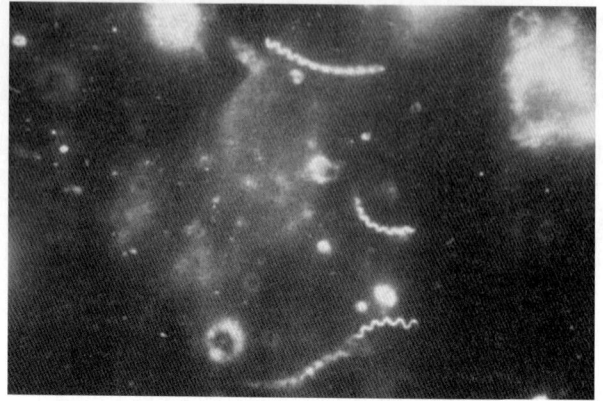

Figure 1 *Treponema pallidum* on darkfield microscopy.

of congenital syphilis are maternal treatment in a woman who is diagnosed with syphilis and timely prenatal care with appropriate syphilis screening. Screening high-risk populations may prevent spread of infection.

Screening

The US Preventive Services Task Force recommends screening people at increased risk for syphilis. This includes women and men who have sex with women who are at increased risk based on incarceration, sex work, geography, race or ethnicity, and age. MSM who have sex with men should be screened annually and more frequently if at increased risk. People with human immunodeficiency virus (HIV) should be screened at their first evaluation and then annually. Gender-diverse people should be screened based on risk factors. All pregnant women should be screened for syphilis at the first prenatal visit. Women at increased risk should be rescreened in the third trimester, at delivery, and after any potential exposure to an infected partner.

Clinical Manifestations

Primary syphilis manifests as a chancre at the site of inoculation. The chancre, a painless ulcer with sharp borders, is usually solitary and associated with regional lymphadenopathy. Atypical presentations include extragenital location (most commonly oral or anal) and the presence of pain or multiple lesions. Secondary syphilis characteristically manifests with a generalized rash with variable features 4 to 8 weeks after onset of primary syphilis (Figure 2). The palms and soles are affected in the majority of patients. Typically, the rash is maculopapular or papulosquamous and nonpruritic. Other clinical manifestations include highly infectious flat lesions (condyloma lata), fever, malaise, sore throat, headache, myalgias, alopecia, and, rarely, renal, bone, eye, or liver involvement. Latent syphilis, by definition, has no clinical manifestations. Neurologic, otologic, and ocular symptoms can occur during any stage of syphilis. People should be screened for neurologic, otologic, and ocular involvement; the presence of any symptoms warrants additional evaluation, which may include cerebral spinal fluid (CSF) examination, ocular examination, or evaluation by otolaryngology.

Tertiary syphilis, which is rare, is a late manifestation in untreated people and includes late neurosyphilis, cardiovascular, and gummatous disease. Gummas are nodular lesions that vary in size and location. They can ulcerate and cause local tissue destruction. Cardiovascular syphilis most commonly manifests as aortitis of the ascending aorta. The clinical manifestations of neurosyphilis are numerous and include meningitis with or without vascular involvement, dementia, tabes dorsalis (posterior column involvement with ataxia and bowel and bladder dysfunction), and ocular or otologic involvement.

Congenital syphilis has early (birth to 2 years) and late (2–20 years) clinical manifestations. Early signs include hepatosplenomegaly, rash, fever, neurosyphilis, pneumonitis, rhinitis, generalized lymphadenopathy, hepatitis, ascites, hematologic disease, renal disease, periostitis, and osteochondritis. Late manifestations

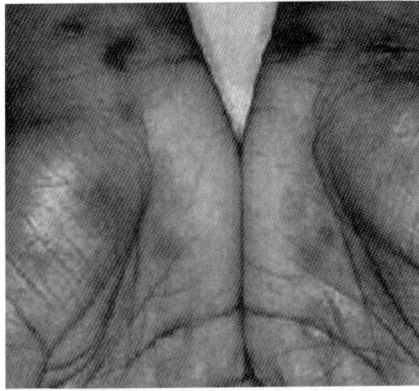
Figure 2 Syphilis skin lesion.

(present in 40% of untreated patients) include skeletal deformities, neurologic disease (deafness), dental abnormalities, and ocular abnormalities.

Diagnosis

Primary syphilis is optimally diagnosed by specific testing of the skin lesion or exudate because it can take several weeks for antibodies to develop. There are three methods for testing of exudate: direct fluorescent antibody testing, PCR testing, and darkfield microscopy; all have limited availability. Serologic testing is done using nontreponemal (Venereal Disease Research Laboratory [VDRL] or rapid plasma reagin [RPR]) and treponemal testing (multiple types, including fluorescent treponemal antibody absorption (FTA-ABS) and *Treponema pallidum* particle agglutination [TPPA]) because both tests have limitations. Nontreponemal testing may be falsely positive with other medical conditions, but antibody titers correlate with disease activity and therefore can indicate response to treatment. Nontreponemal tests usually become nonreactive after successful treatment. A serofast reaction can occur in which the nontreponemal test stays reactive. Treponemal tests are specific for syphilitic infection but stay reactive in the majority of people regardless of treatment or disease status. Treponemal test antibody titers do not match the level of disease activity and therefore cannot be used to monitor treatment response.

Both traditional algorithm testing (nontreponemal testing followed by treponemal specific testing if positive) and reverse sequence testing (treponemal specific testing followed by nontreponemal testing if positive) are acceptable approaches. The majority of laboratories continue to use traditional algorithm testing. Reverse sequence testing has a higher false-positive rate with the initial screening step of testing but identifies more cases of syphilis, particularly early infection, previously treated infection, or long-standing infection. If reverse sequence screening is used with discordant results, a different treponemal specific test should be used to determine true from false positives.

Neurosyphilis is diagnosed based on clinical signs and symptoms using laboratory testing to support a clinical diagnosis. No single test can be used to diagnose all patients with neurosyphilis, which means that neurosyphilis is usually diagnosed by a combination of serologic testing, testing of cerebrospinal fluid (CSF), and clinical evaluation. Laboratory testing includes reactive serologic testing; cerebrospinal fluid (CSF) VDRL (Venereal Disease Research Laboratory) testing, which is specific but not sensitive; and CSF positive for white blood cells or protein, or both. The CSF FTA-ABS (fluorescent treponemal antibody absorption) test is sensitive but less specific than CSF VDRL testing. Patients with latent or tertiary syphilis, or neurosyphilis should be tested for HIV infection.

Congenital syphilis diagnosis is complicated by the presence of maternal antibodies in the infant's bloodstream for up to a year of age which can make treponemal-specific testing inaccurate. Nontreponemal testing is recommended for newborns born to a mother with positive syphilis serology during pregnancy using the same nontreponemal test as used with the mother in order to compare titers.

Differential Diagnosis

Syphilis, which can affect every organ system, has historically been called the great mimicker. Syphilis is on the differential diagnosis of, most commonly, conditions causing genital ulcers or lesions, conditions causing systemic rashes affecting the palms and soles, conditions causing ocular and otologic manifestations (uveitis, sudden visual changes, hearing loss), and conditions causing dementia, meningitis, or ataxia.

Treatment

Penicillin G is the preferred treatment for all stages of syphilis; other forms of penicillin (oral penicillin, combinations of benzathine and procaine [Bicillin CR]) are not effective. The stage and extent of clinical disease determine which preparation is used, the dosage, and the length of treatment (Table 1). In penicillin-allergic patients, antibiotic alternatives exist for all types and stages of syphilis except for syphilis in pregnancy and congenital syphilis. Consider consultation with infectious disease for nonpenicillin treatment regimens for patient with latent, tertiary, ocular, otic, or neurosyphilis.

In people with a penicillin allergy and primary or secondary syphilis, doxycycline (100 mg orally [PO] twice daily for 14 days) or tetracycline (500 mg PO four times per day for 14 days) can be used. Ceftriaxone ([Rocephin] 1 g daily intramuscularly [IM] or intravenously [IV] for 10 days)[1] has also been used, although the optimal dose and duration are not known. Azithromycin (Zithromax)[1] should not be used given the potential for resistance.

The treatment of latent syphilis in penicillin-allergic people can include doxycycline (100 mg twice daily) or tetracycline (500 mg four times daily) for 28 days. Neither ceftriaxone nor azithromycin are indicated.

The Jarisch-Herxheimer reaction is an acute febrile reaction (with accompanying headache, myalgias, and other symptoms) occurring within 24 hours of treatment of syphilis. It is more common in early stages of syphilis and rare in newborns.

Monitoring

No definite criteria exist for either cure of syphilis or treatment failure. It is recommended that nontreponemal antibody titers be followed every 6 months, and patients should be periodically reexamined for clinical signs or symptoms of syphilitic infection. Treatment failure is probable in patients with either persistent or recurrent clinical signs or symptoms or a sustained fourfold increase in nontreponemal antibody titer (compared to maximum titer at time of treatment). Treatment failure is possible if nontreponemal antibody titers fail to decline fourfold within 6 months after treatment. Suspected treatment failure warrants retesting for neurosyphilis and HIV infection. Patients with HIV infection, with congenital syphilis, who are pregnant, or who have neurosyphilis warrant closer and more-specific laboratory and clinical follow-up. Full recommendations can be found in the Centers for Disease Control and Prevention (CDC) treatment guidelines (http://www.cdc.gov/std/treatment-guidelines/syphilis.htm). Additional questions about testing and treatment for syphilis can be directed to the National Network of STD Clinical Prevention Training Centers at https://www.stdccn.org/controller/Public/AddPublicConsultRequestStep1.

Congenital Syphilis

Like other forms of syphilis, congenital syphilis is increasing in prevalence. The majority of cases are associated with late or no maternal testing and/or inadequate maternal treatment.

---

[1] Not FDA approved for this indication.

TABLE 1 Centers for Disease Control and Prevention Recommendations for Treatment of Syphilis

STAGE	RECOMMENDED PENICILLIN TREATMENT	
	PENICILLIN	DOSAGE
Primary and secondary syphilis	Benzathine penicillin G (Bicillin LA)	2.4 million U IM once
Early latent syphilis (acquired within previous 12 mo)	Benzathine penicillin G	2.4 million U IM once
Late latent syphilis	Benzathine penicillin G	2.4 million U IM weekly × 3 doses
Tertiary syphilis	Benzathine penicillin G	2.4 million units IM weekly × 3 doses
Neurosyphilis	Aqueous crystalline penicillin G *or* Continuous infusion *or* Procaine penicillin (Wycillin) *plus* Probenecid	3–4 million U q4h 18–24 U daily IV × 10–14 d (preferred) 2.4 million U IM 500 mg PO qid
Congenital Syphilis		
Proven or highly probable disease	Aqueous crystalline penicillin G *or* Procaine penicillin G	100,000–150,000 U/kg/d (divided 50,000 U/kg/dose) IV q12h × first 7 d of life, then q8h for total of 10 d of treatment 50,000 U/kg/dose IM daily × 10 d
Normal examination but mother inadequately treated	Aqueous crystalline penicillin G *or* Procaine penicillin G *or* Benzathine penicillin G	100,000–150,000 U/kg/d (divided 50,000 U/kg/dose) IV q12h × first 7 d of life, then q8h for total of 10 days of treatment 50,000 U/kg/dose IM daily × 10 d 50,000 U/kg/dose IM once
Normal examination, serologic titers ≤4 × the maternal titer, and mother adequately treated during pregnancy	Benzathine penicillin G	50,000 U/kg/dose IM once

Infection usually reflects transplacental transmission of *T. pallidum;* direct exposure to maternal genital lesions during delivery is a less common route of transmission. Greater than 50% of fetuses exposed to early maternal syphilitic infection will be affected; risk of transmission decreases for maternal infection acquired more than 1 year before pregnancy. Current guidelines recommend screening for syphilis at the first prenatal visit as well as at 28 weeks and delivery for women at increased risk.

Congenital syphilis is most commonly diagnosed with the use of ultrasonography after 18 weeks' gestational age looking for characteristic signs of intrauterine infection (i.e., hepatomegaly, placentomegaly, hydrops, and polyhydramnios). Neonatal diagnosis can be established by evidence of placental infection, nontreponemal titers in the neonate that are greater than four times maternal titers. Treponemal antibodies can be passively transferred from mother to baby so are not useful for diagnosis of neonatal infection.

Symptoms of congenital syphilis include anemia and thrombocytopenia, small for gestational age, bony abnormalities, hepatobiliary dysfunction, and skin or mucus membrane lesions. Neonates with congenital syphilis have a 60% risk of having neurosyphilis. Symptoms of neurosyphilis include seizures, cerebral infarcts, cranial nerve palsies, and eye abnormalities. After 2 years of age, late manifestations can include bony malformations, hearing loss, eye abnormalities, and Hutchinson's teeth.

Complications

Complications of syphilis are primarily related to neurologic involvement, tertiary syphilis, or late manifestations of congenital syphilis.

References

ACOG. Clinical Practice: syphilis resurgence reminds us of the importance of STD screening and treatment during prenatal care. Available at https://www.acog.org/About-ACOG/ACOG-Departments/ACOG-Rounds/May-2017/Syphilis-Resurgence.

Cantor AG, Pappas M, Daeges M, Nelson HD: Screening for syphilis: updated evidence report and systematic review for the US Preventive Services Task Force, *JAMA* 315:2328–2337, 2016.

Centers for Disease Control and Prevention: *Sexually transmitted infections treatment Guidelines,* 2021. Available at: http://www.cdc.gov/std/treatmentguidelines/syphilis.htm.

Centers for Disease Control and Prevention: Clinical advisory: ocular syphilis in the United States. Available at, https://www.cdc.gov/std/syphilis/clinicaladvisoryos2015.htm, 2015.

Centers for Disease Control and Prevention: *National overview of STDs,* 2023. Available at http://cdc.gov/sti-statistics/annual/summary.html.

Centers for Disease Control and Prevention: Discordant results from reverse sequence syphilis screening: five laboratories, United States, 2006–2010, *MMWR Morb Mortal Wkly Rep* 60(5):133–137, 2011.

Kent ME, Romanelli F: Reexamining syphilis: an update on epidemiology, clinical manifestations, and management, *Ann Pharmacother* 42:226–236, 2008.

Koss CA, Dunne EF, Warner L: A systematic review of epidemiologic studies assessing condom use and risk of syphilis, *Sex Trans Dis* 36:401–405, 2009.

Lautenschlager S: Cutaneous manifestations of syphilis, *Am J Clin Dermatol* 7:291–304, 2006.

Marra CM: Update on neurosyphilis, *Curr Infect Dis Rep* 11:127–134, 2009.

New York City Department of Health and Mental Hygiene, and the New York City STD PreventionTraining Center: *The diagnosis and management of syphilis: an update and review,* 2019. www.nycptc.org.

Papp JR, Park IU, Fakile Y, Periera L, et al: CDC laboratory recommendations for Syphilis Testing, United States 2024, *Morb Motal Wkly Rep* 73(1):1–32, 2024.

Stafford IA, Workowski KA, Bachman LH: Syphilis complicating pregnancy and congenital syphilis, *N Engl J Med* 390:242–253, 2024.

Woods CR: Congenital syphilis—persisting pestilence, *Pediatr Infect Dis* 28:536–537, 2009.

USPSTF: *Syphilis infection in nonpregnant adults and adolescents: screening,* 2016.

ACNE VULGARIS

Method of
Linda K. Oge, MD

CURRENT DIAGNOSIS

- Acne vulgaris lesions may occur on the face, chest, upper back, neck, and upper arms.
- Acne vulgaris lesions may be inflammatory (pustules, papules, cysts, and nodules) or noninflammatory (whiteheads and blackheads).
- Acne vulgaris may be classified as clear, almost clear, mild, moderate, or severe.
- No specific microbiological or laboratory testing is routinely indicated to establish the diagnosis of acne vulgaris.

CURRENT THERAPY

- Topical retinoids and benzoyl peroxide may be used as monotherapy in mild acne vulgaris.
- Combination topical therapy is favored over monotherapy for the management of mild to moderate acne vulgaris.
- Topical and oral antibiotics should never be used as monotherapy for the management of acne vulgaris.
- Benzoyl peroxide should be added to topical retinoids, topical antibiotics, and oral antibiotics to reduce the development of resistance.
- Combination therapy with oral antibiotics (preferably doxycycline) and topical therapies is recommended for moderate to severe acne or acne that has failed topical therapy.
- Isotretinoin (Accutane, Claravis) should be considered for severe, recalcitrant nodular acne and acne that has been refractory to other treatment regimens, associated with significant scarring, or caused great psychological distress. Significant potential for adverse reactions, including risk of teratogenicity, must be weighed against the benefit of treatment.
- Combined oral contraceptives may be helpful in patients with acne flares with menses, signs of hyperandrogenism, or acne that does not respond sufficiently to other treatments.
- Therapeutic interventions implemented to treat acne vulgaris should be continued for 6 to 8 weeks before making changes to the intervention unless the patient is experiencing intolerable side effects.

Epidemiology

Globally, acne vulgaris (AV) is the second most common skin disease and the eighth most common disease overall, affecting 9.4% of the world's population. Eighty-five percent of patients aged 12 to 25 will experience some degree of AV. The overall prevalence of AV is slightly higher in boys versus girls, and boys also have a higher prevalence of severe AV. Although the prevalence declines with advancing age, AV occurs into the thirties and forties, affecting women more than men in adulthood. Studies confirm genetic influences on AV. Patients with a family history of AV and oily skin type are more likely to develop AV and to have severe AV.

Prevention

The effect of diet on AV has long been debated; however, currently available literature is limited by study heterogeneity and bias. Although further research is required, evidence exists supporting recommendation for diets with low glycemic index/glycemic load, free of some dairy (milk/ice cream showed causal effect but not cheese/butter), and rich in omega-3 and omega-6 fatty acids. One small study suggests probiotics may be beneficial in AV management.

Pathophysiology

Multiple pathogenetic factors exert an effect on the pilosebaceous unit, influencing the development of AV: complex inflammatory mechanisms involving innate and acquired immunity, excess sebum production, follicular hyperkeratinization, and colonization with *Cutibacterium acnes*.

Clinical Manifestations

AV is characterized by the presence of noninflammatory (comedones) and inflammatory lesions (papules, pustules, and nodules). Noninflammatory lesions include closed comedones (formed by the accumulation of sebum/keratin within the hair follicle and called whiteheads) and open comedones (formed by distension with keratin causing the follicle to open and darken and called blackheads). AV lesions may be distributed on the face, neck, upper back, upper arms, or chest. Skin changes including scarring and hyperpigmentation may also occur. Patients with untreated AV often experience bullying, depression, anxiety, and low self-esteem and are at increased risk for suicide.

Diagnosis

AV has been classified and graded using many systems; however, no method has been universally accepted for clinical use. The American Academy of Dermatology (AAD) has endorsed a 5-point scale from 0 to 4 (clear, almost clear, mild, moderate, and severe) for clinical use, but definitions for each ordinal have not been standardized and validated. Ideally, documentation should include the number and types of primary acne lesions, areas of skin involvement, and presence of hyperpigmentation or scarring. Digital photography may also be helpful in documenting severity and response to treatment. The AAD does not endorse any routine laboratory or microbiological testing for the diagnosis and management of routine AV. Patients with features suggestive of hyperandrogenism or polycystic ovarian syndrome (hirsutism, oligomenorrhea or amenorrhea, infertility, scalp hair loss) may need endocrinologic screening (free and total testosterone, dehydroepiandrosterone sulfate, androstenedione, luteinizing hormone, follicle stimulating hormone, and 17-hydroxyprogesterone levels). Patients with abnormal endocrine testing should be evaluated by an endocrinologist.

Differential Diagnosis

The differential diagnosis of AV includes acneiform eruptions that may be precipitated by topical cosmetic and hair products (acne cosmetica) or certain medications (glucocorticoids, lithium, oral contraceptives, phenytoin, isoniazid, cyclosporine, and androgens). Drug-induced acne tends to be monomorphic (uniform in appearance). Rosacea may be distinguished from AV by the presence of telangiectasias and diffusely distributed erythema affecting the central face, and the absence of comedones. Other differential considerations include folliculitis (monomorphic, no comedones), seborrheic dermatitis (yellow, greasy scales), and perioral dermatitis (papules, pustules, erythema affecting chin/nasolabial folds and sparing area around the vermilion border).

Treatment

Management of AV begins with an assessment of severity and targets the pathogenetic factors that precipitate AV. Agents are available over the counter and by prescription in multiple strengths and combinations. The vehicle used (gel, foam, washes, creams, lotions, or pads) depends on the location and extent of AV involvement and skin type. Creams and lotions may be preferred for combination skin or dry skin, whereas gels may be helpful for oily skin. Foams, washes, and lotions allow coverage of larger surface area and are useful in management of truncal AV. Washes can be applied and rinsed off to reduce skin irritation and improve tolerance. The U.S. Food and Drug Administration (FDA) approved topical treatments for AV include retinoids, topical antibiotics, benzoyl peroxide (BP), a topical antiandrogen (clascoterone [Winlevi]), salicylic acid, dapsone (Aczone), and azelaic acid (Azelex cream).

Topical Retinoids

Topical retinoids are considered a preferred first-line treatment for mild comedonal AV. Topical retinoids are vitamin A derivatives that have antiinflammatory and comedolytic properties. Retinoids may be used alone in mild AV or in combination with topical antibiotics, BP, or other topical agents in mild to moderate AV. Topical retinoids may also be used with oral antibiotics for moderate to severe AV and for maintenance therapy once remission is achieved and oral antibiotics are discontinued. The FDA-approved topical retinoids for use in AV include adapalene (Differin), tretinoin (Retin-A and others), tazarotene (Tazorac), and most recently, trifarotene (Aklief). These retinoids differ in their binding affinity for the different retinoic acid receptors, allowing for subtle differences in tolerability and efficacy. Burning/stinging, dryness, erythema, and photosensitivity are commonly associated with retinoid use. Retinoid formulations should be applied at bedtime because of their photolabile nature. Tretinoin is available in cream (0.02%, 0.025%, 0.0375%, 0.05%, 0.075%, 0.1%), gel (0.01%, 0.025%, 0.05%, 0.1%), and lotion (0.05% [Altreno]). Side effects can be reduced by gradual titration of dosage strength, use of newer microgel formulations of tretinoin (Retin-A Micro 0.04%, 0.06%, 0.08%, 0.1%) and daily use of sunscreens. Coapplication with BP may cause oxidation and inactivation of tretinoin; however, microsphere formulations of tretinoin, tazarotene (Arazlo, Fabior, Tazorac) and trifarotene are not subject to these limitations. Trifarotene (0.005% once nightly)

was approved in 2019 owing to its specificity for the gamma receptor, which confers increased potency and reduction in skin irritation.

Adapalene 0.1% (Differin) gel is the only retinoid available over the counter. Adapalene is also available by prescription in 0.1% (cream, gel, lotion, solution, or swab), 0.3% (gel only), and in combination with BP as Epiduo gel or swab (0.1%/2.5%) and Epiduo Forte gel (0.3%/2.5%). According to AAD guidelines, current research does not suggest superiority of one retinoid over another in efficacy or tolerability; however, a recent network meta-analysis suggests topical tazarotene (available in cream, foam, or gel and strengths of 0.05% and 0.1%) may show slight superiority. Although systemic absorption is minimal, human data are limited, and topical retinoids are not recommended for use in pregnancy based on animal studies and reports of fetal malformations with oral retinoids. Tazarotene is contraindicated in women who are or who may become pregnant.

Benzoyl Peroxide

BP is available over the counter in various formulations (bar, cream, lotion, wash, liquid, gel, foam) and strengths (2.5%–10%). BP has proven efficacy against inflammatory and noninflammatory AV lesions owing to comedolytic and antimicrobial properties. BP can be used as monotherapy or in combination with retinoids, topical and oral antibiotics, and other topical agents. Because no C. acnes resistance to BP has been reported, its use is recommended in combination with other agents to reduce the development of antibiotic resistance. Common side effects of BP use include burning/stinging, dryness, and erythema, and uncommonly patients may experience contact dermatitis (5% of patients). Skin irritation may be minimized by using reduced strength or wash-off formulations. Care should be taken in applying BP as it may cause bleaching of hair and clothing. Co-application of BP with dapsone and over-the-counter sodium sulfacetamide preparations causes orange-brown skin discoloration, which can be avoided by applying these agents at separate times of the day. BP is also safe for use in pregnancy and during lactation.

Topical Antibiotics

Topical antibiotics approved for use in the management of AV include clindamycin 1% (applied daily or twice daily and available in gel, lotion, foam, swab, or solution), erythromycin 2% (applied daily and available in gel, solution, or swab), and minocycline 4% (Amzeeq 4% topical foam applied once daily). Topical antibiotics are efficacious against inflammatory AV because of antimicrobial activity against C. acnes and antiinflammatory effects, but they have minimal effect on comedonal acne.

Topical antibiotic monotherapy should be avoided to reduce antibiotic resistance. Adding BP to topical antibiotic therapy may mitigate development of resistance. Topical antibiotics may be used in combination with BP, retinoids, and other topical agents but not oral antibiotics.

Insufficient data exist to support use of one topical antibiotic over another. Both topical clindamycin and erythromycin are safe in pregnancy, but minocycline is not recommended in pregnancy or during lactation. Rare cases of antibiotic-associated diarrhea and Clostridium difficile colitis have occurred with topical clindamycin use.

Azelaic Acid

Azelaic acid possesses comedolytic, antimicrobial, and antiinflammatory properties and may also lighten hyperpigmentation associated with AV. Azelaic acid is available over the counter in lower dose formulations and by prescription as 20% Azelex cream applied twice daily. Azelic acid foam or gel (Finacea

15%) has an indication for use in acne rosacea but has been used off-label for AV.[1]

Salicylic Acid
Salicylic acid is a comedolytic agent available over the counter in strengths of 0.5% to 2% as a cream, gel, lotion, pad, or wash. Limited evidence supports its use in mild acne.

Topical Dapsone
Topical dapsone (Aczone) has antiinflammatory and antimicrobial properties and is available in doses of 5% and 7.5% gel used once or twice daily. It is safe in patients with glucose-6 phosphate dehydrogenase deficiency and sulfa allergy. It can be used in combination with other topical agents but should not be concurrently with BP because of temporary orange-brown staining of skin.

Topical Androgen Receptor Inhibitor
Clascoterone (Winlevi) 1% cream is a first in class topical androgen receptor inhibitor approved by the FDA in 2020 for the treatment of AV in persons 12 and older. Clascoterone 1% applied twice daily demonstrated a reduction in both inflammatory and noninflammatory AV lesions in two randomized controlled trials. Patients reported side effects of erythema, scaling, and burning/stinging comparable to placebo. Despite its efficacy and safety, concern remains regarding affordability and equitable access.

Combination Topical Therapy
When treating AV with topical therapies, combination therapy is recommended over topical monotherapy with retinoids or BP as it optimizes treatment effectiveness, reduces the development of antibiotic resistance, and may improve adherence. Addition of BP to any topical treatment regimen is AAD guideline recommended to prevent the development of antibiotic resistance. Fixed-dose BP with topical antibiotic (clindamycin/BP 1%/5% gel [BenzaClin], clindamycin/BP 1.2%/3.75% gel [Onexton], clindamycin/BP 1.2%/2.5% gel [Acanya], and erythromycin/BP 3%/5% gel [Benzamycin]), fixed-dose BP with topical retinoid (Epiduo 0.1%/2.5%, Epiduo Forte 0.3%/2.5%), and fixed-dose topical retinoid with topical antibiotic (tretinoin 0.025%/clindamycin 1.2% gel [Ziana, generic]) all have compelling evidence supporting their use. A 2023 network meta-analysis evaluating comparative efficacy of pharmacologic treatment for AV affirmed that combination therapies are more effective than monotherapy. Triple therapy using a topical antibiotic, a topical retinoid and BP ranked second only to isotretinoin in effectiveness. In October of 2023, Cabtreo (clindamycin phosphate 1.2%/BP 3.1%/adapalene gel 0.15%) became the first and only FDA approved fixed-dose triple combination topical treatment for AV for persons over age 12. Cabtreo is not yet covered by many insurance plans and its cost ($935–$1157 per 50-g tube) will limit access for many.

Systemic Antibiotics
Systemic antibiotics are commonly used in managing nodulocystic acne and moderate to severe acne unresponsive to treatment with multimodal topical therapy. Systemic antibiotic use should be limited to less than 3 to 4 months, if possible, to mitigate development of antibiotic resistance and limit side effects. Additionally, systemic antibiotics should never be used as monotherapy because of the risk of developing resistance. The 2024 AAD guidelines recommend oral antibiotics always be used in combination with BP and other topical agents. A recent network meta-analysis comparing therapeutic interventions for the management of acne ranked triple therapy with oral antibiotic, topical retinoid, and BP third (behind isotretinoin oral and triple topical therapy) in overall effectiveness among all treatment regimens for the management of AV. Oral tetracycline class antibiotics have long been the mainstay of antibiotic therapy for AV. Oral tetracycline class antibiotics exert antibiotic effects via the inhibition of protein synthesis and antiinflammatory effects by suppressing cytokines, matrix metalloproteinases, and neutrophil chemotaxis. Doxycycline, minocycline and sarecycline (Seysara) are FDA approved for the management of AV.

Doxycycline is the recommended tetracycline class antibiotic for AV management per AAD guidelines because of documented efficacy, low cost, and fewer serious side effects compared with minocycline. The AAD recommendation has been reinforced in a recent network meta-analysis of comparative efficacy of pharmacologic treatments for AV documenting superiority of doxycycline over sarecycline and minocycline. Low-dose doxycycline (20 mg twice a day or 40 mg delayed release [Oracea] once daily) has proven efficacy in a few randomized controlled trials; however, there is insufficient evidence directly comparing low dose regimens versus standard-dose doxycycline (50 or 100 mg once or twice daily for 2–3 months). Adverse reactions commonly associated with doxycycline include nausea, vomiting, diarrhea, pill esophagitis, and photosensitivity. Taking doxycycline with food and water and remaining erect may prevent esophagitis, and use of sunscreens is strongly encouraged to prevent sunburn. Sarecycline is a narrow spectrum tetracycline dosed by weight (1.5 mg/kg) with less potency for enteric gram-negative bacteria. Consequently, sarecycline may have less effect on the gut microbiome and improved gastrointestinal tolerance compared with doxycycline or minocycline. Sarecycline also causes less photosensitivity and vertigo. Sarecycline use is conditionally recommended by the ADD because of concerns regarding affordability and equitable access. Minocycline use is associated with rare but significant side effects including vertigo, DRESS (drug reaction with eosinophilia and systemic symptoms), autoimmune hepatitis, and minocycline-induced hyperpigmentation (resulting in brown or blue-gray skin discoloration). Tetracycline-class antibiotics are contraindicated in pregnancy, lactation, and children under age 9 because of concern for permanent teeth discoloration and abnormal bone development.

In past iterations of the AAD guidelines for AV management, limited use of oral erythromycin[1] and azithromycin[1] for pregnant patients and restricted use of trimethoprim-sulfamethoxazole[1] or trimethoprim[1] for tetracycline class–intolerant patients was suggested. Because of the absence of adequate evidence supporting their use, the risk of promoting antibiotic resistance, and the potential for severe adverse reactions, the current AAD guidelines discourage broad use of oral erythromycin, azithromycin, trimethoprim-sulfamethoxazole, or trimethoprim for AV in these patient populations. It also does not endorse the use of penicillin or cephalosporins because of lack of supporting evidence.

Oral Isotretinoin
Oral isotretinoin (Accutane, Absorica, Claravis), a vitamin A derivative, was found to be the most effective treatment for AV in a recent network meta-analysis. The mechanism of action is not fully understood, but isotretinoin has activity against all the pathogenetic mechanisms causing AV. Oral isotretinoin is comedolytic, antiinflammatory, reduces sebum production, and inhibits growth of C. acnes.

Oral isotretinoin is FDA approved for the management of severe, recalcitrant nodular acne. The AAD guidelines also endorse the use of isotretinoin for patients with AV who failed standard treatment with topical agents and oral antibiotics, patients who are relapse prone after standard therapy, and patients with severe scarring or psychosocial distress relating to AV. Various isotretinoin dosing schedules have been used including daily versus intermittent dosing and standard-dose (0.5–1.0 mg/kg/day divided in bid dosing) versus low-dose (<0.5 mg/kg/day) regimens. The ADA guideline conditionally recommends the daily dosing schedule over intermittent dosing. Isotretinoin

---

[1]Not FDA approved for this indication.

[1]Not FDA approved for this indication.

may induce acne remission with cumulative treatment dosages between 120 mg to 150 mg/kg, but some studies have treated patients for 2 months after complete resolution of AV lesions. Common but reversible dose-dependent adverse reactions associated with isotretinoin include xerosis, cheilitis, dry eyes, and myalgias. The prescribing information for isotretinoin includes warnings about potential for inflammatory bowel disease and psychiatric disorders (depression, psychosis, suicidal ideation); however, population-based studies have not supported these findings. Studies suggest treatment with isotretinoin reduces AV-associated depression and anxiety, and compelling evidence from a large cohort study reported lower suicide rates in patients treated with isotretinoin compared with the general population. Clinicians should, however, screen for depression, anxiety, and suicidality during treatment. Because of the risk of teratogenicity associated with isotretinoin, all prescribers of isotretinoin, participating pharmacists, and all patients receiving isotretinoin must participate in *iPLEDGE* (an FDA-mandated Risk Evaluation and Mitigation Strategy for preventing isotretinoin exposure in pregnancy). All patients who may become pregnant must adhere to complete abstinence or use two documented methods of contraception for at least 1 month before and after treatment with isotretinoin. Monitoring recommended during isotretinoin treatment includes liver function tests and lipid profile until stable and monthly pregnancy tests in patients with childbearing potential.

Combined Oral Contraceptive

Combined oral contraceptives reduce sebum production due to antiandrogenic properties and are effective in treating inflammatory and noninflammatory acne. Four combined oral contraceptives are currently FDA approved for treatment of AV in women who desire contraception: norgestimate/ethinyl estradiol (Tri-Sprintec), norethindrone acetate/ethinyl estradiol/ferrous fumarate (Estrostep Fe, Tilia Fe, Tri-Legest Fe), drospirenone/ethinyl estradiol (Gianvi, Jasmiel, YAZ), and drospirenone/ethinyl estradiol/levomefolate (Beyaz). Currently available evidence does not support the use of one combined oral contraceptive over another. Combined oral contraceptives should be considered in menstruating patients with inadequate response to or intolerance of other treatments, AV flares temporally related to menses, or signs of hyperandrogenism. Combined oral contraception should be taken for at least 3 to 6 months to ensure maximum clinical benefit. The decision to prescribe combined oral contraceptives should employ a patient-centered approach with shared decision-making and explore the potential benefits of the medication in managing AV versus the risks of adverse events. Venous thromboembolism risk is increased with combined oral contraceptive use (incidence is 3 to 9/10,000 person years compared with 1 to 5/10,000 person years in those not using combined oral contraceptives) but VTE risk significantly less than during pregnancy (5–20/10,000 person years) or the 12-week postpartum period (40–65/10,000 person years). Other potential adverse events include myocardial infarction, stroke, and slight increases in breast cancer and cervical cancer. Consideration should be given to a patient's comorbid conditions and their potential risk evaluated using U.S. Medical Eligibility Criteria for Contraceptive Use via a readily available mobile application.

Spironolactone

Spironolactone[1] has commonly been used as an adjunct in AV management in women with treatment resistant and hormonally mediated acne due its antiandrogenic effects.

Spironolactone is conditionally recommended by the AAD for AV, but its use is not FDA approved. A recent randomized clinical trial reaffirmed efficacy of spironolactone at doses of 50 to 100 mg/day. Start at 25 mg and titrate dose gradually. Co-administration with combined oral contraceptives is recommended because of the risk of fetal antiandrogenic effects and to mitigate menstrual irregularities common with spironolactone use. Other adverse reactions may include breast

---

[1] Not FDA approved for this indication.

tenderness, breast enlargement, dizziness, headache, and rarely, hyperkalemia. Potassium monitoring should be considered in patients based on older age, comorbidities (diabetes mellitus, chronic kidney disease, hypertension) and concurrent use of medications known to cause hyperkalemia (angiotensin converting enzyme inhibitors, angiotensin receptor blockers, nonsteroidal antiinflammatory agents, and others).

Intralesional Corticosteroid Injections

Intralesional corticosteroid injections may be used as adjuvant therapy in patients with nodulocystic acne to reduce pain, inflammation, and scarring.

Physical Treatment Modalities

Laser- and light-based therapies, photodynamic therapy, comedo extraction, microneedling, and chemical peels lack sufficient studies to formulate a recommendation for their use in inflammatory and comedonal acne. Many of these physical modalities have applications in the management of acne scarring.

Monitoring

Patients should be re-evaluated to determine the effectiveness of therapeutic interventions at regular intervals. Measures of effectiveness should include reduction in comedonal and inflammatory lesions, reduction in AV-associated anxiety and depression, and prevention of scarring. Therapeutic interventions should be continued for at least 8 weeks for maximum benefit unless patients have allergic reaction or adverse events. Patients not improving after multiple interventions should be referred to a dermatologist.

References

Baldwin H, Tan J: Effects of diet on acne and its response to treatment, *Am J Clin Dermatol* 22(1):55–65, 2021.
Desai SR, Druby KM, et al: Guidelines of care for the management of acne vulgaris, *J Am Acad Dermatol* 90(5):1006.e1–1006.e30, 2024.
Eichenfield DZ, Sprague J, Eichenfield LF: Management of acne vulgaris: a review, *JAMA* 326(20):2055–2067, 2021.
Heng AHS, Chew FT: Systematic review of the epidemiology of acne vulgaris, *Sci Rep* 10(1):5754, 2020.
Huang CY, Chang IJ, et al: Comparative efficacy of pharmacological treatments for acne vulgaris: a network meta-analysis of 221 randomized controlled trials, *Ann Fam Med* 21(4):358–369, 2023.
Oge LK, Broussard A, Marshall MD: Acne vulgaris: diagnosis and treatment, *Am Fam Physician* 100(8):475–484, 2019.
Stein Gold L, Baldwin H, et al: Efficacy and safety of a fixed- dose clindamycin phosphate 1.2%, benzoyl peroxide 3.1%, and adapalene 0.15% gel for moderate-to-severe acne: a randomized phase II study of the first triple-combination drug, *Am J Clin Dermatol* 23(1):93–104, 2022.

ATOPIC DERMATITIS

Method of
Peck Y. Ong, MD

CURRENT DIAGNOSIS

- Itch must be present for the diagnosis of atopic dermatitis. In addition, the diagnosis must include three or more of the following criteria (U.K. Working Party's Diagnostic Criteria for Atopic Dermatitis):
  - History of generalized dry skin
  - Visible flexural dermatitis
  - Onset of the skin condition before 2 years (not used for patients younger than 4 years)
  - History of itchy skin involving the following areas: elbows, behind knees, front of ankles, or around the neck
  - History of asthma or allergic rhinitis (or for children younger than 4 years, history of atopic disease in a first-degree relative)

- Bathe or shower for 10 to 20 minutes daily and pat dry gently.
- Follow immediately by applying an emollient on unaffected areas and an antiinflammatory medication on affected areas.
- Use topical corticosteroids as a first-line antiinflammatory medication. Alternative medications are topical calcineurin inhibitors, topical phosphodiesterase 4 inhibitors, topical or oral janus kinase (JAK) inhibitors and monoclonal antibodies.
- Avoid environmental triggers such as extreme heat, humidity, or dryness.
- Avoid food allergens that may cause anaphylaxis. Consult an allergist regarding the interpretation of serum-specific IgE tests or food challenge.
- Treat skin infection only when clinical signs are present (e.g., oozing, impetigo).
- Severe, generalized infection or vesicular lesions may indicate herpes simplex virus infection; persistent fever may indicate invasive *S. aureus* infection.

TABLE 1 Differential Diagnoses of Atopic Dermatitis

DISEASE CATEGORY	DIFFERENTIAL DIAGNOSES
Dermatologic diseases	Contact dermatitis, seborrheic dermatitis, psoriasis, dyshidrotic eczema, eosinophilic pustular folliculitis, ichthyosis vulgaris
Neoplastic diseases	Cutaneous T-cell lymphoma, Langerhans cell histiocytosis
Immunodeficiencies	Hyper-IgE syndrome, severe combined immunodeficiency, Omenn syndrome, IPEX (immune dysregulation, polyendocrinopathy, enteropathy X-linked) syndrome
Infectious diseases	Scabies, cutaneous candidiasis, tinea versicolor
Nutritional deficiencies	Acrodermatitis enteropathica (zinc deficiency), essential fatty acid deficiency, biotin deficiency
Multisystemic disorders	Netherton syndrome, dermatitis herpetiformis

Atopic dermatitis (AD) is a chronic inflammatory skin disease that is characterized by itch and a predilection of eczema on extensor areas in young infants or flexural areas in older children and adults. In the United States, AD affects about 15% of children and 7% of adults. For more than 85% of patients, AD begins during the first 5 years, but 50% of the children with AD improve significantly or outgrow the disease by age 7. The persistence of AD depends on various factors: early onset, severity, family history of AD, personal history of asthma, and food or inhalant allergies.

The itch associated with AD causes significant discomfort in these patients and often leads to sleep loss and to poor school or work performance. The quality of life of children with generalized AD is worse than that for children with diabetes, epilepsy, asthma, cystic fibrosis, or renal disease. The maternal stress in taking care of children with moderate to severe AD is equivalent to that associated with care of children with diabetes, Rett syndrome, profound deafness, or the need for enteral feeding.

Pathophysiology

AD is caused by a combination of genetic and environmental factors. Patients with AD have a defective skin barrier. This leads to a loss of skin hydration and susceptibility to environmental triggers. There is evidence that the skin barrier defects of AD are caused by genetic mutations. Studies have shown that many AD patients carry a genetic mutation in filaggrin, a protein with important barrier function.

Potential external triggers of AD include microbial pathogens and environmental allergens. Almost 100% of AD skin lesions are colonized by *Staphylococcus aureus*, which may produce toxins that trigger immune response in the skin. As a result, AD patients produce an increased amount of pro-allergic cytokines, such as interleukin-4 (IL-4), IL-5, and IL-13, in their skin. These cytokines lead to an increased infiltration of inflammatory T cells and eosinophils. IL-4 and IL-13 also are important for the production of serum IgE, the level of which is elevated in AD patients.

Diagnosis and Clinical Assessment

Most AD patients can be diagnosed by clinical history and physical examination. Typical presentation includes itch, dryness, flexural dermatitis, early age of onset, and atopy such as multiple food allergies. Patients with generalized eczema or adult-onset eczema can present as a diagnostic challenge. The differential diagnosis

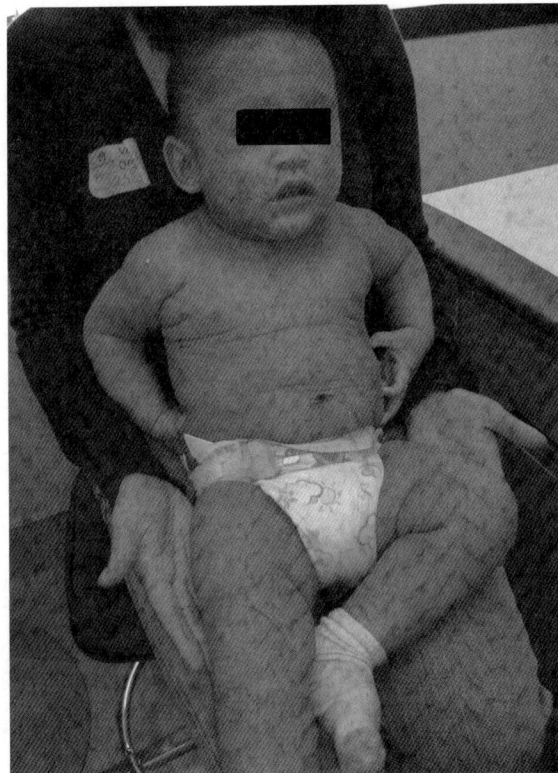

Figure 1 Generalized atopic dermatitis.

includes immunodeficiency (e.g., hyper-IgE syndrome, Omenn syndrome), malignancy (e.g., cutaneous T-cell lymphoma), zinc deficiency (i.e., acrodermatitis enteropathica), and celiac-associated dermatitis (i.e., dermatitis herpetiformis) (Table 1). AD children seldom present with failure to thrive, unless they are under severe dietary restriction. Failure to thrive should therefore prompt further investigation. Punch skin biopsies may be needed when the diagnosis is still unclear.

The prevalence of mild, moderate, and severe AD is 80%, 18%, and 2%, respectively. Most patients with mild to moderate disease have flexural, extensor, or facial involvement, whereas patients with severe disease often present with total-body involvement with or without erythroderma (Figure 1). Validated scales for assessing the severity of AD include validated Investigator Global Assessment (vIGA; https://www.eczemacouncil.org/assets/docs/Validated-Investigator-Global-Assessment-Scale_vIGA-AD_2017.pdf), patient-oriented Eczema Measure (POEM; https://www.nottingham.ac.uk/research/groups/cebd/documents/methodological-resources/poem-for-self-completion-or-proxy-completion.pdf), Scoring of Atopic Dermatitis (SCORAD) and Eczema Area and Severity Index (EASI). These scoring systems or a simplified diagram documenting the extent of dermatitis are useful for more objective follow-up of the patient's progress.

Management of Atopic Dermatitis and Associated Conditions

Daily Maintenance Care

Changes in humidity can adversely affect AD symptoms. Dry conditions lead to increased transepidermal water loss and dry AD skin. Extreme heat, humidity, and sweating may lead to irritation of AD skin. AD patients are at increased risk for contact or irritant dermatitis, which may occur with over-the-counter topical skin medications that contain multiple ingredients. Wool or synthetic acrylic fabrics may also be irritating to AD skin.

To improve barrier function, AD patients should bathe or shower for 10 to 20 minutes once or twice daily, followed immediately by gently drying the skin and applying an emollient on the unaffected areas and a topical antiinflammatory medication on the affected areas. A petrolatum-based emollient is recommended in infants and young children because of its occlusive property. In older children and adults, the ointment may not be tolerated well because of its greasy feel, and another emollient or moisturizer may be chosen based on the patient's preference or experience.

Itch may continue to be a problem even if the rash has improved. The mechanisms of itch in AD are not fully understood but do not appear to be mediated solely by histamine. The use of first-generation antihistamines (diphenhydramine [Benadryl][1] and hydroxyzine [Vistaril]) in AD largely depend on their sedative effects and are best used at bedtime. The second-generation, nonsedating antihistamines such as loratadine (Claritin)[1] and cetirizine (Zyrtec)[1] have not proved helpful in treating AD. Low-dose doxepin[1] has been used anecdotally to treat itching in AD.

Topical and Systemic Medications

The first-line medication for AD is a topical corticosteroid (TCS). For mild AD, a TCS with group VI and VII potency (Table 2) may suffice. However, for moderate to severe AD, a TCS with at least group III to V potency is chosen to increase efficacy and to shorten the duration of need for these medications.

The use of TCS is confronted with various obstacles, including rare side effects such as skin atrophy, but mostly patients' or parents' misunderstanding of TCS. Studies have shown that twice-daily use of fluticasone propionate (Cutivate) 0.05% cream (group V) and desonide (DesOwen, Tridesilon) 0.05% ointment or aqueous gel (group V and VI, respectively) continuously up to 1 month in young children with AD results in no significant adverse effect. It is therefore important to clarify for patients or parents the safety and side effects based on the potency of the TCS.

Topical calcineurin inhibitors (TCI) (pimecrolimus [Elidel] 1% cream and tacrolimus [Protopic] ointment) are alternative nonsteroidal antiinflammatory medications for AD. Elidel is indicated for mild to moderate AD in patients older than 2 years, whereas 0.03% and 0.1% Protopic are indicated for moderate to severe AD in patients 2 to 15 years old and in patients 16 years old or older, respectively. Both Elidel and Protopic have an FDA black box warning saying that their long-term use may be associated with cancer risk. However, a recent meta-analysis concluded that TCI do not increase the risk of cancer. These medications continue to be useful alternatives for skin areas that are prone to atrophy, including the face, axillae, and groins.

---

[1]Not FDA approved for this indication.

TABLE 2	Classification of Topical Corticosteroids Based on Potency
GROUP	**TOPICAL CORTICOSTEROIDS**
I (most potent)	Clobetasol propionate 0.05% (Temovate) (cream, ointment, gel), betamethasone dipropionate, augmented 0.05% (Diprolene) (cream, ointment), diflorasone diacetate 0.05% (Psorcon) (ointment)
II	Amcinonide 0.1% (Cyclocort) (ointment), betamethasone dipropionate 0.05% (Diprosone) (ointment), mometasone furoate 0.1% (Elocon) (ointment), halcinonide 0.1% (Halog) (cream), fluocinonide 0.05% (Lidex) (gel, cream, ointment), desoximetasone (Topicort) (0.05% gel, 0.25% cream, 0.25% ointment)
III	Fluticasone propionate 0.005% (Cutivate) (ointment), amcinonide 0.1% (Cyclocort) (lotion, cream), diflorasone diacetate 0.05% (Florone) (cream), betamethasone valerate 0.1% (Valisone) (ointment)
IV	Flurandrenolide 0.05% (Cordran) (ointment), mometasone furoate 0.1% (Elocon) (cream), triamcinolone acetonide 0.1% (Kenalog) (cream), fluocinolone acetonide 0.025% (Synalar) (ointment), hydrocortisone valerate 0.2% (Westcort) (ointment)
V	Flurandrenolide 0.05% (Cordran) (cream), fluticasone propionate 0.05% (Cutivate) (cream), hydrocortisone butyrate 0.1% (Locoid) (cream), fluocinolone acetonide 0.025% (Synalar) (cream), desonide 0.05% (Tridesilon) (ointment), betamethasone valerate 0.1% (Valisone) (cream), hydrocortisone valerate 0.2% (Westcort) (cream), prednicarbate 0.1% (Dermatop) (cream)
VI	Alclometasone dipropionate 0.05% (Aclovate) (cream, ointment), fluocinolone acetonide 0.01% (Synalar) (solution, cream) (Derma-Smoothe/FS Oil), Desonide 0.05% (Tridesilon) (cream and aqueous gel)
VII (least potent)	Hydrocortisone 1%/2.5% (lotion, cream, ointment).

Data from Stoughton RB. Vasoconstrictor assay—specific applications. In Maibach HI, Surber C, editors. *Topical Corticosteroids.* Basel, Switzerland: Karger, 1992, pp 42–53.

A third class of topical medication, phosphodiesterase 4 inhibitor (crisaborole [Eucrisa] 2% ointment), is approved for patients 2 years and older with mild to moderate AD. Another phosphodiesterase inhibitor, roflumilast [Zoryve] 0.15% cream once daily, has been approved for mild to moderate AD in patients 6 years and older.

A fourth class of topical medication, topical janus kinase (JAK) inhibitor, has been approved for patients with mild to moderate AD. Ruxolitinib cream (Opzelura) is currently approved for patients ≥12 years with mild to moderate AD. The use of this medication is limited to 20% or less of the body surface areas.

Tapinarof [Vtama] 1% cream once daily, which has skin barrier repair effects, has been approved for mild to severe AD in patients 2 years and older.

For patients with moderate to severe AD, there are four recently-approved systemic medications. Dupilumab (Dupixent), a monoclonal antibody that targets IL-4/IL-13, is approved for ≥6 months; Tralokinumab (Adbry), a monoclonal antibody that targets IL-13, is approved for ≥12 years. Other monoclonal antibodies that have been approved for patients ≥12 years with moderate to severe AD are lebrikizumab (Ebglyss) and nemolizumab (Nemluvio), which target IL-13 and IL-31, respectively. All the monoclonal antibodies are administered subcutaneously. Two oral JAK inhibitors, upadacitinib (Rinvoq) and abrocitinib (Cibinqo), are approved for ≥12 years and ≥18 years, respectively. As JAK inhibitors are immunosuppressants, topical ruxolitinib, oral upadacitinib, and oral abrocitinib carry the boxed warnings of serious infections, mortality, malignancy, major adverse cardiovascular events and thrombosis.

Wet-wrap treatment, phototherapy, and systemic immunosuppressive therapies (e.g., cyclosporine [Sandimmune, Neoral],[1] azathioprine [Imuran],[1] methotrexate [Trexall],[1] and mycophenolate mofetil [CellCept])[1] are alternatives, but systemic immunosuppressants are not approved by FDA for AD patients.

Systemic corticosteroids are not recommended for long-term control of AD because of their known adverse effects, including stunted growth in children, adrenal suppression, osteoporosis, and cataracts. A rebound of AD symptoms is common after the medication is stopped. If a systemic corticosteroid is used, it should be tapered over a short period while nonsteroidal antiinflammatory treatment is intensified.

The efficacy and side effects of the following medications have not been established in AD: intravenous immunoglobulin (IVIG),[1] anti-IgE (omalizumab [Xolair]),[1] probiotics,[7] montelukast (Singulair),[1] Chinese medicinal herbs,[7] and fish oils.[1]

Food Allergies

At least 30% of children with moderate to severe AD have one or more food allergies, compared with 4% to 6% of the general population. Accurate diagnosis of food allergies in AD patients is crucial because it can prevent life-threatening anaphylaxis or unnecessary food restriction.

The diagnosis of food allergy involves history taking and food challenge. History taking is helpful in the diagnosis of food allergy in most patients. It is often useful to begin by asking the patients whether they have any problems or reactions with any of the seven food allergens: milk, egg, peanut, wheat, soybean, seafood, and tree nuts. These foods account for more than 90% of food allergies. Almost all food allergic reactions occur in the first hour. AD patients may complain of immediate worsening of itching after ingestion. Symptoms of anaphylactic reactions include throat-clearing, cough, shortness of breath, vomiting, dizziness, fainting, and headache, which may be attributed to hypotension. Most food allergic reactions also manifest with skin symptoms, including hives, swelling, or generalized itching.

Skin tests and serum specific IgE are useful in the context of negative or undetectable test results because they have a negative predictive value of more than 95%. The level of a positive test result (i.e., skin test wheal size or serum-specific IgE level), which correlates with the chance of a reaction, should be interpreted in the context of a clinical reaction. Consider consultation with an allergist regarding food challenge if there are still concerns regarding positive serum-specific IgE. More accurate epitope-specific IgE assays may be available to clinicians in the near future.

Patients with confirmed food allergy should avoid any amount of the food allergen, unless they are supervised by their allergist. Parents or patients should be instructed to read food allergen labels carefully. All packaged foods in the United States are required to label the contents of milk, eggs, peanuts, wheat, soybeans, fish, shellfish, or tree nuts. Organizations, such as the Food Allergy Research & Education, can provide patients and parents with useful information on potential hidden food allergens and alternative food sources.

AD children often have multiple food allergies, including cow's milk and soy, and the use of a hydrolyzed or amino acid–based formula can provide an alternative source of nutrition. For these patients, consultation with a dietitian can be helpful in managing food avoidance and nutrition needs.

Patients or parents of children with anaphylactic reactions should be prescribed and instructed on the use of an epinephrine autoinjector (EpiPen or Auvi-Q 0.15 mg for patients who weigh

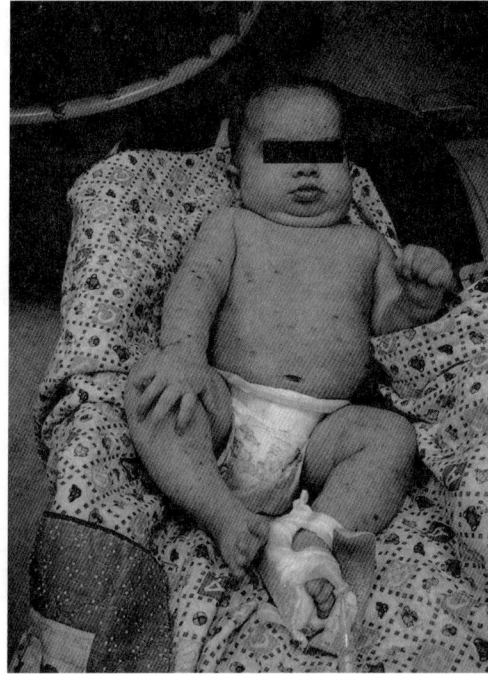

Figure 2 Eczema herpeticum.

more than 15 kg but less than 30 kg; 0.3 mg for patients who weigh 30 kg or more, while Auvi-Q 0.1 mg for patients who weigh 7.5–15 kg). Nasal epinephrine spray (Neffy) is also available as an alternative for patients ≥4 years of age who weigh ≥15 kg.

Infants with severe AD who consume peanut products early have a 86% relative risk reduction in the development of peanut allergy. For any infants with AD under a year, clinicians should consider introducing peanut products early in their diet according to the guidelines of National Institute of Allergy and Infectious Disease, or consult an allergist.

Infections

Most AD patients are colonized by *S. aureus* on their skin lesions or in their nostrils. The frequency of colonization increases with AD severity. Exacerbation of AD is frequently associated with secondary *S. aureus* skin infections. Other common skin pathogens in AD include group A β-hemolytic *Streptococcus* and herpes simplex virus (HSV), which causes eczema herpeticum (Figure 2). Many reports have documented invasive *S. aureus* infections such as bacteremia, septic arthritis, osteomyelitis, and endocarditis in AD patients. Persistent fever or focal limb pain should alert the physician to the possibility of these infections.

The reasons for the high rate of bacterial colonization and skin infections in AD are not completely understood. A defective skin barrier and decreased cutaneous innate immunity (i.e., deficiency in natural skin antibiotics) likely contribute to the frequency of skin infections in patients with AD.

Because of the concern about increasing bacterial resistance, antibiotics are not recommended unless clinical infection is confirmed. The use of dilute bleach in treating AD remains controversial.

Inhalant Allergies and Asthma

Eighty-five percent of AD infants have concurrent respiratory allergies or are at risk for allergic rhinitis or asthma. However, whether inhalant allergens lead to a worsening of AD remains controversial. Randomized, double-blind, placebo-controlled studies have shown positive and negative effects of house dust mites (HDM) as a trigger for AD symptoms. Because there is no serious side effect associated with the use of HDM-proof bed and pillow encasings, unless cost is an issue, these encasings are recommended for AD patients with HDM sensitization.

---

[1]Not FDA approved for this indication.
[7]Available as a dietary supplement.

Further research is needed to confirm the role of inhalant allergens, including furry pets and pollens, as triggers for AD.

Referral to Specialists
Patients who have failed topical treatments or who have been limited by their eczema in daily activities should be considered for referral to specialists in allergy/immunology or dermatology for systemic treatments.

References

Beattie PE, Lewis-Jones MS: A comparative study of impairment of quality of life in children with skin disease and children with other chronic childhood diseases, *Br J Dermatol* 155:145–151, 2006.

Beck LA, Thaçi D, Hamilton JD, et al: Dupilumab treatment in adults with moderate-to-severe atopic dermatitis, *N Engl J Med* 371:130–139, 2014.

Devasenapathy N, Chu A, Wong M, et al: AAAAI/ACAAI Joint Task Force on Practice Parameters for Atopic Dermatitis Guideline Development Group. Cancer risk with topical calcineurin inhibitors, pimecrolimus, and tacrolimus for atopic dermatitis: a systematic review and meta-analysis, *Lancet Child Adolesc Health* 7(1):13–25, 2023.

Du Toit G, Roberts G, Sayre PH, et al: Randomized trial of peanut consumption in infants at risk for peanut allergy, *N Engl J Med* 372:803–813, 2015.

Eichenfield LF, Basu S, Calvarese B, et al: Effect of desonide hydrogel 0.05% on the hypothalamic-pituitary-adrenal axis in pediatric subjects with moderate to severe atopic dermatitis, *Pediatr Dermatol* 24:289–295, 2007.

Elias PM: Barrier-repair therapy for atopic dermatitis: corrective lipid biochemical therapy, *Expert Rev Dermatol* 3:441–452, 2008.

Faught J, Bierl C, Barton B, Kemp A: Stress in mothers of young children with eczema, *Arch Dis Child* 92:683–686, 2007.

Friedlander SF, Hebert AA, Allen DB; for the Fluticasone Pediatrics Safety Study Group: Safety of fluticasone propionate cream 0.05% for the treatment of severe and extensive atopic dermatitis in children as young as 3 months, *J Am Acad Dermatol* 46:387–393, 2002.

Ong PY, Boguniewicz J, Chu DK: Skin antiseptics for atopic dermatitis: dissecting facts from fiction, *J Allergy Clin Immunol Pract* 11(5):1385–1390, 2023.

Suprun M, Sicherer SH, Wood RA, et al: Early epitope-specific IgE antibodies are predictive of childhood peanut allergy, *J Allergy Clin Immunol* 146(5):1080–1088, 2020.

Togias A, Cooper SF, Acebal ML, et al: Addendum guidelines for the prevention of peanut allergy in the United States: report of the National Institute of Allergy and Infectious Diseases-sponsored expert panel, *J Allergy Clin Immunol* 139:29–44, 2017.

Yim HJ, Jean T, Ong PY: Recent advances in immunomodulators for atopic dermatitis, *Curr Opin Pediatr* 35(6):671–679, 2023.

Wang V, Boguniewicz J, Boguniewicz M, Ong PY: The infectious complications of atopic dermatitis, *Ann Allergy Asthma Immunol* 126(1):3–12, 2021.

AUTOIMMUNE BULLOUS DISEASES

Method of
Dominic J. Wu, MD; and Anand Rajpara, MD

CURRENT DIAGNOSIS

- There is a significant overlap between the major autoimmune bullous diseases, which include pemphigus vulgaris, bullous pemphigoid, dermatitis herpetiformis, linear IgA bullous disease, and more.
- Biopsy is usually required for diagnosis, including routine hematoxylin and eosin stain (H&E) histology and other special tests including direct immunofluorescence (DIF), indirect immunofluorescence (IIF), and ELISA.
- Preferred biopsy sites include edge or entire intact blister/bulla (H&E), perilesional "normal" appearing skin (DIF).
- Different staining patterns on DIF, salt-split skin, and IIF can help differentiate between diseases that appear similar on routine histology.
- It is important to evaluate for other causes of blistering disease, including infectious causes such as bullous impetigo, herpes simplex virus, varicella zoster virus, and noninfectious causes such as severe contact allergic dermatitis, poison ivy dermatitis, and others.

CURRENT THERAPY

- Immunosuppressive medications are the mainstay treatment for autoimmune bullous diseases.
- Specific treatments for each diagnosis are listed under each section. Many of the treatment regimens are not Food and Drug Administration (FDA)–approved treatments and should only be attempted by experienced clinicians familiar with each medication and their side effect profiles and monitoring parameters.
- Traditional first-line therapy is with oral corticosteroids to induce remission, with or without adjunctive steroid-sparing therapy.
- Topical corticosteroids should be attempted for milder cases of bullous pemphigoid prior to initiation of systemic corticosteroids because of side effects and risks for systemic steroids and efficacy of topicals.
- Adjunctive steroid-sparing therapy may help clinicians lower and eventually taper the doses of corticosteroids.
- Patients on higher doses of corticosteroids and/or longer courses of treatment with corticosteroids may require prophylaxis or treatment of osteoporosis and peptic ulcer disease.
- Early involvement of relevant specialties is critical given the complex nature of the disease and treatment options.

Epidemiology
The autoimmune bullous diseases are a heterogenous group of diseases, mostly occurring in the elderly. Please see each section for specific epidemiologic comments.

Pathophysiology
Specific antibodies and pathophysiology will be discussed under specific diseases discussed in this chapter.

Diagnosis
There is significant clinical overlap between the major autoimmune bullous diseases. In addition to obtaining a detailed clinical history, biopsies are usually required for diagnosis. Ideal sample sites for routine histology (H&E) are of the blister/bullae (intact if possible, or the edge of the bulla), and normal-appearing perilesional skin for direct immunofluorescence (DIF). Punch biopsies (usually 4 mm punch tool) or deeper shave biopsies are common biopsy methods. Specific staining patterns are noted under each individual disease entity below. Indirect immunofluorescence (IIF) may also be helpful, although it is beyond the scope of this chapter and will not be discussed in detail.

Pemphigus
Pathophysiology
In normal skin tissue, epithelial cells are held together by adherens and desmosome protein junctions. In pemphigus diseases, different desmosomal proteins are targeted by autoantibodies, causing a loss of connection between adjacent cells, resulting in splitting of skin layers. The causes of pemphigus diseases vary, including idiopathic, drug-induced cases (traditionally penicillamine and ACE inhibitors such as captopril), underlying conditions such as thymoma, myasthenia gravis, autoimmune thyroiditis, and more. Epidemiologic studies have shown higher incidence in people of Jewish ancestry. Certain genetic predispositions have also been identified, including HLA-DRB1, HLA-DR4, and HLA-DR6.

The pemphigus group of bullous diseases includes (1) pemphigus vulgaris and pemphigus vegetans, (2) pemphigus foliaceus and pemphigus erythematosus, and (3) paraneoplastic pemphigus. Pemphigus vulgaris and pemphigus vegetans are caused by circulating IgG autoantibodies, primarily against desmoglein 3 (Dsg3), which is mostly found on the lower portion of the epidermis. Desmogleins are desmosomal cadherin proteins that form desmosomes, which join cells together. Patients with pemphigus foliaceus have autoantibodies directed against desmoglein 1 (Dsg1). As its name denotes, paraneoplastic pemphigus is a paraneoplastic syndrome associated with an underlying neoplastic disorder (most frequently non-Hodgkin's lymphoma, CLL, Castleman's disease, thymoma, sarcoma, and Waldenström's macroglobulinemia). In paraneoplastic pemphigus, patients may have circulating autoantibodies against nearly all the different components of the desmosome junction including plakin family proteins and both Dsg1 and Dsg3.

Clinical Manifestations

Pemphigus vulgaris presents with painful flaccid skin blisters/bullae and erosions in the oral cavity. Oral involvement is typically seen in cases of pemphigus vulgaris, which can be quite helpful in distinguishing between pemphigus foliaceus (typically no oral involvement) and other autoimmune bullous diseases such as bullous pemphigoid, in which a smaller subset of patients have oral mucosal involvement. Nikolsky sign (shearing of skin with slight pressure or rubbing of perilesional skin) and Asboe-Hansen (pressure placed on intact bulla results in spreading of bulla to surrounding skin) are both found in cases of pemphigus vulgaris.

Pemphigus foliaceus (including the Brazilian endemic variant Fogo Selvagem and pemphigus erythematosus) typically present with impetigo-like crusted erosions involving the face, scalp, and upper trunk. Blisters tend to be more superficial and fragile, creating what is frequently described as a cornflake-like scale and crust. Nikolsky sign also is typically positive. Pemphigus foliaceus typically spares mucosal surfaces, differentiating it from pemphigus vulgaris.

Paraneoplastic pemphigus presents as a more severe-appearing form of pemphigus. In addition to pemphigus vulgaris-like skin findings, paraneoplastic pemphigus typically presents with severe mucosal involvement with extensive crusted stomatitis extending onto the vermillion lip and scarring conjunctivitis. There may also be erosions in the esophagus, genitalia, and nasopharynx. Palms and soles may also be affected, distinguishing this entity from pemphigus vulgaris.

Diagnosis

In addition to classic clinical findings, biopsy is usually required to confirm diagnosis with routine H&E histology, DIF, and other workup as indicated (including IIF, ELISA, and immunoprecipitation/immunoblotting).

Pemphigus vulgaris biopsies initially show eosinophilic spongiosis, followed by suprabasilar acantholysis without keratinocyte necrosis. Classically, one would also expect to find a tombstoning pattern of vertically oriented keratinocytes of the basal layer attached to the basement membrane zone (BMZ). DIF shows intercellular IgG deposition (with or without C3) in a chicken-wire appearance, with greater concentration in the lower epidermis.

Pemphigus foliaceus and its variants appear similarly to pemphigus vulgaris on histology, but on DIF one would expect to find higher concentration of IgG +/- C3 deposition in the upper epidermis. Pemphigus erythematosus may also have granular to linear IgG and C3 deposition along the BMZ.

Paraneoplastic pemphigus histology demonstrates intercellular IgG and C3 deposition, in addition to linear IgG and C3 deposition along the BMZ. Gold standard of diagnosis of paraneoplastic pemphigus is immunoprecipitation or immunoblotting for antibodies against plakin proteins, and ELISA detection of anti-DsG antibodies.

Treatment and Monitoring

Pemphigus can be a severe and deadly disease requiring immunosuppressive treatment. Because of the complex nature of the disease and treatment, early involvement of relevant specialists including but not limited to dermatology, rheumatology, gastroenterology, otolaryngology, oral medicine, and ophthalmology is critical. Clinicians prescribing immunosuppressive medications must be comfortable and familiar with the medications, including their side effect profile and monitoring parameters.

First-line treatment of pemphigus diseases is systemic corticosteroids for rapid disease control in conjunction with steroid-sparing immunosuppressive medications such as azathioprine (Imuran),[1] mycophenolate mofetil (CellCept),[1] or rituximab (Rituxan only for pemphigus vulgaris). Although numerous systemic steroids may be used, most frequently clinicians use prednisone 1 mg/kg/day. Higher doses of prednisone (100–150 mg daily) may sometimes be needed for more severe diseases, but prolonged use of higher doses may result in greater morbidity and mortality. In our practice, we aim to taper patients completely off of corticosteroids within 3 to 6 months. However, low-dose regimens such as prednisone 5 mg daily may be required for several years. For patients on long-term corticosteroid therapy vitamin D, calcium supplementation, and especially bisphosphonate therapy can help prevent or treat osteoporosis, while H_2 blockers (e.g., famotidine [Pepcid][1], ranitidine [Zactac][2]) or PPIs (e.g., omeprazole [Prilosec][1]) are recommended to prevent or treat peptic ulcer disease in patients taking concomitant nonsteroidal anti-inflammatory drugs (NSAIDs).

Corticosteroid therapy should be initiated in combination with a steroid sparing agent because these agents typically take 3 to 6 months to take full effect. First-line steroid sparing agents include azathioprine[1] (2–3 mg/kg/day based on the patient's thiopurine methyltransferase [TPMT] levels), mycophenolate mofetil[1] (1–1.5 g twice daily), and rituximab (Rituxan only for pemphigus vulgaris). In our practice we dose rituximab IV 1000 mg once every 2 weeks for 2 doses, followed by maintenance dose of 500 mg at months 12 and 18, and every 6 months thereafter based on clinical response. Milder cases may be treated with dapsone[1] (25 mg daily for 1 week, then increase dose in 25 mg increments weekly based on clinical response up to maximum 100 mg daily), niacinamide[1] (nicotinamide), and tetracycline.[1] Topical corticosteroids such as triamcinolone 0.1% ointment or clobetasol 0.05% ointment twice daily may be helpful in milder cases for pruritic or painful skin lesions. Second-line steroid-sparing agents with varying levels of efficacy described include methotrexate[1] (10–25 mg once weekly with folic acid supplementation[1] on days not taking methotrexate), cyclophosphamide,[1] and TNF-a inhibitors.[1] Severe refractory cases may be treated with IV immunoglobulin (IVIG)[1] therapy, or with rituximab or cyclophosphamide,[1] with or without plasmapheresis.

Treatment response should be monitored with IIF or ELISA levels, which can help detect quantitative levels of circulating antibodies.

Patients with paraneoplastic pemphigus may also have improvement in cutaneous lesions with systemic steroids, with or without adjunctive steroid-sparing agents. Excision of benign neoplasms such as thymomas and localized Castleman's disease may lead to resolution within months. Cases of paraneoplastic pemphigus from underlying malignancies are highly recalcitrant to treatment and carry a poor prognosis of up to a 90% mortality rate.

Bullous Pemphigoid
Pathophysiology

Bullous pemphigoid (BP) is the most common autoimmune blistering disorder and typically affects elderly patients. Patients with BP have circulating autoantibodies against different proteins, along the BMZ. The most common and important antigenic targets in BP include IgG autoantibodies targeted against the hemidesmosomal proteins BP180 (also referred to as BPAG2 and type XVII collagen) and BP230 (also referred to as BPAG1). BP180 is the primary mediator of BP. Complement activation causes eosinophilic and neutrophilic infiltration to the tissues, release of mediators and degradatory enzymes resulting in subepidermal blisters. Drug-induced cases of BP are most frequently because of furosemide, ACE inhibitors, NSAIDs, and antibiotics including cephalosporins, beta-lactams, and D-penicillamine.

Clinical Manifestations

BP initially presents as pruritic urticarial papules and plaques on the trunk, abdomen, and flexures of extremities. This progresses

---

[1] Not FDA approved for this indication.
[2] Not available in the United States.

to tense fluid-filled blisters and bullae on a urticarial base. Patients often complain of intense pruritus. After the bullae and blisters rupture, denuded areas of erosions and crusted areas remain.

Diagnosis

In addition to clinical findings and history, biopsy is required for diagnosis. On histology, lesions of the urticarial phase demonstrate eosinophilic spongiosis with eosinophils lining up at the dermoepidermal junction (DEJ). During the bullous phase, lesions demonstrate subepidermal split with numerous eosinophils in the blister cavity and dense inflammation in the dermis. DIF is the most sensitive test for BP and shows linear IgG and C3 deposition along the DEJ. Salt-split skin DIF is a special type of modified DIF study that uses NaCl solution to split the biopsy specimen at the lamina lucida, allowing for localization of the bound antibodies. BP antibodies classically show staining on the top of the blister cavity. Unlike in pemphigus vulgaris, IIF levels do not correlate well with BP disease activity and are not useful for determining treatment response.

Treatment

Although BP carries lower mortality risk compared with pemphigus vulgaris, treatment is indicated for its significant morbidity.

There have not been many controlled trials performed for BP therapies, and recommendations tend to be based on consensus opinion and clinician experience. Most frequently used first-line therapy includes high-potency topical corticosteroids or systemic corticosteroids and steroid-sparing immunosuppressive medications. Some studies have shown that topical clobetasol propionate (Temovate, Clobex) 0.05% may have better response than oral prednisone 0.5–1 mg/kg/day, with fewer side effects. Although prednisone has traditionally been the standard approach to oral therapy, side effects should be weighed highly, and topical steroids should be attempted first in mild to moderate cases. Dapsone[1] (see pemphigus vulgaris section on treatment) or tetracycline[1] (500 mg four times daily) given with niacinamide[1] (500 mg three times daily) may also be efficacious as first-line treatment. There have been increasing reports of successful treatment with dupilumab (Dupixent)[1] (600 mg subcutaneous injection loading dose, followed by 300 mg every other week) and prednisone. We have implemented this successfully in patients with BP in our institution.

Immunosuppressive medications may be necessary in severe or recalcitrant cases. Azathioprine[1] and mycophenolate mofetil[1] have shown similar efficacy. Rituximab,[1] methotrexate,[1] cyclophosphamide,[1] IVIG,[1] and cyclosporine[1] (4–5 mg/kg/day) are potentially effective second-line options. IVIG may be especially helpful in steroid-resistant cases. Dosing regimens for these medications are similar to those of pemphigus. There have been several case reports of omalizumab (Xolair)[1] (monoclonal anti-IgE antibody) showing good response in some patients.

In our practice, for patients with severe bullous pemphigoid and no contraindications, we start prednisone at 0.5 mg/kg/day along with mycophenolate mofetil. We aim to taper the patient off of steroids in 3 to 6 months while increasing mycophenolate mofetil to a max dose of 1.5 gm twice daily if needed. For patients with mild to moderate disease, or in patients with severe disease but contraindications to corticosteroids and/or immunosuppressants, we treat with topical steroids in conjunction with doxycycline/nicotinamide, IVIG, and/or dapsone.

Denuded, eroded areas tend to heal spontaneously and may not require further treatment other than appropriate wound care. BP is considered a chronic condition, although some cases may be self-limited over a period of about 5 years. High levels of BP180 at the time of discontinuing therapy are associated with a higher risk of relapse.

---

[1] Not FDA approved for this indication.

Mucous Membrane Pemphigoid

Pathophysiology

Mucous membrane pemphigoid (MMP), also referred to as *cicatricial pemphigoid*, is a rare autoimmune bullous disease with numerous targets in the anchoring filament zone including epiligrin (also referred to as laminin 332), $\alpha_6\beta_4$ integrin (specifically the β_4 subunit), and c-terminus of BP180. Antiepiligrin MMP has a strong association with underlying malignancy, most frequently adenocarcinoma. Patients with antibodies against the $\alpha_6\beta_4$ integrin may have exclusive ocular involvement. MMP most frequently affects the elderly, with a female predominance.

Clinical Manifestations

As its name denotes, MMP mostly involves the mucosa, most commonly the oral and conjunctival mucosa. Patients with oral involvement present with numerous painful chronic erosions of the oral mucosa including the gingiva, buccal mucosa, palate, and lips. Eye involvement is typically bilateral, initially presenting as a relatively nonspecific conjunctivitis, which progresses to fibrosis and eventual formation of adhesions of the bulbar and palpebral conjunctiva (symblepharon), ectropion, dry eyes, and inward facing eyelashes (trichiasis). Skin involvement is less common and tends to be more limited. The most common extramucosal sites include the scalp, face, neck, and upper trunk. Skin lesions may heal with atrophic scars, which may help distinguish this entity from BP.

Diagnosis

In addition to clinical history[1] and examination findings, biopsy is required for diagnosis including routine histology, DIF, and salt-split skin. IIF may also be helpful. Routine histology findings are similar to BP with fewer eosinophils. DIF staining shows linear IgG, IgA, +/- C3 deposition along the BMZ. Salt-split skin testing shows an epidermal staining pattern, except for antiepiligrin, which shows dermal staining pattern.

Treatment

For patients with mild, limited oral disease, treatment with topical triamcinolone acetonide (Oralone) 0.1% dental paste twice daily to oral lesions can be quite effective. Dapsone[1] (start 25 mg daily and titrate slowly based on response after 1 week) is our first-line systemic treatment for mild-moderate oral mucosal disease. Limited cutaneous disease can be treated with topical corticosteroids such as triamcinolone 0.1% ointment or clobetasol 0.05% ointment twice daily to affected areas on the body. Tetracycline[1] (500 mg four times daily) with niacinamide[1] (500 mg three times daily) may also be effective.

In patients with more severe oral disease and/or ocular disease, treatment with systemic steroids and cyclophosphamide is often needed. Most frequently oral prednisone 1 mg/kg/day is started with cyclophosphamide[1] (1–2 mg/kg/day), and therapy may continue after clinical remission for maintenance. Clinicians should attempt to taper prednisone after remission is achieved if possible, although some patients may continue to require low doses of prednisone to prevent recurrence. Ocular disease may result in scarring, and early involvement of an experienced ophthalmologist is essential.

MMP is a chronic condition which may result in scarring, disfigurement, and even blindness.

Linear IgA Bullous Dermatosis/Chronic Bullous Disease of Childhood

Pathophysiology

Adult-onset linear IgA bullous dermatosis (LABD) is a rare autoimmune subepidermal bullous disease affecting elderly patients greater than 60 years old. Chronic bullous disease of childhood (CBDC) is typically a self-limited bullous disease affecting young children beginning around 2 or 3 years old and may remit by teenage years. Patients with LABD/CBDC have circulating IgA autoantibodies targeting antigens derived from BPAG2, and some patients may have both IgA and IgG autoantibodies. Medication-induced LABD/CBDC is most frequently caused by vancomycin, followed by penicillin and cephalosporin antibiotics, captopril, NSAIDs, phenytoin, and many more offending medications.

Clinical Manifestations
Both adult-onset LABD and CBDC present with tense blisters/bullae and urticarial plaques that may be arranged in an annular or polycyclic formation, often described as *crown of jewels arrangement*. Individual lesions may appear quite similar to that of bullous pemphigoid and dermatitis herpetiformis. The most frequently affected sites include the trunk, flexures of extremities, groin, buttocks, and the face (in children). Patients may or may not have mucosal involvement.

Diagnosis
Biopsies of early urticarial lesions may show diffuse neutrophilic infiltrate along the BMZ. Biopsies of bullous lesions show subepidermal blisters/bullae filled with neutrophils and a neutrophil-predominant infiltrate in the papillary dermis. DIF of perilesional skin is the gold standard for diagnosis and shows linear IgA deposition along the BMZ. Salt-split skin testing may show epidermal staining.

Treatment
Dapsone[1] is considered first-line therapy for cases of LABD and CBDC. We recommend starting at 25 mg daily, which may be increased weekly by increments of 25 mg based on clinical response (maximum dose varies by age). Second-line agents for those who cannot tolerate dapsone include colchicine[1] (up to 0.6 mg two times daily in pediatric patients and up to three times daily in adult patients) and sulfapyridine[2] (500 mg twice daily starting dose, titrated appropriately based on clinical response).

In cases of drug-induced LABD/CBDC, the offending medication should be discontinued. Lesions are expected to resolve within a few weeks of stopping the medication.

Epidermolysis Bullosa Acquisita
Pathophysiology
Epidermolysis bullosa acquisita (EBA) is a very rare acquired bullous disease, most commonly found in adults of East Asian and African American descent. It is frequently associated with inflammatory bowel disease (especially Crohn's disease), multiple myeloma, systemic lupus erythematosus, diabetes mellitus, hepatitis C infection, and other underlying diseases.

Patients may have IgG autoantibodies targeting type VII collagen, which is a major component of anchoring fibrils in the basement membrane zone.

Clinical Manifestations
The noninflammatory, or mechanobullous, variant of EBA is the most commonly recognized subtype. Patients present with hemorrhagic bullae and erosions on trauma-prone sites including the dorsal hands and feet, elbows, and knees. Lesions may heal with scarring, milia, and nail dystrophy. Inflammatory EBA clinically is indistinguishable to BP. Lesions of inflammatory EBA may also heal with scarring and milia. Patients may also have oral and ocular erosions which may appear similarly to MMP.

Diagnosis
In addition to clinical findings, biopsy is required for diagnosis of EBA to distinguish it from other subepidermal bullous diseases. Routine histology shows subepidermal blisters with varying degrees of neutrophilic and eosinophilic infiltrates. DIF of perilesional skin shows linear IgG and C3 deposition along the BMZ. Unlike BP,

DIF of EBA lesions tend to show more linear IgG deposition rather than C3. Salt-split skin technique shows dermal staining.

Treatment Options
Some patients may have good response to prednisone (0.5–1 mg/kg/day), with or without dapsone. Dapsone[1] monotherapy may also be effective for patients (initiated at 25 mg daily and increased appropriately based on clinical response). This dose should be maintained for several months prior to tapering attempts. Colchicine[1] (0.6 mg twice to thrice daily) may be effective. Patients with resistant or severe disease may have more rapid relief with cyclosporine[1] (4–5 mg/kg/day). Other agents with reported success include rituximab,[1] IVIG,[1] infliximab (Remicade),[1] minocycline,[1] plasmapheresis, and PDE-4 inhibitors.[1]

Unfortunately, cases of EBA tend to be quite resistant to treatment relative to BP and other subepidermal bullous diseases. The disease is usually chronic and waxes and wanes. Patients should avoid trauma as much as possible because it may contribute to further blister formation. The inflammatory subtype of EBA may have better response to therapy compared with the mechanobullous noninflammatory subtype.

Dermatitis Herpetiformis
Pathophysiology
Dermatitis herpetiformis (DH) is a chronic and relapsing bullous disease which is strongly associated with celiac disease. People of Northern European descent are most commonly affected, and it is quite rare in patients of Asian and African American descent. More than 97% of patients with DH and celiac disease have one or both HLA-DQ2 and HLA-DQ8 alleles. In addition to celiac disease, DH is also associated with other autoimmune conditions including Hashimoto's thyroiditis, type 1 diabetes mellitus, and pernicious anemia.

Gluten is a grain protein found in many foods containing wheat, rye, and barley. Gluten is broken down into gliadin during digestion, which is then transported across the gastrointestinal (GI) mucosa to the lamina propria, where it binds with tissue transglutaminase 2 (TTG2). This complex is recognized by HLA-DQ2 or HLA-DQ8 on antigen presenting cells (APCs) and activating the T-cell and B-cell activated autoinflammatory cascade to form IgA autoantibodies against TTG2 or the TTG2-gliadin complex. These bound IgA antibodies lead to neutrophil recruitment, resulting in damage to intestinal villi. Epitope spreading (diversification of epitope specificity) results in production of IgA autoantibodies against epidermal transglutaminase (TTG3), which then binds to TTG3 within dermal papillae. Neutrophils recruited by this process release elastase and other proteolytic enzymes, resulting in the formation of subepidermal blisters seen in DH.

Clinical Manifestations
Patients with DH classically present with extremely pruritic herpetiform vesicles on an urticarial base. The vesicles can be ruptured very easily, so excoriations, rather than intact vesicles, are more frequently seen on examination. Lesions are typically distributed on the symmetric extensor extremities (elbows and knees), buttocks, back, neck, face, and scalp. A minority of approximately 20% of patients with DH have symptomatic gastrointestinal disease; however, the majority of patients have evidence of gluten-sensitive enteropathy on gastrointestinal biopsy samples.

Diagnosis
Clinical history can be particularly helpful in cases of DH. A history of worsening of disease with gluten-containing diets is a useful clue, although patients are not always aware of their specific dietary habits unless they keep a careful food diary.

Biopsy samples should be obtained on early blisters if possible. Routine histology shows subepidermal bullae most pronounced above the dermal papillae, and neutrophilic infiltrates in the dermal papillae. These findings can be quite similar to LABD, so DIF testing

---

[1] Not FDA approved for this indication.
[2] Not available in the United States.

and serologic testing can be helpful. DIF of perilesional skin shows granular IgA deposits with or without C3 deposition in the dermal papillae. Serologic testing for DH and celiac disease can be helpful, including serum antitissue transglutaminase or antiendomysial antibodies (present in approximately 80% of patients with DH and greater than 95% of patients with celiac disease); however, it is important to keep in mind that tests can also be falsely negative if the patient has been keeping a gluten-free diet. Patients with IgA deficiency may also have falsely negative testing for anti-TTG antibodies, so IgA levels should be assessed concurrently.

Treatment Options

Dapsone is the treatment of choice in patients with DH. Patients tend to have a rapid response to dapsone (within 2–3 days) with improvement in cutaneous disease. The usual dose of dapsone in DH is to start at 50 mg daily and increase in increments of 25 mg based on clinical response to a maximum of to a maximum of 100–200 mg daily. Typically, patients are well controlled on 50–100 mg daily. Patients do not typically see an effect on their GI disease, if present. Prior to initiating dapsone, it is important to evaluate for G6PD deficiency. Sulfapyridine[2] is an effective second-line therapy with less risk of hemolysis.

Gluten-free diets (avoiding wheat, rye, and barley) can be effective to control both cutaneous and gastrointestinal disease. It may also reduce the risk of development of GI lymphomas associated with celiac disease. DH is typically a lifelong, chronic, relapsing disease. It is important to involve relevant specialties including dermatology, nutrition, and gastroenterology to help manage patients with DH.

---

[2] Not available in the United States.

References

Abdat R, Waldman RA, et al: Dupilumab as a novel therapy for bullous pemphigoid: a multicenter case series, *J Am Acad Dermatol* 83(1):46–52, 2020.
Bolotin D, Petronic-Rosic V: Dermatitis herpetiformis, *J Am Acad Dermatol* 64(6):1017–1033, 2011.
Cizenski JD, Michel P, et al: Spectrum of orocutaneous disease associations: immune-mediated conditions, *J Am Acad Dermatol* 77(5):795–806, 2017.
Feliciani C, Joly P, et al: Management of bullous pemphigoid: the European Dermatology Forum consensus in collaboration with the European Academy of Dermatology and Venereology, *Br J Dermatol* 172(4):867–877, 2015.
Gouveia A, Teixeira A, et al: Linear immunoglobulin A bullous dermatosis, *J Pediatr* 170:338, 2016. e1.
Kirtschig G, Murrell D, et al: Interventions for mucous membrane pemphigoid/cicatricial pemphigoid and epidermolysis bullosa acquisita: a systematic literature review, *Arch Dermatol* 138(3):380–384, 2002.
Murrell DF, Peña S, et al: Diagnosis and management of pemphigus: recommendations of an international panel of experts, *J Am Acad Dermatol* 82(3): 575–585, 2020.
Mutasim DF: Management of autoimmune bullous diseases: pharmacology and therapeutics, *J Am Acad Dermatol* 51:859–877, 2004.
Wojnarowska F, Kirtschig G, et al: Guidelines for the management of bullous pemphigoid, *Br J Dermatol* 147:214–221, 2002.

BACTERIAL DISEASES OF THE SKIN

Method of
Karissa Gilchrist, MD

CURRENT DIAGNOSIS

- The large variety of bacterial skin infections can usually be distinguished by history, physical exam, and clinical presentation.
- Bacterial infections can range from those affecting the superficial layers of skin to the deep layers and soft tissue.
- Many infections are precipitated by a breach in the normal skin barrier.
- Infection can vary in severity depending on how extensive and invasive it is.
- Deep infection can lead to systemic toxicity.
- Necrotizing infection can rapidly progress and cause extensive tissue damage and even death.

CURRENT THERAPY

- Antibiotic therapy is selected based on knowledge of the most likely causative pathogen or based on culture results.
- When a loculated abscess is identified, procedural incision and drainage should be performed.
- Broad-spectrum empiric antibiotic coverage should be initiated when a rapidly progressing necrotizing infection is suspected.
- Delay in surgical consultation and debridement of necrotizing infection may result in tissue damage, limb loss, and/or death.
- Tissue culture of necrotizing infection can guide antibiotic choice.

Bacterial infections of the skin can manifest in a broad range of clinical presentations. Bacterial skin diseases can occur both superficially and in the deep layers. They can also range from mild to aggressive and life-threatening infection. Skin infections have increased in prevalence and severity in part due to the development of resistant bacterial organisms. For this reason, it is critical for clinicians to be able to promptly recognize and manage bacterial infections of the skin.

Common Infections

Cellulitis

Cellulitis is an acute bacterial skin infection that causes poorly demarcated areas of erythema, warmth, tenderness, and edema of the skin involving the deep dermal and subcutaneous layers. Depending on the extent of edema and inflammation, the affected skin may develop bullae, ecchymosis, or maceration. Cellulitis may occur on any area of the skin but is typically found on the lower extremities and is almost always unilateral. Cellulitis develops when there is a break in the skin and pathogens are able to breach the surface. It most commonly arises from infection with streptococci. *Staphylococcus aureus* is a less common cause of cellulitis but should be considered in special circumstances such as bite wounds, penetrating trauma, intravenous drug use, or in immunocompromised patients (Table 1).

Culture or biopsy of the affected skin is not routinely recommended for the diagnosis of cellulitis. Cultures often yield negative or unhelpful results as the rapidly spreading skin manifestations may be more likely related to a strong inflammatory response to the inciting pathogen and may not be representative of the bacterial load. Blood cultures may be considered if there are systemic signs of infection. Diagnosis of cellulitis should be made clinically. Labs and imaging may be obtained to help distinguish cellulitis from other diagnoses and rule out complications such as underlying abscess, deep venous thrombosis, osteomyelitis, or necrotizing fasciitis. Stasis dermatitis is commonly mistaken for cellulitis and can be differentiated by its bilateral appearance and lack of skin trauma.

In the treatment of mild cases of uncomplicated nonpurulent cellulitis without systemic signs of infection, an oral antibiotic agent

TABLE 1 Primary Pathogen for Common Bacterial Skin Infections

DIAGNOSIS	ORGANISM
Cellulitis	Streptococci (*Staphylococcus aureus* less common)
Impetigo	*S. aureus* Group A beta-hemolytic streptococci
Folliculitis	*S. aureus* Gram-negative bacteria
Abscess	*S. aureus*, predominantly MRSA

MRSA, Methicillin-resistant *S. aureus*.

TABLE 2 **Suggested Antibiotic Agents for Common Bacterial Skin Infections**

DIAGNOSIS	ANTIBIOTIC
Cellulitis	• Cephalexin (Keflex) • Dicloxacillin[1] • Amoxicillin/clavulanate (Augmentin) Alternative: • Clindamycin Severe infection: • Cefazolin (Ancef) • Ceftriaxone (Rocephin) MRSA risk factors: • Vancomycin
Impetigo	Mild cases: • Topical mupirocin (Bactroban) Severe or extensive cases: • Cephalexin (Keflex) • Dicloxacillin[1] MRSA risk factors: • Doxycycline • Clindamycin • Trimethoprim/sulfamethoxazole (Bactrim DS)[1]
Folliculitis	Suspected *S. aureus*: • Topical mupirocin (Bactroban)[1] or clindamycin[1] • Cephalexin (Keflex) • Dicloxacillin Suspected *Pseudomonas*: • No treatment • Ciprofloxacin (Cipro)[1]
Abscess	• Trimethoprim/sulfamethoxazole (Bactrim DS)[1] • Clindamycin

MRSA, Methicillin-resistant *S. aureus.*
[1]Not FDA approved for this indication.

that is active against streptococci—such as cephalexin (Keflex), dicloxacillin[1], or amoxicillin/clavulanate (Augmentin)—should be used. If the patient has a penicillin allergy, clindamycin can be used as an alternative. The typical treatment duration is 5 days, but this may be extended in the case of residual symptoms. In patients who fail oral antimicrobial treatment or in those with systemic signs of infection, an intravenous regimen with an agent such as cefazolin (Ancef), ceftriaxone (Rocephin), or clindamycin should be considered. In cases where there is increased risk of methicillin-resistant *S. aureus* (MRSA) infection, such as penetrating trauma or intravenous drug use, intravenous vancomycin should be added (Table 2).

Erysipelas

For some, the term *erysipelas* is synonymous with cellulitis. However, erysipelas refers to infection that is limited to the upper dermis; cellulitis extends into the deeper dermis. The borders of the erysipelas rash are more clearly demarcated than those of cellulitis. Erysipelas is always nonpurulent. The treatment outlined earlier for cellulitis can be applied to erysipelas with antibiotics targeted against streptococci and, if systemic signs or symptoms are present, parental agents can be used.

Impetigo

Impetigo is a common bacterial skin infection that can occur at any age but is most commonly seen in children. It is most prevalent in hot, humid conditions and is highly contagious. It is transmitted by direct contact and may develop secondarily after a disruption of the skin occurs from an insect bite or other underlying disease such as eczema or psoriasis.

Impetigo can be classified into two major categories: bullous and nonbullous. Bullous impetigo is a result of *S. aureus* infection. Strains of this organism produce a factor that cleaves the junction between the epidermal and dermal skin layers. This causes a delicate vesicle to form, which may break open, leaving behind a

crusted erosion. Nonbullous impetigo is most commonly caused by *S. aureus*, group A beta-hemolytic streptococci, or a combination of both (see Table 1). This form of impetigo typically begins as erythematous papules or pustules. These lesions develop a discharge that dries and forms a classic honey-colored crust.

Treatment for both bullous and nonbullous impetigo consists of antibiotic therapy aimed at both staphylococcal and streptococcal organisms (see Table 2). Either topical or oral antibiotics can be used for treatment of impetigo depending on the severity and extent of infection. Topical treatment with mupirocin (Bactroban) ointment 2% three times daily for 5 days can be effective for mild cases of impetigo. Over-the-counter topical bacitracin[1] or triple antibiotic ointments are not as effective as mupirocin in the treatment of impetigo. If an oral agent is desired for more severe or extensive cases, therapy should consist of an antibiotic medication that is active against *S. aureus*, such as cephalexin (Keflex) or dicloxacillin[1] for 7 days. *S. aureus* isolates from impetigo are typically methicillin-susceptible *S. aureus* (MSSA); however, if MRSA is suspected or confirmed with direct culture of an impetiginous lesion or its drainage, treatment with doxycycline, clindamycin, or sulfamethoxazole-trimethoprim (Bactrim DS)[1] for 7 days is recommended.

Ecthyma

Ecthyma is a form of impetigo that infects deeper layers of the skin into the dermis. Lesions appear as "punched out" ulcerations with an overlying crust and surrounding erythematous edema. Ecthyma differs from impetigo in that it heals with scarring due to the deep skin involvement. The principal pathogen causing ecthyma is group A streptococcus (GAS). Treatment of ecthyma differs from that of impetigo and always requires oral antibiotic therapy. Penicillin is the first-line choice of antibiotic agent. With both impetigo and ecthyma, care should be taken to use contact precautions and frequent handwashing to prevent spread.

Ecthyma Gangrenosum

Ecthyma gangrenosum is a skin eruption that classically arises in immunocompromised patients with *Pseudomonas aeruginosa* bacteremia. An ecthyma gangrenosum lesion typically begins as an erythematous macule or pustule and quickly develops into a gangrenous ulcer. This lesion results from bacterial invasion of the vascular wall and subsequent tissue ischemia and necrosis. There may be one single eruption or several. Lesions can occur in any location, with the axilla and genital regions most commonly affected. Although it is possible for lesions to occur in an immunocompetent patient without any signs of systemic illness, the presence of ecthyma gangrenosum should definitely raise the clinician's suspicion for bacteremia, especially with *P. aeruginosa*. Treatment involves empiric antibiotic therapy with an antipseudomonal agent. Blood cultures should be obtained, and lesions can be swabbed for culture to help guide antibiotic narrowing.

Folliculitis

Folliculitis is the infection and inflammation of hair follicles. It typically presents as erythematous papules or pustules in hair follicles. As with most inflammatory skin diseases, pruritus is the most frequent symptom. Lesions may be painful. Folliculitis is typically infectious, with the most common etiology being bacterial. It can also be caused by viral, fungal, or parasitic infection. Bacterial folliculitis is most frequently caused by *S. aureus* but may also result from infection with gram-negative bacteria (see Table 1). Multiple factors may predispose a patient to develop folliculitis; these include underlying immunodeficiency, frequent scratching (from underlying eczema or other pruritic skin disease), nasal colonization with *S. aureus*, shaving in the opposite direction of hair growth, hyperhidrosis, or prolonged use of topical corticosteroids. Exposure to underchlorinated heated water is the classic risk factor for developing "hot tub folliculitis," which is caused by *P. aeruginosa* infection. In this example of gram-negative folliculitis, pustules appear on the areas of hair-bearing skin

[1]Not FDA approved for this indication.

that were exposed to the contaminated water. Onset may occur up to 48 hours after exposure.

Diagnosis is typically made clinically, and the distribution of lesions may be suggestive of a pathogenic etiology. Folliculitis occurring primarily on the face or scalp is most likely due to *S. aureus*. Culture of pustule contents may be considered if the diagnosis is unclear. Pseudomonal folliculitis is often self-limiting but may necessitate treatment with oral ciprofloxacin (Cipro)[1]in the setting of immunodeficiency or in severe cases. Topical mupirocin (Bactroban)[1] or topical clindamycin[1] is an effective treatment for cases of superficial folliculitis thought to be caused by *S. aureus*. In very mild and localized cases of *S. aureus*, lesions may even resolve spontaneously. If the disease is extensive, refractory to topical treatment, or appears to involve the deep areas of the follicles, an oral antibiotic should be used for treatment. First-line agents include cephalexin (Keflex) or dicloxacillin treatment for 7 to 10 days. If MRSA is suspected or confirmed on culture, oral trimethoprim/sulfamethoxazole (Bactrim DS)[1], clindamycin, or doxycycline should be used for treatment (see Table 2). It is important to try to minimize or eliminate any predisposing factors identified in order to prevent recurrence.

Abscess

An abscess is a collection of pus within the skin or soft tissue. It presents as an erythematous, painful nodule that is fluctuant, sometimes with an overlying pustule. *S. aureus* is responsible for the majority of abscesses (see Table 1), with a large portion being due to methicillin-resistant strains (MRSA). Immunosuppression or any disruption of the normal skin barrier may predispose a patient to develop one or multiple abscesses. Procedural incision and evacuation of the abscess debris should be performed for treatment. Care should be taken to probe the cavity and release loculated areas within the abscess. Proper wound care should follow with application of a dry gauze dressing with or without packing of the wound space. Systemic antibiotics should be used in addition to incision and drainage in cases of multiple lesions, abscesses larger than 2 cm, immunosuppression, signs of systemic toxicity, refractory lesions, extensive surrounding cellulitis, or presence of implanted medical devices. It is reasonable to forgo antibiotic therapy in an otherwise healthy patient with a single small abscess, especially in the setting of numerous antibiotic allergies. However, there is now evidence to suggest that treatment with trimethoprim/sulfamethoxazole (Bactrim DS)[1] or clindamycin for any patient who has undergone incision and drainage may improve cure rates and decrease the risk of recurrence (see Table 2).

Furuncle and Carbuncle

When an abscess forms at the base of a hair follicle, it is referred to as a furuncle. This is different from folliculitis, where infection does not extend deeper than the epidermis. A carbuncle develops when several furuncles occur in multiple adjacent follicles and the infection coalesces into a larger mass of pus. Carbuncles commonly occur on the back of the neck and in the axilla. As in the case of cutaneous abscesses, the principal pathogen for furuncles and carbuncles is *S. aureus*. Many furuncles will rupture spontaneously, allowing the pus to drain. The application of moist heat may also help to encourage spontaneous drainage. Carbuncles and larger furuncles should be treated with incision and drainage.

Invasive Infections

Necrotizing Soft Tissue Infection

Necrotizing cellulitis is an aggressive, rapidly spreading life-threatening bacterial infection of the skin. When there is involvement of the fascia or muscle, the descriptive term becomes *necrotizing fasciitis* or *necrotizing myositis*, accordingly. These infections result in significant tissue destruction and have a high mortality rate. Necrotizing infections may be precipitated by varying degrees of disruption of the skin barrier due to anything from insect bites to intravenous

drug use or major penetrating trauma. Diabetes increases the risk of developing a necrotizing soft tissue infection.

Necrotizing infection presents as skin erythema, edema, and warmth with underlying crepitus that develops quickly over the course of hours and progresses rapidly. Skin findings are usually associated with severe pain, which may be out of proportion to findings on examination. Signs of systemic toxicity, such as fever or hemodynamic instability, may also appear. Delayed clinical recognition can result in extensive tissue damage, limb loss, or death. Prompt surgical consultation should be made if a necrotizing soft tissue infection is suspected. If the diagnosis is unclear, a computed tomography scan may be helpful in revealing the presence of gas in the soft tissues, but it should not delay surgical intervention. Treatment should include emergent surgical debridement as well as empiric antibiotic administration. Care should be taken to provide hemodynamic support as needed. Blood cultures would ideally be obtained prior to the administration of antibiotics. Empiric therapy should consist of a polymicrobial approach with a combination of agents aimed at treating MRSA, aerobes, and anaerobes (Table 3). Antibiotic therapy can be tailored according to culture results from tissue obtained during surgical debridement.

Fournier Gangrene

Fournier gangrene is a form of necrotizing soft tissue infection involving the perineal region. It is typically seen in middle-aged adults, particularly those who have diabetes mellitus. Potential predisposing factors may include recent urologic procedures, chronic use of an indwelling urinary catheter, or urethral trauma. However, this condition can develop without these risk factors. Cutaneous and systemic findings are similar to those of other necrotizing soft tissue infections, and prompt surgical debridement with broad-spectrum empiric antibiotic coverage is critical.

Invasive Group A Streptococcal Infection with Toxic Shock Syndrome

GAS is a common cause of superficial skin infections, as outlined earlier in this chapter. However, this pathogen can sometimes lead to invasive disease and result in necrotizing infection. Toxic shock syndrome is a complication that may arise when invasive GAS produces a toxin that induces the subsequent release of inflammatory cytokines. Skin manifestations include induration and erythema of the affected areas, eventually giving rise to hemorrhagic skin

TABLE 3	Suggested Antibiotic Agents for Invasive Bacterial Skin Infections
DIAGNOSIS	**ANTIBIOTIC**
Necrotizing soft tissue infection Group A streptococcal infection with toxic shock syndrome	1. Vancomycin, linezolid (Zyvox), or daptomycin (Cubicin) plus 2. Piperacillin-tazobactam (Zosyn) or a carbapenem or Ceftriaxone (Rocephin) plus metronidazole(Flagyl) or Fluoroquinolone plus metronidazole (Flagyl)
Invasive	1. Clindamycin plus 2. Penicillin
Staphylococcal scalded skin syndrome	Intravenous oxacillin, nafcillin, cefazolin (Ancef), or vancomycin
Tularemia	Mild or moderate disease: • Oral fluoroquinolone or doxycycline Severe disease: • IV/IM gentamicin[1] or IM streptomycin

[1]Not FDA approved for this indication.

[1]Not FDA approved for this indication.

sloughing. It is often associated with signs of systemic toxicity and multiorgan failure. Toxic shock syndrome may also develop as a result of invasive postpartum endometritis. It is a rapidly progressive disease and prompt treatment should be provided along with hemodynamic support. Antibiotic treatment includes coverage with both clindamycin and penicillin (see Table 3). Clindamycin has the additional benefit of helping to suppress the toxin-mediated inflammatory response. Dual coverage with penicillin is important due to potential clindamycin resistance.

Staphylococcal Scalded Skin Syndrome

Staphylococcal scalded skin syndrome is a complication that can arise from any infection caused by *S. aureus*, such as impetigo, for example. It typically occurs in children and develops as a result of exotoxins produced by the bacteria. Skin findings include painful erythema and desquamation; the mucous membranes are spared. Fever and generalized malaise usually accompany the cutaneous findings. Diagnosis can usually be made clinically; however, culture of the suspected primary infection can be collected for confirmation. One should keep in mind that areas of desquamation or bullae in scalded skin syndrome will be sterile, as these lesions are a result of the exotoxins and not direct bacterial infection. Therefore culture of these areas is unlikely to be helpful.

Patients with staphylococcal scalded skin syndrome are typically treated in an inpatient setting with intravenous antibiotics and supportive care. First-line antibiotic agents include oxacillin, nafcillin, cefazolin (Ancef), and vancomycin (see Table 3). Clindamycin is not a recommended first-choice agent due to high rates of resistance.

Tularemia

Tularemia is an uncommon infection caused by *Francisella tularensis*; it occurs after exposure to an infected insect or animal, most commonly a tick or rabbit. Clinical manifestations vary in severity. The most common form of tularemia is ulceroglandular disease. Symptom onset typically occurs within 3 to 5 days following exposure and begins with nonspecific constitutional symptoms such as fever, headache, myalgias, and generalized malaise. Cutaneous manifestations commonly begin with a single erythematous ulceration with or without a central eschar. Location of the skin lesion is based on the site of inoculation, and the anatomic distribution of findings is regional. Rarely, there may be multiple skin lesions. Ulceroglandular tularemia is associated with localized tender lymphadenopathy. Glandular tularemia has the same characteristics as ulceroglandular tularemia without the ulcerations.

When tularemia is suspected clinically, serology should be sent for diagnosis. It generally takes 2 weeks for antibodies to *Francisella* to reach diagnostic levels, and serology may need to be repeated if clinical suspicion is high. Polymerase chain reaction (PCR) testing can be completed more rapidly depending on lab availability of the test. Blood or tissue cultures are rarely positive; if such specimens are collected, laboratory staff should be notified in advance of tularemia suspicion in order to optimize conditions for culture growth as well as for infection control precautions. Treatment consists of selecting an effective antibiotic regimen. In general, an oral fluoroquinolone or doxycycline would be a reasonable initial treatment for patients with mild or moderate disease. If the infection is severe, intravenous or intramuscular gentamicin[1] or intramuscular streptomycin is recommended (see Table 3). Of note, *F. tularensis* has the potential to be used as a bioterrorism agent, as it is easily disseminated and infection can occur at low exposure. In such a case, recognition and reporting are critical.

---

[1]Not FDA approved for this indication.

References

Daum RS, Miller LG, Immergluck L, et al: A placebo-controlled trial of antibiotics for smaller skin abscesses, *N Engl J Med* 376:2545–2555, 2017.
Handler MZ, Schwartz RA: Staphylococcal scalded skin syndrome: diagnosis and management in children and adults, *J Eur Acad Dermatol Venereol* 28:1418–1423, 2014.
Jeng A, Beheshti M, Li J, Nathan R: The role of beta-hemolytic streptococci in causing diffuse, nonculturable cellulitis: a prospective investigation, *Medicine (Baltimore)* 89:217–226, 2010.
Luelmo-Aguilar J, Santandreu MS: Folliculitis: recognition and management, *Am J Clin Dermatol* 5:301–310, 2004.
Pereira LB: Impetigo – review, *An Bras Dermatol* 89:293–299, 2014.
Raff AB, Kroshinsky D: Cellulitis: a review, *JAMA* 316:325–337, 2016.
Snowden J, Simonsen KA: Tularemia. In *StatPearls*. Treasure Island (FL), StatPearls Publishing, 2020.
Stevens DL, Bisno AL, Chambers HF, et al: Practice guidelines for the diagnosis and management of skin and soft tissue infections: 2014 update by the Infectious Diseases Society of America, *Clin Infect Dis* 59:e10–52, 2014.

CONTACT DERMATITIS

Method of
Yul W. Yang, MD, PhD; and James A. Yiannias, MD

CURRENT DIAGNOSIS

- Gather a detailed history on skin exposures, including use of the following items:
  - Irritants
  - Alkalis: soaps, detergents, cleansers
  - Acids
  - Hydrocarbons: petroleum, oils
  - Solvents
  - Potential allergens including:
    - Metals: nickel sulfate; cobalt chloride (e.g., jewelry, makeup, personal products)
    - Fragrances: linalool, balsam of Peru (Myroxylon pereirae; fragrance); fragrance mix; propolis
    - Methylisothiazolinone, methylchloroisothiazolinone, benzisothiazolinone, benzalkonium chloride (preservatives)
    - Formaldehyde and formaldehyde-releasing preservatives such as quaternium-15
    - Topical antibiotics such as neomycin, bacitracin
- Examine the skin for the location and pattern of eruption:
  - Eyelid: nail polish
  - Postauricular scalp: perfume
  - Perioral area: chewing gum, toothpaste
  - Trunk: dyes, clothing finish
  - Wrist: nickel, chrome
  - Waistline: rubber
  - Feet: shoes
  - Wounds: topical antibiotic ointment
- Perform patch testing:
  - T.R.U.E. TEST with 35 allergens (note: two common allergens, benzalkonium chloride and propolis, are not included in this panel)
  - Customized series with 70 or more allergens

CURRENT THERAPY

- Avoid irritants and allergens, using the prepared patient handout.
- Consult the SkinSAFE shopping list of skin care products free from the top 10 most common allergens (if patch testing is not performed).
- Consult a customized SkinSAFE shopping list of skin care products free from the patient's contact allergens, based on patch test results.
- Topical corticosteroids can be applied.
- Hydrocortisone 2.5% (Hytone) can be applied twice daily on the face, neck, axillae, groin, and intertriginous areas.
- Triamcinolone 0.1% (Kenalog) can be applied twice daily on the body.

Continued

- For severe reactions, short-term, higher-potency steroids can be applied (e.g., clobetasol [Clobex] 0.05% twice daily).
- Sedating antihistamines can be taken: doxepin (Sinequan)[1] 10 to 20 mg qhs.
- Steroid-sparing topical agents can be applied twice daily to any skin surface (but may be more expensive than topical corticosteroids): tacrolimus 0.1% (Protopic),[1] pimecrolimus 1% (Elidel),[1] crisaborole 2% (Eucrisa),[1] ruxolitinib 1.5% (Opzelura)[1]
- For severe, acute episodes, systemic corticosteroids can be taken in a several-week tapering course (e.g., prednisone 60 mg for 5 days, 40 mg for 5 days, and 20 mg for 5 days).
- Longer-term systemic therapy is possible for severe or recalcitrant disease.
- Phototherapy with narrow-band ultraviolet B[1] is suggested.
- Azathioprine (Imuran)[1] can be taken 1 to 3 mg/kg qd.
- Mycophenolate mofetil (CellCept)[1] can be taken 2 to 3 g qd.
- Methotrexate[1] can be taken 10 to 25 mg per week.
- Cyclosporine (Neoral)[1] can be taken 2.5 to 5 mg/kg qd short term.
- Dupilumab (Dupixent)[1] can be taken by SQ injection at 600 mg initially and then 300 mg every other week.
- Tralokinumab (Adbry)[1] can be taken by SQ injection at 600 mg initially and then 300 mg every other week.
- Lebrikizumab (Ebglyss)[1] can be taken by SQ injection at 500 mg initally at week 0 and week 2, followed by 250 mg every other week until week 16 or later, and then reduced to 250 mg every 4 weeks.
- Upadacitinib (Rinvoq)[1] can be taken 15 to 30 mg qd.
- Abrocitinib (Cibinqo)[1] can be taken 100 to 200 mg qd.

[1]Not FDA approved for this indication.

BOX 1 Top 10 Most Common Allergens

North American Contact Dermatitis Group
- Nickel sulfate
- Methylisothiazolinone (MI)
- Fragrance mix
- Linalool
- Benzisothiazolinone
- Methylisothiazolinone/methylchloroisothiazolinone (MI/MCI)
- Propolis
- Balsam of Peru
- Cobalt
- Formaldehyde

Mayo Clinic Contact Dermatitis Group
- Nickel sulfate
- Methylisothiazolinone (MI)
- Balsam of Peru
- Linalool
- Methyldibromo glutaronitrile
- Neomycin
- Cobalt
- Fragrance Mix
- Benzalkonium chloride
- Bacitracin

Data from DeKoven JG, Warshaw EM, Reeder MJ, et al: North American contact dermatitis group patch test results: 2019–2020, *Dermatitis* 34(2):90–104, 2023; and Zawawi S, Yang YW, Cantwell HM, et al. Trends in patch testing with the Mayo Clinic Standard Series, 2017–2021, *Dermatitis* 34(5):405–412, 2023.

Dermatitis typically manifests as papules and vesicles with weeping and oozing that can become lichenified and scaly when chronic. When this clinical picture is secondary to an exogenous substance coming into contact with the skin, it is termed *contact dermatitis*. Further delineation leads to irritant versus allergic contact dermatitis, although in practice these often overlap.

Irritant contact dermatitis is not an allergic process. It represents damage to the skin from repeated and cumulative exposure to an agent. Irritants do not require prior sensitization. A decreased barrier function of the skin (e.g., with frequent handwashing) can predispose to the condition or exacerbate it. Examples include alkalis (in soaps, detergents, and cleansers), acids (in germicides, dyes, and pigments), hydrocarbons (in petroleum and oils), and solvents.

Allergic contact dermatitis is an immunologic process classified as a type IV cell-mediated delayed hypersensitivity reaction. Poison ivy is a classic example. It requires an initial exposure to the contactant in which sensitization occurs but without outward physical effect. Subsequent exposure can elicit a striking response that is independent of the amount of the contactant.

Recent studies were performed by the North American Contact Dermatitis Group (NACDG) and the Mayo Clinic Contact Dermatitis Group (MCCDG) to find the the 10 most common allergens (Box 1). Common sources of exposure to nickel include costume jewelry, snaps, zippers, and other metal objects. Linalool, Balsam of Peru, and fragrance mix are markers for fragrance sensitivity. Sources of exposure to formaldehyde include skin care products, household products, and the resins in plastics and clothing. Neomycin and bacitracin are topical antibiotics available alone and in combination with polymyxin (Neosporin), antifungals, and corticosteroids. Cobalt is found with other metals, including zinc, and in items such as jewelry, crayons, hair dye, and antiperspirants. MI is a common preservative found in personal care products and may be used in combination with another preservative, methylchloroisothiazolinone (MCI). Benzalkonium chloride is commonly used in the healthcare field as a cleanser, antiseptic, and preservative, but it is also found in personal care products such as wipes and an increasing number of skin care products.

Others less consistently in the top 10 during that period were methyldibromo glutaronitrile, gold sodium thiosulfate, potassium dichromate, *p*-phenylenediamine, thiuram mix, and propolis. Methyldibromo glutaronitrile is a preservative and can be found in healthcare and personal products. Clinically relevant sources of gold may be found in jewelry and dental appliances. Potassium dichromate is used in cement, leather, and steel surfaces. Permanent hair dyes are the usual source of *p*-phenylenediamine. Thiuram mix is in rubber and some personal products. Propolis is another marker of fragrance sensitivity.

Each year since 2000, the American Contact Dermatitis Society has designated an allergen of the year, designed to spotlight allergens, common or not, that are increasing in significance. For 2025, toluene-2,5-diamine sulfate was chosen. While used in other applications to add color, toluene-2,5-diamine sulfate is primarily found in permanent hair dyes, although less commonly than the more ubiquitous common allergen, p-phenylenediamine.

Other designated allergens of the year have been alkyl glucosides, cobalt chloride, benzophenones, MI, acrylates, dimethyl fumarate, neomycin, mixed dialkyl thioureas, nickel, fragrance, *p*-phenylenediamine, corticosteroids, cocamidopropyl betaine, bacitracin, thimerosal, gold, disperse blue, propylene glycol, nonallergen parabens, isobornyl acrylate, acetophenone azine, and aluminum, lanolin, and sulfates. Alkyl glucosides are surfactants that are pervasive in consumer products, including cosmetics. Benzophenones, such as oxybenzone, are chemical ultraviolet light filters that are found in sunscreens and personal care products. Artificial nails, dentures, and bone cement contain acrylates, but these substances are only allergenic when in the liquid, powder, or paste forms. Dimethyl fumarate is a biocide in furniture, shoes, and textiles. It is often placed in little paper packets with these items. Rubber products and shoe glue are common sources of mixed dialkyl thioureas. Shampoos often contain cocamidopropyl betaine as

Introduction

Eczema, also known as dermatitis, is an inflammation of the skin due to dryness, irritation, or possible external allergy. Eczema/dermatitis is not contagious.

Some skin care products contain fragrance even though the package says "fragrance free" or "unscented." Therefore, please choose the skin care products as listed below by their *exact brand name*.

Suggestions

Soaps/cleansing
- Vanicream soap
- Free and clear liquid cleanser
- Dove Sensitive Skin Fragrance Free Beauty Bar
- CeraVe Eczema Soothing Body Wash
Any of the shampoos listed in this brochure may be used as your hand or body soap.
- Vanicream shave cream for sensitive skin

Moisturizers
- Vanicream, vanicream lite
- Aveeno Active Naturals Daily Moisturizing Lotion, Sheer Hydration
- Plain vaseline, vaniply
- Use moisturizers twice daily.
- All of the above are OK to use on the face.
- After showering, blot excess water with hands and apply cream. Do not use a towel to dry.

Deodorants
- Almay unscented antiperspirants
- Plain cornstarch from the grocer can be used.
- Vanicream Anti-perspirant/Deodorant

Avoid

Soaps/cleansing
- No hot water (use lukewarm).
- Avoid hot tubs.
- No rubbing alcohol.

Moisturizers
- No creams, lotions, oils or powders other than those recommended in this brochure.
- No neosporin, triple antibiotic, or bacitracin antibiotic ointments.

Fragrances
- No perfumes, colognes, after shave, or pre-shave on any part of body/clothing.

Shampoo
- Free and clear shampoo and conditioner
- DHS clear shampoo and DHS conditioner
- DHS sal shampoo, neutrogena T-sal shampoo, or Free and Clear Medicated Anti-Dandruff Shampoo (not T-Gel).
- Conditioners can be used

Hairspray
- Fragrance-free hairspray such as free and clear hairspray
- Caution: Hairsprays labeled as "unscented" may not be fragrance free.

Laundry and home care
- Unscented laundry detergents such as Arm & Hammer Liquid Laundry 2x Concentrate Perfume & Dye Free, All Free Liquid Laundry Detergent with Stainlifters, Tide Free & Gentle HE Liquid Laundry Detergent
- Wash all new clothes and linens five times before using.
- Old clothes and fabrics are preferred.
- Use white vinegar in rinse cycle to help remove soap.

Hand, nail, and general skin care tips
- Wear cotton gloves under rubber/vinyl gloves for any activities where hand-wetting is expected.
- Trim nails short. Long nails are dangerous to skin, especially when sleeping.

Sunscreens
- Vanicream sunscreen #30 or #60

Make-ups/cosmetics
- If you would like a list of make-ups and cosmetics that are free of the most common allergy-causing ingredients, ask your provider about "virtual patch testing" using the Mayo SkinSAFE program, www.SkinSafeProducts.com

Laundry and home care
- No fabric softener in washer.
- Bounce unscented fabric softener sheets in dryer if desired.
- No washing machine water softener such as calgon (in-house water softeners are acceptable).
- White vinegar may be used as a general household cleaner.

Hand, nail, and general skin care tips
- No wetting of hands more than five times a day.
- Avoid tight-fitting clothes unless your doctor has advised you to wear a pressure garment such as support hose.
- No scrubbing! No loofah! No pumice stone!
- Do not pull off dead skin. Snip with scissors instead.
- Avoid prewetted cleansing wipes.

Figure 1 Sample of prepared handout (used at the Mayo Clinic Arizona) with recommendations for the patient on hypoallergenic skin care products.

a lathering agent. Thimerosal is a preservative for medications and personal care products, including contact lens solution. Disperse blue is a fabric dye. Patients with an allergy to disperse dyes may also react to *p*-phenylenediamine. Propylene glycol is a common ingredient in personal care products, topical corticosteroids and other medications, and foods. Parabens are preservatives commonly found in cosmetics, foods, pharmaceuticals, dentifrices, and suppositories. Isobornyl acrylate, an adhesive, is often used in medical devices, such as insulin pumps, and can also be found in acrylic nails. Acetophenone azine is found in shin pads and footwear that contain cushioning foam made of ethyl vinyl acetate. Aluminum is a common metal used both as a metal in industry and everyday life and also as a salt in cosmetics, sunscreen, food, tattoos, medicine, and water purification. Lanolin is a complex wax mixture (historically from wool) that is used not only in personal care products as an emulsifier and emollient/moisturizer but also in industrial products. Sulfites are inorganic compounds used as antioxidants and preservatives, found in personal care products, swimming pool water, medications, gloves, foods, and water, as well as other industrial uses.

Diagnosis

The evaluation of a patient with suspected contact dermatitis begins with the history. Specific questions directed at the patient's occupation, hobbies, and home routine will be helpful. Examination should note the location and pattern of the eruption. Although eyelid dermatitis may be seen in the atopic patient, nail polish may be the source of the offending allergen. Dyshidrotic eczema occurs as vesicles along the lateral aspects of the fingers, whereas eczematous changes along the dorsal hands are more commonly caused by an allergen. Other distributions as clues include postauricular scalp (perfume), perioral area (chewing gum, toothpaste), trunk (dyes or clothing finish), wrist (nickel or chrome), waistline (rubber), feet (shoes), and history or presence of wounds (topical antibiotic ointment).

Patch testing can confirm or reveal a contact allergy. It involves placement of allergens against the skin of the patient's back for 48 hours. An initial reading is then done, with follow-up readings typically at 96 hours. Prepared series include the thin-layer, rapid-use epicutaneous (TRUE) test, which consists of 35 allergens and 1 negative control (https://mytruetest.com/). Customized series, such as the NACDG Standard Series with 70 allergens and the Mayo Clinic's Standard Series with 80 allergens, must be manually assembled. The majority of dermatologists performing patch testing use the TRUE test. Note that benzalkonium chloride, MI, and propolis are not included in this panel. Overall, the NACDG estimates that 25% to approximately 40% of allergic reactions would have been missed by the TRUE test based on their data for 2015 to 2016.

In addition to ascertaining degree of positivity, relevance must be determined. This involves collaborating with patients to assess the likelihood that they are currently exposed to the positive antigen.

Treatment

Ideally, the allergen or allergens will be identified and avoided. Realistically, compliance is a challenge. To assist patients in avoiding antigens in skin care products, SkinSAFE was created in 1999. It includes 17,480 ingredients and 146,874 individual over-the-counter and prescription skin care products as of February 5, 2025. Once the patient's allergens have been identified with patch testing, they can be entered into the database, and a list of products free from those substances is generated. The patient should be reminded that even small and infrequent exposures can perpetuate the eczema.

Topical corticosteroids applied twice daily are helpful in hastening resolution and may also be used for disease control when the allergen is unknown. Low-potency corticosteroids such as 2.5% hydrocortisone (Hytone) are recommended for the thinner skin of the face, neck, axillae, groin, and intertriginous areas. Midpotency steroids such as triamcinolone 0.1% (Kenalog, Kenonel) are appropriate for the thicker skin of the body. Short-term use of higher-potency steroids may be necessary if the reaction is severe. If there is significant pruritus, sedating antihistamines such as doxepin (Sinequan)[1] 10 to 20 mg taken nightly 2 hours before bedtime can provide relief. Steroid-sparing topical immunomodulators such as tacrolimus (Protopic),[1] pimecrolimus (Elidel),[1] crisaborole (Eucrisa)[1] and ruxolitinib 1.5% (Opzelura)[1] may be helpful adjuncts, but they may be more expensive. Treatment for severe acute episodes can entail a several-week tapering course of systemic corticosteroids, especially if the eruption is widespread. Other longer-term systemic therapies for severe or resistant disease include phototherapy or systemic immunosuppressants such as azathioprine (Imuran),[1] mycophenolate mofetil (CellCept),[1] methotrexate,[1] cyclosporine (Neoral),[1] or dupilumab (Dupixent).[1] Newer agents include tralokinumab (Adbry),[1] lebrikizumab (Ebglyss),[1] upadacitinib (Rinvoq),[1] and abrocitinib (Cibinqo).[1]

It may take many weeks before the skin reverts to a normal appearance despite successful avoidance of antigens. A prepared handout with concrete recommendations for the patient on truly hypoallergenic skin care is beneficial. A sample of that used at Mayo Clinic Arizona is shown in Figure 1.

If patch testing is not performed, an initial approach may be to instruct the patient on avoiding the most common contact allergens via a handout and prescribing symptomatic treatment including topical and oral therapies. SkinSAFE can generate a shopping list of products free from the top 10 allergens as identified by the NACDG and the MCCDG. Patients may access SkinSAFE independently (at https://www.skinsafeproducts.com, the Apple App Store, or the Google Play Store under SkinSAFE) to generate this list or build customized lists free from fragrances, common preservatives, parabens, nickel, lanolin, coconut, and topical antibiotics. In 35% of patients, simply using products free from the top 10 allergens can prompt clearance. Some physicians follow these measures for several months, especially if the eruption is mild, before pursuing formal patch testing.

An excellent primer for the physician interested in learning more about contact allergy diagnosis and management is *Contact and Occupational Dermatology*.

---

[1] Not FDA approved for this indication.
[1] Not FDA approved for this indication.

References

Aerts O, Herman A, Mowitz M, et al: Isobornyl acrylate, *Dermatitis*, 2020, https://doi.org/10.1097/DER.0000000000000549. [Epub ahead of print].

Bruze M, Zimerson E: Dimethyl fumarate, *Dermatitis* 22:3–7, 2011.

Castanedo-Tardana MP, Zug KA: Methylisothiazolinone, *Dermatitis* 24:2–6, 2013, https://doi.org/10.1097/DER.0b013e31827edc73.

DeKoven JG, Warshaw EM, Belsito, et al: North American contact dermatitis group patch test results 2013-2014, *Dermatitis* 28:33–46, 2017, https://doi.org/10.1097/DER.0000000000000225.

DeKoven JG, Warshaw EM, Zug KA, et al: North American contact dermatitis group patch test results: 2015-2016, *Dermatitis* 29:297–309, 2018, https://doi.org/10.1097/DER.0000000000000417.

Heurung AR, Raju SI, Warshaw EM: Benzophenones, *Dermatitis* 25:3–10, 2014, https://doi.org/10.1097/DER.0000000000000025.

Jacob SE, Scheman A, McGowan MA: Allergen of the year: propylene glycol, *Dermatitis*, 2017, https://doi.org/10.1097/DER.0000000000000315.

Macneil JS: Henna tattoo ingredient is allergen of the year, *Skin & Allergy News*, 2006. Available at http://www.skinandallergynews.com/index.php?id=372&cHash=071010&tx_ttnews%5Btt_news%5D=559.

Marks JG, Elsner P, DeLeo VA: In *Contact and occupational dermatology*, Mosby, 2002.

Nelson SA, Yiannias JA: Relevance and avoidance of skin care product allergens: pearls and pitfalls, *Dermatol Clin* 27:329–336, 2009.

Raison-Peyron N, Sasseville D: Acetophenone azine, *Dermatitis* 32:5–9, 2021.

Sasseville D: Acrylates, *Dermatitis* 23(3–5), 2012, https://doi.org/10.1097/DER.0b013e31823d5cd8.

Splete H: Dermatologists name isobornyl acrylate contact allergen of the year, *Dermatology News*, 2019. Available at https://www.mdedge.com/dermatology/article/195656/contact-dermatitis/dermatologists-name-isobornyl-acrylate-contact.

Thin-layer rapid-use epicutaneous test (T.R.U.E. TEST), https://www.smartpractice.com/shop/wa/category?cn=Products-T.R.U.E.-TEST&id=508222&m=SPA, 2021.

Veverka KK, Hall MR, Yiannias JA, et al: Trends in patch testing with the Mayo Clinic standard series, 2011-2015, *Dermatitis* 29(6):310–315, 2018, https://doi.org/10.1097/DER.0000000000000411.

Warshaw EM, Belsito DV, Taylor JS, et al: North American contact dermatitis group patch test results: 2009 to 2010, *Dermatitis* 24:50–59, 2013.

Warshaw EM, Maibach HI, Taylor JS, et al: North American contact dermatitis group patch test results: 2011-2012, *Dermatitis* 26(1):49–59, 2015, https://doi.org/10.1097/DER.0000000000000097.

Wentworth AB, Yiannias JA, Keeling JH, et al: Trends in patch test results and allergen changes in the standard series: a Mayo Clinic 5-year retrospective review. January 1, 2006, through December 31, 2010, *J Am Acad Dermatol* 70:269–275.e4, 2014. https://doi.org/10.1016/j.jaad.2013.09.047.

Yiannias J: *Virtual patch testing: data driven empiric contact allergen avoidance*, Baltimore, MD, 2013, American College of Allergy, Asthma and Immunology Annual Scientific Meeting, November 11, 2013.

CUTANEOUS T-CELL LYMPHOMAS, INCLUDING MYCOSIS FUNGOIDES AND SÉZARY SYNDROME

Method of
Gary S. Wood, MD; and Jeanette R. Comstock, MD

CURRENT DIAGNOSIS

For cutaneous T-cell lymphomas, obtain the following:

- History: duration and pace of lesion development
- Skin examination: extent of patches, plaques, tumors, and ulcers
- Extracutaneous examination: status of lymph nodes, liver, and spleen
- Laboratory: complete blood cell count, differential, complete metabolic panel, lactate dehydrogenase, and lesional biopsy results
- Imaging: CT or fused PET/CT scans of the chest, abdomen, and pelvis (not needed for early-stage mycosis fungoides)

CURRENT THERAPY

Guidelines are primarily for mycosis fungoides and Sézary syndrome:

- Stages IA–IIA: skin-directed therapy with potent topical corticosteroids, topical mechlorethamine (Valchlor), or phototherapy; radiation therapy; topical imiquimod (Aldara);[1] topical bexarotene (Targretin) in selected cases
- Stages IIB–IVB: skin-directed therapy plus one or more systemic therapies, such as pegylated interferon alfa-2a (Pegasys),[1] bexarotene (Targretin), methotrexate, or romidepsin (Istodax); targeted antibodies including mogamulizumab, brentuximab vedotin, or extracorporeal photopheresis for erythrodermic cases
- Combination therapies are often used in intermediate- and advanced-stage disease
- Multiagent chemotherapy is usually not an effective long-term treatment strategy

[1]Not FDA approved for this indication.

Cutaneous T-Cell Lymphomas

Classification

Virtually every subtype of T-cell lymphoma involves the skin either primarily or secondarily. The principal types of primary cutaneous T-cell lymphomas (CTCLs) recognized in the World Health Organization and European Organization for Research and Treatment of Cancer classification include mycosis fungoides (MF) and its leukemic variant, the Sézary syndrome (SS); CD30+ large cell lymphoma and lymphomatoid papulosis (LyP); CD30– large cell lymphoma; and pleomorphic CD4+ small or medium cell variants (Table 1). All other primary CTCLs comprise only a few percent of the total. The fifth edition of the *World Health Organization Classification of Haematolymphoid Tumours: Lymphoid Neoplasms*, available in 2024, is an excellent resource for the most contemporary classification schema. This discussion focuses on MF and SS because they account for up to 75% of primary cutaneous cases.

Standard Diagnosis and Staging Methods

The evaluation of CTCL patients begins with a thorough clinical history and physical examination. Key elements of the history include the pace and nature of disease development, the presence or absence of spontaneous regression of lesions, prior therapy, and ingestion of drugs (e.g., anticonvulsants, antihistamines, or other agents with antihistaminic properties associated with lymphoproliferative skin eruptions that can mimic CTCLs). The review of systems should establish the presence of lymphoma-associated constitutional symptoms (e.g., fever of unknown origin, night sweats, weight loss, fatigue). In addition to general aspects, the physical examination should document the type and distribution of skin lesions and whether there is lymphadenopathy, hepatosplenomegaly, or edema of extremities (i.e., potential sign of lymphatic obstruction).

Histopathologic analysis of representative lesional skin biopsy specimens is the primary means of confirming the clinical diagnosis. Biopsy specimens should be deep enough to include the deepest portions of the cutaneous lymphoid infiltrates because these areas often exhibit the most diagnostic features. Putative extracutaneous involvement should be confirmed by biopsy if it is relevant to clinical management.

Routine blood tests include a complete blood cell count, differential review, and general chemistry panel, as well as lactate dehydrogenase. A peripheral blood flow cytometric assay is used to assess peripheral blood involvement.

Internal nodal and visceral involvement by lymphoma usually is assessed with computed tomography (CT) or combined positron emission tomography and CT (PET/CT) scans of the chest, abdomen, and pelvis. These radiologic studies are usually not needed for patients with early forms of MF (i.e., nontumorous skin lesions without evidence of extracutaneous involvement assessed by physical examination); however, they are usually obtained during the workup of other types of CTCLs. The role of immunopathologic and molecular biologic assays in the diagnosis and staging of CTCLs is discussed later.

An algorithm for the diagnosis of early MF has been proposed by the International Society for Cutaneous Lymphomas (ISCL)

TABLE 1	Simplified Classification of Primary Cutaneous T-Cell Lymphomas	
CTCL TYPE	**PROPORTION OF PRIMARY CTCL (%)**	**5-YEAR SURVIVAL RATE (%)**
MF and variants	60	85
SS	3	35*
CD30+ large cell/LyP	25	<95
Pleomorphic small/ medium cell**	8	99
Miscellaneous	<1	Variable

*The 5-year survival rate depends on the criteria used to define SS, and it may be as low as 10%.

**Now regarded as a lymphoproliferative disorder, not lymphoma.

Abbreviations: CTCL = cutaneous T-cell lymphoma; MF = mycosis fungoides; SS = Sézary syndrome.

Complete classification in Willemze R, Cerroni L, Kempf W, et al: The 2018 update of the WHO-EORTC classification for primary cutaneous lymphomas, *Blood* 133(16):1703–1714, 2019.

(see Pimpinelli et al. in References). It relies on a combination of clinical, histopathologic, immunopathologic, and clonality criteria. This differs from former approaches primarily based on histopathologic criteria.

Mycosis Fungoides, Sézary Syndrome, and Variants
Clinical Features
MF classically manifests as erythematous, scaly, variably pruritic, flat patches or indurated plaques, often favoring the most sun-protected areas. The patches or plaques may progress to cutaneous tumors and involvement of lymph nodes or viscera, although this usually does not occur if the skin lesions are reasonably well controlled by therapy. SS manifests as total-body erythema and scaling (i.e., erythroderma), generalized lymphadenopathy, hepatosplenomegaly, and leukemia. Large plaque parapsoriasis is essentially the prediagnostic patch phase of MF. Lesions may exhibit poikiloderma (i.e., atrophy, telangiectasia, and mottled hyperpigmentation and hypopigmentation), which have been referred to as *poikiloderma atrophicans vasculare*.

Follicular mucinosis refers to a papulonodular eruption in which hair follicles are infiltrated by T cells and contain pools of mucin. In hairy areas, this may result in alopecia. Follicular mucinosis may exist as a lesional variant of MF (i.e., follicular MF) or as a clinically benign entity (i.e., alone or associated with other lymphomas). Clinicopathological criteria can distinguish between indolent and aggressive forms of follicular MF. Granulomatous slack skin is a variant of MF that manifests with pendulous skin folds in intertriginous areas. Lesional skin biopsy specimens contain atypical T lymphocytes in a granulomatous background.

Pagetoid reticulosis manifests as a solitary or localized, often hyperkeratotic plaque containing atypical T cells that are frequently confined to a hyperplastic epidermis. Some authorities regard it as a variant of unilesional MF, whereas others believe it is a distinct entity.

Other variants of MF include hypopigmented, palmoplantar, bullous, and pigmented purpuric forms. The latter form shows clinicopathologic overlap with the pigmented purpuric dermatoses.

Histopathologic and Cytologic Features
A well-developed plaque of MF contains a band-like, cytologically atypical lymphoid infiltrate in the upper dermis that infiltrates the epidermis as single cells and cell clusters known as Pautrier's microabscesses. The atypical lymphoid cells exhibit dense, hyperchromatic nuclei with convoluted, cerebriform nuclear contours and scant cytoplasm. The term *cerebriform* comes from the brain-like ultrastructural appearance of these nuclei. In more advanced cutaneous tumors, the infiltrate extends diffusely throughout the upper and lower dermis and may lose its epidermotropism. In the earlier patch phase of the disease, the infiltrate is sparser, and lymphoid atypia may be less pronounced. In some cases, it may be difficult to distinguish early patch-type MF from various types of chronic dermatitis. The presence of lymphoid atypia and absence of significant epidermal intercellular edema (i.e., spongiosis) help to establish the diagnosis of early MF.

Involvement of lymph nodes by MF begins in the paracortical T-cell domain and may progress to complete effacement of nodal architecture by the same types of atypical lymphoid cells that infiltrate the skin. These cells can be seen in low numbers in the peripheral blood of many MF patients; however, those with SS develop gross leukemic involvement, usually defined as at least 1000 tumor cells/mm^3. These cells are known as Sézary cells, and they are traditionally detected by manual review of the peripheral blood smear (the so-called Sézary prep). They may also be defined by various immunophenotypic criteria.

Immunophenotyping
Cellular antigen expression is usually assessed by immunoperoxidase methods for tissue biopsy specimens and flow cytometry for blood specimens. Almost all cases of MF or SS begin as phenotypically and functionally mature CD4+ T-cell neoplasms of skin-associated lymphoid tissue (SALT). MF and SS express homing markers consistent with "effector memory" and "central memory" T cells, respectively. They express the SALT-associated homing molecule cutaneous lymphocyte antigen (CLA) and most mature T-cell surface antigens, with the exceptions of CD7 and CD26, which are often absent. As disease progresses, the tumor cells often dedifferentiate and lose one or more mature T-cell markers, such as CD2, CD3, or CD5.

Cases typically express the α/β form of the T-cell receptor. Early stages of CTCL tend to exhibit T_H1 cytokines such as IL-2 and interferon-γ, but late-stage disease shifts to a cytokine profile consistent with the T_H2 subset of CD4+ T cells (i.e., production of interleukin [IL]-4, IL-5, and IL-10). MF cases that express CD8+ or other aberrant phenotypes occur occasionally but behave like conventional cases. They should not be confused with rare aggressive CTCLs exhibiting cytotoxic T-cell differentiation.

In addition to tumor cells, MF and SS lesions contain a minor component of immune accessory cells (i.e., Langerhans cells and macrophages) and CD8+ T cells with a cytolytic phenotype. This presumed host response correlates positively with survival and tends to decrease as lesions progress. A favorable response to therapy, such as photopheresis, appears to correlate with normal levels of circulating CD8+ cells.

Molecular Biology
Well-developed MF or SS is a monoclonal T-cell lymphoproliferative disorder. Southern blotting or polymerase chain reaction (PCR) assays demonstrate monoclonal T-cell receptor gene rearrangements. The greater sensitivity of PCR assays allows the demonstration of dominant clonality in many early patch-type lesions of MF. These assays sometimes detect dominant clonality in lesional skin showing only chronic dermatitis histopathologically. These cases are called *clonal dermatitis* and may represent the earliest manifestation of MF because several have progressed to histologically recognizable MF within a few years. However, some cases of clinicopathologically defined early-phase MF lack a detectable monoclonal T-cell population until later in their clinical course. Next-generation, high-throughput T-cell receptor sequencing is emerging as a more sensitive and quantitative alternative to other molecular assays of T-cell clonality.

In addition to aiding initial diagnosis, gene rearrangement analysis has facilitated staging and prognosis. Because some patients without MF or SS can have low levels of circulating Sézary-like cells, and because not all cases of peripheral blood involvement in MF or SS exhibit morphologically recognizable tumor cells, the demonstration of dominant clonality that matches the clone in lesional skin has proved to be a useful diagnostic adjunct. The same holds true for assessing lymph node involvement. T-cell receptor gene rearrangement analysis of MF and SS lymph nodes is more sensitive than histopathology and possesses at least some prognostic relevance. Mutations in more than 80 genes can occur in MF/SS, including those involving T-cell receptor related pathways, *TP53* and *PD1*. In addition to providing insights into pathogenesis and prognosis, these mutations will form the basis of future precision medicine–based treatments.

TNMB Staging
Although several proposed methods have used a weighted extent approach to more accurately determine the MF or SS tumor burden, the preferred approach is the tumor–node–metastasis–blood (TNMB) system, which is detailed in Tables 2 and 3. The original tumor (skin), lymph nodes, and metastasis (visceral organs) version of this system has been modified by the ISCL to incorporate the extent of blood involvement (B classification) into the staging process. Table 2 shows the TNMB classification relevant to MF and SS, and Table 3 shows how this information

TABLE 2	TNMB Classification of Mycosis Fungoides and Sézary Syndrome

Skin (T)

T1	Patches and/or plaques; <10% body surface area
T2	Patches and/or plaques; ≥10% body surface area
T3	Tumors with/without other skin lesions
T4	Generalized erythroderma

Lymph Nodes (N)

N0	Not clinically enlarged; histopathology not required
N1	Clinically enlarged; histopathologically negative
N2	Clinically enlarged; histopathologically equivocal
N3	Clinically enlarged; histopathologically positive

Visceral Organs (M)

M0	No involvement
M1	Involvement

Peripheral Blood (B)

B0	Atypical cells ≤5% of lymphocytes
B1	Atypical cells >5% of lymphocytes
B2	Atypical cells ≥1000/mm^3

T1 and T2 can be subclassified as patch only vs. plaque ± patch. N and B categories can be subclassified as clone positive or negative. For updates, see www.nccn.org.

TABLE 3	TNMB Staging System for Mycosis Fungoides and Sézary Syndrome

STAGE	SKIN	LYMPH NODES	VISCERA	BLOOD
IA	T1	N0	M0	B0–1
IB	T2	N0	M0	B0–1
IIA	T1–2	N1–2	M0	B0–1
IIB	T3	N0–2	M0	B0–1
IIIA	T4	N0–2	M0	B0
IIIB	T4	N0–2	M0	B1
IVA-1	T1–4	N0–2	M0	B2
IVA-2	T1–4	N3	M0	B0–2
IVB	T1–4	N0–3	M1	B0–2

Modified from Olsen E, Vonderheid E, et al: Revisions to the staging and classification of mycosis fungoides and Sézary syndrome: A proposal of the International Society for Cutaneous Lymphomas (ISCL) and the cutaneous lymphoma task force of the European Organization of Research and Treatment of Cancer (EORTC), *Blood* 110(6):1713–1722, 2007. For updates, see www.nccn.org.

is used to determine the stage of disease. The prognostic relevance of this staging system has been supported by numerous studies, and use of the TNMB helps to guide the selection of therapies. For example, early-stage MF is the most amenable to control with topically directed treatments, whereas advanced MF or SS with extracutaneous involvement usually requires systemic therapies or topical plus systemic combinations.

Treatment

Treatment guidelines for CTCL published by the National Comprehensive Cancer Network can be found at www.nccn.org. Rather than cure, which is attained in less than 10% of cases, the goal of MF and SS therapy is to reduce the impact of the skin disease on quality of life. For most patients, this is achieved by reducing pain, itch, and infection and improving clinical appearance. Appearance is affected by the disfigurement of the eruption and the profound degree of scale shedding in some patients. Because the natural history of early-stage MF predicts a virtually normal lifespan, the goal of treatment must be directed at quality of life. For more advanced stages, prolongation of life expectancy may be a reasonable treatment goal.

Regardless of presentation, relief of symptoms should be addressed early. For dryness and scaling, the use of emollient ointments is indicated. These include petrolatum, Aquaphor, and commercially available shortening such as Crisco (an inexpensive alternative).[1] For modest dryness, creams (e.g., Nivea, Cetaphil, Eucerin) can be adequate and more acceptable to patients. Mild superfatted soaps such as Dove and Oil of Olay are recommended. Soap substitutes such as Cetaphil are also acceptable.

Pruritus can be a debilitating symptom of MF or SS. Treatment of the lymphoma is the best treatment for pruritus but can also be addressed with oral agents such as hydroxyzine (Atarax) 25 mg three times daily or diphenhydramine (Benadryl)[1] 25 to 50 mg three times daily as tolerated. Mirtazapine (Remeron),[1] at a dose of 7.5 to 15 mg/day, can help with pruritus and can improve appetite. Aprepitant[1] ([Emend], an antagonist of the NK-1 receptor of substance P) has shown efficacy in MF/SS pruritus. Naltrexone[1] or naloxone,[1] antagonists of the μ-opioid receptor, may also relieve symptoms of itch. Measures to reduce dryness also help to reduce pruritus.

There is emerging evidence to suggest that chronic antigenic stimulation, especially by Staphylococcus species, might drive cutaneous lymphoma in some patients. Some patients may benefit from dilute bleach baths or other topical measures to decrease the burden of pathogenic bacteria on the skin. Secondary infection needs to be treated with appropriate antibiotics. Their selection is guided by results of skin cultures but usually involves coverage of gram-positive organisms.

Phototherapy

Two main phototherapeutic regimens are used to treat CTCLs. Ultraviolet B radiation (290–320-nm broad band or 311-nm narrow band) can be used for patients with patches but not those with well-developed plaques or tumors. Seventy percent of patients achieve total clinical remission, usually within about 3 to 5 months. Another 15% achieve partial remission. Narrow-band UVB usually is more effective than broadband UVB and achieves maximal responses more rapidly. A synthetic form of hypericin (HyBryte)[5] applied topically and activated by visible fluorescent light has undergone clinical trials and is being evaluated for approval by the FDA.

Psoralen–ultraviolet A (PUVA) photochemotherapy uses oral 8-methoxypsoralen (8-MOP), 0.6 mg/kg, as a photosensitizer before UVA (320–400 nm) exposure. Sixty-five percent of patients with patch or plaque disease achieve complete remissions, and 30% have partial responses to this modality. For most patients, maximal responses are achieved within 3 months, and after 5 months, it is unlikely that further improvement will be gained. Limitations of these modalities include actinic damage, photocarcinogenesis, retinal damage (if eyes are not protected), and the inconvenience of getting to phototherapy centers. PUVA also has the risk of nausea and a theoretical risk of cataract induction without proper eye protection.

During the clearing phase of treatment, phototherapy treatments usually are administered three times per week. After

---

[1] Not FDA approved for this indication.
[5] Investigational drug in the United States.

resolution of skin lesions, treatment frequency is usually tapered gradually to once weekly for UVB and once every 4 to 6 weeks for PUVA. These maintenance regimens are often continued for months to years because abrupt cessation of phototherapy is commonly associated with rapid relapse, which is probably related to the persistence of microscopic disease after clinical clearing.

Topical Therapy

Like phototherapeutic regimens, topical therapies are appropriate for disease confined to the skin (stage I). Topical corticosteroids are frequently used for CTCLs, often before diagnosis. Low-potency formulations are useful on the face and skin folds. Medium-potency preparations are appropriate for the trunk and extremities. High-potency formulations are useful for recalcitrant lesions; however, prolonged use of such potent agents can cause local atrophy and adrenal suppression. Roughly half of patients achieve complete remissions, and most others have partial remissions. Response duration varies widely with the individual pace of disease and patient compliance. Topical corticosteroids are particularly useful to ameliorate severe signs and symptoms relatively quickly and as an adjuvant therapy in combination with other primary treatments.

Mechlorethamine (nitrogen mustard, HN_2, Mustargen) is applied topically in an aqueous solution or an ointment, such as Aquaphor. Although these forms are not FDA approved for this indication, a 0.016% gel formulation (Valchlor) is now commercially available and FDA approved. The aqueous form is prepared at home and involves a daily dose totaling 10 mg in 60 mL water. The ointment form is prepared by a pharmacist in 1-pound lots at a concentration of 10-mg mechlorethamine per 100-g ointment. Only the amount of ointment needed to apply a thin layer is used. Either formulation is usually applied at bedtime to lesional skin for limited disease or the entire skin surface (excluding the head unless it is also involved) for more extensive disease. It is then showered off every morning using soap and water. Results are similar to those from PUVA. Advantages include therapy at home and availability in all regions of the country. Disadvantages are daily preparation (aqueous form only), daily application, and possible allergic contact dermatitis (more common with the aqueous preparation). Maximal efficacy is expected within 6 months. Mild flare-ups of disease may occur during the first few months of treatment and probably represent inflammation of subclinical skin lesions, analogous to the clinical accentuation of actinic damage during topical therapy with 5-fluorouracil (Efudex). As with phototherapy, topical mechlorethamine is tapered gradually after remission is achieved to delay clinical relapse.

Carmustine (BCNU, BiCNU)[1] is applied to the total skin surface as an alcohol/aqueous solution (10–20 mg in 60 mL).[6] Complete responses are seen in 85% of patients with stage IA disease (<10% involvement) and 50% of patients with stage IB disease (>10% involvement). Another 10% of patients obtain partial responses. Advantages include those described for nitrogen mustard and reports of success with application only to lesional skin. Disadvantages include skin irritation followed by telangiectasia formation and possible bone marrow suppression necessitating blood monitoring.

A topical gel formulation of the retinoid X receptor (RXR)–specific retinoid, bexarotene (Targretin), is useful for localized or limited skin lesions. The principal side effect is local irritation.

Imiquimod (Aldara) 5% cream is an off-label topical with use supported by small case series and reports. Imiquimod exerts antitumoral activity by modifying the local immune response via toll-like receptor 7 agonism. A thin layer of imiquimod 5% cream is applied to affected areas up to five nights weekly. Side effects include dermatitis and rarely, systemic, flu-like symptoms.

Radiotherapy

Conventional radiotherapy for mycosis fungoides therapy has been used for approximately 100 years. It is most useful in the treatment of isolated, particularly problematic lesions such as recalcitrant tumors or ulcerated plaques. In addition to benefit from the photons delivered by radiotherapy, electron beam therapy (12–36 Gy delivered over 8–12 weeks) is also useful for CTCL therapy. An approximately 85% complete response rate of skin disease with a median duration of 16 months is expected with electron beam therapy. Disadvantages include limited access to required equipment and expertise and cutaneous toxic effects, such as alopecia, sweat gland loss, radiation dermatitis, and skin cancers. As with other skin-directed therapy, the benefit for internal disease is limited. Cumulative toxicity also limits the number of courses a patient may receive. Localized electron beam therapy is also useful for treating cases of limited-extent MF and treating selected problematic MF lesions in patients who are otherwise responding to therapy. After completion of total-skin electron beam therapy, patients require maintenance therapy such as topical mechlorethamine[6] or phototherapy to prolong remission. Low-dose radiotherapy is emerging as an effective alternative to conventional regimens.

Apheresis-Based Therapy

Leukapheresis and particularly lymphocytapheresis (6000–7000 mL of blood treated three times per week initially, then according to response) have been used in the treatment of SS patients. Benefit has been reported in several case reports and small case series; however, response rates are variable. Photopheresis (i.e., extracorporeal photochemotherapy) describes an apheresis-based therapy in which circulating lymphocytes are first exposed to a psoralen (orally or extracorporeally) and then exposed to UVA extracorporeally. In contrast to leukapheresis, in which leukocytes are discarded, all cells are returned to the patient's circulation during photopheresis. Response rates in erythrodermic patients are 33% to 50%, and median survival for SS patients is prolonged from 30 months to more than 60 months. In recent years, extracorporeal photochemotherapy has been used increasingly in conjunction with one or more systemic therapies to enhance efficacy. The toxicity of the systemic agents is diminished because they are often used in combination at reduced doses.

Cytokine Therapy

Pegylated interferon alfa-2a (Pegasys)[1] has replaced interferon alfa-2a and alfa-2b, which have been discontinued. 90 to 180 µg is given subcutaneously or intralesionally once weekly. Response rates are approximately 55%, with complete responses occurring in 10% of patients. Advantages include the relative ease of delivery. Disadvantages include side effects of anorexia, fever, malaise, leukopenia, and risk of cardiac dysrhythmia. An alternative treatment is interferon gamma-1b (Actimmune)[1] (1-2 MU) injected three times weekly. Interferon combined with narrow-band UVB or PUVA is effective for many patients with generalized skin lesions unresponsive to phototherapy alone.

Tumor-Associated Antigen-Directed Therapies

Various specific tumor-associated antigens have been targeted with antibody-based therapy. Less specific targets are CD4, CD5, and IL-2 receptor. Alemtuzumab (Campath)[1] is an antibody directed against CD52. It has shown benefit in advanced-stage disease. This agent can be used alone or in conjunction with multiagent chemotherapy. Brentuximab vedotin (Adcetris) is an anti-CD30 antibody linked to the microtubule toxin monomethyl auristatin E. It can be effective in those cases of MF that express sufficient CD30. Mogamulizumab (Poteligeo) is an antibody directed against CCR4. It is approved for relapsed or refractory MF or SS after at least one other systemic therapy. Pembrolizumab (Keytruda)[1] is an antibody directed against PD1. It can be of benefit for relapsed or refractory MF or SS.

Systemic Chemotherapy
Various regimens of single-agent and multiagent chemotherapy have been used in the treatment of MF and SS. Oral methotrexate, chlorambucil (Leukeran)[1] with or without prednisone,[1] and etoposide (VePesid)[1] have shown therapeutic activity. The best response has been in erythrodermic patients treated with methotrexate (5–125 mg weekly),[3] who have shown a 58% response rate. The combination of low-dose methotrexate and interferon alfa[1] has been reported to yield a high response rate in advanced-stage MF and SS.

The use of multiagent regimens is controversial because of the small number of patients treated with any given regimen. There is even some evidence that for some populations of CTCL patients, survival may be reduced. For individual patients with advanced disease, however, cyclophosphamide (Cytoxan),[1] doxorubicin (Adriamycin),[1] vincristine (Oncovin),[1] and prednisone[1] (CHOP regimen) can provide some short-term palliation. In some cases, CHOP has successfully eradicated large cell transformation of MF and returned patients to their more clinically indolent patch or plaque baseline disease. Idarubicin (Idamycin)[1] in association with etoposide, cyclophosphamide, vincristine, prednisone, and bleomycin (Blenoxane)[1] (VICOP-B regimen) has demonstrated response rates of 80% (36% complete response rate) for patients with stage II through IV disease and 84% for MF patients, with a median duration of response longer than 8 months. Other regimens have been used with more modest success.

Several purine nucleoside analogues have been used for CTCL treatment, including erythrodermic variants. These include 2-chlorodeoxyadenosine (cladribine [Leustatin][1], with a response rate of 28%), 2-deoxycoformycin (pentostatin [Nipent],[1] with a response rate of 39%), and fludarabine (Fludara).[1] Toxicities include pulmonary edema, bone marrow and immune suppression, and neurotoxicity.

Retinoids
Retinoids have therapeutic activity against MF and SS alone and in combination with other therapies, such as interferon alfa or PUVA (the latter combination is called Re-PUVA). Bexarotene (Targretin) is an RXR-specific retinoid with 45% to 55% response rates that carries an FDA approval for advanced stage or refractory MF. The recommended initial starting dose is 300 mg/m², though many clinicians prefer starting at low dose (150 mg daily) and titrating up based on response and side effects. Bexarotene is generally well-tolerated though has known toxicities that require careful monitoring. Side effects include central hypothyroidism, hyperlipidemia, and leukopenia. Bexarotene can increase triglycerides into the thousands, placing patients at risk for pancreatitis, so careful monitoring is required. Nearly all patients require thyroid replacement, and this is often started prophylactically (levothyroxine [Synthroid] at 25–50 mcg daily). Omega-3 fatty acids[7] are recommended for all patients, and lipid-lowering agents (rosuvastatin [Crestor] or fenofibrate are favored) are often required to control triglyceride and low-density-lipoprotein levels.

Arotinoid[5], acitretin (Soriatane)[1], and 13-cis-Retinoic acid (isotretinoin [Accutane])[1] have various degrees of efficacy, and they typically are used in conjunction with other modalities. With all retinoids, clinicians should counsel on the well-known side effects including teratogenicity, xerosis, decreased night vision, and photosensitivity (which is particularly relevant in MF and SS patients who may be concurrently treated with phototherapy).

Enzyme Inhibitors
Vorinostat (Zolinza) is the first histone deacetylase inhibitor to be FDA approved for MF and SS. The overall response rate approaches 40% using a standard oral dose of 400 mg/day. Side effects include gastrointestinal symptoms, thrombocytopenia, and cardiac conduction abnormalities. Romidepsin (Isotodax) is an intravenously administered histone deacetylase inhibitor approved by the FDA for MF and SS. Preclinical studies show that treatment of CTCL cells with romidepsin and birabresib[5] (a BET inhibitor) suppresses oncogenic p73 isoforms and kills CTCL cells. Forodesine[5] is a purine nucleoside phosphorylase inhibitor that preferentially affects T cells because they contain relatively high concentrations of this enzyme. Forodesine has undergone clinical trials for MF and SS in the United States and appears to have a response rate of about 40%.

Miscellaneous Therapies
Various other therapies have been tried for MF and SS with modest success. Nonmyeloablative allogeneic stem cell transplantation has led to favorable responses in some patients; however, the total number treated is small. Cyclosporine (Sandimmune)[1] has been tried for MF and SS. Transient improvement is followed by worsened survival due to immunosuppression, and it is not a recommended therapy. Thymopentin[5] has given excellent results in SS patients (i.e., 40% complete response rate and 35% partial response rate, with a median duration of response of 22 months). The lack of follow-up reports in recent decades leaves the status of this therapy in question. Inhibitors of JAK/STAT and other signal transduction pathways may be useful in patients bearing relevant activating mutations.

Selection of Therapy
Initial choices among conventional treatments for MF and SS depend on the types of lesions and the stage of disease. Disease subsets are followed by recommended initial treatments in parentheses: unilesional or localized MF (local radiation therapy), patch MF (broad- and narrow-band UVB, PUVA, mechlorethamine), patch/plaque MF (PUVA, mechlorethamine), thick plaque/tumor MF (electron beam radiation therapy, interferon alfa-2, bexarotene, histone deacetylase inhibitors), erythrodermic MF/SS (photopheresis), and nodal or visceral MF or SS (interferon alfa-2, bexarotene, histone deacetylase inhibitors, experimental systemic therapies, systemic chemotherapy). Targeted monoclonal antibodies are also indicated for patients with stage IIB or greater disease.

Second-line therapeutic choices often involve interferons, retinoids, or histone deacetylase inhibitors, usually in combination with primary modalities. Multimodality combinations, often at reduced doses, are used commonly to treat patients with stage IIB or more advanced disease. Medium-potency topical corticosteroids, such as 0.1% triamcinolone cream or ointment (Kenalog),[1] are useful adjuncts to many different therapies. The optimal use of newer therapeutic agents in various subtypes and stages of MF and SS is still being established. Evidence-based guidelines for MF and SS therapy have been developed by the National Comprehensive Cancer Network (NCCN) (www.nccn.org).

---

[3] Exceeds dosage recommended by the manufacturer.
[1] Not FDA approved for this indication.
[5] Investigational drug in the United States.
[7] Available as dietary supplement.

---

[1] Not FDA approved for this indication.
[5] Investigational drug in the United States.

Lymphoproliferative Disorders Associated with Mycosis Fungoides and Sézary Syndrome

Types and Clinical Features

Patients with MF or SS are at increased risk for large T-cell lymphomas, lymphomatoid papulosis, and Hodgkin's disease. Molecular biologic analysis has shown that these disorders and MF often share the same clonal T-cell receptor gene rearrangement when they arise in the same individual. As a consequence, they are considered to be subclones of the original MF tumor clone. The development of large T-cell lymphoma in a patient with MF or SS is referred to as *large cell transformation of MF*. This occurs in up to 20% of cases in some series and is associated with a median survival of only 1 to 2 years. One-half of these large T-cell lymphomas are CD30+; however, the generally favorable prognosis of primary cutaneous CD30+ anaplastic large cell lymphoma does not seem to extend to these secondary forms of CD30+ lymphoma. These patients may need to be treated with systemic chemotherapy such as CHOP or with experimental systemic therapies appropriate for advanced-stage CTCL.

Lymphomatoid papulosis manifests as recurrent, usually generalized crops of spontaneously regressing, erythematous papules that can exhibit crusting or vesiculation before resolution. It is the clinically benign end of a disease continuum that has primary cutaneous CD30+ anaplastic large cell lymphoma at its other extreme. Intermediate forms of disease can occur. Histopathologically, lesions contain a mixed-cell infiltrate, including large, atypical T cells that resemble Reed-Sternberg cells and their mononuclear variants (so-called type A) or large MF-type cells (so-called type B). Type A cells are CD30+. A type C form is also recognized. It has sheets of type A cells histologically mimicking CD30+ large T-cell lymphoma but is different from it clinically. A type D variant containing CD8+ CD30+ large atypical cells has also been described recently, as well as a few other rare subtypes. All types of lymphomatoid papulosis behave similarly. Patients with lymphomatoid papulosis sometimes respond to tetracycline[1], mumps antigen[1] or erythromycin[1] (500 mg PO bid), presumably on the basis of antiinflammatory activity. Most cases improve within 1 month with low-dose methotrexate (10–20 mg PO every week). PUVA and narrow-band UVB given three times per week are other therapeutic options.

Treatment

In most cases, non-MF/SS CTCLs are treated with radiation therapy (with or without complete surgical excision) if they are localized or with various multiagent systemic chemotherapy regimens if they are generalized. The roles of other agents remain to be defined, except that studies have proved that methotrexate (10–40 mg PO every week) is effective therapy for most cases of primary cutaneous CD30+ anaplastic large cell lymphoma. Therapies being investigated for this lymphoma include anti-CD30 antibodies, alone or conjugated to toxins. One of these antibody conjugates (brentuximab vedotin [Adcetris]) is FDA approved for primary cutaneous anaplastic large cell lymphomas and CD30+ MF. Denileukin diftitox ([Ontak] not currently available) and histone deacetylase inhibitors have been reported to be effective against some subcutaneous panniculitic T-cell lymphomas. The recent discovery of JAK fusion mutations in aggressive epidermotropic cytotoxic CTCL (Berti's lymphoma) suggests that JAK inhibitors might be beneficial in this rare disorder.

---

[1]Not FDA approved for this indication.

References

Dai J, Duvic M: Cutaneous T-Cell Lymphoma: Current and Emerging Therapies, *Oncology (Williston Park)* 37(2):55–62, 2023, https://doi.org/10.46883/2023.25920984. PMID: 36862846.

Jawed SI, Myskowski PL, Horwitz S, Moskowitz A, Querfeld C: Primary cutaneous T-cell lymphoma (mycosis fungoides and Sézary syndrome): part I. Diagnosis: clinical and histopathologic features and new molecular and biologic markers, J Am Acad Dermatol 70(2):205.e1–16, 2014; quiz 221–2. https://doi.org/10.1016/j.jaad.2013.07.049. PMID: 24438969.

Olsen E, Vonderheid E, et al: Revisions to the staging and classification of mycosis fungoides and Sézary syndrome: A proposal of the International Society for Cutaneous Lymphomas (ISCL) and the cutaneous lymphoma task force of the European Organization of Research and Treatment of Cancer (EORTC), *Blood* 110(6):1713–1722, 2007.

Park J, Daniels J, Wartewig T, et al: Integrated genomic analyses of cutaneous T-cell lymphomas reveal the molecular bases for disease heterogeneity, *Blood* 138(14):1225–1236, 2021.

Pimpinelli N, Olsen EA, Santucci M, et al: Defining early mycosis fungoides, *J Am Acad Dermatol* 53(6):1053–1063, 2005.

Richardson SK, Lin JH, Vittorio CC, et al: High clinical response rate with multimodality immunomodulatory therapy for Sézary syndrome, *Clin Lymphoma Myeloma* 7(3):226–232, 2006.

Vonderheid EC, Bernengo MG, Burg G, et al: Update on erythrodermic cutaneous T-cell lymphoma: Report of the International Society for Cutaneous Lymphomas, *J Am Acad Dermatol* 46(1):95–106, 2002.

Willemze R, Cerroni L, Kempf W, et al: The 2018 update of the WHO-EORTC classification for primary cutaneous lymphomas, *Blood* 133(16):1703–1714, 2019.

Wood GS, Greenberg HL: Diagnosis, staging, and monitoring of cutaneous T-cell lymphoma, *Dermatol Ther* 16(4):269–275, 2003.

Zhao L, Xiao T, Stonesifer C, Daniels J, et al: The Robust Tumoricidal Effects of Combined BET and HDAC Inhibition in CTCL Can Be Reproduced by ΔNp73 Depletion, *J Invest Dermatol* 142:3253–3261, 2022.

CUTANEOUS VASCULITIS

Method of
Molly A. Hinshaw, MD; and Susan Lawrence-Hylland, MD

CURRENT DIAGNOSIS

- Cutaneous vasculitis can be limited to skin (leukocytoclastic vasculitis) or associated with systemic disease.
- Perform punch biopsy of intact, nonulcerated skin lesion.
- "Vasculitis" on skin biopsy describes vessel appearance and is not a clinical diagnosis.
- Thorough review of systems and physical examination are necessary to evaluate for systemic vasculitis.

CURRENT THERAPY

Leukocytoclastic Vasculitis
- First identify instigating factors: infection, medications.
- Care is symptomatic. Lesions typically remit without treatment.
- If needed, short course of prednisone may be given and tapered over 3 to 6 weeks.

All Forms of Vasculitis
- Treat underlying systemic vasculitis.

Vasculitis is an inflammatory-mediated destruction of blood vessels. The systemic vasculitides have historically been differentiated by their involvement of small, medium, or large blood vessels. Names used to describe isolated cutaneous vasculitis have included hypersensitivity vasculitis and leukocytoclastic vasculitis (LCV). In 1990, the American College of Rheumatology proposed five criteria for the classification of hypersensitivity vasculitis: age older than 16 years, possible drug trigger, palpable purpura, maculopapular rash, and skin biopsy showing neutrophils around vessel. At least three out of five criteria yield a sensitivity of 71% and specificity of 84%. In 1994, a new nomenclature proposed at the Chapel Hill International Consensus Conference in North Carolina further classified vasculitis (Box 1). The term "hypersensitivity vasculitis" was not used, because most vasculitides that would have previously been in this category fall into either microscopic polyangiitis or cutaneous LCV. LCV is vasculitis restricted to the skin without involvement of vessels in other organs. Cutaneous vasculitis may be a clue to systemic vasculitis and guides the clinician to a comprehensive evaluation (Table 1).

Vasculitis can affect almost any organ, and once affected, end organs can become dysfunctional. Such dysfunction may be as innocuous as cutaneous, tender, transient papules or as devastating as a stroke. A thorough evaluation of the patient with a complete review of systems, physical examination, laboratory evaluation, and clinical follow-up allows a distinction to be made between the different forms of vasculitis.

Leukocytoclastic Vasculitis

Epidemiology
LCV is common. The incidence and prevalence are unknown. Mean age of onset ranges from 34 to 49 years of age. The female-to-male ratio ranges from approximately 2:1 to 3:1.

Risk Factors
LCV is often secondary to a known trigger including infection, drug ingestion, or malignancy. LCV can also be a presenting feature of autoimmune disease.

Pathophysiology
LCV is best characterized as immune complex–mediated inflammatory destruction of the postcapillary venules of any organ. The exact mechanisms of vascular destruction is unknown.

Clinical Manifestations
LCV typically manifests as nonblanchable macules that evolve to papules or, less commonly, pustules and ulcers (Figure 1). Clues to

BOX 1	Chapel Hill Consensus 1994 Classification of Vasculitis

Large-Vessel Vasculitis
Giant cell arteritis
   Takayasu's arteritis

Medium-Vessel Vasculitis
Classic polyarteritis nodosa
   Kawasaki's disease

Small-Vessel Vasculitis
Churg-Strauss syndrome
   Cutaneous leukocytoclastic vasculitis
   Essential cryoglobulinemia
   Henoch-Schönlein purpura
   Microscopic polyangiitis (polyarteritis)
   Wegener's granulomatosis

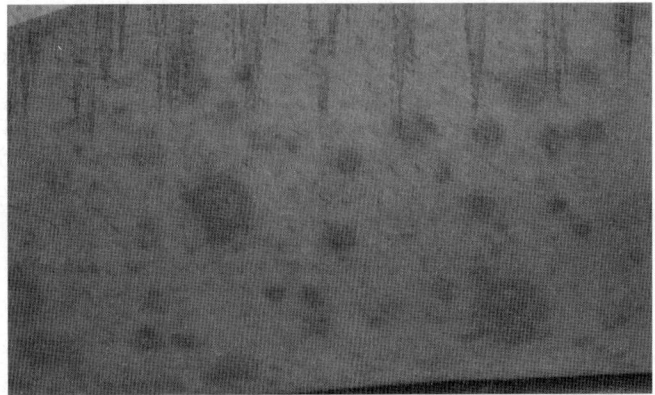

Figure 1 Leukocytoclastic vasculitis: palpable, purpuric, nonblanching, erythematous to ruddy-brown thin papules. Additional secondary changes include small pustules (pustular vasculitis) or shallow, small ulcerations.

TABLE 1	Diseases with Cutaneous Vasculitis as a Component of Their Presentation	
DISEASE	**SKIN LESIONS**	**CLUES AND CONFIRMATION**
Urticarial vasculitis	Individual lesions look like urticaria but last >24 h; typical urticaria last a few hours, always <24 h Pruritus, burning of skin lesions	May be associated with connective tissue disease, medications, low complement, viral infections (e.g., hep B, hep C, EBV) Skin biopsy
Henoch-Schönlein purpura	Wheals progress to petechia, ecchymoses and palpable purpura Lesions are in gravity-dependent or pressure-dependent areas such as legs or the buttocks in toddlers	Arthralgia or arthritis, hematuria, abdominal pain, melena Skin biopsy and DIF for IgA
Essential mixed cryoglobulinemia	Palpable purpura	Peripheral neuropathy, GN Hep C positive Serum cryoglobulins
Wegener's granulomatosis	Palpable purpura, hemorrhagic lesions, petechiae, skin ulcers	c-ANCA >80% Pulmonary hemorrhage, GN Biopsy affected organ
Churg-Strauss syndrome	Maculopapular rash, palpable purpura, hemorrhagic lesions, subcutaneous nodules, livedo reticularis or Raynaud's disease	ANCA (50%) Asthma, allergic rhinitis Eosinophilia >1.5 × 10⁹/L Pulmonary infiltrates, pulmonary neuropathy Biopsy affected organ
Microscopic polyangiitis	Palpable purpura, hemorrhagic lesions, petechiae, skin ulcers, splinter hemorrhages	p-ANCA >60% Pulmonary hemorrhage, GN Biopsy affected organ
Polyarteritis nodosa	Livedo reticularis, tender nodules, skin ulcers, bullae or vesicles	Hypertension, elevated creatinine, abdominal pain, constitutional symptoms (fever) Abnormal angiogram Biopsy affected organ

Abbreviations: c-ANCA = classic antineutrophil cytoplasmic antibody; DIF = direct immunofluorescence; EBV = Epstein-Barr virus; GN = glomerulonephritis; hep = hepatitis; Ig = immunoglobulin; p-ANCA = protoplasmic-staining antineutrophil cytoplasmic antibody.

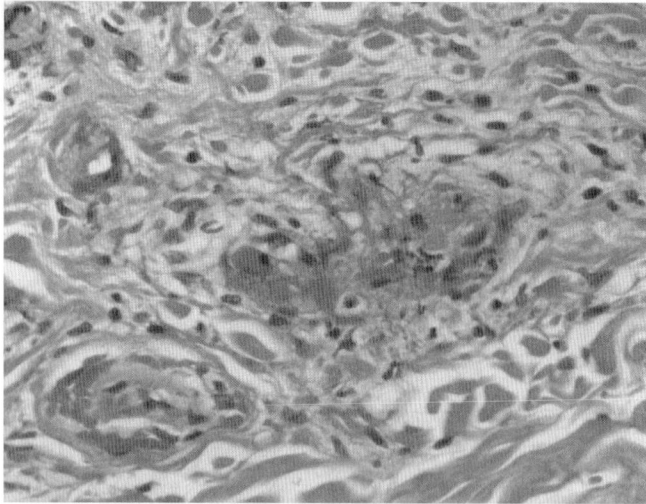

Figure 2 Biopsy of intact clinical lesion of leukocytoclastic vasculitis. Histology shows destruction of postcapillary venules with fibrin deposition, degenerate inflammatory cells, and extravasated erythrocytes.

the diagnosis include a monomorphous, ruddy-brown appearance owing to leakage of hemosiderin pigment from vessels. Lesions measure a few millimeters to a few centimeters in diameter. LCV is often localized to the lower extremities but may be diffuse. Pruritus, pain, or burning of the skin lesions are indicators that the patient might have a vasculitis extending beyond LCV.

Diagnosis
To confirm a clinical impression of LCV, perform a punch biopsy in the center of a nonulcerated cutaneous lesion that is less than 24 to 48 hours old and submit the sample in 10% formalin (standard medium). It is important to biopsy an intact, nonulcerated active lesion (Figure 2) because ulcers can show histologic features simulating vasculitis regardless of whether the patient has true vasculitis or not.

Pathology reveals a mononuclear or polymorphonuclear inflammation of the small blood vessels (called LCV), most prominent in the postcapillary venules. The appearance may be necrotizing or non-necrotizing.

Differential Diagnosis
LCV manifests as erythematous papules or occasionally as papulopustules that can simulate a variety of entities (see Table 1). The review of systems and physical examination should be directed to evaluate for diseases that have cutaneous vasculitis as a component of their presentation (see Table 1). All patients with LCV should have a urinalysis to evaluate for hematuria as a sign of kidney involvement, with subsequent evaluation and management if identified.

Treatment
The primary goal in the management of LCV is to identify and treat instigating factors, including infection and medications. Supportive treatment includes resting, elevating legs, and wearing support hose. When review of systems, physical examination, and urinalysis do not reveal associated systemic diseases, treatment of LCV is generally not necessary. Lesions typically remit without treatment. In rare patients with symptomatic, extensively pustular, or progressive lesions, a short course of prednisone[1] dosed at 1 mg/kg/day initially and tapered over 3 to 6 weeks may be used, although no controlled trials have been performed using oral corticosteroids for isolated LCV. Rapid steroid taper can lead to rebound. Systematic evaluation of the use of other medications,

[1]Not FDA approved for this indication.

such as colchicine[1] or dapsone,[1] to treat isolated LCV has not been performed.

Monitoring
Patients with LCV are at risk for recurrent or chronic vasculitis. In addition, apparent LCV can occur as a systemic disease that is not recognizable at the first episode. Patients with persistent or recurrent LCV require follow-up to ensure disease clearance, to monitor for medication side effects, and to evaluate for evolving disorders known to be associated with cutaneous vasculitis (see Table 1).

Complications
Isolated LCV generally resolves without sequelae. However, pustular or ulcerative LCV may be complicated by local sequelae such as cutaneous ulcerations and scars.

Cutaneous Vasculitis Associated with Systemic Vasculitis
Cutaneous vasculitis may be a component of the presentation of multiple diseases (see Table 1). When a clinician reads a pathology report from a biopsy of a skin lesion that states "vasculitis," it is important to realize that this term is a descriptor of the histopathology. It is the clinician's challenge to determine whether "vasculitis" is as potentially innocuous as LCV or part of a more severe systemic disease. Symptoms that are clues to a systemic process can include fever, arthralgias, myalgias, anorexia, abdominal pain, pulmonary abnormalities, or neurologic symptoms.

Skin biopsy may aid in the diagnosis of a systemic vasculitis (Henoch-Schönlein purpura), but biopsy of an affected end organ may be necessary to confirm a diagnosis. Pathology focuses on the confirmation of vasculitis in a small, medium, or large vessel.

Aside from Henoch-Schönlein purpura, treatment of systemic vasculitis is typically much more aggressive than treatment of LCV and should be pursued in conjunction with involvement of a rheumatologist, nephrologist, or pulmonologist. Systemic disease leads to severe complications including renal failure, pulmonary damage, permanent vascular disease, or neurologic insult depending on the viscera affected.

[1]Not FDA approved for this indication.

References
Gayraud M, Guillevin L, le Toumelin P, et al: Long-term followup of polyarteritis nodosa, microscopic polyangiitis, and Churg-Strauss syndrome: Analysis of four prospective trials including 278 patients, *Arthritis Rheum* 44:666–675, 2001.
Hannon CW, Swerlick RA: Vasculitis. In Bolognia J, Jorizzo J, Rapini R, editors: Dermatology, vol 1. St Louis, 2003, Mosby, pp 381–402.
Hoffman GS, Kerr GS, Leavitt RY, et al: Wegener granulomatosis: An analysis of 158 patients, *Ann Intern Med* 116:488–498, 1992.
Jennette JC, Thomas DB, Falk RJ: Microscopic polyangiitis (microscopic polyarteritis), *Semin Diagn Pathol* 18:3–13, 2001.
Jenette JC, Falk RF, Andrassy K, et al: Nomenclature of systemic vasculitides. Proposal of an international consensus conference, *Arthritis Rheum* 37(2):187–192, 1994.

DISEASES OF THE HAIR

Method of
Dirk M. Elston, MD

CURRENT DIAGNOSIS

- A sudden increase in shedding most commonly represents telogen effluvium.
- Hair thinning is more likely to represent pattern alopecia.
- Scarring alopecia generally requires a biopsy for diagnosis.
- Most medically significant hirsutism results from polycystic ovarian syndrome.
- New-onset virilization suggests the possibility of a tumor.

CURRENT THERAPY

- Pattern alopecia in men is treated with oral finasteride (Propecia), low-dose oral minoxidil[1] or topical minoxidil (Rogaine), or both.
- Pattern alopecia in women is treated with antiandrogens (such as spironolactone [Aldactone][1]) and oral[1] or topical minoxidil. Platelet-rich plasma injections may be of benefit in both men and women.
- Alopecia areata can require intralesional corticosteroid injections, topical immunotherapy, or therapy with agents such as methotrexate (Trexall)[1] or Janus kinase (JAK) inhibitors.
- A scalp biopsy is critical to guide therapy in scarring alopecia.
- Hirsutism may be treated with laser epilation or systemic antiandrogens. Topical eflornithine (Vaniqa) can slow regrowth of hair.

Epidemiology

Hair disorders are common, with more than half of the population affected by pattern alopecia and the prevalence of hirsutism varying significantly by ethnicity.

Risk Factors

Most causes of alopecia and hirsutism are genetically determined.

Pathophysiology

Pattern alopecia relates to increased sensitivity to dihydrotestosterone. Telogen effluvium relates to an alteration in the normal hair cycle, with many hairs shedding synchronously. Alopecia areata represents an inflammatory insult directed against melanocytes in the hair bulb. There is strong evidence that the disease is mediated by Th1 lymphocytes. Polycystic ovarian syndrome is an insulin-resistance syndrome resulting in excess production of androgens.

Prevention

Little can be done to prevent hair disorders, so the focus is generally on diagnosis and treatment.

Clinical Manifestations

Pattern alopecia manifests with apical scalp thinning. In men, receding of the hairline at the temples is typical, whereas women demonstrate widening of the part but retain the anterior hairline. Telogen effluvium manifests with diffuse shedding of telogen hairs (hairs with a nonpigmented bulb). Alopecia areata typically occurs with patchy hair loss. Shed hairs demonstrate tapered fracture at the base. Syphilitic alopecia resembles alopecia areata but often affects smaller areas, with only partial hair loss, resulting in a moth-eaten appearance. Scarring alopecia shows permanent areas of smooth alopecia lacking follicular openings.

Polycystic ovarian syndrome manifests with evidence of anovulation and excess androgen production. Signs of virilization suggesting a possible tumor include new onset of hirsutism, deepening of the voice, change in body habitus, and clitoromegaly.

Diagnosis

Alopecia

The first step is to determine whether a hair shaft abnormality exists (Box 1). This is particularly important in Black patients, in whom trichorrhexis nodosa is a common cause of hair loss. Trichorrhexis nodosa results from overprocessing of the hair. Hair density is normal at the level of the scalp, but hairs break off, leaving patches of short hair.

The next step is to determine whether telogen effluvium exists. Telogen effluvium manifests with increased shedding of hairs with a blunt nonpigmented bulb (Figure 1), and it commonly follows an illness, surgery, delivery, or crash diet by 3 to 5 months. Hairs

---

BOX 1 Diagnosis of Alopecia

Trichodystrophy

Types
- Trichorrhexis nodosa
- Inherited trichodystrophies
- Fractures

Causes
- Alopecia areata
- Chemotherapy
- Heavy metal

Determine Type

Anagen Effluvium
Tapered fractures can be caused by
- Alopecia areata
- Chemotherapy
- Heavy metal
  Loose anagen can be caused by
- Loose anagen syndrome
- Easily extractable anagen in scarring alopecia

Telogen Effluvium
Increased shedding of club hairs can be caused by
- Diet, illness
- Pregnancy
- Medication
- Papulosquamous disorders
- Pattern alopecia

Diagnosis

Laboratory Studies
- Iron
- Thyroid-stimulating hormone
- Endocrine studies in virilized women

Biopsy

Nonscarring types
- Telogen effluvium
- Pattern alopecia
- Alopecia areata

Scarring types
- Lupus erythematosus
- Lichen planopilaris
- Folliculitis decalvans

Other Permanent Alopecia
- Idiopathic pseudopelade
- Morphea

---

can often be easily extracted with a gentle hair pull or 1 minute of combing. The presence of tapered fracture suggests alopecia areata, syphilis, or heavy metal poisoning. Alopecia areata can result in diffuse hair loss, but it more commonly manifests with well-defined round patches of hair loss. The skin is either normal or salmon pink. Syphilis more often shows a moth-eaten pattern of alopecia (Figure 2).

Most patients with hair loss need only limited laboratory testing or none at all. Thyroid disorders and iron deficiency are common, and testing for them is relatively inexpensive. I recommend them when telogen effluvium is present. Their presence can also accelerate the course of pattern alopecia, and it is reasonable to test for them in women with this disorder. Thyroid-stimulating hormone is the best screen for thyroid disorders. The role of iron deficiency in telogen hair loss is controversial, but iron deficiency is common, easily established, and inexpensive to correct. Iron status also serves as an indicator of overall nutritional status. Although a low ferritin level proves iron deficiency, ferritin behaves as an acute phase reactant and a normal level does not

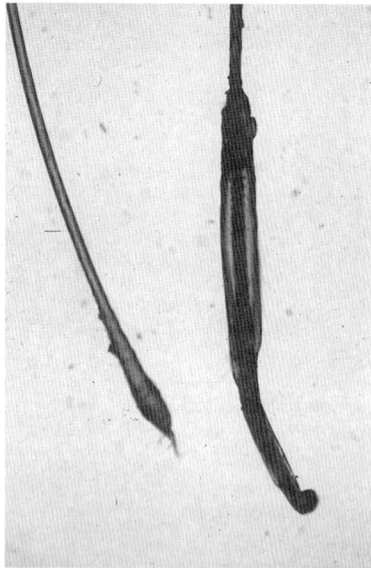

Figure 1 Telogen hair on *left*, anagen hair on *right* for comparison.

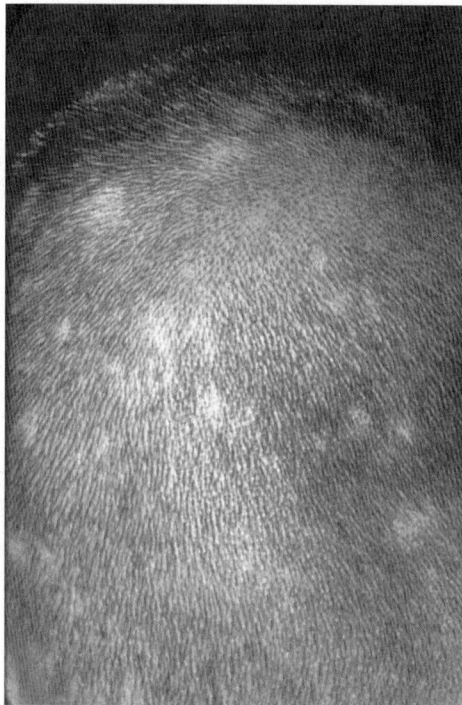

Figure 2 Moth-eaten syphilitic alopecia.

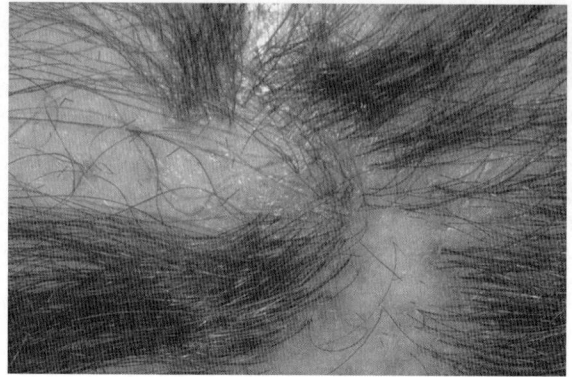

Figure 3 Scarring alopecia secondary to chronic cutaneous lupus erythematosus.

rule out iron deficiency. Therefore, I recommend measurement of ferritin, serum iron, iron binding capacity, and saturation.

A scalp biopsy is required in any patient with scarring alopecia. It may also be necessary in other patients if history and physical examination do not establish a diagnosis and the alopecia is progressive. The scalp biopsy should be performed with a 4-mm biopsy punch oriented parallel to the direction of hair growth. Collagen hemostatic sponge (Gelfoam and others) can be placed into the resulting hole to stop bleeding and eliminate the need for sutures. The biopsy should be done in a well-established but still active area of inflammation if one can be identified. A combination of vertical and transverse sections increases the diagnostic yield and is usually recommended. In patients with scarring alopecia, half of the vertically bisected specimen should be sent for direct immunofluorescence. An additional biopsy of an end-stage scarred area can demonstrate characteristic patterns of scarring with an elastic tissue stain. This can help distinguish among causes of scarring alopecia such as lupus erythematosus (Figure 3), lichen planopilaris, pseudopelade, and folliculitis decalvans.

Hirsutism

Patients with new-onset virilization should be evaluated to rule out an ovarian or adrenal tumor. Ovarian and adrenal imaging studies and a total testosterone level are the best screens. A total testosterone more than 200 ng/dL or dehydroepiandrostenedione sulfate (DHEAS) more than 8000 ng/dL suggests tumor. In patients with physical signs of Cushing disease, a 24-hour urine cortisol should be obtained. Most patients with *chronic* medically significant hirsutism have polycystic ovarian syndrome (PCOS). The diagnosis is established by means of history and physical examination, and the most important laboratory tests are serum lipids and fasting glucose to establish associated cardiac risk factors. A clinical diagnosis of PCOS requires the presence of hirsutism, acne or pattern alopecia, and evidence of anovulation (fewer than nine periods per year or cycles longer than 40 days). Ratios of luteinizing hormone (LH) to follicle-stimulating hormone (FSH) have poor sensitivity and specificity for diagnosing PCOS. Imaging for ovarian cysts seldom affects management.

Differential Diagnosis

Syphilis can mimic alopecia areata, and serologic testing should be performed in any sexually active patient with a new diagnosis of alopecia areata. Correct diagnosis of scarring alopecia depends of a thorough examination for other cutaneous signs of lupus erythematosus or lichen planus as well as the results of a skin biopsy.

Tinea capitis can occur as inflammatory boggy areas with hair loss (kerion) or with subtle seborrheic-type scale and black-dot areas of hair loss. A potassium hydroxide (KOH) examination can be performed by rubbing the affected area with moist gauze and examining broken hairs that cling to the gauze.

Hirsutism should be distinguished from hypertrichosis. Hirsutism is a male pattern of hair growth occurring in a woman and is hormonal in nature. Hypertrichosis is excess hair growth that occurs outside of an androgen-dependent distribution. It can be found in metabolic disorders such as porphyria or may be a sign of internal malignancy (Figure 4).

Nonclassic 21-hydroxylase deficiency accounts for up to 10% of patients with medically significant hirsutism. Screening with a baseline morning 17-OH-progesterone is associated with many false positive results. A stimulated 17-OH-progesterone is more specific, but the results of testing seldom affect management because outcomes with dexamethasone (Decadron)[1] are no better than with spironolactone (Aldactone).[1]

Treatment

Alopecia

Telogen effluvium commonly resolves spontaneously once the cause has been eliminated. Poor diet and papulosquamous diseases of the scalp such as seborrheic dermatitis and psoriasis can perpetuate a telogen effluvium and should be treated. The importance of a diet containing adequate protein and trace minerals should be emphasized. Deficiencies and thyroid abnormalities should be addressed. Seborrheic dermatitis responds to topical corticosteroids. Medicated shampoos containing selenium sulfide

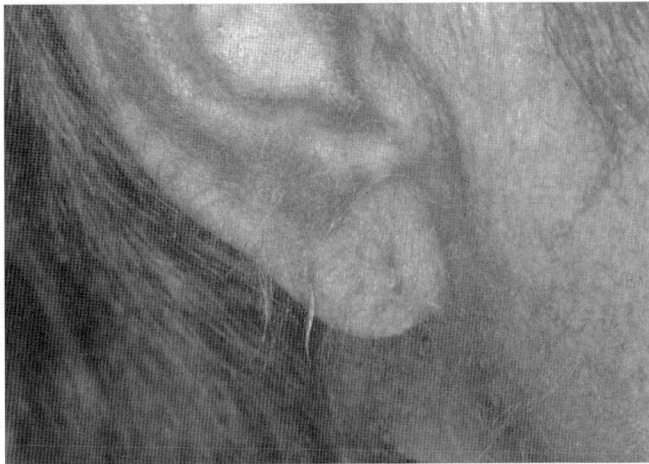

Figure 4 Malignant hypertrichosis secondary to ovarian cancer.

TABLE 1	Treatment of Tinea Capitis	
ANTIFUNGAL AGENT	**DOSAGE**	**USUAL DURATION OF THERAPY**
Griseofulvin (Fulvicin U/F)	Required dosages are often higher than reflected in the product label; 4–10 mg/kg/day is a good starting dosage	1 month or more
Fluconazole (Diflucan)[1]	5–6 mg/kg/day; adult: 200 mg/day	1 month or more
Itraconazole (Sporanox)[1]	3–5 mg/kg/day; adult: 200 mg/day	1 week, repeated monthly until cured
Terbinafine (Lamisil)	Patient <20 kg: 62.5 mg/day Patient 20–40 kg: 125 mg/day Patient >40 kg: 250 mg/day	1 month or more

[1]Not FDA approved for this indication.

(Selsun Blue) or zinc pyrithione (T/Gel Daily Control) can be helpful. Scalp psoriasis can require more potent topical steroids such as fluocinonide solution (Lidex) and calcipotriene (Dovonex) applied on weekends or daily. Systemic agents such as methotrexate (Trexall)[1] at doses of 7.5 to 20 mg once weekly may be required to control severe scalp psoriasis.

Pattern alopecia in men is mediated by dihydrotestosterone (DHT). Men with pattern alopecia may be treated with daily topical minoxidil 2% to 5% (Rogaine), oral minoxidil (Loniten)[1] in doses from 0.5 to 5 mg daily, and oral finasteride (Propecia) at a dose of 1 mg daily. In women, the pathogenesis is complex, and adrenal androgens may play a larger role. Finasteride[1] is of less benefit in the majority of women with pattern alopecia. Spironolactone[1] 100 mg twice daily can be helpful and may be combined with oral minoxidil.[1] In women of childbearing potential, spironolactone should always be used in conjunction with an oral contraceptive. Side effects are uncommon but can include urinary frequency, irregular periods, dyspareunia, and nausea. Most patients demonstrate a minor increase in serum potassium. Those with kidney failure are at risk for life-threatening potassium retention. Topical 2% minoxidil can also be of benefit, and some women derive added benefit from the 5% formulation. All patients with pattern alopecia should be evaluated for superimposed causes of telogen effluvium such as inadequate diet and seborrheic dermatitis.

Tinea capitis is often overlooked in adults and Black children, in whom the manifestations of inflammation can be subtle. Black dot and seborrheic tinea are common in Black children. Patchy hair loss is an important clue to the diagnosis. Treatment is summarized in Table 1.

Localized patches of alopecia areata respond to intralesional injections of triamcinolone hexacetonide (Aristospan) (2.5–5 mg/mL) given once per month. Approximately 0.1 mL/cm² is injected to a maximum of 3 mL during any one session. Minoxidil solution produces slow regrowth in some patients who cannot tolerate other treatments. Anthralin (Dritho-Scalp 0.5%)[1] is sometimes used in children. It is applied 30 minutes before showering. It can stain skin and anything else it touches.

Topical immunotherapy with dinitrochlorobenzene (DNCB),[1] squaric acid dibutylester (SADBE),[1] or diphenylcyclopropenone (DPCP)[1] is more effective than either minoxidil or anthralin. DNCB is mutagenic in the Ames assay and none of the topical immunotherapies are currently approved for human use. A 2% solution of the sensitizer is applied to the arm in acetone to induce initial sensitization. Subsequently, diluted solutions, starting at about 0.001%, are applied weekly to the scalp with a cotton-tipped applicator. Roughly 20% to 60% of patients have responded to this regimen in various studies.

Baricitinib (Olumiant), tofacitinib (Xeljanz)[1] and other JAK inhibitors are often effective in patients with refractory alopecia areata. Biologic agents have shown mixed results. Methotrexate[1] in psoriatic doses (7.5–20 mg weekly for an adult) can be effective. Sulfasalazine (Azulfidine)[1] is sometimes effective in doses ranging from 500 to 1500 mg three times a day.[3] Patients should be encouraged to read about new therapies on the National Alopecia Areata Foundation website (https://www.naaf.org).

Early, aggressive therapy for discoid lupus erythematosus is recommended to prevent permanent scarring. Topical corticosteroids are rarely sufficient. Intralesional injections are performed in a manner similar to that described earlier. Initial control of severe disease can be achieved with a single 3-week tapered course of oral prednisone at a dose of 60 mg daily for the first week, 40 mg daily for the second week, and 20 mg daily for the third week. Intralesional steroid injections or a systemic steroid-sparing agent are required for maintenance therapy. Systemic agents that can be effective include antimalarials, dapsone,[1] methotrexate,[1] mycophenolate mofetil (CellCept)[1], and thalidomide (Thalomid).[1] I generally begin treatment with hydroxychloroquine (Plaquenil)[1] at a dose of 400 mg daily for an adult. Dapsone is used at a dose of 100 mg daily for an average sized adult, not to exceed 5 mg/kg. Thalidomide has been used effectively at doses of 50 to 100 mg daily, but peripheral neuropathy and teratogenicity limit its use. Mycophenolate mofetil is used at a dose of 1 g twice daily, and methotrexate is used at doses of 7.5 to 20 mg weekly. Background pattern (androgenetic) alopecia should be treated as well.

End-stage cicatricial alopecia is best treated by scalp reduction and hair transplantation. The disease can flare up in response to surgery, and it is best to plan a 3-week tapered course of pred-nisone[1] or a month of cyclosporine (Neoral)[1] to help prevent the flare.

Lichen planopilaris is treated in a manner similar to lupus, except that hydroxychloroquine[1] is of less benefit and oral retinoids (acitretin [Soriatane][1] at doses of 25 to 50 mg daily) are more likely to be successful. Topical calcineurin inhibitors can be effective in achieving and maintaining remission. A few months of pioglitazone (Actos)[1] can induce remission in a subset of patients and the frontal fibrosing alopecia variant can respond to dutasteride (Avodart).[1] Patients should be aware of the risks associated with each of these treatments, including bladder cancer and hypospadias in a male fetus. Mycophenolate mofetil (CellCept)[1] 1 g twice daily or a JAK inhibitor may be effective when other treatments fail, and excimer laser can also be effective for lichen planopilaris. It is contraindicated in lupus erythematosus.

Folliculitis decalvans manifests with crops of pustules that result in permanent scarring. Patients respond to weekend applications

[1]Not FDA approved for this indication.

[3]Exceeds dosage recommended by the manufacturer.

of clobetasol (Clobex, Olux) together with prolonged use of antistaphylococcal antibiotics such as doxycycline (Doryx)[1] 100 mg twice daily.

Hirsutism

Treatment options include laser epilation, eflornithine (Vaniqa) cream to reduce the rate of hair growth, or spironolactone[1] at a starting dose of 100 mg twice daily as described for pattern alopecia. Cyproterone acetate is used in some countries but is not available in the United States. Other options that are less commonly used include insulin sensitizers, flutamide (Eulexin),[1] metformin (Glucophage),[1] and leuprolide (Lupron)[1] plus estrogen.[1]

Monitoring

Patients treated with topical or intralesional corticosteroids should be monitored for cutaneous atrophy. Patients on JAK inhibitors should have quarterly evaluations of blood count, chemistries, and lipids. Those on hydroxychloroquine should be monitored for ocular toxicity, including corneal deposits and retinal damage, although these are very rare at usual doses. They should also be monitored periodically for thrombocytopenia, agranulocytosis, and hepatitis. Patients beginning dapsone therapy should be screened for G6PD deficiency. Potential side effects include hemolysis, methemoglobinemia, and neuropathy. Monitoring includes periodic blood count assessment and measurement of strength and sensation. Mycophenolate mofetil can produce pancytopenia, and blood counts should be monitored. Methotrexate is cleared by the kidneys, and kidney function should be assessed at baseline. Periodic assessment of liver-function tests and blood count is warranted, as is a yearly chest radiograph. I also monitor procollagen 3 terminal peptide levels quarterly to assess the risk of hepatic fibrosis. Patients on antiandrogen therapy should be monitored for dyspareunia resulting from vulvar atrophy.

Complications

Patients with pattern alopecia and PCOS have a greater risk of metabolic syndrome with cardiac complications. They should be evaluated for lipid abnormalities and glucose intolerance and treated appropriately.

---

[1] Not FDA approved for this indication.

References

Brown J, Farquhar C, Lee O, et al: Spironolactone versus placebo or in combination with steroids for hirsutism and/or acne, *Cochrane Database Syst Rev* 2:CD000194, 2009.

Buzney E, Sheu J, Buzney C, Reynolds RV: Polycystic ovary syndrome: a review for dermatologists: Part II. Treatment, *J Am Acad Dermatol* 71(5):859.e1–859.e15, 2014.

Durdu M, Ozcan D, Baba M, Seckin D: Efficacy and safety of diphenylcyclopropenone alone or in combination with anthralin in the treatment of chronic extensive alopecia areata: a retrospective case series, *J Am Acad Dermatol* 72:640–650, 2015.

Elston DM, Ferringer T, Dalton S, et al: A comparison of vertical versus transverse sections in the evaluation of alopecia biopsy specimens, *J Am Acad Dermatol* 53(2):267–272, 2005.

Fukumoto T, Fukumoto R, Magno E, Oka M, Nishigori C, Horita N: Treatments for alopecia areata: a systematic review and network meta-analysis, *Dermatol Ther* 25:e14916, 2021, https://doi.org/10.1111/dth.14916. Epub ahead of print 33631058.

Gentile P, Garcovich S, Scioli MG, et al: Mechanical and controlled prp injections in patients affected by androgenetic alopecia, *J Vis Exp* 27(131), 2018.

Giordano S, Romeo M, di Summa P, et al: A meta-analysis on evidence of platelet-rich plasma for androgenetic alopecia, *Int J Trichology* 10(1):1–10, 2018.

Ramadan WM, Hassan AM, Ismail MA, El Attar YA: Evaluation of adding platelet-rich plasma to combined medical therapy in androgenetic alopecia, *J Cosmet Dermatol* 12, 2021, https://doi.org/10.1111/jocd.13935. Epub ahead of print 33438346.

Somani N, Turvy D: Hirsutism: an evidence-based treatment update, *Am J Clin Dermatol* 15(3):247–266, 2014.

Vano-Galvan S, Pirmez R, Hermosa-Gelbard A, et al: Safety of low-dose oral minoxidil for hair loss: a multicenter study of 1404 patients, 00418-7, *J Am Acad Dermatol* S0190-9622(21)00418-7, 2021, https://doi.org/10.1016/j.jaad.2021.02.054. Epub ahead of print 33639244.

Waśkiel-Burnat A, Kołodziejak M, Sikora M, et al: Therapeutic management in pediatric alopecia areata: a systematic review, *J Eur Acad Dermatol Venereol* 25, 2021, https://doi.org/10.1111/jdv.17187. Epub ahead of print 33630354.

DISEASES OF THE MOUTH

Method of
Lisa Simon, MD, DMD; and Hugh Silk, MD, MPH

CURRENT DIAGNOSIS

High-risk conditions
- Ludwig angina: Spread of infection most commonly from a mandibular molar into the sublingual and submaxillary spaces that surround the airway, causing urgent respiratory compromise.
- Cavernous sinus thrombosis: Ascending infection and thrombosis of intracranial vessels that can be caused by a maxillary dental infection. Requires urgent neurologic and neurosurgical evaluation.
- Lesions concerning for oral cancer: Most commonly squamous cell carcinoma (SCC) may present as sessile or fungating, with red or white shading. Usually asymptomatic, may feature fixed, painless lymph nodes. Associated with alcohol and tobacco use.

Common conditions
- Dental caries: Most common infectious disease globally, near 100% prevalence. Dental pain indicates that the tooth will require root canal therapy or extraction to resolve the infection.
- Periodontal disease: Inflammatory loss of the tooth's attachment structure, which can cause pain, tooth mobility, and eventual tooth loss.

Oral ulcers
- Acute ulcers most likely infectious (herpes simplex virus [HSV], Coxsackie) or aphthous ulcers, tend to resolve within 7 to 10 days.
- Chronic ulcers will appear more desquamative and widespread within the oral cavity. They are more likely to be due to a dermatologic condition (pemphigus vulgaris, mucous membrane pemphigoid, lichen planus) and should prompt investigation of other dermatologic findings.

Oral lesions and masses
- Cessation of triggering activity (e.g., use of chewing tobacco) and evaluate for resolution.
- Refer for biopsy if lesions persist for more than 14 days.

Xerostomia
- Perception of dry mouth, which can make speaking and swallowing more difficult and predisposes patients to rampant dental decay.
- Associated with polypharmacy, especially drugs with known anticholinergic properties.
- Can also be due to autoimmune destruction of salivary glands from SICCA syndrome.

Osteonecrosis of the jaw
- Antibiotics for purulent exudate.
- Refer to oral surgeon or oral medicine specialist for monitoring and possible resection of necrotic bone.

Antibiotic prophylaxis for dental procedures
- For infective endocarditis prevention, this is necessary only in individuals with prosthetic valves or implants, unrepaired cyanotic congenital heart disease or repair with residual defect, history of cardiac transplant with valvular regurgitation, or history of infective endocarditis.
- No prophylaxis necessary for individuals with prosthetic joints.
- Prophylaxis necessary only for procedures that involve manipulating the gingiva.
- Prophylaxis can be taken up to 2 h after a procedure with equivalent efficacy.

Caries

Dental caries are the most prevalent infectious disease in the world, affecting more than 90% of the population. Caused primarily by the acidogenic species *Streptococcus mutans* and lactobacilli, fermentation of dietary sugars produces acids that create holes in the teeth. Diets high in sugar—including both fermentable carbohydrates, sugary foods, and sugar-sweetened beverages—increase caries risk.

The prevalence and severity of caries has decreased substantially in the United States since the introduction of fluoride into community water sources. For pediatric patients ages 6 months to 16 years who primarily drink well water or reside in communities without water fluoridation, fluoride supplementation should be offered according to the guidelines set by the American Academy of Pediatrics.

Saliva is basic in nature and can reduce acid in the mouth and remineralize teeth to counteract the caries process. Consequently individuals with xerostomia, a common side effect of many medications, are at higher risk of caries, which are more likely to develop at the base of the tooth (the cervical aspect) in xerostomic mouths (see xerostomia, further on) (Figure 1).

Caries initially appear as chalky white spots on the tooth enamel. Eventually, decay will expand into a visible lesion, which may appear dark yellow, brown, or black. Interproximal decay (caries between the teeth) may be visible only radiologically until quite advanced. Patients may report sensitivity to sweet foods, progressing to sensitivity to hot and cold. Spontaneous pain caused by tooth decay indicates that the bacterial infection has spread to the neurovascular supply within the tooth (the pulp) and should be managed as a dental abscess (see later).

Patients with visibly carious dentition should be urged to visit a dentist as promptly as possible. If available, topical 5% sodium fluoride varnish can be applied off label by a provider to slow the progression of caries. Patients should also be counseled to reduce the quantity and frequency of dietary sugar intake.

Prevention includes twice daily brushing of teeth with proper technique and fluoridated toothpaste, daily flossing, and limiting sugary drinks and snacks. Children should be assisted with brushing until approximately age 8 and should use only a smear of fluoride-containing toothpaste until age 3. Fluoride should be offered (as noted previously) in communities with nonfluoridated water, and fluoride varnish should be offered at medical visits until age 5. Everyone with teeth should visit a dental provider regularly for cleanings, radiographs, and advice, usually twice annually, more or less based on risk. Individuals without teeth should still have regular dental visits to evaluate denture fit.

Periodontitis

Periodontal disease is a polymicrobial infection of primarily anaerobic, gram-negative pathogens within the *periodontium*, the attachment apparatus between the tooth and the alveolar bone. Proliferation of bacteria in the periodontal space causes local inflammation, which leads to sensitive and friable gingival tissue and eventual tooth mobility from inflammatory damage to the periodontal ligament and bone. Periodontal disease is extremely common, present in approximately 40% of all adults worldwide and in 20% of middle-aged US adults, and prevalence increases with age. Patients with diabetes are at especially high risk of periodontal disease. Note that periodontitis is associated with other conditions including worsening heart disease, uncontrolled diabetes, and preterm labor. Severe congenital forms of periodontal disease are known to be caused by disorders of neutrophil adhesion.

Accumulation of bacteria near or within the periodontal space may initially present with gingivitis, or inflammation of the gingiva without bone or attachment loss. Patients may report friable gingiva (bleeding when eating, brushing, or flossing the teeth) and sensitivity. As the disease progresses, the loss of bone will cause the teeth to appear to lengthen. Teeth with reduced attachment may become spaced apart or splayed due to the impact of repeated occlusal forces on unstable teeth. In advanced stages, teeth may be freely mobile on examination. The gingiva will appear boggy and friable, and bleeding or suppuration may be noticed when the teeth or gingiva are manipulated. Patients presenting with an acute onset of new bleeding and expansile gingiva should be evaluated for a hematologic abnormality suggestive of malignancy prior to referral for dental treatment.

Definitive diagnosis, including the severity of the periodontal disease and whether individual teeth can be maintained or must be extracted, must be made by a dentist using clinical exam and radiographic findings. Dental professionals will perform probing to evaluate loss of attachment between bone and tooth. The primary treatment to prevent further attachment loss is *scaling and root planing* to remove the bacterial concretions below the gingiva that are causing the inflammatory response.

Topical and occasionally systemic antibiotic therapy may be prescribed by a dental professional as part of surgical treatment for periodontitis. Patients presenting with an acute abscess (e.g., fluctuant swelling, pain, constitutional symptoms) should be managed in the same manner whether the abscess is periodontal or dental in origin, as noted in the section titled "Odontogenic Infections," later.

Prevention of periodontitis is similar to caries prevention in terms of dental hygiene, diet, and professional dental care. For adults,

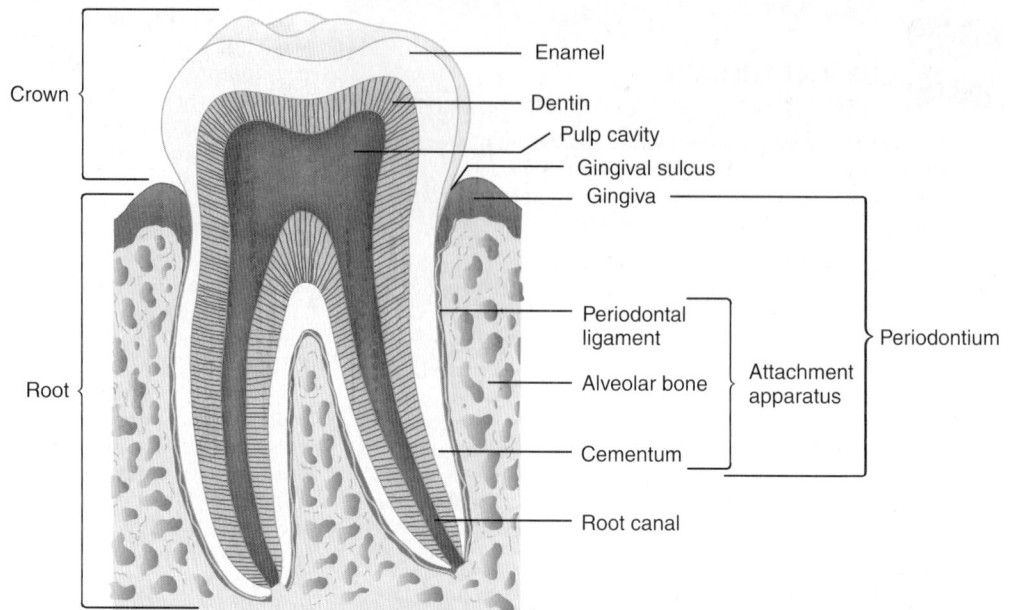

Figure 1 Basic anatomy of the tooth and periodontium. (From Walls R, et al: *Rosen's Emergency Medicine: Concepts and Clinical Practice*, ed 9. Philadelphia, 2018, Elsevier.)

electric toothbrushes may reduce plaque and gingivitis compared with manual toothbrushing, especially for patients with manual dexterity limitations. Tobacco use also contributes to periodontal disease; thus avoidance or cessation should be encouraged.

Necrotizing Ulcerative Gingivitis

An uncommon presentation of gingival disease is necrotizing ulcerative gingivitis (NUG), also referred to as Vincent angina or "trench mouth" for its prevalence among young soldiers during World War I. More common in young people, NUG presents with fever, malaise, and severe gingival pain without loss of bone or attachment. It is caused by mixed bacterial infection that includes anaerobes. Clinical exam will reveal exquisitely tender gingiva throughout the mouth, possibly more severe in the anterior teeth, with inflammation and the appearance of "punched out" gingival papillae between the teeth, with a fetid odor.

Patients require source control in the form of dental scaling, but topical antibiotic treatment with chlorhexidine gluconate (Peridex) as well as empiric treatment with penicillin or metronidazole (Flagyl)[1] can dramatically improve symptoms. Individuals presenting with NUG should be evaluated for a potential underlying source of immunocompromise, such as human immunodeficiency virus (HIV) infection. Other risk factors include nutritional deficiencies and stress.

Odontogenic Infections

Progression of untreated dental disease, both periodontitis and dental caries, can result in focal infection. Infection may be due to a periodontal abscess or spread of infection from a necrotic tooth into the supporting bone. Patients will often have globally poor dentition on exam and report a history of prior dental pain that may have resolved spontaneously.

Patients most often present with severe localized pain that may be worse at night. Involved teeth may be localized by evaluating for focal fluctuance, tooth mobility, or pain produced by percussion of the tooth with a tongue depressor. Visible drainage of exudate through a fistula or the gingival cuff of a tooth may be associated with relief of pain due to reduced buildup of pressure.

Most dental infections do not result in systemic compromise; however, providers should be proactive in ruling out more serious complications. Ludwig angina is a form of airway compromise resulting from spread of infection, most commonly from the mandibular molars, into the submandibular and submaxillary fascial spaces that ring the trachea, causing urgent airway compromise. Patients will appear acutely ill with trismus, submandibular

TABLE 1	Complications of Dental Infection Requiring Emergent Transfer and Their Clinical Presentation
Ludwig angina	• History of toothache in a mandibular molar • Fever and malaise, submandibular swelling, trismus, drooling, muffled voice, elevated floor of mouth, stridor
Cavernous sinus thrombosis	• History of toothache in a maxillary tooth • Fever and malaise, loss of nasolabial fold, periorbital swelling, confusion, obtundation

swelling, and difficulty managing secretions. Patients require imminent transfer to a tertiary care facility for airway management and surgical source control. Cavernous sinus thrombosis, most commonly resulting from the ascending infection from maxillary anterior teeth, initially manifests with loss of the nasolabial fold, periorbital swelling, and ophthalmoplegia; it can lead to vision loss, elevated intracranial pressure, and stroke and requires urgent transfer. Descriptions of these two conditions are given in Table 1.

For stable patients, evidence of systemic spread such as fever, tachycardia, or descending lymphadenopathy are indications for antibiotic treatment. Although not medically indicated, patients who do not have timely access to a dentist may benefit from antibiotic prescription as a palliative measure to reduce infection burden and pain until they can receive definitive treatment. Most infections are polymicrobial, with a predominance of aerobic, gram-positive organisms and a low prevalence of antibiotic resistance. A 1-week course of penicillin VK, amoxicillin, or clindamycin[1] for patients with penicillin allergy should be enough to provide several weeks of pain relief.

For acute pain relief, patients should be offered a local anesthetic injection if possible. Bupivacaine (Marcaine, Sensorcaine, generic) provides the longest-lasting relief, but lidocaine with 1:100,000 epinephrine can also be effective. Combined analgesia with a nonsteroidal antiinflammatory drug (NSAID) and a non-NSAID is effective in reducing dental pain, and adult patients without contraindications may take up to 800 mg tid of ibuprofen and 1000 mg tid of acetaminophen concurrently for relief. Providers may consider short courses (3 days) of opioid analgesia for unremitting pain.

Definitive treatment of all oral infections requires source control, whether from extraction of the involved tooth, root canal treatment, or periodontal therapy. Referral to a dentist as soon as feasible

---

[1]Not FDA-approved for this indication.

should be a primary goal, and it should be emphasized to patients that infection will recur even if their symptoms resolve transiently.

Oral Ulcers

Ulcerated lesions within the oral cavity may be due to multiple possible etiologies, including infectious or autoimmune causes. The likely etiology can often be determined by a careful history and physical exam.

About 90% of the population is ultimately infected with oral herpes simplex virus (HSV), most commonly HSV-1, with rarer infection by HSV-2. Initial presentation of HSV infection (primary herpetic gingivostomatitis) is more likely to involve severe ulceration of the oral mucosa as well as constitutional symptoms such as fever. Adults are more likely to present with nonspecific symptoms such as pharyngitis, whereas children are more likely to have the classic presentation. If ulceration is severe enough to prevent adequate fluid intake, those presenting with more severe symptoms should be evaluated for risk of dehydration. Symptoms generally resolve within 1 to 2 weeks without severe complications such as encephalitis.

Following initial infection, HSV remains dormant in the sensory nerve ganglia, with rate and severity of recurrence varying considerably among individuals. Recurrence may be activated by periods of stress, including local trauma or systemic illness. Recurrent HSV-related ulcerations favor fixed keratinized tissue such as the gingiva or lips (herpes labialis). Symptoms typically present with a prodromal burning or tingling sensation followed by the appearance of painful small vesicles that rupture. The ulcer may appear purple or gray on the periphery, and a yellow layer of keratin overlying the ulcer may be present. Patients who present with prodromal symptoms may have a shortened course if they are prescribed acyclovir (Zovirax), either as a capsule or a topical cream, very early in the presentation of symptoms. Patients with repeat recurrence may benefit from a "pill in pocket" approach to treatment. Recurrence is usually seen one to six times a year and generally becomes less severe and frequent with time. If recurrences are frequent, antivirals can be given orally for suppression with the patient reevaluated annually. Treatment of first episodes requires a longer duration of treatment with oral antivirals.

Aphthous stomatitis is an immune complex–mediated condition that can also result in recurrent oral ulceration. Patients may similarly report that ulcers are induced by stress or local trauma and share a similar prodrome of pain or pruritus at the site of ulcer formation. Ulcers are most commonly less than 10 mm in size, though they can be larger. Aphthous ulcers may be distinguished from HSV-related ulcers due to their predilection for less keratinized oral surfaces such as the buccal, sublingual, and palatal mucosa and for presenting with multifocal lesions. Ulcers resolve within 7 to 10 days without treatment. Aphthous ulcers can be quite painful, and patients may find relief from topical benzocaine 20% (Orabase or Orajel), although patients should be cautioned to forego excessive use in order to avoid the risk of methemoglobinemia. Exceedingly painful ulcers may resolve more quickly with topical corticosteroids. Triamcinolone 0.1% in orabase (Kenalog Orabase) can be applied topically after each meal and at bedtime; if ulcers are extensive, dexamethasone (Decadron)[1] 0.5 mg/5 mL elixir can be prescribed as a rinse for 2 minutes (and then expectorated) after each meal and at bedtime.

Symptomatic relief of oral ulcers from any cause may be obtained from a mouth rinse with a combination of diphenhydramine (Benadryl)[1] and a coating agent such as bismuth subsalicylate (Kaopectate)[1] or aluminum/magnesium antacid (Maalox)[1]. This formulation is sometimes colloquially referred to as "magic mouthwash."[6]

Several other conditions may initially present with oral ulceration. Simple trauma such as biting the buccal mucosa can lead to a local ulceration. Oral lichen planus may present with oral ulcerations or peeling of keratinized gingiva around the teeth as well as reticulated

white "Whickham striae" on the mucosa. Generalized sloughing of the mucous membranes should prompt high concern for a systemic source and demands a more complete dermatologic exam. Onset within weeks of beginning a new medication could indicate the onset of Stevens-Johnson syndrome or toxic epidermal necrolysis, which may present first with mucosal involvement. Mucous membrane pemphigoid or pemphigus vulgaris may also present with mucosal sloughing. Such presentations should be referred for biopsy and further workup. Behçet disease also presents with genital and oral ulcerations; there are usually multiple ulcers and systemic symptoms, including eye inflammation, skin ulcers, and arthralgias. Coxsackie virus presenting as "hand, foot, and mouth disease" is usually more obvious, as many of the lesions are outside of the mouth on and around the lips and the classic round lesions on the hands, feet, and occasionally the buttocks. Coxsackie is also much more common in children and rare in adults.

Last, mucositis may be induced by chemotherapy or head and neck radiation. Such ulcerations are often widespread and exquisitely painful and may impair patients' ability to take in adequate fluids and nutrition. These symptoms should be managed jointly with a patient's oncology team, including prevention, which can involve the following treatments: aloe vera,[7] amifostine (Ethyol),[1] granulocyte colony stimulating factor (G-CSF),[1] honey, keratinocyte growth factor (palifermin, Kepivance), polymyxin/tobramycin/amphotericin (PTA)[1], antibiotic pastille/paste[6], and sucralfate (Carafate)[1].

Oral Soft Tissue Lesions

Lesions within the oral cavity can be extremely heterogenous in appearance, ranging from fungating to sessile, white to red and even pigmented, and ulcerated or smooth. White coloration often indicates increased keratinization, whereas increased red shading indicates increased vascularity. Oral SCC is the most common malignancy of the oral cavity, representing 90% of all intraoral cancers. Malignant lesions are more likely to manifest with raised/irregular borders, be fixed or indurated, be painless, and feature painless lymphadenopathy. The highest-risk sites for malignant transformation are the lateral aspect of the tongue, the floor of the mouth, and the junction of the hard and soft palate. Both alcohol and tobacco use are risk factors, and both behaviors together increase the risk of SCC up to 300-fold. Rising rates of HPV infection have increased the prevalence of HPV-associated SCC of the throat (including tonsils and base of tongue); however, there has not been a similar rise in rates of oral SCC. The HPV vaccine may help to reduce oropharyngeal cancer rates.

Detection of an intraoral lesion should prompt examination for possible traumatic causes (e.g., a recent burn or tongue bite) and removal of potential causative factors (e.g., smoking cessation). Bilateral lesions are more likely to be benign and this can be a reassuring finding. Any lesion that fails to resolve after 2 weeks of observation should be biopsied and/or referred for definitive diagnosis. Note that brush biopsy should be used cautiously due to a positive predictive value of only 58%; tissue biopsy should be used for all all negative biopsies. The differential diagnosis for common oral soft tissue lesions is listed in Table 2.

Treatment of oral squamous cell carcinoma (SCC) is multidisciplinary and often requires both surgical resection/excision as well as chemotherapy and radiation. Five-year survival rates remain around 60%. Unfortunately, no preventive measures have been widely successful, with even routine oral examination being given a designation of insufficient evidence to support implementation ("I") and not recommended by the US Preventive Services Task Force. However, providers should consider periodic thorough examinations of high-risk patients.

Lesions that may appear benign, such as leukoplakia or erythroplakia, should be monitored closely and biopsied if not resolving. Mild forms of these lesions will resolve on their own, whereas persisting lesions can be precancerous. They are often thickened,

[1]Not FDA approved for this indication.
[6]May be compounded by pharmacists.

[1]Not FDA-approved for this indication.
[6]May be compounded by pharmacists.
[7]Available as dietary supplement.

TABLE 2 Differential Diagnosis of Common Oral Soft Tissue Lesions

Red or White Lesions

Traumatic/frictional keratosis	Benign thickening of keratin layer due to repeated trauma
Leukoedema	Variant of normal; bilateral whitening of the buccal mucosa, which disappears when the mucosa is stretched
Oral candidiasis	Fluffy white patches that will reveal an erythematous base when scraped
Oral papilloma	Related to infection with low-risk HPV strain; may be fungating or pedunculated, most commonly on tongue
Oral lichen planus	Reticulations, Wickham striae, and desquamation of buccal mucosa and gingiva
Leukoplakia/ erythroplakia/ erythroleukoplakia	Irregular, usually unilateral change in coloration, risk of malignant transformation, biopsy needed
Squamous cell carcinoma	May appear as white, red, or ulcerative lesion; biopsy any lesion that persists after 2 weeks

Ulcerations

Aphthous ulcers	Immune-mediated ulcers on nonkeratinized oral mucosa
Herpetic ulcers	Ulcers most prominent on gingiva and lips
Angular cheilitis	Ulcerations at corners of the lips; may be associated with nutrient deficiency, ill-fitting dentures, or fungal infection
Mucous membrane pemphigoid	Desquamation of gingiva; associated with desquamation of other body mucosal surfaces
Pemphigus vulgaris	Desquamation of mucosa to vermillion border; may present months or years before presentation on the skin

HPV, Human papillomavirus.

painless, on the buccal mucosa (inside cheek), on the tongue or floor of mouth, and either white or red in color. The smoking of tobacco is a risk factor for these lesions.

Oral Candidiasis

Oral candida infections are heterogenous in presentation. Other than in extremely rare cases, all are caused by *Candida albicans*, which is also a common colonizer of asymptomatic individuals. Recent antibiotic use is a risk factor, as is uncontrolled diabetes and the use of inhaled corticosteroids. Of note, although immunocompromised patients are at higher risk, oral candidiasis is *not* considered indicative of immunocompromise.

Most commonly, patients will report the presence of white patches that may appear on the buccal mucosa and palate. Such patches can be scraped away with a tongue depressor or gauze, and irritated, bleeding tissue will be present beneath. Patients may report some mouth dryness, irritation, or discomfort when swallowing, but they will not be constitutionally ill.

In addition to the more classic presentation of oral thrush, candida may colonize macerated tissue in contact with dentures (atrophic candidiasis), or in the moist regions at the labial corners (angular cheilitis). Atrophic candidiasis may be asymptomatic, or patients may report worsening discomfort with denture use. The candida infection will be evident as a bright red outline in the shape of the patient's dental prosthesis. White patches are usually not present.

Angular cheilitis may cause pain with wide mouth opening and will reveal erythematous, sometimes weeping tissue at the corners of the mouth. Although angular cheilitis is associated with some B vitamin deficiencies, it can also be caused by ill-fitting dentures, causing the collapse of the facial tissues and producing a moist environment suitable for fungal superinfection. A nutritional history and evaluation for other signs or symptoms of nutrient deficiency can rule out the need for further evaluation; regardless, a topical antifungal treatment should be prescribed. New properly fitting dentures and vitamin supplementation are the other necessary treatments.

The choice of anticandidal treatment should be based on the extent of infection. More widespread infection such as thrush or atrophic candidiasis should be treated with clotrimazole (Mycelex) troches or nystatin (Mycostatin) pastilles or rinse. Nystatin rinse is more suitable for patients with xerostomia, who may find the troches difficult to dissolve, and for patients who wear dentures, who should be instructed to soak their dentures overnight in the nystatin solution in addition to receiving intraoral treatment. For patients with angular cheilitis, a nystatin ointment or clotrimazole cream applied to the affected area may be more comfortable. Systemic antifungals such ketoconazole (Nizoral) or fluconazole (Diflucan) should be considered only for immunocompromised patients or those who cannot tolerate topical treatment.

To prevent the development of candidiasis, patients with partial or complete dentures should be advised to brush their dentures twice daily and to remove them during sleep, when they can be soaked in an over-the-counter denture cleansing solution or a mouthwash such as Listerine. Dentures should not be brushed or cleaned with toothpaste, which can scratch the surface. Management of xerostomia can prevent the development of candidiasis in these patients (see later). Individuals using corticosteroid inhalers should be advised to rinse their mouths with water after use and expectorate. There is some evidence that probiotic prescription concurrently with oral antibiotics may reduce risk of candidiasis development, especially for denture wearers.

Xerostomia

Xerostomia refers to the subjective feeling of a dry mouth due to reduced salivary flow. This may be due to autoimmune conditions such as SICCA (e.g., Sjögren syndrome) or a history of head and neck radiation but is more commonly due to the anticholinergic effects of numerous medications, with polypharmacy putting individuals at particularly high risk. Behavioral factors such as tobacco, marijuana, and methamphetamine use can also increase risk.

As saliva plays a critical role in remineralizing the dentition after acidic insults from dietary sugar intake, xerostomia is associated with higher caries risk; widespread caries at the base of the tooth nearest the gingiva is a common finding. Saliva also has antibacterial and antifungal properties, thus xerostomia places patients at higher risk for other oral infections.

Patients may report a feeling of "cotton mouth," which makes it difficult or even painful to eat, swallow, or talk. Physical exam will reveal dry, shiny oral tissues with thickened, ropy white saliva that may aggregate at the corners of the lips. Severity of reported symptoms may not correlate fully with physical findings.

Patients for whom the xerostomia is possibly a pharmacologic adverse reaction should undergo a thorough medication review, with reduction in dose or elimination of any unnecessary medications, especially those with known anticholinergic side effects. Following this and for individuals with a known cause of xerostomia (e.g., head and neck radiation), treatment is symptomatic. Many patients report improvement with frequent small sips of water throughout the day. Symptoms should first be managed with over-the-counter salivary replacement rinses or gels (such as Biotène). Sucking candy can increase salivary flow, although it is essential to select sugar-free candies. Patients should be advised to avoid sugar-rich foods, including sugar-sweetened beverages, if at all possible, given their heightened caries risk.

If this fails to cause improvement, prescription of a cholinergic agonist such as cevimeline (Evoxac), pilocarpine (Salagen), or bethanechol (Urecholine)[1] can be considered. Although these medications successfully increase salivary output, the inevitability of undesired cholinergic agonism causing excessive sweating, gastritis, and other symptoms often results in discontinuation of the medications. Patients considering systemic treatment with a cholinergic agonist should be warned of these adverse effects as well as the increased risk of acute angle-closure glaucoma.

Osteonecrosis of the Jaw

Osteonecrosis of the jaw (ONJ) most commonly occurs in individuals with a history of head and neck radiation or with bisphosphonate exposure. Intravenous bisphosphonates put patients at much higher risk of ONJ (95% of cases) compared with those on an oral bisphosphonate regimen. Because it has a relatively lower vascular supply, the mandible is more prone to osteonecrosis.

Individuals should be warned of the risk of ONJ and advised to complete necessary dental work, especially dental extractions, prior to beginning radiation or bisphosphonate therapy when appropriate. Due to the prolonged half-life of bisphosphonates, drug holidays prior to dental treatment for patients already taking them are not recommended. Patients with a history of head and neck radiation in need of oral surgery, especially in the mandible, may benefit from adjunctive hyperbaric oxygen therapy, which may require close collaboration with the treating dentist or oral surgeon.

Lesions may appear spontaneously due to occlusal forces. Patients may report an area of roughness or mild discomfort, most commonly on the medial aspect of the mandible, near the tongue. Alternately, patients may present with nonhealing sockets after a tooth extraction or other dental procedure. Such areas of necrosis may expand over time. Diagnosis is empiric but may benefit from confirmation by an oral medicine practitioner or oral surgeon.

Management is largely symptomatic. Patients should be prescribed antibiotics if the area is purulent (see the earlier section titled "Odontogenic Infections"), and extensive areas of necrosis may need to be resected. Chlorhexidine gluconate (Peridex) rinses may assist with reducing the bacterial burden within the areas of necrosis, thus reducing rates of superinfection.

Antibiotic Prophylaxis Before Dental Procedures

Changes to guidelines by the American Dental Association and the American Heart Association within the last 7 years have greatly restricted recommendations for the use of antibiotic prophylaxis prior to dental procedures. Currently, the only patients who require antibiotic prophylaxis for the prevention of infectious endocarditis are those with prosthetic valves or prosthetic materials used for valve repair, a history of cardiac transplant with ongoing valvular regurgitation, unrepaired cyanotic congenital heart disease or repaired heart disease with a residual defect or regurgitation adjacent to a prosthetic patch or device, and individuals with a prior history of infective endocarditis. Children within 6 months of repair of a congenital cardiac condition or with a residual defect should also be prescribed prophylactic antibiotics. Patients without these conditions who may have received antibiotic prophylaxis in the past should be reassured that the potential risks of antibiotic prescription (including *Clostridium difficile* infections) outweigh the extremely low risk of infective endocarditis caused by dental procedures.

It is currently not recommended that patients with a history of prosthetic joint replacement receive prophylactic antibiotics.

Only those dental procedures that involve manipulation of the gingiva (e.g., a dental cleaning or dental extraction) require antibiotic prophylaxis. Patients should be advised to discuss the necessity of prophylaxis with their dentist, who may also be the prescriber of any necessary antibiotics. One dose of antibiotic should be taken 30 to 60 minutes before the procedure. In the event they forget to take a dose before a dental appointment, patients should also be informed that the prophylactic efficacy of antibiotics is equivalent up to 2 hours after a dental procedure.

---

[1]Not FDA-approved for this indication.

Amoxicillin[1] is the antibiotic of choice for most patients. For those with an allergy to penicillins, cephalexin (Keflex)[1], clindamycin[1], azithromycin (Zithromax)[1], or clarithromycin (Biaxin)[1] can be used, though care should be taken for potential cross-reactivity of cephalosporins in penicillin-allergic patients. Generally doses are as follows: amoxicillin 2 g; if penicillin allergic, clindamycin 600 mg, cephalexin 2 g, azithromycin or clarithromycin 500 mg.

---

[1]Not FDA approved for this indication.

References

Bui FQ, Almeida-da-Silva CLC, Huynh B, Trinh A, et al: Association between periodontal pathogens and systemic disease, *Biomed J* 42(1):27–35, 2019.

Cochrane Oral Health. Available at: https://oralhealth.cochrane.org/ Accessed January 20, 2020.

Lockhart PB, Tampi MP, Abt E, et al: Evidence-based clinical practice guideline on antibiotic use for the urgent management of pulpal- and periapical-related dental pain and intraoral swelling: A report from the American Dental Association, *J Am Den Assoc* 150(11):906–921, 2019.

Neville BW, Damm DD, Allen CM, Chi AC: *Oral & Maxillofacial Pathology*, ed 4, Missouri, 2015, WB Saunders, Elsevier.

Nishimura RA, Otto CM, Bonow RO, et al: 2017 AHA/ACC focused update of the 2014 AHA/ACC guideline for the management of patients with valvular heart disease: A report of the American College of Cardiology/American Heart Association Task Force on clinical practice guidelines, *Circulation* 135:e1159–e1195, 2017.

Plemons JM, Al-Hashimi I, Marek CL: American Dental Association Council on Scientific Affairs managing xerostomia and salivary gland hypofunction: executive summary of a report from the American Dental Association Council on Scientific Affairs, *J Am Den Assoc* 145(8):867–873, 2014.

Reddy SG, Kanala S, Chigurupati A, et al: The sensitivity and specificity of computerized brush biopsy and scalpel biopsy in diagnosing oral premalignant lesions: a comparative study, *J Oral Maxillofac Pathol* 16(3):349–353, 2012.

Reamy BV, Derby R, Bunt CW: Common tongue conditions in primary care, *Am Fam Physic* 81(5):627–634, 2010.

Sollecito TP, Abt E, Lockhart PB, et al: The use of prophylactic antibiotics prior to dental procedures in patients with prosthetic joints: Evidence-based clinical practice guideline for dental practitioners--a report of the American Dental Association Council on Scientific Affairs, *J Am Den Assoc* 146(1):11–16 e8, 2015.

Stephens MB, Wiedemer JP, Kushner GM: Dental problems in primary care, *Am Fam Physic* 98(11):654–660, 2018.

DISEASES OF THE NAIL

Method of
Jonathon Firnhaber, MD, MAEd, MBA

CURRENT THERAPY

Ingrown nail
- Ingrown nails with mild acute inflammation may be treated with antiseptic soaks and a moderate-potency topical steroid. The distal anterior tip and lateral edges of the ingrown toenail can be elevated with cotton or wool to allow the nail to advance without further penetrating the nail fold.
- Ingrown nails with moderate or greater inflammation generally require surgical intervention. Partial nail plate removal is performed under local anesthesia.
- If the ingrown nail is recurrent, liquid phenol or a radiofrequency surgical electrode can be used to permanently ablate the lateral portions of the nail matrix and germinal tissue.

Onychomycosis
- Physicians should not prescribe oral antifungal therapy for suspected onychomycosis without confirmation of infection.
- Terbinafine (Lamisil) is the preferred agent for onychomycosis. It offers a higher cure rate and fewer drug interactions than alternative antifungal agents.
- Topical agents for onychomycosis offer limited efficacy as primary treatments. Efficacy may be improved by thorough debridement of the affected nail or nails prior to treatment and at multiple points during treatment.
- The risk of recurrent onychomycosis may be reduced by preventing and treating tinea pedis.

CURRENT DIAGNOSIS

Onychomycosis
- The vast majority of onychomycosis is caused by dermatophytes, typically *Trichophyton rubrum* and *Trichophyton mentagrophytes*.
- Dermatophyte onychomycosis typically presents with invasion of the hyponychium or lateral nail folds, causing onycholysis, nail plate thickening, and subungual debris.
- Superficial white onychomycosis is also caused by dermatophytes and presents as a powdery white discoloration of the nail surface.
- Nondermatophyte organisms are responsible for 10% to 20% of cases of onychomycosis but may be clinically indistinguishable from disease caused by common dermatophytes.
- *Candidal* onychomycosis is uncommon and may present as proximal nail changes in association with paronychia.
- Accurate diagnosis of onychomycosis depends on the collection of an adequate sample for evaluation. The affected nail plate and subungual debris should be sent for fungal culture.

Nail Anatomy

The nail unit includes several clinically important components (Figure 1). The nail plate is made of keratin, which is hard and translucent. The skin of the lateral and proximal nail folds surrounds the nail plate, and the proximal nail fold overlies the matrix. The keratin layer of the proximal nail fold extends over the nail plate to form the cuticle. The tip of the proximal nail fold has capillary loops, which are typically inapparent but may become visible in connective tissue diseases such as systemic lupus erythematosus (SLE) and scleroderma.

The nail plate is primarily synthesized by the matrix epithelium. The distal aspect of the nail matrix is visible as the lunula and is continuous with the nail bed. The nail bed extends from the distal nail matrix to the hyponychium and consists of parallel longitudinal ridges. Splinter hemorrhages, which are visible through the nail plate, represent bleeding at the base of these ridges. The hyponychium begins at the distal edge of the nail bed and is a short segment of keratinized skin that is not covered by the nail plate.

Fingernails grow 0.5 to 2 mm per week and thus take approximately 6 months to grow from the proximal matrix to the distal free edge. Toenails grow much more slowly, taking 12 to 18 months for complete replacement of the nail. Although nailsgrow

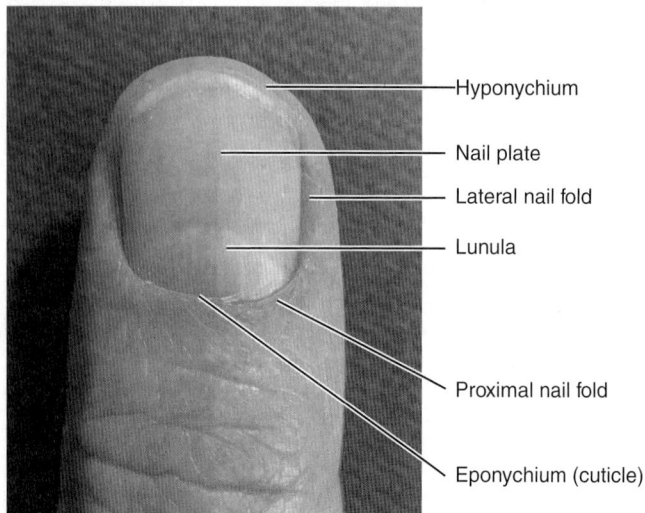

Figure 1 Surface anatomy of the nail unit.

— Hyponychium
— Nail plate
— Lateral nail fold
— Lunula
— Proximal nail fold
— Eponychium (cuticle)

continuously, their growth rate slows with age and with decreased capillary perfusion.

Noninfectious Nail Disorders

Psoriasis

Clinical Features and Diagnosis

Although multiple inflammatory skin diseases may affect the nail unit, nail changes are seen in up to 90% of patients with psoriasis over the course of their disease. Nail involvement typically occurs in conjunction with skin disease and is particularly common in patients with psoriatic arthritis involving the distal digits. Nail changes may, however, occur as an isolated finding and support a diagnosis of psoriasis when skin changes are equivocal or absent.

Nail psoriasis has multiple presentations, depending on the portion of the nail unit that is affected. Most commonly, nail matrix psoriasis presents as nail plate pitting. More extensive nail matrix involvement leads to leukonychia (white discoloration of the nail) and loss of integrity of the nail plate, with crumbling and fragmentation. Psoriasis of the hyponychium leads to an accumulation of scaly yellow debris that may elevate the nail plate. Psoriasis of the nail bed may trigger irregular separation of the nail plate and nail thickening, resulting in yellow discoloration of the nail plate. Both of these changes may be mistaken for onychomycosis, and onychomycosis may occur in psoriatic nails, emphasizing the importance of verifying the presence of a fungal infection prior to treatment.

Treatment

Topical treatments for psoriatic nail disease include high-potency topical steroids, vitamin D analogues, and topical retinoids; however, relatively poor penetration of the nail plate by these agents limits their potential benefit. Systemic therapy is rarely indicated for nail disease without skin or joint involvement.

Onychogryphosis

Onychogryphosis, or "ram's horn nail," affects the great toes and causes marked thickening, discoloration, and curvature of the nail plate. The condition may be triggered by repeated minor trauma from poorly fitting shoes and can eventually make it impossible for the patient to wear shoes. This deformity may be complicated by pain, distal onycholysis, subungual hemorrhage, or onychomycosis. Treatment primarily involves mechanical debridement of the thickened nail plate with a high-speed rotary burr. Surgical removal of the entire nail is associated with prolonged healing of the nail bed, which is generally not well tolerated. Onychogryphosis is more commonly seen in older patients and is also associated with self-neglect, homelessness, dementia, and peripheral vascular disease.

Pincer Nails

Inward deformation of the lateral edges of the nail plate results in a tube- or pincer-shaped nail. The nail bed is drawn into and pinched by the nail, often causing significant pain. Triggers for pincer nails include onychomycosis, psoriasis, and local tumors. Most commonly, however, biomechanical or arthritic changes cause the nail matrix to widen, and the nail ultimately becomes too wide for the nail bed. In extreme cases, removal of the medial, lateral, or both nail margins with ablation of the associated nail matrix, in a manner similar to treatment of an ingrown nail, is indicated to relieve the compression of the nail bed.

Spoon Nails

Spoon-shaped nails, with lateral elevation and a central depression of the nail plate, is termed koilonychia. Although spoon nails may be seen in healthy children and adults, the spontaneous onset of spoon nails is associated with iron deficiency anemia and may be seen in 50% of patients with idiopathic hemochromatosis. The spoon deformity resolves once the anemia has been corrected.

Beau Lines

Beau lines are transverse depressions in the nail plate that arise from the temporary interruption of nail growth within the nail matrix. Acute systemic events may trigger Beau lines in all nails, whereas localized trauma or paronychia will limit the finding to the traumatized nail or nails. The grooves have been associated with multiple systemic conditions including zinc deficiency, pemphigus, Raynaud disease, and myocarditis as well as with illnesses accompanied by high fever, such as rheumatic fever, measles, mumps, hand-foot-and-mouth disease, and malaria. They may also be triggered by chemotherapeutic agents cytotoxic to the nail matrix.

The distance of a Beau line from the proximal nail fold can allow the clinician to estimate the time of the triggering event based on an average growth rate of 3 mm per month for fingernails and 1 mm per month for toenails.

Habit-Tic Deformity

Habit-tic deformity is triggered by chronic biting or picking at a section of the proximal nail fold, usually of the thumb. The resulting nail plate deformity consists of a longitudinal band of horizontal grooves that often extend from the proximal nail fold to the tip of the nail. Habit-tic deformity may be confused with Beau lines associated with chronic paronychia or chronic eczema of the proximal nail fold. Habit-tic deformity produces closely spaced sharp grooves, whereas Beau lines tend to be more smooth and undulating. Formal treatment is not necessary, and the deformity resolves once the chronic irritation ceases and the nail grows out.

Ingrown Nail

Clinical Features and Diagnosis

Ingrown nails (onychocryptosis) are common, painful conditions, most often affecting the great toe. The nail plate of the great toe extends several millimeters beyond the medial and lateral nail folds. In properly trimmed nails, its margin should be apparent at the distal portion of the nail. Excessive or improper trimming of the lateral nail plate will often leave behind a sharp spike of nail that is covered by the lateral nail fold. Lateral pressure from poorly fitted shoes or trauma may exacerbate the problem. The nail pierces the lateral or medial nail fold and enters the dermis, acting as a foreign body. Initial pain and swelling give way to a robust inflammatory response with edema, purulent drainage, and granulation tissue surrounding the penetrating nail.

Treatment

Ingrown nails with mild acute inflammation may be treated conservatively with antiseptic soaks and a moderate-potency topical steroid. If visible, the distal anterior tip and lateral edges of the ingrown toenail can be elevated from the adjacent soft tissue with cotton or wool, which both withdraws the foreign body and allows the nail to advance without further penetrating the nail fold. If collodion is available, it can help fix the cotton or wool in place, so that it will require less frequent replacement. Antibiotics are of limited value, as purulent drainage is associated with the foreign body reaction and is less indicative of an acute bacterial infection.

Ingrown nails with greater-than-mild inflammation generally require surgical intervention. The toe is anesthetized with 1% or 2% lidocaine without epinephrine, either with a digital block or local infiltration of the proximal and lateral nail fold. A narrow periosteal elevator is inserted under the ingrown nail parallel to the lateral nail fold and advanced with upward pressure against the nail plate to minimize risk of damage to the underlying nail bed. The surgeon must ensure that the periosteal elevator is fully advanced to the base of the nail plate, which is 3 to 5 mm proximal to the proximal nail fold. Once the elevator reaches the base of the nail, a sudden decrease in resistance will be noted and care should be taken to not advance it further into the toe. The elevated nail is clipped longitudinally, again taking care to include the most proximal portion of nail, and removed. Residual granulation tissue can be removed with iris scissors or a curette.

If the ingrown nail is recurrent, liquid phenol can be used to permanently ablate the lateral portions of the nail matrix and germinal tissue. Once the nail bed has dried, a phenol-soaked cotton swab is applied for 3 minutes, followed by a thorough wash with 70% isopropyl alcohol, which neutralizes the phenol. Alternatively, a radiofrequency surgical electrode can be used to cauterize the nail matrix and germinal tissue. A flattened tip coated with Teflon on one side is used to protect the proximal nail fold. Regrowth of the nail occurs in up to 25% of patients following phenol cauterization, but the rate of regrowth is less than 5% with radiofrequency cauterization.

Subungual Hematoma

Subungual hematoma is most often caused by direct trauma to the nail plate, which causes bleeding and separation of the nail plate from the nail bed. Hematomas that are fully contained under the nail plate can be exquisitely painful. Drainage, whether spontaneous or by clinician intervention, relieves the pain immediately. The quickest and most effective method of draining the hematoma is by puncturing the nail plate with a hot-tip electrocautery or with a red-hot paperclip tip, taking care not to advance the instrument into the nail bed. Anesthesia is not required for this procedure. Trephination of the nail with a fine-point scalpel blade or large-bore needle tip can be painful, as pressure is required to puncture the nail. Trauma to the proximal nail fold or underlying nail matrix can cause bleeding that is not apparent until the nail plate emerges from the nail fold with blood stains. Staining will be present until the nail fully grows out.

Acute Paronychia

Trauma or manipulation of the proximal and lateral nail fold may trigger acute, painful swelling and erythema of the proximal and/or lateral nail folds, which is termed acute paronychia. Most superficial infections will present with a collection of purulent material about the cuticle or lateral nail fold. These superficial abscesses can quickly be drained with a 1- to 2-mm nick from the tip of an 18- or 21-gauge needle or #11 scalpel blade. Alternatively, the instrument may be inserted between the proximal nail fold and the nail plate, lifting the nail fold to achieve drainage. Neither anesthesia nor oral antibiotics are required. More diffuse erythema and swelling without any superficial abscess suggest a deeper infection. Antibiotics active against *Staphylococcus* and a deeper incision may be required. Acute and chronic paronychias are distinctly different processes.

Chronic Paronychia

Chronic paronychia is triggered by chronic exposure to contact irritants and moisture. Clinically, it presents with tenderness, mild erythema, and mild swelling about the proximal and lateral nail folds of most or all fingers. Typically, many or all fingers are involved simultaneously. The primary pathophysiologic change is separation of the cuticle from the nail plate, which allows bacteria and fungal organisms to colonize the space between the nail plate and proximal nail fold. Manipulation of the cuticle further disrupts the barrier and accelerates the process. Culture of purulent material expressed from the proximal nail fold may show polymicrobial growth and will often include *Candida*. In this case, *Candida* is a colonizer rather than a true pathogenic cause of chronic paronychia, and it disappears once the integrity of the cuticle barrier has been restored. If the colonizing organisms include *Pseudomonas aeruginosa*, the nail plate may develop a green discoloration. The nail plate itself is not infected but may develop Beau lines as a result of the chronic inflammation.

Chronic paronychia is slow to resolve; its treatment hinges on eliminating exposure to contact irritants, limiting exposure to moisture, and treatment of the associated inflammation and infection. Low- to midpotency topical steroid creams may be used for 2 to 4 weeks. Because of the broad polymicrobial colonization typical of chronic paronychia, oral or topical antibiotics are unlikely to affect the time to resolution. Topical

TABLE 1 Oral Antifungal Agents for Onychomycosis

DRUG	DOSING	INDICATIONS	POTENTIAL COMPLICATIONS
Terbinafine (Lamisil)	250 mg daily for 12 weeks (toenails); 6 weeks (fingernails)	First-line treatment for typical dermatophytes	Hepatic toxicity
Itraconazole (Sporanox)	200 mg bid for 7 days, then 21 days off for two courses (8 weeks total) (fingernails); 200 mg daily for 12 weeks (toenails)	Preferred for nondermatophyte molds Treatment option for *Candida*	Hepatic toxicity Multiple drug interactions Lower cure rate than terbinafine
Fluconazole (Diflucan)[1]	150–300 mg weekly for 6 months	Treatment of choice for *Candida*	Hepatic toxicity Multiple drug interactions Lower cure rate than terbinafine

[1]Not FDA approved for this indication.

antifungal agents, such as ciclopirox (Loprox)[1] applied to the proximal nailfold two or three times per day, or oral fluconazole (Diflucan)[1] 200 mg daily for 1 to 4 weeks, may help to mitigate the chronic inflammation.

Myxoid Cysts

Digital mucous, or myxoid, cysts present as solitary dome-shaped nodules 2 to 6 mm in diameter located at the distal interphalangeal joint (DIP) or proximal nail fold. They are contiguous with the DIP joint capsule and contain synovial fluid, which is viscous, gelatinous, and clear to light yellow in color. Myxoid cysts most commonly occur in the 40- to 70-year age group and are twice as common in women as in men. When the lesion extends to the proximal nail fold, it can compress the matrix, causing a longitudinal groove on the nail plate. Myxoid cysts may be triggered by a reactive process or by herniation of the synovium; they are typically associated with a joint affected by osteoarthritis. Although most lesions are asymptomatic and do not require intervention, they may cause pain or decreased range of motion. In those cases, simple incision and drainage with the tip of a large-bore needle often provides relief. Recurrent lesions may require excision by a hand surgeon.

Nail Infections

Fungal Nail Infections

Clinical Features and Diagnosis

Tinea of the nails, or tinea unguium, affects 2% to 14% of the general population; prevalence increases with age.

About 90% of toenail and virtually all fingernail onychomycosis is caused by dermatophytes, typically *Trichophyton rubrum* and *Trichophyton mentagrophytes*. *Epidermophyton* and *Microsporum* species are less frequent causes. The most common clinical presentation of dermatophyte onychomycosis is fungal invasion of the hyponychium or lateral nail folds, which causes onycholysis, nail plate thickening, and subungual debris. Fungus may also invade the nail plate from above; superficial white onychomycosis causes a powdery white patchy discoloration of the nail surface. Least commonly, fungus will invade through the proximal margin, giving the appearance of infection emerging from beneath the nail as it grows. This presentation—proximal subungual onychomycosis—is a marker for lack of resistance to dermatophyte infection and is more prevalent in individuals with immunodeficiency.

Dermatophytes invade normal keratin, whereas molds invade altered keratin. Onychomycosis, therefore, can be caused by other fungal species, including *Candida* and nondermatophyte molds such as *Acremonium*, *Alternaria*, *Aspergillus*, *Fusarium*, *Onycholiza*, *Scopulariopsis*, and *Scytalidium* species. Nondermatophyte organisms are responsible for 10% to 20% of cases of onychomycosis. The distinction is important because treatment may differ from that for dermatophyte infection. Candidal

onychomycosis is uncommon and may present as proximal nail changes in association with paronychia or as onycholysis with typical nail plate thickening and subungual debris. Nondermatophyte infection most commonly presents with distal-lateral subungual onychomycosis and may be difficult to distinguish from typical dermatophyte onychomycosis.

At least half of patients with onychomycosis will experience some degree of pain or discomfort. As a result, patients may choose less than ideal footwear or have difficulty with ambulation, increasing the risk of falls, particularly among the elderly. Additionally, dystrophic nails may disrupt the surrounding cutaneous barrier, creating a point of entry for skin bacteria or leading to toe or foot ulceration.

Accurate diagnosis of onychomycosis depends on the collection of an adequate sample for evaluation. The onycholytic portion of the affected nail plate should be trimmed as far proximally as possible. Subungual debris is then collected from the nail bed using a curette, taking care to sample from different parts (proximal and distal) of the infected nail. Fungi collect in the nail plate and in the cornified cells of the nail bed. Superficial nail samples are unlikely to produce a high fungal yield.

All national guidelines recommend that physicians not prescribe oral antifungal therapy for suspected onychomycosis without confirmation of infection. Direct microscopy of nail scrapings using potassium hydroxide (KOH) can quickly confirm the presence of fungal hyphae, but the procedure does not identify the exact infectious organism. Formal culture may take 4 weeks or longer to produce a result and offers a sensitivity of only about 50%.

Treatment

Oral antifungal agents—including terbinafine (Lamisil), itraconazole (Sporanox), and fluconazole (Diflucan)[1]—penetrate keratinizing tissue and produce higher drug levels in the nail plate than in plasma. Therapeutic levels may remain in the nails for at least a month after the discontinuation of therapy. Periodic debridement of the infected nail during the course of treatment may increase the cure rate. Treatment with systemic antifungals must be weighed against the risk of hepatic toxicity and the potential for interactions with multiple other medications.

Despite adequate treatment, recurrence of onychomycosis is seen in 40% to 70% of patients and is more likely in patients with extensive involvement of the proximal nail, immunosuppression, or peripheral vascular disease. Oral antifungal agents for onychomycosis are outlined in Table 1.

Three topical drugs for onychomycosis are available in the United States: ciclopirox (Penlac), efinaconazole (Jublia), and tavaborole (Kerydin). Fingernails are treated daily for 24 weeks; toenails are treated daily for 48 weeks. Once weekly, the lacquer should be removed with acetone and any residual diseased nail material filed or clipped away. Complete cure rates typically do not exceed 15% but may be enhanced by thorough debridement of a thickened, lytic nail prior to treatment.

[1]Not FDA approved for this indication.

[1]Not FDA approved for this indication.

Toenails take 12 to 18 months to be replaced; fingernails take 4 to 6 months for the same process. Therefore, immediately after completion of therapy, the nail will not appear to be completely normal. Rather, a proximal segment of newly formed, fungus-free, and normal-appearing nail will be present and will gradually extend distally as a new nail is produced.

The risk of recurrent onychomycosis may be reduced by preventing and treating tinea pedis. Prolonged use of a topical antifungal agent, such as terbinafine (Lamisil), may prevent nail reinfection after successful treatment with oral medication. Avoidance of trauma to the tips of the nails from tight-fitting shoes may also decrease the risk of recurrence. Foot powder and the use of moisture-wicking socks can limit the moisture surrounding the foot, preventing the warm, dark, moist environment that is conducive to fungal growth.

Pseudomonas Nail Infection

Pseudomonas is the bacterium that is most likely to infect the nail unit, and such infections are characterized by blue-green discoloration beneath the nail and onycholysis. Typically, only one nail is involved. Risk factors include chronic nail trauma, nail disease such as psoriasis, and chronic paronychia. Topical treatment, such as fluoroquinolone or aminoglycoside solutions, or antiseptic soaks with dilute bleach or chlorhexidine (Hibiclens), are often curative. Response rates are enhanced by trimming away any diseased or lytic nail prior to treatment.

Periungual Verrucae

Verruca vulgaris—common warts—are caused by human papillomavirus infection and can involve the periungual and subungual skin of the nail unit. Fingers are more commonly affected than toes. Periungual verrucae present the same as warts at other cutaneous sites, with a hyperkeratotic papule, associated thrombosed capillaries, and disruption of epidermal architecture. Verrucae do not typically involve the nail matrix, but lesions of the proximal nail fold can compress the matrix and lead to nail plate dystrophy.

Periungual verrucae are notoriously difficult to treat. Topical agents are appropriate initial therapeutic options for periungual verrucae, typically including the use of a keratolytic such as salicylic acid. Success rates with topical agents are enhanced with occlusion of the lesion, but several months of daily treatment may be required. Cryotherapy is an additional first-line option and is more efficacious if the lesion is debulked with scissors or scalpel prior to treatment. Longer freeze times may also improve efficacy. Aggressive cryotherapy at the proximal nail fold may damage the underlying nail matrix and lead to permanent nail dystrophy. Intralesional treatment with candida antigen[1], mumps antigen[1], or bleomycin[1] has demonstrated success in the treatment of refractory periungual verrucae. Surgical approaches such as excision and electrosurgery have a moderate potential for scarring and are associated with higher recurrence rates. Squamous cell carcinoma of the nail unit presents as a hyperkeratotic lesion that may be indistinguishable from a wart. Therefore lesions that are recalcitrant to conventional therapy warrant biopsy.

[1]Not FDA approved for this indication.

References

de Berker D: Clinical practice. Fungal nail disease, *New Engl J Medicine* 360(20):2108–2116, 2009.

de Berker D: Nail anatomy, *Clin Dermatol* 31(5):509–515, 2013.

Biesbroeck LK, Fleckman P: Nail disease for the primary care provider, *Med Clin N Am* 99(6):1213–1226, 2015.

Gupta AK, Versteeg SG, Shear NH: Onychomycosis in the 21st century: an update on diagnosis, epidemiology, and treatment, *J Cutan Med Surg* 21(6):525–539, 2017.

Lipner S, Scher R: Evaluation of nail lines: Color and shape hold clues, *Cleve Clin J Med* 83(5):385–391, 2016.

Maddy AJ, Tosti A: Hair and nail diseases in the mature patient, *Clin Dermatol* 36(2):159–166, 2018.

Westerberg DP, Voyack MJ: Onychomycosis: Current trends in diagnosis and treatment, *Am Fam Physician* 88(11):762–770, 2013.

ERYTHEMA MULTIFORME

Method of
Chad Douglas, MD, PharmD

CURRENT DIAGNOSIS

- Acute cutaneous target-like papules, plaques, and bullae
- Oral mucosal lesions can be present
- Predominance in young adults
- Most often associated with acute or chronic herpes simplex virus (HSV-1) infection
- Less commonly associated with medications such as sulfonamide and penicillin antibiotics

CURRENT THERAPY

- Treat any underlying infection, and discontinue any potential offending medications.
- Mild disease: Provide symptomatic care with oral antihistamines, topical corticosteroids.
- Severe and persistent disease: Treatment includes prednisone, cyclosporine (Neoral and Sandimmune),[1] azathioprine (Imuran).[1]
- Recurrent episodes: Provide prophylaxis with HSV antiviral agents.

Epidemiology

Erythema multiforme (EM) is an acute, mucocutaneous, immune-mediated hypersensitivity disorder. This rare self-limiting disorder has an estimated incidence of 0.01% to 1% and predominately occurs in young adults between 20 and 40 years of age. Up to 20% of cases occur in children and adolescents. The median age of onset of recurrent EM in children is 9 years of age.

Risk Factors

EM is most commonly associated with viral, fungal, and atypical bacterial infections. More than 60% of infection-associated cases of EM occur with herpes simplex virus (HSV), most commonly HSV-1. *Mycoplasma pneumoniae* is the second most common infectious organism associated with EM, and up to 5% of patients with this atypical pneumonia develop EM. Most cases of recurrent EM are associated with acute HSV infection or reactivation of chronic HSV infection. The second most common cause of EM are medications. Medications account for 10% to 20% of EM cases and is referred to as *drug-induced erythema multiforme* (DIEM). The most common medication classes and agents in DIEM are sulfonamides, penicillins, erythromycin, nitrofurantoin, tetracyclines, nonsteroidal anti-inflammatory drugs, and aromatic amine anticonvulsants such as carbamazepine, phenytoin, and phenobarbital. DIEM is considered a separate and distinct entity from hypersensitivity and cutaneous adverse drug reactions such as maculopapular erythema, Stevens-Johnson syndrome (SJS), and toxic epidermal necrolysis (TEN).

Pathophysiology

The pathophysiology of EM has been extensively delineated in herpes-associated erythema multiforme (HAEM). HSV DNA fragments are transported to distant skin sites by peripheral blood mononuclear cells. HSV genes within these fragments express various enzymes including DNA polymerase that leads to recruitment of CD4+ TH1 cells. These CD4+ TH1 cells release interferon-gamma (INF-gamma), which initiates an inflammatory cascade with the sequestration of circulating monocytes, natural killer (NK) cells, and lymphocytes as well as recruitment of autoreactive T cells. This extensive immune response leads to keratinocyte destruction. In contrast, the pathophysiology of DIEM involves tumor necrosis factor α (TNF-α) production that leads to epidermal destruction. Human leukocyte antigen polymorphisms have not been extensively characterized in DIEM as they have been in more classic immune-mediated cutaneous drug hypersensitivity reactions such as SJS and TEN.

Prevention

There is no current prevention for EM; however, the knowledge of infectious agents and medications that can cause EM can help one identify patients who could be at risk for development of this condition. Future studies in the advancement of pharmacogenetics may potentially identify human leukocyte antigen polymorphisms that could predispose patients to HAEM or DIEM.

Clinical Manifestations and Diagnosis

EM is a self-limiting eruption that most often appears in a symmetric distribution on the distal extremities with frequent involvement of dorsal surfaces of the hands and extensor surfaces of the extremities. Prodromal syndrome such as fever, chills, malaise, and arthralgia can occur but are rare. Lesions often burn or itch and progress from distal areas of the body toward proximal regions. Initial lesions are usually sharply demarcated red or pink macules that can resemble hives or early stages of SJS. Unlike hives, these lesions become fixed and do not migrate. Mucosal involvement and skin sloughing is less common than with SJS. The macules become papular and may gradually enlarge into plaques that are several centimeters in diameter. Lesions often contain three concentric zones including a central darker red region, a pale pink edematous zone, and a peripheral red ring. These characteristic "target" or "iris" lesions may only contain a central dark red region with a lighter peripheral ring and may not appear until several days after onset of the eruptions. Lesions of multiple morphology are usually present, thus the name *multiforme*. Mucosal lesions, when present, are red and edematous and often involve blister formation. These lesions are usually limited to the oral cavity and affect the lips, inside of the cheeks, and the tongue. Typically, lips are swollen with hemorrhagic crusting. EM associated with *Mycoplasma pneumoniae* may present with mucosal lesions alone without cutaneous manifestations. Diagnosis is most often made clinically in patients with characteristic lesions and a preceding or concurrent infection that is known to be commonly associated with EM. A clinical diagnosis can also be made in patients with characteristic lesions who are taking a commonly associated medication. Rarely, a skin biopsy is needed to rule out other conditions, although there is no single diagnostic histologic feature or immunofluorescence finding specific to EM. EM usually resolves spontaneously within 3 to 5 weeks.

Differential Diagnosis

Early EM lesions can resemble urticaria, drug eruptions, viral exanthem, maculopapular erythema, and the early stages of SJS and toxic epidermal necrosis. Bullous lesions may resemble bullous pemphigoid, and target lesions may resemble pityriasis rosea or vasculitis.

Treatment

Although EM is self-limiting, early identification and treatment of the causative infectious agent or immediate discontinuation of an offending medication can reduce the severity and duration of the condition. Symptomatic treatment with oral first-generation antihistamines (diphenhydramine [Benadryl] 25 to 50 mg po q 6 hours prn or hydroxyzine [Atarax] 25 to 100 mg po q 6 hours prn) and mid-potency topical corticosteroids (triamcinolone [Kenalog] 0.1% cream) will usually suffice for mild disease. More severe disease including cases with mucosal involvement as well as recurrent EM can be treated with prednisone, cyclosporine (Neoral, Sandimmune),[1] or azathioprine (Imuran).[1] The use of dapsone[1] and antimalarial agents in severe disease has demonstrated varying success. Recurrent EM is most often associated with HSV-1, and herpes viral suppressive therapy with acyclovir (Zovirax)[1] or valacyclovir (Valtrex)[1] has been shown to be effective. Valacyclovir (Valtrex) is given once daily until the patient is recurrence free for 4 months. The valacyclovir dose is then reduced with eventual discontinuation. Although reintroduction of an offending medication

does not frequently cause recurrence of EM, caution should still be advised when considering the future use of such medication or other medications within the same drug class.

Monitoring and Complications

Mucosal involvement may limit a patient's ability to eat or drink, and close monitoring is advised in such cases. This can be of particular concern in pediatric patients. Skin lesions are usually not associated with scarring, but postinflammatory hyperpigmentation can occur and often takes several months to resolve.

References

Anquier-Durand A, Mockenhaupt M, et al: Correlations between clinical patterns and causes of erythema multiforme majus, Stevens-Johnson syndrome, and toxic epidermal necrolysis: results of an international prospective study, *Arch Dermatol* 138(8):1019–1024, 2002 Aug.

Aurelian L, Ono F, Burnett J: Herpes simplex virus (HSV)-associated erythema multiforme (HAEM): a viral disease with an autoimmune component, *Dermatol Online J* 9(I), 2003.

de Risi-Pugliese T, Sbidian E, Ingen-Housz-Oro S, et al: Interventions for erythema multiforme: a systematic review, *J Eur Acad Dermatol Venereol* 33(5):842–849, 2019.

Kokuba H, Aurelian L, Burnett J: Herpes simplex virus associated erythema multiforme (HAEM) is mechanistically distinct from drug-induced erythema multiforme: interferon-gamma is expressed in HAEM lesions and tumor necrosis factor-alpha in drug-induced erythema multiforme lesions, *J Invest Dermatol* 113:808–815, 1999.

Heinze A, Tollefson M, Holland KE, et al: Characteristics of pediatric recurrent erythema multiforme, *Pediatr Dermatol* 35(1):97–103, 2018.

Lamoreux MR, Sternbach MR, Hsu WT: Erythema Multiforme, *Am Fam Physician* 74(11):1883–1888, 2006 Dec 1.

Ono F, Sharma BK, Smith CC, et al: CD34+ Cells in the peripheral blood transport herpes simplex virus DNA fragments to the skin of patients with erythema multiforme (HAEM), *J Invest Dermatol* 124:1215–1224, 2005.

Sokumbi O, Wetter DA: Clinical features, diagnosis, and treatment of erythema multiforme: a review for the practicing dermatologist, *Int J Dermatol* 51:889–902, 2012.

Svensson CK, Cowen EW, Gaspari AA: Cutaneous drug reactions, *Pharmacol Rev* 53(3):357–379, 2001 Sep.

Trayes KP, Love G, Studdiford JS: Erythema Multiforme: Recognition and Management, *Am Fam Physician* 100(2):82–88, 2019.

FUNGAL INFECTIONS OF THE SKIN

Method of
Therese Holguin, MD; Chad Douglas, MD, PharmD; Kriti Mishra, MD; and Sabah Osmani, MD

CURRENT DIAGNOSIS

- Dermatophyte infections
  - Non–hair-bearing (glabrous) skin diagnostic techniques include scraping the leading edge of scale with a glass slide onto glass slide, placing a cover slip, and applying 10% potassium hydroxide (KOH) to the edge of the coverslip. Then the bottom of the slide is slightly heated, cleaned with a tissue, and viewed under a microscope with lowered condenser. Counterstaining with chlorazol black E or Parker blue-black ink may help visualize hyphae.
  - Hair-bearing skin may require a tissue biopsy with special fungal stains to confirm diagnosis.
  - Culture of scale, hair, and nail fragments sent to the laboratory in a sterile urine cup and clearly marked "for dermatophyte culture" is an additional testing method. Nail fragments can be sent in formalin for periodic acid-Schiff (PAS) staining (a quick-turnaround test).
- Tinea versicolor
  - Diagnostic techniques include stratum corneum removal with a glass slide against a glass slide and KOH examination as noted earlier for dermatophyte infections. Cultures require a special media, and the laboratory must be notified that this is the organism suspected.
- Candida cutaneous infections
  - Unroofing a pustule by scraping gently with a No. 15 blade and spreading contents onto a glass slide for KOH evaluation will review the characteristic yeast and pseudohyphae. Culture is usually not necessary.

- Dermatophyte infections
  - Mild non–hair-bearing skin infections are treated with topical agents if severe and widespread; systemic and topical agents together will provide a higher cure rate. Measures to prevent reinfection of feet include wearing sandals when in public places (e.g., swimming pools), alternating shoes, and keeping feet dry. Measures to prevent reinfection of groin infections include drying well after showering and putting socks on before underwear.
  - Hair-bearing skin and hair infections require systemic therapy for cure. Nail infections may be cured with newer topical agents.
- Tinea versicolor
  - Topical treatment with topical agents such as selenium sulfide lotion applied for 10 minutes for 2 weeks, neck to knees, is a cheap and effective treatment. Systemic agents may be needed for resistant cases. Prevention may require maintenance therapy with topical agents during warm and humid months.
- Candida cutaneous infections
  - Topical agents such as nystatin or ketoconazole cream are an effective choice. Prevention of intertrigo is somewhat successful if routine care is taken to dry body fold areas thoroughly after showering. Zinc-talc shake lotion may be used once or twice daily.

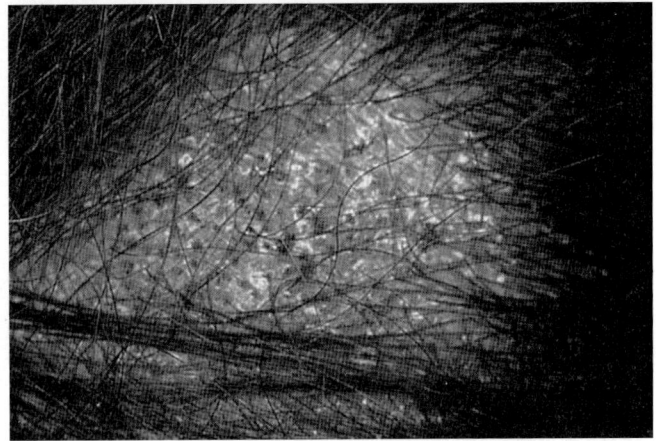

Figure 1 Black dot tinea.

Dermatophyte (tinea) infections are a group of filamentous fungal infections of the skin, hair, and nails and can be noninflammatory or inflammatory. The route of acquisition for dermatophytes is either person-to-person (anthropophilic) or from animals (zoophilic). Geophilic dermatophytes grow in soil and are a rare source of infection in humans. The causative organisms are of three genera: *Microsporum*, *Trichophyton*, and *Epidermophyton*.

Dermatophytoses are the most common fungal infections worldwide, affecting 20% to 25% of the world population. The predominant agents have changed over time by geography and population based on migration of populations, hygiene practices, and therapeutic breakthroughs (griseofulvin [Gris-PEG]). Clinical classification is based on the site of infection. Tinea pedis refers to infection of the feet, tinea manuum to the hands, tinea cruris to the groin, and tinea corporis to the skin excluding the aforementioned sites plus the scalp and nails. Tinea unguium (onychomycosis) refers to nail infection, tinea barbae to the beard area, tinea faciei to the face, and tinea capitis to the scalp and hair. Virulence of the infection is dependent on underlying factors suppressing immunity (diabetes, cancer, HIV infection). Dissemination can be seen in the immunosuppressed. Resistance to griseofulvin may be due to it not being available in certain countries, and terbinafine resistance in *Microsporum* spp. and *Trichophyton* spp. has led to the use of fluconazole and itraconazole instead.

Superficial infections of the skin and mucous membranes caused by yeasts are caused by *Candida* species. Also common are infections caused the lipophilic yeast *Malassezia*.

Superficial Mycoses Dermatophytes
Tinea Capitis
The populations most at risk are children, with boys more commonly affected than girls. Tinea capitis infection in adults is becoming more common, and *T. tonsurans* is the usual pathogen. The onset of puberty and change in the relative composition of unsaturated fatty acids in sebum is protective. African Americans and Hispanics have an increased incidence of *Trichophyton tonsurans*. Pet exposure is associated with infections of *Microsporum canis*. Infection with *Trichophyton schoenleinii (favus)*, still seen in less-developed countries, is of characteristic cup-shaped crusts, or scutula.

The usual presentation of tinea capitis is of scale and itch on the scalp with broken-off hairs with a "black dot" appearance (Figure 1) or an inflamed boggy plaque, referred to as a *kerion*. Inflammatory presentations are most often seen in zoophilic infections. Patches of alopecia are common.

Tools for diagnosis include potassium hydroxide (KOH) preparation of scale or microscopic examination of hair tweezed from the affected patch. Trichoscopy is a useful tool in distinguishing between endothrix and ectothrix infections and can guide treatment. Also, PCR testing can help distinguish between genus and species. A Wood's lamp will show fluorescence with ectothrix infections (organism on outside of the shaft) but not endothrix infections (spores on inside of the shaft). Samples for culture are obtained by rubbing a wet cotton-tipped applicator over the affected area and applying this or pulled hairs onto the dermatophyte test medium or other medium if species identification is required in resistant cases. The differential diagnosis includes seborrheic dermatitis, psoriasis, folliculitis, pediculosis, secondary syphilis, discoid lupus erythematosus, lichen planus, lichen simplex chronicus, trichotillomania, alopecia areata, and other inflammatory follicular conditions.

Tinea Faciei and Barbae
Frequently misdiagnosed, infection of the face or beard is rare. Beard infections (tinea sycosis or barber's itch) can be deep and inflammatory and are seen in agricultural workers, especially those working with farm animals. Discoid lupus is a commonly mistaken diagnosis, and biopsies are sometimes required to differentiate.

Tinea Corporis
Ringworm is the layperson's descriptive term of the characteristic clinical findings of dermatophyte infections. The term accurately portrays the appearance of an erythematous annular plaque with a scaly, raised, leading edge (Figure 2). Severe infections may herald new HIV infection or be secondary to topical immunosuppressants such as calcineurin inhibitors or, more commonly, steroids. KOH examination sampling should be taken from the leading edge. The differential diagnosis includes pityriasis rosea, impetigo, inflammatory dermatoses such as psoriasis and seborrheic dermatitis, and syphilis.

Tinea Cruris
More common in men and when humidity is high, "jock itch" or "crotch itch" involves the upper thigh, intertriginous area, and peripheral spread into the perineum and perianal areas. The scrotum is rarely involved. The usually well-defined border may display scale, papules, or pustules.

The differential diagnosis includes a bacterial infection, erythrasma, candidiasis, intertrigo, psoriasis, and dermatitis. Morphology of the rash and expected involvement of other cutaneous sites is useful to eliminate these possible diagnoses. The origin of

Figure 2 Tinea corporis.

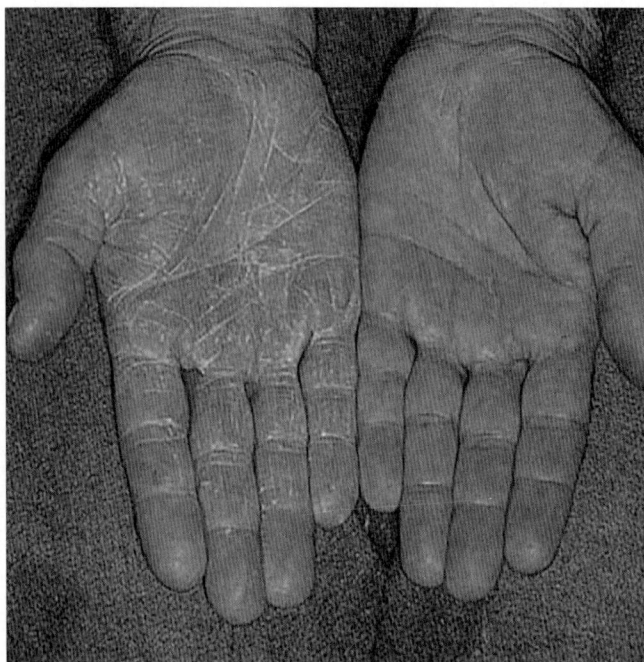

Figure 3 Tinea manuum.

the infection is believed to be autoinoculation from tinea pedis or onychomycosis.

Tinea Manuum and Pedis

A classic finding of "one hand and two feet" involvement is useful to lead one to consider tinea manuum (Figure 3). The organism involved in the infection determines the amount of resultant inflammation. Whereas *Trichophyton rubrum* produces a dry scale with erythema of the hands and feet (moccasin-type), *Trichophyton interdigitale* (previously known as *Trichophyton mentagrophytes*) often leads to a painful, itchy, blistering eruption of the feet. Other signs of *T. interdigitale* include interdigital maceration and superficial infection of the toenails with a distinct white appearance (white superficial onychomycosis). Toe-web infection with gram-negative bacteria may be consequential. Hyperhidrosis is often a precursor to this type of infection. An idiopathic reaction "dermatophytid" is a fairly common pruritic rash of small blisters involving the palms and sometimes the sides of the feet.

Onychomycosis

Fungal infections of the nail are caused by dermatophytes (tinea unguium), yeasts, and nondermatophytic molds. It is common in the general population, accounting for 50% of skin fungal infections. Risk factors include advanced age, diabetes, circulatory disorders, and family history. There are three major subtypes of onychomycosis: *distal lateral subungual onychomycosis, white superficial onychomycosis,* and *proximal subungual onychomycosis.* Distal lateral subungual onychomycosis is the most common subtype and is caused by the anthropophilic dermatophytic fungus, *T. rubrum.* Symptoms include an initial discoloration of the distal corner of the nail that may be white, gray, or brown caused by accumulation of keratinous debris under the nail that eventually spreads to involve the entire nail. Other common features are onycholysis, or splitting of the nail from the bed, nail thickening, and impaired nail growth. The diagnosis typically involves KOH, mycologic laboratory confirmation (culture), and biopsy. Yeast onychomycosis is most commonly caused by *Candida albicans* and typically involves fingernails of hands frequently exposed to moisture. Nondermatophytic molds primarily involve toenails. Though not life-threatening, onychomycosis can significantly impair an individual's quality of life with concerns such as issues cutting the nails and cosmetic disfigurement.

Pityriasis Versicolor

This superficial fungal infection of the skin is caused by the *Malassezia* species, a dimorphic lipophilic fungus that is part of the physiologic skin flora. Certain environmental, genetic, and immunologic factors can predispose the fungus to convert to its pathogenic hyphal form and development of disease. It grows best in warm, humid climates; thus there has been a higher prevalence reported in tropical climates. Furthermore, potential hormonal changes during adolescence can increase sebum production and allow for *Malassezia* to thrive, and the prevalence is even further increased in active adolescents. The pathophysiology may also be related to an impaired immune system.

The diagnosis is usually made clinically, but the presentation may vary; it classically consists of a well-demarcated rash with fine scale and thin plaques. The rash may be hyperpigmented, hypopigmented, or erythematous. Typically, the rash appears on the torso but may become widespread. The lesions may be mildly pruritic or asymptomatic. If KOH is performed on skin scrapings, numerous spores and hyphae can be visualized ("spaghetti-and-meatball" appearance). Treatment options include topical antifungals, including azoles and terbinafine,[1] selenium sulfide (antidandruff), and zinc pyrithione (Vanicream Z-Bar, DHS Body Wash). Topical retinoids may have a role in recalcitrant cases (Cosio et al., 2021). Oral azole antifungals also can be used, however systemic treatment is not first-line therapy because of side effects.

Candidiasis

A dimorphic commensal fungus inhabiting the skin, mouth, and reproductive tract, candidiasis is found in up to 70% of healthy individuals. *Candida* infection of the skin usually involves moist or occluded areas such as the groin, axillae, and diaper area in the young. Candidal intertrigo classically presents as erythematous and macerated plaques with peripheral scaling. Satellite lesions help differentiate candidal lesions from other conditions. Skin lesions are typically nontender but may develop central pallor or become hemorrhagic in patients with thrombocytopenia. Primary treatment consists of topical azole and polyene (nystatin) antifungals that are well tolerated. Adjunct therapy with low-dose topical corticosteroids may be used for associated pruritus and pain. Systemic antifungal therapy is rarely used but may be used for refractory disease.

---

[1] Not FDA approved for this indication.

Treatment
Tinea Capitis
First-line treatment for tinea capitis is systemic griseofulvin, but terbinafine may also be considered. Terbinafine may be more effective than griseofulvin in treating *T. tonsurans*, whereas griseofulvin may be more effective against *Microsporum*. Fluconazole[1] and itraconazole[1] are additional options that have demonstrated less evidence-based efficacy.

Pediatric Dosages (≥2 years)
Griseofulvin

- Microsize ([Grifulvin V, generic] 500-mg tablets): 20 to 25 mg/kg/day × 6 to 12 weeks (daily max 1000 mg/day)
- Ultramicrosize ([Gris-PEG, generic] 125 mg, 250-mg tablets): 10 to 15 mg/kg/day × 6 to 12 weeks (daily max 750 mg/day)
- Griseofulvin microsize suspension ([Grifulvin V, generic] 125 mg/5 mL): 15 to 25 mg/kg/day × 2 to 12 weeks

Terbinafine ([Lamisil, generic] 250-mg tablets)[1]

- 10 to 20 kg: 62.5 mg/day × 4 to 6 weeks
- 20 to 40 kg: 125 mg/day × 4 to 6 weeks
- >40 kg: 250 mg/day × 4 to 6 weeks

Terbinafine (Lamisil granules)[2]

- <25 kg: 125 mg/day × 4 to 6 weeks
- 25 to 35 kg: 165.5 mg/day × 4 to 6 weeks
- >35 kg: 250 mg/day × 4 to 6 weeks

Fluconazole oral suspension ([Diflucan, generic][1] 10 mg/mL, 40 mg/mL)

- Continuous: 6 mg/kg/day × 20 days (daily max 400 mg)
- Pulse: 6 mg/kg/day, once per week × 6 to 12 weeks

Itraconazole (Sporanox)[1]

- Continuous:
- Oral suspension (10 mg/mL): 5 mg/kg/day × 4 weeks
- Pulses (three pulses)
- Oral suspension: 3 mg/kg/day, 1 week/month × 2 to 3 months
- Capsules (100 mg): 5 mg/kg/day, 1 week/month × 2 to 3 months

Adult Dosages
Terbinafine (Lamisil)[1]

- 250 mg/day × 4 to 6 weeks

Fluconazole (Diflucan)[1]

- 50 mg/day × 4 to 7 weeks
  OR
- 150 mg/week × 4 weeks

Itraconazole (Sporanox)[1]

- 100 to 200 mg/day × 4 weeks

Topical therapies can also be helpful when used twice-weekly in conjunction with systemic treatment. These include antifungal shampoos like selenium sulfide (antidandruff), ciclopirox (Loprox), and zinc pyrithione (Head & Shoulders).

Tinea Corporis, Tinea Cruris, Tinea Pedis, Tinea Mannum, Tinea Faciei, and Tinea Barbae
Topical treatments should be used for 2 to 6 weeks once or twice daily. Options include terbinafine (Lamisil), butenafine (Lotrimin-Ultra), naftifine (Naftin), clotrimazole (Lotrimin), econazole (Ecoza), ketoconazole (Nizoral), sertaconazole (Ertaczo), luliconazole (Luzu), and eberconazole (Ebernet).[2] (The use of aforementioned topical products in tinea manuum is off-label). Begin therapy with topical treatment and reserve systemic treatment for widespread, resistant, or severe disease. If necessary:

Pediatric Dosages (all are off-label and not FDA approved)
Terbinafine (tablets)[1]

- <20 kg: 62.5 mg/day × 2 weeks
- 20 to 40 kg: 125 mg/day × 2 weeks
- >40 kg: 250 mg/day × 2 weeks

Itraconazole[1]

- 5 mg/kg/day divided qd-BID × 2 weeks (max 200 mg/day)

Griseofulvin (dosages listed are for age >2 to adolescent)

- Microsize: 10 to 20 mg/kg/day × 2 to 8 weeks
- Ultramicrosize: 5 to 15 mg/kg/day divided qd-BID
- Max: 750 mg/day

Adult Dosages (all are off-label and not FDA approved)
Terbinafine[1]

- 250 mg/day × 2 to 4 weeks

Itraconazole[1]

- 200 mg/day × 1 week

Fluconazole[1]

- 150 to 300 mg/week × 2 to 4 weeks (pulse dosing)

Griseofulvin

- Microsize: 500 to 1000 mg/day × 2 to 4 weeks
- Ultramicrosize: 375 to 500 mg/day × 2 to 4 weeks

Terbinafine

- 250 mg plus itraconazole 200 mg × 3 weeks (resistant cases)[1]

Tinea Unguium
Children may respond completely to antifungal topical lacquer or solutions without systemic therapy. Lacquers, such as amorolfine (Curanail, Loceryl, Locetar, Odenil)[2] are debrided and reapplied daily. Hydrolacquers, such as ciclopirox (Penlac) may also be used and are removable with washing and reapplied daily. Topical solutions, like efinaconazole (Jublia) and tavaborole (Kerydin), are used for 48 to 60 weeks. Topical retinoids may have a role in recalcitrant cases (Cosio et al., 2021).

If systemic therapy is required—and in all adult cases—first-line treatment is terbinafine. Systemic treatment in conjunction with lacquers has been associated with higher cure rates. Additionally, conventional oral therapy followed by topical therapy for maintenance may help prevent recurrence.

If there is no response to treatment or the patient cannot tolerate the medication, itraconazole may be used. Fluconazole[1] has not been shown to be as effective and requires a long duration of treatment (up to 6 months); therefore it is not a preferred treatment. Griseofulvin is not recommended. Lasers and photodynamic therapy if available are considered third-line options. Surgical options include chemical (40% to 50% urea compound) or surgical nail avulsion.

Pediatric Dosages
Terbinafine (≥2 years)

- <20 kg: 62.5 mg/day
- 20 to 40 kg: 125 mg/day
- >40 kg: 250 mg/day × 6 weeks for fingernails, × 12 weeks for toenails

Itraconazole
Daily for 1 week/month (2 months for fingernails, 3 months for toenails)

- <20 kg: 5 mg/kg/day
- 20 to 40 kg: 100 mg/day
- 40 to 50 kg: 200 mg/day
- >50 kg: 200 mg 2x/day

Adult Dosages
Terbinafine

- Continuous: 250 mg/day × 6 weeks for fingernails, × 12 weeks for toenails
- Pulse (for toenails): 250 mg BID × 4 weeks, no treatment × 4 weeks, 250 mg BID × 4 weeks (12 weeks total)

Itraconazole

- Continuous: 200 mg/day × 6 weeks for fingernails, × 12 weeks for toenails
- Pulse: 200 mg BID 1 week/month × 2 months for fingernails, × 3 months for toenails

Additional Comments
Before beginning systemic antifungal therapy, a baseline complete blood count and liver function tests must be obtained.

---

[2] Not available in the United States.
[1] Not FDA approved for this indication.

---

[2] Not available in the United States.

Laboratory tests are repeated if therapy lasts longer than 6 weeks.

Griseofulvin is contraindicated in pregnancy, and there are restrictions for becoming pregnant or fathering after a medication course is complete. Patients should avoid alcohol during treatment. Griseofulvin is more effectively absorbed with fatty foods like peanut butter, yogurt, and ice cream. (Therapeutic failures have been noted as a result of lack of absorption.) Itraconazole has negative inotropic effects and can lead to QT prolongation. Ketoconazole[1] has risks of fatal liver damage and adrenal insufficiency and is generally not recommended.

Acknowledgment

Dr. Holguin would like to recognize Dr. Sabah Osmani and Dr. Kriti Mishra for their past contributions to this chapter.

References

Andersen PL: Treatment adherence and psychosocial impact of tinea capitis in families: qualitative pilot study, *Dermatol Ther* 33(4), 2020.

Bouchara J-P, Nenoff P, Gupta AK, Chaturvedi V, (eds.): *Dermatophytes and dermatophytoses*, Springer International Publishing, New York, 2021.

Asz-Sigall D, Tosti A, Arenas R: Tinea unguium: diagnosis and treatment in practice, *Mycopathologia* 182:95–100, 2017.

Chen X, Jiang X, Yang M, et al: Systemic antifungal therapy for tinea capitis in children: an abridged cochrane review, *J Am Acad Dermatol* 76:368–374, 2017.

Cosio T, Gaziano R, Zuccari G, et al: Retinoids in Fungal Infections: From Bench to Bedside, *Pharmaceuticals (Basel)* 14(10):962, 2021. Published 2021 Sep 24. https://doi.org/10.3390/ph14100962.

Galili E, Goldsmith T, Khanimov I, et al: Tinea capitis caused by *Trichophyton tonsurans* among adults: clinical characteristics and treatment response, *Mycoses* 66(2):144–149, 2023.

Genedy RM: Trichoscopic signs of tinea capitis: a guide for selection of appropriate antifungal, *Int J Dermatol* 60(4):471–481, 2021.

Gupta AK: The growing problem of antifungal resistance in onychomycosis and other superficial mycoses, *Am J Clin Dermatol* 22(2):149–157, 2021.

Gupta A, Foley K, Versteeg S: New antifungal agents and new formulations against dermatophytes, *Mycopathologia* 182:127–141, 2017.

Gupta AK, Kogan N, Batra R: Pityriasis versicolor: a review of pharmacological treatment options: expert opinion on pharmacotherapy, *Expert Opin Pharmacother* 6:165–178, 2005.

Hay R: Tinea capitis: current status, *Mycopathologia* 182:87–93, 2017.

Kyriakis KP, Terzoudi S, Palamaras I, et al: Pityriasis versicolor prevalence by age and gender, *Mycoses* 49:517–518, 2006.

Nenoff P, Krüger C, Ginter-Hanselmayer, et al: Mycology—an update. Part 1: Dermatomycoses: Causative agents, epidemiology and pathogenesis, *J Dtsch Dermatol Ges* 12:188–209, 2014.

Perlroth J, Choi B, Spellberg B: Nosocomial fungal infections: epidemiology, diagnosis, and treatment, *Med Mycol* 45:321–346, 2007.

Priyanka S, Mala B, Gurvinder P, et al: Evaluation of efficacy and safety of oral terbinafine and itraconazole combination therapy in the management of dermatophytosis, *J Dermatol Treat*, 2019, https://doi.org/10.1080/09546634.2019.1612835.

Solís-Arias MP, García-Romero MT: Onychomycosis in children: a review, *Int J Dermatol* 56:123–130, 2017.

KELOIDS AND HYPERTROPHIC SCARS

Method of
Monica Chamorro, MD

CURRENT DIAGNOSIS

- Keloids and hypertrophic scars (HTS) are dermal fibroproliferative disorders characterized by excessive formation of fibrous tissue.
- Keloids manifest as an elevated lesion with borders that extend beyond the original wound.
- Keloids and HTS are more likely to affect young individuals than older individuals.
- Diagnosis of keloids and HTS is based on history and clinical examination.
- Ultrasound and dermoscopy might be used to support the diagnosis.
- A skin biopsy may be necessary if the diagnosis is unclear or malignancy is suspected.

CURRENT THERAPY

- Treatment of keloids and HTS is challenging.
- There are a wide variety of invasive and noninvasive treatment options.
- There is no single therapy that is particularly effective for treatment of keloids or HTS.
- Prevention is always the best approach, whenever possible.
- In most difficult cases, a combination of treatments is usually required.
- Regular follow-up to assess treatment effectiveness and recurrence is highly encouraged.

Keloids and hypertrophic scars (HTS) are dermal fibroproliferative disorders arising from cutaneous injury and irritation. The formation of excessive fibrous tissue characterizes these conditions. Keloids and HTS can be triggered by various factors such as trauma, insect bite, burn, surgery, vaccination, skin piercing, acne, folliculitis, chickenpox, and other skin infections. These conditions' functional and cosmetic implications can negatively impact a person's quality of life and daily activities.

Certain characteristics can help distinguish between keloids and hypertrophic scars. Keloids usually develop up to a year after an injury, are thicker and disorganized, and typically do not resolve on their own. On the other hand, hypertrophic scars typically become noticeable within the first few months after an injury, are organized, and usually resolve without treatment.

Etiology

The wound healing process can be divided into three phases: the inflammatory phase, the proliferative phase, and the remodeling phase. *The inflammatory phase* begins immediately at the time of injury with platelet migration and activation of the hemostasis mechanism. During this phase, inflammation and hemostasis occur. There is an influx of inflammatory cells and neutrophils, activation of clotting factors, and the release of cytokines and growth factors such as interleukin-6 (IL-6) and IL-8, epidermal growth factor, platelet-derived growth factor, and transforming growth factor-beta (TGF-β). The inflammatory phase lasts 1 to 3 days. The next phase is the *proliferative phase*, which lasts from day 4 to day 21, during which macrophages, endothelial cells, and fibroblasts play a crucial role in wound healing. Collagen type III is deposited to form granulation tissue, and keratinocytes differentiate, allowing migration and closure of the wound. During the *remodeling phase*, which can last up to a year after the injury, the extracellular matrix is reorganized, apoptosis of cells that formed granulation tissue occurs, and type III collagen is replaced by type I collagen, which is stronger and more stable. Myofibroblasts will contract to reduce the area of the scar.

Abnormal wound healing can result in a visible scar, especially when the balance between collagen production and breakdown is lost during scar maturation. Keloids and HTS are two types of scars that can result from abnormal wound healing. The borders of HTS remain within the boundaries of the original lesion, while the borders of keloids spread beyond those boundaries and can continue to grow over time. The factors contributing to the formation of keloids are poorly understood. However, the injury must reach the reticular dermis for abnormal scar tissue to form, and local mechanical forces may be the most critical factor in keloid formation. Keloids have been associated with several medical conditions and chronic inflammatory disorders, including hypertension, obesity, atopy, and osteoporosis. This suggests that keloids are a cutaneous inflammatory disorder and a systemic manifestation of chronic inflammation.

TABLE 1 Prevention Strategies for Keloids and Hypertrophic Scars

THERAPEUTIC METHOD	SUGGESTED MECHANISMS	EFFECT	DOSE	EVIDENCE
Tension free closure	Natural orientation of collagen fibers	Reduce inflammation	NA	
Taping/silicon sheeting	Mechanical stabilization	Avoid postsurgical stretching Hydration of stratum corneum	Begin 2 weeks after primary treatment; 12–24 h/d for at least for 2 mo	1
Onion extract[7]	Regulation of expression: of TGF-β, NF-κB Antioxidant response element and nitric oxide	Reduce inflammation. Reduce angiogenesis. Induce reepithelialization Antioxidant properties	Begin 2 weeks after primary injury or treatment; apply twice a day for 4–6 mo	2
Pressure therapy	Local vasoconstriction	Induce hypoxia. Reduce TGF-β1 expression and fibroblast activity.	Begin within 2 mo after injury. Minimal pressure of 15–25 mm Hg for at least 12 mo Preferred 24 h/d	3

[7]Available as a dietary supplement.
Key to evidence base support: Meta-analysis or RCT (1), large series (2), lesser quality series (3), small series (4).

Epidemiology

Hypertrophic scars are more common than keloids, and the prevalence is higher in darker-pigmented skin (Africans, Hispanics, Asians). Keloids are common worldwide, but the prevalence can vary from 0.09% in England to 16% in Zambia. It is estimated that more than 10 million people have this condition, but data are limited. Keloids do not have a sex preference and usually affect young individuals between the ages of 10 and 30, possibly because younger skin has greater tension and a higher collagen synthesis rate. Additionally, younger age groups are more prone to trauma exposure. Keloids tend to occur in specific areas of the body that experience friction and tension, with the chest being the most common site (48.9% of cases), followed by the scapular region (26.9%), and the lower back/neck region (12.1%). Less common areas include the upper arm (4.8%), the dorsal region (2.5%), the lower abdomen (1.9%), the femoral regions (1.7%), and the upper abdomen and knees (0.5%).

Clinical Manifestations and Evaluation

Patients with keloids typically present with an elevated, smooth-surfaced lesion that extends beyond the original wound. They may have a recent history of inflammation or trauma in the affected area.

The color of keloids may vary from pink-purple to dark brown and may be skin-colored in older lesions. Keloids can be painful, pruritic, and sensitive to touch. In some cases, they can restrict the normal movement of adjacent tissues. For example, a keloid in the antecubital fossa may prevent full extension of the elbow.

Diagnosing keloids is usually done by clinical examination—visual inspection and palpation are usually sufficient. A focused history, including the patient's personal and family history, should be collected. In some cases, dermoscopy and/or ultrasound can differentiate keloids from other skin lesions. A skin biopsy may be necessary if the diagnosis is unclear or malignancy is suspected.

The differential diagnosis for keloids includes lobomycosis (subcutaneous mycosis), keloidal forms of scleroderma and morphea, a sclerotic form of xanthoma disseminatum, and fibromatous tumors. Fibromatous tumors include dermatofibrosarcoma protuberans, rare variants of melanoma such as desmoplastic melanoma, and the scar-like variant of squamous cell carcinoma.

Prevention

Prevention of keloid formation is vital (Table 1). Special attention should be paid to patients with a family history and known risk factors. One simple step toward prevention is to avoid nonessential trauma to the skin, such as ear piercing, cosmetic surgery, or tattoos. Preprocedure planning can improve outcomes. Scarring can be reduced by techniques such as making skin incisions that follow the natural orientation of collagen fibers, leading to a better cosmetic outcome. Another technique to decrease the risk of pathologic scarring is to reduce the tension on the edges of the wound, which can be accomplished by hiding sutures in natural skin folds and limiting incisional wounds to a single cosmetic subunit (primary structural areas of the face that are separated by natural folds and borders and which share similar characteristics).

Other preventive strategies include avoiding ultraviolet exposure after a skin injury and applying paper tape or silicone tape or sheeting products (Mederma Silicone Scar Sheet, ScarAway Clear Silicone Scar Sheets, Nuvadermis Scar Sheets). For best results, though the evidence is weak, the silicone product should be applied consistently for 12 to 24 hours a day for at least 2 months after the injury.

Finally, flavonoids such as those present in onion extract[7] (topical onion extract gel [Mederma Skin Care Gel, Contractubex Gel]), that work by inducing matrix metalloproteinases and inflammatory regulation, applied twice a week for 4 to 6 months starting 2 weeks after primary wound treatment, have also been used.

Treatment

Targeting specific symptoms such as pain, itching, and inflammation should be a treatment priority in addition to reducing the size of the lesion. Other factors to consider are the location of the injury, severity of functional impairment, and amount of distress experienced by the patient. Although the approach to treating keloids and HTS is generally the same, it is essential to differentiate between them before starting treatment to determine the prognosis, likelihood of response to therapy, and risk of recurrence.

A wide variety of invasive and noninvasive management options exist. One noninvasive option to reduce scar thickness and redness is to use silicone-based products. However, the regimens are quite intense and require compliance and time for their effects to be seen. As noted previously, the silicone products must be used consistently for a minimum of 12 to 24 hours per day for 2 months.

Intralesional corticosteroid injections have been used for a long time. They work by increasing expression of collagenases (a group of enzymes that break down collagen bonds and promote healthy

[1]Not FDA approved for this indication.

TABLE 2 Summary of Pharmacologic Treatment

THERAPEUTIC AGENT	SUGGESTED MECHANISMS	EFFECT	DOSE	EVIDENCE
Steroids* (Intralesional triamcinolone acetonide (TAC) [Kenalog-10, Kenalog-40][1])†	Reduce TFG-β, IGF-I, VEGF Increases bFGF	Decrease inflammation Decrease collagen Increase collagenase	10–40 mg/mL concentration intralesionally† Sessions vary: from 2–8 injections with 4-to 8-wk interval	1
5-Furacil[1] (Intralesional 5-FU)	Inhibits thymidine synthase Reduce TFG-β and type I collagen gene expression	Reduce fibroblast proliferation Reduce angiogenesis	50 mg/mL Every 1–4 wk (usual) Up to 3 times a week	2‡
ACE inhibitors/ARBs§,[1] (Topical/intralesional)ᵖ,[2,6]	ARBS: AT 1R inhibition AICE: TGF-β/SMAD suppression antifibrotic effect	Inhibits collagen Antifibrotic effect	Varies Captopril[1] cream 5%[6] twice a day for 6 wk Losartan[1] gel 5%[6] twice week for 12 wk 0.2% losartan–urea cream[6]	2
Bleomycin[1] (Multiple puncture technique)	Reduce TFG-β Reduction of lysyl oxidase	Decrease collagen synthesis Induce apoptosis	1.5 IT/mL Max 10 IT per session Monthly	3
Pentoxifylline[1]	Increase collagenase activity	Reduce fibroblast proliferation.	400 mg tid PO 1 mg/mL intralesional[2]	4
Botulinum toxin A (Botox)[1] (intralesional)	Reduce muscle/wound tension	Decrease fibroblast proliferation and collagen activity	20–140 U 2–8 wk interval	1
Imiquimod[1] (topical)	Increases TNF-α, IFN-γ, α	Inhibits inflammatory response Response is usually poor	5% cream (Aldara)[1] applied for 6–8 wk	1
Dupilumab (Dupixent)§,[1]	IL-4 and IL-13 blockade	Reduce inflammation Decrease pruritus	SQ (thighs/buttocks/ abdomen): 600 mg once, followed by 300 mg every 2 wk	4
Interferon[1]	Down regulate TGF-β1	Reduce collagen synthesis Response is usually poor	INF-alpha-2b 1.5 × 10⁶ IU (intralesional)[1] bid × 4 d	1

[1]Not FDA approved for this indication.
[2]Not available in the United States.
[6]May be compounded by pharmacists.
*Ointments, tapes also available.
†Only Kenalog-10 (10 mg/mL) is approved for intralesional administration. Kenalog-40 (40 mg/mL) is used off label and may require further dilution using appropriate diluents to concentrations appropriate for the lesion.
‡Better evidence in combination: TAC/5 FU; laser/TAC/5FU.
§Clinical trial ongoing.
ᵖACE inhibitors and ARBs are available in oral formulation only in the United States and Canada. None of the ACEIs or ARBs are approved for topical or intralesional administration.
ACE, Angiotensin-converting enzyme; *ACEI*, angiotensin-converting enzyme inhibitor; *ARB*, angiotensin receptor blocker; *AT1R*, angiotensin 1 receptor; *bFGF*, basic fibroblast growth factor; *bid*, twice daily; *IL*, interleukin; *PO*, orally; *SQ*, subcutaneously; *TFG*, transforming growth factor; *tid*, three times daily.

tissue growth), reducing inflammation and cell proliferation, and producing vasoconstriction. Among the treatment options, triamcinolone acetonide (TAC) 10 to 40 mg/mL (Kenalog-10, Kenalog-40[1]) intralesional injections can be performed every 4 to 6 weeks with good results. Only Kenalog-10 (10 mg/mL) is approved for intralesional administration. Kenalog-40 (40 mg/mL) is used off-label and may require further dilution using appropriate diluents to concentrations appropriate for the lesion. A triamcinolone injection into keloid tissue is recommended to prevent skin from dimpling or denting (from atrophy) or changing color. To inject, advance the needle to the far end of the keloid and then inject while pulling out, directing the injection into the canal that was created. A Luer-Lok syringe or insulin syringe with a 25- to 30-gauge needle can be used.[1]

For those who want to avoid needles, steroid tape/plasters are a good option. Fludroxycortide tape (also known as flurandrenolide [Cordran Tape]) is approved for corticosteroid-responsive dermatoses in the United States, and plasters with deprodone propionate are only available in Japan. Steroid tapes and plasters are considered the first line of treatment in pediatric populations.

Topical high-potency steroids such as clobetasol propionate 0.05% (Clobex, Clodan, Tovet) are also an option, especially if itching is the main complaint.

The most common side effects of steroid use include telangiectasia and skin atrophy.

Fluorouracil (5-FU) is an antineoplastic agent that has some evidence of effectiveness. The mechanisms suggested for its effectiveness include inhibition of fibroblast proliferation and inhibition of angiogenesis. When treating keloids, 50 mg/mL 5-fluorouracil[1] is injected directly into the scar tissue using a 27- to 30-gauge needle until blanching occurs. The injection can be repeated every 1 to 4 weeks. Ulceration and pain are possible side effects.

Another agent included in this group is bleomycin.[1] Bleomycin is applied using a multiple puncture technique with a usual concentration of 1.5 IU/mL. Bleomycin decreases collagen synthesis and induces apoptosis.

Other medications that may be used include pentoxifylline[1]; immunomodulators such as tacrolimus (Protopic)[1] and 5% imiquimod cream (Aldara),[1] onabotulinumtoxin A (Botox),[1] and insulin.[1] Intralesional injection of interferon (IFN) has been used for the treatment of keloids; IFN-α2b[1] is used more often than IFN-gamma.[1]

[7]Available as a dietary supplement.

TABLE 3	Summary of Nonpharmacologic Treatment			
THERAPEUTIC METHOD	**SUGGESTED MECHANISMS**	**EFFECT**	**DOSE**	**EVIDENCE**
Surgery	Reduce inflammation	Reorientation and construction of multiple tension vectors	NA	2
Radiotherapy*	Destruction of connective stem cells Fibroblast apoptosis	Reduce inflammation Angiogenesis	Begin 24–72 h after surgery Total of 40 Gray or less	1
Cryotherapy	Vascular damage Anoxia	Tissue necrosis	Contact more effective (cryoprobes) Every 4 wk for 1–10 sessions	2
Laser†	Selective photothermolysis Decrease TGF-β	Reduce inflammation. Reduce collagen production	Dose and number of treatments varies; multiple treatments required	1

*Multiple doses and fractions described
†Pulsed dye laser (best evidence), CO2 fractional laser, neodymium-doped yttrium aluminum garne.
Key to evidence base support: Meta-analysis or RCT (1), large series (2), lesser quality series (3), small series (4).

More recently, verapamil[1] injections 2.5 mg/mL every 3 weeks up to 6 sessions, captopril[1] cream (5%)[6] twice a day for 6 weeks and losartan[1] gel 5%[6] twice a day for 12 weeks have shown benefits via their antifibrotic effect inhibiting the TGF-β/Smad pathway and antagonizing the RAS system. There are a limited number of human studies to date but some have shown promising results.

Although surgical excision is the most definitive treatment, it also has the highest rate of recurrence, which can be as high as 100% depending on anatomic location, technique used and individual skin healing factors. Therefore, when appropriate, multimodal therapy is usually suggested. Radiation therapy is frequently used in conjunction with surgical excision to more effectively prevent recurrence than either procedure alone. Doses administered may vary. Recent studies have shown that the maximal biologic effective dose for treating keloids is 30 Gy. It is important to consider the secondary carcinogenic risk associated with radiotherapy.

Cryotherapy is a treatment that causes damage to the blood vessels, resulting in reduced oxygen supply, cellular injury, and eventually tissue necrosis. Cryotherapy treatment may cause local pain, blister formation, and changes in skin color. In cases where specialized needle probes are used for cryotherapy, fewer treatments may be required and the risk of side effects may be reduced.

Different types of lasers (carbon dioxide, neodymium-doped yttrium aluminum garnet [Nd:YAG], and pulse dye laser [PDL]) have been used to treat keloids. The mechanism of action has been described as thermal injury and downregulation of TGF-β. It is important to note that there can be adverse effects of laser therapy, including hyperpigmentation and hypopigmentation, scarring, and pain. Additionally, the treatment can be expensive and may require multiple sessions. For a better outcome, lasers may need to be used in combination with steroids or 5-FU infiltration[1] (Table 3).

Emerging therapies include dupilumab (Dupixent),[1] fat grafting, lipofilling, and stem cell therapy. An innovative approach to developing drugs for keloid treatment involves exploring potential diagnostic and therapeutic targets such as cytokine-based therapy and gene therapy. Among the cytokine-based therapies, the TGF-β signaling pathway is being studied for its ability to inhibit cell proliferation and collagen synthesis. The regulation of gene expression is currently under in vitro testing, following recent studies that have shown dysregulated noncoding RNAs (ncRNAs) as having a significant role in the formation of keloids. Enhancing drug delivery systems, such

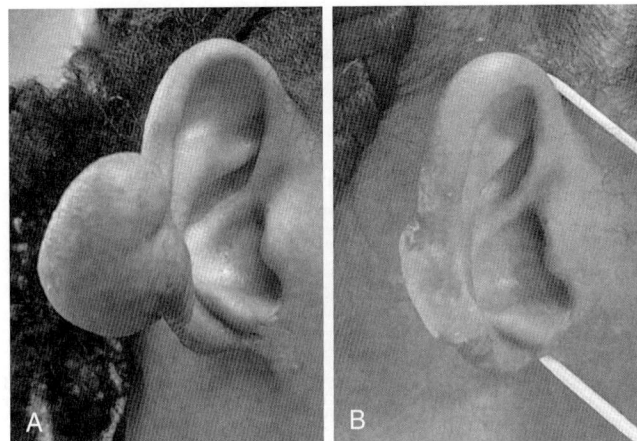

Figure 1 Regression of keloid after treatment. Keloid before (A) and after (B) combination cryosurgery and intralesional steroids. (Knowles, A., & Glass, D. A., 2nd. [2023]. Keloids and hypertrophic scars. *Dermatologic Clinics, 41*[3], 509–517. https://doi.org/10.1016/j.det.2023.02.010 [Fig 5])

as the use of nanoparticles, might provide additional benefits in the future.

Combining different therapies can be more effective than monotherapy, especially in refractory or recurrent cases. Intralesional steroid injections have been used along with other therapies such as surgical excision, cryotherapy, and laser treatment (Figure 1). The first intralesional steroid injection should be administered on the same day as the procedure, with subsequent sessions scheduled every 4 to 6 weeks. A combination of intralesional steroids with 5-fluorouracil (5-FU)[1] has also been reported to have a better response than steroid injections alone. Other combinations that have been described include surgery followed by radiotherapy or cryotherapy. Cryotherapy is administered 2 weeks after the sutures are removed.

Monitoring

It is crucial to evaluate patients regularly and document their progress. Follow-up visits must include a detailed discussion to address treatment adherence, side effects, and the patient's feelings about the treatment. Objective evaluation of treatment is necessary, and a digital photogram is a good option for monitoring treatment progress. This helps to prevent complications and adjust or discontinue treatment if necessary. Because there is a high rate of recurrence, follow-up for at least 1 year after the completion of treatment is recommended. During this period, immediate and aggressive treatment is suggested if there are any signs of recurrence.

[1] Not FDA approved for this indication.
[6] May be compounded by pharmacists.
[1] Not FDA approved for this indication.

[1] Not FDA approved for this indication.

References

Ho JL, Yong JJ: Recent Understandings of Biology, Prophylaxis and Treatment Strategies for Hypertrophic Scars and Keloids. 19(3), 711–711 https://doi.org/10.3390/ijms19030711, 2018, .

Huang C, Wu Z, Du Y, et al: The Epidemiology of Keloids. 2020 Dec 8. In Téot L, Mustoe TA, Middelkoop E, et al: *Textbook on Scar Management: State of the Art Management and Emerging Technologies [Internet]*, Cham (CH), 2020, Springer, https://doi.org/10.1007/978-3-030-44766-3_4. Chapter 4. Available from: https://www.ncbi.nlm.nih.gov/books/NBK586088/.

Knowles A, Glass DA: Keloids and hypertrophic scars, *Dermatol Clin* 41(3):509–517, 2023, https://doi.org/10.1016/j.det.2023.02.010.

Machan S, Molina-Ruiz AM, Requena L: Dermal Hypertrophies. In Bolognia J, Schaffer JV, Cerroni L, editors: *Dermatology*, ed 5, Elsevier, 2024, pp 1730–1740. (98.

Ogawa R: Keloid and hypertrophic scars are the result of chronic inflammation in the reticular dermis, *Int J Mol Sci* 18(3), 2017https://doi.org/10.3390/ijms18030606.

Qi W, Xiao X, Tong J, Guo N: Progress in the clinical treatment of keloids, *Front Med* 10, 2023:1284109, https://doi.org/10.3389/fmed.2023.1284109.

Stanley GHM, Pitt ER, Lim D, Pleat J: Prevalence, exposure and the public knowledge of keloids on four continents, *J Plast Reconstr Aesthet Surg* 77:359–370, 2023, https://doi.org/10.1016/j.bjps.2022.11.017.

Ud-Din S, Bayat A: New insights on keloids, hypertrophic scars, and striae, *Dermatol Clin* 32(2):193–209, 2014, https://doi.org/10.1016/j.det.2013.11.002.

▮ MELANOMA

Method of
Geoffrey T. Gibney, MD; and Arlene M. Ruiz de Luzuriaga, MD, MPH, MBA

CURRENT DIAGNOSIS

- ABCDEs:
  - **A**symmetry of lesion
  - **B**order irregularity, bleeding, or crusting
  - **C**olor change or variegation
  - **D**iameter larger than 6 mm or growing lesion
  - **E**volving: Surface changes or symptomatic
- The "ugly duckling" sign: A mole that looks or feels different compared with surrounding moles
- Total-body photography and dermoscopy
- Excisional biopsy with narrow margins
- Interpretation by physician experienced in the microscopic diagnosis of pigmented lesions
- Molecular analyses (rarely)
- Appropriate staging workup
- Genetic testing when appropriate (rarely)

CURRENT THERAPY

- Early diagnosis and appropriate surgical therapy is the gold standard.
- Complete excision must be achieved with appropriate margins based on tumor thickness.
- Sentinel lymph node biopsy should be offered to patients with melanoma greater than 1 mm thick, with clinically unaffected regional nodes and without distant metastases. Similarly sentinel lymph node biopsy should be considered in patients with melanoma 0.8 to 1 mm thick or less than 0.8 mm thick if ulceration is present.
- Dissection of the lymph node basin is not routinely offered to patients with microscopic nodal metastases, although it can be offered in select patients.
- Dissection of the lymph node basin is considered for most patients with macroscopic nodal metastases.
- Adjuvant therapy is offered for resected stage IIB and IIC disease.
- Neoadjuvant and/or adjuvant therapy is offered for resectable stage III and IV disease.
- Stage IV treatment depends on location and extent of metastatic disease and may include surgical resection, radiation therapy, and/or systemic therapy.

Melanoma is a malignancy of pigment-producing cells (melanocytes). Melanocytes are located predominantly in the skin but are also found in the eyes, ears, gastrointestinal tract, leptomeninges, and oral and genital mucous membranes.

Epidemiology

Even though melanoma accounts for less than 5% of skin cancer cases, it causes the most skin cancer deaths. The American Cancer Society's estimates for melanoma in the United States for 2025 are 104,960 new cases, with 8430 deaths. The prevalence of melanoma in the United States doubled over 3 decades from 1982 to 2011, from 11.2 per 100,000 population to 22.7 per 100,000. From 2009 to 2018 the incidence increased by about 1% annually, with the majority diagnosed at a localized stage. The lifetime risk for developing melanoma is about 1 in 29 for males and 1 in 40 for females. Age-adjusted mortality rates have been decreasing about 2.8% each year between 2014 and 2023. Mortality rates remain higher in Black individuals compared with all races combined.

Risk Factors

A large number of nevi is the strongest risk factor for melanoma in persons of European ancestry. Atypical mole syndrome is another risk factor. Exposure to ultraviolet light is a major risk factor, especially in persons who have fair hair and skin; who have solar damage; who had sunburns and short, sharp bursts of sun exposure in childhood; and who used tanning beds. Tanning beds appear more detrimental when used before the age of 20 years. The International Agency for Research on Cancer has classified indoor tanning devices as "carcinogenic to humans" based on extensive review of scientific evidence. Familial risk factors include mutations in *CDKN2A (p16INK4a)*, which are associated with increased risks for both melanoma and pancreatic cancer; they are transmitted in an autosomal dominant fashion and account for approximately 20% to 50% of familial melanoma cases. Mutations in *BRCA1*-associated protein 1 (BAP1), shelterin complex, microphthalmia-associated transcription factor (MITF), and phosphatase and tensin homolog (PTEN) have also been associated with melanoma and other malignancies. Organ transplant recipients have an increased risk for melanoma. Genodermatoses with a defect in DNA repair (such as xeroderma pigmentosum) increase the risk for melanoma.

Pathophysiology

Transformation of normal melanocytes into melanoma cells likely involves a multistep process of progressive genetic mutations that alter cell proliferation, differentiation, and death and affect susceptibility to the carcinogenic effects of ultraviolet radiation. Primary cutaneous melanoma can develop in pre-existing melanocytic nevi, but more than 60% of cases likely appear de novo.

Melanomas arising in skin that is chronically sun damaged show molecular features that distinguish them from melanomas arising in skin that is not sun damaged. In particular, the tumor mutational burden is highest in melanoma arising from sun-exposed areas, which is associated with response to immunotherapies. In addition, activating somatic mutations in the *BRAF* gene are seen in 40% to 60% of cutaneous melanoma, leading to constitutive activation of the MAPK pathway. Additional common mutations include *NRAS* (28%), *P53* (15%), *NF1* (14%), *CDKN2A* (13%), and *PTEN* (9%). The genetic makeup of non–sun-exposed acral melanoma differs from cutaneous melanoma, with a lower frequency of *BRAF* mutations and the presence of *KIT* mutations in up to 12% of patients. Genetic studies have shown that 50% of familial melanomas and 25% of sporadic melanomas may be associated with mutations in the tumor suppressor gene *p16*. Linkage studies have identified chromosome 9p21 as the site of the familial melanoma gene.

Prevention

Early detection of thin cutaneous melanoma is the best means of reducing mortality. Patients with a history of melanoma should be educated regarding sun-protective clothing and sunscreens, skin self-examinations for new primary melanoma, possible recurrence within the surgical scar, and screening of first-degree relatives, particularly if they have a history of atypical moles.

Clinical Manifestations

Early signs of melanoma include the ABCDEs:
- Asymmetry of lesion
- Border irregularity, bleeding, or crusting
- Color change or variegation
- Diameter larger than 6 mm or growing lesion
- Evolving: Surface changes or symptomatic

The "ugly duckling" sign is also useful to recognize lesions that look or feel different compared with surrounding moles.

Melanoma in situ represents melanoma that is limited to the epidermis. Lentigo maligna is a subtype of melanoma that typically occurs on chronically sun-damaged skin and begins as an irregular tan-brown macule that slowly expands on sun-damaged skin of elderly persons. Long-term cumulative sun exposure confers the greatest risk. It is estimated that 3.5% to 5% of lentigo maligna lesions progress to invasive melanoma (lentigo maligna melanoma), with a 2020 study estimating the risk of progression to be 3.5% per year.

Superficial spreading melanoma, the most common type in light skin tones, represents approximately 70% of all melanomas. Peak incidence is in the fourth and fifth decades. Superficial spreading melanoma can arise in a preexisting melanocytic nevus that slowly changes over several years; it most commonly affects intermittently sun-exposed areas with the greatest nevus density (upper backs of men and women and lower legs of women). Pigment varies from black and blue-gray to pink or gray-white, and the borders are irregular. Absence of pigmentation may represent regression.

Nodular melanoma represents 15% of all melanomas. The median age at onset is 53 years. Clinically, a uniform blue-black, blue-red, or red nodule usually begins de novo and grows rapidly. About 5% are amelanotic. The most common sites are the trunk, head, and neck.

Acral lentiginous melanoma accounts for 10% of melanomas overall but is the most common type among Japanese, African Americans, Latin Americans, and Native Americans. The median age is 65 years, with equal gender distribution. It occurs on the palms or soles or under the nails and is on average 3 cm in diameter at diagnosis. Clinically, the lesion is a tan, brown-to-black, flat macule with color variegation and irregular borders. It does not appear to be linked to sun exposure.

Diagnosis

Excisional biopsy with narrow margins is recommended for diagnosis. Incisional biopsy is acceptable when suspicion for melanoma is low, the lesion is large, or it is impractical to perform a complete excision. It is believed not to be detrimental if subsequent therapeutic surgery is performed within 4 to 6 weeks. Dermoscopy and total body photography are adjunctive noninvasive diagnostic techniques. Routine laboratory tests and imaging studies are not required for asymptomatic patients with primary cutaneous melanoma 1 mm or less in thickness for initial staging or routine follow-up. Indications for such studies are directed by a thorough medical history and complete physical examination, and/or need for surgical planning.

Histologic interpretation should be performed by a physician experienced in the microscopic diagnosis of pigmented lesions. Molecular analyses for evidence of gene mutations, DNA copy-number abnormalities, or changed protein expression are useful adjunctive tools in the assessment of histologically ambiguous primary melanocytic tumors. It is now known that melanomas arising in sun-damaged skin, non–sun-damaged skin, or mucosal or acral surfaces harbor distinct molecular phenotypes.

The new revised American Joint Committee on Cancer (AJCC) staging system was published in 2017. Key changes in the eighth edition of the AJCC Cancer Staging Manual include the following:
- Tumor thickness measurements are to be recorded to the nearest 0.1 mm, not 0.01 mm
- Definitions of T1a and T1b are revised (T1a, <0.8 mm without ulceration; T1b, 0.8–1.0 mm with or without ulceration or <0.8 mm with ulceration), with mitotic rate no longer a T category criterion
- Pathologic (but not clinical) stage IA is revised to include T1b-N0M0 (formerly pathologic stage IB)
- The N category descriptors "microscopic" and "macroscopic" for regional node metastasis are redefined as "clinically occult" and "clinically apparent"
- Prognostic stage III groupings are based on N category criteria and T category criteria (i.e., primary tumor thickness and ulceration) and increased from three to four subgroups (stages IIIA–IIID)
- Definitions of N subcategories are revised, with the presence of microsatellites, satellites, or in-transit metastases now categorized as N1c, N2c, or N3c based on the number of tumor-involved regional lymph nodes, if any
- Descriptors are added to each M1 subcategory designation for lactate dehydrogenase (LDH) level (LDH elevation no longer upstages to M1c)
- A new M1d designation is added for central nervous system metastases

These evidence-based AJCC melanoma staging updates will continue to inform patient treatment, improve prognostic estimates, and enhance stratification of clinical trial participants.

Five-year and 10-year survival rates based on the TNM classification range from 99% and 98% for patients with stage IA melanomas to 82% and 75%, respectively, for patients with stage IIC melanomas based on the AJCC 8th edition (Table 1). This data set included patients dating as far back as 1998, which likely underrepresents the current melanoma-specific survival given the development of highly effective targeted and immune checkpoint therapies since the 2010s.

Differential Diagnosis

The differential diagnosis includes melanocytic nevus, lentigo, angioma, pigmented basal cell carcinoma, pyogenic granuloma, seborrheic keratosis, Kaposi sarcoma, hematoma, and tinea nigra (especially for acral lentiginous melanoma).

Treatment

Early diagnosis combined with appropriate surgical therapy is curative in most patients. For melanoma in situ, wide excision with 0.5- to 1.0-cm margins is recommended; lentigo maligna histologic subtype may require greater than 0.5-cm margins to achieve histologically negative margins because of characteristically broad subclinical extension. Surgical margins for invasive melanoma should be at least 1 cm and up to 2 cm clinically measured around the primary tumor; clinically measured surgical margins do not need to correlate with histologically negative margins. Margins may be modified to accommodate individual anatomic or functional considerations. The recommended margins are described in Table 2.

The recommended deep margin is muscle fascia. Wider margins and Mohs micrographic surgery (MMS) can reduce the risk of contiguous subclinical spread for the desmoplastic variant of melanoma. MMS may also be considered for melanoma in situ, lentigo maligna type on the face, ears, or scalp.

Sentinel lymph node biopsy (SLNB) provides accurate staging information for patients with clinically unaffected regional nodes and without distant metastases. The status of sentinel lymph nodes is widely considered the most important prognostic indicator for disease-specific survival in patients with primary cutaneous melanoma; however, the SLNB has not demonstrated an improvement in overall survival (MSLT1 study). Candidates for SLNB include patients with newly diagnosed primary cutaneous melanoma with a depth of at least 0.8 mm or presence of ulceration and who are clinically node negative and have no clinical evidence of metastatic disease. In cases of positive SLNB, completion lymph node dissection has not demonstrated a survival advantage over observation and nodal surveillance in two large randomized prospective studies (DeCOG-SLT and MLST2). This has been practice changing in that most melanoma patients with positive SLNB are now managed by observation/nodal surveillance along with adjuvant systemic therapy, although completion lymph node dissection may be offered to select patients and remains an option within the National Comprehensive Cancer Network (NCCN) guidelines. In patients with clinically detected regional nodal metastases (palpable and positive cytology or histopathology), therapeutic lymph node dissection of the involved basin has been the standard management in the absence of distant metastases, but its role is now evolving with the use of neoadjuvant therapy.

For resectable local or in-transit recurrences, excision with a clear margin is recommended. For numerous or unresectable in transit metastases, isolated limb perfusion or infusion with melphalan[1], intralesional injection with the oncolytic viral therapy talimogene laherparepvec (TVEC [Imlygic]), or systemic targeted or immune checkpoint therapy is generally considered.

Radiotherapy is indicated in select patients with lentigo maligna melanoma, as an adjuvant in patients where reresection of positive margins/recurrence is not feasible, for management of solitary/oligometastatic metastases (especially for brain metastases), and for palliation of symptomatic tumor sites.

Numerous adjuvant therapies have been investigated for the treatment of locoregional cutaneous melanoma after complete surgical removal. The current U.S. Food and Drug Administration (FDA) approved agents include interferon alfa-2b ([Intron A][2] high-dose and pegylated formulations [Sylatron][2]), anti-cytotoxic T-lymphocyte antigen-4 (CTLA-4) therapy (ipilimumab [Yervoy]), anti–programmed cell death 1 (PD-1) therapy (nivolumab [Opdivo] and pembrolizumab [Keytruda]), and *BRAF* targeted therapy (dabrafenib [Tafinlar] plus trametinib [Mekinist] in *BRAF* V600 mutant melanoma only). Interferon and ipilimumab are no longer recommended since the approval of the anti-PD1 and BRAF targeted therapies which are generally well tolerated and reduce recurrence rates by greater than 40% in patients with resected stage III melanoma. Nivolumab is also approved as adjuvant therapy for resected stage IV melanoma. Additionally, adjuvant anti–PD-1 therapy (pembrolizumab and nivolumab) are FDA approved for patients with resected stage IIB and IIC melanoma after randomized phase III studies demonstrated a relative risk reduction for recurrence of 39% and 58%, respectively, over placebo.

Recent neoadjuvant immunotherapy studies have demonstrated clinical benefit in patients with macroscopic stage III/IV melanoma. In particular, the S1801 study showed a significant improvement in the 2-year event-free survival (EFS) when pembrolizumab was given as a neoadjuvant followed by surgery and adjuvant therapy compared with surgery and adjuvant therapy alone (2-year EFS rates of 72% vs. 49%, respectively). Similarly, the NADINA study showed a significant improvement in the 12-month EFS rate with neoadjuvant nivolumab/ipilimumab followed by surgery compared with surgery followed by nivolumab (12-month EFS rates of 83.7% vs. 57.2%, respectively). Patients with major pathologic responses in the NADINA study did not receive adjuvant treatment; the 1-year recurrence-free survival was 95% in this subgroup. The use of neoadjuvant immunotherapies is now routinely offered to patients in the context of multidisciplinary care teams.

Metastatic melanoma is an aggressive, immunogenic, and molecularly heterogeneous disease. Fortunately, treatment options have dramatically improved with the discovery of targeted therapy aimed at the *BRAF* mutations in the mitogen-activated protein kinase (MAPK) pathway and immune checkpoint inhibitors. In 2011 the FDA approved ipilimumab (Yervoy), an anti–CTLA-4 antibody for metastatic melanoma therapy. Since then, novel

TABLE 1	Melanoma Specific Survival by American Joint Committee on Cancer 8th Edition	
STAGE	5-YEAR SURVIVAL (%)	10-YEAR SURVIVAL (%)
Stage I		
IA	99	98
IB	97	94
Stage II		
IIA	94	88
IIB	87	82
IIC	82	75
Stage III		
IIIA	93	88
IIIB	83	77
IIIC	69	60
IIID	32	24

monoclonal antibody agents that inhibit PD-1 (pembrolizumab [Keytruda] and nivolumab [Opdivo]) were approved in 2014, followed by the nivolumab plus ipilimumab combination therapy in 2015 and, more recently, the nivolumab plus relatlimab combination therapy (anti-PD-1 plus anti-LAG-3 antibodies [Opdualag]) in 2022. Three additional classes of immunotherapy have been FDA approved, including the intralesional oncolytic viral therapy (talimogene laherparepvec [T-VEC, Imlygic]) in 2015 for patients with palpable metastatic melanoma, the bispecific gp100 peptide-HLA–directed CD3 T cell engager (tebentafusp [Kimmtrak]) for HLA-A*02:01–positive patients with metastatic uveal melanoma in 2022, and tumor infiltrating lymphocyte (TIL) therapy (lifileucel [Amtagvi]) for patients post-anti-PD-1 therapy and BRAF-targeted therapy (if BRAF V600 mut disease) in 2024. The selective *BRAF* inhibitor vemurafenib (Zelboraf) was also approved in 2011 for the treatment of patients with advanced *BRAF* V600 mutant melanoma. Additional *BRAF* targeted regimens were subsequently approved, with the combination *BRAF* plus MEK inhibitors now the standard approach based on improvement in survival over monotherapy. The three approved *BRAF* plus MEK inhibitor regimens include dabrafenib (Tafinlar) plus trametinib (Mekinist), vemurafenib (Zelboraf) plus cobimetinib (Cotellic), and encorafenib (Braftovi) plus binimetinib (Mektovi). Long-term survival of patients has dramatically improved with the new classes of *BRAF* targeted and anti-PD-1 therapies. Historically, approximately 10% of patients with advanced unresectable melanoma were alive at 5 years. In frontline prospective studies with dabrafenib plus trametinib, pembrolizumab, nivolumab, and nivolumab plus ipilimumab have shown 5-year survival rates of 34%, 43%, 44%, and 52%, respectively. In the CheckMate 067 study, the 10-year melanoma-specific survival rates were 52% with nivolumab plus ipilimumab and 44% with nivolumab monotherapy.

Although melanoma previously was regarded as a near-uniformly fatal malignancy, more than 50% of patients with stage IV disease are likely now to be long-term survivors with the available treatments. Recent advances in the treatment of melanoma have also expanded our understanding that melanoma is a family of molecularly distinct diseases. Emerging evidence suggests that different melanoma subtypes may each be driven by diverse mechanisms of progression, associated with differing mechanisms of tumor escape and specific immunosuppression, innate immune cell activation, and altered T-cell trafficking into tumor sites that in turn modulate response to immunotherapies.

Monitoring

Most metastases occur in the first 1 to 3 years after treatment of the primary tumor, and an estimated 4% to 8% of patients with a history of melanoma develop another primary melanoma, usually within the first 3 to 5 years after diagnosis. The risk of new

---

[1] Not FDA approved for this indication.
[2] Not available in the United States.

| | CLINICALLY MEASURED | | |
TUMOR THICKNESS	SURGICAL MARGIN	STRENGTH OF RECOMMENDATION	LEVEL OF EVIDENCE
In situ	0.5–1.0 cm	B	II, III
≤1.0 mm	1 cm	A	I, II
1.01–2.0 mm	1–2 cm	A	I
≥2.0 mm	2 cm	A	I

TABLE 2 Strength of Recommendations: A, B, C Level of Evidence: I, II, III

From https://www.aad.org/member/clinical-quality/guidelines/melanoma, accessed May 9, 2024.

primary melanoma increases in the presence of multiple dysplastic nevi and family history of melanoma. Consider cancer genetics consultation in patients with three or more melanomas in aggregate in first- or second-degree relatives on the same side of the family, families with three or more cases of melanoma or pancreatic cancer on the same side of the family, and (in low-incidence countries) patients with three or more primary melanomas.

The frequency of dermatologic monitoring is as follows:

- For patients with stage IA to IIA: every 6 to 12 months for 5 years, then every year as needed
- For patients with stage IIB to IV every 3 to 6 months for 2 years, then every 3 to 12 months for 3 years, then every year as needed

Follow-up visits for all patients should include a thorough medical history, review of systems, complete skin examination, and examination of lymph nodes. In patients at high risk for recurrent metastatic disease (resected stages IIB–IV) or with abnormal examination/symptoms, appropriate imaging studies, laboratory studies, or biopsies may be indicated. Evidence to support the use of routine imaging and laboratory studies in patients who are asymptomatic with low-risk resected stage I to IIA melanoma is limited, so they are not recommended by the NCCN guidelines.

Complications

Metastasis may occur locally in the regional lymph node basins, or it can occur distally in the skin (away from the melanoma scar), the remote lymph node(s), the viscera, and skeletal and central nervous system sites. In patients treated with immune checkpoint inhibitor therapies, immune-related adverse events can occur even after therapy discontinuation.

References

Abbasi NR, Shaw HM, Rigel DS, et al: Early diagnosis of cutaneous melanoma: revisiting the ABCD criteria, *JAMA* 292:2771–2776, 2004.
American Cancer Society: *Lifetime Risk of Developing or Dying From Cancer.* https://www.cancer.org/cancer/risk-prevention/understanding-cancer-risk/lifetime-probability-of-developing-or-dying-from-cancer.html. Accessed September 26, 2025.
Blank CU, Lucas MW, Scoylyer RA, et al: Neoadjuvant nivolumab and ipilimumab in resectable stage III melanoma, *N Eng J Med* 391(18):1696–1708, 2024.
Cancer Genome Atlas N: Genomic classification of cutaneous melanoma, *Cell* 161:1681–1696, 2015.
Cancer Stat Facts: *Melanoma of the Skin.* https://seer.cancer.gov/statfacts/html/melan.html. Last accessed September 26, 2025.
Centers for Disease Control and Prevention: *United States cancer statistics: incidence of malignant melanoma of the skin—United States, 2009–2018,* USCS Data Brief, no. 28. Atlanta, GA, 2022, Centers for Disease Control and Prevention, US Department of Health and Human Services.
Gershenwald JE, Scolyer RA, Hess KR, et al: Melanoma staging: evidence-based changes in the American Joint Committee on Cancer eighth edition cancer staging manual, *CA Cancer J clin* 67:472–492, 2017.
Guy Jr GP, Thomas CC, Thompson T, et al: Vital signs: melanoma incidence and mortality trends and projections - United States, 1982-2030, *MMWR Morb Mortal Wkly Rep* 64:591–596, 2015.
Higgins 2nd HW, Lee KC, Galan A, Leffell DJ: Melanoma in situ: Part I. Epidemiology, screening, and clinical features, *J Am Acad Dermatol* 73(2):181–192, 2015. https://doi.org/10.1016/j.jaad.2015.04.014.
Kwak M, Farrow NE, Salama AKS, et al: Updates in adjuvant systemic therapy for melanoma, *J Surg Oncol* 119:222–231, 2019.
Larkin J, Chiarion-Sileni V, Gonzalez R, et al: Five-year survival with combined nivolumab and ipilimumab in advanced melanoma, *N Engl J Med* 381:1535–1546, 2019.
Luke JJ: *Lancet* 399(10336):1718–1729, 2022. https://doi: 10.1016/S0140-6736(22)00562-1. Epub 2022 Apr 1.
Menzies, Scott W, Liyanarachchi S, Coates E, et al: Estimated risk of progression of lentigo maligna to lentigo maligna melanoma, *Melanoma Res* 30(2)193–197, 2020.
National Comprehensive cancer Network (NCCN) clinical practice guidelines in Oncology. *Cutaneous melanoma.* Version 2.2024. nccn.org.
Patel SP: *N Engl J Med* 388(9):813–823, 2023. https://doi: 10.1056/NEJMoa2211437.
Ran NA, Nugent ST, Veerabagu SA, et al: Desmoplastic melanoma treated with wide local excision or Mohs micrographic surgery: rates of positive margins, local recurrence, and repeat surgeries, *J Am Acad Dermatol* 87(6):1376–1378, 2022.
Robert C, Grob JJ, Stroyakovskiy D, et al: Five-year outcomes with dabrafenib plus trametinib in metastatic melanoma, *N Engl J Med* 381:626–636, 2019.
Siegel RL, et al: *CA Cancer J Clin* 73:17–48, 2023.
Sladden MJ, Balch C, Barzilai DA, et al: Surgical excision margins for primary cutaneous melanoma, *Cochrane Database Syst Rev* CD004835, 2009.
Soura E, Eliades PJ, Shannon K, Stratigos AJ, Tsao H: Hereditary melanoma: update on syndromes and management: genetics of familial atypical multiple mole melanoma syndrome, *J Am Acad Dermatol* 74:395–407; quiz 408-310, 2016.
Wolchok JD, Chiarion-Sileni VC, Rutkowski P, et al: Final, 10-year outcomes with nivolumab plus ipilimumab in advanced melanoma, *N Engl J Med* 392:11–22, 2025.
Wong SL, Faries MB, Kennedy EB, et al: Sentinel lymph node biopsy and management of regional lymph nodes in melanoma: American Society of Clinical Oncology and Society of Surgical Oncology clinical practice guideline update, *J Clin Oncol* 36:399–413, 2018.
Yeh I, Jorgenson E, Shen L, et al: Targeted genomic profiling of acral melanoma, *J Natl Cancer Inst* 111:1068–1077, 2019.

NEVI

Jane M. Grant-Kels, MD; and Michael Murphy, MD

CURRENT DIAGNOSIS

Benign Melanocytic Lesions
- Symmetric
- Sharply demarcated border
- Uniform color
- Diameter usually 6 mm or less and stable

Malignant Melanocytic Lesions
- Asymmetric
- Poorly circumscribed border
- Variegated in color
- Diameter often >6 mm and increasing (changing or evolving)

CURRENT THERAPY

- Acquired melanocytic nevus: No treatment is required unless the lesion is asymmetric or has an irregular border, change or variegation in color, or change in diameter. Symptomatic lesions should be biopsied.
- Recurrent melanocytic nevus: No treatment required if the original biopsy was benign.
- Halo melanocytic nevus: No treatment, but excision is recommended if atypical clinical features are identified.
- Congenital melanocytic nevus: Removal based on melanoma risk, cosmetics, and functional outcome. If not excised, routine follow-up with the use of photography; dermoscopy; and other new technology, like reflectance confocal microscopy, is recommended.
- Blue nevus: No treatment, but excision is recommended if atypical clinical features are identified.
- Spitz nevus: If the patient is > 12 years of age or the lesion is clinically or dermoscopically unusual, a complete excisional biopsy is recommended.
- Dysplastic nevus: If only one lesion is present, excision may be considered. Patients with many dysplastic nevi require close surveillance, with removal of any lesion suspicious for melanoma.

Melanocytic nevi, or moles, are benign neoplasms composed of melanocytes. Compared with normal junctional melanocytes, nevus cells are not dendritic, are larger, and contain more abundant cytoplasm, often with coarse melanin granules. Nevus cells tend to aggregate into groups or nests. Melanocytic nevi are extremely common and can be found on almost everyone, anywhere on the cutaneous surface. The term eruptive melanocytic nevi (EMN) describes an increasing number of nevi that have newly developed within several months. EMN may be associated with other skin diseases in 50% of cases, medications in 41%, and idiopathic causes in 9%. The underlying mechanisms of EMN remain to be elucidated. This article discusses the most common types of melanocytic nevi: acquired melanocytic nevi (AMN), recurrent melanocytic nevi, halo melanocytic nevi, congenital melanocytic nevi (CMN), blue nevi, Spitz nevi, and dysplastic melanocytic nevi.

Most melanocytic nevi show activation of the mitogen-activated protein kinase (MAPK) pathway. A single initiating "driver" oncogenic event results in limited clonal expansion/proliferation of melanocytes but is not sufficient for malignant transformation because uncontrolled growth is inhibited by additional cellular safeguards. Specific initiating alterations are known to correlate with nevus phenotypes. BRAF and NRAS gene mutations are characteristic of conventional (acquired) melanocytic nevi and large congenital nevi, respectively; HRAS mutations and tyrosine/serine-threonine kinase gene rearrangements are associated with Spitz nevi and pigmented spindle cell nevi; and GNAQ and GNA11 mutations are seen in blue nevi. Melanocytes in the skin exist in varied microenvironmental niches, with the spectrum of melanocytic nevi developing from disparate developmental and genetic pathways. It is postulated that melanocyte progenitor cells travel to the skin from the neural crest via two pathways during embryogenesis: dorsolaterally under the epidermis, and ventrally along nerves. Nevus development has been hypothesized to arise from dermal- or epidermal-based stem cells or from phenotypically invisible incipient nevus nests. Conflicting theories suggest that nevi initially develop in the epidermis and progress into the dermis or arise in the dermis and migrate upwards to the epidermis. No current theory completely explains the clinical-histopathological findings of melanocytic nevi. Ongoing molecular studies will continue to elucidate nevogenesis pathways and biology.

An intermediate subset of melanocytic lesions, now classified as "melanocytomas," is known to harbor two oncogenic events: an alteration in the MAPK pathway (similar to nevi) and an additional change involving a separate pathway. Examples of melanocytomas (with their characteristic secondary alterations) include deep penetrating nevus (CTNNB1 or APC mutation), pigmented epithelioid melanocytoma (inactivation of PRKAR1A), BAP1-inactivated melanocytic tumor (BAP1 inactivation, usually with BRAF activating mutations), and proliferative nodule arising in a congenital nevus (gains and losses of entire chromosomes). Some genetic alterations found in melanocytomas lead to distinct cytomorphological features in addition to providing a growth or survival advantage. Melanocytomas are often combined lesions, with a nevus carrying the initial alteration and a phenotypically distinct melanocytic population demonstrating the additional genomic event. The most recent 4th World Health Organization (WHO) Classification of Skin Tumors (2018) describes both low-grade and high-grade melanocytomas, accounting for multiple progression steps between benign nevus and melanoma, with high-grade lesions requiring fewer additional genomic hits for malignant transformation and therefore a higher risk for progression to melanoma. The absolute risk of transformation is not yet known. Most melanocytomas have an indolent biologic behavior but may disseminate to the local lymph node basin. Distant spread is exceptionally rare. Additionally, those melanocytomas consistent with the BAP1-inactivated melanocytic tumor can be associated with a germline mutation. Therefore when a patient reports with several newly acquired 2- to 10-mm flesh-colored or reddish-brown papules, one of the nevi should be biopsied

and stained with BAP-1 immunostain. If the nuclei of the epithelioid melanocytes in the dermis of these lesions do not stain with BAP-1 immunostain, the patient requires surveillance and/or genetic testing (for germline mutation) because they may have an increased risk of malignancies, including cutaneous as well as uveal melanoma, mesothelioma, and renal cell carcinoma.

Only 20% to 30% of melanomas arise in preexisting nevi, and the malignant transformation of an individual nevus has been estimated to occur at a rate of 0.00005% to 0.003% per year. Therefore the routine removal of melanocytic nevi is generally not considered beneficial for most patients. The risk of melanoma development from a melanocytic nevus is related to the number of melanocytes present, explaining the increased risk of melanoma in giant congenital nevi and in patients with increased numbers of acquired melanocytic nevi. Melanomas that arise within nevi (or de novo) accumulate additional genetic/epigenetic alterations that provide a survival or growth advantage and lead to uncontrolled cellular proliferation. These alterations can include inactivation of CDKN2A, PTEN, TP53, or NF1 genes; TERT promoter mutations; and activation of RAC1, ERBB2, MAP2K1, EGFR, or MET oncogenes.

The current classification of melanoma recognizes eight pathways of cutaneous and mucosal melanoma development, some with associated benign (nevus) and intermediate (melanocytoma) precursors. In addition, a revised Melanocytic Pathology Assessment Tool and Hierarchy for Diagnosis (MPATH-Dx) reporting method has been proposed, grouping melanocytic lesions into a four-class schema and providing a robust tool for standardized diagnostic reporting of melanocytic lesions and management of patients.

The majority of melanocytic tumors can be readily classified as nevus (or melanoma) based on histopathologic examination and immunohistochemistry findings (i.e., Ki-67, pHH3, p16 reactivity). The latter includes PRAME immunostaining (most nevi are negative; most melanomas are positive). However, there exists a small subset of melanocytic tumors that cannot be definitively classified as benign or malignant using light microscopy. Several molecular tests have been developed to help refine diagnosis and determine biologic potential of histologically ambiguous melanocytic tumors. These tests include gene expression profiling and assessment of DNA copy number alterations (CNAs). Most melanomas demonstrate unstable genomes with numerous CNAs, whereas nevi lack or have a limited number of CNAs. Molecular tests identifying telomerase reverse transcriptase promoter (TERT-p) mutations or homozygous deletion of CDKN2A have also been used to differentiate a benign nevus from melanoma.

Total Body Photography/Dermoscopy/Reflectance Confocal Microscopy

In addition to visual examination, total body photography, dermoscopy, and reflectance confocal microscopy are important clinical tools in the evaluation of patients with melanocytic lesions.

Total body photography is useful in evaluating clinical changes in melanocytic lesions over time in select patients at high risk for melanoma who require regular, long-term follow-up to aid in detection of early-stage tumors.

All melanocytic lesions of clinical concern should be examined with a dermatoscope—a handheld instrument with a 10× magnified lens and a light source (with or without polarization). This instrument allows evaluation of colors and microstructures not visible to the naked eye, helps determine whether pigmented lesions are melanocytic or nonmelanocytic, and aids in distinguishing whether melanocytic pigmented lesions are likely to be malignant. Used by an experienced physician with proper training, the dermatoscope improves diagnostic accuracy by 20% to 30%. The dermoscopic patterns of nevi are broadly classified as globular (round to oval structures), reticular (net-like pattern), homogenous (structureless pattern), or complex (representing overlapping and other distinct or diverse patterns not otherwise categorized). Globular nevi are more common in children, whereas reticular and/or homogenous nevi are more common in adults. Globular nevi correlate to dermal or dermoepidermal nests of melanocytes, whereas reticular nevi correlate to a lentiginous (single cell) and small nested growth pattern along the dermoepidermal junction. Dermoscopic patterns are known to correlate with underlying genetic events. Serial dermoscopy is a powerful tool to alert the clinician to subtle changes that might suggest an early evolving melanoma.

Another useful technology is reflectance confocal microscopy (RCM) because it safely offers noninvasive imaging of skin lesions at cellular-level magnification and is reported to reduce unnecessary biopsies by 50% to 70%. RCM utilizes a low-energy diode laser light that focuses on a specific area of tissue; the magnitude of back-scattering of light depends on the differences in refractive indices of various structures in the skin. The horizontal images of the skin afford review of a lesion up to 8 mm × 8 mm in diameter and extend 200 to 300 μm into the skin, affording visualization at a cellular level of the epidermis, dermal-epidermal junction, and papillary dermis.

Acquired Melanocytic Nevi

Acquired melanocytic nevi (AMN) are subdivided into junctional, compound, and intradermal types based on the location of the nevus cells. By definition, these lesions are not present at birth but can begin to appear in early childhood, usually after 6 to 12 months of age. Peak ages of appearance of melanocytic nevi are 2 to 3 years of age in children and 11 to 18 years in adolescents. Although nevi can appear at any age, it is relatively unusual for new melanocytic nevi to develop in middle-aged or older adults. With time, nevi can spontaneously regress. Consequently, patients in their ninth decade of life usually demonstrate few melanocytic nevi. An average White adult has 10 to 40 melanocytic nevi, but African Americans have far fewer, averaging only 2 to 8.

Clinically, AMN can be flat, elevated, polypoid, papillomatous, or verrucous and flesh-colored to black, but they are characteristically uniform in color, symmetric, and well marginated. AMN are usually small (<6 mm). The number and location of melanocytic nevi have been shown to be associated with sun exposure, immunologic factors, and genetics. Consequently, melanocytic nevi are most numerous on the sun-exposed skin of the head, neck, trunk, and extremities, but they are only rarely found on covered areas such as the buttocks, female breasts, and scalp. Genome-wide association studies (GWAS) have identified a subset of single nucleotide polymorphisms (SNP) associated with total nevus counts. Most adults have 10 to 40 melanocytic nevi. Evidence suggests that patients with an increased number of melanocytic nevi (especially >100) might have an increased risk of melanoma. These patients can be easily identified without counting all their nevi because they generally have >10 on each arm or >20 nevi on their trunk.

AMN tend to appear in a sequential fashion. Junctional melanocytic nevi arise during childhood as flat, dark macules. Histologically, an increase in single or nested melanocytes is located at the dermoepidermal junction. With time, it is hypothesized that some of the junctional nests of melanocytes migrate into the dermis (compound melanocytic nevi). Clinically, compound melanocytic nevi are elevated and less heavily pigmented than junctional melanocytic nevi. Ultimately, all of the nevus cells migrate into the dermis (intradermal melanocytic nevi), resulting in the development of a tan or skin-colored dome-shaped papule.

It is unnecessary to surgically remove all AMN because they are benign neoplasms of melanocytes. However, indications for removal include ABCDE (asymmetry, irregular border, variegation or change in color, change in diameter, or evolving), symptoms (e.g., pruritus), evidence of inflammation or irritation, cosmetic issues, and patient anxiety. In addition, there are specific dermoscopic changes that alert the clinician to the possibility of a melanoma, including asymmetry of more than two structures,

presence of more than four colors, atypical pigment network, angulated lines, irregular blotches, irregular dots and/or globules, irregular streaks and/or pseudopods, gray-dot granules, blue-white veil, negative pigment network, shiny white structures, and atypical vascular pattern. Melanocytic nevi on acral, genital, or scalp skin that appear benign do not require surgical removal. Shave biopsies are appropriate therapy for lesions considered clinically benign. However, if a lesion is being removed because of concern regarding the possibility of malignancy, an excisional biopsy (biopsy of choice) or incisional biopsy (including a deep scoop) that extends to the subcutaneous tissue is indicated. All melanocytic lesions should be submitted to a dermatopathologist for histologic review. A history of recent sun exposure or trauma should be conveyed to the dermatopathologist because such external trauma can induce reactive atypical histologic findings. Most AMN (~80%) harbor a BRAF V600E mutation in every constituent melanocyte, with a minority harboring an activating NRAS mutation or other genetic alteration. The presence of a BRAF V600E mutation is associated with distinct histopathological features—predominantly nested melanocytes within the epidermis, larger nests of melanocytes within the epidermis, and larger melanocytes.

Nodal nevi aggregates have been described, and the majority are seen as small deposits of melanocytes in the capsule or subcapsular space of lymph nodes. These melanocytes are limited in their ability to proliferate and resemble those of acquired melanocytic nevi.

Recurrent Melanocytic Nevi

Recurrent melanocytic nevi are melanocytic nevi that have previously been incompletely removed (either iatrogenically or traumatically) and have recurred weeks to months later. Irregular brown pigmentation is clinically noted within the scar site. If the original biopsy demonstrated a benign melanocytic nevus, retreatment is unnecessary unless there is suspicion for a malignancy, such as from an extension of pigment clinically beyond the scar. However, these nevi can demonstrate pseudomelanomatous histologic features. Therefore if the repigmented area is excised, the dermatopathologist should be notified of the clinical history and, if possible, the slides from the original biopsy should be obtained and reviewed to ensure that the lesion is not histologically misdiagnosed.

Halo (Melanocytic) Nevi

Halo (melanocytic) nevi are melanocytic nevi in which a white rim or halo has developed. This phenomenon most commonly occurs around compound or intradermal nevi and is histologically associated with a dense, bandlike inflammatory infiltrate. The white halo area is histologically characterized by diminished or absent melanocytes and melanin. Approximately 20% of patients with halo nevi also exhibit vitiligo.

Although a halo can develop around many lesions in the skin, the most important differential diagnosis is between a halo nevus and melanoma with a halo. The halo and the central melanocytic proliferation of halo nevi are symmetric, round or oval, and sharply demarcated. Halo nevi most commonly occur in adolescence as an isolated event, but approximately 25% to 50% of affected persons have two or more.

The clinical course of halo nevi is variable. With time, the halo can repigment while the central nevus persists. Alternatively, the melanocytic nevus can regress completely and leave a depigmented macule that can persist or repigment over months or years.

Halo nevi do not require surgical excision unless atypical features clinically and dermoscopically suggest the possibility of an atypical melanocytic lesion. It is advisable (particularly in adults, in whom halo nevi are less common) to perform a complete cutaneous examination with and without the aid of a Wood's lamp to rule out any associated atypical pigmented or regressed lesions. It is recommended that, if a middle-aged or older adult reports with a sudden appearance of halo nevi and there is no obvious melanoma or history of melanoma, the patient should be referred to an ophthalmologist for an ocular exam to exclude a choroidal halo nevus. All patients should be advised to use sunscreen or protective clothing because of the increased risk of sunburn in the depigmented halo region.

Congenital Melanocytic Nevi

By definition, congenital melanocytic nevi (CMN) are present at birth. CMN can be classified by their clinical features, including size, location, number of satellite lesions, and morphologic characteristics (such as color, rugosity, nodularity, hypertrichosis). This classification can help stratify patients according to their risk for adverse outcomes, including neurocutaneous melanosis and progression to melanoma. Arbitrarily, they have been classified into small (<1.5 cm), medium (1.5 to 20 cm), large (>20 to 40 cm), and giant (>40 cm) lesions. Terms such as *bathing trunk* or *garment-type* nevi refer to CMN that cover a significant portion of the cutaneous surface. The spectrum of initiating mutations typically correlates with the size of the nevus. The majority of large CMN harbor NRAS mutations, with a minority harboring kinase fusions or BRAF mutation. Most small CMN harbor BRAF mutations. Recent studies suggest that pathogenesis of large/giant CMN is associated with deficient mismatch repair (MMR) mechanisms and linked to lesion size and presence of multiple lesions.

The approximate incidence of small congenital nevi is 1% of all live births. Large congenital nevi are rare and reported in only 1 in 20,000 births. Histologically, some congenital nevi have distinguishing histologic features (melanocytic nevus cells that extend into the deeper dermis as well as the subcutis and melanocytic nevus cells arranged periadnexally, angiocentrically, within nerves, and interposed between collagen bundles). However, these features have been identified in some acquired melanocytic nevi and are absent in some congenital nevi (especially small ones). In addition, the history obtained from the patient or their parents is often inaccurate. Consequently, it can be very difficult in some cases to distinguish a small congenital nevus from an acquired nevus.

Congenital nevi can give rise to dermal or subcutaneous nodular melanocytic proliferations. Most of these lesions, particularly in the neonatal period, are biologically benign, despite a worrisome clinical presentation and atypical histologic features. Genetic analysis has shown that benign melanocytic proliferations within congenital nevi harbor aberrations that are qualitatively and quantitatively different from those seen in melanoma.

Patients with multiple CMN (two or more, of any site or size) are at risk for extracutaneous (i.e., endocrine, metabolic, neurologic) manifestations, termed *CMN syndrome*. The primary significance of congenital nevi is related to the potential risk for progression to melanoma. Essentially, the larger the nevus, particularly if accompanied by multiple small CMN, the greater the risk of progression to melanoma. Historically, even small nevi were estimated to exhibit a lifetime melanoma risk of 5%. However, recent prospective studies suggest that small and medium congenital nevi are associated with a low risk that may approximate the risk of acquired nevi. Conversely, large congenital nevi have a lifetime risk of melanomatous progression of approximately 6.3%. Up to two-thirds of melanomas that arise within these giant congenital nevi have a nonepidermal origin (arising mainly in the deep dermis and subcutis with high Breslow thickness on report), thus making clinical observation for malignant change difficult. Approximately 50% of these melanomas occur in the first 5 years of life, 60% in the first decade, and 70% before 20 years of age. Patients with large congenital nevi, especially those that involve posterior axial locations (head, neck, back, or buttocks) and are associated with satellite congenital nevi, are at increased risk for neurocutaneous melanosis (melanosis of the leptomeninges) and primary central nervous system (CNS) melanoma. Recent data suggest that in up to one-third of these patients, the primary melanoma develops within the CNS rather than the skin. The risk of melanoma appears to be higher in those with congenital abnormalities of the CNS (12% vs. 1% to 2% without CNS changes).

For large congenital nevi that involve a posterior axial location, screening magnetic resonance imaging (MRI) is indicated to characterize congenital disease, if any, and act as a baseline should the child report with new neurologic symptoms at a later stage. If clinical symptoms or MRI indicate neurocutaneous melanosis, excision of the large nevus should be postponed until 2 years of age (the median age of neurologic symptoms). Patients with neurocutaneous melanosis have a greater than 50% mortality rate within 3 years. Due to the risk and morbidity of multiple, staged excisions of a large CMN, it is not appropriate in patients with symptomatic neurocutaneous melanosis. All other large CMN are candidates for excision as soon as general anesthesia is considered a relatively safe risk. Other issues that need to be considered before undertaking staged excisions include cosmetic issues, functional outcome, and psychosocial issues. The staged excisions are usually started after 6 months of age for nevi on the trunk and extremities and later for those on the scalp to allow closure of the fontanelle. If removal is not undertaken, follow-up with monthly self-examination, as well as routine follow-up using photography, serial dermoscopy, and reflectance confocal microscopy, is recommended.

For small congenital nevi, routine excision is not always recommended because the risk of melanoma is lower, and if it occurs, it usually arises within the epidermis after puberty. If the lesions are not excised, follow-up by alternating visits to a dermatologist and primary care physician, along with serial photography, is indicated. Inasmuch as small congenital nevi typically enlarge with the growth of the child and can change in appearance with time, educating families on benign, predictable changes in contradistinction to potentially alarming changes is extremely important. If a lesion enlarges or changes suddenly or if parental anxiety or cosmetic issues arise, excision should then be contemplated for even small congenital nevi. Elective excision is best done when the patient is approximately 8 years old. With the use of topical anesthetic cream EMLA (eutectic mixture of local anesthetics: 2.5% lidocaine plus 2.5% prilocaine) or topical 4% lidocaine (ELA-Max), children of this age are usually cooperative and unscathed by the procedure.

Blue Nevi

Blue nevi occur primarily on the face and scalp, in addition to the dorsal surfaces of the hands and feet, as well-circumscribed, slightly raised or dome-shaped bluish papules that are usually less than 1 cm in diameter. Although these lesions are usually acquired in childhood and adolescence, rare congenital lesions have been reported. Histologically, the majority of blue nevi demonstrate a combination of intradermal spindle or dendritic melanin-pigmented melanocytes and melanophages with dermal fibrosis. Hypopigmented variants have also been described. The cellular subtype contains central fascicles of spindled melanocytes with ovoid nuclei. The blue appearance of these lesions is a function of both the depth of the melanin in the dermis and the Tyndall phenomenon: longer wavelengths of light penetrate the deep dermis and are absorbed by the lesional melanin, and shorter wavelengths (e.g., blue) are reflected back. Blue nevi that are clinically stable and that do not demonstrate atypical features do not require removal.

Blue nevi are initiated by activating mutations of the Gαq pathway, typically point mutations in GNAQ or GNA11 (shared with uveal and leptomeningeal melanocytic proliferations). Less commonly, hotspot mutations in CYSLTR2, PLB4, or protein kinase C (PKC) fusions are reported and associated with unique histopathological features. BAP1 inactivation in blue nevus–type lesions suggests malignant transformation and portends a poor prognosis.

Spitz Nevi

According to the 4th WHO Classification of Skin Tumors, the Spitz group of melanocytic proliferations is defined by a combination of distinctive morphologic features and driver molecular genetic events. This group includes benign Spitz nevi, in addition to atypical Spitz tumors and spitzoid melanomas. Morphologically, all of these neoplasms are characterized by large, oval, polygonal, epithelioid, and/or spindled melanocytes with abundant eosinophilic cytoplasm and vesicular nuclei with prominent nucleoli, often in association with epidermal hyperplasia. A lack of interobserver agreement in histopathological classification of skin tumors with spitzoid morphology is well reported.

Spitz nevi are relatively uncommon. In Australia, an annual incidence of 1.4 per 100,000 people has been recorded. Most Spitz nevi are noted in children and adolescents: One-third occur before the age of 10 years, one-third between the ages 10 to 20 years, and one-third past the age of 20 years. Rarely, lesions can occur in patients older than 40 years. Seven percent of Spitz nevi have been reported as congenital.

Four clinical types of Spitz nevi are recognized: light-colored soft Spitz nevi that can resemble a pyogenic granuloma; light-colored hard Spitz nevi that can resemble a dermatofibroma; dark Spitz nevi that must be distinguished from other melanocytic lesions, including melanoma; and disseminated or agminated Spitz nevi. Spitz nevi are typically smaller than 6 mm in diameter and dome shaped, with a smooth pink or tan surface and sharp borders. Although they can occur anywhere on the cutaneous surface except mucosal or palmoplantar areas, they are mostly seen on the face (especially in children) and legs (especially in women). Spitz nevi in adults are usually more heavily melanized than those in children. A Reed nevus or pigmented spindle cell nevus of Reed, a variant of a Spitz nevus, generally presents as an acquired 2- to 8-mm dark-brown to black macule or papule on the leg of a young adult.

Dermoscopy can assist in establishing the clinical diagnosis of some Spitz nevi. Histologically, the lesion can demonstrate features similar to those of melanoma, which earned the lesion its original designation by Sophie Spitz as a melanoma of childhood. Because Spitz nevi can be histologically difficult to distinguish from melanoma in some cases, if a biopsy is performed on a lesion because of parental, cosmetic, transitional, or clinical/dermoscopic concern, complete excision with clear margins is recommended.

Based on the underlying driver genetic aberrations, Spitz melanocytic proliferations can be divided into distinct groups: (1) 11p amplified/HRAS mutated proliferations (20% of cases), (2) proliferations with tyrosine kinase or serine/threonine kinase fusions (50% of cases), and (3) proliferations with Spitz morphology but no driver genetic changes characteristic of other defined melanocytic subgroups. Immunohistochemistry can be used for screening purposes to detect specific fusion proteins. Specific driver aberrations are often associated with distinctive histopathological changes and tumor aggressiveness—11p amplification/HRAS mutation and tyrosine kinase fusions correlate with indolent behavior—whereas serine-threonine kinase (MAP3K8, BRAF) fusions are more frequent in the atypical/malignant spectrum of Spitz melanocytic proliferations with a potential for aggressive biologic behavior. Additional genetic events (biallelic inactivation of CDKN2A and TERT promoter mutations) are often necessary for the development of overt Spitz malignancy.

Dysplastic Melanocytic Nevi

Dysplastic melanocytic nevi, or Clark's nevi, or nevi with architectural disorder and cytologic atypia, can occur sporadically as an isolated lesion or lesions or as part of a familial autosomal dominant syndrome. When such lesions occur sporadically, they are considered a marker for a patient who is at increased risk of melanoma (6% risk vs. an approximate 0.6% risk in the normal White population in the United States). In association with a family history or personal past medical history of melanoma, patients with dysplastic melanocytic nevi should be considered to have a significant risk of melanoma. One first-degree family member with melanoma is associated with a lifetime risk of melanoma of 15% for the patient with dysplastic melanocytic nevi. Two or more first-degree family members with melanoma place a patient with dysplastic melanocytic nevi at a lifetime risk of developing

melanoma that approaches 100%. Less commonly, dysplastic melanocytic nevi can progress to melanoma. Such progression has been documented by serial photography. However, these data are confounded by the fact that, clinically and histologically, dysplastic melanocytic nevi may be difficult to distinguish from an early melanoma.

Dysplastic melanocytic nevi are clinically distinguished from common AMN by a diameter usually larger than 6 mm, an irregular border, asymmetry, and variable color with possible shades of brown, red, pink, and black; dysplastic melanocytic nevi can be flat, with or without a raised center (fried egg appearance). The lesions begin to appear in mid-childhood and early adolescence. New lesions can appear throughout the patient's life. In addition to the back and extremities, these lesions can occur on sun-protected areas, including the scalp, buttocks, and female breasts. Dysplastic melanocytic nevi can be few or numerous, with hundreds of lesions. Dysplastic nevi show significant upregulation of follicular keratinocyte–related genes compared with AMN.

Histologically, dysplastic melanocytic nevi show architectural disorder: extension of the junctional component beyond the dermal component (shouldering), bridging of nests between adjacent rete ridges, papillary dermal concentric and lamellar fibroplasia, and a variable lymphocytic infiltrate with vascular ectasias. They also show cytologic atypia of melanocytes: increased nuclear size, hyperchromasia, dispersion, or variation of nuclear chromatin patterns and the presence of nucleoli. There are no set and universally accepted criteria on the spectrum of melanocytic dysplasia, and cytologic atypia is often reported as mild, moderate, or severe. However, discordance exists in the histologic grading of dysplastic nevi among dermatopathologists. According to the revised MPATH-Dx reporting system and 2018 WHO Classification of Skin Tumors, there is evidence to support the use in clinical practice of a simplified two-tier grading system: low-grade dysplasia and high-grade dysplasia. The probability of having a personal history of melanoma in any given patient with dysplastic melanocytic nevi correlates with the grade of cytologic atypia in melanocytic nevi cells. In addition, the presence of severe cytologic atypia in dysplastic melanocytic nevi correlates with a significantly greater risk of melanoma development (19.7%) compared with moderate (8.1%) or mild (5.7%) cytologic atypia.

Management of these patients is difficult. Dysplastic melanocytic nevi are not uncommon. Reportedly, as many as 4.6 million people in the United States have one or more sporadic dysplastic melanocytic nevi. Familial dysplastic melanocytic nevi are estimated to involve 50,000 patients in the United States. The risk of melanoma for these patients is probably on a continuum and correlated with their family history of melanoma or dysplastic melanocytic nevi, personal history of melanoma, number of acquired and dysplastic melanocytic lesions, and history of sun exposure. Removal of all dysplastic melanocytic nevi is inappropriate inasmuch as the chance of any single lesion becoming malignant is small, and, in addition, most melanomas arise de novo.

In cases of mild and moderate dysplastic nevi with microscopically positive margins and no concerning residual clinical lesion, observation, rather than reexcision, is the recommended form of management. All severely dysplastic nevi should be reexcised. Partial biopsy of any pigmented lesion that is clinically or pathologically suspicious for melanoma can lead to delayed melanoma diagnosis and is discouraged.

Management includes patient education and total body photography for comparison at future skin examinations and sequential dermoscopy. Patients should avoid the sun and use sunscreens and protective clothing. These patients should have regular biannual or quarterly examinations of the entire integument, including the scalp and the oral, genital, and perianal mucosa, and an ophthalmologic examination. Comparison with the previous total body photographs and use of the dermatoscope can be helpful. Any lesions that are suspicious for melanoma should be excised. Examination of first-degree family members (parents, siblings, and children) of patients with melanoma or dysplastic melanocytic nevi is recommended to identify other persons at high risk.

References

Andea AA: Molecular testing for melanocytic tumors: a practical update, *Histopathology* 80:150–156, 2022.

Argenziano G, Catricala C, Ardigo M, et al: Dermoscopy of patients with multiple nevi, *Arch Dermatol* 147:46–49, 2011.

Arumi-Uria M, McNutt NS, Finnerty B: Grading of atypia in nevi: correlation with melanoma risk, *Mod Pathol* 16:764–771, 2003.

Barnhill RL, Elder DE, Piepkorn MW, et al: Revision of the Melanocytic Pathology Assessment Tool and Hierarchy for Diagnosis classification schema for melanocytic lesions: a consensus statement, *JAMA Netw Open* 6:e2250613, 2023.

Bauer J, Bastian BC: Distinguishing melanocytic nevi from melanomas by DNA copy number changes: comparative genomic hybridization as a research and diagnostic tool, *Dermatol Ther* 19:40–49, 2006.

Burian EA, Jemec GBE: Eruptive melanocytic nevi: A review, *Am J Clin Dermatol* 20(5):669–682, 2019.

de Snoo FA, Kroon MW, Bergman W, et al: From sporadic atypical nevi to familial melanoma: risk analysis for melanoma in sporadic atypical nevus patients, *J Am Acad Dermatol* 56:748–752, 2007.

Drozdowski R, Spaccarelli N, Peters MS, Grant-Kels JM: Dysplastic nevus part I: Historical perspective, classification, and epidemiology, *J Am Acad Dermatol* 88:1–10, 2023.

Elder DE, Massi D, Scolyer RA: *WHO classification of skin tumours*, vol 11, ed 4, International Agency for Research on Cancer, 2018.

Ferrara G, Soyer HP, Malvehy J, et al: The many faces of blue nevus: a clinicopathologic study, *J Cutan Pathol* 34:543–551, 2007.

Gelbard AN, Tripp JM, Marghoob AA, et al: Management of Spitz nevi: a survey of dermatologists in the United States, *J Am Acad Dermatol* 47:224–330, 2002.

Goodson AG, Florell SR, Boucher KM, et al: Low rates of clinical recurrence after biopsy of benign to moderately dysplastic melanocytic nevi, *J Am Acad Dermatol* 62:591–596, 2010.

King R, Hayzen BA, Page RN, et al: Recurrent nevus phenomenon: a clinicopathologic study of 357 cases and histologic comparison with melanoma with regression, *Mod Pathol* 22:611–619, 2009.

Kinsler VA, O'Hare P, Bulstrode N, et al: Melanoma in congenital melanocytic naevi, *Br J Dermatol* 176:1131–1143, 2017.

Maher NG, Scolyer RA, Colebatch AJ: Biology and genetics of acquired and congenital melanocytic naevi, *Pathology* S0031-3025(22):00683-3, 2022.

Naeyaert JM, Brochez L: Dysplastic nevi, *N Engl J Med* 349:2233–2240, 2003.

Price HN, Schaffer JV: Congenital melanocytic nevi: when to worry and how to treat: facts and controversies, *Clin Dermatol* 28:283–302, 2010.

Que K, Grant-Kels JM, Longo C, Pellacani G: Basics of confocal microscopy and the complexity of diagnosing skin tumors: new imaging tools in clinical practice, diagnostic workflows, cost-estimate and new trends, *Dermatol Clinics* 34:367–375, 2016.

Roh MR, Eliades P, Gupta S, Tsao H: Genetics of melanocytic nevi, *Pigment Cell Melanoma Res* 28:661–672, 2015.

Šekoranja D, Pižem J, Luzar B: An update on molecular genetic aberrations in spitz melanocytic proliferations: correlation with morphological features and biological behavior, *Acta Med Acad* 50:157–174, 2021.

Sommer LL, Barcia SM, Clarke LE, Helm KF: Persistent melanocytic nevi: a review and analysis of 205 cases, *J Cutan Pathol* 38:503–507, 2011.

Spaccarelli N, Drozdowski R, Peters MS, Grant-Kels JM: Dysplastic nevus part II: Dysplastic nevi: Molecular/genetic profiles and management, *J Am Acad Dermatol* 88:13–20, 2023.

Tetzlaff MT, Reuben A, Billings SD, et al: Toward a molecular-genetic classification of spitzoid neoplasms, *Clin Lab Med* 37:431–448, 2017.

Wei B, Gu J, Gao B, et al: Deficient mismatch repair is detected in large-to-giant congenital melanocytic naevi: providing new insight into aetiology and diagnosis, *Br J Dermatol* 188:64–74, 2023.

Yeh I: Melanocytic naevi, melanocytomas and emerging concepts, *Pathology* S0031-3025(22):00679-1, 2022.

NONMELANOMA CANCER OF THE SKIN

Method of
Jake Lazaroff, MD; and Diana Bolotin, MD, PhD

CURRENT DIAGNOSIS

- Skin cancers are polymorphous in appearance, ranging from small papules and plaques to nodules and tumors of different colors, sizes, and consistencies.
- The surface may be smooth, scaly, ulcerated, or crusted.
- A common feature is that all of these skin neoplasms grow continuously and relapse when superficially treated.
- The distinction between skin cancers and benign neoplasms or inflammatory dermatoses may be difficult for the nondermatologist to make.

CURRENT THERAPY

- For the majority of nonmelanoma skin cancers, localized treatments are sufficient and include cryotherapy, immunotherapy, topical chemotherapy, and photodynamic therapy.
- Surgical techniques include electrodesiccation and curettage, simple excision, and Mohs micrographic surgery, which offers intraoperative confirmation of complete tumor removal and maximal cure rates.
- The Mohs procedure is indicated for more aggressive tumors, for tumors in certain anatomic locations, and in immunosuppressed patients.
- Rarely, sentinel lymph node dissection and adjuvant therapies, such as radiotherapy and chemotherapy, are warranted.

Nonmelanoma skin cancer (NMSC) is a heterogeneous group of skin malignancies that includes basal cell carcinoma (BCC) and squamous cell carcinoma (SCC). These are the most common skin cancers, and NMSC in the stricter sense of the definition (Figure 1). The more-inclusive use of the term *NMSC* also includes malignant neoplasms of adnexal, fibrohistiocytic, and vascular origin as well as Merkel cell carcinoma and metastatic tumors. The vast majority of NMSCs are slowly growing and locally invasive neoplasms that are often diagnosed and treated by dermatologists. Management of the more aggressive tumors often requires a team approach to diagnosis, treatment, and clinical follow-up (Table 1).

Basal Cell Carcinoma

BCC accounts for the majority of NMSCs in the United States and is increasingly diagnosed in younger patients. Light skin complexion and history of ultraviolet (UV) light exposure are the predominant risk factors for BCC in the majority of the population. Intermittent intense UV light exposures early in life, but not cumulative UV light exposure, pose the highest risk factor for developing BCC later in life. Other risk factors for BCC include exposure to ionizing radiation, psoralen photochemotherapy, arsenic, and smoking. A history of BCC also increases one's risk for developing a subsequent BCC. Immunosuppression, especially in recipients of solid-organ transplants, presents a significant risk factor for BCC. Inherited genodermatoses such as Gorlin, Bazex, and Rombo syndromes; xeroderma pigmentosum; and some forms of albinism are predisposing factors for BCC as well. Mutations in *PTCH1* that are found in Gorlin syndrome have been shown to be an early event underlying BCC pathogenesis.

Clinically, BCC is most commonly found on the head and neck region, though any part of the body can develop this tumor. The presentation varies depending on the histologic subtype of the tumor. Although many histologic variants of BCC exist, the most common subtypes are superficial, nodular and micronodular, morpheaform, and metatypic. The histologic heterogeneity results in variable clinical findings. Superficial BCC typically forms an erythematous scaly patch or plaque. Nodular BCC is the more classic-appearing lesion, a pink pearly nodule with or without central crust or ulcer. Unlike these subtypes, morpheaform BCC clinically resembles an ill-defined scar; it is the most histologically aggressive variant with a tendency for deep local invasion. Metatypic BCC is also known as *basosquamous carcinoma* because it has histologic features of both BCC and SCC, though it is distinguished from the latter by molecular markers. This subtype also has a tendency for more aggressive growth.

Although it is potentially locally destructive, BCC rarely metastasizes. Successful treatment of this tumor involves its local eradication. A number of treatment options exist and depend on the histologic subtype of the tumor. For small, superficial tumors, a

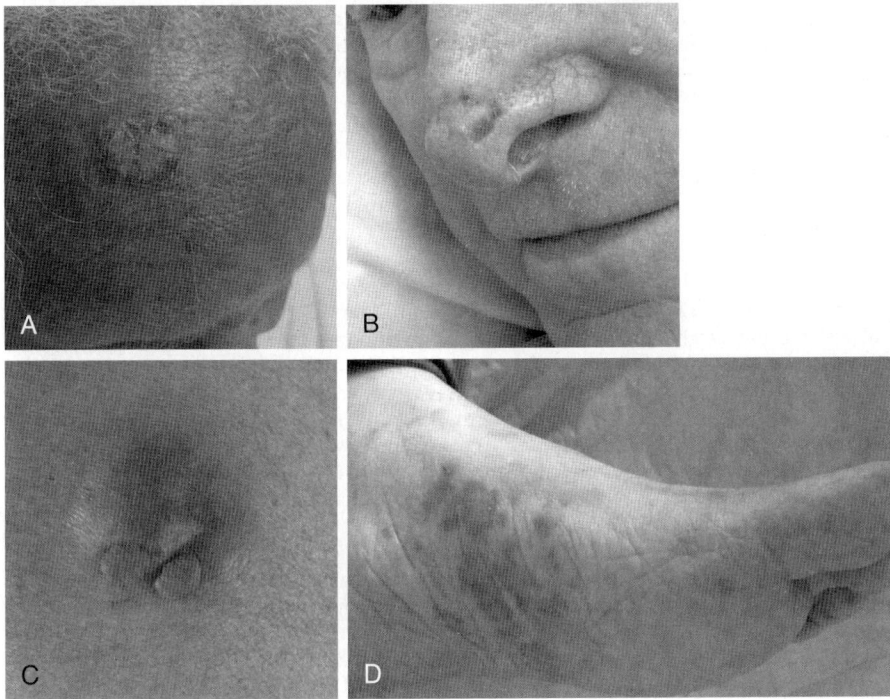

Figure 1 Clinical images of skin cancers. A, Squamous cell carcinoma in sun-exposed skin of a 102-year-old African American woman. B, Depressed scarlike appearance of a morpheaform basal cell carcinoma on the nose. C, This firm tumor on the abdomen is a dermatofibrosarcoma protuberans. D, Violaceous plaques on the instep in an elderly Greek man typical for endemic Kaposi's sarcoma.

TABLE 1	Overview of Therapeutic Modalities for the Management of Skin Cancers		
THERAPEUTIC MODALITY	**NEOPLASM**	**COMMENT**
Cryotherapy	AK, SCC in situ Superficial BCC Kaposi's sarcoma	Versatile, but operator dependent
Topical 5-fluorouracil (Efudex)	AK, SCC in situ[1] Superficial BCC	Will treat preclinical AK
Topical imiquimod (Aldara)	AK Superficial BCC	Flulike adverse effects can occur
Photodynamic therapy	AK, SCC in situ Superficial BCC	SCC and BCC are off-label uses
Electrodesiccation and curettage	AK, SCC BCC	
Excision	All	
Mohs micrographic surgery	BCC, SCC MAC, sebaceous carcinoma DFSP, AFX Angiosarcoma EMPD, MCC	Preferred for certain types of invasive tumors (e.g., morpheaform BCC), on high-risk regions (e.g., nose, lip), and settings (e.g., recurrence, immunosuppressed patient)
Radiation therapy	BCC, SCC Kaposi's sarcoma, angiosarcoma MCC Inoperable tumors	Careful risk-to-benefit evaluation

AFX, Atypical fibroxanthoma; *AK*, actinic keratosis; *BCC*, basal cell carcinoma; *DFSP*, dermatofibrosarcoma protuberans; *EMPD*, extramammary Paget's disease; *MAC*, microcystic adnexal carcinoma; *MCC*, Merkel cell carcinoma; *SCC*, squamous cell carcinoma.
[1]Not FDA approved for this indication.

nonsurgical approach can suffice, though nonsurgical treatment often carries a higher risk of recurrence than surgical treatment. Nonsurgical options include topical 5-fluorouracil (Efudex 5%), topical imiquimod (Aldara), liquid nitrogen cryotherapy, photodynamic therapy, and local radiation therapy.

Electrodesiccation and curettage (ED&C) is an option that has a high cure rate for small and superficial tumors (95% to 98%). Standard excision with adequate margins is an appropriate surgical treatment providing good cure rates, especially for tumors with nonaggressive histologic pattern. Mohs micrographic surgery (MMS) offers the advantage of precise margin examination during excision and therefore carries the lowest overall rate of recurrence. This tissue-sparing procedure is also advantageous in terms of reconstruction on cosmetically sensitive regions. MMS is indicated to treat recurrent tumors, those in immunosuppressed patients, aggressive histologic variants, and BCCs located on certain areas of the face known to carry a higher risk of recurrence.

Although locally advanced and metastatic BCCs are uncommon, treatment with targeted molecules such as vismodegib (Erivedge) have demonstrated clinical efficacy.

Squamous Cell Carcinoma

Cutaneous squamous cell carcinoma (SCC) is the second most common skin malignancy. Its incidence is increasing among both men and women in the United States. Development of SCC is intimately linked to the cumulative UV radiation exposure of the patient via a mechanism that combines DNA damage with immunosuppression. History of ionizing radiation exposure is a risk factor as well. Similar to BCC, occupational exposures such as arsenic can also predispose one to SCC. Patients with xeroderma pigmentosum or oculocutaneous albinism also are at higher risk for SCC.

Chronic inflammation or injury can predispose to epidermal malignant transformation. Examples of this phenomenon are SCC developing within scars from burns, in chronic ulcers and skin overlying osteomyelitis, and in persistent lichen sclerosus or lichen planus. These tumors have a more aggressive behavior and higher rates of metastasis.

Human papilloma virus (HPV) predisposes to SCC. Verrucous carcinoma, a well-differentiated subtype of SCC, has a well-documented association with HPV types 6 and 11.

Transplant patients are at high risk for SCC that correlates with the degree of immunosuppression. In fact, SCC development is up to 250 times greater in immunosuppressed individuals compared with the general population, whereas BCC increases to a lesser extent with immunocompromise. A more common association between HPV and SCC has been noted in the immunocompromised population and might account for the disproportional increase of SCC over BCC in this population.

As with BCC, history of previous SCC has been found to be a risk factor for developing a subsequent SCC. This risk appears especially pronounced in smokers.

Unlike BCC, SCC often has a precursor lesion: actinic keratosis. Histologically, actinic keratosis demonstrates partial-thickness atypia of the epidermis, and patients often describe it as waxing and waning. Full-thickness histologic atypia is seen in SCC in situ (Bowen's disease), whereas invasive SCC penetrates the basement membrane to invade the underlying dermis. Histologically, the degree of differentiation of SCC tends to correlate with its clinical behavior. Well-differentiated lesions tend toward local invasion, as opposed to poorly differentiated SCC, which more commonly is infiltrative.

The typical clinical presentation of SCC is that of a hyperkeratotic pink plaque. More advanced lesions may be nodular and can ulcerate. In most cases, SCC shows only local invasion; however, perineural invasion and rarely metastasis are more likely with SCC than with BCC. The central face, temples, and scalp present high-risk zones for recurrence and metastasis.

Treatment of SCC involves modalities similar to those used for BCC. Cryotherapy is the mainstay of treatment for actinic keratosis. Topical treatment with 5-fluorouracil (Carac 0.5%, Fluoroplex 1%, Fluorouracil 2 or 5%, or Efudex 5%)[1] alone or in combination with calcipotriol (Dovonex),[1] imiquimod (Aldara or Zyclara),[1] tirbanibulin (Klisyri),[1] or photodynamic therapy is often used as field therapy to depopulate large regions of the skin of actinic keratosis lesions. Continued sun protection has been shown to be of benefit to prevent progression from actinic keratosis to SCC, especially in the immunocompromised population. Systemic retinoids, such as acitretin (Soriatane)[1] and nicotinamide[7] have also been used for the prevention and reduction of NMSC, particularly in high-risk populations. SCC in situ may be treated with ED&C. Excision with a clear surgical margin is often used in the treatment of SCC on the trunk or extremities, but MMS yields the highest cure rates, especially in high-risk areas such as the face and scalp. Adjuvant radiotherapy, surgical excision, and targeted approaches with anti–PD-1 monoclonal antibodies may be used alone or in combination for more aggressive tumors. Overall, the prognosis for a patient with cutaneous SCC depends heavily on location, degree of histologic differentiation, invasion, and metastasis.

Neoplasms of Adnexal Origin

The adnexal structures of the skin include the pilosebaceous unit as well as apocrine and eccrine glands and ducts. A great number of benign and malignant tumors of adnexal origin occur in the skin. Most of the adnexal malignancies are rare. Sebaceous carcinoma and microcystic adnexal carcinoma (MAC) are two of the more common adnexal carcinomas that have an aggressive nature and may be subtle at presentation.

Sebaceous Carcinoma

Sebaceous carcinoma is an aggressive malignancy that is most commonly found on the head and neck region. More specifically, it is one of the more common tumors of the eyelid and periocular area. Because of its nonspecific clinical presentation, it is often treated as chalazion before biopsy and diagnosis. Population-based risk factors associated with development of sebaceous carcinoma include older age and European ethnicity. History of irradiation and immunosuppression predisposes to sebaceous carcinoma development, similar to BCC and SCC. Sebaceous carcinoma is one of the cutaneous neoplasms characteristic of Muir-Torre syndrome, which results from mutations in DNA mismatch repair genes and is associated with multiple sebaceous neoplasms and internal malignancy.

Clinical diagnosis of sebaceous carcinoma is difficult, therefore progressive or nonresolving eyelid lesions require biopsy. Treatment of sebaceous carcinoma is primarily surgical. Wide local excision with 5- to 6-mm margins or MMS is indicated. A lower rate of recurrence with MMS (11.1%) has been shown compared with local excision (32%). Close follow-up is indicated to monitor for recurrence and metastasis.

Microcystic Adnexal Carcinoma

MAC is another adnexal malignancy with predilection for the head and neck. In the United States, it is most prevalent in the white population and on the left side of the body, suggesting UV irradiation as a risk factor. Although it can be seen in a wide age range of patients, older adult patients have a higher risk of developing MAC. The low incidence of this tumor makes it difficult to evaluate other risk factors, though cases have been reported in immunosuppressed patients and those with a history of radiation therapy.

Clinically, MAC occurs as a slowly growing, pink- to flesh-colored ill-defined plaque. Paresthesia and/or numbness are common complaints and have been attributed to the high degree of perineural invasion by this tumor. MAC is a locally aggressive tumor with an unpredictable pattern of infiltrative growth. Histologically, MAC exhibits both pilar and sweat duct differentiation, deep invasion with a desmoplastic stromal response, and perineural invasion.

Surgical excision is the standard of care treatment for MAC, and radiation as an adjunct therapy is reported in a few cases. Because this tumor can extend for centimeters subclinically, MMS is favored as the first-line surgical treatment because it allows complete examination of the surgical margins intraoperatively and has been reported to have a lower recurrence rate than standard excision.

Fibrohistiocytic Malignancies

Fibrohistiocytic tumors of the skin are derived from the mesenchymal tissue and range from those of intermediate malignant potential to aggressive pleomorphic sarcomas. Of these overall rare malignancies, dermatofibrosarcoma protuberans (DFSP) and atypical fibroxanthoma are more frequently encountered.

Dermatofibrosarcoma Protuberans

DFSP is the most common fibrohistiocytic malignancy of the skin. It occurs at various ages ranging from infancy to older adulthood. The pathogenesis of DFSP involves a translocation between chromosomes 17 and 22 that fuses the collagen type 1 α_1 gene (COL1A1) with the platelet-derived growth factor B-chain gene (PDGFB). This fusion gene results in overexpression of PDGFB, which acts as a potent growth stimulant for mesenchymal cells. In general, slowly growing DFSPs are locally invasive and infiltrative rather than metastatic. Therefore treatment of this tumor is primarily surgical.

---

[1] Not FDA approved for this indication.
[7] Available as dietary supplement.

A high recurrence rate has been noted in a number of studies and is attributed to the infiltrative growth of the tumor. MMS reduces recurrence rates and is often recommended. DFSP is thought to be a radiosensitive tumor, and adjunctive radiation therapy has been successful used both preoperatively and postoperatively. The discovery of the *COL1A1-PDGFB* fusion gene has led to trials of imatinib (Gleevec) therapy as an adjunct to surgery for DFSP and is currently approved for use in unresectable, recurrent, or metastatic disease.

Atypical Fibroxanthoma

Atypical fibroxanthoma is a low-grade sarcoma of the skin. This locally invasive tumor favors sun-damaged skin of the head and neck region in older adults. Patients with xeroderma pigmentosum have a higher risk for developing atypical fibroxanthoma. It has a nonspecific clinical presentation, and a biopsy with histopathology is needed for diagnosis. Histologically, this tumor often exhibits marked pleomorphism and frequent mitoses. Often immunohistochemical staining is necessary for definitive diagnosis. Surgery is the treatment of choice for atypical fibroxanthoma. Either wide local excision or MMS may be used, though lower recurrence rates have been reported with MMS. Despite the pleomorphic microscopic appearance, this tumor rarely metastasizes, and the prognosis with appropriate treatment is favorable.

Vascular Malignancies

Vascular neoplasms of the skin are rare. Kaposi's sarcoma (KS) and angiosarcoma, both increasingly encountered in healthy older adults as well as in immunosuppressed patients, are discussed here.

Kaposi's Sarcoma

Controversy exists regarding the nature of cell proliferation seen in KS. Some regard it as a true malignancy, and others view it as a reactive proliferation. Four types of KS exist: KS of older adult men of Jewish and Mediterranean origin, African-endemic KS, immunosuppression-associated KS, and AIDS-associated KS. Infection with human herpesvirus 8 (HHV-8) is involved in the pathogenesis of all types of KS. Clinical findings include nonblanching purpuric patches and plaques that can progress to nodules with ulceration. KS can be isolated to the skin or can become disseminated to the lymph nodes and viscera. Diagnosis is established with histopathology and immunostaining. Management of KS is complex because of the varied clinical course of the four subtypes. In cases of localized lesions, surgery, cryotherapy, or laser treatment may be useful. Radiotherapy can also be used for localized disease. Patients with disseminated KS are generally treated with chemotherapy. In AIDS-associated KS, institution of HIV medications has been shown to effect resolution of KS.

Angiosarcoma

Angiosarcoma is a rarer but more aggressive vascular cutaneous malignancy that tends to metastasize and carries a poor prognosis. Clinically, angiosarcoma favors the head and neck area of older adult men; it can also arise within sites of previous radiation therapy or chronic lymphedema. No association between angiosarcoma and HHV-8 has been found. Patients present with an asymptomatic enlarging purpuric plaque that can eventually develop a nodular component. Angiosarcoma may have multifocal involvement that is often not appreciated clinically. The treatment for angiosarcoma involves wide local excision and postoperative radiotherapy. The overall prognosis is poor, and distant metastasis-free 5-year survival rates range between 20% and 37%.

Other Nonmelanoma Skin Cancers

Merkel Cell Carcinoma

Merkel cell carcinoma (MCC) is a rare but often fatal NMSC that derives from cutaneous neuroendocrine cells. Fair skin and a history of exposure to UV light are risk factors for developing MCC. Like many other NMSCs, MCC favors the head and neck and is much more common in older adults. Immunosuppression appears to be a risk factor for MCC development because its incidence is significantly increased in patients with AIDS and

recipients of organ transplants. Polyomavirus has been implicated in the pathogenesis of MCC.

This malignancy is often metastatic upon presentation. Clinically, it occurs as a nonspecific, red asymptomatic papule or nodule. A biopsy with immunohistochemical analysis is diagnostic. The therapy for MCC involves surgery with wide local excision or MMS. Sentinel lymph node biopsy can be performed for staging purposes but should be considered on a case-by-case basis. MCC is sensitive to radiotherapy, which is a recommended adjuvant treatment for patients with lymph node involvement. Palliative chemotherapy often produces a response; however, recurrence is common. Preliminary data indicate a promising signal with checkpoint immunotherapy in patients with advanced disease, though prognosis remains poor for metastatic disease or lymph node involvement.

Paget's Disease

Paget's disease refers to intraepidermal spread of adenocarcinoma. Two types are seen in the skin: mammary Paget's disease and extramammary Paget's disease (EMPD). Mammary Paget's disease is most commonly seen in women and has a strict association with adenocarcinoma of the breast. The lesions are usually unilateral scaly red plaques that favor the nipple. Often the underlying tumor is not clinically present but is detected through imaging. Other dermatoses of the nipple can resemble mammary Paget's disease, therefore definitive diagnosis requires biopsy and immunohistochemistry. Surgical excision along with appropriate treatment of the breast cancer is the recommended treatment. Prognosis depends on the extent of breast cancer at diagnosis, though it appears to be poorer for breast cancer patients with mammary Paget's disease than those without.

EMPD consists of two types of disease: type I disease is associated with distant adenocarcinoma, and type II disease is a primary cutaneous EMPD. Both are very rare, but, like mammary Paget's disease, they have a female predominance. Most commonly extramammary Paget's disease is found in the genital or perianal region; however, other areas of the skin can be affected less frequently. Clinically, EMPD manifests as a well-demarcated red plaque that can become erosive. Long-standing disease can spread from the groin to the trunk, mimicking an inflammatory dermatosis. Definitive diagnosis is based on biopsy findings, and further workup includes extensive screening for associated internal malignancy. Treatment relies on surgical excision with wide margins. MMS can be used to examine margins intraoperatively. The prognosis for type I EMPD depends on the extent of underlying tumor, but the prognosis for type II is favorable.

Cutaneous Metastases

Metastasis to the skin often heralds the systemic spread of an internal malignancy. Primary malignancy underlying the skin metastasis tends to differ by sex and age. In men, lung cancer is the most common source of skin metastasis, whereas breast cancer is the more common primary tumor in women. The head and neck are favored as sites of skin metastasis in men, but the trunk is favored in women.

The clinical presentation of skin metastasis is varied and often nonspecific. A new, asymptomatic cutaneous or subcutaneous nodule may be the reason for a biopsy that reveals metastasis of an unknown primary tumor. Diagnosis is made by histopathology and appropriate molecular staining. Specific clinical patterns of metastasis may be encountered. Inflammatory carcinoma can be seen with cutaneous breast cancer metastases. Occasionally, neoplastic infiltration leads to localized areas of alopecia. Zosteriform distribution of skin metastasis has been reported with breast cancer, colon cancer, or SCC.

Leukemia cutis refers to skin involvement with acute myelogenous leukemia, chronic myelogenous leukemia, myelodysplastic syndromes, chronic lymphocytic leukemia, or adult T-cell lymphoproliferative diseases. In rare cases, skin involvement precedes bone marrow disease and is termed *aleukemic leukemia cutis*. In chronic leukemias, skin involvement tends to predict disease progression into the acute phase. Children appear to have a higher incidence of leukemia cutis compared with adults but have a more favorable overall prognosis.

Metastatic skin tumors are distinguished from primary cutaneous malignancies histologically. Treatment is always geared toward the primary malignancy. Regardless of the type of neoplasm or site of metastasis, spread of an internal malignancy to the skin carries a poor prognosis.

References

Alam M, Ratner D: Cutaneous squamous-cell carcinoma, *N Engl J Med* 344(13):975–983, 2001.

Billings SD, Folpe AL: Cutaneous and subcutaneous fibrohistiocytic tumors of intermediate malignancy: An update, *Am J Dermatopathol* 26(2):141–155, 2004.

Blauvelt A, Kempers S, Lain E, et al: Phase 3 Trials of Tirbanibulin Ointment for Actinic Keratosis, *N Engl J Med* 384(6):512–520, 2021.

Buitrago W, Joseph AK: Sebaceous carcinoma: The great masquerader: Emerging concepts in diagnosis and treatment, *Dermatol Ther* 21(6):459–466, 2008.

Chen L, Aria AB, Silapunt S, Migden MR: Emerging nonsurgical therapies for locally advanced and metastatic nonmelanoma skin cancer, *Dermatol Surg* 45(1):1–16, 2019.

Cho-Vega JH, Medeiros LJ, Prieto VG, Vega F: Leukemia cutis, *Am J Clin Pathol* 129(1):130–142, 2008.

Christenson LJ, Borrowman TA, Vachon CM, et al: Incidence of basal cell and squamous cell carcinomas in a population younger than 40 years, *JAMA* 294(6):681–690, 2005.

Cumberland L, Dana A, Liegeois N: Mohs micrographic surgery for the management of nonmelanoma skin cancers, *Facial Plast Surg Clin North Am* 17(3):325–335, 2009.

Dasgupta T, Wilson LD, Yu JB: A retrospective review of 1349 cases of sebaceous carcinoma, *Cancer* 115(1):158–165, 2009.

Dubina M, Goldenberg G: Viral-associated nonmelanoma skin cancers: A review, *Am J Dermatopathol* 31(6):561–573, 2009.

Eisen DB, Michael DJ: Sebaceous lesions and their associated syndromes: Part I, *J Am Acad Dermatol* 61(4):549–560, 2009.

Fan H, Oro AE, Scott MP, Khavari PA: Induction of basal cell carcinoma features in transgenic human skin expressing Sonic Hedgehog, *Nat Med* 3(7):788–792, 1997.

Feng H, Shuda M, Chang Y, Moore PS: Clonal integration of a polyomavirus in human Merkel cell carcinoma, *Science* 319(5866):1096–1100, 2008.

Hussein MR: Skin metastasis: A pathologist's perspective, *J Cutan Pathol* 37(9):e1–320, 2010.

Kamino H, Jacobson M: Dermatofibroma extending into the subcutaneous tissue. Differential diagnosis from dermatofibrosarcoma protuberans, *Am J Surg Pathol* 14(12):1156–1164, 1990.

Kanitakis J: Mammary and extramammary Paget's disease, *J Eur Acad Dermatol Venereol* 21(5):581–590, 2007.

Karagas MR, Stukel TA, Greenberg ER, et al: Risk of subsequent basal cell carcinoma and squamous cell carcinoma of the skin among patients with prior skin cancer. Skin Cancer Prevention Study Group, *JAMA* 267(24):3305–3310, 1992.

Lee DA, Miller SJ: Nonmelanoma skin cancer, *Facial Plast Surg Clin North Am* 17(3):309–324, 2009.

Lehmann P: Methyl aminolaevulinate-photodynamic therapy: a review of clinical trials in the treatment of actinic keratoses and nonmelanoma skin cancer, *Br J Dermatol* 156(5):793–801, 2007.

Lemm D, Mugge LO, Mentzel T, Hoffken K: Current treatment options in dermatofibrosarcoma protuberans, *J Cancer Res Clin Oncol* 135(5):653–665, 2009.

Maddox JS, Soltani K: Risk of nonmelanoma skin cancer with azathioprine use, *Inflamm Bowel Dis* 14(10):1425–1431, 2008.

Marcet S: Atypical fibroxanthoma/malignant fibrous histiocytoma, *Dermatol Ther* 21(6):424–427, 2008.

McGuire JF, Ge NN, Dyson S: Nonmelanoma skin cancer of the head and neck. I: Histopathology and clinical behavior, *Am J Otolaryngol* 30(2):121–133, 2009.

Mendenhall WM, Mendenhall CM, Werning JW, et al: Cutaneous angiosarcoma, *Am J Clin Oncol* 29(5):524–528, 2006.

Prieto VG, Shea CR: Selected cutaneous vascular neoplasms. A review, *Dermatol Clin* 17(3):507–520, 1999; viii.

Rockville Merkel Cell Carcinoma Group: Merkel cell carcinoma: Recent progress and current priorities on etiology, pathogenesis, and clinical management, *J Clin Oncol* 27(24):4021–4026, 2009.

Rubin AI, Chen EH, Ratner D: Basal-cell carcinoma, *N Engl J Med* 353(21):2262–2269, 2005.

Schwartz RA, Micali G, Nasca MR, Scuderi L: Kaposi sarcoma: A continuing conundrum, *J Am Acad Dermatol* 59(2):179–206, 2008.

Smeets NW, Krekels GA, Ostertag JU, et al: Surgical excision vs Mohs' micrographic surgery for basal-cell carcinoma of the face: Randomised controlled trial, *Lancet* 364(9447):1766–1772, 2004.

Spencer JM, Nossa R, Tse DT, Sequeira M: Sebaceous carcinoma of the eyelid treated with Mohs micrographic surgery, *J Am Acad Dermatol* 44(6):1004–1009, 2001.

Ulrich C, Jurgensen JS, Degen A, et al: Prevention of non-melanoma skin cancer in organ transplant patients by regular use of a sunscreen: A 24 months, prospective, case-control study, *Br J Dermatol* 161(Suppl. 3):78–84, 2009.

Wetter R, Goldstein GD: Microcystic adnexal carcinoma: a diagnostic and therapeutic challenge, *Dermatol Ther* 21(6):452–458, 2008.

Yu JB, Blitzblau RC, Patel SC, et al: Surveillance, Epidemiology, and End Results (SEER) Database analysis of microcystic adnexal carcinoma (sclerosing sweat duct carcinoma) of the skin, *Am J Clin Oncol* 33(2):125–127, 2010.

PAPULOSQUAMOUS ERUPTIONS

Method of
Tam T. Nguyen, MD

CURRENT DIAGNOSIS

- Psoriasis can be clinically described as erythematous plaques with silvery white scales.
- Severity is rated as mild (< 5% body surface area [BSA]), moderate (5%–10% BSA), or severe (>10% BSA).
- Most cases are mild chronic plaques involving the extensor surfaces.
- Involvement of scalp and palmar and plantar surfaces is classified as severe.
- Psoriasis is commonly comorbid with several conditions, including cardiovascular disease, depression, and metabolic disorders.

CURRENT THERAPY

- Class I/II (super-potent) topical steroid is the mainstream treatment of mild to moderate psoriasis.
- For moderate to severe cases, systemic treatment with methotrexate is the gold standard.
- Narrowband ultraviolet B (UVB) remains a safe treatment option for all patients including children and pregnant women.
- Several immunomodulators or biologicals including etanercept (Enbrel) have been proved very effective therapy. Biologicals can be given as monotherapy or in combination with other modalities for very recalcitrant cases.
- Treatment of comorbid conditions is paramount.

Epidemiology

Psoriasis, a common chronic idiopathic inflammatory disorder, affects 2% to 3% of Americans. The number of persons affected by this condition has more than doubled from 1970 to 2000. It is a chronic disorder that can involve many organ systems including skin, mucosa, the gastrointestinal tract, and joints. Although the onset of psoriasis can occur at any age, there is a bimodal distribution peaking in young adults in their early 20s and again in persons in their 50s. There is an equal prevalence among male and female patients, but the incidence is higher in men among younger adult populations.

Risk Factors

There is a strong family history and association with HLA-Cw6, HLA-B13, and HLA-B27. Psoriatic genes appear to be located on four key genes called pSOR1-4, which show an autosomal dominant pattern. There are more than 60 gene loci associated with psoriasis. The genome-wide association study (GWAS) showed that the genes STAT3 and STAT5 regulate the cytokines associated with psoriasis. In addition to the genetic etiology, environmental triggers, such as drugs, infection, and stress, also have a role in the pathogenesis of the psoriasis. Psychogenic stress from home and school is especially common in pediatric cases. Lithium and β-blockers are two well-known triggers of psoriasis. Certain conditions, such as Crohn's disease and multiple sclerosis, predispose patients to developing psoriasis.

Pathophysiology

Even though the exact mechanism is unknown, psoriasis is a disease of T cells that leads to abnormal epidermal differentiation and hyperproliferation. Normal skin has epidermal turnover of

Plaque-like
Eczema
Fungal infection
Squamous cell carcinoma
Subacute cutaneous lupus erythematous

Guttate
Secondary syphilis
Pityriasis rosea

Erythrodermic
Pityriasis rubra pilaris
Drug eruptions

Pustular
Candidiasis
Acute generalized exanthematic pustulosis

Inverse
Intertrigo
Cutaneous T-cell lymphoma

Figure 2 Chronic plaque psoriasis on the extensor surfaces.

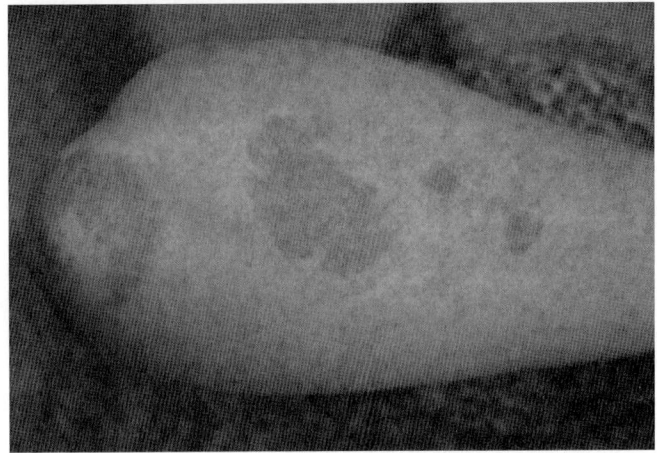

Figure 1 Guttate psoriasis with droplike, discrete papules and small plaques with scales.

about 21 to 28 days, but psoriatic skin turns over every 3 to 4 days. Several cytokines, including TNF-alpha, IL-17, IL-12, and IL-23, are part of the immune-mediated disease.

Diagnosis

Although most psoriatic lesions have characteristic scaly and silvery plaques, the lesions can be misleading. Refer to Box 1 for the differential diagnosis. Psoriasis has several subtypes including erythrodermic, pustular, and vulgaris. Psoriasis vulgaris has several subtypes including chronic plaque, guttate (Figure 1), and inverse psoriasis. More than 80% to 90% of psoriasis cases are the chronic plaque psoriasis. Therefore this chapter focuses on this subtype.

Severity of psoriasis is classified based on the body surface area (BSA) involved. There are several severity instruments, such as Koo-Menter Psoriasis, for assessing the severity. One of the best validated tools is the Psoriasis Area Severity Index (PASI). These instruments are used to classify the condition according to coverage of body surface area (BSA) as either mild (< 5% of BSA), moderate (5%–10% of BSA), or severe (>10% of BSA). BSA can be estimated using the rule of 9s. Each upper extremity and the head is 9%, and the chest, back, and each lower extremity are 18%. For children, similar rules apply, except that each lower extremity is 13.5%. When the lesions involve difficult regions such as hands, feet, face, scalp, and genitalia, they are treated as severe regardless of the amount of BSA they cover.

Fortunately, more than 70% to 75% of cases are classified as mild to moderate, and there is no need for blood work. However, when psoriasis is associated with comorbidities, such as depression and heart disease, or when systemic medications cause serious side effects, it may be reasonable to get basic laboratory tests such as a complete blood count with platelet (CBC), chemistry, liver function tests (LFTs), cholesterol panel, hepatitis B and C, uric acid, and erythrocyte sedimentation rate (ESR). For patients at high risk, consider HIV testing. Also, consider evaluating for tuberculosis with a PPD test. These laboratory tests are even more crucial when considering treating with immunosuppressants like methotrexate (Trexall) and biological agents. Liver biopsy should be done if methotrexate is used at a cumulative dose of 3.5 to 4g. Equally important, patients' quality of life needs to be assessed, which can be done with an instrument called the Dermatology Life Quality Index (DLQI).

Differential Diagnosis

The differential diagnosis of psoriasis is lengthy and can be tricky. Box 1 lists the differential diagnosis of psoriasis.

Clinical Manifestations

Most presentations of psoriasis are asymptomatic. When symptomatic, the most common clinical manifestation is pruritus. Other possible symptoms include fever and malaise, especially for more extensive disease. When psoriasis involves the joints, patients can have pain and stiffness in the involved joints; many of these cases involve the distal interphalangeal joints. On physical examination, the lesions are well-circumscribed dark pink to red plaques with silvery to white scales (Figures 2 and 3). Scales can be absent in certain locations, such as the intertriginous area (gluteal folds) (Figures 4 and 5). The margins are sharp and distinct, especially over extensor surfaces such as the elbows and knees (see Figure 2). Lesions also can involve the sacral area, nails, scalp, and the genitalia. If psoriasis forms under a nail, onycholysis (lifting of the nail plate) can occur with pitting and subungual keratosis.

When the scales are removed, several distinctive minute blood droplets appear, called the Auspitz sign. Use caution when removing the scales because it can be painful. When new lesions form at a site of trauma, it is called the Koebner phenomenon. Diagnosis can be made clinically. However, when in doubt, biopsy the lesion, which will show a thickened epidermis with an absent granular cell layer. The stratum corneum is hyperkeratotic, with classic infiltration of neutrophils.

If this inflammatory process affects the joints, psoriatic arthritis ensues. Although this article does not discuss psoriatic arthritis, it is important to recognize when it occurs. Unlike rheumatoid arthritis, the distal interphalangeal (DIP) joints are regularly involved, but it can affect any joints. Psoriatric arthritis only occurs in 4% to 42% of patients with psoriasis. Diagnosis can

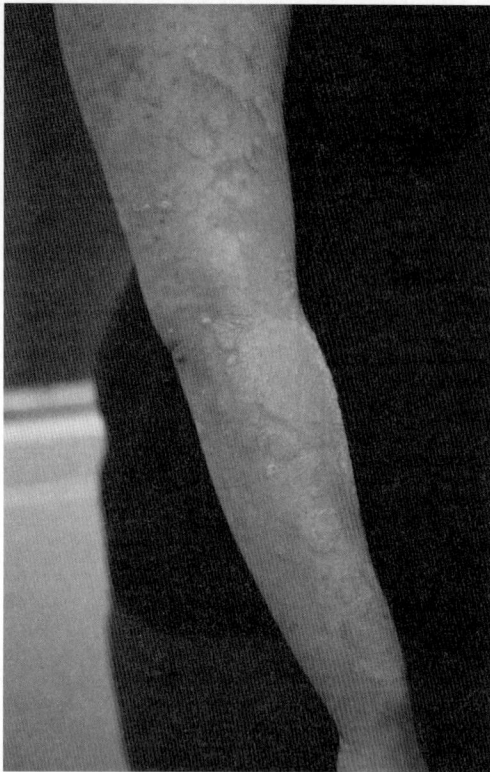

Figure 3 Chronic plaque psoriasis with classic silvery scales.

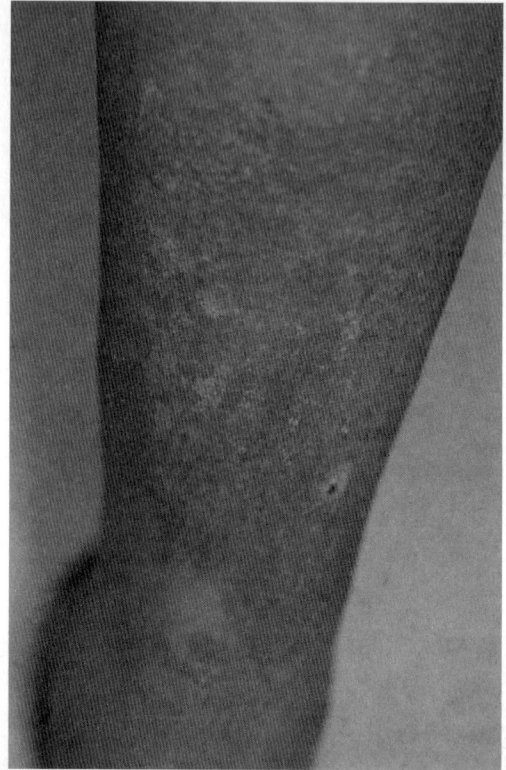

Figure 5 Chronic plaque psoriasis without scales.

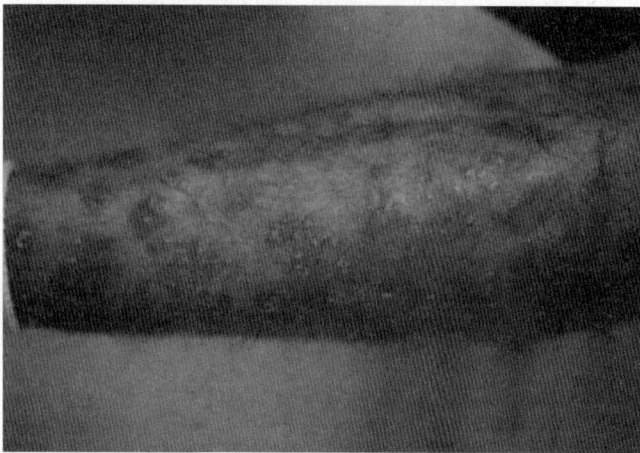

Figure 4 Chronic plaque psoriasis with limited scales.

be made with the CASPAR criteria, which evaluates five possible presentations, including having psoriasis, nail dystrophy, negative rheumatoid factor, dactylitis, and radiographic evidence.

Treatment

Corticosteroids remain the mainstay for psoriasis therapy; they reduce inflammation, decrease mitosis, and reduce erythema. Because most cases are mild to moderate, the first-line therapy to consider is topical corticosteroids. Even for severe cases that require systemic treatment, topical steroids should still be considered as a first-line adjuvant therapy. Because psoriatic lesions are thickened, it is critical to go directly to super-potent steroids (class I), such as clobetasol (Clobex) (refer to Box 2 for steroid potency). When the localized lesions are lichenified and do not respond to potent topical corticosteroids, using steroid-impregnated tapes (flurandrenolide tape [Cordran]), which function as an occlusive wrap, can help. However, for areas of thinner skin, such as mucosa and lesions on the face, use less-potent topical steroids.

Use caution when using class 1 steroids owing to all the potential side effects, including skin atrophy, hypopigmentation, telangiectasis, striae, and potential systemic absorption. In addition to the possible side effects, tachyphylaxis (reduced efficacy with prolonged use) can occur. Therefore it is crucial to limit the use of potent topical steroids to less than 12 weeks. Mild to moderate potency topical steroid can be use safely during pregnancy and by women who are breastfeeding.

One way to reduce the use of topical steroids is by using the vitamin D_3 analogue class, such as calcipotriene (Dovonex). This class of drugs inhibits epidermal proliferation and stimulates cellular differentiation. It is considered as effective as medium-potency corticosteroids, without the side effects. However, one drawback is that it takes about 8 weeks to be effective. Therefore it should not be used for acute psoriatic eruptions. More often it is used in combination with topical steroids, since topical calcipotriene in combination with high dose topical steroids like betamethasone (Enstilar) works better than either alone. It is generally well tolerated topically, but about 10% of patients experience burning and itching or hypercalcemia.

Other topical applications include tazarotene (Tazorac) and anthralin (Dritho-Crème HP 1%, Dritho-Scalp 0.5%). Tazarotene is an acetylenic retinoid and can be as effective as high-potency topical corticosteroids. However, its use is limited owing to the side effects of erythema, burning, pruritus, and peeling. Therefore it is best to combine it with corticosteroids to reduce the irritation. In addition, tazarotene can stain clothing, and it is less popular owing to the side effects (redness and irritation on skin as well as staining) and the feel and smell of the solutions. However, it is a good alternative to topical corticosteroids.

For a limited number of thickened lesions, consider intralesional steroid injections, such as a single intralesional injection of a mid-potency steroid (e.g., triamcinolone acetonide or Kenalog-10, 5–10 mg/mL). Most injected plaques clear completely and remain in remission for months. However, as with other steroid injections, side effects of skin atrophy and telangiectasis can occur. Therefore the face and intertriginous areas should not be injected because of the increased risk of side effects.

BOX 2 Classification of Topical Steroids, With a Few Samples From Each Class

Class 1: Super Potent
Clobex lotion 0.05%, clobetasol propionate
Cormax cream or solution, 0.05%, clobetasol propionate
Diprolene gel or ointment, 0.05%, bethamethasone dipropionate
Olux foam, 0.05%, clobetasol propionate

Class 2: Potent
Elocon ointment, 0.1%, mometasone furoate
Florone ointment, 0.05%, diflorasone diacetate
Halog ointment/cream, 0.1%, halcinonide
Lidex cream, gel, ointment, 0.05%, fluocinonide

Class 3: Upper Mid-Strength
Cutivate ointment, 0.005%, fluticasone propionate
Cyclocort cream/lotion, 0.1%, amcinonide
Lidex-E cream, 0.05%, fluocinonide
Maxivate cream/lotion, 0.05%, betamethasone dipropionate
Valisone ointment, 0.1%, betamethasone valerate

Class 4: Mid-Strength
Aristocort cream, 0.1%, triamcinolone acetonide
Cordran ointment, 0.05%, flurandrenolide
Elocon cream, 0.1%, mometasone furoate
Kenalog cream, ointment, spray, 0.1%, triamcinolone acetonide

Class 5: Lower Mid-Strength
DesOwen ointment, 0.05%, desonide
Diprosone lotion, 0.1%, betamethasone dipropionate
Kenalog lotion, 0.1%, triamcinolone acetonide
Synalar cream, 0.025%, fluocinolone acetonide

Class 6: Mild
Derma-Smoothe/FS Oil, 0.01%, fluocinolone acetonide
DesOwen cream, 0.05%, desonide
Synalar cream/solution, 0.01%, fluocinolone acetonide
Tridesilon cream, 0.05%, desonide

Class 7: Least Potent
Topicals with hydrocortisone, dexamethasone[6], methylprednisolone[6], and prednisolone[6]

[6]May be compounded by pharmacists.

BOX 3 Other Treatment Modalities for Moderate to Severe Psoriasis

Fumaric acid esters[2]: First-line therapy in a couple of European countries
Hydroxyurea (Hydrea)[1]: A good option because there is no liver or kidney toxicity; however, be cautious of bone marrow suppression
Leflunomide (Arava)[1]
Mycophenolate mofetil (Cellcept)[1]: good choice for HIV patients and patients with immunobullous disorders
Retinoic acid metabolism–blocking agents: liarozole[2] and talarozole (Rambazole)[5]
Alitretinoin topical (Panretin)[1]
Sulfasalazine (Azulfidine)[1]
Tacrolimus (Prograf)[1]
6 thioguanine (Tabloid)[1]

[1]Not FDA approved for this indication.
[2]Not available in the United States.
[5]Investigational drug in the United States.

For severe and recalcitrant cases, systematic medications are needed. One of the gold standards in the United States and many other countries is methotrexate (Trexall) because it is available as a generic. Its exact mechanism is unknown; initially it was believed to inhibit proliferation, but more-recent studies describe an antiinflammatory property. The most common serious side effect of this drug is hepatotoxicity (as many as 33% of patients show some liver disease). Therefore it is crucial to screen for alcohol dependency, liver disease, and obesity. Standard practice is to check baseline CBC and liver function enzymes, and then repeat these laboratory tests after 1 month of therapy. Methotrexate is highly teratogenic; hence it is absolutely contraindicated in pregnancy. After stopping the medication, men should wait at least 3 months and women should wait one ovulatory cycle before attempting to conceive.

There are two methods for initiating methotrexate. Most patients start at an initial dose of 7.5mg (3 tabs of 2.5mg) weekly; in pediatric cases dosage[1] is 0.2 to 0.7 mg/kg weekly. Others start at a higher dosage of 0.4 to 0.5 mg/kg weekly. Unfortunately, there is no current study to compare the two methods. With either dosing regimen, do not exceed 30 mg per week. Methotrexate depletes the body's storage of folic acid, so it is important to supplement folic acid[1] 1mg daily except the day when methotrexate is taken. The methotrexate can be titrated upward every 2 to 4 weeks. Methotrexate is contraindicated in pregnancy because it is teratogenic and can cause abortion.

Unlike methotrexate, which can take several weeks before it becomes effective, cyclosporine (Neoral), a calcineurin inhibitor, is rapidly effective for severe cases. It is dosed at a low dose of 2 to 5 mg/kg/day[3] divided into two doses and increased slowly every 2 to 4 weeks. Maintenance dosage is about 3 to 5 mg/kg/day.[3] A main concern for this drug is nephrotoxicity. As long as the use of cyclosporine is limited to 1 year, it is generally safe. However, kidney function still needs to be monitored regularly. Cyclosporine has been associated with an increased risk of squamous cell carcinoma, especially when the patient has a history of psoralen plus ultraviolet A (PUVA) therapy.

Although not FDA-approved, azathioprine (Imuran) has been a successful systemic medication for psoriasis. Generally, it is initially dosed at 0.5 mg/kg. If there is cytopenia, then the dosage can be increased by 0.5 mg/kg/day every 4 to 6 weeks as needed. Another dosing method is based on thiopurine methyltransferase (TPMT) levels. If the TPMT is less than 5.0 U, do not use azathioprine. If the level is between 5 and 13.7 U, the maximum daily dose should be 0.5 mg/kg/daily. If the TMPT level is between 13.7 and 19.0 U, then the maximum daily dose may be increased to 1.5 mg/kg. There is only one FDA-approved phosphodiesterase type-4 inhibitor (PDE4), apremilast (Otezla). Taken orally twice a day, this drug inhibits PDE4 leading to increased intracellular cAMP levels. In 2023, the FDA approved roflumilast (Zoryve) as the only topical PDE4 inhibitor for use in patients 6 years and older.

Acitretin (Soriatane) and isotretinoin (Claravis)[1] are retinoids, which are vitamin A derivatives. Although acitretin is more commonly used, either may be used and requires a period of 3 to 6 months to achieve results. However, these retinoids are generally less effective than methotrexate and cyclosporine. Though they are less effective and a longer time is required for this class of agents to work, their main benefits include no malignancy potential and no immunosuppression. Therefore these drugs are safe in patients with HIV and other immunosuppressive conditions. Unfortunately, acitretin and isotretinoin are highly teratogenic. Both male and female patients need to be drug free for 1 year for isotretinoin and 3 years for acitretin before they conceive. For other possible treatment agents, refer to Box 3.

In recent years, immunomodulators or biologicals have revolutionized the treatment course of psoriasis. Generally, criteria for this class of therapy are PASI greater than 10 and failure of other

[1]Not FDA approved for this indication.

[1]Not FDA approved for this indication.
[2]Not available in the United States.

therapies or a contraindication to other therapies such as methotrexate. Most agents are limited to 1 to 2 years of use because most studies have not been evaluated beyond 2 years. Tuberculosis should be evaluated (PPD and possibly chest x-ray) before starting these biologics. All the medications in this class should be avoided in pregnancy. Alefacept (Amevive)[2] and efalizumab (Raptiva) are T-cell inhibitors. Efalizumab (Raptiva) was withdrawn from the market in 2009 owing to reported cases of progressive multifocal leukoencephalopathy. Another class is tumor necrosis factor (TNF). Etanercept (Enbrel), one of the first TNF inhibitors, should not be used in patients with multiple sclerosis. Four monoclonal antibodies include infliximab (Remicade), adalimumab (Humira), certolizumab (Cimzia), and golimumab (Simponi)[1], and all are TNF inhibitors. In recent years, a new class of biologics that inhibit interleukin (IL)-12 and IL-23 has shown promising results. Ustekinumab (Stelara) was first approved within this class, followed by guselkumab (Tremfya), tildrakizumab (Ilumya), and risankizumab (Skyrizi) in 2019. Secukinumab (Cosentyx), a new biological for plaque psoriasis is a recombinant, high-affinity, fully humanized IgG monoclonal antibody that selectively binds and neutralizes interleukin-17A (IL-17A). Additional three IL-17A inhibitors, ixekizumab (Taltz), bimekizumab (Bimzelx)[2] and brodalumab (Siliq), have been approved for use. Currently, bimekizumab and mirikizumab are investigational drugs in the US. With increased understanding of TYK2, small molecule inhibitors have been approved for treatment. Deucravabitinib (Sotyktu) selectively binds to the TYK2 regulatory domain. Two other agents (brepocitinib[5] and ropsactimb[5]) are in the pipeline for approval. This class of medication is an oral medication, making it convenient for patients.

Etanercept (Enbrel) blocks TNF-α. It is generally dosed at 50mg SC twice weekly for 12 weeks and then 50mg weekly. Patients can self-administer the drug; laboratory monitoring is not required. There are limited data beyond 2 years. Etanercept is the preferred drug for children. Infliximab (Remicade) blocks both soluble and bound TNF-α. Its dosage is 3 to 5 mg/kg IV on weeks 0, 2, and 6, and then every 6 to 8 weeks. Medication generally is infused over 2 hours. It is approved for 1 year. In a comparative study, infliximab was found to be superior to methotrexate. TNF does not appear to increase the risk of herpes zoster but could be associated with an increase in melanoma.

Adalimumab (Humira) blocks both soluble and bound TNF-α. Initiate the dose at 40mg SC every 2 weeks, although some patients require dosing every 7 to 10 days. Alternatively, the initial dose may be 80mg followed by 40mg. Patients may self-administer the

injections. As with infliximab, before initiating treatment, obtain a PPD (and consider chest x-ray as well). Antibodies can develop within the first 28 weeks, which will decrease the efficacy of the drug. Both infliximab, which has been in use for many years, and adalimumab have limited long-term safety data beyond 1 year. Some data suggest an increase in cancer risk beyond 1 year. Adalimumab is FDA approved for psoriatic arthritis.

Alefacept (Amevive)[2], a T-cell inhibitor, is dosed at 15mg IM or IV once a week for 12 weeks. Its efficacy follows the rule of thirds: It works well in about one-third of cases, does not work at all in one-third of cases, and the rest fall in between. After a cycle of 12 weeks, the courses may be repeated as needed. However, it is crucial initially to monitor T-cell counts biweekly. A newer agent, ustekinumab (Stelara), has been shown to improve lesions in 66% to 76% of cases. It is initially dosed at 45 to 90mg SC at weeks 0 and 4, depending on body weight. Maintenance is every 12 weeks. Besides ustekinumab, another Il-12/IL-23 inhibitor, guselkumab (Tremfya), was approved in 2017 and is dosed at 100 mg/mL SC in weeks 0 and 4, then every 8 weeks.

When these therapies are contraindicated, one alternative is phototherapy. This is the reason many patients report decreased symptom severity during the summer months due to the natural UV light. Phototherapy started with photochemotherapy with oral or topical psoralens combined with UVA light (PUVA). Although phototherapy is very effective for psoriasis, even in very thick lesions, recent studies have shown an increased risk of skin cancer. Therefore PUVA has become less popular since the advent of UVB radiation treatment, especially with narrow-band UVB (NB-UVB). NB-UVB is equally effective as PUVA and does not have the risk of skin cancer. The exact mechanism is unknown, but it is believed to affect DNA and to suppress IL-17 and IL-23, creating photoproducts that interfere with cell cycle progression. NB-UVB is first-line course of therapy for pregnant and pediatric patients. There are two methods for initiating NB-UVB phototherapy: the skin type protocol, which is easier to execute; and the minimum erythema dose (MED), which is more detailed but more accurate. Refer to Table 1 for treatment protocols. Both protocols generally require 30 to 35 treatments with the optimal frequency of three times a week.

Given all the treatment options (refer to Box 4), the choice of the treatment regimen depends on several factors. First, the severity of the psoriasis must be determined as well as the social and emotional impact of the condition. Another consideration is financial, including the insurance coverage, copayment, and deductibles. The lowest-cost treatment is methotrexate, and alefacept is the highest. The patient's conveniences and preferences should be discussed. If the severity is

[3]Exceeds dosage recommended by the manufacturer.
[5]Investigational drug in the United States.

[2]Not available in the United States.

TABLE 1 Methods for Initiating Narrow-Band Ultraviolet B (NB-UVB) Therapy and Subsequent Dosing of Phototherapy

THERAPY	MED NB-UVB PROTOCOL						MED NB-UVB PROTOCOL
	TYPE 1	TYPE 2	TYPE 3	TYPE 4	TYPE 5	TYPE 6	
Initial dose	130 mJ/cm²	220 mJ/cm²	260 mJ/cm²	330 mJ/cm²	350 mJ/cm²	400 mJ/cm²	Start with 50%–70% MED The starting dose should be based on the provider's comfort and the patient's history of response to light; e.g., start closer to 70% if the patient has a history of tanning and start closer to 50% if the patient has a history of burning; most centers start at 70%

SUBSEQUENT DOSES

Severe erythema	No treatment. When burn resolves, decrease by 50% of last dose and then increase dose by 10%

THERAPY	MED NB-UVB PROTOCOL						MED NB-UVB PROTOCOL
	TYPE 1	TYPE 2	TYPE 3	TYPE 4	TYPE 5	TYPE 6	
Mild erythema	Same dose	Same dose	Same dose	Same dose	Same dose	Same dose	Decrease dose by 20%
Barely perceptible erythema	—	—	—	—	—	—	Same (erythmogenic) or slight decrease (suberythmogenic)
No erythema: increase dose by	15 mJ/cm^2	25 mJ/cm^2	40 mJ/cm^2	45 mJ/cm^2	60 mJ/cm^2	65 mJ/cm^2	20%

DOSING SCHEDULE

Optimal schedule	3 ×/wk (M, W, F) is the optimal schedule because less is not as effective and more does not improve the resolution. Subsequent treatments should not be less than 24 hours from the last treatment. For the treatment of eczema, no clear guideline to the frequency. Some use 5 ×/wk.

DOSE ADJUSTMENTS FOR MISSED DAYS

MISSED DAYS	DOSE ADJUSTMENT
1–7	Increase doses per skin type
8–11	Same dose
12–14	Decrease by 2 treatments' worth
15–20	Decrease by 25%
21–27	Decrease by 50%
28 +	Start over

BOX 4 | Treatment Options for Psoriasis

Topical
Steroid
Tar (e.g., Balnetar, Psoriasin, Scytera)
Anthralin (Dritho-Crème HP, Dritho-Scalp)
Calcipotriene (Dovonex)
Calcitriol (Vectical)
Adapalene (Differin)[1]
Tazarotene (Tazorac)
Tretinoin (Retin-A)[1]
Calcineurin inhibitors (pimecrolimus [Elidel][1], tacrolimus [Protopic][1])

Oral or Systemic
Methotrexate (Trexall)
Acitretin (Soriatane)/Isotretinoin (Claravis)[1]
Cyclosporine (Neoral)
Mycophenolate mofetil (Cellcept)[1]

Immunomodulators
Alefacept (Amevive)[2]
Etanercept (Enbrel)
Infliximab (Remicade)
Adalimumab (Humira)
Ustekinumab (Stelara)
Secukinumab (Cosentyx)
Ixekizumab (Taltz)
Brodalumab (Siliq)

Phototherapy
UVA
UVB

---

[1]Not FDA approved for this indication.
[2]Not available in the United States.

only mild to moderate without much emotional impact, topical steroid and vitamin D analogue should be considered the first options. Other topicals include tar (Balnetar, Psoriasin, Scytera), anthralin

(Dritho-Crème HP, Dritho-Scalp), and tretinoin (Retin-A)[1]. If the degree is severe and/or the patient has emotional impact, systemic medications should be used. Most insurance plans will probably require that the patient try at least one oral medication before employing the biologicals. If systemic therapy is used, consider combining it with phototherapy (if possible). If there is no improvement within 2 to 4 months, the regimen should be changed to biologicals. Other combinations may be employed for better resolution.

For healthy patients, any of these therapies may be tried. Unfortunately, there are limitations with children, pregnant women, and patients trying to conceive. For pediatric patients, topical agents should be tried first, followed by UVB monotherapy. If the plaques are still recalcitrant, add either methotrexate (Trexall) or phototherapy. If phototherapy is not available and topical agents have failed, consider using methotrexate or cyclosporine (Neoral). Other options for pediatric patients include adalimumab (Humira) and etanercept (Enbrel). For pregnant women and patients trying to conceive, first try topical agents followed by UVB (ideally narrowband). This combination remains the safest option. If stronger options are needed, the only class B drugs are systemic steroids, adalimumab (Humira), alefacept (Amevive)[2], infliximab (Remicade), and ustekinumab (Stelara). An absolute contraindication in this population is the retinoid class, such as isotretinoin (Claravis)[1] and acitretin (Soriatane).

Complications

Patients suffering from psoriasis cope with the physical appearance of their lesions as well as the associated mental anguish associated with many other chronic ailments. Furthermore, psoriasis is associated with other chronic diseases, such as abdominal obesity, metabolic syndrome, and atherogenic dyslipidemia. Weight loss can improve the appearance of psoriatic plaques. Patients with psoriasis are more likely to have coronary artery disease, elevated blood pressure, obesity, and insulin resistance. Treating psoriasis decreases the cardiovascular risks. There is an increased risk of malignancy, such as lymphoma. Substance abuse and smoking are common among these patients as well.

---

[1]Not FDA approved for this indication.
[2]Not available in the United States.

References

Ahlehoff O, et al: Cardiovascular disease event rates in patients with severe psoriasis treated with systemic anti-inflammatory drugs: a Danish real-world cohort study, *J Intern Med* 273:197–204, 2012.

American Academy of Dermatology Work Group, Menter A, Korman NJ, Elmets CA, et al: Guidelines of care for the management of psoriasis and psoriatic arthritis: section 6. Guidelines of care for the treatment of psoriasis and psoriatic arthritis: case-based presentations and evidence-based conclusions, *J Am Acad Dermatol* 65(1):137–174, 2011.

Callen JP, Krueger GG, Lebwohl M, et al: AAD: AAD consensus statement on psoriasis therapies, *J Am Acad Dermatol* 49(5):897–899, 2003.

Dubertret L: Retinoids, methotrexate and cyclosporine, *Curr Probl Dermatol* 38:79–94, 2009.

Foulkes AC, Grindlay DJ, Griffiths CE, Warren RB: What's new in psoriasis? An analysis of guidelines and systematic reviews published in 2009–2010, *Clin Exp Dermatol* 36(6):585–589, 2011 Aug quiz 588–9.

Gottlieb A, Korman NJ, Gordon KB, et al: Guidelines of care for the management of psoriasis and psoriatic arthritis: section 2, *Psoriatic arthritis: overview and guidelines of care for treatment with an emphasis on the biologics, J Am Acad Dermatol* 58(5):851–864, 2008.

Herrier RN: Advances in the treatment of moderate-to-severe plaque psoriasis, *Am J Health Syst Pharm* 68(9):795–806, 2011.

Jensen P, Zachariae C, Christensen R, et al: Effect of weight loss on the severity of psoriasis: a randomized clinical study, *JAMA Dermatol* 149:795–801, 2013.

Johnson-Huang LM, Suárez-Fariñas M, Sullivan-Whalen M, et al: Effective narrowband UVB radiation therapy suppresses the IL-23/IL-17 axis in normalized psoriasis plaques, *J Invest Dermatol* 130(11):2654–2663, 2010.

Kalb RE, Strober B, Weinstein G, Lebwohl M: Methotrexate and psoriasis: 2009 National Psoriasis Foundation Consensus Conference, *J Am Acad Dermatol* 60:824–837, 2009.

Kimball AB, Gladman D, Gelfand JM, et al: National Psoriasis Foundation: National Psoriasis Foundation clinical consensus on psoriasis comorbidities and recommendations for screening, *J Am Acad Dermatol* 58:1031–1142, 2008.

Kuhn A, Patsinakidis N, Luger T: Alitretinoin for cutaneous lupus erythematosus, *J Am Acad Dermatol* 67(3):e123–6, 2012.

Menter A, Gottlieb A, Feldman SR, et al: Guidelines of care for the management of psoriasis and psoriatic arthritis: section 1. Overview of psoriasis and guidelines of care for the treatment of psoriasis with biologics, *J Am Acad Dermatol* 58:826–850, 2008.

Ormerod AD, Campalani E, Goodfield MJ: BAD Clinical Standards Unit: British Association of Dermatologists guidelines on the efficacy and use of acitretin in dermatology, *Br J Dermatol* 162:952–963, 2010.

Trueb RM: Therapies for childhood psoriasis, *Curr Probl Dermatol* 38:137–159, 2009.

Tsoi LC, et al: Identification of 15 new psoriasis susceptibility loci highlights the role of innate immunity, *Nat Genet* 44:1341–1348, 2012.

PARASITIC DISEASES OF THE SKIN

Method of

Andreas Katsambas, MD, PhD; and Clio Dessinioti, MD, MSc, PhD

CURRENT DIAGNOSIS

Cutaneous Amebiasis
- Purulent, foul-smelling nodules, ulcers, cysts, sinuses
- Microscopic identification of *Entamoeba histolytica* in stool or biopsy samples
- Molecular methods

Cutaneous Leishmaniasis
- Ulcerated nodule (i.e., volcano sign)
- Identification of *Leishmania* parasites by direct examination or culture from the lesion aspirate or biopsy
- Montenegro skin test
- In vitro lymphocyte proliferation assay
- Polymerase chain reaction

Trypanosomiasis

Chagas' Disease
- Chagoma: painful erythematous nodule
- Regional adenopathy
- Cardiomyopathy, megaesophagus, megacolon
- Microscopic examination of *Trypanosoma cruzi* in blood, lymph node biopsy, or skin biopsy or culture

African Sleeping Sickness
- Trypanosome chancre: painful, inflammatory nodule
- Regional adenopathy
- Fever, generalized pruritic eruption with erythematous annular plaques
- Central nervous system involvement
- Microscopic identification of *Trypanosoma brucei* in chancre fluid, lymph node aspirates, blood, bone marrow, cerebrospinal fluid

Cutaneous Toxoplasmosis
- Roseola, urticaria, prurigo-like nodules
- Isolation of *Toxoplasma gondii* in the skin

Ascariasis
- Urticaria
- Identification of adult worm or eggs in stool

Cutaneous Larva Migrans
- Creeping eruption
- Intense pruritus

Cysticercosis
- Subcutaneous nodules
- Isolation of *Taenia solium* in skin lesion
- Serologic tests

Dracunculiasis
- Ruptured blister with prolapsing worm

Filariasis

Lymphatic Filariasis
- Fever with lymphangitis and lymphadenitis
- Chronic pulmonary infection
- Progressive lymphedema leading to massive tissue thickening, especially of the legs and scrotum (i.e., elephantiasis)
- Microscopic identification of microfilariae in blood

Onchocerciasis (River Blindness)
- Subcutaneous nodules, dermatitis, "leopard skin," "lizard skin," lymphedema
- Identification of microfilariae in skin snips
- Blindness

Loiasis (Calabar Swellings)
- Pruritus, localized subcutaneous swellings
- Serpiginous lesion on the conjunctivae
- Microscopic identification of microfilariae in blood

Schistosomiasis (Snail Fever)
- Pruritic papules, edema
- Fever, lymphadenopathy, diarrhea
- Bilharziasis cutanea tarda: pruritic, grouped papules
- Identification of the eggs in stool, urine, biopsy of affected tissues
- Enzyme-linked immunosorbent assay (ELISA) tests

Cercarial Dermatitis (Swimmer's Itch)
- Extremely pruritic erythematous macules, papules, vesicles on body areas exposed to infested water

Human Scabies
- Pruritus worsening at night
- Papules, excoriations, nodules, burrows on genitals, interdigital spaces, axillae, wrists
- Microscopic identification of mites or eggs or feces from burrows or papules

Pediculosis

Pediculosis Capitis
- Intense pruritus of the scalp
- Nape dermatitis
- Identification of lice and nits on the hair

Pediculosis Corporis (Vagabond's Itch)
- Intense pruritus, erythema, urticarial lesions, papules, nodules, and excoriations
- Identification of lice and nits on clothing

Pediculosis Pubis
- Pruritus
- Blue macules
- Identification of lice and nits on pubic hair

CURRENT THERAPY[a]

Cutaneous Amebiasis
- Metronidazole (Flagyl) 750 mg PO three times daily for 7 to 10 days, or
- Tinidazole (Tindamax) 2 g once PO daily for 5 days, followed by iodoquinol (Aloquin) 650 mg PO three times daily for 20 days or paromomycin (Humatin) 25 to 35 mg/kg/day PO in three doses for 7 days

Cutaneous Leishmaniasis
- Preparations of pentavalent antimony are sodium stibogluconate (Pentostam)[10] or
- Meglumine antimoniate (Glucantime).[2] Dose of pentavalent antimonium: 20 mg/kg/day IV or IM for 20 days, or
- Miltefosine (Impavido) (FDA-approved), for persons 12 years of age and older who weigh at least 45 kg: 150 mg/day for 28 days, or
- Topical paromomycin applied twice daily for 10 days or
- Cryotherapy, topical 5-ALA PDT, intralesional antimonial regimens

Trypanosomiasis
Chagas' Disease (American Trypanosomiasis)
- Nifurtimox (Lampit) 8 to 10 mg/kg/day PO in three divided doses for 60 days, for patients younger than 18 years (weighing at least 2.5 kg), or
- Benznidazole (Radanil, Rochagan)[10] 5 to 7 mg/kg/day PO in two divided doses for 60 days for patients 2 to 12 years of age

East African Sleeping Sickness
- Suramin (Germanin)[10] 4 to 5 mg/kg (day 0) (test dose) IV, then 20 mg/kg IV (max 1 gm/injection) on days 1, 3, 7, 14, 21
- For second stage, melarsoprol (Mel-B)[10] 2.2 mg/kg/day (max 180–200 mg/day) IV for 10 days.

West African Sleeping Sickness
- Fexinidazole can be used for 10 days, with doses depending on age and weight.
- For second stage *T. b. gambiense*, NECT combination therapy: For adults, Nifurtimox[1] 15 mg/kg/day orally in 3 doses for 10 days, and eflornithine[2] 400 mg/kg/day IV in 2 infusions for 7 days

Cutaneous Toxoplasmosis
- It is rare and may be a symptom of disseminated toxoplasmosis, usually in immunosuppressed patients.

Ascariasis
- Albendazole (Albenza)[1] 400 mg PO once, or
- Mebendazole (Vermox) 100 mg PO twice daily for 3 days or 500 mg once, or
- Ivermectin (Stromectol)[1] 150 to 200 μg/kg PO once

Cutaneous Larva Migrans
- Self-limiting skin disease. Albendazole or ivermectin may be used off-label, if needed.

Filariasis
Lymphatic Filariasis
- Diethylcarbamazine (DEC, Hetrazan)[10] 6 mg/kg/day PO as a 1 day or 12 day treatment course for the treatment of active infection. DEC is contraindicated in some patients, and consultation with a tropical medicine specialist is recommended.

Onchocerciasis
- Ivermectin (Stromectol) 150 μg/kg PO once for 6 months
- Patients with Loa loa co-infections should not be treated for onchocerciasis without consulting an expert on loiasis.

Schistosomiasis
- Praziquantel (Biltricide) 40 mg/kg/day orally in two divided doses for 1 day (*S. haematobium* and *S. mansoni*) and 60 mg/kg/day orally in three divided doses for 1 day (*S. japonicum, S. mekongi*)

Human Scabies
- Permethrin (Acticin, Elimite) 5% cream rinse, applied for 10 hours head to toe; a second application 7 to 10 days later, or
- Benzyl benzoate[1,6] 10% to 25% lotion[6] applied once daily at night on 2 consecutive days with re-application at 7 days. or
- Sulfur[1,6] 6% to 30% ointment in petrolatum,[6] or as cream or lotion, applied on three successive days.
- Ivermectin (Stromectol)[1] 200 μg/kg PO as 2 doses taken 1 week apart.

Pediculosis
Pediculosis Capitis
- Permethrin (Nix) 1% lotion, applied and washed off after 10 minutes; second application 7 to 10 days later; approved for children older than 2 years
- Pyrethrins with piperidyl butoxide (RID) applied for 10 minutes
- Benzyl benzoate 25% lotion[1,6]
- Malathion (Ovide) 0.5% lotion, applied for 8 to 12 hours before being washed off; can be used for children older than 6 years, or
- Lindane shampoo: for recalcitrant disease, associated with serious reactions not to be used in children
- Ivermectin 0.5% lotion (Sklice), apply to dry hair and scalp then rinse off after 10 minutes

Pediculosis Corporis
- Disinfection of clothes

Pediculosis Pubis
- Same treatment as pediculosis capitis: three times daily

---

[a]All doses in box and text are recommended for adults unless otherwise indicated. Note that additional contraindications of treatments may apply for children and for women during pregnancy and lactation.
[1]Not FDA approved for this indication.
[2]Not available in the United States.
[3]Exceeds dosage recommended by the manufacturer.
[6]May be compounded by pharmacists.
[10]Available in the United States from the Centers for Disease Control and Prevention.

Parasitic diseases are a common cause of morbidity and mortality, particularly in tropical and developing countries. They may be caused by protozoa, helminths, or arthropods. Because of the immigration of persons from tropical and subtropical countries worldwide and the travel of people from industrialized to tropical regions, parasitic diseases may be found in temperate climates. Skin lesions may provide important diagnostic clues for parasitic infections, and they are reviewed in the following sections, along with updated treatment guidelines.

Diseases Caused by Protozoa
Cutaneous Amebiasis

Intestinal amebiasis is caused by *Entamoeba histolytica*, which may rarely invade the skin and cause cutaneous amebiasis. The disease is transmitted by ingestion of food or water contaminated with cyst forms of the parasite and through fecal exposure during sexual contact.

Cutaneous amebiasis develops at the site of the invasion of the parasites into the skin from an underlying amebic abscess, usually at the perianal area or the abdominal wall. Cutaneous findings include purulent, foul-smelling nodules, cysts, and sinuses, which are associated with regional adenopathy and dysentery. Skin lesions grow rapidly and may lead to death if left untreated.

Diagnosis of cutaneous amebiasis is confirmed by microscopic identification of *E. histolytica* in the stool and in aspirates or biopsy samples obtained during colonoscopy, during surgery, or from the border of an ulcer. Treatment of choice for extraintestinal amebiasis is oral metronidazole (Flagyl) 750 mg PO three times daily for 7 to 10 days or tinidazole (Tindamax). Either treatment should be followed by iodoquinol (Aloquin) 650 mg PO three times daily for 20 days or paromomycin 25 to 35 mg/kg/day PO divided in three doses for 7 days.

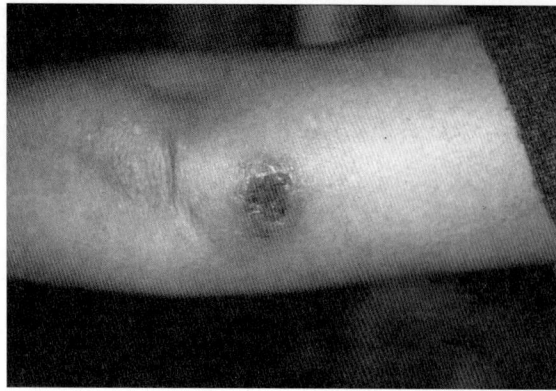

Figure 1 Cutaneous leishmaniasis is characterized by an ulcerated nodule with a raised and indurated border (i.e., volcano sign).

Leishmaniasis

Leishmaniasis results from the infection with intracellular protozoan parasites belonging to the genus *Leishmania*. Leishmania parasites are transmitted to humans and other mammalian hosts (e.g., dogs, rodents) during feeding by infected female phlebotomine sandflies that serve as vectors. The parasites exist as promastigotes in the midgut of sandflies and as amastigotes (i.e., Leishman-Donovan bodies) within macrophages of humans and other mammals. Based on the extent and the severity of involvement in the human host, leishmaniasis may be clinically classified as cutaneous leishmaniasis, diffuse cutaneous leishmaniasis, mucocutaneous leishmaniasis, and visceral leishmaniasis.

Cutaneous leishmaniasis (New World or Old World form) begins as a small erythematous papule at the site of the bite of the sandfly, which evolves into an ulcerated nodule with a raised and indurated border (i.e., volcano sign) (Figure 1). The lesions gradually heal with a depressed scar. Diffuse cutaneous leishmaniasis is characterized by widespread cutaneous involvement without visceralization. Mucocutaneous leishmaniasis (known as espundia in South America) affects the skin, the mucosa, and the cartilages of the upper respiratory tract (especially the nose and the larynx) and may result in severe disfigurement. Visceral leishmaniasis results from the involvement of the bone marrow, spleen, and the liver, and it may lead to death if left untreated. It manifests with fever, splenomegaly, pancytopenia, and wasting. Post–kala azar dermal leishmaniasis may appear within a year after visceral disease independent of treatment, and it is characterized by macules, papules, and nodules, which are usually hypopigmented.

Diagnosis of leishmaniasis is based on finding the parasites in the skin from the lesion aspirate or biopsy by direct examination or culture. The leishmanin (Montenegro) skin test shows past and current infections, and it detects the inflammatory response in the skin after injection of phenol-killed parasites into the dermis. A past or current infection is also documented by an in vitro lymphocyte proliferation assay that requires a drop of blood from a finger prick. Polymerase chain reaction (PCR) techniques may be used to identify different *Leishmania* species. Circulating antibody levels are not considered a useful diagnostic sign.

Cutaneous leishmaniasis is usually self-limited and may not require treatment. Treatment of cutaneous leishmaniasis is indicated in case of numerous lesions or when lesions affect the face to avoid scarring. Therapies include the preparations of pentavalent antimony, such as sodium stibogluconate (Pentostam)[10] 20 mg/kg/day IV or IM for 20 days. Meglumine antimoniate (Glucantime)[2] 20 mg/kg/day IV or IM for 20 days or miltefosine (Impavido) for 28 days may be used. In 2014, FDA approved oral miltefosine for the treatment of cutaneous leishmaniasis caused by *L. braziliensis*, *L. paramensis*, and *L. guyanensis* in adults and adolescents who are not pregnant or breastfeeding. The FDA-approved treatment regimen for persons 12 years of age and older who weigh from 30 to 44 kg is one 50-mg oral capsule of miltefosine twice a day (total of 100 mg per day) for 28 consecutive days. The approved regimen for persons 12 years of age and older who weigh at least 45 kg (99 pounds) is one 50-mg capsule three times a day (total of 150 mg per day) for 28 consecutive days. Miltefosine is contraindicated in pregnant women during treatment and for 5 months thereafter. Alternatively, intralesional injections of antimonials, cryotherapy, local heat, oral ketoconazole (Nizoral)[1], topical amphotericin B[2], pentamidine (Pentam)[1] IM or IV, 5-aminolevulinic acid[1] photodynamic therapy (PDT), or topical paromomycin[2] (applied twice daily for 10–20 days) have been used.

The production of antileishmanial antibodies does not correlate with resolution of the disease. Infection and recovery are associated with lifelong immunity to reinfection by the same species of *Leishmania*, although interspecies immunity may also exist.

Trypanosomiasis

There are three types of trypanosomiasis:
- American trypanosomiasis or Chagas' diseases, caused by *Trypanosoma cruzi*
- East African sleeping sickness, caused by *Trypanosoma brucei rhodesiense*
- West African sleeping sickness, caused by *Trypanosoma brucei gambiense*

American trypanosomiasis (i.e., Chagas' disease) is caused by the parasite *T. cruzi*, and it is endemic in Central and South America. The disease is transmitted by the bite of infected "cone-nosed" insects, by transfusion of infected blood, by organ transplantation, and across the placenta. During the acute stage, Chagas' disease manifests with a painful erythematous nodule, known as chagoma, which is associated with regional adenopathy. The chronic stage manifests with cardiomyopathy, megaesophagus, and megacolon. Diagnosis is confirmed by microscopic identification of the parasite in fresh anticoagulated blood, in blood smears, by lymph node biopsy or skin biopsy, or by culture. Antiparasitic treatment is indicated for all cases of acute or reactivated Chagas' disease and for chronic *T. cruzi* infection in chlidren up to age 18. Physicians should consider factors such as the patient's age, clinical status, and health. Treatment recommended by CDC for pediatric patients includes benznidazole (Radanil, Rochagan) 5 to 7 mg/kg/day PO in two divided doses for 60 days or nifurtimox (Lampit) 8 to 10 mg/kg/day PO in three divided doses for 60 days.

African trypanosomiasis (i.e., East and West African sleeping sickness) occurs in Africa and is transmitted by the bite of infected male and female tsetse flies. It manifests with a highly inflammatory, painful, red or violaceous, indurated nodule surrounded by an erythematous halo, called trypanosome chancre, at the site of the inoculation of the parasites. There is regional adenopathy. Later, the chancre resolves spontaneously, and the patient has fever, malaise, a generalized pruritic eruption with erythematous annular plaques or urticarial lesions, and central nervous system (CNS) involvement with personality changes, apathy, somnolence, coma, and death. Diagnosis is based on the identification of trypanosomes by microscopic examination in chancre fluid, affected lymph node aspirates, blood, bone marrow, or in the late stages of infection, cerebrospinal fluid.

Treatment of first stage *T.b. rhodesiense*, East African sleeping sickness, in adults may include suramin (naphthylamine sulfonic acid, Germanin)[10] 4 to 5 mg/kg (test dose) IV and then 20 mg/kg (max 1 g/injection) IV over several hours on days 1, 3, 7, 14, and 21. For second stage disease (*T. b. rhodesiense*), melarsoprol B (a trivalent organic arsenical, Mel-B)[10] is used 2.2 mg/kg/day (max 180–200 mg/day) IV for 10 days. For West African sleeping sickness, first stage *T.b. gambiense* infection, fexinidazole can be used for 10 days, with doses depending on age and weight. For second stage *T. b. gambiense*, CDC recommends NECT

---

[1]Not FDA approved for this indication.
[2]Not available in the United States.

[10]Available in the United States from the Centers for Disease Control and Prevention.
[1]Not FDA approved for this indication.

(nifurtimox-eflornithine combination therapy): Nifurtimox[1] 15 mg/kg orally in three doses for 10 days, and eflornithine[2] 400 mg/kg/day IV in two infusions for 7 days (adult doses).

Cutaneous Toxoplasmosis

Systemic toxoplasmosis (congenital or acquired) is caused by the protozoan parasite *Toxoplasma gondii*, and transmission can be foodborne, animal-to-human (usually cats), or congenital. Toxoplasmosis in immunocompetent individuals is usually asymptomatic, or it may present clinically as asymptomatic lymphadenopathy. Immunosuppressed patients may develop severe symptoms. Cutaneous involvement is rare. It manifests with punctate macules or ecchymoses in the congenital form, and the acquired form manifests with roseola and erythema multiforme lesions, urticaria, prurigo-like nodules, and maculopapular lesions. Diagnosis is confirmed by PCR and immunohistochemistry detection of the parasite from a skin biopsy specimen. Treatment of lymphadenopathic toxoplasmosis is rarely indicated for healthy nonpregnant patients because symptoms usually resolve in a few weeks. Information regarding management of toxoplasmosis in pregnant women is provided by the CDC.

Diseases Caused by Helminths

Ascariasis

Ascariasis is caused by *Ascaris* species, mainly *Ascaris lumbricoides*. It is transmitted by the ingestion of eggs in soil contaminated with human feces. Skin involvement of ascariasis manifests with urticaria. Diagnosis is based on finding the adult worm or eggs in the feces. Treatment includes albendazole (Albenza)[1] 400 mg PO once or mebendazole (Vermox) 100 mg PO twice daily for 3 days (or 500 mg once) or ivermectin (Stromectol)[1] 150 to 200 µg/kg PO once.

Cutaneous Larva Migrans

Cutaneous larva migrans is also known as creeping eruption, with the first term describing a syndrome and the second a clinical sign found in various conditions. The syndrome cutaneous larva migrans is caused when various nematode larvae (i.e., hookworms, such as *Ancylostoma braziliense*, *Ancylostoma caninum*, *Bunostomum phlebotomum*) of dogs, cats, and other mammals penetrate and migrate through the skin. Cutaneous larva migrans is transmitted by skin contact to soil contaminated with animal feces. In humans, larvae are unable to reach internal organs and eventually die. Cutaneous larva migrans manifests with intensely pruritic, papular lesions, which evolve as the larvae migrate to a characteristic linear, minimally elevated, serpiginous tract that moves forward in an irregular pattern. Diagnosis is easily made clinically and is supported by a travel history or by possible exposure in an endemic area.

Cutaneous larva migrans is self-limiting. Treatment includes off-label use of albendazole[1] and ivermectin.[1] Symptomatic treatment may be advised for severe itching.

Filariasis

Filariasis is caused by nematodes (i.e., roundworms) that inhabit the lymphatics and subcutaneous tissues. The most common filarial infections include lymphatic filariasis, onchocerciasis, and loiasis.

Lymphatic filariasis is caused by *Wuchereria bancrofti*, *Brugia malayi*, and *Brugia timori*, and it is transmitted by mosquitoes. Adult worms result in a chronic inflammatory cell infiltrate around lymphatic vessels, causing their dilatation, hypertrophy, and obstruction. Many patients are asymptomatic, but some may develop fever with lymphangitis and lymphadenitis, chronic pulmonary infection, and progressive lymphedema leading to massive tissue thickening, especially of the legs and scrotum (i.e., elephantiasis). The overlying skin is thickened. Diagnosis is based on microscopic identification of the microfilariae in the blood and affected tissues.

For the treatment of active infection, diethylcarbamazine citrate (DEC)[10] is the recommended treatment by the CDC for adults at a dose of 6 mg/kg/day, as a 1 day or 12 day treatment course. However, DEC is contraindicated in some patients and consultation with a tropical medicine specialist is recommended. Lymphedema and elephantiasis are not indications for DEC therapy because there is usually no active infection.

Onchocerciasis

Onchocerciasis (i.e., blinding filariasis) is caused by the filarial nematode *Onchocerca volvulus*, which is transmitted by the blackflies *Simulium*. It may manifest with subcutaneous onchocercid nodules, acute or chronic dermatitis, depigmentation (i.e., leopard skin), and skin atrophy (i.e., lizard skin), and in later stages, it may manifest with lymphadenopathy and lymphedema. The microfilariae have a predilection for the eyes, and the infection can lead to blindness (i.e., river blindness). Diagnosis is based on identification of microfilariae in skin snips.

Treatment in adults consists of ivermectin (Stromectol) 150 µg/kg in one dose PO every 6 months. DEC is contraindicated as it may accelerate onchocercal blindness. To kill macrofilariae, CDC recommends doxycycline[1] 100 to 200 mg orally daily for 6 weeks. Patients with *Loa loa* co-infection should not be treated for onchocerciasis without consulting an expert on loiasis.

Loiasis

Loiasis (i.e., Calabar swellings) is caused by the parasite *Loa loa*, which is transmitted by deerflies (*Chrysops*). Cutaneous manifestations include pruritus, urticaria, and Calabar swellings, which are erythematous, warm, subcutaneous swellings associated with the migration of the worm through the subcutaneous tissues. Occasionally, there is subconjunctival migration of the adult worm, producing a migrating serpiginous lesion on the conjunctivae. Diagnosis is confirmed by identification of microfilariae in the blood by microscopic examination.

Schistosomiasis

Schistosomiasis (i.e., snail fever) in humans is caused mainly by the trematodes *Schistosoma haematobium*, *Schistosoma japonicum*, and *Schistosoma mansoni*. All trematodes have a life cycle that involves the snail as an intermediate host. The infective cercariae leave the snail, swim, and penetrate the human skin, causing a pruritic papular dermatosis. The disease is transmitted by exposure to contaminated water with live cercariae or by drinking infested water. Skin findings of acute schistosomiasis include pruritic schistosomal dermatitis due to a hypersensitivity response to the cercariae and edema of the face, extremities, genitals, and trunk. Schistosomal fever (i.e., Katayama fever), lymphadenopathy, and diarrhea may also develop. Late skin findings (i.e., bilharziasis cutanea tarda) appear in patients with visceral disease and include firm, pruritic, grouped papules. Secondary infection, ulceration, and development of squamous cell carcinoma may follow. Diagnosis is confirmed by identification of the eggs in the urine or stool, by biopsy of affected tissues, or by enzyme-linked immunosorbent assay (ELISA).

Treatment includes praziquantel (Biltricide) 40 mg/kg/day orally in two divided doses for 1 day (for *S. haematobium* and *S. mansoni*) or 60 mg/kg/day orally in three divided doses for 1 day (for *S. japonicum*).

Cercarial Dermatitis

Cercarial dermatitis (i.e., swimmer's itch) is caused by cercariae (i.e., larvae) of nonhuman schistosomes that penetrate the skin and die without invading other tissues. It is transmitted by contact with fresh or salt water contaminated with cercariae. It manifests with extremely pruritic, erythematous macules of sudden onset, which evolve into papules, vesicles, and urticarial lesions located on parts of the body directly exposed to the water, while sparing clothed areas. Cercarial dermatitis is a self-limited disease, and treatment is symptomatic with topical steroids and oral antihistamines.

[2]Not available in the United States.
[10]Available in the United States from the Centers for Disease Control and Prevention.

[10]Available in the United States from the Centers for Disease Control and Prevention.

Diseases Caused by Arthropoda
Human Scabies

Scabies is a common skin infestation caused by the mite *Sarcoptes scabiei*, which is an obligate human parasite. Scabies is transmitted by direct contact with an infested individual or by contact with bedding and clothing. The incubation period for scabies is about 3 weeks, and reinfestation results in symptoms within 1 to 3 days. Scabies is characterized by pruritus that usually worsens at night. Papules, nodules, excoriations, and burrows may be found. Lesions are usually located on interdigital spaces, wrists, ankles, axillae, waist, and genitals. Scabies manifests as red-brown nodules that represent a hypersensitivity response. In adults, the head is usually spared, whereas the involvement of the scalp, palms, and soles is common in infants.

Crusted or Norwegian scabies manifests with hyperkeratotic papules or plaques of the hands and feet (often with nail involvement) and an erythematous scaly eruption on the face, neck, scalp, and trunk. Because pruritus is often absent, this disease can be misdiagnosed as psoriasis, eczema, or an adverse drug reaction. Lesions contain thousands of mites and are highly contagious. Crusted scabies mainly affects immunocompromised patients (e.g., patients with human immunodeficiency virus infection), mentally retarded persons, or debilitated patients.

Diagnosis is confirmed with the microscopic identification of mites or their eggs or feces from burrows or papules. In sexually active patients, serological screening for sexually transmitted infections is recommended. Treatment should be applied from the neck down in adults, and in infants, application should include the scalp and face (avoiding the eyes and mouth).

Treatment includes 5% permethrin (Elimite) applied head to toe for 10 hours and repeated after 1 week. Benzyl benzoate lotion[1,6] 10% to 25% applied once daily at night on 2 consecutive days with re-application after 7 days, is also a recommended treatment. Sulfur ointments in petrolatum[1,6] or as cream or lotion, at concentrations of 6% to 30% may be used with application on 3 successive days. Ivermectin (Stromectol)[1] 200 µg/kg/dose (taken with food) as two doses 1 week apart, can be used. Regarding treatment of scabies in special situations, the European guidelines 2017 mention that permethrin is safe in pregnancy (grade B recommendation) and lactation and is licensed for use in children from age 2 months onwards. Benzyl benzoate and sulphur are considered safe in pregnancy (grade B recommendation) by the European guideline. Ivermectin should not be used during pregnancy or in children weighing less than 15 kg. Aggressive treatment with ivermectin at a single dose of 200 µg/kg on days 1, 2, and 8 with topical 5% permethrin cream (two applications, 1 week apart) and keratolytics (5% salicylic acid ointment[1] applied twice daily) is the treatment of choice for crusted scabies. All sexual and close personal and household contacts within the preceding 6 weeks should be treated simultaneously. Bedding and clothing towels and other items should be machine washed and dried using the hot cycle or dry cleaned or sealed and stored in plastic bag for 1 week, because the mite dies when separated from the human host. Post-treatment itch should be treated with repeated application of emollients. Oral antihistamines and mild topical corticosteroids may also be useful.

Pediculosis

Pediculosis (i.e., lice) is a contagious dermatosis, caused by lice, which are blood-sucking, wingless insects and are obligate human parasites. Two species of lice infest humans causing three clinical forms of infestation: *Pediculus humanus capitis* (i.e., head louse), *Pediculus humanus corporis* (i.e., body louse), and *Phthirus pubis* (i.e., pubic louse). The body louse is the only louse that can carry human disease, including rickettsioses and epidemic typhus.

Pediculosis Capitis

Pediculosis capitis is caused by *P. humanus capitis*, and it is transmitted by close contact or by fomites with combs, brushes, towels, and hats. It manifests with pruritus (due to the saliva of the louse), excoriations, nape dermatitis, secondary bacterial infection, and cervical and suboccipital lymphadenopathy. Diagnosis is based on identification of lice and eggs or nits on the hair and on fluorescence of nits with Wood's light. Visible nits are deposited on the hair shaft, close to the scalp. After adequate treatment, nits found at 1.0 to 1.5 cm from the scalp are not alive.

Topical pediculicides should be applied according to the package instructions. Treatment includes malathion (Ovide) 0.5% lotion applied for 8 to 12 hours or permethrin (Nix) 1% cream rinse applied to shampooed hair for 10 minutes. A second application with permethrin is recommended 1 week later to kill hatching progeny. Alternatively, pyrethrins with piperidyl butoxide (RID) can be applied and washed off after 10 minutes. Benzyl benzoate 25% lotion[1,6] is mainly a scabicide, but it may also be used as a pediculicide. Ivermectin lotion 0.5% (Sklice) was approved by the FDA in 2012 for treatment of head lice in persons 6 months of age and older, and is used as a single application. Bedding, clothing, and headgear should be decontaminated (as for scabies) or removed from body contact for 2 weeks. The nits must be removed from the hair by combing.

Pediculosis Corporis

Pediculosis corporis (i.e., vagabond's itch) is caused by *P. humanus corporis*, which lives and reproduces in the lining of clothes and leaves the clothing only for feeding from the skin. Transmission occurs mainly through contact with contaminated clothing or bedding. Clinical manifestations include pruritus, excoriations, and small, red macules that usually occur on the back. Clothes should be examined carefully for lice.

Treatment is the same as for pediculosis capitis and is applied on the affected body area. Dry heat or washing in hot water followed by ironing is effective in killing the lice and their ova in clothing. Items that cannot be washed should be removed from body contact for 2 weeks.

Pediculosis Pubis

Pediculosis pubis is caused by *P. pubis* and affects the pubic hair. However, if left untreated, it may also affect very hairy regions of the chest, abdomen, axillary region, and especially in children, the eyelashes, edge of the scalp, and eyebrows. Patients present with pruritus. Useful diagnostic signs include small, blue-gray macules on the trunk, thighs, and axillae (i.e., taches bleuâtres or maculae ceruleae) due to conversion of bilirubin to biliverdin by the saliva of the louse and a brown "dust" found on underclothing due to the excreta of the insects. Nits and/or lice attached to hairs are visible with the naked eye or using a dermatoscope. *P. pubis* is transmitted mainly by sexual contact, but it also may be transmitted by clothing or from parents to children.

Patients with pubic lice should be evaluated for other sexually transmitted diseases. Treatment of pediculosis pubis is the same as for pediculosis capitis and is applied on the affected areas. Bedding and clothing should be decontaminated (as for scabies) or removed from body contact for 2 weeks. Attention should be paid to treating sexual partners within the previous 3 months because they are a common cause of reinfestation. For infested eyelashes and eyebrows, ophthalmic-grade petrolatum ointment may be used two to four times daily for 10 days, and lice and nits should be carefully removed from the eyelashes with forceps.

---

[6]May be compounded by pharmacists.

References

Amir G, et al: Cutaneous toxoplasmosis after bone marrow transplantation with molecular confirmation, *J Am Acad Dermatol* 59:781–784, 2008.

Centers for Disease Control and Prevention (CDC): Disease exposure while traveling, Available at: http://www.cdc.gov/travel/ (accessed August 15, 2014).

Centers for Disease Control and Prevention (CDC): Leishmaniasis, Available at: http://www.cdc.gov/parasites/leishmaniasis/health_professionals/index.html#tx (accessed March 1, 2015).

---

[1]Not FDA approved for this indication.
[6]May be compounded by pharmacists.

Centers for Disease Control and Prevention (CDC): Malathion, Available at: http://www.cdc.gov/parasites/lice/head/gen_info/faqs_malathion.html (accessed March 1, 2015).

Centers for Disease Control and Prevention (CDC): African Trypanosomiasis. Treatment. Available at: https://www.cdc.gov/parasites/sleepingsickness/health_professionals/index.html [accessed March 11, 2023].

Centers for Disease Control and Prevention: American trypanosomiasis. Treatment. Available at: https://www.cdc.gov/parasites/chagas/health_professionals/tx.html (accessed on March 11, 2023).

Centers for Disease Control and Prevention (CDC): Lymphatic filariasis. Guidance for evaluation and treatment. Available at: https://www.cdc.gov/parasites/lymphaticfilariasis/health_professionals/dxtx.html (accessed March 11, 2023).

Centers for Disease Control and Prevention (CDC): Onchocerciasis treatment. Available at: https://www.cdc.gov/parasites/onchocerciasis/health_professionals/index.html#tx (accessed March 11, 2023).

Centers for Disease Control and Prevention: Toxoplasmosis. Available at: https://www.cdc.gov/parasites/toxoplasmosis/health_professionals/index.html (accessed on March 10, 2023).

Gorkiewicz-Petkow A: Scabicides and pediculicides. In Katsambas AD, Lotti TM, Dessinioti C, D'Erme AM, editors: *European Handbook of Dermatological Treatments*, 3rd ed, Berlin, 2015, Springer 2015, pp 1513–1519.

Heukelbach J, Feldmeier H: Epidemiological and clinical characteristics of hookworm-related cutaneous larva migrans, *Lancet Infect Dis* 8:302–309, 2008.

Leder K, Weller PF: Intestinal entamoeba histolytica amebiasis. *UpTodate*. www.uptodate.com (accessed February 20, 2022).

Lucchina LC, Wilson ME: Cysticercosis and other helminthic infections. In Freedeberg IM, Eisen AZ, Wolff K, et al: *editors: Fitzpatrick's Dermatology in General Medicine, 6th ed.*, New York, 2003, McGraw-Hill, pp 2225–2259.

Onder M, Gurer MA: Leishmaniasis. In Katsambas AD, Lotti TM, Dessinioti C, D'Erme AM, editors: *European Handbook of Dermatological Treatments*, 3rd ed, Berlin, 2015, Springer, pp 495–503.

Paller AS, Mancini AJ: Bites and infestations. In *Hurwitz Clinical Pediatric Dermatology*, Philadelphia, 2006, Saunders, pp 479–501.

Salavastru CM, Chosidow O, Boffa MJ, et al: European guideline for the management of scabies, *J Eur Acad Dermatol Venereol* 31:1248–1253, 2017.

Stone SP: Scabies and pediculosis. In Freedeberg IM, Eisen AZ, Wolff K, et al: , *editors: Fitzpatrick's Dermatology in General Medicine*, 6th ed., New York, 2003, McGraw-Hill, pp 2283–2289.

Wadowski L, Balasuriya L, Harper HN, et al: Lice update: new solutions to an old problem, *Clin Dermatol* 33:347–354, 2015.

PIGMENTARY DISORDERS

Method of
Rebat M. Halder, MD; and Ahmad Reza Hossani-Madani, MD, MS

CURRENT DIAGNOSIS

Hyperpigmentation

- Ephelides: Multiple, small (1–4 mm), light- to dark-brown macules with poorly defined margins that occur on sun-exposed areas of the body.
- Solar lentigines: Light- to dark-brown macular hyperpigmented lesions that are induced by natural or artificial sources of radiation and that can coalesce; they are located on face, neck, forearms, and hands.
- Melasma: Arcuate or polycyclic light- to dark-brown macules that coalesce into patches on face, neck, or forearms.
- Postinflammatory hyperpigmentation: Dark patches or macules with indistinct margins at the location of an inciting inflammatory event.

Hypopigmentation

- Pityriasis alba: Round, well-defined, pale macules with fine overlying powdery white scales, ranging in size from 0.5 to 5 cm in diameter, that transition to smooth, hypopigmented macules.
- Vitiligo: Sharply demarcated, depigmented, milky-white macules in a localized or generalized distribution.
- Idiopathic guttate hypomelanosis: Multiple circular, smooth, small macules that are porcelain white, with occasional black dots, found on sun-exposed areas of upper and lower extremities.
- Postinflammatory hypopigmentation: Off-white or tan macules with ill-defined borders at the site of an inciting inflammatory event.

CURRENT THERAPY

Hyperpigmentation

- Ephelides: Hydroquinone cream 4% plus maximum ultraviolet A (UVA)-blocking sunscreen in the morning and tretinoin 0.025% cream (Retin-A)[1] in the evening.
- Solar lentigines: Hydroquinone cream 4% plus tretinoin 0.025% cream (Retin-A)[1] in the evening; cryotherapy; laser therapy.
- Melasma: Monotherapy with hydroquinone cream 4% twice daily or tretinoin cream 0.025%[1] in the evening; double therapy with hydroquinone cream 4% twice daily plus tretinoin 0.025%[1] in the evening; triple therapy with fluocinolone acetonide cream 0.01% plus hydroquinone cream 4% plus tretinoin cream 0.05% (Tri-Luma Cream) in the evening; cysteamine cream (Cyspera)* once daily; azelaic acid gel 15% (Finacea)[1] once daily.
- Postinflammatory hyperpigmentation: Treat inciting event; hydroquinone 4% alone or in combination with low-potency topical steroid; cysteamine cream (Cyspera)* once daily.

Hypopigmentation

- Pityriasis alba: Emollients, lubricants, sunscreen; tacrolimus 0.1% ointment (Protopic)[1] twice daily or low-potency non-halogenated steroid cream for face and medium-potency steroid for body; phototherapy (UVB) for extensive disease.
- Vitiligo: In patients with less than 20% body surface area (BSA) involvement, treat with cover-up cosmetics; topical (potent or very potent steroid or calcineurin inhibitor trial for less than 2 months), phototherapy (UVB), or excimer laser; ruxolitinib cream 1.5% (Opzelura) for limited areas up to 10% body surface area. If local treatment fails, a surgical grafting approach may be used if the patient has less than 20% BSA involvement. For patients with more than 20% BSA involvement, phototherapy (UVB) is preferred. For patients with more than 50% BSA or disfiguring facial involvement, depigment with monobenzyl ether of hydroquinone (monobenzone 20% [Benoquin]), 4-methoxyphenol, or Q-switched ruby laser (694 nm).
- Idiopathic guttate hypomelanosis: Cryotherapy; dermabrasion; surgical minigrafting; intralesional steroids.
- Postinflammatory hypopigmentation: Cosmetics; topical corticosteroids; topical PUVA.

[1]Not FDA approved for this indication.
*Available through dispensing clinics or online.

Definition

The word *chromophore* is defined as elements that impart color to the skin. Hyperchromias describe abnormally darker skin, and hypochromias describe abnormally lighter skin. Pigmentation refers to melanotic causes of skin color change, differentiating it from skin color changes as a result of blood, carotene, bilirubin, or other causes. Hyperpigmentation refers to an increase in melanin production, melanocyte number, or both in the skin. Hypopigmentation refers to decrease of melanin, melanocytes, or both in the skin. Depigmentation refers to the absence of both melanin and melanocytes. Deposition of melanin in the epidermal layers visibly appears as a yellow to brownish hue. Dermal deposition appears as blue or blue-gray, with mixed epidermal and dermal melanin deposition appearing gray or blue-brown.

Evaluation

A thorough history and visual inspection of the pigmentary disorder can provide useful clues to the diagnosis, particularly recognition of pigmentary patterns (diffuse, circumscribed, linear, or reticulated). Further examination may be achieved by using the Wood lamp to differentiate epidermal from dermal melanin.

General Recommendations for All Pigmentary Disorders

Broad-spectrum sunscreen with an SPF of 30 is recommended, in addition to wearing protective clothing. Avoiding prolonged sun exposure is also desired.

Hyperpigmentation

Ephelides

Description

Ephelides (freckles) are multiple, small (1–4 mm), light- to dark-brown macules with poorly defined margins that occur on sun-exposed areas of the body (face, upper back, arms). They are more commonly found in children (fading with age), fair-skinned persons, and those with red or blonde hair (especially those of Celtic ancestry). A relationship has been shown between painful sunburns in youth and development of ephelides, and the macules become darker with greater ultraviolet (UV) exposure. They are thought to be genetic in origin, following an autosomal dominant pattern, and are strongly associated with variants in the melanocortin-1-receptor (MC1R). Ephelides are significant because they are associated with an increased risk of melanoma and nonmelanoma skin cancer, perhaps serving as a marker for sun susceptibility.

Treatment

Although treatment is not necessary, modalities include either hydroquinone cream 4% plus maximum UVA-blocking sunscreen in the morning and tretinoin 0.1% cream (Retin-A)[1] in the evening. Other therapies have included cryotherapy, lasers, and chemical peels.

Solar Lentigo (Lentigo Senilis Et Actinicus)

Description

Solar lentigines are pigmented spots that share morphologic similarities with ephelides, making differentiation difficult. They are defined as light-brown to dark-brown macular hyperpigmented lesions induced by natural or artificial sources of radiation, which can coalesce. The incidence increases with age, and more than 90% of White persons older than 50 years demonstrate lesions. They appear most often on the face, neck, forearms, and hands. They can occur in nonclassic locations in those receiving phototherapy (such as the penis). Histologically, they differ from ephelides by the presence of epidermal hyperplasia, increased melanocyte number, and elongation of the rete ridges.

Treatment

Although treatment is not necessary, two different modalities have been used: physical therapies and topical therapies. Physical therapies include cryotherapy and lasers, and topical treatments include retinoids or combinations of agents. Liquid nitrogen may be used with a cotton swab for 5 to 10 seconds to induce lightening. Recurrence rates may be as high as 55% at 6 months. Side effects include atrophy with longer cryoprobe application, postinflammatory hyper- or hypopigmentation, and pain. The Q-switched Nd:YAG (1064-nm) laser, among others, has been used with success.

Melasma

Description

Melasma is a hypermelanosis of the face, neck, and forearms that occurs with a higher incidence in women of African American, Latin American, and Asian descent. It appears on sun-exposed areas as arcuate or polycyclic macules that coalesce into patches. Epidermal melanin deposition causes a brownish appearance, and dermal melanin appears bluish. Combined epidermal and dermal melanin deposition appears gray. It is distributed in a central facial (65%), malar (20%), or mandibular (15%) pattern. More commonly seen in women and those with darker skin, it can also be found in men. Contributing factors include a genetic predisposition, pregnancy, oral contraceptive use, endocrine dysfunction, hormonal treatment, UV light exposure, cosmetics, and phototoxic drugs.

Treatment

First-line treatment for melasma consists of broad-spectrum sunscreen with greater than SPF 30 coverage in addition to monotherapy with hydroquinone cream 4% twice daily or tretinoin cream 0.025% (Retin A)[1] nightly. Double therapy with hydroquinone cream 4% twice daily plus tretinoin 0.025%[1] nightly may prove efficacious after an unsuccessful trial of monotherapy. If that fails, triple therapy may be attempted, with fluocinolone acetonide cream 0.01%, hydroquinone cream 4%, and tretinoin cream 0.05% (Tri-Luma) once daily being effective. Side effects of triple therapy include erythema, desquamation, burning, dryness, and pruritus at the site of application; telangiectasia; perioral dermatitis; acne breakouts; and hyperpigmentation. Cysteamine cream (Cyspera)* once a day can be used as an alternative to hydroquinone. Chemical peels, superficial and medium depth, and Q-switched 1064-nm Nd:YAG laser or intense pulsed light (IPL) may also be used for patients whose topical treatments have failed.

Postinflammatory Hyperpigmentation

Description

Postinflammatory hyperpigmentation is a very common condition that occurs as a result of a previous or ongoing inflammatory process, most commonly acne vulgaris, atopic dermatitis, infections, and phototoxic reactions, and as a result of treatment with topical medications, chemical peels, and lasers. Postinflammatory hyperpigmentation occurs more commonly in persons with darker skin pigmentation and appears as dark patches or macules with indistinct margins at the location of the inciting inflammatory event.

Treatment

Primary treatment is aimed at treating the inciting cause of the hyperpigmentation. Additional effective therapies include 4% hydroquinone alone or in combination with a topical steroid. Broad-spectrum sunscreen should also be employed. Cysteamine cream (Cyspera)* can be used as an alternative to hydroquinone.

Hypopigmentation or Depigmentation

Pityriasis Alba

Description

Pityriasis alba is a childhood or adolescent condition that affects all races. It begins as an erythematous macule with ill-defined borders. The erythema fades after a few weeks, leaving two or three round, well-defined, paler macules with overlying fine powdery white scale, ranging in size from 0.5 cm to 5 cm in diameter. These eventually transition to smooth, hypopigmented lesions, which are generally located on the face. The pathogenesis of this disorder is unknown.

Treatment

Pityriasis alba is thought to be a self-limited skin disease. However, general treatment guidelines include use of emollients and lubricant, use of sunscreen, and decreasing sun exposure. Lesions limited to the face may be treated with hydrocortisone 1%[1] or other mild, nonfluorinated steroid. More potent steroids may be used for lesions on the body, including hydrocortisone valerate 0.2% (Westcort)[1] or alclometasone dipropionate 0.05% (Aclovate)[1]. However, these can lead to atrophy if used over an extended period. Newer, nonsteroidal, effective alternatives include tacrolimus 0.1% ointment (Protopic)[1] twice daily. Side effects include a burning sensation that fades over time. Extensive disease that is not amenable to topical therapy might benefit from phototherapy (UVB).

Vitiligo

Description

Persons with vitiligo acquire sharply demarcated, depigmented macules in a localized or generalized distribution. These macules appear milky white compared with the surrounding normally pigmented skin. Lesions can increase in size. There is no predilection

---

[1] Not FDA approved for this indication.

---

* Available through dispensing clinics or online.
[1] Not FDA approved for this indication.
* Available through dispensing clinics or online.

for race or sex, and three-quarters of patients generally present before the age of 30 years.

Treatment

General recommendations include the use of sunscreen, avoidance of the sun, and use of protective clothing. Treatments for localized vitiligo (<20% of body surface area) include cover-up cosmetics, a 2-month trial of topical treatment (potent or very potent corticosteroid or calcineurin inhibitor), excimer laser, or topical PUVA. In 2022, an approved treatment for limited areas up to 10% body surface area is a new class of drug, a topical JAK inhibitor, ruxolitinib cream 1.5% (Opzelura). Adults who have failed treatments for localized vitiligo may be considered for narrow-band UVB or surgical treatment, which includes split-skin grafting, transfer of suction blisters, or autologous epidermal suspensions added to dermabraded skin. Surgical candidates should have localized, limited involvement and should not demonstrate lesion enlargement or Koebner phenomenon for 12 months before treatment. Patients with more than 20% body involvement may be considered for narrow-band UVB (311 nm). Those with greater than 50% body involvement or disfiguring facial involvement may be considered for complete depigmentation with monobenzyl ether of hydroquinone 20% (monobenzone 20%)*. Children are generally not offered surgical treatment.

Idiopathic Guttate Hypomelanosis

Description

This is an acquired, asymptomatic leukoderma with multiple, circular, smooth, small macules that have a porcelain-white color. Brown dots are occasionally observed within the macules. The macules increase in number with age, but they generally do not increase in size. They are most commonly located on sun-exposed areas of the upper and lower extremities.

Treatment

Treatments have included cryotherapy, dermabrasion, surgical minigrafting, and intralesional steroids; however, none of these have shown consistent acceptable results. Phototherapy has not been shown to be effective.

Postinflammatory Hypopigmentation

Description

Postinflammatory hypopigmentation is the result of an inciting inflammatory event leading to lesions that are off-white or tan, with ill-defined borders. This entity is noticed more commonly in those with darker skin.

Treatment

Hypopigmentation resolves with treatment of the underlying condition. Cosmetic cover-ups may be useful. Topical corticosteroids, tacrolimus 0.1% ointment (Protopic)[1], and phototherapy may also be used in patients who have lesions in cosmetically distressing areas.

---

* Available through dispensing clinics or online.
[1] Not FDA approved for this indication.

References

Cestari T, Arellano I, Hexsel D, Ortonne JP: Melasma in Latin America: option for therapy and treatment algorithm, *J Eur Acad Dermatol Venereol* 23:760–772, 2009.

Gupta AK, Gover MD, Nouri K, Taylor S: The treatment of melasma: a review of clinical trials, *J Am Acad Dermatol* 55:1048–1065, 2006.

Halder RM, Richards GM: Management of dyschromias in ethnic skin, *Dermatol Ther* 17:151–157, 2004.

Halder RM, Richards GM: Topical agents used in the management of hyperpigmentation, *Skin Therapy Lett* 9:1–3, 2004.

Hexsel DM: Treatment of idiopathic guttate hypomelanosis by localized superficial dermabrasion, *Dermatol Surg* 25:917–918, 1999.

Lin RL, Janniger CK: Pityriasis alba, *Cutis* 76:21–24, 2005.

Nordlund JJ, Boissy RE, Hearing VJ, et al: In *The pigmentary system: physiology and pathophysiology*, Blackwell Publishing, 2007.

Nordlund JJ, Cestari TF, Chan F, Westerhof W: Confusions about color: a classification of discolorations of the skin, *Br J Dermatol* 156(suppl 1):S3–S6, 2007.

Ortonne JP, Pandya AG, Lui H, Hexsel D: Treatment of solar lentigines, *J Am Acad Dermatol* 54:S262–S271, 2006.

Ploysangam T, Dee-Ananlap S, Suvanprakorn P: Treatment of idiopathic guttate hypomelanosis with liquid nitrogen: light and electron microscopic studies, *J Am Acad Dermatol* 23:681–684, 1990.

Rigopoulos D, Gregoriou S, Charissi C, et al: Tacrolimus ointment 0.1% in pityriasis alba: an open-label randomized, placebo-controlled study, *Br J Dermatol* 155:152–155, 2006.

Taylor SC, Burgess CM, Callender VD, et al: Postinflammatory hyperpigmentation: evolving combination treatment strategies, *Cutis* 78:S6–S19, 2006.

PREMALIGNANT SKIN LESIONS

Method of
Daniel Stulberg, MD; and Alicia Julovich, MD

CURRENT DIAGNOSIS

Actinic Keratosis
- Scaly white or flesh-colored lesions often with palpably rough surface
- Risk factors: light skin and hair color
- Most common on sun-exposed skin, including face and hands

Actinic Cheilitis
- Scale or fissure on lips
- Lower lip more commonly affected

Human Papillomavirus–Related Disease
- Verrucous or papular flesh-colored lesions associated with human papillomavirus (HPV) infection
- Genital, perineal, perianal, and oropharyngeal lesions at risk of malignancy

Atypical Nevi
- Multiple irregularly pigmented nevi in the familial atypical mole and melanoma syndrome
- Numerous, often raised nevi, especially with shades of red, brown, and black
- The subtypes atypical lentiginous nevus and orange granular flat nevus exhibited a stronger association with severe atypia and a history of melanoma

CURRENT THERAPY

Actinic Keratosis or Cheilitis
- Cryosurgery first line for limited lesions
- Topical medications for field therapy
- 5-fluorouracil (5-FU; Carac, Efudex) most efficacious topical single-agent therapy in common use at 75% clearance
- Combination 5% 5-FU (Efudex) and 0.005% calcipotriene (Calcitrene, Dovonex)[1], applied twice daily for 4 days has slightly higher clearance rates
- Tirbanibulin 1% ointment (Klisyri), has a higher compliance rate than 5-FU. It is safe during pregnancy, with a 44% to 54% clearance rate, but as a newer medication it is currently expensive
- Imiquimod (3.75% cream [Zyclara])
- Diclofenac (3% gel [Solaraze])
- Less commonly, laser, curettage, photosensitizing medications followed by light therapy

Human Papillomavirus
- Prevention of infection with HPV vaccination
- Topical imiquimod (3.75% cream [Zyclara], 5% cream [Aldara])
- Local destruction of lesions

[1] Not FDA approved for this indication.

Actinic keratoses (AKs) are the most common precancerous skin lesions seen in usual practice. They result from the abnormal proliferation of keratinocytes. A clinically useful estimate is 8% of lesions will progress to squamous cell carcinoma (SCC) over 10 years. Actinic cheilitis represents a similar proliferation of premalignant cells on nonkeratinizing epithelium (the lips). Risk factors for developing AKs and actinic cheilitis include lighter skin colors, ultraviolet radiation exposure from the sun, increased sensitivity to the sun from medications like hydrochlorothiazide, male sex, tanning beds, and immunosuppression. Skin cancer was more common among sexual minority (SM) males than heterosexual males (7.4% vs. 6.8%; AOR 1.16). The difference was especially notable among Hispanic (4.0% vs. 1.6%; adjusted odds ration [AOR] 3.81) and non-Hispanic Black males (1.0% vs. 0.5%; AOR 2.18). There is typically a long lead time between sun exposure and onset of the disease, so patients with a history of treated AKs should be monitored and counseled on their risk of recurrent or new premalignant or malignant lesions. Screening exams are performed every 6 to 12 months for patients with a history of precancerous or cancerous skin lesions and immunosuppressed patients, including patients with solid organ transplant, chronic lymphocytic leukemia, or use of immunosuppressing medications. Patients undergoing treatment are seen more frequently based on risk stratification. Avoiding sun exposure and using broad-brimmed hats, protective clothing, and sunscreen can help reduce the development of AKs.

Beyond AKs and actinic cheilitis, there are many other types of premalignant skin lesions. Actinic porokeratoses may be isolated or diffuse. Diffuse superficial porokeratoses are the result of an autosomal recessive trait. Infection with the human papillomavirus (HPV) can lead to development of verrucous or papular lesions. Those present in the genital, perineal, and oropharyngeal regions are at increased risk for progression to malignancy. The HPV vaccine is highly effective in reducing infections from cancer-causing strains of the virus and provides nearly complete protection against external genital warts. Patients with chronic inflammation are also at risk of developing skin cancers in affected areas. This can include patients with chronic ulceration, burn scars, radiation therapy fields, or underlying inflammatory conditions, such as discoid lupus, lichen planus, lichen sclerosis, and lymphedema. In familial atypical mole and melanoma syndrome, previously called atypical nevus syndrome, patients have multiple abnormal appearing nevi and a family history of melanoma. Patients with atypical nevi and more than one first-degree relative with melanoma have a nearly 100% chance of developing melanoma themselves.

Hereditary genodermatoses are genetic conditions that predispose patients to premalignant and malignant skin lesions, including basal cell carcinomas (BCCs), SCCs, and melanomas. Although rare, early recognition allows for close monitoring for associated malignancies in these patients. The genodermatoses include nevoid BCC syndrome (Gorlin syndrome), xeroderma pigmentosum, dyskeratosis congenita, oculocutaneous albinism, and nevus sebaceous.

Given their prevalence, we will focus on the clinical recognition and treatment of AKs in the remainder of this chapter.

Clinical Manifestations

AKs present as rough or scaly macules that are white or flesh-colored and often have a slightly erythematous base (Figure 1). They are typically found on sun-exposed areas, like the head and scalp, ears, neck, legs, and dorsum of the arms and hands. A combination of visual inspection of the skin and tactile examination is useful to diagnose these lesions. Often, they are easier to identify by gently palpating the patient's skin for their characteristic rough surface on sun-exposed areas. Patients may note that they have scratched off these lesions, only to have them return over time. Patients who have had multiple AKs become very adept at pointing them out to their clinician. Significant underlying erythema and thickened tissue should prompt concern that the lesion has already progressed to SCC (Figure 2). Dermoscopy improves

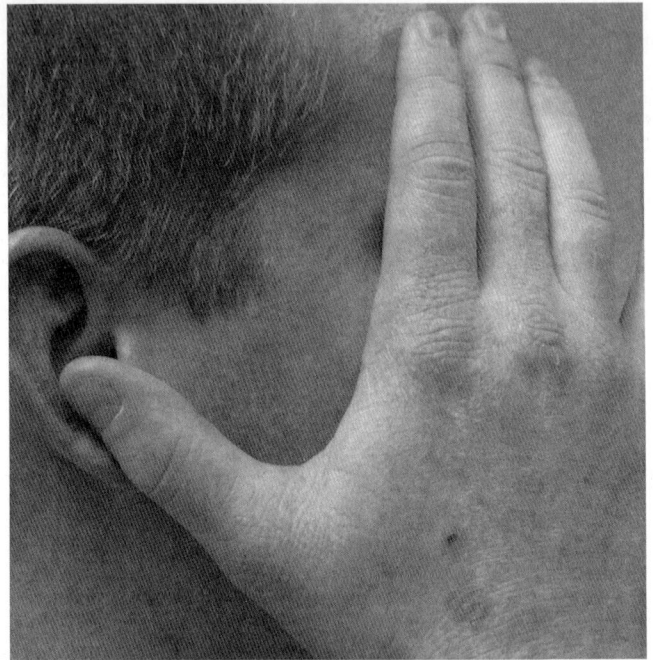

Figure 1 Early onset of actinic keratoses in a young man with high-risk skin type.

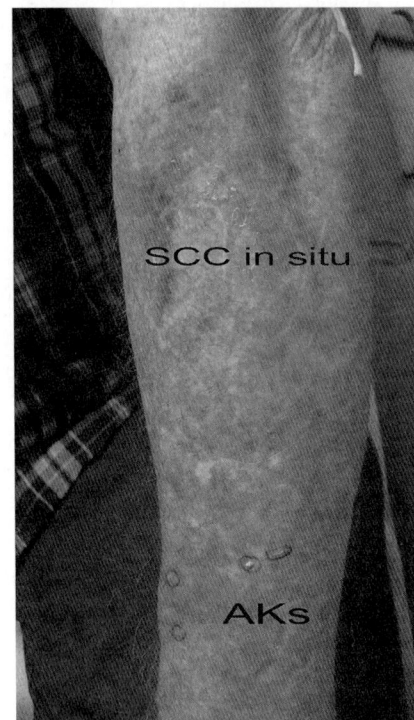

Figure 2 Sun-damaged skin with multiple actinic keratoses and squamous cell carcinoma in situ, also known as Bowen disease.

diagnostic accuracy up to 98.7% sensitivity and 95.0% specificity and can also identify lesions that have progressed to SCC. Common dermoscopic findings in AKs include scaling, follicular openings, erythematous starburst pattern, linear wavy vessels, and rosettes under polarized light. Findings of SCC on dermoscopy include asymmetric coiled tortuous vessels, hyperkeratosis "surface scale," or structureless white to yellow areas.

Actinic cheilitis is the same precancerous process presenting as rough or persistently chapped areas on the lips. It is more common on the lower lip, which catches the sun's rays more directly. Topical lip balm does not resolve the lesion as it would with

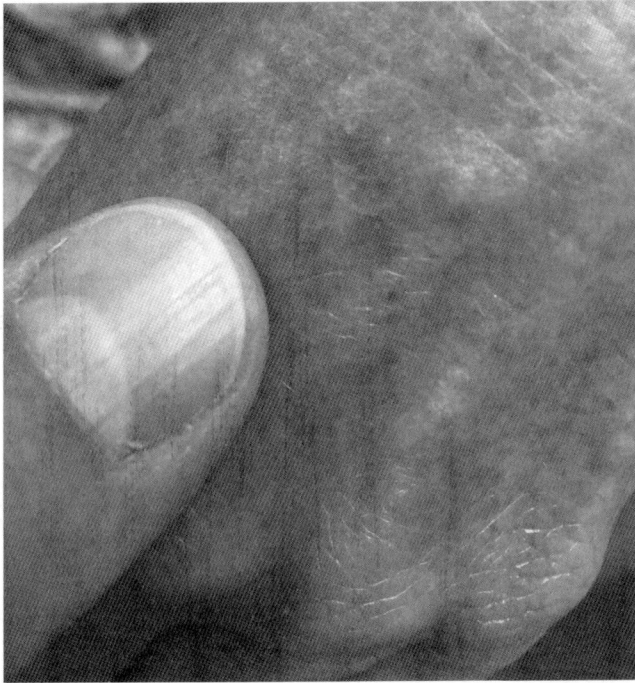

Figure 3 Porokeratosis with rice-paper appearance and peripheral ridge, also known as cornoid lamella.

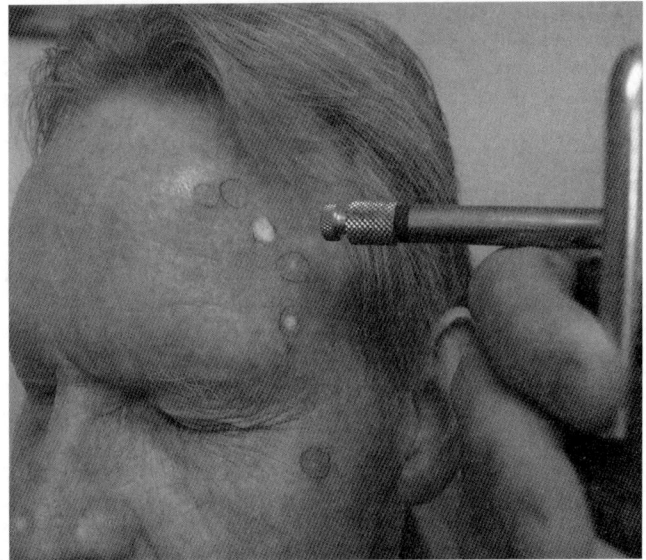

Figure 4 Treating multiple actinic keratoses with cryosurgery.

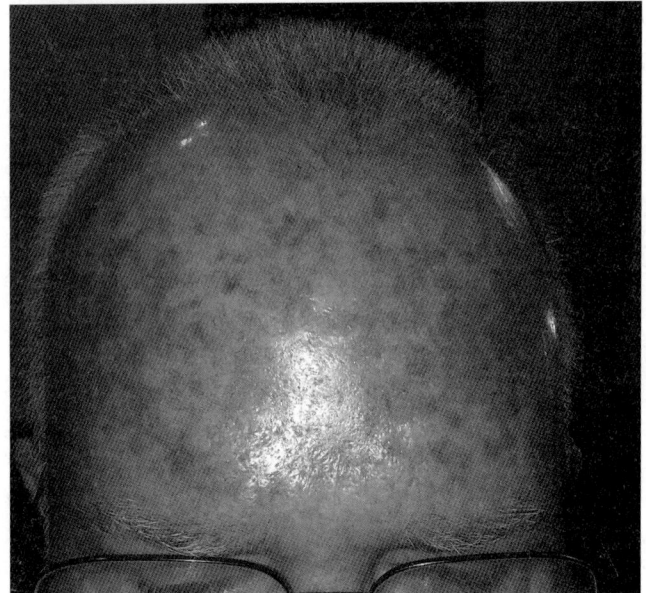

Figure 5 Twice daily 5-fluorouracil at 3 weeks.

dyshidrosis. Ulceration or significant labial thickening should prompt concern for SCC.

Of note, porokeratoses have a similar clinical presentation to AKs and actinic cheilitis and usually appear as atrophic or rice paper–appearing lesions surrounded by a slightly raised border (Figure 3).

Treatment

Lesions that are suspicious for malignant transformation should be biopsied before treatment. In general, it is recommended that all AKs be treated to reduce the risk of progression to SCC. In cases where the discomfort of treatment outweighs the benefit, as in some cases of patients with limited life expectancy, treatment may be avoided.

AKs, actinic cheilitis, and isolated porokeratoses are treated similarly. For patients with a limited number of lesions, destruction with cryosurgery is a quick and effective treatment. Success rates are as high as 95% in treatment of AKs. Cryosurgery can be performed using a variety of tools. Liquid nitrogen spray devices provide the coldest temperatures and fastest treatment in clinical practice. There are multiple-size apertures available for clinician use, and protocols may vary by clinician preference or lesion size. One protocol is to spray the lesion until frozen from a distance of 1 to 2 cm. The lesion should be kept frozen for 6 seconds, allowed to thaw, and then refrozen. A lighter freeze protocol is appropriate for the lips and other sensitive surfaces. For clinical efficiency, it is useful to treat several lesions in succession to allow the earlier lesions to thaw before repeating the freeze (Figure 4). Other useful options include nitrous oxide spray devices, evaporative refrigerant liquids, mechanically cooled probes via refrigerant technology, compressed nitrous oxide or carbon dioxide devices, or a swab dipped in liquid nitrogen. Protocols for the use of each of these options vary. The patient should be counseled that the cold spray does cause discomfort that may feel like a burning or stinging sensation. Patient discomfort varies with the procedure. Most individuals will tolerate treatment of up to 15 lesions. Patients can return for additional cryosurgery at subsequent visits. After treatment, the lesions typically become erythematous, have slight swelling, and may blister. If they blister or erode, topical petrolatum and an adhesive bandage may be used to protect the healing wound. Lesions that do not heal after cryosurgery treatment should raise concern for malignancy and undergo biopsy.

Cryosurgery is usually avoided in patients with dark skin because of the high risk of hypopigmentation. Alternatives include topical therapies or curettage with electrocautery.

Field-directed or blanket therapy may be preferred to lesion-directed therapy in individuals with large, affected areas or multiple lesions. Field therapy may provide a prophylactic effect on development of new lesions in treated areas as they treat subclinical lesions. Topical chemotherapy with 5-fluorouracil (5-FU; Carac, Efudex) is very effective in clearing at least 75% of AK lesions in treated areas. There are multiple formulations and protocols. One protocol calls for application of 5% 5-FU (Efudex) to affected areas twice daily for 2 weeks, which leads to significant inflammation, including erosions and exudate (Figures 5 and 6). If there has been no reaction, treatment can be extended out to 3 weeks. There is significant patient discomfort, which may lead to discontinuation or incomplete adherence to this treatment protocol. Patients should be counseled to expect marked inflammation in affected areas. Treating smaller areas sequentially and allowing them to heal before progressing can lessen discomfort. Treatment of forearm(s) may allow the patient to gain familiarity with the use of the medication before treating the face or scalp. The combination of 5% 5-FU and 0.005% calcipotriene (Calcitrene,

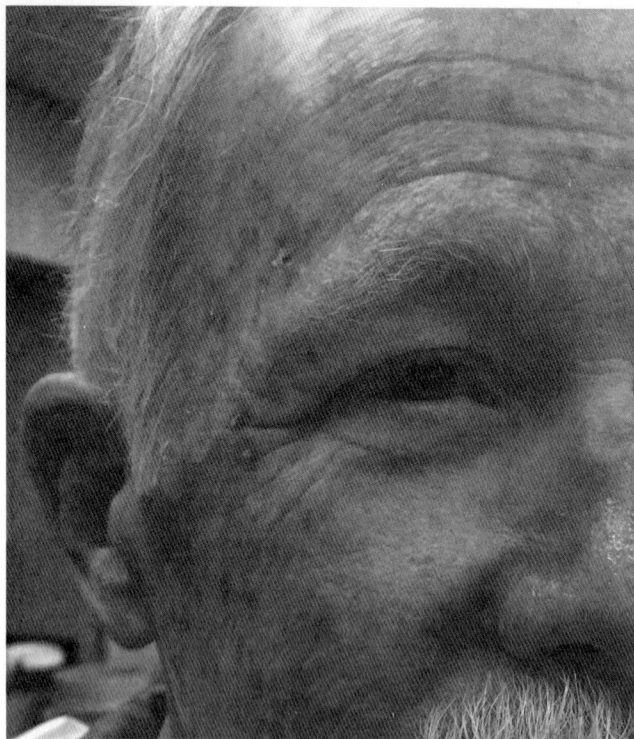

Figure 6 Daily 5-fluorouracil at 5 weeks.

Dovonex)[1], applied twice daily for 4 days, appears to enhance the clearance of AKs more effectively than 5-FU alone, offering better tolerability with fewer local site reactions and adverse effects. The 0.5% 5-FU (Carac) formulation may be better tolerated in treatment of actinic cheilitis. Treatment with 5-FU does lead to photosensitivity and increased risk of sunburn. It is preferable to perform therapy in the winter months when there is less sun exposure or to use strict sun avoidance. It is advisable to manage seborrheic dermatitis before initiating 5-FU treatment, as 5-FU can exacerbate inflammatory responses in areas affected by seborrheic dermatitis.

Given the significant patient discomfort with 5-FU treatment, other topical treatments have been developed. They cause less inflammation than 5-FU but also appear to have lower efficacy rates, including in limited head-to-head trials. These agents include topical imiquimod Aldara 5% twice weekly at bedtime for 16 weeks; Aldara 3.75% or Zyclara 3.75% daily at bedtime for 2 weeks on and 2 weeks off, repeat treatment cycle for a total of 8 weeks, diclofenac (Solaraze gel 3%) twice daily for 8 to 12 weeks, and tirbanibulin 1% ointment (Klisyri) once daily for 5 days. Imiquimod in the 5% formulation has been found to be an effective treatment of AKs in immunosuppressed patients. Tirbanibulin has better tolerability than 5-FU and is now approved for 100 cm^2 (approximately 4 × 4 inches), whereas it was previously approved for only 25 cm^2, a much smaller amount of skin than is typically treated with topical agents. Tirbanibulin has 47% efficacy for complete clearance of AKs.

Outside of typical primary care practices, several other options for treatment exist. Photodynamic therapy can be used after a sensitizing application of aminolevulinic acid (Levulan) or methyl aminolevulinate (Metvixia)[2]. Nonselective chemical peels, dermabrasion, and ablative lasers can be used for field therapy to an entire area. Clinically unaffected skin in the treatment field is treated with these options.

Nicotinamide[7] 500 mg orally twice daily has been shown to reduce the incidence of new nonmelanoma skin cancers (NMSCs) and AKs in individuals with AKs or NMSC. It reduced the rate of developing additional AKs by 15% and NMSC by 23%. The protective effect diminishes upon discontinuation, indicating the necessity for continuous use to maintain its benefits. While nicotinamide has demonstrated efficacy in reducing the incidence of NMSCs and AKs in immunocompetent individuals, it was not found effective in immunocompromised patients, such as organ transplant recipients.

Oral retinoids like acitretin (Soriatane)[1] can help reduce the risk of SCC and AKs in organ transplant recipients. Studies show that low-dose retinoids lower SCC risk within the first 3 years, with benefits lasting up to 8 years. However, side effects such as headaches, rashes, joint pain, and high lipid levels may limit their use. Retinoids are contraindicated in pregnancy due to the risk of birth defects. Pregnancy should be avoided within 3 years of acitretin use according to the American Academy of Dermatology.

[1] Not FDA approved for this indication.

References

Arcuri D, Ramchatesingh B, Lagacé F, et al: Pharmacological agents used in the prevention and treatment of actinic keratosis: a review, Int J Mol Sci 24(5), 2023. https://doi.org/10.3390/ijms24054989.

Azoulay L, St-Jean A, Dahl M, et al: Canadian Network for Observational Drug Effect Studies (CNODES) Investigators: Hydrochlorothiazide use and risk of keratinocyte carcinoma and melanoma: a multisite population-based cohort study, J Am Acad Dermatol 89(2):243–253, 2023. https://doi.org/10.1016/j.jaad.2023.04.035, Epub 2023 Apr 25. PMID: 37105517.

Am Health Drug Benefits 8(Spec Issue):13–14, 2015.

Brodell EE, Smith E, Brodell RT: Exacerbation of seborrheic dermatitis by topical fluorouracil, Arch Dermatol 147(2):245–246, 2011. https://doi.org/10.1001/archdermatol.2010.420.

Cheng B, Veerabagu S, Miller CJ, et al: A comparison of invasive squamous cell carcinoma greater than 1 year after treatment with 5-fluorouracil, imiquimod, or photodynamic therapy with aminolevulinic acid, J Am Acad Dermatol 87(3):592–596, 2022. https://doi.org/10.1016/j.jaad.2022.05.051.

Clauwaert V, Verhaeghe E, De Schepper S, Haspeslagh M, Brochez L: Clinicopathologically defined nevus subtypes and melanoma risk, J Invest Dermatol 145(2):383–392.e3, 2025. https://doi.org/10.1016/j.jid.2024.03.046. Epub 2024 Jun 26. PMID: 38942231.

Camillo L, Zavattaro E, Savoia P: Nicotinamide: a multifaceted molecule in skin health and beyond, Medicina 61(254), 2025.

Cohen JL: Actinic keratosis treatment as a key component of preventive strategies for nonmelanoma skin cancer, J Clin Aesthet Dermatol. 3(6):39–44, 2010. PMID: 20725550; PMCID: PMC2921751.

Christensen RE, Elston DM, Worley B, et al: Dermatopathologic features of cutaneous squamous cell carcinoma and actinic keratosis: consensus criteria and proposed reporting guidelines, J Am Acad Dermatol 88(6):1317–1325, 2023. https://doi.org/10.1016/j.jaad.2022.12.057. Epub 2023 Feb.

Dirschka T, Gupta G, Micali G, et al: Real-world approach to actinic keratosis management: practical treatment algorithm for office-based dermatology, J Dermatolog Treat 28(5):431–442, 2017. https://doi.org/10.1080/09546634.2016.1254328.

Dlott AH, Spencer SA, Di Pasqua AJ: Calcipotriol and 5-fluorouracil combination therapy for the treatment of actinic keratosis in the clinic: a review article, Clin Drug Invest 44(10):733–737, 2024.

Eisen DB, Asgari MM, Bennett DD, et al: Guidelines of care for the management of actinic keratosis, J Am Acad Dermatol 85(4):e209–e233, 2021. https://doi.org/10.1016/j.jaad.2021.02.082.

Gerstenblith MR, Goldstein AM, Tucker MA: Hereditary genodermatoses with cancer predisposition, Hematol Oncol Clin N Am 24:885–906, 2010. https://doi.org/10.1016/j.hoc.2010.06.003. Chapter.

Goldenberg G: Treatment considerations in actinic keratosis, J Eur Acad Dermatol Venereol 31(suppl 2):12–16, 2017. https://doi.org/10.1111/jdv.14152. PMID: 28263018.

George CD, Lee T, Hollestein LM, Asgari MM, Nijsten T: Global epidemiology of actinic keratosis in the general population: a systematic review and meta-analysis, Br J Dermatol 190(4):465–476, 2024. https://doi.org/10.1093/bjd/ljad371.

Jansen MHE, Kessels JPHM, Nelemans PJ, et al: Randomized trial of four treatment approaches for actinic keratosis, N Engl J Med 380(10):935–946, 2019. https://doi.org/10.1056/nejmoa1811850.

Jansen MHE, et al: Randomized trial of four treatment approaches for actinic keratosis, Engl J Med 380(10):935–946, 2019.

Lampley N, Rigo R, Schlesinger T, Rossi AM: Field therapy for actinic keratosis: a structured review of the literature on efficacy, cost, and adherence, Dermatol Surg 49(2):124–129, 2023. https://doi.org/10.1097/DSS.0000000000003677.

Li Pomi F, Vaccaro M, Pallio G, Rottura M, Irrera N, Borgia F: Tirbanibulin 1% ointment for actinic keratosis: results from a real-life study, Medicina (Kaunas) 60(2):225, 2024. https://doi.org/10.3390/medicina60020225. PMID: 38399512; PMCID: PMC10890708.

Mohney L, Singh R, Grada A, Feldman SR: Use of topical calcipotriol plus 5-fluorouracil in the treatment of actinic keratosis: a systematic review, J Drugs Dermatol 21(1):60–65, 2022.

Menter A, Gelfand JM, Connor C, et al: Joint American Academy of Dermatology-National Psoriasis Foundation guidelines of care for the management of psoriasis with systemic nonbiologic therapies, J Am Acad Dermatol 82(6):1445–1486, 2020.

Mirali S, Tang E, Drucker AM, et al: Follow-up of patients with keratinocyte carcinoma: a systematic review of clinical practice guidelines, JAMA Dermatol

[1] Not FDA approved for this indication.
[2] Not available in the United States.
[7] Available as dietary supplement.

159(1):87–94, 2023. https://doi.org/10.1001/jamadermatol.2022.4590. PMID: 36322063.

Nikas IP, Paschou SA, Ryu HS: The role of nicotinamide in cancer chemoprevention and therapy, *Biomolecules* 10(3):1–20, 2020. https://doi.org/10.3390/biom10030477.

Rypka KJ, Wendland ZD, Steele MV, Wehner MR, Yeung H, Mansh MD: Sexual orientation and lifetime prevalence of skin cancer across racial and ethnic groups, *JAMA Dermatol* 160(9):977–983, 2024. https://doi.org/10.1001/jamadermatol.2024.2097. PMID: 39018081; PMCID: PMC11255965.

Shao SC, Lai CC, Chen YH, Lai EC, Hung MJ, Chi CC: *BMC Med*, 2022.

Thamm JR, Welzel J, Schuh S: Diagnosis and therapy of actinic keratosis, *JDDG - J Ger Soc Dermatology* 22(5):675–690, 2024. https://doi.org/10.1111/ddg.15288.

Tirbanibulin 1% ointment (klisyri) for actinic keratosis, *Med Lett Drugs Ther* 63(1623):70–71, 2021.

Nikas IP, Paschou SA, Ryu HS: The role of nicotinamide in cancer chemoprevention and therapy, *Biomolecules* 10(3):477, 2020. https://doi.org/10.1111/ddg.15288. Accessed March 8, 2025.

PRESSURE INJURY

Method of
Rebecca M. Wester, MD

CURRENT DIAGNOSIS

- The National Pressure Injury Advisory Panel redefined the definition: pressure injury replaces the terms "pressure ulcer," "decubitus ulcer," and "bed sores."
- Pressure injury develops from pathologic changes in combination with localized skin and underlying soft tissue damage, typically over a bony prominence or associated with a medical device. Skin can be intact or have an open ulcer. Pressure Injury can occur with shearing.

CURRENT THERAPY

- Treatment is based on the stage and characteristics of the pressure injury.
- Nutrition and pressure relief are important interventions.
- Host-specific factors have profound effects on the healing process and have a greater influence than what is put on the wound.
- Utilize interdisciplinary approach (physical and occupational therapy, and dietary consultation) for optimal outcomes.

Epidemiology

Most pressure injuries develop during acute hospitalizations, in spite of the adoption of national pressure ulcer prevention guidelines. Prevalence rates for pressure injuries have changed little over the past two decades. Hospitalized patients in intensive care or undergoing cardiovascular or hip surgery have higher rates. Hospitalized individuals with COVID-19 and acute respiratory distress syndrome (ARDS) requiring mechanical ventilation have demonstrated increased risk for pressure injury related to prone positioning.

End-stage skin failure occurs when hypoperfusion occurs at the end of life. The prevalence of pressure injuries is 11% to 18% for palliative care patients, nearly double in comparison with hospital rates. Pressure injuries impose a significant burden, not only on the patient but also on the entire health care system. To put it into perspective, the cost of treating 10 pressure injuries is equivalent to 5 knee replacements, 6 hip replacements, 9 pacemakers, or 5 bypass operations.

Risk Factors

External factors that lead to the development of pressure injuries include pressure, shearing forces, friction, and moisture. Interaction of these external factors with host-specific factors such as immobility, sensory loss, incontinence, reduced perfusion, and compromised nutritional status culminates in tissue damage. Decreased skin perfusion resulting from hypotension, anemia, shock, or peripheral artery disease is increasingly recognized as an important cause of pressure ulcers. Hypercoagulation and microvascular occlusion associated with COVID-19 infection affect the skin and cause increased risk of skin discoloration and breakdown. Other risk factors are cerebrovascular disease, cardiovascular disease, recent lower extremity fractures, medications, and diabetes.

Pressure ulcer risk assessment. The Braden and Norton scales are commonly used for pressure risk assessment. These scales assess risk factors such as physical and mental condition, mobility, moisture, continence, and nutrition. However, they are weak predictors of risk of ulcers and may be no better at reducing risk than clinical judgment.

Pathophysiology

Pressure alone is not sufficient to cause an ulcer; it's the addition of the confounding host-specific factors that ultimately leads to tissue damage. Superficial lesions are primarily the result of moisture and friction. Exposure to moisture in the form of perspiration, urine, or feces can lead to skin maceration. Friction occurs when patients are dragged across an external surface. This results in an abrasion with damage to the most superficial layer of skin. Friction contributes mostly to stage 2 pressure injuries, with limited contributions to stage 3 to 4 pressure injuries because it does not cause the necrotic changes associated with deep tissue injury. Pressure injuries are greatest over bony prominences where weight-bearing points come in contact with external surfaces and immobilization devices. Pressure over a bony prominence tends to result in a cone-shaped distribution, with the most affected tissues located deep, adjacent to the bone–muscle interface. Thus the extent of injury to deep tissues is often much greater than perceived from the visible ulcer on the skin surface. Typically, stage 3 to 4 pressure injuries start as a deep tissue injury that may then progress to the surface. There is little evidence to suggest that a stage 4 pressure injury develops as a gradual progression from stage 1 to stage 4.

Differential Diagnosis

Besides pressure injuries, other chronic skin ulcers are arterial ulcers, venous stasis ulcers, and diabetic ulcers: arterial ulcers occur in distal digits or over bony prominences, venous stasis ulcers occur on the lateral aspect of the lower leg in the setting of chronic edema, and diabetic ulcers occur in regions of callous formations. Traumatic injuries such as abrasions, skin tears, or burns are not pressure injuries; nor are surgical incision sites. COVID-19-related skin changes should be considered for purple discoloration found on non–pressure loaded skin surfaces. These areas have been found to lack pressure-shear etiology and should not be classified as a pressure injury. Only pressure injuries are staged; never stage a wound that arises from a different etiology.

Diagnosis

Staging is done according to the National Pressure Ulcer Advisory Panel Pressure Injury Staging System:

Stage 1: Nonblanchable erythema of intact skin. May appear differently in darkly pigmented skin. Color changes do not include purple or maroon discoloration; this indicates deep tissue injury. Changes in skin temperature, sensation, and firmness may be present prior to visual changes in skin color.

Stage 2: Partial-thickness skin loss with exposed dermis. The wound bed is viable, pink or red, and moist, and may also present as an intact or ruptured serum-filled blister. Adipose (fat) is not visible and deeper tissues are not visible. Granulation tissue, slough, and eschar are not present. This stage should not be used to describe moisture-associated skin damage (MASD) including incontinence-associated dermatitis (IAD), intertriginous dermatitis (ITD), medical adhesive–related skin injury (MAR-SI), or traumatic wounds (skin tears, burns, abrasions).

Stage 3: Full-thickness skin loss. Adipose (fat) is visible in the ulcer and granulation tissue and rolled skin edges are often present. Slough or eschar may be visible. The depth of tissue damage varies by anatomic location; areas of significant adiposity can develop deep wounds. Undermining and tunneling may occur. Fascia, muscle, tendon, ligament, cartilage, and bone are not exposed. If slough or eschar obscures the extent of tissue loss, then it is an unstageable pressure injury.

Stage 4: Full-thickness skin and tissue loss. Exposed or directly palpable fascia, muscle, tendon, ligament, cartilage, or bone is in the ulcer. Slough or eschar may be visible. Rolled edges, undermining, and tunneling often occur. Depth varies by anatomic location. If slough or eschar obscures the extent of tissue loss, then it is an unstageable pressure injury.

Unstageable: Obscured full-thickness skin and tissue loss. The extent of tissue damage within the ulcer cannot be determined because it is obscured by slough or eschar. If slough or eschar is removed, a stage 3 or 4 pressure injury will be revealed. Stable eschar (dry, adherent, intact, without erythema or fluctuance) on the heel or ischemic limb should not be softened or removed.

Deep tissue injury: Persistent, nonblanchable, deep red, maroon, or purple discoloration. May appear as a dark wound bed or blood-filled blister. Pain and temperature skin changes often precede skin color changes. Discoloration may appear differently in darkly pigmented skin. The wound may evolve rapidly from intense or prolonged pressure and shear forces at the bone–muscle interface. The wound may evolve rapidly to reveal the actual extent of injury or may resolve without tissue loss. If necrotic tissue, subcutaneous tissue, granulation tissue, fascia, muscle, or other underlying structure is visible, then it is a full-thickness pressure injury (unstageable or stage 3 or 4). Do not use deep tissue injury to describe vascular, traumatic, neuropathic, diabetic, or dermatologic conditions.

Medical device–related pressure injury: Results from the use of devices designed and applied for diagnostic or therapeutic purposes. The resultant pressure injury generally conforms to the pattern or shape of the device. The injury should be staged using the staging system.

Mucosal membrane pressure injury: Found on mucous membranes in patients with a history of a medical device in use at the location of the injury. Owing to the anatomy of the tissue, these ulcers cannot be staged.

Therapy

Pressure relief. Position the patient frequently at fixed intervals to relieve pressure over compromised areas. There is no evidence to suggest an optimal interval at which to reposition patients, although every 2 hours is recommended based on expert opinion. Advanced static support surfaces (mattress overlays and foam, gel, or air mattresses) rather than standardized hospital mattresses should be used to prevent pressure injuries in high-risk patients. Check the pressure-relieving devices for "bottoming out" by inserting your hand (palm up) between the device and the bed under the patient's sacral area. The device is considered ineffective if you are unable to slide your hand freely. For immobile individuals, offload the heels by "floating the heels" with pillows under the patient's legs.

Pain. Dressing changes hurt. Use individualized pain management. Assess pain frequently using a valid and reliable tool when possible. Attention should also be paid to visual cues and signs of pain when determining pain levels, specifically for those patients who are unable to provide pain rating or description. Both pharmacologic and nonpharmacologic interventions should be considered. Physical and occupational therapy consult may be beneficial as E-stim, diathermy, and ultrasound have demonstrated effectiveness in reducing pain associated with pressure injury. Additionally, consider premedication prior to wound dressing changes or other procedures.

Assessment of nutrition/hydration. Pressure injuries occur in sicker individuals in whom overall intake may be reduced by coexisting illness. If adequate dietary intake is compromised, supplemental vitamins/minerals at the recommended daily allowance (RDA) should be considered. Protein supplementation may improve outcomes in the treatment of pressure ulcers, as per

TABLE 1	Débridement Methods

Mechanical: Wet-to-dry dressings; removes both devitalized and viable tissues; causes pain. Cleansing wound with each dressing change is considered mechanical débridement and is beneficial in reducing biofilm and bacteria in wound bed.

Surgical (sharp): Scalpel, scissors, or forceps to remove devitalized tissue; quick and effective by skilled clinician; should be used when infection is suspected; causes pain

Enzymatic: Topical débriding agent to dissolve the necrotic tissue; appropriate when there are no signs or symptoms of local infection

Autolytic: Synthetic dressing to allow the devitalized tissue to self-digest from the enzymes found in the ulcer fluids; recommended for those who cannot tolerate débridement; may take a long time to be effective; commonly used with palliative wounds

Biosurgery: Larvae to digest devitalized tissue; quick and effective; good option for those who cannot tolerate surgical débridement; limited by access to larvae

current guidelines. However, a 2014 Cochrane review concluded that there is no clear evidence that nutritional interventions (i.e., dietary supplementation) reduce the number of people who develop pressure injuries or help the healing of existing pressure injuries. There is no evidence to support the use of vitamin C or zinc to treat pressure injuries in patients who are not deficient in these nutrients. There is no difference in healing rates associated with supratherapeutic doses of vitamin C or zinc. Adequate nutrition and hydration are essential for wound healing. Current guidelines recommend dietary referral for comprehensive nutritional assessment. This includes documentation of food and fluid intake, BMI and weight history, and nutrition focused physical assessments to assess for muscle wasting. Serum protein, serum albumin, prealbumin, and other laboratory values are no longer recommended as they are affected by inflammation, renal function, and other factors and do not correlate well with clinical observation of nutritional status. Protein supplements have demonstrated effectiveness in promoting wound healing and maintaining weight in individuals with pressure injury. Artificial nutrition is considered an option for those patients who cannot meet their nutritional requirements via normal oral intake. The decision to use tube feeding must consider the patient's wishes, overall goal of care, and complications of tube feeding. Recent studies surprisingly observed that the use of tube feedings increased the incidence of pressure injuries and was associated with poorer healing. Tube feeding is associated with agitation, increased use of physical and chemical restraints and worsening of ulcers in individuals with severe dementia.

Removal (débridement) of necrotic tissue. Débridement by any of several methods (Table 1) may improve the time to a clean wound bed, but the effect of débridement on the time to healing remains to be determined.

Promotion of healing (reepithelialization). Pressure injuries should be cleansed with wound cleanser, saline, or tap water in combination with gauze to remove biofilm, slough, or necrotic debris that can be easily removed with each dressing change (see Table 1). The choice of a particular dressing depends on the wound characteristics, such as amount of exudate, dead space, or wound infection. A hydrocolloid, foam, or other nonadherent dressing that promotes a moist wound environment should be used (Table 2). Follow manufacturer recommendations regarding frequency of dressing changes. Negative pressure wound therapy (NPWT), skin grafting, and surgical closure are advanced options for closure of pressure injuries and are effective at reducing infection and heal time. This can greatly improve quality of life for patients with pressure injuries. Consider referral to wound specialist or surgeon for evaluation of these options.

Monitoring

Measurement. After staging the pressure injury, measure the length, width, and depth of ulcers. Document the presence of

TABLE 2	Pressure Injury Dressing Types
DRESSING	**RECOMMENDATIONS**
Hydrocolloid	Light to moderate exudate ulcers
	Clean stage 2 or shallow (noninfected) stage 3 ulcers
	Consider using filler dressing beneath in deep ulcers to fill dead space
Transparent film	Partial thickness with minimal exudate ulcers or closed wounds
	Consider for autolytic débridement
	Consider as secondary dressing with alginate or other wound filler that will likely remain in the ulcer for an extended time (3–5 days)
	Do not use on moderately to heavily exudative ulcers
	Do not use as cover dressing over enzymatic débriding agents
Hydrogel	Full thickness with minimal or no exudate (stage 3 or 4) ulcers
	Consider use on shallow, minimally exudate ulcer
	Consider amorphous hydrogel for granulating noninfected ulcers
	Consider for dry ulcer beds
Alginate	Full thickness with moderate to heavy exudate ulcers with cavities (stage 3 or 4)
	Consider in clinically infected ulcer with concurrent treatment for the infection
Foams	Exudate stage 2 and shallow stage 3 ulcers
	Avoid using single small piece pf foam in exudate ulcer with cavities
	Consider gelling foam in heavily exuding ulcers
Silver impregnated	Clinically infected or heavily colonized. Avoid prolonged use; discontinue when wound infection is controlled

exudate, necrotic tissue, eschar, slough, undermining, and tunneling. Presence of healing tissue (pink granulation or epithelialization) should be recorded as well. Measurement frequency depends onthe patient's care location, whether it's the hospital, a long-term care facility, or home care.

Infection. All pressure ulcers are colonized with bacteria. Never swab a chronic ulcer. The presence of bacteria alone does not indicate active infection, only colonization. Edema, odor, and purulent discharge are nonspecific. Worsening pain, erythema at wound edges, and warmth are signs of advancing cellulitis. Fever or delirium may be the only signs of infection. Systemic rather than topical antibiotics should be used to treat an infected pressure ulcer. Consider osteomyelitis when bone is exposed.

References

The cost of pressure injuries. Available at http://www.cobro.co.nz/cms/the cost of pressure injuries [accessed February 14, 2017].

Don't recommend percutaneous feeding tubes in patients with advanced dementia; instead offer oral assisted feeding. Available at http://www.choosingwisely.org [accessed February 14, 2017].

Black J, Cuddigan J, Members of the National Pressure Injury Advisory Panel Board of Directors. Skin manifestations with COVID-19: the purple skin and toes that you are seeing may not be deep tissue pressure injury. An NPIAP White Paper. Available at https://npiap.com [accessed March 3, 2022].

Langer G, Fink A: Nutritional interventions for preventing and treating pressure ulcers, *Cochrane Database Syst Rev* 6:CD003216, 2014.

Lyder CH: *Pressure ulcers and wound care. Geriatric Review Syllabus: A Core Curriculum in Geriatrics Medicine*, ed 8th, New York, 2013, American Geriatrics Society.

National Pressure Injury Advisory Panel. Available at https://npiap.com [accessed March 3, 2022].

Raetz JG, Wick KH: Common questions about pressure ulcers, *Am Fam Physician* 92(10):888–894, 2015.

Team V, Team L, Jones A, et al: Pressure injury prevention in COVID-19 patients with acute respiratory distress syndrome. Available at https://www.ncbi.nlm.nih.gov [accessed on March 2, 2022].

Thomas DR: Clinical management of pressure ulcers, *Clin Geriatr Med* 29:397–413, 2013.

Thomas DR: Does pressure cause pressure ulcers? An inquiry into etiology of pressure ulcers, *J Am Med Dir Assoc* 11:397–405, 2010.

PRURITUS ANI AND VULVAE

Method of
Muhammad Ahmad Ghazi, MD

CURRENT DIAGNOSIS

- Anogenital pruritis is primarily idiopathic; most secondary etiologies can be divided into dermatologic, anogenital conditions, and systemic causes.
- Good history and physical examination are important for accurate diagnosis.
- Laboratory tests and procedures to diagnose the cause of pruritis ani and vulvae should be tailored to individual patients based on their presentation.

CURRENT THERAPY

- Initial treatment is usually conservative, and clinicians should focus on reassurance, education about hygienic practices, regular bowel movements, avoidance of moisture and irritants, and a trial of topical corticosteroids.
- Anogenital conditions such as hemorrhoids, fissures, skin tags, and fistulas—if present—must be treated first.
- Pruritus vulvae secondary to lichen planus, lichen sclerosus, and lichen simplex chronicus usually require superpotent topical steroid treatment.
- Refractory cases of pruritus ani may benefit from injectable treatments of methylene blue.[1]
- Suspicious lesions of vulva and perineum that are resistant to initial treatment must be biopsied to rule out malignancy.

[1]Not FDA approved for this indication.

Pruritus ani and vulvae is not a disease per se; rather, it is a symptom or manifestation of an underlying disease or the result of poor personal hygienic practices. Pruritus is derived from the Latin *prurire*, which means "to itch." Pruritis ani is literally an unpleasant sensation leading to scratching the skin around the anal opening. Anogenital pruritus is a commonly ignored skin condition. Symptoms range from mild to severe and can be complicated by sleep disturbances, anxiety, depression, and social embarrassment. Pruritus ani and vulvae can be primary, in which case there is no identifiable cause, or be secondary to an underlying condition. Most of the secondary causes are anorectal, including hemorrhoids, fistulas, and fissures. Psoriasis, lichen sclerosus, and lichen simplex chronicus are common secondary dermatological causes of pruritus in the vulvar region.

Epidemiology

Pruritus ani is a common condition with an estimated prevalence of 1% to 5% of the population. It affects all ages and both

BOX 1 Common Causes of Pruritus Ani

Acute
Idiopathic up to 25% of cases
Fecal contamination:
Poor hygiene
Fecal incontinence
Anal sphincter dysfunction
Anorectal pathology: 10% to
50% of cases
Hemorrhoids, perianal
fissures, pilonidal sinus,
perianal abscess, rectal
prolapse, polyps, and
papilloma
Mechanical factors:
Excessive washing, rubbing,
synthetic undergarments
Infectious:
Erythrasma (corynebacterium
infection), Candida,
dermatophytosis, herpes
simplex, human papilloma
virus, HIV, syphilis
Parasitic:
Scabies, pinworm
Dermatoses:
Allergic or contact dermatitis,
psoriasis, drug eruptions
Dietary factors:
Tomatoes, chilis, coffee, beer,
soda, dairy, chocolate, tea,
citrus fruits

Chronic
Dermatoses:
Allergic or contact dermatitis,
psoriasis, lichen planus,
lichen simplex chronicus,
lichen sclerosis, Hailey-
Hailey disease
Inflammatory:
Inflammatory bowel disease
(ulcerative colitis and
Crohn's disease)
Malignant:
Anal squamous cell cancer
Extramammary Paget's
disease
Lymphoma/leukemia
Metabolic:
Diabetes mellitus, chronic
liver disease and chronic
kidney disease, celiac
disease, iron deficiency
anemia, hypovitaminosis A,
B, D, E
Miscellaneous:
Hyperhidrosis
Neuropathic pruritus
Psychogenic (anxiety related)

BOX 2 Common Causes of Pruritus Vulvae in Women

PREPUBERTAL AGE
Poor hygiene
Sensitization
of vulvar
skin: soaps,
deodorants
Contact dermatitis
Parasitic
infestations:
Pinworms
(Enterobius
vermicularis),
pediculosis,
scabies
Bacterial infections
(Group A beta
hemolytic
infections and
Escherichia coli)
Vaginal candidiasis
(rare in this age
group)
Lichen sclerosis
Suspected child
sexual abuse
(based on
evidence of
genital trauma)

REPRODUCTIVE AGE
Vaginitis
Trichomonas
Bacterial vaginosis
Candidiasis
Rarely tinea cruris
Herpes simplex
type II
HIV, syphilis
Dermatitis
Atopic dermatitis
Contact dermatitis
Psoriasis
Lichen planus
Lichen simplex
chronicus
Lichen sclerosis
Seborrheic
dermatitis
Pregnancy
Vulvar itching
is worsened
because of vulvar
engorgement;
pregnancy also
predisposes
women to
vaginal discharge
and candidiasis
Systemic diseases:
Diabetes, renal
and liver
diseases
Miscellaneous
Vulvar
intraepithelial
neoplasia (HPV)
Mechanical
trauma
Idiopathic

POSTMENOPAUSAL AGE
Urinary or fecal
incontinence
Menopause: Lack
of estrogen leads
to loss of skin
elasticity and
makes it prone
to itching
Atrophic vaginitis
Lichen sclerosis
Paget's disease of
vulvae
Vaginal malignancy
(squamous cell
cancer)

genders. Male to female prevalence of pruritus ani is about 4:1. Symptoms are worse at night and in warm, moist climates. Pruritus vulvae is seen in women of all ages. Young females usually present with an infectious etiology while the primary disease is more common in postmenopausal women. Genital pruritus in men is rare and usually presents with balanitis.

Risk Factors
Poor personal hygiene, chronic diarrhea, obesity, high-risk sexual behaviors, and immunodeficiency states predispose a person to pruritus in the anogenital area. Heat, sweating, and tight undergarments may exacerbate the condition. A proposed list of causative factors is included in Boxes 1 and 2.

Pathophysiology
The itching sensations of pruritus ani and vulvae are mediated by unmyelinated C fibers, which are distributed densely in the perineal region at the dermal-epidermical junction of the skin. Irritants in stool (exotoxins, intestinal lysozymes, endopeptidase, trypsins) and increased alkalinity of certain foods such as tomatoes, chocolate, and caffeine contribute to the perianal itching that precedes scratching. The itch-scratch cycle is mediated by several mechanical and inflammatory mediators, including histamine, kallikrein, bradykinin, trypsin, serotonin, and neuropeptides. The resulting nerve impulse is carried via spinothalamic tract to the thalamus, where the itching sensation is perceived. Intestinal transit time and altered anal sphincter pressure are influenced by certain foods that predispose people to perianal seepage and pruritus.

Pruritus vulvae is the result of increased permeability of the dermis resulting from a structurally thin strateum corneum as compared to the rest of the vulvar skin. Factors aggravating the pruritus include constant friction, rubbing, anatomic location, occlusion, moistness, fear of uncleanliness in women, and excessive washing. The most common cause of pruritus vulvae is vulvar dermatitis or eczema, which affects one-third to half of all women presenting with this complaint. Dermatitis or eczema can be endogenous and the result of familial disposition, and it manifests as atopic dermatitis. Exogenous dermatitis such as contact dermatitis can be allergic, given that a trigger (allergen) might induce an immune response or contact irritant dermatitis. Common irritants include soaps, shampoos, vaginal creams, alcohol, tea tree oil,[7] douches, vaginal hygiene products, vaginal contraceptives, sanitary pads, nylon underwear, and toilet paper. Chemical allergens contributing to contact dermatitis in the genital area include benzocaine, neomycin, ethylenediamide, propylene glycol, latex dyes, nickels, semen, lanolin, perfumes, and tampons.

Clinical Manifestations
Perianal and vulvar itching, erythema, excoriations, fissures, hemorrhoids, pinworms, and fecal incontinence may be noticed on inspection of the perineal area. In the acute phase, skin redness of varying degrees is visible. Excoriations from the skin from itching may be present. Fissures in the labial folds may be present. Superinfection with yeast or bacteria may complicate the presentation.

Chronic anogenital dermatitis usually presents as erythema of varying degrees, and papillae appear in the labial folds. Hypo- or hyperpigmentation of the skin or thickening of the labial skin

---

[7]Available as dietary supplement.

might develop over time, causing "lichenification," which leads to lichen simplex chronicus.

Diagnosis of Pruritus Ani and Vulvae

A detailed history of bowel habits and personal hygiene (including products used, such as perfumes); dietary habits (e.g., caffeine consumption); and previous medical, psychiatric, and surgical history help elucidate the cause of pruritus ani. The patient should be asked about personal or family history of hives, asthma, conjunctivitis, or atopy when allergic dermatitis is suspected. Other relevant questions of history include recent use of antibiotics, clothing preferences, family history of cancers, other family members with similar symptoms (pinworms and scabies), rectal bleeding, change in bowel habits, or sexual preference (anal receptive intercourse). For pruritus vulvae, the patient should be asked about any history of itching, burning sensation, vaginal discharge, postcoital bleeding, or dysperunia. Rarely, elderly patients with lumbosacral radiculopathy may experience perianal itching as a result of neurological deficits.

Physical Examination

Inspection with a bright light and a chaperone is recommended. Palpation includes a digital rectal exam and a female pelvic examination in case of pruritus vulvae. Wet preparation of vaginal secretions for Candida, bacterial vaginosis, potassium hydroxide testing, and cultures for *Neisseria gonorrhoeae* and chlamydia are recommended. Microscopic examination of scrapings will help to differentiate the parasitic and fungal infections.

Laboratory Tests

Laboratory tests should not be done routinely in all cases and should be tailored to the patient's history and physical examination. Below is a list of laboratory tests that should be considered when diagnosing possible causes of anogenital pruritus:

1. CBC (complete blood count) helps to differentiate between parasitic and infectious cases and diagnoses anemia (a possible cause of chronic pruritus ani)
2. Chemistry profile (to identify systemic causes such as hepatic and kidney diseases)
3. Urinalysis to screen for infection and systemic diseases such as diabetes
4. DNA polymerase chain reaction probe for gonorrhea and chlamydia
5. Cellophane tape test to look for pinworms
6. Stool for ova and parasites
7. Test for diabetes mellitus and HIV if suspected
8. Anal Pap smear for HPV is indicated if there is a history of anal receptive intercourse

Procedures

Anoscopy and proctoscopy are indicated to diagnose hemorrhoids and perianal fistulae. Colposcopic examination of the perineum may provide a detailed view of local pathology.

Colonoscopy is indicated for patients over 40 with a family history of colon cancers. Patch testing should be performed to diagnose allergic contact dermatitis. A skin biopsy is indicated in case of ulcerated skin lesions, refractory cases, and suspicious lesions to rule out malignancy. A 3 to 6 mm punch biopsy is recommended.

Differential Diagnosis

A broad range of clinical problems can be enumerated in the differential diagnosis, including (but not limited to) allergic skin reactions, infections, parasitic infestations, chronic liver disease, diabetes, and neoplasms; chronic conditions such as psoriasis or dermatitis; infections such as condylomata accuminata; and skin cancers such as Bowen's disease, squamous cell cancer, Paget's disease, or melanoma.

Prevention and Treatment

General Principles of Treatment

The goal of treatment should be the resolution of symptoms, restoration of skin anatomy, and prevention of recurrence. The most important step in the management of pruritus ani and vulvae is reassurance and patient education (Figure 1). An informed and educated patient tends to deal with symptom-related anxiety better. To identify and treat the cause, it should be understood that pruritus ani and vulvae are commonly idiopathic, and conservative measures are usually sufficient to treat the condition. However, secondary causes need to be identified and treated.

Anorectal conditions such as hemorrhoids, fistulas, and fissures may require surgical treatment and consultation. Antidiarrheals should be used in cases of loose stool. A high-fiber diet should be started.

Women presenting with vulvar pruritus should be screened and treated for vaginal infection (e.g., one dose of oral fluconazole [Diflucan] 150 mg for vulvovaginal candidiasis; metronidazole [Flagyl] 500 mg oral twice daily for 7 days for bacterial vaginosis). Dermatological conditions such as psoriasis and dermatitis are treated with topical steroids. Hormone replacement therapy can be used in cases of menopause. Topical estrogen creams are better alternatives for symptomatic relief.

Patients should be instructed to gently cleanse the perianal area twice daily and after each bowel movement. Sitz baths with plain warm water are recommended for perianal pruritus. The perianal area should be patted dry after washing. Patients with vulvar pruritus should avoid tight undergarments, jeans, and panty hose. The use of laundry detergents, bubble baths, feminine douches, or sprays containing protease should be discouraged. Women with a predisposition to vulvar dermatitis should wear loose pants. Panty liners should be avoided and replaced with tampons or cotton cloth. Vulvae should be washed gently; women should avoid vigorous rubbing or cleaning. Patients with vulvar pruritus should use a bland moisturizer as a soap substitute to avoid irritation resulting from chemicals. The vulva should be dried before wearing underwear, and excessive perspiration should be controlled with talcum powder. Patients should be encouraged to manage incontinence and maintain an ideal body weight. Cornstarch should be avoided, as it can lead to bacterial colonization and exacerbation of symptoms.

Dietary modifications (for anal pruritus) are imperative, including limitations on the consumption of chocolate, tea, coffee, citrus fruits, and alcoholic beverages. Eating yogurt is recommended, especially while on antibiotics, to prevent diarrhea and worsening of perianal seepage.

Emollients such as aqueous creams or petrolatum or emulsifying ointments treat itching and dry skin, which can prevent erosion and ulcer formation. These agents can be used irrespective of the etiology of pruritus. Zinc oxide (Desitin) cream is used topically to prevent excoriations in cases of perianal and vulvar pruritus. Combination products such as zinc oxide/bacitracin (rash relief antibacterial), zinc oxide/menthol (Calmoseptine), and zinc oxide/miconazole (Vusion) are available and can be used for symptomatic relief. Topical anesthetics (lidocaine 5% [L-M-X5 Anorectal, Topicaine 5]) may be used twice a day to help with acute symptoms. Topical benzocaine (Vagisil Anti-Itch Creme) should be avoided, as it is a strong irritant and allergen. Cool compresses and gel packs can help. Ice should not be used, as it can cause frostbite.

Antihistamines should be used to improve sleep, and patients should wear cotton gloves at night to prevent itching while asleep. Nails should be cut short, and nail varnish should be avoided. Sedating antihistamines might help (e.g., hydroxyzine [Vistaril] 50 mg PO at bedtime; doxepin [Sinequan][1] 10 to 100 mg at bedtime; citalopram [Celexa][1] 20 to 40 mg during the daytime). Citalopram can also help with underlying anxiety symptoms, but caution is advised in the elderly and patients at risk of

---

[1]Not FDA approved for this indication.

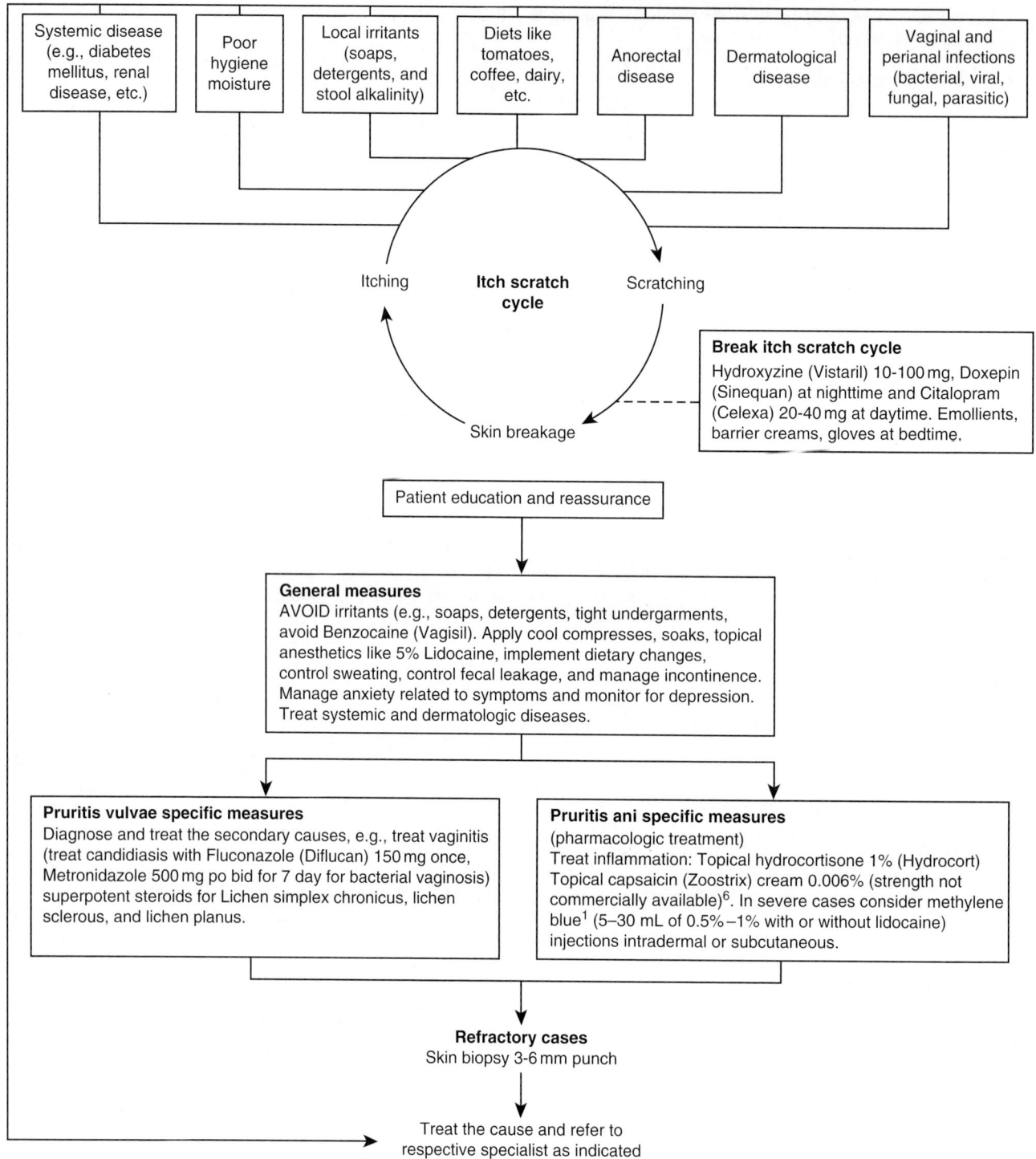

```
┌─────────────┐ ┌──────────┐ ┌──────────────┐ ┌──────────────┐ ┌──────────┐ ┌──────────────┐ ┌──────────────────┐
│Systemic     │ │          │ │Local irritants│ │Diets like    │ │          │ │              │ │Vaginal and       │
│disease      │ │Poor      │ │(soaps,        │ │tomatoes,     │ │Anorectal │ │Dermatological│ │perianal infections│
│(e.g., diabetes│ │hygiene   │ │detergents, and│ │coffee, dairy,│ │disease   │ │disease       │ │(bacterial, viral,│
│mellitus, renal│ │moisture  │ │stool alkalinity)│ │etc.        │ │          │ │              │ │fungal, parasitic)│
│disease, etc.)│ │          │ │              │ │              │ │          │ │              │ │                  │
└─────────────┘ └──────────┘ └──────────────┘ └──────────────┘ └──────────┘ └──────────────┘ └──────────────────┘
```

Itching — **Itch scratch cycle** — Scratching

Break itch scratch cycle
Hydroxyzine (Vistaril) 10-100 mg, Doxepin (Sinequan) at nighttime and Citalopram (Celexa) 20-40 mg at daytime. Emollients, barrier creams, gloves at bedtime.

Skin breakage

Patient education and reassurance

General measures
AVOID irritants (e.g., soaps, detergents, tight undergarments, avoid Benzocaine (Vagisil). Apply cool compresses, soaks, topical anesthetics like 5% Lidocaine, implement dietary changes, control sweating, control fecal leakage, and manage incontinence. Manage anxiety related to symptoms and monitor for depression. Treat systemic and dermatologic diseases.

Pruritis vulvae specific measures
Diagnose and treat the secondary causes, e.g., treat vaginitis (treat candidiasis with Fluconazole (Diflucan) 150 mg once, Metronidazole 500 mg po bid for 7 day for bacterial vaginosis) superpotent steroids for Lichen simplex chronicus, lichen sclerous, and lichen planus.

Pruritis ani specific measures
(pharmacologic treatment)
Treat inflammation: Topical hydrocortisone 1% (Hydrocort) Topical capsaicin (Zoostrix) cream 0.006% (strength not commercially available)[6]. In severe cases consider methylene blue[1] (5–30 mL of 0.5%–1% with or without lidocaine) injections intradermal or subcutaneous.

Refractory cases
Skin biopsy 3-6 mm punch

Treat the cause and refer to respective specialist as indicated

Figure 1 Pathogenesis and management of pruritus ani and vulvae. [1]Not FDA approved for this indication. [6]May be compounded by pharmacists.

arrhythmias, because citalopram can cause QT interval prolongation. Any suspicious lesions of the vulvae and perineum should be biopsied to rule out underlying malignancy.

Pharmacologic Treatments

For mild pruritus ani, 1% to 2.5% hydrocortisone (Hydrocort) topical ointment is effective. Pramoxine (Prax, Senna Sensitive) can also be used alone or in combination with topical hydrocortisone cream (Analpram-HC, Pramosone). 1% Hydrocortisone/1% iodoquinol (Vytone) can be used as an antiinflammatory treatment for external use in the anal and vulvar area. Topical capsaicin cream 0.006%[6] has been used in cases of refractory itching and can be combined with topical hydrocortisone cream to avoid hypersensitivity. This strength of capsaicin cream is not commercially available.[6] Mild topical corticosteroid ointments are sufficient to treat the perianal pruritus, and superpotent steroids should be avoided, as the skin is thin and there is a risk of ulcer formation. Methylene blue[1] injections are reserved for long-standing, intractable pruritus ani. Methylene blue 0.5% to 1% 5 to 30 mL mixed with normal saline and local anesthetics is injected intradermally, subcutaneously, and intracutaneously in the perianal skin to produce hypoesthesia. This treatment may be repeated, and studies report a success rate of 80% to 90%. Possible complications associated with methylene blue injections include cellulitis, transient urinary incontinence, urinary retention, skin abscess and skin necrosis. Long term effectiveness of these injections need further prospective studies.

---

[6]May be compounded by pharmacists.

For moderate vulvar disease, 0.1% triamcinolone (Kenalog) ointment is recommended. For severe cases and thickened skin, the superpotent steroid topical clobetasol (Temovate) or halobetasol (Ultravate) 0.05% ointments can be used. The use of these superpotent steroid creams should be limited and reserved for the resistant cases of pruritus vulvae, lichens simplex chronicus, lichen sclerosus, or resistant lichen planus. Vulvar lichen and lichen planus should be treated over the long term with superpotent steroids for adequate response and treatment. A very thin layer of steroid cream should be used, and patients should be educated about the side effects of the medication before starting the treatment. For vulvar lichen planus and lichen sclerosus, superpotent steroids are used topically once or twice daily for 2 to 3 months; three times a week for 1 month; then once or twice per week for the long term. For lichen simplex chronicus, treatment is twice daily for 2 weeks and then once daily for 2 weeks. It then moves to three times per week.

Topical calcineurin inhibitors 1% pimecrolimus cream (Elidel)[1] or 0.03% to 1% tacrolimus ointment (Protopic)[1] may be used for refractory cases as steroid-sparing agents. A common side effect of these agents is a burning sensation, so their use is controversial in cases of lichen sclerosis and lichen planus. Lichen sclerosis has 2-5% increased risk of developing squamous cell cancer, therefore clinical monitoring is recommended every 6–12 months and suspicious lesions must be biopsied.

In cases of neuropathic pruritus ani and vulvae, amitriptyline (Elavil)[1] 10 to 150 mg at bedtime is suggested. Other options are gabapentin (Neurontin)[1] 300 to 3600 mg up to three times a day (maximum daily dose is 3600 mg); pregabalin (Lyrica)[1] 75 to 400 mg/day; and mirtazapine (Remeron)[1] 7.5 to 15 mg at bedtime. In resistant and rare cases in which none of the above mentioned treatments is effective, radiation treatment may be indicated to destroy nerve endings. Naltrexone[1], an opioid antagonist has shown effectiveness in reducing itching episodes after one week of treatment in a case study. Case reports suggest treatment of perianal atopic dermatitis resistant to other treatments may respond to dupilumab (Dupixent)[1], which is a monoclonal antibody. Treatment should be reserved for biopsy confirmed cases of atopic dermatitis in consultation with dermatologist. Several experimental treatments, such as laser phototherapy, alcohol injection therapy, radiation, and surgery, have not been studied and are not recommended routinely.

Complications
Pruritus ani and vulvae can lead to myriad complications, including lichenification, skin excoriations, ulcers, secondary bacterial infections, and abscess formation.

Referral
For undiagnosed and resistant skin conditions, patients should be referred to a dermatologist. Persistent anal itching, a change in bowel habits, and rectal bleeding should prompt a referral to a gastroenterologist and colorectal specialist. Pruritus vulvae with vaginal bleeding and weight loss are indications for referral to a gynecologist.

Monitoring and Prognosis
Most cases of pruritus ani and vulvae are treated with general measures that lead to a full recovery. Long-term use of corticosteroids should be discouraged, and periodic monitoring for side effects, including skin erosions and bleeding, is advisable based on reported symptoms. The idiopathic disease usually persists and depicts a relapsing remitting course.

[1]Not FDA approved for this indication.

References
Al-Ghnaniem R, Short A, Pullen A: 1% Hydrocortisone ointment is an effective treatment of pruritus ani: A pilot randomized controlled crossover trial, *Int J Colorectal Dis* 22:1463–1467, 2007.
Family Practice Notebook: Pruritus vulvae. Available at http://www.fpnotebook.com/gyn/vulva/vlvrprts.htm, 2013 (accessed December 14, 2013).
Jones DJ: ABC of colorectal disease. Pruritus ani, *BMJ* 1305:575–577, 1992.
Margesson LJ: Overview of treatment of vulvovaginal disease, *Skin Therapy Lett* 16:5–7, 2011.
Margesson L, Danby WF: Pruritus ani and vulvae. In *Conn's Current Therapy 2013*: Philadelphia, 2012, Elsevier, pp 276–278.
Markell KW, Billingham RP: Pruritus ani: Etiology and management, *Surg Clin North Am* 90:125–135, 2010.
Mentes BB: Intradermal methylene blue injection for the treatment of intractable idiopathic pruritus ani: Results of 30 cases, *Tech Coloproctol* 8:11–14, 2004.
Reidy T, Rafferty JF: Management of pruritus ani. In *Current Surgical Therapy*, Philadelphia, 2011, Elsevier Mosby, pp 243–246.
Siddiqi S, Vijay V, Ward M, et al: Pruritus ani, *Ann R Coll Surg Engl* 90:457–463, 2008.
Stermer E, Sukhotnic I, Shoul R: Pruritus ani: An approach to an itching condition, *J Pediatr Gastroenterol Nutr* 48:513–516, 2009.
Weichert GE: An approach to the treatment of anogenital pruritus, *Dermatol Ther* 17:129–133, 2004.
Yang EJ, Murase JE: Recalcitrant anal and genital pruritis treated with dupilumab, *Int J Womens Dermatol* 4:223–226, 2018.

PYODERMA GANGRENOSUM

Method of
Dominic J. Wu, MD; and Anand N. Rajpara, MD

CURRENT DIAGNOSIS

- Pyoderma gangrenosum (PG) is a chronic inflammatory and ulcerative skin disease of uncertain etiology that is commonly mistaken for skin infection.
- Diagnosis of PG is typically a diagnosis of exclusion. Thorough workup to exclude other causes of ulcerative diseases (e.g., infection, malignancy, vascular) is paramount.
- There is no uniformly accepted diagnostic algorithm, and many have been proposed. A recent Delphi consensus set of diagnostic criteria is becoming more widely adopted.
- Recent diagnostic criteria require biopsy of the ulcer edge demonstrating neutrophilic infiltrate as the major criterion, while ruling out infection is no longer an absolute requirement.

CURRENT THERAPY

- There is no established gold standard treatment regimen.
- Goals of therapy should include reducing inflammation, reducing pain, and controlling any contributing underlying diseases.
- Due to the nature of the disease and complex medical treatments, it is important to involve relevant consultants early on, such as dermatology, rheumatology, gastroenterology, rheumatology, ophthalmology, etc.
- For mild, localized disease, consider topical and/or intralesional corticosteroids.
- For moderate to severe cases, the first-line systemic agents are historically systemic corticosteroids and cyclosporine (Neoral, Sandimmune).[1]
- Alternative treatment options that have shown success include tumor necrosis factor-α (TNF-α) inhibitors such as infliximab (Remicade)[1] and adalimumab (Humira),[1] mycophenolate mofetil (CellCept),[1] IVIG,[1] tetracyclines,[1] and more.
- Avoid debridement and surgical procedures due to risk of pathergy.
- Appropriate wound care is essential, including selection of appropriate dressings. Less exudative wounds can be treated with hydrogels and films. More exudative lesions should be managed with more absorptive dressings such as hydrocolloids and alginates. Consider involvement of wound care specialists.

[1]Not FDA approved for this indication.

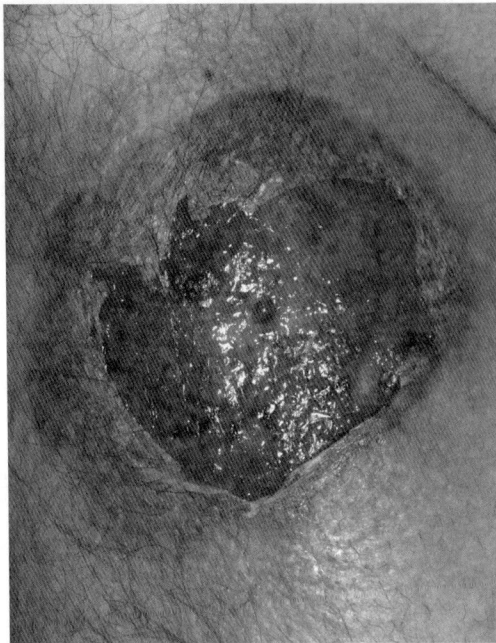

Figure 1 Classic ulcer of pyoderma gangrenosum with dusky to violaceous, irregular, undermined border. From James WD, et al: *Andrews' Diseases of the Skin*. Philadelphia: Elsevier; 2019.

Pathophysiology and Epidemiology

Pyoderma gangrenosum (PG) is a chronic ulcerative inflammatory neutrophilic dermatosis of uncertain etiology that is often misdiagnosed as severe skin infection. It is a relatively rare condition with incidence estimated at approximately 3 to 10 cases per million people per year, but it is not uncommonly encountered in dermatology clinic. It most frequently presents in young to middle-aged female adults between 20 to 50 years of age. Although its exact etiology is unknown and 25% to 50% of patients have idiopathic disease, it is frequently associated with numerous systemic diseases including inflammatory bowel disease (ulcerative colitis, Crohn disease), malignancy, granulomatosis with polyangiitis, Behçet disease, and more. This association suggests a possible underlying immunologic abnormality. PG is also a component of multiple genetic conditions including PAPA (pyogenic arthritis, PG, acne), PASH (PG, acne, hidradenitis suppurativa), and PAPASH (pyogenic arthritis, PG, acne, hidradenitis suppurativa) syndromes. Pathergy, even from minor trauma, may result in initiation and aggravation of PG lesions.

Clinical Manifestations

The clinical appearance of PG can often mimic other skin diseases, especially ulcerative infectious skin diseases, vascular diseases, and malignancies. The classic most characteristic clinical subtype is ulcerative PG. In addition, there are three other main clinical subtypes including pustular, bullous, and vegetative. The initial lesion of classic PG (ulcerative) typically begins as a painful solitary nodule or pustule that ruptures and undergoes necrosis, resulting in the formation of an ulcer. The most frequent location of PG is on the lower extremities (especially the pretibial region); however, it can appear anywhere including mucous membranes. The center of the classic PG ulcer is frequently coated with purulent material and granulation tissue. The edge of the ulcer is characteristically dusky to violaceous, irregular, undermined, and overhanging (Figure 1). Pustular PG is more commonly seen in patients with underlying inflammatory bowel disease and presents with multiple pustules with surrounding erythema to violaceous rim. These pustules may or may not rupture to form a more classic-appearing PG ulcer. Bullous, or atypical PG, is most commonly seen in patients with underlying lymphoproliferative disorders such as leukemia or multiple myeloma. Lastly, vegetative PG presents with more superficial ulcerations without significant central purulence and undermined borders.

Although the ulcer of PG is not infectious in itself, it may become secondarily infected, resulting in increased purulence and malodor.

Diagnosis

The clinical, laboratory, and histologic findings in PG are rather nonspecific; thus a diagnosis of PG is typically a diagnosis of exclusion. A detailed history of the lesion including evolution, pain, pathergy, and any associated underlying conditions are critical. General approach to workup includes biopsy of ulcer edge demonstrating neutrophilic infiltrate, and broad workup should be considered to exclude other causes including complete blood count (CBC; underlying hematologic disorder), bacterial and fungal cultures, herpes simplex virus (HSV)/varicella zoster virus (VZV) PCR, antinuclear antibody (ANA) (underlying autoimmune conditions—systemic lupus erythematosus, collagen vascular disorders), antineutrophil cytoplastic antibodies (ANCA; granulomatous vasculitis), hypercoagulability studies (vascular etiology), rheumatoid factor, urinalysis, serum and/or urine protein electrophoresis, chest imaging, and colonoscopy (evaluate for inflammatory bowel disease [IBD]). Other laboratories including comprehensive metabolic profile, hepatitis panel (which can also be helpful in evaluating for cryoglobulinemia), and tuberculosis screening are also helpful in preparation of potential treatment with immunosuppressive agents. Individual clinicians may choose varying levels of workup, depending on clinical suspicion and patient history.

Numerous diagnostic criteria and algorithms have been proposed, although they have not been uniformly accepted. Previously, diagnostic criteria required excluding all other diagnoses including infection, which is challenging and often results in delayed treatment. A recent Delphi consensus of international experts proposed and validated a set of diagnostic criteria as below:

Major criterion:

- Biopsy of ulcer edge demonstrating a neutrophilic infiltrate

Minor criteria:

- Exclusion of infection
- History of pathergy
- Personal history of IBD or inflammatory arthritis
- History of papule, pustule, or vesicle that rapidly ulcerated
- Peripheral erythema, undermining border, and tenderness at site of ulceration
- Multiple ulcerations (at least one occurring on an anterior lower leg)
- Cribriform or "wrinkled paper" scar(s) at sites of healed ulcers
- Decrease in ulcer size within 1 month of initiating immunosuppressive medication(s)

Diagnosis of PG requires the major criterion and four or more minor criteria. These criteria are becoming more widely adopted in academic institutions.

Differential Diagnosis

It is important to consider and exclude alternative diagnoses when evaluating a patient with possible PG. PG can mimic ulcerative infections such as herpes simplex virus, ecthyma gangrenosum, chancroid, deep fungal infections, sporotrichosis, atypical mycobacterial infection, necrotizing fasciitis, syphilis, and Buruli ulcer. Vascular disorders to consider include venous or arterial ulcerations, vasculitides including granulomatosis with polyangiitis, polyarteritis nodosa, cryoglobulinemia, and so on.

Therapy

There is no one-size-fits-all treatment for PG, and the goal of therapy is primarily to reduce the inflammatory process, promote healing, reduce pain, and treat any contributing underlying medical conditions. Debridement and surgical therapy should be avoided if possible due to pathergy and potential for worsening disease. Surgical therapy in other areas of the body should also be avoided if possible due to risk of developing similar lesions at other sites. It is important to involve relevant consultants as soon as possible based on the patient's case, including dermatology, ophthalmology, rheumatology, oncology, gastroenterology, and so on.

First-line therapy includes local high-potency topical corticosteroids such as clobetasol propionate 0.05% (Clobex, Temovate) twice a day and/or systemic corticosteroids such as prednisone 0.5 to 1 mg/kg/day divided in two to three doses, with slow taper over weeks to months. Colchicine[1] 0.6 mg PO three times a day has shown success as monotherapy or used in conjunction with corticosteroids. Cyclosporine (Neoral, Sandimmune)[1] 2.5 to 5 mg/kg/day divided twice a day has been demonstrated to lead to rapid improvement in pain and improvement in ulceration. Combination therapy with systemic corticosteroids and cyclosporine has also demonstrated success. Milder localized disease can be treated with intralesional corticosteroid injections such as with triamcinolone acetonide (Kenalog) 10 mg/mL into the ulcer edge or high-potency topical corticosteroids.

Alternative therapies utilized with success for moderate to severe disease include infliximab (Remicade)[1] 5 mg/kg IV at weeks 0, 2, and 6; adalimumab (Humira)[1] 80 mg SC loading dose, followed by 40 mg SC weekly or every other week; mycophenolate mofetil (Cellcept)[1] 750 mg to 1.5 g PO twice a day; dapsone[1] 50 to 150 mg daily; sulfasalazine (Azulfidine) 0.5 to 6 g PO daily divided in 3 to 4 doses, methotrexate[1] 2.5 to 25 mg PO, SC, or IM weekly, and more. The authors have also seen success with intravenous immunoglobulin (IVIG)[1] 1.5 to 3 g/kg IV monthly given over 2 to 5 days, although this can be incredibly expensive and is generally used as adjuvant therapy. IVIG is also an option for treatment if there is secondary infection and immunosuppressive therapies with TNF-α inhibitors are contraindicated.

Tetracycline antibiotics such as minocycline (Minocin)[1] 200 to 300 mg/day divided in 2 doses have also been reported to show success in treatment of PG, thought to be related to their antiinflammatory properties by reducing chemotaxis of neutrophils.

Appropriate wound care for PG ulcers is essential, depending on the clinical appearance of the lesion. Wound care specialists should be utilized if possible. Occlusive dressings are often utilized to increase the rate of healing by promoting angiogenesis, promoting collagen synthesis, and acting as a barrier against secondary infection. Hydrogels and films such as Tegaderm may be used in lesions with minimal exudate. In more exudative lesions, more absorptive dressings such as hydrocolloids, foams, and alginates would be more appropriate. Examples of these dressings that are frequently utilized for ulcer management include DuoDERM and SeaSorb. It is important to note that these dressings, especially alginates, may be associated with foul odor due to their reaction with healing tissue and may not actually be an indicator of secondary infection. Avoid wet-to-dry dressings, as this debridement may incite pathergy and cause aggravation of the wound.

Monitoring

PG tends to be a chronic and recurrent disease. Ulcers may take many months to heal, and it is essential to monitor for any signs of developing infection. Patients and clinicians should monitor for increased pain, increased purulence, fevers, increased erythema and/or streaking—all of which can be indicators for secondary infection. Topical and oral antimicrobials may be helpful; however, this may lead to antibiotic resistance and should be utilized only if secondary infection is confirmed.

Adequate control of any contributing underlying conditions is essential, and patients should be advised that trauma and elective surgical procedures may trigger the development of future PG lesions.

Many of the treatments utilized in the management of PG also have their large range of adverse side effects, and it is important to monitor patients closely when they are taking these medications. For example, systemic corticosteroids are the most commonly employed agents in PG. More severe or resistant lesions may require prolonged therapy and at higher doses, which can lead to increased adverse side effects. These patients should be closely monitored, and consider recommending supplemental calcium, vitamin D, proton pump inhibitors if indicated, and even bisphosphonates. The duration of treatment is case-dependent and should be determined based on clinical response and any concerning side effects.

References

Ahronowitz I, Harp J, Shinkai K: Etiology and management of pyoderma gangrenosum: a comprehensive review, *Am J Clin Dermatol* 13(3):191–211, 2012.

Braswell SF, Kostopoulos TC, Ortega-Loayza AG: Pathophysiology of pyoderma gangrenosum (PG): an updated review, *J Am Acad Dermatol* 73(4):691–698, 2015.

Brooklyn T, Dunnill G, Probert C: Diagnosis and treatment of pyoderma gangrenosum, *BMJ* 333(7560):181–184, 2006.

Cummins DL, Anhalt GJ, et al: Treatment of pyoderma gangrenosum with intravenous immunoglobulin, *Br J Dermatol* 157(6):1235–1239, 2007.

Davis MDP, Moschella SL: Neutrophilic Dermatoses: pyoderma gangrenosum. In Bolognia JL, et al: *Dermatology 2018*, ed 4, Philadelphia, 2018, Elsevier, pp 459–463.

Maverakis E, Ma C, et al: Diagnostic criteria of ulcerative pyoderma gangrenosum: a Delphi consensus of international experts, *JAMA Dermatol* 154(4):461–466, 2018.

Neill BC, Seger EW, et al: The 5 P's of pyoderma gangrenosum, *J of Drugs in Dermatol* 18(12):1283, 2019.

Patel F, Fitzmaurice S, et al: Effective strategies for the management of pyoderma gangrenosum: a comprehensive review, *Acta Derm Venereol* 95(5):525–531, 2015.

ROSACEA

Method of
Cassie Scripter, MD

CURRENT DIAGNOSIS

- Rosacea is a chronic dermatologic disease characterized by exacerbations and remissions. It affects the central face.
- Rosacea is a clinical diagnosis based on the phenotype. Diagnosis based on phenotype allows the clinician to tailor the patient's treatment based on patient symptoms and preferences.
- The diagnosis of rosacea is made if one of two diagnostic phenotype or two of four major phenotypes are present. Diagnostic phenotypes are (1) fixed centrofacial erythema that may periodically intensify and (2) phymatous changes, which most commonly affect the nose. Major phenotypes include papules and pustules, flushing/transient erythema, telangiectasia, and ocular manifestations.

CURRENT THERAPY

- Identification and avoidance of triggers is essential. Emphasize the importance of proper skin care when discussing treatment.
- Two topical medications are FDA approved for fixed centrofacial erythema: brimonidine topical 0.33% gel (Mirvaso) and oxymetazoline hydrochloride 1% cream (Rhofade).
- Inflammatory papules/pustules can be treated with topical metronidazole (MetroCream, Noritate, MetroLotion, Rosadan, MetroGel), topical azelaic acid (Finacea 15% foam or gel, Azelex 20% cream[1]), or ivermectin cream (Soolantra). Doxycycline delayed release (Oracea) 40 mg once daily is an option in moderate to severe cases.
- Isotretinoin (Accutane)[1] can be used for severe treatment refractory papules and pustules.
- Phymatous changes typically require ablative laser therapy or surgical intervention if severe and disfiguring.
- Eyelid hygiene is important in the treatment of ocular rosacea.

[1]Not FDA approved for this indication.

TABLE 1	Rosacea Diagnostic Criteria
DIAGNOSTIC PHENOTYPES (1 FOR DIAGNOSIS)	**MAJOR PHENOTYPES (2 FOR DIAGNOSIS)**
Persistent centrofacial erythema	Papules and pustules
Phymatous changes	Flushing/transient erythema
	Telangiectasias
	Ocular manifestations

TABLE 2	Treatment of Persistent Centrofacial Erythema	
TREATMENT		**DOSAGE AND FREQUENCY**
Brimonidine topical (Mirvaso)		0.33% gel once daily
Oxymetazoline hydrochloride (Rhofade)		1% cream once daily
Laser and light therapies		Varies

Epidemiology

Rosacea is a chronic inflammatory dermatologic disease affecting the central face that is characterized by exacerbation and remission of symptoms. It is estimated that up to 5.5% of the population may have rosacea. Rosacea predominantly affects women between 30 and 50 years.

Pathophysiology

The pathogenesis of rosacea is not fully understood but is likely multifactorial. Immune system dysregulation, vascular dysfunction, cutaneous microorganisms, and genetic factors have all been proposed as possible contributors to the development of rosacea.

Clinical Manifestations

Clinical manifestations of rosacea can include flushing, papules, pustules, erythema, telangiectasias, and phymas. Ocular manifestations such as dryness, burning, photophobia, and blurred vision occur in 50% to 75% of patients diagnosed with rosacea. More concerning ocular symptoms including corneal inflammation and scarring, globe perforation, and vision loss are seen in advanced disease. Phymatous skin changes, resulting from hypertrophy of the sebaceous glands and fibrosis, are more likely to affect males and usually involve the nose.

Diagnosis

The diagnosis of rosacea is based on the phenotype (Table 1). Classifying rosacea based on phenotype allows the clinician to individualize care based on patient presentation and preference. The diagnosis is made if one of two diagnostic phenotypes or two of four major phenotypes are present. Patient history and physical exam are key for diagnosis as no laboratory test exists. Biopsy is rarely necessary.

The two diagnostic phenotypes include (1) chronic centrofacial erythema that may periodically intensify and (2) phymatous changes, which most commonly affect the nose. Major phenotypes include papules and pustules, flushing/transient erythema, telangiectasia, and ocular manifestations that include lid margin telangiectasia, interpalpebral conjunctival injection, spade-shaped infiltrates in the corner, scleritis, and sclerokeratitis.

Minor, or secondary, phenotypes may appear with diagnostic or major phenotypes but are not specific to the disorder. These secondary features include burning or stinging sensation, edema, and dryness. Additional secondary manifestations set forth by the National Rosacea Society include "honey crust" and collarette accumulation at the base of the lashes, irregularity of the lid margin, and rapid tear breakup time.

Differential Diagnosis

The differential diagnosis includes acne vulgaris, perioral dermatitis, steroid-induced rosacea, sun-damaged skin, seborrheic dermatitis, dermatomyositis, flushing disorders, and lupus erythematosus.

Therapy

Management is individualized for each patient based on the phenotype and impact on the patient's quality of life. Symptoms can be diminished or controlled through a variety of modalities including appropriate skin care, avoidance of triggers, topical and oral medications, and laser- and light-based therapies.

Nonpharmacologic measures are recommended for all patients diagnosed with rosacea. One such measure includes identifying lifestyle and environmental triggers by keeping a symptom diary and then avoiding those triggers. The National Rosacea Society has a free, downloadable diary available at https://www.rosacea.org/pdf/RosaceaDiary_2021-web.pdf. Commonly identified triggers include sun exposure, stress, temperature extremes, alcohol, and certain foods. Gentle skin care focused on maintaining the skin barrier and daily sunscreen application of at least SPF 30 is also important. Evidence for skin-soothing over-the-counter products containing botanic and sulfur ingredients is lacking. Cosmetics with a green or yellow tint may lessen the erythematous appearance of the skin. More information from the National Rosacea Society regarding skin care and cosmetics can be found at https://www.rosacea.org/patients/skin-care-and-cosmetics.

Two topical medications are FDA approved for fixed centrofacial erythema, which is one of the diagnostic criteria (Table 2). These medications are brimonidine topical 0.33% gel (Mirvaso), an alpha-2 adrenergic receptor agonist, and oxymetazoline hydrochloride 1% cream (Rhofade), an alpha-1A adrenergic receptor agonist. Both are applied once daily. Common adverse effects include application site dermatitis, worsening erythema, and burning. The combination of topical brimonidine 0.33% and ivermectin 1% has shown promising improvement in both erythema and inflammation after 8 weeks of treatment. Laser- and light-based therapies may be used to treat persistent erythema.

Several options for treatment of major features are available. Mild-to-moderate inflammatory papules/pustules of rosacea can be treated with topical metronidazole in various formulations (Metro-Cream 0.75% twice daily, Noritate 1% daily, MetroLotion 0.75% twice daily, Rosadan 0.75% gel twice daily, MetroGel 1% daily), topical azelaic acid (Finacea 15% gel, Azelex 20% cream[1]) twice daily, or ivermectin cream (Soolantra 1%) once daily. Reactions to these topical preparations include irritation, burning, and stinging. Doxycycline delayed release (Oracea) 40 mg once daily can be considered if the patient presents with moderate-to-severe disease or if treatment with topical preparations is ineffective. Potential adverse reactions include gastrointestinal distress and photosensitivity. The lower-dose formulation of doxycycline has fewer adverse effects than the higher dosage of doxycycline used to treat infections. Doxycycline has not been associated with development of bacterial resistance. Other off-label oral antibiotics or isotretinoin (Accutane)[1] using weight-based dosing can also be used for treatment of refractory papules and pustules. Isotretinoin requires clinician and patient enrollment in the iPLEDGE REMS safety program at https://www.ipledgeprogram.com to mitigate the risk of isotretinoin's teratogenicity. In addition to harmful fetal effects, isotretinoin can cause cheilitis, eczema, abdominal pain, myalgias, and dry eyes. Table 3 outlines treatment options for papules and pustules. Laser and light-based therapies are effective treatments for telangiectasias.

Treatment of phyma typically involves combination therapy. Patients may benefit from tetracycline[1] therapy, as well as ablative laser therapy or surgical intervention. Adverse effects of laser ablation and surgical intervention include pain, crusting, scarring, and pigmentation changes. Oral isotretinoin (Accutane, Claravis)[1] with weight-based dosing can be considered.

Treatment of ocular rosacea includes increased eyelid hygiene twice daily with lid scrubs and warm compresses to improve meibomian gland function, as well as elimination of any medications that may cause eye dryness. Oral omega-3 fatty acids[1] have shown benefits in fighting eye dryness. Ophthalmic cyclosporine drops (Restasis)[1], one drop applied twice daily, may decrease inflammation. More severe cases may require an oral tetracycline, such as doxycycline delayed release 40 mg daily. Referral to an ophthalmologist is warranted if eyesight might be affected or if symptoms are not reduced with recommended treatments.

---

[1] Not FDA approved for this indication.

TABLE 3	Treatment of Papules and Pustules
TREATMENT	**DOSAGE AND FREQUENCY**
Metronidazole topical (MetroCream, Noritate, MetroLotion, Rosadan, MetroGel)	Cream (MetroCream) 0.75% twice daily Cream (Noritate) 1% daily Lotion (MetroLotion) 0.75% twice daily Gel (Rosadan) 0.75% twice daily Gel (MetroGel) 1% daily
Azelaic acid topical (Finacea, Azelex)	Gel (Finacea) 15% twice daily Cream (Azelex)[1] 20% twice daily
Ivermectin topical (Soolantra)	Cream (Soolantra) 1% daily
Doxycycline delayed release oral (Oracea)	40 mg daily
Isotretinoin oral (Accutane)[1]	Weight-based

[1]Not FDA approved for this indication.

References

Gold LS, Papp K, Lynde C, et al: Treatment of rosacea with concomitant use of topical ivermectin 1% cream and brimonidine 0.33% gel: a randomized, vehicle-controlled study, *J Drugs Dermatol* 16(9):909–916, 2017. PMID: 28915286.

Hampton PJ, Berth-Jones J, Duarte Williamson CE, et al: British Association of Dermatologists guidelines for the management of people with rosacea 2021, *Br J Dermatol* 185(4):725–735, 2021.

Mohamed-Noriega K, Loya-Garcia D, Vera-Duarte GR, et al: Ocular rosacea: an updated review, *Cornea* 44(4):525–537, 2025. https://doi.org/10.1097/ICO.0000000000003785.

Pakdaman SF, Samadi A, Fattahi M, et al: Fabrication and efficacy assessment of combination of brimonidine and ivermectin for treatment of papulopustular rosacea, *J Cosmet Dermatol* 23:2973–2981, 2024. https://doi.org/10.1111/jocd.16372.

Sajdeh F, Samadi A, Naeimifar A, et al: Efficacy and safety of oxymetazoline 1% cream for the treatment of mild to moderate facial rosacea, *J Cosmet Dermatol* 24(4):e16782, 2025. https://doi.org/10.1111/jocd.16782. PMID: 40165547; PMCID: PMC11959211.

Schaller M, Almeida LMC, Bewley A, et al: Recommendations for rosacea diagnosis, classification and management: update from the global ROSacea Consensus 2019 panel, *Br J Dermatol* 182:1269–1276, 2020.

Schaller M, Almeida LM, Bewley A, et al: Rosacea treatment update: recommendations from the global ROSacea COnsensus (ROSCO) panel, *Br J Dermatol* 176:465–471, 2017.

Thiboutot D, Anderson R, Cook-Bolden F, et al: Standard management options for rosacea: the 2019 update by the national rosacea society expert committee, *J Am Acad Dermatol* 82(6):1501–1510, 2020.

van Zuuren E: Rosacea, *N Engl J Med* 377:1754–1764, 2017.

van Zuuren EJ, Fedorowicz Z, Tan J, et al: Interventions for rosacea based on the phenotype approach: an updated systematic review including GRADE assessments, *Br J Dermatol* 181(1):65–79, 2019.

STEVENS-JOHNSON SYNDROME AND TOXIC EPIDERMAL NECROLYSIS

Method of
Scott Worswick, MD

CURRENT DIAGNOSIS

- A diagnosis of toxic epidermal necrolysis (TEN) can be rendered when the body surface area (BSA) involved contains more than 30% denuded skin.
- A diagnosis of Stevens-Johnson Syndrome (SJS) can be rendered when less than 10% of the BSA involves denuded skin.
- SJS-TEN overlap is diagnosed when the involved BSA is between 10% and 30% BSA.
- Patients with SJS, SJS-TEN overlap, and TEN should have involvement of not only the cutaneous surface but also at least one mucosal region (most commonly the oral mucosa). Cases do exist with no mucosal involvement but this is rare and should prompt consideration of an alternate diagnosis.
- A thorough drug history and skin biopsy (ideally using the fresh-frozen technique) are essential when considering a diagnosis of SJS or TEN.

CURRENT THERAPY

- Conservative therapy is a cornerstone of therapy for all patients. This includes appropriate wound care, monitoring for fluid loss and electrolyte imbalance, thorough daily skin exams, and monitoring of vital signs to rule out concurrent infection.
- A dermatologist should be involved in the care of all hospitalized patients with Stevens-Johnson Syndrome and toxic epidermal necrolysis. In the appropriate clinical context, ophthalmology and OBGYN should also be involved. Depending on hospital resources, ICU and/or plastic surgery and the burn unit should be involved early in the care of these patients.
- Classically, systemic corticosteroids and intravenous immunoglobulin (IVIG)[1] were utilized in the management of these patients. New data suggest either cyclosporine (Neoral, Sandimmune)[1] or etanercept (Enbrel)[1] may improve overall outcomes.

[1]Not FDA approved for this indication.

Epidemiology

Toxic epidermal necrolysis (TEN) is a rare diagnosis, only afflicting approximately one patient per million per year (most studies cite this incidence rate, though one study from the United States did cite an incidence rate as high as 12.7 per year). Stevens-Johnson Syndrome (SJS) and SJS-TEN overlap affect approximately five per million patients per year. The overall mortality varies greatly among different studies but has classically been estimated to be ~25% for TEN. It can affect patients of any age, and most data regarding therapy are stratified by age into pediatric and adult cohorts. There are some experts who feel there may be a viral trigger or co-factor for the disease because prevalence increases in the spring.

Risk Factors

Common implicated agents include sulfonamide antibiotics as well as more recently described penicillin and cephalosporin antibiotics, aromatic anticonvulsants, allopurinol, and nonsteroidal antiinflammatory drugs (NSAIDs). Numerous other medications have been reported to trigger the disease and some other common offending agents include the anti-programmed death-1 and anti-cytotoxic T-lymphocyte-associated protein 4 chemotherapeutic agents, dapsone and nevirapine (Viramune). The most important intervention is to determine and remove the offending agent as some studies cite an increase in mortality of 34% per day if the offending agent is not removed from the patient's regimen.

Certain tests can be performed after hospitalization in selected cases to determine the most likely offending agent if unknown. For example, patch testing can be done, and in the case of carbamazepine-induced SJS-TEN, has a sensitivity greater than 70%. Likewise, if multiple drugs are suspected as potential inciting agents, it may be worth checking the patient's human leukocyte antigen (HLA) types and correlating this with his/her ethnicity to make an educated guess about likely agent (if a patient has three potential inciting agents including allopurinol, the patient is of Asian descent, and HLA-typing reveals positive HLA-B5801, it could be concluded with a higher level of certainty that allopurinol is the most likely agent).

Less common triggers include vaccines such as MMR and less commonly the meningococcal, varicella and influenza vaccines, herpes, and ultraviolet light. These are more likely to be implicated in patients with target lesions or low body surface area (BSA) involvement and are exceedingly rare in patients diagnosed with full-blown TEN. An important trigger to consider in the work-up is mycoplasma, which can be responsible for causing mycoplasma-induced rash and mucositis (MIRM). MIRM is a clinical mimicker common in pediatric patients, which is characterized by lower BSA but worse mucosal involvement (typically involving two sites and usually including the ocular mucosa in dramatic fashion). Other infectious agents have been reported to cause a similar eruption that is called reactive infectious mucocutaneous eruption (RIME). These include COVID-19, influenza B, *C. pneumoniae*, enterovirus, rhinovirus, human metapneumovirus, and human parainfluenza virus 2.

In addition to the causes of SJS and TEN described previously, there are risk factors that seem to predispose patients to the disease. These include: HIV (some studies cite a thousand-times increased chance of developing TEN among HIV-positive patients, even when controlled for the number and type of medications these patients were exposed to), lupus, female gender, Asian or African ethnicity, patients undergoing brain cancer treatment with corticosteroids and radiation, and certain HLA types. For example, one recent meta-analysis found that certain HLA-B subtypes predispose Asian patients to the development of carbamazepine-induced TEN, including HLA-B1502, HLA-B4001, HLA-B4601, and HLA-B5801. Other studies have identified HLA-B1502 as a risk factor for aromatic anticonvulsant-induced TEN among various Asian populations, HLA-B5801 as a risk factor for allopurinol-induced TEN among Asians, HLA-C0401 for nevirapine-induced TEN among patients in Malawi, and HLA types B3802, A29, B12, and DR7 as a risk factor among Europeans for sulfonamide-induced TEN.

Pathophysiology

As described previously, an immunologic basis for the development SJS and TEN is hypothesized given the fact that certain HLA types among certain groups predispose them to development of the disease. There currently exist four theories to explain how small drugs might interact with HLA and T-cell receptors (TCRs) to initiate a chain of events leading to SJS/TEN.

In the hapten theory (which has been validated in the case of penicillin-induced drug reactions), it is presumed that the drug molecule combines with an endogenous peptide and this is presented to the HLA molecule and recognized by the TCR. In the p-i model (pharmacologic interaction with the immune receptors), which has been validated in carbamazepine-HLA-B1502 interactions, the drug itself binds directly, reversibly, and noncovalently to HLA and/or TCR. In the altered peptide repertoire model, it is proposed that the drug binds to the peptide-binding groove of the HLA molecule thereby altering the overall binding ability of the HLA molecule. Lastly, in the altered TCR repertoire model, it is suggested that some drugs (such as sulfamethoxazole) can bind directly to the TCR (but not with the HLA molecule) and thereby alter the conformation of the TCR giving them the ability to bind to self-HLA.

Regardless of the type of interaction that allows a drug to alter the way HLA and TCR react to self, patients with TEN exhibit increased activity of natural killer (NK) cells and specific T lymphocytes (NK T-cells and CD* + cytotoxic T-cells). These cells mediate keratinocyte cell death via a cascade of events including Fas–FasL binding and procaspase-8 activation, increased tumor necrosis factor-α and interferon-γ levels, and activation of the perforin-granzyme-granulysin apoptosis pathway.

Differential Diagnosis

Patients with SJS and TEN typically complain of skin pain before the eruption begins. A prodrome consisting of low-grade fever, malaise, and/or flu-like symptoms is not uncommon. Within days some degree of mucosal involvement (which can take the form of dusky erythema, bullae/vesicles, denuded mucosal surface(s), dysuria, ocular erythema, pain with defecation, or pain with swallowing) is almost universal, while the extent of cutaneous involvement can vary dramatically but should include either a dusky erythema with eventual vesicles, bullae, or denuded skin, or less commonly targetoid lesions. The majority of patients with SJS and TEN present with painful red-purple (dusky) patches or macules that progress over the span of a few days. Areas that began with dusky erythema develop superimposed bullae, vesicles, or denuded skin.

Most patients with SJS and TEN do not present with typical targets on cutaneous exam. Such lesions are characterized by a small red central papule surrounded by a white ring and finally most peripherally by another ring of erythema. These lesions characterize erythema multiforme, which is much more commonly the result of herpes rather than drug allergy. However, there are rare reported cases of SJS and TEN that do include or are even dominated by cutaneous typical or atypical targets.

The main differential diagnosis for patients with classic dusky erythema, mucosal involvement, and skin pain includes acute graft-versus-host disease (GVHD), bullous lupus, generalized fixed drug eruption (FDE), cutaneous burns, and paraneoplastic pemphigus (PNP); in pediatric patients especially MIRM and RIME; and in infants infection with the Chikungunya virus. The majority of these entities can be ruled out by clinical history alone, as patients with acute GVHD should have had a recent transplant and patients with PNP a concurrent malignancy. Dramatic mucosal involvement, in any age group, should prompt work-up for mycoplasma and RIME; when MIRM is suspected it should be treated with empiric antibiotics and in severe cases IVIG[1]. Patients with a known malignancy (particularly chronic lymphocytic leukemia [CLL], lymphoma, Castleman disease, sarcoma, or thymoma) and/or of older age and with significant mucosal disease should have, in addition to a biopsy, a direct immunofluorescence (DIF) performed and serum drawn for indirect immunofluorescence and ELISA performed to rule out PNP. It is important to check a DIF as well in any patients with joint pain or other symptoms suggestive of systemic lupus erythematosus (SLE), as well as antinuclear antibody (ANA), anti-Sjogren's syndrome–related antigen (SSA), and anti-Sjogren's Syndrome Type B (SSB), anti-dsDNA and anti-Smith. Likewise, if you are evaluating an infant who has no medication exposure and is from an endemic area, it is important to check serum titers for the Chikungunya virus.

Diagnosis

Determining the inciting agent is as important as making a quick diagnosis of TEN. A thorough drug history is essential including prn medication usage (frequently patients do not report their NSAID use or a recent antibiotic exposure). If SJS or TEN is suspected and the inciting agent is known, it is important to immediately inform the patient and his/her family of the suspected allergy and add it to the patient's medication allergy list. Dermatology should be consulted and when possible/necessary will ideally perform a skin biopsy to be processed emergently using the fresh-frozen technique (results can be ready within 30 minutes). Hematoxylin and eosin staining will also be done on permanent sections (and these results are available 1 to 3 days later depending on the site/lab).

After making a diagnosis of SJS or TEN, a practitioner can employ a scoring system called SCORTEN to estimate the patient's mortality. In this system a patient receives one point if he/she is aged above 40 years, BSA greater than 10%, history of concurrent malignancy within 2 years, serum blood urea nitrogen greater than 28 mg/dL, glucose greater than 252 mg/dL, bicarbonate level less than 20 mEq/L, and heart rate more than 120 beats per minute during the first 24 hours. With each increasing point, mortality increases such that a score of 2 confers an expected mortality of 12%; a score of 3 equates to a 35% mortality; a score of 4 with a 58% mortality; and a score of 5 or higher with an expected 90% chance of mortality.

Therapy
Medical Therapy

Classic therapy for SJS and TEN was with systemic corticosteroids but this has fallen out of favor in the United States due to recent meta-analyses suggesting no improvement in outcomes. Likewise, IVIG[1] was a mainstay of therapy in the early 21st century, but a large review from Europe found a worsened mortality in patients given IVIG compared with those given steroids or supportive care alone. Other data are conflicting with some studies suggesting that a 4-day dose of daily 1 g/kg IV[1] provides a mortality benefit, with other studies finding no improvement.

More recent success seems to have come from the utilization of etanercept (Enbrel)[1] or cyclosporine (Neoral, Sandimmune)[1] in the treatment of this disease. In 2014 a group from Italy treated

---

[1]Not FDA approved for this indication.
[1]Not FDA approved for this indication.

10 patients with one 50 mg subcutaneous dose and found not only a 0% mortality despite an expected mortality of 47%, but also decreased time to re-epithelialization. Likewise, in 2018 a Taiwanese group found an improved mortality benefit of etanercept over corticosteroids among 96 patients.

Similarly, data emerging in the last decade have suggested that cyclosporine also confers a mortality benefit. In 2010 a British case series found a 0% mortality in patients receiving 3 mg/kg per day orally despite a predicated ~30% mortality based on SCORTEN. Another study cites a significantly decreased time to re-epithelialization (3.67 days) among patients who survived after receiving cyclosporine at a dose of 3 to 4 mg/kg per day.

Adjuvant Mucosal Therapies

Patients with SJS/TEN can suffer from long-term skin/hair/nail complications including post-inflammatory hyperpigmentation, photosensitivity (70% of patients according to one study), chronic pruritus, eruptive nevi, nail changes, hypertrophic scars, and telogen effluvium. They also have a significant morbidity when their mucosal surfaces are severely involved with disease. Ocular complications can include ectropion, trichiasis, ankyloblepharon, corneal scarring, and even blindness. To some extent these complications are minimized by a choice of systemic therapy to mediate disease (i.e., either etanercept or cyclosporine). However, other measures can also be employed including amniotic membrane grafting by ophthalmology (which has been shown in a randomized controlled trial to improve multiple ocular outcome measures), topical steroid application, oxygen therapy, and bronchodilators. Likewise, urogenital sequelae occur in about one in four patients and can include adhesions leading to dyspareunia or even total vaginal fusion. Therefore involvement of gynecology or urology in the care of any patient with genital SJS/TEN is essential.

Monitoring

It is important to remember that the cutaneous examination of a patient with TEN differs greatly depending on the time of exam relative to the onset of eruption. With onset it is possible the patient will only complain of pain and have no skin lesions whatsoever. Within days a typical exam would include florid oral mucosal involvement with areas of skin showing dusky erythematous macules or patches. Over the next few days, most of the cutaneous lesions will evolve and become vesicles, bullae, or entire surfaces will denude. Monitoring for efficacy of chosen therapy means being aware of what is expected in terms of progression (that some or all areas that were dusky will denude), and ensuring that no new dusky areas develop.

The most common cause of death in patients with TEN is infection, so checking daily white blood cell counts and following vitals every 2 to 4 hours if not more frequently is essential. Fevers can occur simply as the result of the disease process itself, but any fever should prompt blood, urine, and sputum cultures. Prophylactic antibiotics have not been shown to improve outcomes but when an infection is suspected it must be treated immediately.

References

Brüggen M-C, Le ST, Walsh S, et al: Supportive care in the acute phase of Stevens-Johnson syndrome and toxic epidermal necrolysis: an international, multi-disciplinary Delphi-based consensus, *Br J Dermatol* 185(3):616–626, 2021.

Canavan TN, Mathes EF, Friedan I, et al: Mycoplasma pneumonia-induced rash and mucositis as a syndrome distinct from Stevens-Johnson syndrome and erythema multiforme: A systematic review, *JAAD* 72(2):239–245, 2015.

Chahal D, Aleshin M, Turegano M, et al: Vaccine-induced TEN: A case and systematic review, *Dermatology, Online Journal* 24(1), 2018.

Chen CB, Abe R, Pan RY, et al: An updated review of the molecular mechanisms in drug hypersensitivity, *Journal of Immunology Research*, 2018.

Conner C, McKenzie E, Owen C: The use of cyclosporine for SJS-TEN spectrum at the University of Louisville: A case series and literature review, *Dermatology Online Journal* 24(1), 2018.

Lee HY, Walsh SA, Creamer D: Long-term complications of SJS/TEN: The spectrum of chronic problems in patients who survive an episode of SJS/TEN necessitates multidisciplinary follow-up, *British Journal of Dermatology* 177:924–935, 2017.

Ortiz EG, Junkins-Hopkins JM: Reactive infectious mucocutaneous eruption due to COVID-19 with erythema-multiforma-like lesions and myeloid cells, *J Cutan Pathol* 50(4):321–325, 2022.

Paradisi A, et al: Etanercept therapy for TEN, *JAAD* 71(2):278–283, 2014.

Schneck J, et al: Effects of treatment on the mortality of SJS and TEN: A retrospective study on patients included in the prospective EuroSCAR Study, *JAAD* 58(1):33–40, 2008.

Valeyrie-Allanore L, Wolkenstein P, Brochard L, et al: Open trial of ciclosporin treatment for SJS and TEN, *British Journal of Dermatology* 163(4):847–853, 2010.

Wang CW, Yang LY, Chen CB, et al: Randomized, controlled trial of TNF-alpha antagonist in CTL-mediated severe cutaneous adverse reactions, *J Clin Invest* 128(3):985–996, 2018.

Wang Q, Sun S, Xie M, et al: Association between the HLA-B alleles and carbamazepine-induced SJS/TEN: A meta-analysis, *Epilepsy Research* 135:19–28, 2017.

SUNBURN

Method of
Kamille S. Sherman, MD

CURRENT DIAGNOSIS

- Typically a first-degree or second-degree burn occurring on sun-exposed or ultraviolet (UV)-exposed (e.g., tanning bed) skin within 4 hours to 2 days of exposure
- May be demarcated from unaffected skin by an obvious boundary where protective clothing prevented the sun or UV exposure, with the burned area having a consistent, continuous appearance

CURRENT THERAPY

- Over the counter nonsteroidal antiinflammatory drugs (NSAIDs) or acetaminophen at doses as directed by the manufacturer on the packaging can relieve pain and decrease inflammation but will not change long-term damage to the skin. Some experts recommend a short-term course of oral steroids if a large area of skin is sunburned.
- Cool the skin, either with a cool bath/shower or apply a cool, damp towel or wear cool, damp flannel clothing over the affected area.
- Drink plenty of water to prevent dehydration or rehydrate if mildly dehydrated.
- Do not break any blisters on the skin.
- Do not apply benzocaine or other "-caine" types of products, as they can irritate the skin, cause allergic reactions, or precipitate methemoglobinemia.
- Apply a soothing moisturizer, such as aloe vera[7] or calamine, PRN. This may be in lotion or gel form.
- As skin heals, apply hydrating moisturizers.
- As healing occurs, avoid reinjury/reexposure of affected skin to sun or UV light.
- Assess for secondary infection and treat if necessary.
- Review patient medication list, as some over-the-counter and prescription drugs and herbal remedies increase sensitivity to UV light.

[7]Available as dietary supplement.

Epidemiology

In a study of 31,162 US adults, using the 2015 National Health Interview Survey (NHIS) Cancer Control Supplement, a total of 34.2% of adults experienced sunburn in 2015. Of those experiencing sunburn, 16.3% experienced one sunburn, 9.9% experienced two sunburns, 3.4% experienced three sunburns, and 4.6% experienced four or more sunburns. There is epidemiologic evidence suggesting that the harmful effects of UV radiation exposure from typical doses of sunlight vary over the course of the life span, with some evidence of a window of biologic vulnerability in childhood that translates into increased skin cancer risk later in life.

Risk Factors

"Sun sensitivity" was assessed using two questions in the 2015 NHIS Cancer Control study. One question asked what would happen to the respondent's skin if, after several months of not being in the sun, the individual went out in the sun for an hour without sunscreen, a hat, or protective clothing (short exposure). The second question asked the individual what would happen if he or she were out in the sun repeatedly, such as every day for 2 weeks, without sunscreen, a hat, or protective clothing (i.e., repeated exposure). About half of individuals who described themselves as "sun sensitive" indicated they would experience sunburn (50.2%).

Non-Hispanic white individuals are more likely to experience sunburn than other racial/ethnic groups. Adults who self-reported skin that tended to burn after repeated sun exposure were more likely to become sunburned as compared with individuals who easily develop tans. Behaviors associated with sunburn include use of self-applied tanning products, aerobic activity, binge drinking in the past 30 days, and overweight or obesity. An increase in the number of sunburns an individual experiences is directly related to an increase in the risk of skin cancer.

Approximately 50.2% of adults aged 18 to 29 years reported having experienced sunburn, as did 14.8% of adults aged 66 years or older.

The level of UV protection afforded by clothing can vary widely based on color, material, and weave of the fabric. The US Preventive Services Task Force (USPSTF) reports that indoor tanning before age 35 years, or more than 10 tanning sessions over a lifetime and for longer than 1 year, have been linked to increased skin cancer risk.

Pathophysiology

UV radiation (both A and B) from both solar and artificial sources has been classified as a human carcinogen by national and international organizations. UVA damage is associated with "aging," whereas UVB is associated with "burning." UVB rays are responsible for directly damaging skin cell DNA by inducing the formation of thymine-thymine cyclobutane dimers. As the body generates a DNA repair response to these dimers, inflammatory markers lead to vasodilation, edema, and pain, which manifest as classic-appearing sunburn. UVB light also activates peripheral nociceptors by causing an increase in chemokines.

Prevention

The most frequently used sun protection behaviors among US adults include staying in the shade (37.1%) and using sunscreen (31.5%). About one-fourth of those engaging in sun-protective behaviors wear long clothing to the ankles (28.4%). Less frequent behaviors include regular use of long-sleeved shirts (12.3%) and wide-brimmed hats (14.2%). Women are more likely to use shade (41.3%) and sunscreen (40.2%) as protective behaviors, whereas men are more likely to wear long clothing to the ankles (34.3%) and to use shade (30.7%).

The sun protection factor (SPF) is a relative measure of the fraction of sunburn-producing UV rays that reach the skin. Assuming correct application, "SPF 20" means that one-twentieth of the burning radiation will reach the skin. The effectiveness of a sunscreen can be calculated by multiplying the SPF by the length of time it takes a user to suffer a burn without sunscreen. For example, if a person develops a sunburn in 20 minutes when not wearing a sunscreen, using an SPF 30 sunscreen would protect the individual for about 10 hours. Because the intensity and wavelength distribution of UVB rays varies throughout the day and by latitude, the effectiveness of sunscreen also varies. Direct exposure to the sun should be avoided between the hours of 10 A.M. and 4 P.M. A broad-spectrum sunscreen with SPF of at least 30 should be applied 30 minutes before sun exposure and every 90 minutes thereafter, even if the product is labeled "water resistant."

There are many suggestions regarding the appropriate use of sunscreen, although the NHIS found that sunscreen users were actually more likely to experience sunburn. This probably happens because sunscreen users are out in the sun more frequently than those who do not use sunscreen regularly.

Along with recommending staying in the shade, the American Cancer Society uses a slogan popularized in Australia as one of that country's skin cancer prevention strategies: "Slip! Slop! Slap! ... and Wrap!" The phrase is a way to remind individuals to slip on a shirt, slop on sunscreen, slap on a hat, and wrap on sunglasses to protect eyes and sensitive skin from the sun's harmful rays.

Clinical Manifestations

Sunburn appears most often as a first-degree burn—an injury affecting the epidermis and associated with erythema, pain, and mild swelling followed by skin peeling. More severe sunburn may lead to second-degree burns, in which blisters accompany the erythema and swelling. Second-degree sunburns hurt more significantly and affect both the epidermis and dermis. These burns can take several weeks to heal.

Diagnosis

The diagnosis is based largely on the history of sun exposure coupled with the classic appearance and distribution of sunburn.

Differential Diagnosis

The differential diagnosis of sunburn includes autoimmune diseases such as systemic lupus erythematosus and dermatomyositis; bacterial infections such as staphylococcal scalded skin syndrome, cellulitis, and erysipelas; and dermatologic diseases such as rosacea, acne, stasis dermatitis, and seborrheic dermatitis. There are also congenital ichthyotic conditions. Other solar reactions caused by the sun's rays include solar urticaria, photoallergic type IV sensitivity reactions, and phototoxic reactions.

Treatment

Treatment for sunburn is largely supportive. Oral analgesics, such as nonsteroidal antiinflammatory drugs and/or acetaminophen, provide some relief. Cool bathing, cool towels, and flannel clothing moistened with cool water can provide some comfort. Moisturizing topical products such as aloe vera or calamine may provide comfort. Some experts recommend steroid usage, either topical or orally, although consensus on their use is mixed and steroids are usually reserved for patients with extensive areas of sunburn. Treatment of secondary skin infections, especially if broken blisters are infected, includes antibiotic usage for common skin pathogens. The avoidance of local anesthetic creams and sprays containing "-caine" derivatives is standard advice. "Caines" can irritate the skin, cause allergic reactions, and precipitate methemoglobinemia. Opioids for pain associated with sunburn should be avoided except in the most unusual circumstances. Adequate water intake to prevent or reverse dehydration is encouraged. In the rare case of extensive sunburn with large areas of blistering accompanied by massive fluid loss and electrolyte imbalances, intravenous rehydration may be considered as well as transfer to a burn unit. Avoiding another sunburn, especially before the first one appears "healed," is important. The DNA damage caused by sunburn is not reversible. There are no topical or systemic agents that are FDA approved to reverse UV damage to the skin.

Monitoring and Complications

Most sunburns are self-limited and will heal over a number of days to weeks, at least appearing "healed" to casual inspection. Patients who suffer severe sunburn should be warned to watch for the development of secondary infections. The underlying DNA changes in the skin are linked to the development of skin cancers, including melanoma. The USPSTF recommends "counseling young adults, adolescents, children, and parents of young children about minimizing exposure to UV radiation for persons aged 6 months to 24 years with fair skin types to reduce their risk of skin cancer."

The USPSTF concludes that current evidence is insufficient to assess the balance of benefits and harms of counseling adults about skin self-examination. Evaluation of suspicious skin lesions should be undertaken by physicians, with monitoring and/or removal of suspicious lesions.

Skin cancer is the most common type of cancer in the United States. Although invasive melanoma accounts for 2% of skin cancer types, it is responsible for 80% of skin cancer deaths. Basal and squamous cell carcinoma, the two predominant types of nonmelanoma skin cancer, represent the vast majority of skin cancers. About 5.4 million basal and squamous cell skin cancers are diagnosed in the United States each year; they occur in an estimated 3.3 million Americans, as some people have more than one. About 8 out of 10 of these are basal cell cancers. About 2000 people die from basal or squamous cell skin cancers in the United States annually. There will be an estimated 100,350 new cases of melanoma skin cancer in 2020. The 5-year survival rate for melanoma, according to the American Cancer Society, is 92%. Treatment for skin cancer can include surgery and radiation therapy, as well as some newer forms of nonsurgical treatment such as novel topical drugs, photodynamic therapy, and laser surgery.

References

Guerra KC, Crane JS: Sunburn. [Updated 2019 Nov 25]. In: StatPearls [Internet]. Treasure Island.

Holman DM, Ding H, Guy GP, et al: Prevalence of sun protection use and sunburn and association of demographic and behavioral characteristics with sunburn among us adults, *JAMA Dermatol* 154(5):561–568, 2018 May, Published online 2018 Mar 14.

US Environmental Protection Agency: Sun safety. Available at https://www.epa.gov/sunsafety. [Accessed 13 January 2020].

US Food and Drug Administration: Sunscreen: how to help protect your skin from the sun. Available at https://www.fda.gov/Drugs/ResourcesForYou/Consumers/BuyingUsingMedicineSafely/UnderstandingOver-the-CounterMedicines/ucm239463. [Accessed 2 December 2019].

U.S. Preventive Services Task Force: Final recommendation statement: skin cancer prevention: behavioral counseling. Available at https://www.uspreventiveservicestaskforce.org/Page/Document/RecommendationStatementFinal/skin-cancer-counseling2. [Accessed 2 December 2019].

URTICARIA AND ANGIOEDEMA

Method of
Joyce M.C. Teng, MD, PhD

CURRENT DIAGNOSIS

- Acute and chronic urticaria have the same features, including erythematous, edematous papules or wheals with central pallor that last less than 24 to 48 hours.
- Laboratory assessments are not recommended for acute urticaria in the absence of evidence suggesting underlying systemic illness.
- Limited laboratory studies are indicated for chronic urticaria only if there are signs of systemic disease.
- Serum measurements of C4 and C1-esterase inhibitor are the recommended initial tests if hereditary or acquired angioedema are suspected.
- Skin biopsy should be considered to rule out urticarial vasculitis if an individual lesion is painful and persists for more than 2 to 3 days with accompanying ecchymosis or petechiae.

CURRENT THERAPY

- Primary treatment of urticaria and angioedema is removal of triggering factors and initiation of therapy for symptomatic relief.
- Oral antihistamines are the cornerstones of therapy. The application of first-generation H_1-antihistamines may be limited by central nervous system and anticholinergic side effects.
- Nonsedating second generation antihistamine are often used as first line therapy. Higher dose can be used when symptoms are not controlled.
- Anti-IgE therapy, omalizumab (Xolair), has been approved for patients over 12 years of age with chronic idiopathic urticaria. Systemic corticosteroids and immunosuppressive therapy, especially cyclosporine (Neoral),[1] have been used successfully in cases that are refractory to the maximum dose of antihistamines.
- Fresh-frozen plasma infusions along with standard airway precautions have been recommended for angioedema patients with laryngeal edema.
- A subcutaneous C1 esterase inhibitor injection (Haegarda) has been used successfully to prevent attack in hereditary angioedema.

[1]Not FDA approved for this indication.

Urticaria, or hives, is a common cutaneous eruption that occurs in up to 25% of the general population sometime during their lives (Bailey, 2008). It is characterized by transient, circumscribed, pruritic, erythematous papules or plaques, often with central pallor. Individual lesions often coalesce into large wheals on the trunk and extremities that may resolve over a few hours without leaving any residual skin changes. The process is mediated by mast cells in the superficial dermis, and skin changes often resolve within 30 min to 24 hr.

Angioedema is a similar process occurring in deep dermis or subcutaneous tissue. Angioedema may occur independently, accompanied by urticaria, or as a component of anaphylaxis. It is characterized by localized swelling that develops over minutes to hours and resolution may take up to 72 hours. Common locations of angioedema include the mucosa and areas with loose connective tissue, such as the face, eyes, lips, tongue, and genitalia. Patients usually do not have pruritus, but they may have pain and a sensation of warmth. Angioedema is usually a benign process that resolves without sequelae unless it involves the larynx. African Americans are disproportionately affected, representing up to 40% of the hospital admissions for angioedema.

Classification

Urticaria can be classified as acute or chronic, depending on the duration. Acute urticaria usually lasts for less than 6 weeks and can be spontaneous or triggered by infection, medication, insect bite, and food (Table 1). The chronic form, lasting more than 6 weeks, accounts for approximately 30% of cases of urticaria, and no clear causes can be identified in more than 80% of these cases. Stress however has been identified as a trigger in some of the cases. Depending on the triggers, chronic urticaria can be classified as cold, heat, solar, delayed pressure, vibratory, cholinergic, contact, or aquagenic urticaria. A significant number of patients with chronic urticaria may have persistent symptoms for more than 10 years. Approximately 40% of patients with chronic urticaria have associated angioedema, although the incidence of laryngeal edema is low.

Diagnosis

Urticaria is diagnosed clinically in most cases. A detailed history, physical examination, and complete review of systems are essential for diagnosing patients with urticaria and angioedema.

TABLE 1	Mechanisms in Urticaria and Angioedema
DISORDER	**CAUSES**
Immunoglobulin-mediated urticaria	Ig-E mediated: food, medication, insect bites, contact allergen, aeroallergens, other causes Urticaria associated with autoimmunity: antinuclear antibodies (ANAs), thyroid autoantibodies, other causes
Direct activation of mast cell degranulation	Physical stimuli: exercise, heat, cold, pressure, aquagenic, solar radiation, etc. Other agents: opiates, antibiotics (e.g., vancomycin [Vancocin]), radiocontrast, ACTH (Cortrosyn), muscle relaxants
Complement-mediated	Viral infections, parasites, blood transfusion
C1-esterase inhibitor deficiency	Genetic and acquired angioedema, paraproteinemia
Reduced kinin metabolism	Angiotensin-converting enzyme (ACE) inhibitors
Reduced arachidonic acid metabolism	Aspirin

The history should include the distribution and characteristics of lesions (e.g., pain, pruritus), duration of skin eruption, accompanying angioedema, airway involvement and other associated systemic symptoms (e.g., fever, arthralgia, swelling joints, refusal to walk by children). Patients should also be questioned about changes in dietary habits, stress, recent exposures, infection, and newly administered medications, including antibiotics, over-the-counter analgesia, and hormones. Patients who suffer from recurrent angioedema should be asked about their use of angiotensin-converting enzyme (ACE) inhibitor medications.

Laboratory assessment is usually not helpful in diagnosing patients with acute urticaria who lack any history or clinical findings to suggest an underlying disease process. A limited number of diagnostic tests are indicated in the evaluation of patients with chronic urticaria when there is sign of systemic disease associated, such as a complete blood cell count with differential white blood cell count, an erythrocyte sedimentation rate (ESR) or C-reactive protein (CRP) determination, a thyroid-stimulating hormone (TSH) level, antithyroglobulin and antimicrosomal antibodies, antinuclear antibodies (ANA), folate, B12, ferritin, liver function test, and hepatitis B and C serologies. A detailed review of systems may help to narrow the focus of the screening test.

A skin biopsy of an early lesion should be performed to rule out urticarial vasculitis if the affected individual has skin lesions that are painful and last for more than 2 to 3 days with residual ecchymosis or petechiae. In patients with angioedema, prominent edema of the interstitial tissue may be demonstrated by biopsy. It is associated with antibodies against C1q, which leads to persistent complement activation and low serum C3, C4. Serum measurements of C4 and C1-esterase inhibitor are recommended initial tests if hereditary or acquired angioedema is suspected. Hereditary angioedema is caused by deficiency (type I) or dysfunction (type II) of C1-esterase inhibitor protein. A C1q level should be obtained to screen for the acquired form of angioedema if the affected individual is middle-aged. Additional constitutional symptoms and extracutaneous manifestations are often present in patients with autoinflammatory syndromes such as Schnitzler's syndrome, cryopyrin-associated periodic syndrome (CAPS), Muckle-Wells syndrome (MWS), neonatal-onset multisystem inflammatory disease (NOMID) and, rarely, hyper-IgD syndrome (HIDS) and tumor necrosis factor receptor alpha-associated periodic syndrome (TRAPS).

Treatment

More than two thirds of cases of urticaria are self-limited. Spontaneous remission of chronic urticaria and angioedema is also common. The primary objective of management is to identify and discontinue the offending trigger. A patient presenting with angioedema must first be assessed for signs of airway compromise. Medical therapy is indicated for those who are symptomatic.

Antihistamines remain the first-line therapy for most patients with urticaria, because the primary complaint of pruritus is predominantly mediated by histamine released from mast cells. First-generation antihistamines such as hydroxyzine (Atarax or Vistaril 1 mg/kg (max 25 mg/dose) for children and 25–50 mg every 6 hours in adults), diphenhydramine (Benadryl 25–50 mg every 6 hours), cyproheptadine (Periactin 4 mg three times daily), and chlorpheniramine[1] (Chlor-Trimeton 4 mg every 6 hours) are potent and have the quickest onset of action. However, the treatments are often limited by their sedating and anticholinergic side effects. Many first-generation antihistamines are available over the counter, providing accessible first-line therapy for patients. Patients with urticaria that lasts for several days should be considered for treatment using second-generation antihistamines such as loratadine (Claritin[1] 10 mg twice daily[3]), desloratadine[1] (Clarinex 5 mg twice daily[3]), cetirizine[1] (Zyrtec 10 mg twice daily[3]), levocetirizine[1] (Xyzal 5 mg daily), and fexofenadine[1] (Allegra 180 mg twice daily[3]). If urticaria is not adequately controlled, the second generation antihistamine dosage can be at least doubled. Doxepin (Sinequan),[1] an H_1- and H_2-receptor antagonist, is seven times more potent than hydroxyzine in suppression of wheal and flare responses. Because of its central nervous system side effects, combined use of doxepin with a first-generation antihistamine should be restricted. Topical 5% doxepin cream (Zonalon)[1] may help to suppress pruritus in patients with localized urticaria. Anti-IgE treatment using omalizumab ([Xolair] 150–300 mg per month) for chronic urticaria refractory to high-dose antihistamine therapy has been approved by the FDA for patients over 12 years of age with chronic urticaria in US. While the treatment is highly effective, safe, and suitable for long-term use, it has a high cost. Several additional biologics have been used in recent years for the treatment of chronic idiopathic urticaria, including dupilumab ([Dupixent] blocking IL-4), benralizumab ([Fasenra] blocking IL-5), mepolizumab ([Nucala] blocking IL-5) and secukinumab ([Cosentyx] anti-IL-17A). However, none of these treatments have received FDA approval.

Systemic prednisone at 30 to 40 mg in a single morning dose is sufficient to suppress acute urticaria in adults. Tapering should be gradual over a 3- to 4-week period by decreasing the dosage 5 mg every 3 to 5 days to minimize rebound. Alternate-morning dosing when reaching 20 mg daily may help to minimize the steroid side effects. Methylprednisolone (Solu-Medrol 40 mg) should be given intravenously as initial therapy to patients with angioedema. This may be followed by a tapering oral course. Chronic therapy with systemic steroids is to be avoided. Three months of off-label treatment with cyclosporine (Neoral)[1] at 3 to 5 mg/kg can be given safely to patients who are refractory to corticosteroid or omalizumab therapy. Close monitoring for hypertension and renal insufficiency is necessary during the treatment.

Leukotriene inhibitors such as zileuton (Zyflo[1] 600 mg four times daily), zafirlukast (Accolate[1] 20 mg twice daily), and montelukast (Singulair[1] 10 mg once daily) may be effective for patients with autoimmune urticaria.

Proper management of underlying autoimmune thyroid disease or autoimmune collagen vascular diseases has been beneficial for patients with associated urticaria. Life-threatening angioedema triggered by angiotensin-converting enzyme (ACE) inhibitors has been successfully treated with infusion of fresh-frozen plasma. Hereditary angioedema can be prevented with tranexamic acid[1] or modified androgens. Intravenous C1-esterase inhibitor (Cinryze) or icatibant (Firazyr), a bradykinin B2 antagonist, can be administered to prevent acute attacks. Subcutaneous injection of C1-esterase inhibitor

---

[1]Not FDA approved for this indication.
[3]Exceeds dosage recommended by the manufacturer.

(Haegarda) has been approved by FDA in 2017 to prevent hereditary angioedema attacks. In addition, lanadelumab (Takhzyro) has also been approved as prophylactic treatment by the FDA for patients age 2 years and older with types 1 and 2 hereditary angioedema. Treatments with methotrexate[1], warfarin (Coumadin),[1] plasmapheresis, colchicine,[1] hydroxychloroquine (Plaquenil),[1] anti-TNF-alpha,[1] interferon,[1] and intravenous immunoglobulin (Baygam)[1] have been reported for severe, refractory[1] urticaria. Vitamin D[1] supplementation can also be beneficial in reducing symptoms in patients with a deficiency. These treatments are administered only by specialists on an individual basis. Non-pharmacotherapeutic means such as frequent use of skin emollients, avoidance of hot shower, scrubbing, and excessive sun exposure should also be recommended as part of management plans.

---

[1]Not FDA approved for this indication.

References

American Academy of Allergy, Asthma and Immunology response to the EAACI/GA 2 LEN/EDF/WAO guideline for the definition, classification, diagnosis, and management of Urticaria 2017 revision, 74(2):411–413, 2019.

Bailey E, Shaker M: An update on childhood urticaria and angioedema, *Curr Opin Pediatr* 20(4):425–430, 2008.

Champion RH, Roberts SO, Carpenter RG, Roger JH: Urticaria and angio-oedema. A review of 554 patients, *Br J Dermatol* 81(8):588–597, 1969.

Joint Task Force on Practice Parameters: The diagnosis and management of urticaria: A practice parameter. Part II. Chronic urticaria/angioedema, *Ann Allergy Asthma Immunol* 85(2):521–544, 2000.

Kaplan AP, Joseph K, Maykut RJ, et al: Treatment of chronic autoimmune urticaria with omalizumab, *J Allergy Clin Immunol* 122(3):569–573, 2008.

Lin RY, Cannon AG, Teitel AD: Pattern of hospitalizations for angioedema in New York between 1990 and 2003, *Ann Allergy Asthma Immunol* 95(2):159–166, 2005.

Longhurst H, Cicardi M, Craig T, et al: Prevention of hereditary angioedema attacks with a subcutaneous C1 inhibitor, *N Engl J Med* 376(12):1131–1140, 2017 Mar 23.

Maurer M, Rosen K, Shieh HJ: Omalizumab for chronic urticaria, *N Engl J Med* 386:2530, 2013, https://doi.org/10.1056/JEJMc1305687.

Maurer M, Rosen K, Hsieh HJ, et al: Omalizumab for the treatmentof chronic idiopathic or spontaneous urticaria, *N Engl J Med* 368:924–935, 2013.

Nizami RM, Baboo MT: Office management of patients with urticaria: An analysis of 215 patients, *Ann Allergy* 33(2):78–85, 1974.

Powell RJ, Du Toit GL, Siddique N, et al: BSACI guidelines for the management of chronic urticaria and angio-oedema, *Clin Exp Allergy* 37(5):631–650, 2007.

Saini SS, Bindslev-Jensen C, Maurer M, et al: Efficacy and safety ofomalizumab in patients with chronic idiopathic/spontaneous urticaria who remain symptomatic on H1 antihistamines: a randomized, placebo-controlled study, *J Invest Dermatol* 135:67–75, 115, 2015.

VENOUS ULCERS

Method of
Marita Yaghi, MD; Jose A. Jaller, MD; and Robert S. Kirsner, MD, PhD

CURRENT DIAGNOSIS

- Venous ulcers are the most common cause of lower-extremity ulceration.
- Valvular incompetence, vein distention, muscular weakness, and/or a decrease in the range of motion of the ankle may lead to venous insufficiency.
- The mechanism of cutaneous ulceration resulting from venous insufficiency remains unclear.
- The typical location for a venous ulcer is on the medial malleolus.
- Complications of chronic venous ulcers are cellulitis and less often squamous cell carcinoma.
- Compression is the gold standard of treatment of venous disease.

CURRENT THERAPY

- Compression therapy is used to deliver a graded compression of 30 to 40 mm Hg at the ankle. Arterial disease should be excluded before full compression.
- Systemic medications as adjuvant therapy to compression bandages include aspirin[1], pentoxifylline (Trental)[1], or micronized purified flavonoid fraction (Daflon 500 mg)[7].
- Other treatments, along with compression, include debridement, engineered skin, placental or skin grafting, electrical stimulation, locally derived growth factors, and venous surgery.
- The lifelong use of elastic compression stockings (30–40 mm Hg) is the mainstay of prevention.

---

[1]Not FDA approved for this indication.
[7]Available as a dietary supplement.

Ulcers resulting from venous insufficiency are the most common cause of leg ulceration. The Wound Healing Society classifies wounds as *acute* if they sustain restoration of anatomic and functional integrity in an orderly and timely process and *chronic* if they do not. Venous leg ulcers (VLUs) are more frequently seen in the elderly population; however, about 1 in 5 primary VLUs occur in patients under 40 years of age. Personal or family history of venous disease, obesity, smoking, advanced age, female sex, hypertension, and leg injuries are strong risk factors to the development of VLUs.

Epidemiology

Venous insufficiency affects approximately 5% of the world's population and about 2% of the American population. VLUs affect 1% to 2% of adults in the United States, accounting for over 2 million lost workdays annually. The associated pain, inability to perform daily activities, and social stigma because of the appearance and odor of the wounds drastically diminish patients' quality of life. Moreover, the high cost of treatment, time off work, and hospital admissions forge a massive economic burden in the healthcare system. Seventy percent of all leg ulcers result solely from venous disease, and an additional 20% of patients have mixed arterial and venous disease. A recent report that used claims data from 2013 private and governmental insurance companies revealed that wounds and ulcers had the highest direct U.S. healthcare cost of all skin diseases ($12 billion), a considerable increase from the $1 billion estimate in 1990, and caused approximately 21% of all deaths related to skin condition, second only to cutaneous cancers. Additionally, it is estimated that 2 million workdays per year are lost because of VLU-related disability, and more than 12% of affected workers retire prematurely.

Pathophysiology

In the lower extremities, the venous system comprises the deep and superficial veins. Blood flows from the superficial to the deep veins through the communicating or perforating veins to ultimately reach the heart. Veins contain unidirectional valves that prevent blood return or reflux. During calf muscle relaxation, the pressure difference (high pressure in the superficial veins) allows blood flow from the superficial to deep veins. When a healthy individual contracts the calf muscles, a high pressure develops in the deep vein system, allowing blood to flow from the deep veins to the heart. If the calf muscle contraction is restricted or the one-way valves are deficient, the system fails to adequately return venous blood to the heart, leading to venous hypertension (also known as sustained ambulatory high pressure).

The pathway to developing an ulcer due to venous insufficiency is unclear, albeit several hypotheses have been considered since the beginning of the 20th century. Patients with chronic venous disease can develop ulcers in their lower extremities for a different reason (e.g., trauma), but given their venous disease and suboptimal wound healing capacity, these lesions can develop into VLUs. In the early 1980s, Browse and Burnard suggested that venous hypertension could lead to endothelial distention, causing extravasation of fibrinogen into the interstitial fluid, which results in "pericapillary fibrin cuff" formation around the capillary vessels. Fibrin cuffs act as a barrier to diffusion of oxygen and nutrients, causing ischemia and ulcer formation. A few years later, Coleridge-Smith and colleagues suggested that venous hypertension could lead to decreased capillary perfusion, resulting in leukocyte trapping. The trapped leukocytes release proteolytic enzymes, which result in free radical formation and capillary damage. The increased capillary permeability causes extravasation of fibrinogen and other metabolites, which leads to the formation of a fibrin cuff around the capillaries and ultimately ischemia.

Further studies supported the presence of increased levels of monocyte aggregation. Claudy and colleagues showed that leukocyte activation caused release of tumor necrosis factor alpha (TNF-α), ultimately leading to pericapillary fibrin cuff formation. In 1993, Falanga and Eaglstein observed that fibrin cuffs were discontinuous around capillaries and therefore did not form a barrier to oxygen and nutrients causing ischemia. They also postulated the "trap" hypothesis, which suggests that venous hypertension causes endothelial cell distention leading to extravasation of macromolecules (i.e., α_2-macroglobulin and fibrinogen) into the dermis. Moreover, α_2-macroglobulin can bind to growth factors, such as TNF-α and transforming growth factor beta (TGF-β), making them unavailable for wound repair. Patients with venous disease may have other factors that contribute to venous ulcer formation, such as systemic alteration in fibrinolysis and arteriovenous shunting. Despite all previously conducted studies and hypotheses, further research is needed to explain the mechanism of cutaneous ulceration resulting from venous insufficiency. An ongoing longitudinal cohort study from our group is prospectively tracking the development of the first VLU among a population of subjects with chronic venous insufficiency (CVI), aims to describe the natural history of CVI leading to the development of VLUs and identify specific risk factors, ultimately allowing for the development of predictive models for VLU occurrence.

Evaluation and Diagnosis

VLUs are diagnosed clinically; however, blood flow imaging, pathology, and microbiologic cultures can aid in ruling out other conditions. The CEAP classification was developed in 1994 by the American Venous Forum (AVF) to standardize the diagnosis and treatment of venous disease. It was based on clinical manifestations (C), etiologic factors (E), anatomic distribution of disease (A), and underlying pathophysiologic findings (P).

Clinical signs, such as wound location, associated venous disease, and past personal history of venous ulcers, are paramount for the diagnosis. VLUs are typically located on the lower leg, particularly in the medial lower third leg or medial malleolus, what is referred to as the "gaiter area." The ulcer usually begins as a blister or erosion on the skin that hinders healing and develops into a full-thickness lesion, or ulcer. Ulcer borders are irregular and usually smooth. The base of the ulcer may be covered with granulation tissue, yellow slough, or both. Venous ulcers are associated with the presence of pigmentation, erythema, dermatitis, edema, and induration (i.e., lipodermatosclerosis) of the surrounding skin and with varicose veins in the lower leg. Variable amounts of exude and pain might be appreciated. Hemosiderin deposition resulting from red blood cell extravasation and iron-related stimulation of melanocytes cause the surrounding hyperpigmentation.

Lipodermatosclerosis is caused by sclerosis of the dermis and subcutaneous tissue. The presence of lipodermatosclerosis has been associated with a greater impairment of fibrinolysis in

patients with venous ulcers and may be a poor prognostic factor for restriction of leg movement. Other known prognostic factors are duration and size of the ulcer and history of venous surgery. Ulcers present for longer than 6 months and larger than 5 cm in diameter tend to be more refractory to therapy.

A diagnosis of venous ulcers may be based on clinical presentation. The findings of a lower leg ulcer associated with lipodermatosclerosis or varicose veins, or both, suggest a venous ulcer. Other common findings include atrophie blanche (i.e., porcelain white scars with telangiectasia and dyspigmentation) and dermatitis. Venous dermatitis is associated with erythema, eczema, pruritus, and scaling of the skin. It should be distinguished from contact dermatitis in the periwound area, which may result from the use of topical agents. A study from our group has identified its prevalence to be as high as 7.2% in patients with confirmed CVI, with a predilection for patients over the age of 75. The presence of venous dermatitis (C4a) and/or lipodermatosclerosis (C4b) is recognized as a precursor to VLUs (C6) as per the CEAP classification system since 1994. Recent consensus revisions in 2020 have recognized corona phlebectatica (C4c) to be an early sign of advanced venous disease, as its presence is 5.3 times more likely to result in VLU development, a risk of similar magnitude to other C4 skin changes. Hence, findings of fan-shaped intradermal telangiectasias on the medial or lateral aspects of the foot in a patient with a lower extremity ulcer are highly indicative of a VLU.

Even though venous insufficiency can be confirmed with a variety of techniques, including duplex ultrasound or plethysmography, the presence or absence of arterial disease is a more important factor dictating treatment and prognosis. Compression should be used with caution in patients with peripheral arterial disease (PAD). Also, sharp debridement should be avoided as much as possible in patients with PAD because of the associated risk of further ischemia and larger ulcer formation. These patients might need evaluation by a vascular surgeon for possible revascularization of the affected vessel.

A simple, noninvasive measurement to assess peripheral arterial disease is the ankle brachial index (ABI). This value is calculated by dividing the systolic pressure in the ankle by the systolic pressure in the arm. An ABI of less than 0.9 indicates peripheral vascular disease and represents an independent risk factor for vascular disease in other vascular beds, such as the coronary arteries. Care must be taken with diabetic or elderly patients who may have a falsely negative ABI value. All patients with an abnormal ABI value should be further evaluated. Consider a vascular consultation, magnetic resonance angiography (MRA), angioplasty, and stent bypass.

To aid in the exclusion of any underlying disease (e.g., hematologic disease, diabetes), initial laboratory tests should include complete blood cell (CBC) count with a differential count, chemistry panel, hemoglobin A1C, liver function tests, and levels of homocysteine, proteins C and S, antithrombin III, and factor V Leiden. The presence of malnutrition should also be evaluated (prealbumin and albumin determinations), as well as the use of immune suppressive medications.

Several vascular studies help in the diagnosis and severity of venous disease. Color duplex ultrasound is usually the initial study done to assess venous reflux in the lower extremities. Continuous-wave Doppler studies may yield false-negative results because it may be difficult to differentiate between the superficial and deep venous system. Air plethysmography and photoplethysmography are helpful in evaluating venous reflux and calf muscle dysfunction. Invasive venography is the gold standard to assess venous reflux, but it is used only as a last resort because of its invasive properties.

Complications

Main complications of long-term or chronic venous ulcers are cellulitis, osteomyelitis, and squamous cell carcinoma. A finding of exposed tendon or bone, in addition to suggesting an underlying osteomyelitis, suggests an ulcer with a nonvenous cause.

Assessment for the presence of skin erythema, excessive warmth, qualitative or quantitative change in the amount exuded, or odor associated with the ulcer should be performed first. Radiographs and biopsy for histology and culture are appropriate next steps in evaluation. Ideally, biopsies of the wound border and including normal skin are to be sent for both atypical bacterial (for example, mycobacterial organisms) and fungal culture, to rule out the presence of atypical organisms. In cases of high suspicion of bone involvement, advanced imaging (MRI) should be sought even in the absence of changes on plain radiography, which is unable to showcase bone marrow edema, the earliest pathological feature of osteomyelitis. If the latter is confirmed, the next step would be to consult an orthopedic surgeon for further analysis and treatment, which may include a bone biopsy and bone debridement.

Treatment

Compression is the gold standard of treatment of venous disease. After arterial disease has been excluded, reversal of the effects of venous hypertension through compression bandages and leg elevation is the cornerstone of therapy.

The goal of compression therapy is to deliver sustained graded compression with 30 to 40 mm Hg at the ankle. These bandages are applied circumferentially from the toes to the knees (involving the heel) with the foot dorsiflexed. The optimal method to deliver this pressure is through multilayered elastic compression dressings. Elastic compression dressings deliver compression during ambulation (i.e., walking) and at rest, accommodate to reduction in edema, and are superior to single-layered dressings. Inelastic compression (short-stretch compression) may deliver similar results but appear to require greater sophistication by those applying them to accomplish this. Inelastic bandages, which do not deliver compression at rest, may be advantageous in patients with arterial disease or patients who do not tolerate full compression (e.g., elderly). Highly pressured compression stockings are as effective as compression wrappings; however, patients' compliance is a significant limitation. Additionally, studies have reported that any leg exercise or physical activity, in addition to compression therapy, may lead to increased VLU healing outcomes.

Increasingly, it is being shown that integrating intermittent pneumatic compression as a complement to compression therapy could accelerate wound healing rates, primarily by reducing the total surface area of the wound. Other mechanical physical therapies, such as radial and focal extracorporeal shockwave therapies, have demonstrated lesser effectiveness in comparison. Nonetheless, all these interventions appear to outperform conventional compression therapy alone in terms of efficacy.

Systemic medication as adjuvant therapy to compression bandages, such as Trental[1] (pentoxifylline 400 to 800 mg three times daily[3]), aspirin[1], or micronized purified flavonoid fraction (MPFF, Daflon 500 mg[7] [diosmin[7] 90% and hesperidin[7] 10%]) have shown to be superior to compression bandages alone with regard to the rate of healing. The use of pentoxifylline as adjuvant therapy to compression in venous ulcers has been shown to be very beneficial.

Wound bed preparation, which often involves debridement, was proposed as a way to help the healing process. It is a multistep process that improves the wound bed by removing necrotic and fibrinous wound tissue, increasing the amount of granulation tissue, and decreasing edema, chronic wound fluid (i.e., exudate), and bacterial burden. It also increases the likelihood that wound edge keratinocytes can respond to prohealing stimuli. There are five types of debridement. *Surgical* debridement, using sharp instruments, remains the fastest method to remove unhealthy tissue and is highly effective. *Mechanical* debridement, such as wet-to-dry dressing, removes both necrotic and viable tissue and is highly associated with resultant infections.

Autolytic debridement relies on the action of enzymatic agents secreted by the wound itself, whereas *enzymatic* debridement involves the use of topical enzymatic agents to debride the wound. Finally, *biologic* debridement, historically used, employs maggots, which secrete necrotic tissue-digesting collagenases and trypsin-like enzymes.

A novel approach integrates the advantages of enzymatic and biologic debridement methods by employing a recombinant topical gel containing tarumase. Derived from medical maggots, this naturally occurring trypsin serine protease enzyme exhibits selective activity against fibrin, collagen, and elastin. Phase II studies have demonstrated the well-tolerated application of tarumase topically to wounds. Additionally, there is evidence suggesting dose-dependent trends toward faster and more effective wound debridement, particularly notable in patients with significant slough at baseline, along with a propensity for accelerated healing rates.

The decision of which wound dressing to use will depend on the amount of wound drainage. Occlusive dressings should be used for dry to mildly exudative wounds, providing a moist environment for healing. These facilitate wound *autolytic* debridement. A variety of types of occlusions may be used, and the choice depends on several factors, including the location of the wound and the amount of fibrinous slough and exudate present. Foam, gel, and calcium alginate dressings are highly absorbent dressings and should be used for moderate-to-severe exudating wounds. Fear of excessive infection with the use of occlusive dressings is unfounded. Additionally, the antiquated notion that the wound should be allowed "to breathe" has been dispelled.

Topical antiseptics and cleansing agents should be used with caution because they may increase the time required for healing. Topical agents such as cadexomer iodine (Iodosorb), silver-impregnated dressings, and topical anesthetics are alternatives that do not prolong healing. These topical agents should be considered when the wound appears contaminated, but not infected. Wound infections should be treated like cellulitis, with systemic antibiotics.

Up to 50% of venous ulcers may be refractory to compression therapy alone. This refractory subset may be predicted by baseline characteristics (size and duration) and by a decrease in size with 2 to 4 weeks of treatment (Figure 1). Other available treatments include tissue-engineered skin, autologous skin, electrical stimulation, treatment with locally delivered growth factors, and venous surgery. Three categories exist for skin grafts: autologous, allogeneic (cultured), and artificial (tissue-engineered skin). Three different techniques have been used for autologous skin grafts: epidermal skin graft (only epidermis and no dermis), split-thickness skin graft (all the epidermis and a portion of the dermis), and full-thickness skin graft (complete dermis and epidermis). The use of artificial, or bioengineered grafts, has risen in the past decades.

Apligraf is a bilayered engineered living skin composed of keratinocytes and fibroblasts from neonatal foreskin that is approved by the U.S. Food and Drug Administration for treatment of venous leg and diabetic neuropathic foot ulcers. Likewise, other synthetic skin grafts have used animal tissue to generate this sophisticated dressing. Surgical treatment of incompetent superficial and perforator veins along with standard of care (i.e., compression) reduce the risk of recurrence. Xenogeneic dermal grafts (Oasis) and placental grafts (EpiFix) are also available alternatives.

After healing occurs, patients with venous insufficiency are at risk for recurrence (60% to 70%) especially in the first 3 months after healing. The lifelong use of elastic compression stockings (30 to 40 mm Hg) is the mainstay of therapy, but early intervention after recurrence is critical. Adjustable compression hook-and-loop wraps are emerging as an alternative to classic elastic compression stockings and provide an alternative to patients with movement limitations due to age or other factors. In addition to compression therapy throughout

---

[1] Not FDA approved for this indication.
[3] Exceeds dosage recommended by the manufacturer.
[7] Available as dietary supplement.

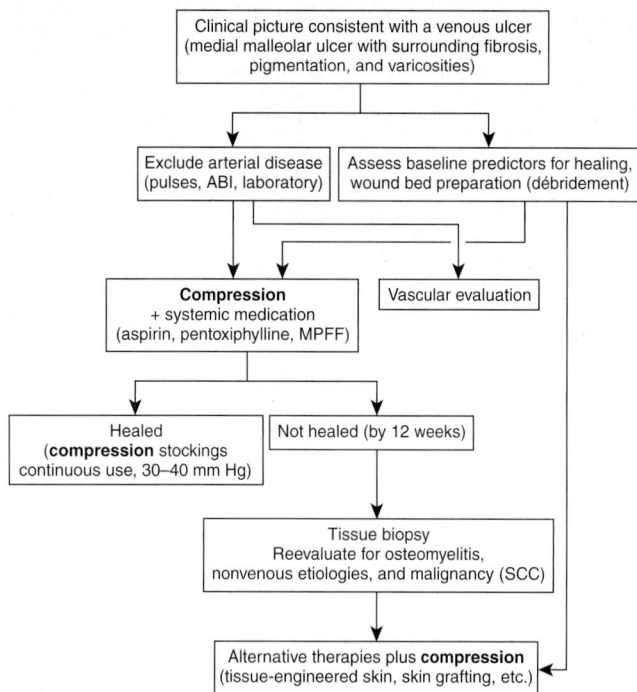

Figure 1 Simplified algorithm for the diagnosis and treatment of patients with venous ulcers. *ABI,* Ankle-brachial index; *MPFF,* micronized purified flavonoid fraction; *SCC,* squamous cell carcinoma.

life, a recent meta-analysis suggested that prescribed exercise therapy, health education, and self-care as supplementary measures have the potential to reduce VLU recurrence. Health professionals need to understand the importance of further research to ultimately minimize the psychological, physical, and socioeconomic impact that ulcers caused by venous insufficiency have on patients and society.

References

Abbade LP, Lastória S: Venous ulcer: Epidemiology, physiopathology, diagnosis and treatment, *Int J Dermatol* 44:449–456, 2005.

Alvarez OM: Healing wounds: Occlusion or exposure, *Inf Surg* 173–181, 1984.

Browse NL, Burnand KG: The cause of venous ulceration, *Lancet* 2:243–245, 1982.

Claudy AL, Mirshahi M, Soria C, et al: Detection of undegraded fibrin and tumor necrosis factor alpha in venous leg ulcers, *J Am Acad Dermatol* 25:623–627, 1991.

Coleridge-Smith PD, Thomas P, Scurr JH, et al: Causes of venous ulceration: A new hypothesis? *Br Med J* 296:1726–1727, 1988.

Da Silva A, Navarro MF, Batalheiro J: The importance of chronic venous insufficiency. Various preliminary data on its medico-social consequences, *Phlebologie* 45(4):439–443, 1992.

Dolibog PT, Dolibog P, Bergler-Czop B, Grzegorczyn S, Chmielewska D: The Efficacy of Extracorporeal Shockwave Therapy Compared with Compression Therapy in Healing Venous Leg Ulcers, *J Clin Med* 13(7):2117, 2024.

Fairlamb DM, Szepeshazi K, Goldsmith D, et al: First clinical evaluation of the safety and efficacy of tarumase for the debridement of venous leg ulcers, *Int Wound J* 21(3):e14805, 2024.

Falanga V, Eaglstein WH: The trap hypothesis of venous ulceration, *Lancet* 341:1006–1008, 1993.

Finlayson K, Edwards H, Courtney M: Factors associated with recurrence of venous leg ulcers: a survey and retrospective chart review, *Int J Nurs Studies* 46(8):1071–1078, 2009.

He B, Shi J, Li L, Ma Y, Zhao H, Qin P, Ma P: Prevention strategies for the recurrence of venous leg ulcers: A scoping review, *Int Wound J* 21(3):e14759, 2024.

Jull A, Arroll B, Parag V, Waters J: Pentoxifylline for treating venous leg ulcers, *Cochrane Database Syst Rev* 3:CD001733, 2007.

Jull A, Slark J, Parsons J: Prescribed exercise with compression vs compression alone in treating patients with venous leg ulcers: a systematic review and meta-analysis, *JAMA Dermatol* 154(11), 2018.

Kirsner R: Wound bed preparation, *Ostomy Wound Manage* (Feb. Suppl)2–3, 2003.

Kirsner RS: Exercise for leg ulcers: "working out" the nature of venous ulcers, *JAMA Dermatol* 154(11), 2018.

Kirsner RS, Falanga V: Techniques of split-thickness skin grafting for lower extremity ulcerations, *J Dermatol Surg Oncol* 19:779–783, 1993.

Kirsner RS, Pardes JB, Eaglstein WH, Falanga V: The clinical spectrum of lipodermatosclerosis, *J Am Acad Dermatol* 28:623–627, 1993.

Lazarus GS, Cooper DM, Knighton DR, et al: Definitions and guidelines for assessment of wounds and evaluation of healing, *Arch Dermatol* 130:489–493, 1994.

Lim HW, Collins SAB, Resneck Jr JS, et al: The burden of skin disease in the United States, *J Am Acad Dermatol* 76(5):958–972.e952, 2017.

Lurie F, Passman M, Meisner M, et al: The 2020 update of the CEAP classification system and reporting standards, *J Vasc Surg Venous Lymphat Disord* 8(3):342–352, 2021.

Mervis JS, Kirsner RS, Lev-Tov H: Protocol for a longitudinal cohort study: determination of risk factors for the development of first venous leg ulcer in people with chronic venous insufficiency, the VEINS (venous insufficiency in South Florida) cohort, *BMJ Open* 3;9(1):e023313, 2019.

Moffatt CJ, Dorman MC: Recurrence of leg ulcers within a community ulcer service, *J Wound Care* 4(2):57–61, 1995.

Olin JW, Beusterien KM, Childs MB, et al: Medical costs of treating venous stasis ulcers: Evidence from a retrospective cohort study, *Vasc Med* 4:1–7, 1999.

Phillips TJ, Machado F, Trout R, et al: Prognostic indicators in venous ulcers, *J Am Acad Dermatol* 43:627–630, 2000.

Singer AJ, Tassiopoulos A, Kirsner RS: Evaluation and management of lower-extremity ulcers, *N Engl J Med* 377(16):1559–1567, 2017.

Trent JT, Falabella A, Eaglstein WH, Kirsner RS: Venous ulcers: Pathophysiology and treatment options, *Ostomy Wound Manage* 51:38–54, 2005.

Yaghi M, Hargis A, Maskan Bermudez N, Chopra D, Lev-Tov H: Prevalence of venous dermatitis: results of a regional cohort study of patients with confirmed chronic venous insufficiency, *Int J Dermatol* 62(10):e550–e551, 2023.

VIRAL DISEASES OF THE SKIN

Method of
Cheryl A. Armstrong, MD

CURRENT DIAGNOSIS

Herpes Simplex Viruses 1 and 2
- Clinical: Grouped vesicles or erosions, especially in perioral or anogenital location
- Laboratory: Tzanck smear, viral culture, antigen detection, PCR, gG-based type-specific serology

Varicella-Zoster Virus
- Clinical: Papules, pustules, vesicles in diffuse (varicella) or dermatomal (herpes zoster) distribution
- Laboratory: Tzanck smear, antigen detection, viral culture, PCR

Hand-Foot-and-Mouth Disease
- Clinical: Papulovesicles on oral mucosa, hands, feet following fever, constitutional symptoms
- Laboratory: PCR

Parvovirus B19
- Clinical: "Slapped cheeks" reticular erythema on trunk or extremities following fever, constitutional symptoms; arthralgias, arthritis, purpuric eruptions; transient aplastic crisis, fetal hydrops
- Laboratory: B19 specific IgM serology, PCR

Molluscum Contagiosum
- Clinical: Few to multiple 1- to 4-mm umbilicated flesh-colored papules
- Laboratory: Histopathology if clinical appearance atypical

Orf
- Clinical: One to several solid to vesicular nodules on hands, forearms; history of exposure to sheep, goats, cattle
- Laboratory: Histopathology if clinical appearance atypical; PCR

Abbreviation: NSAID = nonsteroidal antiinflammatory drug.

Herpes Simplex Viruses 1 and 2

Herpes simplex virus types 1 and 2 (HSV-1 and HSV-2) are the most closely related members of the human herpesvirus family, and the skin lesions they produce are clinically indistinguishable. Clusters of tense blisters on an erythematous base often quickly evolve into erosions or ulcerations with associated crusting. Lesions can develop at any mucocutaneous site but are typically found in the perioral or anogenital regions. Both HSV-1 and HSV-2 are transmitted by direct mucocutaneous contact with an infected host. Following viral replication in the skin or mucosa, intact viral nucleocapsids travel via sensory neurons to the corresponding dorsal root ganglia to establish latency. Later, a variety of stimuli can trigger reactivation. The virus travels back along the sensory neurons to the mucocutaneous surface to replicate and induce active or subclinical infection. In the case of subclinical infection, no active skin lesions are evident, but infectious particles are present, a state known as asymptomatic shedding. Although the viral titer is much lower than during clinically active disease, asymptomatic shedding of the virus in oral and genital secretions is thought to be responsible for the majority of cases of HSV transmission.

Primary, initial nonprimary (also known as first episode), and recurrent are terms used to further define the nature of the HSV infection. A *primary* infection refers to a patient's first infection with either type of HSV at any site. These patients are seronegative initially but subsequently develop HSV type-specific antibodies. A patient who is already infected with one HSV type and then develops an infection with the alternate type experiences an *initial nonprimary* or first-episode infection (e.g., the first episode of genital herpes in a patient with a prior history of orofacial herpes). These patients are seropositive for one type-specific HSV antibody (e.g., HSV-1) and later develop antibodies specific for the alternate HSV type (e.g., HSV-2). A *recurrent* infection is one that occurs at a site of prior infection. These patients are seropositive for HSV-1 or HSV-2, or both. Because most primary infections, whether oral or genital, are asymptomatic, the first evidence of disease often represents a recurrent or initial nonprimary infection.

Orofacial Herpes Simplex Virus Infection

Orofacial HSV, also known as herpes labialis, fever blisters, or cold sores, is commonly acquired during childhood or adolescence. Symptomatic primary disease usually takes the form of gingivostomatitis with or without additional lesions on the cutaneous perioral surfaces. Fever, malaise, and tender lymphadenopathy may also be present. In recurrent episodes, clusters of blisters erupt along the vermillion border of the lips, and subsequent erosions and crusting persist for several days up to 2 weeks. Lesions can develop anywhere in the perioral area, especially on the cheeks. In men, a viral folliculitis of the beard area (herpetic sycosis) may be mistaken for a bacterial process because it is often pustular. The presence of a prodrome and recurrence in the same site are clues to the correct diagnosis. Although recurrent intraoral lesions of HSV can occur, they are uncommon in immunocompetent persons. Exposure to ultraviolet light is a common trigger factor for herpes labialis, as is fever or intercurrent infection.

Genital Herpes Simplex Virus Infection

When symptomatic, primary genital herpes often involves bilaterally distributed lesions in the anogenital area with associated fever, inguinal adenopathy, and dysuria or urinary retention. Aseptic meningitis can also occur. The lesions often persist for 2 to 3 weeks or longer. Nonprimary infections are usually less severe and have fewer constitutional symptoms. Recurrent episodes tend to be milder and shorter in duration. Often, there is a prodrome of tingling or burning followed by the development of localized vesicles that can quickly rupture, leaving nonspecific erosions or ulcerations. The lesions may be anywhere within the anogenital region but tend to recur close to the same area in subsequent episodes. The time between exposure and development of primary disease is estimated to be from 3 to 14 days. However, more often the first clinical indication of disease is a recurrence, which can occur weeks to years after the initial infection. Prior infection with HSV-1 provides some protection against acquisition of HSV-2.

Based on seroepidemiologic evidence, it is estimated that approximately 17% of the United States population aged 14 to 49 years are infected with HSV-2. In most of these persons, this disease has not been officially diagnosed and they are unaware that they are infected. Nevertheless, they experience asymptomatic shedding and unknowingly transmit the disease to sexual partners. Interrupting this cycle of transmission has become a major focus among health care providers who work with these patients. A combination of patient education and appropriate use of systemic antiviral agents may be gradually having some impact on this epidemic. Recommendations for patients with genital herpes include avoiding sex with uninfected partners when active lesions or prodromal symptoms are present and routinely using latex condoms to minimize transmission during periods of asymptomatic shedding. Chronic suppressive doses of oral antiviral agents (Table 1), including acyclovir (Zovirax), valacyclovir (Valtrex), and famciclovir (Famvir), significantly reduce the frequency of clinical recurrences as well as the rate of asymptomatic shedding and may be recommended together with these other practices to reduce the risk of transmission.

Although HSV-2 is the etiologic agent in a majority of cases of genital herpes infections, an increasing number of genital herpes infections are caused by HSV-1. Symptomatic recurrences and asymptomatic shedding are less frequent with genital HSV-1 infection than with genital HSV-2 infection, and this distinction becomes important for patient counseling and prognosis.

Other Mucocutaneous Herpes Simplex Virus Infections

Eczema herpeticum, also known as Kaposi's varicelliform eruption, represents a cutaneous dissemination of HSV usually seen in patients with atopic dermatitis or other underlying skin disease. Herpetic vesicles develop over an extensive mucocutaneous surface, most often the face, neck, and upper trunk, presumably spreading from a recurrent oral HSV infection or asymptomatic shedding from the oral mucosa. Eczema herpeticum can also develop in the presence of genital HSV. As with other HSV infections, eczema herpeticum may be recurrent. In addition, patients can develop localized, recurrent HSV in previously

TABLE 1 Recommendations for Systemic Antiviral Treatment of Mucocutaneous Herpes Simplex Virus Infection

EPISODE	DRUG	DOSAGE
Genital Herpes Simplex Virus		
Primary or first episode	Acyclovir	Mild to moderate: 400 mg PO tid[3] or 200 mg PO 5 ×/d × 7–10 d Severe: 5 mg/kg IV q8h × 5 d
	Valacyclovir	1 g PO bid × 7–10 d
	Famciclovir[1]	250 mg PO tid × 10 d
Recurrent episode (start at prodrome)	Acyclovir	400 mg PO tid × 5 d[3] or 800 mg PO bid × 5 d[3] or 800 mg PO tid × 2 d[3]
	Valacyclovir	500 mg PO bid × 3 d or 1 g daily × 5 d
	Famciclovir	1 g PO bid × 1 d or 125 mg PO bid × 5 d
Chronic suppression	Acyclovir	>6 outbreaks per year: 400 mg PO bid or 200 mg PO tid Adjust up or down according to response
	Valacyclovir	6–10 outbreaks per year: 500 mg PO qd ≥10 outbreaks/year: 1 g PO qd
	Famciclovir	≥6 outbreaks/year: 250 mg PO bid
Orofacial Herpes Simplex Virus		
Primary or first episode	Acyclovir[1]	15 mg/kg 5 ×/d × 7 d
	Valacyclovir[1]	1 g bid × 7 d
	Famciclovir[1]	500 mg bid × 7 d
Recurrent episode (start at prodrome)	Acyclovir[1]	400 mg PO 5 ×/d × 5 d
	Valacyclovir	2 g PO bid × 1 d
	Famciclovir	1500 mg in 1 dose
Chronic suppression	Acyclovir[1]	400 mg PO bid-tid
	Valacyclovir[1]	500 mg–1 g PO qd
Orolabial or Genital Herpes Simplex Virus in Immunosuppressed Patients		
Recurrent or suppressive	Acyclovir[1]	400 mg PO tid or 5–10 mg/kg IV q8h
	Valacyclovir	500 mg–1 g PO bid
	Famciclovir	500 mg PO bid

[1]Not FDA approved for this indication.
[3]Exceeds dosage recommended by the manufacturer.

involved areas. Because of the extensive and inflammatory nature of the process and the possible secondary bacterial infection, the underlying viral etiology may be obscured. A history of eczema and recurrent HSV in the patient and careful observation for the grouped vesicles or erosions can be key to the correct diagnosis.

Herpetic whitlow refers to HSV infection of the hand, usually one or more distal digits. Previously thought to be limited to health care professionals with exposure to oral secretions of their patients, it is now recognized that autoinoculation from orolabial or genital HSV contributes to a significant number of cases.

Herpes gladiatorum is a problem seen most commonly in athletes who participate in close contact sports such as wrestling. Typically transmitted from active herpes labialis or asymptomatic shedding in oral secretions of an infected opponent, herpes gladiatorum often affects the head, neck, or shoulders and may be recurrent. In the wrestler with frequent outbreaks, chronic suppressive therapy may be recommended.

Diagnosis

Viral culture remains a common and acceptable method for diagnosing HSV infection. This method is sensitive when specimens are obtained from lesions that have not yet become too dry or crusted, usually during the first 2 to 3 days after onset. An adequate sample, obtained by unroofing the blister and swabbing the base, increases the likelihood of an accurate result. Antigen detection tests can remain positive even after lesions have dried, as long as the specimen includes epithelial cells and not just debris. For this method, a scraping from the lesion is usually smeared on a glass slide to be sent to the laboratory. Not all antigen detection methods are designed to distinguish HSV-1 from HSV-2.

Polymerase chain reaction (PCR) is highly sensitive and has become routinely available for diagnosis of mucocutaneous HSV infections. PCR may also be useful for detection of asymptomatic shedding.

The Tzanck smear (cytologic detection) is both insensitive and nonspecific but may be of use in some clinical settings. It does not differentiate HSV types or HSV from varicella-zoster virus (VZV). Immunohistochemical staining of biopsy specimens can help differentiate between VZV and HSV within 1 to 2 days in laboratories with these techniques available.

Serologic testing for HSV was previously of limited use because it could not reliably differentiate HSV-1 from HSV-2. Because they share significant genetic homology, HSV-1 and HSV-2 code for a number of common proteins that are not antigenically distinct. However, they also code for type-specific proteins that can be used to differentiate them. Current tests based on detecting type-specific viral glycoprotein G (gG-based, type-specific assays) are accurate and should be requested for this purpose. A positive HSV-2 serology may be useful in confirming the diagnosis of genital herpes in a patient with a negative viral culture or with unrecognized or asymptomatic disease. Alternatively, a negative serology can help exclude the diagnosis of HSV in a patient with chronic, nonspecific oral or genital symptoms.

Varicella Zoster Virus

VZV, another member of the human herpesvirus family, produces two specific patterns of disease in the skin. The primary infection results in varicella, also known as chickenpox, a widespread vesicular eruption usually seen in the pediatric population. Since the attenuated chickenpox vaccine was introduced in 1995, there has been a progressive decline in this disease. Following the primary infection, VZV establishes latency in the dorsal root ganglia until some later point, when reactivation can occur. The ensuing unilateral dermatomal distribution of blisters, often preceded by neuralgic pain, is known as herpes zoster or shingles. Herpes zoster is especially common in patients older than 50 years, but it may be seen at any age. It is also seen more commonly in immunocompromised patients, such as organ transplant recipients or patients infected with HIV. Herpes zoster is no longer considered a marker for underlying cancer, and evaluation for occult malignancy in an otherwise asymptomatic patient is not indicated. A single recurrence of herpes zoster, usually in the same dermatome, may occur, but this is uncommon in immunocompetent individuals. Additional recurrences, however, suggest a dermatomal form of HSV, and laboratory assessment for this possibility may be indicated.

The most common dermatomes involved with herpes zoster are in the thoracolumbar (T3-L2) and trigeminal (V1) regions. Skin lesions typically evolve from papules to vesicles and pustules, and then to crusted erosions, before healing approximately

TABLE 2 Recommendations for Systemic Antiviral Treatment of Herpes Zoster

DRUG	DOSAGE	
	IMMUNO-COMPETENT PATIENTS	IMMUNO-SUPPRESSED PATIENTS
Acyclovir	800 mg PO 5 × per d × 7–10 d	800 mg PO 5 × per d × 10 d* 10 mg/kg/dose IV q8h × 7–10 d*
Valacyclovir	1 g PO tid × 7 d	1 g PO tid × 10 d*
Famciclovir	500 mg PO tid × 7 d	500 mg PO tid × 10 d*

*Continue until there are no new lesions for 48 h.

TABLE 3 Topical Treatment Options for Mucocutaneous Herpes Simplex Virus and Varicella Zoster Virus Infections

TREATMENT	COMMENT
Cool, moist compresses using tap water or aluminum acetate 1:20 to 1:40 (Burow's solution, Domeboro, Bluboro)	Good for moist, oozing lesions to accelerate drying Apply wet dressing to involved skin and cover with a dry cloth to allow evaporation
Calamine lotion or similar shake lotion containing alcohol, menthol, and/or phenol; Aveeno colloidal oatmeal	Useful as drying and antipruritic agent May be applied after wet dressing
Bacitracin,[1] Polysporin, mupirocin[1] (Bactroban)	Use if there is concern for localized secondary bacterial infection
2% Viscous lidocaine, compounded suspensions[1,6] (e.g., Kaopectate[1] or Maalox,[1] diphenhydramine,[1] lidocaine)	Useful for temporary pain relief of oral or genital mucosal involvement
Acyclovir ointment	Used together with systemic antiviral agents, may be of benefit to immunocompromised individuals for localized HSV
Penciclovir (Denavir) cream	Can decrease the duration of lesions in herpes labialis by half a day if applied every 2 h while awake for 4 days beginning at the first sign of disease
Acyclovir buccal tablet (Sitavig) 50 mg	Can decrease the duration of herpes labialis by 0.8 days if single tablet is applied within 1 hour of prodromal symptom

[1]Not FDA approved for this indication.
[6]May be compounded by pharmacists.
Abbreviation: HSV = herpes simplex virus.

2 to 4 weeks after onset. The associated neuropathic pain commonly persists after the lesions have healed. Pain that continues for more than 3 months after the skin lesions resolve is referred to as postherpetic neuralgia, one of the most common and debilitating complications of this infection.

Several clinical presentations of herpes zoster deserve additional attention. Ophthalmic zoster, with lesions along the tip, side, or base of the nose indicating involvement of the nasociliary branch of the trigeminal nerve (Hutchinson's sign), may be associated with increased risk for ocular complications. Prompt initiation of a systemic antiviral agent (Table 2) and evaluation by an ophthalmologist are recommended. Disseminated zoster, with more than a few lesions outside the primary and immediately adjacent dermatomes, can indicate visceral involvement and its associated complications. The term *zoster sine herpete* describes patients with neuropathic pain resembling zoster but without any skin lesions. The diagnosis can be supported by demonstration of increased IgG antibody titers between the acute and convalescent phases. Chronic zoster is seen predominantly in HIV-infected persons. Single or multiple warty growths can persist for weeks or months in areas of skin previously involved by typical lesions of varicella or herpes zoster. Chronic zoster is often resistant to acyclovir. Tissue biopsy and viral cultures, with further testing for antiviral resistance, may aid in assessment.

Herpes Zoster
Diagnosis
Diagnosis of herpes zoster is often made on clinical grounds alone. A Tzanck smear can provide additional support of the viral etiology. With atypical presentations, however, the diagnosis is best confirmed by real time PCR. An antigen detection method can be used if active blisters are present. Both are rapid and differentiate VZV from HSV. Viral cultures are insensitive but may be required if there is a need to assess possible antiviral resistance. Basic VZV serology is rarely useful for diagnosis.

Treatment
There are three systemic antiviral agents routinely used for the treatment of HSV and VZV infections: acyclovir, valacyclovir, and famciclovir. All three are highly effective and generally well tolerated. Because they inhibit only actively replicating viral DNA, they have no impact on latent infection. Recommendations for antiviral treatment of mucocutaneous HSV infections and herpes zoster, localized topical measures, and available formulations are outlined in Tables 1 to 5. Optimal antiviral dosage schedules for less-common HSV infections, such as herpetic whitlow, have not been determined. The doses outlined in Table 1 for either episodic or chronic suppressive therapy can be used as a guideline in these cases.

Acyclovir became available more than 25 years ago and continues to be widely used. Inside an infected host cell, acyclovir must be phosphorylated—first by a virally encoded enzyme (thymidine kinase) and then by host-cell enzymes—to the active form of the drug, acyclovir triphosphate. As a nucleotide analogue, acyclovir triphosphate is incorporated into replicating viral DNA, abruptly terminating further synthesis of that viral DNA chain. Acyclovir triphosphate also interferes with viral DNA replication by directly inhibiting viral DNA polymerase. Valacyclovir is an oral prodrug of acyclovir and has a much higher bioavailability. After ingestion, valacyclovir is rapidly

TABLE 4 Formulations of Acyclovir, Valacyclovir, and Famciclovir

DRUG	ORAL	TOPICAL	INTRAVENOUS
Acyclovir	200, 400, 800 mg 50 mg buccal tablet	5% Ointment (5g, 15g, 30g) 5% cream (5 g)	Yes
Valacyclovir	500 mg, 1 g	No	No
Famciclovir	125, 250, 500 mg	No	No
Penciclovir (Denavir)	No	1% cream (1.5 g, 5 g)	No

TABLE 5 Recommended Antiviral Dose Modification in Patients with Impaired Renal Function

CREATININE CLEAR-ANCE (ML/MIN)	GENITAL HERPES SIMPLEX VIRUS			HERPES ZOSTER	HERPES LABIALIS
	INITIAL	RECURRENT	SUPPRESSION		
Acyclovir (Zovirax)					
>25	200 mg 5 ×/d	200 mg 5 ×/d	400 mg q12h	800 mg 5×/d	
10–24	200 mg 5 ×/d	200 mg 5 ×/d	400 mg q12h	800 mg q8h	
<10	200 mg q12h	200 mg q12h	200 mg q12h	800 mg q12h	
Valacyclovir (Valtrex)					
>50	1 g q12h	500 mg q12h	500 mg-1 g q24h	1 g q8h	2 g PO bid for 1 d
30–49	1 g q12h	500 mg q12h	500 mg-1 g q24h	1 g q12h	1 g PO bid for 1 d
10–29	1 g q24h	500 mg q24h	500 mg q24-48h	1 g q24h	500 mg bid for 1 d
<10	500 mg q24h	500 mg q24h	500 mg q24-48h	500 mg q24h	500 mg single dose
Famciclovir (Famvir)					
>60		125 mg q12h	250 mg q12h	500 mg q8h	
40–59		125 mg q12h	250 mg q12h	500 mg q12h	
20–39		125 mg q24h	125 mg q12h	500 mg q24h	
<20		125 mg q24h	125 mg q24h	250 mg q24h	
>60	1 g bid × 1 d				1500 mg single dose
40–59	500 mg bid × 1 d				750 mg single dose
20–39	500 mg single dose				500 mg single dose
<20	250 mg single dose				250 mg single dose

metabolized to acyclovir, and the subsequent mechanism of action is as just described. Famciclovir is an oral prodrug of penciclovir (Denavir), designed for greater bioavailability. Similar to acyclovir, penciclovir must first be phosphorylated by viral thymidine kinase and then by cellular enzymes to penciclovir triphosphate. In this active form, penciclovir triphosphate interferes with viral DNA synthesis and replication by inhibiting viral DNA polymerase. Famciclovir has greater bioavailability and a longer intracellular half-life than acyclovir. For all three agents, the required activation by viral thymidine kinase and the preferential inhibition of viral DNA synthesis contribute to the highly specific antiviral activity.

If taken as recommended, acyclovir, valacyclovir, and famciclovir are generally comparable in their safety and effectiveness. Valacyclovir and famciclovir offer the convenience of less-frequent dosing. Dosing for all three should be adjusted in the presence of renal insufficiency (see Table 5).

Although antiviral therapy does not decrease the incidence of postherpetic neuralgia, all three agents decrease the time for lesion healing and shorten the overall duration of pain if initiated within 48 to 72 hours after the onset of herpes zoster. Valacyclovir and famciclovir appear to be more effective than acyclovir for this purpose, presumably because of easier dosing. An otherwise healthy person younger than 50 years who has discrete involvement on the trunk

and mild to moderate pain might benefit minimally or not at all from this intervention, especially if it is initiated after 72 hours of lesion onset. However, patients who are older than 50 years, are immunosuppressed, have involvement in the ophthalmic distribution, or have more-extensive lesions or severe pain should receive systemic antiviral therapy, even if the 72-hour deadline has expired. Adequate pain control, often requiring opiates, is also important.

The addition of systemic corticosteroids to the antiviral regimen is not recommended for uncomplicated herpes zoster. Corticosteroids may be of benefit in herpes zoster complicated by facial paralysis, cranial polyneuropathy, or acute retinal necrosis. Corticosteroids should not be used without concomitant systemic antiviral therapy.

Vaccination with a herpes zoster vaccine substantially reduces the incidence of both herpes zoster and postherpetic neuralgia. There are two herpes zoster vaccines available. The live attenuated vaccine (ZVL/Zostavax) has been in use since 2006 and is given as a single intramuscular injection. The Zoster Vaccine Recombinant, Adjuvanted (RZV/Shingrix) received FDA approval in October 2017, for immunocompetent adults 50 years and older. RZV is a non-live recombinant glycoprotein E vaccine and requires 2 doses given intramuscularly 2–6 months apart. The U.S. Advisory Committee on Immunization Practices (ACIP) currently recommends the use of RZV for immunocompetent adults aged 50 years or older for the prevention of herpes zoster and related complications. The ACIP also recommends RZV for adults aged 50 years or older who previously received the live-attenuated herpes zoster vaccine (ZVL/Zostavax) and either RZV or ZVL for adults aged 60 years or older (RZV is preferred).

Despite widespread use of these antiviral agents, antiviral resistance is rarely a problem in the immunocompetent population. However, it does arise in the setting of immunosuppression. The basis for the resistance is most commonly a mutation in the gene coding for thymidine kinase. Less often there is a mutation in the viral DNA polymerase. In either case, all three standard drugs become ineffective. Alternative antiviral agents available for treatment of acyclovir-resistant HSV and VZV infections include foscarnet (Foscavir)[1] and cidofovir (Vistide).[1]

Hand-Foot-and-Mouth Disease

Hand-foot-and-mouth disease is typically a disease of childhood. The most common etiologic agent is a nonpolio enterovirus, Coxsackie A16, and transmission is via the oral–oral or fecal–oral route. It is highly contagious. Several days after exposure, a prodrome of low-grade fever, malaise, abdominal pain, or respiratory symptoms can develop, followed by the appearance of papulovesicles on the palate, tongue, or buccal mucosa. Similar lesions can subsequently develop on the feet and hands. The eruption persists for 7 to 10 days and then resolves. Treatment is symptomatic. Nail dystrophies including onychomadesis (separation of the proximal portion of the nail plate from the nail bed) and Beau's lines (horizontal grooves in the nail plate) may be seen 2–4 weeks later.

Since 1997, outbreaks of hand-foot-and-mouth disease caused by enterovirus 71 have been reported in Asia and Australia. Although hand-foot-and-mouth disease associated with Coxsackie A16 infection is typically a mild illness, hand-foot-and-mouth disease caused by enterovirus 71 has shown a higher incidence of neurologic involvement, including fatal cases of encephalitis.

An atypical hand-foot-and-mouth disease with more widespread cutaneous involvement has been reported as associated with Coxsackievirus A6. There is a predilection for areas commonly involved in atopic dermatitis, such as the antecubital and popliteal fossae and this presentation may be confused with eczema herpeticum or VZV infection. Diagnosis of these more atypical cases may require laboratory assessment. This could include antigen detection or PCR to exclude HSV and VZV. Reverse Transcription PCR (RT-PCR) of vesicle fluid, oropharyngeal swab or stool specimen may be used to confirm the enterovirus infection.

Parvovirus B19

Cutaneous manifestations of parvovirus B19 infection include the childhood exanthem known as erythema infectiosum (fifth disease) and, less commonly, petechial or purpuric eruptions. The virus is transmitted primarily via respiratory secretions and, to a much lesser extent, through blood or blood products. The host cells for viral replication are erythroid progenitor cells, which subsequently undergo cell lysis.

A child with erythema infectiosum typically develops a low-grade fever and nonspecific upper respiratory symptoms approximately 2 days before the onset of rash. The rash has been described as having a slapped-cheeks appearance, with prominent redness over the malar eminences. This is followed by a pink-to-red lacy or reticular eruption over the trunk and extensor surfaces of the arms and legs. The rash usually lasts a week to 10 days but can transiently recur over months in response to precipitating factors such as sunlight, exercise, and bathing. Diagnosis of erythema infectiosum is usually made on clinical grounds, and treatment is symptomatic. By the time the rash appears and the diagnosis has been made, the child is no longer infectious. Much less commonly parvovirus B19 infection may manifest as a papular-purpuric eruption with edema, erythema, and patecchiae in a "gloves and socks" distribution on the hands and feet.

Infection with parvovirus B19 in older adolescents and adults often manifests with arthralgias or arthritis rather than a rash. In certain patient populations, parvovirus B19 infections may be

TABLE 6	Treatment Options for Molluscum Contagiosum
TREATMENT	**COMMENT**
Cryotherapy (liquid nitrogen)	Freeze individual lesions for 5–10 sec Repeat PRN in 2–3 wk
Curettage	Entire lesion may be removed using a curette; this results in bleeding Removal of central core with toothpick or other pointed instrument is also effective
Cantharidin (Cantharone)[1]	Blister-inducing agent: Apply to lesion with toothpick, air dry Cover with tape or adhesive bandage Patient to wash area after 24 h (or sooner if significant pain)
Podophyllin (25% in tincture of benzoin)[1]	Cytotoxic agent: Apply to lesion with toothpick Patient to wash off after 4–6 h Contraindicated in pregnancy
Podofilox (Condylox 0.5% gel or solution)[1]	Done by patient: Apply bid for 3 consecutive d/wk × 2–4 wk Contraindicated in pregnancy
Salicylic acid/lactic acid (Occlusal, Duofilm)[1]	Done by patient: Apply daily
Imiquimod (Aldara) 5% cream[1]	Done by patient: Apply daily 5 consecutive d/wk Leave on overnight Continue for 8–12 wk
Cimetidine (Tagamet)[1]	30 mg/kg/d PO × 6–12 wk Can boost cell-mediated immunity
Candida antigen (Candin)[1]	Intralesional injection 0.3 mL[3]

[1]Not FDA approved for this indication.
[3]Exceeds dosage recommended by the manufacturer.

associated with complications including transient aplastic crisis, chronic anemia, and hydrops fetalis. In these less-typical presentations, serology (anti-B19 IgM or documented seroconversion) may be needed for diagnosis. Intravenous immunoglobulin (IVIg [Gamimune N][1]) is used successfully for treatment of chronic or persistent infection in immunosuppressed patients.

Molluscum Contagiosum

Molluscum contagiosum are benign umbilicated papules caused by infection with the *Molluscipoxvirus*, a member of the poxvirus family. Lesions are limited to the mucocutaneous surface and typically appear in clusters on the face, trunk, and skin fold areas in children and on thighs, lower abdomen, and suprapubic areas in sexually active adults. Large numbers of lesions in an extensive distribution may be seen in the immunosuppressed population.

Transmission routinely occurs by skin-to-skin contact with an infected host, but transmission from contaminated fomites has been reported. Autoinoculation commonly occurs. Diagnosis is usually based on clinical examination, but histopathology of atypical lesions may be used for confirmation.

Because molluscum contagiosum tends to be self-limited, treatment is not always recommended, but it can reduce the risk of autoinoculation and transmission to others. Treatment modalities are primarily aimed at destroying the lesions, similar to those used for verruca vulgaris (Table 6). In the case of sexual transmission, evaluation for other sexually transmitted diseases may be indicated.

Orf and Milker's Nodules

Orf (also known as ecthyma contagiosum) and milker's nodules are caused by the closely related *Parapoxvirus*, a member of the poxvirus family. The virus responsible for orf is widespread in

[1]Not FDA approved for this indication.

sheep and goats, whereas the virus causing milker's nodules is found in cattle. Transmission to humans is by direct contact with infected animals or recently vaccinated animals and is usually seen several days and up to 2 weeks after exposure. Preexisting skin trauma or other disruption of the normal cutaneous barrier enhances the risk of transmission. Barrier precautions and proper hand hygiene are important preventive measures.

Orf and milker's nodules most commonly appear as one to several nodules on the dorsal aspect of the hands or forearms. Lesions evolve through several clinical stages over a period of 3 to 5 weeks, ranging from solid red nodules to vesicular, exudative, or wartlike tumors. As with other poxvirus infections, lesions of orf often demonstrate central umbilication. Regional lymphadenopathy and lymphangitis are commonly seen.

Diagnosis is based on a history of exposure and clinical examination. Tissue biopsy for histopathology or electron microscopy may also be used. Orf virus infection can resemble skin lesions associated with potentially life-threatening zoonotic infections such as tularemia, cutaneous anthrax, and erysipeloid. Should this be a concern, definitive diagnostic testing using PCR is available through the Centers for Disease Control and Prevention (CDC).

In general, the lesions of orf are self-limited, resolving within 4 to 6 weeks, and treatment is not routinely required. However, immunocompromised persons can develop more progressive and destructive lesions requiring therapeutic intervention such as topical cidofovir[1,6] or imiquimod (Aldara).[1]

---

[1] Not FDA approved for this indication.
[6] May be compounded by pharmacists.

References

Advisory Committee on Immunization Practices Recommended Immunization Schedule for Adults Aged 19 Years or Older—United States, 2018, *MMWR* 67(5):158–160, 2018.

Bergqvist C, Kurban M, Abbas O: Orf virus infection, *Rev Med Virol* 27(4), 2017.

Centers for Disease Control and Prevention: Sexually Transmitted Diseases Treatment Guidelines, 2010. MMWR 59(RR-12), 2010, http://www.cdc.gov/STD/treatment/2010.

Cernik C, Gallina K, Brodell RT: The treatment of herpes simplex infections: an evidence-based review, *Arch Intern Med* 168(11):1137–1144, 2008.

Dayan RR, Peleg R: Herpes zoster - typical and atypical presentations, *Postgrad Med* 129(6):567–571, 2017.

Gnann JW, Whitley RJ: Genital herpes, *N Engl J Med* 375:666–674, 2016.

Nassef C, Ziemer C, Morrell DS: Hand-foot-and-mouth disease: a new look at a classic viral rash, *Curr Opin Pediatr* 27(4):486–491, 2015.

Qiu J, Soderlund-Venermo M, Young NS: Human parvoviruses, *Clin Microbiol Rev* 30(1):43–113, 2017.

Sacks HS: Review: Adjuvant recombinant subunit vaccine prevents herpes zoster more than live attenuated vaccine in adults ≥ 50 years, *Ann Intern Med* 170(4), 2019.

van der Wouden JC, van der Sande R, Kruithof EJ, et al: Interventions for cutaneous molluscum contagiosum, *Cochrane Database Syst Rev* 17(5):CD004767, 2017.

WARTS (VERRUCAE)

Method of
M. Chantel Long, MD

CURRENT DIAGNOSIS

- Common warts: rough, hyperkeratotic, firm papules usually found on the extremities.
- Flat warts: small, flat, pink or flesh-colored papules on the face, arms, or legs.
- Plantar and palmar warts: callus-like lesions that disrupt skin lines on the soles or palms.
- Mosaic warts: large clusters of warts.
- Filiform warts: small, finger-like lesions on the face.
- Genital warts: flesh to brown colored, flat or exophytic, found in the anogenital region.
- Differential diagnoses: seborrheic keratoses, molluscum contagiosum, keratoacanthoma, squamous cell carcinoma, acrochordon, amelanocytic melanoma, calluses, and corns.

CURRENT THERAPY

- Approximately 20% of warts spontaneously resolve within 3 months and 60% within 2 years in a healthy person.
- Salicylic acid and dimethyl ether.
- Cryotherapy.
- Cantharidin (Cantharone).[1,6]
- Surgical removal.
- Pulsed-dye laser.
- Immunotherapy: topical imiquimod (Aldara),[1] intralesional *Candida* antigen (Candin).[1]
- Photodynamic therapy.

[1] Not FDA approved for this indication.
[6] May be compounded by pharmacists.
Note: Cantharidin and Candin are not FDA approved. Aldara is approved for genital and perianal warts only.

Verrucae, commonly known as cutaneous warts, are benign skin growths caused by the human papillomavirus (HPV). Cutaneous warts are divided into common warts, plantar warts, flat warts, and genital warts. Common warts account for 70% of all cutaneous warts. Two-thirds of untreated common warts spontaneously regress within 2 years, but previously infected individuals have a higher rate of developing new warts than those who were never infected.

Epidemiology

It is estimated that 10% of the general population has cutaneous warts, and warts are one of the most common reasons for dermatologic visits. Transmission occurs through direct contact with an infected person. As a result, warts are seen with greater frequency among groups of people in close contact, such as schoolchildren. Thus, warts are more common in adolescents with a frequency estimated as high as 20%. Since the extent of infection is determined by the immune response, warts are also more common in immunocompromised patients. Autoinoculation is possible by scratching the lesions, often leading to a linear pattern.

Pathophysiology

Warts are caused by HPV. More than 200 genotypes of HPV have been identified, and the virus is prevalent. HPV causes both clinical and subclinical infections and plays a role in certain cutaneous malignancies, including squamous cell carcinoma. It is found in the basal layer of the epidermis but replicates in the superficial, well-differentiated layer of the skin. The cellular proliferation gives rise to thick, hyperkeratotic lesions generally known as warts. The warts can occur anywhere on the skin or mucous membranes.

Clinical Manifestations

Most warts are asymptomatic, though patients often present with complaints of a "bump." Usually, the warts appear flesh-colored, brown, or gray and can be flat to exophytic, giving them the classic "cauliflower" appearance. The lesions may be single or multiple and may range in size from miniscule to several centimeters in diameter. Localized irritation, pruritus, pain, or bleeding may occur. Symptoms vary based on the location and size of the lesions.

Several types of warts occur with variations in appearance, site of infection, and the specific type of HPV involved. Common warts (verrucae vulgaris) are white to flesh-colored, rough, hyperkeratotic, raised, and firm, usually found on the extremities. They disrupt normal skin lines on the fingers and toes and are most associated with HPV types 1, 2, and 4. Flat warts (verrucae plana) are caused by HPV types 3, 10, or 28 and are tan to flesh colored. They are small, 1 to 3 mm in diameter, flat, sharply demarcated growths that appear in large numbers on the face, arms, or legs. They usually occur in a linear arrangement related to local trauma, such as shaving. Butcher warts are associated with HPV type 7 and have a thick, raised, exophytic appearance. They are most common in workers who regularly handle raw meat or fish. Plantar and palmar warts (verrucae plantaris and verrucae palmaris) are hard, thickened, callus-like lesions that disrupt skin lines on the soles or palms. They are associated with HPV types 1, 2, 4, 27, and 57. They are usually flesh colored, covered with callus, and can be painful, especially when located on pressure points. If warts coalesce into a plaque, this is termed a *mosaic* wart. Filiform warts are slender, finger-like growths most commonly seen on the face, especially around the eyelids, nose, and mouth. Periungual warts are common warts impinging on and growing under toenails or fingernails. Genital warts (condyloma acuminatum) are flesh colored to brown, flat or exophytic lesions, occurring in anogenital regions. Mucosal papillomas are warts that occur on mucous membranes, usually in the mouth or vagina, and tend to be white in color.

Epidermodysplasia verruciformis is a rare, autosomal recessive disorder that leads to widespread reddish brown, flat papules on the trunk, hands, face, and extremities. These warts have malignant potential, especially on sun-exposed areas. It is estimated that one-third may become malignant. These patients present in childhood. Chronically infected with multiple types of HPV, including types 3, 5, 8, 9, 12, 14, 15, 17, 19 to 25, 36 to 38, 47, 49, and 50, the warts have lifelong persistence. Another related disease is verrucous carcinoma. This is a slow-growing variant of squamous cell carcinoma that occurs in the oral mucosa, anogenital region, or plantar surface. These warts are associated with HPV types 6 and 11.

Risk Factors

Risk factors most associated with verrucae include immunosuppression and close contact. Due to their decreased immune response, immunocompromised hosts are at increased risk not only for infection, but also for malignant transformation of the warts. Pregnancy, previous wart infection, and handling raw meat or fish are also known risk factors.

Differential Diagnosis

The differential diagnosis of warts includes seborrheic keratoses, molluscum contagiosum, keratoacanthoma, squamous cell carcinoma, acrochordon, amelanocytic melanoma, porokeratosis, calluses, corns, and cutaneous malignancy.

Diagnosis is based on clinical findings. When the clinical appearance of the lesion is typical, no other confirmatory tests are usually necessary. Paring down the stratum corneum, or outer layer of skin, may reveal black dots, which are thrombosed or bleeding capillaries, and helps confirm the diagnosis. If needed, tissue biopsy can provide histopathologic confirmation. In immunocompromised patients, biopsy is recommended to rule out squamous cell carcinoma in any suspicious lesions, which includes large or rapidly growing, pigmented, atypical, friable, bleeding, or ulcerated lesions.

Treatment

Approximately 20% of warts spontaneously resolve within 3 months and 60% within 2 years in a healthy person. Therefore, treatment is not always necessary. Current treatments do not eradicate the virus and do not guarantee resolution. Most patients seek treatment because of the physical appearance, discomfort, or interference with daily and social functioning, especially if located on the palms, digits, or soles. The American Academy of Dermatology established reasoning for wart treatment, including the desire of the patient; for symptoms of pain, bleeding, itching, or burning; for disabling or disfiguring lesions; for large numbers or large size of lesions; for a desire to prevent spread to unblemished skin; and because of a concomitant immunocompromised condition. Immunosuppressed patients are at higher risk for developing numerous warts and require treatment to prevent progression to squamous cell carcinoma. It is often more difficult to eradicate warts in an immunosuppressed host.

Many therapeutic modalities are available for the treatment of warts. No single therapy is universally effective. Warts can resolve, recur, shrink, or grow despite therapy. It is likely that all wart therapies work by triggering an immune response to the presence of papillomavirus in the skin. Treatment of warts must be individualized and often more than one modality is needed to achieve resolution. Conservative, less painful, and less expensive treatments are preferred.

Treatment methods are divided into the categories of home remedies, over-the-counter treatments, and office-based therapies. Office-based treatments include destructive methods, surgical or laser procedures, immunologic intervention, and combination therapy.

Home Remedies

Home remedies include applications of tea tree oil,[7] garlic extract,[7] duct tape,[1] and hyperthermic therapy. One study comparing cryotherapy with duct tape occlusion of common warts showed resolution in 85% of the children treated by occlusion, compared with 60% in the liquid nitrogen group. Proper protocol involves covering the wart with duct tape, which is left in place for 6 days. Then the site should be soaked, pared down with an emery board, and left uncovered overnight. This is repeated for a total of eight cycles. Another common home remedy is hyperthermic therapy. This involves immersing the affected area in a 45°C water bath for 30 minutes three times per week. It is a safe and inexpensive option.

Over-the-Counter Treatment

The most common over-the-counter option used by patients is one of the salicylic acid products, such as Compound W, Duofilm, WartStick, and Mediplast. These keratolytic products are offered as a solution, gel, cream, or pad in concentrations from 10% to 60%. They can be quite successful when used consistently and as directed in motivated patients. Repeated application, with pumice stone or callus file use, results in cure rates of 60% to 80%, but takes several weeks to work.

More recently, several over-the-counter wart-freezing therapies have become available. One such option is dimethyl ether, marketed as Compound W Freeze Off or Dr. Scholl's Freeze Away. These are available in aerosol form for wart treatment, which can be repeated every 2 weeks. Dimethyl ether achieves a temperature of −57°C, which is markedly higher than the −196°C temperature obtained with liquid nitrogen. This results in a more shallow depth of destruction. Because salicylic acid and dimethyl ether treatments destroy the infected epidermis and cause an immune reaction, they can be irritating and tedious, prompting many patients to seek medical care.

Office-based Treatment

Office-based treatments are largely destructive, immunomodulating, or both. Destructive treatments include cryosurgery, surgical excision, laser therapy, or repeated application of topical chemotherapy agents, such as salicylic acid, cantharidin (Cantharone),[1,6] podophyllin (Podocon),[1] or 5-fluorouracil (Efudex).[1] The most commonly used physician office-based treatment is cryotherapy with liquid nitrogen. It can be applied by a cotton-tipped applicator or cryogun. The wart and a 1 to 2 mm margin are frozen for 10 to 30 seconds. The freeze should be repeated once after a thaw of 20 seconds. If the warts are thick, they can initially be pared down. The patient is told that a blister will result and should be left intact if possible. Treatment should be repeated every 3 to 4 weeks until normal skin markings return. Cryotherapy has demonstrated a 60% to 80% cure rate. If warts persist beyond 3 months of therapy, another method of treatment should be selected.

Another option is cantharidin (Cantharone) in a 0.7% colloidal solution. It is a chemical derived from blister beetles that is painless on application and well tolerated by children. It causes epidermal necrosis with blistering after application and occlusion for 8 hours. It is applied in the office and repeated every 4 weeks. Although not Food and Drug Administration (FDA) approved, it is a commonly used technique and can be compounded by a pharmacist. It is useful for treatment of common, periungual, and plantar warts in children,

---

[1]Not FDA approved for this indication.
[7]Available as dietary supplement.
[1]Not FDA approved for this indication.

and the cure rate approaches 80%. Unfortunately, an occasional "donut wart," a ring of new warts surrounding the cleared original site, occurs.

Surgery is used for large, solitary warts, and is more direct. Large common warts of the hands or extremities are more easily treated if they are debulked surgically. This method is not recommended for plantar warts because of scarring. Surgical removal followed by electrodesiccation and curettage is effective but requires local anesthesia and can result in scarring.

Other destructive methods of wart removal usually are reserved for resistant, multiple lesions, or recalcitrant warts in immunosuppressed patients. This often requires specialty referral. Acids, including bichloroacetic and trichloroacetic acid (Tri-Chlor),[1] should be applied by a skilled practitioner because they are known to cause pain on application, ulceration, and even scarring. Laser therapy, most often with a pulsed-dye laser (PDL) or carbon dioxide (CO_2) laser, provides selective photothermolysis of blood vessels within the wart, which compromises blood supply and results in necrosis. The PDL method is less aggressive and less painful than CO_2 vaporization. These treatments cause minimal damage to normal skin. Overall, both therapies are generally well tolerated, but local anesthesia may be necessary. Although more expensive, these methods have cure rates ranging from 45% to 90%. Photodynamic therapy (PDT) is useful for patients with multiple recalcitrant warts, especially patients who are immunosuppressed. PDT involves a topical photosensitizer applied by a trained provider. It is activated by visible light, resulting in tissue destruction. Studies of this method have been promising.

Immune modulation alone or in combination with destructive methods is helpful in treating resistant warts. The self-applied immunomodulator imiquimod (Aldara) was initially approved for treatment of genital warts. It is also used anecdotally to treat flat and common warts[1] by inducing cytokines, including interferon production, at the site of application. A thin coat is applied at bedtime and then washed off after 6 to 10 hours. It is usually applied three times weekly and combined with cryotherapy or salicylic acid.

Intralesional immunotherapy, which includes *Candida* antigen (Candin),[1] interferon alfa-2b (Intron A),[1] bleomycin,[1] and MMR vaccine,[1] is an effective option for treatment in some patients. *Candida* antigen injection (Candin) is considered a first-line therapy in children with large or multiple warts and a second-line therapy for patients with resistant warts. It is well tolerated. *Candida* antigen is commercially available as a 1:1000 dilution. Using a 30-gauge needle and tuberculin syringe, one can inject 0.2 to 0.3 mL directly into the wart and repeat every 3 weeks. Pretesting is unnecessary, side effects are minimal, and more than 75% of patients treated with a series of three injections have clearing of the injected and distant warts. Intralesional interferon alfa-2b (Intron A) has been used successfully to treat genital warts and warts that have not responded to conventional therapies. The clearance rate varies from 36% to 62%, but it requires multiple injections in a physician's office, is expensive, and can cause systemic adverse effects such as flu-like symptoms. Intralesional bleomycin is effective but expensive and causes severe pain. The MMR vaccine is used off-label for intralesional injection and often combined with lidocaine for comfort.

Other topical immunomodulators, such as squaric acid dibutylester (SADBE)[1,6] or diphencyprone,[1,7] are contact sensitizers that induce an allergic dermatitis through type IV hypersensitivity reactions. Although time consuming, treatment with SADBE is well tolerated and a good choice for recalcitrant warts in children. Other topical products available for off-label treatment include retinoids, formaldehyde compounds, and 5-fluorouracil (Efudex).[1] These agents interfere with epidermal proliferation, effect a nonspecific antiviral action, or inhibit mitosis, leading to keratinocyte and viral death. All of these choices usually require specialty referral.

Oral immunomodulation with high-dose cimetidine (Tagamet)[1] has been proposed. It is postulated to enhance cell-mediated immune response. Evidence has been anecdotal. Daily doses of 30 to 40 mg/kg have been used divided twice a day to four times a day for 8 to 12 weeks.

To ensure resolution and no recurrence of warts, the patient and practitioner must often make compromises in regard to convenience, discomfort, and scarring. The factors to consider when deciding on treatment include wart location and size, patient tolerance and preference, cost, convenience, and clinician preference. Patient-applied options allow the patient greater control; however, this requires good compliance and the warts must be accessible by the patient or caregiver. Provider-applied treatments are good choices for large treatment areas. Data regarding the efficacy of using more than one modality at a time are lacking. It is common practice for health care providers to combine treatment modalities. Table 1 outlines current therapy regimens.

Patient Education

Counseling of patients regarding the goal and length of treatment is necessary. Patients should be educated that current treatments do not eradicate HPV, and therefore the objective of therapy is elimination of symptoms. They also need to understand that a repeated course of therapy is often required and it may take weeks to months to achieve desired results. Each treatment should be reviewed in detail, including risks and benefits. Subsequently, the management should be tailored depending on the wart, patient, and practitioner.

---

[6]May be compounded by pharmacists.

[1]Not FDA approved for this indication.
[6]May be compounded by pharmacists.
[7]Available as dietary supplement.

TABLE 1	Treatment Regimens			
DRUG	**AVAILABLE AS**	**MECHANISM OF ACTION**	**DISADVANTAGES**	**INSTRUCTIONS**
Patient Applied				
Salicylic acid (Compound W, Duofilm, or Mediplast)	Solution, gel, lotion, cream, plaster, pad 10%–60% concentration	Keratolytic that destroys the infected epidermis while irritation stimulates an immune response	Local irritation Requires multiple applications Requires compliance Wart may need to be pared down to increase penetration	Apply nightly until clear, usually for weeks to months
Dimethyl ether (Compound W, Freeze Off, Dr. Scholl's Freeze Away)	OTC in spray canister	As above	Local irritation Requires compliance Blistering may occur	May treat every 2 weeks Total of four treatments per wart advised
Retinoids (Accutane, Retin-A, Soriatane)[1]	Soriatane (10 and 25 mg tabs), Accutane (10, 20, and 40 mg tabs), Retin-A cream/gel	Antimitotic that interferes with epidermal proliferation	Systemic with mucocutaneous dryness, elevated triglycerides, abnormal liver enzymes Avoid use in pregnancy Local irritation and dryness	Take PO daily If topical form, apply nightly
Imiquimod (Aldara)[1]	Cream 5%	Immunomodulator that mediates cytokines	Irritation, erythema, pruritus, scarring, hyperpigmentation	Apply 3 times/wk on mucosal skin Apply daily on keratinized skin
Cimetidine (Tagamet)[1]	Tablets (200, 300, 400 mg) Liquid (300 mg/5 mL)	Immunomodulator that may enhance immune response	Unclear efficacy Diarrhea Many drug-drug interactions	30–40 mg/kg daily, divided bid–qid for 8–12 weeks
Provider Applied				
Cryotherapy	Cryogun or cotton-tip application	Destroys infected dermis, induces inflammation, and leads to stimulated immune response	Pain, erythema, blistering, hypopigmentation, scarring Onychodystrophy if not careful with periungual warts	Freeze for 10–30 seconds with a 1–2 mm border, allow to thaw, then repeat May offer/need local anesthesia May repeat every 3–4 weeks
Candida antigen injections (Candin)[1]	1:1000 dilution	Immunomodulator	Discomfort	Intralesional injection of 0.2–0.3 mL
Trichloroacetic acid (TCA)[1]	Solution, up to 80%	Destroys infected epidermis; best for mucosal surfaces	Pain	Apply sparingly with cotton tip, air dry Repeat weekly to every other week Do not allow to "run" on normal skin Neutralize with soap or sodium bicarbonate
Cantharidin (Cantharone)[1]	Colloidal solution 0.7%, compounded	Destroys epidermis, leads to blister formation Is painless, good for kids	Avoid on face Blistering will occur	Apply with fine applicator to wart only and have patient wash off after 6–8 hr
Surgery		Surgical removal	Avoid if bleeding disorder Often requires anesthesia Scarring	Surgical excision followed by curettage and cauterization
Interferon alpha-2b (Intron A)[1] injections		Immunomodulator	Expensive Flu-like side effects	Multiple intralesional injections several times a week Often requires specialty referral
Laser vaporization		Destroys epidermis	Expensive Requires local anesthesia	Requires specialty referral

[1]Not FDA approved for this indication.

Abbreviations: bid=twice a day; OTC=over-the-counter; PO=orally; qid=four times a day.

References

Cockayne S, Hewitt C, Hicks K, et al: Cryotherapy versus salicylic acid for the treatment of plantar warts: a randomized controlled trial, *BMJ* 342:d3271, 2011.

Kwok CS, Holland R, Gibbs S: Efficacy of topical treatments for cutaneous warts: a meta-analysis and pooled analysis of randomized controlled trials, *Br J Dermatol* 65:233–246, 2011.

Leung L: Recalcitrant nongenital warts, *Aust Fam Physician* 40–42, 2011.

Simonart T, De Maertelaer V: Systemic treatments for cutaneous warts: a systematic review, *J Dermatolog Treat* 23:72–77, 2012.

Yelverton CB: Warts. In *Manual of dermatologic therapeutics*, Philadelphia, 2007, Lippincott Williams & Wilkins, pp 233–240.

ACUTE KIDNEY INJURY

Method of
Sarah Burns, DO, MS, FACP, SFHM

CURRENT DIAGNOSIS

- Acute kidney injury (AKI) is a common diagnosis seen in the outpatient setting, in the emergency department, and in hospitalized patients.
- AKI is defined by increase in serum creatinine by ≥0.3 mg/dL within 48 hours, increase ≥1.5 times the baseline creatinine within 7 days, or oliguria.
- Identify the underlying cause of AKI, denoted by pathophysiologic etiology (prerenal, intrinsic, and postrenal) to determine therapy.

CURRENT THERAPY

- Treat any reversible causes identified.
- Ensure hemodynamic stability.
- Correct any imbalances in electrolytes or in acid-base standing.
- Avoid nephrotoxins and renally dose all medications if glomerular filtration rate (GFR) is decreased.
- Prompt consultation to specialists to determine whether renal replacement treatment is appropriate.

Background/Definitions

Acute kidney injury (AKI) is a diverse syndrome defined by a sudden decrease in kidney function shown by a rise in serum creatinine and/or decrease in urine output. This sudden decrease in renal function affects fluid balance, electrolyte balance, acid-base balance, and waste elimination. The older term *acute renal failure* has been supplanted by AKI. The term *AKI* reflects a lack of strict separation between normal renal function and complete failure of the kidneys.

Previously there was no standard definition for diagnosing AKI, and there were more than 30 different definitions in the literature. In 2004 Risk, Injury, Failure, Loss, and End Stage Kidney Disease (RIFLE) criteria were proposed, evolving into the AKI Network (AKIN) criteria in 2007. In 2012 these validated criteria were adapted into international clinical practice guidelines released by Kidney Disease: Improving Global Outcomes (KDIGO). Although KDIGO criteria are widely used in research, there are parts of the definition that have not been validated. However, most experts endorse the use of KDIGO criteria for the diagnosis and management of AKI.

KDIGO criteria denote AKI when there is an increase in serum creatinine greater than or equal to 0.3 mg/dL within 48 hours, or an increase greater than or equal to 1.5 times the baseline creatinine within 7 days, or a decrease in urine volume to less than 0.5 mL/kg/h over 6 hours. To further describe the severity of AKI, there are stages (Table 1) describing the amount of change in serum creatinine from baseline. Multiple studies have demonstrated that increasing severity of AKI is associated with increased mortality and worse kidney function in the future.

Epidemiology

AKI is commonly found in hospitalized patients, and the incidence appears to be increasing over time in the United States. A 2013 meta-analysis for all hospitalized patients worldwide showed an overall incidence of AKI in 21.6% of patients. With the KDIGO definition, this study showed that one in five adults and one in three children worldwide experience AKI during a hospital stay. A 2015 multinational cross-sectional study of AKI in patients in the intensive care unit (ICU) showed AKI occurred in 57.3% of patients in the ICU. Additionally, it has been observed that rises in serum creatinine are associated with adverse patient outcomes, increased mortality, longer length of hospital stay, and higher healthcare costs. AKI also has been shown to be an independent risk factor for mortality.

There are multiple factors, based on several observational studies, that may affect the chance of developing AKI. These factors vary between individuals, and it is not clear why one factor would cause an individual to develop an AKI and another not to. As delineated by KDIGO clinical practice guidelines, the following increase the risk of AKI: critical illness, sepsis, shock, burns, trauma, major surgery including cardiac surgery, nephrotoxic drugs, iodinated radiocontrast agents, and poisonous animals and plants. KDIGO clinical practice guidelines indicate that certain patient populations are susceptible to AKI, and they include the following: volume depletion, older age, female sex, Black race, chronic kidney disease (CKD), other chronic diseases (including heart, lung, and liver), diabetes mellitus, cancer, and anemia.

Etiology

The causes of AKI can be broadly divided by the pathophysiologic etiology, specifically prerenal, intrinsic, and postrenal causes (Box 1). Prerenal AKI from renal hypoperfusion is the most common cause of AKI in the community setting. Acute tubular necrosis (ATN; an intrinsic etiology) is the most common cause of hospital-acquired AKI. Although the cause of AKI is traditionally classified by the portion of the kidney affected, it should be

1199

TABLE 1	Staging of Acute Kidney Injury (Based on Kidney Disease: Improving Global Outcomes)	
STAGE	**SERUM CREATININE**	**URINE OUTPUT**
1	≥0.3 mg/dL increase OR 1.5–1.9 times baseline	<0.5 mL/kg/h for 6–12 h
2	2–2.9 times baseline	<0.5 mL/kg/h for ≥12 h
3	3 times baseline OR Increase in creatinine to ≥4 mg/dL OR Starting renal replacement therapy	<0.3 mL/kg/h for ≥24 h OR Anuria for ≥12 h

BOX 1 Etiology of Acute Kidney Injury by Pathophysiology

Prerenal Causes

- Hypovolemia caused by true or effective intravascular volume depletion
  - Hemorrhage of any cause, gastrointestinal (GI) losses (diarrhea, vomiting), diuretics, burns, cirrhosis, nephrotic syndrome
- Diminished cardiac output or pump failure
  - Shock, pericardial disease, heart failure, pulmonary embolism, pulmonary hypertension, and sepsis
- Systemic vasodilation
  - Sepsis, cirrhosis, anaphylaxis, and drugs
- Vasoconstriction of renal vessels
  - Sepsis (initially), hepatorenal syndrome, iodinated contrast, medications such as norepinephrine (Levophed) and vasopressin, nonsteroidal antiinflammatory drugs, and angiotensin-converting enzyme inhibitors
- Increased abdominal pressure
  - Abdominal compartment syndrome

Intrinsic Causes

- Intrinsic renal vascular disease
  - Small: vasculitides, thrombotic thrombocytopenic purpura, scleroderma, atheroembolic disease, and malignant hypertension
  - Large: infarct from aortic dissection, systemic thromboembolism, renal artery aneurysm, and renal vein thrombosis
- Intrinsic renal glomerular disease
  - Nephritic: proliferative glomerulonephritis (e.g., rapidly progressive glomerulonephritis)
  - Nephrotic: nonproliferative glomerulonephritis
- Intrinsic tubular and interstitial disease
  - Acute tubular necrosis
  - Angiotensin-converting enzyme inhibitors/angiotensin II receptor blockers plus nonsteroidal antiinflammatory drugs, radiocontrast or other nephrotoxins, after cardiac surgery, sepsis/shock or prerenal state, and rhabdomyolysis
- Acute interstitial nephritis
  - Nonsteroidal antiinflammatory drugs, aspirin, omeprazole (Prilosec), thiazide diuretics, furosemide, allopurinol (Zyloprim), penicillin, vancomycin, and cephalosporins
- Cast nephropathy
  - Multiple myeloma
- Acute urate nephropathy
  - Tumor lysis syndrome
- Crystalline nephropathy
  - IV acyclovir (Zovirax)
- Acute phosphate nephropathy after phosphate bowel prep

Postrenal Causes

- Extrinsic
  - Benign prostatic hyperplasia
  - Metastatic cancer
  - Retroperitoneal fibrosis
  - Neurogenic bladder
- Intrinsic
  - Calculi
  - Crystals
  - Blood clots

noted that diseases may cross these pathophysiologic boundaries. Therefore AKI may be multifactorial.

Prerenal

Prerenal AKI is caused by renal hypoperfusion caused by a decrease in the arterial volume. Recall that autoregulation will help maintain the kidney's glomerular filtration rate (GFR) by blunting changes in blood flow by various mechanisms. Ultimately, autoregulation can only compensate for a degree in decreased renal perfusion. For example, in those with CKD, these autoregulatory mechanisms are diminished, which increases the susceptibility of developing an AKI on CKD. Decreased arterial volume occurs in renal vasoconstriction, which is caused by sepsis (early in course), hepatorenal syndrome, iodinated contrast, medications such as norepinephrine or vasopressin, nonsteroidal antiinflammatory drugs, and angiotensin-converting enzyme inhibitors. Intravascular volume depletion reduces the arterial volume to the kidneys and is caused by gastrointestinal losses, hemorrhage, diuretic use, cirrhosis, nephrotic syndrome, and burns. Renal hypoperfusion is also caused by reduction in cardiac output, which is seen in shock, pericardial disease, heart failure, pulmonary embolism, pulmonary hypertension, and sepsis. Systemic vasodilation is another cause of renal hypoperfusion and is caused by sepsis, cirrhosis, anaphylaxis, and drugs. Increased abdominal pressure as seen in abdominal compartment syndrome can be another cause of prerenal AKI.

The clinical presentation of prerenal AKI is variable and dependent on the cause. The cause should be investigated first with an excellent history and physical examination. Prerenal causes may be suspected in patients with dehydration, gastrointestinal losses such as vomiting or diarrhea, sweating, other insensible losses, increased ostomy output, bleeding, dizziness, or syncope. Prerenal causes should be suspected in patients with chronic medical conditions, such as heart failure or cirrhosis. All medications (current, recently used, prescribed, over-the-counter) should be investigated in every patient suspected to have an AKI from any cause. Further work-up is discussed below. Prerenal AKI may improve rapidly if the underlying cause is treated, if the volume status is improved, and/or if the offending medication is removed.

Intrinsic

Intrinsic AKI can be divided into the component of the kidney that is affected, which includes diseases of the vasculature, the glomeruli, the tubules, and the interstitium. Vascular causes are uncommon and include those that affect the small vessels and those that affect the large vessels. Small vessels are affected by vasculitides, scleroderma, and malignant hypertension. Large vessels are affected by aneurysms, infarct from aortic dissection, venothrombosis, and atheroembolism especially in the setting of recent vascular surgery or arterial catheterization.

Glomerular diseases originate from inflammation of the vessels and the glomeruli and may be a manifestation of an infection, of a vasculitis, or of a rheumatologic disorder. Glomerular diseases are divided into nephritic and nephrotic diseases, determined by less than 3 g of proteinuria per day or more than 3 g of proteinuria per day, respectively. Rapid progressive glomerulonephritis (RPGN) is an acute cause of AKI that may be seen in the hospital and always presents with a nephritic pattern. Nephrotic patterns of AKI are rarely encountered in hospitalized patients.

Tubular and interstitial diseases commonly cause AKI specifically from damage caused by ischemia, endogenous or exogenous nephrotoxins, medications, or infections. Tubulointerstitial diseases include ATN, acute interstitial necrosis, cast nephropathy, acute urate nephropathy, crystalline nephropathy, and acute phosphate nephropathy. The most common AKI in hospitalized patients is caused by ATN. ATN occurs from prolonged renal hypoperfusion and tissue ischemia or from endogenous or exogenous nephrotoxic exposure. Common endogenous nephrotoxins include hemolysis, rhabdomyolysis, tumor lysis syndrome, and multiple myeloma. Common exogenous nephrotoxins include radiocontrast, aminoglycosides, ethylene glycol, cisplatin, and methotrexate. Common nephrotoxins associated with AKI are listed in Box 2. Cast nephropathy is attributable to excess immunoglobulin light chains in multiple myeloma. Excess cellular contents released into circulation after chemotherapy can cause acute urate nephropathy in tumor lysis syndrome, less common nowadays with the prophylactic use of allopurinol (Zyloprim) or rasburicase (Elitek) prior to chemotherapy administration.

BOX 2 Common Nephrotoxic Medications Associated With Acute Kidney Injury

- Vancomycin
- Aminoglycosides
- Penicillin
- Piperacillin and tazobactam (Zosyn)
- Cephalosporins
- Heme pigments
- Cisplatin
- Radiocontrast
- Pentamidine (Pentam)
- Foscarnet (Foscavir)
- Cidofovir (Vistide)
- Tenofovir (Viread)
- IV immunoglobulin
- Mannitol
- Synthetic cannabinoids
- Nonsteroidal antiinflammatory drugs
- Angiotensin-converting enzyme inhibitors
- Aspirin
- Omeprazole (Prilosec)
- Thiazide diuretics
- Furosemide (Lasix)
- Allopurinol (Zyloprim)

Intravenous acyclovir (Zovirax) causes crystalline nephropathy. Oral sodium phosphate solution (Fleet) given for a bowel preparation for colonoscopy can cause acute phosphate nephropathy through an unclear mechanism.

The clinical presentation of intrinsic AKI is variable and dependent on the cause. The cause should be investigated first with an excellent history and physical examination. Vascular causes of intrinsic AKI should be suspected in recent vascular surgery, recent arterial catheterization, anticoagulation, atheroembolic disease, flank pain, or trauma. Glomerular causes of intrinsic AKI should be suspected in patients with systemic lupus erythematosus, systemic sclerosis, rash, arthritis, HIV infection, hepatitis C viral infection, cough, sinusitis, hematuria, hemoptysis, or weight loss. ATN should be suspected in patients with exposure to nephrotoxins, hypotension, trauma, or exposure to radiocontrast agents. AIN should be suspected in medication use or if there is a rash, fever, infection, or arthralgias. Further work-up is described in the following. Management and prognosis are variable and depend on the underlying cause.

Postrenal

Postrenal AKI is caused by obstruction of any cause in the urinary tract, within the kidney itself, or from the ureter, bladder, bladder neck, or urethra. The most common cause is caused by obstruction of the bladder neck, either structural or functional, such as seen in benign prostatic hyperplasia. Other causes include extrinsic compression from metastatic cancer, neurogenic bladder, or retroperitoneal fibrosis, or intrinsic obstruction from calculi, crystals, or blood clots.

The clinical presentation of postrenal causes of AKI with variable urine output from anuria to polyuria, hematuria (if clots are present or malignancy is suspected), dysuria, urgency, increased frequency, weak stream, nocturia, spinal cord injuries, or long-standing poorly controlled diabetes. An excellent history and physical examination will start the investigation of the cause. It is important to diagnosis and treat postrenal causes promptly to avoid long-term damage and improve the chance for recovery.

Approach to Diagnosis

The cause of AKI should always be approached in a patient-centered manner. The diagnostic work-up will depend on clinical context, severity, and duration of AKI in addition to comorbid conditions. For patients in the outpatient setting with new onset or rapidly worsening GFR, close follow-up is warranted, and these patients should likely be hospitalized for daily monitoring of laboratory studies and clinical status, especially if urgent or emergent treatment is warranted.

Careful review of the medical record can aid in determining trends in serum creatinine, assisting in the determination of an acute, acute on chronic, or chronic process. Once an acute process is identified, the evaluation of AKI should be categorized into prerenal, intrinsic, or postrenal cause to determine further work-up and ultimately treatment. At minimum, the clinician should obtain urinalysis, urine microscopy, laboratory studies including complete blood count, and metabolic panel with creatinine and electrolytes. Prerenal causes are more suggestive when blood urea nitrogen (BUN):creatinine ratio is greater than 20, when urine specific gravity is elevated, or when urine sodium is low. A renal ultrasound may be useful to obtain to assess for postrenal causes including obstruction and can specifically give information on cortical thickness, differences in densities in cortex and medulla, integrity of the collecting system, and kidney size. Postvoid residual may be considered and placement of urinary catheter if obstruction is suspected. Although a patient's urine output is an important clinical indicator, it is not necessarily kidney specific. Urine output may increase, decrease, or maintain irrespective of the insult affecting the kidneys. Trends in urine output can be useful when determining possible causes of AKI.

Measurements of fractional excretion of sodium (FeNa) or urea (FeUr) have not consistently been shown to have clear clinical correlations. FeNa is defined by the following formula:

$$FE_{Na} = \frac{U_{Na} \times P_{Cr}}{P_{Na} \times U_{Cr}} \times 100$$

FeNa <1% suggests prerenal and FeNa >2% suggests ATN. Despite the claims that a FeNa calculation can determine prerenal AKI versus ATN, there is no absolute FeNa value that is always diagnostic of prerenal disease. There are many limitations in using FeNa, including that there are other causes of AKI that have a calculated FeNa <1% (including some occasions of ATN). Additionally, single measurements of creatinine may be misleading, given that serum creatinine can vary even in a given day. Patients with CKD have impaired sodium handling and in the setting of prerenal disease will have a FeNa that is greater than 1%. However, this FeNa value should not preclude the clinician from addressing the underlying issue (for example, hypovolemia causing prerenal AKI in a patient with known CKD) solely based on a FeNa percentage. FeNa is not sensitive or specific enough in the inpatient population and therefore is not generalizable to the average hospitalized patient. *The entirety of a patient's presentation should allow the clinician to determine the cause of AKI.*

Approach to Treatment

The cause of AKI will determine the treatment. If history and examination are indicating prerenal volume depletion as the mechanism of AKI, intravenous fluids should be administered. This does not apply to prerenal AKI from heart failure or cirrhosis. Hypovolemia and hypotension should be addressed with balanced crystalloid solutions (for example, lactated Ringer's), which will reduce the risk of severe hyperchloremic metabolic acidosis that can occur with saline solutions. The optimal rate of infusion of fluids depends on the clinical status of the patient and comorbidities with expert recommendation to consider 1 to 3 L of fluid to start and to avoid volume overload. Concern for sepsis or infection should be treated appropriately, including cultures as indicated, intravenous fluid resuscitation (30 mL/kg for initial resuscitation), and antibiotics. Urinary obstruction should be treated and depending on the site of obstruction, a patient may need placement of a urinary catheter or percutaneous nephrostomy tube. Depending on the patient's GFR, any medication given should be renally dosed. All nephrotoxic insults should be avoided. Diuretics should be used in the setting of volume overload, such as in acute decompensated heart failure causing AKI, and it should be noted that diuretics do not specifically affect AKI recovery or have a survival benefit. If there are life-threatening abnormalities or imbalances caused by

AKI including volume overload, hyperkalemia, acidemia, or uremia, prompt consultation is warranted with a nephrologist and likely with a critical care specialist. In these cases, renal replacement therapy or another hemodialysis modality will likely be considered. The ideal timing to starting dialysis in patients with AKI is unknown, and the mortality benefit to early initiation of dialysis also is unclear. As already mentioned, in patients with acute decompensated heart failure, diuretics are used and inotropes may also be necessary to achieve improvement in renal perfusion in the setting of decreased cardiac output. In patients with liver disease and concomitant AKI, hepatorenal syndrome (HRS) may be considered as the underlying cause of AKI and is a diagnosis of exclusion. Type 1 hepatorenal syndrome (HRS-AKI) is the more serious disease with the recommended treatment of terlipressin (Terlivaz) and albumin[1] for patients on the general medical floor rather than midodrine (Proamatine),[1] octreotide (Sandostatin),[1] and albumin.[1] Acute interstitial nephritis should be treated with the withdrawal of the inciting medication or agent, and if there is no improvement in some days, patients may benefit from glucocorticoids. ATN has no one specific treatment, because it is dependent on the underlying cause (ischemia or nephrotoxins).

Prognosis and Outcomes

AKI is associated with adverse patient outcomes, increased mortality, longer length of hospital stay, and higher healthcare costs. The duration of AKI tends to vary between 7 and 21 days. Some patients with AKI recover kidney function within days and some require dialysis for months. After an episode of AKI, patients are at increased risk for CKD and end-stage renal disease (ESRD). Patients with CKD who experience AKI are more likely to advance to ESRD. Some patients may never return to their baseline kidney function. Irreparable decline in kidney function is more likely in patients of advanced age, those with CKD, and those with heart failure. Mortality rates range from 16% to 50% according to stage of AKI and also depend on cause of AKI, concurrent comorbid conditions such as sepsis, lung or liver failure, and cerebrovascular events. Patients who are discharged after a hospitalization during which AKI occurred warrant close follow-up. The KDIGO clinical practice guideline, in their expert opinion, recommended that clinicians evaluate patients 3 months after AKI for resolution of AKI or new-onset CKD or worsening of preexisting CKD.

Developing Issues—Biomarkers

The aim of AKI biomarkers is to excel in early diagnosis, to assess risk accurately, to assess treatment response, and to evaluate prognosis. There are over 20 biomarkers available to date that can be divided into functional biomarkers, tubular enzymes, damage biomarkers, and preinjury phase biomarkers in the evaluation of AKI. Nearly all biomarkers can be affected by at least one factor. The urine biomarker NephroCheck (insulin-like growth factor-binding protein [IGFBP7] and tissue-inhibitor of metalloproteinases 2 [TIMP2]) is FDA approved and commercially available. Despite validation in the prediction of onset of severe AKI in the critical care setting, this test has limitations including that it can commonly lead to false positive results (especially if used in patients that are low risk for AKI) and cannot be used in the outpatient setting. Given the heterogeneity of AKI, it is evident that no one biomarker is entirely specific for AKI. Biomarkers are but one factor in risk assessment in AKI, and there are newer developments related to monitoring and evaluating AKI risk progression. These include electronic alert systems and machine learning algorithms and artificial intelligence, in addition to models based on renal angina index, furosemide stress test, or biomarkers. Additional study is needed to validate and to standardize risk models to better intervene in AKI to improve outcomes.

[1] Not FDA approved for this indication.

References

Alge JL, Arthur JM: Biomarkers of AKI: a review of mechanistic relevance and potential therapeutic implications, *Clin J Am Soc Nephrol* 10(1):147–155, 2015, https://doi.org/10.2215/CJN.12191213.

Balogun R: Fractional excretion of sodium, urea, and other molecules in acute kidney injury - UpToDate. https://www.uptodate-com.libproxy.unm.edu/contents/fractional-excretion-of-sodium-urea-and-other-molecules-in-acute-kidney-injury?search=fena&source=search_result&selectedTitle=1~40&usage_type=default&display_rank=1#H791015361.

Cooper CM, Fenves AZ, Cooper CM: Before you call renal: acute kidney injury for hospitalists, *J Hosp Med* 10(6), 2015. Available at: 10.1002/jhm.2325.

Hoste EAJ, Bagshaw SM, Bellomo R, et al: Epidemiology of acute kidney injury in critically ill patients: the multinational AKI-EPI study, *Intensive Care Med* 41(8):1411–14232015. Available at: https://doi.org/10.1007/s00134-015-3934-7.

Levey AS, James MT: Acute kidney injury, *Ann Intern Med* 167(9):ITC66, 2017, https://doi.org/10.7326/AITC201711070.

Oh DJ: A long journey for acute kidney injury biomarkers, *Ren Fail* 42(1):154–165, 2020, https://doi.org/10.1080/0886022X.2020.1721300. PMID: 32050834; PMCID: PMC7034110.

Ostermann M, Bellomo R, Burdmann EA, et al: Conference participants. Controversies in acute kidney injury: conclusions from a kidney disease: improving global outcomes (KDIGO) conference, *Kidney Int* 98(2):294–309, 2020, https://doi.org/10.1016/j.kint.2020.04.020. Epub 2020 Apr 26. PMID: 32709292.

Ostermann M, Joannidis M: Acute kidney injury 2016: diagnosis and diagnostic workup, *Crit Care* 20(1):299, 2016, https://doi.org/10.1186/s13054-016-1478-z.

Ostermann M, Lumlertgul N, Jeong R, et al.: Acute kidney injury, Lancet 405(10474):241–256, 2025, https://doi.org/10.1016/S0140-6736(24)02385-7.

Pahwa AK, Sperati CJ: Urinary fractional excretion indices in the evaluation of acute kidney injury: urinary excretion indices in AKI, *J Hosp Med* 11(1):77–80, 2016, https://doi.org/10.1002/jhm.2501.

Rahman M, Shad F, Smith MC: Acute kidney injury: a guide to diagnosis and management, *Acute Kidney Injury* 86(7):9, 2012.

Section 2: AKI definition, *Kidney Int Suppl* 2(1):19–36, 2012, https://doi.org/10.1038/kisup.2011.32.

Sharfuddin AA, Weisbord SD, Palevsky PM, Molitoris BA: *Acute kidney injury. Brenner and Rector's the Kidney*, Philadelphia, PA, 2016, Elsevier, pp 958–1011. e19. http://www.clinicalkey.com/#!/content/book/3-s2.0-B9781455748365000031X.

Susantitaphong P, Cruz DN, Cerda J, et al: World incidence of AKI: a meta-analysis, *CJASN* 8(9):1482–1493, 2013, https://doi.org/10.2215/CJN.00710113.

Wald R: Changing incidence and outcomes following dialysis-requiring acute kidney injury among critically ill adults: a population-based cohort study-clinical key, *Am J Kidney Dis* 65(6):870–877, 2015.

Wasung ME, Chawla LS, Madero M: Biomarkers of renal function, which and when? *Clin Chim Acta* 438:350–357, 2015, https://doi.org/10.1016/j.cca.2014.08.039.

Wong F, Pappas SC, Curry MP, CONFIRM Study Investigators, et al: Terlipressin plus albumin for the treatment of type 1 hepatorenal syndrome, *N Engl J Med* 384(9):818–828, 2021, https://doi.org/10.1056/NEJMoa2008290. PMID: 33657294.

Yu MK, Kamal F, Chertow GM: Updates in management and timing of dialysis in acute kidney injury, *J Hosp Med* 7, 2019. Available at: https://doi.org/10.12788/jhm.3105.

CHRONIC KIDNEY DISEASE

Method of
Mark Unruh, MD; and Darren Schmidt, MD

CURRENT DIAGNOSIS

- Chronic kidney disease (CKD) is defined as reduced kidney function and/or evidence of kidney damage for more than 3 months, with implications for health (i.e., associated with morbidity or decreased longevity).
- The estimated glomerular filtration rate (eGFR) is the generally accepted best index of kidney function. Normal eGFR varies according to age, sex, and body size; in young adults it is approximately 125 mL/min/1.73 m^2 and declines with age.
- The most common method used to assess glomerular filtration rate is the CKD-EPI equation based on serum creatinine.
- In line with recommendations from the Task Force on Reassessing the Inclusion of Race in Diagnosing Kidney Diseases, a joint effort by both the National Kidney Foundation and American Society of Nephrology, a modified version of the CKD-EPI equation without race has been published (2021) and has been adopted by major labs and many centers as the preferred equation.
- The most common marker of kidney damage is urine albumin, most often expressed as the urine albumin/creatinine ratio.

- Presently, there are three cornerstones of therapy to limit progression of chronic kidney disease (CKD): (1) blood pressure (BP) control, (2) renin-angiotensin system (RAS) blockade, and (3) sodium glucose cotransporter type 2 inhibitor (SGLT2i) therapy.
- A BP target of less than 130/80 mm Hg has been a well-established goal for most kidney outcomes, though tighter BP control is thought to have additional benefits, especially for cardiovascular outcomes, and targets are being lowered in new guidelines.
- RAS blockade involves using angiotensin-converting enzyme inhibitors or RAS blockade, and it should be employed in patients with CKD and hypertension and/or proteinuria.
- SGLT2 inhibitors reduce progression of CKD and the risk of developing end-stage kidney disease in both diabetic and nondiabetic kidney disease with proteinuria, and in more recent studies this benefit appears to extend to patients without proteinuria.
- In CKD, prevention and treatment of biochemical or clinical abnormalities, including serum potassium, bicarbonate, calcium, phosphorus, parathyroid hormone, and hemoglobin, become increasingly important with lower levels of kidney function. An evaluation for the presence of comorbid conditions such as hypertension, diabetes, and cardiovascular disease should be undertaken in patients with CKD.

Chronic kidney disease (CKD) is the term used to describe patients with evidence of persistent (>3 months) kidney damage or reduced kidney function with implications for health. The formal definition, which comes from international guidelines, includes the phrasing "implications for health" to prevent minor lab abnormalities or other findings (e.g., radiographic evidence of simple cysts) that are unlikely to have such an association with significant morbidity or reduced longevity, leading to the label of a disease state in the otherwise healthy. Kidney function is most commonly assessed with a calculated estimate of the glomerular filtration rate (eGFR). *Kidney damage* is defined as structural or functional abnormalities of the kidney. Markers of kidney damage include certain abnormalities in the composition of the urine or blood and structural abnormalities identified in imaging tests or pathology. CKD should be classified by cause, kidney function, and severity of albuminuria. *End-stage kidney disease (ESKD)* is the term used to describe patients who have advanced kidney failure; whose kidney function is reduced to the point where initiation of renal replacement therapy (RRT) (i.e., either hemodialysis/peritoneal dialysis or transplantation) has become necessary. Progression in CKD is quite variable and depends on a number of factors, including the cause or causes of CKD, the extent of damage, and the degree of proteinuria. The rate of decline can be as rapid as 7 to 10 mL/min/year in those with untreated diabetic nephropathy, but other forms of CKD may not show such rapid progression. Electrolyte homeostasis, causes of progressive kidney function decline, and manifestations of kidney failure are similar enough across the different pathologies that we can think in terms of common underlying routes to progression, symptoms, and hopefully amelioration of CKD. These interventions often do not reverse kidney disease; rather, they slow its progression. Therefore earlier diagnosis and treatment may delay kidney death so a patient can avoid undergoing dialysis, transplantation, and the complications of kidney failure.

Prevalence of Chronic Kidney Disease

Approximately 14.7% of the U.S. adult population is thought to have some form of CKD. Unfortunately, most people with stage 1 to 3 kidney disease may not even be aware of their kidney disease.

Furthermore, more than 75 million of the U.S. adult population are thought to have an increased risk of developing CKD. Only a fraction of patients understand that they have CKD, so it is crucial to convey this to them so they can take steps to slow the progression. The high frequency of kidney disease is now seen in almost all parts of the world, which has triggered an international effort to address the problem. This effort has, in part, taken shape in the Kidney Disease Improving Global Outcomes (KDIGO) guidelines issued by the International Society of Nephrology. The guidelines cover a variety of topics relevant to the care of patients with kidney disease and are intended for both nephrologists and primary care clinicians.

Risk Factors for Chronic Kidney Disease

Nonmodifiable risk factors, such as age and ethnicity, are important for risk stratification by screening and for understanding the pathophysiology of CKD progression (Box 1). For example, Black patients with diabetes have a two- to threefold higher risk of developing kidney failure compared with White patients. Modifiable risk factors are important for understanding both disease progression and possible options for prevention or therapy. For example, heavy consumption of nonsteroidal analgesics has been associated with the development of kidney failure. The number of patients who develop kidney disease and are at risk for developing kidney disease will increase with the increasing prevalence of diabetes and obesity. As the population ages, the number of individuals with eGFR below 60 becomes increasingly common; however, there is some debate on the implications of this reduced eGFR among older adults on health in the absence of an accelerated decline in renal function or other forms of kidney damage.

Approach to the Diagnosis of Chronic Kidney Disease

In clinical practice, the serum creatinine and blood urea nitrogen (BUN) concentrations are commonly used as indicators of glomerular filtration rate (GFR). The laboratory measurement of creatinine and urea is accurate and reliable, although normal values may vary slightly among laboratories. Creatinine production varies with muscle mass; therefore changes in lean body weight influence the serum creatinine level. For example, a young bodybuilder may have an elevated creatinine but normal renal function and vice versa for a cachectic older adult with muscle atrophy. When using plasma creatinine to assess GFR, it is also important to keep in mind the relationship between the serum creatinine concentration and GFR is nonlinear, and small changes in creatinine with normal and near normal creatinine reflect larger changes in GFR than a similar change in creatinine from a creatinine value elevated at baseline.

There are additional biomarkers available to estimate kidney function. The most widely used is cystatin C. Cystatin C is a low-molecular-weight cysteine protease inhibitor produced in all nucleated cells. It generally has a constant level of production,

---

BOX 1 Risk Factors for the Development or Progression of Chronic Kidney Disease

Albuminuria
Hypertension
Episodes of acute kidney injury
Underlying cause of kidney disease (e.g., diabetic nephropathy)
Obesity
Hyperlipidemia
Smoking
High-protein diet
Metabolic acidosis
Hyperphosphatemia
Hyperuricemia
Hyperglycemia

and levels increase with decrements in kidney function; hence cystatin C may serve to improve the estimates of GFR in a number of clinical settings. Importantly, it does not share creatinine's tendency to vary significantly with muscle mass. That being said, thyroid disease, cancer, and inflammation can affect cystatin C levels, so providers should interpret this biomarker with caution in these settings.

Over time, there have been ongoing efforts to use serum creatinine and cystatin C along with other clinical markers to estimate kidney function to increase accuracy of CKD evaluation. Earlier formulas derived from pooled data, such as those by Cockroft and Gault and the Modification of Diet in Renal Disease (MDRD), in which GFR was correlated with other factors (e.g., body weight, age, and serum albumin), are sufficiently accurate to use for clinical purposes. However, the CKD-EPI equation has largely taken their place in clinical practice as encouraged by the KDIGO guidelines. In recent years, the inclusion of a race adjustment in creatinine-based GFR equations has been questioned as race is a social construct and not a biologic variable; therefore its inclusion in GFR calculations is nonscientific. The Task Force on Reassessing the Inclusion of Race in Diagnosing Kidney Diseases, a joint effort by both the National Kidney Foundation and American Society of Nephrology, advised the removal of the race adjustment in GFR equations in 2021 because its inclusion led to higher GFR estimations in individuals identified as Black and led to delays in CKD diagnosis and kidney care. Therefore, in 2021 the CKD-EPI equation was updated to remove race.

The task force also recommended more widespread use of serum cystatin C for CKD confirmation in addition to use of creatinine-based equations. There is a cystatin-C based CKD-EPI equation that was introduced in 2012 which did not have a race component, so it remains unchanged. There is also a 2021 CKD-EPI equation that uses both creatinine and cystatin C, which is felt to be the most accurate overall. It does not use a race variable.

In 2012 the KDIGO guideline recommended the classification of CKD include a measure of albuminuria. A spot urine albumin/creatinine ratio serves as a very important biomarker. Higher levels of albuminuria are linked to CKD progression, higher frequency of acute kidney injury, higher rates of dialysis, and higher risk of death. A urine protein/creatinine ratio can be used if a urine albumin/creatinine ratio is not available. Some labs are not able to report albumin/creatinine ratio when the urine albumin is above a certain threshold; in these cases, the spot urine protein/creatinine ratio is the best option. In most cases it is not necessary to obtain a 24-hour urine collection to quantify proteinuria, and, overall, these collections are more cumbersome for patients and not more accurate. However, there can be cases where it can still be helpful to obtain a 24-hour urine collection, such as at the extremes of the typical range of creatinine production (e.g., very large or very small body size).

If CKD is diagnosed, it is important to define the underlying etiology. As part of this evaluation, a thorough history is an important initial step to identify underlying medical problems that pose a risk of kidney disease (e.g., diabetes mellitus [DM] or systemic lupus erythematosus) or to identify family histories of kidney disease (e.g., autosomal dominant polycystic kidney disease [ADPKD]). A careful review of all medications, whether they are prescribed, over the counter, or herbal/traditional, is critical so that potential nephrotoxins can be identified and withdrawn. The physical exam can also provide clues to the nature of the condition; blood pressure (BP) measurement is an essential example, and findings, such as the presence and amount of peripheral edema, help shape the differential. Additionally, the microscopic appearance of the urine (e.g., presence of hematuria and/or casts) and the quantity of proteinuria can help focus the differential diagnosis. There are many serologies and other specialized lab tests that can be employed to help make a specific diagnosis in the appropriate clinical setting. Imaging studies can also be important to establish certain diagnoses (e.g., ADPKD or obstructive nephropathy) and also in assessing chronicity.

The role of genetic testing for the evaluation of chronic kidney disease is evolving. The cost has become less of a barrier and utilization seems likely to increase. Still, many question remain around how best to incorporate this new tool into clinical practice. Finally, in some cases a kidney biopsy will be necessary to fully characterize the underlying etiology and to guide subsequent treatment.

Management of Chronic Kidney Disease
Staging
The purpose of CKD staging is to guide management, including stratification of risk for progression and complications of CKD. Staging of CKD should be done according to Figure 1 and Table 1 based on (1) the cause of kidney disease, (2) six categories of eGFR (G stages), and (3) three levels of albuminuria (A stages).

Therefore to properly stage CKD, one needs to know the eGFR and degree of albuminuria, which collectively produce a G score (G1–5) and an A score (A1–3). Note that stage G3 is divided into 3a and 3b, with eGFR of 45 to 59 being G3a and eGFR 30 to 44 being 3b. The schema is reflected in the heat map reproduced in Figure 1. The risk of renal failure increases with both lower eGFR and greater albuminuria. This risk mapping can be used not only to determine the likelihood of progression and complications but also can aid in consideration for initiation of certain therapies and the referral to nephrology. The provider can use the CKD classification system shown in Figure 1 to educate patients and highlight the need for adhering to strategies to slow the rate of CKD progression. There are additional tools for assessing risk more precisely that can be easily employed in clinical practice. The Kidney Failure Risk Equation is one such tool, which can be accessed online (https://kidneyfailureriskequation.com) by providers or the patients themselves and can prove useful in further refining the timing of referrals or other interventions.

General Approach to Treatment of Chronic Kidney Disease
The physician treating the patient with CKD has three primary goals: preventing or delaying CKD progression, alleviating the electrolyte and hormonal abnormalities that can lead to symptoms or complications, and initiating targeted therapies focusing on cardiovascular risk reduction.

Strategies to Slow Chronic Kidney Disease Progression
Because we have a better understanding of the progression of kidney disease, we can effectively slow progression. Rather than losing 10 mL/min/year of kidney function with untreated type 1 DM, those with adequate disease control can markedly forestall the need for dialysis by slowing the rate of progression. The U.S. Food and Drug Administration (FDA) has accepted that altering the slope of decline in eGFR is an appropriate end point for clinical trials in CKD, and, as such, the slope also makes a suitable therapeutic target in clinical practice. Providers can treat the underlying cause by identifying the underlying etiology in certain cases and reversible factors such as volume depletion, uncontrolled hypertension, obstructive uropathy, and nephrotoxins. This makes a dramatic difference to individuals and society in terms of quality of life and costs to the healthcare system.

Blood Pressure Control
BP targets continue to evolve; a goal BP less than 130/80 mm Hg has generally been accepted in CKD as a suitable target to lower the risk of progression and reduce proteinuria. However, the most recent KDIGO BP guidelines, based largely on data from the SPRINT trial, recommend a target systolic BP of less than 120 mm Hg for all patients with CKD (with the exception of children and transplant patients). However, somewhat controversially, these guidelines also extended the BP target (<120 mm Hg) to patients with diabetes. The ACCORD trial failed to show a clear benefit of the lower BP target. However, in that study they were looking at both standard and intensive blood sugar control.

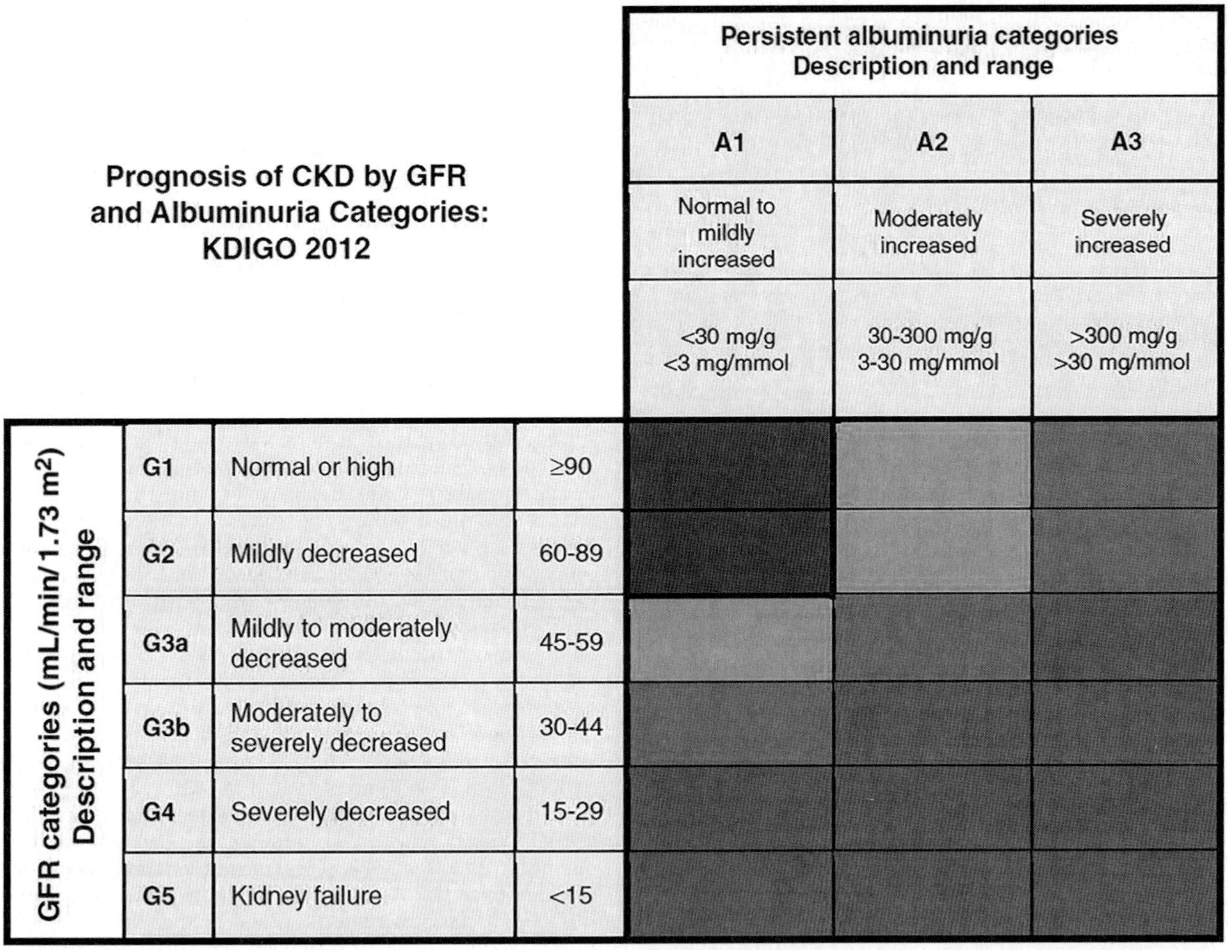

Prognosis of CKD by GFR and Albuminuria Categories: KDIGO 2012

				Persistent albuminuria categories Description and range		
				A1	**A2**	**A3**
				Normal to mildly increased	Moderately increased	Severely increased
				<30 mg/g <3 mg/mmol	30-300 mg/g 3-30 mg/mmol	>300 mg/g >30 mg/mmol
GFR categories (mL/min/1.73 m²) Description and range	**G1**	Normal or high	≥90			
	G2	Mildly decreased	60-89			
	G3a	Mildly to moderately decreased	45-59			
	G3b	Moderately to severely decreased	30-44			
	G4	Severely decreased	15-29			
	G5	Kidney failure	<15			

Very dark gray (G1/G2 and A1): low risk (if no other markers of kidney disease, no CKD); Light gray (G3a and A1; G1/G2 and A2): moderately increased risk; Medium gray (G3b and A1; G3a and A2; G1/G2 and A3): high risk; Medium dark gray (G4/G5 and A1; G3b/G4/G5 and A2; G3a/G3b/G4/G5 and A3): very high risk.

Figure 1 Prognosis of chronic kidney disease by glomerular filtration rate and albuminuria.

TABLE 1	Chronic Kidney Disease Classification Based on Glomerular Filtration Rate and Albuminuria

GFR STAGES	eGFR (mL/min/ 1.73 m²)	TERMS
G1	>90	Normal or high
G2	60–89	Mildly decreased
G3a	45–59	Mildly to moderately decreased
G3b	30–44	Moderately to severely decreased
G4	15–29	Severely decreased
G5	<15	Kidney failure (add *D* if treated by dialysis)

ALBUMINURIA STAGES	ALBUMIN-TO-CREATININE RATIO (mg/g)	TERMS
A1	<30	Normal to mildly increased
A2	30–300	Moderately increased
A3	>300	Severely increased

Chronic kidney disease is defined as either GFR ≤ 60 mL/min/1.73 m² for ≥3 months or structural or functional abnormalities manifested by the presence of markers of kidney damage in blood, urine, or imaging studies.

eGFR, Estimated glomerular filtration rate; *GFR*, glomerular filtration rate.

In the subgroup of patients with standard blood sugar control, intensive BP control was associated with better outcomes. Nonetheless, this BP target of 120/80 mm Hg for those with diabetes is not universally embraced. However, all guidelines agree that it is important to individualize targets and optimize technique in BP measurement. Finally, there is a real opportunity to improve care because of gaps in awareness, treatment, and control of BP among patients with CKD. Although BP treatment has been shown to slow CKD progression, a substantial number of CKD patients have poor BP control. Around 30% of CKD patients are not aware of their BP. Even among those who are aware, substantial portions are untreated, and few of those that are treated are controlled. Only one-fifth of patients with CKD stages 3 and 4 have awareness, treatment, and control of BP even to more modest goals.

Renin-angiotensin system (RAS) blockade is thought to be first-line therapy for patients with hypertension and CKD, particularly in patients with proteinuria/albuminuria (as discussed further in the next section). In addition to the use of an angiotensin-converting enzyme inhibitor (ACEI) or angiotensin receptor blocker (ARB), management of hypertension in CKD also entails therapy with a salt-restricted diet and often diuretic therapy (Table 2). Historically, it was felt that thiazide diuretics lost their efficacy in patients with eGFR below 30; however, a recent study showed that chlorthalidone maintained marked efficacy for BP control in CKD down to eGFRs of 15 mL/min/1.73 m². It is not uncommon for patients with hypertension and CKD to require multiagent regimens for BP

TABLE 2 Recommendations for the Treatment of Patients With Chronic Kidney Disease

BLOOD PRESSURE CONTROL IN CKD	MAINTAIN BLOOD PRESSURE < 130/80 mm Hg OR < 140/90 mm Hg FOR DIABETIC CKD
Reduce proteinuria by administering ACEIs or ARBs.	Decrease urine protein excretion to as low as possible, at least to <1 g/day.
Control phosphate concentration with phosphate binders, using non–calcium-containing binders, when possible.	Maintain serum phosphate toward the normal range in CKD.
Maintain vitamin D level by administration of vitamin D analogs.	Maintain 1,25(OH)2D$_3$ levels at 30 ng/mL by administration of cholecalciferol (D$_3$) or ergocalciferol (D$_2$).
Prevent hyperparathyroidism with vitamin D analogs or calcimimetics.	Maintain parathyroid levels between 150 and 600.
Correct anemia with erythropoiesis-stimulating agents and iron replacement, as needed.	Maintain hemoglobin between 10 and 11 mg/dL. Keep iron saturation (iron/TIBC) > 20%.
Administer diuretics to control hypertension and volume overload.	Maintain euvolemia, when possible.
Control serum potassium with dietary restriction, diuretics, and/or potassium exchange resin, as necessary.	Maintain serum potassium < 5.0 mEq/L.
Prevent malnutrition with adequate calorie and protein intake.	Maintain protein intake between 0.6 and 1 g/kg in CKD and between 1 and 1.3 g/kg on dialysis.
Control metabolic acidosis with administration of sodium bicarbonate or sodium citrate.	Maintain serum bicarbonate >22 mEq/L but <26 mEq/L.

1,25(OH)2D3, 1,25(OH)2–Vitamin D$_3$; *ACEI*, angiotensin-converting enzyme inhibitor; *ARB*, angiotensin receptor blocker; *CKD*, chronic kidney disease; *TIBC*, total iron-binding capacity.

control. Dihydropyridine calcium channel blockers are frequently part of these regimens as they are effective vasodilators that are generally simple to take (daily dosing) and have favorable side effect profiles. If a fourth agent is needed, mineralocorticoid blockade (spironolactone [Aldactone]/eplerenone [Inspra]) may be a good option, but caution is needed with regard to hyperkalemia especially when paired with RAS blockade.

RAS Blockade: Angiotensin-Converting Enzyme Inhibitors and Angiotensin Receptor Blockers

Angiotensin II (Ang II) plays a key role in the progression of glomerulosclerosis, and there is a large amount of experimental data in both animals and humans that blocking Ang II mitigates progression. This is thought to be caused by a reduction in glomerular capillary hypertension, reduction in proteinuria, and a diminution of the Ang II fibrosing effects. ACEIs and ARBs both are likely to delay progression of kidney disease and have cardiovascular benefits. Some studies have examined the possibility of using both together in treatment of CKD, with results suggesting more harm than benefit because of higher rates of hyperkalemia and acute kidney injury among patients receiving dual therapy. There appears to be equipoise as to whether ACEI/ARB medications should be discontinued in advanced CKD (eGFR < 30). When an ACEI or ARB causes an increase in creatinine greater

than 30%, the agent should be held to investigate potential renal artery stenosis or volume depletion.

The Effect of Sodium-Glucose Cotransporter-2 Inhibitors on Progression of Chronic Kidney Disease

Sodium-glucose cotransporter-2 inhibitors (SGLT2i) have expanded the pharmacotherapeutic options for the treatment of CKD, not only with type 2 DM but also in many forms of nondiabetic CKD. SGLT2 receptor expression is limited to the renal proximal tubule. These receptors reabsorb filtered urinary glucose and sodium. SGLT2i lower serum glucose by preventing renal reuptake of glucose, producing a diuresis. This mechanism improves glycemic control in diabetics, but to a moderate degree (e.g., hemoglobin A$_{1c}$ improvement in treatment of naïve patients ~0.9%). Nevertheless, in what were initially intended as safety trials, significant cardiovascular benefits and then renal benefits have been observed. This was subsequently confirmed in numerous studies in patients with type 2 diabetes for all the available agents on the market. This observed benefit in diabetic CKD, despite only limited impact on glycemic control, prompted subsequent studies in nondiabetic patients that have similarly demonstrated significant benefits reducing the risk of progression of CKD and the development of ESKD. SGLT2i include canagliflozin (Invokana), empagliflozin (Jardiance),[1] dapagliflozin (Farxiga), and ertugliflozin (Steglatro).[1] A small reduction in eGFR will frequently occur after starting an SGLT2i and should be followed; it is generally not a reason to discontinue the drug. Evidence for benefit is more robust in patients with significant albuminuria, but there are increasing data showing benefit in those with lesser amounts of albuminuria. Similarly, early studies focused on patients with eGFR at least 30 mL/min/1.73 m^2. However, there have been some reports supporting their benefits extend to patients with lower levels of kidney function, even though the glucose-lowering effects diminish with lower eGFR. These medications are generally well tolerated, though there is an increased risk for genitourinary infections (bacterial urinary tract infections and candida vulvovaginitis). One rare but serious complication is euglycemic diabetic ketoacidosis; the best way to mitigate this rare complication remains uncertain. Some advocate holding SGLT2i when a patient is acutely ill, in the hope of reducing risk. Active peripheral arterial disease, particularly with ulceration, is a relative contraindication to initiating SGLT2i; in a single study to date, there was an increased risk of amputation. Even as evidence of SGLT2i renal benefits has been extended to nondiabetic nephropathy, there is a concern that it would be potentially harmful in ADPKD and could potentially accelerate cyst growth and renal progression; so, at this this point it would be best to avoid these agents in this subgroup.

Disease-Specific Therapy

Depending on the etiology of the kidney disease, specific therapy may be available. In the setting of autoimmune kidney disease, there is an increasing array of agents that might be employed. A kidney biopsy is generally necessary to make a definitive diagnosis of these disorders to employ these agents appropriately and optimally. Effective therapy in primary glomerulonephritis has often been steroid based; however, alternative and adjunctive therapies are being increasingly utilized with greater success and reduced dependence on steroids. Similarly, secondary autoimmune kidney diseases (e.g., lupus nephritis, renal vasculitis) have a broader array of therapeutic options. A more detailed discussion of these disorders can be found elsewhere in Conn's.

In the setting of diabetic nephropathy, there is expansive literature on how to reduce the risk of progression. As for general CKD, a holistic approach using both lifestyle and pharmacologic intervention is likely best. In type 2 diabetes, weight loss is particularly of importance for obese patients, and the cardiovascular risk of tobacco use is further magnified in the setting of diabetes so that smoking cessation gains additional importance. Glycemic control is key for reducing risk of onset and progression of microvascular complications (including diabetic

---

[1] Not FDA approved for this indication.

nephropathy); however, this must be balanced by an increasing risk of hypoglycemia with advanced CKD. Hemoglobin A_{1c} targets should be individualized based on risks and benefits in diabetic CKD. For type 2 diabetes, metformin is a cornerstone of therapy, though concerns for its continued risk and potential implications for lactic acidosis increase with eGFR below 30 (consistent with stage 4 and 5 CKD). SGLT2i have expanded their role in increasing the number of patients with type 2 DM, largely based more on the cardiorenal benefits than their contribution to glycemic control. Glucagon-like peptide receptor agonists are another class of antiglycemic agents with added benefits beyond glucose control, with certain agents having demonstrated cardiovascular benefit, renal outcomes, and weight loss. Finerenone (Kerendia), a nonsteroidal antialdosterone agent, has been found to reduce the risk of kidney failure and slow the rate of progression in patients at a wide range of stages of CKD by about 18% in patients with type 2 diabetes. The most common side effect is hyperkalemia, and, though it was used as an adjunct to RAS blockade in the relevant studies, there are concerns that the rate of hyperkalemia in community use may be greater than what was observed in clinical trials. There is hope that this benefit might extend to nondiabetic CKD, and this is currently being studied.

In the setting of ADPKD, there is also disease-specific therapy in the form of tolvaptan (Jynarque), an agent that blocks the effect of antidiuretic hormone (ADH) in the kidney. ADH stimulates cyst growth in ADPKD. Patient selection is based on the risk of progression, most frequently as defined by the Mayo ADPKD classification system. Kidney volume as calculated from cross-sectional imaging (computed tomography [CT] or magnetic resonance imaging) along with apparent rate of decline determine who is an appropriate candidate for therapy. Tolvaptan has been found to reduce the slope of decline by approximately 1 to 1.5 mL/min/year. A natural consequence of therapy and expected side effects is polyuria. In addition, though rarely seen, there is concern for severe liver injury. Therefore to use this agent in the United States, patients and providers have to be enrolled in the FDA-mandated Risk Evaluation and Mitigation Strategy program and adhere to close monitoring of liver enzymes.

Dietary Protein Restriction and Plant-Based Diets

The role of dietary protein restriction in renoprotective strategies for CKD patients remains controversial. KDIGO guidelines suggest daily restriction in protein intake to 0.8 g/kg for CKD patients, although a very-low-protein diet has been associated with increased mortality over the long term. Some focus has shifted to protein source, with plant-based proteins showing advantages in CKD over proteins derived from animal products and in particularly heavily processed meat.

Although there were inconclusive results in the MDRD study, the largest controlled clinical trial performed to investigate protein restriction in CKD (comparing moderate- and low-protein diets), a benefit of greater protein restriction was suggested by long-term follow-up analysis. Several prior and subsequent studies and metaanalyses appear to support the role of low protein in slowing CKD progression and delaying initiation of maintenance dialysis therapy.

Overall, most experts believe that despite the absence of observed benefit in the MDRD trial, systematic reviews suggest that protein restriction may be beneficial, and the balance of evidence suggests a benefit of moderate dietary protein restriction. Limiting protein intake is also associated with favorable laboratory and metabolic effects, including reduction of BUN levels, uremic toxins, and acid load, in addition to reduced phosphorus load with better control of metabolic bone disorders. Protein restriction may be particularly effective in diseases characterized by hyperfiltration, such as diabetes and certain glomerulopathics. In patients with CKD, a balanced and individualized dietary approach based on a low-protein diet should be carefully monitored, with periodic follow-up for adequate caloric intake and surveillance to identify protein malnutrition through measurement of body weight and serum albumin.

Other Lifestyle Interventions

Tobacco use has been associated with a more rapid decline in renal function in CKD and can be seen as a primary etiology of certain kidney diseases including nondiabetic nodular sclerosis and secondary focal segmental glomerulosclerosis. In addition, as patients with CKD are at increased risk of cardiovascular disease (CVD), reducing reversible risk factors, including smoking, is important. Obesity is both a cause of CKD (most commonly secondary focal segmental glomerulosclerosis) and a risk factor for progression. As such, interventions for weight loss in patients with obesity are important with CKD to reduce progression. In contrast, with advanced CKD, loss of appetite and involuntary weight loss raise additional concerns. There are likely benefits for regular exercise in patients with CKD, though it is not well established that this affects progression of CKD, but ideally it would be a component of a generalized approach to improving renal, cardiovascular, and functional outcomes.

Avoiding Nephrotoxic Medications

Note that patients must avoid nephrotoxins, and both prescription and over-the-counter medications can have deleterious kidney effects. The most concerning nephrotoxins are nonsteroidal antiinflammatory drugs, proton pump inhibitors, and a number of herbal medications (e.g., licorice, cat's claw). Several prescription medications can be deleterious to the kidney. Noteworthy are the calcineurin inhibitors such as cyclosporine (Neoral, Sandimmune, Gengraf) and tacrolimus (Prograf, Envarsus XR, Astagraf XL), which cause progressive renal insufficiency. We know this, in part, because nonrenal solid-organ transplants have a high rate of kidney dysfunction where these agents are employed. Other medications, such as aminoglycosides and amphotericin, and intravenous (IV) contrast have detrimental effects on the hospitalized patients. There has been some reassuring data on the safety of IV contrast; when used for diagnostic CTs the risk of nephrotoxicity appears to be significantly lower than previously thought. Nevertheless, arterial procedures (e.g., cardiac catheterization) and high volumes of contrast continue to pose a risk for acute kidney injury and subsequent progression or development of CKD.

Clinical Manifestations of Kidney Failure

Piorry coined the word *urémie* in 1847 to indicate problems caused by "contaminating the blood with urine." The basic abnormality is the presence of waste products that are not being eliminated by the kidney. In current use, the term *uremia* reflects a clinical syndrome associated with loss of kidney function. Uremic symptoms in advanced CKD result both from kidney excretory failure (e.g., retention of waste such as urea, and larger molecular waste products/so-called middles molecules) and from the loss of metabolic and endocrine functions normally performed by the kidney. Uremia is thought to be, in part, caused by protein intake because a low-protein diet mitigates some of the symptoms. Although we know that some of the uremic toxins are partially dialyzable, the exact etiology of uremia remains unknown.

Uremia also relates to a loss of metabolic and endocrine functions normally performed by the intact kidney. Hence, kidney failure is a multisystem disorder (Box 2). The precision of the measures of kidney function can be variable, and this degree of variability makes it difficult to use as the only factor in clinical decision-making. Therefore, as CKD progresses, clinicians tend to regularly assess the subjective symptoms associated with uremia. In particular, uremia has been described in the following systems: neurologic (sleep, memory), gastrointestinal (appetite, nausea, dysgeusia), and dermatologic (itching). If the severity of these symptoms cannot be managed by symptomatic therapy, this would be an indication for starting dialysis. Furthermore, if a dialysis patient has these symptoms, it may reflect inadequate treatment, and the dialysis dose will need to be increased. Of note, the usual physical signs of kidney failure can be rapidly assessed during an examination: BP, pericardial rub, edema, and crackles on lung examination.

BOX 2	Signs and Symptoms of Kidney Failure

Cardiovascular Complications
Hypertension
Ischemic cardiac disease
Pericardial disease
Congestive heart failure

Endocrine Disorders
Secondary hyperparathyroidism
Glucose intolerance (uremic diabetes)
Hyperlipidemia
Sexual dysfunction/infertility

Hematologic Abnormalities
Anemia
Bleeding tendency

Immunologic Defects
Lymphocytopenia, leukopenia
Decreased antibody responses
Decreased cell--mediated response
Increased susceptibility to infection

Neuropsychiatric Abnormalities
Peripheral neuropathy
Central nervous system disturbances
Seizures
Sleep disorders

Dermatologic Abnormalities
Pruritus, uremic pigmentation
Uremic frost, calciphylaxis, nail changes

Musculoskeletal Abnormalities
Bone disease
Myopathies
Carpal tunnel syndrome

Gastrointestinal Abnormalities
Anorexia, nausea, vomiting
Upper tract disease: gastritis, duodenitis

BOX 3	Factors to Consider in the Management of Patients With Chronic Kidney Disease

Contributors to the Loss of Kidney Function
Hypertension
Diabetes mellitus
Dietary salt intake
Proteinuria
Metabolic acidosis

Complications of Chronic Kidney Disease
Anemia
Platelet dysfunction
Abnormal bone and mineral metabolism (e.g., secondary hyperparathyroidism)
Lipid abnormalities (elevated cholesterol and triglycerides)
Metabolic acidosis
Volume overload
Electrolyte disturbances (e.g., hyperkalemia)
Cardiovascular disease

There is increasing recognition that there is a role for active conservative management of advanced CKD (kidney failure) to reduce morbidity and mortality in individuals who elect against or are not good candidates for more aggressive treatment of ESKD (RRT). This approach involved practicing the same objectives of CKD care as earlier-stage CKD, with an increased awareness of symptoms of advanced CKD and their management. Outcomes in the elderly with this approach, particularly when there is a significant burden of comorbidity, approaches more aggressive models of care (i.e., dialysis).

Measures Designed to Treat Comorbidity in Kidney Disease
Anemia
Anemia (Box 3) may be managed in patients with CKD by first ruling out other causes of anemia such as gastrointestinal bleeding and iron deficiency. Iron deficiency is common in patients with CKD and may be evaluated with a total iron saturation (TSAT) and ferritin. Low ferritin (<100 ng/mL) and TSAT (<20%) in patients with moderate to advanced CKD indicate an absolute iron deficiency. Iron deficiency may be treated using the oral or IV route. After iron stores are restored, if the anemia persists and other causes are ruled out, then an erythropoiesis-stimulating agent (ESA) such as erythropoietin (epoetin alfa [Procrit, Epogen]) may be used. For CKD patients, the use of ESAs has been shown to reduce the need for blood transfusions and modestly improve quality of life. The risks associated with ESA use include an increase in cardiovascular events, hypertension, and cancer progression. For CKD patients, the recommendations are to initiate therapy if Hgb is less than 10 g/dL with an individualized decision for a target based on risks and benefits. In many cases, providers target a hemoglobin between 10 and 11 mg/dL and avoid levels greater than 12 mg/dL.

Metabolic Acidosis
Metabolic acidosis develops in CKD when the eGFR decreases below 30 mL/min. Recent studies have linked metabolic acidosis in CKD to protein wasting, loss of bone, and sympathetic activation. Observational studies have also linked metabolic acidosis to a higher rate of CKD progression and increased risk of death. There are a large number of ongoing studies testing whether oral sodium bicarbonate supplementation in CKD preserves renal function, and bicarbonate supplementation has been widely adopted for metabolic acidosis in CKD. A standard dose used in clinical trials for CKD patients has been sodium bicarbonate 0.5 to 1 mEq/kg/day. The supplemental bicarbonate may be titrated up or down depending on serum bicarbonate and symptoms. If bicarbonate is not tolerated by patients, then clinicians could try Shohl solution (citric acid/sodium citrate [Oracit]), as citrate is converted to bicarbonate by the liver. Currently, a reasonable target serum bicarbonate for patients with moderate to advanced CKD would be greater than 18 mEq/L and less than 26 mEq/L.

Divalent Ion Metabolism
CKD is associated with abnormalities of divalent ions (Ca^{+2}, P^-) and of the hormones that regulate the concentration of these minerals in body fluids. The dysregulation of these divalent ions has also attracted attention as a possible source of CVD because individuals with CKD are found to have calcium deposition and a calcification of heart valves. A low-phosphorus diet is recommended for most patients with advanced CKD (CKD 4 and 5), but it is most important to avoid nonnutritive sources of dietary phosphorus (e.g., phosphate-based preservatives, cola). Serum phosphorus is controlled by administration of phosphate binders, usually starting with calcium citrate (Citracal)[1] or calcium acetate (PhosLo). If these are not successful or if patients have elevated serum calcium levels, then sevelamer carbonate (Renvela) or lanthanum (Fosrenol) can be used alone or in combination with calcium binders. Physicians should aim to maintain serum phosphorus levels between 2.7 and 4.6 mg/dL in CKD stages 3 and 4 and between 3.5 and 5.5 mg/dL in CKD stage 5. Low 25-hydroxyvitamin D levels have been documented in many patients, both with and without renal failure. In patients with renal impairment, this can contribute to the abnormal $1,25(OH)2D_3$ levels. Measurement of 25-hydroxyvitamin D levels should be obtained in all patients with CKD and eGFR below 60 mL/min/1.73 m^2. If 25-hydroxyvitamin D levels are below 30 ng/mL, ergocalciferol (D_2) or cholecalciferol

---

[1] Not FDA approved for this indication.

(D_3) should be given at sufficient doses to maintain it above this level. Defining the target parathyroid hormone (PTH) level in the setting of CKD remains a challenge because of end organ resistance to PTH. PTH levels should be maintained between 150 and 600 pg/mL (2–9 times normal) in patients with ESKD and those on dialysis. However, in pre-ESKD, CKD-specific PTH targets are not specified. Suppression of PTH secretion can be achieved by administration of various vitamin D analogs in combination with calcimimetic agents such as cinacalcet (Sensipar) and etelcalcetide (Parsabiv). Serum calcium levels should be monitored closely. Finally, failed management of divalent ions may lead to calcific uremic arteriolopathy or to calciphylaxis. Calciphylaxis is a rare syndrome characterized by the development of painful nodules in the soft tissue that indurate and ulcerate. This disorder has no uniformly effective treatment and has a high mortality rate.

Hyperkalemia

The clinical consequence of hyperkalemia includes cardiac toxicity, muscle weakness, and death. The target potassium concentration for patients with CKD should remain in the normal range, and patients should be monitored during treatment with ACEIs/ARBs or mineralocorticoid receptor antagonists. Management of high serum potassium in patients with CKD should include a low-potassium diet. If there is a sudden increase, it may be caused by the use of salt substitutes, large amounts of juice, or eating high-potassium foods. It may be helpful to obtain a nutrition consult to help the patient maintain a low-potassium diet. In addition, it is recommended to review medications for those associated with hyperkalemia and consider decreasing the dose of the ACEI or ARB. Diuretics also may be used to decrease serum potassium levels in CKD, loop diuretics being the most widely used for patients with an eGFR below 30 mL/min, but new data suggest chlorthalidone[1] continues to be effective at eGFR down to 15 mL/min. Finally, potassium-binding agents may be used to control serum potassium levels in patients with advanced CKD. The potassium exchange resin, sodium polystyrene sulfonate (Kayexalate), or one of the newer exchange resins, patiromer (Veltassa) or sodium-zirconium cyclosilicate (Lokelma), will decrease serum potassium levels.

Volume Overload

Sodium retention contributes to hypertension and edema among patients with CKD. To adequately address volume overload, both the intake and sodium excretion may need to be addressed in patients with CKD. Patients should adhere to a low-sodium diet, which is often complicated by other dietary restrictions (low-potassium, low-phosphate, American Diabetes Association diet). Given the complexity of diet in CKD, use of a registered dietician with expertise in kidney-related diets can help both volume overload and the other complications of CKD. In addition to sodium restriction, patients may need to use a diuretic for BP and volume management. Loop diuretics are often used to address volume overload. The loop diuretics such as furosemide (Lasix) should be dosed frequently enough to maintain a negative sodium balance. If the loop diuretic at higher doses is not adequately addressing volume overload, then an additional distal tubule diuretic such as metolazone (Zaroxolyn) may be used to increase urinary sodium excretion. It should be noted that increasing sodium excretion may cause acute kidney injury in CKD patients, particularly in the setting of ACEIs/ARBs and other diuretics. In this case patients will often respond to reducing the diuretic dose with close monitoring.

Chronic Kidney Disease–Mineral Bone Disorder

Chronic kidney disease–mineral bone disorder (CKD-MBD) is a systemic disorder of mineral and bone metabolism. CKD-MBD is associated with CKD and results from hyperphosphatemia caused by diminished kidney phosphorus excretion and hypocalcemia caused by impaired kidney production of active $1,25(OH)2D_3$, which leads to secondary hyperparathyroidism. Elevations in serum fibroblast growth factor 23, metabolic bone disease, soft tissue calcifications, and other metabolic derangements are associated with morbidity and mortality in CKD. The management of CKD-MBD is complex because of the influence of the homeostatic system and the availability of multiple treatment options without definitive randomized trials. The ideal strategy should be normalizing serum calcium, phosphate, PTH, and metabolic acidosis while minimizing the risks associated with the therapies. The various treatment options for hyperphosphatemia and secondary hyperparathyroidism include dietary phosphorus restriction, phosphate binders, calcitriol (Rocaltrol) or other active vitamin D analogs, calcimimetic agents, adequate hemodialysis, and parathyroidectomy. The optimal PTH level in the setting of CKD remains a challenge and has not been prospectively determined. KDIGO guidelines recommend that PTH be kept between 2 and 9 times the upper limit of normal for the assay in patients with ESKD.

Cardiovascular Disease

Although more than 10 million American adults are estimated to have CKD 3 or worse (i.e., GFR < 60 mL/min), far fewer are on dialysis or have received a transplant. Why is there a disparity between the number receiving RRTs and the number with CKD? Most patients with CKD die of CVD before requiring dialysis or transplantation. On dialysis, the risk of death from CVD remains 10 to 100 times higher than in the general population. A 25-year-old male patient on hemodialysis has approximately the same risk of dying from heart disease as an 80-year-old patient without CKD. Traditional risk factors account for only a portion of the CVD risk associated with CKD. Traditional risk factors include age, diabetes, lipids, hypertension, and smoking, among others. Many nontraditional risk factors are believed to play a role in increasing CVD risk in patients with CKD. Some of these risk factors are anemia, volume overload, hyperparathyroidism, calcium/phosphate disturbances, uremia, and malnutrition/inflammation often associated with CKD. The exact role these nontraditional risk factors play is an actively researched area. In general, one should consider patients with CKD high-risk patients for CVD, and CKD is considered by some to be a coronary equivalent. Data indicate that patients with a lower GFR (<45 mL/min) and microalbuminuria/proteinuria carry a very high CVD risk (approximately equivalent to a prior history of coronary disease). This is important when assessing a patient in the emergency department for chest pain or evaluating a patient preoperatively for surgery, and so on.

Treatment focuses on optimizing management of known CVD risk factors and being alert for harbingers of active CVD. Those caring for CKD patients must address CVD risk management. Primary prevention focuses on BP, diet, exercise, and, in some cases, aspirin and/or statins. Furthermore, SGLT2i have demonstrated significant benefits with regard to cardiovascular events and mortality in this high-risk group that are driven, in large part, by a reduction in congestive heart failure events. Similarly, specific to patients with diabetic kidney disease, finerenone also reduces the frequency of adverse cardiovascular events. The data available for cardiovascular risk management in CKD are limited in part because of the exclusion of patients with significant CKD in many large cardiovascular studies. Hence the utility of aspirin and statins (if any) in this setting is not well established. CKD patients often present with atypical symptoms of CVD; therefore a high index of suspicion is important.

References

Agarwal R, Sinha AD, Cramer AE, et al: Chlorthalidone for hypertension in advanced chronic kidney disease, N Engl J Med 385(27):2507–2519, 2021.

Bakris GL, Agarwal R, Anker SD, et al: Effect of finerenone on chronic kidney disease outcomes in type 2 diabetes, N Engl J Med 383(23):2219–2229, 2020.

Chebib FT, Perrone RD, Chapman AB, et al: A practical guide for treatment of rapidly progressive ADPKD with tolvaptan, J Am Soc Nephrol 10:2458–2470, 2018.

Cheung AK, Chang TI, Cushman WC, et al: Executive summary of the KDIGO 2021 clinical practice guideline for the management of blood pressure in chronic kidney disease, Kidney Int 99(3):559–569, 2021.

Herrington WG, Staplin N, Wanner C, et al: Empagliflozin in patients with chronic kidney disease, N Engl J Med 388(2):117–127, 2023.

Inker LA, Eneanya ND, Coresh J, et al: New creatinine- and cystatin C-based equations to estimate GFR without race, N Engl J Med 385(19):1737–1749, 2021.

Joshi S, McMacken M, Kalantar-Zadeh K: Plant-based diets for kidney disease: a guide for clinicians, Am J Kidney Dis 77(2):287–296, 2021.

KDIGO: Clinical practice guideline update for the diagnosis, evaluation, prevention, and treatment of chronic kidney disease–mineral and bone disorder (CKD-MBD), *Kidney Int Suppl (2011)* 7(1):1–59, 2017.

Kidney Disease: Improving Global Outcomes (KDIGO) CKD Work Group: KDIGO 2024 clinical practice guideline for the evaluation and management of chronic kidney disease, *Kidney Int* 105(4s):s117–s314, 2024.

Kidney Disease: Improving Global Outcomes (KDIGO) Diabetes Work Group: KDIGO 2020 clinical practice guideline for diabetes management in chronic kidney disease, *Kidney Int* (4S) S1–S115, 2020.

Mottl AK, Alicic R, Argyropoulos C, et al: KDOQI US Commentary on the KDIGO 2020 clinical practice guideline for diabetes management in CKD, *Am J Kidney Dis* 79:457–479, 2022.

Pitt B, Filippatos G, Agarwal R, et al: Cardiovascular events with finerenone in kidney disease and type 2 diabetes, *N Engl J Med* 385(24):2252–2263, 2021.

Raphael K: Metabolic acidosis in CKD: core curriculum 2019, *Am J Kidney Dis* 74(2):263–275, 2019.

Tangri N, Grams ME, Levey AS, et al: Multinational assessment of accuracy of equations for predicting risk of kidney failure: a meta-analysis, *JAMA* 315(2):164–174, 2016.

Toyama T, Neuen BL, Jun M, et al: Effect of SGLT2 inhibitors on cardiovascular, renal and safety outcomes in patients with type 2 diabetes mellitus and chronic kidney disease: a systematic review and meta-analysis, *Diabetes Obes Metab* 21(5):1237–1250, 2019.

Wright Jr JT, Williamson JD, Whelton PK, et al: A randomized trial of intensive versus standard blood pressure control, *N Engl J Med* 374(23):2284, 2016.

MALIGNANT TUMORS OF THE UROGENITAL TRACT

Method of
Danica May, MD; and Moben Mirza, MD

CURRENT DIAGNOSIS

Prostate cancer

- Prostate cancer is the most common cancer diagnosis for men in the United States.
- Screening with prostate-specific antigen (PSA) should be offered starting at age 45 to 50 and ending at age 70 for the average risk patient. For higher risk patients (African American patients or strong family history of prostate cancer), screening should be discussed starting between 40 and 45.
- Prostate cancer risk factors include African ancestry, family history, as well as Lynch syndrome and other genetic mutations.
- Transrectal ultrasound (TRUS)-guided biopsy is the diagnostic test for prostate cancer and may be indicated for patients with elevated PSA or abnormal DRE.
- Staging involves cross-sectional abdominal and pelvic imaging as well as bone scan for patients with high risk cancer.

Benign and malignant renal rumors

- Most patients with renal cell carcinoma (RCC) are diagnosed incidentally on imaging work-up for other symptoms or complaints. The classic triad of a palpable mass, hematuria, and flank pain is a relatively rare presentation.
- Risk factors for RCC are smoking, obesity, hypertension, and genetic syndromes such as von Hippel-Lindau disease, Birt-Hogg-Dube syndrome, and tuberous sclerosis complex.
- Most malignant renal masses are renal cell carcinoma, but lymphoma, metastases from other malignancies, and other renal malignancies should be considered in the differential as treatment options will vary.
- Benign masses include oncocytoma, angiomyolipoma (AML), renal cysts, and adenomas among others.
- Staging of renal masses involves abdominal imaging with CT scan or MRI. Chest imaging should be obtained. Laboratory analysis should include a CBC, CMP, and urinalysis. CT-guided core renal mass biopsy may be obtained after urologic consultation.

Urothelial cell carcinoma

- Urothelial cell carcinoma can affect the renal pelvis, ureter, bladder, or urethra, though most cases occur in the bladder.
- The average patient is older than age 60 and may have significant medical comorbidities.
- Risk factors include smoking, radiation, certain chemical exposures, and Lynch syndrome.
- Microscopic or gross hematuria is the most common presentation. Patients may also present with urgency, frequency, dysuria, flank pain, or have hydronephrosis discovered on imaging.
- Work-up involves a CT urogram for patients with adequate renal function and cystoscopy.
- Tumors discovered in the bladder should be resected endoscopically for diagnosis and staging. Tumors in the renal pelvis or ureters can be biopsied ureteroscopically.

Primary carcinoma of the prostate and urethra

- Primary urethral malignancies typically consist of urethral or squamous cell carcinoma.
- Patients often present with hematuria, and overall survival remains poor.
- Studies are lacking on this rare disease state, but treatment depends on stage, disease location, and histology.

Penile cancer

- Penile cancer is a rare malignancy with poor prognosis for men with advanced stage disease.
- Presentation often involves an ulceration or palpable mass, and biopsy is the key to diagnosis.
- The vast majority of penile lesions are squamous cell carcinomas.
- Risk factors for penile cancer involve chronic inflammation, tobacco use, lack of neonatal circumcision, STDs, HPV infection specifically with subtypes 6, 16, and 18, and phimosis.
- Staging scans involve chest, abdomen, and pelvis imaging with attention paid to the inguinal lymph nodes.

Testicular cancer

- Testicular cancer is diagnosed in men with a median age of 33 years and has excellent outcomes at 5 years.
- Risk factors for testicular cancer include undescended testis and a personal or family history of testicular cancer.
- The majority of testicular cancers are germ cell tumors, which include seminoma and non-seminoma.
- Germ cell tumors can also present in extra-testicular locations such as the retroperitoneum or mediastinum.
- Men with a testicular mass should undergo an ultrasound and intratesticular masses that are concerning for malignancy should be removed via radical orchiectomy. Sperm banking should be offered.
- Serum tumor markers include beta-hCG, AFP, and LDH. Staging, pathology, and tumor markers dictate next management steps.

CURRENT THERAPY

Prostate cancer

- Treatment options depend on PSA, Gleason grade, clinical stage, and the patient's overall health and life expectancy. Men with limited life expectancy may be good candidates for watchful waiting. Active surveillance is an option for men with low-risk and some men with favorable intermediate risk prostate cancer.
- Treatment options for clinically localized prostate cancer include radical (typically robotic) prostatectomy and radiation therapy in the form of external beam or brachytherapy with or without androgen deprivation therapy.
- The cornerstone of treatment for men with nodal or metastatic disease involves androgen deprivation therapy.
- Other treatment options include chemotherapy, immunotherapy, or newer secondary hormone therapies.

- Following definitive therapy, follow up for men treated for prostate cancer involves regular PSA monitoring every few months for 5 years and then yearly after that.

Benign and malignant renal tumors

- Surgery remains a mainstay of treatment for localized renal cell carcinoma. Partial or radical nephrectomy can be performed taking into consideration the clinical stage, tumor location, patient's overall health, renal function, presence or absence or a contralateral kidney, and genetic syndromes predisposing the patient to future malignancies.
- Ablative therapy and active surveillance are options for small renal masses.
- Simple renal cysts do not require treatment. Complex or enhancing cysts should be treated based on their risk of malignancy.
- Follow up for patients treated for renal cell carcinoma involves periodic laboratory analysis as well as cross-sectional abdominal and chest imaging.
- Systemic therapy options for patients with metastatic renal cell carcinoma have increased drastically with the newest treatments including immune checkpoint inhibitors.
- The treatment of angiomyolipomas (AMLs) is often based on size and is directed toward prevention of the complication of retroperitoneal hemorrhage. Embolization or surgical removal has traditionally been proposed at a 4-cm size, although larger AMLs can be safely observed.

Urothelial cell carcinoma

- Treatment options depend on stage, grade, and tumor location.
- Superficial low-grade bladder tumors can be managed with resection and periodic surveillance cystoscopy.
- Patients with superficial high-grade cancer or cancers invasive into the lamina propria (T1) diagnosed on initial resection may be offered a repeat resection. Treatment following this often involves induction and maintenance intravesical Bacillus Calmette-Guérin (BCG) therapy. Patients with high-grade T1 bladder cancer should be counseled and offered radical cystectomy. These patients should have periodic cystoscopy and upper tract imaging as indicated.
- The standard of care for patients with muscle invasive (T2) bladder cancer is cisplatin-based neoadjuvant chemotherapy followed by radical cystectomy. Patients ineligible for cisplatin-based chemotherapy should undergo immediate radical cystectomy.
- For patients who are unwilling or unfit for radical cystectomy, chemoradiation therapy can be offered.
- Upper tract tumors of the renal pelvis or ureter are managed by grade as well as clinical stage. The pathologic stage may not be accurately established prior to definitive treatment.
- Nephroureterectomy should be offered for patients with upper tract urothelial cell carcinoma. Other options can include endoscopic management with tumor ablation or partial resection of the ureter if tumor location is amenable. Cisplatin-based neoadjuvant or adjuvant chemotherapy should be considered.

Primary urothelial carcinoma of the prostate and urethra

- Superficial urothelial tumors (Tis, Ta, T1) of the urethra can be resected or biopsied followed by intravesical BCG therapy.
- The surgical treatment for men with T2 proximal urethral cancer involves removal of the bladder and prostate with urethrectomy. More distal disease involving the pendulous urethra can be managed with a distal urethrectomy or partial penectomy.
- Women are often treated with cystectomy and urethrectomy.
- Patients with higher stage urethral cancer may be offered neoadjuvant or adjuvant chemotherapy or radiation therapy.

Penile cancer

- Organ sparing approaches include topical therapy, laser therapy, Mohs surgery, glansectomy, radiation therapy, or wide local excision and are most utilized in patients with superficial or properly selected penile cancer patient with T1 disease.
- More aggressive tumors should be treated with partial or total penectomy.
- Higher risk patients need to undergo inguinal node dissection and pelvic node dissection should be considered for highly selected patients.
- Neoadjuvant chemotherapy should be considered for bulky, bilateral, or fixed inguinal lymphadenopathy.

Testicular cancer

- Following radical orchiectomy, imaging of the chest, abdomen, and pelvis is key for staging. Repeat tumor markers should also be collected as persistent tumor marker elevation after orchiectomy changes treatment.
- Patients with localized seminoma with normal tumor markers can undergo surveillance, chemotherapy, or radiation therapy.
- For patients with more advanced disease, treatment options should include chemotherapy or radiation therapy.
- In patients with pure seminoma and a residual retroperitoneal mass, further work-up with a PET/CT scan can aid in characterization of residual disease.
- Radiation therapy is not a standard treatment for men with non-seminoma testicular cancer.
- Patients with localized non-seminoma with normal tumor markers can undergo observation, chemotherapy, or retroperitoneal lymph node dissection (RPLND).
- For patients with more advanced disease, treatment options should include chemotherapy and/or surgical resection.
- Residual retroperitoneal masses in the patient treated for non-seminoma testicular cancer should be removed via RPLND.
- Follow up for all patients with testicular cancer includes surveillance with chest, abdominal, and pelvic imaging as well as periodic tumor markers.

Prostate Cancer

Background

Prostate cancer is the most common cancer diagnosis among men in the United States. It accounts for over 268,490 new cases in 2022 and is the second most common overall malignancy after breast cancer. It is a relatively indolent cancer with 96.8% 5-year relative survival. Family history of prostate cancer, particularly among first-degree relatives, is a well-known risk factor for developing prostate cancer. Known genetic alterations include both germline as well as somatic mutations. Common mutations include BRCA1/2, ATM, MLH1, MSH2, MSH6, and PMS2, among many others. Syndromes linked to prostate cancer include Lynch syndrome and hereditary breast and ovarian cancer (HBOC) syndrome. Other risk factors for development of prostate cancer include increasing age, African American ancestry, smoking, and Ashkenazi Jewish heritage.

Diagnosis

Prostate cancer is most often diagnosed in a localized and asymptomatic state via screening. Rarely, prostate cancer is detected at a locally advanced state with symptoms of pelvic pain, urinary retention, or ureteral obstruction with hydronephrosis. The minority of men are diagnosed in the metastatic state, with the most frequent complaint being bone pain from metastases. The utilization of prostate-specific antigen (PSA) blood testing has drastically changed the diagnosis of prostate cancer from a historically predominantly metastatic state to a localized and potentially curable state in the current era. In 2012, the US Preventive Services Task Force released a grade D recommendation against the use of PSA-based screening for any man. This recommendation was modified in 2018 to allow for informed decision making for prostate cancer screening in men aged 55 to 69. The American Urological Association recommends individualized prostate cancer screening for men aged 40 to 54 who are at higher risk, shared decision-making for men aged 45 to 69, and cessation of screening for men aged 70 or older or those men with life expectancy less than 10 to 15 years. Screening of prostate cancer with PSA should not be dismissed with the assumption that prostate cancer is an indolent cancer. Screening can lead to diagnosis and appropriate risk stratification.

The basis of prostate cancer screening is serum PSA. While PSA is only produced by the prostate, it is not specific to malignant versus benign cells, and there are a variety of causes of elevated PSA. Benign causes of elevated PSA include benign prostate hypertrophy, prostatitis, instrumentation of the urethra such as catheterization or utilization of cystoscopy, and urinary tract infections. One of the difficulties of PSA utilization is that there is no cutoff normal level. In fact, 6.6% of men with a PSA of 0.5 ng/mL or less were found to have prostate cancer with rates increasing to 26.9% in men with PSA of 3.1 to 4.0 ng/mL. In general, PSA increases with age. Some men may have an abnormal DRE, which can prompt further work-up. Worrisome findings include induration or nodules palpable within the prostate.

Following screening with PSA, further work-up includes prostate biopsy. The vast majority of prostate biopsies are performed with transrectal ultrasound (TRUS) to help with volumetric and anatomical surveys. The majority of prostate cancer is detected in the peripheral zone, so the standard 12-core biopsy template targets this area in a systematic fashion. Prostatic volume as well as anatomy such as large intravesical lobes should be noted as this information can be helpful in surgical planning.

Prostate MRI is an increasingly utilized tool in men with various clinical situations including elevated PSA with a prior negative biopsy, performance of active surveillance (AS; further discussed below), staging, and surgical planning, as well as in men whose pathology appears discordant with their rectal examination or PSA level. Multiparametric MRI gives not only detailed anatomic information, but also functional assessment of various tumor regions.

This information can then be used for an MRI-guided biopsy or more commonly fusion biopsy via platforms that fuse concerning MRI findings with real-time TRUS biopsy for improved lesion targeting.

The vast majority of prostate cancers are adenocarcinomas. Prostate biopsy pathology is based on Gleason grading system 1 to 5, with 5 reflecting poorly differentiated and most aggressive cells. The grading system is translated into a score that adds the most common and second most common grading pattern to yield a score between 2 and 10. Further classification into a Gleason group between 1 and 5 informs appropriate risk classification. In general, low-risk prostate cancer consists of Gleason 6 prostate cancer (Gleason group 1), while intermediate risk prostate cancer consists of Gleason 7 prostate cancer (Gleason group 2 and 3). High-risk prostate cancer includes Gleason sums 8, 9, and 10 prostate cancer (Gleason groups 4 and 5). Risk groups also take into account clinical stage, PSA levels, and biopsy core positivity. TNM staging is used for prostate cancer. Prostate cancer diagnosed either surgically via a transurethral resection of the prostate or via TRUS biopsy is stage T1. T2 is organ-confined prostate cancer, while T3 is defined as extra-prostatic extension. Finally, T4 involves invasion of surrounding structures including the bladder, pelvic floor or sidewall, or rectum (Table 1). Grade, stage, and risk group are instrumental in treatment decisions.

Current recommendations include germline testing for patients with positive family history of prostate cancer; high-risk, regional, or metastatic prostate cancer; Ashkenazi Jewish ancestry; or intraductal histology. Various genetic alterations necessitate genetic counseling as well as change some treatment options. Staging imaging should be carried out for certain men diagnosed with prostate cancer. Current recommendations include pelvic imaging with or without abdominal imaging via CT or MRI as well as a radionuclide bone scan in men with unfavorable intermediate, high risk, and very high-risk disease.

Treatment

Treatment decisions for men diagnosed with prostate cancer depend on a series of factors including risk group, staging, and

---

TABLE 1 | Risk Stratification and Staging Workup

NCCN RISK GROUP	CLINICAL/PATHOLOGIC FEATURES	IMAGING
Very low	T1c AND Gleason score ≤6/grade group 1 AND PSA <10 ng/mL AND Fewer than 3 prostate biopsy fragments/cores positive, ≤50% cancer in each fragment/core AND PSA density <0.15 ng/mL/g	Not indicated
Low	T1–T2a AND Gleason score ≤6/grade group 1 AND PSA <10 ng/mL	Not indicated
Favorable intermediate	T2b–T2c OR Gleason score 3 + 4 = 7/grade group 2 OR PSA 10–20 ng/mL AND Percentage of positive biopsy cores <50%	Bone imaging: not recommended for staging Pelvic ± abdominal imaging: recommended if nomogram predicts >10% probability of pelvic lymph node involvement
Unfavorable intermediate	T2b–T2c OR Gleason score 3 + 4 = 7/grade group 2 or Gleason score 4 + 3 = 7/grade group 3 OR PSA 10–20 ng/mL	Bone imaging: recommended if T2 and PSA >10 ng/mL Pelvic ± abdominal imaging: recommended if nomogram predicts >10% probability of pelvic lymph node involvement
High	T3a OR Gleason score 8/grade group 4 or Gleason score 4 + 5 = 9/grade group 5 OR PSA >20 ng/mL	Bone imaging: recommended Pelvic ± abdominal imaging: recommended if nomogram predicts >10% probability of pelvic lymph node involvement
Very high	T3b–T4 OR Primary Gleason pattern 5 OR >4 cores with Gleason score 8–10/grade group 4 or 5	Bone imaging: recommended Pelvic ± abdominal imaging: recommended if nomogram predicts >10% probability of pelvic lymph node involvement

NCCN, National Comprehensive Cancer Network; *PSA,* prostate-specific antigen.
From Partin AW: *Campbell-Walsh-Wein Urology,* ed 12, Elsevier, 2021.

clinical node status on imaging, as well as the patient's overall health and life expectancy. In patients with limited life expectancy, observation may be utilized. Observation of known prostate cancer involves monitoring the patient with eventual initiation of palliative androgen deprivation therapy (ADT) for symptomatic or imminently symptomatic disease. On the other hand, AS may be utilized for patients with very low risk or low risk disease, and the properly selected favorable intermediate risk disease patient with adequate life expectancy. AS involves periodic assessment of PSA, DRE, and surveillance biopsies. Prostate MRI may also be utilized in an AS algorithm. AS aims to allow for early disease reclassification with ability to perform definitive treatment at that point. Approximately two-thirds of men on AS will be able to avoid treatment and the associated side effects. Another effect of AS is less overtreatment of small, indolent prostate cancers.

The preferred treatment for very low risk and low risk prostate cancer patients with adequate life expectancy is AS. Other options in the properly selected patient population include external beam radiation therapy (EBRT) or brachytherapy, radical prostatectomy (RP), or observation. As previously mentioned, AS remains an option for patients diagnosed with favorable intermediate risk prostate cancer. This cohort of men may also be treated with EBRT or brachytherapy as well as RP. Treatment recommendations for men with unfavorable intermediate risk prostate cancer include RP, EBRT combined with ADT, or EBRT and brachytherapy boost with ADT. For men with high risk or very high risk prostate cancer, treatment recommendations include EBRT and ADT with or without abiraterone (Zytiga), EBRT with brachytherapy and ADT, or RP. In men with regional lymphadenopathy, the cornerstone of treatment is ADT. This may be combined with EBRT or abiraterone (Zytiga).

Following definitive treatment, patients should be monitored with PSA and DRE every 3 to 6 months. Following RP, PSA should be undetectable as all prostate and prostate cancer tissue has theoretically been surgically removed. Men treated with EBRT or brachytherapy should have a decline in PSA to a low, steady level. In men with detectable or rising PSA after RP, repeat imaging including bone imaging, CT, MRI, C-11 choline, F-18 fluciclovine PET/CT, or PET/MRI may be utilized to assess for sites of disease recurrence. If no metastases are detected, observation or EBRT with or without ADT are treatment options. When metastases are detected, ADT combined with apalutamide (Erleada), docetaxel (Taxotere), abiraterone (Zytiga), enzalutamide (Xtandi), darolutamide (Nubeqa), or EBRT to the primary tumor in the setting of low volume metastases are treatment options. Most men with metastatic prostate cancer initially have castration-naïve prostate cancer and respond to medical or surgical (orchiectomy) castration. A rising PSA in the setting of castrate level testosterone indicates the advent of castration-resistant prostate cancer (CRPC), and ADT should be continued indefinitely. Once castration resistance has been identified, bone health should be prioritized with utilization of denosumab (Xgeva) or zoledronic acid (Zometa) in the setting of bone metastases. Therapy options include abiraterone (Zytiga), docetaxel (Taxotere), enzalutamide (Xtandi), sipuleucel-T (Provenge), radium Ra 223 dichloride (Xofigo) for symptomatic bone metastases, or mitoxantrone (Novantrone) for palliation in men who cannot tolerate other therapies. Painful bony metastases can be palliated with EBRT.

Benign and Malignant Renal Tumors
Background
Kidney and renal pelvis cancers account for 4.1% of all new cancer cases at more than 79,000 cases in the United States in 2022 leading to 13,920 deaths. The 5-year relative survival from 2010 to 2016 is approximately 76.5%. The majority of kidney masses are detected incidentally on cross-sectional imaging for other chief complaints, and the median age at diagnosis is 65 years. These tumors can be primary renal cell carcinoma (RCC), metastases from second primaries such as breast, lung, ovarian, or melanoma as well as lymphoma deposits, or benign renal tumors such as oncocytoma,

angiomyolipoma (AML), renal cysts, leiomyoma, and adenomas. RCC subtypes include clear cell, chromophobe, papillary, collecting duct, translocation, and medullary carcinoma. The majority of tumors are clear cell RCC, which comprise 70% of RCC subtypes.

Hereditary syndromes predisposing patients to RCC include von Hippel-Lindau (VHL) disease, hereditary papillary renal carcinoma (HPRC), hereditary leiomyomatosis and renal cell carcinoma (HLRCC), tuberous sclerosis complex (TSC), and Birt-Hogg-Dube (BHD) syndrome, among others. Other risk factors include smoking, obesity, and hypertension.

Diagnosis
Rarely patients with RCC present with a triad of symptoms including hematuria, a flank mass, and flank pain. More commonly, patients are found to have a renal mass on imaging performed for other indications and the frequency of incidental detection has increased with widespread abdominal imaging. In the patient with a renal mass, laboratory analysis should include a CBC, CMP, and urinalysis. Cross-sectional abdominal imaging with CT or MRI with contrast should be obtained if not already performed. A chest x-ray is required to complete staging but chest CT, bone scan, brain MRI, and core-needle biopsy may also be obtained. Patients who present with multiple renal masses or young age (<46 years old) may be referred for genetic evaluation. Core-needle biopsy of renal masses may be indicated in patients with unclear etiology of their renal mass such as concern for an infiltrating mass like lymphoma, AS guidance, or in combination with ablation strategies.

TNM stage and histologic grade are important for prognosis and treatment guidance in the patient with RCC. Stage T1 tumors are tumors ≤7 cm in greatest dimension and are limited to the kidney. T2 tumors are greater than 7 cm but ≤10 cm and are limited to the kidney. T3 disease involves invasion into major veins including the renal vein or vena cava or invasion into perinephric tissue, while T4 disease is invasion beyond Gerota's fascia. Histologic grade is graded as G1 through G4 with increasing dedifferentiation.

Renal cysts are a very common benign finding and are graded via Bosniak classification with scores ranging from I to IV. Simple cysts are defined as thin-walled cysts without septa, calcifications, or solid component and lack enhancement. As the Bosniak score increases, so does the complexity and malignancy risk of the cyst with Bosniak IV cysts defined as cysts with enhancing soft tissue components and thick or irregular walls or septa. Oncocytomas are the most common benign, enhancing mass and are associated with BHD syndrome. They are often diagnosed on pathology as diagnosis via imaging characteristics can include hypervascularity with a central scar but are not definitive findings. AMLs are common manifestations in patients with TSC but are often easily diagnosed on CT or MRI due to the presence of macroscopic fat, which has negative Hounsfield units. While benign, AMLs are the leading cause of spontaneous retroperitoneal hemorrhage and intervention is targeted toward prevention of this outcome. A cutoff size of 4 cm has been suggested, at which point treatment via surgery or embolization may be offered and discussed. Treatment should be tailored to patient circumstances. Patients with TSC and multiple or enlarging AMLs may be offered everolimus (Afinitor), an mTOR inhibitor for size reduction. While other benign renal lesions do occur, they are relatively rare and beyond the scope of this chapter.

Treatment
Surgery remains a mainstay of treatment for localized RCC. Surgical options include removal of the whole kidney via radical nephrectomy or removal of the mass with preservation of the remaining healthy parenchyma via partial nephrectomy. In general, partial nephrectomy is the approach of choice for stage T1 tumors, especially if tumors are less than 4 cm with a favorable location within the kidney. Radical nephrectomy may be indicated based on tumor size, clinical stage, and anatomy but can be associated with decreased renal function. Concomitant lymph node dissection has not been shown to improve oncologic outcomes. The adrenal

gland should be removed for large upper pole tumors or abnormal appearance on staging imaging. Other treatment options include AS or ablative techniques. AS is preferable for elderly patients with comorbidities and small renal masses or in patients who prefer to avoid intervention. Periodic imaging is performed with intervention for enlarging masses. Ablative techniques involve microwave, cryoablation, or thermal ablation and are again most utilized in small renal masses less than 3 cm. Advanced RCC can extend into the renal vein, vena cava, or even the right atrium. Depending on the level of tumor thrombus, cardiothoracic surgery may need to be involved with resection to allow for utilization of vascular bypass. Follow up for patients is dependent on stage but involves periodic laboratory analyses as well as chest and abdominal imaging.

Some patients who present with metastatic disease may ultimately undergo a cytoreductive nephrectomy with resection of the primary tumor followed by systemic therapy. In general, this is offered to patients with lung-only metastases, good performance status, and good prognostic features. Patients who do not fit these criteria should undergo a biopsy and be evaluated for systemic therapy. In addition, some patients with localized disease treated with a partial or radical nephrectomy will develop systemic disease and should also consider systemic therapy. Tumor histology determines treatment options with clear cell being the most common histology. Systemic therapy for RCC is rapidly evolving with a shift from the cytokine era to targeted therapies consisting of tyrosine kinase inhibitors (TKIs), mammalian target of rapamycin inhibitors (mTORs), and immune checkpoint inhibitors. Systemic therapy for kidney cancer are evolving rapidly based on new therapies, prior therapy, and cellular subtype.

Urothelial Cell Carcinoma

Background
Urothelial cell carcinoma is a malignancy that can affect the renal pelvis, ureter, bladder, and urethra, although the majority of cases are bladder cancer. In 2022, in the United States an estimated 81,180 new cases of bladder cancer will be diagnosed with nearly 17,100 deaths. Urothelial cell cancer is a male predominant disease and affects the elderly with a median age of diagnosis of 73 with many patients having significant medical comorbidities. Modifiable risk factors include smoking, pelvic radiation, chemical exposure, obesity, and diabetes mellitus. Lynch syndrome is associated with upper tract urothelial cell carcinomas.

Diagnosis
The most common presenting sign of urothelial cell carcinoma is microscopic or gross hematuria but can also include lower urinary tract complaints, hydronephrosis on imaging, or flank pain. Work-up for hematuria involves upper tract imaging frequently with a CT urogram, a CT of the abdomen and pelvis with pre-contrast, post-contrast, and delayed images, as well as cystoscopy. If tumors are found in the bladder and cross-sectional imaging has not been performed, a CT or MRI of the abdomen and pelvis should be obtained. Next steps involve endoscopic resection of the tumors for pathological analysis and staging. Upper tract, which includes renal pelvis or ureteral tumors, may be visualized during ureteroscopy with biopsy allowing for differentiation of low versus high grade tumor cells as well as identification of location and volume of tumor for future treatment guidance. Chest imaging as well as laboratory tests complete staging.

Stage and grade are key to guide treatment decisions for patients with urothelial cell carcinoma with grade designated as low or high. TNM staging of bladder cancer is broken up into Ta, Tis, T1, T2, T3, and T4. Ta is noninvasive while Tis is urothelial carcinoma in situ. T1 involves invasion into lamina propria, T2 invades muscularis propria, T3 invades perivesical tissue, and T4 invades prostatic stroma, uterus, vagina, pelvic wall, abdominal wall, or seminal vesicles. TNM staging is similar for the renal pelvis and ureter with T3 defined as invasion into peripelvic fat, renal parenchyma, or periureteral fat and T4 defined as invasion into adjacent organs or through the kidney into perinephric fat.

Most bladder, ureter, and renal pelvis tumors are urothelial cell carcinomas. Subtypes also known as variant histology include nested, microcystic, micropapillary, plasmacytoid, clear cell, sarcomatoid, squamous, and lymphoepithelioma-like. Distinct and more rare types of genitourinary tract malignancies of the urothelium include squamous cell, adenocarcinoma, and small cell carcinoma.

Treatment
Bladder
Once bladder cancer has been diagnosed, appropriate pathologic and radiologic staging should be completed. Pathology determines need for repeat transurethral resection of bladder tumor (TURBT) with recommendations for second resection for Ta high-grade tumors and any T1 tumors. Patients with Ta low-grade tumors may be observed. For patients with high-grade T1 disease, a radical cystectomy should be offered. Patients with Tis, Ta high-grade, and T1 disease should be offered intravesical therapy usually with Bacillus Calmette-Guérin (TICE BCG) or BCG therapy (Figure 1). Treatment options for muscle invasive or T2 disease are quite different and the gold standard is platinum-based neoadjuvant chemotherapy followed by radical cystectomy (Figure 2). Prior to treatment for muscle invasive bladder cancer (MIBC), a CBC, CMP, and chest imaging should be obtained. A bone scan is indicated if concern for bony metastases exists. A radical cystectomy involves removal of the bladder, prostate, and seminal vesicles for men. A radical cystectomy in females involves removal of the bladder often with concomitant removal of the uterus, ovaries, anterior vagina, and urethra. A urinary diversion is then formed with the majority of patients receiving an ileal conduit with abdominal stoma. Continent diversions are also options. Cisplatin-based neoadjuvant chemotherapy with dose dense methotrexate[1], vinblastine[1], doxorubicin (Adriamycin), and cisplatin (ddMVAC) or gemcitabine (Gemzar)[1] with cisplatin (GC) are the current recommendations. If patients are unable to tolerate chemotherapy, immediate radical cystectomy should be performed. Adjuvant chemotherapy is recommended for adverse pathologic features including stage T3-T4 or node positive disease if not given in a neoadjuvant fashion. Finally, chemoradiotherapy with bladder preservation may be selected by some patients. Ideal candidates should not have hydronephrosis or extensive carcinoma in situ. Concurrent radiation therapy with radio sensitizing chemotherapy such as cisplatin and 5-FU (fluorouracil)[1] are administered. The patient's bladder should be reassessed after 2 to 3 months with surgical consolidation as a consideration for residual muscle invasive disease. In patients who present with concern for nodal involvement or metastases, options include neoadjuvant therapy followed by consolidative cystectomy or systemic therapy alone. In the locally advanced or metastatic patient population who are cisplatin ineligible, gemcitabine (Gemzar)[1] with carboplatin (Paraplatin), atezolizumab (Tecentriq)[1], or pembrolizumab (Keytruda)[1] are the preferred regiments.

Upper Tract Urothelial Cell Carcinoma
The treatment of upper tract urothelial cell carcinoma follows the same basic principles as treatment of bladder cancer. As previously mentioned, ureteroscopy with biopsy of tumor allows for grade determination though is much less likely to accurately diagnose stage due to the limited ability to obtain specimens via a ureteroscope. The gold standard for nonmetastatic upper tract disease involves a radical nephroureterectomy with bladder cuff removal. Platinum-based neoadjuvant chemotherapy should be considered for patients with lymphadenopathy, large high-grade tumors, sessile tumors, or concern for parenchymal invasion. For some small, papillary, unifocal, low-grade tumors, management may involve endoscopic management with laser ablation of tumor and periodic surveillance ureteroscopy or cross-sectional imaging. Distal ureteral tumors can at times be managed with a distal ureterectomy with ureteral reimplant.

---

[1]Not FDA approved for this indication.

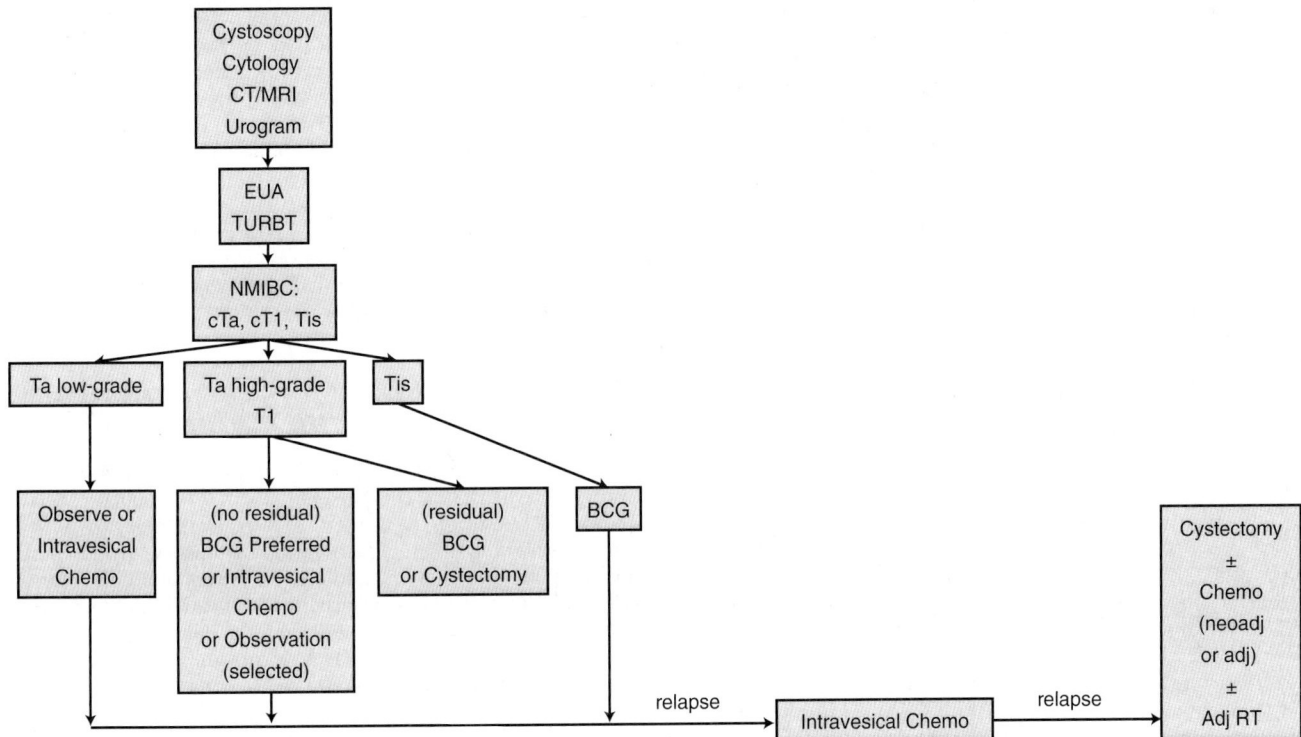

Figure 1 Management algorithm for non-muscle-invasive bladder cancer. *BCG,* Bacillus Calmette-Guerin; *Chemo,* chemotherapy; *CT,* computed tomography; *EUA,* examination under anesthesia; *NMIBC,* non-muscle-invasive bladder cancer; *MRI,* magnetic resonance imaging; *RT,* radiotherapy; *TURBT,* transurethral resection of bladder tumor. From LaRiviere MJB, Brian C, Christodouleas JP: Bladder cancer. In *Gunderson & Tepper's Clinical Radiation Oncology,* 2020, Elsevier.

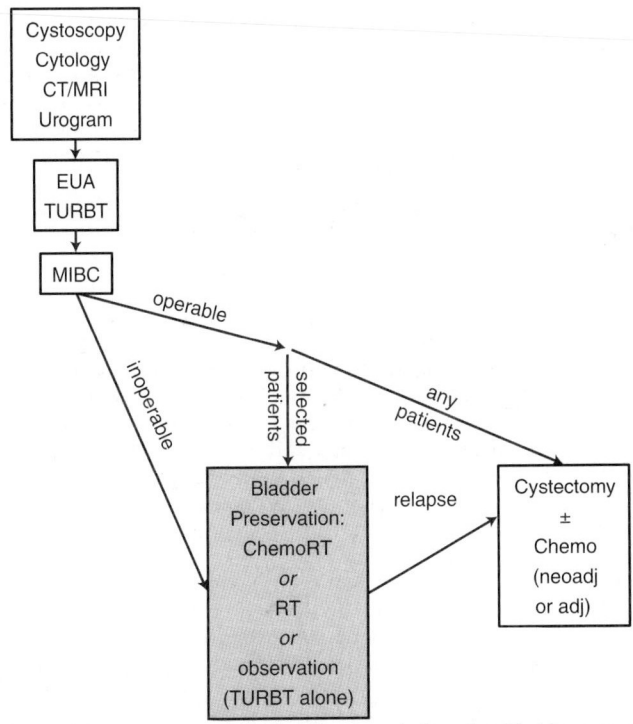

Figure 2 Management algorithm for muscle-invasive bladder cancer. *adj,* Adjuvant; *Chemo,* chemotherapy; *ChemoRT,* chemoradiotherapy; *CT,* computed tomography; *EUA,* examination under anesthesia; *MIBC,* muscle-invasive bladder cancer; *MRI,* magnetic resonance imaging; *neoadj,* neoadjuvant; *RT,* radiotherapy; *TURBT,* transurethral resection of bladder tumor. From LaRiviere MJB, Brian C, Christodouleas JP: Bladder cancer. In *Gunderson & Tepper's Clinical Radiation Oncology,* 2020, Elsevier.

Primary Carcinoma of the Prostate and Urethra

Background

Primary carcinoma of the prostate or urethra is quite rare. Prostatic urethral histology is most often urothelial in origin while the remaining urethral primary malignancies are predominantly squamous cell carcinoma. Overall survival is relatively poor at 42% at 5 years. Due to the low incidence, a lack of data and studies of ideal management for these patients are lacking. Stage, disease location, histology, and tumor size remain important prognostic factors.

Diagnosis

Initial work-up involves DRE in men with cystoscopy and transurethral or transvaginal resection or biopsy of the tumor. Cross-sectional imaging with MRI or CT of the pelvis assists with tumor staging as well as assesses for concomitant lymphadenopathy, while chest imaging assesses for metastases.

Treatment

As with urothelial malignancies of the bladder, Tis, Ta, or T1 urothelial cell carcinoma of the male prostate or urethra and female urethra should be followed by a repeat resection and subsequent BCG treatment[1]. In men, proximal urethral disease (prostatic or bulbar urethra) stage T2 or higher is ideally managed with a urethrectomy with cystoprostatectomy. T2 urothelial disease of the pendulous urethra can be managed with a distal urethrectomy or partial penectomy. Adverse pathology or positive margins may be further managed with chemotherapy or chemoradiotherapy. In women, T2 urethral urothelial malignancies should be managed with chemoradiotherapy, urethrectomy with cystectomy, or distal urethrectomy if tumor location is amenable. In more advanced disease stages including T3–T4 or palpable inguinal lymphadenopathy, systemic therapy with or without concomitant radiation followed by consolidative surgery are guideline recommendations.

---

[1]Not FDA approved for this indication.

Penile Cancer

Background

Penile cancer remains a rare disease in North America and Europe, with approximately 2200 cases diagnosed and 440 deaths in 2020 in the United States. It remains a highly lethal disease if not caught at a very early stage. Once disease has spread to pelvic lymph nodes, 5-year survival rates are less than 10%. As with prostate and bladder malignancies, increasing age is a risk factor for penile cancer with a median age of diagnosis of 68 years in the United States. Other risk factors include phimosis, which also limits examination and early detection as well as tobacco use, chronic inflammation, balanitis, lichen sclerosis, poor hygiene, STDs (specifically HIV and HPV), and lack of neonatal circumcision. Key HPV types include 6, 16, and 18. Histology of penile cancer is overwhelmingly squamous cell carcinoma with subtypes including verrucous, papillary squamous, warty, and basaloid. Verrucous histology carries the most favorable prognosis with more aggressive variants including sarcomatoid and adenosquamous. Tumor grade is designated as grade 1 to 4 with 1 being well differentiated and grade 4 being poorly or undifferentiated.

Diagnosis

A careful physical examination is key for men who present with penile lesions, while care should be taken to observe lesion characteristics including location, size, and consistency, as well as perform an inguinal lymph node examination to assess for lymphadenopathy. Staging utilizes the TNM staging system with Tis defined as carcinoma in situ, Ta as non-invasive squamous cell carcinoma, T1 as superficial invasion substratified based on lymphovascular/perineural invasion and high versus low grade, T2 with corpus spongiosum or urethral invasion, T3 with corpora cavernosal invasion, and T4 as invasion into surrounding structures such as the bony pelvis, prostate, or scrotum. Tissue should be obtained for pathologic analysis. MRI or ultrasound can assess with anatomic characterization of the tumor.

Treatment

Organ sparing approaches for management of penile cancer include topical therapy, laser therapy, Mohs surgery, glansectomy, and wide local excision. Topical therapies include imiquimod (Aldara)[1] and 5-FU (Efudex)[1]. Organ sparing approaches can be primary treatment options for patients with Tis, Ta or the properly selected patient with T1 penile cancer. Low-grade T1 tumors can also be treated with radiation therapy. If location or size preclude less aggressive therapies, partial penectomy may be necessary. Higher-grade T1 tumors often necessitate partial or total penectomy with intraoperative frozen sections to ensure negative margins. T2 tumors or greater should be treated aggressively with partial or total penectomy, although radiotherapy or chemoradiotherapy are also options. Patients with low risk pathology, Tis-T1a penile cancer, should undergo inguinal lymph node surveillance while higher risk pathology, T1b or greater penile cancer, necessitates cross-sectional imaging of the chest, abdomen, and pelvis with inguinal lymph node dissection or dynamic sentinel node biopsy. In low risk patients with palpable lymphadenopathy, biopsy should be performed with node dissection performed for positive nodes with or without neoadjuvant chemotherapy. For palpable inguinal lymphadenopathy larger than 4 cm, fixed lymph nodes smaller than 4 cm, or bilateral lymphadenopathy, patients should receive neoadjuvant chemotherapy if medically suitable

followed by inguinal lymphadenectomy with or without pelvic lymphadenectomy. Other treatment options include radiation therapy or chemoradiotherapy. Adjuvant chemotherapy should be offered for patients with multiple positive nodes or extranodal extension. Finally, adjuvant radiation therapy should be offered to the patient with positive pelvic nodes. For patients who present with metastases, systemic chemotherapy, radiation therapy, or chemoradiotherapy are options. The preferred chemotherapy regimen is TIP with paclitaxel (Taxol)[1], ifosfamide (Ifex)[1], and cisplatin (Platinol)[1]. Patients with recurrence should be referred for a clinical trial or treatment with pembrolizumab (Keytruda)[1].

Testicular Cancer

Background

Testicular cancer is predominantly a disease of younger men with median age at diagnosis of 32 years of age. An estimated 9,910 new cases will be detected in 2022 with 460 deaths. Testicular cancer has a high 5-year survival rate of 95%. Risk factors include a family history of testicular cancer, personal history of testicular cancer, or undescended testicle. The majority of testicular tumors are germ cell tumors consisting of seminoma and nonseminoma. Seminomas are the more common subtype and carry a more favorable prognosis. Nonseminomas can be comprised of choriocarcinoma, embryonal carcinoma, yolk sac tumors, and teratoma. Germ cell tumors that originate outside the testicle may be located in the retroperitoneum or mediastinum and follow similar treatment recommendations.

Diagnosis

Men with testicular cancer often present with painless testicular enlargement or a mass. They may at times experience pain, which can be confused with epididymitis or orchitis. Ultrasound examination is the next step with findings of an intratesticular mass necessitating collection of serum tumor markers including AFP, beta-hCG, and LDH.

Staging follows the TNM classification. Tis tumors are germ cell neoplasia in situ, T1 tumors are limited to the testis without lymphovascular invasion (LVI), T2 tumors are limited to the testis with LVI or invade hilar soft tissues or epididymis, T4 tumors invade the spermatic cord, and T4 tumors involve scrotal invasion. Nodal metastases are classified based on size, and metastases are divided into non-retroperitoneal nodal disease/pulmonary metastases or non-pulmonary metastases. Finally, the S stage is based on post-orchiectomy tumor markers.

Treatment

Once an intratesticular mass is identified on physical exam or trans-scrotal ultrasound, radical inguinal orchiectomy is the next step (Figure 3). Sperm banking should be offered to any patient who wishes to preserve future fertility before radical orchiectomy and certainly prior to any systemic therapy or retroperitoneal lymph node dissection. Following orchiectomy, chest imaging and a CT scan of the abdomen and pelvis should be obtained with repeat post-operative tumor markers. For patients with T1 to T4 localized pure seminoma with normal tumor markers, treatment following orchiectomy can include surveillance (which is preferred), carboplatin (Paraplatin)[1], or radiation therapy. For patients with pure seminoma and retroperitoneal lymphadenopathy less than 5 cm in maximum dimension, options include chemotherapy with a regimen of bleomycin, etoposide (Toposar), and cisplatin (Platinol) or etoposide (Toposar) with cisplatin, as

---

[1]Not FDA approved for this indication.

[1]Not FDA approved for this indication.

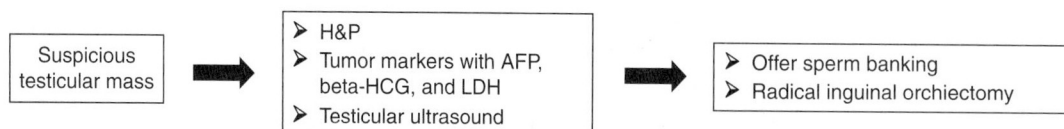

Figure 3 Management algorithm for suspicious testicular mass.

well as radiation therapy to the retroperitoneum. For patients with bulkier retroperitoneal lymphadenopathy, non-regional lymphadenopathy, or metastases, chemotherapy is recommended. PET/CT scans may be obtained in the patient with residual post-chemotherapy masses with resection if PET positive.

Non-seminomatous testicular cancer is managed differently than seminoma, and radiation therapy is not indicated. For patients without lymphadenopathy and normal tumor markers, options include surveillance, chemotherapy regimens as previously described for pure seminoma, and RPLND. For patients with enlarged lymph nodes in the retroperitoneum, treatment options include chemotherapy or RPLND. Treatment should be focused on chemotherapy for patients with bulky retroperitoneal lymphadenopathy, non-retroperitoneal lymphadenopathy, or metastases. Patients who undergo chemotherapy with residual masses larger than one centimeter on follow up CT scans should undergo surgical resection. Follow up for patients treated for testicular cancer can include periodic tumor markers, CT scan of the abdomen and pelvis, and chest x-ray.

Early urologic consultation should be considered for several common clinical conditions to prevent delayed diagnosis. Patients with elevated PSA or hematuria may frequently be treated with antibiotics for presumptive prostatitis or urinary tract infections. These patients should instead be promptly referred to a urologist to prevent delayed diagnosis of prostate cancer or urologic malignancy. In addition, patients with testicular masses may not seek work-up and treatment in a timely fashion. Upon presentation, a prompt ultrasound should be obtained. Initial empiric treatment with antibiotics for presumed orchitis or epididymitis can be avoided for intratesticular masses seen on ultrasound to allow for expedient orchiectomy.

References

"Cancer Stat Facts." Retrieved 6/12/2020, 2020, from https://seer.cancer.gov/stat-facts/.
LaRiviere MJB, Brian C, Christodouleas John P: Bladder Cancer. *Gunderson & Tepper's Clinical Radiation Oncology. ClinicalKey*, Elsevier, 2020.
"NCCN Guidelines." NCCN Guidelines for Treatment of Cancer by Site. Retrieved 6/25/20202, 2020.
Thompson IM, et al: "Prevalence of prostate cancer among men with a prostate-specific antigen level < or =4.0 ng per milliliter, *N Engl J Med* 350(22):2239–2246, 2004.
Taneja SSB, Marc A: In *Active Management Strategies for Localized Prostate Cancer. Campbell-Walsh-Wein Urology. A. W. Partin. ClinicalKey*, Elsevier, 2020.
Wei JT, Barocas D, Carlsson S, et al: Early detection of prostate cancer: AUA/SUO guideline part I: prostate cancer screening, *J Urol* 210(1):45-53, 2023.

NEPHROLITHIASIS

Method of
Rajan Ramanathan, MD

CURRENT DIAGNOSIS

- Many renal calculi are asymptomatic and are often discovered as an incidental finding on an unrelated radiologic study. Nonobstructing renal calculi can infrequently present with symptoms of flank pain, caused by intermittent obstruction or from inflammation.
- Renal calculi can move and drop into the ureter causing obstruction. Such ureteral calculi typically present with severe flank pain. The pain level does not correlate with the size of the stone or the severity of obstruction.
- Pain can radiate from the flank, wrapping around the side, to the lower abdomen, groin, or testicle.
- Many patients with a ureteral colic will present to the emergency department (ED). Nausea and vomiting are common accompanying symptoms. Fever is an uncommon finding, and temperature over 101°F suggests serious infection and is an acute urologic emergency.

- Physical examination will reveal a patient having intermittent sharp, excruciating costovertebral pain, without significant abdominal tenderness. Pain commonly is described as colicky. Percussion of the costovertebral angle may elicit tenderness.
- The differential diagnosis should include other causes of abdominal pain like cholecystitis, appendicitis, or ovarian conditions such as torsion or ruptured ovarian cysts.
- Urinalysis may demonstrate either microscopic or gross hematuria. Presence of leukocytes on urine microscopy in the absence of bacteriuria is common and does not always indicate infection.
- Mild elevation of serum creatinine is also a common finding. However if the patient has an obstruction to the dominant functioning kidney or in a solitary kidney, the patient can become oligoanuric, and the creatinine can rise significantly. This would be a reason to admit for observation and/or treatment.
- Mild leucocytosis between 11,000 to 14,000 white blood cells (WBC)/μL is a common finding in many patients presenting to the ED with a ureteral colic and is often an acute phase reaction to the pain and inflammation, arising out of a reaction to the colic, WBC demargination, and production of colony-stimulating factors.
- Computed tomography without intravenous contrast (CT kidney stone protocol) is the definitive diagnostic study. Abdominal plain film radiography and renal ultrasonography are not as accurate as CT, but may be offered when following up patients with known ureteral stones, and in patients who have had an initial CT performed within the last 3 to 6 months.

CURRENT THERAPY

- Asymptomatic renal stones can be managed with observation or with surgical intervention.
- The decision for treatment of asymptomatic stones is based on medical and social considerations. Recurrent visits to the ED, presence of infected stones, repeated obstructions causing deterioration of kidney function, stones associated with hematuria, presence of stones in patients with anatomic abnormalities (e.g., ureteropelvic junction obstruction), and continued increase in size of the stone could be some medical factors driving therapy. Sometimes patient's social factors (e.g., an airline pilot may need to get the stones treated before they are cleared to fly again) also need to be taken into consideration.
- During an acute episode in the ED, the goals of therapy include adequate pain control, hydration, and triaging to assess if the patient needs emergency or urgent treatment, and to assess the likelihood of spontaneous stone passage.
- Stones 4 mm or less in size have an over 90% probability of spontaneous passage. Stones 6 mm or greater have a less than 20% probability of spontaneous passage.
- Studies have shown the superiority of nonsteroidal antiinflammatory drugs (NSAIDs) in the management of acute pain from ureteral stones. Opioid analgesia can be used as second line or as adjunctive treatment.
- If the pain is not well controlled in the ED, or if this is the second or third visit for the same stone, a urology consult should be obtained and/or the patient should be admitted for a possible urologic intervention.
- Once an acute episode is well controlled, the patient is discharged from the ED, with oral analgesics, advice regarding liberal oral fluid intake, alpha blockers like tamsulosin (Flomax)[1], and instructions to strain the urine to try and collect the stone for chemical analysis. This approach is called medical expulsive therapy (MET).

- A follow-up renal ultrasound examination should be obtained 3 to 4 weeks after the first presentation of symptoms. If hydronephrosis persists but the patient is asymptomatic and urine is not infected, a repeat CT could be ordered or the patient can be referred to a urologist for consideration for an endoscopic procedure.
- Fever greater than 101°F and/or leukocytosis, regardless of a negative urine, indicates possible infected hydronephrosis or pyonephrosis; this is a urologic emergency, as is oligoanuria secondary to calculus. The patient should be admitted for treatment.

[1]Not FDA approved for this indication.

Pathophysiology

In general, a solution is said to be undersaturated until the concentration of its cation and anion exceed the solubility product, at which point the salt tends to crystallize.

Under some conditions, some salts can be held in solution even after the solubility product is exceeded, but only until it reaches a threshold level called *formation product*. Calcium oxalate is considered sparingly soluble, but urine is a complex solution and has many inhibitors, which prevent crystallization of calcium oxalate. Once the concentration of salts has exceeded the solubility product, but is still below that of the formation product, the solution is said to be in a metastable state.

After the concentration exceeds the formation product, the urine is in an unstable state and the salt can no longer be held in solution, even in the presence of protective agents; the salt will then crystallize. Once formed, crystals tend to grow. They do this by addition of other crystals of the same kind or of a different kind (a process called *epitaxy*).

When calcium oxalate or other type of crystals form and grow, the concretions eventually become kidney stones. Most clinically significant stones typically tend to form at the confluence of the many collecting ducts on the renal papillae. However, crystals can also form and clog the flow of urine in the collecting ducts (e.g., uric acid nephropathy). This happens when the flow of urine is sluggish from dehydration, or when there is dilatation of the ducts (as in medullary sponge kidney).

Stones that form in the different calyces can stay attached to the site where they initially formed and continue to grow, or they can detach and move to other parts of the kidney or drop into the ureter where they can cause obstruction to the flow of urine from that kidney.

Inhibitors that protect against stone formation include citrate, magnesium, glycoproteins (e.g., nephrocalcin, Tamm-Horsfall protein), and pyrophosphates. Citrate is the major inhibitor. Citrate complexes with calcium, reducing the availability of calcium to bind with oxalates, and also by inhibiting crystal nucleation. Magnesium binds to oxalate, thus reducing the availability of oxalate to combine with calcium.

Randall plaques have often been described as the major promoter of stone formation. The mechanism is believed to be an abnormal ulcerated plaquelike base that forms the nidus for easy crystal depositions. Any foreign body (e.g., retained stent, residual stone fragments) can also do the same, and this author has also seen one case of an extruded metal coil used to angioembolize a kidney serving as the nidus for the stone formation.

Chemical Basis of Stone Formation
Calcium and Oxalate Metabolism

Calcium levels in the blood need to be maintained, and this is ensured by regulating calcium transport at three sites: intestine, bone, and kidney. A decrease in serum calcium causes an increase in levels of parathyroid hormone (PTH). PTH regulates the conversion of 25-hydroxyvitamin D to the active form of vitamin D (1,25-dihydroxyvitamin D_3 or calcitriol). PTH also stimulates the mobilization of calcium from bone through the action of osteoclasts and increases the absorption of calcium from renal tubules.

The dietary calcium is handled in the intestines with approximately 30% to 40% of calcium being absorbed in the small intestine. If there is less calcium in the diet, relatively more of it is absorbed (increased fractional absorption) due to a vitamin D–dependent process, which is not activated when there is excess dietary calcium. Because the absorption of dietary calcium is in its ionic form, many anions that combine with calcium (e.g., phosphate, citrate, oxalate, and sulfate) can reduce calcium absorption. About 60% of phosphorus is absorbed in the intestines, and active transport is regulated by 1,25-dihydroxyvitamin D_3.

In the kidney, most of the calcium (98%) that is filtered is reabsorbed: renal proximal tubule (~60%), thick ascending limb of the loop of Henle (~30%), and distal convoluted tubule (~10%). Approximately 80% to 90% of phosphorus is absorbed, and PTH enhances renal calcium reabsorption and reduces renal tubular reabsorption of phosphate.

Hypercalciuria is a common finding in many calcium stone formers, and can be seen in over 50% of the patients with calcium stones. Hypercalciuria is defined as a calcium excretion of >250 mg/day in women or >300 mg/day in men. A more precise way to assess is to check for a calcium excretion >200 mg/day while on a 1-week restricted diet of 400 mg/day of calcium and 100 mEq/day sodium (2300 mg/day).

Because calcium that reaches the urine is regulated at three sites, hypercalciuria is broadly classified into the three types based on this. However, mechanisms of hypercalciuria may be more complex in many patients.

1. Absorptive hypercalciuria is the most common cause of hypercalciuria (30%–40%) and is due to increased intestinal absorption of calcium. Restricting dietary calcium normalizes urinary excretion of calcium in some patients (type 2) but not in others (type 1). Hypercalciuria is the main finding in such patients.

   Absorptive hypercalciuria and renal calculi can also occur from an increased synthesis of active form of vitamin D that is seen in patients with renal phosphate wasting (e.g., hereditary hypophosphatemia with rickets and hypercalciuria), and this occurs in <3% of patients).

2. Renal hypercalciuria, seen in approximately 5% to 8% of patients, is due to a decreased ability to reabsorb the filtered calcium load by the kidneys. This causes a compensatory rise in PTH, active form of vitamin D synthesis and maintenance of a normal serum calcium level arising out of increased intestinal absorption of calcium, or bone resorption. High fasting urine calcium levels, a reactive increase in PTH required to maintain serum calcium, and normal serum calcium levels are the typical findings in such patients.

3. Resorptive hypercalciuria is relatively uncommon (3%–5%) and is due to a primary increase in PTH. The rise in PTH causes increased production of the active form of vitamin D and results in mobilization of calcium from the bones, as well as increased absorption in the intestines. The hypercalcemia and the resultant hypercalciuria are responsible for stone formation. Such patients have an elevated PTH, hypercalcemia, hypophosphatemia, and hypercalciuria.

   However, not all patients with hypercalciuria can be classified into these 3 broad subgroups.

Some patients have idiopathic hypercalciuria, and others could have hypercalciuria secondary to hypercalcemia from other conditions. Hypercalcemia is seen patients with sarcoidosis, granulomatous diseases, malignancy, and glucocorticoid use. Of the malignancies, lung and breast are the common causes, but hypercalcemia can also be seen in renal, hematologic, and other malignancies. Glucocorticoids stimulate the release of PTH, and nephrolithiasis is common in patients with Cushing syndrome.

Treatment of hypercalciuria can help decrease stone recurrence, and persistent hypercalciuria is often a finding in patients failing medical treatment.

Oxalate

Less than 10% of the dietary oxalate is absorbed in the intestines; this varies widely between individuals, and some studies suggest that oxalate stone formers tend to have higher levels of oxalate absorption compared with non–stone formers. Oxalate absorption is also markedly increased in patients with intestinal disease or after intestinal resection. Other factors can modify oxalate absorption, including the presence of oxalate-binding cations such as calcium or magnesium and oxalate-degrading bacteria. Ingestion of calcium along with oxalate-containing foods causes calcium to bind with oxalate in the intestines, and this reduces the availability of free oxalate ions for absorption. In patients aggressively restricting calcium in their diets (with an aim to reducing the incidence of calcium stones), lower levels of dietary calcium result in more oxalate being available for absorption, and this can paradoxically lead to more stones.

Hyperoxaluria

Hyperoxaluria is defined as oxalate excretion of >40 mg/day.

Primary hyperoxaluria is an autosomal recessive disorder and there is a defect in the conversion of glyoxylate to glycine, thereby increasing conversion of glyoxylate to oxalate. Three forms of primary hyperoxaluria exist, and the most severe type is the type 1 primary hyperoxaluria, which if left untreated can cause end-stage renal failure before 15 years of age in 50% of young patients.

Enteric hyperoxaluria is the commonest form of acquired hyperoxaluria. It is associated with chronic diarrheal conditions, loss of bowel segments due to resection, or from inflammatory bowel disease. Fat malabsorption in these patients results in decreased intestinal calcium availability, with resultant increased oxalate absorption in the intestines.

Dietary hyperoxaluria is seen in patients who consume oxalate-rich foods such as nuts, brewed tea, spinach, beets, and rhubarb. Hyperoxaluria can also occur in patients who severely restrict dietary calcium, and a decrease in intestinal binding of oxalate and increased intestinal oxalate absorption is said to be the cause. Excessive ascorbic acid supplementation has also been shown to cause hyperoxaluria by in vivo conversion to oxalate.

Uric Acid Metabolism

Uric acid is the end product of purine metabolism. Humans lack the enzyme uricase, which converts the relatively insoluble uric acid to the soluble compound allantoin. Uric acid typically has a pKa1 of around 5.4 and tends to crystallize in acidic environment with pH less than 5.4.

Hyperuricosuria is defined as urinary uric acid exceeding 600 mg/day.

Hyperuricosuria can result in uric acid stones, but by a complex process they can also increase the crystallization of calcium oxalate. When stones are analyzed, it is not uncommon to find uric acid as a minor component in some calcium stones. Hyperuricosuria is often due to an increased dietary purine intake. However, other conditions may also be accompanied by hyperuricosuria: gout, hematologic conditions like myeloproliferative malignancies, polycythemia, lymphoproliferative disorders, multiple myeloma, and Lesch-Nyhan syndrome.

Uric acid stones form when patients have hyperuricosuria, low urine volumes, and low urinary pH. The low urinary pH is suspected to be from an apparent deficit in excretion of ammonium, and this is linked to the metabolic syndrome and insulin resistance state. Urinary alkalinization is a treatment option for asymptomatic uric acid renal stones.

Citrate Metabolism

Citrate is an important inhibitor of stone formation. It forms a complex with calcium and thus reduces the calcium saturation in urine. It also prevents crystal formation and crystal growth.

The bulk of filtered citrate is reabsorbed in the proximal tubule. Citrate excretion can be affected by the acid-base state. Acidosis results in increased utilization of citrate in the citric acid cycle, and the decreased availability of citrate causes an enhanced renal tubular reabsorption. Acidosis therefore results in hypocitraturia.

Hypocitraturia is defined as a level <320 mg/day, although different labs may use other cut points that are similar. Although hypocitraturia can present as an isolated abnormality, it is also seen in any condition that can result in systemic acidosis like renal tubular acidosis type 1, excessive animal protein load, or from mechanisms related to combinations including intracellular acidosis like use of thiazide diuretics, carbonic anhydrase inhibitors, angiotensin converting enzyme inhibitors, and topiramate (Topamax).

Cystine

Cystine is a dibasic amino acid and is filtered and freely absorbed by the nephron. Patients with cystinuria lack the ability to transport cystine and other dibasic amino acids across the tubular cell, and thus the fractional excretion of cystine (and other dibasic amino acids like cystine ornithine, lysine and arginine [COLA]) increases. Among these amino acids, only cystine crystallizes as the concentrations rise. Cystine crystallizes more readily in acidic urine (therefore urinary alkalinization helps dissolve cystine stones), and also when there is hypercalciuria, hyperuricosuria, or hypocitraturia.

Renal Tubular Acidosis

Renal tubular acidosis (RTA) describes a defect in urinary acidification resulting in a metabolic acidosis. Hypokalemia, elevated urine pH, hypocitraturia, and hypercalciuria can lead to stone formation.

Type 1 (distal) RTA is the commonest type of RTA, and patients have a defect in H^+ ion excretion (distal nephron) despite acidosis. They develop a hyperchloremic, hypokalemic, non–anion gap acidosis with urine pH >6, and nephrocalcinosis and nephrolithiasis. Hypercalciuria, a high urine pH, and hypocitraturia (from acidosis) are common urinary findings. Calcium phosphate stones are often seen in this clinical setting.

Type 2 (proximal) RTA is due to a defect in reabsorption of bicarbonate. As metabolic acidosis progresses, there is bicarbonate depletion and the filtered bicarbonate can be reabsorbed, leading to urinary pH <5.5. Because of relatively normal urinary citrate, nephrolithiasis is uncommon.

Type 4 RTA is seen with chronic kidney damage. An overall decrease in renal function renders a global reduction in filtered salts, thus nephrolithiasis is uncommon.

Types of Stones

Calcium is the most consistent component and is seen in almost 80% of kidney stones. Calcium stones can be calcium oxalate stones and these can be in the monohydrate [$CaC_2O_4 \cdot H_2O$ (Whewellite)] or dihydrate [$CaC_2O_4 \cdot 2H_2O$ (Weddellite)] form. They can also complex with phosphates to form calcium phosphate [hydroxyapatite crystal unit, $Ca_{10}(PO_4)_6(OH)_2$] or calcium phosphate dihydrate (brushite, $CaHPO_4 \cdot 2H_2O$) stones.

The noncalcium stones are uric acid stones, ammonium magnesium phosphate (struvite, [$NH_4MgPO_4 \cdot 6H_2O$]) and cystine stones. Other rarer stones like triamterene or valproic acid stones can be from precipitation of medications.

Uric acid stones tend to form in acidic urines with pH <5.4.

Mono- and dihydrogen phosphate buffers have a pKa of around 6.8, and these stones tend to crystallize in alkaline pH, which is commonly seen when there is alkaline urine (e.g., RTA).

Diagnosis

Diagnostic studies for stones are usually offered in two settings: (1) the acute presentation in the ED and (2) as part of the long term follow-up for stone disease.

In the acute setting, a good history and physical examination should be followed by labs including a urine analysis. A past history of stone disease is a good predictor that the patient's symptoms could be again from a new stone episode. Presence of gross hematuria also points to the urinary tract as the source of pain.

Mild leucocytosis between 11,000 and 14,000 white blood cells (WBC)/μL is a common finding in many patients presenting to the ED with ureteral colic, and it is often an acute phase reaction to the pain and inflammation arising out of a reaction to the colic, WBC demargination, and production of colony-stimulating factors. However, if the leucocytosis is considered significant (e.g., >15,000 WBC/μL), or if it accompanied by shaking chills, rigors, or fever >101°F, the patient should be considered to have an infected hydronephrosis or pyonephrosis and should be admitted for treatment.

Mild elevation of serum creatinine is also a common finding. However, if the patient has an obstruction to the dominant functioning kidney or in a solitary kidney, the creatinine can rise significantly. Patients with known obstruction to a solitary or dominant functioning kidney should be admitted for observation and/or treatment.

Urinalysis may demonstrate either microscopic or gross hematuria. A high leukocyte count in the urine in the absence of bacteriuria is common and does not always indicate infection.

When the differential diagnosis points to a kidney or ureteral stone as possibility, a CT without contrast (referred to as low-dose stone protocol CT) should be ordered. This is a CT that visualizes the entire urinary system, typically using 1.25- to 3-mm axial reconstructions, and results in a radiation exposure of around 3.0–3.8 mSv. A CT stone protocol has an overall diagnostic accuracy (both sensitivity and specificity) of around 98%.

A CT can also predict the composition of the stone. Softer stones like uric acid stones have an attenuation value of 300 to 700 Hounsfield units (HU), while harder stones like calcium oxalates are in the range of 800 to 1200 HU.

Abdominal plain film radiography, also called an x-ray KUB (kidney, ureter, bladder), or an intravenous urogram (IVU) can be used in select situations. Small (<3–4 mm) stones and radiolucent stones (uric acid, cystine) are difficult to see on plain film radiographs. A plain film KUB results in a radiation exposure of around 0.8 mSv and in general has lower diagnostic accuracy, in the range of 60% to 75%.

Renal ultrasonography is a good tool to identify and follow hydronephrosis. Its sensitivity for stones is low (~60%), but specificity is high (>95%). Some signs that are helpful in improving the diagnostic accuracy include postacoustic shadowing effect, twinkle artifact, and loss of ureteral jet on the affected side. It could be a good first-line screening study in pregnant patients. There is no ionizing radiation with renal ultrasonography.

MRI has been used as a second-line study to diagnose ureteral stones in pregnant patients. Its capacity to identify stones as such is limited, and interpretation is often based on surrogate markers like a signal void effect and hydronephrosis; this interpretation is dependent on the radiologist's experience and familiarity with the technique. There is no ionizing radiation from an MRI.

In the follow-up setting, very often it is the urologist who drives the imaging and the treatment. Radiation exposure to the patient is a real risk, and the cumulative radiation dose can build up very quickly unless a conscious effort is made to keep this to an "as low as reasonably achievable" level. Therefore our approach is to restrict the use of imaging that involves ionizing radiation only to when it is likely to change the management.

In general, for long-term follow-up, an ultrasonogram and an x-ray KUB are considered appropriate and can be done at 6- to 12-month intervals. A CT is the preferred imaging when there is a change in status (e.g., recurrence of pain) or when a plan for surgical intervention is made on a patient previously being managed conservatively.

Differential Diagnosis

Asymptomatic nephrolithiasis is usually discovered as an incidental finding on a CT scan done for another condition, and the diagnosis is straightforward.

In the acute setting, a good history and physical examination often help in identifying the source of the pain and in planning the evaluation and treatment.

In patients with a history of recurrent kidney stones who present with a dramatic onset of excruciating flank pain, the diagnosis of a ureteral stone is fairly straightforward. However, not all patients with ureteral stones have severe pain, and not all of them will present in the classic fashion; thus it behooves the astute clinician to keep in mind atypical presentations of other conditions that can mimic renal stone disease. The differential diagnosis should include cholecystitis (right-sided upper abdomen or flank pain), acute appendicitis (right lower quadrant pain), ovarian conditions (e.g., cyst rupture, ectopic pregnancy, torsion), incarcerated inguinal hernia, testicular torsion, and diverticulitis (left side).

Treatment
Renal Stones

The incidence of stone disease is rising, but this could be partly due to the detection of asymptomatic stones from use of imaging for other conditions. However, in a study from Iceland, this rise in detection of stones did not lead to a corresponding increase in acute stone episodes. Asymptomatic renal stones can be managed conservatively. In a study, about 60% of stone remained asymptomatic on follow-up.

Stones 4 mm or less tend to pass spontaneously (>90%), and stones more than 6 mm will pass spontaneously <20% of the time. Lower pole stones are more likely to stay asymptomatic and can be managed conservatively.

Larger stones (>10 mm) or staghorn stones are more likely to require treatment and should be offered a urologic procedure, after weighing the risks and benefits of the procedure against the risks of possible complications due to the patient's comorbidities.

The following treatment options are used:

Medical expulsive therapy (MET): MET is the name given to a nonsurgical management comprising hydration (high urine output >2.5 L/day), good pain relief, and use of α-blockers like tamsulosin (Flomax)[1] for ureteral stones. Tamsulosin has not consistently been shown to improve stone clearance rates in some randomized trials but is still widely used. It is less effective for proximal ureteral stones than for distal ureteral stones.

Extracorporeal shockwave lithotripsy (ESWL): ESWL uses shock waves generated by a machine that are transmitted into the patient's body and brought to focus on the stone. ESWL should not be offered to patients who are pregnant or have an uncorrected coagulopathy. Because the patient has to pass the stone fragments, they should also not be offered to patients with obstruction distal to the stone. ESWL has an overall efficacy of around 50% to 80%.

Ureterorenoscopy (URS): In this technique the urologist places a fine endoscopic instrument into the upper urinary tract. The approach is transurethral and involves entry into the ureter through the ureteral orifice. When kidney stones are treated this way, it is customary to use a flexible ureteroscope. The technique is also called retrograde intrarenal surgery (RIRS). A holmium or thulium laser device is used to fragment stones, and the fragments can be flushed out or removed using a grasper or a wire basket. When used in the right clinical setting, URS/RIRS is a safe and efficacious procedure with stone clearance rates in excess of 90%.

Percutaneous nephrolithotomy (PCNL): This approach involves placement of a tract into the kidney. The tract is dilated, and a working sheath is used to pass an endoscope called a nephroscope. This technique is typically used for larger stones (>2–2.5 cm). An ultrasonic, pneumatic, or laser energy source is used to fragment the stones. The fragments are suctioned out or extracted using graspers. The stone clearance rates are over 85%; however, this procedure is invasive and can have more serious complications.

Pyelolithotomy is rarely offered these days but may sometimes be necessary; this can be done by a surgical approach or by using a laparoscopic (robot-assisted laparoscopic) technique. Stone clearance rates are over 95%; however, these are more invasive procedures.

---

[1] Not FDA approved for this indication.

Chemodissolution for stones has variable results. Urinary alkalinization can help manage stones that form in an acidic medium (e.g., uric acid stones/cystine stones); acetohydroxamic acid (AHA [Lithostat] 250 mg three times a day), an oral urease inhibitor, has been shown to be effective in treatment of struvite stones. However, AHA is recommended as a treatment option only when surgical options have been exhausted. Hemolytic anemias and deep vein thrombosis are some of the side effects that can be seen with the use of AHA.

When deciding on the best-fit treatment for a patient, the following considerations are reviewed: size of the stone, stone composition, location, number of stones, body habitus, presence of infection, presence of obstruction, kidney function, and patient's personal preference. Combinations of treatment can be used (e.g., PCNL followed by ESWL for small residual stones), and sandwich therapy refers to a change in modality between two sessions of the same treatment modality (e.g., URS followed by ESWL followed by URS).

Ureteral Stones
Ureteral stones can be managed by MET or surgical intervention.

Rigid and/or flexible ureteroscopy with holmium laser disintegration of stones is rapidly replacing ESWL for ureteral calculi. The success rate for stone destruction and removal is higher than for ESWL.

Patients with certain symptoms or signs are considered to have a urologic emergency and should be admitted. Fever and leukocytosis, or signs of sepsis, are suggestive of a severe infection in an obstructed kidney, or even pyonephrosis. Such patients should receive intravenous antibiotics. Other emergent situations include anuria or oliguria secondary to an obstructing stone in a solitary kidney or bilateral ureteral stones. Patients with severe pain, vomiting, and electrolyte abnormalities or significant worsening of renal function also need to be admitted. The obstructed kidney in many such patients will need to be drained by either a percutaneous nephrostomy tube or a double J stent placement.

A patient that is discharged is asked to strain urine to try and catch the stone. Once the patient collects the stone, it should be sent for analysis. A follow-up renal sonogram should be obtained 6 to 8 weeks after passage to identify any residual silent hydronephrosis. If hydronephrosis is present, urologic consultation should be obtained.

Complications
Some patients with acute severe obstruction can get perirenal urinary collections. These could be from urinary leaks and extravasations. Uninfected collections will resolve spontaneously once the obstruction is relieved. Rarely they get infected, or if they are large collections, they may need to be drained percutaneously.

Acute infections like acute pyelonephritis, infected hydronephrosis, and pyonephrosis can be seen with stone disease. They require admission and intravenous antibiotics in addition to possible surgical drainage.

Chronic infections like xanthogranulomatous pyelonephritis (XGP) are rare, and are seen in patients with a combination of infected stones, recurrent obstructions, and diabetes. Most patients with severe XGP end up requiring a nephrectomy.

Loss of function in the renal unit is from ongoing silent obstruction, intermittent severe obstruction with cortical atrophy, or combinations of obstruction and infection. Loss of function in one or both kidneys predisposes patients to develop chronic kidney disease.

Monitoring, Follow-Up, and Prevention of Recurrences
When available, the stone should be analyzed to provide a diagnosis and a specific plan tailored to the type of stone and underlying pathologic cause if present.

A complete medical history and appropriate evaluation should be carried out to identify an underlying cause such as hyperparathyroidism, Cushing syndrome, or type 2 diabetes. Imaging will help identify anatomic factors like ureteropelvic junction (UPJ)

obstruction, or horseshoe kidney. The list of medications should be reviewed, as some medications like diuretics, antiretroviral medications, and medications used for migraine and headaches can cause stones.

Stone patients should have annual radiologic studies for at least the first 3 to 5 years after they present with a stone. CT is the most accurate test, but because of the risk of cumulative radiation exposure, abdominal plain film radiography is useful if the stone(s) are radiopaque. Renal ultrasonography can also be used in specific situations, to screen for hydronephrosis, especially if the patient complains of a recurrence of symptoms and a CT has been done within the previous 6 months.

If the stone burden increases over time, a urologic consultation should be obtained.

Metabolic evaluation should be offered to all high-risk stone formers. These include a very young patient with a first stone episode, recurrent stone formers, patients with strong family history of stones, patients with chronic diarrhea or inflammatory bowel disease, pathologic skeletal fractures, solitary kidney/anatomic abnormalities, or if stones are composed of cystine, uric acid, or struvite.

If a 24-hour urine collection is obtained and dietary or medical treatment is recommended, the metabolic evaluation should be repeated 6 months later to follow up on the effectiveness of treatment and patient compliance. It is also good practice to repeat the evaluation again in 1 to 2 years.

Stones tend to recur. The risk of recurrence is estimated to be around 50% in the next 5 to 10 years.

Recurrent stone disease poses a very high financial burden, both in terms of ER visits as well loss of work from patients taking sick days off. Prevention of recurrences is therefore an important goal in the management of renal stones.

Diet Therapy
The strategies for the prevention of recurrence hinge around increasing oral intake of fluids to produce at least 2.5-L daily urine output (American Urological Association [AUA] guidelines). The fluid intake reduces the dwell time, and small crystals that form will get flushed out. Our response to patients asking about the kind of fluid starts with emphasizing that water is the most readily available and the cheapest source of fluid. We also recommend limiting caffeinated drinks like coffee and colas.

The role of healthy diet and exercise cannot be overemphasized. Patients with obesity tend to also have a metabolic syndrome and are at risk for stone formation

Recurrent stone formers should be managed using a multidisciplinary approach. and urology, nephrology and nutritionist consultations are recommended.

Patients with calcium stones and hypercalciuria should be advised to restrict the sodium in the diet to 100 mEq or less (2300 mg). A low-sodium diet has been shown to decrease urinary calcium excretion. Patients with oxalate stones and hyperoxaluria should also be advised to avoid oxalate-rich foods, to be on low-oxalate diets, and to have a normal calcium intake (1000–1200 mg/day). Aggressive calcium restriction can result in increased oxalate absorption from the gut leading to higher levels of urinary oxalate.

Patients with low citrate should be encouraged to add fruits and vegetables to their diet and limit animal protein (as should hyperuricosuric patients), as excess animal protein can cause hyperuricosuria, and also hypocitraturia through an acid load effect. Patients with cystine stones should also be asked to restrict animal protein and sodium.

Patients deficient in vitamin D should receive supplements enough to normalize levels.

Pharmacologic Therapy
Thiazide diuretics are the gold standard for treatment of recurrent calcium stones. They should be offered to patients with recurrent calcium stones having hypercalciuria and should also be offered along with potassium citrate to patients without hypercalciuria.

Chlorthalidone[1] 25 mg daily, hydrochlorothiazide[1] 50 mg daily, and indapamide[1] 2.5 mg daily are all well tolerated. (Patients should be monitored for hypokalemia.)

Potassium citrate (Urocit-K) 10 to 20 mEq daily can be prescribed for patients with recurrent calcium oxalate stones demonstrating hypocitraturia, uric acid stones, and cystine stones. Sodium citrate is an alternate choice but risks creating a higher urinary calcium load.

A baseline 24-hour urinary citrate level and follow-up study 6 months later will determine whether therapy is effectively increasing urinary citrate levels.

Chemodissolution can be attempted for small uric acid stones by urinary alkalinization using potassium citrate. Allopurinol should not be offered as first-line treatment for uric acid stones. However, patients with uric acid stones and hyperuricosuria should be offered allopurinol (Zyloprim) 300 mg daily (or a renal dosage depending on glomerular filtration rate). Patients with recurrent calcium oxalate stones, hyperuricosuria, and normal urinary calcium should also be treated with allopurinol.

Patients with cystine stones should be managed with high fluid intake, urinary alkalinization with potassium citrate, and reduction in sodium and protein intake. Thiol drugs should be prescribed if dietary measures fail. α-Mercaptopropionylglycine (tiopronin [Thiola] 800 mg daily in three divided doses) is the standard treatment. An alternative preparation, D-penicillamine (Cuprimine), is associated with more severe side effects and should be a second-line choice.

Struvite stones occur in the presence of chronic urinary infection. Surgical management of the stone along with sterilization of the urinary tract offers the best long-term results. Acetohydroxamic acid (Lithostat), an oral urease inhibitor, can be offered (250 mg three times daily) for residual or recurrent stones only after surgical options have been exhausted.

---

[1] Not FDA approved for this indication.

References

Pearle MS, Antonelli JA, Lotan Y: Urinary lithiasis: etiology, epidemiology, and pathogenesis. In Partin AW, Dmochowski RR, Kavoussi LR, Peters CA, Wein AJ, editors: *Campbell-walsh urology*, 12th ed., Philadelphia, 2016, Elsevier Saunders, ([2005-35].

Assimos D, Krambeck A, Miller NL, et al: Surgical management of stones: American urological association/endourological society guideline, part I, *J Urol* 196:1153–1160, 2016.

Assimos D, Krambeck A, Miller NL, et al: Surgical management of stones: American urological association/endourological society guideline, part II, *J Urol* 196:1161–1169, 2016.

Pearle MS, Goldfarb DS, Assimos DG, et al: Medical management of kidney stones: AUA guideline, *J Urol* 192:316–324, 2014.

Jiang P, Xie L, Arada R, et al: Qualitative review of clinical guidelines for medical and surgical management of urolithiasis: consensus and controversy 2020, *J Urol* 205(4):999–1008, 2021.

Somers, WJ: Nephrolithiasis. In Kellerman RD, Heidelbaugh JJ, Lee EM, eds: *Conns Current Therapy 2025*, Elsevier: Philadelphia; 2025;1213–1216.

PRIMARY GLOMERULAR DISEASE

Method of
Saeed Kamran Shaffi, MD, MS

CURRENT DIAGNOSIS

- Hematuria, proteinuria, hypoalbuminemia, hyperlipidemia, and elevated blood urea nitrogen and creatinine levels are the main laboratory abnormalities seen in patients with primary glomerular diseases.
- Our ability to diagnose some of the glomerular diseases and to monitor their disease-activity has improved with the recent discovery of disease-specific serum and kidney biopsy markers.

CURRENT THERAPY

- The goals of management of a patient with a primary glomerular disease are:
- To diagnose the glomerular abnormality
- To slow the progression of chronic kidney disease and subsequent development of end-stage kidney disease
- To manage and ameliorate the glomerular disease symptoms
- To prevent complications of glomerular diseases and the therapies used for their management, such as infection, thrombosis, coronary vascular disease, osteoporosis, and trace metal deficiencies

Clinical Presentation

The clinical presentation of the primary glomerular diseases can be grouped into syndromes, which are listed in Box 1.

Nephrotic syndrome: The disease-defining symptoms of the nephrotic syndrome are >3.5 g/day of proteinuria in adults, serum albumin of <3 g/L, and edema. Hyperlipidemia and thrombophilia are often present.

Sub-nephrotic proteinuria: These patients have proteinuria of <3.5 g/day without hypoalbuminemia, edema, and hyperlipidemia.

Acute nephritic syndrome: Nephritic syndrome presents as microscopic hematuria, which is defined as >3 red blood cells (RBC) per high-power field (HPF). Patients with the nephritic syndrome also have a varying amount of proteinuria and may have an elevated creatinine level indicating a decline in the glomerular filtration rate (GFR).

Asymptomatic microhematuria: Hematuria is seen on urinalyses; however, these patients do not develop progressive kidney dysfunction.

Rapidly progressive glomerulonephritis (RPGN): Rapidly progressive glomerulonephritis is a syndrome associated with a rapid decline in renal function over the course of a few days, weeks, or months. On the kidney biopsy, RPGN presents as glomerular crescents which form due to the disruption of the glomerular basement membrane with fluid spillage in the Bowmans space resulting in extracapillary cellular proliferation and crescent formation.

Slowly progressive nephritic syndrome: Some of the glomerular diseases have a smoldering course with persistent hematuria and proteinuria that may eventually lead to CKD and end-stage kidney disease.

Causes of primary glomerular diseases: Table 1 lists the causes of primary glomerular diseases.

Diagnosis of the Primary Glomerular Diseases

A glomerular disease is suspected when a clinician notices hematuria, proteinuria, or an abnormal blood urea nitrogen or creatinine level. It is paramount to rule out other conditions which can present with similar abnormalities.

Hematuria: It is imperative to differentiate between the glomerular and nonglomerular hematuria (Box 2 and Figure 1).

Proteinuria: Proteinuria is often seen in primary glomerular diseases. Urinary protein and albumin excretion in an adult should not exceed 150 mg/day, and 30 mg/g, respectively. Reduction in proteinuria—especially when sustained longitudinally—is associated with better clinical outcomes. In clinical practice, a spot urine protein to creatinine (P/C) ratio or albumin to creatinine ratio is often used for the assessment of the proteinuria; however, the concordance between the spot and the 24-hour urine collection is poor. On the other hand, 24-hour urine collection is cumbersome, is not feasible in children, and is associated with significant

BOX 1	Clinical Presentation of Glomerular Diseases

Nephrotic syndrome
Sub-nephrotic proteinuria
Acute nephritic syndrome
Asymptomatic microhematuria
Rapidly progressive glomerulonephritis
Slowly progressive chronic nephritis

TABLE 1	Causes and Clinical Presentation of the Primary Glomerular Diseases

CAUSES OF PRIMARY GLOMERULAR DISEASE	PRESENTATION
Minimal change disease	Nephrotic syndrome
Primary focal segmental glomerulosclerosis	Usually nephrotic syndrome, rarely nephritic syndrome
Primary membranous glomerulonephritis	Nephrotic syndrome
IgA nephropathy	Usually nephritic syndrome, sometimes microscopic hematuria or gross hematuria
Postinfectious glomerulonephritis	Nephritic syndrome
Membranoproliferative glomerulonephritis due to alternate complement pathway abnormalities (dense deposit disease and C3 glomerulonephritis)	Nephritic syndrome
Fibrillary glomerulonephritis	Nephritic or nephrotic syndrome
Thin basement membrane disease	Asymptomatic microscopic hematuria

BOX 2	Signs of Glomerular Hematuria

>22% dysmorphic* RBCs on optical and >40% on phase contrast microscopy
   In the setting of hematuria and dysmorphic RBCs, an immunoreactive albumin excretion of >0.59 mg/mg total protein excretion is strongly suggestive of glomerular hematuria
   The newer generation of the urinalysis machines (sediMAX) automate the phase-contrast microscopy detection of dysmorphic RBCs without loss of precision

*Red blood cells (RBCs), originating from the glomeruli, develop characteristic membrane abnormalities and are called dysmorphic. A certain type of dysmorphic RBC, with membrane blebs called acanthocytes, are strongly correlated with glomerular hematuria (Figure 1).

under- and overcollection even in highly motivated patients. Therefore, a morning first void spot urine (P/C) ratio is adequate for proteinuria surveillance; however, a 24-hour urine collection for proteinuria assessment should be considered when the use of therapeutic agents that can cause significant morbidity is being contemplated.

GFR assessment: The best method to estimate GFR in patients with glomerular diseases is not known. Assessment of the longitudinal trends in the estimated GFR (eGFR) in this population may provide the clinicians with a better guide of renal status than a single value in isolation.

Kidney biopsy: Apart from a few situations such as serum anti-phospholipase A 2 receptor positivity in a high biopsy risk patient and steroid responsive nephrotic syndrome in children, which is almost always due to minimal change nephropathy, a kidney biopsy is essential for the diagnosis of primary glomerular diseases. Kidney biopsy not only provides a definitive diagnosis of the primary glomerular abnormality in most of the patients but also informs the clinician of the prognosis by quantifying the degree of the irreversible changes such as glomerulosclerosis, interstitial fibrosis, and tubular atrophy.

General Management of Primary Glomerular Diseases
Primary glomerular diseases may manifest as signs and symptoms (Box 3) which can be debilitating.

Treatment of Primary Glomerulonephritis
Edema: Dietary sodium restriction (1.5 to 2 g or 60 to 80 mmol/day) is the first step for edema management due to nephrotic syndromes. Oral loop diuretics (Table 2) should be used if the sodium restriction does not ameliorate the symptoms. Use of diuretics with better oral bioavailability and longer half-life may be more effective in edema management (see Table 2). Gut wall edema in patients with severe nephrotic syndrome may preclude effective diuresis with orally administered diuretics in which case intravenous loop diuretics alone or combined with a thiazide diuretic (e.g., metolazone [Zaroxolyn]) may be tried. Use of loop diuretics with intravenous albumin (Albuminar)[1] to maximize diuresis is controversial with some reports showing beneficial while others showing equivocal results; this strategy can be considered in patients with severe diuretic resistance.

Hypertension: Optimal control of hypertension in patients with a glomerular disease may decrease cardiovascular morbidity and mortality, and slow CKD progression. Sodium restriction and maximum-tolerated dose of angiotensin-converting enzyme inhibitors (ACEi) or angiotensin receptor blockers to achieve a BP target of <125/75 mm Hg in patients with >1 g/day of proteinuria is recommended.

Hyperlipidemia: Patients with primary glomerular diseases are at risk of developing hyperlipidemia and cardiovascular events. Hyperlipidemia should be treated aggressively to the same targets as the general population.

Hypercoagulable states: Patients with glomerular diseases are at significant risk of thromboembolism due to the alterations in the pro-coagulant and anticoagulant factors. The incidence of thromboembolism has been reported as high as 8% to 44%, and 5% to 62% in nephrotic syndrome and membranous glomerulonephritis, respectively. Anticoagulation should be considered in patients with a low serum albumin (below 2 to 2.5 g/dL) along with one of the following: >10 g/d of proteinuria; BMI of >35 kg/m^2; family history and genetic disposition of thromboembolism; New York Heart Association Class III or IV congestive heart failure; recent abdominal or orthopedic surgery; prolonged immobilization. The Chapel Hill group has devised an online calculator (https://www.med.unc.edu/gntools/) to aid the clinicians in deciding about the use of anticoagulation in patients with membranous glomerulonephritis.

Case-reports have described aspirin[1], warfarin (Coumadin)[1], low-molecular–weight heparin,[1] or direct-acting oral anticoagulant (DOAC) use for thromboembolism prevention in patients with nephrotic syndrome. Expert opinion suggests starting anticoagulation with low-dose, low-molecular–weight heparin, followed by introduction of warfarin; heparin should be discontinued when a therapeutic INR is achieved. Alternatively, low-molecular–weight heparin with aspirin has been suggested for a period of 3 months before introducing warfarin if proteinuria does not resolve.

Chronic kidney disease: Studies have shown that complete remission of proteinuria is associated with preservation of renal

---

[1] Not FDA approved for this indication.

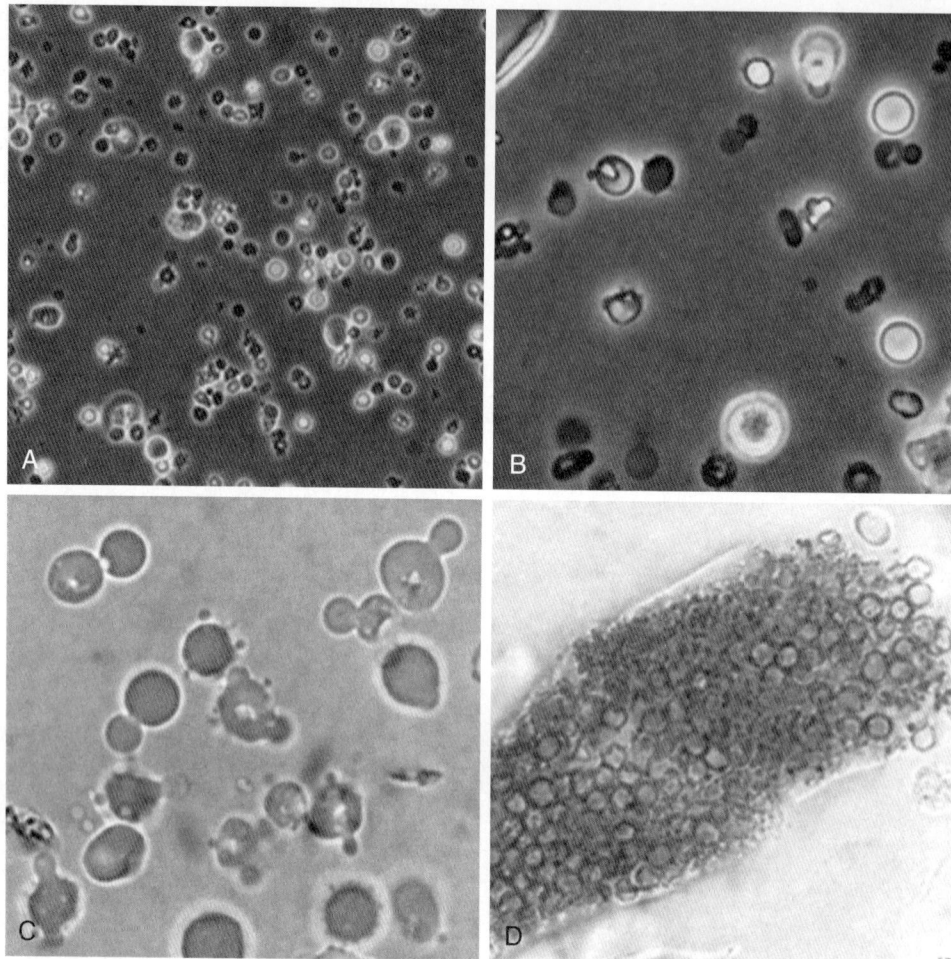

Figure 1 A and B. Acanthocytes: phase contrast microscopy, unstained; C. Acanthocytes: brightfield microscopy, unstained; D. RBC cast: brightfield microscopy, unstained. (Courtesy of Jay R. Seltzer, M.D. Chief of Nephrology - Missouri Baptist Medical Center - St. Louis Missouri.)

| BOX 3 | Abnormalities Seen in the Primary Glomerular Diseases |

Edema, if severe anasarca
Hypertension
Hyperlipidemia
Hypercoagulable state
Chronic kidney disease
Trace mineral and vitamin deficiencies
Endocrine hormonal abnormalities
Immunocompromised state

function and end-stage kidney disease. Disease-modifying therapies, which will be described later, should be used to prevent the development of renal fibrosis which is irreversible.

Trace mineral and vitamin deficiency: Patients with primary glomerular diseases who have nephrotic syndrome may have deficiencies of iron, copper, zinc, and selenium. Twenty-five hydroxyvitamin D [25-(OH)D] deficiency, which is extremely common in patients with nephrotic syndrome, is due to urinary loss of 25(OH)D, and is often difficult to treat unless the patient achieves complete remission. Treatment of 25(OH)D deficiency is outlined in Box 4 and is similar to that in the general population.

Endocrine abnormalities: Loss of hormone-binding proteins and albumin in patients with proteinuric glomerular diseases leads to various endocrine abnormalities. Low T4 levels are seen in approximately 50% of nephrotic syndrome patients with preserved renal function due to urinary loss of thyroid-binding globulin; however, these patients are usually euthyroid due to their preserved ability to convert T4 to T3. On the other hand,

patients with primary glomerular diseases with advanced CKD have a diminished T3 due to decreased conversion of T4 to T3; however, unlike other chronic illnesses, the conversion of T4 to metabolically inactive reverse T3 (rT3) is not enhanced.

Risk of infections: Chronic kidney disease, nephrotic syndrome, and use of the immunosuppressive medications are some of the risk factors that increase the propensity to develop infections in patients with primary glomerular diseases. Patients should be up to date on their vaccinations to mitigate infection risk (Box 5).

Pneumocystis jirovecii prophylaxis should be administered to patients who are on >20 mg of prednisone and/or on immunosuppressive medications that affect the T cells such as corticosteroids and cyclophosphamide (Cytoxan).

Therapy of Specific Glomerular Diseases

Minimal-Change Disease

Minimal-change disease is the most common cause of nephrotic syndrome in children (90%) and is rare adults (10%). No abnormality is detected on light microscopic evaluation of the kidney; however, the electron microscopy shows diffuse foot process effacement. A child presenting with nephrotic syndrome is assumed to have a minimal-change disease and does not require a kidney biopsy. In adults, minimal-change disease is a rare occurrence and is usually diagnosed with a kidney biopsy. Most cases of minimal-change disease are idiopathic, although secondary causes such as drugs (nonsteroidal antiinflammatory drugs [NSAIDs]), hematological malignancies, and thymoma are associated with this condition. Therapy of minimal-change disease is shown in Box 6.

Primary Focal Segmental Glomerulosclerosis

Primary focal segmental glomerulosclerosis is a pathological term denoting patchy glomerulosclerosis and is thought to be due to

TABLE 2 Pharmacokinetics of Loop Diuretics

NAME	RELATIVE POTENCY	ORAL BIOAVAIL-ABILITY	HALF-LIFE (HOURS)	ELIMINATION ROUTE	COMMENTS
Furosemide (Lasix)	1	~60%	~1.5	~65% renal, 25% metabolism	Renal disease prolongs half-life
Bumetanide (Bumex)	40	~80	~0.8	~62% renal, 38% metabolism	Liver disease prolongs half-life
Torsemide (Demadex)	20	~80%	~3.5	~20% renal, 80% metabolism	Liver disease prolongs half-life

---

BOX 4 Treatment of Vitamin D Deficiency in Primary Glomerular Diseases

25(OH)D level less than 12 ng/mL: treat with 50,000 international units (IU) of vitamin D2 (ergocalciferol)[1] or vitamin D3 (cholecalciferol)[1] orally once a week for 6 to 8 weeks followed by 800–1000 IU/day of vitamin D3 for maintenance therapy. Higher doses of daily vitamin D3 may be necessary if the levels remain low (<30 ng/mL) 3 months after therapy initiation.

25(OH)D levels between 12 and 20 ng/mL: treat with 800–1000 IU/day of vitamin D3. Repeat levels in 3 months. Higher vitamin D3 doses may be necessary if the levels are below the normal range (30–50 ng/mL).

25(OH)D level between 20 and 30 ng/mL: treat with 600–800 IU of vitamin D3 daily.

[1]Not FDA approved for this indication.

BOX 5 Recommended Immunization in Patients With Glomerular Diseases

- Hepatitis A vaccine (Havrix, VAQTA)
- Hepatitis B vaccine (Engerix-B, Recombivax HB)
- *Haemophilus influenzae* type B conjugate vaccine (Hib [ActHIB, Hiberix])
- Annual trivalent inactivated influenza vaccine
- Pneumococcal vaccination, series, and vaccine type based on the most up-to-date ACIP/CDC recommendations for condition
- COVID-19 vaccination series and further COVID-19 boosters based on the most up-to-date ACIP/CDC recommendations for condition
- Meningococcal Vaccine against sero-group (A, C, W and Y; Menactra, Menveo)[1]

[1]Not FDA approved for this indication.

BOX 6 Minimal-Change Disease Therapy

Prednisone 1 mg/kg (maximum 80 mg) or alternate-day single dose of 2 mg/kg (maximum 120 mg) for 4–16 weeks. Taper slowly in 6 months if complete remission (proteinuria <300 mg/g) is achieved in 4 weeks.

Most patients respond to corticosteroids but 25% of treated patients have frequent relapses and 30% become steroid dependent (two relapses during or within 2 weeks of completing steroid therapy). No response to steroids in 8–16 weeks should be considered steroid resistance.

Second-line agents are calcineurin inhibitors, oral cyclophosphamide (Cytoxan), or rituximab (Rituxan)[1]

[1]Not FDA approved for this indication.

BOX 7 Primary Focal Segmental Glomerulosclerosis Therapy

- First line: Prednisone 1 mg/kg q day or 2 mg/kg every alternate day. Continue high-dose steroids for 4–16 weeks until complete remission is achieved, followed by a taper in 6 months.
- Second line: Calcineurin inhibitors for patients who cannot tolerate prednisone.
- Third line: Patients with frequently relapsing primary FSGS may respond to rituximab (Rituxan)[1]
- Fourth line: Mycophenolate mofetil (MMF [CellCept]).[1]
- Adrenocorticotropic hormone (ACTH) gel (Corticotropin [HP Acthar]).[1]

[1]Not FDA approved for this indication.

an unknown permeability factor which causes proteinuria, hypertension, and kidney dysfunction. This condition should be differentiated from the secondary glomerulosclerosis (focal or global) which is a sequela of acute or chronic kidney injury. Reduction in proteinuria is associated with better renal survival and is the goal of therapy. Box 7 shows the therapies used for the management of primary focal segmental glomerulosclerosis.

Primary Membranous Glomerulonephritis

Idiopathic membranous glomerulonephritis is the second most common cause of nephrotic syndrome in the US adults. This condition is characterized by diffuse subepithelial deposits seen on kidney biopsy. Our understanding of the pathophysiology of the idiopathic membranous glomerulonephritis was revolutionized in 2009 with the discovery of elevated M-type phospholipase-A(2) receptor [PLA2R], an antigen expressed in the human podocytes, antibody in the serum and the immune deposits in the glomeruli of the vast majority of patients. Since then, numerous other antigens have been identified in patients with primary or secondary membranous glomerulonephritis. Antibodies against thrombospondin type 1 domain-containing

7A (THSD7A) have been found in PLA2R negative idiopathic membranous patients (2% to 4%). Serum anti-PLA2R and THSD7A antibody levels are measured by commercial laboratories and are used to monitor idiopathic membranous glomerulonephritis disease activity—a rise in titer is associated with relapse while a fall is associated with remission. Box 8 details the treatment strategies used for the management of primary membranous glomerulonephritis.

IgA Nephropathy

IgA nephropathy is the leading cause of glomerulonephritis worldwide. A multi-hit hypothesis has been proposed in the pathogenesis of IgA nephropathy, with mistracking of the poorly O-glycosylated galactose deficient IgA1 (Gd-IgA1) into the circulation—thought to be derived from the mucosal B cells—production of IgG and IgA antibodies against Gd-IgA1, formation and deposition of mesangial immune complexes, and activation of the complement system resulting in immune-mediated kidney injury. The antigen-antibody complexes deposit in the kidneys and cause a mesangial (M) and endocapillary (E) proliferative glomerulonephritis which can lead to glomerulosclerosis (S) and tubular atrophy (T). At times, IgA nephropathy can also present as crescentic glomerulonephritis (C). The MEST-C classification of the kidney

BOX 8 | Primary Membranous Glomerulonephritis Therapy

Watchful waiting for 6 months with maximization of ACEi or ARB. Factors associated with low likelihood of achieving spontaneous remission are persistence of >4 g/day of proteinuria with no response to antihypertensive/antiproteinuric therapy in 6 month; presence of life threatening nephrotic syndrome; greater than 30% increase in serum creatinine; and a high anti-PLA2R antibody titer.

Rituximab[1] has similar rates of complete remission as cyclophosphamide, however, the complete remission rate is lower. Furthermore, rituximab-treated patients are less likely to develop adverse events than cyclophosphamide-treated groups. Therefore, rituximab is the first-line therapy for the management of primary membranous glomerulonephritis.

Oral cyclophosphamide[1] and prednisone with or without intravenous methylprednisolone (Solumedrol) pulses in alternate months for 6 months. Some centers use cyclophosphamide and prednisone together for 3 months.

Calcineurin inhibitors are as effective as cyclophosphamide in inducing remission; however, the risk of relapse after medication discontinuation is high.

[1]Not FDA approved for this indication.
ACEi, Angiotensin-converting enzyme inhibitors; *ARB*, angiotensin receptor blockers.

BOX 9 | IgA Nephropathy Therapy

Antifibrotic Therapy
Maximal dose ACEi/ARB, as tolerated, should be prescribed to optimize blood pressure control and to decrease the proteinuria to <1 g/day. An SGLT2 inhibitor should be added to this regimen, which can improve proteinuria and renal outcomes.

Sparsentan (Filspari 200 mg or 400 mg), a dual endothelin A1 and angiotensin II receptor antagonist, was approved by the FDA to decrease proteinuria in patients with IgA nephropathy (IgAN). Due to a risk of hepatotoxicity and birth defects, the prescribing physicians, patients, and dispensing pharmacies must enroll in a Risk Evaluation and Mitigation Strategies (REMS) program.

Atrasentan (Vanrafia), another endothelin A1 receptor antagonist, was approved by the FDA to decrease proteinuria. Unlike sparsentan, it has not been associated with hepatotoxicity.

Immunosuppression
Patients who continue to have >1 g/day of proteinuria, despite antifibrotic therapy for ≥3 months, with a BP of <125/75 mm Hg, should receive a course of an immunosuppressive agent.

Budesonide delayed-release capsule (Tarpeyo), used for 9 months, decreases proteinuria and stabilizes eGFR in the short term in adults with primary IgAN.

Iptacopan (Vanrafia), a factor B inhibitor that targets the alternative complement pathway, was approved by the FDA in 2024 for the treatment of severe primary IgAN. It has been shown to reduce proteinuria. Due to a significantly increased risk of infection due to encapsulated organisms such as *N. meningitidis*, *S. pneumoniae*, and *H. influenzae* type b, the prescribers, dispensing pharmacies, and patients require enrollment in a REMS program and vaccination against these organisms (MenACWY with MenB for *N. meningitidis* and PCV20 or PCV15 with PPSV23 for *S. pneumoniae*; Hib vaccination against *H. influenzae* type b is strongly suggested) before starting therapy. If vaccines cannot be administered, antibiotic prophylaxis with Penicillin V[1] 250 mg twice a day should be started until 2 weeks after vaccination.

Low dose oral methylprednisolone[1] (0.4 mg/kg/day) tapered in 6 to 9 months with PJP prophylaxis for 12 weeks decreased proteinuria and improved renal outcomes; this regimen can be tried if budesonide or iptacopan cannot be prescribed.

Immunosuppressive therapy should be prescribed if the eGFR is >50 mL/min/1.73 m². Immunosuppressive therapy may be of benefit if the eGFR is between 30 and 50 mL/min/1.73 m² but is associated with increased risk of adverse events, which should be discussed with the patient.

Patients with IgA nephropathy in whom >50% glomeruli show crescents should be treated with corticosteroids and cyclophosphamide.[1]

Clinical Trials
If eligible, patients should be provided information about the currently ongoing clinical trials for IgA nephropathy.

[1]Not FDA approved for this indication.
ACEi, Angiotensin-converting enzyme inhibitors; *ARB*, angiotensin receptor blockers; *eGFR*, estimated GFR; *PJP*, *Pneumocystis jirovecii* pneumonia.

biopsy provides useful information regarding disease prognostication. The secondary cause of IgA nephropathy such as HIV and cirrhosis should be ruled out. IgA nephropathy often has a smoldering course presenting as a nephritic syndrome with progressive loss of kidney function that may lead to end-stage kidney disease. Recently, it has been shown that decreasing proteinuria to <1 g/day results in better renal survival and has become one of the goals of therapy. Box 9 shows the therapeutic options for IgA nephropathy.

There is a paradigm shift in the management of IgA nephropathy, with a two-pronged approach targeting renal fibrosis and immune-mediated kidney injury.

Postinfectious Glomerulonephritis

Acute postinfectious glomerulonephritis presents as nephritic syndrome, acute kidney injury, and low serum complement levels and is more common in children and young adults. This condition was classically described in the convalescence of scarlet fever, but other bacteria, viruses, and protozoa can also cause this condition. Kidney biopsy shows diffuse proliferative glomerulonephritis with prominent mesangial and subepithelial deposits that on immunofluorescence microscopy show positivity for C3 and IgG. It can also present as crescentic glomerulonephritis which portends a poor prognosis. The treatment of renal failure due to postinfectious glomerulonephritis is symptomatic. The primary infection that caused postinfectious glomerulonephritis should be treated appropriately if present at the time of diagnosis. Children have an excellent prognosis with the recovery of kidney function in the vast majority of the patients. However, adults with this condition have a poor renal prognosis with 30% of the patients developing CKD. The outcomes are particularly worse for patients with severe proteinuria with two out of three patients developing progressive kidney dysfunction.

Membranoproliferative Glomerulonephritis due to Alternate Complement Pathway Abnormalities

Membranoproliferative glomerulonephritis (MPGN) is a pathological phenotype seen on kidney biopsy characterized by endocapillary proliferative glomerulonephritis, increased mesangial matrix, and thickening of the glomerular basement membranes. Various infectious, autoimmune, vascular, and neoplastic processes can lead to this type of glomerular injury. MPGN is now classified on the basis of disease mechanism rather than the

histological findings with an emphasis on staining intensity of C3 and IgG on immunofluorescence microscopy. Presence of both C3 and IgG point toward an immune-complex-mediated process. Predominant C3 staining on immunofluorescence with minimal IgG staining indicates abnormalities in the alternate complement pathway that manifest as dense deposit disease (DDD) or C3 glomerulonephritis (C3GN). These are rare conditions affecting children and young adults and present as nephritic syndrome, renal function abnormalities, and hypertension. Laboratory data abnormalities include low C3 levels with normal C4 levels (alternate complement pathway abnormality), presence of antibodies

(C3 nephritic factor, anti-factors H, B, or I), gene mutations of the alternate complement pathway proteins (complement factor H and I-related protein gene mutations), diminished serum factors that regulate the alternate complement pathway (serum factor H, B, I, and serum membrane cofactor protein [MCP]), and elevated terminal complement pathway constituents (C5b-9). Treatment options for DDD and C3GN are listed in Box 10.

Fibrillary Glomerulonephritis

Fibrillary glomerulonephritis is an uncommon condition primarily affecting adults. Kidney biopsy shows amyloid-like deposits; however, they are Congo-Red negative and thus are not truly amyloid. Electron-microscopy shows characteristic findings of randomly organized fibrils sized 10 to 30 nm. One-third of the patients with fibrillary glomerulonephritis have another disorder such as autoimmune disease, malignancy, and monoclonal gammopathy. Recently, our understanding of the pathophysiology of idiopathic fibrillary glomerulonephritis improved significantly with the identification of DnaJ homolog subfamily B member 9 (DNAJB9)—a member of the molecular chaperone gene family—in fibrillary deposits. Almost all the patients with fibrillary glomerulonephritis showed positive immunohistochemistry to DNAJB9 while all the patients with amyloidosis were negative. The disease usually presents as nephritic syndrome. The prognosis is generally poor with most of the patients developing end-stage kidney disease. Antiproteinuric therapy with ACEi/ARB and immunosuppression have been tried with variable results with the patients with milder disease (non-nephrotic range proteinuria and preserved eGFR) more likely to achieve complete remission.

References

Agrawal S, Zaritsky JJ, Fornoni A, Smoyer WE: Dyslipidaemia in nephrotic syndrome: mechanisms and treatment, *Nat Rev Nephrol* 14(1):57–70, 2018 Jan.

Cattran DC, Kim ED, Reich H, et al: Membranous nephropathy: quantifying remission duration on outcome, *J Am Soc Nephrol JASN* 28(3):995–1003, 2017 Mar.

Floege J, Barbour SJ, Cattran DC, et al: Management and treatment of glomerular diseases (part 1): conclusions from a Kidney Disease: Improving Global Outcomes (KDIGO) Controversies Conference, *Kidney Int* 95(2):268–280, 2019 Feb.

Harris RC, Ismail N: Extrarenal complications of the nephrotic syndrome, *Am J Kidney Dis Off J Natl Kidney Found* 23(4):477–497, 1994 Apr.

Lee T, Biddle AK, Lionaki S, et al: Personalized prophylactic anticoagulation decision analysis in patients with membranous nephropathy, *Kidney Int* 85(6):1412–1420, 2014 Jun.

Nasr SH, Vrana JA, Dasari S, et al: DNAJB9 is a specific immunohistochemical marker for fibrillary glomerulonephritis, *Kidney Int Rep* 3(1):56–64, 2017 Aug 8.

Ponticelli C, Glassock R: *Treatment of primary glomerulonephritis*, North America, 2009, ESCCO eBook Subscription Academic Collection.

Radice A, Trezzi B, Maggiore U, et al: Clinical usefulness of autoantibodies to M-type phospholipase A2 receptor (PLA2R) for monitoring disease activity in idiopathic membranous nephropathy (IMN), *Autoimmun Rev* 15(2):146–154, 2016 Feb.

Reich HN, Troyanov S, Scholey JW, Cattran DC: Remission of proteinuria improves prognosis in IgA nephropathy, *J Am Soc Nephrol* 18(12):3177–3183, 2007 Dec 1.

Rovin BH, Alder SG, Barratt J, et al.: KDIGO 2021 clinical practice guideline for the management of glomerular diseases, *Kidney Int* 100(4): S1–S276, 2021.

Rovin BH, Caster DJ, Cattran DC, et al: Management and treatment of glomerular diseases (part 2): conclusions from a Kidney Disease: Improving Global Outcomes (KDIGO) Controversies Conference, *Kidney Int* 95(2):281–295, 2019 Feb.

PYELONEPHRITIS

Method of
Mark Wirtz, MD; Julia R. Lubsen, MD; and Melissa Stiles, MD

CURRENT DIAGNOSIS

- Clinical manifestations of pyelonephritis include systemic signs and symptoms (fever, chills, sweats, malaise), urinary symptoms (frequency, urgency, dysuria), flank pain, costovertebral angle (CVA) tenderness, nausea, and vomiting.
- Up to 20% of patients do not have urinary symptoms.
- Signs and symptoms such as malaise and altered mental status may be atypical in older adults and immunocompromised patients.
- Urinalysis shows pyuria, bacteriuria, or both. A urine culture growing >10,000 colony-forming units (CFU) of uropathogenic bacteria confirms pyelonephritis in the appropriate clinical context.
- Computed tomography (CT) of the abdomen/pelvis should be considered in patients who have known or suspected nephrolithiasis, acute kidney injury, or concern for complicated pyelonephritis.
- Imaging and repeat urine culture and blood cultures should be considered in patients who worsen or do not improve after 24 to 48 hours of appropriate antibiotic therapy.

CURRENT THERAPY

- Evaluate the risk for antimicrobial resistance based on local antibiograms and patient risk factors.
- Empiric outpatient treatment
  - Fluoroquinolones or trimethoprim-sulfamethoxazole (TMP-SMX [Bactrim]) are reasonable oral antibiotics.
  - Strongly consider a single dose of a long-lasting empiric intravenous antibiotic such as ceftriaxone (Rocephin) or gentamicin in addition to starting an oral agent.
- Empiric inpatient treatment
  - Ceftriaxone is recommended as empiric coverage.
  - Cefepime (Maxipime), a carbapenem, or an aminoglycoside can be considered if there is concern for ceftriaxone resistance.

Epidemiology

Pyelonephritis is a common, severe urinary tract infection (UTI) with an annual incidence in the United States of 459,000 to 1,138,00 cases. Pyelonephritis is more common in women than in men, and women are five times more likely to be hospitalized. The highest-risk group for hospitalization are adults older than 65 years of age. In the United States, costs related to pyelonephritis (direct and indirect) are around $2 billion per year. Recurrent pyelonephritis is uncommon (<10%) and should prompt evaluation for predisposing conditions.

Pathophysiology and Microbial Etiology

Pyelonephritis is usually caused by an ascending enteric bacterial infection from the bladder but can also be caused by direct seeding via bacteremia. The result is inflammation of the renal pelvis and kidney. Uropathogenic *Escherichia coli* (UPEC) strains

TABLE 1	Differential Diagnosis of Acute Pyelonephritis

- Appendicitis
- Cholangitis
- Cholecystitis
- Cystitis
- Diverticulitis
- Gastroenteritis
- Herpes zoster
- Musculoskeletal pain
- Ovarian cysts, ovarian torsion, ovarian tumors, ectopic pregnancy
- Pancreatitis
- Perforated viscus
- Pelvic inflammatory disease
- Pneumonia
- Prostatitis
- Renal vein thrombosis, renal infarction
- Nephrolithiasis

account for as much as 80% of all outpatient pyelonephritis in women. Other bacteria implicated include other *Enterobacteriaceae* (*Klebsiella pneumoniae*, *Proteus mirabilis*), *Staphylococcus saprophyticus*, *Candida* species, *Pseudomonas aeruginosa*, *Enterococcus* species, and *Ureaplasma* species. The likelihood of these pathogens increases with male sex, increasing age, hospitalization, and complicated infections, although UPEC still predominates.

Risk Factors

Risk factors for pyelonephritis include the following:
- Risk factors for cystitis (personal or maternal history of cystitis, spermicide exposure, new sexual partner, recent sexual intercourse)
- Urinary tract obstruction
- Incontinence in women older than 30 years of age
- Diabetes mellitus
- Genetic predisposition (low *CXCR1* expression resulting in altered immunity)
- Pregnancy

Clinical Manifestations

Clinical manifestations of pyelonephritis can include systemic signs and symptoms such as fever, chills, sweats, and malaise. Typical urinary symptoms (e.g., urinary frequency, urgency, and dysuria) may be present, but up to 20% of patients do not have any bladder-related symptoms. Other symptoms can include flank pain, CVA tenderness, nausea, and vomiting. Depending on disease severity, signs and symptoms of sepsis may be present. It is important to note that certain groups (older adults, immunocompromised patients) may not have typical systemic or urinary symptoms and can present with only vague symptoms (e.g., malaise) and/or mental status changes.

Diagnosis

Pyelonephritis should be suspected in patients with flank pain or tenderness and a urinalysis that shows pyuria (2 to 5 white blood cells per high-power field), bacteriuria, or both. As discussed earlier, presenting signs and symptoms may be atypical, especially in older adults and immunocompromised patients. The differential diagnosis of acute pyelonephritis is listed in Table 1.

In the correct clinical context, the diagnosis is confirmed by a urine culture that grows ≥10,000 CFU of a uropathogenic bacteria. A urine culture should be ordered in all patients suspected of having pyelonephritis. Blood cultures are not recommended for uncomplicated pyelonephritis. Although bacteremia is common, pathogens isolated from blood cultures are usually concordant with pathogens isolated from urine cultures, and blood culture results rarely change management. Blood cultures should be considered in patients with complicated pyelonephritis (see the "Complications" section later in this chapter) and in all patients presenting with severe sepsis and septic shock.

Abdominal imaging is not always needed to diagnose pyelonephritis, but it can identify complications such as urinary tract obstruction, renal or perinephric abscess, and emphysematous pyelonephritis. Initial imaging should be considered in patients

who have known or suspected nephrolithiasis, significant acute kidney injury, or concern for complicated pyelonephritis. Imaging and repeat urine culture and blood cultures should be considered in patients who worsen or do not improve after 24 to 48 hours of appropriate antibiotic therapy. In most cases, the preferred imaging test is CT of the abdomen/pelvis with and without contrast enhancement. Renal ultrasonography is more sensitive than CT for diagnosing hydronephrosis and urinary tract obstruction. Noncontrast CT of the abdomen/pelvis is preferred for detecting nephrolithiasis. A CT of the abdomen/pelvis with contrast is best for detecting abscesses and emphysematous pyelonephritis, but contrast may be contraindicated in patients with acute kidney injury.

Treatment Considerations

The most appropriate empiric treatment and disposition of a patient with pyelonephritis requires consideration of several factors including antimicrobial resistance, ability for close-interval follow-up, host vulnerability, and severity of illness.

Antimicrobial resistance is a significant concern that drives decisions regarding treatment and disposition. Fluoroquinolone resistance (ciprofloxacin, 5.1% to 39.8%) is now as common as TMP-SMX resistance (14.6% to 37.1%) in developed countries. Local antimicrobial resistance may not be known, and hospital antibiograms may not accurately reflect the setting in which the clinician practices. Patient markers for antimicrobial resistance include prior history of a resistant infection or same antibiotic class use in the past year, older age, long-term care or hospitalization, diabetes, and recurrent pyelonephritis. If an appropriate oral antibiotic is not available, hospital admission is warranted until culture data are available.

The ability of close interval follow-up is crucial in the management of pyelonephritis, especially if the outpatient setting is being considered. It is not uncommon for symptoms such as fever, flank pain, and nausea to persist for the first few days of appropriate antibiotic treatment. Hence a patient with stable housing, reliable transportation, and a supportive psychosocial environment would be best suited for outpatient management.

Several risk factors related to host vulnerability can increase morbidity and mortality. Anatomic risk factors include stones, neoplasms, and anomalies that may impair drainage of the urinary tract. Interventional factors can be related to bladder catheters, nephrostomy tubes, or recent instrumentation. Immunologic risks include immunosuppression, older age, and diabetes. Pyelonephritis in pregnancy is dangerous to both the mother and fetus, and it should be treated in an inpatient setting with intravenous antibiotics.

Hospitalization should be considered for patients who have severe pain, intractable nausea and vomiting, and hypovolemia. Patients with complicated pyelonephritis, severe sepsis, or septic shock would warrant hospital admission.

Outpatient Management

Supportive care is important for all patients. Antiemetics, antipyretics, and analgesics should be given for symptom relief. Patients with hypovolemia, nausea, and vomiting may require intravenous fluid resuscitation.

Antibiotics should be administered quickly, cover the organisms of concern, and have activity in the urine, kidneys, and bloodstream (Table 2). Earlier practice guidelines, including those from the Infectious Diseases Society of America (IDSA), strongly favored fluoroquinolones. However, increasing rates of resistance and the significant adverse effects of fluoroquinolones have led to subsequent guidelines recommending either a fluoroquinolone *or* TMP-SMX. Additionally, most guidelines also recommend using clinical judgment in escalating therapy beyond a single oral agent to include a supplemental parenteral, long-lasting antibiotic at time of diagnosis if resistance of an organism to the proposed oral antibiotic chosen is greater than a threshold of 10%. Prompt follow-up should be arranged to reevaluate the patient's response and review culture data. Oral beta-lactams (including

| **TABLE 2** | Antimicrobial Therapy for Acute Pyelonephritis |

Oral

- Ciprofloxacin (Cipro) 500 mg twice daily for 5–7 days
- Ciprofloxacin extended-release (Cipro XR) 1000 mg daily for 5–7 days
- Levofloxacin (Levaquin) 750 mg daily for 5–7 days
- Trimethoprim-sulfamethoxazole DS (Bactrim DS) 160/800 mg twice daily for 10–14 days
- Amoxicillin-clavulanate (Augmentin) 875–125 mg twice daily for 10–14 days
- Cefixime (Suprax) 400 mg daily for 10–14 days
- Cefpodoxime (Vantin)[1] 200 mg twice daily for 10–14 days

Intravenous

- Ceftriaxone (Rocephin) 1 g IV/IM every 24 hours
- Cefepime (Maxipime) 1–2 g IV every 8–12 hours
- Piperacillin-tazobactam 3.375 g IV every 6 hours
- Ertapenem (Invanz) 1 g IV every 24 hours
- Meropenem (Merrem)[1] 1 g IV every 8 hours
- Gentamicin 5 mg/kg of body weight IV every 24 hours

Switch to appropriate oral regimen once symptoms improve based on culture and susceptibility results. Total duration of therapy ranges from 5 to 14 days depending on clinical response and oral antibiotic chosen.

is initially managed with antibiotics, glycemic control, and percutaneous drainage, and some cases may require partial or total nephrectomy. Severe pyelonephritis can lead to septic shock and death. Treating these complications may involve consultations with urology, nephrology, interventional radiology, surgery, and critical care.

Prevention

At this time, there are no specific preventive measures for pyelonephritis above those for prevention of recurrent cystitis. Of note, long-term studies of antimicrobial prophylaxis demonstrated that breakthrough urinary tract infections were resistant to the prophylactic antibiotic utilized, which should inform treatment of pyelonephritis in this setting. In pregnant patients, treatment of asymptomatic bacteriuria significantly lowers the risk of pyelonephritis.

References

Choong FX, Antypas H, Richter-Dahlfors A: Integrated Pathophysiology of Pyelonephritis, *Microbiol Spectr* 3(5):1–15, 2015.
Johnson JR, Russo TA: Acute Pyelonephritis in Adults, *N Engl J Med* 378(1):48–59, 2018.
Kamei J, Yamamoto S: Complicated urinary tract infections with diabetes mellitus, *J Infect Chemother* 27(8):1131–1136, 2021.
Kolman KB: Cystitis and Pyelonephritis: Diagnosis, Treatment, and Prevention, *Prim Care* 46(2):191–202, 2019.
Kot B: Antibiotic Resistance Among Uropathogenic *Escherichia coli*, *Pol J Microbiol* 68(4):403–415, 2019.
Long B, Koyfman A: Best Clinical Practice: Blood Culture Utility in the Emergency Department, *J Emerg Med* 51(5):529–539, 2016.
Neumann I, Fernanda Rojas M, Moore P: Pyelonephritis in non-pregnant women, *Clin Evid* 14:2352–2357, 2005.
Schneeberger C, Holleman F, Geerlings SE: Febrile urinary tract infections: pyelonephritis and urosepsis, *Curr Opin Infect Dis* 29(1):80–85, 2016.

amoxicillin-clavulanate [Augmentin], cefdinir [Omnicef][1], and cefpodoxime [Vantin])[1] have inferior efficacy compared with the fluoroquinolones and TMP-SMX. Their use should be restricted to situations in which sensitivities are known and clear contraindications to fluoroquinolones and TMP-SMX exist.

Inpatient Management

Intravenous antibiotics should be administered promptly for hospitalized patients. Ceftriaxone (Rocephin) is an acceptable option for empiric coverage of uncomplicated pyelonephritis (see Table 2). Other antibiotics such as cefepime (Maxipime), piperacillin-tazobactam (Zosyn), a carbapenem, or an aminoglycoside can be considered if there are risk factors for ceftriaxone resistance or if there is worsening or no improvement after 24 to 48 hours of empiric therapy with ceftriaxone. Multidrug-resistant organisms need special consideration and may warrant consultation with infectious disease. Antibiotic therapy should be tailored based on urine culture and susceptibilities. If the patient is clinically improving, antibiotics can be switched from intravenous to oral administration if there is an acceptable oral option.

Complications

The treatment of pyelonephritis may be complicated by urinary tract obstruction, renal abscess, emphysematous pyelonephritis, renal failure, and septic shock. Obstruction usually requires drainage for source control, either percutaneous drainage, ureteral stent placement, or Foley catheter placement depending on the location. Urinary tract obstruction can be associated with significant renal failure. Renal abscess formation is often associated with obstruction and may also require drainage. Emphysematous pyelonephritis is a rare, life-threatening, gas-producing, necrotizing kidney infection often associated with diabetes (95% of cases). Emphysematous pyelonephritis

---

[1]Not FDA approved for this indication.

TRAUMA TO THE GENITOURINARY TRACT

Method of
Amelia Khoei, MD, MPH; and Yooni Blair, MD

The genitourinary tract is involved in about 10% of trauma cases. The kidney, followed by the bladder and urethra, are the most commonly involved genitourinary organs. In most cases, injury to the genitourinary tract is not isolated, and the initial evaluation of urologic injuries should consider the context of the patient's associated injuries and triage more pressing or life-threatening issues. Still, early involvement of the urologist is prudent to help plan further interventions. The spectrum of genitourinary injuries is widespread, and management can range from immediate repair to temporization with delayed reconstruction. The goal of a urologist in the trauma setting is to establish urinary drainage in order to optimize kidney function, minimize hemorrhage, and control urinary extravasation to reduce associated complications such as infection or ileus.

Renal Trauma

Renal injury occurs in 1% to 5% of all trauma cases. Blunt impact accounts for the majority of renal injuries (82% to 95%) and causes damage secondary to direct organ injury or disruption of the kidney from its attachments (e.g., renal hilum and ureteropelvic junction). Penetrating trauma most commonly is caused by stabbing or gunshot wounds. The damage from penetrating injury can be limited to the tract of the stab wound, or it can be more extensive secondary to necrosis from energy transfer and the blast effect of high-velocity bullets. The history is crucial in the diagnosis of renal injury and should include the mechanism of trauma as well as any preexisting kidney disease or condition that might contribute to worsening renal function. Hematuria has a very poor correlation with degree of injury because disruption of the ureteropelvic junction, arterial disruption or thrombosis, and other severe injuries can exist in a setting with no hematuria.

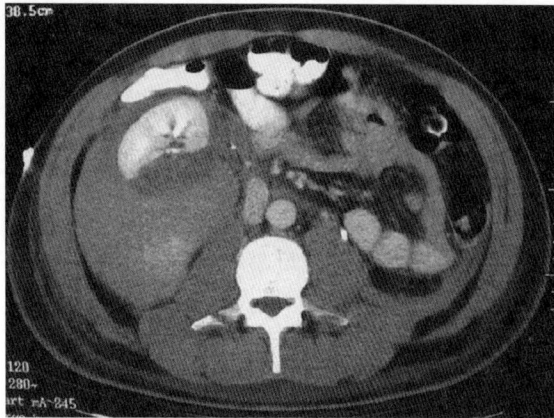

Figure 1 Computed tomography scan demonstrating large right perirenal hematoma and thrombosed posterior segmental artery. This was classified as a grade IV renal injury.

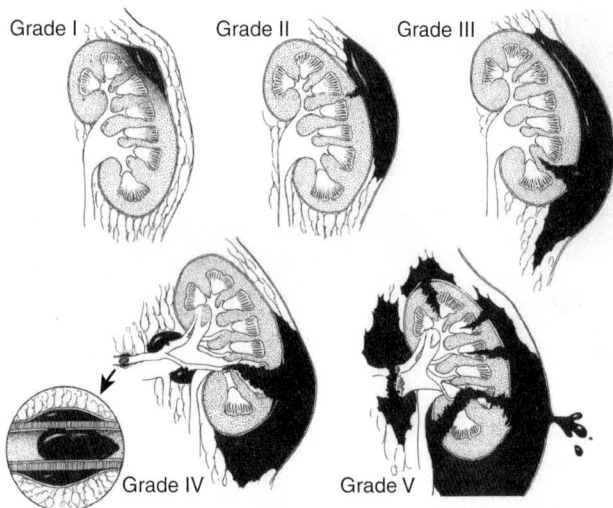

Figure 2 American Association for the Surgery of Trauma grading system for traumatic renal injuries: grade I, renal contusion and subcapsular hematoma; grade II, cortical laceration and perirenal hematoma; grade III, laceration into medulla or segmental renal artery thrombosis without a parenchymal injury; grade IV, laceration involving the collecting system, with or without a devascularized segment and contained vascular injury; grade V, renal artery thrombosis, avulsion of the renal pedicle, and shattered kidney. (From McAninch JW [ed]: Traumatic and Reconstructive Urology. Philadelphia, WB Saunders, 1996.)

The American Association for the Surgery of Trauma (AAST) classifies renal injuries into five grades (Figs. 1 and 2):

- Grade 1: Nonexpanding subcapsular hematoma/contusion with absence of parenchymal injury
- Grade 2: Less than 1 cm laceration into the renal cortex, not extending into the collecting system, with a nonexpanding hematoma confined to the perirenal fascia
- Grade 3: Greater than 1 cm laceration, extending through the renal cortex and medulla but not the collecting system
- Grade 4: Laceration extending to the collecting system with urinary extravasation or a segmental vascular injury with contained hematoma; renal artery thrombosis
- Grade 5: Shattered kidney or renal pedicle avulsion

With evolving imaging technology and endovascular management techniques, one group attempted to simplify injury severity grades 4 and 5 as follows:

- Grade 4: Parenchymal laceration involving the collecting system, lacerations of the collecting system with urinary extravasation, renal pelvis laceration and/or complete ureteral pelvic disruption; vascular segmental injuries

- Grade 5: Vascular compromise of the main renal arteries or veins such as laceration, avulsion, or thrombosis

Renal injury should be suspected in any trauma patient who has a penetrating injury with flank ecchymosis, broken ribs, gross or microscopic hematuria ($\geq$3 red blood cells per high-power field), a blunt injury with gross hematuria, or a blunt injury with microscopic hematuria and shock (systolic blood pressure <90 mm Hg). In addition, imaging of the urinary tract should be obtained in children who have more than 50 red blood cells per high-power field even in the absence of hypotension.

In a stable patient with concern for renal injury (e.g., rapid deceleration, flank ecchymosis, rib fracture), radiographic evaluation should consist of computed tomographic (CT) scanning with intravenous contrast and delayed images showing opacification of the collecting system and ureters (CT urogram). In the absence of CT imaging in a patient who is transported directly to the operating room for exploration, an intraoperative single-film intravenous pyelogram (IVP) can be performed to confirm that two functioning kidneys are present; however, the poor quality of the images makes IVP unreliable for staging purposes.

In contemporary renal trauma management, there have been increasing rates of conservative management (>80%, if not higher), resulting in decreased rates of nephrectomy. The factors that are most predictive of nephrectomy are grade of injury and penetrating injury.

Nonoperative management consists of supportive care with intravenous hydration, antibiotics, bedrest, and serial measurements of hemoglobin and hematocrit. Patients can ambulate after they are clinically stable, gross hematuria has resolved, and the hemoglobin and hematocrit have been relatively constant over 24 hours.

Kidney exploration is indicated for the patient who is hemodynamically unstable despite resuscitation in whom renal injury is thought to be the reason for life-threatening and persistent hemorrhage. If there are findings of large perirenal hematoma (>4 cm) and/or notable vascular contrast extravasation in the setting of a grade 3–5 injury and hemodynamic instability, intervention should be performed. Another absolute indication for renal exploration and revascularization is renal artery hilar avulsion or renal artery thrombosis when bilateral or in a solitary kidney. In patients undergoing exploratory laparotomy for associated injuries, renal exploration should be performed only in the presence of an expanding or pulsatile hematoma. Exploration of a nonexpanding, nonpulsatile hematoma is associated with a higher rate of nephrectomy and should be avoided. Almost all other injuries can be managed conservatively or with minimally invasive methods. Patients with bleeding specifically limited to segmental renal vessels and who are stable can be taken for angioembolization. This minimally invasive procedure is only appropriate at institutions with skilled and available interventional radiologists.

Routine early follow-up imaging for grades 1 to 3 blunt renal injury is unnecessary. Any imaging should be motivated by a change in the patient's clinical situation or laboratory values. However, follow-up imaging is indicated within 48 hours of initial injury for patients with grade 4 or 5 injuries. Imaging is also prudent if there is concern for worsening urinoma or hematoma that might require further intervention. Clinical signs such as worsening flank or abdominal pain, abdominal distension, fevers, and/or continued drop in blood counts can alert clinicians to such complications. Additionally, there should be periodic monitoring of blood pressure following renal trauma.

Ureteral Trauma

Trauma to the ureter is rare (1% of all genitourinary trauma). This is most likely because of its position in the retroperitoneum and bony pelvis protection, its relatively small caliber, and its mobility. The etiology of ureteric trauma is mostly iatrogenic occurring secondary to gynecologic, general surgery, and urologic procedures. Ureteral injury should be suspected in all cases of

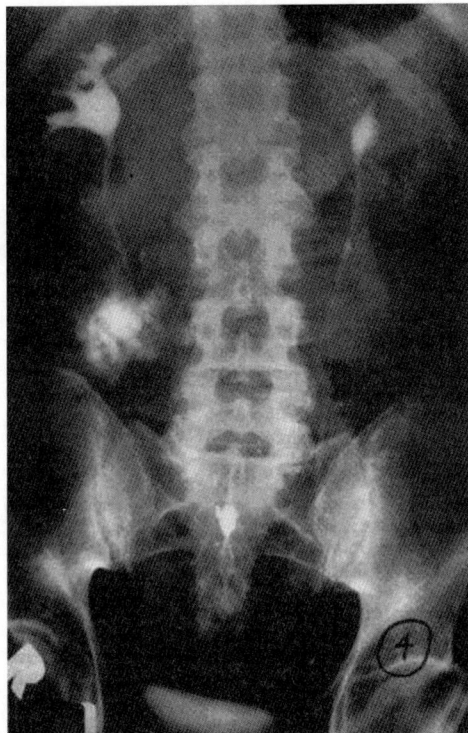

Figure 3 Intravenous pyelogram demonstrating extravasation of urine from right mid-ureter.

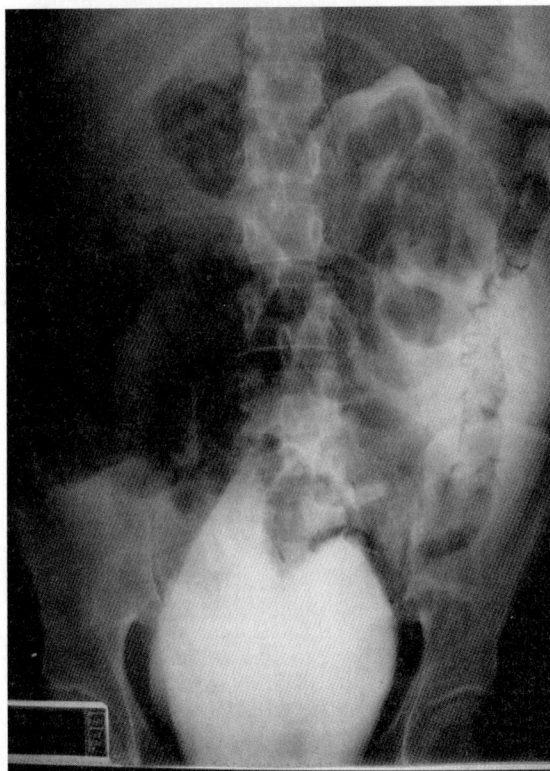

Figure 4 Intraperitoneal bladder rupture. Note contrast extravasating from the dome of the bladder and outlining the small intestine as well as the left colon.

penetrating trauma to the abdomen, especially with high-velocity projectiles, because of the blast effect.

The AAST has classified ureteric injuries into five grades of severity:

- Grade 1: Hematoma only
- Grade 2: Injury involving less than 50% of the circumference of the ureter
- Grade 3: Injury involving greater than or equal to 50% of the circumference of the ureter
- Grade 4: Complete transection with less than 2 cm of devascularization
- Grade 5: Complete transection with more than 2 cm of devascularization

The diagnosis usually is made intraoperatively if a high suspicion of ureteric injury is present or postoperatively by imaging obtained for investigation of fistula formation or clinical signs of upper tract obstruction. Hematuria is not a sensitive marker for ureteral injury; therefore, lack of hematuria does not portend a lack of ureteral injury. For non-iatrogenic injuries, imaging should be obtained in patients who experienced rapid deceleration or penetrating injuries to the flank. Imaging modalities used are usually intravenous pyelography, CT scanning with intravenous contrast and delayed images (CT Urogram), and retrograde pyelography. Findings indicative of ureteral injury include contrast extravasation, ureteral narrowing, and delayed peristalsis (Fig. 3). Alternatively, the ureters may be interrogated intraoperatively through direct inspection, injection of intravenous methylene blue[1], or by passing a ureteral catheter (if it passes easily, an injury is unlikely).

Grade 1 and 2 injuries can be managed initially by placement of a ureteral stent. If grade 2 or 3 injuries are identified immediately during exploration for a suspected ureteric injury, they can be managed by primary closure of the ureteric injury over an internal stent and placement of an abdominal drain as long as there is no associated thermal injury or necrosis. Grade 3 through 5 injuries usually require debridement of nonviable ends with re-anastomosis over an internal ureteral stent or more complicated surgical procedures involving mobilization of the

bladder and reimplantation of the ureter into the bladder. In an unstable patient, ureteral repair may be managed with temporary urinary drainage and a definitive repair in a delayed fashion. If internal ureteral stent placement is not possible, percutaneous nephrostomy tubes can be placed. An additional drain may be required if the urine leak is not contained by nephrostomy tubes alone. The type of ureteral repair depends on the amount of devitalized tissue and the location of the injury (proximal, mid, or distal ureter). Ureteroureterostomy, transureteroureterostomy, ureterocalicostomy, renal autotransplantation, ureteroneocystostomy with or without Boari flap or psoas hitch, and bowel interposition are all treatment options for various degrees of ureteral injuries.

Bladder Trauma

Blunt trauma accounts for 51% to 86% of bladder injuries resulting from external trauma, and approximately 70% (35% to 90%) of those patients have associated pelvic fractures. The most common cause of blunt trauma is motor vehicle crashes. Penetrating trauma accounts for 14% to 49% of traumatic bladder injuries. The incidence of iatrogenic injury varies by procedure but is highest for hysterectomy and other obstetric and gynecologic procedures. In cases of blunt trauma, injury should be suspected in patients who have pelvic fractures, suprapubic pain, inability to void, ileus or abdominal distention. In cases with iatrogenic injuries, urine in the field, visible laceration of the bladder, or gas distention of the urinary drainage bag in laparoscopic surgery warrants further investigation. Most importantly, clinicians must delineate whether a bladder injury is an intraperitoneal or extraperitoneal rupture (Figs. 4 and 5). Intraperitoneal rupture often occurs at the level of the bladder dome, where the muscular support is weakest.

The diagnostic test of choice is retrograde cystography, in which the bladder is filled with contrast to capacity (350 to 400 mL instilled by gravity). Passive filling of the bladder by clamping of the catheter is associated with unacceptably high rates of false-negative tests. With cystography, it is important to obtain scout

---

[1] Not FDA-approved for this indication.

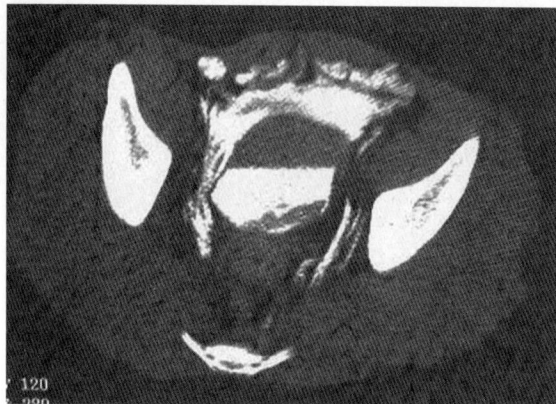

Figure 5 Extraperitoneal bladder rupture seen on computed tomographic cystogram.

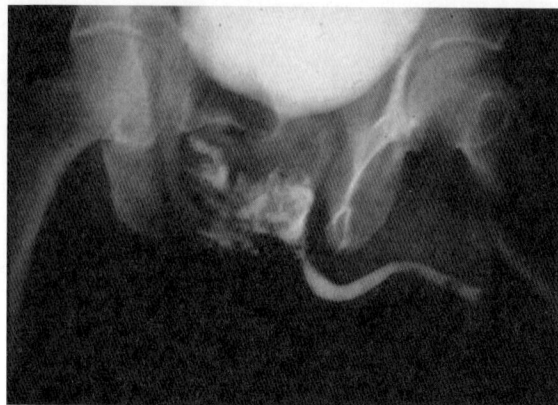

Figure 6 Retrograde urethrogram diagnostic of partial bulbar urethral transaction resulting from straddle injury.

imaging prior to fill and post-drainage films (if obtaining plain film cystography, may consider oblique views). Before placement of a foley catheter, retrograde urethrography should be performed if there is a suspicion of urethral injury

Most extraperitoneal bladder ruptures can be managed with Foley catheter drainage for 7 to 10 days. However, bladder neck involvement, concomitant vaginal or rectal injuries, presence of bone fragments in the bladder, or bladder wall entrapment necessitate surgical intervention. Intraperitoneal ruptures should be managed with surgical exploration because of the associated ileus and peritonitis caused by urine leak. It is recommended that penetrating bladder injuries are explored and repaired because of the risk of necrosis. Bladder repair is performed with a multiple-layer closure and catheter drainage for 7 to 10 days.

Urethral Trauma

Traumatic injury to the urethra occurs in 1.5% to 10% of patients who sustain a pelvic fracture. Female urethral injuries are very rare. The male urethra is anatomically divided into a posterior portion (prostatic and membranous urethra) and an anterior portion (bulbous urethra, penile/pendulous urethra, and fossa navicularis). Injury to the anterior urethra occurs mostly from blunt trauma, penetrating injuries, or instrumentation. Posterior urethral injuries are usually associated with pelvic fractures but can occur secondary to blunt, penetrating, or iatrogenic injury.

Classic signs of urethral injury include blood at the meatus, a high-riding prostate on rectal examination, inability to void, or perineal or scrotal ecchymosis. Imaging is indicated with any of these signs. The imaging study of choice is a retrograde urethrogram, and it should be performed before placement of a urethral catheter. In the absence of any signs, the diagnosis is most frequently made if retrograde urethrography is performed to investigate difficulty with urethral catheter placement (Fig. 6).

The AAST grading system does not distinguish between anterior or posterior injury but classifies urethral injuries as follows:

- Grade 1: Contusion and blood at the meatus with normal urethrogram
- Grade 2: Stretch injury with no extravasation of contrast
- Grade 3: Partial disruption with contrast extravasating at the injury site but still reaching the bladder
- Grade 4: Complete disruption with contrast not reaching the bladder; urethral defect of less than 2 cm
- Grade 5: Complete disruption with urethral defect greater than 2 cm or complex injury involving the bladder neck, prostate, rectum, or vagina

Grade 1 and 2 injuries can be managed conservatively by the placement of a urethral catheter. Management of grade 3 urethral injury should initially emphasize stabilization of the patient because extensive bleeding could be present in cases of severe injury to the pelvis. Placement of a catheter may be attempted even if there is a suspicion of partial urethral injury. If this is met

with difficulty, a suprapubic tube may be placed. Notably, suprapubic tubes may be placed in patients undergoing open reduction internal fixation procedures with orthopedic surgery.

In cases of complete disruption, prompt urinary drainage should be established by placement of a suprapubic tube catheter. This can help facilitate a primary realignment or repair with delayed urethroplasty. Primary realignment involves endoscopic passage of a guidewire across the defect and placement of a catheter over the guidewire. Immediate open repair is rarely indicated unless complex injury extends into the bladder neck, rectum, or vagina. Immediate exploration is recommended for anterior urethral injuries associated with penetrating trauma or penile fractures. Female urethral injuries are optimally treated at initial presentation to decrease the risk of incontinence. Physicians should continue to follow patients for at least 1 year, monitoring for complications such as incontinence, erectile dysfunction, and stricture formation.

Trauma to the External Genitalia

Injury to the scrotum is most frequently secondary to blunt trauma and can cause a hematoma, ecchymosis, or testicular injury. Scrotal swelling and patient discomfort can make separation of testicular injury from extratesticular scrotal trauma difficult on physical examination. In the case of blunt scrotal injuries, a scrotal ultrasound should be performed in most patients with suspicion of testicular rupture. A heterogeneous echo pattern in the testicular parenchyma on ultrasonography suggests testicular injury (Fig. 7). Visualization of a tear in the tunica albuginea is less accurate. Ultrasound studies with Doppler additionally provide information about any compromise in testicular blood flow. In the setting of penetrating scrotal injury, surgical exploration is recommended.

Scrotal exploration should be performed whenever testicular injury is suspected. If the tunica is ruptured and there is extrusion of seminiferous tubules, the extruded tubules should be debrided, hemorrhage controlled, and the tunica closed. Testicular salvage rates are highest when the scrotum is explored acutely compared to delayed exploration. Another possible indication for scrotal exploration is a large hematoma; evacuation of the hematoma can decrease the morbidity associated with protracted recovery and resolution of the hematoma and can occasionally identify a manageable source of bleeding. Scrotal exploration should also be performed in cases of inconclusive ultrasound findings or whenever the clinical suspicion for testicular injury is high.

Trauma to the penis can range in severity from a contusion to complete amputation. In cases of penile amputation, stabilization of the patient is important, and the need for transfusion should be addressed. Immediate microreimplantation is the management technique of choice if available. The severed penile segment should be immediately placed in a normal saline bag over ice to help preserve the fragment for reimplantation.

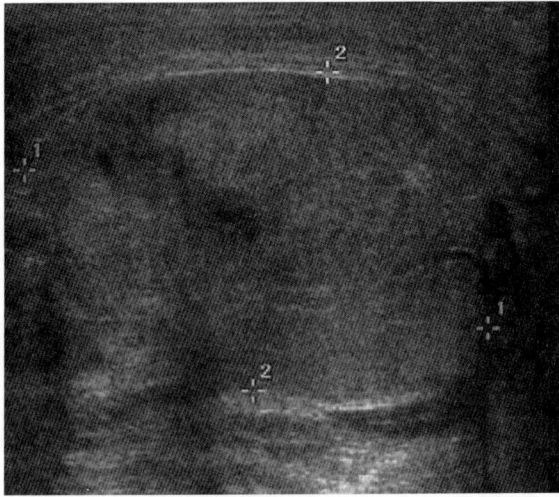

Figure 7 Testis ultrasound image demonstrating heterogeneous architecture characteristic of testicular rupture.

A penile fracture occurs after blunt injury to the erect penis rupturing the tunica albuginea. Such injuries are usually incurred during sexual intercourse and patients often report a "crack" or a "pop" followed by pain and detumescence. The hematoma is usually limited to the penis, unless the injury also involves Buck fascia, causing ecchymosis and bruising that involves the scrotum as well. Surgical exploration, closure of the fascial defect, and repair of any associated urethral injury should be done acutely. In cases of unclear history or physical examination, the provider may consider penile ultrasound or penile MRI for more conclusive evidence of a penile fracture. It is also important to rule out associated urethral injury, which occurs in 10% to 22% of the cases.

In females, blunt trauma to the vulva is rare. Injuries to genitalia can be associated with sexual assault and must be evaluated in that context. Consequently, vaginal smears should be taken, and the vagina should be thoroughly inspected under anesthesia with a speculum.

Trauma resulting in skin loss, such as burns, large abrasions, and avulsions, should be explored and debrided in an effort to stage the injury and decrease the risk of complications such as Fournier gangrene. Delayed reconstruction can be performed after stabilization and proper delineation of viable versus nonviable tissues. The reconstructive options include mobilization of local flaps or skin grafts.

Conclusion

Critical considerations when treating urogenital trauma include patient stability, mechanism of injury, and maintaining broad differentials for organ involvement. Appropriate imaging in the hemodynamically stable patient is crucial to avoid missing injuries that can risk severe complications such as uncontrolled bleeding, urine leaks, and infections. Guidelines have migrated towards more conservative treatments demonstrating success in select cases such as decreased nephrectomy rates and improved urethral healing without strictures. Early involvement of a urologist to guide proper workup and management can help optimize recovery outcomes.

References

Coccolini F, Cremonini C, Chiarugi M: Kidney and urotrauma. In: Cremonini C, Chiarugi M, eds: *Textbook of Emergency General Surgery*, Springer: Cham, Switzerland; 2023, pp 1461–1482.

Keihani S, Yizhe MS, Presson AP, et al: Contemporary management of high-grade renal trauma, *J Trauma Acute Care Surg* 84(3):418–425, 2018.

Kitrey ND, Campos-Juanatey F, Hallscheidt P, et al: *EAU Guidelines on Urological Trauma*. Presented at the EAU Annual Congress Milan March 2023. EAU Guidelines Office, Arnhem, the Netherlands.

Kozar RA, Crandall M, Shanmuganathan K, et al: Organ injury scaling 2018 update: spleen, liver, and kidney, *J Trauma Acute Care Surg* 85:1119–1122, 2018.

Lumen N, Kuehhas FE, Djakovic N, et al: Review of the current management of lower urinary tract injuries by the, *EAU Trauma Guidelines Panel* 67(5):925–929, 2015.

Matta R, Keihani S, Hebert K, et al: Proposed revision of the American Association for Surgery of Trauma Renal Organ Injury Scale: secondary analysis of the multi-institutional genitourinary trauma study. *J Trauma Acute Care Surg* 97(2):205-212.

McGeady JB, Breyer BN: Current epidemiology of genitourinary trauma, *Urol Clin North Am* 40(3):323–334, 2013.

Morey AF, Brandes S, Dugi DD, et al: Urotrauma: AUA guideline, *J Urol* 192(2):327–335, 2014.

Phonsombat S, Master VA, McAninch JW: Penetrating external genital trauma: A 30-year single institution experience, *J Urol* 180(1):192–195, 2008, discussion 195–196.

URETHRAL STRICTURE DISEASE

Method of
Hadley Wyre, MD; and Sable Shew, MD

CURRENT DIAGNOSIS

- Perform a thorough history and physical examination, delineating past trauma, instrumentation, and sexual history, as well as a complete genitourinary examination.
- Patients with urethral stricture will commonly present with obstructive symptoms of weak urinary stream, straining to urinate, and even frank urinary retention.
- In-office testing consists of urinalysis and urine culture for evaluation of infection, as well as uroflowmetry and postvoid residual bladder ultrasound to evaluate urine flow rate and emptying ability.
- Retrograde urethrogram remains the gold standard for diagnosis of urethral stricture disease.

CURRENT THERAPY

- In the acute setting of urinary retention, the ideal management would be placement of a suprapubic tube to avoid manipulation of the stricture; however, dilation and catheter placement may be appropriate or necessary in some patients.
- Depending on the patient, goals of care should be delineated regarding treatment of stricture disease; that is, definitive therapy versus chronic management of stricture symptoms.
- Endoscopic treatments are available and include urethral dilation and direct visualization internal urethrotomy; however, repeat attempts at these approaches have a low long-term success rate.
- Surgical management includes both anastomotic and augmentation urethroplasty—both of which are more invasive than endoscopic approaches but are known to have improved long-term patency rates.

Urethral stricture disease affects 0.6% of the male population and can be classified in multiple ways: anterior versus posterior, benign versus malignant, extrinsic versus intrinsic, and congenital versus acquired. The urethra is a conduit for urine from the bladder to outside of the body. In males, the anterior urethra (region encircled by corpus spongiosum) begins at the meatus and includes the fossa navicularis, penile urethra, and bulbar urethra—strictures here are the result of scarring of the urethral epithelium and surrounding spongy tissue, termed spongiofibrosis. As this scarring narrows the urethral lumen, symptoms become noticeable. Typically, the urethral lumen must narrow to less than 14 French for this scarring to be the cause of any voiding

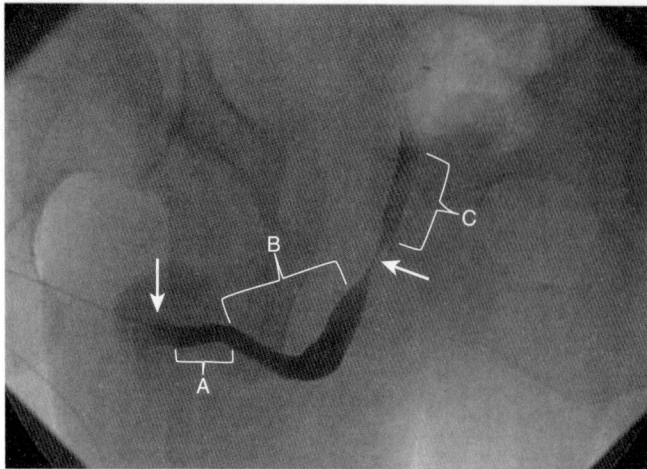

Figure 1 Anatomy of male urethra. (A) Penile urethra. (B) Bulbar urethra. (C) Prostatic urethra. White arrow by A=fossa navicularis; white arrow between B and C=membranous urethra.

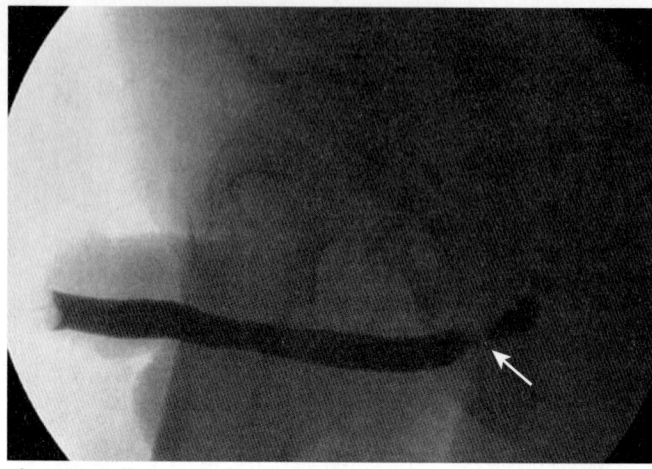

Figure 2 Bulbar urethral stricture visualized on retrograde urethrogram.

symptoms. Anterior urethral stricture can be secondary to iatrogenic injury, infections, penile/perineal trauma, pelvic fractures, and self-instrumentation. In the posterior urethra, including the membranous urethra, prostatic urethra, and bladder neck, narrowing is termed contracture or stenosis and is the result of a distraction injury sustained during pelvic trauma or prior surgical procedures of the prostate (Figure 1).

Diagnosis
Often patients with strictures will present with obstructive voiding symptoms including weak or intermittent stream, postvoid dribbling, straining to urinate, or overt urinary retention. Nonobstructive symptoms include postvoid fullness, urinary tract infections, and pelvic pain. A thorough history, including a detailed social/sexual history, and physical examination should be done, and any prior trauma to or instrumentation of the genitourinary tract noted. The physical examination should be comprehensive, with the genital examination examining for palpable strictures in the anterior urethra.

Laboratory workup should include urinalysis and urine culture for evaluation of infection, as well as a basic metabolic panel to evaluate for any renal function compromise. It is possible to perform an assessment of voiding symptoms in a clinic setting with the use of postvoid ultrasound and uroflowmetry. Once the patient has voided to completion, an ultrasound measurement of postvoid residual urine volume can objectively estimate the patient's ability to evacuate and alert the provider to overt retention. Uroflowmetry is the measurement of flow rate of urine—findings that suggest significant stricture include an elongated voiding time and a low maximal flow rate, essentially flattening the flow curve to a plateau appearance.

The gold standard in urethral stricture diagnosis remains the retrograde urethrogram. Radiocontrast is administered via catheter in a retrograde fashion, filling the urethra and opacifying it—this study is especially helpful for evaluating the length, location, and severity of strictures in the anterior urethra. Additionally, an antegrade study, or voiding cystourethrogram, can be performed to allow for visualization of the bladder neck, prostatic urethra, and membranous urethra. In addition to cystoscopic evaluation for direct visualization of the stricture, ultrasound of the penis/perineum can be used to further delineate characteristics of the stricture. Biopsy is occasionally performed to rule out malignancy as a cause of the stricture (Figure 2).

Acute Treatment
Acutely, the main complication from a urethral stricture is frank urinary retention, which may be associated with a decline in renal function. Typically a urethral catheter cannot be placed because of obstruction from the stricture. In the setting of overt urinary retention, a suprapubic tube is often placed at the bedside or in the operating room to allow for rapid decompression of the urinary system without manipulating the stricture. There are times where suprapubic tube placement may not be possible, and it is therefore reasonable to dilate the stricture and place a urethral catheter to drain the urine. However, manipulation of the stricture can lead to an increase in the length of the stricture and complexity of the eventual repair.

Long-Term Treatment
Multiple modalities exist for the treatment of urethral stricture disease, with varying success rates and complication rates. A thorough discussion between the patient and provider, considering the patient's goals for either cure or symptom management, life expectancy, and stricture qualities, is vital to ensuring that an appropriate care plan is developed. Prior to proceeding with any treatment, it is essential to evaluate the urethra proximal to and distal to the stricture with the modalities mentioned earlier; this is to ensure removal of all affected tissue and prevent recurrence.

Conservative management with urethral dilation is appropriate as a first attempt at treatment of a short stricture with minimal spongiofibrosis, with the ultimate goal of stretching rather than tearing tissue to open the lumen without increasing the scarring present. Direct visualization internal urethrotomy (DVIU) is opening of a stricture—by laser, cold knife, or hot knife—to release the scar and allow the urethra to heal at a larger diameter over a catheter. Long-term success rates for DVIU have been reported at 20% to 30% for short strictures with minimal spongiofibrosis. It is important to note that the success rate of repeat DVIU is close to 0%, and after failure, the patient should be referred for definitive surgical repair.

Surgical management includes operations to excise the scar and perform urethral anastomosis, and tissue transfer reconstruction with harvesting of distant tissue—typically oral mucosa—for urethral augmentation. Anastomotic urethroplasty is best for short strictures, 1 to 2 cm in length, while augmentation urethroplasty can be utilized for much longer defects. For any type of urethral reconstruction, restricture is the most common complication, as well as sexual dysfunction and ejaculatory dysfunction. Other treatment options include long-term suprapubic tube drainage, perineal urethrostomy, and urinary diversion, depending on each patient's individual case and discussion with the patient's surgeon. Regardless of modality, clinicians should monitor patients for symptomatic recurrence of strictures.

References
Albers P, Fichtner J, Bruhl P, et al: Long-term results of internal urethrotomy, *J Urol* 156:1611–1614, 1996.
Andrich DE, Mundy AR: The nature of urethral injury in cases of pelvic fracture urethral trauma, *J Urol* 165:1492–1495, 2001.

Bhargava S, Chapple CR, Bullock AJ, et al: Tissue-engineered buccal mucosa for substitution urethroplasty, *BJU Int* 93:807–811, 2004.

Fichtner J, Filipas D, Fisch M, et al: Long-term outcome of ventral buccal mucosa onlay graft urethroplasty for urethral stricture repair, *Urology* 64:648–650, 2004.

Hudak SJ, Atkinson TH, Morey AF: Repeat transurethral manipulation of bulbar urethral strictures is associated with increased stricture complexity and prolonged disease duration, *J Urol* 187(5):1691–1695, 2012.

Kellner DS, Fracchia JA, Armenakas NA: Ventral onlay buccal mucosal grafts for anterior urethral stricture: Long-term followup, *J Urol* 171:726–729, 2004.

McCallum RW, Colapinto V: The role of urethrography in urethral disease. Part I. Accurate radiological localization of the membranous urethra and distal sphincters in normal male subjects, *J Urol* 122:607–611, 1979.

McCammon KA, Zuckerman JM, Gerald HJ: Surgery of the penis and urethra. In Wein A, et al: 11th ed, Campbell-Walsh UrologyPhiladelphia, 2016, Elsevier, pp 907–945.

Rosen MA, Nash PA, Bruce JE, et al: The actuarial success rate of surgical treatment of urethral strictures, *J Urol* 151:370, 1994.

URINARY INCONTINENCE

Method of
Simon Patton, MD; and Renee M. Bassaly, DO

CURRENT DIAGNOSIS

- Urinary incontinence is broadly categorized as stress urinary incontinence or urgency urinary incontinence.
- The diagnosis can often be determined by a careful history and physical examination but can be aided with noninvasive methods such as a bladder diary.
- It is important to rule out any other potential causes of incontinence including urinary tract infection, urinary retention, or medication side effect.

CURRENT THERAPY

- Modest weight loss has been shown to help both forms of incontinence and is an important first-line therapy.
- Urgency urinary incontinence can initially be managed with lifestyle modifications including timed voiding and avoidance of bladder irritants, as well as physical therapy. Further options include medications (anticholinergics or B$_3$ agonists).
- Third-line therapy for urgency urinary incontinence includes sacral neuromodulation, botulinum toxin injections, and tibial nerve stimulation.
- Stress urinary incontinence can be managed conservatively with home Kegel exercises or formal pelvic floor training with physical therapy. Mechanical urethral support using a disposable tampon-like device or incontinence pessary is another non-invasive option.
- Surgical management of stress urinary incontinence is midurethral slings, principally using synthetic mesh.

Epidemiology

Urinary incontinence is a very common problem particularly in the female population, with incidence roughly twice that of male patients (30% vs. 17%). The exact incidence may be difficult to know, however, because this is a sensitive subject that patients may not volunteer unless solicited. The annual cost of treating incontinence is estimated to be $24 billion, and annually 260,000 women undergo surgery for stress incontinence.

Risk Factors

Risk factors vary between genders. Women are at greater risk due to anatomic differences, principally a shorter urethral length. Other risk factors include increased age, parity, obesity, diabetes, smoking, and pelvic radiation. In male patients a history of prostate surgery or an enlarged prostate are potential risk factors. Urinary tract symptoms including incontinence may represent manifestations of neurologic disorders including history of stroke, multiple sclerosis, or spinal cord injury.

Pathophysiology

The bladder consists of a smooth muscular reservoir (the detrusor muscle), two inlets (the ureters), and an outlet (the urethra). Urine from the kidneys enters the bladder via the ureters and exits via the urethra, which is itself a muscular tube consisting of smooth and striated muscle. Bladder function has two phases: storage and emptying. During the storage phase, the bladder collects urine; this phase involves relaxation of the detrusor muscle and contraction of the urethral muscle, all of which is under sympathetic and voluntary control. The emptying phase involves relaxation of the urethral muscles and contraction of the detrusor, which is mediated by the parasympathetic system. Under normal circumstances, emptying is voluntarily initiated in the adult.

In women, the bladder and urethra are supported by the anterior vaginal wall, which, in turn, is suspended by connective tissue attachments from the pelvic floor muscles. Continence is maintained when the urethral closure pressure exceeds the detrusor pressure. Adequate support from the anterior vaginal wall is required to maintain this relationship during periods of increased intraabdominal pressure. Consequently, urinary continence depends on the relative relaxation of the detrusor, the contraction of urethral muscles, and the support of the anterior vaginal wall. Incontinence can ensue when these relationships are disrupted.

Prevention

The pelvic floor musculature plays an important role in the maintenance of continence, and as such, pelvic floor physical therapy directed at these muscles has been shown to improve continence in both postmenopausal women and younger postpartum women, at least in the short term. Physical therapy in the male population has not been studied as a prevention strategy. One modifiable risk factor for incontinence is obesity, and even a modest weight loss of 10% has been shown to help improve continence status.

Clinical Manifestation

Urinary incontinence can be a sign, symptom, as well as a diagnosis. Urinary incontinence falls into two broad categories: stress incontinence and urge incontinence. Stress urinary incontinence occurs when urethral closure pressure cannot increase sufficiently to compensate for a sudden increase in intraabdominal pressure, as from laugh, cough, or Valsalva maneuver. Urgency urinary incontinence occurs when an unintended bladder contraction creates an insuppressible urge to void, leading to urinary leakage. When patients have signs or symptoms of both stress and urge incontinence, it is referred to as *mixed urinary incontinence*.

Diagnosis

Diagnosis rests principally on a careful history and physical examination. A thorough history is important to solicit what causes a patient to leak. Leakage with laughing, coughing, sneezing, exercise, or similar exertion would likely be stress urinary incontinence. Leakage associated with an urge that is difficult to defer is likely urgency urinary incontinence. If patients have both symptoms, then they likely have mixed urinary incontinence. If a patient complains of symptoms of mixed incontinence, a careful history to determine which is most bothersome is important. If the patient has difficulty knowing what has caused their leakage, a 3-day bladder diary recording liquid consumed, times and amounts voided, and leakage events with associated symptoms can help with diagnosis and treatment.

Other pertinent components to a thorough history include surgery to the spinal cord, bladder neck, or pelvic floor, which may lead to obstruction; neurologic disease (e.g., multiple sclerosis or a spinal cord lesion); or psychiatric disease (e.g., dementia, which may limit the ability to recognize a need to void). Musculoskeletal function, with emphasis on mobility, should be reviewed. A detailed medication history will identify any medications that may affect urine output or bladder function. It is important to also elicit any other symptoms that may coexist with incontinence and signal pelvic floor dysfunction, including nocturia, fecal incontinence, or constipation.

After a thorough history, a detailed physical examination is necessary. A focused genitourinary examination includes inspection of the external genitalia. Eliciting reflexes from the S2-S4 nerve roots will help determine whether there is any neurologic component. In female patients, perform a pelvic examination and look for any prolapse or pelvic masses and note whether any atrophy is present. Palpation of the urethra allows for evaluation of any urethral masses or possible diverticula. Lastly, assessment of pelvic floor musculature is important, evaluating for any pain or discomfort in the levator ani muscles and assessing the patient's ability to perform a proper Kegel exercise. In males, performance of a digital rectal examination is recommended to evaluate for any prostatic masses or hypertrophy.

The physical examination provides an opportunity for diagnosis as well; asking the patient to cough or perform a Valsalva maneuver allows for the direct visualization of stress incontinence if present. Additionally, this provides an opportunity in female patients to evaluate for prolapse and assess urethral mobility. Historically, this was done by placing a cotton swab in the urethra to observe for hypermobility seen with >30 degrees of mobility on strain from baseline. However, because of patient discomfort, this test is not routinely performed. After completing the physical examination, one must perform a urinalysis to rule out any infectious etiology and at times perform a post-void residual (either with a bladder scan or with catheterization) to evaluate for any possible voiding dysfunction. If the patient has a more complex history because of prior urologic surgery, neurologic disease, or is difficult to diagnose on history and physical alone, then complex urodynamic testing may be indicated.

Differential Diagnosis

The differential diagnosis for urinary incontinence includes stress urinary incontinence, urgency urinary incontinence, and a mixture of the two as mentioned above. Other causes of undesired leakage of urine include overflow (due to urinary retention), functional (due to impaired mobility or mental capacity), as well as a fistula or diverticulum. A patient with a fistula most commonly presents with the complaint of constant persistent urinary leakage. In the industrialized world these generally form after genitourinary surgery, whereas in developing countries trauma from childbirth is the primary cause. A diverticulum may present with a painful anterior vaginal wall mass as well as irritative voiding symptoms such as urinary frequency, urgency, dysuria, and postvoid dribbling. Other causes of lower urinary tract symptoms such as urgency, frequency, and dysuria include urinary tract infection, uncontrolled diabetes, or urinary tract malignancy.

Therapy

Stress Urinary Incontinence

Nonsurgical options for treatment of stress urinary incontinence include strengthening of the pelvic musculature through Kegel exercises and mechanical support of the urethra. Kegel exercises may be performed by the patient at home, although some patients may have difficulty identifying the muscles to perform them properly. Formal training with a pelvic floor physical therapist can help the patients learn to identify the muscles (sometimes using biofeedback devices) and contract them appropriately. Proper contraction of the levator ani muscles provides improved support for the bladder and urethra and helps decrease leakage.

Mechanical support of the urethra and bladder neck can be accomplished using an incontinence pessary or a disposable incontinence tampon. Pessaries are ring-shaped silicone devices with a knob that is meant to sit under the urethra. Patients are fitted for the correct size in the office. Patients must be followed up for at 3 to 6 month intervals to ensure the pessary has not caused any erosions or excoriations. This can be avoided by teaching patients how to insert and remove the pessary themselves or prescribing a vaginal estrogen cream in postmenopausal patients. A disposable option is available over the counter as well. It comes in three sizes, and the patients can fit themselves at home with the starter pack. Once they find the correct size, it can be placed when the patient desires and may be kept in place for up to 8 hours. Some patients choose this option if they only have stress incontinence during certain times (i.e., exercise).

If conservative therapies do not adequately address their complaints, surgical options are available. The general principle of restoring support to the urethra is the same as in conservative therapies. This can be accomplished by placing a sling under the urethra. The sling material can be lightweight polypropylene mesh or fascia (either autologous or cadaveric). The most commonly used type is the synthetic mesh and it is placed either retropubically or through the obturator membrane. Both methods have been shown to have a high rate of satisfaction with a low complication rate.

Stress incontinence in men is much less common but can also be treated with slings placed at the bulbar urethra. Artificial urinary sphincters can also be implanted that compress the urethra and can be controlled by the patient.

Urgency Urinary Incontinence

Lifestyle modifications are a good first-line therapy for patients with urgency urinary incontinence. Drinking an appropriate amount of fluids and avoiding foods and beverages that are known to irritate the bladder can provide significant relief. Additionally, performing timed voiding can help retrain the bladder. Formal training with a pelvic floor physical therapist has also been shown to significantly decrease incontinence episodes. It is important to note, however, that just performing Kegel exercises is often not adequate in these patients and can in fact worsen their symptoms if they already have tightly held, nonrelaxing pelvic floor musculature.

Pharmacologic therapy consists of anticholinergic medications or beta 3 agonists. Anticholinergic medications target the muscarinic receptors on the bladder; however, they are not specific and can cause significant dry mouth, dry eyes, and constipation, side effects that lead to a high discontinuation rate. Patients are unable to take this class of medication if they have closed-angle glaucoma. Additionally, there have recently been some concerns raised about long-term use leading to cognitive decline. The beta 3 agonists also work to slow down detrusor contractions but do so by targeting a different receptor. They have been shown to raise blood pressure and so are precluded in patients with uncontrolled severe hypertension; all patients should routinely check their blood pressure after starting one of these medications.

Third-line therapies for urgency urinary incontinence include sacral neuromodulation, tibial nerve stimulation, and intradetrusor injection of botulinum toxin A. Sacral neuromodulation has been approved by the Food and Drug Administration for this indication, as well as fecal incontinence and voiding dysfunction. It consists of a lead placed in the S3 foramen and connected to a pacemaker-like device that is implanted in the adipose of the buttocks. Patients are then able to control some of the settings (including program and amplitude) from an external device. The sacral nerve roots can also be stimulated via the tibial nerve. Treatments involve a small, acupuncture-sized needle placed in the tibial nerve followed by 30 minutes of stimulation. These are carried out at weekly treatments for 12 weeks followed by monthly maintenance therapy. Botulinum toxin A, a neurotoxin that works by decreasing the presynaptic release of acetylcholine, can be injected directly into the detrusor muscle. A risk of this treatment is urinary retention, which requires that patients be able to perform self-catheterization.

Mixed Urinary Incontinence

If a patient presents with components of both stress and urgency, eliciting first which symptom is the most bothersome allows for appropriate tailoring of treatment. It is important to remind patients that even a modest weight loss of 10% can help reduce bothersome urinary symptoms by up to 60%. As noted above, physical therapy can help address both type of incontinence as a valuable first-line therapy.

Overflow Incontinence

If a patient is diagnosed with overflow incontinence, then management is directed at maintaining an empty bladder through self-catheterization. In male patients, if the retention is due to prostatic hypertrophy, then pharmacologic therapy with α-agonists or 5α reductase inhibitors may be warranted. If medication fails to improve their symptoms, then surgical treatment with ablation (microwave or radiofrequency) or resection is indicated.

Complications

Urinary incontinence can cause significant morbidity in terms of financial as well as psychological burdens on patients. In addition to causing rashes and skin breakdown, incontinence also leads to depression, isolation, anxiety, depression, and increased risk of falls. Incontinence is one of the leading causes of institutionalization in the elderly. As the population ages, the incidence of incontinence will continue to increase, making its diagnosis and treatment increasingly important.

References

Abrams P, Cardozo L, Fall M, et al: The standardisation of terminology of lower urinary tract function: report from the Standardisation Sub-committee of the International Continence Society, *Neurourol Urodyn* 21:167–178, 2002.

AUGS: Consensus Statement: Association of Anticholinergic Medication Use and Cognition in Women With Overactive Bladder, *Female Pelvic Med Reconstr Surg* 23:177–178, 2017.

Hay-Smith EJ, Herderschee R, Dumoulin C, Herbison GP: Comparisons of approaches to pelvic floor muscle training for urinary incontinence in women, *Cochrane Database Syst Rev*, 2011;12: CD009508.

Hersh L, Salzman B: Clinical management of urinary incontinence in women, *Am Fam Physician* 87:634–640, 2013, Review. Erratum in: Am Fam Physician 2013;88:427.

Hu TW, Wagner TH, Bentkover JD, et al: Costs of urinary incontinence and overactive bladder in the United States: a comparative study, *Urology* 63:461–465, 2004.

16 Men's Health

BENIGN PROSTATIC HYPERPLASIA

Method of
Judd W. Moul, MD; and Chad M. Gridley, MD

CURRENT DIAGNOSIS

- Benign prostatic hyperplasia (BPH) is an extremely common condition in aging men, characterized by prostate gland growth that can obstruct the flow of urine and cause urinary symptoms.
- Diagnosis of BPH is usually based on symptoms of weak urine stream, hesitancy, intermittent stream, nocturia, and dribbling. These symptoms are generally called *lower urinary tract symptoms* (LUTS).
- Additional diagnostic aids include digital rectal examination (DRE), urinary flow rates and post void residual (PVR) measurements, PSA blood test, cystoscopy, and sometimes urodynamic testing.

CURRENT THERAPY

- Medical therapies include α-blocker agents (most commonly tamsulosin [Flomax]) and 5α-reductase inhibitors (finasteride [Proscar] or dutasteride [Avodart]), sometimes used individually or together.
- Surgical therapy includes transurethral resection of the prostate (TURP), photoselective vaporization of prostate (PVP), laser enucleation, and open or robotic simple prostatectomy.
- More recent minimally invasive surgical approaches include UroLift, REZUM, iTind, and prostate artery embolization (PAE).
- Therapy is individualized based on degree of urinary symptoms, patient bother, side effect profile, and the size of the prostate.

Benign prostatic hyperplasia (BPH) is a disease process characterized by the increased growth of the number of prostatic cells within the prostate gland, which sits at the base of the bladder and surrounds and fuses with the urethra. These glandular changes may result in changes in urinary flow, collectively known as lower urinary tract symptoms (LUTS). The presence of LUTS, such as weak stream, increased frequency, and urgency of urination, nocturia, and the feeling of incomplete bladder emptying occurring secondary to prostate enlargement, are more accurately characterized as benign prostatic obstruction (BPO); however, most clinicians routinely and acceptably apply the BPH diagnosis. Although many other disease processes (congestive heart failure, poorly controlled diabetes, renal failure, and many others) can contribute to LUTS in males, BPH is a leading contributor to urinary dysfunction in older males and is known to significantly affect quality of life.

Epidemiology

BPH is generally considered a disease of the aging male, with associated symptoms uncommon before the age of 40 years. By ages 60 years and 85 years, the histologic prevalence of BPH at autopsy is 50% and 90%, respectively. Likewise, the associated LUTS increase with age. At age 70 years, about 40% of men report LUTS; by age 75 years, the incidence of LUTS increases to 50%.

Pathophysiology

Although BPH is common, we know very little about its true pathophysiology. Current thought attributes BPH to an "awakening" of senescent epithelial and smooth muscle cells of the prostatic transition zone. Before the 1980s, BPH was generally thought of as a static condition of a gradually growing prostate gland causing progressive bladder outlet obstruction, following the "donut hole" analogy that the prostate is like a donut surrounding the bladder neck and outlet. With aging and prostate growth, the donut hole gets smaller, causing progressive obstruction. In the era when surgical treatment via transurethral resection of the prostate (TURP) was the only effective treatment, this simple static explanation was sufficient. We now know that BPH has both a static obstructive and a dynamic component under neural control. In addition, the contribution of the bladder to LUTS has been well recognized as a key contributor to the dynamic component of BPH and LUTS.

Specifically, the static growth and proliferation of the periurethral tissue in BPH is thought to be driven by androgens, as men castrated before puberty do not develop BPH. Testosterone, the main male hormone, is converted to the more active metabolite dihydrotestosterone (DHT) by the enzyme 5α-reductase in the prostatic stromal and epithelial cells. 5α-Reductase occurs in two forms, types 1 and 2. However, only type 2 is present in the prostate and genitalia. This is critical for understanding one of the two main classes of medical therapy for BPH—the 5α-reductase inhibitors (5-ARIs), medications that block the conversion of testosterone to DHT.

The dynamic component of BPH and LUTS is attributed to autonomic input to the smooth muscles in the lower urinary tract, including the bladder, prostate, and urethra. These areas have a large concentration of α_1-adrenergic receptors that, when stimulated, cause increased smooth muscle tone. This physiology then leads to increased urethral resistance and contributes to the obstructive symptoms of BPH, leading to the basis for the other main class of drugs to treat BPH—the α_1-adrenergic blockers.

Symptoms

LUTS include urinary frequency, decreased force and caliber of the urinary stream, hesitancy, straining to void, urgency, and nocturia. The degree of impact may range from minimal "bother" to frank urinary retention with renal failure. Most urologists now use a standardized self-administered questionnaire, such as the International Prostate Symptom Score (IPSS) (Figure 1), designed to elicit symptoms and bother in a typical male population with suboptimal health-seeking behavior.

It is now very common for men to be referred to urology for a collection of age-related issues including elevated prostate-specific

International Prostate Symptom Score (I-PSS)

Patient Name: _____ Date of birth: _____ Date completed _____

In the past month:	Not at all	Less than 1 in 5 times	Less than half the time	About half the time	More than half the time	Almost always	Your score
1. Incomplete emptying How often have you had the sensation of not emptying your bladder?	0	1	2	3	4	5	
2. Frequency How often have you had to urinate less than every two hours?	0	1	2	3	4	5	
3. Intermittency How often have you found you stopped and started again several times when you urinated?	0	1	2	3	4	5	
4. Urgency How often have you found it difficult to postpone urination?	0	1	2	3	4	5	
5. Weak stream How often have you had a weak urinary stream?	0	1	2	3	4	5	
6. Straining How often have you had to strain to start urination?	0	1	2	3	4	5	
	None	1 Time	2 Times	3 Times	4 Times	5 Times	
7. Nocturia How many times did you typically get up at night to urinate?	0	1	2	3	4	5	
Total I-PSS score							

Score 1–7: *Mild* 8–19: *Moderate* 20–35: *Severe*

Quality of life due to urinary symptoms	Delighted	Pleased	Mostly satisfied	Mixed	Mostly dissatisfied	Unhappy	Terrible
If you were to spend the rest of your life with your urinary condition just the way it is now, how would you feel about that?	0	1	2	3	4	5	6

Figure 1 The International Prostate Symptom Score (IPSS) questionnaire. Available from the Urological Sciences Research Foundation at: http://www.usrf.org/questionnaires/AUA_SymptomScore.html. Accessed September 16, 2024.

antigen (PSA), LUTS, BPH, and erectile dysfunction (ED). Commonly, the PSA or ED brings the patient to the attention of the healthcare system for the first time in years and may be the first opportunity to influence men on healthy living and health maintenance as they enter their middle or older age. Recognizing this, all healthcare providers should keep this in mind and try to perform a broader men's health assessment while the patient is available.

Diagnosis

The diagnosis of BPH is generally made based on symptoms or the IPSS standardized questionnaire, self-administered by the patient, combined with a digital rectal examination, PSA blood test, urinalysis, and, in some cases, a transrectal ultrasound or cystoscopy. The differential diagnosis can include urinary tract infection (UTI), prostatitis, urinary stones in the lower urinary tract, urethral stricture disease, neurogenic or overactive bladder, prostate or bladder cancer, and even congestive heart failure.

Some common medications, such as over-the-counter cold medicines containing α-adrenergic agents, can exacerbate LUTS and can even put a man into acute urinary retention if he has underlying BPH.

A properly performed digital rectal examination is critical to master in the diagnosis of BPH. Because the posterior prostate gland is located adjacent to the rectum and about 3 to 5 cm internal to the anus, the experienced clinician can gain valuable information from this examination. We prefer the patient to bend over the examining table with toes pointed slightly inward, the knees bent slightly forward and the forehead and arms/elbows resting on the table. The examiner uses a liberally lubricated gloved index finger to palpate the posterior side of the prostate for size estimate and for any induration or nodularity that might indicate the presence of prostate cancer. In such a case, referral to a urologist would be mandatory.

The size of the prostate is measured either by estimating the weight in grams or the volume in cubic centimeters. Models have been developed to teach clinicians how to gauge size and consistency. In general, a normal-size prostate is 20 to 25 g (or cm^3) in middle-aged men. A size of 25 to 30, 30 to 50, and greater than 50 g (or cm^3) is a general guide to mild, moderate, and severe BPH, respectively. However, size does not necessarily correlate with symptoms, and both symptom score and size estimate should be reported. The size gauges the histologic condition and the symptoms indicate the LUTS and the bother index, which are both important for individualized treatment.

The laboratory assessment should include a urinalysis to rule out hematuria. Like an abnormal digital rectal examination, a urinalysis that shows persistent red blood cells should prompt referral to a urologist for cystoscopic and upper urinary tract assessment. A urinalysis suggesting UTI should be followed up with a urine culture. If the patient presents in acute or chronic urinary retention and especially if there is a high postvoid or post-catheter removal residual bladder volume, a serum creatinine and blood urea nitrogen should be obtained. Severe BPH sometimes causes hydronephrosis and renal insufficiency; rarely, it causes renal failure. In-office bladder ultrasound scanners are very useful to quickly assess residual urine.

Contemporary diagnosis of BPH involves obtaining a PSA result. The latest guidelines from the American Urological Association (AUA) (https://www.auanet.org) regarding the use of PSA testing are very helpful. Although the traditional upper limit of normal for PSA testing has been 4.0 ng/mL, recent guidelines are based more on changes in PSA levels over time, considering that most men with BPH will have prior PSA results. In the specific setting of using PSA to help manage BPH, the best data come from the Proscar Long-Term Efficacy and Safety Study (PLESS), where a PSA of 0 to 1.3 ng/mL, 1.4 to 3.2 ng/mL, and greater than 3.2 ng/mL was associated, respectively, with small, medium, and large prostate glands (assuming that prostate cancer has been ruled out) and predicted therapeutic response to finasteride (see later).

Treatment

Treatment of BPH is always individualized to the patient and involves evaluation of symptoms and bother along with objective findings from examination and laboratory results. Current treatments range from periodic monitoring with a surveillance-only approach to the treatment of extreme cases with open or robotic enucleation surgery.

Active Surveillance and Watchful Waiting

For many men, especially those with lower symptom scores and little bother, annual monitoring with digital rectal examination, PSA, urinalysis, and symptom assessment are all that is required. Many men are happy to be reassured that they do not have clinically significant prostate cancer and are glad to hear that no immediate treatment is necessary.

Complementary and Alternative Medicine

The use of complementary and alternative medicine supplements is very common, and physicians should ask patients about their use, just as they ask about prescription medications. There are now many "prostate" and "men's health" supplements containing a variety of chemicals, including zinc[1], saw palmetto[7], vitamin E[1], vitamin D[1], and selenium[7], among others. Aside from a few European clinical trials of saw palmetto, the use of supplements to help BPH is speculative. One challenge is quality assurance of dose and ingredients of these agents, which are not regulated by the U.S. Food and Drug Administration (FDA). Although it was not done to investigate BPH, the NIH-funded Selenium and Vitamin E Cancer Prevention Trial (SELECT) to determine whether vitamin E or selenium, or both, would prevent prostate cancer, is illustrative. Neither supplement had any

effect on prostate cancer (or BPH to our knowledge). With the lack of robust trial data for the plethora of supplements, the answer from evidence-based medicine is clear.

Medical Therapy
α-Blocker Medications

The use of oral α-adrenergic blocking agents to treat BPH has been commonplace since the 1980s. These agents are directed at the dynamic component of BPH and LUTS by relaxing the smooth muscle tissue in the bladder neck and prostate. In simple terms, they relax the bladder outlet, resulting in better urinary flow. Initial agents, such as prazosin (Minipress)[1], were not selective blockers and were also used to treat hypertension. Furthermore, these early agents were not long acting and had to be taken multiple times per day, which severely limited their practical clinical utility. The next generation in the class included doxazosin (Cardura) and terazosin (Hytrin), which were longer-acting agents dosed only once a day. However, they were not selective and also lowered blood pressure, so titration was necessary. The current, third-generation agents are selective blockers that treat BPH but do not lower blood pressure when used at recommended doses. The three in this class are tamsulosin (Flomax), alfuzosin (Uroxatral), and silodosin (Rapaflo).

In general, clinicians use α-blockers in men with smaller prostate glands (≤30–35 g or cm^3), in younger men, and in patients where rapid effect is needed. Side effects of this class can include headache, dizziness, asthenia, drowsiness, and retrograde ejaculation, with alfuzosin reported to have the lowest rate of retrograde ejaculation among these drugs. Silodosin is reported to have the lowest risk of affecting blood pressure, reducing the risk of dizziness. This is an important consideration when considering α-blockers for elderly patients at risk of falls. The α-blockers are also now frequently used to relieve the dysfunctional voiding, which is believed to contribute significantly to some cases of prostatitis.

5α-Reductase Inhibitors

The 5α-reductase inhibitors have been available since the early 1990s. Finasteride was the first agent in this class (5 mg/day) and is a type 2 inhibitor. Dutasteride (Avodart; 0.5 mg/day) is a type 1 and type 2 inhibitor that was approved in 2002. Both drugs prevent the conversion of testosterone to the more active metabolite DHT in the prostate. This inhibition results in involution of BPH tissue and prostatic shrinkage. On average, most men achieve a reduction of 20% to 40% in prostate size after at least 6 months of use. In general, these agents are most effective in men with prostate glands more than 30 g (or cm^3) in size. Both drugs are expected to result in lower PSA levels by about 50% after 6 months of use. It is critical to take this into account when a patient is being screened for prostate cancer. If the PSA level does not fall by about half and the patient has been compliant with medication, he should be referred for urologic evaluation. In following up on men taking finasteride or dutasteride, PSA is generally doubled in assessing risk for prostate cancer. However, the PSA velocity or doubling time and other prostate cancer screening tools are still valid as long as the effect on PSA is appreciated.

Two key clinical trials are important. The Medical Therapy of Prostate Symptoms (MTOPS) trial showed that the combination of an α-blocker (doxazosin) and a 5α-reductase inhibitor (finasteride) was more effective than either alone or than placebo in treating BPH and LUTS. The Prostate Cancer Prevention Trial (PCPT), in a large 7-year study, showed that finasteride lowered the rate of prostate cancer by 25% over placebo. The Reduction by Dutasteride of Prostate Cancer Events (REDUCE) trial confirmed the prostate chemoprevention benefit of this class of drugs, showing that dutasteride also lowered the rate of prostate cancer by 23% over placebo. In 2010, the FDA ruled that dutasteride would not be approved for prostate cancer prevention, citing safety concerns in this prevention setting. In 2013, the long-term follow-up of the PCPT showed that there was no excess mortality

[1] Not FDA approved for this indication.
[7] Available as dietary supplement.

associated with long-term finasteride use compared with placebo, proving the long-term safety of this therapy.

Urologists frequently use 5α-reductase inhibitors to treat chronic hematuria due to an enlarged prostate after exclusion of more worrisome etiologies such as renal or bladder cancer; they may also prescribe these agents before prostate surgeries or procedures for BPH to lessen surgical bleeding.

Minimally Invasive Procedures

In the past 35 years, a series of minimally invasive surgical therapies (MISTs) have appeared in practice with the goals of reducing prostatic obstruction while preserving sexual function with normal erections and ejaculation. Balloon dilation, transurethral microwave therapy (TUMT), and transurethral needle ablation (TUNA) have all fallen from favor due to lack of durable effect in improving LUTS. Two newer minimally invasive procedures have, however, shown durability in multiyear randomized clinical trials. The prostatic urethral lift procedure (UroLift) uses small, permanently implanted anchors placed cystoscopically that physically retract and compress the obstructing lobes of the prostate and can provide almost immediate improvement in flow rates and symptom scores. Alternatively, water vapor thermal therapy (Rezum) uses radiofrequency-generated water vapor (103°C) injected cystoscopically into the prostate tissue, resulting in gradual resorption of the treated tissue and significant improvements in flow rates and symptom scores over the course of weeks after the procedure. Both procedures carry the benefits of very low rates of ED and retrograde ejaculation; however, whether either procedure will provide long-lasting relief of LUTS, similar to more invasive surgical procedures remains unknown but will be discovered as long-term follow-up studies are completed. Prostatic artery embolization (PAE) has shown promise in several studies as a minimally invasive therapy for BPH; however, the AUA guidelines on BPH, which were amended in 2023, were unable to find substantial evidence to recommend this treatment over other minimally invasive BPH therapies. This is due to the challenging nature of the procedure, steep learning curve, and prolonged fluoroscopy times. Continued investigation was recommended by the panel. High-intensity focused ultrasound was granted FDA approval in 2015 for ablation of prostate tissue but has not gained wide use for BPH management and is more frequently used in the treatment of prostate cancer. The iTind (Temporary Implanted Nitinol Device) is another FDA-approved MIST for BPH that expands the prostatic opening. Several other MISTs are in development.

Surgical Therapy

TURP remains the gold standard treatment for men who have failed to improve on medical therapy, who dislike or are intolerant of medication side effects, or who have developed urinary retention, renal failure secondary to BPH, recurrent urinary tract infection, or large bladder calculi. TURP is associated with relatively low rates of incontinence and ED; however, retrograde ejaculation is an expected and permanent outcome for most men undergoing this surgery. Evolutions of the traditional TURP procedure now use saline irrigation, thereby reducing the risk of "TURP syndrome" (dilutional hyponatremia) during the procedure. Several laser technologies (Greenlight, Holmium, or Thulium) used for the enucleation or vaporization of prostate tissue have resulted in reduced hospital stays, transfusion rates, and duration of catheterization compared with TURP and are recommended treatment options for medically complex cases calling for anticoagulant therapy. Aquablation uses a transurethral water jet to ablate prostate tissue under ultrasound guidance. Recent research is also showing promise for the use of Aquablation in large prostates. Finally, for men with severe BPH and large (>80 g) or very large glands (>150 g), laser prostatectomy (enucleation using Holmium or Thulium) and simple prostatectomy performed robotically or via a small suprapubic incision are valuable and highly effective surgical treatments. As with radical prostatectomy used for the treatment of prostate cancer, laser and simple prostatectomy for BPH should be performed by urologic surgeons who are highly experienced in this area.

Summary

With the widespread acceptance of medical therapies for BPH in the 1980s and 1990s, treatment paradigms rapidly shifted away from surgical treatment for bothersome voiding symptoms. A growing number of studies have suggested an association between medical therapies for LUTS and the development of adverse effects including heart failure, psychiatric disorders, and dementia. These studies are controversial and preliminary; however, it is common in our practice to encounter elderly men who are using two or three medications for the management of symptoms. With increasing awareness of the risks of polypharmacy and with the advent of new minimally invasive, office-based procedures that continue to expand, the pendulum seems to be swinging back toward the earlier consideration of surgical treatment for BPH.

References

Barkin J: Benign prostatic hyperplasia and lower urinary tract symptoms: evidence and approaches for best case management, *Can J Urol*(Suppl 18)14–19, 2011.

Biester K, Skipka G, Jahn R, et al: Systematic review of surgical treatments for benign prostatic hyperplasia and presentation of an approach to investigate therapeutic equivalence (non-inferiority), *BJU Int* 109:722–730, 2012.

Dahm P, Brasure M, MacDonald R, et al: Comparative effectiveness of newer medications for lower urinary tract symptoms attributed to benign prostatic hyperplasia: a systemic review and meta-analysis, *Eur Urol* 71:570–581, 2017.

Djavan B, Kazzazi A, Bostanci Y: Revival of thermotherapy for benign prostatic hyperplasia, *Curr Opin Urol* 22:16–21, 2012.

Gravas S, Bachmann A, Reich O, et al: Critical review of lasers in benign prostatic hyperplasia (BPH), *BJU Int* 107:1030–1043, 2011.

Lepor H, Kazzazi A, Djavan B: α-Blockers for benign prostatic hyperplasia: the new era, *Curr Opin Urol* 22:7–15, 2012.

Nicholson TM, Ricke WA: Androgens and estrogens in benign prostatic hyperplasia: past, present and future, *Differentiation* 82:184–199, 2011.

Roehrborn C, Barkin J, Gange S, et al: Five year results of the prospective randomized controlled prostatic urethral L.I.F.T. study, *Can J Urol* 24(3):8802–8813, 2017.

Roehrborn C, Gange S, Gittelman M, et al: Convective thermal therapy: durable 2-year results of randomized controlled and prospective crossover studies for treatment of lower urinary tract symptoms due to benign prostatic hyperplasia, *J Urol* 197(6):1507–1516, 2017.

Sandhu JS, Bixler BR, Dahm P, et al. Management of lower urinary tract symptoms attributed to benign prostatic hyperplasia (BPH): AUA Guideline amendment 2023. *J Urol* 023;10.1097/JU.0000000000003698.

Slater S, Dumas C, Bubley G: Dutasteride for the treatment of prostate-related conditions, *Expert Opin Drug Saf* 11:325–330, 2012.

EPIDIDYMITIS AND ORCHITIS

Method of
Robin A. Walker, MD

CURRENT DIAGNOSIS

- Subacute or gradual onset of scrotal pain and swelling that occasionally radiates to the lower abdomen. Typically unilateral; however, inflammation can spread to the opposite testicle.
- Fever and urinary tract symptoms (e.g., dysuria, frequency, urgency, hematuria) may be present.
- The testicle should be in normal position with the cremasteric reflex intact (rule out torsion).
- Pain is relieved by elevation of the testicle (Prehn sign).
- Ultrasonography with Doppler is readily available and has high sensitivity and specificity for ruling out testicular torsion; however, referral to urology should not be delayed if torsion is suspected.
- Urinalysis should be obtained, preferably on a first-void urine specimen.
- Urine is sent for culture, especially when sexually transmitted disease (STD) is not suspected.
- Urine is the preferred specimen for nucleic acid amplification assays for *Gonorrhea* and *Chlamydia*.

- Acute epididymitis most likely caused by chlamydia or gonorrhea: ceftriaxone (Rocephin)[1] 500 mg IM once PLUS doxycycline (Vibramycin)[1] 100 mg twice daily for 10 days. Use 1 g of ceftriaxone if patient weights ≥150 kg.
- Acute epididymitis mostly likely caused by chlamydia, gonorrhea, or enteric organisms (men who practice insertive anal intercourse): ceftriaxone (Rocephin)[1] 500 mg IM once PLUS levofloxacin (Levaquin)[1] 500 mg once daily × 10 days. Use 1 g of ceftriaxone if patient weights ≥150 kg.
- Acute epididymitis most likely caused by enteric organisms alone: levofloxacin (Levaquin)[1] 500 mg once daily × 10 days
- Oral cephalosporins and fluoroquinolones are no longer recommended for gonococcal infections.
- Cultures, if obtained, should be followed and treatment adjusted accordingly.
- Patients should follow up in 2 to 3 days. Pain should improve in 1 to 3 days with treatment. Failure to improve should elicit reevaluation of the diagnosis and therapy, and consideration should be given to other causes such as a testicular tumor/cancer, abscess, infarction, and tuberculosis (TB) or fungal pathogens.
- Sexual partners should be referred for evaluation and treatment if there was intercourse in the preceding 60 days from onset of symptoms.
- Education should occur regarding prevention of STDs.

[1]Not FDA approved for this indication.

Epidemiology

Epididymitis is most common in males 18 to 35 years of age, but it can occur in all ages.

In men 35 years of age or younger who are sexually active, the most common pathogens are *Chlamydia trachomatis* and *Neisseria gonorrhoeae*. In those older than 35 years of age, the cause is most likely urinary tract pathogens such as *Escherichia coli*. In men who perform insertive anal intercourse, coliform bacteria are common causative agents. Other less common pathogens include TB, fungal infections, and viruses. Cytomegalovirus has been identified as a cause in HIV patients.

In boys 2 to 13 years of age, the incidence is approximately 1.2 per 1000 individuals and is most commonly a postinfectious inflammatory reaction to pathogens such as enteroviruses, adenoviruses, and mycoplasma pneumonia. If a bacterial pathogen is isolated, a urologic workup for any anatomic abnormalities is warranted.

Other uncommon noninfectious causes of epididymitis include vasculitides and medications such as amiodarone (Pacerone).

Orchitis is less common than epididymitis and is most often associated with concurrent epididymitis, occurring in approximately 60% of men with epididymitis. In prepubertal boys, orchitis is usually a sequela of mumps infection. Between 20% and 30% of men with mumps develop orchitis.

Risk Factors

The predominant risk factor for epididymitis is unprotected sexual intercourse. Additionally, trauma from strenuous physical activity, bicycle or motorcycle riding, and prolonged sitting can predispose to epididymitis. Risk factors in prepubertal boys and men older than 35 years of age are related to anatomic abnormalities (e.g., prostatic obstruction, posterior urethral valves, meatal stenosis), recent instrumentation, or urogenital tract surgery (e.g., vasectomy). In prepubertal boys, recent infections can predispose to a postinfectious inflammatory reaction in the epididymis.

Pathophysiology

Infective epididymitis is usually caused by retrograde ascent of pathogens, most commonly bacterial. Noninfectious epididymitis can be autoimmune or can be associated with known syndromes (e.g., Behçet disease) or a side effect of medications, most notably amiodarone (Pacerone). If symptoms last longer than 3 months, the patient meets the diagnostic criteria for chronic epididymitis.

Clinical Manifestations

The typical presentation is subacute onset of unilateral scrotal pain. Any acute onset of pain requires careful consideration of possible testicular torsion. The pain in epididymitis can radiate to the lower abdomen. Fever and urinary tract symptoms such as increased frequency, dysuria, and hematuria are frequently present. The cremasteric reflex is preserved and the testicle should be in its normal anatomic position. The epididymis is tender, swollen, and often indurated. Pain is relieved on testicular elevation (Prehn sign). Over time, scrotal wall erythema and a reactive hydrocele may appear, and infection can spread from the epididymis to the testicle (orchitis) as well as to the opposite testicle.

Epididymitis secondary to noninfectious causes tends to have a more gradual onset of symptoms.

Viral orchitis from mumps is characterized by abrupt onset of unilateral testicular pain with swelling that typically occurs 4 to 7 days after the development of parotitis. About 75% of patients with orchitis will also have fever, and one-third will complain of dysuria.

Diagnosis

Diagnosis can be made by a careful history and physical examination; however, laboratory testing can help confirm epididymitis.

All suspected cases should undergo point-of-care evaluation for urethral inflammation by one of three tests. (1) Gram, methylene blue, or gentian violet stain of urethral secretions demonstrating ≥2 white blood cells (WBCs) per oil immersion field; (2) positive leukocyte esterase on first-void urine; (3) Microscopic examination of sediment spun from first-void urine demonstrating ≥10 WBCs per high-power field. The presence of inflammation helps differentiate it from testicular torsion.

Nucleic acid amplification tests for *N. gonorrhoeae* and *C. trachomatis* should be run on all sexually active men, and urine is the preferred specimen. Gonococcal infection is established by the presence of WBCs containing intracellular gram-negative diplococci. Urine should be obtained for analysis and culture, preferably from a first-void sample. All men with acute epididymitis should be tested for HIV and syphilis.

Color Doppler ultrasonography is a readily availability study with a sensitivity and specificity for testicular torsion ranging between 89% and 100%. However, imaging should not delay immediate referral to a specialist if torsion is clinically suspected.

Differential Diagnosis

- Testicular torsion: duration less than 6 hours, absence of cremasteric reflex, diffuse testicular tenderness. Elevation of the testis usually exacerbates discomfort.
- Orchitis: testicular tenderness and swelling, normal cremasteric reflex.

Therapy/Treatment

In sexually active men 14 to 35 years of age, empiric treatment should be started for suspected epididymitis before laboratory results are available. The current recommended regimen is ceftriaxone (Rocephin)[1] 500 mg IM once plus doxycycline (Vibramycin)[1] 100 mg orally twice daily for 10 days. For sexually

[1]Not FDA approved for this indication.

active men who practice insertive anal intercourse, the recommended treatment is ceftriaxone (Rocephin)[1] 500 mg IM once plus levofloxacin (Levaquin)[1] 500 mg orally once daily for 10 days. The dose of ceftriaxone (Rocephin) should be increased to 1 g IM for patients who weigh ≥150 kg. The Centers for Disease Control and Prevention (CDC) no longer recommends fluoroquinolones or oral cephalosporins for the treatment of gonococcal infections.

When enteric pathogens alone are suspected, treatment consists of levofloxacin (Levaquin)[1] 500 mg orally for 10 days.

Most patients can be treated in the outpatient setting. Inpatient treatment is recommended for suspicion of abscess, intractable pain, signs of sepsis, or failure of outpatient care. Symptomatic care consists of pain control with supportive garments, nonsteroidal antiinflammatory drugs (NSAIDs), rest, and cold packs.

Men whose epididymitis was confirmed or suspected to be caused by gonorrhea or chlamydia should be instructed to refer all sexual partners over the previous 60 days from the onset of symptoms for evaluation and treatment. Patients and their partners should be advised to abstain from sexual intercourse until they have been treated and symptoms have resolved.

Orchitis, when not associated with epididymitis infection, is typically treated in a supportive manner with hot or cold packs, rest, NSAIDs, and scrotal elevation. Symptoms from viral associated orchitis typically resolve in 3 to 10 days.

Complications
Complications include sepsis, abscess, formation, extension of infection, and infertility.

References

Centers for Disease Control and Prevention: STI Treatment Guidelines 2021, Epididymitis. Available at https://www.cdc.gov/std/treatment-guidelines/epididymitis.htm [accessed 02.28.22].
Centers for Disease Control and Prevention: Update to CDC's sexually transmitted diseases treatment guidelines, 2010; oral cephalosporins no longer recommended treatment for gonococcal infections, *MMWR Morb Mortal Wkly Rep* 61:590–594, 2012.
Centers for Disease Control and Prevention: Update to CDC's sexually transmitted diseases treatment guidelines, 2006; fluoroquinolones no longer recommended for treatment of gonococcal infections, *MMWR Morb Mortal Wkly Rep* 56:332–336, 2007.
Kaver I, Matzkin H, Braf ZF: Epididymo-orchitis: a retrospective study of 121 patients, *J Fam Pract* 30:548–552, 1990.
Remer EM, Casalino DD, Arellano RS, et al: ACR appropriateness criteria; acute onset of scrotal pain—without trauma, without antecedent mass, *Ultrasound Q* 28:47–51, 2012.
Trojian TH, Lishnak TS, Meiman D: Epididymitis and orchitis: an overview, *Am Fam Physician* 79:583–587, 2009.

ERECTILE DYSFUNCTION

Method of
Aleksandr Belakovskiy, MD; Joel J. Heidelbaugh, MD; and Karl T. Rew, MD

CURRENT DIAGNOSIS

- Questionnaire
- Sexual Health Inventory for Men (SHIM) [also called International Index of Erectile Function (IIEF-5)] https://www.usrf.org/questionnaires/AUA_SymptomScore.html
- Assessment of risk factors
- Tobacco use
- Diabetes
- Hypertension
- Hyperlipidemia
- Obesity
- Iatrogenic causes
- Psychogenic causes
- Physical exam including vitals, body mass index (BMI), genital exam, and assessment for secondary sex characteristics
- Relationship between erectile dysfunction, endothelial dysfunction, and coronary heart disease

CURRENT THERAPY

- Lifestyle modifications including tobacco cessation, weight-loss, increased exercise
- Sexual health counseling
- Medication modification if taking medications known to contribute to erectile dysfunction
- Pharmacotherapy (Table 1)
- Oral phosphodiesterase type 5 (PDE-5) inhibitors: avanafil (Stendra), sildenafil (Viagra), tadalafil (Cialis), and vardenafil (Levitra, Staxyn)
- Prostaglandin: alprostadil; either by intracavernosal injection (Caverject, Edex) or as an intraurethral suppository (Muse)
- Requires a test dose in the office and instruction on technique for proper administration
- Vacuum erectile devices
- Penile implants

Erectile dysfunction is the inability to attain or maintain a penile erection sufficient for sexual satisfaction.

Epidemiology
Numerous studies have investigated the prevalence of erectile dysfunction in men of various ages. Based on the most recent studies, worldwide prevalence increases with age. For men under age 40 the prevalence is 1% to 10%; for ages 40 to 49 it is 2% to 15%; for men ages 50 to 59 it is mixed, ranging from 15% to 40%; for ages 60 to 69 it is 20% to 40%; and for men 70 and older it is 50% to 100%. Among men in the United States the prevalence is 22% overall. This is higher than the 16% prevalence for seven other countries found in a study comparing the United States to Brazil, Mexico, United Kingdom, Germany, France, Italy, and Spain. Accurate diagnosis of erectile dysfunction has varied over time, with current literature favoring the use of validated questionnaires such as the Sexual Health Inventory for Men (SHIM; https://www.baus.org.uk/_userfiles/pages/files/Patients/Leaflets/SHIM.pdf).

Risk Factors
A number of medical conditions can predispose to erectile dysfunction. Numerous studies have demonstrated the correlation between cardiovascular disease and the incidence of erectile dysfunction. Risk factors that predispose to cardiovascular disease also play similar roles in erectile dysfunction, including increasing age, diabetes, hypertension, hyperlipidemia, tobacco use, and obesity.

Certain classes of medications can contribute to the development of erectile dysfunction. One of the most common is the antidepressants, specifically selective serotonin reuptake inhibitors (SSRIs) and serotonin norepinephrine reuptake inhibitors (SNRIs). Common antihypertensive medications can also contribute to or exacerbate erectile dysfunction, including beta blockers, alpha blockers, calcium channel blockers, and thiazides. Other medication classes that should be considered in patients with erectile dysfunction include opiates, first-generation antihistamines, and benzodiazepines.

Risk factors for psychogenic erectile dysfunction should also be evaluated. Psychogenic erectile dysfunction can occur at any age, but it is frequently seen in men under age 40, and it often occurs in men with anxiety, stress, depression, or a history of sexual abuse. Assess for healthy sexual partnerships by asking about performance anxiety and sexual desire discrepancy, both of which are common contributors to erectile dysfunction. Clues that erectile dysfunction may have a psychogenic component include the ability to have normal erections with masturbation, and the continued presence of nocturnal erections. If needed for evaluation, nocturnal tumescence testing can be performed.

Tobacco, alcohol, opioids, and substances such as marijuana and cocaine can cause erectile dysfunction. All substance use should be assessed. Many other health issues can contribute to erectile dysfunction, including a history of prostate or pelvic surgery, radiation therapy, or trauma; gonadal, thyroid, or other diseases that affect hormone levels; testicular pain; and chronic diseases that affect general health and well-being.

Pathophysiology

The pathophysiology of erectile dysfunction depends on the etiology of the condition. Many men have multiple potential causes. Psychogenic erectile dysfunction is due to nonorganic causes, while individuals with risk factors for cardiovascular disease primarily have etiologies stemming from vascular disease. Iatrogenic erectile dysfunction due to medication use or prior surgery may be caused by inhibition of the parasympathetic nervous system or other mechanisms of action.

Erectile dysfunction can be a warning sign of silent cardiovascular disease. The relationship between erectile dysfunction and the risk factors for coronary heart disease was noted in the Massachusetts Male Aging Study. The endothelial dysfunction that can precede the clinical stage of atherosclerotic disease is recognized as an additional risk factor for erectile dysfunction in men without symptoms of cardiovascular disease. Endothelial function is mediated by nitric oxide, which is also the mechanism responsible for the vascular dilatation required to obtain and maintain an erection. A man with erectile dysfunction should be considered at risk for cardiovascular disease until proven otherwise.

Prevention

Erectile dysfunction prevention is centered around treating modifiable risk factors. Treatment of overweight and obesity with dietary changes and increased aerobic exercise can aid in the prevention of erectile dysfunction. For tobacco users, cessation should be strongly encouraged. Bupropion (Zyban) and varenicline (Chantix) can be used for smoking cessation with limited risk of exacerbating erectile dysfunction. Nicotine replacement therapy can be used as a bridge to help with tobacco cessation. Appropriate treatment of comorbid diseases, including diabetes, hypertension, and hyperlipidemia can also aid in prevention. Sexual health counseling that focuses on good partner communication and healthy relationship dynamics can help prevent psychogenic erectile dysfunction.

Clinical Manifestations

Many men are uncomfortable mentioning problems of sexual function. Some men will report erectile dysfunction without providing information on the specifics of their concern. It is important for physicians to proactively ask about sexual function, and to clarify if a patient's concern is with achieving or maintaining an erection, or if it may be related to ejaculation or low libido. Low libido can be secondary to stress, mood disorders, hypogonadism, or other causes. The evaluation and potential treatments will differ based on the specific concern. Questionnaires such as the SHIM (https://www.baus.org.uk/_userfiles/pages/files/Patients/Leaflets/SHIM.pdf) can provide additional information to help distinguish the specific clinical manifestation.

Diagnosis

The history provides the majority of information needed for the diagnostic evaluation, including a review of known medical and surgical history, use of medications and substances, an assessment of current relationship satisfaction, and a questionnaire such as the SHIM. The history should include risk factor evaluation, assessment for any history of cardiovascular disease, diabetes, hypertension, hyperlipidemia, or mood disorders, as well as a review of medications that might contribute to erectile dysfunction. A physical exam should also be performed, including evaluation of blood pressure, body mass index, secondary sex characteristics, and a genital exam.

The role of laboratory studies is limited. In individuals who lack secondary sex characteristics, as well as those with refractory symptoms despite PDE-5 inhibitor use, check a morning total testosterone to assess for hypogonadism. Limited evidence supports obtaining a morning total testosterone in all men with erectile dysfunction. If the initial morning total testosterone is low, it should be repeated at least once in several months to confirm the diagnosis. If morning testosterone levels are normal in a patient with high likelihood of hypogonadism, a free testosterone or bioavailable testosterone can be checked to help account for the effects of sex hormone–binding globulin. If evidence of hypogonadism is found, additional testing to distinguish primary versus secondary hypogonadism should be done. Hemoglobin A1c and a lipid panel may be helpful if there is a suspicion for underlying diabetes, hyperlipidemia, or cardiovascular disease contributing to erectile dysfunction. If a review of symptoms elicits a suspicion for hypothyroidism, checking a thyroid stimulating hormone level may be indicated. Consultation with a urologist, endocrinologist, or men's health specialist may be helpful when the etiology is unclear.

Differential Diagnosis

In men presenting with concern for erectile dysfunction, the differential diagnosis is geared toward deciphering the underlying cause. As previously mentioned, there are numerous potential contributing factors to erectile dysfunction. It is important to assess for both organic and psychogenic causes. The history should include asking about nocturnal tumescence, as well as the ability to achieve and maintain an erection with and without a partner. If erectile dysfunction occurs regardless of situation, this is more likely to indicate an organic etiology. If it occurs primarily with a partner, further evaluation of the relationship is indicated. As mentioned above, numerous factors can predispose to erectile dysfunction, and related diagnoses may include cardiovascular disease, tobacco use, diabetes, hypertension, hyperlipidemia, obesity, and metabolic syndrome. Medications should also be reviewed, because they can cause iatrogenic erectile dysfunction in some patients.

Therapy (or Treatment)

Lifestyle modifications play an important role in both the prevention and treatment of erectile dysfunction. Weight reduction for overweight or obese men (BMI >25 kg/m²) and increased exercise for all men can improve SHIM scores. Underlying illnesses such as hyperlipidemia, hypertension, and diabetes should be adequately controlled in order to decrease their potential impact on erectile dysfunction. Another important consideration is tobacco cessation; current or former smoking increases the risk of erectile dysfunction. Sexual health counseling is often helpful for individuals and couples dealing with erectile dysfunction, no matter what the etiology is. Referral to a mental health professional or sexuality expert may be beneficial.

Pharmacologic treatment begins with oral PDE-5 inhibitors. They prevent the breakdown of cyclic guanosine monophosphate (cGMP) and allow increased nitric oxide levels, causing smooth muscle relaxation of the corpora cavernosa, and helping to sustain an erection. This requires a functional libido as well as intact vasculature in order to achieve an erection. There are four PDE-5 inhibitors currently approved in the United States for treatment of erectile dysfunction: avanafil (Stendra), sildenafil (Viagra), tadalafil (Cialis), and vardenafil (Levitra, Staxyn) (see Table 1). There are no significant differences in safety or benefit among these medications. Tadalafil has a longer duration of action than the others.

PDE-5 inhibitors are usually taken on an as-needed basis, with onset of effects typically within about 1 hour of ingestion. The lowest effective dose should be used to reduce the risk of

TABLE 1	Pharmacotherapy for Erectile Dysfunction			
GENERIC NAMES	**BRAND NAMES**	**SIZES**	**TYPICAL DOSING**	**COMMENTS**
Oral Phosphodiesterase Type 5 (PDE-5) Inhibitors				
avanafil	Stendra	50-, 100-, 200-mg tablet	50–200 mg by mouth once daily as needed, 1 h before sexual activity	Use lowest effective dose. Contraindicated with nitrates.
sildenafil	Viagra	25-, 50-, 100-mg tablet	25–100 mg by mouth once daily as needed, 1 h before sexual activity	Use lowest effective dose. Contraindicated with nitrates.
tadalafil	Cialis	2.5-, 5-, 10-, 20-mg tablet	5–20 mg by mouth once daily as needed, 1 h before sexual activity OR 2.5–5 mg by mouth once daily without regard to sexual activity	Use lowest effective dose. Contraindicated with nitrates. Has a longer duration of action than other PDE-5 inhibitors.
vardenafil	Levitra Staxyn	5-, 10-, 20-mg tablet 10-mg oral dissolving tablet	5–20 mg by mouth once daily as needed, 1 h before sexual activity	Use lowest effective dose. Contraindicated with nitrates. Available as a 10 mg oral dissolving tablet (Staxyn)
Prostaglandin				
alprostadil injectable	Caverject Caverject Impulse Edex	20 mcg/mL, 40 mcg/mL vials 10 mcg/0.5 mL, 20 mcg/0.5 mL prefilled syringes 10 mcg/mL, 20 mcg/mL, 40 mcg/mL cartridges	Initiate dose at 1.25 or 2.5 mcg intracavernosally and titrate does with no more than 2 doses per 24 hours (maximum dose: 40 mcg [Edex], 60 mcg [Caverject]). Self administration: maximum 3 times/week with 24 hours between doses	Provide an in-office test dose and instruction in proper technique for administration. Use lowest effective dose.
alprostadil intraurethral	Muse	125-, 250-, 500-, 1000-mcg urethral suppositories	Initiate dose at 125 or 250 mcg intraurethrally and titrate dose on separate occasions in physician's office. Maximum 2 suppositories per 24 hours for self-administration	Provide an in-office test dose and instruction in proper technique for administration. Use lowest effective dose.

adverse reactions. Higher doses do not lead to a linear increase in beneficial effect, but can increase the risk of adverse reactions. Tadalafil, because of its longer duration of action, can be taken daily at a lower dose with similar efficacy to as-needed dosing. The duration of adverse effects may be longer with daily use.

The most common adverse reactions to PDE-5 inhibitors include headache, flushing, dyspepsia, dizziness, nasal congestion, visual disturbance, and myalgias. Overall, these adverse reactions tend to be mild to moderate in nature and are similar across all four medications. Special consideration should be given to individuals who take nitrate-containing medications; the combination of a PDE-5 inhibitor with nitrates can cause severe hypotension that may be life threatening.

Testosterone is not an effective monotherapy for erectile dysfunction. However, for men with confirmed hypogonadism, the combination of a PDE-5 inhibitor with testosterone replacement may be effective.

On June 13, 2023, the US Food and Drug Administration authorized the marketing of an over-the-counter nonmedicated hydro-alcoholic gel, MED3000 (Eroxon), for the treatment of erectile dysfunction in adult males aged 22 years and older. The proposed mechanism of action relies on topical temperature changes that begin with a cooling effect and then a slower warming effect resulting in tumescence. No peer reviewed publications were available for further insight into effectiveness or safety.

If patients do not have adequate symptom relief with lifestyle modification, sexual health counseling, and oral PDE-5 inhibitor use, the prostaglandin alprostadil (Caverject, Edex, Muse) can be considered. Alprostadil works by relaxing arterial smooth muscle and is available in intraurethral and injectable preparations (see Table 1). The intraurethral formulation (Muse) is a dissolvable suppository placed in the urethra with an applicator. The injectable form (Caverject, Edex) is injected directly into one side of the corpora cavernosa. Alprostadil can be used as a single agent or in combination with a PDE-5 inhibitor. If the patient is amenable to a trial of alprostadil, an in-office test dose should be administered to find the lowest effective dose and to teach proper administration technique. Some patients may not be suitable candidates if they are not comfortable with injections or intraurethral insertion. Alprostadil should be avoided in patients who have sickle cell anemia or other risk factors for priapism.

If pharmacological therapies are ineffective or contraindicated, patients may elect to use a vacuum erectile device. These prescription devices are placed over the penis and a vacuum pump removes air from inside the device, creating an influx of blood into the penis and leading to an erection. A ring is then slid from the base of the vacuum tube onto the penis to constrict the outflow of blood and maintain the erection. To avoid ischemic injury, the ring should only be used for up to 30 minutes. Adverse effects of vacuum erectile devices may include the erect penis feeling cool or cold to the touch due to the restricted blood flow, and bending at the base of the penis due to the application of the constricting ring. Overall, these devices have a fairly high satisfaction rate. Caution should be used when considering a vacuum erectile device for patients who are taking anticoagulants or have bleeding disorders.

For patients with erectile dysfunction refractory to the above treatments, surgical implantation of a penile prosthesis can be offered. Penile prostheses come in several forms, including inflatable devices and persistently semirigid implants. Patients and their partners should be counseled regarding risks and benefits to ensure realistic postsurgical expectations. Risks include scarring, penile shortening, recurrent infections, and mechanical failure requiring removal.

Monitoring

A validated questionnaire such as the SHIM (https://www.baus.org.uk/_userfiles/pages/files/Patients/Leaflets/SHIM.pdf) is a simple and reliable tool for monitoring ongoing symptoms. A periodic clinical evaluation, including a review of all supplements and medications, can be helpful to identify potential causes of symptoms and any adverse reactions.

Management of Complications

The majority of adverse reactions with PDE-5 inhibitors are mild to moderate in nature and can be limited by using the lowest effective dose. PDE-5 inhibitors are contraindicated in patients taking nitrates because of the significant risk of life-threatening hypotension. If accidentally ingested, the patient should be monitored by healthcare professionals. The risk also depends on which specific agent was ingested, as the duration of action differs between medications. While the risk of prolonged erection (priapism) is low with PDE-5 inhibitors, men with erections lasting greater than 4 hours should seek emergency attention.

The major potential complication of alprostadil is a prolonged erection lasting greater than 4 hours, which will require emergent urological treatment. Penile fibrosis is also a risk that has been reported in 4.9% of patients using alprostadil at 4 years.

Treatment with exogenous testosterone impairs spermatogenesis and should be avoided in men who are trying to conceive or are interested in future fertility.

The major complication of vacuum erectile devices is ischemic injury, generally when the constricting ring is left in place for greater than 30 minutes at a time. Any suspicion for ischemic injury should also prompt emergent urologic intervention.

Patients with penile implants are prone to recurrent infections or mechanical failure, potentially requiring removal of the device.

References

Burnett AL, Nehra A, Breau RH, et al: Erectile dysfunction: AUA Guideline, *J Urol* 200(3):633–641, 2018 Sep, https://doi.org/10.1016/j.juro.2018.05.004. Epub 2018 May 7.

Buvat J, Büttner H, Hatzimouratidis K, et al: Adherence to initial PDE-5 inhibitor treatment: randomized open-label study comparing tadalafil once a day, tadalafil on demand, and sildenafil on demand in patients with erectile dysfunction, *J Sex Med* 10(6):1592–1602, 2013.

Costa P, Grandmottet G, Mai HD, Droupy S: Impact of a first treatment with phosphodiesterase inhibitors on men and partners' quality of sexual life: results of a prospective study in primary care, *J Sex Med* 10(7):1850–1860, 2013.

Ghanem HM, Salonia A, Martin-Morales A: SOP: physical examination and laboratory testing for men with erectile dysfunction, *J Sex Med* 10(1):108–110, 2013.

Khayyamfar F, Forootan SK, Ghasemi H, Miri SR, Farhadi E: Evaluating the efficacy of vacuum constrictive device and causes of its failure in impotent patients, *Urol J* 10(4):1072–1078, 2014.

Martin-Morales A, Haro JM, Beardsworth A, Bertsch J, Kontodimas S: Therapeutic effectiveness and patient satisfaction after 6 months of treatment with tadalafil, sildenafil, and vardenafil: results from the erectile dysfunction observational study (EDOS), *Eur Urol* 51(2):541–550, 2007.

Mccabe MP, Sharlip ID, Lewis R, et al: Incidence and prevalence of sexual dysfunction in women and men: a consensus statement from the Fourth International Consultation on Sexual Medicine 2015, *J Sex Med* 13(2):144–152, 2016.

Mulhall JP, Trost LW, Brannigan RE, et al: Evaluation and management of testosterone deficiency: AUA Guideline, *J Urol* 200(2):423–432, 2018 Aug, https://doi.org/10.1016/j.juro.2018.03.115. Epub 2018 Mar 28.

Rosen RC, Fisher WA, Eardley I, et al: The multinational Men's Attitudes to Life Events and Sexuality (MALES) study: I. Prevalence of erectile dysfunction and related health concerns in the general population, *Curr Med Res Opin* 20(5):607–617, 2004.

Selvin E, Burnett AL, Platz EA: Prevalence and risk factors for erectile dysfunction in the US, *Am J Med* 120(2):151–157, 2007.

PROSTATE CANCER

Method of
William G. Nelson, MD, PhD

CURRENT DIAGNOSIS

- Serum prostate-specific antigen (PSA) testing, with or without digital rectal examination (DRE), can be used for prostate cancer screening for men beginning at 50 years of age until 70 years of age.
- Prostate cancer screening carries significant risks of overdiagnosis and overtreatment of clinically insignificant prostate cancers.
- The diagnosis of prostate cancer is usually made via ultrasound-guided transrectal core needle biopsies that sample the prostate; magnetic resonance imaging (MRI) is increasingly used to direct core biopsies to regions of the prostate suspicious for harboring aggressive prostate cancers.
- Histologic grade (Gleason score) and anatomic stage provide the prognosis needed for treatment decision making. Several different tumor-based molecular biomarker tests can add further prognostic information.
- Metastatic prostate cancer can be evaluated using ^{99m}Tc-methylene diphosphonate (MDP) or ^{18}F-sodium fluoride (NaF) bone scans, abdominopelvic computed tomography (CT) or MRI scan, and ^{11}C-choline, ^{18}F-fluciclovine, ^{68}Ga-PSMA, or ^{18}F-piflufolastat positron emission tomography (PET) studies.
- Germline genetic testing for DNA repair gene variants along with tumor testing for DNA repair gene defects tends to accompany diagnosis of high-risk localized, locoregionally advanced, and metastatic prostate cancer.

CURRENT THERAPY

- Options for management of localized prostate cancer include active surveillance, radical prostatectomy, external-beam radiotherapy (EBRT), brachy therapy, and proton-beam radiotherapy.
- Androgen-deprivation therapy (ADT) using gonadotrophic hormone-releasing hormone analogues is a mainstay of systemic prostate cancer treatment.
- CYP17 inhibitors and androgen receptor antagonists can be added to further ablate androgen signaling.
- CYP17 inhibitors, androgen receptor antagonists, and taxane chemotherapy can improve survival when given along with ADT for hormone-sensitive metastatic prostate cancer or upon progression to castration-resistant prostate cancer (CRPC).
- Stereotactic bone radiation therapy (SBRT) can be directed at metastatic lesions in the setting of oligometastatic disease progression to prolong progression-free survival.
- The α-particle–emitting calcium mimetic ^{223}Ra can palliate painful bony metastases.
- Lutetium Lu 177 vipivotide tetraxetan improves survival for castration-resistant prostate cancer (CRPC).
- Poly(ADP-ribose) polymerase (PARP) inhibitors may be effective in up to 20% of men with CRPC who carry germline and/or somatic mutations in homologous recombination repair genes (*BRCA1*, *BRCA2*, *ATM*, and others).
- Immune checkpoint blockade may be of benefit for patients with mismatch repair–deficient prostate cancer.
- Platinum-based chemotherapy can be used to treat small cell/neuroendocrine prostate cancer.

Prostate cancer comprises the most commonly diagnosed cancer among men in the United States, with an estimated 313,780 new cases and 35,770 deaths expected for 2025. At some point during life, 1 in 8 men can expect to be diagnosed with prostate cancer, though the risk of dying from the disease is less than 1 in 40. African-American men suffer disproportionately with the disease, exhibiting more than twice the age-adjusted mortality as Caucasians.

The prostate gland itself is a male sex accessory gland located adjacent to the rectum in the pelvis and surrounding the urethra to supply secretions to the ejaculate. Why it should spawn so many cancers has proven enigmatic. The prostate can be divided into three zones: a *peripheral zone*, where most prostate cancers arise; a *transition zone* near the urethra that is prone to benign enlargement (benign prostatic hyperplasia/hypertrophy [BPH]); and a *central zone*. Under the influence of the male androgenic hormones testosterone (T) and dihydrotestosterone (DHT), normal epithelial cells produce the serine protease prostate-specific antigen (PSA; encoded by the *KLK3* gene). The appearance of PSA in the bloodstream tends to indicate epithelial barrier dysfunction within the prostate gland, attributable to three highly prevalent conditions in aging men in the United States: inflammation (prostatitis), BPH, or prostate cancer. Blood testing for PSA has emerged as a common screening tactic for prostate cancer, necessarily confounded by the near-ubiquitous coexistence of prostatitis and BPH.

Most patients present with prostate cancer apparently confined to the prostate gland, often detected by PSA screening. Though usually indolent, when aggressive, prostate cancer tends to spread to bony sites, causing pain by undermining bone architecture through stimulating osteoblastic activity, a phenomenon readily evident via NaF bone scanning. Patients dying of prostate cancer also manifest metastasis to lymph nodes, liver, the dura, and elsewhere.

Patients who are diagnosed with prostate cancer today confront a large and often confusing array of treatment options. The typical patient diagnosed with the disease is at least 65 years of age or older; the risks and benefits associated with different treatment choices in this age range are relevant not only for prostate cancer specialty care, but for general medical care as well. The 5-year survival for a man with localized prostate cancer is >95%, underscoring the need for balancing prostate cancer treatment selection with other health priorities.

Epidemiology

Heredity plays as significant a role in prostate cancer development as for any other common cancer. Analyses of concordance for prostate cancer between monozygotic (identical) versus dizygotic (fraternal) twins have consistently found excess prostate cancers among the identical twins despite similar environmental exposures, leading to the estimate that as many as 42% of prostate cancer cases may be attributable to inheritance. Two sets of inherited susceptibility genes merit special attention for prostate cancer treatment. Germline defects in DNA double-strand break repair genes, such as *BRCA1*, *BRCA2*, *ATM*, *PALB2*, *FANCA*, *RAD51D*, and *CHEK2*, or in DNA mismatch repair genes, such as *MSH2*, *MLH1*, *MSH6*, and *PMS2*, may increase the risk of developing prostate cancer or of exhibiting metastatic prostate cancer progression. Defective DNA repair in prostate cells has important treatment implications. When germline DNA repair gene defects are accompanied by somatic alterations at the remaining allele, crippling of DNA double-strand break repair can serve as an indication for treatment with poly(ADP-ribose) polymerase (PARP) inhibitors, while loss of DNA mismatch repair constitutes an indication for treatment with immune checkpoint inhibitors. With a growing role in prostate cancer treatment decision making, both germline testing and tumor tissue testing for DNA repair gene defects has become increasingly common for patients with the disease. Of course, the detection of defective DNA repair genes in the germline of a patient with prostate cancer should also alert his physician to consider cascade genetic testing of relatives as abnormal repair gene carriers could be at risk for breast, ovarian, colorectal, or other cancers.

Evidence for a critical contribution of the environment to prostate cancer is as strong as is the case for an impact of heredity. Prostate cancer incidence and mortality vary widely throughout the world, and migrants from low-risk regions to high-risk regions tend to adopt higher prostate cancer predilection within a single generation. It has not been established whether the high rates of prostate cancer in the United States reflect ingestion of food carcinogens (such as the heterocyclic amines and polycyclic aromatic hydrocarbons in overcooked meats, which are known to cause prostate cancer in rodents) or inadequate intake of tomatoes and cruciferous vegetables (which contain antioxidant micronutrients known to protect against prostate cancer in model studies). Whatever the etiology of the disease, prostate glands removed at autopsy from high-risk parts of the world display an astonishing abundance both of chronic inflammation and of undiagnosed prostate cancers. Also, in rodent models, exposures that cause prostate cancer also trigger chronic prostatic inflammation, connecting the two disease processes. In the United States, asymptomatic prostatitis arises in nearly all men as they age, leading to the appearance of proliferative inflammatory atrophy (PIA) lesions, the earliest histologic precursors to prostate cancer. In turn, small prostate cancers ultimately appear in as many as 64% of men 60 to 70 years of age. Fortunately, the majority of these cancers pose little threat to health or to life. Nonetheless, this reservoir of indolent asymptomatic disease in the midst of chronically inflamed prostates complicates prostate cancer screening, early detection, and treatment, leading to significant overdiagnosis and overtreatment of the disease.

Risk Factors

Key risk factors for prostate cancer include age, family history, African ancestry, a diet rich in saturated fats and red meats, and a sedentary lifestyle, all features that may motivate the use of prostate cancer screening as a part of routine primary care. The most widely used screening strategies feature blood testing for PSA with or without DRE, usually beginning at 50 to 55 years of age or earlier for African-American men, for men with a strong family history, or for men known to be carriers of prostate cancer risk genes. Unfortunately, even though the benefits of screening for reducing prostate cancer progression to metastasis and prostate cancer mortality have been demonstrated in a large randomized trial, prostate cancer screening remains highly controversial. The U.S. Preventive Services Task Force (USPSTF) formally recommends that men 55 to 69 years of age discuss the potential benefits and harms of prostate cancer screening with their physician before pursuing PSA testing and rectal examination (assigning a grade C). For men 70 years of age and older, the USPSTF recommends against prostate cancer screening (grade D).

Pathophysiology

Nearly all of the exposures that can cause prostate cancers in laboratory mice and rats, ranging from charred meat carcinogens to estrogens to various "hit-and-run" infectious agents, trigger chronic inflammatory changes in prostate tissues that lead to PIA. Some fraction of PIA lesions, likely those exhibiting morphologic atypia and containing somatic genome alterations, in turn progress to prostatic intraepithelial neoplasia (PIN) and to prostate cancer.

The normal prostate contains an epithelium able to contribute secretions to the ejaculate. The epithelium features (1) basally located cells expressing cytokeratins K5 and K14, and p63; (2) columnar secretory cells expressing the androgen receptor (AR), PSA, cytokeratins K8 and K18, and prostate-specific membrane antigen (PSMA); and (3) neuroendocrine cells producing chromogranin A, neuron-specific enolase, and synaptophysin. PIA lesions arising in response to epithelial damage give rise to "intermediate cells" that express markers characteristic of both basal and luminal cells. The cellular target of transformation is likely such an "intermediate cell"; the resultant PIN or prostate cancer cells exhibit many of the phenotypic characteristics of columnar secretory cells, including the expression of AR, PSA, and PSMA, and acquire expression of new gene products, such as α-methylacyl-CoA racemase (AMACR). For this reason, many prostate pathologists use immunohistochemical staining for basal cells (antibodies against cytokeratins K5/K14 and p63) and for neoplastic prostate cells (antibodies against AMACR) to aid in prostate cancer diagnosis; prostate cancer cells tend to be cytokeratin K5/K14 negative, p63 negative, and AMACR positive.

Prostate cancer cells tend to over-express MYC, activate telomerase, and acquire a number of somatic genome and epigenome alterations. Fusion translocations of an androgen-regulated gene, TMPRSS2, to genes encoding various members of the E26 transformation-specific (ETS) family of transcription factors are the most common somatic genetic changes in prostate cancers. Somehow, these gene fusions allow prostate cancer cells to coopt androgen signaling to drive neoplastic transformation and malignant progression. As a result, interference with androgen signaling forms the foundation for most advanced prostate cancer treatments. When such translocations are not present, other somatic alterations, such as mutations in SPOP, are more frequent. Hypermethylation of GSTP1, encoding detoxification enzyme for carcinogens and oxidants, can be detected in >90% of cases. DNA methylation changes at other loci are also very common. The somatic defects in genes and gene function somehow allow prostate cancer cells to proliferate, escape terminal differentiation, and survive to grow in ectopic sites, such as in bones, lymph nodes, and other organs. Two notable somatic gene defects, mutations or deletions in TP53 and in PTEN, have been consistently associated with malignant prostate cancer progression.

Prevention

There are no established drugs that prevent prostate cancer, although there have been three very large randomized clinical trials of agents for prostate cancer prevention. One such trial aimed to test predictions from epidemiologic studies and earlier small clinical trials that inadequate intake of the micronutrients selenium and vitamin E might lead to increased prostate cancer risk. The trial, called the Selenium and Vitamin E Cancer Prevention Trial (SELECT), enrolled men 55 years of age or older (50 years or older for African Americans) with an unremarkable DRE and a serum PSA of 4.0 ng/mL or less to treatment with the micronutrients for 7 to 12 years (randomized to 200 μg selenomethionine[7] daily, 400 IU α-tocopherol[7] daily, the combination, or neither). Unfortunately, the study failed to show any reduction in prostate cancer, instead revealing a slight increase in prostate cancer incidence among men taking vitamin E. As a result, high-level intake of selenium, vitamin E, and other nutritional supplements for the purpose of prostate cancer prevention should be discouraged.

The two other large randomized trials tested the propensity for the 5α-reductase inhibitors finasteride (Proscar)[1] and dutasteride (Avodart)[1] to prevent prostate cancer development. In one of the studies, called the Prostate Cancer Prevention Trial (PCPT), finasteride (5 mg daily or a placebo) was given to healthy men 55 years of age and older, with a normal DRE and a serum PSA of 3.0 ng/mL or less, for 7 years. During the trial, men with increasing PSA values or an abnormal DRE were subjected to prostate biopsy. At the end of the trial, biopsies were planned for all of the men. The results were a decrease in prostate cancer detection from 24.4% of men receiving a placebo to only 18.4% of men treated with finasteride, but an increase in more aggressive high-grade prostate cancers in men receiving finasteride versus placebo from 6.4% to 5.1%.

Similar results were encountered with dutasteride in the other trial, the Reduction by Dutasteride of Prostate Cancer Events (REDUCE) trial, in which men with an elevated serum PSA between 2.5 and 10.0 ng/mL and a recent negative prostate biopsy were given dutasteride (0.5 mg daily) or a placebo for 4 years, with prostate biopsies obtained after 2 and 4 years on study. Overall, prostate cancer was reduced from 25.1% to 19.9% for men taking dutasteride, but high-grade prostate cancer was increased in these men from <0.1% to 0.5%. Data from the PCPT and REDUCE trials clearly indicated that 5α-reductase inhibitors are better at preventing low-grade cancers than high-grade cancers. Whether the development of high-grade cancers was actually increased in either trial or these cancers were just more easily detected has been controversial, and the U.S. Food and Drug Administration (FDA) has not approved either finasteride or dutasteride for prostate cancer prevention. In 2019, long-term follow-up of participants in the PCPT revealed no increases in prostate cancer mortality accompanying finasteride treatment, likely affirming the general safety of 5α-reductase inhibitor treatment for BPH and male pattern baldness, and reanimating discussions about how 5α-reductase inhibitors might be used to lower the overall burden of prostate cancer in some way.

Clinical Manifestations

Most patients present for prostate cancer care after a diagnosis triggered by prostate cancer screening and are thus initially asymptomatic. Local progression of the disease can result in lower urinary tract symptoms of voiding obstruction or irritation; urinary tract infections and urosepsis; erectile dysfunction; hematospermia; and diminished ejaculate volume. Metastatic prostate cancer dissemination most often involves the skeleton, resulting in bone pain and low blood counts, and involves pelvic lymph nodes and nearby lymphatics, resulting in lower extremity edema or retroperitoneal fibrosis, respectively.

Diagnosis

Prostate cancer diagnosis is typically made using transrectal ultrasound (TRUS)-guided prostate biopsy. The technique involves the repeated firing of an 18-gauge needle from a spring-loaded gun through a port on the TRUS probe. To sample prostate tissue, the biopsy needle passes through the rectum into the prostate, and fluoroquinolone antibiotics are typically administered before the biopsy procedure. Hematuria and/or hematospermia occur commonly after prostate biopsy. Hospital admissions, usually the result of an infection, are rare but can occur in up to 7% of men with significant comorbidities. Importantly, TRUS does not delineate the locations of prostate cancers within the prostate. For this reason, the numbers and sites of biopsies placed during a prostate biopsy procedure, typically 10 to 12 directed laterally into the peripheral zone of the gland, are designed to minimize the chance of missing life-threatening high-grade cancers.

Increasingly, magnetic resonance imaging (MRI) has been employed to better direct prostate biopsies, hoping to reduce detection of low-grade cancers that pose little threat to life and to more accurately sample high-grade disease. Multiparametric MRI (mpMRI) incorporates T2-weighted anatomic imaging, diffusion-weighted imaging, and contrast enhancement to highlight suspicious areas in the prostate for biopsy. The technique generates a standardized "suspicion" score for individual lesions, using the Prostate Imaging–Reporting and Data System (PI-RADS). The MR image itself can then be used to direct TRUS biopsies via coregistration (or "fusion") of the acquired mpMRI data with real-time TRUS. Biopsies obtained by MRI/TRUS fusion are becoming more widespread, especially for patients who need a repeat biopsy because of a persistently elevated or increasing serum PSA. At the time of initial diagnosis, MRI-guided biopsies may result in less detection of clinically insignificant cancers.

The histologic grade and anatomic stage of newly diagnosed prostate cancer carry important prognostic information useful for treatment planning. Recently, prostate cancer grade "groups" (1 most favorable prognosis and 5 poorest prognosis) have been introduced into clinical practice as risk tools for localized prostate cancer. These "groups" are derived from Gleason scoring as conducted by an expert genitourinary pathologist. The Gleason score represents the sum of the two most common histologic patterns of growth exhibited by the cancer within the prostate; the pattern designations range from pattern 3 to pattern 5 (there are no patterns 1 or 2), providing Gleason scores from 6 to 10. The disease stage focuses on the extent of tumor in the prostate itself (T1, not palpable by DRE; T2, palpable by DRE; T3, extending outside the prostate itself; and T4, invading adjacent pelvic structures), in regional lymph nodes (N0, no lymph node metastases; N1, lymph node metastases), and in distant sites (M0, no distant metastases; M1, metastases). Staging tools include a number of imaging modalities, including abdominopelvic CT or MR images and nuclear medicine scans for soft tissue and for bone, using ^{11}C-choline, ^{18}F-fluciclovine, and ^{18}F-sodium fluoride. Positron emission tomography (PET)-CT (or PET-MRI) scanning now features prostate-specific membrane antigen (PSMA) targeting tracers such as ^{68}Ga-PSMA and ^{18}F-piflufolastat.

---

[1] Not FDA approved for this indication.
[7] Available as dietary supplement.

Differential Diagnosis

The critical issue surrounding the diagnosis and staging of many patients with prostate cancer is whether the disease is at risk to progress to threaten life or whether it is so indolent as to not need treatment. Most patients with indolent disease indicated by a Gleason score of 6 (grade group 1) do not need immediate treatment, and many may never need treatment. Instead, these patients can be monitored using *active surveillance*, with serum PSA tests twice yearly, DREs each year, and MRI and/or prostate biopsies as necessary or after 2 to 4 years. This surveillance strategy aims to detect higher Gleason score prostate cancer if it appears. A Gleason score of 7 or higher (grade groups 2 to 5) tends to be an indication for curative local disease treatment with surgery or radiation therapy. Deferring aggressive local therapy as part of active surveillance appears safe, and as a result, active surveillance has become a common approach to prostate cancer care. By avoiding aggressive intervention until and unless necessary, active surveillance is distinct from observation or watchful waiting approaches, which are typically reserved for patients with significant comorbidities and limited life expectancy. Biopsy tissue-based molecular classifiers are increasingly used to inform decision making about pursuit of active surveillance.

Therapy

For localized prostate cancer with a Gleason score of 7 or higher (grade groups 2 to 5), curative treatments include radical prostatectomy, interstitial brachytherapy, and external beam radiation therapy (EBRT). Most radical prostatectomies these days are performed using a robot-assisted laparoscopic approach. Urinary incontinence and erectile function after the procedure vary greatly among surgeons, with as many as 20% of patients describing some level of urine leakage 2 years after radical prostatectomy and at least 26% reporting significant sexual dysfunction 1 year after surgery. Ideally, following surgery, the serum PSA should decrease to an undetectable level and remain so in perpetuity if the procedure resulted in prostate cancer cure. Two-thirds of patients subjected to radical prostatectomy remain free from PSA recurrence 15 years after surgery. An increasing serum PSA after surgery is a sign that prostate cancer has recurred or persisted somewhere. Nonetheless, such a PSA increase may not herald imminent overt metastasis or death. In one analysis, only 30% of men with an increasing postsurgery serum PSA had suffered with metastatic prostate cancer by 8 years after the initial PSA increase. The rate of serum PSA increase can be informative; a rapid doubling of serum PSA values is usually associated with a greater threat of symptomatic disease progression.

Prostate brachytherapy provides for direct irradiation of localized prostate cancer via implantation of radioactive sources into the prostate using image guidance. The procedure itself is fairly convenient and can be completed as an outpatient within a couple of hours using spinal anesthesia. The most common radioactive sources used are ^{125}I (iodine) and ^{103}Pd (palladium); as many as 100 seeds might be implanted. Although the ^{125}I seeds generally decay more slowly than the ^{103}Pd seeds, prostate brachytherapy implants are essentially inert by 10 months after insertion into the prostate. Complications of brachytherapy for prostate cancer differ from those of radical prostatectomy and of EBRT, with irritative voiding symptoms reported by at least one-half of patients in the first few months after implant placement. These symptoms tend to abate after 1 year or so, persisting in some 15% to 20% of patients. Long-term side effects can include urethral stricture, incontinence, erectile dysfunction, and rectal irritation. Relative contraindications to prostate brachytherapy include large prostate size (requires a lot of seeds or use of androgen deprivation to shrink the prostate), preimplant obstructive urinary symptoms (greatly worsen after implantation), and history of transurethral surgery for symptomatic BPH (tends to lead to incontinence).

A series of technical innovations have improved both the efficacy and safety of EBRT, including CT-based treatment planning, the use of multileaf collimators in modern linear accelerators, and improvements in treatment planning software. Three-dimensional conformal radiation therapy (3D-CRT) allows creation of more accurate target volumes using reconstructions of pelvic CT images and better sparing of vulnerable structures such as the bladder and the rectum. Intensity-modulated radiotherapy (IMRT) even further optimizes dose distribution for prostate cancer treatment by controlling the intensity of radiation dose in addition to the shape of the volume designated for treatment. Finally, the delivery of EBRT using fewer treatment fractions, with a higher dose/fraction and referred to as stereotactic body radiotherapy (SBRT), has been found to be noninferior to conventional fractionation schemes. Despite more accurate deposition of radiation doses to the prostate, side effects of EBRT remain mostly rectal toxicity (early irritation and late rectal bleeding), late urethral strictures, and erectile dysfunction. EBRT can also be used as adjuvant therapy for prostate cancer with positive surgical margins after radical prostatectomy or as salvage therapy for local prostate cancer recurrence after surgery.

Proton-beam radiotherapy has become available at a limited number of treatment centers. The physical properties of protons allow them to deposit energy very precisely, with little radiation dose to skin and little radiation scatter to nearby tissues. This behavior is ideal for cancers located in close proximity to sensitive structures in the body, such as at the base of the skull, near the eye, and elsewhere. For prostate cancer, proton-beam radiotherapy has emerged as an effective treatment for localized disease, but whether this approach offers an improvement over conventional EBRT using 3D-CRT with IMRT awaits the results of an ongoing randomized clinical trial.

Systemic approaches to prostate cancer include agents targeted at androgen signaling, taxane chemotherapy, radiopharmaceuticals, PARP inhibitors, and immune checkpoint inhibitors. Disruption of androgen signaling has been a mainstay of advanced prostate cancer care for seven decades. Originally accomplished by surgical removal of the testes and later by the administration of estrogens, ADT, involving a reduction in circulating testosterone levels to <50 ng/mL, is now more commonly achieved by inhibition of pituitary gonadotropin production, using luteinizing hormone–releasing hormone (LHRH) analogues that cause suppression of testosterone production. Injectable LHRH analogues are all available in long-acting depot formulations, including agonists (goserelin [Zoladex LA] 10.8-mg depot every 3 months, leuprolide [Lupron Depot] 22.5-mg depot every 3 months, and triptorelin [Trelstar] 3.75-mg depot monthly) and antagonists (degarelix [Firmagon] 240 mg depot initially followed by 80 mg depot monthly). An oral LHRH antagonist, relugolix [Orgovyx or Relumina] 360 mg initially followed by 120 mg daily, is also available. LHRH agonists are frequently administered along with first-generation AR antagonists (nilutamide [Nilandron, Anandron] 150 mg twice daily for the first 4 weeks and then 150 mg daily thereafter, flutamide [Eulexin] 250 mg three times daily, and bicalutamide [Casodex] 50 mg daily). The benefits of ADT are evident in most patients by a decrease in serum PSA, a shrinkage of metastatic cancer deposits, and improvements in symptoms, such as bone pain, that accompany metastatic prostate cancer progression. Side effects often include hot flashes, bone loss, reduced libido, decreased muscle mass, increased fat, and fatigue. An increased risk for cardiovascular disease is also suspected, and ADT may prolong the QT/QT$_c$ interval by electrocardiography.

Ultimately, most male patients on ADT for advanced prostate cancer progress to CRPC. Nonetheless, the prostate cancers in many patients with CRPC remain addicted to androgen signaling and continue to produce PSA, which requires an activated AR. In this setting, two strategies have emerged to ablate androgen signaling more completely. One involves the use of the AR antagonists enzalutamide ([Xtandi] 160 mg daily), apalutamide ([Erleada] 240 mg daily), and darolutamide ([Nubeqa] 600 mg twice daily). Each is approved by the FDA for CRPC; enzalutamide is approved for CRPC with or without overt metastases, while apalutamide and darolutamide are approved for CRPC without overt metastases (enzalutamide and apalutamide are also approved to give along with ADT for castration-sensitive metastatic prostate cancer). A second approach involves inhibition of adrenal steroid biogenesis to further reduce circulating levels of androgenic hormones. Abiraterone ([Zytiga] 1000 mg daily with 5 mg prednisone twice daily), a CYP17 inhibitor, suppresses extragonadal androgen production and provides an effective treatment for CRPC. Abiraterone must be administered along with replacement corticosteroids (5 mg prednisone twice daily). Blood testing for circulating prostate cancer cells expressing the *AR* mRNA splice variant V7 (AR-V7) for patients with CPRC can predict resistance to AR antagonists and abiraterone, steering them instead toward taxane chemotherapy. Also, both AR antagonists and abiraterone are being explored in combination with LHRH analogues in clinical trials as initial systemic hormone treatment for high-risk localized prostate cancer.

ADT can be used as adjuvant therapy along with prostate radiotherapy, as initial treatment for prostate cancer recurrence manifest as a rapidly increasing serum PSA in the absence of overt metastases following surgery or radiotherapy, and as treatment for established metastatic prostate cancer, with or without taxane chemotherapy. Of these three indications, the use of ADT for patients with disease recurrence after primary therapy remains somewhat controversial. The concern is that the benefits may not be much better than waiting to initiate ADT until overt metastases can be detected, while the hazards, including bone loss, possible risk for cardiovascular complications, and poor quality of life are significant. Careful monitoring of PSA increases and periodic use of imaging studies may allow for introduction of ADT before symptoms of metastatic prostate cancer appear. PET-CT or PET-MRI scanning with ^{68}Ga-PSMA or and ^{18}F-piflufolastat for prostate recurrence in the setting of a increasing serum PSA can aid in treatment planning and timing. For men found to have 1 to 3 bone metastases, stereotactic ablative radiotherapy (SABR) can be delivered to improve progression-free survival, delaying the need for ADT. Another tactic for ADT in this setting has been intermittent administration. Intermittent ADT appears to control prostate cancer progression as well as continuous ADT and provides some minor improvement in quality of life. Finally, a novel strategy now in clinical trials for patients with advanced prostate cancer exposed to ADT for at least 6 months is the administration of androgenic hormones. This approach can lower serum PSA levels in more than one-half of treated patients and improve quality of life.

Of all the cytotoxic chemotherapy drugs used for advanced prostate cancer, agents targeting intracellular microtubules have exhibited disproportionate activity. Prostate cancer cells tend to have low growth rates, rendering most antineoplastic drugs that interfere with cell replication less effective than for other cancers. Taxane drugs, including docetaxel (Taxotere) and cabazitaxel (Jevtana), disrupt microtubule function in both replicating and nonreplicating cells. In nonreplicating prostate cancer cells, the taxane drugs may hinder the trafficking of AR and other critical gene regulatory proteins into the cell nucleus, triggering apoptosis. Both docetaxel (75 mg/m² every 3 weeks given along with prednisone 10 mg daily) and cabazitaxel (25 mg/m² every 3 weeks given along with prednisone 10 mg daily) are effective treatments for CRPC, able to lower serum PSA, reduce measurable volumes of cancer seen on imaging studies, and prolong disease survival. Docetaxel toxicity includes significant neutropenia, ankle edema, peripheral neuropathy, hair loss, and nail changes. Cabazitaxel, which was more effective than docetaxel for multidrug-resistant tumor cells in preclinical studies and better able to penetrate the blood-brain barrier, was initially used to treat docetaxel-resistant CRPC. In that setting, cabazitaxel caused more substantial neutropenia than docetaxel and was associated with more diarrhea and asthenia. A randomized trial comparing docetaxel to cabazitaxel as first-line treatment for metastatic CRPC revealed similar overall survival for either treatment, and docetaxel remains the preferred first-line chemotherapy option. Six doses of docetaxel given every 3 weeks is now frequently used along with ADT for patients with metastatic hormone-sensitive prostate cancer, significantly prolonging overall survival when compared with ADT alone in two large randomized clinical trials. In addition to the taxanes docetaxel and cabazitaxel, the topoisomerase poison mitoxantrone (Novantrone) is approved by the FDA as an agent capable of improving quality of life for patients with CRPC.

Palliation of symptomatic bone metastases in patients with CRPC can be achieved using the α-particle–emitting calcium mimetic ^{223}Ra. The agent has a brief half-life ($t^{1/2}$ = 11.4 days) and a marked proclivity for skeletal uptake; an estimated 40% to 60% of administered ^{223}Ra ends up in bones. ^{223}Ra (50 kBq/kg) is typically given in six injections at 4-week intervals. Side effects include nausea, vomiting, diarrhea, leg swelling, and low blood counts. More recently, Lu-Labeled PSMA ligand (lutetium Lu 177 vipivotide tetraxetan [Pluvicto] 7.4 GBq every 6 weeks for up to 6 doses) has been introduced into the care of patients with CRPC, delivering improvements in overall survival. Toxicity includes fatigue, dry mouth, nausea, anemia, thrombocytopenia, and rare acute kidney injury.

The up to 20% of patients with CRPC who carry germline and/or somatic mutations in homologous recombination repair genes (*BRCA1*, *BRCA2*, *ATM*, and others) may derive significant benefit from treatment with PARP inhibitors. PARPs are enzymes that contribute to several steps in DNA repair. Inhibition of PARP in cells with homologous recombination deficiency results in "synthetic lethality" and apoptosis. This phenomenon has been exploited successfully for the treatment of ovarian and breast cancers carrying defective homologous recombination repair genes. The PARP inhibitors olaparib ([Lynparza] 300 mg twice daily), rucaparib ([Rubraca] 600 mg twice daily), talazoparib ([Talzenna] 0.5 mg daily), and niraparib ([Zejula][1] 300 mg daily) have all shown early evidence of activity in the treatment of CRPC with deficient homologous recombination repair; olaparib and rucaparib are FDA approved for CRPC in the setting of homologous recombination repair gene defects. Common side effects of PARP inhibitors include gastrointestinal symptoms and fatigue.

Two additional systemic treatment approaches merit attention. First, for CRPC arising in the setting of DNA mismatch repair deficiency, like other cancers with DNA mismatch repair defects, the immune checkpoint inhibitor pembrolizumab ([Keytruda][1] 200 mg every 3 weeks) can be effective at achieving significant and durable treatment responses. Major side effects include "autoimmune breakthrough events" such as colitis, pneumonitis, and hypophysitis. Immune checkpoint inhibitor therapy otherwise shows very little activity against prostate cancers. Second, for patients with CRPC manifest as small cell neuroendocrine cancer, treatment with chemotherapy doublet regimens like cisplatin[1] or carboplatin[1] and etoposide[1] may be helpful.

Monitoring

Patients treated for clinically localized prostate cancer by surgery or radiation therapy are monitored for cancer recurrence principally by serum PSA testing every 6 to 12 months and by DRE yearly. A newly detectable or increasing serum PSA can trigger a more complete evaluation using abdominopelvic CT or MRI and nuclear medicine scanning with ^{11}C-choline, ^{18}F-fluciclovine, ^{68}Ga-PSMA, or ^{18}F-piflufolastat. ^{18}F-deoxyglucose PET imaging is not helpful. If necessary, a prostate biopsy may be undertaken in the setting of disease recurrence after radiation therapy.

Metastatic prostate cancer treatment can be monitored using serial serum PSA determinations and repeated imaging at known and/or symptomatic sites of disease. In addition, whether used for nonmetastatic or metastatic prostate cancer, ADT carries a substantial risk of osteoporosis. As such, patients should be subjected to dual-energy x-ray absorptiometry (DEXA) scanning. For patients with a low fracture risk, calcium (1000 mg) and vitamin D (400 IU) supplements may suffice, but for patients facing a higher probability of bone fracture, treatment with agents such as denosumab ([Prolia] 60 mg every 6 months), zoledronic acid ([Reclast][1] 4 mg no more often than monthly), or alendronate ([Fosamax][1] 70 mg once weekly) should be considered along with calcium and vitamin D. Patients receiving ADT should also be screened for diabetes and for cardiovascular disease, conditions that are common among men in the age range for prostate cancer.

Management of Complications

Men who are survivors of prostate cancer face a number of health challenges that comprise long-term side effects of the treatment(s)

---

[1]Not FDA approved for this indication.

they received. Surgery tends to disrupt urinary and sexual functions. Stress incontinence may be the most common urinary problem, though more severe incontinence can occur. Urinary symptoms, such as urgency, frequency, and nocturia can arise; sometimes these symptoms herald the appearance of a urethral stricture at the site of the anastomosis of the bladder neck to the urethra during surgery. Urethral strictures related to scarring can be distinguished from cancer recurrence and treated via dilation by a urologist. Sexual problems include difficulties achieving erections sufficient for intercourse and a change in sexual experience attributable to lack of ejaculation and to differences in orgasms. Frank discussions about sexual function after primary prostate cancer treatment can aid in sexual recovery. Some urologists have attempted to use phosphodiesterase type 5 inhibitors (sildenafil [Viagra][1] 50 mg, vardenafil [Levitra][1] 10 mg, and tadalafil [Cialis][1] 5 mg) early after surgery to augment restoration of erectile function. These drugs have also been used successfully by some patients to improve erections months and years after surgery. Radiation therapy late effects can also include urinary and sexual difficulties, and they can involve the rectum in inflammation, pain, bleeding, and incontinence. Minor rectal symptoms can be alleviated using stool softeners, but more severe complications require the attention of a gastroenterologist or colorectal surgeon. Hyperbaric oxygen may help some patients with radiation proctitis as a late effect of prostate cancer treatment.

ADT causes a diverse collection of long-term side effects, including loss of libido, erection problems, hot flashes, weight gain and obesity, mood changes/depression, anxiety/distress, gynecomastia, anemia, osteoporosis (see previously), diabetes/metabolic syndrome, and decreased lean muscle mass. Increased physical activity and dietary changes appropriate for obesity can be helpful. Careful attention and screening for psychological stress and depression should be a routine aspect of prostate cancer survivorship care. Even patients likely cured of prostate cancer by surgery or radiation therapy frequently suffer with significant "PSA anxiety" around the time of follow-up vigilance to detect disease recurrence. Hot flashes, which occur in as many as 40% of patients on ADT, can be treated using selective serotonin reuptake inhibitors such as paroxetine ([Paxil][1] 10 to 20 mg daily), serotonin and norepinephrine uptake inhibitors such as venlafaxine ([Effexor XR][1] 75 mg daily), or the anticonvulsant gabapentin ([Neurontin][1] 600 mg or more daily).

[1] Not FDA approved for this indication.

References

Antonarakis ES, Feng Z, BJet al. Trock, et al: The natural history of metastatic progression in men with prostate-specific antigen recurrence after radical prostatectomy: long-term follow-up, *BJU Int* 109:32–39, 2012.

De Marzo AM, Platz EA, Sutcliffe Set al, et al: Inflammation in prostate carcinogenesis, *Nat Rev Cancer* 7:256–269, 2007.

Mateo J, Carreira S, Sandhu S, et al: DNA repair defects and olaparib in metastatic prostate cancer, *N Engl J Med* 373:1697–1708, 2015.

Nelson WG, Antonarakis ES, Carter HB, De Marzo AM, DeWeese TL: Prostate cancer. In Niederhuber JE, Armitage JO, Doroshow JH, Kastan MB, Tepper JE, editors: *Abeloff's Clinical Oncology*, 6th edition, Philadelphia, 2018, Churchill Livingstone.

Nelson WG, Brawley OW, Isaacs WB et al.: Health inequity drives disease biology to create disparities in prostate cancer outcomes, *J Clin Invest* 132: e155031, 2022.

Nelson WG, De Marzo AM, Isaacs WB: Prostate cancer, *N Engl J Med* 349:366–381, 2003.

Nuhn P, De Bono JS, Fizazi K, et al: Update on systemic prostate cancer therapies: management of castration-resistant prostate cancer in the era of precision oncology, *Eur Urol* 75:88–99, 2019.

Sanda MG, Dunn RL, Michalski J, et al: Quality of life and satisfaction with outcome among prostate-cancer survivors, *N Engl J Med* 358:1250–1261, 2008.

Siegel RL, Kratzer TB, Giaquinto AM, et al: Cancer statistics, 2025, *CA Cancer J Clin* 75:10–45, 2025.

Viswanathan SR, Ha G, Hoff AM, et al: Structural alterations driving castration-resistant prostate cancer revealed by linked read genome sequencing, *Cell* 174:433–447, 2018.

PROSTATITIS

Method of
Charles Powell, MD

CURRENT DIAGNOSIS

- The workup for prostatitis begins with a thorough history and physical examination as well as a urinalysis and urine culture. Diagnosis is based on symptoms (Figure 1) and tenderness on digital rectal examination. There is a controversial role for prostate massage and culture of expressed prostatic secretions.
- Urinalysis and midstream urine culture are important to distinguish bacterial from nonbacterial causes, but it is not necessary for the diagnosis of prostatitis.
- Prostatitis is categorized as *acute* or *chronic*. It has been further grouped by the National Institute of Diabetes, Digestive, and Kidney disorders (NIDDK), part of the National Institutes of Health (NIH) into four categories: *acute bacterial, chronic bacterial, chronic pelvic pain syndrome* (also called *chronic nonbacterial prostatitis*), and *asymptomatic* (Table 1).
- Chronic prostatitis is defined as duration longer than 3 months and typically manifests with pelvic pain and lower urinary tract symptoms.

CURRENT THERAPY

- The majority of prostatitis falls under the category of chronic prostatitis/chronic pelvic pain syndrome, and monotherapy has not proven effective.
- Fluoroquinolone antibiotics are the first-line therapy for acute and chronic *bacterial* prostatitis, which are thought to comprise <10% of all cases. Ciprofloxacin (Cipro) and levofloxacin (Levaquin) demonstrated cure rates of 73% to 75% in one randomized controlled trial (RCT) with culture-proven prostatitis.
- Trimethoprim/sulfamethoxazole (Bactrim)[1] can be considered first-line therapy, but local antibiotic resistance patterns should be considered before initiating empiric treatment.
- First-generation cephalosporins, doxycycline,[1] tetracycline[1] (not available in most areas), azithromycin (Zithromax),[1] and clarithromycin (Biaxin)[1] are all second-line agents.
- Acute prostatitis may require inpatient admission and intravenous (IV) antibiotics depending on severity and presence of sepsis. Urinary retention may require suprapubic tube urinary drainage as a Foley catheter may worsen prostate inflammation.
- The role of antibiotics in the treatment of *chronic pelvic pain syndrome* is less clear. Treatment directed at *specific phenotypes* has improved outcomes. The UPOINT treatment philosophy (*urinary symptoms, psychosocial dysfunction, organ-specific findings, infection, neurologic/systemic*, and *tenderness of muscle*) has garnered much interest in the urologic community and is used to phenotype subjects and to direct multimodal therapy.

[1] Not FDA approved for this indication.

Epidemiology

The prevalence of prostatitis is approximately 8.2% (range: 2.2% to 9.7%). It accounts for 8% of visits to urologists and up to 1% of visits to primary care physicians. In 2000, the estimated cost

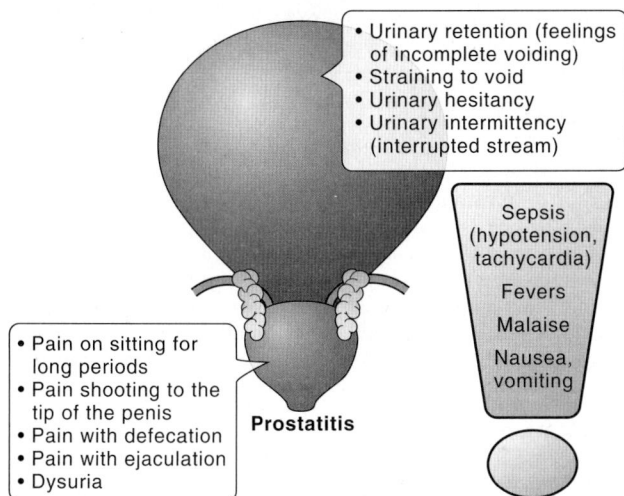

• Urinary retention (feelings of incomplete voiding)
• Straining to void
• Urinary hesitancy
• Urinary intermittency (interrupted stream)

Sepsis (hypotension, tachycardia)
Fevers
Malaise
Nausea, vomiting

Prostatitis

• Pain on sitting for long periods
• Pain shooting to the tip of the penis
• Pain with defecation
• Pain with ejaculation
• Dysuria

Figure 1 Symptoms associated with prostatitis.

TABLE 1	National Institutes of Health Consensus Classification of Prostatitis
CATEGORY	**DESCRIPTION**
I. Acute bacterial prostatitis	Acute infection of the prostate gland with positive urine or semen cultures. Symptoms present for less than 3 months
II. Chronic bacterial prostatitis	Chronic infection of the prostate gland with positive urine or semen cultures. Symptoms present for longer than 3 months
III. Chronic pelvic pain syndrome	Chronic pelvic pain in the absence of bacterial infection localized to the prostate. Symptoms present for longer than 3 months
A. Inflammatory	Significant WBC count in the prostatic secretions, urine, or semen
B. Noninflammatory	Insignificant WBC count in the prostatic secretions, urine, or semen
IV. Asymptomatic prostatitis	WBC count elevated and/or bacteria in the prostatic secretions, urine, semen, or histologic specimens of prostate tissue

to diagnose and treat prostatitis was $84 million, not including pharmaceutical spending.

Risk Factors
The risk factors for prostatitis include urinary tract infection, elevated postvoid residual (urinary retention), recent history of prostate biopsy, urinary catheterization, unprotected anal intercourse, recent urethral instrumentation such as cystoscopy, and condom catheter use.

Pathophysiology
Prostatitis is commonly associated with infection but can also describe non-infectious chronic pelvic pain as well as asymptomatic histologic evidence of sterile inflammation. The causes for acute and chronic *bacterial* prostatitis include prior genitourinary infections such as epididymitis/orchitis, infection resulting from prostate needle biopsy, and recent urinary tract infection. Other predisposing factors include obstruction of urine from urethral stricture, benign prostatic hyperplasia (BPH), or neurogenic causes. A causative organism can be found in <10% of prostatitis cases. The causative organisms include *Escherichia coli* (most common at 65% to 80% of infections), *Pseudomonas aeruginosa*, *Serratia* species, *Klebsiella* species, and *Enterobacter aerogenes*. Gram-positive organisms include enterococci. Organisms isolated from patients with a recent history of lower urinary tract instrumentation or manipulation exhibit more resistance to ciprofloxacin and cephalosporins. For these patients, ciprofloxacin is often inadequate. A combination of cephalosporins and aminoglycosides is appropriate. Patients with a history of HIV infection should prompt investigation for atypical pathogens. The cause of chronic pelvic pain syndrome/chronic nonbacterial prostatitis (NIH category 3) is less well understood, as is asymptomatic prostatitis (NIH category 4).

Prevention
Prophylactic antibiotic dose is appropriate before urologic procedures, particularly prostate needle biopsy according to the American Urological Association Best Practice Statement for Urologic Surgery (http://www.auanet.org). Preprocedure rectal swabs to assess resistance patterns are now considered in select cases in which resistance is more likely.

Clinical Manifestations
Figure 1 details some of the symptoms of prostatitis, separated by domain.

Diagnosis
Diagnosis of acute and chronic bacterial prostatitis is primarily based on history, physical examination, urine culture, and urine specimen testing pre– and post–prostatic massage. If acute bacterial prostatitis is suspected, prostatic massage should not be performed as this might be harmful. Sexually active men younger than 35 years of age and older men who engage in high-risk sexual behaviors should be tested for *Neisseria gonococcus* and *Chlamydia trachomatis* as well. The presence of leukocytes in the semen, first-void urine, midstream urine, expressed prostatic secretions, or post-prostatic massage urine did not correlate with symptoms when studied in a prospective manner. Bacterial localization studies, such as the Meares-Stamey four-glass test, are useful in subcategorizing type 3 chronic pelvic pain syndrome but have unclear significance in the acute clinical setting.

Differential Diagnosis
The differential diagnosis of prostatitis includes acute cystitis, BPH, prostate cancer, urinary tract stones, bladder cancer, prostatic abscess, enterovesical fistula, foreign body within the urinary tract, voiding dysfunction, and inflammatory conditions of the bladder such as interstitial cystitis/painful bladder syndrome.

Therapy (or Treatment)
Treatment depends on the NIH-NIDDK Prostatitis Classification Category. For those with acute prostatitis, oral ciprofloxacin (Cipro)[1] 500 mg orally, twice daily for 4 to 6 weeks or levofloxacin (Levaquin)[1] 500 mg orally, once daily for 4 to 6 weeks is appropriate for nonseptic-appearing patients. Trimethoprim/sulfamethoxazole (Bactrim, Septra),[1] 160 mg/800 mg orally twice daily for 4 to 6 weeks is also appropriate, depending on local antibiotic resistance patterns. Patients who appear septic (hypotension, tachycardia, high fevers) should be admitted to the hospital and started on broad-spectrum antibiotics such as ampicillin 2 g IV every 6 hours and

---

[1] Not FDA approved for this indication.

an aminoglycoside such as gentamicin 1 mg/kg IV every 8 hours. Aminoglycosides should be monitored and adjusted based on serum peak and trough levels. Aminoglycosides should be used cautiously in patients with azotemia. Prostatic abscess should be considered if patients do not improve within 24 to 48 hours. Prostatic abscesses are urologic emergencies and can be drained with transurethral resection of the prostate, ultrasound-guided transrectal needle drainage, or CT-guided needle drainage. Urinary retention should be treated with suprapubic catheter drainage in cases of acute prostatitis. Chronic bacterial prostatitis (CBP) is treated with the same oral agents as acute bacterial prostatitis. For the treatment of chronic pelvic pain syndrome (CPPS) antibiotics play a less clear role, but fluoroquinolone antibiotics used empirically for 4 to 6 weeks have been effective in previously untreated patients. There is little value to repeated courses of antibiotics if the first course is not effective. There is conflicting evidence for alpha blockers such as tamsulosin (Flomax 0.4 mg orally once per night)[1]. The interested reader is referred to a 2010 review by Nickel wherein a multidisciplinary approach is advocated, taking into account a more detailed six-domain phenotype with therapy directed at the relevant phenotype(s). This is known as UPOINT. These phenotype domains include *u*rinary symptoms (divided into voiding and storage symptoms), *p*sychosocial dysfunction (divided into depression and catastrophizing), *o*rgan-specific findings (divided into bladder and prostate), *i*nfection (noted in the urine or expressed prostatic secretions), *n*eurologic (divided into focal and systemic), and *t*enderness (of muscle). Categorizing patients according to these domains may allow clinicians to personalize treatment using a multimodal approach involving physical therapy, psychiatry, and medication.

Other therapies have been described with low-quality evidence for efficacy. These are included here as an alternative treatment option for patients who do not respond to the interventions and strategies outlined earlier. The 5-alpha reductase inhibitors (finasteride [Proscar][1]) have demonstrated slight improvement over placebo in two underpowered RCTs, but carry a 10% to 15% risk of adverse events including "partial impotence." Chronic opioid therapy (COT) is appealing to some, but as the U.S. Centers for Disease Control and Prevention (CDC) has noted, the harms outweigh the benefits for most causes of chronic pain, and its use should be discouraged. Celecoxib (Celebrex)[1] has demonstrated no benefit over placebo in one RCT utilizing the National Institutes of Health Chronic Prostatitis Symptom Index (NIH-CPSI) as the validated endpoint. Allopurinol (Zyloprim)[1] has demonstrated a slight benefit versus placebo in an underpowered RCT that utilized a nonvalidated questionnaire as the clinical endpoint. Pentosan polysulfate (Elmiron)[1] has demonstrated a slight benefit in the NIH-CPSI quality-of-life domain compared with placebo, but not in other endpoints. In this study, 22 of 100 men (22%) withdrew from the study because of adverse events such as diarrhea, headache, and nausea. Transurethral microwave therapy (TUMT) of the prostate, a treatment for BPH, has been noted in one very small RCT (*n* = 20) comparing sham treatment versus TUMT. This study reported 7 of 10 patients having at least 50% improvement, measured by a nonvalidated "global assessment" endpoint. Transurethral resection of the prostate (TURP) has also been discussed, but no RCT exists with the intent to treat men with chronic prostatitis. It is an untested option for men in whom all other treatment modalities have failed, but it has a long history of ameliorating obstructive and irritative lower urinary tract symptoms (LUTS) that often accompany CP/CPPS. Investigators have noted some non-randomized benefit to administration of 200 units onabotulinumtoxin A (Botox)[1] directly into the prostate. They report that 72% of 42 nonrandomized men responded at 3 months compared with 0% who underwent cystoscopy alone.

[1] Not FDA approved for this indication.

The improvement decreased to 37% at 12 months, which is not surprising because the medication loses efficacy 6 to 12 months after administration.

Monitoring

Monitoring is based on symptoms. In cases of acute prostatitis treated with appropriate antibiotics, persistent fevers should prompt a workup for prostatic abscess. The NIH-CPSI patient-reported questionnaire can be used to quantify symptoms over time. It is available online at https://www.ncbi.nlm.nih.gov/pmc/articles/PMC2736311. PSA testing plays no role in the treatment or monitoring of prostatitis, but it should be considered if risk factors for prostate cancer are present such as a prostate nodule or family history. PSA testing is affected by acute inflammation and should be postponed until a few months after the symptoms of prostatitis have resolved.

Complications

Acute prostatitis can progress to urosepsis and hypotension. Chronic bacterial prostatitis might have the ability to progress to chronic pelvic pain syndrome and become a source of pain for years.

References

Abdel-Meguid TA, Mosli HA, Farsi H, et al: Treatment of refractory category III nonbacterial chronic prostatitis/chronic pelvic pain syndrome with intraprostatic injection of onabotulinumtoxinA: a prospective controlled study, *Can J Urol* 25(2):9273–9280, 2018.

Bowen DK, Dilubanza E, Schaefer A: Chronic Bacterial Prostatitis and Chronic Pelvic Pain Syndrome, *Clinical Evidence* 8:1802, 2015.

Bundrick W, Heron SP, Ray P, et al: Levofloxacin versus ciprofloxacin in the treatment of chronic bacterial prostatitis: a randomized double-blind multicenter study, *Urology* 62:537–541, 2003.

Collins M, Stafford RS, O'Leary MP, et al: How common is prostatitis? A national survey of physician visits, *J Urol* 159(4):1224–1228, 1998.

Ha US, Kim ME, Kim CS, et al: Acute bacterial prostatitis in Korea: clinical outcome, including symptoms, management, microbiology and course of disease, *Int J Antimicrob Agents* 31(Suppl 1):S96–101, 2008.

Krieger JN, Lee SW, Jeon J, et al: Epidemiology of prostatitis, *Int J Antimicrob Agents* 31(Suppl 1):S85–90, 2008.

Leskinen M, Lukkarinen O, Marttila T: Effects of finasteride in patients with inflammatory chronic pelvic pain syndrome: a double-blind, placebo-controlled, pilot study, *Urology* 53:502–505, 1999.

Litwin MM, Fowler FJ, Nickel JC, et al: *Prostatitis: The National Institutes of Health Chronic Prostatitis Symptoms Index (NIH-CPSI)*. Retrieved 12/26/2012, 2012, from http://www.prostatitis.org/nih-cpsi.html, 2002.

Litwin M, McNaughton-Collins M, Fowler FJ, et al: The National Institutes of Health chronic prostatitis symptom index: development and validation of a new outcome measure. Chronic Prostatitis Collaborative Research Network, *J Urol* 162(2):369–375, 1999.

Nickel JC, Shoskes DA: Phenotypic approach to the management of the chronic prostatitis/chronic pelvic pain syndrome, *BJU Int* 106(9):1252–1263, 2010.

Nickel JC, Downey J, Pontari MA, et al: A randomized placebo-controlled multicentre study to evaluate the safety and efficacy of finasteride for male chronic pelvic pain syndrome (category IIIA chronic nonbacterial prostatitis), *BJU Int* 93:991–995, 2004.

Nickel JC, Forrest JB, Tomera K, et al: Pentosan polysulfate sodium therapy for men with chronic pelvic pain syndrome: a multicenter, randomized, placebo-controlled study, *J Urol* 173:1252–1255, 2005.

Nickel J, Sorensen R: Transurethral microwave thermotherapy for nonbacterial prostatitis: a randomized double-blind sham controlled study using new prostatitis specific assessment questionnaires, *J Urol* 155:1950–1955, 1996.

Persson B, Ronquist G, Ekblom M: Ameliorative effect of allopurinol on nonbacterial prostatitis: a parallel double-blind controlled study, *J Urol* 155:961–964, 1996.

Pontari MA, Joyce GF, Wise M, et al: Prostatitis, *J Urol* 177(6):2050–2057, 2007.

Roberts RO, Lieber MM, Rhodes T, et al: Prevalence of a physician-assigned diagnosis of prostatitis: the Olmsted County study of urinary symptoms and health status among men, *Urology* 51:578–584, 1998.

Schaeffer AJ, Knauss JS, Landis JR, et al: Leukocyte and bacterial counts do not correlate with severity of symptoms in men with chronic prostatitis: the National Institutes of Health Chronic Prostatitis Cohort Study, *J Urol* 168(3):1048–1053, 2002.

Sharp VJ, Takacs EB, Powell CR: Prostatitis: diagnosis and treatment, *Am Fam Physician* 82(4):397–406, 2010.

Wolf JS, Carol J, Dmochowski RR, et al: Urologic Surgery Antimicrobial Prophylaxis. *Transrectal prostate biopsy*. Retrieved 12/26/2012, 2012, from http://www.auanet.org/content/media/antimicroprop08.pdf, 2008.

Zhao WP, Zhang ZG, Li XD, et al: Celecoxib reduces symptoms in men with difficult chronic pelvic pain syndrome (Category IIIA), *Braz J Med Biol Res* 42:963–967, 2009.

URINARY TRACT INFECTIONS IN THE MALE

Method of
Donald A. Neff, MD

CURRENT DIAGNOSIS

- Urinary tract infection (UTI) can involve any portion of the urinary tract.
- Infection at any site in the urinary tract places the entire system at risk.
- UTIs can be broadly categorized as uncomplicated or complicated.
- Although uncommon, men can have uncomplicated UTI.
- Urologic evaluation is recommended for UTI in young boys.
- Detailed workup of uncomplicated UTI in the adult male is usually not needed.
- Urinalysis is useful to establish presumptive diagnosis.
- Urine culture with sensitivities is helpful to document infection and guide therapy.
- Repeat urine culture after treatment is unnecessary in uncomplicated infections.
- Screening urine cultures in asymptomatic individuals should be avoided.

CURRENT THERAPY

- The goal of treatment is elimination of infection from the urinary tract.
- Prompt initiation of treatment can prevent the spread of infection to other portions of the urinary tract.
- Management of complicated UTI should include imaging of the upper urinary tract.
- Efforts should be made to control underlying risk factors in patients with complicated UTI.
- For complicated UTI, repeat culture after treatment may be helpful to document clearance of infection.

Definitions

Standardized terminology is helpful for communications between providers.

Bacteriuria: Presence of bacteria in the urine. This may be symptomatic or asymptomatic. Asymptomatic bacteriuria may not require treatment.

Pyuria: Presence of white blood cells (WBCs) in the urine. Suggests infection or inflammatory response of the urothelium. Sterile pyuria is lack of bacterial growth in presence of WBCs in the urine and should warrant further investigation to determine the underlying cause.

Urinary tract infection (UTI): Inflammatory response of urothelium to bacterial invasion

Uncomplicated UTI: Infection in a healthy patient with anatomically and functionally normal urinary tract. These infections respond promptly to appropriate treatment.

Complicated UTI: Infection associated with an anatomically or functionally abnormal urinary tract. The host may be immunocompromised. Risk factors for complicated UTI include male gender, advanced age, diabetes, immunosuppression, recent antibiotic use, the presence of an indwelling urinary catheter, recent instrumentation, and recent hospitalization.

Colonization: Presence of bacteriuria in the urine and absence of inflammatory response. Often seen in patients with indwelling urinary catheters. Generally, colonization does not require treatment. Overtreatment of the colonized urinary tract will select for bacterial resistance.

Isolated UTI: Infection in patient with no or remote prior history

Recurrent UTI: Infection that occurs after successful treatment of a prior infection. May be bacterial persistence or reinfection. Persistence is suggested by growth of the same organism. Reinfection usually shows growth of different types of organisms.

Unresolved UTI: Generally due to bacterial persistence. Repeated infection with same organism with similar resistance profile.

Introduction

Urinary tract infections (UTIs) are one of the most common bacterial infections in humans. UTI is defined as an inflammatory response of the urothelium to bacterial invasion. Infections of the urinary tract encompass a wide variety of diagnoses depending on the specific anatomic site of infection, the common denominator being bacterial invasion of genitourinary organs and tissues. Any site within the urinary tract may be involved including the kidney (pyelonephritis), ureters (ureteritis), bladder (cystitis), prostate (prostatitis), epididymis (epididymitis), and urethra (urethritis). Once any part of the urinary tract is infected, the remaining portions of the system are placed at risk for further bacterial invasion. Due in part to the relative rarity of UTI in adult males, evaluation and management of UTI in this population is hampered by lack of high-quality empirical data with which to guide treatment decisions.

Incidence and Epidemiology

UTI in males is not a reportable disease. Therefore, true incidence is difficult to assess in the United States. For both sexes, UTI accounts for 7 million office visits and 400,000 hospitalizations annually. In men, UTI accounts for 0.6% of all office visits. During infancy, the incidence of symptomatic UTIs is higher in boys than in girls, primarily related to circumcision status. Bacteria adhere to the inner prepuce, allowing easier access to the meatus followed by ascending infection. Neonatal circumcision reduces the rate of UTI in boys by over 90%. After the neonatal period, symptomatic UTI is uncommon until middle age. The incidence then increases to approach 10% by age 61, 14% in ages 61 to 70, 26% in ages 71 to 80, and 42% over age 81.

Pathophysiology

In the modern era most infections of the urinary tract occur via the ascending route. This begins with colonization of the perineum, most commonly with fecal bacteria. These bacteria then move from the perineal area to the urethra and to the bladder, ureter, and eventually the kidney. Fecal flora is a common source with *Escherichia coli* being the most common cause of UTIs. *E. coli* accounts for 85% of community acquired and 50% of hospital acquired infections. Hematogenous seeding does occur; however, this is much less likely in anatomically and physiologically normal individuals. The kidney may be secondarily infected by *Staphylococcus aureus* or *Candida fungemia* in this manner. In certain geographic areas, tuberculosis of the urinary tract is still seen and reaches these organs hematogenously. These types of infection are facilitated by prior renal damage or obstruction of the urinary tract.

Adherence of bacteria to the uroepithelium is an essential step in the pathogenesis of UTI. Bacterial virulence factors such as adhesins, type-1 pili, and P pili facilitate adherence to receptors on uroepithelial cells. Some individuals are genetically predisposed to infection, with increased uroepithelial receptivity to adherence of bacteria resulting in increased susceptibility to infection. Once within the bladder, uropathogenic bacteria are internalized into the intracellular space of superficial urothelial cells. In this space, the bacteria are more protected from the immune response and form intracellular bacterial communities, eventually forming protective biofilms. Bacteria then escape from the intracellular space into the urinary lumen, where they readhere and reinvade the uroepithelium. Once the inoculum is sufficient, a host immune response occurs. This response involves multiple cell types including neutrophils, macrophages, and other immunocytes along with associated cytokines. This inflammatory response results in the symptoms of UTI. Indeed, the levels of certain inflammatory factors have been correlated with the severity of symptoms.

The urinary tract has natural defenses in place to resist adherence and ascension of bacteria. Normal urogenital flora form a barrier to colonization by uropathogenic bacteria. Inhibitory urinary factors include osmolality, urea, organic acid concentration, and pH. Uromodulin is a protein present in the urine that binds to type-1 pili, preventing binding of bacteria to the urothelium. Regular and complete emptying of the bladder helps to expel bacteria and keep bacterial inoculum low.

Clinical Manifestations

The specific clinical symptoms of UTI depend on the anatomic site of infection. Urethritis presents with dysuria, urinary urgency and frequency, and penile discharge. The penis may be tender or swollen. Associated inguinal lymphadenopathy may be present. Epididymitis usually presents as unilateral testicular pain that is gradual in onset. The scrotum is swollen, warm, and erythematous. Scrotal cellulitis may be present. Acute prostatitis includes fevers, chills, dysuria, and pelvic pain. Urinary hesitancy and weak stream are often seen due to swelling of the prostate gland and increased resistance of flow through the prostatic urethra. Cystitis is associated with dysuria, urinary urgency, and urinary frequency. There may be associated suprapubic pain or gross hematuria. Pyelonephritis is associated with the classical triad of fevers, chills, and flank pain. In older adults, symptoms may not be as clear. Generalized abdominal pain, increased confusion, and altered mental status may be the presenting signs of UTI in these individuals.

An important consideration is the entity of asymptomatic bacteriuria. In this instance bacteria are able to be identified in a noncontaminated urine culture. However, there is no associated immune response, or the clinical symptoms mentioned above. Indeed, urine is not sterile as has been previously thought, with a normal urinary microbiome present that is difficult to detect on routine culture media.

Prevalence of asymptomatic bacteriuria increases with age and can be seen in up to 15% of men over age 75. In general, asymptomatic bacteriuria should not be treated. The 2019 guidelines of the Infectious Diseases Society of America (IDSA) recommend screening and treatment of men for asymptomatic bacteria only in patients undergoing invasive urologic procedures. Inappropriate treatment of asymptomatic bacteria contributes to antimicrobial resistance.

Differential Diagnosis

The differential diagnosis of UTI should be focused on the anatomic location of symptoms. Urethritis can be caused by multiple organisms, and sexually transmitted diseases should be considered. Lower urinary tract symptoms (urgency, frequency) associated with cystitis can also be seen with bladder stones or bladder tumors. Flank pain may result from urinary tract obstruction due to stone, trauma, or musculoskeletal sources. Sterile pyuria should prompt investigation for stone, tuberculosis, and malignancy. Sterile pyuria may also be associated with nonurologic diagnosis such as appendicitis, diverticulitis, or autoimmune diseases.

Clinical Evaluation

The foundation for evaluation of a patient with UTI remains a thorough history and physical examination. A detailed surgical history is helpful to determine risk factors for complicated UTI. A urinalysis is essential in the evaluation of urinary symptoms and can provide information for a preliminary diagnosis. Normal urine should be free of bacteria and inflammation. False negatives can occur early in the clinical course or when a patient has taken antimicrobial therapy prior to obtaining the urine specimen. False positives may be caused by contamination or over-the-counter remedies such as phenazopyridine (positive nitrites). The decision to send a urine culture should be based on the overall clinical picture. For an uncomplicated UTI, a urine culture is helpful but not required unless the patient fails to improve with treatment. If symptoms fail to improve, or if the patient has risk factors for complicated UTI, a culture is strongly recommended to determine the underlying organism and antimicrobial sensitivities. Proper collection and storage of the urine specimen can minimize the potential for false results.

Localization of bacteria to differentiate the source of an infection within the lower urinary tract of males can be challenging. The Meares-Stamey four-glass urinary tract localization test has been well described. First, the patient is asked to void 5 to 10 cc into a sterile container (VB1). A second, midstream specimen is then obtained (VB2). A prostatic massage is then performed by digital rectal examination (DRE), and the expressed fluids are collected (EPS). Finally, the postprostate massage urine is collected. The four specimens are then sent separately for culture and sensitivity. VB1 represents urethral flora, VB2 represents bladder urine flora, EPS and VB3 represent prostatic flora. The four-glass test can be expensive, cumbersome, and is often of low diagnostic yield. An alternate approach is a modified Meares-Stamey two-glass test, which is easier and less costly to perform. This is performed by collecting a urine specimen premassage and then a second specimen post-massage. The premassage specimen represents bladder flora, and the post-massage specimen represents the prostatic flora.

Due to the rarity of urinary infection in boys outside of the neonatal period, urologic investigation is essential for the evaluation of UTI in the pediatric population to rule out structural abnormalities. These include vesicoureteral reflux, posterior urethral valves, congenital ureteropelvic junction obstruction, ureterocele, and megaureter. Referral to a pediatric urologist should be considered. Early diagnosis and therapy will help prevent scarring and preserve renal function. A history of constipation should be elucidated, as bowel-bladder dysfunction places boys at risk of UTI. The optimal imaging approach to the pediatric patient is controversial. The combination of renal-bladder ultrasound and voiding cystourethrogram (VCUG) has traditionally been used to assess both the upper and lower urinary tracts. In the modern era, provided the renal bladder ultrasound is normal, VCUG may be safely deferred. A nuclear medicine scan can be useful to determine differential renal function and identify the presence of obstruction of the upper urinary tract.

For adults, the use of radiographic investigations is again based on the unique clinical picture of a given patient. For uncomplicated UTI, particularly in otherwise healthy men whose infections resolve easily, detailed investigations, including imaging, are often not necessary. Complicated infections require further investigation to search for a nidus or anatomic abnormality. These include patients with a recurrent or unresolved infection or patients with aforementioned risk factors. Computed tomography (CT) urography is a complete study of the upper urinary tract and includes a noncontrast phase, a nephrographic phase, and delayed images to evaluate the upper urinary drainage system. This study allows for assessment of renal stones, masses, impaired or altered drainage, and is the imaging study of choice in patients with normal renal function. For patients with poor renal function, renal-bladder ultrasound is a reasonable alternative. Measurement of post-void residual is helpful to determine whether retention of urine is causing urinary stasis.

Treatment

Elimination of the infecting organism from the urinary tract is the goal of therapy for UTI. There is limited data to guide duration of treatment of UTI in males, with many treatment strategies extrapolated from studies done in females. Although traditionally men have been considered to always have complicated UTIs, an afebrile man with a first UTI and no complicating factors can be considered to have an uncomplicated UTI.

In general, empirical selection of antimicrobial therapy should be selected to target the pathogen being treated, with local resistance patterns taken into consideration. Uncomplicated infections should be anticipated to resolve promptly with appropriate therapy. Duration of therapy for these types of infections in men is not well established, but 5 to 7 days of treatment is reasonable depending on the agent chosen. Prompt initiation of broad spectrum therapy in complicated UTIs will help prevent further dissemination of the infection and the development of sepsis. Treatment can later be tailored to the results of culture and sensitivities. These infections require longer duration of therapy, 10 to 14 days. In the setting of multidrug-resistant isolates, parenteral therapy may be required for the duration of treatment. For patients with bacterial persistence after treatment, a thorough urologic evaluation should be made, followed by an attempt to eliminate the source of bacteria if possible.

Monitoring and Prevention

In most patients with UTI, routine repeat culture of urine after therapy is not indicated. However, if patients thought to have uncomplicated UTI do not improve as expected, a urine culture should be obtained to guide therapy. Similarly, rapid recurrence of symptoms after initial improvement should prompt repeat urine culture. Antibiotic prophylaxis in males is generally not warranted, and prevention should be directed at elimination or treatment of the underlying cause if possible. For example, initiation of medications in patients with incomplete bladder emptying due to BPH, or treatment of an infected urinary stone would be of higher yield than suppressive antibiotics.

Management of Complications

Complications in patients with UTI should be managed according to the clinical setting. The decision to admit a patient to the hospital is dictated by multiple factors. Nontoxic patients who can take PO medications may be safely managed as outpatients. Immunosuppressed or diabetic patients may warrant admission for observation. These patients and those with other risk factors for complicated UTI may progress rapidly to sepsis, and admission to the intensive care unit (ICU) may be necessary. Patients who develop perinephric or prostatic abscess will require either percutaneous or surgical drainage.

Special Considerations

Patients with chronic indwelling catheters will nearly always be colonized. Screening cultures are not indicated and should be avoided. In general, bacterial colonization of the urinary tract should not be treated unless symptoms develop. It is often counterproductive to attempt clearance of bacteria in this population as overtreatment will select for bacterial resistance. Further, elimination of benign colonizing bacteria from the urinary tract in these individuals often allows more virulent bacteria to establish residence. Antimicrobial prophylaxis is not indicated. Treatment strategies in these individuals should be focused on the underlying factors leading to the need for catheter drainage. These include institution of clean intermittent catheterization when possible, or more frequent changing of the catheter if necessary.

Another special consideration is the presence of a bacterial UTI in an obstructed urinary system. This most commonly occurs when a kidney stone causes ureteral obstruction in the setting of pyelonephritis. These patients can rapidly progress to sepsis. Prompt drainage of the affected renal unit either by ureteral stent or by percutaneous nephrostomy tube, along with institution of appropriate antimicrobial therapy, is essential in the management of these patients.

References

Detweiler K, et al: Bacteria and urinary infections in the elderly, *Urol Clin North Am* 42(4):561–568, 2015.

Foxman B: Epidemiology of urinary tract infections: incidence, morbidity, and economic costs, *Am J Med* 113(Suppl 1A):5S–13S, 2002.

Nicolle L: Asymptomatic bacteriuria: when to screen and when to treat, *Infect Dis Clin North Am* 17(2):367–394, 2003.

Nicolle L: Uncomplicated urinary tract infection in adults including uncomplicated pyelonephritis, *Urol Clin North Am* 35:1–12, 2008.

Nicolle L, et al: *Clinical Practice Guideline for the Management of Asymptomatic Bacteriuria: 2019 update by the Infectious Diseases Society of America*, Available at: https:// https://www.idsociety.org/practice-guideline/asymptomatic-bacteriuria/. Accessed February 28, 2021.

Schappert SM: Ambulatory care visits of physician offices, hospital outpatient departments, and emergency departments: United States, 1995, *Vital Health Stat* 13:1–38, 1997.

Simmering JE, et al: *The increase in hospitalizations for urinary tract infections and the associated costs in the United States, 1998–2011 open forum infectious diseases. 2017 winter*, 4(1). Available at: https://www.ncbi.nlm.nih.gov/pmc/articles/PMC5414046/. Accessed February 28, 2021.

Subcommittee on Urinary Tract Infection: Reaffirmation of AAP Clinical Practice Guideline: the diagnosis and management of the initial urinary tract infection in febrile infants and young children 2–24 months of age, *Pediatrics* 138(6), 2016.

Schaeffer MD Anthony J, et al: Infections of the urinary tract. In Wein AJ, editor: *Campbell-Walsh Urology* Elsevier, pp 237–303, 2015.

17 Women's Health

ABNORMAL UTERINE BLEEDING

Method of
Sarina Schrager, MD, MS

CURRENT DIAGNOSIS

- Anovulation and pelvic structural abnormalities are the most common causes of abnormal vaginal bleeding in reproductive-age women.
- All women with abnormal bleeding should have a pregnancy test.
- A pelvic ultrasound will detect many structural causes of abnormal bleeding.
- Either a pelvic ultrasound or endometrial biopsy is appropriate for evaluation of postmenopausal bleeding.

CURRENT THERAPY

- Unstable women with acute heavy vaginal bleeding should be admitted to hospital for intravenous (IV) estrogen therapy (Premarin) or surgical intervention.
- Treatment of anovulatory bleeding includes ovulation induction if a woman desires pregnancy and hormonal cycle control if she does not.
- Anovulatory women are at risk for endometrial hyperplasia or carcinoma due to unopposed estrogen and should have regular progesterone-induced withdrawal bleeds.
- Treatment of menorrhagia can include nonsteroidal anti-inflammatory drugs (NSAIDs), tranexamic acid (Lysteda), or insertion of a levonorgestrel IUD.

TABLE 1	Causes of Abnormal Uterine Bleeding (ACOG)
PALM (structural causes) Polyp Adenomyosis Leiomyoma Malignancy and hyperplasia	**COEIN (non-structural causes)** Coagulopathy Ovulatory dysfunction Endometrial Iatrogenic Not yet classified

TABLE 2	Signs and Symptoms of Ovulatory Cycles
Regular cycle length	Presence of premenstrual syndrome (PMS)
Dysmenorrhea	Mittelschmerz (pain at ovulation)
Changes in cervical mucus	Biphasic temperature curve
Premenstrual breast tenderness	Positive test result from luteinizing hormone (LH) predictor kit

Epidemiology

Abnormal vaginal bleeding is a common complaint in primary care. The prevalence of some type of abnormal bleeding is between 10% and 30% among women of reproductive age. Anovulatory bleeding is more common in women who are perimenopausal and who are overweight. The estimated direct and indirect costs of abnormal bleeding are $1 billion and $12 billion annually, respectively. Abnormal bleeding is also a common reason for women to be referred to gynecologists and is an indication for up to 25% of all gynecologic surgery.

Pathophysiology

Normal menstrual bleeding is defined as regular vaginal bleeding that occurs at intervals from every 21 to 35 days. A normal menstrual cycle is ovulatory, with two distinct phases: the follicular phase and the luteal phase. The follicular phase is the first half of the cycle. The luteal phase occurs after ovulation, when the corpus luteum develops in anticipation of a possible pregnancy. Table 1 defines vocabulary to describe different patterns of abnormal bleeding.

The pathologic abnormality in anovulatory cycles is a lack of ovulation, which produces an unopposed estrogen state. The luteal phase of the menstrual cycle is dominated by progesterone, which is only produced after ovulation. This lack of progesterone contributes to irregular endometrial growth and nonuniform bleeding. In a normal cycle, the entire endometrium sloughs off during menstruation. In an anovulatory cycle, different sections of endometrium outgrow their blood supply at different times and bleed erratically. Anovulatory bleeding (also referred to as dysfunctional uterine bleeding) is unpredictable in timing and amount of bleeding.

The most common structural abnormalities that cause abnormal bleeding are endometrial polyps, leiomyomas, adenomyosis, and hyperplasia or malignancy.

Abnormal bleeding is also common in women who use hormonal contraception, usually due to endometrial abnormalities from exogenous hormones. Women who take combination estrogen/progestin contraception often have intermenstrual bleeding for the first 3 months of treatment. Missed pills are a very frequent cause of abnormal bleeding. In women using progestin-only methods, the abnormal bleeding usually is caused by progestin-induced endometrial atrophy.

Diagnosis

All women with abnormal bleeding should have a thorough history and physical examination and a pregnancy test. If the pregnancy test is negative, the next step is to determine whether her cycles are ovulatory or anovulatory. Table 2 describes characteristics of ovulatory cycles. Laboratory evaluation includes looking for causes of anovulation (Table 3), assessing for anemia with a hemoglobin and hematocrit level, and consideration of getting a pelvic ultrasound to look for structural abnormalities.

In menorrhagia, evaluation for a coagulation disorder (most commonly von Willebrand disease), liver failure, or chronic renal failure is also indicated. Evaluation in an acute bleeding episode (usually due to anovulatory bleeding) should include a hemoglobin and hematocrit if the bleeding is heavy, assessment of volume status, and an endometrial biopsy. Postmenopausal bleeding is

1259

TABLE 3	Causes of Anovulatory Cycles

Hypothalamic
- Weight loss
- Eating disorders
- Relative energy deficiency in sport (RED-S)
- Chronic illness
- Stress
- Excessive exercise

Polycystic ovary syndrome

Thyroid disorders

Hyperprolactinemia

Idiopathic chronic anovulation

Medication-induced (i.e., after discontinuation of hormonal contraceptives)

TABLE 4	Clinical Evaluation of a Woman With Abnormal Bleeding

OVULATORY BLEEDING	ANOVULATORY BLEEDING
History, physical examination, pregnancy test	History, physical examination, pregnancy test
In menorrhagia: • Consideration of liver function tests, BUN/Cr, CBC, coagulation profile • Pelvic ultrasound or pelvic MRI to exclude uterine fibroids • Sonohysterogram to exclude polyps or adenomyosis • Endometrial biopsy (especially if age >45) to exclude endometrial hyperplasia	Laboratory studies: • TSH • Prolactin • CBC (if acute bleeding episode or frequent heavy bleeding) • Consideration of endometrial biopsy (especially if age >45) to exclude hyperplasia or malignancy • Evaluation for other symptoms of PCOS
In intermenstrual bleeding: • Pap smear, cervical cultures	Screen for eating disorder, stress, female athlete triad

BUN/Cr, Blood urea nitrogen/creatinine; CBC, complete blood count; Pap, Papanicolaou smear; PCOS, polycystic ovary syndrome; TSH, thyroid-stimulating hormone.

TABLE 5	Treatment Options for Abnormal Vaginal Bleeding

Anovulation: cycle control with estrogen/progestin contraception, DMPA, levonorgestrel IUD (Mirena), or scheduled progestin-induced withdrawal bleeds, ovulation induction with clomiphene citrate (Clomid) or letrozole (Femara)[1], and referral to gynecologist if pregnancy desired

Acute bleeding episode—outpatient: administration of high-dose OCPs (up to 4 per day) for 5–7 days with subsequent continuous cycling with OCPs for at least 1 month, administration of oral estrogen to acutely stop bleeding, or administration of oral progesterone to acutely stop bleeding

Acute bleeding episode—inpatient: IVF, supportive care, IV estrogen therapy, consultation for surgical intervention

Menorrhagia—treatment with NSAIDs, tranexamic acid (Lysteda), insertion of levonorgestrel IUD, referral for endometrial ablation or surgical treatment of structural abnormality

On combination estrogen/progestin contraception: supportive care for first 3 months, assessment of adherence to pill regimen, add supplemental estrogen, change to a method with a higher dose of estrogen or a different class of progestin, or consider changing to patches or vaginal ring.

On progestin-only contraception: add supplemental estrogen or combination oral contraceptive pill and NSAID to decrease bleeding

[1]Not FDA approved for this indication.
DMPA, Depot medroxyprogesterone acetate (Depo-Provera); IUD, intrauterine device; IV, intravenous; IVF, intravenous fluids; NSAID, nonsteroidal antiinflammatory drug; OCP, oral contraceptive pill.

levonorgestrel IUD [Kyleena, Liletta, Mirena, Skyla]) are all effective treatments (Table 5).

Treatment of women with abnormal bleeding on OCPs involves education and support to try to get them through the first 3 months on the pills. After that, consideration of supplemental estrogen, changing to a higher dose of an estrogen pill, changing to a pill with a different class of progestin, use of a supplemental NSAID to decrease the amount of bleeding, decreasing the hormone free interval, or changing to a nonhormonal type of contraception are all potential treatments.

related to an increased risk of endometrial hyperplasia and cancer and should be evaluated with a transvaginal ultrasound to look at the endometrial thickness (under 4 mm is reassuring) or an office endometrial biopsy. Table 4 describes the steps in evaluation of a woman with abnormal bleeding.

Treatment

If a woman presents with heavy bleeding and exhibits any signs or symptoms of hypovolemia, she should be admitted to the hospital and either treated with IV conjugated estrogen (Premarin) to stop the bleeding or have a surgical procedure (such as dilation and curettage). If the bleeding is heavy but the woman is stable and her hemoglobin and hematocrit are close to normal, outpatient treatment with high-dose oral contraceptive pills (OCPs), estrogen, cyclic progesterone, NSAIDs, or tranexamic acid (Lysteda) is indicated. Women with structural abnormalities causing menorrhagia should be referred for possible surgical treatment.

Treatment of women with ovulatory bleeding is indicated if the woman is anemic or is bothered by her bleeding pattern. However, treatment of anovulation with some type of progesterone is necessary to reduce the risk of endometrial hyperplasia or carcinoma. All women with chronic anovulation should have regular progesterone-induced withdrawal bleed. OCPs, monthly cycling of progesterone, and continuous administration of progestin contraception (e.g., depot medroxyprogesterone acetate [Depo-Provera] or

References

Abdel-Aleem H, d'Arcangues C, Vogelsong KM, et al: Treatment of vaginal bleeding irregularities induced by progestin only contraceptives, *Cochrane Database Syst Rev*(4), 2007. CD003449.

ACOG: Practice bulletin no 128: Diagnosis of abnormal uterine bleeding in reproductive-aged women, *Obstet Gynecol* 120:197–206, 2012.

ACOG: Practice bulletin no. 136. Management of abnormal uterine bleeding associated with ovulatory dysfunction. *Obstet Gynecol* 122(1):176–185, 2013.

Bofill Rodriguez M, Dias S, Jordan V, et al: Interventions for heavy menstrual bleeding; overview of Cochrane reviews and network meta-analysis, *Cochrane Database Syst Rev* 31;5(5):CD013180, 2022.

Bofill Rodriguez M, Lethaby A, Low C, Cameron IT: Cyclical progestogens for heavy menstrual bleeding. *Cochrane Database Syst Rev* 8(8):CD001016, 2019. https://doi.org/10.1002/14651858.CD001016.pub3.

Bryant-Smith AC, Lethaby A, Farquhar C, Hickey M: Antifibrinolytics for heavy menstrual bleeding. *Cochrane Database Syst Rev* 4(4):CD000249, 2018. https://doi.org/10.1002/14651858.CD000249.pub2.

Creinin MD, Barnhart KT, Gawron LM, et al: Heavy menstrual bleeding treatment with a levonorgestrel 52-mg intrauterine device. *Obstet Gynecol* 141(5):971–978, 2023.

Ely JW, Kennedy CM, Clark EC, et al: Abnormal uterine bleeding: a management algorithm, *J Am Board Fam Med* 19:590–602, 2006.

Lethaby A, Wise MR, Weterings MA, et al: Combined hormonal contraceptives for heavy menstrual bleeding, *Cochrane Database Syst Rev* 11;2(2):CD000154, 2019.

Liu Z, Doan QV, Blumenthal P, et al: A systematic review evaluating health-related quality of life, work impairment, and health-care costs and utilization in abnormal uterine bleeding, *Value Health* 10:183–194, 2007.

Naoulou B, Tsai MC: Efficacy of tranexamic acid in the treatment of idiopathic and non-functional heavy menstrual bleeding: a systematic review, *Acta Obstet Gynecol* 91:529–537, 2012.

Sangkomkamhang US, Lumbiganon P, Pattanittum P: Progestogens or progestogen-releasing intrauterine systems for uterine fibroids (other than preoperative medical therapy). *Cochrane Database Syst Rev* 11(11):CD008994, 2020. https://doi.org/10.1002/14651858.CD008994.pub3.

Schrager S, Fox K, Lee R: Abnormal uterine bleeding associated with hormonal contraception, *Am Fam Physician* 109(2):161–166, 2024.

Sweet MG, Schmidt-Dalton TA, Weiss PM, et al: Evaluation and management of abnormal uterine bleeding in premenopausal women, *Am Fam Physician* 85:35–43, 2012.

Wouk N, Helton M: Abnormal Uterine Bleeding Premenopausal Women. *Am Fam Physician* 99(7):435–443, 2019.

AMENORRHEA

Method of
Colleen Loo-Gross, MD, MPH

CURRENT DIAGNOSIS

- In the absence of physiologic causes (e.g., pregnancy, lactation, and menopause), four conditions account for the majority of amenorrhea cases: polycystic ovary syndrome, hypothalamic amenorrhea, hyperprolactinemia, and primary ovarian insufficiency.
- Most causes of amenorrhea can be identified through a detailed history, physical examination, and laboratory evaluation.
- Müllerian agenesis is the most common cause of anatomic malformations associated with amenorrhea.
- In the evaluation of amenorrhea, it is important to exclude physiologic causes such as pregnancy and lactation, as well as potential iatrogenic causes (e.g., hormonal contraception, chemotherapy and radiation therapy, and medications that may cause hyperprolactinemia).
- Initial laboratory evaluation should include follicle-stimulating hormone (FSH), thyroid-stimulating hormone (TSH), and prolactin levels.
- In amenorrheic women less than 40 years of age, an elevated FSH level in the menopausal range indicates primary ovarian insufficiency.
- A low or normal FSH value in amenorrhea without evidence of anatomic cause suggests chronic anovulation, most commonly attributed to hypothalamic amenorrhea or polycystic ovary syndrome.
- In cases of elevated prolactin level (with no evidence of thyroid disease), MRI is warranted to assess for a possible pituitary tumor.

CURRENT THERAPY

- The underlying cause of amenorrhea should be treated accordingly.
- For those with an estrogen deficient state, cyclic hormone therapy may be indicated, and adequate calcium and vitamin D intake are essential to reduce the risk of osteoporosis.
- Fertility considerations should be addressed in all causes of amenorrhea.
- Psychosocial support, such as counseling services and peer support groups, is an important aspect of management.

Amenorrhea is defined as the absence of menses. Its prevalence, when not related to pregnancy or lactation, is approximately 3% to 4% among premenopausal women. Amenorrhea is further categorized into primary amenorrhea (prior to menarche) and secondary amenorrhea (following menarche). Evaluation for primary amenorrhea should be initiated when menarche has not occurred by 15 years of age, or sooner for females without onset of menses within 5 years of thelarche. Evaluation should also be considered when thelarche has not occurred by 13 years of age. Secondary amenorrhea is the lack of menses for 3 months in females with preceding regular cycles or 6 months in those with irregular menstrual cycles.

Etiology

There are a number of potential etiologies of amenorrhea. In the absence of physiologic causes (e.g., pregnancy, lactation, and menopause), four conditions account for the majority of amenorrhea cases: polycystic ovary syndrome (PCOS), hypothalamic amenorrhea, hyperprolactinemia, and primary ovarian insufficiency. The approximate frequency of common causes of primary and secondary amenorrhea are shown in Tables 1 and 2. Other considerations may also include adrenal disease, adrenal hyperplasia, chronic disease, Cushing syndrome, androgen-secreting tumors, central nervous system infections, and a history of trauma (such as traumatic brain injury).

With primary amenorrhea, anatomic defects and chromosomal abnormalities (with associated primary ovarian insufficiency) are often causative factors. Anatomic abnormalities may cause amenorrhea due to obstruction along the genital outflow tract. With Müllerian agenesis, incomplete development of the Müllerian duct embryologically results in a range of defects due to agenesis or atresia of the uterus and/or vagina, though ovarian function is usually unaffected. Müllerian agenesis is a common cause of primary amenorrhea among females who present with normal signs of adrenarche and breast development. In primary ovarian insufficiency, amenorrhea occurs as the result of ovarian follicle depletion or dysfunction. It comprises 2% to 10% of cases of amenorrhea.

Excluding pregnancy, the most common causes of secondary amenorrhea are hypothalamic amenorrhea and PCOS. Functional hypothalamic amenorrhea occurs in the presence of hypothalamic-pituitary-ovarian axis suppression, without evidence of organic cause. In these cases, the regulatory pulsatile secretion of gonadotropin-releasing hormone (GnRH) is affected, leading to abnormally low levels of estrogen.

Evaluation

Most causes of amenorrhea can be identified through a detailed history, physical examination, and laboratory evaluation. It is important to exclude physiologic causes of amenorrhea such as pregnancy and lactation, as well as potential iatrogenic causes (for example, hormonal contraception, chemotherapy and radiation therapy, and medications that may cause hyperprolactinemia such as antipsychotics, antidepressants, opiates, and metoclopramide [Reglan]). The incidence of amenorrhea is approximately 12% in women taking antipsychotic medications, due to the resultant increase in prolactin levels.

History

Obtaining a detailed history is an important component in the evaluation of amenorrhea. The presence of vasomotor symptoms, such as hot flashes, may be indicators of primary ovarian insufficiency, whereas reports of headache or vision changes may prompt further evaluation for possible central nervous system tumor or empty sella syndrome. Women with anatomic causes of amenorrhea, such as transverse vaginal septum, imperforate hymen, and isolated absence of the vagina or cervix, may report cyclic pelvic pain, which occurs due to blood accumulation behind the outflow tract obstruction and in some cases, associated endometriosis. Anosmia may be an indication of the rare Kallmann syndrome, which presents with amenorrhea due to GnRH deficiency and is associated with abnormal development of the olfactory bulb.

Additional history details should include assessment of mood and stress, weight changes, nutrition and eating patterns, and exercise routines, with evaluation for a possible eating disorder or other cause of an overall energy deficit. Abnormal historical findings such as these may be suggestive of functional hypothalamic amenorrhea. It is also important to assess for signs or symptoms of thyroid disease and of other potential chronic medical conditions.

Family history may also provide useful information. A positive family history for delayed menarche may suggest constitutional delay of puberty as the cause of amenorrhea, though this is considered a diagnosis of exclusion. A family history of primary ovarian insufficiency is also worth noting, given the related genetic predisposition. Moreover, early menopause in family members is a risk factor associated with primary ovarian insufficiency.

TABLE 1	Common Causes of Primary Amenorrhea	
CATEGORY	**APPROXIMATE FREQUENCY (%)**	
Breast development present	30	
Müllerian agenesis	10	
Androgen insensitivity	9	
Transverse vaginal septum	2	
Imperforate hymen	1	
Constitutional delay of puberty	8	
No breast development: high FSH	40	
46,XX	15	
46,XY	5	
Abnormal karyotype	20	
No breast development: low FSH	30	
Constitutional delay of puberty	10	
Prolactinoma	5	
Kallmann syndrome	2	
Other CNS etiology	3	
Stress, weight loss, eating disorders	3	
Polycystic ovary syndrome	3	
Congenital adrenal hyperplasia	3	
Other	1	

CNS, Central nervous system; FSH, follicle-stimulating hormone.
Adapted from Practice Committee of American Society for Reproductive Medicine. Current evaluation of amenorrhea. *Fertil Steril.* 2008;90:S219–S225.

TABLE 2	Common Causes of Secondary Amenorrhea	
CATEGORY	**APPROXIMATE FREQUENCY (%)**	
Low or normal FSH	66	
Stress, weight loss, eating disorders		
Non-specific hypothalamic causes		
Chronic anovulation, including PCOS		
Hypothyroidism		
Cushing syndrome		
Pituitary tumor, empty sella, Sheehan syndrome		
Gonadal failure: high FSH	12	
46,XX		
Abnormal karyotype		
Hyperprolactinemia	13	
Anatomic	7	
Asherman syndrome (intrauterine synechiae)		
Other hyperandrogenic states	2	
Ovarian tumor		
Non-classic congenital adrenal hyperplasia		
Undiagnosed		

FSH, Follicle-stimulating hormone; PCOS, polycystic ovary syndrome.
Adapted from Practice Committee of American Society for Reproductive Medicine. Current evaluation of amenorrhea. *Fertil Steril.* 2008;90:S219–S225.

Physical Examination

About 15% of those with primary amenorrhea have an abnormality noted on genital examination. Both internal and external genitalia should be examined. A shortened vagina is associated with conditions such as Müllerian agenesis (which may present with a range of defects resulting from incomplete embryologic development of the Müllerian duct), imperforate hymen, transverse vaginal septum, cervical atresia, or other uterine anomalies. In some cases, the vagina may appear as no more than a small dimple.

Additional physical findings may also help guide the evaluation of amenorrhea. Dysmorphic features should be noted, such as a webbed neck or short stature, which may be suggestive of Turner syndrome. Galactorrhea may warrant evaluation for a pituitary tumor. Clinical evidence of self-induced vomiting may be suggestive of a hypothalamic etiology of amenorrhea.

The physical examination should further assess for secondary sexual characteristics, such as the presence of pubic hair and also breast development, which is an indicator of endogenous estrogen effect. Conversely, the presence of thin vaginal mucosa is a sign of low endogenous estrogen level. Signs of hirsutism, acne, and male pattern alopecia are indicators of androgen excess, which may suggest hyperandrogenic etiologies of amenorrhea such as PCOS. Body mass index (BMI) also helps to differentiate PCOS from other causes of amenorrhea (such as functional disorders of the hypothalamus) given its typical presentation with obesity.

Laboratory Studies

When the etiology of amenorrhea is not evident after completing a thorough history and physical examination, additional assessment is warranted. Initial laboratory evaluation should include levels of follicle-stimulating hormone (FSH), thyroid-stimulating hormone (TSH), and prolactin. Abnormal thyroid levels should be managed accordingly. An elevated prolactin level without apparent cause necessitates further investigation with diagnostic imaging of the pituitary gland.

In amenorrheic women less than 40 years of age, an elevated FSH level in the menopausal range indicates primary ovarian insufficiency. The FSH level should be repeated at least 1 month following the initial result for confirmation. For women less than 30 years of age with identified primary ovarian insufficiency, a karyotype should be obtained to assess for possible chromosomal abnormality. Karyotype analysis may be considered for those over 30 years of age as well. In cases when the cause is not identified, particularly in women who also have a family history of primary ovarian insufficiency, premutation carrier testing for the fragile X gene (*FMR1*) should be considered.

A low or normal FSH value in amenorrheic women without evidence of anatomic cause suggests chronic anovulation, most commonly attributed to hypothalamic amenorrhea or PCOS. In principle, hypothalamic amenorrhea would be associated with low estradiol levels, and PCOS would more often be associated with normal estradiol levels. However, estradiol levels fluctuate and testing is not recommended to help distinguish between these diagnoses. Similarly, the progesterone challenge test for withdrawal bleeding is not considered a reliable indicator of estrogen levels, given both high false positive and false negative rates.

Imaging Studies

In certain situations, further evaluation with imaging may be indicated, such as the use of ultrasound, magnetic resonance imaging (MRI), or hysteroscopy to assess for a potential anatomic abnormality. Examples include the absence of the uterus in primary amenorrhea, as may be seen with Müllerian agenesis and 46,XY conditions like androgen insensitivity syndrome, or the presence of intrauterine synechiae (Asherman syndrome) in those with prior procedural instrumentation of the uterus. In cases of an elevated prolactin level (with no evidence of thyroid disease), MRI is warranted to assess for a possible pituitary tumor, which is present in 50% to 60% of women with hyperprolactinemia.

Diagnoses and Management

Anatomic Causes

Müllerian agenesis is the most common cause of anatomic malformations associated with amenorrhea, comprising approximately 10% of primary amenorrhea cases. In addition to malformations along the genital tract, over half of Müllerian agenesis cases may also present with other congenital abnormalities, such as urinary tract or skeletal defects (e.g., scoliosis, vertebral arch anomalies, and wrist hypoplasia). Thus, it is important to assess for the presence of coexisting congenital anomalies in those with Müllerian agenesis. Renal ultrasound and spinal X-ray imaging should be considered in these women.

A less common cause of anatomical defects in the uterus or vagina is complete androgen insensitivity, which accounts for 5% of primary amenorrhea. Other anatomic defects leading to primary amenorrhea include transverse vaginal septum (2% of cases), imperforate hymen (1% of cases), and isolated absence of the vagina or cervix. In women with prior history of procedural interventions involving the uterus or cervix, intrauterine synechiae (Asherman syndrome) and cervical stenosis should also be considered as potential etiologies of amenorrhea. In cases of Asherman syndrome, treatment often involves hysteroscopy for lysis of the intrauterine adhesions.

Women with Müllerian agenesis typically present with normal secondary female sexual characteristics, in the setting of anatomic defects in all or some aspects of the uterus and vagina. Women with complete androgen insensitivity may also present with vaginal defects, though in addition they have a family history suggestive of androgen insensitivity, lack of pubarche, and may present with inguinal hernias or masses containing testes. Complete androgen insensitivity is an X-linked recessive condition and is confirmed by an elevated serum testosterone level in the male range and karyotype analysis (46,XY). Of note, complete androgen insensitivity confers an increased risk of gonadal malignancy, and treatment includes gonadal removal, typically after completion of growth and breast development. Hormonal replacement therapy is indicated following prophylactic gonadal removal for the maintenance of bone health.

The first-line treatment for Müllerian agenesis includes vaginal dilation to achieve elongation, a nonsurgical, patient-controlled therapy that has a success rate above 90%. Surgery to create a vagina is much less commonly required and reserved for rare cases. Psychosocial support is another important aspect of treatment for these individuals. Fertility considerations should also be addressed. In those with Müllerian agenesis who desire children, options may include assisted reproductive technology with gestational surrogacy or adoption. With regard to ongoing care, routine cervical cancer screening is not typically indicated given the absence of a cervix in these women.

Primary Ovarian Insufficiency

Persistently elevated FSH levels in the menopausal range indicate impaired ovarian function, consistent with primary ovarian insufficiency. Other terms to describe this condition have been previously used, including premature ovarian failure, premature menopause, and primary ovarian failure. This condition may affect 1% to 5% of women, though the etiology is not always known.

Congenital causes are a factor in some cases of primary ovarian insufficiency, with certain chromosomal abnormalities leading to gonadal dysgenesis, an example being Turner syndrome (45,X). Chromosomal abnormalities are identified in 50% of adolescents without comorbidities who present with primary amenorrhea and in 13% of women 30 years of age or younger who present with secondary amenorrhea. With regard to management, it is important to remember that the incidence of gonadal malignancy is up to 25% for women with a Y chromosome. Accordingly, in 46,XY women with lack of gonadal function as evidenced by elevated FSH levels and absence of hormone secretion, gonadal removal is indicated at the time of diagnosis.

Primary ovarian insufficiency has shown associated genetic predisposition, and premutation carrier testing for fragile X syndrome should be considered in these women when another cause has not been identified. Among those with a normal karyotype, 6% of women with primary ovarian insufficiency are found to have premutation of the *FMR1* (fragile X) gene. Additionally, primary ovarian insufficiency may also be seen with various endocrinopathies, such as hypoparathyroidism and hypoadrenalism, or autoimmune disease. Specifically, approximately 4% of cases have adrenal or ovarian antibodies, and autoimmune disorders may be found in up to 40% of women with primary ovarian insufficiency, most commonly thyroid disease.

For women with primary ovarian insufficiency, infertility should be addressed, though up to 10% may have temporary remission with spontaneous conception. It is unclear whether oral contraceptives are as effective in this population, so alternative methods such as barrier contraception or intrauterine device options are more appropriate for pregnancy prevention. Genetic predisposition for this condition should also be addressed. Consultations with reproductive endocrinology and fertility specialists are indicated when pregnancy is desired, as options are limited beyond donor *in vitro* fertilization. Psychosocial counseling and support should be offered as well.

Annual visits are recommended in those with primary ovarian insufficiency. Given the increased cardiovascular risk associated with the early estrogen deficient state, steps should be taken to ensure optimized cardiovascular health, including routine screening for hypertension and a lipid panel at least every 5 years. Furthermore, hormonal treatment until the typical age of menopause is appropriate both to support bone health as well as to develop and maintain secondary sexual characteristics. The estrogen deficient state in this condition poses risk to the attainment of peak bone mass. Thus, weight-bearing exercise as well as adequate calcium (1300 mg per day) and vitamin D (400 to 1000 IU per day) intake are also important aspects of management to reduce the risk of osteoporosis. With regard to hormone therapy in these cases, additional potential benefits include decreased risk of ischemic heart disease, less cardiovascular mortality, and vasomotor symptom control. Of note, combined oral contraceptives provide higher levels of hormones than are necessary for this purpose and are not recommended in this setting. A more appropriate regimen would include daily estradiol (e.g., 100 µg dose in transdermal [Alora, Dotti, Minivelle, Vivelle] or oral form [Estrace], though the latter confers a relatively higher thromboembolism risk), with 12 days of cyclic progesterone monthly (e.g., medroxyprogesterone acetate [Provera] 10 mg). For those still undergoing pubertal growth and maturity, specialized care is recommended, as hormone therapy should begin with estrogen before the introduction of progesterone, with the purpose of mimicking hormonal levels associated with development.

Hyperprolactinemia and Pituitary Causes

Another potential etiology of amenorrhea or oligomenorrhea is an elevated prolactin level, which inhibits the release and thus the effect of gonadotropins. Specifically, the presence of hyperprolactinemia suppresses GnRH secretion. When hyperprolactinemia is identified, in the absence of other potential causes such as medications or thyroid disease, an MRI of the head is warranted for further evaluation. Among women who present with amenorrhea and elevated prolactin, 50% to 60% are associated with a pituitary tumor. Additionally, pituitary disorders including Sheehan syndrome, pituitary gland necrosis, and empty sella syndrome may also be causes of anovulation and amenorrhea, as well as other pituitary or central nervous system tumors and organic diseases.

Regarding treatment for hyperprolactinemia, dopamine agonists may be used to aid in decreasing prolactin levels, regardless of the presence of pituitary tumor. This has an effect on the subsequent restoration of menses. In cases of pituitary adenoma, surgical resection may be warranted.

Hypothalamic Amenorrhea

The most common cause of chronic anovulation is functional hypothalamic amenorrhea, often associated with stress, weight loss, poor nutrition, and strenuous exercise. In these cases, suppression of the normal hypothalamic-pituitary-ovarian axis occurs as a result of an overall energy deficit, though the exact pathophysiology remains unclear. A much less common cause of hypothalamic amenorrhea is isolated gonadotropin deficiency, such as that seen in Kallmann syndrome (primary GnRH deficiency).

Multidisciplinary care should be considered in the approach to treatment of functional hypothalamic amenorrhea. Appropriate nutrition rehabilitation and reduction of strenuous exercise are important aspects of management for these women, and restoration of menses usually occurs following correction of the energy deficit. Furthermore, treatment should address stress reduction and psychosocial health, which may also play a role in the resumption of menses. As for pharmacologic management, evidence suggests that the use of leptin may help restore GnRH pulsatility and thus ovulation and menses, given its regulatory role in hypothalamic dysfunction. For those with hypothalamic amenorrhea desiring pregnancy, treatment options for ovulation induction may be pursued, typically with GnRH or gonadotropin therapy.

Similar to primary ovarian insufficiency, hypothalamic amenorrhea is associated with an estrogen deficient state, so affected women are at increased risk for osteoporosis. Bone density screening may be considered. In addition to nutrition rehabilitation and a decrease of strenuous activity, it is important to ensure adequate calcium and vitamin D intake with supplementation. Cyclic hormone therapy at physiologic doses may be considered for optimizing bone health, such as in cases where correction of the underlying cause of hypothalamic amenorrhea is not easily achieved. However, the potential beneficial effects on bone density in these cases are limited in the absence of appropriate nutrition rehabilitation. Furthermore, the use of bisphosphonates in the premenopausal population is not recommended given the limited data available and concern for potential teratogenic risks. Thus, treatment should primarily focus on addressing the underlying cause of hypothalamic amenorrhea.

Polycystic Ovary Syndrome

Chronic anovulation and amenorrhea may also occur with PCOS, though these women are more likely to present with oligomenorrhea. The presence of obesity and concomitant signs of androgen excess help distinguish PCOS from hypothalamic amenorrhea. Typically, a higher BMI is associated with PCOS, while normal or low BMI is more often associated with functional hypothalamic amenorrhea. According to the Rotterdam Consensus Criteria from 2003, the diagnosis of PCOS requires at least two of the following: (1) signs of androgen excess, (2) the presence of polycystic ovaries, and (3) ovulatory dysfunction. However, the 2006 Androgen Excess Society criteria for PCOS differ slightly from these guidelines, specifically requiring hyperandrogenism as one of the diagnostic conditions, along with ovarian dysfunction (oligo-anovulation and/or polycystic ovaries) and exclusion of other androgen excess or related disorders. The evidence of hyperandrogenism may be established by clinical findings (e.g., hirsutism, acne, male pattern alopecia) or laboratory measurement. Generally, serum androgen levels in those with PCOS do not exceed twice the upper limit of normal range, so further investigation for other etiologies of hyperandrogenism would be warranted in these cases.

The management of women with PCOS includes monitoring for insulin resistance and glucose intolerance, dyslipidemia, and cardiovascular risk, with subsequent interventions as indicated for any identified comorbidities. Treatment also involves healthy lifestyle modifications directed at dietary changes, exercise, and weight loss, given the association of PCOS with obesity. Furthermore, low-dose combined oral contraceptives are recommended to reduce the risk for endometrial cancer in the setting of chronic anovulation. Pharmacotherapy with metformin (Glucophage)[1] is another important treatment consideration, which may provide beneficial effects on ovulation, menstrual abnormalities, and androgen levels, in addition to its known effects on improving glucose tolerance.

---

[1]Not FDA approved for this indication.

References

American College of Obstetricians and Gynecologists: Committee Opinion No. 728. Müllerian agenesis: diagnosis, management, and treatment, *Obstet Gynecol* 131:e35–42, 2018.
American College of Obstetricians and Gynecologists: Committee Opinion No. 605. Primary ovarian insufficiency in adolescents and young women, *Obstet Gynecol* 123:193–197, 2014.
Gordon CM: Clinical practice: Functional hypothalamic amenorrhea, *N Engl J Med* 363(4):365–371, 2010.
Klein DA, Poth MA: Amenorrhea: An approach to diagnosis and management, *Am Fam Physician* 87(11):781–788, 2013.
Practice Committee of American Society for Reproductive Medicine: Current evaluation of amenorrhea, *Fertil Steril* 90:S219–S225, 2008.

BACTERIAL INFECTIONS OF THE URINARY TRACT IN WOMEN

Method of
Kinder Fayssoux, MD

CURRENT DIAGNOSIS

- Acute cystitis is the most common urologic disorder in women.
- *Escherichia coli* and *Staphylococcus saprophyticus* are the causative agents for 80% of community acquired urinary tract infections (UTIs).
- *E. coli* is also the most common uropathogen in the nosocomial setting.
- Anatomic risk factors include short urethra, the proximity of the urethra to the anus, and the colonization of the periurethral mucosa with bowel flora.
- Other risk factors include previous UTI, sexual intercourse, and, separately, the use of spermicide, pregnancy, diabetes, incontinence, cystocoele, and incomplete emptying of the bladder and dysfunctional voiding (defined as abnormal bladder emptying in the absence of neurologic disease).
- Postmenopausal women are also at increased risk if they are estrogen deficient.
- Acute cystitis typically presents with abrupt onset of dysuria, increased frequency, and/or urgency. Less frequently a patient will present with hematuria, suprapubic discomfort, or back/costovertebral angle pain. If a fever is present, it is usually less than 38.9°C (102°F).
- Acute pyelonephritis can evolve from either asymptomatic bacteruria or from an ascending bladder infection.
- Symptoms usually include fever usually greater than 38.9°C (102°F) with chills, nausea/vomiting, dysuria, increased frequency, urgency, and costovertebral angle (CVA) tenderness (usually unilateral).
- *E. coli* is the major pathogen in acute pyelonephritis and treatment depends on severity and pregnancy status.

CURRENT THERAPY

- Empiric therapy for uncomplicated UTIs should be dependent on the most recent antibiotic guidelines and the uropathogen resistance patterns in a community.
- In a community with >20% incidence of resistant *E. coli*, nitrofurantoin (Macrobid) 100 mg bid for 7 days is the treatment of choice with quinolones as second-line therapy.
- In a community with <20% *E. coli* resistance, trimethoprim/sulfamethoxazole 160/800 (Bactrim DS) PO twice daily for 3 days is also acceptable as first-line therapy with quinolones still considered as second-line therapy.
- Phenazopyridine (Pyridium), a smooth muscle relaxant, can be prescribed for spasm relief.
- Fungal UTIs or candiduria should be treated with fluconazole (Diflucan) 200 mg daily for 2 weeks.
- Outpatient treatment guidelines for acute pyelonephritis are the same as for uncomplicated UTI except the duration of antimicrobial therapy is longer (10–14 days).
- Inpatient treatment for acute pyelonephritis is typically IV levofloxacin (Levaquin) (750 mg daily) or ampicillin (1 g every 6 h).
- Acute pyelonephritis should resolve in 48 to 72 hours, if patients are not getting better, imaging should be undertaken with ultrasound or CT scan to assess for renal abscess or urethral obstruction.

Acute Cystitis (Urinary Tract Infection)

Acute cystitis is the most common urologic disorder among women. It represents 4% of all outpatient visits. Of these visits, 52% present to a primary care clinic and 23% to the emergency department. The annual health care costs associated with urinary tract infections (UTIs) are roughly 1.6 billion and climbing. Antimicrobial prescriptions for UTIs account for 15% of all outpatient prescriptions. One-third of all women will have at least one symptomatic UTI by age 24, with more than half of all women having at least one during their lifetime.

Acute cystitis can be defined as uncomplicated or complicated. Uncomplicated cystitis is defined as a UTI in patients with normal urinary tract anatomy without a contributing medical condition such as diabetes mellitus, neurogenic bladder, pregnancy, renal insufficiency, immune deficiency, recent antibiotic use, recent genitourinary instrumentation, spinal cord injury, ureteral obstruction, or nephrolithiasis. Complicated cystitis is defined as a UTI in patients with abnormal urinary tract anatomy or with one of the aforementioned medical conditions. These patients generally require urine culture as part of the initial work-up to guide antimicrobial therapy and often additional condition specific evaluation and treatment.

Acute cystitis is caused by ascending bacteria of perineal/urethral/fecal origin through the urethra into the bladder and renal systems. *Escherichia coli* and *Staphylococcus saprophyticus* are the causative agents for 80% of community acquired UTIs (complicated and uncomplicated). *E. coli* is also the most common uropathogen in the nosocomial setting. Other known uropathogens include *Pseudomonas spp*, *Klebsiella spp*, *Proteus*, *Corynebacterium urealyticum*, and *Providencia*. Fungal UTIs caused by *Candida spp*, *Aspergillus spp*, and *Cryptococcus neoformans* are also increasingly encountered. These are usually caused by indwelling urinary devices and seen more frequently in diabetics. Other populations prone to fungal UTIs include patients who are immunocompromised, hospitalized, or elderly.

There are numerous risk factors for acute cystitis, several specific to women. Risk factors unique to women include several related to their anatomy. These anatomic differences are the primary reason for the increased incidence of UTI in women when compared to men and include the female's relatively short urethra (when compared to the male counterpart), the proximity of the urethra to the anus, and the colonization of the periurethral mucosa with bowel flora.

Other risk factors include previous UTI, sexual intercourse, and, separately, the use of spermicide, pregnancy, diabetes, incontinence, cystocoele, and incomplete emptying of the bladder and dysfunctional voiding (defined as abnormal bladder emptying in the absence of neurologic disease). Postmenopausal women are also at increased risk if they are estrogen deficient.

Dysfunctional voiding has an unknown etiology and results in increased external sphincter activity during voluntary voiding which results in reflux, increasing chances of UTI.

Commonly advised behavioral modifications thought to decrease the risk of UTI (e.g., postcoital voiding, increased fluid intake, avoidance of urinary holding, douching, front-to-back wiping, proper tampon/sanitary napkin use, and loose/cotton underwear) have been supported by the literature.

Acute cystitis typically appears as an abrupt onset of dysuria, increased frequency, and/or urgency. Less frequently a patient will present with hematuria, suprapubic discomfort, or back/costovertebral angle pain. If a fever is present, it is usually less than 38.9°C (102°F).

Obtaining a good history that assesses for risk factors and symptoms is important in diagnosing acute cystitis. In a woman who presents with one or more symptoms of UTI (dysuria, frequency, urgency, hematuria), the probability of infection is already 50%. A urine dipstick is a useful diagnostic test, with a positive (+) nitrite or leukocyte esterase result increasing the chances of infection. The combination of positive nitrite *and* leukocyte esterase results has the highest diagnostic correlation with UTI. Physical examination findings may include suprapubic tenderness or costovertebral angle tenderness, although these are unlikely in an uncomplicated UTI scenario.

The gold standard for diagnosis of acute cystitis is a culture that has 10^2 to 10^3 colony-forming units of a single uropathogen from a clean catch or catheterized urine specimen. However, research has shown that, for uncomplicated cystitis, ordering cultures and sensitivities makes little difference in treatment while increasing cost of care. Thus, it is reasonable to start empiric treatment without a culture and sensitivities in a patient presenting with uncomplicated UTI.

The differential diagnosis for an uncomplicated UTI includes:
- Vaginitis/vaginal infections: can cause dysuria
  - *Gardnerella*, *Candida albicans*, and *Trichomonas*
- Urethritis: can cause dysuria/frequency
  - STDs (*Chlamydia trachomatis*, gonorrhea, herpes simplex)
  - Pelvic floor spasm (leads to urethral spasm/irritability)
- Interstitial cystitis
- Malignancy
- Renal tuberculosis

Differentiating between sexually transmitted infections (STI), vaginal infections, and UTIs can be difficult because symptoms and signs commonly overlap. History elements that should prompt a pelvic examination and laboratory evaluation for pathogens are complaints of a vaginal discharge or vaginal irritation/pruritus. Persistent hematuria should raise the concern for underlying malignancy or renal tuberculosis, and further evaluation should be done.

Empiric therapy for uncomplicated UTIs should be dependent on the most recent antibiotic guidelines and the uropathogen resistance patterns in a community. In a community with >20% incidence of resistant *E. coli*, nitrofurantoin (Macrobid) 100 mg bid for 7 days is the treatment of choice with quinolones as second-line therapy. In a community with <20% *E. coli* resistance, trimethoprim/sulfamethoxazole 160/800 (Bactrim DS) PO twice daily for 3 days is also acceptable as first-line therapy with quinolones still considered as second-line therapy. Phenazopyridine (Pyridium), a smooth muscle relaxant, can be prescribed for spasm relief and is usually only necessary for the first 24 hours after treatment is initiated. Fungal UTIs or *candiduria* should be treated with fluconazole (Diflucan) 200 mg daily for 2 weeks.

For a complicated UTI, a culture must always be obtained and the patient should be evaluated in the context of his or her specific comorbid condition before treatment.

Acute Pyelonephritis

Acute pyelonephritis can evolve from either asymptomatic bacteriuria or from an ascending bladder infection. Although it can progress from an uncomplicated cystitis, it more commonly presents from a complicated cystitis in the setting of other medical conditions such cholelithiasis, urinary obstruction, malformations, or pregnancy.

Symptoms usually include fever usually greater than 38.9°C (102°F) with chills, nausea/vomiting, dysuria, increased frequency, urgency, and CVA tenderness (usually unilateral). These symptoms can present on a spectrum from mild to severe. *E. coli* is the major pathogen, and treatment depends on severity and pregnancy status. Pregnant patients or patients with moderate to severe nausea/vomiting that would interfere with oral antibiotic treatment should be hospitalized and have blood cultures done in addition to urine culture. Patients with mild symptoms and the ability to tolerate oral antibiotics can be treated as on an outpatient basis with a urine culture obtained before initializing treatment. Outpatient treatment guidelines are the same as for uncomplicated UTI, except the duration of antimicrobial therapy is longer (10–14 days). Inpatient treatment is typically IV levofloxacin (Levaquin 750 mg daily) or ampicillin (1 g every 6 h). Once the inpatient is able to tolerate oral antibiotics and the infection is felt to be controlled, he or she can be switched to oral antibiotics and discharged to complete a 14-day course of treatment as an outpatient.

Symptoms should resolve in 48 to 72 hours; if patients are not getting better, imaging should be undertaken with ultrasound or CT scan to assess for renal abscess or urethral obstruction.

Urethritis

Urethritis usually has a gradual onset and is accompanied with milder symptoms of dysuria, frequency, urgency, or hematuria. It can also occur with a vaginal discharge and complaints of dyspareunia and vaginal pruritus depending on cause. Chalmydial, gonorrheal, candidal and trichomonal urethritis is usually accompanied by a vaginal discharge. Candidal urethritis can also be associated with pruritus and dyspareunia. If urethritis is suspected, a pelvic examination and further laboratory work-up is necessary.

Asymptomatic Bacteriuria

Asymptomatic bacteriuria is defined as the presence of 100,000 microorganisms/milliliter of urine without any symptoms of cystitis.

No screening should be performed in healthy nonpregnant women, elderly living in the community, diabetic women, institutionalized elderly, or persons with spinal cord injury. Pregnant women are the exception. They should be screened; positive cultures need to be treated, as there is an increased likelihood of asymptomatic bacteriuria turning into UTI or pyelonephritis because of vesicoureteral reflux and urinary stasis resulting from increased progesterone levels.

Recurrent Cystitis

Recurrent cystitis is defined as at least three episodes of uncomplicated UTI with one or more documented positive (+) cultures in 12 months. It can be due to relapse or reinfection. Relapse is defined as infection occurring with the same organism as a previous UTI. Reinfection is when symptoms return after treatment and a completely symptom-free interval along with a negative urine culture or when the second infection is caused by a different organism. Most recurrent cystitis tends to be caused by reinfection.

In patients presenting with recurrent cystitis, an age-based evaluation is a good place to start. Adolescents who are not sexually active should be evaluated for congenital abnormalities. Premenopausal females should be questioned about the temporal relationship of the onset of UTI to increased frequency/recent sexual intercourse, spermicide use (with or without condom or diaphragm), or renal stones. Postmenopausal females should be evaluated for decreased estrogen/vaginal atrophy, incontinence, incomplete bladder emptying, cystocoeles, and prolapse.

If a complete and thorough evaluation is done, complicating factors are ruled out, modifiable factors are treated, and recurrent cystitis still remains a problem, then treatment should be considered. Treatment options include continuous antibiotics, postcoital therapy, or self- initiated treatment at the first sign or symptom of an infection.

Gross hematuria or persistent microscopic hematuria should increase suspicion for an underlying malignancy. Also, recurrent cystitis symptoms in a setting of negative cultures may suggest mycobacterial infection or interstitial cystitis.

Catheter Associated Urinary Tract Infection

Catheter-associated UTI is defined as a UTI in a patient who had an indwelling urethral catheter within 48 hours of onset of infection. Indwelling urinary catheters and clean intermittent catheterization are associated with the highest rates of bacteriuria; after 1 month of either there is almost 100% risk of bacteriuria. Formation of a bacterial biofilm on the catheter is thought to be the mechanism of infection in this setting.

No treatment is recommended for asymptomatic patients, and neither prophylactic antibiotics nor routine UA and culture are recommended for this population. For symptomatic patients, the first step is to determine whether the catheter can be removed. If it cannot, then it should be replaced. In addition, a blood and urine culture (taken from a new catheter) should be obtained. Initial treatment is the same as for an uncomplicated UTI as discussed earlier. Confirmation of susceptibility should be confirmed with culture results.

References

Litza JA, Brill JR: Urinary tract infection, *Primary Care Clinical Office Practice* 37:491–507, 2010.
Minardi D, d'Anzeo G, Cantoro D, et al: Urinary tract infections in women: Etiology and treatment options, *Int J Gen Med* 4:333–343, 2011.
Finer G, Landau D: Pathogenesis of urinary tract infections with normal female anatomy, *Lancet* 4:631–634, 2004.
Foster RT: Office gynecology uncomplicated urinary tract infections in women. Obstet Gynecol Clin 35:235–48.
Berek JS: *Berek and Novak's Gynecology*, Philadelphia, 2012, Lippincott. p. 570–71.
Essentials evidence plus: Urinary tract infection (adults), Available at http://essentialevidenceplus.com, accessed August 16, 2016.
Essentials evidence plus: Urethritis (female), http://essentialevidenceplus.com, Accessed August 16, 2016.
Bent SN, Nallamothu BK, Simel DL, et al: Does this woman have an acute uncomplicated urinary tract infection? *JAMA* 287:2701–2710, 2002.
Wagenlehner F, Weidner W, Naber K: An updated on uncomplicated urinary tract infections in women, *Curr Opin Urol* 19:368–374, 2009.
Dielubaza EJ, Schaeffer AJ: Urologic issues for the internist- urinary tract infections in women. Med Clin North Am 95:27–41.
Giesen LG, Cousins G, Dimitrov BD, et al: Predicting acute uncomplicated urinary tract infections in women: A systematic review of the diagnostic accuracy of symptoms and signs, *BMC Fam Pract* 11:78, 2010. Available at http://www.biomedcentral.com/1471-2296/11/78, accessed August 16, 2016.

BENIGN BREAST DISEASE

Method of
Lauren Nye, MD

CURRENT DIAGNOSIS

- Mammography is used for breast cancer screening, and it is recommended to begin screening in women at average risk for breast cancer between ages 40 and 50.

- Benign breast disease may present with an abnormality on screening breast imaging or with a breast symptom such as a breast mass or nipple discharge.
- Nonproliferative breast lesions are not associated with an increased risk of breast cancer.
- Proliferative breast lesions without atypia are associated with a slightly increased risk for breast cancer, whereas proliferative lesions with atypia are associated with a significantly increased risk for breast cancer.
- Factors contributing to a woman's breast cancer risk include family history, personal health history, and modifiable lifestyle factors.

CURRENT THERAPY

- Some benign breast lesions do not need any further intervention after diagnosis; others may require surgical excision to rule out malignancy.
- Women at high risk for breast cancer may warrant additional breast screening or begin screening at an earlier age.
- Women at high risk for breast cancer should be counseled on risk reduction strategies, including lifestyle modification.
- Chemoprevention agents include tamoxifen, raloxifene (Evista), and aromatase inhibitors.

Breast health is an important aspect of women's health care; it includes breast cancer screening and evaluation of breast concerns. Benign breast disease can be identified on a biopsy done for an abnormal screening test, a palpable breast mass, nipple discharge, or other breast concerns. Benign breast disease may be associated with an increased risk for breast cancer. Women at high risk for breast cancer should be considered for additional breast cancer screening recommendations and risk reduction strategies.

Presentation and Workup

Patients can present with benign breast disease after an abnormality detected on screening imaging or after workup for breast symptoms such as a palpable mass, breast pain, or spontaneous nipple discharge. In women who are considered at average risk for breast cancer based on medical and family history, screening includes history and physical examination by their health care provider, clinical breast examination, and breast imaging. Breast awareness should be encouraged, but formal breast self-examinations in average-risk women have not been shown to have a breast cancer mortality benefit, although in women who performed self-breast examinations, a greater number of benign breast lesions were detected.

Breast Cancer Screening

Women at average risk for breast cancer should be considered for screening mammography at age 40. The US Preventive Services Task Force (USPSTF) is currently updating recommendations for breast cancer screening. Updated USPSTF drafts and recommendations can be found at: https://www.uspreventiveservicestaskforce.org/uspstf/draft-recommendation/breast-cancer-screening-adults. The 2015 American Cancer Society (ACS) breast cancer screening guidelines for women at average risk include a strong recommendation to begin screening mammography at age 45 and a qualified recommendation to begin at age 40, continuing as long as the woman is in good overall health and life expectancy is 10 years or greater. The most updated recommendation from the National Comprehensive Cancer Network (NCCN) and the American College of Radiology (ACR) is for annual screening mammography beginning at age 40. The standard for breast cancer screening is the digital mammogram; however, in recent years digital breast tomosynthesis has become more prevalent and available to women at breast imaging centers. Digital breast tomosynthesis has both a higher breast cancer detection rate and a lower recall rate compared with the digital mammogram for breast cancer screening. In women with heterogeneously dense breast or dense breast tissue on screening mammogram, the risks and benefits of supplemental screening with bilateral breast screening ultrasound or breast MRI should be discussed as high breast density limits mammogram sensitivity.

Normal and abnormal findings on breast imaging are reported using the universal classification system by the ACR's classification: the Breast Imaging Reporting and Data System (BI-RADS). Table 1 includes the BI-RADS categories, the risk of malignancy, and the recommended follow-up. BI-RADS 0 indicates an incomplete assessment and that further workup is needed, typically with additional imaging recommendations. BI-RADS 3 lesions are considered probably benign based on appearance; a mammogram and/or ultrasound in 6 months is recommended for follow-up. BI-RADS 4 and BI-RADS 5 lesions are suspicious or highly suggestive of malignancy, respectively, and a biopsy of the lesion is recommended.

Palpable Breast Mass

In patients who present with a palpable breast mass, workup is determined by patient age, menopausal status, and degree of suspicion of breast mass. Fig. 1 outlines the algorithm for evaluation of a woman with a breast mass. In women younger than age 30 with a mass of low clinical suspicion, it would be appropriate to consider observation over one to two menstrual cycles prior to moving on to ultrasound imaging if the mass persists. If no mass is detected on ultrasound, short-term clinical follow-up is recommended. Diagnostic mammography with ultrasound may be considered in women younger than age 30 who have a mass of high clinical suspicion or increased breast cancer risk. In postmenopausal women and women 30 years of age and older, a clinically palpable breast mass should be evaluated with a diagnostic mammogram and ultrasound. A clinically suspicious mass without a radiographic correlate on imaging should be evaluated for palpation-guided biopsy of the mass. A patient identified to have a simple cyst on imaging can return to age-appropriate breast screening. A solitary complicated cyst should be aspirated or be followed in short-term follow-up for stability. Multiple complicated cysts are considered a benign finding and do not require aspiration or short-term follow-up. Routine cytology of aspirated fluid is not recommended. If the mass persists after aspiration of a complicated cyst or if initial imaging shows a mass of high clinical suspicion or a complex cystic and solid mass, ultrasound-guided biopsy of the mass is recommended.

The sonographic description of a simple cyst is a round or oval circumscribed mass with acoustic enhancement and lacking any solid components or Doppler signals. A nonsimple cyst may be complicated or a complex cystic and solid mass. A complicated cyst is round or oval and circumscribed but may show low-level internal echoes without demonstrating vascular flow, whereas a complex cystic and solid mass may have thick septations, thick and irregular walls, and an internal solid component; it may display internal echoes, internal blood flow, and lack of posterior wall enhancement.

Nipple Discharge

Some women may present with nipple discharge without a palpable mass. Concerning features for pathologic nipple discharge include a spontaneous unilateral single-duct discharge that is reproducible on examination and discharge that is clear, serous, sanguineous, or serosanguineous. Nonspontaneous nipple discharge or multiduct discharge is likely physiologic and the most common cause is duct ectasia. Women should be educated on avoiding further breast compression to elicit the discharge, ensure that they are up to date on age-appropriate breast cancer screening, and review potential medications that could cause nipple discharge. In women with spontaneous pathologic single-duct nipple discharge, the most common etiology is an intraductal papilloma.

TABLE 1	Breast Imaging Reporting and Data System Mammography Classification		
BI-RADS CATEGORY	**DEFINITION**	**RISK FOR MALIGNANCY**	**RECOMMENDED FOLLOW-UP**
0	Incomplete assessment	N/A	Further imaging
1	Negative study	N/A	Routine mammogram screening
2	Benign	N/A	Routine mammogram screening
3	Probably benign	≤ 2%	Repeat imaging in 6 months
4	Suspicious	>2%–95% depending on degree of suspicion	Biopsy recommended
5	Highly suggestive of malignancy	≥ 95%	Biopsy recommended
6	Known biopsy-proven malignancy	N/A	Appropriate action should be taken

BI-RADS, Breast Imaging Reporting and Data System.

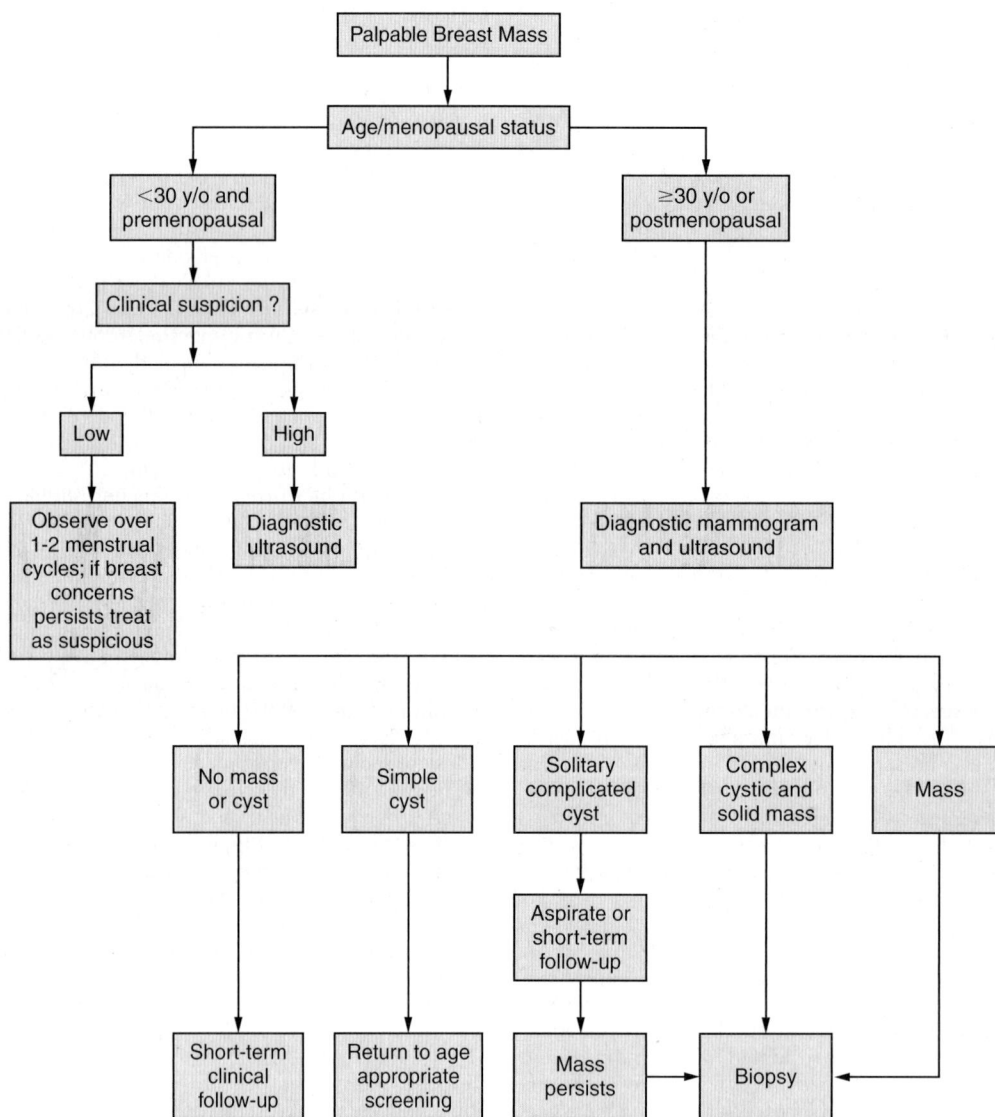

Figure 1 Algorithm for the evaluation of a woman with a breast mass.

The most common malignant explanation would be ductal carcinoma in situ (DCIS). The workup should include diagnostic mammography and ultrasound for women 30 years of age or older and at least a diagnostic ultrasound in women younger than age 30. Suspicious or highly suspicious imaging findings warrant biopsy. If initial imaging does not explain the nipple discharge, a ductogram or magnetic resonance imaging (MRI) may be considered for further evaluation. In some cases duct excision may be recommended; otherwise the patient should have short-term follow-up with clinical breast examination and imaging.

Benign Lesions

Benign breast diseases can be categorized as nonproliferative, proliferative without atypia, proliferative with atypia, and

TABLE 2	Benign Breast Lesions	
NONPROLIFERATIVE LESIONS	**PROLIFERATIVE LESIONS WITHOUT ATYPIA**	**PROLIFERATIVE LESIONS WITH ATYPIA**
Apocrine metaplasia	Fibroadenomas	Atypical ductal hyperplasia
Breast cysts	Microglandular adenosis	Atypical lobular hyperplasia
Columnar cell change	Moderate or florid usual ductal hyperplasia	
Duct ectasia	Papilloma	
Fibrosis	Radial scar	
	Sclerosing adenosis	

miscellaneous other conditions such as fat necrosis, various types of mastitis, pseudoangiomatous stromal hyperplasia, fibrous mastopathy, amyloid deposits, and dermatologic conditions. Table 2 outlines the benign breast lesions. A study by Dupont and Page in the 1980s and a review by Hartmann et al. in 2005 found that nonproliferative breast disease was not associated with an increased risk for breast cancer. Proliferative breast disease without atypia is associated with a slightly increased risk for breast cancer but less than two times the average population risk. Proliferative breast disease with atypia is associated with a significantly increased breast cancer risk that can be four to five times higher than the average population risk.

Nonproliferative Lesions

Nonproliferative breast lesions are also known as fibrocystic disease or change and include duct ectasia, fibrosis, and apocrine metaplasia. In women without a significant family history of breast cancer, nonproliferative breast lesions are not associated with an increased breast cancer risk. In the study by Dupont and Page including 3303 patients with benign breast disease, only 2.2% of the patients with nonproliferative lesions had breast cancer at a mean follow-up of 17 years. The Hartmann study of 9087 women followed for a median of 15 years found that the strength of family history was an independent risk factor; in women with nonproliferative lesions, the relative risk of breast cancer was 1.27. No increased risk was found in women with no family history.

Ductal ectasia and breast cysts are common findings. Occasionally the ectatic ducts are surrounded with periductal inflammation, which can occur in nonlactating women when the duct becomes congested with debris. This can lead to periductal mastitis that requires treatment with antibiotics. Breast cysts are most common in perimenopausal women but can occur in premenopausal women and postmenopausal women on hormone replacement therapy. Breast cysts may present in women with fibrocystic breast disease, which women may report as nodular breast tissue and is caused by microcystic formation and stromal proliferation of the breast. Apocrine metaplasia, in which acini and cysts are lined with large columnar cells that resemble the apocrine sweat glands, is not an uncommon finding. The individual cells are large, with abundant granular eosinophilic cytoplasm. The apical aspects of these cells have a rounded protrusion into the cyst spaces. Columnar cell change is characterized by enlargement of the terminal duct lobular units and dilated acini without atypia.

Proliferative Lesions Without Atypia

Proliferative breast lesions without atypia include fibroepithelial lesions such as fibroadenomas, moderate or florid usual ductal hyperplasia, microglandular and sclerosing adenosis, papillomas, and radial scars. Proliferative breast lesions without atypia are

associated with a slightly increased risk of breast cancer compared with the average risk of the population, with the relative risk estimated between 1.8 and 1.9. These lesions are not currently considered to put a woman at high risk for breast cancer unless other risk factors are present, such as family history.

Fibroadenomas are benign processes containing glandular and fibrous tissue. Fibroadenomas were originally classified as nonproliferative lesions (including in the Hartmann study) but are now typically considered proliferative breast lesions. Simple fibroadenomas without associated proliferative disease are not associated with an increased risk for breast cancer, while complex fibroadenomas and those with coinciding proliferative disease are associated with a slight increase in breast cancer risk. Fibroadenomas are most common in young premenopausal women and can fluctuate in size with changes in hormones. They do not routinely need to be excised unless they are enlarging or have associated symptoms, such as tenderness.

The normal number of epithelial linings within the breast is two. Epithelial hyperplasia has a spectrum of changes from mild to severe, presenting with an escalating scale of complexity. Usual ductal hyperplasia (UDH) is an increased number of cells within the duct that will vary in size and shape but will appear benign and without atypia. Microglandular adenosis and sclerosing adenosis are lesions with an increased number of glandular elements within fibrous stroma. Microglandular and sclerosing adenosis may be associated with microcalcifications and/or a mass on mammography.

Classic papillomas are masslike lesions that occur within large ducts close to the subareolar area. Histologically, they are composed of arborizing fronds of fibrovascular stroma lined by epithelial cells with a stalk attaching the mass to the wall of the cyst within which they arise. They can appear as a mass on mammography or present with unilateral nipple discharge. Papillomas can be associated with hyperplasia with and without atypia or DCIS; in those cases, surgical excision is recommended to rule out malignancy.

Radial scars or complex sclerosing lesions are a pathologic diagnosis but can cause abnormalities on breast imaging including mass, nonmass enhancement, or architectural distortion. Histologically, they have a central fibroelastic core with radiating and branching ducts and lobules at the periphery. The etiology of these lesions is unknown. Depending on the size and presentation, surgical excision may be recommended to rule out underlying malignancy.

Proliferative Lesions with Atypia

Proliferative lesions with atypia include atypical ductal hyperplasia (ADH) and atypical lobular hyperplasia (ALH). These atypical hyperplasia lesions are characterized by an abundance of monotonous-appearing epithelial cells partially filling a duct and/or lobule. The presence of atypical hyperplasia is a risk factor for future breast cancer and is associated with a relative risk of breast cancer between four and five times the general population risk. The risk of breast cancer over the 25 years following a biopsy demonstrating atypical hyperplasia is estimated at 30%. The number of foci of atypia present in the specimen can stratify the risk, with one focus being a lower risk compared to three or more foci of atypia. These patients should be managed in a multidisciplinary fashion to include assessment of concordance between radiology and pathology. The standard management for atypical hyperplasia including ADH and ALH is surgical excision to rule out underlying malignancy; however, select patients who have concordance with imaging may be appropriate for screening in lieu of surgical excision.

Miscellaneous Benign Breast Conditions

Pseudoangiomatous stromal hyperplasia (PASH) is a lesion of a stromal proliferation with anastomosing spaces, with the dense hyalinized stroma intermixed with glandular components. These spaces could appear as vascular structures to the untrained pathologist. PASH may appear similar to an angiosarcoma but can be differentiated by the lack of atypia and mitosis. PASH can present with a palpable mass, with a mammogram abnormality, or as an incidental finding. Historically this lesion commonly underwent excision; however, depending on the size of the lesion, concordance with imaging, and other risk factors, PASH may be appropriately monitored with follow-up imaging.

Fat necrosis is secondary to trauma or injury to the breast. Fat necrosis typically presents with a painless breast mass and appears as an ill-defined dense mass on breast imaging. A biopsy is recommended to rule out malignancy; however, no further treatment is necessary.

High-Risk Evaluation and Management
The lifetime risk of breast cancer for women in the United States is approximately one in eight. There are elements of a woman's personal or family history that may increase her risk for breast cancer and potentially warrant additional screening and management. Risk factors that contribute to a women's lifetime risk of breast cancer include family history of breast and/or ovarian cancer, genetic mutations associated with hereditary breast cancer, reproductive history, personal history of multiple breast biopsies or a breast biopsy showing atypical hyperplasia or lobular carcinoma in situ (LCIS), and dense breast tissue on mammography. Women who received thoracic radiation prior to age 30 are also at an increased risk for breast cancer. Modifiable risk factors for breast cancer include increased body mass index, sedentary lifestyle, alcohol intake, and hormone replacement therapy with estrogen and progesterone. Breast cancer risk assessment tools are available to estimate a woman's risk and include the Breast Cancer Risk Assessment Tool (previously referred to as the Gail model) and family history–based models such as, BRCAPRO, and Tyrer-Cuzick. In 2019, the USPSTF updated recommendations for BRCA-related cancer risk and recommended women with a family history of breast, ovarian, tubal, or peritoneal cancer and previously treated survivors of any of those cancers should be assessed for genetic risk.

Women considered at high risk for breast cancer include those with a Gail Model 5-year breast cancer risk of greater than or equal to 1.7%, a lifetime risk of breast cancer of greater than 20% based on a family history–based model, or a history of thoracic radiation prior to age 30, as well as women harboring a deleterious genetic mutation associated with breast cancer or a personal history of atypical hyperplasia or lobular carcinoma in situ. Women at high risk for breast cancer may be eligible for additional screening including earlier age at initiation of screening/imaging and consideration of an annual breast MRI.

Women at high risk for breast cancer should be counseled on screening recommendations and risk reduction strategies. Lifestyle modifications associated with decreased breast cancer risk include breastfeeding, achieving a healthy body mass index, limiting alcohol consumption, and exercising regularly. Some women may be considered for risk-reducing surgery. Chemoprevention may also be an option for women at high risk for breast cancer.

Chemoprevention
Risk-reducing agents, also known as chemoprevention, are appropriate to consider in women with atypical hyperplasia, LCIS, or a 5-year breast cancer risk of greater than or equal to 1.7%. Risk-reducing agents include tamoxifen, raloxifene (Evista), and the aromatase inhibitors (exemestane [Aromasin][1] and anastrozole [Arimidex][1]). Chemoprevention is taken daily for 5 years and associated with a potential risk reduction of 40% to 65%. No survival benefit has been demonstrated in women who take chemoprevention, and the risks and benefits of each therapy should be discussed. Tamoxifen is a selective estrogen receptor modulator (SERM) and is the only agent available for premenopausal women. Tamoxifen should not be recommended to women who

are currently pregnant or considering future pregnancy owing to potential teratogenic effects. The National Surgical Adjuvant Breast and Bowel Project (NSABP) Breast Cancer Prevention Trial (NSABP P-1) of tamoxifen 20 mg daily for 5 years verses placebo included both pre- and postmenopausal women at high risk for breast cancer and demonstrated a reduced risk of invasive breast cancer of 49%. In this study tamoxifen was associated with an increased rate of endometrial cancer, deep vein thrombosis, pulmonary embolism, and stroke, and these events were more frequent in women over the age of 50. Low-dose tamoxifen (5 mg per day for 3 years) can be considered for women with atypical hyperplasia, especially those unable to tolerate full-dose tamoxifen (20 mg per day). Raloxifene is a second-generation SERM. The STAR trial (NSABP P-2) randomized postmenopausal women at high risk for breast cancer to 5 years of tamoxifen 20 mg daily versus raloxifene 60 mg daily. Raloxifene was demonstrated to be as effective as tamoxifen at reducing the risk of invasive breast cancer but not noninvasive breast cancer. Raloxifene was associated with a lower rate of venous thromboembolic events and endometrial cancer. Aromatase inhibitors were studied in postmenopausal women for breast cancer prevention in the MAP.3 (exemestane) and IBIS-II (anastrozole) trials. Exemestane 25 mg daily for 5 years was associated with a 65% relative reduction in annual incidence of breast cancer compared with placebo. Anastrozole 1 mg daily for 5 years reduced the incidence of estrogen receptor–positive breast cancers by over 50% compared with placebo with a hazard ratio (HR) of 0.47. In both trials, musculoskeletal complaints and vasomotor symptoms were more common in the aromatase inhibitor groups. Vaginal dryness and decreased libido are also common side effects of aromatase inhibitors. There is potential for a decrease in bone mineral density while taking an aromatase inhibitor; however, no increased fracture rate was seen in either trial. In postmenopausal women, age and comorbidities along with bone health should be considered when a risk-reducing agent is being selected.

References
Ciatto S, Houssami N, Bernardi D, et al: Integration of 3D digital mammography with tomosynthesis for population breast-cancer screening (STORM): a prospective comparison study, Lancet Oncol 14(7):583–589, 2013, https://doi.org/10.1016/S1470-2045(13)70134-7. 23623721.

Cuzick J, Sestak I, Forbes JF, et al: Investigators I-I. Anastrozole for prevention of breast cancer in high-risk postmenopausal women (IBIS-II): an international, double-blind, randomised placebo-controlled trial, Lancet 383(9922):1041–1048, 2014, https://doi.org/10.1016/S0140-6736(13)62292-8. 24333009.

Dupont WD, Page DL: Risk factors for breast cancer in women with proliferative breast disease, N Engl J Med 312(3):146–151, 1985, https://doi.org/10.1056/NEJM198501173120303, PubMed PMID: 3965932.

Fisher B, Costantino JP, Wickerham DL, et al: Tamoxifen for prevention of breast cancer: Report of the National Surgical Adjuvant Breast and Bowel Project P-1 Study, J Natl Cancer Inst 90(18):1371–1388, 1998, PubMed PMID: 9747868.

Goss PE, Ingle JN, Ales-Martinez JE, et al: Investigators NCMS. Exemestane for breast-cancer prevention in postmenopausal women, N Engl J Med 364(25):2381–2391, 2011, https://doi.org/10.1056/NEJMoa1103507. 21639806.

Hartmann LC, Sellers TA, Frost MH, et al: Benign breast disease and the risk of breast cancer, N Engl J Med 353(3):229–237, 2005, https://doi.org/10.1056/NEJMoa044383. 16034008.

Lazzeroni M, Puntoni M, Guerrieri-Gonzaga A, et al.: Randomized placebo controlled trial of low-dose tamoxifen to prevent recurrence in breast noninvasive neoplasia: a 10-year follow-up of TAM-01 study, J Clin Oncol 41(17):3116–3121, 2023.

Oeffinger KC, Fontham ET, Etzioni R, et al: American Cancer Society. Breast cancer screening for women at average risk: 2015 guideline update from the American Cancer Society, JAMA 314(15):1599–1614, 2015, https://doi.org/10.1001/jama.2015.12783, PMCID: PMC4831582. PubMed PMID: 26501536.

Siu AL, USPST Force: Screening for breast cancer: US Preventive Services Task Force Recommendation Statement, Ann Intern Med 164(4):279–296, 2016, https://doi.org/10.7326/M15-2886. PubMed PMID: 26757170.

Thomas DB, Gao DL, Ray RM, et al: Randomized trial of breast self-examination in Shanghai: final results, J Natl Cancer Inst 94(19):1445–1457, 2002. PubMed PMID: 12359854.

Vogel VG, Costantino JP, Wickerham DL, et al: National Surgical Adjuvant Breast and Bowel Project. Effects of tamoxifen vs raloxifene on the risk of developing invasive breast cancer and other disease outcomes: the NSABP Study of Tamoxifen and Raloxifene (STAR) P-2 trial, JAMA 295(23):2727–2741, 2006, https://doi.org/10.1001/jama.295.23.joc60074. 16754727.

---

[1]Not FDA approved for this indication.

BREAST CANCER

Method of
Lauren Nye, MD

CURRENT DIAGNOSIS

- Mammography is used for breast cancer screening, and it is recommended to begin screening in women at average risk for breast cancer between ages 40 and 50.
- Women with an elevated risk for breast cancer may be considered for additional high-risk screening that can include breast magnetic resonance imaging (MRI) or other supplemental screening in addition to annual mammography.
- Individuals with a palpable breast mass or breast symptom concerning for malignancy and those with an abnormal screening mammogram need diagnostic breast imaging.
- Women with diagnostic breast imaging that is suspicious or highly suggestive of malignancy should undergo core needle biopsy.

CURRENT THERAPY

- Breast cancer is a heterogeneous disease and requires a multidisciplinary approach and multimodality therapy.
- The treatment of early-stage breast cancer may include local therapy such as surgery and radiation as well as systemic therapy including chemotherapy, endocrine therapy, and biologic therapy.
- Metastatic breast cancer is treated with systemic therapy; the goal of treatment is disease control and preserving quality of life.
- Breast cancer survivors may have multiple long-term complications of therapy that need to be addressed, including vasomotor symptoms, osteoporosis, lymphedema, and increased cardiac risk factors as well as psychosocial distress and financial toxicity.

Overview

Breast cancer is the most common cancer and the third leading cause of death among women in the United States. It is a heterogeneous disease for which a personalized approach is important in the evaluation and treatment of each individual. Furthermore, the multidisciplinary team is vital in the management of breast cancer and can include a medical oncologist, surgical oncologist, plastic surgeon, radiation oncologist, pathologist, supportive services, and the patient's personal physician. At the conclusion of treatment and active surveillance, the patient typically returns to his or her primary care physician for continued survivorship care.

Epidemiology

It is estimated that there were 310,720 new cases of breast cancer in 2024. The estimated deaths from breast cancer in the same year were 42,780. Female breast cancer is most commonly diagnosed among women from 55 to 64 years of age, with the median age at diagnosis of 62. Although rare, male breast cancer comprises 1% of all breast cancer cases in the United States. The incidence of breast cancer has risen slowly by 0.3% annually, whereas the mortality rate has been falling by 1.8% each year. The 5-year relative survival rate improved by 16% over 30 years, from 74% in 1980 to 90.9% in 2010. Despite the improvement in mortality for most individuals, there remains a breast cancer mortality disparity for African American women diagnosed with breast cancer.

Risk Factors

Well-recognized risk factors for breast cancer include older age, female sex, white race, obesity, high exposure to hormones (either exogenous or endogenous), personal and family history of breast cancer, inherited genetic mutations, benign breast disease (e.g., atypical hyperplasia and LCIS), previous history of radiation therapy to the chest, as well as lifestyle factors such as alcohol consumption and obesity.

Individuals who carry a *BRCA1* or *BRCA2* mutation are at a significantly higher risk for developing breast cancer. In a 2017 case-control study by Couch et al. of more than 65,000 women with breast cancer, genetic mutations associated with an increased risk of breast cancer were identified in 10.2% of cases. The most common gene mutations identified included *BRCA1, BRCA2, ATM, CHEK2, PALB2, BARD1,* and *RAD51D.* Individuals with a strong family history of cancer should be considered for genetic counseling and testing for appropriate risk stratification.

Risk Reduction

For women at an average risk for breast cancer, lifestyle modifications including regular aerobic exercise, maintaining a healthy weight, and limiting alcohol are most important for breast cancer risk reduction. In addition, complying with breast cancer screening recommendations provides an opportunity for early detection and decreased mortality. Women at average risk for breast cancer should be considered for screening mammography at age 40. The US Preventive Services Task Force (USPSTF) is currently updating recommendations for breast cancer screening. Updated USPSTF drafts and recommendations can be found at: https://www.uspreventiveservicestaskforce.org/uspstf/draft-recommendation/breast-cancer-screening-adults. The 2015 American Cancer Society (ACS) breast cancer screening guidelines for women at average risk include a strong recommendation to begin screening mammography at age 45 and a qualified recommendation to begin at age 40 and continue as long as the patient remains in good overall health and has a life expectancy of 10 years or greater. The most updated recommendations from the National Comprehensive Cancer Network (NCCN) and the American College of Radiology (ACR) are for annual screening mammography beginning at age 40. The standard for screening breast imaging is the digital mammogram; however, in recent years digital breast tomosynthesis has become more prevalent and available to women at breast imaging centers. Digital breast tomosynthesis has both a higher breast cancer detection rate and lower recall rate compared with the digital mammography for breast cancer screening.

Women who are at an increased risk for breast cancer may be considered for additional screening and risk reduction measures. Factors that increase a women's risk include having a known genetic mutation associated with hereditary breast cancer, having a family history of breast cancer in a first- or second-degree relative, especially premenopausal breast cancer or male breast cancer, having a personal history of a breast biopsy with atypical hyperplasia or lobular carcinoma in situ, having a personal history of chest radiation before age 30, or having a high breast density. Several breast cancer assessment tools are available for the evaluation of personalized breast cancer risk (e.g., Breast Cancer Risk Assessment Tool, Tyrer-Cuzick, BRCAPRO models). Women with a lifetime risk of breast cancer greater than 20% on a family history–based model or women with a genetic mutation or prior chest radiation may be eligible for additional annual screening with breast MRI. Certain high-risk populations may benefit from risk-reducing therapies such as chemoprevention and risk-reducing mastectomy, especially for carriers of high-penetrance mutations.

Clinical Manifestations

Women with ductal carcinoma in situ (DCIS) and early-stage breast cancer may be asymptomatic. The most common symptoms of breast cancer include the following:

- New palpable mass in the breast or axilla
- Skin changes such as dimpling, erythema, irritation, edema, thickening, peau d'orange (Fig. 1)
- Nipple retraction

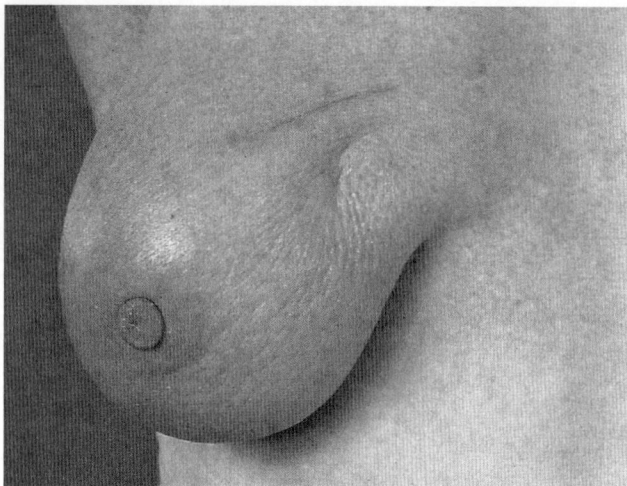

Figure 1 Peau d'orange of the breast.

- Abnormal nipple discharge
- New asymmetric appearance of breast

Differential Diagnosis

Differential diagnoses include benign conditions such as fibroadenoma, papilloma, breast cyst, and mastitis as well as malignant conditions such as breast lymphoma, sarcoma, neuroendocrine tumors, leukemia, and skin metastasis from breast or other primary tumors.

Diagnosis

Once breast malignancy is suspected clinically, either by palpation or breast imaging (Fig. 2), further evaluation is warranted. Women with an abnormal mammogram should undergo further diagnostic imaging, which may include diagnostic mammography, ultrasonography, or breast MRI. Normal and abnormal findings on breast imaging are reported using the universal classification system of the American College of Radiology (Breast Imaging Reporting and Data System [BI-RADS]). BI-RADS 0 indicates an incomplete assessment and that further workup is needed, typically with additional imaging. BI-RADS 1 and BI-RADS 2 lesions are negative or benign, respectively. BI-RADS 3 lesions are considered probably benign based on appearance; a mammogram or ultrasound scan in 6 months is recommended for follow-up. BI-RADS 4 and BI-RADS 5 lesions are suspicious or highly suggestive of malignancy, respectively, and a biopsy of the lesion is recommended. Core needle biopsy is the recommended approach for tissue sampling. The pathology report from a biopsy of a primary breast cancer will typically include the histology and tumor prognostic markers. These histologic subtypes of breast cancer include ductal, lobular, mixed, metaplastic, as well as the more favorable histologic subtypes of tubular, mucinous, and papillary.

Once breast cancer has been diagnosed, appropriate clinical staging is done, directed by a medical oncologist or surgical oncologist. This may include further breast imaging to characterize the extent of the tumor, axillary staging with ultrasound to assess for abnormal-appearing lymph nodes, and clinical examination with consideration of whole-body staging with computed tomography (CT) scan of the chest, abdomen, and pelvis depending on the size and lymph node involvement of the primary lesion. Bone scanning or positron emission tomography (PET/CT) may also be considered in some circumstances. Staging of the breast cancer is done in accordance with the American Joint Committee on Cancer (AJCC) staging system. The most updated version, the *AJCC Cancer Staging Manual*, Eighth Edition, was published in December 2017 and includes anatomic stage groups, clinical prognostic stage groups, and pathologic prognostic stage groups. All patients should have a clinical prognostic stage documented as part of their treatment plan, and those with surgery as initial treatment may also have a pathologic prognostic stage. The updated staging guidelines also include biomarker testing results within the staging system.

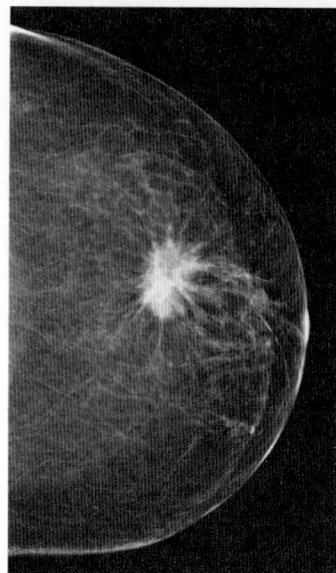

Figure 2 Breast cancer on mammogram.

Pathophysiology

Breast cancer is a heterogeneous disease. Malignant cells arise from neoplastic proliferation of epithelial cells in the ducts or lobules of the breast. If neoplastic cells are confined within the duct or lobule, the lesion is termed *ductal* or *lobular in situ*, respectively. DCIS is a precursor lesion that can potentially develop into invasive carcinoma. Invasive carcinoma is classified into four distinct molecular subtypes: luminal A, luminal B, basal-like, and HER2 enriched. More frequently we use the tumor receptor markers of the breast cancer to guide therapy, namely estrogen receptor (ER), progesterone receptor (PR), and HER2 overexpression. Hormone receptor–positive breast cancer (meaning progesterone- or estrogen receptor–positive) is the most common type of breast cancer, comprising more than 65% of all breast cancers. In general it has a less aggressive course with a long survival, even in the metastatic setting. In contrast, hormone receptor–negative and HER2-negative breast cancer—also known as triple negative breast cancer (TNBC)—tends to be more aggressive and has a much poorer outcome, especially in the advanced setting. Although the natural course of HER2-overexpressed disease tends to be aggressive, HER2-positive breast cancer now has a longer survival time since the advent of effective HER2-directed therapies.

Treatment

Breast cancer is a complex disease that requires multidisciplinary management as well as a tailored therapy plan depending on the stage, histologic subtype, and prognostic tumor marker status. Current modalities for treating breast cancer include local therapy such as surgery and radiation therapy as well as systemic therapy including chemotherapy, endocrine, and biologic therapy.

Early-stage breast cancer is treated with surgery (lumpectomy or mastectomy) with or without radiation therapy. Women who undergo lumpectomy and radiotherapy have equivalent survival outcomes to those receiving mastectomy. Axillary lymph nodes are typically evaluated by sentinel lymph node biopsy and/or axillary lymph node dissection depending on initial clinical findings and lymph node involvement with metastases on pathologic review. For selected cases, preoperative (neoadjuvant) treatment with chemotherapy or endocrine therapy are used. Neoadjuvant chemotherapy is indicated for inoperable or locally advanced breast cancer such as inflammatory breast cancer, extensive primary tumor extending to the chest wall or skin, bulky or matted axillary lymph nodes, and extra-axillary lymph node involvement. In the setting of operable breast cancer, neoadjuvant systemic treatment may be recommended to optimize surgical outcomes or to allow for assessment of tumor response on surgical pathology to guide adjuvant systemic therapy.

After definitive surgical management, adjuvant systemic therapy may be offered to reduce the risk of local and distant recurrence.

Chemotherapy is considered for those at high risk for recurrence, characterized by large tumor size, positive lymph nodes, high-grade histology, or a triple negative (hormone receptor–negative, HER2-negative) breast cancer. For hormone receptor–positive, HER2-negative, axillary node–negative breast cancer, the 21-gene recurrence score is widely used to evaluate for the potential benefit of adjuvant chemotherapy. HER2-positive breast cancer is treated with HER2-directed biologic agents along with chemotherapy followed by maintenance therapy with anti-HER2 agents such as trastuzumab (Herceptin), pertuzumab (Perjeta), and ado-trastuzumab emtansine (Kadcyla). When an anthracycline chemotherapy or HER2 antibody therapy is indicated, baseline cardiac function evaluation by either echocardiogram or multigated acquisition scan must be obtained before treatment and will be regularly monitored during the treatment with HER2-directed therapies. In high-risk triple negative breast cancer, chemotherapy may be combined with immunotherapy for systemic treatment. Radiation therapy, if indicated, is typically offered after chemotherapy.

After local treatment of hormone receptor–positive breast cancer with or without chemotherapy, adjuvant endocrine therapy is recommended for a minimum of 5 years with either a selective estrogen-receptor modulator (SERM) such as tamoxifen (Nolvadex), an aromatase inhibitor such as anastrozole (Arimidex), letrozole (Femara), or exemestane (Aromasin). In general, the choice of endocrine therapy agents is based on the menopausal state and side-effect profiles. Aromatase inhibitors need to be combined with ovarian suppression in premenopausal women. Adjuvant endocrine therapy is associated with an approximate 50% reduction in breast cancer recurrence.

Locally recurrent disease without distant metastasis can be managed with a curative intent. Combination of local therapies and systemic treatment may be used depending on the clinical scenario. Metastatic (stage IV) breast cancer with distant metastasis is not curable and is managed with the intent of disease control while maintaining quality of life and requires systemic therapy. Local therapies such as surgery and radiation therapy are indicated for palliative purposes when appropriate. Hormone-positive metastatic breast cancer can be treated with endocrine therapy as first-line treatment. Cyclin-dependent kinase (CDK4/6) inhibitors have emerged as promising agents for hormone receptor–positive, metastatic disease. In combination with endocrine therapy, CDK inhibitors demonstrated longer progression-free survival, and in some cohorts an overall survival benefit.

Metastatic HER2-positive breast cancer is treated with HER2-directed agents and chemotherapy. Additional strategies include drug antibody conjugates (ado-trastuzumab emtansine [Kadcyla], fam-trastuzumab deruxtecan-nxki [Enhertu]) or dual HER2 blockade such as trastuzumab (Herceptin) and pertuzumab (Perjeta) or lapatinib (Tykerb) or neratinib (Nerlynx) with chemotherapy, which demonstrate superior progression-free survival compared with a single HER2 agent added to chemotherapy. Biosimilars for trastuzumab are now available. For HER2-positive and hormone receptor–positive disease, dual HER2-targeted therapy combined with an aromatase inhibitor may be beneficial.

In the setting of metastatic triple negative breast cancer, systemic therapy can include the immunotherapy drug pembrolizumab (Keytruda) combined with chemotherapy, chemotherapy alone, antibody drug conjugates such as sacituzumab govitecan-hziy (Trodelvy), or targeted agents. Immunotherapy overall is better tolerated than chemotherapy but has a unique profile of potential toxicities including colitis, pneumonitis, dermatologic reactions, and endocrinopathies along with less common immune mediated adverse events.

Although single chemotherapy is preferred for metastatic disease, combined chemotherapy may be indicated for diseases with high tumor burden or in visceral crisis. Management of metastatic breast cancer may also include germline genetic testing for a BRCA1 or BRCA2 mutation and/or genomic testing of the tumor to identify potential molecular targets unique to the individual or tumor. In 2018, the US Food and Drug Administration (FDA) approved olaparib (Lynparza) and talazoparib (Talzenna), which are a poly-ADH ribose polymerase inhibitors, for the treatment of metastatic HER2-negative, BRCA-associated breast cancer. Additional therapies targeting somatic mutations such as PI3K, ESR1, AKT, PTEN, and HER2 are also available. Further targeted therapies may be explored in the setting of a clinical trial.

For patients with bone metastasis, bone-targeted therapies such as denosumab (Xgeva) and intravenous bisphosphonates are given to reduce skeletal-related events, such as pathologic fractures. Patients with poor dentition or oral hygiene who need future dental procedures during treatment are at increased risk for osteonecrosis of the jaw; thus dental evaluation is important before bone-directed therapy is initiated.

Monitoring and Survivorship

The majority of breast cancer patients are treated with curative intent and gain long-term survival. The risk of recurrence, however, is a realistic concern for many years after definitive therapy, especially for women with locally advanced or node-positive disease. Once the patient has completed definitive treatment, careful history taking and physical examination become the most important aspects of surveillance. Patients are advised to schedule an office visit up to four times yearly for the first 5 years and then annually. Monitoring for recurrence by laboratory and radiologic tests should be kept minimal in the nonmetastatic setting unless clinically indicated otherwise.

Women should continue to undergo annual screening mammography for their remaining breast tissue. If they were receiving high-risk screening with a breast MRI based on a genetic mutation, this may also be continued after breast cancer treatment. Annual gynecologic assessment is recommended for women on tamoxifen because of the associated increased risk of uterine cancer, which typically presents with abnormal bleeding in postmenopausal women. Patients on an aromatase inhibitor should have a bone mineral density completed at baseline and then annually while receiving treatment. Bone-modifying agents such as intravenous bisphosphonates or RANK ligand inhibitors may be used for management or prevention of osteoporosis while on aromatase inhibitor therapy.

In addition, women receiving adjuvant endocrine therapy may experience menopause-related symptoms such as vasomotor symptoms, vaginal dryness, and sexual dysfunction. Patients are encouraged to discuss these symptoms with their physicians because they can frequently be managed with nonhormone-based approaches. Venlafaxine (Effexor)[1], oxybutynin (Ditropan)[1], and gabapentin (Neurontin)[1] have demonstrated efficacy in management of hot flashes, as well as cognitive behavioral therapy acupuncture and avoiding triggers. Vaginal moisturizers and lubricants can be applied to help alleviate symptoms of vaginal dryness. Laser therapy may also be considered in some circumstances.

Long-term complications after definitive treatment may include lymphedema and self-image issues after surgery, skin changes after radiation therapy and persistent neuropathy, prolonged hair loss, fatigue, cognitive impairment, and a small risk of developing leukemia and myelodysplastic syndrome after chemotherapy.

Heart disease remains the leading cause of death among US women. Those who have undergone treatment for breast cancer may be at a higher risk for myocardial events depending on their baseline risk factors and the treatment they received. Accumulating evidence suggests that lifestyle modifications including regular exercise, achieving a healthy body mass index, limiting alcohol intake, and abstaining from tobacco products lead to optimal outcomes for breast cancer survivors.

---

[1] Not FDA approved for this indication.

References

American Cancer Society: Cancer Facts & Figure 2024. Atlanta: American Cancer Society; 2024.

Baselga J, Cortes J, Kim SB, et al: Pertuzumab plus trastuzumab plus docetaxel for metastatic breast cancer, N Engl J Med 366:109–119, 2012.

Couch FJ, Shimelis H, Hu C: Associations between cancer predisposition testing panel genes and breast cancer, JAMA Oncol 3(9):1190–1196, 2017.

Davies C, Pan H, Godwin J, et al: Long-term effects of continuing adjuvant tamoxifen to 10 years versus stopping at 5 years after diagnosis of oestrogen receptor-positive breast cancer: ATLAS, a randomized trial, Lancet 381(9869):805–816, 2013.

Finn RS, Crown JP, Lang I, et al: The cyclin-dependent kinase 4/6 inhibitor palbociclib in combination with letrozole versus letrozole alone as first-line treatment of oestrogen receptor-positive, HER2-negative, advanced breast cancer (PALOMA-1/TRIO-18): a randomized phase II study, *Lancet Oncol* 16(1):25–35, 2015.

Fisher B, Anderson S, Bryant J, et al: Twenty-year follow-up of a randomized trial comparing total mastectomy, lumpectomy, and lumpectomy plus irradiation for the treatment of invasive breast cancer, *N Engl J Med* 347:1233–1241, 2002.

Noone AM, Howlander N, Krapcho M, et al: SEER Cancer Statistics Review, 1975-2015, National Cancer Institute. Bethesda, MD, https://seer.cancer.gov/csr/19 75_2015/, based on November 2017 SEER data submission, posted to SEER website, April 2018.

Slamon DJ, Leyland-Jones B, Shak S, et al: Use of chemotherapy plus a monoclonal antibody against HER2 for metastatic breast cancer that overexpresses HER2, *N Engl J Med* 344:783–792, 2001.

Sparano JA, Gray RJ, Makower DF, et al: Prospective validation of a 21-gene expression assay in breast cancer, *N Engl J Med* 373:2005–2015, 2015.

Verma S, Miles D, Gianni L, et al: Trastuzumab emtansine for HER2-positive advanced breast cancer, *N Engl J Med* 367:1783–1791, 2012.

CANCER OF THE ENDOMETRIUM

Method of
Locke Uppendahl, MD; and Boris Winterhoff, MD

CURRENT DIAGNOSIS

- The high incidence of uterine cancer in developed countries reflects increased obesity rates.
- The progression from atypical hyperplasia to adenocarcinoma is a consequence of prolonged, unopposed estrogen exposure.
- Approximately 90% of women with uterine cancer report abnormal uterine bleeding, with postmenopausal bleeding the most common.
- Over 95% of uterine cancers are diagnosed in women 40 years or older.
- In most uterine cancer cases, the tumor is confined to the uterine corpus at the time of diagnosis and portends a good prognosis.
- Uterine carcinomas are classified into two broad histologic categories: the estrogen-related endometrioid (type I) and non–estrogen-related (type II) tumors.
- The FIGO staging system, updated in 2023, reflects improved understanding of prognosis and treatment.

CURRENT THERAPY

- Comprehensive surgical staging with total hysterectomy, bilateral salpingo-oophorectomy, and bilateral pelvic and paraaortic lymphadenectomy remains a critical component for the diagnosis and management of all endometrial cancers.
- The utility and extent of lymph node dissection in endometrial cancer is controversial.
- The decision for adjuvant therapy is based on the risk of relapse and persistent disease.
- Surgery alone is usually curative for women with early-stage, low-risk disease.
- Adjuvant vaginal brachytherapy is recommended for early-stage endometrial cancers that demonstrate pathologic features known to increase risk of vaginal cuff recurrence, such as high-grade, deep myometrial invasion, cervical involvement, or presence of lymphovascular space invasion.
- Women with advanced-stage (stage III or IV) or recurrent endometrial cancer are frequently treated with systemic, platinum-based chemotherapy plus immunotherapy.

Epidemiology

In the United States, uterine cancer is the most common gynecologic malignancy of the female genital tract, with an estimated 67,880 new cases and 13,250 deaths expected for 2024. Approximately 1 in 32 (3.1%) women will develop invasive cancer over their lifetime, with an average age of diagnosis of 62 years old. Uterine cancer incidence rates have been increasing by about 1% per year since the mid-2000s among women age 50 years and older and by nearly 2% per year since the mid-1990s among younger women. The high incidence observed in developed countries has been attributable to increased obesity rates, decreased fertility rates, and other risk factors.

Uterine cancer is one of the few malignancies in which survival has not improved since the mid-1970s. In fact, death rates for uterine cancer rose in 2011 through 2015 by 2% per year. Despite being the fourth most common cancer diagnosed in women, it ranked twenty-fourth in the National Cancer Institute research funding in 2018. Uterine cancer has one of the highest Black-White survival differences. The 5-year survival rate for all stages is 22% lower for Black women compared to White women. This large disparity likely reflects a delay in diagnosis in this population.

Classification

Uterine cancers arising from the lining of the uterus are called endometrial carcinoma and are classified into two broad histologic categories: the estrogen-related endometrioid (type I) and non–estrogen-related (type II) tumors.

Type I Tumors

Type I tumors are the predominant form of endometrial cancer, comprising approximately 80% of new diagnoses. The average age at diagnosis is approximately 63 years old, with nearly 70% of the tumors confined to the uterus at time of diagnosis. They include tumors of endometrioid histology (grade 1 and 2) and often arise in the background of atypical and/or complex endometrial hyperplasia. Type I tumors are more indolent, diagnosed at an earlier stages, occur in younger women, and overall portend a favorable prognosis. Patients with high-grade (grade 3) endometrioid adenocarcinoma have a less favorable prognosis.

Comprehensive genomic characterization has identified a number of genetic alterations associated with type I tumors. The loss of function in the DNA mismatch repair (MMR) enzymes MLH1, MSH2, MSH6, and PMS2 results in the inability to properly detect and repair abnormal DNA sequences. This leads to mutations in genes that have microsatellite repeats. Microsatellite instability (MSI) is found in approximately one-third of type I tumors and can be as a result of germline or sporadic mutations. Other commonly mutated genes include *PTEN*, *CTNNB1*, *PIK3CA*, *ARID1A*, and *KRAS*. These distinct molecular subtypes offer an opportunity for targeted therapies.

Type II Tumors

In contrast to type I tumors, other endometrial cancers are unrelated to unopposed estrogen exposure. Type II cancers include clear cell, carcinosarcoma, undifferentiated/dedifferentiated, serous, and some grade 3 endometrioid histology tumors. They are diagnosed more frequently among older, nonobese, non-White women and portend an unfavorable prognosis because of the later stage in diagnosis and the aggressive nature of the tumor.

Serous carcinoma of the endometrium represents approximately 5% to 10% of endometrial carcinomas, but account for 40% of all endometrial cancer-related deaths. They often deeply invade into the myometrium and demonstrate the ability for early peritoneal spread. Uterine serous carcinomas are molecularly distinct and are characterized by high genomic instability (high copy number alterations), low mutational burden, and *TP53* mutations. Newer evidence demonstrates dysregulation of the *Her2/neu* oncogene in 27% of cases. Clear cell carcinomas, another rare but aggressive subtype, represent approximately 5% of endometrial carcinomas. The 5-year overall survival rates for serous and clear cell carcinomas are 41% and 65%, respectively. Recently, genomic characterization identified approximately 25% of grade 3 endometrioid tumors that cluster with serous carcinomas, with very high somatic copy-number alterations. Nearly 90% of these tumors have *TP53* mutations. Novel mutations in *TAF1* have been implicated in a subset of clear cell carcinomas.

Risk Factors

Type I tumors are strongly linked to long-term, unopposed exposure to estrogen. Therefore risk factors include any excessive exogenous (hormonal therapy, tamoxifen) or endogenous (obesity, chronic anovulation, estrogen-secreting tumors) estrogen exposure to the uterine lining. In the United States, the high prevalence of obesity has increased the incidence of uterine cancer over the past two decades. A body mass index (BMI) of 25 to less than 30 kg/m^2 confers a relative risk of 1.5 to develop endometrial cancer compared to 7.1 for BMI greater than 40 kg/m^2. Other risk factors for type I tumors include nulliparity, diabetes mellitus, and hypertension.

Tamoxifen is a selective-estrogen receptor modulator (SERM) used in the treatment and prevention of breast cancer. The drug functions as an antagonist in the breast, but has agonist effects on the endometrium. The risks of endometrial cancer associated with tamoxifen, although very low, are well documented in the literature.

Lynch/hereditary nonpolyposis colorectal cancer (HNPCC) syndrome is caused by mutations in DNA mismatch-repair genes *MLH1, MSH2, MSH6,* and *PMS2.* The lifetime risk of developing colorectal and endometrial cancer is 9% to 61% and 13% to 54% (depends on mutated gene), respectively.

Pathophysiology

The World Health Organization (WHO) has clarified the classification of endometrial hyperplasia, differentiating between only two categories: (1) hyperplasia without atypia and (2) atypical hyperplasia/endometrioid intraepithelial neoplasia. Multiple studies have demonstrated the progression of atypical hyperplasia to adenocarcinoma is a consequence of prolonged, unopposed estrogen exposure.

Prevention

Over 95% of uterine cancers are diagnosed in women 40 years or older. Therefore abnormal uterine bleeding in these women should prompt evaluation with endometrial biopsy or dilatation and curettage (D&C). Depending on age and reproductive desire, women with endometrial hyperplasia may be treated with removal of estrogen stimulus, the periodic use of progestins, or by hysterectomy to prevent the onset of uterine cancer. For women with atypical hyperplasia, hysterectomy is the treatment of choice for because coexistent adenocarcinoma may be present in 40% of cases. In addition, this group of women carries a 30% risk of developing invasive carcinoma later in life. Finally, women with a uterus should never receive estrogen-only hormone replacement therapy (HRT). The addition of a progestin to HRT can prevent endometrial hyperplasia and subsequent endometrial cancer.

Despite no current scientific evidence, women diagnosed with Lynch syndrome should consider annual screening with endometrial sampling and transvaginal ultrasound annually, beginning between ages 30 and 35. Hysterectomy with or without oophorectomy is an option after childbearing to deter the risk of endometrial cancer.

Clinical Manifestations

Abnormal uterine bleeding is often the only presenting symptom in women diagnosed with endometrial cancer. Upward of 90% of women diagnosed with endometrial cancer report abnormal uterine bleeding, with postmenopausal bleeding the most common. However, postmenopausal bleeding has many causes and only approximately 15% of these women will have endometrial cancer.

For premenopausal and perimenopausal women, the diagnosis is more challenging and often delayed. For this group of women, intermenstrual bleeding; prolonged, heavy bleeding; or the absence of menses for several months interrupted with episodes of bleeding warrants investigation.

Finally, Papanicolaou smears demonstrate malignant cells in only approximately 50% of women with underlying endometrial cancer. This highlights the ineffectual screening method of indirectly sampling the endometrium. To date, no screening method for the general population is recommended.

Diagnosis

Diagnosis of endometrial cancer is confirmed with a histologic specimen. All women suspected of having uterine cancer due to abnormal uterine bleeding should have their endometrium sampled by biopsy. Most often, this can be done in the clinic with a rigid or flexible catheter. With this technique, reported detection rates for postmenopausal and premenopausal women are 99.6% and 91%, respectively. However, there is approximately a 10% false-negative rate with endometrial biopsy. Therefore a negative biopsy result in women highly suspicious for endometrial cancer should undergo examination under anesthesia and curettage. Finally, transvaginal ultrasound demonstrating an endometrial thickness of 5 mm or more in a postmenopausal woman requires endometrial sampling.

Women taking tamoxifen should be counseled about the increased risk of endometrial cancer and to report any abnormal vaginal bleeding so they can be thoroughly evaluated. However, no evidence supports the screening of asymptomatic women with ultrasound or serial endometrial sampling.

Staging

Increased understanding of the pathogenesis and molecular profile of endometrial cancers prompted the Cancer Committee of the International Federation of Gynecology and Obstetrics (FIGO) to update the staging of endometrial cancer in 2023. The updated staging system incorporates various histologic subtypes, tumor patterns, and molecular classifications to provide improved prognosis and treatment recommendations. This staging system replaced the 2009 FIGO surgical staging system.

Treatment

Comprehensive surgical staging with exploration of the abdominal cavity, total hysterectomy with bilateral salpingo-oophorectomy, and bilateral pelvic and para-aortic lymphadenectomy remains a critical component for the diagnosis and management of all endometrial cancers. For type II tumors, meticulous surgical staging with the addition of collection of peritoneal washings for cytology, omentectomy with or without peritoneal biopsies is required because metastatic disease is often identified only microscopically. In cases with gross metastatic disease, cytoreductive surgery may be required. Surgical staging can be performed by laparotomy, laparoscopy, or robotically assisted approach.

The utility and extent of lymph node dissection in endometrial cancer is controversial. Different strategies, including universal, selective, and sentinel lymph node mapping are currently used. The universal method performs uniform comprehensive surgical staging for nearly all patients with endometrial cancer. This method allows for the most complete information postoperatively to make adjuvant decisions, but a significant percentage of women will develop lymphedema secondary to the nodal dissection. A selective approach involves intraoperative diagnosis and deferring lymph node dissection in patients with low risk of nodal metastases. Finally, a more popular approach is using sentinel lymph node mapping with indocyanine green dye.

After surgical management, women are stratified by age and pathologic features to determine their risk for recurrence and adjuvant therapy is offered if necessary.

Adjuvant Therapy

The decision for adjuvant therapy is difficult and is based on the risk of relapse and persistent disease. In general, women with stage IA, grade 1 or 2 endometrioid adenocarcinoma have a favorable prognosis and no adjuvant therapy is necessary after surgery. Early-stage endometrial carcinomas with risk factors for recurrence, stage II to IV cancers, and all serous and clear cell carcinomas often require adjuvant therapy in the form of radiation, chemotherapy, or a combination of both.

Early-Stage Disease

Surgery alone is usually curative for women with early-stage, low-risk disease. Women with early-stage, high-risk, or high-intermediate risk factors are often recommended adjuvant radiation. The treatment can be in the form of external beam radiation therapy or vaginal brachytherapy. All serous and clear cell carcinomas of the uterus are recommended to receive adjuvant platinum-based combination chemotherapy regardless of stage. Adjuvant systemic therapy in patients with high-risk, early-stage endometrioid carcinoma remains controversial and is an active area of research.

Advanced-Stage Disease

Approximately 15% to 25% of patients will present with metastatic disease at presentation. Surgical cytoreduction is the preferred treatment approach if complete resection is achievable because it is associated with improved progression-free and overall survival. This would be followed by adjuvant therapy due to the increased risk for recurrence. The optimal form of adjuvant therapy is controversial. Extrauterine disease confined to lymph nodes may be treated with pelvic radiation therapy alone or with combination chemotherapy. However, systemic therapy with platinum-based combination chemotherapy is regarded as the foundation for extrauterine disease. The most common regimen is carboplatin (Paraplatin)[1] plus paclitaxel (Taxol).[1]

In 2023 the National Comprehensive Cancer Network Guidelines added immune-checkpoint inhibitors (pembrolizumab [Keytruda] and dostarlimab [Jemperli]) upfront as preferred, primary therapy options in combination with chemotherapy based on data from two large, phase III randomized, placebo-controlled trials. Both trials significantly improved progression-free survival in patients with primary advanced or recurrent endometrial cancer.

Patients who are not candidates for surgical cytoreduction because of either grossly metastatic disease or being too poor a surgical candidate have a poor prognosis, with 5-year relative survival of less than 20%. These patients should be offered systemic chemotherapy generally with palliative intent. Radiation therapy to achieve local control in the pelvis to palliate bleeding, discharge, and pain is often performed.

Recurrent Disease

Local recurrences, distance metastases, and simultaneous local and distant metastases are found in 50%, 29%, and 21%, respectively. Isolated vaginal recurrences are often salvaged with either surgery or radiation. Distant recurrent endometrial cancer portends a poor prognosis. Systemic chemotherapy with immunotherapy is given with a palliative intent.

Hormone Therapy

Before endometrial cancer, the risk of endometrial hyperplasia and the development into carcinoma can be significantly reduced with administration of a progestin. After the development of carcinoma, patients whose tumors test positive for estrogen receptor (ER) and progesterone receptor (PR) are associated with longer survival, with PR being a stronger predictor than ER. However, the role of adjuvant progestins in stage I or II endometrial cancer has not been demonstrated to be of value and may worsen cardiovascular disease. Progestins are commonly used in advanced or recurrent well-differentiated endometrial cancers. Oral megestrol acetate (Megace) and medroxyprogesterone acetate (Provera)[1] are two of the most commonly used progestins.

The SERM tamoxifen[1] has been used to treat patients with recurrent endometrial cancer, with response rates seen in approximately 22% of patients. The aromatase inhibitors anastrozole (Arimidex)[1] and letrozole (Femara)[1] were investigated in recurrent and metastatic endometrial cancer and demonstrated minimal activity.

Targeted Therapy

Multiple novel agents are being evaluated in clinical trials for use in treatment against endometrial cancer. Bevacizumab (Avastin)[1] is a monoclonal antibody directed against vascular endothelial growth factor that is active in endometrial cancer. Pembrolizumab (Keytruda) and dostarlimab (Jemperli) are immune checkpoint inhibitors that are often used after progression on platinum-based chemotherapy in women with MMR or MSI tumors. However, immunotherapy is now the preferred option for primary, systemic therapy in advanced stage or recurrent endometrial cancer. Trastuzumab (Herceptin)[1] and lapatinib (Tykerb)[1] are anti–human epidermal growth factor 2 (HER2) being tested as single agents and in combination with chemotherapy in some endometrial cancers. Chemotherapy with the addition of trastuzumab is now the preferred regimen for advanced-stage HER2-positive uterine serous or carcinosarcomas. The mechanistic target of rapamycin (mTOR) inhibitors everolimus (Afinitor)[1] and ridaforolimus[5] have been used to treat advanced-stage and recurrent endometrial cancers with mixed response.

Monitoring

Surveillance recommendations for endometrial cancer are stratified by risk of recurrence, and most women diagnosed and treated for endometrial cancer will fall into the low risk category. High risk for recurrence is defined as advanced stage III or grade 3 endometrioid, serous, or clear cell histology. Follow-up recommendations for women at low risk involve a history and physical examination, including a speculum and pelvic examination, scheduled every 6 months for the first 2 years, then yearly. Women with high risk of recurrence should have the same follow-up recommendations at intervals of 3 months for the first 2 years, every 6 months in years 2 to 5, then yearly. Pap test/cytology, CA-125, and routine radiographic imaging are not recommended. Women suspected of recurrence should have imaging performed.

---

[1] Not FDA approved for this indication.
[5] Investigational drug in the United States.

References

Berek JS, Matias-Guiu X, Creutzberg C, et al: FIGO staging of endometrial cancer: 2023, *Int J Gynaecol Obstet* 162(2):383–394, 2023, https://doi.org/10.1002/ijgo.14923.

Eskander RN, Sill MW, Beffa L, et al: Pembrolizumab plus Chemotherapy in Advanced Endometrial Cancer, *N Engl J Med*. 10, 2023.

Kandoth C, et al: Integrated genomic characterization of endometrial carcinoma, *Nature* 497(7447):67–73, 2013.

Mirza MR, Chase DM, Slomovitz BM, et al: Dostarlimab for Primary Advanced or Recurrent Endometrial Cancer, *N Engl J Med* 10, 2023.

Salani R, et al: An update on post-treatment surveillance and diagnosis of recurrence in women with gynecologic malignancies: Society of Gynecologic Oncology (SGO) recommendations, *Gynecol Oncol* 146(1):3–10, 2017.

Siegel RL, Giaquinto AN, Jemal A: Cancer statistics, 2024, *CA Cancer J Clin* 74(1):12–49, 2024, https://doi.org/10.3322/caac.21820.

The American College of Obstetricians and Gynecologists Committee Opinion no. 631: Endometrial intraepithelial neoplasia, *Obstet Gynecol* 125(5):1272–1278, 2015.

---

[1] Not FDA approved for this indication.

CANCER OF THE UTERINE CERVIX

Method of
Chandler Sparks, DO, MPH

CURRENT DIAGNOSIS

- Cervical cancer screening by cytology or more recently endorsed primary HPV testing is recommended for all patients with a cervix starting at age 21; frequency of follow-up is risk stratified.
- High-risk human papillomavirus (HPV) and high-risk cytology raise concern for cervical intraepithelial neoplasia (CIN3) and require an urgent biopsy.
- After discovery of CIN3+, squamous cell carcinoma (SCC), or adenocarcinoma in situ (AIS), an urgent evaluation by CT, MRI, and/or positron emission tomography (PET) scan guides therapy.

CURRENT THERAPY

- Early detection and treatment are the hallmarks of improved survival. Prevention by vaccination against HPV is safe and effective.
- Combined approaches with radiation, surgery, and chemotherapy are effective and customized to the patient's needs.
- Early referral to a specialized regional cancer center improves patient outcomes and satisfaction.

Epidemiology

Cervical cancer is relatively rare but is diagnosed most frequently in women aged 35 to 44 years. It is the fourth most common cancer in women worldwide for both incidence and mortality, with 661,021 new cases and 348,189 deaths in 2022. Most cases of cervical cancer are preventable with routine screening and treatment of precancerous lesions. As a result, most cervical cancer cases are diagnosed in women who live in regions with inadequate screening protocols.

The NIH estimates 13,360 new cases of cervical cancer in the United States in 2025, with 4320 deaths due to the disease.

Pathophysiology

Cervical carcinoma begins at the squamocolumnar junction. It can involve the outer squamous cells, inner glandular cells, or both. The precursor lesion is dysplasia: cervical intraepithelial neoplasia (CIN) or adenocarcinoma in situ (AIS), which can subsequently become invasive cancer. This process can be quite slow. Longitudinal studies have shown that in patients with untreated in situ cervical cancer, 30% to 70% will develop invasive carcinoma over a period of 10 to 12 years. However, in about 10% of patients, lesions can progress from in situ to invasive in less than 1 year. As it becomes invasive, the tumor breaks through the basement membrane and invades the cervical stroma. Extension of the tumor in the cervix may ultimately manifest as ulceration, exophytic tumor, or extensive infiltration of underlying tissue, including the bladder or rectum.

The primary risk factor for cervical cancer is infection with human papillomavirus (HPV), and it far outweighs other risk factors in development of preinvasive and invasive carcinomas. HPV infection is very common (≥60% of the population) and is often cleared spontaneously without causing cell dysplasia or preinvasive lesions, especially in young women. Two subtypes of HPV are most closely associated with high-grade dysplasia (HSIL) and cancer. HPV subtypes 16 and 18 may confer an approximately 11-fold to 17-fold increased risk of rapid development of high-grade CIN. Secondary risk factors for invasive lesions are early age at first parity, greater number of lifetime sex partners (especially >6), earlier age at first intercourse, current oral contraceptive pill (OCP) use with duration >5 years, low socioeconomic status, and smoking (squamous cell carcinoma [SCC]). HIV infection and immunosuppression, whether infectious or therapeutic (solid organ transplant, rheumatologic disorders), increase a patient's risk for all cervical cancers, which is likely due to impaired immune clearance of HPV.

Prevention and Screening

Vaccination against HPV subtypes 16 and 18 has been shown to reduce incidence of cervical cancer and decrease other HPV-related disease. There are several FDA-approved vaccines; the most recently developed vaccine is the 9-valent HPV (9vHPV [Gardasil 9]) vaccine, which includes the four primary HPV subtypes associated with cervical cancer and genital warts (6, 11, 16, and 18), as well as five other cancer-causing subtypes (31, 33, 45, 52, and 58).

The Centers for Disease Control and Prevention (CDC) recommends any form of the HPV vaccine be administered as a two-dose regimen at least 6 months apart, under the age of 15 years. If the vaccine series is *initiated* after the 15th birthday, a three-dose regimen is recommended. The vaccination course does not need to be restarted even after a long gap between doses. The greatest reduction in cancer risk is achieved by administering the vaccine series before exposure to anogenital HPV (before the onset of sexual activity).

Screening guidelines endorsed by the American College of Obstetricians and Gynecologists are summarized in Table 1.

TABLE 1 Cervical Cytologic Screening Guidelines from the American College of Obstetricians and Gynecologists

AGE (YEAR)	RECOMMENDATION FOR CYTOLOGIC SCREENING	COMMENTS
Younger than 21	Avoid screening	
21–29	Screen every 3 years	
30–65 or 70	May screen every 3 years	This recommendation applies only to women with 3 consecutive cytologic tests; exceptions include women with HIV infection, compromised immunity, a history of cervical intraepithelial neoplasia grade 2 or 3, or exposure to DES in utero
	Screen every 5 years	FDA approved primary hrHPV testing alone or Pap + HPV cotesting
65 and older	May discontinue screening	This recommendation applies only to women with ≥3 consecutive negative cytologic tests and no abnormal tests in the preceding 10 years; exceptions include women with multiple sexual partners

DES, Diethylstilbestrol; *HPV,* human papillomavirus; *hrHPV,* high-risk human papillomavirus.
Adapted from American College of Obstetricians and Gynecologists (ACOG). Cervical cancer screening and prevention. American College of Obstetricians and Gynecologists (ACOG); (ACOG practice bulletin; no. 168); 2016. (Reaffirmed April 2023)

Primary high-risk HPV (hrHPV) testing is commercially available for use in the clinical setting and endorsed by the American Society for Colposcopy and Cervical Pathology (ASCCP). Examples of such tests include Onclarity (Becton Dickinson) and Roche Cobas 4800 HPV Test. Patient's may self-collect these swabs, and results have been found to be reliable with this modality. At-home tests are available, but these are not recommended by professional societies at this time. Self-collection is not recommended for patients who experience abnormal bleeding or discharge, take medication that suppresses the immune system, or have had a recent abnormal HPV or Pap test result. Out of an abundance of caution, self-collection frequency is recommended at a 3-year follow-up interval.

Diagnosis and Staging

Preinvasive lesions and even early-stage cervical cancers may be present without any symptoms or warning signs at all, which is why screening is so important to reduce morbidity and mortality. Diagnosis is made with cervical cytology and HPV testing, or cytology alone. After a positive HPV test or high-risk cytology result, colposcopy is performed to visualize the cervix and obtain biopsies. If CIN2 or lower preinvasive disease is detected, excision is recommended by loop electrosurgical excision procedure (LEEP) or cold-knife conization. These procedures seek to remove the lesion, the transition zone, and obtain clear margins. Subsequent surveillance is risk based and can be easily determined by using the ASCCP algorithm or electronic application. Thermoablation is a satisfactory option in resource-limited settings and does reduce progression to cancer, but it is not the standard of care where LEEP or conization is available.

If CIN3+ is detected, management will advance based on FIGO classification (Table 2). Ninety percent of cervical cancers are squamous cell in origin, and 10% are glandular (adenocarcinomas). These cancers can spread by local invasion, hematogenous spread, or lymphatic spread. Extent of the disease should be evaluated with CT scan, pelvic ultrasound, and chest x-ray initially, possibly followed by positron emission tomography (PET) scan, MRI, or cystoscopy.

Management

Prognosis is closely associated with the extent of disease at the time of diagnosis. Pap smears with HPV testing allow early detection of more than 90% of cervical cancer cases. Features that confer a worse prognosis include positive HIV status, MYC oncogene overexpression, HPV-18 DNA, and alterations in enzymes that affect specific chemotherapies. Adenocarcinoma at any stage is almost always managed with hysterectomy, though excisional procedure with clear margins is acceptable in those who desire future childbearing, so long as postoperative surveillance is rigorous.

Treatment is customized depending on disease stage. Modalities include radiation, surgery, immunotherapy, and chemotherapy, each alone or in combination with one another. Stages IA, IB1, and selected IIA1 (Table 2) may be amenable to surgical intervention alone. Whether or not the patient desires fertility may dictate the operative approach. Simple, modified, or radical hysterectomy may be undertaken based on the extent of disease. In general, stage IB are treated with radical hysterectomy. If the disease has become locally invasive (stage II), platinum-containing agents concurrently with radiation are preferred. In metastatic or recurrent disease, multiagent chemotherapy is preferred. Bevacizumab (Avastin), an anti–vascular endothelial growth factor (anti-VEGF) monoclonal antibody, should be considered as an adjunct in patients with recurrent, persistent, or metastatic cervical cancer because it has been shown to improve overall survival. Pembrolizumab (Keytruda), an anti–PD-1 immune checkpoint inhibitor, is effective for patients whose tumors express this specific biomarker. Emerging therapies with other checkpoint inhibitors (cemiplimab [Libtayo][1],

---

[1] Not FDA approved for this indication.

TABLE 2 Revised FIGO Staging for Carcinoma of the Cervix

STAGE	CRITERIA
Stage I	
I	The carcinoma is strictly confined to the cervix
IA	Invasive carcinoma, which can be diagnosed only by microscopy, with deepest invasion ≤5 mm and largest extension ≥7 mm
IA1	Measured stromal invasion of ≤3 mm in depth
IA2	Measured stromal invasion of >3 mm in depth and extension of >5 mm
IB	Clinically visible lesions limited to the cervix or preclinical cancers greater than stage IA
IB1	Lesion >5 mm depth of stromal invasion and <2 cm greatest dimension
IB2	Lesion 2 cm to <4 cm in greatest dimension
1B3	Lesion >4 cm in dimension
Stage II	
II	Cervical carcinoma invades beyond the uterus, but not to the pelvic wall or to the lower third of the vagina
IIA	Without parametrial invasion
IIA1	Clinically visible lesion ≤4 cm in greatest dimension
IIA2	Clinically visible lesion >4 cm in greatest dimension
IIB	With obvious parametrial invasion
Stage III	
III	The tumor extends to the pelvic wall and/or involves lower third of the vagina and/or causes hydronephrosis or nonfunctioning kidney
IIIA	Tumor involves lower third of the vagina, with no extension to the pelvic wall
IIIB	Extension to the pelvic wall and/or hydronephrosis or nonfunctioning kidney
IIIC1	Pelvic lymph node metastasis only
IIIC2	Para-aortic lymph node metastasis
Stage IV	
IV	The carcinoma has extended beyond the true pelvis or has involved (biopsy proven) the mucosa of the bladder or rectum; a bullous edema, as such, does not permit a case to be allotted as stage IV
IVA	Spread of the growth to adjacent organs
IVB	Spread to distant organs

Adapted from Bhatla N, et al.: Revised FIGO Staging for carcinoma of cervix uteri, *Int J Gynaecol Obstet* 155(Suppl 1):28–44, 2021.

nivolumab [Opdivo][1]) and targeted agents like PARP inhibitors (olaparib [Lynparza][1], rucaparib [Rubraca][1]) may expand treatment in the near future. Referral to a regional cancer center with centralized services is also shown to improve outcomes. Common complications include secondary malignancies, especially in adjacent organs near to the radiation of the cervix, and obstructive uropathy.

Guidelines for follow-up recommendations after cervical cancer treatment are lacking. Routine imaging for surveillance is not recommended. Recurrence is most likely to occur within 2 years from treatment, so increased surveillance during this time is recommended. Most recurrences are discovered due to new signs and symptoms expressed by the patient, so a thorough review of systems and physical exam is important. Symptoms to ask about include abdominal pain, back pain, swollen leg, urinary problems, fatigue, and cough. Cervical cancer screening annually for the remainder of a patient's life after treatment is advisable, weighing risks and life expectancy appropriately.

References

American Cancer Society: *Cancer facts and figures 2025*. 2025, Available at https://www.cancer.org/research/cancer-facts-statistics/all-cancer-facts-figures/2025-cancer-facts-figures.html. Accessed October 14, 2025.

American College of Obstetricians and Gynecologists (ACOG): Cervical cancer screening and prevention. Practice bulletin #168, *ACOG, Obstet Gynecol* 128:e111–e130, 2016.

American Society for Colposcopy and Cervical Pathology. *New guidelines released for self-collected HPV screening*. Press release. February 21, 2025.

Cantillo E, et al: Less is more: minimally invasive and quality surgical management of gynecologic cancer, *Obstet Gynecol Clin North Am* 46:55, 2019.

Cervical Cancer Treatment (PDQ®). 2025. Available at https://www.ncbi.nlm.nih.gov/books/NBK66058/. Accessed October 14, 2025.

Management of premenstrual disorders: ACOG clinical practice guideline No. 7, *Obstet Gynecol* 142(6):1516–1533, 2023, https://doi.org/10.1097/AOG.0000000000005426.

Teoh D, Musa F, Salani R, Huh W, Jimenez E: Diagnosis and management of adenocarcinoma in situ: a society of gynecologic oncology evidence-based review and recommendations, *Obstet Gynecol* 135(4):869–878, 2020.

Wipperman J, Neil T, Williams T: Cervical cancer: evaluation and management, *Am Fam Physician* 97(7):449–454, 2018. PMID: 29671552.

CONTRACEPTION

Method of
Rachel A. Bonnema, MD, MS

CURRENT THERAPY

- Long-acting reversible contraception (LARC) such as an implant or intrauterine device (IUD) is safe and extremely effective and should be considered in all women, including nulliparous women.
- Combined estrogen and progesterone methods (e.g., pills, patch, ring) are effective and commonly used. They provide excellent cycle control and decreased rates of ectopic pregnancy, pelvic inflammatory disease, and endometrial and ovarian cancer, and they can be used in extended-cycle methods for patients who desire fewer than 12 periods per year.
- The use of estrogen has been associated, albeit rarely, with the development of deep venous thrombosis, myocardial infarction, and stroke; estrogen should not be used in smokers older than 35 years of age and in patients with diabetes with end organ damage, coronary artery disease, migraines with aura, or a known hypercoagulable condition.
- For women with a contraindication to estrogen, progestin-only methods are safe to use.

Nearly one-half of all pregnancies in the United States are unplanned, a rate higher than the rate in other developed countries. Primary care physicians need up-to-date knowledge on contraceptive counseling for women to provide the best match between patient and contraceptive method, in part because providers frequently need to supply contraceptives to women who have particular medical comorbidities. Newer contraceptive preparations are now available, including a vaginal ring that can be reused for up to 1 year and a progestin-only pill (POP) with a wider window for missed doses.

Nonhormonal Methods

Nonhormonal methods of contraception include barrier methods and the copper intrauterine device (IUD). These methods are safe, easily available, inexpensive, and reversible. Common barrier methods include male and female condoms, spermicides, vaginal sponges, diaphragms, and cervical caps (Table 1). Only condom use has been consistently found to protect against sexually transmitted infections (STIs) including HIV, and condom use may reduce the risk of cervical cancer as well. Of note is a novel pH-buffering spermicide, Phexxi, that is available by prescription only. Although it is not more effective than non-oxynol-9 spermicides, further studies are planned to evaluate Phexxi as a novel STI prevention method. Barrier methods have the lowest efficacy rates of all contraceptive methods, and users should also be counseled about emergency contraception (EC). The copper IUD is an extremely effective form of long-acting reversible contraception (LARC) and is a particularly attractive option for women who have contraindications to hormone use and desire effective contraception.

Combined Hormonal Contraception

Combined hormonal contraception (CHC) contains estrogen and a progestin and work primarily by preventing the surge of luteinizing hormone and thereby preventing ovulation. The majority of CHCs contain ethinyl estradiol (EE), though a new contraceptive has been approved with a novel endogenous estrogen, estetrol (E4). CHC can be delivered as an oral contraceptive pill (OCP), as a vaginal ring (NuvaRing, Annovera), or as a transdermal patch (Xulane, Twirla). Risks, benefits, side effects, and contraindications of CHC are thought to be largely similar across delivery methods.

There are many noncontraceptive benefits to CHC, including first-line treatment for dysfunctional uterine bleeding, dysmenorrhea, and menorrhagia. Benefits in addition to menstrual control include reduction in the risk for and symptoms of endometriosis, ovulatory pain, ovarian cysts, benign breast disease, premenstrual syndrome, and premenstrual dysphoric disorder. CHCs also reduce the risk of ovarian and endometrial cancers; these risk reductions extend for years after discontinuing CHC. The most common side effects of CHC are outlined in Table 2. The risk of venous thromboembolism (VTE) may be higher in obese patients, smokers, and those who use certain progestins such as desogestrel or drospirenone. This risk is lower, however, than the risk of VTE associated with pregnancy, and the absolute risk of VTE among CHC users remains small. The novel OCP with E4 (E4 plus drospirenone [Nextstellis]) has demonstrated more neutral effects on the liver, with preliminary findings suggesting lower VTE risk compared with other CHC.

CHCs can be used safely by those with a range of medical conditions, including well-controlled hypertension, uncomplicated diabetes, migraines *without* aura when younger than 35 years of age, and a family history of breast cancer, to name a few. CHC use is contraindicated in patients who have a history of migraine headache with aura at any age or in those older than 35 years of age with any migraine because of an elevated risk for stroke. CHC is also contraindicated in patients with diabetes with end organ damage, those with known cardiovascular disease, and individuals who smoke after 35 years of age because of an elevated risk for cardiovascular disease. Other contraindications include a personal history of breast cancer, an estrogen-dependent tumor, unexplained vaginal bleeding, stroke, known thromboembolic disorder, or known VTE. Elevated risk of VTE and negative effect on lactation restrict the use of CHC in the first 6 weeks after delivery.

Combined Oral Contraceptive Pills

There are dozens of formulations of OCPs that differ by their estrogen type and dosage, progestin type and dosage, and hormone delivery schedule. OCPs can be monophasic in which each pill contains the same amount of hormones, or multiphasic in which pills contain different amounts of hormones throughout the monthly cycle. The different formulations offer patients options in cycle length, hormone levels, duration of withdrawal bleeding, and side-effect profile. Education should include taking the pill at the same time each day. If a pill is missed, it should be taken as soon as remembered. If 2 days of pills are missed,

TABLE 1	Nonhormonal Contraception				
	BARRIER METHODS				**INTRAUTERINE DEVICE**
	CONDOM (MALE/FEMALE)	**DIAPHRAGM OR CERVICAL CAP**	**SPONGE**	**SPERMICIDE**	**COPPER IUD**
Duration	Female condom can be inserted up to 8 h before intercourse; male condoms must be changed with each act of intercourse	Can be placed up to 6 h before intercourse and should be removed within 6 h after	Can be left in for 30 h and through multiple acts of intercourse	Placed 30–60 min before intercourse; proper instructions should be followed according to product directions	Approved for up to 10 years
Typical-use failure rate*	15%	15%	15%	10%–22%†	Less than 0.1%
Side effects and considerations	High failure rates: condom can break or slip Acceptability by partner may be limited	Requires expert fitting Must be refitted after childbirth Requires dexterity and self-placement by patient Use with spermicide increases efficacy but can lead to risk of UTIs, increased risk of toxic shock syndrome, and potential increased risk of HIV transmission	May increase risk of UTIs Use with spermicide increases efficacy but can lead to risk of UTIs, increased risk of toxic shock syndrome, and potential increased risk of HIV transmission	Vulvovaginal burning/itching can occur Phexxi is a novel spermicide available only with prescription; nonoxynol-9 formulations are commonly available over the counter	Bleeding and cramping with menses initially Low risk of ectopic pregnancy, premature delivery, perforation, or expulsion Avoid with active infection, undiagnosed genital bleeding, cervical cancer, or Wilson disease
Consider in:	Patients at risk for STIs Patients without access to medical care and who are looking for nonhormonal, reversible, and convenient methods of contraception	Women who are looking for nonhormonal, reversible, and convenient methods of contraception	Women who are looking for nonhormonal, reversible, and convenient methods of contraception Patients without access to medical care	Women using other barrier methods or looking for moderately effective contraception	Women with contraindication to hormones or who desire hormone-free, long-acting, reversible contraception Women in need of EC followed by long-term effective contraception

*Trussell J. Contraceptive failure in the United States. *Contraception.* 2011;83(5):397–404.
†Varies according to product, Wong JC, Creinin MD. 2021 update on contraception. *OBG Manag.* 2021;33(10):23–25, 30–32, 34, e1.
EC, Emergency contraception; *HIV,* human immunodeficiency virus; *IUD,* intrauterine device; *UTI,* urinary tract infection.

the regimen includes two pills daily for 2 days in a row with a backup method utilized. If 3 days of pills are missed, the pill pack should be discarded and a backup method utilized. At that point, it should be discussed whether to start a new pack or to change contraceptive methods.

For those who desire fewer days of menses or fewer than 12 menses per year, extended-cycle OCP regimens can be offered that offer a placebo week every 4 months or eliminate the placebo week altogether. Extended-cycle regimens have other benefits, including decreased hormone withdrawal symptoms such as headaches, tiredness, bloating, excessive bleeding, or menstrual pain. In addition to estrogen dose and scheduling, it is also important to consider the progestin component, which theoretically may affect libido, weight gain, acne, and hirsutism.

Contraceptive Patch

Norelgestromin/EE (Xulane) is a thin transdermal patch delivering a daily dose of 35 µg/day EE and 150 µg/day norelgestromin. Levonorgestrel/EE (Twirla) is a newly approved patch delivering a daily dose of 30 µg/day EE and 120 µg/day levonorgestrel. Both patches are administered similarly: changed weekly for 3 weeks on "patch change day" followed by a patch-free week during which menses occur. Only one patch should be worn at a time, and no more than 7 days should pass during the patch-free week. Both have decreased efficacy in obese women and are contraindicated in patients with a BMI >30 kg/m². Most of the noncontraceptive benefits, side effects, cardiovascular risks, and contraindications are similar to those of other forms of CHC, but there may be an increased risk of VTE in patch users compared with OCP users, though studies are controversial as to the actual increase in associated risk. Of note, the VTE risk associated with patch use is lower than that associated with pregnancy.

Vaginal Ring

Contraceptive vaginal rings (CVRs) deliver hormones directly through the vaginal epithelium for highly effective contraception without the need for daily dosing. There are currently two CVRs that are approved by the U.S. Food and Drug Administration (FDA) for use in the United States. Etonogestrel/EE (NuvaRing) is a soft plastic ring that is inserted vaginally by the patient, usually for 3 weeks and then removed for 1 week, at which time menses occur. A new ring is inserted 7 days after

TABLE 2 Hormonal Contraception

| | COMBINATION ESTROGEN-PROGESTIN | | PROGESTIN-ONLY | | | |
| | TRADITIONAL (OCPS, PATCH, SA/EE RING) | EXTENDED CYCLE (OCPS, ENG/EE RING) | PILL | | INJECTION | IMPLANT/IUD |
			NORETHINDRONE	DROSPIRENONE		
Duration	Daily pill	Daily pill or monthly ring	Daily pill with no hormone-free interval	Daily with 4 day hormone-free interval	3 months	3–8 years
Reversibility	Immediate	Immediate	Immediate	Immediate	Variable	Immediate
Typical-use failure rate*	9%	9%	9%		6%	0.05%–0.8%
Side effects†	Spotting, nausea, headache, breast tenderness, VTE, stroke, MI	Similar to traditional with increased risk for unpatterned bleeding	Unpatterned bleeding, or absence of bleeding; headaches, nausea, mood changes, breast tenderness		Unpatterned bleeding or absence of bleeding; weight gain, depression, reversible decrease in BMD	Unpatterned bleeding, or absence of bleeding
Consider in:	Women with dysmenorrhea, menorrhagia, irregular menstrual periods, acne, hirsutism, or polycystic ovary syndrome	Women who do not desire monthly periods. Offers particular benefit for women with estrogen withdrawal symptoms, dysmenorrhea, or endometriosis	Women with contraindication to estrogen, hypercoagulable states, dysmenorrhea, migraine with aura, or breast-feeding		Women with contraindication to estrogen, seizure disorder, hypercoagulable states, dysmenorrhea, migraine with aura, or breast-feeding	Women with contraindication to estrogen, seizure disorder, hypercoagulable states, dysmenorrhea, migraine with aura, or breast-feeding

*Trussell J. Contraceptive failure in the United States. *Contraception.* 2011;83(5):397–404.
†Note: For all combination methods, must have no contraindication to estrogen.
BMD, Bone mineral density; *IUD*, intrauterine device; *MI*, myocardial infarction; *OCP*, oral contraceptive pill; *VTE*, venous thromboembolism.

the last one was removed, even if bleeding is not complete. The ring releases 15 µg of ethinyl estradiol and 0.12 mg of etonogestrel daily for 3 to 5 weeks, so it can be kept in longer than 3 weeks for those desiring the benefits of extended-cycling use discussed previously. Each ring releases approximately one-half the level of hormones as the average OCP without affecting efficacy. If the ring falls out (as occurs rarely), it can be rinsed and reinserted without a change in efficacy. Most find the ring easy to insert and remove and comfortable to retain during intercourse.

A newer ring containing a year's contraception with segesterone acetate (SA) and EE is now available. The SA/EE ring (Annovera) is used for 21 days followed by a 7-day use-free interval for up to 13 consecutive cycles. Unlike the NuvaRing, no data are available on extended periods of continuous use with the same SA/EE ring; during counseling, special emphasis should be placed on the increased pregnancy risk for patients who remove the ring for more than 2 hours. Both rings available are highly effective, similar to other combined hormonal methods, and have excellent cycle control. The vaginal ring has been associated with an increase in leukorrhea. Otherwise, its noncontraceptive benefits, side effects, cardiovascular risks, and contraindications are similar to those of other forms of CHC.

Progestin-Only Contraceptives

Progestin-only contraceptives are particularly beneficial for those with a contraindication to estrogen because progestin-only methods have decreased associated medical risks, including no increased risk of stroke, myocardial infarction, or VTE. All progestin-only methods have a similar method of action: Ovulation is variably inhibited, cervical mucus is thickened, and the endometrial lining undergoes histologic alterations, making implantation less likely.

Because many of the progestin-only methods are long acting, they tend to have lower failure rates as opposed to CHCs (see Table 2). All progestin-only methods are appropriate for breast-feeding.

Pill

There are now three POPs available in the United States. Norethindrone pills as prescription and norgestrel pills now available as Opill over the counter, are taken without a hormone-free interval, and fertility returns immediately on discontinuation. In fact, most experts believe fertility can return in as little as 3 hours after a missed dose; thus patients should be counseled to use a backup method if 3 or more hours late in taking her dose. Given this small window for error, this method should be prescribed only to patients who can adhere closely to a daily pill schedule. Additionally, counseling should include that while taking norethindrone pills or Opill, normal menstrual patterns may include anything from amenorrhea to menometrorrhagia. This unpatterned bleeding is likely one of the greatest obstacles to wider use of progestin-only oral contraception.

A new POP contraceptive contains drospirenone 4 mg (Slynd) and is available in a 24-day supply of hormone and a 4-day supply of placebo, allowing for a timed withdrawal bleed. The drospirenone-only pill maintains contraceptive efficacy, even with 24-hour delayed or missed-pill errors; patients can be counseled to take a missed pill as soon as remembered if within 24 hours or with the next scheduled dose if more than 24 hours late. Although intermenstrual bleeding rates are still high, the menstrual profile may be more tolerable compared with other POPs.

Because POPs have demonstrated no significant negative effects on breast-feeding, POPs can be prescribed immediately postpartum. POPs may have similar effects as other progestin-only methods in decreasing the frequency of sickle cell crises; however, unlike depot medroxyprogesterone acetate (DMPA,

Depo-Provera) injections, certain anticonvulsants may lower the effectiveness of the POP, so other methods may be more beneficial in patients with seizure disorders.

Injectable

The intramuscular DMPA injection (Depo-Provera 150 mg) is given every 12 weeks and has a typical-use failure rate of 6%. A lower dose of DMPA (104 mg in Depo-SubQ Provera) has been approved for subcutaneous injection. Patients with seizure disorders are particularly good candidates for DMPA injections because, unlike other forms of contraception, the efficacy of DMPA is not affected by enzyme-inducing antiepileptic drugs. Depo-Provera may also decrease seizure frequency, providing additional benefit. DMPA reduces serum estradiol levels, which can adversely affect bone health. There is a clear association between DMPA use and decreased bone mineral density (BMD); however, data have shown the BMD loss to be reversible with discontinuation of use, and there is no increased risk of fracture with the use of DMPA. The World Health Organization has recommended that there be no restriction on the use of Depo-Provera in patients who are 18 to 45 years of age. According to recent consensus guidelines, clinicians should advise patients about the risk for BMD loss but can reassure them about reversibility with discontinuation.

Intrauterine System

The levonorgestrel intrauterine system (LNG-IUS) is a highly effective contraceptive method long considered to be reversible sterilization because of its excellent efficacy in preventing pregnancy and quick return to fertility after its removal. There are now multiple formulations of LNG IUS that prevent pregnancy for 3 to 8 years (Skyla, Kyleena, Mirena, Liletta), categorized by the amount of levonorgestrel that they contain: 52 mg in Mirena and Liletta, 19.5 mg in Kyleena, or 13.5 mg in Skyla. The LNG-IUS is ideal for those who require highly effective contraception and is particularly beneficial for patients requiring a progestin-only contraception. Its relatively low cost over time is another factor for patients to consider. Numerous studies have confirmed the effectiveness of the LNG-IUS for reduction of menstrual blood loss in menorrhagia, leiomyomas, and pain caused by endometriosis; Mirena received FDA approval for the indication of menorrhagia and has been shown to decrease menorrhagia for those on anticoagulation. Insertion of the LNG-IUS requires a trained provider. At the time of placement, cramping and pain may occur; a rare complication of placement is uterine wall rupture. Many will likely develop amenorrhea, though they may experience initial irregular bleeding and spotting.

Implant

There is one single-rod subdermal implant available in the United States called Nexplanon that is a highly effective long-term contraceptive containing the progestin etonogestrel (ENG). The rod is implanted in the upper arm and remains active for 3 years. ENG does not cause a hypoestrogenic state and thus is not considered to have any significant effect on BMD. ENG implantation can be done as a simple procedure by a trained provider under local anesthesia with a preloaded, disposable applicator. Patients experience a quick return to normal cycles after implant removal, and there have been no reports of infertility after removal. Similar to other progestin-only forms of contraception, irregular bleeding is the major side effect of the ENG implant. The most common bleeding pattern associated with the implant is infrequent, irregular bleeding. This remains an important counseling point because the highest rate of discontinuation is during the first 8 to 9 months of use, primarily as a result of frequent bleeding.

Permanent

Permanent birth control methods include vasectomy and female sterilization by various procedures. These methods are highly effective (typical failure rate 0.15% to 0.5%); however, they are permanent. Each sterilization procedure has advantages and disadvantages that should be considered by the patient before choosing which one to use.

Emergency Contraception

Familiarity with EC is critical both for those having unprotected sex and for those who are using methods with higher failure rates. EC use has not been shown to reduce compliance with other first-line methods. EC primarily acts by inhibiting or delaying ovulation and works before implantation; if a fertilized egg has already implanted, EC will not work. EC includes pills (composed of estrogen plus progestin, progestin only, and antiprogestins) and copper or Mirena IUD placement (inserted up to 5 days after unprotected intercourse). Neither IUD has FDA labeling for emergency contraception, though they have long-term use. EC pills are most effective when taken in the first 12 hours but have gradually decreasing effectiveness for up to 120 hours after intercourse. The most accessible form of EC in the United States contains levonorgestrel only (Plan B One Step) and is available over the counter without age restrictions.

Counseling

When counseling patients about their contraceptive choices, it is important that providers are aware of their role in giving information and allowing patients to make informed decisions. The only effective contraceptive is one that a patient is willing to use consistently and correctly, and the choice of contraception is ultimately the patient's decision. Providers must educate patients regarding the advantages and disadvantages of each method that is medically appropriate for them. Discussing patient preferences for menstrual frequency and tolerance for scheduled and unscheduled bleeding is important in deciding which contraceptive best fits a patient's needs. Providers should counsel patients on expected side effects as well as expectant management strategies. Every effort should be made to remove barriers to initiation, including having no requirement for a pelvic examination or Pap smear before initiation. Using the conversation about contraceptives to also discuss safe sex is ideal.

References

ACOG Committee on Practice Bulletins—Gynecology: ACOG practice bulletin. No. 73: use of hormonal contraception in women with coexisting medical conditions, *Obstet Gynecol* 107:1453–1472, 2006.

Baker C, Creinin MD: Contraception update, *OBG Manage* 32(10):10–18, 2020.

Baker CC, Creinin MD: Long-acting reversible contraception, *Obstet Gynecol* 140(5):883–897, 2022.

Curtis KM, Tepper NK, Jatlaoui TC, et al: U.S. Medical eligibility criteria for contraceptive use 2016, *MMWR Recomm Rep* 65(RR-3):1–104, 2016, https://doi.org/10.15585/mmwr.rr6503a1.

Finer LB, Zolna MR: Unintended pregnancy in the United States: incidence and disparities, *Contraception* 84:478–485, 2006. 2011.

Lanza LL, McQuay LJ, Rothman KJ, et al: Use of depot medroxyprogesterone acetate contraception and incidence of bone fracture, *Obstet Gynecol* 121:593–600, 2013.

Parkin L, Sharples K, Hernandez RK, et al: Risk of venous thromboembolism in users of oral contraceptives containing drospirenone or levonorgestrel: nested case control study based on UK General Practice Research Database, *BMJ* 340:d2139, 2011.

Petitti DB: Combination estrogen-progestin oral contraceptives, *N Engl J Med* 349:1443–1450, 2003.

Spencer AL, Bonnema RA, McNamara MC: Helping women choose appropriate hormonal contraception: update on risks, benefits, and indications, *Am J Med* 122:497–506, 2009.

Trussell J: Contraceptive failure in the United States, *Contraception* 83:397–404, 2011.

Turok DK, Gero A, Simmons RG, et al: Levonorgestrel vs. copper intrauterine devices for emergency contraception, *N Engl J Med* 384(4):335–344, 2021.

DYSMENORRHEA

Method of
Linda Speer, MD

CURRENT DIAGNOSIS

- Primary dysmenorrhea (painful menses without underlying pathology) is common among adolescents and young women. It usually begins shortly after menarche.
- Diagnosis of primary dysmenorrhea can be made based on typical history of crampy pelvic pain during the first 1 to 3 days of the menstrual cycle. Pelvic examination is not required.
- Secondary dysmenorrhea (with underlying pathology) should be considered in cases that do not match the typical history, begin later in life, and/or are refractory to treatment.
- The most common cause of secondary dysmenorrhea is endometriosis. The clinical standard for diagnosis of endometriosis is laparoscopic confirmation. Ultrasound imaging is useful in some cases.

CURRENT THERAPY

- Nonsteroidal antiinflammatory drugs (NSAIDs) are well-established first-line therapy for treatment of primary dysmenorrhea. None has been confirmed as superior to others.
- Cyclooxygenase-2 (COX-2) inhibitors are effective and have fewer gastrointestinal side effects but may be less effective than NSAIDs.
- Oral contraceptives and the levonorgestrel intrauterine system (Mirena)[1] reduce dysmenorrhea.
- Other effective therapies include topical heat, high-frequency transcutaneous electrical nerve stimulation (TENS), and several herbal preparations.
- Treatments for endometriosis as a secondary cause of pelvic pain and dysmenorrhea include hormonal suppression of the endometrial tissue, conservative laparoscopic surgical debulking, and hysterectomy in selected cases.

[1]Not FDA approved for this indication.

Dysmenorrhea is defined as painful menses. Primary dysmenorrhea occurs without underlying pathology, typically beginning soon after menarche. It is common in adolescent girls, with prevalence ranging from 20% to 90% depending on measurement methods; about 15% of adolescents describe their dysmenorrhea as severe. The median duration of each episode is 2 days beginning with the onset of menses. During adolescence, dysmenorrhea leads to high rates of school absence and activity nonparticipation. According to representative national survey data in the United States, 14% of adolescent girls aged 12 to 17 years frequently miss school because of menstrual cramps.

A prospective cohort study showed that the prevalence and severity of dysmenorrhea was lower at 24 years of age than at 19 years of age. At 24 years of age, 67% of the women still experienced dysmenorrhea, and 10% reported pain severity that limited daily activity. The prevalence and severity of dysmenorrhea were reduced in women who were parous at 24 years and nulliparous at 19 years, but they were unchanged in women who were still nulliparous or women who had had a miscarriage or abortion.

There is a significant correlation between the severity of dysmenorrhea and the amount of menstrual flow. Survey data demonstrate that depression and anxiety are associated with menstrual pain and suggest that loss of social support is a significant contributor to menstrual symptoms. The severity of dysmenorrhea is not associated with height, weight, or regularity of the menstrual cycle. A relationship to smoking has been found inconsistently.

Secondary dysmenorrhea typically starts later in life after the onset of an underlying causative condition, most often endometriosis. The association between dysmenorrhea and endometriosis is uncertain for women with minimal disease. However, based on a study of more than 1000 women with laparoscopically confirmed endometriosis, chronic pelvic pain, dyspareunia, and dysmenorrhea are in fact related to the extent of endometriosis.

Diagnosis

For adolescents who present with complaints typical for primary dysmenorrhea, treatment may be started empirically without a pelvic examination or diagnostic studies. Sexually active adolescents and young women should be screened for chlamydia and gonorrhea, which can be done with either urine or a genital sampling.

For adolescents and women who do not have a history consistent with primary dysmenorrhea or who are refractory to treatment, endometriosis may be suspected. The gold standard for diagnosis is laparoscopy and biopsy. Ultrasound may also be useful, especially to identify endometriomas.

Treatment

Nonsteroidal Antiinflammatory Drugs

A Cochrane review of randomized, controlled trials (RCTs) concluded that among women with primary dysmenorrhea, NSAIDs were significantly more effective for pain relief than placebo or acetaminophen (Tylenol). No specific NSAID was shown to be superior to others for either pain relief or safety. However, the available evidence had little power to detect such differences, because most individual comparisons were based on few small trials. In one study in which diclofenac (Voltaren) 100 mg was compared with placebo for treatment of primary dysmenorrhea, the authors found that leg strength and aerobic capacity were maintained at the level found during luteal phase when women took diclofenac for dysmenorrhea, but they were reduced during menses in the placebo group.

COX-2 Inhibitors

Several COX-2 inhibitors have been evaluated for treatment of dysmenorrhea in RCTs. Celecoxib (Celebrex) 200 mg was compared with naproxen sodium (Naprosyn) 550 mg and placebo for treatment of dysmenorrhea and found to be superior to placebo but not as effective as naproxen. Etoricoxib (Arcoxia)[5] 120 mg daily was found to be better than placebo and equivalent to mefenamic acid (Ponstel) for treatment of primary dysmenorrhea with less nausea and epigastric pain than mefenamic acid.

Oral Contraceptives

In a systematic review of NSAIDs and oral contraceptives (OCs) for treatment of dysmenorrhea that included 10 placebo-controlled RCTs of NSAIDs, two RCTs of OCs and six prospective observational studies of OCs, the authors concluded that both are effective. In a study of women with laparoscopically proven endometriosis, low-dose ethinyl estradiol and norethisterone (norethindrone) decreased dysmenorrhea associated with endometriosis as compared with placebo (with pain assessment on a verbal rating scale from 0 to 3). There was also a significant reduction in volume of endometriomas with OCs but not placebo.

Levonorgestrel Intrauterine System

The levonorgestrel intrauterine system (LNG-IUS), Mirena, reduces menstrual bleeding and dysmenorrhea, which can be a desirable side effect for women desiring long-term contraception. In an uncontrolled case series of women treated with LNG-IUS for adenomyosis, dysmenorrhea diminished continuously during

---

[5]Investigational drug in the United States.

the 3-year study from a mean 78 mm to a mean 12 mm on a 100-mm visual analog scale. Overall satisfaction with treatment was 73%. Depot medroxyprogesterone acetate[1] (Depo-Provera) is similarly effective, but it is less likely to be well tolerated owing to unpredictable bleeding, weight gain, and mood changes.

Transcutaneous Electrical Nerve Stimulation
A small randomized controlled trial demonstrated that transcutaneous electrical nerve stimulation (TENS) applied to low abdomen and/or low back significantly reduced dysmenorrhea compared with sham treatment. High-frequency TENS has been found to be effective for the treatment of dysmenorrhea in a number of small trials. Low-frequency TENS does not appear to be effective.

Topical Heat and Infrared Light
Two meta-analyses have concluded that topical heat is likely an effective therapy based on several small low-to-moderate-quality studies. In a trial comparing far-infrared emitting belt versus placebo belt for treatment of primary dysmenorrhea, both with concurrent application of topical heat, both groups improved, and the duration of the analgesic effect was significantly longer in the group treated with the infrared belt.

Complementary and Alternative Medicine Approaches
Herbal
Several herbal remedies have been studied in RCTs for treatment of dysmenorrhea and found to be effective as compared with placebo or NSAIDs. They include *Psidii guajava* extract[7] 6 mg/day, French maritime pine bark extract (pycnogenol),[7] ginger root powder[7] 250 mg 4 times daily, salix extract[7] (willow bark) 400 mg daily, turmeric[7] 500 mg, fennel,[7] and cinnamon[7] one 1000 mg capsule daily. A pilot study of oral lactobacillus capsules (probiotic)[7] suggests that it may also be helpful.

Acupressure and Acupuncture
The evidence for the effectiveness of acupuncture is not conclusive. In unblinded studies women experience clinically relevant reduction in pain scores, a mean of more than 10 points on a 100-point scale, which could be due to placebo effect. In fact, in a well-designed RCT of electro-acupuncture at the Sanyinjiao point (the point expected to be related to uterine pain) compared to an unrelated nonacupoint or no acupuncture, the only significant differences were with the no-acupuncture group as measured with a visual analogue rating scale.

Adequate blinding is also an issue among studies of acupressure. For example, in an RCT comparing auricular seed acupressure versus adhesive tape only for treatment of primary dysmenorrhea the acupressure group (but not the tape only group) had instructions to massage the seed 15 times, three times daily for 20 days. Menstrual pain decreased significantly in the acupressure group. Several other studies suggest that acupressure at the Sanyinjiao point or Taichong point is more effective than no intervention or inadequately blinded control groups. Because acupressure is a low-cost and harmless intervention, it may be worth considering even if the pain reduction is a placebo response. It appears to be less effective than analgesics.

Yoga and Other Physical Activity
Yoga is another alternative approach with low cost and little risk that may be worth considering despite weak evidence for effectiveness. In one unblinded RCT, three yoga poses (cat, cobra, and fish) were studied for treatment of primary dysmenorrhea. Participants randomized to the intervention group were told to do the yoga poses during luteal phase and complete a questionnaire regarding menstrual characteristics. The control group was asked to complete the questionnaire only. There was significant reduction in intensity and duration of pain in the yoga group compared with baseline and with the control group.

Two meta-analyses have concluded limited quality evidence suggests that physical activity interventions reduce the duration and intensity of primary dysmenorrhea, perhaps more than oral analgesics. Further study is needed to determine what physical activity regimens are most beneficial.

Spinal Manipulation
Overall there is no evidence to suggest that spinal manipulation is effective in the treatment of primary and secondary dysmenorrhea.

Surgical Treatment
Surgical treatment may be considered in severe and refractory cases of pelvic pain including dysmenorrhea. Laparoscopic uterosacral nerve ablation (LUNA, $n=35$) alone has been compared with LUNA plus presacral neurectomy ($n=32$). There were no differences between groups for relief of dysmenorrhea at 3-, 6-, and 12-month follow-up, but more surgical complications were experienced with neurectomy.

Treatment of Endometriosis
Treatment of endometriosis may start with use of NSAIDs, hormonal contraceptives, and/or LNG-IUS.[1] However, often endometriosis is diagnosed after those first-line therapies have failed. Debulking of the ectopic endometrial tissue during laparoscopy can relieve pain.

Other treatments involve hormonal suppression of endometrial tissue. Danazol is a 19-nortestosterone derivative with a long history of use for treatment of endometriosis pain at a dosage of 400 to 800 mg daily for 6 months, but it is often poorly tolerated owing to androgenic side effects. Progestin regimens (medroxyprogesterone acetate[1] [Depo-SubQ Provera 104]) 104 mg SQ every 3 months or norethindrone ([Aygestin] up to 15 mg PO daily) may be used to suppress menses for a 6-month course. Other accepted therapies include gonadotropin-releasing hormone (GnRH) agonist analogues such as leuprolide (Lupron). Aromatase inhibitors have been shown to be effective in a systematic review of several small RCTs. Etonogestrel subdermal implant[1] (Nexplanon) has been evaluated in an uncontrolled case series and found to be associated with pain relief.

In severe refractory cases, hysterectomy may be considered.

---

[1]Not FDA approved for this indication.

References
Alonso C, Coe CL: Disruptions of social relationships accentuate the association between emotional distress and menstrual pain in young women, *Health Psychol* 20:411–416, 2001.

Andersch B, Milsom I: An epidemiologic study of young women with dysmenorrhea, *Am J Obstet Gynecol* 144:655–660, 1982.

Armour M, Smith CA, Steel KA, Macmillan F: The effectiveness of self-care and lifestyle interventions in primary dysmenorrhea: a systematic review and meta-analysis, *BMC Complement Altern Med* 19:22, 2019.

Bazarganipour F, Lamyian M, Heshmat R, et al: A randomized clinical trial of the efficacy of applying a simple acupressure protocol to the Taichong point in relieving dysmenorrhea, *Int J Gynaecol Obstet* 111:105–109, 2010.

Brown J, Crawfort TJ, Datta S, Prentice A: Oral contraceptives for pain associated with endometriosis, *Cochrane Database Syst Rev* CD001019, 2018.

Brown J, Pan A, Hart RJ: Gonadotrophin-releasing hormone analogues for pain associated with endometriosis, *Cochrane Database Syst Rev* (12):CD008475, 2010.

Carroquino–Garcia P, Jimenez–Rejano JJ, Medrano–Sanchez E, et al: Therapeutic exercise in the treatment of primary dysmenorrhea: A systematic review and meta-analysis, *Phys Ther* 99:1371-80, 2019.

Celik AS, Apay SE: Effect of progressive relaxation exercises on primary dysmenorrhea in Turkish students: A randomized prospective controlled trial. *Complement Ther Clin Pract* 42:101280, 2021.

Chantler I, Mitchell D, Fuller A: Diclofenac potassium attenuates dysmenorrhea and restores exercise performance in women with primary dysmenorrhea, *J Pain* 10:191–200, 2009.

Cote P, Hartvigsen J, Axen I, et al: The global summit on efficacy and effectiveness of spinal manipulative therapy for prevention and treatment of non-musculoskeletal disorders: a systematic review of the literature. *Chiropr Man Therap* 29:8, 2021.

Daniels S, Robbins J, West CR, Nemeth MA: Celecoxib in the treatment of primary dysmenorrhea: Results from two randomized, double-blind, active- and placebo-controlled, crossover studies, *Clin Ther* 31:1192–1208, 2009.

---

[1]Not FDA approved for this indication.
[7]Available as dietary supplement.

Doubova SV, Morales HR, Hernández SF, et al: Effect of a *Psidii guajavae folium* extract in the treatment of primary dysmenorrhea: A randomized clinical trial, *J Ethnopharmacol* 110:305–310, 2007.

Guy M, Foucher C, Juhel C et al: Transcutaneous electrical neurostimulation relieves primary dysmenorrhea: a randomized, double-blind clinical study versus placebo, *J Prog Urol* 32:487–97, 2022.

Harlow SD, Park M: A longitudinal study of risk factors for the occurrence, duration and severity of menstrual cramps in a cohort of college women, *Br J Obstet Gynaecol* 103:1134–1142, 1996.

Hesami S, Kavianpour M, Rashidi Nooshabani M, et al: Randomized, double-blind, placebo-controlled clinical trial studying the effects of turmeric in combination with mefenamic acid in patients with primary dysmenorrhea. *J Gynecol Obstet Hum Reprod* 50:101840, 2021.

Jahangirifar M, Taebi M, Dolatian M: The effect of cinnamon on primary dysmenorrhea: A randomized, double-blind clinical trial, *Complement Ther Clin Pract* 33:56–60, 2018.

Jensen JT: Noncontraceptive applications of the levonorgestrel intrauterine system, *Curr Womens Health Rep* 2:417–422, 2002.

Juang CM, Chou P, Yen MS, et al: Laparoscopic uterosacral nerve ablation with and without presacral neurectomy in the treatment of primary dysmenorrhea: A prospective efficacy analysis, *J Reprod Med* 52:591–596, 2007.

Jo J, Lee SH: Heat therapy for primary dysmenorrhea: A systematic review and meta-analysis of its effects on pain relief and quality of life, *Sci Rep* 8:16252, 2018.

Khodaverdi S, Mohammedbeigi R, Khaled M, et al: Beneficial effects of oral lactobacillus on pain severity in women suffering from endometriosis: A pilot placebo-controlled randomized clinical trial, *Int J Fertil Steril* 13:178–183, 2019.

Klein JR, Litt IF: Epidemiology of adolescent dysmenorrhea, *Pediatrics* 68:661–664, 1981.

Lee CH, Roh JW, Lim CY, et al: A multicenter, randomized, double-blind, placebo-controlled trial evaluating the efficacy and safety of a far infrared-emitting sericite belt in patients with primary dysmenorrhea, *Complement Ther Med* 19:187–193, 2011.

Lopez-Liria R, Torres-Alamo L, Vega-Ramirez FA, et al: Efficacy of physiotherapy treatment in primary dysmenorrhea: a systematic review and meta-analysis. *Int J Environ Rs Public Health* 18:7832, 2021.

Matthewman G, Lee A, Kaur JG, Daley AJ: Physical activity for dysmenorrhea: a systematic review and meta-analysis of randomized controlled trials, *Am J Obstet Gynecol* 219, 2018. 255e.1–e.20.

Marjoribanks J, Ayeleke RO, Farquhar C, Proctor M: Nonsteroidal anti-inflammatory drugs for dysmenorrhoea, *Cochrane Database Syst Rev* (7): CD001751, 2015.

Mirbagher-Ajorpaz N, Adib-Hajbaghery M, Mosaebi F. The effects of acupressure on primary dysmenorrhea: A randomized controlled trial. Complement Ther Clin Pract 2011;17:33–26.

Moen MH, Stokstad T: A long-term follow-up study of women with asymptomatic endometriosis diagnosed incidentally at sterilization, *Fertil Steril* 78:773–776, 2002.

Momoeda M, Taketani Y, Terakawa N, et al: Is endometriosis really associated with pain? *Gynecol Obstet Invest* 54(Suppl. 1):18–21, 2002.

Nawathe A, Patwardhan S, Yates D, et al: Systematic review of the effects of aromatase inhibitors on pain associated with endometriosis, *BJOG* 115:818–822, 2008.

Ozgoli G, Goli M, Moattar F: Comparison of effects of ginger, mefenamic acid, and ibuprofen on pain in women with primary dysmenorrhea, *J Altern Complement Med* 15:129–132, 2009.

Raisi Dehkordi Z, Rafaieian-Kopaei M, Hosseina-Baharanchi FS: A double-blind controlled crossover study to investigate the efficacy of salix extract on primary dysmenorrhea, *Complement Ther Med* 44:102–109, 2019.

Rakhshaee Z. Effect of three yoga poses (cobra, cat and fish poses) in women with primary dysmenorrhea: A randomized clinical trial. J Pediatr Adolesc Gynecol 2011;24:192–6.

Ranong CN, Sukcharoen N: Analgesic effect of etoricoxib in secondary dysmenorrhea: A randomized, double-blind, crossover, controlled trial, *J Reprod Med* 52:1023–1029, 2007.

Selak V, Farquhar C, Prentice A, Singla A: Danazol for pelvic pain associated with endometriosis, *Cochrane Database Syst Rev* (4):CD000068, 2007.

Shahrahmani H, Ghazanfarpour M, Shahrahmani N, et al: Effect of fennel on primary dysmenorrhea: a systematic review and meta-analysis. *J Complement Integr Med* 18:261–269, 2021.

Sheng J, Zhang WY, Zhang JP, Lu D: The LNG-IUS study on adenomyosis: A 3-year follow-up study on the efficacy and side effects of the use of levonorgestrel intrauterine system for the treatment of dysmenorrhea associated with adenomyosis, *Contraception* 79:189–193, 2009.

Strinić T, Buković D, Pavelić L, et al: Anthropological and clinical characteristics in adolescent women with dysmenorrhea, *Coll Antropol* 27:707–711, 2003.

Sundell G, Milsom I, Andersch B: Factors influencing the prevalence and severity of dysmenorrhoea in young women, *Br J Obstet Gynaecol* 97:588–594, 1990.

Suzuki N, Uebaba K, Kohama T, et al: French maritime pine bark extract significantly lowers the requirement for analgesic medication in dysmenorrhea: A multicenter, randomized, double-blind, placebo-controlled study, *J Reprod Med* 53:338–346, 2008.

Tahir A, Sinrong AW, Jusuf EC, et al: The influence of macronutrient intake, stress and prostaglandin levels (pgf2alpha) of urine with the incidence of dysmenorrhea in adolescents. *Gac Satit* 35:S298–S301, 2021.

Telimaa S, Puolakka J, Rönnberg L, Kauppila A: Placebo-controlled comparison of danazol and high-dose medroxyprogesterone acetate in the treatment of endometriosis, *Gynecol Endocrinol* 1:13–23, 1987.

Tugay N, Akbayrak T, Demirtürk F, et al: Effectiveness of transcutaneous electrical nerve stimulation and interferential current in primary dysmenorrhea, *Pain Med* 8:295–300, 2007.

Vahidi M, Hasanpoor-Azghady SB, Amiri-Farahani L, Khaki I: Comparison of auriculotherapy and mefenamic acid on the severity and systemic symptoms of primary dysmenorrhea: a randomized clinical trial. *Trials* 22:655, 2021.

Yisa SB, Okenwa AA, Husemeyer RP: Treatment of pelvic endometriosis with etonogestrel subdermal implant (Implanon), *J Fam Plann Reprod Health Care* 31:67–70, 2005.

ENDOMETRIOSIS

Method of
Zachary Kuhlmann, DO

CURRENT DIAGNOSIS

- Clinical symptoms associated with endometriosis include chronic pelvic pain, dysmenorrhea, dyspareunia, and infertility.
- A pelvic sonogram may be helpful to aid in diagnosis of endometriosis. Care should be taken to exclude other gynecologic and non-gynecologic etiologies of pain.
- Diagnostic laparoscopy may reveal powder burn–like lesions, adhesions, endometriomas, or other signs of endometriosis on inspection.
- The gold standard to make a pathologic diagnosis of endometriosis requires a tissue biopsy of a suspected lesion.

CURRENT MANAGEMENT

- Initial therapy for endometriosis includes NSAIDs, progesterones, combined OCPs, danazol (Danocrine), GnRH agonists, and GnRH antagonists.
- Diagnostic laparoscopy with excision or ablative techniques are often used to treat endometriosis.
- It is reasonable to consider empiric medical therapy with a GnRH agonist before surgery in some situations.
- Hysterectomy with bilateral salpingo-oophorectomy is definitive surgical treatment for endometriosis.

Endometriosis is a common and benign gynecologic condition diagnosed when endometrial tissue is found outside the uterus. Common places for endometrial tissue to implant include the peritoneum and ovaries, although endometriosis can occur outside the pelvis as well. Other locations for endometriosis to be found include the rectovaginal septum, bowel, bladder, pleura, abdominal wall, and even the brain in rare cases. Endometriosis is an estrogen-dependent, inflammatory disorder.

Epidemiology

Endometriosis affects between 5% to 10% of women of reproductive age. Women who experience infertility may have a prevalence of endometriosis of up to 50%, and women with chronic pelvic pain may experience a prevalence of endometriosis well over 80%.

Risk Factors

There appears to be an inheritable component for endometriosis. Women who have a first-degree relative affected by endometriosis may have a 6 to 7 times higher incidence than women without an affected relative. Other risk factors for endometriosis include menarche before age 11 and extremes of cycle length (either short or long cycles). Women who breastfeed for long durations, women who have more children, and women who exercise regularly may see a reduction in their risk of endometriosis.

Pathophysiology

There are many theories regarding the origin of endometriosis. Perhaps the most popular hypothesis proposes that retrograde menstruation allows for endometrial tissue to be passed back through the fallopian tubes and implant into the pelvis. Another theory suggests that coelemic metaplasia occurs. In this theory, it is thought that the differentiation of mesothelial cells into endometrial cells results in endometriosis lesions. It is also thought that hematogenous or lymphatic spread is a plausible explanation for endometriosis. Endometrial cells may be deposited from the vascular or lymphatic vessels onto tissues outside the uterus. One final theory for the etiology of endometriosis involves bone marrow. Cells originating from the bone marrow may differentiate into endometrial tissue outside the uterus.

No matter how endometriosis originates, the immune system plays a pivotal role in the disease process. Endometriosis is associated with an overproduction of estrogen, prostaglandins, and cytokines. Estrogen is overproduced by an increase in aromatase activity. Cyclooxygenase-2 (COX-2) activity is also increased, which stimulates prostaglandin production. Endometriosis is also associated with progesterone resistance, and that magnifies the effect of estrogen in an already estrogen-rich environment. This inflammatory cascade leads to an increase in cytokines and macrophages. The cytokines increase the presence of macrophages and lymphocytes in the peritoneum.

The chronic inflammation identified in endometriosis may cause pain by stimulating the nerve endings or affect the neural innervations of the uterus. Fallopian tube function and sperm function may be adversely affected by the inflammatory cytokines. Also, the fallopian tubes may be completely blocked in some cases of endometriosis.

Clinical Manifestations

Many clinical symptoms have been associated with endometriosis. Cyclical pain is often described with endometriosis. Some of the more commonly recognized symptoms include dysmenorrhea, chronic pelvic pain, dyspareunia, and infertility. Dysmenorrhea can be described as primary or secondary. The dysmenorrhea with endometriosis is classically described as secondary dysmenorrhea because it is associated with a pathologic diagnosis. Primary dysmenorrhea is when there is painful menstruation in the absence of pelvic pathology. Examples of chronic pelvic pain with endometriosis may include other visceral symptoms such as dyschezia or dysuria. Hematuria, diarrhea, constipation, and chronic back pain may all be symptoms associated with endometriosis.

Interestingly, the extent of disease may not necessarily correlate with the severity of symptoms. Some women with a small foci of endometriosis may have excruciating symptoms, whereas others with extensive endometriosis may only experience mild symptoms.

Exam findings consistent with a diagnosis of endometriosis may include uterosacral ligament nodulartiy/tenderness and presence of an adnexal mass. Tenderness in the cul-de-sac with a fixed and immobile uterus may also indicate presence of endometriosis. Cyclical hemoptysis has been reported with endometriosis. Endometriotic implants have also been located in scars, so the presence of cyclical pain in an abdominal incision may lead to suspicion of endometriosis.

Diagnosis/Differential Diagnosis

The diagnosis of endometriosis is made surgically. The gold standard to make a diagnosis of endometriosis is to have a pathologic specimen from a tissue biopsy of a suspected lesion. Histology will reveal endometrial glands and stroma and inflammation. If a biopsy is not performed, surgical findings consistent with an endometriosis diagnosis include lesions that look like black powder burns and nonclassical red or white lesions. Endometriomas have also been described as a classic surgical finding of endometriosis. Endometriomas are an ovarian structure filled with endometriosis and are colloquially described as chocolate cysts because when they rupture, it appears as though chocolate syrup flows out of the cyst. Endometriomas appear on sonographic imaging as cysts with homogenous internal echoes. Although rare, endometriosis can sometimes be found in the bladder. If bladder involvement is suspected, such as the case of cyclical hematuria, a cystoscopy may be of benefit for diagnosis. Although surgery remains the mainstay of diagnosis

for endometriosis, some studies suggest there is a low correlation between the severity of symptoms, the amount of endometriosis visualized on surgical inspection, and diagnostic histologic findings.

Pelvic imaging may be helpful in the evaluation of endometriosis, especially in the presence of an adnexal mass. In patients with pelvic pain or disorders of menstruation, a sonogram is usually the preferred imaging modality for the pelvis. Computed tomography (CT) may help delineate the size and characteristic of an adnexal mass and is likely most useful to rule out other pathology or surrounding organ involvement. The usefulness of magnetic resonance imaging (MRI) is limited in the evaluation of endometriosis and should be reserved for extreme cases where specific organ involvement such as the bladder or bowel is suspected. MRI may also be useful in evaluating specific musculoskeletal conditions.

There is no good serum marker to make the diagnosis of endometriosis. CA-125 levels may be elevated in endometriosis, but there are many other inflammatory conditions that cause an elevation in CA-125 levels.

When initially evaluating for endometriosis, one should consider a thorough differential diagnosis for causes of chronic pelvic pain. Table 1 lists the differential diagnosis for chronic pelvic pain. A basic approach to the patient with chronic pelvic pain should include a detailed history and physical, urinalysis, gonorrhea/chlamydia cultures, consideration of pelvic sonogram, and serum or urine beta human chorionic gonadotropin (Bhcg). If after careful evaluation, endometriosis is at the top of the differential diagnosis for the patient's pelvic pain, then discussion with the patient regarding empiric treatment or diagnostic workup should occur.

Medical Therapy

The goal of medical intervention for endometriosis is the treatment of pain. A reasonable approach to treating the patient with suspected endometriosis is to give a trial of empiric medical therapy. Although endometriosis is a surgical diagnosis, some patients with suspected endometriosis may wish to avoid surgery. Medical therapy is usually preferred for those patients who would like to preserve fertility and who are interested in delaying childbearing while managing their symptoms.

The combined oral contraceptive pill (OCP) is a usual first-line therapy for the treatment of suspected or diagnosed endometriosis. A 3- to 6-month trial with empiric treatment with OCPs is a reasonable time frame to assess effectiveness of medical treatment. OCPs should be avoided in patients that have contraindications to OCPs including pregnancy, history of thrombosis, liver disease, migraine with aura, uncontrolled hypertension, and those patients that smoke and are over the age of 35 years.

Other medications used to treat endometriosis include danazol (Danocrine), nonsteroidal anti-inflammatory drugs (NSAIDs), progestins, and gonadotropin releasing hormone (GnRH) agonists and antagonists. NSAIDs may improve the pain and dysmenorrhea associated with endometriosis. Danazol is an effective treatment for endometriosis. The side effect profile for danazol limits its use. Danazol has been associated with masculinizing symptoms, which can include acne and hair growth. Danazol should be avoided in pregnancy because the masculinizing effects could be detrimental to a female infant.

Physicians commonly prescribe progestins in three different ways to treat endometriosis: injectable, oral, or intrauterine. Injectable medroxyprogesterone (Depo-SubQ Provera 104) is approved by the Food and Drug Administration (FDA) for the treatment of endometriosis. Depo-Provera's side effects may include weight gain, bleeding, amenorrhea, and slow return to fertility. Patients using Depo-Provera may initially experience irregular bleeding but often develop amenorrhea after the second dose is administered. Return to fertility after Depo-Provera is discontinued can also pose a problem. Oral agents such as norethindrone acetate (Aygestin) have also been approved by the FDA for the treatment of endometriosis. The levonorgestrel-containing intrauterine device (IUD) (Mirena)[1] is approved only for contraception and the treatment of menorrhagia, but it may still be an effective treatment for endometriosis.

---

[1]Not FDA approved for this indication.

TABLE 1	Differential Diagnosis for Chronic Pelvic Pain Based on Organ Systems		
GYNECOLOGIC	**GASTROINTESTINAL**	**URINARY**	**MUSCULOSKELETAL**
Endometriosis	Irritable bowel syndrome	Urinary tract infection	Fibromyalgia
Adenomyosis	Diverticuli	Interstitial Cystitis	Ankylosing spondylitis
Cervicitis	Crohn's	Malignancy	Arthritis
Leiomyoma	Ulcerative Colitis	Renal lithiasis	Muscle strains
Ovarian cysts	Gastroenteritis		
Pelvic adhesive disease	Hemorrhoids		
Hydrosalpinx/tubal disease			
Pelvic congestion syndrome			

The GnRH agonists are among the most effective medications available to treat endometriosis. The side effects of GnRH agonists include menopausal-like symptoms such as vaginal dryness, hot flashes, and osteopenia. The addition of add-back therapy may help ameliorate some of the GnRH agonist symptoms. Typically, add-back therapy involves the use of progestins concurrently with a GnRH agonist. Practice patterns vary; some providers may start add-back therapy immediately when a patient is started on a GnRH agonist. It is recommended that add-back therapy be initiated after 6 months of GnRH agonist use if it was not started previously. In addition to progestins, the combination of progestins and estrogen have been used for add-back therapy. The maximum duration of GnRH agonist treatment is typically 12 months. Another class of medication to treat endometriosis is the GnRH antagonist, currently available as elagolix (Orilissa). Advantages to this medication are that it is in an oral form and available in multiple doses. Studies showed estradiol suppression in a dose dependent manner. Common side effects include hot flashes, headaches, and nausea. When using elagolix, a nonhormonal contraception would be recommended. Relugolix is another GnRH receptor antagonist which has been studied in combination with estradiol and norethisterone to treat endometrosis associated pain. The relugolix/estradiol/norethindrone combination (Myfembree) can be offered as a long-term treatment option for endometriosis-associated pain. Potential advantages to the relugolix/estradiol/norethindrone combination are decreased vasomotor symptoms and bone mineral density that can be associated with GnRH antagonists.

Surgical Therapy

The goal of surgery for endometriosis is to relieve pain and/or infertility. One of the first questions the provider must answer is when to perform surgery. Surgery may be indicated if medical treatment has failed. Other times, the severity of symptoms or presence of large endometriomas may direct a provider to consider surgery sooner.

Laparoscopy is a common surgical approach for patients with confirmed or suspected endometriosis. At the time of laparoscopy, the surgeon can assess the uterus, ovaries, and surrounding viscera for pathology. When endometriosis is encountered on laparoscopy, common approaches are to excise or ablate the lesions. Excision of endometriosis allows for a pathologic diagnosis. If the provider elects to ablate the lesions, this can be performed through electrocautery or laser. In addition to diagnosing and treating endometriosis, further evaluation of patients with infertility can be done at the time of laparoscopy. Tubal function can be assessed through a chromotubation where dye is passed through the fallopian tubes to prove the tubes are patent. Although laparotomy allows for thorough evaluation of the pelvis, it is usually reserved for cases of confirmed endometriosis where the extent of adhesions and distorted anatomy makes laparoscopy unsafe.

Endometriomas present an array of challenges when noted at the time of surgery. The decision to drain the cyst versus perform a cystectomy during surgery must be made by the surgeon. A general approach is to use a "3-centimeters (cm) rule" to help guide management decisions. Patients with an endometrioma greater than 3 cm may benefit from cystectomy, whereas endometriomas less than 3 cm may be managed by drainage and ablation. Although removing the endometrioma through cystectomy may confer a decreased risk or recurrence, the risk of damaging healthy ovarian tissue is ever present. Other confounders to consider are future fertility plans of the patient, severity of symptoms, and previous treatments for endometriosis.

In a patient who has completed childbearing or has no desire for future fertility, hysterectomy with a bilateral salpingo-oophorectomy (BSO) may be considered for treatment of endometriosis. Studies suggest that hysterectomy alone is less effective at curing pain than hysterectomy with a BSO. Although hysterectomy with BSO offers definitive treatment for endometriosis, surgery does not guarantee resolution of pain. Many routes may be considered for surgery, including laparoscopic, robotic-assisted laparoscopic, or laparotomy with a total abdominal hysterectomy/BSO. Although vaginal hysterectomy is a common and preferred route of surgery, the distorted anatomy and presence of adhesions often associated with endometriosis tends to discourage many surgeons from performing vaginal hysterectomies for endometriosis.

Monitoring

Patients diagnosed with endometriosis may require frequent monitoring of symptoms. Routine visits with a physician may help determine the effectiveness of current treatment regimens. Physicians should consider what the patient's goals of treatment are: Does the patient want resolution of pain or infertility or both? Individualized plans may help each patient achieve their goals of treatment. As with any diseases involving chronic pain, care should be taken to regularly assess patients with endometriosis for depression.

References

ACOG Practice Bulletin Number 114. Management of Endometriosis. 2010.
Bulun SE: Endometriosis, *N Engl J Med* 360:268–279, 2009.
Cramer DW, Missmer SA: The epidemiology of endometriosis, *Ann N Y Acad Sci* 955:11–22, 2002.
Davis L, Kennedy SS, Moore J, Prentice A: Oral contraceptives for pain associated with endometriosis, *Cochrane Database Syst Rev* 2007;(3):Cd001019.
Dlugi AM, Miller JD, Knittle J: Lupron depot (leuprolide acetate for depot suspension) in the treatemnt of endometriosis: a randomized, placebo-controlled, double-blind study, *Fert Steril* 54:419–427, 1990.
Guidance LC, Kao LC: Endometriosis, *Lancet* 364:1789–1799, 2004.
Giudice LC, Sawsan AS, et al: Once daily oral relugolix combination therapy versus placebo in patients with endometriosis-associated pain: two replicate phase 3, randomised double-blind studies (SPIRIT 1 and 2), *Lancet* 399:2267–2279, 2022.
Olive DL, Pritts EA: The treatment of endometriosis: a review of the evidence, *Ann N Y Acad Sci* 955:360–372, 2002.
Pittaway DE, Fayez JA: The use of CA-125 in the diagnosis and management of endometriosis, *Fertil Steril* 46:790–795, 1986.
Rawson JM: Prevalence of endometriosis in asymptomatic women, *J Reprod Med* 36:513–515, 1991.
Ripps BA, Martin DC: Endometriosis and chronic pelvic pain, *Gynecol Clin North Am* 20:709–717, 1993.
Surrey E, Taylor HS: Long-term outcomes of elagolix in women with endometriosis, *Obstetrics and Gynecology* 132:147–160, 2018.
Sutton CJ, Ewen SP, Whitelaw N, Haines P: Prospective, randomized, double blind, controlled trial of laser laparoscopy in the treatment of pelvic pain associated with minimal, mild, and moderate endometriosis, 62:696–700, 1994.
Walter AJ, Hentz JG, Magtibay PM, Cornella JL, Magrina JF: Endometriosis: correlation between histologic and visual findings at laparoscopy, *Am J Obstet Gynecol* 184:1407–1411, 2001.

FEMALE SEXUAL CONCERNS

Method of
Kiersten A. Wulff, DNP; and Cathleen E. Morrow, MD

CURRENT DIAGNOSIS

- Sexual concerns are common, and definitions for specific sexual disorders are evolving. Patients do not need to meet the criteria diagnosis for sexual disorder to benefit from attention to concerns.
- Screen for sexual concerns during routine care with open-ended questions. Offer validation regarding concerns, provide any initial education, and plan for follow-up for more in-depth discussion and evaluation as needed.
- Clinicians should be particularly attuned to the potential for sexual concerns among those with chronic health conditions such as cancer, history of pelvic surgery, or radiation exposure.
- More research is needed to better understand both prevalence and health impacts of sexual concerns among non-heterosexual and gender diverse people.
- Cultural factors such as sex-negativity, religious influences, restricted access to reliable contraception, chronic stress due to discrimination, and limited access to sex education all represent potential barriers to healthy sexual function.

CURRENT TREATMENT

- A biopsychosocial framework is best to understand the origins of sexual concerns as well as to plan treatment.
- A multidisciplinary team approach can be very helpful and may include pelvic floor physical therapists, sex therapists, and colleagues in gynecology/urogynecology.
- Comprehensive history collection is key to determining the origins of a given sexual concern, and physical exam may also be helpful for certain conditions. Lab testing has a limited role in evaluation.
- Effective pharmacotherapy options for bothersome low sexual desire are limited.
- Pain is an important source of sexual distress with many potential causes.
- Sex therapists are licensed psychotherapists who are skilled at addressing the cognitive and interpersonal aspects of sexual function.

Introduction

Sexual concerns are common across the lifespan, and estimates suggest that almost half of women will experience concerns related to sexual function. The clinician's responsibility to a patient with a concern about sexual function is to offer validation, non-judgmental listening, and thorough history collection while taking care to normalize concerns about sex, provide basic education regarding normal variation of sexual response, move efficiently to evaluate sources of pain, offer simple and straightforward suggestions for initial self-care, and provide additional resources and referrals as needed. Gender identity and experience is diverse, and the heterogeneity of human sexuality is vast. Using definitions of female sexual concerns common to the medical literature compels the use of a gender binary, which may be limiting to clinician and patient alike. To discuss sexual concerns within the confines of this chapter, we will use the term "women" and "female" to indicate persons born with reproductive organs including ovaries, uterus, vagina, and vulva. We tend to use the term "concern" rather than "dysfunction" or "disorder" except when referring to specific diagnoses given the commonality of sexual concerns that exist within expected and normal sexual function (i.e., reduced interest in sex with a partner when there is relationship discord).

Origins and Etiologies of Sexual Concerns

Healthy sexual function, briefly, is the ability to engage in desired sexual activity that is non-painful and non-coerced; is satisfying to individual and interpersonal pursuits whether that of pleasure, connection, or relaxation; and may include orgasmic sensations. There are four main categories of sexual concerns affecting sexual function: desire, arousal, orgasm, and sexual pain. While a concern may arise in isolation, these concerns are often co-occurring, sometimes overlapping, may arise from similar contextual factors, and can require a multidisciplinary approach to sufficiently address. A biopsychosocial framework is used to best understand the etiologies of sexual concerns. Table 1 depicts the internal and external factors that influence sexual function including the physiologic, psychologic/emotional, sociocultural, and interpersonal domains. These factors are implicated in most, if not all, sexual complaints and bear consideration for any patient presenting with a sexual concern. Take time to familiarize yourself with these etiologies as they are useful in guiding evaluation and understanding approach to care.

Clinical Manifestations and Diagnoses

There are no outward signs to indicate sexual wellbeing, and clinicians should avoid making assumptions about sexual function based on age, gender, sexual orientation, or relationship status. Some patients present to the clinic ready to voice their sexual concern, and many will not. Studies indicate that the vast majority of patients do wish to speak to their provider about sexual health, and almost all prefer that the clinician bring up the topic in discussion. Clinicians should routinely (e.g., as part of a review of systems) offer an opportunity for patients to talk about their sexual concerns and then offer a follow-up discussion and evaluation. While screening tools and questionnaires for sexual function and related distress have been developed and validated for use in some scenarios, the available tools may lack appropriateness for diverse populations, so an open-ended question with a normalizing statement may be more effective in the clinical setting. For example: "Many people have concerns about sex at some point. If you have any concerns related to your sexual health, is there anything that you'd like to discuss?" This question can create an

TABLE 1 Origins of Sexual Function Concerns: Biopsychosocial Framework

INTERNAL FACTORS	
BIO-PHYSIOLOGIC	**PSYCHO-EMOTIONAL**
<ul><li>Neurobiology</li><li>Reproductive phase (peripartum, menopause)</li><li>Hormonal changes</li><li>Chronic health conditions (cardiovascular, neurologic, endocrinologic, cancer)</li><li>Medication/treatments</li><li>Urogenital disorders (prolapse, pain, incontinence, atrophy)</li></ul>	<ul><li>Self- or body-image</li><li>Substance use/disorder</li><li>Mood disorders (anxiety, depression)</li><li>Trauma history (intimate partner violence, toxic stress, discrimination, medical trauma including childbirth)</li></ul>

EXTERNAL FACTORS	
SOCIOCULTURAL	**INTERPERSONAL**
<ul><li>Sexual education</li><li>Values/views about sex and relationships</li><li>Religious beliefs</li><li>Societal taboos, norms</li><li>Gender and sex expectations</li><li>Sex negativity</li></ul>	<ul><li>Relationship status and quality</li><li>Partner communication</li><li>Logistics, privacy</li></ul>

environment of openness, normalizes sexual concerns, indicates that the clinician understands sexual wellbeing as part of overall health, and positions the clinician as a future resource as needed.

Defining sexual disorders and applying the definitions in clinical practice presents multiple challenges. Updated definitions and criteria from *Diagnostic and Statistical Manual of Mental Disorders*, 5th ed (DSM-V) are cited in most clinical guidelines written within the past several years but have been met with significant critique, and we find they are not especially useful for clinical practice. The evolution over time of definitions of sexual disorders is fascinating but overall beyond the scope of this chapter. Given these present issues of clarity and consensus about what exactly constitutes a specific type of sexual disorder, it is our opinion that primary care clinicians may offer evaluation, followed by any relevant resources and referrals to patients expressing a specific sexual concern regardless of whether a patient appears to meet criteria for a disorder as defined by any major medical society. Brief summaries of the main categories of sexual function issues follow.

Libido/desire: It is normal for sexual desire to evolve throughout the lifespan and in response to a host of biophysiologic, psycho-emotional, social, cultural, and interpersonal factors as listed in Table 1. Fluctuating levels of desire are commonly relatable to modifiable individual or partner factors, but without education regarding the basics of sexual function or exploration of context, a person may be quick to worry that a change in pattern of desire represents a personal shortcoming. The DSM-V and International Society for the Study of Women's Sexual Health (ISSWSH) definitions of desire disorders are described as a persistent significant decrease or complete lack of at least three of the following: interest in sexual activity, sexual fantasies or erotic thoughts, enjoyment or excitement during sexual activity, initiation of sexual activity or responsiveness to initiation, interest or arousal in response to erotic or sexual cues, genital and non-genital arousal, and sensations during sexual activity. Using the DSM criteria, a sexual desire disorder can only be diagnosed when the symptoms can be attributed to another non-sexual mental health use disorder, are not occurring within a context of relationship distress, or are not better explained by the presence of health condition, medication use, or substance use.

Arousal: Arousal disorders are defined by significant decrease in or lack of genital sexual arousal including engorgement, vaginal lubrication, and pleasurable sensations in response to stimulation that are persistent despite attention to internal and external factors (e.g., relationship difficulty, stressors, medication use)

Orgasm: Disorders related to orgasm are defined as marked delay in, infrequency of, or absence of orgasm and/or reduced intensity of orgasmic sensations. Some orgasm disorders occur with "normal" sexual desire function. Often, an acquired orgasm disorder will occur with symptoms of desire/arousal difficulties, genito-pelvic pain symptoms, and frequently in relation to a biologic influence (such as medication, medical treatment, medical condition) and/or psychosocial influence (relationship stressors, psychologic stress).

Pain: Genito-pelvic pain disorder is defined by the presence of pain or fear of pain that accompanies or interferes with desired sexual activity. Genito-pelvic pain/penetration disorders as denoted in the DSM as psychologic condition are not attributable to "organic disease," but ISSWSH asserts that the neurobiology of chronic/persistent pain almost always includes expectations and experience in a way that implicates both mental and physical domains. Outside of these definitions, concerns about genital or pelvic pain that interfere with sex can include a wide array of conditions including vulvodynia, vulvovaginal injury (e.g., obstetric injury), myofascial pain, dermatological problems, postmenopausal changes, or bladder or bowel pain disorders. Experiencing pain with sex, either once or repeatedly, may be an important factor in a person's decreased desire or experience of mental or physical arousal.

Generally, to be considered a sexual dysfunction or disorder, the problem as described by the patient must occur either episodically or persistently over a period of several months and be accompanied by significant distress. If the individual is satisfied with their sexual experience, no sexual dysfunction or disorder should be diagnosed. Conversely, some women will present with distress without clear locus of dysfunction, and this may be more related to the cognitive aspects of sexual function (e.g., thoughts and beliefs regarding sexuality and sexual expectations).

Evaluation

Approach to the conversation: Given prevalent cultural sex-negativity, many people have difficulty discussing sex without embarrassment. The clinician can help overcome this by using a welcoming and nonjudgmental tone while remaining sensitive to patient boundaries around the conversation. The clinician can empower the patient at the outset of the discussion by offering permission to choose to discontinue the conversation at any point for any reason. Generally we find it helpful to ask the patient what terms they use to describe genitalia and sexual functions and adopt the same; in some cases, providing language for a very uncomfortable patient may be indicated. Additionally, clinicians need to take care to avoid assumptions due to sexual orientation and gender expression and approach each patient as a unique individual.

History: History collection is often the most valuable component of an evaluation for a sexual concern. General history includes the nature, onset, and duration of the symptoms; the presence of distress and level thereof; and any efforts made or self-care undertaken to alleviate the issue(s). Asking about temporality of the symptoms and the evolution of symptoms over time can discern whether an issue in one domain has triggered an issue in another domain (e.g., pain and then decreased desire). Regardless of category, the nature of the concern can be further classified as to whether it is acquired or lifelong, generalized or situational, episodic or constant. See Table 2 for suggestions for specific questions that can help clarify the nature of a given complaint. It is very valuable to ask, "What do you think is causing

---

TABLE 2	Pertinent History Questions for Specific Sexual Concerns

When the Chief Concern Is Sexual Desire or Arousal

When did you last feel satisfied with the level of your arousal/desire, and what was different then compared to now? Do you believe stress, logistics, lack of privacy are contributing to your concern? Do you feel your level of sexual desire is different from your partner's, and have you discussed this with them? Which measures have you taken with your partner to try to help with this, and were any of the measures helpful? When you first started to notice this, were there any changes in your health, your medical treatments, your reproductive health, or your life circumstances that happened around the same time?

When the Chief Concern Is Pain

Has sex always been painful or is this a new occurrence?
If new, has there been a change in partner or change in sex activities that preceded the pain?
Do you only have pelvic/genital pain during sex or between encounters as well?
Do you notice the pain externally or internally? Does the pain happen immediately with touch/penetration or over time? Does the pain happen with deep penetration only? Have you comfortably used a tampon/menstrual cup before? Does the pain occur only with partnered sex versus masturbation/a specific partner versus all of your partners?
Is there any bleeding after sex?

When the Chief Concern Is Reduced/Absent Orgasms

Are you bothered by reduced, absent, or difficult to reach orgasm sensations?
Has this been a lifelong concern or a recent concern?
Does the difficulty occur during partnered sex, masturbation, or both?

the problem?" as an approach to gain deeper insight into the patient's understanding and experience.

Comprehensive history collection for any sexual concern should consider the topics in Table 1 with an emphasis on the domains of the biophysiologic, psychologic, and interpersonal issues. Biophysiologic factors include recent reproductive events like childbirth or menopause; injuries or overall health status changes (e.g., new cardiovascular disease or worsening arthritis pain); related medical history including neurologic disorders such as spine injuries; signs and symptoms of genitourinary disorders including sexually transmitted infections, incontinence, prolapse, pelvic masses, and bladder pain; and bowel disorders including constipation. External relational factors for initial consideration include partner's sexual function, relationship, and communication quality. Associated external psychologic factors include history of past or current abuse or violence, presence of mood disorder, substance use disorder, and body image concerns. Review of medications that can impact sexual desire, mental or genital arousal, or orgasm is important. See Table 3 for a list of known agents that impact sexual function.

Physical exam: Complaints related to sexual pain call for excellent pelvic exam skills, as many times concerns about discomfort have clear physiologic causality and can be readily remedied once identified. Use of a trauma-informed approach to the pelvic exam is recommended universally. The pelvic exam should include full inspection of external genitalia and anorectal regions with attention to any visible injuries or skin abnormalities. Localization of the pain origin, whether external, internal, or deep within the vaginal vault, are potential clues to the etiology of the source of the pain, and the clinician should seek direct feedback from the patient through each phase of the exam. Observation of tissue integrity, presence of adhesions or structural changes of the vulva, presence of vaginismus, pelvic floor muscle spasm or tenderness, and lesions within the vagina or cervix are important clues in diagnosis. Presence or absence of signs of infection—whether sexually transmitted or otherwise—are part of standard assessment. It is useful to remember that, beyond a pelvic exam, when evaluating for pelvic pain or pelvic floor muscle dysfunction, it is often relevant to perform a careful abdominal exam to evaluate for bowel sounds, abnormal masses or distension, and abdominal muscle tenderness. In the case of orgasm or genital arousal difficulties, a relevant neurologic examination includes lower extremity muscle tone, reflexes, strength, and sensation.

Laboratory evaluation: Common sexual complaints rarely call for such laboratory testing. Patients may have read that they "need" these values for evaluation. Hormonal and other laboratory evaluation should be reserved for specific indications for suspected individual disease states (e.g., PCOS; hypothyroidism) rather than as a scan to "make sure" nothing is amiss. If symptoms of menopause are premature or the patient is experiencing abnormal uterine bleeding, this should be evaluated with the appropriate lab workup. Measuring testosterone levels in females has not been proven to predict or reliably explain sexual function issues.

Radiologic evaluation: The results of pelvic exam may, at times, call for imaging of the pelvis typically by trans-vaginal ultrasound to evaluate palpable adnexal masses or unexpected uterine enlargement discovered while examining a patient with pelvic pain.

Therapy or Treatment

Libido/arousal/desire: Distressing and persistent reduced or lack of desire for sex often necessitates a multidisciplinary approach that includes the primary care or gynecologic clinician, occasionally pelvic floor physical therapist, and occasionally psychotherapist. If an evaluation suggests that a patient is primarily distressed by an experience of reduced spontaneous desire, primary care clinicians can provide helpful basic education regarding current understandings of sexual response cycle. Explaining the differences between "spontaneous desire" versus "responsive desire" as variations of normal is a helpful starting point for the patient to then pursue an active cultivation of the desire style that works for them. Education about dual-control model of desire

(as mediated by excitatory factors and inhibitory factors) with a focus on identifying possible modifiable inhibitors that may be impacting a person's interest in sex can be helpful and can also help to frame the external/contextual factors as important and reassure a patient that they are not "broken." Sexual therapists are licensed psychotherapists that address the cognitive belief

TABLE 3	Medications Associated With Female Sexual Dysfunction		
MEDICATION	**DESIRE DISORDER**	**AROUSAL DISORDERS**	**ORGASM DISORDERS**
Anticholinergics	–	+	–
Antihistamines	–	+	–
Amphetamines and related anorexic drugs	–	–	+
Cardiovascular and antihypertensive medications			
Anti-lipid medications	+	–	–
β-Blockers	+	–	–
Clonidine	+	+	–
Digoxin	+	–	+
Spironolactone	+	–	–
Methyldopa	+	–	–
Hormonal preparations			
Danazol	+	–	–
GnRH agonists	+	–	–
Hormonal contraceptives	+	+	–
Antiandrogens	+	+	+
Tamoxifen	+	+	+
GnRH analogues	+	–	–
Narcotics	+	–	+
Psychotropics			
Antipsychotics	+	+	+
Barbiturates	+	+	+
Benzodiazepines	+	+	–
Lithium	+	+	+
SSRIs	+	+	+
TCA	+	+	+
MAO inhibitors	–	–	+
Venlafaxine	+	+	+
Other			
Histamine 2 receptor blockers and promotility agents	+	–	–
Indomethacin	+	–	–
Ketoconazole	+	–	–
Phenytoin sodium	+	–	–
Aromatase inhibitors	+	+	–
Chemotherapeutic agents	+	+	–

+ = yes; – = no.

Adapted from Buster JE: Managing female sexual dysfunction, *Fertil Steril* 100(4):905–915, 2013.

TABLE 4	Additional Helpful Resources

Find a licensed sexual therapist: American Association of Sexuality Educators www.ASSECT.org

Find a sexual medicine clinician: International Study for the Science of Women's Sexual Health www.ISSWSH.org

Popular press books:
- *Come as You Are* by Dr. Emily Nagoski
- *Better Sex Through Mindfulness* by Dr. Lori Brotto
- *When Sex Hurts* by Drs. Goldstein, Pukall, Goldstein, and Krapf

and sociocultural aspects of sexual identity and desire. We also find recommendations for further reading useful and strongly encourage patients in this direction (see Table 4). Physiologic factors that can be addressed include urogenital disorders causing pain or self-image issues, identifying and treating neurologic or endocrine conditions, reviewing and addressing medications that reduce desire or make orgasm difficult, and offering appropriate treatment for psychologic/behavioral/emotional conditions such as substance use disorder or depression. Pharmacotherapeutics for low sexual desire are limited, and for most patients, the risk/benefit profile and lack of available long-term safety data would discourage medication use as a primary approach. Expert consensus guidance from the Endocrine Society and North American Menopause Society provides a review of the available options as well as their uses and limitations.

Bupropion[1] (150-400 mg SR nightly) – For women experiencing low sexual desire or orgasm difficulty related to SSRI use, the addition of bupropion has been demonstrated among women and men alike to improve sexual dysfunction compared to placebo, as measured by female sexual dysfunction rating scale scores.

Flibanserin (Addyi) (100 mg nightly) is a serotonin antagonist/agonist that was approved by the FDA in 2015 for treatment of hypoactive sexual desire dysfunction among premenopausal women who do not have depression nor relationship problems causing the reduced desire. Its effectiveness in clinical trials was minimal, resulting in an average of less than one additional satisfying sexual encounter per month. Following postmarketing studies, in 2019, the FDA required relabeling the medication with a black box warning for hypotension that occurs with concomitant alcohol use. The prescribing physician and the dispensing pharmacist must complete a risk evaluation and mitigation strategy certification (REMS). While some studies demonstrate similar minimal effectiveness among postmenopausal women, flibanserin is not currently FDA approved for postmenopausal women.

Androgen therapy (1/10 of standard male dose or less); Transdermal testosterone has been studied for short-term use for treatment of low sexual desire in postmenopausal women and have demonstrated effectiveness compared to placebo. There are no FDA-approved formulations of testosterone for use in women. It is recommended testosterone levels be monitored before and during treatment due to risk for androgen excess. Long-term safety and efficacy of transdermal testosterone for low desire among postmenopausal women is not known. Measuring serum testosterone outside of monitoring during androgen therapy has not been proven clinically useful and therefore is not recommended. We recommend reviewing the most up-to-date guidelines from the Endocrine Society and Menopause Society if the clinician is considering prescribing testosterone. Androgen treatments lacking sufficient effectiveness and safety data that should not be prescribed based on current evidence includes testosterone "pellets," compounded hormones, and systemic DHEA (dehydroepiandrosterone).[1] As a non-hormonal agent, sildenafil citrate is also not recommended.

Orgasm: Depending on the origin of the issue, treatment for an orgasm concern varies considerably. First, normalizing non-penetrative orgasms is helpful education for a patient who is distressed about how they do or do not experience orgasm. Patients who present with a worry that they have never experienced orgasm may benefit from sex therapist referral for masturbation training or counseling on sensate focus/mindfulness therapy. In the absence of genito-pelvic pain which may significantly inhibit pleasurable sensations during partnered or solo-sex, patients who notice reduced or absent orgasmic sensations or difficulty achieving orgasm benefit from a review of potentially causative medications, addressing any concomitant mental health condition, trauma history, substance use disorder, and/or treatment for any vulvovaginal conditions discovered on physical exam that affect clitoral structure and sensitivity including postmenopausal vaginal atrophy. External factors to address may include sex-negative cultural or religious messaging or interpersonal factors such as communication with a partner regarding sexual technique; sex therapists can be very helpful in these situations.

Sexual pain: A treatment plan for sexual pain is based upon the differential formed during evaluation. For a history of sexual trauma, trauma-focused therapy is the standard, and co-existing vaginismus or myofascial pain could be addressed with a trauma-sensitive pelvic floor physical therapist. Dermatologic conditions of the vulva, including vulvovaginal atrophy, lichen sclerosis, and lichen simplex chronicus, can all be managed with topical treatments. Vulvodynia that is nerve- or hormone-mediated can be treated with neuralgia-reducing medications, whether topical or systemic, or removing the agent causing low estrogen (i.e., combined hormonal contraceptives) if present. Low-dose vaginal estrogen is safe and effective for treating the effects of estrogen loss among peri- and postmenopausal women. Pelvic floor dysfunction or myofascial pelvic pain is best treated by a pelvic floor physical therapist. Refractory or severe cases including myofascial or nerve pain can include trigger point injections or pudendal nerve treatments performed by a urogynecologist or female reconstructive medicine specialist. Self-care counseling around reducing contact irritants including soaps, scented products, douches, and wipes can also eliminate common sources of external discomfort.

Monitoring and Follow-up

A primary care provider with an established trusting relationship and rapport is well positioned to follow up regarding the effect of any education, treatment, or referral. The persistence of symptoms despite basic interventions may lead to further evaluation or illustrate the need for referral. Many women feel their symptoms are minimized or dismissed by the medical system and, essentially, give up seeking care. It should be emphasized that, for persistent or refractory sexual concerns, a team approach is beneficial; we work closely with our colleagues in behavioral medicine, psychiatry, pelvic floor therapy, and urogynecology.

Complications

Distress related to sexual function can have a significant impact on quality of life, can contribute to depression, be source of low self-image, and contribute to relationship discord. Dismissing or missing sexual function concerns or attempting to adhere to rigid diagnostic models can lead to under-identification of patients who would benefit from addressing an underlying health issue, making a medication adjustment, and/or referral to a sexual therapist, mental/behavioral health counselor, or pelvic floor physical therapist. Certain aspects of sexual concerns fall into the realm of "do not miss." This includes a history of sexual trauma/abuse, active/ongoing intimate partner violence, or reactive distress to sexual function that is severe.

References

American College of Obstetricians and Gynecologists' Committee on Practice Bulletins—Gynecology: Female sexual dysfunction: ACOG practice bulletin clinical management guidelines for obstetrician gynecologists, Number 213, *Obstet Gynecol* 2019 134(1):e1–e18, 2019.

Clayton AH, Goldstein I, Kim NN, et al: The International society for the study of women's sexual health process of care for management of hypoactive sexual desire disorder in women, *Mayo Clin Proc* 93(4):467–487, 2018, https://doi.org/10.1016/j.mayocp.2017.11.002.

[1] Not FDA approved for this indication.

Faubion SS, Rullo JE: Sexual dysfunction in women: a practical approach [published correction appears in Am Fam Physician. 2016 Aug 1;94(3):189], *Am Fam Physician* 92(4):281–288, 2015.

Parish SJ, Cottler-Casanova S, Clayton AH, McCabe MP, Coleman E, Reed GM: The Evolution of the Female Sexual Disorder/Dysfunction Definitions, Nomenclature, and Classifications: a review of DSM, ICSM, ISSWSH, and ICD, *Sex Med Rev* 9(1):36–56, 2021.

Robison K, Kulkarni A, Dizon DS: Sexual Health in Women Affected by Gynecologic or Breast Cancer, *Obstet Gynecol* 143(4):499–514, 2024.

The North American Menopause Society (NAMS): The 2020 genitourinary syndrome of menopause position statement of The North American Menopause Society, *Menopause* 27:976–992, 2020.

INFERTILITY

Michael P. Diamond, MD; and Jessica Rachel Kanter, MD

CURRENT DIAGNOSIS

- Infertility is defined as the inability to conceive with regular intercourse after 12 months in couples in which the female partner is younger than 35 or after 6 months in couples in which the female partner is 35 or older.
- The incidence of infertility is increasing.
- Consideration should be given to expedited evaluation, including possible referral to a reproductive endocrinologist, in couples in which the female partner is 40 years of age or older. Immediate evaluation should be undertaken if a woman has a condition known to cause infertility.

CURRENT THERAPY

- Assisted reproductive technologies are being used with increasing frequency and with increasing success rates.

Epidemiology

Infertility is defined as the failure to conceive after 12 months of regular, unprotected intercourse. In couples where the female partner's age exceeds 35 years, evaluation may begin after just 6 months of infertility, and in those over 40 years, more immediate evaluation may ensue, owing to the time-sensitive nature of the problem. In some circumstances, including in those in which the woman has a condition known to cause infertility, such as anovulation or advanced-stage endometriosis, diagnostic evaluation and therapeutic intervention are warranted at an earlier time. Infertility affects approximately 15% of couples. Many of these patients present to their primary care physician. Timely evaluation and potential referral to an infertility subspecialist are prudent.

Risk Factors

There are numerous risk factors that contribute to infertility. The most common is female partner age. However, it is necessary to evaluate other potential contributing factors to infertility because this may help narrow the differential diagnosis and achieve a more targeted subsequent treatment plan. For example, a history of sexually transmitted infections (STIs), especially chlamydia, and episodes of pelvic inflammatory disease have been associated with tubal factor infertility in women. Metabolic disorders such as obesity and polycystic ovarian syndrome, which may lead to anovulation, are an increasingly more prevalent concern and a major risk factor for infertility. Endocrinopathies such as thyroid disease and diabetes are common modifiable risk factors for infertility. Finally, certain genetic diseases such as fragile X, Turner syndrome, cystic fibrosis, and Klinefelter disease may also lead to inability to conceive or difficulty in conceiving.

Pathophysiology

The pathophysiology of infertility should be grouped first by male and female factors and then by the component of their respective reproductive tracts. One must not discount the fact that multiple factors may coexist, including etiologies of infertility in both partners of a heterosexual couple. Unexplained infertility has been reported to be accountable for 8% to 28% of infertility in couples; however, in intensively evaluated couples, the rate is likely to be 25%.

Prevention

Some etiologies of infertility may be preventable. Many cases of tubal factor infertility may be prevented by protecting against the transmission of STIs. Barrier contraception is essential to prevent STIs, particularly in high-risk individuals with an early age of coitarche and/or those with multiple sexual partners. Even with highly efficacious forms of contraception such as intrauterine devices, long-acting injectable progestins, and progestin-containing subdermal implants, providers must counsel their patients that barrier contraception is still of the utmost importance in preventing STI transmission.

There are also various medical therapies, particularly those related to cancer treatment, that may be detrimental to fertility. In these cases, oncofertility consultation prior to treatment will optimize fertility preservation. For men, sperm cryopreservation is a relatively easy, noninvasive method. Oocyte or embryo preservation, experimental approaches to medically induce ovarian suppression, ovarian transposition, and experimental ovarian tissue cryopreservation are all helpful tools for women undergoing gonadotoxic chemotherapy or radiation therapy.

Finally, fertility should also be considered when managing tubal ectopic pregnancy in women. Medical therapy, when not contraindicated, is an excellent option in the compliant patient with an ectopic pregnancy. When surgery is necessary, salpingostomy may be considered, when possible, in lieu of salpingectomy, in an attempt to preserve tubal function—particularly in the setting of a damaged or absent contralateral fallopian tube. It should be noted that, although these approaches may allow for preservation of a fallopian tube, these patients are at increased risk of subsequent ectopic pregnancy.

Clinical Manifestations

Infertile patients generally present with failure to conceive after a variable time of home intercourse. The definition of infertility is subdivided into primary and secondary infertility. Primary infertility means the patient has not conceived in the past. Secondary infertility means the patient has a history of prior successful conception, regardless of pregnancy outcome.

Diagnosis

The diagnosis of infertility begins with a thorough history and physical examination. It is important to remember that a history must be obtained from both partners during this evaluation. The male partner assessment begins with a semen analysis. Semen analysis should be performed after 2 to 5 days of abstinence for optimal results. If abnormal parameters are noted, a second semen analysis may be warranted, preferably separated in time by at least 1 month.

Female partner assessment should focus on ovulatory function, ovarian reserve, and structural abnormalities. Initial evaluation should include determination of estradiol levels and of ovarian reserve by hormonal evaluation of antimüllerian hormone (AMH) or cycle day 2 to 5 follicle-stimulating hormone (FSH). A thyroid-stimulating hormone (TSH) may also be considered as thyroid dysfunction is common in women of reproductive age. Ovulation may be confirmed with a midluteal progesterone level, with a result greater than 3 ng/mL demonstrating evidence of ovulation. Other labs may be ordered if clinically indicated, such as androgens in women with hirsutism or prolactin in the setting of oligomenorrhea with or without galactorrhea. Tubal patency is assessed by sonohysterosalpingogram or hysterosalpingogram.

These imaging tests also allow assessment of the uterine cavity for uterine contour and abnormalities, including fibroids or polyps. Sonography may also be useful in identifying müllerian anomalies or anomalies of the basic structure of the uterus. Magnetic resonance imaging remains the gold standard for identifying müllerian anomalies; however, 3D ultrasonography has demonstrated promising and more cost-effective results in recent literature. In cases where other pelvic pathologies such as endometriosis and adhesions are suspected, diagnostic laparoscopy may be considered. Chromotubation during laparoscopy may be performed to assess fallopian tube patency. Finally, in the setting of recurrent pregnancy loss, karyotype analysis may be considered for both partners in addition to antiphospholipid antibody testing for the female partner.

Differential Diagnosis

When determining a differential diagnosis, both male and female factors must be considered.

Male Factors

Male factor infertility is a component of infertility in approximately 40% to 50% of couples. The most common etiologies of male factor infertility are oligospermia and azoospermia. The etiologies leading to these diagnoses are broad and varied and include genetic conditions such as cystic fibrosis (leading to congenital absence of the vas deferens).

Female Factors

Female factors for infertility are numerous and most easily subdivided by system.

Ovulatory Dysfunction

Inability to produce a viable oocyte each month can be related to several factors. First, anovulation may occur, meaning that oocytes are present in the ovaries but none are released on a regular basis. This can be related to hormonal ovarian suppression or metabolic disturbances. Alternatively, an oocyte may not be produced secondary to a paucity of oocytes owing to age, genetic factors, or prior insults to the ovaries, such as radiation therapy. In addition to the aforementioned AMH and day 2 to 5 FSH and serum estradiol to assess ovarian function, ultrasound may be employed to evaluate antral follicle count—another marker of ovarian reserve.

Tubal Factor

The fallopian tubes are responsible for transporting the oocyte from the ovaries to the uterine cavity. For this to occur, at least one fallopian tube must be patent. Perhaps the most common etiology of tubal factor infertility is a history of pelvic inflammatory disease, most frequently secondary to *Chlamydia trachomatis*. *C. trachomatis* is particularly problematic in women because the initial infection may be asymptomatic. Other tubal infertility may arise from prior tubal ligation, other tubal surgery, history of ectopic pregnancy, or scarring of the tubal lumen.

Uterine Factor

Irregularities within the uterine cavity may also lead to infertility, generally secondary to poor implantation of the fertilized embryo. Some such etiologies may be present from birth—namely, müllerian anomalies. The abnormally shaped uterine cavity in these anomalies reduces the opportunity for normal implantation and embryo growth.

During the course of a woman's life, she may develop benign intrauterine growths, including polyps and leiomyomas, that can reduce the opportunity for normal embryo implantation. Finally, prior uterine surgery may damage the endometrium and myometrium, as in Asherman syndrome, or cause uterine cavity scarring, known as *synechiae*.

Combined

One must not forget that multiple etiologies in a wide variety of combinations may be at play in female factor infertility.

Unexplained

Perhaps the most frustrating of all diagnoses is unexplained infertility. In couples who have had a negative fertility workup, a specific etiology of infertility may never be revealed. There is new, burgeoning research in the area of sperm microRNA that may identify male factor infertility in men with otherwise normal semen analyses. Although not currently in wide use, such studies may be of great utility in the future.

Prior Diagnosis

As the field of infertility is becoming understood to an increasingly greater degree, there are prior diagnoses that have fallen out of favor. One such diagnosis is cervical factor insufficiency. It was previously evaluated by the postcoital test, in which a sample of cervical mucus was taken after intercourse and was evaluated for the presence of motile sperm. This test has fallen out of favor owing to subjectivity, lack of reproducibility, and poor correlation with future fertility.

Also out of favor is the prior diagnosis of luteal phase deficiency (LPD), previously defined as inadequate endogenous progesterone production during the luteal phase of the menstrual cycle. No clinical tests have proven reliable for LPD, nor have any treatments demonstrated any significant improvement in treating infertility.

Treatment

The mainstay of therapy is first treating underlying disorders such as obesity, thyroid disease, and so forth. Other known causes of infertility that require surgical management may include intrauterine pathology (e.g., polyps, fibroid tumors) or removal of a hydrosalpinx—a distally blocked fallopian tube filled with serous fluid.

With at least one patent fallopian tube and a normal male partner semen analysis, the first step in intervention is generally an oral agent to induce ovulation combined with intrauterine insemination. Options for induction include clomiphene citrate (Clomid) and off-label use of letrozole (Femara), an aromatase inhibitor. If this fails, therapy can proceed to treatment with in vitro fertilization. Various additional procedures may be considered if in vitro fertilization is pursued, including intracytoplasmic sperm injection to increase fertilization rates of the oocytes, particularly in the setting of male factor infertility, and preimplantation genetic testing for aneuploidy to evaluate for embryonic genetic anomalies, particularly in women of advanced maternal age.

Monitoring

To reduce the risks associated with ovarian stimulation and ovarian stimulation, monitoring of serum estradiol and follicular development is performed. Monitoring provides the ability to minimize the occurrence of multiple gestation and complications associated with ovarian hyperstimulation syndrome.

References

Gelbaya TA, Potdar N, Jeve YB, Nardo LG: Definition and epidemiology of unexplained infertility, *Obstet Gynecol Surv* 69(2):109–115, 2014.

Infertility Workup for the Women's Health Specialist: ACOG committee opinion summary, number 781, *Obstet Gynecol* 133(6):e377–e384, 2019.

Jodar M, Sendler E, Moskovtsev SI, et al: Absence of sperm RNA elements correlates with idiopathic male infertility, *Sci Transl Med* 7(295):295–296, 2015, https://dx.doi.org/10.1126/scitranslmed.aab1287.

Practice Committee of American Society for Reproductive Medicine: Fertility evaluation of infertile women: a committee opinion, *Fertil Steril* 116(5):1255–1264, 2021.

Practice Committee of American Society for Reproductive Medicine: Diagnosis and treatment of luteal phase deficiency: a committee opinion, *Fertil Steril* 115(6):1416–1423, 2021.

Sharlip ID, Jarow JP, Belker AM, et al: Best practice policies for male infertility, *Fertil Steril* 77(5):873–882, 2002.

Schlegel PN, Sigman M, Collura B, et al: Diagnosis and treatment of infertility in men: AUA/ASRM guideline, *J Urol* 205(1):36–43, 2020.

MENOPAUSE

Method of
Andrew M. Kaunitz, MD, MSCP; and
JoAnn E. Manson, MD, DrPH, MSCP

CURRENT DIAGNOSIS

- In women who meet clinical criteria for menopause and present for management of vasomotor symptoms (VMS), checking follicle-stimulating hormone and estradiol levels is not necessary. However, if no recent level is available, checking the thyroid-stimulating hormone level to rule out thyroid disease is appropriate.
- Occasionally, nonmenopausal conditions can masquerade as menopausal VMS.
- Although genitourinary syndrome of menopause (GSM) can be presumptively diagnosed based on a characteristic history, a pelvic examination can help exclude other vulvovaginal conditions that can present with similar symptoms.
- Although laboratory assessment is not necessary to establish that GSM is present, vaginal pH is typically higher than 5.0.

CURRENT THERAPY

- Estrogen represents the most effective therapy for VMS and related symptoms.
- Oral and transdermal estrogen have similar efficacy in treating menopausal VMS.
- Estrogen-progestin therapy (EPT) is appropriate when treating menopausal symptoms in women with an intact uterus.
- For healthy women with bothersome symptoms who are younger than 60 years of age and/or within 10 years of menopause onset, the benefits of systemic hormone therapy (HT) are likely to outweigh the risks.
- Randomized trial data clarify that estrogen-only therapy, including conjugated equine estrogens and estradiol, does not elevate risk of breast cancer, and in fact, reduces breast cancer risk.
- Observational studies suggest that in contrast with oral estrogen, transdermal estradiol does not increase risk of venous thromboembolism. Randomized clinical data addressing this issue, however, are not available.
- Observational studies suggest that, in contrast with synthetic progestins (including medroxyprogesterone acetate), use of micronized progesterone does not increase risk of breast cancer. Randomized clinical trial data, however, are not available.
- Conjugated estrogens 0.45 mg combined with the selective estrogen receptor modulator bazedoxifene 20 mg formulation (Duavee) (without concomitant use of a progestational agent) are approved to treat VMS and prevent osteoporosis in women with an intact uterus.
- The two nonhormonal formulations approved to treat menopausal VMS are fezolinetant 45 mg (Veozah) and low-dose paroxetine mesylate 7.5 mg (Brisdelle). Off-label use of venlafaxine (Effexor), desvenlafaxine, (Pristiq), escitalopram (Lexapro), citalopram (Celexa), gabapentin (Neurontin), and pregabalin (Lyrica) are also effective in treating VMS. However, these agents, along with low-dose paroxetine mesylate, are less effective than standard-dose HT.
- Arbitrary discontinuation of systemic HT when women turn 65 is not evidence based. Extended use of systemic HT in well-counseled women for treatment of persistent VMS, prevention of bone loss, and prevention/treatment of atrophic genital changes may be appropriate. Women considering extended use of systemic HT should be aware that with a longer duration of EPT, the risk of breast cancer increases. If GSM/atrophic changes represent the only indication for HT, local low-dose vaginal estrogen is appropriate and highly effective.

Epidemiology

Menopause, the permanent cessation of menstruation caused by loss of ovarian function, occurs at a mean age of 51 to 52 years. With increases in life expectancy, currently more than 50 million women in the United States are 50 years of age or older.

Risk Factors

Spontaneous menopause represents a natural event. Spontaneous menopause occurs at a younger age in women who smoke or undergo hysterectomy with ovarian conservation. Chemotherapy, radiotherapy, or bilateral oophorectomy can induce menopause.

Clinical Manifestations and Pathophysiology

Often described by women as hot flushes, or night sweats, vasomotor symptoms (VMS) represent the most bothersome symptoms of menopause and the most common reason women present for care at the time of the menopausal transition. VMS often include a sudden sensation of heat in the face, neck, and chest and persist for several minutes or less. VMS may cause flushing, chills, anxiety, and sleep disruption. VMS are caused by estrogen withdrawal and are associated with pulsatile luteinizing hormone secretion, decreased endorphin concentration in the hypothalamus, and increased release of norepinephrine and serotonin. VMS occur in almost three-fourths of women during the late perimenopausal transition and are more prevalent among the groups listed in Box 1. The median duration of moderate-to-severe VMS is approximately 10 years.

Genitourinary syndrome of menopause (GSM), also known as *vulvovaginal* or *genital atrophy*, signifies the progressive changes in the vulva, vagina, and urethra resulting from estrogen deficiency. GSM, which characteristically causes vaginal dryness and pain with sex, represents a common condition that adversely affects health, sexuality, and quality of life in women in menopause.

Diagnosis

Although follicle-stimulating hormone levels increase and estradiol levels decrease in women in menopause, assessing serum levels of these hormones is not necessary when perimenopausal or postmenopausal women report characteristic VMS as described previously. Because thyroid disease is common in women and can cause symptoms that mimic VMS, checking the thyroid-stimulating hormone level is appropriate in women seeking treatment for VMS.

Although GSM can be presumptively diagnosed based on a characteristic history, a pelvic examination can help exclude other vulvovaginal conditions that can present with similar symptoms (see the next section). Physical examination findings characteristic of GSM are listed in Box 2. Although laboratory assessment is not necessary to establish that GSM is present, vaginal pH is typically higher than 5.0.

Differential Diagnosis

Nonmenopausal conditions that can masquerade as menopausal VMS include anxiety disorders, thyroid disease, autoimmune conditions, carcinoid syndromes, diabetic autonomic dysfunction/hypoglycemia, insulinoma/pancreatic tumors, epilepsy, infections, tuberculosis, mast cell disorders, and new-onset hypertension, as well as the use of certain selective serotonergic reuptake inhibitors or serotonin-norepinephrine reuptake inhibitors.

Lichen sclerosus, chronic candidiasis, contact dermatitis, and lichen planus represent vulvar/vaginal conditions that might be confused with GSM.

Therapy

Estrogen represents the most effective therapy for VMS and related symptoms. Higher doses are more effective; oral and transdermal formulations have comparable efficacy. Many estrogen formulations/doses are also approved for the prevention of osteoporosis. Because estrogen-only therapy (ET) in women with an intact uterus increases the risk of endometrial neoplasia, estrogen-progestin therapy (EPT) is appropriate when treating VMS in women with a uterus. In the United States the most commonly used oral estrogens for systemic treatment of VMS are estradiol (E2; Estrace [generics available]) and conjugated equine estrogens (CEE; Premarin). Standard doses of these estrogens are 1.0 and 0.625 mg, respectively; lower and higher doses are available. Weekly and twice-weekly skin patches and other transdermal E2 formulations are available; estradiol patches releasing 0.05 and 0.0375 mg daily are considered standard dose; lower- and higher-dose patches are available. A 3-month vaginal systemic E2 ring (Femring) for treatment of VMS is also available; the ring that releases 0.05 mg E2 daily is considered the standard dose.

In the United States progestational agents commonly prescribed to accompany systemic ET in women with an intact uterus include medroxyprogesterone acetate (MPA; Provera and generics, available in 2.5-, 5-, and 10-mg doses) and micronized progesterone (Prometrium and generics) in 100- and 200-mg capsules. Micronized progesterone is formulated with peanut oil. With standard-dose estrogen, an appropriate daily dose of MPA or micronized progesterone used continuously is 2.5 and 100 mg, respectively. Because micronized progesterone has a hypnotic effect, it should be taken at bedtime. A variety of oral estrogen-progestin formulations, all of which have demonstrated endometrial safety, are available in different doses and combine CEE with MPA (Prempro), E2 or ethinyl E2 with norethindrone acetate (Activella, Femhrt [generics available for both formulations]), or E2 with drospirenone (Angeliq), norgestimate (Prefest and generics), or progesterone (Bijuva). Transdermal estrogen-progestin combination formulations combine E2 with norethindrone acetate (CombiPatch) or levonorgestrel (Climara Pro).

Although off-label use of testosterone can increase sexual desire in menopausal women, efficacy is achieved only with supraphysiologic doses, which may cause hyperandrogenic adverse effects.

Conjugated estrogens 0.45 mg combined with the selective estrogen receptor modulator bazedoxifene 20 mg (Duavee) is approved to treat VMS and prevent osteoporosis in women with an intact uterus without the concomitant use of a progestational agent and does not increase the incidence of uterine bleeding or endometrial hyperplasia. This novel combination formulation may be useful for women with an intact uterus who choose not to use progestin, including those intolerant of progestin side effects.

Among U.S. women using systemic menopausal hormone therapy (HT), approximately one-third are using compounded HT; most users are not aware that these formulations are not evaluated or approved by the U.S. Food and Drug Administration (FDA). FDA-approved HT is preferable to compounded HT, unless a specific FDA-approved formulation is not available.

Nonhormonal therapy with paroxetine (Paxil)[1], escitalopram (Lexapro)[1], citalopram (Celexa)[1], venlafaxine (Effexor)[1], desvenlafaxine (Pristiq)[1], gabapentin (Neurontin)[1], pregabalin (Lyrica)[1], and fezolinetant (Veozah) is more effective than placebo but less effective than HT in treating VMS. Low-dose paroxetine mesylate 7.5 mg (Brisdelle) and fezolinetant 45 mg once daily are the only nonhormonal formulations approved to treat VMS. Fezolinetant is the first neurokinin 3 receptor antagonist used for the treatment of moderate-to-severe VMS. Its most common side effects include insomnia, diarrhea, hot flushes, abdominal and back pain, and elevated hepatic transaminase levels.

Lowering the ambient temperature, using fans, wearing layered clothing, and avoiding tobacco, alcohol, and caffeine represent commonsense measures for women bothered by VMS. In a clinical trial, clinical hypnosis was found more effective than placebo in addressing VMS. Although over-the-counter herbal formulations, including soy and black cohosh, have been widely used to treat VMS, these have not been found to be more effective than placebo.

When clinicians identify GSM, they should advise women that (unlike VMS) without proactive management, GSM progresses. If severe symptoms are not present, recommending use of over-the-counter lubricants (or substances such as coconut oil or olive oil) for sexual activity, as well as regular use of vaginal moisturizers, is helpful. Such women should also be advised that regular sexual activity that includes penetration may help improve symptoms and prevent progression. If other indications for systemic HT such as treatment of VMS or prevention of osteoporosis are present, systemic HT is effective in treating GSM. However, if GSM represents the only indication for HT, local low-dose vaginal estrogen is appropriate and highly effective. Vaginal estrogen also reduces the risk of recurrent urinary tract infections and overactive bladder symptoms in menopausal women. In the United States, two low-dose creams, estradiol and CEE, are available. Although package labeling provides instructions for patients regarding dose and schedule, in practice, most women apply a fraction of an applicator vaginally (and often also benefit from digital application to vestibular tissues) 1 to 3 nights weekly. Some women find the use of vaginal estrogen creams to be messy. Vaginal tablets (Vagifem and generics) equivalent to 10 mcg E2 are inserted vaginally with an applicator nightly for 2 weeks and then twice weekly for maintenance. Vaginal 4 or 10 mcg E2 inserts (Imvexxy) are placed digitally nightly for 2 weeks and then twice weekly for maintenance. The 3-month low-dose E2 vaginal ring (Estring) releases 7.5 mcg E2 daily. An oral systemic selective estrogen receptor modulator, ospemifene (Osphena), improves symptoms of GSM; some users report VMS. In addition, vaginal dehydroepiandrosterone (prasterone [Intrarosa]) is approved for the treatment of GSM.

Monitoring

For most women using systemic HT, monitoring of serum estrogen levels is not indicated. However, when women continue to report bothersome symptoms despite escalating HT doses, monitoring can be useful. In contrast with fluctuating serum estrogen levels in women using oral estrogen, transdermal ET results in relatively steady-state levels; serum E2 levels of 40 to 100 pg/mL represent a reasonable target range for menopausal women 50 years of age or older. Serum E2 levels as high as 120 pg/mL may be appropriate for younger menopausal women. Because hepatotoxicity may occur with use of fezolinetant, the FDA recommends testing liver function tests at baseline and at months 1, 2, 3, 6, and 9 after initiating this medication.

Side Effects of Systemic Hormone Therapy

Breast tenderness, bloating, and uterine bleeding represent common side effects of ET. Although lowering the ET dose may reduce side effects, this may cause VMS to increase. Progestins cause dysphoria in some women. Prescribing a different progestin, prescribing progestins sequentially, off-label use of a progestin intrauterine device (Skyla, Kyleena, Mirena, Liletta), or use

---

[1] Not FDA approved for this indication.

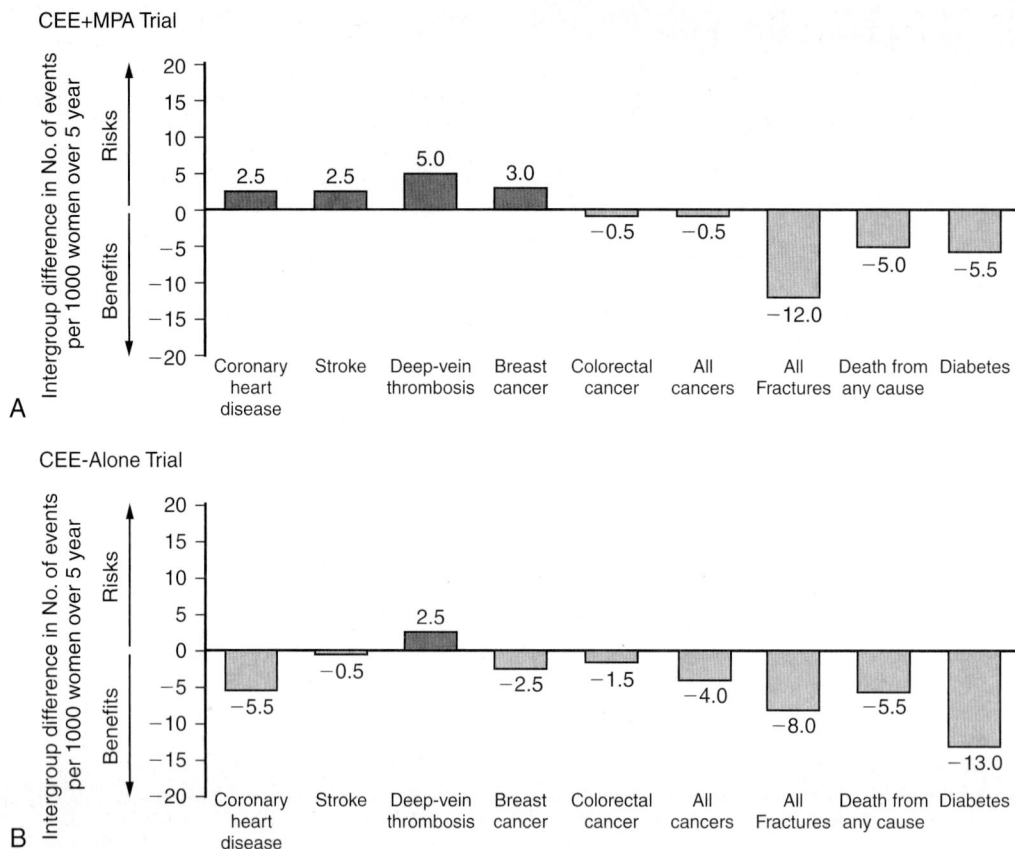

Figure 1 Benefits and risks of the two hormone therapy formulations evaluated in the Women's Health Initiative. Results are shown for the two formulations, CEEs alone (B) or in combination with medroxyprogesterone acetate (A), for women 50–59 years of age. Risks and benefits are expressed as the difference in the number of events (number in the hormone therapy group minus the number in the placebo group) per 1000 women over 5 years. (Data from Manson JE, Chlebowski RT, Stefanick ML, et al: Menopausal hormone therapy and health outcomes during the intervention and extended poststopping phases of the Women's Health Initiative randomized trials, *JAMA* 310[13]:1353–1368, 2013.)

of the CEE/bazedoxifene combination formulation (Duavee) or antidepressant therapy may be helpful in this setting.

Safety of Hormone Therapy

Findings from the Women's Health Initiative (WHI) study of oral CEE and MPA, as well as CEE alone, have helped clarify the benefits and risks of combination EPT and estrogen-alone therapy. A 2013 WHI report detailed findings from the two HT trials with a median 13 years of cumulative follow-up. Since initial findings of the WHI were first published in 2002, use of systemic HT has dramatically decreased as a result of misinterpretation of WHI findings, which has generated anxiety and confusion among clinicians and women. Importantly, absolute risks of adverse events related to HT were much lower for younger women (50–59 years of age) than for older women (Figure 1). Overall, for healthy women with bothersome VMS younger than 60 years of age and/or within 10 years of menopause onset, the benefits of initiating HT outweigh the risks.

With respect to coronary heart disease (CHD), the effect of HT varies by age of users. Among women who initiate HT before 60 years of age and/or within 10 years of menopause, HT does not increase (and may reduce) risk. In contrast, among women older than 60 years of age and/or more than 10 years after menopause onset, initiating HT appears to increase CHD risk.

With respect to stroke, the WHI found that CEE alone or with MPA increased risk; however, for women younger than 60 years of age, the absolute increase in risk was small (see Figure 1).

With respect to venous thromboembolism (VTE), including pulmonary embolism, oral estrogen with or without progestin increases risk, particularly during the first 2 years of HT initiation. Absolute risks of VTE are higher for women initiating HT more than 10 years after menopause onset. Most observational

studies have found that in contrast with oral HT, HT with transdermal (e.g., skin patch) estrogen elevates VTE risk less (if at all). Because oral estrogen and body mass index represent independent risk factors for VTE, transdermal estrogen is preferable for most women at elevated baseline VTE risk, including women with obesity. Personal and familial risk of cardiovascular disease, stroke, and VTE should be considered when initiating HT. Low-dose vaginal estrogen has not been found to elevate the risk of CHD, stroke, VTE, breast cancer, or endometrial cancer.

With respect to breast cancer risk, WHI results diverged, with increased risk in the CEE-plus-MPA group and borderline reduced risk in the CEE-alone group. A meta-analysis aggregating data from the WHI and nine smaller randomized trials found that use of estrogen-alone (conjugated equine estrogen or estradiol) in women posthysterectomy significantly reduces risk of breast cancer (relative risk [RR] 0.77; 95% confidence interval [CI], 0.65–0.91). In WHI, with 13 years of follow-up, a modest elevation of risk (hazard ratio [HR] = 1.28) persisted in the CEE-plus-MPA group in all participant age strata. To put the elevated risk of breast cancer observed among women randomized to CEE plus MPA into perspective, the attributable risk with combination HT is less than one additional case of breast cancer diagnosed per 1000 users of combination HT annually. Another way to put this elevated HR into perspective is to recognize that the HR of 1.28 is slightly higher than that seen with one daily glass of wine and less than that noted with two daily glasses. With long-term follow-up of WHI participants randomized to CEE alone, a significantly reduced risk of breast cancer (HR = 0.79) emerged. During a cumulative 18-year follow-up of all participants in the WHI hormone therapy trials, all-cause mortality rates did not differ appreciably between the intervention and placebo groups in the overall cohort. The HR for all-cause mortality among women assigned HT compared with those assigned placebo was 0.99 (95% CI, 0.94–1.03) in the overall pooled cohort; HRs were 1.02 (95% CI, 0.96–1.08) with CEE plus MPA and 0.94 (95% CI, 0.88–1.01) with CEE alone. In a 2019 report, women with prior bilateral oophorectomy and randomized to estrogen alone in their 50s, compared with those randomized to placebo, were found to have a statistically significant 32% reduction in all-cause mortality during long-term follow-up. With more than 20 years of follow-up of WHI participants in the two randomized trials, prior randomized use of CEE alone, compared with placebo, among women who had a previous hysterectomy was associated with a significantly lower breast cancer incidence and lower breast cancer mortality. In contrast, prior randomized use of CEE plus MPA, compared with placebo, among women who had an intact uterus was associated with a significantly higher breast cancer incidence but no significant difference in breast cancer mortality. Although randomized clinical trial data are not available, observational studies suggest that in contrast with synthetic progestins (including medroxyprogesterone acetate and norethindrone acetate), use of micronized progesterone does not increase risk of breast cancer.

Although trials up to 2 years in duration found that CEE plus bazedoxifene did not increase the risk of breast cancer, long-term trials are needed. In women with *BRCA1* or *BRCA2* mutations who have intact breasts but have undergone risk-reducing bilateral salpingo-oophorectomy before age 45, observational data suggest that use of HT does not increase breast cancer risk and that safety concerns regarding HT treatment should not cause mutation carriers to defer risk-reducing salpingo-oophorectomy.

Low-dose vaginal ET may be used as long as needed, including indefinitely; routine use of concomitant progestin therapy for endometrial protection is not recommended. In the absence of reported spotting or bleeding, routine endometrial surveillance during the use of vaginal ET is not recommended. However, clinicians should recognize that endometrial safety data for currently marketed formulations are based on 1-year trials, with no trials assessing the safety of longer-term administration available.

Current package labeling for low-dose vaginal estrogen, as for all systemic HT formulations, includes a boxed warning that refers to endometrial cancer, myocardial infarction, stroke, invasive breast cancer, pulmonary emboli, and dementia. This warning reflects safety concerns associated with findings from clinical trials of systemic HT and does not reflect current evidence regarding local low-dose vaginal estrogen.

A personal history of breast cancer is listed as a contraindication to use of all systemic and local low-dose vaginal HT (other contraindications to the use of HT are listed on the package labeling). However, a systematic review and meta-analysis of observational data found that, with the exception of women using aromatase inhibitors, use of vaginal estrogen among breast cancer survivors does not appear to elevate risk of breast cancer recurrence or death from breast cancer. In package labeling for vaginal dehydroepiandrosterone, a personal history of breast cancer is not listed as a contraindication, although current or past history of breast cancer is listed in the Warning and Precautions section.

Early/Induced Menopause

Whether spontaneous or induced by surgery, radiation, or chemotherapy, early menopause is associated not only with an adverse effect on quality of life but also with cardiovascular, neurologic, and skeletal morbidity and mortality. Clinicians caring for women with early surgical menopause should recognize that in addition to effectively treating menopausal symptoms, HT may mitigate the potential long-term adverse effects of early estrogen deprivation on bone mineral density, cognitive health, and cardiovascular health. Accordingly, unless a contraindication is present, use of HT is appropriate for women with early menopause at least up to the normal age of spontaneous menopause (51–52 years of age).

Extended Use/Discontinuation of Systemic Hormone Therapy

Arbitrary discontinuation of systemic HT when women turn 65 is not evidence based. Although controversial, extended use of systemic HT may be appropriate for the treatment of persistent VMS, prevention of bone loss, and prevention/treatment of GSM in selected, well-counseled women. Extended use of systemic HT should not be confused with the initiation of systemic HT by women older than 60 years of age or more than 10 years after menopause onset—a practice that is known to be associated with an elevated risk of CHD (see the "Safety of Hormone Therapy" section). Women considering extended use of systemic HT should be aware that with longer duration of EPT using synthetic progestins, the risk of breast cancer increases. Because older age is an independent risk factor for VTE, the use of transdermal estrogen formulations should be considered in this setting.

When women discontinue systemic HT, a loss of bone mass and progression of GSM/atrophic genital changes occur. The likelihood of recurrent VMS in this setting appears similar with abrupt and gradual (dose-tapering) discontinuation of HT.

Financial Disclosure

Dr. Kaunitz's department receives research funding from Bayer and Mylan. He previously served as a consultant for Estetra and Mylan. Dr. Manson does not report any potential conflicts of interest.

References

Abenhaim HA, Suissa S, Azoulay L, et al: Menopausal hormone therapy formulation and breast cancer risk, *Obstet Gynecol* 139:1103–1110, 2022.

Beste ME, Kaunitz AM, McKinney JA, Sanchez-Ramos L: Vaginal estrogen use in breast cancer survivors: a systematic review and meta-analysis of recurrence and mortality risks, *Am J Obstet Gynecol* 232:262–270, 2025.

Bhupathiraju SN, Grodstein F, Stampfer MJ: Vaginal estrogen and chronic disease in the nurses' health study, *Menopause* 26(6):603–610, 2019.

Chlebowski RT, Anderson GL, Aragaki AK, et al: Association of menopausal hormone therapy with breast cancer incidence and mortality during long-term follow-up of the Women's Health Initiative randomized clinical trials, *J Am Med Assoc* 324:369–380, 2019.

Chlebowski RT, Aragaki AK, Pan K, et al: Randomized trials of estrogen-alone and breast cancer incidence: a meta-analysis, *Breast Cancer Res Treat* 206:177–184, 2024.

Kaunitz AM, Kapoor E, Faubion S: JAMA Insights Women's Health: treatment of women after bilateral salpingo-oophorectomy performed prior to natural menopause, *JAMA* 326:1429–1430, 2021.

Kaunitz AM, Manson JE: Clinical expert series: management of menopausal symptoms, *Obstet Gynecol* 126:859–876, 2015.

Kaunitz AM, Reese C, Pinkerton JV: Menopausal symptom management in patients after risk-reducing oophorectomy, *Obstet Gynecol* 146:223–232, 2025.

Lederman S, Ottery FD, Cano A, et al: Fezolinetant for treatment of moderate-to-severe vasomotor symptoms associated with menopause (SKYLIGHT 1): a phase 3 randomised controlled study, *Lancet* 401(10382):1091–1102, 2023.

Manson JE, Aragaki AK, Bassuk SS, et al: For the WHI Investigators. Menopausal estrogen-alone therapy and health outcomes in women with and without bilateral oophorectomy: a randomized trial, *Ann Intern Med* 171:406–414, 2019.

Manson JE, Aragaki AK, Rossouw JE, et al: Menopausal hormone therapy and long-term all-cause and cause-specific mortality: the Women's Health Initiative randomized trials, *J Am Med Assoc* 310:927–938, 2017.

Manson JE, Chlebowski RT, Stefanick ML, et al: Menopausal hormone therapy and health outcomes during the intervention and extended poststopping phases of the Women's Health Initiative randomized trials, *JAMA* 310:1353–1368, 2013.

Manson JE, Kaunitz AM: Menopause management: getting clinical care back on track, *N Engl J Med* 374:803–806, 2016.

Melisko ME, Goldman ME, Hwang J, et al: Vaginal testosterone cream vs estradiol vaginal ring for vaginal dryness or decreased libido in women receiving aromatase inhibitors for early-stage breast cancer: a randomized clinical trial, *JAMA Oncol* 3:313–319, 2017.

North American Menopause Society: The 2020 genitourinary syndrome of menopause position statement of the North American Menopause Society, *Menopause* 27:976–992, 2020.

North American Menopause Society: The 2022 hormone therapy position statement of the North American Menopause Society, *Menopause* 29:767–794, 2022.

Pan K, Lavasani S, Aragaki AK, Chlebowski RT: Estrogen therapy and breast cancer in randomized clinical trials: a narrative review, *Menopause* 29:1086–1092, 2022.

Trabuco EC, Moorman PG, Algeciras-Schimnich A, et al: Association of ovary-sparing hysterectomy with ovarian reserve, *Obstet Gynecol* 127:819–827, 2016.

Vinogradova Y, Coupland C, Hippisley-Cox J: Use of hormone replacement therapy and risk of venous thromboembolism: nested case-control studies using the QResearch and CPRD databases, *BMJ* 371:m3873, 2020.

OVARIAN CANCER

Method of
Mihae Song, MD; and Zenas Chang, MD, MS

CURRENT DIAGNOSIS

- The U.S. Preventive Services Task Force, the American College of Obstetricians and Gynecologists, and the Society of Gynecologic Oncologists recommend against the routine screening of low-risk asymptomatic women with transvaginal ultrasonography (TVUS) or serum tumor marker testing.
- Women at high risk (previously identified *BRCA* gene mutation or a family cancer history of suggestive of a hereditary cancer syndrome) should be referred for formal genetic counseling and testing. Current National Comprehensive Cancer Network guidelines recommend screening this population with TVUS and serum CA 125 levels every 6 months.
- Patients with persistent and progressive abdominal symptoms should be evaluated for ovarian cancer. A pelvic exam and imaging studies (TVUS) may be helpful in identifying a pelvic mass. Findings such as an elevated CA 125 (in a postmenopausal woman), a nodular or fixed pelvic mass, ascites, or evidence of abdominal or distant metastasis warrant referral or consultation with a gynecologic oncologist.

CURRENT THERAPY

- Asymptomatic women at high risk for ovarian cancer because of a hereditary cancer syndrome should be referred for consideration of a prophylactic bilateral salpingo-oophorectomy. The timing of this procedure may depend on the cancer syndrome and the patient's reproductive wishes. Referral to a gynecologic oncologist for this discussion may be appropriate.
- Ovarian cancer is treated with a combination of surgical resection and chemotherapy. The sequence of treatment depends on the clinical status of the patient and whether the disease can be resected (debulking). Conventional chemotherapy remains the backbone of adjuvant treatment; myelosuppression, fatigue, and neuropathy are some of the most common side effects during treatment.

Epidemiology

Ovarian cancer is the second most common type of female reproductive cancer but the leading cause of death from gynecologic cancer. There are approximately 22,000 new cases of ovarian cancer per year in the United States, with almost 14,000 deaths yearly. There are several histologic subtypes of ovarian cancer, including epithelial (arising from the surface epithelium of the ovary), sex cord stromal (arising from the cells that support and surround the oocytes), and germ cell tumors (derived from primordial oocytes). In women under 20 years of age, germ cell tumors are the most common, whereas epithelial ovarian cancer occurs most commonly in women over 50 years of age. The stage at diagnosis and prognosis varies significantly based on histology. Epithelial tumors account for most cases and deaths from ovarian cancer.

Epithelial ovarian cancer has a low prevalence of approximately 1 case per 2500 women per year, with an approximate 1.3% lifetime risk for developing ovarian cancer. The average age at diagnosis is approximately 63 years. Approximately 75% of patients are diagnosed with advanced-stage disease because of a lack of accurate screening tests and vague reporting symptoms; as

a result, average 5-year survival ranges from 20% to 30%. White women have the highest incidence rate of ovarian cancer.

In contrast to epithelial ovarian cancer, most patients with malignant sex cord-stromal neoplasms are diagnosed at an earlier stage and age. Incidence is as low as 0.2 per 100,000 women. Germ cell tumors occur predominantly in young women between 10 and 30 years of age. These neoplasms are primarily limited to one ovary but tend to grow rapidly compared with epithelial or sex cord-stromal tumors. Young women of Asian/Pacific Islander and Hispanic descent are more likely to develop germ cell tumors than White women.

Risk Factors

Significant risk factors for epithelial ovarian cancer are age, early menarche, late menopause, hereditary cancer syndromes, nulliparity, endometriosis, and asbestos. Age and each additional year of ovulation (early menarche/late menopause, nulliparity) are hypothesized to increase risk because of trauma to the ovarian epithelium, which can lead to malignant transformation. Other factors are controversial and include menopausal hormone therapy, obesity, polycystic ovary syndrome, intrauterine devices, talc, cigarette smoking, diet, or infertility and infertility treatments. Systemic reviews of these factors do not currently show clear associations with an increased risk of ovarian cancer.

Approximately 15% to 20% of ovarian cancer cases may be due to hereditary cancer syndromes. More than half of women with an inherited ovarian cancer will have a deleterious mutation in *BRCA1/2* or have Lynch syndrome (mutations in *MLH1, MSH2, MSH6, PMS2*). Other rare hereditary syndromes, such as Li-Fraumeni *(TP53)*, Cowden *(PTEN)*, or Peutz-Jeghers *(STK11)*, also can increase the risk for ovarian cancer. The lifetime risk of ovarian cancer can vary significantly by mutation, with an estimated 40% risk with *BRCA1*, 15% risk with *BRCA2*, and 11% to 24% risk with Lynch syndrome (depending on genotype). As medical genetic counseling and testing rates increase, additional genes *(BRIP1, RAD51C, RAD51D, PALPB2)* continue to be identified that may increase the risk for ovarian cancer.

BRCA1/2 mutations are inherited in an autosomal dominant pattern and markedly increase susceptibility to breast and ovarian cancer, with some increased risk for tumors in prostate, male breast, and pancreas. Certain ethnic groups such as Ashkenazi Jewish (2.5%), Icelandic (0.6%), and French Canadian have increased rates of *BRCA* mutations, although *BRCA* mutations have also been identified in Hispanic and African American populations as well. The risk for ovarian cancer under 40 years is low; however, women with *BRCA* mutations tend to have a younger average age at the time of diagnosis (age 50 for *BRCA1*; age 60 for *BRCA2*). Discussion of risk-reducing bilateral salpingo-oophorectomy (BSO) in these women is recommended (see Prevention) to reduce ovarian and breast cancer risk.

Lynch syndrome is also inherited in an autosomal dominant fashion and is similarly associated with the development of multiple cancer types—primarily colon and endometrial cancer. Ovarian cancer is less common than endometrial cancer in these women, but surveillance for gynecologic malignancies is recommended, with risk-reducing surgery indicated at the completion of childbearing and/or by a certain age (see Prevention).

Pathophysiology

Approximately 95% of malignant ovarian cancers are epithelial ovarian cancers. The most common subtype of epithelial ovarian cancers is high-grade serous carcinoma, which represents approximately 70% of cases. The remaining 30% are considered rare and include histologic types such as low-grade carcinoma, mucinous carcinoma, clear cell carcinoma, and endometrioid carcinoma. High-grade serous carcinomas are more likely to present at an advanced stage (stage III or IV, with intrabdominal spread), whereas the rare subtypes are more likely to present in early stages (stage I or II, limited to the pelvis).

High-grade serous ovarian cancer, fallopian tubal carcinoma, and primary peritoneal carcinoma are considered a single clinical entity because of shared clinical behavior and treatment. Embryologically, the coelomic epithelium differentiates into a variety of cell types, including those found in the fallopian tube, uterus, cervix, and ovarian stroma. Historically, the ovary was the presumed source, as most patients would report with large ovarian masses at the time of diagnosis. Current evidence suggests that there may be more than one mechanism for carcinogenesis, including malignant transformation of the ovarian surface epithelium, tubal neoplasia that leads to metastasis to the ovary, or malignant transformation from endometriosis or endosalpingiosis. These carcinomas generally demonstrate genetic instability, grow and metastasize rapidly, but are more chemo-sensitive. Even though most patients with high-grade serous ovarian cancer are diagnosed at an advanced stage, the majority will respond to chemotherapy and enter remission. Unfortunately, many of these patients will then recur and eventually succumb to their disease.

Low-grade serous tumors account for less than 5% of all cases of ovarian carcinoma and are typically diagnosed at advanced stages as well. However, they share characteristics with borderline ovarian neoplasms (tumors of low malignant potential). Borderline tumors are intermediate lesions between benign cysts and malignant tumors, with characteristics of atypical proliferation, and can recur but are noninvasive. Low-grade tumors may arise from a prior borderline tumor, are invasive, but are relatively indolent. Once diagnosed, primary surgery is the recommended approach, as low-grade serous ovarian cancers are more chemo-resistant.

Clear cell and endometrioid carcinoma differ from serous tumors in that they may arise from foci of preexisting endometriosis. Mucinous carcinomas of the ovary may arise from a mucinous borderline tumor. These subtypes are generally diagnosed at earlier stages but generally behave more aggressively if metastatic. At advanced stages, there is worse overall survival compared with high-grade serous carcinoma; this is generally thought to be due to resistance to chemotherapy.

Sex cord-stromal neoplasms include granulosa cell and Sertoli-Leydig cell neoplasms. Compared with epithelial neoplasms, they are more likely to produce sex steroid hormones, present with early-stage disease, and rarely metastasize to the lymph nodes. Prognosis for early-stage disease is generally favorable.

Germ cell tumors include a variety of benign and malignant neoplasms. The most common germ cell tumor is a mature cystic teratoma (dermoid), which is benign. Dysgerminomas are the most common malignant ovarian germ cell tumor, but other malignant subtypes include yolk sac tumors, immature teratomas, and embryonal carcinomas. These subtypes are often chemo-sensitive, with an excellent prognosis if diagnosed early.

Prevention

No routine screening for ovarian cancer in the general population is recommended. The sensitivity, specificity, positive predictive value, and negative predictive value of transvaginal ultrasonography (TVUS) and serum tumor markers (CA 125) have been unreliable due to the low prevalence of ovarian cancer and do not reduce ovarian cancer mortality. Given the high false-positive rate, this can lead to moderate to substantial harm from unnecessary surgical interventions in women who do not have cancer (U.S. Preventive Services Task Force recommendations). This was recently evaluated by the large, randomized Prostate, Lung, Colorectal, and Ovarian Cancer Screening Trial, which found that annual screening of postmenopausal women with both CA 125 and TVUS compared with usual care did not reduce mortality in the general population. The incidence of ovarian cancer was not different for women who were screened, and a majority of women who developed ovarian cancer were still diagnosed with advanced-stage disease.

Factors that may decrease the risk of epithelial ovarian cancer include BSO, tubal ligation/salpingectomy, hysterectomy, oral contraceptive use, breastfeeding, and parity. BSO is the most effective risk-reducing strategy; however, women may still develop peritoneal carcinoma at a rate of approximately 1%. With the role of tubal neoplasia in the development of epithelial ovarian cancer, tubal ligation (regardless of the technique used) has been associated in large epidemiologic studies with an approximate 20% decrease in risk of ovarian cancer. Studies on the effect of opportunistic salpingectomy (removal of fallopian tubes in average-risk women undergoing pelvic surgery for another indication) without oophorectomy are currently ongoing. A meta-analysis of hysterectomy without BSO similarly showed a 20% reduction in the risk of ovarian cancer. Prolonged oral contraceptive use has also been shown to reduce the risk of ovarian cancer, with a meta-analysis showing more than 50% reduction in risk among average-risk women with greater than 10 years of use. Protective factors are less clear for sex cord-stromal and germ cell tumors given their rarity.

Women with a significant family history for breast cancer (notably male breast cancer), uterine, ovarian, or colon cancer should be referred for genetic counseling and possible genetic testing. Expert opinion suggests screening for women at high risk for a hereditary ovarian cancer with TVUS and CA 125 every 6 months, starting at age 30 for patients with *BRCA* mutations or 5 to 10 years before the earliest age of first diagnosis of ovarian cancer in the family for those with family history of ovarian cancer. Screening for patients with Lynch syndrome may begin at age 30 to 35 or 5 to 10 years before the earliest age of first diagnosis of any Lynch-related cancer in the family.

In women with a known *BRCA* mutation, risk-reducing BSO is recommended at completion of childbearing, between 35 and 40 years in women with *BRCA1*, or 40 to 45 years in women with *BRCA2*. BSO has been shown to decrease ovarian cancer risk and mortality in these patients; however, there remains a baseline 1% risk for developing primary peritoneal cancer. Hysterectomy is not routinely recommended as part of the risk-reducing procedure. Although general gynecologists may be able to perform this procedure, consider referral to a gynecologic oncologist, if available. There are specific protocols for pathologic review, as well as for the management of abnormal findings. In women who have not completed childbearing, oral contraceptive use has been shown to have potentially up to a 5% decrease in ovarian cancer risk per year of use. There is some theoretical concern that hormonal contraception may increase the risk of breast cancer in these patients; however, in the large meta-analysis available, there is no evidence supporting increased risk in current users or in the first 10 years after cessation of use. Use of other contraceptives, such as the patch or vaginal ring, have not yet been studied in this context.

The American College of Obstetricians and Gynecologists, the Society of Gynecologic Oncologists (SGO), and the American College of Gastroenterology recommend risk-reducing total hysterectomy with BSO for women with Lynch syndrome after completion of childbearing or by age 40 to 45. The remaining risk for peritoneal cancer of 1% after BSO is extrapolated from studies in women with *BRCA* mutations.

Clinical Manifestations

Patients with ovarian cancer may present with a wide variety of symptoms (Box 1). Most commonly, women will report in the outpatient setting with vague symptoms such as pelvic or abdominal pain, or gastrointestinal symptoms such as abdominal enlargement (from ascites or from mass effect), bloating, early satiety, or changes in bowel habits. Occasionally, incidental findings of a pelvic mass or signs of more advanced disease (peritoneal spread, lymphadenopathy) may be identified at the time of imaging performed for other indications. Acute symptoms are typically due to widely metastatic disease, causing conditions such as bowel obstruction or pleural effusions that may require prompt intervention. Postmenopausal bleeding may be a reporting symptom but is more likely to be associated with uterine pathology. Of note, young patients with signs of precocious puberty, abnormal vaginal bleeding, or hirsutism (likely due to

BOX 1 — Presenting Symptoms

Nausea
Abdominal fullness or early satiety
Pelvic/back pain
Abdominal mass or umbilical mass (Sister Mary Joseph nodule)
Bowel dysfunction (diarrhea, constipation)
Urinary dysfunction (urinary frequency, new incontinence, or obstruction due to mass effect)
Bowel obstruction
Shortness of breath (pleural effusions)

BOX 2 — Indications for Referral

CA 125 > 200 in a premenopausal woman
CA 125 > 35 in a postmenopausal woman
Nodular or fixed pelvic mass on exam
Ascites seen on imaging
Evidence of abdominal or distant metastasis on imaging

BOX 3 — Differential Diagnosis of an Adnexal Mass

Functional cyst
Endometrioma
Tuboovarian abscess
Benign neoplasms (mature teratomas, cystadenomas)
Hydrosalpinx
Pedunculated leiomyoma
Malignant neoplasms (epithelial, germ cell, sex cord-stromal tumors)
Diverticular abscess
Appendiceal abscess
Metastatic cancer (breast, gastrointestinal)
Colorectal malignancy
Retroperitoneal sarcoma

---

abnormal hormone production) should be evaluated for possible sex cord-stromal neoplasms. Rarely, patients may report paraneoplastic syndromes with neurologic findings, hemolytic anemia, or nephrotic syndromes.

Diagnosis

Patients with persistent and progressive abdominal symptoms should be evaluated for ovarian cancer. A pelvic exam and imaging studies (TVUS) may be helpful in identifying a pelvic mass. Composition of the mass (mixed cystic and solid), as well as the presence of thick septations, mural nodules, or papillary excrescences on imaging, would increase suspicion for malignancy. Other diagnostic findings (Box 2), such as an elevated CA 125 (in a postmenopausal woman), a nodular or fixed pelvic mass on exam, or evidence of ascites, abdominal, or distant metastasis on imaging, warrants referral or consultation with a physician trained to stage and debulk ovarian cancer, such as a gynecologic oncologist. Aspiration or biopsy of a cystic pelvic mass is not generally recommended. Needle biopsy of a solid metastatic lesion or paracentesis for cytology may be considered for diagnosis.

Differential Diagnosis

Ovarian cancer may present with varied and nonspecific symptoms; therefore, the differential diagnosis is broad. Even if an adnexal mass is identified, different gynecologic as well as gastrointestinal or urologic causes should still be considered. These may include benign or malignant conditions (Box 3).

Therapy

Historically, ovarian cancers have been treated, regardless of histology, with a combination of chemotherapy and surgery. Referral to a gynecologic oncologist for management is recommended. The backbone of chemotherapy is a platinum agent such as carboplatin (Paraplatin) in combination with a taxane like paclitaxel (Taxol), or doxcetaxel (Taxotere). Maintenance therapy should be considered, with bevacizumab (Avastin) for high-risk patients or poly(ADP-ribose) polymerase (PARP) inhibitors for women with germline or deleterious somatic mutations in *BRCA1* or *BRCA2*. Options for PARP inhibitors include olaparib (Lynparza) for 2 years or niraparib (Zejula) for 3 years. For those who have homologous recombination deficiency (HRD) positive status, either olaparib with bevacizumab or niraparib are options. In recurrence, surgery may

be considered for platinum-sensitive recurrent ovarian cancer patients who have isolated sites of recurrent disease. Systemic treatment with chemotherapy, antibody drug conjugates (targeting *FOLR1* or *HER2*), or combination therapy with checkpoint inhibitors can be considered. All patients with diagnosed ovarian cancer should also be referred for genetic counseling and for genetic testing.

Monitoring

During chemotherapy, myelosuppression, fatigue, and neuropathy (from a combination of a taxane and platinum agent) are some of the most common side effects. Management of these symptoms will be in coordination with the treating oncologist or potentially with palliative care. Neuropathy, difficulties with memory and concentration ("chemo brain"), and fatigue may improve in the first year after completion of therapy, but some symptoms may persist in the long term, with effects on quality of life. The etiology of cognitive dysfunction and fatigue is not well understood, but these patients may respond to cognitive behavioral therapy and exercise.

Current SGO recommendations for posttreatment surveillance include a thorough evaluation of symptoms and physical examination. For years 0 to 2 after completion of treatment, surveillance visits are scheduled every 3 to 4 months. For years 2 to 3, visits are every 4 to 6 months; and for years 3 to 5, they are every 6 months. After 5 years, yearly visits with a gynecologic oncologist or general gynecologist are appropriate. No Pap tests or cytology studies are indicated during this time, and routine CA 125 levels upon each visit are optional. No routine radiographic imaging (chest x-ray, positron emission tomography, or computed tomography [CT] scans, magnetic resonance imaging, or ultrasound) is recommended during surveillance because there is insufficient data to support this use. If recurrence is suspected because of symptoms, CT scans or CA 125 may be useful before repeat consultation with a gynecologic oncologist.

References

Buys SS, Partridge E, Black A, et al: Effect of screening on ovarian cancer mortality: the Prostate, Lung, Colorectal and Ovarian (PLCO) cancer screening randomized controlled trial, *JAMA* 305(22):2295, 2011.

Eskander R, Berman M, Keder L: Practice Bulletin No 174: Evaluation and management of adnexal masses, *Obstet Gynecol* 128(5):e210–e226, 2016.

Matteson KA, Gunderson C, Richardson DL: Committee Opinion No. 716: The role of the obstetrician-gynecologist in the early detection of epithelial ovarian cancer in women at average risk, *Obstet Gynecol* 130(3):e146–e149, 2017.

Salani R, Khanna N, Frimer M, et al: An update on post-treatment surveillance and diagnosis of recurrence in women with gynecologic malignancies: Society of Gynecologic Oncology (SGO) recommendations, *Gynecol Oncol* 146(1):3–10, 2017.

Schorge JO, Modesitt SC, Coleman RL: SGO white paper on ovarian cancer: etiology screening and surveillance, *Gynecol Oncol* 119(1):7–17, 2010.

Yoon SH, Kim SN, Shim SH, et al: Bilateral salpingectomy can reduce the risk of ovarian cancer in the general population: a meta-analysis, *Eur J Cancer* 55:38–46, 2016.

PELVIC INFLAMMATORY DISEASE

Method of
Amy Curry, MD

CURRENT DIAGNOSIS

- Pelvic inflammatory disease is a clinical diagnosis based on suspicious clinical findings in a woman who is at risk.
- Patients may be asymptomatic. Symptoms may range from nonspecific complaints including lower abdominal pain, vaginal discharge, dyspareunia, and irregular uterine bleeding to high fever, vomiting, and lower abdominal tenderness with rebound tenderness.
- Physical examination findings may include vaginal and endocervical discharge as well as cervical motion, uterine and adnexal tenderness, and adnexal fullness.
- Cultures should be performed for *Chlamydia trachomatis* and *Neisseria gonorrhoeae,* the two most commonly implicated organisms, though a variety of infectious agents may be causative.

CURRENT THERAPY

Empiric treatment for pelvic inflammatory disease (PID) should be initiated in any woman at risk for sexually transmitted infections if:
- Pelvic or lower abdominal pain is present
- Cervical motion tenderness *OR* uterine tenderness *OR* adnexal tenderness is found on pelvic examination
- No other cause for the pain can be identified

Recommended inpatient treatment for PID:
- Ceftriaxone (Rocephin) 1 g IV every 24 hours *PLUS* doxycycline (Vibramycin)[1] 100 mg PO/IV every 12 hours *PLUS* metronidazole (Flagyl) 500 mg PO/IV every 12 hours.
  OR
- Cefotetan (Cefotan) 2 g IV every 12 hours *OR* cefoxitin (Mefoxin) 2 g IV every 6 hours *PLUS* doxycycline (Vibramycin)[1] 100 mg PO/IV every 12 hours.

Alternative inpatient treatment for PID:
- Ampicillin/sulbactam (Unasyn) 3 g IV every 6 hours *PLUS* doxycycline (Vibramycin)[1] 100 mg PO/IV every 12 hours.
  OR
- Clindamycin (Cleocin) 900 mg IV every 8 hours *PLUS* gentamicin (Garamycin)[1] 2 mg/kg of body weight loading dose followed by 1.5 mg/kg of body weight IV/IM every 8 hours. A single daily dose of 3 to 5 mg/kg of body weight IV/IM can also be used.

Outpatient treatment for PID:
- Ceftriaxone (Rocephin) 500 mg (1 g if weight ≥150 kg) IM single dose *PLUS* doxycycline (Vibramycin)[1] 100 mg PO every 12 hours for 14 days *WITH* metronidazole (Flagyl) 500 mg PO every 12 hours for 14 days.
  OR
- Cefoxitin (Mefoxin) 2 g IM and probenecid (Benemid)[1] 1 g PO both given concurrently as a single dose *PLUS* doxycycline (Vibramycin)[1] 100 mg PO every 12 hours for 14 days *WITH* metronidazole (Flagyl) 500 mg PO every 12 hours for 14 days.
  OR
- Other parenteral third-generation cephalosporins: either ceftizoxime (Cefizox)[2] 1 g IM single dose *OR* cefotaxime (Claforan) 1 g IM single dose *PLUS* doxycycline (Vibramycin)[1] 100 mg PO every 12 hours for 14 days *WITH* metronidazole (Flagyl) 500 mg PO every 12 hours for 14 days.
- Alternative treatment options are available for those who have penicillin or cephalosporin allergies.

[1]Not FDA approved for this indication.
[2]Not available in the United States.

Pelvic inflammatory disease (PID) is a polymicrobial infection of any or all of the upper genital tract organs in women. It is initiated by a community-acquired sexually transmitted agent and can involve the uterus, fallopian tubes, ovaries, and adjacent pelvic structures.

Epidemiology
In the United States, the diagnosis of PID accounted for 90,000 initial visits to physician offices between 2007 and 2016, and 4.4% of women (2.5 million) 18 to 44 years of age reported a history of PID based on 2013 to 2014 survey data.

Risk Factors
The single greatest risk factor for PID is a history of multiple sex partners. Other risk factors include 15 to 25 years of age, a male partner with symptoms of a sexually transmitted infection (STI) such as dysuria or urethral discharge, history of previous STI or PID, inconsistent use of condoms, African American ethnicity, and use of vaginal douching. Any phenomenon that disrupts the mucus barrier of the endocervical canal can also potentially facilitate PID, such as menses, bacterial vaginosis, or intrauterine instrumentation. Accordingly, the risk of an intrauterine device (IUD) causing PID usually occurs during the first 3 weeks following insertion and rarely thereafter.

Pathophysiology
PID occurs when bacteria from the vagina ascend into the normally sterile environment of the upper genital tract. This often occurs in the setting of a *Neisseria gonorrhoeae* or *Chlamydia trachomatis* infection, although this is occurring less frequently. Ascending bacteria can include anaerobes, especially those implicated in bacterial vaginosis, group A and B *Streptococcus, Escherichia coli, Klebsiella, Proteus mirabilis, Haemophilus influenzae, Peptococcus,* genital *Mycoplasma, Actinomycosis,* and cytomegalovirus. Methicillin-resistant *Staphylococcus aureus* has been reported to cause PID, but rarely. Once present, this polymicrobial infection can remain asymptomatic or cause endometritis, salpingitis, oophoritis, peritonitis, perihepatitis, or tubo-ovarian abscesses.

Clinical Presentation
PID may be asymptomatic. It may have an indolent presentation of low-grade fever, weight loss, and nonspecific abdominal pain. A more symptomatic presentation of PID includes bilateral lower-quadrant abdominal pain, recent onset of dyspareunia, abnormal vaginal bleeding, and vaginal discharge. On physical examination, the patient may have fever, decreased bowel sounds, diffuse lower abdominal tenderness with rebound tenderness, and/or right upper quadrant tenderness. During the pelvic examination, purulent vaginal or endocervical discharge, vaginal mucosa redness, and cervical irritation or friability may be noted. Cervical motion pain or tenderness of the adnexa or uterus during the bimanual examination is strongly suggestive of PID.

There are several diagnostic findings that support the diagnosis of PID: the presence of abundant white blood cells or clue cells in vaginal or cervical mucus; the presence of an STI, especially gonorrhea or chlamydia; an elevated erythrocyte sedimentation rate or C-reactive protein; an elevated serum white blood cell count; evidence of endometritis on endometrial biopsy; findings of thickened, fluid-filled fallopian tubes, free fluid in the pelvis, or a tubo-ovarian abscess on transvaginal ultrasonography or magnetic resonance imaging; or evidence of pelvic organ inflammation on laparoscopic exploration.

Diagnosis
Unfortunately, no single element of the history, finding on physical examination, laboratory test result, or diagnostic procedure has both the sensitivity and the specificity to help the clinician accurately diagnose PID. Consequently, PID remains a diagnosis based primarily on clinical suspicion in at-risk women.

Differential Diagnosis

The differential diagnosis of PID includes ectopic pregnancy, inflammatory bowel disorders, ovarian cysts and cyst rupture, ovarian torsion, appendicitis, endometriosis, proctitis, urinary tract infections, diverticulitis, constipation, or functional pain related to current or past abuse.

Treatment

The 2021 Centers for Disease Control and Prevention (CDC) treatment guidelines for PID are outlined in the Current Diagnosis and Current Therapy boxes. These guidelines recommend empiric treatment for PID in all at-risk women who meet the criteria listed, as "prevention of long-term sequelae is dependent on early administration of recommended antimicrobials."

Treatment guidelines are based on the patient's need for inpatient versus outpatient care. The Pelvic Inflammatory Disease Evaluation and Clinical Health (PEACH) trial demonstrated no difference in the reproductive outcomes of women with mild-to-moderate PID who were randomized to inpatient treatment versus those randomized to outpatient treatment.

Indications for inpatient treatment of PID include the following: pregnancy; failed trial or intolerance to oral medications; signs of severe PID such as high fever, nausea, vomiting, or intractable abdominal pain; complicated PID (e.g., peritonitis, perihepatitis); and pelvic abscess. The need for surgical intervention or diagnostic exploration to rule out other abdominal pathology would also mandate inpatient treatment. In patients who require inpatient treatment, any one of the parenteral antibiotic regimens as outlined earlier may be administered, depending on the patient's history of allergies and the cost and availability of treatment options. When possible, the use of oral doxycycline (Vibramycin)[1] and metronidazole (Flagyl) is preferred over intravenous (IV) infusion as they both have similar oral bioavailability compared with IV infusion, and infusion of IV doxycycline (Vibramycin) can be painful. Treatment should also include appropriate analgesia, antiemetics, antipyretics, IV fluids, and rest. Patients may be transitioned from parenteral to oral therapy after 24 to 48 hours of sustained clinical improvement including lack of fever. Further completion of a total of 14 days of treatment with oral medications is recommended. Patients who are treated with any of the recommended inpatient regimens should be transitioned to oral doxycycline (Vibramycin)[1] 100 mg every 12 hours and metronidazole (Flagyl) 500 mg PO every 12 hours to complete 14 days of total treatment.

Those treated with clindamycin (Cleocin) and gentamicin (Garamycin)[1] should be transitioned to oral doxycycline (Vibramycin)[1] 100 mg every 12 hours or oral clindamycin (Cleocin) 450 mg every 6 hours to complete 14 days of total treatment. If a tubo-ovarian abscess is present, in addition to surgical consultation and at least 24 hours of inpatient monitoring, the patient should be transitioned to oral clindamycin (Cleocin) 450 mg every 6 hours or oral metronidazole (Flagyl) 500 mg every 12 hours plus doxycycline (Vibramycin)[1] 100 mg every 12 hours for a total of 14 days of treatment.

In patients who do not meet the criteria for inpatient treatment, any of the outpatient treatment regimens as outlined earlier may be used, the choice being again dependent on the cost and availability of treatment options. The addition of metronidazole (Flagyl) is recommended because of cephalosporin limitations in anaerobic coverage and in the case of Trichomonas or bacterial vaginosis infections. The addition of metronidazole (Flagyl) is also recommended if there is a history of recent uterine instrumentation.

Routine use of quinolones is no longer recommended in empiric treatment of PID because of increasingly resistant N. gonorrhoeae. If a cephalosporin allergy exists and inpatient treatment with clindamycin (Cleocin) and gentamicin (Garamycin)[1] is not available, risk for gonorrhea is low, cultures are obtained, and follow-up is available, levofloxacin (Levaquin)[1] 500 mg PO every 24 hours or moxifloxacin (Avelox)[1] 400 mg PO every 24 hours with metronidazole (Flagyl) 500 mg PO every 12 hours for 14 days may be used. Azithromycin (Zithromax) 500 mg IV every 24 hours for one to two doses followed by 250 mg PO every 24 hours with metronidazole 500 mg PO every 12 hours for 12 to 14 days total can also be used.

In patients with a history of penicillin allergy, a careful reaction history should be taken to assess the risk of using a cephalosporin in the empiric treatment of PID. There is negligible cross-reactivity between penicillins and third-generation cephalosporins. If a cephalosporin cannot be safely used, the patient can be admitted for treatment with parenteral clindamycin (Cleocin) and gentamicin (Garamycin).[1]

Regardless of the treatment regimen used, patients should be advised to abstain from intercourse until treatment is completed and they are free from symptoms. In patients with an IUD, there is inconclusive data to recommend its removal, unless clinical improvement does not occur, but close clinical follow-up is warranted. There is no difference in the treatment regimens for PID in women with a history of HIV.

Patient Monitoring and Counseling

Patients treated with an outpatient regimen should be evaluated for clinical improvement within 48 to 72 hours. If no improvement is noted, the patient should be hospitalized for parenteral antibiotics and further diagnostic evaluation. All patients should be counseled on the need to complete the full course of antibiotic treatment to decrease the potential complications of PID. Patients should be informed of the cause of their infection, if known, and the need for any sexual partners to be tested and treated. Patients with PID caused by N. gonorrhoeae or C. trachomatis infections should be retested 3 months after completing treatment. Testing for HIV, syphilis, and hepatitis B and C should also be offered. If the patient is an appropriate candidate, immunization against hepatitis B (Engerix-B, Recombivax HB) and human papillomavirus (Gardasil 9) should also be offered. To decrease future PID episodes, patients should be advised on the need for safe sex practices and the recommendation for future routine screening for chlamydia and gonorrhea.

Complications

Complications of PID include recurrence of the infection, infertility secondary to fallopian tube scarring, chronic pelvic pain, and ectopic pregnancy. Extension of the infection can also occur, potentially causing pelvic abscess, peritonitis, and perihepatitis (Fitz-Hugh–Curtis syndrome).

---

[1]Not FDA approved for this indication.

References

Campagna JD, Bond MC, Schabelman E, Hayes BD: The use of cephalosporins in penicillin-allergic patients: a literature review, *J Emerg Med* 42(5):612–620, 2012.

Curry A, Williams T, Penny M: Pelvic inflammatory disease: diagnosis, management, and prevention, *Am Fam Physician* 100(6):357–364, 2019.

Kreisel K, Torrone E, Bernstein K, Hong J, Gorwitz R: Prevalence of pelvic inflammatory disease in sexually experienced women of reproductive age United States, 2013–2014, *MMWR Morb Mortal Wkly Rep* 66(3):80–83, 2017.

Ness RB, Soper DE, Holley RL, et al: Effectiveness of inpatient and outpatient treatment strategies for women with pelvic inflammatory disease: results from the pelvic inflammatory disease evaluation and clinical health (PEACH) randomized trial, *Am J Obstet Gynecol* 186:929–937, 2002.

Tepper NK, Steenland MW, Gaffield ME, Marchbanks PA, Curtis KM: Retention of intrauterine devices in women who acquire pelvic inflammatory disease: a systematic review, *Contraception* 87(5):655–660, 2013.

Workowski KA, Bachmann LH, Chan PA, et al: Sexually Transmitted Infections Treatment Guidelines, 2021, *MMWR Recomm Rep* 70(4):1–187, 2021.

---

[1]Not FDA approved for this indication.

PREMENSTRUAL DYSPHORIC DISORDER

Method of
**Stephanie Trentacoste McNally, MD; and
Kristina M. Deligiannidis, MD**

CURRENT THERAPY

- SSRIs are the first-line treatment. SNRIs may have some benefits.
- Certain combined oral contraceptives have been shown to help alleviate symptoms of PMDD.
- Hormonal interventions with progesterone or estrogen or GnRH antagonists have varied effects.
- Surgery that removes the ovaries improves symptoms of PMDD; however, it will lead to surgical menopause, which has other risk factors for women's health.
- Complimentary medicine, lifestyle changes, and herbal treatments provide supportive options.

CURRENT DIAGNOSIS

- PMS and PMDD are within the spectrum of PMD.
- PMS refers to the physical and emotional symptoms that some women experience in the lead up to menstruation.
- PMDD is a narrowly defined DSMV diagnosis. Symptoms must be present during the luteal phase of most menstrual cycles for 2 months.

Introduction

Premenstrual dysphoric disorder (PMDD) refers to the psychological, cognitive, and physical changes that affect women during the luteal phase of their menstrual cycle. It is on the spectrum of premenstrual disorders (PMDs) and can have significant impact on daily living. This chapter will provide an overview of the diagnosis, sequelae, and treatment options for PMDD.

Diagnosis

The International Society for Premenstrual Disorders (ISPMD) is a consensus group that has defined a spectrum of PMDs, including core and variant PMDs as outlined in Table 1.

Core PMDs are defined as the psychological or somatic symptoms that arise during the luteal phase of the menstrual cycle, affect normal daily function, including changes in mood, and resolve with the onset of menstruation. Premenstrual syndrome (PMS) and premenstrual dysphoric disorder (PMDD) are considered core PMDs. PMDD is a more severe form of PMD than PMS. *Variant PMDs* include premenstrual exacerbations of underlying psychiatric disorders, symptoms occurring in response to exogenous progesterone, and symptoms arising from ovarian activity other than ovulation including those that occur when ovulation has been suppressed.

PMS refers to the physical and emotional symptoms that some women experience in the lead up to menstruation. The definition of PMS is focused on the presence of symptoms but does not specify the frequency or intensity of those symptoms. On the other hand, *PMDD* is narrowly defined by the *Diagnostic and Statistical Manual of Mental Disorders*, 5th Edition (DSM-5). The diagnosis of PMDD requires one core symptom plus a minimum of 5 of 11 possible symptoms (Table 2). To meet the criteria for a diagnosis of PMDD, symptoms must be present in the luteal phase of most menstrual cycles during the prior year and must result in clinically significant distress or interference in daily life.

The diagnosis of PMDD is made using validated tools, most commonly the Daily Record of Severity of Problems (DRSP).

The DRSP is used prospectively to characterize luteal phase symptoms over two cycles. Prospective evaluation is the standard for diagnosis. In the past, the diagnosis of PMDD often relied on a retrospective assessment of a woman's symptoms during the luteal phase. While screening tools, structured clinical interviews, and self-report scales are available, these retrospective assessments have limited value due to their subjectivity and potential for recall bias. Thus, prospective monitoring with the DPSP is the gold standard of diagnosis.

The prevalence of PMDD, according to the American Psychiatric Association, is 1.8% to 5.8% of menstruating people in the United States, though researchers acknowledge this may not reflect the true prevalence due to inconsistencies in following the DSM-5 and ICD-11 diagnostic and coding criteria.

Pathophysiology

During the menstrual cycle, there is a complex hormonal interaction involving the hypothalamic-pituitary-ovarian axis. A normal menstrual cycle is 21 to 35 days with the average cycle being 28 days. The first half of the cycle, the follicular phase, is associated with an increase in estradiol which peaks at ovulation, release of follicle stimulating hormone (FSH) and luteinizing hormone (LH), maturation of an ovarian follicle, and ovulation. This leads to the second half of the cycle known as the luteal phase. During the luteal phase, the ovulated follicle becomes the corpus luteum which secretes progesterone. If pregnancy does not occur, the corpus luteum degenerates and progesterone levels drop leading to menstruation.

Progesterone is lipophilic and can cross the blood-brain barrier. PMS and PMDD result from an abnormal brain response to hormonal fluctuations of estradiol, progesterone and progesterone metabolites, especially allopregnanolone, during a normal menstrual cycle. Recent neuroimaging studies suggest that PMS is related to cyclic differences in brain serotonin levels. With less serotonin in the synapse, rates of depression during the luteal phase for women with PMDD are higher. Across the menstrual cycle, patients with PMDD have abnormalities in serotonin transporter binding and impaired interactions between the gamma-aminobutyric acid (GABA) receptor and progesterone metabolites, including allopregnanolone. Women with PMDD have an increased sensitivity to allopregnanolone in the luteal phase, which may be due to abnormal GABA receptor plasticity.

Data have shown that women with PMDD have the same level of estrogen and progesterone compared with the cycles of women without the diagnosis. Since the absolute hormone levels are consistent for women with and without PMDD, a theory behind the occurrence of PMDD is related to differences in hormone receptor uptake and hormone interaction. This is most significant with the progesterone metabolite isomers in women with PMS.

Though no definite genes have been associated with PMDD, there are studies in identical twins that show a familial predisposition to PMDD. A family history of PMDD may exist. Some gene polymorphisms for estrogen and serotonin receptors may play a role in how hormones interact. Different receptor sensitivity responses may trigger more symptoms in women with PMDD. Smoking and elevated body mass index are associated with an increased risk of PMDD. Stress and inflammation have also been associated with PMDD.

Currently, there are no known preventive measures for women with PMDD. Making the appropriate prospective diagnosis, monitoring, and treatment should be the focus of clinical care.

Clinical Manifestations

Ninety percent of women will have a premenstrual symptom during their reproductive life; 20% to 30% of women have symptoms during their cycles that are severe enough to qualify for PMS; while 2% to 6% of women have PMDD. PMDD may be difficult to diagnose. It can start as early in menarche. It may present differently in women from different cultural and socioeconomic backgrounds and therefore may be underdiagnosed. PMDD is complex and patients may present with a myriad of

TABLE 1   ISPMD Classification of Premenstrual Disorders

Core PMDs

Premenstrual syndrome and premenstrual dysphoric disorder	Symptoms occur in ovulatory cycle
Subclassified according to nature of symptoms • Predominantly physical • Predominantly emotional • Mixed	Symptoms can be physical or psychological Symptoms absent after menstruation and before ovulation Symptoms must be prospectively rated for at least 2 cycles Symptoms must cause functional impairment

Variant PMDs

Premenstrual exacerbation	Exacerbation of an underlying somatic (e.g., asthma, migraine) or psychological disorder that is present throughout the month but worsens in the luteal phase
Non-ovulatory PMD	Poorly understood and rare; symptoms arise from follicular activity of the ovary
Progestogen-induced PMD	PMD symptoms arise from exogenous sources of progestogen in the COC or HRT
PMD with absent menstruation	PMD arises from cyclical ovarian activity even though menstruation has been suppressed (e.g., in women who have had endometrial ablation, have IUS or have had a hysterectomy)

COC, Combined oral contraceptives; HRT, hormone replacement therapy; ISPMD, International Society of Premenstrual Disorders; IUS, intrauterine device; PMD, premenstrual disorder.
From Ismaili E, Walsh S, O'Brien PMS, et al: Fourth consensus of the International Society for Premenstrual Disorders (ISPMD): auditable standards for diagnosis and management of premenstrual disorder, Arch Womens Ment Health 19:953–958, 2016.

TABLE 2   Symptoms of PMDD—DSM-5

Criteria

Must have at least 5 out of the 11 symptoms below, with at least one core symptoms

Core Symptoms

Marked affective lability (e.g., mood swings; feeling suddenly sad or tearful or increased sensitivity to rejection)

Marked irritability or anger or increased interpersonal conflicts

Marked depressed mood, feelings of hopelessness, or self-deprecating thoughts

Marked anxiety, tension, and/or feelings of being keyed up or on edge

Additional Symptoms

Decreased interest in usual activities

Poor concentration

Lethargic, reduced stamina

Marked change in appetite; overeating or food cravings

Sleep changes (e.g., hypersomnia or insomnia)

A sense of being overwhelmed or out of control

Physical symptoms such as breast tenderness, joint pains, bloating

DSM-5, Diagnostic and Statistical Manual of Mental Disorders, 5th Edition; PMDD, premenstrual dysphoric disorder.

physical and emotional symptoms. The most common symptoms are related to anxiety and depression exacerbations during the luteal phase of the menstrual cycle. These symptoms abate during pregnancy and menopause when there are no progesterone peaks post ovulation.

Pharmacologic Treatments

Selective Serotonin Reuptake Inhibitors

Selective serotonin reuptake inhibitors (SSRIs) are the first-line treatment for PMDD. Multiple randomized controlled trials (RCTs) have established that SSRIs, dosed continuously or only in the luteal phase of the menstrual cycle, are the gold standard of treatment for PMDD.

The mechanism by which SSRIs treat PMDD is unknown, though it likely involves both serotonergic and non-serotonergic mechanisms. One non-serotonergic mechanism that may lead to affective symptom relief is that SSRIs act as selective brain steroidogenic stimulants, increasing the conversion of progesterone to allopregnanolone. In a recent study, treatment with sertraline (50 mg) during the luteal phase significantly increased serum pregnanolone levels, increased the serum pregnanolone:progesterone ratio, decreased 3 alpha, 5 alpha androsterone levels, and improved psychologic symptoms. SSRIs more effectively treat the affective symptoms of PMDD compared to the physical symptoms. SSRIs have rapid onset within 24 hours and peak within 48 hours. Only fluoxetine (Sarafem), sertraline (Zoloft), and paroxetine (Paxil CR) are approved by the Food and Drug Administration (FDA) for treatment of PMDD.

Serotonin-Norepinephrine Reuptake Inhibitors

Some data have shown potential benefits of serotonin-norepinephrine reuptake inhibitors (SNRIs) for PMDD. In open-labeled studies of venlafaxine[1] and duloxetine[1] and small single blinded trials of duloxetine, with continuous and luteal phase dosing, SNRIs have shown efficacy for the treatment of PMDD. Placebo-controlled trials are warranted for further investigation of these agents for the treatment of PMDD, but it is reasonable to use them as a second-line agent if tolerability limits use of SSRIs.

Combined Oral Contraceptives (COCs)

Combined oral contraceptives (COCs) are an effective treatment for somatic symptoms of the menstrual cycle, including but not limited to dysmenorrhea, gastrointestinal changes, and menorrhagia. Data concerning the effect of COCs on affective premenstrual symptoms have been inconsistent.

Drospirenone, a progesterone derivative, combined with ethinyl estradiol (EE) is the only current FDA-approved COC (Gianvi, Jasmiel, Nikki, Vestura, Yaz) for the treatment of PMDD. Trials lasting up to 3 months indicate that the maximum efficacy is achieved with a 24 days active/4 days placebo schedule of drospirenone and 20 mcg of ethinyl estradiol (EE) measured by the DRSP score. A randomized controlled trial using drospirenone and 30 mcg of EE with a 21 day active/7 day placebo schedule versus 28 days of placebo for women with PMDD found significant improvement in the active treatment arm only for acne, appetite, and food craving. Though results trended toward improvement in affective symptoms, they did not reach significance. A recent meta-analysis of COCs for PMDD or PMS concluded that while COCs were shown to be effective for symptom reduction overall, they were not effective for depressive symptoms specifically. To date, no specific formulation has shown superiority over others.

Gonadotropin Releasing Hormone (GnRH) Receptor Agonists

GnRH receptor agonists act to suppress ovulation. Suppression of ovulation has been shown to treat PMS as it inhibits increases in estrogen and progesterone during the luteal phase in a chemical induced menopause.

---

[1] Not FDA approved for this indication.

Leuprolide (Lupron)[1], a GnRH agonist, and danazol (Cyclomen)[1], an anti-gonadotropic derivative of ethisterone, show some efficacy in treatment-resistant *PMDD*. These medications have side effects so they should be used with caution. GnRH agonists suppress ovarian function, medically inducing menopause. Secondary to the long-term effects on cardiovascular and bone health with an early menopause, GnRH agonist should not be used for long periods of time without additional hormone therapy such as progesterone and estrogen. Moreover, danazol has significant negative somatic and mood side effects secondary to its anti-androgenic properties precluding long-term use.

Investigational GABA-ergic Neuroactive Steroids
Sepranolone is a synthetic allopregnanolone antagonist that interacts with the GABA receptors. A post-hoc analysis of placebo-controlled and double-blind RCTs showed low-dose sepranolone improved PMDD symptoms in the 9 days before menses. The medication is not FDA approved and remains investigational as the initial trial did not meet the primary endpoints.

Estrogens
Estrogen[1] treatment is not a mainstay for treatment of PMDD. There are data to indicate that elevated levels of luteal phase estrogen may contribute to more severe symptoms of PMDD. This relationship may be due to interactions of estrogen with other neurotransmitters rather than estrogen being a direct cause of PMDD. Therefore, estrogen is not a direct treatment option.

Androgens
Dutasteride (Avodart) inhibits 5 alpha-reductase and the conversion of progesterone to allopregnanolone thereby stabilizing the levels throughout the menstrual cycle. A small double-blind placebo-controlled study evaluating daily doses of dutasteride[1] demonstrated significant efficacy for the 2.5 mg dose in ameliorating anxiety, sadness, bloating, irritability, and food cravings.

Progesterone
To date, progesterone-only interventions have not consistently demonstrated reduction of PMS and PMDD symptoms. One open label study of 37 women given 100 mg of sublingual micronized progesterone (Prometrium)[1] on day 11 to day 25 of their cycles across three cycles reported significant efficacy of treatment over placebo. The authors hypothesized that increased bioavailability of sublingual dosing was more significant than oral progesterone 5 mg daily over 28 days resulting in a significant increase in remission of PMDD, a promising result warranting further study.

Selective Progesterone Receptor Modulator
Ulipristal acetate (Ella)[1], used and marketed as emergency contraception, has been shown to treat the emotional and depressive symptoms of PMDD. Ulipristal acetate interacts with progesterone receptors in the pituitary gland to inhibit ovulatory triggers.

Anxiolytics
Although benzodiazepines have a history of clinical use in the treatment of PMDD, the literature assessing their efficacy is sparse and clinically out of date. While benzodiazepines may be useful during the symptomatic phase of PMDD, the evidence to recommend their use is weak, and they should be considered for adjunctive treatment only in refractory cases.

Clonidine
One randomized-placebo controlled study of clonidine[1], an alpha-2 adrenergic agonist, for PMDD failed to show efficacy over placebo on any collected mood or premenstrual symptom scale.

Nonpharmacologic Treatment Options
Psychotherapy
Several psychotherapeutic modalities have been shown to be efficacious in the treatment of PMS and PMDD with cognitive behavioral therapy (CBT) being the most efficacious.

In terms of comparative efficacy, one meta-analysis concluded that CBT showed the same small to moderate effect size as antidepressants in the treatment of PMS and PMDD and hypothesized that improved outcomes could be achieved with combination treatment. An additional study assessing CBT versus fluoxetine versus combined treatment for women with PMDD demonstrated similar efficacy between treatment groups.

Neurofeedback
For women diagnosed with PMDD, patients were trained in neurofeedback techniques targeting the limbic system. Emotional symptoms, specifically anger and mood liability related to PMDD were improved by using neurofeedback techniques.

Surgery
Hysterectomy with bilateral salpingectomy/oophorectomy (BSO) has been successfully utilized as a definitive treatment option for women with PMDD. The reported remission rate is 93.6%.

Novasure is a procedure to thermally ablate the endometrial lining. For the treatment of menorrhagia, a prospective cohort study of 36 women undergoing the procedure found significant improvement in symptoms of PMS. The mechanism of the effect on PMS is not clear and further research is needed to validate these preliminary findings. Novasure was only studied in patients diagnosed with PMS and was not studied in patients with PMDD.

Complementary and Integrative Medicine Approaches
A 2019 systematic review of RCTs assessing safety and efficacy of acupuncture or acupressure for PMS or PMDD found greater but limited reductions in physical and psychological symptoms compared to sham treatment. Reflexology and yoga may provide benefits for symptomatic reduction but are not proven in larger RCTs.

Herbal Preparations
Chasteberry's extract (Vitex Agnus castus) has been studied as a treatment option for PMDD in a variety of trials. Overall, when administered orally during the luteal phase, it has been shown to be superior to placebo in reduction of symptoms.

Other herbal preparations including chamomile, Kami-shovo-san (TJ-24), Saffron, and Hypericum perforatum (St. John's wort), are thought to have anxiolytic, anti-inflammatory, or antispasmodic effects. They are not mainstay treatment options but may be considered as complementary to prescribed medications for PMDD symptoms.

Vitamins
Vitamin B6 (pyridoxine)[1], a cofactor in the synthesis of monoamines and gamma-aminobutyric acid (GABA), has more than twice the effectiveness of decreasing PMDD symptoms compared to placebo. Tested doses ranged from 50 mg/day to 150 mg/day. There was no change in efficacy with higher doses. Therefore, lower doses should be prescribed given evidence of adverse effects such as peripheral neuropathy. Magnesium[1] supplementation may have some protective effects particularly during the luteal phase. Omega-3 polyunsaturated fatty acids (PUFAs)[1] have been shown to be effective for reducing the severity of symptoms of PMS, particularly in older women and with increased length of treatment. Calcium[1] and vitamin D[1] supplementation have not shown consistent results in studies to reduce PMDD symptoms.

---

[1] Not FDA approved for this indication.

[1] Not FDA approved for this indication.

Physical Activity

Though the most effective type of exercise and the exact duration of exercise recommended is not well-defined, aerobic physical exercise and its ability to increase endorphins has been shown to regulate the synthesis of estrogen and progesterone and improve psychologic, physical, and behavioral symptoms of PMDD.

Diet

Increased carbohydrate intake during the luteal phase may have beneficial effects on the symptoms of PMDD. This is likely related to increased tryptophan and serotonin availability. Vitamin B1 (thiamine)[1] as a treatment for PMS remains unclear, although its function as a cofactor in the metabolism of carbohydrates and amino acids is of interest.

Monitoring

There are not consistent algorithms in terms of monitoring a patient's frequency and length of follow-up visits. A multidisciplinary team should be in place with an individualized treatment plan for each patient. The following should be done:

1. Make an appropriate diagnosis using DSM-5 prospective criteria.
2. Provide treatment based on patient-centered care.
3. Incorporate multiple modalities into care plans to achieve the best results and improvement of patient quality of life.

Complications

PMDD and its associated PMDs have varied consequences for patients. As listed in the diagnostic criteria, emotional and psychologic affects are the key findings. Women with PMDD have a higher rate of unipolar, bipolar, and perinatal depression. These women are at increased risk for suicide with some studies reporting up to a 28.1% suicide risk with 40% of women reporting a suicidal ideation sometime in their life. Risk factors for suicide include panic disorder, non-white skin color, greater severity of depressive symptoms, and history of childhood trauma. There are economic ramifications as well. Physical and emotional symptoms may be debilitating, affecting one's activities of daily living, including the ability to work.

---

[1] Not FDA approved for this indication.

References

American Psychiatric Association: *Diagnostic and statistical manual of mental disorders*, ed 5, Washington, DC, 2013, America Psychiatric Association.

Backstrom T, Haage D, Lofgren M, et al: Paradoxical effects of GABA-A modulators may explain sex steroid induced negative mood symptoms in some persons, *Neuroscience* 191:46–54, 2011.

Carlini SV, Lanza di Scalea T, McNally ST, Lester J, Deligiannidis KM: Management of premenstrual dysphoric disorder: a scoping review, *Focus (Am Psychiatr Publ)* 22(1):81–96, 2024.

Cary E, Simpson P: Premenstrual disorders and PMDD - a review, *Best Pract Res Clin Endocrinol Metab* 38(1):101858, 2024.

Comasco E, Kopp Kallner H, Bixo M, et al: Ulipristal acetate for treatment of premenstrual dysphoric disorder: a proof-of-concept randomized controlled trial, *Am J Psychiatry* 178(3):256–265, 2021.

Hantsoo L, Jagodnik KM, Novick AM, et al: The role of the hypothalamic-pituitary-adrenal axis in depression across the female reproductive lifecycle: current knowledge and future directions, *Front Endocrinol (Lausanne)* 14:1295261, 2023.

Kaltsouni E, Fisher PM, Dubol M, et al: Brain reactivity during aggressive response in women with premenstrual dysphoric disorder treated with a selective progesterone receptor modulator, *Neuropsychopharmacology* 46(8):1460–1467, 2021.

Li DJ, Tsai SJ, Bai YM, et al: Risks of major affective disorders following a diagnosis of premenstrual dysphoric disorder: A nationwide longitudinal study, *Asian J Psychiatr* 79:103355, 2023.

Liguori F, Saraiello E, Calella P: Premenstrual Syndrome and Premenstrual Dysphoric Disorder's Impact on Quality of Life, and the Role of Physical Activity, *Medicina (Kaunas)* 59(11), 2023.

Management of Premenstrual Disorders: *ACOG Practice Bulletin* 142(6), 2023.

Miller KN, Standeven L, Morrow AL, Payne JL, Epperson CN, Hantsoo L: GABAergic neuroactive steroid response to sertraline in premenstrual dysphoric disorder, *Psychoneuroendocrinology* 160:106684, 2024.

Reilly TJ, Patel S, Unachukwu IC, et al: The prevalence of premenstrual dysphoric disorder: Systematic review and meta-analysis, *J Affect Disord* 349:534–540, 2024.

Sacher T, Zsido R, Barth C, Zientek F, Rullman M, et al: Increase in serotonin transporter binding in patients with premenstrual dysphoric disorder across the menustral cycle: a case-control longitudinal neuroreceptor ligand positron emission tomography imaging, *J Biol Pyschiatry* 93(12):1081–1088, 2023.

UTERINE LEIOMYOMA

Method of
Jamie Peregrine, MD, MS; and Laura Tatpati, MD

CURRENT DIAGNOSIS

- Uterine leiomyomas (fibroids) are both the most common and the most symptomatic pelvic tumor in people with a uterus.
- These noncancerous, smooth muscle tumors may be causal OR incidental to common gynecologic/obstetric manifestations: abnormal uterine bleeding (AUB) and subsequent anemia, pelvic pain/pressure, dysmenorrhea, dyspareunia, bowel/bladder complaints, infertility, pregnancy loss, and other obstetric complications.
- LOCATION, LOCATION, LOCATION: As in real estate, fibroid location and size are critical! Careful assessment aids in (1) determining the probability that fibroids are the true cause of symptoms, (2) differentiating from alternate diagnoses, and (3) selecting the most efficacious treatment. Systematic documentation properly conveys the nature of the fibroids to other care providers.

CURRENT THERAPY

- Shared patient decision-making should balance goals of (1) diagnostic certainty, (2) treating symptoms and quality of life, (3) minimizing complications of the therapeutic approach, and (4) optimizing future fertility and obstetric outcomes, when applicable.
- Medical therapies, the most effective of which cause ovarian suppression, may be used for longer term symptom relief or to provide short-term benefits to optimize the patient condition for surgery.
- Excisional/ablative procedures are most ideal for fibroids with intracavitary endometrial involvement and in cases where there is concern for malignancy, conservative treatment fails, or when more aggressive emergent treatment is warranted.

Pathophysiology

Fibroids are sex hormone sensitive, monoclonal, smooth muscle tumors with excessive extracellular matrix and angiogenesis. The leading model for fibroid pathogenesis centers on the transformation of a single myometrial stem cell into a tumor-initiating cell that supports clonal tumor growth. Genetic, environmental, hormonal, and other "hits"/pathways are involved in this conversion and sustaining fibroid growth.

Many theories explain how fibroids cause bleeding, bulk symptoms, and adverse reproductive outcomes. While certainty regarding exact mechanisms requires further research, whether a fibroid causes symptoms does correlate to fibroid location and size. The International Federation of Gynecology & Obstetrics organization (FIGO) leiomyoma subclassification system (Figure 1; part of the PALM-COEIN classification of abnormal uterine bleeding [AUB] in reproductive years) is useful in clinical practice. Using the PALM-COEIN system should decrease the likelihood that symptoms are misattributed to incidental fibroids.

Epidemiology/Prevention

Numerous risk factors for fibroid burden have been identified by epidemiologic studies of varying strengths. The most consistent associations are between fibroid burden and Black race, lower parity, and increasing age until menopause. The relationship between Black race and fibroid burden is complex, and treatment disparities have been identified in this patient population. No

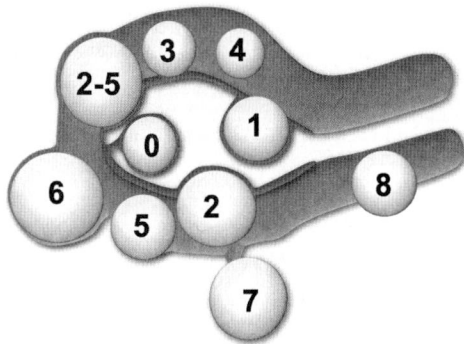

FIGO Leiomyoma Subclassification System

Polyp		
Adenomyosis		Submucous
Leiomyoma		Other
Malignancy & hyperplasia		

Coagulopathy
Ovulatory dysfunction
Endometrial
Iatrogenic
Not otherwise classified

SM - Submucous	0	Pedunculated intracavitary
	1	<50% intramural
	2	≥50% intramural
O - Other	3	Contacts endometrium; 100% intramural
	4	Intramural
	5	Subserous ≥50% intramural
	6	Subserous <50% intramural
	7	Subserous pedunculated
	8	Other (specify e.g., cervical, parasitic)
Hybrid (contact both the endometrium and the serosal layer)		Two numbers are listed separated by a hyphen. By convention, the first refers to the relationship with the endometrium while the second refers to the relationship to the serosa. One example is below.
	2-5	Submucous and subserous, each with less than half the diameter in the endometrial and peritoneal cavities, respectively.

© Malcolm G. Munro MD

Figure 1 The FIGO leiomyoma subclassification system. *FIGO*, International Federation of Gynecology and Obstetrics.

primary or secondary prevention strategies (i.e., modification of diet, lifestyle, body composition, or environmental exposures) for fibroids have yet been sufficiently investigated.

Clinical Manifestations

Abnormal Uterine Bleeding and Anemia

Hypotheses for how fibroids cause heavy menstrual bleeding include (1) enlargement of the uterine cavity and subsequent endometrial surface area, (2) stiff, extracellular matrix-heavy fibroids leading to dysfunctional myometrial contractions and increased bleeding from denuded spiral arteries during menses, and (3) overall angiogenesis integral to fibroid growth. Increased quantity, volume, and lower FIGO type increase the likelihood leiomyomas will cause AUB. Acute and chronic anemia, mild and severe, and subsequent iron deficiency can result. Appropriate treatment of anemia includes iron replacement, judicious blood transfusion, and ·addressing the underlying source of bleeding with appropriate medical or surgical treatment.

Bulk Symptoms

Increased size, number, and higher FIGO types are associated with increased risk of bulk symptoms: pelvic pain, pelvic pressure, back pain, leg pain, dysmenorrhea, dyspareunia, bloating, constipation, tenesmus, and hydronephrosis, in addition to urinary incontinence, frequency, and hesitancy. On the other hand, even very large fibroids may be present without apparent symptoms. Bulk symptoms are more likely to respond to surgical treatment than medical treatment.

Reproductive and Pregnancy Impact

Data regarding the impact of fibroids and fibroid treatment on fertility and pregnancy loss are difficult to interpret. In their 2017 review of the literature, the American Society of Reproductive Medicine (ASRM) recommends that in women with cavity-distorting myomas (FIGO types 0-2), myomectomy (removal of the fibroid itself) may be considered to improve pregnancy rates. They also conclude there is fair evidence that myomectomy does not impair clinical pregnancy or live birth after assisted reproductive technology, such as in vitro fertilization. While fibroids have been hypothesized to impact fertility and pregnancy loss by impairing uterine contractility necessary for gamete transport, altering endometrial receptivity and implantation of embryos, and impairing blood supply to early pregnancy, the literature is too limited to substantiate evidence-based conclusions in support of these hypotheses.

Obstetric outcomes research also has limitations, commonly omitting one of the clinically important comparison groups: those without fibroids, with fibroids (untreated), and those after myomectomy/treatment. Pregnant patients with fibroids are associated with higher rates of preterm birth, cesarean section, and placenta previa, and these risks appear to persist with a history of myomectomy. Myomectomy does introduce higher risk of uterine rupture, and potentially associated outcomes of abruption, postpartum hemorrhage, and low birth weight have not been compared between treated and untreated pregnant patients with fibroids. Fibroids can undergo degeneration and necrosis due to loss of blood supply, which can be very painful. If this occurs during pregnancy, it can be difficult to diagnosis and manage. Other pregnancy-associated risks include fibroid-related uterine entrapment in the pelvis as the uterus grows beyond the first trimester, labor dystocia at the time of vaginal delivery, and complications with the cesarean uterine incision. Myomectomies are typically avoided at the time of cesarean delivery due to the potential increased difficulty with removal and repair and increased risk of hemorrhage, but may be unavoidable.

Diagnosis

History and Physical Exam

The patient history should include gynecologic, abdominal/pelvic, gastrointestinal and genitourinary, hematologic, and obstetric history that may reveal symptoms associated with fibroids. Careful abdominal, bimanual pelvic examination, and rarely speculum examination may detect discrete fibroids, uterine enlargement, and/or asymmetry of the uterus.

Imaging

The purpose of imaging is to identify, localize, and classify fibroids in a systematic way. FIGO subtype, location relative to uterine plane, and size of the fibroids (particularly the large and/or most likely impactful) should be documented, regardless of imaging modality. Pelvic ultrasound (transabdominal and transvaginal) is standard in diagnosis; saline infusion sonohysterogram and pelvic MRI have selective use and may guide procedural planning. When AUB, infertility, or recurrent pregnancy loss are present, 3D ultrasound and/or saline infusion sonohysterography help exclude alternative etiologies and specify whether fibroids are cavity-distorting. With distorting, extensive, or large fibroids, and/or concern for leiomyosarcoma, pelvic MRI with and without contrast is useful but not perfectly sensitive/specific.

Treatment

Choosing the optimal treatment includes shared decision-making that should balance goals of (1) diagnostic certainty, (2) treating

TABLE 1 Medical Treatment of Uterine Leiomyoma

METHOD	TREATS BLEEDING	TREAT BULK SYMPTOMS
Expectant management	No	No
Nonsteroidal anti-inflammatory drugs (NSAIDs)	Modest: no specific AUB-L studies	May treat dysmenorrhea
Tranexamic acid (Lysteda)	Yes, more than NSAIDs	No
Progestin-only (pills like Slynd, Micronor, Aygestin; Depo-Provera; levonorgestrel containing IUDs)	Yes, especially LNG-IUD	May treat dysmenorrhea Depo-Provera temporarily reduces size
Combined hormonal contraceptives (pills, patch, ring)	Yes, more than NSAIDs, less than LNG-IUD	May treat dysmenorrhea
GnRH agonist (IM:Lupron)	Yes, consistent reduction in bleeding and anemia	Yes, consistently but temporarily reduces size
GnRH antagonist without addback (pills: Orlissa)	Yes	Yes, more than with add-back
GnRH antagonist with addback (pills: Oriahnn, Myfembree)	Yes	Yes, temporarily reduces size

AUB-L, Abnormal uterine bleeding (AUB) associated with leiomyomata; *GnRH,* gonadotropin-releasing hormone; *LNG-IUD,* levonorgestrel intrauterine device.

symptoms and quality of life in a method the patient finds acceptable, (3) minimizing complications of the therapeutic approach, and (4) optimizing future fertility/obstetric outcomes, when applicable. With the potential for symptomatic improvement following menopause, anticipated time to menopause may also influence treatment choice.

The following are resources that are useful for shared decision-making and patient education.
- https://familydoctor.org/condition/uterine-fibroids/
- https://www.acog.org/womens-health/faqs/uterine-fibroids
- https://www.highriskpregnancyinfo.org/fibroids-in-pregnancy
- https://www.reproductivefacts.org/browse-all-topics/fibroids-topic/

Medical Treatment

Medical treatments (Table 1) are primarily chosen for symptoms associated with heavy bleeding including dysmenorrhea and anemia with some having potential for improvement in bulk symptoms as well. Options for heavy menses with or without anemia include tranexamic acid (Lysteda) and hormonal suppression medications including progestin only (pill, depot medroxyprogesterone acetate [Depo-Provera][1], levonorgestrel IUD [Mirena, Liletta]), combined estrogen/progestational agents, GnRH agonists with or without the addition (add-back) of estrogen and/or progestin therapy, and most recently GnRH antagonists with add-back of estrogen and/or progestin. If iron deficiency anemia is present, traditional therapy with oral or IV iron should be utilized, and in life-threatening circumstances, appropriate resuscitation including red blood cell transfusion may be indicated.

The oral gonadotropin antagonists with add-back of estrogen and progestin mark a significant development in medical treatment of symptomatic fibroids. Elagolix (300 mg twice daily) has been combined with estradiol (1 mg) and norethindrone acetate (NETA) (0.5 mg) in a formulation known as Oriahnn, as the first in its class to be approved by the U.S. Food & Drug Administration (FDA) for fibroid indications. Relugolix (40 mg daily) combined with add-back estradiol (1 mg) and NETA (0.5 mg) is a once daily tablet (Myfembree) and is also FDA-approved for fibroid related bleeding. For both agents: improvement in pain symptoms (including pressure/bulk symptoms), objective decrease in bleeding, and improvement in clinically significant anemia are demonstrated by multiple clinical trials with highly generalizable populations. The add-back of estrogen and progestin results in

vasomotor side effects near placebo levels and preservation of bone density with an FDA advisory for up to 24 months of treatment. There is not a similar advisory limit on therapy in European countries. When add-back of estrogen and progestin is included, decrease in fibroid volume/size is modest to none, but again, pain/pressure symptoms are significantly decreased, and quality of life scores increased. These medications do come with an FDA warning regarding thrombosis; however, this complication was not seen in clinical trials. Unplanned pregnancies were seen in clinical trials; thus, non-hormonal contraception is indicated. Starting these medications with a period can help to avoid exposure to unrecognized pregnancy and improve time to treatment effect.

Procedural Treatment

Procedural treatment options (Table 2) are commonly categorized as surgical versus interventional radiographic procedures, although newer minimally invasive approaches include a combination of the two. As anemia and size of the fibroids can affect modality choice and risk for transfusion, pretreatment intervention with GnRH agonists or antagonists may improve surgical outcomes, with improved preoperative hemoglobin and reduced intraoperative blood loss and fibroid volume. For hysterectomy, reduced operative time was also demonstrated in GnRH agonist pretreatment groups.

Myomectomy may be performed in a variety of surgical approaches. Hysteroscopic myomectomy is considered the optimal treatment option for Types 0 and 1 submucosal myomas as it is minimally invasive, safe and highly effective. For Types 2 to 8 myomas: laparoscopic, robotic-assisted, or open laparotomy myomectomy are options for patients who have not completed childbearing and/or desire to retain their uterus. The approach is chosen taking into account fibroid size, location, number and surgeon experience. Although typically quite effective, this therapy is associated with risk of intraoperative hemorrhage with large or abundant myomas, risk for incomplete resolution of symptoms, and risk of recurrence.

Hysterectomy is considered a suitable surgical option for properly consented patients who (1) desire definitive therapy, (2) have completed childbearing (if desired), and (3) are candidates for major surgical intervention and accept the surgical risks and potential sequelae of the procedure. Oophorectomy is not required for the management of fibroids.

Various radiologic-assisted interventions are available for additional minimally invasive treatment options for myomas. Pregnancy outcome data remain somewhat limited for each of

[1] Not FDA approved for this indication.

TABLE 2 Interventional and Surgical Treatment of Uterine Leiomyoma

METHOD	TREATS BLEEDING	TREATS BULK SYMPTOMS	FERTILITY PRESERVED	TYPE
Uterine artery embolization	Yes	Yes	Yes	
High-intensity focused ultrasound ablation	Yes	Yes	Yes	
Radiofrequency ablation	Yes	Yes	Yes	
Myomectomy	Yes	Yes	Yes, first line for future intended pregnancy	Hysteroscopic: 0, 1 Laparoscopic with or without robotic: 2–7 Open/abdominal: 2–8
Hysterectomy	Yes (100%)	Yes	No	0–8

these options. Uterine artery embolization (UAE) and magnetic resonance-guided focused ultrasound (MR-FUS) are both incisionless approaches that are generally well tolerated. With UAE, there is a small risk of reintervention for post-procedural pain related to fibroid necrosis. Both have a higher risk of reintervention than traditional surgical approaches but offer a reasonable alternative in the carefully selected patient. Pregnancy data with UAE suggest subsequent pregnancies have increased risk of pregnancy loss and postpartum hemorrhage. Radiofrequency ablation (laparoscopic, transvaginal, or transcervical) is another minimally invasive approach. UAE may also be considered as an emergency therapeutic option in the event of severe acute hemorrhage due to fibroids. Availability of these radiologic options may be more geographically limited than the more traditional surgical options.

Monitoring

As these are typically benign tumors, asymptomatic or mildly symptomatic patients can be managed expectantly. That said, it is important for patients to know that current fibroid treatments have been shown to improve symptom severity, mental health metrics, and quality of life, and they should seek care to consider treatment if symptoms arise. Potential impact on fertility or pregnancy should be assessed and counseled upon for these patients due to the high rates of unplanned pregnancy. Surveillance guidelines have not been established; however, patients should be counseled to return for concerning symptoms or if pregnancy is being contemplated.

Complications

One remaining consideration is the risk of misdiagnosis, both benign and malignant. Adenomyomas, a confluent mixture of endometrial glands, stroma, and myometrium, can be mistaken for leiomyoma particularly on ultrasound imaging. These masses can be more difficult to treat medically and surgically.

The two major concerns for malignancy include endometrial cancer and leiomyosarcoma. Endometrial malignancy is the most prevalent gynecologic cancer with 3.1% of women estimated to be diagnosed with uterine cancer in their lifetime. As such, women with fibroids should undergo appropriate diagnostic testing for this condition if signs and symptoms and clinical risk factors for endometrial cancer are present to avoid missing a life-threatening but highly treatable diagnosis when identified early. Comparatively, leiomyosarcomas occur much less frequently. The underlying risk of identifying a leiomyosarcoma at surgery in symptomatic uterine masses presumed to be leiomyoma is estimated to occur in 1 in 770 to 1 in 10,000 surgeries. MRI shows some promise in identifying leiomyosarcoma prior to surgery and may be helpful for surgical planning.

References

American College of Obstetrics and Gynecology: Management of symptomatic uterine leiomyomas: ACOG Practice Bulletin No. 228, *Obstet Gynecol* 137(6):e100–e115, 2021.

American College of Obstetrics and Gynecology: Uterine morcellation for presumed leiomyomas: ACOG Committee Opinion No. 822: *Obstet Gynecol* 137(3):e64–e74, 2021.

Ascher S, Wasnik A, Robbins J, et al: ACR appropriateness criteria fibroids, *J Am Coll Radiol* 19(11s):s319–s328, 2022.

Lee SJ, Ko HS, Na S, et al: Nationwide population-based cohort study of adverse obstetric outcomes in pregnancies with myoma or following myomectomy: retrospective cohort study, *BMC Pregnancy Childbirth* 20(1):716, 2020.

Makary M, Zane K, Hwang G, et al: ACR appropriateness criteria management of uterine fibroids: 2023 update, *J Am Coll Radiol* 21(6s):s203–s218, 2024.

Munro M, Critchley H, Fraser I: The two FIGO systems for normal and abnormal uterine bleeding symptoms and classification of causes of abnormal uterine bleeding in the reproductive years: 2018 revisions, *Int J Gynaecol Obstet* 143(3):393–408, 2018.

National Cancer Institute. Cancer Stat Facts: Uterine Cancer. Available at https://seer.cancer.gov/statfacts/html/corp.html. [Accessed 19/03/25].

Neblett 2nd M, Stewart E: Oral gonadotropin-releasing hormone antagonists for the treatment of uterine leiomyomas, *Obstet Gynecol* 141(5):901–910, 2023.

Neumann B, Singh B, Brennan J, et al: The impact of fibroid treatments on quality of life and mental health: a systematic review, *Fertil Steril* 121(3):400–425, 2024.

Practice Committee of the American Society for Reproductive Medicine: Removal of myomas in asymptomatic patients to improve fertility and/or reduce miscarriage rate: a guideline, *Fertil Steril* 108(3):416–425, 2017.

Yang Q, Ciebiera M, Bariani M, et al: Comprehensive review of uterine fibroids: developmental origin, pathogenesis, and treatment, *Endocr Rev* 43(4):678–719, 2022.

VULVAR NEOPLASIA

Method of
Christine Conageski, MD

CURRENT DIAGNOSIS

- Most cystic lesions are benign. Excision is reserved for symptomatic cysts and suspicious Bartholin's gland cysts, especially in women older than 40 years of age.
- All solid lesions should be biopsied for diagnostic purposes.
- Multifocal disease requires multiple biopsies to rule out invasive disease.
- Most premalignant and malignant lesions cause pruritus, discomfort, or a noticeable lesion.
- The vagina and cervix in women with dysplastic or malignant vulvar lesions should be evaluated.

CURRENT THERAPY

- Benign solid lesions should be excised.
- After ablative treatment of vulvar intraepithelial neoplasia (VIN), excise any residual lesions to rule out occult invasive disease.
- Avoid podophyllin and 5-fluorouracil in women of reproductive potential.
- Rule out synchronous neoplasms in women with Paget's disease.
- Invasion more than 1 mm requires radical excision and lymph node evaluation.

The female external genitalia includes the mons pubis, labia majora, labia minora, clitoris, perineal body, and the structures of the vaginal introitus or vestibule. Whether benign or malignant, vulvar neoplasms are uncommon, occur at all ages, and have varying characteristics. Therefore liberal use of biopsies is usually required for diagnosis and treatment decisions.

Benign Cystic Neoplasms

Benign cystic lesions of the vulva include Bartholin's duct cyst, sebaceous and epidermal inclusion cysts, mucinous cysts, Skene duct cysts, and cysts of the canal of Nuck. Bartholin's duct cyst, located in the posterior labia near the vaginal introitus, is most common. Treatment is usually not required in asymptomatic young women (<40 years). If the cyst is symptomatic or infected, however, drainage, marsupialization or use of a Word catheter, is indicated. Bartholin's gland carcinomas are rare, especially in women younger than 40 years of age. But if the mass feels firm or nodular, it should be biopsied.

Sebaceous and epidermal inclusion cysts are also common. They are prone to infection but rarely malignant. If an infection develops, they should be incised and drained. Mucinous cysts are rare and possibly arise from the minor vestibular glands. They are located anteriorly on the vulva, typically on the inner labia minora. Skene duct cysts are located next to the urethra. Excision of these cysts is necessary only if symptomatic.

Cysts of the canal of Nuck are located in the anterior portion of the labia majora at the termination of the insertion of the round ligament. These cysts represent herniation of the peritoneum through the inguinal canal and contain peritoneal fluid. If symptomatic, excision must be accompanied by closure of the fascial defect to prevent recurrence.

Benign Solid Neoplasms

The benign solid tumors of the vulva include fibromas, myomas, lipomas, hidradenomas, syringomas, myoblastomas, vestibular adenomas, and angiomas, among others. Benign pigmented lesions, such as nevi and seborrheic keratoses, may occasionally be found. Malignancy is rare, but most should be excised for diagnostic and therapeutic purposes.

Condyloma Acuminatum

Vulvar condyloma acuminatum is a sexually transmitted verrucous lesion of the vulva caused by human papilloma virus (HPV), most frequently types 6 and 11. These lesions are warty growths that frequently cover large areas of the vulva. Smoking and immunosuppression are risk factors. Representative biopsies should be obtained to document disease and rule out malignancy. Wide local excision can be used for small lesions, although these growths are usually best treated by ablation to avoid morbdity associated with excision.

Chemical ablative techniques include self or provider-administered medications. Self-administered medications include topical podofilox (0.5%, Condylox) or imiquimod (5%, Aldara). Podofilox is applied twice daily for 3 days, repeated weekly for 4 weeks and imiquimod is applied three times per week for up to 16 weeks. It is primarily an immune modulator. Providers may instead choose in-office application of trichloroacetic acid (Tri-Chlor), 5-fluorouracil[1] (1%, Fluoroplex or 5%, Efudex),[1] or podophyllin. Podophyllin and 5-fluorouracil should not be used in women who could become pregnant. Surgical ablative therapies include CO_2 laser vaporization and use of the Cavitron ultrasonic aspirator (CUSA), especially for extensive disease.

Intraepithelial Neoplasms of the Vulva

Vulvar Intraepithelial Neoplasia

Vulvar intraepithelial neoplasia (VIN) is a dysplastic condition of the squamous epithelium whose incidence is increasing, especially in younger women. There are two pathologically distinct types of VIN, usual and differentiated types.

The usual type has a strong association with HPV infections and thus shares similar risk factors with cervical intraepithelial neoplasias (CIN). These risk factors include early first intercourse, multiple sexual partners, smoking, and immunosuppression. Up to 22% of women have concurrent CIN lesions and up to 71% have had a previous, concominant or subsequent history of vaginal intraepithelial neoplasia. Differentiated VIN is not associated with HPV and is found in relation to vulvar dermatoses such as lichen sclerosus. Differentiated VIN typically occurs in older women with a mean age of 67 years compared to 47.8 years in usual type VIN. Symptoms of both types include pruritus (most common), pain, a noticeable lesion, and discoloration. Most patients with HPV-related disease have multifocal lesions. Typical findings are raised white, gray, red, or mottled lesions; application of 4% acetic acid for several minutes can help identify faint lesions and outline abnormal vascular patterns. Diagnosis of VIN is made by punch biopsies through full thickness of the epithelium to rule out invasion. Usual and differentiated VIN have very different cancer progression risks, 5.7% for HPV-mediated VIN and 32.8% for differentiated VIN. Differentiated VIN, also, has a shorter time to progression, 22.8 months compared to 41.4 months.

Treatment of VIN can be categorized into excisional and ablative therapies. Management should be individualized to each patient taking into account risk of progression, distribution of disease and histologic features on biopsy. Often a combination of medical and surgical management is appropriate. Patients at risk for microinvasion (unifocal disease, raised lesions, older age, and prior radiation) should have the lesion excised completely if possible. Skinning vulvectomy is rarely used because of psychological and sexual consequences related to scarring and disfigurement.

The ablative therapies can be divided into mechanical and chemical. The mechanical method most commonly used is the CO_2 laser, although use of the CUSA is also described. Both can ablate large or multifocal lesions successfully with an excellent cosmetic and functional outcome. The chemical method most commonly used is topical 5-fluorouracil (5%, Efudex).[1] Because of its teratogenic potential, it should not be used in women who could become pregnant. It canbe applied on two consecutive nights weekly for 10 weeks. An alternative ablative therapy is use of imiquimod[1] (Aldara), as described earlier. Because of the irritation caused by these topical therapies, many patients have problems with treatment compliance. Residual disease should be excised to rule out invasion.

Patients with VIN frequently have recurrent disease, regardless of the treatment method used (Table 1). Continued smoking increases this risk, so patients should be counseled in smoking cessation. In those patients whose cancers recur and are retreated, subsequent 5-fluorouracil prophylaxis, with a single application biweekly, is used successfully to minimize further recurrences.

Paget's Disease

Paget's disease of the vulva is an uncommon condition characterized by a patchy, eczematoid lesion that frequently covers much of the vulva. Most patients are postmenopausal and present with complaints of pruritus. Although Paget's disease is an in situ disease process, 15% to 25% of patients have an underlying malignancy, usually an adenocarcinoma of the apocrine glands but occasionally an invasive Paget's. In addition, up to 30% of patients have a synchronous adenocarcinoma of the breast,

---

[1]Not FDA approved for this indication.

TABLE 1	Recurrence of Vulvar Intraepithelial Neoplasia III
TREATMENT METHOD	**% RECURRENCE**
Chemical ablation	20–40
Mechanical ablation	20–40
Wide local excision	
Negative margin	15–25
Positive margin	30–45

TABLE 2	Incidence of Regional Node Metastases by Tumor Diameter
TUMOR DIAMETER (CM)	**% POSITIVE INGUINAL NODES**
<1	1–15
5–20	
25–35	
35–50	
≥50	≥50

TABLE 3	Incidence of Regional Node Metastases by Depth of Tumor Invasion
DEPTH OF INVASION (MM)	**% POSITIVE INGUINAL NODES**
<1	1–5
1–3	10–15
3–5	15–30
5–10	30–45

colon, rectum, or upper genital tract. Screening for these cancers is therefore recommended. To assess for invasion, the lesion should be excised via wide local excision or simple vulvectomy with at least 5 mm of the adjacent subcutaneous tissue. Achieving negative margin status is frequently difficult. However, the risk of recurrence is approximately 30% whether margins are negative or positive. Thus expectant management, reserving treatment for symptomatic recurrences, is usually recommended.

Invasive Vulvar Lesions

Less than 5% of gynecologic cancers arise on the vulva. Over 90% are squamous cell carcinomas. The etiology of this type appears mixed. The differentiated type is more common, occurs in older women (age 60–69, mean age 65) and is associated with vulvar dystrophies. The classic or usual type is predominantly associated with HPV-16. These women are slightly younger (age 45–52 years) and present with earlier stage disease. Other histologic types are melanomas (5%–10%), basal cell carcinomas (2%–3%), adenocarcinomas (1%), and sarcomas (1%–2%). Most patients present with a combination of symptoms, including pruritus, discomfort, and complaints of a mass. Examination frequently reveals a suspicious lesion, which should be biopsied for diagnosis. Vulvar cancers typically spread by local extension and lymphatic dissemination. Factors that influence dissemination include tumor size (Table 2), depth of invasion (Table 3), lymphovascular space invasion, and tumor grade. Staging is surgical and classified using the tumor, nodes, and metastasis (TNM) system as well as the International Federation of Gynecology and Obstetrics (FIGO) system (Table 4).

Squamous Cell Carcinomas and Adenocarcinomas

Surgical management of squamous cell carcinomas and adenocarcinomas depends on the size, depth of invasion, and location of the lesion. The vulvar lesion is managed with a radical excision. Management of the groins is based on depth of invasion. Lesions with invasion of less than 1 mm (Stage IA) have minimal risk of lymphatic spread (<1%) and do not require lymphadenectomy. All others require surgical assessment of the lymph nodes. Lesions less than 2 cm in size of the primary tumor, greater than 2 cm from the vulvar midline and are of squamous histology require only unilateral lymphadenectomy. Those without these characteristics or have palpable lymph nodes of the contralateral side require bilateral assessment. This surgical approach is associated with significant morbidity including disfigurement, wound breakdown, and problems with lymphocysts and chronic lymphedema. For patients with very large lesions or lesions in sensitive areas such as the clitoris, preoperative radiation, followed by less radical excision of residual disease, may minimize problems with the vulvar wound. Current investigations are ongoing in the use of sentinel lymph node dissections as a method of minimizing the groin morbidity without sacrificing survival. Positive vulvar margins or metastases to lymph nodes are managed with postoperative radiation. Survival depends on stage at diagnosis (Table 5).

Verrucous Carcinoma

Verrucous carcinoma is a large exophytic tumor that resembles giant condyloma acuminatum. It is a variant of squamous carcinomas but has an excellent prognosis because of the lack

TABLE 4	Staging Vulvar Carcinoma
STAGE	**DESCRIPTION**
I	Tumor confined to the vulva
IA	Tumor size ≤2 cm and stromal invasion ≤1 mm
IB	Tumor size >2 cm or stromal invasion >1 mm
II	Tumor of any size with extension to lower one-third of the urethra, lower one-third of the vagina, lower one-third of the anus with negative nodes
III	Tumor of any size with extension to upper part of adjacent perineal structures or with any number of nonfixed nonulcerated lymph nodes
IIIA	Tumor of any size with disease extension to upper two-thirds of the urethra, upper two-thirds of the vagina, bladder mucosa, rectal mucosa, or regional lymph node metastases ≤5 mm
IIIB	Regional lymph node metastases >5 mm
IIIC	Regional¶ lymph node metastases with extracapsular spread
IV	Tumor of any size fixed to bone, or fixed, ulcerated lymph node metastases, or distant metstases
IVA	Disease fixed to pelvic bone, or fixed or ulcerated regional¶ lymph node metastes
IVB	Distant metastases

FIGO Staging 2021.

of metastases. Verrucous carcinomas have a high tendency to recur and should be managed with radical local excision.

Malignant Melanoma

Malignant melanoma is the second most common vulvar malignancy. Most patients have disease on the mucosal surfaces of the vulvar introitus, clitoris, and labia minora. The vulvar lesion is treated by radical excision, but management of the groins is controversial. The risk of spread is significant with a tumor thickness greater than 0.75 mm, but survival at 5 years is only approximately 10% with groin node metastases. Some argue against node dissection for this reason. However, given some long-term survivors with modern melanoma therapy,

TABLE 5	Survival Rate by FIGO Stage for Patients With Invasive Squamous Cell Vulvar Cancer		
FIGO STAGE	**OVERALL SURVIVAL (PERCENT)**		
	One year	Two years	Five years
I	96.4	90.4	78.5
II	87.6	73.2	58.8
III	74.7	53.8	43.2
IV	35.3	16.9	13.0

Abbreviation: FIGO = International Federation of Gynecology and Obstetrics.

either lymphadenectomy or sentinel lymph node dissection, as is done for other cutaneous melanomas, appears indicated.

Basal Cell Carcinoma

Basal cell carcinomas typically occur in elderly white women, are commonly located on the labia majora, and have characteristics similar to basal cell carcinomas at other sites. Treatment is wide local excision only because metastases are rare. Basal cell carcinomas are prone to local recurrence, however. A malignant squamous component must be ruled out because it should be managed as a squamous cell carcinoma.

Sarcomas

Leiomyosarcoma is the most common vulvar sarcoma and usually arises in the labia majora. Malignant fibrous histiocytoma is the second most common. Management of these lesions is radical vulvar excision.

References

Beller U, Quinn MA, Benedet JL, et al: Carcinoma of the vulva, *Int J Gynaecol Obstet* 95:S7, 2006.

Garland SM: Imiquimod, *Curr Opin Infect Dis* 16:85–89, 2003.

Homesley HD, Bundy BN, Sedlis A, et al: Prognostic factors for groin node metastasis in squamous cell carcinoma of the vulva (a Gynecologic Oncology Group study), *Gynecol Oncol* 49:279–283, 1993.

Hording U, Junge J, Lundvall F: Vulvar intraepithelial neoplasia III: a viral disease of undetermined progressive potential, *Gynecol Oncol* 56(2):276, 1995.

Krebs HB: The use of topical 5-fluorouracil in the treatment of genital condylomas, *Obstet Gynecol Clin North Am* 14(2):559–568, 1987.

Modesitt SC, Waters AB, Walton L, et al: Vulvar intraepithelial neoplasia III: Occult cancer and the impact of margin status on recurrence, *Obstet Gynecol* 92(6):962–966, 1998.

Phillips GL, Bundy BN, Okagaki T, et al: Malignant melanoma of the vulva treated by radical hemivulvectomy, a prospective study of the Gynecologic Oncology Group, *Cancer* 73:2626–2632, 1994.

Tebes S, Cardosi R, Hoffman M: Paget's disease of the vulva, *Am J Obstet Gynecol* 187:281–284, 2002.

Trimble CL, Trimble EL, Woodruff JD: Diseases of the vulva. In Hernandez E, Atkinson BE, editors: *Clinical Gynecologic Pathology*, Philadelphia, 1995, WB Saunders, pp 1–90.

Van de Nieuwehnof, et al. Vulvar squamous cell carcinoma development after diagnosis of VIN increases with age. *Eur J Canc* 45:851, 2009.

Wright VC, Chapman WB: Colposcopy of intraepithelial neoplasia of the vulva and adjacent sites, *Obstet Gynecol Clin North Am* 20(1):231–255, 1993.

VULVOVAGINITIS

Method of
Heather L. Paladine, MD, MEd; and Joanne Dempster, MD, MHA

CURRENT DIAGNOSIS

- The most common causes of vulvovaginitis are bacterial vaginosis (BV), candidal vulvovaginitis, and *Trichomonas* infection.
- Vulvovaginitis should be diagnosed by a combination of patient history, physical examination findings, and office-based or laboratory testing. Patients should not be treated presumptively based on history and physical examination.

- BV is diagnosed based on at least three of four of the Amsel criteria: fishy vaginal odor spontaneously or with potassium hydroxide (KOH) testing; vaginal pH above 4.5; thin, homogeneous vaginal discharge; and clue cells on saline microscopy.
- Vulvovaginal candidiasis is diagnosed based on symptoms of a thick whitish discharge, itching, and/or discomfort together with budding or pseudohyphae on KOH microscopy or positive fungal culture.
- The gold standard for *Trichomonas* diagnosis is nucleic acid amplification testing.

CURRENT TREATMENT

- Treatment of bacterial vaginosis (BV) is recommended for patients who are symptomatic, and both oral and topical metronidazole (Flagyl tablet 500 mg[1] as well as MetroGel [0.75%]) or topical clindamycin (Cleocin 2%) are first-line treatments for both pregnant and nonpregnant people.
- First-line treatment for symptomatic people with vulvovaginal candidiasis includes either oral fluconazole (Diflucan) or topical azole therapy for nonpregnant individuals; for pregnant people, topical azole therapy is preferred.
- First-line therapy for *Trichomonas* vaginal infection includes a 1-week course of metronidazole.
- Patients should be adequately counseled about treatment regimens for vaginitis, including potential weakening of condoms by oil-based topical therapies and the importance of avoidance of sexual intercourse until treatment of BV or *Trichomonas* is complete. The Centers for Disease Control and Prevention no longer recommends that patients abstain from drinking alcohol while taking oral metronidazole.

[1]Not FDA approved for this indication.

Epidemiology

The term *vulvovaginitis* includes conditions that result in irritation of the vagina or vulva, causing symptoms of itching, burning, pain, odor, or discharge. Vulvovaginitis is a common condition in primary care, accounting for about 10% of office visits each year and affecting almost every person with a vagina at some point in their life. The three most common causes of vulvovaginitis are bacterial vaginosis (BV, accounting for up to 50% of cases in which a diagnosis is made), vulvovaginal candidiasis (VVC, accounting for 30% of cases), and *Trichomonas* (accounting for 15% to 20% of cases). The remaining diagnoses include genitourinary syndrome of menopause (GSM, formerly called *atrophic vaginitis*), inflammatory vaginitis, and allergic/irritant vaginitis. A specific cause is not found in up to 30% of patients.

Risk Factors

Risk factors for vulvovaginitis vary by condition. Although BV is not a sexually transmitted infection, it occurs almost exclusively in people of reproductive age with vaginas who are sexually active and more commonly in individuals with new or multiple sexual partners. BV is found more often in people with vaginas who smoke cigarettes or douche.

VVC is more common in patients who are immunosuppressed, such as those who have HIV or diabetes or are pregnant. Recent antibiotic use is also a risk factor.

Trichomonas is a sexually transmitted infection and is more likely to occur in people who have other sexually transmitted infections, who have multiple sexual partners, or who have had unprotected intercourse. As with many sexually transmitted infections, disparities exist in the prevalence of *Trichomonas*, with infections more commonly occurring in non-White, low-income, and formerly incarcerated people.

Pathophysiology
Prevention
Although previous studies have defined risk factors for BV, it is not known whether avoiding these risk factors (e.g., douching, unprotected intercourse) will reduce the risk. Studies that have looked at the prevention of recurrent BV through treatment with probiotics such as lactobacilli or other methods to maintain an acidic vaginal pH have not been conclusive.

Routine testing for conditions such as HIV or diabetes is not recommended in people with VVC unless they have other risk factors. Patients who are prone to develop VVC after taking antibiotics can use topical or oral antifungal medications during their treatment with antibiotics. Although probiotics are commonly used for the prevention and treatment of VVC, they have not been well studied.

Trichomonas is a sexually transmitted infection; therefore, prevention includes condom use or being in a monogamous relationship.

Clinical Manifestations
Table 1 includes symptoms and physical examination findings for the common causes of vulvovaginitis. These symptoms can cause significant feelings of shame, distress, and decreased quality of life, especially in people with recurrent infections.

Diagnosis
The diagnosis of vulvovaginitis is unreliable based on history and physical examination findings alone and should include office-based or laboratory testing to confirm. There is a risk of misdiagnosis or delay in diagnosis with presumptive treatment, as patients may get temporary relief of vulvovaginal symptoms with topical antifungals even if they do not have a fungal infection. Although newer laboratory tests have become available for the diagnosis of BV and VVC, the American College of Obstetricians and Gynecologists continues to recommend testing with history, examination, microscopy, and pH testing unless microscopy is not available. The newer tests include DNA testing for *Gardnerella vaginalis* or for the presence of vaginal sialidase activity for the diagnosis of BV, as well as DNA testing for *Candida* species. The newer tests are also less cost effective. Table 1 also includes pH and microscopy findings for causes of vulvovaginitis.

BV is traditionally diagnosed via the Amsel criteria (Table 2), although Gram stain is considered the gold standard. A positive diagnosis requires three out of four criteria: fishy vaginal odor or positive odor on testing of vaginal discharge with 10% potassium hydroxide (KOH); vaginal pH above 4.5; a thin, homogeneous vaginal discharge; and clue cells (epithelial cells with adherent bacteria (Figure 1) on microscopic examination of vaginal discharge with normal saline (wet mount).

VVC is diagnosed based on the combination of clinical signs and symptoms and either microscopy or fungal culture of vaginal discharge. Microscopy has a sensitivity of 50% to 70% for candidal vulvovaginitis; therefore, fungal culture is recommended when microscopy is negative in a patient with typical symptoms. Figure 2 demonstrates microscopy results with KOH that are positive for yeast. Fungal culture can also identify non-*albicans* species of *Candida*, which may be more difficult to treat.

Nucleic acid amplification testing is recommended for the diagnosis of *Trichomonas* as microscopy is only 50% to 60% sensitive. Commercial DNA probe tests and a point-of-care antigen detection test are also available. Sensitivities may be lower with the newer tests, although this varies by test. Figure 3 shows positive saline microscopy for *Trichomonas*.

Differential Diagnosis
In addition to BV, VVC, and *Trichomonas*, other less common conditions can result in vulvovaginal symptoms. GSM was formerly known as *atrophic vaginitis* and results from a decrease in estrogen levels after menopause. People who are breastfeeding or using progestin-only contraception also have a relative estrogen deficiency and may experience similar symptoms. GSM is characterized by vaginal dryness and discomfort and may also include urinary tract symptoms and clear vaginal discharge. GSM is a presumptive diagnosis made on characteristic examination

TABLE 1	Diagnosis of Vulvovaginitis			
CONDITION	**SYMPTOMS**	**EXAMINATION FINDINGS**	**PH**	**MICROSCOPY FINDINGS**
Normal	Discharge changes with menstrual cycle	Thin, clear or whitish discharge	Normal (4–4.5)	Epithelial cells, lactobacilli
Bacterial vaginosis	Fishy odor, vaginal discharge, vaginal discomfort/dyspareunia	Homogenous gray/white discharge	Elevated (≥4.6)	Clue cells on wet mount
Vulvovaginal candidiasis	Vulvar irritation or itching, vaginal discharge	Vulvar excoriations or erythema Thick, clumpy white discharge	Normal (4–4.5)	Pseudohyphae or budding yeast on potassium hydroxide examination
Trichomonas	Foul-smelling discharge, vaginal pain or discomfort	Cervical inflammation with "strawberry cervix," yellow-green frothy vaginal discharge	Elevated (≥4.6)	Mobile trichomonads on wet mount, white blood cells
Genitourinary syndrome of menopause (formerly *atrophic vaginitis*)	Vulvar itching, vaginal pain or discomfort, dyspareunia, vaginal dryness	Vulvar excoriations, clear vaginal discharge, thin friable mucosa with loss of vaginal rugae	Elevated (≥4.6)	May have white blood cells, parabasal cells, decreased lactobacilli
Irritant/allergic vaginitis	Vulvar or vaginal discomfort or pain	Vulvar or vaginal erythema, fissures, lichenification	Elevated (≥4.6)	May have white blood cells, parabasal cells, decreased lactobacilli
Inflammatory vaginitis	Vulvar or vaginal discomfort, pain, or burning Vaginal discharge	Purulent vaginal discharge Vaginal erythema or rash	Elevated (≥4.6)	Many white blood cells, parabasal cells, decreased lactobacilli

TABLE 2	Amsel Criteria	
CRITERION	**POSITIVE RESULT**
Vaginal discharge	Thin homogeneous discharge
Odor of discharge	Fishy odor on testing with potassium hydroxide
Vaginal pH	pH ≥4.6
Microscopy	Clue cells on saline microscopy

Three positive criteria are needed for a diagnosis of bacterial vaginosis.

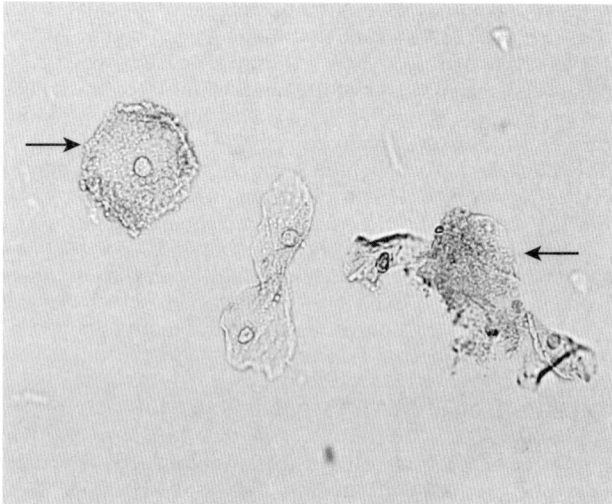

Figure 1 Clue cells on saline microscopy. (From Brunzel NA. *Fundamentals of Urine & Body Fluid Analysis.* 4th ed. Elsevier; 2018.)

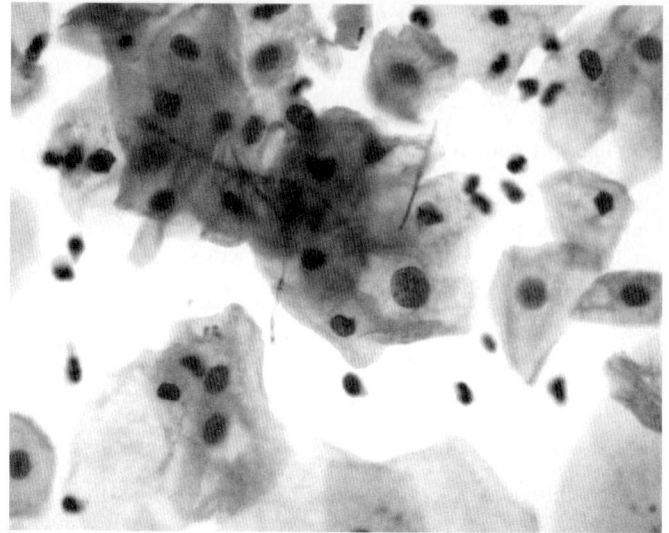

Figure 2 Candidal pseudohyphae on potassium hydroxide microscopy. (From Herran CP, Nucci MR: *Gynecologic Pathology: A Volume in the Series Foundations in Diagnostic Pathology.* 2nd ed. Elsevier; 2021.)

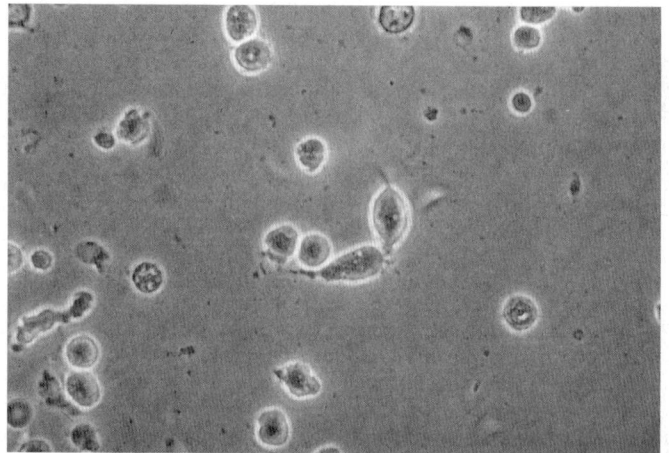

Figure 3 *Trichomonas* on saline microscopy. (From Mandell GL, Bennett JE, Dolin R: *Principles and Practice of Infectious Diseases.* 7th ed. Churchill Livingstone Elsevier; 2010.)

findings in a postmenopausal woman once other causes of vaginitis have been excluded.

Vulvovaginitis may be caused by a reaction to irritant or allergen exposure. Triggers can include latex (used in condoms), spermicides, and chemicals in sanitary pads or toilet paper. This is also a diagnosis of exclusion. In unclear cases, referral to an allergist for patch testing may be helpful.

Inflammatory conditions are thought to be underdiagnosed and may be responsible for many of the cases of vulvovaginitis that were not previously given a diagnosis. They occur more commonly in individuals who are perimenopausal. The patient has a purulent vaginal discharge with vulvovaginal erythema or rash, and microscopy characteristically demonstrates many white blood cells. The etiology is thought to be autoimmune.

Treatment
Bacterial Vaginosis
Treatment of BV is recommended to alleviate symptoms but may also be helpful in reducing susceptibility to other sexually transmitted diseases including HIV and those caused by *Chlamydia trachomatis, Neisseria gonorrhoeae,* and *Trichomonas vaginalis.* Treatment also reduces the risk of recurrence. Additionally, in pregnant people, treatment has been associated with potential decreases in adverse outcomes including late miscarriages and poor neonatal outcomes, although it may not have a significant effect on the prevention of preterm labor, as may have been thought in the past. Treatment is recommended for all people who are symptomatic. Both initial oral and topical therapies are acceptable treatments in pregnancy.

Initial and alternative treatment regimens are presented in Table 3; considerations in choosing regimens include patient preference and cost. Of note, secnidazole (Solosec) is a newer oral agent that provides for one-time dosing; however, it may be cost-prohibitive for patients. The Centers for Disease Control and Prevention (CDC) no longer recommends avoidance of alcohol while patients are taking oral metronidazole. The previous warning was based on laboratory experiments and not on clinical data. Patients should also be counseled that oil-based topical therapies including clindamycin may weaken latex condoms or diaphragms for 5 days after use. Additionally, to prevent recurrent infection, patients should be counseled to avoid sexual intercourse until after completion of therapy and to avoid douching. The CDC does not recommend the use of probiotics[7] as an adjunctive or replacement therapy for women with BV. A systematic review and meta-analysis of probiotic use in non pregnant women by Huey-Sheng et al. showed an increase in normal vaginal flora after probiotic treatment for BV and a lower recurrence rate of vaginitis when probiotics combined with antibiotics was compared to antibiotics with placebo. For patients who are interested in probiotics as an adjunct there is promise for use with antibiotics for BV.

Vulvovaginal Candidiasis
The rationale for the treatment of VVC is relief of symptoms. Treatment regimens for VVC are listed in Table 4 for initial treatment and treatment of recurrence. In nonpregnant patients, the choice between oral and topical azoles can be based on patient preference. Those patients who are prescribed topical therapies

---

[7] Available as dietary supplement

TABLE 3 · Treatment of Bacterial Vaginosis

Initial regimens	Metronidazole (Flagyl)[1] 500 mg PO twice daily for 7 days OR metronidazole 0.75% gel (MetroGel), one full applicator (5 g) intravaginally daily for 5 days OR clindamycin 2% cream (Cleocin), one full applicator (5 g) intravaginally at bedtime for 7 days
Alternative regimens	Secnidazole (Solosec) 2 g PO once Tinidazole (Tindamax) 2 g PO daily for 2 days OR Tinidazole 1 g PO once daily for 5 days OR clindamycin[1] 300 mg PO bid for 7 days OR clindamycin ovules 100 mg intravaginally at bedtime for 3 days
Pregnancy	Either oral or vaginal regimens suggested in initial treatment section
Treatment of recurrence	First recurrence: retrial of same regimen or trial of alternative initial regimen Multiple recurrences: metronidazole 0.75% gel, intravaginally twice weekly for 4–6 months[3]

[1]Not FDA approved for this indication.
[3]Exceeds dosage recommended by the manufacturer.
PO, Orally.

TABLE 4 · Treatment of Vulvovaginal Candidiasis

Initial regimens	*Topical azole therapy:* clotrimazole (Gyne-Lotrimin) 1% cream 5 g intravaginally daily for 7–14 days OR clotrimazole 2% cream 5 g intravaginally daily for 3 days OR miconazole 2% cream 5 g intravaginally daily for 7 days OR miconazole 4% cream 5 g intravaginally daily for 3 days OR miconazole 100 mg vaginal suppository, one suppository daily for 7 days OR miconazole 200 mg vaginal suppository, one suppository for 3 days OR miconazole 1200 mg vaginal suppository, one suppository for 1 day OR tioconazole (Monistat 1-Day) 6.5% ointment 5 g intravaginally in a single application *Prescription intravaginal agents:* Butoconazole (Gynazole–1) 2% cream (single-dose bioadhesive product), 5 g intravaginally in a single application OR terconazole (Terazol 7) 0.4% cream 5 g intravaginally daily for 7 days OR terconazole (Terazol 3) 0.8% cream 5 g intravaginally daily for 3 days OR terconazole 80 mg vaginal suppository, one suppository daily for 3 days OR fluconazole (Diflucan) 150 mg PO once
Alternative regimens	N/A
Pregnancy	Topical azole therapy applied intravaginally for 7 days
Treatment of recurrence	Topical azole therapy for 7–14 days OR fluconazole 150 mg every 3 day for three doses[3] *For maintenance:* oral fluconazole (100, 150, or 200 mg) weekly for 6 months;[3] consider topical treatment if oral is not feasible

[3]Exceeds dosage recommended by the manufacturer.

TABLE 5 · Treatment of Trichomonas Infection

Initial regimens	For vaginitis: metronidazole (Flagyl) 500 mg PO twice daily for 7 days For urethritis: metronidazole 2 g PO in a single dose
Alternative regimens	Tinidazole 2 g PO in a single dose
Pregnancy	Metronidazole 500 mg PO twice daily for 7 days
Treatment of recurrence	Trial of metronidazole, 500 mg twice daily for 7 days *If metronidazole 500 mg twice daily for 7 days fails:* trial of metronidazole, 2 g daily for 7 days *If above regimens fail:* susceptibility testing considered (contact Centers for Disease Control and Prevention)

PO, Orally.

should be counseled that topical azole preparations may be oil based and can weaken latex condoms. Topical therapies may cause local irritation or hypersensitivity reactions, although systemic effects are not of concern. Oral azoles can cause nausea, abdominal pain, headache, and rarely elevations in liver function tests. For pregnant patients, only topical therapies should be prescribed.

For those with severe VVC or with immunocompromise, longer treatment may be necessary, such as a 7- to 14-day course.

For recurrent VVC (four or more episodes within a year), longer duration of initial therapy followed by maintenance therapy is recommended. Non-*albicans* VVC should also be considered and appropriate diagnostic testing performed to guide treatment, which may include a 7- to 14-day course of an azole topical or oral regimen (other than fluconazole [Diflucan]) and potentially a 2-week course of treatment with boric acid[1] if recurrent. The CDC does not recommend use of probiotics or homeopathic medications for treating VVC. Systematic reviews of probiotic use concurrently with antifungals show some promise with improving recurrence rates of vaginitis; however, there was no significant increase in normal vaginal flora when compared to antifungal/placebo.

Trichomonas

The rationale for the treatment of *Trichomonas* infection includes a decrease of symptoms and reduced transmission to sexual partners. *Trichomonas* infection in pregnant patients is associated with adverse outcomes including preterm birth and low-birth-weight infants; however, treatment has not shown a definite reduction in these outcomes. For patients with HIV, *Trichomonas* infection is associated with pelvic inflammatory disease; thus, screening and treatment can help prevent this complication. Regimens for initial therapy and treatment of recurrence are listed in Table 5. The CDC no longer recommends single-dose treatment for *Trichomonas* infection for vaginitis; a 7-day course has been shown to be more effective.

Persistent or recurrent *Trichomonas* infection is often caused by reinfection. When patients are being counseled about treatment, they should be advised to avoid intercourse until treatment is completed, symptoms have resolved, and partners have been treated. All patients diagnosed with *Trichomonas* should be asked to inform partners of the need for presumptive treatment. Additionally, patients should be retested within 3 months of diagnosis

to ensure adequate treatment and address potential reinfection. In cases in which treatment-resistant infection is suspected, a 1-week regimen should be attempted. If the infection persists, further testing should be implemented according to guidance from the CDC.

Noninfectious Vaginitis

Treatment of GSM includes low-dose vaginal estrogen therapy or topical lubricant therapy for less severe symptoms. Inflammatory vaginitis is still not well understood, although long-term maintenance therapy with topical clindamycin[1] or steroids may be helpful.

[1]Not FDA approved for this indication.

References

American College of Obstetricians and Gynecologists: Vaginitis in nonpregnant patients, ACOG practice bulletin no. 215, *Obstet Gynecol* 135:e1–e17, 2020.

Anderson MR, Klink K, Cohrssen A: Evaluation of vaginal complaints, *JAMA* 291(11):1368–1379, 2004.

Centers for Disease Control and Prevention: Sexually transmitted diseases treatment guidelines, *MMWR Recomm Rep* 70(4):1–187, 2021.

Jeng H-S, Yan T-R, Chen J-Y: Treating vaginitis with probiotics in non-pregnant females: a systematic review with meta-analysis, *Exp Ther Med* 20:3749–3765, 2020.

Rahn DD, Carberry C, Sanses TV, et al: Vaginal estrogen for genitourinary syndrome of menopause: a systematic review, *Obstetr Gynecol* 124(6):1147, 2014.

Reichman O, Sobel J: Desquamative inflammatory vaginitis, *Best Prac Res Clin Obstetr Gynaecol* 28(7):1042–1050, 2014.

Sobel JD: Recurrent vulvovaginal candidiasis, *AJOG* 214(1):15–21, 2016.

18 Pregnancy and Antepartum Care

ANTEPARTUM CARE

Method of
Matthew K. Cline, MD; and Natawadee Young, MD

CURRENT DIAGNOSIS

- Pregnancy evaluation should begin 3 to 6 months before conception with optimization of underlying medical conditions, update of immunizations, and commencement of prenatal vitamins with 400 µg of folic acid.[1]
- Preconception counseling with a specialist in high-risk pregnancies should be considered in all patients with underlying medical conditions, such as diabetes and hypertension.
- Early ultrasound (< 13 weeks) assists with establishment of accurate estimated date of confinement and is an essential task in the first prenatal visit.
- The first prenatal visit should include a review of the medical and obstetric histories, current medications, allergies, herbal remedies, supplements, and tobacco, alcohol, and drug use.
- Prenatal laboratory studies should be done at the first visit after a pregnancy is confirmed with a urine pregnancy test. These studies include hemoglobin, platelet count, blood and Rh type and antibody screening, rubella status, hepatitis B and C screening, syphilis screen, and a urine culture. All women should be screened for HIV. High-risk patients should be screened for gonorrhea and chlamydia.
- Genetic screening should be offered based on ethnic history.
- Offer aneuploidy screening to all women in the first trimester along with counseling about risks and benefits. These tests aid in diagnosis of chromosome abnormalities. If a patient opts for a first-trimester screen, it is important to perform an alpha-fetoprotein (AFP) screen in the second trimester to screen for neural tube defects. All women should be offered amniocentesis or chorionic villous sampling for genetic testing with appropriate counseling.
- Appropriate weight gain in pregnancy depends on maternal body mass index (BMI) before pregnancy. In patients with a normal BMI, a 25- to 30-pound weight gain is recommended. Underweight patients are encouraged to gain 30 to 35 pounds, and overweight patients are encouraged to gain no more than 20 pounds.
- Prenatal visits should begin at 8 to 12 weeks' gestation and continue monthly until 28 weeks. Visits should then be every 2 weeks until 36 weeks and then weekly. Each visit should include assessment of maternal weight, blood pressure (BP), fundal height measurement, documentation of fetal heart tones, and review of symptoms of preterm labor and preeclampsia.
- All patients should undergo a glucose challenge test at 24 to 28 weeks. This is done nonfasting by administering a 50-g load of glucose and obtaining a serum sample 1 hour after administration. A level greater than 140 mg/dL is considered abnormal, and a 3-hour glucose tolerance test is indicated (which is done after a 12-hour fast with a 100-g oral glucose load). If a woman demonstrates abnormalities in two of the four values, gestational diabetes is diagnosed.

[1]Not FDA approved for this indication.

CURRENT THERAPY

- Administration of the inactivated influenza vaccine (Fluzone, FluLaval, Fluarix) is recommended in all pregnant patients, regardless of trimester, who will be pregnant (or up to 3 months postpartum) during the flu season.
- Additionally, administer Tdap vaccine (Adacel, Boostrix) in each pregnancy given between 27 and 36 weeks or immediately postpartum in order to decrease rates of pertussis in this age group.
- Vaccination during pregnancy for protection against Covid-19 and RSV is a rapidly changing area of preventive therapy. The most updated recommendations can be accessed at the CDC website https://www.cdc.gov/vaccines-pregnancy/hcp/vaccination-guidelines/index.html.
- Folic acid supplementation[1] should begin before conception. The recommended dose is 400 µg daily and is usually given as a prenatal vitamin. In patients with a previous pregnancy complicated by a neural tube defect, 4 mg daily[3] is recommended to decrease the chance of recurrence of a neural tube defect.
- All patients with HIV should be treated with appropriate HAART (highly active anti-retroviral therapy) for the patient and her HIV viral type throughout the pregnancy.
- Intrapartum zidovudine (Retrovir) is recommended for all patients with HIV whose HIV RNA load is ≥ 50 copies/ml or who have concerns with adherence to HAART therapy. Consideration of cesarean delivery is appropriate based on viral load evaluation.

[1]Not FDA approved for this indication.
[3]Exceeds dosage recommended by the manufacturer.

Antepartum Care

Ideally, antepartum care commences 3 to 6 months before conception with the recommendation that women who are sexually active and not using contraception should begin taking daily multivitamin or folic acid supplements. The most convincing trials of this were performed in Europe and China when it was concluded that women of reproductive age should take multivitamin supplements containing 0.4 mg of folate daily to reduce the incidence of neural tube defects. Women with histories of children with neural tube defects or other anomalies should increase this dose to 4 mg[3] of folate in the periconceptional period to reduce risks of recurrence.

Preconception counseling should also include an accurate assessment of preexisting maternal medical conditions. This is the ideal time to stress changes in factors that respond to early intervention: quitting smoking, refraining from alcohol or drug abuse, treating gum disease, and avoiding teratogens. Alcohol is a known teratogen. Immunization status should be reviewed and vaccines should be administered as appropriate. Special consideration is given to patients with thyroid disease. Concern focuses on associations with low intelligence quotients (IQs) in children conceived by hypothyroid mothers. Patients with diabetes should

[3]Exceeds dosage recommended by the manufacturer.

XVIII Pregnancy and Antepartum Care

BOX 1   Potential Indications for High-Risk Referral

- Current disease involving renal, cardiac, or endocrine systems
- Fetal anomalies (in previous pregnancies or first-degree family relatives)
- History of preterm delivery
- Incompetent cervix or recurrent miscarriages
- Isoimmunization
- Known carrier of genetic disorder
- Multiple gestation
- Placenta previa after 28 weeks
- Prior intrauterine fetal demise or stillbirth
- Systemic diseases such as hypertension, diabetes, or asthma
- Third-trimester bleeding

be counseled that the increased risk of birth defects is directly related to the level of glucose control at conception.

High-risk obstetric referrals may be offered to women with potential for obstetric complications suggested by conditions listed in Box 1. Identification of the high-risk patient is critical to minimizing adverse outcomes.

In most cases, a woman's pregnancy is a normal event that is complicated by potentially dangerous disease in a minority of cases. The physician who manages pregnant patients must follow the normal changes that occur during antepartum care, so that abnormalities can be recognized and treated appropriately. Additionally, routine prenatal care offers multiple opportunities for patient education, primary intervention, and appropriate monitoring of the low-risk pregnancy in the setting of the family and community. For some women, antepartum care is part of their own continuum in a long-term primary care relationship with caregivers.

Timeline of Routine Antepartum Care

First Visit and Early Care

History

After pregnancy is confirmed, it is extraordinarily important to determine the duration of pregnancy and the estimated date of confinement (EDC). Further care is heavily predicated on this estimate. The history begins with ascertaining the first day of the last normal menstrual period and calculating the EDC by assuming duration of pregnancy averages 280 days (40 weeks). Because a first-trimester dating ultrasound (US) is accurate to within 5 days at confirmation or determination of an accurate EDC, its value cannot be overestimated.

The documentation of prior obstetric history includes prior complications, route of delivery, and estimated birth weights. Maternal medical disorders are often exacerbated by pregnancy; cardiovascular, renal, and endocrine disorders require evaluation and counseling concerning possible treatments required. A history of previous gynecologic surgery, including cesarean delivery, is important to consider. A family history of twinning, diabetes mellitus, familial disorders, or hereditary disease is relevant.

Current medications (prescription and nonprescription) are reviewed, along with any herbals or supplements. Certain prescription medications are known teratogens and should be discontinued. Examples include isotretinoin (Accutane), tetracycline (Sumycin), quinolone antibiotics (ciprofloxacin [Cipro], levofloxacin [Levaquin]), "statin" cholesterol-lowering medications such as atorvastatin (Lipitor) and rosuvastatin (Crestor) and warfarin (Coumadin). Angiotensin-converting enzyme (ACE) inhibitors and angiotensin receptor blockers (ARBs) should not be used in pregnancy because they can be associated with fetal renal agenesis.

It is important to determine the pregnant patient's risks for developing preeclampsia during the first trimester prenatal visit because starting low dose aspirin[1] (81 mg) between 12 to 28

weeks (ideally before 16 weeks' gestation) can prevent morbidity and mortality from preeclampsia. One or more of the following high-risk factors is an indication for beginning low dose aspirin after 12 weeks: a history of previous preeclampsia, multifetal gestation, renal disease, autoimmune disease, diabetes, and chronic hypertension. Consideration of low dose aspirin should be given for patients with more than one of moderate-risk factors for preeclampsia including obesity, advanced maternal age, history of low birth weight infants or adverse birth outcomes, and low socioeconomic status or African American race.

Open discussion of substance abuse (alcohol, tobacco, and illicit drugs) is an integral part of the patient interview. Counseling patients about smoking cessation is vital in early pregnancy. Smoking increases the risk of fetal death or damage in utero. It is also associated with increased risk of placental abruption and placenta previa, each of which put both mother and child at risk, along with premature birth. The interest that pregnant women have in delivering a healthy infant can be a potent motivator for change at this point.

Opioid use in pregnancy has escalated in the last decade. Early screening for opioid use, misuse, and for opioid use disorder along with brief intervention and referral is recommended for all pregnant women. Pregnant women with opioid use disorder should be referred to psychosocial resources and to a qualified clinic or treatment center that is able to assist in managing the patient with methadone or buprenorphine throughout the pregnancy and postpartum period. Medically assisted withdrawal is currently not recommended in pregnancy due to the high risk for relapse and the associated harms that occur with addiction. Patients and care teams should be prepared for the risk of neonatal abstinence syndrome if there is continued opioid or other illicit drug use during pregnancy.

Domestic Violence Screening and Counseling

Pregnancy is also a time of increased incidence of domestic or intimate partner violence, and because of this, it is appropriate to screen patients about the safety of their homes and relationships starting at the first prenatal visit. The United States Preventive Services Task Force (USPSTF) gives screening for domestic or intimate partner violence a "B" rating, supporting its use in routine prenatal care. A large evidence review supports benefit to patients being screened with one of many possible screening tools. The Personal Violence Screen consists of three "Yes" or "No" questions that can be quickly administered to a patient in private, and a positive result is one or more "Yes" responses:

1. Have you been hit, kicked, punched, or otherwise hurt by someone in the past year?
2. Do you feel unsafe in your current relationship?
3. Is there a partner from a previous relationship who is making you feel unsafe now?

A positive screen should be followed by specific referral to local resources for the patient to reach a safe environment and continued support. Each office should evaluate local resources and have a prepared contact list for these patients to use as their next step to safety.

Examination

Physical examination begins with a thorough general examination to assess maternal well-being, including BMI and BP. The BMI is calculated by dividing weight in kilograms by height in meters squared. The BMI of a patient is categorized as underweight (under 19.8), normal weight (19.8 to 25), overweight (25 to 30), or obese (over 30).

Breast examination may be significant for changes in pregnancy that result from hormonal responses by the mammary ducts. These changes include engorgement and vascular prominence, occasionally resulting in mastodynia. Enlargement of areolar sebaceous glands occurs between 6 and 8 weeks' gestation.

A pelvic examination is performed with attention to the adequacy of pelvis and evaluation for adnexal masses. Numerous changes in the pelvic organs occur in pregnancy. For example, congestion of the pelvic vasculature (Chadwick's sign) causes bluish discoloration of the vagina and cervix. Softening of the cervix

---

[1]Not FDA approved for this indication.

TABLE 1 · U.S. Preventive Services Task Force Recommendations for Pregnancy

Grade A = The USPSTF recommends the service. There is high certainty that the net benefit is substantial. Screening/actions in pregnancy in this category include the following:
- Screen for hepatitis B infection in all pregnant women.
- Screen for HIV infection in all pregnant women.
- Screen for syphilis in all pregnant women.
- Screen for cervical cancer in all women between 21 and 65 who have a uterus.
- Ask about smoking and provide augmented, pregnancy-tailored counseling for those who smoke and are pregnant.
- All women planning or capable of pregnancy should take 400–800 μg of folic acid daily.
- Screen all women at the first visit by Rh(D) typing and antibody screen.

Grade B = The USPSTF recommends the service. There is high certainty that the net benefit is moderate or there is moderate certainty that the net benefit is moderate to substantial. Screening/actions in pregnancy in this category include the following:
- Screen for asymptomatic bacteriuria at 12 to 16 weeks or at first prenatal visit.
- Screen for chlamydia and gonorrhea in pregnant women 24 and younger or at high risk.
- Screen for Hepatitis C in all persons aged 18–79.
- Provide intervention during pregnancy and after birth to support breast-feeding.
- Screen for alcohol misuse and provide behavioral counseling interventions to reduce its misuse.
- For women at high risk of preeclampsia, start low-dose aspirin[1] at 81 mg/day after 12 weeks of gestation.
- Screen for gestational diabetes mellitus (GDM) in asymptomatic pregnant women after 24 weeks of gestation.
- Screen for depression in pregnant and postpartum women.
- Screen women of childbearing age for intimate partner violence (IPV), such as domestic violence, and provide or refer women who screen positive to intervention services.
- Screen throughout pregnancy for preeclampsia by blood pressure measurement.
- Repeat Rh(D) antibody testing for all unsensitized women at 24-28 weeks.

Grade C = Clinicians may provide this service to selected patients depending on individual circumstances. However, for most individuals without signs or symptoms there is likely to be only a small benefit from this service.

Grade D = The USPSTF recommends against the service. There is moderate or high certainty that the service has no net benefit or that the harms outweigh the benefits.
- Screen for bacterial vaginosis in asymptomatic pregnant women at low risk for preterm birth.
- Screen for herpes simplex with serology in asymptomatic pregnant women.

Grade I = The USPSTF concludes that the current evidence is insufficient to assess the balance of benefits and harms of the service.
- Screen for iron deficiency anemia in asymptomatic pregnant women.
- Screen for illicit drug use in pregnancy.
- Screen for elevated blood lead levels in asymptomatic pregnancy women.

Listing of all topics is available at https://www.uspreventiveservicestaskforce.org/BrowseRec/Index/browse-recommendations.
Abbreviation: USPSTF = U.S. Preventive Services Task Force.
[1]Not FDA approved for this indication.

due to increased vascularity of the cervical tissue (Goodell's sign) can occur as early as 4 weeks.

Portable devices using Doppler will reliably detect fetal heart tones at a normal rate of 120 to 160 beats per minute as early as 11 weeks.

Laboratory Studies

Routine laboratory studies and screenings in pregnancy are listed in Table 1, along with their USPSTF level of recommendation.

Other Studies

Aneuploidy screening for common chromosomal abnormalities should be offered to all women, with counseling about risks and benefits. Current strategies include either cell free DNA aneuploidy screening or the more traditional maternal serum biomarker tests (PAPP-A/b-HCG) with or without nuchal translucency measurement. Invasive diagnostic testing for fetal chromosomal disorders through either chorionic villus sampling or amniocentesis is offered to all women, but especially if patients have increased risk or if the screening tests are abnormal. Second trimester screening for neural tube defects with maternal serum alpha fetoprotein is offered to all women. Second trimester fetal anatomy ultrasound evaluation is also offered around 20 weeks of gestation. Women may decline all screening and testing options after informed counseling.

Cell-free DNA screening was utilized primarily after 10 weeks in high-risk women such as those with prior aneuploidy, or older than age 35. However, there is now evidence using cell-free DNA screening in the general population, and results appear to be comparable. It has the highest detection rate (DR) for Down syndrome in high-risk women (98% DR with positive screening rates of less than 0.5%, positive predictive value of 93%). Positive predictive values are lower for trisomy 18 (64%), trisomy 13(44%), and sex chromosome aneuploidies (39%). However, it must be emphasized that for younger or low-risk women, false positive rates will be higher because of a lower pretest probability in these populations. In addition, the test cannot distinguish between fetal and maternal DNA, and causes of false positive screening tests can include placental mosaicism, a resorbing twin, or even maternal malignancy or aneuploidy. For this reason, ACOG recommends diagnostic testing with CVS or amniocentesis after a positive cell-free DNA screen prior to decisions about termination of the pregnancy. Cell-free DNA screening testing after a positive first trimester screen can also add additional information prior to diagnostic invasive tests. Appropriate pre and posttest counseling is important due to these evolving issues.

Chorionic villus sampling (CVS) (done at 10–12 weeks' gestation) or amniocentesis (performed at 14–16 weeks' gestation) should be offered to women older than 35 years, to those with abnormal first-trimester screens or second trimester "quad" screens, and to those with significant family history of genetic disease. From either test, fetal cells grown in culture may be subjected to chromosomal, metabolic, or DNA study for trisomy 13, 18, or 21 or abnormal numbers of sex chromosomes. CVS cannot be used for diagnosis of neural tube defects, but amniocentesis can accurately diagnose open neural tube defects or open abdominal defects by measuring amniotic fluid AFP.

Patients with tuberculosis exposure may be assessed for active tuberculosis with skin testing (if not vaccinated with Bacillus Calmette-Guérin [BCG]) and chest x-ray with abdominal shielding. Serologic assessment for toxoplasmosis, cytomegalovirus, and varicella immunity are not routinely indicated.

Currently it is recommended that all pregnant couples of Caucasian background be screened for being carriers of cystic fibrosis genes. Additionally, screening for genetic disorders should be undertaken if concern exists based on racial or ethnic background (hemoglobinopathies, β-thalassemia, α-thalassemia, Tay-Sachs disease) or familial background (cystic fibrosis, fragile X, Duchenne's muscular dystrophy).

Education

Several areas are appropriate for routine education during the first prenatal visit, and may be provided by handouts, nursing instruction, or directly by the physician. These will vary based on the patient's individual knowledge and prior experience, but at a minimum should include discussions of the following:
- Common discomforts of pregnancy and safe methods to relieve them
- Foods to avoid during pregnancy and safe food preparation
- Avoidance of tobacco, ethanol, and nonprescribed drugs throughout pregnancy

- Limitations on travel and importance of proper seatbelt use
- Danger signs of pregnancy and reasons to call or be seen after hours
- Availability of birth education classes, tours, and other educational resources

Follow-up

Follow-up visits are scheduled once monthly until 28 weeks' gestation, and then patients are followed twice monthly until 36 weeks. Visits are then scheduled at weekly intervals until delivery. At each visit, weight, BP, fetal heart tones, and fundal height are noted. In the last 6 weeks of pregnancy, assessing fetal position is also appropriate.

Interval history includes questions about diet, sleeping patterns, and fetal movement. Warning signs such as bleeding, contractions, leaking of fluid, headache, or visual disturbances are reviewed.

15 to 20 Weeks' Gestation

Interval History

At each visit, it is appropriate to ask about specific symptoms: headache, dysuria, swelling, vaginal discharge, any bleeding, pelvic pain, and nausea or vomiting. The nausea and vomiting of the first trimester usually begins to decrease after 12 to 14 weeks. By this point in the pregnancy, the patient is usually feeling well. The other items above, if present, may indicate reasons for a targeted examination to evaluate for the cause, such as a speculum examination with wet prep for an increased symptomatic discharge (though the physiologic discharge of pregnancy has often become evident by this point, it should be asymptomatic).

Alpha-Fetoprotein and Aneuploidy Testing

For patients who received first-trimester aneuploidy screening, maternal serum AFP testing should be offered for all pregnancies at 16 to 20 weeks as a means of screening for open neural tube defects. High levels of AFP are associated with various fetal anomalies, including neural tube defects, multiple gestations, and ventral wall defects. Unexplained elevation of AFP has been associated with poor fetal growth, fetal loss, and preeclampsia. In cases with unexplained elevation of AFP, maternal and fetal surveillance should be increased. Low levels of AFP are associated with increased risk of Down syndrome.

For those who did not have the first trimester screen, a "quad screen" with multiple analytes can be done at this time to screen for aneuploidy such as trisomy 21, 18, and 13 as well. The interpretation of this test depends on the gestational age; even if timed correctly, it is known to have a moderate level of false-positive results. Therefore the first step after an abnormal AFP or quad screen is to refer for a detailed ultrasound to confirm gestational age and assess fetal anatomy. If the results of the screening remain abnormal, definitive testing via amniocentesis is recommended.

Physical Findings

Interval changes in the physical examination now include the start of colostrum secretion, which can begin as early as 16 weeks' gestation. The mother might detect fetal movements (quickening) at around 18 to 20 weeks. The uterus is palpable at 20 weeks at the umbilicus.

Chloasma is darkening of the skin over the forehead, bridge of the nose, or cheekbones and is more obvious in those with dark complexions. It can begin to manifest at this time, and is intensified by exposure to sunlight. Darkening of the skin in the areolae and nipples becomes more accentuated. A darkened line appears in the lower midline of the abdomen from the umbilicus to the pubis (linea nigra). The basis of these changes is stimulation of melanophores by increased melanocyte-stimulating hormone.

At 15 to 20 weeks, abdominal enlargement can appear more rapid as the uterus rises out of the pelvis and into the abdomen.

Ultrasonography

Sonography has long established itself as the single most useful technology in monitoring pregnancy and diagnosing complications. It is for this reason that an anatomic US is offered at 18 to 20 weeks to evaluate growth, placentation, amniotic fluid volume, and fetal anatomy. If earlier dating of the pregnancy is uncertain, this is an opportunity to confirm or refute prior estimates. If anomalous conditions are discovered or the patient has a history of diabetes, advanced maternal age, or has prior children with anomalies, more comprehensive US becomes necessary.

20 to 35 Weeks' Gestation

Interval History

This period in the middle trimester of the pregnancy is often the time when patients feel their best: the challenges of nausea and vomiting from the first trimester are usually past. Patients should be asked about diet and activity, fetal activity (which should continue to increase throughout this period), and any symptoms that might suggest preeclampsia, such as hand or face swelling, visual changes, or severe headaches. Vaginal secretions do increase during this period but any bleeding or leakage of a large amount of fluid, along with any uterine rhythmic contractions, should also prompt a call or evaluation of the patient.

Physical Findings

The uterus should be palpable at the umbilicus at 20 weeks, and from this period until 34 weeks the measurement in centimeters from the fundus to the symphysis pubis should correspond to the gestational age in weeks. Measurements that are more than 2 cm below the expected size should raise suspicion for oligohydramnios, intrauterine growth restriction, fetal anomalies, or an abnormal fetal position. Conversely, measurements more than 2 cm larger than expected may indicate multiple gestation, polyhydramnios, or fetal macrosomia. These rules apply for the gestational ages of 20 to 34 weeks. Either situation can be evaluated with maternal US examination and consultation with a maternal-fetal-medicine specialist.

New physical examination findings at this time include the onset of stretch marks (striae) of the breasts and abdomen. These are caused by separation of underlying collagen tissue, a response to increased adrenocorticosteroid. The ligamentous structures of the pelvis also undergo slight but definite relaxation of the joints, a progesterone effect. As the uterus enlarges, it often rotates to the right. Braxton-Hicks contractions, characterized as painless uterine tightening, increase in regularity. The fetal outline can be easily palpated through the maternal abdominal wall.

Laboratory Studies

Increased surveillance for preeclampsia should occur in any patient with a previous history of preeclampsia or chronic hypertension predating the pregnancy. Newer guidelines require only two blood pressures 4+ hours apart that are 140/90 or greater for the diagnosis of preeclampsia along with 1+ urinary protein, a urinary protein to creatinine ratio of 0.3 or greater, or >300 mg of protein in a 24-hour urine collection. Further evaluation for patients with elevated BP (>140/90) should include evaluation for symptoms or findings that are consistent with severe features: headaches, visual changes, pulmonary edema, RUQ pain or epigastric pain, BP of 160 or higher systolic or 110 or higher diastolic on two occasions 4 hours apart, or laboratory evidence of thrombocytopenia (platelets below 100,000), liver transaminases elevated to at least twice the normal level, a serum creatinine that has doubled or is greater than 1.1. If any severe feature is present, the diagnosis of preeclampsia does not require proteinuria. Once the diagnosis of preeclampsia is made, management will be based on gestational age as well as presence of severe features. For additional details, please see chapter "Hypertension in Pregnancy."

A complete blood count (to screen for anemia) and a nonfasting 1-hour glucose tolerance test (after ingestion of 50 g of glucose) are scheduled to detect patients at risk for developing gestational diabetes at 24 to 28 weeks. If the screening test is abnormal, a

3-hour test is performed with 100 g of glucose to confirm the diagnosis. Two or more abnormal values on this test are considered diagnostic of gestational diabetes mellitus.

A repeat Rh antibody is checked at 28 weeks' gestation in Rh-negative mothers. Those who remain unsensitized at 28 weeks' gestation receive a first dose of Rho(D) immune globulin (Rho-GAM) of 300 μg to prevent maternal isoimmunization to fetal red blood cells. (This should also be given at any point after the first 12 weeks of pregnancy in the setting of significant maternal trauma in an Rh-negative mother. If there is suspicion of a significant fetal-maternal hemorrhage, a Kleihauer-Betke test can be used to quantitate the amount of fetal blood in the maternal circulation in order to increase the dose of RhoGAM appropriately.)

Given the increase in rates of syphilis and the resultant rise in cases of congenital syphilis in the last decade, current guidelines recommend retesting those at high risk for syphilis at 28 weeks and again at delivery.

Follow-up

Return visits at 2-week intervals are initiated beginning at 28 weeks, and the patient is oriented to the labor and delivery ward. Precautions are given regarding the onset of conditions listed in Box 2. The onset of any of these should prompt immediate medical attention.

36 to 41 Weeks' Gestation
Physical Findings

Patients often note increased vaginal discharge at this time in their pregnancy, a physiologic consequence of hormone stimulation. The discharge consists mainly of epithelial cells and cervical mucus and is treated with reassurance. Discharge accompanied by itching, burning, or malodor should be evaluated with a wet prep and any abnormalities treated.

Laboratory Studies

Vaginal and rectal rapid molecular tests are collected to evaluate for the presence of group B streptococci (GBS) at 36 0/7 to 37 6/7 weeks. GBS organisms are implicated in preterm labor, amnionitis, endometritis, and wound infection. If tests are positive, the patient will be given antibiotic prophylaxis during active labor to protect the newborn against vertical transmission and the resulting infection that could occur. If a patient has a positive urine testing during the pregnancy of over 100,000 colony-forming units of GBS, she is treated at the time of that culture but also assumed to be heavily colonized and given intrapartum antibiotics without performing the vaginal/rectal cultures at 36 0/7 to 37 6/7 weeks.

Follow-up

Follow-up visits are planned on a weekly basis with emphasis on weight gain, BP, and signs of preeclampsia. Review of precautions regarding infection, pregnancy loss, and symptoms of preeclampsia completes the visit. Elective induction of labor after 39 completed weeks gestation may be offered for low-risk singleton pregnancies.

Late Term and Postterm Gestation

About 6% of pregnancies continue beyond 42 weeks and are considered postterm. The period between 41 0/7 and 41 6/7 weeks is named late term pregnancy. Due to increased perinatal morbidity and mortality beginning at 41 0/7 weeks, guidelines recommend elective induction of labor at 41 weeks after shared decision-making with patients. Should the patient decline induction, then experts recommend fetal surveillance twice weekly between 41 and 42 weeks gestation with nonstress testing, amniotic fluid measurement, or the biophysical profile, followed by induction of labor at 42 weeks gestation.

Common Concerns of the Antenatal Period
Bleeding

About one-half of pregnant women experience some form of bleeding during the pregnancy; often this is benign. Patients also have a heightened awareness of symptoms that previously may have gone unnoticed in the nonpregnant state. Efficient and competent evaluation, followed by compassion and reassurance when prudent, allays many fears and provides clear direction. Spotting due to bleeding at the implantation site occurs from the time of implantation (about 6 days after fertilization) until 29 to 35 days after the last menstrual period in many women. Usually, cardiac activity on US and appropriate β-hCG levels confirm a viable early pregnancy. First-trimester bleeding may be a sign of spontaneous miscarriage or ectopic pregnancy and deserves further evaluation, often with a pelvic examination and US. Vaginal bleeding in late pregnancy is covered in other chapters.

Nausea

Nausea is a common symptom that occurs in most pregnancies. It is heightened before 14 weeks' gestation and is largely benign. The etiology is not well understood but likely is related to elevating levels of β-hCG. Nausea of pregnancy can occur at any time during the day. Aggravating factors vary with the individual patient; success varies with interventions designed to reduce symptoms.

Uncomplicated nausea may be responsive to small nonfatty portions at mealtime. Pyridoxine (vitamin B_6)[1] tablets 12.5 mg three times daily with 12.5 mg of doxylamine (Unisom)[1] twice a day are safe in pregnancy and may be helpful. A combination product of doxylamine 10 mg and pyridoxine 10 mg (Diclegis) is approved by the FDA for the treatment of nausea and vomiting of pregnancy in women who do not respond to conservative management. Antiemetic drugs in the outpatient setting are the next step; ondansetron (Zofran, FDA category B)[1] 4 to 8 mg up to three times a day and meclizine (Antivert, FDA category B)[1] 12.5 to 25 mg three times a day are agents with the best safety profile.

Inability to control protracted vomiting in conjunction with clinical dehydration can require hospitalization for IV fluids and treatment of hyperemesis gravidarium. Extreme nausea and vomiting that persists beyond 18 to 20 weeks' gestation may be a sign of multiple gestation, thyroid disease, molar pregnancy, or liver or pancreatic disease.

Nutrition and Weight Gain

The mother's nutrition is a vital factor in the development of the fetus from preconception through the postpartum period. Therefore, the pregnant woman should be advised to eat a balanced diet and should be informed of the additional 300 kcal/day needed during pregnancy. The American College of Obstetricians and Gynecologists (ACOG) recommends a target weight gain of 22 to 27 pounds (10–12 kg) during pregnancy. It also advises that underweight women might need to gain more and obese women should gain less. Nutritional requirements for protein are 80 g/day, for calcium are 1500 mg/day, for iron are 30 mg/day, and for folate are 0.4 mg/day (4 mg/day in some cases, such as those patients with previous baby with neural tube defects). Patients with seizure disorders managed with valproic acid (Depakene)

---

[1]Not FDA approved for this indication.

or carbamazepine (Tegretol) are also at risk for birth defects and might benefit from the higher dose of folate.

Heartburn

Heartburn in the form of reflux esophagitis is caused by the enlarging uterus displacing the stomach and by progesterone's relaxation of the lower esophageal sphincter. Treatment consists of taking antacids, decreasing exacerbating factors such as spicy foods, eating more frequently but in smaller quantities, limiting eating before bedtime, and taking H_2-blockers.

Urinary Symptoms

Urinary frequency, nocturia, and bladder irritability are common complaints due to progesterone-mediated relaxation of smooth muscle and subsequent altered bladder function. Later in pregnancy, urinary frequency becomes even more prominent from pressure on the bladder by the enlarging uterus and the fetal presenting parts, such as when the fetal head descends into the pelvis.

Dysuria, however, is often a sign of infection that requires antibiotic treatment. Bacteriuria combined with urinary stasis from altered bladder function predisposes the patient to pyelonephritis. Although simple urinary tract infections are treated on an outpatient basis, pyelonephritis remains the most common nonobstetric cause for hospitalization during antenatal care.

Patients with a diagnosis of pyelonephritis require hospitalization, aggressive fluid replacement, and IV antibiotics until they remain afebrile for longer than 24 hours. Close monitoring of maternal respiratory status is important because these women are at risk for acute respiratory distress syndrome (ARDS) and renal failure as well as a significant increase in preterm labor and delivery. All patients should complete a 14-day course of antibiotic treatment. After treatment has been completed, suppressive therapy should be continued until delivery.

Infection

Two infections of special note are HIV and bacterial vaginosis (BV). HIV transmission to the newborn can be reduced significantly with appropriate infectious disease and maternal-fetal medicine specialty management. Although all symptomatic pregnant women with BV should be treated, evidence is inconclusive for screening and treating asymptomatic women, even those with a high risk history of prior preterm delivery or PPROM. Because of well-documented safety and efficacy of oral[1] and vaginal metronidazole, and vaginal clindamycin cream, any of these three are considered first-line for treatment in pregnancy.

Chlamydia trachomatis is an obligate intracellular bacterium and is the most common sexually transmitted bacterial infection in women of reproductive age. It may be associated with urethritis, mucopurulent cervicitis, and acute salpingitis, or it may be clinically silent. Perinatal transmission is clearly associated with neonatal conjunctivitis (leading to blindness) and pneumonia and is likely associated with preterm delivery, premature rupture of membranes, and perinatal mortality. Diagnosis is confirmed by nucleic acid amplification testing (NAAT) during routine screening. Doxycycline should be avoided in pregnancy, and erythromycin is associated with gastrointestinal upset, so treatment with azithromycin (Zithromax 1000 mg as single dose) is often the best choice in pregnancy.

Gonococcal infection is associated with concomitant chlamydia infection in about 40% of infected pregnant women. It is usually limited to the lower genital tract, including the cervix, urethra, and periurethral or vestibular glands. Because of an association between gonococcal cervicitis and septic spontaneous abortion, and because preterm delivery, premature rupture of membranes, and postpartum infection are more common with gonococcal infection, routine cultures are appropriate at the first antenatal visit. Because some strains have rendered some β-lactam drugs ineffective for therapy, uncomplicated gonococcal infections should be treated with a single IM dose of 500 mg of ceftriaxone

(Rocephin) for patients under 150 kg; for patients who weigh 150 kg or more, the dose should be 1000 mg of ceftriaxone IM.

Syphilis cases have been on the rise since 2012, with rates higher now than in the 1950s. This has resulted in more than 3800 cases of congenital syphilis in the United States in 2023. Congenital syphilis can result in devastating consequences to the fetus, including stillbirth. Consequently, ACOG has issued a Practice Advisory to universally re-test for syphilis in pregnancy at 28 weeks and at delivery. Early syphilis is treated with IM benzathine pencillin G (Bicillin LA) 2.4 million units as a single does. Late latent syphilis requires a total of 7.2 million units of benzathine penicillin G, administered as 3 doses of 2.4 million units IM each at 1-week intervals.

Vaginosis due to *Candida albicans* can become symptomatic with caseous white discharge and vaginal itching or burning, and it may be associated with red satellite lesions on the vulva. Marked inflammation of the vagina and introitus may be noted. Topical application of over-the-counter antifungal creams such as miconazole nitrate (Monistat) or nystatin (Mycostatin) is generally helpful in controlling the imbalance of vaginal flora, but this requires a 7-day regimen to achieve adequate cure rates. A single dose of fluconazole (Diflucan), 150 mg by mouth, is another appropriate choice, but only after the first trimester.

Trichomonas vaginalis can be found in 20% to 30% of pregnant patients, but only a small number complain of discharge or irritation. This flagellated, oval, motile organism can be seen on normal saline wet prep and is evident clinically by presence of a foamy or greenish discharge accompanied by multiple cervical petechiae. The CDC now recommends highly sensitive and specific nucleic acid amplification test (NAAT) in testing for trichomonads (95.3–100% sensitive, 93.2–100% specific for the APTIMA T. vaginalis test), as wet prep microscopy is rather insensitive (51–65%). There are also several new point-of-care tests that are now FDA-approved using antigen detection or DNA hybridization probe technology that have results available in as little as 10 minutes (OSOM Trichomonas rapid test) to 45 minutes (Affirm VP III). Treatment is oral metronidazole (Flagyl) as a single 2-g dose for the patient and her partner (though most states support expedited partner treatment, each practitioner will need to individualize this approach).

Rubella, also known as German measles, is directly responsible for spontaneous miscarriage and severe congenital malformations. Although large epidemics of rubella are nonexistent in the United States because of immunization, the disease can still affect up to 25% of susceptible women. Absence of rubella antibody indicates susceptibility. Vaccination involves an attenuated live virus (MMR) and therefore is avoided in pregnancy. Vaccination of nonpregnant susceptible women (including those during the postpartum period) and hospital personnel continues to be the mainstay of therapy. Detection by immunoglobulin M (IgM)–specific antibody confirms recent infection.

Varicella-zoster virus, the etiologic agent of childhood chickenpox, is a DNA herpes virus that remains latent in the dorsal root ganglia and may be reactivated years later to cause herpes zoster or shingles. Infection early in pregnancy can lead to severe congenital malformations, including chorioretinitis, cerebral cortical atrophy, hydronephrosis, and cutaneous and bony leg defects. Varicella-zoster immunoglobulin (VariZIG) (30–40 kg: 500 U; ≥40.1 kg: 625 U) can attenuate varicella infection if given to an exposed, nonimmune pregnant woman within 96 hours of her exposure to a patient with active varicella.

Genital herpes simplex virus (HSV) can present at any gestational age and is characterized by multiple, painful genital ulcers or vesicles; the diagnosis can be confirmed (if not in labor) through use of PCR laboratory testing. If active genital lesions are noted in labor, cesarean delivery is indicated because the fetus is at risk for acquiring the virus during passage through the birth canal. For HSV outbreaks remote from term, acyclovir (Zovirax) and its derivatives can shorten the course of an outbreak. For those with a history of active herpes during or preceding pregnancy, prophylaxis with acyclovir or similar approved antiviral

---

[1]Not FDA approved for this indication.

medications from 36 weeks onward can decrease the chance of an outbreak at term and the need for a cesarean delivery.

Influenza can occur during pregnancy, and because the risk of secondary complication such as pneumonia is increased during the antepartum period, influenza vaccination is recommended for all patients in any trimester who are pregnant or up to 3 months postpartum during the local influenza season. Rapid testing of nasal or throat swabs can ascertain the diagnosis of influenza. Though oseltamivir (Tamiflu) and zanamivir (Relenza) are both FDA category C in pregnancy, no toxic effects have been observed in animal trials, so these are the preferred agents. These agents need to be started as soon as possible to provide the most benefit in symptom duration and severity. Similarly, Covid-19 (SARS-CoV2) infection can confer a higher risk of severe illness to pregnant patients. Current CDC guidelines recommend vaccination (preferably with mRNA vaccines) due to data demonstrating vaccine safety and efficacy.

Varicose Veins

Pressure by the enlarged uterus on venous return from the legs and progesterone-mediated vasodilation can lead to prominent varicosities and edema of the legs or vulva. Any concern for deep vein thrombosis should be ruled out with duplex ultrasound imaging. Benign varicosities almost invariably return to normal after delivery, thus limiting the need for intervention in the antepartum period, though their symptoms may be decreased through the wearing of support hose. Edema of the lower extremities is common, responds to elevation, and must be differentiated from facial or hand edema accompanying preeclampsia. Hemorrhoids are manifestations of the varicosities of the rectal veins. Treatment focuses on stool softeners, sitz baths, and over-the-counter topical preparations. If a hemorrhoid becomes firm and tender, evaluation for possible treatment by opening and removing the thrombus can provide immediate relief.

Constipation

Bowel transit time and relaxation of intestinal smooth muscle are both increased due to progesterone effects, resulting in overall slowing of bowel function. If pronounced, this can lead to constipation. Dietary management of this condition is centered on recommendations for increased fluids and high-fiber foods; stool softeners, such as docusate (Colace), can also be used in pregnancy. Enemas and laxatives are not recommended.

Upper Extremity Discomfort

Periodic numbness and tingling of the fingers is due to exacerbations of carpal tunnel compression exacerbated by tissue edema. Splinting of the affected hand at night may help, along with stretching exercises of the wrist and neck that can be done throughout the day. Most of these symptoms resolve after delivery.

Backache and Pelvic Discomfort

Endocrine relaxation of ligamentous structures coupled with an offset center of gravity create exaggerated lordotic spinal curve, joint instability, and back pain. Most women experience some form of this discomfort as pregnancy progresses. Advice given for improvements in posture, local heat, acetaminophen (Tylenol), and massage may be helpful. Minimizing the time spent standing can have a positive effect. Round ligament pain usually occurs during the second trimester and is described as sharp bilateral or unilateral groin pain. It may be exacerbated by change in position or rapid movement and might respond to similar measures. These routine aches and pains of pregnancy must be differentiated from rhythmic cramping pains originating in the back or uterus. The latter may be a sign of preterm labor requiring appropriate evaluation.

Leg Cramps

Leg cramps in the form of recurrent muscle spasms in pregnancy are believed to be due to lower levels of serum calcium or higher levels of serum phosphorus. The calves are most commonly involved and attacks are more frequent at night and in the third trimester. There are no data from controlled trials to show benefit over placebo for

treatment targeted toward reduced phosphate and increased calcium or magnesium intake. Local heat, putting the affected muscle on stretch, acetaminophen, and massage can be helpful in acute events.

Intercourse

In general, intercourse is considered safe in pregnancy. The exception to this rule is found in patients who have a known placenta previa, are experiencing uterine bleeding, or have postcoital cramps and spotting. It may be wise to avoid intercourse in couples who are at risk for special circumstances. Firmer recommendations can be made in instances of placenta previa or known rupture of membranes; in these instances intercourse should not occur.

Dental Care

Ideally, women should have dental care completed before conception. However, dental procedures under local anesthesia may be carried out at any time during the pregnancy. Use of nitrous oxide inhalants is to be avoided, however. Long procedures should be postponed until the second trimester. Antibiotics are appropriate as needed for dental infections and in cases of rheumatic heart disease or mitral valve prolapse with regurgitation.

X-rays, Ionizing Radiation, and Imaging

The adverse effects of ionizing radiation are dose dependent, but there is no single diagnostic procedure that results in a dose of radiation high enough to threaten the fetus or embryo. Diagnostic radiation of less than 5000 mrad is considered by ACOG to have minimal teratogenic risk, and if medically indicated, x-ray imaging may be performed safely (with appropriate abdominal shielding). Patients receiving dental x-rays are additionally protected by a lead apron. Still, the need for x-ray films should be evaluated for risks and potential benefits in the individual pregnant patient to conservatively protect the mother and fetus from theoretical genetic or oncogenic risk. Magnetic resonance imaging (MRI) is considered safe due to its mechanism of action, which is a nonionizing form of radiation. Radioactive iodine (^{131}I) is contraindicated in pregnancy.

Immunization

Live virus vaccines must be avoided during pregnancy because of possible effects on the fetus. These include measles, mumps, rubella (MMR), yellow fever (YF-Vax), and varicella (Varivax) vaccinations. The risks to the fetus from the administration of rabies vaccine (RabAvert, IMOVAX) are unknown.

Diphtheria and tetanus toxoid with pertussis (Tdap) is recommended between 27 and 36 weeks by the CDC and ACIP to decrease the risk of whooping cough in the newborn infant. The hepatitis B vaccine (Engerix B, Recombivax HB) series is safe and may be given in pregnancy to women at risk. The inactivated influenza vaccine (Fluzone, FluLaval, Fluarix) is also recommended in all women during any trimester they will be pregnant during the flu season (or up to 3 months postpartum during flu season).

Vaccination recommendations during pregnancy for protection against Covid-19 and RSV are rapidly changing areas of preventive therapy. Updated recommendations can be accessed at the CDC website at https://www.cdc.gov/vaccines-pregnancy/hcp/vaccination-guidelines/index.html.

Tests of Fetal Well-Being

A primary goal in antepartum care is the competent management of patient care extended to both mother and baby in order to reduce the risk of fetal demise after 24 weeks, ensure optimal conditions for term delivery after 37 weeks, and intervene for evolving conditions threatening the well-being of either patient. Any pregnancy that may be at increased risk for antepartum fetal compromise is a candidate for tests of fetal well-being performed weekly, beginning at 28 to 32 weeks. Some conditions requiring antepartum testing are listed in Box 3.

Nonstress Test

The nonstress test (NST) consists of fetal heart rate monitoring in the absence of uterine contractions. A reactive tracing is one in

BOX 3	Conditions That Prompt Enhanced Fetal Surveillance

- Decreased fetal movements
- Fetal growth restriction
- Hypertensive disorders
- Insulin-dependent diabetes mellitus
- Multiple gestation with discordant fetal growth
- Oligohydramnios or polyhydramnios
- Postterm pregnancy
- Prior loss or stillbirth

which heart rate accelerations of 15 beats/min above the baseline of 120 to 160 beats/min are of at least 15 seconds' duration. Two of these accelerations must be observed in a 20-minute period. False-positive nonreactive tracings are more common before 28 weeks' gestation.

Biophysical Profile

The biophysical profile (BPP) consists of an NST with ultrasound observations. A total of 10 points is given for the following elements (2 points each):

- Reactive NST
- Presence of fetal breathing movements of 30 seconds or more in 30 minutes
- Fetal movement defined as three or more discrete body or limb movements within 30 minutes
- Fetal tone defined as one or more episodes of fetal extremity extension and return to flexion
- Quantification of amniotic fluid volume, defined as a pocket of fluid that measures at least 2 cm by 2 cm

The results of a BPP are usually reported out of 8 points if done without the NST, and out of 10 points if done with an NST. Scores of 8 or 10 points (out of 10) are considered reassuring, with retesting indicated in 4 to 7 days depending on the original indication for the testing. A score of 6 points is borderline; testing should be repeated in 24 hours. Scores of 4 or 2 points are nonreassuring and should prompt additional testing, treatment, or planning for delivery depending on the setting.

References

ACOG Committee Opinion No: 743. Low-dose aspirin use during pregnancy, *Obstet Gynecol* 132(1):44–52, 2018.

ACOG Committee Opinion No: 797. Prevention of group B streptococcal early-onset disease in newborns, *Obstet Gynecol* 35(2):51–72, 2020.

ACOG Practice Advisory: COVID-19 Vaccination Considerations for Obstetric-Gynecologic Care. Last updated October 16, 2024 [accessed March 23, 2025].

ACOG Practice Advisory: Screening for Syphilis in Pregnancy. April 2024 [accessed March 23, 2025]

American College of Obstetricians and Gynecologists: *Compendium of selected publications*, Atlanta, 2012, American College of Obstetricians and Gynecologists.

American College of Obstetricians and Gynecologists: Screening for fetal aneuploidy. Practice Bulletin 163, *Obstet Gynecol* 127(5):e123–e137, 2016.

American College of Obstetricians and Gynecologists' Committee on Obstetric Practice; Society for Maternal-Fetal Medicine: Medically indicated late-preterm and early-term deliveries; committee opinion, no. 831, *Obstet Gynecol* 138(1):e35–e39, 2021.

Centers for Disease Control and Prevention: Sexually Transmitted Infections Treatment Guidelines 2021. Available at: https://www.cdc.gov/std/treatment-guidelines/default.htm. [accessed March 23, 2025].

Committee Opinion No: 711. Opioid use and opioid use disorder in pregnancy, *Obstet Gynecol* 130(2):81–94, 2017.

Grobman WA, Rice MM, Reddy UM: Eunice Kennedy Shriver National Institute of Child Health and Human Development Maternal-Fetal Medicine Units Network. Labor induction vs. expectant management in low-risk nulliparous women, *N Engl J Med* 379(6):513–523, 2018.

McParlin C, O'Donnell A, Robson SC, et al: Treatments for hyperemesis gravidarum and nausea and vomiting in pregnancy: a systematic review, *JAMA* 316(13):1392–1401, 2016.

Middleton P, Shepherd E, Crowther CA: Induction of labour for improving birth outcomes for women at or beyond term, *Cochrane Database of Systematic Reviews* 5:CD004945, 2017, https://doi.org/10.1002/14651858, CD004945.pub4.

Nelson HD, Bougatsos C, Blazina I: Screening women for intimate partner violence: a systematic review to update the U.S. Preventive Services Task Force Recommendation, *Ann Intern Med* 156:796–808, 2012, W279–82.

Ramirez SI: Prenatal care: an evidence-based approach, *Am Fam Physician* 108(2):139–150, 2023.

ECTOPIC PREGNANCY

Method of
Christina M. Kelly, MD

CURRENT DIAGNOSIS

- Vaginal bleeding and abdominal pain in the first trimester of pregnancy raise concern for ectopic pregnancy, but a normal intrauterine pregnancy (IUP) or early pregnancy loss (EPL) could exist.
- High-resolution transvaginal ultrasound (TVUS) and measurement of serum β–human chorionic gonadotropin (hCG) are the best initial steps in determining whether a pregnancy is ectopic.
- A single hCG value is not diagnostic of pregnancy location, viability, or gestational age. It can determine whether the level is in the discriminatory zone.
- If the hCG is above the discriminatory zone (3000–3500 mIU/mL), absence of a gestational sac with a yolk sac or embryo visualized in the uterus is highly suggestive of a nonviable gestation, either an early pregnancy loss or an ectopic pregnancy.
- If the initial hCG is below the discriminatory zone and there is no ultrasound evidence of ectopic pregnancy, patients should be followed up with repeat hCG levels every 48 hours. There is no universal method to predict an expected minimal rise for serial hCG levels for a viable IUP. Rather, it is dependent on the initial hCG level. Updated guidelines about the appropriate hCG patterns help guide decision making and determine whether additional diagnostic interventions are needed.
- If definitive findings of an intrauterine or ectopic pregnancy are not present on TVUS in a pregnant patient with a positive hCG level, a pregnancy of unknown location exists. Serial monitoring is needed to either establish a definitive diagnosis or reasonably exclude an IUP before an ectopic pregnancy is diagnosed and treated. Uterine aspiration can be considered to confirm the diagnosis of early pregnancy loss or ectopic pregnancy based on the presence or absence of chorionic villi.

CURRENT THERAPY

- Surgical management of ectopic pregnancy is indicated when a patient is hemodynamically unstable, exhibits signs of intraperitoneal bleeding, reports symptoms concerning for a ruptured ectopic mass, or has a contraindication to methotrexate.
- For a patient who is clinically stable and has a nonruptured ectopic pregnancy, either surgical or medical management of ectopic pregnancy are safe and effective options. A shared decision-making model can be used to help patients make informed decisions, which reviews the risks and benefits of both approaches and considers the clinical features of the ectopic pregnancy, stability of the patient, future fertility plans, and additional patient characteristics that would preclude one approach or the other.
- Medical management with systemic methotrexate (not approved by the Food and Drug Administration) requires regular patient follow-up for laboratory and office visits until hCG levels are undetectable.
- Medical management with methotrexate is most effective when ectopic pregnancies are less than 4 cm on TVUS, pretreatment hCG levels are less than 5000 mIU/mL, and fetal cardiac activity is not detected on TVUS.
- Expectant management of ectopic pregnancy may be considered in special circumstances, such as an asymptomatic and informed patient with reliable social resources in the setting of decreasing hCG levels that indicate pregnancy resolution.

An ectopic pregnancy is a potentially serious threat to the general and reproductive health of a pregnant person. Despite vast improvements in the clinical care of patients with ectopic pregnancy over recent years, diagnostic challenges and therapeutic controversies regarding this condition still exist. The objective of this chapter is to provide an overview of the epidemiology, diagnosis, and contemporary management of ectopic pregnancy. The chapter focuses on ectopic pregnancies that implant in the fallopian tube, which represent greater than 95% of all ectopic pregnancies.

Epidemiology

Of all pregnancies in the United States, approximately 1% to 2% are diagnosed as ectopic. Ectopic pregnancy incidence is difficult to calculate accurately due to insufficient hospital and outpatient data tracking, but recent studies estimate that over the last 25 years, it has increased sixfold. This rise may be the result of enhanced diagnostic capabilities, increased incidence of sexually transmitted infections and other risk factors, expanded use of infertility treatments, and heightened awareness of health professionals.

Ectopic pregnancy is the leading cause of maternal mortality in the first trimester of pregnancy in the United States, accounting for 2.7% of pregnancy-related deaths, and there should be continued high suspicion for at risk patients. However, the ectopic-related mortality rate is declining despite the increase in incidence. Between 1980 and 2007, 876 deaths were attributed to ectopic pregnancy, which represented a 56.6% decline in mortality rate between 1980 to 1984 and 2003 to 2007. However, age and racial disparities still persist. The ectopic pregnancy mortality ratio was 6.8 times higher for Black people compared with whites and 3.5 times higher for patients over 35 years old compared with those younger than 25 years old.

Pathophysiology

Damage to the fallopian tube and fallopian tube dysfunction are the primary factors associated with development of ectopic pregnancy. Normal embryo transport can be disrupted by damage to the structural integrity of the mucosal portion of the fallopian tube. Intratubal scarring secondary to infection or trauma could lead to trapping of a conceptus within intratubal adhesions or diverticula. Alteration of the hormonally mediated events leading to implantation, which can occur during infertility treatments, offers another mechanism for consideration. A change in the estrogen-to-progesterone ratio could theoretically affect smooth muscle activity in the fallopian tube, immobilizing ciliary activity.

Risk Factors

Half of all patients with ectopic pregnancy will not report any known risk factors; therefore the absence of risk factors should not decrease clinical suspicion. However, identification of clinical and historical risk factors for ectopic pregnancy could aid in early diagnosis. The most significant historical risk factors include prior ectopic pregnancy, prior fallopian tube surgery, infertility treatment, and hospitalization for pelvic inflammatory disease (PID). History of prior ectopic pregnancy is the strongest of these. Major clinical risk factors include pain or moderate-to-severe vaginal bleeding at presentation. Less significant risk factors are tobacco use and age >35 years old. Up to 53% of pregnancies that occur with a copper or progestin-releasing intrauterine device (IUD) in place are ectopic; however, the overall failure rate of IUDs is less than 1%.

Diagnosis and Clinical Manifestations

Although some patients present acutely with a ruptured ectopic pregnancy and hemoperitoneum, the vast majority (up to 80%) of ectopic pregnancies are diagnosed in stable patients who can be managed in the outpatient setting. Therefore reproductive-age people who present with symptoms of vaginal bleeding or abdominal discomfort need to be tested for pregnancy. If a patient is found to be pregnant, then their pregnancy needs to be differentiated as an ectopic pregnancy, an intrauterine gestation at risk for EPL, or a normally developing IUP. The use of TVUS and hCG assays represent the current standard for this differentiation and for accurate and timely diagnosis of ectopic pregnancy.

Transvaginal Ultrasonography

Proper evaluation of a patient with suspected ectopic pregnancy with TVUS requires an understanding of the typical findings for normal and abnormal pregnancies. The earliest ultrasonographic finding of a normal IUP is the gestational sac surrounded by a thick echogenic ring, located eccentrically within the endometrial cavity. On average, the gestational sac is seen on TVUS 5 weeks after the first day of the last menstrual period. The gestational sac grows and follows an approximate developmental timeline, which is represented by the following findings on TVUS: a yolk sac seen within the gestational sac at 5.5 weeks of gestation, an embryonic (fetal) pole at 6 weeks gestation, and cardiac activity at 6.5 weeks gestation.

A definitive IUP can be diagnosed by TVUS when a gestational sac with a yolk sac or embryo with or without cardiac activity is seen. A normal-appearing gestational sac should not solely be used to diagnose an IUP because it can be simulated by a pseudo-gestational sac, which occurs in 8% to 29% of patients with ectopic pregnancy. The pseudogestational sac likely represents bleeding into the endometrial cavity by the decidual cast. The presence of an adnexal gestational sac with a fetal pole and cardiac activity is the most specific but least sensitive sign of ectopic pregnancy, occurring in only 10% to 17% of cases. Adnexal rings (fluid sacs with thick echogenic rings) that have a yolk sac or nonliving embryo are accepted as specific signs of ectopic pregnancy and are visualized in ectopic pregnancies 33% to 50% of the time.

A critical concept in the evaluation of early pregnancy by TVUS is that of the hCG discriminatory zone—the level at or above which an examiner should see a normal intrauterine gestation, if present. In the setting of an hCG level above the discriminatory zone and no IUP on ultrasound, an ectopic pregnancy or an abnormal intrauterine pregnancy is highly likely. The exact hCG discriminatory value varies based on the institution, ultrasound machine, ultrasonographer's experience, and hCG assay used. The value used should be conservatively high—at least 3000 mIU/mL and up to 3500 mIU/mL—to minimize the risk of misdiagnosing a desired IUP as an ectopic pregnancy and treating it as such.

Hormonal Assays

Many patients with suspected ectopic pregnancy will present with a pregnancy of unknown location (PUL), where a hCG is below the discriminatory zone and a TVUS does not definitively diagnosis an intrauterine or extrauterine gestation (7%–20%). Serial monitoring is needed for PUL to establish a definitive diagnosis. Repeat hCG measurements are indicated at least every 48 hours to evaluate the appropriateness of hormonal trends along with serial TVUS studies. Comparing serial measurements of hCG from an individual patient to accepted patterns of hCG trends in early pregnancy helps distinguish an ectopic pregnancy from a viable IUP or a spontaneous EPL.

When evaluating serial hCG levels and predicting an expected minimal rise between values for a viable IUP, current evidence demonstrates there is not a universal trend that applies to all pregnancies at all gestations. Rather, it depends on the initial hCG level. Previous data showed that approximately 99% of viable intrauterine pregnancies are associated with a ≥53% increase in β-hCG values every 2 days. For pregnancies with an initial hCG value below 1500 mIU/mL, this calculation could apply. However, for pregnancies with higher initial hCG values, a laxer calculation should be used. One study suggests the following for an expected minimal rise for different initial hCG levels: 49% for levels <1500 mIU/mL, 40% for levels 1500 to 3000 mIU/mL, and 33% for levels >3000 mIU/mL. This represents a more conservative approach to incorporating invasive diagnostic procedures when following hCG values and preventing the interruption of normal IUPs.

Patients with symptomatic first-trimester pregnancies, nondiagnostic ultrasound, and a hCG level that is declining (when the initial value is below the discriminatory zone) should also be followed with serial hCG levels until resolution to distinguish a resolving

EPL from an ectopic pregnancy. Fifty percent of patients with ectopic pregnancies will present with declining hCG levels. Research describing the expected elimination of hCG in spontaneous EPL indicate that the minimum rate of decline ranges from 12% to 35% at 2 days to 34% to 84% at 7 days. Faster rates of decline occur with higher initial hCG levels. When the serial decline in hCG is in the range associated with spontaneous EPL, continued surveillance is indicated. If the hCG decline is slower than expected for an EPL, an ectopic pregnancy must be highly suspected.

Uterine Aspiration

The patient presenting with either (1) initial hCG below the discriminatory zone followed by an abnormal rise or decline or (2) initial hCG value at or above the discriminatory zone with no detectable IUP has an abnormal pregnancy. The only exception to the rule for the second scenario would be if a multiple gestation had been conceived. The challenge for the clinician is then to determine whether the pregnancy is nonviable IUP or an ectopic pregnancy. Office uterine vacuum aspiration or dilation and curettage in the operating room can help confirm the diagnosis of EPL or ectopic pregnancy based on the presence or absence of chorionic villi. However, before this is considered, a progressing IUP must be reasonably excluded through serial monitoring with TVUS and hCG levels.

Uterine aspiration may spare some patients from receiving methotrexate[1]. If chorionic villi are present in the uterine aspiration specimen, then a failed IUP is confirmed. No further treatment is indicated. If chorionic villi are absent, hCG levels need to be monitored starting at 12 to 24 hours after the procedure to determine whether they increase, plateau, or decrease appropriately. The hCG trend after uterine aspiration determines whether medical management of ectopic pregnancy with methotrexate should be implemented. The patient's preference, presence of symptoms, and level of clinical suspicion for ectopic pregnancy also play an important role in whether methotrexate is indicated.

There is debate in the literature on whether uterine aspiration is needed before methotrexate is given to treat ectopic pregnancy. Empiric treatment of suspected ectopic pregnancy without the performance of uterine vacuum aspiration or dilation and curettage could result in inappropriate treatment of up to 40% of patients. Performing uterine aspiration could delay treatment of an ectopic pregnancy; however, the risk of tubal rupture for these patients is low (1.7%).

Treatment and Therapeutic Monitoring

Surgery has long been the mainstay of treatment for ectopic pregnancy, but medical management is a widely used alternative. Both are safe and effective treatment options for patients who are clinically stable. The choice of any treatment depends on factors such as clinical presentation, the risks of either surgery or medical management to the patient, and future fertility plans.

Surgical Management

Patients with hemodynamic instability caused by a ruptured ectopic pregnancy require laparotomy and salpingectomy of the involved fallopian tube due to extensive tubal damage. Most patients with ectopic pregnancy who are stable can be safely treated with laparoscopy. For patients with an unruptured ectopic pregnancy, surgical options include tube-sparing salpingostomy or removal of the fallopian tube (salpingectomy).

The decision between salpingostomy and salpingectomy depends on the location of the ectopic pregnancy within the fallopian tube, the extent of the damage to the fallopian tube, and the patient's desire for future fertility. Ideal candidates for salpingostomy include patients who have an ectopic pregnancy in the ampulla or infundibulum of the fallopian tube. Salpingectomy is reserved for patients with isthmic ectopic pregnancies, tubal rupture, or an ipsilateral recurrent ectopic pregnancy. Patients who have completed childbearing might be better candidates for salpingectomy than salpingostomy.

TABLE 1	Contraindications to Medical Management of Ectopic Pregnancy With Methotrexate
Absolute contraindications	Intrauterine pregnancy; breastfeeding; laboratory evidence of immunodeficiency; preexisting blood dyscrasias (bone marrow hypoplasia, leukopenia, thrombocytopenia, or clinically significant anemia); known sensitivity to methotrexate; active pulmonary disease; peptic ulcer disease; clinically significant hepatic, renal, or hematologic dysfunction; hemodynamically unstable patient; inability to participate in follow-up*
Relative contraindications	Ectopic mass >4 cm by TVUS; embryonic cardiac activity by TVUS; high initial hCG concentration (>5,000 mIU/mL); refusal to accept blood transfusion

TVUS, transvaginal ultrasound; hCG, β–human chorionic gonadotropin.
Data are from the American College of Obstetricians and Gynecologists (ACOG).
*A committee opinion published by the American Society for Reproductive Medicine (ASRM) has the same contraindications listed, but the inability to participate in follow-up is listed as a relative contraindication.

With respect to future fertility, subsequent IUP, and repeat ectopic pregnancy, a systematic review and meta-analysis of two randomized controlled trials (RCT) and 16 cohort studies showed that for the RCTs, there was no difference between salpingectomy and salpingostomy. For the cohort studies, salpingectomy was associated with a lower likelihood of subsequent IUP. The cohort studies also found a higher risk for repeat ectopic pregnancy among pregnant people treated by salpingectomy with risk factors for future infertility (previous ectopic pregnancy, endometriosis, history of infertility, history of tubal surgery, pregnancy conceived with in-vitro fertilization, known hydrosalpinx or tubal occlusion, or intraoperative identification of contralateral tubal pathology).

Medical Management

Methotrexate (MTX) is a folic acid antagonist that impairs DNA synthesis and cellular replication targeting rapidly proliferating cells such as trophoblasts. It can be used for medical management of ectopic pregnancy[1] in patients who have a confirmed or high clinical suspicion of ectopic pregnancy, an unruptured mass, and no contraindication to the medication.

Absolute contraindications to medical management of ectopic pregnancy are listed in Table 1. Among the most important of these is the inability of the patient to comply with follow-up after initiation of therapy. Without the ability to monitor the response to MTX and provide additional doses if deemed appropriate, opportunities to prevent ectopic rupture could be missed. To ascertain whether a patient is eligible for MTX therapy, a comprehensive laboratory and medical evaluation should first be performed, including a complete blood count and renal and liver function tests. Treatment failure occurs when the hCG level decline is deemed inadequate and surgery is required. In some cases, medication failure presents as tubal rupture requiring emergent surgery.

Relative contraindications in Table 1 pertain to patient characteristics that reduce the odds of successful treatment. The strongest predictor for the efficacy of MTX treatment is an initial hCG concentration >5000 mIU/mL, and it is associated with a failure rate of at least 14.3%.

Three methotrexate treatment regimens exist: single-dose, two-dose, and multidose regimens (Table 2). These designations refer more to the number of intended doses in the protocol rather than the actual number of doses received by all patients. For any of the protocols, once hCG levels have declined by at least 15% between interval assessments, no additional doses of medication are required, but hCG must still be followed until complete resolution to ensure treatment efficacy. A systematic review and meta-analysis

---

[1]Not FDA approved for this indication.

[1]Not FDA approved for this indication.

TABLE 2 Methotrexate[1] Protocols for Treatment of Ectopic Pregnancy

	SINGLE DOSE	TWO DOSE	MULTIDOSE
Day 1	Check hCG value. Administer first dose of MTX 50 mg/m^2 IM.	Check hCG value. Administer first dose of MTX 50 mg/m^2 IM.	Check hCG value. Administer first dose of MTX 1 mg/kg IM followed by folinic acid (leucovorin)[1] 0.1 mg/kg IM on day 2. Check hCG on day 2.
Day 4	Check hCG value.	Check hCG value. Administer second dose of MTX 50 mg/m^2 IM.	Administer second dose of MTX (day 3) and folinic acid (day 4). Administer third dose of MTX (day 5). Check hCG on day 3 and 5.
Day 7	Check hCG value looking for 15% decrease between days 4 and 7. If >15% fall, check hCG weekly until undetectable. If <15% fall, administer second dose of MTX 50 mg/m^2 IM.	Check hCG value for 15% decrease between days 4 and 7. If >15% fall, check hCG weekly until undetectable. If <15% fall, administer third dose of MTX 50 mg/m^2 IM.	Continue administering alternating doses of MTX and folinic acid until hCG values decline by 15%. Do not exceed 4 doses. If >15% decline, check hCG weekly until undetectable.
Day 11		Check hCG value for 15% decrease between days 7 and 11. If >15% decline, check hCG weekly until not detectable in serum. If <15%, administer fourth dose of MTX 50 mg/m^2 IM.	
Weekly surveillance	If follow-up hCG value plateau or rise, consider surgical intervention or repeat dose of MTX as additional therapy.	If follow-up hCG value plateau or rise, consider surgical intervention or repeat dose of MTX as additional therapy.	If follow-up hCG value plateau or rise, consider surgical intervention or repeat dose of MTX as additional therapy.

hCG, β–Human chorionic gonadotropin; IM, intramuscular; MTX, methotrexate.
[1]Not FDA approved for this indication.

of six RCTs demonstrated that the single-dose and multiple-dose regimens have similar success rates, and the difference between the single-dose and double-dose regimens was not statistically significant. More side effects occurred with the multiple-dose regimen compared with single-dose and double-dose. The definition of successful treatment with MTX is resolution of the ectopic pregnancy without surgery, and the success rate ranges from 70% to 95% depending on the initial hCG level and treatment protocol.

The biggest risk of medical management with MTX is ectopic pregnancy rupture. Additional risks include fetal death or teratogenic effects if an IUP occurs shortly after treatment, and patients should be counseled to wait one ovulatory cycle after hCG levels are undetectable before attempting pregnancy again.

Side effects of MTX therapy occur in up to 30% of patients; however, most resolve rapidly and are mild. Abdominal pain is common early in treatment, possibly due to tubal miscarriage, but it can also be a sign of tubal rupture. Additional potential side effects include nausea, vomiting, diarrhea, gastritis, stomatitis, and liver transaminitis. Serious side effects such as alopecia and neutropenia can occur but are extremely rare.

Reproductive success after successful MTX therapy appears similar to that after salpingostomy. The most critical predictors of fertility after ectopic pregnancy treated by any conservative means are the condition of the contralateral fallopian tube and the presence of additional ectopic risk factors.

Expectant Management

Because numerous ectopic pregnancies resolve spontaneously, there has been great interest in considering expectant management in patients who are asymptomatic, have a plateau or decreasing hCG level, and are willing to accept the risks (spontaneous rupture, hemorrhage, and need for emergency surgery). A systematic review and meta-analysis of four RCTs showed no statistically significant difference between expectant management and MTX for these selected patients when the hCG level is less than 2000 IU/L. Expectant management includes close monitoring of symptoms, determination of hCG levels every 48 hours, serial TVUS. Medical or surgical management is indicated if hCG levels do not sufficiently decrease.

Trauma-Informed Care

Being diagnosed with and treated for an ectopic pregnancy is a traumatic event for many patients, and the psychological implications can be overlooked. A multicenter prospective cohort study found patients with an ectopic pregnancy met criteria for posttraumatic stress (23%), moderate to severe anxiety (21%), and moderate to severe depression (7%) one month after their experience. These psychological sequelae declined over time but were still clinically significant at 9 months. A trauma-informed approach can help clinicians be intentional in supporting patients with an ectopic pregnancy during treatment, posttreatment, and with any future pregnancies.

References

ACOG: Practice bulletin No. 193 interim update: tubal ectopic pregnancy, *Obstet Gynecol* 131:e91–e103, 2018.

Barnhart KT, Guo W, Cary MS, et al: Differences in serum human chorionic gonadotropin rise in early pregnancy by race and value at presentation, *Obstet Gynecol* 128:504–511, 2016.

Barnhart K, van Mello NM, Bourne T, et al: Pregnancy of unknown location: a consensus statement of nomenclature, definitions, and outcome, *Fertil Steril* 95:857–866, 2011.

Connolly A, Ryan DH, Stuebe AM, Wolfe HM: Reevaluation of discriminatory and threshold levels for serum beta-hCG in early pregnancy, *Obstet Gynecol* 121:65–70, 2013.

Farren J, Jalmbrant M, Falconieri N, et al: Posttraumatic stress, anxiety and depression following miscarriage and ectopic pregnancy: a multicenter, prospective, cohort study, *Am J Obstet Gynecol* 222(4):367.e1–367.e22, 2020.

Hendriks E, Rosenberg R, Prine L: Ectopic pregnancy: diagnosis and management, *Am Fam Physician* 101(10):599–606, 2020. PMID: 32412215.

Insogna IG, Farland LV, Missmer SA, Ginsburg ES, Brady PC: Outpatient endometrial aspiration: an alternative to methotrexate for pregnancy of unknown location, *Am J Obstet Gynecol* 217:185.e1–185.e9, 2017.

Naveed AK, Anjum MU, Hassan, A, et al: Methotrexate versus expectant management in ectopic pregnancy: a meta-analysis, *Arch Gynecol Obstet* 305(3):547–553, 2022.

Ozcan MCH, Wilson JR, Frishman GN: A systematic review and meta-analysis of surgical treatment of ectopic pregnancy with salpingectomy versus salpingostomy, *J Minim Invasive Gynecol* 28(3):656–667, 2021. https://doi.org/10.1016/j.jmig.2020.10.014. Epub 2020 Oct 24. PMID: 33198948.

Yang C, Cai J, Geng Y, Gao Y: Multiple-dose and double-dose versus single-dose administration of methotrexate for the treatment of ectopic pregnancy: a systematic review and meta-analysis, *Reprod Biomed Online* 34(4):383–391, 2017. https://doi.org/10.1016/j.rbmo.2017.01.004.

HYPERTENSIVE DISORDERS IN PREGNANCY

Method of
Marc Parrish, DO; and Juliana Bakk, MD

CURRENT DIAGNOSIS

- Hypertensive disorders in pregnancy complicate 2% to 8% of pregnancies and are among the leading causes of maternal and perinatal death worldwide.
- Hypertensive disorders are divided into four categories:
  - Chronic hypertension
  - Chronic hypertension with superimposed preeclampsia (with and without severe features)
  - Gestational hypertension
  - Preeclampsia (with and without severe features)
- Preeclampsia can be diagnosed without proteinuria in the presence of end organ damage.

CURRENT THERAPY

- The only current method for prevention of preeclampsia is administration of aspirin[1] (81 mg/day) to patients who are at risk, optimally prior to 16 weeks' gestation.
- The definition for an elevated blood pressure (BP) during pregnancy is either systolic greater than 140 mm Hg or diastolic greater than 90 mm Hg on two occasions more than 4 hours apart. New-onset hypertensive disease of pregnancy requires these elevations occur after 20 weeks' gestation. If they are prior to 20 weeks' gestation, the patient meets the diagnosis of chronic hypertension.
- Two severe-range BP values (≥160/110 mm Hg), taken 15 to 60 minutes apart, constitute a hypertensive emergency and require intravenous (IV) treatment if the patient has new-onset hypertension in pregnancy.
- Patients with chronic hypertension should receive pharmacologic therapy to keep BP less than 140/90 mm/Hg during pregnancy to decrease adverse events, as reported in the Chronic Hypertension and Pregnancy trial.
- Nifedipine and labetalol are the preferred agents for use during pregnancy. Methyldopa can be used but is typically the second-line because of side effects and lower efficacy.
- Patients diagnosed with gestational hypertension or preeclampsia without severe features can be managed closely as outpatients. They require frequent BP and symptom assessments in addition to laboratory monitoring and fetal testing.
- Delivery is the definitive treatment for preeclampsia, but preeclampsia and eclampsia can present after delivery.
- Hypertensive disorders necessitate earlier delivery. Delivery timing is based off of severity of maternal disease and fetal monitoring.
- IV or intramuscular magnesium sulfate is used for treatment of eclampsia and for prevention of eclampsia in patients diagnosed with preeclampsia with severe features.
- Patients with preeclampsia are at risk for developing hypertension and cardiovascular or renal disease later in life.

[1]Not FDA approved for this indication.

Epidemiology

In the United States, 84% of all maternal deaths have been determined to be preventable. In high-income countries, 16% of maternal deaths are attributed to hypertensive disorders. Chronic hypertension complicates approximately 2% of pregnancies, with the incidence increasing each year because of increasing rates

TABLE 1	Risk Factors for Development of Preeclampsia*
High Risk (incidence ≥8%)	
Chronic hypertension	
History of preeclampsia, especially with adverse outcome	
Autoimmune disease (systemic lupus erythematous, antiphospholipid antibody syndrome)	
Kidney disease	
Pregestational type 1 or 2 diabetes	
Multifetal gestation	
Moderate Risk Factors	
Nulliparity	
Obesity (body mass index > 31)	
First-degree family history of preeclampsia	
Black race	
Low socioeconomic status	
Age ≥ 35 years	
In vitro fertilization	
Personal history factors (low birth weight or small for gestational age, previous adverse pregnancy outcome, >10-year pregnancy interval)	

*Low birth weight or small for gestational age, previous adverse pregnancy outcome, >10-year pregnancy interval.
Data from American College of Obstetricians and Gynecologists. Low-dose aspirin use for the prevention of preeclampsia and related morbidity and mortality. Practice Advisory. ACOG; 2021. Accessed August 22, 2023. https://www.acog.org/clinical/clinical-guidance/practice-advisory/articles/2021/12/low-dose-aspirin-use-for-the-prevention-of-preeclampsia-and-related-morbidity-and-mortality

of advanced maternal age pregnancies and obesity. Approximately 20% to 50% of patients with chronic hypertension will develop superimposed preeclampsia, and 75% of patients with end organ disease prior to pregnancy will develop it. Between 2017 and 2019, the rates of hypertensive disorders of pregnancy among delivery hospitalizations increased from 13.3% to 15.9%, according to the Centers for Disease Control and Prevention. Prevalence is highest among non-Hispanic Black women and women 35 years and older.

Pathophysiology

There are many theories about the development of preeclampsia, but the precise mechanism is still unknown. It is believed that uteroplacental ischemia and inappropriate remodeling of the spiral arterioles within the placenta lead to increased circulating concentrations of antiangiogenic factors and angiogenic imbalances. The complex interaction of vasoactive agents, such as prostacyclin, thromboxane A2, nitric oxide, and endothelins, with opposing effects ultimately results in intense vasospasm. Decreased colloid oncotic pressure causes capillary leak, resulting in increased edema and risk of flash pulmonary edema that is often exacerbated by intravenous (IV) fluid therapy.

Prevention

Low-dose aspirin[1] (81 mg/day) is recommended in women with one high risk factor or more than one moderate risk factor. Table 1 highlights these risk factors. This should be initiated between 12 and 28 weeks' gestation, with the best outcomes resulting from initiation prior to 16 weeks. It should be continued daily until delivery. There is currently no consensus on the optimal dosing of aspirin for the prevention of preeclampsia because some trials have demonstrated a larger impact on prevention with higher doses (100–150 mg/day). No trials have evaluated the efficacy of doses greater than 150 mg, but the higher dose

[1]Not FDA approved for this indication.

TABLE 2 Diagnostic Criteria for Preeclampsia	
Blood pressure	Systolic BP ≥140 mm Hg or diastolic BP ≥90 mm Hg on two occasions at least 4 hours apart after 20 weeks' gestation with previously normal blood pressures Systolic BP ≥160 mm Hg or diastolic BP ≥110 mm Hg (severe hypertension can be confirmed within minutes to ensure timely treatment)
and	
Proteinuria	≥300 mg per 24-h urine collection Protein/creatinine ratio ≥ 0.3 Dipstick reading of 2+ (used only if other methods are not available)

Or in the absence of proteinuria, new-onset hypertension with new onset of any of the following:

Thrombocytopenia (platelet count < 100 × 10⁹/L)	Pulmonary edema
Elevated transaminases more than twice upper limit of normal	Severe headache unresponsive to medication and not accounted for by other diagnoses
Renal insufficiency (creatinine > 1.1 mg/dL or doubling of baseline concentration)	Visual disturbances

Thrombocytopenia (platelet count $< 100 \times 10^9$/L)

Elevated transaminases more than twice upper limit of normal

Renal insufficiency (creatinine > 1.1 mg/dL or doubling of baseline concentration)

Adapted from *ACOG Practice Bulletin #222: Gestational Hypertension and Preeclampsia.*

TABLE 3 Diagnostic Criteria for Preeclampsia With Severe Features*	
Only one criteria is required for diagnosis of severe features as long as it cannot be explained by another cause or diagnosis.	
Symptoms	Severe and persistent right upper quadrant pain or epigastric pain unresponsive to medication Severe headache unresponsive to medication Visual disturbances
Laboratory	Thrombocytopenia (platelet count $< 100 \times 10^9$/L) Elevated transaminases more than twice upper limit of normal Renal insufficiency (creatinine > 1.1 mg/dL or doubling of baseline concentration)
Vitals/Physical Exam	Systolic blood pressure ≥160 mm Hg or diastolic blood pressure ≥110 mm Hg on two occasions 4 hours apart Pulmonary edema

*Of note, fetal growth restriction and significant proteinuria (>5 g/24 h) are no longer considered severe features.

in North America can be achieved by taking two 81-mg tablets daily. The mechanism by which aspirin prevents preeclampsia is not completely understood but is speculated to be due to improvement in the placentation process and antithrombotic/antiinflammatory effect.

A United States Preventive Services Task Force report on low-dose aspirin identified no increased risk of placental abruption, postpartum hemorrhage, mean blood loss, or congenital anomalies. Aspirin should be avoided in patients with known nasal polyps (use may result in life-threatening bronchoconstriction), aspirin-induced bronchospasm, gastrointestinal bleed, active peptic ulcer disease, or hypersensitivity to nonsteroidal antiinflammatory drugs. Bed rest, dietary modification, and salt restriction have been proven not to assist in the prevention of preeclampsia and are therefore not recommended for this purpose.

Diagnosis

Hypertensive disease prior to 20 weeks' gestation or outside of pregnancy is considered *chronic hypertension*. Patients without this diagnosis who present after 20 weeks' gestation with new-onset hypertension, either systolic blood pressure (BP) of 140 mm Hg or greater or diastolic of 90 mm Hg or greater on two occasions more than 4 hours apart, are considered to have *gestational hypertension*.

In 2017, the American College of Cardiology/American Heart Association Hypertension Clinical Practice Guidelines lowered the threshold for diagnosis of stage 1 hypertension outside of pregnancy from 140/90 mm Hg to 130/80 mm Hg. Patients who meet this new definition of hypertension outside of pregnancy should be managed as having chronic hypertension during pregnancy. Observational studies have shown increased risk of adverse pregnancy outcomes with BPs greater than 130/80 mm Hg in early pregnancy with no previous diagnosis of hypertension, but further studies are necessary to lower the threshold for diagnosis of hypertension during pregnancy. A workup for secondary hypertension should be considered when chronic hypertension is refractory to treatment, if it is diagnosed at a young age, or in patients with features favoring secondary hypertension.

Preeclampsia is a disorder that can affect multiple organ systems and can present any time after 20 weeks' gestation, including during the immediate postpartum period. The traditional diagnosis involves new-onset hypertension (as with gestational hypertension), with the additional finding of proteinuria. Clinically significant proteinuria is 300 mg or greater on a 24-hour urine protein collection or a ratio of 0.3 or greater for spot protein/creatinine. The use of a dipstick for diagnosis is discouraged but can be used if neither of the preferred options is available; concerns for preeclampsia are raised if 3+ protein on dipstick is observed. Severity of proteinuria does not typically correlate with worse disease, and serial measurements of proteinuria are therefore not necessary after the diagnosis is made.

It is important to note that some patients can present with signs of end organ damage *without proteinuria* and would thus still meet the diagnosis of preeclampsia. The presence of any severe feature is concerning for severe disease and impending eclampsia. These features include thrombocytopenia, renal insufficiency (serum creatinine > 1.1 mg/dL), impaired liver function (serum aspartate transaminase [AST] and alanine aminotransferase [ALT] double the institutional upper limits of normal), persistent right upper quadrant pain, pulmonary edema, headache unresponsive to medication, or new visual disturbances.

Women with new-onset hypertension in pregnancy who develop severe-range BPs (two BP values ≥160/110 mm Hg taken ≥4 hours apart) should be diagnosed with preeclampsia with severe features. Other criteria for severe features are listed in Table 3. Patients with preeclampsia superimposed on chronic hypertension will meet criteria for severe features with any of these findings as well.

Management

Chronic Hypertension

Chronic hypertension is associated with many complications of pregnancy (fetal growth restriction, placental abruption, medically indicated preterm birth, perinatal death) and is the greatest risk factor for the development of preeclampsia. Patients with chronic hypertension are also at an increased risk for gestational diabetes, pulmonary edema, acute kidney injury, cardiomyopathy or cardiac events, stroke, and maternal mortality. Prior to 2022 treatment of chronic hypertension of pregnancy aimed to keep the blood pressure below 160/100 mm Hg. Studies using lower target blood pressure levels with higher doses and more frequent dosing of antihypertensive medications showed increased rates of fetal growth restriction and a lack of improved maternal outcomes.

The Chronic Hypertension and Pregnancy trial published in 2022 resulted in Society of Maternal-Fetal Medicine and American Congress of Obstetricians and Gynecologists recommending targeting BPs below 140/90 mm Hg during pregnancy. This study

	TABLE 4	Common Dosages for Oral Antihypertensive Agents During Pregnancy

DRUG	DOSE	TYPICAL INITIAL DOSE	TYPICAL MAXIMUM DOSE	CAUTION
Labetalol	200–2,400 mg/d PO, 2–3 times daily	100–200 mg twice daily	800 mg three times daily	Avoid labetalol with history of asthma or heart dysfunction
Nifedipine (extended-release)	30–120 mg/d PO	30 mg once daily	60 mg twice daily[3]	Avoid nifedipine with tachycardia. Sublingual and immediate-release formulations are reserved for treatment of acute elevations
Methyldopa	500–3000 mg/d PO, 2–4 times daily	250 mg twice daily	3 g/d in 2–4 divided doses	Side effects are sedation, depression, and dizziness.

[3]Exceeds dosage recommended by the manufacturer.
Not recommended during pregnancy: angiotensin-converting enzyme inhibitors, angiotensin receptor blockers, renin inhibitors, and mineralocorticoid receptor antagonists.
PO, Orally.
Adapted from American College of Obstetricians and Gynecologists (ACOG): *Chronic Hypertension in Pregnancy. Practice Bulletin #223*, January 2019.

found that patients in this treatment group compared with standard treatment had a lower composite incidence of preeclampsia with severe features, medically indicated preterm birth at less than 35 weeks' gestation, placental abruption, or fetal or neonatal death, (30.2% vs. 37.0% for adjusted risk ratio of 0.82 [95% CI 0.74 to 0.92, $P < 0.001$]) without an increase in the incidence of small-for-gestational-age birth weights or other neonatal morbidity. Patients with underlying renal dysfunction or comorbidities may benefit from a lower threshold for treatment. However, it is recommended to maintain BPs at or above 120/80 mm Hg during pregnancy.

Preferred treatment of hypertension during pregnancy includes nifedipine and labetalol. Methyldopa is less effective and has more adverse side effects. Hydrochlorothiazide can be used but is typically second-line and administered in consultation with maternal fetal medicine (see Table 4 for dosage information). The use of angiotensin-converting enzyme inhibitors, angiotensin receptor blockers, renin inhibitors, and mineralocorticoid receptor antagonists is generally not recommended for use during pregnancy. Nonpregnant women taking these medications who are of childbearing age should be counseled about effective birth control methods or transitioned to a different regimen. Atenolol (Tenormin) is also not recommended because of the increased risk of fetal growth restriction.

Patients with chronic hypertension should have baseline laboratory testing (complete blood count, serum liver function levels, electrolyte levels, creatinine levels, blood urea nitrogen levels, and urine protein/creatinine ratio with 24-hour urine protein if the protein/creatinine ratio is abnormal or borderline) in the first trimester. If there is concern about heart disease or the patient has long-standing hypertension, electrocardiogram with or without transthoracic echocardiogram should be obtained. The fetus should be monitored with serial growth ultrasounds every 4 weeks after 20 weeks' gestation and with weekly antenatal testing after 32 weeks, with nonstress testing or a biophysical profile; the choice is typically institution-dependent because of the lack of definitive data.

Gestational Hypertension

Gestational hypertension is managed expectantly with delivery scheduled no later than 37 weeks' gestation or at diagnosis if after 37 weeks' gestation. Prior to 37 weeks, patients can be monitored as outpatients twice weekly with BP and symptom assessments, laboratory monitoring, and antenatal testing. Fetal growth should be monitored at least every 4 weeks. Patients should be closely monitored for worsening disease, with a low threshold for inpatient observation and administration of corticosteroids (12 mg betamethasone [Celestone Soluspan][1] intramuscularly [IM] every

24 hours for 2 doses OR 6 mg betamethasone every 12 hours for 4 doses) to prompt fetal lung maturity if preterm.

Preeclampsia With and Without Severe Features

Preeclampsia without severe features should be managed similarly to gestational hypertension. If severe features develop (see Table 3) before 34 weeks' gestation, the patient should be managed as an inpatient until delivery at 34 weeks' gestation. If prior to 34 weeks' gestation, the patient should be given corticosteroids to prompt fetal lung maturity, and delivery should be delayed for 48 hours unless there are contraindications to expectant management. The contraindications to expectant management include uncontrolled severe-range BPs not responsive to antihypertensive medication, persistent headache refractory to repeat treatment without other cause, epigastric or right upper quadrant pain without other cause unresponsive to repeat analgesics, stroke, myocardial infarction, HELLP (*h*emolysis, *e*levated *l*iver enzymes, and *low p*latelet count) syndrome, worsening renal dysfunction, eclampsia, pulmonary edema, suspected acute placental abruption, abnormal fetal testing, fetal death, or lethal anomaly/extreme prematurity. If severe features develop later than 34 weeks' gestation, the patient should be delivered without waiting for the corticosteroid window to be complete.

If the patient is able to be expectantly managed until delivery at 34 weeks' gestation, oral antihypertensives can be initiated to increase the time before delivery is necessary (see Table 5 for agents used for acute BP control). It is recommended to start magnesium sulfate (MgSO4) to prevent eclampsia, and this can be discontinued once stability is proven and if the patient is not being delivered. MgSO4 is initiated with a 4 to 6 g IV loading dose given over 15 to 30 minutes, followed by 1 to 2 g/h maintenance infusion. Patients less than 32 weeks' gestation have the added benefit of fetal neuroprotection from magnesium and should be treated with the higher dose if tolerated. Patients on magnesium should be monitored with hourly neurologic exam, vitals and intake/output (see Table 6 for signs and symptoms of magnesium toxicity). If this is suspected, magnesium should be immediately discontinued, and the magnesium level should be obtained. Patients at risk of impending respiratory depression may require intubation and treatment with 10 mL of 10% calcium gluconate IV along with IV furosemide. Patients undergoing inpatient expectant management should have MgSO4 reinitiated prior to anticipated delivery and continued for 24 hours postpartum.

Patients should be counseled on mode of delivery by usual obstetric indications. However, the likelihood of cesarean delivery ranges from 65% to 97% if delivery is occurring at less than 32 weeks' gestation. The decision for mode of delivery should be individualized in these circumstances, as well as in patients with associated fetal morbidities.

Preeclampsia may begin or worsen in the postpartum period, so serum labs (liver function, electrolyte levels, creatinine levels, blood urea nitrogen), symptoms, and BP should be monitored

[1]Not FDA approved for this indication.

TABLE 5 Antihypertensive Agents Used for Acute Blood Pressure Management

The trigger is severe-range BP (SBP ≥160 mm Hg or DBP ≥110 mm Hg) that persists for 15 minutes or more; continue treatment algorithm if BP continues to be severe range on rechecks

DRUG ALGORITHM	CAUTION	FIRST DOSE	SECOND DOSE	THIRD DOSE/ ACTION	FOURTH ACTION
Labetalol (maximum daily dose 300 mg, administer each dose over 2 minutes)	Avoid labetalol with active asthma and heart disease/CHF. It may cause fetal bradycardia.	20 mg IV, BP repeated in 10 minutes	40 mg IV, BP repeated in 10 minutes	80 mg IV, BP repeated in 10 minutes	Move to hydralazine algorithm, and consult.*
Hydralazine[1] (maximum daily dose 20 mg)	Risk of maternal hypotension is higher with frequent dosing.	5–10 mg IV, BP repeated in 20 minutes	10 mg IV, BP repeated in 20 minutes	Move to labetalol algorithm.	Consult.*
Nifedipine[1] (immediate-release, maximum daily dose 180 mg)	Nifedipine may cause reflex tachycardia and headaches.	10 mg PO, BP repeated in 20 minutes	20 mg PO, BP repeated in 20 minutes	20 mg PO, BP repeated in 20 minutes	Move to labetalol algorithm, and consult.*

BP, Blood pressure; *CHF,* congestive heart failure; *DBP,* diastolic blood pressure; *IV,* intravenously; *PO,* orally; *SBP,* systolic blood pressure.
*Consult should be placed emergently to MFM, internal medicine, anesthesia, or critical care.
[1]Not FDA approved for this indication.

closely before discharge. Patients with elevated BP around the time of delivery should have a clinic visit to check for vital signs and undergo a limited physical exam no later than 1 week postpartum. Preeclampsia is a risk factor for the future development of hypertension, cardiovascular disease, and renal disease; the risk is twofold higher in women with preeclampsia and eightfold higher for early-onset preeclampsia requiring delivery earlier than 34 weeks' gestation. Two- to five-year follow-up rates of chronic hypertension can be as high as 50%. Patients should be counseled and encouraged to undergo yearly follow-up with their primary care physician, with the workup including, at a minimum, weight monitoring and assessments of BP, lipids, and fasting glucose.

Complications

HELLP Syndrome

HELLP syndrome is a severe form of preeclampsia because of the increased rate of morbidity and mortality. There is debate about the specific criteria for diagnosis, but many clinicians use lactate dehydrogenase (LDH) of 600 IU/L or greater, AST and ALT greater than twice the upper limit of normal, and platelets less than 100×10^9/L as a threshold guide. Other markers for hemolysis besides LDH can be used (peripheral smear, bilirubin > 1.2 mg/dL). HELLP syndrome can have an atypical or slow onset, with 15% of patients lacking hypertension or proteinuria. Thirty percent can present postpartum. Patients can present with generalized malaise, nausea and vomiting, and right upper quadrant pain.

Patients with HELLP syndrome should have serum lab testing for coagulopathy (prothrombin time, partial thromboplastin time, platelet count and fibrinogen) because patients can progress to disseminated intravascular coagulopathy very quickly. Neuraxial anesthesia is typically contraindicated in patients with platelets less than 70×10^9/L because of the risk of epidural hematoma. Platelet transfusion is indicated for platelet counts less than 20×10^9/L before vaginal delivery and less than 50×10^9/L before cesarean delivery or with active bleeding.

Patients with stable serum labs can be expectantly managed on MgSO4 through the corticosteroid window (48 hours after the first dose) if they are diagnosed prior to 34 weeks' gestation. Management and delivery timing in this situation should occur with consultation of a maternal-fetal medicine specialist.

Eclampsia

Eclampsia is a life-threatening complication of hypertensive disorders of pregnancy involving new-onset tonic-clonic, focal, or multifocal seizures in the absence of other causative conditions. A small proportion of patients with preeclampsia without severe features (1.9%) or preeclampsia with severe features (3.2%) developed eclampsia in the placebo arm of two randomized controlled trials evaluating seizure prophylaxis. Eclampsia is a significant cause of maternal death, especially in low-resource settings, and should be treated as an obstetric emergency. Eclampsia can occur before, during, or after delivery and is typically preceded by neurologic symptoms, such as severe headache or visual changes, suggesting cerebral irritation. As with HELLP syndrome, eclampsia can occur in the absence of hypertension or proteinuria. Seizures are typically shorter than 90 seconds, self-limited, and followed by a postictal state. Patients without an IV can have 5 g of $MgSO_4$ administered IM in each buttock. For those with IV access, a loading dose of 6 g of MgSO4 should be given over a period of 15 to 30 minutes and then the maintenance infusion should be 2 g/h and continued for 24 hours after the last seizure. If seizures persist, the patient should be evaluated for other causes and treated with lorazepam (Ativan) 2 to 4 mg IV (repeated after 10–15 minutes if necessary) or diazepam 5 to 10 mg IV every 5 to 10 minutes (maximum dose of 30 mg). Care should be taken during the seizure to protect the patient's airway, reduce risk of aspiration, and prevent maternal injury. Fetal monitoring should be accomplished when feasible, but delivery should not be undertaken until the mother is stable. If the patient lacks refractory seizures or other factors necessitating emergent delivery, the patient can undergo an induction of labor and have cesarean delivery reserved for usual obstetric circumstances.

TABLE 6 Signs and Symptoms of Magnesium Toxicity

SERUM MAGNESIUM CONCENTRATION (mg/dL)	EFFECT
5–9	Typical therapeutic range
>9	Loss of patellar reflex, double vision
10–12	Somnolence, slurred speech
>12	Respiratory paralysis
>30	Cardiac arrest

Contraindications to magnesium: myasthenia gravis; avoid with pulmonary edema and use caution in renal insufficiency (magnesium sulfate is renally cleared).

References

ACOG Committee Opinion No. 743: Low-dose aspirin use during pregnancy, *Obstet Gynecol* 132:e44–e52, 2018.

American College of Obstetricians and Gynecologists (ACOG): Gestational Hypertension and Preeclampsia, *Practice Bulletin* 222, 2020.

American College of Obstetricians and Gynecologists (ACOG): Chronic Hypertension in Pregnancy, *Practice Bulletin* 223, 2019.

CDC Pregnancy-Related Deaths: Data from Maternal Mortality Review Committees in 36 US States, 2017–2019. Susanna Trost, MPH; Jennifer Beauregard, MPH, PhD; Gyan Chandra, MS, MBA; Fanny Njie, MPH; Jasmine Berry, MPH; Alyssa Harvey, BS; David A. Goodman, MS, PhD

CDC Morbidiy and Mortality Weekly Report. Hypertensive Disorders in Pregnancy and Mortality at Delivery Hospitalization — United States, 2017 2019. Weekly / April 29, 2022 / 71(17);585–591. Nicole D. Ford, PhD[1]; Shanna Cox, MSPH[1]; Jean Y. Ko, PhD[1]; Lijing Ouyang, PhD[1]; Lisa Romero, DrPh[1]; Tiffany Colarusso, MD[1]; Cynthia D. Ferre, MA[1]; Charlan D. Kroelinger, PhD[1]; Donald K. Hayes, MD[2]; Wanda D. Barfield, MD[1]

Creasy & Resnik's Maternal-Fetal Medicine: Chapter 72: Pregnancy as a Window to Future Health; and Chapter 48: Pregnancy-Related Hypertension

Davidson KW, Barry MJ, Mangione CM, et al: Aspirin use to prevent preeclampsia and related morbidity and mortality: US Preventive Services Task Force Recommendation Statement. US Preventive Services Task Force, *JAMA* 326:1186–1191, 2021.

Roberge S, Nicolaides K, Demers S, Hyett J, Chaillet N, Bujold E: The role of aspirin dose on the prevention of preeclampsia and fetal growth restriction: systematic review and meta-analysis, *Am J Obstet Gynecol* 216(2):110–120, 2017.

(The RCT ASPRE Trial), Rolnik DL, Wright D, Poon LC, et al: Aspirin versus Placebo in Pregnancies at High Risk for Preterm Preeclampsia, *N Engl J Med* 377(7):613–622, 2017.

Tita AT, Szychowski JM, Boggess K, et al: Chronic Hypertension and Pregnancy (CHAP) Trial Consortium. Treatment for Mild Chronic Hypertension during Pregnancy, *N Engl J Med* 386(19):1781–1792, 2022.

Whelton PK, Carey RM, Aronow WS, et al: 2017 ACC/AHA/AAPA/ABC/ACPM/AGS/APhA/ASH/ASPC/NMA/PCNA Guideline for the Prevention, Detection, Evaluation, and Management of High Blood Pressure in Adults: A Report of the American College of Cardiology/American Heart Association Task Force on Clinical Practice Guidelines, *Hypertension* 71(6):e13–e115, 2018, https://doi.org/10.1161/HYP.0000000000000065. Epub 2017 Nov 13. Erratum in: Hypertension. 2018 Jun;71(6):e140-e144.

POSTPARTUM CARE

Method of
Tara J. Neil, MD

CURRENT DIAGNOSIS

- The postpartum period consists of the period from delivery of the infant until 6 to 8 weeks postpartum.
- Postpartum hemorrhage is a medical emergency and is usually caused by uterine atony.
- Fever during the postpartum period is typically caused by endometritis or mastitis.

CURRENT THERAPY

- Continue to monitor and check for resolution of any complications or medical conditions that arise during pregnancy.
- Uterine atony responds to massage and medications. Providers should be familiar with the medications and their dosages.
- Postpartum contraception counseling should be started immediately and all forms can be used by 6 weeks postpartum.
- Breastfeeding is the preferred nutrition for newborns and success is dependent on provider counseling and encouragement.

Postpartum care encompasses the period after delivery of infant and placenta until 6 to 8 weeks after delivery. The hormonal and physiologic systems that underwent changes during pregnancy return to normal during this time. During the initial 24 to 48 hours, most patients are monitored in the hospital for possible complications after delivery.

| BOX 1 | Causes of Postpartum Hemorrhage |

- Uterine atony
- Vaginal or cervical laceration
- Coagulation disorder
- Uterine inversion
- Retained placenta/products

Postpartum Hemorrhage

Postpartum hemorrhage is defined as total blood loss of greater than 1000 mL or signs of hypovolemia. It is the major cause of maternal morbidity and mortality worldwide. Practitioners should be prepared to diagnose and treat the cause.

Some common causes of hemorrhage are identified in Box 1, including the most common cause: uterine atony. Once abnormal bleeding is identified, resuscitation measures should be started, including intravenous (IV) access, nursing assistance, starting fluid resuscitation with crystalloids or blood products, and anesthesia if needed. In addition, administration of tranexamic acid (Cyklokapron)[1] 1000 mg IV has been shown to decrease mortality regardless of the cause of bleeding. The uterus should be examined using a bimanual examination and vigorous massage. If the uterus is boggy, the medications listed in Table 1 can be used to improve uterine tone and decrease bleeding. If the bladder is full, a catheter should be placed. Careful inspection of the cervix, vaginal walls, and perineum should be performed to identify other sources of hemorrhage. If bleeding is not slowed or the cause of hemorrhage not identified, manual exploration of the uterus can be performed with proper anesthesia to check for retained products. Surgical treatment with dilation and curettage and hysterectomy can also be used if manual exploration and medical management do not control bleeding. If the patient is hemodynamically stable and the resources are available, embolization of the uterine arteries can also control bleeding.

Postpartum Care After Hospital Dismissal

Clinical care in the postpartum period should be focused on continued care of the mom and baby and not as a single visit. To better facilitate this, the patient should have clinical contact by phone or at appointment with the provider or clinical team in the first 3 weeks. Ongoing care should be provided on an as-needed basis. Ultimately, the postpartum period ends with a comprehensive visit and exam occurring by 12 weeks. This visit should include full physical and psychosocial assessment as well as discussion of interpregnancy spacing and management of any chronic health conditions.

Fever and Infection

Fever greater than 38°C (100.4°F) should be evaluated and a source identified. Box 2 lists the most common causes of postpartum fever. Evaluation should include a physical examination to include the uterus and breasts, with attention to any lacerations or incisions. Laboratory testing should include urinalysis, complete blood count (CBC), and blood cultures if appropriate.

Endometritis, a polymicrobial infection of the endometrium of the uterus, typically causes fever in the first 1 to 2 weeks postpartum. Diagnostic criteria include fever and uterine pain with palpation. Endometritis is treated with IV broad-spectrum antibiotics until fever and uterine pain resolve. If there is no clinical improvement after several days of treatment, imaging with computed tomography (CT) or ultrasound of the pelvis can be used to look for complications, including pelvic abscess and septic pelvic thrombophlebitis.

Mastitis causes fever in breastfeeding mothers. It is caused by the introduction of skin flora through cracks in the nipple and skin and infects milk ducts and surrounding soft tissues in areas of stasis. Treatment includes frequent feeding or pumping to alleviate

---

[1]Available as dietary supplement.

TABLE 1 Medications Used to Treat Uterine Atony

MEDICATION	ADMINISTRATION	FREQUENCY	SPECIAL CONSIDERATIONS
Oxytocin (Pitocin)	10 units IM 10–40 units in 1000 mL of IV solution	Once Continuous to maintain uterine tone	Should not be given directly in IV
Methylergonovine maleate (Methergine)	0.2 mg IM/IV 0.2 mg PO	Repeat every 2–4 h as needed 3–4 times daily for maximum of 7 days	Contraindicated in hypertension
Carboprost tromethamine (Hemabate)	0.25 mg IM	Repeat every 15–90 min. Maximum dose 2 mg	Contraindicated in active cardiac, renal, pulmonary, and liver disease. Use cautiously in asthmatics.
Misoprostol (Cytotec)[1]	800–1000 μg rectally[3]	One-time dose	

[1]Not FDA approved for this indication.
[3]Exceeds dosage recommended by the manufacturer.

BOX 2 Causes of Postpartum Fever

- Mastitis
- Endometritis
- Urinary tract infection
- Wound infection (perineal or abdominal)
- Septic thrombophlebitis
- Deep vein thrombosis

---

the stasis. There is inadequate evidence to support antibiotic use, but if symptoms persist after effectively emptying breasts, most practitioners treat with a 10- to 14-day course of oral narrow-spectrum antibiotics. Complications can include breast abscesses, which are usually diagnosed by ultrasound.

Immunization

Immunizations should be updated during the postpartum period. Rubella status is routinely checked during the prenatal period and immunization should be given if indicated. Tdap (tetanus toxoid, reduced diphtheria toxoid, and acellular pertussis vaccine [Adacel, Boostrix]) should be given to the patient and offered to other members of the family if they have not received a pertussis booster to help protect the infant from contracting pertussis. Influenza vaccine should be given if it was not given during pregnancy. Rh(D)-negative mothers should receive anti-D immune globulin if their infants are Rh(D) positive.

Breastfeeding

Breast milk is universally recognized as the best nutrition for newborns. Infants who are breastfed have fewer ear, lower respiratory, and gastrointestinal infections. They are also less likely to develop asthma, diabetes, and obesity. Contraindications to breastfeeding include human immunodeficiency virus (HIV), active herpetic lesions on breasts, maternal drug abuse, and certain medications. Any medications prescribed during breastfeeding should be checked for safety. It is currently recommended, when possible, for infants to be exclusively breastfed until 6 months and supplemented with foods between the ages of 6 months and 1 year. Clinicians play a crucial role in educating mothers about the importance of breastfeeding and supporting them during breastfeeding.

Contraception

Discussing contraception after delivery is important for healthy birth spacing. Ovulation can occur as early as 3 weeks after delivery. Breastfeeding mothers can use lactational amenorrhea during this period if they are exclusively breastfeeding. They can also use progesterone-only contraception (Micronor, Depo-Provera, Nexplanon) or intrauterine device starting 6 weeks postpartum. Combined estrogen-progesterone formulations can be started as early as 3 weeks postpartum in nonbreastfeeding mothers. Starting estrogen-containing formulations before this can increase the risk for thromboembolism. Intrauterine devices and diaphragms are typically placed at 6 weeks after the uterus has returned to its normal size. Medroxyprogesterone intramuscular (IM) injection (Depo-Provera) and etonogestrel subcutaneous (SC) implant (Nexplanon) may be given in the first 5 days postpartum if a patient is not breastfeeding.

Other Considerations

Close evaluation and continued management of medical conditions that develop during pregnancy, including thyroid disease, gestational diabetes, and preeclampsia, should be continued.

The postpartum period is an important time for new mothers. Open communication with their providers during this time helps support them and helps them to recognize conditions that are important for their health and the health of their newborn.

References

American College of Obstetricians and Gynecologists: *Compendium of selected publications*, Atlanta, 2007, American College of Obstetricians and Gynecologists.

Breastfeeding, Family Physicians Supporting. Available at. http://www.aafp.org/online/en/home/policy/policies/b/breastfeedingpositionpaper.html (accessed February 25, 2020).

Centers for Disease Control: Pertussis (whooping cough) vaccination. Available at http://www.cdc.gov/vaccines/vpd-vac/pertussis/default.htm (accessed February 25, 2020).

Committee on Practice Bulletins-Obstetrics. Practice bulletin no. 183: postpartum hemorrhage, *Obstet Gynecol* 130(4):e168–e186, 2017.

French LM, Smaill FM: Antibiotic regimens for endometritis after delivery, *Cochrane Database Syst Rev* (4):CD001067, 2004.

Jahanfar S, Ng C-J, Teng CL: Antibiotics for mastitis in breastfeeding women, *Cochrane Database Syst Rev* 1:CD005458, 2009.

Optimizing postpartum care. ACOG Committee Opinion No. 736: American College of Obstetricians and Gynecologists, *Obstet Gynecol* 131:e140–e150, 2018.

Truitt ST, Fraser AB, Gallo MFet al, et al: Combined hormonal versus nonhormonal versus progestin-only contraception in lacation, *Cochrane Database Syst Rev* (2):CD003988, 2003.

WOMAN Trial Collaborators: Effect of early tranexamic acid administration on mortality, hysterectomy, and other morbidities in women with post-partum haemorrhage (WOMAN): an international, randomised, double-blind, placebo-controlled trial, *Lancet* 389(10084):2105–2116, 2017.

POSTPARTUM DEPRESSION

Method of
Daniel Stephen Oram, MD; and Lydia U. Lee, MD

CURRENT DIAGNOSIS

- All pregnant and postpartum women should be screened for postpartum depression with a validated tool, such as the Edinburgh Postpartum Depression Scale.
- Care should be taken to exclude bipolar disorder.

CURRENT THERAPY

- Cognitive behavioral therapy and interpersonal therapy are the most well-studied interventions.
- Selective serotonin reuptake inhibitors are modestly effective for postpartum depression and are generally safe, with most data for sertraline (Zoloft).[1]
- Zuranolone (Zurzuvae), an allopregnanolone analogue affecting GABA receptors, has recently been shown in randomized controlled trials to rapidly improve symptoms of postpartum depression.

[1]Not FDA approved for this indication.

Introduction

Postpartum depression is a common mood disorder that carries the potential for substantial morbidity. There is no universally agreed-upon definition. Increasingly, postpartum- and antepartum-onset depression are being considered together as peripartum depression; the *Diagnostic and Statistical Manual of Mental Disorders*, fifth edition (DSM-5) uses the specifier "with peripartum onset" to refer to an episode of major depression that occurs during pregnancy or within 4 weeks of delivery. Clinically, however, postpartum depression is often identified if onset is within 1 year of delivery. There are considerations in management of mood disorders that are unique to the postpartum period. Therefore this chapter will focus on depressive episodes with postpartum onset, in line with much of the primary literature on this topic.

Epidemiology

In developed countries, postpartum depression has an incidence of about 15% (including both major and minor depression) in the first 3 months of the postpartum period. Worldwide prevalence varies widely by country; estimates using most rigorous methods vary from 0.1% to 26%, with culture influencing both maternal mood and how mood symptoms are communicated.

Risk Factors

The most consistently identified risk factors for depression with postpartum onset include history of mental illness before or during the pregnancy (especially prior postpartum depression, recurrent major depression, and bipolar disorder), stressful life events, poor social support, poor partner relationships, and infant medical illness. Abuse is also frequently reported as a risk factor and includes current or lifetime history of physical, psychological, or sexual abuse by intimate partners or family members. A wide range of other risk factors that have been less consistently cited include infant temperament, negative attitude toward pregnancy, low socioeconomic status, young maternal age, unplanned pregnancy, and obstetric complications. Among women who are identified as having postpartum depression, a recent prospective cohort study predicted risk factors for a severe depressive episode with high accuracy. They found that at-risk women had higher Edinburgh Postpartum Depression Scale (EPDS) scores obtained,

higher parity, lower education, and lower Global Assessment of Functioning scores, although this approach will need further validation.

Pathophysiology

Although the etiology of postpartum depression has not been fully elucidated, it is best understood through a biopsychosocial model. Sex hormones fall rapidly after delivery and likely precipitate depressive symptoms. In particular, experimental evidence in postpartum women supports the role of low postpartum levels of estrogen and the progesterone metabolite allopregnanolone (which affects GABA signaling) in contributing to the depressed mood. Genetic variants in hormonal and serotonergic pathways likely place some women at increased risk. This genetic risk is likely potentiated by social stressors. Finally, cultural factors affect both norms of social support provided to new mothers and the language mothers use to express their symptoms.

Prevention

Care teams should identify women at high risk early in pregnancy; this process should include routine use of a mood inventory such as the EPDS. At-risk women should receive multifaceted support throughout pregnancy and the postpartum period. Components can include a longitudinal patient-provider relationship, which may benefit from more frequent visits, social needs assessment, referral to community maternal–infant health resources, and early initiation of therapy. Interpersonal therapy is the best-supported modality for the prevention of postpartum depression. Postpartum home visits and telephone follow-up have been found helpful in decreasing depression incidence. Starting an antidepressant prophylactically has not been effective experimentally in preventing postpartum depression. However, discontinuing antidepressants prescribed before pregnancy increases the risk of depression relapse, even in women whose depression is in remission before pregnancy.

Clinical Manifestations

In general, postpartum depression is similar to other forms of depression. However, the stresses of feeding and caring for a new infant, changes in partner relationship dynamics, and the sometimes traumatic experiences of childbirth add unique themes to the experience of postpartum depression. Depressive symptoms may arise in part from unmet expectations about childbirth or mothering; a sense of loss is common among women with postpartum depression. Compared with other episodes of depression, postpartum depression episodes are less correlated with sleep or appetite disruption, perhaps because these are common experiences among new mothers. Thoughts of harming the infant are extremely common but of varying severity. Effects of depression may be visible in a dysfunctional parenting style. Conversely, new moms may experience recurrent worries and intrusive thoughts about harm befalling their newborn, sometimes accompanied by a need to repetitively check the infant, which can be reminiscent of obsessive-compulsive disorder.

Diagnosis

Screening should be performed at the initial prenatal visit, later in pregnancy, and at the postpartum visit. The EPDS is the most well-studied inventory and has been validated for use in the identification of patients with postpartum depression. It has a sensitivity of about 80% and a specificity of about 90%. Scores of 13 or higher are generally interpreted as a positive screen. Alternatively, it is reasonable to employ a lower score of 10 as a threshold for pursuing further investigation to improve sensitivity for detecting potential cases of postpartum depression. A clinical interview supportive of an episode of major depression then confirms the diagnosis (Table 1).

Differential Diagnosis

"Baby blues" is the most common mood disruption of the postpartum period. Although it lacks formal diagnostic criteria, it is considered to be a mild, self-limited condition characterized by frequent mood swings that does not extend beyond 2 weeks postpartum.

| TABLE 1 | Abbreviated Diagnostic Criteria for Major Depressive Disorder |

Five or more during a 2-week period; must include either depressed mood or anhedonia.

SYMPTOM	ASSESSED IN EPDS?
Depressed mood	Yes
Anhedonia	Yes
Insomnia/hypersomnia	Yes
Weight or appetite decrease or increase	No
Psychomotor agitation or retardation	No
Fatigue or loss of energy	No
Worthlessness or guilt	Yes
Decreased concentration or indecisiveness	No
Thoughts of death, or suicidal plan/attempt	Yes

EPDS, Edinburgh Postpartum Depression Scale.

Depression Postpartum

Depending on how it is defined, depression is present in 20% to 80% of postpartum women. Bipolar disorder should be considered any time postpartum depression is diagnosed. It is associated with increased morbidity, and antidepressants may trigger manic episodes in affected women. Further, up to 25% of women who screen positive on the EPDS meet criteria for bipolar disorder in some studies. Clinicians should consider routine screening for bipolar disorder with a validated questionnaire such as the Mood Disorder Questionnaire (can be completed by patient on single piece of paper, limited by suboptimal test characteristics) or the CIDI-based Screening Scale for Bipolar Spectrum Disorders (requires clinician to administer; positive answers track DSM criteria for bipolar disorder) at the time of identification of a depressive episode. Finally, review of systems should include evaluation for hallucinations, delusions, or disorganized behaviors that would suggest psychosis.

Therapy

Postpartum depression can often be effectively managed in the primary care setting, and should begin with establishing a supportive clinician–patient relationship through frequent visits. Therapy is the cornerstone of treatment. Cognitive-behavioral therapy and interpersonal therapy are the most well-studied interventions. Interpersonal therapy, which focuses on troubleshooting relationships and maximizing social support, may be particularly well suited to the relational transitions of the postpartum period. However, a wide variety of modalities and settings have been found to be effective. In light of this, brief office interventions can enhance patients' early access to care. For instance, clinicians can use motivational interviewing to support behavioral activation. Similarly, problem-solving interventions can assist patients in working through relationship difficulties, and discussion of mindfulness practices can promote more adaptive responses to stress. In contrast to other forms of depression, the evidence base for pharmacotherapy with standard antidepressants is fairly small, and effect sizes are modest. Selective serotonin reuptake inhibitors (SSRIs) are the best-studied drug class, followed by tricyclic antidepressants (Table 2). Limited experimental evidence has not supported concurrent therapy and antidepressant use. However, this remains a clinically reasonable approach. In severe postpartum depression, therapy and medication may be started concurrently, as medication efficacy may be delayed several weeks. Antidepressant safety is a frequent concern. A detailed discussion of use during pregnancy is outside the scope of this article. The most common class-related adverse effect is neonatal withdrawal, a syndrome of irritability and poor feeding, which affects a minority of infants and is usually self-limited. Inconsistent evidence suggests SSRIs may be associated with a small risk of congenital cardiac lesions (possibly higher risk with paroxetine [Paxil]) or persistent pulmonary hypertension. Antidepressants are generally excreted in low levels in breast milk, and evidence of infant toxicity is limited to case reports. In general, breastfeeding is not contraindicated with antidepressants. Consideration should be given to risk for future pregnancy; for instance, paroxetine is generally avoided in pregnancy because of the potentially higher risk for cardiac anomalies.

In 2023, an oral allopregnanolone analogue, zuranolone (Zurzuvae), was approved by the FDA after two randomized, double-blind, placebo-controlled multicenter studies demonstrated its efficacy. In these studies, symptom improvement occurred as soon as 3 days, and the treatment effect lasted at least 42 days after the last dose. Although not a primary endpoint of the studies, depression remission appeared to be increased in the treatment arm, with a number needed to treat of 7 at day 45 in one of the studies. Studies included women with either third trimester or early postpartum (<4 weeks) depression onset; treatment should be limited to these patient populations until further studies are performed. The medication must be administered with a fatty meal to ensure absorption. Similar to other medications that increase GABA signaling, sedation and dizziness are common side effects, so patients should not drive while taking the medication. Breastfed infants receive a very low relative infant dose of zuranolone, although the clinical effects on breastfed infants have not been studied. Zuranolone may cause fetal harm, and women who take it should use effective contraception. Access to the medication will likely be limited by cost and availability in the short term. Another analogue of allopregnanolone, brexanolone (Zulresso) is also available, with similar efficacy. However, clinical use has been limited by cost and the need for a 60-hour, monitored IV infusion.

Among complementary modalities for treating postpartum depression, exercise has most consistently been shown to be beneficial. Yoga may also facilitate recovery. Limited evidence supports light therapy. The use of supplements is generally not evidence based. For instance, omega-3 fatty acids[7] are the most studied supplement and have not been clearly shown to alleviate postpartum depression.

Monitoring

Clinicians should monitor for return to function in self-care, child care, and other interpersonal relationships. Readministering depression inventories, such as the EPDS, can provide further objective evidence of disease course. An EPDS score of less than 10 is often used as evidence of remission. If antidepressants are being used, they should be continued for a minimum of 6 months beyond entrance into remission.

The maternal–infant pair should be assessed in the office for signs of dysfunctional attachment. Women with depression may display decreased responsiveness to infant needs, or conversely an anxiety-driven overresponsiveness. Breastfeeding difficulties may be a sign of impaired attachment. Clinicians should offer nonjudgmental support to women regardless of their preference to continue or discontinue breastfeeding, as this can be a significant source of stress for some mothers while providing therapeutic benefit to others.

Risk for suicide and infanticide should be assessed routinely. Suicide is a leading cause of death in the postpartum period, and postpartum women may be more likely than their peers to attempt suicide with high-lethality methods such as use of a weapon. Similarly, thoughts of infanticide are very common, although rarely acted upon. Risk-increasing factors include the presence of psychosis, mania, or severe cognitive distortions.

Management of Complications

Hospitalization is indicated if a woman demonstrates signs of mania, psychosis, or high-risk thoughts of suicide or infanticide. Expert consultation should be considered if depression is refractory to therapy or medication. Electroconvulsive therapy has

---

[7] Available as dietary supplement.

TABLE 2 Selected Antidepressant Characteristics for Postpartum Depression

CLASS	MEDICATION	RCT SUPPORTING USE?	PREGNANCY CONSIDERATIONS	BREAST MILK LEVELS	POSSIBLE INFANT ADVERSE EFFECTS?	CLINICAL COMMENTS
SSRIs	Sertraline (Zoloft)[1]	Yes	Preferred SSRI	Very low	None known	Most studied; preferred SSRI during breastfeeding
	Paroxetine (Paxil)[1]	Yes	Possibly higher risk of neonatal symptoms, cardiac malformations	Very low	None known	Well-studied in breastfeeding. Avoid in pregnancy. High risk for maternal withdrawal symptoms
	Fluoxetine (Prozac)[1]	Yes	Delayed infant clearance (long half-life)	Low-medium	Possible: poor weight gain. Case reports: colic, sleep disturbance, GI disturbance	Metabolite with long half-life may dose-accumulate in infant
	Citalopram (Celexa)[1]/ escitalopram (Lexapro)[1]	No[a]	Preferred SSRI	Low	Case reports: sleep disturbance, irritability.	Escitalopram is less well studied than citalopram in breastfeeding, although clinical experience supports a similar safety profile
SNRIs	Venlafaxine (Effexor)[1]	No	Less well-studied than SSRIs	Low	None known	Case reports of higher infant levels of active metabolite. High risk for maternal withdrawal symptoms
	Duloxetine (Cymbalta)[1]	No	Minimal data	Low	None known	Less studied in breastfeeding. Case reports of galactorrhea
Tricyclics	Nortriptyline (Pamelor)[1]	Yes	Less well studied than SSRIs	Low	None known	Well studied in breastfeeding
	Amitriptyline (Elavil)[1]	No		Low	Case report: oversedation	
Allopreg-nanolone analogues	Zuranolone (Zurzuvae)	Yes	May cause fetal harm	Low	Unknown; pregnancy registry available	Administer orally
	Brexanolone (Zulresso)	Yes	May cause fetal harm	Low	Unknown; pregnancy registry available	Administer IV
Other	Bupropion (Wellbutrin)[1]	No	Minimal data	Low	Case report: seizure	Case report of galactorrhea
	Mirtazapine (Remeron)[1]	No	Minimal data	Low	None known	Less studied in breastfeeding. Case reports of galactorrhea

[a]Citalopram (Celexa) and escitalopram (Lexapro) were among medications used in a naturalistic open-label RCT.
[1]Not FDA approved for this indication.
GI, Gastrointestinal; *RCT,* randomized controlled trial; *SNRIs,* serotonin/norepinephrine reuptake inhibitors; *SSRIs,* selective serotonin reuptake inhibitors.

been shown to be effective for treatment of refractory postpartum depression.

References

American College of Obstetricians and Gynecologists: Screening and diagnosis of mental health conditions during pregnancy and postpartum: clinical practice guideline no. 4, *Obstet Gynecol* 141(6):1232–1261, 2023.

Association AP: *Diagnostic and statistical manual of mental disorders (DSM-5®)*, American Psychiatric Pub, 2013.

Deligiannidis KM, Meltzer-Brody SM, Maximos B, et al: Zuranolone for the treatment of postpartum depression, *Am J Psychiatry* 180(9):668–675, 2023.

Dennis CL, Dowswell T: Psychosocial and psychological interventions for preventing postpartum depression, *Cochrane Database Syst Rev* (2):Cd001134, 2013.

Field T: Postpartum depression effects on early interactions, parenting, and safety practices: a review, *Infant Behav Dev* 33(1):1–6, 2010.

Larsen ER, Damkier P, Pedersen LH, et al: Use of psychotropic drugs during pregnancy and breast-feeding, *Acta Psychiatr Scand Suppl* 445:1–28, 2015.

Lindahl V, Pearson JL, Colpe L: Prevalence of suicidality during pregnancy and the postpartum, *Arch Womens Ment Health* 8(2):77–87, 2005.

Meltzer-Brody S, Colquhoun H, Riesenberg R, et al: Brexanolone injection in postpartum depression: two multicentre, double-blind, randomised, placebocontrolled, phase 3 trials, *Lancet* 392(10152):1058–1070, 2018.

Molyneaux E, Howard LM, McGeown HR, Karia AM, Trevillion K: Antidepressant treatment for postnatal depression, *Cochrane Database Syst Rev* (9), 2014.

Molyneaux E, Telesia LA, Henshaw C, Boath E, Bradley E, Howard LM: Antidepressants for preventing postnatal depression, *Cochrane Database Syst Rev* 4:Cd004363, 2018.

Nillni YI, Mehralizade A, Mayer L, Milanovic S: Treatment of depression, anxiety, and trauma-related disorders during the perinatal period: a systematic review, *Clin Psychol Rev* 66:136–148, 2018.

Norhayati MN, Hazlina NH, Asrenee AR, Emilin WM: Magnitude and risk factors for postpartum symptoms: a literature review, *J Affect Disord* 175:34–52, 2015.

O'Connor E, Rossom RC, Henninger M, Groom HC, Burda BU: Primary care screening for and treatment of depression in pregnant and postpartum women: evidence report and systematic review for the US preventive services task force, *JAMA* 315(4):388–406, 2016.

Rundgren S, Brus O, Bave U, et al: Improvement of postpartum depression and psychosis after electroconvulsive therapy: a population-based study with a matched comparison group, *J Affect Dis* 235:258–264, 2018.

Sharma V, Doobay M, Baczynski C: Bipolar postpartum depression: an update and recommendations, *J Affect Dis* 219:105–111, 2017.

Venkatesh KK, Zlotnick C, Triche EW, Ware C, Phipps MG: Accuracy of brief screening tools for identifying postpartum depression among adolescent mothers, *Pediatrics* 133(1):e45–e53, 2014.

VAGINAL BLEEDING IN PREGNANCY

Method of
Zachary J. Baeseman, MD, MPH

CURRENT DIAGNOSIS

- There are several diagnoses in the differential of dangerous late pregnancy bleeding and management varies based on the etiology.
- Avoid digital vaginal examination in a patient with late pregnancy bleeding until placenta previa has been excluded by ultrasound.
- Uterine tenderness with vaginal bleeding is consistent with a clinical diagnosis of placental abruption.
- Vaginal bleeding with a rupture of membranes should prompt consideration of vasa previa.
- Early pregnancy bleeding in a hemodynamically stable patient is worked up with a complete history and physical, complete blood count, human chorionic gonadotropin, and a transvaginal ultrasound.

CURRENT THERAPY

- Placenta previa requires cesarean delivery; however, with a placental edge of more than 2 cm from the cervical os, a vaginal delivery may be attempted in a stable patient.
- Antenatal diagnosis of vasa previa by ultrasound, appropriate administration of antenatal steroids, and a planned cesarean delivery between 34 and 36 weeks gestation is associated with significantly reduced perinatal morbidity and mortality.
- Definitive management of a patient with late-pregnancy bleeding who is hemodynamically unstable should not be delayed in order to obtain an ultrasound or other diagnostic testing.
- In early and late pregnancy bleeding, attention must be directed to the Rh status of the pregnant woman.

Vaginal Bleeding in Late Pregnancy

Epidemiology

Bleeding in the second half of pregnancy complicates 2% to 5% of pregnancies. Placental previa, placental insertion into the lower uterine segment covering all or part of the internal cervical os, causes 30% of late-pregnancy bleeds and occurs in 0.5% of all pregnancies. Placental abruption, premature separation of the placenta from the uterine wall, causes 20% of antepartum hemorrhages and occurs in 1% of all pregnancies. The diagnosis of placental abruption is typically clinical; ultrasound can be useful to rule in the diagnosis, but notably, it can miss >50% of diagnoses. Other serious causes include uterine rupture (occurs in approximately 0.7% of women with a history of previous low-transverse cesarean section) and vasa previa (0.5% of late-pregnancy bleeding and approximately 0.0002% to 0.0008% of all pregnancies). Vasa previa occurs when fetal blood vessels are present in the membranes, traversing the cervix beneath the fetal presenting part.

Risk Factors

Higher parity and maternal age, smoking or cocaine use, a prior history of placenta previa or placental abruption, and multifetal gestation are risk factors for both placenta previa and abruption. Risk factors for placenta previa also include uterine abnormalities, assisted reproductive technology (ART), and history of uterine surgery, including cesarean section. Additional risk factors for abruption include blunt abdominal trauma, polyhydramnios,

hypertensive disorders in pregnancy, and external cephalic version. The greatest risk factor for uterine rupture is a trial of labor after cesarean section (TOLAC), particularly with induction and the use of prostaglandins, which are contraindicated in TOLAC. A uterine scar increases risk; spontaneous uterine rupture is rare on an unscarred uterus. Other risk factors include uterine abnormalities, maternal connective tissue disease, abnormal placentation, and uterine hyperstimulation during labor. Shortened interpregnancy interval (less than 18 to 24 months between pregnancies) can also increase risk. Risk factors for vasa previa include artificial reproductive techniques, bilobed or succenturiate lobed placenta (odds ratio [OR] = 22.11), placenta previa (OR = 22.86), certain fetal anomalies, and a velamentous cord insertion.

Pathophysiology

The cause of placenta previa is unknown but may be related to impaired placental attachment in a uterus with a previous scar. Placental abruption, defined as premature separation of the placenta from the uterus, is caused by hemorrhage where the placenta and decidua meet. Abruption is often preceded by vasospasm (such as that induced by cocaine), thrombosis, or shearing forces. Some cases are acute, but many cases could present a chronic process in which abruption is the end result. Uterine rupture most often occurs in a uterus with a previous scar and is a dehiscence of that scar; often the presenting sign is an abnormal fetal heart rate or a regression of fetal station in labor. The pathophysiology of vasa previa is unknown, although it is theorized to be caused by abnormal development or growth of the umbilical cord secondary to a velamentous insertion or reduced intrauterine space.

Prevention

Previous cesarean section is a risk factor for both placenta previa and uterine rupture, therefore reducing unnecessary cesarean sections can prevent these conditions. Patients who have had a cesarean section should be advised to space out their next pregnancy by 18 to 24 months to mitigate the risk of uterine rupture. Uterine rupture may also be prevented by limiting or avoiding certain agents to induce or augment labor. In women undergoing TOLAC, spontaneous labor is preferred due to the lower risk of uterine rupture. Although vasa previa cannot be prevented, fetal morbidity and mortality are significantly reduced by early diagnosis and delivery. Placental abruption is associated with smoking and cocaine use; counseling directed to cessation theoretically reduces risk. Seat belts are recommended for all pregnant women; trauma sustained during a motor vehicle accident is a potential cause of abruption due to shearing forces. Control of hypertension and treatment of thrombophilia have not been proved to prevent abruption, although both interventions are recommended. Magnesium sulfate given intrapartum to women with preeclampsia can reduce the risk of placental abruption.

Clinical Manifestations

Placenta previa classically manifests with painless vaginal bleeding, whereas placental abruption and uterine rupture are typically associated with pain and bleeding. Because these conditions are not mutually exclusive, it is important to consider the possibility of more than one serious cause of antepartum hemorrhage. Bleeding secondary to placenta previa may be heavy or light, can recur, and is not associated with the degree of previa or prognosis. Thirty percent of women with placental abruption may not present with vaginal bleeding and have a retroplacental clot concealing an abruption. Approximately one half of women with placental abruption present in labor, and 30% of cases are complicated by fetal death. Monitoring can reveal uterine irritability or hypertonicity. Uterine rupture can manifest with abnormal fetal heart tracing, loss of fetal station, or palpable uterine defect. Pain and bleeding might not occur until after uterine rupture, when both maternal and fetal status are compromised. Vasa previa is detectable on ultrasound and color Doppler imaging, but it most commonly presents as vaginal bleeding with rupture ofmembranes. Placental abruption, uterine rupture, and vasa previa can manifest with concerning fetal heart tracings.

Diagnosis

Ultrasound can reliably detect placenta previa and vasa previa. Transvaginal ultrasonography (TVU) is recommended to establish placental location because transabdominal ultrasonography has a false-positive rate for placenta previa up to 25%. TVU has a sensitivity of 87.5% and a specificity of 98.8% for placenta previa and is safe in the presence of vaginal bleeding. Vasa previa can be diagnosed using TVU and color Doppler. High-risk women may be screened in order to plan for cesarean delivery at 34 to 36 weeks of gestation. Vasa previa may also be detected on magnetic resonance imaging (MRI; rarely used), amnioscopy, palpitation of vessels during reginal examination, or identifying fetal blood cells in vaginal blood, although tests to detect fetal hemoglobin cannot be performed quickly enough to be clinically useful. Placental abruption is primarily a clinical diagnosis; it can be ruled in by ultrasound, but notably >50% of cases of placental abruption are missed on ultrasound. The diagnosis is made clinically in a patient with bleeding and a hard or tender uterus, uterine irritability, and often a nonreassuring fetal heart tracing; bleeding may be absent in 20% to 30% of presentations.

Differential Diagnosis

In addition to placenta previa, placental abruption, uterine rupture, and vasa previa, diagnostic considerations include bloody show, cervical trauma, cervical polyp, cervical cancer, or infection.

Therapy

Women with placenta previa and active bleeding are managed expectantly in the hospital, although outpatient management may be a reasonable approach in women who are not bleeding, have adequate support at home, and are able to get to the hospital quickly. Women with any degree of placental overlap with the cervical os should be delivered by cesarean section.

Treatment of women with placental abruption depends on multiple factors including severity of clinical presentation, gestational age, fetal status, and maternal status. In the most severe cases in which there has been fetal death, vaginal delivery is acceptable if the maternal status is reassuring. Because of risk for disseminated intravascular coagulopathy (DIC) and blood loss, women should be carefully monitored, proceeding to cesarean section for worsening maternal status or failed vaginal delivery. In mild cases of placental abruption before term, steroids should be administered between 24 and up to 36 6/7 weeks of gestation; preterm birth is the leading reason for perinatal death. With a stable abruption in a preterm patient with reassuring fetal and maternal status, outpatient management may be reasonable after a period of inpatient observation. Antenatal magnesium sulfate in women <32 weeks gestation can reliably decrease cerebral palsy and neonatal gross motor dysfunction, however, tocolysis is not routinely recommended in placental abruption. Labor may progress toward a goal of vaginal delivery if both maternal and fetal status are reassuring, although cesarean section should be performed expeditiously for any fetal or maternal compromise. Longer decision-to-incision intervals are associated with worse perinatal outcomes. When placental abruption is known or suspected in a term patient, delivery should proceed.

Vasa previa is managed with immediate cesarean section if diagnosed during labor and with a planned cesarean section if diagnosed antenatally. Administration of steroids is recommended at 28 to 34 weeks of gestation depending on the timing of planned delivery, and hospitalization should be considered at around 30 to 32 weeks of gestation because approximately 10% of women have premature rupture of membranes and could need an urgent cesarean section. Certain patients are appropriate candidates for outpatient management. Optimal time for planned cesarean section is not definitely established and has been recommended between 34 and 36 weeks gestation. Neonatal resuscitation,

including fluid resuscitation or transfusion, may be required and should be anticipated.

Uterine rupture is associated with high perinatal morbidity and mortality. When rupture is clinically recognized or suspected, cesarean delivery should proceed rapidly. Occasionally a uterine window can be seen antenatally within the previous uterine scar on ultrasound. Scheduled cesarean delivery at 37 weeks is recommended for these patients and labor is contraindicated due to the risk of uterine rupture during labor.

Monitoring

In placenta previa, the distance between the placental edge and cervical os is monitored during pregnancy by ultrasound because the placental location can change with advancing pregnancy. After 35 weeks' gestation, women with a placental edge more than 20 mm from the internal cervical os may be offered a trial of labor because they are likely to achieve vaginal delivery. When the placental edge is greater than 0 mm but less than 20 mm from the internal cervical os, vaginal delivery might still be possible, although the likelihood of cesarean section and intrapartum complications are much higher. Women at increased risk of vasa previa should be screened with TVU and color Doppler. When vasa previa is identified, serial ultrasound is indicated because abnormal vessels regress in up to 15% of women. If a woman has an Rh negative blood type and experiences bleeding in pregnancy, she should receive a standard dose of 300 µg Rho(D) human immune globulin to prevent maternal Rh alloimmunization. For massive maternal-fetal hemorrhage a Kleihauer-Betke test should be performed in Rh negative mothers to assist in confirming maternal-fetal hemorrhage and Rho(D) human immune globulin dosing.

Complications

Maternal risks associated with placenta previa include need for cesarean section, postpartum hemorrhage, and blood transfusion. Women who have history of cesarean section and who have placenta previa are at increased risk for placenta accreta. Fetal risks are primarily associated with prematurity. Placental abruption can cause hypovolemic shock, postpartum hemorrhage, and DIC. Perinatal complications include prematurity, intrauterine growth restriction, anemia, coagulopathy, and death. Uterine rupture can be catastrophic for both mother and baby. Maternal risks include surgical risk associated with cesarean section, hypovolemic shock and hemorrhage, and hysterectomy. Perinatal morbidity can include hypoxic-ischemic encephalopathy. Stillbirth and neonatal death are possible as well. When undiagnosed prior to labor vasa previa carries a fetal mortality rate of greater than 60%. Antenatal diagnosis with planned cesarean section decreases fetal mortality to 2% to 3% and reduces the need for transfusion from 60% to 3%. Because the hemorrhage is fetal blood, maternal risk from vasa previa is primarily associated with complications related to cesarean section.

Vaginal Bleeding in Early Pregnancy
Epidemiology

Vaginal bleeding in early pregnancy is common and has been reported in 20% to 40% of pregnant women. A viable intrauterine pregnancy is the most common diagnosis. The two most common complicating diagnoses of early pregnancy bleeding are threatened abortion and ectopic pregnancy. Threatened abortion, an intrauterine pregnancy with bleeding and pain before 20 weeks gestation that has cardiac activity and a closed cervix, is the cause of 12% to 57% of early pregnancy bleeding. The incidence of ectopic pregnancy is 19.7 cases per 1000 pregnancies and is increasing worldwide. Ectopic pregnancy is the leading cause of morbidity and maternal mortality in the first trimester of pregnancy.

It has been suggested that the rate of miscarriage can be as high as 30% to 50% of all fertilized eggs and often goes undetected. The incidence of miscarriage in an intrauterine pregnancy with confirmed fetal cardiac activity is 2.1% in women under 35 years of age and 16.1% in women greater than 35 years of age. Othercommon causes of early pregnancy bleeding include intercourse, cervicitis, pelvic inflammatory disease, functional placenta hormonal changes, fertilized egg implantation into the uterine wall, and gestational trophoblastic disease.

Pathophysiology

The most common diagnosis of bleeding in early pregnancy is a normal and viable intrauterine pregnancy. Vaginal spotting can commonly occur after implantation of a fertilized egg into the intrauterine wall, usually occurring a few days prior to the expected onset of menstruation (8 to 9 days after ovulation and fertilization). Early pregnancy bleeding may also be caused by the commencement of a hormonally functional placenta, usually at 6 to 7 weeks of gestation. Concerning causes of early pregnancy bleeding are maternal hormonal deficiency, placental dysfunction, subchorionic hemorrhage, extrauterine implantation of the embryo, and nonviability of the pregnancy. The amount of hemorrhage in early pregnancy may be associated with the risk of pregnancy loss.

Management

Early pregnancy bleeding is worked up with a complete set of vital signs, a complete history and physical examination including visualization of the cervix with a speculum, a complete blood count, β-hCG (human chorionic gonadotropin), and a transvaginal ultrasound (TVU) to determine fetal viability and exclude an ectopic pregnancy. Concern for ectopic or early pregnancy loss should be raised if the β-hCG level is greater than the discriminatory level (1500 to 3000 mIU/mL) without intrauterine contents seen on TVU. If the patient is hemodynamically unstable, urgent surgical consultation is paramount as it is possible to have intraabdominal exsanguination from a ruptured ectopic pregnancy. If the patient is hemodynamically stable and the pregnancy is viable, bleeding is most often managed expectantly, provided the fetus has not reached extrauterine viability of 23 to 24 weeks gestation.

If the patient is hemodynamically stable, a miscarriage can be managed expectantly, inducing medical expulsion of the nonviable fetal tissue with a combination of mifepristone and misoprostol, or surgical management with dilation and suction curettage depending on the risk of infection, maternal hemorrhage and anemia, maternal preference, and medical necessity. Medical management has been proven to increase the effectiveness and decrease the time of complete expulsion compared to expectant management. Due to the risk of alloimmunization, it is recommended that women who are Rh negative blood type have surgical management and receive prophylactic Rho(D) human immune globulin to reduce the risk of alloimmunization. Alloimmunization is a devastating complication where an Rh negative mother can develop antibodies to Rh positive fetal blood, placing future pregnancies at risk.

If a woman has an Rh negative blood type and experiences bleeding in pregnancy, she should receive Rho(D) human immune globulin to prevent maternal Rh alloimmunization. Failure to receive Rho(D) human immune globulin can complicate all subsequent pregnancies and ultimately lead to future severe fetal anemia and hydrops fetalis (severe and life-threatening fetal edema secondary to profound fetal anemia). For early pregnancy bleeding in an Rh negative mother of less than 12 weeks of gestation, 150 μg of Rho(D) is sufficient; greater than 12 weeks of gestation, a standard dose of 300 μg should be given. These dosages provide maternal protection from up to 30 mL of fetal whole blood. For massive maternal-fetal hemorrhage a Kleihauer-Betke test should be performed in Rh negative mothers to assist in confirming maternal-fetal hemorrhage and Rho(D) human immune globulin dosing.

If there is recurrent pregnancy loss, defined as greater than 3 total pregnancy losses, two consecutive pregnancy losses, or a pregnancy loss greater than 20 weeks of gestation, secondary causes should be sought including a workup for antiphospholipid antibody disorder, clotting disorders, and maternal or fetal chromosomal testing. The products of conceptions resulting from gestational trophoblastic disease should undergo chromosomal analysis.

References

Antenatal corticosteroid therapy for fetal maturation. Committee Opinion No. 677. American College of Obstetricians and Gynecologists, *Obstet Gynecol* 128:e187–194, 2016.

Deutchman M, Tubay AT, Turok D: First trimester bleeding, *Am Fam Physician* 79(11):985–994, 2009 Jun 1.

Duley L, Guelmezoglu AM, Henderson-Smart DJ, Chou D: Magnesium sulphate and other anticonvulsants for women with pre-eclampsia, *Cochrane Database Syst Rev* 11, 2010.

Early Pregnancy Loss: Practice Bulletin No. 200. American College of Obstetricians and Gynecologists, *Obstet Gynecol*, August 29, 2018. Interim Update.

Gagnon R, Morin L, Bly S, et al: Guidelines for the management of vasa previa, *J Obstet Gynaecol Can* 31:748–760, 2009.

Hasan R, Baird DD, Herring AH, et al: Patterns and predictors of vaginal bleeding in the first trimester of pregnancy, *Ann Epidemiol* 20(7):524–531, 2010, Available at: https://doi.org/10.1016/j.annepidem.2010.02.006.

Hendricks E, et al: First trimester bleeding: evaluation and management, *Am Fam Physician* 99(3):166–174, 2019 Feb 1.

Krywko DM, Shunkwiler SM: Kleihauer Betke Test. [Updated 2019 Jan 27]. In: StatPearls [Internet]. Treasure Island (FL): StatPearls Publishing; 2019 Jan-. Available from: https://www.ncbi.nlm.nih.gov/books/NBK430876/.

Magann EF, Cummings JE, Niderhauser A: Antepartum bleeding of unknown origin in the second half of pregnancy: A review, *Obstet Gynecol Surv* 60:741–745, 2005.

Management of preterm labor. Practice Bulletin No. 171. American College of Obstetricians and Gynecologists, *Obstet Gynecol* 128:e155–164, 2016.

Oppenheimer L, Armson A, Farine D, et al: Diagnosis and management of placenta previa, *J Obstet Gynaecol Can* 29:261–266, 2007.

Oyelese Y, Ananth C: Placental abruption, *Obstet Gynecol* 108:1005–1016, 2006.

Royal College of Obstetricians and Gynaecologists (RCOG): *Antepartum hemorrhage*, London (UK), November 2011, Royal College of Obstetricians and Gynaecologists (RCOG)November 2011.

Sinha P, Kuruba N: Ante-partum hemorrhage: An update, *J Obstet Gynaecol* 28:377–381, 2008.

Smith JG, Mertz HL, Merrill DC: Identifying risk factors for uterine rupture, *Clin Perinatol* 35:85–99, 2008.

Smith KE, Buyalos RP: The profound impact of patient age on pregnancy outcome after early detection of fetal cardiac activity, *Fertil Steril* 65:35–40, 1996.

Tenore J: *Am Fam Physician* 61(4):1080–1088, 2000 Feb 15.

Zlatnik MG, Cheng YW, Norton ME, et al: Placenta previa and the risk of preterm delivery, *J Matern Fetal Neonatal Med* 20:719–723, 2007.

ACUTE LEUKEMIA IN CHILDREN

Method of
Stacy Cooper, MD; and Rachel E. Rau, MD

Leukemias are characterized by a marked proliferation of abnormal blood cells in the bone marrow and blood that may be associated with widespread infiltration in extramedullary sites including the central nervous system (CNS), testes, thymus, liver, spleen, and lymph nodes.

Classification

The first level of classification of leukemia is *acute* versus *chronic*. Acute leukemia is characterized by the predominance of very immature white blood cell precursors, or blasts, and is an aggressive, rapidly fatal disease if left untreated. Conversely, chronic leukemia is characterized by proliferation of relatively mature white blood cells and is typically a more indolent disease. Chronic leukemias are uncommon in pediatrics.

The second level of classification is *lymphoid* versus *myeloid*, depending on whether the leukemic cells display characteristics of lymphocyte precursors or myelocyte (granulocyte, erythrocyte, monocyte, or megakaryocyte) precursors. Acute lymphoblastic leukemia (ALL) and acute myeloid leukemia (AML) account for the overwhelming majority of pediatric leukemias.

ALL and AML are further subclassified by morphology and expression of cell surface antigens using flow cytometry. For ALL, classification is largely based on cell surface and cytoplasmic marker expression (Table 1). AML cases are classified by characteristic chromosomal abnormalities (if present) or by light microscopic morphology in cases where these specific chromosomal changes are absent (Box 1).

Epidemiology

Leukemia accounts for approximately 30% of childhood cancers, making it the most common form of childhood cancer. The distribution of the major forms of leukemia is vastly different in children than in adults (Figure 1). In general, children are far more likely to have acute leukemia, and ALL is much more common than AML. In adults, most cases of leukemia are chronic, and AML is more common than ALL. Specifically, there are approximately 3100 children and adolescents diagnosed with ALL in the United States each year and approximately 700 children and adolescents diagnosed with AML in the United States each year.

The incidence of the various forms of leukemia varies by age in both children and adults (Figure 2). This is especially true for childhood ALL, for which there is a marked incidence peak in the 2- to 4-year-old age group. This ALL age peak is primarily found in children living in industrialized nations, leading to speculation that a common environmental exposure, coupled with age-related immunologic susceptibility, is at least partially responsible for many cases of ALL. Except for a small peak in infants, the incidence of AML is fairly constant in childhood but rises quickly in later adulthood.

Prognosis

One of the most dramatic success stories in modern medicine is the improvement in survival of children with ALL over the past four decades. Leukemia was once a uniformly fatal diagnosis, with less than a 5% to 10% cure rate until the mid- to late 1960s. Today, approximately 90% of children with ALL are cured. The improved prognosis has been built on pioneering observations on the efficacy of multiagent systemic therapy and the importance of CNS treatment in the late 1960s and early 1970s. Further successive, incremental improvements in outcome have been achieved due to clinical trials conducted by large single centers and national and international cooperative groups that have successfully enrolled a high percentage of eligible children.

Similar approaches have unfortunately not been quite so successful in improving the prognosis of children with AML. Although approximately one half of children with AML are cured today, this has been accomplished by intensifying therapy to the point that the toxic death rate in the early phases of therapy is about 10%. Current research in AML is therefore focusing on developing novel molecularly targeted agents that hold the promise of improving efficacy and limiting toxicity.

TABLE 1	Classification of Childhood Acute Lymphoblastic Leukemia					
	PHENOTYPIC MARKER					
ALL SUBTYPE	**CD19**	**CD10**	**CLG**	**SLG**	**%**	**COMMENT**
Pre-pre B	+	−	−	−	5	Mostly infants, poor prognosis, frequent *KMT2A* 11q23 rearrangements
Early pre-B	+	+	−	−	63	Common ALL, young children, good prognosis
Pre-B	+	+	+	−	16	Older children, good prognosis with intense therapy
B-cell	+	+	+	+	4	Burkitt leukemia, *MYC/Ig* fusion genes, good prognosis with lymphoma-type therapy
T-cell	−	−	−	−	12	Adolescents, anterior mediastinal mass, CNS involvement, good prognosis with intense therapy

ALL, Acute myeloid leukemia; *clg*, cytoplasmic immunoglobulin; *CNS*, central nervous system; *slg*, surface immunoglobulin.

BOX 1 | Classification of Childhood Acute Myeloid Leukemia (World Health Organization Criteria)

Acute Myeloid Leukemia With Recurrent Genetic Abnormalities

Acute myeloid leukemia with t(8;21)(q22;q22), *(RUNX1/RUNX1T1)*

Acute myeloid leukemia with abnormal bone marrow eosinophils and inv(16)(p13q22) or t(16;16)(p13;q22), *(CBFβ/MYH11)*

Acute promyelocytic leukemia with t(15;17)(q22;q12), *(PML/RARA),* and variants

Acute myeloid leukemia with 11q23 *(KMT2A)* abnormalities

Acute Myeloid Leukemia, Not Otherwise Categorized

Acute myeloid leukemia, minimally differentiated (FAB M0)

Acute myeloid leukemia without maturation (FAB M1)

Acute myeloid leukemia with maturation (FAB M2)

Acute myelomonocytic leukemia (FAB M4)

Acute monoblastic/acute monocytic leukemia (FAB M5)

Acute erythroid leukemia (FAB M6)

Acute megakaryoblastic leukemia (FAB M7)

FAB, French–American–British classification.

Etiology

The question "What is the cause of leukemia?" can be considered on a few different levels. First, what is wrong with *this child* that caused the child to develop leukemia? Second, what is wrong with *the leukemia cell* that causes it to behave so badly? Third, what is wrong with *the leukemia cell's genes* that cause the cell to behave that way?

Predispositions

The answer to the first question is unknown in the vast majority of cases. Attempts to correlate various genetic features or environmental or infectious exposures with risk of childhood leukemia have been largely uninformative. It is presumed that children are particularly susceptible to ALL because of the marked expansion and genetic rearrangement of lymphocytes that occurs during early childhood as the result of exposure to a multitude of immunogenic antigens for the first time. The proliferation required to meet the constant demand for granulocytes, erythrocytes, and platelets is likely a setup for the development of AML in children.

Although a number of constitutional and single-gene disorders confer an increased risk of childhood leukemia (Table 2), in total, these are known to be involved in only a minority of cases. However, with a growing list of recognized genetic disorders predisposing to myeloid malignancies in particular, a careful

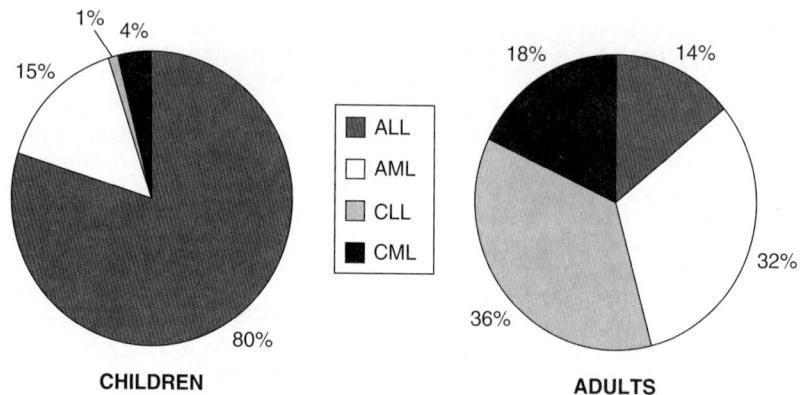

Figure 1 Relative incidence of four major leukemia subtypes in children and adults. *ALL,* Acute lymphoblastic leukemia; *AML,* acute myeloid leukemia; *CLL,* chronic lymphoblastic leukemia; *CML,* chronic myeloid leukemia.

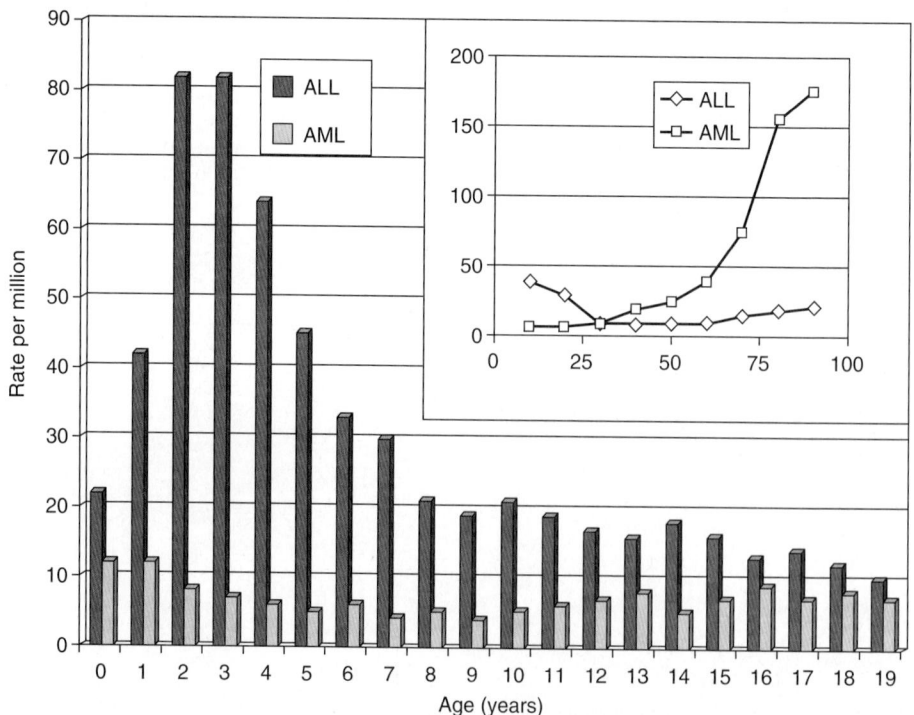

Figure 2 Age-specific incidence of acute lymphoblastic leukemia *(ALL)* and acute myeloid leukemia *(AML)* in children and in adults *(inset).*

TABLE 2 Summary of Known Constitutional and Heritable Childhood Leukemia Predispositions

DISORDER	INHERITANCE	MALIGNANCY TYPE	COMMENTS
Ataxia-telangiectasia	AR	ALL, NHL	ATM gene mutations lead to defective DNA repair
Bloom's syndrome	AR	AML, ALL	Chromosomal instability, sister chromatid exchanges
Down syndrome	Sporadic	AML, ALL	See text
Li-Fraumeni syndrome	AD	AML, ALL, many others	p53 mutations; leukemias less common than solid tumors
Fanconi's anemia	AR	AML	Chromosomal instability, increased sensitivity to DNA damage
Kostmann's syndrome	AR	AML	G-CSF receptor mutations lead to agranulocytosis
Neurofibromatosis type 1	AD	AML, JMML, MPNST	NF1 gene mutations lead to enhanced RAS signaling
Familial platelet disorder with associated myeloid malignancy	AD	MDS, AML, ALL	Loss of function mutations of the myeloid transcription factor RUNX1 lead to abnormal myeloid development Individuals have platelet defects and ~35% risk of myeloid malignancy development
Germline CEBPA mutations	AD	AML	Estimated penetrance of AML development ~90% in affected individuals. Approximately 10% of patients with biallelic CEBPA mutant AML have a germline CEBPA mutation. AML in those with germline CEBPA mutations are chemosensitive, but individuals have high rates of second primary AMLs.
MonoMAC syndrome; germline GATA2 mutations	AD	MDS, AML	MonoMAC is an immunodeficiency with risk for mycobacterial, fungal, and human papilloma virus infections with monocytopenia and risk for MDS/AML, often with monosomy of chromosome 7
MIRAGE syndrome, ATXPC/MLSM7 syndrome; Germline mutation of SAMD9 and SAMD9L	Mostly de novo		MIRAGE syndrome (myelodysplasia, infection, restriction of growth, adrenal hypoplasia, genital phenotypes, enteropathy); ATXPC, ataxia-pancytopenia syndrome and MLSM7, myelodysplasia and leukemia syndrome with monosomy 7 caused by gain of function mutation of SAMD9 or SAMD9L
CBL syndrome	AD	JMML	Impaired growth, developmental delay, cryptorchidism, deafness, and predisposition to JMML caused by loss of function mutation of rumor suppressor gene CBL. JMML that develops can be self-resolving. Vasculitis risk later in life after JMML resolution.

AD, Autosomal dominant; *ALL,* acute lymphoblastic leukemia; *AML,* acute myeloid leukemia; *AR,* autosomal recessive; *G-CSF,* granulocyte colony-stimulating factor; *JMML,* juvenile myelomonocytic leukemia; *MPNST,* malignant peripheral nerve sheath tumor; *NHL,* non-Hodgkin lymphoma.

past medical history, family history, and examination for dysmorphisms and low threshold for genetic referral is warranted for any child with a myeloid malignancy. The most common of these is Down syndrome. Children with Down syndrome have a 10- to 20-fold increased risk of leukemia, with an approximately equal incidence of ALL and AML. The peak age at onset of leukemia for children with Down syndrome is earlier than for other children. In the newborn period, patients with Down syndrome can present with transient myeloproliferative disease (also known as transient abnormal myelopoiesis), which can manifest with hepatomegaly and peripheral blasts, that appears indistinguishable from congenital AML but usually resolves spontaneously within 3 to 6 months. These children have an increased risk of megakaryoblastic leukemia (AMKL, FAB classification M7) within the first 4 years of life. Children with Down syndrome tend to present with leukemia that is particularly susceptible to chemotherapy agents (e.g., cytarabine [Cytosar], methotrexate), but they also suffer increased toxicity from therapy. On balance, the prognosis of leukemia in Down syndrome patients with ALL is inferior to those without Down syndrome, whereas in AML, children with Down syndrome have favorable outcomes compared with children without Down syndrome.

The only environmental exposures that are known to predispose to leukemia are ionizing radiation (such as was seen with atomic bomb survivors) and prior exposure to certain chemotherapy drugs (e.g., cyclophosphamide [Cytoxan], etoposide [Toposar, VePesid]). There is also evidence that in utero exposure to maternal diagnostic radiation also increases the risk of childhood cancer (including leukemia), particularly if the exposure is in the first trimester. Other environmental or infectious exposures remain unproven as risk factors for childhood leukemia, including electromagnetic fields from power lines.

Cellular Pathogenesis

Three major characteristics of leukemia cells distinguish them from normal hematopoietic cells. They proliferate rapidly, they do not differentiate, and they have defects in apoptosis. This results in a growth advantage for leukemia cells, leading to progressive replacement of the normal bone marrow with a massive clonal population of poorly differentiated leukemic blasts.

TABLE 3	Summary of Common Leukemogenic Genetic Events

ACUTE LYMPHOBLASTIC LEUKEMIA	ACUTE MYELOID LEUKEMIA
Chimeric Transcription Factors	
t(12;21): *ETV6-RUNX1* fusion	t(8;21): *RUNX1-RUNX1T1* fusion
t(1;19): *TCF3-PBX1* fusion	t(15;17): *PML-RARA* fusion
t(4;11), et al: *KMT2A* fusions	t(9;11), et al: *KMT2A* fusions
t(8;14), t(8;22), t(2;8): *Ig-MYC* fusions	inv(16): MYH11-CBFB
T-cell receptor fusions	
Mutationally Activated Oncogenes	
t(9;22): *BCR-ABL1* fusion	*FLT3* mutation
JAK2 mutation	*RAS* mutation
CRLF2 fusion	*KIT* mutation
Altered Tumor-Suppressor Genes	
CDKN2A deletion	*NPM1* mutation
IKZF1 mutation	*WT1* mutation
TP53 mutation	*CEBPA* mutation

BOX 2	Summary of Clinical Manifestations of Childhood Leukemia*

Bone Marrow
Pancytopenia, bone pain

Reticuloendothelial System
Lymphadenopathy
Hepatosplenomegaly

Thymus
Anterior mediastinal mass (T-cell leukemia)

Bones
Bone pain is common
Fractures and chloromas are rare

Gums
Gingival hypertrophy (M4 and M5 AML)

Skin
Leukemia cutis and chloromas (M2, M4, and M5 AML, infant ALL)

Central Nervous System
Meningitis
Cranial nerve palsies
Rarely intracranial epidural or orbital chloromas (M4 and M5 AML, T-cell ALL)

Kidneys
Often infiltrated or enlarged
Rarely acute renal failure (except in tumor lysis syndrome)

Genitourinary
Testicular enlargement (T-cell ALL)

*See Box 1 for descriptions of classifications.
ALL, Acute lymphoblastic leukemia; *AML,* acute myeloid leukemia; *TBSA,* total body surface area.

Another characteristic of leukemia cells is their tendency to spread throughout the body and infiltrate organs other than the bone marrow. This is discussed in more detail in the section on clinical presentation.

Molecular Pathogenesis

As is true of most human cancers, development of leukemia is a multihit process. The initiating mutation (first hit) in childhood ALL often occurs in utero or early infancy, which is the peak of lymphocyte expansion and recombinase activity for the normal immune system.

The initiating events are typically chromosomal rearrangements that activate expression of cellular proto-oncogenes by fusing them to transcriptionally active immunoglobulin or T-cell receptor genes or alternatively by joining two genes from different chromosomes to create a new fusion gene that encodes a chimeric protein with unique functional properties. The most common of these sentinel chromosomal rearrangements are translocations (exchanges of genetic material between chromosomes), which can serve as a unique marker of the malignant clone. Retrospective studies of blood obtained at birth and preserved on filter paper used for diagnosis of genetic disorders (Guthrie cards) of children who developed leukemia in early childhood have shown that leukemia-associated fusion genes were present at birth in a large percentage of children, including some who did not develop leukemia for one or more years.

In ALL, the promotional mutation (second hit) likely occurs during the proliferative stress generated by immune responses to exogenous antigens. Because these are maximal in the 2- to 4-year-old age group, this is thought to explain the age peak of childhood ALL during these years. The lack of such a peak in AML suggests that the promotional mutations can occur at any time or are not necessarily triggered by immune stimulation. Examples of specific genetic hits known to be associated with the development of childhood leukemia are summarized in Table 3.

Clinical Presentation

Most symptoms and signs of childhood leukemia are the result of the propensity of leukemia cells to replace the bone marrow and infiltrate multiple other organs throughout the body. It is estimated that approximately 10^9 (1 trillion) leukemia cells are present in the child's body at diagnosis.

The replacement of normal bone marrow is responsible for the characteristic abnormal blood counts, which in most cases include the triad of neutropenia, anemia, and thrombocytopenia. Depending on the number of circulating leukemic blasts in the peripheral blood, the total white blood cell (WBC) count may be low, normal, or high. The neutropenia is often profound (absolute neutrophil count <500/µL) and is associated with an increased risk of serious infection. Blood cultures and broad-spectrum intravenous antibiotic coverage are indicated in any patient with newly diagnosed leukemia and fever. Anemia is often manifested by fatigue, lethargy, headache, pallor, and, in extreme cases, congestive heart failure that may be precipitated by vigorous transfusion or intravenous hydration. Thrombocytopenia often leads to bruising and petechiae; however, clinically significant hemorrhage is uncommon in industrialized countries. Platelet transfusion is indicated for bleeding or for very low platelet counts (<10,000–20,000/µL).

Infiltration of organs other than the bone marrow with leukemia cells is responsible for additional presenting clinical features. Box 2 summarizes the organ systems most often involved in leukemia and the typical clinical manifestations.

Medical Emergencies in Childhood Leukemia

A child with newly diagnosed leukemia needs to be promptly evaluated for several medical emergencies. There are several potentially life-threatening complications that may be present at diagnosis or can develop within a short time after diagnosis, in addition to the need to diagnose and treat potential infection in patients who are febrile and neutropenic, which was discussed earlier.

Tumor lysis syndrome (TLS) is a complication resulting from the rapid breakdown of large numbers of tumor cells, releasing intracellular contents. Although TLS is seen most often after initial treatment with chemotherapy, it can also be present before therapy is initiated due to spontaneous lysis. Risk factors include high WBC count, lymphadenopathy, hepatosplenomegaly, high mitotic index, and specific diagnoses of ALL (especially Burkitt leukemia or lymphoma and T-cell ALL). TLS is characterized by the triad of hyperuricemia (from breakdown of purines by xanthine oxidase), hyperkalemia, and hyperphosphatemia (with secondary hypocalcemia). Renal insufficiency can develop due to the nephrotoxic effects of precipitated urate crystals in the renal tubules; in severe cases, dialysis may be necessary.

Management consists of aggressive hydration to reduce tubular uric acid concentration. The xanthine oxidase inhibitor allopurinol (Zyloprim) is routinely used to decrease uric acid production. Rasburicase (Elitek) (recombinant urate oxidase) is a new agent used in severe cases of TLS to almost instantaneously convert uric acid to the more soluble allantoin. Frequent electrolyte monitoring with standard management of abnormal levels is essential.

Hyperleukocytosis becomes a potential clinical problem and is usually seen with WBC counts above 100,000/µL. Markedly elevated WBCs lead to increased blood viscosity that can produce sludging of blood in the brain, lungs, kidneys, and other organs, causing clinical features such as depressed level of consciousness, stroke, intracranial hemorrhage, respiratory distress, hypoxia, diffuse pulmonary infiltrates, and renal insufficiency. The risk of hyperviscosity is higher with AML than ALL because myeloblasts are generally larger and "stickier" than lymphoblasts (likely due to increased expression of integrins and other mediators of cell–cell adherence on the surface of myeloblasts). Management consists of treating the leukemia as soon as possible. It is also possible to perform exchange transfusion or leukopheresis in cases where symptoms are severe, although this is only a temporizing measure at best.

Life-threatening bleeding is another potential complication of leukemia. Although all patients with thrombocytopenia are at risk, patients with concomitant coagulopathy due to disseminated intravascular coagulation (DIC) are at particularly high risk. The leukemia subtype most commonly complicated by DIC and serious bleeding is acute promyelocytic leukemia (APL). This association results from the release of thromboplastin from the cytoplasmic granules in these promyelocytic blasts. Aggressive blood product support through transfusions and early treatment with the differentiation-inducing agent all-*trans* retinoic acid (ATRA, tretinoin) has been shown to decrease the risk of bleeding in APL. Despite these measures, up to 10% of patients die of bleeding complications during the initial weeks of therapy, and additional patients suffer lasting morbidity from retinal hemorrhages and nonfatal CNS hemorrhages.

Tracheal compression and superior vena cava syndrome can result from large anterior mediastinal masses, which are commonly present in T-cell ALL but are also rarely seen in other forms of leukemia as well. Patients can present with respiratory distress, cough, orthopnea, headaches, syncope, dizziness, facial swelling, or plethora. A chest x-ray should be performed to assess the mediastinum in any patient suspected to have leukemia. If the mediastinum is enlarged, a neck computed tomography (CT) is indicated to assess airway patency. This evaluation must precede any attempts at sedation for diagnostic procedures because even light sedation can precipitate acute airway collapse. Diagnostic material should be obtained by the least invasive method possible before treatment. If necessary, emergent airway compromise can be treated with radiation or steroids, or both, although recognize that the use of steroids prior to diagnostic procedures can impair staging (e.g., CSF involvement at diagnosis, presenting peripheral WBC count).

Differential Diagnosis

Although leukemia should be considered in cases of isolated neutropenia, anemia, or thrombocytopenia, the vast majority of leukemia patients present with decreases in more than one cell line. In suspected cases of immune thrombocytopenic purpura (ITP), for example, a careful review of the peripheral blood smear should be performed to rule out the presence of circulating leukemic blasts or other morphologic abnormalities. Routine bone marrow aspiration is not necessary for children with ITP, but it should be performed in patients with atypical features, such as concomitant anemia or neutropenia, hepatosplenomegaly, bone pain, or significant weight loss. Treatment of ITP with corticosteroids should be instituted only after evaluation by an experienced hematologist.

Pancytopenia can be caused by diseases other than leukemia. Some viral infections have a propensity to suppress bone marrow function and cause low peripheral blood cell counts, including Epstein-Barr virus (EBV), herpes simplex virus (HSV), influenza, hepatitis viruses, and HIV. Infectious mononucleosis from EBV infection can be particularly difficult to differentiate from leukemia because patients often have hepatosplenomegaly and circulating atypical lymphocytes (which can appear very similar to leukemic blasts). Pancytopenia on the basis of bone marrow failure (from acquired aplastic anemia or rare inherited bone marrow failure syndromes) can be distinguished from leukemia by bone marrow biopsy for assessment of overall marrow cellularity. Certain solid tumors have a tendency to metastasize to the bone marrow and cause cytopenias, including neuroblastoma and rhabdomyosarcoma, but it is rare for pancytopenia to be the sole primary presenting feature in these cases.

Joint pain, fever, hepatosplenomegaly, and pallor are common presenting features in both systemic-onset juvenile idiopathic arthritis (JIA) and leukemia. An elevated platelet count should be seen in JIA and can be helpful to distinguish the two, as a low or even normal platelet count is rare in JIA given the inflammation that should cause elevations in acute phase reactants. A bone marrow aspirate should be performed to rule out leukemia before treatment with steroids in suspected cases of systemic-onset JIA.

Risk Stratification

In the last several years, treatment decisions for children with newly diagnosed acute leukemia have been based on the concept of risk stratification. Using factors identified during clinical trials to predict a high or low risk of relapse, patients are separated into risk groups before the start of treatment, at the end of the first month of induction therapy, and at postinduction therapy timepoints for select patients. Based on these features, the treatment plan is tailored to the degree of risk. The desired result is that patients with relatively low-risk disease can be treated with less toxic therapy without compromising cure rates, and patients with high-risk disease receive more-intensive, potentially toxic therapy and/or warrant consideration of experimental options. The risk groups are currently defined based on several criteria and differ for ALL and AML. Different centers and cooperative groups typically employ different risk-stratification strategies.

In ALL, risk assignment is based on a combination of leukemia phenotype (B- versus T-lineage), clinical and genetic features, and early response to therapy. The initial risk assessment for B-ALL is based on two simple clinical parameters that are available immediately at the time of diagnosis (the National Cancer Institute [NCI] or Rome criteria): WBC count (>50,000/µL is high risk), and age (<1 year or >9 years is high risk). Presence or absence of leukemia outside of the bone marrow (extramedullary) including presence and level of disease in the CNS and leukemic involvement of the testes increases the risk of relapse.

For B-ALL, low-risk cytogenetic features include hyperdiploidy (≥50 chromosomes in the leukemia cells) or trisomies of specific chromosomes or the presence of a t(12;21) that results in *TEL/AML1* fusion. High-risk cytogenetic features include hypodiploidy (<44 chromosomes in the leukemia cells), the presence of either an 11q23 (*KMT2A*, formerly *MLL*, gene) rearrangement,

TABLE 4	Summary of Treatment for Childhood Leukemia	
CHARACTERISTICS	**ACUTE LYMPHOBLASTIC LEUKEMIA**	**ACUTE MYELOID LEUKEMIA**
Remission Induction		
Chemotherapy	4 weeks with prednisone or dexamethasone, vincristine, PEG asparaginase, daunorubicin (not all cases)	Two courses (6–8 weeks) with cytarabine (Ara-C), doxorubicin, others (e.g., etoposide,[1] thioguanine)
Toxic death rate	Low (<3%)	High (>10%)
Remission rate	>98%	75%–85%
CNS Preventive Therapy		
Intrathecal Chemotherapy	Methotrexate	Cytarabine
Cranial irradiation	For high risk only (excessive disease in CSF at diagnosis)	None
Consolidation		
Chemotherapy	Combinations of various drugs (not cross-resistant) Intensity/duration based on risk stratification	Based on cytogenic/molecular risk group and minimal residual disease (MRD) Low risk: 2–3 additional courses Intermediate risk: If MRD-negative, treat as low risk; if MRD positive, treat as high risk High risk: BMT for patients with best available donor
Maintenance		
Chemotherapy	Low-dose oral (6-mercaptopurine)[1] and methotrexate) Total duration of therapy 2–3 years	No maintenance therapy (does not improve survival)

BMT, Bone marrow transplant; *CNS,* central nervous system; *CSF,* cerebrospinal fluid; *HLA,* human leukocyte antigen; *WBC,* white blood cell.
[1]Not FDA approved for this indication.

the presence of intrachromosomal amplification of chromosome 21 at the locus containing the gene, *RUNX1* (iAMP21), or a t(9;22), or Philadelphia chromosome, that creates a *BCR/ABL* fusion gene. For T-ALL, cytogenetic features have not been routinely incorporated into risk stratification.

Early response has historically been measured by the response to a prednisone prophase that includes a single dose of intrathecal methotrexate and 7 days of prednisone, or by the percentage of blast cells remaining in the bone marrow after 7 to 14 days of multiagent therapy. Over the past 15 to 20 years, measures of tumor burden remaining in the marrow at the end of induction therapy (minimal residual disease [MRD]) have been shown to be highly predictive of outcome and have been integrated into risk-stratification schemata of all the major leukemia cooperative groups.

In AML, risk stratification is based largely on cytogenetics. Low-risk features include t(8;21), which results in the *RUNX1-RUNX1T1* (formerly *AML1/ETO)* fusion and either inv(16) or a t(16;16), both of which create the *CBFβ/MYH11* fusion. High-risk features include monosomy 7 and abnormalities in the long arm of chromosome 5. More recently, data suggest other cytogenetic features may portend a poor prognosis, such as certain *KMT2A* fusions, t(3;21)(q26.2;q22) resulting in the *RUNX1-MECOM* fusion, and 11p15 rearrangements involving the gene *NUP98,* among others. Most other cytogenetic abnormalities, as well as normal cytogenetics (which are seen in approximately 60% of cases), are considered intermediate risk by most pediatric leukemia consortia. In addition to cytogenetic features, specific molecular lesions are also prognostically relevant in AML. Mutations of the genes *NPM1* and *CEBPA* are associated with a more favorable outcome. Mutations of the receptor tyrosine kinase, *FLT3,* most commonly as internal tandem duplications (ITD) of the juxtamembrane domain, have been historically associated with a poor prognosis, but this risk appears to be dependent on the constellation of co-occuring mutations, as those with both *FLT3*-ITD mutations and either mutation of *NPM1* or *CEBPA* appear to have favorable outcomes. Thus how such mutations are

incorporated into risk stratification schemas varies among pediatric cancer consortia.

Response to therapy has also been incorporated into the risk stratification of AML. Failure to achieve remission with induction chemotherapy is another high-risk feature in AML. Measurement of MRD at the end of induction is now also routinely used for risk stratification of AML.

Treatment

There are significant differences in the specific treatments for ALL and AML, so they will be discussed separately. Table 4 summarizes the most salient features of the treatment for each.

Acute Lymphoblastic Leukemia

Treatment for ALL generally occurs in three phases: remission induction, consolidation, and maintenance with CNS preventive therapy administered throughout each of these phases. Remission induction in ALL typically lasts 4 to 6 weeks and includes three to five systemic agents. Common to almost all regimens are a corticosteroid (either prednisone [Deltasone] or dexamethasone [Decadron]), vincristine (Vincasar), and PEG asparaginase (pegaspargase [Oncaspar]), which compose the three-drug induction. An anthracycline, typically daunorubicin (Cerubidine), is also included in many regimens (four-drug induction), with other agents such as cyclophosphamide (Cytoxan) or etoposide (Toposar, VePesid)[1] used in a small minority of centers. More than 98% of children enter morphologic remission (defined as <5% blasts in the bone marrow) by the end of 4 weeks of induction therapy, and the mortality rate from toxicity during induction therapy is generally less than 2% to 3% in industrialized countries.

The concept that the CNS could be a sanctuary site for leukemia emerged in the mid-1960s when the introduction of multiagent systemic chemotherapy led to high remission rates,

[1]Not FDA approved for this indication.

but a majority of patients relapsed within 6 to 12 months, with many of these recurrences being limited to the CNS. Routine introduction of presymptomatic CNS radiation in the late 1960s and early 1970s led to substantial increases in cure rates to approximately 50%. Modern CNS preventive therapy includes periodic administration of intrathecal chemotherapy (usually methotrexate) starting at the time of the first diagnostic lumbar puncture. Systemic agents with improved CNS penetration (dexamethasone rather than prednisone, higher doses of intravenous methotrexate) might also play an important role in CNS control. Cranial irradiation is currently reserved for patients at the highest risk for CNS relapse (e.g., those with high diagnostic WBC count or leukemic blasts in CSF at diagnosis). Over time, CNS radiation has been given to fewer and fewer ALL patients; some groups believe that it can be eliminated for all patients. With these modern strategies, the risk of isolated CNS relapse is less than 5%.

Following the induction of remission, patients receive additional chemotherapy designed to consolidate the remission. The intensity and duration of the consolidation phase are risk based, and alternating cycles of non–cross-resistant chemotherapy drugs are typically used. These consolidation or intensification phases typically last about 6 months and often include a reinduction phase similar to the first month of treatment.

It has been clearly demonstrated that the risk of relapse in ALL can be reduced with an extended phase of continuous low-dose chemotherapy (maintenance) that lasts until 2 to 3 years from the time of diagnosis. Oral 6-mercaptopurine (Purixan, Purinethol) and methotrexate are used universally, with variable administration of intrathecal chemotherapy. Some centers or groups also employ periodic doses of vincristine and 5- to 7-day pulses of prednisone or dexamethasone. The optimal frequency of intrathecal chemotherapy treatments and vincristine and steroid pulses is uncertain and might depend on the intensity of therapy delivered during the induction and consolidation phases.

Acute Myeloid Leukemia

Remission induction in AML typically consists of two courses of very intensive chemotherapy with cytarabine (Cytosar, Tarabine) and doxorubicin (Adriamycin), often combined with thioguanine (Tabloid) or etoposide.[1] Remission rates are 75% to 85%, with about one half of the failures due to resistant leukemia and the others to mortality from toxicity (usually infection).

Similar to ALL, CNS preventive therapy in AML begins at diagnosis with intrathecal chemotherapy (usually cytarabine) and continues with additional periodic intrathecal treatments during consolidation. High-dose cytarabine, which is a key component of most AML treatment regimens, also contributes to CNS treatment. Cranial radiation is not typically administered by most groups to children with AML, except for treatment of chloromas (solid masses of leukemia cells) that do not resolve with chemotherapy.

Consolidation in AML is risk dependent. High-risk patients can be identified who have less than a 20% to 25% chance of cure with intensive chemotherapy. Most groups consider these patients to be candidates for bone marrow transplant (BMT). If a matched sibling is unavailable, then alternative donor sources (e.g., matched unrelated bone marrow, umbilical cord blood, or haplo-identical transplant from a parent) are usually offered. For low-risk patients, for whom the cure rate with chemotherapy alone approaches 70%, BMT is usually not offered in first remission, even for patients with a matched sibling donor. In addition, relapses in low-risk patients, unlike relapses in intermediate-risk or high-risk patients, can often be successfully treated with BMT in second remission, justifying reservation of BMT for use as a salvage therapy for low-risk patients. Consolidation in these cases consists of two to three additional chemotherapy courses that are slightly less intense and usually consist of cytarabine combined with drugs not used in induction, such as mitoxantrone (Novantrone) and L-asparaginase (Elspar).[1] For intermediate-risk patients, MRD testing at the end of induction is increasingly being used to determine whether to consolidate with chemotherapy or BMT. Unlike ALL, most groups have found no benefit to extended maintenance therapy in children with AML.

Relapse

The most common site of relapsed leukemia is the bone marrow (with or without concomitant CNS involvement). Less common are isolated extramedullary relapses (CNS or testicular relapse in ALL, chloromas in AML). For both ALL and AML, a critical determinant of outcome following relapse is the time from diagnosis to relapse.

ALL patients who relapse within 18 months of initial diagnosis have a dismal outcome, with only about one half able to attain a second remission and less than 10% overall cure rate; the outcome is marginally better for those who relapse between 18 and 36 months after diagnosis. ALL patients with such early relapses are typically treated with 3 to 4 months of intensive therapy to achieve a second remission and attain further cytoreduction, followed by BMT using a matched sibling or unrelated donor. In contrast, children with ALL who relapse more than 3 years after initial diagnosis have an approximately 95% chance of entering a second remission, and 40% to 70% can be cured with intensive chemotherapy without BMT. Notably, with successful introduction of immunotherapeutic agents such as blinatumomab (Blincyto), the CD19-targeting bispecific T-cell engager and CD19-directed chimeric antigen receptor T-cell (CART) tisagenlecleucel (Kymriah), the therapeutic approach for relapsed B-ALL is evolving. Recent data suggest blinatmomab compared with standard chemotherapy is better tolerated and more likely to achieve an MRD-negative remission prior to hematopoietic stem cell transplant (HSCT) in high-risk relapsed B-ALL. Additionally, emerging evidence suggest CD19 CART can achieve durable remissions in some relapsed B-ALL patients without BMT. Thus the approach for the treatment of relapsed ALL is largely shifting away from intensive standard chemotherapy and BMT to a hybrid of chemotherapy and immunotherapy with or without BMT.

Overall, relapsed AML has a dismal outcome (long-term survival approximately 20%), and the approach is to attempt to reinduce remission and then proceed to BMT or investigational treatments. Even in this setting, there is clearly an improved outcome for patients who relapse after a prolonged initial remission (>12 months from the end of remission-induction therapy) compared with patients who have refractory disease or who relapse after a shorter period of remission.

New treatment strategies are urgently needed for patients with relapsed ALL and AML because the current regimens produce poor results and are associated with a great deal of toxicity. The major clinical trial groups are testing novel and targeted therapies in these patient populations.

Late Effects

Approximately 70% of children with leukemia are cured of their disease. As the numbers of long-term survivors of childhood leukemia have grown, there has been increasing interest in assessing the late effects of leukemic therapy. In childhood ALL, with cure rates of 90%, a major effort is being made in ongoing clinical trials to reduce the intensity of therapy for lower-risk patients, with the hope of reducing late effects of therapy without compromising high cure rates. The most common late effects of leukemia therapy, with the known treatment-related risk factors and recommended diagnostic approach for each, are summarized in Table 5. Many pediatric

---

[1]Not FDA approved for this indication.

[1]Not FDA approved for this indication.

TABLE 5   Summary of Late Effects of Leukemia Treatment

LATE EFFECT	TREATMENT-RELATED RISK FACTORS	DIAGNOSTIC APPROACH
Bone	Avascular necrosis, osteonecrosis	X-ray and/or MRI of major joints for persistent pain
Cardiac dysfunction	Anthracyclines: cardiomyopathy (risk related to cumulative dose, higher risk in AML)	ECG or echocardiogram every 3–5 years (cardiomyopathy can occur decades after treatment)
Cataracts	CNS RT	Yearly eye examination
CNS and psychosocial	CNS RT, IT chemotherapy: learning problems, neurocognitive dysfunction	Yearly educational assessment, neurocognitive testing
Dental abnormalities	CNS RT	Yearly dental examinations
Endocrine and reproductive	CNS RT: pituitary dysfunction Alkylators: primary gonadal failure	Yearly growth curves, TSH, LH, FSH LH, FSH, estradiol or testosterone, semen analysis
Hepatic dysfunction	Methotrexate, 6-mercaptopurine, 6-thioguanine: late hepatic fibrosis	Yearly LFTs
Secondary neoplasms	CNS RT: brain tumors Alkylators or epipodophyllotoxins: secondary AML	MRI for symptoms CBC in symptomatic patients

ALL, Acute lymphoblastic leukemia; *AML,* acute myeloid leukemia; *FSH,* follicle-stimulating hormone; *IT,* intrathecal; *LFT,* liver function test; *LH,* luteinizing hormone; *MRI,* magnetic resonance imaging; *RT,* radiation therapy; *TSH,* thyroid-stimulating hormone.

oncology centers have developed late-effects programs to conduct surveillance for the development of these problems and provide follow-up care to patients who develop late complications of therapy.

References

Special section: cancer in children and adolescents. In: American Cancer Society: cancer Facts and Figures 2014. American Cancer Society, 2014, pp 25-42.

Bolouri H, Farrar JE, Triche T, et al: The molecular landscape of pediatric acute myeloid leukemia reveals recurrent structural alterations and age-specific mutational interactions, *Nat Med* 24(1):103–112, 01 2018, https://doi.org/10.1038/nm.4439.

Brown AL, Arts P, Carmichael CL, et al: RUNX1-mutated families show phenotype heterogeneity and a somatic mutation profile unique to germline predisposed AML, *Blood Adv* 4(6):1131–1144, 03 2020, https://doi.org/10.1182/bloodadvances.2019000901.

Brown PA, Ji L, Xu X, et al: Effect of postreduction therapy consolidation with blinatumomab vs chemotherapy on disease-free survival in children, adolescents, and young adults with first relapse of B-cell acute lymphoblastic leukemia: a randomized clinical trial, *J Am Med Assoc* 325(9):833–842, 03 2021, https://doi.org/10.1001/jama.2021.0669.

Buitenkamp TD, Izraeli S, Zimmermann M, et al: Acute lymphoblastic leukemia in children with Down syndrome: a retrospective analysis from the Ponte di Legno study group, *Blood* 123(1):70–77, Jan 2, 2014, https://doi.org/10.1182/blood-2013-06-509463.

Creutzig U, Zimmermann M, Reinhardt D, et al: Changes in cytogenetics and molecular genetics in acute myeloid leukemia from childhood to adult age groups, *Cancer* 122(24):3821–3830, Dec 2016, https://doi.org/10.1002/cncr.30220.

Davidsson J, Puschmann A, Tedgård U, Bryder D, Nilsson L, Cammenga J: SAMD9 and SAMD9L in inherited predisposition to ataxia, pancytopenia, and myeloid malignancies, *Leukemia* 32(5):1106–1115, 05 2018, https://doi.org/10.1038/s41375-018-0074-4.

Gaynon PS, Qu RP, Chappell RJ, et al: Survival after relapse in childhood acute lymphoblastic leukemia: Impact of site and time to first relapse—the Children's Cancer Group Experience, *Cancer* 82:1387–1395, 1998.

Gibson BE, Wheatley K, Hann IM, et al: Treatment strategy and long-term results in paediatric patients treated in consecutive UK AML trials, *Leukemia* 19:2130–2138, 2005.

Greaves MF, Wiemels J: Origins of chromosome translocations in childhood leukaemia, *Nat Rev Cancer* 3:639–649, 2003.

Hunger SP, Mullighan CG: Acute lymphoblastic leukemia in children, *N Engl J Med* 373(16):1541–1552, Oct 15, 2015, https://doi.org/10.1056/NEJMra1400972.

Locatelli F, Zugmaier G, Rizzari C, et al: Effect of blinatumomab vs chemotherapy on event-free survival among children with high-risk first-relapse B-cell acute lymphoblastic leukemia: a randomized clinical trial, *J Am Med Assoc* 325(9):843–854, 03 2021, https://doi.org/10.1001/jama.2021.0987.

Loh ML, Sakai DS, Flotho C, et al: Mutations in CBL occur frequently in juvenile myelomonocytic leukemia, *Blood* 114(9):1859–1863, Aug 27, 2009.

Maude SL, Laetsch TW, Buechner J, et al: Tisagenlecleucel in children and young adults with B-cell lymphoblastic leukemia, *N Engl J Med* 378(5):439–448, 02 2018, https://doi.org/10.1056/NEJMoa1709866.

Möricke A, Zimmermann M, Reiter A, et al: Long-term results of five consecutive trials in childhood acute lymphoblastic leukemia performed by the ALL-BFM study group from 1981 to 2000, *Leukemia* 24(2):265–284, Feb 2010, https://doi.org/10.1038/leu.2009.257.

Pui CH, Campana D, Pei D, et al: Treating childhood acute lymphoblastic leukemia without cranial irradiation, *N Engl J Med* 360(26):2730–2741, Jun 2009, https://doi.org/10.1056/NEJMoa0900386.

Pui CH, Cheng C, Leung W, et al: Extended follow-up of long-term survivors of childhood acute lymphoblastic leukemia, *N Engl J Med* 349:640–649, 2003.

Pui CH, Pei D, Sandlund JT, et al: Long-term results of St Jude total therapy studies 11, 12, 13A, 13B, and 14 for childhood acute lymphoblastic leukemia, *Leukemia* 24(2):371–382, Feb 2010, https://doi.org/10.1038/leu.2009.252.

Ries LAG, Melbert D, Krapcho M, et al: *SEER cancer statistics review, 1975–2004,* Bethesda, Md, 2007, National Cancer Institute2007.

Silverman LB, Stevenson KE, O'Brien JE, et al: Long-term results of Dana-Farber Cancer Institute ALL Consortium protocols for children with newly diagnosed acute lymphoblastic leukemia (1985-2000), *Leukemia* 24(2):320–334, Feb 2010, https://doi.org/10.1038/leu.2009.253.

Stahnke K, Boos J, Bender-Gotze C, et al: Duration of first remission predicts remission rates and long-term survival in children with relapsed acute myelogenous leukemia, *Leukemia* 12:1534–1538, 1998.

Uffmann M, Rasche M, Zimmermann M, et al: Therapy reduction in patients with Down syndrome and myeloid leukemia: the international ML-DS 2006 trial, *Blood* 129(25):3314–3321, 06 2017, https://doi.org/10.1182/blood-2017-01-765057.

Wakeford R, Little MP: Risk coefficients for childhood cancer after intrauterine irradiation: a review, *Int J Radiat Biol* 79:293–309, 2003.

Wlodarski MW, Hirabayashi S, Pastor V, et al: Prevalence, clinical characteristics, and prognosis of GATA2-related myelodysplastic syndromes in children and adolescents, *Blood* 127(11):1387–1397, Mar 2016, https://doi.org/10.1182/blood-2015-09-669937. quiz 1518.

Woods WG, Neudorf S, Gold S, et al: A comparison of allogeneic bone marrow transplantation, autologous bone marrow transplantation, and aggressive chemotherapy in children with acute myeloid leukemia in remission, *Blood* 97:56–62, 2001.

ADOLESCENT HEALTH

Method of
Kari R. Harris, MD

CURRENT DIAGNOSIS

- In addition to general medical care, it is important to identify psychosocial health concerns at all adolescent visits.
- The key components of a psychosocial history are addressed in the HEADS private and confidential interview.
- Conducting a Home/Education/Employment/Activities/Accident Prevention/Diet/Disordered Eating/Drugs/Depression/Suicide/Self-harm/Sex/Sleep/Social Media (HEADS) interview is standard practice for adolescent care: it should be part of all adolescent well-checks and used, as time permits, in acute visits for teens who have high-risk behaviors or have no regular health care.
- High-acuity areas identified from the HEADS interview include substance use, disordered eating, sexual activity, and mental health.
- Anxiety and depression screening should be part of well visits for all adolescents.
- Substance use screening should be included in all adolescent well visits.
- HIV universal screening should be completed initially between 15 and 18 years of age and the need for rescreening reassessed annually.
- Immunization status should be assessed at every visit, with routine and catch-up vaccines provided.

CURRENT THERAPY

- Minor consent and confidentiality laws vary by state and are important to understand when caring for adolescents.
- Long-acting reversible contraception (LARC) provides safe and effective contraception for teenagers.
- Emergency contraception and post-exposure prophylaxis should be considered for adolescents.
- When discussing substance use, consider prescribing naloxone and discussing use.
- Treatment for teens is often multidisciplinary, involving subspecialists, mental health providers, medical or psychiatric inpatient units, and county welfare or health departments.

Setting the Stage for the Adolescent Visit

Comprehensive care for adolescents includes screening for high-risk behaviors in addition to routine medical care. To facilitate open communication, providers should be clear about consent and confidentiality policies in their practices. This can be achieved by discussing policies with patients and parents/caretakers during young adolescent visits (11 to 14 years) and by providing materials documenting the policies and practices, such as a standard letter to parents. Policies can also be displayed in the office, provided in practice newsletters and materials, and made available through patient access portals.

Adolescent visits differ from early childhood visits in several important respects. At the beginning of the visit, time should be spent with both the teen and parent or caregiver clarifying medical history and current concerns. The adolescent should then be offered time without the parent or caregiver present to discuss sensitive issues, including reproductive and mental health. At the end of the visit, the parent/caregiver should be provided with a summary of the visit, limited to the nonconfidential portion,

and including recommendations and arrangements for follow-up appointments.

Consent and Confidentiality Laws—Consent Does Not Equal Confidential

Consent and confidentiality laws vary by state. Most states allow minors to consent for reproductive health care, including testing and treatment for sexually transmitted infections (STIs). Most states also allow physicians and clinicians to prescribe contraceptives to minors. Many states have a "mature minor" statute that allows physicians to provide care if they deem the adolescent patient mature and capable of understanding the medical care. These laws give teens autonomy to consent to their own health care and they also enable care to be provided when a parent is unable to attend the appointment.

While consent and confidentiality laws are related, they are separate entities. Many states allow minors to consent for specific health services but do not prohibit a physician or clinician from informing the teen's parent/caretaker about that service. Even if allowed by law, expert consensus holds that such disclosures should only be made when in the best interest of the minor patient. The disclosure should not compromise future health care. Many teens will not seek reproductive health care if they have to involve a parent, making confidentiality necessary for comprehensive adolescent health care.

Confidentiality is limited when a minor patient is in direct harm, such as intimate partner violence, sexual coercion or rape, certain pregnancy, suicidality, or self-harm. In such instances, a parent/caretaker should become involved, unless he/she is the perpetrator or some other extraordinary circumstances exist. Local authorities or social welfare agencies may also need to be contacted. These necessary breaches in confidentiality to protect safety must be explained beforehand to the patient and be included in written policies. Any breach of confidentiality must be carried out in a professional manner, explained sensitively to the patient and others, and be well documented. Every attempt must be made not to compromise future care.

Information on consent and confidentiality laws for each state is available at the National Center for Youth Law (youthlaw.org).

The HEADS Interview

The HEADS acronym provides a structured psychosocial history-taking tool that also screens for strengths and high-risk behaviors (Table 1). Although several variations of HEADS have been described, they all cover the most common risk categories for adolescents. Progressing from the least invasive topics to the most sensitive issues, HEADS covers all essential categories (see Table 1).

When using the HEADS interview tool, it is important to build rapport with the patient and include a discussion of what will and will not be kept confidential. The teen deserves explanation of why they are being asked personal questions and every attempt should be made to increase patient comfort and trust. The interview begins with questions regarding hobbies, school, and home life. Once rapport is established, questions proceed to more sensitive issues. Questioning should be open-ended, nonassuming, and nonjudgmental. This allows for honest answers and does not discriminate among patients.

Home/Education/Employment/Activities/Accident Prevention

These topics begin the interview with the least risky activities for adolescents. Although grouped together in this text, each category deserves its own time and questions (see Table 1). All adolescents should identify a trusted adult with whom they can discuss concerns. Safety at home and school safety, including any bullying or coercion regardless of site or circumstances, should be discussed and addressed. Current school performance, concerns, grades and post graduation goals should be discussed. After-school employment has benefits but can also negatively impact academic performance, mood, or family dynamics. These should be screened for and addressed if present. Healthy after-school activities should be

TABLE 1	**HEADS Acronym with Sample Questions**	
H	Home	Who lives with you at home? Tell me about your relationships at home. Are you safe at home? Do you have a trusted adult to confide in at home? Do you have your own space at home? Have there been any changes at home?
E	Education	What grade are you in and what school? How do you receive your education (online, in person, at home)? Is your school safe? Tell me about your friends. Does anyone bother you at school? Who is an adult you can trust at school? How are your grades? Do you have any problems with school? How many days of school have you missed this year and why? Do you plan to graduate? What do you want to do after graduation?
	Employment	Are you working? Do you like your job? How do you spend the money you earn from working? Do you feel stressed because of work? Is your family stressed by your work? How many hours a week do you work?
A	Activities	Tell me about your activities. What do you do for fun? Who do you hang out with? Tell me what you do after school. Are you in any organized after-school or summer activities? Tell me about your hobbies. Do you have a religious preference?
	Accident prevention	Do you wear a seatbelt? Do you wear a helmet while biking or using an all-terrain vehicle? Have you ever ridden with someone while they were under the influence of drugs or alcohol, or have you ever driven under the influence? Where is your cell phone while you are driving?
D	Diet/disordered eating	Tell me about your diet. Do you feel like you have enough food at home? Are you ever worried you might not get three meals a day because there is not enough food? Do you eat breakfast daily? How many fruits and vegetables do you eat? How do you feel about your weight? Do you like the way you look? Have you ever not eaten to try to lose weight? Do you ever feel guilty about what you have eaten? Have you ever skipped meals, vomited on purpose, or exercised excessively after you have eaten?
	Drugs	Have you seen drugs at your school? Do any of your friends smoke, vape, drink alcohol, or use other drugs? Have you ever tried drugs? Have you ever taken a pill given to you by someone else? Do you have naloxone available to you, and do you know how and when to use it? Have you ever been in trouble because of drug use?
	Depression/anxiety	Do you ever feel sad, down, or depressed? Have you ever felt like you had nothing to look forward to? Do you still like to do the things you used to do? Do others say you are more irritable than normal? Do you worry much? Do you have trouble sleeping at night? Do you ever feel like you cannot shut off your mind? Have you ever had a panic attack?
S	Suicide/self-harm	Have you ever been so upset you have wanted to hurt yourself? Have you ever cut yourself? Have you ever thought about killing yourself or someone else? Who would you talk with if you did have thoughts like this?
	Sex	Are you in a relationship? Tell me about the type of person you are attracted to. Tell me about your identity. When is the last time you had sex? Did you use a condom? Are you using anything to prevent pregnancy? Have you ever been tested for STIs? How many partners have you had? Tell me about your partner (age, gender, etc.). Do you feel safe with your partner? Have you ever been forced to have sex or do something you were not comfortable with?
	Sleep	What time do you go to bed? Where is your cell phone when you go to sleep? When do you wake up in the morning? Do you feel rested when you wake up?
	Social media	What social media sites do you have profiles on? Are you friends with people you do not know in real life? How much time do you spend on social media? Does this affect your grades? Tell me about your privacy settings. Do you have any trusted adults that can access your social media sites?

STI, Sexually transmitted infections.

Adapted from Klein DA, Goldenring JM: HEEADSSS 3.0: The psychosocial interview for adolescents updated for a new century fueled by media. *Contemporary Pediatrics.* 2014. Available at https://www.contemporarypediatrics.com/view/heeadsss-30-psychosocial-interview-adolescents-updated-new-century-fueled-media. (Accessed February 1, 2024.)

encouraged. Predictably, adolescent illegal activity, drug use, and sexual activity peak during after-school hours. Participation in organized, supervised, extracurricular activities has been shown to decrease these risky behaviors and confer positive health and emotional benefits. Accidents remain the leading cause of death for this age group and prevention should be emphasized. Safety should be assessed at this time, as well as throughout the course of the interview as it applies to each topic.

Diet/Disordered Eating

Nutritional health problems are of concern with adolescents. Many lifestyle habits, especially regarding nutrition, are formed during this period. Asking the teen to describe his/her typical diet provides insight on potential areas for improvement. Limiting portion sizes, avoiding excessive or late night snacking, and replacing sugary drinks with water is common advice for teens. This portion of the interview provides opportunity to screen for body image distortion or disordered eating. The growth chart should be reviewed and any significant weight changes discussed.

Drugs (Substance Use)

When asking about riskier behaviors, it is important to have rapport and trust. Because alcohol, marijuana, electronic vaping, and tobacco use are so prevalent among high school students, an initial question about peer use can help direct the interview to personal use. Personal use should include the above substances and other recreational drugs, prescription medications, and opioid/fentanyl use. The CRAFFT acronym is a brief and effective screening tool designed specifically for use with adolescents. The questions are broken into part A and B. If a patient answers "yes" to any questions in part A, then part B questions are asked. If the patient answers "yes" to two or more questions of part B, the screen is positive and further evaluation is recommended (Table 2). Substance use is a leading cause of morbidity and mortality for teens in the United States, and teens who use substances at an early age are more likely to develop a substance use disorder. If a substance use disorder is suspected or diagnosed, referral should be made to a qualified substance use/addiction medicine therapist. The physician, therapist, patient, and family should work together to determine if pharmacologic intervention is an

TABLE 2

TABLE 2 CRAFFT+N Substance Use Disorder Screening Tool for Adolescents (to be verbally administered by a clinician in a private setting with the teen)

Part A

During the past 12 months did you:

1. Drink more than a few sips of beer, wine, or any drink containing alcohol? Say "0" if none.
2. Smoked any marijuana (weed, oil, or hash by smoking, vaping, or in food) or "synthetic marijuana" (like "K2", "Spice")? Say "0" if none.
3. Used anything else to get high (like other illegal, prescription, or over-the-counter medications, and things that you sniff, huff, or vape)? Say "0" if none.
4. Use any tobacco or nicotine products (for example, cigarettes, e-cigarettes, hookahs, smokeless tobacco)? Say "0" if none.

If all answers in part A are 0, then ask only "CAR" Part B, then stop.
If any answer to part A is >0, then ask all 6 questions of Part B.

Part B

C 1. Have you ever ridden in a **CAR** driven by someone (including yourself) who was high or had been using alcohol or other drugs?

R 2. Do you ever use alcohol or other drugs to **RELAX**, feel better about yourself, or fit in?

A 3. Do you ever use alcohol or other drugs while you are by yourself, **ALONE**?

F 4. Do you ever **FORGET** things you did while using alcohol or drugs?

F 5. Do your **FAMILY** or **FRIENDS** ever tell you that you should cut down on your drinking or drug use?

T 6. Have you ever gotten into **TROUBLE** while you were using alcohol or other drugs?

*Two or more YES answers suggest a serious problem and need for further assessment. See http://crafft.org/get-the-crafft/ for further instructions.

The CRAFFT+N 2.1. John R. Knight, MD: The Center for Adolescent Substance Abuse Research (CeASAR); Boston Children's Hospital; Harvard Medical School Teaching Hospital. 2018. Available at: http://crafft.org (Accessed October 4, 2019).

appropriate component of treatment for a substance use disorder. Additionally, opioid use has drastically increased in recent years; therefore, physicians and clinicians should ask about opioid use and, if disclosed, prescribe and educate on the use of naloxone. While a clear message of non-use should be provided regarding all substances, harm reduction should also be discussed during the visit, especially for those using multiple substances and opioids.

Depression/Anxiety/Suicide/Self-Harm

Depression screening is recommended at all well visits beginning at age 12. Several screening tools are available. Questions covering loss of interest in normal activities and feeling depressed, down, or hopeless open the door to more specific questions regarding signs and symptoms of depression. In addition to depressive feelings, teens should be explicitly screened for suicidal intention, past attempts, plans, self-harm, and safety. If a teen discloses an unsafe environment, law enforcement may need to be included in an immediate plan of care. If a teen is actively suicidal, then immediate inpatient treatment is warranted. Anxiety is common in adolescents and those 8 years and older should be screened. Screening can occur concomitantly with depression screening. History should assess social function, somatic symptoms, and coping strategies. Outpatient treatment for mental health disorders in teens includes cognitive behavioral therapy with or without medication. School accommodations may also be helpful for teens with mental health diagnoses. For most teens, parental involvement is necessary when treating mental health disorders. If the physician or clinician feels the teen is unsafe due to their own actions or those of others, then the caretaker must be included in the next stage of management.

Sex

Nearly half of high school students have had sex. Of those, only about a quarter used reliable contraception at their last intercourse. Adolescents and young adults account for the majority of gonorrhea and chlamydia cases each year. Risk factors for morbidity related to sexual activity include early sexual initiation, increasing number of partners, substance use prior to sex, and unprotected sexual acts. Teenagers and men who have sex with men are the population groups at highest risk for STIs. STI screening should be discussed for those at risk. Recommendations are outlined in Table 3.

When discussing the sensitive issue of sex with teens, it is important to use neutral terms and remain nonjudgmental. Important aspects of a sexual history include age of first sexual encounter, age of partner(s), gender of partner, number of partners, type of sexual activities, date of last sexual activity, and contraceptive and barrier use. Consider assessing gender identity, romantic interest, and quality of relationships, as 7% of high school students report that they have experienced sexual dating violence including sexual coercion and rape.

While prevention remains the best method to prevent morbidity related to sex, physicians and clinicians should be aware of postexposure options to prevent disease and pregnancy. Emergency contraception can be offered up to 5 days postcoital and is around 80% to 90% effective at preventing pregnancy. Postexposure prophylaxis is available for some populations to decrease the risk of sexually transmitted infections such as gonorrhea, chlamydia, syphilis, and human immunodeficiency virus (HIV). Additionally, for those at increased risk for HIV, preexposure prophylaxis is also available. Teens should also be counseled that condoms are an additional method to prevent infections and pregnancy and should be used during all sexual intercourse.

Teens should be counseled on contraceptive options, including abstinence, emphasizing that LARC (intrauterine contraception and implants) is safe and the most reliable contraception available for teens. Quick-start contraception (prescribing or providing contraception at the current appointment) should be strongly considered to improve adherence in sexually active teens. The possibility of pregnancy should be reasonably ruled out prior to providing contraception by taking a careful sexual history, including last menstrual period, date of last sex, and method of contraception; lab work may also be considered (see the US Selected Practice Recommendations for Contraceptive Use for guidance on how to reasonably rule out pregnancy, https://www.cdc.gov/mmwr/volumes/73/rr/rr7303a1.htm). If a patient has been recently sexually active, most non-intrauterine contraceptives have not been shown to harm an existing pregnancy. Nevertheless, counseling regarding this risk is important prior to initiating contraception, and pregnancy testing should be performed 2 to 4 weeks following contraception initiation. For patients who have had unprotected sex in the past 5 days, emergency contraception should be discussed and offered at the time of quick start contraception. Concurrent barrier contraception should be stressed. Aside from abstinence, male condoms are the most effective way of preventing STIs.

Sleep/Social Media

The conclusion of this format of the HEADS interview concerns less sensitive topics and allows for a comfortable close to the interview. Sleep is problematic for many teens and can usually be improved with better sleep hygiene. Encourage all teens to have a consistent sleep and wake time and 8 to 10 hours of sleep daily. Caffeinated beverages should be limited. Daily exercise should be recommended. The teen's bedroom should be free from distractions, including screened electronic devices.

Social media and cell phones are now integral to popular culture. While these offer some benefits to teens, use should be limited. Both social media and cell phones contribute to unintentional injuries, especially with distracted driving. In addition, personal information being shared on the internet through electronic media opens the teen up to vulnerability. Lastly, both can act as significant distractions from academic

TABLE 3 Laboratory Screening and Procedure Recommendations

SCREENING	AGE	TEST/PROCEDURE	COMMENTS
Dyslipidemia	9–11 17–21	Nonfasting lipid profile	Once between 9 and 11 years and again between 17 and 21 years with annual risk assessment (NHLBI, AAP) Insufficient evidence for screening (USPSTF)
Hemoglobin/hematocrit	11–21	Verbally screen for risk	No routine testing recommended
Hepatits B	Adolescents at increased risk	Serology for hepatitis B surface antigen	Screen if increased risk regardless of vaccination status (USPSTF, AAP)
Hepatitis C	18–79	Serology for anti–hepatitis C antibody	Once between 18 and 79 years, with annual reassessment and testing if risk factors are present (USPSTF, CDC, AAP)
Human immunodeficiency virus (HIV)	15–18	HIV 1–2 immunoassay	At least once if >15 years with more frequent screening if high-risk (CDC, USPSTF, AAP) Screen MSM at least annually (CDC)
Chlamydia	Females <25	NAAT at site of potential infection	Screen all sexually active women <25 years at risk (USPSTF) or annually and MSM at least annually (CDC)
Gonorrhea	Females <25	NAAT at site of potential infection	Screen all sexually active women <25 years at risk (USPSTF) and MSM at least annually (CDC)
Syphilis	Adolescents at increased risk	Serology with confirmatory testing if positive	Screen persons at increased risk (USPSTF). Screen MSM at least annually (CDC)
Cervical dysplasia screening	21 years	Pap smear	Other indications for pelvic exam still apply but routine Pap testing <21 years is not recommended (USPSTF, AAP)
Immunizations	All ages	Routine vaccinations per CDC guidelines	Immunization status should be assessed and routine and catch-up vaccines provided at all adolescent visits

AAP, American Academy of Pediatrics; *CDC*, Center for Disease Control and Prevention; *MSM*, Men who have sex with men; *NAAT*, nucleic acid amplification testing; *NIHLB*, National Heart, Lung, and Blood Institute; *Pap smear*, Papanicolaou smear; *USPSTF*, US Preventive Services Task Force.
Data from US Preventive Services Task Force: A & B recommendations. Available at: https://www.uspreventiveservicestaskforce.org/uspstf/recommendation-topics/uspstf-a-and-b-recommendations. [accessed 2-19-23].

work, family time, and sleep. Discuss safe and appropriate use of electronic devices with patients and summarize to parents.

Summary

In addition to providing routine health care to teens, physicians and clinicians should focus on the psychosocial history. The HEADS acronym provides a tool to approach these sensitive topics systematically. This interview should take place privately, respecting the teen's ability to consent for certain care, and when able, keeping care confidential. Physicians and clinicians should be familiar with the laws regarding consent and confidentiality of minors in their state. Although teens should be allowed access to confidential health care, often the best care includes a trusted adult. Parents should be involved in their teen's care when appropriate. Once teens have been assessed for high-risk behaviors, problematic behaviors should be addressed and positive behaviors should be commended and encouraged.

References

2022 recommendations for preventive pediatric health care, *Pediatrics* 150 (1): e2022058044, 2022. doi: 10.1542/peds.2022-058044.

American Academy of Pediatrics. *Performing preventive services: A bright futures handbook*, 2010, AAP. Available at http://brightfutures.aap.org/pdfs/preventive%20services%20pdfs/physical%20examination.pdf [accessed 10.13.14].

Centers for Disease Control and Prevention; Sexually transmitted diseases treatment guidelines, 2021, *MMWR Recomm Rep* 70(4):1–187, 2021. Available at https://www.cdc.gov/std/treatment-guidelines/STI-Guidelines-2021.pdf

Cohen DA, Farley TA, Taylor SN, et al: When and where do youths have sex? The potential role of adult supervision, Pediatrics 110: Available at http://pediatrics.aappublications.org/content/110/6/e66.long [accessed 02.10.18].

Curtis KM, Jatlaoui TC, Tepper NK, et al: 2016 U.S. Selected Practice Recommendations for Contraceptive Use, *MMWR Recomm Rep* 65(No. RR-4):1–66, 2016, https://doi.org/10.15585/mmwr.rr6504a1. [Accessed 14 March 2017]. accessed.

English A, Gudeman R: Minor consent and confidentiality: a compendium of state and federal laws. National Center for Youth Law, August 2024. https://youthlaw.org/sites/default/files/2024-10/NCYLMinorConsentCompendium2024.pdf [accessed 02.27.25].

Expert panel on integrated guidelines for cardiovascular health and risk reduction in children and adolescents: summary report. National Heart, Lung, and Blood Institute. Available at https://www.nhlbi.nih.gov/health-topics/integrated-guidelines-for-cardiovascular-health-and-risk-reduction-in-children-and-adolescents [accessed 02.01.24].

Gregory KD, Chelmow D, Nelson HD: Screening for anxiety in adolescent and adult women: a recommendation from the Women's Preventive Services Initiative, *Ann Intern Med* 173(1):48–56, 2020.

Centers for Disease Control and Prevention. Youth Risk Behavior Surveillance - United States, 2019. MMWR Suppl 2020;69, 2020. Available at https://www.cdc.gov/mmwr/volumes/69/su/pdfs/su6901-H.pdf. Accessed February 8, 2022.

Klein DA, Goldenring JM: HEEADSSS 3.0: the psychosocial interview for adolescents updated for a new century fueled by media, *Contemp Pediatr*, 2014. Available at https://www.contemporarypediatrics.com/view/heeadsss-30-psychosocial-interview-adolescents-updated-new-century-fueled-media [accessed 02.01.24].

The CRAFFT+N 2.1. John R. Knight, MD, The Center for Adolescent Substance Abuse Research (CeASAR); Boston Children's Hospital; Harvard Medical School Teaching Hospital. 2018. Available at: http://crafft.org/. Accessed Oct. 4, 2019.

U.S. Preventive Services Task Force. Recommendations for Primary Care Practice. Available at https://www.uspreventiveservicestaskforce.org/Page/Name/recommendations [accessed 02.10.18].

ASTHMA IN CHILDREN

Method of
Kevin W. Gray, MD

CURRENT DIAGNOSIS

- Recurrent shortness of breath, cough, and wheeze are the hallmark symptoms of asthma.
- Personal and family histories of atopic disease are associated with an increased risk of asthma development.
- Physical examination is frequently normal; however, edematous nasal mucosa, atopic dermatitis, tachycardia, tachypnea, and expiratory wheeze may be present.
- Asthma is diagnosed objectively with variability of lung function and expiratory airflow limitation in the presence of typical symptoms.
- Objective testing under the age of 5 years can be difficult, and initial treatment based on observation and clinical judgment may be reasonable in this population.
- Spirometry is the gold standard for diagnosis showing an obstructive pattern with some evidence of reversibility after bronchodilator therapy.
- Peak expiratory flow may be an appropriate surrogate for formal spirometry when resources for such may not be readily available.
- Chest imaging and serum testing including complete blood count and IgE levels are not required for diagnosis but may provide useful information.

CURRENT TREATMENT

- Asthma treatment is aimed at reduction of impairment in activities and the risk of exacerbation.
- Short-acting β agonist (SABA)-only treatment is not recommended in patients 6 years of age and older.
- Inhaled corticosteroids (ICS) are the most effective controller medication, and much of the benefit is achieved at low dosage.
- Initial controller therapy can be decided by the frequency and severity of symptoms present.
- Antiinflammatory reliever (AIR) therapy and maintenance and reliever therapy (MART) have grown in adoption as initial therapy in many patients.
- AIR therapy includes the addition of a low-dose ICS to as-needed SABA therapy.
- Budesonide-formoterol (Breyna, Symbicort) is the most commonly used MART for patients over the age of 6 years.
- Patients and caregivers should be involved in the development of an asthma action plan as a means of shared decision making and education opportunity on the identification and management of symptom escalation.
- Escalation of therapy can be considered for uncontrolled symptoms after adherence and technique of current therapy has been evaluated.
- De-escalation of therapy should be considered after 3 months of symptom control with current controller therapy.
- Referral to a pulmonologist or allergist should be considered for patients whose symptoms are not controlled by standard therapy.
- Treatment of acute exacerbations includes SABA, inhaled and/or oral corticosteroids, and supplemental oxygen to maintain oxygen saturation of 94% to 98% in the pediatric population.

Epidemiology

Asthma is the most common chronic disease in children, with a prevalence of 6.5% in children under 17 years, and is characterized by chronic airway inflammation. Common symptoms include shortness of breath, cough, wheezing, and chest tightness. The symptoms are often variable and present with variable airflow limitation. Although not necessary for diagnosis, airway hyperreactivity and inflammation are associated with asthma. Expiratory airflow limitation is typically present with symptoms, and its severity can be variable.

Risk Factors

Several factors have been found to increase the likelihood of asthma diagnosis. These include personal or family history of atopic disease including allergic rhinitis, atopic dermatitis, and asthma in addition to childhood symptoms. A prospective cohort study in the United States found an increased risk of early wheeze in children 1 to 2 years of age, in children with parental history of asthma, in children whose mothers smoked during pregnancy, in children of mothers who did not graduate high school, and in children of mothers who did not receive any college education. Additionally, factors increasing risk of persistent wheeze include Black race, Hispanic ethnicity, parental history of smoking, and smoking during pregnancy.

Pathophysiology

Asthma is a heterogeneous disease with complex pathophysiology led by airway hyperreactivity. An exaggerated bronchoconstrictor response is implicated, typically in the presence of irritants. Atopy with an increase in immunoglobulin E (IgE) level and response of type 4 hypersensitivity are implicated in the exacerbation of disease. In a simplistic view, asthma symptoms are caused by airway narrowing, which is variable and leads to airflow limitation by several mechanisms. Bronchial smooth muscle contraction decreases airway diameter and is targeted by bronchodilator therapy. Airway edema related to inflammatory mediated microvascular leakage causes additional narrowing. Because of mucosal thickening and fibroblast mediating, remodeling may occur with prolonged and severe disease and is not easily reversed by current treatments. Mucus plugging results from excess secretion of mucus in the airways, leading to the functional limitation of small airways.

Prevention

Although prevention of asthma is an important topic and many studies have looked specifically at primary prevention of asthma, the data on single interventions remain unclear. The Global Initiative for Asthma (GINA) guidelines encourage vaginal delivery where possible, as exposure to the vaginal microbiome may be beneficial and rates of asthma are higher in children born via cesarean section; discouraging the use of broad-spectrum antibiotics in the first year of life; identification and correction of vitamin D deficiency in women with asthma who are pregnant or planning pregnancy; avoiding exposure to environmental tobacco smoke during pregnancy and in the first year of life; and encouraging breastfeeding for its health benefits regardless of potential impact on development of asthma in the child. Maternal intake of foods commonly seen as allergenic, such as peanuts, tree nuts, shellfish, and milk, may reduce the risk of asthma in the developing child. Some findings suggest that maternal obesity and weight gain increase the risk of asthma and wheezing in their child. Whereas infant respiratory syncytial virus (RSV) immunization increases risk of wheezing in the first year of life, effect beyond that time has not yet been demonstrated. Prenatal and/or infant vaccination to RSV is a more recent recommendation; however, further research is needed to monitor potential long-term effects on incidence of wheeze and asthma. The British Thoracic Society (BTS), Scottish Intercollegiate Guideline Network (SIGN), and National Institute for Health and Care Excellence (NICE) guidelines recommend reduction in utero and early life exposure to air

BOX 1 Asthma Triggers

Allergens
- Animal dander
- Dust mites
- Mold
- Pollen

Chemical Irritants
- Air pollution
- Cleaning chemicals
- Gases
- Tobacco smoke
- Wood stove smoke

Medications
- Aspirin
- β-Blockers
- Nonsteroidal antiinflammatory drugs

Other
- Changes in weather
- Cold air
- Exercise
- Extremes of emotion
- Gastroesophageal reflux
- Respiratory infection
- Stress

allergens such as dust mites, pets, or single food allergen in addition to maternal food allergy and avoidance during pregnancy and lactation.

Clinical Manifestations

Asthma is characterized clinically by recurrent episodes of chest tightness, shortness of breath, and wheezing but also may manifest as a chronic dry cough especially occurring at night. Wheezing in the presence of predictable triggers is common in pediatric asthma (Box 1).

Diagnosis

Many studies have examined the diagnostic accuracy of asthma with findings of overdiagnosis in some populations and underdiagnosis in others. In groups affected by social determinants of health, the cost of objective testing, treatment, and underreporting of respiratory symptoms has been implicated. In patients over 5 years where objective testing can be more reliably performed, diagnosis based on symptoms and response to treatment should be avoided to avoid overdiagnosis. An accurate diagnosis of asthma is important and ideally should be completed with objective testing in most patients before therapy initiation. However, in certain populations, such as those under 5 years of age, this may be logistically difficult. Diagnosis by objective testing avoids unnecessary and over-treatment and enables prompt evaluation for other differential diagnoses in the case of normal values. Additionally, objective testing becomes more difficult to interpret once patients are started on controller treatment.

History

A careful history is important for the initial presentation of patients with respiratory symptoms as several features have been shown to increase or decrease the probability of asthma diagnosis. Additionally, personal history and childhood of allergic rhinitis, eczema, or family history of asthma or allergy increases the probability that respiratory symptoms are related to an asthma diagnosis. It is important to note that although these features are commonly found in patients with asthma, they are not specific to asthma and are not always present in all asthma phenotypes. It is important to inquire about specific respiratory symptoms and patients with allergic rhinitis or eczema.

Features that increase the probability that a patient has asthma include the following:
- Presence of one or more of the following symptoms that worsen at night or in the early morning: wheeze, shortness of breath, cough, and/or chest tightness
- Symptoms that worsen at night or in the early morning
- Symptoms that vary in intensity and over time
- Symptoms that are triggered by viral infections, such as colds, exercise, allergen exposure, changes in weather, laughter, or irritants such as car exhaust fumes, smoke, or strong smells

Features that decrease the probability that a patient has asthma include the following:
- Isolated cough without other respiratory symptoms
- Chronic sputum production
- Shortness of breath associated with dizziness, lightheadedness, or peripheral paresthesia
- Chest pain
- Exercise-induced dyspnea with noisy inspiration

Physical Examination

Lending to its variable nature and symptoms, physical examination is often normal. Expiratory wheezing, or rhonchi, is the most frequent abnormality noted on the examination, although it may be heard only on forced expiration and absent altogether depending on severity of symptoms. It is important to note that wheezing may also be noted in several other differential diagnoses for asthma. Crackles and inspiratory wheezes are not typical features of asthma and may point more toward a cardiac or upper airway pathology, respectively. Examination of the ears, nose, and throat may reveal signs of allergic rhinitis or nasal polyps. Pulse oximetry should be completed in all patients presenting with respiratory complaints, and saturation (SpO_2) less than 90% should signal the need for aggressive treatment. Peak expiratory flow (PEF) testing should be performed for children older than 5 years at each visit.

Imaging

Although imaging studies are not usually necessary for diagnosing asthma, they can be beneficial for patients with challenging-to-treat asthma to explore alternative diagnoses such as infections, inhaled foreign bodies, and cardiac silhouette evaluation. Chest radiography may also be useful for evaluating acute respiratory complaints when the diagnosis of asthma is typically not made. High-resolution computed tomography of the chest can help identify structural pathology and rule out other conditions that can be responsible for wheezing.

Pulmonary Function Testing

The goal of pulmonary function testing in asthma diagnosis is to document expiratory airflow limitation and variability in lung function.

Expiratory airflow limitation can be confirmed in children with a ratio of forced expiratory volume in 1 second to forced vital capacity (FEV_1/FVC) of less than 0.9 at a time where FEV_1 is reduced.

Variability in lung function can be documented objectively by several means:
- An increase in FEV_1 from baseline of greater than 12% of the predicted value 10 to 15 minutes after 200 to 400 μg of albuterol
- Greater than 13% average daily diurnal PEF variability calculated by (highest PEF – lowest PEF)/(mean of highest PEF and lowest PEF)
- Exercise challenge test with a decrease of greater than 12% of predicted FEV_1 or greater than 15% from baseline
- Variation of greater than 12% in FEV_1 or greater than 15% PEF between visits

Testing from spirometry is more reliable in its accuracy when compared with PEF testing.

Bronchial Provocation Testing

Bronchial provocation testing is not required for diagnosis of asthma but may be performed to verify airway

BOX 2 Differential Diagnosis

Upper Airway
- Allergic rhinitis
- Sinusitis

Large Airway Obstruction
- Vocal cord dysfunction
- Laryngotracheomalacia (infants)
- Tracheal stenosis (infants)
- Vascular rings
- Tracheal webs
- Inhaled foreign body
- Tumor or enlarged lymph nodes compressing airway

Small Airway Obstruction
- Viral bronchiolitis
- Pneumonia
- Obliterative bronchitis
- Cystic fibrosis
- Bronchopulmonary dysplasia
- Heart failure

Other
- Gastroesophageal reflux disease
- Swallowing mechanism dysfunction leading to aspiration

hyperresponsiveness in cases where spirometry is not feasible. This testing can be performed with inhaled methacholine (Provocholine), histamine[2], or mannitol (Aridol) and with exercise or eucapnic voluntary hyperventilation. Although this testing can be sensitive for the diagnosis of asthma, this may be technically difficult in the pediatric population, and findings can be masked in patients who are already treated with inhaled corticosteroid (ICS) therapy.

Allergy Testing

Serum or skin-prick testing can be considered for the evaluation of atopy. Specific serum IgE levels to common regional allergens may increase the likelihood that respiratory symptoms are related to an allergic asthma phenotype; however, it is not specific to asthma.

Diagnosis in children 5 years and under can be both clinically and technically challenging. In general, diagnosis in this patient population is made without formal pulmonary testing. The presence of typical symptoms, risk factors, positive therapeutic response, and alternative diagnosis exclusion is typically sufficient for asthma diagnosis. Symptoms typical of asthma in this age group include recurrent wheeze, cough, breathlessness resulting in activity limitation, nocturnal symptoms, or awakenings. Risk factors associated with the development of asthma include family history of atopy, allergic sensitization, allergy or asthma, or a personal history of atopic dermatitis or food allergy. Most patients in this age group have asthma if they develop symptoms for more than 10 days during upper respiratory tract infections (URTI), having more than three episodes of wheezing in a year, severe wheezing, or worsening at night, cough, wheeze, or heavy breathing during play or laughing in between episodes. Fewer patients 5 years and younger have asthma if symptoms associated with URTI last less than 10 days, there are only two to three episodes per year, and no symptoms are present in between episodes.

Differential Diagnosis

Differential diagnosis of wheeze can be divided into upper airway pathology, large airway obstruction, small airway obstruction, and other causes (Box 2).

Treatment

Treatment of asthma within the pediatric population is based on age, severity of symptoms, and disease control. The goals of treatment are to reduce the impairment of the disease and risk of exacerbation of symptoms. Historically, pediatric asthma severity was classified as intermittent or persistent with persistent divided into mild, moderate, and severe. Previously, initial treatment began with short-acting β agonist (SABA) use as needed for symptoms. Newer strategies focused on avoidance of excessive SABA-only treatment with the goal of decreasing exacerbation, acute visit, and hospitalization risk have emerged.

Nonpharmacological treatment includes cessation of environmental tobacco exposure, smoking, and vaping; routine physical activity to improve fitness, symptoms, and quality of life; avoidance of occupational and domestic exposure to allergens and irritants; avoidance of medications that may make asthma worse, including NSAIDs and nonselective β-blockers (such as propranolol, which is used to treat infantile hemangiomas); healthy diet and weight reduction in obese patients; breathing exercises and relaxation techniques for pulmonary fitness and emotional benefit; and, at a higher level, addressing social risk that may predispose patients to suboptimal disease control, morbidity, and mortality. Pharmacologic treatment for asthma typically falls into three categories – rescue medications, controller medications, and add-on treatments, which are typically reserved for severe disease states.

In addition to objective testing (FEV$_1$ and PEF) to guide therapy, several subjective symptom control measures have been developed. The use of these tools can assist in escalation and de-escalation of therapy. The Asthma Control Test has been validated in two groups of patients, 4 to 11 years and 12 years and older (ACT; https://www.asthmacontroltest.com/).

Rescue Medications

The mechanism of action for bronchodilating rescue medications targets the acute bronchoconstriction of asthma pathophysiology. β$_2$ receptor agonists act at the adrenergic receptors of intracellular adenyl cyclase of bronchial smooth muscle by causing conversion of adenosine triphosphate to cyclic adenosine monophosphate (cAMP). Increased levels of cAMP result in bronchial smooth muscle relaxation and inhibit the hypersensitivity of mast cells. There are short-acting and long-acting β$_2$ agonist medications (SABA and LABA). These agents are available commercially in liquid and powder metered dose inhalers (MDI), liquid for use in nebulizers, and oral liquid and tablets. Albuterol (ProAir, Proventil, Ventolin) and levalbuterol (the R-enantiomer [Xopenex]) are the most common SABA formulations. For common dosing, see Table 1.

LABA medications are typically more lipophilic than their SABA counterparts and have a duration of action around 12 to 24 hours compared with 4 to 6 hours, respectively. Examples of LABA products include extended-release albuterol (albuterol ER tablet), salmeterol (Serevent), formoterol (Perforomist)/arformoterol (Brovana), indacaterol (Arcapta), vilanterol, and olodaterol (Striverdi Respimat). More recently, the rapid onset of action and duration of formoterol has encouraged its use as a rescue agent[1] in some age groups, sometimes in combination with ICS as antiinflammatory relievers (AIR) and single maintenance and reliever therapy options (SMART/MART). Other bronchodilating agents include anticholinergic long-acting muscarinic antagonists (LAMA) including ipratropium (Atrovent)[1] and tiotropium (Spiriva Respimat) and methylxanthines such as theophylline; however, the use of these agents is typically not first line and is reserved for add-on therapies.

Controller Medications

ICS are still the hallmark of pharmacologic controller medications. The corticosteroid medications used in the treatment

---

[2]Not available in the United States.

[1]Not FDA approved for this indication.

TABLE 1	Rescue Dose Chart	
DRUG	**BRONCHOSPASM**	**ACUTE EXACERBATION**
Albuterol	1–2 puffs every 4–6 hours prn 0–4 years: 0.63–2.5 mg q4–6h prn ≥4 years: 1.25–5 mg q4–6h prn	4–10 puffs q20 min × 3 doses, then q1–4h prn (via spacer, add mask where appropriate) 0.15 mg/kg (max 2.5 mg) nebulized q20 min × 3 doses, then 0.15–0.3 mg/kg (max 5 mg) q1–4h prn
Levalbuterol (Xopenex)	≥4 years: 1–2 puffs q4–6h prn 0–4 years: 0.31–0.63 mg nebulized q4–6h prn ≥4 years: 0.63–1.25 mg nebulized q8h prn	4–8 puffs q20 min × 3 doses, then q1–4h prn (via spacer, add mask where appropriate) 0.075 mg/kg (min 1.25 mg) q20 min × 3 doses, then 0.075–0.15 mg/kg (max 5 mg) q1–4h prn

prn, As needed.

of asthma represent analogues to cortisol, an endogenous glucocorticoid. These compounds have antiinflammatory and immune-suppressive effects that, over time, result in alteration of gene transcription responsible for asthma pathophysiology. Glucocorticoids inhibit proinflammatory macrophages, eosinophils, mast cells, lymphocytes, and dendritic cells. Additionally, they inhibit phospholipase A2, expression of cycloogygenase-2, inducible nitric oxide synthase, tumor necrosis factor-α, interleukins, prostaglandin, and leukotriene, and reduce neutrophil migration.

ICS are synthetic halogenated analogues of glucocorticoids that increase the local potency in respiratory tissues without significant effect on systemic effects. Their action is primarily intracellular, resulting in effects longer than their plasma presence. ICS therapy has been shown to result in improvement in quality of life; improved lung function testing; reduction of airway hyperreactivity and inflammation, asthma symptoms, asthma-related morbidity and mortality; and reduction in the frequency and severity of acute exacerbations. Adverse effects of the class of medications include oropharyngeal candidiasis, dysphonia, coughing, and dose-related effects on growth velocity, bone mineral density, and hypothalamus-pituitary-adrenal axis function.

Some of these adverse effects can be mitigated by spacer devices and rinsing the mouth with water after use. In their aerosolized form, the use of a spacer or chamber device can reduce the amount of active ingredient compound delivered to the oropharynx or swallowed, further increasing the amount of medication delivered to the pulmonary tissues.

ICS dosing is typically divided into low-, medium-, and high-dose (LD/MD/HD) categories, with most of the clinical benefit achieved at low dosing. Similar dose strength categorization does not imply potency equivalence, however. High-dose ICS are used in few patients as the clinical benefit is often not above lower doses, but local and systemic side effects are dose dependent. In the United States, commercially available ICS formulations include beclomethasone (Qvar RediHaler), budesonide (Pulmicort Flexhaler), ciclesonide (Alvesco), fluticasone (ArmonAir, Arnuity, Flovent), and mometasone (Asmanex). These medications are also found in combination with LABA and/or LAMA ingredients. Recently, a combination product of albuterol and budesonide (Airsupra) has been approved for the use in patients over the age of 18 but is currently not approved for use in pediatric patients (Table 2).

Starting Treatment

When starting treatment for asthma, initial controller treatment and its corresponding treatment step is based on frequency and severity of symptoms. Referral to the age-based stepwise approach to treatment can help with treatment initiation and titration (Table 3):

- If daily symptoms are present and the child is waking at night with symptoms one or more times a week, or if low lung function is present (<65% predicted FEV_1), start controller treatment at **Step 4** with consideration of concomitant short course of oral corticosteroids.

- If symptoms are present most days or the child is waking at night with symptoms once or more a week, start treatment at **Step 3**.
- If symptoms are twice a month or more, start treatment at **Step 2**.
- If symptoms are less frequent than twice a month, start treatment at **Step 1**.

Choice of treatment device in the pediatric population is important as a means of active medication delivery and mitigation of side effects associated with systemic absorption. In general, patients aged 3 and under benefit most from a pressurized MDI combined with dedicated spacer with face mask with an alternative method of delivery via nebulizer with face mask. In patients who are 4 and 5 years old, the preferred device is a pressurized MDI plus spacer with mouthpiece with an alternative of MDI and spacer with face mask or nebulizer with face mask. Several studies have demonstrated similar treatment response with MDI and appropriate spacer and mouthpiece when compared with nebulized treatment; however, when use of an MDI is not feasible because of patient tolerance or prolonged treatment is required, nebulized treatments are a reasonable alternative.

Add-On Treatments

Allergen immunotherapy can be a treatment option for patients whose allergic symptoms result in asthma-associated morbidity and symptomatology. Options for immunotherapy include subcutaneous injections and sublingual administration. There is currently no recommendation for immunotherapy for the treatment of asthma alone in the pediatric population.

Leukotriene modifiers decrease the effects of leukotriene in the pathogenesis of asthma. Agents include the receptor antagonists montelukast (Singulair) and zafirlukast (Accolate) and 5-lipoxygenase inhibitor zileuton (Zyflo). Currently, these oral treatments are reserved as add-ons for patients who are not controlled with daily ICS, but their clinical effects are less than those associated with the addition of LABA treatment. Montelukast carries a black box warning for its association with neuropsychiatric effects including agitation, depression, sleep disturbances, and suicidality.

Newer biologic agents targeting various type-2 inflammatory pathophysiologic compounds in asthma have been developed including those targeting IgE, interleukin 4 (IL-4), interleukin 5 (IL-5), and thymic stromal lymphoprotein. Type-2 inflammation can be evaluated by blood eosinophil count of 150/μL or greater, FeNO of 20 ppb or greater, sputum eosinophils of 2% or greater, and/or clinically allergy-driven asthma defined as elevated blood eosinophil and FeNO on the lowest possible ICS or 1 to 2 weeks after oral corticosteroid treatment). Individual criteria for these agents vary and should be referenced before initiation.

Immunizations that are recommended for patients with asthma include annual influenza and COVID-19 vaccines and RSV monoclonal antibody (nirsevimab [Beyfortus]) within the first 8 months of life if their mother was not vaccinated or their delivery was within 14 days of maternal administration. A second dose may be recommended at 12 to 19 months of age for children who were born prematurely with chronic lung disease (including asthma) because of the risk of severe RSV illness.

TABLE 2	Inhaled Corticosteroid Potency			
INHALED CORTICOSTEROID		**LOW (DAILY μg)**	**MEDIUM (DAILY μg)**	**HIGH (DAILY μg)**
Ages 12+				
Beclomethasone dipropionate standard particle (Clenil)[2]		200–500	500–1000	>1000
Beclomethasone dipropionate extrafine particle (Qvar RediHaler)		100–200	200–400	>400
Budesonide standard particle (Pulmicort Flexhaler)		200–400	400–800	>800
Ciclesonide (Alvesco)		80–160	160–320	>320
Fluticasone furoate (Arnuity Ellipta)		100	100	200
Fluticasone propionate (ArmonAir, Flovent)		100–250	250–500	>500
Mometasone (Asmanex)		200–400	200–400	>400
Ages 6–11				
Beclomethasone dipropionate standard particle (Clenil)[2]		100–200	200–400	>400
Beclomethasone dipropionate extrafine particle (Qvar RediHaler)		50–100	100–200	>200
Budesonide standard particle (Pulmicort)		100–200	400–800	>400
Budesonide nebules (Pulmicort Respules)		250–500	500–1000	>1000
Ciclesonide (Alvesco)[a]		80	80–160	>160
Fluticasone furoate (Arnuity)		50	50	N/A
Fluticasone propionate (ArmonAir,[a] Flovent)		50–100	100–200	>200
Mometasone (Asmanex)		100	100	200
INHALED CORTICOSTEROID		**LOW DOSE IN DAILY MG (AGE APPROVED)**		
Age 5 and Under				
Beclomethasone dipropionate standard particle (Clenil)[2]		100 (≥5)		
Beclomethasone dipropionate extrafine particle (Qvar RediHaler)[b]		50 (≥5)		
Budesonide nebulized solution (Pulmicort Respules)		500 (≥1)		
Ciclesonide (Alvesco)[a]		Not approved		
Fluticasone furoate (Arnuity)[c]		Not approved		
Fluticasone propionate (ArmonAir,[a] Flovent[b])		50 (≥4)		
Mometasone (Asmanex Twisthaler)[b]		100 (≥5)		

[a]FDA-approved use in patients ≥12 years of age.
[b]FDA-approved use in patients ≥4 years of age.
[c]FDA-approved use in patients ≥5 years of age.
[2]Not available in the United States.

Macrolide antimicrobials including azithromycin (Zithromax)[1] are not routinely recommended for chronic use or in acute exacerbations for the treatment of pediatric asthma. Bronchial thermoplasty is not recommended for asthma treatment in pediatric patients.

Asthma Exacerbations

Asthma exacerbations occur when symptoms acutely worsen. This may manifest in subacute or acute worsening of wheezing, cough, or shortness of breath, and these symptoms may be caught earlier in their milder form or later with life-threatening severity. Ideally, these symptoms can be recognized early, and intervention can hinder progression.

The hallmark treatments for acute exacerbations include short-acting bronchodilators, corticosteroids, and oxygen administration if hypoxia is present. SABA may be administered via MDI with appropriate spacer or nebulizer and combined with ipratropium (Combivent, DuoNeb)[1] in severe cases and when initial response to SABA therapy is inadequate. Oral corticosteroid treatment is indicated in children with PEF/FEV$_1$ less than 60% of predicted or best or those who are not improving after 48 hours of treatment with increased reliever and controller treatment. Intravenous corticosteroids are appropriate in patients whose respiratory status precludes swallowing of oral formulation. Intramuscular administration has not been found to be more clinically beneficial than oral administration.

Many episodes of acute worsening of symptoms or objective testing (PEF) may be treated at home without seeking additional medical care.

Patients and caregivers are advised to seek medical attention immediately in the event of acute distress, if symptoms are not relieved promptly by inhaled bronchodilator treatment, if the

[1]Not FDA approved for this indication.

[1]Not FDA approved for this indication.

TABLE 3 Step Chart

AGE	STEP 1	STEP 2	STEP 3	STEP 4	STEP 5
5 and under	SABA ± LD ICS with viral illness	LD ICS	Double LD ICS	Refer	Refer
6–11	AIR	LD ICS	LD ICS/LABA MD ICS Very LD MART	MD ICS/ LABA LD MART	Refer HD ICS/LABA Add-on therapy
12+ with preferred controller and reliever	MART	MART	LD MART	MD MART	LAMA Refer Daily HD MART Add-on therapy
12+ with alternate controller and reliever	AIR	LD ICS	LD ICS-LABA	MD/HD ICS/ LABA	LAMA Refer Daily HD MART Add-on therapy

STEP	AGE	MEDICATION/DEVICE	METERED DOSE (µG)	DELIVERED DOSE (µG)	DOSAGE
AIR/MART Chart					
Steps 1–2 AIR	6–11	No evidence	—	—	—
	12+	Budesonide-formoterol DPI (Breyna, Symbicort)	200/6	160/4.5	1 puff prn
Step 3 MART	6–11	Budesonide-formoterol DPI	100/6	80/4.5	1 puff daily + 1 puff prn
	12+	Budesonide-formoterol DPI	200/6	160/4.5	1 puff 1–2/day + 1 puff prn
Step 4 MART	6–11	Budesonide-formoterol DPI	100/6	80/4.5	1 puff 2/day + 1 puff prn
	12+	Budesonide-formoterol DPI	200/6	160/4.5	2 puffs 2/day + 1 puff prn
Step 5 MART	6–11	No evidence	—	—	—
	12+	Budesonide-formoterol DPI	200/6	160/4.5	2 puffs 2/day + 1 puff prn

AIR, Antiinflammatory reliever; *DPI*, dry powdered inhaler; *HD*, high dose; *ICS*, inhaled corticosteroid; *LABA*, long-acting β agonist; *LAMA*, long-acting muscarinic antagonist; *LD*, low dose; *MART*, maintenance and reliever therapy; *MD*, medium dose; *prn*, as needed; *SABA*, short-acting β agonist.

duration of symptom relief from bronchodilator therapy becomes progressively shorter, or if a child younger than 1 year requires bronchodilator treatment over several hours.

In the primary care setting, a primary survey of airway security, breathing, and circulation should be carried out. Symptoms indicating a severe or life-threatening exacerbation may include inability to speak in full sentences and drink, agitation, central cyanosis, use of accessory respiratory muscles, tachycardia/tachypnea, hypoxia with SpO_2 less than 90%, PEF of 50% or less than predicted or best. In these cases, urgent transfer to a higher level of care is indicated. While awaiting transfer for these patients, administration of SABA, oxygen to achieve a target SpO_2 of 94% to 98%, corticosteroid administration, and consideration of nebulized ipratropium (Atrovent)[1] can be considered.

In the emergency department setting, consideration for additional agents may be appropriate for more severe symptoms. Systemic corticosteroids typically have a 1- to 2-hour onset of action and duration of 18 to 36 hours. Oral administration is faster, less invasive, less expensive, and as effective as intravenous. Typical duration of 1 to 10 days is indicated, with taper not indicated if treatment course is less than a week. When administered within the first hour after presentation, high-dose ICS reduces the need for hospitalization in patients who do not require hospitalization.

Intravenous magnesium sulfate[1] is not routinely recommended for the treatment of asthma exacerbation but may be considered for children with FEV_1 of 60% or less predicted after 1 hour of treatment. Cromolyn is not recommended for treatment because of poor efficacy and risk for gastrointestinal side effects. Intramuscular epinephrine is indicated for acute asthma associated with anaphylaxis and angioedema, but not with other asthma

exacerbations. Helium-oxygen therapy has not been found to be superior to standard therapy. Noninvasive ventilation can be considered with close monitoring if failing to improve with standard therapy; however, sedation must be avoided given the association of sedatives and avoidable asthma-related deaths.

GINA-proposed discharge criteria include symptomatic improvement no longer requiring SABA, improvement of PEF to 60% to 80% of predicted or best, SpO_2 of 94% or greater on room air, and adequate home resources and ability to seek care in the event of symptom regression.

After appropriate treatment of acute asthma exacerbation, follow-up is typically recommended within 1 to 2 working days. At the follow-up visit, a history, physical examination, and objective testing where appropriate can be used to determine the need for continued oral corticosteroid if applicable, presence and mitigation of modifiable risk factors including inhaler technique and adherence, adjustment in controller medication dose, reduction of reliever therapy to as needed, appropriateness of current asthma action plan or possible modification, and scheduling outpatient follow-up visit (Table 4).

Monitoring

Affording the variable nature of asthma-related symptoms and airflow limitation, routine scheduled patient follow-up with their primary care physician is of utmost importance for evaluation of symptom control and therapeutic adjustments. At the time of initial diagnosis, management appointments may need to be as frequent as every 2 to 6 weeks with follow-up frequency in controlled patients extended to every 3 to 6 months. If asthma symptoms remain well controlled over 3 months, clinicians should consider stepping down treatment.

At each visit, clinicians should review interval symptoms, exacerbations, side effects, lung function comorbidities, and

---
[1] Not FDA approved for this indication.

TABLE 4 Usual Dosing of Medications Used in Exacerbations

MEDICATION	DOSING
Corticosteroids	
Methylprednisolone, prednisolone, prednisone	1–2 mg/kg daily for 3–7 days (max 20 mg for 0–2 years, 30 mg for 3–5 years, 40 mg for ≥6 years)
Dexamethasone	0.3–0.6 mg/kg orally daily for 1–2 days (max 16 mg)
Epinephrine (anaphylaxis)	1:1000 concentration (1 mg/mL) 0.01 mL/kg SQ/IM (max 0.3 mL)
Ipratropium bromide inhalation solution[1]	≤5 years: 250 µg nebulized ×2, then q4h prn >5 years: 500 µg nebulized ×2, then q4h prn
Magnesium sulfate[1]	25–50 mg/kg IV up to 2 g over 10–20 minutes

[1]Not FDA approved for this indication.
prn, As needed.

satisfaction of the patient and caregiver; assess the need for diagnosis confirmation, symptom control and modifiable risk factors/comorbidities, inhaler technique/adherence, and patient and caregiver preferences and goals; adjust modifiable risk factors/comorbidities, treatments (both pharmacologic and nonpharmacologic); and educate and train both the patient and caregivers.

Asthma Action Plan

Asthma action plans serve to outline current treatments, help to identify and remind of common irritants, allergens, and triggers, and empower patients to recognize increasing symptoms, escalate treatment, and provide guidance on when to seek additional care. Examples of asthma action plans can be found on the websites of the National Heart, Lung, and Blood Institute (https://www.nhlbi.nih.gov/resources/asthma-action-plan-2020), Centers for Disease Control and Prevention (https://www.cdc.gov/asthma/action-plan/documents/asthma-action-plan-508.pdf), and the Allergy and Asthma Foundation of America (https://aafa.org/asthma/asthma-treatment/asthma-treatment-action-plan/).

Complications

Asthma carries significant morbidity and mortality risk in the pediatric and adult populations. Complications from asthma include reduction in lung function, pneumonia, pneumothorax, and death. Outside of pulmonary-specific complications, symptoms associated with asthma and chronic cough may result in poor sleep, missed school, impaired academic performance, and limitation in participation in physically active activities. Appropriate diagnosis and treatment assist in the reduction and elimination of these complications.

References

Aaron SD, Boulet LP, Reddel HK, Gershon AS: Underdiagnosis and overdiagnosis of asthma, *Am J Respir Crit Care Med* 198(8):1012–1020, 2018, https://doi.org/10.1164/rccm.201804-0682CI.

Asthma: diagnosis, monitoring and chronic asthma management, London, 2021, National Institute for Health and Care Excellence (NICE) (NICE Guideline, No. 80.) https://www.ncbi.nlm.nih.gov/books/NBK560178/.

British Thoracic Society and Scottish Intercollegiate Guidelines Network (BTS/SIGN): *National clinical guideline on management of asthma*, BTS/SIGN, 2019. https://www.sign.ac.uk/media/1773/sign158-updated.pdf.

Cloutier, M. M., et al. 2020 focused updates to the Asthma Management Guidelines: A report from the National Asthma Education and Prevention Program Coordinating Committee Expert Panel Working Group. *J Allergy Clin Immunol*, 146(6), 1217–1270. https://doi.org/10.1016/j.jaci.2020.10.003

Foster J, et al: Perspectives of mild asthma patients on maintenance versus as-needed preventer treatment regiments: a qualitative study, *BMJ Open* 12:e048537, 2022.

Global Initiative for Asthma: *Global Strategy for Asthma Management and Prevention*, 2024. Updated May 2024 www.ginasthma.org.

Graham BL. Standardization of spirometry 2019 update. An Official American Thoracic Society and European Respiratory Society Technical Statement. Available at: https://www.atsjournals.org/doi/10.1164/rccm.201908-1590ST.

Zanobetti A, Ryan PH, Coull B, et al: Childhood asthma incidence, early and persistent wheeze, and neighborhood socioeconomic factors in the ECHO/CREW consortium, *JAMA Pediatr* 176(8):759–767, 2022, https://doi.org/10.1001/jamapediatrics.2022.1446.

ATTENTION-DEFICIT/HYPERACTIVITY DISORDER

Method of
Sophie Robert, PharmD; Erin Hayes, MD; and Jennifer K. Poon, MD

CURRENT DIAGNOSIS

- Attention-deficit/hyperactivity disorder (ADHD) is one of the most common childhood neurodevelopmental disorders affecting not only academic achievement but also well-being and social interactions.
- ADHD is a chronic condition that can continue to cause symptoms and dysfunction into adulthood.
- The primary care provider encountering any child or adolescent 4 years of age and older should evaluate for ADHD when there is a presenting academic or behavioral problem with symptoms of inattention, hyperactivity, or impulsivity.
- The diagnosis of ADHD is a clinical diagnosis that is based on criteria from the *Diagnostic and Statistical Manual of Mental Disorders,* fifth edition, Text Revision *(DSM-5-TR),* documenting symptoms and dysfunction in more than one setting, including parent/patient concerns, as well as collateral information from individuals who have knowledge of how the patient functions in another setting.
- The use of ADHD-specific questionnaires and rating scales is important in data collection and to detect the presence of coexisting conditions.
- All ADHD evaluations should assess for coexisting behavioral conditions, such as oppositional defiant disorder, mood disorders, anxiety, depression, substance use, developmental conditions such as learning and language disorders, and physical conditions including tics and sleep apnea.

CURRENT THERAPY

- The goal of treatment is symptomatic and functional improvement.
- Evidence-based, age-appropriate behavioral and educational interventions may be recommended as initial treatment, or in addition to pharmacotherapy, especially if there are coexisting conditions; psychoeducation is recommended along with pharmacotherapy.
- For preschool-age children, evidence-based parent training in behavior management and/or classroom behavior interventions are the first line of treatment, if available.
- For children 6 years of age and older, first-line treatment includes stimulant medications or nonstimulant alternative medications such as atomoxetine (Strattera) and viloxazine (Qelbree).
- Second-line treatment includes α2 agonists (e.g., clonidine ER [Kapvay], guanfacine ER [Intuniv]), bupropion (Wellbutrin),[1] and venlafaxine (Effexor).[1]

[1]Not FDA approved for this indication.

Pathophysiology

The cited prevalence of attention-deficit/hyperactivity disorder (ADHD) varies throughout the literature as a result of methodologic differences, the diagnostic criteria used, the population studied, and the sources used to make the diagnosis. There are no specific laboratory tests or imaging studies that diagnose ADHD. It is a clinical diagnosis. The prevalence has ranged from 4% to 12%, often higher in community samples, and higher among males. National studies cite that approximately 7% of children meet the *Diagnostic and Statistical Manual of Mental Disorders*, fifth edition Text Revision *(DSM-5-TR)* criteria for ADHD. Males are more commonly diagnosed because they may present with externalizing symptoms such as overactivity and aggression, in contrast with females, who may present with less noticeable internalizing symptoms such as daydreaming and poor school performance. ADHD is considered a chronic condition because data suggest that approximately 50% of cases will persist into adulthood. Follow-up studies indicate that functional impairment persists in approximately 10% to 60% of childhood-onset cases.

ADHD has no single causative factor, and common theories such as allergies to food coloring, poor parenting/discipline, and/or poor schooling have not been supported by research. Rather, the disorder has a complex, multifactorial etiology consisting of genetic and environmental factors. ADHD is familial, and a number of family epidemiologic studies of association of symptoms in twin, adoption, and segregation analyses have supported heritability at 65% to 90%. Neuroimaging studies have demonstrated differences in the basal ganglia, cerebellar vermis, and frontal lobes in individuals with ADHD versus controls. Biologic factors such as prenatal exposure to substances have been associated with ADHD symptomatology. Also, psychosocial problems such as parental psychopathology and poor family cohesion have been cited to be more common in families of children with ADHD than in children without the disorder.

Clinical Manifestations

The life course of ADHD may be variable from person to person, depending on a number of psychosocial factors. However, parents may first notice difficulties in children as toddlers who may be overly active, sometimes posing behavioral issues at daycare, safety issues, or social difficulties. However, at the toddler age, it may be difficult to discern between normative behavior of an active child versus true ADHD before the preschool years. Hyperactivity may be noted more in preschool years if children are having challenges in a structured setting, such as school, or if safety issues emerge. The elementary school years are a common time when ADHD is brought to attention. During these years, inattention may be more prominent, particularly as academics evolve from rote memory activities to second-order thinking. Often in adolescence and adulthood, the motor hyperactivity lessens, but there is persistent restlessness, impatience, inattention, and impulsivity. ADHD has an adverse effect on long-term academic outcomes, which most consistently improve with multimodal treatment.

As with any disorder, ADHD has functional consequences, not only affecting academics in school-age children, but occupational performance as well as interpersonal relationships for adults. There is a greater risk for development of conduct disorder in adolescence and antisocial personality disorder in individuals with ADHD. Furthermore, studies have found that individuals with ADHD have increased rates of substance use disorders (SUDs) and incarceration. Youth prison populations and adult prison populations have a fivefold and 10-fold increase in ADHD prevalence, respectively, compared with prevalence in the general population.

Diagnosis

The American Academy of Pediatrics recommends an evaluation for ADHD in any child or adolescent 4 years of age or older presenting with inattention, hyperactivity, impulsivity, academic underachievement, and/or behavior problems. The diagnostic criteria for ADHD are found in the *DSM-5-TR* within the neurodevelopmental disorders section. The practitioner specifies whether the patient meets criteria for the predominantly inattentive presentation, the predominantly hyperactive/impulsive presentation or combined presentation, as well as whether symptoms are in partial remission and current severity of mild, moderate, or severe.

To diagnose ADHD, several symptoms must be present before 12 years of age and affect the patient in two or more settings such as at home, at school, at work, with friends or relatives, or in other activities. The symptoms have a negative effect on the patient's level of social, academic, or occupational functioning. The symptoms are present to a degree that is inconsistent with the patient's developmental level. Symptoms must not occur exclusively during schizophrenia or another psychotic disorder or be part of another mental disorder. Symptoms must not be completely caused by oppositional behavior, being defiant, or failing to understand instructions and tasks.

Inattentive symptoms are designated in Criterion A1 of the *DSM-5-TR*. To meet criteria for the predominantly inattentive presentation, a patient must have at least six of the following symptoms for the past 6 months: (1) failing to give attention to details or making careless mistakes, (2) having difficulty sustaining attention, (3) appearing to not listen when spoken to directly, (4) not following through on instructions or failing to complete schoolwork, chores, or workplace duties, (5) having difficulty organizing tasks and activities, (6) avoiding or lacking interest in tasks requiring sustained mental effort, (7) losing necessary objects to complete tasks or activities, (8) being distracted easily, and (9) being forgetful in completing daily activities. If older than 17 years of age, the patient must have at least five of the symptoms.

Hyperactive and impulsive symptoms are designated in Criterion A2 of the *DSM-5-TR*. To meet criteria for the predominantly hyperactive/impulsive presentation, a patient must have at least six of the following symptoms for the past 6 months: (1) fidgeting or having trouble sitting still, (2) leaving a seat when it is expected to remain seated, (3) running or climbing in inappropriate situations, (4) having difficulty playing or doing leisure activities quietly, (5) being "on the go" or "driven by a motor," (6) talking excessively, (7) blurting out the answer before a question is completed, (8) having trouble waiting his or her turn, and (9) often interrupting and intruding on others. If older than 17 years of age, the patient must have at least five of the symptoms.

Patients with at least six symptoms in Criterion A1 and at least six symptoms in Criterion A2 are said to have the combined presentation.

To obtain an accurate picture of the effect these symptoms have in various settings, it is helpful to obtain collateral information from individuals who have knowledge of how the patient functions in a given setting. For this reason, it is common to obtain input from current and former teachers, coaches, religious leaders, other relatives, and so on. The use of ADHD-specific questionnaires and rating scales is important in data collection and detection of comorbid conditions. All ADHD evaluations should assess for coexisting conditions such as oppositional defiant disorder, mood disorders, anxiety disorders, trauma, and learning disabilities.

Therapy
Behavioral Interventions

For preschool-age children (48 to 59 months of age) with ADHD, the primary recommended first-line intervention is parent training behavior management, if available. Such training helps parents understand developmentally appropriate expectations, how to strengthen the parent-child relationship, and specific management of disruptive behaviors. The largest multisite study of methylphenidate used in preschool-age children with ADHD with moderate-to-severe dysfunction demonstrated that parent training behavior management alone resulted in symptom improvement. Such therapies may be group programs or dyadic therapy for the parent and child. Schools may also be able to provide behavioral support as well. Box 1 lists patient and parent resources for the management of attention-deficit/hyperactivity disorder.

Parent training behavior management techniques and/or behavioral classroom interventions are also recommended along with medications approved by the U.S. Food and Drug Administration (FDA) for ADHD in children 6 to 12 years of age. Behavioral classroom interventions may include modifying school environment, class placement, instructional placement, and behavior supports. Such supports may include a rehabilitation plan (504 plan) or Individualized Education Program (IEP).

Similarly, adolescents 12 to 18 years of age should be prescribed FDA-approved medications for ADHD with their assent and should also have evidence-based training interventions and/or behavioral interventions if available, as outlined for school-age children. Furthermore, a transitional care plan is important as a part of a chronic care model for ADHD. This transition to adult care should be introduced at around 14 years of age to help identify resources before high school completion.

Behavioral therapy and training interventions have studies supporting their effectiveness for the treatment of ADHD; however, these should be differentiated from other psychological interventions, particularly ones that are designed to change emotional status or thought patterns (e.g., play therapy, talk therapy). The latter have not shown efficacy for the treatment of ADHD core symptoms and do not generalize to the home or classroom. Evidence-based behavior therapies involve training adults to shape the environment in order to improve behavior in a setting and to learn effective responses to symptoms such as interrupting, aggressive behaviors, and noncompliance with requests. Although studies indicate that stimulants have a greater immediate effect on the core symptoms of ADHD, there is greater parental satisfaction with behavior therapy, with the positive effects tending to last.

Pharmacotherapy

Stimulants are considered first-line medications for the treatment of ADHD in patients 6 years of age and older. Nonstimulant alternatives include atomoxetine (Strattera), viloxazine (Qelbree), and α_2 agonists for all age groups, with the exception of α_2 agonists in adults, where information is much more limited but promising for guanfacine ER (Intuniv). Additional options with lesser evidence include bupropion (Wellbutrin),[1] venlafaxine (Effexor),[1] and tricyclic antidepressants (TCAs).[1]

For preschool-age children (3 to <6 years of age), pharmacotherapy with stimulants is generally reserved for patients with moderate to severe ADHD symptoms who have responded insufficiently to behavioral therapies. Although off-label in that age group, methylphenidate (Ritalin) is the preferred stimulant based on its evidence of efficacy, safety, and clinical experience. Methylphenidate medications are listed in Table 1. Amphetamines may be considered as a second-line alternative. Despite FDA-approval of certain formulations, evidence supporting the efficacy and safety of amphetamines has only recently started to emerge. Other off-label alternatives in preschoolers include atomoxetine and α_2 agonists. Atomoxetine has limited evidence of modest efficacy and tolerability in children as young as 5 years old. As for α_2 agonists, emerging favorable published data is supportive of

---

[1] Not FDA approved for this indication.

their widespread clinical use. These agents are recommended by the American Academy of Child and Adolescent Psychiatry's Preschool Psychopharmacology Working Group in cases of nonresponse or intolerance to stimulant medication and by the Society for Developmental-Behavioral Pediatrics Complex ADHD guideline as first-line for those with co-occurring ADHD and severe irritability, oppositional behavior, or both.

Stimulants

The benefits of short-term stimulant therapy on ADHD symptoms are well documented, with large effect sizes ranging from 0.9 to 1.0 in pediatrics, and 0.49 to 0.79 in adults. Evidence suggests that amphetamines may be more efficacious, most notably in adults, yet may have poorer tolerability, particularly in children. Amphetamine medications are listed in Table 2. The subtype of ADHD does not appear to predict response to a specific class. Individual response to methylphenidate versus amphetamine is unpredictable, particularly in adults, but 80 to 90% of patients will ultimately have a beneficial response with trials of various medications from both classes. Beyond symptomatic improvement, stimulant treatment is associated with improved academic outcomes, improved social functioning, and a protective effect on accidents and injuries.

Stimulants are Schedule II controlled drugs because of their potential for misuse and diversion. While SUDs may co-occur with ADHD, treatment with stimulant medication does not increase the risk of developing SUDs; on the contrary, effective treatment of ADHD (even with stimulants) at least delays, and may even reduce, the risk of developing SUDs. If concerns over misuse arise, extended-release formulations (or nonstimulants) should be favored given their slower increase in plasma concentrations resulting in less "likeability" and less potential for misuse. However, for patients with active SUDs, prescribing of stimulants should generally be reserved for mental health specialists. Additionally, diversion is a growing problem, particularly among adolescents and college-age students, thus extended-release stimulants and nonstimulant alternatives can be considered if such concerns arise. Nonstimulant medications are listed in Table 3.

Stimulants are available as short-, intermediate-, and long-acting formulations, and they come in a variety of preparations. These include regular tablets, transdermal patches, liquid/suspension, chewable or orally disintegrating tablets, and capsules that can be opened with contents sprinkled on food. Although overall efficacy is similar, the pharmacokinetic characteristics of individual formulations affect the timeline and duration of action.

Short-acting formulations offer dosing flexibility, which may be especially beneficial for young children; disadvantages include multiple daily dosing and higher risk of abuse/misuse. Intermediate-acting formulations provide a longer duration of action (up to 8 hours) but often require twice daily dosing. Long-acting formulations allow for once daily dosing, which is associated with improved treatment adherence. Disadvantages include potential adverse effects on evening appetite and sleep along with higher cost, especially for branded formulations. Short- or intermediate-acting formulations can be used in combination with long-acting formulations early in the day (e.g., for faster onset in the morning) or later in the day (e.g., management of late afternoon "rebound"). Different formulations of the same stimulant may be tried to optimize response and tolerability. If maximum tolerated doses of a stimulant are inadequate, then another formulation within the same stimulant class or another stimulant class should be considered. When converting from one stimulant to another, the following dose equivalence can be utilized: amphetamines 10 mg = dextroamphetamine 10 mg = lisdexamfetamine 30 mg = dexmethylphenidate 10 mg = methylphenidate 20 mg. Knowledge of dose equivalence can be very helpful in other situations when barriers arise that necessitate a change in stimulant prescription (e.g., insurance coverage, national drug shortages).

Stimulants are usually initiated at low doses and titrated gradually based on response and tolerability (see Table 2). Stimulant

TABLE 1 Methylphenidate Medications*

MEDICATION (BRAND NAME EXAMPLES)	INITIAL DOSE	ONSET (MINUTES)	TMAX (HOURS)	DURATION (HOURS)	FDA MAXIMUM DAILY DOSE	FDA-APPROVED AGES	SPLIT/CRUSH/SPRINKLE	COMMENTS
Short-Acting								
Methylphenidate (Ritalin, Methylin)	5 mg BID–TID	20–30	1.9	3–4	60 mg	6–17, adults	Can split or crush tablet; oral solution (grape flavor); chewable tablet (grape flavor)	High-fat meal increases exposure by 25%, and decreases Tmax by 0.5 h for tabs but delays it by 1 h for solution and chewtabs
Dexmethylphenidate (Focalin)	2.5 mg BID	30	1–1.5	3–6	20 mg	6–17	Can split or crush	High-fat meal delays Tmax by 1.5 h; 2.5 mg = 5 mg methylphenidate
Intermediate-Acting								
Methylphenidate (Methylin ER)	20 mg AM	60–90	4.7	3–8	60 mg	6–17, adults	Do not crush, chew, or split	Preferable to take 30–45 min before meals
Long-Acting								
Methylphenidate (Ritalin LA)	10–20 mg AM	100	First: 1.5 Second: 6.6	7–9	60 mg	6–12	Can open and sprinkle on applesauce	Capsule is 50% IR and 50% DR beads; high-fat meal delays first Tmax
Methylphenidate (Metadate CD)	10–20 mg AM	90	First: 1.5 Second: 4.5	7–9	60 mg	6–15	Can open and sprinkle on applesauce	Capsule is 30% IR and 70% DR beads; high-fat meal delays first Tmax by 1 h
Methylphenidate (Quillivant XR)	10–20 mg AM	45	4	12	60 mg	6+	Oral suspension (banana flavor)	Suspension is 20% IR and 80% DR beads; high-fat meal reduces Tmax by 1 h; shake vigorously for at least 10 sec
Methylphenidate (QuilliChew ER)	10–20 mg AM	45	5	8	60 mg	6+	Chewable tablet (cherry flavor)	Tablet is 30% IR and 70% DR beads
Methylphenidate (Aptensio XR)	10 mg AM	60	First: 2 Second: 8	12	60 mg	6+	Can open and sprinkle on applesauce	Capsule is 40% IR and 60% DR beads; high-fat meal decreases second peak

TABLE 1 Methylphenidate Medications*—cont'd

MEDICATION (BRAND NAME EXAMPLES)	INITIAL DOSE	ONSET (MINUTES)	TMAX (HOURS)	DURATION (HOURS)	FDA MAXIMUM DAILY DOSE	FDA-APPROVED AGES	SPLIT/CRUSH/SPRINKLE	COMMENTS
Methylphenidate (Concerta, Relexxii)	Children: 18 mg AM / Adults: 18–36 mg AM	30–60	First: 1 / Second: 6–10	10–12	6-12 years: 54 mg / ≥ 13 years: 72 mg	6–17, adults	No	Nonabsorbable tablet is 22% IR and 78% DR beads
Methylphenidate (Cotempla XR-ODT)	17.3 mg AM	Within 60 min	5	12	51.8 mg	6–17	Allow to dissolve, do not crush or chew	Tablet is 25% IR and 75% DR beads; 8.6 mg = 10 mg methylphenidate
Methylphenidate (Jornay PM)	20 mg PM	12-13 hours	14	10	100 mg	6+	Can open and sprinkle on applesauce	High-fat evening meal delays Tmax by 2.5 h
Methylphenidate transdermal (Daytrana)	10 mg AM	120–240	8–10	10–12	30 mg	6–17	Transdermal	Remove after 9 h; absorption may continue for several hours after removal; 15 mg approx. = 20 mg methylphenidate
Dexmethylphenidate (Focalin XR)	5 mg AM	30	First: 1.5 / Second: 6.5	9–12	6–17 years: 30 mg / Adults: 40 mg	6–17, adults	Can open and sprinkle on applesauce	Capsule is 50% IR and 50% DR beads; high-fat meal delays Tmax
Serdexmethylphenidate/ Dexmethylphenidate (Azstarys)	39.2/7.8 mg AM	30	2	13	52.3/10.4 mg	6+	Can open and sprinkle on applesauce or added to water	Capsule is 30% IR d-MPH and 70% XR prodrug of d-MPH (ser-d-MPH)

*Pregnancy/lactation: risk of congenital anomalies does not appear to be increased based on animal studies and a limited number of human pregnancies.
DR, delayed release; *ER*, extended release; *IR*, immediate release; *LA*, long-acting; *ODT*, orally disintegrating tablet; *SR*, sustained release; *Tmax*, time to maximum concentration (peak); *XR*, extended release.

Attention-Deficit/Hyperactivity Disorder

TABLE 2   Amphetamine Medications

MEDICATION (BRAND NAME EXAMPLES)	INITIAL DOSE	ONSET (MIN)	TMAX (H)	DURATION (HOUR)	FDA MAXIMUM DAILY DOSE	FDA-APPROVED AGES	SPLIT/ CRUSH/SPRINKLE	COMMENTS
Short-Acting								
Dextroamphetamine (generic, ProCentra, Zenzedi)	3–5 years: 2.5 mg AM ≥6 years: 5 mg AM or BID	20–60	3	4–6	40 mg	3–16	Can split or crush tablet; oral solution (bubblegum flavor)	
Mixed amphetamine salts (Adderall)	3–5 years: 2.5 mg AM ≥6 years: 5 mg AM or BID	30	3	5–8	40 mg	3+	Can split or crush	
Amphetamine (Evekeo)	3–5 years: 2.5 mg AM ≥6 years: 5 mg AM–BID	30	3	4–10	Rarely ≥ 40 mg	Evekeo: 3+ Evekeo ODT: 6–17	Tablet: can split or crush ODT: dissolves	1:1 d:l amphetamine ratio
Intermediate-Acting								
Dextroamphetamine (Dexedrine Spansules)	5 mg AM or BID	60–90	8	6–10	Rarely ≥40 mg	6–16	Can open and sprinkle on applesauce	
Long-Acting								
Dextroamphetamine (Xelstrym transdermal patch)	Children (6-17 years): 4.5 mg/9 hr Adults: 9 mg/9 hr	120	6–9	9	18 mg	6–17, adults	Transdermal	Remove after 9 h; absorption may continue for several hours after removal; 18 mg approx. = 60 mg lisdexamfetamine
Mixed amphetamine salts (Adderall XR)	Children: 5–10 mg AM, ≥13 years: 10–20 mg AM	30	7	10–12	30 mg/day (children 6-12 yrs Rarely ≥40 mg/day for adolescents and adults)	6–17, adults	Can open and sprinkle on applesauce	Capsule is 50% IR and 50% DR beads; food delays Tmax by 2–3 h
Mixed amphetamine salts (Mydayis)	13–17 years: 12.5 mg AM Adults: 12.5–25 mg AM	30	7–10	12–16	13–17 years: 25 mg Adults: 50 mg	13–17, adults	Can open and sprinkle on applesauce	Capsule contains IR and two types of DR beads; high-fat meal delays peak by 5 h
Amphetamine (Dyanavel XR)	≥6 years: 2.5–5 mg AM	60	4	10–13	20 mg	6+	Oral suspension and chewable tablet (both bubblegum flavor)	Ion exchange resin; high-fat meal delays peak by 1 h; 2.5 mg = 4 mg MAS

TABLE 2 Amphetamine Medications—cont'd

MEDICATION (BRAND NAME EXAMPLES)	INITIAL DOSE	ONSET (MIN)	TMAX (H)	DURATION (HOUR)	FDA MAXIMUM DAILY DOSE	FDA-APPROVED AGES	SPLIT/ CRUSH/SPRINKLE	COMMENTS
Amphetamine (Adzenys XR-ODT)	Children: 6.3 mg AM Adults: 12.6 mg AM	30	5	10–12	6–12 years: 18.8 ≥13 years: 12.5	6–17, adults	ODT: allow to dissolve, do not crush or chew (orange flavor)	Tablet is 50% IR and 50% DR beads; 6.3 mg = 10 mg MAS
Lisdexamfetamine (Vyvanse) (capsules)	6–17 years: 20–30 mg AM Adults: 30 mg AM	90–120	3.5	10–12	70 mg	6–17, adults	Can open and dissolve in water, yogurt or orange juice	High-fat meal delays peak by 1 h; lower abuse potential; 70 mg = 30 mg MAS
Lisdexamfetamine (Vyvanse) (chewable tabs)	6–17 years: 20–30 mg AM Adults: 30 mg AM	90–120	4.4	10–12	70 mg	6–17, adults	Chewable tablet (strawberry flavor)	High-fat meal delays peak by 1 h; lower abuse potential; 70 mg = 30 mg MAS

*Pregnancy/lactation: limited human data suggest possible risk of premature delivery/low birth weight/neonatal withdrawal, but no impact on cognitive development at 3 years of age; not considered compatible with breast-feeding.
DR, Delayed release; *IR*, immediate release; *MAS*, mixed amphetamine salts; *ODT*, orally disintegrating tablet; *Tmax*, time to maximum concentration (peak).

Attention-Deficit/Hyperactivity Disorder

TABLE 3　Nonstimulant ADHD Medications*

MEDICATION* (BRAND NAME EXAMPLES)	INITIAL DOSE	ONSET (WEEKS)	TMAX	DURATION	MAXIMUM DAILY DOSE	FDA MAXIMUM DAILY DOSE	FDA-APPROVED AGES	SPLIT/CRUSH/ SPRINKLE	COMMENTS
Atomoxetine (Strattera)	Children ≤70kg: 70 kg: 0.5 mg/kg/day (target 1.2 mg/kg/day) Children >70 kg and adults: 40 mg daily (target 80 mg daily)	2–4	1–2 h	24 h	100 mg	<70 kg: 1.4 mg/kg/day; NTE: 100 mg >70 kg: 100 mg	6–17, adults	No	High-fat meal delays peak by 3 h; no abuse potential
Viloxazine Extended-Release (Qelbree)	Children: 100 mg QD Adolescents, adults: 200 mg QD	1	5 h	24 h	600 mg	6–17 years: 400 mg Adults: 600 mg	6–17, adults	Sprinkle	Can open and sprinkle on applesauce
Clonidine ER (Kapvay, Onyda XR)	0.1 mg PM	2	6.5 h	12 h	0.4 mg	N/A	6–17	Do not crush or chew tablet; oral suspension (orange flavor)	Do not stop abruptly; ER tablet and oral suspension are bioequivalent; relative bioavailability 89% vs. clonidine
Guanfacine ER (Intuniv)	Children, adolescents: 1 mg QD (target 0.05–0.12 mg/kg/day) Adults: 1 mg QD	2–3	6 h	8–14 h; up to 24 h in higher doses	6–12 years: 4 mg 13–17 years: 7 mg QD Adults: 4 mg QD	6–12 years: 4 mg 13–17 years: 7 mg Adults: NA	6–17	No	Do not stop abruptly; high- fat meal increases exposure by 40%; relative bioavailability 58% vs. guanfacine
Bupropion[1] (Wellbutrin [IR], Wellbutrin SR or XL)	Children, adolescents: lesser of 3 mg/kg/day or 150 mg daily Adults: 150–200 mg	2–4	IR: 2 h SR: 3 h XL: 5 h	XL: 24 h	Children, adolescents: lesser of 6 mg/kg or 300 mg Adults: 300–450 mg	N/A	Not for ADHD	IR: Split SR or XL: No	No abuse potential
Venlafaxine[1] (Effexor [IR], Effexor XR)	Children, adolescents: 12.5–25 mg Adults: 75 mg	2–4	IR: 2 h XR: 6 h	IR: 4–6 h XR: 24 h	Children, adolescents: <30 kg: 50 mg; ≥30 kg: 75 mg Adults: 150–225 mg	N/A	Not for ADHD	IR: split XR: No	No abuse potential; discontinuation syndrome

*Pregnancy/lactation: Caution in pregnancy due to limited data; insufficient data for use during breast-feeding.
[1]Not FDA approved for this indication.

onset of effect is rapid; however, a 1-week trial or longer at an adequate therapeutic dose may allow for better assessment of full effect. Medication doses should be maximized as tolerated for an adequate period before changing treatment regimen due to insufficient symptomatic and functional improvement. Of note, effective dose is not closely correlated with age, weight, or symptom severity. Some patients may report tolerance to a specific stimulant medication, which may be addressed with dosage adjustment, drug holidays, or switching stimulant medications.

Selective Norepinephrine Reuptake Inhibitors (NRIs)

Atomoxetine (Strattera) may be considered a first-line medication based on preferences or the presence of comorbidities such as anxiety, tics, or SUDs. Atomoxetine is an effective alternative for patients who experience severe side effects with stimulants. However, evidence suggests that atomoxetine is less efficacious than stimulants, with an effect size of 0.45 in adults and 0.6 in children/adolescents. Onset of action is slower over 1 to 2 weeks, and maximum benefits may not be reached for 4 to 6 weeks. Atomoxetine is best initiated at a low dose and titrated gradually to optimize tolerability (especially gastrointestinal). Although FDA labeling states that doses can be titrated after a minimum of 3 days, stepwise titrations at weekly intervals (e.g., 0.5 mg/kg/day, then 0.8 mg/kg/day, and then 1.2 mg/kg/day) may be better tolerated for patients weighing less than 70 kg.

Viloxazine (Qelbree), recently approved in the United States for the treatment of pediatric and adult ADHD, has a long history of use in Europe for the treatment of depression. Its efficacy is primarily ascribed to its norepinephrine reuptake activity, however serotonergic modulation observed in preclinical studies may also contribute. Evidence suggests that viloxazine is less efficacious than stimulants, with an effect size that ranges from 0.5 to 0.6 in children and adolescents and is approximately 0.3 in adults. Onset of action is 1 to 2 weeks, with full benefits reached after 4 weeks or longer. Dose titration may be considered at weekly intervals based on response and tolerability. Although viloxazine represents a new and interesting option for the management of ADHD, its cost as a brand-only product will likely be a significant barrier to widespread use. Additionally, viloxazine is a strong cytochrome P450 1A2 inhibitor, hence it may reduce the metabolism of several medications; its package label recommends avoiding concomitant use of several different medications such as duloxetine (Cymbalta) and melatonin[7] and cautious use with others such as clozapine (Clozaril) and olanzapine (Zyprexa).

α₂ Agonists

Clonidine and guanfacine are available as immediate-release (IR) and extended-release formulations (ER). IR formulations have been used off-label for pediatric ADHD (including preschool age) for many years, while ER formulations (clonidine ER [Kapvay], guanfacine ER [Intuniv]) were subsequently developed and FDA-approved as ADHD monotherapy or adjunctive therapy to stimulants for children and adolescents. α₂ agonists are less efficacious than stimulants and closer in efficacy to other nonstimulant alternatives, with effect sizes of 0.6 to 0.7. For patients with coexisting tics or stimulant-exacerbated tics, α₂ agonists offer the best combined improvement in both tic and ADHD symptoms, either as monotherapy or as an adjunct to a stimulant. They may also be considered as alternatives to stimulants in the context of comorbid SUDs. While clonidine has not been studied in adults, emerging data support the efficacy of guanfacine ER in this age group, with an effect size of approximately 0.6.

Generally, α₂ agonists are initiated at low doses and titrated gradually based on response and tolerability (see Table 3). Clinical trial data with guanfacine ER suggest increased efficacy with weight-based dosing; clinically meaningful ADHD symptom improvement in pediatrics is seen with doses of 0.05 to 0.08 mg/

kg/day, with further efficacy (but also increased incidence of side effects) at doses up to 0.12 mg/kg/day. Onset of effect on core ADHD symptoms is gradual over 2 to 4 weeks.

Other Agents

Bupropion (Wellbutrin), venlafaxine (Effexor), and TCAs are occasionally used off-label for the treatment of ADHD. The evidence base for these medications is far weaker; effect sizes are smaller than stimulants and more similar to other nonstimulant alternatives. They may be considered in patients with coexisting depression, anxiety (namely venlafaxine), or nicotine use disorder who desire smoking cessation (bupropion).

Side Effects

Both stimulant classes share a common set of side effects that can be transient (e.g., headache, dizziness, anxiety) and minimized with low-dose initiation, gradual titration, and possibly dose reductions. Contrary to popular belief, stimulant treatment of ADHD does not induce aggression but rather can provide strong benefits on associated aggression and antisocial behavior. Clinicians should distinguish between aggression/emotional lability that is present when the stimulant is active (which may indicate excessive dosage) and increased hyperactivity/impulsivity in the evening or at the end of a dosing interval when the medication is no longer effective (commonly referred to as *rebound*). The latter may be addressed by administering a small dose of short-acting stimulant in the late afternoon. Children who experience emotional lability, experience irritability (e.g., feeling too "wired"), or feel too serious, tired, dull, flat, or listless when the stimulants are active may benefit from a dose reduction or a switch to an alternate agent. Side effects that tend to persist in long-term treatment with all stimulants include insomnia, decreased appetite, and/or weight loss. Although controlled evidence does not show an increased risk of tics with stimulants, their use is occasionally associated with unmasking or worsening tics; if this side effect persists and is problematic, an alternative medication (particularly nonstimulant) may need to be considered.

Stimulants and NRIs should generally be avoided in patients with serious cardiac disease given concerns for increased cardiac events and possible sudden cardiac death; a detailed medical history, family history, and physical examination are recommended before initiation, with referral to a cardiologist if risk factors are detected. Both classes of medications are associated with small increases in heart rate and blood pressure overall; however, these may be clinically relevant in a subset of patients.

Growth impairments are linked to stimulant treatment and, to a lesser extent, atomoxetine treatment. Reduced growth velocity is most prominent in the first 1 to 3 years of stimulant treatment, with subsequent attenuation but a possible small negative impact on final adult height. Weight and body mass index (BMI) are also negatively affected by stimulant treatment; longer duration of treatment and higher doses have been linked to greater effects on height and weight suppression. Atomoxetine has also been associated with reduced growth velocity in the first 1 to 2 years of treatment, followed by normalization after 2 to 3 years of treatment. The long-term impact of viloxazine remains to be established.

NRIs have less pronounced effects on sleep and appetite than stimulants but are associated with somnolence and more nausea and vomiting (atomoxetine more than viloxazine). Abdominal pain/discomfort may be improved by dividing the total daily dose of atomoxetine into twice-daily dosing (morning and early evening); however, this may further suppress appetite. Rare cases of hepatotoxicity, including liver failure, have been reported with the use of atomoxetine. Routine monitoring of hepatic function is not required during atomoxetine treatment; however, patients who develop jaundice, dark urine, or other symptoms of hepatic disease should discontinue atomoxetine and seek medical evaluation including liver function test assessment. Atomoxetine and viloxazine carry a black box warning regarding increased suicidality risk in children and adolescents.

---

[7] Available as dietary supplement.

The α_2 agonists are associated with a high rate of drowsiness, headache, dizziness, hypotension, and bradycardia, as well as abdominal pain and dry mouth/constipation. Caution is recommended when discontinuing clonidine and guanfacine; the dose should be gradually decreased to avoid sudden increases in blood pressure.

Monitoring

As mentioned earlier, small increases in blood pressure and heart rate and decelerations in growth can be observed with use of stimulant medication. It is recommended to monitor patient vital signs within 1 to 3 months of medication initiation and then every 6 to 12 months. Vital signs should be closely monitored with dosage titration or discontinuation because α_2 agonists may decrease blood pressure. In cases of poor weight gain secondary to stimulants, it may be beneficial to take a "drug holiday" from the medication over weekends or school breaks. At regular follow-up visits, providers will monitor for adverse drug reactions including insomnia and decreased appetite or weight loss with stimulant administration. If concerns exist for diversion or poor medication adherence, urine drug screens may be administered. To track the patient's response to medication, rating scales from caregivers and teachers should be repeated throughout treatment. Clinicians should also regularly update family history, especially with regard to cardiac disease, and screen for cardiac symptoms.

Complications

Academic underachievement, school problems, and peer neglect are commonly associated with elevated inattentive symptoms; peer rejection and accidental injury are more likely to occur in those with marked hyperactivity and/or impulsivity.

When to Refer

Patients who are younger than 6 years of age; have a comorbid substance use disorder, a conduct disorder, or bipolar disorder; or fail to respond to adequate trials of methylphenidate, amphetamine, or atomoxetine should be considered for referral to a mental health specialist.

References

American Psychiatric Association: *Diagnostic and Statistical Manual of Mental Disorders (DSM-5-TR)*, 5th ed Text Revision, Arlington, VA, 2022, American Psychiatric Association.
Arnold LE, Hodgkins P, Kahle J, et al: Long-term outcomes of ADHD: academic achievement and performance, *J Atten Disord* 24:73–85, 2020.
Barbaresi WJ, Campbell L, Diekroger EA, et al: Society for Developmental and Behavioral Pediatrics clinical practice guideline for the assessment and treatment of children and adolescents with complex attention-deficit/hyperactivity disorder, *J Dev Behav Pediatr* 41:S35–S57, 2020.
Boland H, DiSalvo M, Fried R, et al: A literature review and meta-analysis on the effects of ADHD medications on functional outcomes, *J Psychiatr Res* 123:21–30, 2020.
Cortese S, Adamo N, Del Giovane C, Mohr-Jensen C, Hayes AJ, Carucci S, et al: Comparative efficacy and tolerability of medications for attention- deficit hyperactivity disorder in children, adolescents, and adults: a systematic review and network meta-analysis, *Lancet Psychiatry* 5(9):727–738, 2018.
Evans SW, Owens JS, Wymbs BT, Ray AR: Evidence-based psychosocial treatments for children and adolescents with attention deficit/hyperactivity disorder, *J Clin Adolesc Psychol* 43:157–198, 2018.
Findling RL, Candler SA, Nasser AF, et al: Viloxazine in the management of CNS disorders: a historical overview and current status, *CNS Drugs* 35:643–653, 2021.
Gleason MM, Egger HL, Emslie GJ, et al: Psychopharmacological treatment for very young children: contexts and guidelines, *J Am Acad Child Adolesc Psychiatry* 46:1532–1572, 2007.
Greenhill L, Kollins S, Abikoff H, et al: Efficacy and safety of immediate-release methylphenidate treatment for preschoolers with ADHD, *J Am Acad Child Adolesc Psychiatry* 45:1284–1293, 2006.
Harstad E, Shults J, Barbaresi W, et al: α2-adrenergic agonists or stimulants for preschool-age children with attention-deficit/hyperactivity disorder, *JAMA* 325:2067–2075, 2021.
Jensen PS, Hinshaw SP, Swanson JM, et al: Findings from the NIMH Multimodal Treatment Study of ADHD (MTA): implications and applications for primary care providers, *J Dev Behav Pediatr* 22:60–73, 2001.
Kooij JJS, Bijlenga D, Salerno L, et al: Updated European Consensus Statement on diagnosis and treatment of adult ADHD, *Eur Psychiatry* 56:14–34, 2019. Epub 2018 Nov.
Molina BS, Hinshaw SP, Swanson JM, et al: The MTA at 8 years: prospective follow-up of children treated for combined-type ADHD in a multisite study, *J Am Acad Child Adolesc Psychiatry* 48:484–500, 2009.
The MTA: Cooperative Group. A 14-Month Randomized Clinical Trial of Treatment Strategies for Attention-Deficit/Hyperactivity Disorder, *Arch Gen Psychiatry* 56:1073–1086, 1999.
Vitiello B, Lazzaretto D, Yershova K, et al: Pharmacotherapy of the preschool ADHD treatment study (PATS) children growing up, *J Am Acad Child Adolesc Psychiatry* 54:550–556, 2015.
Wolraich ML, Hagan JF, Allan C, et al: Clinical practice guideline for the diagnosis, evaluation, and treatment of attention-deficit/hyperactivity disorder in children and adolescents, *Pediatrics* 144(4):e20192528, 2019.
Young S, Moss D, Sedgwick O, et al: A meta-analysis of the prevalence of attention deficit hyperactivity disorder in incarcerated populations, *Psychol Med* 45:247–258, 2015.

BRONCHIOLITIS

Method of
Tamara Wagner, MD

CURRENT DIAGNOSIS

- Clinical diagnosis most commonly associated with respiratory distress in a child younger than 2 years of age.
- Symptoms include nasal congestion or rhinorrhea associated with findings of lower respiratory tract involvement, most notably elevated respiratory rate, wheezing, or crackles.
- Diagnostic testing in the form of chest x-ray or viral testing is not recommended.

CURRENT THERAPY

- Standard treatment is supportive care, including clearance of nasal passages, oxygen for saturation less than 90%, fluids for dehydration, and early nutritional support.
- There is no indication for corticosteroids (inhaled or systemic), albuterol, racemic epinephrine, or decongestant drops.
- Nebulized hypertonic saline has recently become a treatment option, but clear benefit has not been established.
- Humidified high-flow nasal cannula (HHFNC) oxygen is used frequently in patients with increased work of breathing to comfortably administer higher percentages of oxygen. Systemic reviews support HHFNC as safe and well tolerated, with a decreased association of intubation in intensive care unit (ICU) patients. Optimal use of HHFNC therapy for mild to moderate bronchiolitis remains unclear.

Background

Clinical bronchiolitis remains one of the most significant diseases within the pediatric population. Bronchiolitis is caused by a viral infection, most often the respiratory syncytial virus (RSV). Bronchiolitis as a clinical disease has a long history of applied medical therapies, which initially showed some promise in small studies and then were abandoned later, when larger studies failed to demonstrate benefit. There remains a high variation in care for patients, which persists despite the development of standardized guidelines. Bronchiolitis is a self-limited disease with a favorable prognosis; recent care guidelines support elimination of therapies without proven benefit.

Epidemiology and Virology

Bronchiolitis follows a seasonal epidemic most closely tied to the spread of the RSV virus. Historically, the incidence of RSV peaks between November and April with regional variation. RSV circulating patterns were significantly disrupted during the emergence of COVID-19. It is unclear when previous seasonal patterns will return. Approximately 800,000 children in the United States require outpatient medical management during the first year of life as a result of bronchiolitis, and approximately 100,000 hospitalizations occur annually. RSV is the most commonly isolated viral pathogen in patients with bronchiolitis. RSV accounts for 50% to 80% of all hospitalizations for bronchiolitis. Other viruses associated with bronchiolitis include human rhinovirus, parainfluenza virus, human meta-pneumovirus, coronavirus, adenovirus, influenza virus, enterovirus, and COVID-19.

Coronavirus Disease 2019

The emergence of the coronavirus disease 2019 (COVID-19) pandemic was associated with a clear epidemiologic shift in clinical bronchiolitis. Measures adopted in response to the pandemic such as masking, social distancing, social isolation, and stay-at-home orders dramatically interfered with the typical seasonal behavior of viral respiratory infections. These measures were associated with disappearance of the typical winter season peak of bronchiolitis followed by an atypical summer peak in many countries coinciding with relaxation of social distancing measures. Previously, theories to explain seasonal bronchiolitis included outside ambient temperature, meteorologic factors, and increased transmission of viruses within indoor structures. The significant disruption of the established pattern of clinical bronchiolitis calls into question the importance of temperature and weather and brings into focus the importance of standard infection prevention measures in preventing RSV infections in young infants. COVID-19 as a pathogen can cause clinical bronchiolitis but does not seem to be associated with severe bronchiolitis symptoms. Pediatric patients admitted with COVID-19 bronchiolitis should receive treatment according to current COVID-19 treatment guidelines, which may include steroids and anti–COVID-19 therapeutics.

Risk Factors

The most significant risk factor for bronchiolitis is age. Up to 90% of children will become infected with RSV before 2 years of age, and nearly one-half of those children will experience bronchiolitis. Since 2020, older toddlers, aged 2 to 4 years, have been described with severe bronchiolitis. It is unclear whether these patients represent patients with decreased immune competency based on less exposure to circulating viruses when they were younger or whether the disease age range is expanding. Infants younger than 3 months of age and those with a history of prematurity have a higher risk of severe bronchiolitis and the complication of apnea. Other risk factors for a severe course include congenital heart disease, chronic lung disease, and poor immune function. Recent studies have demonstrated that environmental factors such as cigarette smoke exposure or air pollution may increase the risk for bronchiolitis.

Pathophysiology

The pathophysiology of bronchiolitis is progressive obstruction of the distal airways caused by mucous production, airway edema, and direct cellular injury of the bronchiolar epithelium. Following viral infection, increased mucous production, airway edema, and impaired ciliary function result in varying degrees of intraluminal obstruction. This obstruction during the positive pressure phase of expiration may cause an audible wheeze. As the disease progresses, virus-induced injury to the bronchiolar lining leads to sloughed cells and distortion of the alveolar structure, resulting in air trapping and atelectasis. With the progression of lung atelectasis, mismatching of ventilation and perfusion occur, resulting in increased work of breathing and hypoxemia.

Prevention

Breast-feeding infants (whether exclusive or partial) have lower hospitalization rates than infants who are not breastfeeding. Additionally, infants receiving breast milk who are hospitalized with bronchiolitis have shorter hospital admissions. Palivizumab (Synagis) is a human-derived immunoglobulin G monoclonal antibody directed against RSV. Use of Synagis has been shown to reduce the rate of hospitalization in premature infants. In 2014, the American Academy of Pediatrics (AAP) released guidelines for patients who should receive Synagis; these are listed in Table 1. Patients receiving prophylactic therapy should receive 1 shot per month, 15 mg/kg per dose, for a maximum of 5 doses. This should be administered

TABLE 1	Guidelines for Use of Palivizumab
DISEASE CONDITION	**PALIVIZUMAB (SYNAGIS) PROPHYLAXIS**
Prematurity	Recommended routinely in first year of life for infants born <29 weeks or <32 weeks with chronic lung disease defined as oxygen therapy for at least 28 days after birth. Recommended within second year of life for children with chronic lung disease who continue to require supplemental oxygen, diuretic therapy, or chronic corticosteroid therapy
Congenital heart disease	May be considered in first year of life for infants with hemodynamically significant heart disease
Congenital pulmonary abnormality	May be considered in first year of life for infants with impaired lung physiology
Neuromuscular disease	May be considered in first year of life for infants with impaired ability to clear secretions
Immunodeficiency	May be considered in first 2 years of life for patients with profound immunosuppression

during the regional RSV season. An RSV-specific vaccine (Arexvy, Abrysvo) has been developed for adults older than 60 years of age, raising the possibility of a successful vaccine strategy to prevent RSV infections in pediatric patients.

Clinical Manifestations

Bronchiolitis begins with upper respiratory findings of congestion or rhinorrhea, which then progresses to involve the lower respiratory tract. An increased respiratory rate is the earliest and most sensitive vital sign change. On physical examination, the most important observation is the work of breathing. All patients should have the shirt lifted and the chest directly observed for retractions. Retractions may be visible in the subcostal, intercostal, or supracostal region. Head bobbing, grunting, "sighing," and "singing" are signs of severe respiratory distress in infants. In very young infants, especially those with a history of prematurity, apnea alone may be the presenting sign as well as a complication of bronchiolitis. Auscultation can reveal a variety of findings, from minimal sounds to a combination of wheezes, crackles, or referred upper airway congestion. Physical examination findings in bronchiolitis are characteristically dynamic, so they may vary from examiner to examiner. There are no robustly supported physical examination findings that have reliably correlated with clinical outcomes such as severity or disposition. Despite fully validated parameters, many institutions use bronchiolitis scoring tools to align resources with patients with more severe clinical symptoms. Respiratory rate, work of breathing, and hypoxia remain the most clinically significant parameters in determining illness severity.

Diagnosis

Bronchiolitis remains a clinical diagnosis based on physical examination and history. Chest x-rays are not recommended for diagnosis. Patients with bronchiolitis often have abnormal appearing radiographs, with findings of hyperinflation, areas of atelectasis, and small infiltrates. These findings do not correlate with disease severity and do not change management. Obtaining chest x-rays has been associated with increased prescription of antibiotics, although a primary or concurrent bacterial pneumonia is rare in bronchiolitis. Viral testing similarly does not change management in the majority of clinical cases and should not be routinely obtained. There are a few clinical situations in which

TABLE 2	Summary of Evidence for Treatment of Bronchiolitis	
MEDICATION	**RECOMMENDATION**	**EVIDENCE QUALITY**
Systemic corticosteroids	Not recommended	Cochrane systematic review shows that corticosteroids do not significantly reduce outpatient admissions when compared with placebo and do not reduce length of stay for inpatient admissions
Epinephrine	Not recommended	Cochrane meta-analysis systematically evaluated the evidence and found no evidence for utility in the inpatient setting
Albuterol	Not recommended	Meta-analyses and systematic reviews have shown that bronchodilators improve clinical symptom scores, but they do not affect disease resolution, need for hospitalization, or length of stay
Hypertonic saline	May consider	Meta-analysis of smaller studies has resulted in differing conclusions as to whether this therapy affects rate of hospitalization or length of stay.
Oxygen therapy	Provide supplemental oxygen if oxyhemoglobin saturation is <90%	
Nutrition and hydration	Administer intravenous or nasogastric fluid for infants unable to maintain hydration orally	

Modified from Ralston SL, Lieberthal AS, Meissner HC, et al.: Clinical practice guideline: the diagnosis, management and prevention of bronchiolitis, *Pediatrics* 134(5):e1474–e1502, 2014.

viral testing may aid management. Young infants (<60 days) may present with fever as a result of bronchiolitis. The risk of serious bacterial infection (SBI) in these infants is low; viral testing may support the provider in decreased additional testing, decreased administration of empiric antibiotics, and avoidance of unnecessary hospitalization. During the seasonal influenza epidemic, influenza testing may identify bronchiolitis secondary to influenza that may benefit from antiviral medications.

Differential Diagnosis

The differential diagnosis for bronchiolitis includes a first episode of asthma, virus-induced wheezing, pertussis infection, chronic aspiration, congenital heart disease, and anatomic thoracic abnormalities. Separating clinical bronchiolitis from a primary asthma exacerbation remains particularly challenging, even for experienced providers. Epidemiologic data support that there is a large burden of virus-induced wheezing in young children, and only a small percentage of this large group will progress to a diagnosis of asthma. It remains unclear whether bronchiolitis causes a lung injury leading to asthma or whether patients with severe bronchiolitis have preexisting differences predisposing them to a severe course and later diagnosis of asthma. Given the high prevalence of virus-induced wheezing in young children, a potential asthma diagnosis (and associated use of albuterol or potentially steroids) should only be considered in patients with risk factors for asthma including eczema, food allergies, or family history of atopy and demonstration of bronchospasm reversed by a bronchodilator. As bronchodilators are not recommended for bronchiolitis, the medical team should carefully assess for efficacy if a trial is performed. Pertussis should be considered in prolonged or atypical courses, especially if the infant has had contact with adults who have not received a booster vaccination. Children with an abnormal neurologic baseline should prompt consideration of chronic aspiration as an etiology or contributor to a prolonged course. Undiagnosed congenital heart defects may present with similar examination findings to bronchiolitis. Other anatomic abnormalities that may be considered include pulmonary malformations, vascular rings, or aspiration of a foreign body.

Treatment

Treatment for bronchiolitis remains supportive therapy and includes the following measures:

- Improve comfort by clearing nasal secretions and administering antipyretics for fever.
- Administer oxygen to maintain oxygen saturations greater than 90%.
- Maintain hydration by administering intravenous fluids or placing a nasogastric tube.
- Support adequate nutrition.
- Educate caregivers on return-to-care precautions.

In 2014, the AAP published "Clinical Practice Guideline: The Diagnosis, Management and Prevention of Bronchiolitis," a revised version of the 2006 guidelines. A summary of the recommended treatments is given in Table 2.

Outpatient Management

Outpatient management centers on parental education in supportive care that can be provided for the child while sick and emphasis on return-to-care precautions. The typical course for bronchiolitis begins with upper respiratory infection (URI) symptoms that will progress to lower respiratory symptoms (cough, increased work of breathing), which peak on days 3 to 5. Cough is the last symptom to resolve, with the majority of patients having some resolving cough for up to 2 weeks and a minority extending to 4 weeks. Parents should be discouraged from administering over-the-counter cough suppressants. Clearance of the nasal passages by bulb syringe or a device of parent choice may increase the comfort of breathing and support feeding in infants. Fever is an expected complication of bronchiolitis and may be treated with antipyretics. Caregivers should monitor comfort with breathing; if persistent retractions are present, patients are unable to feed, or they appear to have distress, they should be evaluated immediately for inpatient supportive care.

Inpatient Management

Inpatient admission to the hospital should be considered for patients with hypoxia, defined as oxygen saturation less than 90% on room air, dehydration, or moderate to severe respiratory distress manifested by tachypnea for age, retractions, grunting, or concern for apnea. Nasal clearance for comfort, oxygen therapy for hypoxia, and nutritional support remain the foundational therapy for inpatient care. Although nasal suction has not been robustly compared with withholding nasal suction, it has become the standard of care in most hospitals. Deep suction is not recommended and may be associated with longer lengths of stay. Medications including albuterol, corticosteroids, and racemic epinephrine are not recommended. Nebulized hypertonic saline has been studied as a therapeutic agent with conflicting trial results. These studies have suffered from design variability both within the United States and internationally. Current evidence does not demonstrate a clear benefit for patients with bronchiolitis. Patients with concurrent dehydration should have volume replacement with isotonic fluids. Bronchiolitis has been described as an independent stimulus for antidiuretic hormone release, placing these patients at risk for inappropriate retention of free water and development of hyponatremia. Isotonic fluid should be used in these patients to decrease the risk of iatrogenic hyponatremia. Aggressive nutritional support should be initiated for infants with poor feeding; nasogastric support should be given to any patient who is not able to meet caloric goals. Oxygen should be administered to maintain saturations greater than 90%. Humidified high-flow nasal cannula (HHFNC) oxygen therapy is frequently used as a safe method of increased respiratory support for hospitalized patients with moderate to severe work of breathing. HHFNC uses blended, humidified, heated air and oxygen at higher flow rates used with nonhumidified oxygen. Systemic reviews support HHFNC as safe and well tolerated, with decreased association of intubation in ICU patients. Which non-ICU patients with bronchiolitis will receive benefit remains unclear. High-flow nasal cannula (HFNC) oxygen support has become a standard tool for respiratory support in hospitalized children (even in non-ICU admissions) despite lack of data for improvement in clinical outcomes and clear indications for initiation. HFNC has become an identified potential low-value intervention for patients with bronchiolitis. Reduction in the overuse of HFNC has become an aim in many children's hospitals. There is high variability in the use and interpretation of pulse oximetry in patients with bronchiolitis. Although pulse oximetry readings are instrumental in determining the need for admission, continuous monitoring has been associated with increased length of stay. Patients should be transitioned to intermittent monitoring as soon as possible, and providers should focus on the clinical course over transient variations in oximetry. Chest physiotherapy is not recommended when managing hospitalized patients with bronchiolitis. Antibiotic therapy should only be used if there is concern for a secondary bacterial infection. Secondary bacterial infections in mild to moderate bronchiolitis are rare, but severe bronchiolitis may have a higher percentage of bacterial co-infection.

Complications

The most common complication of bronchiolitis is acute otitis media, which should be treated according to current guidelines. A small percentage of bronchiolitis patients will progress to respiratory failure requiring intensive care support and mechanical ventilation. These patients may represent a unique cohort with a higher incidence of preexisting comorbid conditions, coinfection from multiple viral agents, or bacterial superinfection. Mortality resulting from RSV in the United States is rare, accounting for fewer than 100 children annually, but worldwide bronchiolitis remains a significant contributor to pediatric mortality in resource-limited countries.

References

American Academy of Pediatrics Committee on Infectious Diseases: American Academy of Pediatrics Bronchiolitis Guidelines Committee: Updated guidance for palivizumab prophylaxis among infants and young children at increased risk of hospitalization for respiratory syncytial virus infection, *Pediatrics* 134:415–420, 2014.
Franklin D, Babl FE, Schlapbach LJ, et al: A randomized trial of high-flow oxygen therapy in infants with bronchiolitis, *N ENgl J Med*, 2018.
Hall CB, Weinberg GA, Iwane MK, et al: The burden of respiratory syncytial virus infection in young children, *N Engl J Med* 360:588–598, 2009.
Hasegawa K, Tsugawa Y, Brown D, et al: Trends in bronchiolitis hospitalizations in the United States, 2000–2009, *Pediatrics* 132:28–36, 2013.
Meissner HC: Viral bronchiolitis in children, *N Engl J Med* 374:62–72, 2016.
Ralston SL, Lieberthal AS, Meissner HC, et al: Clinical practice guideline: the diagnosis, management and prevention of bronchiolitis, *Pediatrics* 134:1474–1502, 2014.
Guitart C, Bobillo-Perez S, Alejandre C, et al: Bronchiolitis, epidemiological changes during the SARS-CoV-2 pandemic, *BMC Infect Dis* 22:84, 2022. https://doi.org/10.1186/s12879-022-07041-x.
Andina-Martinez D, Alonso-Cadenas JA, Cobos-Carrascosa E, et al: SARS-CoV-2 acute bronchiolitis in hospitalized children: neither frequent nor more severe, *Pediatr Pulmonol*, 2021.

DIABETES MELLITUS IN CHILDREN

Method of
Gregory Goodwin, MD

CURRENT DIAGNOSIS

- Random glucose >200 mg/dL
- Fasting glucose >126 mg/dL
- 2-h glucose >200 mg/dL after glucose tolerance test
- Hemoglobin A1c >6.5%
- Diabetic ketoacidosis: pH <7.3, serum bicarbonate <15 mmol/L

CURRENT TREATMENT

Type 1 Diabetes
- Basal/bolus regimen**: rapid-acting insulin* before meals and long-acting insulin[†,‡] at bedtime
- Insulin pump therapy**: infusion of rapid-acting insulin in hybrid closed loop with continuous glucose monitoring (CGM)
- Total daily insulin dose (TDD): 0.15 to 1.2 U/kg per day
  - Basal/bolus: 50% long acting, 50% rapid acting
  - Insulin pump: ~50% basal, ~50% rapid acing bolus insulin

Diabetic Ketoacidosis
- Fluids: 10 to 20 mL/kg normal saline once, repeat if shock/poor perfusion. Ongoing fluids: one-half normal saline with 20 mEq/L potassium acetate and 20 mEq/L potassium phosphate at 1.5 to 2.0 times maintenance fluids
- Regular insulin infusion: 0.05 to 0.1 U/kg per hour
- Add dextrose (5%–10%) when glucose is less than 300 mg/dL
- Urgent consultation with center experienced in treatment of pediatric ketoacidosis (if not available on site)

Type 2 Diabetes
- Aggressive dietary modification
- Metformin (Glucophage): 500 to 1000 mg bid, titrate up to avoid gastrointestinal side effects
- The first two items on this list plus insulin therapy: either as single long-acting insulin at bed or full basal bolus regimen until stable glucose control
- Glucagon-like peptide-1 (GLP-1) agonist in obese pediatric patients older than 10 years

**Preferred treatment.
*Rapid-acting insulin: lispro (Humalog, Admelog), aspart (Novolog, Fiasp), glulisine (Apidra).
[†]Long-acting insulin: glargine (Lantus, Toujeo, Basaglar), detemir (Levemir)[2], degludec (Tresiba).
[2]Not available in the United States.
[‡]75% intermediate-acting insulin, 25% rapid-acting insulin (Humalog 75/25).

Type 1 Diabetes: Introduction

Type 1 diabetes mellitus (T1DM) results from progressive autoimmune destruction of insulin-producing cells (β cells) of the pancreatic islets, ultimately leading to insulin deficiency and resulting in hyperglycemia and in some cases ketoacidosis.

The precise cause or causes of T1DM remains elusive, but a strong association with human lymphocytic antigens (HLAs) has been known for decades. Genome-wide linkage studies have identified up to 60 genes associated with T1DM, and many are related to the immune response. However, identical twin studies show a concordance rate of only 30% to 60%, suggesting that unidentified environmental factors make up the remaining risk. Environmental factors implicated in T1DM risk include viral infections, toxins (nitrosamines), and dietary factors such as exposure to cow's milk and gluten-containing cereals in early infancy. However, prospective studies have shown no advantage of using elemental formulas or delaying the introduction of gluten until 1 year of life in infants at increased risk for development of T1DM. A large meta-analysis of 24 studies of over 4000 participants showed an almost 10-fold risk of reverse transcription polymerase chain reaction (RT-PCR)-determined enteroviral infections in T1DM patients versus controls, whereas the TEDDY study showed an almost 50% conversion of high-risk infants and children to expressing islet cell antibodies when more than five respiratory infections in the preceding 9 months were reported.

Epidemiology
The prevalence of T1DM is about 1 per 300 individuals (0.3%) in the United States, with significant global and racial variations. The presence of a first-degree relative with T1DM, such as a sibling or parent, increases the chances of developing T1DM to 3% to 6%.

The highest incidence rates of T1DM in children are seen in early adolescence (10–14 years), followed by early childhood (5–9 years). The youngest age of onset of T1DM can be seen in infants younger than 1 year, but usually not before 6 months.

The incidence of T1DM has been increasing steadily by 2% to 5% per year over the past several decades in the United States, Europe, and Australia. Interestingly, in some but not all studies, the youngest age group (0–4 years) demonstrates the highest rates of increase.

The onset of T1DM is seasonal. In the Northern Hemisphere, the highest incidence of onset is in the fall and winter and the fewest are in the summer.

Prediction and Prevention of Type 1 Diabetes Mellitus
β-Cell antibodies appear months to years before the clinical diagnosis of diabetes. Screening of family members of patients with T1DM can therefore lead to identification of individuals at high risk for development of diabetes. Screening for β-cell antibodies can be obtained at commercial laboratories or from the type 1 diabetes TrialNet program at no cost. The FDA approved teplizumab (Tzield) in 2022, an anti–T-cell (anti-CD3) antibody for the treatment of individuals with more than 2 β-cell autoantibodies and biochemical dysglycemia. Teplizumab has resulted in delay of onset of T1DM for up to 24 to 32 months in high-risk antibody positive patients. Further research in T1DM prevention will hopefully lead to complete prevention of this disorder in the future.

Presentation
The classic symptoms of diabetes are polyuria, polydipsia, and nocturia, which is the result of an osmotic diuresis induced by hyperglycemia. Symptoms can be present for days to months, but the majority of patients present after 1 to 2 weeks of symptoms. Weight loss is a common finding on presentation because insulin plays an important role in the synthesis of protein and fat; therefore insulin deficiency results in the loss of muscle and fat stores. Weight loss also occurs because calorie loss from high concentrations of glucose in the urine can be substantial.

Abdominal pain, nausea, and vomiting are classic signs of ketoacidosis that can often be misdiagnosed as gastroenteritis. Approximately 70% of patients with new-onset diabetes have hyperglycemia without ketoacidosis at presentation, whereas some 25% to 30% of cases present in diabetic ketoacidosis (DKA), although there can be significant variations from various centers internationally.

Diagnosis
A random glucose greater than 200 mg/dL in the presence of classic symptoms of diabetes is diagnostic of diabetes. A fasting glucose greater than 126 mg/dL is also diagnostic of diabetes; however, a fasting glucose or a glucose tolerance test is rarely necessary in the diagnosis of T1DM.

A venous pH less than 7.3 or a serum bicarbonate less than 15 mmol/L is diagnostic of DKA in the presence of hyperglycemia.

TABLE 1	Suggested Total Daily Insulin Dosage in New-Onset Type 1 Diabetes	
PATIENT CATEGORY	**INSULIN DOSE (U/KG PER DAY)**
Prepubertal without DKA	0.25–0.5 (<6 years, 0.15–0.25)
Prepubertal with DKA	0.5–0.75
Pubertal without DKA	0.5–0.75
Pubertal with DKA	0.75–1.2

DKA, Diabetic ketoacidosis.

Distinguishing type 1 from type 2 diabetes can sometimes be difficult at presentation, particularly in an overweight adolescent. In this circumstance, islet cell autoantibodies are useful in making this distinction. Islet cell autoantibodies include anti–glutamic acid decarboxylase (GAD), antiinsulin, antiinsulinoma autoantigen 2 (IA-2), and anti–zinc transporter 8 (ZnT8). These antibodies are available in most commercial laboratories, but results are usually not available until weeks after initial presentation. The safest course of action in most pediatric patients with new-onset diabetes is to treat with insulin until islet antibodies and other parameters such as endogenous insulin production as assessed by c-peptide levels are available.

Treatment of Type 1 Diabetes Mellitus
Type 1 Diabetes Mellitus (Without Ketoacidosis or After Ketoacidosis Has Resolved)
Insulin is the mainstay of treatment for T1DM. Intensive insulin therapy has become the standard of care for patients with T1DM. Typically a long-acting basal insulin—such as glargine (Lantus, Toujeo, Basaglar), or degludec (Tresiba)—along with premeal boluses of rapid-acting insulin—such as lispro (Humalog, Admelog), aspart (NovoLog,), or glulisine (Apidra)—is instituted.

Required total daily insulin dosing (TDD) is dependent on age at presentation, pubertal stage, and the presence of acidosis at diagnosis. Total daily insulin requirements range from about 0.25 to 1.0 U/kg per day (Table 1). Long-acting or basal insulin is typically 50% of TDD; the remaining 50% is bolus insulin. Bolus rapid-acting insulin dosing is calculated by the following formulas (Figure 1):

To cover meal carbohydrates, a *carbohydrate ratio* is derived from the formula

$$500 \text{ divided by total daily insulin dose}$$

To correct hyperglycemia, a *correction factor* is derived from the formula

$$1500 \text{ divided by total daily insulin dose}$$

Correction doses should not be given more frequently than every 3 hours.

For new-onset patients, a *target glucose* of 150 mg/dL is assigned, whereas more established patients typically use 120 mg/dL. Correction at bedtime or during the night should be less aggressive and a higher target may be assigned—for example, 150 to 200 mg/dL.

Carbohydrate ratios, correction factors, and targets are adjusted on the basis of fasting and postprandial glucose levels. High postprandial glucose levels would require a lower carbohydrate ratio. High blood glucose levels that do not correct after a correction dose has been given would require a lowering of the correction factor. High morning fasting glucose levels would require an increase in the long-acting insulin dose.

Implicit in this recommended treatment regimen is that (1) the patient or family is able to count carbohydrates correctly, and (2) the family is able to calculate insulin dosing correctly using the carbohydrate ratio, correction factor, and target. If the patient or family is unable or unwilling to perform these calculations, a simplified insulin regimen should be devised using fixed doses

Patient Example 1

- 6-year-old girl has 2-week history of polydipsia and polyuria.
- She is otherwise well with a normal exam.
- Serum glucose in the ER is 425 mg/dL, and serum bicarbonate is 20.
- Weight in the ER is 20 kg

- Total daily insulin = – 20 kg × 0.3 U /kg/d = 6 units.
- ˜50% basal = 3.0 units (glargine, degludec)
- Target = 150
- Carbohydrate ratio: 500/6 = 83˜80
- Correction factor: 1500/6 = 250

Figure 1 New-onset type 1 diabetes in a 6-year-old girl who is not in diabetic ketoacidosis (DKA). Total daily insulin dosage is determined by multiplying body weight by recommended dosage requirements for a prepubertal girl who is not in DKA. One-half of the total daily insulin dose is given as long-acting insulin, which is 3.0 units in this example. Carbohydrate ratio and correction factors are calculated using formulas provided in the text. Calculated ratios can be adjusted up to 10% to simplify calculations.

Patient Example 2

- 14-year-old with cognitive delays has 3-week history of polydipsia and polyuria and 10 lb weight loss.
- Glucose 625 mg/dLin ER
- Bicarbonate 19 mEq/L
- Tanner 4 on exam
- Weight 44 kg
- Parents also have cognitive impairments.

- Total daily dose: 44 kg × 0.6 U/kg/d = 26.4 units per day.
- Medical team decides fixed mixed 75/25 insulin regimen may be best.
- 2/3 TDD given before breakfast = 17 units
- 1/3 before dinner = 9 units
- Sliding scale rapid acting: 1 unit per 50 mg/dL over 200 mg/dL

Figure 2 A 14-year-old boy with intellectual impairments presents with new-onset type 1 diabetes without diabetic ketoacidosis. Because of cognitive delays in both the patient and his parents, a simplified two-injection regimen was derived using the previously described calculations. This regimen may be supplemented with a sliding scale of rapid-acting insulin.

of intermediate-acting insulin and a sliding scale of rapid-acting insulin.

In certain challenging cases where there are significant compliance or cognitive deficits, fixed doses of premixed intermediate- and rapid- or short-acting insulin such as Humalog mix (75/25) can be used before breakfast and before dinner (Figure 2). Premixed 75/25 insulin preparations come in vials or pens and consist of 75% intermediate-acting neutral protamine Hagedorn (NPH) and 25% rapid-acting (lispro) insulins.

Treatment of Diabetic Ketoacidosis

There are critical differences in the treatment of DKA between children and adults. A major complication of the treatment of DKA in children is cerebral edema, a complication rarely seen in adults. Although a relatively infrequent complication (<1% of DKA episodes), cerebral edema can be associated with serious morbidity and mortality.

Risk factors for the development of cerebral edema include new-onset diabetes, younger age at diagnosis, longer duration of symptoms before diagnosis, and severity of acidosis—manifested as DKA with hypocapnia, high blood urea nitrogen, bicarbonate boluses, and failure for the corrected serum sodium to rise as treatment for DKA progresses. For these reasons, overly aggressive fluid resuscitation and boluses of bicarbonate are avoided in the treatment of pediatric DKA.

Judicious fluid replacement with a bolus of normal saline—initially 10 mL/kg and, if necessary, a second 10-mL/kg bolus of saline solution—may be given in the first hour of treatment. Thereafter, half normal saline with 40 mEq/L of potassium acetate or potassium phosphate at a fluid rate of no more than 1.5 to 2.0 times maintenance is administered (Table 2). Potassium should not be added to intravenous fluid until the potassium is less than 5 meq/L. The two-bag system for fluid management of DKA—in which two bags contain identical electrolytes but differ in that one bag contains no dextrose and the second bag contains 10% dextrose—can be useful. The relative contribution of each bag is then titrated depending on the blood glucose level. Although estimates of fluid deficit in DKA are between 5% and 10% of body weight, intravascular volume is often preserved in the hyperosmolar state; hence hypovolemic shock is uncommon in DKA. The goal is to replace the fluid deficit slowly over 24 to 48 hours. Frequent neurologic checks are highly recommended in the first 24 hours of treatment. Altered mental status or the development of headaches during treatment for DKA is a potentially serious sign of cerebral edema.

Insulin plays a critical role in the treatment of DKA, not only in lowering serum glucose levels but also in the paramount role of shutting down ketogenesis in the liver. The standard insulin drip for pediatric DKA is 0.1 U/kg per hour; however, treatment with 0.05 U/kg per hour has also been effective. Human regular insulin remains the standard insulin in the intravenous treatment of DKA.

TABLE 2	Formulas for the Calculation of Maintenance Fluids for Infants and Children
For infants 3.5–10 kg, daily fluid requirement = 100 mL/kg	
For children 11–20 kg, daily fluid requirement = 1000 mL + 50 mL/kg for every kg over 10 kg	
For children >20 kg, daily fluid requirement = 1500 mL + 20 mL/kg for every kg over 20, up to a maximum of 2400 mL daily	

Once the acidosis has resolved, as reflected by a normal anion gap and serum bicarbonate greater than 15 mmol/L and pH greater than 7.35, the insulin drip can be discontinued. Hyperchloremic non–anion gap acidosis (HCO3 <15 but normal anion gap <12) can occur during the recovery phase of DKA. Hyperchloremic metabolic acidosis is likely due to a large amount of chloride administered in intravenous fluids as both NaCl and KCl supplementation. For this reason, many centers typically give 50% of the potassium replacement as potassium phosphate. Once the acidosis is resolved and the patient can tolerate oral intake, subcutaneous insulin can be started (see "Treatment of Type 1 Diabetes Mellitus" section). The most convenient time to transition to subcutaneous insulin is just before a meal.

Importantly, treatment of pediatric DKA should ideally occur in centers with experienced pediatric intensivists, endocrinologists, and nursing staff. If referral to a pediatric center is not practical, then early contact with a pediatric endocrinologist for treatment guidance is highly recommended.

Finally, the most common causes of pediatric DKA are (1) new-onset diabetes presenting in DKA and (2) infusion site failure in a patient on an insulin pump or missed long-acting insulin injections in a patient on insulin injections. Infections including gastroenteritis and febrile illnesses are infrequently the exclusive cause of DKA in pediatrics.

Diabetes Self-Management Education

Children and adolescents with type 1 diabetes should receive outpatient care by multidisciplinary teams including an endocrinologist, certified diabetes nurse educator, registered dietitian, and licensed clinical social worker. Provision of comprehensive education at the time of diagnosis is essential because this is the time when the patient and family are most receptive and impressionable. Patients who do not receive proper early education often fall into habits of suboptimal diabetes care, which can be hard to undo once established.

Important educational topics that must be rapidly learned by the family and patient (in addition to glucose monitoring and insulin administration) include diet and carbohydrate counting, prevention and treatment of hypoglycemia, emergency glucagon, exercise and hypoglycemia, prevention of ketoacidosis, and sick day management. Learning to count carbohydrates accurately can be a particular challenge.

Mental Health Considerations in Type 1 Diabetes Mellitus

Diabetes "burnout" issues are common in the treatment of youth with diabetes, particularly during the adolescent years. Conflicts between parents and teens can often arise during this time. It is important for the parents to maintain a healthy supporting role with their child or teenager in a manner appropriate to the child's age and level of development. Recognition of relatively common mental health comorbidities—such as depression, anxiety, and eating disorders—is essential to the overall well-being of the pediatric patient with T1DM.

Goals of Therapy for Patients With Type 1 Diabetes Mellitus

The number one goal of the diabetes healthcare team is to prevent readmission to the hospital for severe hypoglycemia or ketoacidosis. Resumption of the full range of daily activities, including returning to school and work and engaging in essentially all meaningful activities that preceded the diagnosis of diabetes, is to be expected.

The glycemic goal in the pediatric age group is to reduce hemoglobin A1c to less than 7.5%, and for decades children and adolescents had great difficulty in achieving this goal. However, with the availability of "smart" hybrid closed-loop insulin pumps, the ability to achieve target glucose control has improved significantly over the past 5 years.

The Diabetes Control and Complications Trial (DCCT) in 1993 showed convincingly that lowering the hemoglobin A1c from 9% to 7.1% resulted in significantly less diabetes-related retinopathy, nephropathy, and neuropathy.

Sick Day Management

Patients with T1DM who have intercurrent infectious illnesses are prone to develop hyperglycemia with ketosis and also hypoglycemia, depending on the nature of the illness. Blood glucose levels should be monitored every 1 to 3 hours during illnesses. Rapid-acting insulin may need to be administered every 2 to 4 hours for hyperglycemia, especially in the presence of serum or urine ketones. Rapid-acting insulin can be dosed at 0.1 to 0.2 U/kg per dose in this setting. Improvement in hyperglycemia and particularly in ketosis using this treatment regimen can be invaluable in preventing ketoacidosis or hospitalization. Patients with persistent vomiting who are unable to keep fluids down need to be referred to the emergency department for intravenous hydration and assessment for DKA.

For patients on an insulin pump, ketosis with nausea and vomiting is often a sign that the insulin infusion set is not properly functioning. Insulin therefore should be given by syringe or pen device until the ketones have cleared and a new infusion set has been placed.

Poor oral intake during a gastrointestinal illness may result in hypoglycemia. Frequent small volumes of sugar-containing fluids such as juice or sports drinks may be necessary to keep the blood glucose greater than 70 mg/dL, and basal insulin requirements may need to be decreased by 10% to 50%. Low-dose glucagon may be used in the setting of recurrent hypoglycemia and poor oral intake. Glucagon can be dosed at 1 unit on an insulin syringe for every year of age, using a standard 1-mg/mL glucagon preparation. The dose may be repeated every 15 minutes as needed. In some cases, persistent low glucose levels (<70 mg/dL) in the setting of recurrent vomiting may be best managed in an emergency department or hospital setting where intravenous dextrose-containing fluids are readily available.

Risk for Additional Autoimmune Disorders

Patients with one autoimmune disorder are at increased risk for the development of one or more additional autoimmune conditions. Children and adolescents with T1DM are particularly at risk for thyroid and celiac disorders. Screening for thyroid disorders with serum TSH and free T$_4$ should occur in the first 6 months after the T1DM diagnosis and every 1 to 2 years thereafter. Celiac disorder should also be screened in the first year after the T1DM diagnosis. Most cases of celiac disorder are detected within the first 5 years after the diagnosis of T1DM, and the majority of cases are asymptomatic. Recent American Diabetes Association recommendations include screening for celiac disorder at diagnosis and again at 2 and 5 years after diagnosis. Elevated serum tissue transglutaminase levels should be referred to a pediatric gastroenterologist. Because celiac disorder is a lifelong condition, it is advised to obtain a small bowel biopsy. Autoimmune adrenal (Addison) disease rarely occurs with T1DM but has the unique presentation of recurrent hypoglycemia, necessitating significant reductions in daily insulin requirements. Sending simultaneous adrenocorticotropic hormone (ACTH) and cortisol levels on a morning blood specimen will usually render the diagnosis of Addison disease if the condition is present.

Screening for Complications of Type 1 Diabetes Mellitus

Microvascular complications of T1DM are infrequent in the pediatric age group, although background retinopathy and microalbuminuria become more prevalent in the late adolescent and young adult age ranges. Proactive early screening regimens are advocated to detect diabetes complications early so that medical interventions can prevent more serious diabetes-related complications, such as proliferative retinopathy and end-stage renal disease.

Annual screening for microalbuminuria with a random urine specimen should be performed at puberty or at age 10 years and older once the child has had diabetes for 5 years. Elevated urine albumin/urine creatinine (>30 mg/g creatinine) ratios should be repeated two to three times over a 6-month period to confirm the diagnosis because transient microalbuminuria is a common finding. Variables such as exercise or recent illness can lead to microalbuminuria; therefore a repeat study after recovery and on a first morning specimen will often yield a normal result. In addition, individuals with the benign condition of orthostatic albuminuria can be identified by finding completely normal albumin excretion on a first morning voided specimen, whereas a random specimen will often be frankly proteinuric. When urinary albumin/creatinine ratios are found to be consistently elevated, treatment with an angiotensin converting enzyme inhibitor is recommended. Referral to a pediatric nephrologist should be arranged in complex cases.

Annual dilated eye examinations are recommended after age 10 or at pubertal onset (whichever comes first) once the patient has had diabetes for 3 to 5 years. Referral to an eye care professional with expertise in diabetic retinopathy is recommended.

Cardiovascular risk factors including blood pressure and lipid profiles should be monitored in patients with T1DM. Blood pressure should be obtained at each visit.

High blood pressure is defined as systolic or diastolic blood pressure greater than the 90th percentile, and hypertension is defined as greater than the 95th percentile for age, sex, and height. Blood pressure measurements should be obtained using an appropriate cuff size, particularly in the overweight patient. White-coat hypertension can be problematic in the adolescent population. Such patients will often demonstrate an elevated heart rate as a clue to stress-induced hypertension. Monitoring blood pressure in a nonthreatening environment, such as at home, using an accurate home blood pressure monitor, may be helpful. When white-coat hypertension is suspected, 24-hour home blood pressure monitoring can be very useful.

Initial management of high blood pressure includes salt restriction and weight-control measures. For persistent hypertension, treatment with an antihypertensive medication (lisinopril) can be instituted.

Shortly after diagnosis and once glucose control has been established, it is important to obtain nonfasting total and high-density lipoprotein cholesterol readings. If total cholesterol is high, a fasting morning lipid panel should be obtained. If low-density lipoprotein (LDL) cholesterol is less than 100, it would be reasonable to repeat it in 5 years. For LDL cholesterol greater than 100, dietary measures are taken, along with efforts to improve metabolic control. For patients beyond 10 years of age with an LDL cholesterol greater than 130 to 160 in whom lifestyle changes have resulted in inadequate control, statin therapy may be considered. Referral to a pediatric preventive cardiology program would also be appropriate.

Technologic Changes in the Care for Patients With Type 1 Diabetes Mellitus

Since 2015, technological changes have revolutionized the care of patients with T1DM. Continuous glucose monitoring (CGM) has evolved into a very powerful and nearly universally used technology in T1DM. Subcutaneous fluid glucose levels are determined every 1 to 5 minutes, and the user is provided with meaningful feedback to influence diabetes self-management decisions in real time. Particularly useful are alarm functions for impending low glucose levels; these can be invaluable in the prevention of hypoglycemia. The accuracy of glucose determinations by CGM technology is now approaching subcutaneous blood glucose technology, and the improved accuracy has led the US Food and Drug Administration (FDA) to approve insulin-dosing decisions based on CGM data. It is important to remember, however, that subcutaneous sensor glucose levels lag behind whole blood glucose levels by about 15 minutes. This fact is particularly important when glucose levels are changing rapidly, so the user is advised to pay attention to the glucose trend. Alarms for predicting hypoglycemia are very important in this regard.

The most remarkable technologic change in the care of patients with T1DM is the coupling of CGM and real-time adjustments in insulin delivery via insulin pump therapy. Thus insulin delivery is suspended when hypoglycemia has occurred or is likely to occur, and basal insulin can be significantly increased when hyperglycemia is predicted to occur or has occurred. *Hybrid closed loop* refers to the fact that some aspects of management, such as carbohydrate counting and manual bolusing for meals, are still required. The first hybrid closed-loop insulin pump was FDA approved in 2016 (Medtronic 670G). Prevention of postprandial hyperglycemia is particularly problematic, but prebolusing rapid-acting insulin 10 to 15 minutes before eating will help limit postprandial hyperglycemia. Prebolusing of insulin is often difficult in view of modern lifestyles. The Tandem insulin pump with Control IQ technology was FDA approved in 2019. This hybrid closed-loop system is user-friendly, with no calibration requirements or forced exits from automated insulin delivery. Hybrid closed-loop technology can be particularly useful for optimizing glycemic control overnight, the time when many patients and families are most fearful of hypoglycemia. The very popular Omnipod 5 tubeless hybrid closed-loop insulin pump was FDA approved in 2022 and can now be operated by a phone application. Medtronic has made major advances with its newest 780G insulin pump with SMARTGARD technology. Finally, the Beta Bionics iLet insulin pump was FDA approved in 2023 and has the major advantage of not requiring precise carbohydrate counting, which is a significant challenge for many patients with type 1 diabetes.

Type 2 Diabetes in Children

Since the 1990s, the incidence of type 2 diabetes mellitus (T2DM) in patients younger than 18 years of age has risen dramatically. The increased incidence of type 2 diabetes has coincided with the obesity epidemic. Children from minority populations (non-Hispanic Blacks, Hispanics, and Native Americans) and those patients with a positive family history of T2DM are at the greatest risk. The majority of pediatric patients diagnosed with T2DM are adolescents, but children as young as 9 or 10 can be diagnosed with prediabetes or new-onset type 2 diabetes.

Diagnosis of T2DM can be made with a fasting glucose greater than 126 mg/dL, random glucose greater than 200 mg/dL, and

the 2-hour glucose from an oral glucose tolerance test greater than 200 mg/dL. A hemoglobin A1c greater than 6.5% is indicative of diabetes as well and is a particularly convenient test in the outpatient setting. An elevated fasting or random glucose and an elevated hemoglobin A1c are diagnostic of T2DM in high-risk patients.

Pediatric patients with T2DM are often symptom free at diagnosis but can present acutely with classic diabetes symptoms and even ketosis or mild ketoacidosis. Distinguishing the latter group from T1DM can be difficult initially, but the absence of β cell antibodies and very stable glycemic control after diagnosis are often telltale signs of T2DM.

In individuals who present with marked hyperglycemia (hemoglobin A1c >8.5%), ketosis, or both, stabilization with insulin initially may be required. Basal bolus regimens using a combination of long- and short-acting insulins can be instituted. Insulin resistance may be quite significant at the time of diagnosis, and relatively high doses of insulin can be required to achieve target glucose levels.

Metformin (Glucophage) is often the initial recommended treatment for T2DM along with dietary management. Maximal dosing of metformin is 1000 mg bid or 1500 to 2000 mg/day of the extended-release preparation (metformin XR). Gastrointestinal side effects are relatively common, and metformin should be taken with meals. Initial dosing can be 500 mg bid or 750 mg extended-release daily; the dose can be titrated upward as needed and tolerated. Please remember that **dietary modifications such as weight control and exercise are of fundamental importance in the treatment of T2DM.**

Glucagon-Like Peptides (GLP-1) in the Treatment of Type 2 Diabetes in Youth

GLP-1 agonists are associated with early satiety, weight loss, and improved glycemic control in T2DM. GLP-1 agonist have become increasingly popular in the treatment of T2DM in children and adolescents as they promote weight loss, while therapy with insulin may facilitate weight gain. Side effects of GLP-1 agents include nausea, vomiting, and, less commonly, pancreatitis. Prescribers should use caution in patients with a history of suicidal ideation and depression. A family history of medullary thyroid carcinoma is a contraindication to treatment with a GLP-1.

Liraglutide (Victoza) was FDA approved in 2019 for the treatment of type 2 diabetes in patients older than 10 years and is administered as a daily subcutaneous injection. Dulaglutide (Trulicity) is FDA approved for children older than 10 years with type 2 diabetes and is administered as a weekly injection. Semaglutide (Ozempic) and tirzepatide (Mounjaro) are approved for the treatment of type 2 diabetes in patients older than 18 years, and these medications have the advantage of weekly subcutaneous administration. Semaglutide (Ozempic) and tirzepatide (Mounjaro) are associated with greater weight loss then liraglutide (15%–17% vs. 5% weight loss). Semaglutide (Wegovy) is approved for the treatment of obesity in children older than 12 years and may be used in a pediatric patient with type 2 diabetes and obesity (BMI >95%). Patients treated with GLP-1 should be counseled to have small low-fat meals to help mitigate GI complaints. Treatment of nausea and or vomiting with ondansetron (Zofran)[1] is not routinely recommended, as antiemetic therapy may mask serious underlying complications such as pancreatitis. It is the authors opinion that semaglutide[1] and tirazeptide[1] are superior to liraglutide and dulaglutide and should be used preferentially in the treatment of type 2 diabetes and obesity in children, adolescents, and young adults.

Monogenic or Maturity-Onset Diabetes of Youth

Single gene mutations leading to diabetes are referred to as *maturity-onset diabetes of youth (MODY) diabetes* or *monogenic*

---

[1] Not FDA approved for this indication.

diabetes. More than 30 different genes have been identified that are associated with MODY, although some 80% of cases are due to glucokinase and *HNF1A* and *HNF1B* gene mutations. Patients can be diagnosed at any age but are usually diagnosed before 35 years of age. Routine laboratory testing or laboratory testing during an illness may lead to the detection of MODY diabetes incidentally. Patients with MODY are often lean, and the family history may reveal two to three affected generations. Testing for islet cell antibodies is universally negative.

Glucokinase diabetes is a very mild form of MODY diabetes that is nonprogressive and does not require treatment, whereas *HNF1A* and *HNF1B* forms of MODY diabetes are progressive; these patients can develop long-term complications of diabetes. HNF diabetes is uniquely sensitive to sulfonylureas; hence the diagnosis can be life changing in an individual who has been treated with insulin before definitive diagnosis.

Genetic panels for MODY diabetes are available commercially. It is important to test for both mutations and deletions of the most common forms of MODY. A full list of laboratories that offer MODY testing is available at the NCBI Genetic Testing Registry (http://www.ncbi.nlm.nih.gov/gtr/).

Neonatal diabetes can also be due to monogenic forms of diabetes, and these infants are usually diagnosed before 6 to 9 months of age. Testing for monogenetic forms of diabetes should be considered in infants younger than 9 to 12 months of age whose islet cell autoantibodies are negative. Single gene mutations in the K-ATP channel of the β cell leading to neonatal diabetes can be remarkably responsive to oral sulfonylureas. Transient forms of neonatal diabetes in an infant born with intrauterine growth retardation and macroglossia are often associated with imprinting abnormalities on chromosome region 6q24. This type of diabetes usually resolves by 18 months but can recur at adolescence.

References

American Diabetes Association: Children and adolescents: standards of medical care in diabetes—2025, *Diabetes Care* 48 (suppl 1):S283-S305.

Copeland KC, Zeiter P, Geffner M, et al: Characteristics of adolescents and youth with recent-onset type 2 diabetes: the TODAY cohort at baseline, *J Clin Endocrinol Metab* 96:159–167, 2011.

Environmental Determinants of Diabetes Study: Available at: https://teddy.epi.usf.edu/. Accessed 2/28/2025.

Glaser N, et al: ISPAD Clinical Practice Guidelines 2022: diabetic ketoacidosis and hyperglycemic hyperosmolar state, *Pediatr Diabetes* 23:835–836, 2022.

Levitsky L, Misra M: *Epidemiology, presentation and diagnosis of type 1 diabetes in children and adolescents.* Up To Date. Available at Up To Date. Updated Feb 2025, Accessed March 25, 2025.

Miller KM, Foster NC, Beck RW, et al: Current state of type 1 diabetes treatment in the US: updated data from the T1D Exchange Clinic Registry, *Diabetes Care* 38:971–978, 2015.

National Center for Monogenic *Diabetes at the University of Chicago Monogenic Diabetes Registry.* Available at Monogenic https://monogenicdiabetes.uchicago.edu/. Accessed February 28, 2025.

White NH: Long-term outcomes in youth with diabetes mellitus, *Pediatr Clin* 62:889–909, 2015.

Wolfsdorf JI, Garvey K: Diabetes mellitus in children. In Jameson L, DeGroot L, editors: *Endocrinology adult and pediatric,* ed 7, Philadelphia, 2016, Saunders, pp 854–882.

Yeung W, Rawlinson W, Craig M: Enterovirus infection and type 1 diabetes mellitus: systematic review and meta-analysis of observational molecular studies, *BMJ* 342(7794):421, 2011.

ENCOPRESIS

Method of
Sarah Houssayni, MD

CURRENT DIAGNOSIS

- Voluntary or involuntary passage of stools into inappropriate places at least once a month for 3 consecutive months once a chronologic or developmental age of 4 years has been reached.
- Encopresis can be primary when it persists from infancy onward or secondary when it appears after toilet training.
- The behavior is not due to the direct effects of a substance such as a laxative or a general medical condition except those associated with constipation.
- Distinguishing subtypes is essential because treatment differs:
  - Retentive encopresis: occurs as a result of involuntary leakage of liquid stools due to severe constipation and impaction.
  - Nonretentive encopresis: children pass bowel movements into their underwear due to their refusal to use the toilet.
  - Children occasionally fail to wipe after bowel movements and the secondary soiling should be distinguished from encopresis.

CURRENT THERAPY

Retentive Encopresis
Initial Disimpaction
- Hyperphosphate enemas (Pedia-Lax Enema) (one daily for 2 or 3 days):
  - Less than 1 year old: 60mL.[3]
  - Greater than 1 year old: 6mL/kg, up to 135mL twice.[3]
- Glycerin suppositories (Glycerin Pediatric Suppositories) for infants and toddlers.

Older Children—Slow Disimpaction
- Polyethylene glycol with electrolytes (Golytely, Colyte)[1] ingested over 2–3 days: 25mL/kg/hr up to 1L/hr until stooling clear bowel movements. (This is not approved for bowel cleansing for children.)
- Over 5–7 days:
  - Mineral oil[1] 3mL/kg twice a day for 1 week. (Mineral oil is not approved for use in children younger than 6 years of age.)
  - Lactulose[1] 2mL/kg twice a day for 1 week.
  - Magnesium hydroxide (Milk of Magnesia) 2mL/kg twice a day for 1 week.
  - Polyethylene glycol without electrolyte (MiraLax)[1] 1.5g/kg/day for 3 days.

Maintenance Therapy
- Polyethylene glycol 3350 (MiraLax)[1] age greater than 1 month: 0.7g/kg divided into 1–2 doses daily.
- Lactulose or sorbitol 70% solution age greater than 1 month: 1–3mL/kg/day divided into 1–2 doses daily for 1–3 months.
- Sennosides (Senna, Senna-GRX, Senexon) are habit forming, doses vary greatly in the different available formulations, and they can only be used for short-term treatment. Give at bedtime for a morning bowel movement. Dose is 5mL (1 tablet) for 1-[1] to 5-year-olds and 2 tablets for 5- to 15-year-olds for a maximum of three tablets daily. (Sennosides are not approved for use in children younger than 2 years of age.)
- Glycerin enemas and bisacodyl suppositories (Dulcolax) can be used for short-term constipation treatment.
- Glycerin/saline enema in patients greater than 10 years of age: 20–30mL/day (solution of 1/2 glycerin and 1/2 normal saline).
- Bisacodyl suppositories in patients greater than 10 years of age: 10mg daily.

Nonretentive Encopresis
- **NO** medical treatment.
- Clean up soiling immediately, involve the child.
- Ensure adequate water and dietary fiber intake.
- Avoid use of stool softeners and laxatives.
- **STOP** all reminders, make child responsible for own toilet habits.
- Use rewards when child defecates in toilet.

Encopresis is the voluntary or involuntary passage of stools at least once a month for 3 consecutive months once a chronologic or developmental age of 4 years has been reached. Encopresis is classified as primary when it persists from infancy onward or secondary when it appears after toilet training. Retentive encopresis occurs as a result of involuntary leakage of liquid stools due to severe constipation and fecal impaction. Nonretentive encopresis occurs in children who pass stool into their underwear due to their refusal to use the toilet. It is important to distinguish between the types of encopresis, because treatment differs.

Epidemiology

The prevalence of encopresis is reported to be 4% in 5- to 6-year-olds and 1.5% in 11- to 12-year-olds. Affected boys outnumber girls by a factor of anywhere from 3:1 to 5:1 depending on the source. Encopresis tends to decrease with age. A large number of children with encopresis go unreported due to the shame associated with the condition and underdiagnosis of the condition.

Diagnosis

The diagnosis of encopresis includes the following four criteria: (1) Repeated passage of feces into inappropriate places such as in clothing or on the floor, whether intentional or involuntary. (2) At least one event a month for at least 3 months. (3) A chronologic age of at least 4 years or an equivalent developmental level. (4) The behavior is not due exclusively to the direct physiologic effects of a substance such as a laxative or a general medical condition other than constipation.

Differential Diagnosis

Retentive encopresis is organic in less than 5% of the affected patients. Organic causes include hypothyroidism, hypercalcemia, cerebral palsy, abnormal anatomy of the anus, Hirschsprung's disease, cystic fibrosis, and neuropathy with secondary impaired voiding sensation. Spinal cord conditions such as tethered cord, spina bifida occulta, and spinal cord dysplasia affect stooling through diminished bowel sensation and secondary fecal retention.

Pathophysiology

Patients who are severely constipated hold stools back because of the pain associated with defecation. This becomes a vicious cycle of constipation, rectal dilation, and secondary encopresis. Frequently, emotional problems emerge due to the fear and shame associated with the problem. Control issues with parents trying to take the stooling issues at hand may worsen the constipation problem.

From 10% to 20% of encopretic patients are not constipated. They are frequently preschoolers or school-age children who are postponing their bowel movements too long because they are distracted or because they associate the bathroom with an unpleasant experience (i.e., fear or disgust).

Clinical Manifestations

History

The history should assess for size and consistency of stools, as well as stooling intervals. Families often confuse soiling with stooling, leading to inaccurate reporting of the frequency of bowel movements. Characteristic symptoms of retentive and nonretentive encopresis differ (Table 1).

In retentive encopresis the physician may elicit a history of difficult or painful defecation, crying with bowel movements, and

---

TABLE 1 Characteristic Symptoms of Retentive and Nonretentive Encopresis

Retentive Encopresis

- Constipation
- Stained underwear
- Fewer than three bowel movements per week
- Large-caliber or hard stools
- Abdominal pain, reports of bloated sensation
- Odor of feces from leakage onto underwear
- Difficult or painful defecation
- Enuresis
- Overflow incontinence
- Anorexia

Nonretentive Encopresis

- Passage of stools in inappropriate places without presence of constipation
- Refusal to sit on toilet even though old enough to (older than 5 years, even older than 8 years at times)
- Refusal to take medications
- Child may be depressed

---

posturing that suggests the child is deliberately holding back stools due to the pain associated with passage.

Children may suddenly become still or hide during play, cross their legs, grimace, or shift their position in an attempt to retain stools. The physician should assess for a history of enuresis and urinary tract infections, anorexia, sensations of bloating, fullness, and abdominal pain leading to the patient's avoidance of food and weight loss. Obtain a dietary history including fiber, fluid, and dairy intake. The historian needs to inquire about streaks of blood on toilet paper and underwear. With retentive encopresis, when the child does pass stool, it may be of large caliber and hard, indicative of constipation.

With nonretentive encopresis, the history often reveals bowel movements of normal size and consistency passed into the underwear once or twice a day. Symptoms of constipation are usually absent. A history of behavioral problems, child-parent struggles, and history of abuse may be elicited. Toilet avoidance is common.

Patients with encopresis eventually develop secondary emotional problems, which can be elicited from the history taking.

Physical Examination

Retentive Encopresis

In retentive soiling the physical examination should assess for abdominal distention and tenderness on palpation. A mass can be occasionally felt in the midline in the suprapubic area. This mass of hardened fecal matter most commonly involves the rectosigmoid area and can sometimes extend throughout the entire colon. If the patient is anxious or in pain and tightens the rectus abdominis, this mass can be missed. Rectal examination is a must; it can be done with minimal discomfort. Rectal examination assesses the dilation of the rectum, which may be 6 to 10 cm wide. It is usually packed with stools with clay-like consistency. Visually inspect the anal opening for tone, fissure, and hemorrhoids.

Nonretentive Encopresis

The child with nonretentive encopresis typically has a normal abdominal examination, is likely to have a rectal vault that is not dilated, and the stool will be of normal caliber and consistency. The rectal vault may be empty if the child has just passed a bowel movement. The anal opening may reveal protruding fecal material in children who are deliberate stool holders.

Treatment

Encopresis is treated through a multistep approach. First, clearing the colon of fecal material will allow the dilated rectal vault and rectosigmoid colon to return to normal. The rectal cleanout can be achieved in different ways (see Current Therapy). Enemas and stool softeners are often used in combination.

Maintenance is achieved by keeping stools soft and ensuring daily bowel movements with mineral oil and hyperosmolar agents (e.g., Miralax[1]) that are very safe and can be used from a very young age and are not habit forming. The goal is painless stools once or twice a day with no associated withholding behavior.

Education is key for families so that they understand the physiology and process of stool elimination. Frustration is associated with failure, guilt, and depression and should be replaced with a positive attitude if success is to be achieved.

- Patients should sit daily on the toilet for 5 minutes after meals twice a day.
- Families need to keep a record of the events, as well as a record for success.
- Soiled underwear should be changed as soon as noticed and the child should be cleaned and changed in a timely, emotionally neutral fashion.
- As soon as compliance wanes, the problem is expected to return and is sometimes worse than the previous episode.
- The care provider's continued involvement in titrating medication with the patient's symptoms is necessary.
- Pain-related impaction can be cured in the majority of cases with medical management of the initial presentation. The success rate is reported to be about 70% with psychogenic impaction.
- With nonretentive encopresis, behavioral modification is essential. Stress reduction, effective coping techniques, relaxation training, and a combination of individual and family therapy is sometimes indicated.

[1]Not FDA approved for this indication.

References

Baker SS, et al: Clinical practice guideline. Evaluation and treatment of constipation in infants and children: recommendations of the North American Society for Pediatric Gastroenterology, Hepatology and Nutrition, *J Pediatr Gastroenterol Nutr* 43:e1–e13, 2006.
Becker A, Ruby M, El Khatib D, et al: Central nervous system processing of emotions with faecal incontinence, *Acta Paediatr* 100:e267–e747, 2011.
Boris NM, Dalton R, et al: *Encopresis. Nelson Textbook of Pediatrics*, ed 19, Philadelphia, 2011, Saunders.
Brazzelli M, Griffiths P: Behavioral and cognitive interventions with or without other treatments for the management of faecal incontinence in children, Art. No. CD002240 *Cochrane Database Syst Rev*(2), 2006. https://doi.org/10.1002/14651858.CD002240.pub3.
Coelho DP: Encopresis. A medical and family approach, *Pediatr Nurs* 37:107–112, 2011.
Har AF, Groffie JM: Encopresis, *Pediatr Rev* 31:368–374, 2010.
Raghumath N, Glassman MS, Halata MS, et al: Anorectal motility abnormalities in children with encopresis and chronic constipation, *J Pediatr* 158:293–296, 2011.

EPILEPSY IN INFANTS AND CHILDREN

Method of
Adam L. Hartman, MD

CURRENT DIAGNOSIS

- At initial diagnosis, determine whether the event was a seizure or a non-epileptic event.
- If appropriate, diagnose an epilepsy *syndrome*.
- Age of onset aids in the development of a differential diagnosis.

CURRENT THERAPY

- Selection of an antiseizure medicine should be made based on the type of seizure.
- General principles include the use of a single agent at the lowest effective dose with the goal of no side effects.
- Epilepsy can be associated with coexisting conditions, including neurodevelopmental concerns, depression and anxiety. Successful management includes referrals and/or management of these and associated psychosocial issues.

A seizure can be defined as clinical signs or symptoms resulting from abnormal neuronal firing. Epilepsy is defined as either (1) at least two unprovoked seizures occurring >24 hours apart; (2) one unprovoked seizure and a probability of further seizures similar to the general recurrence risk (at least 60%) after two unprovoked seizures, occurring over the next 10 years; or (3) diagnosis of an epilepsy syndrome. There may be associated psychological, social, and cognitive consequences. Approximately 3% to 5% of the US population have had a seizure (mostly febrile seizures). Nearly 1% of the US population are being treated actively for seizures at any given time. Infants and children represent one of the two major peaks in seizure incidence, making this a very common diagnosis in pediatric practice.

Risk Factors

The primary risk factors for epilepsy in any age group include a history of meningitis, encephalitis, brain trauma, complicated perinatal course, and febrile seizures. Other risk factors for seizures include cortical or developmental malformations, certain inborn errors of metabolism or genetic syndromes, congenital infections, stroke, intracranial hemorrhage, acute metabolic abnormalities, and drug withdrawal.

Pathophysiology

Because the primary alteration is abnormal neuron firing, many different types of pathology can lead to seizures. Alterations in neuronal networks (e.g., cortical malformations), structure (e.g., abnormal dendrite structure in trisomy 21), or ion channels (e.g., *KCNQ2*) can lead to seizures. In many cases, an underlying cause of seizures cannot be identified. Some forms of epilepsy have been linked to various pathogenic genetic variants, although the exact relationship between specific genotypes and phenotypes is unclear for most.

Clinical Manifestations

Broadly speaking, the clinical manifestations of seizures vary depending on which brain structures are involved. Although most people think of seizures only as generalized tonic–clonic seizures (GTCS), a wide variety of signs and symptoms can be caused by seizures. Furthermore, a GTCS may be the initial manifestation of a seizure (i.e., as seen in primary generalized epilepsy) or it may be the end result of a seizure that started in one brain location and then spread to the rest of the brain (e.g., a focal-onset seizure with spread to other broad cortical regions of the brain). These two broad categories (generalized versus focal onset) are approached somewhat differently from a diagnostic and therapeutic perspective.

Signs of a generalized seizure (i.e., those involving abnormal neuronal firing in both sides of the brain) include loss of interaction or staring (absence seizures), myoclonus, tonic posturing, and/or tonic–clonic seizures. Signs of focal-onset seizures can involve specific regions controlling motor, sensory, or autonomic function, a loss of interaction and/or awareness, or automatisms (chewing, lip smacking, repetitive hand motions), to name a few. Patients with focal seizures might have an aura (a warning sign just prior to the seizure). The aura is an altered sensory function that can include salty or metallic taste, tingling sensations, rising sensation in the abdomen, déjà vu, jamais vu, sense of fear, or a nonspecific feeling that something is about to happen. After a seizure, patients also can have a period of postictal lethargy, confusion, or irritability. The latter can be misinterpreted by bystanders as disruptive behavior and has led to inappropriate interventions, even by first responders. This becomes a safety issue for the patient. Education about this type of behavior is critical.

The initial symptoms or signs of a seizure are the most important in determining whether a seizure is generalized or focal in origin because they often localize the anatomic site of pathology. Thus, it is the beginning of a seizure, rather than its end, that is most useful in making a specific diagnosis.

Diagnosis and Management
History and Physical Examination
A detailed history is usually more valuable than any expensive test in diagnosing a seizure or epilepsy. In addition to a description of the actual event, it is useful to inquire about subtle signs that might not be recognized by observers as a seizure, including staring spells, myoclonic jerks, loss of time, and unexplained nocturnal tongue biting, enuresis, or emesis. The presence of postictal weakness can help localize the hemisphere of onset after a focal seizure, even if there is bilateral spread. Making the diagnosis of a specific epilepsy syndrome allows the clinician to develop a plan for further diagnosis and treatment and to counsel about prognosis. On physical examination, any signs of focal neurologic deficits can indicate an underlying lesion. A skin examination might identify a neurophakomatosis, such as tuberous sclerosis complex or Sturge Weber syndrome.

Diagnostic Studies
In selected cases, typical clinical findings in the right clinical context strongly support the diagnosis of epilepsy, but an electroencephalogram (EEG) may be required to confirm the diagnosis. Even if the patient does not have a seizure during the EEG recording, interictal findings (when the patient is not having a seizure) can provide enough evidence to make the diagnosis of epilepsy. Under ideal circumstances, a single EEG can detect epileptiform activity in a patient with untreated generalized epilepsy about 75% of the time, making it a very sensitive test. In contrast, an EEG might detect epileptiform activity in a patient with focal-onset seizures only 50% of the time (although this number increases to about 90% after three EEGs have been done). Conversely, a single normal interictal EEG (particularly one that includes sleep and provocative maneuvers such as intermittent photic stimulation and hyperventilation) in an untreated patient suggests, but is not necessarily diagnostic of, a focal rather than generalized onset.

Other ancillary studies can show underlying structural lesions that lead to epilepsy or provide physiologic information. Magnetic resonance imaging (MRI) can be useful in detecting lesions such as tumors, cortical dysgenesis, and strokes (both ischemic and hemorrhagic). Recent advances in image analysis have substantially improved the ability to find subtle regions of cortical dysgenesis that may be the source of seizures. Positron-emission tomography (PET) scans may show regions of abnormal metabolism that might not be evident on MRI. Another nuclear medicine study, single photon emission tomography (SPECT), can be used to identify the region of onset of a seizure. Functional MRI (fMRI) studies show regions involved in a specific task (e.g., motor or language) or identify important structures in certain networks.

Magnetoencephalography, when combined with MRI, can be useful in detecting areas of abnormal electrical activity that might not be evident on a scalp EEG recording. Neuropsychology evaluations can aid in localization of regions of dysfunction and also aid in determining risk for loss of function if surgery is performed. The intracarotid amobarbital (Amytal)[1] test (Wada

test) or intracarotid methohexital (Brevital)[1] test is used to lateralize language function and memory; fMRI is being investigated as a replacement for aspects of this invasive test. Intracranial electrodes can localize the onset of a seizure prior to a surgical resection and identify regions of eloquent neurologic function (regions where critical function would be lost if they were removed).

Specific Epilepsy Syndromes
Some of the more common syndromes are described here, listed by typical age at presentation.

Neonatal Seizures
Seizures in neonates can be caused by any type of neurologic pathology, including infections (prenatal or postnatal), strokes, hemorrhages, electrolyte abnormalities, cortical dysgenesis, inborn errors of metabolism (including vitamin B_6 dependency), genetic syndromes, drug (illicit and licit) withdrawal, and medications. Some neonatal seizure syndromes (self-limited neonatal epilepsy and self-limited familial neonatal epilepsy) are self-limited in terms of resolution of seizures; seizures in early-infantile developmental and epileptic encephalopathy frequently are refractory to medical treatment, and the babies have a poor prognosis for development. Neonatal seizures should be managed in conjunction with specialists.

Febrile Seizures
Febrile seizures are the most common type of seizure, occurring in 3% to 5% of people in the United States. Febrile seizures, even though they can recur, are not diagnostic of epilepsy because they are provoked (i.e., by fever). With an onset between 1 month and 5 years of age (and almost always outgrown by 6 to 7 years of age), these seizures can be generalized or focal in onset. Meningitis and encephalitis also can manifest with seizures and fever and thus are exclusion criteria for febrile seizures because the prognosis and treatment are completely different. Febrile seizures that last longer than 15 minutes, have a focal onset, or occur more than once in a febrile illness are complex febrile seizures (only one of the three criteria are needed to make the diagnosis). Patients with complex febrile seizures are at a higher risk for developing epilepsy, although the overall risk is still low (4%). In patients who lack all three of these factors (i.e., simple febrile seizures), routine imaging, blood work, lumbar puncture, and EEG are not necessary for diagnosing the cause of the seizure. Rather, the workup should be guided by other concerns, such as dehydration, concern for occult bacteremia, or, in the appropriate clinical context, meningitis.

Approximately one-third of patients have a recurrence of a febrile seizure. Factors that increase the recurrence risk include very young age at onset, family history of febrile seizures, low-grade fever at onset of the seizure, frequent febrile illnesses, or the occurrence of the seizure in the first hour of the fever. Febrile seizures always are outgrown, so typically long-term seizure prophylaxis is not used. Oral diazepam (Valium) prophylaxis[1], started at the onset of fever, prevents febrile seizures but can lead to excessive sedation and is not used routinely. Patients who have prolonged febrile seizures can benefit from rectal diazepam gel (Diastat) or other benzodiazepines given soon after the onset of a febrile seizure to prevent additional prolonged seizures or febrile status epilepticus. A similarly good prognosis is seen in infants and children who have febrile seizures in the setting of acute gastroenteritis (whether febrile or not). The risk of epilepsy is increased after a febrile seizure in the setting of a complex febrile seizure, abnormal development, frequent febrile seizures, or a family history of epilepsy.

Infantile Epileptic Spasms Syndrome
With an onset typically around 3 to 12 months of age, infantile epileptic spasms syndrome may include two or more of a triad of typical seizures (head drops and brief flexor and/or extensor spasms occurring in clusters around sleep transitions), a highly disorganized multifocal EEG pattern called hypsarrhythmia, and developmental delays. Between 70% and 90% of patients have

---

[1] Not FDA approved for this indication.

identifiable underlying neurologic pathology associated with this syndrome. This is one of the most medically intractable epilepsy syndromes, and the prognosis for seizure control and development is very poor, except in a small subset of patients with no identifiable underlying pathology. Treatment typically is with corticosteroids (prednisolone [Orapred][1] or ACTH [Acthar HP]), or vigabatrin (Sabril), which is commonly the first-line treatment in infants with tuberous sclerosis complex (Box 1).

Dravet Syndrome

The typical presentation for Dravet syndrome is a prolonged febrile seizure involving one side of the body (hemiclonic) or recurrent GTCS in a previously normal infant. After a relatively quiescent period, seizures (including myoclonic, focal, and absence) may appear in the second year of life. Additional features include developmental abnormalities, ataxia, and extrapyramidal signs. Seizures induced by heat (either with fevers or exogenous) may be noted.

Genetic testing for mutations in the *SCN1A* gene is recommended because this eliminates the need for other extensive testing for an underlying diagnosis and allows the clinician to prognosticate. The EEG may be normal initially but later shows generalized spike-and-wave complexes and may show focal abnormalities. Treatment typically is with antiseizure medications; drugs that block sodium channels are typically avoided because they may exacerbate seizures. The ketogenic diet may be useful. Heated environments might need to be avoided and accommodations (e.g., air-conditioned buses and classrooms) may be recommended in some cases.

Lennox–Gastaut Syndrome

Typically occurring between the ages of 1 and 8 years, Lennox–Gastaut syndrome is characterized by mixed seizure types, a markedly abnormal EEG, and abnormal development. Virtually any type of brain pathology can be seen as an antecedent of Lennox–Gastaut syndrome. Infantile epileptic spasms syndrome is a common antecedent. Patients with Lennox–Gastaut syndrome typically have combinations of tonic, atonic, and absence seizures, although focal-onset seizures and GTCS also occur. The EEG shows slow (less than 2.5 Hz) spike-and-wave complexes and a paroxysmal fast pattern, although background slowing also is very common. The vast majority of patients have developmental delays. Diagnosis is made in the setting of typical findings. Seizures are very difficult to control, but treatment commonly includes medicines and/or nonpharmacologic options (see Box 1). The prognosis for seizure control and development is poor. The differential diagnosis of Lennox–Gastaut syndrome also includes epilepsy with myoclonic-atonic seizures, which is characterized by myoclonic and astatic seizures (although other seizure types can occur). In epilepsy with myoclonic-atonic seizures, patients often have normal development and a good prognosis once seizures are controlled.

Childhood and Juvenile Absence Epilepsy

Most clinicians are familiar with childhood and juvenile absence epilepsy. The typical age of onset is 4 to 13 years, and there is a slight female predominance. The most common type of seizure is an absence seizure, characterized by staring and loss of interaction lasting 3 to 20 seconds, occurring tens to hundreds of times per day. Patients also can have GTCS (particularly if they present later in childhood) and/or myoclonic seizures. There is no aura and there are no postictal behavior changes. Absence seizures can be induced with 3 to 4 minutes of hyperventilation at the bedside. The interictal EEG shows a 3Hz generalized spike-and-wave pattern. Treatment includes ethosuximide (Zarontin) if the patient has not had a GTCS (see Box 1). Valproate (Depakene) is the

---

BOX 1   Recommendations for Treatment

Infantile Epileptic Spasms Syndrome
Oral steroids[1]
Adrenocorticotropic hormone
Ketogenic diet
Topiramate (Topamax)[1]
Valproate (Depakote)[1]
Zonisamide (Zonegran)[1]
Pyridoxine[1]
Benzodiazepines[1]
Surgery (if there is a lesion)
Vigabatrin (Sabril) (may use first if patient has tuberous sclerosis)

Dravet Syndrome
Valproate[1]
Topiramate[1]
Stiripentol (Diacomit)
Cannabidiol (Epidiolex)
Fenfluramine (Fintepla)
Ketogenic diet
Benzodiazepines[1]

Lennox–Gastaut Syndrome
Valproate[1]
Clobazam (Onfi)
Lamotrigine (Lamictal)
Topiramate
Benzodiazepines
Rufinamide (Banzel)
Felbamate (Felbatol)
Ketogenic diet
Vagus nerve stimulator
Surgery

Epilepsy With Myoclonic-Atonic Seizures
Valproate[1]
Clobazam
Ketogenic diet
Clonazepam (Klonopin)[1]
Levetiracetam (Keppra)
Ethosuximide (Zarontin)[1]
Vagus nerve stimulator
Corpus callosotomy

Childhood Absence Epilepsy
Ethosuximide
Valproate
Lamotrigine[1]

Juvenile Absence Epilepsy
Valproate
Ethosuximide
Lamotrigine[1]

Self-Limited Epilepsy With Centrotemporal Spikes
Levetiracetam (Keppra)
Carbamazepine (Tegretol)
Zonisamide
Oxcarbazepine (Trileptal)
Lacosamide (Vimpat)

Juvenile Myoclonic Epilepsy
Valproate[1]
Levetiracetam
Topiramate
Zonisamide[1]
Lamotrigine

---

[1] Not FDA approved for this indication.
Adapted from Muthugovindan D, Hartman AL: Pediatric epilepsy syndromes. *Neurologist* 2010;16:223–237.

first choice if the patient has had a GTCS. Nearly two-thirds of patients grow out of their seizures by young adulthood.

Self-Limited Epilepsy With Centrotemporal Spikes, Self-Limited Epilepsy With Autonomic Seizures, and Childhood Occipital Visual Epilepsy

One of the more common epilepsies in childhood, self-limited epilepsy with centrotemporal spikes (also known commonly as benign rolandic epilepsy), first occurs between the ages of 3 and 14 years. The typical seizure involves the face and/or hand, but GTCS also are common. The most common time for a seizure is within the first few hours of sleep, but a minority of patients only have daytime seizures. The diagnosis is made based on a typical seizure history and EEG (which shows spikes over bilateral central and temporal regions). Learning disabilities, which may be very subtle, are fairly common in patients with this syndrome, so extra vigilance is warranted.

Self-limited epilepsy with autonomic seizures (also known as Panayiotopoulos syndrome or "benign" occipital epilepsy) can occur between the ages of 1 and 14 years (with a peak at 3 to 6 years) with autonomic symptoms such as emesis, pallor, flushing, or tachycardia, as well as focal-onset or generalized seizures. Patients also can have visual symptoms. The EEG can show sharp waves in the occipital regions, but abnormal activity has been reported in other brain regions as well.

Because most patients have fewer than six seizures in both syndromes, medicine usually is not prescribed. Seizures typically are outgrown by adolescence. Patients with frequent seizures are treated with medicine. Childhood occipital visual epilepsy occurs in older children and can require medication treatment because of seizure recurrence.

Juvenile Myoclonic Epilepsy

The most common form of generalized seizures in adolescents, juvenile myoclonic epilepsy first occurs between the ages of 10 and 24 years. Most patients have brief myoclonic seizures that tend to cluster in the early morning hours (but may occur at any time of day). Patients often are unaware that these are seizures but on careful questioning report loss of control of a toothbrush or spoon. Many patients also have absence seizures. The interictal EEG typically shows a 4 to 5Hz generalized spike-and-wave pattern. The prognosis for lifelong remission of seizures is poor, although most patients' seizures are controlled easily with medicines (see Box 1). There is a subgroup of patients (many of whom previously had childhood absence epilepsy) whose seizures are very challenging to control.

Other Epilepsy Syndromes With a Poor Prognosis

Developmental epileptic encephalopathy with spike-and-wave activation in sleep and epileptic encephalopathy with spike-and-wave activation in sleep are syndromes characterized by mild seizures, nearly continuous epileptiform activity during sleep, and neuropsychological deterioration. Progressive myoclonus epilepsy represents a family of disorders characterized by medically intractable epilepsy (commonly including myoclonic seizures) and significant neurologic deterioration. Underlying diagnoses include myoclonus epilepsy with ragged red fibers (MERRF), Unverricht–Lundborg disease, and Lafora disease, among others. Gelastic (laughing) seizures can be caused either by hypothalamic hamartomas or temporal lobe seizures. The prognosis depends on response to medication and/or surgery but is not always bad. Rasmussen syndrome is characterized by medically intractable epilepsy, progressive unilateral neurologic deficits, and cortical atrophy on MRI. Because they are so rare, any suspicion of these diagnoses should prompt referral to a pediatric epilepsy center with expertise in diagnosing and managing these conditions.

Tumors

Brain tumors can manifest with seizures and are covered in a separate chapter. Certain developmental tumors are seen with an increased frequency in pediatric epilepsy clinics, including dysembryoplastic neuroepithelial tumors (DNET) and gangliogliomas.

These tumors typically manifest with seizures and can be associated with malformations of cortical development. EEG can show abnormalities over the involved region but can be falsely localizing as well. MRI shows the location of the tumor but can underestimate the extent of surrounding abnormal tissue. If seizures are not controlled with medicine, or if there is progression in tumor size, resection surgery is recommended.

Cortical Dysgenesis

Abnormal brain development can lead to inappropriately wired brain circuitry, which can be the underlying substrate for seizures. Two forms of abnormal cortical development include lissencephaly (abnormally smooth, or simplified, gyral pattern) and polymicrogyria. Another form of cortical dysgenesis, malformations of cortical development, is graded based on both dyslamination of the normal six-layer neocortex and the occurrence of abnormal cell types (including balloon cells). EEG shows epileptiform abnormalities over the involved region. MRI shows the anatomic location of the involved tissue in more severe cases but may be normal if the abnormality is mild. In patients with focal abnormalities, if seizures are not controlled with medicine, resection surgery is an option. Patients with more extensive abnormalities can try nonpharmacologic options if medicines do not work.

Mesial Temporal Lobe Epilepsy With Hippocampal Sclerosis

The mesial temporal structures (particularly the hippocampus) can become scarred, and the remaining neurons develop abnormal connections. This can lead to medically intractable seizures. EEG shows interictal epileptiform activity over the temporal head regions. Imaging studies show atrophic mesial temporal structures with increased signal on T2-weighted FLAIR (fluid-attenuated inversion recovery) images. A temporal lobectomy should be considered as an option for patients who do not respond to two appropriately chosen and tolerated medications for seizure control.

Coexisting Conditions

The definition of epilepsy includes coexisting conditions, which in turn can have a significant impact on quality of life. Clinicians must actively probe for these underlying conditions in order to optimize outcomes. People with epilepsy have increased rates of depression and anxiety compared to the general population. Developmental disorders and learning disabilities are more common in children with epilepsy, as are attention-deficit/hyperactivity disorder, sleep disorders, and migraines. Once identified, these conditions should be managed by clinicians experienced with their treatment.

Differential Diagnosis

The differential diagnosis of seizures depends largely on age. In infants, opisthotonic posturing can be seen in gastroesophageal reflux disease (Sandifer syndrome). Some infants have benign myoclonus or shuddering attacks. The EEG in all these disorders is normal, but the diagnosis can be made based on the history. Brief resolved unexplained events can appear to be seizures, although apnea rarely is the only manifestation of a seizure. Hyperekplexia is an exaggerated startle response that can be due to abnormal glycine receptor subunits in the spinal cord. Because of potential involvement of the diaphragm, this disorder can be lethal. In children, stereotypies can be paroxysmal and persistent, but the behaviors during these episodes are typical enough that the diagnosis usually is made based on the history.

Breath-holding spells may be associated with an older infant or toddler who is upset, followed by unresponsiveness and either facial pallor or mild cyanosis, lasting less than 1 to 3 minutes. These episodes are typical enough that the history is all that is usually needed to make the diagnosis. Children with pallid breath-holding spells are at higher risk for vasovagal syncope in the adolescent and young adult ages.

TABLE 1 Summary of New Commonly Used Antiseizure Drugs

DRUG	MAINTENANCE DOSAGE*	STARTING DOSAGE*	HALF-LIFE (H)	COMMON SIDE EFFECTS	SERIOUS IDIOSYNCRATIC SIDE EFFECTS
Brivaracetam (Briviact)	> 16y, 25–100mg bid	50mg bid	9	Agitation, behavioral disinhibition, dizziness	Suicidality
Cannabidiol (Epidiolex)	5mg/kg bid (can go up to 10mg/kg bid)	2.5mg/kg bid	56–61	Somnolence, decreased appetite, diarrhea, transaminase elevations (check before initiating therapy), fatigue, rash, sleep disorders, infections	Severe encephalopathy leading to respiratory depression and oversedation, hepatic injury, suicidality
Cenobamate (Xcopri; adults only)	200mg once/day	12.5mg once daily, titrate per manfacturer	50–60	Somnolence, dizziness, aphasia, dysarthria, vertigo, diplopia, vomiting, constipation, diarrhea, transaminase elevations	Hyperkalemia, appendicitis, QTc shortening, DRESS, suicidality
Fenfluramine (Fintepla)	Maintenance >2y, w/o stiripentol: 0.1-0.35 mg/kg/dose bid; >2 y, w/ stiripentol and clobazam, 0.1-0.2 mg/kg/dose bid;	Starting 0.1 mg/kg/dose bid	20	Anorexia, diarrhea, fatigue, echocardiographic abnormalities, weight loss, blood pressure change, behavior changes, tremor, irritability, gastroenteritis, URI, rash	serotonin syndrome, suicidality, hypertension, angle-closure glaucoma
Clobazam (Onfi)	> 2y, < 30kg: 10mg bid > 2y, > 30kg: 20mg bid	> 2y, < 30kg: 5mg/d > 2y, > 30kg: 5mg bid	Parent drug: 36–42 Active metabolite: 71–82	Sedation irritability Needs to be tapered off slowly	Respiratory depression, benzodiazepine withdrawal, Stevens–Johnson syndrome
Eslicarbazepine (Aptiom)	4-17y (11-21kg), 400-600mg once/day 4-17y (22-31kg), 500-800mg once/day 4-17y (32-38kg), 600-900mg once/day 4-17y (>38kg), 800-1200mg once/day >17y, 800-1600mg once/day	4-17y (11-21kg), 200mg once/day 4-17y (22-31kg), 300mg once/day 4-17y (32-38kg), 300mg once/day >4y (>38kg), 400mg once/day	13–20	Somnolence, dizziness, hyponatremia, thyroid dysfunction	Stevens-Johnson, toxic epidermal necrolysis, withdrawal seizures if stopped abruptly
Lacosamide (Vimpat)	4-16y (11-<30kg), 3-6mg/kg bid 4-16y (30-50kg), 2-4mg/kg bid >4y (>50kg), 100–200mg bid	4-16y (<50kg), 1mg/kg bid >4y (≥50kg), 50mg bid	13	Somnolence, fatigue, headache	Cardiac conduction abnormalities, Stevens-Johnson syndrome, cytopenias
Levetiracetam (Keppra)	20–60mg/kg/d	10mg/kg/d, incr in 10-mg/kg increments	6–8	Agitation, behavioral disinhibition, rashes	Suicidal ideation
Oxcarbazepine (Trileptal)	30–60mg/kg/d	8–10mg/kg/d, incr by 10–15mg/kg increments	Parent drug: 2 Metabolite: 9	Hyponatremia, somnolence, lethargy, dizziness, blurred vision	Rash
Perampanel (Fycompa)	> 12y, 8–12mg at bedtime	> 12y, 2–4mg at bedtime	105h	Somnolence, headaches	Serious psychiatric and behavior reactions
Rufinamide (Banzel)	45mg/kg/d	10mg/kg/d	6–10	Nausea, vomiting, somnolence	Seizures, QT shortening
Stiripentol (Diacomit; to be used as a clobazam adjunct)	Up to 3g/day	25mg/kg bid	4.5–13	Somnolence, decreased appetite, agitation, ataxia, tremor, cytopenias, vomiting, weight gain	Suicidality, cytopenias, withdrawal seizures
Vigabatrin (Sabril)	50–150mg/kg/d	50mg/kg/d	7.5 (5.7 in infants)	Headache, dizziness, fatigue, tremor, swallowing problems, T2-weighted or DWI hyperintensities	Vision loss
Zonisamide (Zonegran)	> 16y: 100–600mg/d	> 16y: 100mg once/day	63	Somnolence, irritability, cognitive slowing, weight loss, renal stones, oligohidrosis	Rash

Abbreviations: DWI = diffusion-weighted imaging; incr = increase.
*Dosages should not exceed maximum adult dosages.

Night terrors, one of the parasomnias, occur in toddlers and young children. Persistent screaming (lasting minutes to 1 hour) and lack of memory of the event are seen commonly; the latter raises a question of whether the child had a seizure. Most commonly, these are outgrown by the late preschool years.

Patients with syncope may have a few mild clonic twitches, but this typically does not represent epilepsy. Screening orthostatic blood pressures should be done to rule out one of the orthostatic syndromes. Consideration also should be given to an electrocardiogram or a cardiology consultation in the appropriate clinical context.

Older children and adolescents can have psychogenic nonepileptic events, also known as psychogenic nonepileptic seizures. Cognitive behavioral therapy is helpful in some patients. This is a very important diagnosis to make so that patients receive appropriate treatment and are not exposed to medicines where the risks outweigh the benefits.

In all age groups, focal lesions such as infarctions, hemorrhages, and infections should be considered in the differential diagnosis, although the diagnostic workup should be guided by the history and physical examination.

Treatment

The goals for treatment are to maximize efficacy and minimize side effects. Medication is the first line of therapy for most patients. Nearly 70% to 80% of children are treated successfully by one of the first two medications tried. Practically speaking, neurologists try to use a single agent at the lowest tolerated dosage. Suggested medicines for the epilepsy syndromes discussed previously are listed in Box 1. Details about specific medicines are listed in Table 1. If one of the first two medicines tried does not work, there are three major options.

1. Trials of Additional Medication

Although the first two medicines might not work, new medicines often are introduced into the market. Clinical trials often show that a modest number of patients respond well to newer medicines, although the positive response to newer medicines is no greater overall than response to older medicines, despite lower rates of adverse effects and drug–drug interactions.

2. Surgery

Anyone who fails to respond to two appropriately-selected medications should be assessed for surgery. In patients with a potentially resectable lesion, surgery offers the greatest chance of seizure freedom. Ideal surgical candidates have identifiable lesions on imaging studies and a seizure onset zone that is distinct from eloquent cortex. People with multifocal or generalized seizures are poor candidates for resection surgery. Options for these patients include the vagus nerve stimulator, which has outstanding adherence because it is surgically implanted. Although this device significantly decreases seizure frequency in some patients, it only rarely leads to seizure freedom. Neurostimulation devices, some of which also include seizure detectors, are being introduced into clinical practice for adults and are being investigated in children.

3. Diet Therapy

The concept of fasting to improve seizure control dates back to Hippocrates, but in modern times, dietary management of epilepsy is implemented using a high-fat, low-carbohydrate (adequate protein) ketogenic diet. A modified Atkins diet and a low glycemic index treatment have been used successfully as well. These diets require varying degrees of clinical supervision at centers experienced in their implementation.

Monitoring

Seizure calendars (which can take the form of notebooks or electronic tools) are very useful for tracking frequency of events, especially if they are completed on a daily basis. There has been a recent explosion in wearable devices and other types of biotechnology for monitoring seizures and vital signs during seizures (for home use). Monitoring for medication-related adverse effects and coexisting conditions should continue during treatment. In addition, some coexisting conditions can occur even if seizures have stopped; there is good evidence for this in patients with childhood absence epilepsy, which typically is considered a "benign" syndrome because seizures typically resolve by adulthood. Patients taking certain medicines are screened periodically for evidence of renal and/or hepatic abnormalities and abnormal blood cell counts. Scenarios for testing drug levels include the following:

- Assessing adherence to a prescribed drug regimen
- Testing whether symptoms result from drug toxicity
- Determining whether a patient can benefit from higher amounts of medicine when the administered doses are already high (i.e., fast metabolizers)

Reminders about seizure-related safety should be reinforced periodically. GTCS counseling typically includes instructions about safety for the patient, including protecting the head and airway (putting the patient on his or her side to prevent aspiration) and not putting anything in the patient's mouth. Other safety topics include water safety and wearing helmets, as well as discouraging participation in certain sports (e.g., scuba diving). Periodic assessments of bone health should be considered for patients taking enzyme-inducing or enzyme-inhibiting medicines. Patients of an appropriate age should be counseled about local driving laws. People capable of bearing children should be counseled about the effect of antiseizure medicines on hormonal forms of contraception (and vice versa). Consideration should be given to prescribing folate in this group, as well.

Complications

Single GTCS can lead to trauma (e.g., from a fall), tongue biting, pneumothorax, fractures of the vertebrae or limbs, and joint dislocations. A brief physical examination can rule out the more serious complications of a single GTCS. Adverse effects of medications are listed in Table 1. Surgical resections can lead to a variety of neurologic deficits, depending on which tissue is involved. Vagus nerve stimulator surgery can lead to hoarseness and coughing. Unsupervised diet therapy also can have adverse effects; such therapy should be undertaken only by centers with experience. Rarely, patients with epilepsy can die unexpectedly from no apparent cause, known as sudden unexplained death in epilepsy (SUDEP). The cause is unknown, but most (not all) patients have epilepsy that is resistant to medications. Counseling about this condition should be provided by an epilepsy expert.

Notice

This material does not represent the official view of the National Institute of Neurological Disorders and Stroke (NINDS), the National Institutes of Health (NIH), or any part of the US Federal Government. No official support or endorsement of this article by the NINDS or NIH is intended or should be inferred.

References

Baldin E, Hauser WA, Buchhalter JR, et al: Yield of epileptiform electroencephalogram abnormalities in incident unprovoked seizures: a population-based study, *Epilepsia* 55:1389–1398, 2014.

Fisher RS, Acevedo C, Arzimanoglou A, et al: ILAE official report: a practical clinical definition of epilepsy, *Epilepsia* 55:475–482, 2014.

Grinspan ZM, Knupp KG, Patel AD, et al: Comparative effectiveness of initial treatment for infantile spasms in a contemporary US cohort, *Neurology* 97:e1217–28, 2021.

Rosati A, Ilvento L, Lucenteforte E, et al: Comparative efficacy of antiepileptic drugs in children and adolescents: A network meta-analysis, *Epilepsia* 59:297–314, 2018.

Subcommittee on Febrile Seizures: American Academy of Pediatrics: Neurodiagnostic evaluation of the child with a simple febrile seizure, *Pediatrics* 127:389–394, 2011.

Wirrell EC, Nabbout R, Scheffer IE, et al: Methodology for classification and definition of epilepsy syndromes with list of syndromes: Report of the ILAE Task Force on Nosology and Definitions, *Epilepsia* 63:1333–1348, 2022.

INFANT AND CHILDREN FEEDING PROBLEMS

Method of
Sarah Edwards, DO; and Dana M. Bakula, PhD

CURRENT DIAGNOSIS

- As of 2021, the primary diagnostic code used to describe feeding problems in infants and children is *pediatric feeding disorder (PFD)*.
- PFD is defined as impairments in oral intake that are not age appropriate.
- PFD is caused by medical, nutritional, psychosocial, and/or feeding skill problems.
- As a result of both the broad criteria and the complex multifactorial nature of the condition, the presentation of PFD can vary significantly from child to child, as can treatments.

CURRENT THERAPY

- A thorough assessment of medical, nutritional, psychosocial, and feeding skills issues is needed to optimize treatment planning.
- It is imperative to treat underlying medical conditions that may be contributing to pediatric feeding disorder.
- Nutritional monitoring is necessary to ensure patient safety and guide clinical decision-making.
- If adequate nutrition cannot be achieved orally, enteral nutrition should be considered.
- Feeding therapy is often necessary to treat feeding skill issues that prevent safe or efficient oral feeding.
- Behavioral treatment is often needed to treat parent and/or child factors that prevent oral feeding.

Pathophysiology

As of 2021, pediatric feeding disorder (PFD) is the primary diagnosis used to describe feeding problems of infants and children. PFD is often multifactorial, including medical, nutritional, psychosocial, and skill-based issues, and typically involves concerns in one or more of these domains. The progression of feeding from breastmilk or formula at birth to table foods is a typical pattern of development that occurs without issue for many children. However, when this typical pattern of development is interrupted, PFD can develop.

Medical etiologies: Cow's milk protein allergy, gastroesophageal reflux disease, and eosinophilic esophagitis are the most common gastrointestinal (GI) etiologies of PFD. They can lead to discomfort with feeding that can contribute to the development of a feeding aversion. Although less common, physiologic processes that increase metabolic demand can lead to PFD, as they make it difficult for the infant or child to keep up with their caloric needs. This is most common in children with congenital heart disease. Medical conditions, such as cardiorespiratory compromise during oral feeding and aspiration and recurrent aspiration pneumonitis, may be causes of feeding problems. Underlying syndromes, neuromuscular disabilities, and genetic differences can interrupt the typical progression of feeding, contributing to feeding intolerance, poor oral intake, or oral aversion. Premature infants who spent time in the neonatal intensive care unit have an increased incidence of feeding difficulties that can be, in part, due to delay of development and multiple painful procedures around their mouth and face that can contribute to oral aversion.

Nutritional etiologies: A nutritional deficit may result from inadequate caloric intake, increased metabolic demand, or excessive GI losses. Inadequate caloric intake can be caused by a decreased hunger drive, often from a grazing pattern of eating, which effectively alleviates the child's sensation of hunger. Therefore the child does not eat an adequately sized meal. Increased metabolic demand results from a medical condition that causes the patient to be unable to gain weight even with usually adequate caloric intake as their nutritional needs are greater than typical for age. This can include such etiologies as congenital heart disease, cystic fibrosis, metabolic disorders, or neuromuscular disorders. Excessive GI losses may occur with vomiting or diarrhea, where calories that are taken in are not effectively used. Malnutrition and nutrient deficiencies may result from a lack of dietary diversity.

Psychosocial etiologies: Infants and children can develop aversions to feeding for several reasons. Psychosocial etiologies may interact with medical or feeding skill concerns. For instance, a child may begin refusing all foods because of a cow's milk allergy as they fear that all foods may result in discomfort, or a child may refuse to drink any liquid because they typically choke on thin liquids. Environmental factors, such as distractions present at meals (e.g., iPad) or a lack of mealtime structure can prevent a child from having sufficient time and opportunity to feed. Further, parents and caregivers for children with feeding challenges can feel anxious or stressed at meals. Parental stress or cultural expectations surrounding feeding may impact how parents interact with their child at meals. Some parents may engage in maladaptive strategies, attempting to get their child to eat more by force-feeding or yelling, which only worsens the problem. Underlying psychosocial conditions, such as autism, attention-deficit/hyperactivity disorder, and oppositional defiant disorder can result in behavioral challenges at mealtimes that prevent sufficient oral intake. Even among infants, these psychosocial factors can manifest. For instance, postpartum depression can impact how mothers interact with their infants during feeding.

Feeding skill etiologies: Oral motor skills are a common contributor to feeding problems. Oral motor problems can be secondary to an anatomic cause, such as a laryngeal cleft or underlying muscle weakness due to a neurologic disorder, or may be idiopathic. Oral motor difficulties may result from inefficient and ineffective chewing and swallowing mechanics. When a child struggles to eat effectively, this can result in the child struggling to eat age-appropriate foods or to consume a sufficient volume of food and to have unsafe swallows, which may lead to aspiration and risk of respiratory infections. Oral motor skill problems can also cause a child to eat less efficiently, resulting in fatigue and longer mealtimes, which may exacerbate child frustrations with mealtimes. In addition, the experiences of discomfort and fear that may come with a child struggling to effectively control the food or liquid in their mouth may result in oral aversion.

Prevention

The key to prevention is in identifying feeding concerns early and providing proactive education and treatment. One common pitfall is to assume that a child who is of normal weight does not have PFD; these are not mutually exclusive. Although a significant proportion of patients with PFD have malnutrition, this is not seen in every case and malnutrition is not typically the first symptom of feeding problems. For instance, well before weight loss is identified, the clinician might hear from a parent that they are having to feed their baby around the clock, that each feeding lasts well over 30 minutes, or that a parent is "having to force-feed" their child to make sure they eat enough. In older children the clinician may hear that parents are only giving the child a few preferred foods because the parent has learned that this is the only way the child will eat. These situations can lead to severe micronutrient deficiencies. For infants, key red flags the clinician should be attuned to listen for include infants who are primarily "dream-feeding" (feeding during sleep), falling asleep during all feedings, not waking to feed on their own, sweating with feedings, choking with feedings, and exhibiting fussiness with feedings. With older children, key red flags the clinician should be attuned to identify are the child being unwilling to eat foods the they were once eating, choking on food, fearing feeding, cutting foods into very small pieces, vomiting after every feed, or eating only a few foods until they burn out on that food and then move to another food (food jags). Early identification and evaluations are the key to prevention.

Clinical Manifestations

Patients can present with a wide spectrum of symptoms. Oral motor concerns can manifest as coughing or choking with feeds, feeling fatigued during feeds, or refusing to eat due to insufficient skills. It is important to understand the timing of when the feeding problems began. If the child ate well for the first 2 years of life but then started to lose interest in foods they were once readily taking without the development of any GI symptoms, this can incite concern for an autism spectrum disorder or sensory sensitivity.

Evaluation of weight and linear growth or height is important. Assessment for malnutrition on the age-appropriate growth chart (World Health Organization growth chart for 0 to 2 years of age and Centers for Disease Control and Prevention growth chart for patients older than 2 years) should be routine. Not all patients with PFD present with malnutrition. Some patients may eat a narrow range of foods, yet they eat enough calories that they gain appropriate weight, and it is not until further investigation that micronutrient deficiencies are identified. Additionally, poor linear growth that precedes difficulty with weight gain can indicate a metabolic etiology for malnutrition.

A thorough history, physical examination, and observation of a feeding are key parts of the evaluation. A history of prematurity or chronic medical conditions can increase the risk of PFD. Attention should be given to the respiratory history and any report of recurrent lower respiratory tract infections or chronic congestion. Timing, volume, and length of feeds, as well as how formula is mixed, are key questions for understanding the total amount of calories a patient is ingesting. Children who demonstrate a grazing pattern of eating typically have less hunger drive and subsequently less oral intake than those patients who eat three meals and two snacks with no food in between. Children taking a long time to feed may be fatigued during the feed or averse to feeding. Questions about a history of vomiting, concerns for pain with feeding and stooling pattern can help identify feeding intolerances. The physical exam should include an oral exam to evaluate for dental caries, palatal abnormalities, or oral lesions; a lung exam to evaluate for aspiration pneumonia or respiratory findings; an abdominal exam to listen for bowel sounds and palpate for masses, distension, or any areas of tenderness; and an evaluation of muscle strength for any signs of hypotonia or hypertonia.

Diagnosis

PFD is the primary diagnostic code used for infants and children with feeding problems. PFD involves impairments in oral intake that are not age appropriate. PFD is a multifactorial condition and is associated with medical, nutritional, psychosocial, and/or feeding skills. As a result of both the broad criteria and the complex multifactorial nature of the condition, the presentation of PFD can vary significantly from child to child, as can the necessary treatments. You may also find it helpful to have families answer the Infant and Child Feeding Questionnaire (a six-question screener), which is freely available and distributed by Feeding Matters, an advocacy organization for children with PFD (https://www.feedingmatters.org/what-is-pfd/is-it-pfd/).

Treatment

Treatment depends on the cause and severity of the feeding impairment. For children who are otherwise healthy but are having difficulty gaining weight, starting with a mealtime structure including three meals with two to three snacks is key. Meals and snacks should be separated by 2 to 3 hours, without any grazing in between. Children may have water between meals, but no other foods or caloric beverages because grazing can lead to an overall decrease in oral intake. The clinician should also seek to increase the caloric density of the child's foods. For infants, this typically means concentrating their feeds from 20 calories an ounce to 22 to 24 calories an ounce. In a child who drinks cow's milk, add 1 tablespoon of heavy whipping cream to 4 ounces of whole milk or add in an oral nutrition supplement. Parents can also add oils or other foods that are high in fats to a child's meal to help supplement their caloric intake. Consultation with a dietitian will help determine optimal next steps for supporting a child's weight gain and growth. Dieticians are specially trained to evaluate a child's current diet and how that diet compares to one that would best meet the child's health needs and to make tailored recommendations to the family.

For patients with symptoms concerning for aspiration or oral motor difficulties, a feeding and swallowing evaluation should be considered. A videofluoroscopic swallow study may be indicated. The child may benefit from consultation with a feeding therapist to improve their feeding skills and may need eating modifications to allow them to eat safely. For instance, a swallow study may identify that the patient is aspirating thin liquids. If this is the case, the feeding therapist may recommend a thickener be added to the child's thin liquids. There may also be special feeding utensils or equipment, feeding position modification, or other strategies recommended to help the child eat safely while the therapist works with the child on progressing their oral motor skills.

Medical interventions should be employed to target any underlying conditions that are impacting the child's feeding problems. This can include upper endoscopy to evaluate for eosinophilic esophagitis, upper GI x-ray to evaluate for anatomic abnormalities such as esophageal stricture, tracheoesophageal fistula or pH study to evaluate for gastroesophageal reflux. Special consideration should be taken to use the North American Society for Gastroenterology, Hepatology and Nutrition guidelines on treatment of gastroesophageal reflux. For example, a formula change may help a child with milk protein allergy before performing a trial of acid suppression. It is also essential to treat constipation for children with PFD as poor feeding puts the child at higher risk for constipation, and constipation may increase abdominal discomfort and/or decrease appetite and therefore increase aversion to feeding. Cyproheptadine[1] can be used for appetite stimulation, but we would caution its use in patients with aversion who may have an undiagnosed underlying, painful condition.

Behavioral interventions may be needed to support children with feeding issues, as psychosocial factors play a significant role in the development of PFD. The paramount recommendation is that mealtimes are positive and that parents do not engage in any force-feeding. When children feel pressured to eat, they can feel stressed and eat even less, or act out during the meal. Parents should be encouraged to make mealtimes pleasant and avoid pressuring or forcing their child to eat. Families can be taught to use the feeding "division of responsibility," which is the concept that parents decide what goes on the child's plate at a meal, when the meal starts and ends, and where the child is during the meal, but the child ultimately decides what they eat or do not eat during the meal. Parents should be encouraged to limit distractions present at mealtimes, such as the television or other screens. Families should be encouraged to have a consistent and predictable schedule of meals and snacks, with clear expectations for how long children must stay seated for meals and snacks. When children do not have a predictable and consistent structure at meals, they are much less likely to engage in the meal and notice their internal hunger cues. Finally, parents should be encouraged to offer the child a variety of foods on their plate, including at least one or two items that are foods the child prefers or enjoys. Sometimes families can be tempted to help a child expand the variety of foods they eat by offering a plate full of new foods at a meal. This can lead to more behavioral challenges, so it is important that children have "preferred foods" on their plate in addition to

---

[1] Not FDA approved for this indication.

options that are new or "nonpreferred." Children with significant behavioral concerns at meals, underlying behavioral problems, developmental disabilities, or significant anxiety around feeding may benefit from consultation with a psychologist or other behavioral specialist, such as an applied behavioral analysis specialist. If a psychologist or behavioral specialist is not readily accessible in the clinician's setting, consider consulting a social worker who may help the family identify behavioral treatment options.

In sum, a multidisciplinary approach is paramount to the success of treatment of children with complex or severe PFD. This may include involvement of a medical professional, feeding therapist (occupational therapist or speech pathologist), psychologist, dietitian, and nurse. It is optimal for these specialists to work together as a team, but, when the development of a team is not possible, we recommend developing strong channels of communication between the various healthcare professionals involved to support the treatment of a child's PFD. Further, the treatment approach should always be tailored to the needs of the child and guided by a clear understanding of the etiology of the feeding issues.

Monitoring

Children with feeding issues should be monitored for ongoing medical, developmental, and behavioral concerns. Micronutrient deficiencies should be evaluated regularly. This includes analyzing the child's dietary intake through patient interviews and checking labs, such as complete blood count and ferritin and vitamin D levels. The clinician may consider running labs that are specific to the child's diet, such as checking a B_{12} level if the child is not consuming much meat, fish, or dairy. The child's weight should be checked at regular intervals, with special attention to the trends of their weight and where they fall on the growth curve, to ensure they are gaining weight adequately for their age. For infants who were born prematurely, age-corrected growth charts should be used. Changes to a child's diet, such as a child no longer being willing to eat a food they used to enjoy, should be monitored regularly This is particularly concerning when children eat very few foods and/or begin "dropping" multiple preferred foods.

The clinician should monitor any changes to the child's GI tolerance, paying special attention to any vomiting, changes in stooling pattern, abdominal pain, or discomfort. These symptoms may indicate a concern about an underlying medical condition that may warrant treatment so that the child does not begin to associate eating with painful or uncomfortable experiences. The child's feeding skills should be monitored over time, with special attention to whether the child has an age-appropriate progression of feeding skills. Difficulties meeting age-appropriate benchmarks may warrant treatment and intervention from a feeding therapist.

Behavioral concerns at meals should be monitored regularly. The clinician should ask if the child is coming to meals willingly most of the time, is able to stay seated or stay at the table for the full meal, and is willing to engage during mealtime. The caregiver should not engage in any force-feeding (i.e., putting food into the child's mouth against their will). This can have adverse iatrogenic side effects.

Enteral Feeding

For children who are receiving enteral nutrition, there should be continuous monitoring of their need for tube feeding. Enteral nutrition may be necessary for only a few months for some children or a lifetime for others. Enteral nutrition can be taxing on a child and family's quality of life, so signs of tube-weaning readiness should be regularly monitored. Signs of tube-weaning readiness include improvement in oral motor skills, treatment of the underlying etiology, and improvement in oral aversion. Next steps include a decrease of enteral nutrition to promote improvement in hunger. It is important that these patients are in weekly feeding therapy as studies show that multidisciplinary tube-weaning interventions are most effective.

Complications

Children with feeding problems may begin to lose weight or have insufficient weight gain for their age. This may result in the need for hospitalization or use of enteral nutrition. In general, the least invasive methods for addressing feeding problems should be attempted first (e.g., feeding therapy, behavioral changes, treatment of underlying medical conditions), but hospitalization and enteral nutrition may be required when a child is experiencing significant difficulties with feeding and it is not possible for them to sustain adequate nutrition by mouth. Dehydration may also be a concern when children struggle with feeding, and every attempt should be made to encourage oral intake with feeding therapy and behavior modification. In situations where this is not possible, hospitalization and/or enteral nutrition are sometimes needed, especially when children with feeding issues experience acute illness, causing their oral intake to worsen from their baseline. Micronutrient deficiencies may occur in children who eat a limited variety of foods; thus it is critical to monitor for these complications in addition to monitoring the child's weight. Finally, behavioral escalations and general behavioral challenges may emerge as a result of pediatric feeding issues. Children who struggle with feeding may find mealtime to be a difficult and stressful experience. Parents of these children are also experiencing notable stress, and this can result in additional behavioral challenges, especially at meals. Encouraging parents to follow behavioral mealtime strategies and consult with a behavioral specialist if concerns persist will be helpful in managing this complication.

References

Berlin KS, Davies WH, Lobato DJ, Silverman AH: A biopsychosocial model of normative and problematic pediatric feeding, *Child Health Care* 38(4):263–282, 2009.

Chen TL, Chen YY, Lin CL, Peng FS, Chien LY: Responsive feeding, infant growth, and postpartum depressive symptoms during 3 months postpartum, *Nutrients* 12(6):1766, 2020.

Davies W, Satter E, Berlin KS, et al: Reconceptualizing feeding and feeding disorders in interpersonal context: the case for a relational disorder, *J Fam Psychol* 20(3):409, 2006.

Edwards ST, Glynn EF, Slogic M, et al: Demographics of children with feeding difficulties from a large electronic health record database, *J Parenter Enteral Nutr* 46:1022–1030, 2022, https://doi.org/10.1002/jpen.2379.

Feeding Matters. Feeding Matters.org. Is it Pediatric Feeding Disorder (PFD)? Accessed February 14, 2023. https://www.feedingmatters.org/what-is-pfd/is-it-pfd/. Accessed May 29, 2023.

Goday PS, Huh SY, Silverman A, et al: Pediatric feeding disorder: consensus definition and conceptual framework, *J Pediatr Gastroenterol Nutr* 68(1):124–129, 2019, https://doi.org/10.1097/MPG.0000000000002188.

Kovacic K, Rein LE, Szabo A, Kommareddy S, Bhagavatula P, Goday PS: Pediatric feeding disorder: a nationwide prevalence study, *J Pediatr* 228:126–131.e3,ISSN 0022–3476, 2021, https://doi.org/10.1016/j.jpeds.2020.07.047.

Killian, H. J., Bakula, D. M., Wallisch, A., et al. (in press). Pediatric tube weaning: a meta-analysis of factors contributing to success. *J Clin Psychol Med Settings*.

Milano K, Chatoor I, Kerzner B: A functional approach to feeding difficulties in children, *Curr Gastroenterol Rep* 21:51, 2019, https://doi.org/10.1007/s11894-019-0719-0.

INFANT HYPERBILIRUBINEMIA

Method of
Sheevaun Khaki, MD

CURRENT DIAGNOSIS

- As bilirubin levels rise during the newborn period, jaundice appears and progresses caudally from head to toe.
- Hyperbilirubinemia is classified as conjugated or unconjugated; conjugated hyperbilirubinemia is always considered pathologic.
- Universal screening for hyperbilirubinemia with a total serum bilirubin (TSB) or transcutaneous bilirubin (TcB) should be performed for all newborns within the first 24 hours of life.

TABLE 1	Risk Factors for Developing Significant Hyperbilirubinemia

- Lower gestational age (ie, risk increases with each additional week less than 40 wk)
- Jaundice in the first 24 h after birth
- Predischarge transcutaneous bilirubin (TcB) or total serum bilirubin (TSB) concentration close to the phototherapy threshold
- Hemolysis from any cause, if known or suspected, based on a rapid rate of increase in the TSB or TcB of >0.3 mg/dL per hour in the first 24 h or >0.2 mg/dL per hour thereafter.
- Phototherapy before discharge
- Parent or sibling requiring phototherapy or exchange transfusion
- Family history or genetic ancestry suggestive of inherited red blood cell disorders, including glucose-6-phosphate dehydrogenase (G6PD) deficiency
- Exclusive breastfeeding with suboptimal intake
- Scalp hematoma or significant bruising
- Down syndrome
- Macrosomic infant of a diabetic mother

TcB, Transcutaneous bilirubin; *TSB*, total serum bilirubin.
From Kemper AR, Newman TB, Slaughter JL, et al.: Clinical practice guideline revision: management of hyperbilirubinemia in the newborn infant 35 or more weeks of gestation, *Pediatrics* 150(3):e2022058859, 2022. Copyright © the American Academy of Pediatrics.

Background

Neonatal hyperbilirubinemia is common during the newborn period, with approximately 50% of term newborns developing jaundice in the first week of age. As bilirubin levels increase, clinical signs of jaundice develop due to deposition of bilirubin in the skin and mucous membranes. For the majority of newborns, this is a transient condition that does not require medical intervention. However, a small portion of late preterm and term newborns will develop hyperbilirubinemia that may require close monitoring and/or medical intervention. The goal of treating neonatal hyperbilirubinemia is to prevent bilirubin-induced neurologic dysfunction, acute bilirubin encephalopathy (ABE), and chronic bilirubin encephalopathy (CBE) or kernicterus. Various screening and monitoring strategies exist to prevent these serious outcomes.

Risk Factors

Prior to hospital discharge, all newborns should be systematically assessed for the risk of hyperbilirubinemia requiring intervention. The American Academy of Pediatrics (AAP) has developed a list of risk factors for the development of hyperbilirubinemia (Table 1). As part of this risk assessment, all birthing parents' blood types should be reviewed to determine whether the baby is at risk for hyperbilirubinemia due to ABO or Rhesus factor (Rh) incompatibility. The newborn's gestational age (GA) is particularly important as late preterm infants (GA 34w0d–36w6d) have additional feeding difficulties and relatively immature red blood cells (RBCs) and hepatic cells, which lead to both increased production and decreased clearance of bilirubin. A thorough family history may provide additional information regarding inheritable conditions, such as glucose-6-phosphate dehydrogenase (G6PD) deficiency, that lead to hemolysis and, therefore, hyperbilirubinemia.

Pathogenesis

An understanding of bilirubin metabolism is essential in determining the etiology of neonatal hyperbilirubinemia. Bilirubin results from the breakdown of heme, the majority of which comes from catabolism of hemoglobin from RBCs. There are multiple steps involved in the removal of bilirubin from the bloodstream. Initially, bilirubin is bound to albumin and transported to the liver where it is conjugated by uridine diphosphate glucuronosyltransferase (UGT1A1). Conjugated bilirubin is excreted into the biliary system and ultimately the gastrointestinal system. Finally, conjugated bilirubin is either deconjugated in the intestines by bacteria and reabsorbed back into the circulation or excreted as stool. A disturbance in any of the above steps of bilirubin clearance can lead to hyperbilirubinemia. Hyperbilirubinemia is classified into unconjugated (indirect) and conjugated (direct) forms.

Unconjugated Hyperbilirubinemia

Unconjugated hyperbilirubinemia results from either increased production or decreased clearance of indirect (unconjugated) bilirubin. Physiologic jaundice results from a combination of these processes. In this condition, bilirubin levels rise from increased number and turnover of RBCs due to the shorter life span of fetal RBCs, decreased activity of UGT1A1 in the liver, and increased enterohepatic circulation due to poor feeding and relative gut sterility. Breastfeeding jaundice results from increased enterohepatic circulation and mild dehydration as breastfeeding is established. Additionally, there are many pathologic conditions that may result in unconjugated hyperbilirubinemia. Hemolytic diseases such as isoimmune-mediated hemolysis (ABO or Rh incompatibility), RBC membrane defects (hereditary spherocytosis), or RBC enzyme defects (G6PD deficiency) contribute to significant morbidity. Decreased clearance of bilirubin may result from a defect in UGT1A1 (Crigler-Najjar syndrome types I and II, Gilbert syndrome), increased enterohepatic circulation due to impaired intestinal motility and poor milk intake, and breast milk jaundice.

Conjugated Hyperbilirubinemia

Conjugated hyperbilirubinemia is always considered pathologic. It is defined as a direct bilirubin concentration that is ≥20% of the total serum bilirubin (TSB). Direct bilirubin should be measured when the TSB is not responding appropriately to phototherapy or when jaundice persists past 2 weeks of age. Broadly, cholestatic jaundice can be divided into obstructive and hepatocellular etiologies. Obstructive etiologies include biliary atresia and choledochal cysts. Hepatocellular etiologies include endocrinopathies (thyroid abnormalities), metabolic disorders (galactosemia, tyrosinemia), and infection (sepsis, congenital infections). For newborns with jaundice past 2 weeks of age, total and direct bilirubin levels should be obtained to rule out biliary atresia, a diagnosis that deserves prompt identification and treatment.

Prevention

While mild physiologic jaundice cannot be prevented in most instances, more severe cases of indirect hyperbilirubinemia can be avoided. Starting in the prenatal setting, all pregnant people should be tested for ABO and Rh blood types and red blood cell antibodies to identify birthing parents whose newborns may be at risk of developing isoimmune hemolytic disease. Pregnant people who are Rh-negative should receive Rho(D) immune globulin (RhoGAM) to prevent the development of antibodies after exposure to Rh-positive blood. Pregnant people should receive at least one dose between 26 and 28 weeks of pregnancy and another within 72 hours after delivery if the baby is found to be Rh-positive. All newborns born to Rh-negative birthing parents should have their blood type tested to allow for timely administration of RhoGAM. Additionally, pregnant people should receive RhoGAM after maternal or fetal bleeding during pregnancy, abdominal trauma, an invasive procedure, and with each pregnancy, including an ectopic pregnancy. If administered correctly, the risk of hemolytic disease of the fetus and newborn is significantly reduced. Pregnancies where the birthing parents have an O blood type are considered to be a "setup" for ABO incompatibility. Early identification of ABO incompatibility may prevent more severe cases of hyperbilirubinemia.

Postnatally, provision of adequate nutrition helps prevent readmission for phototherapy. During the newborn hospitalization, parents who intend to breastfeed should receive information and support to establish an adequate milk supply. Early and sustained skin-to-skin contact should be emphasized to promote lactogenesis and dyads should be assessed for risks of delayed lactogenesis. Serial newborn weights should be obtained to document weight loss as an early sign of inadequate intake. The newborn early weight loss tool, NEWT, (https://www.newbornweight.org) may be used to identify newborns 36 weeks of gestation and greater who have lost an excessive amount of weight and incorporated into the decision to initiate supplemental feeds. Prevention of dehydration in the early newborn period may help prevent clinically significant hyperbilirubinemia.

Diagnosis

During the newborn hospitalization, the newborn should be assessed clinically for visible jaundice with all routine vital sign checks, preferably next to a well-lit window. The newborn who is jaundiced within the first 24 hours of age should have a TSB level drawn immediately as this finding is considered to be pathologic. It should be understood that while visual assessments are important to gauge progression of jaundice as it proceeds caudally from head to toe, they are particularly problematic in estimating the degree of hyperbilirubinemia and should not solely be relied upon. Rather, all newborns should undergo routine bilirubin testing either by TSB or transcutaneous (TcB) measurement within the first 24 hours of life. A TcB screening device offers the ability to estimate the bilirubin level quickly and avoids a painful procedure. However, providers must understand the limitations of their specific device (including decreased accuracy at higher bilirubin levels) and decide on thresholds where a serum level should be obtained.

The current AAP guidelines recommend plotting the measured bilirubin level on an hour-specific nomogram based on gestational age and presence of neurotoxicity risk factors (Figure 1). An important neurotoxicity risk factor is a positive direct antiglobin test (DAT) (Table 2). Specifically, a blood type and DAT should be obtained for newborns whose birthing parents are blood type O. If the baby is blood type A, B, or AB, this is referred to as a "setup" for ABO incompatibility. In this setting, a DAT will evaluate the presence of anti-A or anti-B antibodies on the surface of the newborn's red blood cells that may be causing hemolysis. A positive DAT does not automatically result in hyperbilirubinemia and, equally, a positive DAT may not be present in the setting of active hemolysis (e.g., G6PD deficiency).

As bilirubin levels peak around 3 to 5 days of age, determination of the newborn's risk is especially important for those discharged from the hospital prior to 72 hours of age as this will inform the decision regarding timing of outpatient follow-up. In general, newborns discharged prior to 24 hours of age should be seen by 72 hours, while those discharged between 24 and 48 hours of age should be seen by 96 hours. The majority of newborns will be discharged between 48 to 72 hours of age and they should be reevaluated in the outpatient setting by 120 hours of age. Those who have additional risk factors such as significant weight loss or an elevated bilirubin at hospital discharge should be seen earlier in the outpatient clinic. After discharge, it is important for guardians to monitor their newborns for clinical signs of jaundice that may necessitate earlier medical follow-up care.

Both in the inpatient and outpatient settings, the TcB or TSB should be plotted on the hour-specific nomogram (Figures 1 and 2) to determine the level at which phototherapy should be initiated. In the new 2022 hyperbilirubinemia guidelines, there are two nomograms based on the presence or absence of neurotoxicity risk factors with separate curves corresponding to the newborn's gestational age.

Treatment

The treatment of hyperbilirubinemia is focused on effective and efficient removal of bilirubin from the bloodstream to prevent ABE and kernicterus. Guardians should be encouraged to feed their newborns frequently, a minimum of 8 to 12 times per day, especially for those who are breastfed, as frequent feeding will help establish the parent's milk supply. The newborn's weight and urine and stool output should be assessed daily during the inpatient hospitalization to determine adequate milk transfer. Parents who intend to breastfeed but experience delayed lactogenesis should work with a lactation specialist and provide supplemental feeds (either in the form of formula or human donor milk) at appropriate volumes to decrease the enterohepatic circulation of bilirubin caused by low intake.

Phototherapy

When a newborn's TSB surpasses the phototherapy threshold, phototherapy should be administered. Phototherapy removes bilirubin by converting it into lumirubin, a water-soluble molecule that can bypass the liver and be excreted in urine or stool. Phototherapy can be delivered using overhead lights or fiberoptic blankets that provide light in the 430 to 490 nanometer wavelength, which is most strongly absorbed by the bilirubin molecule. The total body surface area that is exposed to light should be maximized for effective phototherapy. To accomplish this, the newborn should receive phototherapy while only wearing eye protection and a diaper. The newborn's temperature and hydration status should be monitored. The manufacturer's instructions should be followed to safely administer phototherapy. It is important to remember that the clinical appearance of jaundice will be affected by phototherapy and thus cannot be used to estimate the degree of hyperbilirubinemia.

Bilirubin levels should be monitored as the newborn is receiving phototherapy. TcB measurements may not be accurate after phototherapy is initiated and the provider must rely on serum levels. For newborns admitted for phototherapy after hospital discharge, the provider should obtain a baseline TSB prior to starting treatment. A repeat serum bilirubin level is typically obtained within 12 hours of phototherapy initiation to ensure that it is not continuing to rise. Subsequent checks can be ordered at the discretion of the clinician. For newborns with ongoing hemolysis or whose bilirubin levels are close to the exchange transfusion threshold, consideration should be given to earlier and more frequent TSB checks. A bilirubin level that continues to rise despite appropriate phototherapy should prompt the provider to consider other etiologies for hyperbilirubinemia. The provider should consider verifying a normal metabolic screen with the state lab and additional laboratory evaluation, including a direct bilirubin.

While the newborn is receiving phototherapy, every effort should be made to optimize feeding. A breastfeeding parent may be encouraged to express milk either manually or using a pump as the newborn may be too inactive for effective milk transfer.

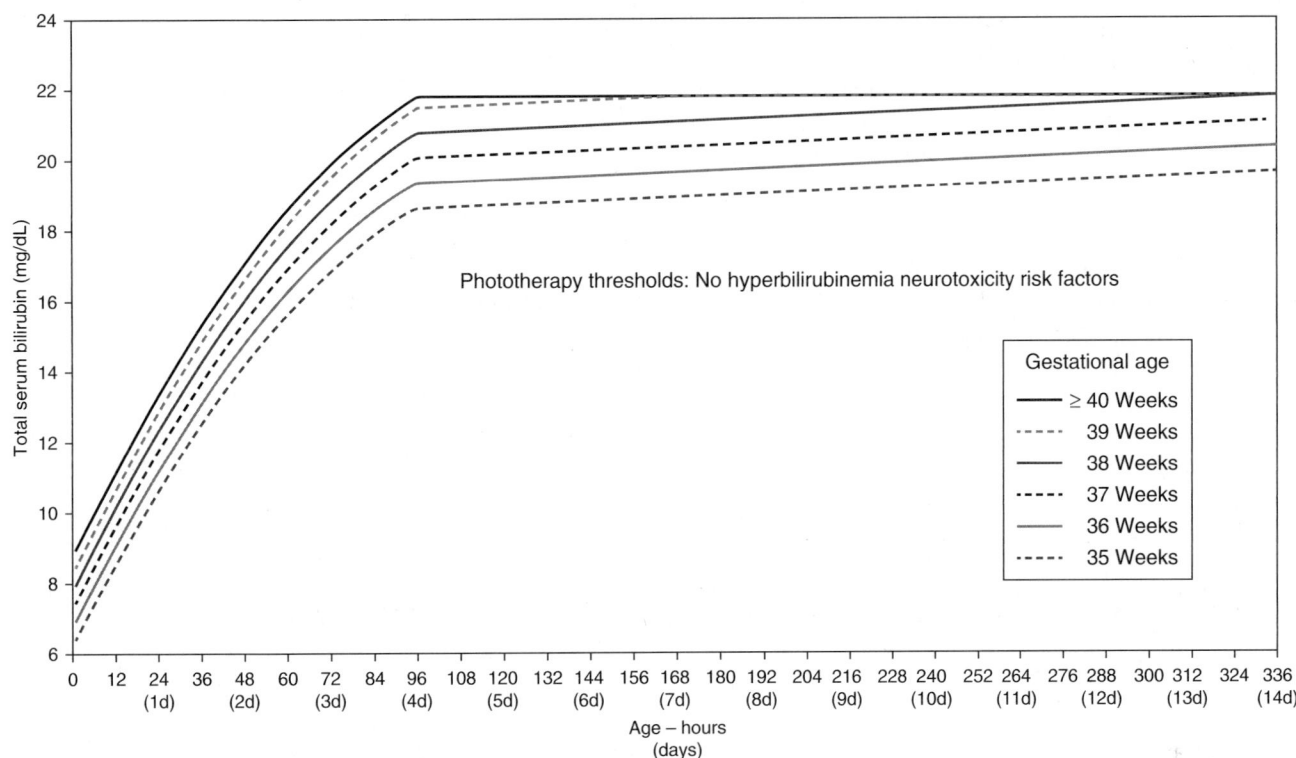

Figure 1 Hour-specific nomogram for phototherapy thresholds based on gestational age in the absence of neurotoxicity risk factors. (From Kemper AR, Newman TB, Slaughter JL, et al.: Clinical practice guideline revision: management of hyperbilirubinemia in the newborn infant 35 or more weeks of gestation, *Pediatrics* 150(3):e2022058859, 2022.)

TABLE 2	Hyperbilirubinemia Neurotoxicity Risk Factors

- Gestational age <38 wk and this risk increases with the degree of prematurity[a]

- Albumin <3.0 g/dL

- Isoimmune hemolytic disease (ie, positive direct antiglobulin test), G6PD deficiency, or other hemolytic conditions

- Sepsis

- Significant clinical instability in the previous 24 h

[a]Gestational age is required to identify the phototherapy thresholds (Figs 2 and 3; Supplemental Tables 1 and 2, and Supplemental Figs 1 and 2) and the exchange transfusion thresholds (Figs 5 and 6; Supplemental Tables 3 and 4, and Supplemental Figs 3 and 4).

From Kemper AR, Newman TB, Slaughter JL, et al.: Clinical practice guideline revision: management of hyperbilirubinemia in the newborn infant 35 or more weeks of gestation, *Pediatrics* 150(3):e2022058859, 2022

The expressed milk can be fed back to the baby and additional supplementation may be offered if needed.

The duration of phototherapy will vary based on the newborn's age, presence of hemolysis, and other risk factors. There is no clear guidance as to when phototherapy should be stopped. Some providers will discontinue phototherapy when the TSB is at least 2 mg/dL below the phototherapy threshold when phototherapy was initiated. However, for those with ongoing hemolysis, an even lower level may be desirable due to concern for rebound hyperbilirubinemia. Rebound hyperbilirubinemia occurs when the TSB returns to or exceeds the AAP phototherapy threshold within 72 hours of terminating phototherapy. A calculator by Chang et al. has been developed(https://pediatrics.aappublications.org/content/139/3/e20162896) to help determine the probability of rebound hyperbilirubinemia for late preterm and term newborns.

Escalation of Care

An escalation of care (EOC) threshold is defined as 2 mg/dL below the exchange transfusion threshold. EOC is a medical emergency, and the newborn should receive emergent intensive phototherapy and IV hydration while the provider consults with a neonatologist and prepares the newborn for transfer to a NICU where an exchange transfusion could be performed. TSB should be measured every 2 hours until the TSB is below the EOC threshold.

Exchange Transfusion

In the current era of universal screening for hyperbilirubinemia, the need for double volume exchange transfusion is rare for late preterm and full-term newborns. Exchange transfusion should be considered when the serum bilirubin exceeds the hour-specific threshold on the exchange transfusion nomogram (Figures 3 and 4).

Exchange transfusion is a procedure where small, calculated aliquots of the newborn's blood are removed and replaced with donated reconstituted RBCs with plasma, preferably through two central lines, in an effort to remove the circulating bilirubin and antibodies. The procedure is continued until the total blood volume has been replaced twice. This is a risky procedure that must only be performed in a neonatal intensive care unit. The procedure carries a complication rate of about 12% and includes coagulopathy, infection, electrolyte imbalance, and even death. The newborn requires close monitoring during and after the procedure.

Pharmacologic Treatment

For newborns with ongoing hemolysis due to ABO or Rh incompatibility whose TSB is continuing to rise despite phototherapy or for those approaching the exchange transfusion threshold, intravenous gamma globulin (IVIG, Gammagard)[1] may be administered. IVIG should be administered at 0.5 to 1 g/kg over 2 hours and repeated after 12 hours if necessary. The effectiveness of IVIG to prevent an exchange transfusion is unclear.

---

[1] Not FDA approved for this indication.

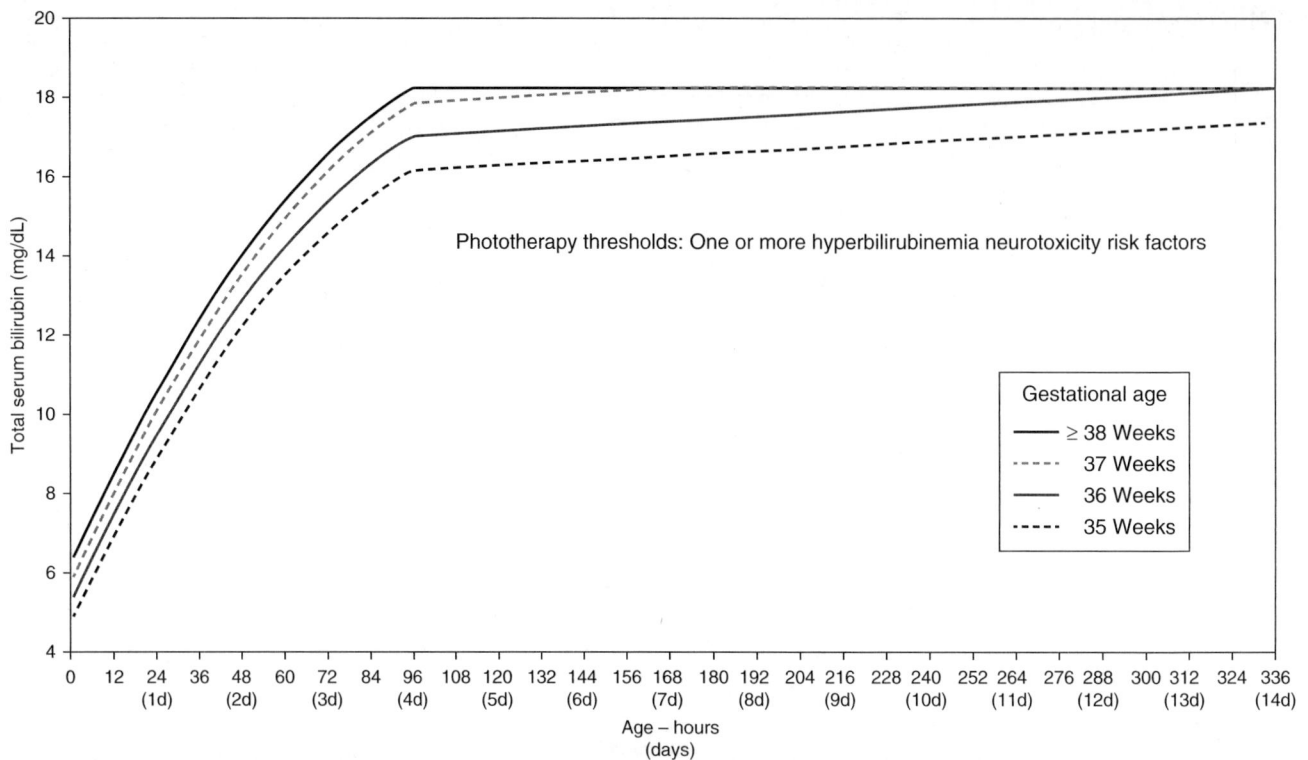

Figure 2 Hour-specific nomogram for phototherapy thresholds based on gestational age in the presence of neurotoxicity risk factors. (From Kemper AR, Newman TB, Slaughter JL, et al.: Clinical practice guideline revision: management of hyperbilirubinemia in the newborn infant 35 or more weeks of gestation, *Pediatrics* 150(3):e2022058859, 2022.)

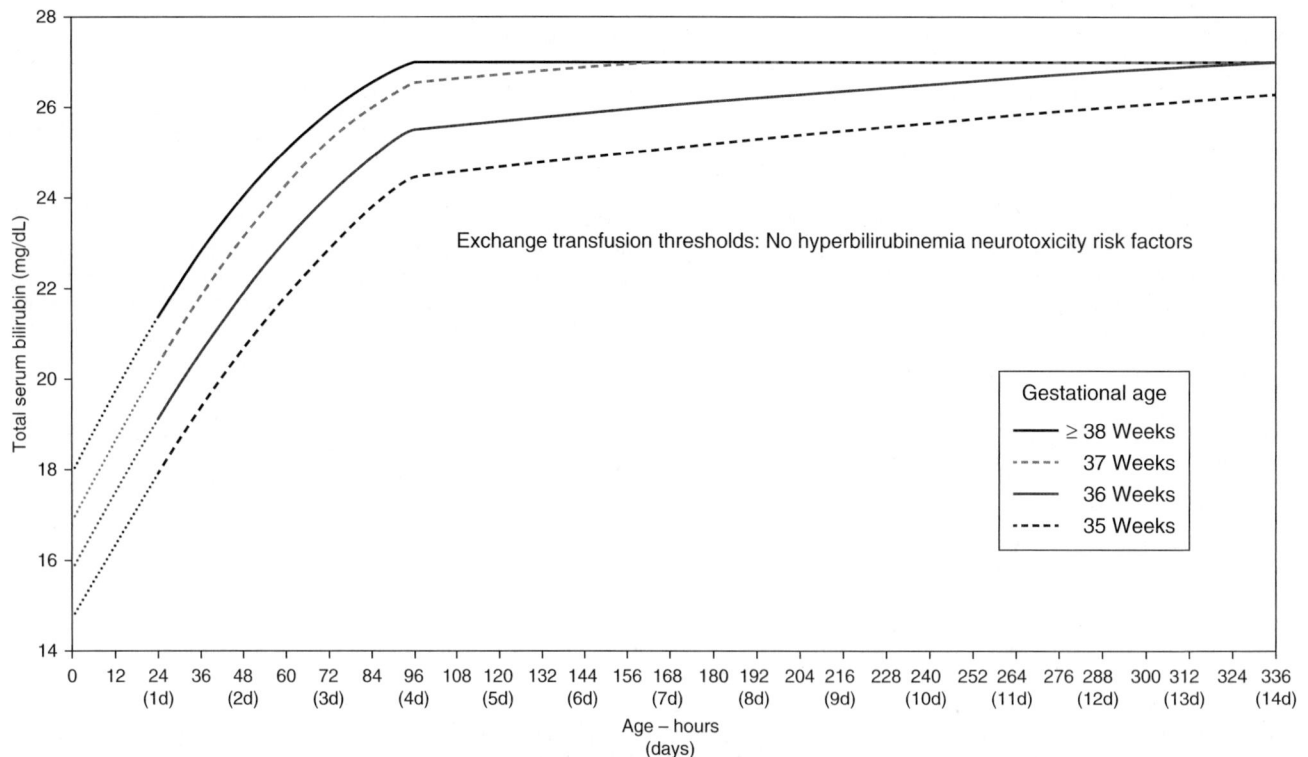

Figure 3 Hour-specific nomogram for exchange transfusion thresholds based on gestational age in the absence of neurotoxicity risk factors. (From Kemper AR, Newman TB, Slaughter JL, et al.: Clinical practice guideline revision: management of hyperbilirubinemia in the newborn infant 35 or more weeks of gestation, *Pediatrics* 150(3):e2022058859, 2022.)

Complications

The spectrum of complications associated with hyperbilirubinemia and its treatments range from mild to severe. Many newborns with hyperbilirubinemia who are approaching the phototherapy threshold may become increasingly tired and not feed effectively. This perpetuates the poor feeding and dehydration that contributed to their hyperbilirubinemia in the first place. Once phototherapy is initiated, efforts are made to maximize exposure to phototherapy, which results in parental-newborn separation and may also compromise the breastfeeding relationship. Phototherapy has been shown to result in a small reduction in breastfeeding at 12 months and exclusivity at 1, 2, and 4 months.

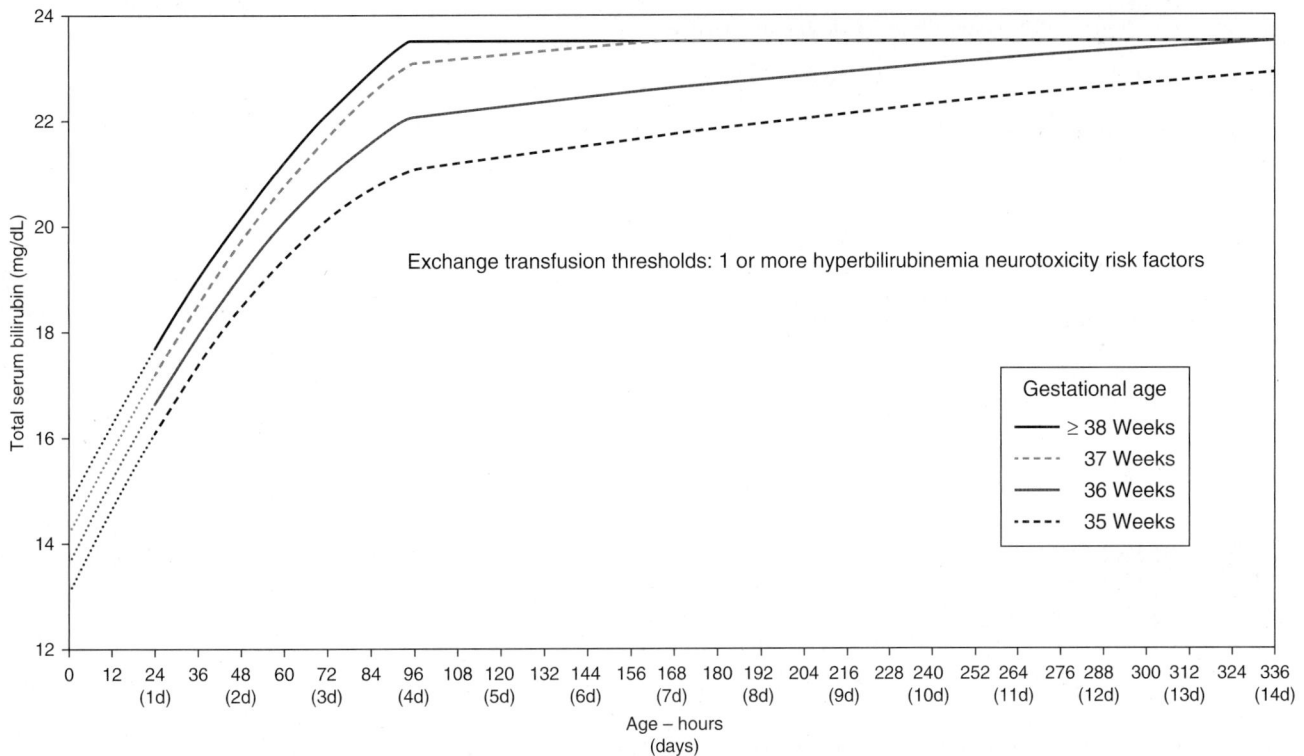

Figure 4 Hour-specific nomogram for exchange transfusion thresholds based on gestational age in the presence of neurotoxicity risk factors. (From Kemper AR, Newman TB, Slaughter JL, et al.: Clinical practice guideline revision: management of hyperbilirubinemia in the newborn infant 35 or more weeks of gestation, *Pediatrics* 150(3):e2022058859, 2022. Copyright © the American Academy of Pediatrics.)

The feared complications of severe hyperbilirubinemia, formerly termed kernicterus, are ABE and CBE. Bilirubin encephalopathy results from unconjugated bilirubin that crosses the blood-brain barrier and deposits in the brain tissue. The exact incidence of ABE is unknown, but in a large cohort of around half a million newborns in Northern California, less than 0.001% presented with ABE and all had TSB levels greater than 35. The symptoms of ABE typically progress through three stages: early, intermediate, and advanced. In the early stage, newborns may present with increased sleepiness, hypotonia, and a high-pitched cry. As symptoms progress to the intermediate stage, the newborn may be lethargic, jittery, and develop backward arching of the neck and trunk (retrocollis and opisthotonos). Finally, in the advanced stage, the newborn develops seizures, hypertonicity, and inconsolability. Death often results from seizures or respiratory failure.

CBE refers to the permanent sequelae of bilirubin-induced neurotoxicity and develops during the first year after birth. In the same cohort in Northern California, newborns who developed cerebral palsy all had TSBs that were at least 5 mg/dL above the exchange transfusion threshold. Additional symptoms of CBE include sensorineural hearing loss, gaze abnormalities, and dental enamel hypoplasia.

Recently, reports have been published regarding potential long-term complications associated with phototherapy. In a study analyzing data of nearly half a million patients, an increased risk of epilepsy was seen, though only in boys. Two studies with very large datasets looked at the potential associations between phototherapy and cancer. After accounting for confounding variables, an association persisted for myeloid leukemia, but this was based on two newborns who received higher doses of phototherapy. For newborns with Down syndrome who have a baseline risk of cancer that is 10 times higher than the general population, extra caution when initiating phototherapy is warranted. Mechanical issues related to phototherapy are rare but do include hypothermia. For patients with porphyria, phototherapy can result in a blistering skin reaction and is therefore an absolute contraindication.

References

Canadian Paediatric Society, Fetus and Newborn Committee: Guidelines for Detection, Management and Prevention of Hyperbilirubinemia in Term and Late Preterm Newborn Infants (35 or More Weeks' Gestation), *Paediatr Child Health* 12:1B–12B, 2007.

Chang P, Newman T: A Simpler Prediction Rule for Rebound Hyperbilirubinemia, *Pediatrics* 144:e20183712, 2019.

Flaherman VJ, Schaefer EW, Kuzniewicz MW, et al: Early Weight Loss Nomograms for Exclusively Breastfed Newborns, *Pediatrics* 135:e16–e23, 2015.

Harb R, Thomas D: Conjugated Hyperbilirubinemia, *Pediatrics in Review* 28:83–91, 2007.

Kemper AR, Newman TB, Slaughter JL, et al.: Clinical practice guideline revision: management of hyperbilirubinemia in the newborn infant 35 or more weeks of gestation, *Pediatrics* 150(3):e2022058859, 2022.

Kuzniewiicz MW, Wickremasinghe AC, Wu YW, et al: Incidence, Etiology, and Outcomes of Hazardous Hyperbilirubinemia in Newborns, *Pediatrics* 134:504–509, 2014.

Lauer B, Spector N: Hyperbilirubinemia in the Newborn, *Pediatrics in Review* 32:341–349, 2011.

Maisels MJ: Transcutaneous Bilirubinometry, *Neoreviews* 7:e217–225, 2006.

Maisels MJ, Bhutani V, Bogen D, et al: Hyperbilirubinemia in the Newborn Infant > 35 Weeks' Gestation: An Update with Clarifications, *Pediatrics* 124:1193–1198, 2009.

MITOCHONDRIAL DISEASE

Method of
Sonal Sharma, MD; Amy Goldstein, MD; and Marni J. Falk, MD

CURRENT DIAGNOSIS

- Mitochondrial disease diagnosis may be a challenge due to their extensive phenotypic and genotypic heterogeneity.
- Biochemical analyses of blood, urine, and cerebrospinal fluid are utilized to evaluate for evidence of mitochondrial dysfunction that may be present in some cases, as well as to evaluate for secondary problems that may develop and be amenable to management approaches. However, there are

- no highly specific or sensitive biomarkers applicable for all forms of mitochondrial disease.
- Diagnosis predominantly relies on next generation sequencing molecular analyses for pathogenic variants in hundreds of genes in both nuclear DNA and mitochondrial DNA (mtDNA). Front-line genomic testing is performed in noninvasive tissues (blood, urine, saliva, etc.).
- Invasive tissue-based diagnostic testing may be beneficial when noninvasive tissue genetic and biochemical testing is inconclusive. Muscle, liver, and/or fibroblast histology, immunohistochemistry, electron microscopy, electron transport chain enzyme activity analyses, fatty acid oxidation analysis, biochemical analyte analyses such as coenzyme Q10 level analysis, mtDNA genome sequencing and deletion quantitation, and mtDNA content analysis are specific tests that may be indicated.

CURRENT THERAPY

- No cures exist for mitochondrial disease.
- Symptom management is the mainstay of mitochondrial disease care.
- Clinicians employ a variety of mitochondrial medicine regimens consisting of vitamins, enzyme cofactors, antioxidants, and metabolic modifiers to enhance electron transport chain enzyme function and reduce toxic metabolites. The use of mitochondrial medicine therapies is based on contemporary understanding of mitochondrial disease pathophysiology to improve resiliency and prevent decompensation, although their clinical efficacy has not been proven in randomized clinical trials. In some cases, mitochondrial medicines may alter disease progression, such as oral arginine[7] to prevent recurrent metabolic strokes.
- Targeted treatment therapies for mitochondrial diseases are increasingly being developed for specific molecular subtypes and improved diagnostic assays to monitor treatment approaches.
- An increasing array of clinical treatment trials evaluating small molecules and genetic therapies are underway or being planned to develop effective treatment strategies that improve health in patients with primary (genetic-based) mitochondrial disease.

[7]Available as dietary supplement.

Epidemiology

Mitochondrial diseases are a clinically heterogeneous group of genetic disorders that are characterized by impaired energy production. Primary mitochondrial disease are caused by pathogenic variants in nuclear DNA (nDNA) or mitochondrial DNA (mtDNA) genes that play a vital role in mitochondrial structure and function. The prevalence of childhood-onset mitochondrial disease (<16 years of age) has been estimated as 5 to 15 cases per 100,000 individuals. A study in North East of England reported the prevalence of mitochondrial disease per 100,000 individuals in adults due to mtDNA mutations as 9.6 cases and those due to nDNA mutations as 2.9 cases. However, prevalence of some mitochondrial disease subtypes may be higher in regions with specific genetic founder effects.

Pathophysiology

Mitochondria are double membrane-bound organelles present in all nucleated eukaryotic cells. The fundamental function of mitochondria is energy production through the process of oxidative phosphorylation (OXPHOS) that occurs in the respiratory chain. In this aerobic process, reducing equivalence generated through the biochemical processing of cellular nutrients enter the electron transport chain (ETC) that is composed of complexes I, II, III, and IV, with oxygen serving as the final electron acceptor (Figure 1).

Electron transfer powers complexes I, III, and IV to generate a proton gradient across the inner mitochondrial membrane, which is dissipated to drive the production of energy by complex V (ATP synthase) in the chemical form of adenosine triphosphate (ATP).

Independent from the nuclear genome, mitochondria have their own mtDNA genome composed of 37 genes. Multiple mitochondria exist per cell, with multiple mitochondrial genome copies in each mitochondrion. Of the 37 genes, 13 encode proteins that are all core structural subunits of ETC complexes, while 22 encode transfer RNAs and two encode ribosomal RNAs to assist in the mitochondrial translation of these 13 protein-coding subunits. Nuclear genes are fundamentally important to mitochondria structure and function, with up to 1500 total proteins comprising mitochondria in different tissues. Thus there exists remarkable heterogeneity in the candidate genes that may directly disrupt mitochondrial dysfunction. Indeed, primary mitochondrial diseases are currently known to result from pathogenic variants in any of the 37 mtDNA genes, single or multiple large-scale deletions of mtDNA involving multiple mtDNA genes, and pathogenic variants in more than 400 nuclear genes. As mtDNA genomes are inherited through the maternal germ cells (oocytes), mtDNA disorders are maternally inherited, or rarely may occur de novo in the affected individual. By contrast, nDNA gene disorders may variably be inherited in an autosomal dominant, autosomal recessive or X-linked pattern. The majority of pathogenic variants cause mitochondrial disease by disrupting OXPHOS, which results in lowered ATP production, increased oxidative stress, and dysfunction of other interlinked metabolic pathways such as fatty acid oxidation. Some nuclear gene pathogenic variants may also cause mitochondrial diseases known as mtDNA depletion syndromes, which result from mtDNA genome instability and reduction in the mtDNA genome content in each mitochondrion.

A pathogenic mtDNA variant is usually present only in a proportion of all mtDNA genomes within a cell or tissue. This phenomenon of harboring healthy or "wild-type" mtDNA genomes as well as affected or "mutant" mtDNA genomes is termed heteroplasmy. Many mtDNA pathogenic variants only cause clinical manifestations when present in a given tissue at a certain level of heteroplasmy, which is known as "threshold effect." The precise threshold for symptom occurrence is not clear for every disease-causing mtDNA pathogenic variant. A general rule-of-thumb is that heteroplasmy levels above 70% are more likely to manifest with severe mitochondrial disease symptoms. However, this depends on the specific pathogenic variant and tissue tested, as some pathogenic variants may cause severe disease at much lower heteroplasmy levels discernible in peripheral tissues, and some may appear at much higher levels even including homoplasmic mutant (with no wild-type copies present) with little to no clinical symptoms. Environmental stressors such as intercurrent infections, fevers, fasting, and lifestyle choices such as nutrition, exercise, and medication or environmental exposures may all influence the onset and progression of clinical symptoms in individuals harboring pathogenic variants in mtDNA.

Clinical Manifestations

Due to impairment of the common pathway of energy production, mitochondrial diseases have wide-ranging variability, even among affected family members, in their age of onset and particular organ system involvement. Secondary mitochondrial dysfunction may also occur in other genetic or complex classes of disease that affect energy production or upon exposure to certain environmental factors and medications. Patients with mitochondrial disease report an average of 16 symptoms involving different organ systems, with a range of 7 to 35 symptoms per patient (Figure 2). Common symptoms include fatigue, exercise intolerance, muscle weakness, developmental delay or regression, poor growth, metabolic strokes, intellectual disability, seizures, dysautonomia, cardiomyopathy, arrhythmia, sensorineural hearing loss, endocrinopathies (diabetes mellitus, thyroid abnormalities, pancreatic, and adrenal dysfunction) as well as impairment of vision, immune, gastrointestinal, liver, and kidney function. Fatigue in mitochondrial myopathy

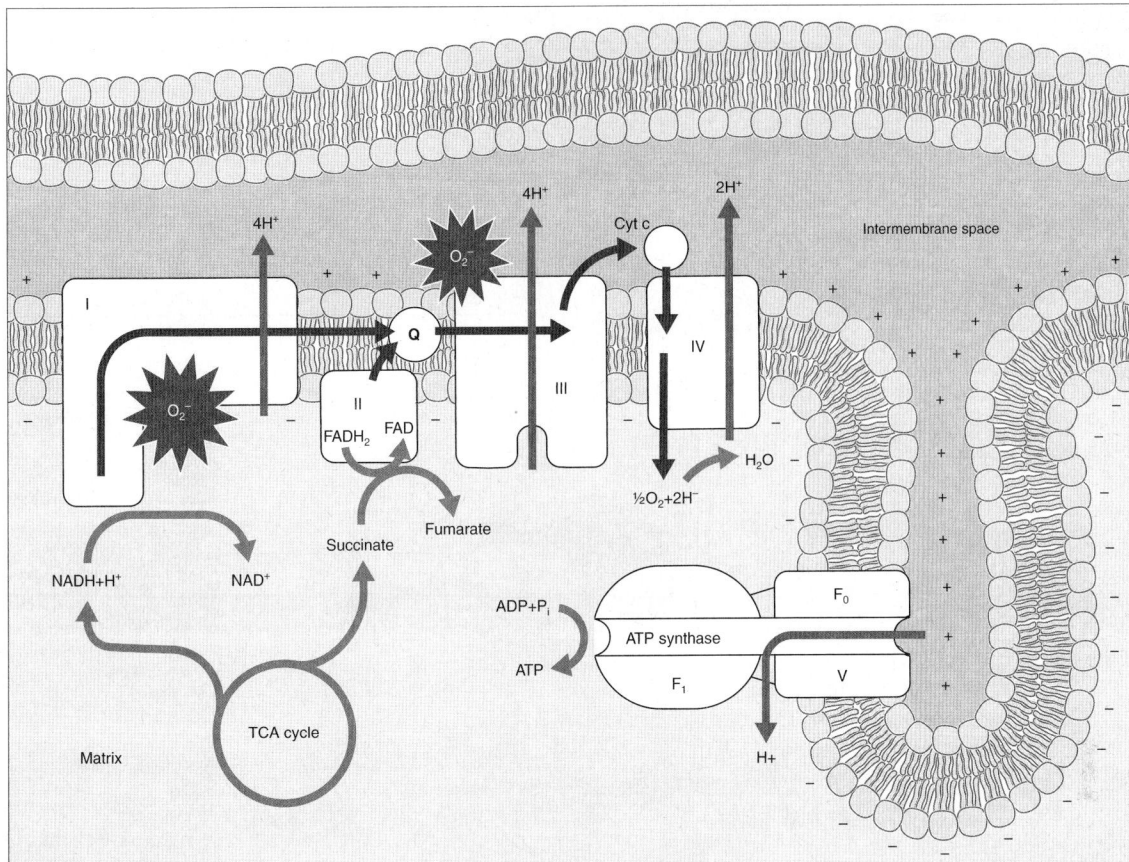

Figure 1 Mitochondrial respiration. The mitochondrial electron transport chain consists of four protein complexes (I–IV) embedded in the inner mitochondrial membrane that are coupled to a fifth (V) unlinked complex, ATP synthase. Reducing equivalents such as NADH and $FADH_2$ generated from other biochemical pathways, mainly the tricarboxylic acid (TCA) cycle and fatty acid oxidation, are oxidized by complex I and II. Electrons from complex I and II are transported to reduce coenzyme Q10 (CoQ10), which transports electrons to complex III, then to cytochrome C and finally to complex IV. The electrons are transferred by complex IV to molecular oxygen in a process that generates water. Complex I, III, and IV pump protons, which result from these reactions from the mitochondrial matrix into the intermembrane space, thereby creating a proton gradient. These protons reenter the matrix through complex V and drive the reaction to synthesize adenosine triphosphate (ATP) from adenosine diphosphate (ADP) and inorganic phosphate. Energy stored in the phosphate bonds of the ATP molecule power multiple cellular reactions. Adapted from Hagberg H, Mallard C, Rousset CI, Thornton C: Mitochondria: hub of injury responses in the developing brain. *Lancet Neurol* 13(2):217–232, 2014.

(MM) is usually accompanied by muscle weakness, exercise intolerance, imbalance, impaired dexterity, and other systemic symptoms. MM-COAST is a valuable clinical assessment tool to quantify key domains of MM. It is prudent for primary care physicians to suspect mitochondrial disease in patients who present with typical "red-flag" symptoms of mitochondrial disease or unexplained symptoms involving three or more unrelated organ systems, although in some cases only single organ dysfunction may be present at presentation. It is also important to recognize that disease onset in a given individual may occur at any age from prenatal to adult, and the severity of symptoms tends to worsen in a nonlinear, progressive manner. There can be episodes of acute decline triggered by infection or other stressors, followed by periods of stability.

Emergencies in mitochondrial disease include acute decompensation that may result from increased metabolic demand secondary to physiologic stressors including ongoing infection, systemic illness, fasting, dehydration, surgery, and/or anesthesia. The presence of neurologic regression, focal neurologic deficits, altered mental status, or seizures should raise concern for acute metabolic stroke. It is also vital to recognize signs of severe metabolic acidosis in patients with primary mitochondrial disease, which include altered mental status, hyperpnea, bradycardia, arrhythmia, hypotension, nausea, vomiting, and severe lethargy.

An additional challenge to the recognition of mitochondrial disease is the complex relationship between genotype and clinical phenotype. A specific gene pathogenic variant can result in different clinical symptoms. A clear example is the m.3243A>G pathogenic variant in *MT-TL1*, which can cause chronic progressive external ophthalmoplegia (CPEO),

mitochondrial encephalopathy, lactic acidosis and stroke-like episodes (MELAS), or maternally inherited diabetes and deafness (MIDD). Similarly, a specific syndrome can result from numerous genetic etiologies such as Leigh syndrome (subacute necrotizing encephalomyelopathy), which can be caused by pathogenic variants in approximately 100 nuclear and mtDNA genes. The clinical symptoms of common mitochondrial diseases are described in Table 1.

Diagnosis

Noninvasive Biochemical Analysis

The diagnosis of mitochondrial disease requires a thoughtful, stepwise approach (Figure 3). Noninvasive laboratory screening using blood and urine samples involves chemistry and biochemistry tests to determine the patient's metabolic stability as well as other organ involvement. Standard biochemistry profiling tests include comprehensive metabolic profile, plasma lactate, plasma pyruvate, lactate to pyruvate ratio, quantitative plasma amino acid analysis, plasma carnitine levels and acylcarnitine profile, ammonia, plasma glutathione level, GDF-15 level, and quantitative urine organic acid analysis. Tests for secondary organ involvement may include complete blood count with differential, creatine kinase, hemoglobin A1c, lipoprotein profile, iron profile and ferritin, thyroid screen, cortisol, adrenocorticotropic hormone, parathyroid hormone, amylase, lipase, fecal elastase, immunoglobulin levels, and urinalysis. However, these tests are not specific for mitochondrial disease and none have sufficiently high sensitivity and specificity to be useful as a biomarker sufficient to confirm or refute the diagnosis of mitochondrial disease. For example, elevated plasma lactate may

Neurological

Seizure related stroke/
metabolic stroke
Epilepsy
Ataxia
Migraine
Dementia
Parkinsonism
Developmental delay
Psychiatric or mood
disorder
Developmental
regression

Ptosis
Progressive external
ophthalmoplegia
Optic atrophy
Retinitis pigmentosa

Sensorineural
hearing loss

Non-neurological

Respiratory failure

Cardiomyopahy
Conduction defect

Liver failure

Fanconi syndrome
Renal tubular
acidosis
Focal segmental
glomerulosclerosis
Renal failure
Adrenal insufficiency

Diabetes mellitus
Pancreatitis

Intestinal pseudo-obstruction
Gastrointestinal dysmotility
Chronic villous atrophy
Failure to thrive

Premature ovarian falure
Male infertility

Kyphoscoliosis
Short stature
Bone marrow failure

Myopathy
Exercise intolerance

Peripheral neuropahy

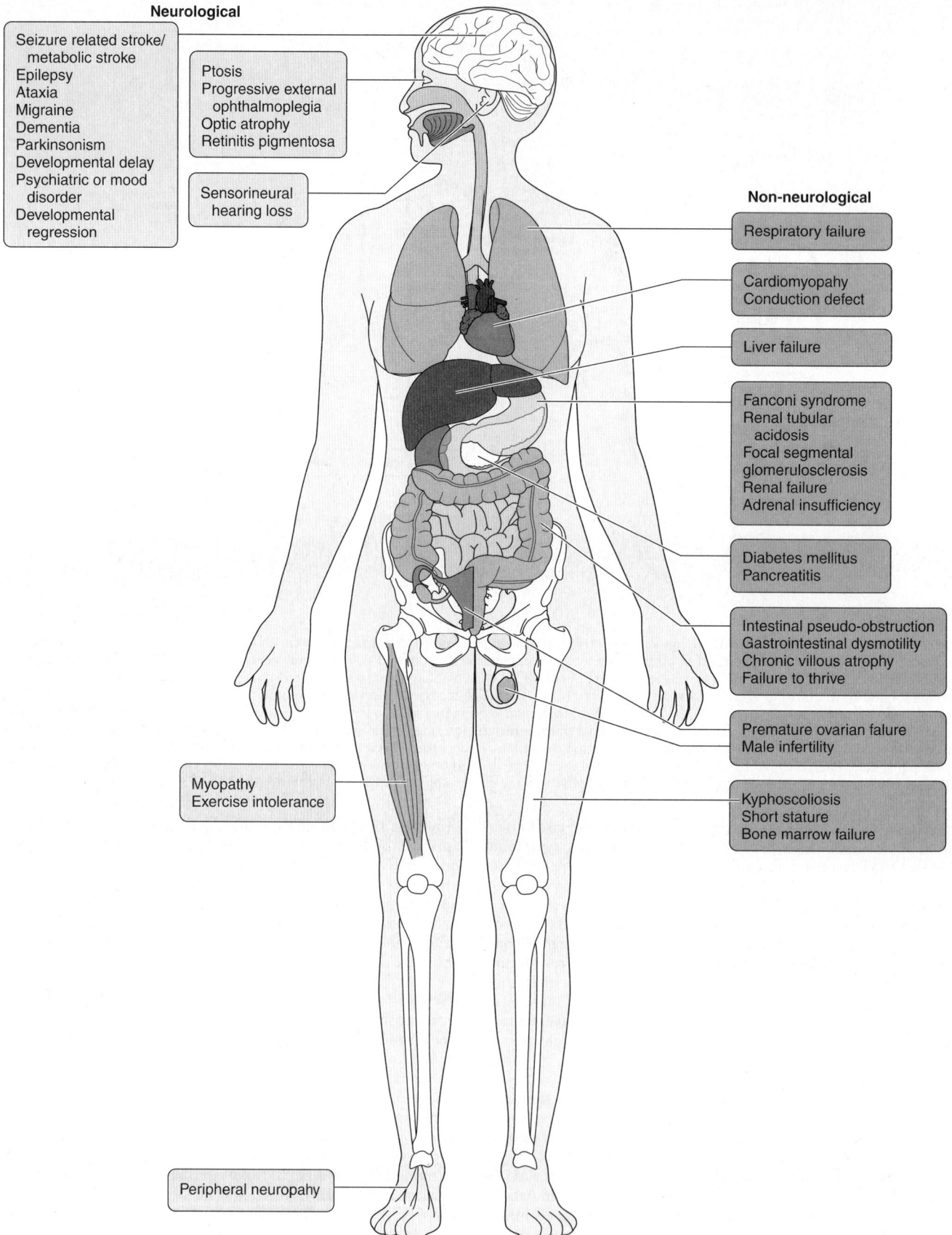

Figure 2 Clinical symptoms in mitochondrial disease are variable and usually involve multiple high-energy demand organ systems. Gorman GS, Chinnery PF, DiMauro S, et al: Mitochondrial diseases. *Nat Rev Dis Primers* 2:16080, 2016.

occur in mitochondrial disease, but levels may also be normal or only intermittently increased under some scenarios or in certain disease subtypes. Further, elevated lactate results in individuals without primary mitochondrial disease from poor tissue perfusion, stroke, sepsis, seizures, or improper handling of the sample.

Neuroimaging

Mitochondrial disease patients with clinical CNS involvement may have nonspecific brain and spine magnetic resonance imaging (MRI) abnormalities. Bilateral, symmetric involvement of deep gray structures in the absence of hypoxia, ischemia, or

TABLE 1 Presentation Overview of Common Mitochondrial Disease Clinical Syndromes

DISEASE	GENETIC ETIOLOGY	CLINICAL FEATURES	OTHER FINDINGS	NEUROIMAGING	SPECIFIC TREATMENT
Mitochondrial encephalomyopathy, lactic acidosis and stroke-like episodes (MELAS)	80%: m.3243A>G variant in MT-TL1; <10%: variants in MT-ND5; less common—15 other mitochondrial disease genes	Seizures, recurrent headaches, stroke-like episodes, cortical vision loss, muscle weakness, recurrent vomiting, short stature, hearing impairment, impaired thinking, diabetes mellitus (type 1 or 2), developmental delay	Lactic acidemia or acidosis in blood and cerebrospinal fluid (CSF), elevated CSF protein, Muscle biopsy: Ragged red fibers, ETC: Low complex I and/or complex IV activities	MRI: asymmetric, T2 hyperintensity not corresponding to specific vascular distribution during stroke-like episodes with predominant posterior cerebrum involvement, slow spreading of stroke like lesion over weeks; MRA: usually normal; MRS: elevated N-acetylaspartate (NAA) and lactate; CT: basal ganglia calcification	Acute or subacute stroke episode: intravenous (IV) arginine[1] 500 mg/kg/day over 60 min for 3–5 days; Prevention of recurrent stroke: oral arginine[7] 150–300 mg/kg/day
Maternally inherited diabetes and deafness (MIDD)	85%: m.3243A>G variant in MT-TL1, MTTE, MTTK genes	Sensorineural hearing loss, impaired vestibular function, diabetes mellitus, dizziness, unsteady gait, dysarthria, seizures, pigmentary retinal degeneration, cardiac conduction defects	Hyperglycemia, glutamic acid decarboxylase (GAD) autoantibody negativity in a nonobese diabetic is a clue		Oral antidiabetic agents and/or insulin; treatment with metformin1 is less effective and avoided due to increased risk of lactic acidosis
Leigh syndrome (subacute necrotizing encephalomyelopathy)	>80 nuclear genes (most common SURF1, in up to 10% of Leigh syndrome cases) 14 mtDNA genes (MT-ATP6 associated with ~50% of all mtDNA-based Leigh syndrome)	Psychomotor retardation or regression, usually provoked by illness followed by a period of stabilization, hypotonia, spasticity, movement disorders, cerebellar ataxia, peripheral neuropathy, hypertrophic cardiomyopathy	Lactic acidosis in blood and CSF during intercurrent illness, ratio of lactate to pyruvate is normal to low in pyruvate dehydrogenase (PDH) deficiency, increased alanine on plasma amino acids reflective of persistent hyperlactic acidemia, respiratory chain complex I, II, III, IV, or V deficiency depending on genetic etiology	MRI: bilateral symmetric T2 signal hyperintensities in the basal ganglia and/or brainstem; spinal cord involvement can appear as demyelinating lesions involving white matter or ischemic/infectious lesions involving gray matter MRS: elevated lactate	Biotin-thiamine responsive basal ganglia disease associated with mutation of SLC19A3: oral biotin[7] (5–10 mg/kg/day) and thiamine1 (in doses ranging from 300–900 mg/day); Biotinidase deficiency: oral biotin 5–10 mg/day; Coenzyme Q10 (CoQ10) deficiency: ubiquinOL7 (reduced) formulation preferred, at dose up to 8 mg/kg/day If ubiquinONE7 (oxidized) formulation is used, oral CoQ10 10–30 mg/kg/day in children, 1,200–3,000 mg/day in adults
Neuropathy, Ataxia, and Retinitis Pigmentosa (NARP)	MT-ATP6	Continuum of clinical spectrum of Leigh syndrome, muscle weakness, neuropathy, ataxia, seizures, retinitis pigmentosa or optic atrophy, learning difficulty	Electromyography (EMG)/Nerve Conduction Velocity (NCV) studies: sensory or sensorimotor axonal polyneuropathy	MRI: cerebral and/or cerebellar atrophy	
Myoclonic Epilepsy associated with Ragged Red Fibers (MERRF)	>80%: m.8344A>G variant in MT-TK, 7 other mtDNA genes also associated with MERRF phenotype	Myoclonus is often the first symptom followed by generalized epilepsy, ataxia, weakness, exercise intolerance, dementia, peripheral neuropathy, hearing loss, short stature, optic atrophy, ptosis, ophthalmoplegia, retinitis pigmentosa, cardiomyopathy, dysrhythmias such as Wolff-Parkinson-White syndrome, multiple lipomas	Lactic acidemia or acidosis in blood and CSF, lactate and pyruvate are elevated at rest and increase excessively after moderate activity, elevated CSF protein, Electron transport chain (ETC) enzyme activity studies: deficiency of respiratory complexes I, III, or IV with mtDNA- encoded subunits Muscle biopsy: ragged red fibers, hyperactive fibers with succinate dehydrogenase stain	MRI: brain atrophy, basal ganglia lesions, bilateral putaminal necrosis, brainstem and cerebellum atrophy	

TABLE 1   Presentation Overview of Common Mitochondrial Disease Clinical Syndromes—cont'd

DISEASE	GENETIC ETIOLOGY	CLINICAL FEATURES	OTHER FINDINGS	NEUROIMAGING	SPECIFIC TREATMENT
Leber's Hereditary Optic Neuropathy (LHON)	>90%: m.3460G>A in MT-ND1, m.11778G>A in MT-ND4, or m.14484T>C in MT-ND6, Six other mtDNA genes may also be causal	Bilateral, painless, subacute visual failure (starts as central visual field blurring in one eye followed by involvement of other eye 2–3 months later), males are four–five times more likely to be affected than females, penetrance 15% in females and 50% in males, with penetrance exacerbated by smoking and alcohol exposure, visual acuity is reduced to counting fingers or worse, optic disc atrophy after acute phase, ataxia, peripheral neuropathy, myopathy, movement disorders, multiple sclerosis–like illness, cardiac arrhythmias	ECG: pre-excitation syndrome, Visual field testing: enlarging dense central or centrocecal scotoma, ETC enzyme activity analysis: m.3460G>A in MT-ND1 associated with severe complex I deficiency	MRI: white matter lesions and/or a high signal within the optic nerves	Treatment of raised intraocular pressure Idebenone (available in Europe, not in the United States) and/or antioxidant vitamin supplementation (N-Acetylcysteine,[1] vitamin E, B12, and C) may be tried to stabilize visual loss and/or accelerate visual recovery to improve final visual outcome
POLG-related disorders	Three most common variants of >200 pathogenic variants (most are autosomal recessive, some can be autosomal dominant): p.Ala467Thr, p.Trp748Ser, p.Gly848Ser	Epilepsy, hepatopathy, neuropathy, ataxia, CPEO, myopathy, parkinsonism	CSF: elevated protein, decreased 5-methyltetrahydrofolate	MRI: Perirolandic signal changes, stroke-like lesions involving occipital lobes	Antiseizure medications, folinic acid (leucovorin)[1], N-acetylcysteine[1] for liver failure
Chronic Progressive External Ophthalmoplegia (CPEO)	Single, large scale mtDNA deletion syndrome (single large-scale deletion ranging in size from 1.1–10 kilobase): can be identified in skeletal muscle, and multiple mtDNA deletions may be seen in POLG	Ptosis, ophthalmoplegia, oropharyngeal weakness, proximal limb weakness, exercise intolerance		MRI: leukoencephalopathy, cerebral or cerebellar atrophy, basal ganglia and brainstem lesions (Leigh syndrome pattern)	Eyelid slings and/or ptosis repair for severe ptosis, eyeglass prisms for diplopia, eye drops for dry eye
Kearns-Sayre syndrome (KSS)	Single large-scale mtDNA deletion syndrome can be identified in blood leukocytes, buccal sample, urine sediment, or muscle	Pigmentary retinopathy, progressive ophthalmoplegia, cerebellar ataxia, impaired intellect, sensorineural hearing loss, oropharyngeal and esophageal dysfunction, muscle weakness, exercise intolerance, cardiac conduction block, endocrinopathy (diabetes mellitus, hypothyroidism, hypoparathyroidism, adrenal insufficiency), renal impairment	Lactic acidemia or acidosis in blood and CSF, elevated CSF protein, Muscle biopsy: ragged red fibers, ETC enzyme activity analysis: reduced activity of complexes I, III, and/or IV	MRI: Leukoencephalopathy, cerebral or cerebellar atrophy, basal ganglia and brainstem lesions (Leigh syndrome pattern)	Prophylactic placement of cardiac pacemakers in individuals with cardiac conduction block, Folinic acid supplementation[1] in individuals with KSS with low CSF 5-methyltetrahydrofolate, Pancreatic enzyme replacement, Hearing aids and/or cochlear implants for sensorineural hearing loss
Pearson syndrome	Single, large scale mtDNA deletion syndrome can be identified in blood leukocytes	Infancy or early childhood onset, sideroblastic anemia typically transfusion-dependent until resolution in early childhood, growth failure, and exocrine pancreatic dysfunction	Macrocytic, sideroblastic anemia with a variable degree of neutropenia and thrombocytopenia (pancytopenia), normocellular bone marrow, hemosiderosis, and ringed sideroblasts	MRI: white matter involvement	Pancreatic enzyme replacement, Transfusion therapy for sideroblastic anemia

[1]Not FDA approved for this indication.
[7]Available as dietary supplement.

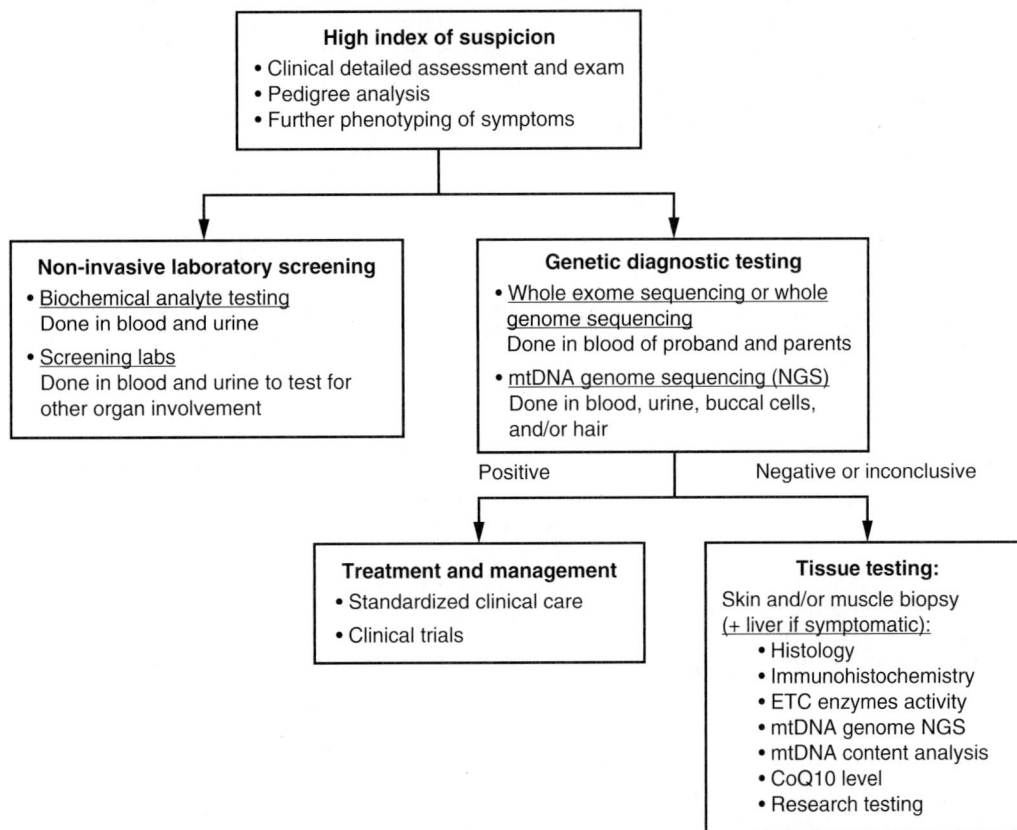

Figure 3 Algorithm for clinical diagnostic evaluation of mitochondrial disease. Muraresku CC, McCormick EM, Falk MJ: Mitochondrial disease: Advances in clinical diagnosis, management, therapeutic development, and preventative strategies. *Curr Genet Med Rep* 6(2):62–72, 2018.

infection should raise suspicion for mitochondrial dysfunction. However, patients with CNS involvement can have a normal MRI depending on the timing of the scan, as some findings may fluctuate, both resolving or newly occurring over time. Certain mitochondrial disease syndromes can be associated with hallmark neuroimaging findings. Leigh syndrome is associated with progressive signal abnormality (T2 hyperintensity, T1 hypointensity) most commonly in the lentiform nuclei (putamen and globus pallidus) and caudate nuclei of the basal ganglia. Signal abnormalities in Leigh syndrome may also involve the thalamus, periaqueductal gray, tegmentum, red nuclei, and dentate nuclei. In some cases, there can also be extensive gliosis and cystic degeneration of white matter and marked global atrophy as the disease progresses. MELAS syndrome is associated with landmark MRI affecting gray matter and not confined to any specific vascular territory. While any cortical location may be involved in MELAS, a predilection for the occipital lobes exists, with clinical correlate of vision loss during a stroke-like episode. Diffuse white matter involvement, particularly in the periventricular and centrum semiovale region, may also occur in multiple mitochondrial disease clinical syndromes such as MELAS, Kearns-Sayre syndrome, and mitochondrial neurogastrointestinal encephalomyopathy (MNGIE) syndrome.

Genetic Diagnostic Testing

Over the past decade, substantial advancements have occurred in the accessibility, affordability, clinical utility, and diagnostic yield of whole exome sequencing (WES) for mitochondrial disease diagnosis. WES is now considered to be the first-line genetic test, with demonstrated improved performance over gene panel-based approaches due to the rapid pace of gene discovery that requires frequent updating of gene panels, as well as the clinically heterogenous nature of mitochondrial disorders that would otherwise require sequential use of multiple different gene panels. Trio-based WES testing is preferred, as this incorporates analysis of proband and both parental samples to allow accurate segregation analysis of multiple variants identified in a proband as well as determination of autosomal dominant disorders with de novo occurrence in the proband. An important application of WES raw data is reanalysis at a future date, which may identify novel gene disorders that were previously not recognized by the diagnostic laboratory at the time of the initial WES report. This is particularly important in pediatric patients, in whom nDNA mutations are the underlying cause of 75% of mitochondrial disease. Appropriate use of WES in the clinical setting requires genetic counselor support for completing informed consent, to understand testing limitations and choices in the type of results that will be returned. Lack of insurance coverage may limit the ability to pursue WES for a specific patient, which may often require insurance preauthorization and escalated coverage requests and justification by the clinician. WES has limitations in the types of genetic errors that may be found, as it may miss certain gene regions not targeted and analyzed, is unable to detect genomic copy number variation, and is unable to be used for triple repeat size analysis. For these reasons, whole genome sequencing (WGS) is emerging as a new clinical test that is able to provide a more comprehensive "exome" than WES, as well as evaluate for these other types of genetic mutations. Further, while WES does not include the mtDNA genome unless it is specifically targeted for capture and analysis, WGS coverage inherently does include the entire mtDNA genome.

The emergence of second-generation chips and improved chemistry has driven down the cost of WGS and made it comparable with other clinical diagnostic procedures. In comparison with WES, WGS detects more variants in the noncoding parts of the genome (introns), as well as in the exons, due to superior mapping quality and captures copy number variations and structural rearrangements. Additionally, RNA-sequencing (RNA-seq) can be employed to understand functional protein expression by investigating the transcriptome (i.e., cellular content of all RNAs, including mRNA, tRNA, rRNA). This can help identify the functional consequences of variants of uncertain significance.

Prenatal testing for prevention of mitochondrial DNA disease is not available in the United States. Females at risk of transmitting an mtDNA pathogenic variant to their offspring can pursue testing internationally at specialized mitochondrial disease centers such as the Newcastle Fertility Centre where research has pioneered mitochondrial donation treatment (MDT). This technique uses mitochondria from eggs of healthy female donors to create embryos that are free from the pathogenic mtDNA mutations that their biological mothers carry.

Commonly, mtDNA genome sequencing is performed by next-generation sequencing (NGS) methodologies, which can be performed in a stand-alone fashion or in many cases ordered concurrently with WES. Approximately 75% of mitochondrial disease among adults result from pathogenic variants in the mtDNA genome. NGS-based tests may accurately detect single nucleotide variants as well as single or multiple large-scale deletions or duplications down in many cases to 1% heteroplasmy levels. NGS testing detects the breakpoints of large-scale rearrangements in mtDNA but is not reliable for their heteroplasmy quantitation due to polymerase chain reaction (PCR)-based overamplification of deleted genomes; thus performance of additional clinical tests such as digital droplet PCR is required to accurately quantify the mtDNA deletion(s) heteroplasmy level in a given tissue. While most mtDNA mutations are detectable in blood, saliva, or urinary sediment, it is important to note that some mutations, such as single large-scale deletions and other mtDNA single nucleotide variants may only be discernible in postmitotic or symptomatic tissues like muscle; thus a normal mtDNA genome sequence test in a peripheral tissue may need to be followed by symptomatic tissue-based mtDNA genome sequencing if clinical suspicion remains. Additionally, the blood heteroplasmy level of some mtDNA point mutations may decline with age, as is known to commonly occur at a rate of 1% per year for the m.3243A>G mutation. mtDNA genome depletion detectable on PCR-based mtDNA content analysis of muscle or liver may also occur, which when found is indicative that any of dozens of known nuclear gene etiology are present that underlies imbalance in the mtDNA genome and nucleotide pools.

If a mtDNA mutation of uncertain significance is identified, heteroplasmy levels of that variant should be tested by ordering clinical testing in as many tissues as possible (e.g., blood, buccal or saliva, fibroblast cells, urine sediment, muscle, etc.). Commonly, pathogenic variants have higher heteroplasmy levels found in clinically symptomatic but are only rarely homoplasmic. Measuring levels of heteroplasmy of the suspected pathogenic variant in tissues of both affected and unaffected maternal relatives may also be beneficial to aide in its pathogenicity assertion determination. The presence of the same or higher heteroplasmy level of a specific mutation in unaffected maternal relatives decreases its likelihood of being pathogenic in the proband.

Invasive Tissue Testing

When genetic diagnostic testing in noninvasive tissues is unrevealing or identifies variants of uncertain significance, tissue biopsies may be useful to obtain sample in which to perform extensive histologic, immunohistochemical, electron microscopy, genetic, and biochemical analysis. Ideally, the most profoundly affected tissue in a patient is the best option. Muscle is commonly affected in mitochondrial disease patients and can be obtained by open biopsy or percutaneous needle biopsy; the right leg vastus lateralis tissue is the standard sample in which normative values have been obtained for biochemical testing of mitochondrial function. While skin is a less metabolically active tissue, skin-derived primary fibroblast cell lines are readily obtainable without general anesthesia and have been widely demonstrated to have utility for a wide array of biochemical analyses that may be informative about mitochondrial function. Liver biopsy can be beneficial in select patients with hepatic involvement.

All three tissues can be clinically tested for respiratory chain enzyme activity spectrophotometric analyses and (where available) high-resolution respirometry studies of integrated OXPHOS capacity. Histologic and immunohistochemical analysis of muscle can reveal evidence of myopathy or lipid or glycogen storage. Ragged-red fibers on modified Gomori trichrome staining may also be seen as red granular deposits of mitochondria in the subsarcolemmal space, which are suggestive of a mitochondrial proliferative response often occurring in response to mtDNA-based disorder. Immunohistochemical analysis of muscle involves several stains to screen mitochondrial enzymatic activities such as NADH dehydrogenase for evaluation of complex I activity, succinate dehydrogenase (SDH) for complex II activity, and cytochrome c oxidase (COX) for complex IV activity. COX-deficient fibers are a nonspecific finding that may be indicative of a mtDNA disorder. Stains are also used to evaluate for a host of other muscle diseases that may aid in the differential diagnosis of mitochondrial disease. Electron microscopy study of muscle in patients with mitochondrial disease may reveal increased mitochondrial number and size, distorted or absent cristae, and paracrystalline or "parking lot" inclusions. Liver histology may reveal microvesicular or macrovesicular steatosis as well as eosinophilic granulations, representing proliferation of mitochondria. Additional biochemical analysis may include quantification of coenzyme Q10 that plays an important role in ETC; while the concentration of coenzyme Q10 varies greatly in tissues, leukocyte Q10 levels have been shown to be most indicative of tissue coenzyme Q10 deficiency.

Quantitative PCR analysis of mtDNA content in liver or muscle tissue is important to identify mtDNA depletion syndromes. mtDNA genome sequencing is also informative, as above, to complete the evaluation for a suspected mtDNA disorder.

Treatment

Acute Symptom Management

Maintenance of adequate hydration through enteral or intravenous (IV) fluids with dextrose to prevent a catabolic state is an important intervention to consider during an episode of acute decompensation. If a stroke-like lesion is identified on brain MRI, treatment should be pursued with IV arginine[1] to aid in vasodilation through its conversion to nitric oxide mediated by nitric oxide synthase. Arginine has proven effective in decreasing severity of stroke like symptoms, reducing frequency of stroke-like episodes, and reducing tissue injury in patients with MELAS and also found to be effective in pediatric Leigh syndrome, particularly those with hemiplegic symptoms, with 50% of patients in a recent study at our center back to their neurologic baseline by hospital discharge. High-dose steroids may also be considered for treatment of vasogenic edema, which can be associated with stroke-like lesions. If severe metabolic acidosis is identified, subspecialty consultation with metabolic medicine, intensive care, or nephrology should be pursued and buffers such as sodium bicarbonate[1] therapy should be considered.

Additional acute symptoms should be managed by organ-based specialists, such as neurology for acute epilepsy or stroke, nephrology for acute renal failure, ophthalmology for acute visual changes, gastroenterology for obstruction or dysmotility, and cardiology for arrhythmia or cardiac failure.

Chronic Management

Unfortunately, no FDA approved treatments exist for mitochondrial disease at this time. Consensus expert opinion has guided the therapeutic dosing of mitochondrial supplemental medicines, colloquially referred to as a "cocktail," based on underlying known pathophysiology of mitochondrial disease, animal or cellular experimental studies, and expert clinical experience. Vitamins and nonvitamin cofactor serve essential roles for several cellular reactions. These include vitamin B1 (thiamine, a cofactor for the pyruvate dehydrogenase complex), vitamin B2 (riboflavin, promotes assembly of complex I), vitamin B3 (niacin or nicotinic acid, a precursor of nicotinamide

---

[1]Not FDA approved for this indication.

adenine dinucleotide that serves as the primary electron donor to complex I), vitamin B7 (biotin, cofactor for mitochondrial carboxylases), and vitamin B9 (folic acid, where cerebral folate deficiency is associated with white matter changes in mitochondrial disease that may be responsive to folinic acid that crosses the blood–brain barrier). Antioxidants are empirically used to reduce oxidative stress both in the mitochondria and throughout the cell that occurs commonly in mitochondrial disease, including vitamin E, alpha-lipoic acid,[1] coenzyme Q10,[1] taurine,[1] and N-acetylcysteine (Acetadote).[1] Amino acid therapies commonly used to prevent stroke-like episodes in mitochondrial disease patients include arginine,[1] citrulline,[1] and/or taurine. High-dose biotin[1] and thiamine[1] may be indicated in biotin-thiamine-responsive basal ganglia disease. L-creatine[1] may be helpful in myopathy to improve phosphocreatine energy stores. Lutein[1] is commonly recommended in individuals with pigmentary retinopathy.

While L-carnitine (Carnitor)[1] has historically been widely used in mitochondrial disease, its use is associated with long-term risk of coronary artery disease in the general population, so is not used in mitochondrial disease patients only for documented carnitine deficiency or in specific fatty acid oxidation disorders. As the molecular basis for specific patient's symptoms are increasingly recognized, additional therapies may be rationally considered to address their unique cellular pathophysiology. Additional, optimizing nutrition, hydration, and exercise are key components of optimizing long-term management and health outcomes in mitochondrial disease. Newer diagnostic tests are being developed at specialized centers to quantify analytes to guide management decisions, including ketone body panels to provide an indicator of cellular NADH/NAD+ redox that may be amenable to NAD+ agonist therapies, leukocyte CoQ10[7] levels to monitor coenzyme Q supplementation therapies, and glutathione (total, reduced GSH, oxidized GSSG) levels to monitor glutathione agonist therapies such as N-acetylcysteine[1].

Preventative Therapies

Preimplantation genetic diagnosis is available for nuclear gene causes of primary mitochondrial disease when the causal gene pathogenic variant(s) are known in advance in a given family. Preimplantation genetic diagnosis for mtDNA pathogenic variants has become increasingly available and reliably performed in several European countries but remains limited in the United States at the time of this writing. Utilizing mitochondrial replacement therapies (MRT) to not just diagnose but actively reduce the heteroplasmy level for a known pathogenic mtDNA variant in oocytes or early-stage embryos remains legally prohibited in the United States at the time of this writing but is being performed under strict government oversight for select patients in the United Kingdom and Australia.

Future Therapies

Therapies under active development for mitochondrial diseases include gene-editing techniques to correct specific pathogenic variants in nuclear and mtDNA genes, intramitochondrial RNA or protein delivery (to replace mutated mitochondrial proteins), cellular therapies to shift mtDNA heteroplasmy levels (selectively damaging mutated mtDNA to increase proportion of wild type mtDNA), and a host of pharmacologic drug or nutrient therapies for a wide range of mitochondrial disease molecular causes, clinical subtypes, and health outcomes. Clinical trials for mitochondrial disease can be explored on https://clinicaltrials.gov.

Monitoring

Annual monitoring with cardiology, audiology, ophthalmology, and endocrinology is recommended to evaluate for the development of often-treatable organ-specific manifestations of mitochondrial disease. Growth and development should be closely monitored in children.

Specialists commonly needed to care for mitochondrial disease patients include a complex care coordinating primary care physician, geneticist or mitochondrial medicine clinician, neurologist, gastroenterologist, cardiologist, ophthalmologist, physiatrist, and therapists with expertise in physical, occupational, and speech/swallowing therapy. Other specific evaluations such as nephrology, neuropsychology, psychiatry, or exercise physiology evaluation may be helpful to pursue based on symptoms present. Laboratory measurement of certain analytes such as glutathione[1] (to support administration and dose optimization of n-acetylcysteine), leukocyte CoQ10 (for dosing of coenzyme Q10), and plasma amino acids (for dosing of arginine or citrulline) is helpful for management of mitochondrial supplements.

Considerations

There are few absolute medication prohibitions in mitochondrial disease, with careful consideration of the health status and potential benefit and risk of each medication the most prudent course. However, some medications are contraindicated in specific mitochondrial disease disorder, such as valproic acid that may induce fulminant liver failure in POLG-related disease and aminoglycosides, which can cause ototoxicity in certain mitochondrial diseases (m.1555A > G and m.1494C > T). Further, statins may induce or exacerbate myopathy by impairing coenzyme Q10 synthesis and inducing mtDNA depletion that may be reversible over time when statin therapy is discontinued. Prolonged use of certain anesthetics such as propofol (Diprivan) (for longer than 30–60 minutes) and volatile anesthetics (sevoflurane [Ultane], isoflurane [Forane, Terrell], etc.) should be carefully administered by knowledgeable clinicians or avoided as they can inhibit complex I activity. Indeed, a recent consortium review found that many medications previously "contraindicated" were being needlessly avoided by the mitochondrial disease patient population and rather, should each be discussed thoroughly with the individual treating clinicians.

Conflicts of Interest

SS and AG have no relevant conflicts of interest to declare. MJF is coinventor on International Patent Application No. PCT/US19/39631 entitled "Compositions and Methods for Treatment of Mitochondrial Respiratory Chain Dysfunction and Other Mitochondrial Disorders and Methods for Identifying Efficacious Agents for the Alleviating Symptoms of the Same," filed in the name of The Children's Hospital of Philadelphia on June 27, 2019. MJF is a scientific advisory board member with equity interest in RiboNova, Inc., and scientific board member as paid consultant with Khondrion and with Larimar Therapeutics.

MJF has previously been or is currently engaged with several companies involved in mitochondrial disease therapeutic preclinical and/or clinical stage development as a paid consultant (Astellas [formerly Mitobridge] Pharma, Inc., Casma Therapeutics, Cyclerion Therapeutics, Imel Therapeutics, Minovia Therapeutics, NeuroVive Pharmaceutical, Precision BioSciences, Primera Therapeutics, Reneo Therapeutics, Sanofi, Stealth BioTherapeutics, Zogenix, Inc.) and/or a sponsored research collaborator (AADI Therapeutics, Astellas [formerly Mitobridge] Pharma, Inc., Cyclerion Therapeutics, Epirium Therapeutics, Khondrion, Imel Therapeutics, Merck, Minovia Therapeutics Inc., Mission Therapeutics, NeuroVive Pharmaceutical, Raptor Therapeutics, REATA, Inc., RiboNova, Inc., Standigm Therapeutics, and Stealth BioTherapeutics), and has served as a paid speaker on mitochondrial disease (Platform Q).

Key Web Resources

Mitochondrial Disease Genes Compendium is a print and/or electronic reference for clinicians on mitochondrial disease from a gene-based perspective. (www.elsevier.com/books/mitochondrial-disease-genes-compendium/falk/978-0-12-820029-2).

Mitochondrial Disease Expert Panel Leigh Syndrome Gene Curation(https://search.clinicalgenome.org/kb/affiliate/10027?page=1&size=25&search=).

Mitochondrial Disease Sequence Resource (MSeqDR) is a publicly accessible bioinformatics resource that provides access to curated knowledge and tools designed to help evaluate nuclear and mtDNA related mitochondrial disease genes and variants(www.mseqdr.org).

Mitochondrial Medicine at Children's Hospital of Philadelphia\(www.chop.edu/centers-programs/mitochondrial-disease-clinical-center).

---

[1]Not FDA approved for this indication.
[7]Available as dietary supplement.

---

[1]Not FDA approved for this indication.

Mitochondrial Medicine Society(www.mitosoc.org/toolkit).
Mitomap is an online database of mitochondrial DNA variants reported to date.
United. Mitochondrial Disease Foundation. (www.umdf.org).

References

Alves CAPF, Teixeira SR, Martin-Saavedra JS, et al: Pediatric leigh syndrome: neuroimaging features and genetic correlations, *Ann Neurol* 88(2):218–232, 2020.

Bagger FO, Borgwardt L, Jespersen AS, et al: Whole genome sequencing in clinical practice, *BMC Med Genomics* 17(1):39, 2024.

Barcelos I, Shadiack E, Ganetzky RD, Falk MJ: Mitochondrial medicine therapies: rationale, evidence, and dosing guidelines, *Curr Opin Pediatr* 32(6):707–718, 2020.

Falk M: In Kliegman R St, Geme J, editors: *Nelson textbook of pediatrics*, ed 21, Elsevier, pp 807–811, 2020.

Flickinger J, Fan J, Wellik A, et al: Development of a mitochondrial myopathy-cdomposite assessment tool, *JCSM Clin Rep* 6(4):109–127, 2021.

Genetics of mitochondrial respiratory chain disease. In Ganetzky R, Falk M, Pyeritz R, Korf B, Korf B, Grody W, editors: *Emery and Rimoin's principles and practice of medical genetics and genomics*, 7 ed, Elsevier, pp 709–737, 2021.

Gorman GS, Chinnery PF, DiMauro S, et al: Mitochondrial diseases, *Nat Rev Dis Primers* 2:16080, 2016.

Muraresku CC, McCormick EM, Falk MJ: Mitochondrial Disease: advances in clinical diagnosis, management, therapeutic development, and preventative strategies, *Curr Genet Med Rep* 6(2):62–72, 2018.

Parikh S, Goldstein A, Koenig MK, et al: Diagnosis and management of mitochondrial disease: a consensus statement from the Mitochondrial Medicine Society, *Genet Med* 17(9):689–701, 2015.

Rahman S, Thorburn D. Nuclear Gene-Encoded Leigh Syndrome Spectrum Overview. 2015 Oct 1 [Updated 2020 Jul 16]. In: Adam MP, Ardinger HH, Pagon RA, et al., editors: GeneReviews® [Internet]. Seattle (WA): University of Washington, Seattle; 1993-2021. Available from: https://www.ncbi.nlm.nih.gov/books/NBK320989/

Schaefer A, Lim A, Gorman GM, Mancuso T: In Klopstock, editor: *Diagnosis and management of mitochondrial disorders*, Springer Nature, pp 63–74, 2019.

Zolkipli-Cunningham Z, Xiao R, Stoddart A, et al: Mitochondrial disease patient motivations and barriers to participate in clinical trials, *PLoS One* 13(5):e0197513, 2018.

NOCTURNAL ENURESIS

Method of
Alexander K.C. Leung, MBBS

Note: This chapter has been published in part in *Common Problems in Ambulatory Pediatrics: Specific Clinical Problems*, volume 1, with permission from Nova Science Publishers, Inc.

CURRENT DIAGNOSIS

- Nocturnal enuresis is defined as involuntary nighttime bedwetting in a child at least 5 years of age.
- Primary nocturnal enuresis is present when the child has never achieved a period of nighttime dryness greater than 6 consecutive months. Secondary nocturnal enuresis is present when the child has experienced a period of nighttime dryness of at least 6 consecutive months.
- The most common causes of primary nocturnal enuresis are a deep sleep pattern, nocturnal polyuria, and a small-capacity bladder or nocturnal detrusor overactivity.
- A urinalysis is warranted to rule out urinary tract infection, glycosuria, and a defect in the ability to concentrate urine.
- Ultrasound examination of the bladder (prevoid and postvoid) can be used to evaluate bladder dysfunction and functional bladder capacity.

CURRENT THERAPY

- Desmopressin (DDAVP, 1-deamino-8-arginine vasopressin) is indicated as a first-line therapy for children with monosymptomatic nocturnal enuresis associated with nocturnal polyuria and normal bladder function.
- Enuretic alarm is indicated as a first-line therapy for children with monosymptomatic nocturnal enuresis associated with a small bladder capacity or in children with severe enuretic symptoms refractory to desmopressin therapy.
- Behavioral therapy such as encouraging the child to urinate frequently during the daytime, emptying the bladder before bedtime, and restricting fluid in the evening may increase the success rate of pharmacologic therapy or enuretic alarm therapy.

Nocturnal enuresis is defined as involuntary nighttime bedwetting in a child at least 5 years of age. Primary nocturnal enuresis is present when the child has never achieved a period of nighttime dryness greater than 6 consecutive months. Secondary nocturnal enuresis is present when the child has experienced a period of nighttime dryness of at least 6 consecutive months. For the majority of children with secondary nocturnal enuresis, the pathogenesis is no different from that of primary nocturnal enuresis.

Nocturnal enuresis is a common problem that is frustrating for children, parents, and physicians alike. The condition may affect the child's self-esteem and may lead to reduced social interaction and behavioral problems.

Epidemiology

It has been estimated that 15% to 25% of 5-year-old children and 5% to 10% of 7-year-old children have nocturnal enuresis. Without specific treatment, approximately 15% of affected children become dry each year. The male-to-female ratio is approximately 3:1.

Risk Factors

Encopresis, daytime wetting (diurnal enuresis), and male gender are significant risk factors. Constipation, emotional stress, developmental delay, bladder dysfunction, sleep deprivation, adenotonsillar hypertrophy, and attention-deficit/hyperactivity disorder also play a role.

Pathogenesis

The most common causes of primary nocturnal enuresis are a high arousal threshold, nocturnal polyuria, and a small-capacity bladder or nocturnal detrusor overactivity. Although these causes may overlap, it is important to conceptualize them separately, because this differentiation will help the physician to understand the problem, to educate both the parents and child, and to plan an appropriate treatment program.

It has been shown that enuretic children have a high arousal threshold and a reduced prepulse inhibition of startle. In most children, arousability from sleep improves with maturation of the central nervous system.

In most circumstances, the rate of secretion of antidiuretic hormone from the posterior pituitary gland is increased at night. This circadian variation is usually established when the child is 3 to 4 years old. Some children with primary nocturnal enuresis have a lack of this circadian variation with an abnormally low nocturnal secretion of antidiuretic hormone with resultant nocturnal polyuria. Other causes of nocturnal polyuria include fluid and solute overload in the evening.

Children with a small-capacity bladder or nocturnal detrusor overactivity often have primary nocturnal enuresis. Conditions that may reduce the functional bladder capacity include cystitis and constipation.

There is a strong genetic component to nocturnal enuresis. The child of parents who were both enuretic has a 77% chance of developing enuresis. If one parent was enuretic, there is up to a 44% occurrence rate. If neither parent was enuretic, the occurrence rate is only 15%. Twin studies also support a genetic basis for nocturnal enuresis: the concordance rate is much higher in monozygotic twins (68%) when compared with dizygotic twins (36%). Linkage studies have suggested possible genetic markers for primary nocturnal enuresis located on chromosomes 12, 13, and 22.

A neurogenic bladder is one of the few anatomic abnormalities that can cause primary nocturnal enuresis. Congenital urethral obstruction is another infrequent anatomic cause of primary nocturnal enuresis. The enuresis in these children is due to an overflow phenomenon from a poorly compliant bladder. The most common cause of urethral obstruction in the male is posterior urethral valves. Girls and boys with significant congenital urethral stenosis may also present with this problem. An ectopic ureter or vesicovaginal fistula is an infrequent anatomic cause of primary nocturnal enuresis in girls.

A defect in the ability of the kidney to concentrate urine can cause primary nocturnal enuresis. The causes of concentrating defects include any cause of chronic renal failure and diabetes insipidus.

Diagnosis
History
Onset and Frequency
The timing of the onset and the frequency of nocturnal enuresis are important historical clues to the etiology. Secondary nocturnal enuresis and intermittent nocturnal enuresis are not usually associated with structural abnormalities in the urinary tract. Nocturnal enuresis due to a structural abnormality of the urinary tract is usually present from birth and is not associated with periods of remission.

Timing, Frequency, and Volume per Episode
A history of soaking absorbent underpants in the morning suggests nocturnal polyuria. Parents of children with nocturnal polyuria often remark that the volume of urine associated with the enuretic episode or the first morning void is very large. Frequent episodes of nocturnal enuresis with a small volume of urine suggest bladder dysfunction such as may occur with a urethral obstruction or a neurogenic bladder. Several episodes of nocturnal enuresis with a large volume suggest diabetes mellitus or diabetes insipidus. Constant wetting suggests an ectopic ureter or vesicovaginal fistula.

Associated Symptoms
Nocturnal enuresis associated with daytime urinary frequency, urgency, incontinence, and difficulties in initiating the urinary stream suggests urethral obstruction. Daytime urinary frequency, urgency, incontinence, squatting behavior, constipation, encopresis, gait disturbance, and a history of spina bifida or spinal trauma suggest a neurogenic bladder. Constant dampness in the underwear by day and night in a female suggests an ectopic ureter or vesicovaginal fistula. Secondary nocturnal enuresis associated with dysuria, urinary frequency, urgency, fever, suprapubic/loin pain, or cloudy, foul-smelling urine suggests a urinary tract infection. Polyuria, polydipsia, polyphagia, and weight loss suggest diabetes mellitus. Polyuria, polydipsia, and episodes of dehydration in a child with a history of central nervous system disease suggest diabetes insipidus. A history of constipation is important because the condition is associated with a reduced functional bladder capacity.

Volume of First Morning Void
Most children with nocturnal enuresis void only a small or average amount of urine in the morning after an enuretic episode. A large volume of urine voided following a significant episode of nocturnal enuresis may be a clue to the presence of low nocturnal secretion of antidiuretic hormone.

Soundness of Sleep
Children with nocturnal enuresis often sleep more deeply than other family members. Some children only wet when they are overtired. Conversely, children who are usually enuretic may be continent during periods of wakeful sleep such as during intercurrent illnesses.

Past Health
A child with a history of a structural abnormality of the urinary tract or neurogenic bladder may have nocturnal enuresis due to these causes. A history of spinal trauma may indicate a neurogenic bladder as a cause of enuresis. A history of central nervous system disorder may indicate neurogenic diabetes insipidus. Certain medications such as methylxanthines and caffeine may be associated with nocturnal enuresis.

Family History
A family history of nocturnal enuresis should be sought because nocturnal enuresis tends to run in the family. A family history of diabetes mellitus, diabetes insipidus, or kidney disease suggests the corresponding disorder. Any stressful events in the family such as birth of a sibling and parental disharmony should be explored, especially in children with secondary nocturnal enuresis.

Physical Examination
Height and weight should be measured and plotted onto standard growth charts. All children should have their blood pressure checked, which, if elevated, might indicate renal disease. A thorough physical examination should include examination of the abdomen and genitalia and a complete neurologic examination. In chronic constipation, fecal masses are often palpable in the left lower quadrant of the abdomen and in the suprapubic area.

In the majority of children with primary nocturnal enuresis, the physical examination is unremarkable. An abnormal physical examination is only present when primary nocturnal enuresis is due to a structural cause. A myelomeningocele is usually obvious at birth; however, subtle spinal defects may also be associated with primary nocturnal enuresis. A midline tuft of hair, an exaggerated dimple, or a birthmark in the area of the lumbosacral spine; a gait abnormality; absence of anal wink; or abnormal motor power, tone, reflexes, or sensation in the lower extremities suggests a neurogenic bladder. A palpably enlarged bladder or kidney and a weak or dribbling urinary stream suggests urinary obstruction, such as may result from posterior urethral valves.

Laboratory and Imaging Studies
A urinalysis is warranted to rule out urinary tract infection, diabetes mellitus, and a defect in the ability to concentrate urine. Ultrasound examination of the bladder (prevoid and postvoid) can be used to evaluate bladder dysfunction and functional bladder capacity.

Treatment
One essential part of the treatment plan of every child with primary nocturnal enuresis should be compassion and support from both the family and physician. It is important to clarify to parents that the child is not at fault and to specify that punishment for bedwetting is inappropriate. The child and family can be reassured that in the absence of structural defect, primary nocturnal enuresis tends to resolve with time.

Simple behavioral strategies such as encouraging the child to urinate frequently during the daytime, emptying the bladder before bedtime, and limiting fluid and solute intake in the evening are often recommended. Caffeinated beverages should be avoided, particularly in the evening. Some authors recommend waking the child 1.5 to 2 hours after bedtime to go to the bathroom. Star charts and reward systems need to reinforce positive behavior. Behavioral therapy may increase the success rate of pharmacologic therapy or enuretic alarm therapy.

Desmopressin (DDAVP, 1-deamino-8-arginine vasopressin) is an analogue of vasopressin that has a profound antidiuretic activity without pressor activity. The medication acts on the V2 receptors of the renal tubules and increases the reabsorption of fluid from the renal tubules, thereby decreasing the amount of urine produced. The medication is indicated as a first-line therapy for children with monosymptomatic nocturnal enuresis associated with nocturnal polyuria and normal bladder function. Desmopressin is available in a sublingual lyophilisate (melt) preparation,[2] as well as a tablet. The bioavailability of the lyophilisate (melt) preparation is approximately 60% greater than that of the tablet formulation. The recommended dose of desmopressin is 120 to 240 µg melt and 200 to 400 µg tablet. The former is usually given 30 minutes to 1 hour before bedtime, and the latter is usually given 1 hour before bedtime. Side effects are rare and include symptomatic hyponatremia with water intoxication. When desmopressin is prescribed, patients should be instructed to avoid high fluid intake in the evening.

Imipramine (Tofranil), a tricyclic agent with antimuscarinic property, may be helpful in children who have not responded to desmopressin alone. Presumably, the medication decreases the amount of time spent in rapid eye movement sleep, stimulates antidiuretic hormone secretion, and relaxes the detrusor muscle. The recommended starting dose is 25 mg for children 6 to 12 years of age and 50 mg for those older than 12 years, given 1 to 2 hours before bedtime. If necessary, the dose may be increased gradually to a maximum of 50 mg in children 6 to 12 years of age and 75 mg for those older than 12 years. However, potential side effects (anxiety, depression, dizziness, headache, drowsiness, lethargy, sleep disturbance, dry mouth, anorexia, vomiting, skin rashes) and serious adverse effects (hepatotoxicity, cardiotoxicity) with overdose limit their use.

Monotherapy with oxybutynin (Ditropan),[1] an anticholinergic and antispasmodic agent that decreases uninhibited bladder contraction, is not effective in treating monosymptomatic nocturnal enuresis. The medication can be added, however, as a second-line drug in the treatment of children with both diurnal and nocturnal enuresis. The dose is 5 mg administered 1 hour before bedtime.

Enuretic alarm is indicated as a first-line therapy for children with monosymptomatic nocturnal enuresis associated with a small bladder capacity or nocturnal detrusor overactivity. Randomized controlled trials have demonstrated that the enuretic alarm has greater efficacy than other forms of treatment. The enuretic alarm is triggered when a sensor in the sheets or night clothes gets wet; a bell or buzzer is thereby activated. Presumably, alarm therapy startles the child and improves arousal from sleep either by classical conditioning or avoidance conditioning. A disadvantage of alarm therapy is that it takes a couple of weeks to take effect. As such, alarms should be used for at least 6 weeks in children who do not respond before discontinuing their use. Because success depends on a cooperative, motivated child, conditioning therapy with an alarm device is generally used in children over 6 years of age.

It has been shown that combination of alarm and desmopressin works better than either treatment alone. Such treatment may be considered for children with refractory nocturnal enuresis.

When an anatomic abnormality or defect in urinary concentration ability is present, the underlying problem may require specific dietary, pharmacologic, or surgical treatment. Any underlying constipation should also be treated.

---

[1] Not FDA approved for this indication.
[2] Not available in the United States.

References

Brown ML, Pope AW, Brown EJ: Treatment of primary nocturnal enuresis in children: a review, *Child Care Health Dev* 37:153–160, 2011.
Glazener CM, Evans JH: Desmopressin for nocturnal enuresis in children, *Cochrane Database Syst Rev* 3:CD002112, 2002.
Glazener CM, Evans JH, Pero RE: Alarm interventions for nocturnal enuresis in children, *Cochrane Database Syst Rev* 2:CD002911, 2005.
Kamperis K, Hagstroem S, Rittig S, et al: Combination of the enuresis alarm and desmopressin: Second line treatment for nocturnal enuresis, *J Urol* 179:1128–1131, 2008.
Leung AK: Nocturnal enuresis. In Leung AK, editor: Common Problems in Ambulatory Pediatrics: Specific Clinical Problems, vol 1. New York, 2011, Nova Science Publishers, pp 161–171.
Lottmann H, Froeling F, Alloussi S, et al: A randomized comparison of oral desmopressin lyophilisate (MELT) and tablet formulations in children and adolescents with primary nocturnal enuresis, *Int J Clin Pract* 61:1454–1460, 2007.
Nevéus T: Nocturnal enuresis—theoretic background and practical guidelines, *Pediatr. Nephrol* 26:1207–1214, 2011.
Robson WL: Evaluation and management of enuresis, *N Engl J Med* 360:1429–1436, 2009.
Robson WL, Leung AK, van Howe R: Primary and secondary nocturnal enuresis: similarities in presentation, *Pediatrics* 115:956–959, 2005.
Robson WL, Leung AK, Norgaard JP: The comparative safety of oral versus intranasal desmopressin in the treatment of children with nocturnal enuresis, *J Urol* 178:24–30, 2007.
Van de Walle J, Rittig S, Bauer S, et al: Practical consensus guidelines for the management of enuresis, *Eur J Pediatr* 171:971–983, 2012.

OBESITY IN CHILDREN

Method of
Mostafa Salama, MBBCh; and Seema Kumar, MD

CURRENT DIAGNOSIS

- Obesity is a serious health problem affecting a large number of children and adolescents in the United States and worldwide. Body mass index (BMI) derived from weight and height is used to classify overweight and obesity. It is calculated as weight in kilograms divided by height (or length) in meters squared (kg/m²).
- A child 2 years of age or older is diagnosed as having overweight if the BMI is at or above the 85th percentile and below the 95th percentile for age and sex, as having obesity if the BMI is at or above the 95th percentile, and as having severe obesity if the BMI is at or above 120% of the 95th percentile or at or above 35 kg/m² (whichever is lower).
- The Centers for Disease Control and Prevention (CDC) recommends using growth curves based on the World Health Organization reference standards for infants and toddlers younger than 2 years of age and using the CDC/National Center for Health Statistics growth reference standards for children 2 years of age or older.

CURRENT THERAPY

- Lifestyle modifications including dietary changes, increased physical activity, and decreased sedentary time are crucial for prevention and treatment of childhood obesity.
- Family-based lifestyle interventions and a multidisciplinary team approach are key components to implement healthy lifestyle changes.
- Pharmacotherapy is recommended as an adjunct to health behavior and lifestyle modification for adolescents aged 12 and older with obesity (BMI ≥ 95th percentile).
- Bariatric surgery has been shown to result in significant weight loss and should be considered for adolescents with severe obesity and those who have significant obesity-related comorbidities.

Introduction

Childhood obesity has emerged as an important public health problem in the United States and across the globe. The increasing prevalence of childhood obesity, severe obesity, and weight-related comorbidities places great risk on affected individuals, societies, and healthcare infrastructure. Moreover, childhood obesity tracks closely with obesity in adulthood, especially those with severe obesity and/or a strong family history of obesity, a relationship that foreshadows bigger problems for future generations. Childhood obesity and evidence-based treatment guidelines are discussed in this chapter.

Diagnosis

Childhood obesity is marked by excess accumulation of body fat. Body mass index (BMI) is considered the most practical method for evaluation of obesity. BMI is calculated from weight in kilograms and the square of the height (or length) in meters, as shown:

$$BMI = \frac{Weight\ (kg)}{Height\ (m^2)}$$

Normal growth and development during childhood results in dynamic changes in weight and height, which vary based on age and sex. Childhood growth parameters, including BMI, may then be plotted against growth curves created from standardized reference populations, normalized by age and sex. The World Health Organization (WHO) has developed growth standards for infants and children up to 5 years of age, and the Centers for Disease Control and Prevention (CDC) has similarly published reference standards for individuals between ages 2 and 20 years. The CDC recommends using the WHO standards from infancy until a child's second birthday and the CDC/National Center for Health Statistics standards for children 2 years of age and older.

Weight status categories for children are generally segregated by BMI percentile by age and sex. Weight status in childhood is categorized as follows: underweight, normal weight, overweight, obese, and severe obesity. Obesity can be further classified as follows: class I obesity, defined as BMI at or above the 95th percentile to less than 120% of the 95th percentile; class II obesity, defined as BMI at or above 120% to less than 140% of the 95th percentile or BMI at or above 35 kg/m² and below 40 kg/m² (whichever is lower); and class III obesity, defined as BMI at or above 140% of the 95th percentile or BMI at or above 40 kg/m² (whichever is lower).

Epidemiology

The prevalence of obesity among children has more than tripled over the last 4 decades. However, it has stabilized in recent years (Figure 1). The prevalence of severe obesity in childhood, on the other hand, continues to increase. According to the 2017 to 2018 National Health and Nutrition Examination Survey, 16.1% of U.S. children have overweight, and 19.3% have obesity. Overweight affects 12.3% of preschool-aged children, 15.4% of school-aged children, and 19.4% of adolescents. Obesity affects 13.4% of preschool-aged children, 20.3% of school-aged children, and 21.2% of adolescents.

The overall prevalence of severe obesity in this survey was 6.1%. Childhood obesity is more common among Black populations, Mexican Americans, and American Indians than in non-Hispanic White populations and Asians. The presence of parental obesity increases the risk of obesity in children. Additionally, higher prevalence of obesity is associated with lower socioeconomic status.

Pathophysiology

Childhood obesity develops as a result of a complex interaction between genetic, metabolic, environmental, and behavioral factors. As such, our historical understanding of "weight equals calories in minus calories out" is an oversimplification of obesity and its pathophysiology. Environmental factors such as family socioeconomic status, wealth, and access to food; neighborhood safety and available community activities; and family dietary patterns are all critical components. Approximately 40% to 85% of variability in adipose tissue deposition may be contributed to heritable factors (polygenic and largely unidentified genetic changes). Having one obese parent increases the risk of childhood obesity by two- to threefold; having two obese parents increases that risk by up to 15-fold. Obesity can rarely (<1% of childhood obesity) result from single gene mutations (e.g., melanocortin 4 receptor deficiency, leptin deficiency, leptin receptor deficiency) and congenital syndromes (e.g., Prader-Willi, Bardet-Biedel, Cohen) (Table 1). As children age and gain more control over their surroundings, individual factors such as lifestyle and dietary choices may also play a role. A host of other etiologic factors include endocrine disorders, neurologic and hypothalamic disorders, and medications.

Environmental factors affecting childhood obesity are diverse and complex. Specific dietary factors that portend risk of childhood obesity include sugar-sweetened beverages, sweet snacks, fast foods, large portion sizes, and maladaptive coping strategies such as eating to suppress negative emotions. Adverse childhood events and emotion and psychological distress increase the risk of childhood obesity. Intrauterine growth restriction and birth size, as well as antibiotic use, may also be predictive factors. Children, adolescents, and adults are also now spending less time being physically active. Time is increasingly spent in sedentary activities such as use of electronic devices: cellular phones, television, tablets, and computers. Evidence suggests that shortened sleep duration and/or decreased quality of sleep also contribute to development of obesity.

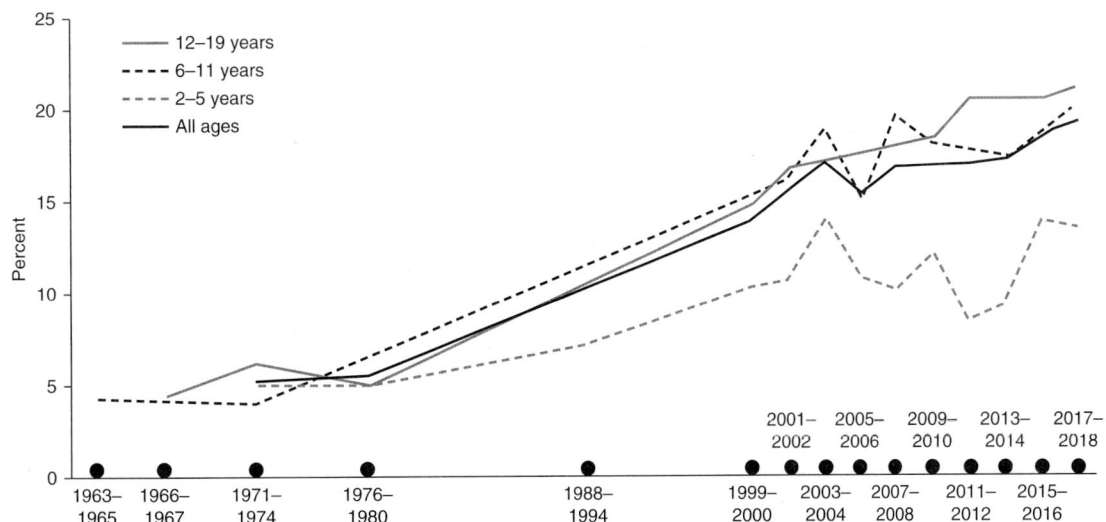

Figure 1 Trends in obesity among children and adolescents aged 2 to 19 years, by age: United States, 1963 to 1965 through 2017 to 2018. National Center for Health Statistics, National Health Examination Surveys II [ages 6–11], III [ages 12–17]; and National Health and Nutrition Examination Surveys [NHANES] I–III, and NHANES 1999–2000, 2001–2002, 2003–2004, 2005–2006, 2007–2008, 2009–2010, 2011–2012, 2013–2014, 2015–2016, and 2017–2018.

TABLE 1 Secondary Causes of Pediatric Obesity

Monogenic Disorders
Leptin deficiency
Leptin dysfunction
Leptin receptor deficiency
Proopiomelanocortin deficiency
Melanocortin 4 receptor
   haploinsufficiency
Melanocortin receptor accessory
   protein 2
Proconvertase 1 deficiency

Syndromes
Prader-Willi
Bardet-Biedl
Cohen
Alström
Albright hereditary
   osteodystrophy
Beckwith-Wiedemann
Carpenter

Neurologic
Brain injury
Brain tumor

Endocrine
Hypothyroidism
Glucocorticoid excess (Cushing
   syndrome)
Growth hormone deficiency
Pseudohypoparathyroidism

Drug Induced
Tricyclic antidepressants
Steroid hormones (e.g.,
   glucocorticoids, birth control
   pills)
Antipsychotic drugs
Antiepileptic drugs
Diabetic medications (e.g.,
   sulfonylureas, insulin,
   thiazolidinediones)
Antidepressants (e.g., tricyclic
   antidepressants, selective
   serotonin reuptake inhibitors)
Beta blockers

Hypothalamic Causes
Tumor
After brain surgery/radiation
   (craniopharyngioma)
ROHHAD/ROHHADNET
   syndrome

ROHHAD, Rapid-onset obesity with hypoventilation, hypothalamic, and autonomic dysregulation; *ROHHADNET,* rapid-onset obesity with hypoventilation, hypothalamic, autonomic dysregulation, neuroendocrine tumor.
Adapted from Kumar S, Kelly AS. Review of childhood obesity: from epidemiology, etiology, and comorbidities to clinical assessment and treatment. *Mayo Clin Proc.* 2017;92(2):251-265.

Clinical Manifestations and Associated Comorbidities

Obesity is categorized as a complex chronic disease by the American Medical Association. Obesity affects essentially every organ system, most notably the endocrine, gastrointestinal, pulmonary, cardiovascular, musculoskeletal, and psychological systems. Importantly, comorbid conditions once thought to be "adult onset"—type 2 diabetes mellitus (T2DM), dyslipidemia, obstructive sleep apnea (OSA), and steatohepatitis—are now commonly encountered in children with obesity.

Cardiometabolic and Cardiovascular

Children with obesity have increased risk of developing prediabetes and T2DM, an association that varies with age and ethnicity. Children with T2DM tend to have higher rates of poor response to metformin therapy and more rapid progression of complications of diabetes, compared with those who present with T2DM later in life. Children with obesity also have a high prevalence of cardiometabolic risk factors, including hypertension (approximately 50% of obese children and adolescents) and associated echocardiographic left ventricular hypertrophy, low levels of high-density lipoprotein cholesterol, and elevated triglycerides. Obesity during childhood is associated with an increased risk for cardiovascular disease during adult life, even after adjusting for BMI during adulthood.

Endocrine

Children with obesity may experience accelerated linear growth and skeletal maturation. Postpubertal females with obesity are also at greater risk of developing hyperandrogenism and polycystic ovarian syndrome, commonly associated with menstrual irregularities, hirsutism, acne, and acanthosis nigricans.

Pulmonary

Obesity during childhood is a significant risk factor for OSA. The severity of OSA and its prevalence are directly related to the severity of obesity. Children with obesity are also at risk for alveolar hypoventilation syndrome, which can result in significant blood-oxygen desaturation and carbon dioxide retention. Childhood obesity is also associated with asthma.

Gastrointestinal

Childhood obesity is associated with a spectrum of liver abnormalities known as nonalcoholic fatty liver disease. This disease spectrum—progressing from nonalcoholic fatty liver to nonalcoholic steatohepatitis to cirrhosis—is the most common cause of liver disease in children in the United States. Children with obesity also are at increased risk for gastroesophageal reflux disease.

Musculoskeletal

Limited mobility, lower extremity joint pain and back pain, genu valgum, lower extremity malalignment, and fractures are more common among obese children than nonobese children. Obesity during childhood is also a predisposing factor to unilateral or bilateral slipped capital femoral epiphysis and tibia vara (Blount disease).

Psychosocial

Psychosocial consequences of childhood obesity are numerous and include poor self-esteem, depression, anxiety, alienation, distorted body image, and low self-reported quality of life. Psychosocial disturbances increase in prevalence and severity with age and are more common in females. Children with obesity are more likely to experience bullying and discrimination. Adult women who were obese during childhood years completed fewer years of advanced education and had greater rates of poverty and lower rates of marriage compared with normal-weight peers. Obesity has also been associated with disordered eating patterns. Overweight or obese adolescents are more likely to engage in self-induced vomiting or laxative use. Weight talk by family members and healthcare providers, and especially weight teasing, is related to disordered eating patterns.

Dermatologic

Obesity is associated with several dermatologic conditions, including acanthosis nigricans, intertrigo, hidradenitis suppurativa, furunculosis, and stretch marks.

Neurologic

Idiopathic intracranial hypertension (pseudotumor cerebri) is rare in childhood but more prevalent among obese children. This risk is further increased among children with severe obesity. Symptoms include headache, vomiting, visual disturbances, and retroocular eye pain. Retinal examination is significant for papilledema.

Clinical Evaluation of the Child With Obesity

Initial evaluation of a pediatric patient with obesity should include a thorough history and physical examination. These components are generally sufficient to determine the cause of the obesity and help the clinician in selecting the children that need further evaluation with laboratory and radiologic testing.

Obtaining an effective history requires identifying factors contributing to obesity and screening for obesity-related comorbid conditions. Dietary history should detail eating habits including frequency, content, and location of meals and snacks. Identifying intake of both calorie-dense foods, such as fruit juices and soda, as well as healthy foods such as fresh vegetables and fruits, is helpful with dietary recommendations and with motivational interviewing. Physical activity assessment should detail time spent in unstructured play, organized sports, school recess, physical education, and recreational screen time. Identifying interest in specific physical activities, regardless of current participation, can be incorporated into motivational interviewing techniques. Medical history should include height, weight, and BMI growth trajectories and use of medications that may cause weight gain such as steroids, antipsychotic drugs, and antiepileptic drugs. Identification of developmental delay during a careful developmental history may suggest genetic or chromosomal causes for obesity. A complete review of systems may be helpful in determining secondary causes of obesity (Table 1) and screening for obesity-related comorbidities such as OSA, musculoskeletal problems, and idiopathic intracranial hypertension. Psychosocial screening should evaluate for bullying, depression, disordered eating habits, and family support and other social support.

Physical examination should include accurate measurement of weight and height and evaluation for dysmorphic features that could represent monogenic or syndromal obesity. Children with obesity and short stature are more likely to have a genetic or syndromic form of obesity. Weight gain in a child with poor linear growth can be indicative of an endocrine cause for obesity such as Cushing syndrome. Physical examination should include evaluation for comorbid features of obesity. A few examples include skin examination for acanthosis nigricans, funduscopic examination to evaluate for papilledema, and musculoskeletal examination for bowing of the legs. Laboratory evaluation is recommended to identify comorbid conditions in children with obesity. These specific recommendations include obtaining fasting lipid profile for all children who have overweight or obesity, and the frequency of follow-up testing should be every 1 to 3 years depending on the child's risk profile. Measurement of serum alanine aminotransferase (ALT) is recommended for screening for fatty liver disease in children who have obesity, with retesting every 2 to 3 years if initial ALT is normal. Screening for T2DM with fasting glucose or hemoglobin A1c is recommended in children with overweight or obesity with one or more risk factors for T2DM. These risk factors include family history of T2DM in a first- or second-degree relative; high-risk race/ethnicity (Native American, African American, Hispanic, Asian American, Pacific Islander); maternal history of diabetes or gestational diabetes mellitus during the child's gestation; small for gestational age; signs of insulin resistance on physical examination such as acanthosis nigricans; and conditions associated with insulin resistance (hypertension, polycystic ovary syndrome, dyslipidemia). Screening for T2DM is recommended starting at 10 years of age or sooner if onset of puberty occurs before age 10. Rescreening should occur every 1 to 3 years depending on the weight trajectory and risk factor profile.

Children in whom a genetic, syndromic, or endocrine cause of obesity is suspected need to undergo specific testing. Children with signs and symptoms of OSA should be evaluated with overnight polysomnography. Children with features suggestive of idiopathic intracranial hypertension require head imaging and referral to appropriate experts.

Treatment

Managing childhood overweight and obesity is challenging but, when conducted properly, can be both effective and rewarding. It is crucial to treat obesity as a chronic disease. Therefore long-term care strategies should be considered. These include ongoing monitoring of obesity and associated comorbidities and ensuring access to treatment. Obesity management requires a primary healthcare team approach. A patient-centered, nonstigmatizing approach should be offered to every child with obesity.

Weight Management Goals

The goals for weight management are dependent on the child's age, the severity of the obesity, and the presence of obesity-related comorbidities. In children with mild obesity who are continuing to grow, maintenance of weight or slower rate of weight gain compared with previous is sufficient as that itself will lead to a decrease in BMI percentile. On the other hand, weight loss is recommended for children with severe obesity. A weight loss of up to 1 lb per month is safe for children between 2 and 11 years of age with obesity and comorbid conditions. More weight loss (up to 1–2 lbs per week) is safe in adolescents with obesity and comorbidities, although this degree of weight loss may not be

feasible with lifestyle interventions only. Very modest reductions in BMI z score have been associated with improvement in cardiometabolic risk factors.

Lifestyle Interventions

Management of obesity should start with identifying the child's and family's motivations to change, which can be achieved by using a motivational interviewing model. This is a nonjudgmental method of interviewing that helps people resolve feelings of ambivalence about wanting to change and not wanting to change and to find the inner motivation to make lifestyle changes. The process involves reflective listening and helps children/families realize their own strengths, values, and motivation to change. This tool has been shown to be useful in treatment of childhood obesity. This can be reinforced by engaging families to change selected behaviors such as increasing physical activity, choosing healthier dietary options, and improving sleep hygiene.

The ongoing relationship between the patient/family and healthcare team should identify challenges that can predispose to treatment failure. Underlying health conditions, mental health issues, and socioeconomic barriers may challenge the achievement of weight loss. Children and their families should identify appropriate behavioral changes and strategies to improve weight status. These strategies include encouraging healthy nutrition, increasing physical activity, and decreasing sedentary behavior. The treatment team should emphasize realistic expectations and develop plans to deal with relapse.

Intensive health behavior and lifestyle change are preferred and recommended for children and adolescents with obesity. This can be facilitated by a multidisciplinary team with dieticians, behavioral counselors (e.g., social workers, psychologists, other mental health practitioners or trained nurse practitioners), an exercise specialist, and a primary care provider who oversees the intervention and manages medical issues. Evidence suggests that delivering 26 hours or more of face-to-face family-based counseling over at least a 3- to-12-month period is effective for weight management for children. Unfortunately, programs with this level of intensity may not be available to each family due to limited resources and financial or transportation challenges. The primary care team can support families by connecting them with community resources to support nutrition and address food insecurity (e.g., food provision programs) and physical activity (e.g., local parks, recreation programs). There is no evidence that intensive lifestyle and behavior interventions cause any serious adverse effects in children or adolescents with overweight or obesity. Evidence-based pediatric obesity treatment has also been shown to reduce the risk for disordered eating.

Specific health behaviors should be recommended to improve energy balance and quality of life. A family-centered approach has been shown to be more effective than a child-centered approach to achieve sustainable weight reduction.

Physical Activity

Enhancing physical activity is an important component of lifestyle change for weight management. Sixty minutes of moderate to vigorous physical activity per day is associated with improved BMI status and cardiometabolic profile. Activities that are fun for children, such as water-based and other non–weight-bearing activities are frequently preferred. Another important component of lifestyle change is reduction in sedentary behavior, including a limitation on screen time. The American Academy of Pediatrics (AAP) recommends no screen time for children younger than 18 months and only 1 hour per day for children ages 2 to 5 years. For older children, parents should have a monitoring plan for media use with a goal of appropriate, non excessive use but without a defined upper limit. Alternative options that are widely accepted by children and adolescents include video "exergames" that require light to moderate physical activity.

Nutrition

Adequate nutrition is a fundamental aspect of lifestyle change for weight management. Consumption of sugar-containing beverages and energy drinks has been associated with increased weight gain in children. Limiting the intake of food made with simple sugar or with a high fat or caloric content is recommended. As nutrition is crucial for children's growth and development, it is important to ensure a balanced meal composition, without caloric restriction, including nutrient-dense but not caloric-dense meals with an adequate mixture of protein and carbohydrates. Some weight management programs use a "traffic light" dietary format, labeling foods as red, yellow, or green on the basis of energy density (red foods indicate high calorie density, green foods indicate low calorie density). Children are encouraged to eat green foods frequently and red foods more sparingly, such as on special occasions. Behavioral modifications, including avoidance of breakfast skipping and maintenance of good sleep hygiene, are associated with better weight reduction outcomes. There is no evidence suggesting greater short-term or long-term efficacy of a specific type of diet for weight loss in children with obesity.

The *5–2–1–0 model* includes multiple aspects of lifestyle modification such as nutrition, screen time and physical activity. The model entails five servings of fruits and vegetables a day in addition to a balanced diet, 2 hours or less of screen time per day, 1 hour or more of moderate to vigorous physical activity per day, and no (or nearly no) sugar-sweetened beverages.

Pharmacologic Therapy

Use of medications for weight loss in children should be done under the care of a physician with expertise in use of these medications. Regular monitoring for efficacy and side effects is essential (Table 2). Pharmacotherapy can be considered as an adjunct to lifestyle interventions, especially in adolescents with severe obesity and associated comorbidities. Continuation of pharmacotherapy is recommended if the medication is felt to be effective, as demonstrated by a 5% or greater BMI reduction from baseline within 12 weeks on the optimal dose, or if slowing down/arrest of weight gain is considered satisfactory due to linear growth in adolescence. Weight-loss medications should be discontinued in the presence of side effects that persist despite adjustment of the dose. Adolescence is defined as ages 10 to 19 years by the WHO and ages 11 to 21 years by the AAP.

Orlistat (Xenical) is approved by the U.S. Food and Drug Administration (FDA) for treatment of obesity in children 12 years of age and older. It is a lipase inhibitor that, when taken at the recommended dose of 120 mg three times a day with meals, blocks absorption of about one-third of fat digested in a meal. Lower doses of 60 mg three times per day with meals are available over the counter (Alli).[1] Side effects include flatulence, oily spotting, fatty stools, diarrhea, and potential for micronutrient deficiencies. Long-term safety data are lacking. The efficacy of orlistat over placebo for treatment of childhood obesity is modest, decreasing BMI by less than 1 kg/m² after 1 year of therapy.

Liraglutide (Saxenda) is a glucagon-like 1 (GLP-1) receptor agonist that is FDA approved for weight management in children and adolescents 12 years and older. It is given subcutaneously at a maximum dose of 3 mg daily. A recent randomized, double-blind, controlled trial in adolescents 12 to less than 18 years of age showed placebo-subtracted BMI reduction of −0.22 kg/m² at 56 weeks; 43% of subjects achieved a BMI reduction of at least 5%. Adverse effects include nausea, vomiting, abdominal pain, diarrhea, and potential hypoglycemia. Semaglutide (Wegovy) is another GLP-1 receptor agonist that is given subcutaneously once weekly and is approved by the FDA for weight management in children at least 12 years of age. In a double-blind, randomized, placebo-controlled trial including 180 adolescents aged from 12 to less than 18 years, semaglutide was associated with a change in mean BMI of −16.1% relative to 0.6% in the placebo group. GLP-1 receptor agonists are contraindicated in patients with a personal or

family history of medullary thyroid cancer or multiple endocrine neoplasia 2A or 2B.

Phentermine (Adipex-P) is a sympathomimetic drug (Schedule IV controlled substance) that potentiates the release of norepinephrine in the hypothalamus, causing decreased appetite. It is approved by the FDA for short-term use in individuals 17 years of age or older. In one study, phentermine was associated with greater reduction in BMI by −1.6% at 1 month of treatment (95% confidence interval [CI] −2.6, −0.6%; $P = 0.001$), −2.9% at 3 months of treatment (CI −4.5, −1.4%, $P < 0.001$), and −4.1% at 6 months (95% CI −7.1, −1%, $P = 0.009$) of treatment compared with standard care consisting of lifestyle interventions only. Adverse effects of phentermine include insomnia, restlessness, dry mouth, anxiety, euphoria, palpitations, hypertension, cardiac arrhythmias, headache, dizziness, visual disturbances, and ocular irritation. Phentermine is contraindicated in patients with hyperthyroidism, glaucoma, cardiovascular disease, or history of drug abuse.

Topiramate (Topamax) is a medication that is used off-label for treatment of obesity in children. The weight-loss effect is likely mediated through modulation of various neurotransmitters. This drug is FDA approved for treatment of epilepsy in children aged 2 years and older and for migraine prophylaxis in children 12 years of age and older. Adverse effects include cognitive dysfunction, paresthesias, metabolic acidosis, kidney stones, and teratogenicity. Adolescents must be counseled about pregnancy because of decreased efficacy of oral contraceptives with treatment. Topiramate has modest efficacy for treatment of obesity. In a small, randomized, placebo-controlled, clinical pilot trial of 30 adolescents, a 2% reduction in BMI at 6 months was noted on topiramate 75 mg daily.

A combination of both topiramate and phentermine (Qsymia) is approved by the FDA for treatment of children with obesity at least 12 years of age. A dose of 15 mg of phentermine and 92 mg of extended-release topiramate was associated with a decrease in BMI of 10.44%, whereas 7.5 mg of phentermine and 46 mg of extended-release topiramate was associated with an 8.11% BMI reduction.

Setmelanotide (Imcivree), a melanocortin 4 receptor agonist, is approved for adults and children age 2 years and older with obesity due to Bardet-Biedl syndrome or due to genetically confirmed proopiomelanocortin (POMC), proprotein convertase subtilisin/kexin type 1 (PCSK1), or leptin receptor (LEPR) deficiency. In a single-arm, open-label, multicenter phase III trial, 80% (8/10) of participants with POMC deficiency and 45% (5/11) of participants with LEPR deficiency achieved at least 10% weight loss at approximately 1 year. Adverse events include injection site reaction, skin hyperpigmentation, nausea, vomiting, and skin discoloration.

Metformin (Glucophage, Glumetza, Riomet) is approved by the FDA for treatment of T2DM in children 10 years of age and older. Use of metformin for weight loss is considered off-label. It may be particularly useful in adolescents with prediabetes,[1] metabolic syndrome,[1] polycystic ovary syndrome,[1] and insulin resistance.[1] Metformin also may be helpful in children with weight gain secondary to treatment with antipsychotic drugs.[1] The dose may be gradually increased as tolerated to a maximum of 2000 mg/day. Improvements in BMI have been modest, with a metaanalysis finding BMI z-score reduction of 0.10 and BMI reduction of 0.86 mg/kg². Adverse effects include abdominal discomfort, diarrhea, flatulence, vitamin B_2 deficiency, and lactic acidosis.

Bariatric Procedures

Bariatric procedures, including bariatric surgery, should be considered for adolescents (≥13 years) with severe obesity and, often, with significant health comorbidities (Table 3). Severe obesity in childhood is a unique subset that has outpaced less severe forms of childhood obesity in prevalence. Importantly, lifestyle modifications alone have not demonstrated significant and lasting weight loss in children with severe obesity.

---

[1]Not FDA approved for this indication.

[1]Not FDA approved for this indication.

TABLE 2	Pharmacologic Agents Used as FDA-Approved and Off-Label Treatments for Childhood Obesity			
DRUG NAME	**MECHANISM OF ACTION**	**FDA INDICATION**	**SIDE EFFECTS**	**ADOLESCENT WEIGHT-LOSS OUTCOMES DATA**
FDA Approved				
Phentermine (Adipex-P)	Sympathomimetic amine	Obesity >16 years of age for short-term treatment	Dry mouth, insomnia, irritability, increased heart rate, blood pressure, constipation, anxiety	Decreased BMI by 4.1% at 6 months
Phentermine/ topiramate (Qsymia)	Sympathomimetic/ Modulation of various neurotransmitters	Obesity in ≥12 years	Phentermine: Insomnia, dry mouth, palpitation, anxiety, increased blood pressure Topiramate: cognitive dysfunction, metabolic acidosis, teratogenicity, and kidney stones	Randomized double-blind clinical trial: 15 mg of phentermine and 92 mg of extended-release topiramate associated with decrease in BMI of 10.44%, whereas 7.5 mg of phentermine and 46 mg of extended-release topiramate associated with an 8.11% BMI reduction
Liraglutide (Saxenda)	GLP-1 receptor agonist	Obesity in ≥12 years	Nausea, vomiting, abdominal pain, diarrhea, potential hypoglycemia	Placebo subtracted BMI reduction of −0.22 kg/m² at 56 weeks
Semaglutide (Wegovy)	GLP-1 receptor agonist	Obesity in ≥12 years	Nausea, vomiting, abdominal pain, diarrhea, potential hypoglycemia	Double blind randomized placebo controlled trial: BMI reduction of 16.1% from baseline relative to 0.6% in placebo-treated group
Setmelanotide (Imcivree)	Melanocortin 4 receptor agonist	Obesity at age ≥2 years due to Bardet Biedl syndrome, genetically confirmed POMC, PCSK1, or LEPR deficiency	Injection site reaction, skin hyperpigmentation, nausea, vomiting, skin discoloration	BMI reduction of at least 5% achieved by 43% of subjects; At least 10% weight loss at approximately 1 year achieved by 80% of participants with POMC deficiency and 45% of participants with LEPR deficiency
Orlistat (Xenical)	Pancreatic and gastric lipase inhibitor	Obesity ≥12 years	Flatulence, diarrhea, oily spotting, fatty stools, micronutrient deficiencies	Weight loss of 2.6 kg more than placebo at 1 year; Placebo subtracted BMI reduction of −0.7 kg/m² at 1 year
Not FDA Approved for Obesity				
Metformin	Activation of protein kinase pathway	≥10 years of age for type 2 diabetes mellitus	Epigastric discomfort, diarrhea, flatulence	Decreased BMI z score by 0.10 and BMI by 0.86
Topiramate	Modulation of various neurotransmitters	Treatment of epilepsy ≥2 years and migraines prevention ≥12 years of age	Cognitive dysfunction, metabolic acidosis, kidney stones, teratogenicity	Decreased BMI by 4.9% on topiramate 75 mg daily for at least 3 months

BMI, Body mass index; FDA, U.S. Food and Drug Administration; GLP-1, glucagon-like peptide-1; LEPR, leptin receptor; PCSK1, proprotein convertase subtilisin/kexin type 1; POMC, proopiomelanocortin.
Adapted from Srivastava G, Fox CK, Kelly AS, et al. Clinical considerations regarding the use of obesity pharmacotherapy in adolescents with obesity. *Obesity.* 2019;27(2):190-204.

TABLE 3	Indications for Bariatric Surgery in Adolescents	
WEIGHT CRITERIA	**COMORBID CONDITIONS PRESENT**	
BMI ≥120% to <140% of the 95th percentile or BMI ≥35 kg/m² and <40 kg/m²	Moderate to severe obstructive sleep apnea, T2DM, idiopathic intracranial hypertension, NASH, Blount disease, slipped capital femoral epiphysis, hypertension, gastroesophageal reflux disease	
BMI ≥140% of the 95th percentile or BMI ≥40 kg/m²	None required, though commonly present	

BMI, Body mass index; NASH, nonalcoholic steatohepatitis; T2DM, type 2 diabetes mellitus.
Adapted from Armstrong SC, Bolling CF, Michalsky MP, Reichard KW. Pediatric metabolic and bariatric surgery: evidence, barriers, and best practices. *Pediatrics* 144(6), 2019.

Eligibility criteria for bariatric surgery include:
1. BMI at least 120% of the 95th percentile for age and gender or BMI at least 35 kg/m², whichever is lower, and a severe comorbidity having significant effects on health (e.g., moderate to severe OSA; apnea-hypopnea index >15), T2DM, idiopathic intracranial hypertension, or severe and progressive steatohepatitis or
BMI at least 140% of the 95th percentile for age and gender or BMI at least 40 kg/m², whichever is lower (obesity-related comorbid conditions are not required);
2. History of previous sustained efforts to lose weight through changes in diet and physical activity;
3. Commitment from the patient and family to adhere to recommended pre- and postoperative treatments, including vitamin and mineral supplementation; and
4. Patient and family understanding of the risks and benefits of bariatric surgery.

Common bariatric procedures

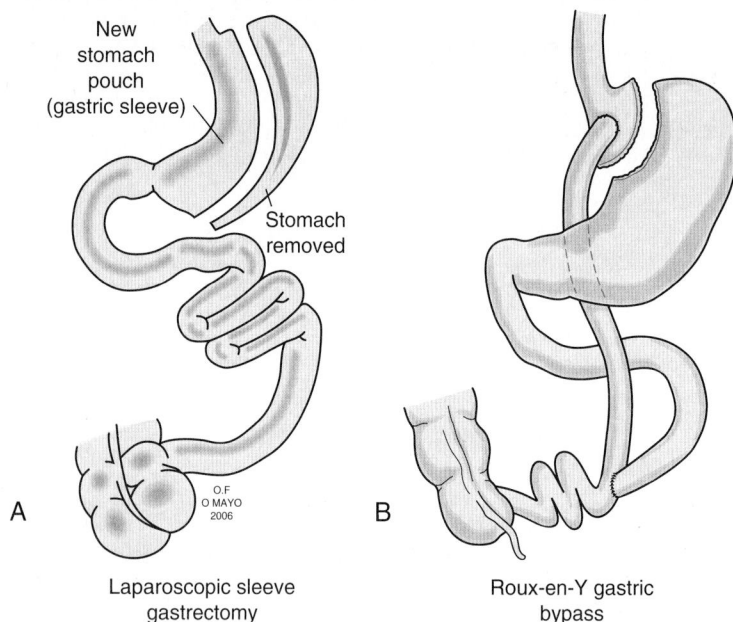

Figure 2 Bariatric surgical procedures commonly used for the surgical treatment of childhood obesity. (A) Laparoscopic sleeve gastrectomy. (B) Roux-en-Y gastric bypass.

The most recent expert guidelines do not recommend withholding surgery in those that have not completed puberty or physical maturity as determined by Tanner stage or skeletal maturation. Contraindications for bariatric surgery include:

1. Medically correctable cause of obesity;
2. An ongoing substance abuse problem (within the preceding year);
3. A medical, psychiatric, psychosocial, or cognitive condition that prevents adherence to postoperative dietary and medication regimens or impairs decisional capacity;
4. Current or planned pregnancy within 12 to 18 months of the procedure; and
5. Inability on the part of the patient or parent to comprehend the risks and benefits of the surgical procedure.

Types of Bariatric Procedures

The sleeve gastrectomy (SG; Figure 2A) is the most commonly performed procedure among adolescents with obesity. SG involves resecting the majority of the greater curvature of the stomach, leaving a tubular structure that serves as the new stomach. SG was initially performed as the first stage of a two-stage procedure in high-risk adults with extreme obesity. The SG procedure is attractive during adolescence and particularly for adolescents with cognitive deficits. The procedure is less complex and can be converted to gastric bypass in the future if there is weight regain. The risk of micronutrient deficiencies is theoretically lower, as it is a purely restrictive procedure.

Roux-en-Y gastric bypass (RYGB; Figure 2B) was previously considered the gold standard of bariatric procedures among adolescents with severe obesity but is now performed less frequently than the SG. The surgery involves creation of a small proximal gastric pouch (<30 mL) and separation of the pouch from the distal stomach and anastomosis to a Roux limb of small bowel that measures 75 to 150 cm in length. Though it is primarily considered a restrictive surgery, some degree of malabsorption does occur that leads to weight loss and places patients at risk for micronutrient deficiencies.

Both bariatric procedures have been shown to result in significant decreases in body weight and BMI in most adolescents undergoing those procedures. In the largest prospective study of bariatric surgery in adolescents (Teen-LABS), 26% reduction in BMI after SG and 28% reduction after RYGB was noted at 3 years. BMI reduction of 29.2% was noted at 5 years in 58 individuals undergoing RYGB. Both procedures have been shown to result in improvement of various comorbid conditions including T2DM, prediabetes, hypertension, dyslipidemia, and renal disease.

Long-term adverse effects include deficiencies of iron, vitamin D, thiamine, and vitamin B_{12}. Adolescents undergoing bariatric surgery need long-term monitoring as long-term safety and efficacy data in this age group are limited.

Conclusion

Childhood obesity presents a growing public health concern in the United States and globally. Weight-related comorbid conditions are common among children with obesity, conferring significant health risks. Treatment of obesity in childhood should be initiated in a timely manner and should begin with lifestyle and behavior change. The list of antiobesity medications for children is increasing, and these medications should be considered as an adjunct to lifestyle changes. Bariatric surgery in adolescents has been associated with significant weight loss and improvement in weight-related comorbid conditions in the short and intermediate term.

References

Armstrong SC, Bolling CF, Michalsky MP, et al: Pediatric metabolic and bariatric surgery: evidence, barriers, and best practices, *Pediatrics* 144, 2019.

Hampl SE, Hassink SG, Armstrong SC, et al: Clinical practice guideline for the evaluation and treatment of children and adolescents with obesity, *Pediatrics* 151, 2023.

Inge TH, Courcoulas AP, Jenkins TM, et al: Weight loss and health status 3 years after bariatric surgery in adolescents, *N Engl J Med* 374:113, 2016.

Kelly AS, Barlow SE, Rao G, et al: Severe obesity in children and adolescents: identification, associated health risks, and treatment approaches: a scientific statement from the American Heart Association, *Circulation* 128:1689, 2013.

Kumar S, Kelly AS: Review of childhood obesity: from epidemiology, etiology, and comorbidities to clinical assessment and treatment, *Mayo Clin Proc* 92:251, 2017.

Srivastava G, Fox CK, Kelly AS, et al: Clinical considerations regarding the use of obesity pharmacotherapy in adolescents with obesity, *Obesity* 27:190, 2019.

PARENTERAL FLUID THERAPY FOR INFANTS AND CHILDREN

Method of
Alan M. Hall, MD; Jimmy Chen, MD; Deval Patel, MD; and Michael L. Moritz, MD

CURRENT DIAGNOSIS

- Maintenance intravenous (IV) fluids are used continuously to maintain extracellular volume and electrolyte homeostasis when intake of enteral fluid (oral or via a feeding tube) is insufficient.
- Resuscitation IV fluids are used for the rapid restoration of intravascular volume.
- Replacement fluids are required to prevent hypovolemia and electrolyte abnormalities when continued excessive fluid losses are present.

CURRENT THERAPY

- Intravenous (IV) fluids should be used only when enteral intake is inadequate and discontinued as soon as safely possible.
- IV fluids should be individualized to each patient, with isotonic fluids recommended for most acutely ill hospitalized patients when maintenance or resuscitation fluids are indicated.
- While a patient receives IV fluids, continuous reassessment is needed, including clinical examination; assessment of vital signs, intake/output, and daily weights; and consideration of laboratory monitoring, especially sodium levels.

Introduction

Intravenous (IV) fluid therapy is an integral component in the care of the acutely ill child. IV fluids may be required as a bolus infusion for resuscitation, as a continuous infusion when sufficient fluids cannot be ingested orally, and to replace excessive ongoing losses from the gastrointestinal (GI) or urinary tract or from serous drains. Fluid therapy aims to provide sufficient fluids to maintain tissue perfusion and normal serum electrolytes. Acutely ill patients frequently have disorders that disrupt normal water and electrolyte homeostasis; therefore choosing the appropriate volume and composition requires great care to prevent impairment in volume or electrolyte balance.

Maintenance Intravenous Fluid Therapy

Maintenance intravenous fluids (MIVFs) are infused continuously to maintain extracellular volume and electrolyte homeostasis when enteral fluid (oral or via a feeding tube) intake is insufficient to meet daily requirements. Crystalloid IV fluids used for maintenance are categorized as isotonic (approximately equal to the plasma sodium concentration) or hypotonic (less than the plasma sodium concentration). Table 1 shows the composition of commonly used IV fluids.

In 1957, Holliday and Segar proposed a theoretical approach to MIVF prescribing; they recommended that hypotonic MIVFs approximating the sodium and potassium concentration of breast milk or cow's milk could provide the water and electrolyte needs for acutely ill children. This led to the widespread use of hypotonic MIVFs; however, the first reports of the syndrome of antidiuretic hormone (SIADH) did not appear until after this publication. SIADH occurs when excess free water is retained, leading to hyponatremia secondary to the nonosmotic and nonhemodynamic triggered release of antidiuretic hormone (ADH).

Virtually all acutely ill hospitalized children have a potential hemodynamic or nonhemodynamic stimulus for ADH production, placing them at risk for hyponatremia (Figure 1). The administration of hypotonic fluids increases their risk of developing hyponatremia, in particular from SIADH, which is the most common cause of hospital-acquired hyponatremia.

Multiple randomized controlled trials and meta-analyses have demonstrated a lower risk of hyponatremia when hospitalized children receive isotonic fluids compared with hypotonic fluids, with an approximate number needed to treat of 7.5. As a result, the American Academy of Pediatrics' Clinical Practice Guideline (AAP CPG) on MIVFs recommends isotonic MIVFs for most patients between 28 days and 18 years of age. In children younger than 28 days of age, the evidence is less clear on the choice between hypotonic and isotonic fluids. The National Institute for Health and Care Excellence guideline recommends isotonic fluids for children 8 days of age or older. A retrospective cohort study showed support for isotonic compared with hypotonic fluids for term newborns. A smaller, prospective randomized trial that included neonates of at least 34 weeks' gestational age showed higher rates of hyponatremia with hypotonic fluids, although this did not reach statistical significance. As a secondary outcome, it did show higher rates of hypernatremia with isotonic fluids that did reach statistical significance. A meta-analysis of randomized controlled trials found a lower risk of hyponatremia but higher risk of hypernatremia with isotonic fluids in neonates. We tend to use this evidence plus extrapolate the evidence from older children and use isotonic fluids in neonates given that they are also at risk for hyponatremia, while being cautious and mindful of potential unique risks for hypernatremia in this population, with consideration of balanced solutions with lower sodium concentrations.

Isotonic fluids can be separated into balanced and unbalanced solutions. Balanced fluids include lactated Ringer solution and Plasma-Lyte 148; they contain a buffer with chloride concentrations close to serum concentrations. A prime example of an unbalanced solution that contains significantly higher chloride concentrations compared with serum without an added buffer is 0.9% saline. Evidence is lacking on the choice between balanced and unbalanced solutions for maintenance in both children and adults. When MIVFs are used for short periods, which is typical for most pediatric patients, either a balanced solution or 0.9% saline is likely reasonable. If MIVFs are needed for long periods or at high doses, it is possible that 0.9% saline could cause a hyperchloremic metabolic acidosis. However, as detailed later (see the "Resuscitation Intravenous Fluid Therapy" section), the evidence regarding whether this could lead to adverse outcomes is equivocal. As a result, 0.9% saline or balanced solutions are both likely sensible options.

Although isotonic MIVFs are indicated for most, the choice of MIVF should be specifically tailored to each patient. Hypotonic fluids may be indicated in a subset of patients, including those with hypernatremia and a free water deficit or ongoing free water losses from a renal concentrating defect such as diabetes insipidus or voluminous watery diarrhea. Dextrose should be added to the MIVF for most children to prevent ketosis. Dextrose is rapidly metabolized upon infusion and does not contribute to the tonicity of the MIVF except in those with uncontrolled diabetes mellitus. There is little guiding evidence, but based on the AAP CPG, it is also recommended to add a potassium additive, typically 20 mEq/L, which can be in the form of potassium chloride. When MIVFs are used for only a short time, a potassium additive may not be needed except in patients with hypokalemia or risk factors for hypokalemia, including severe malnutrition and diuretic use. Hyperkalemia is a potentially serious complication of IV fluids, and potassium should be withheld from fluids if there is any concern for abnormal renal function or decreased or unknown urinary output.

The rate of infusion for MIVFs should be customized to each patient. There is no robust evidence to guide infusion rates, but this can be estimated by body surface area (1500 mL per 1.73 m^2 of body surface area per 24 hours) or weight (the Holliday-Segar

TABLE 1 Composition of Commonly Used Intravenous Fluids

IV FLUID	mmol/L						OSMOLARITY (mOsm/L)
	SODIUM	CHLORIDE	POTASSIUM	CALCIUM	MAGNESIUM	BUFFER	
Human plasma	135–144	95–105	3.5–5.3	2.2–2.6	0.8–1.2	23–30 bicarbonate	308
Isotonic/Near Isotonic Solutions							
0.9% saline	154	154	0	0	0	0	308
Plasma-Lyte 148	140	98	5	0	1.5	27 acetate and 23 gluconate	294
Lactated Ringer solution	130	109	4	1.5	0	28 lactate	273
Hypotonic Solutions							
0.45% saline	77	77	0	0	0	0	154
0.2% saline	34	34	0	0	0	0	78

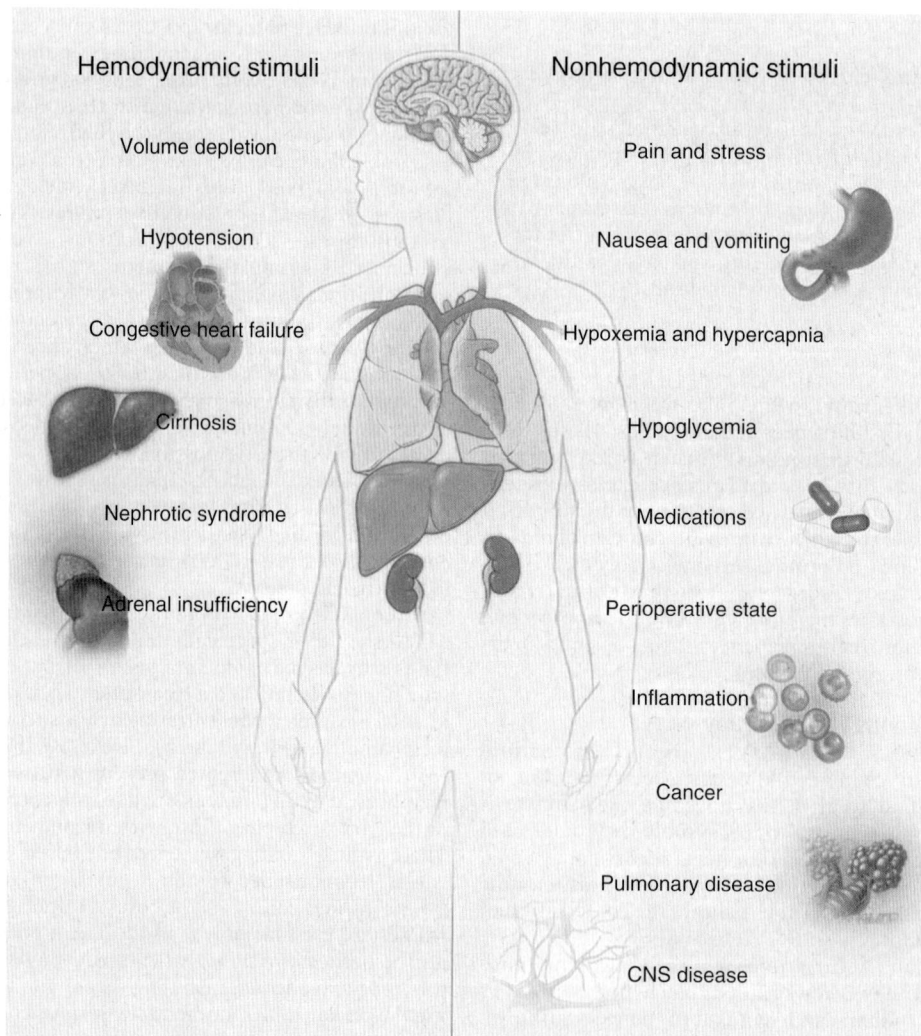

Figure 1 Nonosmotic states of antidiuretic hormone excess. *CNS,* Central nervous system. (From Moritz ML, Ayus JC: Maintenance intravenous fluids in acutely ill patients, *N Engl J Med* 373:1350–1360, 2015. ©2015 Massachusetts Medical Society.)

formula). With the Holliday-Segar formula, fluids are calculated as follows:

100 mL/kg per 24 hours for the first 10 kg of body weight

plus

50 mL/kg per 24 hours for weight between 10 and 20 kg

plus

20 mL/kg per 24 hours for weight above 20 kg

This formula is estimated by what is known as the *4-2-1 rule*. It provides an estimate for the hourly MIVF infusion rate as follows:

4 mL/kg per hour for the first 10 kg of body weight

2 mL/kg per hour for weight between 10 and 20 kg

1 mL/kg per hour for weight above 20 kg

MIVF infusion rates may need to be increased from these estimates in patients with polyuria from renal concentrating defects. Additionally, MIVFs may need to be avoided or used at lower rates of infusion in patients with volume overload states, including oliguric acute kidney injury, chronic kidney disease, cirrhosis, and congestive heart failure. Close monitoring of daily weights, frequent vital signs, strict measurements of intake and output, and serial physical examinations are necessary while a patient is on MIVFs. Laboratory monitoring, specifically to follow sodium levels, should be considered for patients on MIVFs, especially in the initial 24 hours, when rates of hyponatremia are highest. Laboratory tests should also be checked if any neurologic symptoms develop, including unexplained nausea or vomiting, headache, confusion, or altered alertness.

Resuscitation Intravenous Fluid Therapy

Volume depletion, commonly referred to as *dehydration,* occurs whenever water and salt losses exceed intake. Resuscitation IV fluids are used for the rapid restoration of intravascular volume to ensure cellular homeostasis and prevent end organ dysfunction. Children are at risk for developing severe volume depletion when they are unable to keep up with fluid losses, such as from vomiting and diarrhea, traumatic injuries with significant blood loss, renal losses (e.g., hyperglycemia in diabetic ketoacidosis), cutaneous losses (e.g., burns), or third spacing (e.g., pancreatitis and sepsis). Rapid treatment can prevent the development of uncompensated shock while also decreasing morbidity and mortality.

The mainstay in the treatment of mild-to-moderate dehydration is oral rehydration therapy. However, patients presenting with severe dehydration or inadequate enteral intake should receive boluses of IV fluid. Because of their low cost and ready availability, isotonic crystalloids such as 0.9% saline, lactated Ringer solution, or Plasma-Lyte 148 are preferred. Given the high risk of severe hyponatremia, hypotonic fluids should never be administered as boluses. Colloids, such as albumin, have not been shown to be superior to crystalloids in resuscitation.

Resuscitation with large amounts of 0.9% saline without a base equivalent may lead to a hyperchloremic metabolic acidosis. Balanced or buffered solutions with lower chloride concentrations (e.g., lactated Ringer solution or Plasma-Lyte 148) pose a lesser risk of causing a hyperchloremic metabolic acidosis. Since 2018, multiple large prospective controlled trials in adults comparing 0.9% saline to buffered solutions have shown no clear benefit in reducing mortality or acute kidney injury from balanced solutions. A systematic review and individual patient data meta-analysis did find a high probability of a small absolute risk reduction in hospital mortality in adult intensive care units with balanced solutions. Notably, balanced solutions have been associated with increased mortality in patients with traumatic brain injury. If a balanced solution is to be used, Plasma-Lyte 148 is preferred because lactated Ringer solution is a near-isotonic solution and can contribute to a mild decrease in serum sodium.

The clinical signs of dehydration are a manifestation of extracellular volume depletion. Signs of extracellular volume depletion in children include elevated heart rate, delayed capillary refill, diminished tearing, dry mucous membranes, a sunken fontanel, poor skin turgor, decreased peripheral pulses, cool extremities, and ultimately a decrease in blood pressure when volume depletion is severe. Three factors determine the amount of extracellular volume depletion and therefore the severity of dehydration: (1) the fluid deficit, (2) the electrolyte deficit, and (3) the speed at which dehydration occurs. Given the same volume loss, hyponatremic dehydration is clinically more severe than hypernatremic dehydration because fluid shifts intracellularly in hyponatremic dehydration. This is the basis for classifying dehydration according to the serum sodium as hyponatremic, isonatremic, or hypernatremic.

To restore intravascular volume rapidly and provide adequate perfusion to vital organs, resuscitation fluid is given in rapid aliquots of 20 mL/kg followed by clinical reassessment. Patients with preexisting conditions, such as cardiac and renal disease, may require using smaller volumes of fluid (e.g., 5–10 mL/kg). In septic shock, up to 40 to 60 mL/kg may be given, with vasopressors quickly added if hemodynamics are not restored based on frequent clinical reassessments.

Potential harm is associated with excessive fluid resuscitation. Severe illness has been associated with damage to the glycocalyx, which lines the vascular endothelium. Damage to the glycocalyx can contribute to increased permeability of the endothelium and result in an increased risk of interstitial edema and fluid overload with IV fluid administration. Fluid overload has been associated with increased mortality, specifically in patients with acute kidney injury. Additionally, a large randomized controlled trial showed increased mortality when African children were given fluid boluses when they presented with a febrile illness and signs of shock. In contrast, a large randomized trial showed no difference in a restrictive versus liberal approach to fluid boluses in adult patients with hypotension from sepsis. Ultimately, there is likely not a one-size-fits-all approach to resuscitation that is uniformly effective. Instead, an individualized approach with frequent reassessment of each patient is needed during resuscitation.

To stay mindful of these potential adverse effects of resuscitation, an approach to fluid resuscitation with four phases has been proposed in critical care settings. The first phase, rescue, is focused on correcting shock with rapid boluses. In the second phase, optimization, fluid is cautiously titrated to optimize tissue perfusion. The third phase includes stabilization with minimal fluid used only for maintenance, and the fourth phase is deescalation focused on mobilizing and removing any excess fluid.

The fluid deficit can be estimated by using the clinical signs listed in Table 2. As an example, a 10-kg boy presents with vomiting and diarrhea that has lasted for 3 days; he now weighs 9 kg. He is lethargic, tachycardic, and has a sunken fontanel with cool extremities. Capillary refill is greater than 3 seconds. His clinical presentation and the amount of weight loss suggest at least 10% dehydration. The patient's calculated fluid deficit is as follows:

$$0.10 \times 10 \text{ kg} \times 1000 \text{ (mL/kg)} = 1000 \text{ mL (fluid deficit)}$$

Because the patient's preillness weight is known, an alternate method of calculation is to subtract his current weight from his preillness weight (10 kg to 9 kg) and multiply by 1000 (mL/kg), also resulting in 1000 mL of deficit. To start the resuscitation, a 20 mL/kg bolus of isotonic fluids (or 9 kg × 20 mL/kg = 180 mL) is then given over 30 minutes. If vital signs are restored to normal, a residual deficit of 820 mL will need to be replaced with oral or IV fluid therapy. If there is continued hemodynamic compromise after the initial bolus, additional boluses of 20 mL/kg are given.

Replacement Intravenous Fluids

Replacement fluids are required to prevent hypovolemia and electrolyte abnormalities when continued excessive fluid losses

TABLE 2 Clinical Signs to Estimate Dehydration

Older Child

	3% (30 mL/kg)	6% (60 mL/kg)	9% (90 mL/kg)

Infant

	5% (50 mL/kg)	10% (100 mL/kg)	15% (150 mL/kg)
Dehydration	Mild	Moderate	Severe
Skin turgor	Normal	Tenting	None
Skin (touch)	Normal	Dry	Clammy
Buccal mucosa/lips	Dry	Dry	Dry/cracked
Eyes	Normal	Slightly sunken	Sunken
Tears	Present	Decreased	None
Fontanelle	Flat	Soft	Sunken
Mental status	Alert	Alert/altered	Lethargic/obtunded
Pulse rate	Normal	Slightly increased	Increased
Pulse quality	Normal	Weak	Weak/very weak
Capillary refill	Normal	2–3 seconds	>3 seconds
Urine output	Normal/mild oliguria	Mild oliguria	Severe oliguria

TABLE 3 Electrolyte Composition of Body Fluids

FLUID	Na$^+$ (mmol/L)	K$^+$ (mmol/L)	CL$^-$ (mmol/L)	HCO$_3^-$
Gastric	20–60	14	140	60–80
Biliary drain	145	5	105	30
Pancreatic drain	125–138	8	56	85
Diarrhea/colostomy	30–140	30–70	—	20–80
Ileostomy	45–140	4–5	25–125	0–30

are present. Common sources of fluid losses necessitating replacement include emesis, diarrhea, urine, and surgical drain outputs (chest tubes, nasogastric tubes, ileostomies, fistulas). If this fluid is not appropriately replaced, hypovolemia and significant electrolyte derangements can develop. Oral replacement of fluid is preferred when tolerated. IV replacement of fluid is necessary when oral replacement cannot meet ongoing losses.

Before replacing ongoing losses, one must first restore extracellular volume with resuscitation fluids, as outlined previously. Once euvolemia is restored, ongoing fluid losses must be closely replaced. It is important to note that this fluid replacement is in addition to the volume of required maintenance fluid. Replacement fluid therapy should be individually tailored for each patient, with inputs and outputs closely monitored. Existing guidelines recommend using 0.9% sodium chloride containing potassium as the initial fluid for replacement therapy. If fluid loss is ongoing and excessive, serial measurement of serum electrolytes is required to adjust the IV fluid prescription. The measurement of electrolyte concentrations may be helpful, as the electrolyte composition varies between sites of fluid loss. When measurement of electrolyte composition is not feasible, one must be familiar with the electrolyte contents of the fluid loss in varying disease processes to maintain the correct balance of electrolytes. The electrolyte composition of some of the common sites of fluid loss is shown in Table 3.

In GI losses from infectious gastroenteritis, the electrolyte content varies based on the type of infection. Rotavirus enteritis can lead to a mean sodium loss of 50 mmol/L and up to 50 mmol/L of bicarbonate. Secretory diarrheal illnesses, such as cholera, can cause massive loss of fluid, with sodium losses as high as 140 mmol/L and bicarbonate losses several times that of other GI illnesses. If either hypernatremia or a metabolic acidosis is developing, a hypotonic replacement fluid or a buffered solution may be required. In the loss of other bodily fluids, such as emesis, a large amount of chloride is lost (90–150 mmol/L) instead of bicarbonate, and buffered solutions should not be used for replacement. Potassium and magnesium may also have to be replaced in diseases such as renal tubulopathies. In understanding the composition of the fluid lost, the appropriate type of IV fluid can be prescribed (see Table 1).

The management of ongoing fluid losses is a labor-intensive process that requires meticulous monitoring of the patient's total input and output. Close clinical assessment of the patient, daily weight measurements, and routine monitoring of electrolytes are necessary to ensure euvolemia and electrolyte homeostasis.

Sodium Disorders

Disorders in serum sodium are the most frequent electrolyte abnormality in hospitalized patients and can occur on presentation or be hospital acquired. Hyponatremia and hypernatremia are both associated with potential neurologic and systemic complications and increased hospital morbidity and mortality. Careful fluid therapy is needed for both prevention and treatment.

Hyponatremia

Hyponatremia is defined as a serum sodium less than 135 mEq/L. The body's primary defense against developing hyponatremia is the kidney's ability to generate dilute urine and excrete free water. In most cases of hyponatremia there is a stimulus for ADH production that results in impaired free water excretion. There are numerous stimuli for ADH production (see Figure 1) that place virtually all hospitalized children at risk for hyponatremia. A particularly common cause of hyponatremia is SIADH. SIADH refers to euvolemic hyponatremia due to nonphysiologic stimuli for ADH production in the absence of renal or endocrine dysfunction. SIADH can be difficult to diagnose, as volume status is difficult to assess accurately and there are no specific biochemical tests for diagnosing SIADH. Before SIADH can be diagnosed, diseases causing decreased effective circulating volume, renal impairment, adrenal insufficiency, and hypothyroidism must be excluded. The hallmarks of SIADH are (1) mild volume expansion with low to normal plasma concentrations of creatinine, urea, uric acid, and potassium; (2) impaired free water excretion with normal sodium excretion, which reflects sodium intake; and (3) hyponatremia that is relatively unresponsive to sodium administration in the absence of fluid restriction. The biochemical parameters most suggestive of SIADH in adults are a spot urine sodium concentration greater than 30 mEq/L, fractional excretion of sodium greater than 0.5%, fractional excretion of urea greater than 55%, fractional excretion of urate greater than 11%, and plasma uric acid less than 4 mg/dL. These parameters may not apply to young children.

The most serious complication of hyponatremia is hyponatremic encephalopathy, which is a medical emergency that can be fatal or can lead to irreversible brain injury if inadequately treated. The primary symptoms of hyponatremia are those of cerebral edema. The most consistent symptoms are nonspecific and can easily be overlooked: headache, nausea, vomiting, and generalized weakness. Advanced symptoms include seizures, respiratory arrest, noncardiogenic pulmonary edema, and decorticate posturing. Children are at particularly high risk for developing hyponatremic encephalopathy as they have a relatively larger brain-to-intracranial volume compared with adults. There is evidence to suggest that even mild and seemingly asymptomatic hyponatremia has deleterious consequences, being an independent risk factor for mortality.

Hyponatremic encephalopathy is a medical emergency that requires immediate therapy with 3% sodium chloride (3% NaCl, 513 mEq/L). The consensus treatment for hyponatremic encephalopathy is to give repeated intermittent boluses of 3% NaCl (2 mL/kg, maximum 150 mL) to raise the serum sodium acutely by approximately 5 mEq/L and decrease the risk of overcorrection. Fluid restriction is the cornerstone of treatment in asymptomatic hyponatremia. Isotonic saline is effective in treating hypovolemic hyponatremia, although it can aggravate hyponatremia due to SIADH. SIADH is usually of short duration and resolves with treatment of the underlying disorder or discontinuation of the offending medication. For more chronic forms of SIADH, therapies include oral sodium supplementation, oral urea (Ure-Na)[7], or vasopressin V2-receptor antagonist.

Overcorrection of severe and chronic hyponatremia can result in brain injury from cerebral demyelination. Cerebral demyelination is primarily seen in chronically hyponatremic patients of greater than 48 hours' duration with a serum sodium of less than 115 mEq/L. Other risk factors that increase the likelihood of cerebral demyelination independent of the degree of hyponatremia or rate of correction are hypokalemia, thiazide diuretic use, severe liver disease, malnutrition, hypophosphatemia, and hypoxia. Two large studies in 2023 in adults have demonstrated that demyelination is rare with an incidence of 0.3%. The development of demyelination was primarily related to risk factors and not the rate of correction. Rates of correction of 8 mmol/L per 24 hours or less did not prevent demyelination and were associated with increased hospital mortality and length of hospital stay compared with rates greater than 8 mmol/L per 24 hours. Excessive increases in serum sodium should be avoided under all circumstances, not just with hyponatremia. In patients with severe and chronic hyponatremia, the serum sodium should not be corrected by greater than 20 mEq/L in the first 48 hours of therapy.

Hypernatremia

Hypernatremia is defined as a serum sodium greater than 145 mEq/L. Hypernatremia occurs in children in the presence of restricted access to water, such as infants, debilitation by an acute or a chronic illness, neurologic impairment, or in the critically ill. Contributing factors for hypernatremia in the intensive care setting are excess sodium administration, renal concentrating defects, GI fluid losses, increased insensible water losses, restricted access to oral fluids, and dialysis-related complications.

If the thirst mechanism is intact and there is unrestricted access to free water, it is rare for someone to develop sustained hypernatremia from either excess sodium ingestion or a renal concentrating defect. The cause of hypernatremia is usually multifactorial. Measuring urine osmolality and electrolyte concentration can help determine whether the renal concentrating ability is appropriate and to quantify the urinary free water losses. Less than maximally concentrated urine (<800 mOsm/kg) in the face of hypernatremia associated with signs of dehydration is a sign of a renal concentrating defect, as hypernatremia is a maximal stimulus for ADH release. A relatively new and useful clinical lab test for distinguishing central from nephrogenic diabetes insipidus is plasma copeptin testing. Copeptin, the C-terminal segment of the prehormone for arginine vasopressin, can be used as a surrogate marker of ADH as it is easier and more reliable to measure than ADH.

Hypernatremia results in an efflux of fluid from the intracellular space to the extracellular space to maintain osmotic equilibrium. This leads to transient cerebral dehydration with cell shrinkage. Children with hypernatremia are usually agitated and irritable but can progress to lethargy, listlessness, and coma. On neurologic examination, they frequently have increased tone, nuchal rigidity, and brisk reflexes. Myoclonus, asterixis, and chorea can be present; tonic-clonic and absence seizures have been described.

The cornerstone of hypernatremia management is providing adequate free water to correct the serum sodium concentration but doing this at a rate that limits the risk of brain injury. Hypernatremia is frequently accompanied by volume depletion; if hemodynamic instability is present, fluid resuscitation with an isotonic solution should be instituted to establish more normal hemodynamics before slowly correcting the free water deficit. After initial volume expansion, the composition of parenteral fluid therapy largely depends on the etiology of the hypernatremia. Patients with sodium overload or a renal concentrating defect require a more hypotonic fluid than those with volume depletion and intact renal concentrating ability. Oral hydration should be instituted as soon as it can be safely tolerated. Plasma electrolytes should be checked frequently until adequate correction is achieved.

A simple way of estimating the minimum amount of fluid necessary to correct the serum sodium is by the equation:

$$\text{Free water deficit (mL)} = 4 \text{ mL} \times \text{lean body weight (kg)} \times (\text{desired change in serum Na mEq/L})$$

The rate of correction of hypernatremia is largely dependent on the severity of the hypernatremia and the etiology. Because of the brain's relative inability to extrude unmeasured organic substances (idiogenic osmoles), rapid correction of hypernatremia can lead to cerebral edema. Although there are no definitive studies documenting the optimal rate of correction without causing cerebral edema to develop, empiric data have shown that a rate of correction of 0.5 mEq/h or 12 mEq/24 h is reasonable. Recent retrospective studies in 2023 have failed to demonstrate an association between more rapid rates of correction and neurologic complications or morbidity. Sodium chloride 0.45% with appropriate amounts of potassium is usually the most suitable composition of IV fluid to treat hypernatremia in children with hypovolemic hyponatremia and intact renal function.

---

[7] Available as dietary supplement.

References

Amer BE, Abdelwahab OA, Abdelaziz A, et al: Efficacy and safety of isotonic versus hypotonic intravenous maintenance fluids in hospitalized children: an updated systematic review and meta-analysis of randomized controlled trials, *Pediatr Nephrol* 39(1):57–84, 2024.

Dathan K, Sundaram M: Comparison of isotonic versus hypotonic intravenous fluid for maintenance fluid therapy in neonates more than or equal to 34 weeks of gestational age–a randomized clinical trial, *J Matern Fetal Neonatal Med* 35(25):6338–6345, 2022.

Didsbury M, See EJ, Cheng DR, Kausman J, Quinlan C: Correcting hypernatremia in children, *Clin J Am Soc Nephrol* 18(3):306–314, 2023.

Feld LG, Neuspiel DR, Foster BA, et al: Clinical practice guideline: maintenance intravenous fluids in children, *Pediatrics* 142:e20183083, 2018.

Holliday MA, Segar WE: The maintenance need for water in parenteral fluid therapy, *Pediatrics* 19:823–832, 1957.

Moritz ML, Ayus JC: Maintenance intravenous fluids in acutely ill patients, *N Engl J Med* 373:1350–1360, 2015.

Moritz ML, Ayus JC: Preventing neurological complications from dysnatremias in children, *Pediatr Nephrol* 20:1687–1700, 2005.

Moritz ML: Syndrome of inappropriate antidiuresis, *Pediatr Clin N Am* 66:209–226, 2019.

National Clinical Guideline Centre (UK): *IV fluids in children: intravenous fluid therapy in children and young people in hospital*, London, United Kingdom, 2015, National Clinical Guideline Centre. https://www.ncbi.nlm.nih.gov/pubmed/26741016.

National Heart, Lung, and Blood Institute Prevention and Early Treatment of Acute Lung Injury Clinical Trials Network, Shapiro NI, Douglas IS, Brower RG, et al: Early restrictive or liberal fluid management for sepsis-induced hypotension, *N Engl J Med* 388(6):499–510, 2023.

Raman S, Gibbons KS, Mattke A, et al: Effect of saline vs gluconate/acetate–buffered solution vs lactate-buffered solution on serum chloride among children in the pediatric intensive care unit: the SPLYT-P randomized clinical trial, *JAMA Pediatr* 177(2):122–131, 2023.

Seethapathy H, Zhao S, Ouyang T, Passos C, et al: Severe hyponatremia correction, mortality, and central pontine myelinolysis, *NEJM Evidence* 2(10):EVI-Doa2300107, 2023..

Tuzun F, Akcura Y, Duman N, Ozkan H: Comparison of isotonic and hypotonic intravenous fluids in term newborns: is it time to quit hypotonic fluids, *J Matern Fetal Neonatal Med* 35(2):356–361, 2022.

PEDIATRIC FAILURE TO THRIVE

Method of
Gretchen Homan, MD

CURRENT DIAGNOSIS

- Pediatric failure to thrive (PFTT), also known as weight faltering, refers to failure to gain weight at an appropriate rate over time.
- History taking, physical examination, and growth chart data are used to identify PFTT.
- Weight below the fifth percentile with a decreasing trend over time indicates potential PFTT.
- Weight measurements declining across two major percentiles may indicate PFTT.
- Failure to gain or maintain weight is the earliest indication of PFTT, but length and head circumference may be impacted and should always be monitored.

CURRENT THERAPY

- Successful treatment includes addressing all causes, including underlying medical problems.
- Hospitalization is generally not indicated, and serial clinic visits can be used to monitor weight gain and maintenance.
- Growth chart parameters can help set a goal weight. Daily weight gain goals can be identified to monitor treatment over weeks to months.
- The majority of patients respond to generalized techniques for increased calories combined with frequent outpatient monitoring of progress.

- Consulting with a dietitian or using detailed nutrition calculations can provide specific guidance for protein and calorie goals in complicated cases, and any contributing social determinants of health should be addressed by community resources.

In pediatric failure to thrive (PFTT), also known as weight faltering, the child fails to gain weight at an appropriate rate; this failure is documented over time. The concept has been recognized for over a century, but there is still no consensus on terminology or a definition. Historically, the terms *organic* and *nonorganic* were used to classify PFTT, and they were attributed to medical conditions and psychosocial causes, respectively. Insufficient usable nutrition is now regarded as the underlying cause of PFTT. It can be due to problems with calorie intake or absorption or both, and it is not unusual for patients to have more than one contributing factor. Approximately 80% of children with PFTT are diagnosed by age 18 months, during the early months of life when growth rates are normally high. For older children, the preferred term is *poor weight gain*.

Epidemiology

In the United States, PFTT occurs in approximately 5% to 10% of children seen in primary care and in up to 5% of children admitted to the hospital. An estimated 20% to 30% of cases are undiagnosed. PFTT is a condition rather than a specific diagnosis, and imprecise diagnostic criteria complicate estimating its incidence and prevalence. Some children age 6 to 18 months show a decrease in their weight curves followed by weight maintenance on the new curve; although this occurs in approximately 25% of children, it is not considered weight faltering but a correction toward their genetic potential.

Risk Factors

Patient-specific risk factors for PFTT can be medical and/or psychosocial. In up to 80% of cases, no obvious medical etiology is identified. Any disease process has the potential to cause PFTT. Prenatal predisposing factors include exposure to toxins, intrauterine growth retardation, and poor maternal nutrition. Infants born prematurely are at high risk for PFTT. Premature infants need to catch up in growth over months to years and should not be expected to reach normal peer percentiles too quickly, as this could have negative implications for healthy weight in adult life. Any medical problem that interferes with or inhibits calorie intake and absorption of nutrients can cause PFTT, as can any condition that creates increased caloric demand. Leading medical causes include development delay, congenital anomalies such as cleft lip and/or palate, genetic conditions such as cystic fibrosis or celiac disease, and childhood cancers and related treatments.

Environmental risk factors include poverty, which is the most powerful psychosocial risk factor for PFTT, as it limits access to appropriate nutrition. Healthcare providers should be aware of "food deserts" in their communities as well as families within their practice that are food insecure. Of note, "food swamps" in which only unhealthy food options exist could contribute to poor nutrition seen in toddlers. Children of families with increased life stresses, social isolation, poor parenting skills, or substance abuse are at increased risk for PFTT. Personal nutritional beliefs and practices can also limit nutrition, leading to PFTT. Examples include prolonged exclusive breast feeding or avoidance of multiple food categories for cultural or religious reasons or real or perceived food allergy.

Pathophysiology

Inadequate caloric intake, malabsorption, or increased metabolic demand, either as isolated entities or concurrently, can lead to PFTT. Caloric intake may be impaired by use of diluted formula, poor feeding habits, neglect, or mechanical feeding difficulties. Inadequate nutrient absorption can be caused by a range of diseases or conditions that affect the gastrointestinal tract, including celiac disease, cystic fibrosis and other pancreatic diseases, milk protein and other food allergy, inborn errors of metabolism, and chronic infections. Increased energy needs and potential caloric deficit leading to PFTT can occur in children with chronic infections, congenital heart or lung disease, hyperthyroidism, malignancy, renal failure, inflammatory conditions, and HIV.

Prevention

Prevention of PFTT begins with prenatal care and maternal health, especially limiting potential exposure to toxins, optimizing maternal nutrition, and conducting routine pregnancy screenings. Being aware of potential genetic conditions facilitates planning appropriate support for the family. State-mandated newborn screening tests provide opportunities for early intervention in patients at risk for PFTT. Routine well-child visits in the first 2 years of life provide surveillance for growth and anticipatory guidance regarding nutrition to support development. Connecting families with appropriate community resources can help provide high-risk children and families with access to nutritional resources. Supporting overall good health with patient education and general preventive services, including oral health and immunization, is essential to reducing the risk of FTT.

Clinical Manifestations

PFTT is defined by problems with weight as a documented trend over time. The Centers for Disease Control and Prevention (CDC) recommend that the World Health Organization growth charts be used to document growth for children under age 2 years and that the CDC growth charts be used for children ages 2 years and older. The majority of PFTT patients show at least one of three characteristics: weight below the 5th percentiles for age and sex, weight drop of two major percentiles, or weight less than the 80th percentile of ideal body weight. Some infants may benefit from a PFTT evaluation when their daily weight gain is less than expected for age and sex but does not yet meet these criteria. If weight faltering persists, length and then head circumference are impacted, and these indicate severe PFTT.

Patients with PFTT can generally be diagnosed as outpatients. Laboratory evaluation or imaging is not generally required and is low yield in the absence of specific findings. Detailed history taking and physical examination, along with the growth chart information, are sufficient to identify PFTT. If the history or physical exam is concerning, initial laboratory work-up may include a complete blood count with differential, iron studies, lead level, chemistry panel, urine analysis, stool studies, or testing for immune deficiency. A delay in

development coupled with weight faltering noted on the growth chart comprise the clinical presentation of severe or prolonged PFTT. The aim of the physical examination is to identify any underlying or contributing medical condition that could impair nutrition and/or increase metabolic demands. The clinician should observe for any dysmorphic features and look for signs of abuse or neglect. Signs of malnutrition may become evident when PFTT is allowed to persist. The most severely affected children show edema, wasting, hepatomegaly, rash, or skin and hair changes.

Differential Diagnosis

Prematurely born infants, infants with intrauterine growth retardation, and small for gestation age infants may be mistaken for patients with PFTT. These infants and children may meet the diagnostic criteria for delay on standard growth charts (values less than the 5th percentile) for age and sex. Ongoing monitoring for underlying medical conditions, regular developmental assessments, and evaluation of the social support network for each patient can provide reassurance that the child does not have PFTT and is expected to "catch up" in growth parameters within 18 to 36 months.

Genetic short stature and constitutional growth delay should be ruled out by reviewing the midparental height and growth patterns for delays. Radiologic testing for bone age may be helpful when confirming constitutional growth delay. Children with autism spectrum disorder symptoms may have behaviorally restricted diets combined with medical complexities that predispose them to malnutrition and thus should be monitored carefully. A number of genetic conditions are known to contribute to poor growth and should be evaluated according to the history, examination, and response to initial therapy.

Therapy

PFTT can have one or multiple causes or complicating factors. Each issue should be addressed in the context of the overall health of the child and family. Any underlying medical condition must be diagnosed and treated. Children with a history of choking, signs of aspiration, or oral motor dysfunction may benefit from a swallow study and speech therapist evaluation and treatment program. Hospitalization is rarely indicated but may be helpful if there are complicating medical or social problems or if outpatient treatment has failed. Outpatient therapy is centered on increasing calorie intake with appropriate food options (Table 1). Equations can be used to calculate estimated calorie

TABLE 1	Techniques to Increase Calories	
AGE	**CALORIE SOURCE ADJUSTMENT**	**FEEDING TECHNIQUE**
Infant – breast fed	• Increase feeds up to 12 in 24 hours • Pump after feeds and use expressed breast milk (EBM) to supplement nursing; add formula powder to expressed breast milk	• Measure infant weight in grams before and after breast feed to determine milk transfer, milk supply • Evaluate and ensure proper latch/position • Feed both breasts with each feeding • Work to keep baby awake for complete feeding • Do not allow feeds to persist beyond 30 minutes total
Infant – formula fed	• Increase calorie concentration by mixing formula powder with less water, from 19/20 to 24/26 kcal; monitor for tolerance • Evaluate feeding volume and frequency to avoid over- or underfeeding; rule of thumb feeds average 1 oz/h (e.g., 3 oz/3 h) • Formula powder may be added to foods at age >4 months	• Evaluate for intolerance and change formula if needed; consider predigested proteins • Use proper bottle nipple speed • Avoid bottle propping, use reflux precautions
Toddler	• Use high-calorie foods and offer proteins such as cheese, peanut butter, avocados, high-fat yogurts, oils, and heavy creams • Encourage a variety of healthy foods such as fruits, vegetables, proteins, and grains • Consider supplement drinks or shake powders to mix 1–2 times/day	• Structured mealtimes for 20–30 minutes in a high chair with adult supervision and without distractions • Evaluate toddler's ability to self-feed effectively; intervene and teach if needed • Aim for 3 meals with 3 snacks daily • Minimize fruit juices • Offer water with meals and offer foods before milk or supplement drinks • Avoid low nutrition foods such as sweets and fried foods

TABLE 2	Estimated Calorie Needs by Age
AGE	**KCAL/KG/DAY**
Preterm infant	115–130; up to 150 for very low birth weight infants
Full-term infant • 0–2 months • 3–12 months	• 104–107 • 95 • 82
Toddler	70–80

Add 5–20 kcal/kg/day for catch-up growth, depending on tolerance and desired rate of recovery.

and protein needs by age and sex for both normal and catch-up growth. To simplify this process, a generalized list of targets is provided in Table 2. When available, a dietitian can define the required protein and calorie goals for catch-up growth initially and over the remaining treatment period. Alternatively, the primary care physician can use the growth chart to determine the desired weight goal for age and plan for a daily weight gain goal over weeks or months. The techniques described in Table 1 can be used to initiate treatment. Frequent visits are necessary. At each visit, the child's measurements should be done on the same well-calibrated scale to provide reliable data for clinical decision making about appropriate weight gain and maintenance. Patients who are unable to grow with these interventions may benefit from either short-term nasogastric tube feedings or more long-term gastric tube feedings.

Monitoring

Children with PFTT may require more frequent monitoring than the scheduled routine well-child visits. Young infants can be seen weekly or monthly and older patients every 2 to 4 months. At these visits, patients should be weighed and measured, infants in only a dry diaper and older children in light clothing without shoes, by trained staff using routinely calibrated devices and standardized techniques to ensure the most accurate measurements. The clinician should review the patient's growth charts, diet and activity history, any changes in the social and medical history, and perform a physical examination. Recent acute illness may slow or reverse growth progress and should be addressed. It may take months for malnourished patients to show and maintain growth recovery. Patients who were born prematurely or with intrauterine growth retardation may require years to catch up. Depending on the underlying cause of PFTT, relapse is possible.

Complications

Weight loss or deceleration is the earliest clinical indicator for PFTT; if allowed to persist, height and length can be affected. Eventually, head size and brain growth can be impaired. At this level of severity, PFTT puts cognitive development and achievement of milestones in jeopardy. Immune system function may be impaired during a malnourished state, thus putting affected patients at risk for infections. Extremely severe cases of malnutrition may require hospitalization to stabilize and transfer to ongoing outpatient care Social and emotional health may also be impacted. Research is ongoing to understand the long-term effects of PFTT.

References

Black MM, Dubowitz H, Krishnakumar A, Starr Jr RH: Early intervention and recovery among children with failure to thrive: follow-up at age 8, *Pediatrics* 120:59–69, 2007.
Cole SZ, Lanham JS: Failure to thrive: an update, *Am Fam Physician* 83:829–834, 2011.
Engorn B, Flerlage J, editors: *The Harriet Lane Handbook: A Manual for Pediatric House Officers*, 20th ed., Philadelphia, 2014, Elsevier Saunders.
Kleinman RE, Greer FR: Failure to thrive. In *Pediatric Nutrition*, Elk Grove Village, IL, 2014, American Academy of Pediatrics, pp 663–700.
Olsen EM, Petersen J, Skovgaard AM, et al: Failure to thrive: the prevalence and concurrence of enthropometric criteria in a general infant population, *Arch Dis Child* 92:109–114, 2007.
Rybak A: Organic and nonorganic feeding disorders, *Ann Nutr Metab* 66(suppl 5):16–22, 2015.
Shields B, Wacogne I, Wright CM: Weight faltering and failure to thrive in infancy and early childhood, *BMJ* 345:e5931, 2012.
Tang, MN, Adolphe S, Rogers SR, Frank DA: Failure to thrive or growth faltering: medical developmental/behavioral, nutritional, and social dimensions, *Pediatr Rev* 42(11): 590–603, 2021.
Wright CM, Parkinson KN, Drewett RF: How does maternal and child feeding behavior relate to weight gain and failure to thrive? Data from a prospective birth cohort, *Pediatrics* 117:1262–1269, 2006.
Yoo SD, Hwang EH, Lee YJ, Park JH: Clinical characteristics of failure to thrive in infant and toddler: organic vs. nonorganic, *Pediatr Gastroenterol Hepatol Nutr* 16:261–268, 2013.

PEDIATRIC SLEEP DISORDERS

Method of
Julie M. Baughn, MD

CURRENT DIAGNOSIS

- Sleep disorders are common in children.
- Evaluation of pediatric sleep disorders in children begins with a thorough sleep history.
- Overnight polysomnography is most commonly used to evaluate for sleep-disordered breathing
- Other diagnostic tools include the multiple sleep latency test (MSLT), oximetry, sleep logs, and actigraphy.
- Common sleep disorders in children include obstructive sleep apnea, insomnia, restless legs syndrome, and delayed sleep phase syndrome.

CURRENT THERAPY

- For most children tonsillectomy and adenoidectomy are an effective treatment for obstructive sleep apnea.
- Behavioral therapy is essential to treating insomnia.
- Only in select circumstances are medications used to treat children with sleep disorders.

Introduction

Pediatric sleep medicine has grown as the importance of sleep in the developing child has been recognized along with the impact that insufficient or disrupted sleep can have on cognitive development and behavior. The American Academy of Sleep Medicine (AASM) and the American Academy of Pediatrics (AAP) have recently published guidelines and practice parameters addressing several aspects of pediatric sleep medicine. Pediatric sleep disorders have unique societal impact; both the child's and the family's sleep can be affected when a disorder is present. The aim of this chapter is to offer a practical approach to the diagnosis and treatment of the most common pediatric sleep disorders, discuss diagnostic tools available, and discuss recommended treatment.

Developmental Aspects of Sleep

Pediatric sleep disorders also have the unique challenge of dealing with sleep issues that are subject to change based on the child's developmental age. The amount of sleep required by age has been described in a recent AASM consensus statement (Table 1). The sleep architecture of the child characteristically changes as he or she develops. The portion of rapid eye movement (REM) sleep declines from 50% at birth to 25% to 30% in adolescence. The proportion of slow-wave sleep is highest in early childhood and continues to decline throughout life. The pattern of sleep and sleep requirement also change. Neonates may not develop a regular sleep-wake pattern until about 3 months of age. Most infants are capable of sleeping

	AVERAGE SLEEP DURATION IN 24 HOURS (OVERNIGHT AND
AGE	NAPS)
Infants (4 to 12 months)	12 to 16 hours
Children (1-2 years)	11-14 hours
Children (3-5 years)	10–13 hours Most give up naps between 3 and 5 years
Children (6-12 years)	9–12 hours
Teenagers (> 12 years13-18 years)	9 hours8-10 hours

TABLE 1 Sleep Requirements in Children by Age

Paruthi S, Brooks LJ, D'Ambrosio C, et al. Consensus Statement of the American Academy of Sleep Medicine on the Recommended Amount of Sleep for Healthy Children: Methodology and Discussion, *J Clin Sleep Med* 2016; 12(11):1549-1561.

through the night by about 6 months of age, but many may continue to waken. Naps are typically given up somewhere between 3 and 5 years of age. Most adolescents, due to many societal and social constraints, do not get a requisite 8 to 10 hours of sleep at night.

Clinical Approach
Taking a Sleep History
There are several key elements to obtaining a sleep history in children. The mnemonic BEARS (Bedtime problems, Excessive daytime sleepiness, Awakenings during the night, Regularity and duration of sleep, and Sleep-disordered breathing) has been offered as a practical starting point for obtaining a history, tailoring questions to both parent and child where appropriate (Table 2).

The primary sleep complaint should be obtained in the child's or parent's own words. Once the primary complaint is detailed, the presence/absence of snoring, the presence of restlessness at sleep initiation and during sleep, and the child's sleep-wake patterns during school should be gathered. The presence or absence of a bedtime routine and the details of that routine should be noted. A child's sleep environment should be carefully queried. A child who shares his or her bedroom, sleeps in his or her parents' bed, or ends up sleeping on a couch in front of the television may lead to specific sleep complaints. A history of whether there is more than one household involved (i.e., shared custody) is particularly important.

Sleepiness in children can be a particularly challenging symptom to evaluate. It is normal physiologically for children to nap until age 5. Other clues to daytime sleepiness that can be obtained in children include behavior issues, hyperactivity, excessive napping, or napping after age 5 years (intentionally or unintentionally). School-age children often display symptoms of behavioral problems or inattentiveness rather than sleepiness. Sleep-wake patterns on school days, weekends, and vacations need to be detailed. Often the child's most natural sleep pattern will emerge over the summer months.

Determining the child's sleep hygiene or good sleep practices is important in diagnosing and treating sleep disorders. Principles of good sleep hygiene are listed in Table 3.

Past Medical History/Family History
A history of prematurity, trisomy 21, velopharyngeal cleft palate repair, or hypotonia is each associated with an increased risk of sleep-disordered breathing. A past history of adenotonsillectomy for snoring is important information to obtain. Chronic nasal obstruction can cause maxillary hypoplasia. Arnold-Chiari malformation, myelomeningocele, or a brainstem lesion can predispose to central sleep apnea due to impaired central respiratory drive. Chronic health issues can also be associated with sleep disruption and consequently with behavioral problems associated with sleep.

A family history of obstructive sleep apnea (OSA), insomnia, or restless legs syndrome (RLS) is important; a family history of RLS can be used to support a diagnosis of RLS in the child.

In particular, questioning the mother if she had symptoms of RLS during any of her pregnancies can be helpful because this is a common time for RLS to present or worsen. Morning or evening preferences (i.e., "night-owl" or "lark" tendencies) can also have a familial element. In addition, sleepwalking can be found to occur in families.

Focused Physical Examination
The physical examination in a child presenting with a sleep complaint should include a general assessment. Presence/absence of sleepiness, fatigue, and irritability/hyperactivity are all important. Height, weight, and body mass index (BMI) should be recorded. Children with OSA can have poor growth and even failure to thrive. Obesity is a risk factor for OSA. Special attention to a child's craniofacial features is important because these may make a child more at risk for sleep-disordered breathing. Assessment of tonsil size, oropharyngeal crowding (using the Mallampati or Friedman classification systems can be useful), and presence of maxillary/mandibular hypoplasia can all offer clues to an airway that may predispose to OSA. The practitioner should evaluate for evidence of nasal obstruction by noting mouth breathing and signs of allergy (i.e., allergic shiners, nasal crease).

Diagnostic Tools
Polysomnography
The AASM has published practice parameters on both the respiratory and nonrespiratory indications for polysomnography (PSG) in pediatric patients. In this chapter, a sleep study or PSG will refer only to an in-laboratory attended study, because home monitoring currently has not been sufficiently evaluated in the pediatric population. PSG in children entails spending the night at a sleep center. A parent or caregiver must also spend the night. During the night, the child's sleep characteristics, respiratory function, and movement are analyzed. This is done by the following measures: electroencephalography (EEG), electromyography (EMG) of chin and limbs, airflow by thermistor and nasal pressure, end-tidal or transcutaneous carbon dioxide measurements, and induction plethysmography to measure respiratory effort. Scoring of a PSG performed on a child is done using pediatric scoring rules set forth by the AASM.

The most common indication for a sleep study in children is OSA. PSG can be used to both diagnose OSA and treat sleep apnea with continuous positive airway pressure (CPAP). PSG can also be used to evaluate for elevated periodic limb movements of sleep, and in rare cases to characterize abnormal nocturnal behavior such as evaluation of parasomnias or nocturnal seizures.

Overnight Oximetry
The gold standard for diagnosis of pediatric OSA is PSG. Overnight oximetry has been suggested as an alternative screening tool for pediatric sleep-disordered OSA. Although an abnormal oximetry will suggest OSA, a normal oximetry does not rule out OSA. Children can have sleep apnea that is severe and still maintain normal oxygenation. In a study by Brouillette and colleagues (2000), when a positive oximetry graph was present (defined by three or more desaturation clusters and at least three desaturations < 90%) in a referred population, the positive predictive value for OSA on PSG was 97%. A negative or inconclusive oximetry by this definition did not rule out OSA and there was still a 47% chance OSA was present on PSG.

Sleep Logs/Actigraphy
Sleep logs can be effective in demonstrating a child's sleep-wake patterns. Actigraphy is often done in conjunction with a sleep log. Actigraphy is a portable wristband that measures movement. The absence of movement over a certain time period is used as a surrogate marker of sleep, and the presence of movement over a certain time period is used as a surrogate for wakefulness. Some devices also measure ambient light exposure. Used in conjunction with actigraphy sleep logs can be extremely helpful in demonstrating discrepancies between perceived and actual sleep, and are helpful in demonstrating insufficient sleep and circadian rhythm

TABLE 2 BEARS Mnemonic: A Screening Tool for Sleep Disorders in Children

	PRESCHOOL (2–5 YEARS)	SCHOOL-AGE (6–12 YEARS)	ADOLESCENT (13–18 YEARS)
Bedtime problems	Does your child have any problems going to bed? Falling asleep?	Does your child have any problems at bedtime? (P) Do you have any problems going to bed? (C)	Do you have any problems falling asleep at bedtime? (C)
Excessive daytime sleepiness	Does your child seem overly tired or sleepy during the day? Does your child still take naps?	Does your child have difficulty waking in the morning, seem sleepy during the day, or take naps? (P) Do you feel tired a lot? (C)	Do you feel sleepy a lot during the day? In school? While driving? (C)
Awakenings during the night	Does your child wake up a lot at night?	Does your child seem to wake up a lot at night? Any sleepwalking or nightmares? (P) Do you wake up a lot at night? Have trouble getting back to sleep? (C)	Do you wake up a lot at night? Have trouble getting back to sleep? (C)
Regularity and duration of sleep	Does your child have a regular bedtime and wake time? What are they?	What time does your child go to bed and get up on school days? Weekends? Do you think your child is getting enough sleep? (P)	What time do you usually go to bed on school nights? Weekends? How much sleep do you usually get? (C)
Sleep-disordered breathing	Does your child snore a lot or have difficulty breathing at night?	Does your child have loud or nightly snoring or any breathing difficulties at night? (P)	Does your teenager snore loudly or nightly? (P)

Abbreviations: C = child; P = parent.
From Owens JA, Dalzell V: Use of the "BEARS" sleep screening tool in a pediatric residents' continuity clinic: A pilot study. Sleep Med 2005;6:63–69.

TABLE 3 Principles of Sleep Hygiene in Children

The child's bedroom should be dark and quiet.
Bedtime routines should be strictly enforced. Routines should be relaxing and only 20 to 30 minutes in length.
The time of morning awakening should be firmly and consistently structured.
Bedroom temperatures should be kept comfortably cool (< 75 °F).
Environmental noise should be minimized as much as possible. Background music and/or white noise may inhibit extraneous noise.
Children should not go to bed hungry and may have a snack before bedtime.
Excessive fluids before bedtime may result in bladder distention and arousal and disrupt sleep.
Children should learn to fall asleep alone (i.e., without their parents' presence in the room).
Vigorous activity should be avoided before bedtime.
A bath is often a stimulating activity for children. If bedtime struggles are present after a child's bath, it may be moved to the morning or separated from the child's bedtime by at least 2 hours.
Methylxanthine-containing beverages and food (e.g., caffeinated beverages/colas, tea, chocolate) should be avoided several hours before bedtime.
Parents should read labels on all over-the-counter and prescription medications. Some may contain alcohol or caffeine and may disrupt sleep.
Naps should be developmentally appropriate. Brief naps may be refreshing, but prolonged naps or napping too frequently may result in significant accumulation of sleep during the day and make it more difficult to fall asleep at night.

Modified from Sheldon SH, Ferber R, Kryger M (eds): Principles and Practice of Pediatric Sleep Medicine. Philadelphia: Elsevier Saunders, 2005.

disorders. Those that measure light as well can aid in uncovering sleep hygiene issues.

Multiple Sleep Latency Test

The multiple sleep latency test (MSLT) is a daytime study used to objectively measure sleepiness. It is often used to aid in the diagnosis of narcolepsy or hypersomnia. It is a set of four to five scheduled naps that typically occur the day after an overnight sleep study. Often 2 weeks of actigraphy are done before the MSLT to determine sleep-wake patterns.

Common Pediatric Sleep Diagnoses and Treatment
Obstructive Sleep Apnea
Epidemiology

Up to one-fifth of children can have intermittent snoring. Prevalence rates of OSA range from 1.2% to 5.7%. OSA is most common in children 2 to 8 years of age corresponding to the peak age of adenotonsillar hypertrophy. Due to the rise in childhood obesity there is now a corresponding rise in older children diagnosed with OSA.

Pathophysiology

The pharynx has many roles, including swallowing, speaking, and maintaining airway patency. Pharyngeal size is determined by the bones and soft tissue. The soft tissue is affected by the size of the tonsils and adenoids, as well as adipose tissue. Airway patency is maintained during wakefulness; a small airway can become vulnerable during sleep resulting in partial or total closure of the airway, hypoxemia, hypercapnia, and an arousal that results in opening of the airway and termination of the obstructive event. This leads to sleep disruption and daytime consequences. OSA in children likely results from a combination of narrowing of the upper airway, abnormal upper airway tone, and genetic factors.

Clinical Manifestation

OSA in adults is typically associated with daytime sleepiness. Associations have been made with hypertension, stroke, and metabolic syndrome. In children, OSA may not present with daytime sleepiness. Children may present with daytime inattention and/or neurocognitive and behavioral issues. Symptoms include snoring with or without apneic pauses or gasps. Restless sleep or secondary enuresis may also be noted. Parents may comment on increased work of breathing while sleeping. Other associations include poor growth, obesity, hypertension, and systemic inflammation.

Diagnosis

The gold standard for diagnosis of pediatric OSA is an in-laboratory attended PSG by an accredited sleep laboratory. History and physical examination lack sensitivity and specificity in predicting which children with snoring have OSA. However, a history of loud snoring, tonsillar hypertrophy, and abnormal oximetry is strongly suggestive of the diagnosis of OSA (see above). History alone cannot distinguish children with OSA from those with primary snoring. Criteria for the diagnosis of OSA in children are met when there is one or more apnea or hypopnea events per hour identified using scoring criteria by the AASM.

Differential Diagnosis

Other forms of sleep-disordered breathing are not as common as OSA. Sleep-related hypoventilation can occur in patients with neuromuscular weakness. Central hypoventilation syndromes are rare, but should be considered in children with persistent gas exchange abnormalities without additional explanation. Sleep-related hypoxemia can be present in pediatric patients with chronic lung disease. Central sleep apnea should be thought of in patients with brainstem abnormalities or Arnold-Chiari malformation. Sleep-related seizures may be difficult to differentiate from OSA in infants and an extended EEG montage may be necessary during their sleep study. Normal breathing patterns of infants and children should also be identified; brief (less than 10 seconds), central respiratory pauses that are self-resolving (and without significant desaturation) are common in normal children in either REM sleep or post-arousal/post-sigh.

Treatment

Treatment of OSA in most children is adenotonsillectomy. Recent guidelines from the AAP recommend an overnight sleep study in children where the practitioner had a clinical suspicion of OSA before adenotonsillectomy. Children with mild OSA preoperative can be monitored clinically postoperatively. Children with moderate to severe OSA, as well as children with craniofacial abnormalities, neurologic disorders, and obesity, should have a follow-up PSG to demonstrate resolution of OSA after surgery. Recent randomized controlled trials have shown that some children may outgrow their OSA, particularly if it is mild. Children who are not candidates for adenotonsillectomy may be treated with CPAP and use may have an impact on neurobehavioral outcomes. Treatment with CPAP therapy in children requires close follow-up because pressure needs may change with growth. In certain children, treatment with intranasal corticosteroids and/or montelukast may be considered with close follow-up.

Difficulty with Sleep Initiation and Night Wakings
Epidemiology
Bedtime problems and night wakings occur in up to 30% of children.

Clinical Manifestations
The diagnosis of insomnia includes difficulty going to sleep and/or staying asleep, the complaint that sleep is not of good quality, and the report of poor daytime functioning. The sleep complaints of infants and young children are often in the words of their parent or caregiver.

In preschool-age children both bedtime problems and night wakings are common and characterized by two types of behavioral insomnia of childhood: sleep-onset association type and limit-setting type. The definition of the *sleep-onset association type*, as defined in the ICSD-3, includes the following: sleep initiation is an extended process, associations are demanding, if the associations are not present sleep onset is delayed, and awakenings require caregiver intervention. The *limit-setting type* involves difficulty initiating or maintaining sleep, there is bedtime stalling or refusal, and the caregiver does not set sufficient and appropriate limits around this behavior. Children with frequent and prolonged night wakings have the sleep-onset association type. They often require an intervention by the caretaker to reinitiate sleep. Both problems can be present at once. Children who have difficulty going to sleep and provide resistance to bedtime have the limit-setting type. Parents of these children may complain of daytime behavioral issues due to the parent's inability to set limits during the day as well.

Diagnosis
Diagnosis is made from the history in the majority of cases. An overnight sleep study may be indicated in cases where another sleep disorder is suspected.

Differential Diagnosis
The differential diagnosis of insomnia or behavioral insomnia of childhood includes sleep disorders such as OSA, RLS, or nocturnal seizures. These disorders can prompt nocturnal awakenings or make sleep initiation difficult. If there is clinical suspicion of one of these disorders, an overnight sleep study may be indicated.

Treatment
Behavioral interventions have been shown to be effective in treating all forms of insomnia. In older children, primary and secondary insomnia can be effectively treated with cognitive-behavioral therapy. This often includes stimulus control and sleep restriction. Stimulus control includes maintaining a regular sleep-wake pattern and using the bed and bedroom only for sleeping. It involves getting out of bed if sleep is not initiated within about 20 minutes. Sleep restriction includes minimizing the time in bed to be only sleeping. It often includes delaying bedtime to the child's actual sleep onset, and then over time gradually advancing the bedtime. Sleep hygiene should be effectively addressed, including development of a relaxing bedtime routine, maintaining a regular sleep-wake pattern, and eliminating electronic use before bedtime.

There are several treatments of behavioral insomnia of childhood sleep-onset association type. No one treatment has been found to be superior. The goal of all of these methods is for the child to fall asleep in his or her crib or bed on the child's own. These include extinction (i.e., "cry it out"), which is often not palatable to caregivers. There is the graduated extinction method, which has parents ignoring crying or protests for specified periods of increasingly longer intervals. Some prefer an even more gradual approach of sitting next to the child's bed in a chair and over several days to weeks moving that chair across the room and out of the room. A consistent bedtime routine should also be implemented. Use of a transitional object can be helpful. Treatment of the limit-setting type includes firm limit setting. Positive reinforcement and limiting negative reinforcement should be used. The use of a reward system can be helpful. Effectively addressing behavioral treatment of sleep issues can be challenging for the primary care provider because of time constraints.

Restless Legs Syndrome/Willis Ekbom Disease
Epidemiology
Prevalence rates for pediatric RLS/WED have ranged from 1% to 6%.

Risk Factors
Risk factors include a family history and a history of anemia or iron deficiency. Attention-deficit/hyperactivity disorder (ADHD) is associated with RLS.

Pathophysiology
Decreased dopamine has been suggested in the pathophysiology of RLS/WED. Iron is a cofactor in the synthesis of dopamine and treatment of iron deficiency or low ferritin, if present, may improve symptoms.

Diagnosis
Diagnosis of pediatric RLS/WED is a clinical diagnosis. It is made using the adult criteria set forth in the ICSD-3 but with

some modification for children due to developmental issues. It consists of the child reporting an urge to move the legs, usually accompanied by an uncomfortable sensation; this urge or sensation worsens during rest or inactivity; the sensations are improved or resolved by movement; the sensations are present or worsen in the evening or night. If a child cannot express a description in his or her own words, diagnosis can be made using two out of the following three criteria: a sleep disturbance for age, a family history of RLS, and a periodic limb movement index on PSG of > 5 per hour. Because of this last criterion, a sleep study can be helpful in children to make this diagnosis. There can be an association with sleep initiation and maintenance difficulties.

Differential Diagnosis

Differential diagnosis of RLS should include insomnia, sleep-disordered breathing, or neurologic or musculoskeletal etiologies for the discomfort.

Treatment

Nonpharmacologic treatment of RLS includes good sleep hygiene, moderate exercise a few hours before bedtime, and avoidance of substances that are associated with worsening of RLS symptoms, including caffeine, alcohol, antihistamines, and antiemetics. A serum ferritin should be drawn in all children with RLS and if < 50 ng/mL, treatment with 6 mg/kg/day of oral elemental iron should be considered. Oral iron absorption is enhanced by vitamin C and impaired by calcium. Gastrointestinal upset and constipation can be common side effects. Compliance can be difficult. A serum ferritin should be rechecked at 3 months to evaluate therapy. Referral to a sleep medicine specialist should be made if lifestyle and oral iron therapy have been unsuccessful. There are no FDA-approved medications for the treatment of RLS in children. Dopamine agonists, gabapentin (Neurontin),[1] clonazepam (Klonopin),[1] and clonidine (Catapres)[1] have been used to treat pediatric RLS.

Delayed Sleep Phase Syndrome

Epidemiology

Delayed sleep phase syndrome (DSPS) occurs most commonly in adolescents and young adults.

Clinical Manifestations

Symptoms usually present in adolescents but can occur in younger children. Adolescents with DSPS consistently have sleep onset at a later time, typically after midnight. They have difficulty initiating sleep earlier. They do not have difficulty maintaining sleep. They have difficulty waking in the morning unless able to sleep until their preferred time, which is typically after 10 AM. They may have sleepiness during the daytime if forced to rise early (i.e., for school); however, during long vacations or summer breaks when allowed to sleep to preferred wake time they feel refreshed. Children who already have a preferred evening preference may find this exacerbated in adolescence. Poor school performance can be present.

Diagnosis

Diagnosis is made from history; actigraphy and sleep logs are also useful. An overnight sleep study may be indicated if another sleep disorder is suspected (e.g., OSA).

Differential Diagnosis

The differential diagnosis includes insomnia, poor sleep hygiene, insufficient sleep, mood disorder, OSA, and RLS.

Treatment

Treatment is typically behavioral and includes good sleep hygiene. Typically either the patient's sleep-wake schedule

is advanced (if there is less than 3 hours between actual and desired bedtime) by 15 minutes every 2 to 3 days until the goal bedtime is achieved. Rise time is advanced as well and if set at the desired wake time initially it should facilitate the advancement of the bedtime by increasing sleep drive. If the desired bedtime of the adolescent is greater than 3 hours from the current bedtime, phase delay can be considered. Bedtime is delayed by 2 to 3 hours each day until the target bedtime is reached. Timing of this therapy should be considered, because it will interfere with school or other daytime activities. Parental or caregiver support is necessary, as well as commitment by the adolescent.

Once the new pattern is established weekends must not differ from weekdays by more than 1 to 2 hours. This is particularly important for the rise time. Relapse is common if strict sleep-wake patterns are not adhered to, a problem common on vacations.

Both bright light exposure and melatonin have been used to help reset the circadian rhythm. Exposure to bright light in the morning is encouraged and can be as simple as increasing sun exposure in the morning. Light boxes using 2500 to 10,000 lux can be used in the morning for 20 to 30 minutes. Exposure to light in the evening should be limited. A small dose of melatonin[7] (0.5 mg) can be used in the early evening (about 5 hours before desired bedtime) to attempt to physiologically advance sleep onset. If the timing is not optimal for both light and melatonin, the phase delay can be worsened; consultation with a sleep physician should be considered.

Parasomnias

Parasomnias can occur out of both non-REM (NREM) and REM sleep. Those occurring out of NREM sleep include sleepwalking, sleep terrors, and confusional arousals. They typically occur in the first one-third of the night, when NREM-3 sleep is most prevalent, and are not recalled the next day. They can be part of normal development, but depending on their nature, they can be distressing to caregiver and child. Parasomnias occurring out of REM sleep include nightmares and REM-sleep behavior disorder (RBD). Nightmares are commonly recalled and have been associated with anxiety in children. Nightmares typically peak in the school-age child. RBD is rare in children but has been reported; it involves the loss of atonia that occurs in REM sleep and consequently dreams are "acted out."

Risk Factors

Poor sleep hygiene, insufficient sleep, irregular sleep-wake patterns, and a positive family history are all risk factors. Sleep disruption from sleep-disordered breathing or periodic limb movements of sleep can exacerbate parasomnias.

Differential Diagnosis

The differential diagnosis should include nocturnal seizures. In addition, if another sleep disorder is present, parasomnias can be exacerbated.

Treatment

Safety is most important in children with parasomnias, and it is important that the child's sleep environment is kept clear of things that could cause injury. Door alarms can be effective. The child should not be awakened during the episode. The event should not be referred to the next morning because this can cause distress for the child. Maintaining good sleep hygiene and regular sleep-wake patterns is important. If the events occur at a predictable time each night, the caregiver can do planned awakenings 30 minutes before the event typically occurs for several weeks. This may abolish the episodes. It can also have the effect of pushing the episode to later in the night. Pharmacologic treatment with a small dose of a benzodiazepine (e.g., 0.5 mg of clonazepam

---

[1]Not FDA approved for this indication.

[7]Available as dietary supplement.

[Klonopin][1] at bedtime) may be indicated in severe cases with the drug tapered slowly after episodes are suppressed.

Hypersomnias

A full discussion of primary hypersomnias (including narcolepsy) in children is beyond the scope of this chapter. Consideration for a primary hypersomnia should be made in a child who is sleepy after common causes of sleepiness such as insufficient sleep and obstructive sleep apnea have been ruled out. Symptoms of narcolepsy include disrupted nocturnal sleep, hallucinations on going to sleep or waking up, and sleep paralysis. Daytime sleepiness is present with "sleep attacks" both during quiet activities and while active. Cataplexy may also be present and is defined by loss of muscle tone without loss of consciousness. It should be noted that onset of narcolepsy is often in adolescence or as a young adult. Diagnosis is often delayed because the symptoms are attributed to other conditions. Treatment of pediatric hypersomnia is done under the supervision of a sleep specialist and often involves use of stimulants.

---

[1]Not FDA approved for this indication.

References

Aurora RN, Lamm CI, Zak RS, et al: Practice parameters for the non-respiratory indications for polysomnography and multiple sleep latency testing for children, *Sleep* 35:1467–1473, 2012.

Aurora RN, Zak RS, Karippot A, et al: Practice parameters for the respiratory indications for polysomnography in children, *Sleep* 34:379–388, 2011.

Berry RB, Brooks R, Gamaldo C, et al: *The AASM Manual for the Scoring of Sleep and Associated Events*, Westchester, Illinois, 2012, American Academy of Sleep Medicine2012.

Brouillette RT, Morielli A, Leimanis A, et al: Nocturnal pulse oximetry as an abbreviated testing modality for pediatric obstructive sleep apnea, *Pediatrics* 105:405–412, 2000.

Fehrm J, Nerfeldt P, Browaldh N, Friberg D: Effectiveness of adenotonsillectomy vs watchful waiting in young children with mild to moderate obstructive sleep apnea: A randomized clinical trial, *JAMA Otolaryngol Head Neck Surg* 146(7):647–654, 2020.

Kaditis A, Kheirandish-Gozal L, Gozal D: Algorithm for the diagnosis and treatment of pediatric OSA: a proposal of two pediatric sleep centers, *Sleep Med* 13:217–227, 2012.

Kheirandish-Gozal L, Bhattacharjee R, Bandla HP, Gozal D: Antiinflammatory therapy outcomes for mild OSA in children, *Chest* 146(1):88–95, 2014.

Kirk V, Baughn J, D'Andrea L, et al: American Academy of Sleep Medicine Position Paper for the Use of a Home Sleep Apnea Test for the Diagnosis of OSA in Children, *J Clin Sleep Med* 13(10):1099–1203.

Kotagal S, Nichols CD, Grigg-Damberger MM, et al: Non-respiratory indications for polysomnography and related procedures in children: an evidence-based review, *Sleep* 35:1451–1466, 2012.

Kuhle S, Hoffmann DU, Mitra S, Urschitz MS: Anti-inflammatory medications for obstructive sleep apnoea in children, *Cochrane Database Syst Rev* 1(1):Cd007074, 2020.

Lloyd R, Tippmann-Peikert M, Slocumb N, et al: Characteristics of REM sleep behavior disorder in childhood, *J Clin Sleep Med* 8:127–131, 2012a.

Marcus CL, Brooks LJ, Draper KA, et al: Diagnosis and management of childhood obstructive sleep apnea syndrome, *Pediatrics* 130:576–584, 2012b.

Marcus CL, Brooks LJ, Draper KA, et al: Diagnosis and management of childhood obstructive sleep apnea syndrome, *Pediatrics* 130:e714–e755, 2012.

Marcus CL, Moore RH, Rosen CL, et al: A randomized trial of adenotonsillectomy for childhood sleep apnea, *N Engl J Med* 368(25):2366–2376, 2013.

Marcus CL, Radcliffe J, Konstantinopoulou S, et al: Effects of positive airway pressure therapy on neurobehavioral outcomes in children with obstructive sleep apnea, *Am J Respir Crit Care Med* 185:998–1003, 2012.

Mindell JA, Barrett KM: Nightmares and anxiety in elementary-aged children: is there a relationship? *Child Care Health Dev* 28:317–322, 2002.

Mindell JA, Owens J: *A clinical guide to pediatric sleep: diagnosis and management of sleep problems*, Philadelphia, 2003, Lippincott Williams & Wilkins.

Mindell JA, Owens J: *A clinical guide to pediatric sleep: diagnosis and management of sleep problems*, ed 2, Philadelphia, 2010, Lippincott Williams & Wilkins.

Morgenthaler T, Alessi C, Friedman L, et al: Practice parameters for the use of actigraphy in the assessment of sleep and sleep disorders: an update for 2007, *Sleep* 30:519–529, 2007.

Morgenthaler T, Kramer M, Alessi C, et al: Practice parameters for the psychological and behavioral treatment of insomnia: an update. An American Academy of Sleep Medicine report, *Sleep* 29:1415–1419, 2006.

Owens JA, Dalzell V: Use of the "BEARS" sleep screening tool in a pediatric residents' continuity clinic: a pilot study, *Sleep Med* 6:63–69, 2005.

Paruthi S, Brooks LJ, D'Ambrosio C, et al: Consensus Statement of the American Academy of Sleep Medicine on the Recommended Amount of Sleep for Healthy Children: Methodology and Discussion, *J Clin Sleep Med* 12(11):1549–1561, 2016.

Picchietti D, Allen RP, Walters AS, et al: Restless legs syndrome: prevalence and impact in children and adolescents—the Peds REST study, *Pediatrics* 120:253–266, 2007.

Sateia MJ, editor: *The International Classification of Sleep Disorders*, 3rd ed, Westchester, Illinois, 2014, American Academy of Sleep Medicine.

Sheldon SH, Ferber R, Kryger M, editors: *Principles and Practice of Pediatric Sleep Medicine*, Philadelphia, 2005, Elsevier Saunders.

St Louis EK, Morgenthaler TI: Sleep disorders. In Bope E, Kellerman R, editors: *Conn's Current Therapy 2013*, Philadelphia, 2013, Saunders Elsevier.

POST-COVID-19 MULTISYSTEM INFLAMMATORY SYNDROME IN CHILDREN

Method of
Ian D. Ferguson, MD; and Carlos R. Oliveira, MD

CURRENT DIAGNOSIS

- Multisystem inflammatory syndrome in children (MIS-C) is a rare hyperinflammatory complication of severe acute respiratory syndrome coronavirus 2 (SARS-CoV-2) infection that is associated with multiorgan dysfunction and hemodynamic compromise.
- Clinicians should suspect MIS-C in a child or adolescent with a recent SARS-CoV-2 infection or exposure who has a persistent fever and at least two other suggestive clinical features such as cardiovascular dysfunction, gastrointestinal symptoms, peripheral edema, rash, oral mucosal changes, conjunctivitis, or neurocognitive symptoms.
- It is recommended that a tiered approach be used for evaluation. The initial laboratory tests aim to screen for evidence of systemic inflammation and confirm active or recent infection. Subsequent tests aim to evaluate for potential organ-specific dysfunction and include cardiac tests, coagulation tests, and hemophagocytosis tests.

CURRENT THERAPY

- Immunomodulatory treatment with intravenous immunoglobulin (IVIG [Gammagard])[1] and glucocorticoids is considered the mainstay of treatment.
- High-dose glucocorticoids and/or biologic agents, such as interleukin or tumor necrosis factor inhibitors, should be considered in patients with refractory disease.
- Unless there are contraindications, all patients with MIS-C should receive thrombosis prevention with aspirin.[1] Anticoagulation with enoxaparin (Lovenox)[1] should also be considered in patients with documented thrombosis and in those with risk factors for thrombosis.
- Given that treatment guidelines are constantly evolving, management decisions should be made in consultation with a multidisciplinary team of pediatric subspecialists.

The Centers for Disease Control and Prevention (CDC) defines a case of MIS-C as an individual younger than 21 years of age, who was recently infected with SARS-CoV-2 (evidenced by the detection of SARS-CoV-2 antibodies, or RNA/antigen in a clinical specimen up to 60 days prior to presentation), and presents with systemic inflammation (fever and a C-reactive protein ≥3 mg/dL) and multisystem organ disease, evidenced by at least 2 of the following: cardiac manifestations (i.e., left ventricular ejection fraction <55%, coronary artery dilatation, troponin elevation), shock, mucocutaneous findings, gastrointestinal symptoms (i.e., abdominal pain, vomiting, diarrhea), or hematologic abnormalities (thrombocytopenia or lymphopenia). The CDC definition also specifies that children must have a clinically severe illness (requiring hospitalization) and have no plausible alternative diagnosis.

Epidemiology

The first pediatric case of coronavirus disease 2019 (COVID-19), the respiratory disease associated with severe acute respiratory syndrome coronavirus 2 (SARS-CoV-2) infection, was reported in the United States on March 2, 2020. Although children with acute COVID-19 infection fared relatively better than adults, their outcomes have not been universally benign, and some became critically ill. In April 2020, several reports were published describing a more severe clinical phenotype of SARS-CoV-2 in which children presented with systemic hyperinflammation and rapid-onset circulatory shock. This inflammatory phenotype is commonly known as multisystem inflammatory syndrome in children (MIS-C). MIS-C is a relatively rare complication of SARS-Cov-2 in children, occurring in approximately 1 of 3000 infections. Most cases have occurred in previously healthy children 6 to 12 years of age. Black and Hispanic children have been disproportionately affected by MIS-C in the United States, although it remains unclear if these disparities in MIS-C will continue with time. The only known way to prevent MIS-C is by avoiding infection in the first place, which can be effectively accomplished with immunization.

Pathophysiology

The pathophysiology of MIS-C has not yet been established. Although some patients with MIS-C test positive for the virus by polymerase chain reaction (PCR), nearly all have SARS-CoV-2–specific antibodies at the time of presentation, which suggests that MIS-C is a postinfectious process. This is further collaborated by a clear epidemiologic link wherein clusters of MIS-C cases in the community are often observed 2 to 5 weeks following a peak in COVID-19 cases.

The current thinking is that the virus may directly activate cells in the innate immune system, which causes uncontrolled inflammation. Another potential etiology is the generation of autoreactive antibodies during the infection. These autoantibodies could mediate disease by damaging the endothelium and microvasculature. This is a conceivable mechanism as some of the manifestations that are characteristic of MIS-C, like the propensity for myocardial injury and thrombosis, suggest a degree of endothelial involvement.

Clinical Manifestations

There is considerable heterogeneity in the clinical manifestations of MIS-C. Symptoms typically begin 2 to 6 weeks after an acute SARS-CoV-2 infection. Fever is the most common MIS-C symptom and can last for 4 to 6 days. Gastrointestinal symptoms such as abdominal pain and emesis are also common, and this serosal inflammation may resemble appendicitis. Some of the classic Kawasaki disease (KD) findings, like nonpurulent conjunctivitis, edema of the hands and feet, mucous membrane lesions, and diffuse erythematous rash, can also be present in MIS-C. There is no standard pattern for the rash, but morbilliform, maculopapular, or diffuse erythema can be present. Retropharyngeal edema is also commonly associated with MIS-C and can present with severe throat pain, cervical lymphadenopathy, and torticollis. Neurocognitive symptoms like lethargy, confusion, and headaches are frequently noted. Severe neurologic manifestations are rare but have also been reported, including seizures, ataxia, strokes, encephalopathy, and cerebral edema. Myocardial dysfunction can occur in 50% to 90% of cases and often leads to hypotension and shock. Children with MIS-C rarely manifest respiratory symptoms, and chest imaging is usually normal. If pulmonary abnormalities are present on imaging, they are usually patchy opacities or pulmonary edema that can be attributable to cardiovascular dysfunction. Most children with MIS-C will have elevated laboratory markers of inflammation, such as C-reactive protein (CRP), ferritin, or procalcitonin. Other common laboratory abnormalities include lymphopenia, thrombocytopenia, hypoalbuminemia, transaminitis, and hypertriglyceridemia.

Diagnosis

The first step to effectively managing MIS-C is making an accurate diagnosis. There are no specific laboratory tests that are diagnostic of MIS-C, and the diagnosis is largely clinical. However, the initial signs and symptoms of MIS-C are not unique to this illness (Table 1). Thus laboratory investigations must be done to rule out alternative diagnoses. KD and toxic shock syndrome (TSS) are the two clinical entities with the most overlap with MIS-C, though the differential can be considerably larger. A tiered approach to laboratory evaluation for patients suspected of having MIS-C has been recommended by the American College of Rheumatology (ACR) and the American Academy of Pediatrics (AAP). The first step is to determine which children should be evaluated for MIS-C. It is recommended that children with unremitting fever, an epidemiologic link to SARS-CoV-2, and at least two suggestive clinical features (e.g., hypotension, rash, gastrointestinal symptoms, edema of the hands and feet, mucocutaneous changes, conjunctivitis, lymphadenopathy, or neurologic symptoms), undergo the initial tier of laboratory testing for MIS-C (Table 1). The evaluation for MIS-C must include a thorough differential diagnosis to rule out other potential etiologies. Thus these patients should ideally be managed by a multidisciplinary team of specialists, including pediatric rheumatology, cardiology, infectious diseases, and depending on clinical severity and symptom development, intensive care, hematology, nephrology, neurology, and gastroenterology.

Initial Evaluation

Tier 1 includes measuring inflammatory markers, testing for SARS-CoV-2 antibodies, and performing a complete blood count and a metabolic panel. Uncontrolled inflammation is characteristic of MIS-C, and elevations in CRP or erythrocyte sedimentation rate (ESR) are nearly always observed. Patients with inflammatory activation will also often have cytopenias and other marrow abnormalities. The presence of lymphopenia has been consistently reported in the medical literature as a predictor of severity. However, a severe reduction in any cell line can be associated with uncontrolled inflammation and may indicate progression into macrophage activation syndrome (MAS) pathophysiology. The diagnosis of MIS-C also requires an epidemiologic link to SARS-CoV-2. This link can take the form of recent close contact with a confirmed COVID-19 case, a positive PCR or antigen test (suggestive of active infection or recent past infection), or a positive serologic test. In patients who have been vaccinated against SARS-CoV-2, the presence of nucleocapsid antibodies is suggestive of a recent infection, whereas in patients who have not been vaccinated, either spike protein or nucleocapsid antibodies could be used to determine if the patient had a previous infection. Approximately 15% of patients suspected of having MIS-C will have PCR positivity. Because the clinical features of acute SARS-CoV-2 infection can overlap with MIS-C, it is important to rule out acute COVID-19 pneumonia in this group as the treatment approach for active COVID-19 will differ from MIS-C. Serology can be helpful in this context as children with active COVID-19 are less likely to have measurable anti–SARS-CoV-2 immunoglobulin G (IgG) antibodies on presentation.

Subsequent Evaluations

Patients proceed to tier 2 of testing if they are suspected of having MIS-C, have an elevation of CRP or ESR, and have at least one additional laboratory abnormality, such as lymphopenia, thrombocytopenia, hyponatremia, neutrophilia, or hypoalbuminemia. Patients who present with severe manifestations, such as shock, are also recommended to proceed to tier 2 diagnostic evaluations. Tier 2 assessments aim to evaluate for potential organ-specific damage and can be useful for evaluating other diseases in the differential that may also be affected by treatment. These assessments include cardiac tests (troponin, brain natriuretic peptide [BNP],

	MULTISYSTEM INFLAMMATORY SYNDROME IN CHILDREN	TOXIC SHOCK SYNDROME	KAWASAKI DISEASE
Age in years	Most 6–12	Most <2 or >13	Most <5
Fever, >38°C	Common	Common	Common
Ocular findings	Nonexudative conjunctivitis	Occasional conjunctivitis	Limb-sparing conjunctivitis
Oral mucosa	Erythema, edema, strawberry tongue	Occasional erythema	Erythema, edema, strawberry tongue
Extremities	Edema, erythema	Edema	Edema, periungual desquamation
Adenopathy	Occasional	Not common	Common, cervical
Dermatologic	Erythematous, polymorphous	Erythroderma, desquamation	Erythematous, polymorphous
Gastrointestinal	Diarrhea, vomiting, or abdominal pain	Diarrhea, abdominal pain	Not common
Cardiovascular	Reduced EF, CA abnormalities	Shock	CA abnormalities
Neurologic	Headaches, lethargy, confusion, seizures	Headaches, lethargy, confusion	Headaches, lethargy
Laboratory findings	• ↑ Inflammatory markers (CRP,* ESR,* ANC,* LDH, ferritin, IL-6, procalcitonin) • ↓ Albumin,* ALC,* sodium,* platelets,* hemoglobin* • Abnormal cardiac tests (troponin, BNP, ECG) • ↑ Liver enzymes (AST, ALT) • Abnormal coagulation (PT, PTT, fibrinogen, D-dimer)	• ↑ CRP, ANC procalcitonin • ↑ liver enzymes (AST, ALT) • ↓ platelets, hemoglobin • Abnormal coagulation • Renal dysfunction • CK elevation	• ↑ CRP, ESR • ↓ ALC, sodium, hemoglobin • ↑ Liver enzymes (AST, ALT) • ↑ Platelets, triglycerides • Sterile pyuria
Distinguishing features	• COVID-19 exposure • Positive SARS-CoV-2 PCR* or serology*	• Positive cultures from either blood, wound, or mucosa	• Concurrent infections are common

*Tier 1 recommended laboratory study.

ALC, Absolute lymphocyte count; *ALT,* alanine transaminase; *ANC,* absolute neutrophil count; *AST,* aspartate transaminase; *BNP,* brain natriuretic peptide; *CA,* coronary arteries; *CK,* creatine phosphokinase; *CRP,* C-reactive protein; *ECG,* electrocardiogram; *EF,* ejection fraction; *ESR,* erythrocyte sedimentation rate; *IL-6,* interleukin 6; *LDH,* lactic acid dehydrogenase; *PCR,* polymerase chain reaction; *PT,* prothrombin time; *PTT,* partial prothrombin time.

electrocardiogram, and echocardiogram), coagulation tests (fibrinogen, D-dimer, prothrombin time, and activated partial thromboplastin time), and hemophagocytosis tests (ferritin, blood smear, lactate dehydrogenase, triglycerides, and cytokine panel). The signs and symptoms of MIS-C can mimic those of other infectious diseases, such as sepsis or TSS. Thus tier 2 tests should also include microbiologic tests (urine analysis, blood cultures, and other viral tests) based on clinical suspicion and specific symptoms.

Cardiac Tests

The feared complication of MIS-C is the development of coronary artery aneurysms. Although coronary vasculitis can occur in MIS-C, it is less common than myocardial involvement resulting in systolic dysfunction and cardiogenic shock. Cardiac evaluations should be completed as soon as possible. Elevation in the BNP or N-terminal pro-BNP suggests systolic dysfunction, and elevation in troponin suggests damage to cardiac myocytes. Elevation in BNP may continue with fluid resuscitation and medication administration, particularly intravenous immunoglobulin (IVIg), as it has a large infusion volume. Electrocardiogram abnormalities, such as abnormal ST- or T-wave segments or first-degree atrioventricular block, are also not uncommon in MIS-C.

Coagulation Tests

Hypercoagulability and thrombosis risk also must be assessed at the onset. Elevation of the D-dimer greater than five times the upper limit of normal is an independent risk factor for developing thrombosis and may help guide decisions around antithrombotic

therapy. Uncontrolled inflammation in the vasculature is also associated with hyponatremia and hypoalbuminemia. These findings are worth noting as they have been associated with a high risk of IVIG resistance in KD. Transaminase elevation is common in uncontrolled inflammation, and aspartate transaminase (AST) or alanine transaminase (ALT) elevation greater than three times the upper limit of normal suggests liver vasculature involvement.

Hemophagocytosis Tests

MIS-C can occasionally progress to a state in which the patient cannot turn off or reduce the endogenous immune response, leading to further organ damage. This dysregulation of the immune system is termed *macrophage activation syndrome.* Key to the diagnosis of this serious immune condition is pancytopenia and evidence of bone marrow destruction. Associated laboratory findings can include high levels of lactate dehydrogenase (LDH), hyperferritinemia, and hypertriglyceridemia. A blood smear can also show pancytopenia and, importantly, should not show any evidence of peripheral neoplasm, which would require different therapy than that for MIS-C. The cytokine panel can also be used, if available, to determine the level of inflammation (particularly the interleukin-6 level). However, cytokine panels often take several days to return, and treatment should not be withheld for these results.

Treatment

Immune Modulators

Children with moderate to severe disease and who require hospitalization should receive immune-modifying therapy with

TABLE 2 Immunologic, Cardiac, and Hematologic Management Recommendations for Multisystem Inflammatory Syndrome in Children

	INITIAL MANAGEMENT*	INTENSIFICATION TREATMENT[‖]
Immunologic	• IVIG[1] 2 g/kg (max dose 100 g) as single dose[†] • Methylprednisolone[1] 2 mg/kg/day IV, in two divided doses[‡] • Serial monitoring of inflammatory markers	• Methylprednisolone[1] 10–30 mg/kg/day, IV (max dose 1 g) for 1–3 days *AND/OR* • Anakinra[1] 4 mg/kg/day SC or IV divided every 6–12 hours *OR* • Infliximab[1] 5–10 mg/kg/day IV as single dose
Cardiac	• Serial monitoring for arrhythmias and ventricular dysfunction	• Vasopressor and/or inotropic support for fluid-refractory shock or severely low EF • ECMO for fulminant disease
Hematologic	• Aspirin[1] 3–5 mg/kg PO daily (max dose 81 mg/day)[§]	• Therapeutic anticoagulation: Enoxaparin[1] SC 1 mg/kg/dose BID, if thrombosis, low EF, or CA dilation. Titrate dosage to achieve target anti-Xa levels of 0.5–1.0 units/mL • Prophylactic anticoagulation: Enoxaparin[1] SC 0.5 mg/kg/dose BID if does not meet above criteria but at high risk for thrombosis

[1]Not FDA approved for this indication.
*Additional treatment for neurologic, respiratory, and renal abnormalities may also be required.
[†]Can be divided over 2 days if there is concern for fluid overload.
[‡]Consider a 2- to 3-week taper.
[§]Hold other nonsteroidal antiinflammatory drugs while on aspirin, and hold aspirin for active bleeding and thrombocytopenia.
[‖]Coordination with pediatric specialists in cardiology, rheumatology, hematology, and infectious diseases is recommended.
BID, Twice a day; *CA*, coronary arteries; *ECMO*, extracorporeal membrane oxygenation; *EF*, ejection fraction; *IV*, intravenously; *IVIG*, intravenous immunoglobulin; *PO*, by mouth; *SC*, subcutaneously.

intravenous immunoglobulin (IVIG [Gammagard])[1] and corticosteroids (Table 2). The recommended initial dose of IVIG is 2 g/kg, with a maximum dose of 100 g. This medication is infused with a relatively large fluid load; thus the patient's systolic function must be assessed before administration and closely monitored afterward. The immune modulation effects of IVIG are best achieved with a single dose, but if there is a concern for volume overload, the doses may be divided into 1 g/kg aliquots over 2 days with diuresis. We recommend pretreatment with acetaminophen and an antihistamine when IVIG is used, as it can frequently cause infusion reactions. In addition to IVIG, hospitalized patients with MIS-C should receive glucocorticoids. Initial therapy is with methylprednisolone (Solu-Medrol)[1] at a dose of 1 to 2 mg/kg/day. Glucocorticoids should ideally be given before IVIG as they may also help reduce the risk of potential IVIG infusion reactions.

The dose of corticosteroids can be increased to 10 to 30 mg/kg/day in patients who have a persistent fever or ongoing end-organ damage despite initial therapy with IVIG and glucocorticoids. Biologic immune therapies, such as interleukin (IL) blockers or tumor necrosis factor (TNF) inhibitors, should be considered in patients with recalcitrant disease or in those who have a contraindication to corticosteroids. The ACR recommends anakinra (Kineret),[1] an IL-1 receptor antagonist, as first-line therapy for recalcitrant MIS-C. It is administered at a starting dose of 4 mg/kg/day and can be escalated up to 8 to 12 mg/kg/day as needed. An alternative biologic agent is infliximab (Remicade, Inflectra, Renflexis, Ixifi, Avsola),[1] an anti–TNF-alpha monoclonal antibody, which can be given as a single dose of 5 mg/kg/day. Much like IVIG, infliximab doses should be pretreated with acetaminophen and antihistamine to reduce the risk of an infusion reaction. As symptoms improve and inflammatory markers wane, corticosteroids should be carefully tapered over 2 to 3 weeks to avoid rebound inflammation. It is also important to consider withdrawal symptoms from cortisol deficiency in patients who have received high-dose pulse therapy.

Antithrombotic Therapy

In addition to immune modulators, all patients with MIS-C should be given antithrombotic therapy, provided that they have no known contraindications and their risk of bleeding is not high (e.g., no bleeding diathesis, no thrombocytopenia, or active bleeding). Initial thrombosis prophylaxis should be with aspirin[1] (3 to 5 mg/kg/day, maximum 81 mg/day) and continued for at least 4 to 6 weeks. Longer courses of aspirin may be needed for patients who have cardiac abnormalities or those who have reactive thrombocytosis on follow-up evaluation. Aspirin is frequently avoided in pediatrics because of the risk of Reye syndrome. However, this is less of a concern when low doses are used (<81 mg/day). Another important toxicity to monitor when using aspirin is liver toxicity, which can be exacerbated by concurrent hypoalbuminemia.

Therapeutic anticoagulation with enoxaparin (Lovenox)[1] may also be needed in some patients with MIS-C. Our recommendations for treatment dosing of enoxaparin are provided in Table 2. Generally, patients with evidence of thrombosis, coronary artery changes (z-score >10), or severely low systolic function (ejection fraction <35%) require the addition of enoxaparin. Prophylactic-dose enoxaparin should be considered in patients with MIS-C who do not have the aforementioned findings yet remain at high risk for thrombosis, such as those admitted to an intensive care unit, those with a markedly elevated D-dimer (>5 times the upper limit of normal), or those who are older than 12 years of age.

Adjunctive Therapies

The need for additional support varies greatly on the initial clinical presentation. In cases in which there is significant cardiovascular disease, both vasopressors and inotropic supporting medications are commonly required. Fluid resuscitation should be used judiciously in these settings as large boluses can negatively affect respiratory status. Because MIS-C can have a similar presentation to that of sepsis, empiric broad-spectrum antibiotics are also often indicated, pending cultures. However, antivirals are rarely needed as MIS-C is often not an active viral process. However,

[1]Not FDA approved for this indication.

[1]Not FDA approved for this indication.

given the phenotypic overlap of MIS-C and acute SARS-CoV-2, distinguishing patients with an active infection from those with postinfectious MIS-C can sometimes be challenging. When there is uncertainty, such as in cases of severe pulmonary involvement with negative serology, we recommend consultation with an experienced infectious disease specialist.

Monitoring

As children with MIS-C can decompensate quickly, close observation and judicious use of laboratory tests are needed to monitor progression. We recommend follow-up laboratory tests every 6 to 12 hours for patients who are critically ill or those who have severe cardiac dysfunction. For patients who are not critically ill, we encourage daily laboratory tests to ensure that treatment is effectively reducing inflammation and normalizing organ dysfunction. There are no clear discharge criteria, but in general, patients should be afebrile without antipyretics (excluding corticosteroid and aspirin) and have down-trending inflammatory markers. For patients with cardiac manifestations, there should also be an improvement in laboratory markers of cardiac strain and an improvement in imaging studies.

Follow-up with a primary care physician should occur within 2 to 3 days of discharge. At our center, follow-up laboratory tests and cardiac imaging are performed 7 to 14 days postdischarge and again after 4 to 6 weeks to ensure that inflammation does not reaccumulate, assess cardiac function, and trend the size of coronary arteries. Aspirin is typically stopped at the 6-week visit if there is no rebound thrombocytosis and follow-up cardiac imaging is normal. Patients who presented with shock or developed coronary changes may require additional follow-up testing, such as a cardiac MRI to assess for scars, fibrosis, or aneurysms. Cardiac stress testing is also encouraged in patients who had a significant troponin leak during initial hospitalization. Three months postdischarge, after the cardiac function returns to normal, we also encourage SARS-CoV-2 immunization if age-eligible.

Complications

Data on long-term outcomes from MIS-C have been limited. However, existing data suggest a mortality rate between 1% and 2% among those treated. The long-term outcomes among survivors have been generally favorable. Follow-up studies have found that nearly all children completely recover by 8 to 10 weeks. Among the few patients with prolonged posttreatment symptoms, most had complaints such as headaches, fatigue, abdominal distress, and anxiety. Whether these persistent symptoms are causally related to MIS-C remains an open question.

References

Abrams JY, Oster ME, Godfred-Cato SE, et al: Factors linked to severe outcomes in multisystem inflammatory syndrome in children (MIS-C) in the USA: a retrospective surveillance study, *Lancet Child Adolesc Health* 5:323, 2021.

Capone CA, Misra N, Ganigara M, et al: Six month follow-up of patients with multi-system inflammatory syndrome in children, *Pediatrics* 148, 2021.

Consiglio CR, Cotugno N, Sardh F, Pou C, et al: The immunology of multisystem inflammatory syndrome in children with COVID-19, *Cell.* 183(4):968–981.e7, 2020 Nov 12.

Feldstein LR, Rose EB, Horwitz SM, et al: Multisystem inflammatory Syndrome in U.S. children and adolescents, *N Engl J Med* 383:334, 2020.

Fernandes DM, Oliveira CR, Guerguis S, et al: Severe acute respiratory syndrome coronavirus 2 clinical syndromes and predictors of disease severity in hospitalized children and youth, *J Pediatr* 230:23–31.e10, 2021 Mar.

Godfred-Cato S, Abrams JY, Balachandran N, et al: Distinguishing multisystem inflammatory syndrome in children from COVID-19, Kawasaki disease and toxic shock syndrome, *Pediatr Infect Dis J* 41(4):315–323, 2022 Apr 1.

Goldenberg NA, Sochet A, Albisetti M, et al: Consensus-based clinical recommendations and research priorities for anticoagulant thromboprophylaxis in children hospitalized for COVID-19-related illness, *J Thromb Haemost* 18:3099, 2020.

Henderson LA, Canna SW, Friedman KG, et al: American College of Rheumatology clinical guidance for multisystem inflammatory syndrome in children associated with SARS-CoV-2 and hyperinflammation in pediatric COVID-19, *Arthritis Rheumatol* 73(4):e13–e29, 2021 Apr. Version 3.

Oliveira CR, Niccolai LM, Sheikha H, et al: Assessment of clinical effectiveness of BNT162b2 COVID-19 vaccine in US adolescents, *JAMA Netw Open* 5(3):e220935, 2022 Mar 1.

Son MBF, Burns JC, Newburger JW: A new definition for multisystem inflammatory syndrome in children, *Pediatrics* 151(3):e2022060302, 2023 Mar 1.

Son MBF, Murray N, Friedman K, et al: Multisystem inflammatory syndrome in children - initial therapy and outcomes, *N Engl J Med* 385(1):23–34, 2021 Jul 1.

RESUSCITATION OF THE NEWBORN

Method of
David S. Gregory, MD; and Hirenkumar Patel, MD

CURRENT DIAGNOSIS

- The transition from intrauterine to extrauterine life at birth requires effective breathing by the infant to expand the lungs and oxygenate the blood. All newborn infants are at risk for delays in this process, prompting a need for resuscitation.
- The fetal and newborn response to hypoxia is to develop apnea. If primary apnea is diagnosed, it can be corrected by gentle stimulation and oxygen delivery. If hypoxia persists, secondary apnea will occur. It is not readily apparent whether a newborn has primary or secondary apnea, and the approach to resuscitation therefore requires that any apneic event be treated using the same sequence of interventions.
- The initial steps of newborn resuscitation include drying the infant, providing warmth, using gentle stimulation, and clearing the airway if needed. Infants who do not respond to these interventions need more assistance. Establishment of effective ventilation spontaneously by the newborn or with assistance by positive-pressure ventilation (PPV) is the most important step in newborn resuscitation.
- Reassessment of the infant's heart rate, respiratory effort, pulse oximeter reading or color, and tone every 30 seconds during resuscitation is crucial to determine the next appropriate intervention. Apgar scoring should *not* be used to guide newborn resuscitation. Electrocardiographic monitoring is the best method for assessing heart rate. Pulse oximetry in the delivery room should be used to guide oxygen therapy. Temperature of the infant should be monitored.
- If application of PPV does not improve the infant's heart rate, chest compressions or drug therapy, or both, may be required. A team approach is needed to coordinate these interventions, and ongoing reassessment is necessary to determine cardiorespiratory and hemodynamic status. Subsequent assessment and treatment should be performed in an intensive care setting.

CURRENT THERAPY

- Term gestation infants who are breathing and crying with good muscle tone do not need newborn resuscitation.
- Most newborns do not require immediate cord clamping and can be monitored during skin-to-skin contact with their mothers.
- Milking the cord is a method of squeezing the umbilical cord toward the infant, whether the cord is cut or not.
- Initial resuscitation includes drying the infant, providing warmth, giving gentle stimulation, and clearing the mouth and nose, if needed.
- If the infant is apneic, breathing slowly, or gasping, positive-pressure ventilation (PPV) with a mask and bag should be administered. A rise in heart rate is the best indicator of effective ventilation and response to resuscitation.

- When oxygen therapy is needed during resuscitation, pulse oximetry should be used to guide oxygen concentration.
- If the heart rate does not improve with adequate ventilation efforts, implement corrective steps using the MR SOPA acronym, and consider an alternative airway, such as an endotracheal tube or a laryngeal mask.
- If the infant's heart rate drops below 60 beats/min, chest compressions should be initiated using the two-thumb technique. Heart rate should be monitored using electrocardiography.
- If the heart rate remains less than 60 beats/min despite PPV and chest compressions, intravenous epinephrine (adrenaline) may be given using an umbilical venous catheter or via intraosseous catheter.
- Infants who do not improve with epinephrine and have a history consistent with blood loss may improve with fluid expansion.
- Reassessment of the newborn every 30 seconds during resuscitation is required to adjust therapy as indicated. The best indicator of successful resuscitation is an increase in heart rate.

The changes that occur in the transition from fetus to newborn are unmatched in any other time of life. Most newborns manage to make this transition on their own, but about 10% require some assistance. Approximately 1% of newborns require extensive resuscitative measures to survive. The approach to resuscitation in infants is similar to that in adults, consisting of evaluation and intervention when needed for the infant's airway, breathing, and circulation. Every birth should be attended by personnel trained in neonatal resuscitation. Specific training and certification are offered by the American Academy of Pediatrics/American Heart Association's Neonatal Resuscitation Provider (NRP) course. This chapter has been updated based on the American Heart Association 2020 Guidelines, the eighth edition of the NRP dated June 2021, and the 2023 neonatal resuscitation guideline updates (Box 1). Ongoing training and a team-based approach are vital components of newborn resuscitation.

Transition From Fetal to Extrauterine Life

The environment of the fetus differs greatly from that of the infant after birth. The fetus depends on receiving oxygen and nutrients from the mother through the placental circulation. The fetus experiences relative hypoxia and almost constant body temperature in the amniotic fluid. The fetal lungs are filled with fluid and do not participate in the exchange of oxygen and carbon dioxide. Several adaptations in the fetus permit survival in this environment.

Oxygenated blood from the mother enters the fetus by means of the placenta through the umbilical vein. Most of this oxygenated blood bypasses the liver through the ductus venosus and enters the inferior vena cava. On entering the right atrium, this oxygenated blood is directed toward the patent foramen ovale into the left atrium, bypassing the fetal lungs. Fetal blood also passes through the right atrium into the right ventricle and then into the pulmonary artery. The vascular resistance and blood pressure of the pulmonary vessels in the fetal lung are higher than in the aorta and systemic circulation; most of the blood is therefore shunted away from the lungs through the ductus arteriosus into the ascending aorta. Only a small amount of fetal blood passes through the lungs to the left atrium and then to the left ventricle. The umbilical arteries branch off from the internal iliac arteries and return fetal blood to the placenta. The functional organ for gas exchange of oxygen and carbon dioxide in the fetus is the placenta.

At birth, the newborn is no longer connected to the placenta, and the lungs become the only source of oxygen. The first breaths of the infant cause the fluid in the lung alveoli to be replaced with air. The umbilical arteries and veins constrict at birth and

BOX 1 — Summary of Key Points for Newborn Resuscitation Based on Neonatal Resuscitation Program, 8th Edition, and the 2023 Neonatal Resuscitation Guideline Updates

- Individual providers and neonatal resuscitative teams should train, prepare, brief, and check equipment as a team before resuscitative efforts.
- Vigorous newborn infants—whether term or preterm—can be evaluated and monitored while providing skin-to-skin contact with their mother, gentle tactile stimulation and skin drying with a soft and absorbent warm towel, and delayed (30 seconds) cord clamping.
- Regarding delayed cord clamping (>30 seconds) and intact cord milking, the 2023 guideline update suggests:
  - In newborns ≥34 weeks gestation.
    - Not requiring resuscitation: There is benefit from delayed cord clamping compared to immediate cord clamping (as soon as is possible <30 seconds), but there is no added benefit of intact cord milking.
    - Requiring resuscitation: There is benefit from both delayed cord clamping and intact cord milking.
  - In infants 28–34 weeks' gestation.
    - Not requiring resuscitation: There is benefit from delayed cord clamping compared with immediate cord clamping. Intact cord milking is reasonable, especially when delayed cord clamping is not possible.
    - Requiring resuscitation: There is benefit from delayed cord clamping, but the benefit of intact cord milking is unknown.
  - For preterm infants <28 weeks' gestation—whether or not requiring resuscitation—delayed cord clamping has benefit but intact cord milking is not recommended.
- Ventilation of a newborn's lungs is the priority when support is required.
- Routine intubation and tracheal suctioning is not recommended for infants born in meconium-stained amniotic fluid (including those who may be nonvigorous).
- Effective ventilation and proper response to resuscitative efforts is first indicated by a rise in newborn heart rate.
- After initial use of room air for ventilation efforts in term infants, pulse oximetry monitoring guides oxygen concentration adjustment to meet goals at specific minute-based intervals after birth.
- In cases of insufficient heart rate response to ventilation of a newborn's lungs (including corrective steps, such as endotracheal intubation), chest compressions are indicated.
- Electrocardiographic monitoring is necessary to assess the heart rate response to chest compressions and medication.
- When chest compressions do not result in an adequate increase in heart rate, epinephrine, preferably via the intravenous route, is indicated.
- Infants with history or examination consistent with blood loss, and having poor response to epinephrine, may require volume expansion.
- After effective resuscitation, if no heart rate is attained by 20 minutes, cessation of resuscitative efforts should be discussed with team and family.

are eventually clamped. This increases the vascular resistance and blood pressure of the systemic circulation. As the oxygen level in the alveoli increases, the blood vessels in the lung start to relax, decreasing pulmonary vascular resistance. Blood in the pulmonary artery travels toward the lung and away from the ductus arteriosus because the blood pressure in the systemic circulation is higher than that in the pulmonary circulation. Increased blood flow to the lungs allows the oxygen from the alveoli to enter the infant's blood, increasing the Po_2. Oxygenated blood enters the left heart through the pulmonary vein and is delivered to the rest of the infant's tissues through the aorta.

Although the initial steps in this transition occur within a few minutes of birth, the entire process may not be completed for several hours to days. The ductus venosus, foramen ovale, and ductus arteriosus remain potentially patent and do not completely involute for days or weeks. Changes in the infant's systemic and pulmonary pressures can result in blood flow through these channels in the infant.

Transition can be prevented or delayed in several circumstances. The infant may not breathe adequately, in which case the lung fluid is not forced out of the alveoli. Material such as meconium may block air from entering the alveoli. If the lungs do not fill with air, hypoxia will quickly develop. Systemic hypotension caused by excessive blood loss, poor cardiac function, or bradycardia prevents the change in the direction of blood flow that is necessary to promote blood flow into the lungs. Failure of the lungs to expand or hypoxia can prevent relaxation of the pulmonary blood vessels, resulting in a high pulmonary vascular resistance. This leads to decreased blood flow to the lungs and worsening of hypoxia.

Risk Factors for Newborn Resuscitation

A number of prenatal and intrapartum factors are associated with a higher chance that the infant will have a delay in transition and require resuscitation (Table 1). A recent multicenter review of risk factors for resuscitation at 34 weeks' gestation or greater found that the following risk factors were significantly associated with a need for advanced resuscitation: 34 to 37 weeks' gestation, intrauterine growth retardation, gestational diabetes, meconium-stained amniotic fluid (MSAF), vacuum- or forceps-assisted delivery, clinical chorioamnionitis, fetal bradycardia, placenta abruption, general anesthesia, and emergency cesarean section. In preparation for labor and delivery, staff should ask the following questions: (1) What is the expected gestational age of the infant? (2) Is the amniotic fluid clear? (3) Are there additional risk factors? and (4) What is the umbilical cord management plan? However, some infants *with no risk factors* need resuscitation; therefore, preparations for neonatal resuscitation should be made during all deliveries.

Reaction to Hypoxia and Asphyxia

Normally at birth, the newborn makes vigorous efforts to breathe. The process of leaving the warm, dark, and liquid environment in utero is replaced by cold air, dryness, and bright lights. Drying the infant with towels and wiping the mouth and nose are all the assistance that most newborns require. The end result of any mechanism that delays transition is a period of hypoxia for the fetus or newborn infant. Laboratory studies have shown that the first sign of oxygen deprivation in the newborn is a change in the breathing pattern. After an initial period of rapid breathing attempts, cessation of breathing occurs. This is called *primary apnea*. Drying the infant may provide enough stimulation for initiation of breathing. If it does not, consider additional stimulation by gently rubbing the back, trunk, or extremities. If hypoxia continues after primary apnea has occurred, the infant will make attempts at gasping and then stop breathing. This is called *secondary apnea*. Stimulation does not affect secondary apnea. Assisted ventilation is necessary to provide breaths to the newborn to reverse the hypoxia. The infant's heart rate starts to decrease when primary apnea occurs. The heart rate increases with stimulation if the infant has primary apnea, and blood pressure is maintained. With continued hypoxia, the heart rate continues to drop, and hypotension develops. If assisted ventilation is not adequate to increase the infant's heart rate, chest compressions will be required.

When a newborn becomes apneic, it is not readily apparent whether the infant has primary or secondary apnea. The approach to resuscitation therefore requires that any apneic event in a newborn be treated using the same sequence of interventions. If the apneic infant responds to simple stimulation,

TABLE 1	Risk Factors for Newborn Resuscitation
PRENATAL FACTORS	**INTRAPARTUM FACTORS**

PRENATAL FACTORS	INTRAPARTUM FACTORS
Maternal Diabetes, preexisting Chronic hypertension Infection Cardiac, renal, pulmonary, thyroid, or neurologic disease Drug therapy Substance use Lack of prenatal care Age <16 or >35 years Previous fetal or neonatal death **Pregnancy** Bleeding in second or third trimester Pregnancy-induced hypertension Toxemia Gestational diabetes Fetal anemia or isoimmunization Polyhydramnios Oligohydramnios Fetal hydrops Postterm gestation Multiple gestation Size-date discrepancy Diminished fetal activity Fetal malformation or abnormality	**Placental** Placenta previa Abruption of the placenta Premature or prolonged rupture of membranes Chorioamnionitis **Fetal** Macrosomia Low birth weight Breech or other abnormal presentation Persistent fetal bradycardia Nonreassuring fetal heart rate patterns **Labor** Premature labor Precipitous labor Prolonged labor (>24h) Prolonged second stage of labor (>2h) Prolapsed cord Emergency cesarean section Forceps or vacuum-assisted delivery **Other** Meconium-stained amniotic fluid General anesthesia Narcotics given within 4h of delivery Uterine hyperstimulation Severe intrapartum bleeding

the diagnosis is primary apnea, and no further intervention is required. If the infant does not improve with stimulation, secondary apnea has occurred, and more intensive intervention is needed.

Unlike adults, the progression from primary apnea to secondary apnea in newborns results in the cessation of respiratory activity before the onset of cardiac failure. For this reason, neonatal resuscitation should begin with positive-pressure ventilation (PPV) rather than with chest compressions For this reason, in any newborn experiencing apnea or ineffective ventilation, effective positive-pressure ventilation (PPV) is prioritized ahead of performing chest compressions.

Preparation for Newborn Resuscitation

The neonatal resuscitation team, before resuscitative efforts, should attempt to perform a team brief and check all necessary equipment. The team brief should include answers to questions that should be asked of the delivery team to clarify neonatal needs, including gestational age, amniotic fluid color and clarity, known risk factors for cardiopulmonary dysfunction (e.g., congenital heart disease) or infection (e.g., chorioamnionitis), and whether delayed cord clamping or intact cord milking is to be used for the delivery (Box 1). The team brief allows the neonatal team to refocus and organize their team response, while checking all equipment ensures that needed instruments, devices, and medications are at their disposal for the resuscitative efforts

Sequence of Newborn Resuscitation
Initial Steps and Basic Resuscitation
Resuscitation of the newborn starts with the rapid assessment of three characteristics: Is the infant at term gestation? Does the infant have good tone? Is the infant crying and breathing? The answers to these questions will affect the approach to care. Resuscitation when fluid is meconium stained is discussed later in this chapter. The information presented here

refers to term infants with clear amniotic fluid. More information regarding the care of premature infants is discussed in a later section.

The infant at term who is crying and breathing with good muscle tone does not need resuscitation and should not be separated from the mother. Current evidence suggests cord clamping should be delayed for at least 30 seconds for most vigorous term and preterm infants unless there is evidence of placental abruption or bleeding. The baby should be dried, placed skin-to-skin with the mother, and covered with dry linen to maintain temperature. Ongoing observation for breathing, activity, and color should continue while the infant is with the mother. If the infant is not term, is not crying and breathing, or does not have good muscle tone, newborn resuscitation should begin with the initial steps: providing warmth, drying and stimulating the infant, then positioning and clearing (if needed) the airway.

The newborn should be placed under a radiant warmer to prevent heat loss and allow easy observation. Although warm blankets or towels can be used to dry the infant, they should not be left in place to cover the infant. Drying the infant, slapping the feet, and rubbing the back are appropriate forms of stimulation. More forceful methods of stimulation can harm the infant. Primary apnea, if present, will respond to stimulation in less than 30 seconds. Prolonged apnea will require PPV.

The newborn should be placed on the back with the neck slightly extended in the "sniffing" position (Figure 1). This facilitates air entry into the lungs by lining up the posterior pharynx, larynx, and trachea. Hyperextension or hyperflexion of the neck can obstruct air entry into the lungs.

If the newborn is crying vigorously, secretions can be removed by wiping the nose and the mouth with a towel. Routine suctioning should be avoided. Gentle suctioning of the mouth and nose with a bulb syringe or suction catheter is *only* indicated when there is obvious obstruction to spontaneous breathing or when there is a need for PPV. Deep or vigorous suctioning can be detrimental to the infant because of stimulation of the vagus nerve, causing bradycardia or apnea. The mouth should be suctioned before the nose to prevent aspiration if the infant gasps during suctioning.

Evaluating the infant's response to resuscitation is essential. The Apgar score is a traditional method for evaluating newborn status at 1 and 5 minutes after delivery. However, effective resuscitation demands that evaluation of the newborn's status not be delayed until 1 minute of age. Apgar scores therefore should *not* be used to guide resuscitative efforts but are a measure of a patient's response to resuscitation efforts. Within 30 seconds of delivery, the infant's need for PPV must be assessed. Establishment of effective ventilation spontaneously by the newborn or with assistance by PPV is the most important step in newborn resuscitation. The respiratory status, heart rate, and color or oximetry reading should be determined. The chest wall should move with each breath, and the newborn should be breathing spontaneously. Although heart rate can be assessed by feeling for a pulse at the base of the umbilical cord, this method can be unreliable. Auscultation with a stethoscope is the preferred method during initial resuscitation. The heart rate should be greater than 100 beats/min. Placement of 3-lead electrocardiograph (ECG) as soon as possible to monitor the infant's heart rate during resuscitation may be beneficial. Monitoring of heart rate using ECG is more reliable than palpation and auscultation and is faster than using the pulse oximeter. Peripheral cyanosis (i.e., blueness of the hands and feet) is acceptable in the initial period after delivery. Central cyanosis in which the lips and trunk are blue indicates hypoxemia and the need for more resuscitation efforts. Pulse oximetry should be used to confirm the perception of central cyanosis. A pulse oximeter can provide continuous assessment of the oxygen saturation and is the optimal method for monitoring the infant's state of oxygenation. The oximeter probe should be placed on the newborn's

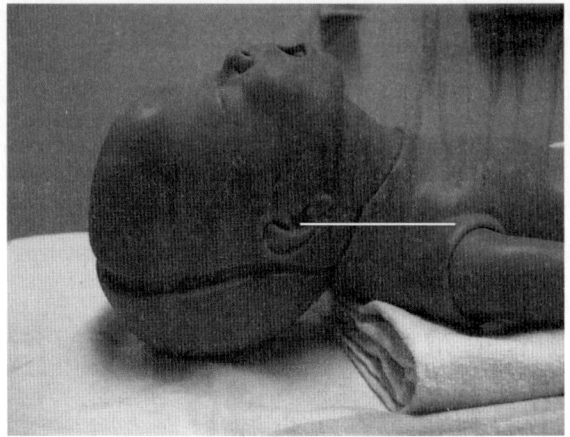

Figure 1 The sniffing position. Positioning the infant on the back with the neck slightly extended brings the posterior pharynx, larynx, and trachea in line (*white line*) to facilitate air entry into the lungs.

right wrist or hand to detect preductal saturation. Temperature should be monitored during newborn resuscitation. The normal range is an axillary temperature of 36.5°C to 37.5°C. The initial steps of stabilization, reassessment, and establishing ventilation should be completed within the first minute of life (the "golden minute").

Respiratory Support and Positive-Pressure Ventilation

If the infant is breathing with a heart rate higher than 100 beats/min but has central cyanosis and below-target oxygen saturation, free-flowing oxygen delivery is indicated. This can be administered with a facemask or by holding oxygen tubing or a flow-inflating bag and mask close to the infant's face. *A self-inflating bag and mask cannot be used to give free-flowing oxygen.* If the newborn is apneic, not breathing effectively, or has a heart rate less than 100 beats/min, PPV using a self-inflating bag (Figure 2), flow-inflating (or anesthesia) bag, or a T-piece resuscitator is required. Use of a flow-inflating bag or T-piece resuscitator requires a compressed gas source. The T-piece resuscitator requires less practice for effective use and is a preferred technique to the use of a self-inflating bag. In case of compressed gas failure, however, a self-inflating bag should be available. Self-inflating bags are easy to use and can be fitted with a pressure-release valve to decrease overinflation. A reservoir must be used with a self-inflating bag to provide 100% oxygen. For free-flow oxygen or PPV, the flow meter on the oxygen source should be set to 10 L/min.

PPV should begin using room air for term newborns. The facemask should cover the infant's nose, mouth, and tip of chin, but not the eyes (Figure 3). Multiple sizes should be available. A tight seal between the infant's skin and the facemask is needed, but excessive pressure can bruise the face. The mask can be held in place using the thumb and index finger in a C-shaped position on top of the mask, with the remaining fingers in an E-shaped position below the infant's chin (Figure 4). Inspiratory pressures of 20 to 25 cm H_2O are usually needed when squeezing the bag to make the infant's chest rise; peak inspiratory pressures in a term newborn of 30 cm H_2O may be required. A pressure gauge can be connected to the self-inflating bag for monitoring inspiratory pressure. The heart rate and color of the infant should rapidly improve if enough pressure is being given. An assistant can also use a stethoscope to listen to breath sounds for air movement. Breaths should be given at a rate of 40 to 60 breaths/min.

Traditionally, 100% oxygen has been used in newborn resuscitation. However, several randomized controlled studies enrolling term and near-term infants have shown that room air can be used initially with oxygen as a backup if room air fails. A metaanalysis of these trials showed a benefit for the use of room air. Providing oxygen at concentrations between room air and 100% requires

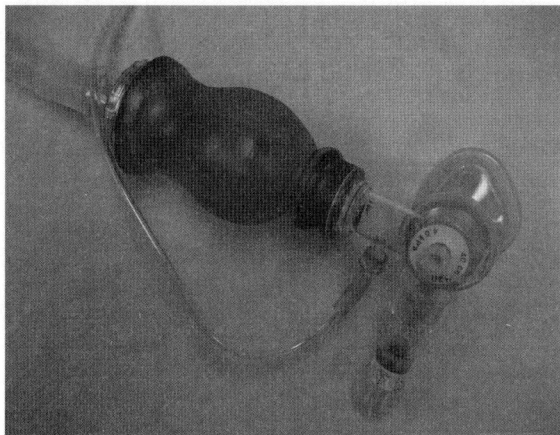

Figure 2 Self-inflating bag with infant mask and reservoir. This type of device is available in most delivery rooms.

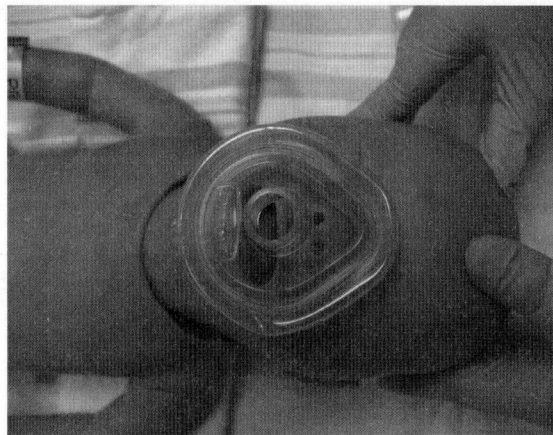

Figure 3 Facemask. Choose a size that covers the infant's mouth and nose.

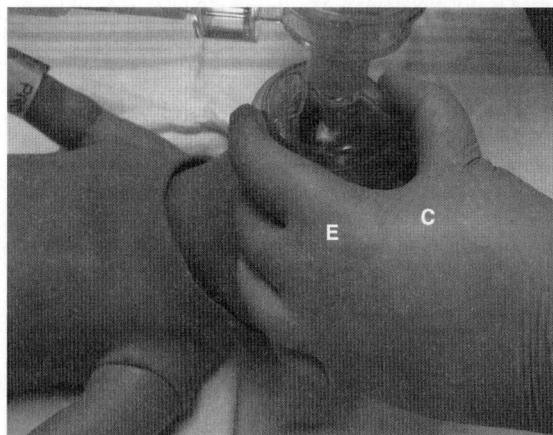

Figure 4 Facemask placement. The thumb and index finger are held in a C-shaped position on top of the mask, and the remaining fingers are held in an E-type position under the chin.

the use of compressed air, oxygen, and blenders by experienced personnel. A pulse oximeter with a probe designed for use in newborns can be used to guide oxygen administration during newborn resuscitation. It will take 1 to 2 minutes to apply the pulse oximeter probe to the infant's right palm or wrist (preductal site) and get a consistent reading. Pulse oximetry often displays lower-than-actual heart rate readings during the first 2 minutes of life. The pulse oximeter may not function during states of very poor cardiac output or perfusion. In these situations, observation for central cyanosis will be necessary. The infant's oxygen saturation may remain in the 70% to 80% range for several minutes after birth. Oxygen may be titrated to the interquartile range of preductal saturations measured in healthy babies after vaginal birth at sea level (Table 2). If blended oxygen is not available, room air should be used for resuscitation. If the infant's heart rate does not respond to PPV with room air after 90 seconds, 100% oxygen should then be used.

After 30 seconds of PPV, the infant should be reevaluated. Once PPV is started, an electronic cardiac monitor is the preferred method to measure heart rate. Ventilation with a bag and mask can be stopped when the newborn has a heart rate higher than 100 beats/min and has sustained spontaneous breathing. If the newborn is not improving, he or she may not be receiving adequate ventilation. When appropriate ventilation is delivered, expect the heart rate to increase within 15 seconds. If the heart rate is not improving, implement corrective steps with the use of the acronym MR SOPA:

- M = Mask adjustment to check seal
- R = Reposition head in sniffing position
- S = Suction mouth and nose
- O = Open mouth with infant's jaw lifted forward
- P = Increase pressure up to 30 to 40 cm H_2O
- A = An alternative airway approach, such as endotracheal [ET] intubation, is worth considering

If corrective steps are applied and the newborn remains apneic or has a heart rate less than 100, consider an alternative airway, such as intubation or laryngeal mask.

ET intubation is a technical skill that must be learned and practiced to maintain competency. Effective ventilation can be given with a bag and mask approach to most newborns. This skill is easily mastered and maintained. If an infant is responding well to bag and mask ventilation, it can be continued for longer periods; however, some air may escape into the esophagus and into the stomach. This may cause gastric distention, which can prevent full expansion of the lungs and cause vomiting and aspiration. An orogastric tube can be placed in the stomach and left open to air to vent any air introduced into the infant's stomach during bag and mask ventilation. In the event a newborn is not responding to PPV via face mask and support is not available for intubation, a supraglottic airway may be considered to provide PPV for babies born ≥34 weeks' gestation.

If the newborn has a heart rate at or greater than 100 with spontaneous respirations but has labored breathing or oxygen saturations levels below the target range, consider administering continuous positive airway pressure (CPAP). CPAP should be used judiciously due to the risk of developing a pneumothorax. For effective CPAP, a flow-inflating bag or a T-piece resuscitator via a facemask may be used. A self-inflating bag does not provide CPAP.

Chest Compressions

Before beginning chest compressions, intubation is strongly recommended to provide effective ventilation. After 30 seconds of effective PPV, the heart rate should be assessed. If the heart rate dips below 60 beats/min, chest compressions are needed to support the circulation. The two-thumb technique (Figure 5) is recommended. The two-thumb technique generates higher blood pressure and coronary perfusion with less rescuer fatigue. It can also be continued with the rescuer at the head of the bed if access to the abdomen is needed. If chest compressions are required, 100% oxygen should be given by PPV. Two people are required to give PPV and chest compressions effectively. To coordinate the breaths and chest compressions, three compressions are given followed by one breath, and this sequence is repeated to give the infant 90 compressions and 30 breaths/min. The thumbs are placed on the lower third of the infant's sternum but above the xyphoid process. The sternum is depressed to a depth of one-third of the infant's anteroposterior chest diameter. The purpose of chest compressions is to squeeze the heart between the sternum and the spine, forcing blood in and out of the heart and to the body. The direction of the compressions should be perpendicular to the chest surface, and

TABLE 2	Titrated Oxygen Saturations After Birth
1 minute	60%–65%
2 minutes	65%–70%
3 minutes	70%–75%
4 minutes	75%–80%
5 minutes	80%–85%
10 minutes	85%–95%

the thumbs should not be lifted off of the chest after the correct placement is obtained. Incorrect methods during chest compressions can cause rib fracture and liver laceration.

After 60 seconds of chest compressions, the infant's heart rate, breathing, pulse oximeter reading or color, and tone are reassessed. If the heart rate is higher than 60 beats/min, chest compressions can be stopped, although PPV may still be needed. If the heart rate is not improving, the following problems must be considered: ventilation is not adequate, 100% oxygen concentration is not being given, or the compressions may not be deep enough or well-coordinated with the breaths.

Medications for Newborn Resuscitation

If the newborn heart rate remains below 60 beats/min despite 30 seconds of effective PPV and 60 seconds of chest compressions, epinephrine (Adrenalin) can be used to stimulate the newborn heart. Fewer than 2 of 1000 infants will require this step in resuscitation. *Intravenous (IV) administration of epinephrine is preferred.*

In the delivery room, a catheter can be quickly inserted into the umbilical vein for IV access. A 3.5 or 5F catheter prefilled with saline and connected to a three-way stopcock is inserted about 2 to 4 cm into the umbilical vein using sterile technique. After blood is aspirated, insertion of the catheter is stopped, and the epinephrine is given rapidly, followed by a 3 mL saline flush. The concentration of epinephrine used in neonatal resuscitation is 1:10,000 (0.1 mg/mL). The IV dose is 0.01 to 0.03 mg/kg (0.1–0.3 mL/kg) (Table 3). The eighth edition of the NRP recommends an initial dose of epinephrine as 0.02 mg/kg (0.2 mL/kg). The intraosseous route can be used if needed. A dose of epinephrine may be considered through the ET tube during the umbilical vein catheterization process, but there is no evidence of benefit. The ET dose of epinephrine is 0.05 to 0.1 mg/kg (0.5–1 mL/kg).[1] The eighth edition of the NRP recommends giving 0.1 mg/kg (1 mL/kg) via the ET tube if needed while establishing vascular access. *These higher doses are for ET use only.* Because lung absorption of epinephrine varies, the IV route using the umbilical vein or intraosseous catheter is preferred.

During umbilical vein cannulation, PPV and chest compressions are continued. More personnel will be needed to place the catheter and draw up the medications and saline flushes. After an IV dose of epinephrine, the infant's heart rate, respirations, color or oximeter reading, and tone are reevaluated. The heart rate should increase to more than 60 beats/min. If the heart rate does not respond, the dose of epinephrine can be repeated every 3 to 5 minutes. The effectiveness of ventilation and compressions should be reassessed. If the infant appears pale, has delayed capillary refill, or has decreased pulses, shock may be present. Infant blood loss might have occurred during delivery from placental problems or other sources. Administration of an isotonic crystalloid solution such as normal saline or type O negative blood at 10 mL/kg over 5 to 10 minutes can improve circulation. Lactated Ringer solution is no longer recommended for newborns. Volume expansion should be used cautiously because there is evidence from animal studies for poorer outcomes when it is used in the absence of

---

[1] Not FDA approved for this indication.

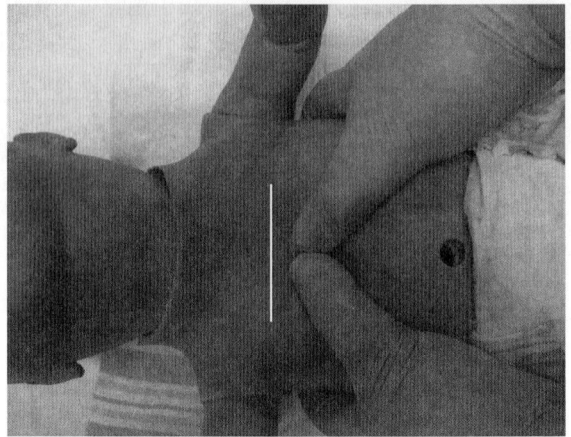

Figure 5 Two-thumb technique. The hands encircle the torso, and the thumbs are placed on top of the lower sternum above the xyphoid process and below a line drawn between the nipples *(white line)*.

hypovolemia. Rapid infusion of large volumes has been associated with intraventricular hemorrhage in premature infants.

Hypoglycemia is common in newborns who have required resuscitation. Blood from the infant's heel or the umbilical vein can be tested at the bedside and IV 10% dextrose (2–5 mL/kg) given for low blood glucose. No specific glucose level has been associated with a poorer outcome. There is no evidence that use of sodium bicarbonate benefits the neonate, and its use during resuscitation in the delivery room is not recommended.

After resuscitation, newborns should be monitored in an intensive care setting. These infants are at risk for several complications, such as infection, metabolic abnormalities, and seizures. Infants of 36 weeks' gestation or older with moderate to severe hypoxic-ischemic encephalopathy may benefit from induced hypothermia under clearly defined protocols.

Special Considerations

Some newborns do not respond to resuscitation because of specific problems. Infants with upper airway obstruction from micrognathia can be helped by a nasopharyngeal airway and placement of the infant in the prone position. Choanal atresia can be treated by placing an oral airway. Absence of breath sounds on one side of the chest can indicate a pneumothorax, requiring needle aspiration of the chest. An infant with a scaphoid abdomen and decreased breath sounds may have a diaphragmatic hernia. These infants should be intubated, and PPV by mask and bag should not be used. Narcotics, magnesium, or general anesthesia administered to the mother shortly before the delivery may be the cause of respiratory depression in the infant. These infants need PPV and respiratory support. Naloxone is no longer recommended as part of initial resuscitative efforts in the delivery room. Heart rate and oxygenation should be supported by PPV.

Endotracheal Intubation

During neonatal resuscitation, ET intubation may be indicated in the following circumstances: where bag and mask ventilation is ineffective or prolonged, where chest compressions are performed, and in special situations, such as congenital diaphragmatic hernia or extremely-low-birth-weight infants. Intubation of the newborn requires preparation that can be performed while the infant is being ventilated by bag and mask. The ET tube should not be placed unless the glottis is visualized by direct laryngoscopy. To ensure that the tube is in the trachea, a CO_2 detector should be used. Listening for equal breath sounds and looking for vapor condensation in the ET tube during exhalation can help, but an increase in the infant's heart rate or a positive detection of CO_2 is most reliable. It should be noted that poor or absent pulmonary blood flow may result in the absence of CO_2 detection despite tube placement in the trachea. The best indicator for effective ventilation is an increase in the newborn's heart rate.

TABLE 3	Drugs for Newborn Resuscitation			
DRUG	**CONCENTRATION**	**DOSE**	**INDICATIONS**	**COMMENTS**
Epinephrine	1:10,000 (0.1 mg/mL)	0.01–0.03 mg/kg IV = 0.1–0.3 mL/kg IV route preferred initial dose: 0.02 mg/kg = 0.2 mL/kg* ETT dose: 0.05–0.1 mg/kg Recommended dose: 0.1 mg/kg = 1 mL/kg*,1	Asystole Bradycardia that does not improve with PPV and chest compressions Shock	May repeat every 3–5 min No evidence for giving epinephrine via ETT
Volume expanders	Normal saline O negative blood	10 mL/kg IV	Hypovolemia	Crossmatch blood to mother if possible Repeat if needed
Glucose	10% dextrose	2 mL/kg IV	Hypoglycemia	Monitor glucometer or venous glucose levels

ETT, Endotracheal tube; *IV*, intravenous.
*Neonatal Resuscitation Program (NRP). 8th ed. 2021.
[1]Not FDA approved for this indication.

Intubation should be performed as quickly as possible, with a goal of 30 seconds from insertion of the laryngoscope to the connection of the ET tube to the resuscitation bag. Complications of intubation include worsening of hypoxia and bradycardia, pneumothorax, contusions, perforation of the trachea or esophagus, and infection. After the infant has been intubated, deterioration in the infant's status should prompt an organized sequence to assess the adequacy of ventilation using the mnemonic DOPE:
- *Dislodged* (D): Is the tube in the right bronchus or out of the trachea?
- *Obstructed* (O): Is the tube obstructed by secretions or blood?
- *Pneumothorax* (P)
- *Esophagus* (E): Is the tube in the esophagus?

An alternative to intubation for infants of at least 34 weeks' gestation and at least 2000 grams is placement of a laryngeal mask airway. This type of airway does not require laryngoscopy. A soft, inflatable mask that is attached to a flexible airway tube is placed in the hypopharynx such that the air in the tube is directed into the larynx and away from the esophagus. However, this type of airway cannot be used to suction the trachea or to give ET drugs. Its use has not been evaluated during chest compressions. For infants who require an alternative airway, cardiac monitoring is recommended to assess the heart rate and whether chest compressions are needed.

Premature Infants
Infants born before 37 weeks' gestation are at increased risk for complications and the need for resuscitation. Premature lungs may lack surfactant, making ventilation difficult. Very-low-birth-weight (less than 1500 g) infants will need additional warming techniques such as prewarming the delivery room, covering the baby in plastic wrapping, and placing the baby under a radiant warmer and/or an exothermic mattress; however, iatrogenic hyperthermia (axillary temperature >38°C) should be avoided. Immature brain development may decrease the drive to breathe. Weak muscles make respiratory efforts less effective. Thin skin and decreased subcutaneous fat make temperature regulation a challenge. Premature infants may have infections such as pneumonia or sepsis. The blood vessels in their brains are fragile and can easily bleed during periods of blood pressure variation. The lower birth weights of premature newborns also require smaller sizes of equipment for resuscitation such as facemasks, suction catheters, ET tubes, and umbilical catheters. Initial oxygen concentrations between room air and 30% should be used to protect premature infants of less than 35 weeks' gestation from oxygen toxicity. The use of CPAP in premature infants who are breathing spontaneously but with difficulty after birth may reduce the need for intubation, mechanical ventilation, and surfactant use. If PPV is needed, it is preferable to use a device that can deliver positive end-expiratory pressure. More than one

person trained in newborn resuscitation should be present at the delivery of a high-risk premature infant.

Meconium Staining of the Amniotic Fluid
Meconium is formed in the newborn gastrointestinal system during gestation. Intrauterine stress can cause release of meconium into the amniotic fluid. Aspiration of MSAF into the lungs can result in severe pneumonitis and lung injury. The approach to resuscitation for an infant born in MSAF has been revised. There is no evidence that the consistency of MSAF (i.e., thick or thin) has an effect on the outcome of the newborn.

Crying and Vigorous Infant
If the newborn born in MSAF has normal respiratory effort and muscle tone with a heart rate higher than 100 beats/min, routine care including delayed cord clamping and skin-to-skin time with the mother is appropriate. Secretions can be wiped from the baby's mouth and nose. *Gentle* mouth and nose suctioning can be performed using a bulb syringe or suction catheter *only if needed*. Deep and prolonged suctioning should be avoided. ET intubation is not required for vigorous infants with MSAF.

Nonvigorous Infant
Routine ET intubation and tracheal suctioning is no longer recommended for nonvigorous newborns born in MSAF; however, the resuscitation team should include someone skilled in ET intubation. If the newborn is gasping or apneic and has poor muscle tone, the initial steps of routine resuscitation should be started: provide warmth, dry the infant, position the airway, and clear the mouth and nose. Tactile stimulation should be limited to drying the infant and rubbing the back and soles of the feet. If there is visible fluid obstructing the airway or a concern about obstructed breathing, the mouth and nose may be suctioned. If there is no response, PPV should be started using a bag and mask. Suction may also be considered if there is evidence of airway obstruction during PPV. If bag and mask ventilation is not effective, intubation should be performed. There is no evidence that suctioning the trachea of nonvigorous newborns born in MSAF prevents morbidity or mortality. It is possible that the main cause of meconium aspiration into the lungs is intrauterine fetal gasping.

Newborn Resuscitation Outside of the Delivery Room
Resuscitation of infants born at home, in an emergency room, in an ambulance, or otherwise outside of a delivery room setting should proceed according to the same principles as in the delivery room. Providing warmth with stimulation and wiping the airway are usually adequate measures. Establishing effective ventilation using a bag and mask is the most important step if the infant fails to breathe on

TABLE 4	Equipment for Newborn Resuscitation
TYPE OF USE	**EQUIPMENT**
General	Warmed towels
	Radiant warmer or heat lamps
	Pulse oximeter
	Cardiorespiratory monitor
	Sterile gowns, gloves
Airway	Bulb syringe
	Suction catheters (5, 8, 10, 12, 14F)
	Suction source with manometer
	Oral and nasopharyngeal airways (newborn sizes)
	Laryngoscope and straight blades sizes 0 and 1
	Endotracheal tubes (sizes 2.5, 3.0, 3.5)
Ventilation	Facemasks (premature, newborn, and infant sizes)
	Self-inflating bag (450–750 mL) with oxygen reservoir and manometer
	Oxygen source
	Orogastric tubes (8, 10F)
	Carbon dioxide (CO_2) indicator
	Chest tubes (8 and 10F)
Circulation	Umbilical catheters (3.5 and 5F)
	Umbilical catheter tray (sterile scissors, scalpel, forceps, umbilical tape)
	Three-way stopcock
	Syringes (1, 3, 5, 10 mL)
	Normal saline
	Epinephrine 1:10,000
	10% dextrose

its own. Emergency providers should be familiar with resuscitation of the newborn, and basic equipment (Table 4) should be available.

Withholding and Withdrawing Newborn Resuscitation

Newborns should be offered resuscitation at delivery except in extreme circumstances. Newborn resuscitation should not be used if the infant has a condition that is incompatible with survival, such as a confirmed gestational age of less than 22 completed weeks, birth weight less than 400 g, or congenital anomalies associated with certain death or extreme morbidity.

In most situations, initial resuscitation can provide time to observe the infant's response to interventions and to discuss the infant's condition with the parents. Techniques for obstetric dating of pregnancies are accurate only to approximately 1 to 2 weeks, and estimates of fetal weight are accurate only to approximately 100 to 200 g. Care must be taken before deciding to withhold resuscitation from a newborn. Ongoing conversation between parents and medical caregivers allows mutual decision-making. Withdrawal of care is indicated if continued support is futile. After 20 minutes of asystole (heart rate of 0), newborns are very unlikely to survive, at which point cessation of resuscitative efforts may be considered, based upon patient-specific factors.

References

American Academy of Pediatrics Committee on Fetus and Newborn, Bell EF: Non-initiation or withdrawal of intensive care for high-risk newborns, *Pediatrics* 119:401, 2007.

Aschner JL, Poland RL: Sodium bicarbonate: basically useless therapy, *Pediatrics* 122:831, 2008.

Berazategui JP, Aguilar A, Escobedo M, et al: Risk factors for advanced resuscitation in term and near-term infants: a case-control study, *Arch Dis Child Fetal Neonatal Ed* 102:F44–F50, 2017.

Chettri S, Adhisivam B, Bhat V: Endotracheal suction for nonvigorous neonate born through meconium stained amniotic fluid: a randomized controlled trial, *J Pediatr* 166:1208–1213, 2015.

Field DJ, Dorling JS, Manktelow BN, et al: Survival of extremely premature babies in a geographically defined population: prospective cohort study of 1994–99 compared with 2000–05, *BMJ* 336:1221, 2008.

Halling C, Sparks JE, Christie L, Wyckoff MH: Efficacy of intravenous and endotracheal epinephrine during neonatal cardiopulmonary resuscitation in the delivery room, *J Pediatr* 185:232–236, 2017, https://doi.org/10.1016/j.jpeds.2017.02.024.

Neonatal Resuscitation 2020 American Heart Association guidelines for cardiopulmonary resuscitation and emergency cardiovascular care, *Pediatrics* 147(s1):e2020038505E, 2021. Downloaded from www.aappublications.org/news, on February 18, 2021.

Weiner GM, Zaichkin J, Kattwinkel J: *Textbook of neonatal resuscitation*, ed 7, Elk Grove Village, IL, 2016, American Academy of Pediatrics and American Heart Association.

Weiner GM, Zaichkin J: *Textbook of neonatal resuscitation*, ed 8, Elk Grove Village, IL, 2021, American Academy of Pediatrics and American Heart Association.

Welsford M, Nishiyama C, Shortt C, et al: Room air for initiating term newborn resuscitation: a systematic review with meta-analysis, *Pediatrics* 143(1), 2019.

Wiswell TE, Gannon CM, Jacob J, et al: Delivery room management of the apparently vigorous meconium-stained neonate: results of the multicenter, international collaborative trial, *Pediatrics* 105(1), 2000.

Yamada NK, Szyld E, Strand ML, et al: 2023 American Heart Association and American Academy of Pediatrics focused update on neonatal resuscitation: an update to the American Heart Association guidelines for cardiopulmonary resuscitation and emergency cardiovascular care, *Circulation* 2;149(1):e157–e166, 2024.

URINARY TRACT INFECTIONS IN INFANTS AND CHILDREN

Method of
Ellen R. Wald, MD

CURRENT DIAGNOSIS

- Urine culture is the gold standard.
- Before urine culture is available, 10 or more white blood cells per cubic millimeter, leukocyte esterase, and nitrites in urine suggest infection.
- Urine culture (significant bacteriuria) depends on how the specimen was collected to diagnose infection:
  - Clean catch = At least 10^5 colony-forming units (CFU)/mL
  - Urethral catheterization = At least 5×10^4 CFU/mL
  - Suprapubic aspiration = Any bacteria in urine

CURRENT THERAPY

- Outpatient treatment: Amoxicillin potassium clavulanate (Augmentin) 30 mg/kg/dose given every 12 hours,[3] a second- or third-generation cephalosporin such as cefuroxime (Ceftin) 50 mg/kg/dose twice daily,[3] cefpodoxime (Vantin)[1] 5 mg/kg/dose given twice daily, cefdinir (Omnicef)[1] 7 mg/kg/dose given twice daily or cefixime (Suprax) 10 mg/kg/dose once daily,[3] or sulfamethoxazole-trimethoprim (Bactrim) 6 to 12 mg/kg/day of trimethoprim in two divided doses.
- Inpatient treatment: Ceftriaxone (Rocephin) 50 mg/kg/day given once daily or ceftazidime (Fortaz) 50 mg/kg/dose every 8 hours.

[1]Not FDA approved for this indication.
[3]Exceeds dosage recommended by the manufacturer.

The urinary tract is the most common site for serious bacterial infections in infants and young children. Urinary tract infections (UTIs) are more common than bacterial meningitis, bacterial pneumonia, and bacteremia.

Infection of the urinary tract may involve only the bladder, only the kidney, or both. In general, infections of the bladder (cystitis), although causing substantial morbidity, are not regarded as serious bacterial infections. In contrast, infections that involve the kidney (pyelonephritis) can cause acute morbidity and lead to scarring with rare consequences of hypertension, preeclampsia, and chronic renal disease.

Clinical Diagnosis

Distinction between cystitis and pyelonephritis is primarily important for determining duration of antimicrobial therapy and potential complications. Clinically, cystitis is characterized by suprapubic discomfort and often symptoms of urethral irritation including dysuria, urinary frequency and urgency. It is most likely to be appreciated in children beyond 2 to 3 years of age. If fever is present at all, it is usually low grade. In contrast, infants and children with pyelonephritis usually have substantial fever (>38.5°C), with or without symptoms of bladder involvement. In addition, flank tenderness may be present in older children and adolescents with pyelonephritis. However, in young infants ages 2 months to 2 years, fever may be the only sign of pyelonephritis. Although about 10% of young infants with pyelonephritis have bacteremia, these infants cannot be distinguished clinically from those without bacteremia, and outcomes are generally excellent in both groups. Fortunately, urosepsis is very uncommon in children with anatomically normal urinary tracts who are immunocompetent. When present, it is signaled by high fever and unstable vital signs in concert with an abnormal urinalysis and a positive urine culture.

Laboratory Diagnosis

The diagnosis of UTI may be suggested by certain signs and symptoms, but culture of the urine is the gold standard. In infants and young children, the probability of UTI and the decision to send a sample of urine for culture may be facilitated by the use of a UTI calculator based on age, maximum temperature, previous history of UTI, being female or an uncircumcised male, duration of fever, and the presence of another source for fever. Because culture results are not available for at least 24 hours, there has been considerable interest in evaluating tests that may predict the results of urine culture, so that appropriate therapy can be initiated at the first encounter with the symptomatic patient. The tests that have received the most attention are urine microscopy for white blood cells (WBCs) and bacteria and biochemical analysis of leukocyte esterase and nitrite, which can be assessed rapidly by dipstick.

Several studies have concluded that both the presence of any bacteria on Gram staining of an uncentrifuged urine sample and dipstick analysis for leukocyte esterase perform similarly in children from birth through 12 years of age and are helpful in identifying individuals with UTI. Other recent studies done involving young infants (<2 months of age) and older infants (<12 months and 1 to 24 months) concluded that a hemocytometer WBC count of 10 or more cells/μL provides the most valuable cutoff point for identifying infants for whom urine culture is warranted.

The definition of a positive urine culture depends on the method used to collect the specimen. This variable definition of significant bacteriuria reflects the fact that urine that has passed through the urethra may be contaminated by bacteria present in the distal urethra. Contamination may occur in a urine sample collected by both the clean-catch method and by urethral catheterization. Contamination of urine samples obtained by catheter can be reduced if the first milliliter of urine is allowed to fall outside the collecting vessel. Unfortunately, the most common bacteria to contaminate a urine sample (*Escherichia coli*) is the same as the most common pathogen found in children with UTI. If the urine is obtained by the clean-catch method, a positive culture is defined as at least 10^5 colony-forming units (CFU)/mL. If the specimen is obtained by catheterization of the urethra, a positive culture is defined as at least 5×10^4 CFU/mL. In symptomatic children the lower bound of significant bacteriuria in urine samples obtained by catheter may be 1×10^4 CFU/mL if there is evidence of inflammation in the urine (i.e., pyuria or a positive leukocyte esterase). Finally, if a urine culture is obtained by suprapubic aspiration, a method that bypasses the potential source of contamination, a positive culture is defined as recovery of any bacteria from the urine. A sample of urine obtained by suprapubic aspiration is easiest to interpret. Use of point of care ultrasound can ensure a positive aspirate, and topical anesthetic, applied to the suprapubic area, can reduce discomfort of the procedure.

The challenge in defining significant bacteriuria is as follows: if contaminating bacteria contribute to a significant colony count,

unnecessary treatment may be initiated. On the other hand, if a low colony count is interpreted as insignificant, there is a risk of an untreated infection.

Although there has been substantial interest in identifying a urine or blood biomarker that will distinguish between patients with pyelonephritis and those with cystitis, there are no satisfactory recommendations at the present time.

Imaging

Imaging studies have been the standard of care for young children with a first UTI for the past decade. Commonly, a renal ultrasound study is performed to evaluate the gross anatomy of the urinary tract (size and shape of the kidneys, duplication or dilatation of the ureters). A voiding cystourethrogram (VCUG) is done to determine whether vesicoureteral reflux is present. This practice has rested on the assumption that continuous prophylactic antimicrobial therapy is effective in reducing the incidence of reinfection of the kidney and renal scarring that may occur in children with vesicoureteral reflux. The 2016 reaffirmation of the 2011 guideline on diagnosis and management of urinary tract infection in infants and children 2 to 24 months of age issued by the American Academy of Pediatrics recommends postponing performance of the VCUG until the second infection (unless there is a major abnormality of the renal ultrasound).

Treatment

In general, there are many choices for the antibiotic treatment of UTIs in children. *E. coli* is by far the most common cause of UTI, whereas *Klebsiella, Proteus, Enterobacter,* and *Enterococcus* species account for 10% to 15% of cases. If a child is toxic in appearance or vomiting (thereby precluding oral antimicrobials and suggesting a diagnosis of pyelonephritis or urosepsis), admission to the hospital for parenteral therapy is appropriate. Many would recommend a third-generation cephalosporin, such as ceftriaxone (Rocephin) 50 mg/kg/day given once daily or ceftazidime (Fortaz) 50 mg/kg/dose every 8 hours, until the emesis has resolved and the patient can be treated orally. Otherwise, children, even those with presumed pyelonephritis, do well on oral therapy.

For the child who is to receive oral therapy, the choices are amoxicillin potassium clavulanate (Augmentin) 30 mg/kg/dose given every 12 hours,[3] a second- or third-generation cephalosporin such as cefuroxime (Ceftin) 50 mg/kg/dose twice daily,[3] cefpodoxime (Vantin)[1] 5 mg/kg/dose given twice daily, cefdinir (Omnicef)[1] 7 mg/kg/dose given twice daily or cefixime (Suprax) 10 mg/kg/dose once daily,[3] or sulfamethoxazole-trimethoprim (Bactrim) 6 to 12 mg/kg/day of trimethoprim in two divided doses. There has been a tendency during the past several years for the prevalence of antimicrobial resistance to increase. The overall resistance to antibiotics varies geographically, and it is essential for the practitioner to be familiar with local antibiotic resistance patterns. In patients with suspected acute pyelonephritis, amoxicillin (Amoxil), cephalexin (Keflex), and sulfamethoxazole-trimethoprim should be avoided as presumptive therapy because of the potentially high rate of antibiotic resistance.

The optimal duration of therapy for children with UTI has been somewhat controversial. If the diagnosis of pyelonephritis is known or suspected, 10 days of treatment is conventional. Shorter courses of therapy have been successful in adult women with infection of the lower urinary tract. A recent meta-analysis conducted by the Cochrane Database of Systematic Reviews evaluated 10 trials (652 children) with lower tract UTI. There was no significant difference in frequency of positive urine cultures between short-term (2 to 4 days) and standard (7 to 14 days) duration of oral antibiotic therapy for cystitis in children, either early after treatment or at 1 to 15 months after treatment. Furthermore, there was no difference between groups in the development of resistant organisms at the end of treatment or in the incidence of recurrent UTIs. Accordingly, in cases in which the

---

[1] Not FDA approved for this indication.
[3] Exceeds dosage recommended by the manufacturer.

diagnosis of cystitis is assured, 4 days of antimicrobial therapy is sufficient.

Voiding Dysfunction

Voiding dysfunction is a broad term indicating a voiding pattern that is abnormal for the child's age. This is a condition that should be considered in all children who are diagnosed as having a UTI after toilet training has been accomplished. Constipation plays a significant role in some children with voiding dysfunction, and attention to this comorbidity often results in resolution of recurrent UTIs. While addressing bowel and voiding dysfunction, this group of children may benefit from prophylaxis for UTI.

Prophylaxis

For children who are thought to be at very high risk for recurrent UTIs and potential scarring, prophylactic treatment with sulfamethoxazole-trimethoprim or nitrofurantoin (Macrodantin) should be considered. These groups include children with high degrees of vesicoureteral reflux (grades 4 and 5), those with frequent and closely spaced UTIs without reflux, children with bowel and bladder dysfunction (while constipation is being addressed), and, occasionally, those who have urologic abnormalities.

The RIVUR (Randomized Intervention for Children with Vesicoureteral Reflux) study was undertaken in 2007 to determine whether antimicrobial prophylaxis with sulfamethoxazole-trimethoprim is effective in preventing recurrent UTI in infants and children with reflux of any grade. The study showed a modest benefit of prophylaxis with regard to febrile episodes of UTI with an approximately 50% reduction; however, there was no difference in scarring. There is no question of the biologic plausibility of prophylactic antimicrobial therapy in preventing recurrent UTI; however, adverse effects, emergence of antimicrobial resistance, and difficulties with long-term adherence to prophylactic strategies present barriers to effectiveness. The choice as to whether to prescribe antibiotic prophylaxis is an opportunity for shared decision making with the family.

In search of a nonantimicrobial intervention that may prevent recurrent UTI in children, probiotics[7] and cranberry juice (proanthocyanidins are the active ingredient) emerge as considerations. Although there is literature supportive of these as preventive strategies, their lack of availability, standardization of dose, and optimal recipient group prevent a recommendation at this time.

References

Kriger O, Belausov N, Gefen-Halevi S, et al: Optimizing the yield of in-and-out urinary catheter cultures by applying a "midstream-like" approach in pediatric patients, *Pediatr Infect Dis J* 43(3):e108, 2024.

Mattoo TK, Shaikh N, Nelson CP: Contemporary management of urinary tract infection in children, *Pediatrics* 147(2):e2020012138, 2021.

Michael M, Hodson EM, Craig JC, et al: Short versus standard duration oral antibiotic therapy for acute urinary tract infection in children, *Cochrane Database Syst Rev* 1:CD003966, 2009. [First published in 2003].

RIVUR Trial Investigators, Hoberman A, Greenfield SP, Mattoo TK, et al: Antimicrobial prophylaxis for children with vesicoureteral reflux, *N Engl J Med* 370:2367–2376, 2014.

Shaikh N, Lee S, Krumbeck JA, Kurs-Lasky M: Support for the use of a new cutoff to define a positive urine culture in young children, *Pediatrics* 152(4):e2023061931, 2023.

Shaikh N, Hoberman A, Hum SW, et al: Development and validation of a calculator for estimating the probability of urinary tract infection in young febrile children, *JAMA Pediatr* 172(6):550–556, 2018.

Shaikh KJ, Osio VA, Leeflang MM, Shaikh N: Procalcitonin, C-reactive protein, and erythrocyte sedimentation rate for the diagnosis of acute pyelonephritis in children, *Cochrane Database Syst Rev* 9(9):CD009185, 2020.

Shortliffe LMD: The beginning of the end: the dilemma of obtaining a reliable urinary specimen in children under 2 years old, *J Urol* 206:1359–1360, 2021.

Subcommittee on Urinary Tract Infection: Reaffirmation of AAP clinical practice guideline: the diagnosis and management of the initial urinary tract infection in febrile infants and young children 2 to 24 months of age, *Pediatrics* 138(6):e20163026, 2016.

Subcommittee on Urinary Tract Infection: Steering Committee on Quality Improvement and Management, Roberts KB: Urinary tract infection: clinical practice guideline for the diagnosis and management of the initial UTI in febrile infants and children 2 to 24 months, *Pediatrics* 128:595–610, 2011.

Wald ER, Eickhoff JC: Determining the best definition of a positive urine culture in young children, *Pediatrics* 152(4):e2023062883, 2023.

Williams G, Hahn D, Stephens JH, Craig JC, Hodson EM: Cranberries for preventing urinary tract infections, *Cochrane Database Syst Rev* 4(4), 2023:CD001321, .

Zhao B, Ivanova A, Shaikh N: Antimicrobial prophylaxis for vesicoureteral reflux: which subgroups of children benefit the most? *Pediat Nephrol* 39(6):1859–1863, 2024.

---

[7] Available as dietary supplement.

20 Physical and Chemical Injuries

BURNS

Method of
Allyson M. Briggs, MD; and Bradley E. Barth, MD

CURRENT DIAGNOSIS

- Perform primary and secondary survey to assess for concomitant injuries.
- Calculate percentage of burns—use a diagram.
- Chemical burns—be aware of treatment difference based on the substance involved.
- Ocular injury—assess for injury and consult ophthalmology.
- Carbon monoxide—check CO-oximetry on burn patients from enclosed fires or with prolonged smoke exposure.

CURRENT THERAPY

- The first, immediate treatment is to stop the burning.
- Use cool water irrigation (NOT ice or ice water); avoid hypothermia.
- Perform standard airway, breathing, and circulation (ABC) resuscitation.
- Calculate resuscitation fluids on the basis of surface area of deep partial and deeper burns—do not include superficial burns.
- Update tetanus vaccination if needed.
- Consult poison control center for chemical injuries.
- Hyperoxia is the treatment of choice for carbon monoxide exposure.
- Hydroxocobalamin (CYANOKIT) is the treatment of choice for cyanide exposure.
- Develop transfer relationship with burn center.

Epidemiology

Annually in the United States there are nearly 500,000 burns that are significant enough to require emergency treatment with 30,000 hospital admissions. The vast majority of the injuries that require admission are treated at a specialized burn center. Fire and fire-related inhalations injuries are responsible for nearly 3300 deaths. Worldwide incidence of burn death from all causes of burns is difficult to estimate due to a lack of centralized reporting, but 180,000 deaths occur annually from fire alone, with 95% of these occurring in low- and middle-income countries.

Risk Factors

Burns are distributed across the spectrum of age, although their types and mechanisms vary. Overall, burn injury tends to be more common in males. Males tend to get burned by flames, while females are more likely to sustain scald or heat contact wounds. Older and pediatric patients are more likely to sustain injury due to inability to get away from heat sources or flame. Use of alcohol and other substances is associated with increased risk of burn injury. Burns tend to have higher incidence in lower socioeconomic groups and are much more common in countries with lower incomes.

Prevention

Public safety initiatives have decreased the risk of burn injury in the developed world. Patient visits provide opportunities for educational interventions, especially if a patient is seen for a minor burn. Campaigns to decrease hot water heater temperatures in homes have helped reduce scald injuries. Safety plugs for electrical outlets decrease the risk of electrical injury in children. Smoke detectors and planned and practiced escape routes increase the likelihood of escaping from structure fires. Reminders to check smoke detectors and to change the batteries with the seasonal clock change ensure that devices are functional. Child-resistant lighters and safety matches increase fire safety, especially when stored out of reach of children. Keeping screens or safety devices around fireplaces and fire pits may decrease injuries as well. Avoiding activities with potential fuel sources and flames, especially while intoxicated, will also decrease fire injuries.

Pathophysiology

The injuries that result from burns are due to a combination of immediate tissue injury and resulting inflammation. This includes the activation of an inflammatory cascade, immediate and delayed cellular and humoral effects, and the delayed effects of changes in gene expression induced by the earlier injuries. The immediate injury is classically divided into three zones. The most severely injured is the central zone of necrosis; this area is surrounded by the zone of stasis, which is surrounded by the zone of hyperemia (Figure 1). The zone of necrosis is composed of coagulated tissue that will progress to rapid cell death and eschar formation. The outer zone of hyperemia has increased blood flow and minimal tissue damage and will almost certainly heal. The middle zone of stasis is the region where blood flow has ceased within the capillary bed. Depending on subsequent actions over the next 24 to 48 hours, this area either will worsen to necrotic tissue or may reepithelialize to healing. The immediate postinjury efforts are focused on salvaging this area.

Burning Tissue

As heat transfers to tissue, damage begins to occur as cellular temperature rises above 44°C. Once the internal cellular temperature reaches 60°C, the cell will die. Generally, once the heat source is removed from the skin, the tissue temperature rapidly returns to normal, but the tissue injury does not stop at that point. Within seconds of the injury, arterioles begin to spasm, and red blood cells aggregate within the tissues. Histologic changes are visible within 15 minutes, and tissue edema begins. Tissue edema typically peaks 6 to 12 hours postinjury.

It is much easier for a burn injury to penetrate through the dermal layers in thin skin than in thick skin, leading to more severe injury in the former with a similar degree of heat transfer. These injuries pose a particular risk in infants and children as well as the elderly.

Shortly after the burning stops, processes of both inflammation and healing begin. There is a complex interplay of inflammatory mediators, immune cell action, and changes in gene expression that will continue over the following weeks to months and will play a role in how the wound heals.

Clinical Manifestations

Descriptions of burns are based on the depth of the injury and the extent of coverage. They are divided into superficial, partial

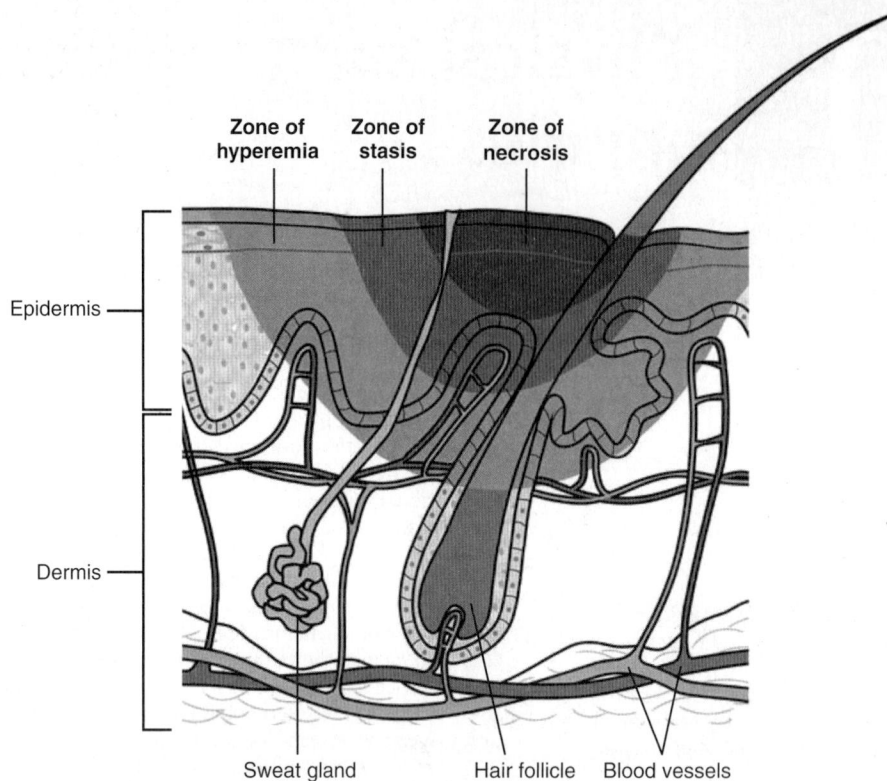

Figure 1 Burn injury.

TABLE 1	Types of Burns				
DEPTH	**ANATOMY**	**APPEARANCE**	**SENSATION**	**TIME**	**TREATMENT**
Superficial	Epidermis only	Pink or red and dry, blanches	Painful	Days	Topical
Superficial partial thickness	Epidermis and upper papillary dermis	Pink, clear blisters, moist surface, blanches	Painful	14–21 days	Debride and topical medication
Deep partial thickness	Epidermis, papillary dermis, and lower reticular dermis	Pink or red, moist surface, blisters, may be hemorrhagic, does not blanch	Painful, may have decreased sensation	Weeks or may progress to full thickness	Debride, topical medication, possible surgery
Full thickness	Epidermis, dermis, and into underlying tissue	White or brown, dry, leathery, does not blanch	Insensate	Weeks, and heals by contraction and scarring	Surgical

(which is further characterized as superficial partial or deep partial), and full thickness (Table 1). Superficial burns involve the epidermis alone. These injuries are typically painful and erythematous, and they will heal without scarring. These injuries are not included in calculations of the percentage total body surface area (TBSA) burned. Superficial partial thickness burns involve the entire epidermis and extend down to the papillary region of the upper dermis. These injuries are painful, erythematous, and moist, and they form blisters. Deep partial thickness burns involve the entire epidermis and extend deeper into the lower reticular dermis. These wounds are typically painful and whitish, and they have less weeping and blanching than superficial partial thickness wounds. These may have less pain than expected depending on the extent of damage to nerve endings in the skin. Full-thickness burns extend through the epidermis and entire dermis and destroy nerves and other deep structures. These wounds are insensate, stiff, white or tan in color, and they do not blanch. Wounds of this depth cannot heal spontaneously and will have significant scarring and contracture if not surgically managed.

Areas of burn that have extensive or circumferential deep partial thickness or full-thickness burns are at risk for development of restrictive eschars. Eschars can restrict circulation, leading to compartment syndrome in extremities and can decrease respiration if on the chest or neck. Ideally, burn patients can reach burn centers before these complications arise, but an escharotomy could be required urgently in some cases.

Inhalation injury is a source of significant morbidity in burn patients. The initial injury may not seem particularly severe, but edema can develop rapidly in the airway, which makes delayed airway management perilous. Early intubation may be necessary.

Special Situations
Ocular Injuries
Patients with any signs of burns to the face, complaints of eye pain, or inability to communicate should undergo eye examinations with fluorescein staining. If corneal burns are identified, appropriate antibiotic ointment should be started, and consultation with an eye specialist should be obtained.

Nonaccidental Trauma
Clinicians should have a high index of suspicion for nonaccidental trauma (NAT) in burns occurring in pediatric patients. NAT has been shown to be present in up to 25% of pediatric burn

cases. Burns caused by NAT are more likely to occur in males and children with developmental delays and may result in a delay in seeking care. Other concerning findings are burns that have clear lines of demarcation (e.g., cigarette burns, dunking, radiator, grill, curling iron), that are symmetric on both extremities, or spare the flexor creases with deep surrounding burns. If NAT is suspected, it must be reported, and the child must be kept in a safe place until authorities have cleared the child to go home.

Chemical Burns

The risk and degree of injury caused by chemical burns vary greatly, depending on the substance involved as well as on the concentration of the material and the duration of exposure. The Centers for Disease Control and Prevention has a pocket guide on chemical hazards that can be found at https://www.cdc.gov/niosh/npg/default.html (accessed March 25, 2025). General precautions for chemical burns are to decontaminate as quickly as possible while avoiding rescuer contamination or injury. For dry or powdered chemicals, remove as much chemical as possible while it is still in the dry form by brushing or other mechanical removal. After mechanical removal, or for liquid contamination, dilute the chemical and continue the removal process by using water. Water should be used via copious, high-flow, low-pressure irrigation for at least 20 minutes. If feasible, check the pH of the contaminated area and continue irrigation until it returns to normal. In most cases, removal and irrigation are more important to neutralizing the chemical because using neutralizing agents can make the injury worse. Evaluate the patient for possible inhalation or ocular injury as well. Ocular chemical exposures should be irrigated with water or lactated Ringer's solution, starting as early as possible after exposure, until a normal pH is obtained. There are important exceptions to typical management, some of which are listed in Table 2.

Electrical Injuries

Injuries with electrical sources vary based on the type of circuit (alternating vs. direct current), amperage, voltage, tissue resistance, duration of exposure, and path of current through the body. High voltage ($\geq 1000V$) tends to cause more thermal tissue injury and often causes concomitant traumatic injuries. Depending on the path of electricity, there may be significant internal injuries beneath normal-appearing skin, especially in high-voltage cases. Significant injuries should be treated more like crush injuries, as the extent of the internal injuries is difficult to assess. Cutaneous burns due to electrical injury can be treated similarly to thermal burns. During the initial evaluation of electrical injury, patients should undergo assessment for other injuries, electrocardiography, and cardiac monitoring. In patients with injury from high-voltage sources, obtaining serum levels of electrolytes, renal function studies, creatine kinase, troponin, and coagulation studies should be considered.

Special circumstances include multivictim injuries and oral commissure burns. In cases of multiple victims of a lightning strike, a reverse triage process occurs whereby care is provided first to the patients who appear to be in cardiac arrest, as cardiopulmonary resuscitation and defibrillation may save their lives if applied early enough. Oral commissure burns occur most often in young children who have chewed through electrical cords. Caregivers should be warned about delayed bleeding from the labial artery that can occur during wound healing. Due to risk of scar contracture and concern for aesthetic outcomes, these patients should be referred to a plastic or oral surgeon.

Therapy and Treatment
First Aid and Office Management

The initial management for burn injuries consists of stopping further injury by removing the heat source and providing cooling. Remove the patient from the burning area in the event of flame injury. If the patient's clothing is on fire, it is important to stop the burning and remove hot clothing as quickly as possible. Hot liquid or scald injuries especially require prompt removal of overlying clothing, as the clothing will trap the heat, which can continue the tissue damage. After the heat source is removed, copious cool water should be used to irrigate the injured area, and any constricting jewelry should be removed immediately. The ideal temperature for cool water irrigation is not clear, but it is likely between 15°C and 25°C (59°F–77°F); colder temperatures can be damaging. The cooling irrigation should be continued for 20 minutes. Early wound cooling decreases the temperature of the injured area quickly to halt the burning process, but irrigation has been shown to be beneficial even after the wound has returned to a normal temperature. Cooling the wound is thought to be effective up to 3 hours after the injury. It is unclear why cool water irrigation improves burn outcomes; heat removal and edema prevention play a role, but it may also lead to alterations in gene expression that decrease injury and improve healing. After cooling the injured area, the initial treatment is to cover the wounds with a clean, thin cloth or sterile sheets while the patient awaits further care. Ensure that the patient's tetanus vaccination is up to date. Check

TABLE 2	Chemical Burns*	
CHEMICAL	**TREATMENT**	**SPECIAL NOTES**
Dry chemical	Brush or remove as much chemical as possible, then copious irrigation	Obtain material safety data sheet information on exposure
Liquid chemical	Copious irrigation	
Ocular injury	Copious irrigation with lactated Ringer's solution, measure pH early and repeat frequently	
Elemental metals (e.g., sodium, magnesium)	Cover with mineral oil if available, physically remove as soon as possible, irrigate with water if no other options	Water causes an intense exothermic reaction, but tissue damage occurs with continued contact
Strong alkalis (pH 10–12; e.g., lye, bleach, cement [calcium oxide], ammonia)	Copious irrigation, continue until pH normalizes but at least 1 hour; may require 12 or more hours	Current recommendations are not to try to neutralize, but research is continuing
Petroleum	Irrigation, mild soap solution	May be seen in vehicle trauma patients
Hydrofluoric acid	Irrigation, topical calcium gluconate (Calgonate)[1] mixed with water-based lubricant (e.g., K-Y jelly), intradermal or intravenous calcium gluconate[1]	Associated with pain out of proportion to appearance, fluoride ion can cause hypocalcemia and death
Phenol	Polyethylene glycol (PEG) (Miralax)[1] stops phenol burn more quickly than water; if PEG is not available, use high-flow, low-pressure, copious irrigation	

*Consider contacting a burn center or poison control center for assistance with chemical injury treatment.
[1]Not FDA approved for this indication.

the patient's temperature and provide warm blankets or a warm air environment to avoid hypothermia.

Superficial burns or superficial partial thickness burns can generally be treated on an outpatient basis, with important exceptions: >10% TBSA, extremes of age, circumferential injury, or burns on the head, face, or genital areas. Debride any ruptured blister tissue. Clean the wounds with mild soap and water or dilute antiseptic solutions and dress the wound. It is unclear whether there is a role for antiseptic dressings in preventing infection. Silver sulfadiazine cream 1% (Silvadene) is now generally discouraged as it may delay healing and can lead to pigmented scarring. Wound dressings may include topical antibiotic cream or ointment, silver impregnated nylon, bismuth tribromophenate and petrolatum impregnated gauze (Xeroform), or various specialized products to form occlusive dressings (including polyurethane films and foams, hydrocolloid, hydrogel, alginate, and chitin in various forms). The management of intact blisters is controversial; however, if a blister appears fragile or likely to rupture, unroof and debride the wound before dressing the wound. If the blister is in thicker skin or appears stable, most recommendations are to aspirate the blister fluid and dress the wound.

Burns are painful injuries and often require early, aggressive pain control, such as with nonsteroidal antiinflammatory drugs (NSAIDs), opioid medications, and acetaminophen. It is important to remember to provide additional analgesia as needed for dressing changes and wound care. Pruritus and neuropathic pain may occur as the wound heals. These are often treated with adjunct pain medications such as gabapentin (Neurontin),[1] and diphenhydramine (Benadryl).[1]

Deep partial thickness or deeper wounds usually require some form of surgical management and should be referred for specialized care. Early surgical management has been demonstrated to be beneficial. Prophylactic antibiotics should not be used for burn management, as they have been shown to be harmful. If burns have not healed within 2 weeks, they should be referred to a specialist.

Initial Hospital Management

For patients with more severe injuries, follow the traditional algorithm of assessing and stabilizing the respiratory and circulatory system first, then proceeding with a complete history and physical examination, including comorbid conditions, allergies, medications, and other past medical history. If possible, identify the mechanisms and circumstances surrounding the injury, including agents involved, duration of exposure, and situation, including possibility of inhalation injury or enclosed space involvement. Assess whether there are chemical or electrical burns and any associated trauma. The social history may play an important role in disposition and management decisions.

Management of Inhalation Injury

Patients who were in an enclosed space or structure fire or who were otherwise exposed to high levels of smoke or toxins should be assessed for carbon monoxide and cyanide injuries. Lactate, troponin, and carboxyhemoglobin levels should be checked in patients at risk for carbon monoxide or cyanide exposure. Patients at risk for cyanide exposure with decreased level of consciousness, hypotension, or a lactate level greater than 9 should receive 5 g (or 70 mg/kg to a maximum of 5 g) of hydroxocobalamin (Cyanokit) intravenously. If the patient is in cardiac arrest or does not improve with the initial dose, a total of 10 g should be given.

A patient with carbon monoxide exposure should have a carboxyhemoglobin level obtained and be placed on 100% oxygen as soon as possible, typically delivered via a nonrebreather face mask. Carbon monoxide binds tightly to hemoglobin, and by increasing the oxygen concentration in the lungs and blood, the half-life of carboxyhemoglobin is greatly reduced. With oxygen levels typically delivered by nonrebreather face mask, the half-life of carboxyhemoglobin is 74 minutes. After 6 hours on 100% oxygen, if the patient is asymptomatic, treatment can be stopped.

[1]Not FDA approved for this indication.

It is unnecessary to use arterial blood or to repeat carboxyhemoglobin levels. Patients with carbon monoxide poisoning may experience delayed neurologic sequelae. Hyperbaric oxygen therapy may reduce the risk of delayed neurologic sequelae in appropriately selected patients. Although controversial, this therapy is thought to be most helpful if it occurs within 12 hours after the end of the patient's exposure, but patients may benefit up to 24 hours after exposure. If possible, consult with a physician capable of providing hyperbaric oxygen therapy or with a poison control center for patients with carboxyhemoglobin levels greater than 10, symptoms consistent with carbon monoxide exposure, or pregnant patients (Box 1).

Patients with inhalation injuries can develop rapidly progressing airway swelling. The initial evaluation of burn patients should include assessment for perioral injury, singed facial or nasal hair, and soot or swelling in the oral or hypopharyngeal cavities. These findings, extensive neck burns, other indications of airway swelling, or difficulty breathing should prompt early placement of a definitive airway. Delay may make placement of an endotracheal tube difficult or impossible.

Burn Management

After evaluation and stabilization of the respiratory and circulatory status of the patient, and after stabilizing acute traumatic injuries, the next step is to evaluate the extent of the burn injuries. Removing the heat source and cooling the injured areas remain a priority. Burned areas can be cooled with cool water irrigation or saline-soaked gauze. Because patients with extensive wounds can be at risk of developing hypothermia during this phase, it is important to raise the ambient temperature in the resuscitation room or use warm blankets to maintain normothermia. The extent of the burns should be determined. The "rule of nines" diagram is an accepted mechanism for approximating the percentage of TBSA burned in adults, but it tends to overestimate. Because children have a proportionally larger head and torso, diagrams have been adapted for use in pediatric populations. The Lund-Browder chart can be utilized with patients of all ages (Figure 2). It can also be useful to diagram the areas of burn by estimated depth. For determination of burn severity, calculation of transfer criteria, and fluid resuscitation, only the areas of partial thickness and deeper burns are added together to determine TBSA. Use of a diagram is recommended because TBSA is frequently overestimated when providers estimate the extent of burned areas. Overestimating TBSA burned leads to excessive fluid administration and the complications that accompany fluid overload.

Fluid Resuscitation and Monitoring

Critically ill burn patients should be monitored in an intensive care setting while awaiting transfer to a burn center. In addition to monitoring respiratory and circulatory status, a Foley catheter should be placed to monitor urinary output and for intermittent assessment of bladder pressure to evaluate for the development of intraabdominal compartment syndrome.

Because burned tissue increases insensible fluid losses, burn victims have increased fluid requirements. Various formulas are available for calculating approximate fluid requirements, but all require

| BOX 1 | Symptoms of Carbon Monoxide Exposure* |

Headache
Dizziness
Nausea
Vomiting
Confusion
Fatigue
Chest pain
Shortness of breath
Loss of consciousness

*It is important to note that carboxyhemoglobin levels do not correlate well with symptoms or with severity of exposure.
Arterial blood gas samples are not superior to venous blood samples.

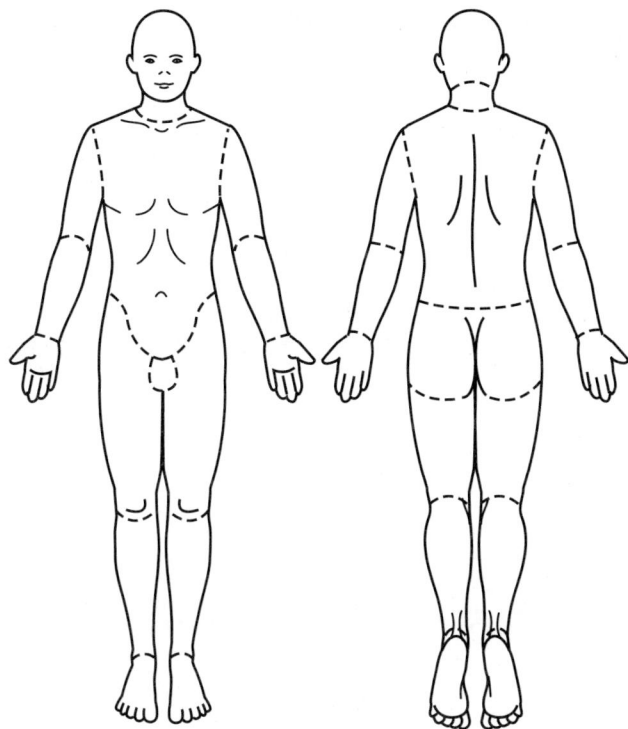

	Birth 1 yr.	1–4 yrs.	5–9 yrs.	10–14 yrs.	15 yrs.	Adult	Burn size estimate
Head	19	17	13	11	9	7	
Neck	2	2	2	2	2	2	
Anterior trunk	13	13	13	13	13	13	
Posterior trunk	13	13	13	13	13	13	
Right buttock	2.5	2.5	2.5	2.5	2.5	2.5	
Left buttock	2.5	2.5	2.5	2.5	2.5	2.5	
Genitalia	1	1	1	1	1	1	
Right upper arm	4	4	4	4	4	4	
Left upper arm	4	4	4	4	4	4	
Right lower arm	3	3	3	3	3	3	
Left lower arm	3	3	3	3	3	3	
Right hand	2.5	2.5	2.5	2.5	2.5	2.5	
Left hand	2.5	2.5	2.5	2.5	2.5	2.5	
Right thigh	5.5	6.5	8	8.5	9	9.5	
Left thigh	5.5	6.5	8	8.5	9	9.5	
Right leg	5	5	5.5	6	6.5	7	
Left leg	5	5	5.5	6	6.5	7	
Right foot	3.5	3.5	3.5	3.5	3.5	3.5	
Left foot	3.5	3.5	3.5	3.5	3.5	3.5	

Total BSAB ――――――――

Figure 2 Lund-Browder classification of burn size.

careful monitoring of the results and progress of fluid resuscitation. Patients who receive more than 250 mL/kg in the first 24 hours are at increased risk of developing fluid-related complications. The American Burn Association Consensus Statement formula is used to guide initial fluid management. The starting fluid requirements are 2 mL/kg of lactated Ringer's solution per TBSA percent value, with half given in the first 8 hours and the rest over the next 16 hours (Box 2). Urine output should be monitored hourly and maintained between 0.5 and 1 mL/kg/h. If a patient's urine output is greater than 1 mL/kg/h, the rate of fluid administration should be decreased by 20% and continued to be monitored hourly. If the urine output is less than 0.5 mL/kg/h, the rate of fluid administration should be increased by 20% and continued to be monitored.

Unfortunately, ensuring adequate urine output does not necessarily guarantee adequate fluid resuscitation. In addition to using urine output as an indicator of resuscitation adequacy, other modes of monitoring can be used to help guide fluid resuscitation (hemodynamic monitoring, echocardiography, gastric tonometry, or other devices). Whether they lead to any increased improvement or survivability is not clear, however.

Burn Center Referral Criteria and Transfer

It is important to identify the closest regional burn referral center and to establish a line of communication with it before a burn patient is encountered in order to know of the center's suggested criteria for transfer (Box 3). Burn centers typically manage more than 200 burn patients annually and have specially trained physicians, nurses, and ancillary personnel who are focused on treating burn patients. Severely burned patients who are treated at specialized centers have better outcomes. It is recommended that hospitals and clinics have

---

BOX 2 Fluid Administration and Calculation

80-kg male patient with a burn of 35% TBSA full-thickness and partial thickness burns:

80 kg × 35 × 2 mL/kg = 5600 mL in first 24 hours

5600 mL/24 hours ÷ 2 = 2800 mL in first 8 hours, 2800 mL in next 16 hours

Initial rate of 350 mL/h over first 8 hours, then switching to a rate of 175 mL/h over next 16 hours

Expected urine output is 0.5–1 mL/kg/h

80 kg × 0.5 mL/kg/h = 40 mL/h

80 kg × 1 mL/kg/h = 80 mL/h

So, for our 80-kg patient, we would expect 40–80 mL of urine every hour. In hours 1 and 2 of resuscitation, the patient has 65 mL of urine per hour. In hour 3 of resuscitation, the patient has 90 mL of urine per hour. We would then decrease the fluid administration rate by 20%, or

350 mL/h–(0.20 × 350) = 280 mL/h

Thus, the rate of administration of lactated Ringer's solution would change from 350 mL/h to 280 mL/h and continue to be monitored and recorded hourly, with continued adjustments based on hourly urine output.

TBSA, Total body surface area.

BOX 3 Burn Center Referral Criteria

Partial thickness burns greater than 10% TBSA

Full-thickness burns

Burns to high-risk areas, such as the face, hands, feet, genitals, perineum, or major joints

Circumferential burns

Electrical burns, including lightning strikes

Chemical burns

Inhalation injury

Preexisting conditions known to impair healing and increase risk of mortality

Burns in combination with traumatic injury (e.g., fracture, traumatic brain injury) whereby the burn is the leading risk for patient mortality

Burn injury in patients who will require special social, emotional, or long-term rehabilitative intervention

All burns in children warrant burn center consultation and consideration for transfer

TBSA, Total body surface area.
Available from https://ameriburn.org/resources/burnreferral/. Accessed March 20, 2025.

---

agreements with burn centers for the management of complicated patients and patients who meet criteria for burn center transfer.

In general, the following criteria are recommended for transfer to a burn center: burns greater than 10% of TBSA; inhalation injury; burns with significant associated mechanical injury; burns of the face, hands, feet, perineum, or genitalia or across major joints; full-thickness burns of any size; and circumferential burns. Burns that warrant a discussion with a burn center for possible transfer or outpatient follow-up include all burns in children; patients with comorbid conditions that will impact healing; and patients with special social, emotional, psychological, or rehabilitative needs.

Complications

Pain management for burns may require multiple modalities because the type of pain varies, depending on where the patient is in the cycle of treatment and healing. There are four types of pain that need to be treated during the care of a burn patient: background pain, breakthrough pain, procedural pain, and long-term pain. Background pain is present from the onset of the injury, and the pain is typically intensified during procedures. There will also be episodes of breakthrough pain. Depending on the severity of the injury, initial pain and background pain may be treated with multimodal therapy including acetaminophen, NSAIDs (e.g., ibuprofen,

naproxen sodium), or opioids. Low-dose ketamine (Ketalar)[1] is increasingly used in addition to opioids for background and breakthrough pain. Procedural pain may require bolus dosing of opioids or other adjunctive medications such as ketamine (0.1–0.2 mg/kg IV). Long-term pain may respond to medications such as gabapentin (Neurontin),[1] clonidine (Catapres),[1] or others.

Psychosocial recovery from burns is impacted by the preexisting conditions and the resilience of the patient. Preexisting mental health, substance abuse, and other medical and psychosocial issues complicate the patient's recovery from burns. Risk factors for burn injury include poverty, a history of abuse or neglect, substance abuse, serious mental illness, and risk for suicide or assault. Psychiatric recovery is negatively affected by posttraumatic stress disorder, depression, learning disorders, substance abuse, stigma, and disability. Individual resilience, social support, and education or occupation also impact patient outcomes.

The patient's age and stage of life at the time of injury impact recovery as well. Younger victims have a longer remaining lifespan to live with persistent scarring and disfigurement. Pediatric patients often have fewer comorbid medical conditions, which can speed their recovery and limit disability, and they tend to heal more quickly. However, their injuries may have a significant impact on their body image development, self-confidence, and interpersonal relationship building. The family may be of assistance in recovery from the injury, but family members, too, may experience stress and psychological concerns related to the child's injury. Adults and older patients have to deal with the impact of the injury on their identity and their ability to return to their preinjury roles.

Some patients and caregivers may develop posttraumatic stress disorder related to the injury or to postinjury treatment. It is thought that early multidisciplinary interventions may decrease this risk, but the research is unclear. Some patients will require long-term, continued outpatient treatment.

Hypertrophic scarring is the most common complication related to healing of burn wounds, but scar contracture and pruritus are common complications as well. It is thought that hypertrophic scarring may be decreased with early, appropriate surgical repair, but it still can occur.

Scar contracture results from tissue loss at the time of injury and tissue-healing properties. Burn injuries are more complicated than other traumatic wounds because the destroyed tissue is surrounded by profoundly damaged tissue. Hypertrophic scars tend to form within the first month after injury and may improve over the first 6 months but then tend not to show significant changes after that time. Burn treatment and scar prevention consist of tissue replacement, tissue rehabilitation, and tension release. Early and existing scars are often treated with compression garments and silicone sheets. It is thought that these may alter and improve remodeling of the extracellular matrix and thereby improve scarring. In some cases, surgical release of tension may be necessary.

References

Akelma H, Karahan ZA: Rare chemical burns: review of the literature, *Int Wound J* 16(6):1330–1338, 2019, https://doi.org/10.1111/iwj.13193.

Barrett W, Buxhoeveden M, Dhillon S: Ketamine: a versatile tool for anesthesia and analgesia, *Curr Opin Anaesthesiol* 33(5):633–638, 2020, https://doi.org/10.1097/aco.0000000000000916.

Bitter CC, Erickson TB: Management of burn injuries in the wilderness: lessons from low-resource settings, *Wilderness Environ Med* 27(4):519–525, 2016, https://doi.org/10.1016/j.wem.2016.09.001.

Bizrah M, Yusuf A, Ahmad S: An update on chemical eye burns, *Eye* 33(9):1362–1377, 2019, https://doi.org/10.1038/s41433-019-0456-5.

Burn Incidence and Treatment in United States: 2016, American Burn Association, 2016.

Carboni RM, Santos GL, Carboni Júnior IC, et al: Therapy for patients with burns—an integrating review, *Rev Assoc Med Bras* 65:1405–1412, 2019.

Cartotto R, Greenhalgh DG, Cancio C: Burn state of the science: fluid resuscitation, *J Burn Care Res* 38(3):e596–e604, 2017, https://doi.org/10.1097/bcr.0000000000000541.

Culnan DM, Craft-Coffman B, Bitz GH, et al: Carbon monoxide and cyanide poisoning in the burned pregnant patient: an indication for hyperbaric oxygen therapy, *Ann Plast Surg* 80(3 Suppl 2):S106–S112, 2018, https://doi.org/10.1097/sap.0000000000001351.

---

[1]Not FDA approved for this indication.

Culnan DM, Farner K, Bitz GH, et al: Volume resuscitation in patients with high-voltage electrical injuries, *Ann Plast Surg* 80(3 Suppl 2):S113–s118, 2018, https://doi.org/10.1097/sap.0000000000001374.

Dyamenahalli K, Garg G, Shupp JW, Kuprys PV, Choudhry MA, Kovacs EJ: Inhalation injury: unmet clinical needs and future research, *J Burn Care Res* 40(5):570–584, 2019, https://doi.org/10.1093/jbcr/irz055.

Friedstat J, Brown D, Levi B: Chemical, electrical, and radiation injuries, *Clin Plast Surg* 44(3):657–659, 2017, https://doi.org/10.1016/j.cps.2017.02.021.

Gigengack RK, Cleffken BI, Loer SA: Advances in airway management and mechanical ventilation in inhalation injury, *Curr Opin Anaesthesiol* 33(6):774–780, 2020, https://doi.org/10.1097/aco.0000000000000929.

Griggs C, Goverman J, Bittner EA, Levi B: Sedation and pain management in burn patients, *Clin Plast Surg* 44(3):535–540, 2017, https://doi.org/10.1016/j.cps.2017.02.026.

Hall AH, Mathieu L, Maibach HI: Acute chemical skin injuries in the United States: a review, *Crit Rev Toxicol* 48(7):540–554, 2018, https://doi.org/10.1080/10408444.2018.1493085.

ISBI Practice guidelines for burn care, Part 2, *Burns* 44(7):1617–1706, 2018, https://doi.org/10.1016/j.burns.2018.09.012.

Jeschke MG, Peck MD: Burn care of the elderly, *J Burn Care Res* 38(3):e625–e628, 2017, https://doi.org/10.1097/bcr.0000000000000535.

Jeschke MG, Shahrokhi S, Finnerty CC, Branski LK, Dibildox M: Wound coverage technologies in burn care: established techniques, *J Burn Care Res* 39(3):313–318, 2018, https://doi.org/10.1097/BCR.0b013e3182920d29.

Jeschke MG, van Baar ME, Choudhry MA, Chung KK, Gibran NS, Logsetty S: Burn injury, *Nat Rev Dis Primers* 6(1):11, 2020, https://doi.org/10.1038/s41572-020-0145-5.

Kim DE, Pruskowski KA, Ainsworth CR, Linsenbardt HR, Rizzo JA, Cancio LC: A review of adjunctive therapies for burn injury pain during the opioid crisis, *J Burn Care Res* 40(6):983–995, 2019, https://doi.org/10.1093/jbcr/irz111.

Partain KP, Fabia R, Thakkar RK: Pediatric burn care: new techniques and outcomes, *Curr Opin Pediatr* 32(3):405–410, 2020a, https://doi.org/10.1097/mop.0000000000000902.

Porter C, Tompkins RG, Finnerty CC, Sidossis LS, Suman OE, Herndon DN: The metabolic stress response to burn trauma: current understanding and therapies, *Lancet* 388(10052):1417–1426, 2016, https://doi.org/10.1016/s0140-6736(16)31469-6.

Shah A, Pedraza I, Mitchell C, Kramer GC: Fluid volumes infused during burn resuscitation 1980–2015: a quantitative review, *Burns* 46(1):52–57, 2020, https://doi.org/10.1016/j.burns.2019.11.013.

Shpichka A, Butnaru D, Bezrukov EA, et al: Skin tissue regeneration for burn injury, *Stem Cell Res Ther* 10(1), 2019, https://doi.org/10.1186/s13287-019-1203-3.

Smolle C, Cambiaso-Daniel J, Forbes AA, et al: Recent trends in burn epidemiology worldwide: a systematic review, *Burns* 43(2):249–257, 2017, https://doi.org/10.1016/j.burns.2016.08.013.

Sofia J, Ambardekar A: Pediatric burn resuscitation, management, and recovery for the pediatric anesthesiologist, *Curr Opin Anaesthesiol* 33(3):360–367, 2020, https://doi.org/10.1097/aco.0000000000000858.

Soussi S, Dépret F, Benyamina M, Legrand M: Early hemodynamic management of critically ill burn patients, *Anesthesiology* 129(3):583–589, 2018, https://doi.org/10.1097/aln.0000000000002314.

Stapelberg F: Challenges in anaesthesia and pain management for burn injuries, *Anaesth Intensive Care* 48(2):101–113, 2020, https://doi.org/10.1177/0310057x20914908.

Walls R, Hockberger R, Gausche-Hill M: *Rosen's emergency medicine—concepts and clinical practice E-Book*, Vol 2, 9 ed, Elsevier Health Sciences, 2018.

Yeroshalmi F, Sidoti EJ, Adamo AK, Lieberman BL, Badner VM: Oral electrical burns in children—a model of multidisciplinary care, *J Burn Care Res* 32(2):e25–e30, 2011, https://doi.org/10.1097/bcr.0b013e31820ab393.

Yoshino Y, Ohtsuka M, Kawaguchi M, et al: The wound/burn guidelines—6: guidelines for the management of burns, *J Dermatol* 43(9):989–1010, 2016, https://doi.org/10.1111/1346-8138.13288.

DISTURBANCES DUE TO COLD

Method of
Jerrold B. Leikin, MD; Scott Leikin, DO; Frederick Korley, MD; and Ernest Wang, MD

CURRENT DIAGNOSIS

- Accidental hypothermia may be classified as mild, moderate, or severe.
- The temperature measured should be core body temperature.
- The method of rewarming depends on the severity of the temperature drop.
- Complications of rewarming include arrhythmias, rewarming-related hypotension, core temperature after drop, and rhabdomyolysis.
- Patients can be declared dead only after they are warm.

CURRENT THERAPY

Mild Hypothermia: 32.2°C to 35°C (90°F to 95°F)
- Begin passive external rewarming; remove wet clothing.
- Ambient temperature should exceed 21°C (70°F).
- Cover the patient with insulating material.

Moderate Hypothermia: 28°C to 32.2°C (82.4°F to 90°F)
- Begin active external rewarming; use radiant heat.
- Use thermal mattresses and electric heating blankets.
- Use forced-air heating blankets.
- Perform active core rewarming; use warmed humidified oxygen.
- Give warmed intravenous saline solution.
- Give bladder, colonic, and gastric irrigation.
- Start pleural cavity lavage.
- Avoid alcohol, caffeine, and nicotine (tobacco).

Severe Hypothermia: Less than 28°C (82.4°F)
- Begin aggressive active core rewarming; use warmed, humidified oxygen.
- Give warmed intravenous saline solution.
- Give bladder, colonic, and gastric irrigation.
- Begin pleural cavity lavage.
- Perform peritoneal lavage or dialysis.
- Perform extracorporeal warming or heated cardiopulmonary bypass.

Frostnip
- Begin gentle rewarming, generally in a water bath of 104°F to 108°F (40°C to 42°C).
- It is usually self-resolving.

Frostbite
- Immerse in warm (not hot) water.
- Débride broken vesicles.
- Do not débride hemorrhagic or intact blisters.
- Apply topical aloe or antibiotic ointment.
- Use nonsteroidal antiinflammatory drugs (NSAIDs) for pain.
- Update tetanus status.
- Do not rub or massage the affected area.
- Do not use a heating pad or heat lamp; affected areas can be easily burned.
- Avoid alcohol and tobacco products.

Chilblain
- Rewarm gently.
- Nifedipine (Procardia)[1] may be useful.

Trench Foot
- Dry the foot.
- Rewarm gently.
- Use NSAIDs for pain.

[1]Not FDA approved for this indication.
[7]Available as dietary supplement.

Accidental Systemic Hypothermia

Hypothermia is classically defined as a reduction in the body's core temperature below 95°F (35°C). Most reported cases of hypothermia are caused by environmental exposure to low ambient temperatures (accidental hypothermia). Other causes of hypothermia include sepsis, severe hypothyroidism (myxedema coma), acute spinal cord injury, diabetic ketoacidosis, multisystem trauma, and prolonged cardiac arrest. Episodic hypothermia can be encountered in patients with advanced secondary progressive multiple sclerosis, subarachnoid hemorrhage, HIV-1 infections, and brain contusion. Shapiro syndrome is episodic hypothermia associated with hyperhidrosis caused by agenesis or lesions of the corpus callosum.

| BOX 1 | Factors Predisposing to Hypothermia or Frostbite |

Physiologic
Decreased Heat Production
- Age extremes (infants, older adults)
- Dehydration or malnutrition
- Diaphoresis or hyperhidrosis
- Endocrinologic insufficiency
- Hypoxia
- Insufficient fuel
- Overexertion
- Physical conditioning
- Prior cold injury
- Trauma (multisystem or extremity)

Increased Heat Loss
- Burns
- Dermatologic malfunction
- Cold infusions
- Emergency resuscitation
- Poor acclimatization or conditioning
- Shock
- Vascular diseases

Impaired Thermoregulation
- Central nervous system trauma or disease
- Metabolic disorders
- Pharmacologic or toxicologic agents
- Sepsis
- Spinal cord injury

Psychological
- Fatigue
- Fear or panic
- Hunger
- Intense concentration on tasks
- Intoxicants
- Mental status or attitude
- Peer pressure

Environmental
- Altitude with or without associated conditions
- Ambient temperature or humidity
- Duration of exposure
- Heat loss (conductive, evaporative, radiative, convective)
- Quantity of exposed surface area
- Wind chill factor

Mechanical
- Constricting or wet clothing or boots
- Inadequate insulation
- Immobility or cramped positioning

Epidemiology

Risk factors for developing hypothermia include extremes of age (older adults might not be able to remove themselves from cold environments, and young children lose heat more rapidly because of their increased total body surface area), major trauma, homelessness, psychiatric illness, and drug and alcohol abuse (Box 1). Cold-related deaths also are reported in military combatants and outdoor winter sports participants. Several drugs and chemicals can predispose to hypothermia. Alcohol is the most common intoxicant associated with hypothermia because of its ability to cause cutaneous vasodilation, impair shivering, and impair adaptive behavior.

Between 1999 and 2011 in the United States, 16,911 deaths (an average of 1301 per year) were attributed to exposure to low environmental temperatures. In 2002, of the 646 hypothermia-related deaths reported, 66% occurred in male patients, 52% occurred in patients who were 65 years of age or younger, 45% occurred among White male patients, and 14% occurred among Black male patients. The state of Alaska (age-adjusted mortality of 2 deaths per 100,000), followed by Montana and New Mexico, had the largest overall age-adjusted death rates from hypothermia from 1999 to 2015. From 2018 to 2020, death rates attributed to excessive cold or hypothermia were generally three to four times higher in more rural areas than urban localities. The incidence of accidental hypothermia in Europe and New Zealand ranges from 0.13 to 6.9 cases per 100,000 annually. The lowest recorded core temperature in a pediatric survivor of accidental hypothermia is 57.9°F (14.4°C), and the lowest temperature in an adult survivor is 56.7°F (13.7°C).

Pathophysiology

The normal range of human core temperature is 97.5°F to 99.5°F (36.4°C to 37.5°C). Humans are thus warm-blooded and are normally able to maintain their body temperature by heat-generating mechanisms and heat-conserving behavior. These compensatory responses, however, can be overwhelmed under extreme environmental conditions, leading to hypothermia.

The anterior hypothalamus coordinates nonshivering heat conservation and dissipation mechanisms, and the posterior hypothalamus coordinates shivering thermogenesis. Heat loss usually occurs by four mechanisms: About 55% to 65% of heat is lost by radiation, 25% to 30% by evaporation from the skin and respiratory tract, and 10% to 15% by conduction and convection. The amount of heat lost via conduction is markedly increased in cold-water immersion (by about 32-fold). Each organ system is affected uniquely by hypothermia.

Skin

Cutaneous blood flow is regulated by the individual's thermoregulatory needs, modulated by neural control through the arteriovenous anastomoses located in the extremities. Sympathetic tone is increased, which leads to arteriovenous constriction, which is maximum at 59°F (15°C). Cold-induced dermal vasodilation can occur at 50°F (10°C). Cold-induced dermal vasodilation can occur at 50°F (10°C) but can be abolished when hypothermia occurs.

Cardiovascular System

One of the initial heat-conserving mechanisms is peripheral vasoconstriction to decrease blood flow to the skin. There are also initial increases in heart rate and blood pressure caused by a catecholamine surge. At core temperatures below 82.4°F (28°C), bradycardia can result from a decrease in spontaneous depolarization of the pacemaker cell firing. Cold water (<59°F or 15°C) immersion can result in cardiac arrest within 30 minutes. The myocardium also becomes irritable, predisposing it to bradyarrhythmia and hypotension. Cardiac output decreases to approximately 45% at a core temperature of 77°F (25°C), and cardiac arrest can occur in a young, healthy individual at a core temperature of 86°F (30°C).

Atrial arrhythmias can occur with a slow ventricular response, and they can precede ventricular arrhythmias and asystole at core temperatures below 77°F (25°C). Moderate hypothermia (82.4°F or 28°C) does not significantly alter ventricular conduction but can result in prolongation of repolarization, leading to arrhythmia. The characteristic Osborn or J waves (a hump seen at the QRS-ST junction) may be seen on an electrocardiogram at core temperatures below 89.6°F (32°C). The development of the Osborn wave appears to be related to lower blood pH, low serum bicarbonate, and higher serum creatinine levels. Orthostasis also commonly occurs. Risk factors for development of cardiac arrest include core temperature less than 82.4°F (28°C), ventricular arrhythmia development, and systolic blood pressure less than 90 mm Hg.

Renal System

Renal blood flow is affected by peripheral vasoconstriction, causing the glomerular filtration rate to fall and contributing to metabolic acidosis. Antidiuretic hormone activity is usually inhibited. This can result in intravascular volume depletion, subsequent vasodilation, increased renal blood flow, and, ultimately, acute renal failure. Urinary output can increase threefold, and this may be accentuated with concomitant ethanol use.

Respiratory System
At core temperatures below 82.4°F (28°C), minute ventilation, tidal volume, respiratory rate, and thoracic elasticity all are reduced; bronchorrhea can occur with a loss of cough and gag reflexes, leading to an increased risk for aspiration. Carbon dioxide production drops by one-half for every 14°F (8°C) drop in temperature, and oxygen consumption is reduced by 75% at 72°F (22°C). Apnea can then result.

Central Nervous System
Cerebral metabolism and brain oxygen requirements are depressed 6% to 7% per 1°C decrease in core temperature. Cerebrovascular autoregulation remains intact until below 77°F (25°C), which helps maintain cortical blood flow. Electroencephalographic activity is clearly not prognostic, but it is abnormal below 92°F (33°C); burst suppression can occur at 71.6°F (22°C), and it silences at around 66.2°F to 68°F (19°C to 20°C). Most patients are unconscious at a core temperature of 82.4°F to 86°F (28°C to 30°C).

Coagulation
Because of depression of enzymatic activity of the activated clotting factors, clotting time (particularly partial thromboplastin time) is prolonged. At 84°F (29°C), a 50% increase of partial thromboplastin time can be expected. Thrombocytopenia also commonly occurs as a result of bone marrow suppression along with splenic and hepatic platelet sequestration, which can be exacerbated by cryoglobulinemia.

Clinical Presentation
Accidental hypothermia is classified as mild at body temperatures of 90°F to 95°F (32.2°C to 35°C), moderate at body temperatures of 82.4°F to 90°F (28°C to 32.2°C), or severe at body temperatures less than 82.4°F (28°C).

In general, a patient's symptoms depend on the severity of the temperature drop. Patients with mild hypothermia can develop vigorous shivering and cold diuresis. Shivering (which is not consistently encountered) is usually not seen with core temperatures under 86°F (30°C). Those with moderate hypothermia can have a paradoxical decrease in shivering, slurred speech, hyporeflexia, and confusion. They are also at risk for intravascular thrombosis. Splanchnic vasoconstriction, gastric erosions, hepatic necrosis, and pancreatitis can occur. Prominent laboratory abnormalities include leukopenia (from splenic sequestration), thrombocytopenia (during rewarming), hypoglycemia, respiratory or metabolic acidosis, and hyperkalemia. In pregnant patients, fetal bradycardia can occur in response to maternal hypothermia, but long-term sequelae are unknown. It should be noted that hypothermia (core temperature below 96.5°F or 35.8°C) portends a poorer prognosis (a longer period of intubation, longer intensive care unit stay, and approximately double the risk of mortality) in patients with coronavirus disease 2019 (COVID-19) infection.

During severe hypothermia, shivering gives way to rigor, minute ventilation decreases, and heart rate and cardiac output decrease. Cardiac instability can be seen at this stage and can manifest in the form of arrhythmias, heart blocks, and eventually asystole. Neurologically, the patient's mental status declines. The patient might attempt to undress (paradoxical undressing) and might respond only to painful stimuli, have decreased gag reflexes, and eventually become apneic. Generally, at about 68°F (20°C), patients become totally neurologically unresponsive, lose corneal and ocular reflexes, and can have a flat electroencephalogram.

Emergency Department Evaluation
Typically, the source of hypothermia is revealed from the patient's history; however, it is very important to rule out secondary causes of hypothermia, such as sepsis, hypothyroidism, central nervous system lesions, and hypoglycemia, among others. All patients arriving in the emergency department with hypothermia need a complete evaluation to rule out traumatic injuries and drug or toxin ingestion or overdose.

As in all resuscitation, attention should be paid to the ABCs (airway, breathing, and circulation). The mean decrease of vital signs associated with a 1°C drop in core temperature in moderate to severe hypothermia is estimated to be 0.5 breaths per minute (respiratory rate), 2.5 beats per minute (heart rate), 4.36 mm Hg (systolic blood pressure), and 0.88 on the Glasgow Coma Scale. Successful neurologic recovery has been documented following 5 hours of cardiopulmonary resuscitation (CPR) in the setting of profound accidental hypothermia (62.4°F or 16.9°C). Ideally, in patients in cardiac arrest, CPR should be maintained throughout the prehospital period. In a patient with a core temperature of less than 28°C, evidence supports alternating 5 minutes of CPR with less than or equal to 5 minutes without CPR, if feasible. With a core temperature less than 20°C, data support alternating 5 minutes of CPR with less than or equal to 10 minutes without CPR. Respiratory failure should be treated with endotracheal intubation and mechanical ventilation. Hypotension can be treated initially with warmed fluids. Placing the patient in a warm environment, removing all cold and wet clothes, and remembering to cover the patient after exposure should help prevent further heat loss.

The temperature should be confirmed by checking a core temperature (e.g., rectal, bladder, or esophageal) using a thermometer capable of recording very low temperatures. Patients should be placed on a cardiac monitor, and an electrocardiogram should be obtained. Laboratory testing is especially useful in the post resuscitative period when complications begin. Laboratory tests should include a complete blood count, a chemistry panel with liver function tests, creatine phosphokinase to evaluate for rhabdomyolysis, a coagulation profile, blood type and screen, arterial blood gas, and drug screen. A Foley catheter should be placed to assess urinary output.

Rewarming Strategies
There are several methods of rewarming. The method of choice usually depends on the severity of hypothermia. During rewarming, the patient should be placed on a cardiac monitor with frequent measurements of blood pressure and temperature (via a rectal probe) for easy detection of complications of rewarming, such as rewarming-related hypotension, arrhythmias, and core temperature after-drop. It should be noted that the human body is capable of raising the body temperature through heat generation by approximately 1°C per hour.

Passive External Warming
Passive external warming is ideal for patients with mild hypothermia (greater than 93°F or 34°C) who are otherwise healthy. It uses the patient's endogenous heat production for rewarming, and it involves simple, logical passive maneuvers that minimize heat dissipation. All wet clothing should be removed when using this method, and the patient should be covered with insulating materials. Patients who are warmed easily using this method can be safely discharged.

Active External Rewarming
Active external rewarming should be considered for patients with core temperatures between 86°F and 92°F (30°C to 34°C). It involves exposing the patient's skin to exogenous heat sources. Radiant heat, thermal mattresses, electric heating blankets, and forced-air heating blankets are some available techniques. Heat applied externally is most effective if concentrated on the axillae, chest, and back, which exhibits the greatest potential for conductive heat transfer. Additionally, heat can be applied to the neck region to prevent heat loss. Extremity placement of heat should be avoided. Also, localized pressure to skin that is cold should be avoided. Chemical heat packs do not provide sufficient heat transfer to increase core temperature and should not be used. The rate of temperature rise is approximately 2.7°F to 7.2°F (1.5°C to 4°C) per hour.

This method has several disadvantages. First, burn injuries can occur to the vasoconstricted skin. Second, any sort of immersion can hinder monitoring and other resuscitative activities. Finally, and most important, active external rewarming produces a phenomenon called *core temperature after-drop*. This refers to a drop in core temperature resulting from sudden peripheral vasodilation. This causes cold, acidic blood to return to the core. Hypotension and potentially fatal dysrhythmias can result. Focusing on rewarming the trunk only (rather than the trunk and extremities) can prevent these temperature gradients. In general, active external rewarming is used in conjunction with active core rewarming.

Active Core Rewarming

Active core rewarming involves techniques to deliver direct heat internally. It should be used in patients with moderate to severe hypothermia (less than 86°F or 30°C). The simplest method entails administration of heated, humidified oxygen at 107.6°F to 114.8°F (42°C to 46°C), which can be used as adjunctive therapy, and intravenous saline solution warmed to 109.4°F (43°C). Saline should be administered via a central line at 150 to 200 mL/h. Gastric, bladder, and colonic irrigations have been used, but their relatively small surface areas usually limit their effect. Urinary bladder or gastric lavage (which is rarely used because of aspiration potential and electrolyte shifts) can rewarm at an hourly rate of 0.9°F to 1.8°F (0.5°C to 1°C).

Another method of active core rewarming is pleural irrigation using two large-bore (36°F or greater) thoracostomy tubes. One tube is placed at the midclavicular line and is connected to saline at 107.6°F (42°C). The other tube is placed at the posterior axillary line and connected to a chest tube drainage kit.

A more aggressive method of active core rewarming is via peritoneal lavage and dialysis, especially as adjunctive therapy. This can be accomplished using a standard diagnostic peritoneal lavage kit and introducing an 8-F catheter into the peritoneum using the Seldinger technique. This method affords the added advantage of allowing the serum potassium level and fluid status to be adjusted. Use of continuous or intermittent renal replacement therapy with local anticoagulation using citrate can achieve rewarming rates of about 2°C per hour.

The most efficient and physiologic active core rewarming method is via extracorporeal warming or heated cardiopulmonary bypass. This is the method of choice for the most severe cases, patients with severe rhabdomyolysis, and patients who require CPR. Survival rates with no chronic neurologic sequelae as high as 75% have been documented. Excellent recovery has been documented from a nasopharyngeal temperature of 13.8°C (and a serum potassium of 11.3 mmol/L) caused by drowning with a submersion time of at least 83 minutes in icy seawater with slow rewarming with extracorporeal membrane oxygenation. Extracorporeal life support can be an effective rewarming tool in patients with prolonged cardiac arrest from accidental hypothermia, particularly in the absence of asphyxia, trauma, or severe hyperkalemia. Veno-arterial extracorporeal membrane oxygenation is increasingly used for its ability to gradually increase core body temperature while providing respiratory and hemodynamic support. Rewarming rates up to 6°C per hour can be achieved via this modality. It should be considered especially in pediatric patients or in individuals requiring prolonged support.

Most arrhythmias are corrected by rewarming. Atrial dysrhythmias often occur during rewarming and generally resolve without treatment. Atropine is typically ineffective for cold-associated bradydysrhythmias. Ventricular tachycardia and fibrillation require electrocardioversion; automated external defibrillator devices can be used as directed for pulseless ventricular tachycardia or ventricular fibrillation. Dopamine, epinephrine (1 mg IV),[1] and vasopressin (Pitressin; 40 units IV)[1] may be effective vasopressors for core temperatures above 30°C (86°F). External pacing may be ineffective. Empiric antibiotics may be given. However, the empiric use of levothyroxine (Synthroid)[1] and corticosteroids may be hazardous. Phenytoin (Dilantin)[1] might have cardiac-depressant qualities in the moderately hypothermic patient. Box 2

---

[1] Not FDA approved for this indication.

- Atropine
- Digoxin
- Fentanyl (Sublimaze, Duragesic)
- Gentamicin (Garamycin)
- Lidocaine (Xylocaine)
- Phenobarbital
- Procaine
- Propranolol (Inderal)
- Sulfanilamide (AVC cream)
- Suxamethonium (succinylcholine, Anectine)
- d-Tubocurarine
- Brain natriuretic peptide

demonstrates drugs with possible decreased metabolism or clearance with resultant increase in toxicity in hypothermia.

For hypothermia caused by myxedema coma, levothyroxine (Synthroid) should be administered intravenously (at a dose of 250 to 500 µg over 30 to 60 seconds). Daily intravenous injections of 100 µg may be required for up to 7 days. Hydrocortisone (Solu-Cortef)[1] (200 to 400 mg IV daily) administration should also be considered. Other active core rewarming techniques are usually not required. Treatment of episodic, spontaneous hyperhidrosis hyperthermia or Shapiro syndrome often responds to clonidine (Catapres)[1] (up to 0.6 mg daily) through its actions on hypothalamic thermoregulation.

Indicators of grave prognosis include development of profound hyperkalemia (serum potassium greater than 10 mEq/L); elevated serum creatinine, serum sodium, or serum lactate concentration; lower prothrombin time; underlying medical conditions; intravascular thrombosis (fibrinogen less than 59 mg/dL); pH less than 6.5; and core temperature less than 82.4°F (28°C). Elevated serum potassium in a hypothermic patient may indicate that hypoxia preceded the onset of hypothermia. Submersion in cold water for over ten minutes is associated with a poor prognosis; if the water is less than 43°F (6°C), survival is unlikely to occur if submerged for over 90 minutes.

Peripheral Cold Injuries

Peripheral cold injuries span a spectrum ranging from minimal to severe tissue damage. Freezing and nonfreezing syndromes can cause these injuries. About 500 patients with frostbite are hospitalized yearly in the United States, with about an 80% male demographic and lower-extremity predominance. The average length of stay in critical care units and total hospital stay is approximately 7 and 10 days, respectively. Frostnip and frostbite are caused by exposure to freezing temperatures. *Frostnip* refers to the numbness and blue-white discoloration of the face and extremities that occur during exposure to freezing temperatures. It is a precursor to frostbite. It is characterized by reversible skin changes, including blanching and numbness with no permanent tissue damage, unlike frostbite. Nonfreezing injuries depend on whether the ambient environment during exposure was wet (trench or immersion foot) or dry (pernio or chilblain).

Pathophysiology

During exposure to cold temperatures, the core body temperature is preserved to the detriment of the extremities. Frostbite occurs in four stages: prefreeze, freeze-thaw, vascular stasis, and late ischemic stages. The prefreeze phase occurs when the temperature of the extremities falls below 50°F (10°C) and cutaneous sensation is lost. Vasoconstriction also occurs along with leakage of intracellular fluid into the interstitium.

The freeze-thaw phase begins at the freezing point of water (32°F or 0°C) with the formation of ice crystals extracellularly. This further enhances the exit of water from the intracellular space under osmotic forces, resulting in cell shrinkage and, ultimately, damage. During the vascular stasis phase, plasma leakage and formation of ice crystals continue. Arachidonic acid breakdown products are then released from underlying damaged tissue. Both prostaglandin $F_2\alpha$ and thromboxane A_2 produce platelet aggregation, leukocyte immobilization, and vasoconstriction.

Endothelial cells are sensitive to cold injury, and the microvasculature becomes distorted and clogged, leading to tissue ischemia. The late ischemic phase is characterized by ischemia, thrombosis, continued shunting, gangrene, autonomic dysfunction, and denaturation of tissue proteins. The tissue can eventually mummify and demarcate more than 60 to 90 days later.

Clinical Presentation of Local Extremity Issues

Frostnip and Frostbite
The skin is particularly sensitive to cold temperatures under 31°F (−0.55°C); dermal blood flow is increased only 10-fold as opposed to over 35-fold when exposed to heat. With cold water exposures under 59°F (15°C), alternating vasoconstriction and vasodilation in the extremities can occur (termed as the Hunting response or Lewis reaction); finger vasculature may remain at a continuous state of vasoconstriction. The face and ears are the most common sites prone to cold injury, followed by the hands and feet. Patients with frostnip usually have blanching and numbness of their fingertips. The skin has a firm or waxy texture. Often the patient is unaware of these changes. Frostnip is usually reversible. Frostbite has been classified as *superficial*, affecting the skin and subcutaneous tissue, or *deep*, affecting the bones, joints, and tendons. After rewarming an area with superficial frostbite, a clear blister may form; however, after rewarming an area with deep frostbite, a hemorrhagic blister may form. This classification, however, has no therapeutic or prognostic value given that frostbites can initially appear benign. Many weeks can pass before the demarcation between viable and nonviable tissue becomes apparent. Facial frostbite, with skin blistering, can also occur following halogenated (especially fluorinated) hydrocarbon inhalation abuse. This can appear initially as angioneurotic edema if it involves the oral mucosa membranes. Acute compartment syndrome of the foot and ankle, associated with gangrenous toe changes, has been described.

Although no prognostic factors can be entirely predictive, favorable factors include retained sensation, normal skin color, and clear rather than cloudy fluid in the blisters, if present. Poor prognostic features include nonblanching cyanosis, firm skin, and dark, fluid-filled blisters. Patients can present with pain, numbness, and a clumsy "chunk of wood" sensation in the affected extremity. The pain is initially described as a dull ache and evolves to become a throbbing sensation in about 48 to 72 hours.

Chilblain
Chilblain, also referred to as *perniosis,* results from repetitive exposure to cold, dry air. It manifests as painful erythematous nodules or cyanotic lesions often referred to as *cold sores.* These lesions usually develop on exposed surfaces after a delay of 12 to 14 hours and are characterized by pruritus and burning paresthesias. Young women, especially those with Raynaud phenomenon and/or a low body mass index, are at risk.

Chilblains are located on acral skin associated with cold exposure. They are usually located on the dorsum of the fingers, toes, and thighs, where blisters or ulcerations can develop in very severe cases. Perivascular lymphocytic infiltration with vacuolation of the basal layer is often seen on histologic analysis, especially when it is associated with an autoimmune disease (particularly lupus erythematosus). Chilblain (usually lasting for 1 to 2 weeks and quite pruritic in nature) has also been associated with COVID-19 infections and post COVID-19 vaccination exposure. Susceptibility to chilblains increases when the ambient temperature is less than 10°C and relative humidity is 60%.

Trench Foot and Immersion Foot
Trench foot occurs as a result of prolonged exposure (about 10 to 15 hours) to a damp, cold, nonfreezing environment (with temperature as high as 15°C or 59°F). It has been classically described among soldiers in World War I, many of whom were confined to cold and damp trenches for prolonged periods. Symptoms include numbness and painful paresthesias that can progress to a throbbing and burning sensation. Initial evaluation reveals a cold, pale extremity, with or without vesicles or bullae. Inflammatory serum markers, such as erythrocyte sedimentation rate or C-reactive protein, may be elevated.

Immersion foot may be considered the sailor's counterpart to trench foot. It occurs after prolonged immersion in cold water at temperatures above freezing. Patients usually present with painless, wrinkled, white feet along with profound sensory loss; arterial thrombosis may cause extremity gangrene.

Treatment
Treatment of frostbite should begin with removing all wet or frozen clothing. For patients with moderate or severe hypothermia, initial resuscitative efforts should be geared toward raising their core temperature. The patient should be moved to a warm environment, and all wet clothing should be removed. The frozen extremity should initially be elevated and rewarmed by immersion in circulation water at 98.6°F to 102.2°F (37°C to 39°C) for about 15 to 30 minutes. Given the risk of thermal injury, the frozen parts should not be exposed to direct or dry heat (such as hair dryers, heating pads, or heat lamps). Do not rub or massage the affected area. The process should be continued until the extremity appears warm and well perfused. Following rewarming, the extremity should be air-dried and remain elevated. Because of the pain associated with reperfusion, there may be the temptation to abruptly abort the rewarming process. This can, however, promote further tissue damage.

Oral or intravenous fluid should be administered to prevent dehydration and vascular stasis. Because the pain is usually prominent at night, amitriptyline (Elavil)[1] at an initial dosage of 10 to 25 mg and a maximum of 100 mg may be helpful. Gabapentin (Neurontin)[1] also may be an alternative therapy. Parenteral analgesic medications—nonsteroidal antiinflammatory drugs (NSAIDs) and opioids—may be administered as needed to make the process more tolerable. Ibuprofen at a dose of 12 mg/kg twice daily (400 mg in adults twice daily, which can be increased to a maximum of 2400 mg daily) may be helpful for its analgesic and antiinflammatory effects.

Almost all authors agree that hemorrhagic blisters should not be débrided because of the risk of secondary desiccation of deep dermal layers, extending the injury. Débriding broken vesicles or bullae is also widely accepted; however, clear, intact vesicles may be broken and débrided or left intact. Topical aloe vera ointment (Dermaide Aloe)[7] or topical antibiotic ointments may be applied. Cold extremity wounds are not considered tetanus prone.

The injured tissue should be loosely covered with sterile, dry, bulky, nonadherent dressing. If possible, elevate the extremity above the cardiac level to decrease dependent edema. Hands and feet may be splinted and elevated to reduce edema. Because the damaged tissue is tetanus prone, patients whose tetanus status has not been updated may require a tetanus booster (Td).

Adjunctive agents that have been used for their antithrombotic and vasodilative properties with varying success include heparin,[1] steroids,[1] NSAIDs,[1] dimethylsulfoxide (Rimso-50)[1] nonionic detergents[1] dipyridamole (Persantine),[1] calcium channel blockers,[1] thrombolytics,[1] pentoxifylline (Trental)[1] and phenoxybenzamine (Dibenzyline).[1] Iloprost (Ventavis)[1] is a prostacyclin analog that is a potent vasodilator that can inhibit platelet aggregation. It may also have fibrinolytic activity. The intravenous dosing is 2 ng/kg/min, 6 hours/day, for 5 days. Although not yet approved by the U.S. Food and Drug Administration (FDA), it has been suggested for severe frostbite within 72 hours of injury. Hyperbaric oxygen with thrombolytic therapy has been used to treat severe frostbite of the hand. Negative pressure wound therapy, following blister excision, has been demonstrated to be beneficial

---

[1] Not FDA approved for this indication.
[7] Available as dietary supplement.

in treating infant frostbite hand injures. Following rewarming, intravenous tissue plasminogen activator (Activase)[1] Following rewarming, intravenous tissue plasminogen activator (Activase)[1] within 48 hours of injury with angiographic evidence of thrombosis with an initial 3-mg bolus followed by a 6- to 12-hour infusion of 1 mg/mL (10 mL/hour) heparin[1] at a dose of 500 units/hour administered concurrently has been utilized effectively (especially for frostbitten hands with no flow distal to the proximal phalanx) with systemic anticoagulation and/or antiplatelet therapy to follow. with an initial 3-mg bolus followed by a 6- to 12-hour infusion of 1 mg/mL (10 mL/hour) heparin[1] at a dose of 500 units per hour administered concurrently has been utilized effectively (especially for frostbitten hands with no flow distal to the proximal phalanx) with systemic anticoagulation and/or antiplatelet therapy to follow. Intraarterial catheter-directed thrombolytic therapy with the concomitant use of angiography has also been used with concurrent intravenous heparin therapy (titrated to a goal of a partial thromboplastin time of 40 to 60 seconds) along with a daily 81 mg oral dose of aspirin.[1] Surgical consultation is appropriate for guiding long-term management because some patients might need débridement of infections or skin grafts for nonhealing wounds. A sympathetic nerve block (sympathectomy) can relieve painful and refractory vasospasms.

A familial association of chilblain (associated with contractual arachnodactyly) has been described in Italy. Chilblain (pernio) may be treated with nifedipine[1] at an oral dose of 20 mg three times daily. Topical 5% minoxidil solution/gel (Rogaine)[1] has been used with minimal success. Oral prednisolone (Millipred),[1] 0.5 mg/kg in two divided doses over 2 weeks, and topical glucocorticoids have been used to treat perniosis; pentoxyfylline[1] (1200 mg/day in three divided doses for 2 weeks) has also been demonstrated to be effective. Acupuncture treatment (once weekly for 12 weeks) has been used to decrease cold sensitivity caused by second-degree frostbite in the fingertips.

Sequelae

Late sequelae of frostbite include cold hypersensitivity, arthritis, numbness, chronic pain, ulceration, decreased sensation, and functional loss of the extremity. This is a result of early neuronal damage and abnormal sympathetic tone. Patients with chronic symptoms should be advised to avoid nicotine and cold exposure while using NSAIDs. Tissue demarcation can occur 60 to 90 days after initial injury. Amputation decisions should be deferred unless there is supervening sepsis or gangrene. The ultimate tissue salvage after a spontaneous slough usually far exceeds the most optimistic initial estimates. A medical simulation flow diagram is presented in Figure 1.

[1] Not FDA approved for this indication.

[1] Not FDA approved for this indication.

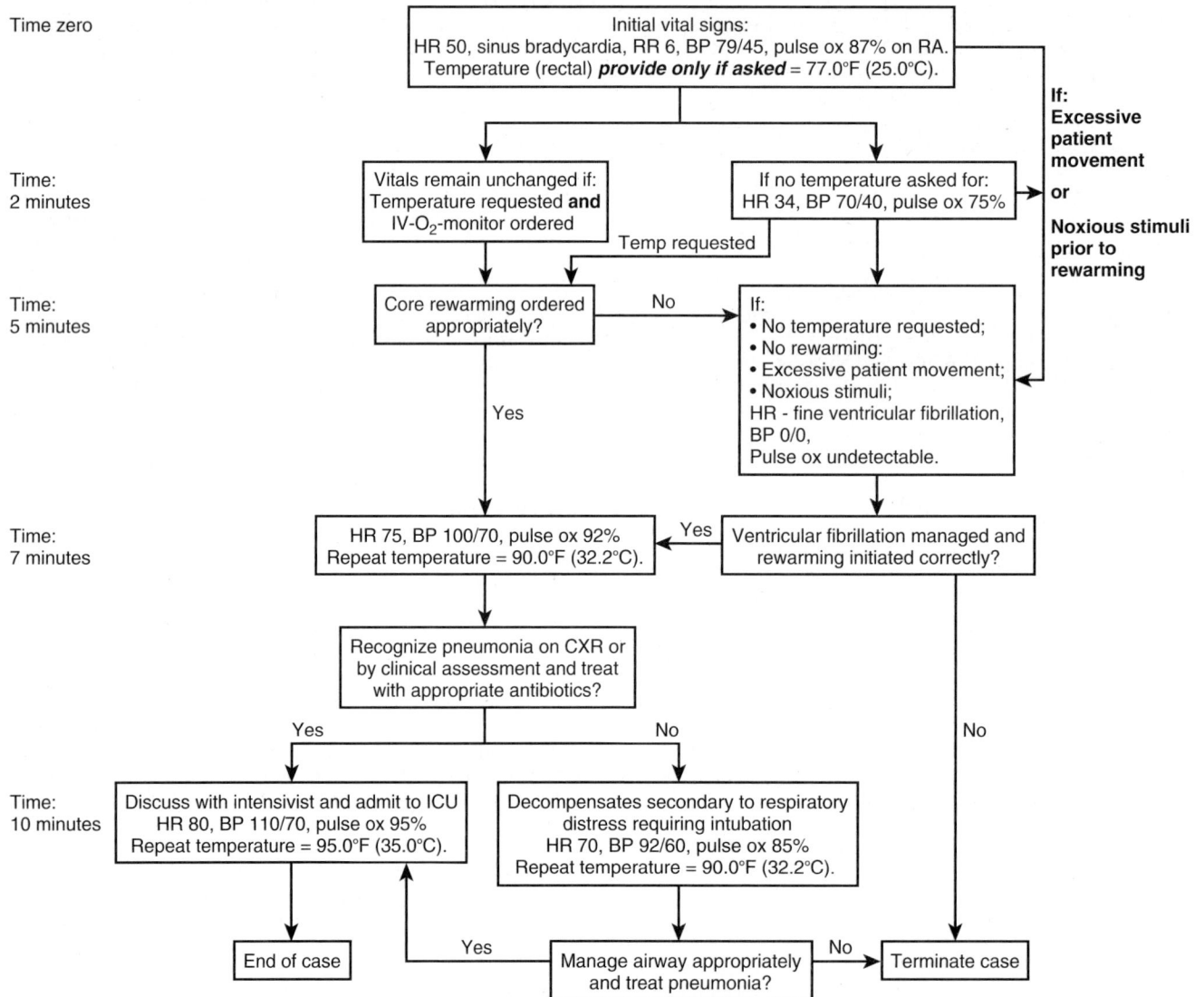

Figure 1 Hypothermia simulation flow diagram.

References

McIntosh SE, Freer L, Grissom CK, et al: Wilderness Medical Society Clinical practice guidelines for the Prevention and treatment of frostbite: 2024 update, *Wilderness Environ Med* 35(2):183–197, 2024.

Poole A, Ahmed Y, Davidson M: The occasional frostbite, *Can J Rural Med* 29(1):30–36, 2024.

QuickStats: death rates attributed to excessive cold or hypothermia, by urbanization level and sex–National Vital Statistics System, 2018-2020, *MMWR Morb Mortal Wkly Rep* 71:282, 2022.

Regli IB, Oberhammer R, Zafren K, et al: Frostbite treatment: a systematic review with meta-analyses, *Scand J Trauma Resusc Emerg Med* 31(1):96, 2023.

Zafren K, Hollis S, Weiss EA, et al: Prevention and treatment of nonfreezing cold injuries and warm water immersion tissue injuries: supplement to Wilderness Medical Society clinical practice guidelines for the prevention and treatment of frostbite. Wilderness Environ Med 34(2):172-181.

HEAT ILLNESS

Method of
Paul Cleland, MD

CURRENT DIAGNOSIS

- Heat illness is a spectrum of disorders caused by environmental exposure to heat and is usually seen among athletes in hot and humid environments.
- Children, older adults, and poorly acclimatized individuals are at increased risk for developing exertional heat illness (EHI).
- Exercise-associated cramps are intense, prolonged, painful muscle spasms that occur during physical activity.
- Heat exhaustion is an elevation in core body temperature (<104°F) without central nervous system (CNS) dysfunction resulting in a collapse or difficulty continuing activity.
- Heat stroke is a life-threatening illness characterized by elevation in core body temperature (≥104°F) with CNS dysfunction (altered consciousness, seizure, coma) and usually end-organ damage.

CURRENT THERAPY

- Acclimatization is key for prevention of EHI.
- Heat illness is most effectively managed by immediate recognition of the signs and symptoms and proper diagnosis.
- Core body temperature measurement *must* be done with a rectal thermometer
- Exercise-associated collapse
  - Continue walking after race to prevent development
  - Position the patient in the supine or Trendelenburg position, and start fluid administration
- Heat exhaustion
  - Provide rapid cooling with ice bags to areas adjacent to large vasculature (groin, neck, axilla).
  - Administer oral or intravenous (IV) fluid to correct for hydration deficit.
- Heat stroke
- Ensure the ability to maintain adequate circulation, airway, and breathing.
  - Ice-water immersion is the most effective way to provide rapid cooling.
  - The goal of cooling is to reduce and maintain a temperature below 101°F (38.3°C).
  - Transport to the hospital may be required if the patient's temperature is not reduced effectively or the patient does not return to normal mental status after 30 minutes of medical treatment.

Heat illness is a continuum of disease that can affect a wide array of individuals including athletes, firefighters, construction workers, soldiers, and others. Exertional heat illness (EHI) is a leading cause of death among young athletes and may be on the rise with possible climate change and increasing popularity of mass events such as marathons. Knowledge of the risk factors presented by the patient and the environment can provide clinicians with a better understanding toward prevention of heat illness. Early recognition and treatment of EHI can lead to significant reduction in the morbidity and mortality associated with this disease.

In the United States, most cases of EHI occur in summer months. Elevations in the ambient temperature and humidity as well as athletic deconditioning are predominant contributing factors. There is an increasing incidence of heat illness associated with decreased heat acclimation and an increase in the wet-bulb globe temperature (WBGT) index. The WBGT index is a tool used to assess the overall environmental conditions and can accurately predict the development of EHI in a particular setting to allow for modification of work or athletic events. High school and collegiate athletic programs that have protocols in place to stop practice, limit the duration of practice, or reduce the frequency of practice in high-heat situations have shown a decreased incidence of heat illness compared with those that do not.

It is important to understand the pathophysiology of heat regulation within the body to gain an accurate picture of heat illness. The human body has a great capacity to withstand drastic reductions in temperature to tolerate cold. However, only mild increases in core body temperature can result in severe consequences. Heat is generated by normal metabolic processes that occur continuously in our bodies and is also absorbed from the environment. Exercise generates additional heat from the skeletal muscles. When the hypothalamus detects a core body temperature increase, it sends signals to induce sweating and cutaneous vasodilation. Blood is then shunted to the skin and exercising skeletal muscle. Under normal conditions, the body is able to dissipate heat through evaporation, radiation, convection, and conduction. Evaporation is the primary means of heat dissipation and occurs as water is converted from its liquid form to its vapor form, but it becomes ineffective above a relative humidity of 75%. Radiation, convection, and conduction are also methods to dissipate heat but are decreasingly effective as the ambient temperature approaches the skin's temperature. When physiologic cooling mechanisms fail, heat is continually produced, and the core body temperature increases. As the temperature increases, cell damage occurs, and a systemic inflammatory response ensues, releasing cytokines throughout the body. Blood is shunted to the peripheral circulation, leading to organ hypoperfusion and ischemia. Organ failure and disseminated intravascular coagulation (DIC) eventually develop and result in death.

The injury caused by heat illness can be mitigated by acclimatization of the patient and is the most important factor to thrive in hot and humid conditions. Acclimatization occurs as the body is repeatedly exposed to certain levels of stress and then makes compensatory changes to allow for better performance the next time the body is under duress. This process occurs over 1 to 2 weeks of exposure to new conditions and appears to be lost with reexposure to the previous climate for about the same period. Several key changes occur as the body is exposed to heat, including production of heat shock proteins that give cells the ability to resist heat stress, decreased sweat temperature threshold, increased sweat production, decreased salt concentration in sweat, and increased skin blood flow. These factors all serve to aid the athlete under high-risk heat conditions to improve performance and alleviate potential heat illness. It is recommended that the athlete spend at least 2 weeks acclimatizing to the environment mimicking both temperature and humidity for maximal outcome. When athletes return to a more temperate environment after training, such as an air-conditioned room, they do not see the same benefit as they would with 24-hour exposure to the conditions. If possible, air-conditioning should be restricted to nighttime only when the athlete is resting.

Risk Factors

Although each person has unique genetic traits that determine how his or her body reacts to specific conditions, there are known

TABLE 1	Substances That May Increase the Risk of Heat Illness

- Amphetamines
- Anticholinergic agents
- Antiepileptic agents
- Antihistamines
- Benzodiazepines
- Beta blockers
- Calcium channel blockers
- Cocaine
- Decongestants
- Diuretics
- Ergogenic stimulants
- Ethanol
- Laxatives
- Lithium
- Phenothiazines
- Tricyclic antidepressants

Data from Bouchama A, Knochel JP. Heat stroke, *N Engl J Med* 346(25):1978–1988, 2002; Wexler RK. Evaluation and treatment of heat-related illnesses, *Am Family Physician* 65(11):2307–2314, 2002.

congenital and acquired risk factors that may preclude an individual toward development of EHI. Exposure to a hot and humid environment may be the most obvious risk factor as ambient heat is transferred to the body and elevated humidity impairs the body's ability to dissipate heat. Poor conditioning, lack of acclimatization, obesity, and dehydration have been shown to increase the incidence of EHI. The use of prescription medications, supplements, and recreational drugs (Table 1) may cause disturbances in the capacity to dissipate or produce heat. Creatine supplementation does not appear to impair heat dissipation or cause a negative impact on hydration.

Children are at increased risk of developing heat illness for several physiologic reasons. A larger surface area–to–mass ratio allows for more heat absorption from the environment. Children also produce more heat compared with their adult counterparts because of higher basal metabolic rates. Fluid is conserved more efficiently in children than in adults, and consequently they have lower sweat rates as they depend more on non-evaporative forms of heat transfer for cooling. Children can make the same physiologic changes of acclimatization that adults can, though it appears to occur at a slower rate.

Environmental characteristics such as heat and humidity may play the largest role in development of heat illness. As mentioned earlier, the WBGT is a tool used to assess the overall environmental conditions and can accurately predict the development of EHI in a particular setting to allow for modification of work or athletic events. The WBGT is a measurement of temperature, relative humidity, and radiant heat from the sun and ground and is recommended over use of the heat index. A dangerous clinical situation is likely to develop when activities are performed with an elevated WBGT. It is recommended that endurance events be adjusted when the WBGT exceeds 82°F (28°C) and that only events that allow adequate rest and recovery are permitted to continue.

Heat Edema

Heat edema is caused by vasodilation of blood vessels resulting in swelling that is typically observed in the hands and feet. The core body temperature of the body is not elevated. Treatment begins with removal from the hot environment, elevation of the extremities, and possible use of compression with stockings or wrapping. Diuretics are not recommended.

Heat Cramps

Also known as *exercise-associated cramps,* heat cramps present as intense pain, spasm, and prolonged muscle contraction as athletes undergo high-intensity activity. Although they are termed *heat cramps,* they are known to occur in cool settings as well, such as swimming and winter sports. The pathophysiology has not been entirely agreed upon but seems to stem from a neurogenic response to muscle fatigue in conjunction with fluid and electrolyte loss. To make the diagnosis, no signs of other illness may be present such as rhabdomyolysis, sickle cell disease or trait, or heat stroke, and it is important to take a thorough medical history to avoid pitfalls in the diagnosis.

Management consists of stretching and massaging the affected muscle and oral replacement of fluid and electrolytes. Intravenous (IV) fluids and benzodiazepines may be used for refractory cases. One study showed that ingestion of pickle juice at 1 mL/kg may cause a faster recovery from electrically induced muscle cramps when compared with deionized water. This would confirm the theory of a neurogenic-mediated process as the recovery occurred before the contents of the pickle juice reached the sites of action in the cramping skeletal muscle, with discontinuation of cramping seen at an average of 85 seconds compared with 134 seconds for deionized water.

Exercise-Associated Collapse

Also termed *exercise-associated postural hypotension,* exercise-associated collapse (EAC) is an inability of the athlete to maintain a standing posture as a result of hypotension that develops commonly *after* an endurance event. Blood in circulation pools in the lower extremities as the athlete finishes the event and discontinues exercising. The skeletal muscles in the lower extremities normally exert a pressure on the corresponding vasculature, but as exercise ceases, the blood pools, causing an unexpected drop in cranial blood pressure, triggering collapse. Heat may play an indirect role in the development of EAC, but the terms *heat syncope* and *heat collapse* are incorrect because there is no elevation in the athlete's core body temperature. Athletes may develop dizziness, nausea, and vomiting as a result of the rapid decrease in blood pressure.

Athletes should be encouraged to continue activity such as walking or light activity at the end of events (rather than abrupt cessation or standing in place) to continue normal blood flow to avoid a sudden collapse, risking injury. If an athlete does collapse, treatment should begin with placing the patient in the supine or Trendelenburg position and keeping the legs and pelvis elevated. Administration of oral fluids containing glucose and electrolytes is helpful. IV fluid administration should be reserved for patients with hypotension (<110 systolic blood pressure) or an elevated pulse (>100 beats/min) who do not respond to oral fluid intake. Generally these athletes will respond favorably within 10 to 30 minutes and should be allowed to leave under their own power.

Heat Exhaustion

Heat exhaustion occurs when the cardiovascular system is unable to provide adequate output to the body to continue to perform activity as a result of fatigue produced by exercise and environmental heat stress. This is clinically manifested most often by collapse or difficulty continuing activity that occurs *before* the event has finished. Core body temperature (rectal) is commonly elevated at 98.6°F to 104°F (37°C to 40°C). It may be accompanied by nausea, vomiting, diarrhea, headache, muscle cramping, tachycardia, hypotension, weakness, dehydration, and electrolyte depletion. Dehydration can be difficult to judge clinically as the only reliable assessment of dehydration is measurement of water loss that occurs through pre-weight and post-weight measurements. A clear distinction between heat exhaustion and heat stroke is the development of central nervous system (CNS) dysfunction such as an altered level of consciousness, delirium, or seizure. Confusion may be present but should be mild and resolve quickly with treatment measures.

Athletes with heat exhaustion should be removed from the heat environment and placed in a cool, shaded, or air-conditioned environment. Vital signs including a rectal temperature should be measured to ensure that the proper diagnosis is made and to be able to monitor cooling status. Any excess clothing should be removed, and the patient should be placed in the supine or Trendelenburg position with the feet elevated. Cooling may be performed initially with placement of ice bags over the groin, axilla, and neck and water or ice-soaked towels over the head, trunk, and extremities. Immersion in an ice bath, tub of cold water, or simply running cold water from a hose over the athlete may be necessary, but these measures tend to be more for comfort as heat exhaustion is not life threatening. Oral administration of an electrolyte-containing solution is helpful to restore adequate hydration and assists in returning the cardiac output to normal. IV fluid administration is beneficial for patients who do not respond or are unable to take oral fluids. Patients who do not respond to these measures should be transported to a hospital to monitor for other developing conditions.

Heat Stroke and Heat Injury

Heat stroke is defined as an elevated core body temperature above 104°F (40°C) with associated CNS dysfunction and end-organ damage. The CNS dysfunction can be observed in several ways including confusion, delirium, aggression or irritability, seizures, altered consciousness, and coma. Heat stroke can occur as classic heat stroke (non-exertional) or exertional heat stroke. Classic heat stroke usually afflicts the older adult population in the summer season and can be related to a lack of access to adequate air conditioning. Heat is continually absorbed from the environment and may be poorly dissipated secondary to other medical conditions and medications that preclude cooling. Exertional heat stroke is seen in a younger and more athletic population and does not necessarily occur in hot and humid environments. Other signs and symptoms are similar to those seen in heat exhaustion, but vital sign abnormalities are more likely to be present. The presence or absence of sweating does not make a diagnosis of heat stroke. Examining a collapsed individual can be difficult, and the differential diagnosis can extend beyond heat exhaustion and heat stroke to include cardiac arrhythmia and exercise-associated hyponatremia. It is important to maintain a degree of suspicion for those athletes who present with collapse but do not have an elevated core body temperature.

The term *heat injury* is not currently recognized by the World Health Organization as a diagnosis but was created by U.S. military physicians to further categorize patients suffering from heat illness. Heat injury is diagnosed as an elevation in core body temperature above 104°F (40°C) with associated end-organ damage, but it lacks the CNS dysfunction seen in heat stroke. Organs most commonly affected with heat stroke or heat injury include the liver, kidneys, and skeletal muscle (rhabdomyolysis).

Patients who present with heat stroke should be assessed beginning with basic life support measures. It is important to secure the airway and ensure that adequate circulation and breathing are maintained. An initial set of vital signs including a rectal temperature should be performed and repeated throughout the course of treatment. If a rectal thermometer is not available, avoid using other methods to determine temperature as they are not accurate to measure core body temperature in athletes who have been exercising. If available, rapid assessment of serum electrolytes including sodium and glucose should be performed, especially with longer-endurance events such as marathons. Rapid cooling should commence as soon as possible after the diagnosis is made because the prognosis worsens the longer the core body temperature is elevated. The most effective cooling measure is cold-water immersion (CWI) with a target water temperature of 35°F to 50°F. Expected cooling rates are about 1°F per 3 minutes or 1°C per 5 minutes of immersion. Measurement with a rectal thermistor allows for continuous monitoring; if this is not available, measurement by a rectal thermometer should be done approximately once every 10 minutes. Cooling should continue until the core body temperature reaches 101°F (38.3°C). If no rectal thermometer is available, cooling should continue until the athlete begins to shiver, or about 15 to 20 minutes. Tarp-assisted cooling oscillation (TACO) is an alternative technique to CWI wherein the athlete is placed on a tarp with at least two individuals holding the edges of the tarp while ice and water are added on top of the patient. If other interventions must be performed (intubation, administration of IV medications or fluid) and CWI or TACO are not available, ice bags should be placed at the groin, axilla, and neck, and ice- or water-soaked towels should be placed over the rest of the body, or a hose can be used to dowse the rest of the body. Fluid resuscitation should be performed, but careful attention should be paid to fluid overload as pulmonary edema can develop with rapid administration of IV fluids. These patients are still at risk for organ damage despite a rapid reduction in core body temperature; therefore it is usually necessary to transport them to the hospital, where appropriate monitoring and laboratory evaluation can be performed. Transport to the hospital is always required in patients who do not regain consciousness within 30 minutes of appropriate cooling and medical intervention or if appropriate response to cooling is not achieved.

Return to Play

The prognosis for returning to physical activity after an episode of EHI is dependent on the individual and the severity of the illness incurred. Athletes who develop heat cramps or EAC should be allowed to return to activity as soon as they feel capable. Decisions about returning those who develop heat exhaustion or heat stroke are more complicated. These athletes should avoid physical activity for at least 7 days. All laboratory abnormalities should be corrected, and the athlete should feel physically and psychologically capable of returning. Once these conditions are met, a gradual progression of activity can begin in a cool or temperate environment. Acclimatization occurs over a period of approximately 2 weeks as activity is increased in duration and intensity and the individual is gradually reexposed to heat. Once the athlete is able to perform full-intensity workouts for 2 to 4 weeks in the heat, he or she may return to competition. For patients who fail to acclimatize at 4 weeks or who have had multiple episodes of EHI, an exercise heat tolerance test should be performed.

References

American College of Sports Medicine, Armstrong LE, Casa DJ, et al: American College of Sports Medicine Position Stand. Exertional heat illness during training and competition, *Med Sci Sports Exerc* 39:556–572, 2007.

Asplund CA, O'Connor FG: Challenging return to play decisions: heat stroke, exertional rhabdomyolysis, and exertional collapse associated with sickle cell trait, *Sports Health* 8(2):117–125, 2016.

Bouchama A, Knochel JP: Heat Stroke, *N Engl J Med* 346(25):1978–1988, 2002.

Boeckmann M, Rohn I: Is planned adaptation to heat reducing heat-related mortality and illness? A systematic review, *BMC Public Health* 14:1112, 2014.

Brukner P, Karim K, Noakes T: Exercise in the heat. *Brukner & Khan's Clinical Sports Medicine*, ed 4, Sydney, 2012, McGraw-Hill, pp 1132–1143.

Cooper ER, Ferrara MS, Casa DJ, et al: Exertional heat illness in American Football Players: when is the risk greatest? *J Athl Train* 51(8):593–600, 2016.

Gaudio FG, Grissom CK: Cooling methods in heat stroke, *J Emerg Med* 50(4):607–616, 2016.

Lopez RM, Casa DJ, McDermott BP, et al: Does creatine supplementation hinder exercise heat tolerance or hydration status? A systematic review with meta-analyses, *J Athl Train* 44(2):215–223, 2009.

Maron BJ, Doerer JJ, Haas TS, et al: Sudden deaths in young competitive athletes: analysis of 1866 deaths in the United States, 1980-2006, *Circulation* 119:1085–1092, 2009.

Miller KC, Mack GW, Knight KL, et al: Reflex inhibition of electrically induced muscle cramps in hypohydrated humans, *Med Sci Sports Exerc* 42(5):953–961, 2010.

Wexler RK: Evaluation and treatment of heat-related illnesses, *Am Fam Physician* 65:2307–2314, 2002.

Yeargin SW, Kerr ZY, Casa DJ, et al: Epidemiology of exertional heat illnesses in youth, high school, and college football, *Med Sci Sports Exerc* 48(8):1523–1529, 2016.

Zurawlew MJ, Walsh NP, et al: Post-exercise hot water immersion induces heat acclimation and improves endurance exercise performance in the heat, *Scand J Med Sci Sports* 26(7):745–754, 2016.

HIGH-ALTITUDE ILLNESS

Method of
**Bethany Howlett, MD, MHS; and
Jill Thein-Nissenbaum, DSC**

CURRENT DIAGNOSIS

Acclimatization
- Symptoms include exertional dyspnea, increased respiratory rate, polyuria, peripheral edema, and insomnia.

High-Altitude Headache
- Occurs within 6 to 10 hours of ascent to altitudes 2500 m (>8200 ft) and resolves within 24 hours of descent to 2500 m (<8200 ft)
- Has at least two of the following characteristics: (1) the headache must be bilateral, (2) mild to moderate in intensity, and (3) aggravated by activities such as exertion, movement, straining or bending.

Acute Mountain Sickness
- Occurs within 6 to 10 hours of ascent to altitudes 2500 m (>8200 ft)
- Symptoms include headache as well as anorexia, nausea, or vomiting; fatigue or weakness; or dizziness or lightheadedness; decreased urine output.

High-Altitude Cerebral Edema
- Appears 3 to 5 days after ascension above 2750 m (9022 ft)
- Neurologic disorder characterized by declining neurologic function, such as altered mental status, slurred speech, cranial nerve palsies, papilledema, and ataxia

High-Altitude Pulmonary Edema
- Presents 2 to 3 days after ascension
- Relative hypoxemia in the setting of at least two signs or symptoms from each of the following lists:
  - Resting dyspnea, cough, weakness, decreased exercise performance, and chest tightness or congestion
  - Wheezing, rales, tachypnea, tachycardia, or central cyanosis

CURRENT THERAPY

High-Altitude Headache
- Ibuprofen (Advil) 600 to 800 mg PO every 8 hours. Acetaminophen (Tylenol) 650 to 1000 mg PO every 6 hours. Enteric-coated aspirin (Ecotrin) 325 to 650 mg PO every 4 hours
- Supplemental oxygen by nasal cannula at 1 to 2 L/min
- Acetazolamide[1] 125 mg PO every 12 hours (adult)

Acute Mountain Sickness
Prophylaxis
- Acetazolamide (Diamox) 125 mg PO every 12 hours (adult); 2.5 mg/kg (maximum single dose 125 mg) PO every 12 hours (children). Begin 24 hours prior to ascent and stop 2 days after maximum altitude has been achieved or once descent has commenced.
- Alternative: dexamethasone (Decadron)[1] 2 mg PO every 6 hours or 4 mg PO every 12 hours (adult); do not use it for prophylaxis in children
- Avoid respiratory depressants (alcohol, sedating medications).

Mild
- Avoid respiratory depressants, strenuous activity, or further ascent until the patient is asymptomatic.
- Acetazolamide 125 to 250 mg PO every 12 hours (adult); 2.5 mg/kg (maximum single dose 250 mg) PO every 12 hours (children). Continue for 24 hours after symptoms resolve.

- Consider therapy for nausea and vomiting. Promethazine (Phenergan) 12.5 to 25 mg PO every 4 to 6 hours (adult). Ondansetron (Zofran)[1] 4 to 8 mg PO every 4 to 8 hours (adult)

Moderate to Severe
- Descend to an altitude lower than that where symptoms began.
- As an alternative to descent, consider supplemental oxygen (1–3 L/min via nasal cannula for 12–48 hours or during sleep only). If available, one can use a manually inflated hyperbaric chamber (1 hour minimum, although 12 hours or more may be required for treatment of severe illness).
- Dexamethasone[1] 4 mg PO every 6 hours (adult); 0.15 mg/kg (maximum single dose 4 mg) PO every 6 hours (children). Continue for 24 hours after symptoms resolve but no more than 7 days total. As an alternative, use acetazolamide 125 to 250 mg PO every 12 hours (adult); 2.5 mg/kg (maximum single dose 250 mg) PO every 12 hours. Continue for 24 hours after symptoms resolve or descent is completed.
- Monitor for mental status changes, confusion, or ataxia and descend immediately at onset.

High-Altitude Cerebral Edema
- Immediately descend (at least 1000 m or 3280 ft) at the first clinical suspicion of high-altitude cerebral edema while the patient remains ambulatory.
- Administer supplemental oxygen to maintain SpO_2 above 90%.
- Dexamethasone[1] 8 to 10 mg PO/IM/IV once followed by 4 mg PO/IM/IV every 6 hours (adult); 0.15 mg/kg (maximum single dose 4 mg) every 6 hours (children). Continue until 24 hours after symptoms resolve but no more than 7 days total.
- Can consider acetazolamide as an adjunct with dexamethasone but not as monotherapy. Acetazolamide[1] 250 mg PO every 12 hours (adult); 2.5 mg/kg (maximum single dose 250 mg) PO every 12 hours. Continue until 24 hours after symptoms resolve or descent is completed.

High-Altitude Pulmonary Edema
Prophylaxis (only in patients with history of prior high-altitude pulmonary edema)
- Nifedipine (Procardia)[1] 30 mg ER PO every 12 hours[3] (adults and children ≥50 kg). Begin 24 hours prior to ascent and continue for 5 days after reaching maximum altitude. Acetazolamide[1] 2.5 mg/kg (maximum single dose 125 mg) PO every 12 hours (children <50 kg). Begin 24 hours prior to ascent and continue 4 to 5 days at maximum altitude.
- Consider the following alternatives for adults, although data are limited:
  - Tadalafil (Cialis)[1] 10 mg PO every 12 hours.[3] Start day of ascent and continue 3 to 5 days at maximum altitude.
  - Sildenafil (Viagra)[1] 50 mg PO every 8 hours.[3] Start day of ascent and continue 3 to 5 days at maximum altitude.
  - Dexamethasone[1] 8 mg PO every 12 hours. Start day of ascent and continue 2 to 3 days at maximum altitude.
  - Acetazolamide[1] 125 to 250 mg PO every 12 hours. Begin 24 hours prior to ascent and continue 2 to 3 days at maximum altitude.

Treatment
- Immediately descend (500–1000 m), particularly in remote high-altitude settings where resources are limited because high-altitude pulmonary edema can progress rapidly.
- Administer supplemental oxygen to maintain SpO_2 above 90%. If available, one can use a manually inflated hyperbaric chamber.
- Rest and avoid cold exposure.
- Nifedipine[1] 30 mg ER PO every 12 hours[3] (adults and children ≥50 kg). Amlodipine (Norvasc)[1] 2.5 to 5 mg PO once daily (children 6–17 years and ≥25 kg); amlodipine 0.1 to 0.6 mg/kg/dose PO once daily (maximum 5 mg/day) (children 1–5 years or <25 kg). Continue until descent is completed, symptoms have resolved, and SpO_2 is normal for altitude.
- Consider the following alternative therapies for adults, although data are limited. Note, it is not advisable to use both

nifedipine and a phosphodiesterase inhibitor; if this becomes necessary, carefully monitor blood pressure and stagger doses to prevent potential cerebral hypoperfusion.

- Tadalafil[1] 10 mg PO every 12 hours.[3] Continue until descent is completed, symptoms have resolved, and SpO_2 is normal for altitude.
- Sildenafil[1] 50 mg PO every 8 hours.[3] Continue until descent is completed, symptoms have resolved, and SpO_2 is normal for altitude.

Concurrent High-Altitude Pulmonary and Cerebral Edema
- Immediate descent and supplemental oxygen therapy are critical.
- Treatment as for high-altitude pulmonary edema with the addition of dexamethasone.[1]

For administration in children, acetazolamide 125 mg and 250 mg tablets can be crushed and suspended in flavored syrup to make an oral suspension.
[1] Not FDA approved for this indication.
[3] Exceeds dosage recommended by the manufacturer.

In today's mobile society, the appeal and ease of traveling to higher altitude abounds. It may stem from an interest in recreational activities, such as skiing, mountaineering, or hiking. Others may experience a temporary rapid ascent due to work-related travel. For others, living at elevation is simply a lifestyle, because over 500 million persons worldwide (6.6% of the population) reside at elevations higher than 1500 m (Denver, Colorado, is 1609 m or 5278 ft). High altitude, whether enjoyed for a weekend visit or as a permanent residence, presents a myriad of environmental stresses that provoke physiologic responses and adaptation and may result in acute sickness or chronic health-related conditions. High-altitude illnesses (HAIs), such as high-altitude headache (HAH), acute mountain sickness (AMS), high-altitude cerebral edema (HACE), and high-altitude pulmonary edema (HAPE), are often preventable (Box 1) and have the potential to cause significant morbidity or death, especially in the individual with risk factors and preexisting comorbidities.

Physiologic Adaptation and Pathophysiology

All altitudes are measured from sea level and are classified as high (1500 to 3500 m or 5000–11,500 ft), very high (3500 to 5500 m or 11,500–18,000 ft), and extreme (above 5500 m or 18,000 ft). At 1500 m (5000 ft), a drop in barometric pressure occurs, resulting in a decrease in the partial pressure of oxygen. Typically, the body responds favorably by triggering a physiologic response that helps the individual adapt to the low oxygen condition. When atmospheric pressure drops, the partial pressure of oxygen (PO_2) decreases in ambient air, inspired air (PiO_2), alveolar air (PAO_2), and arterial blood (PaO_2), and arterial oxygen saturation (SaO_2) decreases with progressive ascent. The physiologic adaptation to the decrease in oxygen pressure in these high-altitude environments is known as acclimatization, and the process of acute acclimatization to high elevation typically takes 3 to 5 days. Acclimatization differs from adaptation, which refers to physiologic changes that take place in response to chronic exposure to hypobaric hypoxia, often occurring over generations. With acclimatization, ventilation will increase (both tidal volume and ventilation) to relieve hypoxemia. This response, known as the hypoxic ventilatory response, causes hyperventilation and results in a simultaneous rapid decrease in the alveolar partial pressure of carbon dioxide (PCO_2) and a proportional increase in alveolar PO_2, causing respiratory alkalosis. After 24 to 48 hours, the kidneys excrete excess bicarbonate, normalizing the elevated pH.

The cardiac response to hypoxia includes an initial increase in heart rate and pulmonary perfusion with a goal to optimize oxygenation in the lungs and supply well-oxygenated blood to the brain, heart, and other tissues. Norepinephrine is released and results in increased cardiac output, heart rate, peripheral

BOX 1   Prevention of High-Altitude Illness

Ascent above 2500 m (8200 ft) should be at a gradual rate of 300 m per 24 hours, with an additional rest day for every 1000 m (3280 ft) gain. With rapid ascent above 2500 m (8200 ft), light activity may be helpful with acclimatization, but strenuous activity should be avoided for at least 48 hours.

Avoid respiratory depressants such as alcohol until acclimatized.

For AMS:
- Acetazolamide (Diamox) 125 mg PO every 12 hours (adult); 2.5 mg/kg (maximum single dose 125 mg) PO every 12 hours (children). Begin 24 hours prior to ascent and stop 2 days after maximum altitude has been achieved or once descent has commenced.
- Alternative: dexamethasone (Decadron)[1] 2 mg PO every 6 hours or 4 mg PO every 12 hours (adult); do not use it for prophylaxis in children.

For persons with a history of HAPE:
- Nifedipine[1] 30 mg ER PO every 12 hours[3] (adult and children ≥50 kg). Begin 24 hours prior to ascent and continue for 5 days after reaching maximum altitude. Acetazolamide 2.5 mg/kg (maximum single dose 125 mg) PO every 12 hours (children ≥50 kg). Begin 24 hours prior to ascent and continue 4 to 5 days at maximum altitude.
- Consider the following alternatives for adults, although data are limited:
  - Tadalafil (Cialis)[1] 10 mg PO every 12 hours.[3] Start day of ascent and continue 3 to 5 days at maximum altitude.
  - Sildenafil (Viagra)[1] 50 mg PO every 8 hours.[3] Start day of ascent and continue 3 to 5 days at maximum altitude.
  - Dexamethasone[1] 8 mg PO every 12 hours. Start day of ascent and continue 2 to 3 days at maximum altitude.
  - Acetazolamide 125 to 250 mg PO every 12 hours. Begin 24 hours prior to ascent and continue 2 to 3 days at maximum altitude.

---

[1] Not FDA approved for this indication.
[3] Exceeds dosage recommended by the manufacturer.
AMS, Acute mountain sickness; *HAPE*, high altitude pulmonary edema.

vascular tone, blood pressure, and pulmonary perfusion. Once acclimatized, heart rate normalizes and plasma volume decreases (diuresis), and cardiac output subsequently decreases. Hypoxia causes generalized pulmonary arterial vasoconstriction and a slight increase in pulmonary arterial pressure independent of the increase in cardiac output. It may initially improve the ventilation-perfusion ratio (V/Q) by redistributing blood flow to less-perfused areas of the lung. Unfortunately, this offers little adaptive advantage over the pathogenesis of HAPE.

Approximately 25% of people who ascend to 3500 m (11,500 ft) and >50% of people who ascend to greater than 6000 m (19,700 ft) develop HAI. The occurrence of HAI relies upon several variables, including the speed of ascent, the overall altitude, sleep quality and quantity, the amount of time spent at high altitude, low temperature, increased ultraviolet radiation, preacclimatization, previous history of HAI, and history of preexisting illnesses. Because of the many factors affecting HAI risk, incidence is highly variable. Globally, the reported incidence for AMS ranges from 10% to 90%; for HAPE and HACE, the range is from <0.01% to 31%. An individual who has a history of HAPE is 10% to 60% more likely to experience a subsequent episode at similar altitude with a similar rate of ascent.

Susceptibility to HAI is highly variable, and there are no reliable measures to predict the risk of developing HAI prior to ascent. Although gender does not appear to be a risk factor, age does play a role. The risk of developing HAI is two times lower in individuals over the age of 50, and HAPE occurs with greater frequency and severity in children and young adults. Fitness level does not appear to be protective against HAI, nor does a high fitness level improve the ability to acclimatize. Conditions that impair ventilation and the ventilatory response can increase the risk of HAI, including sedating medications, alcohol, moderate to severe chronic obstructive pulmonary disease, absence of carotid bodies (radiation, surgical resection), and neuromuscular diseases affecting the diaphragm. Conditions such as interstitial lung disease and cystic fibrosis, congenital cardiac anomalies involving right-to-left shunts, and obstructive sleep apnea are also likely to increase the risk of HAI, although data are limited. Pulmonary hypertension is known to increase the risk of HAPE, and tobacco smoking and asthma do not confer any additional risk. Chronic conditions such as hypertension and diabetes do not appear to be associated with increased risk of HAI.

When evaluating a patient for hypoxemia, it is essential to consider the limitations of current clinical tools. Pulse oximeter devices are widely used to evaluate peripheral blood oxygen saturation; however, there is growing evidence that pulse oximeters are less accurate in patients with dark skin tones at lower saturation (<80%), resulting in overestimation of SpO_2 and higher rates of clinically unrecognized hypoxemia. Awareness of potential limitations of pulse oximeter devices in patients with dark skin tones is essential to avoid treatment delays and mitigate health disparities.

High-Altitude Headache

HAH is recognized as a standalone diagnosis, even though it is a symptom of other AMS. HAH is a result of decreased barometric pressure seen with ascension into higher altitudes. This results in a lower percentage of oxygen molecules per breath. The body's immediate response is to increase respiration. Approximately 80% of people report a headache while ascending to high altitudes, particularly when the ascent is rapid and if altitude is >15,000 ft (4500 m). By definition, HAH can occur within 1 hour after ascent but typically occurs within 6 to 10 hours of ascent to altitudes >8200 ft (2500 m); it resolves within 24 hours of descent to <8200 ft (2500 m). Additionally, the headache should have at least two of the following characteristics: (1) the headache must be bilateral, (2) mild to moderate in intensity, and (3) aggravated by activities such as exertion, movement, straining, or bending. An HAH is often worse in the morning; photophobia and phonophobia are atypical for pure HAH. Treatment of the patient with mild HAH consists of medication, such as acetaminophen or ibuprofen, and implementing descent if the initial strategies are not successful. See the Current Therapy Box and Box 2 for a complete listing.

High-Altitude Syndromes

Acute Mountain Sickness

The most common form of altitude illness is AMS and typically occurs in unacclimatized individuals with rapid ascension to altitudes greater than 2500 m (8200 ft). Similar to HAH, onset can occur within 1 hour but usually begins within 6 to 10 hours after ascent. This condition is a result of exposure to hypobaric hypoxia. Symptoms include headache as well as anorexia, nausea, or vomiting; fatigue or weakness; dizziness or lightheadedness; and decreased urine output.

Early recognition of AMS is essential to promptly initiating treatment that may prevent evolution to the potentially fatal HACE, which exists along the same spectrum. Treatment for mild AMS includes the use of analgesics and antiemetics without further ascent. Acetazolamide is recommended for mild AMS; dexamethasone[1] is recommended for moderate to severe symptoms. For moderate to severe symptoms, low-flow supplemental oxygen and hyperbaric chambers can also be used. Descent is recommended if symptoms do not improve or worsen after 24 hours of rest or treatment. Graded ascent can be resumed once symptoms resolve. However, immediate descent should be undertaken for ataxia, altered mental status, or any signs of pulmonary edema. Refer to the Current Therapy Box and Box 2 for dosing and summary.

High-Altitude Cerebral Edema

HACE is a neurologic disorder characterized by headaches, impaired coordination and muscle weakness as well as

---

[1] Not FDA approved for this indication.

| BOX 2 | Common Medications Used in the Treatment of HAI |

Acetazolamide

Acetazolamide (Diamox) is a central-acting respiratory stimulant that stimulates bicarbonate diuresis and causes a metabolic acidosis to facilitate acclimatization. It is effective in preventing and treating HAI. Patients should be warned about side effects, including paresthesias, flat taste of carbonated beverages, and polyuria. Persons with a history of asthma, sulfonamide allergy, anaphylaxis, or penicillin allergy should try this medication under the supervision of a medical professional prior to departure. It should not be used in patients with type 1 diabetes due to the risk for acidosis and diuresis resulting in dehydration. It also should not be used in chronic lung disease if FEV_1 is less than 25% predicted or in patients on potassium-wasting diuretics or long-term high doses of aspirin.

Dexamethasone

Dexamethasone (Decadron)[1] is also effective in the prevention of AMS and treatment of AMS and HACE, though its mechanism is not completely understood. Unlike with acetazolamide, it does not facilitate acclimatization. It is not recommended for prophylaxis of AMS unless acetazolamide is contraindicated, though it is the drug of choice for treatment of HACE. Use is cautioned in patients with diabetes due to risk of hyperglycemia. Side effects can include insomnia, irritability, gastrointestinal upset, and euphoria.

Nifedipine

Nifedipine (Procardia)[1] is a calcium channel blocker that inhibits pulmonary vasoconstriction secondary to hypoxia at high altitude and is used in prevention and treatment of HAPE.

Caution should be used with other antihypertensives due to the risk for hypotension. Medications that inhibit the cytochrome P450 3A4 pathway, including macrolides, doxycycline, and azoles, may increase plasma concentrations and also precipitate hypotension. Ginkgo biloba[7] may also increase levels of nifedipine and cause hypotension and should be avoided.

Tadalafil (Cialis)[1] and Sildenafil (Viagra)[1]

Phosphodiesterase inhibitors that cause pulmonary vasodilation can be considered in the prevention or treatment of HAPE, although data are limited. They should not be used in conjunction with nitrates due to risk for significant hypotension or with alpha blockers due to orthostatic hypotension. Medications that inhibit the cytochrome P450 3A4 pathway, including macrolides, doxycycline, and azoles, may increase plasma concentrations and also precipitate hypotension.

---

[1] Not FDA approved for this indication.
[7] Available as a dietary supplement.
AMS, Acute mountain sickness; FEV₁, forced expiratory volume; HACE, high altitude cerebral edema; HAPE, high altitude pulmonary edema.

---

impairments of consciousness. It is considered a separate disease from acute mountain sickness and typically progresses over 1 to 3 days. Established risk factors for HACE include rapid ascent, inadequate acclimatization, extreme altitudes, physical exertion, and a prior history of HAI. Clinical signs of HACE typically appear 3 to 5 days after ascension above 2750 m (9022 ft) and include declining neurologic function, such as altered mental status, slurred speech, cranial nerve palsies, papilledema, and ataxia. Truncal ataxia, implying impaired coordination between the trunk and the extremities, is a common sign. If computed tomography or magnetic resonance imaging is available acutely, findings would be consistent with vasogenic edema. If a lumbar puncture is performed, increased opening pressure is typically present. Differential diagnosis is similar to that for AMS but would also include diabetic ketoacidosis, hypoglycemia, electrolyte imbalances, brain tumor, stroke, acute psychosis, and seizure. If symptoms appear when at elevation, early recognition is crucial to prevent evolution to irreversible disease. The most important element of treatment is descent of at least 1000 m (3280 ft). Supplemental oxygen and hyperbaric bags may be used during descent and are imperative if descent is not possible. Dexamethasone[1] should be initiated as soon as possible and continued after descent until symptoms resolve. Currently, there is no evidence to support the use of acetazolamide as monotherapy in treating HACE.[1] Dosages are listed in the Current Therapy Box and details on pharmacology can be found in Box 2.

High-Altitude Pulmonary Edema

HAPE is a potentially lethal pulmonary disorder defined as non-cardiogenic (left ventricular function is preserved) pulmonary edema caused by pulmonary blood gas barrier leak in the lung. It is typically diagnosed with at least two of the following: resting dyspnea, cough, weakness or decreased exercise performance, and chest tightness or congestion, in addition to two of the following: wheezing or rales, tachypnea, tachycardia, or central cyanosis. Cough is initially dry but in late stages is productive of pink or bloody sputum. This condition does not typically manifest itself until 2 to 3 days after ascension and rarely presents after 4 days. The physiologic response includes increased pulmonary arterial pressure, hypoxic pulmonary vasoconstriction, and hypoxemia. Physical examination is significant for rales that can begin in the right axilla and progress diffusely along with low-grade temperature elevation. Hypoxia, often very pronounced, is noted on pulse oximetry; oxygen levels will be disproportionately low for a given elevation. Plain films of the thorax show pulmonary thickening but no cardiomegaly; imaging may also include unilateral or bilateral patchy fluffy opacities predominantly in the dependent zone of the lungs. Differential diagnosis includes heart failure, acute myocardial ischemia, pulmonary embolus, asthma, bronchitis, and pneumonia. Although HAPE is associated with the highest rate of mortality of altitude conditions, it is unlikely to cause long-term sequelae if treated appropriately. Treatment includes immediate descent and supplemental oxygen or a hyperbaric chamber. If available, supplemental oxygen and bedrest may be sufficient. If the pulmonary edema is severe, though, descent is the definitive treatment and should be undertaken without delay. Exertion and cold stress should be avoided during descent. Nifedipine (Procardia)[1] may be of benefit in treatment of HAPE but is not as effective as oxygen or descent and should be used as an adjunct.

High-Altitude Retinopathy

Hypoxia is known to cause hyperemia and engorgement of the retinal vessels at any elevation and will be seen above 2500 m (8200 ft) in the setting of hypobaric hypoxia. Macular or vitreous hemorrhage, disc edema, and cotton wool spots can be seen in more severe high-altitude retinopathy (HAR). There may be a delay between ascent and onset of hemorrhage. The retinopathy is generally asymptomatic; however, scotomas and visual field deficits may occur, particularly with macular hemorrhage. Lower oxygen saturation, higher ascent, strenuous exertion, and longer duration at high altitude are associated with HAR. Higher baseline intraocular pressure, hypercoagulable disorders, and aspirin and nonsteroidal antiinflammatory drug (NSAID) use also appear to be risk factors. Slower ascent and improved acclimatization are protective. Acetazolamide[1] does not appear to affect incidence. Research has not shown a definitive correlation between HAR and AMS or HACE.

Most HAR will resolve within days to weeks of descent. Rarely visual deficits have persisted longer. Descent is recommended for any premacular hemorrhage due to higher risk to central vision and unclear long-term prognosis, as well as any new visual deficits. Given the potential risk of worsening retinopathy, patients with risk for or preexisting retinopathy (including patients with diabetic retinopathy) should avoid travel to elevations greater than 4000 m (13,000 ft) and consult with their physician if such travel is unavoidable.

Upper Respiratory Disorders at High Altitude

Rhinorrhea, chronic cough, and noninfectious pharyngitis and bronchitis are commonly seen at high altitude and very prevalent at extreme altitude. Sputum is often purulent. Onset of high-altitude bronchitis and chronic cough is generally after strenuous activity and use of a balaclava to increase humidification of inhaled air may help diminish symptoms. Cough may become severe enough to cause rib fractures. Comprehensive studies on the most effective treatment are lacking, but symptomatic therapies may be useful, including decongestant nasal sprays, inhaled corticosteroids, and beta agonists. Infectious upper respiratory syndromes should remain in the differential; however, viral etiologies are most common with judicious consideration of antibiotic therapy.

Additional Considerations

Acetazolamide and Sulfa Allergy

Cross-reactivity among sulfonamide antibiotics and sulfa-containing medications is based on theory more so than data. Because the acetazolamide structure lacks the arylamine side chain (aromatic amine group) that all sulfonamide antibiotics possess, the clinical risk of reaction to acetazolamide in a patient with sulfonamide allergy is low. Given the limited options for prevention and treatment of HAI, one could consider administering a clinic drug challenge to a patient with reported sulfa allergy prior to travel. This would include administration of acetazolamide 125 mg by mouth (adult), observation for 1 to 2 hours, and daily treatment for several days to exclude a delayed hypersensitivity reaction. Use clinical judgment and shared decision making to evaluate an individual's risk.

Pregnancy

Although the healthy patient with no pregnancy concerns can safely travel to altitude, high-altitude activities in pregnancy can cause dyspnea and palpitations. The Centers for Disease Control and Prevention suggest that pregnant individuals avoid sleeping at altitudes greater than 3658 m (12,000 ft) due to the risk of hypobaric hypoxia. Many symptoms of HAI (insomnia, nausea, and vomiting) also occur frequently in pregnancy, rendering it difficult to differentiate the origin of symptoms and accurately diagnose HAI. There are limited safety data regarding acetazolamide use in pregnancy; acetazolamide is present in breast milk. When traveling to altitude, the expectant patient should also consider the availability of medical resources, should medical intervention be necessary. For all of these reasons, the pregnant patient should communicate travel plans or concerns to their physician.

Children

There are unique considerations for children and infants when traveling to altitude. Although many symptoms of HAI in children mirror those of adults, assessment of preverbal and nonverbal children requires thoughtful attention. Signs may include a loss of appetite, sporadic or poor sleep patterns, decreased playfulness and engagement with others, and increased fussiness. It is imperative that the healthcare professional educate parents and guardians to remain attentive to these symptoms. If a child has an acute respiratory infection or acute otitis media, additional caution should be exercised during rapid ascent above 8200 feet.

Recommendations to prevent HAI in children include using a very gradual ascent and avoiding ascending more than 1600 ft per day beyond 8200 ft. In addition, it is recommended that an individual spend at least 5 days at an intermediate altitude (~10,000–13,000 ft) before proceeding to higher levels of elevation.

Treatment for the infant or child experiencing HAI is based on severity and includes medications for headache (acetaminophen and ibuprofen), supplemental oxygen, acetazolamide, and dexamethasone.[1] Dosages are listed in the Current Therapy Box.

---

[1]Not FDA approved for this indication.

[1]Not FDA approved for this indication.

Older Adults

Because populations are living longer, there has been an increase in the number of travelers over the age of 60, many of whom are seeking destinations at higher elevations. It is important to consider that the normal aging process may result in a decrease in overall physical activity and fitness as well as an increase in comorbidities affecting the cardiovascular and pulmonary systems. Older persons with impairments in the respiratory system may have diminished ventilatory response to hypoxia and hypercapnia, placing them at risk during high-demand conditions. In addition, the older population may be more prone to infections or injuries related to a fall. Recent research has examined the effect of aging on the risk of AMS and determined that older age does not seem to be a contraindication for traveling to high altitudes. However, an older person with a history of cardiovascular and/or pulmonary conditions who plans to travel to altitude should discuss their plans with their physician well in advance. The use of prophylactic medications, physical preparedness, and risk of falls are important considerations.

Sickle Cell Trait and Altitude

Sickle cell trait (SCT) is a condition (not a disease) resulting from the inheritance of one gene for sickle hemoglobin (S) and one gene for normal hemoglobin (A). Sickle cell trait is found in approximately 8% of African Americans and 0.05% of the Ehite population in the United States. SCT has a risk of increased manifestation at altitude. At altitude, the low oxygen tension allows calcium influx and potassium leakage. This results in the cell membrane to become stiff, viscous, and sickle shaped in the individual with SCT; the sickle-shaped erythrocytes become sticky and adhere to structures in the microvascular system. The spleen appears to be particularly vulnerable. As such, the low oxygen density, especially when combined with exercise exertion (hiking, for example) and dehydration, put the individual with SCT at risk.

Physical manifestations of sickling may include lower extremity muscle weakness, which differs from pain seen with muscle cramps. There is no loss of consciousness, which is distinctly different from the individual experiencing cardiac arrhythmia. Upon presentation with these symptoms, the individual should be examined for splenomegaly. Acutely, the individual should descend and be treated at a hospital for aggressive fluid and electrolyte management, cardiac monitoring, and lab studies. Once the individual is medically stable and has normal organ function, the individual can resume a gradual return to activity.

References

Aksel G, Çorbacıoğlu Ş.K., Özen C: High-altitude illness: management approach, *Turk J Emerg Med* 19(4):121–126, 2019.

Centers for Disease Control and Prevention. High altitude travel and altitude illness. Available at: https://wwwnc.cdc.gov/travel/yellowbook/2020/noninfectious-health-risks/high-altitude-travel-and-altitude-illness.

Centers for Disease Control and Prevention. Pregnant travelers. Available at: https://wwwnc.cdc.gov/travel/yellowbook/2020/family-travel/pregnant-travelers#:~:text=Pregnant%20women%20should%20avoid%20activities,experience%20exaggerated%20breathlessness%20and%20palpitations.

Gianfredi V, Albano L, Basnyat B, Ferrara P: Does age have an impact on acute mountain sickness? A systematic review, *J Travel Med* 27(6):taz104, 2020.

Jamali H, Castillo L, Cosby Morgan C, et al: Racial disparity in oxygen saturation measurements by pulse oximetry: evidence and implications, *Ann Am Thorac Soc* 19(12):1951–1964, 2022.

Marmura MJ, Hernandez PB: High-altitude headache, *Curr Pain Headache Rep* 19(5):483, 2015.

Mikołajczak K, Czerwińska K, Pilecki W, et al: The impact of temporary stay at high altitude on the circulatory system, *J Clin Med* 10(8):1622, 2021.

Savioli G, Ceresa IF, Gori G, et al: Pathophysiology and therapy of high-altitude sickness: practical approach in emergency and critical care, *J Clin Med* 11(14):3937, 2022.

Scordino D, Kirsch T: Splenic infarction at high altitude secondary to sickle cell trait, *Am J Emerg Med* 31(2):446.e1–446.e3, 2013.

Shah T, Moshirfar M, Hoopes Sr P: "Doctor, I have a sulfa allergy": clarifying the myths of cross-reactivity, *Ophthalmol Ther* 7:211–215, 2018.

Villca N, Asturizaga A, Heath-Freudenthal A: High-altitude illnesses and air travel: pediatric considerations, *Pediatr Clin North Am* 68(1):305–319, 2021.

Zelmanovich R, Pierre K, Felisma P, et al: High altitude cerebral edema: Improving treatment options, *Biologics (Basel)* 2(1):81–91, 2022.

MARINE POISONINGS, ENVENOMATIONS, AND TRAUMA

Method of
Allen Perkins, MD, MPH

CURRENT DIAGNOSIS

- History of exposure is necessary for diagnosis.
- Ingested toxins can cause unusual symptoms, predominately gastrointestinal.
- Jellyfish envenomation is very painful but almost always self-limited.
- Trauma management follows principles of dirty wounds.
- Specific marine pathogens should be covered if contamination is suspected.

CURRENT THERAPY

Ingestions
- Avoidance is the best strategy.
- Early decontamination with activated charcoal (Actidose-Aqua) can reduce duration of symptoms.
- Symptomatic care is generally sufficient.

Jellyfish
- Remove visible stingers.
- Control pain with topical analgesia.

Trauma
- Avoiding water at feeding time can help avoid injury.
- If envenomation is suspected, consider hot water immersion.
- Tetanus status should be checked.
- Antibiotic coverage should take marine pathogens into account.

The United States has more than 80,000 miles of coastline, and more people are enjoying water-dependent recreation activities such as scuba diving, snorkeling, and surfing. As a consequence, people are more likely to suffer trauma, envenomation, or poisoning related to an encounter with a marine creature, which will come to the attention of a physician. The science of marine medicine is limited; hence, treatment of these conditions is largely based on case reports and expert opinion; very few randomized, controlled studies are available. Misdiagnosis is common, especially when the patient has returned from vacationing or when the patient has been poisoned by improperly handled seafood. This article describes common ailments and injuries occurring as a consequence of direct contact with sea creatures and discusses management and prevention.

Ingestions

Ciguatera Fish Poisoning

Epidemiology

Ciguatera fish poisoning (CFP) is the most commonly reported marine toxin disease in the world. It is caused by human ingestion of reef fish that have bioaccumulated sufficient amounts of the dinoflagellate *Gambierdiscus toxicus*, either through direct ingestion or through ingestion of smaller reef fish. Although limited to tropical regions, it is heat and cold tolerant, is lipid soluble, and can survive transport to other areas. The toxin becomes more concentrated as it passes up the food chain; fish such as amberjack, grouper, and snapper pose less of a risk than predatory fish such as barracuda and moray eel. Ciguatera fish poisoning affects at least 50,000 people worldwide annually, and there are several thousand cases

> **BOX 1** Symptom Patterns Associated With Ciguatera Fish Poisoning
>
> **Gastrointestinal Pattern**
> Onset 15 minutes to 24 hours, typically worsens, lasts 1–2 days and resolves
> - Nausea and/or vomiting
> - Profuse, watery diarrhea
> - Abdominal pain
>
> **Neurologic Pattern**
> Onset up to 24 hours after ingestion, commonly nonphysiologic pattern, can last several months
> - Numbness and paresthesias
> - Vertigo
> - Ataxia
> - Severe weakness or lethargy
> - Severe myalgia
> - Decreased vibration and pain sensations
> - Diffuse pain pattern
> - Cold sensation reversal
> - Coma
>
> **Cardiovascular Pattern**
> Onset up to 24 hours after ingestion is uncommon but occurs rapidly
> - Bradycardia
> - Hypotension
> - Cardiovascular collapse

of poisoning in Puerto Rico, the U.S. Virgin Islands, Hawaii, and Florida each year.

Clinical Features

Patients can exhibit a primarily gastrointestinal (diarrhea, abdominal cramps, and vomiting), neurologic (parasthesias, diffuse pain, blurred vision), cardiac (bradycardia), or mixed pattern of symptoms. Additionally, a cold sensation reversal, in which a patient perceives the cold temperatures as a hot sensation and vice versa, occurs in 80% of patients and is considered pathognomonic for ciguatera poison (Box 1).

The attack rate is high. As many as 80% to 100% of people who ingest affected fish develop symptoms depending on the size of the fish and the toxin load. Ingestion of internal organs where the toxin accumulates (e.g., liver, roe) is associated with more severe symptoms, but avoiding these organs is not protective. The symptoms are also related to the number of exposures over time, and patients typically have more severe symptoms with subsequent exposures. There is no age-related susceptibility, and no immunity is acquired through exposure.

Symptoms typically begin 1 to 6 hours after ingestion, although a delay of 12 to 24 hours can occur. Duration is 7 to 14 days, and neurologic symptoms occasionally persist for months to years. Chronic ciguatera syndrome can also occur as a constellation of symptoms such as general malaise, depression, headaches, muscle aches, and dysesthesias in the extremities. Patients with chronic disease report recurrences with ingestion of fish, ethanol, caffeine, and nuts up to 6 months after the acute illness resolves.

Diagnosis

The diagnosis should be entertained in any patient who has neurologic, gastrointestinal, or cardiac symptoms and a history of ingesting predatory fish within the past 24 hours. The symptom constellation can be similar to other ingestions, such as certain shellfish toxins, and differentiation requires knowledge of the patient's diet for the previous day. Additionally, scombroid and type E botulinum poisoning should be considered, but these are unlikely if the patient did not ingest ill-appearing game. Other poisonings, such as organophosphates, can produce a similar symptom complex. There are no currently available clinical assays to assist in making the diagnosis, which is based on clinical suspicion and knowledge of the patient's diet history.

Treatment

If CFP is suspected soon after ingestion, I would consider gut decontamination with activated charcoal (Actidose-Aqua) because it can reduce the toxin load and subsequent symptoms. Initial symptomatic treatment typically consists of fluid replacement to replace gastrointestinal losses.

Atropine (AtroPen) is used in patients who have bradycardia. Temporary electrical pacing may be used for refractory symptoms, and pressors may be needed in cases of severe hypotension. Neurologic symptoms are problematic because of their extended course as well as their severity. Mannitol (Osmitrol)[1] is often cited as effective in reducing the duration of neurologic symptoms, but I would use it with caution because the only double-blind trial failed to show any benefit. There are many local remedies used throughout the world that are said to be successful, which likely attests to the self-limited course of the ingestion in most cases. Table 1 offers more details regarding treatments currently used for CFP.

Prevention

Prevention is difficult except by avoiding ingestion of affected reef fish. The toxin is not deactivated by cooking, freezing, smoking, or salting. There are no outward signs of ciguatera: The fish look, taste, and smell normal. Although several commercial assays are available, they are neither sensitive nor specific enough to be relied on to prevent CFP.

To decrease the risk of CFP, I recommend the following steps: Avoid warm-water reef fish, especially those caught where ciguatera poisoning is known to occur; avoid moray eel ingestion; avoid ingesting large game fish; avoid consuming the internal organs; and limit the amount of initial ingestion if you are in an area where ciguatera is known to occur. Additionally, patients travelling to distant locales should be made aware that, although the vast majority of cases result from direct ingestion, there have been cases of CFP passed through sexual contact and through breast milk, so they should be wary of body fluid contact if ciguatoxin is endemic to the area, if for no other reasons.

Scombroid
Epidemiology

Scombroid poisoning (also known as histamine fish poisoning) results from improper handling of certain fish between the time the fish is caught and the time it is cooked. In the United States it is most common in Hawaii and California. Improper preservation and refrigeration lead to histamine and histamine-like substances being produced in the dark meat of certain fish through a conversion of histidine to histamine by bacterial decarboxylases. Members of the family Scombridae, such as tuna and mackerel, contain the highest amounts of this substance, but both scombroid and nonscombroid fish have been associated with the disease. The production of toxins requires the introduction of bacteria during the handling process, primarily during storage at high temperatures. It is the total amount of histamine, the presence of other biogenic amines, and individual susceptibility that determine the severity of the symptoms.

Clinical Features

The patient develops a histamine reaction 20 to 30 minutes after ingestion. Symptoms can be cutaneous, gastrointestinal, neurologic, or hemodynamic, or any combination of these. Cutaneous symptoms include flushing, urticaria and conjunctival injection, and localized edema; gastrointestinal symptoms include dry mouth, nausea, vomiting, diarrhea, and abdominal cramping; neurologic symptoms include severe headache and dizziness; and hemodynamic symptoms include palpitations and hypotension. In severe cases there can be bronchospasm and respiratory distress. These symptoms typically

---

[1] Not FDA approved for this indication.

TABLE 1 Treatment for Ciguatera Fish Poisoning

DRUG	DOSE	INDICATION
Activated charcoal (Actidose-Aqua)	Children <1 y: 1 g/kg	Gut emptying and decontamination
	Children 1–12 y: 25–50 g	
	Adults: 25–100 g	More effective in first hour
Antiemetics (no preference)	Administer per dosing recommendations	Intractable nausea and/or vomiting
Intravenous fluid bolus and infusion (normal saline or lactated Ringer's as initial)	Per volume replacement protocols	Hypovolemia
Atropine (AtroPen)	0.5–1.0 mg IV every 3–5 min to a maximum dose of 0.04 mg/kg per episode	Bradycardia
	Maximum total dose: 3 mg for adults, 2 mg for adolescents, 1 mg for young children	
Pressors: Dopamine (Intropin), dobutamine (Dobutrex), epinephrine	Varies with clinical response	Hypotension, shock
Antihistamines (no preference)	Administer per dosing recommendations	Pruritus
Mannitol (Osmitrol)[1]	1 g/kg of a 20% solution given IV over several h	Neurologic symptoms, double-blind study did not show benefit
	Adult dose: 25–100 g, titrate to urinary output of 100 mL/h	
Amitriptyline (Elavil)[1]	25–75 mg PO bid for patients >25 kg	Pruritus, dysesthesias

[1]Not FDA approved for this indication.

come on rapidly (within several minutes) and last less than 6 to 8 hours. Flushing is the most consistent clinical sign, occurring on exposed areas so it typically resembles sunburn. Diarrhea is also very common, occurring in 75% of symptomatic patients.

Diagnosis
As with ciguatera, the diagnosis is one of history. If the time between ingestion and illness is short and the patient has ingested a type of fish previously implicated in scombroid, then a tentative diagnosis can be made. The diagnosis is often confused with an allergic reaction. It can be distinguished from allergy by the lack of a previous allergic reaction as well as by testing the remaining fish for histamine, although testing is rarely warranted.

Treatment
Treatment is the same as for any histamine reaction, the cornerstone of which is antihistamine. Diphenhydramine (Benadryl) 50 mg for adults and 0.5–1 mg/kg/dose for children, repeated every 4 hours until symptoms abate, is delivered either intravenously or intramuscularly in severe cases and orally for milder cases. For severe cases, cimetidine (Tagamet)[1] 300 mg for adults, 20 mg/kg for children, either orally or intravenously, might be added for more complete histamine-receptor blockade. In cases where ingestion was recent, consider induced emesis using syrup of ipecac: 15 mL for children younger than 12 years or 30 mL otherwise. Most patients require only reassurance, and pharmacologic treatment will be unnecessary. It should be stressed to the patient that this is not an *allergic* reaction to fish, because the histamine is exogenous. Prevention is possible in regions where food storage and preparation are monitored through identification and removal of suspect fish.

Other Ingested Toxins
In addition to the toxins just discussed, ingestion of certain other marine creatures can lead to problems.

Ingestion of bivalves harvested from contaminated waters has been associated with hepatitis A, Norwalk virus, *Vibrio parahaemolyticus* and *Vibrio vulnificans* infections, the latter two particularly problematic and occasionally fatal in immunocompromised

patients. I counsel patients likely to be immunocompromised, including diabetics and those with known liver disease, to avoid uncooked bivalves.

Shellfish are occasionally known to contain one or more of several toxins acquired through bioaccumulation of certain algae. These dinoflagellates tend to bloom in summer months. The symptoms occur immediately after ingestion and last several hours and are typically neurologic or gastrointestinal, or both. The shellfish poisoning syndromes are known as paralytic, neurologic, diarrheal, or amnestic depending on the predominant symptom. The care is typically supportive. Public health officials typically monitor local mollusk populations fairly carefully and alert the public to possible hazards.

Ingestion of the flesh of certain puffer fish has been associated with tetrodotoxin poisoning. The flesh of the fish (fugu) is considered a delicacy. The toxin builds up in internal organs such as the liver and the roe. If the toxin is ingested, it is likely to be fatal, but there are certified chefs who are trained in avoiding the toxin when preparing the dish. Despite this precaution, as many as 50 deaths occur in Japan annually from exposure to this toxin. Avoiding this puffer fish and avoiding the ingestion of certain other exotic animals (such as the blue-ringed octopus) eliminate the risk of acquiring this toxin.

Envenomations
Many marine creatures are venomous, and beachgoers experience clinically significant envenomations with some regularity. Jellyfish and related creatures (Cnidarians), sea urchins (Echinodermata), and stingrays (Chondrichthyes) are some of the more commonly identified marine animals involved with envenomations.

Jellyfish
These invertebrates have stinging cells called *nematocytes*, which carry nematocysts that continue to function when separated from the larger organism. For example, jellyfish nematocysts can sting if the tentacle is separated and after the jellyfish is dead. The venom is antigenic and causes a reaction of a dermatonecrotic, hemolytic, cardiopathic, or neurotoxic nature. The severity of the reaction depends on several variables, including the number of nematocysts that discharge, the

[1]Not FDA approved for this indication.

toxicity of the coelenterate involved, and each patient's unique antigenic response.

Clinical Features
Although occasionally fatal as a consequence of an anaphylactic response in the United States and Caribbean, the primary concern in these areas with contact is pain, which is almost always self-limiting. Other, less common symptoms include paresthesias, nausea, headaches, and chills. The symptoms may last up to 2 to 3 days. Certain Pacific jellyfish primarily found in the waters around Australia have a more potent toxin and are much more likely to cause death (which is still very uncommon). Additionally, the Irukandji syndrome, which occurs in the Pacific, is a suite of symptoms including muscle spasms, vomiting, hypertension, incessant coughing, and occasionally heart failure and brain hemorrhage. Almost all exposed people, regardless of the geographic location, do not have a severe reaction, and the principles of first aid are primarily the same throughout the world.

Treatment
In my experience, treatment is mostly concerned with limiting pain and neurologic symptoms, because anaphylaxis and other severe reactions are rare, and the following general guidelines can be applied. In the field, either the victim or a companion should remove any visible tentacles. To do so requires using care, with gloves or forceps being optimal to prevent further stings. If a towel is used, any nematocysts remaining on the towel can still discharge. Salt water can be used to wash off the nematocysts. Urine, household vinegar, fresh water, and rubbing with sand should be avoided.

Should the victim present to the physician's office or emergency department, topical lidocaine (4%)[1] should be liberally applied for 30 minutes or until the pain subsides, followed by removal of the nematocysts, usually through use of the gloved hand or with forceps. Another method for removing the nematocysts is to apply shaving cream or baking soda slurry to the area and scrape off the nematocysts with a razor. Applications of cold, in the form of an ice pack, and immersion in hot water have variously been shown to improve pain, but because of the self-limited nature of the discomfort, it is hard to gauge an optimum therapy. Either is probably acceptable until the patient is comfortable. Meat tenderizer has been found to be ineffective. Local anesthetics, antihistamines, and steroids are all used to control prolonged symptoms, based on anecdotal experience. Antibiotics are not generally necessary. In the rare cases of cardiovascular collapse, supportive care and principles of treatment of anaphylaxis should be followed. A delayed hypersensitivity reaction can occur 1 to 3 days out, which will almost certainly be self-limited and can be treated with oral antihistamines and topical steroids if symptoms are severe.

Sea bather's itch is a form of jellyfish sting caused by the larvae of the thimble jellyfish. It is characterized by a painful, itchy rash under the edges of the bathing suit or wet suit. It can occasionally progress to a papular rash. Topical steroids can be used to relieve symptoms.

Prevention
Prevention is mostly a matter of common sense. Staying away from the organism (the tentacles can extend several meters from the body of the organism) and staying out of the water when jellyfish are known to be present are the most effective. There is a commercially available product, Safe Sea, which has been shown to reduce the number of nematocyst discharges and thus the severity of the sting should a swimmer need to be in the water when jellyfish are present. Wetsuits and other protective gear are ineffective.

Echinoderms
The Echinoderm family includes sea urchins. Urchins have toxin-coated spines that break off, leaving calcareous material in the wound, which can potentially cause infection. Symptoms include local pain, burning, and local discoloration. The discoloration is thought to be a temporary tattooing of the skin resulting from

dye in the spines; absence of a spine is indicated if the discoloration spontaneously resolves within 48 hours. Theoretically, hot water disables the toxin, although there is no evidence in humans that it is effective. If a spine is present and easily accessible, it should be removed with fingers or forceps. If it is close to a joint or neurovascular structure, it should be surgically removed. If the spines do not cause symptoms, retained pieces will likely reabsorb into the skin.

Stingrays
Although many fish are venomous, stingrays are the most clinically important, accounting for an estimated 1500 mostly minor injuries in the United States annually. These creatures partially bury themselves in the shallow, sandy bottom of the ocean, leading water enthusiasts to accidentally step on them or grab at what they think is a seashell.

Clinical Features
Stingrays have a spine at the base of their tail, which contains a venom gland. The spine, including the venom gland, is broken off and may be left in the resulting wound. The venom has vasoconstrictive properties that can lead to cyanosis and necrosis with poor wound healing and infection. Symptoms can include immediate and intense pain, salivation, nausea, vomiting, diarrhea, muscle cramps, dyspnea, seizures, headaches, and cardiac arrhythmias. Fatalities are rare and mostly a consequence of exsanguination at the scene or penetration of a vital organ.

Treatment
Home care should include rinsing the area thoroughly with fresh water if available (salt water if not) and removing any foreign body. If the damage is minimal, the victim may soak the wound in warm water at home. The victim should watch for signs of infection and seek care for excessive bleeding, retained foreign body, or infection.

For severe wounds that lead the victim to seek medical attention, treatment should include achieving hemostasis followed by submersion of the affected region in hot but not scalding water (42–45 °C, 108–113 °F) for 30 to 90 minutes or until the pain resolves. Spines and stingers are typically radiopaque, so radiographs or an ultrasound should be obtained if a retained spine is suspected. The wound should be thoroughly cleansed, and delayed closure should be allowed. Tetanus immunization status should be reviewed and updated as appropriate. Surgical exploration may be necessary to remove residual foreign bodies. Prophylactic antibiotics are typically not necessary unless there is a residual foreign body or if the patient is immunosuppressed. If the wound becomes infected, *Staphylococcus* and *Streptococcus* species are the most common pathologic organisms. Unique to the marine environment are *Vibrio vulnificus* and *Mycobacterium marinum*, and antibiotic coverage should include coverage for all of these (Table 2).

Other Venomous Sea Creatures
Seasnakes are venomous creatures found most commonly in the Indo-Pacific area. Bites are uncommon (and envenomation is even less common), but should they occur, the toxin is very potent. The care is supportive. There is antivenom, which may be available in areas where the snakes are endemic.

Certain other fish and octopi have been associated with envenomation and occasional death. Most are tropical such as the stonefish, scorpionfish, and rabbitfish and the blue-ringed octopus. Certain varieties of catfish have venom as well. Envenomations are rare, and if they occur, treatment is based on good first-aid principles and antivenom where available (mostly in tropical areas).

Certain cone shells contain a toxin that can be fatal. This toxin is injected by the mollusk into the victim from a proboscis, which it extends from the small end of the cone. Treatment is primarily supportive.

---

[1] Not FDA approved for this indication.

	DOSAGE	
DRUG	**PEDIATRIC**	**ADULT**
Outpatient Management		
Ciprofloxacin (Cipro)[1]	20–30 mg/kg/day PO × 14 d[1]	500 mg PO bid × 14 d
Levofloxin (Levaquin)[1]		750 mg PO qd × 14 d
Doxycycline (Vibramycin, Doryx)[1]	>8 y: 2.2 mg/kg PO qd × 14 d	100 mg bid × 14 d
Inpatient Management		
Preferred		
Ceftazidime (Fortaz, Tazicef)[1] *plus*	150 mg/kg/d q8h	1 g IV q8h
PO or IV quinolone or doxycycline	See outpatient dosing above	See outpatient dosing above
Alternative		
Clindamycin[1] *plus*	25 to 40 mg/kg per day	600 mg IV q 8 hours
PO or IV quinalone or doxycycline	See outpatient dosing	See outpatient dosing

TABLE 2 Antibiotic Choices in Marine Injuries

[1]Not FDA approved for this indication.
Abbreviation: TMP-SMX = trimethoprim-sulfamethoxazole.

Trauma

Abrasions, bites, and lacerations are usually the result of a marine animal's instinct to protect itself against a perceived danger. The most commonly involved marine animals are octopi, sharks, moray eels, and barracuda. The trauma alone creates problems for patients, but the trauma can be further complicated by envenomation. It is often difficult to identify the marine animal involved in the attack. Treatment is for the most part symptomatic, with local cleansing and topical dressing usually sufficing. If the wound becomes infected, antibiotics should cover common organisms (see Table 2).

Environmental Hazards

Abrasions from the ambient environment are also common. These wounds should be thoroughly cleansed with soap and water and a topical antibiotic applied, because the wounds can contain toxins and are commonly contaminated with bacteria. Coral contains nematocysts and also has very sharp edges. Scuba divers in particular suffer from coral cuts in the course of their recreational diving. If these wounds become infected, coverage for *Vibrio* species should be included as well.

Sharks

Although shark attacks receive a lot of publicity, there are only around 50 such attacks worldwide annually and they result in fewer than 10 deaths. The majority of the deaths are in South Africa. Typically these attacks involve the tiger, great white, gray reef, and bull sharks. Attacks occur in shallow water within 100 feet of shore during the evening hours when sharks tend to feed. Common sense dictates avoiding areas where aggressive shark feeding has been noted.

Sequelae of a shark attack range from abrasions to death from hemorrhage. Abrasions and lacerations can occur when sharks brush or aggressively investigate humans. Soft tissue damage, fractures, and neurovascular damage result from such attacks. The majority of attacks result in minor injuries that require simple suturing. Morbidity increases in wounds that are greater than 20 cm or where more than one myofascial compartment is lost. General principles of first aid in marine animal injuries are found in Box 2. Although it would seem self-evident, practices such as urinating on the injury, applying oil or gasoline to injuries, and application of any strong oxidizing agents, such as strong bases or acids, should be counseled against when doing patient education regarding self-care.

BOX 2

Management of Marine Trauma
Remove the victim from the water.
Ensure airway control.
Control bleeding.
Do not remove the wet suit if the victim is wearing one.
Attempt to identify the animal involved in the injury.
If the injury is severe, transport the victim to a hospital.
If envenomation is suspected, consider hot water immersion.
Irrigate the wound with normal saline.
Perform surgical débridement of the wound as appropriate.
If sutures must be placed, place them loosely and allow drainage. Primary suturing should be avoided in puncture wounds, crush injuries, and wounds in the distal extremities.
Start appropriate antibiotics if indicated.

References

Birsa L, Verity P, Lee R: Evaluation of the effects of various chemicals on discharge of and pain caused by jellyfish nematocysts, *Comp Biochem and Physiol Part C: Toxicology & Pharmacology* 151:426–430, 2010.

Centers for Disease Control and Prevention. Vibrio species causing vibrosis. Information for Health Professionals. Available at https://www.cdc.gov/vibrio/healthcare.html (Accessed Februrary 7, 2022).

Edmonds C: Marine animal injuries. In Bove AA, editor: *Bove and Davis' Diving Medicine*, ed 4, Philadelphia, 2004, Saunders, pp 287–318.

Feng C, Teuber S, Gershwin ME: Histamine (scombroid) fish poisoning: a comprehensive review, *Clinic Rev Allerg Immunol* 50:64–69, 2016.

Friedman MA, Fernandez M, Backer LC, et al: An updated review of ciguatera fish poisoning: clinical, epidemiological, environmental, and public health management, *Mar Drugs* 15(3):72, 2017.

Isbister GK: Venomous fish stings in tropical northern Australia, *Am J Emerg Med* 19:561–565, 2001.

Lynch PR, Bove AA: Marine poisonings and intoxications. In Bove AA, editor: *Bove and Davis' Diving Medicine*, ed 4, Philadelphia, 2004, Saunders, pp 287–318.

Petrini B: Mycobacterium marinum: ubiquitous agent of waterborne granulomatous skin infections, *Eur J Clin Microbiol Infect Dis* 25(10):609–613, 2006.

Perkins A, Morgan S: Poisonings, envenomations, and trauma from marine creatures, *Am Fam Physician* 69:885–890, 2004.

Thomas C, Scott SA: *All Stings Considered: First Aid and Medical Treatment of Hawaii's Marine Injuries*, Honolulu, 1997, University of Hawaii Press.

Thomas CS, Scott SA, Galanis DJ, Goto RS: Box jellyfish *Carybdea alata* in Waikiki. The analgesic effect of Sting-Aid, Adolph's meat tenderizer and fresh water on their stings: a double-blinded, randomized, placebo-controlled clinical trial, *Hawaii Med J* 60:205–210, 2001.

MEDICAL TOXICOLOGY

Method of
Howard C. Mofenson, MD; Thomas R. Caraccio, PharmD; Michael McGuigan, MD; Joseph Greensher, MD; Laura Kruger, MD; and Joel J. Heidelbaugh, MD

CURRENT DIAGNOSIS

- Perform initial assessment following Basic Life Support and Advanced Cardiac Life Support principles.
- Primary Survey: Assess airway, breathing, circulation and assess Glasgow Coma Scale Score (GCS).
- Secondary Survey: Assess for injuries that could contribute to or be caused by toxic ingestion including removal of all clothing.
- Initial diagnostic studies should be completed based upon each clinical toxidrome.
- A mnemonic for gathering information is **STATS**:
  - S—substance
  - T—type of formulation
  - A—amount and age
  - T—time of ingestion
  - S—signs and symptoms
- The examiner should attempt to obtain **AMPLE** information about the patient:
  - A—age and allergies
  - M—available medications
  - P—past medical history including pregnancy, psychiatric illnesses, substance abuse, or intentional ingestions
  - L—time of last meal, which may influence absorption and the onset and peak action
  - E—events leading to present condition

CURRENT THERAPY

- Support vital functions including airway, breathing, and circulation with establishing a secure airway, assisted ventilation, intravenous fluids, supplemental oxygen if needed.
- Consider administration of thiamine,[1] glucose (as D50W), and/or naloxone if etiology is unknown.
- Consult your regional Poison Control Center so they can assist with providing the latest management and case-specific recommendations.
- Provide substance-specific management including decontamination and use of antidotes relative to each toxin.

[1]Not FDA approved for this indication.

Introduction

According to the National Poison Data System, in 2022 U.S. Poison Centers responded to over 2 million human exposure cases, resulting in a case of poisoning every 15 seconds on average. The National Poison Data System (NPDS) is the data warehouse for the nation's 55 poison control centers. Each poison center submits de-identified case data to NPDS after providing necessary poison exposure management and information services to callers. Over 24% percent of these cases were reported from a healthcare facility. Over 40% of exposures involved children aged 5 years or younger and the most commonly implicated substance categories were analgesics (11.5%), household cleaning substances (7.2%), antidepressants (5.6%), cosmetics/personal care products (5.2%), and antihistamines (4.8%). The most common substances involved were fentanyl and delta-8 tetrahydrocannabinol. Ninety-three percent of cases occurred in a residence, 76% were unintentional exposures, 19% were intentional exposures, 5% were adverse reactions, and 67% of cases were managed on site where the exposure occurred.

Patients may present with toxic manifestations from medications or illicit substances in the ambulatory care setting including doctor's offices, urgent cares, and emergent care settings. While not exhaustive, this chapter reviews many common elements of medical toxicology to guide clinicians. It is important for clinicians to be aware of clinical manifestations that may suggest toxic ingestion, to stabilize patients, and to know common resources to guide management including local poison control centers and online resources.

Assessment and Maintenance of Vital Functions

Initial assessment of all patients in medical emergencies should follow the principles of Basic and Advanced Cardiac Life Support. These principles include assessing and ensuring adequacy of the patient's airway, degree of ventilation, and circulatory status (ABC's). Vital signs should be measured frequently and should include body core temperature. Level of consciousness should be determined by use of the Glasgow Coma Scale (Table 1). If the patient is comatose, then management requires administering 100% oxygen, establishing vascular access, and obtaining pertinent serologic studies including arterial blood gas (ABG), comprehensive panel, complete blood count with platelets, and serum acetaminophen and salicylate levels, as well as a urine toxicology screen. The administration of glucose, thiamine,[1] and naloxone, as well as intubation to protect the airway, should be considered. An electrocardiogram (ECG), as well as radiography of the chest and abdomen may be useful. The examiner should completely expose the patient by removing clothes and other items that interfere with a full evaluation.

Chest radiographs may be helpful for suspected aspiration pneumonia, pulmonary edema, foreign bodies while abdominal radiographs may detect radiopaque substances.

The mnemonic for radiopaque substances seen on abdominal radiographs is CHIPES:
- C—chlorides and chloral hydrate
- H—heavy metals (e.g., arsenic, barium, iron, lead, mercury, zinc)
- I—iodides
- P—Play-Doh, Pepto-Bismol, phenothiazine (inconsistent)
- E—enteric-coated tablets
- S—sodium, potassium, and other elements in tablet form (e.g., bismuth, calcium, potassium) and solvents containing chlorides (e.g., carbon tetrachloride)

Toxicology Screens

Common urine toxicology screens assay for amphetamines, barbiturates, benzodiazepines, cannabinoids, cocaine, opiates, and phencyclidine including various metabolites. A gas chromatography-mass spectrometry (GCMS) study can more accurately assay for specific drugs, drug metabolites, and toxins; not all drugs may be detected on routine urine toxicology screens due to varying rates of false negative and false positive testing. When a specific drug or toxin is highly suspected, GCMS should be utilized.

Use of Antidotes

Antidotes are available for only a relatively small number of poisons and toxins and should be used in conjunction with appropriate supportive care. Table 2 summarizes commonly used antidotes, their indications, and their methods of administration. Consultation with your regional Poison Control Center can provide further information and education. Table 3 lists common blood chemistry derangements that suggest various common poisonings.

[1]Not FDA approved for this indication.

TABLE 1	Glasgow Coma Scale			
SCALE	**ADULT RESPONSE**	**SCORE**	**PEDIATRIC, 0–1 YEARS**	
Eye opening	Spontaneous	4	Spontaneous	
	To verbal command	3	To shout	
	To pain	2	To pain	
	None	1	No response	
Motor response				
To verbal command	Obeys	6	Localized pain	
To painful stimuli	Localized pain	5	Flexion withdrawal	
	Flexion withdrawal	4	Decorticate flexion	
	Decorticate flexion	3	Decerebrate flexion	
	Decerebrate extension	2	None	
	None	1		
Verbal response: adult	Oriented and converses	5	Cries, smiles, coos	
	Disoriented but converses	4	Cries or screams	
	Inappropriate words	3	Inappropriate sounds	
	Incomprehensible sounds	2	Grunts	
	None	1	Gives no response	
Verbal response: child	Oriented	5		
	Words or babbles	4		
	Vocal sounds	3		
	Cries or moans to stimuli	2		
	None	1		

Data from Teasdale G, Jennett B: Assessment of coma impaired consciousness, *Lancet* 2:83, 1974; Simpson D, Reilly P: Pediatric coma scale, *Lancet* 2:450, 1982; Seidel J: Preparing for pediatric emergencies, *Pediatr Rev* 16:470, 1995.

Approach to the Patient With Suspected Toxic Ingestion Based on Clinical Manifestations

Nervous System Manifestations

Table 4 lists effects of various agents and their central nervous system (CNS) effects. CNS depressants include cholinergic, opioid, sedative-hypnotic, and sympatholytic agents. Signs and symptoms of CNS overdose and intoxication include lethargy, sedation, stupor, and coma. Several key exceptions to those listed in Table 4 include the following: (a) barbiturates may produce an initial tachycardia; (b) convulsions can be produced by codeine, propoxyphene (Darvon),[2] meperidine (Demerol), glutethimide,[2] phenothiazines, methaqualone (Quaalude),[2] and tricyclic and cyclic antidepressants; (c) benzodiazepines rarely produce coma that will interfere with cardiorespiratory functions; and (d) pulmonary edema is common with opioids and sedative-hypnotics. Signs and symptoms of withdrawal from these substances primarily include convulsions and hyperactivity.

Metabolic Abnormalities

Clues From Anion Gap

$$(Na - [Cl + HCO3]) = \text{Anion Gap } (\text{Normal range} = 0 - 12)$$

Table 5 lists common causes of metabolic acidosis, manifested by elevated anion gap. Poisoning from salicylates, methanol, and ethylene glycol cause an increased anion gap, have specific antidotes, and hemodialysis can effectively treat toxic levels. Lactic acidosis can also cause an increased anion gap and may be related to hypoxia, hypoglycemia, infection, and convulsions.

Clues From Serum Osmolal Gap

$$(\text{Sodium} \times 2) + (\text{BUN}/3) + (\text{Glucose}/20)$$
$$(\text{Normal} \leq 10 \text{ mOsm / kg water})$$

Table 6 lists common causes of elevated osmolal gap. Serum osmolality represents the concentration of various solutes in the aqueous phase in plasma. Sodium chloride, sodium bicarbonate, glucose, and urea make up the bulk of solutes in healthy individuals.

Serum osmolality is classically estimated by the following formula:

$$\text{Calculated Serum Osmolality} = (2 \times [Na]) + [\text{glucose, in mg/dL}]/18 + [\text{blood urea nitrogen, in mg/dL}]/2.8$$

or, with SI units (in mmol/L):

$$\text{Calculated Serum Osmolality} = (2 \times [Na]) + [\text{glucose}] + [\text{urea}]$$

If the serum concentration of alcohol or other glycols (acetone, ethanol, ethylene glycol, glycerin, isopropyl alcohol, isoniazid, mannitol, methanol, and trichloroethane) is known, then it may be included in calculation of osmolal gap. Alcohol and glycols may be suspected when additional symptoms are present including vision loss (methanol), metabolic acidosis (methanol and ethylene glycol), or renal failure (ethylene glycol).

A normal osmolal gap may be reported in the presence of toxic alcohol or glycol poisoning if the parent compound is already metabolized. This can occur when the osmolar gap is measured after a significant time has elapsed since the ingestion. In cases of alcohol and glycol intoxication, an early osmolar gap is a result of the relatively nontoxic parent drug and delayed metabolic acidosis, and an anion gap is a result of the more toxic metabolites.

Gastrointestinal Decontamination

Induction of emesis, gastric lavage, and cathartics are no longer routinely recommended. In most cases of toxic ingestion, activated charcoal therapy is the first-line treatment. Oral activated charcoal (single or multidose [MDAC]) adsorbs toxins onto its surface and provides varying levels of absorption depending upon drug or toxin and should be administered within 1 hour of toxic ingestion. Table 7 lists substances that are poorly adsorbed by activated charcoal. Milk, cocoa powder, and ice cream may diminish effectiveness. Contraindications to use of activated charcoal include ingestion of caustics and corrosives, comatose patients prior to securing their airway and patients with absent bowel sounds. The usual initial adult dose is 60 to 100 g and the dose for children is 15 to 30 g. It is administered orally as a slurry mixed with water or by nasogastric or orogastric tube.

---

[2] Not available in the United States.

TABLE 2 Initial Doses of Antidotes for Common Poisonings

ANTIDOTE	USE	DOSE	ROUTE	ADVERSE REACTIONS/COMMENTS
N-Acetyl Cysteine (NAC, Mucomyst): Stock level to treat 70 kg adult for 24 h: 25 vials, 20%, 30 mL	Acetaminophen, carbon tetrachloride (experimental)	Loading dose: 150 mg/kg (max: 15 g) infused over 1 hour. Second dose: 50 mg/kg (max: 5 g) infused over 4 hours. Third dose: 100 mg/kg (max: 10 g) infused over 16 hours.	PO IV	Nausea, vomiting. Dilute to 5% with sweet juice or flat cola. Useful for those who cannot tolerate oral route.
Atropine: Stock level to treat 70 kg adult for 24 h: 1 g (1 mg/mL in 1, 10 mL)	Organophosphate and carbamate pesticides: bradydysrhythmics, β-adrenergics,[1] calcium channel blockers/nerve agents[1]	*Child:* 0.02–0.05 mg/kg repeated q5–10 min to max of 2 mg as necessary until cessation of secretions. *Adult:* 1–2 mg q5–10 min as necessary. Dilute in 1–2 mL of 0.9% saline for ET instillation. *IV infusion dose:* Place 8 mg of atropine in 100 mL D$_5$W or saline. Conc. = 0.08 mg/mL; dose range = 0.02–0.08 mg/kg/h or 0.25–1 mL/kg/h. Severe poisoning may require supplemental doses of IV atropine intermittently in doses of 1–5 mg until drying of secretions occurs.	IV/ET	Tachycardia, dry mouth, blurred vision, and urinary retention. Ensure adequate ventilation before administration.
Calcium Chloride (10%): Stock level to treat 70 kg adult for 24 h: 10 vials 1 g (1.35 mEq/mL)	Hypocalcemia, fluoride,[1] calcium channel blockers,[1] β-blockers,[1] oxalates,[1] ethylene glycol,[1] hypermagnesemia[1]	0.1–0.2 mL/kg (10–20 mg/kg) slow push q10 min up to max 10 mL (1 g). Since calcium response lasts 15 min, some may require continuous infusion 0.2 mL/kg/h up to maximum of 10 mL/h while monitoring for dysrhythmias and hypotension.	IV	Administer slowly with BP and ECG monitoring and have magnesium available to reverse calcium effects. Tissue irritation, hypotension, dysrhythmias from rapid injection. Contraindications: digitalis glycoside intoxication.
Calcium Gluconate (10%): Stock level to treat 70 kg adult for 24 h: 20 vials 1 g (0.45 mEq/mL)	Hypocalcemia, fluoride,[1] calcium channel blockers,[1] hydrofluoric acid;[1] black widow envenomation[1]	0.3–0.4 mL/kg (30–40 mg/kg) slow push; repeat as needed up to max dose 10–20 mL (1–2 g).	IV	Same comments as calcium chloride.
Infiltration of Calcium Gluconate	Hydrofluoric acid skin exposure[1]	Dose: Infiltrate each square cm of affected dermis/subcutaneous tissue with about 0.5 mL of 10% calcium gluconate using a 30-gauge needle. Repeat as needed to control pain.	Infiltrate	
Intra-arterial Calcium Gluconate	Hydrofluoric acid skin exposure[1]	Infuse 20 mL of 10% calcium gluconate (not chloride) diluted in 250 mL D$_5$W via the radial or brachial artery proximal to the injury over 3–4 h.		Alternatively, dilute 10 mL of 10% calcium gluconate with 40–50 mL of D$_5$W.
Calcium Gluconate Gel (Calgonate): Stock level: 3.5 g	Hydrofluoric acid skin exposure	2.5 g USP powder added to 100 mL water-soluble lubricating jelly, e.g., K-Y jelly or Lubifax (or 3.5 mg into 150 mL). Some use 6 g of calcium carbonate in 100 g of lubricant. Place injured hand in surgical glove filled with gel. Apply q4h. If pain persists, calcium gluconate injection may be needed (above).	Dermal	Powder is available from Spectrum Pharmaceutical Co. in California: 800-772-8786. Commercial preparation of Ca gluconate gel is available from Pharmascience in Montreal, Quebec: 514-340-1114.

Continued

TABLE 2 Initial Doses of Antidotes for Common Poisonings—cont'd

ANTIDOTE	USE	DOSE	ROUTE	ADVERSE REACTIONS/COMMENTS
Cyanide Antidote Kit: Stock level to treat 70 kg adult for 24 h: 2 Lilly Cyanide Antidote kits	Cyanide Hydrogen sulfide (nitrites are given only) Do not use sodium thiosulfate for hydrogen sulfide Individual portions of the kit can be used in certain circumstances (consult PCC)	Amyl nitrite: 1 crushable ampule for 30 sec of every min. Use new amp q3 min. May omit step if venous access is established.	Inhalation	If methemoglobinemia occurs, do not use methylene blue to correct this because it releases cyanide.
	Cyanide Hydrogen sulfide (nitrites are given only) Do not use sodium thiosulfate for hydrogen sulfide Individual portions of the kit can be used in certain circumstances (consult PCC)	Sodium nitrite: *Child:* 0.6 mg/kg (0.2 mL/kg) of 3% IV solution if hemoglobin level is not known, otherwise based on tables with product. *Adult:* up to 300 mg (10 mL). Dilute nitrite in 100 mL 0.9% saline, administer slowly at 5 mL/min. Slow infusion if fall in BP.	IV	If methemoglobinemia occurs, do not use methylene blue to correct this because it releases cyanide.
	Do not use sodium thiosulfate for hydrogen sulfide Individual portions of the kit can be used in certain circumstances (consult PCC)	Sodium thiosulfate: *Child:* 1.6 mL/kg of 25% solution, may be repeated q30–60 min to a maximum of 12.5 g or 50 mL in adult. Administer over 20 min.	IV	Nausea, dizziness, headache. Tachycardia, muscle rigidity, and bronchospasm (rapid administration).
Dantrolene Sodium (Dantrium): Stock level to treat 70 kg adult for 24 h: 700 mg, 35 vials (20 mg/vial)	Malignant hyperthermia	2–3 mg/kg IV rapidly. Repeat loading dose every 10 min. If necessary up to a maximum total dose of 10 mg/kg. When temperature and heart rate decrease, slow the infusion 1–2 mg/kg q6h for 24–28 h until all evidence of malignant hyperthermia syndrome has subsided. Follow with oral doses 1–2 mg/kg four times a day for 24 h as necessary.	IV/PO	Hepatotoxicity occurs with cumulative dose of 10 mg/kg. Thrombophlebitis (best given in central line). Available as 20 mg lyophilized dantrolene powder for reconstruction, which contains 3 g mannitol and sodium hydroxide in 70-mL vial. Mix with 60 mL sterile distilled water without a bacteriostatic agent and protect from light. Use within 6 hours after reconstituting.
Deferoxamine (Desferal): Stock level to treat 70 kg adult for 24 h: 17 vials (500 mg/amp)	Iron	IV infusion of 15 mg/kg/h (3 mL/kg/h: 500 mg in 100 mL D₅W) max 6 g/d Rates of >45 mg/kg/h[3] if conc >1000 μg/dL.	Preferred IV: avoid therapy >24 h	Hypotension (minimized by avoiding rapid infusion rates) DFO challenge test 50 mg/kg is unreliable if negative.
Diazepam (Valium): Stock level to treat 70 kg adult for 24 h: 200 mg, 5 mg/mL; 2, 10 mL	Any intoxication that provokes seizures when specific therapy is not available (e.g., amphetamines, PCP, barbiturate and alcohol withdrawal) Chloroquine poisoning[1]	*Adult,* 5–10 mg IV (max 20 mg) at a rate of 5 mg/min until seizure is controlled. May be repeated 2 or 3 times. *Child,* 0.1–0.3 mg/kg up to 10 mg IV slowly over 2 min.	IV	Confusion, somnolence, coma, hypotension. Intramuscular absorption is erratic. Establish airway and administer 100% oxygen and glucose.

TABLE 2 Initial Doses of Antidotes for Common Poisonings—cont'd

ANTIDOTE	USE	DOSE	ROUTE	ADVERSE REACTIONS/COMMENTS
Digoxin-Specific Fab Antibodies (DigiFab, Digibind): Stock level to treat 70 kg adult for 24 h: 20 vials	Digoxin, digitoxin, oleander tea[1] with the following: 1. Imminent cardiac arrest or shock 2. Hyperkalemia >5.0 mEq/L 3. Serum digoxin >5 ng/mL (child) at 8–12 h post ingestion in adults 4. Digitalis delirium 5. Ingestion over 10 mg in adults or 4 mg in child 6. Bradycardia or second- or third-degree heart block unresponsive to atropine 7. Life-threatening digitoxin or oleander poisoning[1]	1. If amount ingested is known total dose × bioavailability (0.8) = body burden. The body burden + 0.6 (0.5 mg of digoxin is bound by 1 vial of 40 mg of Fab) = # vials needed. 2. If amount is unknown but the steady state serum concentration is known in ng/mL: Digoxin: ng/mL: (5.6 L/kg Vd) × (wt kg) = µg body burden. Body burden + 100 = mg body burden/0.5 = # vials needed. Digitoxin body burden = ng/mL × (0.56 L/kg Vd) × (wt kg) Body burden + 1000 = mg body burden/0.5 = # vials needed. 3. If the amount is not known, it is administered in life-threatening situations as 10 vials (400 mg) IV in saline over 30 min in adults. If cardiac arrest is imminent, administer 20 vials (adult) as a bolus.	IV	Allergic reactions (rare), return of condition being treated with digitalis glycoside. Administer by infusion over 30 min through a 0.22-µ filter. If cardiac arrest imminent, may administer by bolus. Consult PCC for more details.
Dimercaprol (BAL in Peanut Oil): Stock level to treat 70 kg adult for 24 h: 1200 mg (4 amps—100 mg/mL 10% in oil in 3 mL amp)	Chelating agent for arsenic, mercury, and lead	3–5 mg/kg q4h usually for 5–10 d	Deep IM	Local infection site pain and sterile abscess, nausea, vomiting, fever, salivation, hypertension, and nephrotoxicity (alkalinize urine).
2,3 Dimercaptosuccinic Acid (DMSA succimer [Chemet]): 100 mg/capsule: 20 capsules	Used as a chelating agent for lead, especially blood lead levels >45 µg/dL. May also be used for symptomatic mercury exposure[1]	10 mg/kg 3 × daily for 5 days followed by 10 mg/kg 2 × daily for 14 days	PO	Precautions: monitor AST/ALT; use with caution in G6PD-deficient patients. Avoid concurrent iron therapy. Relatively safe antidote, rarely severe, uncommon minor skin rashes may occur.
Diphenhydramine (Benadryl): Antiparkinsonian action. Stock level to treat a 70 kg adult for 24 h: 5 vials (10 mg/mL, 10 mL each)	Used to treat extrapyramidal symptoms and dystonia induced by phenothiazines, phencyclidine, and related drugs	Children: 1–2 mg/kg IV slowly over 5 min up to maximum 50 mg followed by 5 mg/kg/24 h orally divided every 6 h up to 300 mg/24 h Adults: 50 mg IV followed by 50 mg orally four times daily for 5–7 d. Note: Symptoms abate within 2–5 min after IV.	IV	Fatal dose: 20–40 mg/kg. Dry mouth, drowsiness.
Ethanol (Ethyl Alcohol): Stock level to treat 70 kg adult for 24 h: 3 bottles 10% (1 L each)	Methanol,[1] ethylene glycol[1]	10 mL/kg loading dose concurrently with 1.4 mL/kg (average) infusion of 10% ethanol (consult PCC for more details)	IV	Nausea, vomiting, sedation. Use 0.22-µ filter if preparing from bulk 100% ethanol.
Flumazenil (Romazicon): Stock level to treat 70 kg adult for 24 h: 4 vials (0.1 mg/mL, 10 mL)	Benzodiazepines (may also be beneficial in the treatment of hepatic encephalopathy[1])	Administer 0.2 mg (2 mL) IV over 30 sec (pediatric dose not established, 0.01 mg/kg), then wait 3 min for a response, then if desired consciousness is not achieved, administer 0.3 mg (3 mL) over 30 sec, then wait 3 min for response, then if desired consciousness is not achieved, administer 0.5 mg (5 mL) over 30 sec at 60-sec intervals up to a maximum cumulative dose of 3 mg (30 mL) (1 mg in children). Because effects last only 1–5 h, if patient responds, monitor carefully over next 6 h for resedation. If multiple repeated doses, consider a continuous infusion of 0.2–1 mg/h.	IV	Nausea, vomiting, facial flushing, agitation, headache, dizziness, seizures, and death. It is not recommended to improve ventilation. Its role in CNS depression needs to be clarified. It should not be used routinely in comatose patients. It is contraindicated in cyclic antidepressant intoxications, stimulant overdose, long-term benzodiazepine use (may precipitate life-threatening withdrawal), if benzodiazepines are used to control seizures, in head trauma.

Continued

TABLE 2   Initial Doses of Antidotes for Common Poisonings—cont'd

ANTIDOTE	USE	DOSE	ROUTE	ADVERSE REACTIONS/COMMENTS
Folic Acid (Folvite): Stock level to treat 70 kg adult for 24 h: 4 100-mg vials	Methanol/ethylene glycol (investigational)	1 mg/kg up to 50 mg q4h for 6 doses	IV	Uncommon
Fomepizole (4-MP, Antizol): Stock level to treat 70 kg adult: 4 1.5-mL vials (1 g/mL)	Ethylene glycol	Loading dose: 15 mg/kg (0.015 mL/kg) IV followed by maintenance dose of 10 mg/kg (0.01 mL/kg) q12h for 4 doses, then 15 mg/kg q12h until ethylene glycol levels are <20 mg/dL. Fomepizole can be given to patients undergoing hemodialysis (dose q4h).	IV	Suggested: co-administer folate 50 mg IV (child 1 mg/kg), thiamine 100 mg/d (child 50 mg), and pyridoxine 50 mg IV/IM q6h until intoxication is resolved. Monitor for urinary oxalate crystals. Adverse reactions include headache, nausea, and dizziness. Antizol should be diluted in 100 mL 0.9% saline or D_5W and mixed well. Antizol should not be given undiluted.
	Methanol			
Glucagon: Stock level to treat 70 kg adult for 24 h: 10 vials, 10 units	β-Blocker,[1] calcium channel blocker[1]	3–10 mg in adult, then infuse 2–5 mg/h (0.05–0.1 mg/kg in child, then infuse 0.07 mg/kg/h) Large doses up to 100 mg/24 h used	IV	Use D_5W, not 0.9% saline, to reconstitute the glucagon (rather than diluent of Eli Lilly, which contains phenol). Vomiting precautions.
Magnesium Sulfate: Stock level to treat 70 kg adult for 24 h: approx 25 g (50 mL of 50% or 200 mL of 12.5%)	Torsades de pointes[1]	Adult: 2 g (20 mL or 20%) over 20 min. If no response in 10 min, repeat and follow by continuous infusion 1 g/h. Children: 25–50 mg/kg initially and maintenance is 30–60 mg/kg/24 h (0.25–0.5 mEq/kg/24 h) up to 1000 mg/24 h. (Dose not studied in controlled fashion.)	IV	Use with caution if renal impairment is present.
Methylene Blue: Stock level to treat 70 kg adult for 24 h: 5 amps (1%, 10 mg/10 mL)	Methemoglobinemia	0.1–0.2 mL/kg of 1% solution, slow infusion, may be repeated q30–60 min	IV	Nausea, vomiting, headache, dizziness.
Naloxone (Narcan): Stock level to treat 70 kg adult for 24 h: 3 vials (1 mg/mL, 10 mL)	Comatose patient; decreased respirations <12;[1] opioids	In postoperative opioid depression reversal, IV 0.1–0.5 µg/kg c2 min as needed and may repeat up to a total dose of 1 µg/kg In suspected overdose, administer IV 0.1 mg/kg in a child younger than 5 years of age up to 2 mg; in older children and adults administer 2 mg every 2 min up to a total of 10–20 mg. Can also be administered into the endotracheal tube. If no response by 10 mg, a pure opioid intoxication is unlikely. If opioid abuse is suspected, restraints should be in place before administration; initial dose 0.1 mg to avoid withdrawal and violent behavior. The initial dose is then doubled every minute progressively to a total of 10 mg. A continuous infusion has been advocated because many opioids outlast the short half-life of naloxone (30–60 min). The naloxone infusion hourly rate to produce a response is equal to the effective dose required (improvement in ventilation and arousal). An additional dose may be required in 15–30 min as a bolus.	IV, ET	Larger doses of naloxone may be required for more poorly antagonized synthetic opioid drugs: buprenorphine (Buprenex), codeine, dextromethorphan, fentanyl, pentazocine (Talwin), propoxyphene (Darvon),[2] diphenoxylate, nalbuphine (Nubain), new potent "designer" drugs, or long-acting opioids such as methadone (Dolophine). Complications. Although naloxone is safe and effective, there are rare reports of complications (<1%) of pulmonary edema, seizures, hypertension, cardiac arrest, and sudden death. The infusions are titrated to avoid respiratory depression and opioid withdrawal manifestations. Tapering of infusions can be attempted after 12 h and when the patient is stable.
Physostigmine (Antilirium): Stock level to treat 70 kg adult for 24 h: 2–4 mg (2 mL each)	Anticholinergic agents (not routinely used, only indicated if life-threatening complications)	Child: 0.02 mg/kg slow push to max 2 mg q30–60 min Adult: 1–2 mg q5 min to max 6 mg.	IV	Bradycardia, asystole, seizures, bronchospasm, vomiting, headaches. Do not use for cyclic antidepressants.

TABLE 2 Initial Doses of Antidotes for Common Poisonings—cont'd

ANTIDOTE	USE	DOSE	ROUTE	ADVERSE REACTIONS/COMMENTS
Pralidoxime (2PAM, Protopam): Stock level to treat 70 kg adult for 24 h: 12 vials (1 g per 20 mL)	Organophosphates/nerve agents	Child ≤12 y, 25–50 mg/kg max (4 mg/min); >12 y, 1–2 g/dose in 250 mL of 0.9% saline over 5–10 min. Max 200 mg/min. Repeat q6–12h for 24–48h. Max adult 6 g/d. Alternative: Maintenance infusion 1 g in 100 mL, of 0.9% saline at 5–20 mg/kg/h (0.5–12 mL/kg/h) up to max 500 mg/h or 50 mL/h. Titrate to desired response. End point is absence of fasciculations and return of muscle strength.	IV	Nausea, dizziness, headache; tachycardia, muscle rigidity, bronchospasm (rapid administration).
Pyridoxine (Vitamin B6): Stock level to treat 70 kg adult for 24 h: 100 mg/mL 10% solution. For a 70 kg patient, 10 g = 10 vials	Seizures from isoniazid[1] or *Gyromitra* mushrooms,[1] ethylene glycol[1]	*Isoniazid: Unknown amount ingested:* 5 g (70 mg/kg) in 50 mL D₅W over 5 min + diazepam 0.3 mg/kg IV at rate of 1 mg/min in child or 10 mg dose at rate up to 5 mg/min in adults. Use different site (synergism). May repeat q5–20 min until seizure controlled. Up to 375 mg/kg have been given (52 g). *Known amount:* 1 g for each gram isoniazid ingested over 5 min with diazepam (dose above). *Gyromitra mushroom:* Child 25 mg/kg or 2–5 g, adults IV over 15–30 min to max 20 g	IV	After seizure is controlled, administer remainder of pyridoxine 1 g/1 g isoniazid total 5 g as infusion over 60 min. Adverse reactions uncommon; do not administer in same bottle as sodium bicarbonate. For *Gyromitra* mushrooms, some use PO 25 mg/kg/d early when mushroom ingestion is suspected.
Sodium Bicarbonate (NaHCO3): Stock level to treat 70 kg adult for 24 h: 10 ampules or syringes (500 mEq)	Tricyclic antidepressant cardiotoxicity (QRS >0.12 sec;[1] ventricular tachycardia,[1] severe conduction disturbances[1]); metabolic acidosis; phenothiazine toxicity[1] *Salicylate:* to keep blood pH 7.5–7.55 (not >7.55) and urine pH 7.5–8.0. Alkalinization recommended if salicylate conc. >40 mg/dL in acute poisoning and at lower levels if symptomatic in chronic intoxication, 2 mEq/kg will raise blood pH 0.1 unit	*Ethylene glycol:* 100 mg IV daily. 1–2 mEq/kg undiluted as a bolus. If no effect on cardiotoxicity, repeat twice a few minutes apart *Adult* with clear physical signs and laboratory findings of acute moderate or severe salicylism: Bolus 1–2 mEq/kg followed by infusion of 100–150 mEq NaHCO₃ added to 1 L of 5% dextrose at rate of 200–300 mL/h *Child:* Bolus same as adult followed by 1–2 mEq/kg in infusion of 20 mL/kg 5% dextrose in 0.45% saline Add potassium when patient voids Rate and amount of the initial infusion, if patient is volume depleted: 1 h to achieve urine output of 2 mL/kg/h and urine pH 7–8 In mild cases without acidosis and urine pH >6, administer 5% dextrose in 0.9% saline with 50 mEq/L or 1 mEq/kg NaHCO₃ as maintenance to replace ongoing renal losses. If acidemia is present and pH <7.2, add 2 mEq/kg as loading dose followed by 2 mEq/kg q3–4h to keep pH at 7.5–7.55. If acidemia is present, recommend isotonic NaHCO₃, 3 ampules to 1 L of D₅W at 10–15 mL/kg/h or sufficient to produce normal urine flow and a urine pH of 7.5 or higher	IV	Monitor sodium, potassium, and blood pH because fatal alkalemia and hyponatremia have been reported. Monitor both urine and blood pH. Do not use the urine pH alone to assess the need for alkalinization because of the paradoxical aciduria that may occur. Adjust the urine pH to 7.5–8 by NaHCO₃ infusion. After urine output established, add potassium 40 mEq/L.
	Long-acting barbiturates[1]: Phenobarbital and primidone (Mysoline). *Note:* Alkalinization is ineffective for the short- or intermediate-acting barbiturates	NaHCO₃: 2 mEq/kg during the first hour or 100 mEq in 1 L of D₅W with 40 mEq/L potassium at a rate of 100 mL/h in adults Adequate potassium is necessary to accomplish alkalinization	IV	Additional sodium bicarbonate and potassium chloride may be needed. Adjust the urine pH to 7.5–8 by NaHCO₃ infusion.
Thiamine: 100 mg/mL, 2 vials	Thiamine deficiency, ethylene glycol poisoning,[1] alcoholism	100 mg IV followed with 100 mg IV/IM for 5–7 days in an alcoholic and followed by 100 mg/d orally	IV/IM	
Vitamin K1 (Aqua Mephyton): 10 mg/1–5 mL; 5-mg tablets	Warfarin anticoagulant or rodenticide toxicity	Usual dose for adults: 1–5 mg PO Usual dose for adults with evidence of bleeding: 2.5–10 mg in combination with 4-factor prothrombin complex concentrate For children without bleeding: 0.03 mg/kg/dose PO For children with significant bleeding: 0.5–5 mg SQ or IV in combination with fresh frozen plasma or 4-factor prothrombin complex concentrate	PO/SC, IV	Give vitamin K daily until PT/INR are normal. Examine stools and urine for evidence of bleeding.

[1]Not FDA approved for this indication.

[2]Not available in the United States.

[3]Exceeds dosage recommended by the manufacturer.

Abbreviations: ALT = alanine aminotransferase; AST = aspartate aminotransferase; amp = ampule; BAL = British anti-Lewisite; BP = blood pressure; conc. = concentration; ECG = electrocardiogram; ET = endotracheal; G6PD = glucose-6-phosphate dehydrogenase; IM = intramuscular; IV = intravenous; PCC = poison control center; PO = oral; PT = prothrombin time; SC = subcutaneous.

TABLE 3 Blood Chemistry Derangements in Toxicology

DERANGEMENT	TOXIN
Acetonemia without acidosis	Acetone or isopropyl alcohol
Hypomagnesemia	Ethanol, digitalis
Hypocalcemia	Ethylene glycol, oxalate, fluoride
Hyperkalemia	β-Blockers, acute digitalis, renal failure
Hypokalemia	Diuretics, salicylism, sympathomimetics, theophylline, corticosteroids, chronic digitalis
Hyperglycemia	Diazoxide, glucagon, iron, isoniazid, organophosphate insecticides, phenylurea insecticides, phenytoin (Dilantin), salicylates, sympathomimetic agents, thyroid vasopressors
Hypoglycemia	β-Blockers, ethanol, insulin, isoniazid, oral hypoglycemic agents, salicylates
Rhabdomyolysis	Amphetamines, ethanol, cocaine, or phencyclidine, elevated creatine phosphokinase

Although repeated dosing with activated charcoal may decrease the half-life and increase the clearance of phenobarbital, dapsone, quinidine, theophylline, and carbamazepine (Tegretol), recent guidelines indicate there is insufficient evidence to support the use of multidose activated charcoal (MDAC) unless a life-threatening amount of one of the substances mentioned is involved. Complications of administration of activated charcoal include vomiting, desorption, and aspiration. Repeated doses of activated charcoal have been associated with pulmonary aspiration, intestinal obstruction or pseudo-obstruction, empyema following esophageal perforation, hypermagnesemia, and hypernatremia.

Whole bowel irrigation with polyethylene glycol (PEG) with electrolytes (e.g., GoLYTELY or Colyte) are used to promote passage of toxins through the gastrointestinal (GI) tract without causing electrolytes disturbances, yet it is not FDA-approved for this indication. Typically, solution is administered orally or via nasogastric tube at a rate of 0.5 L per hour in children less than 5 years old and 2 L per hour in adolescents and adults for 5 hours. The procedure is complete when stools are clear or radiopaque materials are no longer seen on abdominal radiographs. Whole bowel irrigation is contraindicated in cases of hematemesis, ileus, bowel obstruction, perforation, or peritonitis. Whole bowel irrigation can reduce effectiveness of activated charcoal. In cases where bowel irrigation is ineffective and bezoars or foreign bodies (such as body-packers) are present, they may be removed surgically or endoscopically.

TABLE 4 Agents With Central Nervous System (CNS) Effects

AGENTS	GENERAL MANIFESTATIONS	AGENTS	GENERAL MANIFESTATIONS
CNS Depressants		**Hallucinogens**	
Alcohols and glycols (S-H)	Bradycardia	Amphetamines‡	Tachycardia and dysrhythmias
Anticonvulsants (S-H)	Bradypnea	Anticholinergics	Tachypnea
Antidysrhythmics (S-H)	Shallow respirations	Cardiac glycosides	Hypertension
Antihypertensives (S-H)	Hypotension	Cocaine	Hallucinations, usually visual
Barbiturates (S-H)	Hypothermia	Ethanol withdrawal	Disorientation
Benzodiazepines (S-H)	Flaccid coma	Hydrocarbon inhalation (abuse)	Panic reaction
Butyrophenones (Syly)	Miosis	Mescaline (peyote)	Toxic psychosis
β-Adrenergic blockers (Syly)	Hypoactive bowel sounds	Mushrooms (psilocybin)	Moist skin
Calcium channel blockers (Syly)		Phencyclidine	Mydriasis (reactive)
Digitalis (Syly)			Hyperthermia
Opioids			Flashbacks
Lithium (mixed)			
Muscle relaxants			
Phenothiazines (Syly)		**Anticholinergics**	
Nonbarbiturate/benzodiazepine glutethimide, methaqualone, methyprylon, sedative-hypnotics (chloral hydrate, ethchlorvynol, bromide)		Antihistamines	Tachycardia, dysrhythmias (rare)
		Antispasmodic gastrointestinal preparations	Tachypnea
		Antiparkinsonian preparations	Hypertension (mild)
		Atropine	Hyperthermia
Tricyclic antidepressants (late Syly)		Cyclobenzaprine (Flexeril)	Hallucinations ("mad as a hatter")
		Mydriatic ophthalmologic agents	Mydriasis (unreactive) ("blind as a bat")
CNS Stimulants		**Over-the-counter sleep agents**	
Amphetamines (Sy)	Tachycardia	Plants (Datura spp.)/mushrooms	Flushed skin ("red as a beet")
Anticholinergics*	Tachypnea and dysrhythmias		Dry skin and mouth ("dry as a bone")
Cocaine (Sy)	Hypertension	Phenothiazines (early)	Hypoactive bowel sounds
Camphor (mixed)	Convulsions	Scopolamine	Urinary retention

TABLE 4 Agents with Central Nervous System (CNS) Effects—cont'd

AGENTS	GENERAL MANIFESTATIONS	AGENTS	GENERAL MANIFESTATIONS
Ergot alkaloids (Sy)	Toxic psychosis	Tricyclic/cyclic antidepressants (early)	Lilliputian hallucinations ("little people")
Isoniazid (mixed)	Mydriasis (reactive)		
Lithium (mixed)	Agitation and restlessness	**Cholinergics**	
Lysergic acid diethylamide (H)	Moist skin	Bethanechol (Urecholine)	Bradycardia (muscarinic)
Hallucinogens (H)	Tremors	Carbamate insecticides (Carbaryl)	Tachycardia (nicotinic effect)
Mescaline and synthetic analogues		Edrophonium	Miosis (muscarinic)
Metals (arsenic, lead, mercury)		Organophosphate insecticides (Malathion, parathion)	Diarrhea (muscarinic)
Methylphenidate (Ritalin) (Sy)		Parasympathetic agents (physostigmine, pyridostigmine)	Hypertension (variable)
Monoamine oxidase inhibitors (Sy)		Toxic mushrooms (*Clitocybe* spp.)	Hyperactive bowel sounds
Pemoline (Cylert) (Sy)			Excess urination (muscarinic)
Phencyclidine (H)‡			Excess salivation (muscarinic)
Salicylates (mixed)			Lacrimation (muscarinic)
Strychnine (mixed)			Bronchospasm (muscarinic)
Sympathomimetics (Sy) (phenylpropanolamine, theophylline, caffeine, thyroid)			Muscle fasciculations (nicotinic)
			Paralysis (nicotinic)
Withdrawal from ethanol, β-adrenergic blockers, clonidine, opioids, sedative–hypnotics (W)			

*Anticholinergics produce dry skin and mucosa and decreased bowel sounds.
‡Phencyclidine may produce miosis.
‡The amphetamine hybrids are methylene dioxymethamphetamine (MDMA, ecstasy, "Adam") and methylene dioxyamphetamine (MDA, "Eve"), which are associated with deaths.
Abbreviations: H = hallucinogen; S-H = sedative–hypnotic; Sy = sympathomimetic; Syly = sympatholytic; W = withdrawal.

TABLE 5 Etiologies of Metabolic Acidosis

NORMAL ANION GAP HYPERCHLOREMIC	INCREASED ANION GAP NORMOCHLOREMIC	DECREASED ANION GAP
Acidifying agents	Methanol	Laboratory error†
Adrenal insufficiency	Uremia*	Intoxication—bromine, lithium
Anhydrase inhibitors	Diabetic ketoacidosis*	Protein abnormal
Fistula	Paraldehyde,* phenformin	Sodium low
Osteotomies	Isoniazid	
Obstructive uropathies	Iron	
Renal tubular acidosis	Lactic acidosis†	
Diarrhea, uncomplicated*	Ethanol,* ethylene glycol*	
Dilutional	Salicylates, starvation solvents	
Sulfamylon		

*Indicates hyperosmolar situation. Studies have found that the anion gap may be relatively insensitive for determining the presence of toxins.
†Lactic acidosis can be produced by intoxications of the following: carbon monoxide, cyanide, hydrogen sulfide, hypoxia, ibuprofen, iron, isoniazid, phenformin, salicylates, seizures, theophylline.

TABLE 6	Etiologies of Osmolal Gap

- Ethylene glycol ingestion
- Methanol ingestion
- Ethanol or isopropyl alcohol ingestion
- End-stage renal disease without regular dialysis
- Ketoacidosis (diabetic or alcoholic)
- Lactic acidosis
- Formaldehyde ingestion
- Paraldehyde ingestion
- Diethyl ether ingestion
- Infusion of nonconductive glycine, sorbitol, or mannitol solutions
- Severe hyperproteinemia
- Severe hyperlipidemia

TABLE 7	Toxins Poorly Absorbed by Activated Charcoal

C	Caustics and corrosives
H	Heavy metals (arsenic, iron, lead, mercury)
A	Alcohols (ethanol, methanol, isopropanol) and glycols (ethylene glycols)
R	Rapid onset of absorption (cyanide and strychnine)
C	Chlorine and iodine
O	Others insoluble in water (substances in tablet form)
A	Aliphatic hydrocarbons (petroleum distillates)
L	Laxatives (sodium, magnesium, potassium, and lithium)

Enhancement of Elimination

Several methods for elimination include dialysis, hemoperfusion, exchange transfusion, plasmapheresis, enzyme induction, and inhibition. These methods should be reserved for life-threatening cases where definite benefit is expected. Hemodialysis and hemoperfusion should be considered in cases where a potentially lethal amount of a compound was ingested, and rapid removal may improve prognosis. Examples include ethylene glycol 1.4 mL/kg 100% solution and methanol 6 mL/kg 100% solution. Dialyzable substances include alcohol, bromides, ethylene glycol, lithium, methanol, and salicylates.

Dialysis should be considered when there is (a) anticipated prolonged coma and the likelihood of complications; (b) renal compromise (toxin excreted or metabolized by kidneys and dialyzable chelating agents in heavy metal poisoning); (c) laboratory confirmation of lethal blood concentration; (d) lethal dose poisoning with an agent with delayed toxicity or known to be metabolized into a more toxic metabolite (e.g., ethylene glycol, methanol); and (e) hepatic impairment when the agent is metabolized by the liver, and clinical deterioration despite optimal supportive medical management.

Hemoperfusion has been shown to be effective in treating glutethimide, phenobarbital, carbamazepine, phenytoin, and theophylline intoxication. The patient-related criteria for hemoperfusion are (a) anticipated prolonged coma and the likelihood of complications; (b) laboratory confirmation of lethal blood concentrations; (c) hepatic impairment when an agent is metabolized by the liver; and (d) clinical deterioration despite optimally supportive medical management.

Treatment and Monitoring Based Upon Toxin
Acetaminophen
Toxic Dose

A single dose of acetaminophen greater than 150 mg/kg in a child or greater than 7.5–10 g for an adult increases the risk of toxicity. Toxicity is likely for single ingestions greater than 250 mg/kg or greater than 12 g over 24 hours. P450 enzyme inducers including barbiturates, phenytoin (Dilantin), isoniazid, and chronic alcohol use can increase toxicity of acetaminophen. Chronic alcohol use, moderate to severe protein-calorie malnutrition, and human

immunodeficiency virus (HIV) infection can deplete glutathione stores and increase toxicity of acetaminophen. Acetaminophen reaches peak plasma concentrations 2 to 4 hours after an overdose. The half-life of acetaminophen is 1 to 3 hours.

Manifestations

The four phases of the intoxication's clinical course may overlap, and the absence of a phase does not exclude toxicity.
- Phase I occurs within 0.5 to 24 hours after ingestion and may consist of a few hours of malaise, diaphoresis, nausea, and vomiting or produce no symptoms.
- Phase II occurs 24 to 48 hours after ingestion and is a period of diminished symptoms. Serum aspartate aminotransferase (AST) (earliest), and serum alanine aminotransferase (ALT) may increase as early as 4 hours or as late as 36 hours after ingestion.
- Phase III occurs at 48 to 96 hours, with peak liver function abnormalities at 72 to 96 hours. The degree of elevation of the hepatic enzymes generally often correlates with outcome. Recovery begins at approximately 4 days after ingestion unless hepatic failure develops. Less than 1% of patients with a history of overdose develop fulminant hepatotoxicity.
- Phase IV occurs at 4 to 14 days, with hepatic enzyme abnormalities resolving. If extensive liver damage has occurred, sepsis and disseminated intravascular coagulation may ensue. Transient renal failure may develop at 5 to 7 days with or without evidence of hepatic damage. If transaminases do not adequately decline or resolve to normal within this period, consideration of hepatic transplantation is warranted due to significant mortality risk.

Lab Investigations

Serum acetaminophen level, as followed by the Rumack-Matthew nomogram (Figure 1), should be followed longitudinally. If a toxic level is reached, then comprehensive panel, complete blood count with platelets, prothrombin time with international normalized ratio, ECG, and urinalysis should be obtained.

Management

Activated charcoal should be useful within 1 hour of ingestion as ipecac and gastric lavage are no longer recommended. Administration should be separated from administration of N-acetylcysteine (NAC) by 1-2 hours to prevent vomiting and enhance adsorption. Oral or IV NAC should be administered within the first 8 hours after toxic acetaminophen ingestion and can be started while awaiting serum acetaminophen concentration levels, yet there is no advantage to giving it prior to 8 hours. If the acetaminophen level is above the upper line on the nomogram (Figure 1), then maintenance NAC should be continued. Repeat acetaminophen level should be obtained 4 hours after the initial level if the initial level was >20 mg/mL because the peak level may be delayed by food or other ingestions. Extended-release formulations may also delay peak acetaminophen level and repeat levels should be obtained every 4 hours until peak.

In patients with chronic alcohol use, NAC should be administered when acetaminophen level is 50% below the upper toxic line on the nomogram or higher. If emesis occurs within 1 hour after oral NAC administration, then the dose should be repeated. Oral NAC should be diluted from 20% to 5% and served in a palatal solution. If this is unsuccessful, it may be administered over 30 to 60 minutes via nasogastric tube. NAC is less effective if initiated 8 to 10 hours post ingestion, but this loss of efficacy is not complete and there may be benefit to administration of NAC up to 36 hours or more after ingestion. Late treatment initiated 24 hours or more after ingestion decreases morbidity and mortality in patients with fulminant liver failure.

Disposition

Disposition depends on development and management of end-organ damage and need for ongoing psychiatric care. Patients should be evaluated for possible intentional overdose and may require psychiatric evaluation and/or psychiatric hospitalization.

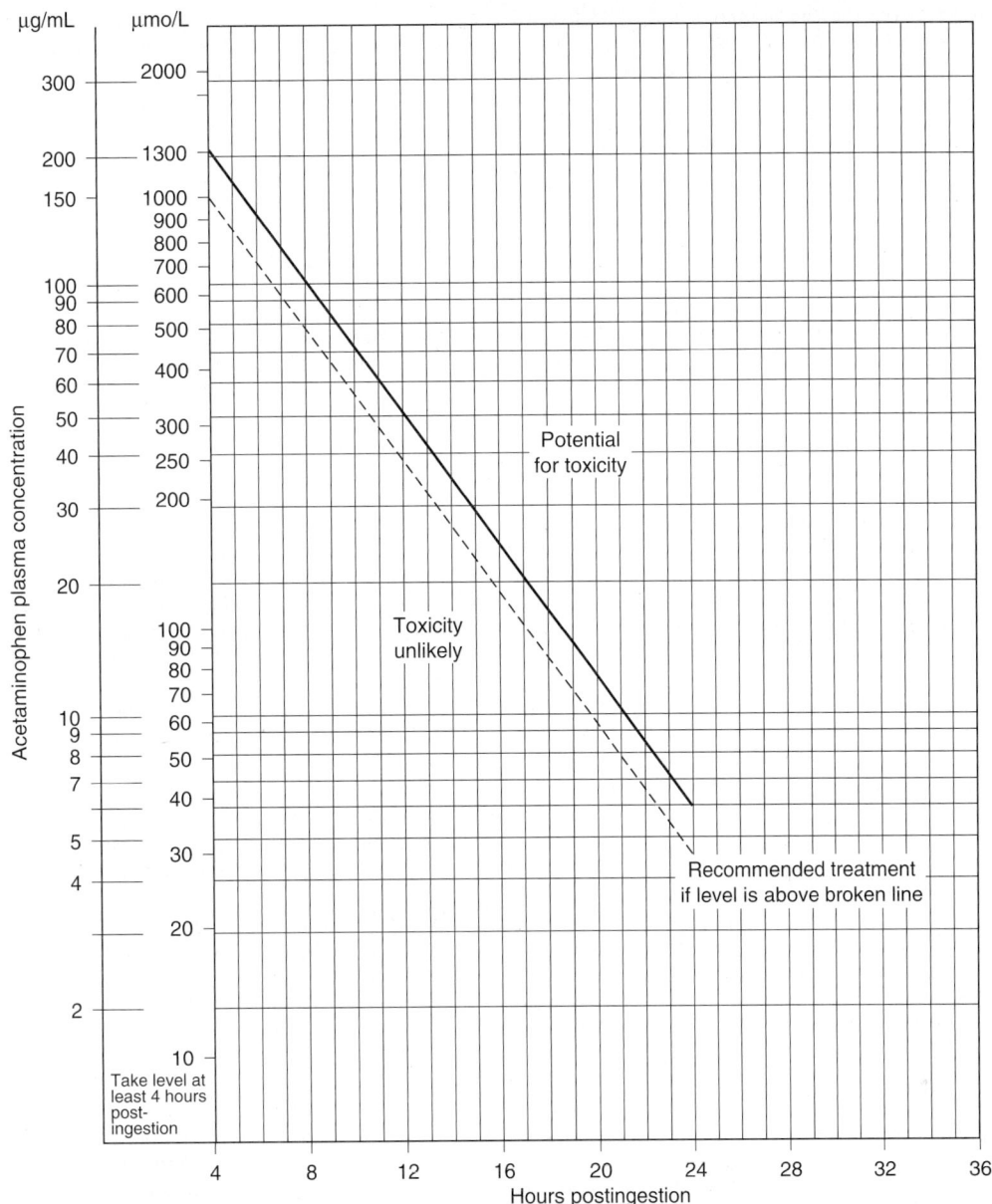

Figure 1 Revised Rumack-Matthew nomogram for acute acetaminophen ingestion. Serum acetaminophen levels should be obtained 4 to 24 hours after ingestion to detect peak serum concentration. Serum concentration is plotted against time since ingestion. This nomogram cannot be used in cases of unknown time of ingestion, chronic ingestion, or presentation longer than 24 hours after ingestion. In these cases, the poison control center should be consulted for guidance. Points on or above the treatment line qualify for treatment with N-acetylcysteine.

Amphetamines

Toxic Dose

Amphetamines are CNS stimulants and sympathetic nervous system stimulants that include methamphetamine, diet pills, MDMA (3,4 methylenedioxymethamphetamine, known as "ecstasy"), MDA (3,4-methylenedioxyamphetamine), phenylpropanolamine,[2] and cocaine. MDMA also causes serotonergic effects including serotonin syndrome, malignant hypothermia and rhabdomyolysis and may be tainted with other substances including cocaine, heroin, and ketamine. Peak effects are typically seen 2 to 4 hours following ingestion. The potentially fatal dose of dextroamphetamine is 20 to 25 mg/kg.

Manifestations

Restlessness, irritation, agitation, tremors, hyperreflexia, auditory and visual hallucination. Hyperpyrexia (fever >41° Celsius) may proceed seizures, paranoia, violence, intracranial hemorrhage, psychosis, and self-destructive behaviors. Dilated reactive pupils, cardiac dysrhythmias (supraventricular and ventricular), tachycardia, hypertension, rhabdomyolysis, and myoglobinuria.

Lab Investigations

In cases of suspected toxicity, ABG, ECG, comprehensive panel, creatine kinase, and cardiac enzymes (if chest pain is present), urine myoglobin, and urine toxicology screen with GCMS should be obtained as false negative testing may occur.

Management

Supportive care including blood pressure control, thermoregulation, cardiac monitoring, and seizure precautions is the mainstay of treatment. Activated charcoal may be administered up to 1 hour after ingestion for GI decontamination. Anxiety, agitation, and convulsions can be treated with diazepam. If this fails to control seizures, then neuromuscular blockers may be used and electroencephalogram (EEG) monitoring should be implemented to assess for non-motor seizures. Neuroleptic phenothiazines including prochlorperazine (Compazine), promethazine (Phenergan), droperidol (Inapsine), and haloperidol should be avoided as these can lower the seizure threshold.

---

[2] Not available in the United States.

Hypertension and tachycardia can be managed by titration of diazepam[1] or other benzodiazepines. For cases of hypertensive crisis, nitroprusside can be infused at a maximum rate of 10 μg/kg/min for 10 minutes followed with a lower infusion rate of 0.3 to 2 mg/kg/min. Myocardial ischemia should be managed with oxygen, nitroglycerin, beta blockers, and cardiac consultation for consideration of procedural therapy when indicated. Aspirin and thrombolytics are not recommended in cases of stimulant ingestion due to the risk of intracranial hemorrhage.

Unstable tachydysrhythmias can be treated with an α-blocker such as phentolamine[1] 5 mg IV for adults or 0.1 mg/kg IV for children and a short-acting β-blocker such as esmolol (Brevibloc) 500 μg/kg IV over 1 minute for adults, or 300 to 500 μg/kg over 1 minute for children. Ventricular dysrhythmias can be treated with lidocaine or synchronized electrical cardioversion in hemodynamically unstable patients. Rhabdomyolysis and myoglobinuria is treated with IV fluids, alkaline diuresis, and diuretics. Hypothermia is managed with external cooling and cool, 100% humidified oxygen.

If the patient develops focal neurologic symptoms, a cerebral vascular accident or intracranial hemorrhage should be suspected and investigated with a noncontrast CT scan of the head and neurology consultation should be sought. Paranoia and agitation should be treated with benzodiazepines.

Disposition

Patients should be observed via telemetry until symptoms of intoxication resolve. Following stimulant ingestion, some patients may experience suicidal ideation and should be placed on suicide precautions with appropriate monitoring and psychiatric care.

Anticholinergics

Anticholinergic drugs include antihistamines (H1 blockers), neuroleptics (phenothiazines), tricyclic antidepressants (TCAs), antiparkinsonism medications (trihexyphenidyl [Artane], benztropine [Cogentin]), atropine (found an ophthalmic products and antispasmodic agents for bladder/bowel control), and common plants (e.g., jimsonweed, deadly nightshade, and henbane). Some antihistamines are sedating including diphenhydramine (Benadryl), dimenhydrinate (Dramamine), clemastine (Tavist), tripelennamine (Pyribenzamine), chlorpheniramine (Chlor-Trimeton), brompheniramine (Dimetane), cyclizine (Marezine), hydroxyzine (Atarax), meclizine (Antivert), and promethazine (Phenergan). Nonsedating antihistamines include astemizole (Hismanal)[2], terfenadine (Seldane),[2] loratadine (Claritin), fexofenadine (Allegra), and cetirizine (Zyrtec). Anticholinergics affect peripheral and CNS muscarinic receptors. Sedating antihistamines can depress or stimulate the CNS. In large overdoses, diphenhydramine can cause cardiac membrane depressant effects and promethazine can cause α-adrenergic receptor blockade effects.

Toxic Dose

In children, more than 2 to 10 mg of atropine can be fatal. The lethal dose in adults is not known. Other anticholinergic agents are less toxic, but in general, an ingestion of 5 times the single dose of an antihistamine is toxic. For diphenhydramine (Benadryl), the toxic dose in a child is 15 mg/kg and the lethal dose is 25 mg/kg. The potential lethal dose of diphenhydramine in adults is 2.8 g.

Manifestations

Hyperpyrexia ("hot as a hare"), mydriasis ("blind as a bat"), flushed skin ("red as a beet"), dry mucus membranes and skin ("dry as a bone"), "Lilliputian type" hallucinations and delirium ("mad as a hatter"), coma, dysphagia, tachycardia, moderate hypertension, and rarely convulsions and urinary retention are key elements to observe in suspected overdose

and toxicity. Cyproheptadine (Periactin) can cause jaundice while diphenhydramine (Benadryl) may cause dystonia and cardiotoxicity in large doses. Doxylamine (Unisom, Sleep Aid) can cause rhabdomyolysis. Non-sedating agents may cause headaches, confusion, nausea, and dysrhythmias (torsades de points).

Laboratory Investigations

ABG (if respiratory depression), comprehensive panel and ECG should be obtained. Urine toxicology screens will not detect this class, yet GCMS can identify specific drugs.

Management

If bowel sounds are present up to 1 hour after ingestion, then activated charcoal may be given for diphenhydramine ingestion. Seizures should be treated with benzodiazepines (diazepam or lorazepam[1]). Physostigmine (Antilirium) is not routinely recommended and is reserved for refractory, life-threatening anticholinergic overdose but should not be given if TCAs are present as it can increase toxicity. Catheterization should be performed to relieve urinary retention. Supraventricular tachycardia should be treated only if the patient is hemodynamically unstable. Ventricular dysrhythmia should be treated with lidocaine or cardioversion. Sodium bicarbonate[1] 1 to 2 mEq/kg IV can be used to treat myocardial depression and QRS prolongation. Torsades de pointes should be treated with magnesium sulfate[1] 4 g or 40 mL 10% solution IV over 10 to 20 minutes. Countershock may be performed for refractory torsades de pointes. Hyperpyrexia is managed by external cooling.

Disposition

Symptomatic patients should be admitted for observation until symptoms resolve and then observed for 3 to 4 hours after resolution for relapse. For nonsedating agents, all asymptomatic children who ingest more than the maximum adult dose and asymptomatic adults who acutely and just more than twice the maximum adult daily dose should be observed for at least 6 hours minimum with cardiac monitoring.

Barbiturates

Barbiturates have multiple uses including as sedatives, anesthetic agents, and anticonvulsants. They act as GABA agonists, which can cause CNS and cardiovascular depression. Their uses have largely fallen out of favor due to increased availability of safer, more effective drugs with fewer adverse effects.

Toxic Dose

The shorter-acting and intermediate-acting barbiturates and their hypnotic doses include amobarbital (Amytal), 100 to 200 mg; aprobarbital (Alurate),[2] 50 to 100 mg; butabarbital (Butisol),[2] 50 to 100 mg; butalbital,[2] 100 to 200 mg; pentobarbital (Nembutal), 100 to 200 mg; secobarbital (Seconal), 100 to 200 mg. They may cause toxicity at lower doses than long-acting barbiturates and have a minimum toxic dose of 6 mg/kg; the fatal adult dose is 3 to 6 g.

The long-acting barbiturates and their doses include mephobarbital (Mebaral),[2] 50 to 100 mg, and phenobarbital, 100 to 200 mg. Their minimum toxic dose is greater than 10 mg/kg, and the fatal adult dose is 6 to 10 g. A general rule is that an amount five times the hypnotic dose is toxic and an amount 10 times the hypnotic dose is potentially fatal. Methohexital (Brevital) and thiopental (Pentothal)[2] are ultrashort-acting parenteral preparations and are not discussed.

Manifestations

Barbiturate intoxication often resembles alcohol intoxication including ataxia, slurred speech, and slowed cognition. Severe

---

[1] Not FDA approved for this indication.
[2] Not available in the United States.

---

[1] Not FDA approved for this indication.
[2] Not available in the United States.

intoxication can cause respiratory depression, coma, and loss of reflexes with the exception of pupillary light reflex. Barbiturates can also cause hypotension due to vasodilation, hypothermia, hypoglycemia, and death due to respiratory arrest.

Laboratory Investigations

Most barbiturates are detected on routine urine toxicology screens. Barbiturate level, ABG, acetaminophen level, comprehensive panel, creatinine kinase levels, and urine pH should be obtained. The minimum toxic plasma levels are greater than 10 μg/mL for short-acting barbiturates and greater than 40 μg/mL for long-acting agents. Fatal levels are 30 μg/mL for short-acting barbiturates and 80 to 150 μg/mL for long-acting agents. Both short-acting and long-acting agents can be detected in urine 24 to 72 hours after ingestion, and long-acting agents can be detected for up to 7 days.

Management

Due to risk of respiratory depression, care should be taken to maintain airway and ventilation. Patients who are obtunded or comatose should be given glucose, thiamine (if concern for chronic alcohol use), and naloxone (in case of suspected or known opioid co-ingestion) intravenously and admitted to an intensive care unit. MDAC (0.5 g/kg) every 2 to 4 hours has been shown to reduce the serum half-life of phenobarbital by 50%, but its effect on clinical course is undetermined. IV fluids may be administered for dehydration and hypotension. Vasopressors may be required for severe hypotension. Sodium bicarbonate, 1 to 2 mEq/kg IV in 500 mL of 5% dextrose in adults or 10 to 15 mL/kg in children during the first hour, followed by sufficient bicarbonate to keep the urinary pH at 7.5 to 8.0, enhances excretion of phenobarbital and shortens the half-life by 50%. Diuresis is not recommended due to the risk of cerebral or pulmonary edema. Hypothermia should be managed with external warming measures.

Disposition

Comatose patients should be admitted to the intensive care unit. Awake and alert patients with an overdose of short-acting agents should be observed until asymptomatic for at least 6 hours. Awake and alert patients with an overdose with long-acting agents should be observed until asymptomatic for at least 12 hours due to risk of delayed absorption. Patients should be assessed for intentional overdose and psychiatric evaluation should be sought if appropriate. Chronic barbiturate use can lead to tolerance, physical dependance, and withdrawal and an appropriate plan should be made for outpatient follow-up.

Benzodiazepines

Benzodiazepines are used as anxiolytics, sedatives, and muscle relaxants. They are also GABA agonists that cause CNS depression. Flunitrazepam (Rohypnol, known as "roofies") is a long-acting benzodiazepine that is not legally available in the United States but is a common "date rape" drug.

Toxic Dose

Table 8 highlights half-lives and dosing of commonly used benzodiazepines. An overdose of short-acting and long-acting benzodiazepines is often 10 to 20 times the therapeutic dose. Fatalities are rare as most patients recover within 24 to 36 hours after overdose. Ultrashort-acting agents have produced respiratory arrest and coma within 1 hour of ingestion. Intravenous injection of midazolam (Versed) and diazepam (Valium) should only be administered in controlled settings as respiratory compromise is common and airway management is imperative. In the elderly, therapeutic doses may cause toxicity and have an additive effect with other CNS depressants.

Manifestations

CNS depression, ataxia, and slurred speech may occur similar to alcohol and barbiturate intoxication. Deep coma and respiratory

TABLE 8	Half Life and Dosing of Benzodiazepines	
LONG-ACTING BENZODIAZEPINES (HALF-LIFE >24 HOURS)	**MAX THERAPEUTIC DOSES**
Chlordiazepoxide (Librium)	50 mg
Clorazepate (Tranxene)	30 mg
Clonazepam (Klonopin)	20 mg
Diazepam (Valium)	10 mg in adults, 0.2 mg/kg in children
Flurazepam (Dalmane)	30 mg
Prazepam[2]	20 mg
SHORT-ACTING BENZODIAZEPINES (HALF-LIFE 10 TO 24 HOURS)	**MAX THERAPEUTIC DOSES**
Alprazolam (Xanax)	0.5 mg
Lorazepam (Ativan)	4 mg in adults, 0.05 mg/kg in children
ULTRASHORT-ACTING BENZODIAZEPINES (HALF-LIFE <10 HOURS)*	**MAX THERAPEUTIC DOSES**
Temazepam (Restoril)	30 mg
Triazolam (Halcion)	0.5 mg
Midazolam (Versed)	0.2 mg/kg
Oxazepam (Serax)	30 mg

*Note that ultrashort-acting benzodiazepines are more toxic than short-acting or long-acting benzodiazepines.
[2]Not available in the United States.

depression suggest use of short-acting benzodiazepines or co-ingestion of other CNS depressants.

Laboratory Investigations

Most benzodiazepines are detected via urine toxicology screens, and GCMS should be used when the aim is to identify a specific drug. Some immunoassays may produce a false-positive benzodiazepine result for use of nonsteroidal anti-inflammatory drugs. If flunitrazepam or other "date rape" drugs are suspected, police or a reference lab should be consulted to conduct confirmatory testing.

Management

Activated charcoal should be used if administered before peak time of absorption occurs. Supportive treatment is the mainstay of management. Benzodiazepine overdose rarely requires intubation or mechanical ventilation. Flumazenil (Romazicon) is a benzodiazepine receptor antagonist that reverses the sedative effect of benzodiazepine, zolpidem (Ambien)[1], and endogenous benzodiazepines produced by hepatic encephalopathy yet is not recommended for reversal of benzodiazepine-induced hypoventilation. In cases where benzodiazepine dependency is suspected, flumazenil should not be used because it can precipitate life-threatening withdrawal. Flumazenil is also contraindicated for patients taking TCAs or if they have a known seizure disorder.

Disposition

Comatose patients should be admitted to the intensive care unit. Patients should be assessed for intentional overdose and psychiatric evaluation should be sought if appropriate. Chronic benzodiazepine use can lead to tolerance, physical dependance, and withdrawal and an appropriate plan should be made for outpatient follow-up.

[1]Not FDA approved for this indication.

Beta Blockers

Toxic Dose

Beta blockers block catecholamine receptors in the bronchi, vascular smooth muscle, and myocardium and are used for a variety of therapeutic applications. Ingestion of doses greater than twice the maximum recommended daily therapeutic dose are considered toxic. For children, ingestion of 1 mg/kg or greater of propranolol can cause hypoglycemia. Fatalities have been reported in adults with 7.5 g of metoprolol. Sotalol is the most toxic beta blocker and atenolol is the least toxic. Most regular-acting agents have a duration of action of 4 to 6 hours. In cases of overdose, this can extend to 24 to 48 hours. Sustained release agents have a duration of action of 24 to 48 hours. Nadolol has the longest half-life of 12 to 24 hours. Esmolol has the shortest half-life of 5 to 10 minutes.

Manifestations

Bradycardia and hypotension can lead to cardiogenic shock. Intrinsic partial agonists can initially cause tachycardia and hypertension. ECG may reveal atrioventricular conduction delay, asystole, and/or QRS and QT prolongation (which may cause torsades de pointes). Sotalol substantially prolongs the QT interval. In patients with reactive airway disease, they may experience bronchospasm because cardioselectivity is lost in an overdose. Beta-blockers can also cause hypoglycemia (due to blocking catecholamine based regulatory mechanisms) and hyperkalemia.

Laboratory Investigations

A comprehensive panel and ECG should be obtained, as well as serum troponin levels if the patient experiences chest pain. If the patient experiences respiratory symptoms, then an ABG may be obtained.

Management

Initial attention should be toward establishing vascular access as well as continuous cardiac and blood pressure monitoring. An external pacemaker should be readily available in case of significant bradycardia or hemodynamic instability. Activated charcoal may be given up to 1 hour after ingestion for GI decontamination. Whole bowel irrigation can be considered in cases of ingestion of sustained release formulations, but this has not been studied to evaluate effectiveness. Cardiology consultation should be considered for cardiovascular abnormalities. Hypotension may be treated with a combination of IV fluids, Trendelenburg position, glucagon,[1] cardiac pacing, amrinone (Inocor),[2] correction of dysrhythmias, or a combination of these elements.

Glucagon is first-line treatment for a beta blocker overdose.[1] It is administered in adults as an initial IV bolus of 5 to 10 mg over 1 minute, followed by a continuous infusion of 1 to 5 mg/h. In children, glucagon is administered as a 0.05 mg/kg IV loading dose over 1 to 2 minutes (not to exceed 1 mg/min). After 10 minutes, if there is inadequate effect, the dose may be repeated once. The loading dose is followed by a continuous infusion of 0.05 to 0.1 mg/kg/h. For large doses and continuous infusions, D5W, sterile water, or saline should be used to reconstitute glucagon instead of phenol provided with some formulations. Glucagon may be used in combination with amrinone. Amrinone (Inocor)[2] is administered as a bolus of 0.15 to 2 mg/kg (0.15 to 0.4 mL/kg) intravenously, followed by infusion of 5 to 10 μg/kg/min. Hypoglycemia is treated with IV glucose. Life-threatening hyperkalemia is treated with IV calcium gluconate[1] for cardiac membrane stabilization (avoid if digoxin is present), bicarbonate,[1] and glucose[1] with insulin.[1] Seizures can be treated with diazepam or phenobarbital. Bronchospasm can be treated with nebulized bronchodilators such as albuterol.

Patients who are unstable (hypotension or high-degree AV block) may be treated with atropine 0.02 mg/kg (up to 2 mg) in adults, glucagon, and/or an external pacemaker. For ventricular tachycardia, overdrive pacing can be used. Class IA antidysrhythmic agents (procainamide, quinidine) and III (bretylium) are not recommended. Sodium bicarbonate may be administered for a wide QRS interval.[1] Torsades de pointes (particularly with sotalol) can be treated with magnesium sulfate[1] and overdrive pacing. For a prolonged QT interval, some have suggested prophylactically giving magnesium sulfate,[1] but there are no data available for the efficacy of this approach. Epinephrine should not be used for hypotension or bradycardia because it can cause an unopposed alpha effect. For refractory hemodynamic compromise, intra-aortic balloon pump can be perused.

Hemodialysis is effective for removal of atenolol, acebutolol, nadolol, and sotalol, particularly when there is renal failure. Hemodialysis is not effective for propranolol, metoprolol, and timolol. Prenalterol[5] has been shown to reverse bradycardia and hypotension associated with beta blocker overdose but is not available in the United States.

Disposition

Asymptomatic patients should be monitored with a baseline ECG and continuous cardiac monitoring for at least 6 hours for regular-release formulations and at least 24 hours for sustained-release formulations. Symptomatic patients should be observed with cardiac monitoring for at least 24 hours. Patients should be admitted to the intensive care unit for seizures, vital sign abnormalities (e.g., hypotension, bradycardia), or arrhythmias. Patients should be assessed for intentional overdose and psychiatric evaluation should be sought if appropriate.

Calcium Channel Blockers

Toxic Dose

Calcium channel blockers are predominantly used for management of hypertension and rate control in patients with arrhythmias, as well as migraines prophylaxis. They cause peripheral, systemic, and coronary vasodilation. Bepridil,[2] diltiazem, and verapamil depress myocardial contractility and cause atrioventricular block.

TABLE 9	Calcium Channel Blocker Dosing	
CALCIUM CHANNEL BLOCKER	**MAXIMUM DAILY ADULT DOSE**	**MAXIMUM DAILY CHILD DOSE**
Amlodipine (Norvasc)	10 mg	<6 y: 0.6 mg/kg/day ≥6 y: ≤10 mg/day
Diltiazem (Cardizem)	360 mg (toxic dose >2 g)	6 mg/kg
Felodipine (Plendil)	10 mg	10 mg
Isradipine (DynaCirc)	10 mg/day	0.6 mg/kg
Nicardipine (Cardene)	120 mg	2 mg/kg
Nifedipine (Procardia)	120 mg	2 mg/kg
Nimodipine (Nimotop)	360 mg	0.85 mg/kg
Nitrendipine (Baypress)[2]	40 mg/day	Undetermined
Verapamil (Calan)	480 mg	8 mg/kg (oral)

[2]Not available in the United States.

Peak action of regular release preparations may be delayed for 6 to 8 hours. Duration of action is up to 36 hours. Peak action of sustained release preparations is 12 to 24 hours. In cases of massive overdose, concretions and prolonged toxicity may develop.

---

[1] Not FDA approved for this indication.
[2] Not available in the United States.

---

[1] Not FDA approved for this indication.
[2] Not available in the United States.
[5] Investigational drug in the United States.

Dosing is outlined in Table 9; any amount greater than the maximum daily dose can potentially cause toxicity.

Manifestations

Hypotension, bradycardia, and conduction disturbances may occur 30 minutes to 5 hours following ingestion. A prolonged PR interval is an early finding and may be seen even with therapeutic doses. All degrees of heart block have been reported but may be delayed up to 16 hours following ingestion. QRS interval is not usually affected, yet torsades de pointes has been reported. Calcium channel blockers may also cause lactic acidosis, hypocalcemia, and hyperglycemia. They may also cause mental status changes, headaches, seizures, hemiparesis, and CNS depression.

Laboratory Investigations

ABG, comprehensive panel, and pulse oximetry should be obtained and monitored. Baseline ECG should be obtained, and ongoing hemodynamic and cardiac monitoring should be implemented.

Management

Initial attention should be paid to establishing vascular access and continuous cardiac and blood pressure monitoring. An external pacemaker should be readily available in case of significant bradycardia or hemodynamic instability. Activated charcoal is recommended for GI decontamination. Whole bowel irrigation can be considered in cases of ingestion of sustained release formulations, but this has not been studied to evaluate effectiveness.

Symptomatic patients should have immediate cardiology consultation and early consideration of pacemaker use. In heart block, atropine is rarely effective, and isoproterenol can cause vasodilation. Hypotension may be treated with a combination of IV fluids, Trendelenburg position, calcium gluconate[1] or calcium chloride,[1] glucagon,[1] ventricular pacing, correction of dysrhythmias, or a combination of these. Calcium gluconate and calcium chloride should be avoided if the patient has taken digoxin. Adult dosing of calcium chloride[1] is 20 mg/kg of 10% solution up to a maximum of 1 to 2 g per dose. Calcium gluconate[1] dosing is 60 mg/kg over 5 to 10 minutes (max: 3–6 g/dose); may repeat every 10 to 20 minutes for 3 to 4 additional doses or initiate a continuous infusion of 60 to 120 mg/kg/h titrated to improve response. Ongoing monitoring of cardiac rhythm, hemodynamics, and serum ionized calcium level should be implemented. The goal is to increase serum calcium by 4 mg/dL above initial level up to a maximum of 13 mg/dL. Calcium response usually lasts 15 minutes and may require repeated doses of continuous infusion of calcium gluconate 0.2 mL/kg/h up to a maximum of 10 mL/h.

If calcium is ineffective, then glucagon[1] can be tried as it has positive inotropic and chronotropic effects. IV fluids, norepinephrine (Levophed), and epinephrine may be required for refractory hypotension. Dobutamine and dopamine are often ineffective. Hemodialysis and charcoal hemoperfusion are not useful. For refractory hemodynamic compromise, intra-aortic balloon pump and cardiopulmonary bypass have been successful.

Disposition

Asymptomatic patients should be monitored for at least 6 hours for regular-release formulation calcium channel blockers and at least 24 hours for sustained-release formulations. Symptomatic patients should be admitted to the intensive care unit. Patients should be assessed for intentional overdose and psychiatric evaluation should be sought if appropriate.

---

[1] Not FDA approved for this indication.

TABLE 10	Carbon Monoxide Exposure and Possible Manifestations
CoHB SATURATION (%)	MANIFESTATIONS
3.5	None
5	Slight headache, decreased exercise tolerance
10	Slight headache, dyspnea on vigorous exertion, may impair driving skills
10–20	Moderate dyspnea on exertion, throbbing, temporal headache
20–30	Severe headache, syncope, dizziness, visual changes, weakness, nausea, vomiting, altered judgment
30–40	Vertigo, ataxia, blurred vision, confusion, loss of consciousness
40–50	Confusion, tachycardia, tachypnea, coma, convulsions
50–60	Cheyne-Stokes, coma, convulsions, shock, apnea
60–70	Coma, convulsions, respiratory and heart failure, death

Carbon Monoxide

Toxic Dose and Manifestations

Carbon monoxide is an odorless, colorless gas produced by incomplete combustion. It can be produced by breakdown of methylene chloride used in paint strippers. Table 10 highlights manifestations of carbon monoxide toxicity. Exposure to 0.5% for a few minutes is lethal. ECG abnormalities, creatinine elevation, rhabdomyolysis, and myoglobinuria may occur. Carboxyhemoglobin (CoHB) indicates the percentage of carbon monoxide bound to hemoglobin. This can be falsely low in patients with anemia. As such, CoHB may not reliably correlate with severity of exposure.

Laboratory Investigations

An ABG may show metabolic acidosis with a normal arterial oxygen pressure. With significant poisoning, ABG, electrolytes, blood glucose, creatine kinase, cardiac enzymes, renal function, and liver function should be monitored. Urinalysis should be obtained and tested for myoglobinuria. Chest radiographs may be helpful in cases of smoke inhalation or if treatment with hyperbaric oxygen is considered. ECG should be obtained for patients older than 40 years, those with a history of cardiac disease, or with moderate to severe symptoms. CoHB should be monitored during and after therapy. Traditional pulse oximetry overestimates oxyhemoglobin saturation in carbon monoxide poisoning. True oxygen saturation is determine by blood gas. Co-oximetry can differentiate CoHB and other hemoglobin binding agents from oxyhemoglobin. Fetal hemoglobin has a greater affinity for carbon monoxide than adult hemoglobin and can falsely elevate the CoHB by up to 4% in young infants.

Management

The patient with suspected carbon monoxide poisoning should be removed from the area of exposure and initial vitals measured. Primary treatment is with 100% oxygen via non-rebreathing mask with an oxygen reservoir or via endotracheal tube and it should be continued until CoHB level is 5% or less. Mechanical ventilation may be necessary in cases of severe hypoxia and ABG and CoHB should be sequentially monitored. A near-normal CoHB level does not exclude carbon monoxide poisoning, particularly if the measurement is taken several hours after exposure or if oxygen has been administered prior to measurement. Pregnant women with carbon monoxide poisoning should be maintained on 100% oxygen for several hours until the CoHB level is almost 0 because fetal hemoglobin has a much stronger affinity to carbon monoxide than adult hemoglobin and carbon monoxide concentrates in the fetus. Therefore, longer maternal oxygen administration is needed to eliminate carbon monoxide from fetal circulation. The fetus should be monitored because carbon monoxide and hypoxia can be teratogenic and/or cause fetal compromise.

Use of a hyperbaric oxygen chamber should be considered if:
- The patient is in a coma or has a history of loss of consciousness or seizures
- The patient experiences cardiovascular dysfunction (clinical ischemic chest pain or ECG evidence of ischemia) or metabolic acidosis
- Symptoms persist despite 100% oxygen therapy
- Initial CoHB is higher than 15% in a child
- The patient is symptomatic with preexisting ischemia
- There are signs of maternal or fetal distress regardless of CoHB

Neurologic evaluation can help determine which patients with a low initial carbon monoxide level may benefit from more aggressive therapy. This includes orientation questions and brief cognitive assessment. Patients with delayed neurologic symptoms or recurrent symptoms for up to 3 weeks may benefit from hyperbaric oxygen treatment. Seizures and cerebral edema should be managed if present. Metabolic acidosis can be treated with sodium bicarbonate if pH is less than 7.2 after correction of hypoxia and hypoventilation. Acidosis shifts the oxygen dissociation curve and aids oxygen delivery to tissues.

Disposition

Patients who are asymptomatic or have mild symptoms and become asymptomatic after several hours of oxygen therapy, have a CoHB level <10%, and have normal physical and neurocognitive exams may be discharged. These patients should be instructed to return if neurologic symptoms occur. Patients who are obtunded or comatose require ICU admission.

Caustics and Corrosives

Toxic Dose

Common acids with corrosive potential include acetic acid (vinegar), formic acid, glycolic acid, hydrochloric acid, mercuric chloride, nitric acid, oxalic acid, phosphoric acid, sulfuric acid (battery acid), zinc chloride, and zinc sulfate. Common alkalis with corrosive potential include ammonia, calcium carbide, calcium hydroxide, calcium oxide, potassium hydroxide (lye), and sodium hydroxide (lye). Acids cause mucosal coagulation necrosis and can be absorbed systemically, but do not penetrate deeply. In particular, injury to gastric mucosa is most likely. Alkalis cause liquefaction necrosis and saponification and penetrate deeply. Oropharyngeal and esophageal mucosa are most likely to be damaged by ingestion. Solids are more likely to damage the oropharynx and esophagus while liquids tend to produce superficial circumferential burns and gastric damage. Toxicity increases with increasing concentration, longer contact time, and extremes of pH (less than 2 or greater than 12).

Manifestations

Findings of ingestion toxicity may include stridor, dysphagia, drooling, oropharyngeal, retrosternal, and epigastric pain, and ocular and oral burns. Alkali burns tend to be yellow, soapy, frothy lesions due to saponification of fats. Acid burns are gray-white initially and later form eschar. Gastric or esophageal perforation can occur returning in retrosternal or abdominal pain or guarding. Formaldehyde causes metabolic acidosis, hydrofluoric acid causes hypocalcemia and renal damage, oxalic acid causes hypocalcemia, phenol causes hepatic and renal damage, and picric acid causes renal damage.

Laboratory Investigations

ABG to determine acid-base status and comprehensive panel to assess electrolytes as well as hepatic and renal function should be obtained. Chest radiograph and pulse oximetry may be indicated if pulmonary symptoms are present. The container of the caustic or corrosive toxin should be examined to determine its identity and its pH should be tested as well as pH of body fluids including vomitus, tears, and saliva.

Management

Inhalation cases should be treated with humidified supplemental oxygen and observation for airway obstruction and pulmonary edema. Radiographic and ABG evaluation may be obtained. Intubation and respiratory support may be necessary.

For ocular exposure, copious water irrigation should be completed immediately after initial stabilization for 15 to 20 minutes with eyelids retracted. Patients should be evaluated with fluorescein dye and by an ophthalmologist. Dermal exposures should be treated with copious water irrigation for 30 minutes. In the case of extensive exposure, the hair, nails, navel, and perineum should be cleansed with soap or shampoo. Caustic (alkali) exposures may require hours of irrigation. A burn specialist should be consulted. For ingestions, GI decontamination is contraindicated with exception of immediate rinsing of the mouth and dilution with small sips of milk or water. Oral dilution is contraindicated with dysphagia, respiratory distress, obtundation, or shock. In cases of acid ingestion, a small nasogastric tube may be placed, and aspiration attempted within 30 minutes of ingestion. Endoscopy is recommended for all patients with intentional ingestion and may be performed immediately but is typically performed 12 to 48 hours following ingestion.

Tetanus prophylaxis is indicated for patients requiring wound care. Antibiotics are not recommended prophylactically. Contrast studies can be used after the first few days to assess severity of damage such as strictures. Contrast studies are not recommended prior to endoscopic evaluation.

Disposition

Infants and small children require medical evaluation and observation. All symptomatic patients should be admitted. If severe symptoms or airway/respiratory compromise are present, patients should be admitted to the ICU. If no damage is detected on endoscopy, then patients may be discharged once able to tolerate oral feeds. Intentional exposures require psychiatric evaluation.

Cocaine

Toxic Dose

Cocaine is a stimulant that causes increased catecholamine and acetylcholine release and increases platelet aggregation. It is used as a local anesthetic and is available as a 4% topical solution in the United States. The maximum therapeutic dose is 200 mg or 2 mL of 10% solution.[2] Most cocaine overdoses occur during recreational use, so ingested doses may be unclear. CNS effects can occur at relatively low doses (50 to 95 mg); they are more common with doses of 1 mg/kg or higher. Cardiac effects can occur with doses greater than 1 mg/kg. The potentially fatal dose is 1200 mg intranasally, but there are reports of fatal cases with parenteral administration of 20 mg.

Manifestations

Cocaine causes euphoria, hyperactivity, agitation, seizures, myocardial infarction, and intracranial hemorrhage. In overdose, cardiac dysrhythmias, hypertension, or hypotension can occur. Vasoconstriction, hyperthermia (resulting in rhabdomyolysis, myoglobinuria, and renal failure), and mydriasis may be observed, and septal perforation can occur, particularly with chronic intranasal use. If ingested orally, cocaine can cause ischemic bowel perforation. Use during pregnancy causes preterm labor and/or

---

[2] Not available in the United States.

placental abruption resulting in fetal compromise. In cases of prolonged toxicity, body cavity packing should be suspected. Mortality is primarily related to cerebrovascular accidents, coronary artery spasm, myocardial injury, and dysrhythmia.

Laboratory Investigations
ABG, oxygen saturation, ECG, comprehensive panel, creatine kinase levels, and urine myoglobin should be obtained. Cardiac enzymes should be monitored for patients with chest pain. Urine toxicology should be performed to test for cocaine and other substances. The cocaine metabolite, benzoylecgonine, can be detected within 4 hours after use and up to 114 hours after use. Some herbal teas, lidocaine, and droperidol (Inapsine) can give false positive results on some immunoassays. If body cavity packing is suspected, abdominal radiographs or ultrasound should be obtained.

Management
Hemodynamic, cardiac, and thermal monitoring along with seizure precautions should be implemented. Diazepam (Valium) is recommended to manage agitation, anxiety, seizures, and dysrhythmias related to cocaine intoxication[1]. Diazepam dosing for adults is typically 2 to 10 mg, up to 20 mg IV. For children, the dose is 0.2 to 0.5 mg/kg at 1 mg/min up to 10 mg.

For ingestions, activated charcoal should be used for GI decontamination. MDAC can adsorb cocaine in body packers. Whole-bowel irrigation with PEG solution has been used for body packers, particularly if in a rigid container. If packages are not visible on plain film radiographs, contrast or CT scan should be obtained to confirm passage of packages. Body packers should be monitored closely until all packages have passed in the stool. Surgical removal may be required if unable to pass the pylorus in cases of intestinal obstruction.

Hypertension and tachycardia are managed by titration of diazepam.[1] Nitroprusside can be used for severe hypertension. Myocardial ischemia is management with oxygen, vascular access, benzodiazepines (diazepam[1]), and nitroglycerin. Aspirin and thrombolytics are not recommended due to risk of intracranial hemorrhage. Dysrhythmias are typically supraventricular and do not require specific management. Adenosine is ineffective. Life-threatening tachydysrhythmias may be treated with phentolamine (Regitine)[1] 5 mg IV bolus in adults or 0.1 mg/kg in children at 5- to 10-minute intervals. Phentolamine also relieves coronary artery spasm and myocardial ischemia[1]. For patients who are hemodynamically unstable, electrical synchronized cardioversion should be considered. Lidocaine may be used after 3 hours for ventricular tachycardia. Wide complex QRS ventricular tachycardia can be treated with sodium bicarbonate[1] 2 mEq/kg as a bolus. Beta blockers are contraindicated due to risk of unopposed alpha-adrenergic stimulation.

If seizures are not controlled with diazepam, then neuromuscular blockers can be used, and EEG activity should be monitored for non-motor seizure activity. Hyperthermia should be managed with external cooling and cool humidified 100% oxygen. Neuromuscular blockers can also help reduce temperature. Dantrolene and antipyretics are not recommended. Rhabdomyolysis and myoglobinuria are treated with fluids, alkaline diuresis, and diuretics. Pregnant women should undergo fetal monitoring for signs of placental abruption or spontaneous abortion.

If the patient develops focal neurologic symptoms, a cerebral vascular accident or intracranial hemorrhage should be suspected and investigated with a noncontrast CT scan of the head and neurology consultation should be sought. Patients may experience severe depression and suicidal ideation following intoxication and may require suicide precautions and psychiatric monitoring and consultation.

Disposition
Patients with mild intoxication or brief seizure who do not require treatment can be discharged after 6 hours provided they are asymptomatic and have appropriate psychosocial follow-up. Cardiac or cerebral ischemic manifestations require ICU admission. Body packers require ICU admission until all material has been eliminated from the GI tract.

Cyanide
Toxic Dose
Cyanide can be produced by burning plastic or wools, metabolism of nitriles (e.g., acetonitrile in nail removers), some fruit seeds (e.g., apricots, peaches, and apples), and in sodium nitroprusside (an antihypertensive vasodilator). Cyanide causes cellular hypoxia and lactic acidosis by inhibiting cellular respiration.

Ingestion of 1 mg/kg or 50 mg of hydrogen cyanide is lethal within 15 minutes. The lethal dose of potassium cyanide is 200 mg. 5 to 10 mL of 84% acetonitrile is lethal. Infusions of nitroprusside above 2 µg/kg per minute can cause cyanide toxicity.

Manifestations
Hydrogen cyanide has a distinctive bitter almond or silver polish odor. Manifestations include hypertension, cardiac dysrhythmias, ECG abnormalities, headache, hyperpnea, seizures, stupor, pulmonary edema, and flushing. Cyanosis is absent or may appear late in cases of toxicity.

Laboratory Investigations
ABG including lactate, oxygen saturation, comprehensive panel and complete blood count with platelets should be obtained. Metabolic acidosis due to increased lactate may be seen along with a decrease in the arterial-venous oxygen difference, and bright red blood. If smoke inhalation is the suspected source, CoHB and methemoglobin (MetHb) concentrations should be measured.

Measurement of cyanide levels in blood are not useful, but approximate levels can be determined by clinical presentation: smokers have less than 0.5 µg/mL; a patient with flushing and tachycardia has 0.5 to 1.0 µg/mL, one with obtundation has 1.0 to 2.5 µg/mL, and one in coma or who has died has more than 2.5 µg/mL.

Management
Patients should be removed from the affected area if cyanide was inhaled. Patients should be administered 100% oxygen, which should be continued during and after administration of the antidote. The antidote kit produces methemoglobinemia and provides a sulfur substrate to detoxify cyanide. Methemoglobin has a greater affinity for cyanide than native enzymes. Methemoglobin and cyanide forms cyanmethemoglobin. Sodium thiosulfate assists with converting cyanide into sodium thiocyanate, which is nontoxic and renally excreted.

The procedure for using the antidote kit is as follows:
- Step 1: Amyl nitrite inhalant Perles[1] are only a temporizing measure (forms only 2% to 5% methemoglobin) and can be omitted once venous access is established. Alternate 100% oxygen and the inhalant for 30 seconds each minute. Use a new perle every 3 minutes.
- Step 2: Sodium nitrite ampule is indicated for cyanide exposures, except for cases of residential fires, smoke inhalation, and nitroprusside or acetonitrile poisonings. It is administered intravenously to produce methemoglobin of 20% to 30% at 35 to 70 minutes after administration. A dose of 10 mL of 3% solution of sodium nitrite for adults and 0.33 mL/kg of 3% solution for children is diluted to 100 mL 0.9% saline and administered slowly intravenously at 5 mL/min. If hypotension develops, the infusion should be slowed.
- Step 3: Sodium thiosulfate is useful alone in cases of smoke inhalation, nitroprusside toxicity, and acetonitrile toxicity and should not be used at all in cases of hydrogen sulfide poisoning. The administration dose is 12.5 g of sodium thiosulfate or 50 mL of 25% solution for adults and 1.65 mL/kg of 25% solution for children intravenously over 10 to 20 minutes.

If symptoms recur, re-treatment is controversial. Some suggest repeating the antidotes for 30 minutes at half the additional dose,

[1]Not FDA approved for this indication.

[1]Not FDA approved for this indication.

but there is not sufficient evidence for its efficacy. One hour after antidote administration, methemoglobin levels should be checked and should not exceed 20%. Methylene blue should not be used for excessive methemoglobin levels.

Activated charcoal is recommended for GI decontamination but has limited efficacy due to rapid absorption of cyanide. Seizures are managed with diazepam. Acidosis may be treated with sodium bicarbonate if not resolved with therapy. Hyperbaric oxygen and hemodialysis are not recommended. Hydroxocobalamin (vitamin B12a) (Cyanokit) can also be used as an effective antidote when given immediately following exposure. Cyanokit dosing is 5 g by IV infusion over 15 minutes. For large exposures, an additional 5 g may be given by IV infusion for a total of 10 g. Dosing for children is 70 mg/kg per dose up to a maximum of 5 g, which may be repeated a second time. Sodium thiosulfate[1] can be given in conjunction with hydroxocobalamin for severe exposures and is typically dosed as 12.5 g IV.

Disposition
Asymptomatic patients should be observed for at least 3 hours. Patients should be observed for at least 24 hours following ingestion of nitrile compounds. Patients requiring antidote administration should be admitted to the ICU.

Digitalis
Toxic Dose
Digitalis and related compounds are found in cardiac medications (e.g., digoxin), yet utilization has decreased dramatically in recent years in favor of other more efficacious drugs. They are also found in common plants (e.g., oleander, foxglove) and skin of the Bufo toad (also known as cane toads). They cause increased cardiac automaticity and ectopy, atrioventricular block, and increased vagal tone.

The therapeutic blood level for digoxin is commonly 0.6 to 2.0 ng/mL. A single toxic dose is greater than 0.07 mg/kg or greater than 2 to 3 mg in an adult. Up to 2 mg in a child and 4 mg in an adult may only produce mild toxicity. A few leaves of oleander and foxglove can contain 1 to 3 mg of digitalis. Fatal doses can be seen with more than 4 mg in a child or more than 10 mg in an adult. Patients with cardiac disease, electrolyte derangements (e.g., hypokalemia, hypomagnesemia, hypercalcemia, decreased thyroxine [T4]), renal impairment, and those taking medications including amiodarone, quinidine, erythromycin, tetracycline, calcium channel blockers, and beta blockers are at increased risk of overdose.

Manifestations
Manifestations can usually be seen within 2 hours but can be delayed for up to 12 hours. Nausea and vomiting are most commonly present in acute ingestion but can be seen with chronic ingestion. Changes on ECG include scooped ST segments and PR prolongation are coined the "digitalis effect". Dysrhythmia, AV block, bradycardia, or supraventricular tachycardia can be seen in overdose. Ventricular tachycardia may be seen in severe poisoning.

CNS manifestations include headache, visual disturbances, and a colored halo vision. Hyperkalemia correlates with digoxin level and outcome in acute overdose. Chronic intoxication is more likely to cause scotoma, color perception disturbances, yellow vision, halos, delirium, psychosis, tachycardia, and hypokalemia.

Laboratory Investigations
Baseline ECG should be obtained, and continuous cardiac and hemodynamic monitoring should be implemented. Blood glucose, electrolytes, calcium, magnesium, BUN, and creatinine levels should be monitored along with an initial digoxin level. Levels should be measured at least 6 hours post-ingestion. Clinical toxicity is typically seen with serum digoxin levels greater than 3.5 ng/mL in adults. Falsely elevated levels may be seen on immunoassay in newborns, women in the third trimester of pregnancy, chronic renal failure, and patients with abnormal immunoglobulins.

Management
Cardiology should be consulted, and a pacemaker should be available in the event of life-threatening cardiac block. Activated charcoal should be administered and induction of emesis and gastric lavage should be avoided due to excessive vagal stimulation.

Digoxin-specific antibody fragments (Digoxin Immune Fab [DigiFab, Digibind]) binds digoxin and is renally excreted. The dose is 40 mg, which binds 0.5 mg of digoxin. The usual dose of digoxin immune fab is 10 vials (40 mg/vial) for adults and children for an unknown quantity ingested. An additional 10 vials may be given for a total of 20 vials. Onset of action is within 30 minutes. Complications are primarily related to digoxin withdrawal include worsened heart failure, hypokalemia, hypoglycemia, and allergic reactions. Digoxin administered after Fab therapy is bound and inactivated for up to 5 to 7 days.

Absolute indications for Fab therapy include the following:
- Life-threatening malignant (hemodynamically unstable) dysrhythmias
- Ventricular dysrhythmias, unstable severe bradycardia, or second- or third-degree blocks unresponsive to atropine or rapid deterioration in clinical status
- Life-threatening digitoxin and oleander poisonings[1]

Relative indications for Fab therapy include the following:
- Ingestions greater than 4 mg in a child and 10 mg in an adult
- Serum potassium level greater than 5.0 mEq/L
- Serum digoxin level greater than 10 ng/mL in adults or children 6 hours after an acute ingestion
- Digitalis delirium and thrombocytopenia response

In emergent situations, Fab can be administered as a bolus through a 22-μm filter. In a non-emergent case, it may be administered over 30 minutes. The usual dose is 10 vials in adults and 5 vials in children for an unknown quantity ingested in a symptomatic patient.

Antiarrhythmic medications or a pacemaker are used if Fab therapy fails. For ventricular dysrhythmias, lidocaine or phenytoin[1] is used. For torsades de pointes, magnesium sulfate[1] 1 to 2 g IV diluted in 50 to 100 mL of D5W over 15 minutes may be given; the dose may be repeated up to a total dose of 4 g in 1 hour. Magnesium should be discontinued if hypotension, heart block, or decreased deep tendon reflexes develop. Magnesium should be used cautiously in patients with renal impairment.

Unstable bradycardia, second-degree, and third-degree block should be treated by Fab first. A pacemaker should be used if this fails. Isoproterenol is contraindicated due to dysrhythmias. Cardioversion may be used with caution with 5 to 10 joules. These patients should be treated with lidocaine because cardioversion may precipitate ventricular fibrillation or asystole.

Antidysrhythmic type Ia medications (e.g., procainamide, quinidine, disopyramide [Norpace], amiodarone [Cordarone]), Ic (propafenone [Rythmol], flecainide [Tambocor]), II (β-blockers), or IV (calcium channel blockers) should never be used, yet class Ib drugs (lidocaine, phenytoin [Dilantin][1], mexiletine [Mexitil], and tocainide [Tonocard][2]) can be used.

Disposition
Patients with significant arrhythmia, symptoms, elevated serum digoxin level, or elevated serum potassium level should be admitted to the ICU. Consultation with cardiology and poison control can help guide duration of monitoring.

Ethanol
Toxic Dose
Ethanol causes CNS depression and anesthetic effects through GABA agonism. It also produces cutaneous vasodilation, inhibits secretion of antidiuretic hormone, inhibits gluconeogenesis (leading to hypoglycemia), and influences fat metabolism. One mL/kg of pure alcohol (100% ethanol or 200 proof) produces a blood

---

[1] Not FDA approved for this indication.

[1] Not FDA approved for this indication.
[2] Not available in the United States.

TABLE 11	Clinical Signs in Ethanol Consumption
ETHANOL BLOOD CONCENTRATION (MG/DL)*	**MANIFESTATIONS**
>25	Euphoria
>47	**Mild incoordination**, sensory and motor impairment
>50	Increased risk of motor vehicle accidents
>100	Ataxia (legal toxic level in many localities)
>150	**Moderate incoordination**, slow reaction time
>200	Drowsiness and confusion
>300	Severe incoordination, stupor, blurred vision
>500	**Flaccid coma**, respiratory failure, hypotension; may be fatal

*Ethanol concentrations sometimes reported in %. Levels may not correlate with clinical manifestations due to tolerance versus intolerance.
Note: mg% is not equivalent to mg/dL because ethanol weighs less than water (specific gravity 0.79). A 1% ethanol concentration is 790 mg/dL and 0.1% is 79 mg/dL. There is great variation in individual behavior at different blood ethanol levels. Behavior is dependent on tolerance and other factors.

ethanol concentration of 100 mg/dL. A potentially fatal dose is 3 g/kg for children or 6 g/kg for adults.

Manifestations

Table 11 lists clinical signs of acute ethanol intoxication. Patients with chronic alcohol use and dependence tolerate higher blood alcohol concentrations and may not exhibit clinical manifestations as a non-chronic alcohol user.

Laboratory Investigations

Blood ethanol concentration should be obtained. Gas chromatography or breathalyzer can give rapid, reliable results if a patient is not belching or vomiting. ABG, comprehensive panel, anion gap, and osmolar gap and serum and/or urine ketones should be obtained. A chest radiograph should be obtained if aspiration pneumonia is suspected depending upon clinical presentation.

Management

Patients may require intubation and mechanical ventilation to provide a secure airway and correct hypoxia. Patients with alcohol intoxication are at increased risk for aspiration. Comatose patients should be treated with IV glucose, 10 to 25 g (20–50 mL of 50% solution) in adults and 0.5 to 1 g/kg per dose (maximum 25 g/dose, 2–4 mL/kg per dose of 25% solution) in children. Thiamine, 100 mg IV, is co-administered for patients with suspected chronic alcohol use, malnutrition, or suspected eating disorders for prevention of Wernicke-Korsakoff syndrome.

Supportive care measures include IV fluids for dehydration and hypotension and correction of electrolyte and acid-base derangements. Vasopressors and plasma expanders may be necessary for severe hypotension. Hypomagnesemia is common with chronic alcohol use and may be corrected with a loading dose of 2 g magnesium sulfate 10% IV over 5 minutes. Cardiac monitoring may be required in cases of hemodynamic instability. Caution should be used with magnesium correction in patients with renal failure.

Hypothermic patients with ethanol intoxication should be warmed. Hemodialysis may be refractory cases when acid-base disturbances cannot be readily corrected. Repeated or prolonged seizures should be treated with diazepam (Valium). Repeated seizures or focal neurologic findings warrant further investigation. Withdrawal symptoms may be treated with a variety of benzodiazepine regimens including chlordiazepoxide, lorazepam[1] or diazepam dosed per hospital protocol based upon severity of symptoms. Patients with delirium tremens may require larger doses of benzodiazepines. In patients with chronic alcohol use, they may experience withdrawal symptoms even with an elevated blood ethanol concentration. Alcohol withdrawal may be fatal if untreated.

Disposition

Severity of withdrawal dictates the level of medical care. Need for intubation, mechanical ventilation, or treatment of severe withdrawal warrants ICU admission. Patients with aspiration pneumonia or uncomplicated withdrawal require inpatient admission. Children should be monitored for hypoglycemia with frequent blood glucose checks for at least 4 hours after ingestion. Intoxicated patients should not be discharged until fully functional (back to baseline cognitive, orientation, and ambulatory status), are evaluated for suicidality, have a safe disposition environment, and a sober escort.

Ethylene Glycol

Toxic Dose

Ethylene glycol is found in solvents, antifreeze, de-icers, and airconditioning units. It is a sweet-tasting colorless water-soluble liquid with a sweet odor. It is metabolized in the body into oxalic acid, which produces a profound metabolic acidosis, increased anion gap, hypocalcemia, and calcium oxalate crystals which deposit in tissues, particularly the kidneys.

Ingestion of 0.1 mL/kg 100% ethylene glycol can result in a toxic serum ethylene glycol concentration of 20 mg/dL. Ingestion of 3.0 mL (less than 1 teaspoonful or swallow) of a 100% solution in a 10-kg child or 30 mL of 100% ethylene glycol in an adult produces a serum ethylene glycol concentration of 50 mg/dL, a concentration that requires hemodialysis. The fatal dose is 1.4 mL/kg of 100% solution.

Manifestations

Phase I: Occurs within 30 minutes to several hours following ingestion. Patients may be inebriated. Hypocalcemia, tetany, calcium oxalate crystals and hippuric acid crystals may be seen in urine within 4 to 8 hours. An elevated osmolal gap may be present prior to metabolism of ethylene glycose. Four to 12 hours following ingestion, metabolism produces an anion gap, metabolic acidosis, coma, seizures, cardiac abnormalities, and pulmonary and cerebral edema.

Phase II: Occurs 12 to 36 hours after ingestion and is characterized by cardiopulmonary deterioration with pulmonary edema and congestive heart failure.

Phase III: Occurs 36 to 72 hours after ingestion with pulmonary edema and oliguric renal failure. Renal failure is caused by calcium oxalate crystal deposition and acute tubular necrosis.

Phase IV: Ranges from 6 to 10 days after ingestion. Characterized by neurologic manifestations including facial diplegia, bilateral vision disturbances, elevated cerebrospinal fluid pressure with or without elevated protein levels and pleocytosis, vomiting, hyperreflexia, dysphagia, and ataxia.

Laboratory Investigations

ABG, blood glucose, electrolytes, ethylene glycol and ethanol levels, plasma osmolarity, hepatic and renal function should be measured. Serum ethylene glycol levels may be spuriously elevated due to the presence of propylene glycol found in many liquids and IV medications. A glycolate level, a metabolite of ethylene glycol, should be obtained if possible. Urinalysis should be obtained to evaluate for oxalate and monohydrate crystals. While some commercial antifreeze products contain fluorescein, urine fluorescence is not a reliable indicator of ethylene glycol ingestion.

---

[1] Not FDA approved for this indication.

Management

Airway protection and mechanical ventilation may be required in some cases to toxic ingestion. Gastric aspiration may be used within 1 hour of ingestion as activated charcoal is not effective. Seizures should be treated with IV diazepam and serum ionized calcium should be obtained. If the patient is hypocalcemic, then they should be treated with 1 to 2 g (10–20 mL) 10% calcium gluconate (29–60 mg/kg in children). The dose may be repeated as needed for correction of hypocalcemia. Metabolic acidosis can be managed with IV sodium bicarbonate.

Fomepizole (Antizol, 4-methylpyrazole) inhibits alcohol dehydrogenase more reliably than ethanol. Fomepizole is available in 1 g/mL vials of 1.5 mL. The loading dose is 15 mg/kg (0.015 mL/kg) IV; maintenance dose is 10 mg/kg (0.01 mL/kg) every 12 hours for four doses, then 15 mg/kg every 12 hours until the ethylene glycol levels are less than 20 mg/dL. The solution is prepared by mixing with 100 mL of 0.9% saline or D5W (5% dextrose in water). Fomepizole can be given to patients requiring hemodialysis but should be dosed as follows:

Dose at the beginning of hemodialysis:
- If <6 hours since last Antizol dose, do not administer dose
- If >6 hours since last dose, administer next scheduled dose

Dosing during hemodialysis:
- Dose every 4 hours

Dosing at the time hemodialysis is completed:
- If <1 hour between last dose and end of dialysis, do not administer dose at end of dialysis
- If 1 to 3 hours between last dose and end of dialysis, administer one half of next scheduled dose
- If >3 hours between last dose and end of dialysis, administer next scheduled dose

Maintenance dosing off hemodialysis:
- Give the next scheduled dose 12 hours from the last dose administered

Hemodialysis is indicated for potentially lethal ingestions, serum ethylene glycol greater than 50 mg/dL, severe acidosis or electrolyte abnormalities refractory to conventional therapy, volume overload, or renal failure. Treatment with fomepizole and hemodialysis should be continued until the serum ethylene glycol level is less than 10 mg/dL, the glycolate level is undetectable, acidosis is resolved, creatinine level is normal, and urine output is adequate.

If fomepizole (Antizol) is not available, then ethanol[1] therapy should be initiated immediately. Ethanol competes with ethylene glycol to bind to alcohol dehydrogenase and blocks metabolism of ethylene glycol into toxic metabolites. Ethanol therapy is indicated if there is a history of ingestion of 0.1 mg/kg of 100% ethylene glycol or more, serum ethylene glycol concentration greater than 20 mg/dL, osmolar gap not accounted for by other alcohols or factors (e.g., hyperlipidemia), metabolic acidosis with an increased anion gap, or oxalate crystals present in the urine. Ethanol is administered intravenously with a loading dose of 10 mL/kg of 10% ethanol along with a maintenance dose of 1.0 mL/kg/h of 10% ethanol to produce a blood ethanol concentration of 100 to 150 mg/dL. In patients with chronic alcohol use, this may be increased to 2 mL/kg/h. Blood ethanol concentration should be monitored hourly and infusion rate adjusted to maintain blood ethanol concentration in the therapeutic range.

Disposition

All patients who have ingested more than 20 mg/dL of ethylene glycol, have a history of a toxic dose, or are symptomatic should be evaluated in the emergency department and admitted. Patients should be monitored for a minimum of 12 hours with serial measures of osmolal gap, acid-base parameters, and electrolytes. Patients should be transferred to another facility if fomepizole or hemodialysis is needed.

---

[1] Not FDA approved for this indication.

Hydrocarbons

Toxic Dose and Manifestations

Hydrocarbons with greater volatility carry higher risk of aspiration. Aliphatic hydrocarbons include gasoline, kerosene, charcoal lighter fluid, mineral spirits, petroleum naphtha, and mineral oil. These produce minimal systemic toxicity; however, aspiration of even small amounts of can cause chemical pneumonitis. Aromatic hydrocarbons such as benzene, toluene, styrene, and xylene can be absorbed through the GI tract to cause CNS depression and multiorgan effects such as leukemia (benzene) and renal toxicity (toluene). The toxic dose of aromatic hydrocarbons is 20 to 50 mL in adults.

Halogenated hydrocarbons contain one or more halogen substitutions. They are well-absorbed by the GI tract, cause CNS depression, and damage the liver and kidneys. Methylene chloride can be converted to carbon monoxide in vivo. Dichloroethylene causes a disulfiram reaction when consumed with ethanol. 1,1,1-trichloroethane (e.g., Glamorene Spot Remover, Scotchgard, typewriter correction fluid) is another example. A lethal oral dose is 0.5 to 5 mL/kg.

Laboratory Investigations

ABG, ECG, serum electrolytes, hepatic and renal function should be obtained and monitored. Serial chest radiographs should be obtained for chemical pneumonitis when clinically indicated.

Management

Dermal absorption can occur with hydrocarbons so removal of clothing and decontamination should be considered. Dermal exposures should be treated with copious water irrigation for 30 minutes. In the case of extensive exposure, the hair, nails, navel, and perineum should be cleansed with soap or shampoo.

Dangerous additives to the hydrocarbons can be assessed with the mnemonic CHAMP:
- C, camphor (demothing agent)
- H, halogenated hydrocarbons
- A, aromatic hydrocarbons
- M, metals (heavy)
- P, pesticides

Asymptomatic patients who ingested small amounts of aliphatic substances can be monitored at home by phone for development of symptoms of aspiration (e.g., cough, wheezing, tachypnea, and dyspnea) for 4 to 6 hours. Ingestion of aliphatic hydrocarbons or heavy hydrocarbons have a low risk for systemic toxicity and GI decontamination is not recommended. Heavy hydrocarbons have high viscosity, low volatility, and minimal GI absorption, so gastric decontamination is not necessary. Examples are asphalt (tar), machine oil, motor oil (lubricating oil, engine oil), home heating oil, and petroleum jelly (mineral oil). Ingestion of aromatic hydrocarbons or halogenated hydrocarbons can cause systemic toxicity even in small amounts. A small-bore nasogastric tube may be placed and aspiration attempted within 2 hours of ingestion provided emesis has not occurred. Inducing emesis is no longer recommended due to risk of aspiration. Activated charcoal has not been proven to be effective but can be useful to adsorb additives such as pesticides or co-ingestants.

Inhalation of any hydrocarbon in an enclosed space can produce intoxication. These patients should receive supplemental oxygen and respiratory support if needed. Intubation may be required for altered mental status due to risk of aspiration. Patients with symptoms of aspiration including coughing, gagging, choking, and wheezing should receive supportive respiratory care and be admitted to the ICU. Chest radiographs may show changes as early as 30 minutes after ingestion, but nearly all are positive for evidence of pneumonitis within 6 hours; an initial negative radiograph does not rule out aspiration. Bronchospasm should be treated with nebulized beta agonists (e.g., albuterol).

Epinephrine should be avoided as it can precipitate arrhythmias. Cyanosis with a normal arterial PaO2 can be the result of methemoglobinemia and should be treated with methylene blue. Corticosteroids and antibiotics have not been shown to be helpful in improving outcomes. Fever and/or leukocytosis can be seen as a reaction to chemical pneumonitis and are not necessarily indicators of infection.

Most cases of aspiration resolve within 1 week, yet lipoid pneumonia can last up to 6 weeks and most pneumatoceles typically resolve spontaneously. Extracorporeal membrane oxygenation (ECMO) has been used in patients with life-threatening respiratory failure to decrease mortality.

Disposition
Asymptomatic patients with small ingestions of aliphatic hydrocarbons can be managed closely at home while symptomatic patients should be admitted for observation. Patients may be discharged once they are asymptomatic, have a normal oxygen saturation, and appear clinically stable.

Iron
Toxic Dose
The toxic dose of iron depends on the amount of elemental iron ingested, not the amount of iron salt (e.g., gluconate, sulfate, fumarate, lactate, chloride). Iron is locally corrosive and can cause fluid loss, hypovolemic shock, and perforation. Unbound iron is directly toxic to blood vessels and causes vasodilation. Iron also causes toxic effects to mitochondria in the liver, kidneys, and myocardium and is thought to be related to free radical damage.

The therapeutic dose of elemental iron is 6 mg/kg/d. An elemental iron dose of 20 to 40 mg/kg can produce mild GI symptoms, 40 to 60 mg/kg causes moderate toxicity, greater than 60 mg/kg causes severe toxicity and is potentially lethal. More than 180 mg/kg is usually fatal without treatment. Children's chewable vitamins and oral drops have 12 to 18 mg of elemental iron per tablet or per 0.6 mL of liquid drops. These have rarely been implicated in toxicity except in extremely large quantities and have never been associated with fatality.

Manifestations
Phase I: GI mucosal injury may occur within 30 minutes to 12 hours following ingestion. Vomiting may start within 30 minutes to 1 hour following ingestion and is often persistent. Hematemesis, hematochezia, and melena may occur. Abdominal cramps, diarrhea, fever, hyperglycemia, and leukocytosis may occur. Enteric coated tablets may pass through the stomach without causing symptoms. Acidosis and shock may occur within 6 to 12 hours.

Phase II: A latent period may occur 8 to 12 hours post ingestion.

Phase III: Systemic toxicity occurs 12 to 48 hours post ingestion with severe metabolic acidosis and cardiovascular collapse due to systemic vasodilation.

Phase IV: Two to 4 days post ingestion, hepatic toxicity may be present with jaundice, elevated liver enzymes, and prolonged prothrombin time. Kidney injury may be seen with proteinuria and hematuria. Pulmonary edema, disseminated intravascular coagulation, and Yersinia enterocolitica sepsis have been reported.

Phase V: Four to 8 weeks post ingestion, pyloric or intestinal stricture may cause obstruction and anemia may occur due to blood loss.

Laboratory Investigations
Iron toxicity causes an anion gap metabolic acidosis. Laboratory evaluation including serum iron with transferrin saturation and ferritin, ABG, comprehensive panel, and complete blood count with platelets should be obtained. Urine output should be monitored. Stools and emesis should be inspected and tested for occult blood. Blood type and screen should be obtained in case of significant GI blood loss.

Serum iron levels should be obtained prior to administering deferoxamine. Serum iron levels less than 350 µg/dL at 2 to 6 hours are typically asymptomatic, 350 to 500 µg/dL usually causes mild GI symptoms, greater than 500 µg/dL have a 20% risk of shock and serious iron toxicity. A repeat serum iron measurement may be useful after 8 to 12 hours to exclude delayed absorption from a bezoar or sustained-release formulation.

Most adult iron tablets are radiopaque initially and dissolve 4 hours post-ingestion. Children's chewable vitamins and liquid iron formulations are not radiopaque. A negative abdominal radiograph more than 4 hours after ingestion does not exclude iron poisoning.

Management
For ingestions of elemental iron greater than 40 mg/kg, induction of emesis with ipecac should be undertaken if vomiting has not already occurred as activated charcoal is ineffective. If radiopaque iron is present after induction of emesis, whole bowel irrigation with PEG[1] can be considered. Endoscopic or surgical removal may be necessary for coalesced iron tablets or in cases of hemorrhagic infarction of bowel or perforation peritonitis.

Deferoxamine (Desferal) is an iron chelating agent; 100 mg of deferoxamine binds 8.5 to 9.35 mg of free iron. Typically, the initial recommended IV dose is 1 g administered at an infusion rate of up to 15 mg/kg/h. If needed, additional doses of 500 mg over 4 hours to 12 hours can be administered. The maximum recommended dose is 6 g daily. Larger daily amounts have been used and tolerated in cases of extreme iron poisoning (>1000 mg/dL). The deferoxamine-iron complex can be removed by hemodialysis in cases of renal failure. Indications for iron chelation include very large symptomatic ingestions, severe clinical intoxication (severe vomiting and diarrhea, abdominal pain, metabolic acidosis, hypotension, shock), symptoms that persist or progress, serum iron level greater than 500 mg/dL. Chelation should be started as early as possible within 12 to 18 hours. The infusion should be started slowly and increased gradually to prevent hypotension. Treatment is completed when the patient is asymptomatic and urine returns to a normal color (if original a positive vin rosé color).

Disposition
Initially asymptomatic patients should be observed for development of symptoms of iron toxicity. Patients with mild GI symptoms who become asymptomatic and have no signs of toxicity for at least 6 hours are unlikely to have serious toxicity and may be discharged after evaluation for intentional ingestion and psychiatric evaluation if indicated. Patients with moderate or severe toxicity require ICU admission.

Isopropyl Alcohol
Toxic Dose
Isopropyl alcohol is found in rubbing alcohol, solvents, and lacquer thinner and is a potent gastric irritant. It is metabolized into acetone, which causes myocardial depression and is twice as effective as ethanol in causing CNS depression. It also inhibits gluconeogenesis similar to ethanol resulting in hypoglycemia. The toxic dose is 0.5 to 1 mg/kg of 70% isopropyl alcohol (equivalent to 1 mL/kg of 70%), which produces a blood isopropanol concentration of 70 mg/dL.

Manifestations
Clinical manifestations are similar to ethanol ingestion but can also cause an acetone odor on the breath, gastritis (sometimes with hematemesis), acetonuria, and acetonemia without anion

---

[1] Not FDA approved for this indication.

gap acidosis. CNS depression can occur with lethargy at levels of 50 to 100 mg/dL, coma at levels of 150 to 200 mg/dL, and potentially death with levels greater than 240 mg/dL. Hypoglycemia and seizures can occur.

Laboratory Investigations

Blood isopropyl alcohol and acetone levels should be obtained. ABG, blood glucose, electrolytes, and hepatic and renal function should be monitored. Serum osmolality should be measured and compared against the calculated osmolality to calculate an osmolal gap. The osmolal gap is increased by 1 mOsm per 5.9 mg/dL of isopropyl alcohol and per 5.5 mg/dL of acetone. If serum acetone does not exceed the normal range (0.3 to 2 mg/dL) within 30 to 60 minutes and urine acetone does not exceed the normal range within 3 hours, this excludes significant isopropyl alcohol ingestion.

Management

In cases of acute respiratory distress, airway should be secured and mechanical ventilation initiated. Glucose should be administered for patients with hypoglycemia. Additional supportive care measures are the same for the patient with ethanol toxicity. Hemodialysis can be used for cases of severe overdose but is rarely needed. Nephrology should be consulted if serum isopropyl alcohol is greater than 250 mg/dL.

Disposition

Symptomatic patients with isopropyl alcohol concentrations greater than 100 mg/dL should be admitted for at least 24 hours of observation. Patients who are severely hypoglycemic, hypotensive, or comatose require ICU admission.

Lead

Toxic Dose

Acute lead intoxication usually occurs through ingestion of lead-based paint or contaminated soil (children) and inhalation of lead-glazed ceramics or workplace exposures (adults). In recent years there have been clustered cases of lead toxicity through consumption of contaminated ground water, for example, in Flint, Michigan. Chronic lead poisoning is most often seen in children between 6 months and 6 years of age and adults with certain high-risk occupations.

In children, a venous blood lead level greater than 10 μg/dL is concerning. In adults a venous blood lead level greater than 40 μg/dL is concerning. At levels greater than 60 μg/dL, adults should be removed from work until levels are below 40 μg/dL. Lead affects neuronal development, heme synthesis, vitamin D conversion, kidney function, osteogenesis, and linear growth.

Manifestations

Common adverse health effects of lead toxicity are highlighted in Table 12. Lead exposure can cause spontaneous abortion, decreased sperm count and/or abnormal sperm morphology, preterm delivery, and teratogenic effects on the fetus.

Laboratory Investigations

In most states lead screening occurs at 1 and 2 years of age, commonly integrated within well child examinations. In cases of suspected toxicity, venous blood lead measurements are taken at presentation, on days 3 and 5 during treatment, and 7 days after chelation therapy, then every 1-2 weeks for 8 weeks, then monthly for 6 months. A CBC, serum ferritin, erythrocyte protoporphyrin (>35 μg/dL indicates lead poisoning and iron deficiency), comprehensive panel, and urinalysis should be obtained. Abdominal and long bone radiographs can identify radiopaque material in the bowel and lead lines on the proximal tibia, which occur after prolonged exposure with lead levels greater than 50 μg/dL.

TABLE 12 Lead-Induced Health Effects in Adults and Children

BLOOD LEAD LEVEL (MG/DL)	AGE GROUP	HEALTH EFFECT
>100	Adult	Encephalopathic signs and symptoms
>80	Adult	Anemia
	Child	Encephalopathy Chronic nephropathy (e.g., aminoaciduria)
>70	Adult	Clinically evident peripheral neuropathy
	Child	Colic and other gastrointestinal symptoms
>60	Adult	Female reproductive effects CNS disturbance symptoms (i.e., sleep disturbances, mood changes, memory and concentration problems, headaches)
>50	Adult	Decreased hemoglobin production Decreased performance on neurobehavioral tests
	Adult	Altered testicular function Gastrointestinal symptoms (i.e., abdominal pain, constipation, diarrhea, nausea, anorexia)
	Child	Peripheral neuropathy*
>40	Adult	Decreased peripheral nerve conduction Hypertension, age 40–59 years Chronic neuropathy*
>25	Adult	Elevated erythrocyte protoporphyrin in males
15–25	Adult	Elevated erythrocyte protoporphyrin in females
>10	Child	Decreased intelligence and growth Impaired learning Reduced birth weight* Impaired mental ability
	Fetus	Preterm delivery

*Controversial.

Management

Since lead does not bind to activated charcoal, abdominal radiographs and whole-bowel irrigation are recommended prior to commencing oral chelation therapy. Chelation therapy should be initiated in children with a venous lead level greater than 45 μg/dL, adults with a level greater than 80 μg/dL, and adults at lower levels who are symptomatic. Consultation with a poison control center or toxicologist is recommended for patients requiring chelation. Edetate calcium disodium is given IV or IM to cause lead elimination in urine. It can cause redistribution of lead to the brain, so typically, dimercaprol (or British anti-Lewisite [BAL]) is given prior to administration for children with levels greater than 55 μg/dL and adults with levels greater than 100 μg/dL. Dimercaprol (BAL) is used for patients with a blood lead level greater than 70 μg/dL. It chelates lead and enhances elimination in urine and bile. It does cross the blood-brain barrier. About 50% of patients have adverse reactions to BAL including metallic taste, injection site pain, sterile abscess, and fever.

Venous blood level greater than 70 μg/dL or presence of clinical symptoms of encephalopathy in children is a life-threatening emergency. These patients should be transferred to a pediatric intensive care unit with a critical care specialist, toxicologist, neurologist, and neurosurgeon available. These patients require monitoring of neurologic, hemodynamic, and fluid status and some may require monitoring of intracranial pressure. Fluids, renal and hepatic function, and electrolytes should be monitored. For severe lead poisoning, intramuscular dimercaprol (BAL) should be given (25 mg/kg/d divided into 6 doses). Four hours later, a second dose of dimercaprol should be given IM concurrently with edetate calcium disodium (CaNa2EDTA) 50 mg/kg/d as a single dose infused over several hours or as a continuous infusion. The double therapy is continued until the venous blood level is less than 40 µg/dL. Therapy is continued for 72 hours as long as venous blood lead level is greater than 40 µg/dL. Following this, parenteral therapy with two drugs (CaNa2EDTA and BAL) is recommended for 5 days or continuation of therapy with CaNa2EDTA alone if a good response is achieved and the venous blood level of lead is less than 40 µg/dL. If a blood lead level is not readily available, BAL and EDTA should be continued for 5 days.

For patients with lead encephalopathy, combination chelation therapy should continue until the patient is clinically stable before changing therapy. Mannitol and dexamethasone can reduce cerebral edema, but their role in lead encephalopathy has not been studied. Surgical decompression is not recommended. If BAL and CaNa2EDTA are used together, a minimum of 2 days with no treatment should elapse before another 5-day course of therapy is considered. The 5-day course is repeated with CaNa2EDTA alone if the blood lead level rebounds to greater than 40 µg/dL or in combination with BAL if the venous blood level is greater than 70 µg/dL. If a third course is required, unless there are compelling reasons, one should wait at least 5 to 7 days before administering the course.

Following chelation therapy, a period of equilibration of 10 to 14 days should be allowed and a repeat venous blood lead concentration should be obtained. If the patient is stable enough for oral intake, oral succimer (Chemet) 30 mg/kg/d in three divided doses for 5 days followed by 20 mg/kg/d in two divided doses for 14 days has been suggested for treatment in adult patients,[1] but there are limited data to support this recommendation. Therapy should be continued until venous blood lead level is less than 20 µg/dL in children or less than 40 µg/dL in adults. In patients with renal failure, chelators bound to lead can be removed by hemodialysis.

Disposition

All patients who are symptomatic or have a lead level greater than 70 µg/dL should be admitted for observation and treatment. Lead poisoning in children should be reported to the local health department. Occupational lead poisoning should be reported to OSHA (Occupational Safety and Health Administration). Sources of lead should be identified and abated prior to the child returning home. Neuropsychological and audiology testing should be considered following treatment.

Lithium
Toxic Dose

Lithium is an alkali metal used in the treatment of bipolar psychiatric disorders. Most cases of toxicity are due to chronic overdose. Lithium impacts brain function by reducing excitatory (dopamine and glutamate) but increases (GABA) neurotransmission. It displaces magnesium which impacts sodium excretion and potassium secretion.

The therapeutic serum lithium concentration in cases of acute mania is 0.6 to 1.2 mEq/L, and for maintenance it is 0.5 to 0.8 mEq/L. Serum lithium concentration levels are usually obtained 12 hours after the last dose. The toxic dose is determined by clinical manifestations and serum levels after the distribution phase. Acute ingestion of 6 g of lithium can produce significant intoxication. Chronic intoxication is caused by conditions that decrease elimination of lithium or increase renal reabsorption of lithium. Sequelae include renal impairment, hyponatremia, hyperkalemia, lithium-induced diabetes insipidus, dehydration, and GI losses.

Manifestations

Side effects can include fine tremors, GI upset, hypothyroidism, leukocytosis, polyuria and frank diabetes insipidus, dermatologic findings (e.g., morbilliform eruption and exfoliative dermatitis), and cardiac conduction defects (e.g., sinoatrial block, intraventricular conduction delay, ST depressions or elevations, Brugada pattern). Lithium is teratogenic and should be avoided in pregnant women or those who plan to become pregnant.

Patients with acute poisoning may be asymptomatic initially but can become symptomatic and deteriorate when the serum lithium concentration decreases by 50% due to lithium distributing to the brain and tissues. Nausea and vomiting can occur within 4 hours, yet it can take up to 3 to 5 days for significant symptoms to develop. Acute toxicity and acute-on-chronic toxicity cause neurologic findings including weakness, fasciculations, altered mental status, myoclonus, hyperreflexia, rigidity, coma, and seizures. Serum lithium levels do not always correlate with symptoms, but higher levels are more predictive of severe intoxication. A serum lithium concentration greater than 3.0 mEq/L with chronic intoxication and altered mental state indicates severe toxicity. Lithium toxicity can result in permanent neurologic abnormalities.

Laboratory Investigations

A comprehensive panel and CBC, renal function, thyroid function, and ECG should be obtained. A serum lithium level, electrolytes, and renal function should be monitored every 2 to 4 hours until levels peak and there is a downward trend close to therapeutic range.

Management

Patients should be placed on seizure precautions and monitored for hypotension and arrhythmias with hemodynamic and cardiac telemetry monitoring. Periodic neurologic monitoring for mental status, rigidity, and hyperreflexia, as well as hydration status, should be performed. Urine output should be monitored. Patients taking diuretics (e.g., thiazides and spironolactone), nonsteroidal anti-inflammatory drugs, salicylates, angiotensin-converting enzyme inhibitors, serotonin reuptake inhibitors, and phenothiazines should hold these medications when possible.

If the patient is on chronic lithium therapy, consideration of discontinuation should be discontinued in favor of other medications with psychiatric consultation. Nephrology consultation is recommended for chronic lithium intoxication, elevated serum lithium concentration (>2.5 mEq/L), large ingestion, or altered mental status. IV fluids may be given for hydration after obtaining initial serum sodium in cases of chronic intoxication due to risk of hypernatremia from diabetes insipidus. Current evidence supports use of 0.9% saline at a rate of 200 mL/h to enhance excretion of lithium. Once urine output, hydration, and normonatremia are achieved, IV fluids should be switched to 0.45% saline at a rate of 100 mL/h.

Gastric lavage is not recommended as activated charcoal is ineffective. Whole-bowel irrigation may be useful for sustained release formulations, but its efficacy has not been proven. Sodium polystyrene sulfonate (Kayexalate)[1] is not recommended. Hemodialysis is the most efficient method for elimination of lithium. It is the recommended treatment for patients with severe intoxication with altered mental status, seizures, and anuric patients. Hemodialysis is continued until serum lithium levels are less than 1 mEq/L. Serum lithium levels should be repeated 4 hours after dialysis to assess for rebound due to extensive re-equilibration.

---

[1] Not FDA approved for this indication.

[1] Not FDA approved for this indication.

Repeated and prolonged hemodialysis may be needed. Neurologic recovery often lags behind improvement in lithium level.

Disposition

Asymptomatic lithium overdose cannot be cleared based on a single lithium level. If patients have any neurologic manifestations, then they should be admitted. They may require ICU admission for dehydration, renal impairment, or for a high or rising lithium level.

Methanol
Toxic Dose

Methanol is metabolized into formaldehyde by alcohol dehydrogenase. This is further metabolized into formate, which causes tissue hypoxia, lactic acidosis, and optic nerve edema.

The minimal toxic amount is 100 mg/kg. In young children, 2.5 to 5 mL of 100% methanol can cause serious toxicity. Ingestion of 5 mL of 100% methanol by a 10 kg child produces a peak blood methanol level of 80 mg/dL. For adults, a fatal oral dose is 30 to 240 mL of 100% methanol (20 to 150 g). Ingestion of 6 to 10 mL of 100% methanol can cause blindness in adults. Blood methanol concentrations greater than 20 mg/dL are toxic; serious toxicity and possibly fatality occur at concentrations higher than 50 mg/dL.

Manifestations

Metabolism delays onset of manifestations by 12 to 18 hours, longer if ethanol is co-ingested. In the first 6 hours following ingestion, patients may experience confusion, ataxia, inebriation, formaldehyde odor on the breath, and abdominal pain, yet some patients may be asymptomatic. During this time, an osmolal gap may be seen, but following metabolism into formate, the osmolal gap disappears and an anion gap metabolic acidosis forms. Therefore, the absence of an osmolar or anion gap does not always exclude methanol intoxication. Within 6 to 12 hours after ingestion patients may experience malaise, headache, abdominal pain, vomiting, or visual symptoms (hyperemia of the optic disc, snow vision, and blindness). More than 12 hours after ingestion, patients may have worsening acidosis, hyperglycemia, shock, and multiorgan failure. Death may result from intractable acidosis and cerebral edema.

Laboratory Investigations

Initial lab investigations should include an ABG, methanol and ethanol levels, a complete blood count with platelets (CBCP), and a comprehensive panel; these tests should be repeated every 4 hours. If available, formate levels should be obtained and monitored as these more closely correlate with severity of intoxication then blood methanol levels.

Management

Initial attention should be paid to airway stabilization, ventilation, and circulation. Nephrology should be consulted early on for possible hemodialysis. Metabolic acidosis should be treated aggressively with sodium bicarbonate 2 to 3 mEq/kg intravenously. Large quantities of sodium bicarbonate may be necessary to treat metabolic acidosis. Ophthalmology consultation is also recommended early in the course.

Antidote therapy is indicated for the patient was ingested greater than 0.4 mL/kg of 100% methanol with a blood ethanol level greater than 20 mg/dL, an osmolar gap not accounted for by other factors, and the patient is symptomatic, has an increased anion gap metabolic acidosis, and/or hyperemia of the optic disc. Either of the following antidote therapies are currently recommended:

1. Ethanol therapy: Ethanol should be initiated immediately if fomepizole is not available. Ethanol blocks metabolism of ethylene glycol and methanol into toxic metabolites. Ethanol should be administered intravenously to produce a blood ethanol concentration of 100 to 150 mg/dL. The oral route of administration is not recommended. The loading dose is 10 mL/kg of 10% ethanol administered intravenously concomitantly with a maintenance dose of 10% ethanol at 1.0 mL/kg/h. This dose may need to be increased to 2 mL/kg/h in patients who are heavy drinkers.

Repeat blood ethanol concentration should be measured hourly, and the maintenance infusion rate should be adjusted to maintain blood ethanol concentration of 100 to 150 mg/dL.

2. Fomepizole (Antizol): Inhibits alcohol dehydrogenase more effectively than ethanol and does not require monitoring of blood ethanol concentration or titration of infusion. Fomepizole is available in 1 g/mL vials of 1.5 mL. The loading dose is 15 mg/kg (0.015 mL/kg) IV, maintenance dose is 10 mg/kg (0.01 mL/kg) every 12 hours for 4 doses, then 15 mg/kg every 12 hours until methanol concentration is undetectable. The solution is prepared by being mixed with 100 mL of 0.9% saline or D5W. See the ethylene glycol section for dosing of omeprazole for patients on hemodialysis.

Hemodialysis can increase clearance of methanol and toxic metabolites 10-fold compared to renal clearance. Previously, hemodialysis was recommended for a blood methanol concentration greater than 50 mg/dL, but some toxicologists recommended early hemodialysis for levels over 25 mg/dL to shorten the course of intoxication. If hemodialysis is used in conjunction with ethanol, then the infusion rate of 10% ethanol should be increased to 2.0 to 3.5 mL/kg/h. Blood ethanol concentration and glucose level should be monitored every 2 hours for these patients. Therapy with hemodialysis and an antidote (ethanol or fomepizole) is continued until blood methanol concentration is undetectable, acidosis has resolved, patient's neurologic or visual changes have resolved.

Disposition

Patients with significant methanol ingestion should be evaluated in the emergency department. Patients requiring hemodialysis or intubation will require ICU admission. Outpatient ophthalmology follow-up should be arranged for all patients.

Opioids
Toxic Dose

Opioids are used for analgesia, as antitussives, and as antidiarrheal agents, and are substances of abuse. Tolerance, physical dependency, and withdrawal symptoms develop commonly. Opioids cause dose-dependent CNS respiratory depression, pulmonary aspiration, and/or cardiac pulmonary edema, all of which may be fatal. Dextromethorphan is found in many over-the-counter cough and cold medicines and can interact with MAOIs to cause hyperthermia or serotonin syndrome.

Toxic dose depends on the drug, route of administration, and tolerance. Table 13 highlights therapeutic and toxic doses. Infants younger than 3 months of age are more susceptible to respiratory depression and therapeutic doses should be reduced by 50%. Fentanyl is 100 times more potent than morphine and is a current national threat.

Manifestations

Mild intoxication can cause miosis, drowsiness, partial ptosis, and head nodding. Larger doses can cause miotic pupils (with exception of dextromethorphan, fentanyl, meperidine, and diphenoxylate), respiratory depression, and depressed level of consciousness. Blood pressure, heart rate, and bowel motility are decreased. Muscle tone is usually decreased, but increased muscle tone can be seen with meperidine and fentanyl. Seizures can occur with codeine, meperidine, propoxyphene,[2] and dextromethorphan. Hallucinations and agitation have been reported with some opioids. Some opioids cause histamine release resulting in pruritus and urticaria. Noncardiac pulmonary edema can occur, particularly after an overdose and especially with IV heroin use. Peripheral vasodilation and hypotension may also occur.

Laboratory Investigations

For patients with overdose, an ABG, comprehensive panel, CBC, coagulation profile, toxicology screen, chest radiograph, urine toxicology with GCMS, and ECG should be obtained initially.

---

[2] Not available in the United States.

TABLE 13 Doses and Onset and Duration of Action of Common Opioids

DRUG	ADULT ORAL DOSE	CHILD ORAL DOSE	ONSET OF ACTION	DURATION OF ACTION	ADULT FATAL DOSE
Camphorated tincture of opium (Paregoric)[2]	2–4 mg morphine/dose	0.1–0.2 mg/dose	15–30 min	4–5 h	NA
Codeine	15–60 mg	0.5–1 mg/kg	15–30 min	4–6 h	800 mg
	>1 mg/kg is toxic in a child; >200 mg is toxic in an adult; >5 mg/kg is fatal in a child; contraindicated in a child <12 yr				
Dextromethorphan	15 mg 10 mg/kg is toxic	0.25 mg/kg	15–30 min	3–6 h	NA
Diacetylmorphine; street heroin is less than 10% pure	60 mg	NA	15–30 min	3–4 h	100 mg
Diphenoxylate atropine (Lomotil)	5–10 mg	NA	120–240 min	14 h	300 mg
	7.5 mg is toxic in a child, 300 mg is toxic in adult				
Fentanyl (Duragesic)	0.1–0.2 mg	0.001–0.002 mg/kg	7–8 min	Intramuscular: ½–2 h	1.0 mg
Hydrocodone with APAP (Lortab)	5–10 mg (hydrocodone)	<50 kg: 0.1–0.2 mg/kg/dose (hydrocodone) >50 kg: 5–10 mg	30 min	3–4 h	100 mg
Hydromorphone (Dilaudid)	1–4 mg	0.03–0.08 mg/kg	15–30 min	3–4 h	100 mg
Meperidine (Demerol)	100 mg	Use not recommended in children	10–45 min	3–4 h	350 mg
Methadone (Dolophine)	2.5–5 mg	0.1 mg/kg	30–60 min	4–12 h	120 mg
Morphine	10–60 mg	0.1–0.2 mg/kg	<20 min	4–6 h	200 mg
	Oral dose is 6 times parenteral dose, MS Contin sustained-release prep				
Oxycodone APAP (Percocet)	5 mg	NA	15–30 min	4–5 h	NA
Pentazocine (Talwin)	50–100 mg	NA	15–30 min	3–4 h	NA
Propoxyphene (Darvon)[2]	65–100 mg	NA	30–60 min	2–4 h	700 mg

[1]Not FDA approved for this indication.
[2]Not available in the United States.

For patients with opioid use disorder, testing for hepatitis B and C, syphilis, and HIV should be considered.

Management

Airway should be secured, and some patients may require assisted ventilation. For reversal of opioids, 0.1 mg of naloxone (Narcan) should be administered immediately. Patients should be placed on a cardiac monitor and IV access established. Induced emesis is not recommended, but activated charcoal can be administered if bowel sounds are present. Patients with opioid use disorder may need to be restrained prior to administering an opioid reversal agent due to risk of agitation. The dose of Narcan should be doubled every 2 minutes until the patient responds or 10 to 20 mg has been given. If opioid use disorder is not suspected, then 2 mg every 2 to 3 minutes for a total of 10 to 20 mg is administered. For naloxone infusions[1], the response dose (dose that produces a complete response to naloxone with mydriasis and improvement in ventilation) should be infused every hour. Methadone ingestions often require naloxone infusions for 24 to 48 hours.

Naloxone lasts 30 to 60 minutes for reversal of respiratory depression and withdrawal affects subside within a short time.

Nalmefene (Revex) is an FDA-approved long-acting (4 to 8 hours) pure opioid antagonist, but its role in acute intoxication is unknown and can produce prolonged withdrawal. Naloxone does not correct noncardiac pulmonary edema. These patients require intubation, mechanical ventilation, positive end expiratory pressure and hemodynamic monitoring. IV fluids should be given judiciously in these patients because opioids may stimulate antidiuretic hormone.

Hypotension caused directly by opioids is rare and other etiologies should be investigated. For agitated patients, hypoxia and hypoglycemia should be excluded. Other complications of opioid use include urinary retention, constipation, rhabdomyolysis, myoglobinuria, hypoglycemia, withdrawal, blood-borne infections, soft-tissue infections, and endocarditis.

Disposition

Following response to naloxone, patients should be admitted for observation for relapse and development of pulmonary edema for at least 6 to 12 hours with cardiac and respiratory monitoring. Patients who require repeated doses of naloxone and/or an infusion or developed pulmonary edema should be admitted to the ICU until they are asymptomatic for at least 12 hours. Patients should be evaluated for intentional overdose and psychiatric evaluation and/or addiction medicine consultation should be considered.

---

[1]Not FDA approved for this indication.

Organophosphates and Carbamates

Toxic Dose

Cholinergic effects can be seen with insecticides (organophosphates or carbamates), some medications (including neostigmine [Prostigmin] and physostigmine [Antilirium]), and nerve gases (e.g., tabun [GA], sarin [GB], soman [GB], and venom X [VX]). Organophosphates cause irreversible inhibition of acetylcholinesterase and pseudocholinesterase while carbamates cause reversible inhibition of these enzymes with rapid return to normal activity. Carbamate toxicity is less and the duration is shorter, and carbamates rarely cause overt CNS effects due to poor CNS penetration, and pralidoxime (Protopam) may not be necessary for mild carbamate intoxication.

Organophosphate insecticides include malathion (low toxicity, median lethal dose [LD50] 2800 mg/kg), chlorpyrifos, which has been removed from the market (moderate toxicity), and parathion (high toxicity, LD50 2 mg/kg). Parathion's minimum lethal dose is 2 mg in children and 10 to 20 mg in adults. The lethal dose of malathion is greater than 1375 mg/kg and that of chlorpyrifos is 25 g; chlorpyrifos is unlikely to be lethal. Carbamate insecticides include carbaryl (low toxicity, LD50 500 mg/kg), propoxur (moderate toxicity, LD50 95 mg/kg), and aldicarb (high toxicity, LD50 0.9 mg/kg).

Manifestations

Organophosphates have a garlic-like odor that can be detected in the breath, gastric contents, and container. Early in the clinical course, cholinergic (muscarinic) signs are present, which can be remembered with the mnemonic DUMBELS: defecation/diarrhea, urinary incontinence, miosis (mydriasis may occur in 20%), bronchospasm/bronchorrhea, excessive secretions/salivation, lacrimation, and seizures. Due to excessive parasympathetic stimulation, bradycardia, pulmonary edema, and hypotension may occur.

Later in the clinical course, sympathetic and nicotinic effects are seen, which are remembered by MATCH: muscle weakness and fasciculation, adrenal stimulation and hyperglycemia, tachycardia, cramping in muscles, and hypertension. Finally, skeletal muscles become paralyzed.

CNS effects include headache, blurred vision, anxiety, ataxia, delirium and psychosis, seizures, coma, and respiratory depression. Cranial nerve palsies have been reported. Delayed hallucinations have been seen. Delayed respiratory paralysis, neurologic disorders, and neurobehavioral abnormalities have been described following ingestion or dermal exposure of some organophosphates. Paralysis of proximal and respiratory muscles that develops 24 to 96 following treatment of organophosphate poisoning is known as "intermediate syndrome". Delayed distal polyneuropathy has been reported with triorthocresyl phosphate, bromoleptophos, and methamidophos.

Laboratory Investigations

Initial studies include ABG, chest radiograph, blood glucose (hyperglycemia is common), pulse oximetry, ECG, coagulation studies, hepatic and renal function, amylase, lipase, and urine alkyl phosphate paranitrophenol level. Red blood cell cholinesterase activity correlates with clinical severity. Mild poisoning is 20% to 50% of normal, moderate is 10% to 20% of normal, and severe is 10% of normal (90% reduction in activity). Postexposure increases in cholinesterase activity of 10% to 15% 10 to 14 days after exposure confirms the diagnosis.

Management

Organophosphates can be absorbed via inhalation, dermal, and enteral routes, therefore care should be taken to decontaminate patients and prevent exposure of healthcare personnel. Healthcare personnel should wear masks, gloves, gowns, and goggles and in some cases may require respirators and/or hazardous material suits. Patients should be kept in isolation until decontamination has been completed. Patients should have continuous cardiopulmonary monitoring. Intubation and mechanical ventilation may be needed. Suctioning should be available for removal of copious secretions.

Contaminated clothing and belongings should be removed and disposed of. Dermal exposures should be treated with copious water irrigation for at least 30 minutes. In the case of extensive exposure, the hair, nails, navel, and perineum should be cleansed with soap or shampoo. Ocular exposures should be irrigated with copious amounts of tepid water or 0.9% saline for at least 15 minutes. Recent oral ingestions may be treated with activated charcoal.

Atropine sulfate can be given as an antidote and is both diagnostic and therapeutic as it primarily improves muscarinic effects but may only partially improve CNS manifestations (coma, seizures). Preservative-free atropine (without benzyl alcohol) should be used. For bradycardia or bronchorrhea, a test dose of 0.02 mg/kg in children or 1 mg in adults, intravenously should be given. If no signs of atropinization occur (tachycardia, drying of secretions, and mydriasis), additional atropine should be administered immediately as follows: 0.05 mg/kg in children or 2 mg in adults, every 5 to 10 minutes as needed to dry the secretions and clear the lungs. Effects are seen within 1 to 4 minutes and maximum effects occur at 8 minutes. The average dose in the first 24 hours is 40 mg, but 1000 mg or more have been required in severe cases. Poisoning with lipophilic agents (e.g., fenthion, chlorfenthion) may require weeks of atropine therapy. In these cases, continuous infusion may be required at the rate of 10% to 20% of the total loading dose (mg) per hour, with additional 5-mg boluses as needed to produce atropinization.

Pralidoxime chloride (Protopam) has antinicotinic, antimuscarinic and possibly CNS affects. Treatment with pralidoxime may reduce dose of atropine needed. Pralidoxime reactivates cholinesterase activity. It should be given early in the clinical course to be most effective but can be beneficial even several days after poisoning. Clinical improvement occurs within 10 to 40 minutes. The initial dose of pralidoxime chloride is 1 to 2 g in 250 mL 0.9% saline over 5 to 10 minutes, maximum 200 mg/min, in adults or 25 to 50 mg/kg, maximum 4 mg/kg/min, in children younger than 12 years of age. The dose can be repeated every 6 to 12 hours for several days. An alternative is a continuous infusion of 1 g in 100 mL 0.9% saline at 5 to 20 mg/kg/h (0.5 to 12 mL/kg/h) up to 500 mg/h and titrated to desired response, as the maximum adult daily dose is 12 g.

Disposition

Asymptomatic patients with a normal exam may be discharged after 6 to 8 hours of observation in the emergency department. Patients should be assessed for intentional poisoning and psychiatric evaluation may be warranted. Symptomatic patients should be admitted to the intensive care unit. For milder cases of carbonate poisoning, patient should be monitored until there asymptomatic for at least 6 to 8 hours. OSHA should be notified of workplace exposures.

Salicylates

Toxic Dose

Salicylates are found in aspirin products, salicylic acid topical products, bismuth subsalicylate, and methyl salicylate (oil of wintergreen). It has multiple mechanisms including stimulating the medullary chemoreceptor trigger zone and respiratory center, uncoupling oxidation, inhibition of clotting factors, alteration of platelet function, and inhibition of prostaglandin synthesis.

Acute mild intoxication occurs at doses of 150 to 200 mg/kg, moderate intoxication at 200 to 300 mg/kg, and severe intoxication at 300 to 500 mg/kg. Salicylate plasma concentrations above 30 mg/dL may be associated with clinical toxicity. Chronic intoxication may occur with ingestions greater than 100 mg/kg/d for more than 2 days. Oil of wintergreen is the most toxic form of salicylate. Fatalities have occurred with ingestion of 1 teaspoonful in children and 1 ounce in adults. It is found in topical ointments and liniments (18% to 30%).

Manifestations

Ingestions of topical salicylic acid preparations may cause mucosal caustic injury to the oropharynx and GI tract. Occult salicylate overdose should be considered in patients with an unexplained acid-base abnormality. Manifestations of acute overdose include the following:

Minimal symptoms: May occur at high therapeutic salicylate plasma concentrations of 20 to 30 mg/dL. Includes tinnitus, dizziness, and deafness. Nausea and vomiting may occur due to gastric irritation.

Phase I: Mild manifestations occur 1 to 12 hours following ingestion with a 6-hour salicylate plasma concentration of 45 to 70 mg/dL. Nausea and vomiting typically occur, followed by hyperventilation within 3 to 8 hours after acute overdose. Hyperventilation causes a mild respiratory alkalosis with a serum pH greater than 7.4 and urine pH greater than 6.0. Patients may also experience lethargy, vertigo, headache, confusion, and diaphoresis.

Phase II: Moderate manifestations occur 12 to 24 hours following ingestion with a 6-hour salicylate plasma concentration of 70 to 90 mg/dL. Marked respiratory alkalosis with anion gap metabolic acidosis, dehydration, and urine pH less than 6.0 may occur. Other abnormalities including hypo or hyperglycemia, hypokalemia, decreased ionized calcium, and increased BUN, creatinine, and lactate may be seen. Confusion, disorientation, and hallucinations may occur. Hypotension and seizures have been reported.

Phase III: Severe intoxication occurs more than 24 hours following ingestion with a 6-hour salicylate plasma concentration of 90 to 130 mg/dL. In addition to the above, seizures develop. Pulmonary edema may occur. Metabolic acidemia (pH less than 7.4) and aciduria (pH less than 6.0) may develop. In adults, alkalosis may persist until terminal respiratory failure. A normalizing pH in any patient with tachypnea is worrisome for impending respiratory failure.

Children less than 4 years of age may develop a mixed metabolic acidosis and respiratory alkalosis within 4 to 6 hours because they have less respiratory reserve and accumulate lactate more quickly. Hypoglycemia is also more common in children.

Fatalities are seen with a 6-hour salicylate plasma concentration greater than 130 to 150 mg/dL and are caused by CNS depression, cardiovascular collapse, electrolyte imbalance, and cerebral edema. Serum salicylate levels may not correlate well for acute or chronic cases of intoxication. Noncardiac pulmonary edema is a common complication in the elderly and is associated with a mortality rate of 25%. Chronic salicylate poisoning in children may mimic Reye syndrome with prominent CNS findings (e.g., hallucinations, delirium, memory loss, papilledema, bizarre behavior, agitation, seizures, and coma). The toxicity course may also be complicated by hemorrhage, renal failure, pulmonary edema, and cerebral edema. Mixed acid-base derangements may be seen often with hypoglycemia. A chronic salicylate plasma concentration greater than 60 mg/dL with metabolic acidosis and altered mental status is a sign of severe chronic intoxication.

Laboratory Investigations

All patients with salicylate overdoses should have both a salicylate and an acetaminophen plasma levels obtained upon presentation. In addition, an ABG, ECG, comprehensive panel, ionized calcium, magnesium, phosphorus, prothrombin time, CBCP, and urinalysis should be obtained. In cases of severe intoxication, an ABG and urine output should be measured every 2 to 4 hours. Pulse oximetry and cardiac telemetry should be monitored.

Management

Salicylate levels do not necessarily correlate with severity of intoxication, particularly for chronic intoxication, thus treatment is based on clinical and metabolic findings. For altered mental status, glucose,[1] naloxone,[1] and thiamine[1] should be administered in standard doses. Bismuth and magnesium salicylate preparations may be radiopaque on abdominal radiographs. For moderate,

severe, or chronic intoxication, consultation with nephrology is recommended.

Activated charcoal is useful for GI decontamination up to 4 hours post ingestion. Concretions may occur with massive (>300 mg/kg) ingestions. If blood salicylate levels fail to improve with standard treatment, contrast radiography should be performed, which may reveal concretions or bezoar that may be removed with whole bowel irrigation, gastric lavage, endoscopy, or gastrostomy.

For acute moderate to severe salicylism, adults should receive a bolus of 1 to 2 mEq/kg of sodium bicarbonate (NaHCO3) followed by an infusion of 100 to 150 mEq NaHCO3 added to 500 to 1000 mL of 5% dextrose and administered over 60 minutes.[1] Children should receive a bolus of 1 to 2 mEq/kg of NaHCO3 followed by an infusion of 1 to 2 mEq/kg added to 20 mL/kg of 5% dextrose administered over 60 minutes[1]. The goal of sodium bicarbonate therapy is to achieve urine output of at least 2 mL/kg/h and urine pH greater than 8. The initial infusion is followed by subsequent infusions (two to three times normal maintenance) of 200 to 300 mL/h in adults or 10 mL/kg/h in children. If the patient is acidotic and has a serum pH of less than 7.15, an additional 1 to 2 mEq/kg of NaHCO3 is given over 1 to 2 hours; persistent acidosis may require 1 to 2 mEq/kg of bicarbonate every 2 hours. The infusion rate, the amount of bicarbonate, and the electrolytes should be adjusted to correct serum abnormalities and to maintain the targeted urine output and urinary pH.

Patients should be monitored for fluid overload due to risk of pulmonary and cerebral edema, particularly in the elderly. A decreased serum bicarbonate with normal or high blood pH indicates predominant respiratory alkalosis and sodium bicarbonate should be administered cautiously. A pH of 7.4 to 7.5 is not a contraindication to bicarbonate therapy because these patients often have a base deficit despite elevated blood pH. If tetany occurs, then sodium bicarbonate should be discontinued, and calcium gluconate 0.1 to 0.2 mL/kg of 10% IV solution should be administered.

Once the patient is producing urine, potassium 20 to 40 mEq/L may be added to fluids. In cases of severe, late, and chronic salicylism, 60 mEq/L may be required. When the serum potassium is below 4.0 mEq/L, 10 mEq/L should be added over the first hour. If the patient has hypokalemia less than 3 mEq/L and flat T waves and U waves, 0.25 to 0.5 mEq/kg up to 10 mEq/h is administered.

Seizures should be managed with diazepam or lorazepam[1] and hypoglycemia and hypocalcemia should be excluded. A CT brain scan should be obtained to evaluate for cerebral edema and hemorrhage. Pulmonary edema is managed with fluid restriction, high FiO2, mechanical ventilation, and positive end-expiratory pressure. Cerebral edema is managed with fluid restriction, elevating the head of the bed, hyperventilation, osmotic diuresis, and dexamethasone. Neurosurgical consultation may be sought.

Prolonged prothrombin time is corrected with parenteral Vitamin K. For active bleeding, patients may require blood products including fresh plasma and platelets due to salicylate inhibition of clotting factors and platelet function. Hyperpyrexia is managed with external cooling measures.

Hemodialysis is the treatment of choice for removal of salicylates and corrects acid-base, electrolyte, and fluid imbalances. Indications for hemodialysis include the following:

- Acute poisoning with salicylate plasma concentration greater than 100 mg/dL without improvement after 6 hours of appropriate therapy
- Chronic poisoning with cardiopulmonary disease and a salicylate plasma concentration as low as 40 mg/dL with refractory acidosis, severe CNS manifestations (coma and seizures), and progressive deterioration, especially in elderly patients
- Impairment of vital organs of elimination
- Clinical deterioration despite good supportive care and alkalinization
- Severe refractory acid-base or electrolyte disturbances despite

---

[1] Not FDA approved for this indication.

[1] Not FDA approved for this indication.

Disposition

Asymptomatic patients should be monitored for at least 6 hours, longer if enteric coated tablets, massive overdose, or suspicion for concretions. All patients should be evaluated for intentional ingestion and receive psychiatric evaluation if indicated. Patients who remain asymptomatic with a salicylate plasma concentration less than 35 mg/dL may be discharged. Patients with acute ingestion, salicylate plasma concentration less than 60 mg/dL, and mild symptoms may be treated in the emergency department. Cases of moderate to severe toxicity, chronic salicylism with acidosis, and altered mental status should be admitted to the ICU.

Selective Serotonin Reuptake Inhibitors
Toxic Dose

Selective serotonin reuptake inhibitors (SSRIs) are used for treatment of depression and anxiety. These include fluoxetine (Prozac), paroxetine (Paxil), sertraline (Zoloft), escitalopram (Lexapro), and citalopram (Celexa). They increase serotonin activity and should not be used within 5 weeks of therapy with monoamine oxidase inhibitors (MAOIs). Likewise, MAOIs should not be initiated within 5 weeks of SSRI therapy.

Manifestations

All SSRIs have the potential to cause serotonin syndrome, which is potentially life-threatening, particularly if administered with an MAOI or in overdose. Serotonin syndrome is caused by cerebral serotonergic stimulation resulting in hyperthermia, myoclonus, rhabdomyolysis, confusion, tremors, and psychiatric disturbances. Serotonin syndrome is diagnosed based on using the Hunter Toxicity Criteria Decision Rules and must include one of the following: (1) Spontaneous clonus, (2) Inducible clonus PLUS agitation or diaphoresis, (3) Ocular clonus PLUS agitation or diaphoresis, (4) tremor PLUS hyperreflexia, or (5) hypertonia PLUS temperature above 38° C PLUS ocular clonus or inducible clonus. Cardiovascular complications and extrapyramidal side effects (e.g., akathisia, dyskinesia, and Parkinsonism) may occur. Suicidal ideation, seizures, sexual dysfunction, and hematologic disorders (due to platelet inhibition) may develop. Syndrome of inappropriate antidiuretic hormone (SIADH) may develop, particularly in elderly patients, resulting in hyponatremia.

Laboratory Investigations

An ABG, CBCP, comprehensive panel, coagulation profile, creatine kinase, and ECG should be obtained.

Management

Initial supportive treatment includes stabilizing vital signs and thermoregulation with external cooling measures. Benzodiazepines should be administered to prevent and control muscle hyperactivity (diazepam [Valium] for seizures, clonazepam [Klonopin] for myoclonus) and assist with thermoregulation. If benzodiazepines are unsuccessful for controlling muscle activity or seizures, then nondepolarizing neuromuscular blockage may be necessary along with EEG monitoring. Patients treated with neuromuscular blockers require intubation and sedation. Electrolyte and acid-base abnormalities should be corrected. Fluids should be given to maintain urine output of at least 2 mL/kg/h if there is risk of myoglobinuria. Cardiac and hemodynamic monitoring should be implemented. Hypertension and tachycardia are often labile and can be managed with short-acting agents including esmolol (Brevibloc), nicardipine (Cardene), or nitroprusside. Citalopram (Celexa) carries an increased risk of QTc prolongation.

Activated charcoal may be used for ingestions within 1 hour. Haloperidol (Haldol) and phenothiazines should be avoided. Serotonin antagonists, such as cyproheptadine (Periactin),[1] may be used to treat serotonin syndrome. When administered as an antidote for serotonin syndrome, an initial dose of 12 mg is recommended, followed by 2 mg every two hours until clinical response

is seen. Cyproheptadine is only available in an oral form, but it may be crushed and given through a nasogastric or orogastric tube. It may produce sedation and transient hypotension.

Disposition

Asymptomatic patients should be observed for at least 6 hours. Symptomatic patients should be admitted until asymptomatic for at least 24 hours. Patients requiring interventions for seizures, hyperthermia, muscle hyperactivity, hemodynamic abnormalities, or cardiac arrhythmias should be admitted to the ICU. All patients should be assessed for suicidal ideation, closely supervised, and receive psychiatric evaluation if indicated.

Tricyclic and Cyclic Antidepressants
Toxic Dose

Tricyclic antidepressants (TCAs) are used for treatment of insomnia, migraine prevention, chronic pain, and disorders of gut-brain interaction. Cyclobenzaprine (Flexeril), a common skeletal muscle relaxant, is structurally related to the TCAs. They have central and peripheral anticholinergic effects, alpha adrenergic blockade, quinidine-like cardiac membrane stabilizing action blockade of fast inward sodium channels, and inhibition of neurotransmitter uptake in the CNS. Toxic levels vary across all drugs within this class based upon dose and renal clearance. Serum levels do not correlate well with toxicity, and clinical signs and symptoms should guide therapy.

Manifestations

Most patients develop symptoms of toxicity within 1 to 2 hours after ingestion of significant quantities, but symptoms may be delayed up to 6 hours after overdose. Small overdoses cause early anticholinergic effects, agitation, and transient hypertension, which is not life-threatening. Large overdoses produce CNS depression, myocardial depression, seizures, and hypotension. Death may occur within 2 to 6 hours following ingestion.

Changes on ECG can be predictive of cardiac or neurologic toxicity from TCA ingestion and include (a) a QRS greater than 0.10 second may produce seizures, and if greater than 0.16 second, 50% of patients may develop ventricular dysrhythmias (20% of these may be life-threatening) and seizures; (b) a terminal 40 msec of the QRS axis greater than 120 degrees in the right frontal plane may be associated with toxicity; or (c) a large R wave greater than 3 mm in ECG lead aVR may predispose the patient to toxicity.

Laboratory Investigations

Patients presenting with altered mental status or ECG abnormalities should have a chest radiograph and have the following checked: blood glucose, serum electrolytes, calcium, magnesium, blood urea nitrogen, creatinine levels, liver profile, and creatine kinase level. Serum levels of tricyclic and cyclic antidepressants may be checked. Levels of the tricyclic and cyclic antidepressants less than 300 ng/mL are therapeutic; levels greater than 500 ng/mL indicate toxicity, and levels greater than 1000 ng/mL indicate serious poisoning and are associated with QRS widening.

Management

In cases of suspected toxicity, IV access should be established, baseline ECG obtained, and cardiac activity, vital signs, and neurologic status should be monitored in all patients for at least 6 hours from admission or 8 to 12 hours after ingestion. Activated charcoal 1 g/kg may be used for GI decontamination up to 1 hour post ingestion. For patients with altered mental status, their airway may need to be secured prior to activated charcoal administration.

Diazepam or lorazepam[1] should be used to control seizures. Status epilepticus may require barbiturates or neuromuscular

---

[1] Not FDA approved for this indication.

[1] Not FDA approved for this indication.

blockers. Refractory seizures may be controlled with paralysis with nondepolarizing neuromuscular blockers, intubation, assisted ventilation, and sedation. Sodium bicarbonate may be used to correct acidosis related to seizures administered in a dose of 1 to 2 mEq/kg undiluted as a bolus and repeated twice a few minutes apart, if needed, for "sodium loading"[1] and alkalinization, which may increase protein binding from 90% to 98%. The sodium loading overcomes the sodium channel blockage and is more important than the alkalinization. Indications include (a) a QRS complex greater than 0.12 second, (b) ventricular tachycardia, (c) severe conduction disturbances, (d) metabolic acidosis, (e) coma, and (f) seizures. Boluses may be repeated as needed; in some cases, infusions may be used. Arterial pH should be monitored frequently with a goal of 7.50 to 7.55. Hyperventilation is not recommended for correction of metabolic acidosis. Potassium, sodium, ionized calcium levels, and pH should be monitored and corrected.

Cardiology consultation should be considered in cases of severe toxicity and when ECG changes are present. Early transient hypertension and sinus tachycardia rarely requires prompt treatment. Hypotension should be treated with IV fluids and in norepinephrine in severe cases. Hemodynamically unstable supraventricular tachycardia should be treated with synchronized electrical cardioversion. Alkalinization may correct ventricular tachycardia. If ventricular tachycardia persists after alkalinization, it may be treated with IV lidocaine or countershock if unstable. Torsades de pointes is treated with magnesium sulfate IV 20% solution,[1] 2 g over 2 to 3 minutes, followed by a continuous infusion of 1.5 mL 10% solution or 5 to 10 mg per minute.

Disposition
All patients should be assessed for intentional overdose and psychiatric evaluation should be sought if applicable. Even if a patient is asymptomatic upon arrival, IV access, vital signs, and baseline and ECG should be obtained, and patients should undergo monitoring of vital signs, neurologic status, and cardiac monitoring for at least 6 hours. In 25% of fatal cases, patients were awake and alert upon presentation.

Patients with any of the following criteria should be admitted to the ICU for 12 to 24 hours: (a) ECG abnormalities except sinus tachycardia, (b) altered mental state, (c) seizures, (d) respiratory depression, and (e) hypotension. Patients who initially present with minor manifestations (e.g., sinus tachycardia, hypertension) who subsequently become and remain asymptomatic for at least 6 hours and asymptomatic patients who remain asymptomatic for at least 6 hours are low risk. Low risk patients may be discharged if their ECG remains normal, they have normal bowel sounds, and have appropriate psychiatric follow-up.

Children with accidental (non-intentional) exposures to amitriptyline (Elavil), desipramine (Norpramin), doxepin (Sinequan), imipramine (Tofranil), or nortriptyline (Aventyl) in a dose less than 5 mg/kg, who are asymptomatic and have a reliable caregiver can be observed at home with poison control follow-up by phone for 6 hours. Parents or caregivers should be educated on signs and symptoms for which to return. Children who are symptomatic or have ingested greater than 5 mg/kg should be referred to the emergency department.

---

[1] Not FDA approved for this indication.

References
Agency for Toxic Substances and Disease Registry: Centers For Disease Control and Prevention. Toxic Substances Portal and Toxicological Profiles. Available at: https://wwwn.cdc.gov/TSP/index.aspx. Accessed June 12, 2024.

Britch SC, Walsh SL: Treatment of opioid overdose: current approaches and recent advances, *Psychopharmacology (Berl)* 239(7):2063–2081, 2022, https://doi.org/10.1007/s00213-022-06125-5.

Chenoweth JA, Albertson TE, Greer MR: Carbon Monoxide Poisoning, *Crit Care Clin* 37(3):657–672, 2021.

Ghanem CI, Pérez MJ, Manautou JE, Mottino AD: Acetaminophen from liver to brain: New insights into drug pharmacological action and toxicity, *Pharmacol Res* 109:119–131, 2016.

Mayans L: Lead Poisoning in Children, *Am Fam Physician* 100(1):24–30, 2019.

National Poison Data System: Available at: https://poisoncenters.org/national-poison-data-system. Accessed June 12, 2024.

Taylor D, Poulou S, Clark I: The cardiovascular safety of tricyclic antidepressants in overdose and in clinical use, *Ther Adv Psychopharmacol* 14, 2024:20451253241243297, .

Taylor JL, Samet JH: Opioid Use Disorder, *Ann Intern Med* 175(1):ITC1–ITC16, 2022.

SPIDER BITES AND SCORPION STINGS

Method of
Anne-Michelle Ruha, MD

CURRENT DIAGNOSIS

Black Widow Bite
- Target lesion, not always present
- Generalized pain and muscle cramps
- Hypertension, regional diaphoresis

Brown Recluse Bite
- Unlikely to occur outside of endemic areas
- Cyanotic or blistering wound within area of pallor surrounded by erythema
- Systemic loxoscelism associated with rash, fever, hemolysis, renal failure

Bark Scorpion Sting
- Absence of lesion or local inflammatory reaction
- Painful paresthesias
- Disconjugate, roving eye movements are characteristic
- Restlessness, agitation, and involuntary jerking of muscles

CURRENT THERAPY

Black Widow Bite
- Opioid analgesics to control pain
- Benzodiazepines to control muscle cramping and anxiety
- Anti-*Latrodectus* antivenom (Antivenin) for persistent severe symptoms

Brown Recluse Bite
- General wound care
- If surgical excision is required, perform after 6 to 8 weeks
- Antibiotics only if infected

Bark Scorpion Sting
- Close attention to airway
- Opioid analgesics to control pain
- Benzodiazepines to control agitation
- *Centruroides* (scorpion) Immune F(ab')$_2$

Spider Bites
The majority of spiders native to the United States are incapable of envenomating humans. Important exceptions are *Latrodectus* and *Loxosceles* spiders, which produce clinical envenomations that, on rare occasion, are life-threatening.

Brown Recluse Spider
The most famous and abundant *Loxosceles* spider in the United States is *Loxosceles reclusa*, known as the brown recluse or fiddleback spider, due to the violin-shaped marking on its cephalothorax. The brown recluse inhabits the midwestern United States, with a range extending from east Texas to west Georgia and reaching north to southern Iowa. Bites from this nonaggressive spider are defensive, and they generally occur when spiders

become trapped in clothes or bedsheets. The risk of a bite, even in heavily infested homes, appears to be very small. Most diagnoses of brown recluse bites, including many published in the medical literature, are likely erroneous, occurring in nonendemic areas without identification of the spider. Other *Loxosceles* species found in the United States are even less likely to bite because they avoid human dwellings. Evidence supporting an association between other native spider species and necrotic wounds is weak.

Although the majority of brown recluse bites do not produce significant injury, some result in loxoscelism, which ranges from minor dermonecrosis to, very rarely, life-threatening illness. The venom component thought responsible for loxoscelism is sphingomyelinase D, which affects platelets and cell membranes and activates inflammatory mediators. The first signs of dermonecrosis are often erythema, pruritus, and pain at the bite site. Over hours the site becomes pale and edematous. Erythema can progress and spread gravitationally. A vesicle can develop, form an eschar, and slough over days to weeks. In the first days after the bite, a sunken bluish wound surrounded by a ring of pallor and then erythema is characteristic. Some patients develop a generalized maculopapular rash. Although most necrotic lesions are not serious, some can enlarge to 40 cm and leave a significant scar. Obese persons are at risk for more-severe lesions.

Very rarely, systemic loxoscelism develops within 48 hours of the bite, characterized by fever, myalgias, and hemolysis. Vomiting and diarrhea can occur, and some patients develop a diffuse erythroderma. Renal failure, disseminated intravascular coagulation, and death can result. Death from massive hemolysis is rare and is more likely to occur in children.

Diagnosis of loxoscelism depends on recognition of signs and symptoms in combination with positive identification of the spider when possible. Alternative etiologies for necrotic wounds are much more common than necrotic arachnidism, especially in nonendemic areas. The differential diagnosis of brown recluse bite is large and includes infectious causes, neoplastic disease, and vascular disease.

Treatment is supportive. Most wounds heal without intervention, although a scar might remain. Early surgical excision, dapsone,[1] hyperbaric oxygen, or prophylactic antibiotics cannot be recommended owing to lack of convincing evidence. Patients should receive tetanus prophylaxis (Td) and general wound care. In severe cases, healing can take months and require surgical intervention, which should occur 6 to 8 weeks following the bite after the wound is fully demarcated. Blood products and corticosteroids are often administered when systemic loxoscelism is associated with severe hemolysis. Patients with hemolysis resistant to steroids have been treated with therapeutic plasma exchange.

Black Widow Spiders

Latrodectus, or widow, spiders are, medically, the most important group of spiders in the world. Native black widow spiders are shiny black with a red hourglass pattern on their ventral surface. They can reside in or near human structures, leading to contact with humans and subsequent bites.

α-Latrotoxin in venom causes neurotransmitters to be released from synaptic vesicles. This results in a combination of neuromuscular and autonomic effects unique to *Latrodectus* bites, termed *latrodectism*. Bites are inconsistently felt, and they might or might not leave visible puncture marks and a target-like lesion. Pain can progress locally or become generalized within several hours. Severe muscle pain, particularly involving the abdomen and back, is common. Other findings include hypertension, tachycardia, tremor, localized or diffuse diaphoresis, periorbital edema, and urinary retention. Less commonly, vomiting, fever, priapism, paresthesias, and fasciculations occur. Rhabdomyolysis can result from increased muscle activity. Rarely, acute cardiomyopathy, cardiac ischemia, and pulmonary edema occur. Deaths are uncommon but reported.

Diagnosis of latrodectism is based on history of a spider bite and consistent clinical findings. In the absence of a witnessed bite, diagnosis can be difficult. Sudden onset and rapid progression of symptoms should raise suspicion. Infectious and surgical etiologies must be considered in a febrile or vomiting patient. Similar neuromuscular and autonomic findings might also be seen with intoxication by stimulant drugs and scorpion envenomations, and these should be considered in the differential.

Latrodectism typically resolves within 2 to 7 days. Opioid analgesics are often required to treat pain. Severe symptoms require intravenous opioids for adequate pain control and benzodiazepines for muscle spasms and anxiety. If symptoms are life-threatening or not controlled with these therapies, antivenom (Antivenin [*Latrodectus mactans*, equine origin], Merck, Boston, Mass.) should be considered. One vial reverses symptoms of envenomation. This whole-immunoglobulin product can produce acute hypersensitivity and should be administered in a monitored setting. Risks and benefits must be weighed before using this product. If antivenom is not an option or the patient is critically ill, care is supportive, including oxygen and airway support as needed, antihypertensives, antiemetics, and other symptomatic treatment.

Tarantulas

Tarantulas are common pets and are generally harmless. Bites may be painful, but envenomation by native species has not been reported. Most injury to humans resulting from interaction with tarantulas is secondary to trauma and inflammation caused by barbed abdominal hairs that the spiders eject defensively when threatened. If the hairs embed in the skin, a rash and pruritus can result. They can also embed in the cornea or be transferred there by rubbing the eyes after handling a tarantula. Ophthalmia nodosa, iritis, and keratouveitis have all been reported following exposure to tarantula hairs.

Treatment of embedded corneal hairs entails referral to an ophthalmologist and removal of the hairs if possible. Topical steroids are generally recommended, and some authors also recommend topical antibiotics.

Scorpion Stings

The bark scorpion, *Centruroides sculpturatus*, is the only native scorpion capable of producing a life-threatening envenomation. This small (<3 inches), yellowish-brown scorpion is found throughout Arizona and in bordering areas of surrounding states.

The scorpion seeks cool, dark environments and commonly enters homes. It injects venom by thrusting its stinger, located at the tip of its tail, toward the victim. The neurotoxic venom increases release of neurotransmitters that act at the neuromuscular junction and autonomic nerve endings.

Most stings are minor, producing local pain and paresthesias. Less than 5% of stings result in neurotoxicity, and the majority of these occur in children. Stings typically do not produce a visible skin lesion, although on rare occasion a small red mark is noted. Pain is immediate, and in a grade 1 envenomation remains local and resolves quickly. Grade 2 envenomations involve pain and paresthesias distal from the sting site, which can persist for days to weeks.

Most severe envenomations affect children younger than 5 years. Symptoms develop within 5 to 45 minutes and can progress for 4 hours. Infants and toddlers can exhibit sudden agitation and crying and transient vomiting, and they might rub their face and ears in response to paresthesias. If the child is verbal, complaints of burning pain and sensation of tongue swelling are common. Sinus tachycardia, hypertension, low-grade fever, and hypersalivation are common, and some children develop stridor. Restlessness, agitation, and twisting of the trunk with thrashing of the extremities is typical, as are tongue fasciculations and dysconjugate eye movements, or opsoclonus. Patients are conscious but often keep their eyes closed owing to diplopia. Presence of cranial nerve findings or neuromuscular agitation constitute a grade 3 envenomation; both are present in grade 4 envenomation. Severe envenomation may be associated with pulmonary edema, rhabdomyolysis, and aspiration pneumonia. Respiratory failure can occur due to several factors, including loss of tongue and respiratory muscle control, hypersalivation, and use of respiratory depressant medications.

Diagnosis often relies on recognition of symptoms, because children might not report a sting. Characteristic findings in regions inhabited by this scorpion usually make diagnosis straightforward.

---

[1]Not FDA approved for this indication.

XX Physical and Chemical Injuries

Differential diagnosis includes seizures or amphetamine toxicity. If a suspected envenomation does not follow the expected clinical course, a urine drug screen should be obtained.

Patients with grade 4 envenomation must be monitored for respiratory compromise in an emergency department or intensive care unit. If available, treatment with the antivenom Centruroides (Scorpion) Immune F(ab′)2 (Equine) Injection (Anascorp) should be considered. Anascorp reverses neurotoxicity within hours and often allows discharge home from the emergency department. In clinical trials Anascorp had an excellent safety profile; however, acute hypersensitivity reactions are possible, so antihistamines and epinephrine (Adrenalin) must be accessible. Serum sickness can also develop up to 3 weeks after receiving antivenom.

If antivenom is not an option, longer-acting medications (morphine and lorazepam [Ativan][1]) may be used to control pain and agitation. Intubation and mechanical ventilation is sometimes necessary owing to venom effects and respiratory depression from the medications used to control symptoms. While the patient is intubated, continuous infusion of sedative, analgesic, and muscle relaxing agents may be necessary until signs and symptoms of envenomation resolve. This typically occurs within 24 hours, although residual medication effects can require prolonged observation.

References

Anascorp package insert: http://www.fda.gov/downloads/BiologicsBloodVaccines/BloodBloodProducts/ApprovedProducs/LicensedProductsBLAs/FractionatedPlasmaProducts/UCM266725.pdf.

Bernardino CR, Rapuano C: Ophthalmia nodosa caused by casual handling of a tarantula, *CLAO* 26(2):111–112, 2000.

Boyer LV, Theodorou AA, Berg RA, et al: Antivenom for critically ill children with neurotoxicity from scorpion stings, *N Engl J Med* 360(20):2090–2098, 2009.

Cain S, Plapp FV, Dasgupta A, Ye Z: Severe complications in a 25-year-old male after brown recluse spider bite treated by therapeutic plasma exchange: a case report and review of other case studies, *J Clin Apher* 38(4):505–509, 2023.

Clark RF, Wethern-Kestner S, Vance MV, Gerkin R: Clinical presentation and treatment of black widow spider envenomation: A review of 163 cases, *Ann Emerg Med* 21(7):782–787, 1992.

Curry SC, Vance MV, Ryan PJ, et al: Envenomation by the scorpion *Centruroides sculpturatus*, *J Toxicol Clin Toxicol* 21(4–5):417–449, 1983-1984.

Furbee RB, Kao LW, Ibrahim D: Brown recluse spider envenomation, *Clin Lab Med* 26:211–226, 2006.

Vetter RS: Spiders of the genus *Loxosceles (Araneae, Sicariidae)*: A review of biological, medical and psychological aspects regarding envenomations, *J Arachnol* 36:150–163, 2008.

Vetter RS, Isbister GK: Medical aspects of spider bites, *Annu Rev Entomol* 53:409–429, 2008.

Vetter RS, Isbister GK: Do hobo spider bites cause dermonecrotic injuries? *Ann Emerg Med* 44(6):605–607, 2004.

Watts P, Mcpherson R, Hawksworth NR: Tarantula keratouveitis, *Cornea* 19(3):393–394, 2000.

VENOMOUS SNAKEBITE

Method of
Christopher Dion, DO; Anne-Michelle Ruha, MD; and †Steven Seifert, MD, MSc

CURRENT DIAGNOSIS

Crotalinae (Rattlesnake, Copperhead, Cottonmouth) Bite
- One or two fang puncture marks
- Dry bites (non-envenomation) may occur in up to 25%; patients should be observed for at least 8 to 12 hours before declaring a dry bite
- Envenomation produces pain and progressive swelling
- Edema and functional deficits may take many weeks to completely resolve
- May include clear or hemorrhagic blisters

---

† The editors of *Conn's Current Therapy 2025* would like to recognize Dr. Steven Seifert's many years of contribution to this text and for sharing his national expertise on this subject. He passed in 2022.

- May include ecchymosis
- Tissue necrosis and infection are rare and usually late (>2 days) complications
- Abnormalities in hematologic clotting elements (platelets, fibrinogen, PT/INR) are variable, may result in significant bleeding, and may persist for more than 2 weeks
- Typical findings in an endemic area are sufficient as an indication for antivenom treatment

Coral Snake Bite
- One or two fang puncture marks
- Dry bites (non-envenomation) may occur in up to 50%; patients should be observed for 24 hours
- Local effects, even with significant systemic envenomation, may be minimal to nil
- Neurologic effects (progressive, descending paralysis) predominate and may require airway support
- Motor effects may be poorly reversible once established and may persist for many weeks

CURRENT THERAPY

Crotalinae Bite
- Opioid-level pain relief may be required
- If signs of envenomation, either Anavip or CroFab may be considered first-line treatment
- Allergic reactions are rare; no pretesting or pretreatments are needed
- Maintenance doses are recommended for CroFab
- Although the incidence of recurrent hematologic effects is low with Anavip, post-discharge hematologic monitoring is needed for all patients treated with CroFab or Anavip
- Wound care follow-up may be required for tissue necrosis
- Serum sickness incidence is low (<5%), and most symptoms are mild

Coral Snake Bite
- Antivenom should be given at the earliest sign of envenomation to prevent progression

Two families of significantly venomous snakes are native to the United States, Viperidae and Elapidae. The Viperidae family (viperids) contains the sub-family Crotalinae (crotalids), which contains all of the New World pit vipers. Native pit vipers from the United States and Canada are from three genera and contain more than 30 species of rattlesnakes, copperheads, and cottonmouths. The native Elapidae family (elapids) is composed of two genera and several species of coral snakes.

Each year, 5000 to 10,000 venomous snakebites by native species are reported to U.S. poison control centers, with fewer than five deaths. At least 97% of these bites are from crotalids.

Currently, there are two antivenoms that are effective against crotalid species: Crotalidae Polyvalent Immune Fab (ovine; CroFab, Boston Scientific/BTG, Farnham, UK) and Crotalidae Immune F(ab′)$_2$ (equine; Anavip; Rare Disease Therapeutics, Inc., Franklin, TN). There is also a single antivenom, Coral Snake *(Micrurus fulvius)* Immune Globulin Antivenin (equine; North American Coral Snake Antivenin [NACSA], Pfizer/Wyeth Laboratories, New York, NY) against coral snakes.

Approximately 50 additional bites per year occur from a wide variety of nonnative venomous species of snakes housed in zoos, academic institutions, serpentariums, and private collections. Identification of the biting species in these cases is usually not an issue.

Diagnostic and Management Overview
Initial Management
There are only a few actions that can be undertaken in the field to reduce morbidity and mortality from a venomous snakebite. Most "treatments" that have been advocated—cutting or sucking, applying tourniquets, heat, cold, or electricity—have no proven efficacy and are much more likely to result in additional tissue injury and delay of definitive therapy. Jewelry should be removed from the affected extremity. Immobilization and a non-constrictive splint in a position of extension may decrease local venom effects in Crotalinae envenomation, but application should not delay transport to a healthcare facility.

Definitive management for native venomous snakebites in the United States is achieved with appropriate local wound care and antivenom, which is composed of antibodies raised in a host animal (horse or sheep) against snake venom components. As native crotalids inhabit every state except Maine, Hawaii, and Alaska, most hospitals should stock or have ready access to one or both antivenoms.

Pfizer/Wyeth coral snake antivenom is not currently being manufactured. Endemic areas such as Florida, Georgia, Texas, Alabama, and Louisiana have stockpiles; however, the stockpiles are currently being depleted. Pfizer has successfully applied for extensions for expiring lots of NACSA; however, new antivenom vials have not yet entered circulation. An experimental F(ab')$_2$ antivenom has completed a phase III clinical trial but is not currently available. Foreign-produced antivenoms against related coral snake species may also have efficacy against U.S. snakes but should be used only when a drug that is approved by the U.S. Food and Drug Administration (FDA) is not available and, ideally, with prior FDA approval.

An even more difficult situation results from exotic envenomations for which the appropriate antivenom (if one exists) is certain to be a non–FDA-approved product and must be located at a zoo or other non-healthcare source potentially distant from the location of the envenomation.

Antivenom, local wound care, and symptomatic and supportive care are the mainstays of envenomation management. A regional poison control center should be contacted for information and assistance in managing any venomous snake exposure, including locating an appropriate antivenom. Poison control centers have personnel who are experienced at assessing and managing envenomations and have access to the Antivenom Index, an updatable online database that lists sources of antivenoms for nonnative species. Poison control centers can be contacted from anywhere in the United States by calling 1-800-222-1222.

Snake Identification
The major branch point in native North American snake envenomation is to determine whether the victim has been bitten by a coral snake or a crotalid. Identification of the specific species can help predict some species-specific challenges; however, more important is to determine if the envenomation was caused by a Crotalinae or Elapidae snake. Crotaline snakes are easily differentiated from coral snakes by virtue of the latter's distinctive color pattern of red, yellow, and black bands. It can be difficult to differentiate a coral snake from nonvenomous snakes that have similar markings. The rhyme "red touches yellow, kills a fellow; red touches black, venom lack," which describes the red band being surrounded on either side by yellow or black, is accurate only for coral snakes in the United States. Mexican and South American coral snakes may have the opposite pattern. Crotalids, or pit vipers, can be distinguished from non-venomous snakes by the presence of vertically elliptical pupils, a triangular-shaped head, and the presence of temperature-sensing pits behind the nostrils.

Physical findings, laboratory evaluation, and geographic location of the envenomation is typically all that is required to determine that the snake is venomous and to guide therapy. Attempting to kill or capture the snake is unlikely to add additional information to treatment decisions and may result in further injury.

Factors Affecting Toxicity and the Severity of Envenomation
Many factors govern whether an envenomation occurs after a bite, the signs and symptoms that develop, and the overall severity of the effects. Up to 25% of crotalid bites and up to 50% of elapid bites do not result in an envenomation. Barriers to fang penetration and other factors may result in no venom being injected. Patients must be watched for a sufficient length of time (i.e., 8 to 12 hours for a crotalid bite and 24 hours for a coral snakebite) to ensure that this is the case.

If an envenomation has occurred, the family and species of snake generally determines the spectrum of symptoms and signs. The amount of venom, specific venom components, and underlying health status of the victim determine severity.

Crotalid Envenomations
Epidemiology
Crotalid snakes are distributed throughout North America. Bites are more common in southern areas during summer months, but they occur year-round and may occur at any time and in any location with captive collections. The various genera and species of crotalids in the United States have relatively stable geographic ranges, with much overlap. Many different species of venomous snakes may inhabit any given area. Nonvenomous or mildly venomous colubrid snakes are also native to the United States.

Pit vipers have large front, mobile fangs through which venom is injected into the victim. As the fangs are curved, venom is usually injected subcutaneously rather than into deeper muscle compartments. Due to anatomic and other physical factors, bite wounds may appear as scratches or as one or more punctures. Envenomation may occur with any break in the skin.

Crotalid venom is complex, consisting of proteolytic enzymes, small peptides, phospholipases, and other elements responsible for the spectrum of clinical effects seen. There is great variability of venom composition among species, within species, and even within a single specimen over the course of a season and its entire life span.

Clinical Effects
The spectrum of clinical effects is based on the specific genus or species of crotalid and is unpredictable, ranging from non-envenomation (a "dry bite"; up to 25% of bites) to life-threatening reactions. Crotalid snake envenomation typically results in tissue injury and hematologic effects. Local effects are typically pain and progressive swelling, and may include ecchymosis, tissue necrosis, or tissue loss. The complete absence of local effects cannot be used as a reliable marker of non-envenomation in a crotalid bite. We recommend a period of observation of 8 to 12 hours with serial blood draws to monitor for coagulopathy or thrombocytopenia.

Systemic effects including hematologic, neurologic, cardiovascular, and nonspecific findings may occur after crotalid envenomations. Rattlesnake (genera *Crotalus* and *Sistrurus*) envenomations are more likely to result in hematologic effects compared with copperhead or cottonmouth (genus *Agkistrodon*) envenomation. Hematologic abnormalities commonly include thrombocytopenia, hypofibrinogenemia, or prolonged prothrombin time (PT). Rattlesnake envenomations are much more likely to produce neurologic effects, such as muscle fasciculation or weakness, compared with copperhead or cottonmouth envenomations; however, these effects can be seen with any crotalid snake. Acute hypersensitivity can occur from any envenomation, which can result in hypotension, airway compromise, ECG changes, and/or coma. Nausea, vomiting, diaphoresis, anxiety, and other nonspecific effects may be seen.

BOX 1   Prehospital Management of Crotalid Envenomation

- Remove jewelry.
- Splint and elevate the extremity in extension.
- Expeditiously transport the patient to a healthcare facility.
- Obtain intravenous access in a non-envenomated extremity.
- Do not use cutting, sucking, tourniquets, heat, cold, or other local "therapies."

BOX 2   Hospital Diagnosis and Initial Management of Crotalid Envenomation

- Remove jewelry.
- Obtain intravenous access in a non-envenomated extremity, and use crystalloid as indicated.
- Obtain CBC with platelet count, PT, and fibrinogen level every 6 to 12 hours until normalizing.
- Determine whether an envenomation has occurred.
- Determine severity based on the family or species of snake, age and health status of the victim, and development and rate of progression of signs and symptoms (e.g., local injury, hematologic abnormalities, hypotension, and other systemic effects).
- Determine the patient's tetanus vaccination status, and update if necessary.
- Seek consultation from a poison control center: 1-800-222-1222.
- Determine whether antivenom is indicated and administer per protocol.
- Provide basic wound care and determine whether local injury requires specific management.
- Determine whether hematologic or other systemic effects require specific management.

Duration of Clinical Effects

Local effects may develop rapidly or may not be apparent for many hours. Progression may occur for days, with resolution of tissue swelling occurring over 1 to 4 weeks. Complications of tissue necrosis may take longer or be permanent. Hematologic effects usually begin within 1 to 2 hours of envenomation. If antivenom is given within this time frame, the detection of these effects may be masked and become apparent only after unbound antivenom has been eliminated from the body, usually within 1 week after treatment. Untreated or recurrent/delayed (after antivenom) hematologic effects may persist for up to 3 weeks after an envenomation. Neurologic and other systemic effects tend to occur within a few hours of envenomation and resolve over 24 to 36 hours.

Severity of Envenomation

Untreated, local injury worsens over time, with proximal progression of tissue injury. Hematologic effects can be profound, resulting in spontaneous hemorrhage. Hypotension may be severe and can result in death. Neurologic and other systemic effects are rarely life-threatening events. As a result of changes in basic medical care and healthcare systems, it is not directly applicable to compare case-fatality rates before the introduction of antivenom (1950) with what can be expected today. Currently, there are approximately five deaths from crotalid snakebites per year in the United States.

Management

Determining Whether Envenomation Has Occurred and Its Severity

Because of the unpredictability of envenomation and the variability of possible clinical effects, each crotalid bite must be assessed and responded to individually (Box 1). It is important to determine whether an envenomation has occurred. If there are no signs or symptoms of envenomation, there is no indication for antivenom or other specific treatment. The severity of the envenomation helps determine the amount of antivenom required to counter and neutralize venom effects, but this may not be immediately apparent because envenomations tend to progress over time, and what may at first appear to be mild venom effects may progress to a severe envenomation.

Initial Hospital Management

On arrival at the hospital, jewelry should be removed and the bitten extremity loosely splinted in an extended position. The wound should be cleansed (Box 2), and tetanus status should be updated if required. The extremity should be elevated to limit distal edema and pain. Patients often require opioid analgesics for pain relief.

At least one large intravenous line should be placed, avoiding the envenomated extremity, and crystalloid should be infused as required. Initial hospital therapy, including a first dose of antivenom, should be provided in an area capable of close monitoring of vital signs and capable of managing life-threatening reactions; this usually is an emergency department. Whether an intensive care unit or similar patient care area is used for subsequent management depends on the clinical situation.

Indications for Antivenom

Because of the safety of the current FDA-approved antivenoms and their ability to stop proximal progression of local tissue injury, all patients with signs of progressive local envenomation effects as well as those with significant systemic effects are candidates for treatment with antivenom.

Depending on the original indication for treatment (local effects, systemic effects, or both), initial control of envenomation effects is the goal of the loading dose of antivenom. Currently, there are two FDA-approved crotalid antivenoms for North American pit viper envenomation: CroFab and Anavip. The incidence of acute hypersensitivity reactions with CroFab and Anavip are low and generally mild and were found to be similar between products in a comparative trial. Pretreatment sensitivity testing is not required or recommended. There are rare reports of IgE-mediated type I hypersensitivity reactions on repeat exposure in individuals who were previously treated with CroFab, but most people who have been previously treated do not develop an adverse reaction to subsequent administration. The incidence of type III hypersensitivity reaction ("serum sickness") with both antivenoms was approximately 2.5% in the comparative trial.

The half-life of CroFab is approximately 18 to 24 hours, which is considerably shorter than IgG or $F(ab')_2$ antivenoms, and it is believed to be responsible for increased late hemotoxicity compared with Anavip. Anavip has a longer half-life (approximately 133 hours) and a lower risk of late coagulopathy or thrombocytopenia.

For treatment of envenomations, antivenom is administered as an intravenous solution, with 4 to 6 vials of CroFab, or 10 vials of Anavip diluted into 250 mL of normal saline. The infusion should start at 25 to 50 mL/hour over the first 5 to 10 minutes, and then the rate is increased to finish by 1 hour if there is no reaction. Acute reactions are usually anaphylactoid (rate-related, not IgE-mediated) in nature, but they may reflect true anaphylaxis (IgE-mediated). Anaphylaxis is usually, but not always, more severe, and distinguishing between them is mostly based on a history of prior exposure or reaction.

If an acute hypersensitivity reaction occurs, the infusion should be slowed or stopped, depending on the severity, and appropriate symptomatic treatment should be started with epinephrine, H_1 and H_2 blockers, corticosteroids, and other supportive measures, as required. It should be determined whether antivenom is still required; if so, it should be restarted at a slower rate or higher dilution, or both, and consideration should be given to using an antivenom from a different source animal. CroFab is raised in sheep, and Anavip is raised in horses. Additionally, Cro-Fab uses papain, an enzyme derived from papaya, during production, which may lead to an allergic reaction in those with papaya allergy.

Treatment of Local Tissue Injury

Monitoring the circumference in three locations along the envenomated extremity is usually sufficient to document progressive local injury. If the antivenom is given exclusively for local findings, the envenomation is deemed to be controlled if measurements stabilize or decrease. Pain in the inguinal or axillary lymph nodes is indicative of spreading envenomation, which may be an indication for further doses of antivenom. There is often some redistribution of existing tissue edema, but uncontrolled proximal progression is usually seen as an indication that the envenomation is not under control. If antivenom is being given for hematologic effects, cessation of worsening or reversal should be seen. Often, thrombocytopenia rebounds dramatically. Hypofibrinogenemia may not rebound as quickly or merely stabilize because the liver must manufacture new fibrinogen. Although an elevated D-dimer value indicates fibrinogenolytic activity, it is not an independent indicator for antivenom treatment; therefore, we do not recommend routinely obtaining this value.

Other systemic effects may serve as indicators for antivenom use, and they should show improvement by the end of the initial infusion. If initial control is not deemed to have occurred, additional doses of antivenom should be administered until initial control is achieved. Most patients achieve initial control with 4 to 12 vials of Fab antivenom and 10 to 20 vials of $F(ab')_2$ antivenom.

Maintenance Doses

A rapid decline of antivenom levels can occur when administering CroFab because of its large volume of distribution. After initial control is achieved, maintenance dosing of two vials every 6 hours for three doses is started. This usually maintains adequate antivenom serum levels to prevent early recurrence of local tissue injury progression; however, late onset of hemotoxicity occurs in about 30% of rattlesnake envenomations after treatment with CroFab. If progression of local effects or hemotoxicity does recur, an additional two vials of antivenom should be administered. Routine maintenance dosing with Anavip is not recommended, but the patient should be observed for an additional 18 hours to ensure that control is maintained. If reemergence of venom effects does occur, an additional four vials of Anavip should be given.

Although significant swelling of limbs may occur and limbs may appear tense, a true compartment syndrome secondary to rattlesnake envenomation is rare. Envenomated extremities may mimic compartment syndrome with symptoms such as paresthesias, swelling, and discoloration. In most cases, the treatment for increased pain, swelling, and other symptoms is more antivenom, as antivenom has been shown to reduce compartment pressure and limit venom-induced decreases in perfusion pressure. If compartment syndrome is suspected, compartment pressures must be directly measured to confirm the diagnosis. If pressures are found to be elevated, an initial trial of additional antivenom and elevation should be undertaken, but fasciotomy may be necessary in rare cases.

Bleb formation at the site of a bite is not an important sign in and of itself, although it may suggest the presence of underlying tissue necrosis. Envenomations to the fingers have significant potential for local necrosis. It is reasonable to unroof blebs at or near the bite site if under significant pressure or to debride obviously necrotic tissue, which usually becomes apparent several days after the bite. The incidence of infection in the United States from crotalid bites is low. There are no data to support the use of prophylactic antibiotics, and it is best to limit the opportunities for adverse drug effects. It is often difficult to distinguish inflammatory venom effects from infection.

| BOX 3 | Management of Hematologic Effects and Recurrence in Crotalid Envenomation |

- CroFab
  - Administer 4 to 6 vials of antivenom (ovine; Crotalidae Polyvalent Immune Fab [CroFab]) in crotalid envenomations for significant abnormalities of platelet count, PT, or fibrinogen.
- Anavip
  - Administer 10 vials of antivenom Crotalidae Immune $F(ab')_2$ (equine; Anavip) in crotalid envenomations for significant abnormalities of platelet count, PT, or fibrinogen.
- Administer additional antivenom in 4- to 6-vial (CroFab) or 10-vial (Anavip) increments until reversal of hematologic abnormalities occurs. Replacement of platelets, clotting factors, or fibrinogen may be gradual, and a positive trend indicates neutralization of venom or replacement in excess of venom effect.
- Patients treated with antivenom are at risk for recurrent hemotoxic effects 2 to 4 days after treatment and should be followed closely, with repeat laboratory tests on days 2 to 3 and days 5 to 7 with CroFab and on days 5 to 7 with Anavip.
- Consider treating recurrent hematologic abnormalities with additional antivenom. Indications include platelets <25,000/mm³; platelets <50,000/mm³ with fibrinogen <80 mg/dL; or any evidence of bleeding or risk factors for bleeding.
- Consider readmission for severe abnormalities, other risk factors (e.g., uncontrolled hypertension, advanced age, other bleeding diatheses), or clinically significant bleeding.
- Administer blood products *plus* additional antivenom for significant bleeding.

Long-Term Local Tissue Effects

The edema and tissue injury produced by most North American crotalid envenomations usually resolve within 1 to 4 weeks, and a return to normal function can be anticipated; however, tissue necrosis or deep tissue injury may result in longer-term or even permanent structural and functional disability. Loss of tissue may occur, including digits and other parts of the extremities, although this is rare and may be associated with prehospital application of tourniquets or other imprudent surgical interventions, delayed care, or complications such as infections. Early antivenom treatment is associated with faster recovery.

Hematologic Abnormalities and Bleeding

One or more hematologic abnormalities may occur with native crotalid envenomation (Box 3). Significant decreases in platelet count or fibrinogen concentrations are independent indications for antivenom treatment. Isolated, mild prolongation of PT does not require antivenom treatment. Crotaline envenomation does not produce a true disseminated intravascular coagulopathy because there is no true intravascular coagulation. Sufficient platelets, fibrinogen, and thrombin are usually available for hemostasis, and clinically significant bleeding is rarely seen; however, severe depletion of individual clotting elements or a combination of hematologic abnormalities can result in bleeding.

The management of initial or persistent laboratory abnormalities is achieved with additional antivenom. Administration of blood products (e.g., fresh-frozen plasma, platelet concentrates, other blood products) should be reserved for clinically significant (life-threatening) bleeding and given in conjunction with additional antivenom because transfused elements are similarly likely to be consumed by venom activity. Bleeding in damaged tissues, expansion of the vascular volume from crystalloid administration, and hemotoxic venom components may produce an anemia that may rarely require a red blood cell transfusion.

Late Hematologic Effects

Although both CroFab and Anavip have similar effects on early manifestations of envenomation, there are significant differences in risk of developing late hemotoxicity. Late hemotoxicity is generally defined as delayed onset or recurrence of thrombocytopenia and/or coagulopathy after completion of antivenom treatment and resolution of early venom toxicity. This usually occurs more than 48 hours after the snakebite occurs. Post-discharge hematologic abnormalities may be severe and may occur, even in patients who did not have initial hemotoxicity.

A study of data reported to a national snakebite registry found that 42% of patients who received CroFab developed late hemotoxicity, but only 4% of patients who received Anavip developed late hemotoxicity ($P \le .001$). One likely mechanism is recurrent unneutralized venomemia after elimination of unbound antivenom. Anavip has a longer half-life and will remain in circulation longer. As a result, Anavip appears to provide longer protection against recurrence. In the same study, 9% of CroFab patients were retreated with antivenom compared with no patients in the Anavip group ($P = 0.049$).

Although the incidence of significant bleeding is low, even with profound laboratory abnormalities, it seems prudent to administer additional antivenom if the platelet count is less than 25,000/mm³ in the setting of a normal fibrinogen; there is multicomponent hemotoxicity with fibrinogen less than 80 mg/dL and platelets less than 50,000/mm³; or there are underlying medical conditions that make hemorrhage more likely, such as pregnancy, advanced age, use of medications that increase risk of bleeding, or a bleeding diathesis.

Disposition

Patients may be discharged if their local effects are regressing, if their pain, hematologic effects, and other systemic effects are controlled and if they do not have complications such as infection or necrosis. Typically, this occurs between 36 and 48 hours after envenomation but may be delayed for up to 1 week. We currently recommend repeat CBC with platelets, PT, and fibrinogen values on days 2 to 3 and days 5 to 7 after envenomation for patients receiving CroFab and on days 5 to 7 in patients receiving Anavip. Ongoing pain relief may be required, with an effort to transition to nonopioid agents during the first week. Acetaminophen is a first-line agent, and in patients considered at low risk for late-onset, new-onset, or recurrent coagulopathy and thrombocytopenia, nonsteroidal antiinflammatory drugs (NSAIDs) may be recommended. Patients should be warned to watch for signs of serum sickness. Occupational or physical therapy should be arranged as needed to maximize return of function, and follow-up for local and systemic effects should be arranged.

Coral Snake Envenomations
Epidemiology

Each year, there are approximately 50 to 100 bites by coral snakes in the United States. Two genera and several species inhabit the United States, with the *Micrurus* genus responsible for bites in Florida, Texas, Georgia, Louisiana, Alabama, and some neighboring states. A smaller genus, *Micruroides*, is found in Arizona and New Mexico, but it is responsible for very few bites, and there have been no reports of serious envenomations. Bites are more common during the warmer months.

Coral snakes belong to the elapid family and have fixed, relatively short fangs, which may decrease the rate of envenomation. Factors that increase the risk of envenomation include more than one puncture, a deep puncture, and a prolonged time of bite with a sensation of "Velcro" as the snake is taken off.

Clinical Effects

Envenomation by the coral snake primarily produces neurologic toxicity from presynaptic toxins, initially producing bulbar muscle weakness, ptosis, diplopia, and dysphagia. These effects can begin within 15 to 30 minutes or may be delayed up to 24 hours

---

BOX 4 Prehospital Management of Elapid Envenomation

- Remove jewelry.
- Expeditiously transport the patient to a healthcare facility.
- Apply a pressure immobilization bandage (e.g., 3- to 4-inch crepe bandage at lymphatic pressure from the tip of the extremity to the trunk) or a lymphatic constriction band (e.g., wide rubber band or blood pressure cuff at 15 to 25 mm Hg proximal to the bite site) only if there will be a significant delay to hospital care.
- Do not delay transport to apply a constriction band.
- Obtain intravenous access in a non-envenomated extremity.
- Do not use cutting, sucking, heat, cold, or other local "therapies."

---

after an envenomation. Muscle weakness and paralysis progress to include respiratory muscles, and they can result in respiratory arrest and death. Typical of presynaptic toxins, effect progression can be arrested with the use of antivenom, but the effects are not rapidly reversed. Typically, there is little or no local tissue injury, and the absence of local injury cannot be used to exclude envenomation. Likewise, there is usually no effect on hematologic function, and other systemic effects are rare. Patients cannot be assumed to have received a dry bite by a coral snake because of lack of symptoms on presentation. Presumed coral snake bites should be observed for at least 24 hours before concluding that an envenomation has not occurred.

Because of changes in basic medical care and healthcare systems, it is not directly applicable to compare case-fatality rates before the introduction of antivenom (1967) with what can be expected today; however, at that time, the case-fatality rate was approximately 10%.

Management

Coral snake envenomation has the potential for rapid progression of motor paralysis and respiratory compromise without significant local tissue injury. It is reasonable to attempt to slow the venom's progression into the circulation in a prehospital setting if the patient will have a prolonged transport time. A pressure immobilization band (i.e., elastic bandage wrapped from an extremity's tip to the trunk with the degree of tension used for sprains) is used for this purpose for elapid envenomations elsewhere in the world (Boxes 4 and 5). In Australian studies, a pressure immobilization bandage has been shown to slow venom absorption. We do not recommend application of pressure immobilization bandages for coral snake envenomation unless there is a significant delay to antivenom administration. We do not recommend routine placement of pressure immobilization bandages once a patient has presented to a hospital.

Standard wound care should be performed, including cleansing the wound and updating the tetanus status, if required. Wound infection is uncommon, and prophylactic antibiotics are not recommended.

Coral snake envenomation can result in progressive neurotoxicity, which may require mechanical ventilation. We recommend the use of antivenom if the patient exhibits any signs of envenomation. North American Coral Snake Antivenin (NACSA) is the only FDA-approved antivenom available for use in the United States. NACSA is equine-derived whole-IgG antivenom that is effective only against two of the North American coral snakes: eastern coral snakes *(Micrurus fulvius)*, and Texas coral snakes *(Micrurus tener)*. The antivenom is not effective against *Micruroides euryxanthus*, the Arizona coral snake; however, this snake does not have any reported medically significant envenomations or deaths reported. At this time, NACSA still remains in short supply, and production has not resumed. Practitioners in coral snake endemic areas have become more conservative with NACSA use. Studies have shown that delaying NACSA use until the patient

BOX 5 | Hospital Diagnosis and Initial Management of Elapid Envenomation

- Remove jewelry.
- If an arterial or a venous tourniquet has been placed, remove the tourniquet.
- Obtain intravenous access in a non-envenomated extremity, and use crystalloid as indicated.
- Determine whether an envenomation has occurred.
- Determine severity based on the family or species of snake, age and health status of the victim, and development and rate of progression of signs or symptoms (e.g., paralysis and other neurologic effects).
- Determine the patient's tetanus vaccination status, and update if necessary.
- Seek consultation from a poison control center: 1-800-222-1222.
- If a pressure immobilization band or lymphatic constriction band has been placed, remove the band.
- Determine whether antivenom is indicated and administer per protocol.
- Provide basic wound care and determine whether local injury requires specific management.
- Determine whether hematologic or other systemic effects require specific management.

shows signs of neurotoxicity was not associated with poor outcomes. Recent case series of Texas coral snake envenomation reported to the North American Snakebite Registry over a 5-year period demonstrated that a "wait and see" approach for NACSA administration was acceptable as no patients received antivenom, and all patients recovered. NACSA stockpiles still exist; however, it does not appear that any new doses of antivenom have been produced. Pfizer has applied to extend the expiration date on lots of antivenom with the FDA.

When paralysis has progressed to significant airway compromise, complete or partial reversal with antivenom may not be possible. Aggressive respiratory support, including intubation and ventilation, may be needed for days or weeks. If an FDA-approved coral snake antivenom is not readily available, there are reports of coral snake antivenoms from Mexico, Costa Rica, and Brazil, and of tiger snake antivenom from Australia, reversing the neurotoxicity of *M. fulvius*. The use of foreign non–FDA-approved antivenoms should be reserved for circumstances in which an FDA-approved product is not available in a timely manner and, if possible, with prior approval by the FDA Center for Biologics Evaluation and Research (240-402-8020; after-hours emergency: 866 300-4374; 301-796-8240; email is industry.biologics@fda.hhs.gov). Because these drugs are imported into the United States as Investigational New Drugs, institutional investigational review boards will also have notification requirements.

Exotic Snakebite

Epidemiology and Clinical Effects

In the United States, most exotic snake envenomations occur in private collections. These are not usually known to authorities or healthcare providers until an envenomation occurs, and they may involve the collection owner or family members, including children. They may occur in any locale, and victims may present to any healthcare facility.

Snakes from the Viperidae and Elapidae families account for the bulk of venomous bites worldwide. Non-US viperids and elapids have patterns of venom activity similar to those of their North American counterparts. Some nonnative elapids, such as cobras, mambas, black snakes, or taipans, produce much higher rates of respiratory paralysis and may produce much greater local tissue injury than U.S. coral snakes. Similarly, envenomation from some nonnative viperids, such as *Bothrops*, *Echis*, or *Bitis* species, or from an African colubrid, such as the booms-lang, results in a greater risk of bleeding. Some of these species may directly activate prothrombin (e.g., *Echis* species, *Bothrops* species) and factor X (e.g., *Vipera* species, *Dispholidus* species), leading to a venom-induced consumptive coagulopathy with intravascular thrombosis, marked organ dysfunction, and, potentially, death.

Management

The specific management of exotic envenomations is beyond the scope of this chapter. Not all venomous exotic snakes have antivenoms. Even for snakes with antivenoms, they may not be available in the United States, although zoos stock antivenoms for snakes in their collections. As discussed earlier, the Antivenom Index lists these antivenoms and is accessible to regional poison control centers. For information on exotic antivenoms and assistance in managing an exotic snake envenomation, the regional poison control center should be contacted.

References

Bush SP, Ruha AM, Seifert SA, et al: Comparison of F(ab')2 versus Fab antivenom for pit viper envenomation: a prospective, blinded, multicenter, randomized clinical trial, *Clin Toxicol (Phila)* 53(1):37–45, 2015.

Greene S, Ruha AM, Campleman S, Brent J, Wax P: Tox ICSSG: Epidemiology, Clinical Features, and Management of Texas Coral Snake (Micrurus tener) Envenomations Reported to the North American Snakebite Registry, *J Med Toxicol* 17(1):51–56, 2021.

Greene SC, Folt J, Wyatt K, Brandehoff NP: Epidemiology of fatal snakebites in the United States 1989-2018, *Am J Emerg Med* 45:309–316, 2021.

LoVecchio F, Klemens J, Welch S, Rodriguez R: Antibiotics after rattlesnake envenomation, *J Emerg Med* 23(4):327–328, 2002.

Ruha AM, Padilla-Jones A, Canning J, Spyres MB, Curry SC: Early Experience with Crotalidae Immune F(ab')2 Antivenom to Treat Arizona Rattlesnake Envenomations, *J Med Toxicol* 18(1):38–42, 2022.

Ruha AM, Kleinschmidt KC, Greene S, Spyres MB, Brent J, Wax P, Padilla-Jones A, Campleman S, Tox ICSSG: The Epidemiology, Clinical Course, and Management of Snakebites in the North American Snakebite Registry, *J Med Toxicol* 13(4):309–320, 2017.

Spyres MB, Skolnik AB, Moore EC, Gerkin RD, Padilla-Jones A, Ruha AM: Comparison of Antivenom Dosing Strategies for Rattlesnake Envenomation, *Crit Care Med* 46(6):e540–e544, 2018.

Spyres MB, Padilla GK, Gerkin RD, Hoyte CO, Wolk BJ, Ruha AM: Late hemotoxicity following North American rattlesnake envenomation treated with Crotalidae immune F(ab')2 (equine) antivenom and Crotalidae immune polyvalent Fab (ovine) antivenom reported to the North American Snakebite Sub-registry, *Clin Toxicol (Phila)*1–5, 2022.

Walter FG, Stolz U, Shirazi F, McNally J: Temporal analyses of coral snakebite severity published in the American Association of Poison Control Centers' Annual Reports from 1983 through 2007, *Clin Toxicol (Phila)* 48(1):72–78, 2010.

Wood A, Schauben J, Thundiyil J: Review of Eastern coral snake (Micrurus fulvius) exposures managed by the Florida Poison Information Center Network: 1998-2010, *Clin Toxicol (Phila)* 51(8):783–788, 2013.

HOME DISASTER PREPAREDNESS

Method of
Tara N. Heagele, PhD, RN

CURRENT DIAGNOSIS

- Climate-related hazards, extreme weather events, and disasters are increasing in frequency and intensity.
- Community members are experiencing extreme weather and disaster-related injuries, illnesses, and deaths in the United States despite the preparedness and mitigation efforts of healthcare professionals, emergency managers, and first responders.
- Home disaster preparedness educational, social support, and community interventions are available in the United States, yet many community members are not aware of these resources.

CURRENT THERAPY

- The home disaster preparedness level of patients can be assessed with a self-administered questionnaire called the Household Emergency Preparedness Instrument. This instrument identifies gaps in preparedness actions or disaster supply kit items of the household.
- Home disaster preparedness educational materials are available in several languages through various sources such as the U.S. Department of Homeland Security's https://www.ready.gov website, the American Red Cross, and state and local offices of emergency management.
- Chronic health condition–specific home disaster preparedness educational materials may also be available through patient advocacy websites.
- Healthcare professionals who discuss the importance of and provide educational materials on home disaster preparedness can improve preparedness levels of patients.
- Adequate home disaster preparedness can reduce climate hazard, extreme weather, and disaster-related morbidity and mortality.

Definitions and Background

Disasters are calamitous events that cause great damage, suffering, or loss to many people, requiring external agencies and resources being brought into the community to assist with response and recovery. Community members with access and functional needs experience disproportionate disaster-related morbidity and mortality compared with others residing in the same geographic location. Broadly, individuals with access and functional needs are defined as people who have a characteristic that may limit their ability to act in an emergency. Specifically, people with access and functional needs can be older adults, children, and those of any age with sensory deficits,

limited mobility, chronic or complex medical conditions, drug or alcohol dependence, physical, psychological, and/or intellectual disabilities, and those who need assistance with activities of daily living or who are experiencing domestic violence. Additional personal characteristics that result in increased risk for disaster-related morbidity and mortality are having a low socioeconomic status, residing in a single parent household, not being able to speak the primary language of the community, undocumented or unhoused status, experiencing marginalization by discrimination, and lacking transportation should an evacuation order be issued.

Epidemiology

Each year, the United Nations Office for Disaster Risk Reduction disseminates disaster-related morbidity and mortality data related to the prior year. For 2024, this organization reported that worldwide there were 393 reported disasters, 16,753 disaster-related deaths, 167.2 million people affected by disasters, and 242 billion U.S. dollars in economic damage. Globally, more than one billion people with disabilities are disproportionately adversely affected by climate-related hazards, including extreme weather events and disasters.

Home Disaster Preparedness Recommendations

Climate-related hazards, extreme weather, and disasters can create similar home and community conditions, no matter the type of event or geographic location. These conditions include living without electricity for an extended period, experiencing limitations on water that is safe to drink, and being unable to gain additional supplies due to shelter-in-place orders or supply chain disruptions. People must prepare to survive the disaster and endure these conditions to minimize their disaster-related risks and maximize their safety and comfort.

Home disaster preparedness consists of planning safe evacuation locations, routes, and transportation, developing an emergency communication plan to contact loved ones in case of separation, and assembling a kit of supplies (Table 1) that can be easily moved during precipitous evacuations. The primary barriers to adequate preparedness of community members are lack of education on how best to prepare and lack of means to purchase disaster supplies. Healthcare professionals can assist their patients with overcoming these barriers.

Assessment

A patient's home disaster preparedness can be assessed with the evidence-based Household Emergency Preparedness Instrument (HEPI), which is free to use for noncommercial research and educational purposes. This questionnaire can be administered via paper and pencil or as an electronic survey. The HEPI (Table 2) is an all-hazards, comprehensive, 50-question, valid, and reliable instrument that asks objective questions about what the patient presently owns or does in relation to their home disaster preparedness. Higher scores on the HEPI indicate higher levels of preparedness, with "no" answers scored as 0 and "yes" answers scored as 1; 2 points are awarded for each disaster supply item stored in an actual kit (measuring purposeful preparedness) versus just being in the home (measuring incidental preparedness).

TABLE 1	Basic Disaster Kit Applicable to All Households

- Portable box or container to store the supplies
- Plastic, water-resistant folder to store important documents
- Water: 1 gallon of water per day for each person in the home for 1 week or water purification tablets or a portable water filter
- Ready-to-eat food: 1 week supply for each person in the home
- Smoke and carbon monoxide detector
- Solar, hand-crank, or battery-operated weather alert radio
- Personal hygiene supplies like hand sanitizer, moist wipes, soap, shampoo, deodorant, comb/brush, toothpaste, toothbrush, and pads/tampons
- Nonelectric portable lighting, such as a battery-operated flashlight, lantern, or light switch
- First aid kit
- Warm blanket or sleeping bag for each person
- Batteries
- Matches or a lighter
- Fire extinguisher
- Wrench, pliers, or a multitool
- Nonelectric can opener
- Dust masks
- Some cash: enough to buy a meal, or firewood, or a tank of gas (banks may be closed and automated teller machines may not work during a power outage)

Note: Additional supplies should be added to meet the unique needs of the family, such as extra prescription glasses or contact lenses, a 2-week supply of medications and medical supplies (with a cooler and cold packs if any medications need to be refrigerated), entertainment for children, bowls and leashes/carriers for pets, and so on.

The HEPI's General Preparedness scale is applicable to all households and consists of two subscales (*Preparedness Actions and Planning* and *Disaster Supplies and Resources*). Two additional subscales (*Special Actions 1* and *Special Actions 2*) are applicable to households with specific characteristics, such as those who have infants, children, pets, prescription corrective lenses, utility connections within the home, or reside in a community that has an emergency alerting system. The Access and Functional Needs subscale is relevant to those who have a disability, are aged 65 years or older, are dependent on at least one prescription medication, pregnant, or are a caregiver of someone with any of those characteristics.

Data has shown that just completing the instrument can serve as a mini intervention, allowing patients to start considering what actions and which supplies are needed in their homes to support their disaster preparedness. This instrument can be self-administered by the patient, after which a discussion with the healthcare professional should occur about plans to address any missing preparedness actions and disaster kit items.

Treatment

Healthcare professionals are trusted members of the community and make excellent risk communicators in the disaster context. Studies have shown that patients who have discussed disaster preparedness with a healthcare professional have higher average preparedness levels than those who have not had this discussion. As a patient safety issue, healthcare professionals should stress the importance of preparing for climate-related hazards, extreme weather, and disaster events to their patients. They should then provide the patient with educational resources to help them overcome any barriers to preparedness they may face.

An evidence-based, effective, inexpensive intervention that has been deployed to community members with access and functional needs by nurses is called Nurses Taking on Readiness Measures (N-TORM). However, it should be noted that the interventionist does not have to be a nurse. This intervention has been done in hospital settings during the patient's admission, in community settings one-on-one, and in group classroom settings. The intervention can take anywhere from 20 to 60 minutes to complete, with one-on-one encounters taking less time than group classroom sessions.

Public health professionals can host the N-TORM intervention at local community events or at community- and faith-based organizations, libraries, and senior centers. They can also train community health workers to provide the intervention.

Healthcare professionals working in outpatient settings like clinics or primary care offices can send the intervention through the patient portal, especially at the start of the hurricane season in June, tornado season, or during National Preparedness Month in September. Healthcare professionals can also disseminate preparedness education as part of the after-visit summary or hang preparedness posters in the waiting and exam rooms. The intervention can also be conducted as a group education session for patients, similar to those held for disease-specific self-management programs.

Healthcare professionals working in in-patient settings can provide the intervention during the patient's hospital stay, or the preparedness information can be included as part of the patient's discharge instructions.

The steps for creating and implementing a home disaster preparedness educational intervention similar to N-TORM (i.e., the "treatment" for preparedness deficiencies) include the following:

1. Identifying any already existing community resources that will provide aid to the patient before, during, and after disasters. Types of resources include agencies that provide evacuation assistance, storm shelters, cooling and warming centers, flood maps, community emergency alert registration, priority utility restoration registries (especially important for those dependent on electronic medical devices), first aid classes, and free distribution of air conditioners. Compile this list of resources into a handout, including contact information of the organizations. If any of these resources do not exist within the community, healthcare professionals should advocate for them to be implemented.

2. Downloading or creating home disaster preparedness educational materials. Many free preparedness resources are offered in multiple languages on the U.S. website http://www.ready.gov. It is also likely that the local emergency management office has educational materials tailored to the disasters for which the community is most at risk. Healthcare professionals can also use these materials as examples/inspiration when creating their own hyperlocal preparedness education.

3. Reviewing the resources with the patient. Assist patients with developing their emergency communication and evacuation plans by having them write their plans in the appropriate sections of the educational materials.

4. Providing a disaster supply kit shopping list (Table 1) that is applicable to all households, while encouraging the patient to further tailor their kit to meet their unique needs. If funding is available, consider providing the kit, or at least some of the supplies, as part of the intervention.

5. Monitoring the preparedness plans at annual visits to make sure that nothing needs to be updated related to a home move, new diagnoses, or decreasing functional status.

There are a few other disaster-related resources that healthcare professionals should be aware of to help meet the needs of their patients before, during, and after extreme weather events and disasters.

The CDC's Heat and Health Tracker provides data collected from emergency department visits for heat-related illnesses and is updated daily. The CDC's online HeatRisk forecast tool provides heat risk by zip code, along with actions that people should take to stay safe. Healthcare professionals can use this data as an early warning system to monitor risk and prepare their patients for dangerous heat by implementing heat alert programs. The website HEAT.gov includes webinars for healthcare professionals, provides shareable infographic materials describing how extreme heat's health impacts compound risk to other hazards, and contains free tools to help practitioners prepare community members for extreme heat events. The CDC and National Institute for Health Care Management also have websites that provide free infographic materials about the warning signs and

TABLE 2 Household Emergency Preparedness Instrument (HEPI)

A. PREPAREDNESS ACTIONS AND PLANNING	NO	YES
1. Do you have a home emergency plan?	0	1
2. Have you practiced or drilled on what to do in an emergency at home?	0	1
3. Have you taken first aid training?	0	1
4. Do you have a fire escape plan for your home?	0	1
5. Do you know the types of disasters that are most likely to occur in your community?	0	1
6. Do you have important documents such as copies of insurance policies, identification, and bank account records in a waterproof, portable container or stored on a flash drive or cloud storage server?	0	1
7. Do you have supplies set aside in your home in a kit to use in case of a disaster?	0	1
8. Do you check your disaster supplies regularly for expired items?	0	1
9. Have you planned for how you would contact important people in your life in an emergency if you were separated?	0	1
10. Do you know if your home is in a designated evacuation zone (e.g., in a flood zone or near a nuclear power plant)?	0	1
11. Do you have a safe place to go if you had to evacuate from your home?	0	1
12. Have you planned what route to take if you evacuate from home?	0	1
13. Have you selected a place to meet important people in your life in case of separation during an evacuation?	0	1
14. Is everyone in your home aware of your evacuation plan?	0	1
15. Do you know where your local emergency shelter is?	0	1
16. Do you have a plan for what you would take if you had to leave your home quickly?	0	1
17. Have you prepared a small kit with emergency supplies to take with you if you had to leave quickly?	0	1
18. Do you have a supply of water that would provide at least 3.8 L (1 gallon) of water per day for each person in your home for 1 week?	0	1

B. DISASTER SUPPLIES AND RESOURCES	I DO NOT HAVE THIS ITEM.	I HAVE THIS ITEM IN MY HOME.	I HAVE THIS ITEM IN MY DISASTER SUPPLY KIT.	THIS DOES NOT APPLY TO ME.
1. Do you have working smoke detectors?	0	1		
2. Do you have a source of transportation to leave your neighborhood quickly in the event of a necessary evacuation of your home?	0	1		
3. If there were no power or telephones, would you have a way to receive information about disasters in your area, such as with a solar, hand-crank, or battery-operated radio?	0	1	2	
4. Do you have a 1-week supply of ready-to-eat food that will not spoil for all those living with you?	0	1	2	
5. Do you have moist wipes, hand sanitizer, and other personal hygiene supplies (e.g., soap, tampons, pads)?	0	1	2	
6. Do you have a flashlight/torch, a headlamp, lanterns, glow sticks, candles, or other nonelectric portable lighting?	0	1	2	
7. Do you have a first aid kit?	0	1	2	
8. Do you have a sleeping bag or warm blanket for each person?	0	1	2	
9. Do you have cash?	0	1	2	
10. Do you have extra batteries?	0	1	2	
11. Do you have matches?	0	1	2	
12. Do you have a fire extinguisher?	0	1	2	

C. SPECIAL ACTIONS PART 1	I DO NOT HAVE THIS ITEM.	I HAVE THIS ITEM IN MY HOME.	I HAVE THIS ITEM IN MY DISASTER SUPPLY KIT.	THIS DOES NOT APPLY TO ME.
1. Do you have a wrench, pliers, or multitool to turn off utilities (e.g., water, gas, propane)?	0	1	2	
2. If you wear prescription glasses or contact lenses, do you have extra glasses or contact lenses?	0	1	2	

Continued

TABLE 2	Household Emergency Preparedness Instrument (HEPI)—cont'd				
C. SPECIAL ACTIONS PART 1		**I DO NOT HAVE THIS ITEM.**	**I HAVE THIS ITEM IN MY HOME.**	**I HAVE THIS ITEM IN MY DISASTER SUPPLY KIT.**	**THIS DOES NOT APPLY TO ME.**
3. If you have a baby, do you have a 1-week supply of formula, bottles, and baby food?		0	1	2	
4. If you have a baby, do you have a 1-week supply of diapers?		0	1	2	
5. If you have a pet, do you have a 1-week supply of pet food and water for each pet?		0	1	2	
6. If your pet takes medications, do you have a 2-week supply of extra medications?		0	1	2	

D. SPECIAL ACTIONS PART 2	**NO**	**YES**	**THIS DOES NOT APPLY TO ME.**
1. Have you signed up for a community emergency alert system?	0	1	
2. If you have shut off valves in your home, do you know how to turn off the utilities (e.g., water, gas, propane)?	0	1	
3. Do you have written contact information of family and friends?	0	1	
4. Do you have family or friends that you could stay with during an emergency?	0	1	
5. If you have a pet, do you have an evacuation plan for your pet?	0	1	

E. ACCESS AND FUNCTIONAL NEEDS SUBSCALE	**NO**	**YES**	**THIS DOES NOT APPLY TO ME.**
1. Do you have your medical history written on paper or stored on a flash drive or cloud storage server?	0	1	
2. Do you have a list of your doctors on paper or stored on a flash drive or cloud storage server?	0	1	
3. Have you asked family or friends if they will be able to help you in a disaster?	0	1	
4. If you take prescription medications, do you have a written list of your medications, including how much you must take?	0	1	
5. If you take medications prescribed to you by your doctor, do you have a 2-week supply of extra medications?	0	1	
6. Do you have a 2-week supply of special diet food, syringes, blood sugar monitoring strips, oxygen cylinders, or other needed medical supplies?	0	1	
7. Do you have a plan for an alternate power source for medical equipment or refrigerated medicine in the event of a power outage?	0	1	
8. Do you have a small cooler or portable ice chest and cold packs/freezer bricks for refrigerated medications?	0	1	
9. Do you have a paper copy of your advanced directives or healthcare professional's order for life-sustaining treatment form, or is it stored on a flash drive or cloud storage server?	0	1	

symptoms of heat-related illnesses, along with solutions to mitigate the risks, that healthcare professionals can share via social media or print and post/provide as educational materials to patients.

As part of their Home Fire Campaign and their Sound the Alarm events, the American Red Cross (ARC) will install smoke alarms in homes free of charge. Individuals can schedule an installation appointment by going to the ARC website. The ARC also operates storm shelters in communities across the United States. To determine where the shelters are located, residents can text the word SHELTER and their zip code to 43362 and the ARC will respond with the closest shelter location. ARC storm shelter sites can also be found in the Federal Emergency Management Agency app.

RX Open is a mapping tool hosted by Healthcare Ready that helps healthcare professionals locate open pharmacies in areas impacted by disasters so that patients may continue obtaining their medications.

Finally, the Substance Abuse and Mental Health Services Administration offers a free Disaster Distress Helpline that patients can call or text when feeling anxious, worried, and angry before, during, and after disasters. It is open 24 hours a day, 7 days a week. By calling 1-800-985-5990, the patient will receive free confidential counseling, and referrals if needed.

Summary
Home disaster preparedness is a shared responsibility of the healthcare team, patient, and community-based and government organizations. As an upstream intervention to reduce disaster-related morbidity and mortality, healthcare professionals can prepare at-risk community members for climate-related hazards, extreme weather events, and disasters. It is plausible that with adequate preparedness, disaster-related morbidity and mortality and the burden placed on disaster responders, emergency services, hospitals, and healthcare professionals will be reduced, thus enhancing disaster-related community resilience.

References

American National Red Cross. Make a Plan: Create and Practice an Emergency Plan So Your Family *Will Know What to Do in a Crisis*. Available at https://www.redcross.org/get-help/how-to-prepare-for-emergencies/make-a-plan.html?srsltid=AfmBOoovVYEfdvAqTQzSaC9S7onDHjEQWSiYHWiwA-ZeO1oyHKfAmylF8. [Accessed 21/5/25].

Centre for Research on the Epidemiology of Disasters: *CRED Crunch: Disaster Year in Review*, 2024. Available at https://www.preventionweb.net/media/106739/download?startDownload=20250521. [Accessed 3/6/25].

Federal Emergency Management Agency. *Glossary: Access and Functional Needs*. Available at https://www.fema.gov/about/glossary. [Accessed 21/5/25].

Heagele TN, Adams LM, McNeill CC, et al: Validation and revision of the household emergency preparedness instrument (HEPI) by a pilot study in the city of New York, *Disaster Med Public Health Prep* 17(e126):1–9, 2022.

Heagele TN, McNeill CC, Adams LM, et al: Household emergency preparedness instrument development: a delphi study, *Disaster Med Public Health Prep* 16(2):570–582, 2020.

Intergovernmental Panel on Climate Change. *Climate Change 2023 Synthesis Report: Summary for Policymakers*. Available at https://www.ipcc.ch/report/ar6/syr/downloads/report/IPCC_AR6_SYR_SPM.pdf. [Accessed 21/5/25].

Killian TS, Moon ZK, McNeill C, et al: Emergency preparedness of persons over 50 Years old: further results from the health and retirement study, *Disaster Med Public Health Prep* 11(1):80–89, 2017.

McNeill CC, Killian TS, Moon Z, et al: The relationship between perceptions of emergency preparedness, disaster experience, healthcare provider education, and emergency preparedness levels, *Int Q Community Health Educ* 38(4):233–243, 2018.

Stein PJ, Stein MA, Groce N, et al: Advancing disability-inclusive climate research and action, climate justice, and climate-resilient development, *Lancet Planet Health* 8(4):e242–e255, 2024.

U.S. Department of Homeland Security. *Ready.gov: Plan Ahead for Disasters*. Available at https://www.ready.gov/. [Accessed 21/525].

IMMUNIZATION PRACTICES

Method of
Beth Damitz, MD

CURRENT DIAGNOSIS

- Single-agent and polyvalent variety vaccines are available in the United States.
- Vaccine-preventable diseases are occurring in the United States despite efforts.
- Vaccine registries and office-based strategies can increase vaccination rates.

CURRENT THERAPY

- Vaccination schedules are available through various sources such as the Centers for Disease Control and Prevention, including catch-up dosing.
- Vaccines can prevent diseases that are still occurring in the United States.
- Vaccination registry participation can increase vaccination rates.
- Each office visit should be used as an opportunity to review and offer vaccines.
- Providers need to be aware of special populations such as breastfeeding and pregnant women, immunosuppressed persons, and healthcare workers who could need different vaccines.

Definitions and Background

Vaccination is one of the most successful and cost-effective ways to prevent infectious diseases. Immunization is the process of inducing immunity artificially by either active immunization or passive immunization. It also occurs naturally through transplacental transmission of antibodies to a fetus, which provides protection against many infectious diseases for the first few months of life.

Physiology of Vaccines

Vaccines prevent disease in the people who receive them and protect those who encounter unvaccinated individuals, such as children too young to receive vaccines, those who cannot be immunized for medical reasons, and those who cannot make an adequate response to vaccination. Vaccines are preparations of proteins, polysaccharides, or nucleic acids of pathogens that are delivered to the immune system as single entities, as part of complex particles, or by live, attenuated agents to induce specific responses that inactivate, destroy, or suppress the pathogen.

Immunization Recommendations

The Advisory Committee on Immunization Practices (ACIP), sponsored by the Centers for Disease Control and Prevention (CDC) (https://www.cdc.gov/vaccines/schedules/hcp/index.html), the American Academy of Pediatrics, and the American Academy of Family Physicians work together to issue a national schedule for routinely recommended vaccinations.

They recommend routine vaccination to prevent 19 vaccine-preventable diseases that occur in infants, children, adolescents, or adults. These recommendations are reviewed and revised periodically. These immunization schedules give ranges of target ages for vaccines to be given (Figures 1–3). They include single and combination vaccine products. Catch-up dosing and schedules for special populations are also available (for updated immunization schedules, see https://www.cdc.gov/vaccines/schedules/downloads/child/0-18yrs-child-combined-schedule.pdf).

Disease Prevention

Since the development of vaccines, we have seen a dramatic decrease in both cases and deaths from vaccine-preventable diseases. For example, in 1950, there were 319,124 cases and 468 deaths from measles. This dramatically decreased to 43 cases and zero deaths in 2007. Obviously, decrease in disease and death is paramount, but it is also important to decrease the cost burden to our healthcare system. For every $1 spent on measles, mumps, and rubella (MMR) vaccine, $21 is saved in direct medical costs of treating a case of measles.

COVID-19 Vaccines

COVID-19 is a respiratory disease caused by SARS-CoV-2, a virus in the coronavirus family, discovered first in China in December of 2019. It spread rapidly across the world, causing a pandemic. Pharmaceutical companies immediately pursued the development of vaccines to COVID-19. Within the next year, several vaccines were authorized for emergency use. In May 6, 2023, Johnson & Johnson/Janssen COVID-19 vaccine (a viral vector vaccine) expired and is no longer available for use in the United States. Currently, three vaccines are available in the United States from these manufacturers: Pfizer-BioNTech (an mRNA type), Moderna (an mRNA type), and Novavax (a protein subunit type).

On September 11, 2023, the U.S. Food and Drug Administration (FDA) amended the emergency use authorization (EUA) of Pfizer-BioNTech COVID-19 vaccine and Moderna COVID-19 vaccine to include the 2023-2024 formula. The Moderna and Pfizer-BioNTech COVID-19 vaccines, 2023-2024 Formula, are available under EUA for all doses administered to individuals 6 months to <12 years of age and are FDA approved for persons 12 years of age and older. The older monovalent and bivalent mRNA COVID-19 vaccines (Moderna and Pfizer-BioNTech) are no longer authorized for emergency use in the United States.

The Pfizer-BioNTech COVID-19 vaccine (2023-2024 Formula), which includes a monovalent component that corresponds to the SARS-CoV-2 Omicron variant XBB.1.5, is authorized for use in children 6 months through 4 years. Individuals who are unvaccinated should receive a three-dose primary series (at 0, 3–8, and 11–16 weeks). Individuals who have received one dose of any Pfizer-BioNTech COVID-19 vaccine should receive 2 doses of the 2023-2024 Formula at 3 weeks after receipt of the previous

Recommended Child and Adolescent Immunization Schedule for Ages 18 Years or Younger, United States, 2025

These recommendations must be read with the notes that follow. For those who fall behind or start late, provide catch-up vaccination at the earliest opportunity as indicated by the green bars. To determine minimum intervals between doses, see the catch-up schedule (Table 2).

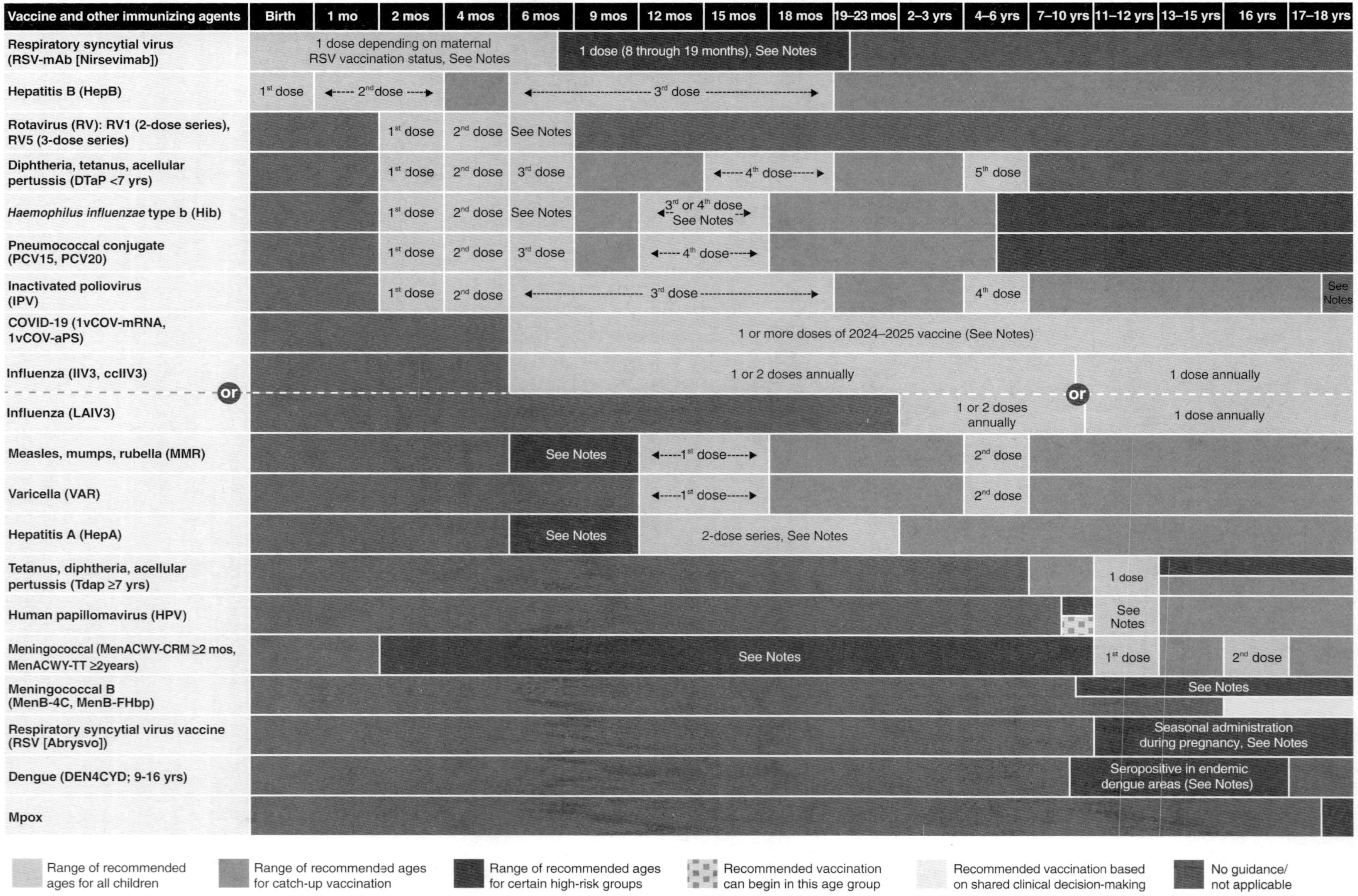

Vaccine and other immunizing agents	Birth	1 mo	2 mos	4 mos	6 mos	9 mos	12 mos	15 mos	18 mos	19–23 mos	2–3 yrs	4–6 yrs	7–10 yrs	11–12 yrs	13–15 yrs	16 yrs	17–18 yrs
Respiratory syncytial virus (RSV-mAb [Nirsevimab])						1 dose depending on maternal RSV vaccination status, See Notes			1 dose (8 through 19 months), See Notes								
Hepatitis B (HepB)	1st dose	←—— 2nd dose ——→			←———————— 3rd dose ————————→												See Notes
Rotavirus (RV): RV1 (2-dose series), RV5 (3-dose series)			1st dose	2nd dose	See Notes												
Diphtheria, tetanus, acellular pertussis (DTaP <7 yrs)			1st dose	2nd dose	3rd dose		←——— 4th dose ———→					5th dose					
Haemophilus influenzae type b (Hib)			1st dose	2nd dose	See Notes		3rd or 4th dose See Notes										
Pneumococcal conjugate (PCV15, PCV20)			1st dose	2nd dose	3rd dose		←——— 4th dose ———→										
Inactivated poliovirus (IPV)			1st dose	2nd dose	←——————— 3rd dose ———————→							4th dose					See Notes
COVID-19 (1vCOV-mRNA, 1vCOV-aPS)					1 or more doses of 2024–2025 vaccine (See Notes)												
Influenza (IIV3, ccIIV3)					←————————————— 1 or 2 doses annually —————————————→							1 or 2 doses annually		1 dose annually			
Influenza (LAIV3)											1 or 2 doses annually			1 dose annually			
Measles, mumps, rubella (MMR)						See Notes	←——— 1st dose ———→					2nd dose					
Varicella (VAR)						See Notes	←——— 1st dose ———→					2nd dose					
Hepatitis A (HepA)							2-dose series, See Notes										
Tetanus, diphtheria, acellular pertussis (Tdap ≥7 yrs)														1 dose			
Human papillomavirus (HPV)													See Notes	See Notes			
Meningococcal (MenACWY-CRM ≥2 mos, MenACWY-TT ≥2years)												See Notes		1st dose		2nd dose	
Meningococcal B (MenB-4C, MenB-FHbp)															See Notes		
Respiratory syncytial virus vaccine (RSV [Abrysvo])														Seasonal administration during pregnancy, See Notes			
Dengue (DEN4CYD; 9-16 yrs)													Seropositive in endemic dengue areas (See Notes)				
Mpox																	

Legend:
- Range of recommended ages for all children
- Range of recommended ages for catch-up vaccination
- Range of recommended ages for certain high-risk groups
- Recommended vaccination can begin in this age group
- Recommended vaccination based on shared clinical decision-making
- No guidance/ not applicable

Figure 1 Recommended immunization schedule for children and adolescents aged 18 years or younger, United States, 2025. All notes may be accessed at https://www.cdc.gov/vaccines/hcp/imz-schedules/downloads/child/0-18yrs-child-combined-schedule.pdf?CDC_AAref_Val=https://www.cdc.gov/vaccines/schedules/downloads/child/0-18yrs-child-combined-schedule.pdf. Please visit the CDC website for their regularly updated information. (From the Center for Disease Control and Prevention.)

Recommended Adult Immunization Schedule by Age Group, United States, 2025

Vaccine	19-26 years	27-49 years	50-64 years	≥65 years
COVID-19	1 or more doses of 2024-2025 vaccine (See Notes)			2 or more doses of 2024-2025 vaccine (See Notes)
Influenza inactivated (IIV3, ccIIV3) Influenza recombinant (RIV3)	1 dose annually			1 dose annually (HD-IIV3, RIV3, or aIIV3 preferred)
Influenza inactivated (aIIV3; HD-IIV3) Influenza recombinant (RIV3)				
Influenza live, attenuated (LAIV3)	1 dose annually			
Respiratory syncytial virus (RSV)	Seasonal administration during pregnancy (See Notes)		60 through 74 years (See Notes)	≥75 years
Tetanus, diphtheria, pertussis (Tdap or Td)	1 dose Tdap each pregnancy; 1 dose Td/Tdap for wound management (See Notes) 1 dose Tdap, then Td or Tdap booster every 10 years			
Measles, mumps, rubella (MMR)	1 or 2 doses depending on indication (if born in 1957 or later)			
Varicella (VAR)	2 doses (if born in 1980 or later)		2 doses	
Zoster recombinant (RZV)	2 doses for immunocompromising conditions (See Notes)		2 doses	
Human papillomavirus (HPV)	2 or 3 doses depending on age at initial vaccination or condition	27 through 45 years		
Pneumococcal (PCV15, PCV20, PCV21, PPSV23)			See Notes	See Notes
Hepatitis A (HepA)	2, 3, or 4 doses depending on vaccine			
Hepatitis B (HepB)	2, 3, or 4 doses depending on vaccine or condition			
Meningococcal A, C, W, Y (MenACWY)	1 or 2 doses depending on indication (See Notes for booster recommendations)			
Meningococcal B (MenB)	19 through 23 years	2 or 3 doses depending on vaccine indication (See Notes for booster recommendations)		
Haemophilus influenzae type b (Hib)	1 or 3 doses depending on indication			
Mpox	2 doses			
Inactivated poliovirus (IPV)	Complete 3-dose series if incompletely vaccinated. Self-report of previous doses acceptable (See Notes)			

Recommended vaccination for adults who meet age requirement, lack documentation of vaccination, or lack evidence of immunity

Recommended vaccination for adults with an additional risk factor or another indication

Recommended vaccination based on shared clinical decision-making

No Guidance/ Not Applicable

For health care personnel (See Notes)

Solid organ transplant (See Notes)

Figure 2 Recommended immunization schedule for adults aged 19 years and older, United States, 2025. All notes may be accessed at https://www.cdc.gov/vaccines/hcp/imz-schedules/downloads/adult/adult-combined-schedule.pdf. Please visit the CDC website for their regularly updated information. (From the Centers for Disease Control and Prevention.)

Recommended Adult Immunization Schedule by Medical Condition or Other Indication, United States, 2025

Figure 3 Recommended immunization schedule for adults aged 19 years or older by medical condition and other indications, United States, 2024 (Table 2). All notes may be accessed at https://www.cdc.gov/vaccines/hcp/imz-schedules/downloads/adult/adult-combined-schedule.pdf. Please visit the CDC website for their regularly updated information. (From the Centers for Disease Control and Prevention.)

a. Precaution for LAIV3 does not apply to alcoholism. b. See Notes for influenza; hepatitis B; measles, mumps, and rubella; and varicella vaccinations. c. Hematopoietic stem cell transplant.

dose and again 8 weeks later. Individuals who have received two to four doses of any Pfizer-BioNTech COVID-19 vaccine should receive a single dose of the 2023-2024 Formula 8 weeks after their previous dose. For individuals 5 years of age though 11 years regardless of immunization status, a single dose of the 2023-2024 Formula should be given. If the individual had received any COVID-19 vaccine, the 2023-2024 Formula should be given 8 weeks after the last previous dose. For immunocompromised individuals 6 months through 11 years, complete at least a 3-dose series with a COVID-19 vaccine each dose 1 month apart, with at least one of the doses being the 2023-2024 Formula.

For individuals 12 years and older, Comirnaty is the licensed Pfizer-BioNTech mRNA COVID vaccine. It is given as a single dose regardless of prior COVID-19 vaccination status.

Moderna COVID-19 vaccine (2023-2024 Formula) is authorized for use in individuals 6 months of age through 4 years. Unvaccinated individuals should receive a two-dose series, with the second dose given 1 month after the first. Individuals who have received one dose of any Moderna COVID-19 vaccine should receive one dose one month after the previous last dose. Individuals who have received two or more doses of any Moderna COVID-19 vaccine should receive one dose 2 months after the previous last dose. Individuals 5 through 11 years, regardless of vaccination status, should receive a single dose of Moderna COVID-19 (2023-2024 Formula). If previously vaccinated with any COVID-19 vaccine, administer at least 2 months after receipt of the last previous dose of any COVID-19 vaccine. Immunocompromised individuals aged 6 months through 11 years should complete a 3-dose series of any COVID-19 vaccine, each one month apart. At least one of those doses should be a 2023-2024 Formula COVID-19 vaccine.

Spikevax is the licensed Moderna COVID-19 (2023-2024 Formula) product for individuals 12 years and older. It is given as a single dose regardless of prior COVID-19 vaccination status.

Novavax is a protein subunit (monovalent) vaccine, available in the United States under FDA EUA. As of October 3, 2023, the 2023-2024 updated Novavax COVID-19 vaccine, Adjuvanted (2023-2024 Formula), was recommended by CDC for use in people aged 12 years and older. This updated version more closely targets the XBB lineage of the Omicron variant and could restore protection against severe COVID-19 that may have decreased over time.

Individuals previously vaccinated with any COVID-19 vaccine: one dose is given at least 2 months after receipt of the last previous dose of any COVID-19 vaccine. Unvaccinated individuals should receive two doses given 3 weeks apart. In immunocompromised individuals an additional dose of Novavax COVID-19 Vaccine, Adjuvanted (2023-2024 Formula), may be administered at least 2 months following the last dose of a COVID-19 vaccine (2023-2024 Formula). Additional doses of Novavax COVID-19 Vaccine, Adjuvanted (2023-2024 Formula) may be administered at the discretion of the healthcare provider, taking into consideration the individual's clinical circumstances. The timing of the additional doses may be based on the individual's clinical circumstances.

See Figures 1 and 2 for COVID vaccine immunization schedules with notes on Figures 4 and 5.

All COVID-19 vaccines can have side effects. Common side effects are minor and include injection site redness, swelling and pain, fever, headaches, fatigue, muscle pain, and nausea. More severe reactions are rare. There have been reports of thrombosis with thrombocytopenia syndrome with the Johnson & Johnson vaccine. Women under the age of 50 seem to be at a higher risk. In addition, there have been reports of myocarditis and pericarditis after the second doses of the mRNA vaccines (Pfizer and Moderna). These reactions are rare, and the CDC has recommended to continue to offer these vaccines as the benefits outweigh the risks.

As with many viruses, COVID-19 can and does mutate. At this time there have been several variants identified. Studies demonstrate that the available vaccines are effective against them. Of note, because COVID-19 is evolving, new information is constantly being obtained. It is advised to explore other resources such as the CDC website (https://www.cdc.gov) for the most up-to-date information.

Pneumococcal Vaccine Update

On October 20, 2021, the ACIP updated its recommendations for pneumococcal vaccination to provide expanded sero-type coverage. For adults 65 years and older who have never received a pneumococcal vaccine or whose vaccination status is unknown, it is recommended they receive one dose of the pneumococcal conjugate vaccine 20 (PCV20) or one dose of the pneumococcal conjugate vaccine 15 (PCV15) followed by a dose of the pneumococcal polysaccharide vaccine 23 (PPSV23) at least 1 year later. Adults 65 years and older with a previous PPSV23 history only should receive either the PCV15 or PCV20 given 1 year or later after they received the PPSV23 with no further doses needed. For adults 65 years and older with a previous pneumococcal conjugate vaccine 13 (PCV13) history or a PCV13 and PPSV23 history, they should complete the PPSV23 series as previously recommended. For adults 19 to 64 years of age with certain medical conditions or risk factors (see Figure 3) who have no or unknown PCV history, they should receive either one dose of the PCV20 or one dose of the PCV15 followed by a dose of the PPSV23 in 1 year.

Respiratory Syncytial Virus Vaccines

Two new respiratory syncytial virus (RSV) vaccines, Abrysvo (by Pfizer) and Arexvy (by GSK), have recently been approved by the FDA to prevent RSV infection in people aged 60 years and older. The ACIP recommends that adults aged 60 years and older may receive a single dose of RSV vaccine based on shared clinical decision-making with a healthcare professional.

Mpox Virus Vaccine

Mpox (formerly known as monkeypox) is caused by a virus that is related to the virus that causes smallpox. JYNNEOS is a 2-dose vaccine developed to protect against mpox and smallpox infections. People need to get both doses of the vaccine for the best protection against mpox. The second dose should be given 4 weeks after the first dose. This vaccine is indicated for a select group of individuals; clinicians should discuss with their patients whether they have risk factors that would advise the administration of this vaccine.

Immunization Responsibility

Appropriate vaccination is the responsibility of the healthcare team and patient (and parents). Education is critical. This can be done through various dissemination techniques such as one-on-one counseling, posters in the office, health fairs, and handouts at school and work. An office-based strategy consists of nursing and physician education of updates and changes in vaccines, the ability to track patient immunization records through registries, sending reminder letters to patients about recommended vaccines, and adopting standing orders to take advantage of appropriate office visits to maximize vaccination opportunities.

There are many sources for keeping current on immunizations and vaccines including the CDC's Morbidity and Mortality Weekly Report (MMWR). For parents and patients, the vaccine information statement (VIS), which is made available by the CDC to inform patients about the risks and benefits of immunizations, is very helpful and by law must be distributed before administering any vaccine. After the patient reads the VIS, the physician can then give any further information or answer questions before administering the vaccine. This discussion should be documented in the patient's medical record, including the refusal to receive certain vaccines (i.e., informed refusal).

**COVID-19 vaccination 6 months to 18 years
(minimum age: 6 months [Moderna and Pfizer-BioNTech COVID-19 vaccines],
12 years [Novavax COVID-19 Vaccine])**

Age 6 months–4 years

All vaccine doses should be from the same manufacturer.

- **Unvaccinated:**
  - 2 doses 2024–25 Moderna at 0, 4–8 weeks
  - 3 doses 2024–25 Pfizer-BioNTech at 0, 3–8, and at least 8 weeks after dose 2
- **Incomplete initial vaccination series before 2024–25 vaccine with:**
  - **1 dose Moderna:** complete initial series with 1 dose 2024–25 Moderna 4–8 weeks after most recent dose
  - **1 dose Pfizer-BioNTech:** complete initial series with 2 doses 2024–25 Pfizer-BioNTech 8 weeks apart (administer dose 1 3–8 weeks after most recent dose).
  - **2 doses Pfizer-BioNTech:** complete initial series with 1 dose 2024–25 Pfizer-BioNTech at least 8 weeks after the most recent dose.
- **Completed initial vaccination series before 2024–25 vaccine with:**
  - **2 or more doses Moderna:** 1 dose 2024–25 Moderna at least 8 weeks after the most recent dose.
  - **3 or more doses Pfizer-BioNTech:** 1 dose 2024–25 PfizerBioNTech at least 8 weeks after the most recent dose.

Age 5–11 years

- **Unvaccinated:** 1 dose 2024–25 Moderna or Pfizer-BioNTech
- **Previously vaccinated before 2024–25 vaccine with 1 or more doses Moderna or Pfizer-BioNTec**h: 1 dose 2024–25 Moderna or Pfizer-BioNTech at least 8 weeks after the most recent dose.

Age 12–17 years

- **Unvaccinated:**
  - 1 dose 2024–25 Moderna or Pfizer-BioNTech
  - 2 doses 2024–25 Novavax at 0, 3–8 weeks
- **Previously vaccinated before 2024–25 vaccine with:**
  - **1 or more doses Moderna or Pfizer-BioNTech:** 1 dose 2024–25 Moderna or Novavax or Pfizer-BioNTech at least 8 weeks after the most recent dose.
  - **1 dose Novavax:** 1 dose 2024–25 Novavax 3–8 weeks after most recent dose. If more than 8 weeks after most recent dose, administer 1 dose 2024–25 Moderna or Novavax or Pfizer-BioNTech.
  - **2 or more doses Novavax:** 1 dose 2024–25 Moderna or Novavax or Pfizer-BioNTech at least 8 weeks after the most recent dose.

Unvaccinated persons have never received any COVID-19 vaccine doses. There is no preferential recommendation for the use of one COVID-19 vaccine over another when more than one recommended age-appropriate vaccine is available. Administer an age-appropriate COVID-19 vaccine product for each dose.

For information about transition from age 4 years to age 5 years or age 11 years to age 12 years during COVID-19 vaccination series, see Tables 1 and 2 at www.cdc.gov/covid/hcp/vaccine-considerations/index.html

For information about interchangeability of COVID-19 vaccines, see www.cdc.gov/vaccines/covid-19/clinical-considerations/interim-considerations-us.html#Interchangeability.

Current COVID-19 schedule and dosage formulation available at www.cdc.gov/covidschedule. For more information on Emergency Use Authorization (EUA) indications for COVID-19 vaccines, see www.fda.gov/emergency-preparedness-and-response/coronavirus-disease-2019-covid-19/covid-19-vaccines.

Figure 4 COVID-19 Vaccine notes for children and adolescents 18 years and under, United States, 2025. https://www.cdc.gov/vaccines/hcp/imz-schedules/downloads/child/0-18yrs-child-combined-schedule.pdf?CDC_AAref_Val=https://www.cdc.gov/vaccines/schedules/downloads/child/0-18yrs-child-combined-schedule.pdf (page 5). Please visit the CDC website for their regularly updated information. (From the Centers for Disease Control and Prevention.)

General Principles for Vaccine Scheduling

Optimal response to a vaccine depends on several factors, including the type of vaccine and the age and immune status of the recipient. Simultaneous administration of vaccines increases the probability that a patient will be vaccinated fully by the appropriate age. Simultaneous administration of all age-appropriate doses of vaccines is recommended by the MMWR for children for whom no specific contraindications exist at the time of the visit. The use of combination vaccine preparations reduces the overall number of injections a child or patient will receive. However, care must be taken to ensure that the individual vaccine entities are not administered too early and too many are not administered at once. This can be a challenge when patients switch clinics or in times of vaccine shortages.

More often, dosing intervals longer than recommended are encountered in the office. Except for oral live typhoid vaccine (Vivotif Berna), an interruption in the vaccination schedule does not require restarting the entire series of a vaccine or toxoid or addition of extra doses. When an unknown or uncertain vaccination status is encountered, every effort should be made to access records. If this cannot be done in a reasonable amount of time, these persons should be considered susceptible and started on the age-appropriate vaccination schedule. Serologic testing for immunity is an alternative to vaccination; however, commercial serologic testing might not always be sufficiently sensitive

---

COVID-19 vaccination

Age 19–64 years

• **Unvaccinated:**

  ◦ 1 dose 2024–25 Moderna or Pfizer-BioNTech

  ◦ 2 doses 2024–25 Novavax at 0, 3–8 weeks

• **Previously vaccinated before 2024–25 vaccine with:**

  ◦ **1 or more doses Moderna or Pfizer-BioNTech:** 1 dose 2024–25 Moderna or Novavax or Pfizer-BioNTech at least 8 weeks after the most recent dose.

  ◦ **1 dose Novavax:** 1 dose 2024–25 Novavax 3–8 weeks after most recent dose. If more than 8 weeks after most recent dose, administer 1 dose 2024–25 Moderna or Novavax or Pfizer-BioNTech.

  ◦ **2 or more doses Novavax:** 1 dose 2024–25 Moderna or Novavax or Pfizer-BioNTech at least 8 weeks after the most recent dose.

  ◦ **1 or more doses Janssen:** 1 dose 2024–25 Moderna or Novavax or Pfizer-BioNTech.

Age 65 years and older

• **Unvaccinated:** follow recommendations above for unvaccinated persons ages 19–64 years and administer dose 2 of 2024–25 Moderna or Novavax or Pfizer-BioNTech 6 months later (minimum interval 2 months).

• **Previously vaccinated before 2024–25 vaccine:** follow recommendations above for previously vaccinated persons ages 19–64 years and administer dose 2 of 2024–25 Moderna or Novavax or Pfizer- BioNTech 6 months later (minimum interval 2 months).

Unvaccinated persons have never received any COVID-19 vaccine doses. There is no preferential recommendation for the use of one COVID-19 vaccine over another when more than one recommended age-appropriate vaccine is available. Administer an age-appropriate COVID-19 vaccine product for each dose.

For information about interchangeability of COVID-19 vaccines, see wcms-wp.cdc.gov/vaccines/covid-19/clinical-considerations/interim-considerations-us. html#Interchangeability.

Current COVID-19 schedule and dosage formulation available at www.cdc.gov/covidschedule. For more information on Emergency Use Authorization (EUA) indications for COVID-19 vaccines, see www.fda.gov/ emergency-preparedness-and-response/coronavirus-disease-2019-covid-19/covid-19-vaccines.

Figure 5 COVID-19 vaccine notes for 19 years and older, United States, 2025. https://www.cdc.gov/vaccines/hcp/imz-schedules/downloads/adult/adult-combined-schedule.pdf (page 4). Please visit the CDC website for their regularly updated information. (From the Centers for Disease Control and Prevention.)

or standardized for detection of vaccine-induced immunity, and research laboratory testing might not be readily available.

Route of Administration

There are three orally administered vaccines in the United States: rotavirus, cholera (Vaxchora), and typhoid vaccines. Rotavirus vaccine (Rotarix, RotaTeq) is licensed for infants and does not need to be repeated if the vaccine is spit up or vomited. Typhoid vaccine capsules (Vivotif) should be taken as directed by the manufacturer. Live, attenuated influenza vaccine (LAIV4, FluMist) is the only intranasal vaccine available. It does not need to be repeated if the person coughs or sneezes immediately after administration. Except for bacille Calmette-Guérin (BCG) vaccine and smallpox vaccine,[10] injectable vaccines are administered by the intramuscular subcutaneous route.

Storage

In general, vaccines need to be stored in a refrigerator or freezer. When vaccines are inappropriately stored, they can lose potency. Refrigerator and freezer storage units must be properly monitored and maintained to ensure vaccine integrity. Temperature logs should be maintained for 3 years unless state or local authorities require a longer time. Vaccines that have been stored at inappropriate temperatures should not be administered. An office protocol should be established with procedures for handling inappropriately stored vaccines, following up when these vaccines are inadvertently given, retrieving and storing emergency vaccines, handling vaccine shipments, maintaining a vaccine inventory log, and rotating vaccine stock to avoid expiration. Care should be taken to store similar vaccine products (sound-alike or look-alike) separately (on different shelves) or by color-coding labels.

---

[10]Available in the United States from the Centers for Disease Control and Prevention.

Vaccines containing diphtheria toxoid, tetanus toxoid, and acellular pertussis are easily confused.

Vaccine Safety

Vaccines in the United States undergo extensive safety and efficacy evaluations through the FDA licensing process. Despite this rigorous process, adverse reactions can and do occur. Adverse reactions are reportable to the Vaccine Adverse Event Reporting System (VAERS). VAERS is a national reporting system created in 1990 to unify the collection of all reports of adverse events after vaccination. Its primary purpose is detecting new or rare vaccine adverse events, increases in rates of known side effects, and risk factors for types of adverse events.

In 1986, the National Childhood Vaccine Injury Act established the Vaccine Injury Compensation Program. It is a no-fault program that covers all routinely recommended childhood vaccines. Those claims may be based on a vaccine injury table, which lists the adverse events associated with vaccines and provides a rebuttable presumption of causation, or by proving by preponderant evidence that the vaccine caused an injury not listed on the table. The table was created to provide swift compensation to those possibly injured by vaccines.

The provider's role to help ensure safety of vaccination includes proper vaccine storage and administration, timing and spacing of vaccine doses, observation of contraindications and precautions, and reporting adverse events to the VAERS.

Contraindications and Adverse Events

A contraindication is a condition in a recipient that increases the chance of a serious adverse reaction. A precaution is a condition in a recipient that might increase the chance or severity of an adverse reaction or compromise the ability of the vaccine to produce immunity. Situations do arise when the benefits outweigh the risks of a side effect. Children who experienced encephalopathy within 7 days after administration of a previous dose of

DTP[2], DTaP (Daptacel, Infanrix), or Tdap (Adacel, Boostrix) not attributable to another identifiable cause should not receive additional doses of a vaccine that contains pertussis. The following are not contraindications to vaccination:

- Minor illness
- Diarrhea
- Mild or moderate local reaction or fever after a prior dose
- Antimicrobial therapy
- Disease exposure or convalescence
- Pregnant or immunosuppressed person in the household
- Premature birth
- Breastfeeding

Vaccination should be deferred for persons with a moderate or severe acute illness. This precaution avoids causing diagnostic confusion between manifestations of the underlying illness and possible adverse effects of vaccination or superimposing adverse effects of the vaccine on the underlying illness.

Vaccine adverse reactions are classified as local, systemic, or allergic. Allergic reactions might be caused by the vaccine antigen, residual animal protein, antimicrobial agents, preservatives, stabilizers, or other vaccine components. Anaphylaxis is rare and usually begins within minutes of vaccine administration. Children who have had an apparent severe allergic reaction to a vaccine should be evaluated by an allergist to determine the responsible allergen and to make recommendations regarding future vaccination.

Barriers

Barriers to appropriate and timely vaccination include patients' misconceptions, false contraindications, complexity of the immunization schedules, religious or philosophic beliefs, and cost. The Vaccines for Children Program is a federally funded program that provides free ACIP-recommended vaccines to adolescents and children younger than 19 years. This program has reduced the barrier of cost.

Recording Vaccinations

Healthcare providers who administer vaccines covered by the National Childhood Vaccine Injury Act are required to ensure that the permanent medical record of the recipient indicates the date the vaccine was administered, the vaccine manufacturer, the vaccine lot number, and the name, address, and title of the person administering the vaccine. In addition, the provider is required to record the edition date of the VIS distributed and the date those materials were provided. Patients should also keep a record of the immunizations their children receive, when they were received, and at what facility they received them. A permanent vaccination record card should be established for each newborn infant and maintained by the parent or guardian.

Immunization information systems (IIS), formerly referred to as immunization registries, are confidential population-based computerized information systems that collect and consolidate vaccination data from multiple healthcare providers within a geographic area. The CDC oversees a network of 64 IIS programs distributed throughout all 50 states, the District of Columbia, and eight U.S. territories. A fully operational IIS can prevent duplicate vaccinations, provide a complete record of immunizations if the patient has received vaccines from multiple sites, and offer catch-up and needed vaccine information. Although participation of a provider is voluntary, it is highly encouraged.

Special Populations
Children

Although infants are born with some level of immunoglobulin (Ig)G that is contributed from the mother via passive immunity,

these levels decrease by 9 months of age, leaving them vulnerable to many infectious diseases. Infants begin developing IgG shortly after birth; these levels continue to increase throughout the first year of life, but children remain susceptible to infection until they achieve adult levels of IgG at 10 years of age. Therefore, this age group is especially important to vaccinate.

Breastfeeding

Neither inactivated nor live virus vaccines administered to a lactating woman affect the safety of breastfeeding for women or their infants. Breastfeeding is a contraindication for smallpox vaccination of the mother because of the theoretical risk for contact transmission from mother to infant. Yellow fever vaccine should be avoided. Breastfed infants should be vaccinated according to the recommended schedule.

Pregnancy

No evidence exists of risk to the fetus from vaccinating pregnant women with inactivated virus or bacterial vaccines or toxoids. Live vaccines, such as smallpox, MMR, and varicella (Varivax), pose a theoretical risk to the fetus and therefore are contraindicated during pregnancy. New recommendations from ACIP advise to give all pregnant women a Tdap vaccine during every pregnancy. New data indicate that maternal antipertussis antibodies are short-lived; therefore, Tdap vaccination in one pregnancy will not provide high levels of antibodies to protect newborns during subsequent pregnancies. Alternatively, if Tdap is not administered during pregnancy, the woman should receive a dose of Tdap as soon as possible after delivery to ensure pertussis immunity and reduce the risk for transmission to the newborn regardless of when she last received a tetanus booster. Routine influenza vaccination is recommended for all women who are or will be pregnant (in any trimester) during influenza season, which usually occurs early October through late March. The live attenuated influenza vaccine (LAIV4) should be avoided because it is contraindicated in pregnancy.

Altered Immunocompetence

Persons with altered immunocompetence include those with primary and secondary causes of immunodeficiency, as well as those with asplenia, chronic kidney disease, treatments with therapeutic monoclonal antibodies, and prolonged administration of high-dose corticosteroids. In general, this population should receive inactivated influenza virus (Afluria, Fluad, Fluarix, Fluzone) and age-appropriate polysaccharide-based vaccines (PCV [Prevnar], PPSV [Pneumovax 23], meningococcal conjugate [MCV4, Menactra], meningococcal polysaccharide [MPSV4, Menomune], and Haemophilus B conjugate [Hib, Act-HIB, PedvaxHIB]). Persons with most forms of altered immunocompetence should not receive live vaccines (MMR, varicella, MMRV [ProQuad], LAIV, zoster [Zostavax], yellow fever, oral typhoid, BCG, and rotavirus).

Healthcare Personnel

Healthcare personnel are at substantial risk for acquiring or transmitting hepatitis B, influenza, measles, mumps, rubella, pertussis, and varicella and should be counseled on appropriate vaccinations.

References

Centers for Disease Control and Prevention. https://www.cdc.gov/vaccines/schedules/downloads/child/0-18yrs-child-combined-schedule.pdf.

Centers for Disease Control and Prevention. https://www.cdc.gov/vaccines/schedules/downloads/adult/adult-combined-schedule.pdf.

Centers for Disease Control and Prevention. https://www.cdc.gov/vaccines/hcp/admin/storage.

Mayo Clinic https://www.mayoclinic.org/diseases-conditions/respiratory-syncytial-virus/symptoms-causes/syc-20353098.

Morris LE: COVID-19 Vaccine updates, *Fam Pract Manag* 30(4):27–30, 2023.

---

[2]Not available in the United States.

TRAVEL MEDICINE

Method of
Kristin Matson, MD, MPH; Matthew Lambert, MD; and Dawd S. Siraj, MD, MPHTM

The affordability and ease of cross-border travel combined with the growing world population is increasing the number of individuals traveling internationally. After a significant drop due to the COVID-19 pandemic, 2024 marked the recovery of international tourism from the worst crisis in the sector's history, with 1.4 billion international tourist arrivals recorded globally, according to the United Nations World Tourism Organization (UNWTO) ((https://www.untourism.int/news/international-tourism-recovers-pre-pandemic-levels-in-2024). This sustained increase in international travel has created a need for the specialty of travel medicine, which focuses on the unique and location-dependent health-related needs of travelers.

An estimated 22% to 64% of travelers report some type of illness while abroad. Most of these illnesses are mild and self-limiting, requiring minimal intervention. Approximately 4% of travelers who seek medical help have an acute, potentially life-threatening disease, and about 1 in 100,000 of these travelers die of complications related to their travel.

The goal of a travel medicine visit is to maximize health and prevent illness while traveling by offering travelers specific structured advice, malaria prophylaxis, and immunization recommendations. Disease risks, current outbreaks, and local health conditions are destination dependent and constantly change; thus the use of current, up-to-date resources is essential for providing travel medicine care (Table 1). Unfortunately, 20% to 80% of international travelers do not undergo a health consultation or receive location-specific pretravel advice before traveling. Travelers visiting friends and relatives in their country of origin, pregnant mothers, children, and travelers who are staying abroad for a long period are at particularly high risk for morbidity and mortality during their trip, requiring special attention to pretravel medical planning. Ideally, pretravel health consultations should take place 4 to 6 weeks before departure to give travelers adequate time to complete the required vaccination series. Pretravel health consultations should be structured and comprehensive. Table 2 lists items that require consideration and discussion during the consultation according to the type of travel and destination. Patients should arrive to their consultation with documentation of their vaccination history. A useful travel history form is available on the Shoreland Travax website (www.shoreland.com).

Vaccinations

Travel clinics often provide travelers with the opportunity to update routine vaccinations that they missed. Additionally, travel medicine provides vaccinations that are recommended or required because of country-specific or ongoing outbreak-specific risks. When deciding which vaccination to recommend, several factors must be considered, including any specific potential risks associated with the travel itinerary, length of stay, and activities. For each vaccine-preventable disease (VPD), one should consider the prevalence and impact of the disease in question.

Routine Vaccines

Routine vaccines are those that are administered at a regular interval for all individuals regardless of travel plans. As the risk of acquisition of these diseases increases during international travel, travel medicine providers should confirm that travelers are up to date on their routine vaccinations before departure. The 2024 importation of measles, which led to outbreaks in travelers' countries of origin, underscores the importance of updating routine vaccinations before international travel. Travelers are advised to bring documentation of all prior vaccinations to confirm vaccination status and determine the need for booster doses.

Measles-Mumps-Rubella Vaccine

Measles remains a serious cause of morbidity and mortality in the non-Western world. Importation of measles by unvaccinated travelers from regions that report endemic disease, such as Europe, Africa, and parts of Asia, remains a concern for countries where disease transmission has been interrupted (like the Americas). Indeed, several cases have been associated with exposure during air travel itself. All travelers born after 1957 (United States) and 1970 (Canada and the United Kingdom) must have two documented vaccinations or evidence of immunity as confirmed by antibody titer. Infants who are 6 to 11 months of age and are traveling to a measles-endemic area should be given one dose of measles-mumps-rubella (MMR) vaccine before departure. Individuals who have no documented vaccination and a negative antibody titer should receive two doses of MMR vaccine at least 4 weeks apart. Those who have two documented doses are considered immune for at least 20 years.

Poliovirus Vaccine

As a result of successful efforts to eradicate poliomyelitis, most of the world is now polio free. As of 2019, a few developing countries, particularly Afghanistan and Pakistan, have reported endemic wild-type poliovirus (WPV) outbreaks. In addition, as of February 2022, a small number of developing countries continue to report cases of circulating vaccine-derived poliovirus (cVDPV; www.polioeradication.org).

The injectable, inactivated poliovirus vaccine (IPV, IPOL) is the only polio vaccine available in the United States. All children must have four doses of IPV. Travelers who are traveling to countries with WPV or cVDPV and who have completed the age-appropriate series are recommended to receive a single lifetime adult booster dose before travel. The recommendation also applies to travelers to bordering countries and those who have a high risk of exposure, such as individuals working in healthcare, refugee camps, or humanitarian aid settings (U.S. Centers for Disease Control and Prevention [CDC] health information for international travel, 2019). As the list of countries with WPV or VDPV circulation changes and recommendations for vaccine is

TABLE 1	Information Resources for Risk Assessment of Travel	
Centers for Disease Control and Prevention	Comprehensive travel reports and travel vaccination and preparation information including the Yellow Book with information on country-specific risks and travel advice	www.cdc.gov/travel/
Travax (Shoreland)	Commercial software–generated reports combining itinerary-specific recommendations on recommended travel vaccines and risks. Requires a fee.	www.shoreland.com
U.S. Department of State	Travel warnings	https://travel.state.gov/content/passports/en/alertswarnings.html
World Health Organization	General travel health information and access to its international travel guide and alerts	www.who.int/ith/en/

TABLE 2 Checklist of Items to Address in the Pretravel Consultation

CATEGORY	ISSUES THAT SHOULD BE ADDRESSED
Patient risk assessment	Obtain history: itinerary, type of travel, personal medical history, age, underlying diseases, allergies, current medications, pregnancy status, previous vaccination status
Immunizations	Update routine immunizations Provide routine travel immunizations Provide destination-specific immunizations
Malaria prophylaxis	If indicated: Provide malaria education and advice; discuss bite-avoidance measures Prescribe antimalaria prophylaxis
Traveler's diarrhea	Prescribe oral rehydration therapy and loperamide (Imodium) 4 mg initially and 2 mg after each loose stool, not to exceed 16 mg/day Prescribe appropriate antibiotic (see Table 4)
Prevention against mosquito bites	Give advice regarding mosquito-borne disease Discuss personal protection measures
Rabies prevention	Give advice regarding behavior near animals Discuss measures to take if bitten or scratched by an animal—seek urgent medical advice Administer vaccine when indicated
Altitude sickness	Provide education Prescribe acetazolamide (Diamox) 125 mg orally twice a day for 1 day before ascent and continuing for 2–3 days on arrival at maximum altitude
Prevention of sexually transmitted diseases	Provide education regarding safe sex
Zika virus	Discuss potential risk of congenital Zika syndrome for pregnant women or women/men planning to conceive after return from an endemic area
Others	Deep venous thrombosis prevention Accident prevention Motion sickness prevention

Some of the recommendations are indicated only for specific destinations or specific at-risk groups.

dynamic, providers are encouraged to refer to the CDC's Travelers' Health web page (https://wwwnc.cdc.gov/travel) for up-to-date advice.

A small number of countries require proof of polio vaccination upon entry or before departure, thus administration should be documented on a vaccination certificate.

Tetanus-Diphtheria-Pertussis Vaccine

Unvaccinated or inadequately vaccinated travelers are at risk of contracting diphtheria in developing countries, as well as tetanus and pertussis anywhere in the world. The potential risk of exposure to pertussis is worldwide, with the highest rates of disease in developing countries where vaccine coverage is low. In recent decades, countries with high vaccination rates, including the United States, have seen a resurgence of pertussis despite adequate vaccination programs. Immunity from natural disease or childhood vaccination wanes over time, thus adolescent and adult travelers who have completed their childhood series should receive a booster dose of tetanus-diphtheria-pertussis (Tdap) vaccine (Adacel, Boostrix). A Tdap booster is recommended for all travelers every 10 years. If the last booster was Td, travelers should get one immediate dose of Tdap, regardless of the interval. If more than 5 years have elapsed since the last booster dose, a tetanus-containing booster should be considered for persons going to remote areas where tetanus boosters may not be readily available after a contaminated trauma.

Varicella Vaccine

Varicella infection remains prevalent worldwide. Infection can occur via inhalation of aerosols or contact of vesicular fluid from a skin lesion. Exposure to active herpes zoster lesions poses a risk of varicella infection to a susceptible traveler. In children, disease is generally mild and self-limiting. However, serious complications can occur in infants, adults, and immunocompromised individuals. Travelers who are age 12 and older and who have not completed age-appropriate vaccination or do not have laboratory evidence of immunity should receive the varicella vaccination (Varivax) before travel. In the U.S., birth before 1980 is considered evidence of immunity. When indicated, travelers should receive two doses at least 4 weeks apart.

Herpes Zoster Vaccine

Herpes zoster, also known as shingles or simply zoster infection, is the reactivation of the varicella virus in a previously infected person. Primary varicella infection (chickenpox) resides permanently in the dorsal root ganglia in a dormant (latent) form. The virus remains suppressed in an immunocompetent host. In the United States, over one million cases of herpes zoster reactivation occur in those over 60 years of age, primarily due to waning immunity. The zoster recombinant vaccine (Shingrix; GSK) is currently recommended as a two-dose schedule for persons aged 50 and older. Taken at least 4 weeks apart, this series reduces the occurrence of shingles by 97%. Immunity is expected to last at least 4 years.

Influenza Vaccine

Influenza is the most common VPD among travelers. Travelers 6 months of age and older should receive the most up-to-date influenza vaccine available in their countries annually if they are traveling to an area where influenza is circulating at the time of their travel (year-round in tropical and subtropical areas and winter months in temperate areas). Travelers who are 65 years of age and older should receive a preferentially recommended vaccine (Fluzone High-Dose, Flublok [recombinant], or Fluad [adjuvanted]) to elicit higher levels of antibody response.

Pneumococcal Vaccine

The prevalence of pneumococcal disease is highest in developing countries. In 2024, the Advisory Committee on Immunization Practices of the CDC recommended administration of pneumococcal conjugate vaccine (PCV15 [Vaxneuvance]) to all individuals 50 years of age and older who did not receive a pneumococcal vaccine in the past or unknown vaccination history, followed by a dose of pneumococcal polysaccharide vaccine (PPSV23 [Pneumovax 23]) given 1 or more years later for immunocompetent patients and 8 or more weeks later for immunocompromised patients. Another alternative is for travelers (≥50 years) to get PCV20 (Prevnar 20) or PCV21 (Capvaxive) once without the need for a follow-up PPSV23.

Recommended Travel Vaccines

Hepatitis A Vaccine

Hepatitis A viral infection is transmitted through ingestion of contaminated food or water. The virus remains viable in ice and frozen foods. Travelers who visit rural areas, trek in the back country, and often eat in a poor sanitary environment are at high risk of hepatitis A infection. Among men who have sex with men, outbreaks have been reported when traveling to endemic areas. Hepatitis A vaccination is recommended for travel to any developing country and some industrialized countries where sanitary conditions are variable.

Two hepatitis A vaccine preparations are available (Havrix, Vaqta), which are approved for administration in those 12 months of age and older. For infants traveling to high-risk endemic countries, vaccination is recommended for all children older than 6 months of age. A combination of hepatitis A and B vaccines (Twinrix) is also available and is approved for travelers 18 years of age and older. For those who are traveling on short notice, an accelerated schedule is approved. A single dose of hepatitis A vaccine given any time before travel will provide adequate protection in an immunocompetent traveler. A booster dose given 6 to 12 months after the first dose will ensure lifetime protection. Infants who received one dose before travel should receive two more doses of the vaccine for long-term protection. Immunoglobulin for hepatitis A virus prophylaxis (GamaSTAN S/D), which can be administered to travelers who are not immune and will be traveling in less than 2 weeks, is rarely recommended considering the immunogenicity of the vaccine and long incubation period of hepatitis A. A study comparing hepatitis A vaccine with immunoglobulin to prevent postexposure hepatitis A infection did not show a difference between the two, suggesting the efficacy of the vaccine as an alternate considering its ease and safety compared with immunoglobulin.

Typhoid Vaccine

Although hepatitis A and typhoid fever are both transmitted through ingestion of contaminated food and water, hepatitis A is 100 times more common than typhoid fever in travelers. The Indian subcontinent seems to be a key focus of typhoid fever in travelers, accounting for more than 80% of travel-related typhoid cases in the United States. The efficacy of typhoid vaccines ranges from 50% to 80% in various published studies.

The typhoid vaccine is protective against *Salmonella enterica* serotype typhi but not against paratyphoid fever, which is caused by strains of *S. enterica* paratyphi A, B, and C. The typhoid vaccine is recommended for long-term travelers to developing countries, short-term travelers to South Asia, and high-risk travelers to other destinations, such as individuals visiting friends and relatives in their country of origin and food adventurers.

Two unconjugated vaccines are available in the United States: the oral live, attenuated typhoid vaccine (Ty21A, Vivotif Berna), which is approved for all travelers older than 6 years of age, and the injectable typhoid Vi polysaccharide vaccine (Typhim Vi) for those older than 2 years of age. The oral vaccine, which consists of four capsules (one taken every other day), is protective for 5 years, whereas the injectable vaccine is only effective for 2 years. Ideally, either vaccine should be given at least 2 weeks before departure.

Hepatitis B Vaccine

The hepatitis B virus (HBV) is endemic worldwide, with a high prevalence in Asia and sub-Saharan Africa. Infection is transmitted through contact with blood, blood products, and body fluids and therefore poses a limited risk to most travelers; however, healthcare professionals traveling to endemic areas are at high risk.

Travelers should be counseled on HBV transmission and minimizing exposure. All patients who are traveling to intermediate to high-prevalence countries (>2% prevalence of HBV surface antigen) should receive the vaccination. The vaccines (Engerix-B, Recombivax HB, Twinrix [hepatitis A and hepatitis B vaccine]) are approved as a series of three doses given at day 0, 1 month, and 6 months. For those traveling on short notice, Twinrix is approved for an accelerated schedule of day 0, 7, and 21 to 30 days. For long-term immunity, a booster dose of Twinrix is recommended at 12 months. Two doses of this regimen completed in a 1-week interval provides adequate immediate protection for travel. A new conjugate recombinant (adjuvanted) vaccine (Heplisav-B) with two doses 1 month apart has been approved for all travelers 18 years of age and older. Protective immunity of Heplisav-B is robust, with over 95% of those who complete the series achieving immunity, and it will likely replace the vaccines that are currently available.

Cholera Vaccine

Most cases of cholera are reported from sub-Saharan Africa, Asia, and the island of Hispaniola (Haiti and the Dominican Republic). The risk of cholera to an average traveler is extremely low. The vaccine is indicated for emergency relief workers, healthcare workers traveling to an endemic area, and travelers going to an area with an active transmission. The vaccine is not required for entry to any country. In 2016 a single dose, oral, live-attenuated vaccine (Vaxchora) is now approved for high-risk travelers 2 through 64 years of age.

Japanese Encephalitis Vaccine

Japanese encephalitis (JE) is a mosquito-borne neurologic disease endemic to China, Korea, the Indian subcontinent, Southeast Asia, and the Western Pacific. The risk varies according to destination, length of stay, season, and activities being undertaken. In early 2022, an outbreak of JE was reported from rural areas of Australia. The risk is highest for travelers to rural areas, especially with nighttime outdoor activities. The overall incidence of JE cases among persons from nonendemic countries traveling to Asia is estimated to be less than 1 per 1 million, though this could be much higher depending on the type, time, and duration of travel. Though less than 1% of those infected develop neurologic illness, the sequela from such infection is devastating. Among those who develop encephalitis, 20% to 30% die, and 30% to 50% of the survivors exhibit long-term neurologic symptoms. Vaccination should be considered for all frequent travelers and those who are planning to stay longer than 1 month in an endemic country.

An inactivated, cell culture–derived vaccine (IXIARO) is licensed in the United States for use in individuals 2 months of age and older. Children 2 months to 2 years of age are given one-half the dose used for adults. The vaccine is given as a two-dose series at 0 and 28 days. An accelerated vaccination schedule of two doses 1 week apart has been approved for travelers who do not have enough time to complete the series before departure.

Rabies Vaccine

Rabies is a fatal viral infection that is transmitted through exposure to saliva of a rabid animal. The virus is neurotropic and results in progressive encephalomyelitis that is often fatal. It has a worldwide distribution with the highest prevalence in Asia, Africa, and South and Central America. Dog bites remain the primary source of infection, though bat exposure is increasingly identified as a common risk factor for disease acquisition. There were 66 cases of rabies documented in travelers from 1990 to 2013 (40% from Asia and 85% after canine exposure). Animal bites are common during travel. Approximately 2700 travelers received care for animal-related exposures and required rabies postexposure prophylaxis at GeoSentinel clinics during a 15-year period (1997–2012). Clinical illness follows a variable incubation period ranging from days to months from exposure. Early symptoms include pain and paresthesia at the site of the bite, which is invariably followed by paresis, paralysis, and fatal encephalitis. Hydrophobia, delirium, and convulsions are classic presentations that often are followed by coma and death. Symptomatic and supportive care, including aggressive wound care and postexposure prophylaxis, may improve survival in patients with this uniformly fatal disease.

Veterinarians, animal handlers, field biologists, laboratory workers who handle animals, and children are at high risk and recommended to receive the preexposure vaccination.

In the event of an exposure, vaccinated individuals require two additional doses of vaccine 3 days apart, whereas unvaccinated travelers require four doses of vaccine and additional human rabies immune globulin (HRIG [HyperRab, Imogam Rabies]), which may be expensive, unavailable, or unreliable in the traveler's locale. In light of the devastating consequences of rabies, the fact that animal bites, scratches, or licks over mucous membranes are common among travelers, even during short trips; the difficulties in receiving rabies immune globulin in the developing world; and the fact that a one-time preexposure vaccination course is likely protective "for life" suggest that the threshold for recommending rabies vaccination to travelers to the developing world should be low.

A two-dose preexposure rabies vaccine (Imovax Rabies, RabAvert), on days 0 and 7, has replaced the old three-dose vaccine and is protective for up to 3 years. High-risk individuals should have their rabies titer checked every 6 months to maintain adequate protection.

Chikungunya Virus Disease Vaccine

Chikungunya is an arboviral infection that is clinically difficult to distinguish from dengue and Zika. It is caused by an alphavirus transmitted by day biting *Aedes* mosquitoes, with peak activity in the early morning and late afternoon. It has a global distribution prevalent in tropical Africa, Asia, Central and South America, and the Caribbean. Chikungunya has a short incubation period with an average of 3 to 7 days from exposure. Presentation is typically characterized by the abrupt onset of fever, rash, and arthralgia. While symptoms usually resolve within a week, about 30% of patient may experience prolonged joint pain for over a year.

Travelers to urban areas of a country where outbreak is identified are at great risk. Personal protective measures, including application of DEET and permethrin during daytime, is the primary method of prevention.

In November 2023, the U.S. Food and Drug Administration (FDA) approved a chikungunya vaccine (IXCHIQ), which is primarily recommended for travelers aged 18 and older who are traveling to a country where there is an ongoing chikungunya outbreak. It may also be considered in persons traveling to a country or territory without an outbreak, but with human transmission in the past 5 years, if that person will be staying for over 6 months, or if they are over 65 years of age and are anticipated to have moderate (>2 weeks cumulative duration) mosquito exposure. IXCHIQ (manufactured by Valneva) is a single-dose IM live attenuated vaccine and contraindicated for those who have severe immunodeficiency disease or who are on a long-term immunosuppressive regimen. Insufficient data exist to establish guidance for pregnant mothers. In general, vaccination should be deferred until after delivery. However, when the risk of infection is high and exposure cannot be avoided, pregnant mothers who are traveling to an area with active outbreak should be considered for vaccination. The need for a booster dose has not yet been determined.

Tick-Borne Encephalitis Vaccine

Tick-borne encephalitis (TBE) is an arboviral zoonosis transmitted primarily through the bite of *Ixodes* species ticks. It is endemic in many popular tourist destinations in Europe, Eastern Europe, and parts of Asia including China, Japan, Russia, and Siberia. Symptoms include fever, body aches, headache, and arthralgia.

Up to 20% to 30% of individuals who are infected will develop encephalitis. Human infections are usually seen in the spring and summer months in temperate zones and in the fall and winter months in the Mediterranean region. A TBE vaccine (TicoVac) is available in Europe, Canada, and now the United States and is considered immunogenic and safe. Vaccination is recommended for travelers with extensive outdoor exposures such as camping in endemic regions during the transmission season. TicoVac is approved by the FDA for travelers aged 1 year and older. The primary vaccine is a three-dose series that takes a minimum of 5 months to finish the series. In addition, travelers should be advised to use insect repellents and avoid tick bites to protect themselves from TBE.

Required Vaccines
Yellow Fever Vaccine

Yellow fever (YF) is a mosquito-borne disease endemic to parts of sub-Saharan Africa and tropical South America. Though most patients with YF are asymptomatic, about 15% develop severe disease, with a reported case fatality rate of 20% to 60%. The YF vaccine (YF-VAX) is a live-attenuated vaccine that travelers should receive at least 10 days before arriving to an endemic country. A large YF outbreak was documented in eastern Brazil in 2016 to 2018, which expanded the previously known endemic area within Brazil. The World Health Organization (WHO) and the CDC are now recommending YF vaccination for all travelers to Brazil except for a few sites around Recife. There has been an ongoing outbreak of YF in parts of Nigeria, and the CDC recommends vaccination to everyone traveling to Nigeria. The risk of a traveler acquiring YF varies with season, location, activities, and duration of travel. Since January 2018, 10 travel-related cases of YF, including 4 deaths, have been reported in travelers returning from Brazil. None of the 10 travelers received the YF vaccination before their travel.

Vaccination is recommended for personal protection of travelers to endemic areas. In addition, under WHO rules, any given country may routinely require YF vaccination for entry into its territory. The aim of the regulation is to protect countries that have the mosquito vector from reintroduction of YF by asymptomatic viremic travelers.

YF-VAX is rarely associated with severe and fatal adverse reactions, which generally follow the first dose. The overall rate of serious adverse reaction is about 1 event per 250,000 doses. The likelihood of serious adverse events increases with age, with patients older than 60 years of age having a much higher risk for a severe adverse reaction.

A change in the International Health Regulations in July 2016 now considers a valid YF vaccination to be effective for life, with no need for booster vaccination at 10-year intervals. This also applies retroactively to YF vaccinations given any time before 2016. The new policy extends the validity of the vaccination for personal protection, with no need for booster doses among healthy, immunocompetent individuals. Per this recommendation, countries cannot require proof of vaccination (booster) against YF as a condition of entry to travelers whose YF vaccination was over 10 years prior. A booster vaccine after 10 years is still recommended for specific high-risk individuals: long-term travelers, travelers to West Africa, and travelers to an area where there is a current outbreak. Travel clinics should confirm the requirements of each country when they advise travelers.

Meningococcal Vaccine

Meningitis is caused by the bacteria *Neisseria meningitidis*. It is acquired by exposure to nasopharyngeal droplets during close contact. The disease spectrum ranges from fever and bacteremia to meningitis. There are eight serogroups of meningococci, but most travel-related diseases are caused by the A, C, X, and W135 serogroups. Disease is endemic worldwide, but the highest risk area is the sub-Saharan region, which is loosely named the *meningitis belt*. There is seasonality to disease incidence, with seasonal epidemics occurring during the dry season (December to June).

TABLE 3 Medication Options for Chemoprophylaxis of Malaria

DRUG	USE IN PROPHYLAXIS	ADULT DOSE	LENGTH OF TREATMENT
Chloroquine	Areas with chloroquine-sensitive *Plasmodium falciparum*	500 mg (300 mg base) weekly	Start 1–2 weeks before exposure. Continue weekly while in the malaria zone and for 4 weeks after leaving.
Mefloquine (Lariam)	Areas with mefloquine-sensitive *P. falciparum*	250 mg weekly	Start ≥2 weeks before exposure. Continue weekly while in the malaria zone and for 4 weeks after leaving.
Atovaquone-proguanil (Malarone)	All malaria zones	250 mg/100 mg once daily	Start 1–2 days before exposure. Continue daily while in the malaria zone and for 7 days after leaving.
Doxycycline	All malaria zones	100 mg daily	Start 1–2 days before exposure. Continue daily while in the malaria zone and for 4 weeks after leaving.
Tafenoquine (Arakoda)	All malaria zones	200 mg	A loading dose is 200 mg taken daily for 3 days before exposure. Then continue 200 mg weekly while in the malaria zone and for 1 week after leaving.
Primaquine[1]	Areas with >90% *P. vivax*	30 mg base daily	Start 1–2 days before exposure. Continue daily while in the malaria zone and for 7 days after leaving.

[1]Not FDA approved for this indication.

Meningococcal disease is rare in travelers (1:100,000 to <1:1,000,000 per month of travel). A quadrivalent conjugated vaccine that protects against serogroups A, C, Y, and W135 (Menactra[2], Menveo, MenQuadfi, and Nimenrix[2]) is recommended for travelers to endemic areas. Travelers to countries in the meningitis belt who anticipate close contact with crowds or the local population, as well as aid workers in refugee camps, are considered at high risk and are recommended to receive the vaccine before travel. Vaccination is required for entry to Saudi Arabia during the Hajj or Umrah seasons. Travelers returning to Saudi Arabia or high-risk zones should receive a booster vaccination every 5 years.

Malaria

Reports of malaria cases in the United States have been steadily increasing over the past few decades, largely due to infection in travelers to geographic areas with ongoing malaria transmission. Over half of the cases reported (59.3%) had a travel history to West Africa. In 2018 there were 1823 cases of malaria reported in the United States. Only 24.5% of U.S. residents who developed malaria that year reported taking any malaria prophylaxis, and 95% did not complete an appropriate chemoprophylactic regimen. Of those who reported a reason for travel, most cases were in travelers visiting friends and relatives (77%) (source: https://www.cdc.gov/mmwr/volumes/71/ss/ss7108a1.htm).

Before travel, a risk assessment should be performed to determine whether malaria chemoprophylaxis is indicated. Malaria transmission can vary greatly, even within a country, based on the region and season of travel. The traveler's specific itinerary should be reviewed for the cities visited, type of accommodations (bed nets, window screens, air conditioning), reason for travel, and special activities while traveling. Mosquito avoidance measures should be recommended in addition to chemoprophylaxis. Up-to-date travel notices and advisories specific to the destination of travel may be found on the CDC website (https://wwwnc.cdc.gov/travel).

The life cycle of malaria in humans involves an initial asymptomatic liver stage followed by a later symptomatic erythrocytic stage. Malaria chemoprophylaxis is used to prevent the development of clinical malaria if a person is infected. Certain chemoprophylactic agents (chloroquine [Aralen], mefloquine [Lariam], and doxycycline [Vibramycin]) only work on the later erythrocytic stage of malaria parasites and are therefore recommended to be taken for a longer time (4 weeks) after leaving a malaria-endemic area. Atovaquone-proguanil (Malarone) can act on the earlier nondormant liver parasite stage; therefore a shorter posttravel duration is recommended (1 week). Unlike other *Plasmodium* species, *Plasmodium vivax* and *Plasmodium ovale* have dormant liver stages known as *hypnozoites,* which are responsible for disease relapse months or years after an acute infection. Tafenoquine (Arakoda) and primaquine[1] are the only available chemoprophylactic medications effective against all liver stages of the malaria parasite, including the liver hypnozoites of *P. vivax* and *P. ovale.*

Malaria Chemoprophylaxis

All malaria chemoprophylactic options should be started before travel, taken throughout travel, and continued for a period posttravel (Table 3). When choosing a chemoprophylactic agent, factors to consider include the traveler's age and medical history, pregnancy status, length of the trip, cost of the drug, drug allergies, drug interactions, and drug resistance at the destination. Up-to-date information regarding local drug resistance in areas of planned travel can be found on the CDC website (https://wwwnc.cdc.gov/travel).

Chloroquine (Aralen) may only be used for malaria prophylaxis in areas of the world with chloroquine-sensitive *Plasmodium falciparum*. Resistance is found worldwide except in Central America west of the Panama Canal, Haiti, and the Dominican Republic, where *P. vivax* is the dominant species. Chloroquine is used once a week for prophylaxis. It should be started 1 to 2 weeks before travel, taken weekly during travel, and continued for 4 weeks after leaving the malaria zone. The most common side effects are gastrointestinal discomfort, nausea, vomiting, or headache. Serious adverse effects are rare and are more likely to occur with prolonged and high doses of therapy. Retinopathy is associated with high doses and when used for more than 5 years. An overdose of chloroquine could be fatal, and the medication should be stored in childproof containers. If a traveler is already taking hydroxychloroquine (Plaquenil) chronically for a rheumatologic condition, they may not have to take additional malaria prophylaxis.

Four potential options are approved by the FDA for malaria chemoprophylaxis in areas with chloroquine-resistant malaria: atovaquone/proguanil (Malarone), doxycycline (Vibramycin), mefloquine (Lariam), and tafenoquine (Arakoda). Primaquine may be used off-label (not FDA approved) for malaria chemoprophylaxis in areas of the world with predominantly *P. vivax* malaria.

Mefloquine should only be used for malaria prophylaxis in areas of the world with mefloquine-sensitive *P. falciparum*. Mefloquine-resistant *P. falciparum* malaria is found in parts of

---

[2]Not available in the United States.

[1]Not FDA approved for this indication.

Southeast Asia (along the borders of Thailand with Cambodia and Myanmar, western Cambodia, eastern Burma, and southern Vietnam), and mefloquine should not be used for malaria prophylaxis in these areas. Mefloquine is used once a week for prophylaxis. It should be started 2 or more weeks before travel, taken weekly during travel, and continued for 4 weeks after leaving the malaria zone. Adverse effects tend to be noted within the first weeks of mefloquine initiation; therefore the medication can be started 2 to 4 weeks before travel to ensure that it will be tolerated during travel. Mefloquine may be associated with sleep disturbances, strange dreams, and insomnia. The FDA also has issued a black-box warning that mefloquine may cause neuropsychiatric adverse effects that can persist after the medication has been discontinued. Mefloquine is contraindicated in those with neurologic and psychiatric disorders and should be avoided in travelers with a significant family history of seizures or major psychiatric disorders. It is also recommended to avoid mefloquine in travelers with cardiac conduction abnormalities. A traveler who is prescribed mefloquine must receive a copy of the FDA medication guide for mefloquine, which can be found online (www.accessdata.fda.gov/drugsatfda_docs/label/2008/019591s023lbl.pdf).

Atovaquone-proguanil (Malarone) can be used for malaria prophylaxis in any malaria zone worldwide. Atovaquone-proguanil is a daily prophylactic drug. It should be started 1 to 2 days before travel, taken daily during travel, and continued for 7 days after leaving a malaria zone. The drug is usually well tolerated, with the most common adverse effect being gastrointestinal upset.

Doxycycline can be used for malaria prophylaxis in any malaria zone worldwide. Doxycycline is a daily prophylactic drug. It should be started 1 to 2 days before travel, taken daily during travel, and continued for 4 weeks after leaving a malaria zone. An added benefit of doxycycline is that it may also provide some protection against rickettsial infections and leptospirosis. However, photosensitivity is a common adverse effect of doxycycline. Patients should also be forewarned about the possibility of pill esophagitis with this medication.

Tafenoquine (Arakoda) can be used for malaria prophylaxis in any malaria zone worldwide. Tafenoquine is used once a week for prophylaxis. It should be started 1 to 2 weeks before travel, taken weekly during travel, and continued for 1 week after leaving the malaria zone. G6PD deficiency must be ruled out by laboratory testing before prescribing this medication because fatal hemolysis could occur in individuals with G6PD deficiency. Tafenoquine should be avoided in those with a history of a psychotic disorder because rare psychiatric events have been observed. The most common adverse events include nonsignificant decreases in hemoglobin, gastrointestinal discomfort, and headache. Tafenoquine is the only FDA-approved medication for malaria prophylaxis that has activity on the hypnozoite stage of the malaria parasite. Note that another tafenoquine-based antimalarial (Krintafel) is approved for radical cure of *P. vivax* infections in those older than 16 years of age.

Primaquine is very effective against *P. vivax* and is an option for travel to areas with greater than 90% *P. vivax* malaria[1]. It is taken daily starting 1 to 2 days before exposure. It is continued daily while in the malaria zone and until 7 days after leaving. It cannot be used in those with G6PD deficiency and may cause gastrointestinal upset.

Posttravel

No prophylaxis is 100% effective. Travelers should be advised to seek medical attention during travel if malaria symptoms occur. They should also be told to notify their physician of their travel history if they develop a febrile illness for up to 1 year posttravel.

COVID-19

Since COVID-19 was identified in late 2019, there have been more than 775 million confirmed cases worldwide with over 7 million deaths (source: https://covid19.who.int/). Travel requirements during this time have been frequently revised. As of June 30, 2022, the CDC no longer requires air passengers traveling from a foreign country to the United States to show a negative COVID-19 viral test or documentation of recovery from COVID-19 before boarding their flight. All nonimmigrant, non–U.S. citizen air travelers to the United States are no longer required to be fully vaccinated and to provide proof of vaccination status before boarding as of May 12, 2023. As of April 27, 2023, the CDC updated the list of accepted vaccine series; it can be found at https://www.cdc.gov/covid/?CDC_AAref_Val=https://www.cdc.gov/coronavirus/2019-ncov/travelers/proof-of-vaccination.html. The CDC continues to recommend, but not require, masks during public transportation and at transportation hubs.

Travelers to other countries should also be aware of travel health notices and arrival restrictions at their destination. Persons should avoid travel if they are sick or experiencing symptoms and may consider returning to normal activities 24 hours after fever and symptoms have ended; during the subsequent 5 days, they should consider additional precautions such as masking, physical distancing, and/or testing. As of March 1, 2024, the CDC released updated guidance incorporating COVID-19 guidance with guidance for other respiratory viruses (https://www.cdc.gov/respiratory-viruses/prevention/index.html?CDC_AA_refVal=https%3A%2F%2Fwww.cdc.gov%2Frespiratory-viruses%2Fguidance%2Findex.html). More information on international travel during COVID-19 can be found on the CDC Travel Recommendations by Destination website (https://wwwnc.cdc.gov/travel/notices).

Personal Protection Measures

Risk for vector-borne disease depends on many factors, including the traveler's destination, season of travel, and length of stay. Viral diseases that may be of concern include JE, Zika virus, dengue, and chikungunya virus. Rickettsial diseases are found worldwide on all continents apart from Antarctica. Malaria is the parasite of greatest concern, but leishmaniasis, trypanosomiasis, and filariasis are other potential parasitic diseases spread by arthropod vectors.

The type of accommodation can affect the traveler's risk of vector-borne diseases. An air-conditioned room for sleeping, effective window screens, and/or bed nets are protective. Wearing long-sleeved shirts, long pants, and socks can also decrease risk. For added protection, a clothing insect repellent, such as permethrin, is recommended. Permethrin activity is maintained on treated clothes despite several wash cycles.

Insect repellents for use on skin have variable efficacy depending on the repellent type and form, concentration, frequency of application, and vector. Typically, a higher concentration of insecticide will provide a longer duration of protection. However, there is a peak at which no further protection is seen, and more toxicity could result. DEET, at a concentration of 20% to 25%, has efficacy against all mosquito species and some tick species, biting flies, chiggers, and fleas. Concentrations of DEET greater than 30% do not appear to provide added benefit. No definitive studies have established what concentration of DEET is safe in children. The American Academy of Pediatrics recommends that repellents should not contain greater than 30% DEET when used on children. Products containing picaridin (icaridin outside the United States) may also be good options. Potential benefits of picaridin over DEET are that it is odorless and does not damage plastic and may be less irritating to the skin. The lowest concentration possible should be used on children. Products containing IR3535 are another option and appear to have particularly good activity against *Ixodes scapularis* ticks (commonly known as *deer ticks* or *black-legged ticks*); it may be equivalent to ~20% DEET.

Traveler's Diarrhea

During a 2-week trip, traveler's diarrhea has an incidence between 10% and 40%. Higher-risk areas include parts of Asia and Central/West Africa. Certain behaviors may affect the risk of developing diarrhea. Practicing hand hygiene measures before eating has been shown to reduce the incidence of diarrhea. Other

---

[1] Not FDA approved for this indication.

ANTIBIOTIC	ADULT DOSE	DURATION	COMMENTS
Rifaximin (Xifaxan)	200 mg tid	3 days	Not recommended in patients with fever or bloody diarrhea
Rifamycin SV (Aemcolo)	388 mg bid	3 days	Not recommended in patients with fever or bloody diarrhea
Azithromycin (Zithromax)[1]	1000 mg	Single dose (or two divided doses on the same day to reduce nausea)	Preferred empiric option in Southeast Asia, and preferred treatment for dysentery
	500 mg daily	3 days	
Ciprofloxacin (Cipro)[1]	750 mg	Single dose	
	500 mg bid	3 days	
Levofloxacin (Levaquin)[1]	500 mg daily	1–3 days	

[1]Not FDA approved for this indication.
bid, Twice daily; *tid,* three times daily.

potentially beneficial measures include avoiding food that has not been properly cooked, avoiding ice, and drinking only bottled or treated water in resource-poor settings.

Traveler's diarrhea is predominantly caused by bacterial pathogens. However, antibiotic prophylaxis to prevent traveler's diarrhea is rarely indicated, given both the cost and potential for adverse events. Bismuth subsalicylate (BSS [Pepto-Bismol])[1] has shown efficacy in decreasing the risk of traveler's diarrhea and may be considered for prevention. However, BSS requires frequent dosing, causes blackening of the tongue, and has the potential for drug-drug interactions.

Treatment

Treatment recommendations for traveler's diarrhea depend on the severity of illness. Ensuring adequate hydration is always a mainstay of treatment. In the case of severe diarrhea, the WHO recommends oral rehydration therapy, which is available at most pharmacies. An antimotility agent such as loperamide (Imodium) can also provide symptomatic benefits for mild to severe traveler's diarrhea. Loperamide is not recommended to be used alone in travelers with dysentery.

When antibiotics are used for self-treatment of traveler's diarrhea, they may reduce the duration of diarrhea by 1 to 3 days. Several effective antibiotic options are available (Table 4). A combination of an antibiotic with loperamide further shortens the duration of diarrhea. However, the benefits of antimicrobial treatment of traveler's diarrhea must be weighed against the potential risks. Each antibiotic option has the potential for specific side effects, such as tendinopathies in the case of fluoroquinolones. Antibiotic use also increases the risk of developing *Clostridioides difficile* diarrhea. Further, multiple studies have shown that antibiotic use for the self-treatment of traveler's diarrhea increases the risk of developing colonization with antibiotic-resistant bacteria, including extended-spectrum β-lactamase–producing Enterobacteriaceae and carbapenemase-producing Enterobacteriaceae.

Given the potential risks, antimicrobial therapy is not recommended for acute diarrhea that is tolerable and does not interfere with planned activities. Loperamide or BSS can be used alone for these mild cases. Loperamide, with or without an antibiotic, may be used in the case of moderate diarrhea that is distressing or interferes with planned activities. An antibiotic is recommended to treat severe traveler's diarrhea, which includes all dysentery cases, as well as diarrhea that is incapacitating or prevents planned activities. Single-dose antibiotic treatment regimens are as effective as 3-day regimens for most cases of traveler's diarrhea.

Fluoroquinolones, such as ciprofloxacin (Cipro)[1] and levofloxacin (Levaquin)[1], have long been used to treat traveler's diarrhea. However, there has been increasing resistance to fluoroquinolones among diarrheal pathogens, especially *Campylobacter* isolates in South and Southeast Asia. In this area of the world, azithromycin (Zithromax)[1] is preferred for empiric treatment of traveler's diarrhea. Azithromycin is also the preferred treatment for dysentery[1]. Rifaximin (Xifaxan) is approved to treat traveler's diarrhea caused by noninvasive strains of *Escherichia coli*. Rifamycin SV (Aemcolo) is a nonabsorbable antibiotic with an enteric coating, and it has the same mechanism of action as rifaximin. Because rifamycin SV and rifaximin are not recommended for treatment of invasive diarrhea, their role in the self-treatment of diarrhea is limited.

High-Altitude Illness

High-altitude illnesses (HAIs) caused by hypoxia can occur during travel to high-elevation areas, typically areas with an elevation greater than 8000 feet above sea level. There are three syndromes that may comprise altitude illness: acute mountain sickness (AMS), high-altitude cerebral edema (HACE), and high-altitude pulmonary edema (HAPE).

AMS is the most common form of HAI, and symptoms may include headache, nausea, and fatigue. If left untreated, AMS can progress to HACE, which is a more serious condition. Manifestations of HACE can include ataxia, drowsiness, confusion, and even death. Acute hypoxia may also lead to HAPE. The pathophysiology of HAPE is different from that of AMS/HACE and is presumably caused by pulmonary vasoconstriction that leads to pulmonary edema. Cough, dyspnea on exertion, and pulmonary congestion can progress to death if ascent is continued.

Prevention of High-Altitude Illnesses

Certain individuals are more susceptible to HAI, but it is not possible to reliably predict who may develop symptoms. Rate of ascent, ultimate elevation, underlying medical conditions, and degree of physical exertion are all potential factors in determining risk of developing HAI. The body's ability to acclimate to a high elevation typically takes 3 to 5 days. A slow ascent that allows time for acclimatization is helpful in preventing the development of all forms of HAI; however, this is not always possible. There are several popular high-altitude tourist destinations that may be reached via direct flights from areas of low elevation. Examples include Cuzco, Peru, located at 11,000 feet; La Paz, Bolivia, at 12,000 feet; and Lhasa, Tibet, at 12,000 feet.

Acetazolamide (Diamox) is a nonantibiotic sulfonamide that was developed as a diuretic to treat hypertension. Its efficacy for this purpose was limited. However, multiple studies have since

---

[1]Not FDA approved for this indication.

---

[1]Not FDA approved for this indication.

shown that the preemptive use of acetazolamide can decrease the risk of developing AMS. Acetazolamide blocks carbonic anhydrase, primarily in the kidney. This decreases reabsorption of bicarbonate and leads to the development of metabolic acidosis, compensating for the respiratory alkalosis associated with high elevations. Acetazolamide is associated with an increased risk of paresthesia and diuresis. The recommended dose of acetazolamide to prevent AMS while minimizing adverse effects is 125 mg orally twice a day. It is generally recommended to start 1 day before ascent and continue through the first 2 days at peak elevation.

A number of other medications have been studied to prevent AMS, but the benefits of alternative therapies are less clear. Dexamethasone (Decadron)[1] is one of the more commonly used alternatives. The typical dose for prophylaxis is 2 mg every 6 hours or 4 mg every 12 hours. Inhaled budesonide (Pulmicort)[1] was found to be ineffective in preventing AMS in 2017 and 2020 published studies and is not recommended.

Treatment

Symptomatic travelers should not continue to ascend further until all symptoms resolve, and they should descend to a lower elevation immediately if symptoms progress. Acetazolamide can be considered for treatment of AMS, but it is better at preventing than treating this disorder. Dexamethasone[1] is more reliable for treatment

---

[1] Not FDA approved for this indication.

of moderate to severe AMS. However, descent is the most effective therapy and should occur immediately in cases of HACE or HAPE.

Summary

A pretravel consultation should include a health assessment, interventions, and counseling to decrease travel-related risks and improve the likelihood of a safe and enjoyable travel experience.

References

Agudelo Higuita NI, White BP, Franco-Paredes C, McGhee MA: An update on prevention of malaria in travelers, *Ther Adv Infect Dis* 8:20499361211040690, 2021.

Angelo KM, Libman M, Caumes E, et al: Malaria after international travel: a GeoSentinel analysis, 2003-2016, *Malar J* 16:293, 2017.

Centers for Disease Control and Prevention: Advisory committee on immunization Practices (ACIP): ACIP recommendations, 2024. https://www.cdc.gov/acip/vaccine- recommendations/index.html.

Centers for Disease Control and Prevention: *CDC yellow book 2024: health information for international travel*, New York, 2024, Oxford University Press.

Freedman DO: Protection of travelers. In Bennett JE, Raphael D, Blaser MJ, Mandell D, editors: *Bennett's principles and practice of infectious diseases*, 8. Philadelphia, 2020, Saunders Elsevier, pp 3818–3827.

Hills SL, Poehling KA, Chen WH, Staples JE: Tick-borne encephalitis vaccine: recommendations of the advisory committee on immunization Practices, United States, 2023, *MMWR Recomm Rep* 72:1, 2023.

Hyle EP, Rao SR, Bangs AC, et al: Clinical Practices for measles-mumps-rubella vaccination among US pediatric international travelers, *JAMA Pediatr* 174:e194515, 2020.

Shlim David R: The use of acetazolamide for the prevention of high-altitude illness, *J Trav Med* 1–6, 2020.

ARTIFICIAL INTELLIGENCE AND PRIMARY CARE

Method of
Vincent Morelli, MD

Introduction

As with humans living in every era, we exist in a time of expanding knowledge and paradigm-shifting breakthroughs—the agricultural revolution, the industrial revolution, the information revolution. We now stand on the verge of another breakthrough, the artificial intelligence (AI) revolution. With it will come exciting opportunities, enhanced efficiencies, unimagined insights, as well as unique challenges and ethical considerations. This chapter explores the AI revolution as it relates to the practice of medicine.

First, we will define terms and offer a brief history of the evolution and development of AI. Next, we will provide an overview of the inner workings of AI so that the practitioner may appreciate its potential and recognize its inherent shortcomings. After this, we will review the literature as it relates to the current use of AI in medical practice—in assisting with screening, prevention, diagnosis, and treatment. We will then give an overview of AI's ability to improve medical administrative tasks and comment on its evolving utility in impacting wider healthcare systems. Finally, we will briefly look at some of the current concerns associated with the use of AI in medicine.

Defining Terms, Evolution, and Development

Defining Artificial Intelligence, Machine Learning, and Deep Learning

AI encompasses computer systems that emulate human intelligence, learning, and problem-solving. Within AI, machine learning (ML) refers to algorithms enabling computers to enhance their performance on tasks, such as predicting heart attacks, through exposure to data without human intervention. ML forms the foundation of fields such as robotics and natural language processing. Deep learning (DL), a subset of ML, simulates the human brain's structure with interconnected nodes or neurons. It processes input data through layers of nodes, adjusting and making corrections as the data runs through the system, thereby improving accuracy and ability to make predictions.

- AI: Computer systems performing tasks requiring human-like intelligence
- ML: Algorithms enabling computers to learn without explicit programming
- DL: A subset of ML using neural networks, mimicking brain neurons' interaction

Evolution and Development of Artificial Intelligence

AI's history traces back to Alan Turing's 1950 paper, followed by the 1956 Dartmouth conference setting AI standards. An initial surge in AI research gave way to the "AI Winter" in the mid-1970s, but advancements in algorithms, processors, and data sparked an "AI Spring" in the mid-1980s. The current AI revolution witnesses widespread AI applications across various domains because of technological progress and data availability.

How Artificial Intelligence Works: An Example

This section illustrates how AI processes patient medical records to identify heart attack risk factors.

1. *Pretraining:* AI learns word to word associations through statistical techniques like Word2Vec and GloVe.
2. *Data collection and processing:* Patient electronic medical record (EMR) data undergoes cleaning and feature engineering to standardize and enhance algorithm comprehension.
3. *Pattern recognition:* AI algorithms analyze EMR data for risk factor patterns, even identifying previously unknown associations (unsupervised learning).
4. *Model selection:* Statistical models like linear regression (LR) or neural networks are chosen based on data suitability.
5. *Supervised training:* Models are trained with "labeled" data to correct errors and refine predictive accuracy.
6. *Testing and validation:* Trained models are tested with separate data sets to ensure accurate predictions.
7. *Deployment:* Finalized models are used to clinically predict heart attacks. In summary, AI's evolution from inception to practical application involves continual refinement of algorithms and models, driven by advancements in technology and data availability. This process illustrates AI's transformation from theoretical concept to real-world utility in various industries.

Artificial Intelligence in Screening, Prevention, Diagnosis, and Treatment

Artificial Intelligence in Screening and Prevention

As noted in the previous section, unsupervised learning may find new risk factors or combinations of risk factors that enable improved screening and preventive strategies. For example, combining demographic data (e.g., age, BMI) with genetic markers has been explored in screening for depression in type 2 diabetics. Many similar "unintuitive" risk factors may be found by AI systems analyzing EMRs in an unsupervised manner or by combining EMRs with data from social media (e.g., use patterns, language choices, posting activity), motor activity monitoring, sleep and exercise data, or inputs from various other sources.

In this manner, many other maladies of aging may be screened for in advance and (hopefully) prevented. Examples include screening for Alzheimer disease, predicting patients who will likely experience atrial fibrillation, monitoring biomarkers that may influence the onset of arthritis, screening for colorectal cancer, fibromyalgia, other types of heart disease, mental health issues, and prostate cancer. For example, one prospective study of a prediction model built using AI and statistical analysis was able to predict which hypertensive patients were most likely to have their high blood pressure caused by adrenal hyperplasia or adenoma. This kind of prediction is significant because the prevalence of adrenal hypertension is estimated at 5% to 20%, yet only 3% are screened for the dysfunction. A more detailed example of the use of AI in screening is presented later to give the reader a clearer idea of AI's overall utility.

1515

Screening for Suicide Risk: An Example

Of the many issues facing modern U.S. society, the current trend in youth suicide is one of the most distressing. In 2000 there were roughly 30,000 suicides in the United States. By 2023 that number had increased to over 50,000, with suicide becoming the second leading cause of death in those under age 35. Various reasons, risk factors, and stressors have been postulated as contributory, but as of yet, analysis has not yielded an effective method of screening or intervention. In fact, a recent 2017 meta-analysis noted that conventional suicide screening tools were barely better than chance at predicting suicide with no change in predictive capability occurring over the previous 50 years.

With this in mind, AI-related research has begun to explore models to improve screening and facilitate early intervention. In 2024 a Canadian study created an AI model to explore the issue. The model recorded a combination of 103 evidence-based individual, community, and systemic risk factors in its analysis. Individual risk factors included variables such as age, sex, urban versus rural domicile, as well as prior diagnosis of depression, bipolar disorder, or schizophrenia; visits to primary care, mental health, or emergency room services; and substance abuse. Community risk factors included neighborhood deprivation, availability of mental health services, and the availability of addiction or primary care services. Finally, system-level risk factors such as per capita regional spending for substance use disorders were included.

These risk factors were collected for 5 years for both cases and controls (suicides vs. nonsuicides), after which researchers trained and tested an AI model in the fashion discussed earlier. The researchers then tried several different statistical frameworks—LR random forest, extreme radiant boost, multilayer perception—and noted the LR model to best fit the outcome data (suicide vs. no suicide). This model was still suboptimal, identifying only 31% to 38% of males who committed suicide and 40% to 47% of females. Despite this lack of sensitivity, the model did prove successful at ranking those who were at higher risk of suicide versus those who were low risk. (Statistically speaking, the area under the curve was roughly .78 for men and .85 for women, indicating an adequate ability to rank high vs. low risk.) Thus this AI-enhanced screener, after combining data from EMRs and various other sources, could at least predict and flag patients who might be at higher risk and enable contact by providers for early intervention.

In the future, it is not hard to imagine that such AI-augmented screening, using similar but even more extensive inputs (e.g., search histories, social posting habits, language analysis, self-reported dietary inputs, mobility monitoring), will become increasingly useful not only in suicide screening but with screening for many other afflictions.

Artificial Intelligence in Diagnosing

As with screening, reviewing all of AI's applications in diagnostics would certainly fill more than the pages allocated for this chapter. But again, just a few examples will give the reader a sense of the utility of AI and hopefully spark curiosity and impel the reader to explore other ways in which AI systems may assist in their particular field of clinical practice or research.

Image Analysis in Pulmonology: An Example

CT screening for lung cancer in smokers and former smokers has been noted to decrease mortality by 20% relative to x-ray screening. The enhanced utility of low-dose CT screening lies in its ability to better visualize, estimate nodule size and density, and follow nodule growth rates—all significant predictors of malignancy. However, because radiologist readings have a documented tendency to misread size by 1 to 5 mm and often to omit density readings, there is definite room for improvement in image analysis. To address this, AI systems have been developed and have demonstrated high sensitivity (83%–97%) and accuracy (82%–98%) for lung nodule detection. Although such systems are improving and are often better at detecting nodules

than radiologists, even the best AI systems are still reading at least one false positive nodule per scan because of the misinterpretation of benign lymph nodes or noncalcified granulomas. Obviously, such overreads, unless subjected to human oversight, could lead to unnecessary patient anxiety, unwarranted procedures, excess patient morbidity, and increased health system costs.

Currently, ongoing development of AI models will further enhance the reliability of image analysis. These developmental models are using a radiomic approach to CT/MR/PET analysis (i.e., using algorithms to simultaneously extract and analyze multiple features such as shape, size, volume, diameter, uptake intensity, smoothness, coarseness, image, density) to develop more accurate prediction models.

Image Analysis in Gynecology: An Example

It is not hard to imagine possible uses for AI image recognition systems in gynecology (e.g., reading Pap smears, colposcopic images, hysteroscopy). For example, Pap smear readings have long been shown to suffer from inter- and intraobserver inconsistencies (different readers coming up with different results or the same reader coming up with different results if read at different sittings).

AI systems have been developed to help address these inconsistencies and improve accuracy. At the time of writing (February 20, 2025), only one FDA-approved AI assisted Pap reading system is commercially available (Hologic's Genius Digital Cytology System). Its role lies in digitizing Pap smear slides and identifying cells of interest for further review by pathologists. This is a time-saving approach that quickly identifies possible abnormal cells, thus reducing pathologist "slide search" time. Studies (done by the company but not yet published in peer-reviewed journals) have also noted a 28% lower false negative rate (resulting in an increased sensitivity) with the AI-powered system.

Similar systems are currently being developed for colposcopic and hysteroscopic image analysis and diagnosis. Even in the early stages of development, these systems are approaching or bettering that of experienced pathologists in terms of sensitivity, specificity, and predictive values.

Similar AI image analyses and diagnostic assistance exist in dermatology, gastroenterology, ophthalmology, hematology, laboratory medicine, and others.

Electrocardiogram Image Analysis in Cardiology: A Final Example

A meta-analysis published in 2020 found that the median accuracy of physicians' ECG interpretations was only 54% and that traditional computerized ECG (using static rule-based algorithms) analysis has been noted to miss up to 30% of myocardial infarctions (MIs).

Other studies have noted traditional computerized analysis to misdiagnose 9% of even simple arrythmias and to poorly identifying specific coronary artery involvement in MI. Such shortcomings can lead to delayed diagnosis, inappropriate treatment, or suboptimal planning when considering intervention such as percutaneous coronary intervention.

AI-assisted ECG analysis, on the other hand, has been shown to improve this situation with better-than-human detection of subtle ECG abnormalities leading to improved detection of MIs (especially non–ST elevation MIs), arrhythmias, structural heart disease (valvular abnormalities), hypertrophic cardiomyopathy, amyloidosis, pulmonary hypertension, and earlier detection of heart failure. The accuracy and expediency of AI systems can particularly impact prevention, early clinical intervention, and emergent situations where quick evaluation, diagnosis, and therapeutic action are necessary.

Triaging and Treating Patients With Vague/Subjective Complaints

Despite the great potential of AI to assist with diagnosis as discussed earlier, making the diagnosis in clinical practice is often not difficult. Rather, it is the treatment where the difficulty lies. For example, it is not difficult to make a diagnosis of musculoskeletal low back pain, but it is challenging to stratify which patients will do well with usual care versus those who will need a more extensive multidisciplinary, biopsychosocial intervention.

Because extensive multidisciplinary treatment is resource intensive, early prediction of which patients might benefit from such treatment would be valuable. This approach is already being explored by pain management apps with AI analysis. These algorithms have been found to accurately predict (68%) which patients could be expected to develop chronic pain necessitating more comprehensive treatment. One early pain management application/prediction model included 130 variables including patient demographics, pain scores, medications, and others in their patient survey. AI analysis was subsequently able to reduce the number of impacting variables to just nine significant predictors of chronic pain,* thus making the model easier to understand and simpler to administer without compromising accuracy.

Taking a closer look at how AI algorithms might assist with treatment stratification in these types of vague, syndrome-type diagnoses (e.g., low back pain, fibromyalgia, irritable bowel syndrome [IBS]), we can look at AI's ability to analyze patient-reported outcome measurements (PROMs). These are patient surveys that are commonly used to monitor patient response in such vague conditions. Using musculoskeletal low back pain as an example, what follows is an explanation of how AI, using PROMs, might assist in treatment stratification.

The process occurs as follows: first, variables that may influence low back pain are chosen and incorporated into a PROM (e.g., concomitant depression, BMI, smoking, abdominal obesity, activity level, pain volatility). The survey is then statistically evaluated for reliability and validity** before it is fitted with a statistical model (e.g., LR, decision tree, random forest, neural network) and trained on patients with known outcomes (which patients did well with standard care vs. which required more extensive psychosocial team intervention). During training, the AI model uses backpropagation to adjust the "weights" of each risk factor; for example, adjusting for the fact that BMI or depression might be stronger risk factors for needing extensive intervention than pain volatility or smoking. Training and testing errors are corrected as described earlier to further improve accuracy. Finally, after training, the model is ready to use in the real world—ready to make stratification predictions and aid in treatment decisions.

Several other AI-assisted treatment models for difficult-to-treat maladies are in development or have already proven beneficial. For example, in depression and anxiety, AI-assisted intervention has been shown to improve depressive symptoms by over 50% compared with usual non–AI-assisted therapy. In fibromyalgia, similar advancements are being explored with some indications of improved diagnosis and treatment outcomes.

Similar AI analysis of PROMs might be used in other "subjective" maladies, such as IBS or chronic fatigue, and may also lead to improved treatment stratification and better patient outcomes, and then to more realistic prognostic expectations, clearer provider-patient communication, improved patient satisfaction, better patient outcomes, and improved allocation of resources.

Administrative Medicine and Health Systems Impact

Artificial Intelligence, Time Demands, and Physician Burnout

Half of U.S. physicians report occupational burnout, attributing it to time restraints, inefficient EMRs, and medical bureaucracy. Studies show primary care physicians spend significant time on EMRs, impacting patient care and significantly increasing major medical errors. Addressing these challenges is crucial, and AI can offer promising solutions.

Artificial Intelligence and Electronic Medical Record Progress Notes

Programs like DeepScribe and DeepCura streamline note writing by converting recorded patient encounters instantaneously into structured notes, improving efficiency and accuracy and ceding time back to the clinician. These "scribe apps" integrate seamlessly into popular EMRs, further enhancing data standardization, and billing accuracy.

Patient Education/Patient Handouts

AI-generated patient educational materials show mixed results in studies, demonstrating high accuracy but limited readability for patients with lower literacy levels. Although AI can assist in generating drafts, final review by humans is essential to ensure readability and effectiveness.

Billing and the Full-Function Electronic Medical Record

Although just two of the top five EMR companies (Oracle Health and eClinicalWorks) currently offer fully integrated billing capabilities, improvements in all EMR billing capability is under development—including those incorporating social determinants of health (SDoH). Such systems will help in preventing overbilling, underbilling, and improve reimbursement accuracy. Fully integrated EMRs will streamline patient encounters, note creation, billing, and follow-up, enhancing efficiency and patient care.

Prior Authorization

Prior authorization requirements (PARs) pose significant administrative burdens, contributing to physician burnout and care delays. AI systems currently in development will streamline PAR processes, improving patient care and reducing administrative strain.

Improving Patient Scheduling With Artificial Intelligence Assistance

Although still early in development, AI-assisted scheduling assistants including products such as Zocdoc, TalonMD, Intouch, Veradigm, and others will soon help predict appointment no-shows, double-book or reschedule as needed—thus allocating appropriate appointment times based on real-time patient data. Reducing this type of scheduling inefficiency will help alleviate stress for physicians, staff, and patients.

Artificial Intelligence and Health System Impact

AI holds great potential to improve individual and community health by providing insights for policymakers and public health workers. Its ability to detect and address SDoH in real-time data offers opportunities for targeted interventions and long-term risk-factor mitigation programs.

AI's role in detecting and addressing SDoH factors, combined with its potential to optimize resource allocation and improve healthcare delivery to underserved populations, makes it a key player in transforming health systems. By making systems more efficient and equitable, AI contributes to improved individual and community health outcomes.

---

*The nine relevant predictors used were (1) the number of days with at least one pain record; (2) the number of pain records; (3) the mean pain severity rating; (4) the standard deviation of the pain severity ratings; (5) the mean of the absolute changes between consecutive pain ratings (pain volatility scores); (6) the standard deviation of the absolute changes between consecutive pain ratings; (7) the change between the start and end of the trend line fitted through the severity ratings; (8) the absolute value of the change between the start and end of the trend line fitted through the severity ratings; and (9) the pain volatility levels in the predictor period.

** *Reliability* refers to the consistency of results when the measurement is repeated. *Validity* refers to the survey's ability to capture what it is designed to measure.

Concerns Associated With Artificial Intelligence
Energy Use in Artificial Intelligence
Although the energy used in AI can be difficult to gauge, rough estimates should include the energy needed to manufacture and maintain a supercomputer's hardware, the energy used to train the AI model, and the energy used to run and maintain AI models after they have been deployed. Despite the uncertainty of estimates, we can confidently say that the total CO_2 produced by a large language model (LLM) is not insignificant. For example, the training of ChatGPT has been estimated to create 500 tons of CO_2. Adding to this the cost of maintaining the model (keeping the model up, running, and responding to user inquiries)—about a quarter ton per day—brings the annual CO_2 produced to around 600 tons/year:

$$500 \text{ tons} + (0.25 \text{ tons} \times 365) = 500 + 91 = 591 \text{ tons}$$

This is roughly equivalent to driving an average car 1.4 million miles.

Keep in mind that these figures are very rough estimates, and that larger models, such as ChatGPT4 and Llama, require larger supercomputers, more offline learning and processing time, and more energy to maintain themselves, thus generating carbon footprints significantly greater than smaller models. The CO_2 footprint estimates will be further altered depending on the energy source. For example, a model trained in France, where nuclear power is more frequently used, will have a much smaller carbon footprint than one trained in the United States or China, where fossil fuels are more commonly used.

In sum, one concern with the use of AI in medicine is that improved individual health and healthcare systems may come with a significant cost in terms of planetary health.

Bias and Other Concerns
As we become more dependent on AI-enhanced systems in medicine, other incumbent hazards must also be kept in mind. There is a potential for error and bias along every step of model development. Choosing an optimal AI architecture, deciding on a best-fit statistical model, insuring transparency of data sources and algorithmic construction in pretraining, and training and testing these models without racial, ethnic, gender, sexuality, age, or other hidden structural biases is crucial. Vested interests, such as corporate, political, or religious bias, also must also be kept out of model development, as their influence—indeed, their mere presence in development—may affect a programmer's unconscious need to please/approval-seeking bias and compromise the veracity of model outputs. A full discussion of each type of concern—various biases, inequity in computational resources, data privacy, scalability issues, security concerns, implementation challenges, algorithmic drift corporate creep, and surveillance capitalism—is beyond the scope of this text, but several well-written reviews can be found in the literature. Awareness of these issues is growing, however, and such concerns are slowly being integrated in AI model development. Recently several reputable organizations, including the Brookings Institution; the University of California, Berkeley; and others have publicly proclaimed that at every step of AI development, stakeholder inclusion must be paramount to help prevent these types of concerns and biases.

Conclusion
Concerns aside, continued AI development and implementation is set to play an increasingly important role in healthcare—mining published data for research insights, integrating data from multimodal sources (e.g., genomics, epigenomics, proteomics, metabolomics, medical imaging), and improving disease prediction, prevention, and management. It will also soon integrate public health and social determinant data into clinical practice, streamline administrative processes, incite health systems change, impact medical education, and inspire the imaginations of administrators, educators, learners, practitioners, and ancillary personnel. AI is set to power the next great leap forward in medicine—and perhaps to power the next great leap forward for humanity.

References
Deo RC: Machine learning in medicine, *Circulation* 132(20):1920–1930, 2015.

Franklin JC, Ribeiro JD, Fox KR, et al: Risk factors for suicidal thoughts and behaviors: a meta-analysis of 50 years of research, *Psychol Bull* 143(2):187–232, 2017.

Gajjar AA, Kumar RP, Paliwoda ED, et al: Usefulness and accuracy of artificial intelligence chatbot responses to patient questions for neurosurgical procedures, *Neurosurgery*, 2024.

Gholi Zadeh Kharrat F, Gagne C, Lesage A, et al: Explainable artificial intelligence models for predicting risk of suicide using health administrative data in Quebec, *PLoS One* 19(4):e0301117, 2024.

Irvin JA, Kondrich AA, Ko M, et al: Incorporating machine learning and social determinants of health indicators into prospective risk adjustment for health plan payments, *BMC Public Health* 20(1):608, 2020.

Kino S, Hsu YT, Shiba K, et al: A scoping review on the use of machine learning in research on social determinants of health: trends and research prospects, *SSM Popul Health* 15:100836, 2021.

Lin W, Gan W, Feng P, et al: Online prediction model for primary aldosteronism in patients with hypertension in Chinese population: a two-center retrospective study, *Front Endocrinol* 13:882148, 2022.

McCarthy BD, Beshansky JR, D'Agostino RB, et al: Missed diagnoses of acute myocardial infarction in the emergency department: results from a multicenter study, *Ann Emerg Med* 22(3):579–582, 1993.

Muzammil MA, Javid S, Afridi AK, et al: Artificial intelligence-enhanced electrocardiography for accurate diagnosis and management of cardiovascular diseases, *J Electrocardiol* 83:30–40, 2024.

Pehrson LM, Nielsen MB, Ammitzbøl Lauridsen C: Automatic pulmonary nodule detection applying deep learning or machine learning algorithms to the LIDC-IDRI database: a systematic review, *Diagnostics* 9(1):29, 2019.

Rahman QA, Janmohamed T, Pirbaglou M, et al: Patterns of user engagement with the mobile app, manage my pain: results of a data mining investigation, *JMIR Mhealth Uhealth* 5(7):e96, 2017.

Timmons AC, Duong JB, Simo Fiallo N, et al: A call to action on assessing and mitigating bias in artificial intelligence applications for mental health, *Perspect Psychol Sci* 18(5):1062–1096, 2023.

US Environmental Protection Agency. *Greenhouse Gas Equivalencies Calculator.* Available at: https://www.epa.gov/energy/greenhouse-gas-equivalencies-calculator#results. [Accessed 05/03/24].

GENOMIC TESTING

Method of
Gregory A. Plotnikoff, MD, MTS, FACP

In 2021 the National Institutes of Health's (NIH) National Human Genomic Research Institute (NHGRI) proclaimed that, by the year 2030, "The regular use of genomic information will have transitioned from boutique to mainstream in all clinical settings, making genomic testing as routine as complete blood counts (CBCs)." Today, we are well on our way to fulfilling this bold prediction. Affordable testing now exists that strengthens our diagnostic capacities and optimizes our therapeutic strategies. Testing that cost $100 million in 2001 can now be done for less than $1000. As costs continue to plummet, several trends have emerged. First, genomic innovations in oncology, hematology, and infectious disease are blurring the traditionally separate topics of diagnosis and therapy. Second, polygenic risk scores are expanding the traditional assessment of risk by family history to include genetic assessment of risk. And third, direct-to-consumer advanced genomic testing is redefining the physician-patient relationship.

Our challenge as clinicians is to keep up with the implications for prescribed therapies. To support this goal, this chapter will describe the ongoing genomic revolution and identify new clinician competencies that accompany three categories of technological breakthroughs: (1) genotyping, (2) cell-free DNA (cfDNA) analyses (blood tests), and (3) whole exome sequencing (WES)/whole genome sequencing (WGS). Each section will address both the current and future implications for enhanced clinical management. The chapter concludes with key resources for further study.

Genotyping
The new world of clinical genomics refers to the study of the entire genome of an organism. Genotyping is the clinical application of genomics where molecular assays are used to detect the presence or absence of a specific variant (or variants) in DNA. Variants in coding DNA is the key operative term here. Three types of genomic variations exist: (1) single nucleotide variants (SNVs) (1 base pair [i.e., A to G]), (2) indels (small, <50 base pair

insertions [i.e., GC to GAAC] and deletions [i.e., ATGC to AC]), and (3) structural variants (SVs). Of the latter, two types occur: copy-number variability (CNV) and others (non-CNV). Two subcategories of genotyping apply to current clinical practice: pharmacogenomic testing and widely advertised direct-to-consumer genetic testing.

Pharmacogenomics

Pharmacogenomics is the study and clinical application of genetic determinants of both drug efficacy (dose response) and drug toxicity including reactions due to impaired or rapid clearance, as well as drug-drug, drug-herb, or drug-nutrient interactions. Pharmacogenomic testing identifies clinically important genetic variations that may affect the safety and effectiveness of any prescribed medication. Knowledge of a patient's baseline variation in the metabolism of pharmaceuticals can guide both optimal drug choice and optimal dosing and thus minimize both toxicity and time to effect.

Pharmacogenomic testing results demonstrate that standard doses may not be appropriate for all patients. Clinically meaningful genetic variations can occur in any of the genes involved in absorption, distribution, metabolism, translocation, binding, or clearance (excretion). This leads to a new clinical competency. Prescribers now need to understand how genetic variations influence both pharmacokinetics and the pharmacodynamics of drug effects and responses.

Without results of pharmacogenomic testing, commonly seen examples of pharmacogenomic variability include the genetically determined variation in INR responses to warfarin dosing, the variable risk of chemotherapy associated side effects, excessively rapid or excessively slow activation of codeine and hydrocodone, and the variation in antidepressant drug response by ethnicity. Additional pharmacogenomic concerns include the additive epigenetic induction or inhibition of drug clearance by such commonly prescribed medications such as clarithromycin (Biaxin), diltiazem (Cardizem), erythromycin, fluconazole (Diflucan), or verapamil or uncommonly prescribed medications such as rifampin (Rifadin) or ritonavir (Norvir).

The US Food and Drug Administration (FDA) has identified over 60 medications where existing data supports therapeutic management recommendations and nearly two dozen more where data indicates a potential safety or response concern. Identified safety concerns include commonly understood adverse side effects and increased risk of suicide and/or harm to others. In 2023, the Clinical Pharmacogenomics Implementation Consortium (CPIC) published guidelines for CYP2D6, CYP2C19, CYP2B6, SLC6A4 (serotonin transporter), and HTR2A (serotonin-2A receptor) testing for assessment of serotonin reuptake inhibitor antidepressant dosing, efficacy, and tolerability. Today, physicians can order pharmacogenomic testing in their patients. Testing companies include focused pharmacogenomic laboratories such as OneOme, GenoMind, GeneSight, or ClarityxDNA. Their reports provide guidance on drug selection and avoidance of adverse effects. Today, all health professionals can readily access evidence-based guidelines that synthesize information relevant to genomic/pharmacogenomic tests and selection of drug therapy (see resources at the end of the chapter).

To navigate effectively requires a fluency in both genetic concepts and nomenclature. To begin, genotype refers to the combination of the two alleles (one maternal, one paternal) of a gene at a particular location on a chromosome. The nonvariant or usual type of allele is referred to as the wild type. Most variations are in a single nucleotide. If this variant is found in more than 1% of the population, this is termed a *single nucleotide polymorphism* (SNP, pronounced "snip"). Variants found in less than 1% of the population are termed *mutations*. One variant allele is termed a heterozygous variant. When both alleles are variants, the patient is deemed to have a homozygous variant.

Variations and mutations are described by either the "rs" identifying number (for the reference SNP) or by the "star" nomenclature for one or both alleles. To illustrate the importance of nomenclature, for the cytochrome P450 enzyme termed CYP2C19, approximately 25 genetic variants in the exonic region of the CYP2C19 gene have been identified. Of these 25 variations, a change in guanine (G) to adenine (A) at position 681 in exon 5 will result in an aberrant splice site that will alter metabolism of several medications including the antiplatelet medication clopidogrel (Plavix). For precise communication, this variation can be described by its rs identifying number rs4244285 or by its star identifying CYP2C19*2. In pharmacogenomic reporting for cytochrome P450 genes, the star nomenclature is most often used. However, the genomic nomenclature is not always so easy as nucleotide position and nucleotide change is often used to report other pharmaceutical metabolizing genes. Examples of the nomenclature complexity include the ATP-binding cassette, subfamily B, member 1 variation termed ABCB1 3435C>T. This is also known as multidrug resistance gene 1 (MDR1) and encodes for P-glycoprotein (P-gp). Likewise, catechol O-methyltransferase (COMT) rs4680 is also reported as COMT Val158Met. To further the nomenclature challenge, haplotypes refer to a simultaneously linked set of SNPs in an individual. For example, for the thiopurine s-methyltransferase gene, TPMT*3A refers to a haplotype comprising two nonsynonymous SNPs rs1800460 and rs1142345.

Within the human genome, several million SNPs have been identified. Of these, most are termed synonymous and do not alter the protein products of the gene expression and have no measurable effects. The consequences of other sequence variants can result in altered structure and function of the encoded proteins or altered level of gene expression. Inheritance of these alleles means that standard doses of a drug therapy can lead to an adverse drug reaction or chemotherapy failure. Several types of polymorphisms can adversely affect drug metabolism. Examples are illustrated in Table 1.

Reported pharmacogenomic cytochrome P450 data is often presented as one of four phenotypic categories: (1) ultrarapid, (2) extensive (normal), (3) intermediate, and (4) poor. To illustrate, variations in CYP2D6 can result in a 200-fold different effect in drug metabolism. The amplified activity with copy number variants such as in CYP2D6*2XN results in faster clearance. The N refers to the number of copies of the gene on a single chromosome. For CYP2D6*2, this can range from 2 to 13.

A tragic example of ultrarapid CYP2D6 metabolism of the prodrug codeine into its active metabolite morphine has been seen in

TABLE 1	Examples of Polymorphisms That Can Affect Drug Metabolism		
POLYMORPHISM	**STAR NAME**	**ACTIVITY CHANGE**	**EXAMPLE MEDICATIONS AFFECTED**
Premature stop codon	CYP2C19*2, CYP2C19*3	Blocked enzyme activity	Clopidogrel (Plavix), omeprazole
Variable number tandem repeats	TMPT*2, TMPT*3	Enhanced active metabolite production	Mercaptopurine (Purinethol)
Gene deletion	CYP2D6*5	Gene absence	Antidepressants, beta blockers, antihistamines, numerous prodrugs, others
Copy number variants	CYP2D6*2XN	Gene amplification and ultrarapid function	Antidepressants, beta blockers, antihistamines, numerous prodrugs, others

children who received codeine after a routine tonsillectomy. The rapid transformation of codeine to morphine has resulted in a rapid systemic delivery of a morphine bolus. As a result, children have died from the sudden onset of opioid-induced central respiratory depression, increased sedation, and decreased supraglottic airway tone.

Another tragic example of poor CYP2D6 metabolism is the impaired transformation of the prodrug hydrocodone into its active metabolite hydromorphone. Patients with this variation have suffered from insufficient analgesia and have been labeled drug-seekers inappropriately. Importantly, risk of insufficient analgesia despite "normal" dosing would be worsened with concomitant administration of common CYP2D6-inhibiting medications such as bupropion (Wellbutrin), fluoxetine (Prozac), paroxetine (Paxil), quinidine, or terbinafine (Lamisil).

Today, prescribers need to know that numerous medications and natural products can modify existing pharmacogenomic function via either induction or inhibition of the genetically determined CYP P450 drug metabolizing enzymes or drug transporters. The presence of clinically significant adverse drug-drug interactions (DDIs) may be exceptionally high in cardiology, oncology, and psychiatry. This risk includes natural product-drug interactions (NPDIs). For example, medicinal cannabis (THC) and cannabidiol (CBD)[7] appear to inhibit multiple CYP P450 enzymes including CYP2D6. St. John's wort (Hypericum perforatum)[7] induces, and grapefruit juice inhibits, CYP3A4 activity, the liver enzyme responsible for metabolizing the vast majority of currently available prescription medications. Berberine[7], an active ingredient in several herbal medicines such as goldenseal (Hydrastis canadensis L)[7], and also sold as an isolated, purified, and concentrated ingredient, can inhibit CYP2D6, CYP3A4, and increase p-glycoprotein function. The FDA provides helpful information here: https://www.fda.gov/drugs/drug-interactions-labeling/drug-development-and-drug-interactions-table-substrates-inhibitors-and-inducers#table5-2.

In addition to cytochrome P450 metabolism, several other variations are important. NAT2 enzyme gene variations can affect an individual's acetylation capacity. For example, slow acetylators of sulfasalazine (Azulfidine) are more likely to experience abdominal pain, nausea, skin rashes, and headaches. Variations in the transporter SLC19A1 gene predict methotrexate efficacy and toxicity. Variations in in the serotonin transporter gene, SLC6A4, affects response to selective serotonin reuptake inhibitors (SSRIs). Variations in the HTR2A gene that encodes the postsynaptic serotonin-2A receptor (5-HT2A) predict SSRI drug response. Variations in the DPYD gene can result in life-threatening increased systemic drug exposure to the anticancer fluoropyrimidines (fluorouracil, capecitabine [Xeloda], and other analogs). Persons with TMPT impairment prescribed mercaptopurine (Purixan, Purinethol) will have reduced production of a nonactive metabolite, which in turn results in enhanced active metabolite production and a significantly increased risk of toxicity including leukopenia. Hypersensitivity to the antiviral abacavir (Ziagen) is closely associated with HLAB*5701, and reactivity to carbamazepine (Tegretol) is strongly linked to HLA-B*1502.

Future clinical practice will undoubtedly bring pharmacogenomic data to the point of service either by the electronic medical record and/or further incorporation of specially trained pharmacists. The future will likely see calls for each person, perhaps starting at birth, to be tested for clinically relevant variations relevant to optimal prescribing and dosing. To support enhanced clinician competency in pharmacogenomics, several excellent resources are noted later in this chapter.

Direct-to-Consumer Genotyping

At this time, the primary genotyping service used in clinics is for pharmacogenomic data to guide therapy. However, since at least

2006, the lay public has seen advertising for home genetic testing for genealogic purposes. Indirectly, direct-to-consumer genomic testing, initially offered by 23andme.com and Ancestry.com, introduced to the public microarray genotyping and SNVs. Soon after, clinicians and others recognized the potential value of the information found in the common (>1% of the population) SNVs known as SNPs found in the unreported raw data in the genomic testing. Consumer empowering websites that could upload 23andme.com raw data and then sort, organize, and prioritize SNPs for interpretative health reasons quickly appeared (e.g., MTHFRsupport.com, livewello.com, geneticgenie.com). Suddenly, consumers had access to their genetic information outside of their physicians' offices. And, suddenly, patients had the capacity to ask very sophisticated health questions that could overwhelm unprepared physicians.

Today, 23andme.com and related consumer-directed SNP analysis services have been eclipsed by much broader testing noted in the next section. Physicians should recognize the difference between testing that generates answers versus testing that generates questions. The limited value of consumer-directed SNP analyses means that, at best, the value of such testing is in generating hypotheses relevant to therapeutic decisions. Clinically relevant categories that can be addressed include the following:

1. Vitamin activation (e.g., BC01 for vitamin A, VKORC1 for vitamin K)
2. Neurotransmitter production impairment (e.g., DDC for dopamine and serotonin; GAD1 for GABA)
3. Metabolic pathway analyses (e.g., genes for methylation, genes for transsulfonation, genes for NAD+ production)
4. Detoxification capacity (e.g., PON1, glucuronidation capacity, glutathione production genes)
5. APOE status (genetic risk of Alzheimer's disease)

The predictive value and clinical utility of such genotyping services has yet to be validated. This is especially true for the infotainment services, which provide very limited and very incomplete data. The future will likely see growth in direct-to-consumer expanded next generation sequencing testing. This may include nutrigenomics (the study of the bidirectional interaction of nutrition and genes), WGS of intestinal microbiomics, and a creative combination of the two perspectives. The NIH has acknowledged how poorly understood the intestinal microbiome, metabolism, nutritional status, genetics, and the environment interact to affect health. In 2024 the NIH announced plans to fund significant new initiatives to generate an evidence base beyond "one-size-fits-all diets" toward precision in dietary guidance for optimal health.

Cell-Free DNA

cfDNA refers to nonencapsulated DNA fragments released into the blood or other bodily fluids because of secretion, apoptosis, and/or necrosis. Technology now allows separation of circulating fetal DNA, mitochondrial DNA, tumor DNA, or microbial DNA. This breakthrough has resulted in profound changes in diagnostic capacities. In obstetrics, noninvasive prenatal testing (NIPT) represents an alternative to amniocentesis and chorionic villus sampling (CVS). In primary care, patients at low risk for colon cancer can now opt for an FDA-approved blood test rather than a colonoscopy. Patients now also have access to blood tests for multicancer early detection (MCED) that go far beyond current US Preventive Services Task Force (USPSTF) recommendations for single-cancer screening (breast, cervical, colorectal, lung).

For oncologic therapy guidance, the capacity to separate tumor DNA from germline DNA from a simple blood draw (referred to as a liquid biopsy) means that surgery is no longer required to obtain tumor tissue for tumor mutation profiling with any solid advanced-stage malignant neoplasm. Such testing can reliably and rapidly determine clinically pertinent DNA point mutations, indels, amplifications, and fusions. Identification of tumor genomic status (e.g., EGFR, ALK, BRAF) can guide optimal selection of targeted chemotherapy for non–small cell lung cancer or

---

[7] Available as dietary supplement.

colon cancer. At this time, Medicare covers this testing for all advanced solid tumors. In the future, the simultaneous mapping of multiple biomarkers of genomic alterations will drive deeper understanding of multitarget therapies and resistance mechanisms. Additionally, I believe this data will lead us to understand better the optimal use of off-label pharmaceuticals and specific dietary interventions as adjunctive therapies for persons with cancer.

In infectious disease, another form of liquid biopsy is available for microbial cell-free DNA sequencing on plasma. This has revolutionized the noninvasive and rapid identification of more than 1000 pathogens including bacteria, fungi, DNA viruses, and protozoans. In this process, cell-free DNA fragments are extracted from the specimen, converted to shotgun DNA sequencing libraries, and then sequenced. The concentration of cell-free DNA molecules from any potential pathogen is then calculated.

A 2022 case record of the Massachusetts General Hospital demonstrated the great value of this testing for targeted and precise treatment of an unknown pathogen. The authors described the clinical challenges of diagnosing a 56-year-old man with myalgias, fever, bradycardia, and inflammatory changes in the epicardial fat abutting the noncoronary sinus of the aortic valve. In this case, testing detected *Listeria monocytogenes* at a concentration of 42 cell-free DNA molecules per microliter (reference value <10). This finding confirmed the diagnosis of listeriosis. The authors noted that these results were associated with 95% sensitivity (at 41 molecules per microliter) and 98% to 99.99% specificity for the diagnosis of listeriosis.

Today, the advantages are clear in terms of identifying difficult-to-culture pathogens, the time to results, and the noninvasive sampling. The advantage over rapid multiplex polymerase chain reaction (PCR) tests is that a presumptive diagnosis of a single pathogen is not needed. The bottom-line implication of microbial cfDNA testing is that presumptive or empiric antipathogen therapies will be less necessary for acute illness. Likewise, such testing, similar to interferon-γ release assays, may clarify the length of treatment required for clearance. And, to speculate boldly, microbial cfDNA testing may help define the presence of an unexpected chronic infectious disease driving perplexing chronic illness.

The cfDNA breakthrough has also led to identification of cell-free mitochondrial DNA (cf-mtDNA) as a marker of trauma, inflammation, acute psychological distress, and physiologic distress. Elevated levels are clearly linked to increased in-hospital mortality. Elevated levels also appear to be linked to cognitive and neurodegenerative disorders. Unlike NIPT and MCED, however, meaningful translation to clinical therapies has yet to be defined.

Whole Exome Sequencing/Genome Sequencing

Due to the profound reduction in cost and the markedly increased capacity to manage huge databases, advanced sequencing is now readily available for diagnostic purposes in clinical settings and direct-to-consumer screening. Of the approximately 20,000 genes in our genome, 1% are protein coding and are termed the exome. WES only tests this portion of the DNA. Of the exome, approximately 4700 genes are associated with a mendelian disorder. This group is termed the Mendeliome or medical exome. And of the Mendeliome, subsets are associated with specific disease categories such as connective tissue disorders or cardiac disorders. Now readily available are panels that represent a focused list of genes for a phenotype such as peripheral neuropathy, familial cancer, or chronic kidney disease.

WGS reports on all of the genome including both the coding and noncoding variants. This includes the SNVs, the indels, and the structural variants but also RNA alterations such as transcriptional abundance and fusion transcripts. Three challenges exist with WGS after cost. First is the management of the massive amount of data generated. Second is the process of annotation, the intensive process of linking specific features in a DNA, RNA, or a protein sequence with descriptive information about structure or function. Third is the interpretation of

both incidental findings unrelated to the initial reason for which the sequencing tests were ordered, as well as variants in a gene of phenotypic significance but of unknown clinical significance (VUOS).

Of great interest is the potential presence or absence of incidentally found "actionable" gene mutations relevant to the avoidance of significant morbidity or mortality. The American College of Medical Genetics and Genomics (ACMG) has identified nearly 100 known pathogenic or expected pathogenic constitutional variants representing numerous conditions with well-known guidelines for prevention or treatment. Each of these should be reported to patients sequenced in a clinical setting. Examples include mutations in the RYR1 gene causally linked to malignant hyperthermia with administration of halothane gas anesthesia or succinylcholine or BRCA1, BRCA2, or PALB2 genes demonstrably connected with breast and ovarian cancers.

Most important for future therapies will likely be the creation of genome-wide polygenic risk scores for an individual's susceptibility to disease. The focus on mendelian single-gene causality appears to have blinded us to the networked or polygenic nature of most noncommunicable disease including cancer and heart disease. Single variants are too often insufficient for assessing disease risk. Even traits thought be the result of single genes, such as eye color, are actually highly polygenic. And for a trait such as height, approximately 80% of one's height requires the contribution of more than 700 genomic variants. To move beyond single-variable science with a polygenic risk score requires the merger of classic genomic sequencing for monogenic variants with artificial intelligence programming. The goal is to enable early recognition and treatment of high-risk individuals before the onset of disease. An additional benefit may be to uncover new causal disease pathways. The future will bring us deeper understanding of the clinical utility of such scores.

Conclusion

In the past, physicians struggled with the apparently random interindividual differences in drug efficacy and toxicity, including DDIs. Practice required patience with trial-and-error approaches for numerous medications. Today, we have the capacity for personalized patient medication choice and dose adjustment. Likewise, both noninvasive diagnostic testing and therapeutic decision making have been greatly enhanced via cell free DNA testing. And the advent of relatively inexpensive WES and WGS tests support more rapid diagnoses of complex illnesses.

In the future, genomic testing will be as common as ordering a CBC. Advances in genotyping, cfDNA, and WGS will clearly transform multiple dimensions of patient care in every subspecialty. With such changes will also come new insights into the multiple forms of noncoding RNA, as well as the role of imprinting and transgenerational epigenetic changes. And whereas current genomic testing may only describe what cards one has been dealt, the secondary "-omics" revolution in transcriptomics, metabolomics, and proteomics, among others, will allow us to know not only what cards one has been dealt but also how they are being played. This will undoubtedly completely transform the practice of medicine.

Genomic Resources
General
ClinGen
- http://clinicalgenome.org
- This is an NIH-funded resource that defines the clinical relevance of genes and variants for use in medicine and research.

ClinVar
- http://www.ncbi.nlm.nih.gov/clinvar/
- This is a public archive of reports about the relationship between specific genetic variants and associated phenotype (symptoms).

dbSNP
- https://www.ncbi.nlm.nih.gov/snp/

- dbSNP is the database for human single nucleotide variations, microsatellites, and small-scale insertions and deletions along with publication, population frequency, molecular consequence, and genomic and RefSeq mapping information for both common variations and clinical mutations.

GeneReviews
- http://www.ncbi.nlm.nih.gov/books/NBK1116/
- This is a collection of chapters, each focused on an individual genetic condition or disease,
- written for healthcare providers by experts in the field.

OMIM
- https://www.omim.org/ or https://www.ncbi.nlm.nih.gov/omim
- OMIM provides information on genes and diseases. The entries on genes are particularly useful. All the entries for a particular gene can also be accessed through ClinGen through the "External Genomic Resources."

PharmGKB (PharmacoGenomicsKnowledgeBase)
- http://www.pharmgkb.org/
- This is the database of pharmacogenomic research findings. This includes free access to the peer-reviewed Clinical Pharmacogenetics Implementation Consortium (CPIC) Guidelines (https://www.pharmgkb.org/page/cpic) for prescribing decisions from genetic laboratory results with supplemental information and updates. Also available at https://www.cpicpgx.org.

Education

Genetics/Genomics Competency Center
- https://genomicseducation.net/
- Categorized educational resources in generics/genomics and pharmacogenomics for healthcare educators and clinicians.

National Human Genome Research Institute
- https://www.genome.gov/For-Health-Professionals/Provider-Genomics-Education-Resources
- Information for healthcare professionals and patients on genetics, pharmacogenomics, direct-to-consumer testing, and more including terminology, videos, and illustrations.

PharmGenEd
- https://pharmacogenomics.ucsd.edu/
- Free educational materials (including recorded lectures and handouts) focused on clinical applications of pharmacogenomics for healthcare students and practitioners.

Med-Legal

GeneReviews: Resources for Genetics Professionals-Direct-to-Consumer Genetic Testing
- https://www.ncbi.nlm.nih.gov/books/NBK542335/#dtc_testing.For_general_predictions_about

Anticipate and Communicate: Ethical Management of Incidental and Secondary Findings in the Clinical, Research, and Direct-to-Consumer Contexts, from the Presidential Commission for the Study of Bioethical Issues
- http://bioethics.gov/sites/default/files/FINALAnticipateCommunicate_PCSBI_0.pdf

Coalition for Genetic Data Protection: Privacy Best Practices for Consumer Genetic Testing Services
- https://fpf.org/wp-content/uploads/2018/07/PrivacyBest-Practices-for-Consumer-Genetic-Testing-Services-FINAL.pdf

Genetic Alliance: Genetic Discrimination
- http://www.geneticalliance.org/advocacy/policyissues/genetic discrimination

National Human Genome Research Institute: Genetic Discrimination
- https://www.genome.gov/about-genomics/policy-issues/Genetic-Discrimination

References

Botton MR, Whirl-Carrillo M, Del Tredici AL, et al. PharmVar GeneFocus: CYP2C19. Clin Pharmacol Ther. 2021 109(2):352–366.

Bousman CA, Stevenson JM, Ramsey LB, et al: Clinical pharmacogenetics Implementation Consortium (CPIC) guideline for CYP2D6, CYP2C19, CYP2B6, SLC6A, and HTR2A genotypes and serotonin reuptake inhibitor antidepressants, Clin Pharmacol Ther 114(1):51–68, 2023.

Doohan PT, Oldfield LD, Arnold JC, Anderson LL: Cannabinoid interactions with cytochrome P450 drug metabolism: a full-spectrum characterization, AAPS J 23(4):91, 2021.

Guo Y, Chen Y, Tan ZR, Klaassen CD, Zhou HH: Repeated administration of berberine inhibits cytochromes P450 in humans, Eur J Clin Pharmacol 68(2):213–217, 2012.

Honeycutt DC, Blom TJ, Ramsey LB, et al: Pharmacogenetic factors influence escitalopram pharmacokinetics and adverse events in your with a family history of bipolar disorder: a preliminary study, J Child Adolescent Psychopharmacol 34(1):42–51, 2024.

Miller, D.T, Lee K, Abul-Husn NS, et al. ACMG SF v3.2 list for reporting of secondary findings in clinical exome and genome sequencing: a policy statement of the American college of Medical Genetics and Genomics (ACMG).

Nasrin S, Watson CJW, Perez-Paramo YX, Lazarus P: Cannabinoid metabolites as inhibitors of major hepatic CYP450 enzymes, with implications for cannabis-drug interactions, Drug Metab Dispos 49(12):1070–1080, 2021.

National Institutes of Health/National Human Genome Research Institute: Bold Predictions for Human Genomics by 2030: An NHGRI Seminar Series. https://www.genome.gov/event-calendar/Bold-Predictions-for-Human-Genomics-by-2030. Accessed March 27, 2022. https://www.genome.gov/about-genomics/fact-sheets/Sequencing-Human-Genome-cost. Accessed March 27, 2022.

National Institutes of Health/Office of Strategic Coordination--The Common Fund. Nutrition for Precision Health, powered by the All of Us Research Program. April 2025. https://commonfund.nih.gov/nutritionforprecisionhealth Accessed September 14, 2025.

Para ML, Khurshid S, Folding B, et al: Case 13-2022: a 56-Year-old man with myalgias, fever, and bradycardia, N Engl J Med 386:1647–1657, 2022.

Rahikainen A-L, Vauhkonen P, Pett H, et al: Completed suicides of citalopram users—the role of CYP genotypes and adverse drug reactions, Int J Leg Med 13(2):353–363, 2019.

US Food and Drug Administration: Table of Pharmacogenetic Associations. https://www.fda.gov/medical-devices/precision-medicine/table-pharmacogenetic-associations. Accessed March 17, 2024.

MONOCLONAL ANTIBODIES

Method of
Michael Dougan, MD, PhD; and Crystal M. North, MD, MPH

CURRENT DIAGNOSIS

- Monoclonal antibodies are unique, specific, and homogeneous antibodies manufactured by immortalizing and copying an antibody secreting B cell of interest.
- Monoclonal antibodies have a wide variety of applications in diagnostic medicine including identification of pathogens, tissue typing, cancer diagnosis, enzyme-linked immunosorbent assay, radioimmunoassay, and other laboratory testing methods.

CURRENT THERAPY

- Monoclonal antibodies have tremendous applications in the field of therapeutic medicine for treatment of numerous diseases affecting every organ system in the body.
- Monoclonal antibodies can be used alone or to carry drugs, cytotoxic agents, or radioactive substances to targeted cells.
- Monoclonal antibodies are useful as drug-reversal agents (e.g., digoxin and dabigatran).
- Monoclonal antibodies are far superior to polyclonal antibodies because of their highly specific and reproducible affinity for target antigens as well as their controlled manufacturing processes.
- The "humanization" of monoclonal antibodies significantly reduces drug side effects.
- Monoclonal antibodies are delivered via injection or infusion.
- Because of the proliferation of monoclonal therapeutic agents, full prescribing information should be reviewed before administration.

Introduction

Antibodies are key components of the adaptive immune system and are produced by B cells. Antibodies provide protection from infections in two broad ways. They bind tightly to their targets, sometimes inhibiting or neutralizing target activity, and they activate other components of the immune system that can recognize antibody-bound structures.

In the setting of a typical infection, the natural immune response develops dozens of antibodies that recognize the invading microbe. These antibodies typically bind at multiple sites and with varying levels of affinity. As an immune response evolves over the course of weeks or on subsequent exposure to the same infection, these antibodies are further refined, typically targeting a distinct region of the infectious organism with increasingly higher-affinity antibodies. This response, termed a *polyclonal response,* is also what happens in the setting of a vaccine.

Each antibody is genetically encoded at the DNA level and produced by a distinct B cell (termed a *clonotype*). These B cells can proliferate and produce multiple progeny cells that manufacture the antibody that we detect in the blood. B cells can also differentiate into plasma cells, which reside in the bone marrow and are responsible for the production of the most high-affinity antibodies.

By isolating specific B cells and determining the affinity and binding specificity of the antibodies they make, genomic technologies can be used to produce unique antibodies that have medically useful binding properties. These are termed *monoclonal antibodies.* After the DNA encoding them is sequenced and cloned into an expression vector that introduces the specific gene into a target cell that directs the cell's ability to synthesize proteins, large quantities of antibodies can be produced at pharmaceutical grade. These antibodies can be used for the diagnosis and treatment of disease.

Properties of Antibodies as Drugs

Antibodies have several features that make them excellent drugs. The first is that they naturally evolve to bind to their targets with exquisite specificity and high affinity, generally exceeding that of typical receptor-ligand interactions. In theory, antibodies can bind to any structure, including carbohydrates, proteins, DNA, and small-molecule drugs that are covalently bound to proteins. This means that they can be used to selectively bind to any target of interest including human proteins, drugs and other small molecules, or infectious organisms. Their high affinity means that they are unlikely to dissociate from their target after binding. Antibodies have two binding arms, increasing their avidity for targets with recurrent structural motifs or with multiple copies of the binding target.

Monoclonal Antibody Structure

Classic antibodies are composed of four polypeptides, two heavy chains, and two light chains that are bound to the N-terminal region of the heavy chains (Figure 1A). The complex of two heavy chains and two light chains produces two broad structural domains: the target (antigen)-binding regions that are fixed at the ends of the antibody arms and the antibody stalk, which attaches to each binding arm through a flexible linker (see Figure 1A). The antibody arms are referred to as *Fab domains* and are made up of a variable region that binds the target and a constant region that connects to the stalk. The heavy chain and the light chain both contribute to the Fab domains. The amino acid sequence in each arm of a naturally occurring antibody is identical to the sequence in the other arm, but the sequence within the variable region differs from all other antibody clones. The unique sequences in these antibody arms confer the binding properties of the antibody. Antibodies can be bioengineered to have nonidentical arms, generating synthetic bispecific antibodies, an area of increasing therapeutic interest.

The antibody stalk is referred to as the *Fc domain* and is responsible for most antibody effector functions through interactions with Fc receptors. The effector functions conferred by the Fc domain include activation of complement, facilitated phagocytosis (opsonization), activation of NK cells, secretion across mucosal barriers (IgA in particular), and activation of mast cells and eosinophils (IgE in particular). The Fc domain is part of the constant region of the antibody, but it comes in multiple classes that define the distinct "isotypes" of antibodies: IgM, IgG1 to IgG4, IgA, and IgE. For IgG, the Fc domain also dramatically extends the half-life of antibodies through interactions with the serum protein FcRn. This half-life extension can be modified

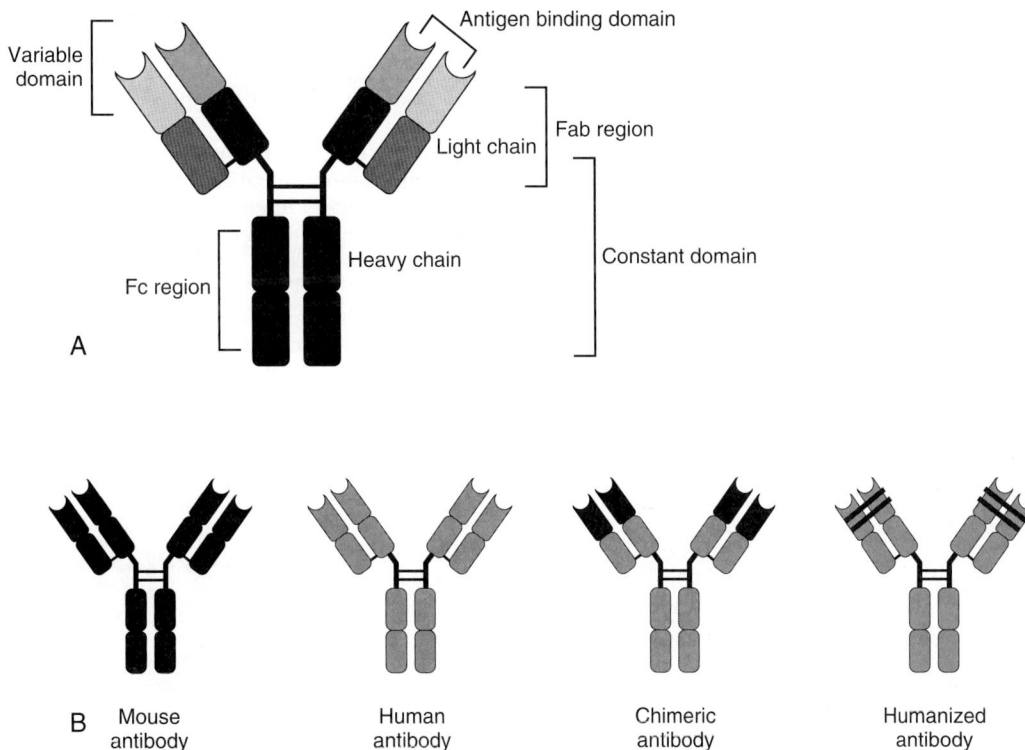

Figure 1 Structure of classic antibodies.

through point mutations, allowing for infrequent dosing of antibody drugs.

The size of monoclonal antibodies prevents efficient absorption across mucosal barriers or the skin. Consequently, all monoclonal antibodies are administered either as injections or as infusions.

Antibodies are produced as part of a normal immune response in all vertebrates, and much of their sequence is highly conserved. Although some important differences exist between human antibody genes and the coding sequence of other animals, modification of antibody sequences to generate "humanized" antibodies is now routinely used to generate drugs from antibodies that were initially identified in other animals. These humanized antibodies have been generated in model organisms such as mice and in culture systems using viruses and bacteria such as *Escherichia coli*. More recent pharmaceutical-grade antibodies have been identified directly in patients. These newer techniques have replaced older techniques for generating antibodies such as the construction of animal-human chimeric antibodies (see Figure 1B), where significant sections of animal sequence remained in the therapeutic antibody, increasing the risk of hypersensitivity reactions during infusion or loss of function caused by antidrug antibodies. Antibodies are recycled from the serum through protein turnover in a process that is independent of hepatic and renal clearance mechanisms. Consequently, antibodies rarely interact with other drugs.

Interestingly, a subset of antibodies produced by camelids (e.g., alpacas, llamas, and camels) are formed without a light chain. These heavy-chain-only antibodies still retain the same variable antigen-binding domains and constant regions found in conventional antibodies, and they demonstrate approximately the same binding affinities for their targets.

Therapeutic Uses of Monoclonal Antibodies

Monoclonal antibodies have been used for a wide variety of therapeutic purposes. Most antibodies in clinical use neutralize the activity of their target, which is often a protein. This has been especially successful when targeting circulating self-proteins that have been dysregulated as part of a disease process. Most of these neutralizing monoclonal antibodies belong to the IgG4 isotype. This isotype retains the ability to bind to FcRn, but lacks engagement with other Fc receptors, reducing the risk of unintended side effects as discussed in more detail later in this chapter.

Cytokines and their receptors are the targets of many monoclonal antibodies that are used for the treatment of autoimmune and allergic diseases. These targets are particularly amenable to monoclonal antibody targeting because they are secreted and are often present in the interstitial fluid and in circulation, making them accessible to infused antibodies. Multiple other immune receptors have been successfully targeted by monoclonal antibodies, resulting in inhibition of receptor-ligand interactions and blockade of essential functions such as cell trafficking (e.g., to treat autoimmunity) or immune regulation (e.g., to treat cancer).

Monoclonal antibodies are also used to inhibit several serum proteins including components of the complement cascade, receptors involved in platelet activation, and more recently a key regulator of the low-density lipoprotein (LDL) receptor. Similar to cytokines, these factors are ideally suited to monoclonal antibody neutralization because of the accessibility of the target in circulation.

Multiple monoclonal antibodies have been developed that enhance phagocytosis of target-expressing cells and activation of cell-mediated immunity and/or complement. These monoclonal antibodies are often IgG1 antibodies and are often used in cancer treatments, binding directly to the malignant cells. Antitumor antibodies are now incorporated into standard treatment regimens for a wide variety of hematologic and solid tumors, resulting in substantial improvements in outcomes. Similar depletion strategies can be used to treat a variety of autoimmune diseases by depleting the immune cells responsible for the disease.

Although the majority of monoclonal antibody therapies target self proteins, an important class of therapeutics has been developed against infectious targets. These antibodies can be highly specific for their targets with minimal or no effects in uninfected people. Antibodies have been developed against viral and bacterial infections, target cell surface proteins, and secreted toxins. Monoclonal antibodies have had some important successes in viral therapy, as discussed later, but they are generally used less frequently than small-molecule antimicrobial drugs.

Monoclonal Antibody Side Effects

Most side effects associated with monoclonal antibodies relate directly to their mechanism of action. Inhibition of self proteins can lead to deficiencies in function that may overcorrect the disease process; this is most evident with antibodies that inhibit the immune system to treat autoimmunity. The infection-related side effects are common, though often less severe than with broader forms of immune suppression such as systemic glucocorticoids. Antibodies can also improve a disease in one organ system while damaging another. Antibodies that deplete target cells can lead to side effects related to the loss of those cells or to damage to the tissues that express the target. This can occur with some of the antitumor antibodies in which the targets are often expressed on healthy cells in addition to malignant ones.

Because of their specificity and target affinity, off-target side effects of monoclonal antibodies are rare. This is a considerable advantage when comparing monoclonal antibodies to other classes of drugs, such as small-molecule inhibitors. Side effects related to hepatic metabolism or renal clearance are also unlikely with monoclonal antibodies because they are not eliminated through these organs, leading to a relatively good safety profile in patients with multiple comorbid conditions.

Infusion reactions and the formation of antidrug antibodies are significant limitations to all monoclonal antibody treatments. The risk of these reactions is related to the fraction of nonhuman sequence present in the antibody structure. The highest-risk monoclonal antibodies currently in use are the few drugs that are chimeric mouse-human antibodies with human constant regions and mouse variable regions. As a result, few chimeric antibodies are still being developed. Most next-generation antibodies are either humanized, with the animal sequence mutated to resemble the human sequence, or human, the result of antibody identification techniques that start from the human antibody genes either inserted into the mouse genome or produced through in vitro techniques. Monoclonal antibodies have been identified directly in patients, and these antibodies have substantial clinical safety value.

Monoclonal Antibody Nomenclature

The naming of monoclonal antibodies is determined by the World Health Organization International Nonproprietary Names (INN) program, which was established in 1991. Each name consists of a prefix, a target substem (also called an *infix*), a source substem (if named before 2018), and a stem (Figure 2). The prefix does not carry any specific meaning. It is a combination of letters that, when combined with the stem and substems, results in an easily

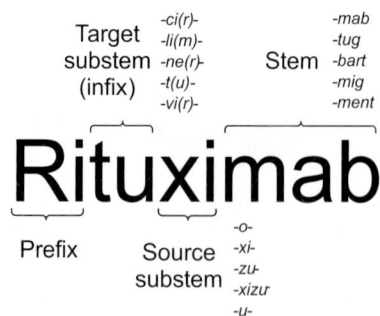

Figure 2 An example of the nomenclature used to name a monoclonal antibody.

pronounced name. The target substem, also called the infix, indicates the target of the monoclonal antibody. It is composed of a consonant, a vowel, and a final consonant that is sometimes dropped if the name of the monoclonal antibody would otherwise not be easily pronounced. Examples include -ci- for agents that target the cardiovascular system and -vi- for agents that target viral products. The source substem indicates the animal from which the antibody was derived but was removed from the nomenclature starting in 2017. Examples include -u- for human-derived antibodies, -o- for mouse-derived antibodies, and -xi- for chimeric antibodies composed of both human and nonhuman components. The stem for all monoclonal antibodies named before 2021 is -mab. Starting in late 2021, monoclonal antibodies are given one of four stems: -tug (**u**nmodified immuno**g**lobulins) -bart (anti**b**ody **art**ificial), -mig (**m**ulti-**i**mmuno**g**lobulin), or -ment (frag**ment**).

Examples of Monoclonal Antibodies Used in Clinical Practice

Monoclonal antibodies have been developed for an ever-expanding number of clinical conditions. Included in the following sections are representative examples of monoclonal antibodies used in a variety of disease processes. This list is not meant to be exhaustive; the pace of monoclonal antibody production would make a comprehensive list outdated by the time of publication. We have grouped these examples by body system or shared mechanism, but many monoclonal antibodies are used for several clinical indications. Not all of the clinical uses described are approved by the U.S. Food and Drug Administration (FDA), but they represent common clinical practice. Side effects that are common to most monoclonal antibodies are highlighted in the previous section, and additional side effects that are of special interest for a given monoclonal antibody are highlighted here. The list of side effects is also meant to be illustrative rather than comprehensive, and full prescribing information should be reviewed before administration of these drugs clinically.

Oncology
Rituximab (Rituxan)
Target: The CD20 antigen on the surface of B cells, leading to depletion of these cells

Similar monoclonal antibodies: Ocrelizumab (Ocrevus), ofatumumab (Arzerra, Kesimpta), obinutuzumab (Gazyva)

Adverse effects of interest: Infusion reactions are quite common, particularly during the first infusion; new and reactivated infections caused by immunosuppression

Initial clinical indication: Relapsed or refractory low-grade or follicular, B-cell non-Hodgkin lymphoma. Rituximab was one of the first monoclonal antibodies developed clinically and the first monoclonal antibody used in oncology.

Other clinical indications: Various lymphomas (non-Hodgkin lymphoma, diffuse large B-cell lymphoma, follicular lymphoma), chronic lymphocytic leukemia, various autoimmune conditions (e.g., rheumatoid arthritis, systemic lupus erythematosus,[1] granulomatosis with polyangiitis)

Bevacizumab (Avastin)
Target: Vascular endothelial growth factor (VEGF), impairing microvascular growth

Similar monoclonal antibodies: Ranibizumab (Lucentis)

Adverse effects of interest: Hemorrhage, gastrointestinal perforation (rarely)

Initial clinical indication: First-line treatment, in combination with 5-fluorouracil, of metastatic colon and rectal carcinoma

Other clinical indications: Macular degeneration,[1] diabetic retinopathy[1]

Cetuximab (Erbitux)
Target: Epidermal growth factor receptor (EGFR), impairing cell growth and proliferation, depletion of target-expressing cells

[1] Not FDA approved for this indication.

Similar monoclonal antibodies: Panitumumab (Vectibix)

Adverse effects of interest: IgE-mediated allergic reactions, dermatologic reactions

Initial clinical indication: EGFR-expressing metastatic colorectal carcinoma

Other clinical indications: *BRAF* V600E+ metastatic colorectal carcinoma, squamous cell carcinoma of the head and neck

Ipilimumab (Yervoy)
Target: Cytotoxic T lymphocyte antigen (CTLA)-4, an immune checkpoint receptor

Similar monoclonal antibodies: Ipilimumab is considered a "checkpoint inhibitor" along with drugs targeting PD-1 and PD-L1

Adverse effects of interest: Multiple inflammatory toxicities referred to as *immune-related adverse events* (irAEs); these resemble autoimmune diseases and most commonly affect the skin, gastrointestinal tract, and endocrine organs

Initial clinical indication: Metastatic or unresectable melanoma

Other clinical indications: Malignant mesothelioma, hepatocellular carcinoma, metastatic colorectal carcinoma, metastatic non–small cell lung cancer, renal cell carcinoma

Nivolumab (Opdivo)
Target: Programmed cell death-1 (PD-1) receptor, blocking the ligands PD-L1 and PD-L2 from binding with the receptor, enhancing T-cell–mediated antitumor responses

Similar monoclonal antibodies: Pembrolizumab (Keytruda), cemiplimab (Libtayo), atezolizumab (PD-L1, Tecentriq), durvalumab (PD-L1, Imfinzi), avelumab (PD-L1, Bavencio)

Adverse effects of interest: Multiple inflammatory toxicities (irAEs); these resemble autoimmune diseases as most commonly affect the skin, gastrointestinal tract, and endocrine organs

Initial clinical indication: Metastatic or unresectable melanoma

Other clinical indications: Metastatic mismatch repair deficient/microsatellite instability high (MMRd/MSI-H) colorectal carcinoma, Merkel cell carcinoma, metastatic gastric or gastroesophageal junction carcinoma, squamous cell head and neck cancer, hepatocellular carcinoma, Hodgkin lymphoma, malignant mesothelioma, non–small cell lung cancer, renal cell carcinoma, urothelial cell carcinoma

Trastuzumab (Herceptin)
Target: Human epidermal growth factor receptor 2 (HER2; a member of the EGFR receptor family), depleting target-expressing cells, inhibiting cell growth and proliferation

Similar monoclonal antibodies: Margetuximab (Margenza), pertuzumab (Perjeta)

Adverse effects of interest: Cardiac toxicity, teratogenic

Initial clinical indication: Metastatic HER2-expressing breast cancer

Other clinical indications: Metastatic HER2-expressing gastric or gastroesophageal junction adenocarcinoma

Rheumatologic/Autoimmune Diseases
Nipocalimab (Imaavy)
Target: Neonatal Fc receptor (FcRN), preventing the receptor from binding the Fc region of antibodies

Similar monoclonal antibodies: None

Adverse effects of interest: None

Initial clinical indication: Early-onset severe hemolytic disease of the fetus and newborn (HDFN)[1]

Other clinical indications: Myasthenia gravis

Infliximab (Remicade)
Target: Tumor necrosis factor alpha (TNFα)

Similar monoclonal antibodies: Adalimumab (Humira), certolizumab (Cimzia), golimumab (Simponi)

Adverse effects of interest: Immunodeficiency, reactivation of mycobacterium tuberculosis, reactivation of hepatitis B virus

Initial clinical indication: Treatment of moderate to severe Crohn's disease

Other clinical indications: Ulcerative colitis, rheumatoid arthritis, psoriasis (plaque, arthritis, pustular[1]), ankylosing spondylitis, pyoderma gangrenosum[1]

Tocilizumab (Actemra)

Target: Membrane-bound and soluble interleukin 6 receptor (IL-6R), preventing IL-6 cytokine activity
Similar monoclonal antibodies: Sarilumab (Kevzara), satralizumab (Enspryng)
Adverse effects of interest: Immunodeficiency, reactivation of mycobacterium tuberculosis
Initial clinical indication: Moderate to severe rheumatoid arthritis
Other clinical indications: Cytokine release syndrome, rheumatoid arthritis, hospitalized patients with COVID-19,[1] giant cell arteritis, systemic sclerosis-associated interstitial lung disease, juvenile idiopathic arthritis

Belimumab (Benlysta)

Target: Soluble human B-lymphocyte stimulator (BLyS) protein, also known as BAFF
Similar monoclonal antibodies: None
Adverse effects of interest: Impaired humoral immunity
Initial clinical indication: Systemic lupus erythematosus
Other clinical indications: None

Basiliximab (Simulect)

Target: Alpha chain of interleukin 2 receptor on activated T lymphocytes
Similar monoclonal antibodies: None
Adverse effects of interest: Severe immunodeficiency
Initial clinical indication: Prophylaxis of acute renal transplant rejection
Other clinical indications: Graft-versus-host disease,[1] prophylaxis of acute transplant rejection in heart, liver, and lung transplantation[1]

Gastrointestinal Diseases
Ustekinumab (Stelara)

Target: The shared p40 component of interleukin 12 and interleukin 23, preventing binding to their target receptors and reducing differentiation of TH1 and TH17 cells, potential reduced activation of NK cells
Similar monoclonal antibodies: None
Adverse effects of interest: Immunodeficiency
Initial clinical indication: Plaque psoriasis
Other clinical indications: Psoriatic arthritis, Crohn's disease, ulcerative colitis

Vedolizumab (Entyvio)

Target: α4β7 integrin, blocking binding with MAdCAM-1, inhibiting lymphocyte migration into the gut
Similar monoclonal antibodies: None
Adverse effects of interest: Minimal
Initial clinical indication: Ulcerative colitis
Other clinical indications: Crohn's disease

Hematology
Emicizumab (Hemlibra)

Target: Binds and bridges activated factor IXa and factor X, acting in place of factor VIII to initiate hemostasis
Similar monoclonal antibodies: None
Adverse effects of interest: Minimal
Initial clinical indication: Hemophilia A
Other clinical indications: None

Caplacizumab (Cablivi)

Target: A1 domain of von Willebrand factor, preventing binding to platelet glycoprotein Ib-X-V and reducing platelet adhesion and consumption; single-domain antibody
Similar monoclonal antibodies: None
Adverse effects of interest: Bleeding
Initial clinical indication: Acquired thrombotic thrombocytopenic purpura
Other clinical indications: None

Cardiovascular Disease
Alirocumab (Praluent)

Target: Binds to proprotein convertase subtilisin/kexin type 9 (PCSK9), which then prevents degradation of hepatocyte LDL receptors, increasing LDL uptake and decreasing plasma LDL levels
Similar monoclonal antibodies: Evolocumab (Repatha)
Adverse effects of interest: Minimal
Initial clinical indication: Familial hypercholesterolemia or atherosclerotic cardiovascular disease with elevated LDL-C
Other clinical indications: Hyperlipidemia

Pulmonary Disease
Omalizumab

Target: Inhibits IgE binding to IgE receptors on mast cells and basophils, thereby reducing the allergic response
Similar monoclonal antibodies: None
Adverse effects of interest: Rare hypersensitivity/anaphylactoid reactions
Initial clinical indication: Moderate to severe persistent asthma
Other clinical indications: Chronic spontaneous urticaria, nasal polyps

Allergic Conditions
Mepolizumab (Nucala)

Target: Inhibits binding of interleukin-5 (IL-5) to the IL-5 receptor, reducing eosinophil production, activation, and survival.
Similar monoclonal antibodies: Benralizumab (anti-IL-5R, Fasenra), reslizumab (anti-IL-5R, Cinqair)
Adverse effects of interest: Potential increased susceptibility to parasitic infections
Initial clinical indication: Severe eosinophilic asthma
Other clinical indications: Eosinophilic granulomatosis with polyangiitis, hypereosinophilic syndrome, rhinosinusitis with nasal polyps

Dupilumab (Dupixent)

Target: Binds to the interleukin 4 receptor alpha (IL-4Rα) subunit, inhibiting IL-4 and IL-13 signaling
Similar monoclonal antibodies: None
Adverse effects of interest: conjunctivitis, potential increased susceptibility to parasitic infections
Initial clinical indication: Atopic dermatitis
Other clinical indications: Moderate to severe asthma, eosinophilic esophagitis, rhinosinusitis with nasal polyps

Neurologic Conditions
Natalizumab (Tysabri)

Target: Alpha-4 integrin subunit, blocking binding to vascular receptors and thereby reducing leukocyte adhesion and transmigration from circulation into the gut and brain
Similar monoclonal antibodies: None
Adverse effects of interest: Increased risk of progressive multifocal leukoencephalopathy
Initial clinical indication: Multiple sclerosis
Other clinical indications: Inflammatory bowel disease (essentially supplanted by the development of the more specific antibody, vedolizumab [Entyvio])

Infectious Diseases
SARS-CoV-2 (COVID-19)

Note: Multiple monoclonal antibodies were selected against the parent SARS-CoV-2 virus and have variable activity against

---

[1] Not FDA approved for this indication.
[1] Not FDA approved for this indication.

subsequent novel variants of concern. By 2022, most monoclonal antibodies were no longer active against the dominant SARS-CoV-2 variants in circulation. At the time of this writing, only one SARS-CoV-2 reactive monoclonal antibody has active Early Use Authorization from the FDA.

Pemivibart (Pemgarda)

Target: Spike protein receptor binding domain of SARS-CoV-2, blocking virus attachment to the ACE2 receptor

Adverse effects of interest: None

Initial clinical indication: Preexposure prophylaxis among those wtih moderate/severe immunocompromise[1]

Other clinical indications: None

Respiratory Syncytial Virus (RSV)

Palivizumab (Synagis)

Target: RSV F glycoprotein

Similar monoclonal antibodies: None

Adverse effects of interest: None

Initial clinical indication: Preexposure prophylaxis against respiratory syncytial virus in pediatric patients at high risk of RSV disease

Other clinical indications: None

Bacillus Anthracis (Anthrax)

Raxibacumab

Target: The free protective antigen component of *Bacillus anthracis* toxin, inhibiting toxin delivery to host cells via the anthrax toxin receptor

Similar monoclonal antibodies: Obiltoxaximab

Adverse effects of interest: None

Initial clinical indication: Treatment of inhalational anthrax, prophylaxis against inhalational anthrax following exposure to *Bacillus anthracis*

Other clinical indications: None

Clostridium difficile

Bezlotoxumab (Zinplava)

Target: *Clostridium difficile* toxin B, causing neutralization and preventing toxic effects

Similar monoclonal antibodies: None

Adverse effects of interest: None

Initial clinical indication: Prevent recurrence of *C. difficile* infection in patients on antimicrobial therapy and at high risk for recurrence

Other clinical indications: None

Drug-Reversal Agents

Digoxin Immune Fab (Digifab)

Target: Free digoxin; digoxin-specific antibody fragments (Fab) form digoxin-immune fragment complexes, decreasing circulating free digoxin concentrations and facilitating the dissociation of digoxin bound to the Na-K-ATPase.

Similar monoclonal antibodies: None

Adverse effects of interest: None

Initial clinical indication: Life-threatening or potentially life-threatening digoxin toxicity

Other clinical indications: None

Idarucizumab (Praxbind)

Target: Free dabigatran and acyl glucuronide metabolites with a binding affinity much greater than that of thrombin, neutralizing the anticoagulant properties

Similar monoclonal antibodies: None

Adverse effects of interest: None

Initial clinical indication: Dabigatran reversal in the setting of uncontrolled bleeding or urgent/emergent surgical procedures

Other clinical indications: None

---

[1] Not FDA approved for this indication.

References

Coiffier B, Lepage E, Briere J, et al: CHOP chemotherapy plus rituximab compared with CHOP alone in elderly patients with diffuse large-B-cell lymphoma, *N Engl J Med* 346:235–242, 2002.

De Benedetti F, Brunner HI, Ruperto N, et al: Randomized trial of tocilizumab in systemic juvenile idiopathic arthritis, *N Engl J Med* 367:2385–2395, 2012.

Dougan M, Azizad M, Chen P, et al: Bebtelovimab, alone or together with bamlanivimab and etesevimab, as a broadly neutralizing monoclonal antibody treatment for mild to moderate, ambulatory COVID-19, *medRxiv*, 2022.

Dougan M, Nirula A, Azizad M, et al: Bamlanivimab plus Etesevimab in Mild or Moderate Covid-19, *N Engl J Med* 385:1382–1392, 2021.

Feagan BG, Rutgeerts P, Sands BE, et al: Vedolizumab as induction and maintenance therapy for ulcerative colitis, *N Engl J Med* 369:699–710, 2013.

Gupta A, Gonzalez-Rojas Y, Juarez E, et al: Early Treatment for Covid-19 with SARS-CoV-2 Neutralizing antibody sotrovimab, *N Engl J Med* 385:1941–1950, 2021.

Hodi FS, O'Day SJ, McDermott DF, et al: Improved survival with ipilimumab in patients with metastatic melanoma, *N Engl J Med* 363:711–723, 2010.

Miller DH, Khan OA, Sheremata WA, et al: A controlled trial of natalizumab for relapsing multiple sclerosis, *N Engl J Med* 348:15–23, 2003.

Murphy K, Travers P, Walport M: *Janeway's Immunobiology*, ed 10. Chapter 4: Antigen Recognition by B-cell and T-cell Receptors, New York, 2022, Garland Science.

Peyvandi F, Scully M, Kremer Hovinga JA, et al: Caplacizumab for acquired thrombotic thrombocytopenic purpura, *N Engl J Med* 374:511–522, 2016.

Shima M, Hanabusa H, Taki M, et al: Factor VIII-Mimetic function of humanized bispecific antibody in Hemophilia A, *N Engl J Med* 374:2044–2053, 2016.

Stein EA, Mellis S, Yancopoulos GD, et al: Effect of a monoclonal antibody to PCSK9 on LDL cholesterol, *N Engl J Med* 366:1108–1118, 2012.

Targan SR, Hanauer SB, van Deventer SJ, et al: A short-term study of chimeric monoclonal antibody cA2 to tumor necrosis factor alpha for Crohn's disease. Crohn's Disease cA2 Study Group, *N Engl J Med* 337:1029–1035, 1997.

Weinreich DM, Sivapalasingam S, Norton T, et al: REGEN-COV antibody combination and outcomes in outpatients with covid-19, *N Engl J Med* 385:e81, 2021.

Wenzel S, Ford L, Pearlman D, et al: Dupilumab in persistent asthma with elevated eosinophil levels, *N Engl J Med* 368:2455–2466, 2013.

STEM CELL THERAPY

Method of
Sunil Abhyankar, MD; and Rupal Soder, PhD

The two words "stem cell" evoke a vision of a multipotent cell that can develop into different kinds of tissue cells. Only *embryonic stem cells* fit this definition and they are guided in their development by external growth factors and environmental events in their final path to form a particular tissue and ultimately a body organ.

The progeny of the embryonic stem cells function as *differentiated stem cells* that are capable of forming new cells for the tissue in which they reside. These are *tissue-specific stem cells*. Such is the case, for example, with hematopoietic stem cells, which reside in the bone marrow (BM) space and are responsible for producing all the cells that make up the blood components. Most of the tissue stem cells have the capacity to regenerate tissue and, under certain growth conditions, can be coaxed to produce related tissues. An example of the latter is the *mesenchymal stem cell* (MSC), also located in the bone marrow, which under certain growth conditions can form cartilage, bone, and other connective tissue cells.

Another category of stem cell is the one artificially produced in the laboratory termed the *induced pluripotent stem cell* (iPSC). These are generally derived from tissue cells (e.g., fibroblasts) and made to grow in selective conditions into the cell of interest, hence the term induced pluripotent cells. iPSCs are finding increasing uses in cellular therapy in the cancer arena.

This review will focus on the committed stem cells that harbor in our tissues and are responsible for healing and replenishing cells of that tissue that are naturally dying (Figure 1).

In the United States, the US Food and Drug Administration (FDA) has the authority to approve cellular therapies. The FDA lists approved cellular and gene therapy products on their website, https://www.fda.gov/vaccines-blood-biologics/cellular-gene-therapy-products/approved-cellular-and-gene-therapy-products.

The list includes cellular therapies with chimeric antigen receptor technology utilized in cancer therapy, autologous cultured chondrocytes on a porcine collagen membrane, and mesenchymal cells used in treatment of severe nasolabial folds defects. The stem cell–based products that are FDA-approved for use in the United States consist of blood-forming stem cells (hematopoietic progenitor cells) derived from cord blood and autologous hematopoietic stem cell–based gene therapy for sickle cell anemia and thalassemia. The blood stem cells are approved for use in patients with disorders that affect the body system that is involved in the production of blood (i.e., the hematopoietic and the immune system). Bone marrow also is used for these treatments but is generally not regulated by the FDA for this use and is considered "grandfathered" for FDA approval. In December 2024, the FDA approved remestemcel-L (Ryoncil), making it the first MSC therapy authorized in the United States for treating steroid-refractory acute graft-versus-host disease (SR-aGVHD) in pediatric patients aged 2 months and older. The use of bone marrow–derived MSC has also been approved for use in Canada, New Zealand, and Japan for the treatment of graft versus host disease in pediatric patients who have undergone a bone marrow transplant.

Transplantation of Hematopoietic Stem Cells

The first report of the use of hematopoietic stem cells from the bone marrow for transplant was in 1957 by E. Donell Thomas, when he and colleagues performed a bone marrow transplant (BMT) in monozygotic twins, one of whom had acute leukemia. This is considered a *syngeneic* (i.e., genetically identical) transplant. Although the procedure was successful, the patient subsequently relapsed. Dr. Thomas continued his pioneering work in BMT and was the recipient of the Nobel Prize in Medicine in 1990.

Utilization of *allogeneic* (genetically dissimilar) bone marrow stem cells in transplant was first described in the 1960s in pediatric patients with congenital immune deficiency (SCID). Subsequently allogeneic BMT has been used to treat a host of hematologic and immunologic conditions including aplastic anemia, hemoglobinopathies (sickle cell anemia and thalassemia), acute and chronic leukemias, lymphoma, and myelodysplastic syndromes. Success of allogeneic BMT has improved over the past decades as shown by data from the Center for International Blood and Marrow Transplant Research registry (CIBMTR). This has been due to several factors including improvements in human leukocyte antigen (HLA) typing resulting in better matched donors, improved supportive care, and an improved understanding of the immune process at play in allogeneic BMT. Thus young patients with idiopathic aplastic anemia can expect a 90% or higher long-term survival with an HLA matched related bone marrow stem cell donor. Despite these advances, the long-term success after an allogeneic BMT in adults is typically in the 50% range; survival is higher in younger compared with older adult patients. A major cause of the lower success in older patients is due to the risk of relapse of the underlying malignancy as well as acute and chronic graft versus host disease (GvHD) occurring after transplantation and the risk of opportunistic infections, usually viral and fungal. Newer approaches to mitigate and treat GvHD (e.g., the use of MSC in acute GvHD), measures to prevent relapse after transplant (e.g., use of targeted therapeutic agents for maintenance therapy after transplant), and the use of viral specific T cells to treat viral infections post-BMT are being investigated. The outcomes of allogeneic BMT continue to improve.

Hematopoietic stem cells can be obtained from the bone marrow, the peripheral blood, and from umbilical cord blood. BM stem cells to be used in transplantation can be harvested surgically from the donor's bone marrow under general anesthesia or from the peripheral blood when stem cells can be mobilized from the BM with high doses of granulocyte colony-stimulating factor (G-CSF). These peripheral blood stem cells are BM stem cells isolated from the blood, making it easier on the donor. Umbilical cord blood (UCB) is also rich in hematopoietic stem cells and can be easily obtained after the birth of the baby after the cord has been cut. The leftover blood from the umbilical cord and placenta can be banked for use in transplantation.

Which source of stem cells is to be used in hematopoietic transplantation? This is dependent on the patient diagnosis and age. In patients who have malignant hematologic diseases, stem cells obtained from the peripheral blood of the donor are often preferred as these stem cell collections are accompanied by a higher number of T lymphocytes, which can improve a patient's ability to fight off their cancerous cells. In contrast, in patients with aplastic anemia or sickle cell anemia, bone marrow harvested stem cells are preferred due to the lower amount of T cells in this product causing less GvHD.

With advances in hematopoietic transplantation, almost every person who will benefit from an allogeneic transplant will be able to find a donor. The choice for finding a donor includes searching for sibling matches and donors in the National Marrow Donor Program (NMDP) database, which contains the HLA typing results of more than 25 million volunteers. For those patients with rare HLA genotypes or for whom a matched donor is not readily available, a half (haplo) matched donor from a family member (e.g., sibling, parent, child, nephew, niece) can often be identified. The use of haploidentical donors in transplantation has been pioneered in the last decade from the BMT team at Johns Hopkins University.

UCB can also serve as the donor source for hematopoietic cells with the advantage that they are readily available and do not need a complete HLA matching for the transplant. BMT teams in Minnesota and Memorial Sloan Kettering have pioneered the use of UCB for transplant. UCB as a source of hematopoietic stem cells for transplant is more often used in the pediatric age group than in adults due to the paucity of the stem cells in UCB samples, which is adequate for engraftment in a child but insufficient for an adult who will either need two cord blood units or the use of UCB stem cells that are expanded by growing them in the laboratory.

In contrast to allogeneic BMT, *autologous* hematopoietic stem cell transplantation uses the patient's own BM stem cells collected from their blood to treat myeloma, lymphoma, and certain autoimmune conditions like severe systemic sclerosis, lupus, certain types of multiple sclerosis, and diabetes. In autologous transplant the stem cells are harvested from the patient's own blood and cryopreserved. The cells are then infused after high-dose chemotherapy to "rescue" the patient. In this situation the benefit from the procedure is mainly due to the effect of the high-dose chemotherapy on the underlying malignancy or autoimmune lymphocytes. In the future it is likely that chimeric antigen receptor (CAR) cell therapy may supplant the need for the high-dose chemotherapy and autologous stem cell rescue.

In December 2023 the FDA approved exagamglogene autotemcel (Casgevy) and lovotibeglogene autotemcel (Lyfgenia) as the first cell-based gene therapies for the treatment of sickle cell disease in patients 12 years and older. In these therapies, bone marrow stem cells are harvested from the blood of the recipient and genetically modified either by CRISPR technology (Cashgevy) or by using a lentiviral vector (Lyfgenia) and then transplanted after high dose chemotherapy. This has shown success in reducing the incidence of painful vasoocclusive crises by >90%. A similar gene therapy–modified stem cell therapy (Casgevy) has also been approved for thalassemia.

Mesenchymal Stem Cell Therapy for Acute Graft Versus Host Disease

Acute graft versus host disease (aGvHD) is a complication that occurs in about 50% of patients undergoing a donor hematopoietic stem cell transplant. The donor T cells attack and try to reject the recipient patient's body. aGvHD results in skin rash, diarrhea, and liver damage. MSCs, because of their immunoregulatory properties, have been used to treat severe forms of aGvHD. The use of bone marrow–derived MSCs (BM-MSCs) has been

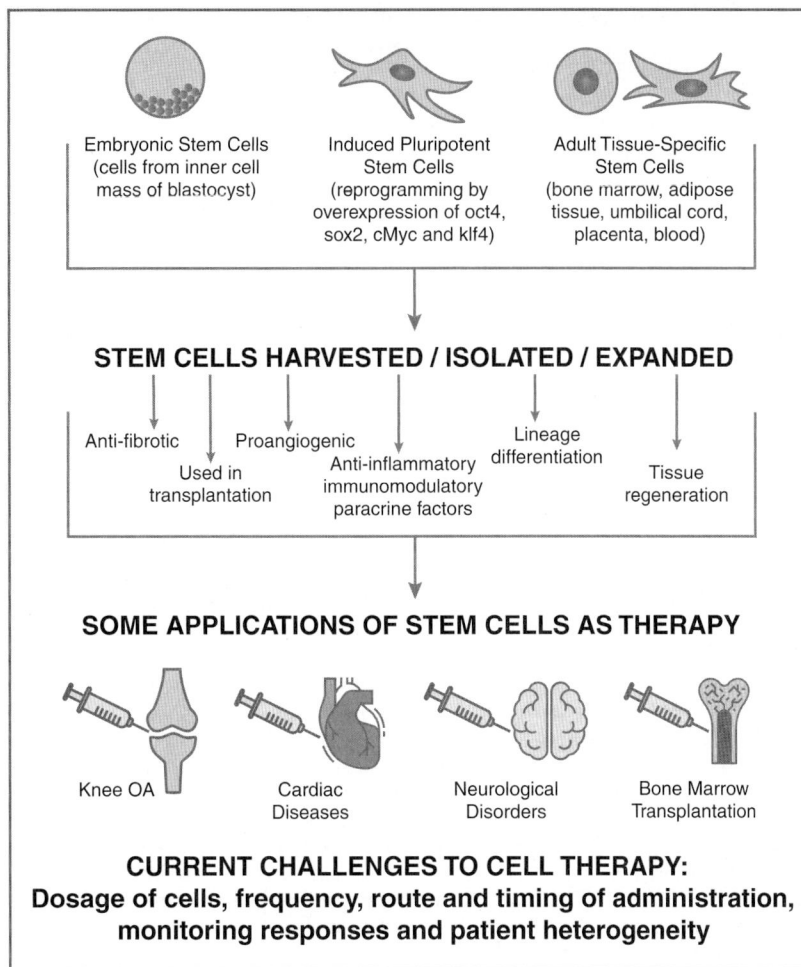

Figure 1 Current stem cell therapies.

approved for use in Canada, New Zealand, and Japan for the treatment of aGvHD in pediatric patients who have undergone a bone marrow transplant. Umbilical cord tissue derived MSCs (Wharton's jelly MSC) have been studied in a Phase I clinical trial. In January 2025, China approved amymetose (Ruibosheng),[2] an umbilical cord–derived MSC therapy, for the treatment of GvHD.

Stem Cell Therapy in Knee Osteoarthritis (OA)

Knee osteoarthritis (OA), the most common form of arthritis, is characterized by loss of articular cartilage, osteophyte formation, and inflammation of the synovial membrane. The main therapeutic approach for knee OA is to improve joint function by cartilage repair, reduction of inflammation, and control of pain. Using cartilage tissue or chondrocytes to replace damaged articular cartilage is one of the potential therapeutic approaches in treating knee OA. In 1997 the FDA approved implantation of autologous chondrocytes, which are allowed to divide and proliferate in vitro, in a process known as expansion, and then injected into the defective cartilage tissue.

Currently, the third generation of this technology, matrix-induced autologous cultured chondrocytes implantation on porcine collagen membrane (MACI), is used where chondrocytes are amplified on a three-dimensional scaffold system before introduction into the joint for the repair of symptomatic cartilage defects of the knee in adult patients. This technology has demonstrated positive results in a 20-year follow-up compared with bone cartilage transplantation. However for autologous chondrocyte transplantation, the number of healthy chondrocytes that can be harvested from older adults are limited in number, and cartilage repair takes a long time after the implantation of

chondrocytes. Hence for cartilage repair, several cell sources are under investigation.

Based on the in vivo and in vitro potential of the MSC to differentiate into chondrocytes and osteocytes and their immuno-modulatory and immunosuppressive potential, the employment of MSCs for the treatment of OA is a rapidly growing area of clinical research. The use of MSC therapies in the treatment of OA has been determined to be feasible and safe in several different studies; however, there are differences in types of cells used, harvesting techniques, cell yield, and chondrogenic potential. The most used MSCs for the clinical use of the treatment of OA are bone marrow–derived mesenchymal stem cells (BMMSC) and adipose-derived stem cells (ASCs), with bone marrow being the gold standard source for musculoskeletal tissue engineering approaches. Various preclinical animal experiments revealed that MSCs, when injected intraarticularly into joints, inhibited synovial lining thickening, inhibited induction of ligament damage, and protected the joint from destruction by both anabolic and metabolic mediators.

Clinical feasibility, safety, and efficacy of allogenic human BMMSC was studied in a randomized controlled trial of 30 patients with chronic knee OA. Patients who received intraarticular injection of 40 million cells displayed improved cartilage quality posttreatment based on MRI imaging and reported improved knee function and a significant decrease in knee pain. There were no adverse events reported. A multinational meta-analysis report of use of MSC therapy in knee OA involving 582 patients suggested that MSC therapy is safe with low rates of adverse events and improved pain and functional scores after 24-month follow-up compared with controls. ASCs have also been studied in the treatment of OA. Intraarticular injection of ASC exhibited a dose-response effect with significant improvement in knee pain and

---

[2] Not available in the United States.

function in the patients who received a higher dose (i.e., 1×10^8 cells).

Due to invasiveness of harvesting procedures for BMMSC and ASCs, various allogeneic MSC products are now available commercially. Park et al. reported the results of a first-in human clinical trial utilizing a stem cell–based product called Cartistem, a composite of allogenic human UCB-derived MSCs and HA hydrogel. A single dose of Cartistem was demonstrated to be safe with no detectable immunologic issues, improved joint function, and improved quality of life over 7 years of follow-up. The South Korean government approved the sale of Cartistem produced by Medipost Inc. in 2012, as the world's first allogenic, off-the-shelf stem cell drug for the treatment of degenerative arthritis and knee cartilage defects. Though current clinical trials have demonstrated the safety of allogeneic MSCs, there is still a debate about whether there is benefit. Larger randomized controlled trials with large sample sizes utilizing standardized and established outcome scores are required. The combination of MSCs with scaffolds, platelet rich plasma (PRP), and growth factors is also being investigated to determine the optimal therapeutic effect.

Overall, for OA of the knee, there is limited availability of strong clinical effectiveness data, a lack of study comparability, and a lack of standardization associated with patient selection and assessment parameters, making it difficult to justify recommendation for the use of this therapy.

Stem Cell Therapy for Cardiac Diseases

Cardiovascular diseases are the most common cause of death, accounting for approximately one-third of deaths worldwide. It has been nearly two decades since the first encouraging preclinical studies reported the repair of infarcted cardiac tissue utilizing bone marrow stem cell transplantation in a model of myocardial infarction. Various studies over the years hypothesize multiple mechanisms by which transplanted cells contribute to repair. The proposed modes of actions include differentiation of cells into cardiomyocytes and paracrine signaling via secretion of cytokines, growth hormones, exosomes, and mitochondrial transfer.

Fueled by the preclinical findings, randomized clinical studies were conducted utilizing BMMSCs and demonstrated safety and improved left ventricular function in patients with acute myocardial infarction. The POSEIDON-DCM study was designed to test the safety and efficacy of allogenic versus autologous BMMSCs in patients with nonischemic dilated cardiomyopathy. The data indicated that allogenic BMMSCs were superior at providing a greater magnitude of clinical efficacy, improved endothelial function, and reduction in the proinflammatory cytokine tumor necrosis factor (TNF)-α in the study population. A recent meta-analysis report that included data between 2017 and 2019 in patients with advanced heart failure suggested that stem cell therapy was safe and was associated with moderate improvement in cardiac function. BOOST, REPAIR-AMI, and REEGENERATE-AMI are some of the other trials that aimed to investigate BMMSC therapy for myocardial infarction (MI) and reported significant improvements in left ventricle (LV) function and emphasized the importance of the timing of cell delivery post-MI.

In contrast to these findings, the SWISS-AMI, Late TIME, and TIME trial showed no improvement in LV function, LV volumes, or infarct size in the treatment group leading to discordant conclusions. These inconsistencies can be attributed to patient variability, heterogenous population of bone marrow–derived cells, different processing procedures, timing of cell delivery, study endpoints, and the unpredictable dynamic course of MI. BioCardia is currently conducting the Phase III CardiAMP Heart Failure (HF) trial using autologous bone marrow cells in patients who developed heart failure post-MI. The study is designed to apply a personalized medicine approach by selecting patients and tailoring treatment to those who are most likely to benefit. The largest trial of MSC therapy for HF to date is by far DREAM-HF, with a total of 537 patients randomized for transendocardial injection of BM-MSCs or sham control catheterization procedure. A single injection of MSC improved LVEF from baseline to 12 months in all patients, with maximal benefit in patients with active inflammation. The risk of MI, stroke, and cardiovascular death was reduced in all treated patients.

ASCs have been evaluated for their usability, safety, and beneficial effects in a few clinical trials in patients with chronic ischemic heart disease and refractory angina. The initial results from the Precise Trial showed improved left ventricular mass and improved exercise capacity at 18-month follow-up. Intracardiac infusion of two doses of autologous ASCs (40 million and 80 million) were assessed in the Athena trial. While the findings supported the feasibility, safety, and scalability for the treatment of ischemic cardiomyopathy, the efficacy was limited with benefits observed on symptoms, quality of life, and VO_2max. These findings clearly require confirmation in additional trials.

Safety and efficacy of Wharton's jelly (WJ) MSC was evaluated for the first time in 2015 in patients with ST-elevation MI (STEMI). In this randomized multicenter trial with 116 patients, Gao et al. reported reductions in scar size, improved LVEF, and increased cardiac function after intracoronary infusion of WJ MSCs in patients with ST-elevation acute MI.

Cardiac stem cells (CSCs), a heterogenous cell population in the heart representing multipotent, self-replicating, c-kit+ cells expressing cardiac markers, have an effective capacity to differentiate into cardiomyocytes. CSCs were first tested in humans in the SCIPIO phase I clinical trial in which c-kit+ CSCs were isolated from biopsies obtained from patients with ischemic cardiomyopathy undergoing coronary artery bypass grafting and administered via intracoronary infusion 4 months later. The results showed improved LVEF and decreased infarct size at 12-month follow-up. Similarly, the CADUCEUS trial reported that intracoronary infusion of autologous CDCs after MI led to scar reduction, an increase in viable heart mass, and improved cardiac contractility. Advantages and disadvantages of stem cells evaluated for the treatment of cardiovascular disorders is outlined in Table 1.

Cellgram-AMI[2] (autologous BM-MSC) product was approved in South Korea in 2011 for improving LVEF in patients with AMI by intracoronary artery infusion. Whereas lessons learned from more than 200 trials of cardiovascular diseases demonstrated the safety and feasibility of the addition of various stem cell types to the routine of care, efficacy studies only showed marginal improvements in cardiac function. The limited clinical success of stem cell therapy in heart disease has been attributed to the low retention and poor survival of transplanted cells.

In 2023, Mesoblast published the results of the DREAM-HF Phase III trial, a randomized, double-blind, controlled study that involved 537 patients with advanced chronic heart failure. The trial demonstrated that a single endomyocardial injection of rexlemestrocel-L (Revascor)[5] led to a significant reduction in cardiovascular death, myocardial infarction, or stroke over a mean follow-up of 30 months. Then in 2024, the FDA granted the regenerative medicine advanced therapy (RMAT) designation to rexlemestrocel-L for the treatment of children with congenital heart disease. This designation is intended to expedite the development and review of regenerative medicine therapies, reflecting growing confidence in regenerative treatments for heart conditions.

Stem Cell Therapy for Neurologic Disorders

Several clinical trials have been conducted to evaluate the safety and efficacy of stem cell therapy for central nervous system disorders. MSCs were shown to be able to cross the blood–brain barrier through paracellular pathways despite the presence of tight junctions. Stem cells can be transplanted into the brain directly intracerebrally or intrathecally or can be delivered by blood infusion. Several mechanisms by which stem cell therapy may offer therapeutic potential in patients with neurologic disorders include:
- Transplantation of stem cells and differentiated neuronal or glial cells to replace damaged neural cells with new, viable cells

[2] Not available in the United States.
[5] Investigational drug in the United States.

TABLE 1 Advantages and Disadvantages of Stem Cells Evaluated for the Treatment of Cardiovascular Disorders

CELL TYPES	ADVANTAGES	DISADVANTAGES
Bone marrow mononuclear cells (BMMNCs)	Extensively studied in clinical trials; safe; some trials showed improved LV functions and contractility.	Heterogenous cell population; inconsistent results regarding therapeutic action; lack of standard methodologies between trials; recent trials showing no improvement.
Mesenchymal stem cells (MSCs)	Autologous and allogeneic sources used; safe; no evidence of tumorigenicity; low risk of rejection; ease of isolation and expansion; immunomodulatory and immunoprivileged ability.	Lack standard study methodologies; limited differentiation potential; inconsistent reports of efficacy; need long-term follow-up.
Cardiac stem cells (CSCs)	Autologous transplantation; safe; immunomodulatory and immunosuppressive ability.	Invasive isolation procedure; limited cell quantity; poor cell quality from older donors; costly expansion.
Embryonic stem cells (ESCs)	Pluripotent; off-the-shelf products; differentiate into cardiomyocytes that can integrate with cardiac muscle.	Ethical concerns; tumorigenic potential; genetic instability; risk of immune rejection; availability issues.
Induced pluripotent stem cells (iPSCs)	Pluripotent; derived from adult somatic cells; no ethical concerns; unlimited quantity; superior functional integration into host cardiac tissue.	Tumorigenic potential; genetic instability; possible risk of immune rejection; lack of efficient procedures to induce pluripotency; no clinical translation yet.

- Transplanted cells may promote angiogenesis and neuroprotection by secreting several neurotropic and growth factors
- Induction of neurogenesis by activating endogenous stem cells accelerating new nerve growth in proliferative niches
- Immunomodulation by reducing the local inflammatory response and promoting remyelination in damage nervous system

Over the past few decades, safety and feasibility of stem cell therapy have been demonstrated in experimental animal models and in phase I/II clinical trials of neurologic diseases such as Alzheimer's disease, stroke, spinal cord injury, amyotrophic lateral sclerosis (ALS), multiple sclerosis, traumatic brain injury, cerebral infarction, and Parkinson's disease. Cell sources for these studies include autologous or allogeneic umbilical cord blood, autologous bone marrow, fetal neural stem cells, embryonic stem cells, and mesenchymal stromal cells derived from adipose tissue or umbilical cord tissue. Most of these trials are registered for ALS, stroke, multiple sclerosis, and spinal cord injury. Neuronata-R[2] was approved as an orphan drug for the treatment of ALS by South Korean authorities in 2014. Neuronata-R[2] contains autologous BM-MSCs mixed with cerebrospinal fluid and is administered by intrathecal injection. The proposed mechanism of action is based on several effects (such as an action on regulatory T lymphocytes, neuroprotective effect by the expression of growth factors, and increased anti-inflammatory cytokines) that can prevent motor-neuron death and slow the progression of ALS. Use of MSCs in early stage clinical trials (phase I/II) for ischemic stroke and multiple sclerosis has demonstrated improvements in motor impairment scales and signs of clinical stabilization. The Phase III MESEMS trial demonstrated positive results for stroke. Results from the study indicated that treatment with MSCs led to improvements in functional recovery, including better motor function and reduced neurologic deficits compared with a placebo group. This trial contributed to the growing evidence supporting the potential of MSCs in neuroprotection and recovery following stroke. Intrathecal and/or intravenous infusion of MSCs following expansion in patients with spinal cord injury demonstrated that MSC administration is safe and well tolerated, with apparent and subtle improvements in sensory (e.g., light touch and pin prick) and bladder functions. However, relative to rehabilitation therapy, no significant improvements in motor function were reported. Japanese authorities have recently granted approval of stem cell therapy (Stemirac) for spinal cord injury based on positive outcomes of a 13-patient study, which was not placebo controlled. Independent researchers warn of the premature nature of this approval and that the trial design cannot claim definitive efficacy.

Bone marrow stem cells have been used in an autologous stem cell transplant setting after high-dose chemotherapy for select patients with multiple sclerosis as reported by Burt and colleagues from Chicago. This needs to be validated by other centers before being accepted as the standard.

Whereas the future of stem cell therapy for neurologic disease appears to be promising, the variables to be determined include the optimal type of stem cell, dosage, route and timing of administration, and the stage of the patient's disease. Evidence is also accumulating on advantages of combined administration of different stem cells/progenitor cells along with various scaffolds. Since complex disease requires complex therapies, it is unlikely that stem cell therapy could be administered as a monotherapy but rather will form part of a more holistic approach that aims to significantly improve the quality of life of affected patients.

Other Promising Indications for Stem Cell Therapy

The future of stem cell therapies looks promising with ongoing clinical research trials for macular degeneration, Crohn disease, rheumatoid arthritis, muscular dystrophy, wound healing, and baldness. Recently in Europe and Japan the regulatory authorities have approved Alofisel)[2] (expanded allogeneic adipose derived MSCs) for the treatment of complex anal fistulas in adult patients with Crohn's disease.

Recently, MSCs (BM or umbilical cord derived) have undergone clinical investigation for the treatment of COVID-19-related complications, especially ARDS pneumonia and inflammation in critically ill ICU patients. Lanzoni et al reported beneficial effects of umbilical cord MSCs in a randomized study of patients with COVID-19 complicated by ARDS. This use does not have FDA-approval.

[2] Not available in the United States.

References

Beltrami AP, et al: Adult cardiac stem cells are multipotent and support myocardial regeneration, *Cell* 114(6):763–776, 2003.

Burt RK, et al: Effect of nonmyeloablative hematopoietic stem cell transplantation vs continued disease-modifying therapy on disease progression in patients with relapsing-remitting multiple sclerosis: a randomized clinical trial, *J Am Med Assoc* 321(2):165–174, 2019.

Center for International Blood and Marrow Transplant Research: https://www.cibmtr.org/ReferenceCenter/SlidesReports/SummarySlides/pages/index.aspx.

[2] Not available in the United States.

Stem Cell Therapy

Chen SL, et al: Effect on left ventricular function of intracoronary transplantation of autologous bone marrow mesenchymal stem cell in patients with acute myocardial infarction, *Am J Cardiol* 94(1):92–95, 2004.

Chugh AR, et al: Administration of cardiac stem cells in patients with ischemic cardiomyopathy: the SCIPIO trial: surgical aspects and interim analysis of myocardial function and viability by magnetic resonance, *Circulation* 126(11 suppl 1):S54–S64, 2012.

Cyranoski D: Japan's approval of stem-cell treatment for spinal-cord injury concerns scientists, *Nature* 565(7741):544–545, 2019.

FDA: https://www.fda.gov/vaccines-blood-biologics/cellular-gene-therapy-products/approved-cellular-and-gene-therapy-products, F.a.s.c.t.

Fisher SA, et al: Stem cell therapy for chronic ischaemic heart disease and congestive heart failure, *Cochrane Database Syst Rev* (4):CD007888, 2014.

Gao LR, et al: Intracoronary infusion of Wharton's jelly-derived mesenchymal stem cells in acute myocardial infarction: double-blind, randomized controlled trial, *BMC Med* 13:162, 2015.

Hare JM, et al: Randomized comparison of allogeneic versus autologous mesenchymal stem cells for nonischemic dilated cardiomyopathy: POSEIDON-DCM trial, *J Am Coll Cardiol* 69(5):526–537, 2017.

Henry TD, et al: The Athena trials: autologous adipose-derived regenerative cells for refractory chronic myocardial ischemia with left ventricular dysfunction, *Catheter Cardiovasc Interv* 89(2):169–177, 2017.

Henry TD, Moye L, Traverse JH: Consistently inconsistent-bone marrow mononuclear stem cell therapy following acute myocardial infarction: a decade later, *Circ Res* 119(3):404–406, 2016.

Jayaraj JS, et al: Efficacy and safety of stem cell therapy in advanced heart failure patients: a systematic review with a meta-analysis of recent trials between 2017 and 2019, *Cureus* 11(9):e5585, 2019.

Jo CH, et al: Intra-articular injection of mesenchymal stem cells for the treatment of osteoarthritis of the knee: a proof-of-concept clinical trial, *Stem Cell* 32(5):1254–1266, 2014.

Lanzoni G, et al: Umbilical cord mesenchymal stem cells for COVID-19 acute respiratory distress syndrome: a double-blind, phase 1/2a, randomized controlled trial, *Stem Cells Transl Med* 10(5):660–673, 2021.

Lee JW, et al: A randomized, open-label, multicenter trial for the safety and efficacy of adult mesenchymal stem cells after acute myocardial infarction, *J Korean Med Sci* 29(1):23–31, 2014.

Makkar RR, et al: Intracoronary cardiosphere-derived cells for heart regeneration after myocardial infarction (CADUCEUS): a prospective, randomised phase 1 trial, *Lancet* 379(9819):895–904, 2012.

Orlic D, et al: Bone marrow cells regenerate infarcted myocardium, *Nature* 410(6829):701–705, 2001.

Perin EC, et al: Randomized trial of targeted transendocardial mesenchymal precursor cell therapy in patients with heart failure, *J Am Coll Cardiol* 81(9):849–863, 2023.

Park YB, et al: Cartilage regeneration in osteoarthritic patients by a composite of allogeneic umbilical cord blood-derived mesenchymal stem cells and Hyaluronate hydrogel: results from a clinical trial for safety and proof-of-concept with 7 Years of extended follow-up, *Stem Cells Transl Med* 6(2):613–621, 2017.

Pelletier JP, Martel-Pelletier J, Abramson SB: Osteoarthritis, an inflammatory disease: potential implication for the selection of new therapeutic targets, *Arthritis Rheum* 44(6):1237–1247, 2001.

Perin EC, et al: Adipose-derived regenerative cells in patients with ischemic cardiomyopathy: the PRECISE Trial, *Am Heart J* 168(1):88–95.e2, 2014.

Richter DL, et al: Knee articular cartilage repair and restoration techniques: a review of the literature, *Sports Health* 8(2):153–160, 2016.

Robinton DA, Daley GQ: The promise of induced pluripotent stem cells in research and therapy, *Nature* 481(7381):295–305, 2012.

Schachinger V, et al: Intracoronary bone marrow-derived progenitor cells in acute myocardial infarction, *N Engl J Med* 355(12):1210–1221, 2006.

Soder RP, et al: A phase I study to evaluate two doses of Wharton's jelly-derived mesenchymal stromal cells for the treatment of De Novo high-risk or Steroid-refractory acute graft versus host disease, *Stem Cell Rev Rep* 16(5):979–991, 2020.

Stamm C, et al: Autologous bone-marrow stem-cell transplantation for myocardial regeneration, *Lancet* 361(9351):45–46, 2003.

ter Huurne M, et al: Antiinflammatory and chondroprotective effects of intraarticular injection of adipose-derived stem cells in experimental osteoarthritis, *Arthritis Rheum* 64(11):3604–3613, 2012.

Thomas ED, et al: Intravenous infusion of bone marrow in patients receiving radiation and chemotherapy, *N Engl J Med* 257(11):491–496, 1957.

Thomson JA, et al: Embryonic stem cell lines derived from human blastocysts, *Science* 282(5391):1145–1147, 1998.

Wollert KC, et al: Intracoronary autologous bone-marrow cell transfer after myocardial infarction: the BOOST randomised controlled clinical trial, *Lancet* 364(9429):141–148, 2004.

Yubo M, et al: Clinical efficacy and safety of mesenchymal stem cell transplantation for osteoarthritis treatment: a meta-analysis, *PloS One* 12(4):e0175449, 2017.

BIOLOGIC AGENTS REFERENCE CHART

Method of
Laurie A.M. Hommema, MD; and Kevin Hommema, BSME

Biological weapons are devices used intentionally to cause disease or death through dissemination of microorganisms or toxins in food and water, by insect vectors, or by aerosols. Potential targets include human beings, food crops, livestock, and other resources essential for national security, economy, and defense. Unlike nuclear, chemical, and conventional weapons, the onset of a biological attack will probably be insidious. For some infectious agents, secondary and tertiary transmission could continue for weeks or months after the initial attack. In the United States, anthrax has been used in 2001 and ricin in 2003, 2004, and 2013 to target individuals. The Department of Homeland Security leads a national strategy to prevent, detect, respond to, and recover from acts of bioterrorism.

Initial detection of an unannounced biological attack will likely occur when an astute health professional notices an unusual case or disease cluster and reports his or her concerns to local public health authorities. Due to the incubation period of most biologic agents, subjects may have traveled from site of exposure to other geographic locations. Physicians and other health professionals should be alert to the following:

- Unusual temporal or geographic clustering of illnesses in humans, as well as animals
- Increase in specific lab testing or prescription drugs
- Sudden increase of illness in previously healthy persons
- Sudden increase in nonspecific illnesses such as pneumonia; flulike illness; bleeding disorders; unexplained rashes, particularly in adults; neuromuscular illnesses; and gastrointestinal syndromes

To enhance detection and treatment capabilities, physicians and other health professionals in acute care settings should be familiar with the clinical manifestations, diagnostic techniques, isolation precautions, treatment, and prophylaxis for likely causative agents (e.g., smallpox, pneumonic plague, anthrax, viral hemorrhagic fevers). Table 1 provides a quick summary of diagnostic and treatment considerations for various infectious and toxic biological agents. For some of these agents, delay in medical response could result in a potentially devastating number of casualties. To mitigate such consequences, early identification and intervention are imperative. Frontline physicians must have an increased level of suspicion regarding the possible intentional use of biological agents as well as an increased sensitivity to reporting those suspicious to public health authorities, who, in turn, must be willing to evaluate a predictable increase in false-positive reports.

Medical response efforts require coordination and planning with emergency management agencies, law enforcement, health care facilities, and social services agencies. Due to the criminal nature of the act, samples need to be collected and handled as evidence. Healthcare agencies should ensure that physicians know whom to call with reports of suspicious cases and clusters of infectious diseases, and they should work to build a good relationship with the local medical community. Resource integration is absolutely necessary to:

- Establish adequate capacity to initiate rapid investigation of an outbreak
- Establish and ensure decontamination protocols are in place
- Educate and protect healthcare workers and the public
- Coordinate mass distribution of antibiotics and vaccines
- Address psychological consequences

In an epidemic, overwhelming numbers of critically ill patients will require acute and follow-up medical care. Both infected persons and the worried well will seek medical attention, with a corresponding need for medical supplies, diagnostic tests, and hospital beds. The impact—or even the threat—of an attack can elicit widespread panic and civil disorder, overwhelm hospital resources, and disrupt social services.

Any suspicious or confirmed exposure to a biological weapons agent should be reported immediately to the local health department, local Federal Bureau of Investigation office, National Response Center (800-424-8802), and the Centers for Disease Control and Prevention Operation's Center (770-488-7100).

1533

TABLE 1 Quick Reference Chart on Biological Weapon Agents

DISEASE AND AGENT	DIAGNOSTIC CONSIDERATIONS				TREATMENT CONSIDERATIONS*		
	SIGNS AND SYMPTOMS	INCUBATION PERIOD	DIAGNOSIS	LETHALITY	TREATMENT	PROPHYLAXIS	COMMENTS
Bacteria							
Anthrax *Bacillus anthracis* (all forms)		1–6 days (perhaps ≤60 days)†	Gram stain and culture of blood, pleural fluid, cerebrospinal fluid, ascitic fluid, vesicular fluid, or lesion exudate. Confirmatory serologic and PCR tests are available through public health laboratory network.		Steroids may be considered for severe edema and for meningitis. Penicillin G should be considered if strain is susceptible and does not possess inducible β-lactamases.	Ciprofloxacin or doxycycline with or without vaccination If strain is susceptible, penicillin VK[1] or amoxicillin[1] (Amoxil) should be considered. Anthrax Vaccine Adsorbed (BioThrax) Preexposure (PrEP): 5 IM injections given at day 0, 1 month, and 6 months, then 12 and 18 months; and annually thereafter for persons who remain at risk. Postexposure (PEP): SC injection given at 0, 2, and 4 weeks combined with po ciprofloxacin or doxycycline for up to 60 days. Raxibacumab (ABthrax) is approved for PEP if no other options are available.	If meningitis is suspected, doxycycline may be less optimal because of poor CNS penetration. Sporicidal decontamination is necessary, such as sodium hypochlorite (chlorine bleach).
Cutaneous	Evolving *painless* skin lesion (face, neck, arms), progresses to vesicle, depressed ulcer, eschar with edema and regional lymphadenopathy		Gram stain and culture of unroofed vesicle, or under eschar	20% if untreated, otherwise rarely fatal	Ciprofloxacin[1] or doxycycline		
Gastrointestinal	Oropharyngeal: fever, severe pharyngitis, oral ulcers with patches and pseudo-membranes Intestinal: Nausea, vomiting, abdominal pain, bloody diarrhea, sepsis Widened mediastinum on chest radiograph is occasionally seen‡.		Gram stain and culture of throat lesions or stool culture	Approaches 100% if untreated, but data are limited. Rapid, aggressive treatment can reduce mortality.			

TABLE 1 Quick Reference Chart on Biological Weapon Agents—cont'd

	DIAGNOSTIC CONSIDERATIONS				TREATMENT CONSIDERATIONS*		
DISEASE AND AGENT	SIGNS AND SYMPTOMS	INCUBATION PERIOD	DIAGNOSIS	LETHALITY	TREATMENT	PROPHYLAXIS	COMMENTS
Inhalational	Abrupt onset of flulike symptoms, fever with or without chills, sweats, fatigue or malaise, non- or minimally productive cough, nausea, vomiting, dyspnea, headache, chest pain, followed in 2–5 days by severe respiratory distress, mediastinitis, hemorrhagic meningitis, sepsis, shock§ Widened mediastinum on chest radiograph or CT is characteristic‡.		Routine blood culture, CSF, and pleural effusions. Sputum is rarely positive.	Once respiratory distress develops, mortality rates approach 90%. Begin treatment when inhalational anthrax is suspected; do not wait for confirmatory testing∥.	Combination therapy of ciprofloxacin[1] or doxycycline plus one or two other antimicrobials should be considered¶. Raxibacumab (a human monoclonal antibody) and Anthrasil (an anthrax immune globulin IV [AIGIV]) are also available as FDA-approved drugs to treat inhalational anthrax.		
Brucellosis *Brucella abortus, B. canis, B. melitensis, B. suis*	Nonspecific flulike symptoms, fever, headache, profound weakness, profuse sweats, chills, weight loss, malaise. Abdominal pain, nausea, vomiting, and diarrhea are common. Hepatomegaly and splenomegaly may be found on exam, as well as osteoarticular findings.	5–60 days, usually 1–2 months	Blood and bone marrow culture (can require 6 weeks to grow *Brucella*) Confirmatory culture and serologic testing	Fatality is rare; morbidity is often significant.	Doxycycline plus rifampin[1] *Alternative therapies:* Ofloxacin[1] plus rifampin[1] Doxycycline plus gentamicin (Garamycin)[1] TMP-SMX[1] plus gentamicin	Doxycycline plus rifampin[1] for high-risk exposure. No approved human vaccine; livestock vaccines are available.	Osteoarticular complications are common, including sacroiliitis, bursitis, tenosynovitis, paravertebral abscess, or discitis.
Glanders *Burkholderia mallei* Melioidosis *Burkholderia pseudomallei*	Fever, sweats, myalgias, headaches, cough, lymphadenopathy. Can progress to hepatosplenomegaly with pustular eruptions. CXR with infiltrates, cavitation, abscess, or military lesions. Imaging with splenic or hepatic abscesses.	Glanders: days to weeks Melioidosis: days to decades	Gram stain, culture, and PCR	Fatal if untreated	IV ceftazidime (Fortaz)[1], meropenem (Merrem)[1] or imipenem (+ cilastatin [Primaxin][1] and prolonged oral TMP-SMX[1]	No approved PEP or vaccines available. TMP-SMX[1] can be considered.	One of the first bacterial agents to be weaponized. Prostatic abscess may be seen. Life-long follow-up for melioidosis as risk of relapse is 10%.

Biologic Agents Reference Chart

Continued

TABLE 1   Quick Reference Chart on Biological Weapon Agents—cont'd

DISEASE AND AGENT	DIAGNOSTIC CONSIDERATIONS			TREATMENT CONSIDERATIONS*			
	SIGNS AND SYMPTOMS	INCUBATION PERIOD	DIAGNOSIS	LETHALITY	TREATMENT	PROPHYLAXIS	COMMENTS
Typhoidal tularemia *Francisella tularensis*	Sudden onset of acute febrile illness, weakness, chills, headache, generalized body aches, elevated WBCs Pulmonary symptoms such as dry cough, chest pain, or tightness with or without objective signs of pneumonia Progressive weakness, malaise, anorexia, and weight loss, potentially leading to sepsis and organ failure. Temperature/pulse mismatch may be seen.	3–5 days' range, 1–21 days	Largely clinical Culture of blood, sputum, biopsies, pleural fluid, bronchial washings; notify laboratory if suspected as culturing poses risk in standard lab.	~30%–60% Fatal if untreated	Streptomycin or gentamicin[1] *Alternative therapies:* Ciprofloxacin[1] Doxycycline Chloramphenicol (Chloromycetin)[1]	Tetracycline Doxycycline Ciprofloxacin[1] Live, attenuated vaccine (USAMRIID, IND) given by scarification; currently under FDA review, limited availability	Ulceroglandular forms with regional lymphadenopathy may also be seen.
Pneumonic plague *Yersinia pestis*	Acute onset of flulike prodrome: fever, myalgia, weakness, headache; within 24 h of prodrome, chest discomfort, cough with bloody sputum, and dyspnea By day 2–4 of illness, symptoms progressing to cyanosis, respiratory distress, shock, and bleeding diathesis.	1–6 days	Gram stain and culture of blood, CSF, sputum, lymph node aspirates, bronchial washings Confirmatory serologic and bacteriologic tests available through public health laboratory network	Almost 100% if untreated 20%–60% if appropriately treated within 18–24 h of symptoms	Streptomycin, gentamicin[1] *Alternative therapies:* Doxycycline Tetracycline Ciprofloxacin[1] Chloramphenicol[1] (Chloromycetin) is first choice for meningitis except for pregnant women.	Tetracycline Doxycycline Ciprofloxacin[1] Previous licensed vaccine not effective against aerosol exposure	Pneumonic plague is expected outcome of biological agent attack, as opposed to the presentation of Bubonic plague with swollen lymph nodes. Begin treatment when diagnosis of plague is suspected; do not wait for confirmatory testing.
Rickettsia Q-fever *Coxiella burnetii*	Nonspecific febrile disease, chills, cough, weakness and fatigue, pleuritic chest pain Pneumonia is possible.	10–17 days, up to 5 weeks	Isolation of organism may be difficult; IgG antibody testing by IFA is gold standard. Confirmatory testing via serology or PCR available through public health laboratory network.	1%–3% Fatalities are uncommon, except in cases of endocarditis. Pregnancy loss if infected in first trimester.	Tetracycline Doxycycline	Tetracycline doxycycline, not endorsed by CDC. Inactivated whole-cell vaccine (Q-Vax) is available in Australia and Europe, but only available in USA for investigational basis (IND).	Chronic disease may occur, including endocarditis. Skin test to determine prior exposure to *C. burnetii* is recommended before vaccination.

TABLE 1 Quick Reference Chart on Biological Weapon Agents—cont'd

| DISEASE AND AGENT | DIAGNOSTIC CONSIDERATIONS | | | TREATMENT CONSIDERATIONS* | | |
	SIGNS AND SYMPTOMS	INCUBATION PERIOD	DIAGNOSIS	LETHALITY	TREATMENT	PROPHYLAXIS	COMMENTS
Viruses							
Smallpox Variola major virus	Prodrone of high fever, malaise, prostration, headache, vomiting, delirium followed in 2–3 days by maculopapular rash uniformly progressing to pustules and scabs, mostly on extremities and face	7–17 days	Clinical pharyngeal swab, vesicular fluid, biopsies, scab material for electron microscopy and PCR testing through public health laboratory network	30% in unvaccinated persons	Supportive care Tecovirimat (Tpoxx) was approved for the treatment of smallpox under the FDA's Animal Rule; however, its efficacy in humans has not been determined. Other IND products are available including cidofovir (Vistide).	ACAM2000 (live smallpox and mpox vaccine) and APSV (Aventis Pasteur smallpox vaccine)[5] are replication-competent vaccines given by multiple puncture technique (limited restricted supply). Vaccination given within 3–4 days following exposure can prevent or decrease the severity of disease. JYNNEOS is an attenuated live vaccine used for prevention of smallpox and monkeypox and can be used in those with immune deficiencies.	Requires astute clinical evaluation; may be confused with chickenpox, erythema multiforme with bullae, or allergic contact dermatitis. Strict airborne and contact precautions. Notify CDC Poxvirus Section at 404-639-2184.
Viral Encephalitis							
All forms	Systemic febrile illness, with encephalitis developing in some populations Generalized malaise, spiking fevers, headache, myalgia		Clinical and epidemiologic diagnosis WBC count can show striking leukopenia and lymphopenia. Confirmatory test and viral isolation available through public health laboratory network.		Supportive care Analgesics, anticonvulsants as needed	No accepted PEP. Several IND vaccines available.	Incidence of seizures and/or focal neurologic deficits may be higher after biological attack.
Eastern equine encephalitis		5–15 days		50%–75%			
Western equine encephalitis		5–10 days		10%			
Venezuelan equine encephalitis		2–6 days		<10%			

Continued

Biologic Agents Reference Chart

TABLE 1   Quick Reference Chart on Biological Weapon Agents—cont'd

| DISEASE AND AGENT | DIAGNOSTIC CONSIDERATIONS | | | | TREATMENT CONSIDERATIONS* | | |
	SIGNS AND SYMPTOMS	INCUBATION PERIOD	DIAGNOSIS	LETHALITY	TREATMENT	PROPHYLAXIS	COMMENTS
Viral Hemorrhagic Fevers							
Arenaviruses (Lassa, Junin, and related viruses) Bunyaviruses (Hanta, Congo–Crimean, Rift Valley) Filoviruses (Ebola, Marburg) Flaviviruses (yellow fever, dengue, various tick-borne disease viruses)	Fever with facial flushing, mucous membrane bleeding, petechiae, thrombocytopenia, and hypotension. Malaise, myalgias, headache, vomiting, diarrhea possible	4–21 days	Clinical diagnosis. Confirmatory testing and viral isolation available through BSL-4 laboratories.	Variable depending on viral strain; 15%–25% with Lassa fever to ≤90% with Ebola	Supportive therapy Ribavirin (Virazole)[1] may be effective for Lassa fever, Rift Valley fever, Argentine hemorrhagic fever, and Congo–Crimean hemorrhagic fever.	Ribavarin (Virazole)[1] is suggested for Arenaviruses and Bunyaviruses. Yellow fever vaccine (YF-VAX) is the only licensed vaccine available for yellow fever prevention. Ebola live virus vaccine (Ervebo) is available for those at high risk of exposure.	Strict airborne, droplet, and contact precautions. Call CDC Special Pathogens Office at 404-639-1115.
Biological Toxins							
Botulism *Clostridium botulinum* toxin	Cranial nerve palsies including diplopia, dry mouth, ptosis, dysphagia. As disease progresses, acute bilateral descending flaccid paralysis, respiratory paralysis resulting in death	1–5 days, typically 12–36 h	Clinical Serum and stool should be assayed for toxin by mouse neutralization bioassay, which can take several days. NCV or EMG.	60% without ventilatory support	Intensive and prolonged supportive care; ventilation may be necessary. Heptavalent Botulism Antitoxin (HBAT) is available.	Pentavalent toxoid (A–E), no longer available. Antitoxin may be sufficient to prevent illness following exposure but is not recommended until patient is showing symptoms.	Anaphylaxis and serum sickness are potential complications of antitoxin. Aminoglycosides and clindamycin (Cleocin) must not be used.
Enterotoxin B *Staphylococcus aureus*	Inhaled: acute onset of fever, chills, headache, nonproductive cough Ingested: nausea, vomiting, cramps diarrhea	3–12 h inhaled, 1–6 h ingested	Clinical Normal chest radiograph Serology on acute and convalescent serum can confirm diagnosis.	Probably low (few data available for respiratory exposure)	Supportive care	No vaccine available. Use of mask to prevent inhalation.	
Ricin toxin *Ricinus communis*	Weakness, nausea, chest tightness, fever, cough, pulmonary edema, respiratory failure, circulatory collapse, hypoxemia resulting in death (usually within 36–72 h)	≤6–24 h	Clinical and epidemiologic Confirmatory serological testing available through public health laboratory network.	Mortality data are not available, but likely to be high with extensive exposure.	Supportive care Treatment for pulmonary edema Gastric decontamination if toxin is ingested. NSAIDs.	No vaccine or antitoxin available. Use of mask to prevent inhalation.	Hypochlorite inactivates.

TABLE 1 Quick Reference Chart on Biological Weapon Agents—cont'd

DISEASE AND AGENT	DIAGNOSTIC CONSIDERATIONS				TREATMENT CONSIDERATIONS*		
	SIGNS AND SYMPTOMS	INCUBATION PERIOD	DIAGNOSIS	LETHALITY	TREATMENT	PROPHYLAXIS	COMMENTS
T-2 Mycotoxins *Fusarium Myrothecium Trichoderma Stachybotrys*	Skin pain, pruritis, erythema, vesiculation, and sloughing. Throat pain, rhinorrhea, cough, and hemoptysis. Weakness, ataxia, shock can occur in severe exposure.	Minutes to hours	Suspect if "yellow rain" with oily pigmented fluids staining close and environment.	Can be seen in severe exposures.	Clinical support	No vaccine available.	Soap and water washing within 4–6 h reduces dermal toxicity; washing within 1 h can eliminate toxicity entirely.
Other filamentous fungi			Confirmation requires testing blood, tissue, and environmental samples.	Severe exposure can cause death in hours to days.			Consult with local health department regarding specimen collection and diagnostic testing procedures.

[1] Not FDA approved for this indication.

[§] Investigational drug in the United States.

*Different situations can require different dosage and treatment regimens. Please consult other references and an infectious disease specialist for definitive dosage information, especially dosages for pregnant women and children.

[†] Data from 22 patients infected with anthrax in October and November 2001 indicate a median incubation period of 4 days (range, 4–7 days) for inhalational anthrax and a mean incubation of 5 days (range, 1–10 days) for cutaneous anthrax.

[‡] Chest radiograph abnormalities include paratracheal and hilar fullness and may be subtle. Consider chest computed tomography if diagnosis is uncertain.

[§] Limited data from the October and November 2001 anthrax infections indicate hemorrhagic pleural effusions to be strongly associated with inhalational anthrax; rhinorrhea was present in only 1/10 patients.

[‖] Limited data from the 2001 terrorist-related anthrax infections indicate that early treatment significantly decreased the mortality rate.

[¶] Other agents with in vitro activity suggested for use in conjunction with ciprofloxacin or doxycycline for treatment of inhalational anthrax include rifampin[1], vancomycin (Vancocin)[1], imipenem (Primaxin)[1], chloramphenicol (Chloromycetin)[1], penicillin G and ampicillin[1], clindamycin (Cleocin)[1], and clarithromycin (Biaxin)[1].

CDC, Centers for Disease Control and Prevention; *CNS*, central nervous system; *CSF*, cerebrospinal fluid; *GI*, gastrointestinal; *IND*, investigational new drug; *PEP*, post-exposure prophylaxis; *PCR*, polymerase chain reaction; *TMP-SMX*, trimethoprim-sulfamethoxazole; *USAMRIID*, U.S. Army Medical Research Institute of Infectious Diseases; *VHF*, viral hemorrhagic fever; *WBC*, white blood cell.

Adapted from "Blue Book" USAMRIID's Medical Management of Biological Casualties, 8th edition, September 2014; and Lyznicki JL: AMA quick reference guide: exposure to toxic chemical agents. In: American Medical Association: *Management of Public Health Emergencies, A Resource Guide for Physicians and Other Community Responders*, Chicago, American Medical Association, 2005.

Popular Herbs and Nutritional Supplements

HERB OR NUTRITIONAL SUPPLEMENT	COMMON USES	REASONABLE ADULT ORAL DOSAGE*	PRECAUTIONS AND DRUG INTERACTIONS
Aloe vera	Commonly found in skin products as a moisturizer Used topically to treat burns, wounds, skin infections, and inflammation Approved in Germany to use orally as a laxative Used orally for a variety of conditions, including diabetes, asthma, epilepsy, and osteoarthritis	For external use, apply aloe gel on the skin tid to qid For constipation, 40–170 mg of dried aloe juice or latex (corresponds to 10–30 mg hydroxyanthracene derivatives) taken in the evening For other conditions, no established dosage documented	Aloe gel is generally well tolerated and safe when used topically Aloe gel taken orally can cause hypoglycemia in patients who are concomitantly taking antidiabetic drugs Aloe juice or latex contains anthraquinone, a cathartic laxative and should not be taken by people with intestinal obstruction, acute intestinal inflammation, and ulcers Pregnant women should not take aloe latex because it may cause uterine contractions Oral use of aloe latex can cause abdominal cramps and diarrhea. Long-term use or abuse can cause electrolyte imbalances, albuminuria, hematuria, and pseudomelanosis coli. Prolonged use of high doses (≥ 1 g/d) can cause nephritis, acute renal failure, and death In 2002, the FDA banned the sale of aloe-containing laxative products in the United States because of the lack of safety data Aloe can decrease platelet aggregation and should be avoided at least 2 weeks before surgery
Astragalus	Used in combination with other herbs to support and enhance the immune system Used to prevent and treat common colds and upper respiratory infections Used for heart disease Widely used in China for chronic hepatitis and as an adjunctive therapy in cancer	Extract: 250–500 mg tid to qid standardized to 0.4% 4-hydroxy-3-methoxyisoflavone 7-sug Powdered root: 500–1000 mg tid Tincture (1:5) in 30% ethanol: 3–5 mL tid Decoction: 3–6 g of dried root per 12 oz water tid	Avoid using astragalus in organ transplant patients and those with autoimmune disorders Side effects include mild stomach upset and allergic reactions Astragalus can decrease the effects of cyclophosphamide and other immunosuppressants
Bilberry fruit	Often used orally to improve visual acuity and to treat degenerative retinal conditions Used orally to treat chronic venous insufficiency, varicose veins, and hemorrhoids Approved in Germany to use orally for acute diarrhea and topically for mild inflammation of the mucous membranes of mouth and throat	For eye conditions and circulation, 80–160 mg tid of the extract standardized to at least 25% anthocyanosides For diarrhea, 20–60 g/d of the dried, ripe berries or as a tea preparation (5–10 g of crushed dried berries in 150 mL water, brought to a boil for 10 min, then strained) For external use, 10% decoction	No known side effects reported with bilberry fruit and extract However, bilberry leaf taken in large quantities or used long term has been shown to cause wasting, anemia, jaundice, acute excitation, disturbances of tonus, and death in animals The anthocyanidin extracts from bilberry can increase the risk of bleeding in those taking warfarin or other blood thinners
Black cohosh root	Commonly used to relieve hot flashes and other menopausal symptoms Used to treat premenstrual discomfort and dysmenorrhea	20 mg bid of the rhizome extract standardized to triterpene glycosides Remifemin is the proprietary brand used in a number of clinical trials The German guidelines do not recommend its use for > 6 months	Black cohosh may have an estrogen-like effect and should be avoided in women with breast cancer Large doses may induce miscarriage and it is contraindicated during pregnancy It may cause GI disturbances, headache, and hypotension Black cohosh is one of the most frequently used herbal supplements that is associated with liver injury
Black haw	To relieve uterine cramps and painful periods To prevent miscarriage and ease pain that follows childbirth	For menstrual pain, 5 mL of tincture in water, taken 3–5 times daily For prevention of miscarriage, 1–2 cups of tea per day (1 tsp of dried herb in 1 cup of boiling water, steeped for 10 min)	Black haw should not be used in pregnancy because of its uterine relaxant effects The salicylate constituent in black haw could trigger allergic reactions in individuals with aspirin allergies or asthma Black haw may aggravate tinnitus Large doses of black haw can prolong bleeding time The oxalic acid component of black haw can increase kidney stone formation in susceptible individuals Black haw can interact with warfarin and increase risk of bleeding

HERB OR NUTRITIONAL SUPPLEMENT	COMMON USES	REASONABLE ADULT ORAL DOSAGE*	PRECAUTIONS AND DRUG INTERACTIONS
Cat's claw	Used primarily to reduce pain in osteoarthritis and rheumatoid arthritis Used for a variety of health conditions, including viral infections (e.g., herpes, HIV), Alzheimer disease, and cancer Used to support the immune system and promote kidney health Used to prevent and abort pregnancy	For osteoarthritis, 100 mg/d of the dry encapsulated extract For rheumatoid arthritis, 20 mg tid of the dry extract standardized to 1.3% pentacyclic oxindole alkaloids free of tetracyclic oxindole alkaloids For general uses, 1–3 cups of tea per day (1 g root bark boiled for 15 min in 250 mL of water) or 1 mL of tincture 2–3 times/d	Avoid using cat's claw during pregnancy or breastfeeding People with autoimmune diseases and transplant recipients should avoid cat's claw because of its immune stimulating effects Side effects include headaches, dizziness, and vomiting Cat's claw can lower blood pressure and cause hypotension when used with antihypertensive drugs Cat's claw can inhibit CYP3A4 enzyme and increase levels of drugs metabolized by this enzyme
Cannabidiol (CBD) (A cannabinoid extracted from the hemp plant and often made into an oil for use)	For relieving anxiety, insomnia, chronic pain, and many common ailments Epidiolex, a purified CBD solution, is the only prescription CBD approved by the FDA to treat Lennox-Gastaut syndrome, Dravet syndrome, or tuberous sclerosis complex in patients aged 1 year and older Various CBD products (oils, gummies, capsules, sprays, drinks, vapes, topical lotions, and creams) are sold as dietary supplements and CBD-infused foods While the 2018 Farm Bill legalized CBD oil derived from the hemp plant containing ≤ 0.3% tetrahydrocannabinol (THC) at the federal level, all 50 states have laws legalizing CBD with varying degrees of restriction. CBD products are readily obtainable in most parts of the United States and have become the hot new products in states that have legalized medical marijuana Currently, the FDA does not allow CBD to be added in foods and it does not approve CBD to be sold as dietary supplements	No established dosage documented for CBD supplement In general, start CBD at a low dose and titrate dose slowly. The usual daily dose is 200 mg or less. Doses of 300–600 mg have been used for anxiety There are concerns about the quality and purity of CBD products. Many have shown to be mislabeled and contain THC (>3%) and other contaminants (e.g., toxic chemicals including heavy metals and pesticides). Consumers should look for the US Hemp Authority seal that certifies the quality of CBD products. A product's certificate of analysis (COA) if available can also be used to determine labeling accuracy and presence of contaminants	Marijuana contains THC and CBD. Unlike THC, pure CBD does not cause a "high" CBD may cause nausea, diarrhea, fatigue, and irritability CBD is associated with elevated liver enzymes and liver dysfunction. No cases of liver injury were reported in adults using CBD doses <300 mg/day. High doses of CBD (≥1000 mg/day) and concomitant use of antiepileptic medications were identified as risk factors for hepatotoxicity Effects of cumulative CBD exposure are unknown Avoid CBD in infants and children, and in pregnant or breastfeeding women Many potential drug interactions: Worsening sedation when combining with CNS depressants CBD inhibits CYP2C8, 2C9, and 2C19 enzymes and can increase levels of drugs such as carbamazepine, warfarin, amitriptyline, citalopram, phenytoin, and valproic acid CBD levels can be increased by CYP3A4 inhibitors, such as clarithromycin, ritonavir, and verapamil Increased sedation when CBD is taken with herbal supplements, including kava, melatonin, and St. John's wort
Chamomile flower	Used orally to calm nerves and treat GI spasms and inflammatory diseases of the GI tract Used topically to treat wounds, skin infections, and skin or mucous membrane inflammation	1 cup of freshly made tea 3–4 times daily (1 tbsp or 3 g of dried flower in 150 mL boiling water for 5–10 min)	Chamomile can cause an allergic reaction, especially in people with severe allergies to ragweed or other members of the daisy family (e.g., echinacea, feverfew, and milk thistle) It should not be taken concurrently with other sedatives, such as alcohol or benzodiazepines
Chaste tree berry (Chasteberry, Vitex)	For normalizing irregular menstrual periods and relieving premenstrual complaints For relieving menopausal symptoms For restoring fertility in women For treating acne associated with menstrual cycles For increasing breast milk production in lactating women	For menstrual irregularities and premenstrual complaints, 30–40 mg/d of the dried berries or an equivalent amount of aqueous-alcoholic extracts (50%–70% v/v) Dried fruit extract, standardized to 0.6% agnusides, is used in doses of 175–225 mg/d For other conditions, no established dosage documented	Chaste tree berry can have uterine stimulant properties and should be avoided in pregnancy Women with hormone-dependent conditions (e.g., breast, uterine, and ovarian cancers, and endometriosis and uterine fibroids) and men with prostate cancer should avoid chaste tree berry because it contains progestins Side effects include intramenstrual bleeding, dry mouth, headache, nausea, rash, alopecia, and tachycardia High doses (≥480 mg/d extract) can paradoxically decrease lactation Chaste tree berry is thought to have dopaminergic effects and can interact with dopamine antagonists, such as antipsychotics and metoclopramide Chaste tree berry can decrease the effects of oral contraceptives and hormone therapy

Continued

HERB OR NUTRITIONAL SUPPLEMENT	COMMON USES	REASONABLE ADULT ORAL DOSAGE*	PRECAUTIONS AND DRUG INTERACTIONS
Chondroitin	Orally, used frequently in combination with glucosamine for osteoarthritis Topically, in combination with sodium hyaluronate, as a viscoelastic agent in cataract surgery	Oral: 200–400 mg tid	Occasional mild side effects include nausea, indigestion, and allergic reactions Chondroitin derived from bovine cartilage carries a potential risk of contamination with diseased animals
Chromium	For diabetes For hypercholesterolemia Commonly found in weight-loss products Also promoted for body building	For diabetes, 100 µg bid for ≤4 months or 500 µg bid for 2 months For hypercholesterolemia, 200 µg tid or 500 µg bid for 2–4 months For body building, 200–400 µg/d Chromium picolinate has been used in most studies, even though the chloride form is also available	Adverse effects are rare, but they include headaches, insomnia, sleep disturbances, irritability, and mood changes; some patients may also experience cognitive, perceptual, and motor dysfunction Long-term use of high doses (600–2400 µg/d) can cause anemia, thrombocytopenia, hemolysis, hepatic dysfunction, and renal failure Interstitial nephritis has been reported A few studies suggest that chromium can cause DNA damage Chromium competes with iron for binding to transferrin and can cause iron deficiency Antacids, H_2 blockers, and proton pump inhibitors can decrease the absorption of chromium
Coenzyme Q10	As adjunctive treatment for congestive heart failure, angina, hypertension, and diabetes Used for reducing cardiotoxicity associated with doxorubicin Used to treat statin-induced myopathy	For heart failure, 100 mg/d in 2 or 3 divided doses For angina, 50 mg tid For hypertension, 60 mg bid For diabetes, 100–200 mg/d	Mild adverse events include gastric distress, nausea, vomiting, and hypotension Doses >300 mg/d can cause elevated liver enzyme levels Coenzyme Q10 can reduce the anticoagulation effects of warfarin Oral hypoglycemic agents and HMG-CoA reductase inhibitors can reduce serum coenzyme Q10 levels
Cranberry	To prevent and treat UTIs or *Helicobacter pylori* infections that can lead to stomach ulcers To prevent dental plaque As an antioxidant to prevent cardiovascular disease and cancer	For UTIs, 150–600 mL of cranberry juice daily or 300–400 mg of standardized extract bid For other conditions, no dosage determined	Drinking excessive amounts of juice could cause GI upset or diarrhea Prolonged use of cranberry juice in large doses increases the risk of kidney stone formation because of its high oxalate content Cranberry can interact with warfarin and cause an increase in INR The effectiveness of proton pump inhibitors can be reduced by cranberry because of its acidity
Creatine	To enhance muscle performance, especially during short-duration, high-intensity exercise	Loading dose of 20 g/d for 5–7 d followed by a maintenance dose of ≥2 g/d An alternative dosing of 3 g/d for 28 d has been suggested	Creatine can cause gastroenteritis, diarrhea, heat intolerance, muscle cramps, and elevated serum creatinine levels Creatine is contraindicated in patients taking diuretics Concurrent use with cimetidine, probenecid, or nonsteroidal antiinflammatory drugs increases the risk of adverse renal effects Caffeine can decrease creatine's ergogenic effects
Dehydroepiandrosterone (DHEA)	Replace low serum DHEA levels in adrenal insufficiency Treat SLE Reverse aging Used in many other conditions, including Alzheimer disease, depression, diabetes, menopause, osteoporosis, impotence, and AIDS Used to promote weight loss Used by bodybuilders to increase muscle mass	For replacement therapy, 25–50 mg/d For SLE, 200 mg/d For antiaging and osteoporosis, 50 mg/d For other conditions, no established dosage documented	Most common side effects are androgenic in nature and include acne, hair loss, hirsutism, and deepening of the voice Cases of hepatitis have been reported When used in high doses, DHEA can cause insomnia, manic symptoms, and palpitations DHEA at physiologic doses increases circulating androgens in women, but not in men; it also increases circulating estrogen in both men and women Avoid use of DHEA in individuals with a history of sex hormone–dependent malignancy Safety of DHEA in individuals aged < 30 years is unknown DHEA inhibits CYP3A4 enzyme and could increase serum concentrations of drugs metabolized by this enzyme (e.g., lovastatin, ketoconazole, itraconazole, and triazolam)
Dong quai root	Commonly used for the relief of premenstrual and menopausal symptoms Used as a "blood tonic" and a strengthening treatment for the heart, spleen, liver, and kidneys	For premenstrual and menopausal symptoms, 3–4 g/d in 3 divided doses For other conditions, no established dosage documented	Dong quai should not be used in pregnant women because of its uterine stimulant and relaxant effects Women with hormone sensitive conditions (e.g., breast, uterine, and ovarian cancers, and endometriosis and uterine fibroids) should avoid dong quai because of its estrogenic effects Drinking the essential oil of dong quai is not recommended because it contains a small amount of carcinogenic constituents Dong quai contains psoralens that can cause photosensitivity and photodermatitis Dong quai contains natural coumarin derivatives that can increase the risk of bleeding in those who are taking anticoagulant or antiplatelet drugs

HERB OR NUTRITIONAL SUPPLEMENT	COMMON USES	REASONABLE ADULT ORAL DOSAGE*	PRECAUTIONS AND DRUG INTERACTIONS
Echinacea	As an immune stimulant, particularly for the prevention and treatment of the common cold and influenza Supportive therapy for lower urinary tract infections Used topically to treat skin disorders and promote wound healing	300 mg tid of *Echinacea pallida* root or 2–3 mL tid of expressed juice of *Echinacea purpurea* herb Do not use for >8 weeks because echinacea may suppress immunity if used long term	Echinacea should not be used in transplant patients and those with autoimmune disease or liver dysfunction Allergic reactions have been reported Adverse events are rare and include mild GI effects It should be discontinued as far in advance of surgery as possible Echinacea can decrease effectiveness of the immunosuppressants
Ephedra (ma huang)	For diseases of the respiratory tract with mild bronchospasm Promoted for weight loss and performance enhancement	1 tsp or 2 g of dried herb (15–30 mg of ephedrine) in 240 mL boiling water for 10 min In Canada, the maximum allowable dosage of ephedrine is 8 mg per dose or 32 mg/d	Ephedra contains ephedrine, which has sympathomimetic activities; consequently, it should not be used in patients who have cardiovascular disease, diabetes, glaucoma, hypertension, hyperthyroidism, prostate enlargement, psychiatric disorders, or seizures Serious adverse effects, including seizures, arrhythmias, heart attack, stroke, and death, have been associated with the use of ephedra; as a result, the FDA banned the sale of ephedra-containing products in the United States. The ban does not apply to traditional Chinese herbal remedies Because of the cardiovascular effects of ephedrine, patients taking ephedra should discontinue use at least 24 h before surgery Concurrent use of ephedra and digitalis, guanethidine, monoamine oxidase inhibitors, or other stimulants, including caffeine, is not recommended
Evening primrose oil	For PMS, especially if mastalgia is present For treatment of atopic eczema Used for other medical conditions, including rheumatoid arthritis, menopausal symptoms, Raynaud phenomenon, Sjögren syndrome, and diabetic neuropathy	For PMS, 2–4 g/d For atopic eczema, 6–8 g/d For rheumatoid arthritis, 2.8 g/d These doses are based on products standardized to 9% γ-linolenic acid Daily dose can be given in divided doses	Evening primrose oil can increase the risk of pregnancy complications Side effects include indigestion, nausea, soft stools, and headache Seizures have been reported in patients with schizophrenia who were taking phenothiazines and evening primrose oil concomitantly Evening primrose oil can interact with anesthesia and cause seizures Concomitant use of evening primrose oil with anticoagulant and antiplatelet drugs can increase the risk of bleeding
Fenugreek seed	For diabetes and hypercholesterolemia For constipation, dyspepsia, gastritis, and kidney ailments Approved in Germany for use orally for loss of appetite and topically as a poultice for local inflammation	For loss of appetite, 1–2 g of the seed tid or 1 cup of tea (500 mg seed in 150 mL cold water for 3 h) several times a day Maximum 6 g/d For other conditions, no established dosage documented For topical use, 50 g powdered seed in 0.25 L of hot water to form a paste	Fenugreek can cause uterine contractions and should be avoided in pregnancy Individuals who have allergies to peanuts or soybeans might also be allergic to fenugreek Fenugreek can cause diarrhea and flatulence; it can also make urine smell like maple syrup Hypoglycemia can occur if fenugreek is taken in large amounts Repeated external applications can result in undesirable skin reactions Fenugreek contains small amounts of coumarins and can interact with anticoagulants and antiplatelet drugs High mucilage content of fenugreek can affect the absorption of oral drugs; therefore, fenugreek should not be taken within 2 h of other drugs
Feverfew	For migraine headache prophylaxis For treatment of fever, menstrual problems, and arthritis	Migraine prevention: 25–75 mg bid of the encapsulated dried leaf extract standardized to 0.2% parthenolide, for up to 4 months 2.08–18.75 mg tid for MIG-99 preparation (a carbon dioxide extract enriched with parthenolide) for 3–4 months For other conditions, no established dosage documented	Feverfew can induce menstrual bleeding and is contraindicated in pregnancy Fresh leaves can cause oral ulcers and GI irritation Sudden discontinuation of feverfew can precipitate rebound headache Feverfew can interact with anticoagulants and potentiate the antiplatelet effect of aspirin

Continued

HERB OR NUTRITIONAL SUPPLEMENT	COMMON USES	REASONABLE ADULT ORAL DOSAGE*	PRECAUTIONS AND DRUG INTERACTIONS
Fish oils (omega-3 fatty acids)	Commonly used in the treatment of hypertriglyceridemia Used to prevent CHD and stroke Used in many noncardiac conditions, including depression, diabetes, dysmenorrhea, rheumatoid arthritis, and IgA nephropathy Used to reduce the risk of developing age-related maculopathy, Alzheimer disease, and cancer Promotes visual and mental development in children Used to decrease inflammation in acne	For hypertriglyceridemia, 3–5 g/d For cardioprotection, 1 g/d for patients with CHD; oily fish at least twice a week, or about 0.5 g/d for people with no known heart disease For other conditions, no established dosage documented Fish oils are composed of EPA and DHA; fish oil capsules vary widely in amounts and ratios of EPA and DHA; the most common fish oil capsules in the United States provide 180 mg of EPA and 120 mg DHA per capsule, and three capsules will provide about 1 g/d of omega-3 fatty acids	Common side effects include fishy aftertaste, GI disturbances, belching, halitosis, and heartburn High doses can cause nausea and loose stools Doses > 3 g/d can inhibit platelet aggregation, suppress immune function, worsen glycemic control, and raise LDL cholesterol levels A large prospective cohort study suggested that regular use of fish oil supplements for primary prevention of cardiovascular disease was associated with an increased risk of atrial fibrillation and stroke Long-term use may be associated with weight gain Less well-controlled preparations can contain appreciable amount of organochloride contaminants Fish oil can increase the risk of bleeding in patients taking warfarin, an antiplatelet agent, or herbs that have antiplatelet constituents (e.g., garlic, ginkgo, and red clover) Fish oils can lower blood pressure and can have additive effects with antihypertensive agents Oral contraceptives can interfere with the triglyceride lowering effects of fish oils
Flaxseed	Orally, approved in Germany for chronic constipation, irritable bowel, and other colon disorders Often used orally for hypercholesterolemia and atherosclerosis Topically, approved in Germany for painful skin inflammation	For constipation, 1 tbsp (5 g) of whole or "bruised" seeds (not ground) in 150 mL of liquid 2–3 times daily For bowel inflammation, 2–3 tbsp of milled flaxseed soaked in 200–300 mL water and strain after 30 min For hypercholesterolemia, 1–2 tbsp flaxseed oil daily Topical: 30–50 g flaxseed flour as poultice or compress for a moist-heat direct application directly to the skin	Flaxseed should be taken with plenty of water to prevent possible intestinal blockage Patients with ileus should not take flaxseed High mucilage content of flaxseed can delay absorption of other drugs taken at the same time
Garlic	To lower blood pressure and serum cholesterol To prevent atherosclerosis	Fresh clove: one 4 g clove per day Tablet: 300 mg bid to tid standardized to 0.6%–1.3% allicin	Intake of large quantities can lead to stomach complaints Garlic has antiplatelet effects, so patients should discontinue use of garlic at least 7 d before surgery Concomitant use of garlic and anticoagulants can increase the risk of bleeding
Ginger root	As an antiemetic For prevention of motion sickness	Fresh rhizome: 2–4 g/d Powdered ginger: 250 mg 3–4 times daily Tea: 1 cup of tea tid (0.5–1 g dried root in 150 mL boiling water for 5–10 min)	Ginger should not be used by patients with gallstones because of its cholagogic effect It can inhibit platelet aggregation; cases of postoperative bleeding have been reported Large doses of ginger can increase bleeding time in patients taking antiplatelet agents
Ginkgo biloba leaf	To slow cognitive deterioration in dementia To increase peripheral blood flow in claudication To treat sexual dysfunction associated with the use of SSRIs	60–120 mg bid of extract Egb761 standardized to 24% flavonoids and 6% terpenoids	Adverse effects are rare and can include mild stomach or intestinal upset, headache, or allergic skin reaction Ginkgo can inhibit platelet aggregation; reports of spontaneous bleeding have been published Patients should discontinue ginkgo at least 36 h before surgery Concurrent use of ginkgo and anticoagulants, antiplatelet agents, vitamin E, or garlic can increase the risk of bleeding
Ginseng root	As a tonic during times of stress, fatigue, disability, and convalescence To improve physical performance and stamina	Root: 1–2 g/d Tablet: 100 mg bid of extract standardized to 4%–7% ginsenosides A 2- to 3-week period of using ginseng followed by a 1- to 2-week "rest" period is generally recommended Ginseng is commonly adulterated, especially Siberian ginseng (eleuthero) products	Ginseng has a mild stimulant effect and should be avoided in patients with cardiovascular disease Tachycardia and hypertension can occur Overdosages can lead to ginseng abuse syndrome, characterized by insomnia, hypotonia, and edema Ginseng has estrogenic effects and can cause vaginal bleeding and breast tenderness Ginseng has been shown to inhibit platelets, so patients should discontinue ginseng use at least 7 d before surgery Ginseng should not be used with other stimulants Patients taking antidiabetic agents and ginseng should be monitored to avoid the hypoglycemic effects of ginseng Ginseng can interact with warfarin and cause a decreased INR Siberian ginseng can increase digoxin levels Ginseng can interact with phenelzine (a MAOI) resulting in insomnia, headache, tremulousness, and manic-like symptoms

HERB OR NUTRITIONAL SUPPLEMENT	COMMON USES	REASONABLE ADULT ORAL DOSAGE*	PRECAUTIONS AND DRUG INTERACTIONS
Glucosamine	For osteoarthritis	500 mg tid with meals Glucosamine is available in the form of sulfate, hydrochloride, or N-acetyl salt; glucosamine sulfate is the form that has been used in most clinical studies	Side effects are generally limited to mild GI symptoms, including stomach upset, heartburn, diarrhea, nausea, and indigestion Glucosamine derived from marine exoskeletons may cause reactions in people allergic to shellfish Glucosamine may raise blood glucose level in patients with diabetes
Goldenseal	Often combined with echinacea to treat colds and other upper respiratory infections Used for diarrhea, dyspepsia, and gastritis Used topically as an eyewash, mouthwash, feminine cleansing product, and skin remedy	Oral: 0.5–1 g of the dried rhizome/root or 2–4 mL tincture (1:10, 60% ethanol) or 0.3–1 mL fluid extract (1:1, 60% ethanol) tid Eyewash: For trachoma infections, 2 drops of a 0.2% aqueous berberine solution tid × 3 week	Avoid using goldenseal during pregnancy and breast feeding; berberine, the principle constituent in goldenseal, can cause uterine contractions and neonatal jaundice Avoid using goldenseal in kidney failure because of inadequate urinary excretion of its alkaloids High dosages or long-term usage can lead to nausea, vomiting, headache, hypotension, bradycardia, leucopenia, and mucosal irritation Berberine can increase the risk of bleeding in patients taking warfarin or an antiplatelet agent Be aware that other herbs containing berberine, including Chinese goldthread and Oregon grape, are sometimes substituted for goldenseal
Grape seed	For conditions related to the heart and blood vessels, such as atherosclerosis, high blood pressure, high cholesterol, and poor circulation For vision problems, diabetic neuropathy or retinopathy, and swelling after an injury or surgery For cancer prevention and wound healing	For general health purposes, 100–300 mg daily of a standardized extract (95% oligomeric proanthocyanidin complexes)	Side effects include headache, dizziness, nausea, and dry, itchy scalp Concomitant use with warfarin or antiplatelet agents can increase risk of bleeding because of the tocopherol content of grape seed oil
Hawthorn leaf with flower	Commonly used in Germany to increase cardiac output in patients with New York Heart Association stage I and II heart failure	160–900 mg water-ethanol extract (30–169 mg procyanidins or 3.5–19.8 mg flavonoids) divided into 2–3 doses	Side effects include GI upset, palpitations, hypotension, headache, dizziness, and insomnia Concomitant use with CNS depressants can have additive CNS effects Hawthorn can potentiate effects of digoxin and vasodilators
Hops	For mood disturbances such as restlessness and anxiety For sleep disturbances Commonly found in combination products with other herbal sedatives	0.5 g of cut or powdered strobile in a single dose; can be taken as tea (0.5 g in 150 mL water), fluid extract 1:1 (0.5 mL), tincture 1:5 (2.5 mL), or dry extract 6–8:1 (60–80 mg) The preparation contains at least 0.35% (v/w) essential oil	Side effects are rare but include drowsiness and allergic reactions Hops is not recommended for use during pregnancy and lactation It can potentiate the sedative effect of CNS depressants (e.g., benzodiazepines, alcohol) and other herbal tranquilizers
Horse chestnut seed	To relieve symptoms of chronic venous insufficiency	250 mg bid of extract standardized to 50 mg aescin in delayed-release form Unsafe to ingest the raw seed, which contains significant amounts of the most toxic constituent, esculin	Mild GI symptoms, headache, dizziness, and pruritis have been reported Ingestion of high doses can cause renal, hepatic, and hematologic toxicity Concomitant use with anticoagulants can increase the risk of bleeding Horse chestnut can potentiate the effects of hypoglycemic drugs
Kava kava	As an anxiolytic for nervous anxiety, stress, and restlessness As a sedative to induce sleep	Herb and preparations equivalent to 60–120 mg/d of kava pyrones Most clinical trials have used 100 mg tid of extract standardized to 70% kava pyrones for anxiety disorders	Kava should not be used by patients with depression Kava should be avoided in pregnant or nursing women Kava can affect motor reflexes and judgment, so it should not be taken while driving and/or operating heavy machinery Accommodative disturbances have been reported; kava can exacerbate Parkinson disease Extended use can cause a temporary yellow discoloration of skin, hair, and nails Reports have linked kava use to at least 25 cases of severe liver toxicity; sale of products containing kava has been banned in Canada and several European countries Kava has been shown to have additive CNS depressant effects with benzodiazepines, alcohol, and herbal tranquilizers Kava can potentiate the sedative effects of anesthetics, so kava should be discontinued at least 24 h before surgery

1545

Continued

HERB OR NUTRITIONAL SUPPLEMENT	COMMON USES	REASONABLE ADULT ORAL DOSAGE*	PRECAUTIONS AND DRUG INTERACTIONS
Lutein	Commonly used to prevent AMD and cataracts Used to prevent skin cancer, breast cancer, and colon cancer Used to protect against cardiovascular disease	For AMD and cataracts, 6–20 mg/d of lutein from diet For other uses, no established dosage documented Foods containing high concentrations of lutein include kale, spinach, broccoli, and romaine lettuce Not known if supplemental lutein is as effective as natural lutein Supplemental lutein in the form of esters might require a higher fat intake for effective absorption than purified lutein	No major adverse effects and drug interactions have been reported
Lycopene	Commonly used to prevent and treat prostate cancer Used for cancer prevention, arthrosclerosis prevention, and reduction of asthma symptoms	For decreasing the growth of prostate cancer, 15 mg supplement bid For prostate cancer prevention, at least 6 mg/d from tomato products (or ≥10 servings/wk) For other uses, no established dosage documented Heat processing converts lycopene in fresh tomatoes from the *trans-* to the *cis-* configuration. The *cis* isomer has better bioavailability Lycopene supplements usually do not specify the type and amount of isomers in their product labeling	Lycopene, when consumed in amounts found in foods, is generally considered to be safe Concomitant ingestion of beta-carotene can increase lycopene absorption Lycopene may reduce cholesterol levels and potentiate the effects of statins
Melatonin	For jet lag, insomnia, shift-work disorder, and circadian rhythm disorders For other medical conditions, including depression, multiple sclerosis, tinnitus, headache, and cancer	For jet lag, 5 mg at bedtime for 2–5 d beginning the day of return For sleep disorders, 0.3–5 mg taken 2 h before bedtime Avoid melatonin from animal pineal gland because of the possibility of contamination.	Avoid use in pregnancy because melatonin decreases serum luteinizing hormone concentrations and increases serum prolactin levels The common adverse reactions include headache, transient depressive symptoms, daytime fatigue and drowsiness, dizziness, abdominal cramps, irritability, and reduced alertness The increasing availability and use of melatonin has put children at risk for potential adverse events; the CDC reported that pediatric hospitalizations and serious outcomes increased during 2012–2021, primarily because of a significant increase in unintentional melatonin ingestions in children aged ≤5 years Concomitant use of melatonin with alcohol, benzodiazepines, or other CNS depressants can cause additive sedation Melatonin can affect immune function and may interfere with immunosuppressive therapy Concomitant use with other herbs that have sedative properties (e.g., chamomile, goldenseal, hop, kava, valerian) can produce additive CNS-impairing effects
Milk thistle fruit	As a hepatoprotectant and antioxidant, particularly for treatment of hepatitis, cirrhosis, and toxic liver damage Used in Europe for the treatment of hepatotoxic mushroom poisoning from *Amanita phalloides*	Average daily dose is 12–15 g of crude drug or formulations equivalent to 200–400 mg of silymarin	Adverse effects are rare but include diarrhea and allergic reactions Milk thistle can potentiate the hypoglycemic effect of antidiabetic agents
Peppermint	Commonly used for indigestion and irritable bowel syndrome (IBS) Used externally for myalgia and neuralgia	Indigestion: 1 tsp dried leaves in 1 cup of boiling water, steeped for 10 min; drink 4–5 times/d between meals IBS: 1–2 enteric coated cap (0.2 mL of peppermint oil/cap) 2–3 times/d. Take peppermint ≥2 h before or after an acid-reducing drug to ensure adequate absorption	Peppermint, in amounts normally found in food, is likely to be safe Larger supplemental amounts can cause side effects including heartburn, flushing, headache, and mouth sores Hypersensitivity reactions, contact dermatitis, and exacerbations of asthma may occur Peppermint can exacerbate symptoms in patients with gastroesophageal reflux disease (GERD) because it can relax the lower esophageal sphincter Peppermint tea has been shown to reduce free testosterone levels in men Peppermint can decrease the blood levels of cyclosporine and drugs that metabolized by the CYP3A4 isoenzyme

HERB OR NUTRITIONAL SUPPLEMENT	COMMON USES	REASONABLE ADULT ORAL DOSAGE*	PRECAUTIONS AND DRUG INTERACTIONS
Probiotics	Prevent and treat antibiotic-associated diarrhea and acute infectious diarrhea Relieve symptoms of IBS Treat atopic dermatitis for at-risk infants Used orally or topically to improve skin condition in people with acne	Dosage varies based on preparations *Lactobacillus* sp., *Bifidobacterium* sp., *Saccharomyces boulardii* are the most widely used organisms For *Lactobacillus* sp., 10 billion CFUs/d For *Lactobacillus* sp./*Bifidobacterium* sp., 100 million to 35 billion CFUs/d For *Saccharomyces boulardii*, 250–500 mg/d Quality of products varies among brands Refrigeration is required to maintain potency	Avoid use in short-gut syndrome and severe immuno-compromised condition Common adverse effects include flatulence, mild abdominal discomfort, and, rarely, septicemia
Red clover flower	Commonly used for conditions associated with menopause, such as hot flashes, cardiovascular health, and osteoporosis Used for PMS, benign prostate hyperplasia, and cancer prevention Used topically to treat psoriasis, eczema, and other rashes	For hot flashes, 40 mg/d of the isoflavones extract (Promensil) For other conditions, no established dosage documented	Red clover has estrogenic activity and should be avoided during pregnancy and lactation Women with hormone-dependent conditions (e.g., breast, uterine, and ovarian cancer, and endometriosis and uterine fibroids) and men with prostate cancer should also avoid taking red clover Side effects include headache, myalgia, nausea, and rash Red clover contains coumarin derivatives and can increase the risk of bleeding in those who are taking anticoagulants or antiplatelet drugs Preliminary report suggests that red clover might antagonize the effects of tamoxifen Some evidence suggests that red clover can increase the levels of drugs that metabolized by the cytochrome P450 3A4 isoenzyme (e.g., lovastatin, ketoconazole, itraconazole, fexofenadine, and triazolam)
SAMe (S-adenosyl-L-methionine)	For treatment of osteoarthritis, depression, fibromyalgia, and liver disease	For osteoarthritis, 200 mg tid For depression and fibromyalgia, 800 mg bid For liver disease, 600–800 mg bid	Common side effects include flatulence, nausea, vomiting, and diarrhea SAMe can cause anxiety in people with depression and hypomania in people with bipolar disorder Concurrent use of SAMe and other antidepressants can cause serotonin syndrome
Saw palmetto berry	To treat symptomatic benign prostatic hyperplasia and irritable bladder	160 mg bid of extract standardized to 85%–95% fatty acids and sterols	Adverse effects are rare but include headache, nausea, and upset stomach High doses can cause diarrhea
Soy	Commonly used for cholesterol reduction in combination with a low-fat diet Used for menopausal symptoms and for prevention of osteoporosis and cardiovascular disease in postmenopausal women	For lowering cholesterol, 25–50 g/d of soy protein For hot flashes, 20–60 g/d of soy protein For osteoporosis, 40 g/d of soy protein containing 90 mg isoflavones	Soy, when consumed as whole foods (e.g., tofu or soy milk), has minimal adverse effects Consumption of large amounts of soy can cause gastric complaints such as constipation, bloating, and nausea Long-term use of soy tablets containing isoflavones (150 mg/d for 5 years) has been shown to cause endometrial hyperplasia
St. John's wort	Used for treatment of mild to moderate depression May have antiinflammatory and antiinfective activities	300 mg tid of hypericum extract standardized to 0.3% hypericin	St. John's wort should not be used in pregnancy Side effects include dry mouth, GI upset, dizziness, fatigue, and constipation St. John's wort can induce photosensitivity, especially in fair-skinned individuals It can cause serotonin syndrome if used with other antidepressants, including SSRIs, or other serotonergic drugs It has been shown to induce CYP3A4 and decrease blood levels of many drugs such as indinavir, nevirapine, cyclosporine, digoxin, theophylline, simvastatin, oral contraceptive pills, and warfarin St. John's wort should be discontinued at least 5 d before surgery to avoid any potential drug interactions
Stinging nettle root	Approved in Germany for difficulty in urination in BPH stage 1 and 2	4–6 g/d of cut root; can be taken as tea (1.5 g in 150 mL boiling water for 10–20 min, tid), fluid extract 1:1 (1.5 mL tid), tincture 1:5 (5–7.5 mL tid), or dry extract 5.4–6.6:1 (0.22–0.33 g tid)	Occasionally, mild GI upsets may occur No known interactions with drugs

Continued

HERB OR NUTRITIONAL SUPPLEMENT	COMMON USES	REASONABLE ADULT ORAL DOSAGE*	PRECAUTIONS AND DRUG INTERACTIONS
Turmeric root	Approved by the German Commission E for dyspeptic conditions Used extensively in Ayurveda medicine for its antiinflammatory and antiarthritic effects Other uses include allergic rhinitis, depression, nonalcoholic fatty liver disease, osteoarthritis and cancer	For dyspeptic conditions: 1.5–3 g/d of cut root as tea infusion or equivalent preparations (e.g., powder, extract, tincture) The Commission E monograph requires turmeric to contain not less than 3% curcuminoids, calculated as curcumin and not less than 3% volatile oil	Side effects are uncommon and are generally limited to mild stomach distress Topical curcumin can cause allergic contact dermatitis Individuals with bile duct obstruction or gallstones should avoid curcumin due to its stimulating effects on the gallbladder Turmeric supplements, especially those concentrated forms for better absorption, have been linked to rare cases of liver injury. People with preexisting liver conditions should avoid taking the supplements
Valerian root	Used as a mild sedative for insomnia and anxiety	2–3 g of dried root or 1–3 mL of tincture, qd to several times per day Two clinical trials found 400–450 mg of the root extract effective for insomnia	Valerian has a bad odor and can cause morning drowsiness Long-term administration can lead to paradoxical stimulation, including restlessness and palpitations Because of the risk of benzodiazepine-like withdrawal, valerian should be tapered over a period of several weeks before surgery It can potentiate the sedative effect of CNS depressants (e.g., benzodiazepines, alcohol) and other herbal tranquilizers

*Doses presented in the table are adapted from the German Commission E Monographs and/or data from clinical trials. Products from different manufacturers vary considerably. A reliable product should have a label clearly stating the botanical name of the herb and milligram amount contained in the product. Standardized extracts should be used whenever possible and are often disclosed on the label of quality products.

AMD, Age-related macular degeneration; *BPH,* benign prostatic hyperplasia; *CFU,* colony-forming unit; *CHD,* coronary heart disease; *CNS,* central nervous system; *CYP3A4,* cytochrome P450 3A4; *DHA,* docosahexaenoic acid; *EPA,* eicosapentaenoic acid; *FDA,* Food and Drug Administration; *GI,* gastrointestinal; *HMG-CoA,* 3-hydroxy-3-methylglutaryl coenzyme A; *INR,* international normalized ratio; *LDL,* low-density lipoprotein; *MAOI,* monoamine oxidase inhibitor; *PMS,* premenstrual syndrome; *SLE,* systemic lupus erythematosus; *SSRIs,* selective serotonin reuptake inhibitors; *UTIs,* urinary tract infections.

References

Ang-Lee MK, Moss J, Yuan C: Herbal medicines and perioperative care, *JAMA* 286:208–216, 2001.

Bent S: Herbal medicine in the United States: Review and efficacy, safety, and regulation, *J Gen Intern Med* 23:854–859, 2008.

Blumenthal M, editor: *Herbal Medicines: Expanded Commission E monographs,* Austin, TX, 2000, American Botanical Council.

Blumenthal M, editor: *The ABC Clinical Guide to Herbs,* Austin, TX, 2003, American Botanical Council.

Chen G, Qian ZM, Zhang J, et al.: Regular use of fish oil supplements and course of cardiovascular diseases: prospective cohort study, *BMJ Med* 21;3(1):e000451, 2024.

Ernst E: The risk-benefit profile of commonly used herbal therapies: Ginkgo, St John's wort, ginseng, Echinacea, saw palmetto, and kava, *Ann Intern Med* 136:42–53, 2002.

Gregory PJ, Worthington M, Shkayeva M, et al, editors: Natural Medicines (database online), Stockton, CA: 2018 Therapeutic Research Center. Available at https://naturalmedicines.therapeuticresearch.com/. (Assessed July 7, 2019).

Gudushauri N, Navarro VJ, Halegoua-De Marzio D: A comprehensive update in herbal and dietary supplement–induced liver injury, *Clin Liver Dis* 23(1):e0185, 2024.

Holland S, Silberstein SD, Freitag F, et al: Evidence-based guideline update: NSAIDs and other complementary treatments for episodic migraine prevention in adults: report of the Quality Standards Subcommittee of the American Academy of Neurology and the American Headache Society, *Neurology* 78(17):1346–1353, 2012.

Kligler B, Cohrssen A: Probiotics, *Am Fam Physician* 78:1073–1078, 2008.

Kronenberg F, Fugh-Berman A: Complementary and alternative medicine for menopausal symptoms: A review of randomized controlled trials, *Ann Intern Med* 137:805–813, 2002.

Lelak K, Vohra V, Neuman MI, et al: Pediatric melatonin ingestions—United States, 2012–2021, *MMWR Morb Mortal Wkly Rep* 71:725–729, 2022.

Lo LA, Christiansen A, Eadie L, Strickland JC, Kim DD, Boivin M, et al. Cannabidiol-associated hepatotoxicity: A systematic review and meta-analysis. *J Intern Med.* 2023; 293: 724–752.

National Center for Complementary and Integrative Health: Herbs at a Glance. Available at https://nccih.nih.gov/health/herbsataglance.htm. Accessed 19 March 2018.

Smet P: Herbal remedies, *N Engl J Med* 347:2046–2056, 2002.

TOXIC CHEMICAL AGENTS REFERENCE CHART

Method of
Laurie A.M. Hommema, MD; and Kevin Hommema, BSME

Toxic chemical agents are poisonous vapors, aerosols, gases, liquids, or solids that have toxic effects on people, animals, or plants. Most of these agents are liquid at room temperature and are disseminated as vapors and aerosols. They may be released as bombs, sprayed from aerosolizing devices, through ventilation systems or introduced to food or water supply. Some of these agents are highly toxic and persistent, features that can render a site uninhabitable and require costly and potentially hazardous decontamination and remediation. Health effects range from irritation and burning of skin and mucous membranes to rapid cardiopulmonary collapse and death.

Efficient deployment of hazardous materials (HazMat) teams is critical to control a chemical agent attack. Although all major cities and emergency medical systems have plans and equipment in place to address this situation, physicians and other health professionals must be aware of principles involved in managing a patient or multiple patients exposed to these agents. Chemical weapon agents have a high potential for secondary contamination from victims to responders. This requires that medical treatment facilities have clearly defined procedures for handling contaminated casualties, many of whom will transport themselves to the facility. Precautions must be used until thorough decontamination has been performed or the specific chemical agent is identified. Healthcare professionals must first protect themselves (e.g., by using protective suits, respiratory protection, and chemical-resistant gloves) because secondary contamination with even small amounts of these substances (particularly nerve agents such as VX) may be lethal.

Primary detection of exposure to chemical agents is based on the signs and symptoms of the potential victim (Table 1). Confirmation of a chemical agent, using detection equipment or laboratory analyses, takes considerable time and will not likely contribute to the early management of mass casualty victims. Several patients presenting with the same symptoms should alert physicians and hospital staff to the possibility of a chemical attack. If a chemical attack occurs, most victims will likely arrive within a short time. This situation differentiates a chemical attack from a biological attack involving infectious microorganisms, which can take days for symptom onset. Additional diagnostic clues include the following:
- Unusual temporal or geographic clustering of illness
- Any sudden increase in illness in previously healthy persons
- Sudden increase in nonspecific syndromes (e.g., sudden unexplained weakness in previously healthy persons; dimmed or blurred vision; hypersecretion, inhalation, or burn-like syndrome)

A coordinated communication network is critical for transmitting reliable information from the incident scene to treatment facilities. Any suspicious or confirmed exposure to a chemical weapons agent should be reported to the local health department, local Federal Bureau of Investigation office, National Response Center (800-424-8802), and the Centers for Disease Control and Prevention (770-488-7100).

TABLE 1   Quick Reference Chart on Chemical Weapon Agents

	DIAGNOSTIC CONSIDERATIONS				TREATMENT CONSIDERATIONS*			
CHEMICAL AGENT	**SIGNS AND SYMPTOMS**	**SYMPTOM ONSET**	**ODOR**	**ACTION**	**TESTING**	**TREATMENT**	**ANTIDOTE**	**COMMENTS**
Cyanides—Asphyxiant/Blood								
Cyanogen chloride (CK) Hydrogen cyanide (AC)	"Cherry red" skin Resp: SOB, chest tightness, hyperventilation, resp arrest GI: nausea, vomiting CV: ventricular arrhythmias, hypotension, cardiac arrest, shock CNS: anxiety, headache, drowsiness, weakness, apnea, convulsions, seizure, coma Metabolic acidosis and increased concentration of venous oxygen (possibly also cyanosis)	Rapid, seconds to minutes	Bitter almond, musty, or chlorine-like	Binds cellular cytochrome oxidase, causing chemical asphyxia	Cyanide, thiocyanate, serum lactate levels Venous and arterial partial oxygen pressure	Immediate treatment of symptomatic patients is critical. Hydroxocobalamin (vitamin B$_{12a}$) [Cyanokit] administered IV with sodium thiosulfate^{S,†} Activated charcoal[1] for oral exposure Mechanical ventilation as needed Circulatory support with crystalloids and vasopressors Metabolic acidosis corrected with IV sodium bicarbonate Seizures controlled with benzodiazepines	Sodium nitrite and sodium thiosulfate (Nithiodote); repeat one-half initial doses of both agents in 30 min if inadequate clinical response; amyl nitrite[1] capsules are available for first aid until intravenous access is achieved. Hydroxocobalamin (vitamin B$_{12a}$, Cyanokit)	Cyanide antidote kits are commercially available. CNS effects may be confused with carbon monoxide and hydrogen sulfide poisoning. Non-persistent, not contact hazard.
Incapacitating Agents								
Agent 15 3-quinuclidinyl benzilate (BZ)	May appear as drug intoxication with erratic behaviors, hallucinations. Mydriasis, blurred vision, dry mouth, dry skin, possible atropine-like flush, initial rise in heart rate, hyperthermia, decreased level of consciousness, confusion, disorientation, impaired memory.	Hours—up to 36 h if only on skin 0–4 h: parasympathetic blockade and mild CNS effects 4–20 h: stupor with ataxia and hyperthermia 20–96 h: full-blown delirium Resolution phase: paranoia, deep sleep, reawakening, crawling, climbing automatisms, eventual reorientation	Odorless	Competitive inhibitor of acetylcholine muscarinic receptor		Support, intravenous fluids	Physostigmine salicylate (Antilirium)[1]	Persistent in soil and water and on contact surfaces. Contact hazard.

Toxic Chemical Agents Reference Chart

Continued

TABLE 1 Quick Reference Chart on Chemical Weapon Agents—cont'd

	DIAGNOSTIC CONSIDERATIONS					TREATMENT CONSIDERATIONS*			
CHEMICAL AGENT	SIGNS AND SYMPTOMS	SYMPTOM ONSET	ODOR	ACTION	TESTING	TREATMENT	ANTIDOTE	COMMENTS	
Nerve Agents									
Cyclohexyl sarin (GF) Sarin (GB) Soman (GD) Tabun (GA) VX	Most toxic of known chemical agents May be confused with organophosphate and carbamate pesticide poisoning Eyes: excessive lacrimation, miosis may be present and blurred vision Resp: rhinorrhea, bronchospasm, resp failure GI: hypersalivation, nausea, vomiting, diarrhea Skin: localized sweating Cardiac: sinus bradycardia Skeletal muscles: fasciculations followed by weakness, flaccid paralysis CNs: loss of consciousness, convulsions, apnea, seizures	Vapor: seconds Liquid: minutes or hours Symptom onset may be delayed up to 18 h, particularly for localized exposures.	GB, VX: none GA: fruity GD: camphor-like	Irreversible acetylcholinesterase inhibitors	Erythrocyte or serum cholinesterase activity to confirm exposure	Rapid establishment of patent airway Early administration of 2-PAM (pralidoxime [Protopam]) is critical to minimize permanent agent inactivation of acetylcholinesterase (i.e., "aging"). Benzodiazepines to control nerve agent–induced seizures Airway and ventilatory support as needed	Atropine and 2-PAM Additional doses until bronchial secretions are cleared and ventilation improved	Atropine, 2-PAM, and diazepam[1] are available in autoinjector kits through the US military. VX is a contact hazard.	

TABLE 1   Quick Reference Chart on Chemical Weapon Agents—cont'd

	DIAGNOSTIC CONSIDERATIONS				TREATMENT CONSIDERATIONS*			
CHEMICAL AGENT	SIGNS AND SYMPTOMS	SYMPTOM ONSET	ODOR	ACTION	TESTING	TREATMENT	ANTIDOTE	COMMENTS

Pulmonary or Choking Agents

CHEMICAL AGENT	SIGNS AND SYMPTOMS	SYMPTOM ONSET	ODOR	ACTION	TESTING	TREATMENT	ANTIDOTE	COMMENTS
Acrolein Ammonia (NH_3) Chlorine (Cl) Chloropicrin (PS) Diphosgene (DP) Nitrogen oxides (NO_x) Perfluoroisobu-tylene (PFIB) Phosgene (CG) Sulfur dioxide (SO_2)	Degree of water solubility of the agent influences onset and severity of respiratory injury. Eye and airway irritation, dyspnea, chest tightness, rhinorrhea, hypersalivation, cough, wheezing High-dose inhalation can cause laryngospasm, pneumonitis, and acute lung injury with delayed onset (≤ 48 h) of acute resp distress syndrome. Chest radiograph: hyperinflation, noncardiogenic pulmonary edema	Rapid or delayed 1–24 h; rarely up to 72 h	CG: freshly mown hay or grass			Supportive measures Specific treatment depends on the agent IV fluids for hypotension; no diuretics Ventilation with or without positive airway pressure Bronchodilators for bronchospasm Methylprednis-olone[1] may be effective in preventing noncardiogenic pulmonary edema.	No specific antidote	Easily absorbed via mucous membranes of eyes, nose, oropharynx. May be confused with inhalation exposure to industrial chemicals (e.g., HCl, Cl_2, NH_3). Not contact hazard.

Riot Control Agents

CHEMICAL AGENT	SIGNS AND SYMPTOMS	SYMPTOM ONSET	ODOR	ACTION	TESTING	TREATMENT	ANTIDOTE	COMMENTS
Mace (CN) Tear gas (CS)	Metallic taste Burning and pain on mucosal membranes and skin Eyes: irritation, pain, tearing, blepharospasm Airways: burning in nose and mouth, respiratory discomfort, bronchospasm (may be delayed 36 h) Skin: tingling, erythema	Immediate	CN: apple blossom CS: pepper	SN2 alkylating agents	No specific laboratory tests	Supportive care Irrigation as necessary Persons with asthma, emphysema might need oxygen, inhaled bronchodilators, steroids, assisted ventilation. Lotions, such as calamine[1] for persistent erythema		Not contact hazard

Continued

Toxic Chemical Agents Reference Chart

TABLE 1   Quick Reference Chart on Chemical Weapon Agents—cont'd

| | DIAGNOSTIC CONSIDERATIONS | | | | TREATMENT CONSIDERATIONS* | | |
CHEMICAL AGENT	SIGNS AND SYMPTOMS	SYMPTOM ONSET	ODOR	ACTION	TESTING	TREATMENT	ANTIDOTE	COMMENTS
	Nausea and vomiting are common. CN can cause corneal opacification.							
Vesicant or Blister Agents								
General	Clinical effects depend on extent and route of exposure.	Effects may be delayed, appearing hours after exposure		Intracellular enzyme and DNA alkylating agents		Immediate decontamination within 2 min if able Supportive care Thermal burn-type treatment Symptomatic management of lesions		Primary liquid hazard. May be confused with skin exposure to caustic irritants (e.g., NaOH, NH₃). Persistent contact hazard.
Sulfur mustard (H) Distilled mustard (HD)	Skin: erythema and blisters (may be delayed ≤ 8 h), pruritus Eye: irritation, conjunctivitis, corneal damage, lacrimation, pain, blepharospasm Resp: mild to marked acute airway damage, pneumonitis within 1–3 days, respiratory failure GI effects (nausea, vomiting diarrhea) may be present Bone marrow stem cell suppression leading to pancytopenia and increased susceptibility to infection Fever, sputum production	Delayed 2–48 h	Garlic, horseradish, or mustard			Skin: silver sulfadiazine¹ Eye: homatropine¹ ophthalmic ointment Pulmonary: antibiotics, bronchodilators, steroids Colony-stimulating factor may be helpful for leukopenia. Systemic analgesic and antipruritics Early use of PEEP or CPAP Maintain fluid and electrolyte balance (do not excessively fluid resuscitate as in thermal burns).	No specific antidote	Combination with lewisite (called mustard-Lewisite or HL) results in rapid effects of lewisite and delayed effects of mustard agents.

TABLE 1 Quick Reference Chart on Chemical Weapon Agents—cont'd

	DIAGNOSTIC CONSIDERATIONS					TREATMENT CONSIDERATIONS*			
CHEMICAL AGENT	SIGNS AND SYMPTOMS	SYMPTOM ONSET	ODOR	ACTION	TESTING	TREATMENT	ANTIDOTE	COMMENTS
Lewisite (L)	Skin: gray area of dead skin within 5 min, erythema within 30 min, blistering 2–3 h, immediate irritation or burning pain on contact, severe tissue necrosis Eye: pain, blepharospasm, conjunctival and lid edema Airway: pseudomembrane formation, nasal irritation Intravascular fluid loss, hypovolemia, shock, organ congestion, leukocytosis	Immediate	Fruity or geranium				British anti-lewisite (BAL or dimercaprol)	More volatile than mustard. Damages eyes, skin, and airways by direct contact.
Phosgene oxime (CX)	Burning, irritation, wheal-like skin lesions, eye and airway damage, conjunctivitis, lacrimation, lid edema, blepharospasm	Immediate	Freshly mown hay	Urticant, nonvesicant agent	No distinctive laboratory findings	Parenteral methylpredniso-lone[1] may be effective in preventing noncardiogenic pulmonary edema. Experimental: aerosolized dexamethasone[1] and theophylline[1] for pulmonary involvement	No antidote	Vapor extremely irritating; vapor and liquid cause tissue damage upon contact.

Continued

Toxic Chemical Agents Reference Chart

TABLE 1 Quick Reference Chart on Chemical Weapon Agents—cont'd

CHEMICAL AGENT	DIAGNOSTIC CONSIDERATIONS				TREATMENT CONSIDERATIONS*			
	SIGNS AND SYMPTOMS	SYMPTOM ONSET	ODOR	ACTION	TESTING	TREATMENT	ANTIDOTE	COMMENTS

Vomiting (Arsine-Based) Agents

CHEMICAL AGENT	SIGNS AND SYMPTOMS	SYMPTOM ONSET	ODOR	ACTION	TESTING	TREATMENT	ANTIDOTE	COMMENTS
Adamsite (DM) Diphenylchlor-arsine (DA) Diphenylcyano-arsine (DC)	Eyes: conjunctival irritation, tearing, and blepharospasm Airways: sneezing, mucosal lung irritation, edema, progressive cough, wheezing Cardiac: tachypnea, tachycardia GI: intestinal cramps, emesis, diarrhea Skin: erythema, edema at the site of dermal contact CNS: depression, syncope	All rapidly acting within minutes	DA: none DC: garlic DM: burning fireworks	Arsine gas depletes erythrocyte glutathione and causes hemolysis.	Chest radiograph to rule out chemical pneumonitis	Supportive care Monitor for hemolysis Wheezing or dyspnea: may need albuterol inhalation Eye irrigation (water, normal saline, lactated Ringer's) in patients with ocular exposure Treat repetitive emesis with IV hydration and antiemetics. Blood transfusion may be required. Exchange transfusion may be required. Hemodialysis may be useful in decreasing arsenic level and treating renal failure.		Primary route of absorption is through respiratory system.

*Different situations can require different treatment and dosage regimens. Please consult other references as well as a regional poison control center (800-222-1222), medical toxicologist, clinical pharmacologist, or other drug information specialist for definitive dosage information, especially dosages for pregnant women and children.

†Available in Europe.

¶Not FDA approved for this indication.

§Investigational drug in the United States.

CNS, Central nervous system; *CPAP*, continuous positive airway pressure; *CV*, cardiovascular; *GI*, gastrointestinal; *2-PAM*, pralidoxime (2-pyridine aldoxime methyl chloride); *PEEP*, positive end-expiratory pressure; *resp*, respiratory; *SOB*, shortness of breath.

Adapted from Lyznicki JL: AMA quick reference guide: Exposure to toxic chemical agents. In American Medical Association: Management of Public Health Emergencies A Resource Guide for Physicians and Other Community Responders, Chicago, American Medical Association, 2005.

U.S. Department of Health and Human Services Chemical Hazards Emergency Medical Management Acute Patient Care Guidelines. 2020. https://chemm.nlm.nih.gov/mmghome.htm

Index

Index